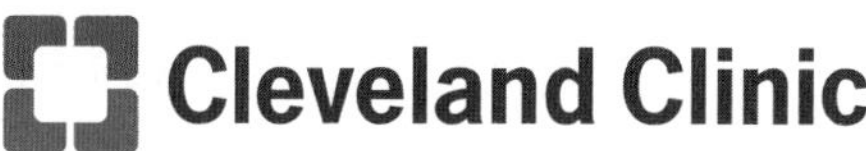

CURRENT CLINICAL MEDICINE

Section Editors

Section 1: Allergy and Immunology
David M. Lang, MD
Head, Allergy/Immunology Section,
Director, Allergy/Immunology Fellowship Program,
Co-Director, Asthma Center,
Respiratory Institute
Cleveland Clinic

Section 2: Cardiology
Robert Hobbs, MD
Associate Professor of Medicine
Cleveland Clinic Lerner College of Medicine of Case Western Reserve University
Heart and Vascular Institute
Cleveland Clinic

Section 3: Dermatology
Kenneth J. Tomecki, MD
Vice Chairman
Department of Dermatology
Cleveland Clinic

Section 4: Endocrinology
Mario Skugor, MD FACE
Associate Professor of Medicine
Cleveland Clinic Lerner College of Medicine of Case Western Reserve University
Associate Director—Endocrinology, Diabetes and Metabolism Fellowship Program
Endocrine and Metabolic Institute
Cleveland Clinic

Sections 5 and 6: Gastroenterology; Hepatology
William D. Carey, MD
Professor of Medicine
Cleveland Clinic Lerner College of Medicine of Case Western Reserve University
Digestive Disease Institute
Cleveland Clinic

Section 7: Hematology and Oncology
Mikkael A. Sekeres, MD, MS
Associate Professor of Medicine
Cleveland Clinic Lerner College of Medicine of Case Western Reserve University
Director, Leukemia Program
Department of Hematologic Oncology and Blood Disorders
Cleveland Clinic

Section 8: Infectious Diseases
Steven Gordon, MD
Associate Professor of Medicine
Cleveland Clinic Lerner College of Medicine of Case Western Reserve University
Chairman, Department of Infectious Disease
Cleveland Clinic

Section 9: Nephrology
Saul Nurko, MD
Staff Physician
Glickman Urological and Kidney Institute
Cleveland Clinic

Section 10: Neurology
Jinny Tavee, MD
Staff Neurologist
Neuromuscular Center
Neurological Institute
Cleveland Clinic

Section 11: Psychiatry and Psychology
George E. Tesar, MD
Associate Professor of Medicine
Cleveland Clinic Lerner College of Medicine of Case Western Reserve University
Director, Psychiatric Residency Training Program
Department of Psychiatry and Psychology
Cleveland Clinic Foundation

Section 12: Pulmonary
Raed A. Dweik, MD
Associate Professor of Medicine
Director, Pulmonary Vascular Program
Department of Pulmonary and Critical Care Medicine
Respiratory Institute
Cleveland Clinic

Section 13: Rheumatology and Immunology
Abby Abelson, MD
Assistant Professor of Medicine
Cleveland Clinic Lerner College of Medicine of Case Western Reserve University
Interim Chair
Department of Rheumatic and Immunologic Diseases
Vice Chair for Education
Orthopedic and Rheumatology Institute
Rheumatology Education Program Director
Director, Education, Center for Osteoporosis and Metabolic Bone Disease
Cleveland Clinic

Section 14: Women's Health
Shakuntala Kothari, MD, FACP
Assistant Professor of Medicine
Cleveland Clinic Lerner College of Medicine of Case Western Reserve University
Primary Care Women's Health
Department of Internal Medicine
Cleveland Clinic

Section 15: Preventive Medicine
Raul J. Seballos, MD, FACP
Vice Chairman, Preventive Medicine
Wellness Institute
Cleveland Clinic

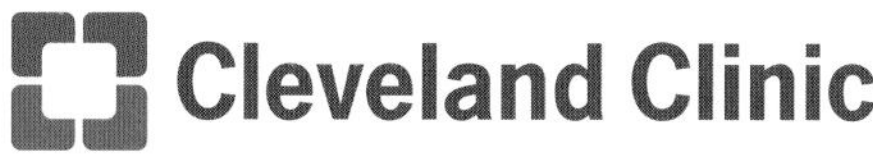

CURRENT CLINICAL MEDICINE

SECOND EDITION

Online + Print

William D. Carey, MD
The Cleveland Clinic
Cleveland, OH

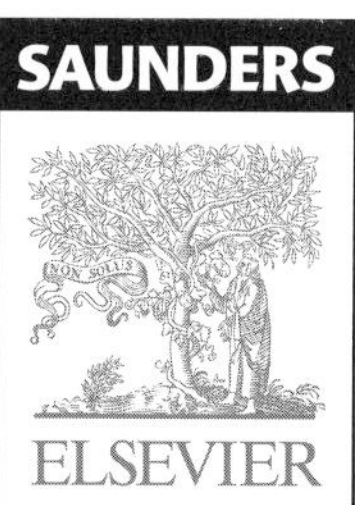

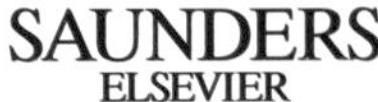

1600 John F. Kennedy Blvd.
Ste 1800
Philadelphia, PA 19103-2899

CURRENT CLINICAL MEDICINE 978-1-4160-6643-9

Notice

Knowledge and best practice in this field are constantly changing. As new research and experience broaden our knowledge, changes in practice, treatment and drug therapy may become necessary or appropriate. Readers are advised to check the most current information provided (i) on procedures featured or (ii) by the manufacturer of each product to be administered, to verify the recommended dose or formula, the method and duration of administration, and contraindications. It is the responsibility of the practitioner, relying on their own experience and knowledge of the patient, to make diagnoses, to determine dosages and the best treatment for each individual patient, and to take all appropriate safety precautions. To the fullest extent of the law, neither the Publisher nor the Authors assumes any liability for any injury and/or damage to persons or property arising out of or related to any use of the material contained in this book.

The Publisher

Library of Congress Cataloging-in-Publication Data

Current clinical medicine / Cleveland Clinic ; [edited by] William D. Carey. —2nd ed.
p. ; cm.
Rev. ed. of: Current clinical medicine 2009 / Cleveland Clinic [edited by] William D. Carey … [et al.]. c2009.
Includes bibliographical references and index.
ISBN 978-1-4160-6643-9
1. Clinical medicine—Handbooks, manuals, etc. I. Carey, William D. (William Dahill) II. Cleveland Clinic Foundation. III. Current clinical medicine 2009.
[DNLM: 1. Clinical Medicine—methods—Handbooks. WB 39 C9746 2010]
RC55.C766 2010
616—dc22

2010019237

Acquisitions Editor: Dolores Meloni
Developmental Editor: Julia Bartz
Publishing Services Manager: Frank Polizzano
Senior Project Manager: Peter Faber
Design Direction: Steve Stave

Printed in China

Last digit is the print number: 9 8 7 6 5 4 3 2 1

To the memory of Eileen Cawley
A generous family gift in her memory made this work possible.

Contributors

Joseph B. Abdelmalak
Abby Abelson
Ahmed Absi
Edgar Achkar
David J. Adelstein
Talal Adhami
Kamal Adury
Anjali Advani
Feyrouz Al-Ashkar
Amjad AlMahameed
Antoine Amado
Sheila Armogida
Wendy S. Armstrong
Mercedes E. Arroliga
Alejandro C. Arroliga
Kathleen Ashton
Arman Askari
Natasha Atanaskova
Marjan Attaran
Federico Aucejo
Joseph Austerman
Robin Avery
H. Nail Aydin
David Barnes
John R. Bartholomew
Pelin Batu
Rachid Baz
Wilma Bergfeld
Deepak Bhatt
Swati Bharadwaj
Laura K. Bianchi
Allan Boike
Michael H. Bolooki
Brian Bolwell
Corinne Bott-Silverman
Andrew Boyle
Linda Bradley
William E. Braun
Yvonne Braver
Sorin J. Brener
Stacy Brethauer
Marie M. Budev
Matthew Bunyard
Carol Burke
Saud Butt
Leonard Calabrese
Charles Camisa
Darwin L. Caldwell
John Carey
William D. Carey
Karin Cesario
Nathaniel Cevasco
Jeffrey T. Chapman
Soumya Chatterjee
Michael C. Chen
Neil Cherian
Priya Chinnappa
Anuja Choure
Jeffrey Y. Chung
Gregory B. Collins
Edward C. Covington
Daniel A. Culver
Ronan Curtin
Mellar Davis
Steven Deitcher
Sevag Demirjian
Robert Dreicer
Thomas J. Dresing
Raed A. Dweik
Bijan Eghtesad
Julie A. Elder
Peter J. Embi
Kristin Englund
Serpil Erzurum
Ronan Factora
Kyrsten Fairbanks
Esteban Faith-Fernandez
Tatiana Falcone
Tommaso Falcone
Gary W. Falk
Suzanne R. Fanning
Richard Fatica
Omar Fattal
Michael Faulx
Elizabeth File
Maria Fleseriu
Fetnat Fouad-Tarazi
Adele Fowler
Robert Fox
Kathleen N. Franco
Thomas G. Fraser
Benjamin J. Freda
Katherine Freeman
John J. FungJorge Garcia
Thomas R. Gildea
Joseph A. Golish
Anil Gopinath
Steven Gordon
Lisa Grandinetti
Adam Grasso
Brian Griffin
Richard Grimm
Rula A. Hajj-Ali
Philip Hall
Amir H. Hamrahian
Shannon Harrison
Teresa Hermida
José Hernández-Rodriguez
Robert Heyka
Gary S. Hoffman
Robert Hobbs
Sandra Hong
Byron Hoogwerf
Fred Hsieh
Julie Huang
M. Elaine Husni
Adriana G. Ioachimescu
Octavian C. Ioachimescu
Harry J. Isaacson
Carlos M. Isada
Naim Issa
Wael A. Jaber
Ron Jacob
Fredrick J. Jaeger
Fred Jaeger
Xian Wen Jin
Georges Juvelekian
Sangeeta Kashyap
Irene Katzan
Gurjit Kaur
Mani Kavuru
Thomas F. Keys
Sami Khalife
Mazen K. Khalil
Atul Khasnis
Esther S.H. Kim
Richard Kim
Alice Kim
R. Koelsch
Curry L. Koening
Ann R. Kooken
Shakuntala Kothari
Richard A. Krasuski
Robert Kunkel
Milton Lakin
David M. Lang
Steven P. LaRosa
Martin E. Lascano
Bret Lashner
Anthony K. Leung
Harry Lever
David S. Lever

Kerry H. Levin
Alan Lichtin
Oren H. Lifshitz
Li Ling Lim
Daniel Logan
Jennifer Lucas
Marina Magrey
Michael Maier
Donald Malone
Judith Manzon
Anjli Maroo
Manu Mathews
Steven D. Mawhorter
Mark Mayer
Ken Mayuga
Peter J. Mazzone
Mark S. McAllister
Kevin McCarthy
Kathleen Maksimowicz-McKinnonn
Adi Mehta
Atul C. Mehta
Tarek Mekhail
Charles M. Miller
Donald Moffa
Asma Moheet
Eamonn Molloy
Halle Moore
Thomas Morledge
Sherif B. Mossad
Preetha Muthusamy
David J. Muzina
Dileep Nair
Joseph Nally
Christian Nasr
Thomas P. Noeller
Gian M. Novaro
Saul Nurko
Robert S. O'Shea
Ravindran Padmanabhan
Velma L. Paschall
Lily C. Pien
Melissa Piliang
Ronnie Pimental
Emilio D. Poggio
Jeannette M. Potts
Leo Pozuelo
Gary W. Procop
Mohammed Qadeer
Christine Radojicic
Mohammed Rafey
Justin L. Ranes
Russell Raymond
Feza Remzi
Thomas Rice
Cristina Rodriguez
Jess Rowney
Camille Sabella
Ronald M. Sabecks
Mandi Sachdeva
Nancy Foldvary-Schaefer
Philip Schauer
Raymond Scheetz
Steven Schmitt
Martin Schrieber
Raul J. Seballos
Robert A. Schweikert
Mikkael A. Sekeres
Bo Shen
Robert W. Shields, Jr.
Anita Shivadas
Laura Shoemaker
Nabin K. Shrestha
Rabin K. Shrestha
Bernard J. Silver
Rishi P. Singh
Vivek Singh
Mario Skugor
Stephen Smith
Edy Soffer
Firas Al Solaiman
Apra Sood
Brian R. Stephany
Tyler Stevens
Glen H.J. Stevens
James K. Stoller
David Streem
Patrick Sweeney
James F. Swiencicki
Alan Taege
Rachel M. Taliercio
Thomas Tallman
Jinny Tavee
Anthony Tavill
David Taylor
James S. Taylor
George E. Tesar
Holly L. Thacker
Karl Theil
Sharon Longshore Thornton
Kenneth J. Tomecki
Walton J. Tomford
Rebecca Tung
Marisa Tungsiripat
Allison Vidimos
Nicola M. Vogel
Jamile Wakim-Fleming
Teo Boon Wee
Christopher Whinney
Anna Wieckowska
Herbert P. Wiedemann
William Wilke
Justin G. Woodhouse
Bridget Wright
Mohamad Yamani
Kristine Zanotti
Claudia O. Zein
Robert Zimmerman
Matthew J. Zirwas

Acknowledgments

Special thanks to original authors:

Christopher T. Bajzer (Acute Myocardial Infarction)

David S. Barnes (Primary Biliary Cirrhosis, Primary Sclerosing Cholangitis, and Other Cholestatic Liver Diseases)

Susan M. Begelman (Venous Thromboembolism)

Divya Singh-Behl (Common Skin Infections)

Robert Dreicer (Prostate Cancer)

Mani Kavuru (Asthma)

Bo Shen (Irritable Bowel Syndrome)

Edy Soffer (Irritable Bowel Syndrome)

David Tschopp (Complications of Acute Myocardial Infarction)

Donald Vidt (Hypertension)

Preface

Cleveland Clinic Current Clinical Medicine springs from a web-based textbook of medicine that has met with success for more than a decade. Two attributes characterize the chapters in this book: authors are either current or past members of the Cleveland Clinic staff; wherever appropriate, chapters reference, expand, and elaborate on nationally produced clinical practice guidelines. I am extremely pleased with the reception of the book's first edition. There have been many positive reviews, some with helpful suggestions for improvement. And we listened. In this edition are 18 new chapters and 61 substantially updated ones. More than ever, it covers topics most likely to be seen by a generalist. It retains simplicity and practicality, as well as the beautiful artwork, photographs, tables, and figures. It seeks to be your daily medical guide.

The book rests on the shoulders of the Section Editors. I owe them special gratitude for their commitment to the project. The Section Editors are recognized experts with considerable clinical and editorial experience. They have assembled the best experts from their respective specialty areas to produce a work that will be of maximum benefit to the practicing clinician. Although most current Section Editors have been present since the inauguration of the web-based virtual textbook, *Disease Management Project*, some have moved on. Brian Bolwell, MD, a longtime member of the Cleveland Clinic Taussig Cancer Institute, holds many important posts; he may best be known for his development of the highly successful bone marrow transplant program. Brian served as the first Section Editor for the Hematology and Oncology Section. Donald Vidt, MD, served as the inaugural Section Editor for the Renal Section. He retired after devoting more than 40 years to an active consulting practice in hypertension and renal disease, combined with medical education and clinical research. David Longworth, MD, was the first Infectious Disease Section Editor. Dr. Longworth served for many years as Chairman of the Department of Infectious Diseases at the Cleveland Clinic. He has published numerous articles in scientific journals and book chapters; he has also edited four textbooks. He is currently Professor and Deputy Chairman, Department of Medicine, Tufts University School of Medicine. Since publication of the 2009 edition of this book, Patrick Sweeney, MD, and Herbert Wiedemann, MD, have moved to Emeritus Section Editor status. I welcome aboard new Section Editors, Jinny Tavee, MD (Neurology) and Raed Dweik, MD (Pulmonary).

The lion's share of thanks goes to the chapter authors. Each is inundated with requests for intellectual contributions—no surprise given their stature in their respective fields. That so many would agree to support this book is a source of tremendous satisfaction. I am beholden to each and every one.

As important as authors and editors, the daunting task of publishing a textbook requires an extended family of publishers, editors, and project managers, and a legion of support staff invisible to the Editor-in-Chief. This book relied on the willingness of Rolla Couchman, Acquisitions Editor at Elsevier, to see promise in this work. His encouragement and good cheer were invaluable. His successor, Druanne Martin, was a tireless advocate. Rolla and Druanne have since left Elsevier to be replaced by the equally capable and encouraging Dolores Meloni. Elsevier's Developmental Editors, Julia Bartz and Mary Beth Murphy, and Project Managers, Jeffrey Gunning and Pete Faber, all played major roles in making this work come to life, and I thank each of them. At the Cleveland Clinic, Ronna Romano deserves special thanks for having ably served as the first manager of this work. Donna Miller and her team did a superb job of crafting each chapter into a unified website.

Finally, it is appropriate to recognize the Cleveland Clinic as an environment that fosters excellence in medicine and urges its faculty to be the best. The founding fathers of this organization urged its creation more than 90 years ago "… to act as a unit." More than words, the Cleveland Clinic culture provides an environment of mutual support for development of best clinical practices and for education of those within and outside our walls.

William D. Carey, MD
Editor-in-Chief

Contents

Section 3 Dermatology

Section 4 Endocrinology

Section 10 Neurology

Section 11 Psychiatry and Psychology

Section 12 Pulmonary

Section 1

ALLERGY AND IMMUNOLOGY

Asthma

David M. Lang, Serpil C. Erzurum, and Mani Kavuru

Although much progress has been made in our understanding of bronchial asthma in recent years, asthma remains a commonly encountered condition that challenges physicians in the office setting as well as in acute care settings.[1-3] Although the 1980s were characterized by increases in asthma morbidity and mortality in the United States, these trends reached a plateau in the 1990s, and asthma mortality rates have declined since 1999. In recent decades, a surge in asthma prevalence also occurred in the United States and other Western countries; data suggest this trend may also be reaching a plateau. Tremendous progress has been made in our fundamental understanding of asthma pathogenesis by virtue of invasive research tools such as bronchoscopy, bronchoalveolar lavage, airway biopsy, and measurement of airway gases, although the cause of airway inflammation remains obscure.

The knowledge that asthma is an inflammatory disorder has become fundamental to our definition of asthma. Evidence-based practice guidelines have been disseminated with a goal of encouraging more frequent use of anti-inflammatory therapy to improve asthma outcomes. To this extent, there has been much emphasis on early diagnosis and longitudinal care of patients with asthma, along with ensuring adherence to recommended therapies. In this context, there have been advances in our pharmacologic armamentarium in both chronic and acute therapy with the development and approval of novel medications. Yet, as exciting as this revolution has been in asthma research and practice, a number of controversies persist, and further fundamental developments in novel therapeutics are imminent.

This review of asthma for the practicing clinician summarizes these developments, including an update on the definition of asthma, its epidemiology, natural history, cause, and pathogenesis. In addition, there is a discussion of the appropriate diagnostic evaluation of asthma and co-occurring conditions, management of asthma, and newer therapies for the future.

DEFINITIONS

Asthma is a chronic, episodic disease of the airways that is best viewed as a syndrome. In 1997, the National Heart, Lung, and Blood Institute (NHLBI) included the following features as integral to the definition of asthma[4]: recurrent episodes of respiratory symptoms; variable airflow obstruction that is often reversible, either spontaneously or with treatment; presence of airway hyperreactivity; and, importantly, chronic airway inflammation in which many cells and cellular elements play a role, in particular, mast cells, eosinophils, T lymphocytes, macrophages, neutrophils, and epithelial cells. All of these features need not be present in any given asthmatic patient. The Expert Panel Report (EPR) 3 guidelines,[5] issued in 2007, state that the immunohistopathologic features of asthma include inflammatory cell infiltration involving neutrophils (especially in sudden-onset, fatal asthma exacerbations; occupational asthma; and patients who smoke), eosinophils, and lymphocytes, with activation of mast cells and epithelial cell injury. Heterogeneity in the pattern of asthma inflammation has been recognized, consistent with the interpretation that phenotypic differences exist that influence treatment response. The inflammation of asthma leads to an associated increase in the existing bronchial hyperresponsiveness to a variety of stimuli. Although the absolute minimum criteria to establish a diagnosis of asthma are not widely agreed on, the presence of airway hyperreactivity can be regarded as a sine qua non for patients with current symptoms and active asthma.

EPIDEMIOLOGY AND NATURAL HISTORY

Several government agencies have been charged with surveillance for asthma, including the NHLBI's National Asthma Education and Prevention Program (NAEPP), the Department of Health and Human Services (Healthy People 2010), and the Centers for Disease Control and Prevention (CDC). Data published by the CDC indicate that approximately 20 million Americans have asthma. Estimates of 12-month period prevalence have found that approximately 3.0% of the U.S. population had asthma in 1970; more recent estimates indicated that the 12-month period prevalence had increased to 5.5% in 1996.[6] In association with rising prevalence, patient encounters—via outpatient visits, emergency department use, and hospitalizations for asthma—also increased during this period. Asthma surveillance data in recent decades have revealed that a disparate burden of asthma exists in certain demographic subgroups: in children compared with adults, in women compared with men, in blacks compared with whites, and among Hispanics of Puerto Rican heritage compared with those of Mexican descent.[6] The trend for increasing asthma mortality that began in 1978 and continued through the 1980s reached a plateau in the 1990s, and since 1999 annual rates in the United States have declined.[6] These trends are reassuring, and they have been correlated with increasing rates of dispensed prescriptions for inhaled corticosteroids (ICS), implying that improved treatment of asthma may be responsible for these favorable developments. The overall annual economic burden for asthma care in the United States exceeds $11 billion.[7]

ETIOLOGY AND PATHOGENESIS

Clinicians have long known that asthma is not a single disease; it exists in many forms. This heterogeneity has been well established by a variety of studies that have demonstrated disease risk from early environmental factors and susceptibility genes, subsequent disease induction and progression from inflammation, and response to therapeutic agents (Fig. 1).

Asthma is an inflammatory disease and not simply a result of excessive smooth muscle contraction. Increased airway inflammation follows exposure to inducers such as allergens or viruses, exercise, or inhalation of nonspecific irritants. Increased inflammation leads to exacerbations characterized by dyspnea, wheezing, cough, and chest tightness. Abnormal histopathology including edema, epithelial cell desquamation, and inflammatory cell infiltration are found not only in autopsy studies of severe asthma cases but even in patients with very mild asthma. Reconstructive lesions, including goblet cell hyperplasia, subepithelial fibrosis, smooth muscle cell hyperplasia, and myofibroblast hyperplasia can lead to remodeling of the airway wall. Many studies have emphasized the multifactorial nature of asthma, with interactions between neural mechanisms, inflammatory cells (mast cells, macrophages, eosinophils, neutrophils, and lymphocytes), mediators (interleukins, leukotrienes, prostaglandins, and platelet-activating factor), and intrinsic abnormalities of the arachidonic acid pathway and smooth muscle cells. Although these types of descriptive studies have revealed a composite picture of asthma (Fig. 2), they have failed to identify a basic unifying defect.

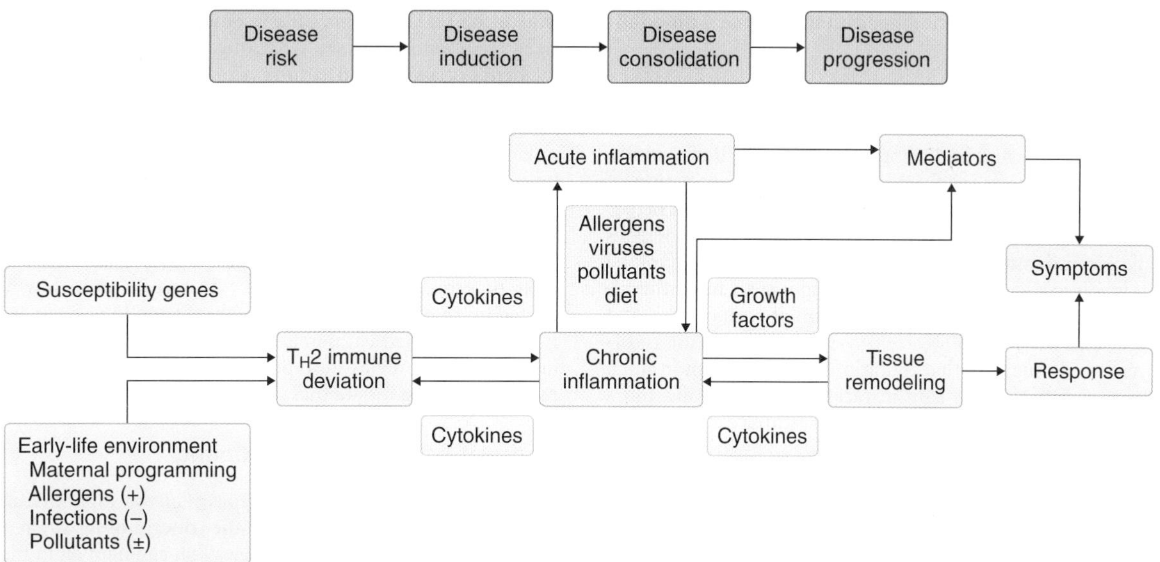

Figure 1 **Natural history of asthma.** *(Reproduced from Holgate ST: The cellular and mediator basis of asthma in relation to natural history. Lancet 1997;350[suppl 2]:5-9. Reprinted in Szefler SJ: The natural history of asthma and early intervention. J Allergy Clin Immunol 2002;109:S550.)*

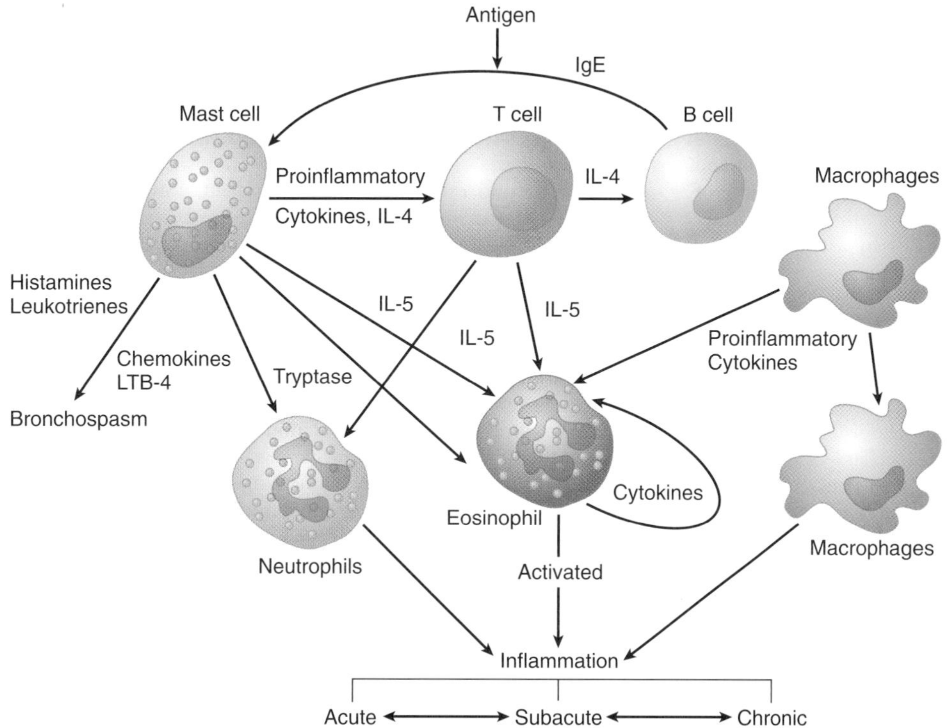

Figure 2 **Schematic showing airway inflammation in patients with asthma.** *(Reproduced from Spahn J, Covar R, Stempel DA. Asthma: Addressing consistency in results from basic science, clinical trials, and observational experience. J Allergy Clin Immunol 2002;109:S492.)*

Advances have been made in our understanding of asthmatic airway inflammation through the use of invasive technology, such as bronchoscopy with airway sampling at baseline state,[8] and with experimental provocation (e.g., allergen challenge) and following administration of interventions, such as anti-inflammatory pharmacotherapy. Further insights have been obtained through transgenic murine models with deletion, or knockout, of specific genes (i.e., those for immunoglobulin E [IgE], CD23, interleukin-4 [IL-4], or IL-5) or overexpression of other putative genes. Also, specific monoclonal antibodies or cytokine antagonists have been used in various asthma models. A number of limitations have hindered our understanding of asthma obtained from these model systems: There are important differences between animal models of asthma and human disease, there are few longitudinal studies of human asthma with serial airway sampling, and it is often difficult to determine cause and effect from multiple mediator studies.

Despite the explosion of information about asthma, the nature of its basic pathogenesis has not been established. Studies suggest a genetic basis for airway hyperresponsiveness, including linkage to chromosomes 5q and 11q. Asthma clearly does not result from a single genetic abnormality; rather it is a complex multigenic disease with a strong environmental contribution. For example, allergic potential to inhaled allergens (e.g., dust mites, mold spores, cat dander) is found more commonly in asthmatic children or asthmatic adults whose asthma began in childhood than in those with adult-onset asthma.

Immunopathogenesis and the Th2 Phenotype

Based on animal studies and limited bronchoscopic studies in adults, the immunologic processes involved in the airway inflammation of asthma are characterized by the proliferation and activation of helper T lymphocytes ($CD4^+$) of the subtype Th2. The Th2 lymphocytes mediate allergic inflammation in atopic asthmatics by a cytokine profile that involves IL-4 (which directs B lymphocytes to synthesize IgE), IL-5 (which is essential for the maturation of eosinophils), and IL-3 and granulocyte-macrophage colony-stimulating factor (GM-CSF).[9] Recent study suggests that mutations in IL-4 receptor alpha (IL4Rα) are associated with a gain in receptor function and more IL-4 functional effect, which is associated with asthma exacerbations, lower lung function, and tissue inflammation, in particular to mast cells and IgE.[10] Eosinophils are often present in the airways of asthmatics (more commonly in allergic but also in nonallergic patients), and these cells produce mediators that can exert damaging effects on the airways.

Knockout studies and anticytokine studies suggest that lipid mediators are products of arachidonic acid metabolism. They have been implicated in the airway inflammation of asthma and have been the target of pharmacologic antagonism by antileukotriene agents. Prostaglandins are generated by the cyclooxygenation of arachidonic acid, and leukotrienes are generated by the lipoxygenation of arachidonic acid. The proinflammatory prostaglandins (prostaglandin [PG]D_2, PGF_2, and TXB_2) cause bronchoconstriction, whereas other prostaglandins are considered protective and elicit bronchodilation (PGE_2 and PGI_2, or prostacyclin). Leukotrienes C_4, D_4, and E_4 compose the compound formerly known as *slow-reacting substance of anaphylaxis,* a potent stimulus of smooth muscle contraction and mucus secretion. Ultimately, mediators lead to degranulation of effector or proinflammatory cells in the airways that release other mediators and oxidants, a common final pathway that leads to the chronic injury and inflammation noted in asthma.

The Hygiene Hypothesis, Airway Hyperresponsiveness, and Disease Progression

Most studies of airway inflammation in human asthma have been conducted in adults because of safety and convenience. However, asthma often occurs in early childhood, and persistence of the asthmatic syndrome into later childhood and adulthood has been the subject of much investigation. The *hygiene hypothesis* has been proposed to explain the epidemiologic observation that asthma prevalence is much greater in industrialized Western societies than in less technologically advanced societies.[11,12] This hypothesis maintains that airway infections and early exposure to animal allergens (e.g., farm animals, cats, dogs) is important in affecting the propensity for persons to become allergic or asthmatic. Specifically, early exposure to the various triggers that can occur with higher frequency in a rural setting might protect against the allergic diathesis that is characteristic of the Th2 paradigm. In a "cleaner" urban Western society, such early childhood exposure is lacking, and this encourages a higher incidence of allergy and asthma. The hygiene hypothesis has become the basis for a number of emerging therapies.

Whether airway hyperresponsiveness is a symptom of airway inflammation or airway remodeling, or whether it is the cause of long-term loss of lung function, remains controversial. Some investigators have hypothesized that aggressive treatment with anti-inflammatory therapies improves the long-term course of asthma beyond their salutary effects on parameters of asthma control and rates of exacerbation over time.[13] This contention has been supported by an observational study[14] that found long-term exposure to ICS was associated with an attenuation of the accelerated decline in lung function previously reported in asthmatics; more studies are required to substantiate these findings.

Concept of Airway Remodeling

The relation between the several types of airway inflammation (early-phase and late-phase events) and the concept of airway remodeling, or the chronic nonreversible changes that can happen in the airways, remains a source of intense research.[4] The natural history of airway remodeling is poorly understood, and although airway remodeling occurs in some patients with asthma, it does not appear to be a universal finding.

Clinically, airway remodeling may be defined as persistent airflow obstruction despite aggressive anti-inflammatory therapies, including ICS and systemic corticosteroids. Pathologically, airway remodeling appears to have a variety of features that include increases of smooth muscle mass, mucous gland hyperplasia, persistence of chronic inflammatory cellular infiltrates, release of fibrogenic growth factors along with collagen deposition, and elastolysis.[15] Increased numbers and size of vessels in the airway wall is a long-recognized characteristic and one of the most consistent features of asthma remodeling occurring in mild, moderate and severe asthmatic lungs.[16-19] (Fig. 3). Many biopsy studies show these pathologic features in the airways of patients with chronic asthma. However, there are many unanswered questions, including whether features of remodeling are related to an inexorable progression of acute or chronic airway inflammation or whether remodeling is a phenomenon separate from inflammation altogether (Figs. 4 and 5).

Research has confirmed that the airway epithelium is an active regulator of local events, and the relation between the airway epithelium and the subepithelial mesenchyma is believed to be a key determinant in the concept of airway remodeling. A hypothesis by Holgate and colleagues[20] proposes that airway epithelium in asthma functions in an inappropriate repair phenotype in which the epithelial cells produce proinflammatory mediators as well as transforming growth factor (TGF)-β to perpetuate remodeling. On the other hand, one of the most striking features reported in early detailed histopathologic studies of asthmatic lungs was the increased amount and size of submucosal vessels, and this has been repeatedly confirmed in other, more recent, reports.[17,19,21-24]

Although understanding of new vessel formation and its genesis in asthma is still in its early stages, it has been suggested that

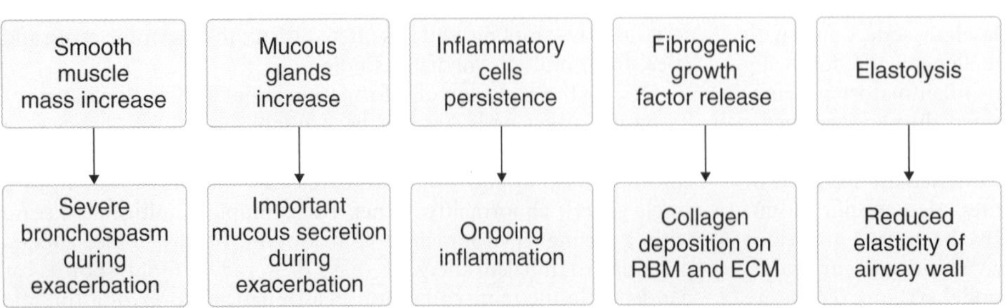

Figure 3 Clinical consequences of airway remodeling in asthma. RBM, respiratory bronchiolar mucosa; ECM, extracellular mucosa. *(Reproduced from Bousquet J, Jeffery PK, Busse WW, et al: Asthma: From bronchoconstriction to airways inflammation and remodeling. Am J Respir Crit Care Med 2000;161:1720-1745.)*

vascular remodeling may be a critical component in the pathophysiology of asthma and a determinant of asthma severity. Asosingh and colleagues showed that angiogenesis is a very early event, with onset during the initiation of acute airway inflammation in asthma.[21] It is linked to mobilization of bone marrow–derived endothelial progenitor cells, which, together with Th1 and Th2 cells, lead to a proangigogenic lung environment in asthma, which is sustained long after acute inflammation is resolved.[21] The enlarged airway vascular bed may contribute to the airflow limitation either through the vascular tissue's itself increasing airway wall thickness or through edema formation. Angiogenesis itself may play a role in the disease progression through recruitment of inflammatory cells, effects that alter airway physiology, or by secretion of proinflammatory mediators.

Exhaled Gases and Oxidative Stress

Asthma is characterized by specific biomarkers in expired air that reflect an altered airway redox chemistry, including lower levels of pH and increased reactive oxygen and nitrogen species during asthmatic exacerbations.[25-29] Reactive oxygen species (ROS) such as superoxide, hydrogen peroxide, and hydroxyl radicals cause inflammatory changes in the asthmatic airway. In support of this concept are the high levels of ROS and oxidatively modified proteins in airways of patients with asthma.[26] High levels of ROS are produced

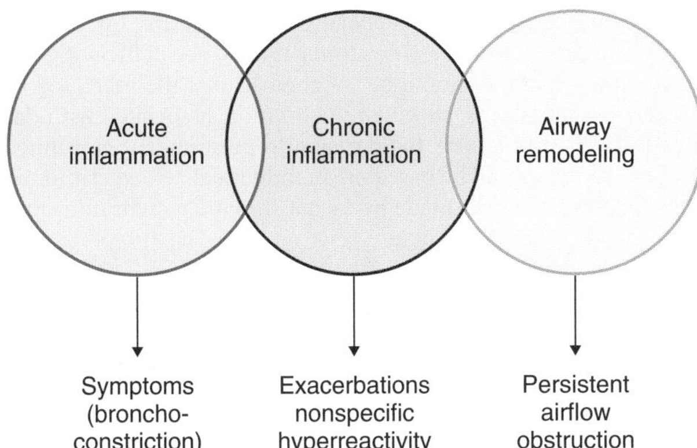

Figure 4 Links between pathologic mechanisms and clinical consequences in asthma. *(Reproduced from Bousquet J, Jeffery PK, Busse WW, et al: Asthma: From bronchoconstriction to airways inflammation and remodeling. Am J Respir Crit Care Med. 2000;161:1720-1745.)*

in the lungs of asthmatic patients by activated inflammatory cells (i.e., eosinophils, alveolar macrophages, and neutrophils).[27] The increased ROS production of neutrophils in asthmatic patients correlates with the severity of reactivity of airways in these patients; severe asthma is associated with neutrophilic airway infiltrates. Other investigators have measured products of arachidonic acid metabolism in exhaled breath condensate.[30] Specifically, 8-isoprostane, a PGF_{2a} analogue that is formed by peroxidation of arachidonic acid, is increased in patients with asthma of different severities, and leukotriene E_4 (LTE_4)-like immunoreactivity is increased in exhaled breath condensate of steroid-naïve patients who have mild asthma, with levels about threefold to fourfold higher than those in healthy subjects. Concomitant with increased oxidants, antioxidant protection of the lower airways is decreased in lungs of asthmatic patients.[28,29]

Another reactive species, nitric oxide (NO), is increased in the asthmatic airway.[26] Nitric oxide is produced by nitric oxide synthase (NOS), all isoforms of which—constitutive (neuronal, or type I, and endothelial, or type III enzymes) and inducible (type II enzymes)—are present in the lung. Abnormalities of NOS I and NOS II genotype and expression are associated with asthma. Recent studies have suggested cytotoxic consequences associated with tyrosine nitration induced by reaction products of NO.[31] Based on the high levels of NO in exhaled breath of asthmatics and the decrease of NO that occurs in response to treatment with corticosteroids, measurement of NO has been proposed as a noninvasive way to detect airway inflammation, diagnose asthma, and monitor the response to anti-inflammatory therapy.[32-34] The development of NHANES (National Health and Nutrition Examination Survey) normative levels for the fractional excretion of NO (FE_{NO}) will facilitate more widespread application of this exhaled gas measure in the clinical care of asthmatics.

The β-Agonist Controversy

Short-Acting β Agonists

Much controversy has surrounded the excessive or regular use of β-agonist preparations and the contention that this could lead to worsening of asthma control and pose a risk for untoward outcomes, including near-fatal and fatal episodes of asthma.

Several studies from New Zealand suggested that the use of inhaled β agonists increases the risk of death in severe asthma.[6,35-37] Spitzer and coworkers conducted a matched, case-controlled study using a health insurance database from Saskatchewan, Canada, of a cohort of 12,301 patients for whom asthma medications had been

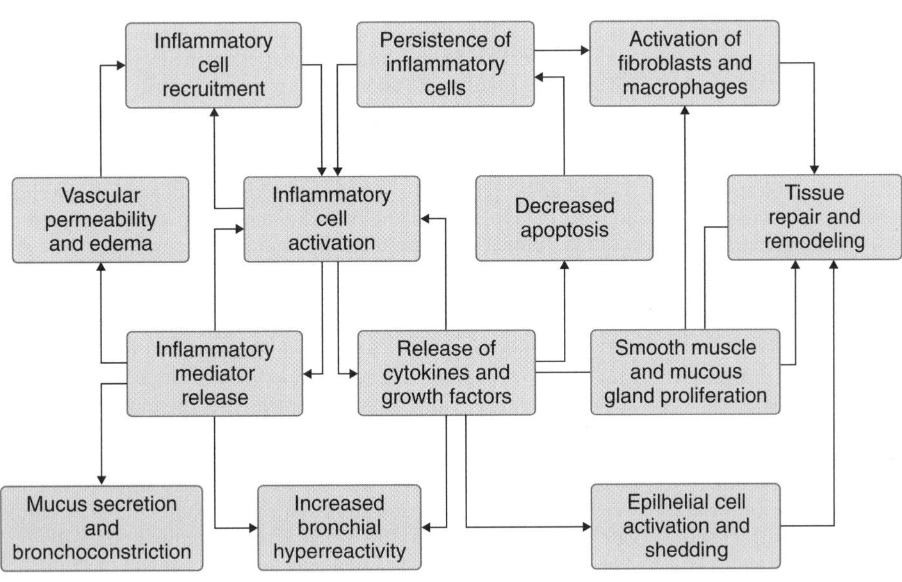

Figure 5 Mechanisms of acute and chronic inflammation in asthma and remodeling processes. *(Reproduced from Bousquet J, Jeffery PK, Busse WW, et al: Asthma: From bronchoconstriction to airways inflammation and remodeling. Am J Respir Crit Care Med 2000;161:1720-1745.)*

prescribed.[38] Data were based on matching 129 case patients who had fatal or near-fatal asthma with 655 controls. The use of a β agonist administered by a metered-dose inhaler (MDI) was associated with an increased risk of death from asthma, with an odds ratio of 5.4 per canister of fenoterol, 2.4 per canister of albuterol, and 1.0 for background risk (e.g., no fenoterol or albuterol). The primary limitation of these data, and a number of other case-controlled studies, relates to the comparability of cases and controls in terms of severity of their underlying disease.

Sears and coworkers conducted a placebo-controlled, crossover study in patients with mild stable asthma to evaluate the effects of regular versus on-demand inhaled fenoterol therapy for 24 weeks.[39] In the 57 patients who did better with one of the two regimens, only 30% had better asthma control when receiving regularly administered bronchodilators, whereas 70% had better asthma control when they employed the bronchodilators only as needed.

Drazen and coworkers randomly assigned 255 patients with mild asthma to inhaled albuterol either on a regular basis (two puffs four times per day) or on an as-needed basis for 16 weeks.[40] There were no significant differences between the two groups in a variety of outcomes, including morning peak expiratory flow, diurnal peak flow variability, forced expiratory volume in 1 second (FEV_1), number of puffs of supplemental as-needed albuterol, asthma symptoms, or airway reactivity to methacholine. Because neither benefit nor harm was seen, it was concluded that inhaled albuterol should be prescribed for patients with mild asthma on an as-needed basis.

A meta-analysis of pooled results from 22 randomized, placebo-controlled trials that studied at least 1 week of a regularly administered β_2 agonist in patients with asthma compared with a placebo group (that did not permit as-needed β_2-agonist use) concluded that regular use results in tolerance to bronchodilator and nonbronchodilator effects of the drug and may be associated with poorer disease control compared with placebo.

Long-Acting β Agonists

The Salmeterol Multiple-Center Asthma Research Trial (SMART) was an observational 28-week study comparing salmeterol 42 μg metered-dose inhaler twice a day with placebo, in addition to usual asthma therapies.[41] More than 26,000 subjects were enrolled.

SMART found that in the salmeterol group there was a statistically significant increase in risk for asthma-related deaths and life-threatening experiences compared with placebo. There were statistically significant differences for respiratory-related deaths (relative risk [RR], 2.16; 95% confidence interval [CI], 1.06-4.41) and asthma-related deaths (RR, 4.37; 95% CI, 1.25-15.34) and in combined asthma-related deaths or life-threatening experiences (RR, 1.71; 95% CI, 1.01-2.89) in subjects randomized to salmeterol compared with placebo. There were 13 asthma-related deaths and 37 combined asthma-related deaths or life-threatening experiences in the salmeterol group, compared with 3 and 22, respectively, in those randomized to placebo.

Of the 16 cases of asthma fatality in subjects enrolled in the study, 13 (81%) occurred in the initial phase of SMART, when subjects were recruited via print, radio, and television advertising; following this, subjects were recruited directly by investigators. These differences in outcomes occurred largely in African American subjects. In African Americans not taking ICS before randomization, salmeterol was associated with statistically significant increases in the risk for combined respiratory-related deaths or life-threatening experiences (RR, 5.61; 95% CI, 1.25-25.26) and combined asthma-related deaths or life-threatening experiences (RR, 10.46; 95% CI, 1.34-81.58).

Medication exposures were not tracked during the study, and allocation to ICS combined with a long-acting β agonist (LABA) was not randomized, so the effect of concomitant ICS use cannot be determined from these data. Whether the statistically significant risk in untoward outcomes reflects genetic predisposition, risk associated with LABA monotherapy, or health maintenance behavior cannot be determined definitively at this time. Based on findings of SMART, the U.S. Food and Drug Administration (FDA) issued a black box warning, public health advisory, and subsequent label changes for LABA and LABA-containing medications.

Data from SMART, combined with other recent reports,[42] have fueled a controversy regarding the role of LABAs in asthma management, such that an honest difference of opinion currently exists regarding the appropriate level of asthma severity at which regular use of LABA combined with ICS is favorable from a risk-to-benefit standpoint. This will require additional studies to fully clarify; however, asthma care providers should also be mindful that use of a LABA in combination with ICS has been associated with a range of favorable outcomes: reduction of symptoms (including nocturnal awakening), improvement in lung function, improvement in quality of life, reduced use of rescue medication, and reduced rate of exacerbations and severe exacerbations compared with ICS at the same or higher dose.[43]

Previously published meta-analyses have shown that low-dose ICS combined with LABA is associated with superior outcomes compared with higher-dose ICS.[44-46] These data led to the recommendation in the EPR-2 update of the NAEPP guidelines to prescribe the combination of ICS and LABA for patients with moderate persistent asthma and severe persistent asthma. The update categorized this management recommendation as based on level A evidence.[2] Based on safety concerns, the EPR-3 guidelines[5] recommend that medium-dose ICS be regarded as equivalent to adding LABA to low-dose ICS, and state "the established, beneficial effects of LABA for the great majority of patients who have asthma that is not sufficiently controlled with ICS alone should be weighed against the increased risk for severe exacerbations, although uncommon, associated with daily use of LABA." At this time, the decision to prescribe, or continue to prescribe, LABA should be based on an individualized determination of risk relative to benefit made by each asthmatic patient in partnership with his or her physician.

Pharmacogenetics

Polymorphisms of the $ADR\beta_2$ gene for the β_2-adrenergic receptor can influence clinical response to β agonists. For the *ADRB2*, single nucleotide polymorphisms (SNPs) have been defined at codons 16 and 27. The normal, or wild-type, pattern is arginine-16-glycine and glutamine-27-glutamic acid, but SNPs have been described with homozygous pairing (e.g., Gly16Gly, Arg16Arg, Glu27Glu, and Gln27Gln). The frequency of these polymorphisms is the same in the normal population as in asthmatics. Presence of a gene variant itself does not appear to influence baseline lung function.

In the presence of a polymorphism, the acute bronchodilator response to a β agonist, or protection from a bronchoconstrictor, may be affected. Studies indicate that in patients with Arg16Arg variant, the resulting β_2-adrenergic receptor is resistant to endogenous circulating catecholamines (i.e., receptor density and integrity are preserved), with a subsequent ability to produce an acute bronchodilator response to an agonist. In patients with Gly16Gly, the β_2-adrenergic receptor is downregulated by endogenous catecholamines; therefore, the acute bronchodilator response is reduced or blunted. In relation to prolonged β-agonist therapy (e.g., >2 weeks) patients who are homozygous for Arg16 were found to exhibit a decline in lung function and an increase in exacerbation rates in association with regular inhaled short-acting β agonists. These same patients, when switched to as-needed albuterol, had no decrease in lung function, as is the case for homozygous Gly16. Polymorphisms at the 27 loci are of unclear significance. Also, the impact of haplotypes (e.g., variant genes linked at >2 loci) is currently unclear. There are conflicting data regarding whether Arg/Arg homozygotes are prone to experience reflex morbidity with inhaled LABA,[43] but the weight of evidence, particularly from more-recent studies,[47,48] indicates that response to LABA when used in combination with ICS does not vary based on β_2-adrenergic genotypes at codon 16.

There are limited data on mutations involving the leukotriene cascade or corticosteroid metabolism. Polymorphisms of the 5-lipoxygenase (5-LO) gene promoter and the LTC_4 synthase gene *(LTC4S)* have been described. Asthmatics with the wild-type allele at 5-LO have a greater response with 5-LO inhibitor therapy compared with asthmatics with a mutant gene. However, mutations of the 5-LO gene promoter occur only in about 5% of asthmatic patients; for this reason, it is unlikely to play an important role in most patients. An SNP in *LTC4S* is associated with increased leukotriene production and has a lower response to leukotriene-modifying agents.

Far less is known about genetic variability in the corticosteroid pathway. Polymorphisms in the glucocorticoid receptor gene have been identified that appear to affect steroid binding and downstream pathways in various in vitro studies. However, polymorphisms in the glucocorticoid pathways have not been associated with the asthma phenotype or clinical steroid resistance.

DIAGNOSTIC EVALUATION, COMORBID DISEASE, AND PEAK EXPIRATORY FLOW MONITORING

The history and physical examination are important to confirm a diagnosis and exclude conditions such as hyperventilation syndrome, vocal cord adduction, heart failure, and others that can masquerade as asthma; to assess the severity of airflow obstruction and the need for aggressive intervention including inpatient management; to identify risk factors for poor outcomes; and to identify comorbid conditions that can make asthma refractory to treatment, including sinusitis, gastroesophageal reflux, and ongoing aeroallergen exposure.

The cardinal symptoms of asthma include chest tightness, wheezing, episodic dyspnea, and cough. Some patients present with atypical symptoms, such as cough alone (cough-equivalent asthma) or primarily dyspnea on exertion. The most objective indicator of asthma severity is the measurement of airflow obstruction by spirometry or peak expiratory flow (PEF). The FEV_1 and the PEF yield comparable results. For initial diagnostic purposes in most patients, spirometry rather than a simple PEF should be performed, although PEF may be a reasonable tool for long-term monitoring.

The NAEPP has set forth the grading of asthma severity into four categories based on frequency of daytime and nocturnal symptoms, peak flows, and as-needed use of inhaled short-acting β agonists: intermittent, mild persistent, moderate persistent, and severe persistent.[5] The mildest category, designated mild intermittent in EPR-2, was changed to intermittent in EPR-3 to emphasize that even patients with this level of asthma severity may have serious or even life-threatening asthma exacerbations.[5]

Hyperinflation, the most common finding on a chest radiograph, has no diagnostic or therapeutic significance. A chest radiograph should not be obtained unless complications of pneumonia, pneumothorax, or an endobronchial lesion are suspected. The correlation of severity between acute asthma and arterial blood gases is poor. Mild-to-moderate asthma is typically associated with respiratory alkalosis and mild hypoxemia on the basis of ventilation-perfusion mismatching. Severe hypoxemia is quite uncommon in asthma. Normocapnia and hypercapnia imply severe airflow obstruction, with FEV_1 usually less than 25% of the predicted value. Hypercapnia in the setting of acute asthma does not necessarily mandate intubation or suggest a poor prognosis.[49] Spirometry in an asthmatic patient typically shows obstructive ventilatory impairment with reduced expiratory flows that improve with bronchodilator therapy. Typically, there is an improvement in either FEV_1 or forced vital capacity (FVC) with acute administration of an inhaled bronchodilator (12% and 200 mL). However, the absence of a bronchodilator response does not exclude asthma. The shape of the flow volume loop can provide insight into the nature and location of airflow obstruction.

In patients with atypical chest symptoms of unclear etiology (cough or dyspnea alone), a variety of challenge tests can identify airway hyperreactivity as the cause of symptoms. By far, the most commonly used agents are methacholine or histamine, which give comparable results. Exercise, cold air, and isocapnic hyperventilation—other approaches that require complex equipment—have a lower sensitivity. In a patient with clinical features typical for asthma, along with reversible airflow obstruction, there is no need for a provocation procedure to establish a diagnosis. The use of measures of airway hyperreactivity has been proposed as a tool to guide anti-inflammatory therapy, but it is not recommended for routine clinical practice. The methacholine challenge test, which is most commonly used in the United States, is very sensitive; a positive test result is defined as a 20% decline in FEV_1 during incremental methacholine aerosolization. However, methacholine responsiveness is nonspecific, and it can occur in a variety of other conditions, including allergic rhinitis, chronic obstructive pulmonary disease, and airway infection. For practical purposes, a negative inhalation challenge with methacholine (or histamine) excludes active, symptomatic asthma. Measurement of FE_{NO} has been associated with a negative predictive value of 92%[50] for ruling out presence of asthma; however, additional studies are required for this more-convenient and less-costly test to supplant methacholine challenge, which is still regarded as the gold standard for the diagnosis of asthma.

PEF monitoring has been advocated as an objective measure of airflow obstruction in patients with chronic asthma. Despite a sound theoretical rationale for PEF monitoring, as advocated by all published asthma guidelines, clinical trials that examined the use of PEF monitoring in ambulatory asthma patients show conflicting results.[49] Over the past decade, 6 of 10 randomized trials have failed to show an advantage for the addition of PEF monitoring beyond symptom-based intervention for the control group.[51] Regular PEF monitoring allows early detection of worsening airflow obstruction, which may be of particular value in a subset of poor perceivers—persons with a blunted awareness of ventilatory impairment. PEF monitoring also has value for risk stratification. Excessive diurnal variation and a morning dip of PEF imply poor control and a need for careful re-evaluation of the management plan. PEF alone is never appropriate; rather, PEF should be part of a comprehensive patient education program.

ASTHMA MANAGEMENT ALGORITHMS

General Concepts Regarding Guidelines

There are many organizational and social barriers to optimal asthma care. Studies suggest that a small subset of patients uses a large percentage of health care resources. A major challenge in improving outcomes for asthma is implementing basic asthma management principles widely at the community level. Key issues include:

- Education of primary health care providers
- Education programs for asthma patients
- Longitudinal outpatient follow-up with easy access to providers
- Emphasis on chronic maintenance therapy rather than acute episodic care
- Emphasis on daily anti-inflammatory therapy

Organized approaches to improving care have included dissemination of clinical practice guidelines, disease state management, and case management.[52]

The thesis of disease state management is a global approach to chronic diseases such as asthma by integrating various components of the health care delivery system. It is hoped that managing all costs of care comprehensively, rather than seeking to minimize the costs of each component, will improve health outcomes and be cost beneficial. This approach relies on information technology to identify patients, monitor care, and assess outcomes and costs. Asthma is viewed as an ideal disease for the disease management approach because it is a chronic disease suitable for self-management and patient education; it can be managed largely on an outpatient basis, thus avoiding costly inpatient care; there is a consensus on what constitutes optimal care; and optimal care implementation can promptly lead to measurable reduction in costs and improved outcomes.

Although many studies have reported interventions that reduce costs and improve outcomes, there are limitations to published asthma disease management studies because a prestudy and poststudy design has typically been employed, usually with no control group; the choice of outcome measures varies; and several interventions have often been performed at the same time and it is difficult to identify the essential components linked with success. These studies have often used proprietary data systems and algorithms that make reproducing them difficult. Other design limitations include control of cofactors such as severity and season.

Practice Guidelines

Guidelines for medical practice have been disseminated for a wide range of conditions. The overall goal of practice guidelines is to improve quality of care, reduce costs, and enhance health care outcomes. These guidelines are of interest to many groups including specialty medical societies, state and federal government, insurers and managed care organizations, commercial enterprises, and hospitals. Possible mechanisms by which practice guidelines can improve patient care include improved clinician knowledge, encouraging clinicians to agree with and accept the guidelines as standard of care, and influencing clinician asthma care behavior.

There is limited evidence, however, that practice guidelines achieve favorable clinical outcomes.[53] Some clinicians have advocated additional strategies to include removing disincentives, adding a variety of incentives, and including the guidelines in a broader program that addresses translation, dissemination, and implementation in the local community.

Asthma Practice Guidelines: Expert Panel Report 3

In 1991, the coordinating committee of NAEPP, along with the NHLBI, convened an expert panel to develop extensive and detailed guidelines for the diagnosis and management of asthma.[1] The EPR-2 was published in 1997[2] and EPR-3 guidelines were released in 2007.[5] Overall, the published guidelines highlight the significant role of airway inflammation in the pathogenesis of asthma, an emphasis on the role of anti-inflammatory maintenance therapy for persistent asthma, and a focus on establishing risk factors for the development of asthma and identifying appropriate programs for control and prevention.

The NAEPP outlined four goals of therapy for asthma: maintain normal activity level, including exercise; maintain near-normal parameters of pulmonary function; prevent chronic and troublesome exacerbations of asthma by maintaining a chronic baseline maintenance therapy; and avoid untoward effects of medications used to treat asthma. To facilitate these goals, the NAEPP outlined a number of key components for management. First, patient education and self-management skills are critical. This education includes knowledge of the disease, proper use of medications, including appropriate metered-dose inhaler technique, and a written action plan for managing exacerbations. A second component involves measures to minimize or avoid exposure to clinically relevant aeroallergens and irritants that can exacerbate asthma. A third component is pharmacotherapy.

The NAEPP guidelines recommend that asthma should be managed in an algorithmic manner, based on asthma severity; EPR-3 guidelines introduced the concept of asthma control and its importance in management. Patients are to be classified as having intermittent, mild persistent, moderate persistent, or severe persistent asthma, based on assessment of the level of symptoms (day or night), reliance on reliever medication, and lung function at time of presentation, with pharmacologic management (see later) then being prescribed in an evidence-based fashion according to each respective categorization. In an ideal world, this recommendation, described in EPR-2 would have resulted in patients with asthma receiving pharmacotherapeutic agents associated with favorable asthma care outcomes that are also appropriate from both cost and risk-to-benefit standpoints. In the real world, however, this paradigm was imperfect, because it relied on the correct categorization of patients for pharmacotherapy to be prescribed appropriately. Both health care providers and patients are prone to underestimate asthma severity,[54] and for this reason, many patients managed based on this paradigm were undertreated.

A new paradigm was proposed in EPR-3 guidelines, based on the assessment of asthma control.[55] Asthma severity and asthma control are not synonymous. Asthma severity is clearly a determinant of asthma control, but its impact is affected by a variety of factors, including patterns of therapeutic adherence and the degree to which recommended avoidance measures for clinically relevant aeroallergens are pursued. Patterns of health service use, including hospitalization and emergency department visits, correlate more closely with asthma control than with asthma severity.[55] This follows from the understanding that a patient with severe persistent asthma who is treated appropriately with multiple controllers and who adheres to orders regarding medications and recommended avoidance strategies can achieve well-controlled (or totally controlled) asthma. This patient will not require hospitalization or emergency department management, will not miss school or work days, and will not experience nocturnal awakening or limitation in routine activities because of asthma. This patient has *severe persistent asthma that is well controlled.* In contrast, a patient with mild-persistent to moderate-persistent asthma who either does not receive appropriate instructions for avoidance measures and controller medications, or both, or who is poorly adherent to therapy, will likely have poor control of asthma. This patient is more likely to require hospitalization or emergency department management, miss school or work days, and experience nocturnal awakening or limitation in routine activities because of asthma. This patient has *mild-to-moderate persistent asthma that is poorly controlled.*

Another limitation of EPR-2 was that the categorization of asthma severity was proposed at a time before long-term therapy was initiated; however, many patients are already taking controller medications when they are initially seen. EPR-3 guidelines[5] stipulate that the asthma severity level can be *inferred*, based upon response, or lack thereof, to asthma pharmacotherapy. This concept, *responsiveness*, is defined as the ease with which asthma control can be achieved by therapy.

EPR-3 guidelines recommend that asthma should be categorized based on level of severity at the initial visit, and at subsequent visits the focus of providers should be on asthma control (Fig. 6). At the initial visit, severity is assigned based on assessment of both impairment and risk domains, as illustrated in Table 1, for patients who are not taking regular controller medication, and for patients on regular pharmacotherapy for asthma.

For all patients with asthma, regardless of severity classification, the goal of asthma management as described in EPR-3[5] is the same: to achieve control by reducing both impairment and risk (see Table 2). The impairment domain is focused on the present and entails assessments of frequency and intensity of asthma symptoms, functional limitation, lung function, and meeting expectations of, and satisfaction with, asthma treatment. The risk domain is focused on the future and includes preventing asthma exacerbations and severe exacerbations, minimizing the need for using health services (emergency department visits or hospitalization), reducing the tendency for progressive decline in lung function, and providing pharmacotherapy that offers minimal or no risk for untoward effects. The impairment and risk domains might respond differently to treatment.

Asthma control is a multidimensional construct. Asthma control can be assessed by use of validated instruments, including the Asthma

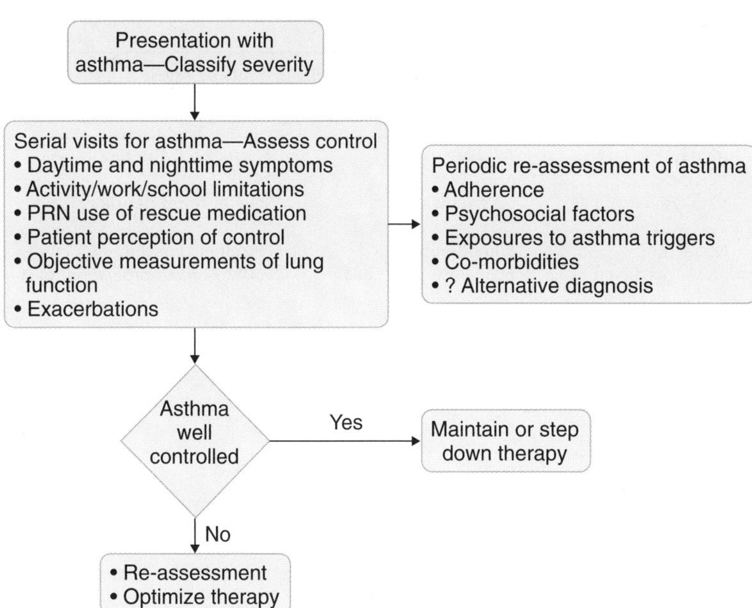

Figure 6 **Revised paradigm for asthma management.** *(Modified from Li JT, Oppenheimer J, Bernstein IL, et al: Attaining optimal asthma control: A practice parameter. J Allergy Clin Immunol 2005;116: S3-S11.*

Table 1 Categorization of Asthma Severity According to Impairment and Risk Domains

Components of Severity		Classification of Asthma Severity ≥12 Years of Age			
			Persistent		
		Intermittent	Mild	Moderate	Severe
Impairment	Symptoms	≤2 days/wk	>2 days/wk but not daily	Daily	Throughout the day
Normal FEV1/FVC: 8-19 yr: 85% 20-39 yr: 80% 40-59 yr: 75% 60-80 yr: 70%	Nighttime awakenings	≤2×/mo	3-4×/mo	>1×/wk but not nightly	Often 7/wk
	Short-acting $\beta_2$agonist use for symptom control (not prevention of EIB)	≤2 days/wk	>2 days/wk but not daily and not >1× on any day	Daily	Several times per day
	Interference with normal activity	None	Minor limitation	Some limitation	Extremely limited
	Lung function	Normal FEV_1 between exacerbations			
		FEV_1>80% predicted	FEV_1>80% predicted	FEV_1>60% but <80% predicted	FEV_1<60% predicted
		FEV_1/FVC normal	FEV_1/FVC normal	FEV_1/FVC reduced 5%	FEV_1/FVC reduced >5%
Risk	Exacerbations requiring oral systemic corticosteroids	0-1/yr*	≥2/yr*	≥2/yr*	≥2/yr*
Recommend Step for initiating treatment		Step 1	Step 2	Step 3†	Step 4 or 5†

*Consider severity and interval since last exacerbation. Frequency and severity may fluctuate over time for patients in any severity category. Relative annual risk of exacerbations may be related to FEV_1.

†And consider a short course of oral systemic corticosteroids.

EIB, exercise-induced bronchospasm; FEV_1, forced expiratory volume in 1 sec; FVC, forced vital capacity.

Adapted from National Heart, Lung, and Blood Institute: Guidelines for the Diagnosis and Management of Asthma (EPR-3) (available at http://www.nhlbi.nih.gov/guidelines/asthma/index.htm).

Control Questionnaire (ACQ), Asthma Therapy Assessment Questionnaire (ATAQ), and the Asthma Control Test (ACT). These instruments include assessment of asthma symptoms, frequency of use of as-needed rescue medication, the impact of asthma on everyday functioning, and, in the case of the ACQ, the impact of asthma on lung function. The ACT is highlighted herein as an example of a validated instrument that can be used in routine asthma management as a gauge of asthma control. The ACT is reliable and responsive to asthma control over time.[56,57] The process of accomplishing the ACT entails a patient's accurately responding to five questions (using a 1-5 scale) pertaining to the previous 4 weeks: activity restriction at work, school, or home; frequency of shortness of breath episodes; frequency of nocturnal awakening; as-needed use of rescue bronchodilator; and overall assessment of asthma control. The lowest possible score is 5 and the highest possible is 25. The higher the score, the better the control of asthma; however, using a cut point of 19 yields the best balance of sensitivity (71%) and specificity (71%) for classifying asthma as poorly controlled or well controlled.[57] Use of

Table 2 Classification of Asthma Control by Impairment and Risk Domains

	Components of Control	Classification of Asthma Control ≥12 Years of Age: Well Controlled	Not Well Controlled	Very Poorly Controlled
Impairment	Symptoms	≤2 days/wk	>2 days/wk	Throughout the day
	Nighttime awakenings	≤2×/mo	1-3×/wk	≥4×
	Short-acting β_2 agonist use for symptom control (not prevention of EIB)	≤2 days/wk	>2 days/wk	Several times per day
	Interference with normal activity	None	Some limitation	Extremely limited
	FEV_1 or peak flow	>80% predicted	60%-80% predicted	<60% predicted/personal best
	Validated Questionnaires*			
	ATAQ	0	1-2	3-4
	ACQ	≤0.75	≥1.5	N/A
	ACT	≥20	16-19	≤5
Risk	Exacerbations requiring oral systemic steroids	0-1/yr	≥2/yr[†]	≥2/yr[†]
	Progessive loss of lung function	Evaluation requires long-term follow-up care.		
	Treatment-related adverse effects	Medication side effects can vary in intensity from none to very troublesome and worrisome. The level of intensity does not correlate to specific levels of control but should be considered in the overall assessment of risk.		

*ATAQ = Asthma Therapy Assessment Questionnaire; ACQ = Asthma control Questionnaire; ACT = Asthma Control Test.
[†]Consider severity and interval since last exacerbation.
Adapted from National Heart, Lung, and Blood Institute: Guidelines for the Diagnosis and Management of Asthma (EPR-3) (available at http://www.nhlbi.nih.gov/guidelines/asthma/index.htm).

serial ACT scores in asthma management can objectify the degree to which the goals of management as described in NAEPP guidelines are being achieved, which can encourage optimal asthma care outcomes. A randomized, controlled trial demonstrated that asthma management guided by assessment of asthma control leads to improved control of asthma over time.[58]

The current paradigm for asthma management (see Fig 6), recommends that asthma care providers categorize asthma severity at the initial visit based on the criteria mentioned earlier, and subsequent visits should proceed with assessment of asthma control. If asthma is well controlled (ACT = 20), the provider, in collaboration with the patient, may consider maintaining current management or a step down. If asthma is not well controlled, it is appropriate to step up management or carry out an assessment to determine whether factors such as poor adherence or a comorbid condition is present that is complicating response to therapy. If asthma is not well-controlled, data indicate that such patients are at elevated risk for exacerbation of asthma, and on this basis they are clearly candidates for intervention.[59]

Although the concept of expert practice guidelines that have become increasingly evidence based merits widespread support, specific treatment regimens must be determined by the physician and patient based on consideration of risk relative to benefit and tailored to individual patient needs. Because asthma research is rapidly evolving and new pharmacotherapeutics are anticipated, continued periodic revision of guidelines for asthma can be anticipated.

Allergy, Allergen Avoidance, and Allergen Immunotherapy

Sensitization to inhalant allergens such as dust mites; mold spores; cat, dog, or other animal proteins; cockroach and other insect allergens; and outdoor pollens is common among asthmatic patients. The 1997 Expert Panel Report 2: Guidelines for the Diagnosis and Management of Asthma differed from the 1991 Expert Panel Report in recommending cutaneous or in vitro testing "for at least those patients with persistent asthma exposed to perennial indoor allergens."[1,2] EPR-3 guidelines[5] point out that "sensitivity to a perennial indoor allergen is usually not possible with a patient's medical history alone."

Box 1 Inhalant Allergens

- Dust mites
- Trees
- Cockroaches
- Grass
- Pets (cats, dogs, etc.)
- Ragweed and other weeds
- Mold spores

Clinical relevance of inhalant allergens can be demonstrated by immediate hypersensitivity skin testing or radioallergosorbent (RAST) assay. Of these, skin testing is more sensitive, is less costly, and entails no delay in yielding results; for these reasons, skin testing is preferred. The information that these diagnostic tests provide, whether the asthmatic patient exhibits IgE-mediated (allergic) potential to inhalant allergens, and which allergens the patient can be said to be allergic to, is used to direct relevant avoidance measures. EPR-3[5] also recommends that diagnostic allergy testing may be indicated for "selected patients who have asthma at any level of severity ... as a basis for education about the role of allergens for avoidance and for immunotherapy." Avoidance of clinically relevant allergens can lead to substantial reduction of symptoms and medication reliance, and for some patients this can be the most important element of asthma management. The inhalant allergens that can provoke and perpetuate asthma symptoms are listed in Box 1. Persons with asthma are usually sensitized to more than one allergen.

Air conditioning can be associated with a dramatic reduction in exposures to outdoor pollens and mold spores while indoors. Because we now spend the majority of our time indoors,[60] the usefulness of air conditioning for improving asthma symptoms should not be underestimated.

Dust mites are microscopic, and they rely on heat and humidity to survive and proliferate.[61] Allergy to dust mites is common in patients with asthma. Recommended avoidance measures to reduce exposures to dust mite allergen include encasing the mattress, box spring, and pillows in impermeable covers; reducing indoor relative humidity; washing bedding weekly in the hot cycle (130°F);

and, if possible, removing carpets in favor of tiled or hardwood flooring.[61]

For patients who are allergic to cat or dog dander and who own pets, no avoidance strategy can rival the benefit that will occur with eliminating the pet from the home. If a cat or dog is removed from the home, however, the allergen can persist for several months. For this reason, clinical benefit cannot be expected promptly.[62] When it is not possible to eliminate pets from the homee, second-best measures include restricting the pet from the bedroom, using high-efficiency particulate or electrostatic air cleaners, and removing carpets and other furnishings that otherwise serve as an allergen reservoir. Washing the cat or dog, if recommended as an avoidance strategy, needs to be carried out frequently—at least twice a week.[63]

When a regimen of avoidance measures combined with appropriate pharmacotherapy is undesirable, not feasible, or ineffective to achieve optimal asthma control, administration of allergen immunotherapy vaccines (allergy shots) can be considered.[64,65] As shown in Figure 7, the EPR-3 guidelines recommend considering allergen immunotherapy for patients who have mild or moderate persistent asthma (steps 2-4) and who have a clinically relevant component of allergic potential to inhalant allergens. Allergen immunotherapy entails the incremental administration of inhalant allergens for the purpose of inducing immune system changes in the host response with natural exposure to these allergens. Numerous studies carried out since 1954 have shown statistically and clinically significant dose-dependent benefits with administration of allergen immunotherapy in properly selected patients with asthma.[64]

The immunologic changes that develop with administration of allergen immunotherapy are complex. Successful immunotherapy results in generation of a population of $CD4^+/CD25^+$ T lymphocytes producing IL-10 and/or TGF-β. Allergen immunotherapy has been shown to block the immediate and late-phase allergic response; decrease recruitment of mast cells, basophils, and eosinophils upon provocation or natural exposure to allergens in the skin, nose, eye, and bronchial mucosa; blunt the seasonal rise in specific IgE; and suppress late-phase inflammatory responses in the skin and respiratory tract.[66] However, the efficacy of immunotherapy in relation to these immunologic changes is not completely understood.

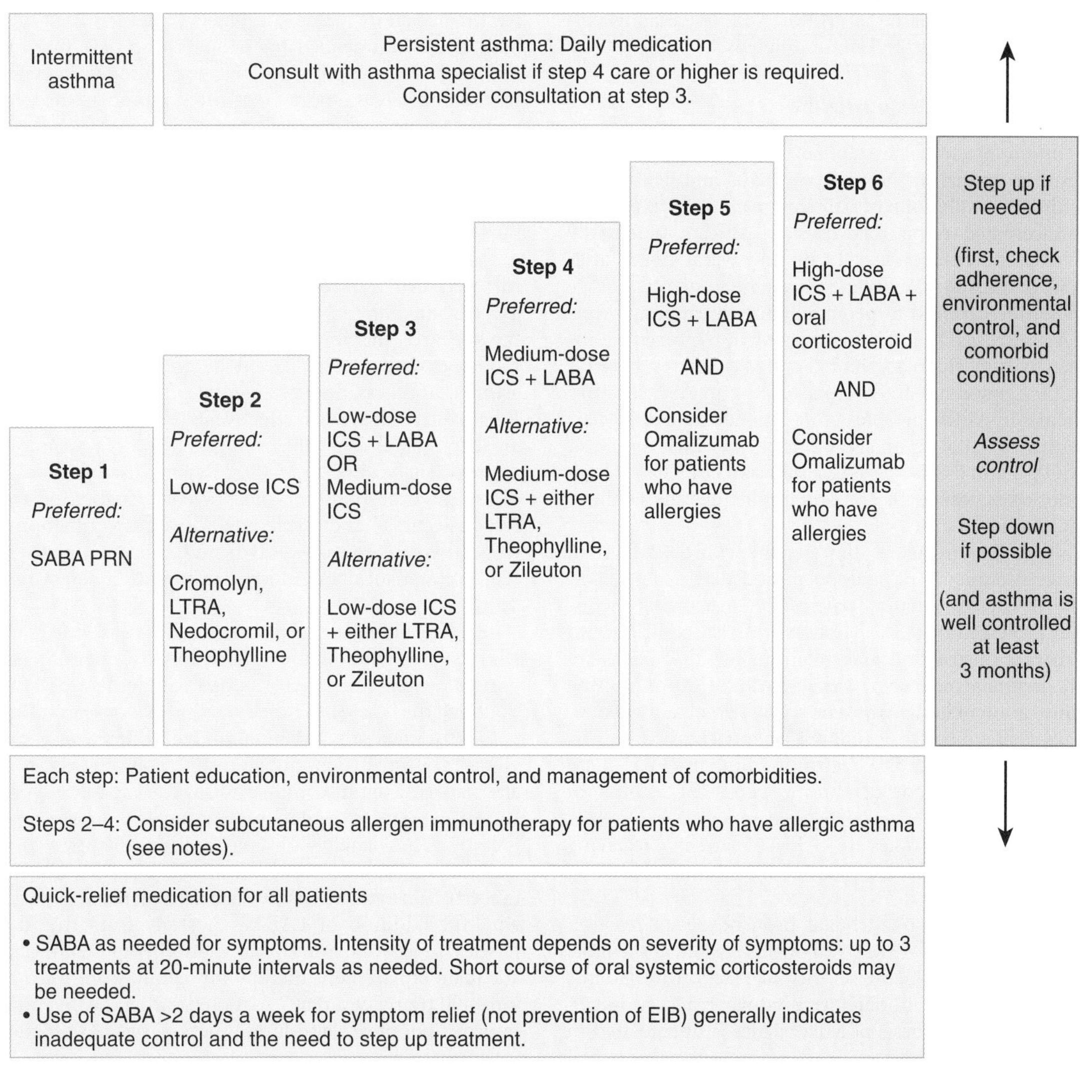

Figure 7 **Stepwise treatment approach for managing asthma in adults and children older than 12 years.** EIB, exercise-induced bronchospasm; ICS, inhaled corticosteroids; LABA, long-acting β agonists; LTRA, leukotriene receptor antagonists; SABA,short-acting β agonists. *(Adapted from National Heart, Lung, and Blood Institute: Guidelines for the Diagnosis and Management of Asthma (EPR-3). Available at http://www.nhlbi.nih.gov/guidelines/asthma/index.htm.)*

In contrast to medication that affects only symptoms, immunotherapy can favorably affect the disease process that underlies asthma symptoms. Numerous randomized, double-blind, placebo-controlled trials have shown that allergen immunotherapy is associated with benefit for reducing symptoms and reducing reliance on medication.[66] A meta-analysis of 75 randomized, placebo-controlled studies confirmed the effectiveness of immunotherapy in asthma, with a significant reduction in asthma symptoms and medication, and with improvement in bronchial hyperreactivity.[67]This meta-analysis included 36 trials for dust mites, 20 for pollens, and 10 for animal dander. Immunotherapy is efficacious for pollen, mold, dust mite, cockroach, and animal allergens; however, its effectiveness is more established for dust mite, animal dander, and pollen allergens, because fewer studies have been published demonstrating efficacy using mold and cockroach allergens.

In the United States, 7 to 10 million immunotherapy injections are administered annually. Because systemic reactions are not uncommon, immunotherapy should be given only in a setting in which adequate precautions are taken and life-threatening anaphylaxis can be treated.[55] The decision to begin allergen immunotherapy should be individualized and based on severity of symptoms, relative benefit with pharmacotherapy, and whether the patient has comorbid conditions such as cardiovascular conditions or is using beta blockers.[68] These factors increase the risk for (serious) anaphylaxis, which is the major risk of allergen immunotherapy.

Aspirin Intolerance and Desensitization

Aspirin (ASA) and nonsteroidal anti-inflammatory drugs (NSAIDs) can provoke bronchospasm (with or without nasal and ocular congestion or flushing) in a subgroup of asthmatic patients.[69] In patients with aspirin-exacerbated respiratory disease (AERD), potentially serious bronchospastic reaction occurs up to several hours after exposure to ASA or an ASA-like drug; even a subtherapeutic dosage of ASA in this setting can lead to potentially life-threatening bronchospasm. ASA and NSAIDs, including ibuprofen, naproxen, sulindac, indomethacin, and etodolac, inhibit cyclooxygenases 1 and 2 (COX-1 and COX-2) and are 100% cross-reactive in ASA-sensitive asthmatic patients. In AERD patients, cross-reaction can also occur with higher doses of salsalate or acetaminophen, which are weak inhibitors of COX-1 and COX-2. Selective inhibitors of COX-2 (e.g., celecoxib) do not cross-react with ASA and can be tolerated without bronchospastic reaction.[69]

COX inhibition downregulates the enzyme PGE_2, leading, in turn, to excessive production of sulfidopeptide leukotrienes (LTC_4, LTD_4, and LTE_4). These mediators participate in acute bronchospastic reaction provoked by ASA ingestion and also contribute to the ongoing airways obstruction and inflammation that persist in AERD patients despite avoidance of ASA and other COX-inhibiting drugs.[69] Administration of antileukotriene agents, which either selectively block leukotriene receptors or inhibit leukotriene synthesis by blocking 5-LO or its activator, 5-LO activating protein (FLAP), are efficacious in the management of chronic persistent asthma in patients with AERD. Added benefit has been reported in double-blind, placebo-controlled studies in AERD patients receiving inhaled (and oral) corticosteroids treated with montelukast[70] or zileuton.[71]

Antileukotriene agents also attenuate bronchospastic reaction provoked by ASA challenge in AERD.[72,73] For this reason, antileukotriene drugs are useful for reducing severity of reaction in patients undergoing desensitization, although respiratory reaction is not blocked completely.[69] Biosynthesis of leukotrienes is upregulated in AERD; a key enzyme, LTC_4 synthase, is overexpressed in bronchial mucosa.[69] AERD patients have increased expression of the Cys-LT_1 receptor on inflammatory leukocytes,[74] thereby enhancing their ability to respond to leukotrienes. Downregulation of Cys-LT_1 receptor expression might explain the mechanism for benefit with ASA desensitization treatment.[74]

Desensitization can be performed for patients who require administration of ASA or ASA-like drugs for management of co-occurring conditions (e.g., arthritis, thromboembolism, or coronary artery disease). Clinical benefit in patients with AERD—particularly for polypoid rhinosinusitis—was observed in 87% of patients who were desensitized and then took ASA regularly for more than 1 year.[75] Improvement included reduced level of symptoms, lower reliance on medication, and less morbidity (as reflected in fewer annual episodes of upper respiratory infection or sinusitis and reduced rates of sinus surgery procedures). Based on these findings and previous experience with ASA desensitization[50] this intervention can also be considered for patients with corticosteroid dependency, poorly controlled asthma, or refractory rhinosinusitis who require repeated sinus surgery procedures. Because of potentially serious bronchospastic reaction that can occur during desensitization, this procedure should only be carried out in settings with experienced physicians and appropriate equipment to treat such reactions.

Pharmacotherapy

The pharmacotherapy for asthma, as recommended by current NAEPP guidelines, is summarized in Figure 7 and Tables 3 through 5. The overall strategy is a stepwise approach based on level of severity. Inhaled short-acting β agonists (relievers) used on an as-needed basis are recommended for patients who have intermittent asthma and who are asymptomatic between episodes. Patients with persistent asthma, with more frequent symptoms, are treated with the addition of an anti-inflammatory agent (controller) used on a scheduled basis in addition to an inhaled short-acting β agonist on an as-needed basis. For patients with more-severe disease and during acute exacerbations, addition of oral corticosteroids as a short-term burst is appropriate.

Inhaled Corticosteroids. With the current paradigm of asthma as a chronic inflammatory disorder of the airways, ICS have become the preferred therapy for all patients with persistent asthma—mild, moderate, and severe. Recent data indicate that ICS do not cure asthma, and cessation of therapy often results in prompt relapse. Inhaled steroids are cost effective in the management of asthma, with an incremental cost-effectiveness ratio for a symptom-free day of approximately $5.00 to $6.00.[76] Regular use of ICS can reduce rates of asthma exacerbation[77] and prevent increases in bronchial hyperresponsiveness[78] and accelerated loss of lung function.[14] A large retrospective case-control study from Canada associated regular use of ICS with statistically significant reductions in rates of mortality from asthma.[79]

Evidence indicates that patients with moderate persistent asthma who remain symptomatic on low-dose ICS monotherapy experience greater benefit from LABA added to low-dose ICS compared with doubling the dose of ICS.[43] Several studies have examined the usefulness of ICS taken in combination with other agents such as theophylline[80] and leukotriene antagonists.[81] These agents are also a rational alternative, taken in combination with ICS, to doubling the dose of ICS in patients who remain symptomatic on low-dose ICS monotherapy. The benefits of combination therapy—as measured by symptom scores, as-needed use of β agonists, lung function, and exacerbation rates—with these other agents are not as dramatic as with the addition of LABA.[82] A study from the Asthma Clinical Research Network found that monotherapy with salmeterol is not adequate replacement therapy for asthma controlled on triamcinolone 400 μg twice a day.[83] As noted earlier, LABA monotherapy can improve symptoms and lung function, but has no effect on airways inflammation.[43]

The molecular mechanism of action of glucocorticoids involves binding to a specific intracellular glucocorticoid receptor (GCR). This binding dissociates heat-shock proteins and creates an active glucocorticoid and receptor (GC-GCR) complex. The GC-GCR complex translocates to the nucleus and binds to specific GCR-

Table 3 Usual Dosages for Long-Term-Control Medications

Medication	Dosage Form	Adult Dose	Child Dose
Inhaled Corticosteroids (See Estimated Comparative Daily Dosages for Inhaled Corticosteroids—Table 4)			
Systemic Corticosteroids			
Methylprednisolone	2,4,8,16, and 32 mg tabs	7.5-60 mg qd in a single dose in A.M. or qod as needed for control	0.25-2 mg/kg qd in single dose in A.M. or qod as needed for control
Prednisolone	5 mg tabs, 5 mg/5 mL, 15 mg/5 mL	Short-course burst to achieve control: 40-60 mg/d as single or two divided doses for 3-10 d (with/without taper)	Short-course burst: 1-2 mg/kg/d, max 60 mg/d for 3-10 d
Prednisone	1, 2.5, 5, 10, 20, and 50 mg tabs; 5 mg/mL, 5 mg/mL	Short-course burst to achieve control: 40-60 mg/d as single or two divided doses for 3-10 d (with/without taper)	Short-course burst: 1-2 mg/kg/d, max 60 mg/d for 3-10 d
Long-Acting Inhaled β_2 Agonists *(Should Not Be Used for Symptom Relief or for Exacerbations; Use with Inhaled Corticosteroids)*			
Salmeterol	MDI, 21 µg/puff	2 puffs q12hr	1-2 puffs q12hr
	DPI, 50 µg/blister	1 blister q12hr	1 blister q12hr
Formoterol	DPI, 12 µg/single-use capsule	1 capsule q12hr	1 capsule q12hr
Combined Medication			
Fluticasone/Salmeterol			
Fluticasone/Salmeterol	DPI 100, 250, or 500 µg/50 µg	1 inhalation bid; dose depends on severity of asthma	1 inhalation bid; dose depends on severity of asthma
Budesonide/ Formoterol		2 puffs bid; dose depends on severity of asthma	2 puffs bid; dose depends on severity of asthma
Cromolyn and Nedocromil			
Cromolyn	MDI, 1 mg/puff nebulizer MDI, 20 mg/ampule	2-4 puffs tid-qid 1 ampule tid-qid	1-2 puffs tid-qid 1 ampule tid-qid
Nedocromil	MDI, 1.75 mg/puff	2-4 puffs bid-qid	1-2 puffs bid-qid
Leukotriene Modifiers			
Montelukast	4 or 5 mg chewable tab, 10 mg tab	10 mg qhs	2-5 yr: 4 mg qhs 6-14 yr: 5 mg qhs >14 yr: 10 mg qhs
Zafirlukast	10 or 20 mg tab	40 mg qd (20 mg tab bid)	7-11 yr: 20 mg qd (10 mg tab bid)
Zileuton	300 or 600 mg tablet	2400 mg daily (give tabs qid)	
Methylxanthines (Serum monitoring is important [serum concentration of 5-15 µg/mL at steady state]).			
Theophylline	Liquids, sustained-release tabs, caps	Starting dose 10 mg/kg/day up to 300 mg max; usual max 800 mg/day	Starting dose 10 mg/kg/day Usual max: <1 yr: 0.2 × (age in wk) + 5 = mg/kg/day >1 yr: 16 mg/kg/day

cap, capsule; DPI, dry powder inhaler; max, maximum; MDI, metered-dose inhaler; qod, every other day; tab, tablet.
Data from the National Asthma Education and Prevention Program.[5]

responsive elements on genomic DNA that induce specific gene expression (i.e., β-adrenergic receptors). The GC-GCR complex might also suppress gene expression by interfering with the interaction of transcription factors (i.e., nuclear factor-κB) with promoter regions of proinflammatory cytokines. Through these mechanisms, glucocorticoids inhibit the production of a wide range of cytokines important in asthma. In addition to inhibiting cytokine production, glucocorticoids also inhibit production of inflammatory leukotrienes and eicosanoids through effects on phospholipase A_2. In contrast, genes for anti-inflammatory or bronchodilatory products (i.e., β receptors and lipocortin) are increased by corticosteroids. Lipocortin, a protein that inhibits phospholipase A_2, further dampens inflammation.

The concept of resistance to corticosteroids has received much attention, although the exact molecular mechanisms remain poorly understood. There is likely only one type of human glucocorticoid receptor; therefore, polymorphisms of the human steroid receptor have not been established. Two discrete types of relative steroid resistance have been described. Type 1 steroid resistance is a relative lack of steroid responsiveness in the airways, although there is evidence for steroid effect in other tissues of the body, usually manifesting as clinical steroid side effects (i.e., cushingoid effects). Type 1 steroid resistance is acquired and more common. Type 2 steroid resistance is caused by a generalized lack of steroid responsiveness in the airways and other organ systems on a genetic basis. Patients with type 2 resistance have poor asthma control despite systemic corticoste-

Table 4 Estimated Comparative Daily Dosages for Inhaled Corticosteroids

	Low Daily Dose		Medium Daily Dose		High Daily Dose	
Drug	**Adult**	**Child***	**Adult**	**Child***	**Adult**	**Child***
Beclomethasone CFC 42 or 84 µg/puff	168-504 µg	84-336 µg	504-804 µg	336-672 µg	>840 µg	>672 µg
Beclomethasone HFA 40 or 80 µg/puff	80-240 µg	80-160 µg	240-480 µg	160-320 µg	>480 µg	>320 µg
Budesonide DPI 200 µg/inhalation	200-600 µg	200-400 µg	600-1,200 µg	400-800 µg	>1200 µg	>800 µg
Budesonide inhalation suspension for nebulization (child dose)		0.5 mg		1.0 mg		2.0 mg
Flunisolide 250 µg/puff	500-1000 µg	500-750 µg	1000-2000 µg	1000-1250 µg	>2000 µg	>1250 µg
Fluticasone MDI: 44, 110, or 220 µg/puff	88-264 µg	88-176 µg	264-660 µg	176-440 µg	>660 µg	>440 µg
Fluticasone DPI: 50, 100, or 250 µg/inhalation	100-300 µg	100-200 µg	300-600 µg	200-400 µg	>600 µg	>400 µg
Triamcinolone acetonide 100 µg/puff	400-1000 µg	400-800 µg	1000-2000 µg	800-1,200 µg	>2000 µg	>1200 µg

*Children ≤12 years of age.
CFC, chlorofluorocarbon [propellant]; DPI, dry powder inhaler; HFA, hydrofluoroalkane [propellant]; MDI, metered-dose inhaler.
Data from the National Asthma Education and Prevention Program.[5]

roids and no systemic steroid side effects. Type 2 steroid resistance is rare. The relative contribution of this concept of steroid resistance in suboptimal asthma control and poor outcomes remains unknown. Patients with such a molecular basis for steroid resistance may be a subset who would benefit from alternative anti-inflammatory approaches.

Steroid "phobia," or excess concern over the systemic effects of ICS by both patients and clinicians, remains a barrier to wider use of these agents despite several reassuring long-term studies and recommendations from evidence-based practice guidelines. One landmark study[84] included 1041 children from ages 5 years through 12 years with mild-to-moderate asthma for a study duration of 4 to 6 years. The children were randomized into three groups: 200 µg of budesonide twice a day, 8 mg of nedocromil (Tilade) twice a day, or placebo. This robust study noted that the asthma clinical outcomes improved most for the budesonide group (fewer hospitalizations, fewer urgent visits, and decreased airway hyperresponsiveness to methacholine). However, there was no significant difference in the degree of change in FEV_1 after bronchodilator use among any of the three groups. Long-term budesonide was well tolerated, and although there was a 1.1 cm smaller increase in height compared with the placebo group during the first year, this reduction in linear growth velocity was absent by the second year, and the projected height in the budesonide-treated group was no different than in the nedocromil or placebo groups. Also, there were no significant differences in bone density or the incidence of cataracts between the three groups. Although a number of other short-term studies have noted a reduction in height and linear growth velocity over 6 to 12 months with ICS, longer-term studies have consistently noted that the final adult height is not influenced by ICS.[85]

Practical approaches to minimize or eliminate systemic toxicity from ICS include using the lowest dose needed by proactively stepping down the dose after several months of optimal asthma control, routinely using a spacer extension device (if metered-dose inhalers are used) or a dry-powder device and rinsing the oropharynx after each use, and adding LABA or another controller agent to facilitate dose reduction of ICS.

Antileukotrienes. The sulfidopeptide or cysteinyl leukotrienes (LTC_4, LTD_4, and LTE_4) are formed by the lipoxygenation of arachidonic acid by the enzyme 5-LO. These compounds, released by mast cells, eosinophils and airway epithelial cells, have a variety of potent effects including bronchoconstriction, increased permeability, and enhanced airway reactivity. Cysteinyl leukotrienes are involved in the pathogenesis of human asthma. Leukotrienes can be recovered from nasal secretions, bronchoalveolar lavage fluid, and urine of patients with asthma. Potent leukotriene antagonists attenuate asthmatic responses to allergens, exercise, cold dry air, and aspirin.[69,73] Placebo-controlled clinical trials have shown salutary effects in asthmatics treated with antileukotriene drugs.[86]

Churg-Strauss vasculitis (CSS) has been reported in patients receiving antileukotriene drugs. In most cases, patients with severe asthma who improved and were able to suspend or taper oral corticosteroids developed CSS.[87,88] It appears that rather than a causal association, this likely reflects an unmasking of extrapulmonary features of preexisting CSS with a tapering of oral steroids following symptomatic improvement on a trial of an antileukotriene drug. Similar cases of CSS have also been reported in association with other asthma drugs, including cromolyn, fluticasone, and omalizumab.

Antileukotrienes have been associated with statistically significant improvement in mild-to-moderate asthma compared with placebo.[89,90] A 3-month, double-blind, parallel-group study of 681 subjects with FEV_1 50% to 80% showed significant improvement with montelukast. Asthma exacerbation decreased by 31%, and asthma-free days increased by 37%.[89] Another randomized trial involving 226 adults with moderate-to-severe asthma showed that montelukast 10 mg allowed significant tapering of inhaled steroids in patients requiring moderate to high doses.[90] A 4-week controlled trial in 80 AERD patients with high medication reliance at baseline showed that montelukast 10 mg given at bedtime significantly improved asthma control.[71]

A current scientific controversy surrounding antileukotrienes is whether they affect the natural history of asthma and can prevent airway remodeling. Data from animal models indicate an effect on eosinophilia and collagen deposition.[91] Whether these findings are relevant to human disease awaits performance of additional studies.

EPR-3[5] guidelines recommend a role for antileukotrienes for mild persistent asthma as an alternative to ICS (or cromolyn or nedocromil). These agents have effects on early and delayed asthma responses; therefore, they act as bronchodilators within 1 to 3 hours after administration as well as anti-inflammatory agents with a response in 2 to 4 weeks. The magnitude of increase in FEV_1 at 4 weeks is about 14% above that of placebo. In comparator trials in patients with mild persistent asthma who were randomized to ICS or antileukotrienes,

Table 5 Pharmacologic Agents for the Treatment of Asthma

Generic Name	Brand Name (Manufacturer)	Delivery Route/Device	Suggested Dosage (Adults)	Comments
Anticholinergics				
Atropine sulfate	[Many]	Sol'n 0.2% (1 mg/0.5 mL) 0.5% (2.5 mg/0.5 mL)(1.25 mg)	0.025 mg/kg diluted with 3-5 mL NS q 6-8hr	Minimal side effects with ipratropium
Ipratropium bromide	Atrovent (Boehringer)	MDI (18 g/puff) Sol'n 0.02% (500-μg unit dose vial)	2-4 puffs qid; max 12 puffs/day 500 μg/tid, qid	Approved for COPD only
Tiotropium	Spiriva (Boehringer)	DPI 8 mg/puff	1 puff per day	Approved for COPD only
β_2-Adrenergic Agents				
Albuterol sulfate	Airet (Medeva)	Sol'n (0.83%)	2.5-10 mg q6-8hr	Inhaled agents have fewer systemic side effects; β_2 selective agents are albuterol, bitolterol, metaproterenol, pirbuterol, terbutaline
	Albuterol (various generic)	Sol'n (0.83%, 0.5%)	2.5-10 mg q6-8hr mL (0.5 mL)	
	Proventil (Schering)	MDI (90 μg puff)	Acute: 2-4 puffs q4-6hr; max 16-20 puffs/day	
		Sol'n for nebulizer	Prophylaxis: 2 puffs 15 min before exercise	
		Tabs (2,4 mg)	2.5-10 mg q6-8hr	
			0.083% (3 mL) or 0.5% (0.5 mL)	
			2-4 mg q6-8hr; max: 32 mg/day	
	Pro Air HFA	Same dose as Proventil or Ventolin	2-4 puffs q4-6hr, max 16-20 puffs/day	
			4 mg q12hr	
	Proventil HFA (Schering)	MDI (90 μg/puff)	2 puffs q4-6hrs, max 16-20 puffs/day	
		Repetab (sustained-release tabs), 4 mg	4 mg q12hr	
	Ventolin HFA (Glaxo)	MDI (90 μg/puff)	2 puffs Hthrs, Max 16-20 puffs/day	
		Rotohaler (200 μg/Rotacap)	200-400 μg q6-8hr; max dose, 2.4 mg/day	
		Sol'n for nebulizer (0.083% μg mL, 0.5% 20 mL)	2.5-10 mg q6-8hr	
		Tabs (2, 4 mg)		
	Volmax (Muro)	Sustained-release tabs (4, 8 mg)	4-8 mg q12hr	
Epinephrine	EPI PEN (Dey) TWINJECT (Sciele)	IM injection 1:1000 (1 mg/mL)	0.2-0.5 mg SC (0.2-0.5 mL SC) q20min	
Formoterol	Foradil (Novartis)	DPI	1 cap q12hr	
Levalbuterol	Xopenex (Sepracor)	Sol'n for nebulizer (0.63 mg)	0.63 mg q6-8hr	
Metaproterenol	Alupent (Boehringer)	MDI (650 μg/puff)	2-3 puffs q3-4hr, max 12 puffs/day	
		Sol'n (0.4%, 0.6%)	0.3 mL in 2.5 mL NS q4-6hr	
		Tabs (10, 20 mg)	10 mg q6-8hr, 10 mg up to 20 mg	
	Metaprel (Sandoz)	MDI (650 μg/puff)	2 puffs q4hr; max 12 puffs	
		Sol'n (0.5%)	0.3 mL in 2.5 mL NS q4-6hr	
		Tabs (10, 20 mg)	10 mg q6-8hr, max 20 mg	
Pirbuterol acetate	Maxair (3M Pharm)	MDI (200 μg/puff)	2 puffs q4-6hr; max 12 puffs/day	
		AutoHaler	2 puffs q6hr	
Salmeterol	Serevent (Glaxo)	MDI (46 μg/puff) Diskus (DPI 50 μg/puff)	2 puffs q12hr 1 inhalation q12hr	

Continued

Table 5 Pharmacologic Agents for the Treatment of Asthma—cont'd

Generic Name	Brand Name (Manufacturer)	Delivery Route/Device	Suggested Dosage (Adults)	Comments
Terbutaline sulfate	Brethaire (Geigy)	MDI (200 μg/puff)	1-2 puffs q4-6hr	
		Sol'n for SC injection	0.25 mg SC q15-30 min; max 0.50 mg/4hr	
		injection or nebulizer (1 mg/mL)	0.75-2.5 mg nebulized with NS	
		Tabs (2.5, 5 mg)	2.5-5 mg tid; max 15 mg/24hr	
	Bricanyl (Marion Merrell Dow)	MDI (200 μg/puff)	2 puffs q6hr	
		Tabs (2.5, 5 mg)	2.4-5 mg tid, max 15 mg/24hr	
Cromoglycates				
Cromolyn sodium	Intal (Fisons)	Spinhaler (20 mg caps)	20 mg qid	Contraindicated in acute asthma
		MDI (800 μg/puffs)	2 puffs qid	
		Sol'n (20 mg/2 mL ampule)	1 ampule qid	
Inhaled Corticosteroids				
Nedocromil sodium	Tilade (Aventis)	MDI (1.75 mg/puff)	2 puffs bid, tid, qid	
Beclomethasone dipropionate	Beclovent (Allen & Hanburys)	MDI (42 μg/puff)	2 puffs tid-qid; max 20 puffs/day	Need more than 400 μg/day to maintain off oral steroids, no adrenal suppression if <800-1200 μg/day
	Qvar (3M) (HFA-BDP formula)	MDI (40 or 80 μg/puff)	2-8 puffs bid	
	Vanceril (Schering)	MDI (42 μg/puff)	2 puffs tid-qid; max 20 puffs/day	
	Vanceril DS (Schering)	MDI (84 μg/puff)	2 puffs tid-qid; max 20 puffs/day	
Budesonide	Pulmicort (AstraZeneca)	Turbuhaler (200 μg/puff)	400-1600 μg in divided doses bid-qid	Approved for 12 mo-8 yr
	Pulmicort Respules (AstraZeneca)	Sol'n (0.25 mg/2 mL or 0.50 mg/2 mL)	0.25 mg to 1 mg qd-bid	
Flunisolide	AeroBid (Forest)	MDI (250 μg/puff)	2 puffs bid; max 8 puffs/day	
Fluticasone propionate	Flovent (Glaxo)	MDI (44, 110, 220, μg/puff)	100-800 μg/day	
		Diskus powder inhaler (50, 100, 250 μg/puff)		
Mometasone furoate	Asmanex (Schering)	Twisthaler (220 μg/puff)	220-880 μg/day	
Triamcinolone acetonide	Azmacort (Rhone-Poulenc Rohrer)	MDI (100 μg/puff)	2-4 puffs qid; max 16 puffs/day	
Combination Products				
Albuterol/ ipratropium	Combivent (Boehringer-Ingelheim)	MDI (18 μg ipratropium/103 μg albuterol per puff)	2 puffs qid	
Salmeterol/ fluticasone	Advair (Glaxo)	Diskus (DPI)	50/100, 50/250, 50/500: 1 puff bid	
Fomoterol/ budesonide (investigational)	Symbicort (AstraZeneca)	Turbuhaler	4.5/80, 4.5/160-2puffs BID	
Antileukotrienes				
Montelukast	Singulair (Merck)	Tabs (5, 10 mg)	10 mg qd in the evening	Take on empty stomach
Zafirlukast	Accolate (Zeneca)	Tab (20 mg)	20 mg bid	Need to follow LFTs, drug interactions
Zileuton	Zyflo (Abbott)	Tab (600 mg)	600 mg qid	Need to follow LFTs, drug interactions

Table 5 Pharmacologic Agents for the Treatment of Asthma—cont'd

Generic Name	Brand Name (Manufacturer)	Delivery Route/Device	Suggested Dosage (Adults)	Comments
Methylxanthines				
Aminophylline	Various	IV	Load: If not on theophylline at home, 5-6 mg/kg over 20 min; if on theophylline, level pending, 3 mg/kg over 20 min; a bolus of 0.5 mg/kg will increase level by 2 in the average adult Maintenance 0.5-0.9 mg/kg/hr; 200-400 mg bid	Decreased clearance with cirrhosis, CHF, erythromycin, cimetidine, troleandomycin Increased clearance with smoking, young age, and phenobarbital Need to follow serum levels
Anti-IgE				
Omalizumab	Xolar (Genentech/ Novartis)	Subcutaneous	0.016 mg × body wt (kg) × IgE level (IU/mL); also see nomogram	See text for details; anaphylaxis 0.1%

BDP, beclomethasone dipropionate; cap, capsule;
CHF, congestive heart failure; COPD, chronic obstructive pulmonary disease;
DPI, dry powder inhaler; IgE, immunoglobulin E; LFTs, liver function tests; max, maximum; MDI, pressurized metered-dose inhaler; N/A, not available; NS, normal saline; sol'n, solution; tab, tablet.

Data from the National Asthma Education and Prevention Program.[5]

ICS have been associated with superior efficacy.[92] Antileukotrienes facilitate reduction in the need for inhaled β agonists and ICS, and they may be associated with improved compliance compared with inhaled medications. Antileukotriene agents also have been shown to attenuate exercise-induced bronchospasm.

Patients with AERD, compared with aspirin-tolerant asthmatics, release higher levels of leukotrienes with aspirin-provoked respiratory reaction, and exhibit greater end-organ responsiveness to leukotrienes. On this basis, patients with AERD warrant a trial of antileukotriene pharmacotherapy, although the rate of response in this subgroup is similar to rates reported among aspirin-tolerant asthmatics. That the data show about the same rate of benefit in AERD compared with ASA-tolerant asthmatics is consistent with the hypothesis that it is the balance between PGE_2 and $PGF_{2\alpha}$ that is critical in this subgroup.[69]

Anti-IgE Therapy. Omalizumab (Xolair), is a humanized monoclonal anti-IgE antibody that binds with high affinity to the FcεRI receptor-binding site on IgE. Omalizumab reduces the amount of free IgE available to bind to FcεRI receptors on mast cells and basophils. This agent is administered subcutaneously every 2 or 4 weeks for asthmatic patients with objective evidence of IgE-mediated (allergic) potential to perennial allergen(s) with serum IgE levels of 30 to 700 IU/mL.

Humbert and colleagues[93] studied 419 patients whose asthma was not adequately controlled on high-dose ICS combined with LABA. The subjects were 12 to 75 years old and had reduced lung function and history of recent asthma exacerbation. These subjects were randomized to treatment with omalizumab or placebo. Omalizumab was associated with a statistically significant reduction in the rate of asthma exacerbations and severe asthma exacerbations, as well as statistically significant improvements in asthma-related quality of life, morning peak expiratory flow rate, and asthma symptom scores. These data provide support for the recommendation to consider a trial of omalizumab in properly selected patients with severe persistent allergic asthma.

In pivotal trials,[94,95] omalizumab was associated with a substantial rate of local reactions. A rate of anaphylaxis of slightly less than 1 in 1000 was observed, and this has been confirmed by surveillance data recorded since approval of the drug in June 2003. Based on the observed risk of anaphylaxis, in July 2007 the FDA added a black box warning to the omalizumab label. The warning states that health care providers administering omalizumab should be prepared to manage anaphylaxis, and patients should be closely observed for an appropriate period after omalizumab administration.

A numerical, but not statistically significant, increase in the rate of malignancy in patients receiving omalizumab was also observed. Malignancies developed in 0.5% of patients receiving omalizumab compared with 0.2% of patients who received placebo. Because these malignancies were diagnosed over a shorter period than the time oncogenesis requires to develop (i.e., 6 months in 60% of cases), and because a heterogeneity of tumors was observed, there is reason to suspect these tumors were not causally related to omalizumab. Postmarketing surveillance studies are in progress that will provide more definitive data on the possible relationship between malignancy and omalizumab.

The EPR-3[5] guidelines state that omalizumab is the only adjunctive therapy to demonstrate added efficacy to high-dose ICS plus LABA in patients with severe persistent allergic asthma and to stipulate that evidence does not support use of certain agents, which in some cases are FDA-approved for management of other conditions and have been advocated for management of severe, refractory asthma. These agents include methotrexate, soluble IL-4 receptor, anti–IL-5, anti–IL-12, cyclosporine A, intravenous immune globulin, gold, troleandomycin, and colchicine. The data supporting use of macrolides were characterized as "encouraging but insufficient to support a recommendation."

EXPERIMENTAL THERAPIES

Inhaled drugs administered by some form of a handheld device (most often a dry-powder device or a pressurized metered-dose inhaler) are generally acceptable, adequate, and effective. This will likely be the therapy for the majority of asthmatics for the foreseeable future. However, certain limitations to these approaches warrant continued development of new therapeutics. Poor adherence with inhaled devices can contribute to poor asthma care outcomes.

Despite evidence to the contrary, patients, parents, and clinicians have lingering questions about the long-term safety of ICS. There are insufficient data for the concept that chronic long-term therapy with the existing agents, including ICS, has a disease-modifying effect or an effect that prevents or reverses airway remodeling. A small subset of patients have inadequately treated asthma despite maximal doses of ICS, and these patients likely have some form of relative steroid resistance. Finally, older nonspecific, systemic, alternative anti-inflammatory agents (methotrexate, gold, cyclosporine) have significant and unacceptable side effects.[96] For these reasons, the pharmaceuticals industry and various investigators have been aggressively pursuing novel therapies for asthma.

Anticytokine Therapies

Th2 cells and their derived cytokines IL-4, IL-5, and IL-13 play a critical role in orchestrating eosinophilia and asthmatic airway inflammation in various models of asthma. Over the past few years, there have been several early-phase human studies with pharmacologic approaches to antagonize these pathways, with mixed results.[97,98] Although the animal studies had been promising, an important study using intravenous humanized monoclonal antibody to IL-5 (SB-240563) at doses of 2.5 mg/kg or 10 mg/kg was disappointing in a double-blind, placebo-controlled trial using an inhaled allergen-challenge model.[97] Even though a single intravenous dose of anti–IL-5 decreased blood eosinophilia for 16 weeks and sputum eosinophilia for 4 weeks, there was no significant effect on the late asthmatic response or airway hyperresponsiveness to allergen challenge.

Several studies with an inhaled soluble IL-4 receptor antagonist, altrakincept (Nuvance) found modest benefit, but further development was discontinued by the manufacturer. In a placebo-controlled, parallel-group study of 62 moderate-persistent asthmatics dependent on moderate doses of ICS, subjects were randomized to placebo or three different doses of IL-4R by once-weekly nebulization for 12 weeks.[98] There were modest improvements in symptom scores and FEV_1 in the highest-dose group, but the asthma exacerbation rate was not significantly different than in the placebo group. An IL-13 antagonist has also shown promise in a primate model of asthma, and clinical studies are being initiated in human patients.

Novel Steroids

Steroids, either systemic or inhaled, are exquisitely active and effective in asthma, but their mechanism of action is broad, and concern for toxicity—even with topical steroids—has limited their wider use. A variety of approaches are being pursued to maximize local activity within the airways and at the same time to minimize systemic absorption and toxicity.[99] One approach is development of on-site-activated steroids such as ciclesonide, which is a nonhalogenated ICS prodrug that requires endogenous cleavage by esterases for activity. Soft steroids are also being developed; these have improved local, topical selectivity and have much less steroid effect outside the target area. They may be inactivated by esterases or other enzymes (for example a lactone–glucocorticosteroid conjugate). Another approach is using dissociated steroids, or agents that favor monomeric glucocorticoid receptor complexes (i.e., they produce transrepression) and avoid dimerization or transactivation, which is undesirable in asthma. Agents from each of these categories are undergoing clinical trials.

CONCLUSION

Further progress in asthma care will require better understanding of the molecular and genetic basis for the clinical heterogeneity seen in this disorder. The relation between acute and chronic inflammation as well as airway hyperresponsiveness and airway remodeling is still unclear. Research in exhaled noninvasive markers of inflammation might eventually translate into practical and clinically useful tools at point of care. The availability of such tools will encourage more precise management of anti-inflammatory therapy. Further development of pharmacogenetics might identify subsets of patients who may preferentially respond to one class of anti-inflammatory agents as opposed to others, thereby eliminating some of the trial and error that often occurs in normative asthma management. Finally, the specific pharmacotherapeutic approaches to block unique pathways offer hope for major new advances in the next 5 to 10 years.

Summary

- Asthma is a chronic, episodic disease of the airways, which is best viewed as a syndrome.
- Prevalence and severity of asthma have increased dramatically in recent decades.
- There is no cure for asthma, but in the overwhelming majority of cases, well-controlled asthma can be achieved with proper management.
- Pharmacogenetics holds promise for identifying subsets of patients who might preferentially respond to select asthma medications and encourage more favorable asthma care outcomes.
- Specific pharmacotherapeutic approaches to block unique pathways involved in asthma inflammation offer hope for major new advances in asthma management in the near future.

Suggested Readings

Bateman E, Boushey H, Bousquet J, et al: Can guideline-defined asthma control be achieved? Am J Resp Crit Care Med 2004;170:836-844.

Bousquet J, Jeffery PK, Busse WW, et al: Asthma: From bronchoconstriction to airways inflammation and remodeling. Am J Respir Crit Care Med 2000;161:1720-1745.

Cox L, Li J, Nelson H, et al: Allergy immunotherapy: A practice parameter second update. J Allergy Clin Immunol 2007;120: S25-S85.

Li JT, Oppenheimer J, Bernstein IL, et al: Attaining optimal asthma control: A practice parameter. J Allergy Clin Immunol 2005;116:S3-S11.

Moorman J, Rudd R, Johnson C, et al: National Surveillance for asthma—United States, 1980-2004. MMWR Surveill Summ 2007; 56:1-14.

National Heart, Lung, and Blood Institute: Guidelines for the Diagnosis and Management of Asthma—Update on Selected Topics 2002. Bethesda, Md, National Institutes of Health, 2002. NIH Publication No. 02-5075 (available at http://www.nhlbi.nih.gov/guidelines/asthma/index.htm).

National Heart, Lung, and Blood Institute: Guidelines for the Diagnosis and Management of Asthma (EPR-3) (available at http://www.nhlbi.nih.gov/guidelines/asthma/index.htm).

National Heart, Lung, and Blood Institute: National Asthma Education and Prevention Program. Expert panel report guidelines for the diagnosis and management of asthma. J Allergy Clin Immunol 1991;88:425-534.

National Heart, Lung, and Blood Institute: National Asthma Education Program Expert Panel Report II: Guidelines for the diagnosis and management of asthma, 1997, Bethesda, Md, NIH Publication No. 97-4051A, 1997.

Sin DD, Man J, Sharpe H, et al: Pharmacological management to reduce exacerbations in adults with asthma. A systematic review and meta-analysis. JAMA 2004;292: 367-376.

References

For a complete list of references, log onto www.expertconsult.com.

Allergic Rhinitis

David M. Lang

DEFINITION

Allergic rhinitis may be defined as an inflammation of the nasal mucous membranes caused by immunoglobulin E (IgE)-mediated (allergic) reaction to aeroallergens.

PREVALENCE

The first recorded case of allergic rhinitis (catarrhus aestivus) was described by Sir John Bostock, who presented himself as a case report to the Medical and Surgical Society of London in 1819.[1] At the dawn of the 20th century, there were only several thousand members of the U.S. Ragweed Association. One hundred years later, allergic rhinitis has become the most common allergic or immunologic disorder in the U.S. population[2-4] and it now affects an estimated one in seven Americans. Allergic rhinitis is acknowledged as a significant health challenge on a global scale.[3] Allergic rhinitis is a major cause of patient visits to physicians in the United States, commonly complicates management of other conditions (e.g., asthma, chronic sinusitis), and if untreated or undertreated can lead to considerable morbidity including missed work or school, sleep disruption, diminished daytime performance, and impaired quality of life.[2,5] The economic burden of allergic rhinitis is substantial.[4]

A rising prevalence of allergic rhinitis has been found not only in children[4] but also in adults.[5] The peak in incidence of allergic rhinitis occurs during the young adult years. Although prevalence declines with age, allergic rhinitis is also an important health concern in older adults.[6] Incidence of allergic rhinitis is equal in male and female patients.

Epidemiologic studies have consistently demonstrated that allergic rhinitis and asthma commonly coexist.[2] Allergic rhinitis is often associated with asthma and is a risk factor for developing asthma; in addition, many patients with allergic rhinitis demonstrate increased bronchial hyperresponsiveness to inhalation challenge with histamine or methacholine.

PATHOPHYSIOLOGY

Persons who have inherited the potential to develop IgE-mediated, or allergic, responses to otherwise innocuous inhalant allergens, with sufficient exposure, generate allergen-specific IgE after T-cell release of interleukins (ILs) 4 and 13 and B-cell switching to produce IgE antibody, thereby becoming sensitized. The allergic reaction that underlies allergic rhinitis results from subsequent exposure to the allergen to which sensitization has occurred, which cross-links at least two IgE antibodies bound to the high-affinity IgE receptor on presensitized effector cells, mast cells, or basophils.[7]

The allergic response includes an early and a late phase.[2,7] The early phase occurs promptly and has a duration of approximately 1 hour. The late phase typically begins in 3 to 6 hours, peaks at 6 to 8 hours, and subsides in 12 to 24 hours. Almost one half of subjects studied in laboratory settings exhibit this dual response.[8] The symptoms of the early phase generally include sneezing, pruritus, and clear rhinorrhea; symptoms characterizing the late phase may be indistinguishable but typically entail more prominent congestion.[2,7] The late phase is promoted by factors generated in the early phase, which encourage release of inflammatory mediators and the activation and recruitment of cells to the nasal mucosa.[2,3,8]

Whereas histamine appears to be the major mediator of the early phase, the late phase is more closely associated with other mediators, chemokines, and cytokines that have inflammatory and proinflammatory effects leading to recruitment of inflammatory cells such as eosinophils and basophils. Eosinophils play an important role in the late phase,[7] including release of leukotrienes, which, data suggest, are of greater importance than histamine for nasal congestion.[9,10] During a clinically relevant exposure in a sensitized person (e.g., outdoors during the ragweed season or indoors with cats), aeroallergens enter the nasal passages on a virtually continual basis. Therefore, it is often difficult to separate the early and late phases of the allergic response in the real-world setting. One can imagine that in many cases, based on the incessant nature of aeroallergen exposure, affected persons experience a perpetual late-phase response.

SIGNS AND SYMPTOMS

There are four major symptoms of allergic rhinitis: sneezing, pruritus, congestion, and drainage; however, many patients with allergic rhinitis do not complain of the entire symptom complex.[11] Patients with allergic rhinitis commonly also experience ocular symptoms, so much so that the term *allergic rhinoconjunctivitis* is often used as an alternative to *allergic rhinitis.*[2]

An appropriate history for allergic rhinitis includes questions to elicit information regarding onset and duration of symptoms, provoking factors or situations, concomitant ocular symptoms, and associated pruritus of other facial structures (e.g., throat, ears, palate). Of the four major symptoms, pruritus and sneezing are more specific for allergic rhinitis compared with conditions in the differential diagnosis of allergic rhinitis, which are shown in Box 1. The propensity for sneezing can entail paroxysms of 5 to 10 or more in rapid succession. Congestion is a bothersome symptom, as it is commonly described by patients with allergic rhinitis, and compared with other symptoms it tends to be less responsive to currently available medications. Rhinorrhea is typically clear; purulent discharge might reflect a secondary infection.

Physical examination can reveal pale, boggy nasal mucous membranes and infraorbital congestion (allergic shiners) but can be relatively unremarkable unless patients are seen when symptoms are prominent. At such times, subtotal or complete nasal obstruction may be present, along with suffusion of conjunctivae.

DIAGNOSIS

Proper recognition of patients with allergic rhinitis requires a careful history and physical examination. The key components of the history that favor allergic rhinitis, as opposed to other causes of rhinitis (see Box 1), include seasonality of symptoms, occurrence of symptoms with certain exposures or situations (e.g., walking into a pet store), improvement of symptoms during spring, summer, and fall when in air-conditioned environments (buildings or automobiles), and the experience of prominent itching of the nose, eyes, ears, throat, or palate. As opposed to younger patients with chronic rhinitis, in older adults allergic rhinitis is less commonly confirmed, and alternative diagnoses for perennial rhinitis, including cholinergic hyperactivity, pharmacologic causes (e.g., α-adrenergic effects of antihypertensive drugs), and chronic sinusitis are found more often.[6]

Box 1 Differential Diagnosis of Allergic Rhinitis

- Vasomotor or irritant rhinitis
- Chronic sinusitis
- Nonallergic rhinitis with eosinophilia
- Gustatory rhinitis
- Atrophic rhinitis
- Rhinitis medicamentosa
- Rhinitis associated with drugs (e.g., antihypertensive agents, oral contraceptives)
- Rhinitis associated with systemic disease (e.g., hypothyroidism, Wegener's granulomatosis, Sjögren's syndrome)
- Structural factors (septal deviation, nasal polyposis, nasopharyngeal carcinoma)

Box 2 Inhalant Allergens

- Cockroaches
- Dust mites
- Grasses
- Mold spores
- Pets (e.g., dogs, cats)
- Trees
- Weeds

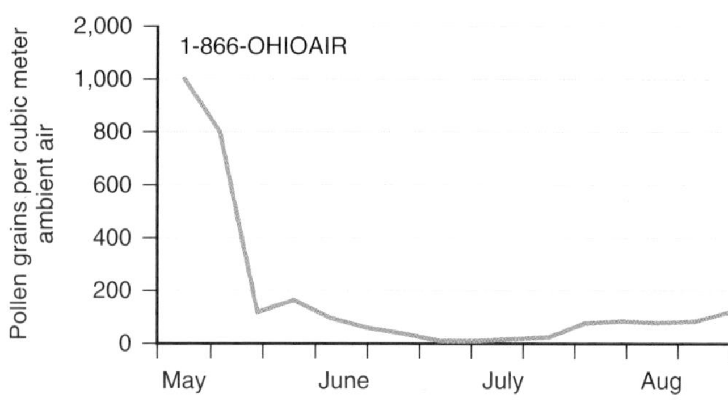

Figure 1 Pollen counts for the Cleveland vicinity, pollen season 2004. The number of pollen grains per cubic meter of ambient air varies from spring to fall. Counts are highest in the spring, in association with the tree pollen season, lowest during the summer, and rise again in early fall during the grass and weed seasons. During the pollen season, these counts are made available three times each week as a public service [866-OHIOAIR]. *Compiled by Dottie Vasas, RN, Nurse Coordinator, Cleveland Clinic Allergy/Immunology.*

The diagnosis of allergic rhinitis requires a positive history, demonstration of IgE-mediated potential to inhalant allergens by cutaneous (or in vitro) testing, and correlation between history and cutaneous (or in vitro) test findings. Immediate hypersensitivity skin testing is recommended as the preferred diagnostic study, because it is associated with lower cost, is more sensitive, and entails no delay in obtaining results.[2,12] Patients who have skin disorders or who are unable to suspend antihistamine medications, such that skin testing would be uninterpretable, are candidates for in vitro testing to detect elevated levels of specific IgE to inhalant allergens.[2,12]

TREATMENT

Once a diagnosis of allergic rhinitis is confirmed, treatment strategies include avoidance, medications, and allergen immunotherapy.

Avoidance

The results of cutaneous (or in vitro) testing can be used to direct specific avoidance measures. Avoiding clinically relevant allergens can substantially reduce symptoms and reliance on medication,[2] and it is arguably the most important aspect of managing allergic rhinitis. The inhalant allergens that can account for allergic rhinitis are listed in Box 2. Persons with allergic rhinitis are often sensitive to more than one allergen.

The occurrence and severity of symptoms among patients with seasonal allergic rhinitis caused by outdoor pollens and mold spores parallel the exposure to and levels of these factors in ambient air. Monitoring pollen and mold counts in one's vicinity is often of benefit, because the knowledge of these counts can be useful for planning outdoor activities. The pollen counts for the Cleveland vicinity during the pollen season of 2004 (May to October) are displayed in Figure 1. A predictable sequence of pollination is observed each year, such that trees predominate in the spring, grasses in the summer, and weeds in the late summer and early fall. Ragweed pollen (Figure 2) is the dominant weed in the midwestern and northeastern United States. Ragweed typically appears in ambient air during the second week of August, peaks in early September (usually Labor Day weekend), and then persists until the frost. Mold spore counts and counts of pollen grains, recorded simultaneously for 3 days each week in the Cleveland vicinity throughout the 2004 season, are shown in Figure 3. Molds are present in samples of ambient air at much higher levels than pollens; however, pollens are more efficient aeroallergens: Grass pollen counts in single digits may be sufficient to provoke symptoms in sensitized persons, whereas mold counts of several thousand are still considered low.

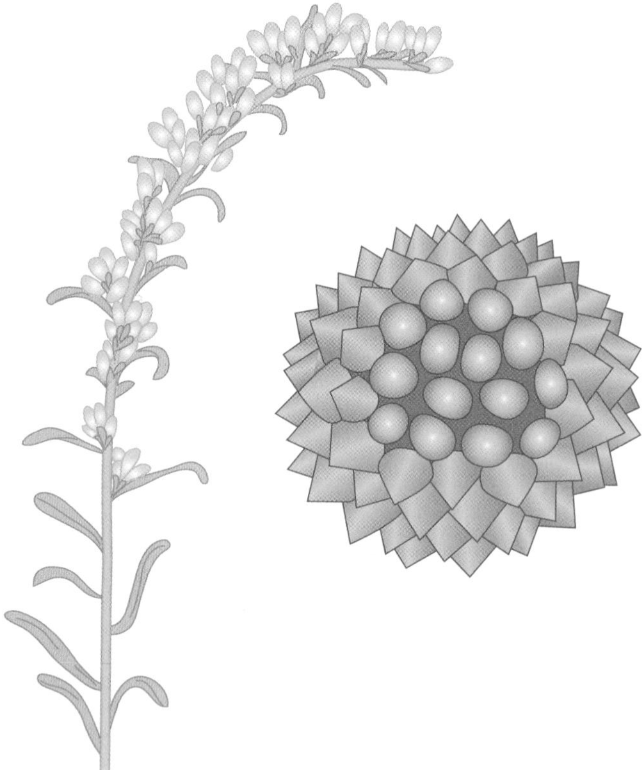

Figure 2 Ragweed is the dominant weed pollen in the Midwestern United States. Flowering spike *(left)*; pollen *(right)*.

For persons who are allergic to outdoor pollens, air conditioning can dramatically relieve symptoms.[2] By reducing indoor relative humidity, air conditioning also significantly reduces mold spore and dust mite allergen levels.[13] We now spend most of our time indoors,[14]

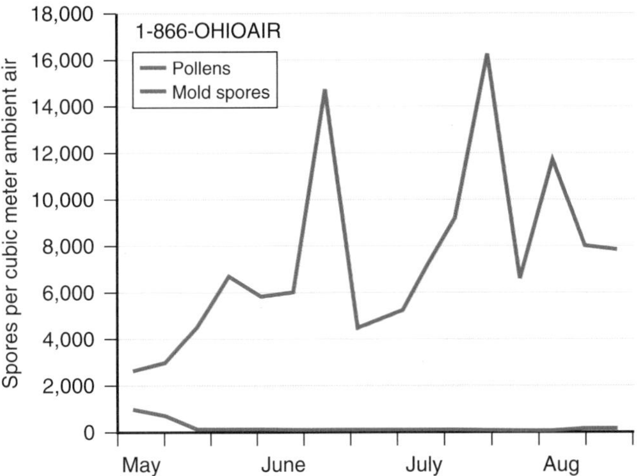

Figure 3 Counts of mold spores from spring through the frost for the Cleveland vicinity, 2004. Mold spore counts are displayed (spores per cubic meter of ambient air). Pollen counts are also shown (pollen grains per cubic meter of ambient air). Mold spores far exceed the levels of airborne pollens in samples of ambient air and peak in association with maximum heat and humidity in the late summer.

and the usefulness of air conditioning for reducing symptoms should not be underestimated.

Dust mites are a major source of allergens in house dust.[2,13] Dust mites have been isolated in dust samples taken from Africa, Asia, Europe, and North and South America. They are microscopic and rely on heat and humidity to survive and proliferate.[2] Allergy to dust mites is common in patients with allergic rhinitis. Recommended avoidance measures to reduce exposure to dust mites include encasing the mattress, box spring, and pillow in impermeable covers; reducing indoor relative humidity; washing bedding weekly in hot water (55° C, 130° F); and removing carpets (if possible) in favor of tiled or hardwood flooring.[13]

For persons who are allergic to cat or dog dander and who have pets, no avoidance strategy can approach the benefit of removing the pet from the home.[15] In view of emotional attachments to pets, as well as the potential therapeutic value of pets,[16] the decision to remove a pet from the home must be discussed openly with allergic patients and considered carefully from an individualized risk-to-benefit standpoint. Removing a cat or dog from the home might not have immediate clinical benefit because the allergen can persist for several months. When it is not possible to remove pets from the home, second-best measures include excluding the pet from the allergic person's bedroom, using high-efficiency particulate air (HEPA) cleaners or electrostatic air cleaners, and removing carpets and other upholstered items that can serve as a reservoir for allergens.[15] Although allergen reduction may be transient and the potential for clinical benefit has not been clearly established, bathing the pet (cat or dog) also might help.

Pharmacotherapy

Because avoidance measures will likely be incomplete, and patients with allergic rhinitis will continue to be exposed to clinically relevant levels of aeroallergens, virtually all patients with allergic rhinitis benefit from medication.

Antihistamines

The most commonly prescribed medications for allergic rhinitis are H_1 antihistamines.[2] These drugs antagonize the action of histamine by blocking receptor sites on target cells. Antihistamines were introduced more than 50 years ago and continue to be widely used.

Table 1 Second-Generation Antihistamines

Medication (Proprietary)	Daily Dose
Azelastine (Astelin)	2 sprays in each nostril bid
Cetirizine (Zyrtec)	5 or 10 mg qd
Fexofenadine (Allegra)	180 mg qd or 60 mg bid
Levocetirizine (Xyzal)	2.5 or 5 mg qd
Loratidine (Claritin)	10 mg qd
Desloratidine (Clarinex)	5 mg qd

Although conventional or first-generation antihistamines are efficacious, they can be associated with drowsiness and performance impairment.[2] Impaired driving performance has been documented with use of conventional antihistamines, even in persons with no subjective awareness of drowsiness.[17] Older adults may be more sensitive to the psychomotor impairment promoted by antihistamines and are at increased risk for complications such as fractures and subdural hematomas caused by falls.[6] Prominent anticholinergic effects, including dryness of the mouth and eyes, constipation, inhibition of micturition, and potential provocation of narrow-angle glaucoma, can occur. Because of concomitant comorbid conditions (e.g., increased intraocular pressure, benign prostatic hypertrophy, preexisting cognitive impairment) that can increase the potential risk associated with regular or even intermittent use, first-generation antihistamines should be prescribed or recommended cautiously in older adults.

Second-generation antihistamines (Table 1), which lack the prominent central nervous system or anticholinergic properties of conventional antihistamines, are generally preferred.[2] Second-generation antihistamines include oral fexofenadine, oral levocetirizine, oral loratidine (available without a prescription), oral desloratidine, oral cetirizine (available without a prescription), and intranasal azelastine.

Decongestants

Oral decongestants primarily reduce nasal congestion and can attenuate drainage, but they do not affect sneezing or itching. They are often helpful taken in combination with an antihistamine. These agents are available without a prescription. Use of these drugs can be problematic,[2] especially in older adults,[6] in view of their propensity for promoting adverse central nervous system effects (e.g., tremor, irritability, insomnia, nervousness) and cardiovascular effects (palpitations, blood pressure elevation). These drugs can also raise intraocular pressure and provoke obstructive urinary symptoms.

Topical decongestants effectively relieve congestion. Benefit is usually prompt and dramatic; however, rebound congestion can follow as the vasoconstrictive action of these agents diminishes. A paradoxical effect then tends to occur with continuing use: The decongestive action lessens, but the sense of nasal obstruction increases. The pathophysiology of this condition, rhinitis medicamentosa, is not fully understood but is believed to entail down-regulation of α-adrenergic receptors, making them less responsive to endogenously released norepinephrine and exogenously applied vasoconstrictors. Because rebound congestion can occur as soon as 3 days from beginning of treatment,[18] use of these agents is most favorable from a risk-to-benefit standpoint for this period, and patients should be advised to stop using topical decongestants after 3 days. Treatment of rhinitis medicamentosa consists of suspending topical decongestant use to permit the nasal mucosa to recover.

Intranasal Corticosteroids

Intranasal corticosteroids are the most efficacious agents for managing allergic rhinitis.[2] Given the understanding that symptoms of allergic rhinitis reflect an inflammatory response promoted by aeroallergen exposure, use of an agent that can achieve a broad range of anti-inflammatory effects and acts through multiple mechanisms would be expected to be associated with maximal relief of allergic rhinitis symptoms compared with other agents.

The therapeutic effects of intranasal corticosteroids include vasoconstriction and reduction of mucosal edema, inhibition of mediator release, suppression of cytokine production, and inhibition of inflammatory cell infiltration.[2] Intranasal corticosteroids are effective for reducing nasal congestion, rhinorrhea, and sneezing, and they can also relieve ocular symptoms.[11] Systemic effects are minimal at recommended doses.[2] The major adverse effect of intranasal corticosteroids is local irritation or epistaxis; patients should be instructed to stop using intranasal corticosteroids at the first sign of bleeding or irritation and to direct the nasal spray laterally, away from the nasal septum.

Other Drugs

Intranasal ipratropium is efficacious for rhinorrhea, but it has little benefit with respect to other allergic rhinitis symptoms.[2] This medication may be helpful if rhinorrhea is refractory to other medications or for persons with vasomotor or irritant rhinitis.[2] Potential adverse effects include local irritation or epistaxis.

Intranasal cromolyn is available over the counter. This medication is well tolerated, but it appears to be more efficacious for preventing inflammation than for reversing it once it occurs.[2] Although its frequency of use limits its usefulness, it poses no risk for systemic adverse effects and may be preferred for select patients (e.g., pregnant women, young children, older adults) based on this safety advantage. As with other topical agents, there is a risk of local irritation or epistaxis.

Oral antileukotrienes have been associated with statistically significant improvement in symptom scores and quality of life compared with placebo in patients with allergic rhinitis.[19] The degree of therapeutic benefit is equivalent to that of loratidine (a second-generation antihistamine), but antileukotrienes are not associated with wheal-and-flare suppression. Therapeutic benefit with intranasal corticosteroids is statistically superior.[20] Many patients with allergic rhinitis have concomitant asthma, and antileukotrienes can treat both of these conditions with a single agent.[21]

Therapeutic Usefulness

Table 2 displays the therapeutic usefulness of these pharmacotherapeutic agents for addressing the four major symptoms of allergic rhinitis in addition to ocular symptoms.[2,11,18] In clinical practice, combination treatment with more than one of these agents is often required to achieve and maintain control of allergic rhinitis.

Evidence-based medicine aids the clinician in making data-driven treatment decisions. Number needed to treat (NNT) and number needed to harm (NNH) calculations have been derived to estimate the magnitude of treatment effects of these medications for allergic rhinitis.[22] NNT is the average number of patients who need to receive a treatment for one patient to benefit, and NNH is the average number of patients who need to receive a treatment for one patient to be harmed. The lower the NNT and higher the NNH, the more effective and favorable a treatment is. NNT and NNH calculations for several of these medications are displayed in Table 2.

Allergen Immunotherapy

Allergen immunotherapy is commonly administered for patients with allergic rhinitis (and/or asthma). Its efficacy is well established for patients with allergic rhinitis[2,23] and for patients with asthma (see the chapter "Asthma," elsewhere in this section).[24]

Allergen immunotherapy entails the incremental administration of inhalant allergens to induce immune system changes in host response with natural exposure to these allergens.[23] Numerous randomized, double-blind, placebo-controlled trials have shown that allergen immunotherapy is associated with reducing symptoms and reducing reliance on medication.[23,25] In a published trial of immunotherapy, 37 of 44 patients randomized to injections of timothy grass pollen or placebo completed a 3-year study[26]; statistically significant reduction in symptoms and medication use for rhinitis and asthma in association with allergen immunotherapy was found, and NNH was 417. This estimate indicates that 417 allergen immunotherapy

Table 2 Medications for Allergic Rhinitis

	Symptoms						
Medication	**Sneezing**	**Rhinorrhea**	**Congestion**	**Pruritus**	**Ocular**	**NNT**	**NNH**
Antihistamine, oral	++	++	+	+++	++	15.2	51
Antihistamine, intranasal	++	++	+	++	0	5	22
Intranasal steroid	+++	+++	+++	++	++	4.4	48
Intranasal cromolyn	+	+	+	+	0		
Decongestant, oral	0	0	+	0	0		
Decongestant, intranasal	0	0	++++	0	0		
Anticholinergic, intranasal		0	++	0	0	0	
Antileukotriene	0	+	++	0	++	14.3	167

NNH, number needed to harm; NNT, number needed to treat.

Adapted from Bousquet J, van Cauwenberge P, Khaltaev N, et al: Allergic rhinitis and its impact on asthma (ARIA). Allergy 2002;57 841-55.

NNT and NNH estimates from Portnoy JM, Van Osdol T, Williams PB: Evidence-based strategies for treatment of allergic rhinitis. Curr Allergy Asthma Rep 2004;4:439-466.

injections were given for 1 person to experience a systemic reaction. Because of the risk of anaphylaxis from allergen immunotherapy, injections should only be given in a setting where adequate precautions are taken and life-threatening anaphylaxis can be treated.[23] A wait of 30 minutes after administration of immunotherapy is also recommended[23] to be certain a systemic reaction has not occurred.

A trial of immunotherapy merits consideration for allergic rhinitis patients who have secondary complications (e.g., sinusitis, otitis), who have concomitant (mild to moderate) asthma for which inhalant allergy is relevant, or for whom a program of optimal avoidance measures and medications is not effective, not feasible, or not preferred.[2,23,25] Allergen immunotherapy also may be desirable for patients with allergic rhinitis who do not tolerate or are disinclined to take regular medications.

The decision to begin allergen immunotherapy should be individualized and is based on symptom severity, relative benefit with pharmacotherapy, and comorbid conditions such as cardiovascular disease or exposure to β_1-adrenergic blockers.[27] The latter conditions are associated with heightened risk for more serious anaphylaxis, the major hazard of allergen immunotherapy.[23]

Summary

- Prevalence of allergic rhinitis has increased dramatically.
- Allergic rhinitis can be managed successfully with a regimen of avoidance measures and regular medication.
- In properly selected patients with allergic rhinitis (or asthma, or both), allergen immunotherapy is efficacious and can reduce symptoms and reliance on medication.
- Much of the morbidity associated with untreated or undertreated allergic rhinitis can be prevented with proper diagnosis and management.

Further Readings

Abramson M, Puy R, Weiner J: Allergen immunotherapy for asthma. Cochrane Database Syst Rev 2003;(4):CD001186.

Arlian LG, Platts-Mills TAE: The biology of dust mites and the remediation of mite allergens in allergic disease. J Allergy Clin Immunol 2001;107:S406-S413.

Bousquet J, van Cauwenberge P, Khaltaev N, et al: Allergic rhinitis and its impact on asthma (ARIA). Allergy 2002;57:841-855.

Calderon M, Alves B, Jacobson M, et al: Allergen injection immunotherapy for seasonal allergic rhinitis. Cochrane Database Syst Rev 2007;(1):CD001936.

Chapman MD, Wood RA: The role and remediation of animal allergens in allergic diseases. J Allergy Clin Immunol 2001;107:S414-S421.

Dykewicz M, Fineman S, Skoner D, et al: Diagnosis and management of rhinitis: Complete guidelines of the Joint Task Force on Practice Parameters in Allergy, Asthma, and Immunology. Ann Allergy Asthma Immunol 1998;81:478-518.

Joint Task Force on Practice Parameters: Allergen immunotherapy: A practice parameter. American Academy of Allergy, Asthma and Immunology. American College of Allergy, Asthma and Immunology. Ann Allergy Asthma Immunol 2003;90:1-40.

Lang DM: Management of allergic rhinitis. Geriatric Times 2002;3(2):41-48.

Naclerio R: Pathophysiology of perennial allergic rhinitis. Allergy 1997;52:7-13.

Spector S, Nicklas RA, Chapman J, et al: Symptom severity assessment of allergic rhinitis. Ann Allergy Asthma Immunol 2003;91:105-116.

References

For a complete list of references, log onto www.expertconsult.com.

Anaphylaxis

Fred Hsieh

DEFINITION AND ETIOLOGY

Anaphylaxis is a serious allergic reaction that has a rapid onset and can cause death. *Anaphylactic reactions* are triggered by immunoglobulin (Ig) E–dependent activation of immune effector cells, whereas *anaphylactoid* reactions are clinically similar to anaphylactic reactions but are not mediated by antigen-specific IgE. Anaphylactic and anaphylactoid reactions are discussed as a single entity in this chapter.

PREVALENCE AND RISK FACTORS

Published incidence and prevalence data are likely inaccurate because anaphylaxis is underdiagnosed and underreported. It is estimated that up to 1000 fatalities caused by anaphylaxis occur every year in the United States. In-hospital anaphylaxis complicates roughly one of every 5000 admissions, and anaphylaxis occurs more frequently in community than in health care settings. Risk factors affecting the incidence of anaphylaxis have been identified (Box 1).

PATHOPHYSIOLOGY

The clinical symptoms of anaphylaxis derive from the mediators (Table 1) released by the activation of sensitized mast cells and basophils. Anaphylactic reactions are triggered by the cross-linking of the high-affinity IgE receptor by receptor-bound IgE that recognizes antigens such as food, drug, or insect venom. Complement protein anaphylatoxins such as C3a and C5a can also trigger anaphylaxis, and nonsteroidal anti-inflammatory agents can trigger anaphylaxis by altering arachidonic acid metabolism. These mediators directly contribute to increased airway resistance, fall in Po_2, and vasodilation with hypotension seen during anaphylaxis.

The most common antigenic triggers of anaphylactic reactions are listed in Box 2. Food-triggered anaphylaxis can occur from any food at any age. Patients allergic to eggs might have an increased frequency of reactions to the egg-containing influenza vaccine, so patients with egg-induced anaphylaxis should not receive the influenza vaccine unless under the guidance of an allergy specialist. Egg-allergic children are not at increased risk for anaphylaxis with the measles–mumps–rubella (MMR) vaccine because sensitivity to this vaccine is likely triggered by sensitivity to gelatin.

Exercise-induced anaphylaxis occurs during or immediately after physical exercise and often after eating a meal. Specific foods have been linked to exercise-induced anaphylaxis. Often, target foods can be tolerated without anaphylaxis in the absence of exercise, and exercise can be tolerated without ingestion of these foods. If specific foods are ingested followed by exercise, however, anaphylaxis can occur. A subset of patients with exercise-induced anaphylaxis can develop anaphylaxis when exercising before or after ingestion of any food, not only a specific food.

If foods, drugs, venoms, or other triggers have not been identified as a cause, then the patient may be classified as having idiopathic anaphylaxis.

SIGNS AND SYMPTOMS

After exposure to an antigenic trigger, symptoms generally develop within 5 to 30 minutes, although symptoms can occur up to several hours after the exposure (Table 2). From 5% to 20% of patients who suffer an anaphylactic event can experience biphasic anaphylaxis during which symptoms can recur up to 8 hours after the initial event, and less than 1% of patients experience protracted anaphylaxis during which symptoms persist for up to 48 hours.

Cutaneous manifestations in anaphylaxis are most common, with respiratory symptoms next most frequent. Death from anaphylaxis results from cardiovascular collapse, bronchospasm, or upper airway edema causing airway obstruction. Gastrointestinal and neurologic manifestations can also occur.

DIAGNOSIS

When considering anaphylaxis in the differential diagnosis, it is important to exclude other clinical disorders that can masquerade as anaphylaxis (Box 3).

Summary

Diagnosis of Anaphylaxis

Anaphylaxis is likely when any one of the following three criteria is fulfilled:

- Acute onset (within minutes to hours) of an illness with skin or mucosal involvement with respiratory compromise and/or reduced blood pressure with associated target-organ sequelae.
- Two or more of the following occur rapidly (minutes to hours) after exposure of a likely allergen: involvement of the skin, respiratory compromise, reduced blood pressure, or persistent gastrointestinal symptoms.
- Reduced blood pressure occurs after exposure to a known allergen for the specific patient; for infants and children, decreased age-specific systolic blood pressure or a greater than 30% decrease from baseline; for adults, systolic blood pressure of less than 90 mm Hg or greater than a 30% decrease from baseline.

Measurement of serum tryptase may be useful in confirming the diagnosis of anaphylaxis. Tryptase is a relatively mast cell–specific protease released upon degranulation. If serum specimens can be obtained between 1 and 6 hours after the event, an elevated serum tryptase level compared with a baseline level obtained when the patient is asymptomatic can confirm that symptoms were caused by an anaphylaxis. Tryptase might not be elevated consistently in patients with food-induced anaphylaxis. An elevated serum histamine level obtained within 1 hour of the event can also suggest anaphylaxis.

Diagnostic testing, if possible, is critical in identifying the triggering antigen. This may be done with cutaneous or serum radioallergosorbent testing overseen by an allergy specialist. Often, a detailed history that reviews over-the-counter medications, ingested foods and drugs, insect stings, and physical activities before the event is the best test. Unfortunately, no clear trigger can be documented in many cases. Diagnostic skin testing should be delayed for at least 6 weeks after the event to obtain an accurate skin test.

Box 1 Risk Factors for the Development of Anaphylaxis

Age
Children: Higher incidence of food-related anaphylaxis
Adults: Higher incidence of anaphylaxis related to antibiotics, radiocontrast media, anesthetic agents, and insect stings

Gender
Females: Anaphylaxis is more common with latex, aspirin, radiocontrast media, and muscle relaxants
Males: Anaphylaxis is more common with insect venom

Socioeconomic Status
Increased frequency of anaphylaxis with higher socioeconomic status

Route of Administration
Oral antigens are less likely to trigger anaphylaxis than parenteral antigens
Oral antigens are less likely to trigger severe symptoms than parenteral antigens

Timing of Administration
Interrupted therapy is more likely to predispose to anaphylaxis

Atopy
Risk factor for anaphylactic and anaphylactoid reactions

Exposure History
The longer the interval since previous antigen exposure, the less likely a reaction will occur

Geography
Prescription rates for self-injection epinephrine devices greater in northern than in southern states

Comorbid Conditions
asthma, cardiovascular disease, substance abuse, mastocytosis

Drugs
Beta blockers and ACE inhibitors can increase anaphylaxis severity
Omalizumab can lead to delayed onset and protracted progression of anaphylaxis

ACE, angiotensin-converting enzyme.

Table 1 Relevant Mediators Released by Mast Cells and Basophils in Anaphylaxis

Mediator	Action
Arachidonic Acid Metabolites	
Cysteinyl leukotrienes Prostaglandins Platelet activating factor	Bronchoconstriction, coronary vasoconstriction, increased vascular permeability, mucus hypersecretion, eosinophil activation and recruitment
Chemokines	
IL-8 MIP-1α	Neutrophil chemotaxis, inflammatory cell recruitment, activation of NADPH oxidase
Cytokines	
GM-CSF IL-3, -4, -5, -6, -10, and -13 TNF-α	Eosinophil chemotaxis and activation; inflammatory cell activation and recruitment, induction of IgE-receptor expression, induction of apoptosis
Proteases	
Chymase Tryptase	Cleavage of complement proteins and neuropeptides, inflammatory-cell chemoattractant, conversion of angiotensin I to angiotensin II, activation of protease-activated receptor-2
Proteoglycans	
Chondroitin sulfate Heparin	Anticoagulation, complement inhibition, eosinophil chemoattractant, kinin activation
Other	
Histamine	Vasodilation, bronchial and gastrointestinal smooth muscle contraction, mucus hypersecretion
Nitric oxide	Vasodilation, increased vascular permeability

GM-CSF, granulocyte-macrophage colony-stimulating factor; NADPH, reduced nicotinamide adenine dinucleotide phosphate; TNF-α, tumor necrosis factor α.

TREATMENT

Rapid recognition of an acute anaphylactic event is essential to prevent an adverse outcome. Initial steps to stabilize the patient should begin with an assessment of the patient's airway and cardiopulmonary status (Box 4). The airway may be secured by intubation or emergent cricothyroidotomy if angioedema from anaphylaxis leads to airway compromise. Intravenous access should be obtained, and any obvious triggering antigen (for example, an insect stinger or an IV medication) should be removed if identified. Vital signs should be monitored, and Trendelenburg positioning and oxygen should be used if necessary. Patients should be kept in the supine position, because deaths have occurred when moving a patient in the midst of an anaphylactic event from the supine to the upright position. The patient should be immediately transported to a facility experienced in managing anaphylaxis.

Epinephrine is the drug of choice in the treatment of anaphylaxis and should be administered immediately on diagnosis. Fatality rates are highest in cases where epinephrine administration is delayed. Adult patients should receive 0.3 to 0.5 mL epinephrine 1:1000 (0.3 to 0.5 mg) IM every 5 to 15 minutes, because up to 16% of patients requiring epinephrine for anaphylaxis require a second dose. Itramuscular administration in the lateral thigh is the recommended site of delivery. If there is no response and the patient is developing signs of shock or cardiovascular collapse, then 0.5 to 1.0 mL of epinephrine 1:10,000 (0.1 mg) IV every 10 to 20 minutes can be given. If IV access cannot be obtained, then epinephrine may be administered by the endotracheal tube. Continuous IV epinephrine infusions have also been used, but its titration should be done in an intensive care unit (ICU) setting.

Other vasopressor medications such as dopamine, norepinephrine, or phenylephrine have also been used in conjunction with colloids or crystalloids for persistent hypotension. H_1 antagonists (e.g., diphenhydramine 25 to 50 mg given PO, IM, or IV) and H_2 antagonists (e.g., ranitidine 50 mg IM or IV) can be useful as adjuncts. Corticosteroids (e.g., hydrocortisone 100 mg to 1 g IV or prednisone 30 to 60 mg PO) used as adjuncts may have a role in preventing the late-phase response. If a patient taking beta blockers experiences anaphylaxis, an IV bolus of glucagon 1 mg may be useful to prevent refractory hypotension and relative bradycardia. Inhaled β-adrenergic aerosols may be useful in treating anaphylaxis-associated bronchospasm.

Summary

- Epinephrine is the treatment of choice for anaphylaxis and should not be withheld even in patients with cardiovascular disease.

Box 2 Triggers of Anaphylactic Reactions

Drugs
Antibiotics
Antisera
Aspirin and other nonsteroidal anti-inflammatory drugs
Opiates
Perioperative medications
Topical benzocaine
Vaccines

Hormones
Insulin
Progesterone

Blood and Blood Products
Antithymocyte globulin
Intravenous immunoglobulins

Enzymes
Streptokinase

Foods*
Egg
Milk
Peanuts
Shellfish
Soy
Tree nuts
Wheat

Venom
Hymenoptera
Fire ant
Snake

Other
Dialysis membranes
Human seminal fluid
Latex
Protamine
Radiocontrast media
Therapeutic allergen extracts
Topical disinfectants

**Any food can cause anaphylaxis.*

Table 2 Signs and Symptoms of Anaphylaxis

Organ	Symptom
Skin	Urticaria and angioedema, flushing, pruritus
Respiratory	Dyspnea, wheezing, airway angioedema, rhinitis
Gastrointestinal	Nausea, vomiting, diarrhea, cramping, pain
Cardiovascular	Tachycardia, hypotension, chest pain, cardiac arrest
Neurologic	Headache, dizziness, seizures, sense of impending doom

Box 3 Masqueraders of Anaphylaxis

Cardiovascular
Cardiogenic shock
Hypovolemic shock
Vasovagal syncope

Endocrinologic
Carcinoid syndrome
Medullary carcinoma of the thyroid
Pheochromocytoma

Pulmonary
Status asthmaticus
Pulmonary embolism
Airway foreign body

Neurologic
Autonomic epilepsy
Seizure disorder
Stroke

Toxic or Metabolic
Drug overdose
Monosodium glutamate ingestion or other restaurant syndromes
Red man syndrome after vancomycin infusion
Scombroid fish poisoning
Sulfite ingestion

Systemic Disorders
Acute promyelocytic leukemia
Basophilic leukemia
Hereditary or acquired angioedema
Systemic mastocytosis

Psychiatric
Globus hystericus
Munchausen syndrome
Panic attack
Vocal cord dysfunction

Box 4 Medical Management of Anaphylaxis

Epinephrine
Recumbent positioning
Vasopressor agents
Airway management with intubation if necessary
Intravenous fluids
Glucagon (in the case of beta-blocker therapy)
H_1 antagonists
H_2 antagonists
Steroids
Inhaled or aerosolized beta agonists

A patient who has had an anaphylactic event should be given specific recommendations based on diagnostic testing to prevent and treat future episodes (Box 5). Patients should wear medical alert jewelry identifying their risk for anaphylaxis and should be prescribed self-injectable epinephrine and instructed in its use. If an etiologic trigger has been identified, then specific instructions should be given to avoid future episodes. In some cases, further risk reduction can be achieved under the care of an allergy specialist, which can include allergen immunotherapy to selected insect venoms, drug desensitization for beta-lactam antibiotics, and premedication regimens for radiocontrast media reactions. Beta-blocker and angiotensin-converting enzyme inhibitors should be discontinued, if possible.

If exercise-induced anaphylaxis is diagnosed and diagnostic testing has identified a specific food trigger, then the patient must refrain from eating that food for 4 to 6 hours before or after exercise. If no specific food is identified, then the patient should limit physical exercise or stop immediately on development of prodromal symptoms. Pretreatment with H_1 blockers is not considered effective. The patient should always exercise with a partner and should carry self-injectable epinephrine at all times.

In the case of idiopathic anaphylaxis, the patient might benefit from long-term prednisone therapy to induce remission. Patients

Box 5 Prevention of Anaphylaxis

Post-event evaluation and identification of specific triggers
Avoidance of potentially cross-reactive antigens
Medical alert jewellery
Self-injectable epinephrine
Avoid beta-blockers, angiotensin-converting enzyme inhibitors if possible*
Education for preventive measures*
Pretreatment, desensitization, or immunotherapy as indicated*

**Specific recommendations need to be individualized for each patient based on risk-to-benefit analyses.*

may be prescribed prednisone 40 to 60 mg PO daily in conjunction with hydroxyzine, albuterol, and self-injectable epinephrine followed by conversion after 1 to 6 weeks of prednisone to alternate-day dosing and reduction of the prednisone dose by 5 to 10 mg/dose each month until the taper is complete. The diagnosis and management of idiopathic anaphylaxis should be performed by an allergy specialist.

OUTCOMES

The most feared outcome of anaphylaxis is death. Although deaths resulting from anaphylaxis are rare, many are potentially preventable. Many of the deaths from anaphylaxis are iatrogenic, and the presence of asthma is a risk factor. The delayed use of epinephrine is a risk factor for a poor outcome, and physicians often inappropriately wait until after cardiac arrest has occurred before administering epinephrine. Nevertheless, some patients still die despite receiving epinephrine. Poor outcomes can occur regardless of the antigenic trigger, and death can occur even in idiopathic anaphylaxis.

Further Readings

Castells MC, Horan RF, Sheffer AL: Exercise-induced anaphylaxis (EIA). Clin Rev Allergy Immunol 1999;17:413-424.

Hare ND, Ballas ZK: Effectiveness of delayed epinephrine in anaphylaxis. J Allergy Clin Immunol 2007;120:716-717.

Lieberman P, Kemp SF, Oppenheimer J, et al: The diagnosis and management of anaphylaxis: An updated practice parameter. J Allergy Clin Immunol 2005;115:S483-S523.

Limb SL, Starke PR, Lee CE, Chowdhury BA: Delayed onset and protracted progression of anaphylaxis after omalizumab administration in patients with asthma. J Allergy Clin Immunol 2007;120:1378-1381.

Lin RY, Schwartz LB, Curry A, et al: Histamine and tryptase levels in patients with acute allergic reactions: An emergency department-based study. J Allergy Clin Immunol 2000;106:65-71.

Sampson HA, Mendelson L, Rosen JP: Fatal and near-fatal anaphylactic reactions to food in children and adolescents. N Engl J Med 1992;327:380-384.

Sampson HA, Munoz-Furlong A, Campbell RL, et al: Second symposium on the definition and management of anaphylaxis: Summary report—Second National Institute of Allergy and Infectious Disease/Food Allergy and Anaphylaxis Network symposium. J Allergy Clin Immunol 2006;177:391-397.

Simons FER: Anaphylaxis, killer allergy: Long-term management in the community. J Allergy Clin Immunol 2006;117:367-377.

Simons FER: Anaphylaxis: Evidence-based long-term risk reduction in the community. Immunol Allergy Clin N Am 2007:27:231-248.

Simons FER, Frew AJ, Ansotegui IJ, et al: Risk assessment in anaphylaxis: Current and future approaches. J Allergy Clin Immunol 2007;120:S2-S24.

Hymenoptera Venom Allergy

Velma L. Paschall

DEFINITION

Hymenoptera venom allergy is an immunoglobulin E (IgE)-mediated hypersensitivity to the venom of insects in the insect order Hymenoptera. This allergic reaction may be caused by stings from a number of species in this insect order, occurring only in epersons who have previously been sensitized to Hymenoptera venom.

EPIDEMIOLOGY

Insect sting allergy can develop at any age and usually manifests after several uneventful stings. The incidence of systemic reactions to Hymenoptera venom is approximately 3% in adults. Although children are stung more often than adults, systemic reactions occur in only about 1% of children younger than 17 years, and many of these reactions are relatively mild. Large local reactions to Hymenoptera stings are more common in children, with an estimated incidence of 20% and 10%, respectively, for children and adults. The prevalence of insect sting allergy is twice as high in male as in female patients and may be a result of increased exposure rather than inherent susceptibility. There is no clear association with other allergies, and only 30% of patients with venom allergy are atopic. In addition, insect sting allergy is statistically not more likely to occur in persons with a family history of sting reactions.

At least 50 deaths per year occur in the United States from insect sting reactions, and many other sting fatalities may be unrecognized. Approximately one half of deaths occur in victims with no history of a prior sting reaction. Most fatalities (80%) occur in adults older than 40 years, and only 2% occur in persons younger than 20 years.

Hymenoptera Stinging Insects

All the stinging insects belong to the insect order Hymenoptera, of which there are 16,000 species in North America. Less than 1% are responsible for human stings (Fig. 1). All the species that are medically important belong to three families: Apidae, Vespidae, and Formicidae. Only the females of each species have stingers, which are ovipositors that have lost their egg-laying function and have been modified for stinging and envenomization. Most species sting in defense of themselves and their nests, although some species also sting as a means of capturing their prey.

Apidae Family

Honeybees are found throughout the United States and live in colonies of up to 65,000 bees. Feral honeybees are less common than domestic honeybees and build their nests inside hollow trees or logs. Domestic honeybees live in human-made hives and are commercially managed for honey production and pollination. They are relatively docile insects and usually sting only when provoked. When a honeybee stings, it leaves a barbed stinger with an attached venom sac in the victim's skin, resulting in evisceration of the bee and its subsequent death. Most honeybee stings, other than in beekeepers, occur in people walking barefoot on lawns or handling flowering plants. Africanized honeybees, commonly referred to as "killer bees," migrated into the United States in 1990 from Mexico and have become a major stinging threat in southern Texas. These bees were brought to Brazil from Africa in 1956 in an attempt to replace the European honeybee with a more productive tropical-climate honeybee. Africanized bees look like domestic honeybees and deliver the same venom, but they mount an aggressive response when they perceive a threat to their hive. The tendency to swarm and then sting in very large numbers has resulted in deaths in cattle and humans because of toxic reactions.

Vespidae Family

Yellow jackets, hornets, and wasps are the stinging insects in the Vespidae family that are of medical importance in the United States. Vespids make nests of masticated wood containing layers of combs with many individual cells. The comb layers are arranged vertically and, except for wasp nests, are encased in an outer layer of paper. Unlike honeybees, vespids have relatively smooth stingers and can sting repeatedly. Some species of yellow jackets occasionally leave their stingers in the skin, however.

Yellow jackets account for most stings overall in the United States. They are especially prevalent in the Northeast and Midwest. They prefer to build their nests underground or in human-made structures low to the ground. They are notorious scavengers and often seek food in picnic areas and around trash containers. They are the most aggressive of all the vespids and sting with little or no provocation during the late summer and early fall, when their colony numbers are largest and food supplies are somewhat limited.

New World hornets are closely related to yellow jackets; they are slightly larger but have similar coloring. Yellow hornets and white-faced (or bald-faced) hornets are actually aerial yellow jackets. They build large nests in trees or shrubs. Like yellow jackets, they are aggressive insects, particularly in the vicinity of their nests. Old World hornets, also known as European hornets, were accidentally introduced into the Eastern United States in the mid-1800s. These hornets usually build their nests in hollow trees and, unlike the other members of the Vespidae family, they typically fly at night and are attracted to bright lights. Although they are much larger and more fearsome in appearance than the New World hornets, they are less aggressive. The population of these insects is gradually increasing, but they are still minor stinging threats.

Paper wasps can be found throughout the United States, most commonly in the southern states. Wasp colonies are relatively small, and wasps are less aggressive than yellow jackets and hornets. Wasps tend to build their nests near human habitation (e.g., under the eaves of houses, on porches, and below deck railings), and stinging encounters with these insects are, therefore, common.

Formicidae Family

Fire ants are the medically important members of the Formicidae family, and several species of both native and imported fire ants exist in the United States. Both can cause severe allergic reactions, but imported fire ants are much more aggressive and prolific and inflict the most stings. Imported fire ants were introduced in 1940 through the port of Mobile, Alabama, by cargo ships from South America. They have spread through the surrounding states and Gulf coast. Imported fire ants build large nests (mounds) in the soil, and when their nests are disturbed, the ants attack in mass and sting their victims repeatedly. A characteristic sterile pustule typically forms at the site of each sting after 24 hours.

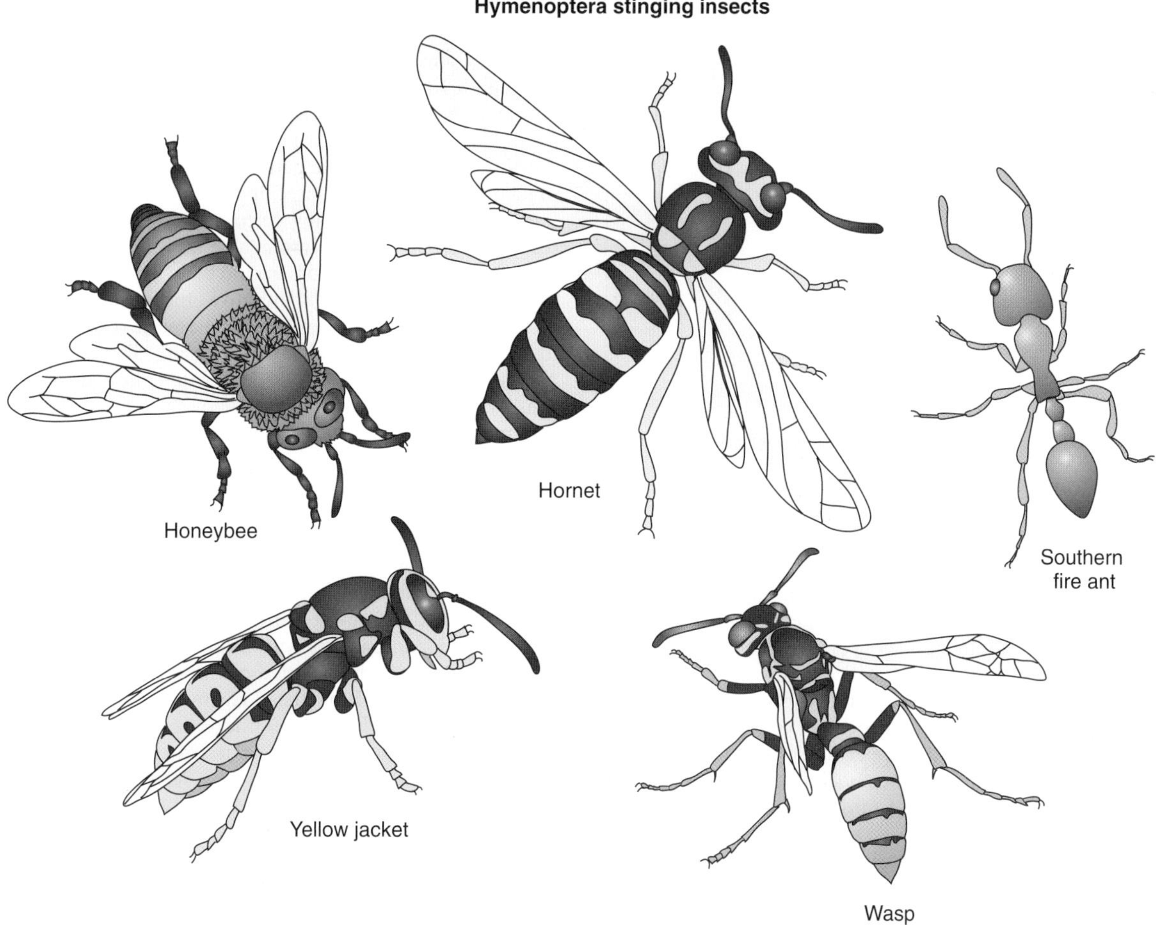

Figure 1 Hymenoptera causing stings in humans include honeybees, wasps, yellow jackets, hornets, and fire ants.

Hymenoptera Venoms

Venoms of the flying Hymenoptera are largely aqueous solutions containing proteins, peptides, and vasoactive amines. The toxic properties of the venom are caused by these components collectively, and several of the venom proteins are allergenic. Immunologic cross-reactivity exists among the Hymenoptera venoms and is extensive between yellow jackets and hornets, moderate between wasps and other vespids, and minimal between honeybees and vespids. Imported fire ant venom is distinctly different from the other venoms and consists of a mixture of piperidine alkaloids and a small aqueous component containing allergenic proteins. One of these proteins is similar to one of the vespid allergens, and cross-reactivity between fire ants and vespids occasionally occurs.

PATHOPHYSIOLOGY

Both systemic and large local reactions to stinging insects are usually caused by IgE-mediated reactions to Hymenoptera venom. At least one prior sting is required to sensitize a person to venom, and sensitization is more likely to occur following multiple simultaneous stings or subsequent stings occurring over a relatively short period of time. Once sensitization has occurred, a sting can cause mast cell and basophil degranulation, resulting in release of the histamine and other inflammatory mediators responsible for the signs and symptoms of anaphylactic and some large local reactions. See the article "Anaphylaxis," for further information on the pathophysiology of anaphylaxis.

SIGNS AND SYMPTOMS

Most Hymenoptera stings cause *small local reactions* of no significant medical consequence. These normal sting reactions are characterized by pain, itching, redness, and swelling at the sting site that resolve within several hours and are caused by the pharmacologic properties of the venom. Some *large local reactions* are caused by a late-phase IgE-dependent reaction that is mild initially but progresses after 12 to 24 hours to a diameter of more than 5 cm; these usually peak in intensity at 48 to 72 hours. These reactions are contiguous with the sting site and occasionally involve an entire extremity. In rare cases, massive swelling causes local anatomic compression. Large local sting reactions typically resolve gradually over 5 to 10 days. Virtually all patients with large local reactions continue to have similar reactions with subsequent stings. This tendency is not modified with venom immunotherapy; therefore, patients with large local reactions are not candidates for further diagnostic evaluation (see later).

Systemic reactions cause signs and symptoms in one or more organ systems and are almost always IgE-mediated. Systemic reactions cause a spectrum of manifestations, ranging from cutaneous signs (*pruritus*, *flushing*, urticaria, angioedema) to respiratory involvement (cough, throat and/or chest tightness, dyspnea, wheezing) and cardiovascular compromise (dizziness, hypotension, unconsciousness), depending on the severity of the reaction. Gastrointestinal manifestations (nausea, vomiting, diarrhea) and uterine cramping also occur occasionally. Cardiac anaphylaxis with manifestations of coronary vasospasm, arrhythmias, or bradycardia can also

Table 1 Symptoms and Signs of Insect Sting Anaphylaxis in Adults and Children

Symptom or Sign	Frequency (%)	
	Adults	Children
Cutaneous only	15	60
Urticaria/angioedema	80	95
Dizziness/hypotension	60	10
Dyspnea/wheezing	50	40
Throat tightness/hoarseness	40	40
Loss of consciousness	30	5

From Golden DBK, Lichtenstein LM. Insect sting allergy. In Kaplan AP (ed): Allergy. New York, Churchill Livingstone, 1985, pp 507-524.

occur following stings, even in persons with no underlying cardiac disease. Systemic reactions usually cause signs and symptoms starting within minutes following a sting. In general, the sooner the symptoms occur, the more severe the reaction. Cutaneous signs and symptoms occur in 80% of adults and 95% of children with systemic reactions, but they are the sole manifestation of the reaction in only 15% of adults. Isolated cutaneous reactions occur in 60% of children, however, who tend to have a more benign course than adults. Although symptoms involving the upper and lower airways occur with approximately the same frequency in children and adults, children have a much lower incidence of cardiovascular manifestations (Table 1).

Systemic reactions also occur occasionally as a result of the toxic properties of Hymenoptera venom. They are most often associated with multiple simultaneous stings or underlying mastocytosis. These reactions may be indistinguishable from acute, systemic IgE-mediated reactions. Large numbers of stings can cause other serious reactions including rhabdomyolysis with renal failure, hemolysis, acute respiratory distress syndrome, and diffuse intravascular coagulation. Delayed reactions of unknown mechanism that rarely occur following stings include serum-sickness–like reactions, neuropathies, Guillain-Barré syndrome, myocarditis, and glomerulonephritis.

DIAGNOSIS

History

The diagnosis of Hymenoptera venom allergy is based primarily on a convincing history, inasmuch as positive skin test results occur in 15% to 20% of persons who are clinically nonreactive. Physicians should ask about serious sting reactions when obtaining a medical history, because many affected persons fail to mention them during a routine history and examination. Details of the history that might help distinguish the type of reaction (toxic or allergic, local or systemic) include the number of stings and their locations on the body, the nature and timing of prior stings, the time course of the reaction, and the symptoms and treatment.

Skin Testing

Positive skin tests to Hymenoptera venom extracts confirm IgE-mediated hypersensitivity in the context of a positive sting reaction history and help identify specific insects to which a patient is allergic. Venom protein extracts are used for diagnostic testing because whole-body extracts do not contain sufficient venom to distinguish allergic from nonallergic persons. Whole-body extracts are currently still being used for the diagnosis of fire ant allergy, because commercial fire ant venom extracts are not yet available. Fire ant whole-body extracts, unlike those of the flying Hymenoptera insects, have sufficient sensitivity and specificity to be useful diagnostically, although fire ant venom extracts, which are still under development, appear to be superior. Hymenoptera venom testing is usually performed with each of the five commercial venom extracts available in the United States, because patients are often inaccurate with regard to identification of the sting culprit.

Venom testing is usually performed initially with prick tests. If results are negative, intradermal skin tests are performed beginning with a venom concentration around 0.001 μg/mL. If the skin tests at this concentration are still negative, the venom concentration is increased by 10-fold increments until a positive skin test occurs, up to a maximum concentration of 1.0 μg/mL. Skin testing with higher concentrations is not performed because they are more likely to cause false-positive reactions caused by the irritant properties of the venom. Because of the known cross-reactivities among the vespid venoms, skin tests are often positive to several venoms even when there has been a reaction to only a single insect sting.

Although most patients with convincing histories of sting reactions have positive skin test results, some skin tests are negative. Skin test findings may be negative during the first 6 weeks after a sting because of a refractory period or anergy, and skin testing in these patients should be repeated after 1 or 2 months. Negative skin tests can also occur in patients with a positive history who had remote sting reactions and have lost their sensitivity and in persons who had systemic non–IgE-mediated reactions as a result of toxic effects of the venom or underlying mastocytosis. Some patients with a positive history and a negative skin test do have venom-specific IgE antibodies in the serum that can be detected by serologic testing using a radioallergosorbent test (RAST). Venom skin tests do not correlate perfectly with serologic venom-specific IgE assays, which are negative in approximately 20% of patients with positive skin tests. On the other hand, venom skin tests are negative in approximately 10% of subjects with detectable venom-specific IgE antibodies.

Venom skin tests and RAST should be considered complementary because neither test alone detects all patients with insect sting allergy. In a 2003 rostrum paper, the Insect Committee of the American Academy of Allergy, Asthma, and Immunology recommended that the published 1999 practice parameter for stinging insect allergy revise the diagnostic algorithm for insect sting allergy to include IgE antivenom serologic testing in patients with positive histories and negative skin tests. The updated 2004 practice parameter for stinging insect hypersensitivity recommends that for patients who have had a severe systemic reaction to an insect sting and who have negative venom skin test, repeat skin testing or in vitro testing for venom-specific IgE antibodies should be performed before concluding that venom immunotherapy is not necessary.

The level of sensitivity of venom skin testing or serologic testing does not accurately predict the severity of subsequent sting reactions. Low sensitivity on skin tests or RAST may be present in some persons who have had near-fatal anaphylactic reactions, and the strongest reactions on skin tests are often in patients who have had only large local reactions to stings.

In most cases, skin testing is not necessary in patients with histories of only large local reactions or in children who have had only mild systemic reactions limited to the skin (flushing, urticaria, angioedema) because their risk of having a more serious reaction subsequently is relatively low (Table 2).

TREATMENT

Treatment of Acute Reactions

Local reactions to insect stings are usually treated with cold packs, oral antihistamines, analgesics, and topical corticosteroids, all of which can help alleviate the associated itching and the local pain and

Table 2 Indications for Insect Venom Skin Testing

Patient	Local Reaction	Cutaneous Systemic Reaction	Anaphylaxis
Child	No	No	Yes
Adult	No	Yes	Yes

swelling. A short course of an oral corticosteroid may be given for very large local reactions and is most effective within the first few hours after a sting. Occasionally, large local reactions are mistaken for cellulitis, and lymphangitic streaks can occur on the extremities as a result of drainage of inflammatory mediators. When these reactions occur in the 24 to 48 hours after a sting, infection is extremely unlikely, and treatment should include cold packs and an oral corticosteroid given for 4 to 5 days.

Treatment of Systemic Reactions

Mild systemic reactions manifested only by cutaneous symptoms may respond to antihistamines alone. Most systemic reactions, however, require treatment with epinephrine. Patients with any signs or symptoms of upper or lower airway obstruction or hypotension should immediately receive aqueous epinephrine intramuscularly, emergency medical attention and treatment, and close observation for 4 hours or longer depending on the reaction severity. Some patients require additional doses of epinephrine and/or other treatment for severe anaphylactic reactions. The recommended dose of epinephrine is 0.3 to 0.5 mg (0.3-0.5 mL of 1:1000 weight/volume solution) for adults, and 0.01 mg/kg (maximum 0.3 mg) or 0.01 mL/kg of 1:1000 weight/volume solution (maximum 0.3 mL) for children. Delay in the use of epinephrine has contributed to fatalities, and some patients with anaphylactic shock are resistant to epinephrine. Patients who are taking beta blockers can also be resistant to epinephrine and can require large amounts of intravenous fluids and glucagon to reverse anaphylaxis. See the article "Anaphylaxis," for additional information on the treatment of anaphylaxis.

FUTURE STING REACTIONS

Prevention

After acute care of a sting reaction, patients should be given a prescription for an epinephrine autoinjector, referral to an allergist or immunologist, and instructions on preventing insect stings. Epinephrine autoinjectors are available in only two strengths (EpiPen 0.3 mg and EpiPen Jr. 0.15 mg). The EpiPen Jr. is usually preferred in children weighing less than 25 kg. Patients and their caregivers should be given instructions on the correct technique for use of the device and reminded to replace it at expiration. Patients should be advised to minimize high-risk exposure to stinging insects that can occur through lawn and garden work, working near trash bins, and eating and drinking outdoors. Stings to the mouth and tongue can occur from ingesting food or flavored drinks that are being scavenged by yellow jackets. Additional information on avoidance and on identification of insects is available at www.aaaai.org/patients/publicedmat/tips/stinginginsect.stm.

Natural History

The risk that a future sting will cause an allergic reaction depends on the history and on the person's immunologic status. For adults who have had a severe systemic reaction and who have positive skin tests or RAST, the risk of a subsequent systemic reaction is approximately 60%, but it is significantly less, approximately 20%, if the prior reaction caused only cutaneous symptoms (flushing, urticaria, angioedema). The outcomes of subsequent stings can vary within an individual patient because of variations in the insect species, the amount of allergen delivered, and fluctuation in the patient's immunologic and physiologic status. The risk of a recurrent systemic sting reaction is higher in patients with honeybee allergy than in those allergic to vespids. Patients who have had severe reactions have a higher risk of recurrent sting reactions than do those who have sustained milder reactions, and adults have a higher risk of recurrent systemic reactions than children.

In general, individuals have a stereotypical response to stings that does not vary greatly from one sting to another; despite popular opinion, it is unusual for patients to have increasingly severe reactions with each subsequent sting. Children who have had mild systemic reactions limited to the skin have only a 10% risk of subsequent systemic reaction, and less than 1% risk of having a reaction more severe than the prior one. The risk of recurrence of a severe systemic reaction in a child is significantly higher, approximately 40%, although it is still lower than for a comparable reaction in an adult.

Adults and children who have had only large local reactions have a relatively low risk (5%-10%) of having a systemic reaction with a subsequent sting, although most of them will continue to have large local reactions.

Venom Immunotherapy

Indications

Venom immunotherapy is the treatment of choice for preventing allergic sting reactions in patients who have a significant risk of a serious reaction to a future sting. Children who have had systemic reactions limited to the skin do not require immunotherapy because they have a very low risk of anaphylaxis from future stings. Adults who have had only mild systemic sting reactions and who have positive skin tests and/or positive RAST results are usually advised to undergo immunotherapy, however, because of their increased risk (compared with children) of having systemic reactions that progress from isolated cutaneous symptoms to anaphylaxis. Immunotherapy is indicated for children and adults who have had severe systemic reactions and have positive skin tests and/or RAST results. Fig. 2 illustrates a clinical algorithm of evaluation and management of insect sting anaphylaxis. Venom immunotherapy is not required for either adults or children who have had only large local reactions because of their low risk of anaphylaxis with subsequent stings.

Selection of Venoms and Dosing

The selection of venom extracts used for immunotherapy is based on the results of the skin tests to the individual venoms. Therapy usually includes all venoms that are positive on skin testing, and mixed vespid venom (containing equal parts of yellow jacket, yellow hornet, and white-faced hornet venoms) is most often used in patients with vespid allergy. Although yellow jacket venom may protect against reactions to hornet stings because of their extensive cross-reactivity, the clinical protection is less reliable with single vespid venom than with mixed vespid venom therapy. Separate injections of honeybee venom and wasp venom extracts are given if skin tests are positive to either or both of these venoms. Immunotherapy with whole-body extracts of fire ants is available for patients with histories of systemic IgE-mediated reactions to fire ant stings.

Venom immunotherapy is initiated at a very small dose of venom that is increased to the full maintenance dose according to a schedule recommended by the laboratory that prepared the venom extract

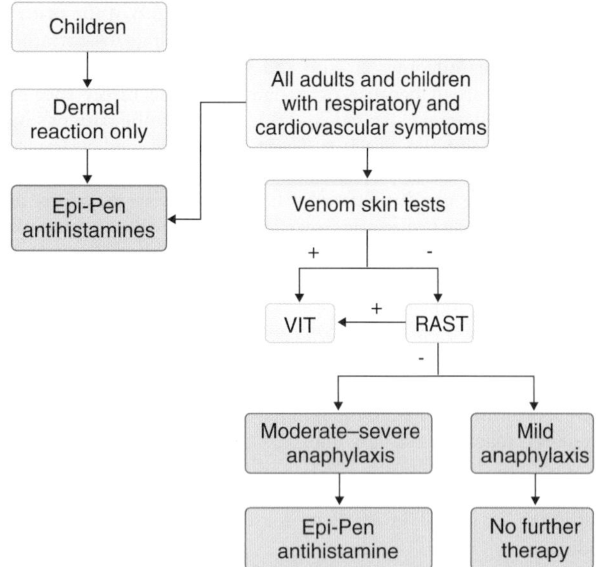

Figure 2 A clinical algorithm of evaluation and management of insect sting anaphylaxis. *(From Reisman RE. Insect sting anaphylaxis. In Leung DYM, Sampson HA, Geha RS, et al, eds: Pediatric Allergy: Principles and Practice. St. Louis, Mosby, 2003, pp 633-642.)*

and/or by the prescribing physician. Adverse reactions are usually no more common with rapid dosage regimens that can achieve maintenance doses in days or weeks than with traditional regimens that take 4 to 6 months. The standard recommended maintenance dose is 100 μg for each venom to which the patient has a positive skin test. This dose was originally selected because it was approximately twice the amount of venom in a single honeybee sting (50 μg). The amount of venom injected by a vespid varies significantly, with estimates ranging from 2 to 20 μg per sting.

Maintenance venom immunotherapy is usually administered at 4-week intervals for at least 1 year. Several studies have shown that the maintenance interval may be extended to 6 to 8 weeks over several years in most patients. Some physicians elect to repeat skin tests every 2 to 3 years while patients are receiving maintenance therapy, although only 50% to 60% of patients have a negative skin test even after 7 to 10 years of therapy.

Efficacy

Venom immunotherapy is extremely efficacious in preventing subsequent systemic reactions in patients with stinging insect allergy. Efficacy is highest with mixed vespid venom; it is 98% effective in preventing subsequent systemic reactions with a maintenance dose of 300 μg (100 μg per venom). For therapy with individual venoms (i.e., honeybee, yellow jacket, or wasp) at a dose of 100 μg per venom, immunotherapy is 75% to 95% effective in preventing systemic reactions to future stings. Those few patients who continue to have systemic reactions usually have milder reactions than before beginning treatment. Increasing the maintenance dose of immunotherapy to 200 μg provides full protection for most patients who have had systemic reactions while receiving treatment with single venoms at a dose of 100 μg.

Safety

Adverse reactions to venom immunotherapy are no more frequent than reactions to immunotherapy for inhalant allergens (i.e., pollen, mold, dust mites). Systemic reactions occur in 5% to 15% of patients, most commonly during the first few weeks of treatment and while receiving maintenance doses, and are more likely to occur in patients receiving honeybee venom than in those being treated with yellow jacket venom. Most systemic reactions to venom immunotherapy are mild and do not require epinephrine. Large local reactions occur in up to 50% of patients receiving venom immunotherapy and are not predictive of systemic reactions to subsequent injections. Pretreatment with antihistamines given before injections decreases both local and systemic reactions and does not interfere with the efficacy of immunotherapy.

Patients who are taking beta blockers are at increased risk for more serious anaphylaxis if they have a systemic reaction during venom immunotherapy in part because they are more likely to be refractory to treatment with epinephrine. An effort should be made to substitute alternative medication (e.g., diuretic or calcium channel blocker for treatment of hypertension) before initiating immunotherapy in these patients. As with inhalant immunotherapy, maintenance venom immunotherapy can be continued during pregnancy, although it is not recommended that it be initiated during pregnancy. Venom immunotherapy should be performed only in an office or clinic that is prepared to give immediate treatment of anaphylaxis, and patients must remain in the office for at least 30 minutes before going home after an injection.

Box 1 Duration of Venom Immunotherapy

In most patients venom immunotherapy can be stopped after 5 years of treatment.

Patients with higher frequencies of anaphylaxis recurrence after immunotherapy is stopped include:

- Those with honeybee allergy
- Those who had a systemic reaction during treatment (sting or venom injection)
- Those who received treatment for less than 5 years
- Those who had severe (nearly fatal) sting reactions before treatment

Patients with any of these high-risk characteristics should probably receive venom immunotherapy indefinitely.

Duration and Outcomes

Since 1979, when the U.S. Food and Drug Administration approved Hymenoptera venom extracts for venom immunotherapy, the product package inserts have recommended that therapy be continued indefinitely. Some experts have suggested that venom immunotherapy can be stopped if venom skin test or venom-specific IgE antibody levels become negative on retesting. However, most patients continue to have positive skin tests and/or venom-specific IgE antibodies after 5 years of therapy. More recent studies have shown that venom immunotherapy can be discontinued after 5 years of therapy in most patients. Although there is usually no reaction to a sting during the first 2 years after stopping treatment, the risk of relapse increases during the third year and does not disappear even up to 15 years after discontinuation. Golden and colleagues reported that after stopping immunotherapy, the chance of a systemic reaction is approximately 10% with each future sting for 10 or more years after treatment is discontinued, even if venom skin tests become negative. Most reactions that occur are less severe than those occurring before venom immunotherapy, although some patients who have had life-threatening reactions before treatment can have very severe reactions after stopping treatment. Patients with honeybee allergy and those who had a systemic reaction while receiving immunotherapy, from either an injection or a field sting, also appear to have higher frequencies of anaphylaxis after discontinuing venom immunotherapy. These patients, as well as those who had very severe reactions before starting therapy, appear to have a higher risk of relapse and should, therefore, probably receive venom immunotherapy indefinitely (Box 1). Extension of immunotherapy beyond 5 years' duration may be considered in other patients who are unwilling to accept the 10% risk of systemic reaction with each future sting.

Summary

- Hymenoptera venom allergy is an IgE-mediated hypersensitivity to the venom of stinging insects in the insect order Hymenoptera.
- Large local reactions from insect stings tend to recur after subsequent stings, with relatively low risk (5% to 10%) of developing anaphylaxis.
- Adults who have had a severe systemic reaction to an insect sting and who have positive skin tests have approximately a 60% risk of anaphylaxis with each subsequent sting.
- The diagnosis of Hymenoptera allergy is based on a convincing history and positive skin tests and/or radioallergosorbent test (RAST).
- People at risk of insect sting anaphylaxis should be educated regarding measures to avoid insect stings, have an epinephrine autoinjector immediately available, and be advised to receive venom immunotherapy.

Further Readings

Barnard JH: Studies of 400 Hymenoptera sting deaths in the United States. J Allergy Clin Immunol 1973;52:259-264.

Golden DB: Insect allergy. In Adkinson NF Jr, Yunginger JW, Busse WW, et al (eds): Middleton's Allergy: Principles & Practice, 6th ed. Philadelphia, Mosby, 2003, pp 1475-1486.

Golden DB, Kagey-Sobotka A, Lichtenstein LM: Survey of patients after discontinuing venom immunotherapy. J Allergy Clin Immunol 2000;105:385-390.

Golden DB, Kagey-Sobotka A, Norman PS, et al: Sting Challenge Trial I: Spectrum of a population with insect sting allergy. J Allergy Clin Immunol 1998;101:S159.

Golden DB, Marsh DG, Kagey-Sobotka A, et al: Epidemiology of insect venom sensitivity. JAMA 1989;262:240-244.

Golden DB, Tracy JM, Freeman TM, Hoffman DR: Insect Committee of the American Academy of Allergy, Asthma and Immunology. Negative venom skin test results in patients with histories of systemic reaction to a sting. J Allergy Clin Immunol 2003;112:495-498.

Lockey RF, Turkeltaub PC, Baird-Warren IA, et al: The Hymenoptera venom study I, 1979-1982: Demographics and history—sting data. J Allergy Clin Immunol 1988;82:370-381.

Lockey RF, Turkeltaub PC, Olive ES, et al: The Hymenoptera venom study. III: Safety of venom immunotherapy. J Allergy Clin Immunol 1990;86:775-780.

Moffitt JE, Golden DB, Reisman RE, et al: Stinging insect hypersensitivity: A practice parameter update. J Allergy Clin Immunol 2004;114:869-886.

Portnoy JM, Moffitt JE, Golden DB, et al: Stinging insect hypersensitivity: A practice parameter. J Allergy Clin Immunol 1999;103:963-980.

Urticaria and Angioedema

Sandra Hong and Sheila Armogida

DEFINITION

Urticaria, also known as hives, is defined as raised, erythematous skin lesions that are pruritic and evanescent. They typically last less than 24 hours without leaving residual marks or bruising. Urticaria can be divided into two categories. *Acute urticaria* is defined as outbreaks of urticarial lesions that do not persist beyond 6 weeks. *Chronic urticaria* is defined as the recurrence of hives on a near daily basis for more than 6 weeks.

Angioedema, deeper asymmetrical swelling of the lower dermal and subcutaneous or submucosal tissue, may be associated with or independent of hives.

PREVALENCE

Urticaria is a common disorder that has been described in the writings of Hippocrates, Pliny the Elder, and Celsus.[1] The term *urticaria* was first used in the late 18th century; however, most of the research describing the different subtypes and pathophysiology has evolved over the last century or so.

Urticaria continues to be a prevalent skin disorder worldwide. Epidemiologic studies show that approximately 15% to 25% of the population experience at least one episode of urticaria in their lifetime.[2,3] Hives affect 6% to 7% of preschool children and 17% of children with atopic dermatitis.[4] In all age groups, 49% have a combination of urticaria and angioedema, 40% have urticaria only, and 11% have isolated angioedema.[3]

Urticaria and angioedema are considerable health care burdens in the United States. They are common causes of patient visits to physicians. Evaluation for the underlying cause can lead to extensive laboratory screening, on average more than 20 laboratory tests.[5] Despite thorough evaluation, 80% of patients with chronic urticaria have no identifiable cause of hives, commonly called *chronic idiopathic urticaria.* Although hives rarely cause mortality, patients with chronic urticaria experience significant impairments in quality of life at home, school, and work from loss of sleep, loss of energy, social isolation, and altered emotional reactions.[6,7]

PATHOPHYSIOLOGY

Urticaria results from activation of cutaneous mast cells.[8] Mast cell stimulation induces vasopermeation and vasodilation, leading to dermal edema and recruitment of cellular and humoral immune effectors. In many cases, the pathogenesis of mast cell activation is incompletely understood and still requires further elucidation. Three metabolic consequences occur with mast cell activation: degranulation (immediate release of mediators including histamine, serotonin, tumor necrosis factor [TNF]-α, proteases, and proteoglycans); cytokine and chemokine synthesis (leading to late-phase inflammation); and leukotriene and prostaglandin synthesis. Depending on the stimulus, mast cell activation can involve any or all three of the metabolic processes in the production and persistence of hives.[9]

Mast cell stimulation leading to acute and chronic urticaria can be caused by IgE-mediated reaction, autoimmunity, direct mast cell activation, arachidonic acid metabolism, infections, physical urticarias, and systemic diseases (Box 1).

IgE-mediated reactions to foods, medications, stinging insects, aeroallergens, and contactants are common causes of acute urticaria.

Direct mast cell stimulation by medications, such as opioid narcotics, vancomycin, neuromuscular blocking agents, and radiocontrast media can cause urticaria and angioedema by a non-IgE-mediated process.

Autoimmunity accounts for 30% to 50% of cases of chronic urticaria in adults and children.[8,10] Autoantibodies against IgE and FcεRI (high-affinity receptor for IgE) have been shown to stimulate histamine release in vitro.[11-14] Additionally, thyroid autoantibodies, such as antithyroglobulin and thyroid peroxidase antibodies, have been found to be significantly elevated in patients with chronic urticaria compared with the normal population (15%-24% versus 3%-6%, respectively).[15-18] Although there is a significant correlation between the presence of thyroid antibodies and chronic urticaria, thyroid function does not necessarily correlate with severity of urticaria. Signs of thyroid autoimmunity in patients who are euthyroid appears to reflect an underlying tendency to develop autoantibodies.[8,15,19]

Arachidonic acid metabolism can be blocked by nonsteroidal anti-inflammatory medications (NSAIDs) that inhibit cyclooxygenase 1, such as aspirin. These medications can cause acute urticaria in susceptible persons and can also cause flares in patients with chronic urticaria.[20] Aspirin-induced urticaria in patients with chronic idiopathic urticaria is reported to be between 21% and 30%.[3,20,21]

Infections have been implicated in both acute and chronic urticaria. Infections, especially those affecting the upper respiratory and gastrointestinal tracts, have been associated with up to 62% of cases of acute urticaria in the general population[22,23] and 80% of cases in the pediatric population.[24] Implicated viruses include cytomegalovirus, Coxsackievirus A and B, and infectious hepatitis.[23,25] A large number of helminthic parasites have also been clearly associated with urticaria, although this is a rare cause in developed countries.[25,26] *Helicobacter pylori* infection has been proposed as a cause of chronic urticaria; however, recent data indicate this association is more likely coincidental than causal.[27,28]

Physical urticarias are chronic urticarias triggered by physical stimulus.

Systemic diseases, such as autoimmune disorders, cryoglobulinemia, and neoplasia, have rarely been implicated in chronic urticaria.

SIGNS AND SYMPTOMS

Urticaria is characterized by the appearance of wheals that have three typical features: central swelling, pruritus, and evanescent nature. The combination of pruritus and transient lesions are more specific for urticaria than the other conditions in the differential diagnosis (Box 2). The skin lesions often involve the trunk and extremities but can occur anywhere on the body.[29] Pruritus is almost always present with urticaria, although some patients complain of pain, tenderness, or burning instead of pruritus.[30] Individual urticarial lesions resolve within 24 hours without residual bruising or hyperpigmentation of the skin. As lesions resolve, others might appear.[31] Although the lesions of acute and chronic urticaria are virtually identical, individual wheals can persist longer in patients with chronic urticaria (4-36 hours).

Physical Urticarias

The physical urticarias are common causes of chronic urticaria. With the exception of delayed pressure urticaria, the lesions of the physical urticarias typically occur within minutes of exposure to the appropriate stimulus and fade within 1 to 2 hours.[30] The physical urticarias are described here in decreasing order of frequency.

The most common physical urticaria is cholinergic urticaria, which is characterized by small pinpoint hives associated with exer-

Box 1 Mechanisms of Urticaria

IgE Mediated
- Foods (e.g., peanuts, tree nuts, wheat, soy, milk, egg, shellfish, fish)
- Inhalants (e.g., animal dander, pollen)
- Insect sting or bite (Hymenoptera venom, fire ants, *Triatoma*)
- Medications (e.g., beta-lactam antibiotics, sulfa-containing medications)
- Contactants (e.g., latex, animal saliva)

Autoimmune Mediated
- Anti-FcεRI antibody
- Anti-IgE antibody

Direct Mast Cell Activated
- Neuromuscular blocking agents (e.g., succinylcholine, pancuronium, atracurium)
- Opioid narcotics (e.g., morphine)
- Radiocontrast media
- Vancomycin

Arachidonic Acid Metabolism
- Aspirin
- NSAIDs

Infections
- Helminthic
- Viral

Physical Urticarias
- Cholinergic urticaria
- Dermatographism
- Delayed pressure urticaria
- Cold urticaria
- Solar urticaria
- Aquagenic urticaria
- Local heat urticaria
- Vibratory urticaria

Systemic Diseases
- Autoimmune disorders (e.g., systemic lupus erythematous)
- Cryoglobulinemia
- Neoplasia

IgE, Immunoglobulin E; NSAID, nonsteroidal anti-inflammatory drug.

Box 2 Differential Diagnosis of Urticaria

Auriculotemporal syndrome
Contact dermatitis
Erythema multiforme minor
Insect bites
Pityriasis rosea
Sweet's syndrome
Urticaria pigmentosa (mastocytosis)
Vasculitis (including urticarial vasculitis and Henoch-Schönlein purpura)
Viral exanthems

cise, hot showers, sweating, or stress. It occurs in up to 11.2% of young adults (16-35 years of age) and is often unnoticed in milder forms.[26,32]

Dermatographism is diagnosed by the development of a wheal-and-flare response after stroking or scratching the skin. About 10% of patients with chronic idiopathic urticaria have symptomatic dermatographism.[33]

Delayed pressure urticaria develops 4 to 12 hours after a significant amount of pressure has been applied to the skin.[34] The lesions of delayed pressure urticaria are often more painful than pruritic. This form of urticaria is invariably associated with chronic idiopathic urticaria.[32,33]

In cold urticaria, symptoms occur after exposure to a cold stimulus including air or water. Fatalities have been reported due to anaphylactoid reactions in extremely cold-sensitive patients swimming in lakes or oceans.[25,32]

Solar urticaria is caused by exposure to sunlight or certain wavelengths of artificial light. Other rare types of physical urticaria include aquagenic urticaria, local heat urticaria, and vibratory urticaria triggered by contact with water, a warm substance, or vibratory stimulus, respectively.

Angioedema

Patients with acute or chronic urticaria can also experience angioedema. Angioedema typically affects areas of loose connective tissue, such as the periorbital region, lips, extremities, and genitals (e.g., scrotum). Occasionally, the tongue and pharynx are involved.[35] Angioedema involving the oropharynx can cause life-threatening airway obstruction. The edema of subcutaneous tissue may be more painful than pruritic. Swelling can take up to 72 hours to resolve. Isolated angioedema, especially laryngeal edema, requires consideration for hereditary or acquired C1-inhibitor deficiency.

DIAGNOSIS

Proper diagnosis of urticaria requires a detailed history and physical examination. Characteristics of the lesions are important for accurate diagnosis, especially if there is no evidence of rash at the time of evaluation. Questions regarding appearance (round or linear, raised, erythematous), duration (more or less than 24 hours), symptoms (pruritic, burning, or painful), and accompanying angioedema can help establish the diagnosis.

A detailed history is important for identifying potential causes of urticaria (see Box 1). Key components of the history include current and recent medication use, including herbals, over-the-counter medications, and hormone replacement; food exposures associated with the onset of symptoms; physical triggers such as pressure, physical exertion, or cold temperatures; symptoms of a concurrent infection, such as hepatitis, mononucleosis, or an upper respiratory infection; contact or inhalant exposure to allergens, including occupational exposures; and recent insect sting or bite.[29] A complete review of systems is necessary to screen for symptoms of systemic diseases, such as collagen vascular disease or malignancy.

Immunoglobulin E

The history might suggest an underlying cause of acute urticaria. A temporal history of an insect sting or bite, contactant, or food exposure followed by the development of urticaria suggests possible IgE-mediated hypersensitivity. Cutaneous testing or serum radioallergosorbent testing (RAST), usually overseen by a specialist in allergy and immunology, may be performed to identify a cause. Foods are a common cause of acute urticaria but a rare cause of chronic urticaria. The most frequently implicated foods eliciting generalized urticaria in children include milk, soy, wheat, eggs, peanuts, tree nuts, shellfish, and fish. Peanuts, tree nuts, shellfish, and fish are common causes in adults. Occasionally, foods cause hives through a non–IgE-mediated reaction. For example, scombroidosis, which occurs after ingesting contaminated scombroid fish such as tuna or mackerel, can cause urticaria with flushing, nausea, and vomiting.[36]

Physical Stimulus

A complete history for evidence of a physical stimulus eliciting a wheal-and-flare or angioedematous response is necessary for a diagnosis. Questions regarding causal relation to heat, exercise, stress, pressure, cold temperatures (air or water), or sun exposure are essential in diagnosing a physical urticaria. Dermatographism can be diagnosed by observing the skin after stroking it with a blunt object (e.g., tongue blade) or dermatographometer. Typically, these patients describe a history of scratching that precipitates linear hives and pruritus. Other specific provocation tests, such as an ice cube test (cold urticaria) or an intradermal injection of methacholine (cholinergic urticaria), may be completed when the history and physical examination suggest a physical urticaria.

Systemic Disease

Chronic urticaria has been uncommonly associated with systemic diseases such as collagen vascular disease or malignancy. In a meta-analysis by Kozel and colleagues, an underlying disease was considered to be the cause of chronic urticaria in only 1.6% of patients.[5] For patients with chronic urticaria, screening laboratory tests may be completed to help detect underlying illness. These tests can include a complete blood count with differential, erythrocyte sedimentation rate, urinalysis, and liver function tests.[29] Because thyroid autoimmunity has been associated with chronic urticaria, thyroid function tests including antimicrosomal and antithyroglobulin antibodies may be obtained.[35] If a connective tissue disease is suspected, antinuclear antibody and other serologic tests may be warranted.[35] A C4 level should be obtained in patients who experience angioedema without urticaria. If the C4 level is low, then C1 inhibitor level and function should be checked to evaluate further for possible hereditary or acquired angioedema.

Autoimmune

Most often, chronic urticaria is not caused by an external trigger or an underlying illness and is classified as idiopathic. Chronic urticaria seems to be an autoimmune process in 40% to 50% of patients.[11] These patients develop a localized wheal and pruritus after intradermal injection of autologous serum. Autoantibodies directed against the high-affinity IgE receptor or, less commonly, IgE itself have been identified in these patients.[11]

Atypical

Palpable and purpuric lesions, the persistence of individual lesions for longer than 24 hours, or the presence of systemic symptoms such as fever or arthralgias, suggest possible urticarial vasculitis. A skin biopsy should be performed when urticarial vasculitis is suspected or when urticaria is particularly difficult to treat.[29] Despite a thorough evaluation, 80% of patients with chronic urticaria have no identifiable underlying cause.

TREATMENT

Urticaria and Angioedema

Nonspecific triggers of urticaria including NSAIDs, alcohol, and overheating should be avoided.[37] Angiotensin-converting enzyme (ACE) inhibitors can cause angioedema; therefore, this class of antihypertensive medications should be avoided, as feasible, in patients with angioedema.[38] If a specific cause of the urticaria is identified, such as a food or medication, avoidance is crucial for treatment success. For physical urticarias, decreasing exposure to the provoking stimulus alleviates symptoms. For example, wearing warm and protective clothing outdoors during cold weather helps prevent exacerbations of cold urticaria.[39]

Antihistamines

H_1 antihistamines are the mainstay of treatment for urticaria.[40] First-generation antihistamines, such as hydroxyzine and diphenhydramine, are effective but cause sedation and anticholinergic side effects (Table 1). The sedation can impair driving, increase the risk for occupational accidents, and adversely affect academic performance and workplace productivity.[29] Anticholinergic effects include dry mouth, constipation, urinary retention, and blurred vision. Second-generation antihistamines—loratidine (Claritin), desloratidine (Clarinex), fexofenadine (Allegra), cetirizine (Zyrtec), and levocetirizine (Xyzal)—are generally preferred as first-line treatment (see Table 1). Loratidine, desloratidine, fexofenadine, and levocetirizine are relatively nonsedating when used at standard recommended doses. Cetirizine causes sedation in a minority of patients. The second-generation antihistamines have few or no anticholinergic side effects.

Table 1 Pharmacologic Treatment for Urticaria

Medication	Dose*
First-Generation H_1 Antihistamines	
Chlorpheniramine	4 mg q4-6h prn, max 24 mg/day
Cyproheptadine (Periactin)	Start 4 mg tid, max 0.5 mg/kg/day
Diphenhydramine (Benadryl)	25 to 50 mg q6h prn
Hydroxyzine (Atarax, Vistaril)	10 to 100 mg q 6 h prn, max 600 mg/day
Second-Generation H_1 Antihistamines	
Cetirizine (Zyrtec)	5 to 10 mg daily
Desloratidine (Clarinex)	5 mg daily
Fexofenadine (Allegra)	180 mg daily or 60 mg bid
Loratidine (Claritin)	10 mg daily
Levocetirizine (Xyzal)	5 mg daily
H_2 Antagonists	
Cimetidine (Tagamet)	400 mg bid or 400 to 800 mg qhs
Famotidine (Pepcid)	20 mg bid or 20 to 40 mg qhs
Nizatidine (Axid)	150 mg bid or 300 mg qhs
Ranitidine (Zantac)	150 mg bid or 300 mg qhs

*Standard recommended doses for adults. Some physicians use higher doses when treating patients with severe urticaria.

Patients should be instructed to take antihistamines on a regular basis, not simply as needed, because treatment failure is more likely when a patient takes an antihistamine intermittently instead of continuously.[41] If patients continue to experience symptoms despite regular use of a second-generation antihistamine, many physicians use a combination of first- and second-generation antihistamines. A commonly used regimen is a nonsedating antihistamine on awakening and a sedating antihistamine before going to bed.[39]

Although the majority of histamine receptors in the skin are of the H_1 subtype, about 15% are of the H_2 subtype.[39] The use of a H_2 receptor antagonist such as ranitidine (Zantac) or cimetidine (Tagamet) in conjunction with H_1 antihistamines can provide additional clinical benefit for treatment of chronic urticaria (see Table 1).[42] Doxepin, a tricyclic antidepressant, has potent H_1 and H_2 antihistamine activities and is effective for treating chronic urticaria.[43] Side effects of this medication include sedation and increased appetite.

Corticosteroids

Systemic corticosteroids are efficacious for treating urticaria, but use should be limited because of potential side effects.[40] In treating acute urticaria, a short course of oral steroids has been shown to provide symptomatic relief earlier than loratidine.[22] In chronic urticaria, corticosteroids should be used only in highly selective situations, such as during a significant exacerbation of symptoms or in severe cases refractory to other treatments.[40] Side effects of systemic corticosteroids include osteoporosis, edema, hypertension, peptic ulcers, glaucoma, and cataracts. Some patients experience a significant flare of urticaria after tapering or discontinuing steroids.[39] Corticosteroids should be prescribed at the lowest effective dose and therapy should be tapered and discontinued as soon as possible to minimize potential side effects.[40]

Epinephrine

Epinephrine can be lifesaving for patients who experience laryngeal edema or anaphylaxis.[37] The proper dose for adults is 0.3 mL to 0.5 mL of intramuscular epinephrine in 1 : 1000 concentration. Pediatric dosing is 0.01 mL/kg of intramuscular epinephrine in 1 : 1000 concentration, up to 0.3 mL. The lateral thigh is the preferred injection site.[44] The dose may be repeated if necessary. Epinephrine should be used with caution in patients with hypertension or ischemic heart disease.[37] Patients with a history of laryngeal edema or anaphylaxis, and patients with a history of food allergy, stinging insect hypersensitivity, or latex allergy should have self-injectable epinephrine (Epipen, Twinject) available at all times.[29] The patient should be instructed on the proper use of this medication and told to seek emergency medical care immediately after use, because symptoms can recur or worsen as the medication wears off. Patients should also be instructed to wear a medical alert bracelet.

Other Medications

The antileukotriene drugs, montelukast (Singulair), zafirlukast (Accolate), and zileuton (Zyflo), although not FDA approved for this indication, can provide clinical benefit in treating chronic urticaria.[45,46] These medications appear to be more effective when used in combination with antihistamines rather than as monotherapy.[47]

Mast cell-stabilizing agents have been used to treat urticaria. Nifedipine, a calcium-channel blocker, has been effective for treating chronic urticaria when used as an adjunct to antihistamines.[48] Oral sympathomimetic agents such as terbutaline occasionally provide relief, but the overall efficacy is low. Side effects of terbutaline include tachycardia and insomnia.[35]

Other interventions have been used to treat refractory urticaria. Thyroxine treatment can lead to remission of symptoms in patients with chronic urticaria and evidence of thyroid autoimmunity.[19] Dapsone and hydroxychloroquine (Plaquenil) have been used to treat severe cases of urticaria.[38,49] Cyclosporine, an immunosuppressant used in organ transplant recipients, has been effective at a low dose for treatment of urticaria.[50] Cyclosporine is contraindicated in patients with a history of malignancy or impaired renal function.[38] Plasmapheresis and intravenous immunoglobulin have been used to treat small numbers of patients.[51,52] Other agents used include colchicine, sulfasalazine, warfarin, and methotrexate.[39]

Hereditary and Acquired Angioedema

Treatment of hereditary and acquired angioedema differs from treatment of idiopathic urticaria and angioedema and is typically supervised by a specialist in allergy and immunology. Danazol, an attenuated androgen, has been used to treat hereditary angioedema. Danazol appears to work by upregulating hepatic synthesis of C1 inhibitor. Abnormal liver function, lipid abnormalities, weight gain, amenorrhea, and hirsutism are side effects of danazol.[53] Antifibrinolytic agents, such as tranexamic acid and ε-amino caproic acid, have also been used to treat hereditary and acquired angioedema. Clinical trials are investigating the use of recombinant C1 inhibitor to treat hereditary angioedema.[54]

Specialist referral should be considered if urticaria might be caused by an IgE-mediated reaction; if the lesions last longer than 6 weeks; if there is evidence of urticarial vasculitis; if the hives respond poorly, there is an impairment on quality of life, or there is increased absenteeism from work or school despite an adequate regimen of antihistamine therapy; if there is evidence of angioedema involving the oral-pharyngeal region; or if there is isolated angioedema (without a history of ACE inhibitor use).

OUTCOMES

In a study by Aoki and colleagues regarding the natural course of acute urticaria, 86% experienced remission of symptoms within 2 weeks, and 6% experienced remission between 2 weeks and 1 month. Symptoms persisted for longer than 6 weeks in 8% of the patients.[23] In those with chronic urticaria, symptoms resolve for 50% of patients within 1 year and for an additional 20% within 1 to 5 years. Symptoms persist for 20 years for 10% to 20% of patients.[3] Physical urticarias tend to persist longer than chronic idiopathic urticaria.[3] Patients who have had one episode of chronic urticaria might experience a later recurrence of symptoms.[39]

Summary

- Urticaria is a common skin disorder that causes significant morbidity.
- Most cases of urticaria are self-limited.
- When there is an identifiable cause such as an immediate hypersensitivity reaction, avoidance is effective in preventing a recurrence.
- A small percentage of patients have symptoms that persist longer than 6 weeks.
- After a thorough evaluation, a significant portion of these patients have no identifiable cause.
- Treatment can be extremely effective in mitigating or resolving the symptoms.

Further Readings

Aoki T, Kojima M, Horiko T: Acute urticaria: History and natural course of 50 cases. J Dermatol 1994;21(2):73-77.

Baxi S, Dinakar C: Urticaria and angioedema. Immunol Allergy Clin North Am 2005;25(2):353-367, vii.

Casale TB, Sampson HA, Hanifin J, et al: Guide to physical urticarias. J Allergy Clin Immunol 1988; 82(5 Pt 1):758-763.

Dibbern DA Jr: Urticaria: Selected highlights and recent advances. Med Clin North Am 2006;90(1):187-209.

Dibbern DA Jr, Dreskin SC: Urticaria and angioedema: An overview. Immunol Allergy Clin North Am 2004;24(2):141-162, v.

Greaves MW: Chronic urticaria. N Engl J Med 1995;332(26):1767-1772.

Hide M, Francis DM, Grattan CE, et al: Autoantibodies against the high-affinity IgE receptor as a cause of histamine release in chronic urticaria. N Engl J Med 1993;328(22):1599-1604.

Joint Task Force on Practice Parameters: The diagnosis and management of urticaria: A practice parameter. Part I: Acute urticaria/angioedema. Part II: Chronic urticaria/angioedema. Ann Allergy Asthma Immunol 2000; 85(6 Pt 2):521-544.

Kaplan AP: Chronic urticaria: Pathogenesis and treatment. J Allergy Clin Immunol 2004;114(3):465-474.

Zuberbier T: Urticaria. Allergy 2003;58(12):1224-1234.

References

For a complete list of references, log onto www.expertconsult.com.

Sinusitis

Christine Radojicic

DEFINITION

Sinusitis is inflammation of the sinuses, which are air-filled cavities in the skull. The etiology can be infectious (bacterial, viral, or fungal) or noninfectious (allergic) triggers. This inflammation leads to blockade of the normal sinus drainage pathways (sinus ostia), which in turn leads to mucus retention, hypoxia, decreased mucociliary clearance, and predisposition to bacterial growth.

Sinusitis can be divided into the following categories:[1]

- *Acute sinusitis,* defined as symptoms of less than 4 weeks' duration (Fig. 1);
- *Subacute sinusitis,* defined as symptoms of 4 to 8 weeks' duration;
- *Chronic sinusitis,* defined as symptoms lasting longer than 8 weeks (Fig. 2);
- *Recurrent acute sinusitis,* often defined as three or more episodes per year, with each episode lasting less than 2 weeks.

PREVALENCE

The prevalence of acute sinusitis is on the rise, based on data from the National Ambulatory Medical Care Survey (from 0.2% of diagnoses at office visits in 1990 to 0.4% of diagnoses at office visits in 1995[2]). In 2001, sinusitis represented 13.6 million outpatient visits according to the U.S. Centers for Disease Control and Prevention (CDC).[3] Approximately 40 million Americans are affected by sinusitis every year, and 33 million cases of chronic sinusitis are reported annually to the CDC.[4]

When sinusitis is considered together with commonly associated comorbid conditions such as allergic rhinitis, asthma, and chronic bronchitis, exacerbation of these diseases affects more than 90 million people—nearly one in three Americans.[5] The socioeconomic impact of this translates to more than $5.8 billion dollars spent on the treatment of sinusitis.[6]

PATHOPHYSIOLOGY

The most common cause of acute sinusitis is an upper respiratory tract infection (URTI) of viral origin. The viral infection can lead to inflammation of the sinuses that usually resolves without treatment in less than 14 days. If symptoms worsen after 3 to 5 days or persist for longer than 10 days and are more severe than normally experienced with a viral infection, a secondary bacterial infection is diagnosed. The inflammation can predispose to the development of acute sinusitis by causing sinus ostial blockage. Although inflammation in any of the sinuses can lead to blockade of the sinus ostia, the most commonly involved sinuses in both acute and chronic sinusitis are the maxillary and the anterior ethmoid sinuses.[7] The anterior ethmoid, frontal, and maxillary sinuses drain into the middle meatus, creating an anatomic area known as the *ostiomeatal complex* (Fig. 3).

The nasal mucosa responds to the virus by producing mucus and recruiting mediators of inflammation, such as white blood cells, to the lining of the nose, which cause congestion and swelling of the nasal passages. The resultant sinus cavity hypoxia and mucus retention cause the cilia—which move mucus and debris from the nose—to function less efficiently, creating an environment for bacterial growth.

If the acute sinusitis does not resolve, chronic sinusitis can develop from mucus retention, hypoxia, and blockade of the ostia. This promotes mucosal hyperplasia, continued recruitment of inflammatory infiltrates, and the potential development of nasal polyps. However, other factors can predispose to sinusitis (Box 1).[8]

When bacterial growth occurs in acute sinusitis, the most common organisms include *Streptococcus pneumoniae, Haemophilus influenzae,* and *Moraxella catarrhalis.*[9] In chronic sinusitis, these organisms, plus *Staphylococcus aureus,* coagulase-negative *Staphylococcus* species, and anaerobic bacteria, are the most likely involved organisms. Organisms isolated from patients with chronic sinusitis increasingly are showing antibiotic resistance. In fact, penicillin resistance rates for *S. pneumoniae* are as high as 44% in parts of the United States.[10] These resistant organisms commonly occur in patients who have received two or more recent courses of antibiotics.

A distinct entity, allergic fungal sinusitis (AFS), occurs in immunocompetent patients and results from an immunologic reaction to fungi that colonize the sinuses.[11] Most people tolerate exposure to mold spores in the air because they are ubiquitous in our environment. However, people with AFS develop a hypersensitivity reaction involving an intense eosinophilic inflammatory response to the fungus that has colonized the sinuses. Common fungi associated with this syndrome include *Bipolaris specifera* and *Aspergillus, Curvularia,* and *Fusarium* species.[11] This is an allergic noninvasive response to the fungus that should be distinguished from invasive fungal sinusitis, which is more common in diabetic and immunocompromised patients. The diagnostic criteria for AFS include findings of chronic sinusitis on computed tomography (CT) of the sinuses (such as mucosal thickening, opacification, polyps, and high-intensity signaling from the high protein content in the mucus) or low signaling of fungal concretions in sinus cavities on MRI. On sinus culture, fungi can be isolated with associated allergic mucin, which is mucus loaded with degranulated eosinophils. Allergy skin testing can verify that these patients have an immunoglobulin E (IgE)-mediated reaction to molds.

SIGNS AND SYMPTOMS

Acute bacterial sinusitis in adults most often manifests with more than 7 days of nasal congestion, purulent rhinorrhea, postnasal drip, and facial pain and pressure, alone or with associated referred pain to the ears and teeth. There may be a cough, often worsening at night.[12] Children with acute sinusitis might not be able to relay a history of postnasal drainage or headaches, so cough and rhinorrhea are the most commonly reported symptoms.[13] Other symptoms can include fever, nausea, fatigue, impairments of smell and taste, and halitosis.

Chronic sinusitis can cause more indolent symptoms that persist for months. Nasal congestion and postnasal drainage are the most common symptoms of chronic sinusitis. Chronic cough that is described as worse at night or on awakening in the morning is also a commonly described symptom of chronic sinusitis. Clinical evidence of chronic sinusitis may be subtle and less overt than in acute sinusitis unless the patient is having an acute sinusitis exacerbation. Because this diagnosis may be more difficult to make in the primary care setting or in a setting without radiographic or rhinoscopic capabilities, Lanza and Kennedy have proposed[14] a major and minor classification system to define chronic sinusitis by the manifesting symptoms (Box 2).

Physical Findings

Typical physical signs include bilateral nasal mucosal edema, purulent nasal secretions, and sinus tenderness (however, this is not a

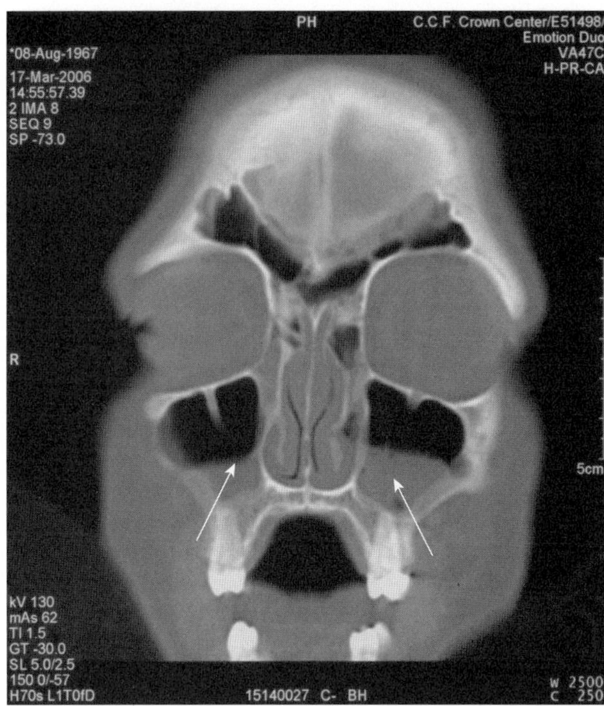

Figure 1 Computed tomography scan showing acute sinusitis. Note the fluid levels in the maxillary sinuses *(arrows)*.

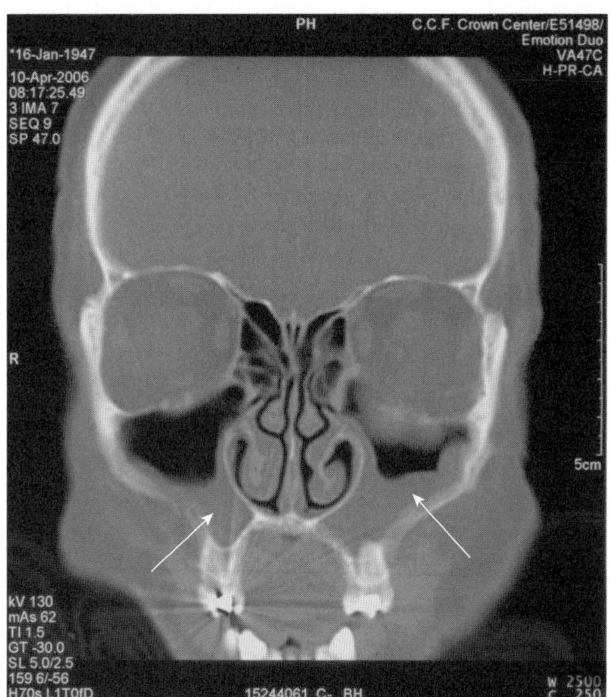

Figure 2 Computed tomography scan showing chronic sinusitis. Note the mucosal thickening in the maxillary sinuses.

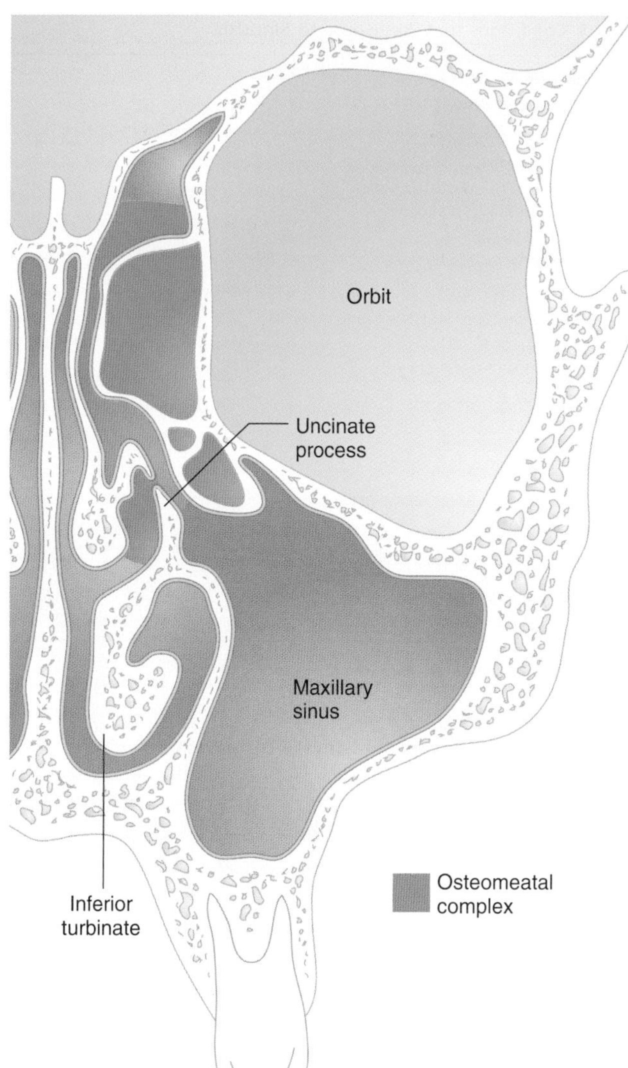

Figure 3 The anterior ethmoid, frontal, and maxillary sinuses drain into the middle meatus. This creates an anatomic area known as the *ostiomeatal complex*.

sensitive or specific finding). The location of sinus pain depends on which sinus is affected. Pain on palpation of the forehead over the frontal sinuses can indicate that the frontal sinuses are inflamed; however, this is also a very common area for tension headaches. Infection in the maxillary sinuses can cause upper jaw pain and tooth sensitivity, with the malar areas tender to the touch. Because the ethmoid sinuses are between the eyes and near the tear ducts, ethmoid sinusitis may be associated with swelling, tenderness, and pain in the eyelids and tissues around the eyes. The sphenoid sinuses are more deeply recessed, and sinusitis there can manifest with vague symptoms of earaches, neck pain, and deep aching at the top of the head.

However, in most patients with a suspected diagnosis of sinusitis, pain or tenderness is found in several locations, and the perceived area of pain usually does not clearly delineate which sinuses are inflamed. Purulent drainage may be evident on examination as anterior rhinorrhea or visualized as posterior pharyngeal drainage with associated clinical symptoms of sore throat and cough.

The nose should be examined for a deviated nasal septum, nasal polyps, and epistaxis. Foreign bodies and tumors can mimic symptoms of sinusitis and should be in the differential diagnosis, especially if the symptoms are unilateral. The ears should be examined for signs of associated otitis media and the chest for the presence of asthma exacerbation, a common comorbid condition.

DIAGNOSIS

In a primary care setting, a good history and physical examination to detect the presence of most or all of the commonly manifesting

Box 1 Conditions that Predispose to Sinusitis

Allergic rhinitis
Nonallergic rhinitis
Anatomic factors:

- Septal deviation
- Paradoxical middle turbinate
- Ethmoid bulla hypertrophy
- Choanal atresia
- Adenoid hypertrophy

Hormonal conditions (e.g., progesterone-induced congestion of pregnancy, rhinitis of hypothyroidism)
Gastroesophageal reflux
Primary immune deficiency:

- Selective IgA deficiency
- Common variable Immune deficiency

Acquired immune deficiency

- Human immunodeficiency virus
- Transplantation
- Chemotherapy
- Cystic fibrosis
- Primary ciliary dyskinesia
- Kartagener's syndrome

Box 2 Symptoms Associated with the Diagnosis of Chronic Sinusitis

Facial pain or pressure
Facial congestion or fullness
Nasal obstruction or blockage
Nasal discharge, purulence, or postnasal drip
Hyposmia or anosmia
Headache
Fever
Halitosis
Fatigue
Dental pain
Cough
Ear pain, pressure, fullness

Reprinted from Otolaryngology-Head and Neck Surgery, Vol 117, Donald C. Lanza, MD and David K. Kennedy, MD, Adult rhinosinusitis defined, pp S1-S7. Copyright 1997, with permission from the American Academy of Otolaryngology—Head and Neck Surgery Foundation, Inc.

signs and symptoms can provide a reliable diagnosis of acute sinusitis. The presence of purulent secretions has the highest positive predictive value for diagnosing sinusitis clinically.

Differentiating it from a common viral URTI is most important. Mucus in URTIs is typically not described as persistently purulent. Nasal congestion is a predominant symptom without persistent or worsening head congestion, headache, or facial pain or fatigue. URTI symptoms would be expected to peak on about day 3 to 5 and resolve within 7 to 10 days. Most other diagnostic modalities, described later, aid in the differential diagnosis of persistent nasal symptoms.

Radiographic Evaluation

The two modalities most commonly used include the plain radiograph and CT scan. Plain radiography does not adequately represent the individual ethmoid air cells, the extent of mucosal thickening in chronic sinusitis, or visualization of the ostiomeatal complex. Magnetic resonance imaging can be considered for evaluation of suspected tumors but is not recommended for acute sinusitis because it does not distinguish air from bone. For these reasons, CT scanning

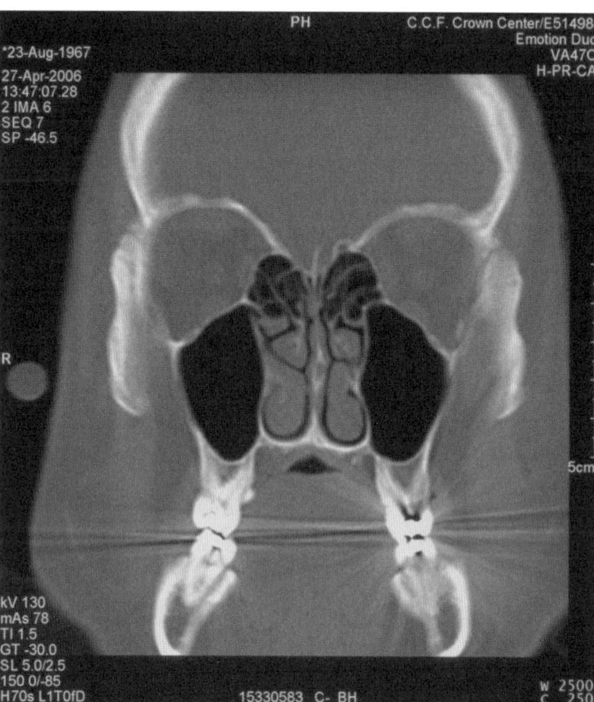

Figure 4 Computed tomography scan of a normal sinus anatomy.

of the sinuses is the imaging procedure of choice (Fig. 4). In many centers, the cost is similar to that of plain radiographs because of the availability of limited coronal views (usually comprising approximately six coronal views of the maxillary, ethmoid, sphenoid, and frontal sinuses) that are optimally sufficient for ruling out sinusitis. More detailed coronal slices are useful for viewing the ostiomeatal complex and for surgical mapping.

Transillumination

A common practice before plain radiographs and CT scans were widely available, transillumination is of limited use and ahs a high rate of error.

Ultrasonography

Ultrasonography has not been proved accurate enough to substitute for a radiographic evaluation. However, it may be considered to confirm sinusitis in pregnant women, for whom radiographic studies could pose a risk.

Nasal Smear

By examining the cellular contents of the nasal secretions, one might find polymorphonuclear cells and bacteria in sinusitis. In a viral infection, these would not be found, and in allergic disease, one would expect to find eosinophils.

Sinus Puncture

The most accurate way to determine the causative organism in sinusitis is a sinus puncture. After anesthetization of the puncture site, usually in the canine fossa or inferior meatus, the contents of the maxillary sinus are aspirated under sterile technique, and bacterial cultures are performed to identify the organism. Culture specimens obtained from nasal swabs correlate poorly with sinus pathogens found by puncture because of contamination of the swab with normal nasal flora. However, because sinus puncture is an invasive procedure, it is not routinely performed. More recently, studies have shown a close correlation between organisms found by sinus puncture and by endoscopically guided aspiration of the sinus cavities through the middle meatus. Although this needs to be done by an otolaryngologist trained in the procedure, it may be necessary for defining the pathogenic organism when standard therapy has failed or in an immunocompromised patient who is at high risk for sequelae of untreated sinusitis, such as orbital or central nervous system complications.

Summary

- Differentiating bacterial sinusitis from a common viral URTI is most important.
- The presence of purulent secretions has the highest positive predictive value for clinically diagnosing sinusitis.
- CT of the sinuses is the imaging procedure of choice.

THERAPY

Treatment of Acute Sinusitis

Antibiotics, such as amoxicillin for 2 weeks, have been the recommended first-line treatment of uncomplicated acute sinusitis. The antibiotic of choice must cover *S. pneumoniae, H. influenzae,* and *M. catarrhalis.* Because rare intracranial and orbital complications of acute bacterial sinusitis are caused by *S. pneumoniae* (most commonly in the immunocompromised host), adequate coverage for this organism is important. Amoxicillin-clavulanate (Augmentin) is also an appropriate first-line treatment of uncomplicated acute sinusitis. The addition of clavulanate, a beta-lactamase inhibitor, provides better coverage for *H. influenzae* and *M. catarrhalis.*[15] Because of *S. pneumoniae* resistance, higher doses of amoxicillin (90 mg/kg/day to a maximum of 2 g/day) should be considered. These higher doses are effective against *S. pneumoniae* because resistance is related to alteration in penicillin-binding proteins, a mechanism distinct from the beta-lactamase enzymatic inactivation of *H. influenzae* and *M. catarrhalis.*

Other options include cephalosporins such as cefpodoxime proxetil (Vantin) and cefuroxime (Ceftin). In patients allergic to beta-lactams, trimethoprim-sulfamethoxazole (Bactrim), clarithromycin (Biaxin), and azithromycin (Zithromax) may be prescribed but might not be adequate coverage for *H. influenzae* or resistant *S. pneumoniae.*[16] Penicillin, erythromycin (Suprax), and first-generation cephalosporins such as cephalexin (Keflex, Keftab) are not recommended for treating acute sinusitis because of inadequate antimicrobial coverage of the major organisms.

If treatment with one of these first-line agents has not shown a clinical response within 72 hours of initial therapy, more broad-spectrum antibiotics should be considered. These include the fluoroquinolones, gatifloxacin (Tequin), moxifloxacin (Avelox), and levofloxacin (Levaquin), especially if amoxicillin-clavulanate, cefpodoxime proxetil, and cefuroxime were previously prescribed.

Treatment of Chronic Sinusitis

Antibiotic therapy for chronic sinusitis is controversial and may be most appropriate for acute exacerbation of chronic sinusitis. Medical therapy should include both a broad-spectrum antibiotic and a topical intranasal steroid to address the strong inflammatory component of this disease. Antibiotic therapy might need to be continued for 4 to 6 weeks.[12] The antibiotics of choice include agents that cover organisms causing acute sinusitis but also cover *Staphylococcus* species and anaerobes. These include amoxicillin-clavulanate, cefpodoxime proxetil, cefuroxime, gatifloxacin, moxifloxacin, and levofloxacin. Currently used topical intranasal steroids such as fluticasone (Flonase), mometasone (Nasonex), budesonide (Rhinocort AQ), and triamcinolone (Nasacort AQ) have a favorable safety profile and indications for the pediatric age group. A short course of oral steroids may be used for extensive mucosal thickening and congestion or nasal polyps.

Adjunctive Therapy

To temporarily alleviate the drainage and congestion associated with sinusitis, decongestant nasal sprays oxymetazoline (Afrin) and phenylephrine hydrochloride (Neo-Synephrine) may be used for 3 to 5 days. Long-term use of topical decongestants can cause rhinitis medicamentosa, which is rebound congestion caused by vasodilatation and inflammation. Oral decongestants (pseudoephedrine) may be a reasonable alternative if the patient has no contraindication such as hypertension. Mucolytic agents (guaifenesin) can help to decrease the viscosity of the mucus for better clearance and are often found in combination with decongestants. Some mucolytics are now available over the counter. Saline spray or irrigation can help clear secretions. Topical corticosteroids are not indicated for acute sinusitis but may be helpful for chronic sinusitis, nasal polyps, and allergic and nonallergic rhinitis. Antihistamines are not indicated for sinusitis but may be helpful for underlying allergic rhinitis.

Surgery

If medical therapy fails or if complications are suspected, an otolaryngology consultation is warranted. This may begin with a nasal endoscopy for better visualization of the nasal cavity and ostiomeatal complex. The otolaryngologist can also perform endoscopically guided sinus culture. If surgical therapy is being contemplated, newer techniques of functional endoscopic sinus surgery are performed to clear sinuses of chronic infection, inflammation, and polyps. This may be combined with somnoturboplasty (i.e., shrinkage of the turbinate using radiofrequency waves). Endoscopic sinus surgery is commonly performed on an outpatient basis using local anesthesia and has less morbidity than traditional open surgery for chronic sinus disease.[1] Special consideration should be given to patients who have chronic sinusitis and nasal polyps and who also have aspirin-induced asthma. This is commonly referred to as the aspirin triad of aspirin sensitivity, asthma, and polyposis. Although most of these patients undergo sinus surgery and polypectomy, additional therapy with nasal steroids, leukotriene modifiers, and aspirin desensitization, followed by 650 mg aspirin twice daily, should be considered.[17]

Additional Evaluations

Laboratory Evaluation

Laboratory evaluation may be necessary to look for an underlying disorder that can predispose to sinusitis. The evaluation may include a sweat chloride test for cystic fibrosis, ciliary function tests for immotile cilia syndrome, blood tests for HIV, or other tests for immunodeficiency, such as immunoglobulin levels.

Allergy Consultation

Any patient with recurrent acute or chronic sinusitis should have an allergy consultation to rule out allergy to dust mites, mold, animal dander, and pollen, which can trigger allergic rhinitis. An allergy consultation will provide immediate hypersensitivity skin testing to delineate which environmental aeroallergens exacerbate allergic rhinitis and predispose to sinusitis. Medical management and environmental control measures are discussed. Treatment options such as medications, immunotherapy, or both (allergy shots) are considered. Additional evaluation for comorbid conditions such as asthma, sinusitis, and gastroesophageal reflux are addressed and treated. Allergists are also trained in aspirin desensitization for treatment of patients with the aspirin triad.

Treatment of Complications of Sinusitis

Orbital extension of sinus disease is the most common complication of acute sinusitis. This complication is more common in children. Immediate management includes broad-spectrum intravenous antibiotics, a CT scan to determine the extent of disease, and possibly surgical drainage of the infection if there is no response to antibiotics. Extension to the central nervous system can also occur. The most common intracranial complications are meningitis (usually from the sphenoid sinus, which is anatomically located closest to the brain) and epidural abscess (usually from the frontal sinuses).

Treatment of Allergic Fungal Sinusitis

Because of the extent of sinus blockage and the strong association with polyps, surgery is usually indicated to remove the inspissated allergic mucin and polyps, followed by systemic corticosteroids to decrease the inflammatory response.[7] Treatment guidelines are based on the use of systemic steroids in allergic bronchopulmonary aspergillosis, in which steroids are tapered to daily or every-other-day dosing to control the disease. Commonly, nasal steroids are also added for topical treatment. Studies are currently being conducted to establish the role of antifungal agents or inhalant allergen immunotherapy for the treatment of AFS.

Summary

- The antibiotic of choice for acute sinusitis must cover S. pneumoniae, H. influenzae, and M. catarrhalis.
- The antibiotics of choice for chronic sinusitis include agents that cover organisms causing acute sinusitis but that also cover Staphylococcus species and anaerobes.
- Medical therapy for chronic sinusitis should include a topical intranasal steroid to address the strong inflammatory component of this disease.
- Allergy consultation should be considered in any patient with recurrent acute or chronic sinusitis to rule out allergy as a contributing factor for sinusitis.
- If medical therapy fails or if complications are suspected, an otolaryngology consultation is warranted.

Outcomes

URTIs of viral origin should run their course, with gradual improvement in symptoms daily until complete resolution of symptoms occurs by day 7 to 10, with supportive treatment only and no antibiotics.

When a secondary bacterial infection is suspected and antibiotics are given for acute sinusitis, the expected clinical outcome would be resolution of the infection and associated symptoms. This was shown in a study by Wald, in which symptoms resolved in 79% of patients who had clinically and radiographically diagnosed sinusitis and who had been treated with amoxicillin or amoxicillin plus clavulanic acid.[18]

The data on outcomes of medical management of chronic sinusitis are showing that we can control symptoms to a degree, although with a high rate of recurrence. Hamilos reported a retrospective series of patients treated medically for chronic sinusitis. Treatment included systemic steroids for 10 days, antibiotic coverage for aerobic and anaerobic organisms for 4 to 6 weeks, nasal saline irrigation, and topical steroid nasal spray. There were symptomatic and radiographic improvements in 17 of 19 patients, but 8 of 19 had persistent ostiomeatal complex abnormalities. In addition, relapse of sinusitis has been significantly associated with nasal polyposis and a history of prior sinus surgery.[7]

Overall, we have many treatment options for the sinusitis patient: antibiotics for the bacterial infection; steroids, systemic or topical, for the inflammatory component; and surgery for the anatomic and structural abnormalities that can predispose to sinusitis. Although these have helped with initial improvement, we still see a high rate of recurrence of sinus disease. This forces us to address the role of comorbid conditions such as allergic rhinitis, environmental irritants (e.g., cigarette smoke), or the need for newer and better treatment modalities for this disease.

Further Readings

American Academy of Pediatrics, Subcommittee on Management of Sinusitis and Committee on Quality Improvement: Clinical practice guideline: Management of sinusitis. Pediatrics 2001;108:798-808.

deShazo RD, Swain RE: Diagnostic criteria for allergic fungal sinusitis. J Allergy Clin Immunol 1995;96:24-35.

Dykewicz MS: The microbiology and management of acute and chronic rhino-sinusitis. Curr Infect Dis Rep 2001;3:209-216.

Hamilos DL: Chronic sinusitis. J Allergy Clin Immunol 2000;106:213-227.

Sinus and Allergy Health Partnership: Antimicrobial treatment guidelines for acute bacterial rhinosinusitis: Executive summary. Otolaryngol Head Neck Surg 2000;123(1 Pt 2):5-31.

Slavin RG: The diagnosis and management of sinusitis: A practice parameter update. J Allergy Clin Immunol 2005:116(6 Suppl):S13-S47.

Spector SL, Bernstein IL, Li JT, et al: Parameters for the diagnosis and management of sinusitis. J Allergy Clin Immunol 1998;102:S107-S144.

Szczeklik A, Stevenson DD: Aspirin-induced asthma: Advances in pathogenesis and management. J Allergy Clin Immunol 1999;104:5-13.

Wald ER: Microbiology of acute and chronic sinusitis in children and adults. Am J Med Sci 1998;316:13-20.

Winstead W: Rhinosinusitis. Prim Care 2003;30:137-154.

References

For a complete list of references, log onto www.expertconsult.com.

Approach to and Management of Adverse Drug Reactions

Mercedes E. Arroliga and Nicola M. Vogel

Adverse reactions to drugs are unintended or undesired effects of a drug therapy that may significantly influence management decisions.[1] The incidence may be as high as 15% in hospitalized patients.[2,3] Budnitz and colleagues, in a study of emergency department visits for outpatient adverse drug reactions, reported that such reactions accounted for 2.5% for all unintentional injury and 0.6% of the estimated visits for all causes.[4]

Predictable adverse drug reactions are common. These reactions are dose dependent or related to the pharmacology of the drug and include overdose, side effects, secondary or indirect effects, secondary effects related to underlying disease, and drug-drug interactions.[1,5] Unpredictable drug reactions are less common and occur in a small subset of patients. These reactions are not related to the dose or the pharmacology of the drug. Unpredictable reactions include drug intolerance, idiosyncratic reactions, pseudoallergic reactions, and immunologic reactions.[1,5]

Based on the mechanism involved, immunologic reactions can be classified as immunoglobulin E (IgE)-mediated (type 1) and non–IgE-mediated reactions. IgE-mediated reactions usually develop within minutes following the administration of the drug but can occur up to 72 hours later. These reactions include but are not limited to anaphylaxis, urticaria, asthma, angioedema, and hypotension. Non–IgE-mediated reactions can be further classified into antibody-mediated (type 2), immune complex-mediated (type 3), and T-lymphocyte-mediated (type 4) reactions. Non–IgE-mediated reactions include erythema multiforme, serum sickness, hemolytic anemia, drug fever, Stevens-Johnson syndrome, thrombocytopenia, and toxic epidermal necrolysis.[6]

This chapter summarizes current understanding of drug reactions, with emphasis on IgE-mediated reactions to penicillins and cephalosporins, adverse reactions to local anesthetics, and angioedema due to angiotensin-converting enzyme (ACE) inhibitors and angiotensin receptor blockers (ARBs).

PENICILLIN

Penicillin is commonly prescribed because of its effectiveness and low toxicity.[7] However, adverse reactions to penicillin are common and often complicate medical therapy. Up to 20% of patients admitted to the hospital claim to have penicillin allergy.[1] These patients are usually treated with more expensive, more toxic, and sometimes less effective antibiotics. Although the exact prevalence of allergic reactions to penicillin is unknown, allergic reactions are estimated to occur in approximately 2% of patients treated with penicillin.[1] Most of these reactions are skin rashes, such as maculopapular or urticarial eruptions.[1] However, the penicillins are one of the most common causes of drug-induced anaphylactic reactions,[8] and fatalities have been reported.[9]

Penicillin is a chemical hapten, with a low molecular weight of 300 daltons, that needs to bind to a tissue macromolecule, usually a protein, to become immunogenic.[7] The major breakdown product of penicillin is the penicilloyl group (approximately 85%-90%), known as the *major determinant.*[7] The reminder of the breakdown products are *minor determinants,* so called because they are formed in smaller quantities.[7] The minor determinants include penicilloate, penicilloylamine, penilloate, and other simple chemical products of penicillin.[7] Immediate reactions following penicillin administration are mediated through IgE antibodies against the major determinants, the minor determinants, or both.

Risk Factors

The risk of penicillin sensitization is increased with multiple short courses of antibiotics and can occur with any route of administration.[7] Anaphylactic reactions to penicillin occur most commonly in persons between 20 and 49 years old. However, they can occur in children and in the elderly. Race, gender, personal or family history of atopic disease, and allergy to other drugs or to the mold *Penicillium* are not predisposing factors.[7]

Testing for Penicillin Allergy

The presence of IgE antibodies to penicillin can be detected through a skin test to penicillin, a radioallergosorbent test (RAST) to penicillin, or the enzyme-linked immunosorbent assay (ELISA). The skin test for penicillin is the most reliable way to demonstrate the presence or absence of specific IgE antibodies to major and minor penicillin determinants. However, it does not predict the future development of IgE-mediated reactions during subsequent courses of penicillin or the development of non-IgE-mediated reactions caused by other immune mechanisms, such as cytotoxic antibody-mediated reactions, antibody-antigen immune complex-mediated reactions, and delayed-type cell-mediated reactions.[10]

Penicillin skin testing is performed using benzylpenicilloyl polylysine (Pre-Pen), penicillin G, and minor determinants (if available) to detect the presence of IgE antibodies to the major and minor determinants. Because the minor determinant mixture is not commercially available, penicillin G at a concentration of 10,000 U/mL has been recommended as a partial source of minor determinants. Methods of preparation of the minor determinants have been published elsewhere.[11,12] Unfortunately, Pre-Pen, the source of major determinants, has been withdrawn from the market and is not available.

Both percutaneous and intradermal tests are performed using diluted penicillin G at a concentration of 10,000 U/mL, Pre-Pen at full strength, and minor determinant mixture (if available). Histamine and saline skin tests are used as positive and negative controls, respectively. Percutaneous testing is done, and the results are read at 15 minutes. If the percutaneous test findings are negative, intradermal testing is performed. The skin test is positive if it produces a wheal more than 3 mm larger than the wheal produced by the negative saline control (Fig. 1).

Up to 99% of patients tolerate penicillin if skin testing is negative for penicillin using major determinants (benzylpenicilloyl) and a mixture of minor determinants and penicillin G. Approximately 97% of patients tolerate penicillin if skin testing is negative using benzylpenicilloyl and penicillin G (as the sole source of minor determinants).[13] However, a few patients who are at risk for anaphylactic reaction are missed with this testing method because penicillin G does not contain all the minor determinants.[13] Patients with a history of penicillin allergy and negative penicillin skin test have a low risk

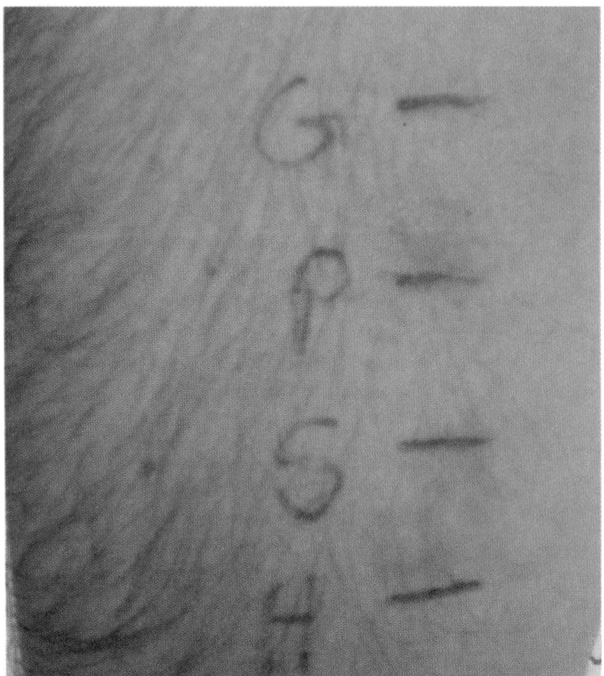

Figure 1 **Positive skin test to Pre-Pen.** *G* indicates penicillin G result; *P* indicates Pre-Pen result; *S* indicates saline result; *H* indicates histamine result.

of developing an IgE-mediated reaction following administration of penicillin. At our institution, we found a reaction rate of 1.7% in a group of 596 patients with a history of penicillin allergy and negative skin tests.[14] Similar to the findings in our study, low rates of adverse reactions also have been reported by other clinicians.[15-17]

The RAST and the ELISA detect only IgE antibodies to the major penicillin determinant. Therefore, these tests are less sensitive than the skin test.[13] If a patient has a positive history and a positive skin test to penicillin, there is a 50% or greater chance of an immediate IgE-mediated reaction if penicillin is received again.[13] Similarly, a positive RAST or ELISA demonstrates the presence of IgE antibodies to penicillin, and these patients should be considered at risk for immediate IgE-mediated reactions to penicillin.[15] These patients should receive an equally efficacious alternative antibiotic or be desensitized.

The detection of IgE antibodies to penicillin by a skin test is affected by the amount of time between the original allergic drug reaction and the skin test. Many patients with documented IgE antibodies to penicillin by skin test lose the sensitivity with time. It is estimated that up to 80% of patients with a history of immediate reactions to penicillin will have a negative skin test at 10 years.[18] However, these patients may be at increased risk of sensitization to penicillin on subsequent administration compared with the rest of the population.[17]

Safety of the Skin Test

If done properly, the skin test is safe, with a rate of systemic reaction of less than 1%.[14,19] Nevertheless, severe reactions such as anaphylaxis and death have occurred. Serious reactions to the penicillin skin test are usually a result of violations of the skin test protocol, such as administering a dose that is too high or performing intracutaneous testing without prick or puncture testing beforehand.[13]

Additional Uses of the Penicillin Skin Test

Penicillin skin testing can also serve as a way to decrease the necessary dose of broad-spectrum antibiotics such as vancomycin and fluoroquinolones.[20,21] These antibiotics, when used extensively, are associated with the emergence of multidrug-resistant pathogens and increased morbidity and mortality.

Evaluation

Most patients labeled allergic to penicillin do not have penicillin-specific IgE antibodies as detected by skin test and can safely be given penicillin. However, patients with a history of penicillin allergy are more likely to experience a reaction on subsequent courses than those without such history.[10]

The evaluation of adverse drug reactions begins with a detailed history. However, many patients do not clearly recall the drug to which they reacted, the type of reaction that occurred, or the duration of drug exposure. In addition, up to 33% of patients with a vague history of penicillin allergy have a positive penicillin skin test.[18] Therefore, it is recommended that even patients who have a vague history of penicillin allergy and who require penicillin have skin testing to determine the presence of penicillin-specific IgE antibodies before it is assumed that the patient will tolerate penicillin.[13] Some clinicians suggest that the penicillin skin test needs to be repeated before each course of penicillin, especially for patients with a history of IgE-mediated reaction who received intravenous penicillin, because of the risk of resensitization.[1] However, Solensky and colleagues have reported that none of 46 patients with a history of penicillin allergy and a negative penicillin skin test were resensitized after receiving three courses of oral penicillin V.[22]

Because of the lack of commercially available penicillin minor determinants for skin testing, some authorities recommend a test-dose challenge in patients with a history of penicillin allergy and negative skin tests to major determinants and penicillin G.[6] A test-dose challenge might be done using 0.01 of the therapeutic dose (0.001 of the therapeutic dose if the previous reaction was severe), followed by 0.1 of the dose, and then the full therapeutic dose if there is no reaction.[6] If a reaction occurs during the test-dose challenge and the drug is essential for treatment, penicillin desensitization is recommended.[6]

Treatment

If the penicillin skin test is positive and the treatment with a penicillin antibiotic is essential, desensitization is needed. Oral and intravenous protocols for penicillin desensitization have been published.[5,6,8,23] Oral desensitization is safer than parenteral desensitization.[23]

The basic principle for oral or parenteral (intravenous) desensitization is similar. The initial dose is very small, usually 0.0001 of the recommended dose. The dose is usually doubled every 15 minutes until the full therapeutic dose is achieved.

Adverse reactions can occur during and after the desensitization procedure.[22] Most of these reactions are mild, such as pruritus, rhinitis, wheezing, and urticaria.[23] These reactions require symptomatic treatment, and the dose of penicillin should be repeated until tolerated. Severe reactions, such as laryngeal edema, require rapid treatment until the patient is stable and a reduction of the next penicillin dose by one third or more of the previous provoking dose.[6] When desensitization is achieved, continuous treatment with penicillin is required to avoid the return of the IgE-sensitive state. A time lapse greater than 12 to 48 hours can allow such sensitivity to return.[6]

CEPHALOSPORINS

Like penicillins, cephalosporins are commonly used. Cephalosporins share a common beta-lactam ring with the penicillin (Fig. 2). However, they have a dihydrothiazide ring instead of the thiazolide ring of the penicillin molecule. Various adverse reactions to cephalosporin have been described including eosinophilia, serum sickness, febrile reactions, interstitial nephritis, and hemolytic anemia.[24] Urti-

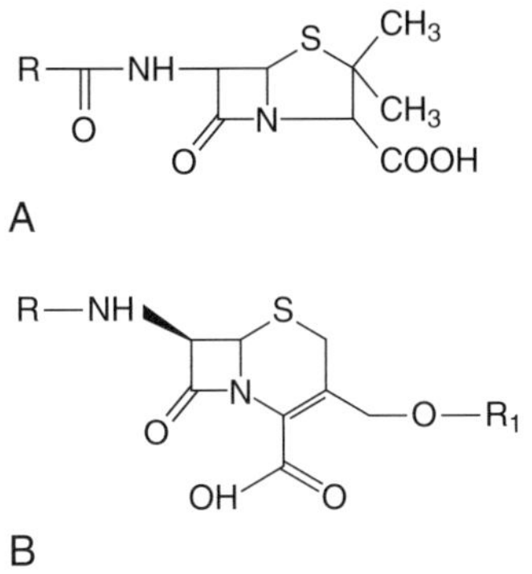

Figure 2 **A,** Penicillin molecule. **B,** Cephalosporin molecule.

caria, rash, exanthema, and pruritus are estimated to occur in approximately 1% to 2.8%.[24] Although anaphylactic reactions after cephalosporin administration are rare,[25] death has been reported.[26,27]

Unlike penicillin, cephalosporin determinants have not been well identified or studied. Therefore, the positive and negative predictive values of cephalosporin skin testing are unknown. A negative skin test does not rule out the presence of IgE antibodies to these drugs. On the other hand, a positive skin test suggests the presence of drug-specific IgE antibodies. These patients should be considered at increased risk for IgE-mediated reaction on administration of the specific drug. They should receive an alternative antibiotic or undergo desensitization. Nonirritant concentrations of commonly used antimicrobial drugs that can be used for skin testing have been published.[8,28]

If the patient needs a cephalosporin and has a history of cephalosporin allergy, the treating physician can choose one of the following approaches: choose a non–beta-lactam antibiotic, give a graded dose challenge with a cephalosporin with a different side chain from the one to which the patient reacted, or perform a cephalosporin skin test with a nonirritating concentration.[24] If the skin test is positive, the patient can be desensitized or tested for another cephalosporin with a different structure.[1] Protocols for cephalosporin desensitization are published elsewhere.[24] Because the negative predictive value of a cephalosporin skin test is unknown, it is preferable that a negative skin test be followed by a provocative graded-dose challenge, if a challenge is favorable from a risk-to-benefit standpoint.[1]

CROSS-REACTIVITY BETWEEN PENICILLINS AND CEPHALOSPORINS

The rate of cross-reactivity between penicillins and cephalosporins is unknown. Clinical cross-reactivity between penicillins and cephalosporins appears to be low, especially for second- and third-generation cephalosporins.[10] However, patients with a history of penicillin allergy appear to be at increased risk for severe IgE-mediated reactions to cephalosporin, including anaphylaxis.

A penicillin skin test can help to determine which patients are at increased risk for severe IgE-mediated reactions when receiving a cephalosporin. A review of 11 studies concluded that the risk for reaction when receiving cephalosporin in a patient with a positive skin test to penicillin was approximately 4.4%.[25] Pumphrey and David reported that 3 of 12 anaphylactic deaths following administration of cephalosporin occurred in patients known to be allergic to penicillin.[29]

Some patients who react to beta-lactam antibiotics other than penicillin have antibodies directed to side-chain structures rather than to the beta-lactam ring, and cross-reactivity among cephalosporins could be explained by the presence of these antibodies.[1] Such antibodies can cause anaphylaxis.[13] Figure 3 shows an extensive list of cephalosporins and their structures, including similarities and differences of side-chain structures (indicated by R_1 and R_2).[30] Cefamandole, cefalothin, cepaloridine, cephalotin, and penicillin G have similar side chains. Similar side chains are present in cefadroxil and amoxicillin, ceftazidime and aztreonam, and cephalexin and amoxicillin.[24] It can be appreciated that reactions to cephalosporin can occur even with a negative penicillin skin test.

If a patient has a history of penicillin allergy and needs a cephalosporin antibiotic, the following approaches have been recommended[10]: First, use a non–beta-lactam antibiotic. Next, consider administration of a cephalosporin (preferably second or third generation) if the patient has a history of mild reaction. Although the risk of life-threatening reaction is low, severe adverse reactions can occur. This approach has been discouraged in published guidelines on the diagnosis and management of drug hypersensitivity.[10] Finally, perform a penicillin skin test. If the skin test is negative, the patient may receive the cephalosporin with a low risk of developing an allergic reaction.

If a patient in need of a penicillin antibiotic has a history of a cephalosporin allergy, the penicillin skin test can identify those at risk for IgE-mediated reaction to penicillin. If the skin test is negative, penicillin may be given. If the skin test is positive and penicillin is needed, the patient should undergo desensitization.

Carbapenems (e.g., imipenem) should be considered cross-reactive with penicillin and cephalosporin because of the presence of a similar beta-lactam ring.[10,13] On the other hand, aztreonam (a monobactam) rarely cross-reacts with penicillin, possibly because of the lack of a second nuclear ring structure.[10,13] However, ceftazidime and aztreonam share the same side chains, and clinical cross-reactivity can occur.[1]

The presence of IgE antibodies to penicillin can be determined by the use of the penicillin skin test. This test can help us to identify patients who have a history of penicillin allergy and can receive penicillin or cephalosporin with a low risk for immediate hypersensitivity reactions, and it can identify patients who should avoid using these drugs. In spite of the importance of penicillin skin testing, Pre-Pen was withdrawn from the market because of manufacturing problems. Without this preparation, a reliable diagnostic test for managing drug hypersensitivity has been lost.

ALLERGIC REACTIONS TO LOCAL ANESTHETICS

Local anesthetics have been used worldwide in different medical procedures since procaine (Novocaine), the first synthetic local anesthetic agent, was developed.

Local anesthetics reversibly block the generation and conduction of nerve impulses by decreasing the permeability of excitable membranes to sodium through interaction with one or more specific binding sites within sodium channels.[31] The duration of anesthesia depends on plasma protein binding and the addition of vasoconstrictors such as epinephrine. Vasoconstrictors decrease the rate of absorption of local anesthetics, localizing the anesthetic to the desired site and allowing its rate of destruction to keep pace with its rate of absorption into the circulation.[31]

The structure of local anesthetics has three segments: a lipophilic or aromatic group, an intermediate chain linkage, and a hydrophilic or amine group. Based on their intermediate chain linkage, local anesthetics are classified into two major groups: the benzoic acid esters or group 1 and the amides and miscellaneous or group 2. Group 1 anesthetics include benzocaine, butamben picrate, cocaine, procaine, tetracaine, proparacaine. Group 2 anesthetics include bupivacaine, dibucaine, dyclonine, etiodocaine, levobupivacaine, lidocaine, mepivacaine, prilocaine).[31,32]

Different types of adverse reactions to local anesthetics have been reported. Most of these appear to be vasovagal, anxiety, and toxic reactions.[33] Case reports have suggested that adverse reactions to the preservatives in local anesthetics, including methylparaben and sulfites, can also occur.[34,35]

Following absorption, local anesthetics may be associated with central stimulation manifested by restlessness, tremor, and seizures. Central stimulation is followed by depression, and death is due to

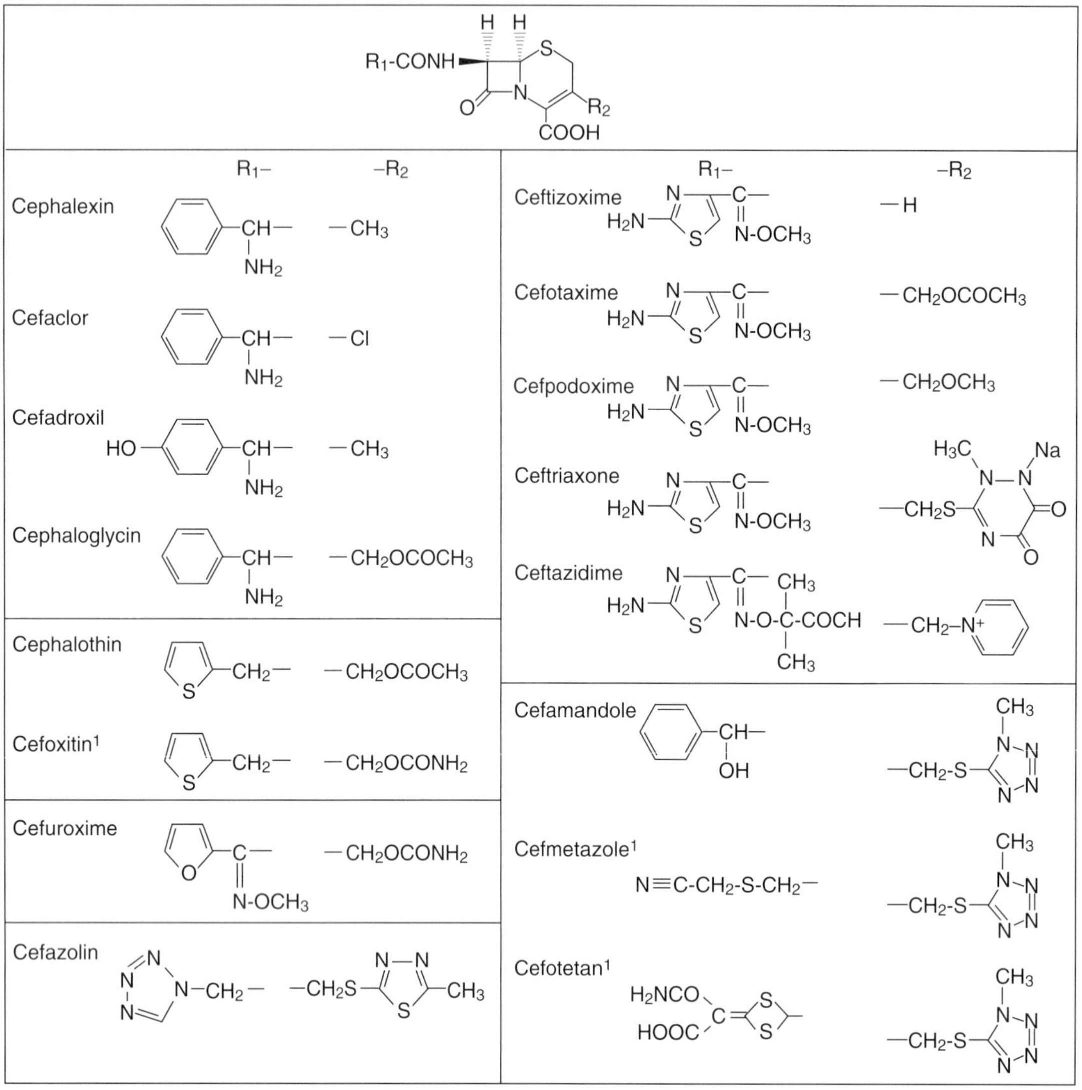

R_1-CONH … COOH … R_2

Cephalosporin	R_1–	–R_2
Cephalexin	CH— NH$_2$	—CH$_3$
Cefaclor	CH— NH$_2$	—Cl
Cefadroxil	HO— CH— NH$_2$	—CH$_3$
Cephaloglycin	CH— NH$_2$	—CH$_2$OCOCH$_3$
Cephalothin	S CH$_2$—	—CH$_2$OCOCH$_3$
Cefoxitin[1]	S CH$_2$—	—CH$_2$OCONH$_2$
Cefuroxime	O C— N-OCH$_3$	—CH$_2$OCONH$_2$
Cefazolin	N N N N-CH$_2$—	—CH$_2$S— N—N S —CH$_3$
Ceftizoxime	N C— H$_2$N— S N-OCH$_3$	—H
Cefotaxime	N C— H$_2$N— S N-OCH$_3$	—CH$_2$OCOCH$_3$
Cefpodoxime	N C— H$_2$N— S N-OCH$_3$	—CH$_2$OCH$_3$
Ceftriaxone	N C— H$_2$N— S N-OCH$_3$	H$_3$C Na N—N —CH$_2$S— =O N O
Ceftazidime	N C— CH$_3$ H$_2$N— S N-O-C-COCH CH$_3$	—CH$_2$–N$^+$
Cefamandole	CH— OH	CH$_3$ N-N —CH$_2$-S— N-N
Cefmetazole[1]	N≡C-CH$_2$-S-CH$_2$—	CH$_3$ N-N —CH$_2$-S— N-N
Cefotetan[1]	H$_2$NCO C= S S HOOC	CH$_3$ N-N —CH$_2$-S— N-N

[1]Cephamycin with an α-methoxy group (-OCH$_3$) at the 7-position.

Figure 3 Similarities in the side chains of different cephalosporins. *From Baldo BA: Penicillins and cephalosporins as allergens-structural aspects of recognition and cross-reactions. Clin Exp Allergy 1999;29(6):744-749. Used with permission.*

respiratory failure.[33] Palpitations, tachycardia, diaphoresis, and ventricular arrhythmias have also been described.[31,32,36]

Hypersensitivity reactions to local anesthetics are uncommon. Contact dermatitis mediated by sensitized lymphocytes is the most common, and it accounts for up to 80% of reactions reported to local anesthetics.[37] Patch testing is available for patients with a history of contact dermatitis. Although IgE-mediated reactions to local anesthetics are extremely rare, cases have been reported.[37] de Shazo and Nelson evaluated 90 patients with a history of adverse reaction to local anesthetics, and only one patient had a positive test by the intradermal method; the other 89 had a negative challenge.[38] Gall and colleagues reported negative skin-test results in 177 patients evaluated for adverse reactions to local anesthetics. Three patients reacted after a provocative dose challenge with the causative drug, two patients had immediate-type reactions to articaine and lidocaine, and one patient had a delayed reaction to mepivacaine.[39] In a large series of 236 patients reported by Berkun and colleagues, all subjects had negative skin test results, and only one patient had a positive provocative dose challenge.[40]

Patients with a history of adverse reactions to local anesthetics are usually advised to avoid them in the future. When surgery is indicated, they must decide whether to undergo surgery without anesthesia, have a procedure with general anesthesia, or forgo benefits of the surgical procedure.

The role of the allergist or immunologist is to rule out IgE-mediated (allergic and anaphylactic) potential to group 1 and group 2 agents. Different protocols for evaluating patients with a history of adverse reactions to local anesthetics have been described.[6,32,40,41] Based on the information obtained from patch-test studies, the benzoic acid esters usually cross-react with each other but not with the amides and the other agents in group 2. The amides and the other agents in group 2 do not appear to cross-react with each other.[6]

One approach to managing these patients begins with identifying the agent that caused the previous untoward reaction. If the drug is a benzoic acid ester (group 1), an amide or a drug from group 2 may be used. If the drug is an amide, another amide may be used and no further evaluation is needed. If the drug is unknown, skin-prick testing with the undiluted local anesthetic to be used can be performed. A negative test can be followed by intradermal testing with 0.1 mL of a 1 : 100 dilution of the same agent. If both tests are negative, the next step is a provocative dose challenge with 1 mL subcutaneous injection of the undiluted agent.

Positive and negative controls should be used with all prick and intradermal testing. Local anesthetics used for skin testing should not contain epinephrine, because false-negative results can occur.[41] Skin testing may be performed with preservative-free local anesthetics or with local anesthetics containing preservatives. However, if the result is positive with a local anesthetic containing preservative , skin testing should be repeated with a preservative-free agent. Another positive skin test might indicate the presence of IgE antibodies, and a different local anesthetic should be considered.

True IgE-mediated reactions to local anesthetics are extremely rare. Allergy and immunology evaluation is useful for patients with suspected local anesthetic allergy, because it can identify local anesthetic agents that can be tolerated without elevated risk of IgE-mediated reaction.

ANGIOTENSIN-CONVERTING ENZYME INHIBITORS AND ANGIOTENSIN II RECEPTOR BLOCKERS

Adverse drug reactions to ACE inhibitors are common and include cough in up to 35% of patients and angioedema in approximately 0.1% to 2.2%.[42-45] Angioedema has also been reported in association with angiotensin II receptor blockers (ARBs).

Cough

Cough associated with ACE inhibitors often develops within the first 2 weeks of starting an ACE inhibitor and generally is a dry, nonproductive cough. Cough may be accompanied by bronchospasm, although this does not occur more often in asthmatics than in nonasthmatics.[46] Cough is more common in women and nonsmokers.[47]

The pathogenesis of ACE inhibitor–associated cough is not completely understood. The mechanism might involve increased levels of prostaglandins, kinins (including bradykinin), and substance P. Bradykinin and substance P are degraded by ACE, and prostaglandin production may be increased by bradykinin. Potential mechanisms involve bradykinin-induced sensitization of airway sensory nerves or activation of bradykinin receptors.[48,49]

Treatment options include discontinuing the medication and using alternative medications. The American College of Chest Physicians (ACCP) Evidence-Based Clinical Practice Guidelines recommend discontinuing the ACE inhibitor.[44] Cough associated with ACE inhibitors usually resolves within a few days of discontinuing the medication but can take up to several weeks.[44,50] Cough often recurs with the same or different ACE inhibitor. Cough has not been reported in association with ARBs, and the ACCP guidelines recommend ARBs as a treatment alternative.[44] In patients in whom the benefits of treatment with an ACE inhibitor outweigh the risks of a recurrence of the cough, a repeat trial of ACE inhibitor might also be indicated.[44]

Angioedema

Although the onset of angioedema associated with ACE inhibitors often occurs during the first week or first month after initiating treatment in 25% to 60% of patients, it can occur at any time.[42,51] This unpredictable characteristic of ACE inhibitor–associated angioedema can lead to a delay in identifying the association. The newer ARBs, often used as an alternative to ACE inhibitors, have also been associated with angioedema.[51-53] Studies estimate that the incidence of ARB-associated angioedema varies from 0% to 32% in patients with a history of ACE inhibitor–associated angioedema.[51,54-56]

Women, African Americans, and patients with a history of either idiopathic angioedema or C1 inhibitor deficiency are at higher risk for angioedema.[42,57] Angioedema associated with either ACE inhibitors or ARBs generally affects the head and neck, and pruritis and urticaria generally do not occur.

Similar to the pathogenesis of ACE inhibitor–induced cough, the pathogenesis of ACE inhibitor–associated angioedema may be related to the accumulation of bradykinin and other vasoactive peptides. ACE catalyzes the conversion of angiotensin I to angiotensin II, which is a vasoconstrictor that can increase blood pressure. ACE also degrades bradykinin, a vasodilator that opposes the effects of angiotensin II. With ACE inhibition, subsequently increased levels of bradykinin can induce angioedema through vasodilation and increased vascular permeability. In some patients with ACE inhibitor–associated angioedema, an active metabolite of bradykinin, des-Arg^9-BK, may be abnormally degraded and lead to increased bioavailability of bradykinin.[58] Dipeptidyl peptidase IV might also play a role in angioedema. Decreased levels of this enzyme can lead to increased amounts of substance P, which can be associated with increased vascular permeability and leakage of plasma proteins.[59]

Evaluation

The approach to a patient with a history of an adverse reaction to an ACE inhibitor or ARB should begin with a detailed medical history including a list of all medications, indication for each medication, dose, date of initiation, and duration of therapy. The clinical manifestations of the reaction, including associated symptoms, should also be reviewed. Additional history to obtain is whether the patient had a prior exposure to the same or other ACE inhibitor or ARB medications, the effect of drug discontinuation, and the treatment of the prior reaction. Other factors that may be related to the development of urticaria and angioedema should be considered, including infections; collagen vascular diseases; malignancy; physical factors such as pressure, vibration, or exposure to heat, cold, or sunlight; and family history of angioedema suggesting C1-inhibitor deficiency.

Treatment

Treatment of angioedema should be tailored to each patient and may include antihistamines, oral or intravenous corticosteroids, or intramuscular or subcutaneous epinephrine for severe airway compromise. No studies support the effectiveness of treatment with antihistamines or corticosteroids. Symptoms generally resolve within 48 hours after treatment is initiated and the ACE inhibitor or ARB is discontinued.

There is no valid skin or blood test to establish a diagnosis of ACE inhibitor–associated or ARB-associated angioedema. Desensitization, a process of administering incremental doses of a drug over hours to days and conversion of a drug allergy to a state of drug tolerance, is not indicated for patients who have angioedema associated with ACE inhibitors or ARB because the reaction is not an IgE-mediated process.

All ACE inhibitors carry the same risk of developing angioedema. Patients who experience angioedema related to one ACE inhibitor are at risk for more severe and frequent episodes with other ACE inhibitors.[60] The best approach for a patient with ACE inhibitor–associated angioedema is to avoid other ACE inhibitors and use alternative, equally efficacious, medications.

Although patients with ACE inhibitor–associated angioedema might tolerate ARBs, ARBs should be used with caution because these patients can also develop angioedema associated with ARB. Studies estimate that the incidence of experiencing ARB-associated angioedema varies from 0% to 32% in patients with a history of ACE inhibitor–associated angioedema.[51,54-56] The largest of these studies involved more than 2000 patients with congestive heart failure. Either an ARB (candesartan) or placebo was given to patients with a history of adverse reaction to ACE inhibitors. In the treatment group, 39 of 1013 patients previously experienced angioedema or anaphylaxis from an ACE inhibitor. Of these 39 patients, only 3 (7.6%) developed angioedema associated with candesartan. More studies are needed to evaluate the incidence of developing ARB-associated angioedema in patients with ACE inhibitor–associated angioedema. Any patient with a history of ACE inhibitor–associated angioedema prescribed an ARB should be counseled regarding the possible risk of developing angioedema.

Summary

- The incidence of adverse drug reactions may be as high as 15% in hospitalized patients.
- Adverse reactions to penicillins and cephalosporins are common and complicate medical therapy.
- Penicillin skin testing can reliably identify patients with a history of penicillin or cephalosporin allergy who can safely take penicillin.
- Patients with positive skin tests can use equally effective alternative antibiotics or undergo desensitization.
- Penicillin skin testing can decrease the use of broad-spectrum antibiotics such as vancomycin and fluoroquinolones.
- Hypersensitivity reactions to local anesthetics are uncommon.
- A board-certified allergist or immunologist can identify local anesthetics that can be used without elevated risk of immunoglobulin E-mediated reaction in patients with a history of allergy to local anesthetics.
- Common adverse drug reactions to ACE and ARBs include cough and angioedema.
- Alternative medications should be considered.

Further Readings

Alvarez del Real G, Rose ME, Ramirez-Atamoros MT, et al: Penicillin skin testing in patients with a history of β-lactam allergy. Ann Allergy Asthma Immunol 2007;98:355-359.

Berkun Y, Ben-Zvi A, Levy Y, et al: Evaluation of adverse reactions to local anesthetics: Experience with 236 patients. Ann Allergy Asthma Immunol 2003;91:342-345.

Joint Task Force on Practice Parameters, American Academy of Allergy, Asthma and Immunology, the American College of Allergy, Asthma and Immunology, and the Joint Council of Allergy, Asthma and Immunology: Executive summary of disease management of drug hypersensitivity: A practice parameter. Ann Allergy Asthma Immunol 1999;83:665-700.

Joint Task Force on Practice Parameters, American Academy of Allergy, Asthma and Immunology, the American College of Allergy, Asthma and Immunology, and the Joint Council of Allergy, Asthma and Immunology: The diagnosis and management of anaphylaxis. J Allergy Clin Immunol 1998;101 (Pt 2):S465-S528.

Kelkar PS, Li JT: Cephalosporin allergy. N Engl J Med 2001;345:804-809.

Mendelson LM: Adverse reactions to β-lactam antibiotics. Immunol Allergy Clin North Am 1998;18:745-757.

Sogn DD, Evans R III, Shepherd GM, et al: Results of the National Institute of Allergy and Infectious Diseases Collaborative Clinical Trial to test the predictive value of skin testing with major and minor penicillin derivatives in hospitalized adults. Arch Intern Med 1992;152:1025-1032.

Soto-Aguilar MC, de-Shazo RD, Dawson ES: Approach to the patient with suspected local anesthetic sensitivity. Immunol Allergy Clin North Am 1998;18:851-865.

References

For a complete list of references, log onto www.expertconsult.com.

Latex Allergy

Lily C. Pien

The dramatic surge in the incidence of latex allergy in the 1980s is believed to be related to increased use of latex gloves after the adoption of universal precautions and to manufacturing changes that might have exposed health care workers and patients to latex gloves with higher latex content. Recognition of latex allergy as a public health concern led to identification of populations at risk, defined clinical symptoms, and recommendations for evaluation and management.[1] In addition, guidelines for preventing new cases of latex allergy and for safety of latex-allergic patients were established.[2] The major thrust of these policies is the restricted use of latex gloves, and the promotion of the use of nonpowdered sterile latex gloves to establish latex-safe environments in the hospital setting. Manufacturers of medical and commercial products have responded by labeling latex products and by developing latex-free items. These efforts to decrease latex exposure appear to have been successful in decreasing rates of sensitization and allergic reactions to latex.[3]

DEFINITION

Latex allergy is defined as the presence of specific immunoglobulin E (IgE) antibody to latex proteins in persons who have a variety of clinical symptoms to latex-containing products. The cause of latex allergy involves exposure and sensitization to the latex, which is derived from the sap of the rubber tree (*Hevea brasilienses*) and is harvested primarily in Malaysia, Indonesia, and Thailand.

PREVALENCE AND RISK FACTORS

Exposure to latex can occur by contact with skin, mucous membranes, or blood. Sensitization to latex proteins depends on the amount and duration of exposure and the predisposition to atopy, and it is defined as identification of specific IgE antibody to latex proteins, with or without clinical symptoms. Allergy is defined by sensitization and clinical symptoms. Prevalence rates of latex allergy or sensitization have varied from population to population. The highest rates are found in patients with spina bifida and other congenital urogenital anomalies (24%-60%), moderate rates are found in health care workers and employees in the rubber industry (5%-15%), and the lowest rates are found in the general population (1%).[4] Irritant dermatitis may be another risk factor for the development of immunologic reactions to latex because the protective skin barrier is altered and allergen exposure and absorption may be increased, leading to possible IgE sensitization.

PATHOPHYSIOLOGY

Latex allergy is caused by latex allergens cross-linking specific IgE antibodies located on allergic effector cells, mast cells, and basophils. This action activates the cells to release preformed mediators, such as histamine, which cause immediate clinical symptoms of allergy, notably sneezing and itching. Activated mast cells also are responsible for the production of newly formed mediators (prostaglandins and leukotrienes) and cytokines (interleukin [IL]-4, IL-13, and tumor necrosis factor [TNF]-α), which contribute to more chronic symptoms of allergy such as nasal congestion and swelling of tissues. More severe clinical manifestations of latex allergy, such as anaphylaxis, are also related to the release of these allergic cell mediators and their effects on vasculature, leading to vasodilation and subsequently to hypotension.

SIGNS AND SYMPTOMS

Signs and symptoms of latex allergy depend on the type of latex product, the route of exposure, the amount of latex proteins, and the level of individual allergic sensitivity. Symptoms can vary from mild itching and urticaria, to rhinitis and asthma, to anaphylaxis. Latex gloves are probably the primary source of exposure, because they are used in many professions, including medicine, dentistry, housekeeping, daycare, and beauty and food services. This wide range of use can cause symptoms not only in persons wearing gloves but also in persons exposed to those wearing the gloves.

The most common adverse reactions experienced by persons wearing latex gloves are irritant reactions, typically erythema, cracking, dryness, and chapping of the skin. These reactions occur without an immunologic mechanism. Damage to the skin can occur by physical trauma with glove wearing, prolonged contact with solvents trapped underneath the gloves, extremes of skin temperature, and sweating.

Allergic contact dermatitis from latex gloves requires lymphocyte sensitization to chemical additives or accelerators that are used in the manufacturing process. The onset of symptoms is typically 24 to 48 hours after contact, and the symptoms are representative of contact dermatitis, including pruritus, erythema, blisters, or vesicles. Chronic symptoms include scaling, dryness, cracking, and thickening of the skin. Thiurams, carbamates, and benzothiazoles can be confirmed as allergens by patch testing.[5]

Immediate hypersensitivity reactions to latex allergens, otherwise known as latex allergy, are IgE-mediated reactions. These reactions occur within minutes of exposure to latex and can cause pruritus, urticaria, angioedema, and rhinoconjunctivitis. More severe symptoms are bronchospasm, hypotension, and anaphylaxis. Contact urticaria is most commonly reported with latex glove use. Facial and periorbital urticaria and angioedema can occur if latex gloves directly contact the face. Rhinitis, conjunctivitis, and asthma occur if latex proteins become airborne.

It is now known that latex allergens bind to cornstarch powder used in glove manufacturing and that significant levels of airborne latex proteins are found in medical and dental offices. Extensive studies performed at the Mayo Clinic demonstrate high levels of latex aeroallergens in operating rooms on days when many powdered latex gloves were used in the area, in contrast to minimal levels of airborne latex on weekend days and holidays when no gloves were used.[6] This information has led to intervention policies to decrease levels of latex in operating rooms and hospitals.

Latex exposure to mucosal surfaces can be associated with systemic symptoms of hypotension, tachycardia, and bronchospasm, leading to anaphylaxis. Unfortunately, even limited mucosal exposure to latex has caused anaphylaxis; generalized reactions have occurred with toy balloons, urinary catheters, condoms, dental surgery, and rectal procedures.[7]

Another IgE-mediated reaction is the cross-reactivity between latex and several foods and fruits. Latex proteins share similar protein structures with other protective plant proteins found in fruits and foods. Latex-allergic persons have had oral symptoms of itching, swelling, and anaphylaxis with exposures to avocado, banana, and chestnuts. There have also been some reported reactions to potato, tomato, and kiwi.[8] For this reason, latex-allergic patients should be questioned and informed about possible food reactions.

DIAGNOSIS

A pertinent history for symptoms related to latex exposures, tests to confirm the presence of IgE antibody, are necessary determine latex allergy. Provocative challenges can be completed if needed.

History

Essential in the workup of latex allergy is the clinical history. Clarification of symptoms that occur with exposure to latex gloves and with other common latex products, such as latex balloons or condoms, is critical. Onset of symptoms after latex exposure should be immediate, usually occurring within minutes to 1 hour. Patients commonly report symptoms of itching, redness, and hives with direct handling of latex products, itching of nose and eyes and wheezing with exposure to powdered latex gloves, and lip swelling when inflating latex balloons. Persons with histories of idiopathic urticaria, food allergy, and idiopathic anaphylaxis have been found to be latex allergic with hidden sources of latex exposure.

Diagnostic Tests

The two most common methods used to identify specific IgE antibody are the percutaneous (prick) skin test and radioallergosorbent test (RAST). Skin testing to identify latex-specific IgE antibody is convenient, sensitive, and fast. Current latex skin testing is problematic because there is no commercially available FDA-approved latex extract, and latex reagents in the United States vary in their preparation, potency, content, and reliability.

Three FDA-approved in vitro serologic tests for latex specific IgE antibody are the Immuno-CAP (Pharmacia-Upjohn, Uppsala, Sweden), AlaSTAT FEIA (Diagnostic Products Corp, Los Angeles, Calif.) and HYTEC-EIA (Hycor Biomedical, Garden Grove, Calif.). Immuno-CAP and AlaSTAT have comparable diagnostic sensitivity (76% and 73%) and specificity (96% and 97%), whereas HY-TEC has more sensitivity (93%), but lower specificity (73%).[9]

Allergists can perform an in vivo provocation test with latex gloves to establish latex allergy if the patient's history and latex skin test or serologic test are discordant. The latex glove use test, when a latex glove is worn for 10 to 15 minutes and symptoms are then noted, is commonly used.[10]

Additional identification of food-specific IgE (either by skin test or RAST, if available) should be performed for persons who report allergic symptoms with fruits and vegetables that can cross-react with latex proteins.

TREATMENT

The latex-allergic person must avoid natural rubber products to the best of his or her knowledge and ability, because there is no cure for latex allergy. It is appropriate to provide lists of latex-containing products as well as to advise about suitable alternative products. Complete latex avoidance is unreasonable to implement and may be unnecessary except for patients who demonstrate the most severe anaphylactic reactions. Reports of outcomes of latex-allergic health care workers show that nonpowdered latex gloves, low-allergen latex gloves, and nonlatex gloves allow some health care workers with latex allergy to continue to work with lessened clinical symptoms in latex-safe environments.[11,12]

Latex-allergic persons should wear medical-alert devices, carry self-injectable epinephrine if there have been prior systemic symptoms, and have latex allergy listed on medical and dental records.

Special considerations are needed for latex-allergic persons who have spina bifida, work in medical or dental settings and in the industrial rubber companies, and are undergoing surgery. Surgical operating rooms can be made latex-safe to decrease risk of anaphylaxis from latex exposure. Stringent latex avoidance measures are needed to prevent latex sensitization and worsening of clinical symptoms. All children with spina bifida are at high risk for latex allergy and should avoid latex in the home and hospital settings. Additional issues for workers with latex allergy include disability and workers' compensation, development of latex-safe environments, and guidance in career options.

Medical management of latex allergy is identical to the treatment of other IgE-mediated reactions. Removal of the allergen should occur first, followed by administration of antihistamines and other medications (including corticosteroids) depending on the severity of symptoms. Epinephrine may be needed if there is progression to systemic reactions of anaphylaxis. Latex immunotherapy and omalizumab (Xolair) have also been administered in the treatment of latex allergy.[13,14]

Summary

- Clinical history and identification of latex-specific IgE antibody are needed to confirm latex allergy.
- Avoidance of latex products is the mainstay of treatment at this time.
- Institutional policies and manufacturing efforts are helping to decrease latex exposure, sensitization, and, ideally, latex allergy.

Further Readings

Beezhold DH, Sussman GL, Liss GM, Chang NS: Latex allergy can induce clinical reactions to specific foods. Clin Exp Allergy 1996:26:416-422.

Bernstein DI, Karnani R, Biagini RE, et al: Clinical and occupational outcomes in health care workers with natural rubber latex allergy. Ann Allergy Asthma Immunol 2003;90(2):209-213.

Hamilton RG, Biagini RE, Kreig EF: Diagnostic performance of Food and Drug Administration–cleared serologic assays for natural rubber latex–specific IgE antibody. J Allergy Clin Immunol 1999;103:925-930.

Hunt LW, Kelkar P, Reed CE, Yunginger JW: Management of occupational allergy to natural rubber latex in a medical center: The importance of quantitative latex allergen measurement and objective follow-up. J Allergy Clin Immunol 2002;110:S96-S106.

Kelly KJ, Kurup VP, Reijula KE, Fink JN: The diagnosis of latex allergy. J Allergy Clin Immunol 1994;47:579-587.

Leynadier F, Doudou O, Gaouar H, et al: Effect of omalizumab in health care workers with occupational latex allergy. J Allergy Clin Immunol 2004;113:360-361.

National Institute for Occupational Safety and Health (NIOSH): NIOSH alert: Preventing allergic reactions to natural rubber latex in the workplace. June 1997. Available at http://www.cdc.gov/Niosh/latexalt.html#sum (accessed February 28, 2009).

Poley GE, Slater JE: Latex allergy. J Allergy Clin Immunol 2000;105:1054-1062.

Pumphrey RS, Duddridge M, Norton J: Fatal latex allergy. J Allergy Clin Immunol 2001;107:558.

Sastre J, Fernandez-Nieto M, Rico P, et al: Specific immunotherapy with a standardized latex extract in allergic workers: A double-blind placebo-controlled study. J Allergy Clin Immunol 2003;111:985-994.

Tarlo S, Easty A, Eubanks K, et al: Outcomes of a natural rubber latex control program in an Ontario teaching hospital. J Allergy Clin Immunol 2001;108 628-633.

Taylor JS: Latex allergy. Am J Contact Dermatitis 1993;4:114-117.

Turjanma K: Incidence of immediate allergy to latex gloves in hospital personnel. Contact Dermatitis 1987;17:270-275.

Turjanma K, Kanto M, Kautianinen H, et al: Long-term outcome of 160 adult patients with natural rubber latex allergy. J Allergy Clin Immunol 2002;110:S70-S74.

References

For a complete list of references, log onto www.expertconsult.com.

Food Allergy

R. Koelsch

DEFINITION

An allergic reaction is but one kind of adverse reaction to food. Other reactions include intolerance to compounds such as lactose, reactions to toxins in cases of food poisoning, and nonallergic immune reactions such as celiac disease. As is the case for any allergy, true food allergy is a reaction mediated by immunoglobulin E (IgE) (allergic) antibodies. Such antibodies are directed at protein allergens in food items. Food allergy is much less common than other kinds of adverse food reactions.

EPIDEMIOLOGY

Food allergy is not as prevalent as commonly believed, given the sizeable proportion of the population who react adversely to various kinds of foods. As much as 25% of the population report adverse reactions to foods. Many of these people, and even some of their physicians, call these reactions an "allergy," but the overwhelming majority are not. Only 4% of the general population and 6% to 7% of children younger than 3 years have a true food allergy.[1]

As seen in Box 1, prevalence of a specific food allergy depends on the patient's age. In children, the most common foods are milk, soy, eggs, wheat, and peanuts. Peanuts are a particular concern from a public health standpoint, because the prevalence of peanut allergy in American children has doubled in the past decade.[1] Most children lose their allergies to egg, soy, milk, and wheat by school age, but they usually retain their allergies to peanuts, tree nuts (walnut, pecan, brazil nut, cashew, hazelnut, pistachio), and seafood throughout their lives. Recent studies of peanut allergy show that although about 20% of children lose this condition with avoidance,[2-4] some reacquire it.[5] Currently, no validated method has been established to predict either outcome.

In adults, the most common food allergies are those to peanuts, tree nuts, and seafood. Many of these adults have retained their allergy since childhood. Some with tree nut allergy have reactions to all tree nuts; others react to only one or two nuts and consume other nuts without problems.

PATHOPHYSIOLOGY

IgE antibodies are generated against food allergens after exposure through the gastrointestinal tract, respiratory tract, or nonintact skin. The clinical manifestations depend upon the characteristics of the offending proteins, the genetic susceptibility of the person, and the route of sensitization. Food allergy is more common in patients who have other allergic conditions, such as atopic dermatitis and allergic rhinitis, and who have a family history of atopy.

SIGNS AND SYMPTOMS

IgE-mediated (allergic) reactions occur promptly, in many cases within minutes of ingesting the offending agent. Typical symptoms include itching or burning of the mouth or lips, swelling of the mouth or face, hives, itching, flushing, vomiting, diarrhea, lightheadedness, loss of consciousness, anxiety, and dyspnea. The allergic person might experience one or several of these symptoms. Sometimes the food allergy manifests as a worsening of eczema instead of with systemic or anaphylactic symptoms.

DIAGNOSIS

Diagnosis of food allergy relies on a history consistent with IgE-mediated reaction to a particular food or foods. Important details include the patient's age, route of exposure, amount of food needed to cause symptoms, timing between the exposure to the food and the onset of symptoms, clinical manifestations of the reaction, duration of symptoms, treatment of the symptoms and response to the treatment, and whether the reaction occurs consistently with exposure to the suspected food. Physical examination is also important because it can reveal other conditions associated with food allergy, such as atopic dermatitis or allergic rhinitis.

Allergists detect food-specific IgE antibodies by percutaneous skin tests and serum assays. Skin tests commonly use commercial extracts. However, the labile nature of some food proteins (e.g., fruits or vegetables) can require use of the actual food for skin testing: The food is pricked, and then the skin is pricked with the same instrument. Intracutaneous skin testing for foods is not recommended because it has been associated with greater risk for systemic reactions; moreover, this method is overly sensitive and can lead to false-positive results. Various serum assays exist for measuring IgE antibodies to specific foods. Prick skin tests and serum detection of IgE antibodies are highly sensitive; however, skin testing is preferred based on its more favorable negative predictive value. A negative skin test indicates a 95% (or higher) probability that food allergy is not present. However, a positive skin test result is clinically significant only 50% of the time.[6] For this reason, skin and serum tests for IgE antibodies to specific foods should be done only after a proper history has been taken and the clinician is able to generate a pretest probability of food allergy.

Trial elimination diets and oral food challenges are also used to diagnose food allergy. Elimination diets can be used to determine whether foods are contributing to chronic conditions such as gastrointestinal disorders or atopic dermatitis. However, many factors can cloud the results of an elimination diet. For instance, not eliminating the food or foods completely, not allowing enough time to achieve improvement, and selecting the wrong foods will give false results.

The gold standard for confirming food allergy is a double-blind, placebo-controlled challenge procedure. However, because this is time and labor intensive, an open challenge is often carried out. This challenge occurs under the direct supervision and observation of the physician. The patient consumes graded doses of the suspected food over time and is observed carefully for signs of reaction. An oral food challenge is the definitive way to assess or rule out allergy to a food, but it carries the risk of inducing anaphylactic reaction. For this reason, such challenges should only be performed under the care of a board-certified allergist.

Summary

- History
- Physical examination
- Prick skin testing
- Serum testing
- Elimination diet
- Oral food challenge

Box 1 Most Common Food Allergies

Children
Milk
Egg
Soy
Wheat
Peanut

Adults
Peanuts
Tree nuts
Seafood

RELATED TOPICS

Oral allergy syndrome is a condition in which patients with a pollen allergy experience oropharyngeal symptoms, when eating raw fruits and vegetables, minutes after the foods come in contact with the oral mucosa. Patients typically experience itching or burning, and occasionally swelling, of the lips, palate, tongue, and throat. Affected persons usually tolerate the cooked versions of these foods, due to the labile nature of the proteins causing symptoms. Oral allergy syndrome is caused by shared proteins between pollens and foods. See Box 2 for some examples of foods that elicit symptoms in this condition.

TREATMENT

Patients with food allergy should be counseled to avoid the offending food completely. They should have access to self-injectable epinephrine at all times in case of accidental ingestion and subsequent reaction. There are no medications that will reliably prevent an allergic reaction to the food.

Summary

- Avoidance
- Self-injectable epinephrine
- No prophylaxis available

FUTURE DIRECTIONS

Immunotherapy is under investigation as a potential treatment for food allergy. Possible routes of administration include sublingual and subcutaneous. However, immunotherapy to foods is considered neither safe nor effective at this time.

Omalizumab is a humanized monoclonal anti-IgE antibody that is FDA-approved for management of moderate to severe allergic asthma refractory to combination controller therapy (see "Asthma" elsewhere in this section). Omalizumab may prove beneficial for patients with food allergy for preventing anaphylaxis during accidental exposure to an offending food or, at least, decreasing the severity of the reaction. Omalizumab is theoretically of interest for patients with food allergy, but it currently is not indicated.

It is hoped that allergists will have more than avoidance to offer to patients with food allergy in the future.

Box 2 Common Foods that Elicit Symptoms in Oral Allergy Syndrome

Birch (Tree) Pollen
Almonds
Apples
Apricots
Carrots
Celery
Cherries
Coriander
Fennel
Fig
Hazel nuts and walnuts
Kiwifruit
Nectarines
Parsley
Parsnips
Peaches
Pears
Peppers
Plums
Potatoes
Prunes
Soy
Wheat

Grass Pollen
Fig
Melons
Oranges
Peaches
Potatoes
Tomatoes

Mugwort (Weed) Pollen
Carrots
Celery
Coriander
Fennel
Parsley
Peppers
Sunflower

Ragweed Pollen
Banana
Cantaloupe
Cucumber
Honeydew melon
Watermelon
Zucchini

Further Readings

Adkinson NF, Busse WW, Bochner BS, et al (eds): Middleton's Allergy: Principles and Practice, 7th ed. St Louis: Mosby, 2008.

Chapman JA, Bernstein L, Lee RE, et al: Food Allergy: A Practice Parameter. Ann Allergy Asthma Immunol 2006;96(3):54-56.

Grammer LC, Greenberger PA (eds): Patterson's Allergic Diseases: Treatment and Prevention, 6th ed. Philadelphia: Lippincott Williams & Wilkins, 2002.

References

For a complete list of references, log onto www.expertconsult.com.

Occupational Asthma

Mark Aronica

DEFINITION

The definition of occupational asthma, much like the definition of asthma itself, has changed over the years; therefore, it is difficult to determine the prevalence of the disorder. According to the current consensus definition,[1] patients with occupational asthma have variable airflow limitation or airway hyperresponsiveness, or both. It occurs in response to a specific work environment and not to stimuli encountered elsewhere.

There are two types of occupational asthma. One is immunologic, occurs after a latency period, and is caused either by agents with a known immunoglobulin E (IgE) reaction or by agents with no known IgE reaction. The other is nonimmunologic and is also known as *irritant-induced asthma* (IrIA) or *reactive airways dysfunction syndrome* (RADS). The irritant type can occur after one or more exposures to high concentrations of irritants (no latency period). A related form of occupational asthma has been termed *work-aggravated asthma.* In this instance, preexisting asthma is aggravated by a workplace exposure. Although work-aggravated asthma is not specifically addressed in this chapter, evaluation of all cases of asthma should include a detailed environmental history regarding exposures in both the home and the workplace.

PREVALENCE

Occupational asthma is a part of a larger category of diseases known as occupational respiratory diseases and includes occupation-induced rhinitis and laryngitis, tracheitis, bronchitis and bronchiolitis, chronic obstructive pulmonary disease, lung cancer, and interstitial diseases such as fibrosis and granuloma formation.[2] Physicians and the lay public are aware of other occupational lung disorders such as silicosis and asbestosis (see "Occupational Lung Disease" in Section 12), but occupational asthma is the most prevalent occupational lung disease in industrialized countries.

Findings regarding the significance of occupation as a cause of asthma vary based on the definition used and the methods of patient selection. In addition, persons who develop occupational asthma often leave the industry in which the illness began (a bias known as the *healthy worker effect*), even when occupational asthma has not yet been diagnosed. In general, asthma affects 5% to 10% of people worldwide, and it is estimated that 2% to 15% of asthma is occupational in origin.

The incidence of occupational asthma also varies with specific exposures. Occupational asthma has been reported in 8% to 12% of laboratory animal workers, 7% to 9% of bakers, and 1.4% of health care workers exposed to natural rubber latex. Even these percentages vary significantly depending on the study cited. Farmers, painters, plastic and rubber workers, and cleaners (window cleaners, chimney sweepers, and road sweepers) are at greatest risk for developing asthma.[3]

PATHOPHYSIOLOGY

Like childhood asthma, occupational asthma is the result of interactions between multiple environmental and genetic factors. Some of the known environmental factors include the route, duration, and intensity of exposure and the substance (or agent) to which the person is exposed. Using the definition of Mapp and coworkers,[1] occupational asthma can be divided into immunologic causes (associated with a latency period) and nonimmunologic causes. Agents associated with an immunologic cause can be further divided into high-molecular-weight (HMW) agents, usually allergens such as proteins from laboratory animals, flour, or plants, and low-molecular-weight (LMW) agents, usually chemicals such as isocyanates, biocides, or drugs.

Occupational Asthma with a Latency Period

HMW agents can induce an IgE response in susceptible persons and can cause asthma by an IgE-mediated mechanism, similar to that seen in a patient with atopic asthma. The bridging of IgE molecules by antigen leads to mast-cell degranulation and the initiation of an inflammatory cascade that results in airway inflammation and airway hyperresponsiveness. It is therefore not surprising that patients with atopic asthma or patients with a family history of atopy are at increased risk for developing occupational asthma from exposure to HMW agents. Smoking is also a risk factor for sensitization.

The pathogenic mechanisms of LMW agents are less well understood; however, there appear to be several mechanisms, both immunologic and nonimmunologic, that can lead to occupational asthma. LMW agents probably act as haptens, combining with human proteins in the respiratory tract to become complete immunogens. Atopy and smoking are not risk factors for occupational asthma caused by LMW agents, as they are for occupational asthma caused by HMW agents. Some of the better-studied agents include isocyanates and plicatic acid. Isocyanates are found in paints and are involved in the manufacture of plastics, rubber, and foam, and plicatic acid is the causative agent in asthma caused by western red cedar. Specific IgE for isocyanates or plicatic acid is found in only a small percentage of patients with documented disease. However, the detection of specific IgE may be a marker of exposure and not of disease.[4]

Activated T cells also play an important role in the pathogenesis and in the inflammation of occupational asthma as they do in other forms of asthma. Bronchial biopsies of patients with occupational asthma induced by isocyanate or red cedar show many activated T cells.[5,6] Several recent studies have also shown associations between HLA class II antigens and various types of occupational asthma.[7]

LMW agents also cause occupational asthma by direct pharmacologic action. Isocyanates can block β_2-adrenergic receptors, and high concentrations of plicatic acid can activate complement. Isocyanates and other agents can stimulate sensory nerves, leading to the release of substance P and other neuropeptides. They can also inhibit the neutral endopeptidases that normally inactivate these substances. This affects a variety of cells in the airways, resulting in cough, smooth muscle contraction, and mucus production.

Box 1 shows some of the more common causes of occupational asthma associated with a latency period.

Occupational Asthma Without Latency

The mechanisms of IrIA or RADS are also poorly understood. IrIA is a nonimmunologically induced asthma that occurs without a latency period. It typically occurs after a brief, high-intensity inhalation exposure followed by the acute onset of persistent respiratory symptoms and ongoing airway hyperresponsiveness. It is postulated that extensive denudation of the airway epithelium occurs, resulting in airway inflammation due to the loss of epithelium-derived relaxing factors, exposure of nerve endings leading to neurogenic inflammation, and nonspecific activation of mast cells with release of

Box 1 Common Agents that Cause Occupational Asthma with Latency

Acrylate
Amines
Anhydrides
Animal-derived allergens
Cereals
Chloramine-T
Drugs
Dyes
Enzymes
Formaldehyde, glutaraldehyde
Fluxes
Gums
Isocyanates
Latex
Metals
Persulfate
Seafood
Wood dusts

inflammatory mediators and cytokines.[8] Ammonia, chlorine, and sulfur dioxide are the most common causes of IrIA, although the list is extensive.

SIGNS AND SYMPTOMS

The signs and symptoms of occupational asthma may be identical to those of other forms of asthma. In patients whose occupational asthma is caused by HMW agents, rhinitis or rhinoconjunctivitis often precedes the onset of asthma symptoms by 1 year or more. In contrast, IrIA or RADS has a characteristically distinct presentation. The exposure is typically acute, singular, and extreme, often involving some type of accident or chemical spill. There is no latency period, and symptoms of airway obstruction are immediate or develop within a few hours of exposure.

In patients with occupational asthma with a latency period, symptom improvement has been noted over a weekend with 24 to 48 hours of work absence in about 70% of patients and in up to 90% of workers with vacation leaves of 7 to 10 days.[9] Symptom patterns can also be very similar to those seen in nonoccupational asthma and include early, late, and dual responses. Early responses are seen within minutes of exposure, reach maximal severity within 30 minutes, and resolve within 1 to 2 hours. Late responses can occur after 4 to 6 hours, peak around 8 hours, and resolve after 24 hours. Dual responses involve both early response with complete or near-complete recovery followed by a late phase.

DIAGNOSIS

Occupational asthma should be considered in all working-age patients with new-onset asthma or worsening asthma. A detailed history of occupational and potential occupational exposures is just as important as identifying environmental triggers when evaluating an asthmatic patient. Although many patients themselves relate their symptoms to the workplace, many other cases of occupational asthma are recognized only because the physician performed a detailed environmental history. Common screening questions include the following: What are your workplace exposures? When during the work shift or work week do symptoms develop? Do symptoms improve during the weekend and over vacations? Do other workers have similar symptoms? The history can be supplemented with material safety data sheets from the workplace and can be compared with agents known to cause occupational asthma. A worksite visit by the physician or by an occupational hygienist might also provide helpful information.

A useful tool can be found at www.asmanet.com. This website provides a list of agents known to cause occupational asthma and the occupations in which they are encountered, and it can be searched by specific occupation.

Although taking a good occupational history is important in establishing a link between symptoms and potential workplace exposures, a history by itself is inadequate to make the diagnosis of occupational asthma. Algorithms and information on the diagnosis of occupational asthma can be found below and in Figure 1. More detailed information can be found elsewhere.[10-12] If possible, skin testing or specific IgE assessment should be performed. This is generally most useful for diagnosing occupational asthma caused by HMW agents.

A determination of nonspecific bronchial hyperresponsiveness (NSBH) with methacholine or histamine challenge should be performed in all patients with suspected occupational asthma. A negative challenge does not exclude occupational asthma if the patient left the workplace some time ago and is now free of symptoms. However, a negative challenge performed when the patient is working and symptomatic can reasonably exclude the diagnosis of occupational asthma.

Serial measurements of NSBH can also be useful. NSBH is typically worse after a period of exposure and can lessen after cessation of exposure. A minimum of 10 to 14 days after removal from the workplace is recommended before retesting. A minimum threefold improvement in PC_{20} (dose of methacholine or histamine needed to cause a 20% decrease in the forced expiratory volume in 1 second [FEV_1]) while the patient is off work is significant; however, a lack of improvement in PC_{20} does not exclude occupational asthma.[13]

Serial peak expiratory flow (PEF) self-monitoring with the subject at work and away from work for the same period is useful in obtaining objective information to confirm occupational asthma. Current recommendations are for four daily measurements; the subject should perform three forced-expiratory maneuvers, and at least two should be within 20 L/min of each other. All three readings should be recorded, but the best should be used for analysis. If a patient is taking inhaled corticosteroids, the dose should not be changed during the PEF monitoring period. All readings should be made before using bronchodilators. Readings should be performed for 2 weeks at work during exposure to the suspected agent and for 2 weeks away from the suspected agent.[13,14] A motivated and compliant patient is essential for PEF monitoring to be useful.

The gold standard for the diagnosis and confirmation of occupational asthma is a specific inhalational challenge with the suspected agent. However, this requires specialized facilities and is available at only a few centers. In general, specific challenge tests are useful when the diagnosis of occupational asthma remains in doubt after serial monitoring of PEF or NSBH, when a patient clearly has occupational asthma but it is necessary to confirm the causative agent for correct management, and when a new agent is suspected of causing occupational asthma.

TREATMENT

The most important aspect in the treatment of occupational asthma is environmental control. Continued exposure can lead to persistent and irreversible airway obstruction, whereas early removal offers the best chance at complete recovery. Other than environmental control, the management of occupational asthma is no different than that for nonoccupational asthma. However, pharmacologic treatment is not effective in preventing deterioration of lung function in sensitizer-induced occupational asthma when subjects remain exposed to the causing agent. (For additional information on the management of asthma, see "Asthma" elsewhere in this section).

In contrast, patients with RADS or IrIA without concurrent sensitization can usually return to the workplace if they have adequate pharmacologic control of their asthma and if there are appropriate

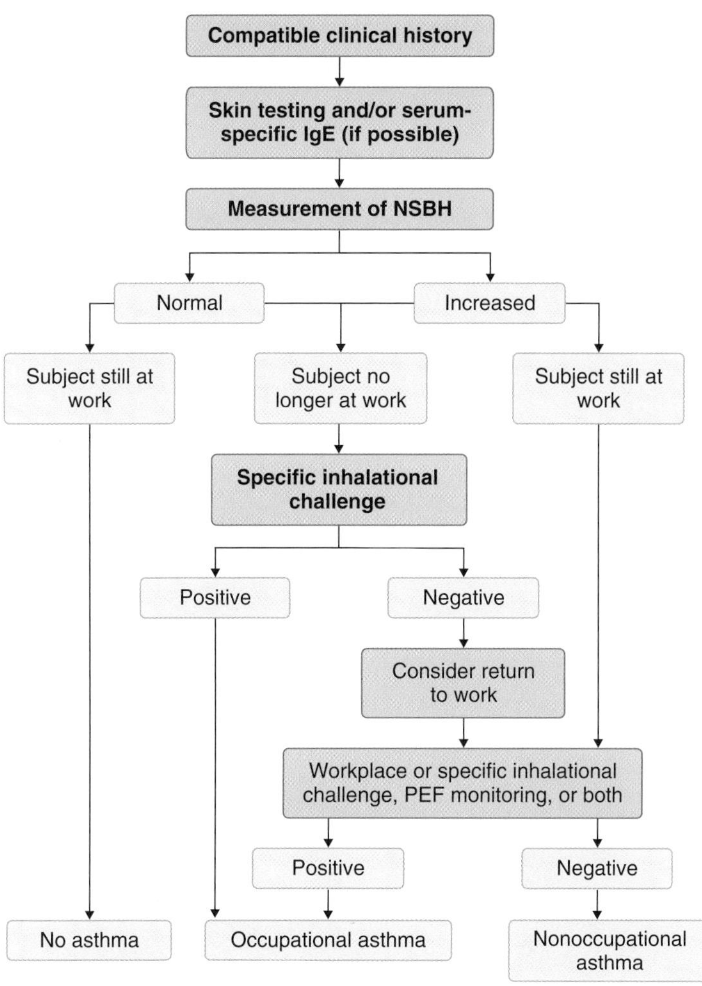

Figure 1 Algorithm to aid in the diagnosis of occupational asthma. IgE, immunoglobulin E; NSBH, nonspecific bronchial hyperresponsiveness; PEF, peak expiratory flow. *(Adapted from Chan-Yeung M, Malo JL: Occupational asthma. N Engl J Med 1995;333:107-112, with permission.)*

occupational hygiene controls in place to prevent the likelihood of a repeat high-level respiratory irritant exposure.

OUTCOMES

The outcome in occupational asthma depends on many of the same elements that are involved with initial sensitization and include the nature of the agent, the concentration of exposure, the duration of exposure, and the smoking history as well as host-dependent factors. Factors predicting a worse outcome are lower PC_{20} at baseline, longer duration of exposure, and the interval since removal of the patient from exposure. Early removal offers the best chance at recovery. However, most patients with occupational asthma with latency do not recover, even after several years away from exposure. In addition, subjects with occupational asthma due to HMW agents seem to have a less favorable outcome. The typical plateau for improvement in spirometry is around 1 year, whereas the plateau for improvement in NSBH occurs around 2 years.

The socioeconomic outcomes of occupational asthma also vary significantly. For example, a patient in Quebec with occupational asthma is provided with a full salary for up to 2 years, which is the estimated time required for retraining for a new occupation. A survey of 134 workers with occupational asthma examined 2 years after diagnosis found that 41 (31%) had found jobs with the same employer in which they were no longer exposed to the causal agent, and only 11 (8%) of workers were still unemployed.[15] In contrast, a survey of 55 patients in the United States with occupational asthma who were assessed an average of 31 months after removal from exposure found that 69% were still unemployed.[16]

Once the diagnosis of occupational asthma is made, that worker is 100% impaired for the job that caused the problem or for jobs with exposure to the same causative agent. It is recommended that long-term assessment of impairment should be performed 2 years after removal from exposure, when improvement tends to plateau. Guidelines for the assessment of permanent impairment due to asthma have been proposed by the American Thoracic Society.[17]

Summary

- Occupational asthma should be considered in any new or worsening case of asthma in working-age persons.
- There are still many controversies regarding the diagnosis, pathophysiology, prognosis, and appropriate compensation for patients with occupational asthma.
- Prompt recognition, diagnosis, and removal from the work environment are necessary to ensure the best possible outcome.
- Additional information on occupational asthma can also be found at www.osha-slc.gov/sltc/occupationalastham/.

Further Readings

American Thoracic Society: Guidelines for the evaluation of impairment/disability in patients with asthma. Am Rev Respir Dis 1993;147:1056-1061.

Banks DE, Jalloul A: Occupational asthma, work-related asthma and reactive airways dysfunction syndrome. Curr Opin Pulm Med 2007;13(2):131-136.

Beckett WS: Occupational respiratory diseases. N Engl J Med 2000;342:406-413.
Boulet LP, Lemiere C, Gautrin D, Cartier A: New insights into occupational asthma. Curr Opin Allergy Clin Immunol 2007;7(1):96-101.
Chan-Yeung M, Malo JL: Occupational asthma. N Engl J Med 1995;333:107-112.
Chan-Yeung M, Malo JL, Tarlo SM, et al: Proceedings of the first Jack Pepys Occupational Asthma Symposium. Am J Respir Crit Care Med 2003;167:450-471.
Henneberger PK: Work-exacerbated asthma. Curr Opin Allergy Clin Immunol 2007;7(2):146-151.
Holness DL, Tabassum S, Tarlo SM, et al: Practice patterns of pulmonologists and family physicians for occupational asthma. Chest 2007;132(5):1526-1531.
Mapp CE, Boschetto P, Maestrelli P, Fabbri LM: Occupational asthma. Am J Respir Crit Care Med 2005;172(3):280-305.
Nicholson PJ, Cullinan P, Taylor AJ, et al: Evidence based guidelines for the prevention, identification, and management of occupational asthma. Occup Environ Med 2005;62(5):290-299.

References

For a complete list of references, log onto www.expertconsult.com.

Section 2

CARDIOLOGY

Coronary Artery Disease

Curtis M. Rimmerman

DEFINITION

Coronary artery disease is characterized by atherosclerosis in the epicardial coronary arteries. Atherosclerotic plaques, the hallmark of atherosclerosis, progressively narrow the coronary artery lumen and impair antegrade myocardial blood flow. The reduction in coronary artery flow may be symptomatic or asymptomatic, occur with exertion or at rest, and culminate in a myocardial infarction, depending on obstruction severity and the rapidity of development.

PREVALENCE

According to the American Heart Association and American Stroke Association's 2006 publication on heart disease and stroke statistics, cardiovascular disease (CVD) remains the leading cause of mortality in the United States in men and women of every major ethnic group. It accounts for nearly 1.4 million deaths per year as of 2002 and was responsible for one in almost three deaths in the United States in 2003. Approximately 13 million persons have a history of coronary artery disease and 7.2 million have suffered a myocardial infarction. Almost 2500 Americans die of CVD each day, an average of one death every 35 seconds. CVD claims more lives each year than the next four leading causes of death combined—cancer, chronic lower respiratory diseases, accidents, and diabetes mellitus.

PATHOPHYSIOLOGY

Coronary artery disease is a chronic process that begins during adolescence and slowly progresses throughout life. Independent risk factors include a family history of premature coronary artery disease, cigarette smoking, diabetes mellitus, hypertension, hyperlipidemia, sedentary lifestyle, and obesity. These risk factors accelerate or modify a complex and chronic inflammatory process that ultimately manifests as fibrous atherosclerotic plaque.

The most widely accepted theory of atherosclerosis states that the process represents an attempt at healing in response to endothelial injury. The first step in the atherosclerotic process is the development of fatty streaks, which contain atherogenic lipoproteins and macrophage foam cells. These streaks form between the endothelium and internal elastic lamina. Over time, an intermediate lesion made up of an extracellular lipid core and layers of smooth muscle and connective tissue matrix eventually forms a fibrous cap. The edge of the fibrous cap (the *shoulder region*) plays a critical role in the development of acute coronary syndromes. The shoulder region is the site where most plaques lose their integrity, or rupture. Plaque rupture exposes the underlying thrombogenic core of lipid and necrotic material to circulating blood. This exposure results in platelet adherence, aggregation, and progressive luminal narrowing, which are associated with acute coronary syndromes.

Inflammation is emerging as a critical component of atherosclerosis genesis, activity, and potential plaque instability. Patients with established coronary artery disease who possess a confluence of risk factors known as the metabolic syndrome remain at particularly high risk for a future vascular event, such as an acute myocardial infarction or cerebrovascular accident. Biochemical markers such as elevated levels of C-reactive protein signal a higher likelihood of vascular inflammation and portend a higher risk of vascular event rates. This marker may also signal more rapidly advancing coronary artery disease and the need for aggressive preventive measures.

SIGNS AND SYMPTOMS

Patients with coronary artery disease present with stable angina pectoris, unstable angina pectoris, or a myocardial infarction. They may seek medical attention with their first symptomatic episode of chest discomfort. Many of these patients suffer from unrecognized coronary artery disease and may experience an acute plaque rupture or acute myocardial infarction. Electrical instability can ensue, including potentially lethal cardiac dysrhythmias. Identifying high-risk persons before their first myocardial event is a multifaceted process that involves patient and physician education efforts. Screening for coronary artery disease is not sufficient. Risk factor modification, from an early age, inititates primary prevention efforts, forestalling the development of symptomatic coronary artery disease. Severe coronary artery disease can be detected before a patient develops symptoms.

Angina pectoris is a perceived symptom resulting from a mismatch of myocardial supply and demand. The compromised myocardial blood flow caused by obstructive coronary artery disease is not able to meet the metabolic demands of the myocardial tissue. The anaerobic threshold is crossed and the patient develops symptomatic angina pectoris. Angina pectoris is typically categorized according to the Canadian Cardiovascular Society's functional classification system (Table 1).

Stable Angina

Angina pectoris is said to be stable when its pattern of frequency, intensity, ease of provocation, or duration does not change over several weeks. Identification of activities that provoke angina and the amount of sublingual nitroglycerin required to relieve symptoms are helpful indicators of stability. A decrease in exercise tolerance or an increase in the need for nitroglycerin suggests that the angina is progressing in severity or accelerating.

Accelerating Angina

Angina pectoris is said to be accelerating when there is a change in the pattern of stable angina. This may include a greater ease of provocation, more prolonged episodes, and episodes of greater severity, requiring a longer recovery period or more frequent use of sublingual nitroglycerin.

Unstable Angina

Unstable angina pectoris occurs when the pattern of chest pain changes abruptly. Signs of unstable angina are pains at rest, a marked increase in the frequency of attacks, discomfort that occurs with minimal activity, and new-onset angina of incapacitating severity. Unstable angina usually is related to the rupture of an atherosclerotic plaque and the abrupt narrowing or occlusion of a coronary artery, representing a medical emergency.

DIAGNOSIS

The initial diagnostic approach for coronary artery disease encompasses a detailed patient history, a complete physical examination, and an electrocardiogram. Once the initial evaluation is performed, laboratory blood tests, stress testing, and cardiac catheterization may be necessary to obtain further diagnostic insight.

Table 1 Canadian Cardiovascular Society Functional Classification of Angina Pectoris

Class	Definition	Specific Activity Scale
I	Ordinary physical activity (e.g., walking and climbing stairs) does not cause angina; angina occurs with strenuous, rapid, or prolonged exertion at work or recreation.	Ability to ski, play basketball, jog at 5 mph, or shovel snow without angina
II	Slight limitation of ordinary activity. Angina occurs on walking or climbing stairs rapidly, walking uphill, walking or stair climbing after meals, in cold, in wind, or under emotional stress, or only during the few hours after awakening, when walking more than two blocks on level ground, or when climbing more than one flight of stairs at a normal pace and in normal conditions.	Ability to garden, rake, roller skate, walk at 4 mph on level ground, have sexual intercourse without stopping
III	Marked limitation of ordinary physical activity. Angina occurs on walking one to two blocks on level ground or climbing one flight of stairs at a normal pace in normal conditions.	Ability to shower or dress without stopping, walk 2.5 mph, bowl, make a bed, play golf
IV	Inability to perform any physical activity without discomfort.	Anginal symptoms may be present at rest. Inability to perform activities requiring 2 or fewer metabolic equivalents without angina

Adapted from Goldman L, Hashimoto B, Cook EF, Loscalzo A: Comparative reproducibility and validity of systems for assessing cardiovascular functional class: Advantages of a new specific activity scale. Circulation 1981;64:1227-1234.

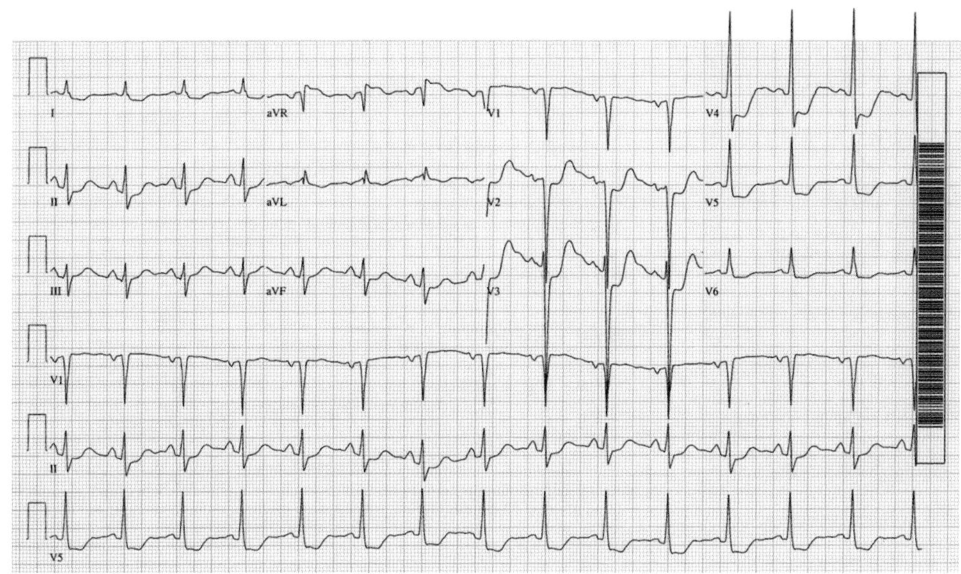

Figure 1 A 12-lead electrocardiogram example of ischemic anterolateral ST-segment depression in a patient with known coronary artery disease.

History

The history should include any current symptoms, a complete inventory of comorbid conditions, including cardiac risk factors, and a complete family history. The history should include information about the character and location of discomfort, radiation of discomfort, associated symptoms, and precipitating, exacerbating, or alleviating factors.

Physical Examination

The results of the physical examination of a patient with stable or unstable angina may be entirely normal. The presence of multiple risk factors or atherosclerosis in the carotid or peripheral arteries increases the likelihood that a chest pain syndrome is related to myocardial ischemia. Evaluation should include measurements of blood pressure and the ankle–brachial index. Examination of the carotid arteries should evaluate upstrokes and auscultation for bruits. Examination of the chest wall, neck, and shoulders for deformities and tenderness may be helpful in diagnosing musculoskeletal chest discomfort. Cardiac auscultation may detect murmurs caused by aortic stenosis or hypertrophic cardiomyopathy, either of which can cause angina in the absence of coronary artery disease. Assessment of the abdominal aorta for an aneurysm or bruits and palpation of lower extremity pulses are necessary to rule out peripheral vascular disease. Careful palpation of all peripheral pulses and assessment of symmetry versus diminution are also valuable noninvasive approaches for assessing the integrity of the arterial circulation. Finally, examination for xanthelasmas, tendon xanthomas, retinal arterial abnormalities, and peripheral neuropathy can be helpful.

Diagnostic and Imaging Studies

Electrocardiography

A resting 12-lead electrocardiogram should be obtained on all patients with suspected coronary artery disease. Electrocardiographic results are normal in approximately 50% of patients with chronic stable angina, and they can remain normal during an episode of chest discomfort. Importantly, a normal electrocardiogram does not exclude coronary artery disease (Fig. 1).

Chest Radiography

The usefulness of a routine chest radiograph in a patient with chest discomfort has not been established. Calcification of the aortic knob is a common finding in older patients and is a nonspecific indicator of flow-limiting obstructive coronary disease. Infrequently, coronary calcification is present.

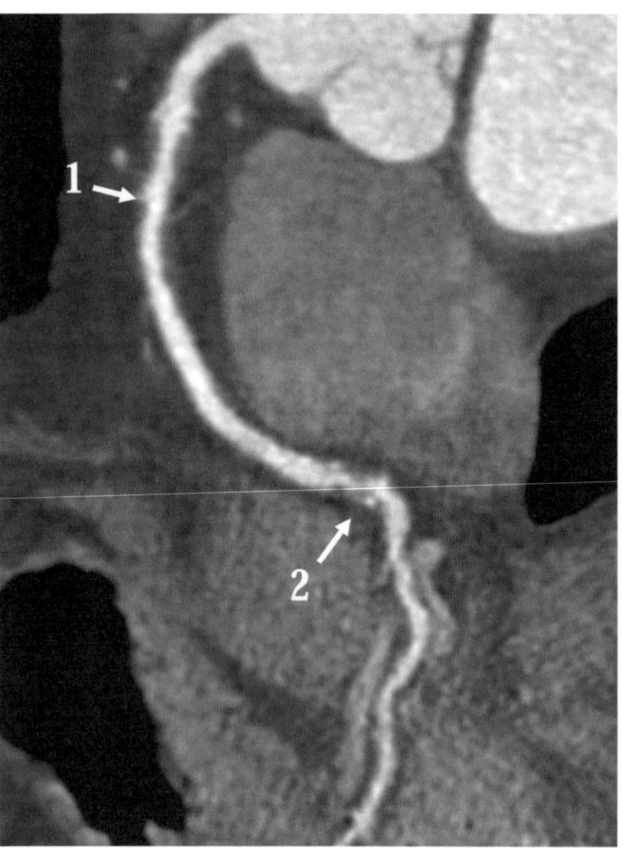

Figure 2 Computed tomography angiogram of the right coronary artery. *1,* Mild proximal stenosis with expansive remodeling and predominantly nonexpansive plaque. *2,* Partially calcified advanced mid to distal stenosis.

Cardiac Computed Tomography Angiography

A noninvasive imaging assessment of coronary atherosclerosis is now possible. When negative, this test possesses a high negative predictive value. The positive predictive value is also high, but exact stenosis quantification can be complicated. Associated calcification can cause a blooming artifact, resulting in an overestimation of stenosis severity (Fig. 2).

Echocardiography

Echocardiography is recommended for patients with stable angina and physical findings suggesting concomitant valvular heart disease. It is invaluable for assessing the patient with suspected hypertrophic cardiomyopathy. It is also recommended for the assessment of global and regional left ventricular systolic function in patients who have congestive heart failure, complex ventricular arrhythmias, or a history of a past myocardial infarction.

Laboratory Studies

Routine laboratory measurements recommended as a part of the initial evaluation of patients with coronary artery disease should include determination of fasting glucose and fasting lipid levels (total cholesterol, high-density lipoprotein [HDL] cholesterol, triglycerides, and calculated low-density lipoprotein [LDL] levels). Other markers such as lipoprotein(a) (Lp[a]) and high-sensitivity C-reactive protein, may be useful in assessing cardiac risk. High-sensitivity C-reactive protein is gaining greater prominence in assessing the inflammatory level of vascular disease and predicting future risk of vascular events, such as myocardial infarctions and cerebrovascular accidents.

Once all these initial evaluations are complete, it is possible to estimate a patient's probability of existing coronary artery disease before proceeding with stress testing or coronary angiography (Table 2).

Stress Testing

Stress testing is another method for determining the presence of flow-limiting, functionally significant coronary artery disease. All stress testing techniques include electrocardiography and blood pressure monitoring. The absolute and relative contraindications to exercise stress testing are outlined in Box 1.

Cardiovascular stress testing takes two forms, exercise and pharmacologic administration. The preferred method of cardiovascular stress testing is exercise, using a treadmill or bicycle. Through aerobic exercise, a higher rate pressure product (peak systolic blood pressure

Table 2 Pretest Probability of Coronary Artery Disease (CAD) by Age, Gender, and Symptom Status*

Age, yr†	Gender	Typical or Definite Angina Pectoris	Atypical or Probable Angina Pectoris	Nonanginal Chest Pain	No Symptoms
30-39	Male	Intermediate	Intermediate	Low	Very low
	Female	Intermediate	Very low	Very low	Very low
40-49	Male	High	Intermediate	Intermediate	Low
	Female	Intermediate	Low	Very low	Very low
50-59	Male	High	Intermediate	Intermediate	Low
	Female	Intermediate	Intermediate	Low	Very low
60-69	Male	High	Intermediate	Intermediate	Low
	Female	High	Intermediate	Intermediate	Low

*High probability, >90%; intermediate, 10%-90%; low, <10%; very low, <5%.

†No data exist for patients younger than 30 yr or older than 69 yr, but it can be assumed that the prevalence of CAD increases with age. In a few cases, patients at the extremes of each decade may have probabilities slightly outside the high or low range.

Adapted from Gibbons RJ, Balady GJ, Beasley JW, et al: ACC/AHA guidelines for exercise testing: Executive summary. A report of the American College of Cardiology/American Heart Association Task Force on Practice Guidelines (Committee on Exercise Testing). Circulation 1997;96:345-354.

Box 1 Absolute and Relative Contraindications to Exercise Stress Testing

Absolute Contraindications

Acute MI within 2 days
Symptomatic or severe aortic stenosis
Decompensated heart failure
Symptomatic or hemodynamically significant cardiac arrhythmias
Unstable angina not previously stabilized by medical therapy
Acute aortic dissection
Acute myocarditis or pericarditis
Acute pulmonary embolus or pulmonary infarction

Relative Contraindications

Left main coronary artery stenosis
Electrolyte imbalance
Systolic blood pressure ≥200 mm Hg
Diastolic blood pressure ≥110 mm Hg
Tachyarrhythmias or bradyarrhythmias
Hypertrophic cardiomyopathy, other forms of outflow tract obstruction
High-degree atrioventricular block
Moderate stenotic valvular heart disease
Mental or physical impairment leading to inability to exercise adequately
MI, myocardial infarction.

Adapted from Gibbons RJ, Balady GJ, Beasley JW, et al: ACC/AHA guidelines for exercise testing: Executive summary. A report of the American College of Cardiology/American Heart Association Task Force on Practice Guidelines (Committee on Exercise Testing). Circulation 1997;96:345-354.

multiplied by peak pulse rate), and therefore greater cardiovascular stress, can be obtained. This permits an assessment of a patient's functional capacity, providing prognostic data using the sole parameter of attained metabolic equivalents or oxygen uptake. Heart rate recovery—how fast the heart rate decreases after exercise cessation—is also an important prognostic parameter.

The most common pharmacologic agents used for nonexercise stress testing are dobutamine, dipyridamole, and adenosine. Dobutamine echocardiography is useful for determining the presence of functionally significant obstructive coronary artery disease and assessing a post–myocardial infarction patient. Using echocardiography, whether it is combined with exercise or dobutamine, the physician interpreter is focusing on the global and regional endocardial thickening responses to cardiovascular stress.

Nuclear stress testing is an equally important modality for assessing the coronary circulation. Unlike stress echocardiography, in which the endocardial thickening response to cardiovascular stress is the marker for inducible myocardial ischemia, nuclear stress testing relies on the concept of coronary flow reserve and differential myocardial blood flow. In the presence of exercise or the administration of a pharmacologic coronary vasodilator, the normal response is hyperemia, with a significant increase in myocardial blood flow. If there is no coronary obstructive disease, the pattern of hyperemia and blood flow is reflected as a symmetrical increase, with a homogeneous distribution of the blood flow tracer. In the presence of a severe coronary artery stenosis, dipyridamole or adenosine induces coronary macrovascular and microvascular vasodilation, which results in differential myocardial blood flow that can be detected by radionuclide imaging with thallium 201 or technetium 99m (Tc 99m)-labeled radiopharmaceuticals (Tc 99m sestamibi or Tc 99m tetrofosmin). Functionally significant coronary artery disease can be suspected on nuclear perfusion imaging when an area of relative hypoperfusion is detected on peak stress images compared with resting images. Resting nuclear cardiac images may also be abnormal (Fig. 3).

Combining imaging with the electrocardiographic stress test adds approximately 15 percentage points to the sensitivity and specificity. In certain cases, electrocardiographic stress testing is of borderline

Box 2 Indications for Cardiac Stress Imaging

Resting ST-segment depression >1 mm
Complete left bundle branch block
Ventricular paced rhythm
Ventricular pre-excitation syndrome
Previous revascularization with PCI or CABG
Inability to exercise

Adapted from Gibbons RJ, Balady GJ, Beasley JW, et al: ACC/AHA guidelines for exercise testing: Executive summary. A report of the American College of Cardiology/American Heart Association Task Force on Practice Guidelines (Committee on Exercise Testing). Circulation 1997;96:345-354.

Table 3 Duke Treadmill Scoring System*

Risk Group	Annual Mortality Rate
Low (>4)	0.25%
Intermediate (–10 to 4)	1.25%
High (<–10)	5.0%

*The Duke treadmill score is calculated according to the following formula:

$$\text{Exercise time (min)} - 5(\text{max ST-segment deviation [in mm, during or after exercise]}) - \text{angina score}$$

where the score is 0 if there is no angina, 4 if angina occurs, and 8 if angina is the reason for stopping the test.

Adapted from Mark DB, Shaw L, Harrell FE Jr, et al: Prognostic value of a treadmill exercise score in outpatients with suspected coronary artery disease. N Engl J Med 1991;325:849-853.

help, particularly in the presence of an abnormal resting electrocardiogram. The indications for cardiac stress imaging are outlined in Box 2.

Cardiac stress imaging is useful for determining the extent, severity, and location of ischemia. The exercise portion of the test also provides prognostic information. Prognostic markers include the Duke treadmill score, heart rate recovery (HRR) score, and the chronotropic response index (CRI). The Duke treadmill scoring system is summarized in Table 3.

The HRR score is calculated according to the following formula:

$$\text{HRR score} = \text{HR(at peak exercise)} - \text{HR(1 min postexercise)}$$

where HR is in beats per minute. A normal HRR score (>12 beats/min) is associated with a low risk of death, whereas a low HRR score (<8 beats/min) is associated with a high risk. HRR scores of 8 to 12 beats per minute indicate an intermediate risk.

The CRI is calculated according to the following formula:

$$(\text{Peak HR} - \text{resting HR})/([220 - \text{patient's age}] - \text{resting HR})$$

where HR is in beats per minute. A normal CRI (>0.8) is associated with a decreased probability of coronary artery disease and a lower risk of death. A low CRI (<0.8) in a patient who is not on beta blocker therapy is associated with an increased likelihood of coronary artery disease and a higher risk of death.

Coronary Arteriography

Cardiac catheterization is currently the gold standard for determining the presence of obstructive coronary artery disease. A cardiac catheterization yields a two-dimensional rendering of the coronary artery circulation. To assist in circumventing the limitations of a two-dimensional depiction of three-dimensional anatomy, multiple views from varying angles are obtained as a standard.

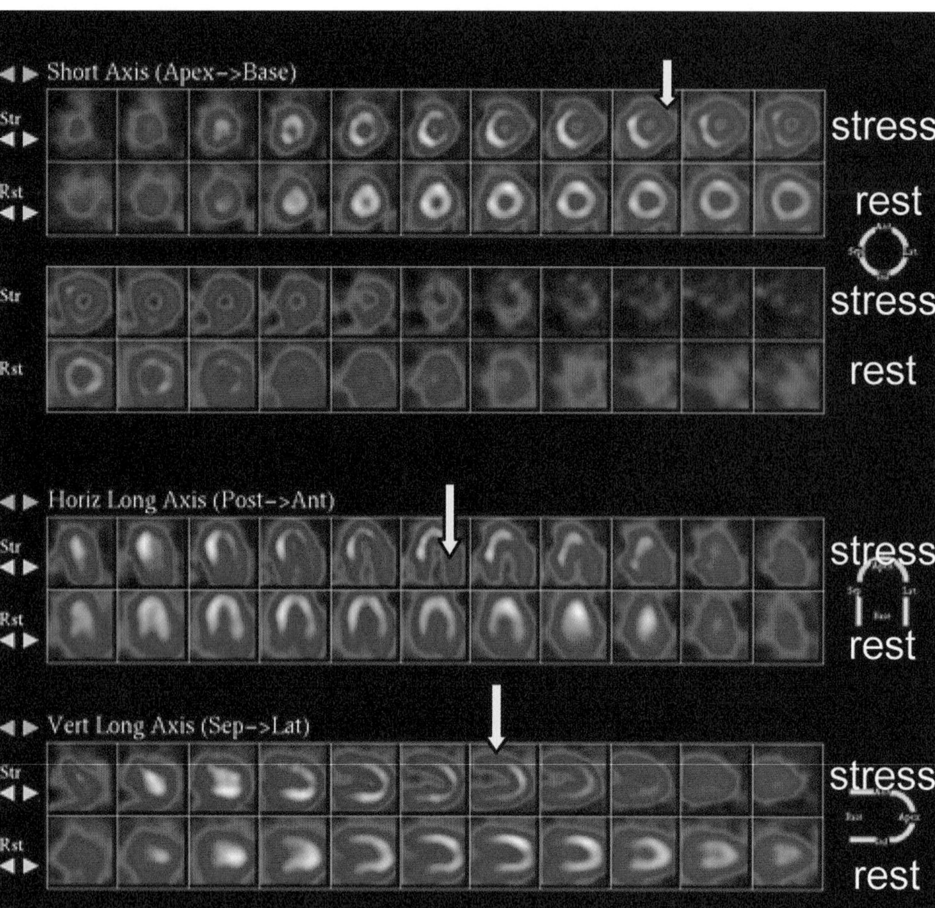

Figure 3 Mycardial perfusion scan. Stress images *(arrows)* demonstrate inferolateral and anterolateral (left circumflex) ischemia.

TREATMENT

Once a cardiac catheterization has been performed, the three most common therapeutic options are medical therapy, percutaneous coronary intervention (PCI), and coronary artery bypass grafting (CABG).

Lifestyle Modification

Patients with documented coronary artery disease should actively pursue lifestyle modifications that reduce the risk of future cardiovascular events.

Smoking

Tobacco use is one of the most important contributors to recurrent cardiovascular events. Tobacco use induces endothelial dysfunction, reduces coronary vasoreactivity, increases circulating carbon monoxide levels, impairs functional status, and raises blood pressure.

Exercise

Functional capacity is a strong predictor of major adverse cardiac events. Functional capacity can be improved by following an exercise program that includes at least 30 minutes of exercise 3 or 4 days a week; a daily regimen is optimal.

Weight Control

The best weight management strategy is diet and exercise. Ideal benchmarks are a body mass index between 19 and 25 kg/m^2 and a waist circumference of no more than 40 inches for men and 35 inches for women. Weight loss has a favorable metabolic syndrome impact on many cardiac risk factors, including hypertension, high LDL level, low HDL level, and glucose intolerance.

Pharmacologic Therapy

Antiplatelet Agents

Aspirin is the mainstay of antiplatelet therapy for patients who have known coronary artery disease or symptoms suggestive of coronary artery disease. Aspirin inhibits both cyclooxygenase and the synthesis of thromboxane A_2.

Clopidogrel (Plavix), a thienopyridine derivative, blocks adenosine diphosphate–induced platelet activation. Clopidogrel is indicated as an alternative for patients who cannot take aspirin.

Antianginal Agents

Beta blockers, calcium channel blockers, and nitrates are the mainstays of antianginal therapy. Unless contraindications exist, all patients who have a history of angina pectoris should carry sublingual nitroglycerin. Beta blockers are recommended as first-line therapy for the management of stable angina in all patients with established coronary artery disease.

Patients who have a history suggestive of vasospastic angina should be treated with a calcium channel blocker or a long-acting nitrate as an initial therapy. Either treatment option can also serve as a substitute for a beta blocker in the presence of traditional angina when intolerable beta blocker effects ensue.

Nitrates improve exercise tolerance and prolong the time to onset of angina in patients with exertional angina. They are contraindicated in patients who have severe aortic stenosis or hypertrophic cardiomyopathy because they can adversely alter hemodynamics and exacerbate symptoms. Ranolazine may be useful for treating refractory angina pectoris.

Risk Factor Management

Hypertension

Management of hypertension in patients with coronary artery disease is exceedingly important. Control of blood pressure reduces myocardial oxygen consumption and thereby reduces angina, and it also lowers the incidence of cardiovascular events.

Beta blockers devoid of intrinsic sympathomimetic activity represent first-line antihypertensive therapy for patients with a history of myocardial infarction or coronary artery disease with angina. Angiotensin-converting enzyme (ACE) inhibitors are indicated for all patients with diabetes mellitus or a history of myocardial infarction, particularly those with impaired left ventricular systolic function. In the Heart Outcomes Prevention Evaluation (HOPE) study, high-risk patients without a history of a myocardial infarction treated with the ACE inhibitor ramipril experienced a significant reduction in major cardiac events.

Calcium channel blockers are useful for patients with hypertension and angina despite maximum tolerable administration of beta blockers. The long-acting dihydropyridines are preferred; short-acting preparations should be avoided because they might increase the risk of cardiac events via precipitous blood pressure reduction and induction of the coronary steal phenomenon, diverting coronary arterial blood flow from flow-limited myocardial regions.

Hyperlipidemia

Guidelines of the National Cholesterol Education Program (NCEP) have recommended an LDL level lower than 70 mg/dL for all patients with coronary artery or other atherosclerotic disease. Patients whose LDL levels are higher than 100 mg/dL should start drug therapy. 3-Hydroxy-3-methylglutaryl coenzyme A (HMG-CoA) reductase inhibitors (statins) are the recommended first-line agents for patients who have coronary artery disease and elevated total and LDL cholesterol levels.

The NCEP also recommends a target HDL level higher than 45 mg/dL for men with coronary artery disease and higher than 55 mg/dL for women. Patients with the metabolic syndrome (obesity, hypertension, and insulin resistance) often have HDL levels lower than 35 mg/dL. These patients are at especially high risk for arterial vascular disease. Their recommended lifestyle changes include regular exercise and weight loss, which are two of the most effective ways to raise HDL levels. If lifestyle changes fail to increase HDL levels to their target, drug treatment with a fibrate or niacin should be considered, particularly in patients whose triglyceride levels are higher than 200 mg/dL.

Diabetes Mellitus

Diabetics with coronary artery disease have a particularly high risk for recurrent cardiovascular events, and they should be targeted for aggressive risk-factor modification. The American Diabetes Association recommends a hemoglobin A_{1c} level lower than 7%.

Surgical Management: Revascularization

The primary revascularization options are PCI and CABG surgery. The most common PCI techniques are percutaneous transluminal coronary angioplasty and coronary stenting. A major limitation of PCI is restenosis at the intervention site. This represents the body's response to local injury with an exaggerated neointimal proliferative response. The use of stents, aspirin, clopidogrel, and glycoprotein IIb/IIIa inhibitors lowers the rate of restenosis to less than 10% at 6 months in optimal circumstances.

The most common conduits for CABG are the saphenous vein and the internal thoracic (mammary) artery. The long-term patency rates of internal thoracic artery grafts are superior to those of venous grafts.

OUTCOMES

Percutaneous Coronary Intervention Versus Medical Therapy

Percutaneous coronary intervention is more effective than medical therapy in relieving angina, but it confers no greater survival benefit. Aggressive lipid-lowering therapy appears to be as effective as percutaneous coronary intervention plus usual medical care for preventing ischemic events.

Coronary Artery Bypass Grafting Versus Medical Therapy

CABG produces better survival rates compared with medical therapy and is recommended for symptomatic patients with left main coronary artery disease, three-vessel coronary artery disease, or two-vessel coronary artery disease marked by stenosis of the proximal left anterior descending artery. CABG is more effective than medical therapy for the relief of angina, although this benefit narrows after 5 to 10 years.

Percutaneous Coronary Intervention Versus Coronary Artery Bypass Grafting

Outcomes following percutaneous coronary intervention and coronary artery bypass grafting have been compared in high-risk patients. The two largest studies in the United States were the Emory Angioplasty versus Surgery Trial (EAST) and the Bypass Angioplasty Revascularization Investigation (BARI). In both trials, percutaneous coronary intervention was limited solely to angioplasty. Similarly, current CABG techniques, including the more frequent use of arterial conduits, were not included in either trial. EAST results have demonstrated that the long-term survival rates following percutaneous coronary intervention and coronary artery bypass grafting are comparable. BARI results have indicated that coronary artery bypass grafting produces better long-term survival rates than percutaneous coronary intervention. However, the benefit of CABG in BARI was not apparent until 7 years postoperatively, and it was largely attributable to the significantly higher survival rate in the subgroup of patients with diabetes mellitus. Both trials have shown that CABG is superior to PCI in relieving angina and obviating the need for repeat revascularization procedures. With the introduction of drug-eluting stents, coupled with improved catheterization techniques, coronary artery disease treatment is shifting away from bypass surgery toward a percutaneous approach. Restenosis rates have been lowered significantly and acute thrombotic complications are rare given the advances in antiplatelet therapy.

Summary

The diagnostic and treatment options for coronary artery disease are changing rapidly.

- New pharmaceuticals are being developed and introduced into the treatment armamentarium.
- Biologic markers are now used to track coronary artery disease activity at the vascular level, guiding medication selection and dose titration.
- Procedures are less invasive and offer percutaneous treatment options, such as drug-eluting stents, that were previously unavailable.
- Despite these advances, coronary artery disease and its deleterious manifestations represent the number one killer in the United States. This is largely caused by poor dietary choices, sedentary lifestyles, and continuance of tobacco use.
- Efforts at primary and secondary prevention of obstructive coronary artery disease among the general public are still lacking.
- Public awareness campaigns are a partial success.
- It is imperative for the physician to allocate time to address the importance of lifestyle modification efforts.
- The genetic basis of coronary artery disease is slowly being unraveled.
- In the future, a genetic assessment of a person's risk for developing atherosclerotic vascular disease may be possible at a young age.
- These findings can guide lifestyle modification prescription and the choice and dosage of select pharmaceuticals.
- A preemptive approach is the best way to tackle the immensity of coronary artery disease.

We must erase the myth that medications, stenting, and bypass surgery are curative approaches. Instead, the patient must meet the health care team at least halfway to achieve a successful health outcome.

Suggested Readings

American College of Cardiology: ACC/AHA 2002 Guideline Update for Exercise Testing. Available at http://www.acc.org/qualityandscience/clinical/guidelines/exercise/exercise_clean.pdf.

ACC/AHA 2002 Guideline Update for the Management of Patients With Chronic Stable Angina. http://www.acc.org/qualityandscience/clinical/guidelines/stable/stable_clean.pdf.

American Heart Association; American Stroke Association: Heart Disease and Stroke Statistics-2006 Update. Available athttp://www.americanheart.org/downloadable/heart/1140534985281Statsupdate06book.pdf.

Antiplatelet Trialists' Collaboration: Collaborative overview of randomized trials of antiplatelet therapy-I: Prevention of death, myocardial infarction, and stroke by prolonged antiplatelet therapy in various categories of patients. BMJ 1994;308:81-106.

Chobanian AV, Bakris GL, Black HR, et al: National Heart, Lung, and Blood Institute Joint National Committee on Prevention, Detection, Evaluation, and Treatment of High Blood Pressure; National High Blood Pressure Education Program Coordinating Committee: The Seventh Report of the Joint National Committee on Prevention, Detection, Evaluation, and Treatment of High Blood Pressure: The JNC 7 report. JAMA 2003;289:2560-2572.

Cole CR, Blackstone EH, Pashkow FJ, et al: Heart-rate recovery immediately after exercise as a predictor of mortality. N Engl J Med 1999;341:1351-1357.

Comparison of coronary bypass surgery with angioplasty in patients with multivessel disease. The Bypass Angioplasty Revascularization Investigation (BARI) Investigators. N Engl J Med 1996;335:217-225.

EPISTENT Investigators: Randomized placebo-controlled and balloon-angioplasty-controlled trial to assess safety of coronary stenting with use of platelet glycoprotein-IIb/IIIa blockade. Evaluation of Platelet IIb/IIIa Inhibitor for Stenting. Lancet 1998;352:87-92.

Hannan EL, Racz MJ, Walford G, et al: Long-term outcomes of coronary-artery bypass grafting versus stent implantation. N Engl J Med 2005:352:2174-2813.

Heart Protection Study Collaborative Group: MRC/BHF Heart Protection Study of cholesterol lowering with simvastatin in 20,536 high-risk individuals: A randomised placebo-controlled trial. Lancet 2002;360:7-22.

King SB 3rd, Lembo NJ, Weintraub WS, et al: A randomized trial comparing coronary angioplasty with coronary bypass surgery. Emory Angioplasty versus Surgery Trial (EAST). N Engl J Med 1994;331:1044-1050.

National Heart, Lung, and Blood Institute: Detection, Evaluation, and Treatment of High Blood Cholesterol in Adults (Adult Treatment Panel III), 2004. Available at http://www.nhlbi.nih.gov/guidelines/cholesterol.

National Institutes of Health: Calculate Your Body Mass Index, 2007. Available at http://www.nhlbisupport.com/bmi.

Roiron C, Sanchez P, Bouzamondo A, et al: Drug-eluting stents: An updated meta-analysis of randomized controlled trials. Heart 2006;92:641-649.

Snader CE, Marwick TH, Pashkow FJ, et al: Importance of estimated functional capacity as a predictor of all-cause mortality among patients referred for exercise thallium single-photon emission computed tomography: Report of 3,400 patients from a single center. J Am Coll Cardiol 1997;30:641-648.

Yusuf S, Sleight P, Pogue J, et al: Effects of an angiotensin-converting-enzyme inhibitor, ramipril, on cardiovascular events in high-risk patients. The Heart Outcomes Prevention Evaluation Study Investigators. N Engl J Med 2000;342:145-153.

Yusuf S, Zhao F, Mehta SR, et al: Effects of clopidogrel in addition to aspirin in patients with acute coronary syndromes without ST-segment elevation. N Engl J Med 2001;345:494-502.

Acute Myocardial Infarction

H. Michael Bolooki and Arman Askari

DEFINITION AND ETIOLOGY

Acute myocardial infarction (MI) remains a leading cause of morbidity and mortality worldwide. Myocardial infarction occurs when myocardial ischemia, a diminished blood supply to the heart, exceeds a critical threshold and overwhelms myocardial cellular repair mechanisms designed to maintain normal operating function and homeostasis. Ischemia at this critical threshold level for an extended period results in irreversible myocardial cell damage or death.

Critical myocardial ischemia can occur as a result of increased myocardial metabolic demand, decreased delivery of oxygen and nutrients to the myocardium via the coronary circulation, or both. An interruption in the supply of myocardial oxygen and nutrients occurs when a thrombus is superimposed on an ulcerated or unstable atherosclerotic plaque and results in coronary occlusion.[1] A high-grade (>75%) fixed coronary artery stenosis caused by atherosclerosis or a dynamic stenosis associated with coronary vasospasm can also limit the supply of oxygen and nutrients and precipitate an MI. Conditions associated with increased myocardial metabolic demand include extremes of physical exertion, severe hypertension (including forms of hypertrophic obstructive cardiomyopathy), and severe aortic valve stenosis. Other cardiac valvular pathologies and low cardiac output states associated with a decreased mean aortic pressure, which is the prime component of coronary perfusion pressure, can also precipitate MI.

Myocardial infarction can be subcategorized on the basis of anatomic, morphologic, and diagnostic clinical information. From an anatomic or morphologic standpoint, the two types of MI are transmural and nontransmural. A transmural MI is characterized by ischemic necrosis of the full thickness of the affected muscle segment(s), extending from the endocardium through the myocardium to the epicardium. A nontransmural MI is defined as an area of ischemic necrosis that does not extend through the full thickness of myocardial wall segment(s). In a nontransmural MI, the area of ischemic necrosis is limited to the endocardium or to the endocardium and myocardium. It is the endocardial and subendocardial zones of the myocardial wall segment that are the least perfused regions of the heart and the most vulnerable to conditions of ischemia. An older subclassification of MI, based on clinical diagnostic criteria, is determined by the presence or absence of Q waves on an electrocardiogram (ECG). However, the presence or absence of Q waves does not distinguish a transmural from a nontransmural MI as determined by pathology.[2]

A consensus statement was published to give a universal definition of the term myocardial infarction. The authors stated that MI should be used when there is evidence of myocardial necrosis in a clinical setting consistent with MI. Myocardial infarction was then classified by the clinical scenario into various subtypes. Type 1 is a spontaneous MI related to ischemia from a primary coronary event (e.g., plaque rupture, thrombotic occlusion). Type 2 is secondary to ischemia from a supply-and-demand mismatch. Type 3 is an MI resulting in sudden cardiac death. Type 4a is an MI associated with percutaneous coronary intervention, and 4b is associated with in-stent thrombosis. Type 5 is an MI associated with coronary artery bypass surgery.[3]

A more common clinical diagnostic classification scheme is also based on electrocardiographic findings as a means of distinguishing between two types of MI, one that is marked by ST elevation (STEMI) and one that is not (NSTEMI). Management practice guidelines often distinguish between STEMI and non-STEMI, as do many of the studies on which recommendations are based. The distinction between STEMI and NSTEMI also does not distinguish a transmural from a nontransmural MI. The presence of Q waves or ST-segment elevation is associated with higher early mortality and morbidity; however, the absence of these two findings does not confer better long-term mortality and morbidity.[4]

PREVALENCE AND RISK FACTORS

Myocardial infarction is the leading cause of death in the United States and in most industrialized nations throughout the world. Approximately 450,000 people in the United States die from coronary disease per year.[5] The survival rate for U.S. patients hospitalized with MI is approximately 95%. This represents a significant improvement in survival and is related to improvements in emergency medical response and treatment strategies.

The incidence of MI increases with age; however, the actual incidence is dependent on predisposing risk factors for atherosclerosis. Approximately 50% of all MIs in the United States occur in people younger than 65 years. However, in the future, as demographics shift and the mean age of the population increases, a larger percentage of patients presenting with MI will be older than 65 years.

Six primary risk factors have been identified with the development of atherosclerotic coronary artery disease and MI: hyperlipidemia, diabetes mellitus, hypertension, tobacco use, male gender, and family history of atherosclerotic arterial disease. The presence of any risk factor is associated with doubling the relative risk of developing atherosclerotic coronary artery disease.[1]

Hyperlipidemia

Elevated levels of total cholesterol, LDL, or triglycerides are associated with an increased risk of coronary atherosclerosis and MI. Levels of HDL less than 40 mg/dL also portend an increased risk. A full summary of the National Heart, Lung, and Blood Institute's cholesterol guidelines is available online.[6]

Diabetes Mellitus

Patients with diabetes have a substantially greater risk of atherosclerotic vascular disease in the heart as well as in other vascular beds. Diabetes increases the risk of MI because it increases the rate of atherosclerotic progression and adversely affects the lipid profile. This accelerated form of atherosclerosis occurs regardless of whether a patient has insulin-dependent or non–insulin-dependent diabetes.

Hypertension

High blood pressure (BP) has consistently been associated with an increased risk of MI. This risk is associated with systolic and diastolic hypertension. The control of hypertension with appropriate medication has been shown to reduce the risk of MI significantly. A full summary of the National Heart, Lung, and Blood Institute's JNC 7 guidelines published in 2003 is available online.[7]

Tobacco Use

Certain components of tobacco and tobacco combustion gases are known to damage blood vessel walls. The body's response to this type of injury elicits the formation of atherosclerosis and its progression, thereby increasing the risk of MI. A small study in a group of volunteers showed that smoking acutely increases platelet thrombus formation. This appears to target areas of high shear forces, such as stenotic vessels, independent of aspirin use.[8] The American Lung Association maintains a website with updates on the public health initiative to reduce tobacco use and is a resource for smoking-cessation strategies for patients and health care providers.

Male Gender

The incidence of atherosclerotic vascular disease and MI is higher in men than women in all age groups. This gender difference in MI, however, narrows with increasing age.

Family History

A family history of premature coronary disease increases an individual's risk of atherosclerosis and MI. The cause of familial coronary events is multifactorial and includes other elements, such as genetic components and acquired general health practices (e.g. smoking, high-fat diet).

PATHOPHYSIOLOGY AND NATURAL HISTORY

Most myocardial infarctions are caused by a disruption in the vascular endothelium associated with an unstable atherosclerotic plaque that stimulates the formation of an intracoronary thrombus, which results in coronary artery blood flow occlusion. If such an occlusion persists for more than 20 minutes, irreversible myocardial cell damage and cell death will occur.

The development of atherosclerotic plaque occurs over a period of years to decades. The two primary characteristics of the clinically symptomatic atherosclerotic plaque are a fibromuscular cap and an underlying lipid-rich core. Plaque erosion can occur because of the actions of matrix metalloproteases and the release of other collagenases and proteases in the plaque, which result in thinning of the overlying fibromuscular cap. The action of proteases, in addition to hemodynamic forces applied to the arterial segment, can lead to a disruption of the endothelium and fissuring or rupture of the fibromuscular cap. The loss of structural stability of a plaque often occurs at the juncture of the fibromuscular cap and the vessel wall, a site otherwise known as the *shoulder region*. Disruption of the endothelial surface can cause the formation of thrombus via platelet-mediated activation of the coagulation cascade. If a thrombus is large enough to occlude coronary blood flow, an MI can result.

The death of myocardial cells first occurs in the area of myocardium most distal to the arterial blood supply: the endocardium. As the duration of the occlusion increases, the area of myocardial cell death enlarges, extending from the endocardium to the myocardium and ultimately to the epicardium. The area of myocardial cell death then spreads laterally to areas of watershed or collateral perfusion. Generally, after a 6- to 8-hour period of coronary occlusion, most of the distal myocardium has died. The extent of myocardial cell death defines the magnitude of the MI. If blood flow can be restored to at-risk myocardium, more heart muscle can be saved from irreversible damage or death.

The severity of an MI depends on three factors: the level of the occlusion in the coronary artery, the length of time of the occlusion, and the presence or absence of collateral circulation. Generally, the more proximal the coronary occlusion, the more extensive the amount of myocardium that will be at risk of necrosis. The larger the myocardial infarction, the greater the chance of death because of a mechanical complication or pump failure. The longer the period of vessel occlusion, the greater the chances of irreversible myocardial damage distal to the occlusion.

STEMI is usually the result of complete coronary occlusion after plaque rupture. This arises most often from a plaque that previously caused less than 50% occlusion of the lumen. NSTEMI is usually associated with greater plaque burden without complete occlusion. This difference contributes to the increased early mortality seen in STEMI and the eventual equalization of mortality between STEMI and NSTEMI after 1 year.

SIGNS AND SYMPTOMS

Acute MI can have unique manifestations in individual patients. The degree of symptoms ranges from none at all to sudden cardiac death. An asymptomatic MI is not necessarily less severe than a symptomatic event, but patients who experience asymptomatic MIs are more likely to be diabetic. Despite the diversity of manifesting symptoms of MI, there are some characteristic symptoms.

- Chest pain described as a pressure sensation, fullness, or squeezing in the midportion of the thorax
- Radiation of chest pain into the jaw or teeth, shoulder, arm, and/or back
- Associated dyspnea or shortness of breath
- Associated epigastric discomfort with or without nausea and vomiting
- Associated diaphoresis or sweating
- Syncope or near syncope without other cause
- Impairment of cognitive function without other cause

An MI can occur at any time of the day, but most appear to be clustered around the early hours of the morning or are associated with demanding physical activity, or both. Approximately 50% of patients have some warning symptoms (angina pectoris or an anginal equivalent) before the infarct.

DIAGNOSIS

Identifying a patient who is currently experiencing an MI can be straightforward, difficult, or somewhere in between. A straightforward diagnosis of MI can usually be made in patients who have a number of atherosclerotic risk factors along with the presence of symptoms consistent with a lack of blood flow to the heart. Patients who suspect that they are having an MI usually present to an emergency department. Once a patient's clinical picture raises a suspicion of MI, several confirmatory tests can be performed rapidly. These tests include electrocardiography, blood testing, and echocardiography.

Diagnostic Procedures

The first diagnostic test is electrocardiography (ECG), which may demonstrate that a MI is in progress or has already occurred. Interpretation of an ECG is beyond the scope of this chapter; however, one feature of the ECG in a patient with an MI should be noted because it has a bearing on management. Practice guidelines on MI management consider patients whose ECG does or does not show ST-segment elevation separately. As noted earlier, the former is referred to as ST elevation MI (Fig. 1) and the latter as non-ST elevation MI (Fig. 2). In addition to ST-segment elevation, 81% of electrocardiograms during STEMI demonstrate reciprocal ST-segment depression as well.

Laboratory Tests

Living myocardial cells contain enzymes and proteins (e.g., creatine kinase, troponin I and T, myoglobin) associated with specialized cellular functions. When a myocardial cell dies, cellular membranes lose integrity, and intracellular enzymes and proteins slowly leak into

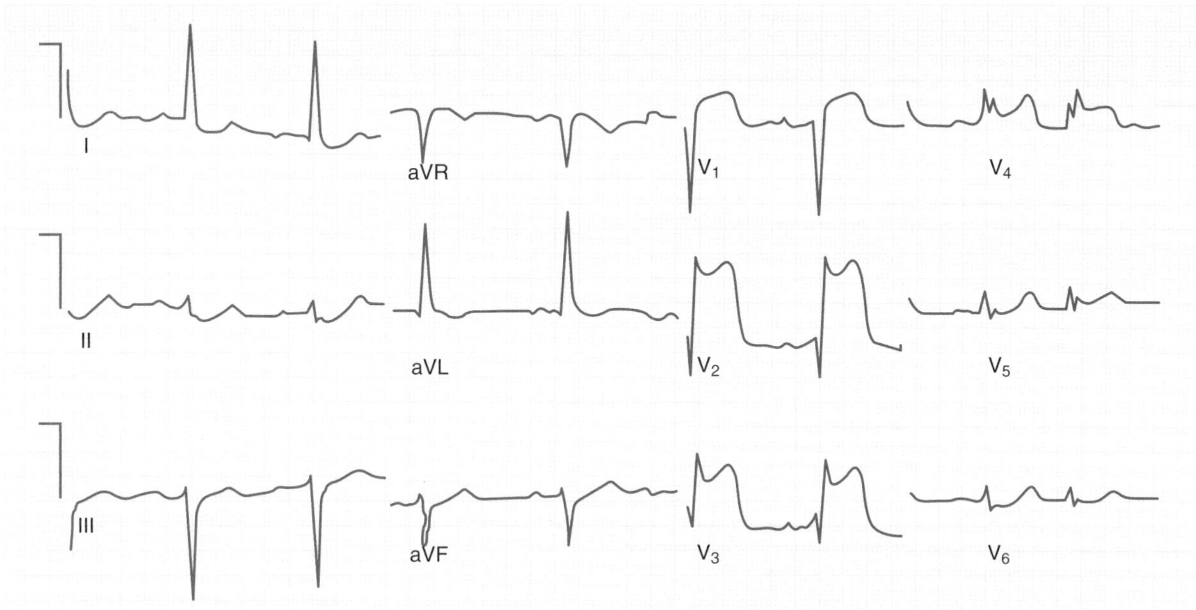

Figure 1 Twelve-lead electrocardiogram showing ST-segment (V_1 to V_4) elevation myocardial infarction. *(Courtesy of Dr. Donald Underwood, Cleveland Clinic Foundation)*

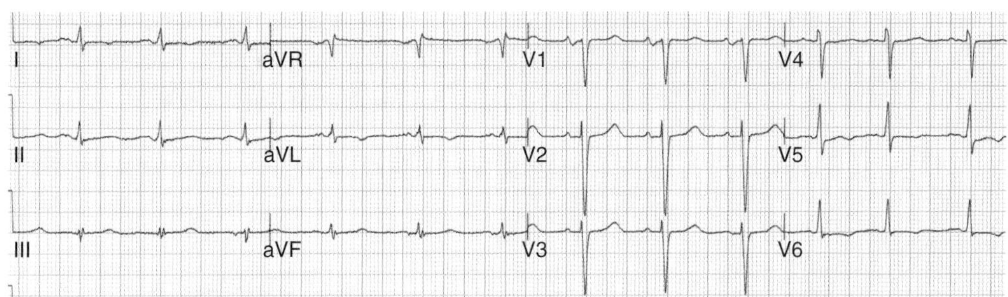

Figure 2 12-lead electrocardiogram showing non-specific ST-segment and T-wave changes as might be seen in non-ST segment elevation myocardial infarction. *(Courtesy of Dr. Michael Bolooki, University of Minnesota)*

the blood stream. These enzymes and proteins can be detected by a blood sample analysis. These values vary depending on the assay used in each laboratory. Given the acuity of a STEMI and the need for urgent intervention, the laboratory tests are usually not available at the time of diagnosis. Thus, good history taking and an ECG are used to initiate therapy in the appropriate situations. The real value of biomarkers such as troponin lies in the diagnosis and prognosis of NSTEMI (Fig. 3).

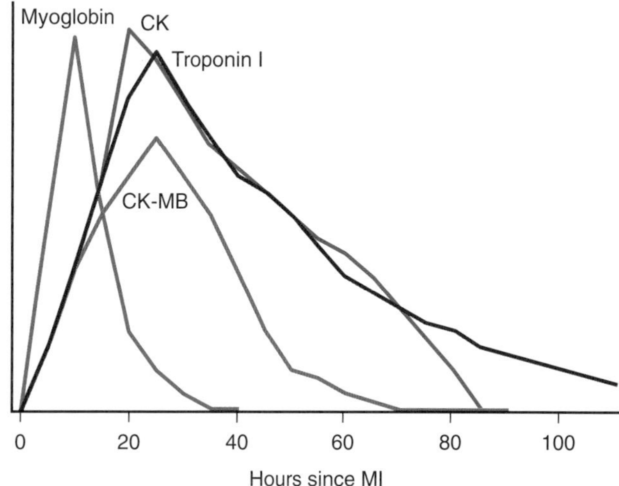

Figure 3 Typical rise and fall of cardiac biomarkers following myocardial infarction.

Imaging

An echocardiogram may be performed to compare areas of the left ventricle that are contracting normally with those that are not. One of the earliest protective actions of myocardial cells used during limited blood flow is to turn off the energy-requiring mechanism for contraction; this mechanism begins almost immediately after normal blood flow is interrupted. The echocardiogram may be helpful in identifying which portion of the heart is affected by an MI and which of the coronary arteries is most likely to be occluded. Unfortunately, the presence of wall motion abnormalities on the echocardiogram may be the result of an acute MI or previous (old) MI or other myopathic processes, limiting its overall diagnostic utility.

TREATMENT

The goals of therapy in acute MI are the expedient restoration of normal coronary blood flow and the maximum salvage of functional myocardium. These goals can be met by a number of medical interventions and adjunctive therapies. The primary obstacles to achieving these goals are the patient's failure to recognize MI symptoms quickly and the delay in seeking medical attention. When patients present to a hospital, there are a variety of interventions to achieve treatment goals. "Time is muscle" guides the management decisions in acute STEMI, and an early invasive approach is the standard of care for acute NSTEMI.[4]

Medical Options

Antiplatelet Agents

The use of aspirin has been shown to reduce mortality from MI. Aspirin in a dose of 325 mg should be administered immediately on recognition of MI signs and symptoms.[4,9] The nidus of an occlusive coronary thrombus is the adhesion of a small collection of activated platelets at the site of intimal disruption in an unstable atherosclerotic plaque. Aspirin irreversibly interferes with function of cyclooxygenase and inhibits the formation of thromboxane A2. Within minutes, aspirin prevents additional platelet activation and interferes with platelet adhesion and cohesion. This effect benefits all patients with acute coronary syndromes, including those with amyocardial infarction. Aspirin alone has one of the greatest impacts on the reduction of MI mortality. Its beneficial effect is observed early in therapy and persists for years with continued use. The long-term benefit is sustained, even at doses as low as 75 mg/day.

The Clopidogrel and Metoprolol in Myocardial Infarction Trial/ Second Chinese Cardiac Study (COMMIT-CCS 2) trial evaluated the use of clopidogrel versus placebo in patients who were taking aspirin but not undergoing reperfusion therapy. It demonstrated a benefit in favor of clopidogrel when used with aspirin.[10] The Clopidogrel as Adjunctive Reperfusion Therapy—Thrombolysis in Myocardial Infarction 28 (CLARITY-TIMI 28) study compared clopidogrel versus placebo in patients receiving fibrinolytics within 12 hours of STEMI and showed a benefit in favor of clopidogrel as well.[11] The current recommendations for antiplatelet agents is summarized in Table 1.

Supplemental Oxygen

Oxygen should be administered to patients with symptoms or signs of pulmonary edema or with pulse oximetry less than 90% saturation.[4] The rationale for using oxygen is the assurance that erythrocytes will be saturated to maximum carrying capacity. Because MI impairs the circulatory function of the heart, oxygen extraction by the heart and by other tissues may be diminished. In some cases, elevated pulmonary capillary pressure and pulmonary edema can decrease oxygen uptake as a result of impaired pulmonary alveolar-capillary diffusion. Supplemental oxygen increases the driving gradient for oxygen uptake.[1]

Table 1 Antiplatelet Medications

Treatment Modality	Aspirin	Clopidogrel
Medical management	75-162 mg/day indefinitely	Optional: 75 mg/day × 1 month
Bare Metal stent	162-325 mg/day × 1 month, then 75-162 mg/day indefinitely	300 mg loading dose,* then 75 mg/day × 1 month
Sirolimus eluting stent (Cypher)	162-325 mg/day × 3 months, then 75-162 mg/day indefinitely	300 mg loading dose,* then 75 mg/day × 1 year
Paclitaxel eluting stent (Taxus)	162-325 mg/day × 6 months, then 75-162 mg/day indefinitely	300 mg loading dose,* then 75 mg/day × 1 year

*Note: No loading dose in patients older than 75 years.

Arterial blood that is at its maximum oxygen-carrying capacity can potentially deliver oxygen to myocardium in jeopardy during an MI via collateral coronary circulation. The recommended duration of supplemental oxygen administration in a MI is 2 to 6 hours, longer if congestive heart failure occurs or arterial oxygen saturation is less than 90%. However, there are no published studies demonstrating that oxygen therapy reduces the mortality or morbidity of an MI.

Nitrates

Intravenous nitrates should be administered to patients with MI and congestive heart failure, persistent ischemia, hypertension, or large anterior wall MI.[4,9] The primary benefit of nitrates is derived from its vasodilator effect. Nitrates are metabolized to nitric oxide in the vascular endothelium. Nitric oxide relaxes vascular smooth muscle and dilates the blood vessel lumen. Vasodilatation reduces cardiac preload and afterload and decreases the myocardial oxygen requirements needed for circulation at a fixed flow rate. Vasodilatation of the coronary arteries improves blood flow through the partially obstructed vessels as well as through collateral vessels. Nitrates can reverse the vasoconstriction associated with thrombosis and coronary occlusion.

When administered sublingually or intravenously, nitroglycerin has a rapid onset of action. Clinical trial data have supported the initial use of nitroglycerin for up to 48 hours in MI. There is little evidence that nitroglycerin provides substantive benefit as long-term post-MI therapy, except when severe pump dysfunction or residual ischemia is present.[4] Low BP, headache, and tachyphylaxis limit the use of nitroglycerin. Nitrate tolerance can be overcome by increasing the dose or by providing a daily nitrate-free interval of 8 to 12 hours. Nitrates must be avoided in patients who have taken a phosphodiesterase inhibitor within the previous 24 hours.[4]

Pain Control

Pain from MI is often intense and requires prompt and adequate analgesia. The agent of choice is morphine sulfate, given initially IV at 5 to 15 minute intervals at typical doses of 2 to 4 mg.[4] Reduction in myocardial ischemia also serves to reduce pain, so oxygen therapy, nitrates, and beta blockers remain the mainstay of therapy. Because morphine can mask ongoing ischemic symptoms, it should be reserved for patients being sent for coronary angiography. This was downgraded to a IIa recommendation in the latest STEMI guidelines.

Beta Blockers

Beta blocker therapy is recommended within 12 hours of MI symptoms and is continued indefinitely.[4,9] Treatment with a beta blocker decreases the incidence of ventricular arrhythmias, recurrent ischemia, reinfarction, and, if given early enough, infarct size and short-term mortality. Beta blockade decreases the rate and force of myocardial contraction and decreases overall myocardial oxygen demand. In the setting of reduced oxygen supply in MI, the reduction in oxygen demand provided by beta blockade can minimize myocardial injury and death (Table 2).

The use of a beta blocker has a number of recognized adverse effects. The most serious are heart failure, bradycardia, and bronchospasm. During the acute phase of an MI, beta blocker therapy may be initiated intravenously; later, patients can switch to oral therapy for long-term treatment. The COMMIT-CCS 2 trial raised safety concerns about the use of early intravenous beta blockers in high-risk patients.[10] In some patients who are considered high risk due to age or hemodynamic instability, it may be reasonable to hold off on early intravenous therapy.

According to the 2007 guideline updates, anticoagulation should be added to standard medical therapy for most patients after myocardial infarction.[4]

Table 2 Beta Blocker Therapy

Agent	Dosing	Original Trial
Metoprolol	15 mg IV × 1 then 200 mg/day PO in divided doses	MIAMI[19]
Atenolol	5-10 mg IV × 1, then 100 mg/day PO	ISIS-1[20]
Carvedilol	6.25 mg bid titrated to 25 mg BID	CAPRICORN[21]

ISIS-1, International Studies of Infarct Survival-1; MIAMI, Metoprolol in Acute Myocardial Infarction.

Box 1 Unfractionated Heparin Dosing

Loading Dose
60 U/kg IV bolus
Max 5000 U if >65 kg or 4000 U if <65 kg

Maintenance Dose
12 U/kg/hr IV
Max 1000 U/hr if >65 kg or 800 U/hr if <65 kg

Titration Goal
PTT 50-70 sec

PTT, prothrombin time.

Unfractionated Heparin

Unfractionated heparin is beneficial until the inciting thrombotic cause (ruptured plaque) has completely resolved or healed. Unfractionated heparin has been shown to be effective when administered intravenously or subcutaneously according to specific guidelines. The minimum duration of heparin therapy after MI is generally 48 hours, but it may be longer, depending on the individual clinical scenario. Heparin has the added benefit of preventing thrombus through a different mechanism than aspirin (Box 1).

Low-Molecular-Weight Heparin

Low-molecular-weight heparin (LMWH) can be administered to MI patients who are not treated with fibrinolytic therapy and who have no contraindications to heparin. The LMWH class of drugs includes several agents that have distinctly different anticoagulant effects. LMWHs are proved to be effective for treating acute coronary syndromes characterized by unstable angina and NSTEMI.[4] Their fixed doses are easy to administer, and laboratory testing to measure their therapeutic effect is usually not necessary (Table 3).

Warfarin

Warfarin is not routinely used after MI, but it does have a role in selected clinical settings. The latest guidelines recommend the use of warfarin for at least 3 months in patients with left ventricular aneurysm or thrombus, a left ventricular ejection fraction less than 30%, or chronic atrial fibrillation.

Fibrinolytics

Restoration of coronary blood flow in MI patients can be accomplished pharmacologically with the use of a fibrinolytic agent. Fibrinolytic therapy is indicated for patients who present with a STEMI within 12 hours of symptom onset without a contraindication. Absolute contraindications to fibrinolytic therapy include history of intracranial hemorrhage, ischemic stroke or closed head injury within the past 3 months, presence of an intracranial malignancy, signs of an aortic dissection, or active bleeding. Fibrinolytic therapy is primarily used at facilities without access to an experienced interventionalist within 90 minutes of presentation.[9]

As a class, the plasminogen activators have been shown to restore normal coronary blood flow in 50% to 60% of STEMI patients. The successful use of fibrinolytic agents provides a definite survival benefit that is maintained for years. The most critical variable in achieving successful fibrinolysis is time from symptom onset to drug administration. A fibrinolytic is most effective within the first hour of symptom onset and when the door-to-needle time is 30 minutes or less.[9]

Table 3 Low-Molecular-Weight Heparin

Generic name	$t_{1/2}$ (after SC dosing)	Dosing in ACS	FDA Approved Indications
Dalteparin	3-5 hr	120 U/kg SC bid	Prevention of ischemic complications in UA and NSTEMI
Enoxaparin	4.5 hr	100 U/kg (1 mg/kg) SC q12h	Prophylaxis of ischemic complications of UA and NSTEMI when administered with aspirin

UA, unstable angina; NSTEMI, non–ST segment elevation myocardial infarction.

Table 4 ACE Inhibitors

Agent	Dosing (PO)	Original Trial
Captopril	6.25 mg tid titrated to 50 mg tid	SAVE: 3-16 days post-MI in asymptomatic patients with EF <40%[22]
Ramipril	1.25 mg bid titrated to 5 mg bid	AIRE: 3-10 days post-MI with symptoms of heart failure[23]
Captopril	6.25 mg bid titrated to 50 mg bid	ISIS-4: started within 24 hr of MI[24]
Lisinopril	5 mg/day titrated to 10 mg/day	GISSI-3: started within 24 hr of MI[25]

AIRE, Acute Infarction Ramipril Efficacy; EF, ejection fraction; GISSI-3, Gruppo Italiano per lo Studio della Sopravvivenza nell'Infarto Miocardico; ISIS-4, International Studies of Infarct Survival-1; MI, myocardial infarction; SAVE, Survival and Ventricular Enlargemen.

Angiotensin-Converting Enzyme Inhibitors and Angiotensin Receptor Blockers

Angiotensin-converting enzyme (ACE) inhibitors should be used in all patients with a STEMI without contraindications. ACE inhibitors are also recommended in patients with NSTEMI who have diabetes, heart failure, hypertension, or an ejection fraction less than 40%. In such patients, an ACE inhibitor should be administered within 24 hours of admission and continued indefinitely. Further evidence has shown that the benefit of ACE inhibitor therapy can likely be extended to all patients with an MI and should be started before discharge.[4,9] Contraindications to ACE inhibitor use include hypotension and declining renal function. The most commonly used ACE inhibitors are summarized in Table 4.

ACE inhibitors decrease myocardial afterload through vasodilatation. One effective strategy for instituting an ACE inhibitor is to start with a low-dose, short-acting agent and titrate the dose upward

Table 5 Glycoprotein IIb/IIIa Inhibitors

Agent	Loading Dose (IV)	Maintenance Dose (IV)	Duration of Infusion	FDA Approved Indications
Abciximab	0.25 mg/kg	0.125 μg/kg/min max 10 μg/min	12-24 hr	Coronary intervention
Eptifibatide	180 μg/kg	2 μg/kg/min	Up to 72 hr	Acute coronary syndrome Coronary intervention
Tirofiban	0.4 μg/kg/min for 30 min	0.1 μg/kg/min	12-24 hr	Acute coronary syndrome Coronary intervention

toward a stable target maintenance dose at 24 to 48 hours after symptom onset. Once a stable maintenance dose has been achieved, the short-acting agent can be continued or converted to an equivalent-dose long-acting agent to simplify dosing and encourage patient compliance. For patients intolerant of ACE inhibitors, angiotensin receptor blocker (ARB) therapy may be considered.

Glycoprotein IIb/IIIa Antagonists

Glycoprotein IIb/IIIa receptors on platelets bind to fibrinogen in the final common pathway of platelet aggregation. Antagonists to glycoprotein IIb/IIIa receptors are potent inhibitors of platelet aggregation. The use of glycoprotein IIb/IIIa inhibitors during percutaneous coronary intervention (PCI) and in patients with MI and acute coronary syndromes has been shown to reduce the composite end point of death, reinfarction, and the need to revascularize the target lesion at follow-up. The current guidelines recommend the use of a IIb/IIIa inhibitor for patients in whom PCI is planned. For high-risk patients with NSTEMI who do not undergo PCI, a IIb/IIIa inhibitor may be used for 48 to 72 hours (Table 5).[4]

Evidence is less well established for the direct thrombin inhibitor, bivalirudin. The 2007 American College of Cardiology (ACC) and the American Heart Association (AHA) guidelines recommend bivalirudin as an alternative to heparin therapy for patients who cannot receive heparin for a variety of reasons (e.g., heparin-induced thrombocytopenia).[4,9]

Statin Therapy

A statin should be started in all patients with a myocardial infarction without known intolerance or adverse reaction prior to hospital discharge. Preferably, a statin would be started as soon as a patient is stabilized after presentation. The Pravastatin or Atorvastatin Evaluation and Infection—Thrombolysis in Myocardial Infarction 22 (PROVE IT-TIMI 22) trial suggested a benefit of starting patients on high-dose therapy from the start (e.g., atorvastatin 80 mg/day).[12]

Aldosterone Antagonists

In the Epleronone Post-Acute Myocardial Infarction Heart Failure Efficacy and Survival Study (EPHESUS) trial, a mortality benefit was seen with eplerenone administration in all post-MI patients, provided multiple criteria were met. The criteria included concomitant use of an ACE inhibitor, ejection fraction less than 40%, symptomatic heart failure or diabetes, a creatinine clearance greater than 30 mL/min, and a potassium level less than 5 mEq/dL.[13] In patients that meet these criteria, the use of eplerenone has a Class I indication.

Other Treatment Options

Percutaneous Coronary Intervention

Patients with STEMI or MI with new left bundle branch block should have PCI within 90 minutes of arrival at the hospital if skilled cardiac catheterization services are available.[9] Patients with NSTEMI and high-risk features such as elevated cardiac enzymes, ST-segment depression, recurrent angina, hemodynamic instability, sustained ventricular tachycardia, diabetes, prior PCI, or bypass surgery are recommended to undergo early PCI (<48 hours). PCI consists of diagnostic angiography combined with angioplasty and, usually, stenting. It is well established that emergency PCI is more effective than fibrinolytic therapy in centers in which PCI can be performed by experienced personnel in a timely fashion.[14] An operator is considered experienced with more than 75 interventional procedures per year. A well-equipped catheterization laboratory with experienced personnel performs more than 200 interventional procedures per year and has surgical backup available. Centers that are unable to provide such support should consider administering fibrinolytic therapy as their primary MI treatment.

Restoration of coronary blood flow in a MI can be accomplished mechanically by PCI. PCI can successfully restore coronary blood flow in 90% to 95% of MI patients. Several studies have demonstrated that PCI has an advantage over fibrinolysis with respect to short-term mortality, bleeding rates, and reinfarction rates. However, the short-term mortality advantage is not durable, and PCI and fibrinolysis appear to yield similar survival rates over the long term. PCI provides a definite survival advantage over fibrinolysis for MI patients who are in cardiogenic shock. The use of stents with PCI for MI is superior to the use of PCI without stents, primarily because stenting reduces the need for subsequent target vessel revascularization.[15]

Surgical Revascularization

Emergent or urgent coronary artery bypass grafting (CABG) is warranted in the setting of failed PCI in patients with hemodynamic instability and coronary anatomy amenable to surgical grafting.[9] Surgical revascularization is also indicated in the setting of mechanical complications of MI, such as ventricular septal defect, free wall rupture, or acute mitral regurgitation. Restoration of coronary blood flow with emergency CABG can limit myocardial injury and cell death if performed within 2 or 3 hours of symptom onset. Emergency CABG carries a higher risk of perioperative morbidity (bleeding and MI extension) and mortality than elective CABG. Elective CABG improves survival in post-MI patients who have left main artery disease, three-vessel disease, or two-vessel disease not amenable to PCI.

Implantable Cardiac Defibrillators

The results of a multicenter automatic defibrillator implantation trial have expanded the indications for automatic implantable cardioverter-defibrillators (ICDs) in post-MI patients. The trial demonstrated a 31% relative risk reduction in all-cause mortality with the prophylactic use of an ICD in post-MI patients with depressed ejection fractions.[16] The current guidelines recommend waiting 40 days after an MI to evaluate the need for ICD implantation. ICD implantation is appropriate for patients in NYHA functional class II or III with an ejection fraction less than 35%. For patients in NYHA functional class I, the ejection fraction should be less than 30% before considering ICD placement. ICDs are not recommended while patients are in NYHA functional class IV.[17]

Treatment Outcomes

An individual patient's long-term outcome following an MI depends on numerous variables, some of which are not modifiable from a clinical standpoint. However, patients can modify other variables by complying with prescribed therapy and adopting lifestyle changes.

Stress Testing

Cardiac stress testing after MI has established value in risk stratification and assessment of functional capacity.[4] The timing of performing cardiac stress testing remains debatable. The degree of allowable physiologic stress during testing depends on the length of time from MI presentation. Stress testing is not recommended within several days after a myocardial infarction. Only submaximal stress tests should be performed in stable patients 4 to 7 days after an MI. Symptom-limited stress tests are recommended 14 to 21 days after an MI. Imaging modalities can be added to stress testing in patients whose electrocardiographic response to exercise is inadequate to confidently assess for ischemia (e.g., complete left bundle branch block, paced rhythm, accessory pathway, left ventricular hypertrophy, digitalis use, and resting ST-segment abnormalities).[4]

From a prognostic standpoint, an inability to exercise and exercise-induced ST-segment depression are associated with higher cardiac morbidity and mortality compared with patients able to exercise and without ST-segment depression.[4] Exercise testing identifies patients with residual ischemia for additional efforts at revascularization. Exercise testing also provides prognostic information and acts as a guide for post-MI exercise prescription and cardiac rehabilitation.

Smoking Cessation

Smoking is a major risk factor for coronary artery disease and MI. For patients who have undergone an MI, smoking cessation is essential to recovery, long-term health, and prevention of reinfarction. In one study, the risk of recurrent MI decreased by 50% after 1 year of smoking cessation.[18] All STEMI and NSTEMI patients with a history of smoking should be advised to quit and offered smoking cessation resources, including nicotine replacement therapy, pharmacologic therapy, and referral to behavioral counseling or support groups.[4,9] Smoking cessation counselling should begin in the hospital, at discharge, and during follow-up. The American Lung Association maintains a website (http://www.lungusa.org) with updates on public health initiatives to reduce tobacco use; it is a resource for smoking cessation strategies for patients and health care providers. Other public and private sources of smoking cessation information are available online as well.

Long-Term Medications

Most oral medications instituted in the hospital at the time of MI will be continued long term. Therapy with aspirin and beta blockade is continued indefinitely in all patients. ACE inhibitors are continued indefinitely in patients with congestive heart failure, left ventricular dysfunction, hypertension, or diabetes.[4,9] A lipid-lowering agent, specifically a statin, in addition to diet modification, is continued indefinitely as well. Post-MI patients with diabetes should have tight glycemic control according to earlier studies. The latest ACC/AHA guidelines recommend a goal HbA_{1c} of less than 7%.

Cardiac Rehabilitation

Cardiac rehabilitation provides a venue for continued education, reinforcement of lifestyle modification, and adherence to a comprehensive prescription of therapies for recovery from MI including exercise training. Participation in cardiac rehabilitation programs after MI is associated with decreases in subsequent cardiac morbidity and mortality. Other benefits include improvements in quality of life, functional capacity, and social support. However, only a minority of post-MI patients actually participate in formal cardiac rehabilitation programs because of several factors, including lack of structured programs, physician referrals, low patient motivation, noncompliance, and financial constraints.

Summary

- MI results from myocardial ischemia and cell death, most often because of an intra-arterial thrombus superimposed on an ulcerated or unstable atherosclerotic plaque.
- Despite advances in therapy, MI remains the leading cause of death in the United States.
- MI risk factors include hyperlipidemia, diabetes, hypertension, male gender, and tobacco use.
- Diagnosis is based on the clinical history, ECG, and blood test results, especially creatine phosphokinase (CK), CK-MB fraction, and troponin I and T levels.
- Outcome following an MI is determined by the infarct size and location, and by timely medical intervention.
- Aspirin, nitrates, and beta blockers are critically important early in the course of MI for all patients. For those with STEMI and for those with new left bundle branch block, coronary angiography with angioplasty and stenting should be undertaken within 90 minutes of arrival at facilities with expertise in these procedures. Fibrinolytic therapy should be used in situations in which early angiographic intervention is not possible.
- Postdischarge management requires ongoing pharmacotherapy and lifestyle modification.

Further Readings

Anderson J, Adams C, Antman E, et al: ACC/AHA 2007 Guidelines for the Management of Patients with Unstable Angina/NSTEMI. J Am Coll Cardiol 2007;50:e1.

Antman EM, Hand M, Armstrong PW, et al: 2007 Focused Update of the ACC/AHA 2004 Guidelines for the Management of Patients with ST-Elevation Myocardial Infarction. J Am Coll Cardiol 2008;51:210-247.

Moss AJ, Zareba W, Hall WJ, et al; Multicenter Automatic Defibrillator Implantation Trial II Investigators: Prophylactic implantation of a defibrillator in patients with myocardial infarction and reduced ejection fraction. N Engl J Med 2002;346:877-883.

National Heart, Lung, and Blood Institute: The Seventh Report of the Joint National Committee on Prevention, Detection, Evaluation, and Treatment of High Blood Pressure (JNC 7). Available at http://www.nhlbi.nih.gov/guidelines/hypertension (accessed February 28, 2009).

National Heart, Lung, and Blood Institute: Third Report of the Expert Panel on Detection, Evaluation, and Treatment of High Blood Cholesterol in Adults (Adult Treatment Panel III), 2004. Available at http://www.nhlbi.nih.gov/guidelines/cholesterol (accessed February 28, 2009).

References

For a complete list of references, log onto www.expertconsult.com.

Complications of Acute Myocardial Infarction

Adam W. Grasso and Sorin J. Brener

Complications of acute myocardial infarction (MI) include ischemic, mechanical, arrhythmic, embolic, and inflammatory disturbances (Table 1). Nevertheless, circulatory failure from severe left ventricular (LV) dysfunction or one of the mechanical complications of MI accounts for most fatalities.

ISCHEMIC COMPLICATIONS

Ischemic complications can include infarct extension, recurrent infarction, and recurrent angina.

Prevalence

Infarct extension is a progressive increase in the amount of myocardial necrosis within the infarct zone of the original MI. This can manifest as an infarction that extends and involves the adjacent myocardium or as a subendocardial infarction that becomes transmural.

Reocclusion of an infarct-related artery (IRA) occurs in 5% to 30% of patients following fibrinolytic therapy. These patients also tend to have a poorer outcome.[1] Reinfarction is more common in patients with diabetes mellitus or prior MI.

Infarction in a separate territory (recurrent infarction) may be difficult to diagnose within the first 24 to 48 hours after the initial event. Multivessel coronary artery disease is common in patients with acute myocardial infarction. In fact, angiographic evidence of complex or ulcerated plaques in noninfarct-related arteries is present in up to 40% of patients with acute MI.

Angina that occurs from a few hours to 30 days after acute MI is defined as postinfarction angina. The incidence of postinfarction angina is highest in patients with non–ST-elevation MI (approximately 25%) and those treated with fibrinolytics compared with percutaneous coronary intervention (PCI).

Pathophysiology

Reinfarction occurs more often when the IRA reoccludes than when it remains patent; however, reocclusion of the IRA does not always cause reinfarction because of abundant collateral circulation. After fibrinolytic therapy, reocclusion is found on angiograms of 5% to 30% of patients and is associated with a worse outcome.

The pathophysiologic mechanism of postinfarction angina is similar to that of unstable angina and should be managed in a similar manner. Patients with postinfarction angina have a worse prognosis with regard to sudden death, reinfarction, and acute cardiac events.

Signs and Symptoms

Patients with infarct extension or postinfarction angina usually have continuous or recurrent chest pain, with protracted elevation in the creatine kinase (CK) level and, occasionally, new electrocardiographic changes.

Diagnostic Testing

The diagnosis of infarct expansion, reinfarction, or postinfarction ischemia can be made with echocardiography or nuclear imaging. A new wall motion abnormality, larger infarct size, new area of infarction, or persistent reversible ischemic changes help substantiate the diagnosis. CK-MB is a more useful marker for tracking ongoing infarction than troponin, given its shorter half-life. Re-elevation and subsequent decline in CK-MB levels suggest infarct expansion or recurrent infarction. Elevations in the CK-MB level of more than 50% over a previous nadir are diagnostic for reinfarction.

Treatment

Medical therapy with aspirin, heparin, nitrates, and beta blockers is indicated in patients who have had a myocardial infarction and have ongoing ischemic symptoms. An intra-aortic balloon pump (IABP) should be inserted promptly in patients with hemodynamic instability or severe LV systolic dysfunction. However, it must be borne in mind that severe peripheral vascular disease (PVD) of the aortoiliac and femoral arteries is a contraindication to IABP placement, due to increased risk of lower extremity ischemia. IABP use is also contraindicated in patients with severe aortic valve insufficiency (AI), because their AI will be worsened by the balloon pump. Coronary angiography should be performed in patients who are stabilized with medical therapy, but emergency angiography may be undertaken in unstable patients. Revascularization, percutaneous or surgical, is associated with improved prognosis.

MECHANICAL COMPLICATIONS

Mechanical complications of acute MI include ventricular septal defect, papillary muscle rupture or dysfunction, cardiac free wall rupture, ventricular aneurysm, LV failure with cardiogenic shock, dynamic LV outflow tract (LVOT) obstruction, and right ventricular (RV) failure.

Ventricular Septal Defect

Independent predictors of ventricular septal defect (VSD) are shown in Box 1.

Prevalence

VSD formerly occurred in 1% to 2% of patients after acute MI in the prethrombolytic era (Figs. 1 and 2). The incidence has dramatically decreased with reperfusion therapy.[2] The GUSTO-I (Global Utilization of Streptokinase and Tissue Plasminogen Activator for Occluded Coronary Arteries) trial has demonstrated an incidence of VSD of approximately 0.2%.[3,4]

VSD can develop as early as 24 hours after MI but was commonly seen 3 to 7 days after MI in the prefibrinolytic era and 2 to 5 days currently. Fibrinolytic therapy is not associated with an increased risk of VSD.[2,5]

Pathophysiology

The defect usually occurs at the junction of preserved and infarcted myocardium in the apical septum with anterior MI and in the basal posterior septum with inferior MI. VSD almost always occurs in the setting of a transmural MI and is more often seen in anterolateral MIs. The defect might not always be a single large defect; it can be a

Table 1 Complications of Acute Myocardial Infarction

Complication Type	Manifestations
Ischemic	Angina, reinfarction, infarct extension
Mechanical	Heart failure, cardiogenic shock, mitral valve dysfunction, aneurysms, cardiac rupture
Arrhythmic	Atrial or ventricular arrhythmias, sinus or atrioventricular node dysfunction
Embolic	Central nervous system or peripheral embolization
Inflammatory	Pericarditis

Box 1 Independent Predictors of Ventricular Septal Defect

Older age
Female gender
Nonsmoking status
Anterior infarct
Worse Killip class on admission
Increasing heart rate on admission

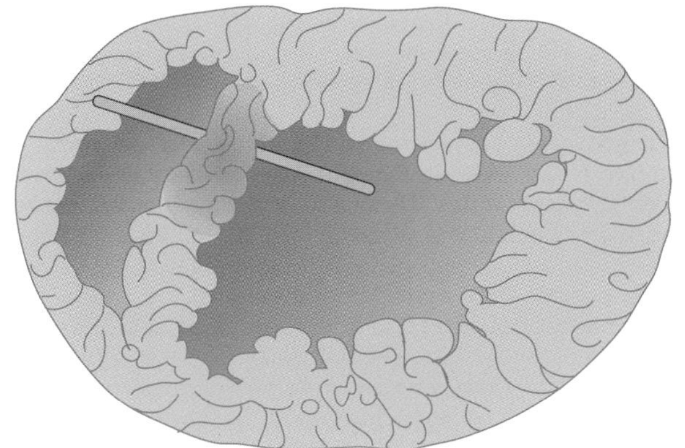

Figure 1 Ventricular septal defect occurred in 1% to 2% of patients after acute myocardial infarction in the prethrombolytic era.

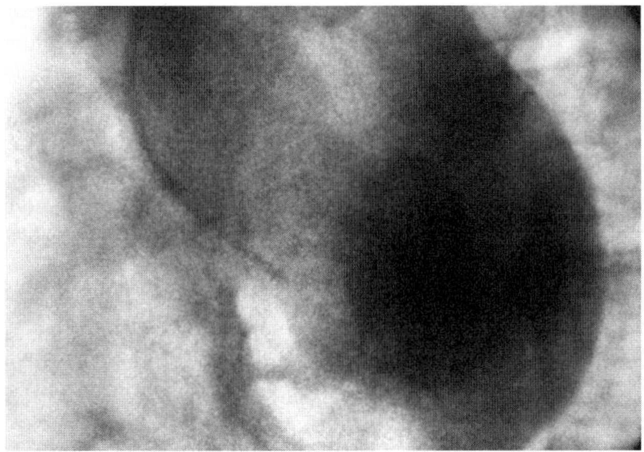

Figure 2 Ventricular septal defect can be seen on this left ventriculogram (left anterior oblique projection).

meshwork of serpiginous channels that can be identified in 30% to 40% of patients.

Signs and Symptoms

Early in the disease process, patients with VSD may appear relatively comfortable, with no clinically significant cardiopulmonary symptoms. Rapid recurrence of angina, hypotension, shock, or pulmonary edema can develop later in the course.

Diagnosis

Rupture of the ventricular septum is often accompanied by a new harsh holosystolic murmur best heard at the left lower sternal border. The murmur is accompanied by a thrill in 50% of cases. This sign is generally accompanied by a worsening hemodynamic profile and biventricular failure. Therefore, it is important that all patients with MI have a well-documented cardiac examination at presentation and daily thereafter.

An electrocardiogram (ECG) may show atrioventricular (AV) nodal or infranodal conduction delay abnormalities in approximately 40% of patients. Echocardiography with color flow imaging is the best method for diagnosing VSD. There are two types of VSD, which can best be visualized in different echocardiographic planes. A posterobasal VSD is best visualized in the parasternal long axis with medial angulation, apical long axis, and subcostal long axis. An apical-septal VSD is best visualized in the apical four-chamber view. Echocardiography can define LV and RV function—important determinants of mortality—as well as the size of the defect and degree of left-to-right shunt by assessing flow through the pulmonary and aortic valves. In some cases, it may be necessary to use transesophageal echocardiography to assess the VSD.

VSD can also be diagnosed by demonstrating an increase in oxygen saturation in the right ventricle and pulmonary artery (PA) on PA catheterization. The location of the increase is significant, because there have been case reports of peripheral PA increases due to acute MR. Diagnosis involves fluoroscopically guided measurement of oxygen saturation in the superior and inferior vena cava, right atrium, right ventricle, and pulmonary artery. An increase in oxygen saturation of more than 8% occurs between the right atrium and right ventricle and pulmonary artery, with a left-to-right shunt across the ventricular septum. A shunt fraction can be calculated as follows:

$$\dot{Q}_p/\dot{Q}_s = (Sao_2 - Mvo_2)/(Pvo_2 - Pao_2)$$

where $\dot{Q}_p$ is the pulmonary flow, $\dot{Q}_s$ is the systemic flow, Sao_2 is the arterial oxygen saturation, Mvo_2 is the mixed venous oxygen saturation, Pvo_2 is the pulmonary venous oxygen saturation, and Pao_2 is the pulmonary arterial oxygen saturation. A calculated $\dot{Q}_p/\dot{Q}_s > 2$ suggests a large shunt, which is likely to be poorly tolerated by the patient.

Treatment

Early surgical closure is the treatment of choice, even if the patient's condition is stable. Initial reports have suggested that delaying surgery is likely to result in improved surgical mortality.[6] These benefits were probably the result of selection bias,[7] because the mortality rate in patients with VSD treated medically is 24% at 72 hours and 75% at 3 weeks. Therefore, patients should be considered for urgent surgical repair.

A high surgical mortality is associated with cardiogenic shock and multisystem failure. This further supports earlier operation before complications develop.[8] Mortality is highest in patients with basal septal rupture associated with inferior MI (70%, compared with 30% in patients with anterior infarcts). The mortality rate is higher because of increased technical difficulty and the frequent need for mitral valve repair or replacement in the patients with mitral regur-

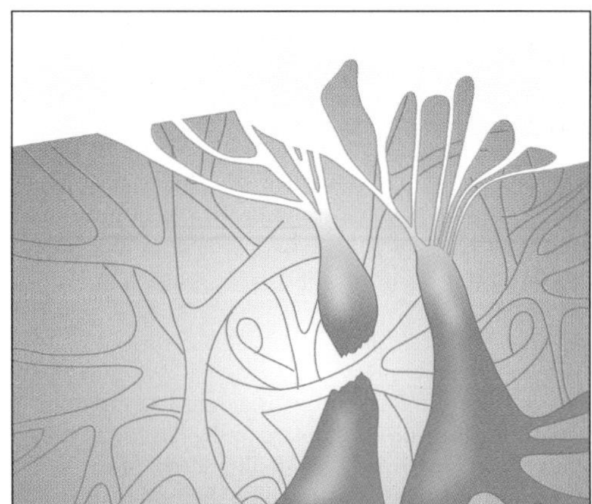

Figure 3 Most mitral regurgitation is transient in duration and asymptomatic. However, mitral regurgitation caused by papillary muscle rupture is a life-threatening complication of acute myocardial infarction.

gitation.[9] Regardless of the location and patient's hemodynamic condition, surgery should always be considered, because it is associated with a lower mortality rate than conservative management.[10]

Intensive medical management should be started to support the patient before surgery. Unless there is significant aortic regurgitation, an IABP should be inserted urgently as a bridge to a surgical procedure. The IABP will decrease the systemic vascular resistance (SVR) and shunt fraction while increasing coronary perfusion and maintaining blood pressure. After the IABP is inserted, vasodilators can be used, with close hemodynamic monitoring. Vasodilators can also reduce left-to-right shunting and increase systemic flow by reducing SVR. Caution should be exercised to avoid a greater decrease in pulmonary vascular resistance than in SVR and a consequent increase in shunting. The vasodilator of choice is intravenous nitroprusside, which is started at 0.5 to 1.0 μg/kg/min and titrated to a mean arterial pressure (MAP) of 60 to 75 mm Hg.

Mitral Regurgitation

Prevalence

Mitral regurgitation (MR) after acute MI predicts poor prognosis, as demonstrated in the GUSTO-I trial. MR of mild to moderate severity is found in 13% to 45% patients following acute MI.[11-14] Whereas most MR is transient in duration and asymptomatic, MR caused by papillary muscle rupture (Fig. 3) is a life-threatening complication of acute MI. Fibrinolytic agents decrease the incidence of rupture; however, when present, rupture can occur earlier in the post-MI period than in the absence of reperfusion. Although papillary muscle rupture was reported to occur between days 2 and 7 in the prefibrinolytic era, the SHOCK (SHould we emergently revascularize Occluded Coronaries in cardiogenic shocK?) Trial Registry demonstrated a median time to papillary muscle rupture of 13 hours.[15] Papillary muscle rupture is found in 7% of patients in cardiogenic shock and contributes to 5% of the mortality after acute MI.[16,17]

Pathophysiology

Mitral regurgitation can occur as a result of a number of mechanisms, including mitral valve annular dilatation secondary to LV dilatation, papillary muscle dysfunction with associated ischemic regional wall motion abnormality in close proximity to the insertion of the posterior papillary muscle, and partial or complete rupture of the chordae or papillary muscle.[16]

Papillary muscle rupture is most common with an inferior MI. The posteromedial papillary muscle is most often involved because of its single blood supply through the posterior descending coronary artery.[18] The anterolateral papillary muscle has a dual blood supply, being perfused by the left anterior descending (LAD) and left circumflex coronary arteries. In 50% of patients with papillary muscle rupture, the infarct is relatively small.

Signs and Symptoms

Complete transection of the papillary muscles is rare and usually results in immediate pulmonary edema, cardiogenic shock, and death. Physical examination demonstrates a new pansystolic murmur, which is audible at the cardiac apex and radiates to the axilla or the base of the heart. If there is a posterior papillary muscle rupture, the murmur radiates to the left sternal border and may be confused with the murmur of VSD or aortic stenosis (intensity of the murmur does not always predict the severity of MR). In patients with severe heart failure, poor cardiac output, or elevated left atrial pressures, the murmur may be soft or absent.

Diagnostic Testing

The ECG usually shows evidence of a recent inferior or posterior MI. The chest radiograph shows evidence of pulmonary edema. Focal pulmonary edema can occur in the right upper lobe when flow is directed at the right pulmonary veins.

The diagnostic test of choice is two-dimensional echocardiography with Doppler and color flow imaging. In severe MR, the mitral valve leaflet is usually flail. Color flow imaging can be useful in distinguishing papillary muscle rupture with severe MR from VSD. Transthoracic echocardiography might not fully appreciate the amount of MR in some patients with posteriorly directed jets. In these patients, transesophageal echocardiography (TEE) may be particularly useful.

Hemodynamic monitoring with a PA catheter can reveal large (>50 mm Hg) V waves in the pulmonary capillary wedge pressure (PCWP). Patients with VSD can also have large V waves as a result of augmented pulmonary venous return in a left atrium of normal size and decreased compliance. Further complicating the diagnostic picture, patients with severe MR and reflected V waves in the PA tracing may have an increase in oxygen saturation in the PA.[19] Mitral regurgitation can be distinguished from VSD with a Swan-Ganz catheter by two characteristics. First, prominent V waves in the PCWP tracing preceding the incisura on the PA tracing are almost always secondary to severe MR. Second, blood for oximetry should be obtained with fluoroscopic control from the central PA rather than from more distal branches to identify a significant increase in oxygen content associated with VSD.

Treatment

Patients with papillary muscle rupture should be rapidly identified and receive aggressive medical treatment while being considered for surgery. Medical therapy includes vasodilator therapy. Nitroprusside is useful in the treatment of patients with acute MR. Nitroprusside directly decreases SVR, thereby reducing the regurgitant fraction and increasing the forward stroke volume and cardiac output. Nitroprusside can be started at 0.5 to 1.0 μg/kg/min and titrated to a MAP of 60 to 75 mm Hg. An IABP should be inserted to decrease LV afterload, improve coronary perfusion, and increase forward cardiac output. Patients with hypotension might tolerate vasodilators after an IABP is inserted.

Patients with papillary muscle rupture should be considered for emergency surgery, because the prognosis is dismal in medically treated patients. Coronary angiography should be performed before surgical repair, because revascularization during MVR is associated with improved short-term and long-term mortality.[17,20] Additional surgical candidates include patients with moderate MR who do not improve with afterload reduction.

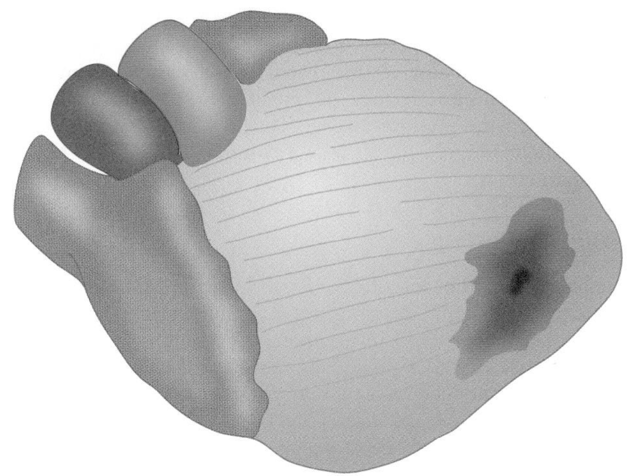

Figure 4 Free wall rupture occurs in 3% of myocardial infarction (MI) patients and accounts for approximately 10% of mortality after MI.

Free Wall Rupture

Prevalence

Free wall rupture occurs in 3% of MI patients and accounts for approximately 10% of mortality after MI (Fig. 4). The timing of cardiac rupture is within 5 days in 50% of patients and within 2 weeks of MI in 90% of patients. Free wall rupture occurs only among patients with transmural MI. Risk factors include advanced age, female gender, hypertension, first MI, and poor coronary collateral vessels.

Pathophysiology

Free wall rupture accounts for part of the early hazard in patients treated with fibrinolytic agents. The overall incidence of free wall rupture is not higher in patients treated with fibrinolytics, however.[21-23] Although any wall can be involved, cardiac rupture most commonly occurs at the lateral wall.

Free wall rupture occurs at three distinct intervals, with three distinct pathologic subsets. Type I increases with the use of fibrinolytics. It occurs early (within the first 24 hours) and is a full-thickness rupture. Type II rupture occurs 1 to 3 days after MI and is a result of erosion of the myocardium at the site of infarction. Type III rupture occurs late and is located at the border zone of the infarction and normal myocardium.

The reduction in type III ruptures as a result of the advent of fibrinolytics has resulted in no change in the overall free wall rupture rate. It has been postulated that type III ruptures can occur as a result of dynamic LVOT obstruction and the resultant increased wall stress.[24]

Signs and Symptoms

Sudden onset of chest pain with straining or coughing can suggest the onset of myocardial rupture. Acute rupture patients often have electromechanical dissociation and sudden death. Other patients may have a more subacute course as a result of a contained rupture, or pseudoaneurysm. They might complain of pain consistent with pericarditis, nausea, and hypotension. In a study evaluating 1457 patients with acute MI, 6.2% of patients had free wall rupture. Approximately one third of these patients presented with a subacute course.[22]

Jugular venous distention, pulsus paradoxus, diminished heart sounds, and a pericardial rub suggest subacute rupture. New to-and-fro murmurs may be heard in patients with subacute rupture or pseudoaneurysm. A junctional or idioventricular rhythm, low-voltage complexes, and tall precordial T waves may be evident on the ECG. Additionally, a large number of patients have transient bradycardia just before rupture, as well as other manifestations of increased vagal tone.

Diagnostic Testing

Although there is generally insufficient time for thorough diagnostic testing in the management of patients with acute rupture, transthoracic echocardiography is the urgent test of choice. Echocardiography demonstrates a pericardial effusion with findings of cardiac tamponade. These findings include right atrial (RA) and RV diastolic collapse, dilated inferior vena cava, and marked respiratory variations in mitral and tricuspid inflow. Additionally, a Swan-Ganz pulmonary artery catheter may reveal hemodynamic signs of tamponade, with equalization of the RA, RV diastolic, and pulmonary capillary wedge pressures.

Treatment

The goal of therapy is to diagnose the problem and perform early emergency open heart surgery to correct the rupture. Emergency pericardiocentesis may be performed immediately on patients with tamponade and severe hemodynamic compromise while arrangements are being made for transport to the hospital. The procedure may be dangerous because of reopening of communication with the pericardium as the intrapericardial pressure is relieved. Medical management has no role in the treatment of these patients, except for the use of vasopressors to maintain blood pressure temporarily as the patient is rushed to the operating room.

Pseudoaneurysm

Pathophysiology

Pseudoaneurysm is caused by contained rupture of the LV free wall. The aneurysm may remain small or undergo progressive enlargement. The outer wall is formed by the pericardium and mural thrombus. The pseudoaneurysm communicates with the body of the left ventricle through a narrow neck whose diameter is by definition less than 50% of the diameter of the fundus.

Signs and Symptoms

Some pseudoaneurysms remain clinically silent and are discovered during routine investigations. However, some patients have recurrent tachyarrhythmia, systemic embolization, and heart failure. Some patients have systolic, diastolic, or to-and-fro murmurs related to the flow of blood across the narrow neck of the pseudoaneurysm during LV systole and diastole. A chest radiograph may show cardiomegaly, with an abnormal bulge on the cardiac border. There may by persistent ST-segment elevation on the ECG. The diagnosis may be confirmed by echocardiography, magnetic resonance imaging (MRI), or computed tomography.

Treatment

Spontaneous rupture occurs without warning in approximately one third of patients with a pseudoaneurysm. Therefore, surgical intervention is recommended for all patients, regardless of symptoms or the size of the aneurysm, to prevent sudden death.

Left Ventricular Failure and Cardiogenic Shock

Prevalence

Some degree of LV dysfunction is to be anticipated after an acute MI. The degree of dysfunction correlates with the extent and location of myocardial injury. Patients with small, more distal infarctions may

Table 2 Incidence of Heart Failure in Acute Myocardial Infarction

Killip Class	Characteristics	Patients (%)
I	No evidence of congestive heart failure	85
II	Rales, ↑jugular venous distention, or S_3	13
III	Pulmonary edema	1
IV	Cardiogenic shock	1

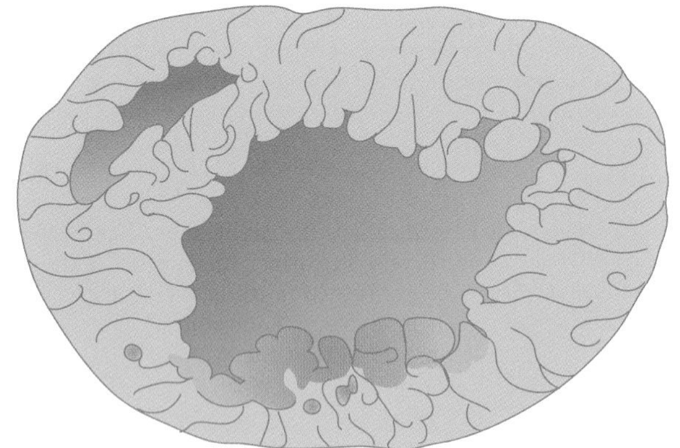

Figure 5 In patients with prior myocardial infarctions and depressed left ventricular function, a smaller acute insult can result in cardiogenic shock.

have discrete regional wall motion abnormalities with preserved overall LV function because of compensatory hyperkinesis of the unaffected segments.[25] Prior MI, older age, female gender, diabetes, and anterior infarction are risk factors for development of cardiogenic shock.[26,27]

Killip and Kimball[28] have developed a classification scheme to categorize patients' prognosis based on their hemodynamic profile. Patients were classified into four hemodynamic subsets, from no evidence of congestive heart failure (CHF) to cardiogenic shock (Table 2). The authors reported an 81% mortality rate in patients presenting in cardiogenic shock.

Forrester and collleagues[29,30] classified patients by their hemodynamic profile with a pulmonary artery catheter using PCWP and cardiac index. They reported a 50% mortality rate in the most compromised subset (PCWP >18 mm Hg; cardiac index <2.2 L/min/m^2). Results of the GUSTO-I trial have indicated that 7% to 8% of patients develop cardiogenic shock clinically. Fibrinolysis did not materially affect mortality, which remains high at 58%.[31,32]

Pathophysiology

Patients can develop cardiogenic shock in association with an acute MI of multiple causes, including large LV infarction, severe RV infarction, VSD, free wall rupture, acute mitral regurgitation, or pharmacologic depression of LV function (beta blockers in proximal left anterior descending MI). Patients who have cardiogenic shock as a result of acute MI typically have severe multivessel disease, with significant involvement of the LAD artery.[33,34] Generally, at least 40% of the LV mass is affected in patients who present in cardiogenic shock as a result of a first MI.[35,36] In patients with prior MIs and depressed LV function, a smaller acute insult can result in cardiogenic shock (Fig. 5).

Signs and Symptoms

Patients who present in Killip class III often have respiratory distress, diaphoresis, and cool, clammy extremities in addition to the typical signs and symptoms of acute MI. Patients in Killip class IV (cardiogenic shock) can have severe orthopnea, dyspnea, and oliguria and may have altered mental status, as well as multisystem organ failure from hypoperfusion. It may be possible to palpate an area of dyskinesia on the precordium. An S_3 gallop, pulmonary rales, and elevated jugular venous pressure are common findings on physical examination.

Diagnostic Testing

Patients with cardiogenic shock caused by acute MI generally have extensive electrocardiographic changes demonstrating a large infarct, diffuse ischemia, or several prior infarcts. If these changes are absent, another cause of shock should be considered. Chest radiography reveals pulmonary edema. Laboratory tests may demonstrate lactic acidosis, renal failure, and arterial hypoxemia.

The patient in cardiogenic shock should be monitored with a pulmonary artery catheter and an arterial line. These can help distinguish between primary LV failure and other mechanical causes of cardiogenic shock (see earlier).

Transthoracic echocardiography helps determine the extent of dysfunctional myocardium. It also helps identify other mechanical complications of MI that may be contributing to cardiogenic shock.

Treatment

A patient in cardiogenic shock should have an IABP placed urgently to reduce afterload, improve cardiac output, and enhance coronary perfusion. Medical therapy with vasodilators (e.g., nitroglycerin, nitroprusside, and angiotensin-converting enzyme [ACE] inhibitors) and diuretics should be used as tolerated. Intravenous nitroglycerin is the first-line drug of choice among vasodilators because it is less likely to produce coronary steal than nitroprusside and protects against ischemia. The starting dose is 10 to 20 μg/min and it may be increased by 10 μg/min every 2 to 3 minutes to a goal MAP of 70 mm Hg. Intravenous nitroprusside can be added if further reduction in afterload is necessary. Nitroprusside is started at 0.5 to 1.0 μg/kg/min and is also titrated to a MAP of approximately 70 mm Hg. Patients with low blood pressures (MAP <70 mm Hg) might not tolerate vasodilators.

ACE inhibitors improve LV performance and decrease myocardial oxygen consumption by reducing the cardiac preload and afterload of patients with heart failure and acute MI. ACE inhibitors can reduce infarct expansion if started in the first 12 hours of an MI if the patient is not already in cardiogenic shock. It is recommended that captopril be started early, at 6.25 mg every 8 hours, with each dose subsequently doubled as tolerated to a maximum dose of 50 mg every 8 hours. Patients with mild pulmonary edema can be treated with diuretics such as IV furosemide, adjusted for creatinine and history of diuretic use. β-Adrenergic agonists such as dobutamine or dopamine may be needed for patients with severe heart failure and cardiogenic shock. This therapy should generally be reserved for those who have failed IABP and maximal vasodilator therapy or for those with a RV infarct. Phosphodiesterase inhibitors such as milrinone may be beneficial for some patients. The bolus may be omitted in patients with marginal blood pressures. Patients without adequate MAP might not tolerate milrinone. Some patients may need norepinephrine to maintain arterial pressure. Norepinephrine is started at 2 μg/min and titrated to maintain the MAP at approximately 70 mm Hg.

PCI or emergency coronary bypass surgery has been associated with an improved prognosis in patients in cardiogenic shock, reducing the mortality rate from 80% to 50%. Multivessel revascularization should be attempted in shock patients.[10]

Emergency surgical revascularization is indicated for patients with severe multivessel disease or substantial left main coronary artery stenosis. Other surgical modalities that may be considered include LV or biventricular assist devices or extracorporeal mem-

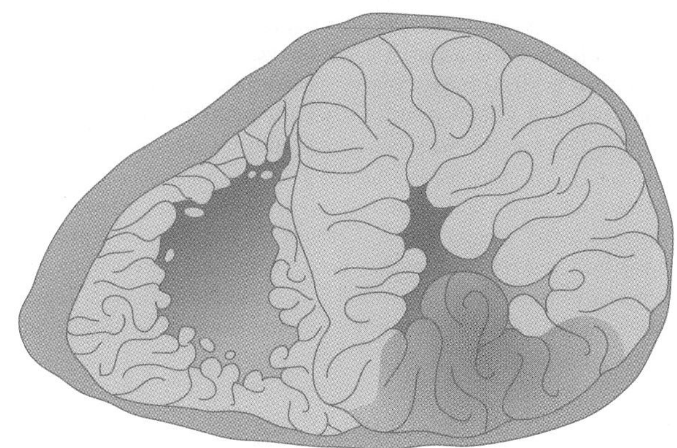

Figure 6 Mild right ventricular (RV) dysfunction is common (approximately 40%) after myocardial infarction (MI) of the inferior or inferoposterior wall. However, hemodynamically significant RV impairment occurs in only 10% of patients with inferior or inferoposterior wall MI.

brane oxygenation as a bridge to heart transplantation. Some patients may be gradually weaned from assist devices after the stunned portion of myocardium recovers, without the need for cardiac transplantation.

Right Ventricular Failure

Prevalence

Mild RV dysfunction is common (approximately 40%) after MI of the inferior or inferoposterior wall; however, hemodynamically significant RV impairment occurs in only 10% of patients with inferior or inferoposterior wall MI (Fig. 6).

Pathophysiology

The degree of RV dysfunction depends on the location of the right coronary artery (RCA) occlusion. Only proximal occlusions (proximal to the acute marginal branch) of the RCA result in marked dysfunction.[37] The degree of RV involvement also depends on the amount of collateral flow from the LAD and the degree of blood flow through the thebesian veins. Because the right ventricle is thin-walled and has lower oxygen demand, there is coronary perfusion during the entire cardiac cycle; therefore, widespread irreversible infarction is rare.

Signs and Symptoms

The triad of hypotension, jugular venous distention with clear lungs, and absence of dyspnea has high specificity but low sensitivity for RV infarction.[38] Severe RV failure can manifest with symptoms of a low cardiac output state, including diaphoresis, cool clammy extremities, and altered mental status. Patients often have oliguria and hypotension. Other causes of severe hypotension in the setting of an inferior MI include bradyarrhythmia, acute severe mitral regurgitation, and VSD.

Patients with isolated RV failure have elevated jugular venous pressure and RV S_3 heart sound in the setting of a normal lung examination. The presence of jugular venous pressure greater than 8 cm H_2O and Kussmaul's sign is highly sensitive and specific for severe RV failure. A rare but clinically important complication of RV infarction is right-to-left shunting secondary to increased pressures in the RA and RV and opening of the foramen ovale. This should be considered in patients with RV infarction and hypoxemia.

Electrocardiographically, patients present with inferior ST elevation in conjunction with ST elevation in the V_4R lead. These findings have a positive predictive value of 80% for RV infarction.[39] The chest radiograph is usually normal.

Diagnostic Testing

Echocardiography is the diagnostic study of choice for RV infarction. It will demonstrate RV dilation and dysfunction and usually LV inferior wall dysfunction. It is also helpful in excluding cardiac tamponade, which can mimic RV infarction hemodynamically. The hemodynamic profile of acute RV infarct can also be diagnostic of an acute pulmonary embolism in the absence of an ischemic event.

Hemodynamic monitoring with a pulmonary artery catheter reveals high right atrial pressures with a low PCWP, unless severe LV dysfunction is also present, because RV failure results in underfilling of the left ventricle and a low cardiac output. In some patients, RV dilatation can cause decreased LV performance on the basis of flattening or bowing of the septum into the left ventricle and restriction of ventricular filling, with elevation of the PCWP. A right atrial pressure of higher than 10 mm Hg and a right atrial pressure-to-PCWP ratio of 0.8 or greater strongly suggest RV infarction.[40]

Treatment

Volume loading to increase LV preload and cardiac output is key to the management of RV infarction. Some patients require several liters in 1 hour to reach a target PCWP of 15 mm Hg. It is important to have hemodynamic monitoring with a pulmonary artery catheter in these patients, because overzealous fluid administration can further decrease LV output. This occurs as a result of septal shift toward the left ventricle and an intrapericardial pressure shift. The target central venous pressure for fluid administration is approximately 15 mm Hg. When volume loading is insufficient to improve cardiac output, inotropes are indicated. Administration of dobutamine increases cardiac index, improves RV ejection fraction, and is better than afterload reduction with nitroprusside.[1]

Patients may benefit from reperfusion therapy, because patients who undergo successful reperfusion of RV branches have enhanced RV function and a lower 30-day mortality rate.[41,42] Patients with RV infarction and bradyarrhythmias or loss of sinus rhythm may have significant improvement with AV sequential pacing. Optimal pacer settings tend to be longer AV delays (approximately 200 msec) and a heart rate of 80 to 90 beats per minute.

Although there have only been case reports of IABP improving the cardiac index (CI) in combination with dobutamine, an IABP may be useful, even though it acts primarily on the left ventricle. Pericardiectomy may be considered for patients with refractory shock because it reverses the septal impingement on LV filling. Most patients with RV infarction improve after 48 to 72 hours. An RV assist device is indicated for patients who remain in cardiogenic shock in spite of these measures.

Ventricular Aneurysm

Prevalence

Patients with apical transmural MIs are at higher risk for aneurysmal formation, followed by those with posterior-basal infarcts. Patients who do not receive reperfusion therapy are at greatest risk for developing this complication (10%-30%).

Pathophysiology

The early open artery hypothesis states that early reperfusion results in improved myocardial salvage and prevents infarct expansion. Even late reperfusion limits infarct expansion through a number of mechanisms, including immediate change in infarction characteristics, preservation of small amounts of residual myofibrils and interstitial collagen, accelerated healing, the scaffold effect of a blood-filled

Table 3 Differences Between True and False Ventricular Aneurysms

Parameter	True Aneurysm	False Aneurysm
Cause	Infarction	Rupture
Incidence	1%-5%	Rare
Neck	Wide	Narrow
Wall	All three layers—scar	Pericardium and thrombus
Rupture	Very rare	Common

vasculature, and elimination of ischemia in viable but dysfunctional myocardium. Infarct expansion and progressive LV dilation are associated with persistent occlusion of an IRA. The aneurysm consists of a stretched portion of the myocardium, containing all three layers and connected to the ventricle by a wide neck. The differences between a pseudoaneurysm (false aneurysm) and true aneurysm are highlighted in Table 3.

Signs and Symptoms

Congestive heart failure and even cardiogenic shock can develop as a result of a large LV aneurysm. Because acute aneurysms expand during systole, contractile energy generated by a normal myocardium is wasted and puts the entire ventricle at a mechanical disadvantage. Chronic aneurysms persist for more than 6 weeks after the acute event and are less compliant than acute aneurysms and less likely to expand during systole. Patients with chronic aneurysms may have heart failure, ventricular arrhythmias, and systemic embolization, or they may be asymptomatic. Palpation of the precordium can reveal a dyskinetic segment of the ventricle. An S_3 gallop may be heard in patients with poor ventricular function.

Diagnostic Testing

Typical electrocardiographic findings include ST elevation, which can persist despite application of reperfusion therapy and Q waves. When electrocardiographic changes (ST elevation) persist for more than 6 weeks, patients might have a chronic ventricular aneurysm. A chest radiograph may reveal a localized bulge in the cardiac silhouette. Echocardiography is the gold standard and accurately identifies the aneurysmal segment. It may also demonstrate the presence of a mural thrombus. Additionally, echocardiography is useful in differentiating true aneurysms from pseudoaneurysms. MRI may also be useful and diagnostic for delineating the aneurysmal section.

Treatment

Congestive heart failure with acute aneurysms is managed with IV vasodilators. ACE inhibitors have been shown to reduce infarct expansion and unfavorable LV remodeling. ACE inhibitors are best started within the first 12 to 24 hours of onset of acute MI, because infarct expansion starts early. Corticosteroids and nonsteroidal anti-inflammatory drugs (NSAIDs) should be avoided in the acute setting because they have been shown to induce infarct expansion and aneurysm formation in experimental models. Heart failure with chronic aneurysms can be managed with ACE inhibitors, digoxin, and diuretics.

Anticoagulation with warfarin sodium is indicated for patients with a mural thrombus. Patients should be treated initially with IV heparin, with a target partial thromboplastin time (PTT) of 50 to 70 seconds. Warfarin is started simultaneously. Patients should be treated with warfarin at a target international normalized ratio (INR) of 2 to 3 for 3 to 6 months. It is controversial whether patients who have large aneurysms without thrombus should receive anticoagulants. Many clinicians prescribe anticoagulants for 6 to 12 weeks after the acute phase. Patients with LV aneurysms and a low global ejection fraction (<40%) have a higher stroke rate and should take anticoagulants for at least 3 months after the acute event. They may be subsequently observed with echocardiography. Anticoagulation may be reinitiated if a new thrombus develops.

Refractory heart failure or refractory ventricular arrhythmias in patients with aneurysms is an indication for surgical resection. Surgical resection may be followed by conventional closure or newer techniques to maintain LV geometry. Revascularization is beneficial for patients with a large amount of viable myocardium around the aneurysmal segment.

Dynamic Left Ventricular Outflow Tract Obstruction

Prevalence

Dynamic LVOT obstruction is an uncommon complication of acute anterior MI and was first described in a case report by Bartunek and associates.[43]

Pathophysiology

This event is dependent on compensatory hyperkinesis of the basal and midsegments of the left ventricle in patients with distal infarcts. Predictors of enhanced regional wall motion in noninfarct zones are the absence of multivessel disease, female gender, and higher flow in the infarct-related vessel. The increased contractile force of these regions decreases the cross-sectional area of the LVOT. The resulting increased velocity of blood through the outflow tract can produce decreased pressure below the mitral valve and result in the leaflet's being displaced anteriorly toward the septum (Venturi effect). This results in further LVOT obstruction and in mitral regurgitation resulting from systolic anterior motion (SAM) of the anterior mitral valve leaflet.

It has been postulated that this complication can play a role in free wall rupture. LVOT obstruction leads to increased end-systolic intraventricular pressure. This in turn leads to increased wall stress of the weakened, necrotic, infarcted zone. This fatal complication occurs most often in women, in older patients (older than 70 years), and in persons without prior MI.

Signs and Symptoms

Patients may have respiratory distress, diaphoresis, and cool, clammy extremities in addition to the typical signs and symptoms of acute MI. Patients with severe obstruction might appear to be in cardiogenic shock with severe orthopnea, dyspnea, and oliguria and may have altered mental status from cerebral hypoperfusion. Patients present with a new systolic ejection murmur heard best at the left upper sternal border, with radiation to the neck. Additionally, a new holosystolic murmur can be heard at the apex, with radiation to the axilla as a result of systolic anterior motion of the mitral leaflet. An S_3 gallop, pulmonary rales, hypotension, and tachycardia can also be present.

Diagnostic Testing

Echocardiography is the diagnostic test of choice and accurately depicts the hyperkinetic segment, the LVOT obstruction, and mitral leaflet SAM.

Treatment

Treatment centers on decreasing myocardial contractility and heart rate while expanding intravascular volume and increasing afterload (modestly). Beta blockers should be added slowly and with careful monitoring of heart rate, blood pressure, and Svo_2. Patients can receive gentle IV hydration with several small (250 mL) aliquots of saline to increase preload and decrease LVOT obstruction and SAM. The patient's hemodynamic and respiratory status should be monitored closely during this therapeutic intervention with a pulmonary artery catheter. Vasodilators, inotropes, and IABP should be avoided because they can increase LVOT obstruction.

Arrhythmic Complications

Ventricular arrhythmia is a common complication of acute MI, occurring in almost all patients, even before monitoring is possible. It is related to the formation of re-entry circuits at the confluence of the necrotic and viable myocardium.

Premature ventricular contractions (PVCs) occur in approximately 90% of patients. The incidence of ventricular fibrillation is approximately 2% to 4%. Although lidocaine has been demonstrated to reduce the rate of primary ventricular fibrillation in patients with MI to some extent, there is no survival benefit and there may be excess mortality. Therefore, it is not recommended that patients receive prophylactic therapy.[44] Amiodarone may be used in patients with MI and frequent PVCs, in patients with nonsustained ventricular tachycardia after MI, or after defibrillation for ventricular fibrillation. The recommended dosing is a bolus of 150 mg and then administration of 1 mg/min for 6 hours, followed by 0.5 mg/min. When starting this medication for ventricular fibrillation or pulseless ventricular tachycardia (VT), the bolus should be increased to 300 mg (the 150-mg bolus can be repeated in 10 minutes). Ventricular arrhythmias not responding to amiodarone may be treated with lidocaine (1-mg/kg bolus to a maximum of 100 mg, followed by a 1- to 4-mg/min drip)[45] or procainamide. Polymorphic VT is a rare complication of acute MI and can be treated with amiodarone, lidocaine, or procainamide, or a combination, as described for monomorphic VT. It is usually associated with recurrent ischemia.

The importance of ventricular fibrillation in the setting of MI has been re-evaluated in the context of the interaction between severe systolic dysfunction and the potential for sudden cardiac death. Implantable defibrillators have been shown to reduce mortality in post-MI patients with an ejection fraction (EF) lower than 30%, regardless of the presence of ventricular dysrhythmia.[45]

Supraventricular arrhythmias occur in less than 10% of patients with acute MI. Because patients who develop these arrhythmias tend to have more-severe ventricular dysfunction, they have a worse outcome. Although isolated right atrial infarction or small inferior infarcts leading to atrial arrhythmias are not associated with higher mortality rates, the appearance of atrial arrhythmias usually heralds the onset of heart failure in the setting of acute MI.

Bradyarrhythmias, including AV block and sinus bradycardia, occur most commonly with inferior MI. Complete AV block occurs in approximately 20% of patients with acute RV infarction. Infranodal conduction disturbances with wide complex ventricular escape rhythms occur most often in large anterior MIs and portend a very poor prognosis.

Temporary transvenous pacing is indicated in patients who present with asystole, Mobitz type 2 second-degree AV block, or complete AV block. Consideration for transvenous pacing should be given to patients with bifascicular or trifascicular block in the setting of acute MI.[46] Pacing is not indicated for the patient in sinus bradycardia or AV dissociation with a slow sinus rate and a more rapid ventricular escape rhythm as long as the patient is maintaining adequate hemodynamics. If mild symptoms exist, the initial treatment for these rhythm disturbances is IV atropine, 0.5 to 1.0 mg. This may be repeated every 5 minutes, to a maximum dose of 2 mg.

Embolic Complications

Prevalence

The incidence of clinically evident systemic embolism after MI is less than 2%. The incidence increases in patients with anterior wall MI. The overall incidence of mural thrombus after MI is approximately 20%. Large anterior MI may be associated with mural thrombus in as many as 60% of patients.[47,48]

Pathophysiology

Most emboli arise from the left ventricle as a result of wall motion abnormalities or aneurysms. Atrial fibrillation in the setting of ischemia can also contribute to systemic embolization.

Signs and Symptoms

The most common clinical manifestation of embolic complications is stroke, although patients may have limb ischemia, renal infarction, or intestinal ischemia. Most episodes of systemic emboli occur in the first 10 days after acute MI. Physical findings vary with the site of the embolism. Focal neurologic deficits occur in patients with central nervous system emboli. Limb ischemia manifests with limb pain in a cold, pulseless extremity. Renal infarction manifests with flank pain and hematuria. Mesenteric ischemia manifests with abdominal pain out of proportion to physical findings and bloody diarrhea.

Treatment

IV heparin should be started immediately with a target PTT of 50 to 70 seconds and continued until the INR is in the therapeutic range. Warfarin sodium therapy should also be started immediately, with a goal INR of 2 to 3, and continued for at least 3 to 6 months for patients with mural thrombi and for those with large akinetic areas detected by echocardiography.

Pericarditis

Prevalence

The incidence of early pericarditis after acute MI is approximately 10%. The inflammation usually develops between 24 and 96 hours after MI.[50,51] Dressler's syndrome, or late pericarditis, occurs with an incidence between 1% and 3%, 1 to 8 weeks after MI.

Pathophysiology

The pathogenesis of acute pericarditis is an inflammatory reaction in response to necrotic tissue. Acute pericarditis thus develops more often in patients with transmural MI. The pathogenesis of Dressler's syndrome is unknown, but an autoimmune mechanism has been suggested.

Signs and Symptoms

Most patients with early pericarditis report no symptoms. Patients with symptoms from early or late pericarditis describe progressive, severe chest pain that lasts for hours. The symptoms are postural—worse in the supine position—and are alleviated by sitting up and leaning forward. The pain tends to be pleuritic in nature and is therefore exacerbated with deep inspiration, coughing, and swallowing. Radiation of pain to the trapezius ridge is almost pathognomonic for acute pericarditis. The pain also can radiate to the neck and, less commonly, to the arm or back.

A pericardial friction rub on examination is pathognomonic for acute pericarditis; however, it can be ephemeral. The rub is best heard at the left lower sternal edge with the diaphragm of the stethoscope. The rub has three components: atrial systole, ventricular systole, and ventricular diastole. In about 30% of patients, the rub is biphasic, and in 10% it is uniphasic. A pericardial effusion can cause fluctuation in the intensity of the rub.

Table 4 Electrocardiographic Changes of Pericarditis

Stage	Electrocardiographic Change
I	ST elevation, upright T waves
II	ST elevation resolves, upright to flat T waves
III	ST isoelectric, inverted T waves
IV	ST isoelectric, upright T waves

Evolving MI changes can mask the diagnosis of pericarditis. Pericarditis produces generalized ST-segment elevation, which is concave or saddle-shaped. As pericarditis evolves, T waves become inverted after the ST segment becomes isoelectric. Conversely, in acute MI, T waves can become inverted when the ST segment is still elevated. Four phases of electrocardiographic abnormalities have been described in association with pericarditis[51] (Table 4).

A pericardial effusion on echocardiography strongly suggests pericarditis, but the lack of an effusion does not rule out pericarditis.

Treatment

Aspirin is the therapy of choice for post-MI pericarditis, 650 mg every 4 to 6 hours. NSAIDs and corticosteroids should be avoided less than 4 weeks after the acute event. These agents can interfere with myocardial healing and contribute to expansion of the infarct. In late pericarditis, NSAIDs and even corticosteroids may be indicated if severe symptoms persist beyond 4 weeks after MI. Colchicine may be beneficial for patients with recurrent pericarditis.

Suggested Readings

Antman EM, Anbe DT, Armstrong PW, et al: American College of Cardiology/American Heart Association Task Force on Practice Guidelines (Writing Committee to Revise the 1999 Guidelines for the Management of Patients With Acute Myocardial Infarction): ACC/AHA guidelines for the management of patients with ST-elevation myocardial infarction-executive summary: A report of the American College of Cardiology/American Heart Association Task Force on Practice Guidelines (Writing Committee to Revise the 1999 Guidelines for the Management of Patients With Acute Myocardial Infarction). Circulation 2004;110:588-636.

Brouwer MA, van den Bergh PJ, Aengevaeren WR, et al: Aspirin plus coumarin versus aspirin alone in the prevention of reocclusion after fibrinolysis for acute myocardial infarction: Results of the Antithrombotics in the Prevention of Reocclusion In Coronary Thrombolysis (APRICOT)-2 Trial. Circulation 2002;106:659-665.

Bueno H, Martinez-Selles M, Perez-David E, et al: Effect of thrombolytic therapy on the risk of cardiac rupture and mortality in older patients with first acute myocardial infarction. Eur Heart J 2005;26:1705-1711.

Crenshaw BS, Granger CB, Birnbaum Y, et al: Risk factors, angiographic patterns, and outcomes in patients with ventricular septal defect complicating acute myocardial infarction. GUSTO-I (Global Utilization of Streptokinase and TPA for Occluded Coronary Arteries) Trial Investigators. Circulation 2000;101:27-32.

Dell'Italia LJ: Reperfusion for right ventricular infarction. N Engl J Med 1998;338:978-980.

Filsoufi F, Salzberg SP, Adams DH: Current management of ischemic mitral regurgitation. Mt Sinai J Med 2005;72:105-115.

Forrester JS, Diamond G, Chatterjee K, et al: Medical therapy of acute myocardial infarction by application of hemodynamic subsets (second of two parts). N Engl J Med 1976;295:1404-1413.

Hasdai D, Topol EJ, Kilaru R, et al: Frequency, patient characteristics, and outcomes of mild-to-moderate heart failure complicating ST-segment elevation acute myocardial infarction: Lessons from four international fibrinolytic therapy trials. Am Heart J Jan 2003;145:73-79.

Moss AJ, Zareba W, Hall WJ, et al: Prophylactic implantation of a defibrillator in patients with myocardial infarction and reduced ejection fraction. N Engl J Med 2002;346:877-883.

Thompson CR, Buller CE, Sleeper LA, et al: Cardiogenic shock due to acute severe mitral regurgitation complicating acute myocardial infarction: A report from the SHOCK Trial Registry. Should we use emergently revascularize occluded coronaries in cardiogenic shock? J Am Coll Cardiol 2000;36(Suppl A):1104-1109.

References

For a complete list of references, log onto www.expertconsult.com.

Lipid-Lowering Strategies and Reduction of Coronary Heart Disease Risk

Byron J. Hoogwerf and *Julie C. Huang*

Observational studies have shown a relation between dyslipidemia and coronary heart disease risk for several decades.[1-3] Intervention trial data over the past two or three decades have demonstrated that cholesterol modification, especially reduction in low-density lipoprotein cholesterol (LDL-C) levels, is associated with favorable effects on reduction in coronary heart disease (CHD) events (in many cases, stroke events), especially in patients at high risk for CHD.[4-26] Two major fibrate trials (Helsinki Heart Study [HHS] and the Veterans Affairs HDL Cholesterol Intervention Trial VA-HIT]) have shown reductions in CHD risk, and risk reduction is associated with favorable effects on the lipid profiles.[5,9-11] The Fenofibrate Intervention and Event Lowering in Diabetes (FIELD) trial in diabetic patients was confounded by a high percentage of statin drop-in.[27,28] Thus, the cholesterol-lowering guidelines have had LDL-C as the primary target for lipid modification.

In 1988, the first National Cholesterol Education Program (NCEP) was begun in an effort to establish targets for cholesterol levels based on assessments of risk.[29] (These guidelines were written by a panel of experts and, in subsequent publications, have been referred to as the Adult Treatment Panel [ATP], with Roman number specification for subsequent sets of guidelines—e.g., ATP II, ATP III). The NCEP guidelines were evidence based, used CHD risk assessment for the recommended LDL-C targets and were relatively simple for health care providers, patients, and payers to understand. Over the past two decades, the NCEP guidelines have changed in terms of lipid targets based on information obtained from clinical trials and observational studies.[30-35] These guidelines have been supported by other organizations, including the American Heart Association (AHA), American College of Cardiology (ACC), American Diabetes Association (ADA), American Association of Clinical Endocrinologists (AACE), and American College of Physicians (ACP).[36-41] Furthermore, nutrition studies and new medications (especially statin therapy) have become available, resulting in accumulating information on lipid-altering strategies.

This chapter reviews the history of the guidelines, how new information has resulted in changing targets, and current approaches to CHD risk assessment and gives a summary of approaches to lowering cholesterol.

HISTORY

The Lipid Research Clinic Coronary Primary Prevention Trial[20,21] was the first large-scale randomized, double-blind, placebo-controlled clinical trial of LDL-C lowering in high-risk men between the ages of 30 and 59. At baseline, LDL-C levels were typically in the 175- to 190-mg/dL range. LDL-C values in the cholestyramine-treated subjects approached the 130-mg/dL range. This trial was the underpinning for the first set of NCEP guidelines, which proposed that patients with and without CHD who had two or more risk factors for CHD have an LDL-C target of 130 mg/dL or lower. Lower risk patients with fewer risk factors had correspondingly higher LDL-C targets. The second set of NCEP guidelines came a few years later.[33] However, over the next decade, a number of clinical end point cholesterol trials in both high-risk primary prevention (no prior known CHD) and secondary prevention (with known CHD) were carried out across a wide range of entry LDL-C levels. Thus, in 2001, NCEP released the third set of guidelines.[34] This set of guidelines incorporated the results of randomized controlled clinical trials into recommendations for the management of high cholesterol levels. Since the publication of the ATP III, several additional five major clinical trials of statin (3-hydroxy-3-methylglutaryl coenzyme A [HMG-CoA] reductase inhibitor) cholesterol-lowering therapy have been published. Consequently, in 2004, an update to the ATP III guidelines was released, suggesting a reset of treatment thresholds and targets.[32]

In contrast to previous versions of ATP (I and II), ATP III placed greater emphasis on the prevention of CHD in patients with multiple risk factors, in addition to treatment for secondary prevention. The ATP III treatment algorithm divided patients into three risk categories based on clinical characteristics and the Framingham 10-year risk score:

1. Established CHD and CHD risk equivalents: High risk (10-year risk higher than 20%)
2. Multiple (two or more) risk factors: Moderately high risk (10-year risk, 10% to 20%); moderate risk (10-year risk lower than 10%)
3. Zero to one (one or none) risk factor: Lower risk (10-year risk lower than 10%)

ATP III greatly expanded the high risk category by defining CHD risk equivalents, including noncoronary atherosclerotic disease, such as peripheral vascular and carotid disease, and abdominal aortic aneurysm; diabetes mellitus; and multiple CHD risk factors conferring an estimated 10-year risk for a cardiovascular event of more than 20%. ATP III major risk factors include the following:

- Age (men, 45 years; women, 55 years)
- Cigarette smoking
- Hypertension (blood pressure = 140/90 mm Hg or patient is on antihypertensive medications)
- Low high-density lipoprotein (HDL) cholesterol level (lower than 40 mg/dL in men, lower than 50 mg/dL in women; HDL cholesterol ≥60 mg/dL is a negative risk factor)
- Family history of premature CHD: Male first-degree relative younger than 55 years *or* female first-degree relative younger than 65 years)

According to the ATP III, the LDL-C goal for high-risk patients is less than 100 mg/dL. For all patients in the high-risk category with LDL-C > 100 mg/dL, LDL-C-lowering dietary therapy should be initiated. In addition, for patients with LDL-C higher than 130 mg/dL, an LDL-C-lowering drug should be started. However, in the LDL-C range of 100 to 129 mg/dL, ATP III guidelines did not mandate drug therapy; rather, therapeutic options included intensified dietary therapy, LDL-C-lowering drugs, or drug therapy for elevated triglyceride or low HDL-C levels. At the time of publication of the guidelines for ATP III, there were not enough data to recommend more intensive drug therapy for this intermediate range of LDL-C.

These recommendations were modified in the ATP III update of 2004, which recommended an LDL-C goal lower than 100 mg/dL for high-risk patients, with an optional goal of lower than 70 mg/dL for very high-risk patients (Table 1). This update also recommended initiating dietary therapy and LDL-C-lowering drugs for all patients over goal, with a planned LDL-C reduction of 30% to 40%. The rationale for these changes was based on several randomized clinical

Table 1 Summary of ATP III Guidelines Update, 2004[32]

Risk Category	LDL-C Goal	Initiate TLC	Consider Drug Therapy
High risk: CHD or CHD risk equivalent (10-year risk >20%)	<100 mg/dL; optional goal, <70 mg/dL	≥100 mg/dL	≥100 mg/dL
Moderately high risk: ≥2 risk factors (10-year risk = 10%-20%)	<130 mg/dL	≥130 mg/dL	≥130 mg/dL
Moderate risk: ≥2 risk factors (10-year risk <10%)	<130 mg/dL	≥130 mg/dL	>160 mg/dL
Low risk: 1 or no risk factors	<160 mg/dL	≥160 mg/dL	≥190 mg/dL

ATP, Adult Treatment Panel; CHD, coronary heart disease; LDL-C, low-density lipoprotein cholesterol; TLC, therapeutic lifestyle changes.

trials whose results were published after the release of the ATP III guidelines. These trials included the Heart Protection Study (HPS), which evaluated the effects of simvastatin, 40 mg daily, versus placebo in a group of 20,536 patients aged 40 to 80 years at high risk for CHD.[4,7] This included patients with coronary disease, other occlusive arterial disease, or diabetes (analogous to the ATP III CHD risk equivalent designation), followed for a 5-year period. Patients treated with simvastatin had a 24% overall reduction in major adverse cardiovascular events compared to placebo; similar propational risk reduction was seen even in subjects with baseline LDL-C <100 mg/dl. The Pravastatin or Atorvastatin Evaluation and Infection—Thrombolysis in Myocardial Infarction 22 (PROVE IT-TIMI 22) was designed to test noninferiority of a less aggressive cholesterol-lowering regimen.[42] Ultimately, it showed that intensive LDL-C level lowering with atorvastatin, 80 mg daily, reduced cardiovascular risk more than standard drug therapy with pravastatin, 40 mg, in a group of high-risk patients hospitalized for acute coronary syndromes. The mean LDL-C level attained was 95 mg/dL with pravastatin and 62 mg/dL with atorvastatin. The study demonstrated a 16% reduction in the composite cardiovascular end point in the atorvastatin group compared with the pravastatin group ($P < 0.005$). Other trials used to support these revised guidelines included the Prospective Study of Pravastatin in the Elderly at Risk (PROSPER),[17] Antihypertensive and Lipid-Lowering Treatment to Prevent Heart Attack Trial-Lipid-Lowering Trial (ALLHAT-LLT),[19] and Anglo-Scandinavian Cardiac Outcomes Trial-Lipid-Lowering Arm (ASCOT-LLA),[24] a trial that evaluated two antihypertensive regimens and a lipid-lowering arm with atorvastatin.

Finally, in the evolution of the cholesterol guidelines, the AHA/ACC guidelines for secondary prevention of CHD released in 2006[40] placed more weight behind the optional goal of LDL-C lower than 70 mg/dL in high-risk patients with CHD, based on data accrued from the Treat to New Targets (TNT) and Incremental Decrease in Endpoints through Aggressive Lipid Lowering (IDEAL) trials.[43,44] It was formulated as a Class IIa recommendation and stated that

> *it is reasonable to treat to LDL <70 mg/dL in such (secondary prevention) patients. When the <70-mg/dL target is chosen, it may be prudent to increase statin therapy in a graded fashion to determine a patient's response and tolerance. Furthermore, if it is not possible to attain LDL-C <70 mg/dL because of a high baseline LDL-C, it generally is possible to achieve LDL-C reductions of >50% with either statins or LDL-C-lowering drug combinations.*[40]

RISK ASSESSMENT

Several variables have been taken into consideration to determine CHD risk. Any patient who has had a CHD event is at markedly increased risk for a subsequent event. Risk models such as the Framingham risk score[1] are used in risk adjustment. Any patient who has a higher than 20% risk for a CHD event based on the Framingham risk score is considered to be at equivalent risk to a patient with established CHD. The Framingham risk score does not take into account family history because of difficulty obtaining this measure in all patients. Furthermore, it does not include some of the newer markers such as high-sensitivity C-reactive protein (hsCRP) or albuminuria (see later)[45-47] or the components of the metabolic syndrome such as waist circumference and trighycerides.[48] Current guidelines and many clinical studies consider diabetes mellitus as a CHD risk equivalent (>20% risk over 10 years) in setting targets for LDL-C and non–HDL-C levels.*

Although many diabetic patients are not CHD risk-equivalent based on models such as the UKPDS risk engine, this approach does ensure that high-risk diabetic patients are treated aggressively. Low HDL-C concentrations are associated with increased CHD risk. Studies such as AFCAPS/TEXCAPS have demonstrated that aggressive LDL-C lowering attenuates much of the adverse risk associated with low HDL-C.[25,26] There are compelling data showing that hs CRP is associated with increased risk for CHD, even when adjustments are made for other risk factors. Current guidelines suggest that hs CRP be used to help in risk assessment in patients who have intermediate risk for CHD.[45,47,56]

Other markers of risk have not been consistently included in guidelines but need to be considered in clinical practice. Renal dysfunction is associated with an increased risk for CHD. This is true for markers of renal disease such as albuminuria, but several studies have shown that impaired renal function is associated with marked increases in CHD risk, especially when associated with the need for renal replacement therapy (dialysis or renal transplantation). Peripheral vascular disease and cerebrovascular disease are also associated with increased risk for CHD events. Furthermore, most statin trials have shown a reduction in risk for stroke, although stroke event rates are consistently lower than CHD event rates in most studies. Several observational studies have suggested that patients who have systemic inflammatory disorders such as rheumatoid arthritis and systemic lupus erythematosus, especially if they are treated with glucocorticoids, are at increased risk for CHD. Similarly, organ transplant recipients, especially renal, heart, and lung transplants, may be at increased risk for CHD. Many CHD risk prevention clinics, including the Preventive Cardiology Clinic at the Cleveland Clinic, have set more aggressive LDL-C targets for such patients, even though intervention trial data are lacking. This approach extends the general concept of more aggressive lipid lowering in patients at increased risk of disease.

LIPID-LOWERING TREATMENT

Diet and Lifestyle

All patients, whether in secondary or primary prevention categories, are strongly recommended to implement lifestyle and dietary recom-

*See references 4, 6, 8, 10, 11, 15, 36, 37, 39, 41, and 49-55.

Table 2 Therapeutic Lifestyle Changes: Diet Recommendations

Nutrient	Recommended Intake
Total fat	25%-35% of total calories
Saturated fat	Less than 7% of total calories
Polyunsaturated fat	Up to 10% of total calories
Monounsaturated fat	Up to 20% of total calories
Trans fat	<1% of total calories
Cholesterol	<200 mg/day
Carbohydrate	50%-60% of total calories
Fiber	20-30 g/day
Protein	Approximately 15% of total calories
Total calories (energy)	Balance energy intake and expenditure to maintain desirable body weight and prevent weight gain.
Other	Consume a diet rich in fruits and vegetables. Choose whole-grain, high-fiber foods. Consume fish, especially oily fish, at least twice a week. Avoid fish with potential for mercury contamination. Minimize intake of beverages and foods with added sugars. Choose and prepare foods with little or no salt. Consume alcohol in moderation. Men, two drinks/day; women, one drink/day When eating food prepared outside the home, follow the American Heart Association diet and lifestyle recommendations.

Adapted from Lichtenstein AH, Appel LJ, Brands M, et al: Diet and lifestyle recommendations, revision 2006: A scientific statement from the American Heart Association Nutrition Committee. Circulation 2006;114:82-96.

mendations as part of a strategy to prevent cardiovascular disease. Healthy eating habits, starting from childhood, are the cornerstone for cardiovascular risk reduction and, together with lifestyle goals, including maintenance of healthy body weight, avoidance of tobacco products, and adherence to a regimen of physical activity, may be termed *elements of primordial prevention.*

Specifically, the American Heart Association recommends a diet low in fat, particularly saturated and *trans* fats, enriched in fruits, vegetables, whole grains, and fish, and low in added sugar and salt (Table 2).[57] This approach, especially regarding fat intake, is supported by other nutrition guidelines.[49,58,59] Controversies regarding the superiority of the Mediterranean diet (including higher proportions of monounsaturated fats and omega-3 fatty acids) over the traditional AHA step II diet may have been settled recently by a study showing their relative equivalence in lipid lowering and risk reduction. In addition, a study of a diet enriched in plant sterols, soy protein, viscous fiber, and almonds has shown comparable reductions in LDL-C and CRP as compared with lovastatin, 20 mg.[60] These findings all highlight the importance of dietary intervention in prevention.

Smoking cessation may have beneficial effects on the lipid profile by increasing HDL-C (mean, 4 mg/dL).[61] Exercise, physical activity, and weight loss may also increase HDL-C and lower triglyceride levels. The AHA recommends 30 minutes of moderate-intensity aerobic exercise on most days of the week. Moderate alcohol intake (one or two drinks per day) is associated with a lower risk of myocardial infarction, possibly because of alcohol's ability to raise the HDL-C level (1 oz/day increases the HDL-C level by a mean of 4 mg/dL) Many studies have been devoted to other potential mediators found in alcoholic beverages, such as polyphenols in red wine. Excessive alcohol consumption is also associated with elevations in triglyceride levels as well as the potential for hepatic dysfunction and addiction; therefore, the recommendation that patients increase or begin consumption is given with several caveats.

Medications

Various medications are currently available for lowering lipid levels; a summary is given in Table 3.

Statins

The introduction in the 1980s of the HMG-CoA reductase inhibitors, also known as the statins, has markedly improved the ability to treat hyperlipidemia and decrease future risk for CHD. The statins are the most effective drugs available for lowering LDL-C and are generally well-tolerated, with an acceptable side effect profile. They are usually the first line of therapy for lipid lowering and attaining ATP III goals.

The mechanism of action of statins has been well characterized. They inhibit HMG-CoA reductase, the rate-limiting step in cholesterol biosynthesis, thus decreasing the hepatic formation of cholesterol. Hepatic LDL-C receptors are upregulated, resulting in further clearance of LDL-C from the systemic circulation.

Statin use results in a 20% to 60% decrease in LDL-C levels, with more modest increases in HDL-C and decreases in triglyceride levels (Table 4). The early landmark trials of statin use in primary and secondary prevention, such as the Scandinavian Simvastatin Survival Study[14,45] and the West of Scotland Coronary Prevention Study (WOSCOPS),[16] have shown that cholesterol lowering resulted in a decreased CHD risk and mortality of approximately 25% to 35%. (Table 5). Later trials, such as the Heart Protection Study (HPS)[7] and PROVE-IT TIMI-22,[42] have shown that risk reduction occurs all along the continuum, including the lower end, of cholesterol lowering, although to a lesser absolute degree. The curve of cholesterol lowering versus risk reduction is therefore probably best understood as a direct logarithmic relationship (Fig. 1).[32,62] To date, the lower limit of cholesterol that still results in risk reduction is unknown, although many experts have theorized that it may be at an LDL-C level of 40 mg/dL.

Not all the cardiovascular risk reduction seen with statin use is attributable to LDL-C lowering. Studies of the pleiotropic effects of statins have suggested that they may also improve endothelial function, have antioxidant and anti-inflammatory effects, and stabilize atherosclerotic plaque. High-dose statin has become part of standard care for patients presenting with acute coronary syndrome, based in part on the results of the PROVE-IT trial.[42]

In addition, the JUPITER trial (Justification for the Use of Statins in Prevention: an Intervention Trial Evaluating Rosuvastatin) (2008) showed significant reductions in cardiovascular events and all-cause mortality in apparently healthy patients with elevated hs CRP ≥ 2.0 mg/L treated with rosuvastatin 20 mg compared to placebo. This study suggests a benefit to statin use in a widely expanded primary prevention population with levels of increased inflammation.

Statins are among the most widely prescribed medications in the United States and, despite the large number of patients taking them, have a remarkably good record of safety. One statin, cerivastatin (Baycol), was removed from the market in 2001 because of excessive muscle toxicity; however, the other statins remain available and safe. The most commonly described side effects are transaminitis, occurring in less than 3% of patients, and myopathy or myositis. Liver enzyme abnormalities are usually reversible when the dose of statin

Table 3 Summary of Lipid-Lowering Medications and Side Effects

	Change in Level (%)			
Drug Class	LDL-C	HDL-C	TGs	Side Effects
Statins	↓20-60	5-15	↓10-20	Myopathy (rarely, rhabdomyolysis); transaminitis
Fibrates	↓10-15	10-15	↓20-50	Dyspepsia, gallstones, myopathy
BARs	↓15-30	3-5	0-20	GI distress, constipation, decreased absorption of other medications and fat-soluble vitamins
Niacin	↓10-25	15-35	↓20-50	Flushing, hyperglycemia, hyperuricemia, GI distress, hepatotoxicity
HRT	↓10-15	2-8	15-20	Hypercoagulability, cholecystitis, increased risk of breast cancer
CAI	↓15-20	No change	No change	Headache, GI distress, myopathy

BARs, bile acid resins; CAI, cholesterol absorption inhibitor; GI, gastrointestinal; HDL-C, high-density lipoprotein cholesterol; HRT, hormone replacement therapy; LDL-C, low-density lipoprotein cholesterol; TGs, triglycerides.
Adapted from Oliver MF, Pyorala K, Shepherd J: Management of hyperlipidaemia. Why, when, and how to treat. Eur Heart J 1997;18:371-375.

Table 4 Approximate Average Lipid Changes By Statin Dosage[63]

	Statin (mg/day)					Lipid Change (%)		
Rosuvastatin*	Atorvastatin	Simvastatin	Lovastatin	Pravastatin	Fluvastatin	LDL-C†	HDL-C	TG
		10	20	20	40	−22	4-8	−10-15
	10	20	40	40	80	−27	4-8	−10-20
	20	40	80			−32	4-8	−15-25
	40	80				−37	4-8	−20-30
	80					−42	4-8	−20-30
5						−38	10	−32
10						−45	11	−7
20						−48	5	−20
40						−56	7	−25

*Rosuvastatin (Crestor) package insert compared with placebo.
†The addition of ezetimibe, 10 mg, to any of these statins will reduce LDL-C by another 12% to 15%.
HDL-C, high-density lipoprotein cholesterol; LDL-C, low-density lipoprotein cholesterol; TG, triglyceride.
Data from Maron DJ, Fazio S, Linton MF: Current perspectives on statins. Circulation 2000;101:207-213.

Table 5 Early Landmark Statin Clinical Trials

Study	No. of Patients in Study	Statin and Daily Dose	Mean Baseline LDL-C (mg/dL)	Mean LDL-C Reduction (%)	Reduction in Coronary Events (%)	NNT
Secondary Prevention						
4S	4444	Simvastatin, 20-40 mg	188	35	34 ($P < 0.0001$)	15
CARE	4159	Pravastatin, 40 mg	139	32	24 ($P = 0.003$)	33
LIPID	9014	Pravastatin, 40 mg	150	25	24 ($P < 0.0001$)	28
Primary Prevention						
WOSCOPS	6595	Pravastatin, 40 mg	192	26	31 ($P < 0.001$)	42
AFCAPS/TEXCAPS	6605	Lovastatin, 20-40 mg	150	25	37 ($P < 0.001$)	24

4S, Scandinavian Simvastatin Survival Study[14]; AFCAPS/TEXCAPS, Air Force/Texas Coronary Atherosclerosis Prevention Study[25]; CARE, Cholesterol and Recurrent Events trial[12]; LIPID, Long-Term Intervention with Pravastatin in Ischemic Disease study[22]; NNT, number needed to treat to prevent one major coronary event; WOSCOPS, West of Scotland Coronary Prevention Study.[16]
Adapted from Maron DJ, Fazio S, Linton MF: Current perspectives on statins. Circulation 2000;101:207-213.

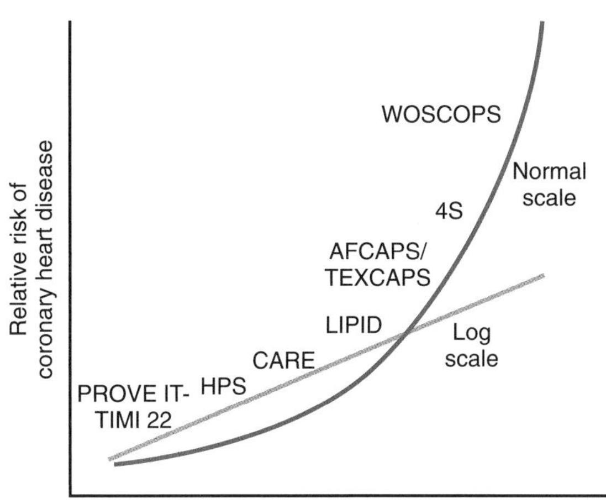

Figure 1 Conceptual graph showing the relation between low-density lipoprotein cholesterol (LDL-C) levels and relative risk and coronary heart disease and baseline LDL-C levels in several recent studies. At the steep end of the curve, a 30-mg/dL decrease in LDL-C decreases the risk of coronary heart disease by about 30%.[7,12,16,25,42] AFCAPS/TEXCAPS, Air Force/Texas Coronary Atherosclerosis Prevention Study; CARE, Cholesterol and Current Events study; 4S, Scandinavian Simvastatin Survival Study; LIPID, Long-Term Intervention With Pravastatin in Ischaemic Disease study; PROVE IT-TIMI 22, Pravastatin or Atorvastatin Evaluation and Infection Therapy-Thrombolysis in Myocardial Infarction 22; WOSCOPS, West of Scotland Coronary Prevention Study. *(From Huang JC, Hoogwerf BJ: Cholesterol guidelines update: More aggressive therapy for higher-risk patients. Cleve Clin J Med 2005;72:253-262.)*

is decreased or the medication is discontinued. Reports of the prevalence of muscular side effects have differed; muscular aching varies in degree of severity, from mild muscle aching or cramps, with or without associated elevations in the creatinine kinase level, to frank rhabdomyolysis, with creatinine kinase elevations higher than 40 times the upper limit of normal, and association with renal dysfunction. Unfortunately, these effects are idiosyncratic and may occur at any point during therapy. In the largest statin trial to date, the Heart Protection Study of 20,536 patients randomized to either simvastatin 40 mg daily or placebo, the incidence of muscle complaints at any time during the study was 32.9% in the drug group and 33.2% in the placebo group; rhabdomyolysis occurred in 0.05% of those in the simvastatin group.[7] The occurrence of adverse side effects increases with concurrent use of the lipid-lowering agents fibrates and niacin, with cyclosporine, antifungal agents, antiretroviral protease inhibitors, verapamil, amiodarone, and grapefruit juice, and in patients with hepatic or renal insufficiency.

The choice of statin may depend on the degree of LDL-C lowering needed to attain ATP III goals, side effect profile, and cost. Among the statins, pravastatin, fluvastatin, and rosuvastatin are hydrophilic and may be associated with fewer muscle side effects. It is commonly noted that side effects encountered with one of the medications in this class may not necessarily be reproduced with another statin medication, and therefore we recommend a trial of another statin whenever possible. We have also found that intermittent statin dosing, from every other day to once weekly, may reduce symptoms.

Ubiquinone (CoQ_{10}) supplementation, 100 to 400 mg daily, is widely used to reduce muscle symptoms, but no robust placebo-controlled trials have confirmed the benefits of this approach.

Fibrates

The lipid-lowering medications known as the fibrates (e.g., gemfibrozil, fenofibrate, bezafibrate, clofibrate) are an important part of the armamentarium for lipid lowering but are rarely used as monotherapy, except in cases of primary prevention with metabolic syndrome profile, in which the goal of the LDL-C level has already been attained.

Fibrates activate the peroxisome proliferator-activated receptor-α (PPAR-α), which ultimately results in increased lipolysis and elimination from plasma of triglyceride-rich particles and increased synthesis of apolipoproteins A-I, A-II, and HDL-C. Fibrates can therefore lower triglyceride levels by 20% to 50% and increase HDL-C levels by 10% to 15%, along with a possible 10% to 15% decrease in LDL-C levels. Although no large randomized clinical trial to date has shown an improvement in mortality with use of the fibrates, the HHS, using gemfibrozil in primary prevention,[5] and VA-HIT, using gemfibrozil in secondary prevention, have shown a significant risk reduction in cardiovascular events, especially in subgroups with high triglyceride and low HDL-C levels.[9-11] The FIELD study in more than 9000 people with diabetes could not confirm these data, but the trial results were confounded by very high rates of statin drop-in.[27,28]

Safety concerns regarding fibrates include the possibility of transaminitis or cholelithiasis and caution must be used when combining a fibrate with a statin (increased risk of myopathy, especially with gemfibrozil) or warfarin (increased risk of bleeding). Because fibrates are primarily excreted renally, caution must be used in the setting of renal insufficiency. If fibrate therapy is indicated, dose reduction with decreased renal function is advisable.

Niacin

One of the older lipid-lowering medications, niacin is commonly prescribed for its ability to raise HDL-C levels by up to 35%. It also lowers triglyceride levels by 20% to 50% and lowers LDL-C levels by 10% to 25%, making it a useful medication for monotherapy or in combination with statins or fibrates. It decreases hepatic production of very low-density lipoproteins (VLDLs) and apolipoprotein (apo) B-100, inhibits free fatty acid release from adipose tissue, and stabilizes apo A-I from HDL-C, maintaining the structure and function of HDL-C.

In addition to the lipid modifications noted earlier, niacin is one of the few medications available to lower the lipoprotein (a)—Lp(a)—level, a modified and highly atherogenic form of LDL-C. The usefulness of this capability is unclear, however. Although an elevated Lp(a) level is associated with increased cardiovascular mortality and morbidity, no randomized clinical trials have shown a benefit in targeting its lowering.

The use of niacin has increased with the introduction of the long-acting forms (e.g., Niaspan), designed to attenuate the most bothersome side effect associated with niacin, an intense feeling of warmth or flushing occurring shortly after ingestion of the medication. Release of a niacin formulation compled with laropiprant, a prostaglandin D_2 blocker, designed to reduce flushing, has been delayed in the United States. Other potential effects include hyperglycemia, hyperuricemia, and the risk of interaction with statins, causing hepatotoxicity or myopathy.

Bile Acid Resins

Bile acid resins act in the small intestine to block the reabsorption of bile acids, thereby decreasing their enterohepatic circulation and upregulating hepatic LDL-C receptors. Although long-term use is considered to be safe because they are not systemically absorbed, the bile acid resins are rarely used in the current era of lipid lowering because of their inferiority compared with statins in LDL-C-lowering capability, approximately 15% to 30%. They may be useful in patients who cannot tolerate statins because of side effects or in patients in whom the risk of statin therapy might outweigh the benefit—for example, during pregnancy when statins are contraindicated because of concerns about a possible teratogenic effect. Whereas bile acid resins are usually well tolerated, they may be associated with gastrointestinal side effects, such as constipation or bloating, and long-term use may cause malabsorption of the fat-soluble vitamins A, D, E, and K. They require administration two or three times daily.

Cholesterol Absorption Inhibitor

Ezetimibe is currently the only available drug in the class of cholesterol absorption inhibitors. It localizes to the epithelial brush border of the small intestine to block uptake of cholesterol, resulting in decreased delivery of cholesterol to the liver and subsequent upregulation of LDL-C receptors. Ezetimibe's glucuronide metabolite is also active and results in a long half-life as the two are circulated enterohepatically. It is usually administered in conjunction with a statin, and may lower LDL-C levels by an additional 15% to 20%, slightly less when used with a statin. Because there is little systemic absorption, ezetimibe is generally well tolerated and side effects are rare. Gastrointestinal symptoms and muscle aches have been reported. Enthusiasm for use of ezetimibe has decreased since publication of ENHANCE (Effect of combination Ezetimibe and High-Dose Simvastation vs. Simvastatin Alone on the Atherosclerotic Process in Patients with Heterozygous Familial Hypercholesterolemia) (2008) showing no difference in progression of cantid intinal-medial thickness between groups treated with simvastation with and without ezetimibe.[64]

Summary

- Guidelines for cholesterol lowering are based on assessment of cardiovascular risk with progressively lower LDL-C goals in patients at higher risk. Currently, patients with CHD or CHD risk equivalents (e.g., stroke, aortic aneurysm, peripheral arterial disease, diabetes mellitus, metabolic syndrome) or multiple CHD risk factors conferring an estimated 10-year risk for a cardiovascular event higher than 20% have a recommended target LDL-C of lower than 100 mg/dL, and optimally lower than 70 mg/dL.
- Framingham risk score, family history, and lifestyle factors are important in the assessment of cardiovascular risk. Additional risk markers, such as microalbuminuria and high-sensitivity C-reactive protein, may be helpful to establish LDL-C targets.
- Statin medications are the most effective and widely used agents for cholesterol lowering and have the most robust clinical trial data to support their use in lowering cardiovascular risk. Statins are generally well tolerated but use may be limited by hepatotoxicity or muscle side effects.
- Lifestyle and dietary interventions are integral parts of primary and secondary cardiovascular prevention and are recommended for all patients.

Suggested Readings

Buse JB, Ginsberg HN, Bakris GL, et al: American Heart Association; American Diabetes Association: Primary prevention of cardiovascular diseases in people with diabetes mellitus: A scientific statement from the American Heart Association and the American Diabetes Association. Diabetes Care 2007;30:162-172.

Expert Panel on Detection, Evaluation and Treatment of High Blood Cholesterol in Adults: Executive Summary of The Third Report of The National Cholesterol Education Program (NCEP) Expert Panel on Detection, Evaluation, And Treatment of High Blood Cholesterol In Adults (Adult Treatment Panel III). JAMA 2001;285:2486-2497.

Fortmann SP, Ford E, Criqui MH, et al: CDC/AHA Workshop on Markers of Inflammation and Cardiovascular Disease: Application to Clinical and Public Health Practice: Report from the population science discussion group. Circulation 2004;110:e554-e559.

Grundy SM, Cleeman JI, Merz CN, et al: Implications of recent clinical trials for the National Cholesterol Education Program Adult Treatment Panel III Guidelines. J Am Coll Cardiol 2004;44:720-732.

Grundy SM, Howard B, Smith S Jr, et al: Prevention Conference VI: Diabetes and Cardiovascular Disease: Executive summary: Conference proceeding for health-care professionals from a special writing group of the American Heart Association. Circulation 2002;105:2231-2239.

Klein S, Sheard NF, Pi-Sunyer X, et al: American Diabetes Association; North American Association for the Study of Obesity; American Society for Clinical Nutrition: Weight management through lifestyle modification for the prevention and management of type 2 diabetes: Rationale and strategies: A statement of the American Diabetes Association, the North American Association for the Study of Obesity, and the American Society for Clinical Nutrition. Diabetes Care 2004;27:2067-2073.

Lichtenstein AH, Appel LJ, Brands M, et al: Diet and lifestyle recommendations revision 2006: A scientific statement from the American Heart Association Nutrition Committee. Circulation 2006;114:82-96.

Smith SC, Jr., Allen J, Blair SN, et al: AHA/ACC; National Heart, Lung, and Blood Institute: AHA/ACC guidelines for secondary prevention for patients with coronary and other atherosclerotic vascular disease: 2006 update: Endorsed by the National Heart, Lung, and Blood Institute. Circulation 2006;113:2363-2372.

Snow V, Aronson MD, Hornbake ER, et al: Lipid control in the management of type 2 diabetes mellitus: a clinical practice guideline from the American College of Physicians. Ann Intern Med 2004;140:644-649.

References

For a complete list of references, log onto www.expertconsult.com.

Cardiac Risk Stratification for Noncardiac Surgery

Mazen K. Khalil and Wael A. Jaber

One of the most common questions posed to physicians is about assessment of the cardiac risks of noncardiac surgery. Once the physician estimates the risk of a patient, he or she will be able to apply measures to decrease the risk for the patient and improve the outcome. Often in these cases, an opportunity is created for the first time to address cardiac risk factors in the patient undergoing surgery. This opportunity often is limited by time constraints and short contact with the patient, especially if the surgery is semiurgent or prescheduled at short notice. The major goal is to assess the risk of myocardial infarction, heart failure, or both, the most common causes of morbidity and mortality with noncardiac surgery. The mortality rate among patients with perioperative myocardial infarction ranges from 30% to 50%.

Conversely, there are very few cases in which the surgical outcomes and treatments are affected by extensive preoperative cardiac testing. Although preoperative testing is indicated in some cases, it does not always lead to a scientifically tangible improvement in outcome. Indiscriminate and extensive preoperative cardiac testing is an ineffective way of using health care funds and can lead to more unwarranted and risky procedures. In addition to the loss of resources, unnecessary testing might cause harm to the patient by delaying surgery. For a test to be considered useful it should be accurate, influence outcome, and have a favorable risk-to-benefit ratio. Therefore, it is essential for the physician to identify patients who will benefit most from an in-depth preoperative evaluation. It is important for the physician to explore noncardiac issues (e.g., lung disease, coagulopathy, anemia, renal disease, cerebrovascular events, diabetes) that can negatively affect the outcome of the surgery. A preoperative evaluation should be considered as an opportunity for a thorough medical evaluation in patients who might not have been in contact with the medical system.

There are various factors to be considered when assessing anesthesia and surgical cardiac risks. These are generally divided into patient-related and surgery-specific risks, as well as test-specific considerations (Box 1).

CARDIAC RISK INDICES

Goldman Risk Index

About 3 decades ago, Goldman and coworkers developed a user-friendly point system that identified perioperative fatal and nonfatal cardiac events. This system created four classes of risk, depending on the total points accumulated (Table 1).

Patients in the lowest risk quartile (0 to 5 points) had less than a 1% risk of postoperative major cardiac complications. In the two quartiles with 6 to 25 points, the major cardiac event risk was 9%, and 22% of the patients in the highest risk group (≥26 points) had a major perioperative cardiac event.

Eagle's Cardiac Risk index

One of the limitations of the Goldman criteria was the inability to predict the operative risk for patients undergoing vascular surgery because of the low number of patients with vascular operations included in the study population. This limitation was addressed by Eagle and colleagues in a study of patients undergoing vascular surgery. Multivariate analysis has shown that the following factors predict an adverse event following vascular surgery:

- Q waves on the electrocardiogram (ECG)
- History of angina pectoris
- History of ventricular ectopy requiring treatment (most specific for predicting events)
- Diabetes mellitus requiring therapy other than diet
- Age older than 70 years
- Thallium redistribution (most sensitive for predicting events)
- Ischemic electrocardiographic changes during or after dipyridamole infusion

Combining both the clinical data and thallium imaging was more sensitive and specific than either alone in predicting postoperative complications. In this model, the following can be noted:

- No clinical predictors of risk factors: 3.1% risk of perioperative ischemic cardiac complications
- Thallium redistribution in addition to one or two clinical predictors: 29.6% risk of perioperative complications
- Three clinical predictors: 50% risk of perioperative cardiac complications

Detsky's Cardiac Risk Index

A modified cardiac index that included a change in the scores allocated to risk factors such as type of operation, age, frequency of premature ventricular contractions (PVCs), and aortic stenosis was published by Detsky and associates in 1986. However, heart failure was defined in this study as pulmonary edema determined by chest radiograph or by history of severe respiratory distress and resolution of the symptoms by use of diuretics. In addition, angina was subdivided into four classes according to the Canadian Cardiovascular Society classification. The score obtained from the patient's risk factors, along with the risk associated with the type of surgery, were used to calculate the probability of a cardiac event.

Revised (Lee's) Cardiac Risk Index

The modified cardiac index was revised by Lee and coworkers, who devised a six-point index score for assessing the risk of complications with noncardiac surgery. The Revised Cardiac Risk Index (RCRI) includes the following variables and risks:

- High-risk surgery (intrathoracic, intra-abdominal. or suprainguinal vascular)
- Ischemic heart disease (defined as a history of myocardial infarction [MI], pathologic Q waves on the ECG, use of nitrates, abnormal stress test, and chest pain secondary to ischemic causes)
- Congestive heart failure
- History of cerebrovascular disease
- Insulin therapy
- Preoperative serum creatinine level higher than 2 mg/dL

Each of the six risk factors was assigned one point. Patients with none, one, or two risk factor (s) were assigned to RCRI classes I, II, and III, and patients with more than two risk factors were considered Class IV. The risk associated with each class was 0.4%, 1%, 7%, and 11% for patients in Classes I, II, III, and IV, respectively. We recommend the use of this index because it is simple, has been extensively validated, and provides a good estimate of the preoperative risk.

Table 1 Goldman Multifactorial Cardiac Risk Index

Risk Factor	Points
Preoperative third heart sound or jugular venous distention indicating active heart failure	11
Myocardial infarction in the past 6 months	10
≥5 premature ventricular complexes/min before surgery	7
Rhythm other than sinus	7
Age >70 years	5
Emergency surgery	4
Significant aortic stenosis	3
Intraperitoneal, intrathoracic, or aortic surgery	3
Markers of poor general medical condition (e.g., renal dysfunction, liver disease, lung disease, electrolyte imbalance)	3

Box 1 Factors to be Considered When Assessing Cardiac Risk

Patient-Related Factors
Age
Chronic diseases (e.g., coronary artery disease, diabetes dellitus, hypertension)
Functional status
Medical therapy
Implantable devices
Previous surgeries

Surgery-Related Factors
Type of surgery (e.g., vascular, endoscopic, abdominal)
Urgency of the operation (e.g., emergent, urgent, elective)
Duration of the operation, possibility of blood loss and fluid shifts

Test-Related Factors
Sensitivity and specificity of a test
Effect on management

Box 2 Clinical Predictors of Increased Perioperative Cardiovascular Risk*

Major Predictors
Unstable coronary syndromes

- Acute or recent MI[†] with evidence of important ischemic risk by clinical symptoms or noninvasive study
- Unstable or severe[‡] angina (Canadian Class III or IV)

Decompensated heart failure
Significant arrhythmias

- High-grade atrioventricular block
- Symptomatic ventricular arrhythmias in the presence of underlying heart disease
- Supraventricular arrhythmias with uncontrolled ventricular rate

Severe valvular disease

Intermediate Predictors
Mild angina pectoris (Canadian Class I or II)
Previous MI by history or pathologic Q waves
Compensated or prior heart failure
Diabetes mellitus (especially insulin-dependent type)
Renal insufficiency

Minor Predictors
Advanced age
Abnormal ECG (e.g., left ventricular hypertrophy, left bundle branch block, ST-T abnormalities)
Rhythm other than sinus (e.g., atrial fibrillation)
Low functional capacity (e.g., inability to climb one flight of stairs with a bag of groceries)
History of stroke
Uncontrolled systemic hypertension
ECG, electrocardiogram; MI, myocardial infarction.

**Myocardial infarction, heart failure, death.*
[†]The American College of Cardiology National Database Library has defined recent MI as >7 days but ≤1 month (30 days); acute MI is within 7 days.
[‡]May include "stable" angina in patients who are unusually sedentary.
Adapted from Campeau L: Grading of angina pectoris. Circulation 1976;54:522-523.

American College of Cardiology Cardiac Risk Classification

The American College of Cardiology (ACC) has divided predictors of perioperative risks into three categories: major, intermediate, and minor (Box 2). Patients presenting with major predictors of risk need extensive investigation and postponement or cancellation of elective surgery, or urgent noncardiac surgery might ensue. Minor predictors of risk are not known to influence the perioperative course of patients. Patients with intermediate risk need careful assessment to decide on the need for noninvasive cardiac testing.

FACTORS AFFECTING CARDIAC RISK

Patient-Related Factors

Patients with Known Coronary Artery Disease

Patients with known coronary artery disease (CAD) should be classified into a specific risk class according to one of the risk indices cited previously, preferably Lee's revised cardiac risk index. For patients classified into the low-risk group, we recommend a preoperative ECG and chest radiograph. Postoperative care should include monitoring for ischemia (serial ECGs, cardiac enzyme levels), especially if the patient has had intraoperative hemodynamic instability. We also recommend an ECG before discharge.

If the patient belongs to the intermediate risk group, he or she should be managed aggressively with beta blockers, lipid-lowering agents, and tight blood pressure control. Much debate is ongoing concerning the use of noninvasive stress testing in this patient subgroup. In any case, there is not much evidence supporting the use of revascularization before noncardiac surgery.

Retrospective data analyses of patients who have undergone coronary artery bypass grafting (CABG) or percutaneous coronary intervention (PCI) months to years before noncardiac surgery have shown a lower incidence of perioperative complications compared with patients who had medical therapy alone. However, the average mortality rate of CABG in the United States in 2002 was 2.6%, which exceeds the risk of surgery in these patients. Furthermore, one study has shown that percutaneous angioplasty performed on stable CAD patients undergoing vascular surgery, with at least one coronary artery having more than 70% stenosis, resulted in no survival benefit over 2.7 years of follow-up.

Another study has revealed that in-stent restenosis might complicate noncardiac surgery if PCI is done within 6 weeks of surgery. In addition, some reports have suggested that the benefit of PCI might not be evident until 90 days after the procedure. To preserve the stent placed during PCI, the patient has to take aspirin and clopidogrel (Plavix) for at least 1 month, which might delay noncardiac surgery further.

More-recent data suggest that with drug-eluting stents, risks of stent thrombosis are high, even 1 year after stent placement, if antiplatelet drugs are stopped. In addition, the percentage of patients who needed revascularization by CABG or PCI was relatively small in most studies. Performing extensive testing to identify these patients is not a cost-effective strategy. Therefore, we recommend managing intermediate-risk patients with extensive medical therapy (see later discussion of medical therapy).

In high-risk patients (RCRI >2 or signs and symptoms of CAD), diagnostic catheterization should be carried out, followed by revascularization if indicated, irrespective of the noncardiac surgical plans.

Patients with Diabetes

Silent myocardial ischemia occurs commonly in diabetic patients because of diabetic neuropathy, even in patients with well-controlled glycemia. In addition, diabetic patients are more predisposed to infection, poor wound healing, and episodes of hypoglycemia and hyperglycemia, which might negatively affect the outcome of noncardiac surgery. Thus, the diabetic patient needs more aggressive evaluation than the euglycemic patient. A study of diabetic patients undergoing noncardiac surgery has concluded that diabetic patients are at high risk for perioperative mortality, mostly because of cardiovascular causes. Assessment should include history, physical examination, and noninvasive testing, depending on the patient's risk factor profile (ECG, noninvasive imaging stress test, and creatinine level). It is recommended that an adequate glucose level be maintained perioperatively by insulin infusion to decrease the risk of wound infection.

Patients of Advanced Age

The association of age with cardiac and noncardiac complications with noncardiac surgery was significant in an analysis done by Polanczyk and colleagues. Advanced age adversely affects the rate of complications, mortality, and the length of stay. Perioperative mortality risk was low (0.3% in patients 50-59 years of age vs. 2.6% in patients >80 years; $P = .002$). However, it is unclear from this study whether older patients were excluded from surgery and that therefore the population studied was a low-risk cohort. It is also unclear from the literature whether the criteria of Goldman and Eagle and associates are sufficient to risk-stratify these patients or whether additional testing and triage will lead to improved outcomes.

The revised cardiac risk index predicts major adverse cardiac events (MACE) more reliably in patients younger than 55 years as compared to patients older than 75 years. Welten and colleagues, in a study on vascular surgery patients older than18 years (60% of the patients were >66 years and 20% were >75 years) showed that addition of age and the type of surgical procedure to the RCRI improves its predictive value; older patients were at higher risk for MACE, with the highest risk being in the 66 to 75 years age group.[1]

Likewise, Feringa and colleagues found that advanced age is an independent predictor of hospital and long-term mortality in patients older than 65 years undergoing major vascular surgery.[2] In addition, the use of aspirin, beta blockers, and statins was associated with 47%, 68%, and 65% relative risk reduction of in-hospital mortality, respectively.[2] The aforementioned drugs and ACE inhibitors were associated with reduced incidence of long-term mortality in the same study as well.[2] Despite the benefit seen in this study, we recommend extreme caution when using beta blockers, diuretics, and other antihypertensive drugs given the reduced clearance of drugs and their metabolites in this age group.

Patients with Hypertension

The main issue with hypertensive patients is whether they have uncomplicated hypertension or hypertension with end-organ damage (e.g., renal dysfunction, cerebrovascular disease, left ventricular hypertrophy, systolic dysfunction, diastolic dysfunction, or coronary artery disease). Patients with hypertension with no evidence of end-organ damage are at no increased risk for major perioperative cardiovascular complications; they can be cleared for surgery without further investigations with tight blood pressure control.

Preoperative cardiac testing (e.g., stress echocardiography, scintigraphy) should be considered if hypertensive patients are undergoing high-risk procedures. If the blood pressure is above 180/110 mm Hg, it is recommended to delay surgery until the blood pressure is normalized. Blood pressure control can take days to weeks, which is acceptable in the setting of elective surgery. However, if the surgery is urgent, blood pressure can be controlled by infusion of IV antihypertensive medications, such as nitroprusside or labetalol. Blood pressure should be lowered slowly because of the risk of cerebral ischemia.

Hypertensive patients with end-organ damage should be considered for preoperative testing (electrocardiography, noninvasive imaging stress test), especially if they are scheduled for moderate- to high-risk surgery. In patients with hypertension and left ventricular hypertrophy, ischemia might ensue because of rapid reduction of coronary perfusion in the thickened ventricle rather than from CAD. Kidney dysfunction is a known sequela of hypertension. An elevated creatinine level is an independent predictor of worse outcome in patients undergoing noncardiac surgery. The serum creatinine level should be determined preoperatively in these patients; testing is indicated if it would change the patient's treatment. Hypertensive medications should be continued, even on the day of surgery. Withdrawal of beta blockers and clonidine may be associated with adverse operative and postoperative complications.

Patients with Valvular Disease

All patients with prosthetic valves should receive antibiotic prophylaxis before noncardiac surgery. Patients with mitral valve prolapse can undergo surgery without antibiotics. The decision to repair or replace a diseased valve should be made in the context of indications for valve surgery, independently of whether the patient is to undergo noncardiac surgery.

Aortic Stenosis. Patients with severe aortic stenosis (AS) are at risk for fatal and nonfatal complications during noncardiac surgery, as has been shown in many observational studies. Proceeding with noncardiac surgery with uncorrected severe AS might have a mortality rate of 10%. Therefore, patients with symptomatic severe AS should undergo aortic valve replacement before noncardiac surgery. Valvuloplasty is a palliative option in patients who are not candidates for cardiac surgery. This approach is often risky, however, and provides only minimal and temporary benefit. Patients manifesting signs of both CAD and AS should undergo appropriate testing (e.g., cardiac catheterization, echocardiography) followed by coronary revascularization and valve replacement before noncardiac surgery. Patients with isolated asymptomatic severe AS and no evidence of CAD can proceed with minor noncardiac surgery; however, care should be taken to avoid hemodynamic instability and blood pressure fluctuations.[1]

Mitral Stenosis. Patients with severe mitral stenosis should undergo percutaneous or surgical correction of the stenosis before undergoing noncardiac surgery. For patients with mild to moderate mitral stenosis, care should be taken to avoid tachycardia postoperatively induced by blood loss or surges in catecholamine level. Tachycardia causes decreased filling time of the left ventricle, which can lead to a decreased cardiac output, pulmonary congestion, and congestive heart failure (CHF). If the patient with mitral stenosis is asymptomatic has no evidence of pulmonary hypertension or atrial fibrillation, the risk of noncardiac surgery is not substantially higher than for normal patients.

Aortic and Mitral Regurgitation. The presurgical management of patients with regurgitant aortic and mitral valves depends on the severity and chronicity of the regurgitation. Patients with preserved left ventricular ejection fraction (LVEF) and volumes by echocardiography, as well as good functional capacity, can undergo noncardiac surgery without excess risk. For patients with severe regurgitant valvular lesions, few guidelines are available to describe the indications and appropriateness of valve repair or replacement before noncardiac surgery.[1] In patients with aortic regurgitation, hemodynamic intraoperative assessment with a pulmonary artery catheter is recommended to monitor afterload and to prevent hypotension, which can adversely affect these patients.[1] Patients with severe mitral regurgitation may be treated with ACE inhibitors and diuretics. Any reduction in the ejection fraction should be considered abnormal and signals increased risk for CHF.[1]

Prosthetic Valves. Patients with prosthetic valves pose a special problem with anticoagulation. Stopping anticoagulation preoperatively can increase the risk of thromboembolic events. Patients with mitral valve mechanical prostheses are at a higher risk than patients with aortic valve mechanical prostheses because of slower flow. However, the risk is increased in both groups.[1] Warfarin should be stopped 72 hours before the procedure; if the patient is on aspirin, it should be stopped 1 week before the procedure. In high-risk patients, anticoagulation is interrupted before the procedure for 4 hours if unfractionated heparin is used and for 12 hours if low-molecular-weight heparin is used. High-risk patients include those with mechanical mitral valve replacement, Björk-Shiley valves (old-generation valves), history of thromboembolic event in the past year, or at least three of the following four risk factors: atrial fibrillation, embolus at any time, hypercoagulable state, and mechanical prosthesis with LVEF of less than 30%, Resumption of anticoagulation in the postoperative period is recommended with heparin; heparin should be continued until warfarin anticoagulation reaches therapeutic target.[1] If the patient is to undergo a minimally invasive procedure, anticoagulation can be withheld to maintain the international normalized ratio (INR) at the low therapeutic range and then resumed after the procedure.[1]

Patients with Arrhythmias and Heart Conduction Defects

The presence of supraventricular and ventricular arrhythmias preoperatively is considered an independent risk factor for adverse postoperative cardiac events. Patients with these arrhythmias are at risk for intraoperative and postoperative arrhythmias. However, they are not at risk for fatal or nonfatal MIs in the perioperative period. Therefore, in patients with no evidence of cardiac disease (structural or coronary) and no risk factors for arrhythmias (e.g., electrolyte abnormalities, acid-base disturbances, drug toxicities), perioperative monitoring or treatment is unnecessary.

In high-risk patients, beta blocker therapy is recommended; it decreases mortality and the risk of cardiac complications. The benefit of preoperative beta blocker therapy, along with a postoperative course of beta blockers, has been shown to last for up to 2 years postoperatively. However, the issue of beta blockade was studied mostly in high-risk patients, especially patients undergoing vascular surgery. Whether the benefit can be extrapolated to low-risk patients is questionable and needs further investigation.

To decide on the use of beta blockade preoperatively, patients should be stratified using the RCRI:

- Low-risk patients (RCRI = 1, with postoperative cardiac complication rate <1%) can undergo surgery without the use of beta blockers.
- Moderate-risk patients (RCRI 1-2) have a risk of cardiac complications of approximately 7%. The ACC update recommends beta blockers, but the level of evidence for recommendation is not well supported.
- High-risk patients (RCRI >2; risk of postoperative cardiac complications without beta blockers >10%) and moderate-risk patients and patients at high risk with normal noninvasive (stress echocardiography, scintigraphy) testing will need to start beta blockers before surgery if not already included in their medications. Patients in the high-risk category should undergo preoperative noninvasive cardiac testing modalities. Beta blockers should be started 1 month before surgery, if possible, to reach a target heart rate. A beta blocker should be restarted postoperatively as soon as possible. If the patient cannot take oral medications, short-acting IV medications are preferable.

Although beta blockers have been shown to decrease postoperative complications, mortality, and increased costs, there is no randomized, controlled trial on their use in the perioperative period. All the studies supporting their use perioperatively were small and involved relatively high-risk patients; in addition, no study used consecutive patients.

Conduction disturbances should be dealt with preoperatively. If the patient has delayed conduction (left bundle branch block [LBBB], right bundle branch block [RBBB], first-degree atrioventricular [AV] block), it is unlikely to progress to complete heart block perioperatively. Patients with delayed conduction and heart block, if they are asymptomatic and ahve no history of syncope, do not require implantation of a temporary or permanent pacemaker. Patients with advanced heart blocks (second-degree Mobitz 2, third-degree) need a temporary or permanent pacemaker.

Patients with Permanent Pacemakers and Implantable Cardioverter-Defibrillators

The issue of utmost importance when assessing patients with pacemakers is the identification of the type, mode, and indication for implantation of an implantable cardioverter-defibrillator (ICD). Other pacemaker-related and patient-related information should also be collected preoperatively (Box 3). A pacemaker check is recommended preoperatively.

The issue of concern in patients with permanent pacemakers or ICDs is the potential for electromagnetic interference. The most common causes of interference in the hospital are listed in Box 4. The most common source of electromagnetic interference in patients undergoing noncardiac surgery is electrocautery (electrocutting

Box 3 Issues to be Addressed in Patients with Pacemakers

Identification of the type of pacemaker
Determination of pacing mode
Knowledge of primary indication for pacing
Details of when device was implanted
When and where pacemaker was last checked
Anatomic position of current active generator
Battery status
Reset mode information
Confirmation of satisfactory thresholds

Box 4 Most Common Causes of Interference with Pacemaker in the Hospital

Electrocautery
External cardioversion-defibrillation
Magnetic resonance imaging
Transcutaneous electrical nerve stimulation
Drugs that interfere with pacemaker thresholds
Therapeutic radiation

Box 5 Possible Problems with Implantable Cardioverter-Defibrillators During Surgery

Resetting to a backup, reset, or noise reversion pacing mode
Temporary or permanent inhibition of pacemaker output
Increasing pacing rate
Firing
Myocardial injury at the lead tip, causing failure to sense or capture, or both
Damage to the pacemaker's circuitry, resulting in failure of pacing

more than electrocoagulation). The intensity of electromagnetic interference from cauterization is related to the distance and direction of the current to the pacemaker generator and leads. If the cautery is to be used in close proximity to the generator, care should be taken to avoid loss of ventricular pacing, causing asystole. In such cases, temporary transcutaneous or transvenous pacing should be used preoperatively. It is advised that a telemetric programmer be present during surgery. If possible, the surgeon should use bipolar cautery, which, unlike unipolar cautery, disperses energy over a small surface area. She or he should use the lowest possible amplitude and apply the current in bursts rather than continuously. If the patient has an implanted defibrillator, arrangements for external defibrillation should be made as soon as the device is disabled; defibrillation patches are preferred over paddles. Postoperatively, a telemetric review of the pacemaker settings should be carried out and it should be returned to the original settings. Antiarrhythmic medications should also be resumed.

Cardioversion-defibrillation, because of the large amounts of energy delivered, is another common source of electromagnetic interference in patients undergoing noncardiac surgery. Distinct problems with the operation of pacemakers and ICDs have been reported (Box 5). However, because of the isolation of the circuitry in titanium pacemakers, the introduction of noise protection algorithms, and the use of bipolar leads, the incidence of these complications is decreasing over time, although they can still occur.

Some pacemakers need to be inactivated (rate-responsive pacemakers, ICDs) before procedures; other pacemakers need to be reprogrammed before procedures (e.g., in pediatric patients, patients with hypertrophic cardiomyopathy [HCM], patients with heart failure). In patients with heart failure, echocardiography, along with pacemaker interval programming, is advisable before surgery. It has been recommended that patients with slow or absent rhythms be switched to VOO (ventricular pacing, no sensing, no response to sensing that is absent in the first place) or DOO (atrial and ventricular pacing, no sensing, no response to sensing, which is absent in the first place), depending on whether they have single- or dual-chamber pacemakers. Others have suggested reprogramming only pacemaker-dependent patients to asynchronous mode. Once the patient finishes the surgery, the device should be reprogrammed back to the original mode. In patients undergoing lithotripsy, the shock waves might inhibit pacemaker output if they are administered asynchronously. Therefore, shock waves should be synchronized with QRS complexes. The same pacemaker management as for other noncardiac surgeries applies to lithotripsy. Reprogramming dual-chamber pacemakers out of DDD mode is recommended in patients who are to undergo lithotripsy.

Patients with Congestive Heart Failure

Patients with congestive heart failure are at increased risk for perioperative complications. Goldman and colleagues have assigned the highest score in the cardiac risk index to signs of heart failure: jugular venous distention and the presence of S_3. However, the challenge remains, not only in the preoperative management of patients with known CHF, but also in identifying patients with undiagnosed CHF. In addition to diagnosing CHF and assessing its severity, the ACC and American Heart Association (AHA) guidelines stress the need for identifying the cause of the heart failure, even though no study has proved a survival difference from heart failure of different causes. The criteria for CHF in the various risk indices include clues from the history, physical examination, and chest x-ray findings.

Echocardiographic Assessment. The utility of echocardiography as a means of screening for CHF in patients undergoing noncardiac surgery has been investigated.[1] It was found that after adjusting for all confounding variables, parameters measured by echocardiography (e.g., LVEF, wall motion score) were not independent predictors of adverse cardiovascular outcomes. In addition, the LVEF had low sensitivity, low positive predictive values, and a likelihood ratio close to 1 for the end points examined. Thus, echocardiography does not add much to the risk-assessment tools used by clinicians to clear a patient for a noncardiac procedure.[1] Dobutamine stress echocardiography (DSE) adds to the clinical predictors of risk used for a patient's assessment preoperatively. However, it detects a measure of inducible ischemia in addition to left ventricular function. An abnormal DSE finding has high sensitivity for detecting postoperative cardiac complications in patients undergoing nonvascular surgery. The LVEF was also shown to be a statistically significant predictor (odds ratio, 0.96; P = .001) of adverse outcome in this study.[1]

Drug Therapy. Some authors have advocated the use of beta blockers in patients with heart failure undergoing noncardiac surgery, despite the limited number of CHF patients involved in studies investigating the effect of beta blockade on perioperative complications.[3] In addition, the need for noninvasive stress testing for CHF patients having a score of 3 points or more on the RCRI index is recommended. In terms of drug management, we recommend continuing the same medications in asymptomatic CHF patients. If patients have symptoms of CHF, optimization of therapy should be attempted[1]; symptomatic patients have twice the complication rates of asymptomatic patients.[4] CHF patients using beta blockers should be kept on this type of medication before surgery. However, we recommend not starting beta blockers immediately before surgery in CHF patients if they have not used this type of therapy beforehand. Therapy might take months to achieve its benefits.[1] As for digoxin, its use preoperatively is not recommended and should be determined by individual circumstances. Patients with NYHA Class III or IV CHF benefit from chronic spironolactone treatment; however, its use preoperatively remains optional because the evidence is nonexistent. In patients undergoing noncardiac surgery, the use of ACE inhibitors the morning of surgery has resulted in more episodes of hypotension, whereas patients who skipped their ACE inhibitor dose before surgery had bouts of hypertension after surgery. We recommend continuing the ACE inhibitors preoperatively; however, in patients with a low baseline blood pressure, it is recommended to skip the dose of ACE inhibitors the morning of surgery to prevent hypotension during the operation.[1]

Pulmonary Artery Catheter. The utility of pulmonary artery catheters in patients undergoing high-risk surgery has been investigated by Sandham and associates.[5] No benefit was found in patients who underwent surgery with the use of a pulmonary artery catheter (PAC) as opposed to patients without one. Of patients who had surgery with a PAC, 7.8% died versus 7.7% of those with no PAC[5]; 13.4% of patients in the standard care group and 12.4% in the catheter group had a NYHA classification of III or IV. We advise against the preoperative use of PACs in noncardiac surgery patients.[6]

Pulmonary Arterial Disease and Congenital Heart Disease

Studies assessing the risk of patients with pulmonary arterial hypertension undergoing surgery are lacking. The risk increases with higher NYHA classification. The optimal and safe type of anesthesia suitable for this population has not been determined, but expert opinion seems to favor epidural anesthesia whenever possible. Anesthesia should be administered by an experienced cardiovascular anesthesiologist in a center experienced with these high-risk patients. Patients receiving oral or inhaled treatment for pulmonary hypertension should be shifted to IV treatment if the expected withholding period of the drug is more than 12 to 24 hours. Early ambulation is preferable after surgery, and deep vein thrombosis (DVT) prophylaxis is advised in case of prolonged immobilization.

Patients with Eisenmenger's syndrome should be followed up routinely at a tertiary care center. Perioperative mortality associated with noncardiac surgery in patients with Eisenmenger's syndrome has approached 19%. The perioperative management of these patients avoids fasting, volume depletion, and hypotension. In case of hypotension, the patient should receive an α-adrenergic agonist (e.g., methoxamine, phenylephrine) or IV fluids if the patient is volume depleted. Endocarditis antibiotic prophylaxis should be carried out. All IV lines should be equipped with air filters to avoid paradoxical air embolism. The hematocrit level should be above normal, because a normal hematocrit value might not provide adequate oxygenation. An intra-arterial cannula should be used to monitor blood pressure and oxygenation. The anesthetic technique should avoid hypotension. Blood loss should be replaced to avoid relative anemia. The patient should be monitored closely in an intensive care setting after surgery. If early ambulation cannot be achieved, thromboembolism prophylaxis should be initiated.

Patients with congenital heart disease were found to have a higher risk of postoperative complications when undergoing noncardiac surgery compared with their peers without congenital heart disease; however, this risk is low (5.8%). As part of the preoperative assessment of patients with congenital heart disease, care should be taken to ensure that the cardiac defect is limited to the heart or is part of a systemic syndrome. Syndromes involving the heart can involve the airway, gastrointestinal (GI) tract, or neurologic system. The patient's course in the hospital should be managed carefully to ensure the absence of any prolonged intubation, subglottic stenosis, difficult vascular access, or thrombosed vessels. Patients with congenital heart disease are predisposed to erythrocytosis because of the chronic cyanotic state that characterizes some conditions. As a result, hyperviscosity might ensue, leading to cerebrovascular complications. Proper preoperative hydration, lowering the transfusion threshold, minimizing the fasting preoperative period, allowing water sips up to 2 hours before the operation, and scheduling the patient as the first case are some measures that can be taken to minimize complications in congenital heart disease patients.

Hypertrophic Cardiomyopathy

The amount of data discussing the preoperative complications of HCM patients undergoing noncardiac surgery is small. A study investigating the outcomes of patients with HCM undergoing noncardiac surgery has revealed that 31 patients (40%) had at least one adverse cardiac event (e.g., death, MI, arrhythmias). Multivariate analysis in this study has revealed that the type and duration of surgery are significant predictors of adverse outcomes in patients undergoing noncardiac surgery. However, the incidence of death or MI was low in this patient population. In hypertrophic obstructive cardiomyopathy (HOCM) patients, care should be taken to avoid hypovolemia, decreased vascular resistance, increased venous capacitance, and use of catecholamines, because they increase outflow obstruction.

Patients with Morbid Obesity

The prevalence of obesity has increased since the 1980s years in the United States. In 2005, 31% of all Americans older than 20 years had a BMI greater than 30. The use of bariatric surgery as an option for weight loss has increased 10 times from the 1990s to 2004 (140,000 bariatric surgeries done in 2004). Given the risks inherent in bariatric surgery, some investigators classify this surgery as a moderate-risk to high-risk surgery.[7] Elevated BMI itself was not found to portray a higher risk of cardiovascular complications or mortality in a case-control study in non–cardiac surgery patients with morbid obesity.[8] However, given the increased number of risk factors that might be associated with morbid obesity and the risks inherent in the surgery itself, careful preoperative assessment of the morbidly obese patient should be preformed to reduce the mortality and morbidity of these patients.[7]

We recommend a detailed history (angina, paroxysmal nocturnal dyspnea, orthopnea, and palpitations), including evaluation of the functional capacity of the patient. Given the challenging auscultation in such patients, the physical examination should be focused on gathering evidence of cor pulmonale, left ventricular dysfunction, pheripheral arterial disease, and venous insufficiency. In addition, the morbidly obese patient should be evaluated for obstructive sleep apnea (OSA) routinely by history (occurrence of apneic episodes, daytime sleepiness) and by physical examination findings (neck circumference, waist-to-hip ratio). Some investigators recommend routine evaluation with polysomnography before bariatric surgery. OSA increases complications (arrhythmias, MI, ICU admissions), cost of postoperative care, and length of hospital stay. Some investigators recommend the use of CPAP in these patients in the perioperative period. This is proven to decrease the rate of postoperative complications.[9]

We recommend appropriate use of medical therapy to control all the comorbidities the patient suffers from; use of CPAP is recommended preoperatively. In addition, the patient should be managed by a multidisciplinary team including an anesthesiologist, a nutritionist, a surgeon and a cardiologist. In patients with OSA, cautious use of analgesic should be exercised postoperatively because some agents induce respiratory depression. The second most common complication postoperatively in such patients is pulmonary embolism; therefore, we recommend prophylactic anticoagulation in this population, taking into account the weight, the renal function of each individual patient, and the patient's risk of bleeding.[10]

Type of Surgery

In addition to assessing the risk imposed by the various medical conditions of the patient, the context in which the patient undergoes the surgery (elective vs. urgent vs. emergent), as well as the type of surgery itself, need to be taken into consideration to assess risk and minimize it. In the development of a predictive model for operative risk, patients undergoing various types of surgeries (except cardiac surgery and cesarean section) were enrolled. Multivariate analysis has revealed that the complexity of the surgical procedure (low, moderate, or high risk) according to the modified Johns Hopkins surgical criteria (Box 6) and the mode of surgery (elective, urgent, or emergent) were two of the four predictors of in-hospital death. This is secondary to the fact that the more urgent the surgery, the less time is available to adequately reduce the patient's risk by medical interventions. The other two factors were age and American Society of Anesthesiologists' (ASA) grade (Table 2).

In patients undergoing elective surgery, two risk factors have been found to significantly influence cardiovascular mortality within 30 days of the operation: prior myocardial infarction and renal failure. In a case-control study on patients who underwent urgent or emergent surgical procedures, a history of congestive heart failure was the only significant predictor of 30-day mortality on multivariate analysis.

The ACC and AHA have jointly classified different types of surgeries into different categories of risk (Box 7). High-risk procedures have a cardiac risk higher than 5% and include emergent major procedures, major vascular surgeries (except carotid endarterectomy, which is intermediate risk), and prolonged procedures, with fluid shifts and possible blood loss. Low-risk procedures have a risk lower than 1% and include all endoscopic procedures, superficial

Box 6 Modified Johns Hopkins Surgical Criteria

Grade I

Minimal to Mild Risk Independent of Anesthesia

Includes

- Breast biopsy

Excludes

- Open exposure of internal body organs

Minimal to Moderately Invasive Procedure

Includes

- Removal of minor skin or subcutaneous lesions

Excludes

- Repair of vascular or neurologic structures

Potential Blood Loss Less than 500 mL

Includes

- Myringotomy tubes
- Hysteroscopy
- Cystoscopy, vasectomy
- Circumcision
- Fiberoptic bronchoscopy
- Diagnostic laparoscopy dilatation and curettage
- Fallopian tube ligation, arthroscopy
- Inguinal hernia repair
- Laparoscopic lysis of adhesion
- Tonsillectomy, rhinoplasty

Excludes

- Placement of prosthetic devices
- Postoperative monitored care setting
- Open exposure of abdomen, thorax, neck, cranium
- Resection of major body organs

Grade II

Moderately to Significantly Invasive Procedures

Includes

- Thyroidectomy

Excludes

- Open thoracic or intracranial procedure

Potential Blood Loss of 500-1500 mL

Includes

- Hysterectomy

Excludes

- Major vascular repair (e.g., aortofemoral bypass)

Moderate Risk to Patient Independent of Anesthesia

Includes

- Myomectomy
- Cystectomy
- Cholecystectomy, laminectomy
- Hip, knee replacement, nephrectomy
- Major laparoscopic procedures
- Resection, reconstructive surgery of the digestive tract

Excludes

- Planned postoperative monitored care setting (ICU, PACU)

Grade III

Highly Invasive Procedure

- Major orthopedic-spinal reconstruction

Potential Blood Loss More than 1500 mL

- Major reconstruction of the gastrointestinal tract

Major to Critical Risk to Patient Independent of Anesthesia

- Major genitourinary surgery (e.g., radical retropubic prostatectomy)

Usual Postoperative ICU Stay with Invasive Monitoring

- Major vascular repair without postoperative ICU stay
- Cardiothoracic procedure Intracranial procedure
- Major procedure on the oropharynx
- Major vascular, skeletal, neurologic repair

ICU, intensive care unit; PACU, postanesthesia care unit.

Table 2 American Society of Anesthesiologists' (ASA) Physical Status Classification

Class	Description
I	Healthy patient
II	Mild systemic disease; no functional limitation
III	Severe systemic disease; definite functional limitation
IV	Severe systemic disease that is constant threat to life
V	Moribund patient; unlikely to survive 24 hr with or without operation

From Donati A, Ruzzi M, Adrario E, et al: A new and feasible model for predicting operative risk. Br J Anaesth 2004;93:393-399.

Box 7 Cardiac Risk* Stratification for Noncardiac Surgical Procedures

High Risk (reported cardiac risk often >5%)

Emergent major operations, particularly in older patients
Aortic and other major vascular surgeries
Peripheral vascular surgery
Anticipated prolonged surgical procedures associated with large fluid shifts, blood loss, or both

Intermediate Risk (reported cardiac risk generally <5%)

Carotid endarterectomy
Head and neck surgery
Intraperitoneal and intrathoracic surgery
Orthopedic surgery
Prostate surgery

Low Risk (reported cardiac risk generally <1%)†

Endoscopic procedures
Superficial procedure
Cataract surgery
Breast surgery

**Combined incidence of cardiac death and nonfatal myocardial infarction.*
†Does not generally require further preoperative cardiac testing.

procedures, and cataract and breast surgeries. The rest of the procedures are classified as intermediate risk, less than 5%. In addition to this stratification, the operative experience of the surgeon and volume of the medical center influence the cardiovascular outcomes, especially in vascular surgeries.

MINIMIZATION OF RISK USING MEDICAL THERAPY

A considerable number of studies have dealt with the appropriate medication that should be started to minimize the risk of patients undergoing noncardiac surgery. These studies involved beta blockers, lipid-lowering agents, clonidine, and other drugs (verapamil, diltiazem).

Beta Blockers

Studies of the use of beta blockade before noncardiac surgery had many limitations in the design, dosing, and titration to target heart rate. Studies assessing the appropriate dose, route, and type of beta blocker, as well as studies comparing different beta blockers, are lacking. However, several studies have shown a decreased incidence of death and MI during and after noncardiac surgery in patients who had used beta blockers. This benefit was most accentuated in patients who were intermediate or high risk. The benefit was not found in the low-risk group. Some studies even reported harm from the use of beta blockers in low-risk populations.

Studies that started therapy hours before surgery did not find benefit from beta blockers.[3,11] The benefit was mostly found in studies that carefully titrated the dose of beta blockers over many days to a target heart rate close to 65 beats/min.[12,13] In addition, a study comparing a long-acting beta blocker (atenolol) to a short-acting beta blocker (metoprolol) found that patients on long-acting beta blockers had lesser complications as compared to those on the short-acting medication (1.6% vs. 2% had MI, and 1.2% vs. 1.6% died, respectively). However, the design of this study was retrospective.[14]

Therefore, we recommend the use of β_1-selective long-acting beta blockers for patients at intermediate to high risk according to the RCRI (risk of postoperative complications >7%). The dosage of the beta blocker should be titrated over many days to keep the heart rate between 60 and 65 beats/min preoperatively and less than 80 beats/min intraoperatively and postoperatively. Beta blockers should be started a few days before surgery and continued for 1 week to 1 month (preferably longer) after surgery. Patients with indications for a beta blocker should be kept on it indefinitely. Those with severe reactive airways disease or advanced heart block should not be prescribed beta blockers before surgery.

Lipid-Lowering Agents

The use of lipid-lowering agents has been advocated by some investigators as a means to reduce perioperative cardiac complications. One retrospective study of patients undergoing vascular surgery found that statin use reduced the incidence of the composite end point of death, myocardial infarction, and ischemia. However, this did not result in a statistically significant difference in myocardial infarction or death. This study was limited by a retrospective design and nonspecified dose and duration of statins.

Another study has retrospectively reviewed the preoperative use of statins in patients undergoing infrainguinal vascular surgery and found that patients who were prescribed statins preoperatively have fewer composite vascular and cardiac end points. Statin use decreased hospital stay. A 5-year follow up of patients taking statins showed better survival.

A recent study on elderly patients undergoing major vascular noncardiac surgery showed evidence of benefit of statin use which increases as age advances.[2] However, the evidence supporting the use of statins in the perioperative period is not solid; therefore, we recommend the use of statins preoperatively in patients who require statins based on their medical profile, regardless of surgical plans. This medication should be continued after surgery.

α_2-Adrenergic Agonists

The evidence of benefit of α_2 agonists in the perioperative setting has been shown in two meta-analyses and one randomized trial, in which it was found that clonidine given before noncardiac surgery reduces the incidence of perioperative ischemia and mortality. However, this benefit was only found in one subgroup of patients (vascular surgery) and not in others; thus, we cannot extrapolate the findings in this study to other surgical patients. The benefit of clonidine use perioperatively is still uncertain; until the evidence of benefit of this medication preoperatively has been established, we do not recommend using it preoperatively unless the patient had been using it previously.

Preoperative Laboratory Tests for Risk Assessment

B-Type Natriuretic Peptide and N-Terminal Pro–B-Type Natriuretic Peptide

Some patients may be leading a sedentary lifestyle secondary to orthopaedic conditions, rheumatologic conditions, or morbid obesity; this lifestyle prevents the clinicians from properly assessing the occurrence of symptoms related to cardiac supply-and-demand mismatch. In addition to the use of the RCRI to risk stratify these patients, some laboratory tests provide an idea about the presence of ventricular overload.

One such test is B-type natriuretic peptide (BNP). BNP measurement in patients undergoing noncardiac surgery was done before surgery in 1590 consecutive patients. The authors used a cutoff value of 189 pg/mL to stratify the patients into low-risk and high-risk groups. Five percent of the patients who had a BNP level less than 189 pg/mL had a postoperative cardiac complication as compared to 13% in the patients who had BNP level between 200 and 300 pg/mL and 81% in the patients whose BNP level was greater than 300 pg/mL. High BNP was more reliable to predict the occurrence of postoperative cardiac events than the Goldman index used in this study.[15]

In addition to its use to predict the occurrence of short term postoperative complications, other investigators used N-terminal pro–B-type natriuretic peptide (NT proBNP) to predict the long-term occurrence of cardiac complications after major vascular surgery (abdominal aortic aneurysm repair or lower-extremity bypass surgery).[16] In this study, patients with NT proBNP value more than 319 pg/dL had a higher risk of cardiac events and mortality at 6 months of follow-up.[16]

Feringa and colleagues found that elevated levels of NT proBNP are associated with high levels of troponin T release and myocardial ischemia in patients undergoing major vascular surgery.[17] In this study, the optimal value of NT proBNP to predict the risk of myocardial ischemia and troponin T release was 270 ng/L. The association found in this study between NT proBNP and cardiac complications and mortality was independent of comorbidities, medication use, and cigarette smoking.[17]

The main limitation of the aforementioned studies is that they mainly included patients undergoing major vascular surgery; hence the applicability of these results on other patient populations is questionable. In patients undergoing major vascular surgery, we recommend stratifying patients according to the RCRI and measuring NT proBNP. Patients with elevated NT proBNP should be managed aggressively with lifestyle modifications and medications both before the surgery and during the long-term follow up. (Table 3)

Glucose and Hemoglobin A_{1c} Measurement

Diabetes mellitus and impaired glucose tolerance are associated with increased risk of cardiovascular events. The occurrence of glucose disturbances before noncardiac surgery was shown by many investigators to be a marker of a poor outcome in the postoperative period.

In one study dealing with patients undergoing major vascular surgery, patients with impaired glucose tolerance and diabetic patients had higher incidence of myocardial infarction, troponin T release, 30-day cardiac complications, and higher mortality as compared to patients with normal glucose level in the blood.[18] Patients who had HbA_{1c} higher than 7% had a similarly worse outcome as compared to patients with HbA_{1c} lower than 7%.[18]

A similar study was done in patients who are subjected to noncardiac nonvascular surgery to assess the effect of baseline glucose elevation on the risk of perioperative complications after surgery.[19] Impaired glucose tolerance was associated with three-fold increased mortality in patients undergoing nonvascular surgery as compared to normoglycemic controls. Patients who had glucose levels in the diabetic range had four-fold increased cardiovascular mortality as compared to normoglycemic patients.[19] However, this study was retrospective in design; the results need to be confirmed by a prospective study.[19]

In one study, an oral glucose tolerance test (OGTT) was done for vascular surgery patients to diagnose new cases of diabetes and

Table 3 Laboratory Tests to Risk Stratify Patients Undergoing Noncardiac Surgery

Study	Test	Cutoff Value	OR/HR of Myocardial ischemia	OR/HR of Death/ nonfatal MI	OR/HR of all cardiac complications
Dernellis et al[15]	BNP	>189 pg/ml	NA	NA	28.78
Feringa et al[17]	NT proBNP	>270 ng/L	1.49*	1.59*	NA
Feringa et al[16]	NT proBNP	>319 ng/L	NA	4†	10.9‡
Feringa et al[18]	HbA_{1c}	>7%	2.8	3.6	5.6
Feringa et al[18]	IGT	5.6-7 mmol/L§	2.2	2	1.9
Feringa et al[18]	DM	>7 mmol/L§	2.6	2.7	3.1

*Odds ratio for each 1 ng/L rise in the natural logarhithm of baseline NT proBNP.
†Hazard ratio for all-cause mortality.
‡Hazard ratio for major adverse cardiac events.
§Fasting glucose values.
BNP, B-type natriuretic peptide; DM, diabetes mellitus; HbA_{1c}, hemoglobin A_{1c}; HR, hazard ratio; IGT, impaired glucose tolerance; MI, myocardial infarction; NA, not available; NT proBNP, pro–B-type natriuretic peptide; OR, odds ratio.

impaired glucose tolerance (IGT) as well as to investigate the relationship of the OGTT with perioperative complications following surgery.[20] Impaired glucose tolerance and diabetes mellitus were detected in 25.7% and 10.6%, respectively, in the population studied. The patients who had a positive OGTT had a higher rate of myocardial ischemia and myocardial infarction and higher mortality as compared to normoglycemic subjects.[20]

We recommend taking a blood glucose level in all patients with cardiac risk factors (e.g., hypertension, dyslipidemia) undergoing noncardiac surgery. If the level is abnormal, then it should be confirmed by another fasting glucose test. If the patient is found to have diabetes, he or she should be reclassified according to the RCRI and managed accordingly. In patients with no risk factors, we recommend taking random glucose measurement by finger stick. Patients who show abnormal results should be subjected to fasting blood glucose measurement. Patients with impaired glucose tolerance or diabetes should have extensive lifestyle modifications, and insulin treatment, if needed, depending on the blood glucose levels. Therapy should preferably be initiated in the hospital. However, antidiabetic drugs should be withheld the morning of the surgery to prevent intraoperative hypoglycaemia. In addition, blood sugar should be monitored closely during the course of the operation; hyper- and hypoglycemic episodes should be treated appropriately (see Table 3).

Summary

Cardiac events are the most common complications of noncardiac surgeries. Fortunately, a few steps can minimize the risks.

- Consider patient-related factors: history of cardiac disease, renal insuffiency, diabetes mellitus, and older patients
- Consider surgery-related factors: vascular surgeries, thoracic and abdominal surgeries, urgent surgeries
- Consider medications and devices: Which medications to continue and which medications to withhold? Could ICDs and pacemakers be affected?

Suggested Readings

Auerbach A, Goldman L: Assessing and reducing the cardiac risk of noncardiac surgery. Circulation 2006;113:1361-1376.

Detsky AS, Abrams HB, Forbath N, et al: Cardiac assessment for patients undergoing noncardiac surgery. A multifactorial clinical risk index. Arch Intern Med 1986;146:2131-2134.

Donati A, Ruzzi M, Adrario E, et al: A new and feasible model for predicting operative risk. Br J Anaesth 2004;93:393-399.

Eagle KA, Berger PB, Calkins H, et al: American College of Cardiology; American Heart Association: ACC/AHA guideline update for perioperative cardiovascular evaluation for noncardiac surgery-executive summary: A report of the American College of Cardiology/American Heart Association Task Force on Practice Guidelines (Committee to Update the 1996 Guidelines on Perioperative Cardiovascular Evaluation for Noncardiac Surgery). J Am Coll Cardiol 2002;39:542-553.

Eagle KA, Coley CM, Newell JB, et al: Combining clinical and thallium data optimizes preoperative assessment of cardiac risk before major vascular surgery. Ann Intern Med 1989;110:859-866.

Fleisher LA, Beckman JA, Brown KA, et al: American College of Cardiology/American Heart Association Task Force on Practice Guidelines Writing Committee to Update the 2002 Guidelines on Perioperative Cardiovascular Evaluation for Noncardiac Surgery; American Society of Echocardiography; American Society of Nuclear Cardiology; Heart Rhythm Society; Society of Cardiovascular Anesthesiologists; Society for Cardiovascular Angiography and Interventions; Society for Vascular Medicine and Biology: ACC/AHA 2006 guideline update on perioperative cardiovascular evaluation for noncardiac surgery: Focused update on perioperative beta blocker therapy: A report of the American College of Cardiology/American Heart Association Task Force on Practice Guidelines (Writing Committee to Update the 2002 Guidelines on Perioperative Cardiovascular Evaluation for Noncardiac Surgery): Developed in collaboration with the American Society of Echocardiography, American Society of Nuclear Cardiology, Heart Rhythm Society, Society of Cardiovascular Anesthesiologists, Society for Cardiovascular Angiography and Interventions, and Society for Vascular Medicine and Biology. Circulation 2006;113:2662-2674.

Galli KK, Myers LB, Nicolson SC: Anesthesia for adult patients with congenital heart disease undergoing noncardiac surgery. Int Anesthesiol Clin 2001;39:43-71.

Goldman L, Caldera DL, Nussbaum SR, et al: Multifactorial index of cardiac risk in noncardiac surgical procedures. N Engl J Med 1977;297:845-850.

Polanczyk CA, Marcantonio E, Goldman L, et al: Impact of age on perioperative complications and length of stay in patients undergoing noncardiac surgery. Ann Intern Med 2001;134:637-643.

Sandham JD, Hull RD, Brant RF, et al: A randomized, controlled trial of the use of pulmonary-artery catheters in high-risk surgical patients. N Engl J Med 2003;348:5-14.

Vongpatanasin W, Brickner ME, Hillis LD, Lange RA: The Eisenmenger syndrome in adults. Ann Intern Med 1998;128:745-755.

Wesorick DH, Eagle KA: The preoperative cardiovascular evaluation of the intermediate-risk patient: New data, changing strategies. Am J Med 2005;118:1413.

References

For a complete list of references, log onto www.expertconsult.com.

Aortic Valve Disease

Gian M. Novaro

The cardiac valves have two functions. By opening, they control the direction in which blood flows and, by closing, they allow pressure differentials to exist in a closed system. Abnormal valve function produces either pressure overloading caused by restricted opening or volume overloading caused by inadequate closure. Valvular heart disease can be approached on the basis of the pathologic lesion-aortic stenosis or aortic regurgitation-or pathophysiologically, as pressure overloading versus volume overloading.

In this chapter, I summarize my current approach to aortic valve disease, aortic stenosis and regurgitation, with particular emphasis on the indications for valve surgery. In general, I adhere to the recommendations given by the American College of Cardiology-American Heart Association (ACC/AHA) 2006 guidelines for the management of patients with valvular heart disease.[1]

AORTIC STENOSIS

Definition

Aortic stenosis refers to obstruction of flow at the level of the aortic valve and does not include the subvalvular and supravalvular forms of this disease. Aortic valve stenosis is usually defined by restricted systolic opening of the valve leaflets, with a mean transvalvular pressure gradient of at least 10 mm Hg. The cause of the stenosis can be further defined based on the anatomy and disease process affecting the valve.

Prevalence and Etiology

Calcific aortic stenosis and congenital bicuspid aortic valve stenosis account for the overwhelming majority of aortic stenosis cases, followed by less common conditions, such as rheumatic aortic stenosis and congenital aortic stenosis. In older adults, mild thickening, calcification, or both of a trileaflet aortic valve without restricted leaflet motion (i.e., aortic sclerosis) affects about 25% of the population older than 65 years. Calcific aortic stenosis, however, affects approximately 2% to 3% of those older than 75 years. Thus, not all patients with aortic sclerosis go on to develop obstructive aortic valve disease. Congenital bicuspid aortic valve stenosis is a major common cause of aortic stenosis; the approximate overall incidence of an anatomic bicuspid aortic valve is 1% to 2% of the population. Of these, about one half will develop aortic stenosis and up to one third will develop aortic regurgitation. Aortic stenosis caused by a congenital bicuspid aortic valve affects men more often than women, but later life calcific disease of a trileaflet valve involves both genders equally. Rheumatic valve disease has declined dramatically in the United States during the past 50 years, and isolated rheumatic aortic stenosis is unusual in any event. Finally, congenital aortic stenosis usually results from failure of the valve commissures to develop fully and manifests with aortic stenosis in childhood or young adulthood.

The most common forms of aortic valve disease (calcific disease of a trileaflet aortic valve, calcification of a congenital bicuspid aortic valve, congenital aortic stenosis) can be distinguished clinically by age at onset and by their characteristic echocardiographic findings. Calcific aortic stenosis (Fig. 1), usually referred to as "degenerative" or "senile type," affects trileaflet aortic valves, often in patients with other risk factors for atherosclerotic disease.[2] The aortic valve disease is an active process, with lipid deposition, inflammation, and calcification. This form of aortic stenosis progresses slowly, and patients often present between the ages of 70 and 90 years. Echocardiographic examination typically reveals varying degrees of nodular thickening and calcification of the three leaflets with restricted systolic motion. Adults with congenital bicuspid aortic valves are predominantly men, often have known of a heart murmur for many years, and usually experience the onset of symptoms between the ages of 40 and 60 years.[3] Bicuspid valves (Fig. 2) usually have fusion of one of the three commissures, most commonly the left and right and, echocardiographically, can be distinguished by the presence of a raphe, leaflet doming, eccentric closure, and fish mouth orifice during systole. Congenital aortic stenosis usually presents in childhood, even in infancy, and the echocardiographic examination will show a unicuspid or bicuspid valve. Other less common causes of aortic stenosis include rheumatic disease, homozygous hypercholesterolemia, and radiation heart disease.

Pathophysiology

Valvular aortic stenosis results in chronic left ventricular pressure overloading. At any stage of life, however, the natural history of aortic stenosis largely reflects the functional integrity of the mitral valve. As long as adequate mitral valve function is maintained, the pulmonary bed is protected from the systolic pressure overloading imposed by aortic stenosis. In contrast to mitral valve disease, in which the pulmonary circuit is directly involved, compensatory concentric left ventricular hypertrophy allows the pressure-overloaded ventricle to maintain stroke volume with modest increases in diastolic pressure, and patients remain asymptomatic for many years.

Eventually, however, left ventricular hypertrophy causes either diastolic dysfunction with the onset of congestive symptoms or myocardial oxygen needs in excess of supply with the onset of angina. Some patients might also experience exertional syncope, probably reflecting the inability to increase cardiac output and maintain blood pressure in response to vasodilation. Vasodepressor (neurocardiogenic) syncope, however, may be an operative mechanism in a portion of these syncopal episodes.

Signs and Symptoms

Most patients with calcific aortic stenosis have known of their heart murmur for many years. The critical points in defining the cardiac history in men include the results of athletic, military, insurance, or employment physical examinations. In women, pregnancy and childbearing history are important to define functional status.

Patients with typical findings of aortic stenosis should have a detailed history-taking session with inquiry about habitual activity levels and any changes in exercise tolerance. The onset of any of the classic symptoms of left ventricular outflow obstruction—angina, syncope, or heart failure—in a patient with valvular aortic stenosis indicates advanced valve disease and should be carefully and promptly evaluated.

On physical examination, the harsh systolic murmur of aortic stenosis, loudest at the base of the heart and radiating to the carotids, is often but not always prominent. Low output states, obesity, or chronic lung disease may mask the findings. The murmur may radiate toward the cardiac apex, in which case the harsh component is lost; this finding may be mistaken for a second murmur. Other hallmarks of significant aortic valve stenosis include a single (pulmonic) component of the second heart sound and a sustained left ventricular apical impulse with a fourth heart sound. The slowly rising, low-volume carotid arterial pulse of severe aortic stenosis may be noted in younger patients, but changes in arterial compliance often mask these findings in older adults.

Diagnosis

The electrocardiogram often shows changes of left ventricular hypertrophy. The chest radiograph is seldom helpful, although occasionally heavy calcification of the valve or ascending aortic dilation may be seen. With their widespread availability, two-dimensional and Doppler echocardiography have become the tests of choice in the evaluation of patients with suspected valvular disease. Echocardiography allows assessment of the valve anatomy as well as of chamber size and ventricular function. Doppler studies permit estimation of pressure gradients and estimations of aortic valve area by using the continuity equation.

With good-quality echocardiography, cardiac catheterization is usually not required to make the diagnosis of aortic stenosis. I generally perform preoperative coronary angiography in men older than 35 years, women older than 35 years with risk factors, and all postmenopausal women, to exclude coronary artery disease. The classic catheterization laboratory studies of transvalvular gradients and cardiac output have been largely superseded by hemodynamic assessment in the echocardiography laboratory.

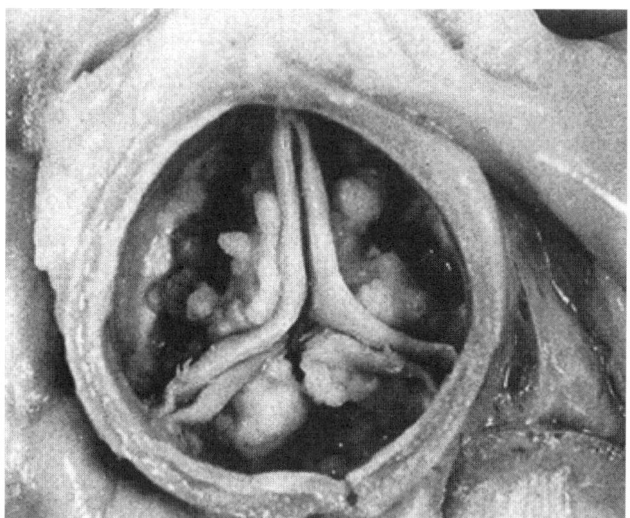

Figure 1 Pathologic specimen of a severely stenotic trileaflet aortic valve. Gross nodular atherocalcific changes on the aortic sides of the leaflets can be seen.

Treatment

Patients with aortic stenosis fall into one of four categories of severity: mild, moderate, severe, or critical (Table 1). Asymptomatic patients with aortic stenosis should have medical follow-up with regular inquiry about changes in exercise tolerance or other symptoms. Serial echocardiographic examinations should be based on an understanding of the natural history of the lesion. Current evidence indicates that calcific aortic stenosis progresses, on the average, at a rate of about 0.1 cm^2 per year decline in valve area. Asymptomatic patients should have an echocardiographic re-evaluation every 2 to 3 years for mild aortic stenosis, every 1 to 2 years for moderate stenosis, and every 6 to 12 months for severe stenosis. Patients with moderate to severe asymptomatic aortic stenosis should avoid strenuous or competitive activity, particularly postprandial exertion. Infective endocarditis precautions following new ACC/AHA guidelines are no longer required.

To date, no medical therapy exists for the treatment of calcific aortic stenosis. The possible impact of secondary prevention measures, particularly lipid lowering with statins, on the progression of aortic stenosis has been investigated.[5,6] Hypertension occurs in up to 40% to 50% of patients with calcific aortic stenosis and should be managed appropriately, because untreated hypertension may lead to earlier onset of symptoms. Antihypertensive medications should be

Table 1 Classification of Aortic Stenosis Severity

Severity	Valve Area (cm^2)	Maximum Aortic Velocity (m/sec)	Mean Pressure Gradient (mm Hg)
Mild	1.5-2.0	2.5-3.0	<25
Moderate	1.0-1.5	3.0-4.0	25-40
Severe	0.6-1.0	>4.0	>40
Critical	<0.6	—	—

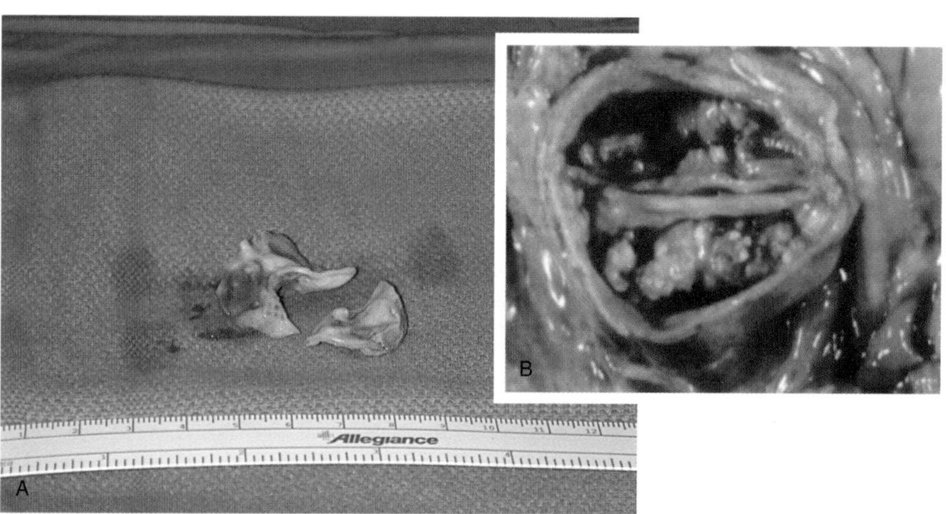

Figure 2 Gross specimens of congenital bicuspid aortic valves. A, Note the larger conjoined leaflet and the smaller noncoronary cusp. **B,** Note the atherocalcific deposits on the surfaces of the leaflets.

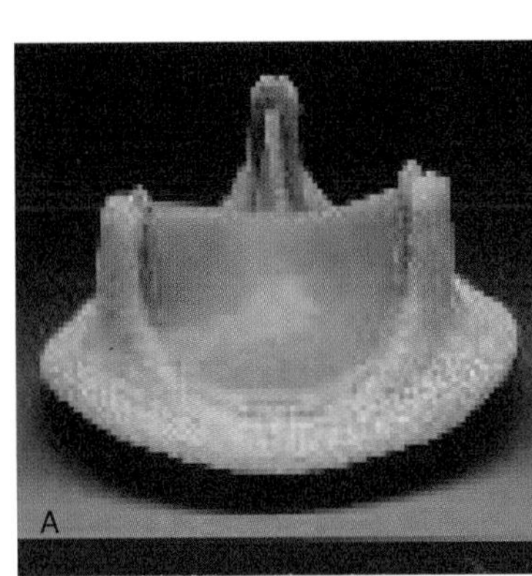

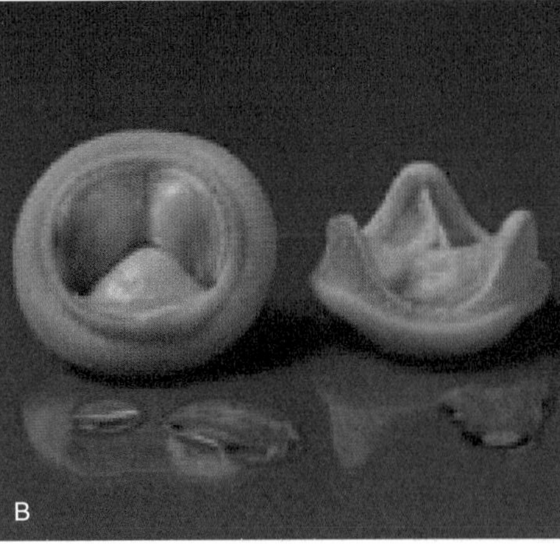

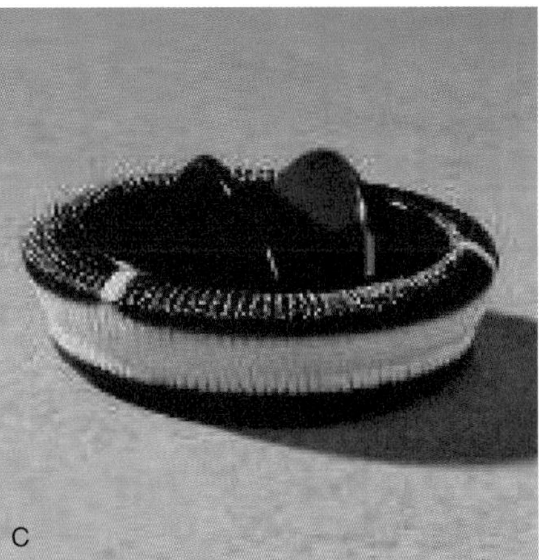

Figure 3 **Prosthetic heart valves. A** and **B,** Bioprosthetic valves. **C,** Mechanical valve.

titrated slowly, and vasodilators should be used with caution with severe aortic stenosis. I do not hesitate to use concomitant beta blockers for select patients.

A supervised exercise tolerance test can provide helpful objective assessment for patients with echocardiographic evidence of moderate to severe aortic stenosis who report atypical symptoms, minimal complaints, or are sedentary and do not experience exercise intolerance. Stress testing performed with caution and under physician supervision can be done with relative safety in those with aortic stenosis. Functional limitation with an inability to exercise to levels more than 6 metabolic equivalents or a blunted blood pressure response (<20 mm Hg) may be viewed as a "symptom." Nevertheless, I rarely encounter truly asymptomatic individuals with critical aortic stenosis, and do not advocate stress testing for patients with severe left ventricular outflow obstruction.

Symptomatic patients (i.e., those with angina, syncope, or dyspnea) with severe aortic stenosis should undergo valve replacement (Class I indication).[1,7] Additional indications for aortic valve surgery include patients with severe aortic stenosis undergoing coronary artery bypass grafting or surgery on the aorta or other heart valves (Class I indication); patients with severe aortic stenosis and left ventricular ejection fractions less than 0.50 (Class I indication); and patients with moderate aortic stenosis undergoing coronary artery bypass grafting or surgery on the aorta or other heart valves (Class IIa indication). Aortic valve surgery may be considered in asymptomatic patients who exhibit an abnormal response to exercise (e.g., drop in blood pressure, abnormal symptoms, or poor functional capacity; Class IIb indication). The preoperative evaluation should address any major comorbid conditions and optimize their management. A carotid duplex examination should be performed, because distinguishing a carotid bruit from a radiating murmur is difficult clinically. Coronary angiography is indicated to evaluate the need for coronary revascularization, because about one half will have significant coronary disease as indicated by the preoperative angiogram. Patients scheduled for valve surgery should not have percutaneous angioplasty if the preoperative catheterization shows obstructive coronary disease, because surgical revascularization adds little to the risk of aortic valve replacement. Smoking cessation is strongly encouraged, and diabetic control to achieve hemoglobin A_{1c} ($HgbA_{1c}$) levels close to 6% may reduce postoperative infection risk. Thyroid disease and the need for thyroid hormone replacement should be assessed. Dental care should be completed before surgery.

The consulting cardiologist, cardiac surgeon, or both should discuss the advantages and drawbacks of mechanical versus bioprosthetic valves (Fig. 3) with the patient and family during the presurgical evaluation. Often, the choice of prosthesis is straightforward, but younger patients in particular may have special needs, which should be addressed. Bioprosthetic valves offer the advantage of not requiring long-term oral anticoagulation, but have the drawback of relatively limited durability. In contrast, mechanical valves offer long-term durability but require lifelong warfarin therapy. The generally accepted risk of serious bleeding with warfarin is about 1% to 2% per year. Childbearing age (in women) and engaging in vigorous sports activities are factors that are relative contraindications to chronic oral anticoagulation with warfarin and may influence the choice of valves. In general, I favor bioprosthetic valves in patients older than 60 years and mechanical valves in those younger than 50 years. For male patients in their 50s, clinical outcomes with bioprosthetic valves are good; in this group, current estimates place the likelihood of reoperation for late (after 10 years) deterioration of a bioprosthesis at about 1 in 10, using competing outcomes analysis. In contrast, healthy women in their 50s should probably receive mechanical valves, because many can expect another 30 years of life. Homograft aortic valve replacement with a cryopreserved cadaveric valve may offer specific advantages for patients with infective endocarditis or diseases of the aortic root.

Patients and physicians should bear in mind that valve replacement is palliative, not curative. A prosthetic heart valve commits a patient to continued infective endocarditis prophylaxis, regular cardiac follow-up, and often continued medical therapy, including anticoagulation with warfarin for those with mechanical prostheses. Reoperation may be required for malfunction of the prosthetic valve. In addition, a small but not insignificant subset of patients may require implantation of a permanent pacemaker after aortic valve surgery. Patients should clearly indicate their willingness to accept the limitations that valve replacement imposes before surgery. In addition, patients must understand that surgical risks include wound infection and stroke, as well as perioperative mortality.

AORTIC REGURGITATION

Definition

Aortic regurgitation is defined by incompetence of the aortic valve, in which a portion of the left ventricular forward stroke volume returns to the chamber during diastole. The cause of the regurgitation, as for aortic stenosis, can be further defined based on the anatomy of the valve and aortic root and the disease process affecting the valve.

Causes and Pathophysiology

Aortic regurgitation can occur because of leaflet pathology or aortic root disease.[8,9] As an isolated lesion, aortic regurgitation usually occurs because of a congenital bicuspid aortic valve, often resulting from leaflet prolapse. Infective endocarditis involving the aortic valve may result in aortic regurgitation because of loss of coaptation, leaflet retraction, or perforation (Fig. 4). However, any pathologic process that results in aortic root dilation and loss of leaflet coaptation can also result in aortic regurgitation. Examples include diseases of the aortic root, such as annuloaortic ectasia (Fig. 5), long standing hypertension, familial aortic aneurysmal disease, and hereditable diseases of connective tissue, such as Marfan syndrome. Additionally, ascending aortic dissections and congenital diseases, such as ventricular septal defects as seen in tetralogy of Fallot, can lead to aortic regurgitation. Other less common conditions include radiation heart disease, Ehlers-Danlos syndrome, and inflammatory aortitis and/or aortic valvulitis caused by giant cell aortitis, reactive arthritis, syphilitic aortitis, ankylosing spondylitis, and rheumatoid arthritis.

Regardless of cause, chronic aortic regurgitation results in volume overloading of the left ventricle and, in contrast to mitral regurgitation, also causes a component of pressure overload. The volume overload usually is well tolerated for long periods, possibly even decades. The sequelae of aortic regurgitation reflect the severity of the diastolic leak; these include left ventricular dilation and hypertrophy, with remodeling of the left ventricle to a more spherical shape. The ejection fraction usually is preserved until the late stages of the disease.

Because patients may tolerate severe aortic regurgitation with minimal symptoms, management should include careful monitoring of left ventricular dimensions and systolic function. In addition, because aortic root and proximal ascending aortic dilation can coexist, careful monitoring of aortic enlargement is warranted in these patients. Surgical intervention is indicated, even in asymptomatic individuals, when left ventricular dilation reaches critical dimensions or ventricular dysfunction occurs.[1]

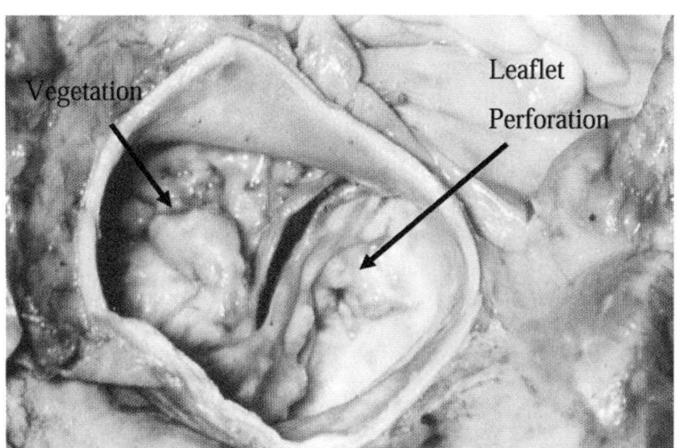

Figure 4 Gross specimen of a bicuspid aortic valve damaged by infective endocarditis. There is a perforation in the body of the leaflet *(arrow)* as well as vegetations on the conjoined leaflet *(arrow)*.

Signs and Symptoms

Patients with chronic aortic regurgitation caused by congenital bicuspid valve, hypertension, or annuloaortic ectasia often have little clinical history other than a known cardiac murmur noted on routine auscultation. In contrast, patients with aortic regurgitation caused by infective endocarditis or certain aortic root diseases, may recount rather dramatic illness or systemic complaints. Nonetheless, cardiac complaints are unusual until the later stages of volume overloading, when effort intolerance becomes a problem. Symptoms of aortic regurgitation often begin with nonspecific fatigue. Patients might relate that their ability to get through a day's work is maintained, but they are exhausted after returning home. Palpitations, or awareness of a forceful heartbeat, is an early complaint, sometimes noted by spouses. With further progression, typical heart failure symptoms follow. Angina pectoris and syncope are much less common with aortic regurgitation than with aortic stenosis. In contrast, palpitations and ventricular premature beats are much more frequent, and nonsustained ventricular tachycardia has often been reported. Overt heart failure and cardiac chest pain are infrequent but, if present, may reflect a more acute process.

Careful physical examination may yield a host of eponymous signs (e.g., Hill's sign, Corrigan's pulse), almost all of which reflect a high stroke volume and wide pulse pressure. The wide pulse pressure, bounding arterial pulses, and hyperdynamic circulation of chronic moderately severe aortic regurgitation are easily noted. In contrast, the soft, blowing, diastolic murmur may be subtle, requiring careful auscultation, with the patient sitting forward in fully held expiration. The murmur is almost always best heard using the diaphragm of the stethoscope applied firmly to the upper right parasternal area of the anterior chest. A systolic murmur may be audible because of increased stroke volume. The duration of the diastolic murmur should be noted, because this reflects the severity of the leak until the late stages of disease, when the left ventricular diastolic pressure increases and shortens the diastolic murmur. An Austin-Flint apical diastolic murmur may also be present. This mid-diastolic murmur, best heard at the apex and often preceded by an S_3 heart sound, occurs in the absence of organic mitral valve disease. It is likely the result of an antegrade flow across an incompletely opened mitral valve caused by the aortic regurgitant jet's effect on the anterior mitral leaflet. An Austin-Flint murmur usually indicates significant aortic regurgitation.

Diagnosis

The electrocardiogram of patients with aortic regurgitation commonly demonstrates voltage consistent with left ventricular hypertrophy, but often without the ST segment depressions and T inversion of the strain pattern. The generous voltage and upright T waves in the lateral chest leads have been referred to as "volume overload left

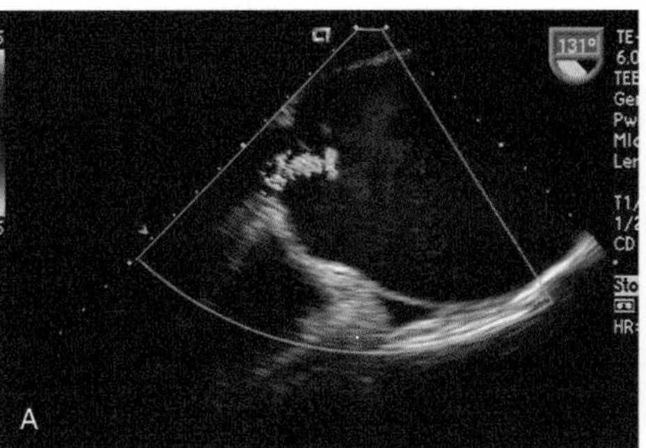

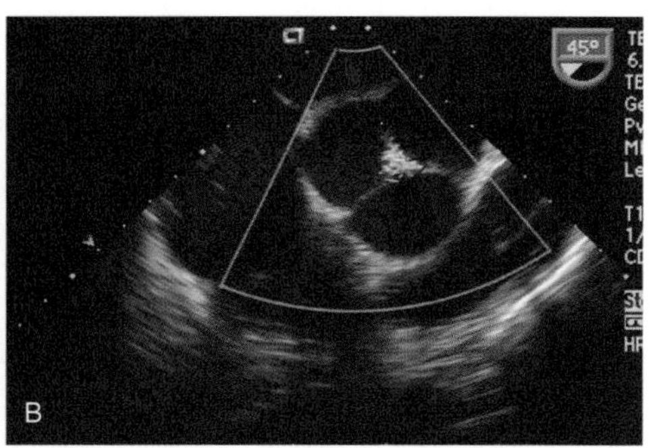

Figure 5 Transesophageal echocardiogram. Long-axis (**A**) and short-axis (**B**) views show an example of a dilated aortic root resulting from annuloaortic ectasia, with secondary aortic regurgitation caused by reduced leaflet coaptation.

ventricular hypertrophy." In addition, premature ventricular contractions may be present.

Echocardiography will, in almost all cases, define the functional anatomy of the valve and aortic root, and Doppler imaging will help assess the severity of the diastolic leak (see Fig. 5). In addition, the echocardiogram documents left ventricular diastolic dimensions, ejection fraction, and wall thickness. If transthoracic echocardiographic imaging is not adequate to define the pathoanatomy, transesophageal echocardiography should be performed. The anatomic consequences of aortic regurgitation include, as noted above, both left ventricular hypertrophy and dilation. Serial echocardiographic measurements of left ventricular systolic function and end-diastolic dimensions provide excellent objective parameters for long-term follow-up of asymptomatic patients.

I no longer use cardiac catheterization as the primary diagnostic imaging modality for aortic regurgitation. Angiographic assessment of regurgitant valve lesion severity is subjective and dependent on technical factors, such as catheter position and the rate and volume of contrast injection. Diagnostic coronary angiography should be performed as part of the presurgical evaluation when valve repair or replacement is planned.

Treatment

In theory, patients with aortic regurgitation should benefit from long-term administration of a direct-acting vasodilator. Angiotensin-converting enzyme inhibitors or angiotensin receptor blockers might not be effective until the renin-angiotensin system is activated, so there may be a role for long-acting dihydropyridine calcium channel antagonists, such as nifedipine and amlodipine, in an attempt to reduce the regurgitant fraction.[10] Such agents may be considered for long-term therapy in asymptomatic patients with severe aortic regurgitation who have ventricular dilation but preserved systolic function (Class IIb indication).[1] In addition, although beta blockers theoretically prolong diastole, many clinicians use modest doses of beta blockers because of the known association between aortic regurgitation and aneurysmal diseases of the aorta.

Patients with aortic regurgitation should have detailed counseling about physical activity. Isometric exercise, weight lifting, and heavy exertional activities, which involve strenuous arm work, should be specifically prohibited because of the reflex increase in peripheral vascular resistance that occurs with arm exercise. In contrast, rhythmic, low-resistance, large muscle group exercise such as bicycling reduces peripheral resistance, and should be encouraged for fitness and a sense of well-being. Infective endocarditis prophylaxis is no longer required based on the new ACC/AHA guidelines.[4]

As noted earlier, most patients with chronic aortic regurgitation have a protracted clinical course, despite evidence of severe regurgitation. Nevertheless, long-term care of the asymptomatic individual with aortic regurgitation consists of carefully monitoring for the onset of symptoms or, more often, of left ventricular dysfunction or dilation. Asymptomatic patients with chronic severe aortic regurgitation and normal left ventricular systolic function should be assessed clinically and echocardiographically approximately every 6 to 12 months. Current guidelines suggest aortic valve surgery for chronic severe aortic regurgitation for patients with symptom onset (Class I indication), asymptomatic patients with left ventricular ejection fraction lower than 0.50 (Class I indication), patients undergoing coronary artery bypass grafting or surgery on the aorta or other heart valves (Class I indication), and patients with preserved ventricular function but left ventricular end-systolic dimension more than 55 mm or end-diastolic dimension more than 75 mm (Class IIa indication). Aortic valve surgery may be considered in asymptomatic patients with preserved ventricular function but left ventricular end-systolic dimension more than 50 mm or end-diastolic dimension more than 70 mm, patients with declining exercise tolerance, and patients with moderate aortic regurgitation undergoing coronary artery bypass grafting or surgery on the aorta or other heart valves (Class IIb indications).[1]

When concerns arise about the physiologic significance of aortic regurgitation and possible indications for surgery, maximal cardiopulmonary exercise testing and stress echocardiography may be useful. Patients who can achieve high levels of activity with evidence of good contractile reserve can generally be managed conservatively. Impaired functional capacity under stress should prompt consideration of valve surgery.

The issues involved in the choice of a prosthetic valve and in postsurgical care are similar for patients with aortic regurgitation, as described earlier for aortic stenosis. A notable distinction is the select group of patients with pliable congenital bicuspid valves and aortic regurgitation, for whom valve repair may be a viable option. However, clinicians should remember the association between aortic root diseases (i.e., aneurysm formation and risk of dissection) in patients with bicuspid aortic valve or connective tissue diseases. I favor maintaining these patients who undergo aortic valve repair or replacement on long-term beta blockade. Concomitant aortic repair should be performed at the time of valve surgery when the aortic size reaches >4.5 cm.

Summary

- Calcific aortic stenosis and congenital bicuspid aortic valve stenosis account for most aortic stenosis cases.
- Two-dimensional and Doppler echocardiography represent the gold standard in the evaluation of patients with suspected aortic valvular disease.
- Symptomatic patients with severe aortic stenosis should undergo valve replacement, as well as those with severe aortic stenosis undergoing cardiac surgery, severe aortic stenosis and left ventricular dysfunction, and moderate aortic stenosis undergoing cardiac surgery.
- Chronic aortic regurgitation may be caused by leaflet pathology, such as a congenital bicuspid aortic valve, or may be related to any pathologic process that results in aortic root dilation.
- Aortic valve surgery for chronic severe aortic regurgitation is indicated for those with symptom onset, asymptomatic patients with left ventricular dysfunction, patients undergoing cardiac surgery, and patients with preserved ventricular function but a left ventricular end-systolic dimension more than 50 to 55 mm or end-diastolic dimension more than 70 to 75 mm.

Suggested Readings

American College of Cardiology; American Heart Association Task Force on Practice Guidelines (Writing Committee to revise the 1998 guidelines for the management of patients with valvular heart disease); Society of Cardiovascular Anesthesiologists, Bonow RO, Carabello BA, Chatterjee K, et al: ACC/AHA 2006 guidelines for the management of patients with valvular heart disease: A report of the American College of Cardiology/American Heart Association Task Force on Practice Guidelines (writing Committee to Revise the 1998 guidelines for the management of patients with valvular heart disease) developed in collaboration with the Society of Cardiovascular Anesthesiologists endorsed by the Society for Cardiovascular Angiography and Interventions and the Society of Thoracic Surgeons. J Am Coll Cardiol 2006;48:e1-e148.

Bekeredjian R, Grayburn PA: Valvular heart disease: Aortic regurgitation. Circulation 2005;112:125-134.

Dajani AS, Taubert KA, Wilson W, et al: Prevention of bacterial endocarditis. Recommendations by the American Heart Association. Circulation 1997;96:358-366.

Enriquez-Sarano M, Tajik AJ: Aortic regurgitation. N Engl J Med 2004;351:1539-1546.

Novaro GM, Tiong IY, Pearce GL, et al: Effect of hydroxymethylglutaryl coenzyme a reductase inhibitors on the progression of calcific aortic stenosis. Circulation 2001;104:2205-2209.

Otto CM: Valvular aortic stenosis: Disease severity and timing of intervention. J Am Coll Cardiol 2006;47:2141-2151.

Rajamannan NM, Gersh B, Bonow RO: Calcific aortic stenosis: From bench to the bedside-emerging clinical and cellular concepts. Heart 2003;89:801-805.

Roberts WC, Ko JM: Frequency by decades of unicuspid, bicuspid, and tricuspid aortic valves in adults having isolated aortic valve replacement for aortic stenosis, with or without associated aortic regurgitation. Circulation 2005;111:120-125.

Scognamiglio R, Rahimtoola SH, Fasoli G, et al: Nifedipine in asymptomatic patients with severe aortic regurgitation and normal left ventricular function. N Engl J Med 1994;331:689-694.

Stewart BF, Siscovick D, Lind BK, et al: Clinical factors associated with calcific aortic valve disease. Cardiovascular Health Study. J Am Coll Cardiol 1997;29:630-634.

References

For a complete list of references, log onto www.expertconsult.com.

Mitral Valve Disease: Stenosis and Regurgitation

Ronan J. Curtin and Brian P. Griffin

The mitral valve is made up of the annulus, anterior and posterior leaflets, and chordae, which attach the leaflets to their respective papillary muscles. A normally functioning valve allows blood to flow unimpeded from the left atrium to the left ventricle during diastole and prevents regurgitation during systole. Normal mitral valve function is dependent not only on the integrity of the underlying valvular structure, but on that of the adjacent myocardium as well.

This chapter reviews three types of mitral valve disease: mitral stenosis, mitral regurgitation, and mitral valve prolapse. Practice guidelines published jointly by the American College of Cardiology (ACC) and the American Heart Association (AHA) for the management of patients with valvular heart disease are referenced in this chapter.[1] Where relevant, we refer in the text to the ACC/AHA evidence grading for diagnostic and therapeutic procedures, as follows:

Class I: There is evidence and/or general agreement in favor of a given procedure or treatment.
Class II: There is conflicting evidence and/or a divergence of opinion about the efficacy of a given procedure or treatment.
Class IIa: The weight of evidence or opinion is in favor of efficacy.
Class IIb: Efficacy is less well established by evidence or opinion.
Class III: There is evidence and/or general agreement that the procedure or treatment is not useful and in some cases may be harmful.

MITRAL STENOSIS

Definition and Etiology

Mitral stenosis (MS) refers to narrowing of the mitral valve orifice, resulting in impedance of filling of the left ventricle in diastole. It is usually caused by rheumatic heart disease. Less common causes include severe calcification of the mitral annulus, infective endocarditis, systemic lupus erythematosus, rheumatoid arthritis, and carcinoid heart disease.

Prevalence and Risk Factors

Although the incidence of rheumatic heart disease has steeply declined during the past four decades in the United States, it is still a major cause of cardiovascular disease in developing countries. It is estimated that 15.6 million people suffer from rheumatic heart disease worldwide, with approximately 282,000 new cases and 233,000 related deaths each year.[2]

Pathophysiology and Natural History

Patients with MS typically present more than 20 years after an episode of rheumatic fever. Single or recurrent bouts of rheumatic carditis cause progressive thickening, scarring, and calcification of the mitral leaflets and chordae. Fusion of the commissures and chordae decreases the size of the mitral opening. This obstruction results in the development of a pressure gradient across the valve in diastole and causes an elevation in left atrial and pulmonary venous pressures. Elevated left atrial pressures lead to left atrial enlargement, predisposing the patient to atrial fibrillation and arterial thromboembolism. Elevated pulmonary venous pressure results in pulmonary congestion and pulmonary edema. In advanced mitral stenosis, patients develop pulmonary hypertension and right-sided heart failure.

Signs and Symptoms

Patients with mitral stenosis may present with exertional dyspnea, fatigue, atrial arrhythmias, embolic events, angina-like chest pain, hemoptysis, or even right-sided heart failure. Previously asymptomatic or stable patients may decompensate acutely during exercise, emotional stress, pregnancy, infection, or with uncontrolled atrial fibrillation.

The characteristic findings of MS on auscultation are an accentuated first heart sound, an opening snap, and a mid-diastolic rumble. The first heart sound may be diminished in intensity if the valve is heavily calcified, with limited mobility. If the patient is in sinus rhythm, there is presystolic accentuation of the murmur during atrial contraction. With increasingly severe stenosis, the duration of the murmur increases and the opening snap occurs earlier during diastole as a result of higher left atrial pressure. There is accentuation of P_2 when pulmonary hypertension is present. If flow across the mitral valve is reduced because of heart failure, pulmonary hypertension, or aortic stenosis the murmur of mitral stenosis may be reduced in intensity or may be inaudible.

Left atrial myxoma may be distinguished from MS by the presence of a "tumor plop" versus an opening snap in early diastole.

Diagnosis

On chest radiography, the characteristic findings of mitral stenosis are pulmonary congestion, enlargement of the main pulmonary arteries, and enlargement of the left atrium without cardiomegaly (Fig. 1). An electrocardiogram (ECG) may reveal evidence of left atrial enlargement, atrial fibrillation or, in advanced disease, right ventricular hypertrophy consistent with pulmonary hypertension (Fig. 2).

Two-dimensional (2D) and Doppler echocardiography is indicated for all patients with suspected MS to confirm the diagnosis and determine its severity (Class I indication).[1] Characteristic findings of MS include valve thickening, restricted valve opening, anterior leaflet doming, and fusion of the leaflets at the commissures. The mean pressure gradient across the mitral valve on Doppler echocardiography (echo) in MS is at least 5 mm Hg; in severe stenosis, it is usually higher than 10 mm Hg. Because the gradient across the mitral valve is flow dependent, the severity of MS is more accurately defined by the mitral valve area (MVA). The normal valve area is 4 to 5 cm^2. In mild mitral stenosis, the MVA is 1.5 to 2 cm^2, in moderate stenosis it is 1 to 1.5 cm^2, and in severe stenosis it is less than 1 cm^2. The valve area may be measured by tracing the mitral valve opening in cross section by 2D echo. Alternatively, the MVA is calculated using the pressure half-time ($P \times {}^1/_2t$), which is the amount of time it takes for the transmitral pressure to fall to one half its initial value ($MVA = 220/[P \times {}^1/_2t]$).

Echocardiography also allows assessment of pulmonary artery pressures, detection of other valve disease, visualization of left atrial thrombus, and identification of important differential diagnoses, such as left atrial myxoma. Transesophageal echo is superior to transthoracic echo at identifying left atrial thrombus in patients who are being considered for percutaneous mitral balloon valvotomy or cardioversion (Class I).[1] Stress echocardiography may be helpful if there is a discrepancy between a patient's severity of symptoms and the baseline hemodynamic data. An exercise mean transmitral gradient of more than 15 mm Hg and peak right ventricular systolic pressure

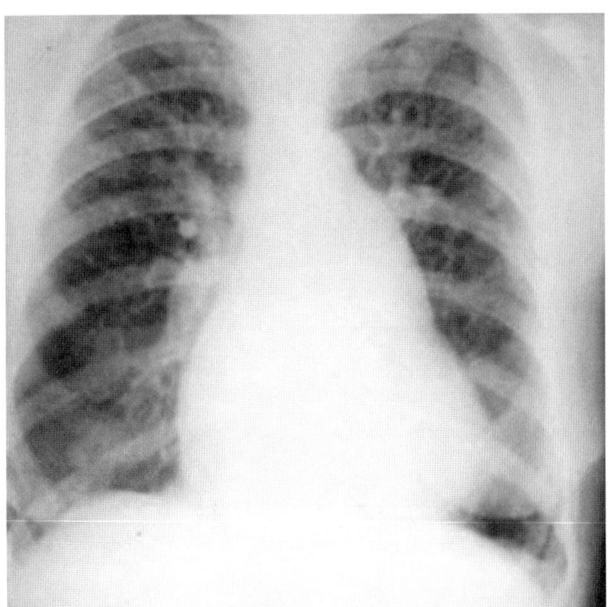

Figure 1 Chest radiograph of a patient with severe mitral stenosis showing pulmonary congestion and left atrial enlargement, with a normal left ventricular silhouette.

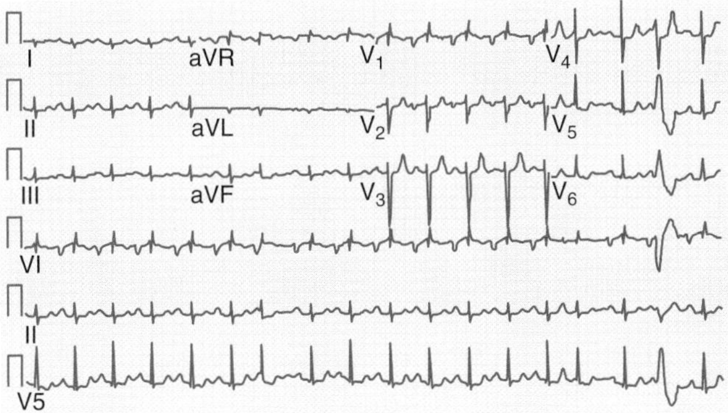

Figure 2 Electrocardiogram of a patient with severe mitral stenosis showing right ventricular hypertrophy and left atrial enlargement.

of more than 60 mm Hg indicate hemodynamically significant MS (Class I).[1]

Cardiac catheterization is not necessary in all cases but, like stress echocardiography, may be helpful in characterizing the severity of mitral stenosis when there is a discrepancy between symptoms and findings on echocardiography (Class I).[1] A more detailed discussion of the diagnosis of mitral stenosis may be found in the AHA/ACC guidelines.[1]

Summary

- Transthoracic echocardiography is necessary to diagnose and determine the severity of mitral stenosis.
- Transesophageal echocardiography is indicated in patients before percutaneous mitral balloon valvotomy or cardioversion.
- Stress echocardiography and cardiac catheterization may be helpful in those cases in which there is a discrepancy between the severity of symptoms and baseline echocardiographic findings.

Treatment

Medical Treatment

Medical therapy has no role in altering the natural history or delaying the need for surgery in patients with MS. Medical treatment is directed toward alleviating pulmonary congestion with diuretics, treating atrial fibrillation, and anticoagulating patients who are at increased risk of arterial embolic events.

Development of atrial fibrillation frequently leads to an acute deterioration in patients with mitral stenosis. The rapid ventricular response results in a decrease in the diastolic filling time. Beta blockers, calcium channel blockers, or digoxin may be used to control ventricular rate. An attempt to restore sinus rhythm with direct current electrical cardioversion or antiarrhythmic drugs may be considered. Anticoagulation with warfarin is indicated to prevent thromboembolism when atrial fibrillation is present, if there is a prior history of thromboembolism, or a thrombus is detected in the left atrium (Class I).[1] Although controversial, anticoagulation may also be considered if the left atrium is markedly dilated (5.0-5.5 mm) or if there is spontaneous contrast on echocardiography (Class IIb).[1,3,4]

Antibiotic therapy is important for the secondary prevention of rheumatic carditis. Patients with a history of rheumatic fever are at high risk of recurrence. Long-term secondary prophylaxis, preferentially with penicillin, is therefore recommended for all patients with a history of rheumatic fever or suspected rheumatic valve disease. The duration of prophylaxis depends on a number of factors, including the time lapsed since the last attack, the age of the patient, the presence or absence of cardiac involvement, and the patient's risk of exposure to streptococcal infections.[1,5] Routine antibiotic prophylaxis for endocarditis is no longer recommended for patients with mitral stenosis.[6]

Surgery

Three invasive options are available for patients with MS: percutaneous mitral balloon valvotomy (PMBV), surgical mitral commissurotomy, and mitral valve replacement (MVR). In experienced centers, PMBV is the initial procedure of choice and should be considered for (1) symptomatic patients (NYHA functional Classes II to IV) with moderate or severe MS (Class I) and (2) asymptomatic patients with moderate or severe MS and pulmonary hypertension (Class I).[1] PMBV is a catheter-based technique in which a balloon is inflated across the stenotic valve to split the fused commissures and increase the valve area. The MVA typically doubles in size, and hemodynamic as well as clinical improvements are seen immediately (Fig. 3).[7] The results are comparable with those achieved with open mitral commissurotomy, but it is less invasive and less costly.[7,8] The mitral valve morphology is an important predictor of successful balloon valvotomy. Severe valve calcification or significant involvement of the subvalvular apparatus on echocardiography before PMBV is associated with a higher complication rate and a greater risk of recurrence. In addition, balloon valvotomy should not be performed in patients who have left atrial thrombus or more than 2^+ (moderate) mitral regurgitation, because the degree of mitral regurgitation usually increases following the procedure. Complications of balloon mitral valvotomy include severe mitral regurgitation (3%), thromboembolism (3%), and residual atrial septal defect with significant shunting (<5%). Mortality with the procedure is lower than 1% in experienced hands. At 7 years after balloon valvotomy, 50% to 69% of patients remain free of cardiovascular events and up to 90% of patients remain free of reintervention.[8,9] However, both balloon valvotomy and surgical commissurotomy are palliative procedures and, in most cases, further intervention is eventually required, usually in the form of a mitral valve replacement.

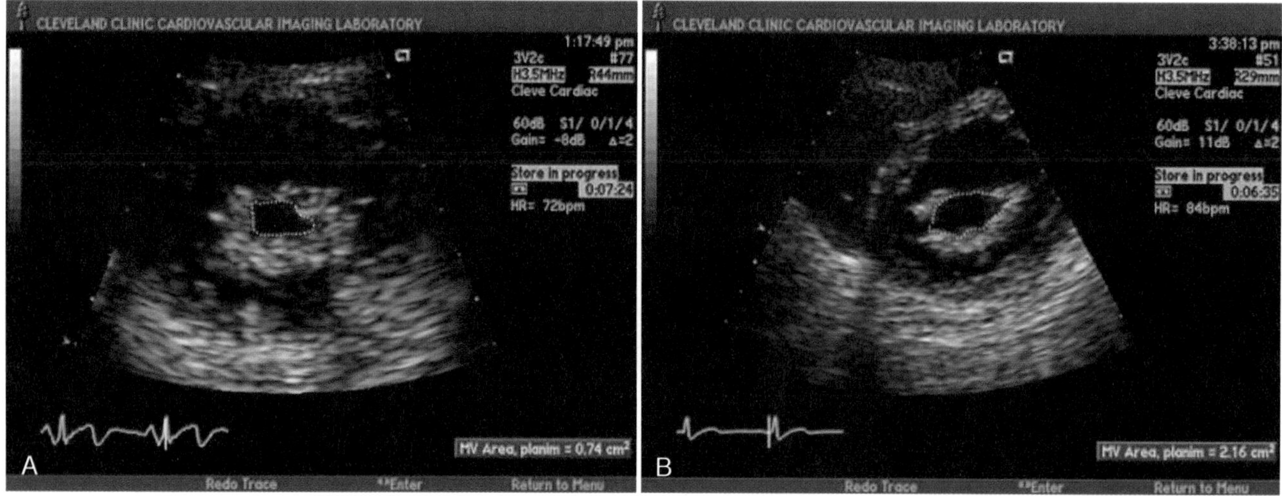

Figure 3 Echocardiogram (parasternal short-axis view) shows the mitral orifice before (**A**) and after (**B**) percutaneous mitral balloon valvotomy (PMBV).

Although closed mitral commissurotomy is still widely used in many developing countries, open mitral commissurotomy is more frequently performed in the United States. It involves the use of cardiopulmonary bypass and the surgical repair of a diseased mitral valve by direct visualization. Open mitral commissurotomy may be considered in the presence of a left atrial thrombus or significant mitral regurgitation if the valve anatomy is suitable. Commissurotomy may also be indicated for patients who have other concomitant valvular disease or coronary artery disease that requires surgery. In patients with calcified valves that cannot be treated by valvotomy or commissurotomy, or in those with significant mitral regurgitation that is not suitable for repair, mitral valve replacement may be necessary. The threshold for mitral valve surgery (commissurotomy or MVR) is higher than for PMBV in patients with mitral stenosis, and commissurotomy or repair is preferable to MVR, if feasible. Surgery for moderate to severe mitral stenosis is indicated for symptomatic patients (New York Heart Association [NYHA] functional Class III or IV) where PMBV is unavailable or contraindicated (Class I).[1] MVR may also be considered for patients with severe MS and severe pulmonary hypertension with NYHA functional Classes I or II symptoms who are not candidates for PMBV or mitral valve repair (Class IIa). Both mechanical and biologic prostheses are used for mitral valve replacement; the choice of valve often depends on factors such as age, need for concomitant anticoagulation, and left ventricular (LV) size. Morbidity and mortality are higher with prosthetic valve replacement than with surgical or balloon valvotomy.

A more detailed discussion of the management of mitral stenosis may be found in the AHA/ACC guidelines.[1]

Summary

- Medical therapy in patients with mitral stenosis includes diuretic therapy, rate control of atrial fibrillation, anticoagulation to prevent thromboembolism, and antibiotic prophylaxis against recurrent rheumatic carditis.
- Invasive therapy should be considered for all patients with symptomatic mitral stenosis. Percutaneous mitral balloon valvotomy and surgical commissurotomy provide equivalent immediate and long-term outcome results and delay the need for mitral valve replacement.

Prevention and Screening

Antibiotic therapy of group A streptococcal tonsillopharyngitis, even delayed 9 days after the onset of symptoms, can prevent rheumatic fever and rheumatic carditis.[10] Antibiotic therapy also reduces transmission to contacts. Routine screening or treatment of asymptomatic contacts of persons with group A streptococcal tonsillopharyngitis is not recommended.

Special Populations

Patients with asymptomatic moderate to severe mitral stenosis may decompensate during periods of increased physiologic stress, such as pregnancy or surgery. Surgical intervention, preferably percutaneous valvotomy, should be considered before a planned pregnancy or surgical procedure in these patients. Balloon valvotomy can also be performed with abdominal or pelvic shielding during pregnancy if symptomatic mitral stenosis does not respond to medical therapy.

MITRAL REGURGITATION

Definition and Causes

Mitral regurgitation (MR) is leakage of blood from the left ventricle into the left atrium during systole. It is caused by various mechanisms related to structural or functional abnormalities of the mitral apparatus, adjacent myocardium, or both. The most common causes of mitral regurgitation in the United States are myxomatous degeneration, chordal rupture, rheumatic heart disease, infective endocarditis, coronary artery disease, and cardiomyopathy.

Prevalence and Risk Factors

Significant mitral valve regurgitation occurs in about 2% of the population with a similar prevalence in males and females.[11] Myxomatous disease is the most common cause of nonischemic mitral regurgitation in the United States (Fig. 4).

Pathophysiology and Natural History

Significant MR leads to volume overload of the left ventricle, because it has to accommodate both the stroke volume and regurgitant volume with each heartbeat. To compensate, the left ventricle dilates and becomes hyperdynamic. In acute severe MR, the left atrial and

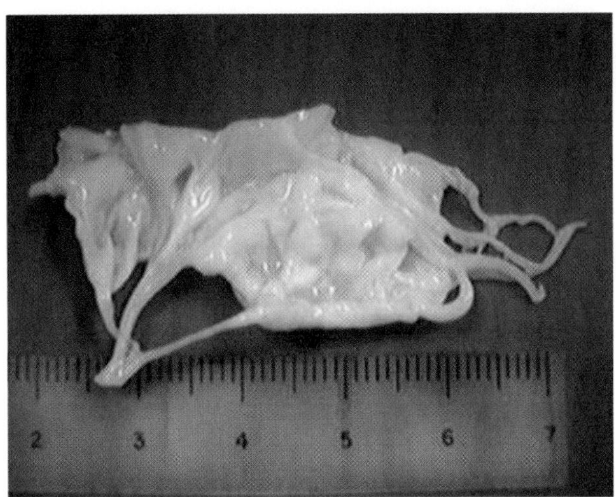

Figure 4 **Myxomatous mitral valve disease.** Note the myxoid appearance of the mitral valve, with leaflet thickening, leaflet redundancy, and interchordal hooding.

pulmonary venous pressures increase quickly, leading to pulmonary congestion and pulmonary edema. In chronic MR, a gradual increase in left atrial size and compliance compensate so that left atrial and pulmonary venous pressures do not increase until late in the course of the disease. Progressive left ventricular dilation eventually leads to an increase in afterload, contractile dysfunction, and heart failure. Left atrial enlargement predisposes the patient to atrial fibrillation and arterial thromboembolism. In long-standing MR, patients may develop pulmonary hypertension and right-sided heart failure.

Signs and Symptoms

Patients with chronic, severe mitral regurgitation may remain asymptomatic for years because the regurgitant volume load is well tolerated as a result of compensatory ventricular and atrial dilation. When symptoms do develop, the most common are dyspnea, fatigue, orthopnea, paroxysmal nocturnal dyspnea, and palpitations caused by atrial fibrillation. Acute severe MR, as occurs with chordal rupture or papillary muscle rupture, is almost always symptomatic because the sudden regurgitant volume load in the nondilated left ventricle and atrium leads to pulmonary venous hypertension and congestion.

The characteristic finding in a patient with MR is a blowing holosystolic murmur heard best at the cardiac apex. When ventricular enlargement is present, the apical impulse may be diffuse and laterally displaced, and a third heart sound may be heard.

Diagnosis

The chest radiograph demonstrates left atrial enlargement and cardiomegaly. Two-dimensional and Doppler echocardiography is indicated for all patients with suspected mitral regurgitation to confirm its presence and determine its severity (Class I).[1] Two-dimensional echocardiography usually reveals the cause (e.g., the presence of myxomatous mitral valve disease and leaflet prolapse or evidence of underlying dilated cardiomyopathy). Evaluation of the severity of mitral regurgitation on echocardiography requires an integrated assessment of several parameters, including regurgitant jet size by color Doppler, regurgitant jet density by continuous-wave (CW) Doppler, and pulmonary vein and mitral valve inflow by pulse-wave (PW) Doppler.[12] Newer applications of Doppler echocardiography allow quantitative measurement of mitral regurgitation, including the regurgitant volume and the regurgitant orifice area (ROA)—that is, the area through which the valve leaks in systole. In asymptomatic patients with significant mitral regurgitation, serial echocardiography every 6 to 12 months to assess LV size and systolic function is important for optimal timing of surgery (Class I).[1] Transesophageal echocardiography is indicated for patients who are not adequately imaged by transthoracic echocardiography and before surgery to assess feasibility for repair (Class I).[1] Stress echocardiography may be useful to assess exercise tolerance and the response of mitral regurgitation severity, pulmonary pressure, and contractile reserve to exercise in asymptomatic patients with significant MR (Class IIa).[1,13]

Cardiac catheterization is no longer routinely performed to evaluate mitral regurgitation severity, but it is indicated for those patients in whom noninvasive test results are inconclusive, and also to detect concomitant coronary artery disease in patients undergoing mitral valve surgery (Class I).[1] A more detailed discussion of the diagnosis of mitral regurgitation may be found in the AHA/ACC guidelines.[1]

Summary

- Determining the severity of mitral regurgitation requires an integrated assessment of several parameters on echocardiography.
- Serial echocardiography with measurement of LV size and function is important for timing surgical intervention in asymptomatic patients.
- Transesophageal echocardiography is necessary before surgery to assess feasibility for repair, as well as for patients who are not adequately imaged by transthoracic echocardiography.

Treatment

Medical Treatment

In patients with acute severe MR, afterload reduction with intravenous nitroprusside and nitroglycerin reduces the regurgitant fraction and pulmonary pressures. Placement of an intra-aortic balloon pump also helps stabilize these patients. However, these are temporary measures before urgent mitral valve repair or replacement. In patients with chronic asymptomatic mitral regurgitation caused by primary valve disease, there is no evidence for the routine use of medication in delaying the need for surgery or preventing left ventricular dysfunction.[14] The management of these patients is focused on deciding on the appropriate timing of surgery, before the development of irreversible left ventricular dysfunction. Patients should be followed up every 6 to 12 months to assess for symptoms and to measure left ventricular size, function, and severity of MR by echocardiography (Class I).[1]

In patients with ischemic heart disease or dilated cardiomyopathy, mitral regurgitation indicates a poor prognosis.[15] MR in these patients is called functional mitral regurgitation and is caused by global or regional changes in left ventricular geometry as well as annular dilation. Functional MR is primarily treated medically with antihypertensive therapy, angiotensin-converting enzyme (ACE) inhibitors, beta blockers, diuretics, and antianginal therapies when mitral regurgitation is worsened by acute ischemia.[16] Biventricular pacing has also been shown to decrease the degree of mitral regurgitation in dilated cardiomyopathy.[17]

Routine antibiotic prophylaxis for endocarditis is no longer recommended for patients with mitral regurgitation.[6]

Surgery

Surgery is indicated for symptomatic patients with severe primary MR (Class I) and asymptomatic patients with severe primary MR and evidence of LV dysfunction (Class I).[1] Optimal timing of mitral valve surgery is challenging in asymptomatic patients because the

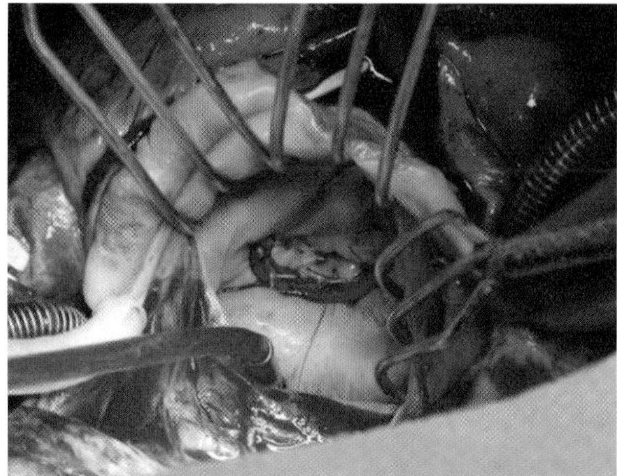

Figure 5 Mitral valve repair for flail mitral valve with insertion of Cosgrove-Edwards annuloplasty ring.

actual contractile function of the left ventricle is difficult to measure. The standard indications for surgery in asymptomatic patients is an LV end-systolic dimension of more than 4.0 cm and a resting LV ejection fraction of less than 60% (Class I).[1] Other indications in asymptomatic patients include pulmonary hypertension or development of atrial fibrillation (Class IIa).[1] In addition, mitral valve repair may be undertaken in experienced surgical centers for asymptomatic patients with severe MR, but without evidence of LV dilation or dysfunction, for whom the likelihood of a successful repair is greater than 90% (Class IIa). Most asymptomatic patients with severe MR develop symptoms, LV dysfunction, or both over long-term follow-up. One retrospective study showed an increased risk of cardiac death (4%/year) in patients with severe mitral regurgitation based on an ROA of more than 0.4 cm^2.[18] However, another recent prospective study has shown that careful follow-up of patients with severe MR and timing of surgery based on symptoms, LV dysfunction, development of atrial fibrillation, or pulmonary hypertension is associated with an excellent patient outcome.[19]

In patients with severe functional mitral regurgitation, surgery may be considered for severe symptoms despite medical therapy. Patients with ischemic MR may improve with coronary bypass surgery if significant ischemia or myocardial viability is present. In many coronary bypass patients with MR, concomitant mitral valve repair with an undersized annuloplasty ring is performed. Patients with severe left ventricular dysfunction and significant MR were once believed to be poor surgical candidates, but recent studies have shown an acceptable operative risk. Symptoms usually improve, although a survival benefit has not been demonstrated.

The two available surgical options are mitral valve repair (Fig. 5) and mitral valve replacement. Mitral valve repair is the procedure of choice in the surgical management of MR caused by degenerative valve disease and in some cases of MR caused by infective endocarditis and ischemic heart disease. Repair offers several advantages over replacement, including lower operative and long-term mortality, better preservation of LV function, a lower risk of subsequent infective endocarditis, and no need for long-term anticoagulation. Reoperation rates for mitral valve repair and replacement are similar, occurring at a rate of 1% to 2% per year. On the other hand, repair is technically more difficult than replacement, and many cases of mitral regurgitation are not amenable to valve repair. Percutaneous mitral valve repair is currently being investigated. The techniques involved include a clip that joins the mitral leaflets at their midpoint and an annuloplasty ring delivered via the coronary sinus.[20,21]

A more detailed discussion of the management of mitral regurgitation may be found in the AHA/ACC guidelines.[1]

Summary

- Medical therapy has no role in the treatment of patients with primary mitral regurgitation but is the mainstay of treatment in patients with functional mitral regurgitation.
- In patients with primary mitral regurgitation, surgery is indicated in the presence of symptoms or, in asymptomatic patients, if there is evidence of secondary LV dysfunction.
- Mitral valve repair is the procedure of choice for the surgical management of mitral regurgitation and is associated with lower mortality and better preservation of LV function.

MITRAL VALVE PROLAPSE

Definition and Causes

Mitral valve prolapse (MVP) is the systolic billowing of one or both mitral leaflets into the left atrium during systole.[22] It may occur in the setting of myxomatous valve disease or in persons with normal mitral valve leaflets.

Prevalence and Risk Factors

MVP is the most common valvular disorder in the United States, occurring in 2.4% of the general population. There is a similar prevalence in men and women, with a greater risk of complications in men.[23]

Pathophysiology and Natural History

Many patients with MVP have normal mitral leaflets, with little or no mitral regurgitation, and a benign prognosis. Survival rates among affected patients are similar to those of age- and gender-matched individuals without MVP.[24] In other patients, MVP is caused by myxomatous valve disease, with typical findings of elongated and thickened leaflets, interchordal hooding, and chordal elongation (see Fig. 4). Patients with myxomatous MVP are at increased risk for cardiovascular complications, particularly when prolapse is associated with at least moderate mitral regurgitation or LV dysfunction. Although most patients with MVP do not develop severe mitral regurgitation, MVP is a common underlying cause of progressive mitral regurgitation, often necessitating mitral valve repair or replacement.[25]

The causes of myxomatous mitral valve disease are not certain, but appear to involve dysregulation of extracellular matrix proteins. Myxomatous mitral valve disease usually occurs sporadically, although there are well-described cases of familial clustering that involve an autosomal dominant mode of inheritance.[22] Three genetic loci for autosomal dominant myxomatous mitral valve disease have been described, but the precise genes and mutations have not yet been identified. Myxomatous MVP also may occur in conjunction with certain connective tissue disorders, such as Marfan syndrome and Ehlers-Danlos syndrome.

Signs and Symptoms

Most patients with MVP are asymptomatic. In the past, multiple nonspecific symptoms (atypical chest pain, dyspnea, palpitations, anxiety, and syncope) and clinical findings (low body weight, low blood pressure, and pectus excavatum) were associated with MVP and termed *mitral valve prolapse syndrome.* Prospective testing has failed to confirm most of these associations.[23] The classic findings of MVP on physical examination are a midsystolic click, with a late systolic murmur, heard best at the cardiac apex.

Diagnosis

Two-dimensional echocardiography is the most important test for diagnosing MVP (Class I).[1] The diagnosis is made when there is displacement of one or both mitral leaflets by 2 mm or more into the left atrium during systole (Fig. 6). Because the mitral annulus is known to have a saddle shape, a normal mitral valve can appear to prolapse in certain echocardiographic views, most notably in the apical two- and four-chamber views. Therefore, the diagnosis of MVP should be based on a long-axis parasternal or apical three-chamber view. In patients with MVP, echocardiography is also useful in determining the presence and severity of MR and assessing left atrial and ventricular chamber size, LV function, and leaflet thickening and redundancy. Unless severe mitral regurgitation is present, findings on the chest radiograph and ECG typically are unremarkable. A more detailed discussion of the diagnosis of mitral valve prolapse may be found in the AHA/ACC guidelines.[1]

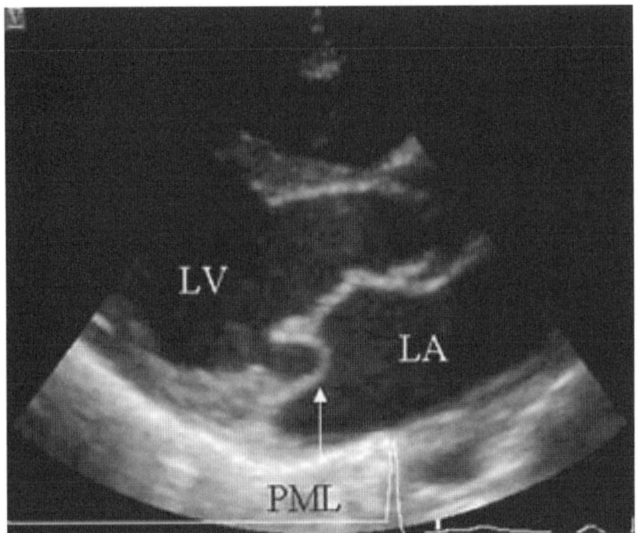

Figure 6 Echocardiogram (parasternal long-axis view) shows severe prolapse of the posterior mitral leaflet (PML) into the left atrium (LA). Prolapse of a mitral leaflet more than 2 mm into the LA during systole in a parasternal long-axis or apical three-chamber view on echocardiography is consistent with mitral valve prolapse. LV, left ventricle.

Summary

- Mitral valve prolapse is present if there is more than 2 mm displacement of the mitral valve leaflets into the left atrium during systole in a parasternal long-axis or apical three-chamber view on echocardiography.

Treatment

Medical Treatment

Asymptomatic patients require no specific treatment and they should be reassured of their excellent prognosis. Although antibiotic prophylaxis for endocarditis was once advocated for certain patients with MVP, more recent guidelines do not recommend antibiotic prophylaxis in this group of patients.[1,6] Beta blockers are useful for alleviating symptoms of palpitations, anxiety, and chest pain in certain patients.

MVP patients without mitral regurgitation should be evaluated every 3 to 5 years. Echocardiography should be performed if the patient has new cardiovascular symptoms or if the physical examination suggests that significant mitral regurgitation has developed. Patients with severe mitral regurgitation or high-risk features should be reviewed with an echocardiogram yearly or more often if their clinical condition warrants it.

Surgery

In MVP patients with severe mitral regurgitation, the indications for mitral valve surgery are similar to those for patients with other causes of severe regurgitation. When surgery is required, mitral valve repair is usually feasible (Fig. 7). Repair is characterized by low mortality and long-lasting durability; the 10-year reoperation-free survival rate ranges between 93% and 96%.[26] A more detailed discussion of the management of mitral valve prolapse may be found in the AHA/ACC guidelines.[1]

Summary

- Mitral valve prolapse is a benign condition in most cases.
- Indications for surgery are the same as those for patients with other causes of primary mitral regurgitation.

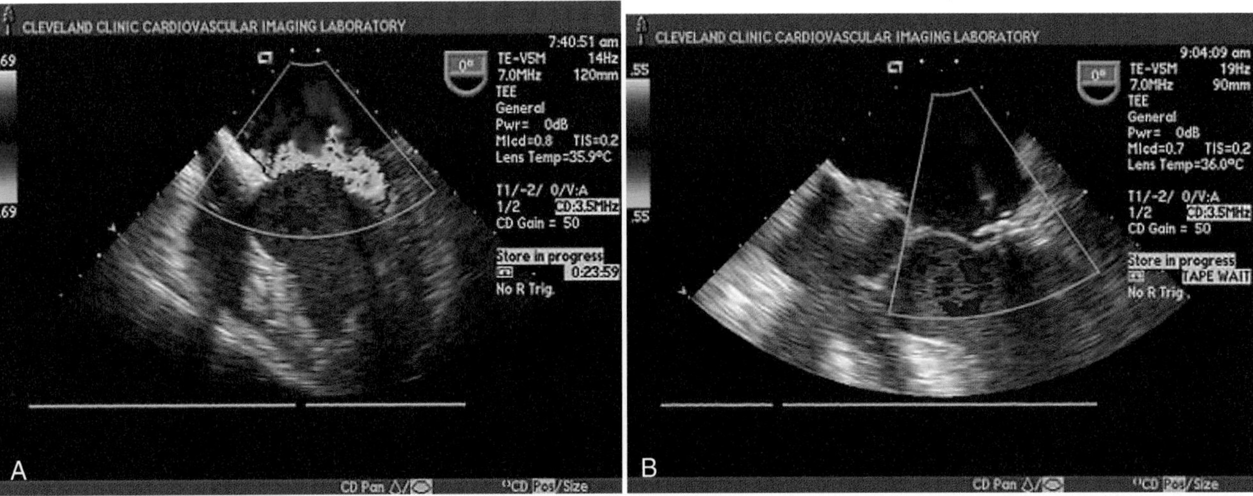

Figure 7 Intraoperative transesophageal echocardiogram shows severe mitral regurgitation before (**A**) and trivial regurgitation after (**B**) the repair of severe mitral valve prolapse.

Suggested Readings

Avierinos JF, Gersh BJ, Melton LJ 3rd, et al: Natural history of asymptomatic mitral valve prolapse in the community. Circulation 2002;106:1355-1361.

Ben Farhat M, Ayari M, Maatouk F, et al: Percutaneous balloon versus surgical closed and open mitral commissurotomy: Seven-year follow-up results of a randomized trial. Circulation 1998;97:245-250.

Bonow RO, Carabello B, Chatterjee K, et al: ACC/AHA 2006 Guidelines for the management of patients with valvular heart disease: A report of the American College of Cardiology/American Heart Association Task Force on Practice Guidelines (Writing Committee to Develop Guidelines for the Management of Patients With Valvular Heart Disease). Circulation 2006;114:e84-e231.

Dajani A, Taubert K, Ferrieri P, et al: Treatment of acute streptococcal pharyngitis and prevention of rheumatic fever: A statement for health professionals: Committee on Rheumatic Fever, Endocarditis, and Kawasaki Disease of the Council on Cardiovascular Disease in the Young, the American Heart Association. Pediatrics 1995;96:758-764.

Enriquez-Sarano M, Avierinos JF, Messika-Zeitoun D, et al: Quantitative determinants of the outcome of asymptomatic mitral regurgitation. N Engl J Med 2005;352:875-883.

Gillinov AM, Cosgrove DM, Blackstone EH, et al: Durability of mitral valve repair for degenerative disease. J Thorac Cardiovasc Surg 1998;116:734-743.

Reyes VP, Raju BS, Wynne J, et al: Percutaneous balloon valvuloplasty compared with open surgical commissurotomy for mitral stenosis. N Engl J Med 1994;331:961-967.

Salem DN, Stein PD, Al-Ahmad A, et al: Antithrombotic therapy in valvular heart disease—native and prosthetic: The Seventh ACCP Conference on Antithrombotic and Thrombolytic Therapy. Chest 2004;126:457S-482S.

Wilson W, Taubert KA, Gewitz M, et al: American Heart Association Rheumatic Fever, Endocarditis, and Kawasaki Disease Committee; American Heart Association Council on Cardiovascular Disease in the Young; American Heart Association Council on Clinical Cardiology; American Heart Association Council on Cardiovascular Surgery and Anesthesia; Quality of Care and Outcomes Research Interdisciplinary Working Group: Prevention of infective endocarditis: Guidelines from the American Heart Association: A guideline from the American Heart Association Rheumatic Fever, Endocarditis, and Kawasaki Disease Committee, Council on Cardiovascular Disease in the Young, and the Council on Clinical Cardiology, Council on Cardiovascular Surgery and Anesthesia, and the Quality of Care and Outcomes Research Interdisciplinary Working Group. Circulation 2007;116:1736-1754.

Zoghbi WA, Enriquez-Sarano M, Foster E, et al: Recommendations for evaluation of the severity of native valvular regurgitation with two-dimensional and Doppler echocardiography. J Am Soc Echocardiogr 2003;16:777-802.

References

For a complete list of references, log onto www.expertconsult.com.

Cardiovascular Emergencies

Hataya Poonyagariyagorn, Matthew Hook, and Deepak L. Bhatt

Cardiovascular emergencies are life-threatening disorders that must be diagnosed quickly to avoid delay in treatment and to minimize morbidity and mortality. Patients may present with severe hypertension, chest pain, dysrhythmia, or cardiopulmonary arrest. In this chapter, we review the clinician's approach to these disorders and their treatments and provide links to other informative resources. Acute coronary syndromes are covered elsewhere in this text.

CARDIOPULMONARY ARREST

Etiology

Cardiopulmonary arrest occurs as a result of a multitude of cardiovascular, metabolic, infectious, neurologic, inflammatory, and traumatic diseases. However, the clinician must be aware of several specific causes, including drug toxicity or overdose, myocardial ischemia or infarction, hyperkalemia, torsades de pointes, cardiac tamponade, and tension pneumothorax. The marked differences in therapeutic intervention among these various causes underscore the need for accurate recognition. The end point of these disorders is commonly pulseless ventricular tachycardia or ventricular fibrillation, pulseless electrical activity, symptomatic bradycardia, or asystole.

Prevalence

An estimated 250,000 people per year in the United States experience sudden cardiac death. However, national statistics on the actual prevalence of cardiopulmonary arrest are unreliable because no single agency collects data relating to the number of patients who receive cardiopulmonary resuscitation (CPR) annually. Ischemic cardiovascular disease underlies many cardiopulmonary arrests in adults.

The value of early CPR and immediate defibrillation has been proved in many community-based studies.[1-4] Additionally, among adults in whom ventricular tachycardia, ventricular fibrillation, or both is more common, the increased use of automated external defibrillators (AEDs) by emergency medical services (EMS), businesses, and airports has improved survival.[5-8] Without defibrillation, mortality from ventricular tachycardia, ventricular fibrillation, or both increases by approximately 10% per minute.[9-12]

Diagnosis and Therapy

The American Heart Association, in collaboration with the International Liaison Committee on Resuscitation, has established guidelines for resuscitation of cardiac arrest patients.[13,14] In each resuscitation scenario, four concepts should always apply:

- Activate EMS or the designated code team.
- Perform basic life support (CPR).
- Evaluate heart rhythm and perform early defibrillation as indicated.
- Deliver advanced life support (e.g., intubation, intravenous [IV] access, transfer to a medical center or intensive care unit).

Ventricular Tachycardia or Ventricular Fibrillation

1. Conduct a primary ABCD survey (***a***irway, ***b***reathing, ***c***irculation, ***d***ifferential diagnosis). Place airway device as soon as possible. Confirm placement, secure device, and confirm oxygenation and ventilation. Establish IV access, identify rhythm, and administer drugs appropriate for rhythm and condition. Search for and treat identified reversible causes, with focus on basic CPR and early defibrillation.
2. On arrival to an unwitnessed cardiac arrest or downtime longer than 4 minutes, five cycles (~2 min) of CPR are to be initiated before evaluation of rhythm. If the cardiac arrest is witnessed or downtime is shorter than 4 minutes, one shock may be administered immediately if the patient is in ventricular fibrillation or pulseless ventricular tachycardia (see later).
3. If the patient is in ventricular fibrillation or pulseless ventricular tachycardia, shock the patient once using 200 J on biphasic (on equivalent monophasic, 360 J).
4. Resume CPR immediately after attempted defibrillation, beginning with chest compressions. Rescuers should not interrupt chest compression to check circulation (e.g., evaluate rhythm or pulse) until five cycles or 2 minutes of CPR have been completed.
5. If there is persistent or recurrent ventricular tachycardia or ventricular fibrillation despite several shocks and cycles of CPR, perform a secondary ABCD survey with a focus on more advanced assessments and pharmacologic therapy. Pharmacologic therapy should include epinephrine (1 mg IV push, repeated every 3-5 min) or vasopressin (a single dose of 40 U IV, one time only).
6. Consider using antiarrhythmics for persistent or recurrent pulseless ventricular tachycardia or ventricular fibrillation. These include amiodarone, lidocaine, magnesium (if there is a known hypomagnesemic state), and procainamide (class indeterminate for persistent and Class IIb for recurrent).
7. Resume CPR and attempts to defibrillate.

Pulseless Electrical Activity

1. Assess the patient and conduct a primary ABCD survey.
2. Review for the most frequent causes of pulseless electrical activity, the five Hs and five Ts: ***h***ypovolemia, ***h***ypoxia, ***h***ydrogen ion (acidosis), ***h***yperkalemia (or ***h***ypokalemia), and ***h***ypothermia and ***t***ablets (drug overdose, accidents), ***t***amponade (cardiac), ***t***ension pneumothorax, ***t***hrombosis (coronary), and ***t***hrombosis (pulmonary embolism).
3. Administer epinephrine (1-mg IV push repeated every 3-5 min) or atropine (1 mg IV if the heart rate is slow, repeated every 3-5 min as needed, to a total dose of 0.04 mg/kg).
4. Conduct a secondary ABCD survey.

Bradycardia

1. Determine whether the bradycardia is slow (heart rate <60 beats/min) or relatively slow (heart rate less than expected relative to underlying condition or cause).
2. Conduct a primary ABCD survey.
3. Check for serious signs or symptoms caused by the bradycardia.
4. If no serious signs or symptoms are present, evaluate for a type II second-degree atrioventricular block or third-degree atrioventricular block.
5. If neither of these types of heart block is present, observe.

6. If one of these types of heart block is present, prepare for transvenous pacing. If symptoms develop, use a transcutaneous pacemaker until the transvenous pacer is placed.
7. If serious signs or symptoms are present, begin the following intervention sequence:
   a. Atropine, 0.5 up to a total of 3 mg IV
   b. Transcutaneous pacing, if available
   c. Dopamine, 5 to 20 μg/kg/min
   d. Epinephrine, 2 to 10 μg/min
   e. Isoproterenol, 2 to 10 μg/min
8. Conduct a secondary ABCD survey.

Asystole

1. Conduct a primary ABCD survey.
2. Perform transcutaneous pacing immediately if needed. Consider transvenous pacing if transcutaneous pacing fails to capture.
3. Administer epinephrine (1 mg IV push, repeated every 3-5 min) or atropine (1 mg IV repeated every 3-5 min, up to a total of 3 mg).
4. Conduct a secondary ABCD survey.
5. If asystole persists, consider withholding or ceasing resuscitative efforts.

HYPERTENSIVE EMERGENCY

Definition

A hypertensive emergency is an acute, severe elevation in blood pressure accompanied by end-organ compromise. In newly hypertensive patients, a hypertensive emergency is usually associated with a diastolic blood pressure higher than 120 mm Hg. Nephrosclerosis that causes acute renal failure frequently complicates hypertensive emergencies, with resultant hematuria and proteinuria. Nephrosclerosis also may perpetuate the elevation of systemic pressure through ischemic activation of the renin-angiotensin system. Ocular involvement with retinal exudates, hemorrhages, or papilledema connotes a worse prognosis.[15,16]

Complications of particular concern include hypertensive encephalopathy, aortic dissection, and eclampsia. Hypertensive encephalopathy signals the presence of cerebral edema and loss of vascular integrity. If left untreated, hypertensive encephalopathy may progress to seizure and coma.[17,18] Aortic dissection is associated with severe elevations in systemic blood pressure and wall stress, requiring immediate lowering of the blood pressure and emergent surgery to reduce morbidity and mortality. Eclampsia, the second most common cause of maternal death, occurs from the second trimester to the peripartum period. It is characterized by the presence of seizures, coma, or both, in the setting of preeclampsia. Delivery remains its only cure.[19]

Etiology

Hypertensive emergencies result from an exacerbation of essential hypertension or have a secondary cause, including renal, vascular, pregnancy-related, pharmacologic, endocrine, neurologic, and autoimmune causes (Box 1).

Box 1 Causes of Hypertensive Emergencies

Essential Hypertension

Renal causes

- Renal artery stenosis
- Glomerulonephritis

Vascular causes

- Vasculitis
- Hemolytic-uremic syndrome
- Thrombotic thrombocytopenia purpura

Pregnancy-related causes

- Preeclampsia
- Eclampsia

Pharmacologic causes

- Sympathomimetics
- Clonidine withdrawal, beta blocker withdrawal
- Cocaine
- Amphetamines

Endocrine causes

- Cushing's syndrome
- Conn's syndrome
- Pheochromocytoma
- Renin-secreting adenomas
- Thyrotoxicosis

Neurologic causes

- Central nervous system trauma
- Intracranial mass

Autoimmune cause

- Scleroderma renal crisis

Prevalence

The prevalence of hypertension rises substantially with increasing age in the United States and is greater among blacks than among whites in every age group.[20,21] Based on the third National Health and Nutrition Examination Survey (NHANES III), the prevalence of hypertension in those older than 70 years was found to be approximately 55% to 60% of the U.S. population.[22,23] A British study has revealed that less than 1% of patients with primary hypertension progress to hypertensive crisis.[24] This study also showed that despite increasingly widespread therapy, the number of patients presenting with hypertensive crises did not decline between 1970 and 1993.

Pathophysiology

Any syndrome that produces an acute rise in blood pressure may lead to a hypertensive crisis. Cerebral vasomotor autoregulation is a key facet of a patient's symptomatic presentation. Patients without chronic hypertension develop hypertensive crisis at a lower blood pressure than those with chronic hypertension. Although the process is not completely understood, an initial rise in vascular resistance mediated by vasoconstrictors such as angiotensin II, acetylcholine, or norepinephrine is responsible for the acute increase in blood pressure. This cascade exceeds the vasodilative response of the endothelium, mediated primarily by nitric oxide. Mechanical destruction of the endothelium by shear stress leads to further vascular obstruction, platelet aggregation, inflammation, and subsequent blood pressure elevation. The rate at which this occurs determines the rate of increase in systemic vascular resistance as well as the acuity of a patient's presentation.

Clinical Evaluation

The symptoms and signs of a hypertensive emergency vary widely. Symptoms of end-organ involvement include headache, blurred vision, confusion, chest pain, shortness of breath, back pain (e.g., aortic dissection) and, in severe end-organ involvement, seizures and altered consciousness.[15,16] Physical examination should assess end-organ involvement, including detailed fundoscopic, neurologic, and cardiovascular examinations, with emphasis on the presence of congestive heart failure and bilateral upper extremity blood pressure measurements. Laboratory evaluation should include measurement of the complete blood count with differential and smear

Table 1 Intravenous Vasodilator Therapy for Hypertensive Crisis

Drug	Dosage	Half-Life
Nitroprusside	2.5-10 μg/kg/min	1-2 min
Labetalol	20- to 80-mg bolus, 2 mg/min maintenance	2-6 hr
Fenoldopam*	0.1-0.5 μg/kg/min	10-20 min
Enalaprilat†	1.25- to 5-mg bolus	4-6 hr

*Recommended starting dose is 0.1 μg/kg/min, with a slow increase to a maximum rate of 0.5 mcg/kg/min and/or target blood pressure.

†Use specifically for angiotensin-converting enzyme-mediated hypertensive crises, such as scleroderma renal crisis. It is contraindicated in pregnancy.

Medical Economics Staff, Physician's Desk Reference, 57th Edition, 2003.

evaluations, measurements of electrolyte, blood urea nitrogen, and creatinine levels, and electrocardiography, chest radiography, and urinalysis.

Treatment

No large randomized clinical trials have assessed therapy in hypertensive emergency; therapeutic intervention is largely a result of expert opinion. All patients with end-organ involvement should be admitted for intensive monitoring and have an arterial blood pressure line placed.[16]

Pharmacologic Therapy

Intravenous vasodilator therapy to achieve a decrease in mean arterial pressure (MAP) of 20% to 25% or a decrease in diastolic blood pressure (DBP) to 100 to 110 mm Hg in the first 2 hours is recommended. Decreasing the MAP and DBP further should be done more slowly because of the risk of decreasing perfusion of end-organs.[16] Several drugs have proved beneficial in achieving this goal (Table 1).

At our institution, we focus on reducing shear forces and combine a beta blocker with sodium nitroprusside (SNP). In cases of marked catecholamine level elevation, large doses of IV beta blockers may be required to achieve blood pressure reduction. One exception to the use of large doses of beta blockers is cocaine overdose, for which vasodilators and benzodiazepines are the mainstays of therapy.

Additional Considerations

In addition to reducing MAP and DBP with medications as described above, early surgical intervention for type A dissection has proved to reduce morbidity and mortality. Reduction in shear stress is best achieved with IV beta blockade and SNP.[25,26]

In addition to delivery, IV magnesium, hydralazine (pregnancy class B drug), and labetalol (pregnancy class B drug) have value in the treatment of preeclampsia and prevention of eclampsia.[19] Angiotensin-converting enzyme inhibitors are strictly contraindicated because of adverse effects to the fetus, although this occurs in the first trimester.

Antihypertensive therapy remains controversial in the presence of stroke because a high cerebral perfusion pressure may be neurologically beneficial. Prompt neurologic consultation should be obtained.

AORTIC DISSECTION

Definition

Aortic dissection is a tear of the aortic intima that allows the shear forces of blood flow to dissect the intima from the media and, in some cases, penetrate the diseased media with resultant rupture and hemorrhage (Fig. 1).[27] Sixty-five percent of dissections originate in the ascending aorta, 20% in the descending aorta, 10% in the aortic arch, and the remainder in the abdominal aorta.[28,29]

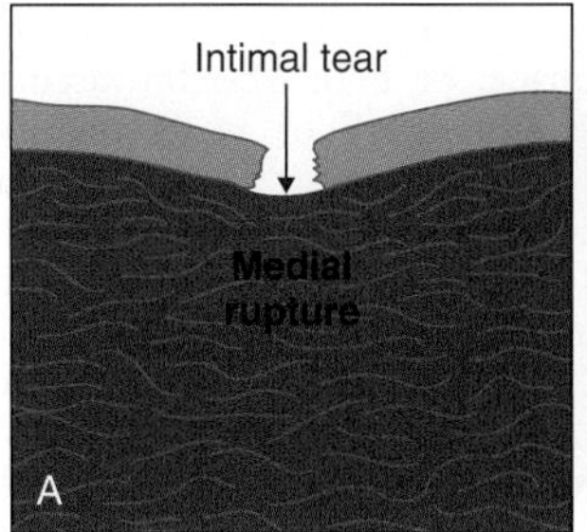

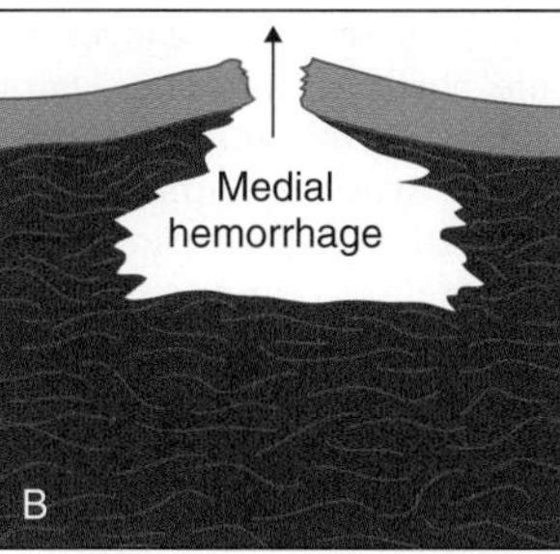

Figure 1 Aortic dissection. The tear has penetrated the diseased media (**A**), with resultant rupture and hemorrhage (**B**).

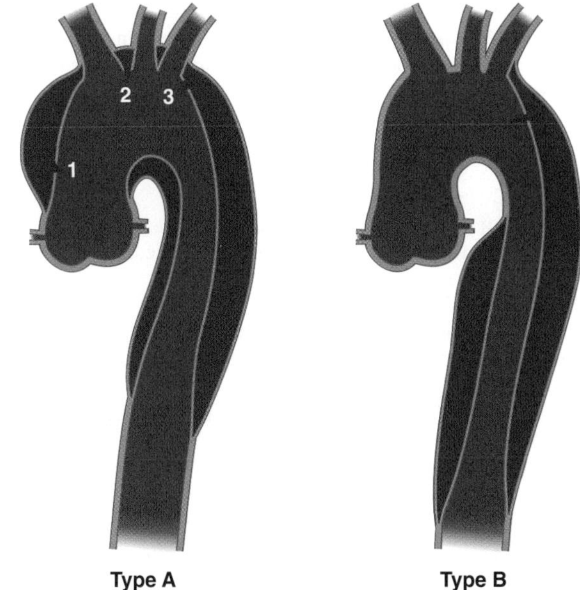

Figure 2 Aortic dissection, types A and B. Type B aortic dissection does not involve the ascending aorta.

By the Stanford system, a dissection that involves the ascending aorta is classified as type A, and one that does not is classified as type B (Fig. 2). Dissections are further classified by chronicity as acute (<2 weeks) or chronic (>2 weeks); mortality peaks at 2 weeks at approximately 80% and then levels off.[28]

Etiology

Any disease that weakens the aortic media predisposes patients to dissection. These include aging, hypertension, Marfan syndrome, Ehlers-Danlos syndrome, bicuspid aortic valve (associated with medial degeneration), coarctation, and Turner's syndrome. Pregnancy poses a unique risk to women with any of these diseases because of increased blood volume, cardiac output, and shear forces on the aorta. Of dissections in women younger than 40 years, 50% occur in the peripartum period.[30] Trauma from catheters or intra-aortic balloon pumps may also dissect the aortic intima.[31] Aortic dissection is infrequently associated with blunt trauma.

Clinical Presentation

Most patients present with acute chest pain that is often tearing or ripping in nature, which peaks in intensity at its onset. Uncommonly, patients present with congestive heart failure (from accompanying acute aortic insufficiency, tamponade, or both), cerebrovascular accident (involvement of the carotid artery or vertebrobasilar system), syncope (tamponade), or cardiac arrest.[32,33] On physical examination, hypertension is usually present, either as the primary cause of dissection or secondary to renal artery involvement. Acute aortic insufficiency with a resultant diastolic murmur may complicate ascending dissections. Loss of pulse, decrease in blood pressure, or both, often asymmetrically, are also found in the many patients.[32] Dissection of the spinal arteries, although rare, may produce secondary paraplegia.

Chest radiographs may reveal an abnormality in approximately 70% to 80% of patients, such as a widened mediastinum or loss of the demarcation of the aortic knob, pleural effusion, or pulmonary edema.[32] Importantly, a normal chest radiograph is not incompatible with an aortic dissection. The electrocardiogram (ECG) may reveal left ventricular hypertrophy, ST depression, T wave inversion, or ST elevation. Electrocardiographic changes indicating inferior territory injury may herald right coronary ostial involvement in 1% to 2% of aortic dissection cases.

Diagnosis

Recognition of several signs is essential in the imaging of aortic dissection because they affect treatment and outcome:

- Involvement of the ascending aorta
- Location of dissection flap, intimal tear
- Presence of pericardial fluid, cardiac tamponade
- Involvement of coronary ostia

Magnetic resonance imaging (MRI) has a sensitivity and specificity of approximately 98% for detection of dissection. Transesophageal echocardiography has a sensitivity of approximately 98%; however, its lower specificity, 77% to 97%, reflects differences in operator experience.[29,35] Computed tomography sensitivity for detecting dissection is approximately 83% to 94%, and its specificity ranges from 87% to 100%, depending on the study.[34,35] Choice of testing should be based on the medical center's expertise, hemodynamic stability of the patient, and access to the imaging modality.[34-36] Although MRI remains the gold standard, its lack of portability, limited access, and long duration of imaging make this a less favorable option in the care of acute aortic dissection in some centers.[36]

Treatment

Surgery

Surgical therapy is the best option for an acute aortic dissection involving the ascending aorta. Studies have shown that delaying surgical intervention, even to carry out left heart catheterization, aortography, or both, results in worse outcomes.[37–39] Surgical repair in patients with type B dissection is generally reserved for those with end-organ compromise or those who do not respond to medical therapy.

Medical Therapy

Medical therapy should be initiated in all patients with acute dissection. Reductions of shear force and blood pressure should be the primary goals. Beta blockers should be given parenterally and titrated to effect (generally, pulse 50-60 beats/min). In our institution, we then add SNP because of its rapid onset and ease of titration, aiming for a MAP of 65 to 75 mm Hg.

In the hypotensive patient, pericardial tamponade, aortic rupture, myocardial infarction, or a combination of these should be suspected. Volume replacement and early surgical intervention should be pursued. Pericardiocentesis should be avoided if tamponade is present, because immediate surgical intervention is the therapy of choice. If hypotension persists, norepinephrine and phenylephrine are the vasopressors of choice because of their limited effects on shear force. Endovascular stenting, a rapidly growing field, remains investigational in this setting.

ACUTE PULMONARY EDEMA

Definition

Acute pulmonary edema is an emergency that necessitates admission to the hospital. It has two major forms, cardiogenic and noncardiogenic. We focus on cardiogenic pulmonary edema, which generally is more reversible than the noncardiogenic form.

Cardiogenic pulmonary edema results from an absolute increase in left atrial pressure, with resultant increases in pulmonary venous and capillary pressures. In the setting of normal capillary permeability, this increased pressure causes extravasation of fluid into the alveoli and overwhelms the ability of the pulmonary lymphatics to drain the fluid, thus impairing gas exchange in the lung.[40,41]

Etiology and Pathophysiology

Left ventricular systolic dysfunction, left ventricular diastolic dysfunction, and obstruction of the left atrial outflow tract are the primary causes of increased left atrial pressure. Left ventricular systolic dysfunction is the most common cause of cardiogenic pulmonary edema.[40] This dysfunction can be the result of coronary artery disease, hypertension, valvular heart disease, cardiomyopathy, toxins, endocrinologic or metabolic causes, or infections.

Diastolic dysfunction results in impaired left ventricular filling and elevation in left ventricular end-diastolic pressure. In addition to myocardial ischemia, left ventricular hypertrophy, hypertrophic obstructive cardiomyopathy, and infiltrative or restrictive cardiomyopathy are all causes of diastolic dysfunction.

Left atrial outflow obstruction is often a result of valvulopathy, such as mitral stenosis or mitral regurgitation, but also can be caused by tumors (atrial myxoma), dysfunctional prosthetic valves, thrombus, and cor triatriatum. It is imperative to distinguish between mitral regurgitation and mitral stenosis, given their very different treatments.

Diagnosis

Pulmonary edema is diagnosed by the presence of various signs and symptoms, including tachypnea, tachycardia, crackles (reflecting alveolar edema), hypoxia (secondary to alveolar edema), and S_3 or S_4 heart sounds, or both. Additionally, if hypertension is present, it may represent diastolic dysfunction, decreased left ventricular compliance, decreased cardiac output, and increased systemic vascular resistance. The presence of increased jugular venous pressure indicates increased right ventricular filling pressure secondary to right ventricular or left ventricular dysfunction. Finally, the presence of peripheral edema indicates a certain chronicity to the patient's condition.

Laboratory data associated with pulmonary edema include hypoxemia on arterial sampling and a chest radiograph showing bilateral perihilar edema and cephalization of pulmonary vascular marking. Cardiomegaly, pleural effusion, or both may be present. Two-dimensional echocardiography may be helpful in the acute setting to assess left ventricular and right ventricular size and function and to look for valvular stenosis or regurgitation and pericardial pathology. The electrocardiogram (ECG) may reflect ongoing ischemia, injury, tachycardia, and atrial or ventricular hypertrophy.

Treatment

Mainstays of immediate therapy include improving oxygen delivery to end organs, decreasing myocardial oxygen consumption, increasing venous capacitance, decreasing preload and afterload, with careful attention to MAP, and avoiding hemodynamic embarrassment. All patients should receive supplemental oxygen to maximize oxygen saturation of hemoglobin. Administration of continuous positive airway pressure provides positive airway pressure, increases gas exchange, and perhaps decreases preload via decreased intrathoracic pressure.[42,43]

Endotracheal intubation and mechanical ventilation should be used immediately if noninvasive supplemental oxygenation proves inadequate. In our experience, repeated attempts to improve oxygenation with noninvasive positive pressure ventilation often prove futile, and restoration of oxygenation is best achieved via endotracheal intubation.

Pharmacologic Therapy

The pharmacologic agents most commonly used in the treatment of acute pulmonary edema are nitroglycerin, SNP, nesiritide, and diuretics.[44]

Nitroglycerin acts immediately to decrease preload and afterload.[45] It should be used for the management of patients with pulmonary edema who are not in cardiogenic shock. Sublingual administration allows rapid delivery of a large dose, which is often required to decrease preload. Parenteral administration also should be used in the nonhypotensive patient and, based on symptoms, titrated to a MAP of approximately 70 to 75 mm Hg.

SNP is an effective vasodilator that is often required for the treatment of the hypertensive patient with pulmonary edema.[46] Its use requires arterial blood pressure monitoring. SNP should be used with caution in the setting of liver dysfunction, although thiocyanate toxicity is uncommon and usually occurs after prolonged infusion at high doses. Concomitant use of nitroglycerin should be strongly considered in the ischemic patient.

A recent addition to the pharmacologic armamentarium, nesiritide is a vasodilator that acts by increasing the level of cyclic guanosine monophosphate, which, in turn, causes smooth muscle cell relaxation. In one trial, it proved superior to low-dose IV nitroglycerin.[47,48] Its serum half-life and blood pressure-lowering effect are much longer than SNP; therefore, it should be used with caution in a patient with a low or low-normal MAP. However, the use of the drug does not require invasive hemodynamic monitoring.

Intravenous diuretics are most helpful for the treatment of volume overload in chronic congestive heart failure. Their vasodilative and diuretic properties also are useful in the management of pulmonary edema. Diuretics should be used with caution in the euvolemic patient to avoid compromising cardiac output and oxygen delivery.

Summary

Cardiovascular emergencies are common in the practice of medicine and quick action is necessary.

- Cardiopulmonary arrest has several causes, all of which require prompt resuscitative efforts.
- Hypertensive emergency warrants admission for intensive monitoring and arterial blood pressure line placement.
- Aortic dissection categorized as type A requires emergent surgery, whereas type B is managed medically.
- Acute pulmonary edema should be treated by improving oxygen delivery to end organs, decreasing myocardial oxygen consumption, increasing venous capacitance, and decreasing preload and afterload.

Suggested Readings

ACOG Committee on Practice Bulletins—Obstetrics: ACOG practice bulletin. Diagnosis and management of preeclampsia and eclampsia. Number 33, January 2002. Obstet Gynecol 2002;99:159-167.

Cigarroa JE, Isselbacher EM, DeSanctis RW, Eagle KA: Diagnostic imaging in the evaluation of suspected aortic dissection. Old standards and new directions. N Engl J Med 1993;328:35-43.

Cotter G, Moshkovitz Y, Milovanov O, et al: Acute heart failure: A novel approach to its pathogenesis and treatment. Eur J Heart Fail 2002;4:227-234.

ECC Committee, Subcommittees, and Task Forces of the American Heart Association: 2005 American Heart Association Guidelines for Cardiopulmonary Resuscitation and Emergency Cardiovascular Care. Circulation 2005;112(Suppl 24):IV1-IV203.

Hazinski MF, Idris AH, Kerber RE, et al: American Heart Association Emergency Cardiovascular Committee; Council on Cardiopulmonary, Perioperative, and Critical Care; Council on Clinical Cardiology: Lay rescuer automated external defibrillator ("public access defibrillation") programs: Lessons learned from an international multicenter trial: Advisory statement from the American Heart Association Emergency Cardiovascular Committee; the Council on Cardiopulmonary, Perioperative, and Critical Care; and the Council on Clinical Cardiology. Circulation 2005:111(21):3336-3340.

Herlitz J, Bang A, Axelsson A, et al: Experience with the use of automated external defibrillators in out-of-hospital cardiac arrest. Resuscitation 1998;37:3-7.

International Liaison Committee on Resuscitation: 2005 International Consensus on Cardiopulmonary Resuscitation and Emergency Cardiovascular Care Science with Treatment Recommendations. Circulation 2005;112:III1-III136.

Larsen MP, Eisenberg MS, Cummins RO, et al: Predicting survival from out-of-hospital cardiac arrest: A graphic model. Ann Emerg Med 1993;22:1652-1658.

Lip GY, Beevers M, Beevers G: The failure of malignant hypertension to decline: A survey of 24 years' experience in a multiracial population in England. J Hypertens 1994;12:1297-1305.

Marwick C: NHANES III health data relevant for aging nation. JAMA 1997;277:100-102.

Penn MS, Smedira N, Lytle B, Brener SJ: Does coronary angiography before emergency aortic surgery affect in-hospital mortality? J Am Coll Cardiol 2000;35:889-894.

Pretre R, Von Segesser LK: Aortic dissection. Lancet 1997;349:1461-1464.

Roberts DA: Magnetic resonance imaging of thoracic aortic aneurysm and dissection. Semin Roentgenol 2001;36:295-308.

Scott C, Burruss N, Kalimi R, et al: Acute ascending aortic dissection during pregnancy. Am J Crit Care 2001;10:430-433.

Shiga T, Wajima Z, Apfel CC, et al: Diagnostic accuracy of transesophageal echocardiography, helical computed tomography, and magnetic resonance imaging for suspected thoracic aortic dissection: Systematic review and meta-analysis. Arch Intern Med 2006;166:1350-1356.

Vaughan CJ, Delanty N: Hypertensive emergencies. Lancet 2000;356:411-417.

References

For a complete list of references, log onto www.expertconsult.com.

Cardiac Arrhythmias

Fredrick J. Jaeger

DEFINITION

Broadly defined, cardiac arrhythmias are any abnormality or perturbation in the normal activation sequence of the myocardium. The sinus node, displaying properties of automaticity, spontaneously depolarizes, sending a depolarization wave over the atrium, depolarizing the atrioventricular (AV) node, propagating over the His-Purkinje system, and depolarizing the ventricle in systematic fashion. There are hundreds of different types of cardiac arrhythmias. The normal rhythm of the heart, so-called normal sinus rhythm, can be disturbed through failure of automaticity, such as sick sinus syndrome, or through overactivity, such as inappropriate sinus tachycardia. Ectopic foci prematurely exciting the myocardium on a single or continuous basis results in premature atrial contractions (PACs) and premature ventricular contractions (PVCs). Sustained tachyarrhythmias in the atria, such as atrial fibrillation, paroxysmal atrial tachycardia (PAT), and supraventricular tachycardia (SVT), originate because of micro- or macro re-entry. In general, the seriousness of cardiac arrhythmias depends on the presence or absence of structural heart disease.

The most common example of a relatively benign arrhythmia is atrial fibrillation (see the chapter "Atrial Fibrillation"). Similarly common are PACs and PVCs, which, although a nuisance, generally are benign in the absence of structural heart disease. In contrast, the presence of nonsustained ventricular tachycardia (VT) or syncope in patients with coronary artery disease (CAD) or severe left ventricular (LV) dysfunction may be a harbinger of subsequent sudden cardiac death and must not be ignored.

PREVALENCE

Cardiac arrhythmias are common. Symptoms such as dizziness, palpitations, and syncope are frequent complaints encountered by family physicians, internists, and cardiologists. In contrast to these ubiquitous complaints, which are generally benign, sudden cardiac death remains an important public health concern. Statistics from the Centers for Disease Control and Prevention (CDC) have estimated sudden cardiac death rates at more than 600,000 per year (Fig. 1).[1] Up to 50% of patients have sudden death as the first manifestation of cardiac disease. Efforts at decreasing this alarming number have obviously focused on primary prevention, such as reducing cardiac risk factors, but have also led to the proliferation of automatic external defibrillators (AEDs). These devices have been shown to reduce mortality when used quickly in the first few minutes after an arrest.

PATHOPHYSIOLOGY

Regardless of the specific arrhythmia, the pathogenesis of the arrhythmias falls into one of three basic mechanisms: enhanced or suppressed automaticity, triggered activity, or re-entry. Automaticity is a natural property of all myocytes. Ischemia, scarring, electrolyte disturbances, medications, advancing age, and other factors may suppress or enhance automaticity in various areas. Suppression of automaticity of the sinoatrial (SA) node can result in sinus node dysfunction and in sick sinus syndrome (SSS), which is still the most common indication for permanent pacemaker implantation (Fig. 2). In contrast to suppressed automaticity, enhanced automaticity can result in multiple arrhythmias, both atrial and ventricular. Triggered activity occurs when early afterdepolarizations and delayed afterdepolarizations initiate spontaneous multiple depolarizations, precipitating ventricular arrhythmias. Examples include torsades de pointes (Fig. 3) and ventricular arrhythmias caused by digitalis toxicity. Probably the most common mechanism of arrhythmogenesis results from re-entry. Requisites for re-entry include bidirectional conduction and unidirectional block. Micro level re-entry occurs with VT from conduction around the scar of myocardial infarction (MI), and macro level re-entry occurs via conduction through (Wolff-Parkinson-White [WPW] syndrome) concealed accessory pathways.

SIGNS AND SYMPTOMS

The signs and symptoms of cardiac arrhythmias can range from none at all to loss of consciousness or sudden cardiac death. In general, more-severe symptoms are more likely to occur in the presence of structural heart disease. For example, sustained monomorphic VT, particularly in a normal heart, may be hemodynamically tolerated without syncope. In contrast, even nonsustained VT may be poorly tolerated and cause marked symptoms in patients with severe LV dysfunction. Complaints such as lightheadedness, dizziness, fluttering, pounding, quivering, shortness of breath, dizziness, chest discomfort, and forceful or painful extra beats are commonly reported with various arrhythmias. Often, patients notice arrhythmias only after checking their peripheral pulses.

Certain descriptions of symptoms can raise the index of suspicion and provide clues about the type of arrhythmia. The presence of sustained regular palpitations or heart racing in young patients without any evidence of structural heart disease suggests the presence of a SVT caused by AV nodal re-entry or SVT caused by an accessory pathway. Such tachycardias are often accompanied by chest discomfort, diaphoresis, neck fullness, or a vasovagal type of response with syncope, diaphoresis, or nausea. It has been shown that the hemodynamic consequences of SVT as well as VT can also have an autonomic basis, recruiting vasodepressor reflexes similar to those observed in neurocardiogenic syncope. Isolated or occasional premature beats suggest PACs or PVCs and are benign in the absence of structural heart disease.

Syncope in the setting of noxious stimuli such as pain, prolonged standing, or venipuncture, particularly when preceded by vagal-type symptoms (e.g., diaphoresis, nausea, vomiting) suggests neurocardiogenic (vasovagal) syncope. Occasionally, patients report abrupt syncope without prodromal symptoms, suggesting the possibility of the malignant variety of neurocardiogenic syncope. Malignant neurocardiogenic syncope denotes syncope in the absence of a precipitating stimulus, with a short or absent prodrome, often resulting in injuries, and is associated with marked cardioinhibitory and bradycardic responses spontaneously or provoked by head-up tilt-table testing.[2] Sustained or paroxysmal sinus tachycardia, frequently associated with chronic fatigue syndrome and fibromyalgia, suggest the possibility of postural orthostatic tachycardia syndrome (POTS). This syndrome, which may be a form of autonomic dysfunction, currently is unexplained. It is characterized by a markedly exaggerated increased chronotropic response to head-up tilt-table testing and stress testing. POTS often has associated systemic signs, such as muscle aches (fibromyalgia), cognitive dysfunction, and weight loss. Inappropriate sinus tachycardia (IST) syndrome is similar in presentation, but it probably represents a separate disorder with another cause—possibly atrial tachycardias in the sinus node area or dysregulation of sinus node automaticity.

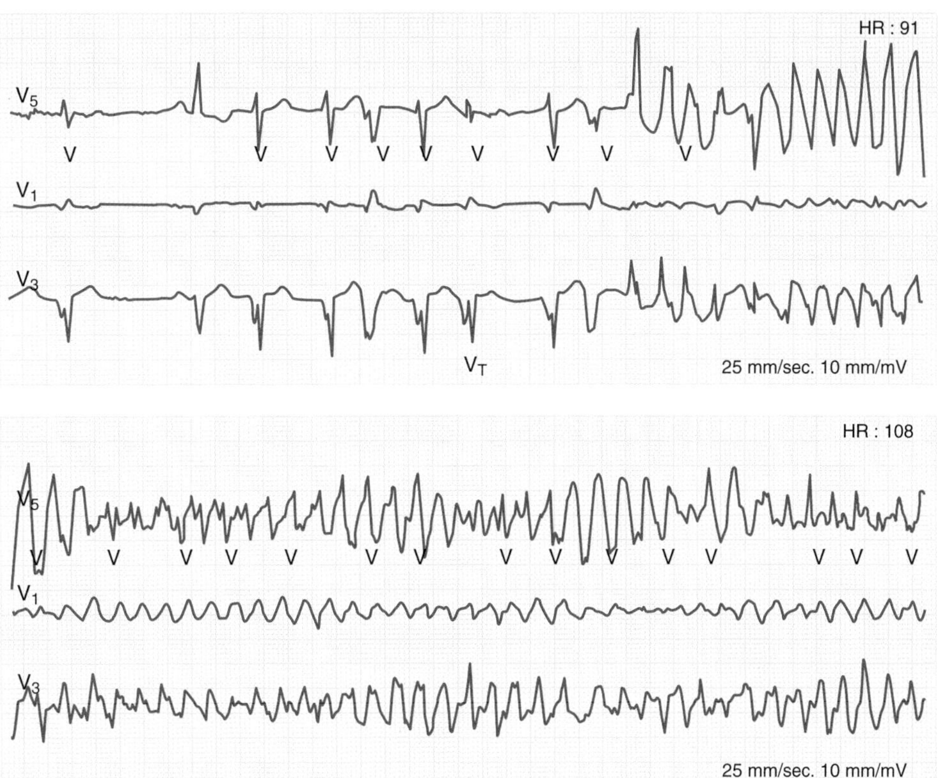

Figure 1 Holter monitor recording showing ventricular tachycardia degenerating to ventricular fibrillation. HR, heart rate.

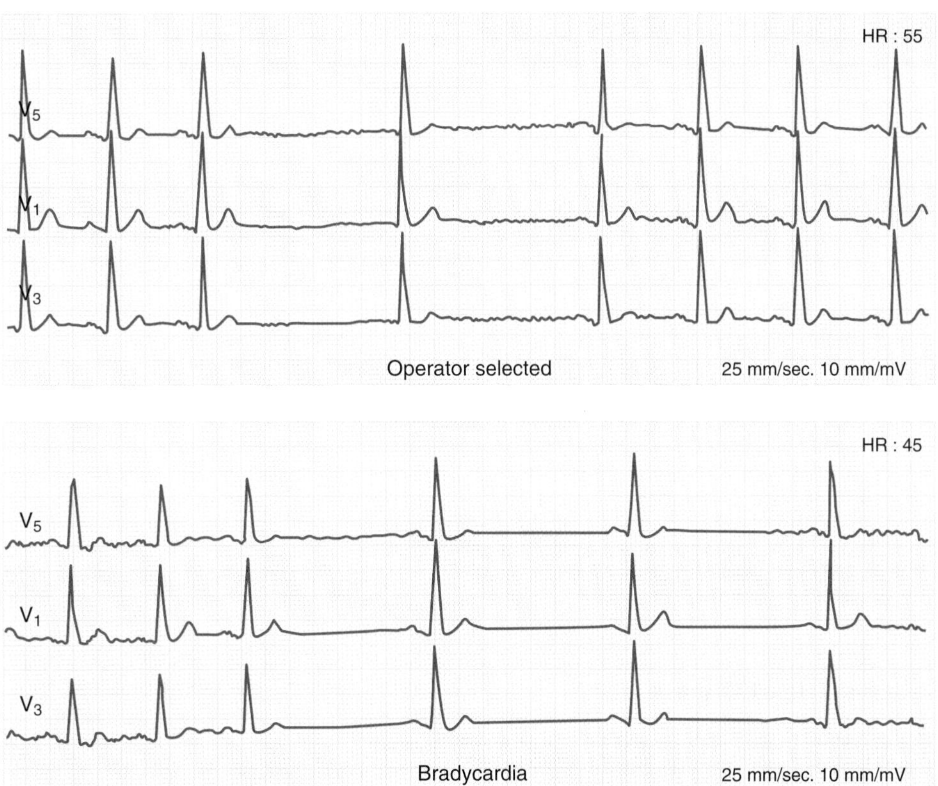

Figure 2 Holter monitor recording in a patient with sick sinus syndrome (SSS) revealing marked abrupt slowing of sinus rate, with symptoms. HR, heart rate.

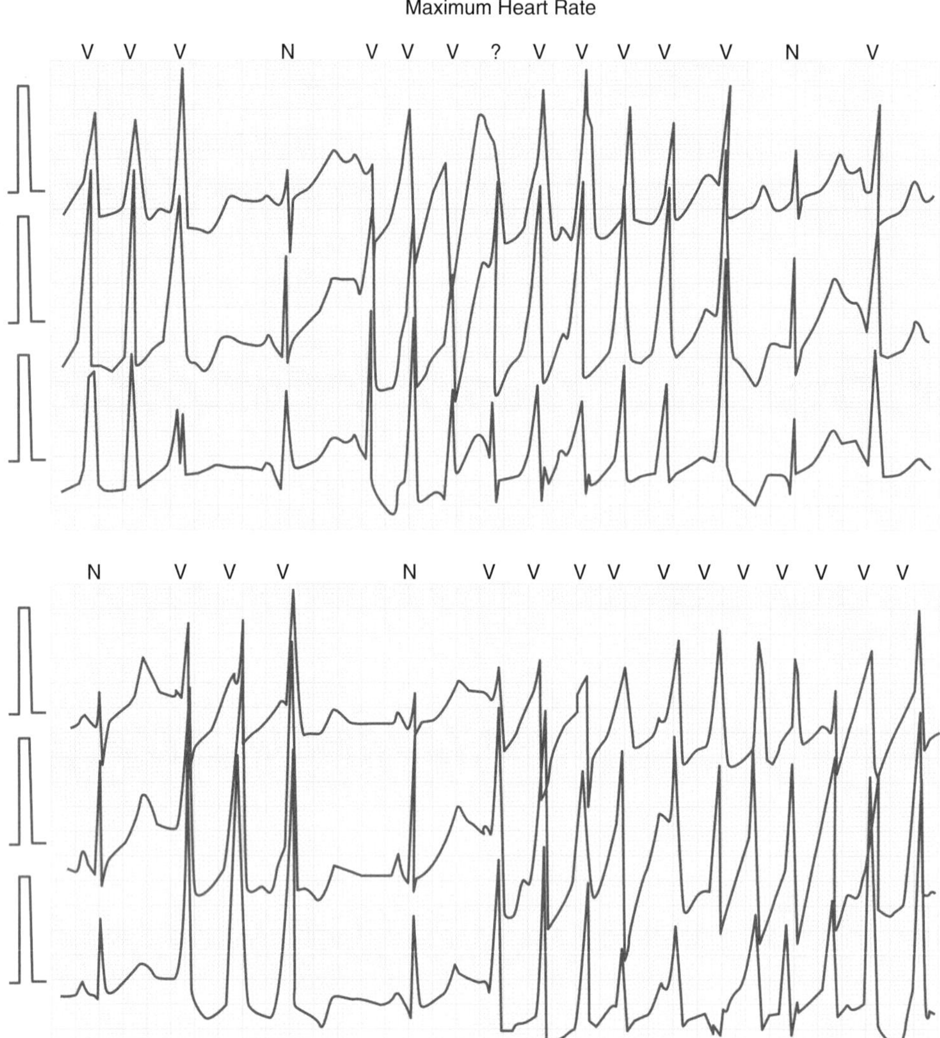

Figure 3 Torsades de pointes in a patient with long QT syndrome.

DIAGNOSIS

Because a number of tests are available for the diagnosis of cardiac arrhythmias, it is important to proceed with a stepwise approach. The goal is to obtain a correlation between symptoms and the underlying arrhythmia and initiation of appropriate therapy. Additional testing is usually advocated to identify patients with arrhythmias caused by ischemia or who are at risk for sudden cardiac death.

This section assumes a basic knowledge of cardiac arrhythmias and will not focus on specific aspects of arrhythmia identification and diagnosis, except to present the various treatment options available for the many commonly encountered arrhythmias. Excellent texts are available that provide core curriculum material for the identification of cardiac arrhythmias, rate determination, interval measurement, and identification of normal and abnormal P, QRS, and T wave morphologies.

Assessment of Structural Heart Disease

The initial assessment of structural heart disease begins with the history and physical examination. Careful attention to CAD or MIs, risk factors for CAD, and family history of sudden cardiac death are extremely important. Careful scrutiny of the electrocardiogram (ECG) is imperative to look for conduction system delays, QRS widening, previous MI, or PVCs. Cardiac auscultation may detect an irregular rhythm or premature beats. Stress testing, usually with imaging (e.g., stress echocardiography or stress thallium and echocardiography) can demonstrate the presence of CAD, LV dysfunction, or valvular heart disease.

Frequently, patients present with a wide complex tachycardia, possibly VT versus SVT with aberrancy. Various algorithms have been described to facilitate the differentiation of wide complex tachycardias. Brugada and colleagues have synthesized the various schemes into one convenient and simple protocol (Fig. 4). The general rule, however, is that sustained or nonsustained wide complex tachycardia in patients with known CAD or previous MI is VT until proven otherwise.[3] Obviously, the initial approach to sustained wide complex tachycardia is to carry out cardioversion if the patient is hemodynamically unstable. In stable patients, assume VT and treat empirically with intravenous medications (e.g., amiodarone, procainamide, lidocaine). If SVT with aberrancy is strongly suspected, diagnostic maneuvers, such as administering adenosine, may be cautiously used.

Holter Monitoring

Ambulatory Holter monitoring has been available for several decades and has proved invaluable in identifying underlying rhythm abnor-

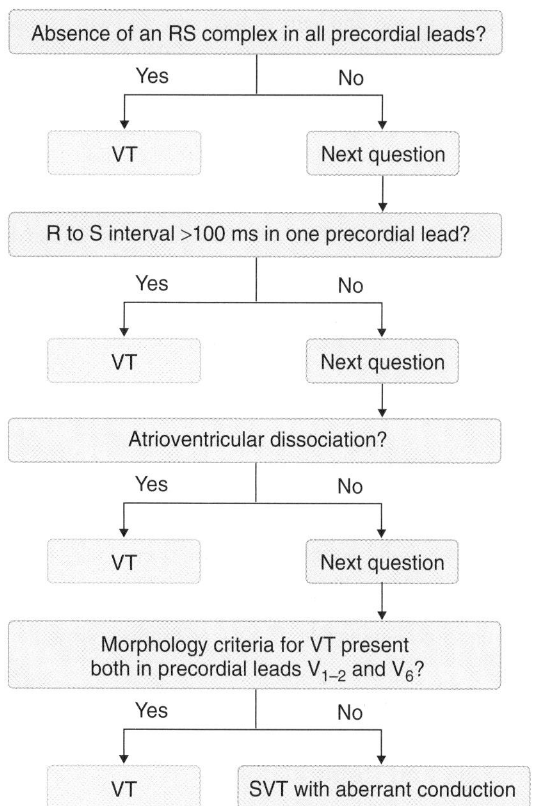

Figure 4 Brugada algorithm for wide complex tachycardia. SVT, supraventricular tachycardia; VT, ventricular tachycardia. *(From Brugada P, Brugada J, Mont L, et al: A new approach to the differential diagnosis of a regular tachycardia with a wide QRS complex. Circulation 1991;83:1649-1659.)*

malities.[4] Generally, 24- to 48-hour baseline Holter monitoring is useful in quantitating and qualifying arrhythmias in patients with frequent symptoms (Fig. 5).

Event Recording

For patients who have symptoms occurring on a weekly or monthly basis, Holter monitoring may not establish the diagnosis unless the patient fortuitously experiences an event during recording. Event recording monitoring systems, also called loop recorders (e.g., King of Hearts, Instromedix, Rosemont, Ill) can be worn for longer intervals (usually a month) and can document infrequent arrhythmia episodes and provide symptom-to-arrhythmia correlation. These devices are automatically activated or patient-activated and use telephone modem technology to transmit the electrocardiographic rhythm strips. They use continuous loop technology (retrograde memory) so that in the event of a symptom, the patient activates the device by pushing a button and records an electrocardiographic rhythm strip several minutes before the event. When prolonged external ambulatory event monitors fail to document an arrhythmia, an implantable device (Reveal, Medtronic, Minneapolis, Minn) can be used in patients with recurrent enigmatic syncope or arrhythmias, in whom conventional testing has not yielded a diagnosis. This device, with a battery life of 14 to 22 months, is implanted subcutaneously and continuously scans for arrhythmias (Fig. 6). The device automatically records and stores tachycardia or bradycardia events and can be patient-activated. Insurance reimbursement for the Reveal device requires extensive conventional diagnostic testing, including negative event monitors, tilt-table testing, and an electrophysiologic study (EPS). Preliminary reports of implantable event monitor studies have shown a significant reduction in time to diagnosis and decreased overall costs when used in patients with syncope and no structural heart disease.

Signal-Averaged Electrocardiogram and T Wave Alternans

Although initially touted as an important screening test for patients with syncope or ventricular arrhythmia risk, the signal-averaged ECG (SAECG) now has a limited role.[5] The presence of low-

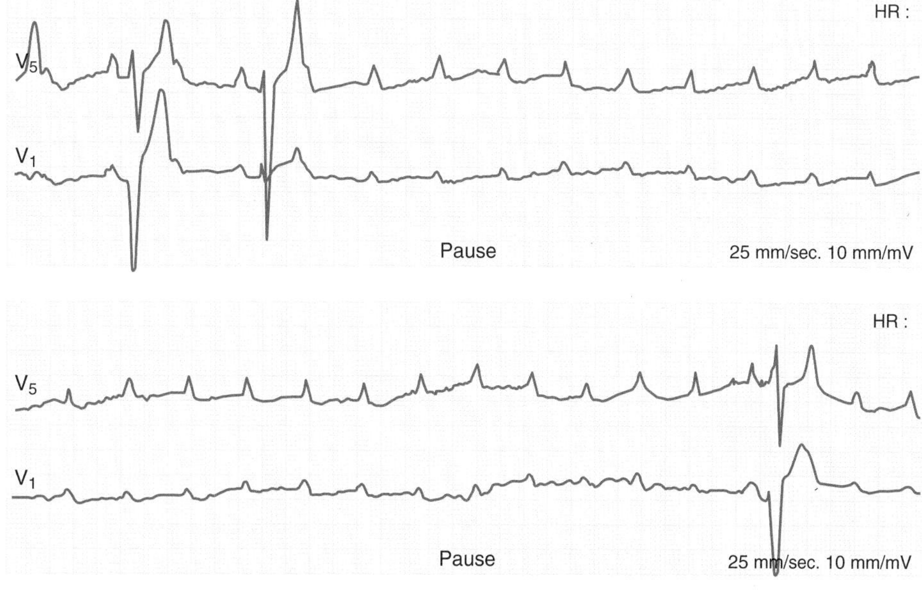

Figure 5 Holter monitor recording demonstrating intermittent complete heart block in a patient with syncope. HR, heart rate.

amplitude late potentials, indicating a positive signal-averaged ECG, suggests an underlying abnormality in ventricular repolarization seen with a discrete scar and can be associated with ventricular ectopy and spontaneous VT (Fig. 7). However, the SAECG may be abnormal in patients with no evidence of structural heart disease and in patients with conduction disturbances (e.g., right bundle branch block [RBBB]) and therefore, a positive study has an uncertain specificity and sensitivity. In contrast, the SAECG can be helpful in screening patients or family members for arrhythmogenic right ventricular dysplasia (ARVD). Similarly, T wave alternans may have an important role for risk stratification in patients with LV dysfunction and complex ventricular arrhythmias. It has long been recognized that abnormalities in the ST segment and T wave may precede the onset of ventricular arrhythmias. Presumably, changes in autonomic activity, as well as repolarization, may facilitate the provocation of lethal ventricular arrhythmias in susceptible patients. Rosenbaum and colleagues[6] have reported that abnormal T wave alternans may be an important marker for assessing patients and determining their risk for sudden cardiac death (SCD). T wave alternans can be measured by stress testing and ambulatory monitors (Fig. 8).

Wireless technologies have now been introduced that are capable of long-term cardiac telemetric monitoring for cardiac arrhythmias, both in the home environment and on an ambulatory basis. External monitoring systems can be worn continuously by the patient and use hard-wired telephone modem connections or wireless cellular network technology. These monitors automatically detect cardiac arrhythmias and transmit the telemetry strip to a central cardiac monitoring station, which alerts the patient, physician, or emergency response systems. These devices are capable of patient activation, but they also have automatic logic algorithms for detecting arrhythmias similar to those incorporated in defibrillators. This wireless technology has become available on implanted devices, such as pacemakers and defibrillators (Biotronik, Lake Oswego, Ore). These devices monitor for arrhythmias and detect pacemaker or defibrillator activity or device malfunction. Ambulatory cardiac monitoring provides an attractive alternative to prolonged hospitalization and may ultimately lower health care costs and reduce mortality.

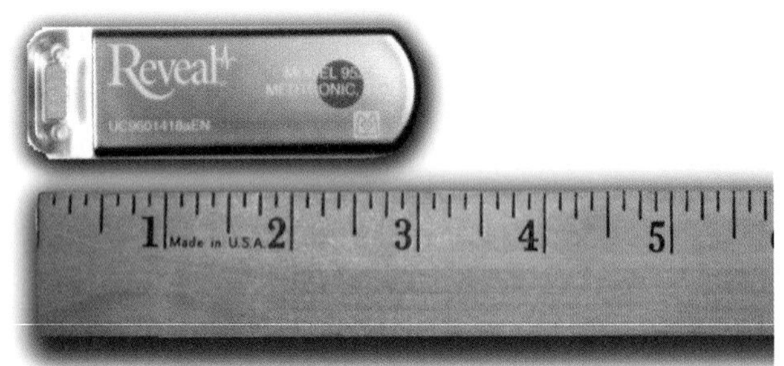

Figure 6 Reveal implantable loop recorder (Medtronic, Minneapolis, Minn). This device is implanted subcutaneously in the left pectoral region and can be patient activated or autoactivated.

Electrophysiologic Testing

Electrophysiologic testing has become an important standard for identifying high-risk patients who have nonsustained VT, such as those with previous MI and LV dysfunction (Fig. 9).[5,7] Inducible, sustained, monomorphic VT predicts substantial risk for subsequent, spontaneous, clinically sustained VT and ventricular fibrillation (VF). Electrophysiologic testing is the gold standard for evaluating patients with recurrent syncope and can help identify underlying His-Purkinje disease, inducible VT, SVT, and sinus node dysfunction (Box 1).[8]

TREATMENT

Pacemakers and Defibrillators

Implantation of a permanent pacemaker requires specific levels of evidence and indications based on American College of Cardiology–American Heart Association (ACC/AHA guidelines.[9] Class I and Class II indications are appropriate for the implantation of a permanent pacemaker (PPM). Correlation of symptoms with underlying bradyarrhythmias or heart block is required. Rarely, intuitive or empirical pacemaker implantation is performed. The implantable cardioverter-defibrillator (ICD) is indicated for sustained VT or VF, survivors of sudden cardiac death (AVID trial [Antiarrhythmics Versus Implantable Defibrillators], secondary prevention),[10] or inducible, sustained, monomorphic VT (MADIT I [Multicenter Automatic Defibrillator Implantation Trial], primary prevention).[11]

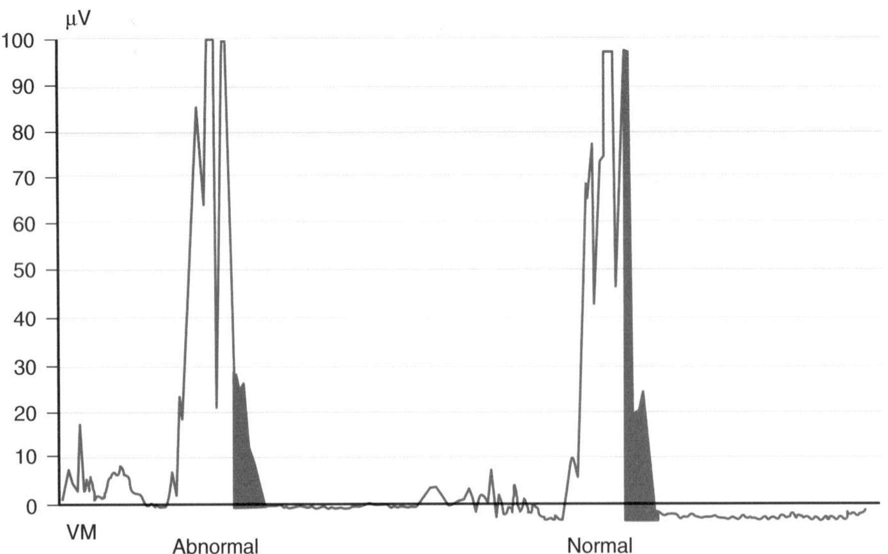

Figure 7 Positive signal-averaged electrocardiogram demonstrating low-amplitude late potentials. VM, vector magnitude.

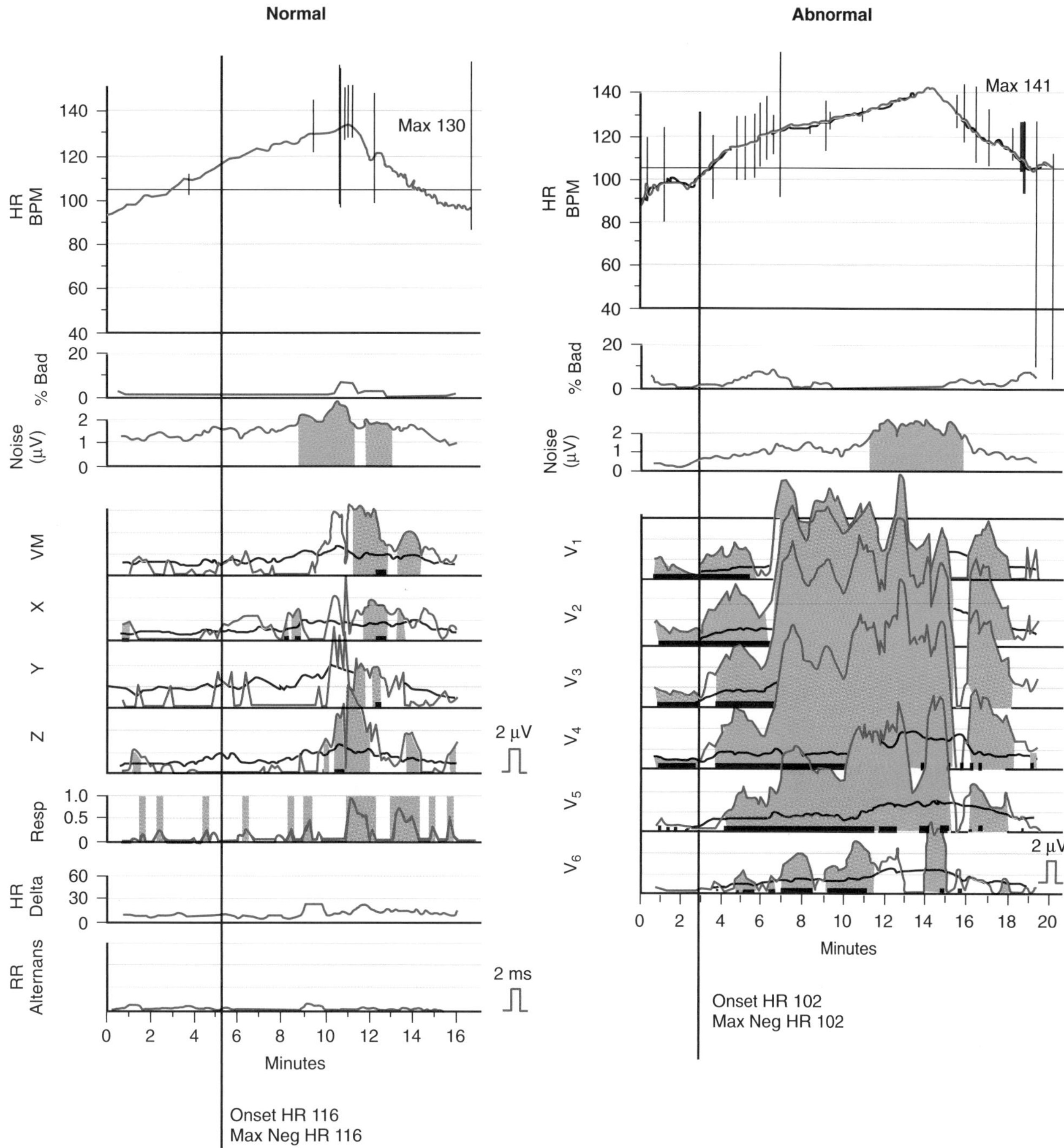

Figure 8 Positive T wave alternans demonstrating marked abnormality of the ST segment *(salmon-pink area)* during exercise testing.

Based on the results of the MADIT II study, ICDs will routinely be implanted in patients with LV dysfunction, ejection fraction (EF) of less than 35%, and a previous MI.[12] Emerging indications for implantation of ICDs include patients with syncope who have dilated cardiomyopathy and patients who have hypertrophic obstructive cardiomyopathy (HOCM) and are believed be at high risk for sudden cardiac death (nonsustained VTs, syncope, and family members who have experienced sudden cardiac death).

Since their introduction 40 years ago, pacemakers have advanced in sophistication, reliability, and longevity. Current pacemakers are expected to last at least 10 years and leads much longer. Although lead technology is continuously undergoing improvement, leads still fail because of material breakdown, fatigue, and manufacturing defects and may require removal and replacement (Fig. 10). Leads and devices may also need to be removed secondary to infection. Chronic leads are often heavily fibrosed by endovascular tissue. Lead extraction requires sophisticated equipment, such as lasers, and experienced operators for safe removal. ICD battery life is currently 5 to 7 years and continues to improve. Follow-ups of PPMs and ICDs are usually every 6 to 12 months, with comprehensive testing of pacing and sensing thresholds. Pacemakers can be dual chamber and have rate-response capability. Rate responsiveness simulates the chronotropic response of the sinus node and uses minute ventilation or, more commonly, motion to estimate the needed heart rate. Pacemakers and ICDs have extensive telemetric capacity, allowing retrieval of event, trend, battery, and lead data. PPMs and ICDs can

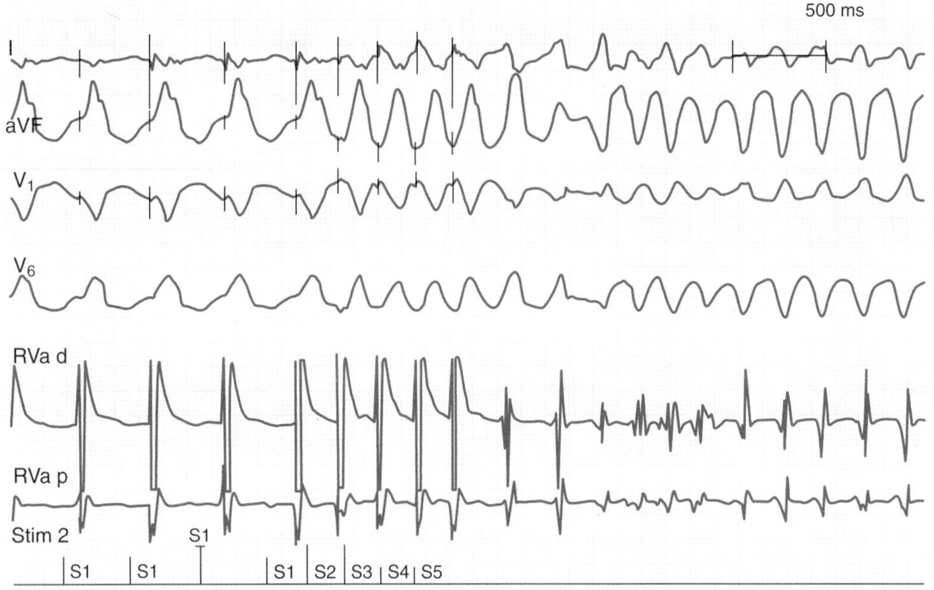

Figure 9 Sustained monomorphic ventricular tachycardia induced during electrophysiologic testing. Following a paced drive train of 150 beats/min (400 msec), four premature ventricular extra beats provoked fast ventricular tachycardia at 240 beats/min.

Box 1 Indications for Electrophysiologic Testing for Syncope

Class I
General agreement and acceptance
Large trials
Patients with suspected structural heart disease and syncope that remains unexplained after appropriate evaluation

Class II
Less certain, but still acceptable
Few studies
Patients with recurrent unexplained syncope without structural heart disease and a negative head-up tilt test

Class III
Not indicated
No data to support testing
Patients with a known cause of syncope for whom treatment will not be guided by electrophysiologic testing

From Zipes DP, DiMarco JP, Jackman WM, et al: Guidelines for clinical intracardiac electrophysiological and catheter ablation procedures. A report of the American College of Cardiology/American Heart Association Task Force on Practice Guidelines (Committee on Clinical Intracardiac Electrophysiologic and Catheter Ablation Procedures), developed in collaboration with the North American Society of Pacing and Electrophysiology. J Am Coll Cardiol 1995;26:555-573.

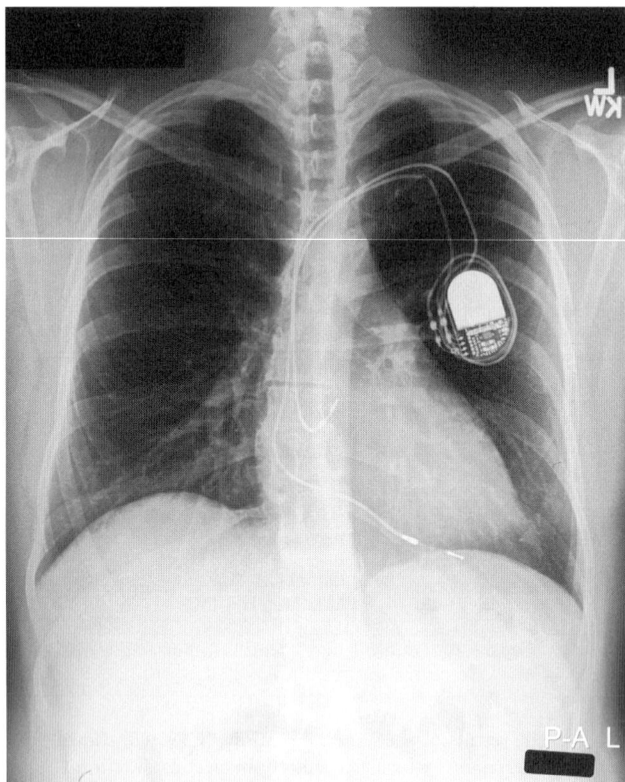

Figure 10 Chest radiograph of pacemaker with atrial and ventricular leads. Note the fracture of the ventricular lead.

also transmit limited data on the telephone. An ICD can obviously terminate VT or VF with a shock (Fig. 11), but it can also terminate sustained VT with antitachycardic pacing (ATP; Fig. 12).

Defibrillators can be single chamber or dual chamber and can have rate responsiveness as well (Fig. 13). The results of the Dual Chamber and VVI Implantable Defibrillator (DAVID) study have demonstrated that dual-chamber pacing ICDs in patients with decreased LV function lead to an increased incidence of congestive heart failure (CHF) and increased mortality.[13] The presumed mechanism is by creating a functional left bundle branch block (LBBB), which can lead to cardiac desynchronization and heart failure. In contrast, restoring cardiac resynchronization with biventricular pacing can improve congestive heart failure symptoms and has led to an explosion of referrals to implant patients with Classes II to IV CHF and severe LV dysfunction.[14] For the primary prevention of sudden death in patients with severe LV dysfunction, normal intact sinus node, AV node, and conduction, and no perceived or anticipated indication for pacing, the preferred ICD device is a single-chamber device (ventricular paced and inhibited [VVI] pacemaker). Dual-chamber ICDs should be reserved for patients with an abnor-

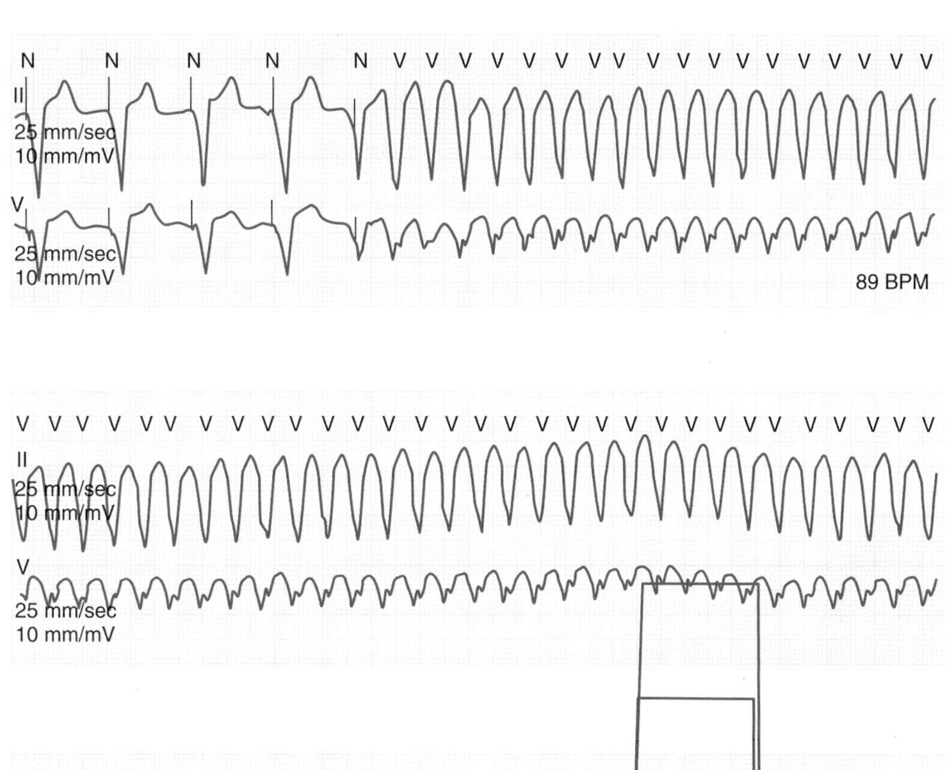

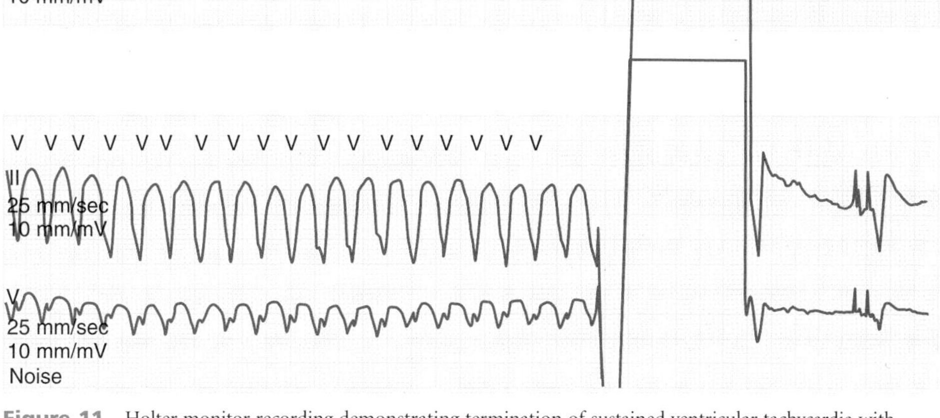

Figure 11 Holter monitor recording demonstrating termination of sustained ventricular tachycardia with a synchronized shock from an implantable cardioverter-defibrillator.

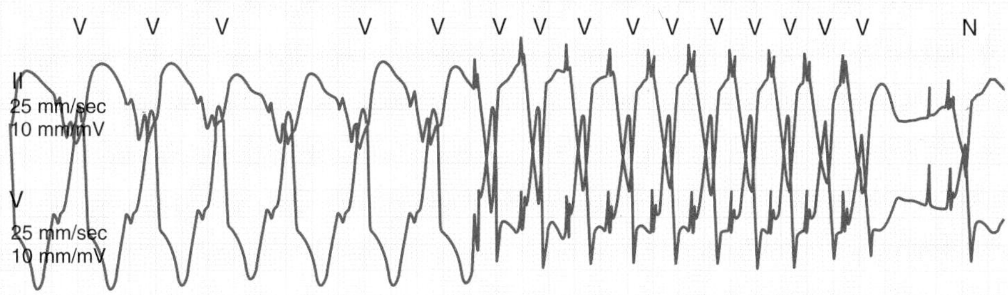

Figure 12 Successful termination of sustained ventricular tachycardia by antitachycardic pacing from an implantable cardioverter-defibrillator.

mal SA or AV node or conduction system or those with frequent supraventricular arrhythmias, such as atrial fibrillation, to avoid spurious shocks secondary to rapid ventricular responses. When dual-chamber pacing is required, and the LV is severely impaired, consideration should be given to a biventricular ICD.

Radiofrequency Ablation

Radiofrequency catheter ablation (RFA) has been a revolutionary advance in the treatment of cardiac arrhythmias.[7,8,15] For the first time, RFA has provided an opportunity to cure a specific cardiac disease completely. Introduced over 2 decades ago as DC ablation, and then again in the late 1980s with radiofrequency, RFA has proved to be a safe, efficacious, and cost-effective treatment for specific cardiac arrhythmias such as atrioventricular nodal re-entry tachycardia (AVNRT), orthodromic reciprocating tachycardia associated with WPW syndrome and concealed accessory pathways, normal heart VT (particularly right ventricular outflow tract tachycardia or fascicular tachycardia), and atrial flutter.[7,8,16] In addition, RFA can provide adjuvant therapy for ischemic VT when the patient is experiencing frequent ICD shocks or failing antiarrhythmic therapy. Finally, pulmonary vein isolation as a treatment option for symptomatic, drug-refractory, paroxysmal, or persistent atrial fibrillation is gaining widespread acceptance and is undergoing intense clinical scrutiny.[17] However, rate control and chronic anticoagulation are acceptable alternatives for asymptomatic or mildly symptomatic patients with atrial fibrillation according to the results of the Atrial Fibrillation Follow-up Investigation of Rhythm Management (AFFIRM) study.[18]

AVNRT is the most common of the SVTs (Fig. 14). Onset is usually in the third to fifth decade of life; the patient may present with a sustained, rapid, tachycardia rate of 180 to 240 beats/min. AVNRT originates from a micro re-entry around the fast and slow pathways of the AV node. Typically, AVNRT shows a narrow complex tachycardia without apparent P waves. Vagal maneuvers or adenosine can terminate AVNRT. Radiofrequency ablation has proved extremely effective at curing AVNRT, with success rates higher than 95%. Complication rates are low and, with successful modification of the AV node, specifically ablation of the slow pathway, the need for a permanent pacemaker is rare.

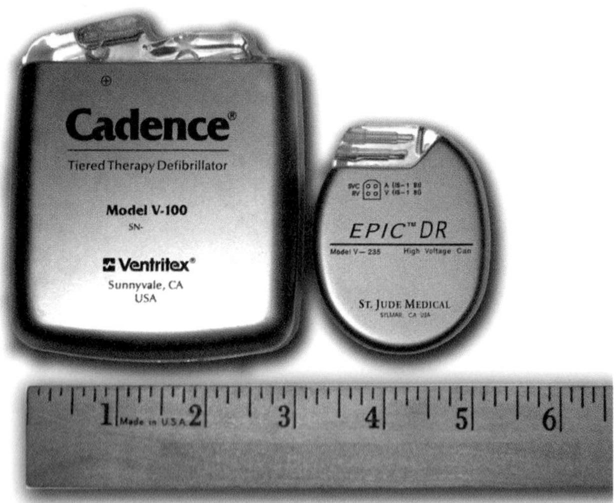

Figure 13 Comparison of implantable cardioverter-defibrillator (ICD) from several years ago *(left)* with a current model from the same manufacturer *(right)*. Note the obvious size reduction. The ICD on the *right*, however, also has more extensive features, enhanced efficacy and reliability, and improved battery life. *(Courtesy of Ventritex, Sunnyvale, Calif.)*

The presence of an accessory pathway (Kent bundle) in various locations around the tricuspid or mitral annulus results in a characteristic delta wave pattern on the ECG (Fig. 15). Macro re-entry tachycardia, called orthodromic reciprocating tachycardia (ORT) or AV reciprocating tachycardia (AVRT), occurs when the AV node is used in an antegrade direction and the accessory pathway is used in a retrograde direction. Typically, AVRT is a narrow complex tachycardia, but it may have small retrograde P waves visible between the QRS and T waves. When the accessory pathway is used in an antegrade direction, antidromic reciprocating tachycardia (ART), a wide complex tachycardia, occurs, which mimics VT. Atrial fibrillation is common with WPW syndrome. It is speculated that constant retrograde re-entry into the atrium during ventricular depolarization is responsible. Because of the potential for rapid conduction over an accessory pathway with atrial fibrillation and WPW, extreme caution must be exercised with AV nodal blocking agents, particularly digoxin, and calcium channel blockers. Although rare, atrial fibrillation with rapid ventricular response over an accessory pathway can initiate ventricular fibrillation, leading to sudden death. Acute treatment of atrial fibrillation and WPW consists of cardioversion and occasionally intravenous procainamide. The most common location for an accessory pathway is in the left ventricular free wall, but it also can be posteroseptal or right sided. Radiofrequency catheter ablation has been successful in ablating and curing WPW. Success rates approaching 97% have been safely achieved in experienced centers. For symptomatic WPW, particularly in young patients, RFA is considered to be the treatment of choice.

Radiofrequency ablation has also been extremely useful in curing typical atrial flutter (Fig. 16), which is identified by an atrial rate of 240 beats/min or higher and characteristic negative sawtooth flutter waves identified on the ECG, typically in inferior leads (II, III, and aVF). Mapping studies have revealed that typical flutter occurs with a counterclockwise rotation of atrial activation descending on the right atrial free wall, traversing the isthmus (zone between the coronary sinus orifice and tricuspid leaflet) and ascending the intra-atrial septum. Disruption of conduction over the isthmus by radiofre-

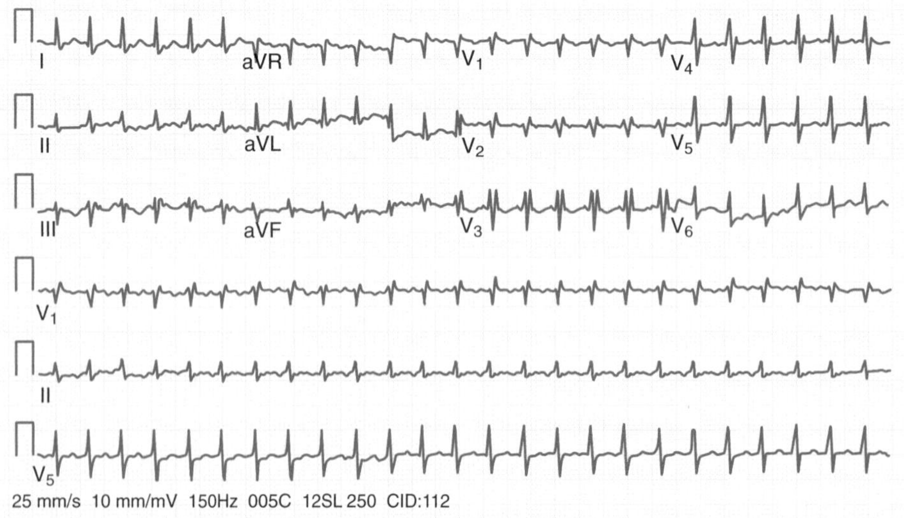

Figure 14 Electrocardiogram taken during an episode of atrioventricular nodal re-entry tachycardia, demonstrating narrow QRS tachycardia and the absence of discernible P waves.

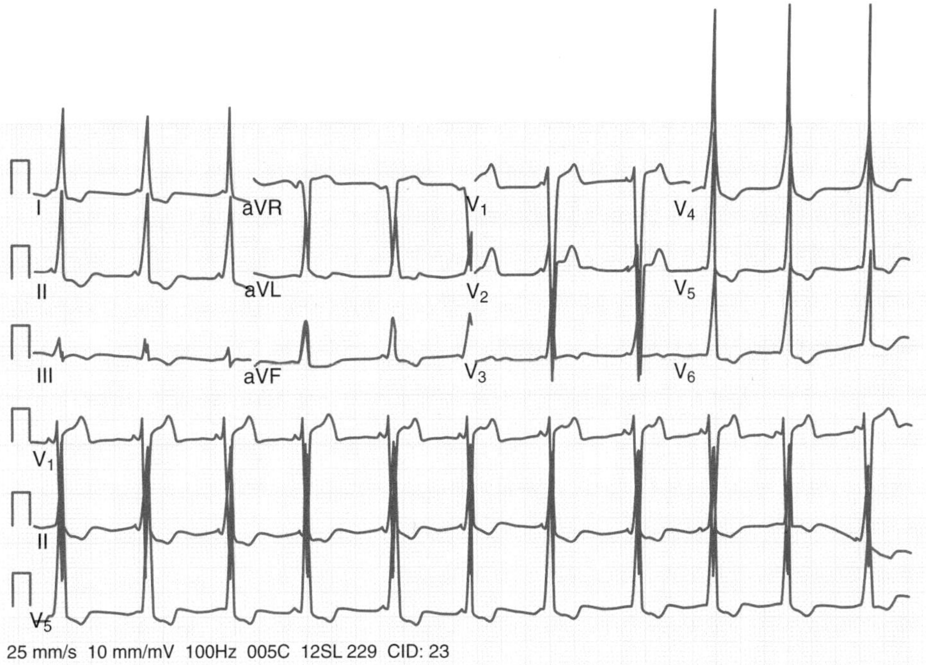

Figure 15 Typical electrocardiogram of Wolff-Parkinson-White syndrome. Note the absence of the PR interval and a broad QRS, with slurring of the initial segment (delta wave).

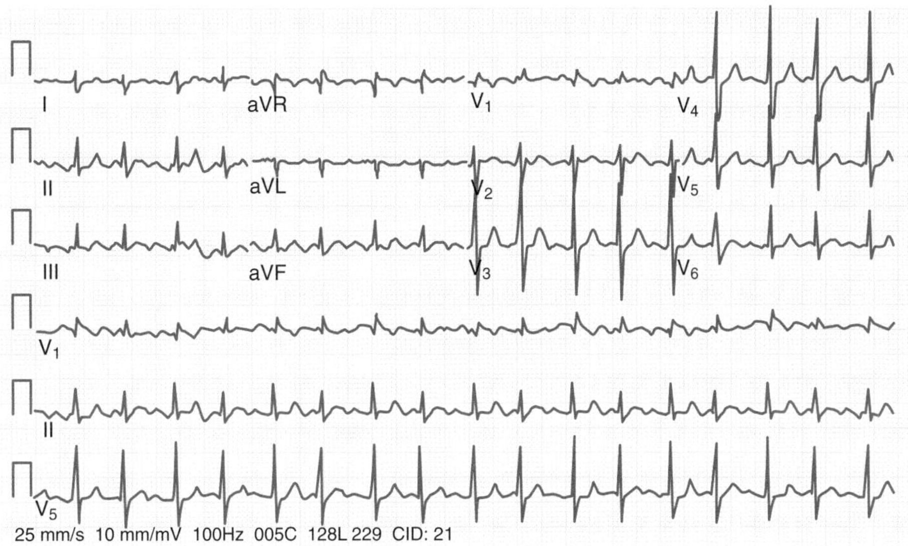

Figure 16 Typical atrial flutter. Note the negative sawtooth flutter waves in leads II, III, and aVF.

quency ablation can successfully eliminate the potential for typical flutter. In up to 25% of cases, patients continue to have atrial tachyarrhythmias, especially atrial fibrillation. Nevertheless, RFA is an acceptable first-line therapy for symptomatic atrial flutter.

Antiarrhythmic Medications

The CAST study (Cardiac Arrhythmia Suppression Trial), published in 1989, radically changed the use of antiarrhythmic medications.[19] CAST was designed to test the hypothesis that antiarrhythmic medication suppression of PVCs and nonsustained VT would improve mortality in patients following an MI who had decreased LV function. The medications selected—moricizine, flecainide, and encainide—were known to have potent ventricular arrhythmia suppression properties. However, CAST demonstrated an increase in mortality in patients treated with antiarrhythmic medications compared with placebo (Fig. 17). It was suspected that the increased mortality resulted from the proarrhythmic effects of these drugs, especially in the presence of ischemia and LV dysfunction.[20] Therefore, type 1C drugs (Table 1) are contraindicated in patients with CAD and ischemia. Because of the CAST findings, there is concern that increased mortality could occur with other antiarrhythmics, especially when administered for relatively benign arrhythmias (e.g., atrial fibrillation, PVCs). Quinidine was subsequently shown to increase mortality when administered to patients with atrial fibrillation.[21]

Since the publication of the CAST study, many other reports have confirmed the proarrhythmic effects of antiarrhythmic medication

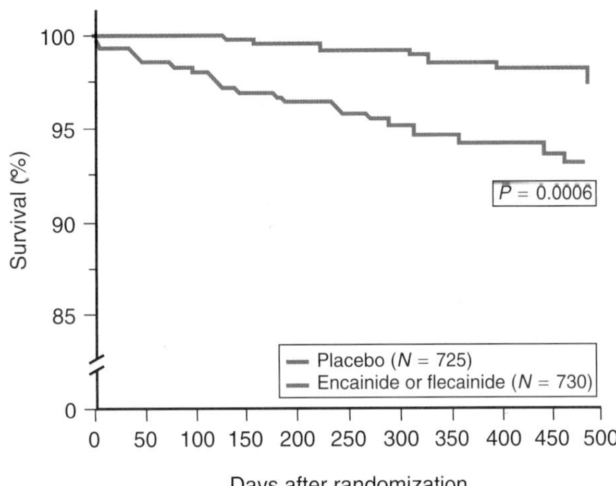

Figure 17 Increased arrhythmic mortality in patients receiving antiarrhythmic medication versus placebo in the Cardiac Arrhythmia Suppression Trial (CAST) study. *(From Cardiac Arrhythmia Suppression Trial [CAST] Investigators: Preliminary report: Effect of encainide and flecainide on mortality in a randomized trial of arrhythmia suppression after myocardial infarction. N Engl J Med 1989;321:406-412.)*

Table 1 Vaughn-Williams Classification of Antiarrhythmic Medications

Class	Actions (Examples)
I	Sodium channel blockers
IA	Depress phase 0 of action potential; delay conduction, prolong repolarization—phase III or IV (quinidine, procainamide, disopyramide)
IB	Little effect on phase 0 of action potential in normal tissues; depress phase 0 in abnormal tissues; shorten repolarization or little effect (lidocaine, tocainide, mexiletine, diphenyl-hydantoin)
IC	Depress phase 0 of action potential; markedly slow conduction in normal tissues (flecainide, propafenone, moricizine)
II	β-Adrenergic blocking agents (acebutolol, atenolol, bisoprolol, carvedilol, metoprolol, nadolol, pindolol, propranolol)
III	Prolong action potential duration by increasing repolarization and refractoriness (amiodarone, sotalol, bretylium, dofetilide, azimilide, ibutilide)
IV	Calcium channel blockers (diltiazem, verapamil)
Others	Digoxin, adenosine

From Chaudhry G, Muqtada MD, Haffajee CI: Antiarrhythmic agents and proarrhythmia. Crit Care Med 2000;28:N158-N164.

when used capriciously. This has led to specific guidelines for the use of antiarrhythmic medications, especially those that prolong the QT interval and increase proarrhythmia. Usually, types IA and III medications are initiated in the hospital with telemetry monitoring. Type IC agents, however, are relatively safe when used in a normal heart. Similarly, amiodarone, because of its long half-life (43 days to months) and low incidence of proarrhythmia, usually can be initiated at low doses in an outpatient setting in the absence of severe LV dysfunction or bradycardia. Based on the results of the CAST study, the U.S. Food and Drug Administration (FDA) and pharmaceutical industry took unprecedented measures to ensure appropriate prescription practices and credentialing of ordering physicians when the new antiarrhythmic medication, dofetilide (Tikosyn), was released for use in patients with atrial fibrillation.

SPECIFIC ARRHYTHMIAS

Normal Heart Ventricular Tachycardia

Occasionally, sustained and nonsustained VT can occur in the absence of structural heart disease, so-called normal heart VT. In general, prognosis is good, with a low risk for sudden cardiac death. Examples include right ventricular outflow tract (RVOT) and left ventricular outflow tract (LVOT) VT, fascicular VT, idiopathic left VT, repetitive monomorphic VT, and sinus of Valsalva VT[22] (Fig. 18). Treatment usually is with beta blockers or calcium channel blockers and, if refractory, RFA. Treatment is aimed at symptom suppression.

Arrhythmogenic Right Ventricular Dysplasia

Arrhythmogenic right ventricular dysplasia (ARVD) is a genetic disease in which right ventricular normal architecture is disrupted by progressive infiltration and transformation into fatty fibrous material. This creates the potential for chaotic depolarization and VT. Symptoms include palpitations, VT, and sudden cardiac death. Diagnosis is suspected by an abnormal ECG showing RBBB, juvenile T wave pattern (inverted precordial T waves), and epsilon waves (prominent deflections in the ST segment, often best seen at higher recording speeds; Fig. 19). The SA ECG is often abnormal, with the presence of low-amplitude late potentials. The ECG reveals RV dysfunction and aneurysms. The diagnosis of ARVD is confirmed with an abnormal computed tomography (CT) or magnetic resonance imaging (MRI) scan showing the typical fatty infiltration (Fig. 20). Symptomatic patients are screened for ventricular arrhythmias with EPS and, if positive, receive an ICD.

Long QT Syndrome

Long QT syndrome (LQTS) is a genetically transmitted disorder causing metabolic abnormalities of cardiac myocyte sodium and potassium channel depolarization (channelopathy), causing prolongation of the QT interval. This prolongation increases susceptibility to spontaneous polymorphic VT, torsades de pointes, and VT (Fig. 21). Treatment consists of atrial pacing, beta blockers, specific antiarrhythmics to improve repolarization, and ICDs in high-risk patients.

Brugada Syndrome

Brugada syndrome is a relatively rare cause of VT and fibrillation. It is characterized by an abnormal ECG exhibiting a right bundle branch block pattern and ST segment elevation in the precordial leads (Fig. 22). Treatment requires implantation of an ICD in patients with syncope and complex ventricular arrhythmias.

Bundle Branch Re-entry Ventricular Tachycardia

Bundle branch re-entry (BBR) VT, in which re-entry around components of the His-Purkinje system and one of the bundle branches results in a VT that resembles the native QRS. This type of VT is often seen in dilated cardiomyopathy. The major prerequisite is a baseline conduction delay, usually LBBB. Confirmation of this type of VT requires an EPS demonstrating His-Bundle participation in the VT. BBR VT can be eliminated by right bundle branch ablation and usually does not result in complete heart block. Patients still require an ICD because other morphologies of VT are usually present or probable.

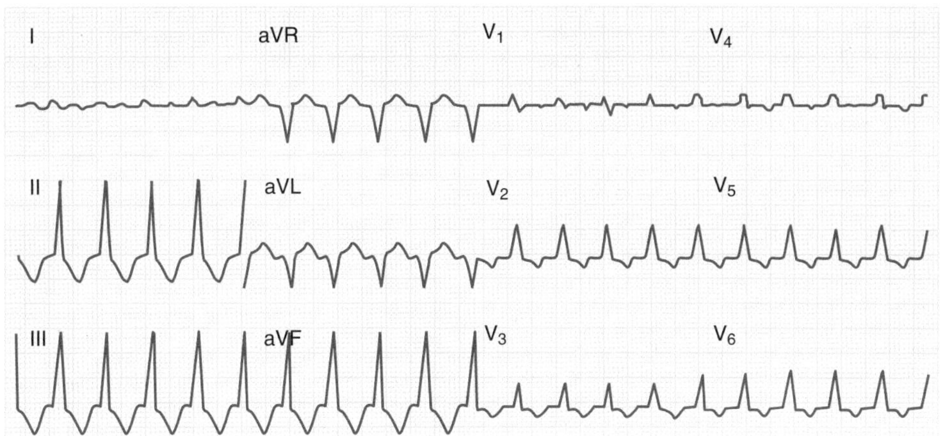

Figure 18 Ventricular tachycardia in a young patient without structural heart arising from the coronary sinus of Valsalva. *(From Kanagaratnam L, Tomassoni G, Schweikert R, et al: Ventricular tachycardias arising from the aortic sinus of Valsalva: An under-recognized variant of left outflow tract ventricular tachycardia. J Am Coll Cardiol 2001;37:1408-1414.)*

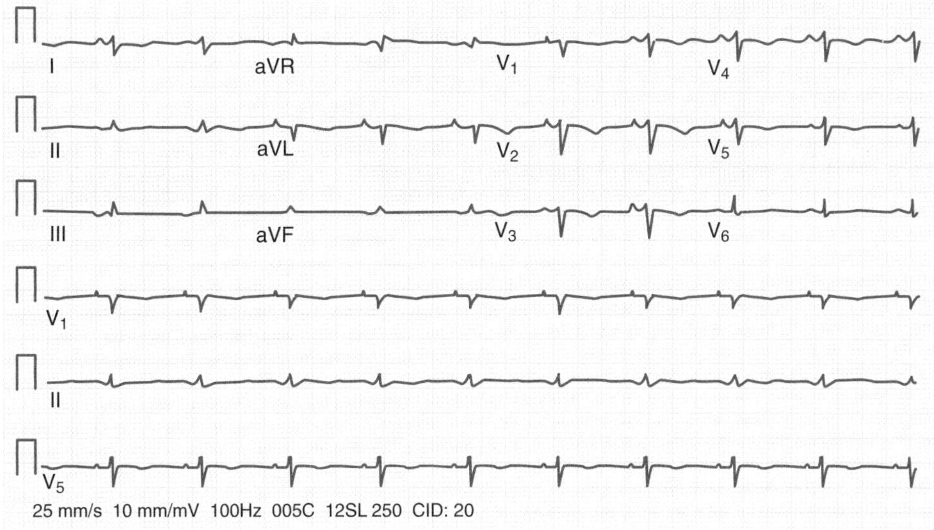

Figure 19 Typical electrocardiographic findings in arrhythmogenic right ventricular dysplasia. Note the presence of incomplete right bundle branch block and anterior T wave changes.

OUTCOMES

In the absence of structural heart disease, benign arrhythmias, such as PACs, SVT, PVCs, and atrial fibrillation, have been shown to have an excellent prognosis.[10] Radiofrequency ablation for SVT has a higher than 95% success rate, with no long-term adverse side effects. The use of ICDs has improved survival in primary and secondary prevention trials. Secondary prevention trials, such as the AVID study, enrolled patients who had a life-threatening arrhythmia and who were successfully resuscitated.[10] The defibrillator proved superior to medical therapy, usually amiodarone, in preventing sudden death. Primary prevention trials have focused on high-risk groups who have not already experienced an untoward ventricular arrhythmia. The MADIT and MUST (Multicenter Unsustained Tachycardia) trials have confirmed superiority of the ICD and survival in patients with inducible, sustained, monomorphic VT during an EPS and a history of CAD and MI.[11,23] The MADIT-II study has suggested that the EPS is superfluous for risk stratification in patients with LV dysfunction (EF <35%) and a history of CAD, regardless of whether ventricular arrhythmias are present or absent.[12] Patients who received an empirical ICD had a significant survival benefit.

Following the publication of MADIT-II results, there was considerable debate about its applicability for clinical practice. A major concern was that widespread adoption of MADIT-II ICD criteria could bankrupt an already stressed health care system. Subsequently, many consensus panels convened to determine the appropriateness of the MADIT-II criteria for ICD therapy. Initially, some insurance carriers required that in addition to the MADIT-II criteria (LV dysfunction, previous MI, EF <35%), the patient should also have a widened QRS interval to qualify for a defibrillator. This was based on ancillary studies showing that a wide QRS could be an independent predictor of mortality. This stringent criterion existed for approximately 1 year, until it was abandoned.

Currently, any patient meeting MADIT-II criteria with an EF lower than 35% and LV dysfunction caused by MI is a candidate for a defibrillator (Box 2). In addition, indications for ICD implantation have been expanded to include patients with a dilated cardiomyopathy and an LV EF of 35% or lower, based on the results of the

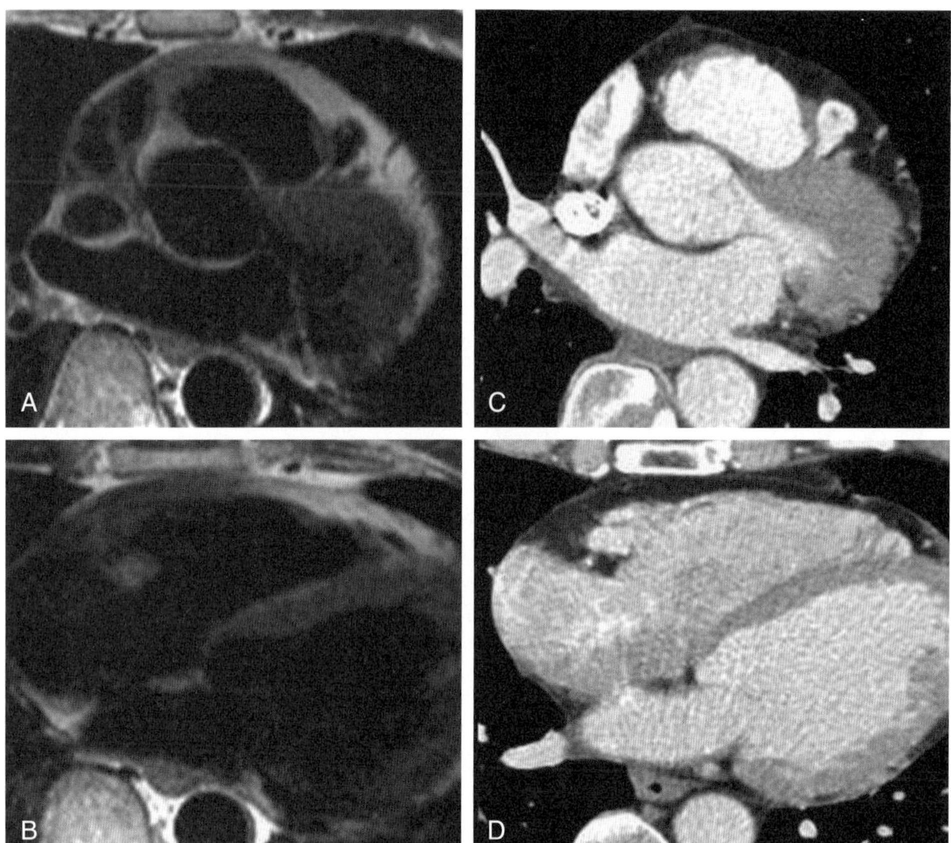

Figure 20 Magnetic resonance imaging (MRI) scans illustrating ventricular fatty infiltration typical of arrhythmogenic right ventricular (RV) dysplasia. **A,** "Black blood" oblique axial cardiac MRI images focused on the right ventricular outflow. Anterior chest wall and right ventricle are at *top*. **B,** "Black blood" MRI four-chamber heart image focused on the right ventricle with anterior chest wall and right ventricle at *top*. Note anterior RV *white areas* indicating fatty infiltration. **C,** "White blood" cine MRI image at similar level as **A.** Note anterior RV darkened myocardium and thinning due to dysplasia. **D,** "White blood" four-chamber cine MRI image showing extensive anterior RV dysplasia and thinning (dark myocardium).

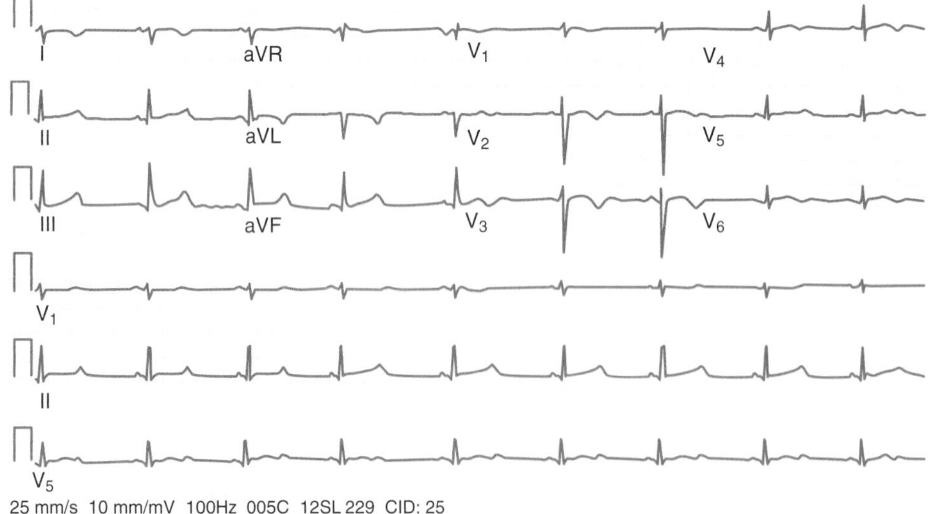

Figure 21 Electrocardiogram showing prolonged QT interval in patient with long QT syndrome, with syncope and torsades de pointes.

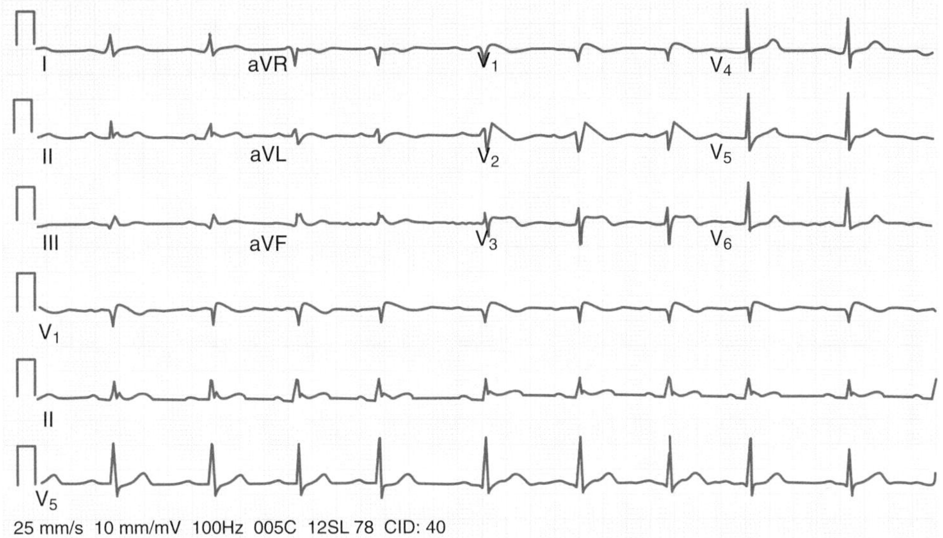

Figure 22 ST elevation and right bundle branch block pattern typical of Brugada syndrome.

Box 2 Indications for Implantable Cardioverter-Defibrillator

Primary Prevention

Dilated or ischemic cardiomyopathy: EF ≤35%, based on MADIT-II, SCD-HeFT, Definite criteria

Secondary Prevention

Survivors of sudden cardiac death or documented hemodynamically unstable or sustained VT or VF

Biventricular ICD

Dilated or ischemic cardiomyopathy, EF <35%, QRS interval >120 msec, functional Class III

Investigational: Biventricular ICD in normal QRS and echocardiographic evidence of biventricular dyssynchrony (Rethinq trial) or biventricular ICD in heart failure, conduction disturbance in functional Class I or II (MADIT-CRT)

Boutique Indications For ICD

Brugada syndrome

Hypertrophic cardiomyopathy

Long QT syndrome

DEFINITE, Defibrillators in Non-Ischemic Cardiomyopathy Treatment Evaluation; EF, ejection fraction; ICD, implantable cardioverter-defibrillator; MADIT-II, Multicenter Automatic Defibrillator Implantation Trial 2; RethinQ, Resynchronization Therapy in Narrow QRS; SCD-HeFT, Sudden Cardiac Death in Heart Failure Trial; VF, ventricular fibrillation; VT, ventricular tachycardia.

SCD-HeFT (Sudden Cardiac Death in Heart Failure Trial) and DEFINITE (Defibrillators in Non-Ischemic Cardiomyopathy Treatment Evaluation) studies.[24,25] Furthermore, patients with dilated and ischemic cardiomyopathies, with a wide QRS (typically >130 msec) and recurrent heart failure, with functional class III or IV symptoms, are ideal candidates for the implantation of a biventricular ICD system. Ongoing studies, such as the RethinQ (Resynchronization Therapy in Narrow QRS) trial and MADIT-CRT, are looking at the role of biventricular pacing in patients with a narrow QRS and those with functional Class I or II symptoms, respectively. If these two studies yield positive results for survival in these subclassifications, it will certainly add to the unprecedented growth of ICD implantation. Anticipating the tremendous need for ICD services, current development is focused on leadless ICD systems, in which a subcutaneous placement of the ICD device could be performed more simply by electrophysiology specialists, as well as by other physicians.

Recently, media attention has been focused on the potential for ICD malfunction or device failure.[26] Most manufacturers have recognized potential design flaws, such as premature battery depletion, oversensing or undersensing of ventricular arrhythmias, and cross-talk. In general, since the introduction of the defibrillator nearly 3 decades ago, the devices have been extremely reliable. The failure rates as reported have been extremely low and have not appreciably increased. However, the burgeoning use of ICDs has led to an awareness of manufacturing defects although, as noted, their incidence has remained relatively low. Many potential device recalls can be managed conservatively with expedited and intensified follow-up of battery status and the use of home telephonic monitoring modalities, such as CareLink (for more information, see www.medtronic.com/carelink).

Summary

- Evaluation of cardiac arrhythmias begins with documentation of the arrhythmia type and investigation for underlying heart disease.
- Radiofrequency ablation is acceptable first-line therapy for many arrhythmias, including SVTs, such as WPW, AVNRT and atrial flutter.
- ICDs should be considered for any patient with an EF of 35% or lower.

Suggested Readings

Bardy GH, Lee KL, Mark DB, et al: Sudden Cardiac Death in Heart Failure Trial (SCD-HeFT) Investigators: Amiodarone or an implantable cardioverter-defibrillator for congestive heart failure. N Engl J Med 2005;352:225-237.

Benditt D, Ferguson D, Grubb B, et al: Tilt testing for assessing syncope. J Am Coll Cardiol 1996;28:263-275.

Buxton AE, Lee KL, Fisher JD, et al: A randomized study of the prevention of sudden death in patients with coronary artery disease. N Engl J Med 1999;341:1882-1890.

Gregoratos G, Abrams J, Epstein AE, et al: American College of Cardiology/American Heart Association Task Force on Practice Guidelines/North American Society for Pacing and Electrophysiology Committee to Update the 1998 Pacemaker Guidelines: ACC/AHA/NASPE 2002 guideline update for implantation of cardiac pacemakers and antiarrhythmia devices: Summary article: A report of the American College of Cardiology/American Heart Association Task Force on Practice Guidelines (ACC/AHA/NASPE Committee to Update the 1998 Pacemaker Guidelines). Circulation 2002;106:2145-2161.

Kadish A, Dyer A, Daubert JP, et al: Defibrillators in Non-Ischemic Cardiomyopathy Treatment Evaluation (DEFINITE) Investigators: Prophylactic defibrillator implantation in patients with nonischemic dilated cardiomyopathy. N Engl J Med 2004;350:2151-2158.

Moss AJ, Zareba W, Hall J, et al: Multicenter Automatic Defibrillator Implantation Trial II Investigators: Prophylactic implantation of a defibrillator in patients with myocardial infarction and reduced ejection fraction. N Engl J Med 2002;346:877-888.

Wilkoff BL, Cook JR, Epstein AE, et al: Dual Chamber and VVI Implantable Defibrillator Trial Investigators: Dual-chamber pacing or ventricular backup pacing in patients with an implantable defibrillator: The Dual Chamber and VVI Implantable Defibrillator (DAVID) Trial. JAMA 2002;288:3115-3123.

Wyse DG, Waldo AL, DiMarco JP, et al: Atrial Fibrillation Follow-up Investigation of Rhythm Management (AFFIRM) Investigators: A comparison of rate control and rhythm control in patients with atrial fibrillation. N Engl J Med 2002;347:1825-1833.

Zipes DP, DiMarco JP, Jackman WM, et al: Guidelines for clinical intracardiac electrophysiological and catheter ablation procedures. A report of the American College of Cardiology/American Heart Association Task Force on Practice Guidelines (Committee on Clinical Intracardiac Electrophysiologic and Catheter Ablation Procedures), developed in collaboration with the North American Society of Pacing and Electrophysiology. J Am Coll Cardiol 1995;26:555-573.

Zipes DP, Wyse G, Friedman PL, et al: A comparison of antiarrhythmic-drug therapy with implantable defibrillators in patients resuscitated from near-fatal ventricular arrhythmias. N Engl J Med 1997; 337:1576-1583.

References

For a complete list of references, log onto www.expertconsult.com.

Atrial Fibrillation

Thomas J. Dresing and *Robert A. Schweikert*

DEFINITION

Atrial fibrillation (AF) occurs when the electrical impulses in the atria degenerate from their usual organized rhythm into a rapid chaotic pattern. This disruption results in an irregular and often rapid heartbeat that is classically described as "irregularly irregular" and occurs because of the unpredictable conduction of these disordered impulses across the atrioventricular (AV) node.

AF may be classified on the basis of the frequency of episodes and the ability of an episode to convert back to sinus rhythm. One method of classification has been outlined in guidelines published by the American College of Cardiology (ACC), American Heart Association (AHA), and European Society of Cardiology (ESC), with the collaboration of the Heart Rhythm Society (HRS).[1] According to these guidelines, if a patient has two or more episodes, AF is considered to be recurrent. Recurrent AF may be paroxysmal or persistent. If the AF terminates spontaneously it is designated paroxysmal and if the AF is sustained, it is designated persistent. In the latter case, termination of the arrhythmia with electrical or pharmacologic cardioversion does not change its designation. The category of persistent AF also includes permanent AF, which refers to long-standing AF (generally >1 year), for which cardioversion was not indicated or attempted.

PREVALENCE

AF is the most common sustained tachyarrhythmia encountered by clinicians. It occurs in approximately 0.4% to 1.0% of the general population and affects more than 2 million Americans annually. Its prevalence increases with age, and it has been diagnosed at some point in up to 10% of the population older than 80 years. With the projected growth of the older adult population, the prevalence of AF will certainly increase.

PATHOPHYSIOLOGY

AF may be associated with physiologic stresses such as surgical procedures, pulmonary embolism, chronic lung diseases, hyperthyroidism, and alcohol ingestion. Disease states commonly associated with AF include hypertension, valvular heart disease, congestive heart failure (CHF), coronary artery disease, Wolff-Parkinson-White (WPW) syndrome, pericarditis, and cardiomyopathy. When no identifiable risk factor for AF is present, the condition is classified as lone AF.

New insights about the factors involved in the initiation and continuation of AF have led some investigators to propose a revised model of this complex arrhythmia. For many years, the focus had been on the substrate in the atria that supports the maintenance of AF. The multiple wavelet model has suggested that AF is sustained by multiple simultaneous wavelets wandering throughout the atria. Therefore, therapy was aimed at making these wavelets less likely to sustain and propagate. Such treatments included antiarrhythmic medications and surgical interruption of the atrial tissue.

More recently, it has been recognized that the initiation of AF in most cases occurs because of premature atrial contractions triggered by beats that arise from the pulmonary veins, usually near the junction with the left atrium. These triggers may also fire repetitively and contribute to the maintenance of AF, essentially becoming drivers of AF.

AF may have hemodynamic consequences. It can decrease cardiac output by as much as 20%, increase pulmonary capillary wedge pressure, and increase atrial pressures. These effects are caused by tachycardia, loss of atrial contribution to left ventricular (LV) filling, increased valvular regurgitation, and irregular ventricular response. Some investigators have suggested that the irregularity of the R-R intervals contributes more to the hemodynamic changes than the mere presence of tachycardia.

AF is associated with important morbidity and even mortality. AF can produce bothersome symptoms that affect quality of life, but patients with AF also have a substantial risk of thromboembolic stroke, as discussed later. It is less apparent, however, that AF is also associated with increased mortality, although the reason for this is unclear. Several studies have demonstrated an association of AF with reduced overall survival.[2,3]

SIGNS AND SYMPTOMS

The clinical manifestation of AF is variable. Often, the symptoms are attributable to the rapid ventricular response. However, even when the ventricular response is controlled, symptoms can occur from loss of AV synchrony. This is particularly important for patients with LV dysfunction. Some patients are completely asymptomatic, even those with rapid heart rates. More often, however, patients report nonspecific symptoms such as fatigue, dyspnea, dizziness, and diaphoresis. Palpitations are a common feature. Occasionally, patients present with extreme manifestations of hemodynamic compromise, such as chest pain, pulmonary edema, or syncope. AF is present in 10% to 40% of patients with a new thromboembolic stroke.

DIAGNOSIS

The clinician must realize that an irregular pulse detected by physical examination or an irregular ventricular rhythm seen on the electrocardiogram (ECG) is not always AF. It is necessary to consider and exclude other types of irregular rhythm disturbances, including atrial or ventricular ectopy, atrial tachycardia or atrial flutter (Fig. 1) with variable AV conduction, multifocal atrial tachycardia (Fig. 2), and chaotic atrial rhythm, or wandering atrial pacemaker. Conversely, a regular pulse or rhythm does not exclude AF. For example, AF can manifest with a regular ventricular response in the presence of AV block or with a ventricular paced rhythm.

An ECG is essential for proper diagnosis. Electrocardiographic findings in AF include the absence of P waves, the presence of chaotic atrial activity and fibrillary waves (f waves), and an atrial rate in the range of 300 to 700 beats/min. In the absence of drug therapy, a patient with normal AV conduction has an irregularly irregular ventricular rhythm and often has a ventricular rate in the range of 120 to 180 beats/min. The baseline on the ECG strip often is undulating and occasionally has coarse irregular activity (Fig. 3). This activity may resemble atrial flutter, but it is not as uniform from wave to wave as atrial flutter.

TREATMENT

Most patients presenting with AF are not in critical condition. However, in some cases, the presence of AF or the way it is treated may be life threatening. It should be emphasized that for any unstable patient presenting with AF—for example, a patient with chest

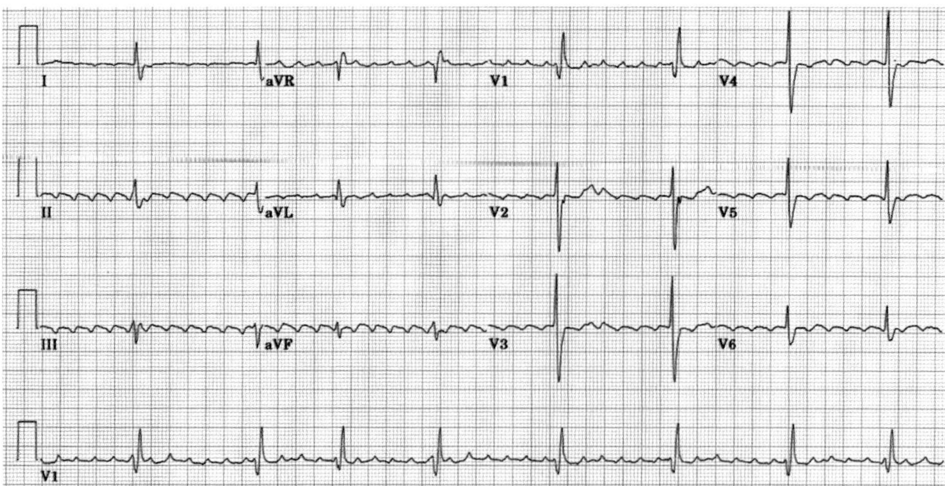

Figure 1 Typical atrial flutter.

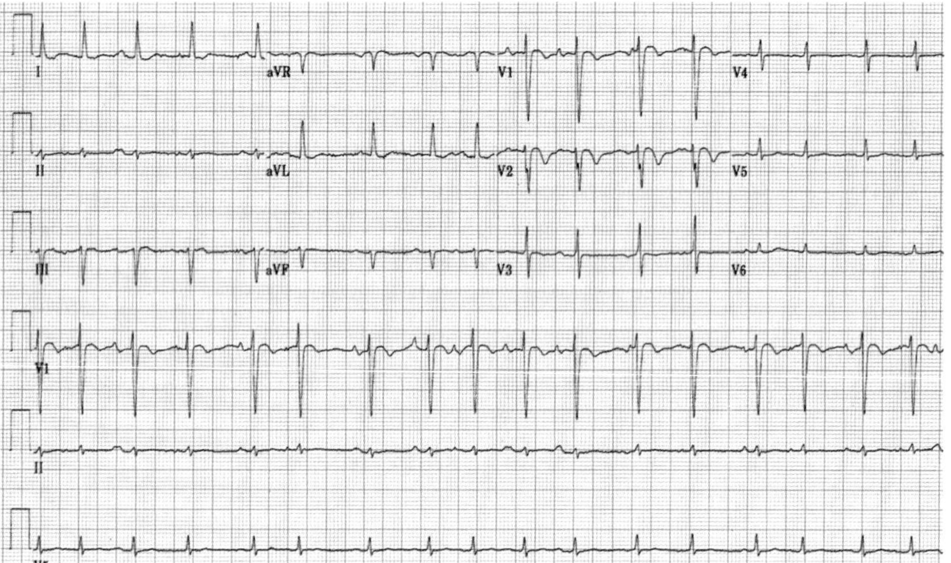

Figure 2 Multifocal atrial tachycardia.

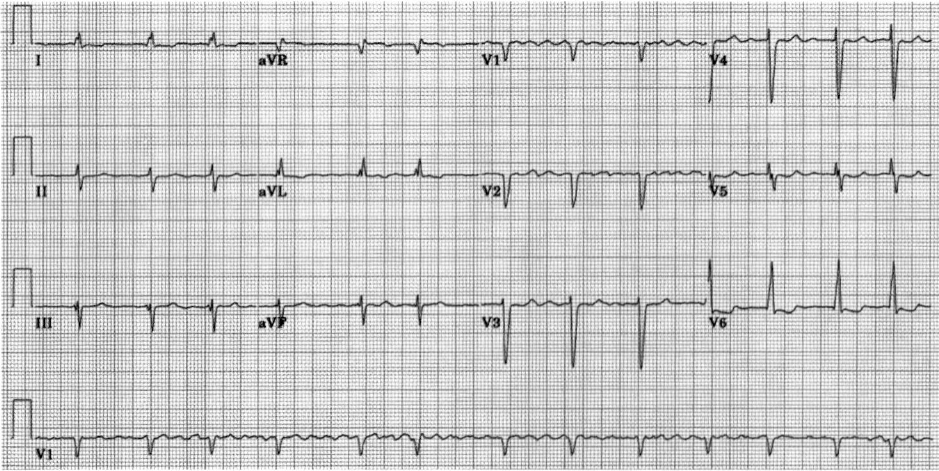

Figure 3 Coarse atrial fibrillation.

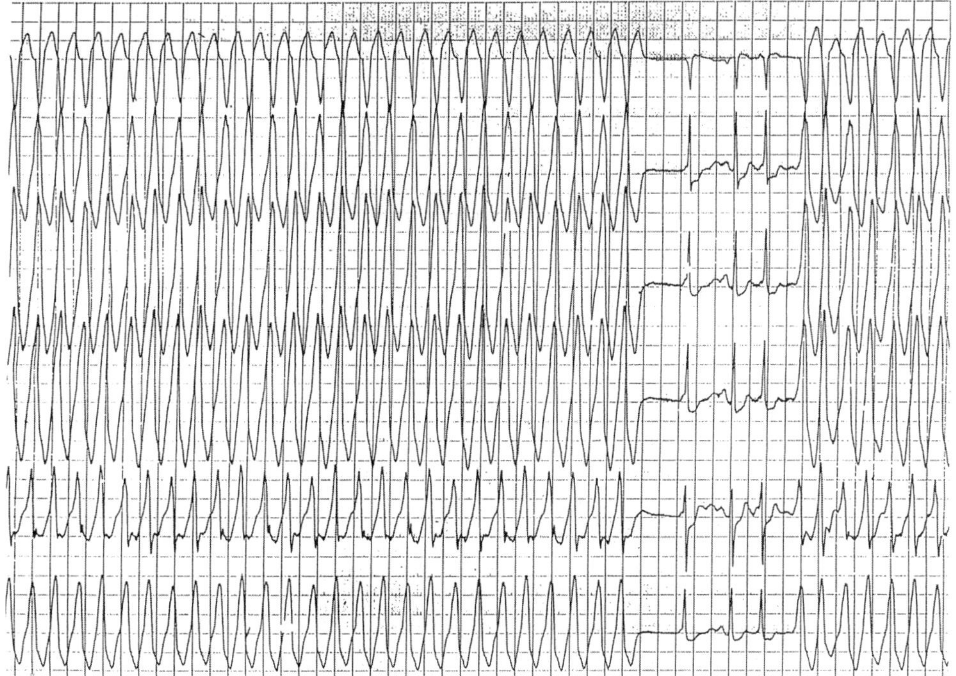

Figure 4 Wide complex tachycardia resulting from atrial fibrillation in a patient with Wolff-Parkinson-White syndrome.

pain, pulmonary edema, or hypotension—the recommended therapy is rapid electrical cardioversion.

AF has particular importance in the setting of the WPW syndrome. Patients with WPW syndrome may be vulnerable to ventricular fibrillation and sudden death because of the development of AF, which can result in extremely rapid conduction over the accessory pathway (Fig. 4). Prompt electrical cardioversion is of utmost importance for these patients. Treatment with AV node–blocking medications such as verapamil or digoxin can facilitate rapid conduction over the accessory pathway and result in ventricular fibrillation. When intravenous (IV) pharmacologic therapy is required, the drug of choice is procainamide or amiodarone.

The management of AF is directed at three basic goals: control of the ventricular rate, minimization of thromboembolism risk (particularly stroke), and restoration and maintenance of sinus rhythm. The first two management goals are essential for most patients, but the third management goal may not be necessary in every patient (see later). The ACC/AHA/ESC guidelines provide a more detailed review of the management of AF.[1]

Control of the Ventricular Rate

The ventricular rate during AF may be rapid and therefore require control. This usually is accomplished with medications that slow conduction through the AV node (Table 1). If these medications are ineffective or their effectiveness is prohibited by the development of excessive bradycardia, then other measures may need to be considered. One option suitable for some patients is catheter ablation of the AV node and pacemaker implantation. A meta-analysis of 21 uncontrolled studies of the ablate-and-pace approach[4] has shown demonstrated improvements in a number of clinical parameters, including symptoms, quality of life, exercise function, and cardiac performance. However, this approach usually results in pacemaker dependence. These patients may be exposed to the risks and complications of the implanted hardware. Pacemaker implantation without AV nodal ablation should be considered if the problem is simply excessive bradycardia that prohibits the effectiveness of rate-controlling medication. Strategies for suppression or cure of AF should be considered for appropriate patients before pursuing ablation of the AV node.

Minimization of Thromboembolism and Stroke Risk

AF carries a considerable risk for thromboembolism and stroke. The Framingham study has shown that during a follow-up period of 30 years, the annual risk of stroke among AF patients is 4.2%; patients with nonvalvular AF had a more than fivefold higher risk of stroke. In the Framingham study, even patients with lone AF had a much higher incidence of stroke than controls over a period of almost 30 years.[5] The annual risk of stroke may be even higher (7%-10%) in patients with AF who have one or more of the following risk factors: age older than 65 years, diabetes mellitus, hypertension, CHF, coronary artery disease, previous stroke, or transient ischemic attack. Findings of left atrial enlargement and reduced LV systolic function on echocardiography indicate an increase in thromboembolic risk.

Antithrombotic therapy for AF generally has consisted of the oral vitamin K antagonist warfarin or of the antiplatelet agent aspirin. A number of trials have studied the reduction of stroke risk in patients with AF, including some that compared the relative benefits and risks of warfarin and aspirin. Overall, warfarin has been shown to reduce the annual average relative risk of stroke by 68%, whereas the reduction with aspirin ranges from 0% to 44% (mean, approximately 20%). The combination of warfarin with aspirin increases the bleeding risk. Studies involving low-dose aspirin and clopidogrel in combination are under way to evaluate their potential efficacy when used as alternatives to warfarin.

Practice guidelines have been published regarding the recommended form of antithrombotic therapy for patients with AF.[1] In general, younger patients with no other risk factors have a low risk of stroke; therefore, aspirin may be an acceptable alternative to warfarin. Patients older than 65 years with or without other risk factors have a greater risk of stroke and should receive anticoagulation with

SECTION 2 CARDIOLOGY

Table 1 Atrial Fibrillation Medications that Slow Conduction Through the Atrioventricular Node

Drug	Advantages	Disadvantages	Usual Dosage	Onset of Action	Elimination Half-Life
Beta Blockers					
Propranolol	Rapid onset of effect, short durations of effect for IV forms; heart rate control at rest and with activity; oral forms available with varying durations of effect	May worsen heart failure in decompensated patient; may exacerbate reactive airway diseases; may cause fatigue, depression; abrupt withdrawal may cause rebound tachycardia, hypertension	IV: 1 mg given as bolus, repeat q5min as needed to achieve goal Oral-10-30 mg/dose q6-8hr	IV: onset of action within 5 min Oral: onset of action within 1-2 hr	IV: duration of effect is 30-60 min Oral: 3-5 hr
Metoprolol			IV: 2.5-5 mg over 2-3 min, repeat q5min as needed to achieve goal Oral: 12.5-100 mg/dose q6-8hr Sustained-release preparations available for once-daily dosing	IV: onset of action within 5 min Oral: onset of action within 1-2 hr	IV: duration of effect is 30-60 min Oral: 3-6 hr
Atenolol			IV: 5 mg over 5 min, repeat q10min to achieve goal Oral: 25-100 mg/dose q8-12hr	IV: onset of action within 5 min Oral: onset of action within 1-2 hr	IV: duration of effect is 30-60 min Oral: 6-9 hr
Esmolol (IV only)			IV: 500 µg/kg over 1 min, then maintenance dose of 25-300 µg/kg/min; titrate by 25-50 µg/kg/min q5-10min to achieve goal	IV: onset of action within 5 min	N/A
Nadolol (oral only)			Oral: 40-80 mg daily initially; increase to 240-320 mg daily as needed to achieve goal; can be given once daily	Oral: onset of action within 1-2 hr	14-24 hr
Calcium Channel Blockers					
Diltiazem	Same as for beta blockers	May worsen heart failure in decompensated patient; may cause fatigue; abrupt withdrawal may cause rebound tachycardia, hypertension	IV: 0.25 mg/kg over 2 min, then infusion at 5-15 mg/hr for up to 24 hr; repeat bolus of 0.35 mg/kg may be necessary Oral: 30-120 mg/dose q6-8hr; sustained-release preparations available as once- or twice-daily doses	IV: onset of action within 5 min Oral: onset of action of 1 hr	5-7 hr
Verapamil	Same as for beta blockers	May worsen heart failure in decompensated patient; may cause fatigue; abrupt withdrawal may cause rebound tachycardia, hypertension	IV: 5- to 10-mg bolus q15-30min to achieve goal Oral: 80-120 mg dose q8-12hr; sustained-release preparations available as once- or twice-daily doses	IV: onset of action within 5 min Oral: onset of action of 1 hr	5-12 hr
Other					
Digoxin	Can be used in patients with heart failure	Slow onset of action; poor control of heart rate with activity; narrow therapeutic margin; long duration of effect	IV loading dose of up to 1.0 mg in first 24 hr, with bolus of 0.25-0.5 mg IV push; then remainder in divided doses 16-8hr; maintenance oral dose, 0.125-0.25 mg qd	IV: up to 30 min Oral: 2-4 hr	36 hr

warfarin, if it is not contraindicated. The goal of warfarin therapy for preventing stroke and thromboembolism from AF generally is an international normalized ratio (INR) between 2.0 and 3.0. Some older patients may be considered poor candidates for warfarin therapy because of excessive risk for bleeding complications, and these patients should be considered for aspirin therapy.

For patients who have been in AF for more than 48 hours and are not adequately anticoagulated, electrical or pharmacologic cardioversion should be delayed until appropriate measures are taken to reduce the thromboembolic risk. There are two approaches for patients being considered for cardioversion of AF longer than 48 hours' duration. The conventional approach is to administer warfarin to achieve an INR value between 2.0 and 3.0 for at least 3 to 4 weeks before electrical or pharmacologic cardioversion. The second approach is the transesophageal echocardiography (TEE)–guided method. In some cases, cardioversion cannot be postponed for 3 or 4 weeks; in other cases, the patient, clinician, or both may prefer an expedited approach to achieving sinus rhythm. In such cases, once a therapeutic level of anticoagulation has been achieved with warfarin or IV heparin, TEE may be performed to rule out the presence of an intracardiac thrombus. If no thrombus is seen, cardioversion may be performed. TEE can detect the presence of a thrombus in the left atrium, particularly in the left atrial appendage, which is poorly seen on transthoracic echocardiography. The TEE-guided approach has been validated in several small multicenter trials as well as in a large, randomized, multicenter trial known as the Assessment of Cardioversion Using Transesophageal Echocardiography (ACUTE) trial.[6]

Warfarin should be continued after cardioversion until sinus rhythm has been maintained for at least 4 weeks to allow the atrial transport mechanism to recover. If the cardioversion was performed using the TEE-guided approach with IV heparin as the method of anticoagulation, it is advisable to continue IV heparin until a therapeutic INR is achieved with warfarin. The decision to initiate and continue anticoagulation for AF shorter than 48 hours' duration should be based on the presence of other risk factors for thromboembolism.

Because of the relatively narrow therapeutic and safety window for warfarin, and the numerous potential drug and food interactions with this medication, there has been substantial interest in the development of an alternative antithrombotic medication. Studies are in progress with oral platelet inhibitors such as clopidogrel and factor Xa inhibitors such as idraparinux. Several studies have been completed regarding the use of ximelagatran, an oral direct thrombin inhibitor with few drug and dietary interactions that does not require anticoagulation monitoring. Ximelagatran has been shown to be not inferior to warfarin, with similar bleeding risks. However, an undefined risk of hepatotoxicity, among other factors, has led the U.S. Food and Drug Administration (FDA) to discontinue grant approval in 2006 for this medication until further study has been completed. At present, a suitable substitute for warfarin for patients requiring more than aspirin therapy has yet to be demonstrated.

Nonpharmacologic methods of stroke prevention for patients with AF are also being studied. Percutaneous left atrial appendage occlusion has shown early clinical promise, but further study is required.

Restoration and Maintenance of Sinus Rhythm

The restoration and maintenance of sinus rhythm have obvious importance for patients with bothersome symptoms. However, this goal for patients with asymptomatic or minimally symptomatic AF has been controversial for many years There are now data from several clinical trials that may provide guidance for certain patients. Unfortunately, the important limitations of these trials have been often overlooked.

The potential benefits of sinus rhythm include reduction of long-term thromboembolism or stroke risk, avoidance of the development of atrial cardiomyopathy from ongoing AF, and improved quality of life. However, this approach often requires the use of antiarrhythmic drugs that may have important and even life-threatening side effects. Some nonrandomized trials have reported an increase in mortality among patients who were on long-term antiarrhythmic therapy for AF, presumably from the proarrhythmic effects of the drugs. In addition, several randomized studies have compared the treatment strategies of ventricular rate control or rhythm control with restoration and maintenance of sinus rhythm, albeit in older patients (mean age, 65-70 years) with minimal or no symptoms during AF.

The largest study, the Atrial Fibrillation Follow-up Investigation of Rhythm Management (AFFIRM) trial, was a large multicenter randomized study that compared these two treatment strategies for patients with AF.[7] Both treatment strategies used appropriate anticoagulation according to established guidelines. This study has demonstrated that a rhythm-control strategy is no better than a ventricular rate control strategy with regard to quality of life, incidence of stroke, or mortality at a follow-up of about 5 years.

A meta-analysis of five randomized, controlled trials of rate control versus rhythm control strategy included more than 5000 patients and demonstrated that a rate-control strategy is not inferior to a rhythm-control strategy for the patients studied.[8] Comparisons of ablation therapies for maintenance of sinus rhythm versus conservative therapies are lacking. A randomized pilot study has shown a reduction of AF recurrence and hospitalization and a greater improvement in quality of life for patients who underwent catheter ablation compared with those who underwent antiarrhythmic drug therapy.[9] These results are encouraging, but larger studies with longer durations of follow-up are needed.

In some cases, the best treatment approach is relatively clear. Patients presenting with an initial episode of paroxysmal AF might not require ventricular rate-controlling or antiarrhythmic drug therapy, particularly if the episode is associated with a treatable or removable physiologic stress, as described earlier. Clinical observation may be an option in some patients, with the decision to treat based on the development of recurrent episodes of AF. Similarly, a patient with an initial episode of persistent AF may be treated with appropriate anticoagulation (see earlier) and, if necessary, a ventricular rate-controlling medication. At the appropriate time, electrical or pharmacologic cardioversion can then be attempted without antiarrhythmic drug therapy. If recurrent AF occurs and restoration and maintenance of sinus rhythm is still desired, antiarrhythmic drug therapy may be considered.

Patients with symptomatic AF after adequate ventricular rate control has been achieved should be considered for a treatment approach that restores sinus rhythm. Such treatment strategies are discussed below. Acutely, restoration of sinus rhythm may be achieved with either pharmacologic or electrical cardioversion. It is important to remember that electrical and pharmacologic cardioversion are no different with regard to the risk of thromboembolic stroke. Therefore, the requirements for anticoagulation outlined earlier apply to either method of cardioversion.

Direct-Current Electrical Cardioversion

Of the two types of cardioversion, electrical cardioversion is more effective. In the past, direct-current electrical cardioversion with a monophasic waveform was acutely successful in approximately 80% of cases. Since the introduction of the biphasic waveform defibrillator, the success rate has increased to almost 95%. Direct-current cardioversion should be administered with the patient under deep sedation, with cardiac and hemodynamic monitoring, and in the presence of personnel skilled in airway management. The administration of an antiarrhythmic drug may promote more successful direct current cardioversion and maintenance of sinus rhythm.

Similarly, it is reasonable to add an antiarrhythmic drug for any patient who fails direct-current cardioversion and to consider a repeat attempt after the drug has been administered.

Table 2 Agents for Immediate Pharmacologic Cardioversion of Atrial Fibrillation

Drug	Advantages	Disadvantages	Guidelines for Dosing	Comments
Procainamide, *N*-acetyl procainamide (NAPA)	Rapid administration may cause hypotension; up to 10% of congestive heart failure patients experience worsened heart failure	10-15 mg/kg given IV up to 50 mg/min, then maintenance drip at 2-4 mg/min	Elimination half-life-2-5 hr for procainamide, 6-8 hr for NAPA; blood levels of both procainamide and NAPA need to be followed to prevent toxicity, especially in the setting of renal or hepatic insufficiency, or both	Can achieve therapeutic levels quickly
Amiodarone	Can be used in patients with severe left ventricular dysfunction	Long-term use associated with many side effects-visual disturbances, tremors and other neurologic sequelae, hepatitis, pulmonary fibrosis, photosensitivity, skin discoloration, thyroid abnormalities, cardiac conduction disturbances	150-300 mg given over 10-120 min, depending on tolerance of blood pressure; maintenance infusion (very expensive) at 0.5-1 mg/min	Half-life is extremely long (up to 120 days)
Ibutilide	Few extracardiac side effects; ease of use	Incidence of torsades de pointes higher than with procainamide or amiodarone	1-mg IV bolus; can repeat after 10 min if no effect	Avoid use in patients with baseline prolongation of QT interval

Pharmacologic Cardioversion

Rates of successful immediate cardioversion by pharmacologic means have ranged from 40% to 90%, with success more likely in patients with AF of shorter duration. However, pharmacologic cardioversion is often chosen as the first line of therapy because of its ease of administration and because there is no need to sedate the patient. Any patient who fails pharmacologic cardioversion should be considered for direct-current cardioversion.

The only IV agents approved in the United States for immediate pharmacologic cardioversion of AF are procainamide, amiodarone, and ibutilide (Table 2). Oral administration of antiarrhythmic medication may also be used for pharmacologic cardioversion. The pill-in-the-pocket treatment may be useful for select outpatients for terminating recent-onset episodes of AF. This approach has the potential to reduce emergency department visits and hospitalizations.

Antiarrhythmic Drug Therapy for Maintenance of Sinus Rhythm

A number of oral agents may be used for long-term maintenance of sinus rhythm for patients with AF (Table 3). Quinidine was once widely prescribed for AF, but its use has decreased in recent years. In fact, all the Class IA antiarrhythmic drugs—quinidine, procainamide, and disopyramide—have become less popular for the long-term treatment of AF. Other antiarrhythmic drugs, such as the Class IC agents flecainide and propafenone, have more favorable side effect profiles. However, the use of these medications does have some degree of risk. The Cardiac Arrhythmia Suppression Trial (CAST) has shown that flecainide and encainide are associated with an increase in mortality when used for the suppression of ventricular arrhythmias in post-MI patients with ventricular dysfunction.[10] As a result, there is much concern about the use of the Class IC antiarrhythmics in patients who have any type of underlying coronary artery or structural heart disease; in these patients, other antiarrhythmic drugs may be better initial choices. Flecainide and propafenone are usually well tolerated and are appropriate first-line options for the treatment of AF in patients without structural heart disease, particularly cardiomyopathy, including hypertrophic cardiomyopathy (HCM). There is a new sustained-release formulation of propafenone that offers the advantage of twice-daily dosing rather than thrice-daily dosing, as for the immediate-release formulation.

Sotalol is a Class III antiarrhythmic that has beta-blocking properties and is generally well tolerated. Patients may have difficulty tolerating the beta blocker side effects, such as fatigue, and there is a potential risk of excessive bradycardia. As with other Class III antiarrhythmic agents, sotalol causes QT prolongation and may result in ventricular proarrhythmia, such as torsades de pointes.

Dofetilide, another Class III agent, is the most recently approved antiarrhythmic drug for the treatment of AF. Its efficacy is similar to that of other agents in its class, and the incidence of proarrhythmia with this drug is acceptably low. Importantly, dofetilide has also been shown to be safe for patients with cardiomyopathy, CHF, and ischemic heart disease. Therefore, dofetilide may be considered as an alternative treatment option to amiodarone for these patients.

Amiodarone, although an effective antiarrhythmic agent, generally is reserved for patients with AF for whom other antiarrhythmic drugs have been contraindicated, ineffective, or poorly tolerated. This is primarily because amiodarone has potential time- and dose-dependent organ toxicities that can affect the liver, thyroid, and lungs and, less frequently, the eyes. It is recommended that baseline studies be performed before initiating this drug. These tests include an ophthalmologic examination, pulmonary spirometry and diffusion capacity tests, and blood tests to assess liver and thyroid function. The blood tests should be repeated at regular intervals, approximately every 6 months, and the ophthalmologic examination should be performed yearly. There is divergence of opinion with regard to routine performance of pulmonary function testing and chest radiography for asymptomatic patients taking amiodarone.

Several new antiarrhythmic medications are under investigation. Particularly promising is the potential for the development of atrium-specific and ion channel-specific antiarrhythmic medications.

Implantable Devices

Implantable devices are being used with increasing frequency for patients with AF. Certainly, there is a substantial incidence of sinus node and AV node dysfunction in the AF population. These devices

Table 3 Oral Medications for Long-Term Maintenance of Sinus Rhythm for Patients With Atrial Fibrillation

Drug	Advantages	Disadvantages	Guidelines for Dosing	Comments
Quinidine	Low cost; less negative inotropic effects	Low toxic-to-therapeutic ratio; interacts with many drugs, including digoxin, warfarin, verapamil; high incidence of side effects (particularly GI intolerance, neurologic side effects, hematologic suppressive effects)	Sulfate: 100-600 mg/dose q4-6hr Gluconate: 324-972 mg/dose q8-12hr	
Procainamide, *N*-acetyl procainamide (NAPA)	Useful in patients with pre-excitation and AF; prolongs refractory period of accessory pathway	Low toxic-to-therapeutic ratio; high incidence of GI, hematologic, immunologic (lupus-like syndrome) side effects; interacts with many medications	250-500 mg/dose q3-6hr Sustained-release: 50 mg/kg/day q6hr or q12hr for twice-daily form	Elimination half-life: 2-5 hr for procainamide, 6-8 hr for NAPA Blood levels of procainamide and NAPA need to be followed to prevent toxicity, especially in the setting of renal and/or hepatic insufficiency
Flecainide	Generally well tolerated	Significant incidence of central nervous system, visual side effects Avoid use in patients with coronary or structural heart disease	50-150 mg/dose q12hr	Shown to increase mortality when used to treat and suppress ventricular arrhythmias in patients after MI May need to combine with an AV nodal blocking agent Single-dose therapy with up to 300-mg doses have been shown to have high efficacy (~65%) for converting acute episodes of AF to SR
Propafenone (immediate-release, sustained-release)	Generally well tolerated; twice-daily dosing; sustained-release form results in more stable blood levels than immediate-release formulation	Three times daily dosing Avoid use in patients with coronary or structural heart disease Cost Avoid use in patients with coronary or structural heart disease	150-300 mg/dose q8hr 225, 325, 425 mg/dose bid	Single-dose therapy with up to 600-mg doses shown to have high efficacy (~75%) for converting acute episodes of AF to SR; cannot be used for acute cardioversion (pill-in-the-pocket)
Disopyramide	May be useful in hypertrophic cardiomyopathy because of its negative inotropic side effects	Anticholinergic effects (e.g., constipation, urinary retention)	150 mg/dose q6hr, 300 mg/dose q12hr for controlled-release preparation (give two thirds of usual dose for adults weighing <50 kg)	
Moricizine	Few drug-drug interactions	Should not be used in patients with coronary or structural heart disease	200-300 mg/dose q8hr	Has properties of Classes IA, IB, and IC drugs; shown to increase mortality when used for treatment and suppression of ventricular arrhythmias in patients after MI
Amiodarone	Can be used in patients with coronary or structural heart disease	Extremely long half-life (≤120 days) Many side effects with long-term use, e.g., visual disturbances, tremors, other neurologic sequelae, hepatitis, pulmonary fibrosis, photosensitivity, skin discoloration, thyroid abnormalities, cardiac conduction disturbances	Oral loading with 400-600 mg/day for 2-4 wk, then 200 mg/day	Baseline eye examination, LFTs, TFTs should be performed before initiating therapy; LFTs and TFTs should be followed 3 or 4 times annually; chest x-ray also advisable Approved only for life-threatening ventricular arrhythmias (but still often used for atrial or supraventricular arrhythmias)
Sotalol	Can be used in patients with coronary structural heart disease; beta-blocking properties allow single-agent therapy for almost all arrhythmias	Causes QTc prolongation; use limited by side effects related to beta-blocking properties (e.g., exacerbation of reactive airway disease, depression, negative inotropy)	80-160 mg/dose q12hr	Inpatient telemetry recommended for initiation of therapy
Dofetilide	Generally well tolerated; few extracardiac effects; can be used in patients with coronary or structural heart disease	Causes QTc prolongation	125-500 µg/dose q12hr	Inpatient telemetry mandated for initiation of therapy; ECG must be checked within 2-3 hr of administration for evidence of QTc prolongation >15% above baseline or >500 msec (550 msec for patients with intraventricular conduction delay)
Azimilide*	Few drug-drug interactions or side effects known to date	Causes QTc prolongation	125 mg/dose bid × 3 days, then 125 mg/day	Preliminary experience indicates efficacy similar to amiodarone; acceptable incidence of side effects

*Not available for use in the United States.

AF, atrial fibrillation; AV, atrioventricular; ECG, electrocardiogram; GI, gastrointestinal; LFT, liver function test; MI, myocardial infarction; SR, sinus rhythm; TFT, thyroid function test.

have several purposes, including bradycardia pacing support, ventricular response regularization, and AF suppression or termination. The ACC, AHA, and HRS have published guidelines for the use of implantable pacemakers and antitachycardia devices.[11] Pacemakers may be implanted simply for pacing support in patients with bradycardia. Sinus node dysfunction, often referred to as *bradycardia-tachycardia syndrome,* is not uncommon in patients with AF. Because this condition can be exacerbated by medications used to control AF, the presence of a pacemaker may allow more aggressive use of rate-controlling or antiarrhythmic medications, or both. However, a few points should be kept in mind. Pauses that occur with conversion to sinus rhythm, some that last as long as several seconds, are common; in the absence of symptoms, these pauses are not an indication for a permanent pacemaker. Even with symptomatic postconversion pauses, a curative approach for the appropriate patient should be considered before implanting a pacemaker.

Pacemakers are also implanted in conjunction with catheter ablation of the AV node. This type of ablation is the ultimate method of ventricular rate control and is often reserved for patients with permanent or paroxysmal AF refractory to medical or curative therapy. The potential benefits of this type of approach extend beyond simply controlling ventricular response, because there is evidence that regularization of the ventricular rhythm also confers hemodynamic or symptomatic benefits. This approach has been shown to be effective and leads to improved quality of life for some patients (see earlier discussion). Even so, this approach does not address the fibrillating atria, and such patients may still require systemic anticoagulation for thromboembolism and stroke prevention.

Several features of pacemaker systems may be useful for patients with AF. A pacemaker that has the capability to change automatically from a dual-chamber to single-chamber pacing mode at the onset of an episode of AF—commonly referred to as *mode switching*—is essential for avoiding the rapid heart rate that might otherwise occur when the pacemaker responds to the sensing of the rapid atrial activity. Other AF suppression algorithms have shown mixed results with regard to effectiveness. Overall, these features have been shown to have modest efficacy at best. Implantable atrial defibrillators have been developed, either as a stand-alone device or in combination with a ventricular defibrillator. However, the atrial defibrillator has not been widely accepted by patients or physicians. In general, patients have difficulty tolerating even the low-energy internal cardioversion shocks without the deep sedation provided during conventional external cardioversion.

Catheter Ablation

The past few years have witnessed a revolution in catheter-based curative strategies for AF. This development is a direct result of the new insights into the critical role of the pulmonary veins as the site of origin for the triggers and drivers of AF. Before these more recent developments, catheter ablation for various forms of atrial arrhythmias, particularly AF, had only limited applications. The best results in terms of success and safety appear to have occurred with catheter ablation of typical right atrial flutter and, to a somewhat lesser degree, atypical atrial flutter and focal atrial tachycardia.

With the recognition of the pulmonary veins as the source of the critical triggering beats of AF in most patients, catheter ablation techniques have shifted to target this substrate. Catheter-based AF ablation techniques have subsequently evolved into several different variations of a pulmonary vein isolation procedure targeting the pulmonary vein–left atrial junction, some of which are purely anatomic approaches and others of which are a combination of anatomic and electrophysiologic mapping approaches. This has led to improved efficacy rates, ranging from about 50% to as high as 90%, and a lower incidence of complications, notably pulmonary vein stenosis. Several experienced centers have reported high rates of successful cure of AF without the need for antiarrhythmic drug therapy.[12]

In spite of the much-improved efficacy and safety of AF catheter ablation, the procedure is still not the first-line treatment for AF. This approach is generally reserved for patients with symptomatic AF refractory to at least two antiarrhythmic drugs. The ideal candidate is a young patient with paroxysmal lone AF, but older patients and those with structural heart disease are not necessarily excluded and may be good candidates for consideration in experienced centers.

Surgical Approaches

The maze surgical procedure for the treatment of AF has substantially evolved from its initial form. In general, it involves a series of incisions or lesions in the atria. These are carefully placed to compartmentalize the atrial tissue to channel atrial activity and prevent the re-entry required for the maintenance of AF. Nonincisional lesions may be placed using radiofrequency, cryothermy, or microwave energy. Reported AF cure rates with the classic Cox maze procedure are high, perhaps more than 90% at some experienced centers.[13,14] However, this approach is invasive and requires a thoracotomy and general anesthesia. The incidence of perioperative complications has been low, and there is a potential need for a permanent postoperative pacemaker in as many as 7% to 10% of cases. This may occur as a result of the procedure itself or underlying sinus node dysfunction. The invasiveness of this approach makes it a less-desirable option for patients with AF alone, but it might be attractive for patients undergoing cardiac surgery for another indication (e.g., valve replacement or coronary bypass surgery).

Surgical approaches have continued to become less invasive, because surgeons are increasingly aware that the invasiveness of the Cox maze procedure is a major obstacle to patient (and referring physician) acceptance, no matter how effective the procedure is. Several centers, such as our own, have been using minimally invasive incisions and even thoracoscopic approaches with robotic equipment.

OUTCOMES

AF is often considered a nuisance arrhythmia because it is not immediately life threatening. However, it is associated with morbidity and mortality. Follow-up data from the Framingham Heart Study[2] and the Antiarrhythmics Versus Implantable Defibrillators (AVID) trial[3] have shown that AF is an independent predictor of increased mortality. It is not clear whether this higher risk is a reflection of the proarrhythmic complications of antiarrhythmic therapy, a failure to comply with prescribed medical therapy, or the presence of other factors such as stroke, worsening CHF, or unknown factors that were not recognized. Furthermore, subgroup analysis of on-treatment patients (versus the trial's overall intention to treat patients) has demonstrated improved survival associated with sinus rhythm in the AFFIRM study.[15] This underscores the importance of completing further studies, including randomized studies of the various treatment options for AF.

FUTURE DIRECTIONS

The prevalence of AF, already at epidemic proportions, is expected to continue to increase as the population ages and more patients with heart disease live longer. This is especially true for the heart-failure population. The rapid growth of curative approaches to AF, as with catheter-based and surgical ablation procedures, is promising and has already relieved many patients of the burden of AF and the side effects and toxicities of antiarrhythmic medications. However, these approaches are invasive and inherently destructive, with a small but important risk of serious complications. Additional refinements to invasive curative treatment approaches are anticipated, but there remains a desperate need for another solution to management of this arrhythmia.

The most beneficial development might be the effective prevention of AF. Research into the underlying molecular and genetic causes of AF may lead to novel methods of treatment targeting specific ion channel, molecular, or genetic defects. The prevention and optimal management of the medical disorders associated with AF, such as heart disease and hypertension, would have an obvious impact. The choice of treatment of such conditions may make a difference. Studies with drugs such as angiotensin-converting enzyme inhibitors, angiotensin receptor blockers, and the beta blocker carvedilol have shown promise as adjunctive therapies for preventing the development of atrial fibrillation.

Further developments in the understanding of atrial fibrillation will lead to advances in optimal therapy and, hopefully, a reduction in the incidence of this ubiquitous arrhythmia.

Summary

- Atrial fibrillation is the most common sustained tachyarrhythmia.
- Therapy for atrial fibrillation is centered around three goals: minimize stroke risk, control ventricular rate, and control the atrial rhythm.
- Any unstable patient presenting with atrial fibrillation should undergo immediate electrical cardioversion.
- Patients who fail pharmacologic conversion to sinus rhythm should be considered for electrical cardioversion, because the success rates for the latter are significantly better. Select patients may safely be treated with long-term anticoagulation and ventricular rate control alone.
- Ablation of atrial fibrillation triggers should be considered for symptomatic patients refractory to standard therapeutic measures.

Suggested Readings

Benjamin EJ, Wolf PA, D'Agostino RB, et al: Impact of atrial fibrillation on the risk of death: The Framingham Heart Study. Circulation. Sep 8 1998;98(10):946-952.

Brand FN, Abbott RD, Kannel WB, Wolf PA: Characteristics and prognosis of lone atrial fibrillation. 30-year follow-up in the Framingham Study. JAMA. Dec 27 1985;254(24):3449-3453.

Fuster V, Ryden Rydén LE, Cannom DS, et al: American College of Cardiology/American Heart Association Task Force on Practice Guidelines; European Society of Cardiology Committee for Practice Guidelines; European Heart Rhythm Association; Heart Rhythm Society: ACC/AHA/ESC 2006 Guidelines for the Management of Patients with Atrial Fibrillation: A report of the American College of Cardiology/American Heart Association Task Force on Practice Guidelines and the European Society of Cardiology Committee for Practice Guidelines (Writing Committee to Revise the 2001 Guidelines for the Management of Patients With Atrial Fibrillation): Developed in collaboration with the European Heart Rhythm Association and the Heart Rhythm Society. Circulation. Aug 15 2006;114(7):e257-e354.

Gregoratos G, Abrams J, Epstein AE, et al: ACC/AHA/NASPE 2002 Guideline Update for Implantation of Cardiac Pacemakers and Antiarrhythmia Devices-summary article: A report of the American College of Cardiology/American Heart Association Task Force on Practice Guidelines (ACC/AHA/NASPE Committee to Update the 1998 Pacemaker Guidelines). J Am Coll Cardiol. Nov 6 2002;40(9):1703-1719.

Klein AL, Murray RD, Grimm RA: Role of transesophageal echocardiography-guided cardioversion of patients with atrial fibrillation. J Am Coll Cardiol. Mar 1 2001;37(3):691-704.

McCarthy PM, Gillinov AM, Castle L, Chung M, Cosgrove D, 3rd., et al: The Cox-Maze procedure: The Cleveland Clinic experience. Semin Thorac Cardiovasc Surg. Jan 2000;12(1):25-29.

Oral H, Knight BP, Tada H, et al: Pulmonary vein isolation for paroxysmal and persistent atrial fibrillation. Circulation. Mar 5 2002;105(9):1077-1081.

Wood MA, Brown-Mahoney C, Kay GN, Ellenbogen KA: Clinical outcomes after ablation and pacing therapy for atrial fibrillation: A meta-analysis. Circulation. Mar 14 2000;101(10):1138-1144.

Wyse DG, Love JC, Yao Q, et al: Atrial fibrillation: A risk factor for increased mortality—an AVID registry analysis. J Interv Card Electrophysiol. Sep 2001;5(3):267-273.

Wyse DG, Waldo AL, DiMarco JP, et al: A comparison of rate control and rhythm control in patients with atrial fibrillation. N Engl J Med. Dec 5 2002;347(23):1825-1833.

References

For a complete list of references, log onto www.expertconsult.com.

Syncope

Fetnat Fouad-Tarazi, Laura Shoemaker, Ken Mayuga, and Fred Jaeger

DEFINITION

Syncope is an abrupt loss of consciousness with a concomitant loss of postural tone. Presyncope, also called near syncope, is the prodrome of syncope, but without loss of consciousness. Syncope is part of a broader clinical network of symptoms that is best described as *postural intolerance,* which is a constellation of symptoms that occur in the upright posture including dizziness, lightheadedness, tremulousness, sweating, nausea, and palpitations. These symptoms improve with the assumption of a recumbent posture.

PREVALENCE AND INCIDENCE

Syncope accounts for 3% of emergency room visits and 1% to 6% of hospital admissions.[1] It happens to men and women of all ages, but it increases in prevalence with age. In our syncope clinic from 1997 to 2007, we treated more women than men; it is unclear if this was due to a higher prevalence in women or to a higher tendency for women to seek medical assistance for this condition. Figure 1 shows the number of tests we performed, broken down by gender.

PATHOPHYSIOLOGY AND NATURAL HISTORY

The autonomic nervous system is vital for maintaining internal homeostasis, including regulation of blood pressure (BP), heart rate, fluid and electrolyte balance, and body temperature.

The hemodynamic response to standing exemplifies the interaction between the circulatory and autonomic nervous systems. When standing, initially the force of gravity pools blood in the distensible veins below heart level. Increased capillary pressure follows, and plasma is lost to interstitial fluid due to ultrafiltration. It is estimated that plasma volume decreases by 15% within 20 minutes of standing. Pooling of blood in the veins decreases venous return to the heart, with subsequent reduction of cardiac output, which in turn, triggers compensatory mechanisms to prevent the fall of arterial pressure.

Normally the physiologic response to standing is gravitational blood pooling in the lower extremities, leading to reduced venous return to the heart. The mean arterial BP and stroke volume decrease, which deactivates strategically located mechanoreceptors that will initiate neural reflexes. These reflexes increase sympathetic outflow, decrease parasympathetic responses, and lead to tachycardia and vasoconstriction. In addition, unloading of the low pressure cardiopulmonary receptors play a role in regulating the release of arginine vasopressin (AVP). The reduction in effective plasma volume and renal blood flow stimulate the postural responses of the renin-angiotensin-aldosterone (RAA) system. Compensatory mechanisms include: increased sympathetic outflow leading to arteriolar vasoconstriction, venoconstriction, and increase in heart rate; increased catecholamine concentration in the plasma and urine; and rise in plasma epinephrine originating from the adrenal medulla.

The autonomic supply to the cardiovascular system is coordinated at the central autonomic network (CAN) in the brainstem. The autonomic nervous system counterbalances postural stressors to maintain mean arterial pressure. During orthostasis, the initial reduction of cardiac filling and stroke volume is sensed by pressure receptors in the heart, carotid sinuses, and aortic arch, which send impulses to the CAN. This initiates sympathetic vasomotor outflow to vascular beds in the skeletal muscles and cutaneous vasculature. Norepinephrine is released, causing vasoconstriction, venoconstriction, and increased heart rate and contractility.

Decreased atrial stretch during postural stress causes increased secretion of AVP and decreased secretion of A-type atrial natriuretic peptide (ANP). This antinatriuresis helps increase extra cellular fluid (ECF) volume and compensates for cardiac filling.

Orthostasis leads to a reflexive decrease of renal blood flow followed by decreased glomerular filtration of sodium. Decreases in renal blood flow and renal perfusion pressure stimulate the RAA system to enhance vasoconstriction.

Sympathetic stimulation plays a major role in the immediate response to upright posture. It maintains mean arterial pressure via constriction of several vascular beds. Venoconstriction causes c orrection of orthostasis by increasing cardiac filling for a given amount of gravitational pooling of blood. Increased cardiac inotropic function augments stroke volume for cardiac filling. Increased heart rate augments cardiac output for stroke volume. Leg pumping of skeletal muscles enhances venous return to the heart. The venoarterial reflex augments arterial vasoconstriction in response to venous distention.

On the other hand, the RAA system plays a minor role in the immediate constrictive response to orthostasis, and its effects are relatively late. In the absence of sympathetic postganglionic outflow, like that seen in cases of spinal cord injury and quadriplegia, orthostatic hypotension occurs despite marked stimulation of the RAA system.

Not every fall in BP leads to brain hypoxia. Syncope or presyncope occurs as a result of brain hypoxia, which is usually secondary to a reduction of cerebral perfusion pressure. This is because the cerebral circulation is autoregulated so brain perfusion is maintained in the face of significant changes in BP. Cerebral autoregulation allows regional cerebral blood flow to remain constant over a range of perfusion pressure (50-140 mm Hg).

ETIOLOGY

In stratifying the etiology of syncope, prospective studies have found that neurally mediated causes account for the largest percentage of events (38%-56%). Cardiovascular causes, separated into cardiac causes (11%-23%) and postural hypotension (2%-24%), account for a smaller percentage of cases. Undetermined causes occur in 14% to 18% of events.

Poor prognosis was reported in syncope patients with underlying heart disease. The etiologies of syncope can be subdivided into those occurring in patients with or without structural heart disease. Hospital admission criteria following emergency department evaluation for a syncope event have been extensively discussed, and decision making about prevention of serious outcomes is critical.[2,3]

Presence of Structural Heart Disease

In patients with structural heart disease, syncope can occur secondary to bradyarrhythmias, tachyarrhythmias, or arrhythmias secondary to medication and electrolyte abnormalities. Cardiac left ventricular outflow obstruction (including aortic stenosis or hypertrophic cardiomyopathy) or right ventricular obstruction (including pulmonary embolus or pulmonary hypertension) can cause syncope. Other cardiac structural abnormalities, such as mitral stenosis, atrial myxoma, or dissecting aortic aneurysm, can also lead to syncope. Finally, the syndromes that accompany cardiac events including myocardial ischemia or infarction, cardiac tamponade, or subclavian steal syndrome can include syncope.

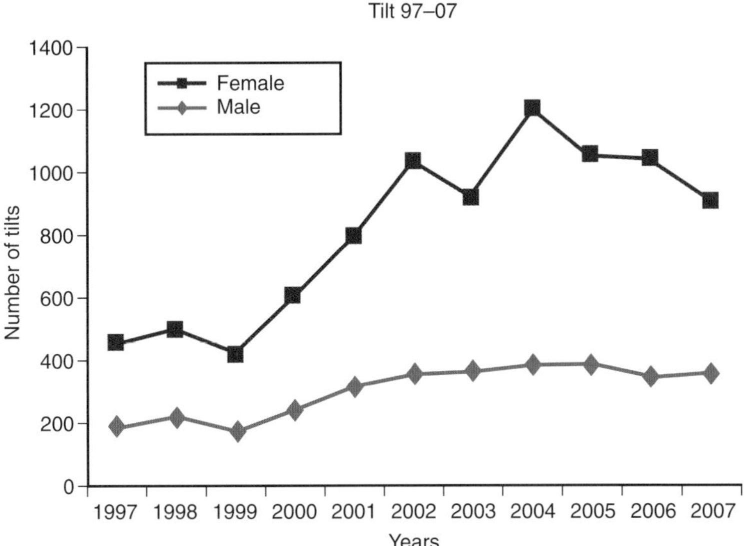

Figure 1 Number of tilt tests from the syncope clinic, 1997-2007, shown according to gender.

Absence of Structural Heart Disease

In the absence of structural heart disease, neurally mediated mechanisms, postural hypotension, postural orthostatic tachycardia syndrome (POTS), metabolic or neurologic abnormalities, and psychogenic causes should be considered as a possible etiology of a syncopal event. For practical purposes, syncope in the absence of heart disease may be grouped into events where the BP declines steadily, those where BP drops only at the endpoint, and those where BP response to upright posture remains normal.

Neurally Mediated Mechanisms

Neurocardiogenic Syncope. Also known as vasovagal syncope and vasodepressor syncope, neurocardiogenic syncope is commonly described using the Bezold-Jarisch reflex model.[2] A reduction in ventricular preload stimulates mechanoreceptors in the inferoposterior part of the left ventricle, leading to a vigorous contraction. This causes an increased afferent discharge of the unmyelinated C fibers from the ventricular mechanoreceptors. The central nervous system responds with reflex sympathetic withdrawal and increased parasympathetic output. These signals cause vasodilation, hypotension, and bradycardia in the vasovagal type, but only vasodilation occurs in the vasodepressor type.

Other potential mechanisms include involvement of central serotoninergic pathways and release of endogenous opioids or catecholamines. Of importance is the report of a monitored vasovagal event in a heart transplant patient.[4]

Carotid Sinus Syncope. Some patients have hypersensitive carotid sinus baroreceptors leading to vagal overstimulation and syncope. The underlying mechanism for hypersensitivity is not known, but it is commonly associated with ischemic heart disease, aging, and hypertension.[5]

Situational Syncope. Situational syncope includes cough, laughter, deglutition, micturition, and defecation syncope. The underlying mechanisms of these events are likely similar to that of neurocardiogenic syncope. Some other situational events may be related to human fear circuitry and sociogenic pseudoneurologic symptoms.[6-8]

Postural Hypotension

Postural hypotension is defined as a drop in systolic BP of at least 20 mm Hg accompanied by a drop in diastolic BP of at least 10 mm Hg with upright posture. It is caused by deviation from the normal physiologic response to upright posture, which leads to postural decline of BP or postural hypotension.

About 16% to 18% patients older than 65 years have postural hypotension, and 2% of these are symptomatic. The value of the clinical history is limited in diagnosing the cause of syncope in older patients (≥65 years) as compared to younger patients (<65 years).[9]

Possible causes of postural hypotension include hypovolemia, autonomic insufficiency, medications or toxins (tricyclic antidepressants, vasodilators, angiotensin-converting enzyme inhibitors, ganglionic blockers, alcohol), metabolic or endocrine causes (Addison's disease, pheochromocytoma, systemic mastocytosis, carcinoid syndrome), or vascular insufficiency (varicose veins, arteriovenous malformations).

Autonomic dysfunction (Box 1) is a disorder of postganglionic noradrenergic transmission. The central nervous system does not appropriately activate efferent sympathetic fibers. Mechanisms of dysfunction include subnormal norepinephrine release, impaired vasoconstriction, and reduced vascular volume from urinary sodium wasting. Autonomic dysfunction is classified as primary or secondary.

Box 1 Autonomic Dysfunction

Primary
- Pure autonomic failure (Bradbury-Eggleston syndrome)
- Multiple system atrophy (Shy-Drager syndrome)
- Autonomic failure with Parkinson's disease

Secondary
- Diabetes mellitus
- Amyloidosis
- Multiple sclerosis
- Spinal tumors
- Carcinomatosis autonomic neuropathy or as a paraneoplastic phenomenon
- Familial dysautonomia (Riley-Day syndrome)

Postural Orthostatic Tachycardia Syndrome

POTS[10,11] is defined by excessive heart rate increments upon upright posture. A person with POTS experiences heart rates that increase 30 beats or more per minute—and that can increase to 120 beats or more per minute—upon standing. These heart rate increases usually occur within 10 minutes of rising. We have described early versus late POTS (accentuated postural tachycardia).[11]

A variety of circulatory and autonomic neural abnormalities occur in association with POTS and can cause accentuated postural tachycardia including hypovolemia, augmentation of postural venous pooling, β-adrenergic hypersensitivity, hyperbradykininemia, and autonomic imbalance. In a substantial number of patients, no definite cause is found. The literature describes this condition as associated with mitral valve prolapse, basilar migraine, chronic fatigue syndrome, and neurocardiogenic (vasovagal) syncope.

Metabolic and Neurologic Conditions

Metabolic disorders include hyperventilation, hypoglycemia, or hypoxia. Neurologic conditions may be due to vertebral-basilar insufficiency or migraine.[12]

Psychogenic Conditions

Psychogenic causes of syncope include anxiety or panic disorder. Cerebral blood flow velocity by ultrasonography of the middle cerebral artery has been assessed in patients with orthostatic intolerance during head-up tilt or during the Valsalva procedure.[12]

COMPLICATIONS AND OUTCOME

The 1-year mortality was 18% to 33% in patients with a cardiac-caused syncope, 0% to 12% for syncope of noncardiac causes, and 6% with syncope of unknown cause.[13]

SIGNS AND SYMPTOMS

Symptoms of postural intolerance are related to brain anoxia or hypoxia resulting from a reduction of BP. Lightheadedness, dizziness, imbalance, tunnel vision, blurriness, spotted visual field, and headache are symptoms related to brain hypoxia. These symptoms may be aborted by assuming a sitting or supine posture. The occurrence and severity of symptoms are influenced not only by the quantitative drop of BP but also by the rapidity of BP decline. However, in elderly patients with chronic postural hypotension, BP can fall extensively without symptoms, possibly due to adaptive mechanisms affecting cerebral autoregulation. Other symptoms of orthostatic intolerance depend on the underlying etiology including palpitations, chest pain or fatigue. Box 2 lists clinical features suggesting specific etiologies.

Box 2 Clinical Features Suggesting Specific Etiologies

Neurocardiogenic syncope

- After unexpected pain, unpleasant smell, or unpleasant sight
- After prolonged standing;
- After exercise in a well-trained athlete

Postural hypotension
Postprandial hypotension
Cardiac syncope

- After exertion
- With a history of significant structural heart disease
- With a family history of sudden death

Carotid sinus syncope

- After neck rotation
- After pressure on neck (i.e., shaving, wearing a tight collar)

Neurologic causes

- Diplopia
- Vertigo
- Ataxia
- Dysarthria

Subclavian steal syndrome (elevation of the ipsilateral arm)

DIAGNOSIS

History

A detailed history from patients and witnesses and a comprehensive physical examination identifies a cause for syncope in up to 50% of cases. It is important to remember conditions simulating syncope such as epileptic seizures, hypoglycemia, or vestibular dysfunction. In a thorough history, questions should cover the event, the week to month before the event, and what happened after the event.

Physical Examination

Careful, comprehensive physical examination is essential. Blood pressure should be checked for both arms and in the supine and standing positions. Signs to look for in the physical examination include dehydration, facial flushing, carotid bruits, cardiac murmurs, abdominal masses, varicose veins, and signs of endocrine disorders in skin, eyes, and thyroid.

Laboratory Testing

Blood work is useful if metabolic disturbance or anemia is suspected, but in general, it has low diagnostic yield.

Electrocardiographic Testing

Although the electrocardiogram (ECG) is often normal on presentation, it is an essential part of the initial evaluation of syncope. Only 5% of initial ECGs are diagnostic. Another 5% suggest an underlying diagnosis. Box 3 lists the European Society of Cardiology Task Force ECG abnormalities, which might suggest an arrhythmia as the etiology of a syncopal event. During the tilt test, T wave changes are common as heart rate increases, and progressive shortening of the PR interval has been observed before cardioinhibitory syncope, but the clinical significance is as yet unclear.[14,15]

Holter monitoring has low diagnostic yield, about 2%, in studies of an unselected syncope population. Symptoms and a recorded arrhythmia are often not correlated. Prolonged Holter monitoring of 48 to 72 hours detects more arrhythmias, but not necessarily correlating with symptoms. A negative Holter monitor recording does not exclude arrhythmia as a cause of syncope, because events may be infrequent and sporadic. Patients with a high pretest probability are those with an abnormal resting ECG or evidence of structural heart disease. In these patients, further evaluation maybe necessary, even if the Holter study is negative. The yield of 24-hour Holter monitoring was found to improve when restricted to high-risk patients.[16] One-month external loop recorders were found to add to the diagnostic yield and considered a help in offsetting the cost.[17]

Event monitors are diagnostically useful, especially in patients with infrequent episodes or symptoms. Transtelephonic event recorders are activated by the patient, who starts recording when symptoms occur. This event can be stored and transmitted at a later

Box 3 Electrocardiographic Abnormalities that Can Cause a Syncopal Event

Bifascicular block
Sinoatrial block
Q waves suggesting myocardial infarction
Right bundle branch block with ST elevation in V_1-V_3, Brugada syndrome
Negative T waves in right precordium, ε wave, and ventricular late potentials suggesting arrhythmogenic right ventricular dysplasia
QRS duration ≥ 120 msec
Prolonged QT interval
Mobitz II second-degree atrioventricular block
Pre-excitation QRS complexes, Wolff-Parkinson-White syndrome

Box 4 Results of Electrophysiology Testing

The results are considered positive if any of the following are induced:

- Sustained monomorphic ventricular tachycardia
- Prolonged sinus node recovery time or corrected sinus node recovery time
- Markedly prolonged H-V interval ≥100 msec at baseline
- Spontaneous or induced infrahisian block during incremental arterial pacing
- Rapid supraventricular tachycardia with symptomatic hypotension

time. A continuous loop event monitor can record up to a few minutes of ECG recording retrospectively when activated by the patient, in addition to recording prospectively. An implantable loop recorder is useful in patients with unexplained syncope and very infrequent events. This device has a life span of 1 to 2 years. It is activated automatically by a rapid heart rate or by the patient or family members applying a magnet.[17]

A signal-averaged ECG can be used to determine late ventricular potentials, which act as a substrate for ventricular arrhythmias. This test has a sensitivity of 63% to 89% and a specificity of 89% to 100% for predicting ventricular tachycardia in patients with syncope. This is a useful screening test if ventricular tachycardia is the only concern, but it does not provide additional information that would be obtained during an electrophysiology study.

Imaging

Cerebral imaging is helpful if a neurologic cause is suspected. Evaluation with echocardiography is a Class I recommendation from the American College of Cardiology and American Heart Association (ACC/AHA) if there is clinical suspicious of structural heart disease, and it is a Class IIb recommendation if there in no evidence of heart disease clinically.

Procedural Tests

Stress testing is appropriate in patients with **a** history of exercise-related arrhythmia or syncope. Stress testing should be avoided in severe patients with symptomatic aortic stenosis and in patients with hypertrophic cardiomyopathy and severe outflow tract obstruction.

Electrophysiology testing has a low yield in patients with a normal ECG, no evidence of structural heart disease, and ejection fraction greater than 40%. Predictors of positive findings include ejection fraction less than 40%, male sex, bundle branch block, history of myocardial infarction, injury, and nonsustained ventricular tachycardia. Overall diagnostic yield is 50% in patients with organic heart disease and 10% in patients without structural heart disease. Electrophysiologic testing is a class I recommendation by the ACC/AHA guidelines for patients with suspected heart disease and unexplained syncope. Criteria for a positive electrophysiology test are listed in Box 4.

Other, more specialized syncope evaluations include an assessment of global autonomic function. This entails a number of maneuvers, pressor testing, Valsalva maneuver, phenylephrine test, and amyl nitrite inhalation. These are performed while heart rate variability and BP are monitored.

Tilt Table Testing

The tilt table test is a provocative test that moves a patient from a supine to an upright position using a tilt table. It is used to examine autonomic neural regulation of cardiovascular orthostatic responses.[18] Indications for the tilt test are shown in Box 5. Figure 2 shows a tilt table laboratory. Evaluations of the tilt test procedure have shown sensitivity of 32% to 85%, specificity of 75% to 93%, reproducibility of 62% to 85%, and false negative rate of 14%.

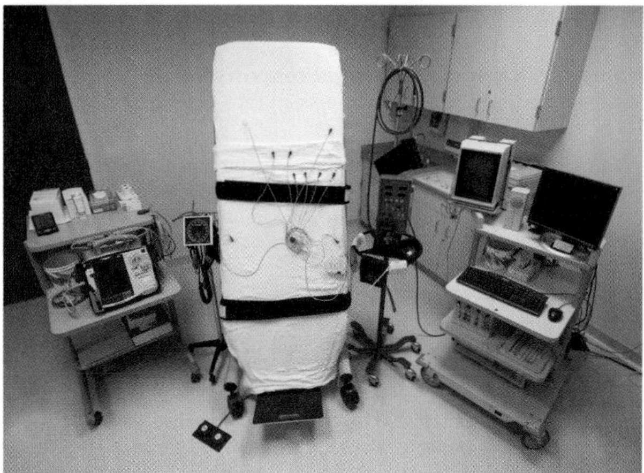

Figure 2 Tilt test laboratory.

Box 5 Indications for Tilt Test

Class I

Unexplained single syncopal episode in a high-risk setting, recurrent syncope episodes with no structural cardiac disease, or presence of structural cardiac disease, after cardiac causes of syncope are excluded

To evaluate exercise-induced or exercise-associated syncope

To demonstrate susceptibility to vasovagal syncope

Class II

To differentiate convulsive syncope from seizures

To evaluate recurrent unexplained falls, especially in older adults

To assess recurrent presyncope or dizziness

When an understanding of the hemodynamic pattern in syncope may alter therapeutic approach

Class III

To assess treatment response

Single episode without injury, not in a high-risk setting

Clear-cut vasovagal syncope; result of tilt test will not alter treatment

Other

Postural hypotension

Postural orthostatic tachycardia syndrome (POTS)

Cerebral syncope

Evaluating chronic fatigue syndrome, basilar migraine

Normally, in response to the tilt procedure, a patient experiences gravitational blood pooling in the lower extremities and reduced venous return to the heart, resulting in a decreased mean arterial BP and stroke volume, which leads to deactivation of various mechanoreceptors and activation of renin-angiotensin system (RAS). This leads to an increase in sympathetic outflow, withdrawal of parasympathetic responses, and tachycardia and vasoconstriction.

Susceptible patients can experience vigorous cardiac contractions with relative central hypovolemia due to peripheral blood pooling.[19] This leads to secondary reflex sympathetic withdrawal and increased vagal output, resulting in bradycardia or hypotension, or both, with symptoms.

During the tilt table procedure, the patient is monitored with continuous ECG recording and an automatic sphygmomanometer or beat-by-beat finger arterial pressure recording. The patient is tilted from the supine position to 70 degrees (range, 60-80 degrees) over a period of 45 minutes. Procedure end-points are induction of syncope or presyncope in association with hypotension or bradycardia; change in BP, heart rate, and symptoms; or completion of planned tilt duration.

Box 6 Induced Abnormal Hemodynamic Patterns During Tilt Test

Neurocardiogenic, vasovagal response
Sudden reduction in blood pressure, heart rate, or both, with symptoms
Three basic responses

- Cardioinhibitory response, including hypotension and bradycardia or asystole
- Vasodepressor response, including hypotension without bradycardia
- Mixed response, in which both elements are present

Postural Hypotension
Reduction in systolic blood pressure >20 mm Hg
Reduction of diastolic blood pressure >10 mm Hg
Increase or decrease in heart rate

Postural Orthostatic Tachycardia Syndrome (POTS)
Sustained increase in heart rate >30 beats/min
Sustained maximum heart rate >120 beats/min
Usually no change in blood pressure

Cerebral Syncope
Syncope occurs in absence of heart rate and blood pressure changes
Syncope is associated with cerebral arteriolar vasoconstriction
Test is performed with transcranial Doppler ultrasound

Psychogenic Response
Symptoms during tilt test without hemodynamic, electroencephalographic, or transcranial Doppler abnormalities

Various BP and heart rate response patterns to the tilt procedure are recognized, and they reflect the underlying pathophysiologic determinants. Additional testing may be planned according to the tilt response pattern, such as hemodynamic evaluation, blood volume, and autonomic reflex testing. The role of blood volume determination was enhanced by research findings.[20] Pharmacophysiologic interventions help differentiation of preganglionic from postganglionic lesions.[21]

Relative contraindications to the tilt test include severe left ventricular outflow tract obstruction, critical mitral stenosis, critical proximal coronary artery stenosis or active angina, and critical cerebrovascular stenosis. Limitations of the head-up tilt test include inability to stand because of leg weakness or pain or because of severe back pain; unstable medical conditions; nability to obtain BP because of incompressible arm arteries, bilateral arm arteriovenous fistulas, or bilateral subclavian artery stenosis; and inability to secure intravenous access.

A normal response to the tilt test is a 10 to 15 beat/min increase in heart rate or a 10% to 15% rise from baseline, a 0 to 10 mm Hg decrease in systolic BP, and a 5 to 10 mm Hg increase in diastolic BP.

Induced abnormal hemodynamic patterns during tilt testing are listed in Box 6.

If the tilt test is negative and the patient's history suggests a neurocardiogenic etiology of syncope, the patient is subjected to the isoproterenol tilt test. The addition of isoproterenol increases the sensitivity of the tilt test for the diagnosis of vasovagal syncope at the expense of a reduction in the specificity of the test for the same diagnosis.[22]

A genetic component in vasovagal syndrome has been considered but is not proved. Pediatric drop attacks with abrupt loss of muscle tone have been described in association with a specific genetic syndrome.[23] Clinical genetic tests to determine patients at high risk for pediatric sudden cardiac death can lead to more aggressive and specific treatment.

TREATMENT

Managing the Acute Episode

Family members should learn to recognize early symptoms. They may notice pallor, sweating, lack of concentration, disorientation, and nausea, which suggest postural hypotension and brain hypoperfusion. Convulsions suggest prolonged or severe brain hypoperfusion. Shakiness, which can accompany hyperadrenergic activity, can simulate seizure. The duration of loss of consciousness as well as the position of the patient during loss of consciousness is important information. Urinary incontinence and tongue biting during a spell favor a seizure event.

Helping the patient sit or lie down quickly and raising the legs above the heart level permit faster recovery in patients with a typical reflex postural hypotension event. Physicians should check the pulse for amplitude and rhythm. When a patient recovers the acute event, ambulation should be resumed with care because recurrence of hypotension may be inevitable at this stage due to circulatory instability. Oral hydration with salty fluids usually is helpful in the early recovery phase if the patient has no known previous history of heart disease. Serious arrhythmogenic events, coronary insufficiency syndromes, pulmonary embolism, strokes or transient ischemic attacks, and blood loss must be recognized for proper immediate medical care. Injuries sustained during a sudden fall require immediate attention.

Admission is necessary for syncope that may be secondary to coronary events, pulmonary embolization, stroke, unstable arrhythmias, and syncope-related injuries. Hospital admission is necessary for status epilepticus, need for detoxication, severe dehydration, or hypertensive crises, which may be part of the autonomic failure syndromes or a complication of the treatment given for syncope.

In patients with syncope secondary to structural heart disease, the underlying causes should be treated. Situational syncope is managed with avoidance of triggers and assumption of a supine position with legs raised at the onset of symptoms.

Some patients continue to have recurrent syncope despite treatment, and the etiology of syncope remains uncertain. Such patients require more specialized laboratory workup to determine the predisposing neurocirculatory factors. In some patients, ambulatory monitoring procedures have proved valuable in determining the heart rate events before and during an episode of syncope or orthostatic intolerance. Patients who have multiple or serious comorbid conditions require special treatment programs that can be monitored in a specialized syncope clinic. See Table 1 for the guidelines for syncope treatment based on pathophysiology.

Pharmacologic Treatment

Anticholinergic Agents

Hyoscyamine is used in patients with neurocardiogenic syndrome who have supine bradycardia and evidence of heightened vagal modulation of heart. Disopyramide possesses a vagolytic effect in addition to its class IA antiarrhythmic action It is rarely used to treat simple syncope without arrhythmias. It requires hospitalization and monitoring of QT interval during the initiation of treatment.

Beta Blockers

Either cardioselective or non-cardioselective beta-blockers can be used to treat syncope and orthostatic intolerance.

Calcium Channel Blockers

Non-dihydropyridine calcium channel blockers have been used to slow heart rate and prevent orthostatic tachycardia in patients who cannot tolerate beta-blockers. Verapamil has been used instead of beta-blockers in asthmatic patients.

Fludrohydrocortisone

Fludrohydrocortisone is a synthetic selective mineralocorticoid when used in small doses; it retains salt and water and promotes plasma volume expansion.

Table 1 Guidelines for Syncope Treatment Based on Pathophysiology

Parameter	Treatment		
	Medications	Diet	Other
Autonomic insufficiency	Fludrocortisone (Florinef), midodrine (ProAmatine)	Salt	Physical therapy; support stockings
Neurocardiogenic syncope	Beta blocker or verapamil, fludrocortisone (Florinef)	Salt	
Hypovolemia	Fludrocortisone (Florinef), clonidine	Salt	
Venous pooling	Midodrine (ProAmatine)		Support stockings, physical therapy
Hyperkinetic heart syndrome, postural tachycardia syndrome	Beta blocker or nondihydropyridine calcium channel blocker (verapamil), midodrine (ProAmatine)		Cardiac rehabilitation program
High vagal tone	Parasympatholytic (atropine, scopolamine patch, hyoscyamine [Levsin, Levbid, NuLev])		

Selective Serotonin Reuptake Inhibitors

Selective serotonin reuptake inhibitors (Paroxetine; Sertraline) can be effective in treating resistant cases of neurocardiogenic syncope.

Vasoconstrictors

Midodrine is an α-adrenergic agonist used for the treatment of autonomic insufficiency and neurocardiogenic syncope. It has been used in combination with beta-blockers and with fludrohydrocortisone. Due to its effect of increasing afterload, it is not advised in hypertension, heart failure, active coronary artery disease, peripheral vascular disease.

Other vasoconstrictors used in the past are sometimes used in the present era such as ephedrine, IM dihydroergotamine, or intra-nasal desmopressin. Other medications tried include ibuprofen with meals, caffeine, and octreotide.

Nonpharmacologic Treatment

Treatment of the individual causes of syncope can be tailored according to the individual diagnosis: neurocardiogenic syncope, carotid sinus syncope, postural hypotension, autonomic failure, and POTS.

Permanent cardiac pacemakers have been tried, but they are rarely used now to treat a vasovagal event. Permanent cardiac pacing is the treatment of choice for the carotid hypersensitivity syndrome.

Compression support stockings help dimish venous pooling. An abdominal binder and small frequent meals are advised in patients with postprandial hypotension.

Physical countermaneuvers and simple postural maneuvers are easy to teach to patients and may be useful in mild orthostatic symptoms, at the very onset of orthostatic symptoms until other interventions are started. During these maneuvers patient should avoid Valsalva straining.

Patients should avoid the triggers such as heat, prolonged standing, decongestants, excess caffeine, large meals, and alcohol. Elevation the head of the bed by 6 to 8 inches can help patients with supine hypertension and postural hypotension.

FOLLOW-UP

Patients with syncope of unknown etiology and without underlying structural heart disease have a favorable outcome compared with those having organic heart disease. These patients should be followed regularly.

Response to treatment can be assessed by noting a patient's overall improvement of symptoms, standing time, the number of syncopal episodes in a predefined period, the extent of drop in BP during standing, and time to drop in BP during standing.

Patients with syncope and underlying structural heart disease need regular and close follow-up due to increased risk of sudden death. Attention should be paid to potential side effects of therapy, such as supine hypertension in susceptible patients taking midodrine and hypokalemia in patients taking fludrocortisone. Pacemakers and implantable cardiac defibrillators should be checked routinely.

PREVENTION AND SCREENING

Recurrence of syncopal episodes may be prevented by patient education and treatment. Patients need to be aware of triggers that can predispose to or precipitate syncopal spells and orthostatic intolerance. There is no definite procedure for screening of subjects for syncope. Practice guidelines are included in the references.

Summary

- Syncope is a part of a broader network of symptoms that is best described as postural intolerance.
- The interaction between the circulatory system and the autonomic nervous system is crucial to understanding the pathophysiology of syncope.
- Syncope or presyncope occurs as a result of brain anoxia, which is usually secondary to reduction of cerebral perfusion pressure and failure of cerebral circulatory autoregulation.
- The tilt test is an important screening test in the evaluation of postural intolerance and syncope.
- Procedural testing other than the tilt test is also used for determining the cause of syncope.

Suggested Readings

Biaggioni I: The sympathetic nervous system and blood volume regulation: Lessons from autonomic failure patients. Am J Med Sci 2007;1(334):61-64.

Blanc J-J, L'Her C, Touiza A, et al: Prospective evaluation and outcome of patients admitted for syncope over a 1-year period. Eur Heart J 2002;23:815-820.

Chapleau MW, Lu J, Hajduczok G, Abboud FM: Mechanism of baroreceptor adaptation in dogs: Attenuation of adaptation by the K^+ channel blocker 4-aminopyridine. J. Physiology [London] 1993;462:291-306.

Goldschlager N, Epstein AE, Grubb BP, et al; Practice Guidelines Subcommittee, North American Society of Pacing and Electrophysiology: Etiologic considerations in the patient with syncope and an apparently normal heart. Arch Intern Med 2003;163:151-162.

Grubb BP, Gerard G, Rousch K, et al: Differentiation of convulsive syncope and epilepsy with head up tilt table testing. Ann Int Med 1991;115:871-876.

Ibrahim MH, Tarazi RC, Dustan HP, et al: Idiopathic orthostatic hypotension: Circulatory dynamics in chronic autonomic insufficiency. Am J Cardiol 1974;34:288-294.

Lipsitz LA, Wei JY, Rowe JW: Syncope in an elderly, institutionalized population: Prevalence, incidence, and associated risk. Q J Med 1985;55:45-55.

Mathias CJ: Role of autonomic evaluation in the diagnosis and management of syncope. Clin Autonom Res 2004;14(Suppl 1):45-54.

Raj S, Robertson D: Blood volume perturbations in the postural tachycardia syndrome. Am J Med Sci 2005;1(334):57-60.

Tarazi RC, Fouad FM: Circulatory dynamics in autonomic failure. In Bannister R (ed): Autonomic Failure: A Textbook of Clinical Disorders of the Autonomic Nervous System. Oxford: Oxford University Press, 1983, pp 96-114.

References

For a complete list of references, log onto www.expertconsult.com.

Pericardial Disease

Ron Jacob and Richard A. Grimm

ACUTE PERICARDITIS

Definition

Acute pericarditis is an inflammatory process involving the pericardium that results in a clinical syndrome with the triad of chest pain, pericardial friction rub, and changes in the electrocardiogram (ECG).[1]

Prevalence

Acute pericarditis is the admitting diagnosis in 0.1% of hospital admissions. It occurs more commonly in men than in women.

Etiology

The most common form of acute pericarditis is idiopathic, which accounts for about 90% of cases (Box 1).[2] Other common causes include infection, renal failure, myocardial infarction (MI),[3] malignancy, radiation, and trauma.[4] These are discussed in more detail later.

Signs and Symptoms

The most common symptom of acute pericarditis is severe, sharp retrosternal chest pain, often radiating to the neck, shoulders, or back. Positional changes are characteristic, with worsening of the pain in the supine position and with inspiration and improvement with sitting upright and leaning forward. Other symptoms can occur, reflecting the underlying disease.

A scratchy, grating, high-pitched friction rub (squeak of leather of a new saddle) caused by fibrinous deposits in the pericardial space (Fig. 1) with three components—atrial systole, ventricular systole, and early ventricular diastole—is classic. It is best heard during inspiration at the left lower sternal border, with the patient leaning forward. The rub may disappear with the development of an effusion and impending cardiac tamponade.[1]

Specific Types

Idiopathic Pericarditis

The cause of acute pericarditis is often difficult to establish, and idiopathic pericarditis remains the most common diagnosis.

Viral Pericarditis

Coxsackievirus B virus and echovirus are the most common viruses, and a fourfold increase in antiviral titers is required for the diagnosis. Patients often experience a prodrome of an upper respiratory tract infection. The prognosis of viral pericarditis is good, the course is usually self-limited, and patients may be treated on an outpatient basis.

Purulent Pericarditis

Before the antibiotic era, pneumonia was the prime cause of purulent pericarditis. Currently, causes include thoracic surgery, chemotherapy, immunosuppression, and hemodialysis. Presentation is usually acute with high fevers, chills, night sweats, and dyspnea, but the classic findings of chest pain or friction rub are rare. Cardiac tamponade is common (42% to 77% of patients in select series), and mortality is high.

If purulent pericarditis is suspected, hospital admission with immediate pericardiocentesis and intravenous broad-spectrum antibiotics is mandatory, followed by early surgical drainage. Findings on pericardial fluid analysis include a high protein level (>6 g/dL), low glucose level (<35 mg/dL), and very high leukocyte count (6,000-240,000/mm^3).[5]

Tuberculous Pericarditis

Tuberculous pericarditis occurs in 1% to 2% of cases of pulmonary tuberculosis. Immunocompromised or human immunodeficiency virus (HIV)-positive patients are at increased risk.[6] Nonspecific symptoms such as dyspnea, fever, chills, and night sweats develop slowly, and a friction rub or chest pain is often absent. The ECG is usually unrevealing, but the chest radiograph may be most useful when findings of pulmonary tuberculosis are present (Figs. 2 and 3). A patient with suspected or diagnosed pericardial tuberculosis should be hospitalized, and antituberculous therapy (e.g., rifampin, isoniazid, streptomycin, ethambutol) started promptly.

Analysis of the pericardial fluid shows high specific gravity, very high protein level (often >6 g/dL), and predominantly lymphocytic cells. A pericardial biopsy with acid-fast bacilli polymerase chain reaction testing is recommended for all patients with suspected tuberculous pericarditis. However, a normal pericardial biopsy does not exclude the diagnosis.

Uremic and Dialysis-Associated Pericarditis

Uremic pericarditis occurs in 6% to 10% of patients with advanced renal failure before hemodialysis is initiated; blood urea nitrogen levels usually exceed 60 mg/dL. The typical ST-segment elevation on the ECG usually is absent. A large hemorrhagic effusion caused by impaired platelet function is common, although tamponade is rare. Dialysis-associated pericarditis is caused by fluid overload, and the fluid is usually serous. With both forms, initiation or intensification of hemodialysis is indicated, usually leading to improvement in 1 to 2 weeks.[7,8]

Pericarditis following Myocardial Infarction

Post-MI pericarditis is a common complication (25%-40% of patients with MI) and occurs early, within 3 to 10 days after the MI. Its development correlates with the extent of necrosis, is more common with anterior than inferior infarcts, and is associated with a higher 1-year mortality rate and incidence of congestive heart failure.[9]

The diagnosis of post-MI pericarditis requires symptoms or a new pericardial friction rub; a pericardial effusion alone is nonspecific. In addition to the typical ST elevation seen with acute pericarditis that may be difficult to differentiate from the actual MI in this setting, findings on the ECG are persistently positive T waves more than 2 days after MI or normalization of previously inverted T waves.[10]

Post–Cardiac Injury Syndrome. Dressler's syndrome typically occurs 2 to 3 weeks after MI or open heart surgery. An autoimmune component and possibly a latent viral infection are believed to be responsible. The fully expressed syndrome consists of pleuritic chest pain, fever, leukocytosis, and a pericardial friction rub. Pleural effusions or pulmonary infiltrates may be seen.[11]

Box 1 Common Causes of Pericarditis and Pericardial Effusion

Idiopathic
Infectious

- Bacterial
- Fungal
- HIV
- Viral

Myocardial infarction
Radiation
Postoperatively after open heart surgery
Chest trauma

- Blunt
- Sharp

Malignancy

- Primary: mesothelioma, angiosarcoma
- Metastatic: lung, breast, bone, lymphoma, melanoma

Collagen vascular diseases

- Rheumatoid arthritis
- Systemic lupus erythematosus

Metabolic

- Hypothyroidism
- Uremia

Pharmacologic

- Cromolyn sodium
- Doxorubicin
- Hydralazine
- Methysergide
- Minoxidil
- Penicillin
- Phenytoin
- Procainamide

HIV, human immunodeficiency virus.

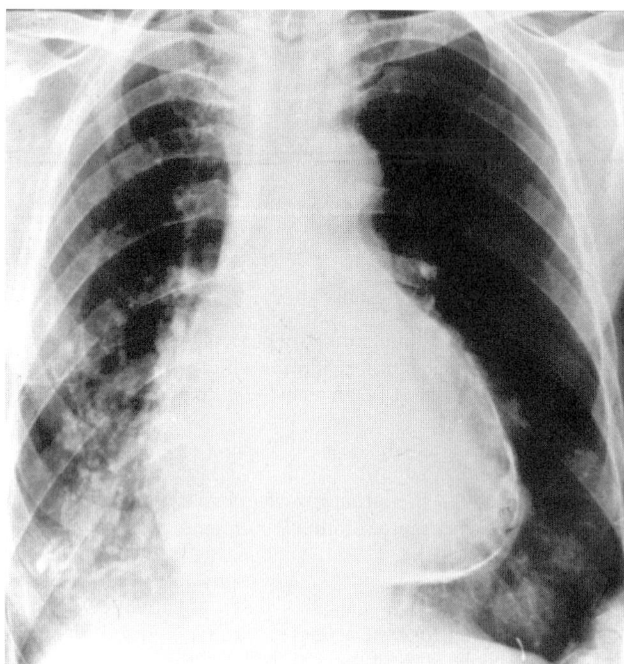

Figure 2 Extensive pericardial calcifications on chest radiograph (posteroanterior projection). Extensive pulmonary infiltrates caused by tuberculosis can be noted (also see Fig. 3).

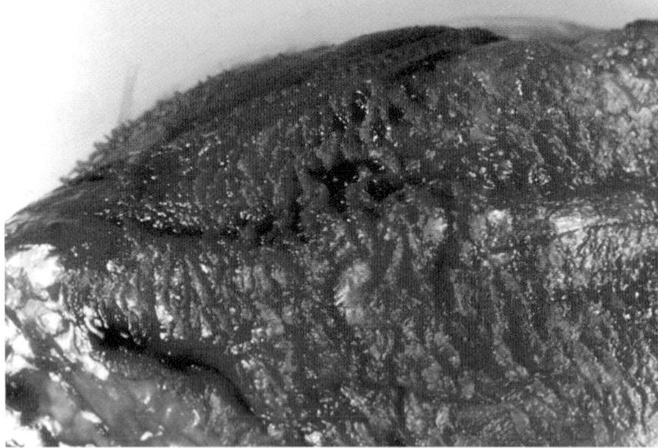

Figure 1 Fibrinous pericarditis. Extensive fibrin deposits in the pericardial space can be seen.

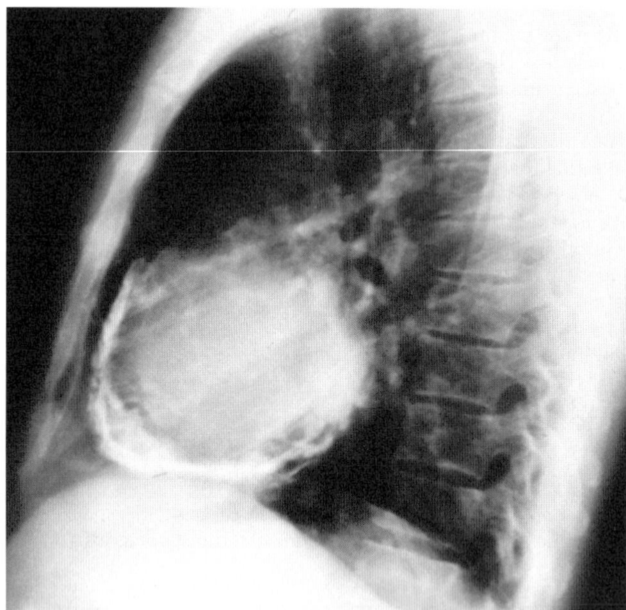

Figure 3 Extensive pericardial calcifications on chest radiograph (lateral projection). These were caused by tuberculosis (also see Fig. 2).

Malignancy

Pericarditis associated with malignancy is caused mostly by metastatic disease. Pericarditis is common in metastasized bronchogenic or breast carcinoma, Hodgkin's disease, and lymphoma (Fig. 4); it is rare in primary mesothelioma and angiosarcoma. Diagnosis is based on analysis of pericardial fluid cytology, which has a sensitivity ranging from 70% to 90% and a specificity of 95% to 100%.[1]

Radiation Pericarditis

Recent or remote mediastinal radiation can cause pericarditis at any time from weeks to months after the exposure.

Traumatic Pericarditis

Sharp or blunt trauma (Figs. 5 to 7) and even a minimally invasive procedure such as cardiac diagnostic or interventional catheterization has been associated with pericardial irritation.

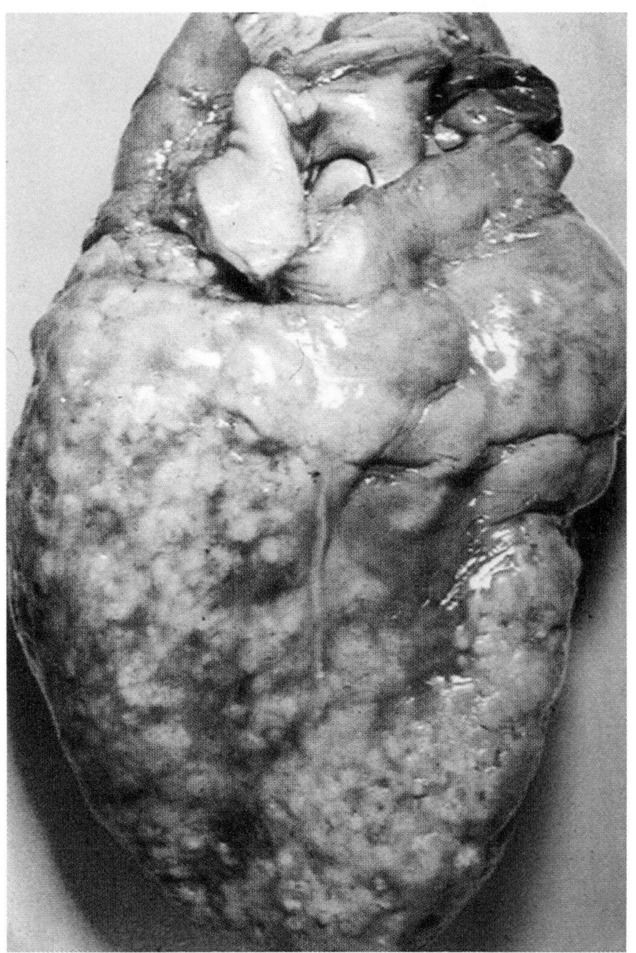

Figure 4 **Metastatic infiltration of the pericardial space.** The primary tumor was a lymphoma.

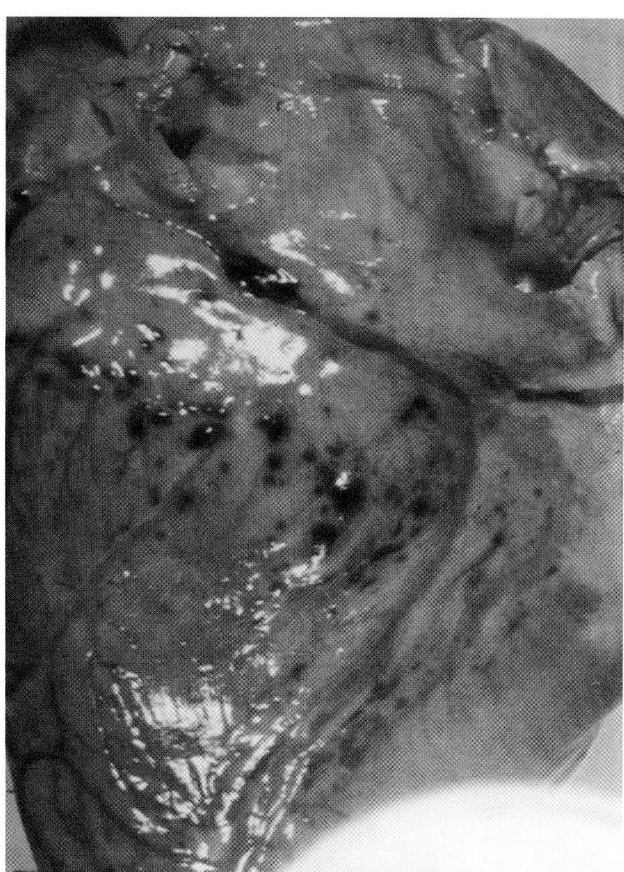

Figure 5 **Hemorrhagic pericarditis.** The patient underwent chest compressions during resuscitative efforts.

Table 1 Stages of Acute Pericarditis by Electrocardiography

Stage	Time	ST Segment	T Wave	PR Segment
1	Hours	Diffuse elevation	Upright	Leads aV_R, V_1: elevation All others: depression
2	Days	Resolution	Flattening	Resolution
3	Days to weeks		Inversion	
4	Days to weeks		Upright	

Table 2 Electrocardiographic Differentiation of Acute Pericarditis and Myocardial Infarction

Parameter	Acute Pericarditis	Acute Myocardial Infarction
ST elevation	Diffuse in I, II, and III Originating from S wave Concave Lead V_6: ST-T amplitude >0.24 mm	Focal—vascular territory Originating from R wave Convex
ST depression	Lead aV_R only	Present; reciprocal changes to ST elevation according to territory
PR segment	Leads aV_R, V_1: elevation frequent	Rare changes if atrial infarction is present

Diagnosis

The diagnosis of acute pericarditis remains a clinical one based on history, physical examination, and the ECG. Other imaging studies, including computed tomography (CT), magnetic resonance imaging (MRI), and echocardiography, may be used in selected cases to investigate the pericardium.

Electrocardiography

The ECG in acute pericarditis has four consecutive stages (Table 1). Stage 1, characterized by diffuse ST elevation, is the most useful stage for the diagnosis of acute pericarditis (Fig. 8). The distinction between pericarditis and acute MI is difficult at times, but there are several clues (Table 2).[12] Troponin levels may be elevated in up to 50% of patients with pericarditis but in the absence of myocarditis, the prognosis remains unchanged.[13]

Chest Radiography

The chest radiograph may be entirely normal unless there is a pericardial effusion causing cardiomegaly (Fig. 9) or there are changes caused by an underlying disease.

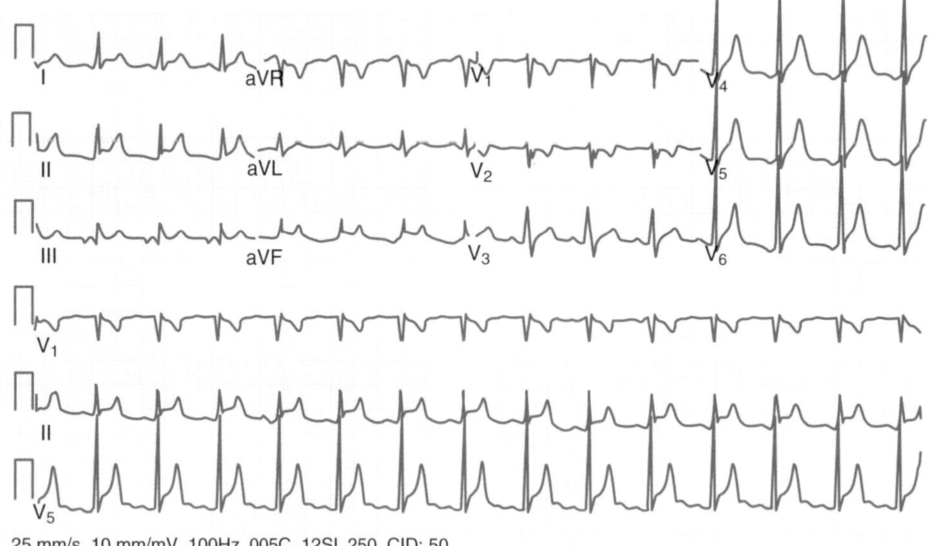

Figure 6 **Hemopericardium.**

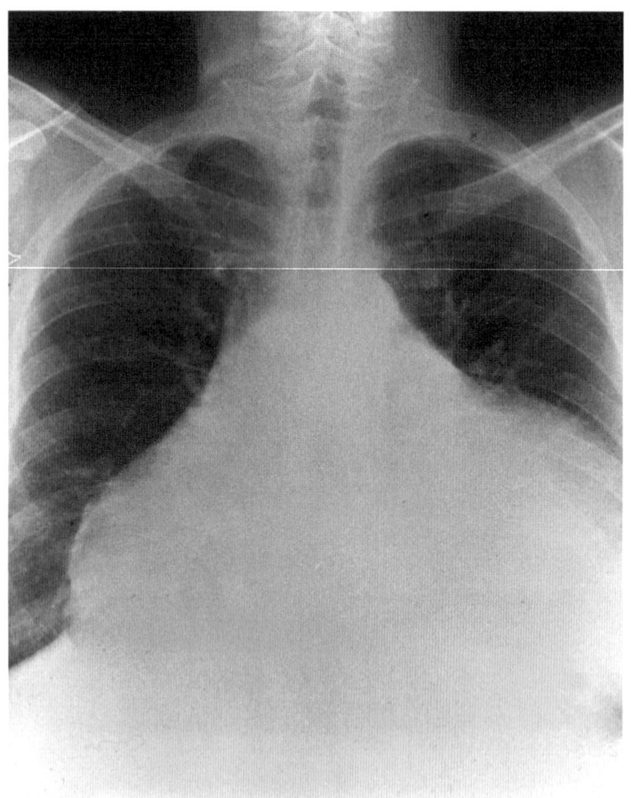

Figure 7 **Hemopericardium after blunt chest trauma.**

Echocardiography

An episode of acute pericarditis that responds well to therapy may be followed clinically. Indications for echocardiography are symptoms persisting for longer than 1 to 2 weeks, the presence of hemodynamic abnormalities, clinical suspicion of a large or increasing pericardial effusion, or recent cardiac surgery.

Treatment

Most cases of acute pericarditis are uncomplicated and self-limited and may be treated on an outpatient basis. Indications for an imaging modality, hospital admission, or both include clinical suspicion of a large effusion, hemodynamic instability, severe pain or other symptoms, suspicion of a serious underlying condition, or any other signs or symptoms of clinical instability or impending deterioration.

Medical Management

Treatment of the underlying disease is the mainstay of therapy.[14] Nonsteroidal anti-inflammatory drugs (NSAIDs) can be used for pain relief; agents such as indomethacin and aspirin have similar efficacy.[15] Ibuprofen may be started at a dose of 400 mg every 8 hours and increased for symptom relief.[15] Ketorolac tromethamine may be used as a parenteral agent for relief of symptoms.[16] NSAIDs are contraindicated in the early period (<7-10 days) after MI (can predispose to cardiac rupture), and aspirin should be used instead.

If pericarditis recurs (20%-30% of patients) or response to NSAIDs is poor, prednisone may be started at high doses and then tapered over 3 weeks. Use of steroids in acute pericarditis can promote a recurrence.[17] As with NSAIDs, steroids should be avoided in post-MI pericarditis because there is an increased incidence of myocardial wall rupture.

Colchicine may be effective for persistent or refractory cases of Dressler's syndrome and idiopathic pericarditis.[18,19] The COPE (Colchicine for Acute Pericarditis) trial found that colchicine in addition to aspirin reduces the recurrence of pericarditis from 32.3% to 10.7%.[20] If they are not mandatory, anticoagulants should be avoided during the acute phase of pericarditis to reduce the risks of bleeding and tamponade.

Pericardiectomy

Indications for pericardiectomy include the development of pericardial constriction and, rarely, recurrent pericarditis. Pericardiectomy is the most definitive procedure, with almost no recurrence; the 30-day perioperative mortality rate is about 5%.

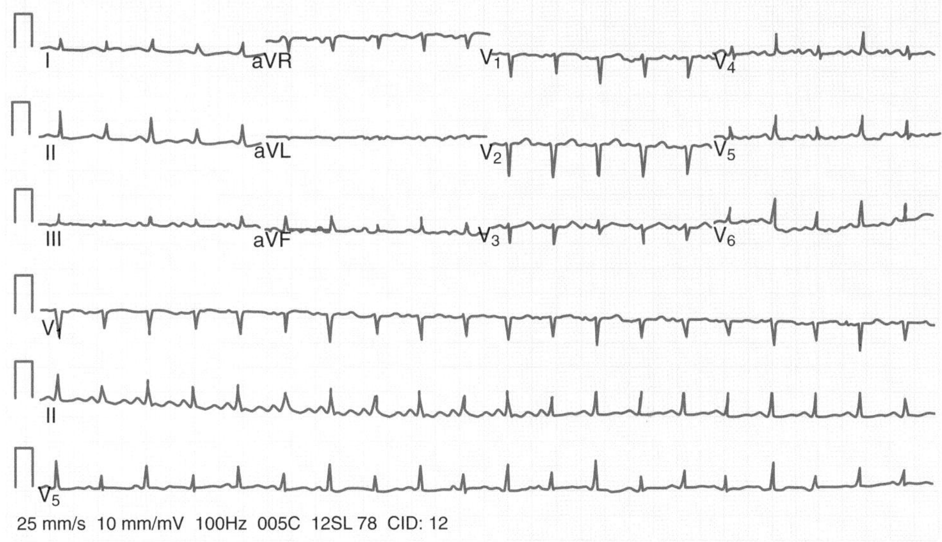

Figure 8 **Stage 1 of acute pericarditis.** There are diffuse concave ST elevation and PR elevation in the aV_R and V_1 leads.

Outcomes

Patients with uncomplicated acute pericarditis should have regular follow-up after the initial visit to ensure resolution of symptoms and rule out the development of constrictive symptoms.

PERICARDIAL EFFUSION

Definition

Pericardial effusion is defined as an increased amount of pericardial fluid.

Etiology

The most common causes of large pericardial effusions (see Box 1) are malignancy (25% of cases), infection (27%), collagen vascular disease (12%), and chest radiation (14%).[21,22] A pericardial effusion is the most common cardiovascular manifestation of acquired immunodeficiency syndrome and is associated with a worse outcome.[23-25]

Pathophysiology

The pericardial sac normally contains 15 to 30 mL of fluid; it can hold 80 to 200 mL of fluid acutely and even up to 2 L if the fluid accumulates slowly. The development of tamponade depends on the rate of accumulation rather than on the volume of the effusion. Typically, signs of right ventricular diastolic failure develop first, followed by left-sided symptoms. As the understanding of tamponade has evolved, it has been shown that cardiac hemodynamics can be altered early, because fluid accumulates without clinical evidence of tamponade.[26]

Signs and Symptoms

Symptoms arise from the compression of surrounding structures (lung, stomach, phrenic nerve) or diastolic heart failure and include chest pressure or pain, dyspnea, nausea, abdominal fullness, and dysphagia. Phrenic nerve irritation can cause hiccup.

With a small effusion, the physical examination is unremarkable. Larger effusions cause muffled heart sounds and, rarely, Ewart's sign (dullness to percussion, bronchial breath sounds, and egophony below the angle of the left scapula). With increasing volume of the effusion, signs and symptoms of cardiac tamponade can occur.

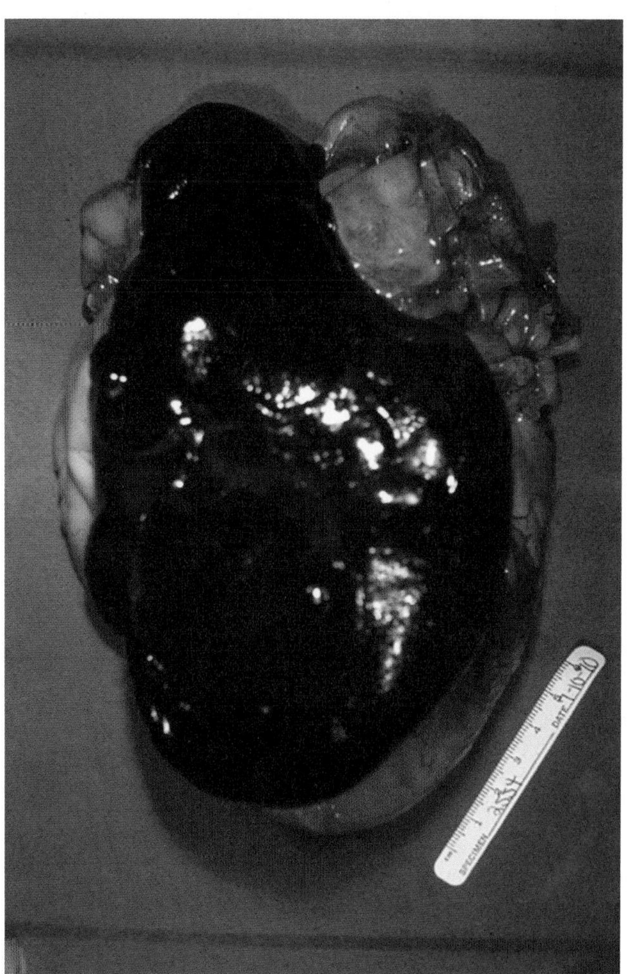

Figure 9 **Chest radiograph of cardiomegaly.** This patient had a very large pericardial effusion.

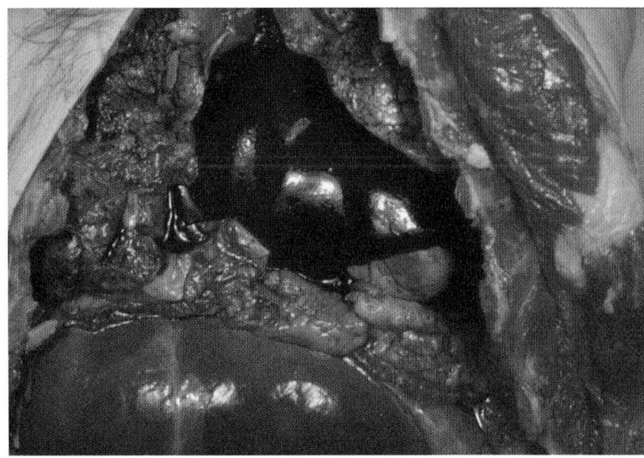

Figure 10 Electrical alternans seen on the electrocardiogram. Note the varying amplitudes of the QRS complexes caused by the swinging of the heart in a large pericardial effusion, which causes variation of the electrical axis with every heartbeat.

Table 3 Sizing of Pericardial Effusion by Echocardiography

Parameter	Small	Medium	Large
Volume (mL)	<100	100-500	>500
Localization	Localized	Circumferential	Circumferential
Width (cm)	<1	1-2	>2

Diagnosis

Electrocardiography

Low-voltage and electrical alternans (Fig. 10) may be seen if the effusion is large.

Chest Radiography

Cardiomegaly occurs if there is more than 250 mL of fluid in the pericardial sac (see Fig. 9). Displacement of the pericardial lining more than 2 mm away from the lower heart border is best seen on lateral film.[27,28]

Echocardiography

A pericardial effusion causes an echo-free space between visceral and parietal pericardium; the extent of the space defines the size of the effusion (Table 3). Large effusions can produce the picture of a swinging heart. Although echocardiography is the imaging modality of choice for diagnosing a pericardial effusion, it can miss small loculated effusions.

Magnetic Resonance Imaging and Computed Tomography

CT is the best imaging modality for assessing the pericardium itself, being slightly superior to MRI in spatial resolution. Both are superior to echocardiography in detecting loculated effusions.

Laboratory Tests

Laboratory analysis in a patient with a pericardial effusion should include a complete blood count, chemistry panel, and erythrocyte sedimentation rate. Further testing should be done according to clinical suspicion.

Table 4 Pericardial Effusion: Exudate Versus Transudate

Parameter	Exudate	Transudate
Cause	Malignancy Infectious, parainfectious Postpericardiotomy syndrome Collagen vascular disease	Radiation Uremia Hypothyroidism Trauma
Specific gravity (g/mL)	>1.015	<1.015
Total protein (g/dL)	>3.0	<3.0
Fluid–to–serum protein ratio	>0.5	<0.5
Fluid–to–serum LDH ratio	>0.6	<0.6
Fluid–to–serum glucose ratio	<1.0	>1.0

LDH, lactate dehydrogenase.

Analysis of Pericardial Fluid

Pericardiocentesis should be performed for diagnostic purposes if the cause is unclear or if malignancy or tuberculous, fungal, or bacterial infection is suspected. Therapeutic pericardiocentesis should be performed for large effusions that are increasing in size or those causing pretamponade or tamponade.

The initial inspection should assess whether the fluid is hemorrhagic, purulent, or chylous. A red blood cell count higher than 100,000/mm^3 is suggestive of trauma, malignancy, or pulmonary embolism (rare). Chylous fluid implies injury to the thoracic duct by trauma or infiltration. The fluid should be sent for a cell count; Gram stain; culture; cytology; acid-fast bacilli; determination of glucose, protein, and lactate dehydrogenase (LDH) levels; and specific gravity. The parameters listed in Table 4 have a high sensitivity for differentiating exudates versus transudates. An elevated protein level higher than 6.0 g/dL often indicates tuberculous, purulent, or parapneumonic effusion. An isolated increased fluid LDH level (>300 U/dL) with a normal serum LDH level is most likely caused by malignancy. A low pericardial fluid glucose level (<60-80 mg/dL) may be caused by parapneumonic, rheumatoid, tuberculous, or malignant effusion. However, no diagnostic test of pericardial fluid is specific for effusion associated with postpericardiotomy syndrome, radiation or uremic pericarditis, hypothyroidism, or trauma. The overall diagnostic yield of pericardial fluid analysis and biopsy is low (about 20%), emphasizing the importance of clinical history and examination.[5]

Treatment

The medical management of pericardial effusion is based on treating the underlying cause.[29] Diuretics may help decrease the intensity of fluid overload symptoms. Effusions causing pretamponade or tamponade require immediate drainage. Volume expansion and inotropic support may be used for hemodynamic stabilization pending drainage. In the immediate postoperative setting, surgical management and open drainage are preferred because of the high incidence of loculated effusions.

Pericardiocentesis

Echocardiographically guided pericardiocentesis is safe and effective. Pericardiocentesis is indicated for a large effusion with hemodynamic compromise or tamponade or for diagnostic purposes.

Surgical Treatment

Percutaneous balloon pericardiotomy is the least invasive of the surgical procedures. It is used mostly for neoplastic effusion with a poor prognosis as a palliative treatment option. The success rate for relieving reaccumulation of pericardial fluid is 85% to 92% at 30 days. It may be performed in the catheterization laboratory under fluoroscopy using a balloon-dilating catheter.

Subxyphoid pericardiostomy, also known as a pericardial window, may be done under local anesthesia. It has a high success rate, with few complications, and recurrence of fluid accumulation is rare.

Outcomes

After drainage, follow-up echocardiography to rule out reaccumulation and constrictive physiology should be performed in all patients. Cardiac tamponade can develop with large or rapidly accumulating effusions.[30]

CARDIAC TAMPONADE

Definition

Cardiac tamponade occurs when fluid accumulation in the finite pericardial space causes an increase in pressure, with subsequent cardiac compression and hemodynamic compromise.

Prevalence

Of patients with large pericardial effusions, 25% to 30% develop tamponade.[31]

Pathophysiology

The elevated intrapericardial pressure leads to progressive limitation of mostly early diastolic ventricular filling, resulting in low cardiac output.[32,33]

Signs and Symptoms

Symptoms

Symptoms resulting from decreased cardiac output and congestion include dyspnea, chest discomfort, weakness, restlessness, agitation, drowsiness, oliguria, and anorexia. If the tamponade develops acutely as a complication of an acute MI (free wall rupture) or trauma, the presentation is usually catastrophic, with sudden death or shock and high mortality (see Figs. 6 and 7).

Physical Examination Findings

The combination of the classic findings known as Beck's triad (hypotension, jugular venous distention, and muffled heart sounds) occurs in only 10% to 40% of patients. Tachycardia, tachypnea, and hepatomegaly are common. Pulsus paradoxus is defined as an inspiratory decline in systolic blood pressure of more than 10 mm Hg resulting from compression and poor filling of the left ventricle caused by increased venous return to right heart. Pulsus paradoxus is nonspecific and insensitive and can occur with extracardiac disease, such as severe chronic obstructive pulmonary disease or asthma.[34]

Diagnosis

Electrocardiography

The ECG may be unremarkable. Abnormal findings on ECG include electrical alternans (see Fig. 10), low voltage, and changes associated with acute pericarditis (see Fig. 8).

Transthoracic Echocardiography

Usually, a moderate-size or large pericardial effusion is present and leads to increasing compression and subsequent diastolic compression of the cardiac chambers, usually in the sequence right atrium, right ventricle, left atrium. The most sensitive finding for tamponade physiology on the echocardiogram is inferior vena cava plethora, with absent inspiratory collapse. Right ventricle inversion is the most accurate finding for diagnosis. Other, less-specific findings include excessive respiratory variations in diastolic mitral valve inflow, which is analogous to pulsus paradoxus.

Right Heart Catheterization

The most typical finding of right heart catheterization is equalization of mean right atrial, right ventricular and pulmonary artery diastolic, and mean pulmonary capillary wedge pressures.

Differential Diagnosis

The symptoms of pericardial tamponade can mimic those of right-sided heart failure, right ventricle infarction, constrictive pericarditis, and pulmonary embolism. However, with the use of echocardiography and right heart catheterization, these may be easily distinguished.

Treatment

Patients with pretamponade and tamponade require immediate hospital admission and prompt pericardial drainage by pericardiocentesis. The drain catheter may be left in place for up to 48 hours if drainage is slow or reaccumulation likely. If follow-up echocardiography documents fluid reaccumulation, a pericardial window should be considered, because the infection risk associated with a pericardial drain increases after 48 hours.[35] Pending drainage, intravenous fluid expansion and inotropic support may be used for hemodynamically unstable patients.

PERICARDIAL CONSTRICTION

Definition

Constrictive pericarditis refers to an abnormal thickening of the pericardium, resulting in impaired ventricular filling and decreased cardiac output.

Etiology

Most cases of pericardial constriction are idiopathic, although a history of acute or chronic pericarditis is occasionally elicited.

Pathophysiology

The initiating event causes a chronic inflammatory pericardial process, resulting in fibrinous thickening, calcification of the pericardium (Fig. 11; also see Figs. 2 and 3), and limitation of intrapericardial volume. This leads to impaired ventricular filling and decreased cardiac output. Ultimately, right and then left ventricular heart failure develop. Distinguishing heart failure caused by constrictive physiology from diastolic restrictive physiology is a classic diagnostic dilemma.

Signs and Symptoms

Clinical Symptoms

Symptoms are often vague and their onset is insidious; they include malaise, fatigue, and decreased exercise tolerance. With progression

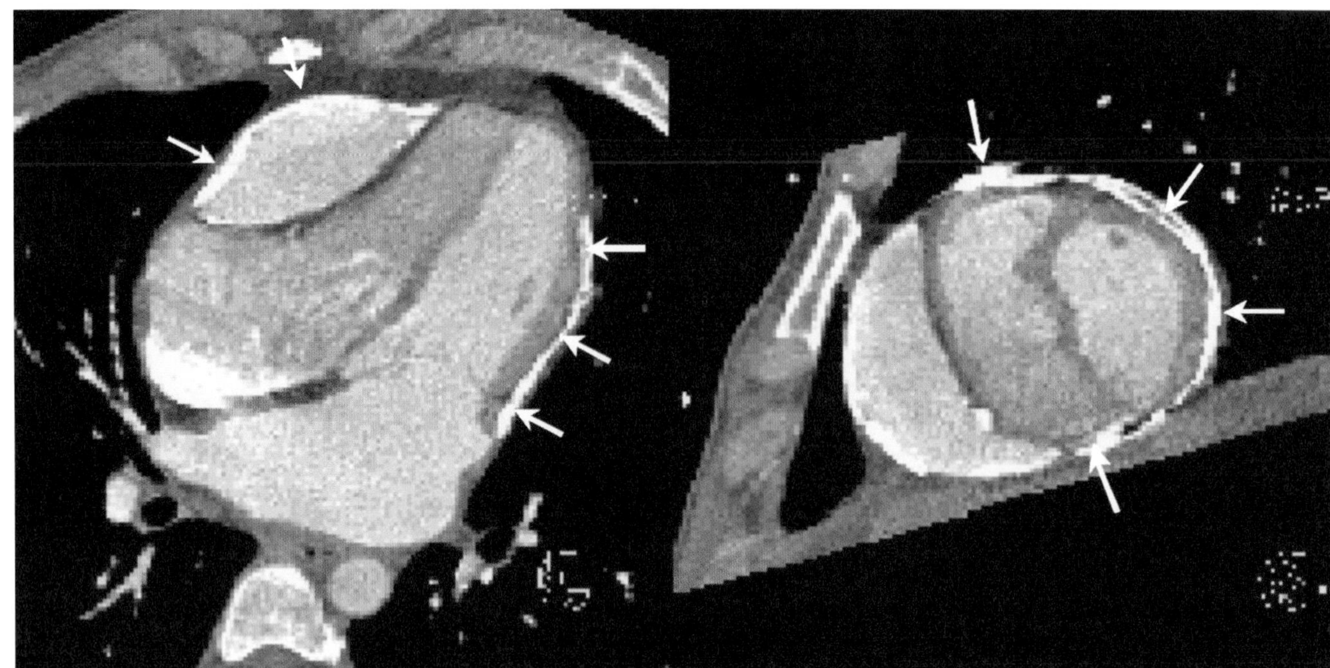

Figure 11 Computed tomographic image showing calcification of the pericardium *(arrows)*.

of constriction, symptoms of right-sided heart failure (e.g., peripheral edema, nausea, abdominal discomfort, ascites) become apparent and usually precede signs of left-sided failure (e.g., exertional dyspnea, orthopnea, paroxysmal nocturnal dyspnea).

Physical Examination Findings

Increased ventricular filling pressures cause jugular venous distention and Kussmaul's sign, (absent inspiratory decline of jugular venous distention), which is sensitive but not specific for constriction.[36] Auscultation reveals muffled heart sounds and occasionally a characteristic pericardial knock (60-200 msec after the second heart sound), which is caused by sudden termination of ventricular inflow by the encasing pericardium.

Constrictive effusive pericarditis consists of a tense pericardial effusion in the presence of pericardial constriction, and both tamponade and constrictive signs and symptoms are present. Therapy includes pericardiocentesis initially, followed by pericardiectomy for long-term management.[37]

Diagnosis

Electrocardiography

The ECG does not show specific findings, but low voltage may be seen.

Laboratory Test Findings

Brain natriuretic peptide (BNP) is a serum biomarker that can help distinguish constrictive pericarditis from restrictive cardiomyopathy. Despite elevated filling pressures in both conditions, levels of BNP are significantly higher in restrictive cardiomyopathy.[38]

Chest Radiography

Pericardial calcifications (see Figs. 2 and 3), pleural effusions, and biatrial enlargement may be noted on the chest radiograph.

Echocardiography

Echocardiography is the best imaging modality for assessing hemodynamic parameters noninvasively. M-mode echocardiography is useful for looking for flattening of the left ventricular free wall. Two-dimensional echocardiography shows septal bounce and inferior vena cava plethora with absent inspiratory collapse, as well as the effects of increased pericardial pressure on the relatively low-pressure right atrial and right ventricular chambers. Doppler echocardiographic findings have the highest sensitivity and specificity for detecting constrictive physiology. Excessive respiratory variations in transmitral, transtricuspid, pulmonary venous, and hepatic vein flow are characteristic.[39,40] More recently developed echocardiographic modalities such as tissue Doppler imaging have enhanced the ability to discriminate between restriction and constriction.[41]

Right Heart Catheterization

Direct pressure measurements are performed if there is doubt about the diagnosis. M- or W-shaped atrial pressure waveforms and square-root or dip-and-plateau right ventricular pressure waveforms reflect impaired ventricular filling. Because of the fixed and limited space within the thickened and stiff pericardium, end-diastolic pressure equalization (typically within 5 mm Hg) occurs between these cardiac chambers. Pulmonary artery systolic pressures are usually normal in pericardial constriction; higher pulmonary pressures suggest a restrictive cardiomyopathy.

Magnetic Resonance Imaging and Computed Tomography

CT is the imaging modality of choice to evaluate the pericardium, being slightly superior to MRI in spatial resolution. Pericardial calcifications can easily be identified on CT. Although the finding of thickened pericardium on the CT or MRI is specific for constriction, up to 18% of patients with constriction confirmed by other modalities do not have pericardial thickening (see Fig. 11).[42]

Treatment

Medical treatment is difficult and does not affect the natural progression or prognosis of the disease. Diuretics and a low-sodium diet may be tried for patients with mild to moderate (New York Heart Association [NYHA] Class I or II) symptoms or contraindications to surgery.[43] For most patients, pericardiectomy is advised; 80% to 90% of patients experience improvement and 50% experience complete relief of symptoms. The 30-day perioperative mortality rate averages 5% to 10%.[44,45]

Outcomes

Recurrence following surgery is caused mainly by incomplete resection. Without surgical treatment, biventricular failure develops.

Transient Constrictive Pericarditis

In a minority of patients, constrictive pericarditis resolves with medical therapy, without surgical intervention. Although most cases are caused by prior cardiovascular surgery, there may be other causes, with the exception of radiation. In select cases, a trial of medical therapy has been reported to be useful in the early stages of pericardial constriction.[46]

Summary

Acute Pericarditis

- Acute pericarditis manifests with the triad of acute chest pain, changes on the ECG, and a pericardial rub.
- Ninety percent of cases are idiopathic, and troponin levels are elevated in about 50% of cases.
- NSAIDs should be used for most patients, except post-MI pericarditis; steroids are an additional option for primary treatment.
- Steroids can increase the recurrence rate of pericarditis.
- Colchicine can reduce the recurrence of pericarditis.

Cardiac Tamponade

- Cardiac tamponade is a clinical diagnosis made by documenting pulsus paradoxus, jugular venous distention, and muffled heart sounds in the presence of a pericardial effusion.
- The signs depend on the volume of fluid in the pericardial sac and the rate at which the fluid accumulates.
- Echocardiography can confirm the diagnosis at an early stage and help with the drainage of the effusion.

Pericardial Constriction

- Pericardial constriction results from an abnormal thickening of the pericardium that causes an impairment of diastolic filling.
- The diagnosis can be made by noting hemodynamic derangements on echocardiography and a thickening of the pericardium on CT or MRI.
- About 20% of patients do not demonstrate thickening of the pericardium by CT.
- The treatment of choice is surgical excision of the pericardium.
- In a minority of patients, transient constriction can occur, which might respond to medical management.

Suggested Readings

Blanchard DG: Pericardial effusion and AIDS. Circulation 1996;94:2312.

Haley JH, Tajik AJ, Danielson GK, et al: Transient constrictive pericarditis: Causes and natural history. J Am Coll Cardiol 2004;43:271-275.

Imazio M, Bobbio M, Cecchi E, et al: Colchicine in addition to conventional therapy for acute pericarditis: Results of the COlchicine for acute PEricarditis (COPE) trial. Circulation 2005;112:2012-2016.

Lange RA, Hillis LD: Clinical practice. Acute pericarditis. N Engl J Med 2004;351:2195-2202.

Leya FS, Arab D, Joyal D, et al: The efficacy of brain natriuretic peptide levels in differentiating constrictive pericarditis from restrictive cardiomyopathy. J Am Coll Cardiol 2005;45:1900-1902.

Little WC, Freeman GL: Pericardial disease. Circulation 2006;113:1622-1632.

Meyers DG, Meyers RE, Prendergast TW: The usefulness of diagnostic tests on pericardial fluid. Chest 1997;111:1213-1221.

Schifferdecker B, Spodick DH: Nonsteroidal anti-inflammatory drugs in the treatment of pericarditis. Cardiol Rev 2003;11:211-217.

Talreja DR, Edwards WD, Danielson GK, et al: Constrictive pericarditis in 26 patients with histologically normal pericardial thickness. Circulation 2003;108:1852-1857.

Zipes DP, Libby P, Bonow RO, Braunwald E (eds): Braunwald's Heart Disease: A Textbook of Cardiovascular Medicine, 7th ed. Philadelphia, WB Saunders, 2005.

References

For a complete list of references, log onto www.expertconsult.com.

Hypertrophic Cardiomyopathy

Michael S. Chen and Harry Lever

DEFINITION AND ETIOLOGY

Hypertrophic cardiomyopathy (HCM) is defined as hypertrophy of the myocardium more than 1.5 cm, without an identifiable cause (Fig. 1). Other causes of left ventricular (LV) hypertrophy, such as long-standing hypertension and aortic stenosis, must be excluded before HCM can be diagnosed. As our understanding of the genetics of HCM progresses, HCM will likely be diagnosed based on genetic testing, with transthoracic echocardiography (TTE) used to assess the phenotypic manifestations and clinical severity of the disease.

PREVALENCE AND RISK FACTORS

HCM is the most common genetic cardiovascular disease. Genetic mutations resulting in HCM primarily involve the cardiac sarcomere but may also involve the connective tissue matrix. The prevalence in the general adult population for people with phenotypic evidence of HCM is 1 per 500. Men are more often affected than women and blacks more often than whites. In young adults, HCM is the most common cause of sudden cardiac death.

Strenuous exercise by increasing afterload, such as heavy weight lifting, could theoretically increase the magnitude of LV hypertrophy and worsen obstruction in subjects with preexisting HCM. Risk factors for the development of end-stage HCM (manifesting as LV systolic dysfunction and LV dilatation) include younger age at onset of HCM, a family history of HCM, greater ventricular wall thickness, and certain genetic mutations.

PATHOPHYSIOLOGY AND NATURAL HISTORY

More than 150 mutations in 10 genes, primarily involving the myosin, actin, or troponin components of the cardiac sarcomere, have been identified as causes of HCM. Five of these mutations are considered especially malignant in light of their propensity for sudden cardiac death. However, a recent study of 293 HCM patients at the Mayo Clinic has assessed the prevalence of these malignant mutations and found that only three patients, or approximately 1%, had one of the malignant mutations for HCM. There are varying expressions of mutations for HCM.

HCM can be considered obstructive or nonobstructive, depending on the presence of a left ventricular outflow tract (LVOT) gradient, either at rest or with provocative maneuvers. Alternatively, HCM can be classified based on location of the hypertrophy, such as the proximal septum or the apex. Finally, there appear to be distinct forms of HCM at different ages. Younger patients often have more diffuse hypertrophy and reversal of septal curvature (Fig. 2), whereas older patients tend to have focal proximal septal hypertrophy, with a sigmoid septal morphology (Fig. 3). These may be two different disease processes, because subjects with reversal of septal curvature were found to have an almost 80% yield for screening for HCM-associated mutations but those with a sigmoid septum had less than a 10% yield. Hypertrophy often develops or worsens during the adolescent growth spurt. An apical variant of HCM also exists (Fig. 4).

LV hypertrophy usually involves thickening of the proximal portion of the interventricular septum, resulting in narrowing of the LVOT. Systolic anterior motion (SAM) of the mitral valve can occur if the mitral valve leaflets are pulled or dragged anteriorly toward the ventricular septum. SAM results in LVOT obstruction and mitral regurgitation. Consequently, the left ventricle has to generate higher pressures to overcome the LVOT obstruction. Premature closure of the aortic valve can occur and is caused by the decline in pressure distal to the LVOT obstruction.

The obstruction that occurs with HCM is dynamic, unlike the fixed obstructions of aortic stenosis and subvalvular aortic membranes. In dynamic obstruction, the degree of obstruction depends more on cardiac contractility and loading conditions than on fixed obstructions. An underfilled left ventricle results in greater obstruction, because there is less separation between the interventricular septum and mitral valve. Augmenting cardiac contractility also increases LVOT obstruction, because a more vigorous contraction is more likely to cause the obstructing components to come together. Most patients with HCM have a favorable prognosis. Complications of HCM include atrial fibrillation, ventricular arrhythmias, congestive heart failure, and sudden cardiac death.

End-stage HCM, which occurs in 5% of those with HCM, manifests as systolic LV dysfunction, thinning of the LV wall, and dilation of the ventricular cavity. Sudden cardiac death tends to occur in younger patients and can occur during heavy exertion, light exertion, or even at rest. In an unselected community-based population with HCM, the estimated incidence of sudden cardiac death is approximately 0.1% to 0.7% per year. HCM can also result in restrictive cardiomyopathy.

SIGNS AND SYMPTOMS

The clinical course of HCM is variable. Most patients with HCM are asymptomatic. For symptomatic patients, the occurrence and severity of symptoms do not necessarily correlate with the magnitude of the LVOT gradient. Symptoms appear to be associated more with the severity of mitral regurgitation and diastolic dysfunction.

Dyspnea on exertion is the most common symptom. Other complaints include chest pain with exertion, syncope or near syncope, or palpitations. Eating can exacerbate symptoms caused by splanchnic vasodilation and the resulting decrease in cardiac preload. Symptoms are often progressive. If patients develop some of the complications of HCM, such as atrial fibrillation or congestive heart failure, symptoms accompanying those particular conditions can occur, such as palpitations and orthopnea, paroxysmal nocturnal dyspnea, or leg edema, respectively.

Physical examination provides several clues suggestive of HCM. Palpation of the carotid pulse aids in distinguishing HCM from aortic stenosis or the presence of a subvalvular aortic membrane. With HCM, the carotid upstroke is brisk, because there is little resistance during early systole in ejecting the blood through the LVOT into the aorta. As systole progresses, LVOT obstruction occurs in HCM, resulting in a collapse in the pulse and then a secondary increase, a finding termed a *bisferiens pulse*. In contrast, because the fixed obstruction of aortic stenosis or subvalvular aortic membranes is present during the entire cardiac cycle, the carotid upstroke in these entities is the classic parvus et tardus pulse (small amplitude and delayed upstroke), a carotid pulse with delayed upstroke and amplitude. Thus, if any patient with a diagnosis of HCM has decreased carotid pulses, one should suspect misdiagnosis and carry out further investigation into fixed obstruction of the LVOT.

The lungs are usually clear and the jugular venous pressure normal. The point of maximal impulse will be forceful and sustained,

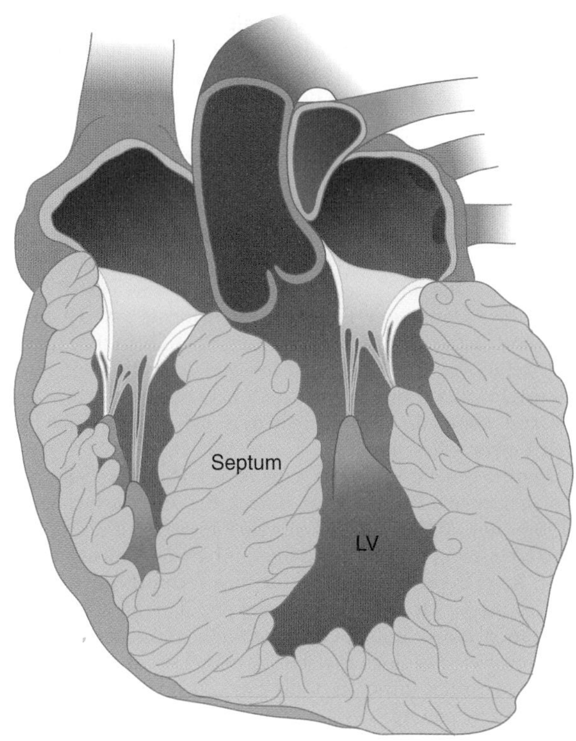

Figure 1 Gross pathology specimen of hypertrophic cardiomyopathy (HCM). Marked septal hypertrophy of the left ventricle (LV) can be seen.

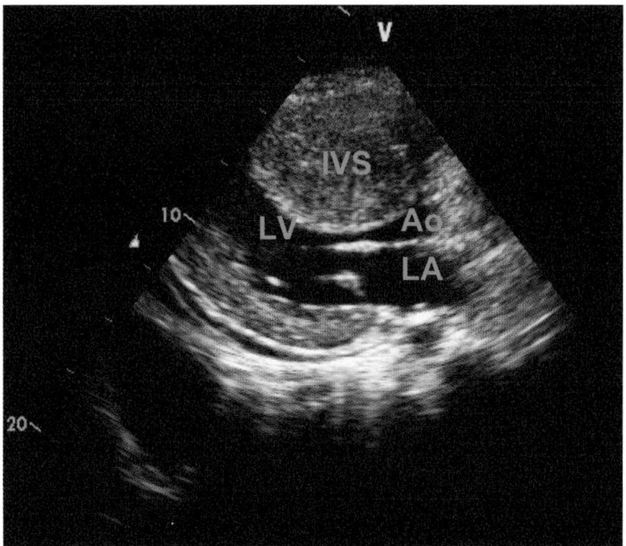

Figure 2 Diffuse hypertrophy variant of hypertrophic cardiomyopathy (HCM). This pattern of hypertrophy is classically seen in younger patients. Ao, aorta; IVS, interventricular septum; LA, left atrium; LV, left ventricle.

and a palpable S_4 gallop may be present. The classic auscultatory finding for HCM is a crescendo–decrescendo systolic murmur along the left sternal border that increases with the Valsalva maneuver. Almost all cardiac murmurs decrease in intensity during Valsalva, with the exception of HCM, so this maneuver is a crucial part of the cardiac examination if HCM is suspected (Table 1). The Valsalva maneuver decreases preload, which results in decreased filling of the left ventricle. An underfilled left ventricle results in an increase in

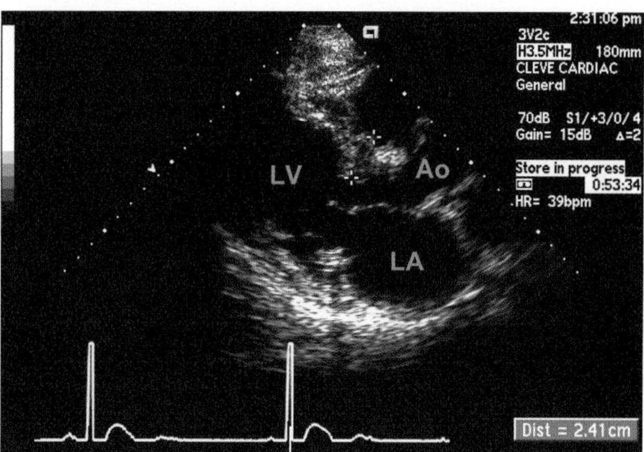

Figure 3 Proximal septal hypertrophy variant of hypertrophic cardiomyopathy (HCM). This pattern of hypertrophy is classically seen in older patients. Ao, aorta; LA, left atrium; LV, left ventricle.

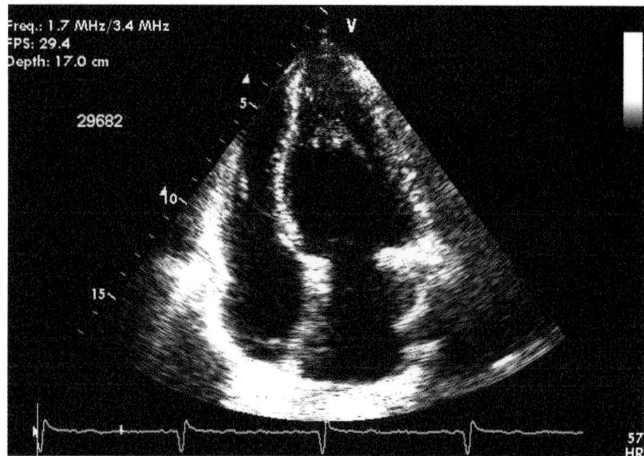

Figure 4 Apical hypertrophy variant of hypertrophic cardiomyopathy (HCM). In this type of HCM the hypertrophy involves mainly the apex.

Table 1 Effects of Physiologic and Pharmacologic Maneuvers on Hypertrophic Cardiomyopathy

Maneuver	Ventricular Volume	Murmur Intensity	LVOT Gradient
Hand grip	Increase	Decrease	Decrease
Valsalva	Decrease	Increase	Increase
Amyl nitrite	Decrease	Increase	Increase
Isoproterenol	Decrease	Increase	Increase
Beta blocker	Increase	Decrease	Decrease
Phenylephrine	Increase	Decrease	Decrease

LVOT, left ventricular outflow tract.

LVOT obstruction. Similarly, rising from squatting to standing decreases left ventricle preload and increases the intensity of the murmur. Finally, amyl nitrite, a profound vasodilator, decreases preload and causes a reflex tachycardia. This results in a louder murmur because of an increased degree of obstruction. In addition, it is imperative to auscultate carefully for a mitral regurgitation murmur; such a finding can indicate systolic anterior motion of the mitral valve, with accompanying mitral regurgitation. The remainder of the examination is generally unremarkable.

DIAGNOSIS

Laboratory Tests

Blood work generally is unremarkable. A chest radiograph may suggest LV hypertrophy but often is normal because the hypertrophy in HCM involves the ventricular septum. The electrocardiogram should show LV hypertrophy and occasionally may also have a pseudoinfarct pattern, in which Q waves are present despite the absence of coronary artery disease. Left atrial abnormality may be present if the patient has had long-standing mitral regurgitation from SAM of the mitral valve. Atrial fibrillation also may be present.

Imaging

Echocardiography is the gold standard for diagnosing HCM (see Figs. 2 to 4). With transthoracic echocardiogram (TTE), the septum can be well visualized and measured in the parasternal long, apical long, apical four-chamber, and parasternal short axis views. On TTE, one should note the septal thickness, location and pattern of hypertrophy, site and degree of left LVOT obstruction, presence of SAM of the mitral valve, presence of premature closure of the aortic valve, and any change in severity of obstruction with provocation. If no LVOT gradient is present in patients with HCM or suspected HCM, patients should undergo provocative testing with squatting, the Valsalva maneuver, or amyl nitrite to determine whether there is latent obstruction. To assess the functional significance of LVOT obstruction further, we often perform stress echocardiography studies in patients with HCM. Some patients have minimal resting gradients but develop large gradients with exercise. In our experience, supervised stress tests in patients with HCM are safe.

Transesophageal echocardiography and magnetic resonance imaging are other potential modalities for diagnosing HCM, particularly in subjects with technically difficult echocardiographic studies. Both modalities have superior resolution to transthoracic echocardiography but are more costly and, in the case of transesophageal echocardiography, more invasive.

Diagnostic Procedures and Differential Diagnosis

HCM should be differentiated from valvular aortic stenosis and a subvalvular aortic membrane. In aortic stenosis, the aortic valve is calcified and has restricted mobility. In HCM, the obstruction occurs below the aortic valve, and the valve structure and function are preserved. However, with aging, degenerative calcific disease of the aortic valve can make it difficult to distinguish between the two entities. A subvalvular aortic membrane is sometimes difficult to visualize on transthoracic echocardiography.

Continuous-wave Doppler imaging is useful in differentiating HCM from fixed obstructions, such as valvular aortic stenosis and a subvalvular membrane. Doppler imaging measures the velocity of blood over time. Fig. 5 illustrates the differences between Doppler signals from HCM and from fixed obstructions. With HCM, the continuous Doppler signal has a late systolic dagger shape; the obstruction is late peaking because of its dynamic nature. During early systole, blood still flows through the LVOT; however, with continued contraction of the left ventricle, exacerbated by systolic anterior motion of the mitral valve, the outflow tract area diminishes and an outflow tract gradient then develops. In contrast, a fixed obstruction is present during all of systole. Thus, the continuous-wave Doppler signal for fixed obstructions is a smoother contour that peaks earlier.

Cardiac catheterization has some value in diagnosing HCM, but advances in echocardiography have made the latter method the predominant means by which HCM is diagnosed. The left ventriculogram demonstrates cavity obliteration and a hyperdynamic left ventricle. LVOT gradients can be assessed by positioning a catheter near the left ventricle apex and recording ventricular pressures during slow catheter pullback. A classic sign of HCM is Brockenbrough's sign, in which the left ventricle-to-aortic gradient increases while the aortic pulse pressure decreases following premature ventricular contraction (PVC) (Fig. 6). Such a phenomenon occurs in HCM because the increased contractility in the post-PVC beat increases the dynamic LVOT obstruction. Patients with HCM often have no obstructive coronary artery disease, although they may have small vessel disease from increased collagen deposition and myocardial ischemia caused by the mismatch between myocardial oxygen supply and demand. This mismatch is driven primarily by the increased myocardial mass.

Currently, genetic testing is expensive and not usually helpful with management. Patients may have a mutation associated with HCM but not display the phenotypic manifestations of HCM. Genetic counseling may be considered for HCM patients and their families. At present, however, we do not recommend widespread genetic testing for HCM for the general population.

Myocardial biopsy is not performed for the purpose of diagnosing HCM. However, histologically, HCM manifests as hypertrophied, disorganized cardiac myocytes. Cells may take on bizarre shapes, and the connections among cells are often in disarray. Myocardial scarring and growth of the collagen matrix also occur. Scarring and disarray may form the substrate for arrhythmias. These pathologic abnormalities are not necessarily confined to the septum, because areas of the heart that appear grossly normal may also have these pathologic features.

Summary

- HCM is hypertrophy of the ventricular septum, generally 1.5 cm, which is not explained by other causes.
- Currently, transthoracic echocardiography is the gold standard for the diagnosis of HCM.
- In the future, genetic testing will allow identification of those possessing mutations associated with HCM; however, diagnosis of HCM as a clinical entity will still require an imaging modality that visualizes myocardial hypertrophy.
- HCM needs to be differentiated from other causes of LVOT obstruction, primarily aortic stenosis or a subvalvular aortic membrane. Brisk carotid upstrokes, a normal or minimally diseased aortic valve, lack of a subvalvular aortic membrane, and a dagger appearance to the Doppler profile of flow through the LVOT all indicate HCM.

Practice Guidelines

Consensus practice guidelines for HCM were published by a joint task force of the American College of Cardiology (ACC) and the European Society of Cardiology (ESC) in 2003. Overall, these guidelines also recommend transthoracic echocardiography as the best modality to make the clinical diagnosis of HCM, and the standard criterion is a LV wall thickness of at least 15 mm in the absence of other causes for hypertrophy. These guidelines also emphasize that *hypertrophic cardiomyopathy* is the preferred terminology for this disease entity because most HCM subjects do not have obstruction under resting conditions. Finally, subjects may have the HCM genotype without the phenotypic manifestations of HCM.

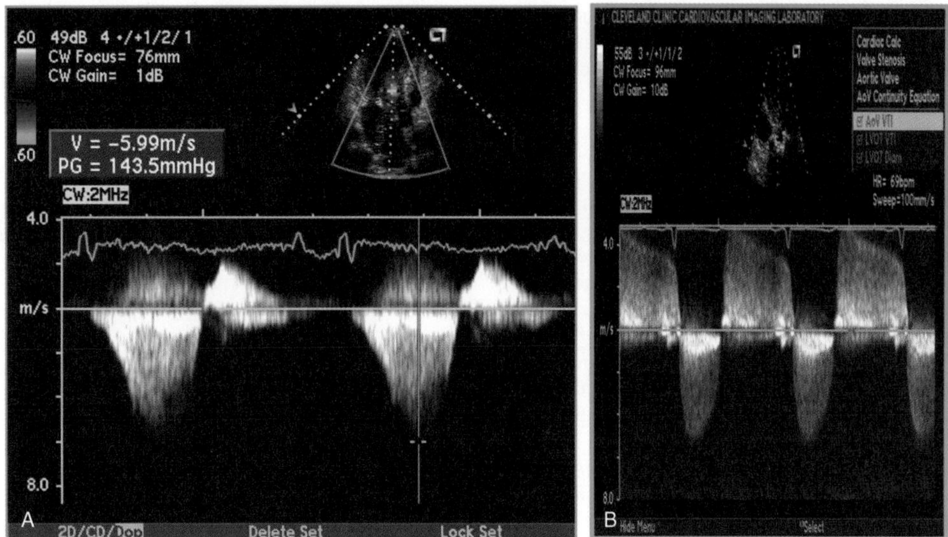

Figure 5 Comparison of Doppler profiles of hypertrophic cardiomyopathy (HCM) (A) and aortic stenosis (B). Because aortic stenosis is a fixed obstruction, a contour of the aortic valve gradient can be seen. In contrast, the Doppler profile of HCM is seen as the classic dagger shape, reflecting the dynamic obstruction.

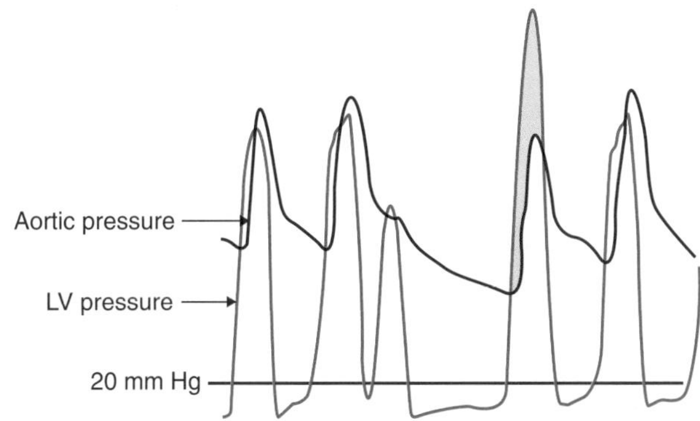

Figure 6 Brockenbrough's response. The Brockenbrough response in the post–premature ventricular contraction (PVC) is classic for hypertrophic cardiomyopathy (HCM). Post-PVC, there is increased preload secondary to a compensatory pause. The increased contractility associated with the post-PVC beat results in increased left ventricular outflow tract (LVOT) obstruction in HCM patients and a subsequent increase in the left ventricular-aortic gradient and decreased aortic pulse pressure during the post-PVC beat. In contrast, in subjects with no LVOT obstruction, a PVC results in increased cardiac contractility, but there is no left ventricle-aortic gradient, either at rest or in the post-PVC beat. The aortic pulse pressure in the post-PVC beat usually increases because of the increased contractility. LV, left ventricular.

TREATMENT

Treatment options for HCM include medical therapy, alcohol ablation, septal myectomy, and heart transplantation. Additionally, pacemaker implantation has been attempted, but results have indicated a substantial placebo effect.

Lifestyle Modifications

To prevent further disease progression, we recommend that HCM subjects avoid strenuous weight lifting, because weight lifting increases the afterload to the myocardium and can worsen hypertrophy. In addition, because of the risk of sudden cardiac death, subjects should avoid competitive athletics. Finally, patients should always remain well hydrated, so that the left ventricle does not become underfilled and result in worsening obstruction.

Medical Options

Beta blockers are considered first-line therapy for symptomatic HCM. By decreasing contractile force, beta blockers decrease the outflow gradient and decrease oxygen demand. Beta blockers also lengthen diastolic filling by slowing the heart rate. We generally start patients on metoprolol tartrate (Lopressor), 50 mg twice daily, or metoprolol succinate (Toprol-XL), 50 mg daily. If symptoms persist, the dose of metoprolol can be increased by 25-mg increments every few weeks. The peak dose is 400 mg/day. Contraindications to beta blockers include severe bronchospasm, marked bradycardia, and severe conduction system disease. Caution should be exercised with beta blocker use in patients with hepatic impairment. Fatigue is a common side effect of beta blockers.

Second-line therapy includes the calcium channel blocker verapamil because of its negative inotropic effect. The extended-release formulation of verapamil (Calan SR, Verelan, Isoptin SR) can be started at 240 mg daily and increased by 60 mg every few weeks. The maximum dose is approximately 480 mg daily. The dose should be decreased and shorter-acting agents should be considered for subjects with hepatic dysfunction. Verapamil should not be used in patients with severe pulmonary hypertension because they can develop excessive vasodilation, which worsens LVOT obstruction and cardiac output, resulting in pulmonary edema. Other contraindications to verapamil use include severe LV systolic dysfunction, conduction system disease, and hypotension. Diltiazem has been used in HCM patients, but there are few data on its effectiveness. Nifedipine, amlodipine, and felodipine should be avoided because they cause peripheral vasodilation, which can result in decreased LV filling and worsening of outflow tract obstruction.

Another second-line agent is disopyramide, a Class IA antiarrhythmic agent that has negative inotropic effects. The extended-release formulation of disopyramide (Norpace CR) may be started at 150 mg twice daily. This can then be increased to 300 mg twice daily in a few weeks if symptoms remain. The maximum dosage is 800 mg/day. The dose of disopyramide should be decreased if there is renal or hepatic dysfunction. Relative contraindications to disopyramide include decompensated congestive heart failure, baseline prolonged QTc interval, or severe conduction system disease.

Disopyramide is also used as an antiarrhythmic, and as such it has both antiarrhythmic and proarrhythmic properties. Common side effects of disopyramide include anticholinergic effects such as dry mouth, urinary retention, and blurred vision.

Atrial fibrillation is a common complication of HCM. In new-onset atrial fibrillation, the clinician should attempt to restore normal sinus rhythm with direct current cardioversion, antiarrhythmic agents, or both. If atrial fibrillation has been present for longer than 48 hours or the duration of atrial fibrillation is uncertain, transesophageal echocardiography (TEE) should be performed to ensure that there is no left atrial or left atrial appendage clot, or an anticoagulant should be given for at least 4 weeks before any electrical or chemical attempts at restoration of sinus rhythm. However, HCM patients often tolerate atrial fibrillation poorly, and TEE followed by electrical cardioversion is generally the preferred approach. Amiodarone or sotalol is the preferred therapy for pharmacologic conversion to or maintenance of sinus rhythm in HCM patients. Digoxin should be avoided in HCM patients, particularly those with resting or latent obstruction, because of its positive inotropic effect.

Treatment of persistent atrial fibrillation in HCM includes anticoagulation with warfarin and rate control, preferably with beta blockers. Atrial fibrillation ablation or a maze procedure may be considered for those with refractory, highly symptomatic atrial fibrillation. In a small number of patients with severe HCM and atrial fibrillation, we have performed combined maze and myectomy procedures.

Patients with HCM should receive prophylactic antibiotics for endocarditis prevention before dental or invasive procedures. Turbulent flow through the LVOT striking the aortic valve, as well as mitral regurgitation from systolic anterior motion of the mitral valve, predispose to endocarditis.

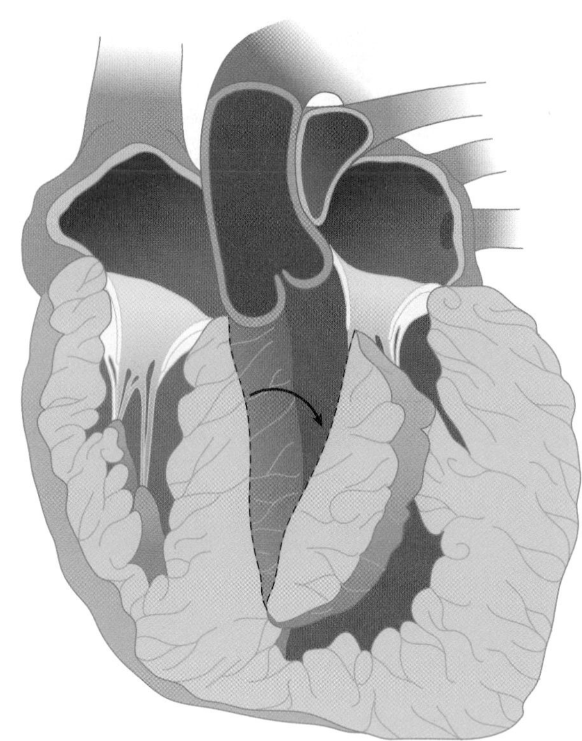

Figure 7 **Septal myectomy.** Septal myectomy involves resecting a portion of the proximal septum.

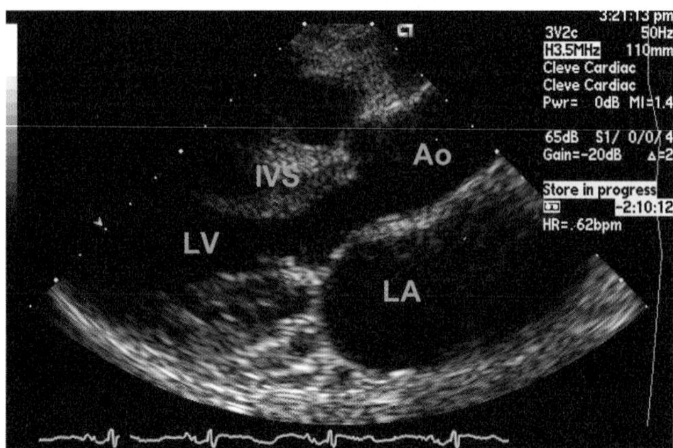

Figure 8 **Premyectomy.** A transthoracic echocardiographic image premyectomy is depicted. Ao, aorta; IVS, interventricular septum; LA, left atrium; LV, left ventricle.

Percutaneous and Surgical Options

Septal Myectomy

Septal myectomy involves resection of part of the proximal septum through an aortotomy (Fig. 7). Pre- and postmyectomy echocardiography images demonstrate a marked reduction in septal thickness after myectomy (Figs. 8 and 9). Abnormalities of the mitral valve, such as redundancy of the anterior or posterior mitral valve leaflet, may predispose to systolic anterior motion of the mitral valve. Thus, myectomy may sometimes be combined with mitral valve repair or replacement if mitral regurgitation or outflow tract obstruction persists on intraoperative TEE after myectomy has been performed. Myectomy may also be combined with coronary artery bypass grafting (CABG).

We recommend septal myectomy as first-line therapy for medically refractory HCM, particularly in young subjects who are otherwise in good health. If a patient remains symptomatic despite optimum medical therapy and has a resting or provocable gradient of 50 mm Hg or higher, septal myectomy should be considered. In contrast, we generally recommend continued aggressive medical management for subjects with gradients above 50 mm Hg if they remain asymptomatic or have only mild symptoms. Myectomy would then be performed for progression of symptoms. One exception is young, otherwise healthy subjects with gradients higher than 75 mm Hg. The low operative risk of these subjects tilts the balance in favor of earlier intervention. Septal myectomy is not indicated in apical hypertrophy.

Operative mortality for isolated myectomy is less than 2%. In one study from the Cleveland Clinic of 323 consecutive myectomy subjects from 1994 to 2004, subjects who underwent myectomy had 0% in-hospital mortality.

Septal myectomy decreases LVOT gradients, improves symptoms, and increases exercise capacity. Both the decrease in LVOT gradient and the decrease in any associated mitral regurgitation are responsible for improvement in symptoms. It is rare to require reoperation for recurrence of LVOT obstruction.

The risk that a myectomy patient will require a permanent pacemaker after myectomy depends on the health of the conduction system. In subjects with normal conduction systems, as noted on the electrocardiogram (ECG), there was a 2% rate of permanent pacemaker implantation after myectomy, whereas for patients with preexisting conduction abnormalities, there was a 10% incidence of permanent pacemaker implantation. Patients at highest risk for requiring a permanent pacemaker are those with preexisting right bundle branch block, because left bundle branch block occurs in more than 90% of patients after myectomy.

Long-term isolated myectomy has had excellent results, with survival rates of 93% to 96% at 5 years and 83% to 87% at 10 years. Factors portending to higher mortality rates include age 50 years or

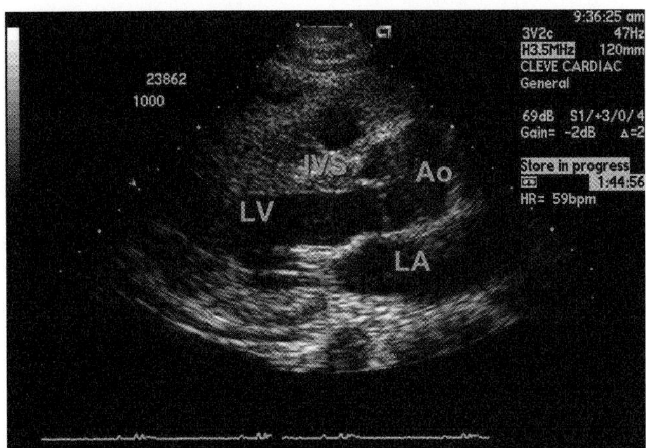

Figure 9 **Postmyectomy.** A transthoracic echocardiographic image postmyectomy is depicted. Note the marked decrease in septal thickness as compared with Figure 8. Ao, aorta; IVS, interventricular septum; LA, left atrium; LV, left ventricle.

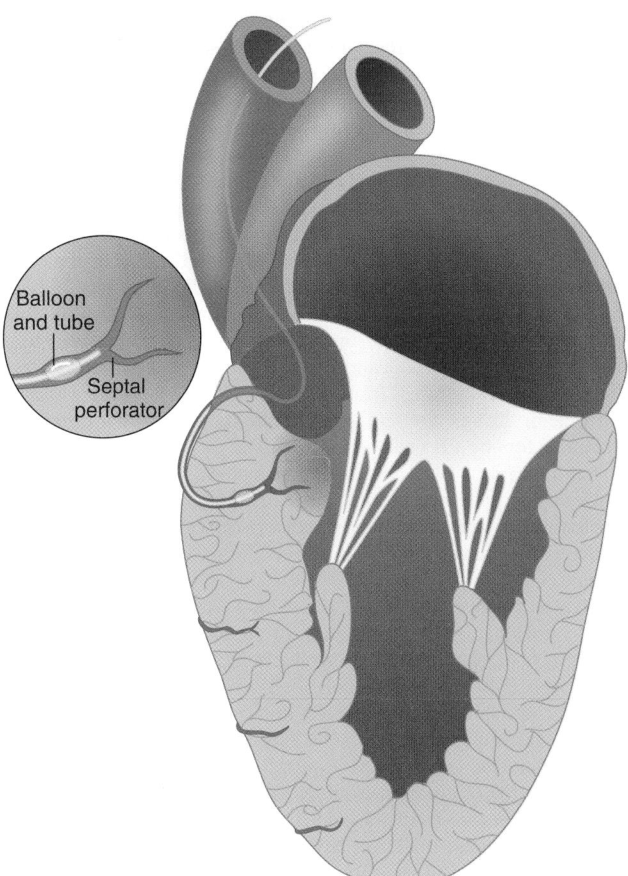

Figure 10 **Alcohol septal ablation.** A balloon is inflated in the proximal septal perforator, and alcohol is then injected into the septal artery through the distal port of the balloon. The goal is to create a controlled myocardial infarction of the proximal septum, resulting in necrosis and shrinkage of the septum and thus a decrease in the left ventricular outflow tract obstruction.

older at time of surgery, female gender, concomitant CABG, history of preoperative atrial fibrillation, and left atrial diameter of at least 46 mm. Concomitant open heart procedures at the time of myectomy are associated with higher long-term mortality rates. Patients undergoing myectomy in conjunction with CABG or valve surgery have demonstrated 5-year survival rates of 80%.

No randomized data exist assessing long-term survival in HCM patients undergoing medical management versus myectomy. However, retrospective, nonrandomized data suggest that HCM patients undergoing myectomy have lower mortality rates than HCM patients with obstruction who did not undergo surgery. It has further been suggested that long-term survival for HCM subjects who have undergone myectomy becomes equivalent to that of the age- and gender-matched general population.

Percutaneous Alcohol Septal Ablation

Alcohol ablation was first reported in 1995, and its popularity subsequently surged. By 2000, more than 3000 alcohol ablations had been performed, more than the number of myectomies performed over 40 years. At the Cleveland Clinic, most alcohol ablations have been performed on older or suboptimal surgical candidates, or both. We prefer that the septum be between 1.8 and 2.5 cm to provide a safety margin; if the septum is too thick, favorable ablation results may be difficult to attain, and if it is too thin, the patient is at higher risk for developing a ventricular septal defect. A septum less than 1.8 cm thick in a patient with the clinical picture of HCM suggests that mitral valve abnormalities, such as long leaflets, abnormal insertion of the papillary muscles, or anterior displacement of the mitral valve apparatus, may be the primary cause for the LVOT obstruction. Such mitral valve abnormalities contraindicate alcohol septal ablation, because the primary cause of LVOT obstruction in these cases is mitral valve abnormalities rather than a thick septum.

We consider alcohol septal ablation as second-line therapy for medically refractory HCM, in part because of concerns about the formation of scar tissue in the myocardium that occurs with ablation, with the accompanying potential arrhythmogenic substrate. In HCM patients with symptoms refractory to optimum medical management and a resting or provocative gradient of 50 mm Hg who are poor surgical candidates or those who refuse open heart surgery, percutaneous alcohol septal ablation is another option. For the most definitive treatment of HCM, we generally do not recommend alcohol septal ablation for reasonable surgical candidates but instead recommend myectomy.

Alcohol septal ablation is performed in the catheterization laboratory. Diagnostic coronary angiography is first performed to assess whether septal ablation is possible, based on the vessel size and area of myocardium subtended by the septal perforators. Echocardiography must also be reviewed to ensure that the LVOT obstruction is a result of contact of the mitral valve with the proximal septum. Because the goal of alcohol ablation is necrosis of part of the proximal septum, alcohol ablation will not benefit the patient if the LVOT obstruction occurs in the mid or distal LV cavity.

First, a temporary pacing wire is placed in the right ventricle to provide protection against complete heart block, which can occur during ablation. Next, through a guide catheter, a coronary guidewire is directed into the first major septal perforator (or the perforator that supplies the proximal septum) of the left anterior descending artery. Rarely, the major septal perforator arises off a diagonal branch of the left anterior descending artery or left circumflex artery. An over-the-wire balloon is then inflated in the septal perforator (Fig. 10). Myocardial contrast echocardiography is performed by injecting contrast through the distal lumen of the coronary balloon into the septal perforator to visualize the size and location of myocardium supplied by the chosen septal perforator. This contrast injection also verifies that no leakage has occurred proximal to the inflated balloon in the septal perforator. Any leakage could be disastrous, because it would result in alcohol flowing antegrade into the left anterior descending artery, causing a myocardial infarction.

After verification of the territory supplied by the septal perforator and ruling out any leaks retrograde in the septal perforator, 1 to 3 mL of desiccated ethanol is instilled into the septal perforator through the distal lumen of the balloon. Alcohol acts as a toxic agent to the coronary artery and surrounding myocardium, resulting in a controlled myocardial infarction of the cardiac muscle supplied by the septal perforator. Consequently, the proximal septum shrinks, LVOT obstruction lessens, and any associated systolic anterior motion is also decreased. In comparison with the effects of septal myectomy on LVOT obstruction, which are instantaneous, the effects of alcohol ablation on LVOT obstruction take longer to manifest because necrosis of the proximal septum needs to occur. After alcohol ablation, the patient is observed in the cardiac intensive care unit for 2 days. Creatine kinase (CK) and CK-MB levels are measured; CK level increases generally range from 400 to 2500 U (3%-10% of the left ventricle or 20% of the septum). Despite the myocardial infarction, global LV function is usually not impaired.

Complications of alcohol ablation include right bundle branch block or complete heart block, anterior myocardial infarction from an incomplete balloon seal in the septal perforator, ventricular tachycardia or fibrillation, and pericarditis. The risks of alcohol ablation include a 2% to 4% procedural mortality rate and a 9% to 27% incidence of patients requiring permanent pacemakers.

Alcohol ablation has not been shown to improve survival because of the lack of randomized controlled trials and a suitable control population. However, alcohol ablation does result in both short-term and long-term significant decreases in the LVOT gradient, as well as a significant improvement in New York Heart Association (NYHA) classification. For example, at 3-month follow-up, we have noted a decrease in LVOT gradient from 64 to 28 mm Hg and an improvement in NYHA class from 3.5 to 1.9. Decreased LV filling pressures and a decrease in septal thickness have also been reported after alcohol ablation. Predictors of suboptimal outcomes after ablation include a residual LVOT gradient of more than 25 mm Hg, measured in the catheterization laboratory, and a peak CK level lower than 1300 U/L.

Unlike septal myectomy, alcohol ablation results in a myocardial scar. Thus, there is a theoretical risk that alcohol ablation will increase the risk of sudden cardiac death, especially because an arrhythmogenic substrate is already present with HCM. One study of 71 HCM patients who already had an implantable cardioverter-defibrillator (ICD) for the primary prevention of sudden cardiac death and were undergoing alcohol ablation reported an 8% appropriate ICD firing rate at almost 2 years after alcohol ablation. Sudden cardiac death has been reported several months after successful alcohol ablation.

Comparison of Septal Myectomy and Alcohol Ablation Treatment Outcomes

Both myectomy and alcohol ablation reduce LVOT gradient and improve symptoms, but septal myectomy is slightly more efficacious (Table 2). A nonrandomized comparison from the Cleveland Clinic of 51 HCM patients who underwent myectomy or alcohol ablation has found larger and more consistent reductions in LVOT gradient with myectomy. Of the 26 patients who underwent septal myectomy, resting LVOT gradient was significantly reduced from 62 mm Hg before myectomy to 7 mm Hg after myectomy. In the 25 alcohol ablation subjects, resting LVOT gradient was significantly reduced from 64 mm Hg before ablation to 28 mm Hg after ablation. Myectomy also demonstrated a more favorable effect in lowering provocable gradients. In those with a resting peak gradient lower than 50 mm Hg, myectomy decreased the amyl nitrite–induced provocable gradient from 86 mm Hg preoperatively to 28 mm Hg at follow-up, whereas alcohol ablation decreased this provocable gradient from 92 mm Hg before ablation to 55 mm Hg at follow-up. NYHA class improved significantly from 3.3 to 1.5 in the myectomy group and from 3.5 to 1.9 in the alcohol ablation group. Additionally, in this study, five patients in the alcohol ablation group later required myectomy secondary to persistent gradients.

Another nonrandomized cohort study of 44 patients found similar improvements in LVOT gradients and NYHA classification after myectomy or ablation, but it found superior results in the myectomy group with respect to exercise parameters, including peak oxygen consumption and peak work rate achieved. A third nonrandomized study compared 41 alcohol ablation patients from Baylor with an age- and gradient-matched cohort of myectomy patients studied at the Mayo Clinic. The functional and hemodynamic changes after 1 year were similar, although alcohol ablation subjects had a significantly higher incidence of permanent pacing.

Practice Guidelines

ACC/ESC guidelines address both medical and surgical treatments for HCM. These guidelines state that the efficacy of medical therapy for asymptomatic subjects with HCM is currently unresolved. For

Table 2 Comparison of Septal Myectomy and Percutaneous Alcohol Septal Ablation

Parameter	Percutaneous Alcohol Septal Ablation	Surgical Myectomy
Invasiveness	Percutaneous groin access	Sternotomy
Onset of reduction in LVOT gradient	Some decrease in gradient instantly, but 6-12 mo for full effect	Instantaneous
Success rate (%)	>80	>95
Procedural mortality (%)	1-2	0-2
Recovery time	2-4 days	1 wk
Effect on LVOT gradient	Decreases to <25 mm Hg	Decreases to <10 mm Hg
Postprocedure conduction abnormality	Right bundle branch block	Left bundle branch block
Need for permanent pacemaker—all patients (%)	12-27	3-10
Need for permanent pacemaker if no preexisting conduction abnormalities (%)	13%	2%
Length of follow-up (yr)	6-8	30-40

LVOT, left ventricular outflow tract.

those who have obstruction with exercise, beta blockers are the preferred therapy. However, little evidence exists for benefit with beta blockers in patients with resting obstruction. The guidelines also state that verapamil is often used as a second-line agent, particularly in those who do not benefit from beta blockers or cannot tolerate them. No evidence exists that combined therapy with beta blockers and verapamil is more advantageous than monotherapy. Finally, disopyramide is regarded as third-line therapy, following beta blockers and verapamil in the guidelines.

In the guidelines, septal myectomy is considered the gold standard for subjects with drug-refractory HCM. Myectomy is not recommended in asymptomatic or mildly symptomatic patients. One exception to this recommendation is the consideration of myectomy for young patients (who are low-risk surgical candidates) with severe (>75 mm Hg) outflow tract obstruction, regardless of whether they are symptomatic. The guidelines regard alcohol septal ablation as second-line therapy for drug-refractory HCM, behind myectomy. It is recommended that septal ablation be confined to older adults.

Our approach to therapy for HCM is similar to that advocated by the guidelines. One slight difference is that although we also favor beta blockers as first-line therapy, we are slightly more aggressive in starting them. For example, we would consider starting beta blockers in patients with resting obstruction, a category for which the guidelines state that benefit is uncertain. We concur that verapamil and disopyramide are second- and third-line therapies, respectively. With respect to interventional therapy for HCM, we absolutely agree that septal myectomy is first-line therapy. We reserve septal ablation for suboptimal surgical candidates, in part because of the scar created by septal ablation and thus the potential for arrhythmias.

Permanent Pacemaker Implantation

Pacemaker implantation has been used to alleviate the symptoms of HCM, but this procedure has fallen out of favor. It has been hypothesized that initiating ventricular contraction at the right ventricular apex and distal septum would alter the sequence of ventricular contraction, such that the outflow gradient would be decreased and symptoms improved.

Although initial, nonrandomized, unblinded studies have reported symptomatic improvement, subsequent double-blind, randomized, crossover trials with dual-chamber pacing have demonstrated no significant change in exercise capacity but a small decrease in LVOT gradient. In addition, patients with and without active pacing have noted subjective improvement in exercise capacity. Thus, a notable placebo effect accounts for the improvement in symptoms attributed to pacemakers. Furthermore, in a nonrandomized concurrent cohort study, 39 patients underwent surgical myectomy or received permanent pacemakers. Surgical myectomy was unquestionably superior in this study, with larger decreases in LVOT gradient (76-9 mm Hg vs. 77-55 mm Hg) and larger improvements in symptoms and exercise duration than permanent pacing.

Practice Guidelines

American College of Cardiology–American Heart Association (ACC/AHA) guidelines consider pacemaker implantation for medically refractory, symptomatic HCM with a significant LVOT gradient to be a Class IIb indication. Class IIb means that there is conflicting evidence for the particular intervention, and its usefulness and efficacy are less well established by the available evidence and expert opinion. We do not recommend a permanent pacemaker specifically for treatment of HCM.

Outcomes

Surgical outcomes for HCM are excellent; operative mortality is lower than 2% for septal myectomy and there is durable symptomatic improvement. Outcomes for alcohol ablation are more limited, with follow-up averaging 3 to 5 years, as compared with decades or myectomy. At 3-month follow-up, both myectomy and alcohol ablation are effective in improving symptoms and reducing LVOT gradients, but myectomy results in larger improvements in LVOT gradients.

Summary

- Beta blockers are first-line therapy for symptomatic HCM, with alternate therapies including verapamil and disopyramide.
- For drug-refractory HCM with severe symptoms (NYHA Class III or IV), septal myectomy is the favored therapeutic approach, with durable improvements in symptoms and exercise capacity.
- Alcohol septal ablation, although also effective for HCM, should be reserved for suboptimal surgical candidates, partly because of the scar formation that accompanies ablation, which increases the potential for malignant arrhythmias.
- Permanent pacemakers are not recommended as therapy for HCM, because randomized controlled trials have demonstrated that their purported benefit in HCM is actually a placebo effect.

PREVENTION AND SCREENING

HCM is a genetic disease. However, given the varying phenotypic expressions of the known HCM mutations, if those with a genetic predisposition for HCM were to limit vigorous exercise, the manifestations of HCM might theoretically be attenuated. Because HCM is the leading cause of death in young athletes, it is recommended in this country that all competitive athletes undergo a history and physical examination before athletic clearance, with consideration for an echocardiogram if a history of syncope is present, a systolic murmur is heard on physical examination, or any other clinical indicator is present that suggests the diagnosis of HCM. Electrocardiographic screening for cardiac disease in competitive athletes is required in Italy but not at this time in the United States. This remains controversial. We do not recommend screening the general population for HCM with transthoracic echocardiography. We do recommend clinical and genetic screening for first-degree relatives of those with HCM. Because HCM is the leading cause of death in young athletes, all competitive athletes should undergo history and physical examination before athletic clearance, with consideration for an echocardiogram if a history of syncope is present, a harsh systolic murmur is heard on physical examination, or any other clinical indicator is present that suggests the diagnosis of HCM.

CONSIDERATIONS IN SPECIAL POPULATIONS

Pregnancy

Patients with HCM generally tolerate pregnancy well. The maternal mortality rate for HCM patients during pregnancy is 1%, which is increased as compared with that of the general population. Maternal morbidity from HCM, generally manifesting as atrial fibrillation, syncope, or congestive heart failure, appears to occur primarily in women who already had similar symptoms and complications of HCM before pregnancy.

Sudden Cardiac Death and Defibrillator Implantation

The most serious complication of HCM is sudden cardiac death (SCD), with an incidence of 0.1% to 0.7% per year. A survivor of an episode of SCD warrants consideration for an ICD. Primary prevention of SCD in HCM patients is not as well defined. Antiarrhythmic therapy for primary prevention is not recommended for asymptomatic patients. HCM patients at higher risk for sudden cardiac death include those with LV wall thickness more than 30 mm, prolonged or repetitive episodes of nonsustained ventricular tachycardia on Holter monitoring, family history of SCD, hypotensive blood pressure response to exercise, and syncope or near syncope. Patients with these risk factors may benefit from automatic ICD implantation for primary prevention of SCD. Assessing the genotype may help ascertain SCD risk in the future, but at present, genetic testing generally does not alter management in regard to the prevention of SCD. Electrophysiologic testing has not been shown to be predictive of SCD in those with HCM.

Nonobstructive Hypertrophic Cardiomyopathy

The treatment of patients with nonobstructive hypertrophic cardiomyopathy is difficult and less effective than those with obstructive disease. Beta blockers may be used to control heart rate, and calcium channel blockers may improve diastolic function. Over time, hypertrophic cardiomyopathy may become burned out and evolve into a picture similar to that of a dilated cardiomyopathy, with decreased LV systolic function and a dilated left ventricle. In patients with symptoms and signs of congestive heart failure, diuretics, angiotensin-converting enzyme inhibitors, and digoxin may be necessary. Heart transplantation is an option for those with end-stage nonobstructive HCM.

Suggested Readings

Ackerman MJ, VanDriest SL, Ommen SR, et al: Prevalence and age-dependence of malignant mutations in the beta-myosin heavy chain and troponin T genes in hypertrophic cardiomyopathy: a comprehensive outpatient perspective. J Am Coll Cardiol 2002;39:2042-2048.

Crawford FA, Killip D, Franklin J, et al: Implantable cardioverter-defibrillators for primary prevention of sudden cardiac death in patients with hypertrophic obstructive cardiomyopathy after alcohol ablation. Circulation 2003;108:386-387.

Elliott P, McKenna WJ: Hypertrophic cardiomyopathy. Lancet 2004;363:1881-1891.

Firoozi S, Elliott PM, Sharma S, et al: Septal myotomy-myectomy and transcoronary septal alcohol ablation in hypertrophic obstructive cardiomyopathy. A comparison of clinical, haemodynamic and exercise outcomes. Eur Heart J 2002;23:1617-1624.

Gregoratos G, Abrams J, Epstein AE, et al: ACC/AHA/NASPE 2002 Guideline Update for Implantation of Cardiac Pacemakers and Antiarrhythmia Devices—summary article: A report of the American College of Cardiology/American Heart Association Task Force on Practice Guidelines (ACC/AHA/NASPE Committee to Update the 1998 Pacemaker Guidelines). J Am Coll Cardiol 2002;40:1703-1719.

Maron BJ: Hypertrophic cardiomyopathy: A systematic review. JAMA 2002;287:1308-1320.

Maron BJ, McKenna WJ, Danielson GK, et al: American College of Cardiology/European Society of Cardiology clinical expert consensus document on hypertrophic cardiomyopathy. A report of the American College of Cardiology Foundation Task Force on Clinical Expert Consensus Documents and the European Society of Cardiology Committee for Practice Guidelines. J Am Coll Cardiol 2003;42:1687-1713.

Maron BJ, Nishimura RA, McKenna WJ, et al: Assessment of permanent dual-chamber pacing as a treatment for drug-refractory symptomatic patients with obstructive hypertrophic cardiomyopathy. A randomized, double-blind, crossover study (M-PATHY). Circulation 1999;99:2927-2933.

Nagueh SF, Ommen SR, Lakkis NM, et al: Comparison of ethanol septal reduction therapy with surgical myectomy for the treatment of hypertrophic obstructive cardiomyopathy. J Am Coll Cardiol 2001;38:1701-1706.

Nishimura RA, Holmes DR Jr: Clinical practice. Hypertrophic obstructive cardiomyopathy. N Engl J Med 2004;350:1320-1327.

Qin JX, Shiota T, Lever HM, et al: Conduction system abnormalities in patients with obstructive hypertrophic cardiomyopathy following septal reduction interventions. Am J Cardiol 2004;93:171-175.

Qin JX, Shiota T, Lever HM, et al: Outcome of patients with hypertrophic obstructive cardiomyopathy after percutaneous transluminal septal myocardial ablation and septal myectomy surgery. J Am Coll Cardiol 2001;38:1994-2000.

Smedira NG, Lytle BW, Lever HM, et al: Current effectiveness and risks of isolated septal myectomy for hypertrophic obstructive cardiomyopathy. Ann Thorac Surg 2008;85:127-134.

Woo A, Williams WG, Choi R, et al: Clinical and echocardiographic determinants of long-term survival after surgical myectomy in obstructive hypertrophic cardiomyopathy. Circulation 2005;111:2033-2041.

Dilated and Restrictive Cardiomyopathies

Corinne Bott-Silverman

Cardiomyopathies are diseases of the myocardium associated with cardiac dysfunction.[1] Table 1 lists the five types of cardiomyopathy: dilated, hypertrophic, restrictive, arrhythmogenic right ventricular, and unclassified. Many conditions manifest as one form of cardiomyopathy and progress to another. For example, hypertensive heart disease can begin with a hypertrophic pattern and subsequently become a dilated cardiomyopathy. Some diseases have features of more than one type of cardiomyopathy (e.g., sarcoidosis can have features of restrictive and dilated cardiomyopathy at different times in the course of the disease).

Cardiomyopathy often results in the heart failure syndrome, with a number of systemic manifestations. On the other hand, many systemic conditions have cardiac involvement and manifest primarily as heart failure. The cardiomyopathies represent a diverse group of conditions whose final common pathway is myocardial dysfunction. With few exceptions, histologic findings are nonspecific and include myocyte hypertrophy, cellular necrosis, and fibrosis.

There are many known causes of cardiomyopathy. Many systemic diseases have myocardial involvement, which can range from mild to severe (Table 2). The most common cause in developed countries is ischemic cardiomyopathy. In other areas, such as equatorial Africa, infiltrative disease is the leading cause.

In this chapter, discussion is confined to the definition, prevalence, signs and symptoms, and diagnosis of cardiomyopathies, with the exclusion of hypertrophic cardiomyopathy. Treatment is discussed in the chapter on heart failure.

DILATED CARDIOMYOPATHY

Definition

This condition may be defined as an ejection fraction of less than 40% in the presence of increased left ventricular dimension (left ventricular end-diastolic size >115% of that calculated for age and body surface area). Increased left ventricular dimensions in the presence of preserved systolic function may be a precursor to the development of systolic dysfunction in certain patients. Pharmacologic intervention with angiotensin-converting enzyme inhibitors and beta blockers might prevent this progression to heart failure in some of these patients.

Prevalence

It is difficult to assess the prevalence of cardiomyopathy accurately. Many cases go undiagnosed and patients with undiagnosed cardiomyopathy can present with sudden cardiac death. Strict diagnostic criteria are lacking. Approximately 5 million Americans have symptomatic heart failure, but it has been estimated that 50 million Americans fulfill American Heart Association–American College of Cardiology definitions of classes A and B heart failure (Table 3)[2] and are either at risk for or have established structural heart disease in the absence of heart failure symptoms. It is unclear how many people fall into stages B, C, and D combined (those with structural heart disease, with or without heart failure symptoms); most of these people have cardiomyopathies.

The estimated prevalence of idiopathic dilated cardiomyopathy is 0.4 per 1000 of the general population. However, in the future, as more causes are elucidated and more patients are found to have genetic or familial cardiomyopathy, the number of patients with idiopathic disease, a diagnosis of exclusion, will decrease.

Pathophysiology

Dilated cardiomyopathy represents the final common morphologic outcome of various biologic insults. It is a combination of myocyte injury and necrosis associated with myocardial fibrosis, which results in impaired mechanical function. Many cases are a result of direct toxicity (e.g., alcohol) or mechanical insults (e.g., chronic volume overload in mitral valvular regurgitation). With myocyte failure and cytoskeletal uncoupling, the chambers become dilated. According to Laplace's law, increased diameter increases wall stress and causes further mechanical disadvantage. Thus, myocardial dysfunction can cause a vicious cycle leading to more myocardial dysfunction in a process termed *adverse ventricular remodeling,* now an important therapeutic target.[3]

Specific Types

Ischemic Cardiomyopathy

Ischemic cardiomyopathy (ICM) is the most commonly identified specific cause of dilated cardiomyopathy, accounting for more than 60% of patients with symptomatic heart failure and many more with asymptomatic left ventricular dysfunction. There are several mechanisms by which coronary artery disease can result in ICM.

Myocardial infarction causes localized myocyte necrosis, with resultant scar formation and loss of contractile function in the ventricular segment perfused by the culprit artery. In addition, the myocardium distal to the area of infarction develops increased wall stress, adverse remodeling, and chamber dilation, so that a cardiomyopathic process occurs in adjacent nonischemic areas.

Another mechanism for myocardial dysfunction is hibernation, in which areas of myocardium are chronically underperfused and metabolically less active. These areas remain metabolically intact but do not contribute to the mechanical activity of the heart. Identification of these areas and restoration of their perfusion through revascularization might improve the ejection fraction and long-term prognosis.

Additional features of ICM include the development of mitral valvular regurgitation, which may be caused by papillary muscle dysfunction or functional factors, such as failure of mitral valve leaflets to coapt in a dilated ventricle. This further increases the volume overload state, increasing myocardial energy demands and causing a vicious cycle of worsening systolic dysfunction.

Atrial and ventricular arrhythmias occur commonly in ICM and include atrial fibrillation, which can further compromise contractile function. The development of atrioventricular conduction delays with the necessity for permanent pacemaker insertion can also cause pacing-induced dyssynchrony when pacing is performed from the right ventricular apex alone.

ICM is generally ascribed to epicardial coronary atherosclerosis, but it can also occur in any vasculitic process (e.g., Takayasu's arteritis), congenital abnormalities (including aberrant coronary arteries), embolic conditions (e.g., atrial fibrillation, endocarditis,

Table 1 World Health Organization Classification of Cardiomyopathies

Type of Cardiomyopathy	Features	Causative Factors
Dilated	Dilated left or both ventricle(s), with impaired contraction	Ischemic, idiopathic, familial-genetic, immune, alcoholic, toxic, valvular
Hypertrophic	Left or right ventricular hypertrophy, or both	Familial, with autosomal dominant inheritance (see elsewhere in this section, "Hypertrophic Cardiomyopathy")
Restrictive	Restrictive filling and reduced diastolic filling of one or both ventricles; normal or near-normal systolic function	Idiopathic, amyloidosis, endomyocardial fibrosis
Arrhythmogenic right ventricular cardiomyopathy	Fibrofatty replacement of right ventricular myocardium, Uhl's anomaly (parchment heart)	Unknown; familial, usually autosomal dominant inheritance, with incomplete penetrance; possible autosomal recessive inheritance; rare forms associated with typical phenotype (e.g., Naxos disease)
Unclassified	Not typical for previous four groups	Fibroelastosis, noncompacted myocardium, systolic dysfunction with minimal dilation, mitochondrial disease

Data from Richardson P, McKenna W, Bristow M, et al: Report of the 1995 World Health Organization/International Society and Federation of Cardiology Task Force on the definition and classification of cardiomyopathies. Circulation 1996;93:841-842.

Table 2 Causes of Cardiomyopathy

Cause	Disorder
Cardiovascular	Ischemic heart disease Hypertension Valvular heart disease Idiopathic dilated cardiomyopathy Idiopathic restrictive cardiomyopathy Cardiac amyloidosis
Metabolic	Starvation, vitamin deficiency Diabetes, hypothyroidism and hyperthyroidism, acromegaly, pheochromocytoma Glycogen storage disease
Infectious, inflammatory	Secondary amyloidosis, sarcoidosis Acute viral (Coxsackie B), HIV, hepatitis C Chagas' disease (protozoal)
Toxic	Alcohol, cocaine, amphetamines, chemotherapy
Genetic	Familial dilated cardiomyopathy Familial cardiac amyloidosis Noncompacted myocardium Systolic dysfunction without dilation Arrhythmogenic right ventricular cardiomyopathy Hemochromatosis
Tachycardia	Tachycardia-induced cardiomyopathy
Pregnancy	Peripartum cardiomyopathy

Table 3 American Heart Association/American College of Cardiology Staging of Heart Failure

Stage	Definition
A	Patients at risk of heart failure, with no structural heart disease
B	Patients with structural heart disease, without symptoms of heart failure
C	Patients with past or present heart failure symptoms
D	Patients with advanced disease (e.g., inotropic support)

Adapted from Hunt SA, Abraham WT, Chin MH, et al; American College of Cardiology; American Heart Association Task Force on Practice Guidelines; American College of Chest Physicians; International Society for Heart and Lung Transplantation; Heart Rhythm Society: ACC/AHA 2005 Guideline Update for the Diagnosis and Management of Chronic Heart Failure in the Adult: A report of the American College of Cardiology/American Heart Association Task Force on Practice Guidelines (Writing Committee to Update the 2001 Guidelines for the Evaluation and Management of Heart Failure): Developed in collaboration with the American College of Chest Physicians and the International Society for Heart and Lung Transplantation: Endorsed by the Heart Rhythm Society. Circulation 2005;112:e154-e235.

thrombophilic states), cardiac allograft vasculopathy, and microvascular ischemia.

Idiopathic Dilated Cardiomyopathy

The term *idiopathic dilated cardiomyopathy* is applied to most patients with nonischemic cardiomyopathy. With progress in the field of gene analysis, it is likely that many patients with idiopathic cardiomyopathy will receive a specific molecular or genetic diagnosis in the future.

Acute myocarditis may be a more common prelude to dilated cardiomyopathy than was once believed. The natural history of acute myocarditis is largely unknown because it is rarely symptomatic. It is most commonly caused by Coxsackie group B viruses. Overall, approximately 50% of patients who receive a diagnosis of acute viral myocarditis develop dilated cardiomyopathy. Up to 76% of patients with nonischemic dilated cardiomyopathy who have had a clinically recognized episode of myocarditis have genomic viral DNA persistence in myocardial samples. Despite this, endomyocardial biopsy (EMB) rarely shows myocarditis in patients with new-onset cardiomyopathy. Most have nonspecific histologic findings by light microscopy. There is significant interobserver variability in the pathologic diagnosis of myocarditis.[4]

No specific genetic abnormality is recognized as causing dilated cardiomyopathy. Numerous abnormalities have been found. There are many putative mechanisms in the development of familial cardiomyopathy beyond the scope of this chapter;

all forms of mendelian inheritance have been observed, including autosomal dominant, recessive, X-linked, and mitochondrial (matrilinear).[5]

Hypertensive heart disease can initially manifest as left ventricular hypertrophy with isolated diastolic dysfunction and preserved systolic function, as assessed by conventional echocardiographic techniques. Because remodeling occurs over time, the hypertrophy can progress to a dilated cardiomyopathy with systolic dysfunction. Atrial fibrillation is a common manifestation of hypertensive heart disease. Hypertensive heart disease is the leading identifiable cause of heart failure in older women.

Valvular Heart Disease

Hemodynamically significant valvular lesions, such as aortic stenosis, aortic regurgitation, and mitral regurgitation, produce pressure and volume overload states that can result in adverse ventricular remodeling and the development of systolic, diastolic, or combined myocardial dysfunction. In valvular disease, excess hemodynamic demands result in myocyte hypertrophy, subsequent chamber enlargement, and myocardial fibrosis. Chamber dilation then creates or exacerbates existing mitral or tricuspid valvular regurgitation, or both. With further chamber dilation, subendocardial ischemia and localized myocyte necrosis develop. In addition, concomitant coronary artery disease, especially with degenerative aortic stenosis, and atrial fibrillation, especially with mitral regurgitation, can cause further deterioration. (Specific valvular lesions are discussed in the chapters on valvular heart disease.)

Toxic Cardiomyopathies

Alcoholic cardiomyopathy may account for approximately 4% of all cardiomyopathies, and men have a significantly worse prognosis.[6] The average duration of heavy drinking (more than 90 g/day) in most cohorts is 15 years. Diastolic dysfunction usually precedes any evidence of systolic dysfunction. Left ventricular dilation is an early finding. Hypertension, atrial fibrillation (holiday heart), and coronary disease are more common in heavy drinkers. Identification of alcohol as a potential cause of cardiomyopathy is vital; abstinence can result in an improved ejection fraction in 50% of patients medically treated for heart failure, and continued drinking can result in further deterioration of cardiac function. The mechanism of alcohol-induced cardiomyopathy is unclear but might involve disturbances in intracellular calcium transients, mitochondrial disruption, decreased myofibrillary proteins, and myocyte apoptosis. Histologic findings are nonspecific.

Cocaine and amphetamines (including 3,4-methylenedioxymethamphetamine, or ecstasy) can result in dilated cardiomyopathy with single and chronic use.[7] The cause is multifactorial and includes direct myocyte toxicity, tachycardia-induced injury, hypertension, and myocardial infarction.

Doxorubicin can cause cardiomyopathy with characteristic histopathologic features. Trastuzumab, used in the treatment of metastatic breast cancer, can cause a cardiomyopathy. Unlike anthracycline-induced toxicity, it usually responds to standard treatment or the discontinuation of trastuzumab.[8] Brain natriuretic peptide (BNP) is proving useful in monitoring cardiac function in patients receiving cardiotoxic chemotherapy, because elevation of the BNP level occurs at an early stage in the condition. Hydroxychloroquine can cause skeletal and cardiac myopathies.

Peripartum cardiomyopathy is dilated cardiomyopathy arising in the last month of pregnancy or within 5 months postpartum.[9] Of these cases, 75% occur in the first 2 months after delivery. Risk factors include age older than 30 years, multiparity, twin pregnancy, African descent, and a family history of peripartum cardiomyopathy.[10] Its cause is unknown but may be related to reduced suppressor T cell activity, which occurs during pregnancy, and can result in an autoimmune type of myocardial inflammation or activation of myocarditis. Recovery, usually within 6 months, occurs in 50% of patients. Patients should be advised not to have more children. (See the chapter "Pregnancy and Heart Disease.")

Infective Cardiomyopathies

In addition to the acute (often presumed viral) myocarditis discussed earlier, various other viral agents have been implicated in the development of cardiomyopathy, including human immunodeficiency virus (HIV) and hepatitis C. *Trypanosoma cruzi* (a protozoan) has infected 20 million people in South and Central America. Infection causes Chagas' disease, a dilated cardiomyopathy (either global or with characteristic apical aneurysm formation) in 20% to 30% of patients, acutely or over many years. Other parasitic infestations that can cause cardiomyopathy in the immunocompetent and immunocompromised patient include *Toxoplasma gondii* and *Trichinella spiralis. Plasmodium falciparum* infection (malaria) can cause parasitic coronary artery occlusion.

Tachycardia-Induced Cardiomyopathy

Prolonged exposure to rapid heart rates can induce myocardial dysfunction. Persistent or permanent atrial fibrillation induces electrical and structural remodeling of the atria. When rapidly conducted, it can cause adverse ventricular remodeling and a dilated cardiomyopathy. The diagnosis is one of exclusion, and rate control or restoration of sinus rhythm can restore systolic function. Sometimes cause and effect can be difficult to determine.

Metabolic Conditions

Malnutrition, as well as selenium, carnitine, phosphate, calcium, and vitamin B deficiencies, can result in dilated cardiomyopathy. Endocrine causes include adrenocortical insufficiency, thyrotoxicosis, hypothyroidism, acromegaly, and pheochromocytoma.

RESTRICTIVE CARDIOMYOPATHIES

Definition

Restrictive cardiomyopathy is a disease of the myocardium characterized by restrictive filling and reduced diastolic volume of either or both ventricles, with normal or near-normal systolic function.[1]

Prevalence

Restrictive cardiomyopathies represent a very small fraction (less than 5%) of cardiomyopathies in the West,[11] but they are more common in certain populations. For example, endomyocardial fibrosis is a relatively common cause of heart failure in equatorial Africa, but ischemic heart disease is not.

Pathophysiology

Restrictive cardiomyopathies result in impaired ventricular filling and primarily diastolic heart failure. They manifest with a clinical heart failure syndrome that is often indistinguishable from that caused by systolic dysfunction. Atrioventricular block and symptomatic bradycardias can be seen, often necessitating pacemaker insertion. Atrial fibrillation is poorly tolerated.

Restrictive cardiomyopathies may be classified as primary (e.g., endomyocardial fibrosis, Löffler's endocarditis, idiopathic restrictive cardiomyopathy) or secondary. Causes of secondary restrictive cardiomyopathy include infiltrative diseases (e.g., amyloidosis, sarcoidosis, radiation carditis) and storage diseases (e.g., hemochromatosis, glycogen storage disorders, Fabry's disease). Fabry's disease, although rare, has assumed a new importance as effective treatment has become available.[12]

Amyloid heart disease is classified as primary, secondary, familial, or senile. Primary amyloid heart disease is caused by overproduction of light chain immunoglobulin from a monoclonal population of plasma cells, usually associated with multiple myeloma. Secondary amyloid heart disease is associated with chronic inflammatory conditions such as Crohn's disease, rheumatoid arthritis, tuberculosis, and familial Mediterranean fever. Familial and senile amyloid heart disease are related to the overproduction of transthyretin. Myocardial amyloid heart disease is confirmed by EMB. The presence of near-normal left ventricular dimensions combined with increased myocardial wall thickness, particularly biventricular thickening, should arouse suspicion of an infiltrative cardiomyopathy, especially if accompanied by low-voltage QRS complexes on the electrocardiogram (ECG). Unfortunately, there is no proven treatment for amyloid heart disease, and the prognosis is poor.[13]

Specific Types

Hemochromatosis

Hemochromatosis (bronze diabetes) is a disease that results in iron overload and deposition of iron in the sarcoplasmic reticulum of many organs, including the heart. It generally follows an autosomal recessive pattern of mendelian inheritance. The use of serum ferritin levels as a screen for this condition is reasonable. Cardiac magnetic resonance imaging (MRI) can be useful for the diagnosis of cardiac involvement. Hemochromatosis can result in a restrictive or dilated cardiomyopathy, with characteristic histologic features. Treatment is by repeated phlebotomy. Family screening is advised.

Sarcoidosis

Sarcoidosis is a systemic disease resulting in the formation of noncaseating granulomas that can infiltrate the myocardium. It is associated with restrictive cardiomyopathy in 5% of patients and can later progress to dilated cardiomyopathy. It is difficult to diagnose unless there is other organ involvement (usually pulmonary). It may be suspected in patients with cardiomyopathy and lymphadenopathy, skin rashes, or splenomegaly. Cardiac sarcoid is associated with ventricular tachycardia and conduction abnormalities (especially complete heart block) that can cause syncope and sudden cardiac death. EMB may show findings specific for sarcoidosis but, because of the patchy nature of the disease, biopsy can miss characteristic lesions, resulting in a low overall sensitivity. Cardiac granulomas occasionally respond to steroids but turn to scar tissue. Sudden death is not prevented by steroids. Regular Holter monitoring is recommended to look for evidence of atrioventricular block, which should be treated with permanent pacemaker insertion, or ventricular arrhythmias, which should be treated with an implantable cardioverter-defibrillator (ICD).

ARRHYTHMOGENIC RIGHT VENTRICULAR CARDIOMYOPATHY

Arrhythmogenic right ventricular cardiomyopathy (ARVC) is a rare but increasingly recognized condition characterized morphologically by apparent patchy apoptosis of the right and, to a lesser extent, left ventricles. It is sometimes called *fat cardiomyopathy* because of fatty infiltration of the right ventricle. It is familial in more than 50% of patients, generally with an autosomal dominant mode of inheritance.[14]

Presentation is usually in early adulthood, with symptoms consistent with supraventricular and ventricular arrhythmias or with right-sided heart failure. It may be discovered during family screening. Often, sudden death is the first sign of ARVC, with the diagnosis made postmortem. EMB is associated with an increased risk of perforation and tamponade. Diagnostic features are summarized in Table 4.

Table 4 Diagnostic Features of Arrhythmogenic Right Ventricular Cardiomyopathy

Diagnostic Modality	Features
Electrocardiography	Epsilon waves (slurred ST segments) V_{1-3}, inverted T waves V_2, V_3*) in absence of right bundle branch block
Echocardiography	Localized RV aneurysm, isolated RV failure
Magnetic resonance imaging	Fatty infiltration of right ventricle
Histology	Fatty infiltration of right ventricle

*In patients older than 12 years.
RV, right ventricular.

Managing these patients is difficult and controversial. Control and prevention of potentially lethal ventricular arrhythmias are of paramount importance and have been approached with antiarrhythmic medications, radiofrequency ablation and, inevitably, ICDs. Control of right heart failure is difficult and sometimes impossible by conventional therapy. Cardiac transplantation provides effective therapy in selected cases.

UNCLASSIFIED CARDIOMYOPATHIES

Noncompacted myocardium manifests in early childhood. It appears to occur as a result of an arrest in endomyocardial morphogenesis. It is often associated with other cardiac abnormalities and extracardiac anomalies. Patchy preservation of the spongy morphology of the embryonic heart occurs, with persisting myocardial sinusoids and prominent ventricular trabeculations seen with echocardiography. It involves the right ventricle and is occasionally biventricular. Clinical presentation includes ventricular arrhythmias, thromboembolism, and progressive systolic or diastolic heart failure, or both. It is a malignant condition with a high mortality. Death usually occurs in childhood. Patients are treated conventionally, and some have successfully undergone heart transplantation.

Systolic dysfunction with minimal dilation, as its name suggests, is characterized by systolic dysfunction, an ejection fraction lower than 30% (with no evidence of restrictive physiology by definition) and preserved left ventricular dimensions. Histologically, there is little myofibrillar loss. It carries a poor prognosis. Patients are treated with conventional approaches. A family history of dilated cardiomyopathy is not uncommon.

Mitochondrial cardiomyopathy, arising from mutations in mitochondrial DNA, with resultant impaired oxidative phosphorylation, is transmitted through the maternal line. The resultant cardiomyopathy is characterized by progressive hypertrophy, dilation, and arrhythmias. Mitochondrial diseases generally are systemic, in tissues with high metabolic activity, and give rise to syndromes. The MELAS syndrome (mitochondrial encephalopathy, lactic acidosis, and strokelike syndrome) can manifest as cardiomyopathy. When a mitochondrial myopathy is suspected, electron microscopy of EMB specimens may reveal giant mitochondria, concentric cristae, and intramitochondrial inclusions. However, skeletal muscle biopsy should be considered first, because it is a safer alternative.

Endocardial fibroelastosis is a rare condition that usually manifests in infancy or early childhood. It is characterized by thickening of the left ventricle and left-sided cardiac valves. Multiple modes of inheritance have been described. Dilated or restrictive cardiomyopathy can result.

GENERAL CONSIDERATIONS

Signs and Symptoms

The cardiomyopathies represent a spectrum of disease and as such have various presentations (Fig. 1). Patients can remain asymptomatic and their cardiomyopathy diagnosed only by screening or postmortem examination. They may present with symptoms of heart failure (see the chapter "Heart Failure"), chest pain, or dysrhythmias. The clinical course can fluctuate. Unfortunately, the most common clinical presentation is one of progressive deterioration, with worsening heart failure and death occurring over a variable time course.

Diagnosis

A careful history is essential, with particular emphasis on family history. A family tree should be constructed to ascertain whether a pedigree exists that is consistent with familial cardiomyopathy. This can necessitate requesting autopsy reports and medical records, because a high index of suspicion is required. Additional features in the history should focus on exposure to cardiotoxins such as alcohol or cocaine. Specific interrogation about a protracted flulike illness or respiratory tract infection can suggest previous myocarditis.

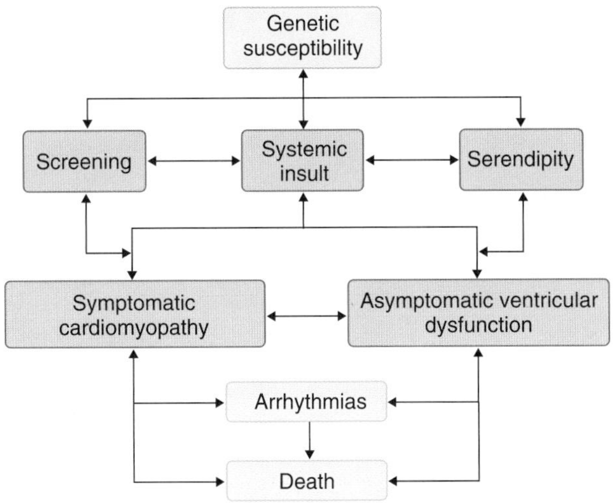

Figure 1 **Clinical presentations of cardiomyopathy.**

Key points to assess in patients with known or suspected cardiomyopathy are as follows:

- Establishing the onset and severity of symptoms of dyspnea, fatigue, fluid retention, and effect on activities of daily living
- Conventional risk factors for vascular disease (e.g., smoking, hypertension, diabetes, hyperlipidemia) or prior cardiac events (e.g., myocardial infarction, coronary artery bypass grafting)
- Family history of heart disease, especially sudden death
- Alcohol, amphetamine, or cocaine use
- Any past or current major medical illness

The use of genetic screening in the management of cardiomyopathy currently is under evaluation in many centers, but it has not yet proved to be clinically useful.

Screening first-degree relatives of patients with known or suspected familial cardiomyopathy is currently best achieved by physical examination, ECG, and echocardiography. The age at which screening should commence and how often it should be continued are unclear.

Examination should focus on whether the heart is palpably dilated, the presence of murmurs, and additional heart sounds (gallops). It is important to look beyond the cardiovascular system to consider a possible systemic disorder that may be contributory or causal, such as hemochromatosis or thyrotoxicosis.

There are five useful clinical signs to establish the presence and severity of cardiomyopathy: general appearance (cachexia and dyspnea at rest indicate severe impairment), hypotension, tachycardia, elevated jugular venous pressure, and displaced left ventricular point of maximal impulse (PMI).

Basic investigations should include a chest radiograph, ECG, and echocardiogram. Screening laboratory investigations include a complete blood cell count and renal, glucose, lipid, liver, and thyroid panels. It is reasonable to measure ferritin levels if hemochromatosis is suspected. The usefulness of viral titers has not been proven, although it may be reasonable to perform specific viral serology, such as for HIV, if indicated by the history.

BNP has been identified as a useful marker for the diagnosis, severity, and prognosis in patients with heart failure. BNP levels correlate with functional class but not with ejection fraction.

The five most common abnormalities seen on the ECG are Q waves (from a previous myocardial infarction), diffuse ST-segment abnormalities, left bundle branch block (or any intraventricular conduction delay), atrial fibrillation, and abnormal P waves (biphasic in leads V_1 and V_2 [left atrial overload]). Fig. 2 shows intraventricular

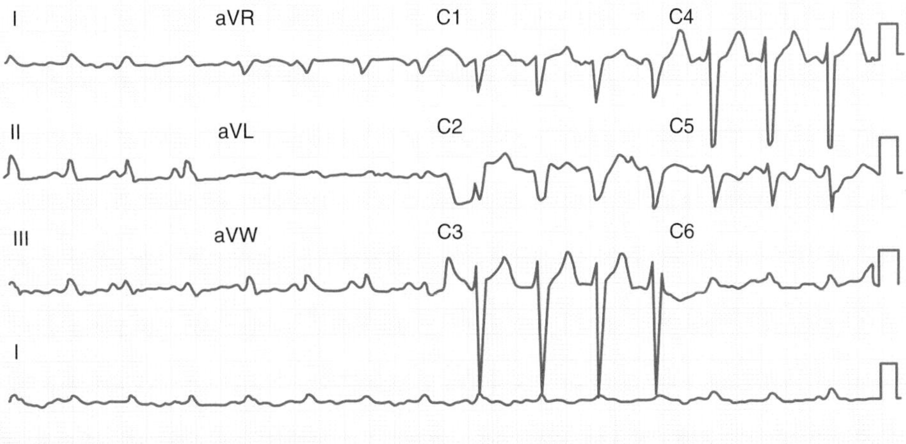

Figure 2 **Electrocardiogram from a patient with dilated cardiomyopathy.** Shown are diffuse ST-segment changes and an intraventricular conduction delay, with a QRS duration of 148 msec.

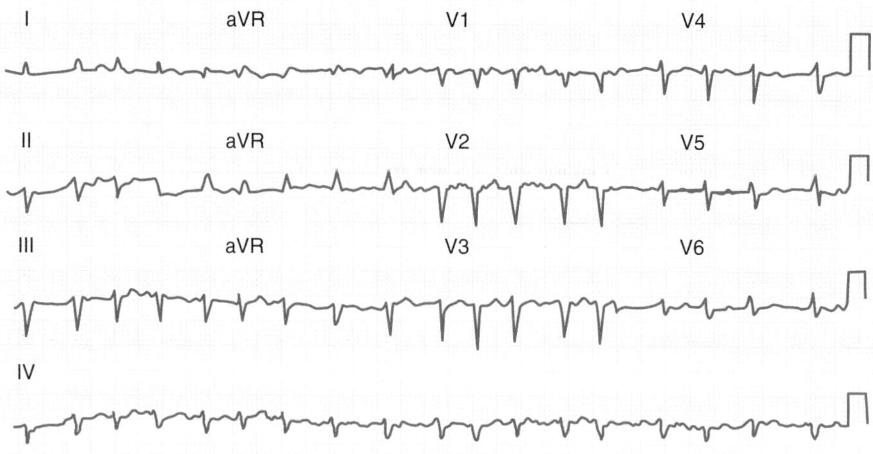

Figure 3 **Electrocardiogram from a patient with ischemic cardiomyopathy.** Atrial fibrillation, poor R wave progression, and nonspecific ST changes can be seen.

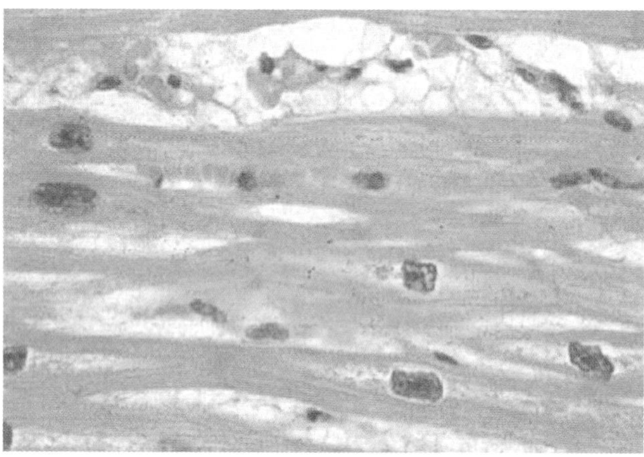

Figure 4 **Histology of dilated cardiomyopathy.** Nonspecific abnormalities, including variations in myocyte size, myocyte vacuolation, loss of myofibrillar material, and fibrosis, can be seen (hematoxylin-eosin stain, ×40). *(Courtesy of N.G. Mahon, MD.)*

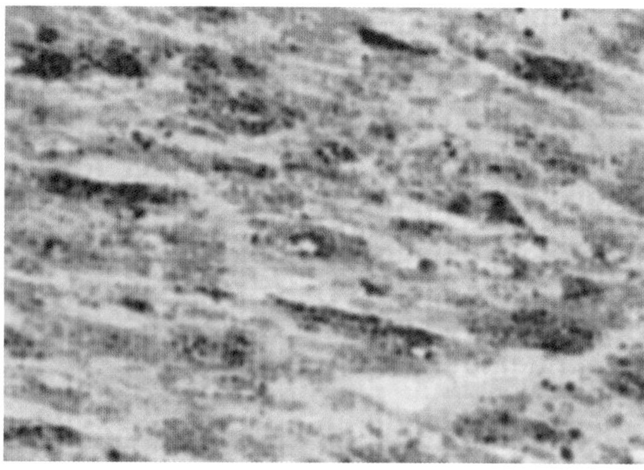

Figure 5 **Endomyocardial biopsy from a patient with hemochromatosis.** The characteristic enhancement of iron deposition can be seen (Perls' stain, ×40). *(Courtesy of N.G. Mahon, MD.)*

delay and diffuse ST-segment abnormalities in an ECG from a patient with dilated cardiomyopathy. Fig. 3 shows atrial fibrillation, poor R wave progression, and diffuse ST-segment abnormalities in an ECG from a patient with ischemic cardiomyopathy.

Common abnormalities seen on the chest radiograph include cardiomegaly, interstitial edema, pleural effusion(s), and evidence of previous sternotomy (sternal wires).

Common abnormalities seen on the echocardiogram include increased chamber dimensions, reduced fractional shortening or ejection fraction, functional mitral and tricuspid valvular regurgitation, regional wall motion abnormalities, and myocardial thickening (hypertrophy or infiltration).

Common abnormalities seen on Holter monitoring include premature ventricular complexes, premature atrial complexes, atrial fibrillation (either sustained or paroxysmal), nonsustained ventricular tachycardia, and first- or second-degree atrioventricular block.

It is important to rule out ischemia as a cause of ventricular dysfunction. This can most definitively be determined by cardiac catheterization and coronary arteriography. Noninvasive modalities such as dobutamine stress echocardiography and nuclear stress testing are available at most centers as screening tests for coronary artery disease. Positron emission tomography and MRI are other noninvasive modalities that are only available at large centers.

Role of Endomyocardial Biopsy in the Diagnosis of Cardiomyopathy

EMB is not indicated in the routine evaluation of cardiomyopathy,[2] even though it has a complication rate of less than 1%.[15] Most histologic specimens demonstrate nonspecific changes of myocyte hypertrophy, cell loss, and fibrosis (Fig. 4) and do not affect medical management. Histologically specific changes do occur in sarcoid (although they are patchy, reducing sensitivity), amyloid, hemochromatosis (Fig. 5), endocardial fibroelastosis, Löffler's endocarditis, and ARVC (Fig. 6). These conditions may be diagnosed with other less invasive tests. In addition, there are no data proving that treatment improves outcome in cardiac sarcoid or amyloid, although some support the use of EMB in suspected cases of amyloid to establish the diagnosis and predict a poor prognosis (mean survival, 6-12 months). Because of recurrent disease, cardiac amyloid generally renders the patient ineligible for cardiac transplantation.

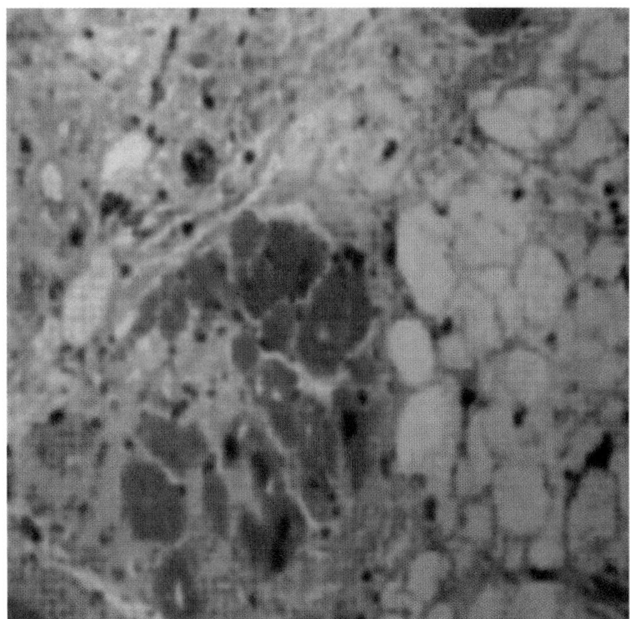

Figure 6 Histologic specimen of arrhythmogenic right ventricular cardiomyopathy. Marked fatty infiltration can be seen (Masson's trichrome stain, ×40). *(Courtesy of N.G. Mahon, MD.)*

EMB in acute myocarditis is not useful because aggressive immunosuppressive regimens, once believed to be efficacious, do not appear to improve outcome. However, the one exception is that giant cell myocarditis, suggested by a rapidly progressive and downhill course, may benefit from aggressive therapy (e.g., intensive hemodynamically guided heart failure therapy, immunosuppression, left ventricular assist device, transplantation). In addition to its use for potential giant cell myocarditis, EMB, combined with cardiac imaging techniques, may be used to document anthracycline toxicity, although BNP level may be a more sensitive marker.

EMB is sometimes useful for distinguishing constrictive from restrictive pathology (the latter being associated with infiltration on EMB).[16] However, this distinction can generally be made with a number of imaging techniques, including echocardiography with diastolic studies (see the chapter "Pericardial Disease"), MRI, computed tomography, and cardiac catheterization.

Treatment and Outcomes of Cardiomyopathies

Therapy for cardiomyopathy generally is the same as for heart failure. However, the usefulness of therapies for specific populations remains to be defined, including those for patients with asymptomatic left ventricular dilation. Neither steroids nor intravenous immunoglobulin are useful in the management of cardiomyopathy.

In the absence of a specific remediable cause (e.g., peripartum, alcoholic, ischemic, or hibernating cardiomyopathy), the overall outcome is poor. The 5-year survival rate of patients with diagnosed heart failure is 50%.[17] This is paralleled by a high morbidity, characterized by polypharmacy and multiple hospital admissions. Several clinical and laboratory features imply a poor prognosis (Table 5).[10,18,19]

Metabolic stress testing is useful to gauge effort tolerance objectively, and a peak $\dot{V}O_2$ uptake of less than 14 mL/kg/min is generally accepted as a criterion for heart transplantation. Heart transplantation provides a median survival of 12 years and is effective palliation for appropriately selected patients.

Table 5 Predictors of Poor Outcome in Dilated Cardiomyopathy

Test	Features
Clinical findings	Increased age, male gender, ischemic heart disease, diabetes, syncope, right heart failure symptoms, symptomatic ventricular arrhythmias, persistent gallop rhythm, persistent jugular venous distention, systemic hypotension, peripheral vascular disease
Laboratory findings	Hyponatremia, persistently elevated B-type natriuretic peptide and A-type natriuretic peptide levels, elevated norepinephrine and renin levels
Electrocardiography	Left bundle branch block, first- and second-degree atrioventricular blocks
Echocardiography	Increased ventricular dimensions, reduced ejection fraction, restrictive diastolic filling pattern, severe mitral or tricuspid regurgitation, or both
Chest radiography	Increased cardiothoracic ratio
Coronary angiography	Multivessel obstructive disease
Hemodynamic data	Pulmonary capillary wedge pressure >20 mm Hg, cardiac index <2.5 L/min/m^2, pulmonary hypertension, elevated central venous pressure
Cardiopulmonary exercise test	Maximal systemic oxygen uptake <12 mL/kg/min
Endomyocardial biopsy	Loss of intracellular myofilaments

Data from Topol E: Textbook of Cardiovascular Medicine. Philadelphia: Lippincott Williams & Wilkins, 2002; Bart BA, Shaw LK, McCants CB, Jr., et al: Clinical determinants of mortality in patients with angiographically diagnosed ischemic or nonischemic cardiomyopathy. J Am Coll Cardiol 1997;30:1002-1008; and Koelling TM, Aaronson KD, Cody RJ, et al: Prognostic significance of mitral regurgitation and tricuspid regurgitation in patients with left ventricular systolic dysfunction. Am Heart J 2002;144:524-529.

"Which patients should I refer to a cardiologist?" Because of the poor prognosis in most cases of cardiomyopathy, all patients for whom active treatment is contemplated should be referred to a cardiologist to ascertain the cause so that an aggressive, tailored treatment plan can be initiated.

Summary

- Cardiomyopathies are diseases of the myocardium associated with cardiac dysfunction, often resulting in the clinical syndrome of heart failure.
- Dilated cardiomyopathy is defined as an ejection fraction of lower than 40% in the presence of increased left ventricular dimensions. There are a number of possible causes.
- Restrictive cardiomyopathy is a disease of the myocardium, characterized by restrictive filling and reduced diastolic volume of the ventricles, with normal or near-normal systolic function.
- Cardiomyopathies are diagnosed by history, physical examination, ECG, chest x-ray, echocardiogram and, in some cases, endomyocardial biopsy.

Suggested Readings

Arbustini E, Morbini P, Pilotto A, et al: Familial dilated cardiomyopathy: From clinical presentation to molecular genetics. Eur Heart J. 2000;21:1825-1832.

Bart BA, Shaw LK, McCants CB, Jr, et al: Clinical determinants of mortality in patients with angiographically diagnosed ischemic or nonischemic cardiomyopathy. J Am Coll Cardiol 1997;30:1002-1008.

Elkayam U, Tummala PP, Rao K, et al: Maternal and fetal outcomes of subsequent pregnancies in women with peripartum cardiomyopathy. N Engl J Med 2001;344:1567-1571.

Falk RH: Diagnosis and management of the cardiac amyloidoses. Circulation 2005;112:2047-2060.

Goldstein S, Ali AS, Sabbah H: Ventricular remodeling. Mechanisms and prevention. Cardiol Clin 1998;16:623-632, vii–viii.

Hunt SA, Abraham WT, Chin MH, et al: American College of Cardiology; American Heart Association Task Force on Practice Guidelines; American College of Chest Physicians; International Society for Heart and Lung Transplantation; Heart Rhythm Society: ACC/AHA 2005 Guideline Update for the Diagnosis and Management of Chronic Heart Failure in the Adult: A report of the American College of Cardiology/American Heart Association Task Force on Practice Guidelines (Writing Committee to Update the 2001 Guidelines for the Evaluation and Management of Heart Failure): Developed in collaboration with the American College of Chest Physicians and the International Society for Heart and Lung Transplantation: Endorsed by the Heart Rhythm Society. Circulation 2005;112:e154–e235.

Koelling TM, Aaronson KD, Cody RJ, et al: Prognostic significance of mitral regurgitation and tricuspid regurgitation in patients with left ventricular systolic dysfunction. Am Heart J 2002;144:524-529.

Levy D, Kenchaiah S, Larson MG, et al: Long-term trends in the incidence of and survival with heart failure. N Engl J Med 2002;347:1397-1402.

Magnani JW, Dec GW: Myocarditis: Current trends in diagnosis and treatment. Circulation 2006;113:876-890.

Piano MR: Alcoholic cardiomyopathy: Incidence, clinical characteristics, and pathophysiology. Chest 2002;121:1638-1650.

References

For a complete list of references, log onto www.expertconsult.com.

Heart Failure

Robert Hobbs and Andrew Boyle

DEFINITION AND ETIOLOGY

Heart failure is a clinical syndrome characterized by systemic perfusion inadequate to meet the body's metabolic demands as a result of impaired cardiac pump function. This may be further subdivided into systolic or diastolic heart failure. In systolic heart failure, there is reduced cardiac contractility, whereas in diastolic heart failure there is impaired cardiac relaxation and abnormal ventricular filling (Fig. 1).

The most common cause of heart failure is left ventricular (LV) systolic dysfunction (about 60% of patients). In this category, most cases are a result of end-stage coronary artery disease, either with a history of myocardial infarction or with a chronically underperfused, yet viable, myocardium. In many patients, both processes are present simultaneously (Fig. 2A). Other common causes of LV systolic dysfunction include idiopathic dilated cardiomyopathy, valvular heart disease, hypertensive heart disease, toxin-induced cardiomyopathies (e.g., doxorubicin, herceptin, alcohol), and congenital heart disease (see Fig. 2B).

Right ventricular systolic dysfunction is usually a consequence of LV systolic dysfunction. It can also develop as a result of right ventricular infarction, pulmonary hypertension, chronic severe tricuspid regurgitation, or arrhythmogenic right ventricular dysplasia. A less-common cause of heart failure is high-output failure caused by thyrotoxicosis, arteriovenous fistulae, Paget's disease, pregnancy, or severe chronic anemia.

Diastolic LV dysfunction (impaired relaxation) usually is related to chronic hypertension or ischemic heart disease. Other causes include restrictive, infiltrative, and hypertrophic cardiomyopathies. Inadequate filling of the right ventricle can result from pericardial constriction or cardiac tamponade.

PREVALENCE AND RISK FACTORS

Heart failure is a common syndrome, especially in older adults. Although more patients survive acute myocardial infarction because of reperfusion therapy, most have at least some residual LV systolic dysfunction, which can lead to heart failure. Currently, 5 million Americans are afflicted with heart failure, approximately 2% of the population.[1] Patients with heart failure account for about 1 million hospital admissions annually, and another 2 million patients have heart failure as a secondary diagnosis. One third of these patients are readmitted within 90 days for recurrent decompensation.

Patients at high risk for developing heart failure are those with hypertension, coronary artery disease, diabetes mellitus, family history of cardiomyopathy, use of cardiotoxins, and obesity.

PATHOPHYSIOLOGY AND NATURAL HISTORY

Although much progress has been made in the treatment of heart failure, there is a high overall annual mortality (5%-20%), particularly in patients with New York Heart Association (NYHA) Class IV symptoms.[2] Many patients succumb to progressive pump failure and congestion, although one half die from sudden cardiac death. Some patients die from end-organ failure resulting from inadequate systemic organ perfusion, particularly to the kidneys. Indicators of poor cardiac prognosis include renal dysfunction, cachexia, valvular regurgitation, ventricular arrhythmias, higher NYHA heart failure class, lower LV ejection fraction (LVEF), high catecholamine and B-type natriuretic peptide (BNP) levels, low serum sodium level, hypocholesterolemia, and marked LV dilation. Patients with combined systolic and diastolic LV dysfunction also have a worse prognosis than patients with either in isolation.[3]

In LV systolic dysfunction, the body activates several neurohormonal pathways to increase circulating blood volume. The sympathetic nervous system increases heart rate and contractility, causes arteriolar vasoconstriction in nonessential vascular beds, and stimulates secretion of renin from the juxtaglomerular apparatus of the kidney. Unfortunately, catecholamines aggravate ischemia, potentiate arrhythmias, promote cardiac remodeling, and are directly toxic to myocytes. Stimulation of the renin-angiotensin system as a result of increased sympathetic stimulation and decreased renal perfusion results in further arteriolar vasoconstriction, sodium and water retention, and release of aldosterone. An increased aldosterone level, in turn, leads to sodium and water retention, endothelial dysfunction, and organ fibrosis.

In heart failure, baroreceptor and osmotic stimuli lead to vasopressin release from the hypothalamus, causing reabsorption of water in the renal collecting duct. Although these neurohormonal pathways initially are compensatory and beneficial, eventually they are deleterious, and neurohormonal modulation is the basis for modern treatment of heart failure.

In contrast, natriuretic peptides are hormones released by secretory granules in cardiac myocytes in response to myocardial stretching. They have a beneficial influence in heart failure, including systemic and pulmonary vasodilation, possible enhancement of sodium and water excretion, and suppression of other neurohormones.

With continuous neurohormonal stimulation, the left ventricle undergoes remodeling consisting of LV dilation and hypertrophy, such that stroke volume is increased without an actual increase in EF. This is achieved by myocyte hypertrophy and elongation. LV chamber dilation causes increased wall tension, worsens subendocardial myocardial perfusion, and can provoke ischemia in patients with coronary atherosclerosis. Furthermore, dilation of the LV chamber can cause mitral annular dilatation and mitral regurgitation, leading to pulmonary congestion.

In diastolic dysfunction, the primary abnormality is impaired LV relaxation, causing high diastolic pressures and poor filling of the ventricle. To increase diastolic filling, left atrial and pulmonary capillary pressures increase and pulmonary edema ensues. As a result, patients are often symptomatic with exertion when increased heart rate reduces LV filling time and circulating catecholamines worsen diastolic dysfunction.

The American College of Cardiology (ACC) and American Heart Association (AHA) have developed a classification of heart failure based on stages of the syndrome (Table 1).[4] Stage A includes patients who are at risk for developing heart failure but who have no structural heart disease at present. The management strategy in this group is prevention of heart failure. Stage B includes patients with structural heart disease but no symptoms. The management goal is prevention of LV remodeling leading to heart failure. Stage C includes patients with structural heart disease with current or prior symptomatic heart failure. Diuretics, digoxin, and aldosterone antagonists may be added to angiotensin-converting enzyme (ACE) inhibitors and beta blockers, depending on the severity of symptoms. Cardiac resynchronization therapy also may be considered. Stage D includes patients with severe refractory heart failure. Physicians should consider either end-of-life care or high-technology therapies such as cardiac transplantation or mechanical circulatory support, based on individual cases.

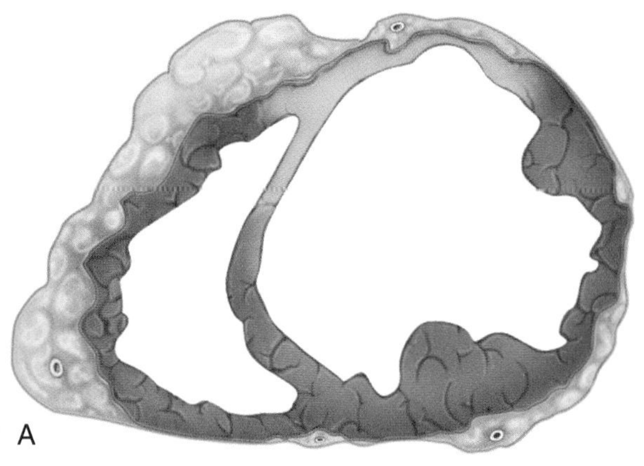

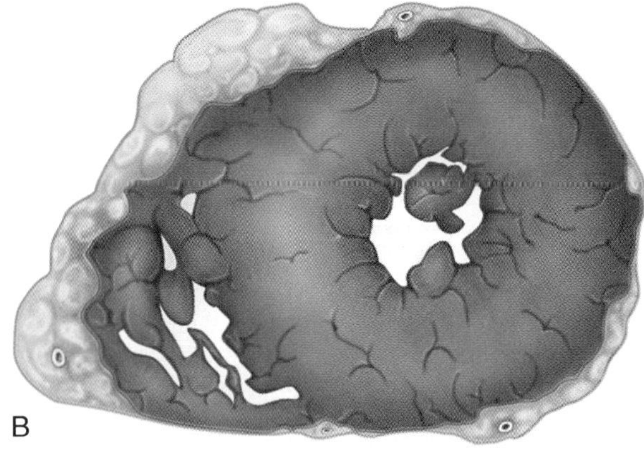

Figure 1 Systolic dysfunction versus diastolic dysfunction. A, This heart had a remote anterior wall infarction, resulting in systolic dysfunction. **B,** This heart has hypertrophic cardiomyopathy and abnormal relaxation.

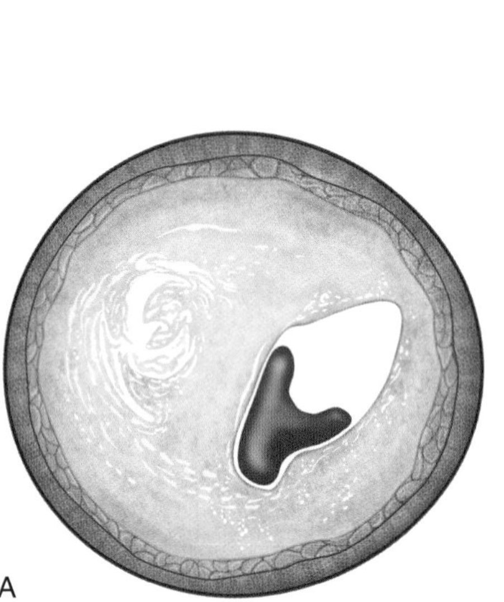

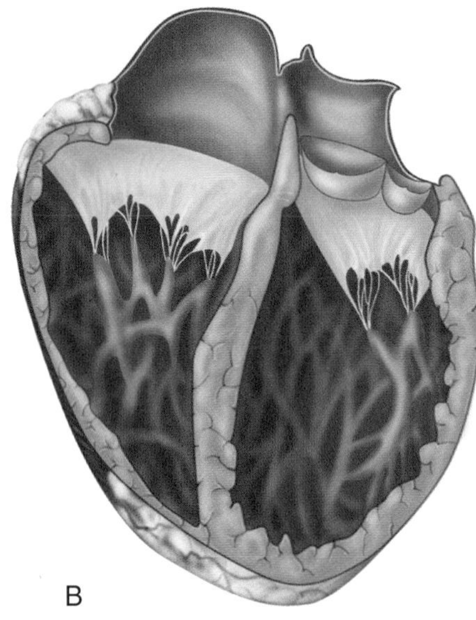

Figure 2 Left ventricular systolic dysfunction. A, Cross section of a coronary artery with severe atherosclerosis. Coronary artery disease is the most common cause of heart failure. **B,** Heart with dilated cardiomyopathy. Here there is biventricular enlargement.

Table 1 American College of Cardiology–American Heart Association Classification of Chronic Heart Failure

Stage	Description
A: High risk for developing heart failure	Hypertension, diabetes mellitus, CAD, family history of cardiomyopathy
B: Asymptomatic heart failure	Previous MI, LV dysfunction, valvular heart disease
C: Symptomatic heart failure	Structural heart disease, dyspnea and fatigue, impaired exercise tolerance
D: Refractory end-stage heart failure	Marked symptoms at rest despite maximal medical therapy

CAD, coronary artery disease; LV, left ventricular; MI, myocardial infarction.

SIGNS AND SYMPTOMS

There is a wide spectrum of potential clinical manifestations of heart failure.[5] Most patients have signs and symptoms of fluid overload and pulmonary congestion, including dyspnea, orthopnea, and paroxysmal nocturnal dyspnea. Patients with right ventricular failure have jugular venous distention, peripheral edema, hepatosplenomegaly, and ascites. Others, however, do not have congestive symptoms but have signs and symptoms of low cardiac output, including fatigue, effort intolerance, cachexia, and renal hypoperfusion. The NYHA functional classification scheme is used to assess the severity of functional limitations and correlates fairly well with prognosis (Table 2).

On physical examination, patients with decompensated heart failure may be tachycardic and tachypneic, with bilateral inspiratory rales, jugular venous distention, and edema. They often are pale and diaphoretic. The first heart sound usually is relatively soft if the patient is not tachycardic. An S_3 and often an S_4 gallop will be present. Murmurs of mitral or tricuspid regurgitation may be heard. Paradoxical splitting of S_2 may be present because of delayed mechanical or electrical activation of the left ventricle. Patients with compensated heart failure will likely have clear lungs but a displaced cardiac apex. Patients with decompensated diastolic dysfunction usually have a loud S_4 (which may be palpable), rales, and often systemic hypertension.

DIAGNOSIS

The initial evaluation of new-onset heart failure should include an electrocardiogram, chest radiograph, and BNP assay. EK6 findings

Table 2 New York Heart Association (NYHA) Heart Failure Symptom Classification System

NYHA Class	Level of Impairment
I	No symptom limitation with ordinary physical activity
II	Ordinary physical activity somewhat limited by dyspnea (e.g., long-distance walking, climbing two flights of stairs)
III	Exercise limited by dyspnea with moderate workload (e.g., short-distance walking, climbing one flight of stairs)
IV	Dyspnea at rest or with very little exertion

of LV hypertrophy, left bundle branch block, intraventricular conduction delay, and nonspecific ST-segment and T wave changes support a diagnosis of heart failure. Q waves in contiguous leads strongly implicate a previous myocardial infarction and coronary atherosclerosis as the cause. Chest radiographic findings of heart failure include cardiomegaly, pulmonary vascular redistribution, pulmonary venous congestion, Kerley B lines, alveolar edema, and pleural effusions.

The single most useful diagnostic test is the echocardiogram, which can distinguish between systolic and diastolic dysfunction. If systolic dysfunction is present, regional wall motion abnormalities or LV aneurysm suggest an ischemic basis for heart failure, whereas global dysfunction suggests a nonischemic cause. Echocardiography is helpful in determining other causes, such as valvular heart disease, cardiac tamponade, or pericardial constriction, and provides useful clues about infiltrative and restrictive cardiomyopathies. Echocardiography can also provide meaningful prognostic information about diastolic function, severity of hypertrophy, chamber size, and valvular abnormalities. In many cases, however, the exact cause of the heart failure cannot be discerned from the echocardiogram.

Cardiac catheterization can detect coronary atherosclerosis as the cause of heart failure. Severe coronary artery disease is so prevalent that coronary angiography routinely should be performed to exclude this cause and, if found, should lead to an assessment of myocardial viability, with a goal of revascularization. Coronary computed tomographic angiography (CTA) might also be a suitable alternative to exclude coronary artery disease in select patients.

Magnetic resonance imaging (MRI) is useful in assessing for arrhythmogenic right ventricular dysplasia, myocardial viability, and infiltrative cardiomyopathies.

Objective information about functional capacity can be obtained from metabolic (cardiopulmonary) exercise testing. This test can distinguish ventilatory from cardiac limitations in patients with exertional dyspnea. A peak oxygen consumption higher than 25 mL/kg/min is normal for middle-age adults, but a value lower than 14 mL/kg/min indicates severe cardiac limitation and poor prognosis.

A useful diagnostic test for the detection of heart failure is the BNP assay.[6,7] BNP levels correlate with severity of heart failure and decrease as a patient reaches a compensated state. This blood test may be useful for distinguishing heart failure from pulmonary disease. Because smokers often have both these clinical diagnoses, differentiating between them may be challenging.

The routine use of invasive hemodynamic monitoring to guide the management of decompensated heart failure has not proved to be beneficial. However, invasive hemodynamic monitoring may be warranted if unanticipated responses to therapies are observed or for diagnostic purposes if the diagnosis is uncertain.

Box 1 Patient Education Guidelines

2-g Sodium diet
Monitoring weight daily
2-L Fluid restriction
Monitoring blood pressure
Medications
Smoking cessation
Light aerobic exercise
Knowing whom to call
Achieving ideal weight
Follow-up visits

Summary

- Jugular venous distention is a useful physical sign of heart failure.
- The lungs usually are clear in chronic heart failure.
- The BNP assay improves the accuracy of diagnosing heart failure.
- Echocardiography is the single most useful diagnostic modality.
- Coronary angiography confirms or excludes coronary artery disease as the cause.

TREATMENT

Lifestyle Modifications

Dietary sodium and fluid restrictions should be implemented in all patients with congestive heart failure. Limiting patients to 2 g/day of dietary sodium and 2 L/day of fluid will lessen congestion and decrease the need for diuretics. Patient education guidelines are listed in Box 1.

Cardiac rehabilitation can improve symptoms and exercise tolerance in patients with heart failure. This will also reduce or prevent skeletal muscle atrophy that could worsen exercise tolerance. Weight loss is encouraged in obese patients. Patients should be counseled about smoking cessation.

Medical Options

Angiotensin-Converting Enzyme Inhibitors

All patients with LV systolic dysfunction should be treated with an ACE inhibitor unless they have a contraindication or intolerance to the drug (stages B to D). ACE inhibitors are useful in preventing heart failure in patients at high risk who have atherosclerotic cardiovascular disease, diabetes mellitus, or hypertension with associated cardiovascular risk factors (stage A). ACE inhibitors and beta blockers should be used for all patients with a history of myocardial infarction, regardless of LVEF. Vasodilation and neurohormonal modulation with ACE inhibitors improve mortality, heart failure symptoms, exercise tolerance, and LVEF as well as reduce emergency room visits and hospitalizations.[8-10]

The dose of ACE inhibitors should be titrated to the maximum tolerated dose[11] or the target dose as listed in Table 3. Approximately 10% to 20% of patients do not tolerate ACE inhibitors. The main side effect from ACE inhibition is a dry hacking cough, which can necessitate change to an angiotensin II receptor blocker (ARB). Most patients who cough on ACE inhibitors have this symptom because of congestive heart failure rather than ACE inhibitor intolerance and might improve with further diuresis. Two uncommon side effects of

Table 3 Angiotensin-Converting Enzyme Inhibitor Dosing

Agent	Target Dose (mg)	Frequency
Captopril*	50	tid
Enalapril*	20	bid
Lisinopril*	40	qd
Ramipril*	5	bid
Quinapril*	20	bid
Fosinopril*	20	bid
Benazepril*	20	qd
Trandolapril†	4	qd

*FDA-approved for treatment of heart failure.
†FDA-approved for treatment of post–myocardial infarction heart failure.

Table 4 Angiotensin Receptor Blocker Dosing

Agent	Initial Dose (mg)	Maximum Dose (mg)
Valsartan*	80	320
Candesartan*	4	32
Losartan	25	100
Irbesartan	75	300
Telmisartan	40	80
Eprosartan	400	800
Olmesartan	20	40

*FDA-approved for treatment of heart failure.

ACE inhibitors are angioedema and acute renal failure (caused by bilateral renal artery stenosis); both necessitate immediate cessation of the drug.

ACE inhibitors should be used in combination with beta blockers in most patients. Either agent may be started first.

Angiotensin Receptor Blockers

ARBs block the effects of angiotensin II at the receptor level (Table 4). In clinical trials, these agents were found to be superior to placebo but no better than ACE inhibitors in improving mortality.[12] ARBs are recommended as second-line therapy in patients who do not intolerate ACE inhibitors because of cough or angioedema (stages B to D). ARBs should not be substituted for ACE inhibitors in cases of hyperkalemia or renal dysfunction. ARBs may have morbidity benefits for patients with diastolic heart failure.[13]

Beta Blockers

Three beta blockers—carvedilol, metoprolol succinate (Toprol XL), and bisoprolol—have been shown to improve survival in patients with heart failure (Table 5).[14-16] Metoprolol tartrate is not U.S Food and Drug Administration (FDA)-approved for heart failure and was less effective than carvedilol in preventing sudden death.[17] The exact mechanism of beta blocker action is unclear, but it likely involves antiarrhythmic, anti-ischemic, antiremodeling, and antiapoptotic properties, as well as improved beta receptor pathway function.

Table 5 Beta Blocker Dosing

Beta Blocker	Initial Dose (mg)	Target Dose
Carvedilol*	3.125 mg bid	50 mg bid if >75 kg 25 mg bid if <75 kg
Metoprolol succinate*	12.5 mg qd	200 mg qd
Bisoprolol	2.5 mg qd	10 mg qd

*FDA-approved for treatment of heart failure.

Myocardial oxygen consumption is reduced with beta blockers, primarily because of a reduction in heart rate.

All stable patients with reduced LVEF should receive a beta blocker unless it is contraindicated (stages B, C and D). Diabetes mellitus, chronic obstructive pulmonary disease, and peripheral arterial disease are not contraindications to beta blocker use, although patients with severe bronchospasm and hypotension might not tolerate the drug. Beta blockers may be used in stable NYHA Class IV patients who are euvolemic.[2] In heart failure patients, a beta blocker should be initiated before hospital discharge or on an outpatient basis at a low dose and titrated slowly to target levels or maximally tolerated doses. Beta blockers usually are given in combination with an ACE inhibitor, but either agent may be initiated first.

Digoxin

Digoxin is a neurohormonal modulating agent that inhibits the enzyme Na^+/K^+-ATPase in various organs. In cardiac cells, this inhibition increases myocardial contractility. In the central nervous system, it reduces sympathetic outflow, and in the kidney, it inhibits renin release. A large, randomized, controlled trial has shown that the use of digoxin reduces the rate of hospitalization for heart failure, but it does not reduce mortality.[18] Digoxin is excreted by the kidneys, so dose adjustment is necessary in cases of renal failure (Table 6). A low dose of digoxin (0.125 mg daily) should be prescribed to most patients. Digoxin may be prescribed for patients with LV systolic dysfunction who remain symptomatic while receiving standard medical therapy, particularly if they are in atrial fibrillation.

Diuretics

Diuretics should be used in combination with an ACE inhibitor (or ARB) and a beta blocker. Most patients with heart failure have some degree of symptomatic congestion and benefit from diuretic therapy.[19] Usually, a loop diuretic is required, with the addition of a thiazide diuretic in patients refractory to the loop diuretic alone (diuretic resistance or cardiorenal syndrome). Although useful for symptomatic relief, diuretics have not been shown to improve survival, and they can cause azotemia, hypokalemia, metabolic alkalosis, and elevation of neurohormone levels (Table 7).

Aldosterone Antagonists

Two aldosterone antagonists have been approved for patients with heart failure: spironolactone and eplerenone. A 30% reduction in mortality and hospitalizations has been reported when spironolactone is added to standard therapy for patients with NYHA Class III or IV heart failure and a serum creatinine less than 2.5.[20] A 15% reduction in the risk of death and hospitalization has been reported in patients who had heart failure and an LVEF lower than 40% after a myocardial infarction and who were treated with eplerenone.[21]

Aldosterone inhibition can prevent sodium and water retention, endothelial dysfunction, and myocardial fibrosis. With aldosterone antagonists, diligent monitoring of serum potassium levels is mandatory, because patients can develop hyperkalemia (see Table 6). These drugs should be avoided in patients with a creatinine level higher than 2.5 mg/dL. Eight percent of men develop gynecomastia with spironolactone but not with eplerenone. Data from studies of mild heart failure are lacking, and so these drugs should be reserved for patients with moderately severe to severe heart failure. Therefore, the addition of an aldosterone antagonist is reasonable for select patients with moderately severe to severe symptoms of heart failure and reduced LVEF who can be carefully monitored for preserved renal function and normal potassium concentration.

Hydralazine and Nitrates

Hydralazine is an arterial dilator and nitrates are venous dilators. Hydralazine also prevents nitrate tachyphylaxis (loss of effect). The combination of hydralazine and nitrate is inferior to an ACE inhibitor in improving survival.[22] Once-daily dosing of ACE inhibitors is easier than giving nitrates three times daily and giving hydralazine four times daily (see Table 6). The combination of hydralazine and nitrate is reasonable for patients who have current or prior symptoms of heart failure and reduced LVEF and who cannot be given an ACE or ARB because of drug intolerance, hyperkalemia, or renal insufficiency. Hydralazine and nitrate also may be added to ACE inhibitors and beta blockers when additional afterload reduction is needed or pulmonary hypertension is present. A fixed-dose combination tablet has been approved for treating heart failure in African Americans.

Other Medical Therapies

Patients with known coronary artery disease should be treated with aspirin and a statin to lower the low-density lipoprotein (LDL) level to 70 mg/dL. Calcium channel antagonists have not been proved beneficial in heart failure patients. Dihydropyridines such as amlodipine have a neutral effect on heart failure and may be useful for treating concomitant hypertension or angina pectoris.[23]

The use of warfarin to prevent cardioembolic strokes remains controversial in the absence of atrial arrhythmias, because the risk appears to be relatively low (1%-3% per year). Warfarin therapy is recommended for patients with atrial arrhythmias, previous embolic event, cardiac thrombi, or LV aneurysms.

Specific therapies for treating atrial fibrillation, sleep apnea, anemia, obesity, and thyroid disease may improve the symptoms and functional limitations of heart failure.

Intravenous Inotropes and Vasodilators

Dobutamine

Dobutamine (Table 8) enhances contractility by directly stimulating cardiac β_1 receptors.[24] Intravenous (IV) dobutamine infusions, sometimes guided by hemodynamic monitoring, may be useful for select patients with acute hypotensive heart failure or shock. The dose of dobutamine should always be titrated to the lowest dose compatible with hemodynamic stability to minimize adverse events. As with many inotropes, long-term infusions of dobutamine can increase mortality, principally because of its arrhythmogenic effect. As a result, chronic dobutamine infusions are reserved for palliative symptom relief or for patients who have an implantable cardioverter-defibrillator (ICD) and are awaiting heart transplantation. Intermittent outpatient infusions of dobutamine are not recommended for routine management of heart failure.

Milrinone

Milrinone (see Table 8) is a phosphodiesterase inhibitor that enhances contractility. Milrinone is useful for patients with low-output heart failure and pulmonary hypertension because it is a more potent pulmonary vasodilator than dobutamine. Milrinone, in contrast to dobutamine, is also useful for patients on chronic oral beta blocker therapy who develop acute heart failure. The OPTIME (Outcomes of a Prospective Trial of Intravenous Milrinone for Exacerba-

Table 6 Other Heart Failure Drugs

Agent	Initial Dose	Maximum Dose	Guidelines
Digoxin	0.125 mg qd	0.25 mg qd	Reduce dose in women with renal dysfunction, with amiodarone
Hydralazine	25 mg qid	100 mg qid	Use concurrently with nitrates to prevent coronary steal
Isosorbide dinitrate	20 mg tid	80 mg tid	Also useful for angina pectoris
Spironolactone	25 mg qd	50 mg qd	Weak diuretic, risk of hyperkalemia, avoid in renal dysfunction; gynecomastia
Eplerenone	25 mg qd	50 mg qd	Risk of hyperkalemia, avoid in renal dysfunction; no gynecomastia

Table 7 Diuretic Dosing

Generic Name	Class	Initial Dose (mg)	Special Considerations
Furosemide	Loop	20	Can be given intravenously; PO equivalent is twice the IV dose
Bumetanide	Loop	0.5	Good oral bioavailability; can be given intravenously; oral and IV doses are the same
Torsemide	Loop	5-10	Best oral availability
Ethacrynic acid	Loop	50	Only diuretic with no sulfhydryl group; used if allergic to furosemide
Hydrochlorothiazide	Thiazide	12.5	Weak diuretic; used mainly for hypertension
Metolazone	Thiazide	2.5	Give ½ hr before furosemide; only available orally; high risk of hypokalemia

Table 8 Intravenous Agents Used for Treatment of Heart Failure

Drug	Dose	Special Considerations
Dobutamine	2-20 μg/kg/min	β receptor agonist; proarrhythmic; heart rate; ischemia
Milrinone	0.25-0.75 μg/kg/min	Phosphodiesterase inhibitor; vasodilator; may improve pulmonary hypertension; used for patients taking beta blockers; proarrhythmic
Nitroglycerin	10-500 μg/min	Anti-ischemic; vasodilator; limited by vascular headache; hypotension, tolerance develops rapidly
Nitroprusside	10-500 μg/min	Thiocyanate accumulation in renal failure; may provoke ischemia by coronary steal; vasodilator; should be given only in intensive care unit
Nesiritide	2-μg/kg bolus; then 0.01 μg/kg/min	Fixed weight-based dose; vasodilator; occasional hypotension

tions of Chronic Heart Failure) study, involving the routine intravenous infusion of milrinone for 48 hours during hospitalization for decompensated heart failure, failed to show clinical benefit and was associated with an increased risk of atrial arrhythmias and hypotension.[25] Similar to dobutamine, intermittent outpatient milrinone infusions are not recommended for routine management of heart failure.

Nitroglycerin

Nitroglycerin (see Table 8) is a nitric oxide donor that causes vasodilation. It is a venodilator at low doses and an arterial dilator at higher doses, lowering intracardiac pressures and alleviating pulmonary congestion.

Nitroglycerin also dilates coronary arteries, making it useful for patients with heart failure and myocardial ischemia. IV nitroglycerin requires dose titration to achieve therapeutic goals. The effectiveness of prolonged infusions is limited by the development of tachyphylaxis (loss of effect) within the first 24 hours.

Sodium Nitroprusside

Sodium nitroprusside (see Table 8) is a nitric oxide donor and a potent short-acting arterial and venous dilator. Nitroprusside infusions generally are reserved for patients in an intensive care unit. During nitroprusside infusions, patients should be converted to oral vasodilators such as ACE inhibitors, ARBs, or hydralazine and a nitrate.

Sodium nitroprusside should be infused for a short duration in patients with severe renal disease to prevent accumulation of thiocyanate, the by-product of hepatic metabolism of nitroprusside, which is excreted by the kidney. Nitroprusside should be avoided in patients with active ischemia because of its potential for coronary steal syndrome, which shunts blood away from the ischemic myocardium to well-perfused muscle.

Nesiritide

Nesiritide (see Table 8), synthetic BNP, is an arterial and venous vasodilator with modest diuretic and natriuretic properties.[26] Nesiritide increases cardiac output by afterload reduction without increasing heart rate or oxygen consumption. It modulates the vasoconstrictor and sodium-retaining effects of other neurohormones. Nesiritide is administered as a weight-based bolus followed by continuous IV infusion in patients who have acutely decompensated heart failure and who have dyspnea at rest or with minimal activity. It may be started in the emergency department and does not require invasive hemodynamic monitoring or frequent titration. Tolerance to the drug does not occur and it is not arrhythmogenic. Intermittent outpatient infusions of nesiritide are not recommended for the routine management of heart failure.

Device Therapies for Heart Failure

Cardiac Resynchronization Therapy

Several clinical trials have shown the potential benefit of cardiac resynchronization therapy (CRT) for patients with severe symptomatic heart failure and a wide QRS complex.[27,28] Symptomatic improvement is achieved in approximately 70% of patients because of improved ventricular contraction, ventricular reverse-remodeling, and reduction of mitral regurgitation. With cardiac resynchronization therapy (biventricular pacing), a third electrode is implanted in a left cardiac vein via the coronary sinus so that the right and left ventricles are paced in a synchronous fashion (Fig. 3). Optimal synchronization of atrial and ventricular contraction is achieved with echocardiographic guidance. Guidelines for resynchronization therapy are listed in Box 2.

Defibrillator Therapy

Approximately 50% of patients with heart failure die suddenly. Implantation of an ICD can improve survival in certain subsets of heart failure patients and has been shown to be superior to antiarrhythmic drug therapy in preventing sudden death.[29-32] Current indications for defibrillator therapy are listed in Box 3. Cardiac resynchronization therapy can be combined with an ICD as a single device if the patient meets criteria for both therapies, as is often the case.

Ultrafiltration Therapy

Ultrafiltration therapy is an effective method for extracting sodium and fluid from volume overloaded heart failure patients with resistance to diuretic therapy. A reduction in rehospitalization has been observed compared with intravenous diuretic therapy.[33]

Surgical Options

Left Ventricular Assist Devices (LVADs)

Certain patients with end-stage heart failure and NYHA Class IV symptoms are referred to a tertiary care center for mechanical circulatory support.[34,35] At present, LV assist devices (LVADs) are used either as a bridge to cardiac transplantation in patients who are appropriate transplantation candidates or as destination therapy in patients ineligible for transplantation. The inflow cannula of an LVAD is connected to the apex of the left ventricle. Blood is mechanically pumped by the device via the outflow cannula to the aorta (Fig. 4). Complications following LVAD implantation are common and often life threatening; these include stroke, infection, perioperative coagulopathy and bleeding, and multisystem organ failure. Newer rotary continuous flow LVADs have proven to be more durable and are associated with fewer complications.[36]

Ventricular Reconstruction Surgery

Ventricular reconstruction surgery, also called ventricular remodeling surgery or a Dor procedure, has been performed for heart failure

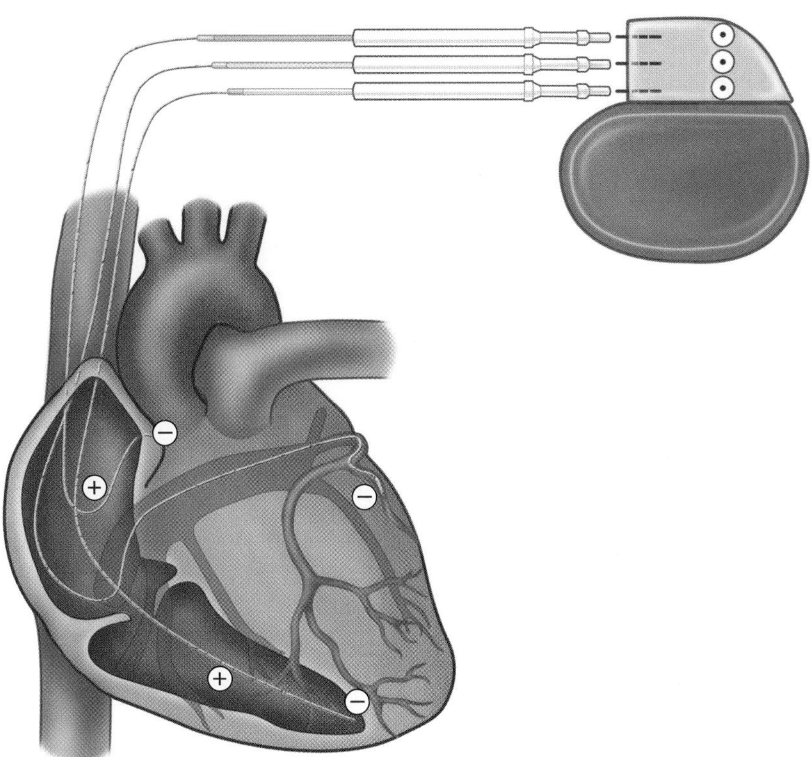

Figure 3 Resynchronization therapy. Pacemaker leads are implanted in the right atrium, right ventricle, and left cardiac vein via the coronary sinus.

Box 2 Guidelines for Resynchronization Therapy

NYHA Class III or IV heart failure symptoms
Symptomatic despite medications
Left ventricular ejection fraction ≤35% (consider cardiac resynchronization therapy-defibrillator)
Wide QRS (>120 msec; left bundle branch block, intraventricular conduction delay)
Evidence of dyssynchrony

Box 3 Indications for an Implantable Cardioverter-Defibrillator

Cardiac arrest survivor
Sustained ventricular tachycardia
Inducible ventricular tachycardia
Ischemic cardiomyopathy,* LVEF ≤35%
Dilated cardiomyopathy†, LVEF ≤35% with symptoms

**40-day waiting period after myocardial infarction, stenting, bypass surgery.*
†9-month waiting period after diagnosis.
LVEF, left ventricular ejection fraction.

secondary to ischemic cardiomyopathy.[37] It consists of several components: coronary artery bypass grafting, mitral and tricuspid valve repair, resection of LV scar or aneurysm, reshaping the left ventricle from a spherical to an elliptic shape, and epicardial LV pacing lead placement (Fig. 5). The STICH trial failed to show benefit over standard bypass or value surgery. Thus, the future of ventricular reconstruction surgery is uncertain.

Cardiac Transplantation

Cardiac transplantation is reserved for otherwise healthy patients who have end-stage heart failure with severely impaired functional capacity despite optimal medical therapy (Fig. 6).[38] Patients are excluded from transplantation if they have chronic medical comorbidities, pulmonary hypertension, active infection, psychosocial contraindications, or medical noncompliance. Survival after cardiac transplantation is about 85% at 1 year, and median life expectancy is approximately 10 years. Complications limiting survival include rejection, infection, transplant coronary vasculopathy, and malignancy. Following cardiac transplantation, patients are subjected to lifelong immunosuppression to prevent rejection, which in turn renders them susceptible to various opportunistic infections and malignancies.

Summary

- All heart failure patients should receive an ACE inhibitor and a beta blocker.
- Diuretics are needed in most patients to manage fluid retention.
- Digoxin is reserved for patients with signs and symptoms of heart failure.
- Aldosterone antagonists are used in patients with Class III or IV heart failure.
- ARBs or a hydralazine plus nitrate may be added to standard therapy for additional benefit.

PREVENTION AND SCREENING

Patients classified as stage A are at high risk for heart failure but without structural heart disease or heart failure symptoms. They include patients with hypertension, diabetes mellitus, obesity, coronary artery disease, or use of cardiotoxins and those with a family history of cardiomyopathy. Preventive therapies include treatment

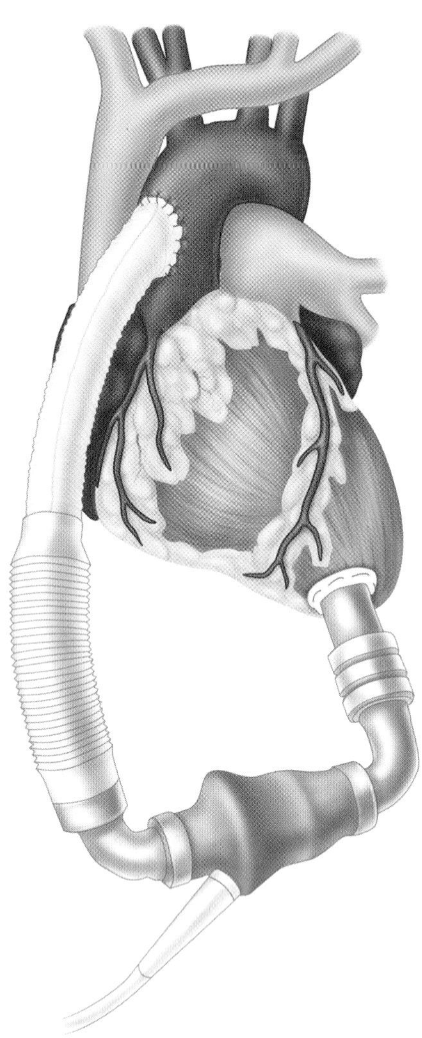

Figure 4 Left ventricular assist device. A HeartMate II is a small continuous flow pump. The inflow cannula is connected to the cardiac apex, and the outflow graft is connected to the ascending aorta.

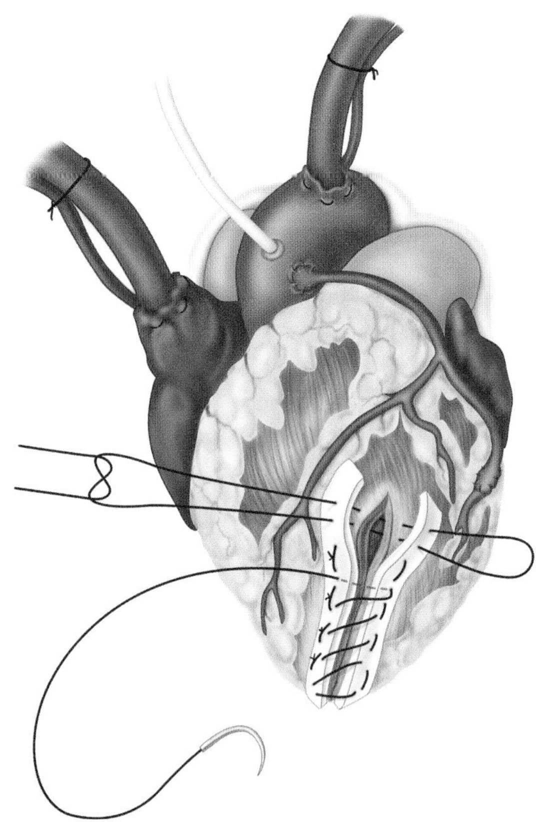

Figure 5 Left ventricular reconstruction. This surgery is also known as a Dor procedure. It consists of the resection of a left ventricular scar or aneurysm, reshaping the left ventricle into an ellipticl chamber, coronary bypass grafting, valve repair, and placement of epicardial pacemaker leads.

of lipid disorders and hypertension, smoking cessation, regular exercise, avoidance of excess alcohol and illicit drugs, and ACE inhibitors in appropriate patients. Patients with stage B heart failure have structural heart disease, but no symptoms of heart failure. These include patients with previous myocardial infarction, LV systolic dysfunction, and asymptomatic valvular disease. Therapies are prescribed to prevent LV remodeling. These include all preventive strategies for stage A, as well as ACE inhibitors and beta blockers for appropriate patients.

CONSIDERATIONS IN SPECIAL POPULATIONS

Heart failure is slightly more common in women than men. In women, heart failure occurs later in life, is often related to hypertension, and is often associated with preserved LV systolic function. Women tend to have more prominent heart failure manifestations and more hospitalizations but better overall survival (except with coronary artery disease) than men. Heart failure therapeutic agents are not gender specific.

African Americans appear to benefit from a combination of hydralazine and nitrates when added to conventional heart failure therapy.[39]

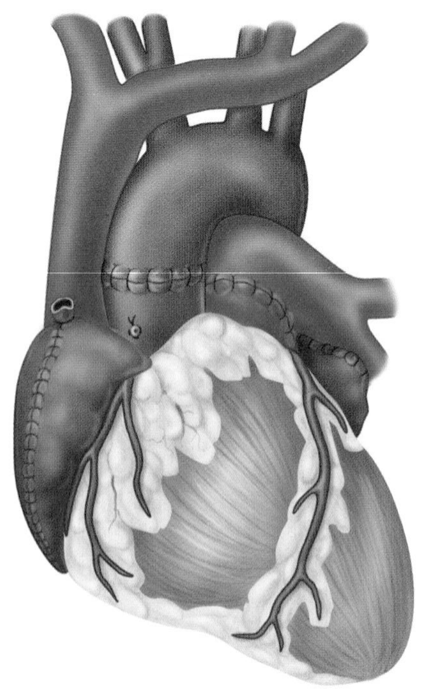

Figure 6 Orthotopic heart transplant. The transplanted heart does not require coronary artery bypass grafting or pacemaker leads.

Suggest Readings

Adams KF, Lindenfeld J, Arnold JMO, et al: Executive summary: HFSA 2006 comprehensive heart failure practice guideline. J Cardiac Failure 2006;12:10-38.

American Heart Association: Heart Disease and Stroke Statistics-2008 Update. Dallas, American Heart Association, 2008.

Bardy GH, Lee KL, Mark DB, et al: Amiodarone or an implantable cardioverter-defibrillator for congestive heart failure. N Engl J Med 2005;352:225-237.

Brater DC: Diuretic therapy. N Engl J Med 1998;339:387-395.

Cleland JGF, Daubert JC, Erdman E, et al: The effect of cardiac resynchronization on morbidity and mortality in heart failure. N Engl J Med 2005;352:1539-1549.

Digitalis Investigation Group: The effect of digoxin on mortality and morbidity in patients with heart failure. N Engl J Med 1997;336:525-533.

Hjalmarson A, Goldstein S, Fagerberg B, et al: Effects of controlled-release metoprolol on total mortality, hospitalizations, and well-being in patients with heart failure: The Metoprolol CR/XL Randomized Intervention Trial in congestive heart failure (MERIT-HF). JAMA 2000;283:1295-1302.

Hunt SA, Abraham WT, Chin MH, et al: American College of Cardiology; American Heart Association Task Force on Practice Guidelines; American College of Chest Physicians; International Society for Heart and Lung Transplantation; Heart Rhythm Society: ACC/AHA 2005 Guideline Update for the Diagnosis and Management of Chronic Heart Failure in the Adult: A report of the American College of Cardiology/American Heart Association Task Force on Practice Guidelines (Writing Committee to Update the 2001 Guidelines for the Evaluation and Management of Heart Failure): Developed in collaboration with the American College of Chest Physicians and the International Society for Heart and Lung Transplantation: Endorsed by the Heart Rhythm Society. Circulation 2005;112:e154-e235.

Mueller C, Scholer A, Laule-Kilian K, et al: Use of B-type natriuretic peptide in the evaluation and management of acute dyspnea. N Engl J Med 2004;350:647-654.

Pitt B, Remme W, Zannad F, et al: Eplerenone, a selective aldosterone blocker, in patients with left ventricular dysfunction after myocardial infarction. N Engl J Med 2003;348:1309-1321.

Pitt B, Zannad F, Remme WJ, et al: The effect of spironolactone on morbidity and mortality in patients with severe heart failure. Randomized Aldactone Evaluation Study Investigators. N Engl J Med 1999;341:709-717.

Swedberg K, Cleland J, Dargie H, et al: Guidelines for the diagnosis and treatment of chronic heart failure: Executive summary (Update 2005). Eur Heart J 2005;26:1115-1140.

References

For a complete list of references, log onto www.expertconsult.com.

Heart Transplantation

Mohamad H. Yamani and David O. Taylor

Cardiac transplantation has emerged as a viable therapeutic strategy for select patients with end-stage heart disease, offering extended survival and improved quality of life. Patients with severe heart failure have a 1- to 2-year mortality rate approaching 50%, despite advanced medical treatment. Approximately 4000 heart transplantation procedures are performed annually worldwide. In the United States, approximately 3000 patients are awaiting transplantation, but only 2000 patients undergo transplantation annually because of lack of donor hearts. Long-term outcomes after transplantation have improved with the advances made in transplant candidate selection, surgical techniques, immunosuppressive modalities, and postoperative care. The current survival rate after heart transplantation has been reported as approximately 50% at 12 years by the International Society for Heart and Lung Transplantation (ISHLT) registry.

INITIAL CONSIDERATIONS

Recipient and Donor Selection

The paucity of the donor pool demands a very careful patient-selection process to ensure appropriate candidacy. A thorough search for reversible or surgically amenable cardiac disease must be completed and optimal medical management implemented before transplantation is considered. Early referral to a heart-failure cardiologist is recommended to evaluate for appropriate candidacy. Certain basic tests are required in the evaluation process and include a right heart catheterization to evaluate hemodynamics and, in particular, to evaluate for any reversible pulmonary hypertension component. A metabolic stress test is also indicated to evaluate peak oxygen consumption. Certain inclusion criteria (Box 1) and exclusion criteria (Box 2) must be met for a successful post-transplantation outcome. Routine blood tests, including screening serology for cytomegalovirus, toxoplasmosis, Epstein virus, hepatitis B, and hepatitis C, are also indicated. Once inclusion and exclusion criteria are met, the patient is listed according to urgency code status (see later).

Donor selection is influenced by many factors, including ABO blood type compatibility, size similarity between the donor and recipient, presence of intrinsic cardiac disease, and presence of transmissible infectious or malignant diseases. The risk of using a specific donor heart is always balanced against the risk of short-term death in a particular recipient. To screen for donor cardiac disease, electrocardiography, echocardiography, and sometimes coronary angiography are used. Some donor hearts with significant coronary artery or valvular disease have been transplanted successfully with simultaneous bypass surgery or valve replacement, but doing so is not yet standard care. Brain death can cause time-dependent changes in left ventricular function that may be related to catecholamine release. Donor heart dysfunction may be reversible, and thyroid hormone is frequently administered to improve donor heart function. Clearly, using an irreversibly damaged donor heart is to be avoided.

Transplantation Urgency Code Status

Once patients are approved for transplantation, they are listed according to the medical urgency status and severity of the illness (Table 1). The median waiting time for transplantation is approximately 9.4 months in the United States. The waiting time to transplantation depends on several factors, including listed status, body weight, blood group, and other differences between recipient and donor. It is estimated that 15% to 20% of patients die while waiting for a transplant.

HEART TRANSPLANTATION SURGERY

Three implantation techniques are available: biatrial technique, bicaval technique, and the rarely used heterotopic technique. The key to successful transplantation is the donor ischemic time, defined as the time from aortic cross-clamping in the donor to release of the aortic cross-clamping in the recipient. An acceptable ischemic time is considered to be less than 4 hours. Concern about the loss of normal atrial anatomy using the biatrial technique has led to the more frequent use of the bicaval technique. The bicaval technique can result in a longer donor heart ischemic time but is associated with lower right atrial pressure, lower incidence of atrial tachyarrhythmias, and less tricuspid valve incompetence. Heterotopic cardiac transplantation can be performed with the donor heart placed in the right lower thorax in parallel to the recipient heart, which is left in place. The indications for heterotopic cardiac transplantation include significant pulmonary hypertension, a small donor heart, and a donor heart with anticipated poor initial function. This technique accounts for only 0.3% of all heart transplantation procedures.

POST-TRANSPLANTATION CARDIAC FUNCTION

The function of the newly transplanted cardiac allograft is influenced by an interplay of several important physiologic factors that include allograft denervation, ventricular loading conditions, hormonal milieu, myocardial injury, donor-recipient size relation, pulmonary performance, and atrial function.

Serial ventricular function evaluation by Doppler echocardiography has suggested the presence of diastolic dysfunction, which is a common phenomenon early after heart transplantation. Prior hemodynamic studies have also noted a restrictive pattern that usually resolves within days or weeks but may persist or recur later because of cell-mediated rejection or hypertrophy.

During the first week after cardiac transplantation, there is generally an increase in the severity of mitral, tricuspid, and aortic regurgitation. These valvular regurgitations are usually asymptomatic at rest, except for tricuspid regurgitation, which is associated with right-sided heart failure in more than 50% of patients in the early postoperative period.

Recently, tissue Doppler imaging has emerged as a technique that permits evaluation of myocardial relaxation velocities and allows estimation of ventricular filling pressures following heart transplantation. Because allograft rejection results in increased myocardial stiffness and abnormal myocardial relaxation tissue, Doppler imaging has been a useful noninvasive tool for the diagnosis of rejection and may have a role as a screening technique if ongoing research confirms its sensitivity and specificity.

Cardiac Allograft Rejection

After heart transplantation, proinflammatory cytokines are elaborated and recipient inflammatory cells are recruited into the cardiac allograft. The sequence of events leading to cardiac allograft rejection encompasses antigen recognition, primary and secondary (costimulatory) signals for T cell activation, and T cell proliferation and dif-

Box 1 Indications for Cardiac Transplantation

Refractory heart failure requiring continuous inotropic support
Cardiogenic shock requiring mechanical assistance (e.g., ventilator, intra-aortic balloon pump, ventricular assist device, total artificial heart) with, at worst, reversible end-organ damage
Congestive heart failure, New York Heart Association (NYHA) Class III or IV symptoms, with objective evidence of impaired functional capacity (peak oxygen consumption <14 mL/kg/min), despite optimal medical therapy
Refractory angina, despite maximal medical therapy, and not amenable to revascularization
Refractory life-threatening ventricular arrhythmias, despite maximal antiarrhythmic therapy by all appropriate conventional medical and surgical modalities (multiple firings from an ICD for documented VT and VF)
Congenital heart disease with progressive ventricular failure that is not amenable to conventional surgical repair
Severe hypertrophic or restrictive cardiomyopathy, with NYHA Class IV symptoms
Cardiac tumors confined to the myocardium, with a low likelihood of metastasis at time of transplantation

ICD, implantable cardioverter-defibrillator; VF, ventricular fibrillation; VT, ventricular tachycardia.

Box 2 Absolute and Relative Contraindications to Cardiac Transplantation

Pulmonary artery systemic pressure >60 mm Hg, mean transpulmonary gradient >15 mm Hg, and/or peripheral vascular resistance >5 Wood units on maximal vasodilator therapy
Active infection (unless associated with left ventricular assist device)
Active peptic ulcer disease
Active diverticulitis
Irreversible severe hepatic disease
Irreversible severe renal disease
Morbid obesity (body mass index >35 kg/m^2)
Severe diabetes mellitus, with end-organ damage
Severe peripheral vascular disease
Recent stroke (unless associated with left ventricular assist device)
Acute pulmonary embolism (<6 wk)
Active neoplasm (must be malignancy-free for at least 5 yr)
Current alcohol or drug abuse
Ongoing tobacco use
Irreversible severe pulmonary disease, with FEV_1 <1 L or FVC <50%
Severe psychiatric or cognitive impairment
Repeated noncompliance with medications or follow-up
Lack of family or social support

FEV_1, forced expiratory volume in 1 sec; FVC, forced vital capacity.

ferentiation. Patients may be asymptomatic or may experience a spectrum of symptoms, ranging from mild exertional dyspnea to overt heart failure symptoms and arrhythmias resulting in syncope, cardiac arrest, or both, depending on the severity of rejection. Echocardiography is helpful to evaluate graft function, but left ventricular function may be preserved in the early stages. Endomyocardial biopsy is the gold standard procedure to establish the diagnosis of rejection (see later).

There are three types of rejection: hyperacute, acute cellular, and acute vascular (antibody-mediated) rejection. Hyperacute rejection is a result of preformed donor-specific antibodies in the recipient. It is a vigorous immune response that takes place within minutes to hours. The outcome, without repeat transplantation or total artificial heart support, is uniformly fatal. The best method for avoiding hyperacute rejection is to avoid transplanting a donor heart into a patient who is sensitized to the donor (a positive donor-specific crossmatch). Acute cellular rejection is the most common form of rejection and occurs at least once in approximately 50% of heart

Table 1 Transplantation Urgency Code Status

Code Status	Description
1A	Patients who are on inotropic support and receiving mechanical support, or on a ventilator or in the intensive care unit, with a pulmonary artery catheter in place for hemodynamic monitoring
1B	Patients who are on inotropic support but not meeting 1A criteria or who have had a ventricular assist device longer than 30 days
2	Patients who are waiting at home on medical therapy
7	Patients who are on hold because of an intervening medical illness, making them inappropriate candidates for transplantation

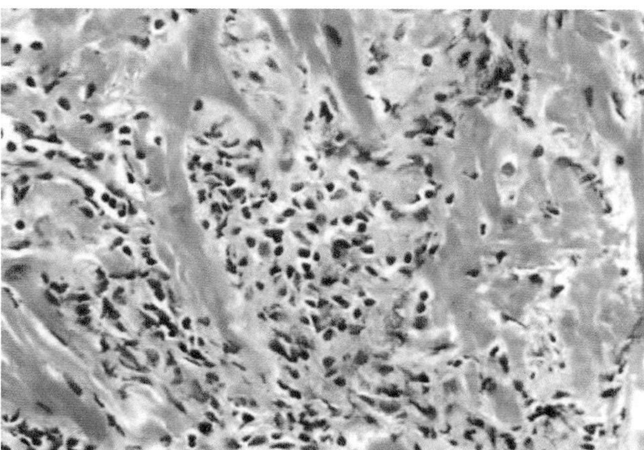

Figure 1 Endomyocardial biopsy showing diffuse lymphocytic infiltrate with myocyte necrosis. These changes correspond to International Society for Heart and Lung Transplantation grade 3B or revised grade 3 cellular rejection.

transplant recipients (Fig. 1). Even though the propensity toward allograft rejection decreases over time and almost 50% of the rejection episodes occur in the first 2 to 3 months, late rejection can and does occur. Vascular rejection may manifest by otherwise unexplained cardiac allograft dysfunction, with or without histologic evidence. Histologic evidence is a scant cellular infiltrate but abundant colocalized immunoglobulin and complement components in the allograft microvasculature seen on one or more biopsy specimens (Fig. 2). In addition, vascular rejection may manifest only histologically in the absence of allograft dysfunction. Vascular rejection is more difficult to treat than acute cellular rejection and is more often accompanied by hemodynamic compromise or instability. As a result, vascular rejection is associated with a worse prognosis and appears to increase the risk of cardiac allograft vasculopathy (CAV) almost tenfold.

Surveillance Endomyocardial Biopsy

Endomyocardial biopsy remains the gold standard for the diagnosis of acute rejection after cardiac transplantation. Recently, molecular gene expression testing in peripheral blood (AlloMap) has been used as a noninvasive tool to detect quiescence and acute rejection. This test has a high negative predictive value, approaching 95%; however, it has low sensitivity. The most commonly used grading scheme for the diagnosis and staging of rejection is that of the ISHLT (Table 2). Rejection is the leading cause of death in the first year after heart

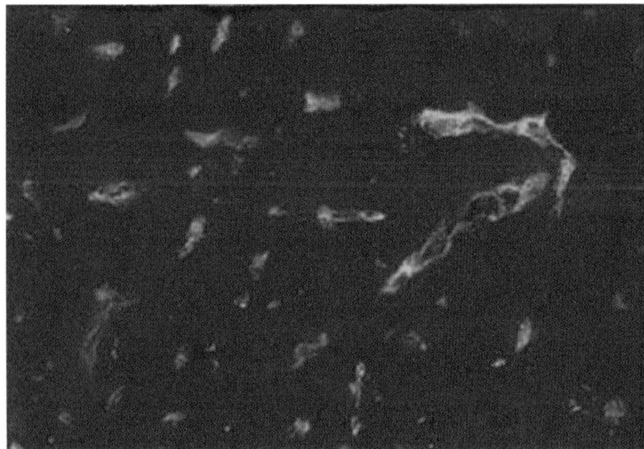

Figure 2 Immunofluorescence in an endomyocardial biopsy. This figure illustrates the deposition of complement C3 in the capillaries, suggesting antibody-mediated rejection.

Table 2 Revised ISHLT Standardized Endomyocardial Biopsy Grading Scheme

Revised Grading	Old Grading	Criteria
0	0	Normal myocardium
1	1A	Focal lymphocytic infiltrate, without myocyte necrosis
	1B	Diffuse but sparse lymphocytic infiltrate, without myocyte necrosis
	2	One focus of aggressive lymphocytic infiltrate, focal myocyte injury, or both
2	3A	Multifocal aggressive lymphocytic infiltrate, focal myocyte injury, or both
3	3B	Diffuse lymphocytic infiltrate with myocyte necrosis
4	4	Diffuse, aggressive, polymorphous infiltrate with necrosis (with or without edema, hemorrhage, vasculitis)

ISHLT, International Society for Heart and Lung Transplantation.

transplantation, and accounts for approximately 20% of all deaths. The frequency of surveillance biopsy varies among centers. In general, routine endomyocardial biopsies are performed weekly for the first month, then every 2 weeks during the second month, and increased to monthly through months 8 to 12. After 1 year, biopsies are done every 4 to 6 months. Following a treated episode of rejection, the endomyocardial biopsy is generally repeated within 14 days to ensure adequate treatment.

Although endomyocardial biopsy is usually considered safe, it entails some procedural risk but has few significant long-term sequelae. Complications during biopsy include hematoma, pneumothorax, hemothorax, cardiac perforation, arrhythmias, and conduction abnormalities, but these complications are rare. Occasional cases of hepatitis B transmission have been reported, and coronary artery fistula formation has been described in 2.9% of patients, most of which close spontaneously without long-term clinical sequelae. Venous thrombosis has also been reported but is unusual. Iatrogenic tricuspid regurgitation is a known but fortunately infrequent complication.

Immunosuppression

Immunosuppression is used to prevent rejection and is generally required for life. Early rejection prophylaxis involves the use of multiple agents (Table 3). Generally, triple therapy is used, consisting of cyclosporine or tacrolimus; azathioprine, mycophenolate mofetil, or sirolimus; and corticosteroids. Triple therapy has proved to be effective for most patients. Drug level monitoring is important to ensure adequacy of immunosuppression and avoid unwanted adverse effects, mainly nephrotoxicity. Therapeutic levels are variable in relation to time since transplantation (Table 4). Because the propensity for rejection decreases over time, dosages of all three drugs may be decreased accordingly. Cyclosporine and tacrolimus are usually maintained long term at levels less than 50% of those used early after transplantation. Long-term dosages of mycophenolate mofetil generally decrease from 3000 to 2000 mg/day. Prednisone can be withdrawn in some patients who demonstrate a low propensity to reject or if they experience steroid-related adverse effects.

The treatment of cardiac allograft rejection depends on several factors, including severity of rejection (ISHLT grade of endomyocardial biopsy specimens), time since transplantation, immunosuppressive history, and hemodynamic status of the patient. In treating rejection, one generally optimizes or increases the dosages of maintenance immunosuppressors. Mild rejection in hemodynamically stable patients—those without evidence of allograft dysfunction—is not treated. Moderate rejection in the absence of hemodynamic instability is usually treated initially with a several-day course of intravenous or high-dose oral corticosteroids. In corticosteroid refractory rejection or in rejection episodes associated with hemodynamic instability, an antilymphocyte antibody such as OKT3 or an antithymocyte globulin is added.

Cardiac Allograft Vasculopathy

CAV is a major cause of morbidity and mortality following heart transplantation. The precise molecular mechanism for the development of vasculopathy is not known. Both immune and nonimmune mechanisms have been implicated in the progression of vasculopathy. Recent studies have focused on different markers related to the extracellular matrix, renin-angiotensin system, fibrinolytic system, adhesion receptors, and markers of inflammation. Angiographic evidence of transplant vasculopathy is seen in 50% to 60% of transplant recipients by 5 years. However, intravascular ultrasound (IVUS) can detect an abnormal coronary intimal thickness in 50% of patients as early as 1 year after cardiac transplantation (Fig. 3). Thus far, the improvements in immunosuppression have not greatly affected the incidence and morbidity associated with CAV development. Various risk factors have been identified for the development of CAV, including donor age, presence of coronary artery disease before transplantation, diabetes mellitus, hypertension, hyperlipidemia, frequency and type of rejection, degree of human leukocyte antigen (HLA) matching, and cytomegalovirus (CMV) infection.

The clinical manifestation of CAV early after transplantation may be silent, occurring as acute myocardial infarction, congestive heart failure, arrhythmias, wall motion abnormalities, or sudden death. Later, typical angina pectoris can occur because of focal, albeit incomplete, reinnervation. Most CAV is diagnosed by routinely scheduled yearly surveillance angiography, although many noninvasive techniques have been evaluated in an attempt to decrease the need for invasive testing. Several studies have explored the role of dobutamine stress echocardiography (DSE) in the detection of coronary vasculopathy. Regional myocardial dysfunction as assessed by DSE was associated with moderate to severe coronary intimal thickening. DSE was also shown to have a significant value in predicting outcome and prognosis following transplantation. The use of thal-

Table 3 Pharmacology of Commonly Used Immunosuppressive Agents

Agent	Mechanism of Action	Administration	Toxicity	Drug-Drug Interactions
Cyclosporine	Binds to cyclophilin, inhibits calcineurin-dependent transcription and translation of cytokine genes, particularly interleukin (IL)-2	PO or IV, oral to IV dose adjustment is 3:1; oral dosage 3-6 mg/kg/day, targeted to level	Renal effects, hypertension, gingival hyperplasia, hirsutism, tremor, headache, paresthesias, flushing	Metabolism decreased by ketoconazole, diltiazem, verapamil, erythromycin, cimetidine, grapefruit; metabolism increased by phenytoin, phenobarbital, isoniazid, rifampin, carbamazepine
Tacrolimus	Binds to FK-binding protein, inhibits calcineurin-dependent transcription and translation of cytokine genes, particularly IL-2	PO or IV, oral to IV dose adjustment is 5:1; oral dosage 0.05-0.15 mg/kg/day, targeted to level	Renal effects, hypertension, tremor, headache, flushing, paresthesias, glucose intolerance	Similar to cyclosporine
Azathioprine	Inhibits purine ring biosynthesis, decreasing synthesis of DNA and RNA	PO or IV, no significant oral to IV adjustment; 1-2 mg/kg/day; white blood cell (WBC) count to remain >4000/mm^3	Macrocytic anemia, leukopenia, pancreatitis, cholestatic jaundice, hepatitis	Allopurinol slows metabolism by inhibiting xanthine oxidase
Mycophenolate mofetil	Inhibits inosine monophosphate dehydrogenase, inhibiting the de novo pathway for guanine nucleotide biosynthesis	PO or IV, no significant oral to IV adjustment; 2000-6000 mg/day	Gastrointestinal distress, leukopenia	No significant interactions
Sirolimus	Binds to FK-binding protein, inhibits IL-2– and IL-6–driven events	PO, loading dose 6 mg, then 2 mg/day	Hypertriglyceridemia, thrombocytopenia, leukopenia	Metabolism decreased by diltiazem and ketoconazole; metabolism increased by rifampin
Corticosteroids	Lymphocytolysis, inhibits release and action of various interleukins, interferes with antigen receptor interactions	PO or IV with methylprednisolone; maintenance dosage of prednisone is 0.0-0.1 mg/kg/day	Cushingoid habitus, glucose intolerance, hyperlipidemia, hypertension, cataracts, myopathy, osteoporosis	Multiple drug interactions, none clinically significant

Table 4 Immunosuppression Drug Level Monitoring

Immunosuppressive Agent	Therapeutic Level
Cyclosporine (ng/mL)	
0-3 mo	300-350
3-12 mo	225-250
After 1 yr	150-175
Tacrolimus (ng/mL)	
0-3 mo	15-20
3-12 mo	10-15
After 1 yr	5-10
Mycophenolate mofetil (mg/L)	2-4

lium-201 (^{201}Tl) imaging has been advocated for the diagnosis of post-transplantation coronary vasculopathy, but its role remains questionable.

The treatment of established CAV appears to be limited to retransplantation and revascularization techniques, because augmented immunosuppression has not been conclusively shown to prevent progression. Retransplantation for CAV can, if performed years after the initial transplantation, result in survival rates of almost 80% at 1 year after retransplantation.

POST-TRANSPLANTATION COMPLICATIONS

Although the patient's primary problem of heart failure is alleviated by a successful transplant, a new set of potential long-term complications may emerge, primarily related to the effects of chronic immunosuppression.

Infectious Complications

Infection is common in organ transplant recipients. The types of infections expected in cardiac transplant recipients vary, depending on the time from transplantation. This is because the intensity of immunosuppression administered varies directly with the propensity for rejection, and the propensity to reject decreases over time. Bacteria and viruses account for more than 80% of infections after transplantation. The most common bacterial infections early after transplantation are nosocomial, caused by infected intravascular catheters or lines, or gram-negative pneumonias. The most common viral infections are caused by the herpesviruses: CMV, herpes zoster, and herpes simplex. Although CMV infection used to be associated with significant morbidity and mortality, the use of ganciclovir has significantly improved the prognosis. The overall incidence of infection is approximately 0.5 infections per patient, although as many as two thirds of patients remain free from serious infections during the first year. Given the potential morbidity and mortality associated with infections during the first post-transplantation year, infection prophylaxis is common (Table 5).

Diabetes Mellitus

Although almost 20% of cardiac transplant survivors develop overt diabetes within the first year, by 5 years after transplantation, only 15% would be classified as diabetic. This is likely related to the use of decreasing dosages of corticosteroids. No evidence exists that cardiac transplant recipients should be managed differently in terms

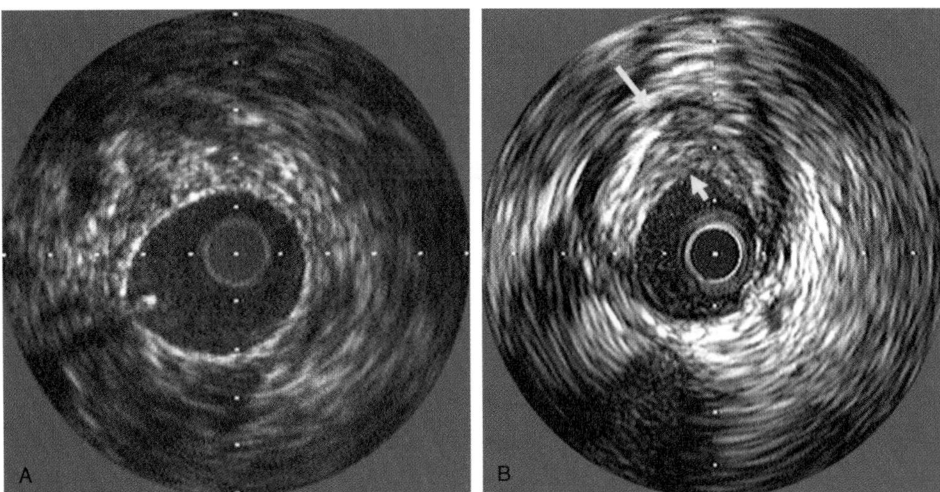

Figure 3 Intravascular ultrasound, 1 year after transplantation. A, Recipient with normal coronaries. **B,** Another recipient with increased coronary intimal thickness (1.2 mm; *arrows*), suggesting severe vasculopathy.

Table 5 Infection Prophylaxis After Cardiac Transplantation

Organism	Regimen
Cytomegalovirus (recipient seropositive)	Ganciclovir, 5 mg/kg IV bid for 2-4 wk, then 1000 mg PO tid until 1 mo post-transplantation, then acyclovir, 800 mg PO qd until 2-3 mo post-transplantation
Cytomegalovirus (recipient seronegative and donor seropositive)	Ganciclovir, 5 mg/kg IV bid for 2-4 wk, then 1000 mg PO tid until 3 mo post-transplantation
Herpes simplex virus	Acyclovir, 200 mg PO qd until prednisone dosage < 20 mg/day
Epstein-Barr virus (recipient seronegative and donor seropositive)	Acyclovir, 800 mg PO qd for 12 mo, then 200 mg PO qd
Toxoplasma gondii (donor or recipient seropositive)	Pyrimethamine, 25 mg PO qd for 6 wk and leucovorin calcium, 5-10 mg PO qd for 6 wk
Pneumocystis carinii	Trimethoprim-sulfamethoxazole, 160 mg-800 mg PO 3-7 times/wk or dapsone, 75-100 mg PO qd if sulfa allergic
Candida albicans	Nystatin, 10 mL swish and swallow qd, or clotrimazole troche, PO qd until prednisone dosage < 20 mg/day

of target levels of blood glucose and glycosylated hemoglobin, or the agents used to treat them.

Hypertension

Hypertension developing after cardiac transplantation is almost universal, occurring in 70% to 90% of cyclosporine-treated and 30% to 50% of tacrolimus-treated patients. This challenging complication reflects the interplay of several pathogenic mechanisms, including altered renal vascular reactivity and sympathetic neuroactivation. Corticosteroids play a minor role in the pathogenesis of cardiac transplantation hypertension, which is described as a salt-sensitive type. Abnormal cardiorenal reflexes secondary to cardiac denervation may contribute to salt-sensitive hypertension and fluid retention.

Generally, blood pressures consistently higher than 140/90 mm Hg should be treated. Titrated monotherapy with angiotensin-converting enzyme (ACE) inhibitors or calcium channel blockers may be effective in about 50% of patients. Some patients are prone to hyperkalemia because of the combined effect of cyclosporine and ACE inhibition. Because of decreased metabolism of cyclosporine, the use of diltiazem and verapamil necessitates the use of lower doses of cyclosporine and, initially, more frequent monitoring of cyclosporine level. Combination therapy with both an ACE inhibitor and a calcium channel blocker is a commonly used strategy. Problematic hypertensives requiring multiple agents often require diuretics as parts of their regimen. Hypertension in some patients is inadequately controlled despite maximally tolerated doses of calcium channel blockers and ACE inhibitors. The final tier of management is to add clonidine, doxazosin, or minoxidil in refractory cases. Beta blockers are usually avoided in the treatment of hypertension because of their known tendency to reduce exercise performance in heart transplant recipients.

Renal Dysfunction

Immunosuppressive therapy with cyclosporine has improved both graft function and survival in heart transplantation. However, cyclosporine-induced nephrotoxicity still remains a serious clinical challenge. Chronic cyclosporine nephrotoxicity is characterized by a decrease in glomerular filtration rate (GFR), afferent arteriolopathy, and striped tubulointerstitial fibrosis. The greatest decline in GFR with cyclosporine occurs in the first 3 to 6 months. In a study of 2088 Medicare beneficiaries, the annual risk of end-stage renal disease was reported to be 0.37% in the first year after transplantation, increasing to 4.49% by the sixth post-transplantation year.

Tacrolimus (FK 506) causes functional and structural abnormalities similar to those caused by cyclosporine. The central mechanism involved is a result of inhibition of calcineurin, which may explain in part the increased systemic vascular resistance because of effects on vascular smooth muscle and indirect effects mediated by increased sympathetic neuroactivation.

Close monitoring of tacrolimus and cyclosporine blood levels is critically important to limit progressive decline in renal function, because there is no known treatment for preventing or reversing nephrotoxicity. At the time of transplantation, initiation of tacrolimus or cyclosporine is delayed postoperatively in patients at high risk for nephrotoxicity, and cytolytic induction therapy (such as monoclonal OKT3 or antithymocyte globulin [Thymoglobulin]) is used for renal-sparing purposes.

Osteoporosis

Cardiac transplantation, with its attendant glucocorticoids and calcineurin inhibitors (cyclosporine and tacrolimus), is associated with rapid bone loss (up to 35% of patients during the first year). Within 2 months after heart transplantation, approximately 3% of whole-body bone mineral density is lost, mostly because of decreases in trabecular bone. Glucocorticoids cause dose-related bone loss, particularly in the first 6 to 12 months. Cardiac transplant recipients lose bone immediately after transplantation at the spine and hip.

The treatment of osteoporosis in heart transplant patients should be directed toward preventing bone loss. Because of the morbidity associated with osteoporosis, patients at highest risk should be treated even before transplantation. Prophylactic administration of calcium carbonate and vitamin D after cardiac transplantation is an effective regimen that reduces bone loss and may decrease osteoporotic complications.

Hyperlipidemia

Hyperlipidemia is one of the most common metabolic disorders after heart transplantation, occurring in 60% to 80% of recipients. It is multifactorial in origin and may be related to preexisting lipid abnormalities, cyclosporine therapy, and corticosteroids. Corticosteroid withdrawal has been associated with lower cholesterol levels.

Coronary vasculopathy has emerged as the main determinant of long-term survival in cardiac transplant recipients. There is controversy as to whether hypercholesterolemia is an important risk factor of allograft vasculopathy. A more consistent observation has been made that an elevated plasma triglyceride level is associated with the development of coronary vasculopathy. Most likely, immune and ischemic mechanisms of endothelial injury in the setting of hyperlipidemia are likely to play a role in the development of coronary vasculopathy.

Lipid-lowering therapy using gemfibrozil, targeted to the modification of triglyceride levels, appears to confer a survival benefit in cardiac transplant recipients beyond the first year. Moderate to severe hypercholesterolemia generally requires the use of a statin agent. In a prospective randomized trial investigating pravastatin use early after heart transplantation, it was observed that pravastatin-treated patients have a decreased incidence of clinically severe acute rejection episodes, resulting in a significant improvement in 1-year survival (94% vs. 78% in the control group; $P = .02$). Follow-up at 5 years has shown continued survival benefit in patients receiving pravastatin (83% vs. 62%). A similar survival benefit result has been observed in a randomized prospective trial with simvastatin. This observed survival benefit probably is a class effect that is shared among all statins. The combination of cyclosporine and a statin increases the risk of rhabdomyolysis over that of a statin alone. Combining lovastatin and gemfibrozil can also predispose to rhabdomyolysis. This combination in general should be avoided. It is thus recommended that periodic creatine kinase and liver enzyme determinations be performed in all transplant recipients receiving statin agents.

Gout

Gouty arthritis is the most common rheumatologic complication among cyclosporine-treated organ transplant recipients. Preexisting gout is observed in 6% of patients before transplantation. Following heart transplantation, gouty arthritis is observed with increasing frequency in 8% to 17% of patients. It is usually polyarticular in nature and often exhibits an accelerated clinical course, with management complicated by the patient's renal insufficiency and interaction with transplant-related medications.

Colchicine is generally effective in treating acute gouty episodes and providing prophylaxis against recurrent episodes. However, cardiac transplant recipients treated with cyclosporine may be at increased risk of developing acute colchicine-induced myoneuropathy, especially in the setting of concurrent renal insufficiency. If colchicine is administered, the dose should be reduced, cyclosporine levels monitored closely, and patients evaluated for signs of neuromuscular toxicity.

Another potential life-threatening drug interaction is the combination of allopurinol and azathioprine, resulting in pancytopenia. Because allopurinol blocks the xanthine oxidase pathway by which azathioprine is metabolized, potentially toxic levels of azathioprine can result. Mycophenolate mofetil metabolism does not involve the xanthine oxidase pathway, but it may be used safely in combination with allopurinol.

Corticosteroids may be the most effective and safest approach in the management of gout in patients with renal dysfunction. As a general rule, nonsteroidal anti-inflammatory drugs are not used because of their propensity to precipitate acute cyclosporine-induced renal toxicity.

Malignancy

Following heart transplantation, malignancy is identified in 3% to 18% of the recipients, with an estimated risk of 1% to 2% per year. It ranks second to coronary vasculopathy as a major cause of mortality, accounting for 10% to 23% of all deaths following heart transplantation. Cutaneous malignancy is the most common type, seen in up to 17% of patients, with a predominance of squamous cell carcinoma.

Post-transplantation lymphoproliferative disorder (PTLD) is a frequently fatal complication, occurring in 1.7% to 6% of cardiac transplant recipients. The peak occurrence of PTLD is 3 to 4 months after transplantation. A strong association of PTLD with Epstein-Barr virus has been observed in several series. The use of OKT3, which may favorably affect the rejection rate, has been shown to increase the risk of lymphoma more than eightfold. This association remains contentious and has been challenged.

The initial management of PTLDs usually involves reduction in immunosuppression, which may be effective in some cases. Nonresponsive patients may require aggressive combination chemotherapy, and mortality of approximately 80% has been reported in these patients.

RETRANSPLANTATION

Many ethical and fiscal issues have been raised concerning the allocation of a scarce organ to a retransplant candidate, who is 20% less likely to survive 1 year after transplantation than a primary candidate. Hence, there is the need for rigorous criteria to select the ideal candidate for retransplantation.

Coronary vasculopathy constitutes the main cause of graft failure, and the most common reason to consider retransplantation, followed by rejection and primary graft failure. Defining the ideal candidate poses a challenging therapeutic dilemma to the transplantation team, and it may not be an easy task to accomplish because of the worldwide shortage of organ donor supply. However, based on the results of some of the major transplant centers' experiences, cardiac retransplantation may be a viable therapeutic strategy for select patients with severe coronary artery disease as the cause of allograft dysfunction. Excluding patients with intractable rejection, primary graft failure, and renal dysfunction may improve survival outcome.

ROLE OF THE PRIMARY CARE PHYSICIAN

Successful long-term care of the transplanted heart is a team effort by the patient, transplantation team, and primary care physician. A knowledge of cardiac transplantation medicine is fundamental for the primary care physician who participates in the ongoing care of the post-transplantation patient.

The primary care physician plays an important role in the management of medical problems that need long-term follow-up, such as diabetes, hypertension, hyperlipidemia, and osteoporosis. Post-transplantation complications such as infection, rejection, coronary vasculopathy, and malignancy pose major threats to the transplanted organ and therefore require a heightened awareness by the primary care physician and appropriate referral to the cardiac transplantation team.

The long-term management of heart transplant patients is continuously evolving with the emergence of new immunosuppressive agents. The key to the safe handling of these agents by the primary care physician requires knowledge of pharmacology, including side effects and various drug-drug interactions. It is recommended that any new medications be given in consultation with the transplantation center. Appropriate antibiotic endocarditis prophylaxis is recommended for cardiac transplant recipients undergoing dental, genitourinary, or gastrointestinal procedures.

Post-transplantation psychological issues are important and often can be addressed by the primary care physician, with appropriate counseling. Hence, the primary care physician assumes a vital role in the management of cardiac transplant patients, and the demand for care continues to grow with the expanding population of long-term heart transplant recipients.

Summary

- Cardiac transplantation has emerged as a viable therapeutic strategy for select patients with end-stage heart disease, offering extended survival and improved quality of life.
- The current survival rate after heart transplantation has been reported as approximately 50% at 12 years by the International Society for Heart and Lung Transplantation (ISHLT) registry.
- The paucity of the donor pool demands a careful patient selection process to ensure appropriate candidacy.
- Patients are listed according to their medical urgency status and severity of their illness.
- Post-transplantation complications include acute rejection, infection, transplant vasculopathy, metabolic complications, renal insufficiency, bone diseases, and malignancy.
- Successful long-term care of the transplanted heart is a team effort by the patient, transplantation team, and primary care physician.

Suggested Readings

Kirklin JK, Pambukian SV, McGiffin DC, Benza RL: Current outcomes following heart transplantation. Semin Thorac Cardiovasc Surg 2004;16:395-403.

Lindenfeld JA, Miller GG, Shakar SF, et al: Drug therapy in the heart transplant recipient. Part I: Cardiac rejection and immunosuppressive drugs. Circulation 2004;110:3734-3740.

Lindenfeld JA, Miller GG, Shakar SF, et al: Drug therapy in the heart transplant recipient. Part II: Immunosuppressive drugs. Circulation 2004;110:3858-3865.

Mehra MR, Uber PA, Uber WE, et al: Allosensitization in heart transplantation: Implications and management strategies. Curr Opin Cardiol 2003;18:153-158.

Sharples LD, Caine N, Mullins P, et al: Risk factor analysis for the major hazards following heart transplantation-rejection, infection, and coronary occlusive disease. Transplantation 1991;52:244-252.

Steward S, Winters GL, Fishbein MC, et al: Revision of the 1990 working formulation for the standardization of nomenclature in the diagnosis of heart rejection. J Heart Lung Transplant 2005;24:1710-1720.

Taylor DO, Edwards LB, Boucek MM, et al: Registry of the International Society for Heart and Lung Transplantation: Twenty-fourth official adult heart transplant report—2007. J Heart Lung Transplantation 2007:26(8):769-781.

Yamani MH, Starling RC: Long-term management issues in heart transplantation. In Norman DJ, Turka LA (eds): Primer on Transplantation, 2nd ed. Mt. Laurel, NJ, American Society of Transplant, 2001, pp 375-381.

Yamani MH, Starling RC: Surrogate markers of transplant vasculopathy. Curr Opin Organ Transplant 2004;9:443-447.

Young JB, Winters WL Jr, Bourge R, Uretsky BF: 24th Bethesda Conference: Cardiac transplantation. Task Force 4: Function of the heart transplant recipient. J Am Coll Cardiol 1993;22:31-41.

Diseases of the Aorta

Gian M. Novaro

Diseases of the aorta account for significant cardiovascular morbidity and mortality worldwide. The incidence of aortic diseases is expected to rise with the increasing age of the population. Diagnostic evaluation of aortic disorders has improved in the last 2 decades, allowing earlier diagnosis and therapeutic intervention. This chapter summarizes the major disease entities affecting the aorta.

ANATOMY

The aorta is the main conduit of blood in the body. A large elastic artery, it is composed of three layers: The intima is the innermost layer and includes the single-layered endothelium. The media is the thickest layer of the aortic wall and is composed of sheets of elastic tissue, smooth muscle cells, and collagen, which provide the aorta with its tensile strength and distensibility. The adventitia is the outermost layer; it is composed of loose connective tissue and contains the vasa vasorum, which constitutes the blood supply to the aortic wall.

Anatomically, the aorta is divided into subcomponents. The thoracic aorta consists of the aortic root, from the aortic annulus, including the sinuses of Valsalva, up to the level just above the sinotubular junction; the ascending aorta, from the sinotubular junction to the innominate artery, with an average diameter of 3 cm; the arch, from the innominate artery to the left subclavian artery; and the descending thoracic aorta, with an average diameter of 2.5 cm, and begins after the origin of the left subclavian artery. The abdominal aorta begins when the descending thoracic aorta passes through the diaphragm. The abdominal aorta (average diameter, 2.0 cm) is further classified as suprarenal or infrarenal.

PATHOLOGIC PROCESSES

Cystic Medial Degeneration

An important predisposing factor to diseases of the aorta, particularly the ascending aorta, is cystic medial degeneration. It is characterized by smooth muscle cell necrosis and apoptosis and by degeneration of elastic fibers within the media of the aortic wall. Cystic spaces form in these areas of degeneration; thus its name. This degenerative process also extends to the elastic components of the adventitial layer. The weakened aortic wall is prone to aneurysm formation and dissection. This degenerative process, which can be genetically determined, is typically seen in connective tissue diseases such as Marfan and Ehlers-Danlos syndromes. However, varying degrees of degeneration can be seen in patients without these disorders, occurring as an idiopathic variant in familial syndromes or as an acquired form. Hypertension and advancing age are associated with the latter. Varying degrees of cystic medial degeneration can also be seen in the genetically inferior aortas seen in association with congenital abnormalities, including bicuspid or unicuspid aortic valves, aortic coarctation, and Turner's and Noonan's syndromes.

Atherosclerosis

Atherosclerosis appears to play a major role in diseases of the aortic arch, descending thoracic, and abdominal aorta. Atherosclerosis can result in weakening of the aortic wall, making it prone to aneurysm formation or dissection. The development of aortic atherosclerosis is associated with traditional cardiac risk factors of smoking, hypertension, hyperglycemia, and atherogenic lipoproteins. Atherosclerosis can also lead to the formation of complex atheromatous plaques, prone to embolization, resulting in cerebral and peripheral arterial occlusive events.

Inflammatory Disorders

Inflammatory disorders represent a third broad category as a predisposing factor causing aortic diseases. These occur in isolation or in the context of systemic disorders. They include infectious and noninfectious causes.

Trauma

Aortic injury from trauma usually occurs because of deceleration injuries. Traumatic dissection or laceration often occurs at the level of the left subclavian artery. Injury can result in the formation of a chronic pseudoaneurysm.

SPECIFIC DISORDERS

Aortic Dissection

Aortic dissection comprises one of the more ominous acute aortic syndromes, also known as *acute thoracic pain syndromes,* which include the dissection variants of penetrating aortic ulcers, intramural hematomas, and symptomatic aneurysms. Aortic dissection involves splitting of the aortic wall, which results in the formation of an aortic false lumen that courses along with a true lumen. The hallmark of aortic dissection is an intimal tear, which allows access of pulsatile high-pressure blood into the aortic media, separating it from the outer layers. Often, the so-called intimal flap (Fig. 1) is usually an intimal-medial flap. The initiating event of dissection may be a tear in the intima. Alternatively, primary rupture of the vasa vasorum can result in an intramural hematoma, which secondarily leads to an intimal tear as blood vents from the intramural space (Fig. 2). Regardless of the initiating event, the force of blood flow propagates the dissection antegrade (and, less commonly, retrograde) for a variable extent along the vessel, splitting the aortic wall, usually along the outer one third of the medial layer.

Classification

Dissections are classified by their location of origin and how far along they extend in the aorta. There are two important classification systems of dissection, the DeBakey and Stanford classifications (Table 1; Fig. 3). Dissections are also classified by their duration. Acute dissections are those of less than 2 weeks' duration after the onset of symptoms; chronic dissections are those that have been present for longer than 2 weeks.

Signs and Symptoms

Dissections typically manifest between the fifth and seventh decades of life, with a male preponderance. Patients typically present with the acute onset of pain, which occurs in up to 96% of cases. Pain is often most severe at its onset and described as a tearing, ripping, or stabbing sensation. Often, the pain is migratory, a crucial component of the history, reflecting propagation of the dissection. Involvement of the ascending aorta results in anterior chest or neck pain, with intrascapular or subscapular pain from involvement of the descending

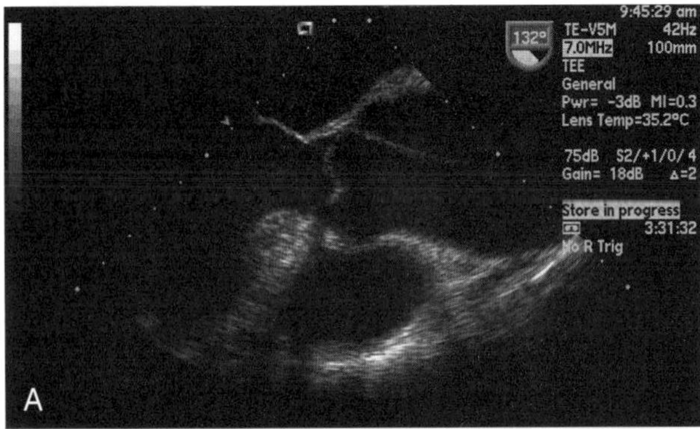

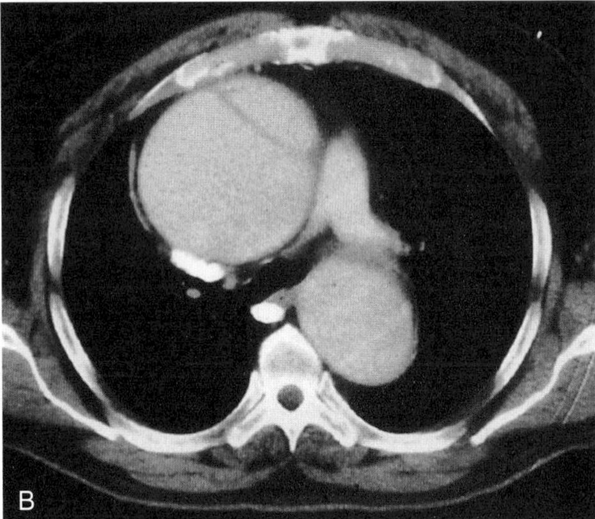

Figure 1 **A,** Transesophageal echocardiography (long-axis view). A large dissection flap in the ascending aorta extending from the level of the aortic sinuses can be seen. **B,** Computed tomography scan of a dissection flap in an aneurysmal ascending aorta. There is contrast filling in both the true and false aortic lumens.

Table 1 Classification of Aortic Dissections

Type	Extent of Aortic Involvement
DeBakey	
I	Originates in ascending aorta, propagates to involve descending aorta
II	Confined to ascending aorta
IIIa	Confined to descending thoracic aorta
IIIb	Involves descending aorta, extending to abdominal aorta
Stanford	
A	Involves ascending aorta
B	Restricted to descending aorta

thoracic aorta, and lower back and left flank pain from thoracoabdominal aortic involvement. Hypertension on presentation is common, more so in distal dissection, although hypotension can be seen if complications have developed, particularly in proximal dissections. The dissection may compromise flow to the great vessels and lead to pulse deficits; these can be transient, because the dissection flap can oscillate. Actual blood pressure may not be appreciated if the arm used has compromise of the brachial circulation (pseudohypotension).

If the dissection involves the aortic root, commissural involvement of the aortic valve can lead to aortic regurgitation. Dilation of the root and aortic annulus, without leaflet involvement, can also lead to aortic valve regurgitation. A diastolic murmur is evident in these cases. Dissections can involve the ostia of the coronary arteries, resulting in acute myocardial ischemia and infarction (2%-3% of cases). The right coronary artery ostium is more commonly affected than the left main. The dissection can extend proximally into the pericardial space, resulting in pericardial effusion and tamponade, a common mechanism of syncope and hypotension in dissection. A pericardial friction rub can be a clue to the presence of hemopericardium. Rupture into the pericardial space represents the most common mode of death in patients with aortic dissection. Acute lower extremity, renal, or mesenteric ischemia can be seen in descending aortic dissections. Focal neurologic deficits can occur with involvement of the great vessels. Compromise of spinal artery perfusion may result in paraparesis. Whereas chest pain and pulse deficits are usually described, it is important to recognize that less than 20% of patients present with these findings. Therefore, a high clinical suspicion for dissection is paramount.

Diagnostic Testing

The chest radiograph may be normal in cases of dissection. A well-recognized finding is mediastinal widening, present in about 60% of cases. Rupture into the pleural or pericardial space manifests as pleural effusions or an enlarged cardiac silhouette; the latter may also be present because of chronic aortic regurgitation. The electrocardiogram can be normal but often shows nonspecific ST-T wave changes. Involvement of the coronary artery ostia can result in ST-segment elevation, representing an acute myocardial injury pattern. Transthoracic echocardiography can on occasion identify a proximal or even distal dissection flap. Even if a flap is not seen, the presence of aortic dilation, aortic regurgitation, or an unexplained pericardial effusion can be important clues in the diagnostic consideration of dissection in a patient with chest pain. More definitive diagnostic modalities include transesophageal echocardiography (TEE), computed tomography (CT), and magnetic resonance angiography (MRA; Fig. 4). Each has relative advantages and disadvantages, but all have excellent sensitivity and specificity (Table 2).

Angiography is less commonly used for the primary diagnosis of aortic dissection. The choice of test is often dependent on expedited availability and expertise at the center in which the patient is evaluated. An important caveat is that in most patients, more than one test may be required. If clinical suspicion is high enough and the initial test is negative or equivocal, consideration should be given to performing another confirmatory test.

Treatment

Anti-impulse medical therapy (i.e., β-adrenergic blockade) should be initiated as soon as the diagnosis of dissection is considered, even while awaiting confirmatory diagnostic testing. In patients who are hypertensive, intravenous beta blockade and sodium nitroprusside are the treatment agents of choice. Beta blockade should be initiated before sodium nitroprusside to prevent a rise in cardiac contractility associated with isolated vasodilator use. In the absence of hypertension, beta blockers can be solely used. In those with ascending aortic dissections, these are temporizing agents while preparing for definitive surgical therapy. In patients with descending dissections, these agents are first-line therapy before longer acting oral agents are initiated. Intravenous nondihydropyridine calcium antagonists such as verapamil and diltiazem are alternatives to those who cannot tolerate beta blockers. Dissections that involve the ascending aorta (proximal, type A) require urgent surgical therapy (Fig. 5) because there is a very

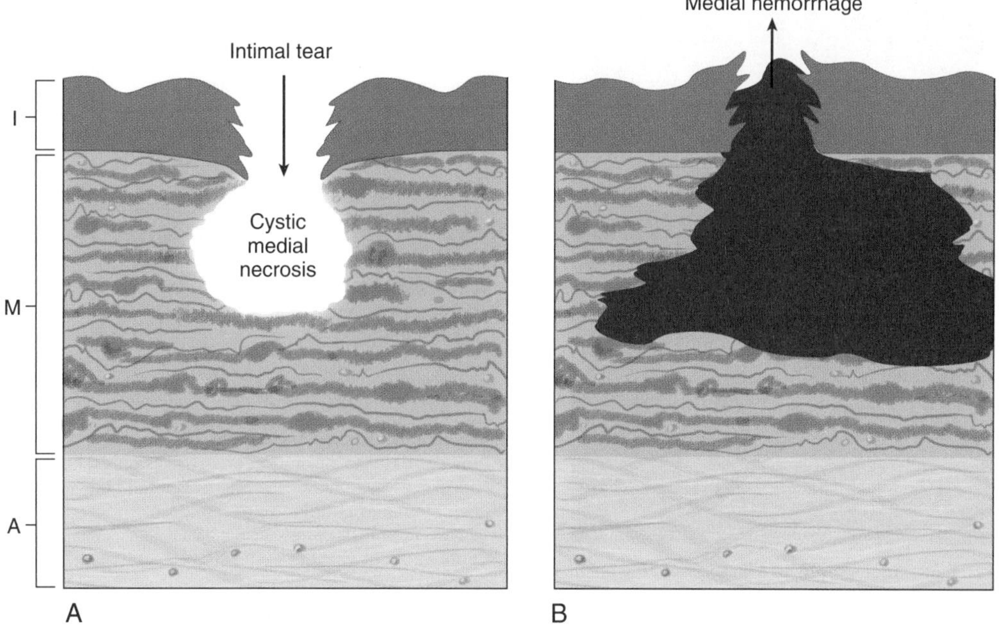

Figure 2 Schematic representation of the initiating event of aortic dissection. A, A tear in the intima. **B,** Primary rupture of the vasa vasorum, secondarily leading to an intimal tear as blood vents from the intramural space.

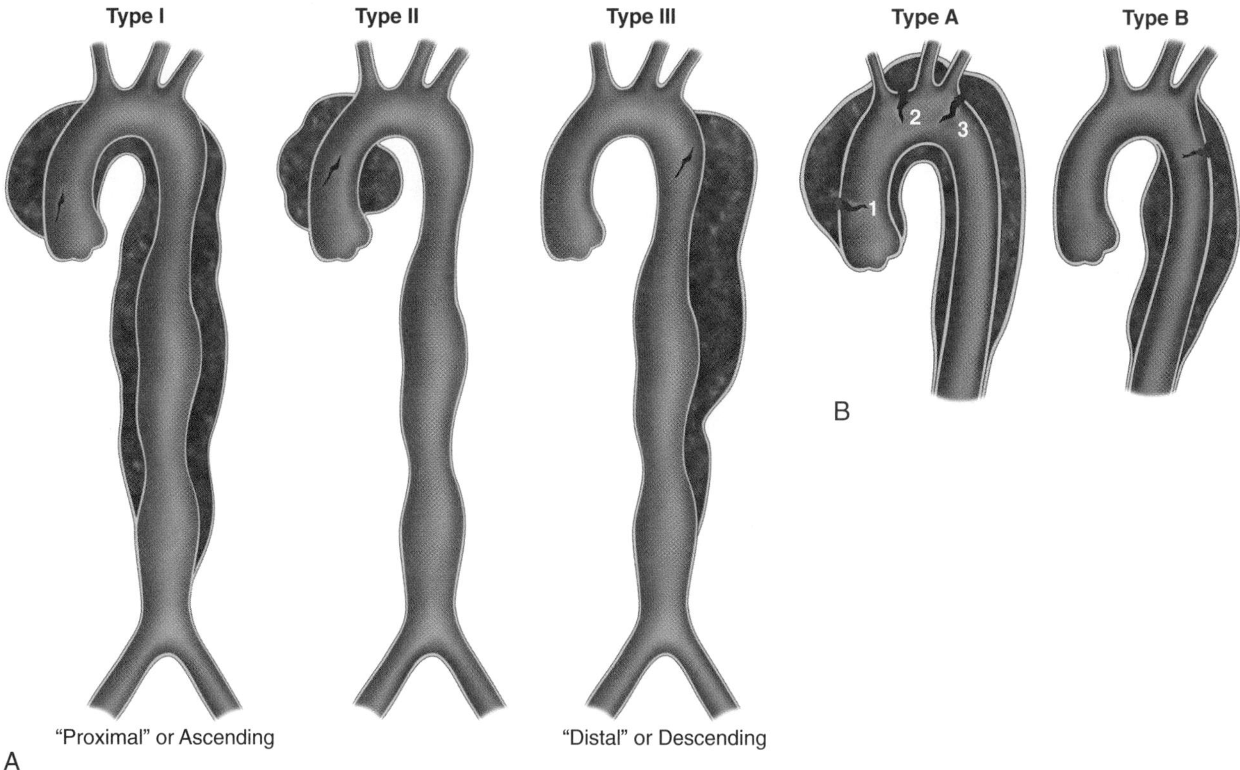

Figure 3 The DeBakey (**A**) and Stanford (**B**) classification systems of aortic dissection.

high early mortality rate (approaching 1%-2%/hour for the first 24-48 hours).

An important management point arises in patients who have pericardial effusion or tamponade in association with a proximal dissection. These patients should not undergo percutaneous pericardiocentesis unless they are in extremis. The evacuation of pericardial blood by such a route has been associated with aortic rupture and increased mortality, perhaps secondary to dissection extension or aortic rupture, or both, because blood pressure and contractility increase after tamponade resolution. Pericardial access should be obtained in the operating room, after the institution of cardiopulmonary bypass.

Dissections that involve the descending aorta (distal, type B) should initially be treated medically. Data suggest that medical therapy is the preferred initial treatment, with surgery guided by a

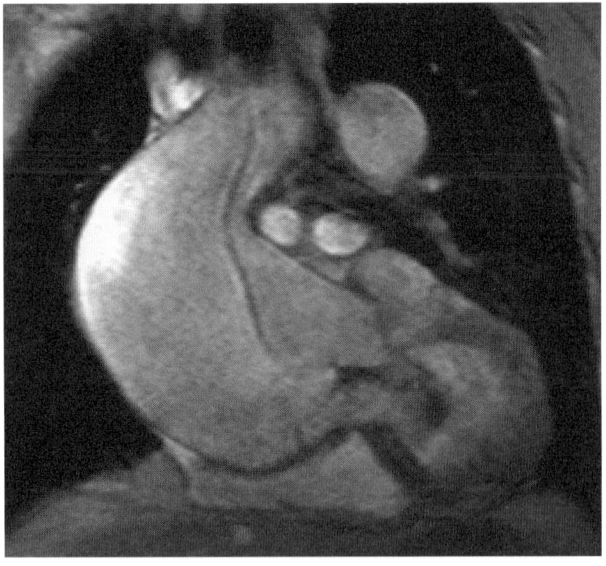

Figure 4 Magnetic resonance angiography of a large ascending aortic aneurysm with a proximal (type A) dissection. There is a dissection flap extending from the aortic sinuses to the arch.

Table 2 Comparison of Imaging Modalities for Aortic Dissection

Advantages	Disadvantages
Transesophageal Echocardiography	
Portability Assesses valvular function Assesses ventricular function No contrast agent	"Blind spot"-ascending aorta where bronchi cross esophagus Difficulty in assessing great vessels Difficulty in diagnosing intramural hematoma Invasive procedure
Spiral Computed Tomography	
Assesses great vessels and branch vessels	Lacks valvular and ventricular function assessment Lacks portability IV contrast agent required
Magnetic Resonance Angiography	
Provides detailed resolution of aorta (i.e., intramural hematoma) in addition to assessing branch vessels Contrast agent without nephrotoxicity	Lacks portability Limited access to scanners Cost
Angiography	
Assesses coronary anatomy (controversial as to whether this should be done before surgery)	Invasive Risk and difficulty in accessing true lumen Contrast agent required

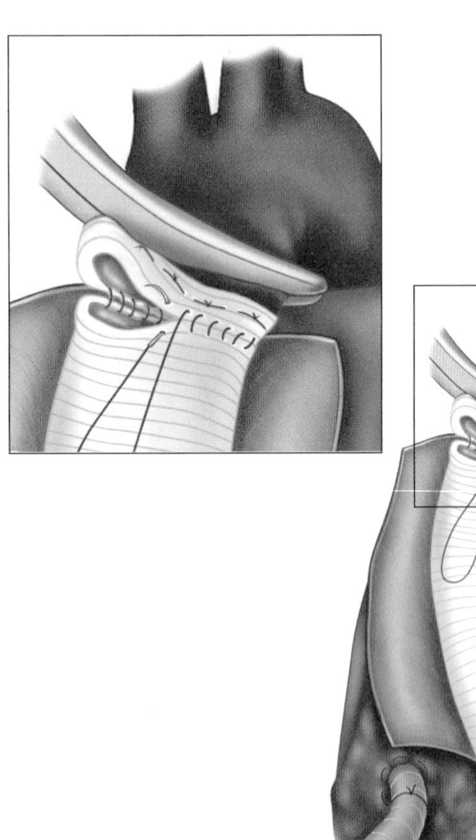

Figure 5 Ascending aortic repair. *Inset,* placement of a supracoronary aortic graft.

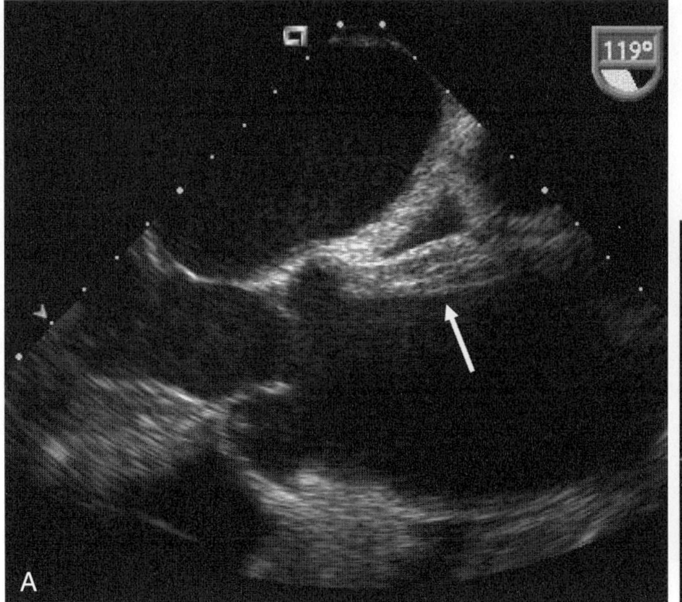

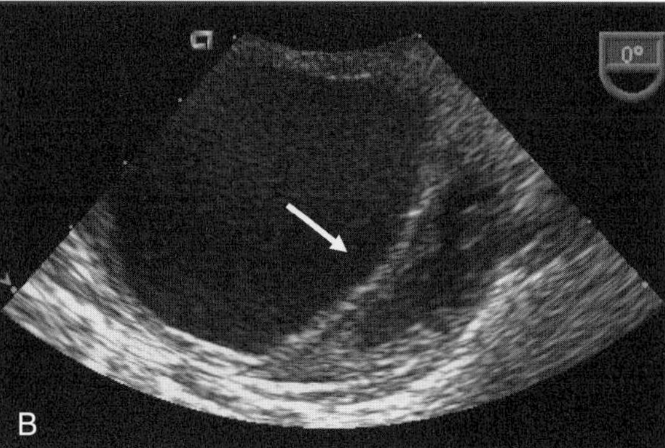

Figure 6 Transesophageal echocardiography in long-axis (**A**) and short-axis (**B**) views. An intramural hematoma is shown (*arrows*), characterized by no dissection flap, a crescent-shaped thickening of the aortic wall, central displacement of intimal calcium, and echolucent intramural pockets of intramural blood.

complication-specific approach. This is because acute aortic surgery is associated with a high mortality and paraplegia rate (inadequate protection of the spinal arteries). Surgery should be considered for the following indications: evidence of organ ischemia secondary to compromise of the branch vessels; persistent pain; aneurysm formation, particularly if saccular; and retrograde dissection to a proximal extent. Alternatively, aortic fenestration, surgical or percutaneous, can also be considered for organ or limb malperfusion in carefully selected patients. Distal (type B) dissections in Marfan syndrome patients carry a poor prognosis and have thus led to recommendations of early aortic surgery.

Aortic Dissection in Younger Adults

Dissections occurring in younger patients (younger than 40 years) typically occur in the context of connective tissue disorders such as Marfan syndrome, congenital bicuspid aortic valve, prior aortic surgery, or the peripartum period. During late pregnancy, it is believed that hormonal changes and a loosening in the ground substance of connective tissue can lead to a heightened risk of dissection.

Chronic Aortic Dissection

Patients with chronic dissection (present for >2 weeks) have survived the period of increased mortality. They can often be managed medically, even in the presence of a proximal dissection. However, their aortas often dilate and are at higher risk for aneurysm formation because of the thinner aortic wall as a result of dissection. A complication-specific approach can be used for chronic dissection patients to guide elective surgical therapy—recurrent pain, aneurysm formation, particularly if saccular, and retrograde dissection extension to the ascending aorta. Serial follow-up imaging (usually CT or MRA), initially at short intervals, is vital in these patients because of their weakened aortic walls.

Iatrogenic Aortic Dissection

Special mention should be made of iatrogenic dissections. Angiographic catheters and guidewires can disrupt the intima and result in dissections anywhere along the aorta's course. These typically result in retrograde dissections, and the false lumens generally thrombose spontaneously. They often can be managed medically unless the dissection is extensive. Dissections can also occur during aortic cross-clamping or cannulation during cardiac surgery. Such dissections are usually diagnosed and treated urgently and successfully at the time of surgery.

Intramural Hematoma and Penetrating Aortic Ulcer

Intramural hematoma and penetrating aortic ulcer differ from classic dissection by the absence of an intimal flap. Recent advances in diagnostic imaging modalities have led to an increased awareness and better understanding of these entities.

Intramural hematoma consists of a noncommunicating blood collection in the aortic wall. Unlike a true dissection, there is no loss of intimal continuity, no entry tear, and thus no intimal flap. The pathophysiology may be related to rupture of the aortic vasa vasorum. By transesophageal echocardiography, intramural hematoma is characterized by the absence of a dissection flap, a regional crescent-shaped thickening of the aortic wall, usually more than 0.7 cm, and central displacement of intimal calcium (Fig. 6). At times, intramural echolucencies representing noncommunicating pockets of blood can be seen. Distinguishing an intramural hematoma from severe atheroma, a thrombosed false lumen, or an aneurysm with mural thrombus can be difficult. Angiography is of limited diagnostic accuracy in the evaluation of hematomas, because it fails to image the aortic wall. If the clinical history is concerning, a negative TEE should not represent the final diagnostic evaluation. CT and MRA are highly accurate imaging modalities and are often used as an initial or complementary study in the evaluation of hematomas. Intramural hematomas can communicate with the adventitial space, lead to rupture, or progress to overt dissection with an intimal tear. However, they may also have a more benign course and gradually resolve with medical therapy and blood pressure control.

Penetrating aortic ulcer develops when an atheromatous plaque erodes inward into the aortic media. The advanced atherosclerotic

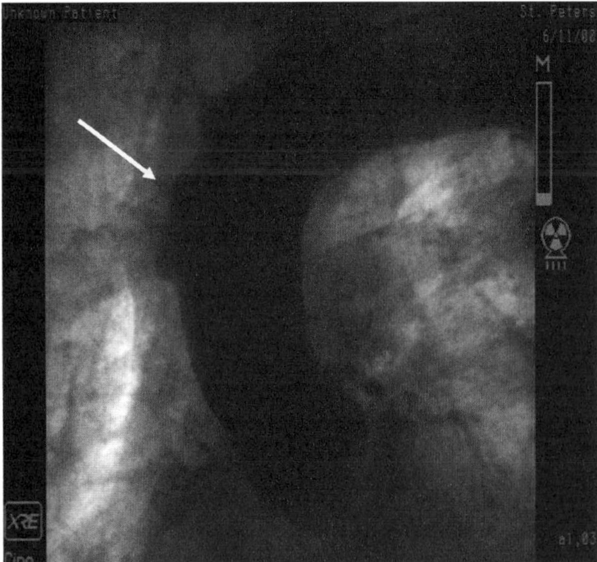

Figure 7 **Aortography of penetrating aortic ulcers in the ascending aorta.** These are characterized as outpouchings of the aortic wall in a region of aortic atheromatous disease (*arrow*).

burden prevents the erosion from extending longitudinally along the vessel wall, as in classic dissection. The ulcer is apparent on imaging modalities as an ulcer crater or contrast-filled outpouching (Fig. 7). Depending how far into the aortic wall the plaque erosion occurs, there can be formation of an intramural hematoma, saccular aneurysm, pseudoaneurysm, or even complete aortic rupture.

Clinical Presentation

Patients with these acute aortic syndromes often present with the same chest or back pain, or both, as patients with classic dissection. There may be a higher incidence of rupture than that seen with classic dissections. Compared with intramural hematomas, patients with penetrating ulcers are usually older and tend to have more aortic atherosclerosis. Isolated intramural hematomas tend to occur more often in the ascending aorta, whereas intramural hematomas associated with penetrating aortic ulcers are located more commonly in the descending aorta, where atherosclerosis is more prevalent.

Treatment

As with aortic dissection, anti-impulse medical therapy should be initiated as soon as the diagnosis of a dissection variant is considered. Intravenous beta blockade and, if needed for blood pressure control, sodium nitroprusside are the treatment agents of choice. For the dissection variants involving the ascending aorta, prompt surgical intervention is considered the treatment of choice. However, there are data indicating that certain patients with intramural hematomas in the ascending aorta may be managed medically. Recent data suggest that penetrating ulcer-like findings in an area of intramural hematoma can identify high-risk patients. Symptoms of sustained or recurrent pain or findings of an increasing pleural effusion are suggestive of disease progression and favor surgical intervention. Guidelines and management strategies are still evolving in this patient population.

For the dissection variants involving the descending aorta, especially intramural hematomas without penetrating ulcers, medical therapy is the preferred initial treatment. However, some have argued that there should be a lower threshold for surgical intervention than for classic distal dissection, particularly when clinical signs of instability are present. The presence of a severely bulging hematoma or a deeply penetrating ulcer may warrant surgical repair. The development of a saccular aneurysm or pseudoaneurysm should merit consideration for surgical repair. For those treated medically, serial imaging studies are warranted to assess for progression or increase in aortic diameter, in which case surgical repair or stent-graft placement may be considered.

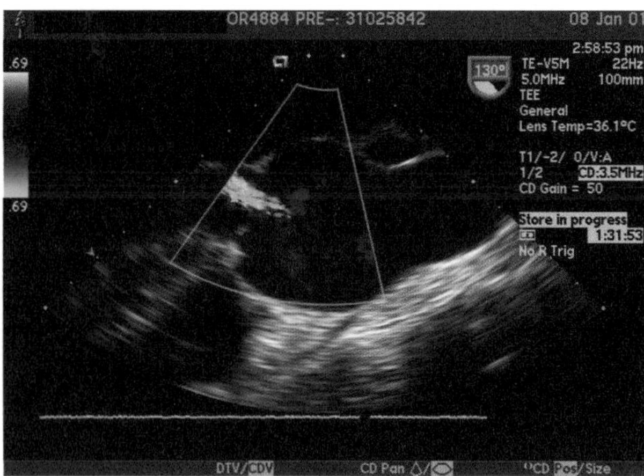

Figure 8 **Transesophageal echocardiography (long-axis view).** This illustrates an ascending aortic aneurysm, with dilation at the level of the sinuses (onion bulb appearance) in a patient with Marfan syndrome.

Thoracic Aortic Aneurysm

An aortic aneurysm is present when there is dilation of the aorta, typically at least 1.5 times its normal reference diameter in an adjacent segment. This dilation can involve the entire circumference of the aortic wall (fusiform) or a localized protrusion of one of the walls (saccular). Ectasia is characterized by dilation less than 1.5 times the normal reference diameter.

The incidence of thoracic aortic aneurysm (TAA) is estimated at 5.9 cases per 100,000 person-years. The leading causes include congenital bicuspid aortic valve, Marfan syndrome (Fig. 8), idiopathic annuloaortic ectasia (Fig. 9), familial thoracic aortic aneurysm syndrome, inflammatory aortitis, acquired because of increased age and hypertension, syphilis, and trauma. Descending TAA may extend distally and involve the abdominal aorta, creating a thoracoabdominal aneurysm. Patients are often asymptomatic at time of presentation, and the TAA may be diagnosed by an imaging modality ordered for other clinical indications. Physical findings may also be absent. When signs and symptoms occur, they are often the result of mass effect. The enlarging aorta can compress nearby structures, such as the superior vena cava, trachea, esophagus, and recurrent laryngeal nerve. This can result in the superior vena cava syndrome, stridor, dysphagia, and hoarseness, respectively. Progressive dilation of the aortic root can lead to aortic regurgitation, which may produce symptoms of congestive heart failure. Enlargement of the aortic sinuses can lead to narrowing of the coronary artery ostia, which may lead to myocardial ischemia and even infarction. Blood flow can be static in large aneurysms, predisposing to thrombus formation and distal embolization.

Noninvasive Imaging

TAAs are often noted incidentally on chest x-ray as mediastinal widening or a prominent aortic knob. Transthoracic echocardiography is the most common modality for initial diagnosis and monitoring dilation of the aortic root. CT scanning and MRA are the preferred techniques to define the entire thoracic aorta and its branch vessels accurately and measure the TAA precisely. Because the thoracic aorta may be tortuous, care must be taken not to measure off-axis axial

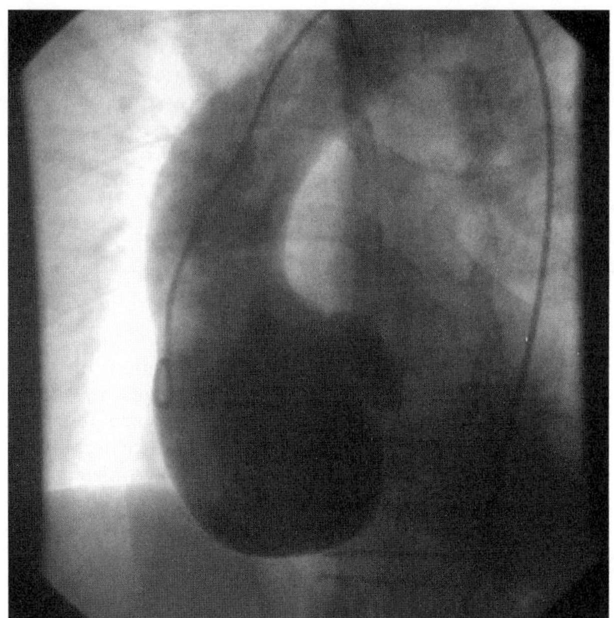

Figure 9 Aortography of an ascending aortic aneurysm in a patient with an idiopathic aortic aneurysm. Dilation is predominating at the aortic sinuses.

cuts; these can overestimate the true cross-section as compared with the actual orthogonal diameter.

Medical Treatment

There are data indicating that beta blockade can slow the rate of thoracic aneurysm expansion in patients with Marfan syndrome, resulting in improved survival. Although the data are extrapolated to those without Marfan syndrome, it would seem reasonable to recommend such therapy while TAA patients are being medically followed. Recognizing that patients treated with β-adrenergic blockade can still present with aortic dilation is important, because serial evaluation and imaging are required.

Marfan Syndrome, Thoracic Aortic Aneurysms, and Pregnancy

Women with Marfan syndrome have an increased risk of aortic dissection during pregnancy, particularly during the third trimester. The risk of dissection greatly increases if the aortic root diameter is more than 4.0 cm or if there is evidence of rapid aortic root dilation during pregnancy. If elective prepartum surgical repair is not performed, beta blockade should be used during pregnancy. Close echocardiographic follow-up and cesarean delivery should be considered if the aortic root size exceeds 4.0 cm or rapid aortic dilation is evident.

Indications for Surgical Treatment

Dissection and rupture are the feared complications of TAA, and prevention of these conditions is the purpose of elective surgical aortic repair. Size is clearly a risk factor and the principal harbinger for dissection and rupture. In one series, the annual rate of dissection or rupture was 2% for TAAs smaller than 5 cm, 3% for TAAs 5.0 to 5.9 cm, and 7% for those larger than 6 cm. Therefore, prophylactic surgical intervention should be considered before the TAA reaches a size that predisposes to aortic instability. Although the optimal timing of prophylactic aortic surgery remains uncertain, recommendations for surgical repair are 5.5 cm for an ascending TAA and 6.0 cm for a descending TAA. Patients with Marfan syndrome, bicuspid aortic valve, or family history of premature aortic instability should be considered for earlier repair (perhaps at 5.0 cm and 5.5 to 6.0 cm for ascending and descending TAAs, respectively). Rapid enlargement of the aorta (>0.5-1.0 cm/year) or symptom development has also been advocated as indications for surgery. The decision for operative repair must take into account the patient's medical comorbidities, and a risk-to-benefit ratio must be individualized for each patient. Patients who are otherwise low medical risks may be considered for elective intervention at smaller aortic sizes.

Abdominal Aortic Aneurysm

The incidence of abdominal aortic aneurysm (AAA) is estimated at 36.5/100,000 person-years. AAA represents the most common form of arterial aneurysm. Seventy-five percent of AAAs are infrarenal. Atherosclerosis is the dominant risk factor in the development of an AAA. Additional risk factors associated with AAA are male gender (four to five times more common in men), increasing age, smoking, and hypertension. There is a clear familial predisposition to AAA, and relatives of affected patients have a 30% increased risk for developing an AAA. Asymptomatic AAA is often diagnosed on physical examination by abdominal palpation. The most common symptom is pain, which is usually steady. The pain may be a localized abdominal pain or may radiate to the back, flank, or groin. Sudden onset of severe abdominal and back pain suggests rupture, representing a surgical emergency. Fewer than one third of patients with rupture present with the classic triad of pain, pulsatile abdominal mass, and hypotension. Atheroemboli may be the first manifestation of an AAA.

Noninvasive Imaging

Ultrasonography, CT scanning, aortography, and MRA have all been used in the initial diagnosis, sizing, and monitoring of AAA. Ultrasonography represents the most practical method of screening and serial monitoring, whereas CT scanning and MRA remain superior for accurately detailing the morphology and extent of the AAA. When AAA is initially diagnosed, the rate of dilation cannot be determined; therefore, the next serial study should be performed in 6 months. In general, for an AAA smaller than 4.0 cm, yearly surveillance imaging is recommended, for an AAA 4.0 to 5.0 cm, imaging every 6 to 12 months, and for an AAA larger than 5.0 cm, imaging every 3 to 6 months. Although predictors of dilation are lacking, a baseline AAA size seems to be the best predictor. Larger aneurysms expand at higher rates than smaller ones.

Medical Treatment

Beta blockade with careful control of hypertension appears to have an impact on delaying the rate of AAA expansion. Smoking should be discontinued, because rupture risk is greater in active smokers.

Indications for Surgical Treatment

Mortality from an AAA is primarily related to rupture. As with thoracic aneurysms, increasing size is the harbinger of rupture risk. Aneurysms smaller than 4 cm have a 0% to 2% risk of rupture over 2 years, those larger than 5 cm have a 22% risk of rupture over 2 years, and those larger than 6 cm show the sharpest rise in risk. An aortic diameter of 5.0 to 5.5 cm is recommended as an indication for prophylactic surgery in asymptomatic AAA patients. Although AAAs are less common in women, when present, they are at greater risk of rupture and have a smaller aortic diameter than in men. Thus, it is recommended that women undergo prophylactic AAA repair at 4.5 to 5.0 cm. Aneurysms that expand rapidly (>0.5-1.0 cm/year) are also associated with an increased risk of rupture and are thus considered for elective surgical repair. Inflammation is present in up to 10% of

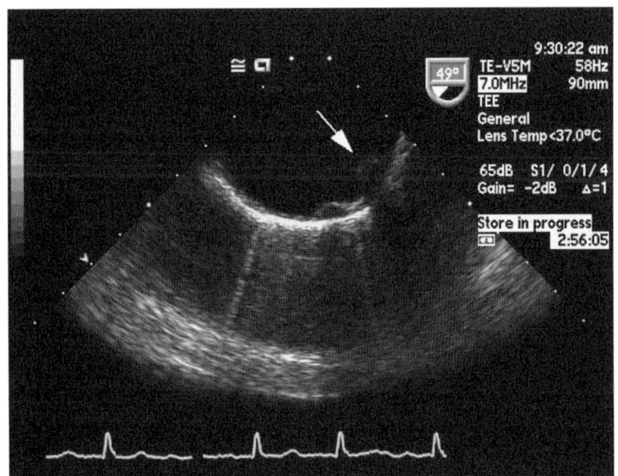

Figure 10 Transesophageal echocardiography (short-axis view). A protruding thick (>4 mm) atheroma can be identified in the descending thoracic aorta (*arrow*).

AAAs. There appears to be a familial tendency, and inflammation often occurs in the context of smoking. Patients present with constitutional symptoms and have an elevated sedimentation rate in addition to the classic symptoms of pain. CT scanning or MRA can identify the inflammatory component. Treatment is aortic surgery.

Endovascular Stent-Graft Repair

A relatively recent therapeutic option for AAA repair is the percutaneous placement of an endovascular stent-graft. The endovascular stent-graft is placed within the aneurysmal segment of the aorta, bridging the normal segments and excluding the aneurysm. However, just over 50% of all AAAs have anatomy suitable for stent-graft placement. Data are still forthcoming on the long-term success of endovascular stent-grafting, and long-term surveillance imaging is currently required after stent graft placement. Nonetheless, the procedure remains an attractive alternative to conventional surgical repair, but it is usually limited to patients with significant comorbid medical conditions who are at high surgical risk.

Atheromatous Aortic Disease

Atherosclerotic plaques (Fig. 10) in the aorta can give rise to cerebral and peripheral embolic events. TEE, in particular, has been a valuable imaging modality for assessing the presence and extent of these plaques. Plaques thicker than 4 mm, or those with mobile components, appear to be strongly associated with subsequent embolic events. Treatment strategies for patients with such plaques have not been evaluated in sufficient numbers in a prospective randomized fashion. However, there is the suggestion that lipid-lowering therapy and anticoagulation with warfarin may have benefit for some patients. Earlier reports of a potential association between warfarin and the cholesterol embolization syndrome have produced some reluctance to use such anticoagulant therapy in these patients, and further study is needed. The potential role of aortic replacement or removal of an atheroma remains to be defined. It has become increasingly common for cardiac surgeons to assess the aorta before instituting cardiopulmonary bypass. The presence of significant plaque may alter the cross-clamp site or may even lead to endarterectomy or aortic replacement at the time of surgery.

Cholesterol Embolization Syndrome

This syndrome represents a distal showering of atheromatous emboli, typically from the descending aorta. The syndrome can be seen in patients undergoing diagnostic angiography, but it can also occur spontaneously. There is a reported association between warfarin anticoagulation and these events. Patients most often present with livedo reticularis and blue toes in the presence of palpable pulses. Renal insufficiency can occur, and may not be reversible. Transient eosinophilia is often present. Treatment is supportive. If the atheroma arose from an AAA, then surgical intervention can help prevent future events.

Inflammatory Aortitis

Giant Cell Arteritis

Giant cell arteritis is an inflammatory disease that affects the temporal arteries, producing local tenderness and headaches. Patients affected are typically older than 55 years, and women are affected twice as often. The most devastating consequence is blindness. Although temporal arteritis is the hallmark of this disorder, there can be involvement of the thoracic aorta and the great vessels. This can lead to branch vessel occlusion, aneurysm formation, or even dissection. Corticosteroid treatment is the mainstay of therapy. With the development of advanced aortic involvement, surgical treatment may be required.

Takayasu's Arteritis

Takayasu's arteritis is an inflammatory disorder of the aorta that typically affects women younger than 40 years. Its prevalence is higher in Asian and African populations than in those of European or North American descent. A subacute inflammatory phase of the illness is manifested by constitutional symptoms. Later, there is occlusive inflammation of the aorta and branch vessels, with segmental narrowing apparent. Symptoms of arterial insufficiency may be present, depending on the vessels involved. Acquired coarctation can occur, leading to hypertension, as can aneurysm formation. Treatment is corticosteroids. For occlusive lesions not responsive to steroids, surgical bypass is warranted.

Syphilitic Aortitis

Syphilitic aortitis represents a manifestation of tertiary syphilis, which can occur 10 to 30 years after the initial infection. This inflammation results in a weakening of the vessel wall and can lead to aneurysm formation, usually saccular. Syphilitic aortitis most commonly affects the ascending aorta and hence can result in aortic regurgitation. The arch may also be affected. Involvement of the descending aorta occurs less often.

Other Types of Inflammatory Aortitis

Aortitis can also be seen in other systemic inflammatory diseases, such as reactive arthritis, ankylosing spondylitis, rheumatoid arthritis, Wegener's granulomatosis, and enteropathic arthropathies. A common genetic underpinning of these conditions is the HLA-B27 genotype, which often plays a role in cases of lone aortic regurgitation, ascending aortic dilation, and conduction system disease. Treatment involves addressing the underlying disorder, with surgery as needed for aneurysmal or aortic valvular complications.

Mycotic Aneurysms

Bacteremia (from endocarditis, trauma, intravenous drug abuse) can result in infection within a weakened aneurysmal arterial wall. Persistent fevers after treatment of the inciting event should raise concern for an infected aneurysm. Mycotic aneurysms more commonly involve the abdominal aorta. Atheromatous plaques can also become infected (bacterial aortitis), serving as a nidus for infection and requiring prolonged antibiotic therapy.

Summary

- An important predisposing factor to diseases of the aorta, particularly the ascending aorta, is cystic medial degeneration.
- Aortic dissection is one of the more ominous acute aortic syndromes, which also include the dissection variants of penetrating aortic ulcer, intramural hematoma, and symptomatic aneurysm.
- Dissections that involve the ascending aorta (proximal, type A) require urgent surgical therapy, whereas dissections that involve the descending aorta (distal, type B) should be initially treated medically with surgery, guided by a complication-specific approach.
- In thoracic aortic aneurysm, recommendations for surgical repair are 5.5 cm for an ascending TAA and 6.0 cm for a descending TAA. Patients with Marfan syndrome, bicuspid aortic valve, or family history of aortic disease should be considered for earlier repair (5.0 and 5.5-6.0 cm for ascending and descending TAAs, respectively).
- In abdominal aortic aneurysms, an aortic diameter of 5.0 to 5.5 cm is recommended as an indication for prophylactic surgery in asymptomatic patients. In shorter women and men, prophylactic AAA repair is recommended at 4.5 to 5.0 cm.
- Atherosclerotic plaques in the aorta can give rise to cerebral and peripheral embolic events. Plaques thicker than 4 mm, or those with mobile components, appear to be strongly associated with subsequent embolic events.

Suggested Readings

Coady MA, Rizzo JA, Elefteriades JA: Developing surgical intervention criteria for thoracic aortic aneurysms. Cardiol Clin 1999;17:827-839.

Coady MA, Rizzo JA, Elefteriades JA: Pathologic variants of thoracic aortic dissections. Penetrating atherosclerotic ulcers and intramural hematomas. Cardiology Clin 1999;17:637-657.

Coady MA, Rizzo JA, Goldstein LJ, Elefteriades JA: Natural history, pathogenesis, and etiology of thoracic aortic aneurysms and dissections. Cardiol Clin 1999;17:615-635.

Daily PO, Trueblood HW, Stinson EB, et al: Management of acute aortic dissections. Ann Thorac Surg 1970;10:237-247.

Hagan PG, Nienaber CA, Isselbacher EM, et al: The International Registry of Acute Aortic Dissection (IRAD): New insights into an old disease. JAMA 2000;283:897-903.

Isselbacher EM, Eagle KA, DeSanctis RW: Diseases of the aorta. In Braunwald E (ed): Heart Disease: A Textbook of Cardiovascular Medicine, 5th ed. Philadelphia, WB Saunders, 1997, pp 1546-1581.

Isselbacher EM: Thoracic and abdominal aortic aneurysms. Circulation 2005;111:816-828.

James KB, Healy BP: Heart disease arising during or secondary to pregnancy. Cardiovasc Clin 1989;19:81-96.

Johnston KW, Rutherford RB, Tilson MD, et al: Suggested standards for reporting on arterial aneurysms. J Vasc Surg 1991;13:452-458.

Milewicz DM, Dietz HC, Miller DC: Treatment of aortic disease in patients with Marfan's syndrome. Circulation 2005;111:150-157.

Pyertiz RE, McKusick VA: The Marfan's syndrome: Diagnosis and management. N Engl J Med 1979;300:772-777.

Schoen FJ, Cotran RS: Blood vessels. In Kumar V, Collins T, Robbins S, Cotran RS (eds): Robbins Pathologic Basis of Disease, 6th ed. Philadelphia, WB Saunders, 1999, pp 493-554.

Spittell PC: Diseases of the aorta. In Topol EJ (ed): Comprehensive Cardiovascular Medicine. Philadelphia, Lippincott-Raven, 1998, pp 3031-3051.

Peripheral Arterial Disease

Firas Al Solaiman, Amjad Almahameed, and John R. Bartholomew

DEFINITION

Peripheral arterial disease (PAD) refers to atherosclerotic and thromboembolic pathophysiologic processes that affect the aorta, its visceral arterial branches, and arteries of the lower extremities.[1] PAD is a marker of systemic atherosclerosis and is found more often among persons with well-known cardiovascular risk factors, especially older age, smoking, and diabetes mellitus, or those with atherosclerosis in other vascular beds. It is associated with a decrease in functional capacity, decreased quality of life, and increased cardiovascular morbidity and mortality, mainly myocardial infarction and stroke.

EPIDEMIOLOGY

In 2000, it was estimated that 8.5 million Americans (7.2% of the population) had PAD.[2] As our population ages, however, the prevalence could reach 9.6 to 16 million in those age 65 years and older by 2050 (Box 1).[3] The prevalence increases with age, and approximately 12% of Americans 60 years and older and 14.2% of those older than 70 years have PAD.[4]

The prevalence of PAD is believed to be slightly higher in men than women across most age groups, although some studies have shown equal distribution.[2,4,5] Recent studies suggest, after adjusting for age, that PAD was more common among African American men and women and Latin American women compared to Latin American men and non–Latin American white men and women.[2,4] This ethnic propensity is independent of susceptibility to known cardiovascular risk factors such as diabetes, hypertension, and obesity.[4,6-8] (Fig. 1 and Fig. 2).

The major impediments to improving care of patients with PAD are related to the lack of recognition of the disease, poor understanding of its impact on the patient, and the gross underuse of safe, effective, and widely available therapies. The PARTNERS (Peripheral Arterial Disease Awareness, Risk, and Treatment: New Resources for Survival) program evaluated 7000 at-risk patients seen in primary care practices.[9] The program uncovered several important facts related to PAD epidemiology. First, PAD is common (29%) in high-risk persons (age >70 years without additional risk factors, or age 50-69 years with a history of cigarette smoking or diabetes) attending primary care clinics. Second, PAD remains poorly recognized (it was diagnosed in 44% of subjects by the time of enrollment in the program) and even when prior diagnosis of PAD was documented in the medical records, only 49% of primary care providers knew about it. Third, diagnosis was more likely in patients who had both PAD and CAD than in patients with PAD alone. Fourth, despite being an independent risk factor for cardiovascular morbidity and mortality, patients with PAD were less intensively managed.[10-12] Specifically, lipid-lowering therapies, antihypertensive treatment, and adequate antiplatelet therapy were less commonly prescribed compared with CAD patients (Fig. 3).[9,13,14]

Emerging evidence suggests that patients with PAD continue to be undertreated with standard therapy such as beta blockers and antiplatelet agents even when CAD is present.[12] The profound lack of public knowledge about PAD's definition, causes, relation to risk of acute MI and stroke, and risk of amputation was also shown in a recent national PAD public awareness survey.[15]

RISK FACTORS

The risk factors for PAD are the same risk factors for atherosclerosis elsewhere (Fig. 4). The three risk factors most strongly associated with PAD are advanced age (>60 years), cigarette smoking, and diabetes mellitus (DM).[6,7,9,16-18] PAD is more common in older adults, with a one-and-a-half-fold to two-fold increase in risk for every 10-year increase in age.[16,17] Smoking or DM increases the risk of PAD independently by approximately three-fold each.[16-18] In addition, smoking has a synergistic effect on other risk factors, and the number of pack-years has been associated with disease severity. Smokers have at least double the risks of mortality, disease progression, and limb amputation rates compared with nonsmokers.[19-22] Although diabetics often have extensive involvement, diffuse and advanced PAD appear to be related to the duration of diabetes rather than glycemic control.[23] Other important risk factors include genetics predisposition, hypertension, chronic kidney disease (CKD), hyperhomocysteinemia, and dyslipidemia; elevations of total cholesterol, low-density lipoprotein (LDL), triglyceride (TG), and lipoprotein(a) levels are all independent risk factors for PAD.[9,16,24,25]

More recently, a number of novel risk factors have been implicated with PAD. These include carotid artery intima media thickness (CIMT), an abnormal waist-to-hip ratio, elevations in D dimer, and markers of inflammation including C-reactive protein (CRP), fibrinogen, and interleukin-6 (IL-6). Baseline CRP, a known marker of systemic inflammation and subclinical atherosclerosis, has been shown to predict the risk of developing PAD in healthy men.[26] In a recent cross-sectional study, elevated high-sensitivity CRP levels were associated with the presence of PAD in healthy men and women older than 40 years without a previous history of DM, hypertension, or known CAD. These findings were independent of the other major cardiovascular risk factors such as hyperlipidemia and smoking.[27] Other proposed risk factors including a high total fat and low-fiber intake have been associated with PAD independent of other classic cardiovascular risk factors.[28]

PATHOPHYSIOLOGY

Atherosclerosis accounts for more than 90% of cases of PAD in the United States, and uncommon vascular syndromes (including popliteal artery entrapment syndrome, cystic adventitial disease, and fibromuscular dysplasia and thromboangiitis obliterans) account for most of the remaining 10%.

Atherosclerosis is a complex process that involves endothelial dysfunction, lipid disturbances, platelet activation, thrombosis, inflammation, oxidative stress, vascular smooth muscle activation, altered matrix metabolism, remodeling, and genetic factors.

Atherosclerotic plaques are composed of a central lipid core, connective tissue, inflammatory cells, and smooth muscle cells, all covered by a fibrous cap. Plaques tend to localize at the bifurcations or proximal segments of large and medium-size arteries. The femoral and popliteal arteries are affected in 80% to 90% of symptomatic PAD patients, the tibial and peroneal arteries in 40% to 50%, and the aortoiliac arteries in 30%.

SIGNS AND SYMPTOMS

Most patients with PAD are asymptomatic or present with atypical symptoms beyond those of classic intermittent claudication (Box 2). Therefore, the diagnosis may be overlooked in up to 90% of patients if intermittent claudication—and not an abnormal ankle-brachial index (ABI)—is used as the sole criterion for diagnosis.[29] In addition to leg symptoms, symptomatic patients often report poor quality of life related to their limited mobility and a subsequent decline in their overall functional capacity.[30,31]

Box 1 Epidemiology of Peripheral Arterial Disease

Affects men more than women
African Americans have a higher incidence than whites
Highest risk for older adults, diabetics, and former smokers (present or remote)
High incidence in patients with chronic kidney disease
High incidence in transplant recipients
Poor public and physician awareness of the disease epidemiology
More than 90% of cases are secondary to atherosclerosis

Box 2 Clinical Presentation of Peripheral Arterial Disease

Most cases are asymptomatic.
In symptomatic patients:

- Most have atypical exertional leg pain.
- Only 10% to 30% present with classic intermittent claudication.
- A minority of patients progress to rest pain or ischemic ulcers (critical limb ischemia).

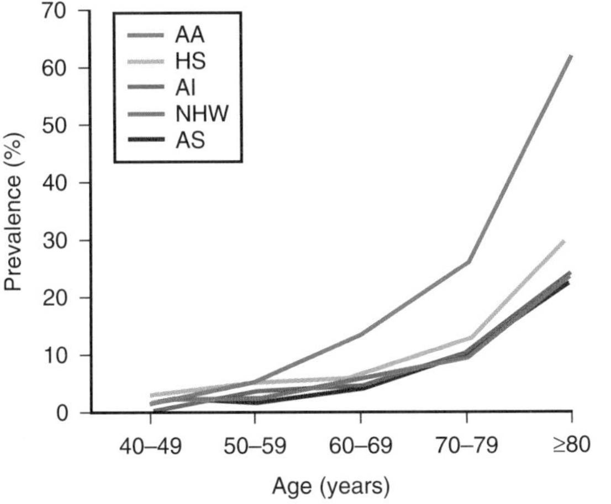

Figure 1 Prevalence of peripheral arterial disease by age and ethnicity in men. AA, African American; AI, American Indian; AS, Asian American; HS, Hispanic; NHW, non-Hispanic white. *Data from Allison MA, Ho E, Denenberg JO, et al: Ethnic-specific prevalence of peripheral arterial disease in the United States. Am J Prev Med 2007;32(4):328-333.*

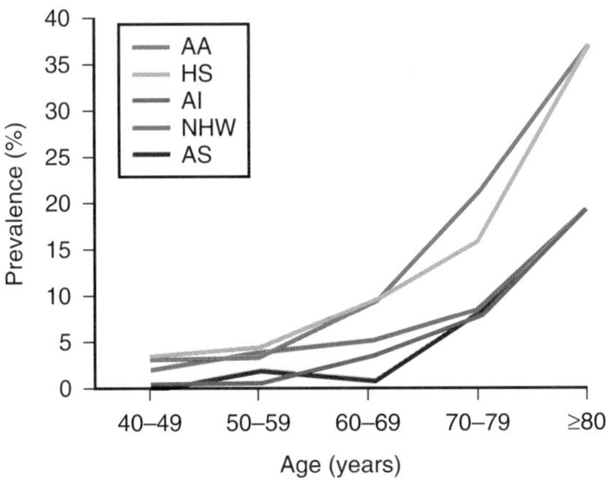

Figure 2 Prevalence of peripheral arterial disease by age and ethnicity in women. AA, African American; AI, American Indian; AS, Asian American; HS, Hispanic; NHW, non-Hispanic white. *Data from Allison MA, Ho E, Denenberg JO, et al: Ethnic-specific prevalence of peripheral arterial disease in the United States. Am J Prev Med 2007;32(4):328-333.*

Patients with classic intermittent claudication typically describe pain, aching, tightening, cramping, or a sense of fatigue in one or more of the lower extremity muscle groups. The symptoms are usually triggered by ambulation and are relieved by rest including standing without the need to sit down. In contrast, patients with pseudoclaudication that results from spinal stenosis (often mistaken for PAD) report that their leg pain improves only with sitting down and not with standing, and their walking distance can vary from day to day. The site of claudication is distal to the diseased arterial segment. For example, buttock, hip, and thigh claudication are seen with aortoiliac disease, and calf claudication is seen with femoral-popliteal disease.

With severe PAD, patients may present with signs and symptoms of critical limb ischemia (CLI). These include rest pain and nonhealing ulcers or gangrene. Rest pain usually occurs at night (because of the horizontal position, which deprives the patient of the effect of gravity on blood flow through the tight lesions) and improves when the legs are in the dependent position. Superimposed edema of the affected leg(s) is occasionally seen in those who tend to dangle their legs overnight. Rest pain is a sign of more severe or multilevel arterial occlusions.

Physical examination should include evaluation of the entire vascular system. The presence of bruits might reflect stenotic lesions in arteries that are not readily amenable to palpation (e.g., iliac, aorta, renal, and mesenteric). Inspection of the lower extremities for skin lesions is also indicated. Patients with intermittent claudication might also have a normal physical examination at rest, including palpable peripheral pulses. Acute limb ischemia (ALI) results from sudden decrease in limb perfusion that causes a potential threat to limb viability. The clinical features of ALI (commonly referred to as the *Ps*) include pain, pallor, pulselessness, paresthesia, paralysis, and poikilothermia (i.e., coldness). Paresthesia and paralysis imply irreversible ischemia, and muscle rigidity is a sign of a nonsalvageable limb.

Laboratory studies are ordered to detect the presence of dyslipidemia, DM, and major metabolic derangement (e.g., renal or hepatic insufficiency). A baseline electrocardiogram (ECG) should be obtained at the time of diagnosis, and for select patients cardiac stress testing may be indicated.

DIAGNOSIS

Peripheral arterial disease can be easily and accurately diagnosed by calculating the ABI. The ABI is the ratio of the higher systolic blood pressure measured at the ankle of each leg by Doppler ultrasound to the higher systolic blood pressure at the brachial arteries (Fig. 5). The ABI test is helpful because of the following:

- Most PAD patients are asymptomatic or have atypical leg symptoms.
- Among symptomatic patients, 11% to 33% report classic intermittent claudication, and up to one third fail to communicate their symptoms to their health care provider.[32]
- Those with asymptomatic PAD have a risk of cardiovascular events (e.g., MI, stroke, cardiovascular mortality) comparable with that of patients with symptomatic CAD.[32-34]
- The severity of PAD (as determined by a lower ABI value or presentation with symptomatic disease) predicts limb outcome and patient survival (Fig. 6).[5,35,36]
- The ABI is an accurate measure (ABI <0.9 has a sensitivity of 95% and specificity of 100% in detecting PAD) that is noninvasive, inexpensive, and office-based and that can be reliably performed by primary care providers and other health care personnel.[1,9,10]
- A high ABI greater than 1.4 (which reflects calcified arteries) also has been correlated with an increased risk of all-cause and CVD mortality (Fig. 7).[37] An ABI greater than 1.4 was also associated with the presence of foot ulcers, neuropathy, and a lower quality of life independent of the other traditional cardiovascular risk factors.[38]

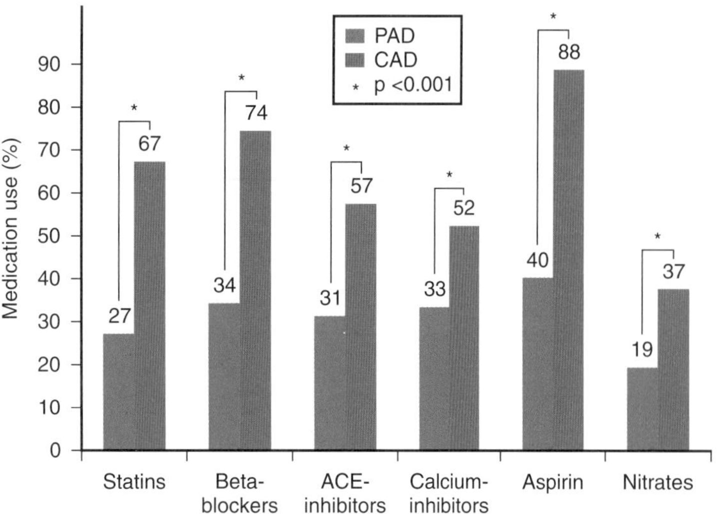

PAD
CAD
* p <0.001
Medication use (%)
0
10
20
30
40
50
60
70
80
90
27
67
34
74
31
57
33
52
40
88
19
37
Statins
Beta-blockers
ACE-inhibitors
Calcium-inhibitors
Aspirin
Nitrates
Medication use according to PAD and CAD patients
ACE_angiotensin-converting enzyme;
PAD_peripheral arterial disease; other abbreviation as in Figure 1.

Figure 3 Medication use by PAD and CAD patients. ACE, angiotensin-converting enzyme; CAD, coronary artery disease; PAD, peripheral arterial disease. *Data from Welten G, Schouten O, Hoeks SE, et al: Long-term prognosis of patients with peripheral arterial disease. J Am Coll Cardiol 2008;51:1588-1596.*

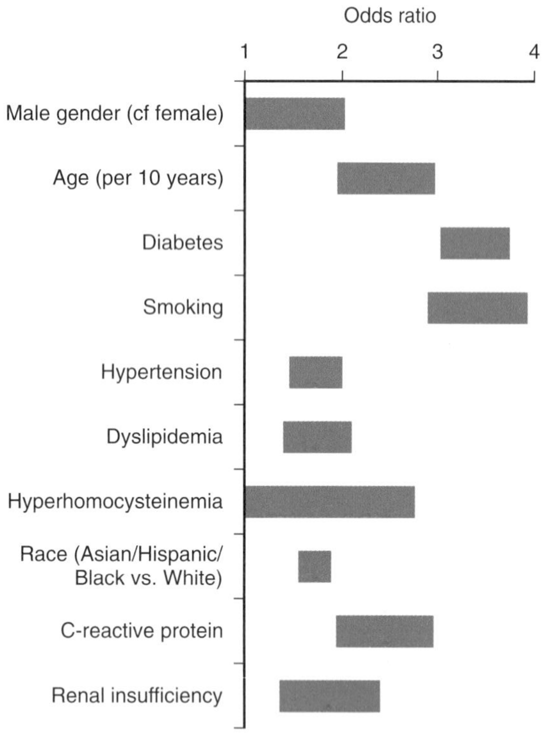

Odds ratio
1
2
3
4
Male gender (cf female)
Age (per 10 years)
Diabetes
Smoking
Hypertension
Dyslipidemia
Hyperhomocysteinemia
Race (Asian/Hispanic/Black vs. White)
C-reactive protein
Renal insufficiency

Figure 4 Odds ratios for risk factors for symptomatic peripheral arterial disease. *Data from Norgren L, Hiatt WR, Dormandy JA, et al; TASC II Working Group: Inter-society consensus for the management of peripheral arterial disease (TASC II). J Vasc Surg J Vasc Surg 2007;45(Suppl S):S5-S67.*

Table 1 compares ABI values with the severity of PAD.

Based on these characteristics, the most recent American College of Cardiology–American Heart Association (ACC/AHA) guidelines advocate ABI measurement for high-risk persons (Box 3).[1] It is hoped that this strategy will facilitate early detection and the institution of management strategies (e.g., risk factor modification, exercise rehabilitation, limb revascularization) that will help prevent disability, decrease cardiovascular events, and lower early mortality.

The shortcomings of the ABI test include the potential to miss mild proximal disease of the aorta and iliac arteries and in patients

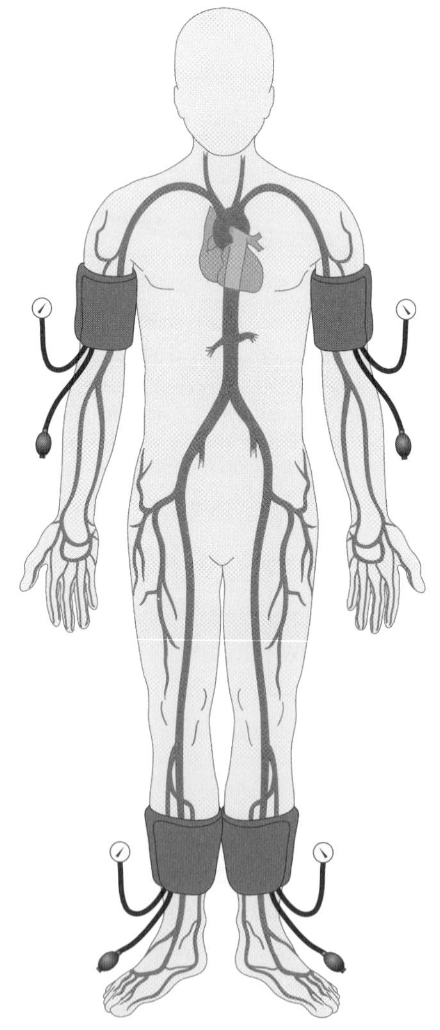

Figure 5 The ankle-brachial index. *Data from Lyden SP, Joseph D: The clinical presentation of peripheral arterial disease and guidance for early recognition. Cleve Clin J Med 2006;73(Suppl 4):S15-S21.*

with significant medial artery calcification. Thus, an exercise ABI should be determined when the resting ABI value is normal if the pretest probability of PAD is high. The exercise ABI also provides significant information regarding the functional limitation of the patient and confirms the relationship between a drop in the ABI and exertional symptoms, when present. Obtaining a complete pulse volume recording (PVR) study and toe brachial index (TBI) is also helpful in patients with calcified vessels (e.g., older persons; those with long standing DM or end-stage renal disease) in whom PAD is suspected but the resting ABI is falsely elevated above 1.3.

Other diagnostic tests including duplex ultrasonography (DUS), magnetic resonance angiography (MRA), and computed tomography angiography (CTA) are indicated if revascularization is considered or when the diagnosis of PAD is ambiguous. Duplex ultrasonography does not require any radiation or contrast exposure and provides homodynamic information by measuring the velocities through the area of stenosis; however, it is labor intensive and operator dependent. Both MRA and CTA provide better details than DUS. CTA was found to be more cost effective than MRA and DUS in a recent randomized, controlled trial.[39] The use of multidetector CTA (up to 64 detectors) has remarkably improved the imaging quality.[40] It is a resonable alternative to conventional digital subtraction angiography (DSA) in evaluating PAD of the entire lower extremity.[40,41] CTA and MRA have the advantage over DSA by allowing three-dimensional reconstructions, which provides helpful anatomic information. The use of conventional DSA is largely limited to patients considered for revascularization procedures. Table 2 lists the recommended noninvasive vascular laboratory tests for lower extremity PAD by clinical presentation.

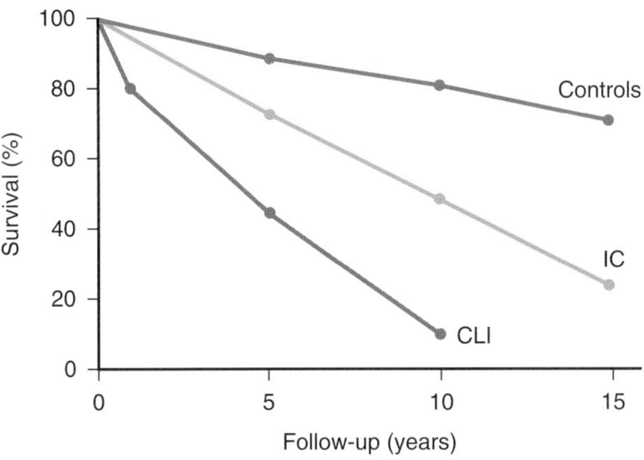

Figure 6 Survival of patients with peripheral arterial disease. CLI, critical limb ischemia; IC, intermittent claudication. *Data from Norgren L, Hiatt WR, Dormandy JA, et al; TASC II Working Group: Inter-society consensus for the management of peripheral arterial disease (TASC II). J Vasc Surg J Vasc Surg 2007;45(Suppl S):S5-S67.*

TREATMENT

The goals of PAD management are limb salvage, symptom relief, improving functional status, and preventing cardiovascular events (acute MI, stroke, and vascular death). All PAD patients require intensive modification of cardiovascular risk factors. Those with lifestyle-limiting intermittent claudication should be referred to a supervised exercise program, and limb revascularization procedures should be offered to select patients. Box 4 summarizes the therapeutic interventions for patients with PAD.

Treatment of Underlying Conditions and Risk Factors

Smoking Cessation

Smoking is the most important preventable risk factor for PAD. Smoking cessation leads to improvement in leg symptoms, lowers the amputation risk, improves long-term patency after revascularization, and reduces the cardiovascular event rate.[42,43] Patients who continue to smoke after lower extremity bypass surgery have a three-fold increased risk of graft failure regardless of the type of graft used.[44] Nicotine is one of the most potent addictive substances known to humans. Data from the PARTNERS program has shown that only 50% of enrolees received advice on smoking cessation.[9] Further analysis has revealed that PAD patients who are taught behavioral modification techniques and receive a physician's advice have a limited abstinence rate (15% per year).[19,45] Thus, physicians should play an active and ongoing role in their patients' smoking cessation efforts; this can be achieved by repeated counseling, referral to a smoking cessation program, and pharmacotherapy.[45]

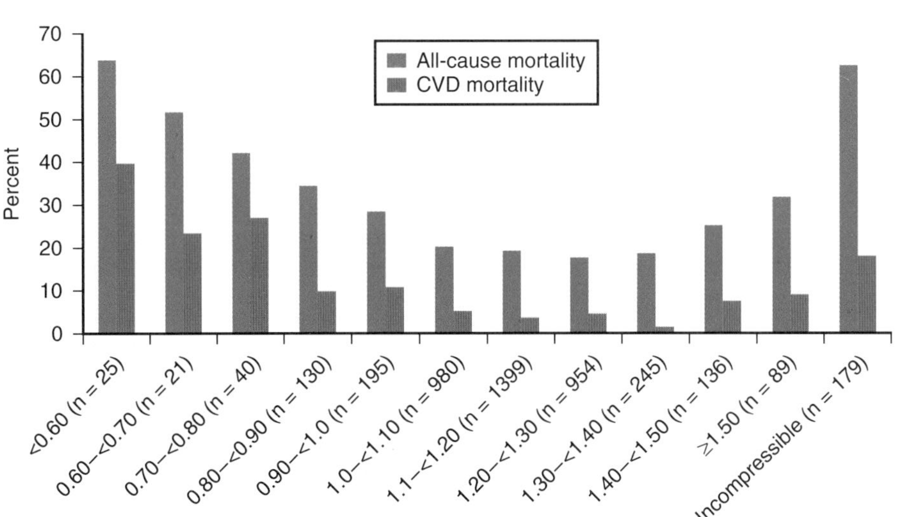

Figure 7 All-cause and cardiovascular disease (CVD) mortality by ankle-brachial index group. *Data from Risnick HE, Lindsay RS, McDermott MM, et al: Relationship of high and low ankle brachial index to all-cause and cardiovascular disease mortality: The strong heart study. Circulation 2004;109:733-739.*

SECTION 2 CARDIOLOGY

Table 1 Ankle-Brachial Index and Severity of Peripheral Arterial Disease

Ankle-Brachial Index	Severity
>1.30	Noncompressible (calcific vessel; diabetes, chronic renal insufficiency, and older age)
0.91-1.30	Normal
0.70-0.90	Mild
0.40-0.69	Moderate
0-0.39	Severe

Table 2 Noninvasive Vascular Laboratory Tests for Lower Extremity Peripheral Arterial Disease Patients by Clinical Presentation

Clinical Presentation	Noninvasive Vascular Test
Asymptomatic lower extremity PAD	ABI
Claudication	ABI, PVR or segmental pressures
	Exercise test with ABI to assess functional status
Possible pseudoclaudication	Exercise test with ABI
Postoperative vein graft follow-up	Duplex ultrasound
Femoral, iliac or popliteal aneurysm or pseudoaneurysm	Duplex ultrasound
Suspected aortic aneurysm	Abdominal aortic ultrasound, Serial AAA follow-up Abdominal ultrasound , CTA or MRA
Candidate for revascularization	CTA, MRA or Duplex ultrasound

AAA, indicates abdominal aortic aneurysm; ABI, ankle-brachial index; CTA, computed tomography angiography; MRA, magnetic resonance angiography; PAD, peripheral arterial disease; PVR, pulse volume recording.

Adapted from Hirsch AT: Recognition and management of peripheral arterial disease. In Braunwald E, Goldman L (eds): Primary Cardiology, 2nd ed. Philadelphia, WB Saunders, 2003, pp 659-671. © 2003, with permission from Elsevier.

Box 3 Who Should Undergo Ankle-Brachial Index Testing?

Patients with overt clinical lower extremity PAD who present with claudication or more severe limb ischemic symptoms:

- Age ≥70 years
- Age 50-69 years with a history of diabetes or smoking
- Age <49 years with diabetes and one additional risk factor (smoking, hypertension or elevated cholesterol levels)
- Abnormal lower extremity pulse examination
- Known atherosclerotic disease elsewhere (coronary, carotid or renal arteries)

Pharmacotherapeutic products—bupropion (Zyban), and the more recently U.S. Food and Drug Administration (FDA)-approved smoking-cessation product varenicline (Chantix)—are effective, but varenicline has shown more favorable results compared with placebo and bupropion.[46] The FDA has recently issued a warning regarding the use of varenicline in patients with serious psychiatric illness. Patients who develop new neuropsychiatric symptoms while taking it should stop and contact their health care provider.

Box 4 Therapeutic Interventions in Patients with Peripheral Arterial Disease

Lifestyle Changes

Complete smoking cessation
Supervised walking exercise program
Weight loss (target BMI, 18.5-24.9 kg/m^2)
Healthy diet
Foot and skin care, other protective measures

Pharmacotherapy

Treat hyperlipidemia

- Use statin to target LDL <100 mg/dL
- If low HDL, high TG, add fibrate or niacin
- If high Lp(a), add niacin

Control hypertension

- ACEIs, ARBs, diuretics preferred
- Add medications as needed to achieve target BP <140/90 mm Hg (<130/80 mm Hg for patients with diabetes or renal insufficiency)
- Consider renal artery stenosis with uncontrolled hypertension
- Beta blocker can be used, especially with coexistent CAD
- Low-dose ACEI may be considered for normotensive patients

Antiplatelet therapy: Use ASA (75-325 mg/day) or clopidogrel (75 mg/day)
Optimize diabetes management
Treat claudication with cilostazol unless patient has history of CHF

Limb Revascularization (Percutaneous or Surgical)

Indicated for:

- Acute limb ischemia
- Critical limb ischemia
- Lifestyle-limiting claudication

ACEI, angiotensin-converting enzyme inhibitor; ARB, angiotensin receptor blocker; ASA, acetylsalicylic acid; BMI, body mass index; BP, blood pressure; CAD, coronary artery disease; HDL, high-density lipoprotein; LDL, low-density lipoprotein; Lp(a), lipoprotein a; TG, triglyceride.

Adapted from Dormandy JA, Rutherford RB: Management of peripheral arterial disease (PAD). TASC Working Group. TransAtlantic Inter-Society Concensus (TASC). J Vasc Surg 2000;31(Suppl):S1-S296. © 2000, with permission from Elsevier.

Managing Diabetes Mellitus

The current Inter-Society Consensus for the Management of Peripheral Arterial Disease (TASC II) recommendations advise targeting a hemoglobin A_{1c} (HbA_{1c}) to less than 7% and as close to 6% as possible in hopes of decreasing macro- and microvascular complications related to DM. Two major recent trials published in 2008, the Action to Control Cardiovascular Risk in Diabetes (ACCORD) trial[47] and the Action in Diabetes and Vascular disease (ADVANCE) trial,[48] however, failed to show a decrease in cardiovascular major events or death when targeting HbA_{1c} targets of less than 6.0% and equal to 6.5%, respectively, in patients with type 2 DM (T2DM). The ACCORD trial was stopped prematurely because of an increased mortality in the arm with intensive glucose control. In line with the United Kingdom Prospective Diabetes Study (UKPDS), the ADVANCE trial showed a decrease in microvascular complications (nephropathy) with intensive glucose control.[48,49] Current recommendations are that HbA_{1c} target in high-risk T2DM patients should remain 7%.[50,51] Lowering HbA_{1c} level to less than 7% could decrease the micorvascular complications; however, this benefit should be looked at in the context of a increased rate of adverse events. Intensive efforts to bring blood glucose levels near normal should be abandoned unless those levels come with ease and without the risk of hypoglycemia. The ACCORD and ADVANCE trials should not lead to the conclusion that blood glucose control in T2DM patients is not important.[50]

Dyslipidemia Treatment

Lipid-lowering therapy reduces the risk of new or worsening symptoms of intermittent claudication.[52] The hyperlipidemia associated with PAD is commonly that of the metabolic syndrome (elevated triglyceride [TG], low high-density lipoprotein [HDL], and normal or slightly elevated LDL levels). The 2001 National Cholesterol Education Program Adult Treatment Panel (NCEP) III has identified PAD patients as being the highest risk group for future coronary events and recommended intensive lipid-lowering therapy to attain a target LDL level of lower than 100 mg/dL and a TG level of lower than 150 mg/dL.[53] A goal of an LDL lower than 70 mg/dL is currently felt to be reasonable in patients with documented evidence of vascular disease in other vascular beds.[5] Statins should be the first-line lipid-lowering therapy, and the evidence supporting their use dates back to the Scandinavian Simvastatin Survival Study (4S), which documented a 38% reduction in new or worsening claudication.[52] The Heart Protection Study (HPS) has also published evidence that supports the routine use of statins in patients with PAD regardless of their cholesterol levels.[54] In this study, simvastatin significantly reduced the cardiovascular ischemic event rate by 23%. More recently, a prospective observational study of 515 patients with severe PAD suggested improved survival with statin therapy[55] (Fig. 8). Several reports have also indicated that statins improve pain-free walking distances and ambulatory activity in claudicants through a mechanism independent of their cholesterol-lowering properties.[56] Niacin or fibrate compounds may be considered for patients with elevated TG or lipoprotein(a) and low HDL levels once the target LDL level is reached.

Hypertension Treatment

The target blood pressure in hypertensive PAD patients is similar to that for patients who have CAD.[57] Special attention should be directed to hypertensive PAD patients who are also diabetic.

The Appropriate Blood Pressure Control in Diabetes (ABCD) trial found a marked improvement in the risk of MI, stroke, or vascular death in the group that received intensive blood pressure-lowering therapy; this benefit was independent of the ABI value.[58] The choice of antihypertensive agents should be individualized. Thiazide diuretics, beta blockers, angiotensin-converting enzyme inhibitors (ACEIs), angiotensin receptor blockers (ARBs), and calcium channel blockers are all effective. The use of beta blockers (once considered contraindicated in patients with PAD) is safe and effective; it reduces the incidence of new coronary events by 53% in those with a prior MI and concurrent symptomatic PAD.[59,60]

The Heart Outcomes Prevention Evaluation (HOPE) trial documented a 22% reduction in the composite end points of MI, stroke, or cardiovascular death in patients with vascular disease or DM randomized to receive an ACEI (ramipril) compared with placebo.[61] A more recent analysis of this trial has concluded that the benefits of ramipril extend to symptomatic and asymptomatic PAD patients (the number needed to treat to prevent one ischemic event during the study treatment period of 4.5 years was 18 and 17 for symptomatic and asymptomatic patients, respectively).

In addition to reducing the risk of fatal and nonfatal ischemic events, an ACEI can also increase peripheral perfusion and lead to improvement in walking distance.[62,63] Given the increased risk of renal artery stenosis in this population, renal function should be monitored closely when starting a PAD patient on an ACEI or ARB.

Antiplatelet Treatment

Given the proven benefit in reducing the risk of MI, stroke, and vascular death in patients with vascular disease by about 25%, the ACC/AHA guidelines have given the strongest recommendation (IA) to the use of antiplatelet therapy (aspirin [acetylsalicylic acid, ASA] 75-325 mg daily, or clopidogrel 75 mg daily) in those with atherosclerotic lower extremity PAD.[1,64-66]

The CAPRIE (Clopidogrel versus Aspirin in Patients at Risk of Ischaemic Events) trial compared clopidogrel (Plavix, 75 mg daily) with aspirin (325 mg daily) in a study of 19,185 patients with atherosclerotic vascular disease, more than 6400 of whom were enrolled on the basis of symptomatic PAD.[66] Clopidogrel provided an 8.7% reduction in the composite end points of fatal or nonfatal ischemic

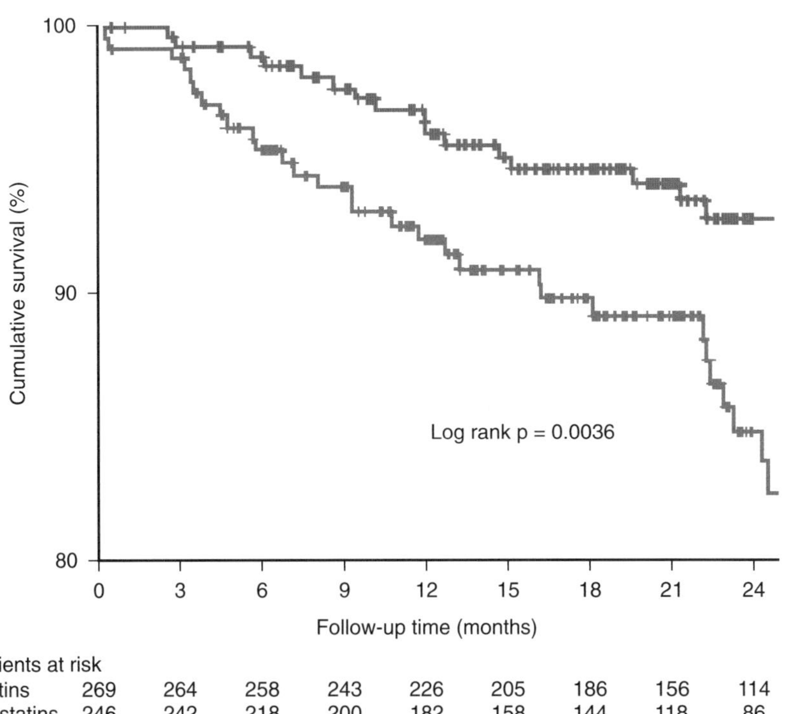

Figure 8 Cumulative survival of 515 patients with and without statin pretreatment. *Data from Schillinger M, Exner M, Mlekusch W, Amighi J. Statin therapy improves cardiovascular outcome of patients with peripheral artery disease. Eur Heart J 2004;25(9):742-748.*

stroke, MI, or other vascular deaths compared with ASA. Importantly, patients in the PAD subgroup manifested a greater benefit from clopidogrel (relative risk reduction, 23.8%). However, the number of patients needed to treat with clopidogrel versus ASA to prevent one event was 87. Clopidogrel can be considered as alternative mainly in patients who cannot tolerate ASA.

Recent data from the CHARISMA (Clopidogrel for High Atherothrombotic Risk and Ischemic Stabilization, Management, and Avoidance) trial did not show any benefit from dual antiplatelet therapy (ASA and clopidogrel) over single antiplatelet agents among patients with stable cardiovascular disease or multiple cardiovascular risk factors.[67] Further subgroup analysis of the CHARISMA trial data suggested a statistically significant reduction in ischemic events in the dual antiplatelet therapy arm within the higher-risk group of patients (documented MI, stroke, or symptomatic PAD).[68] These finding represent results from a post hoc subgroup analysis and therefore should be interpreted with caution. At the current time, the use of dual antiplatelet therapy can not be recommended routinely in stable symptomatic PAD patients.

Ticlopidine (Ticlid) is another antiplatelet agent that received FDA approval for use in PAD earlier than clopidogrel. Its use has declined markedly because of adverse hematologic effects (e.g., thrombocytopenia, neutropenia, thrombotic thrombocytopenic purpura), which occur in 2% to 3% of treated patients.

The controversy regarding the use of oral anticoagulation in combination with antiplatelet therapy in patient with PAD was recently addressed in a major clinical outcomes trial. The WAVE trial demonstrated no benefit from combination therapy versus antiplatelet agents alone in patients with PAD. At the same time, there was an increased risk of major bleeding in the combination therapy group.[69]

The use of oral anticoagulation should be limited to selected cases such as lower extremity recurrent bypass graft thrombosis despite appropriate antiplatelet therapy, or when it is indicated for other concomitant reasons like atrial fibrillation prosthetic heart valves or venous thromboembolism.

Treatment of Leg Symptoms and Improving Walking Distance

Exercise, pharmacotherapy, and invasive (surgical or percutaneous) procedures are strategies that relieve exertional leg symptoms, increase ambulatory distance, and improve quality of life. Revascularization procedures might also be required to prevent tissue loss, facilitate wound healing, and preserve the limb.

A structured exercise rehabilitation program is one of the most effective strategies to improve claudication symptoms. This is recommended by the ACC/AHA and TASC II guidelines as initial treatment for claudication (grade IA).[1,70-74] A meta-analysis of 21 published studies has shown that PAD rehabilitation programs increase pain-free walking time by as much as 179% and maximal walking time by up to 122%.[70] The greatest benefit is obtained when the patient participates in three to five sessions per week, each lasting 30 to 45 minutes, for a minimum of 12 weeks. Maintenance of such a program should be considered indefinitely or the benefit may eventually be lost. The limitations of exercise rehabilitation programs are patient motivation and compliance, lack of availability, and insurance coverage and cost.

Pharmacotherapy

Cilostazol (Pletal) is a reversible phosphodiesterase inhibitor that inhibits platelet aggregation, thrombin formation, and vascular smooth muscle proliferation; promotes vasodilation; and increases HDL and lowers TG levels.[75-77] Cilostazol is the only FDA-approved medication to demonstrate consistent benefits on objective measures of exercise capacity and subjective measures of daily functioning and quality of life. In randomized, placebo-controlled trials, cilostazol has been found to be superior to placebo and pentoxifylline (Trental), which is also an FDA-approved medication for relieving claudication.[78] On average, cilostazol increases pain-free and maximal walking distance by 50% to 60%. The ACC/AHA guidelines have given cilostazol a grade IA recommendation for patients with intermittent claudication.[1] Common side effects of cilostazol include headache (30% of patients), diarrhea and gastric upset (15%), and palpitations (9%). Most of these side effects, however, are short lived and rarely require discontinuation of the medication. Given the increased incidence of sudden cardiac death with other phosphodiesterase inhibitors (e.g., milrinone, vesnarinone) cilostazol is contraindicated in patients with heart failure of any severity.[79,80]

Pentoxifylline is a methylxanthine derivative that decreases blood viscosity and has hemorheologic (improves erythrocyte and leukocyte deformability), anti-inflammatory, and antiproliferative effects. It is also reported to improve pain-free and maximal treadmill walking distance, community-based ambulation, and quality of life. Since its approval for intermittent claudication in 1984, two meta-analyses and two systematic reviews, however, have concluded that its effect on improving walking capacity is small, if any. Thus, it has lost its status as a widely used medication for this indication. The ACC/AHA guidelines have given pentoxifylline a grade IIB recommendation.[1]

Naftidrofuryl, a 5-hydoxytrptamine receptor antagonist, has been shown to improve pain-free treadmill walking distance by 25%.[81-83] Naftridrofuryl has been available in Europe for more than 20 years but is not available in United States.

Revascularization

At present, the absolute indications for lower extremity revascularization are acute limb ischemia, critical limb ischemia (usually manifested as rest pain, nonhealing lower extremity ulcers), and lifestyle, vocational, or economically limiting claudication. In general all patients with lifestyle-limiting intermittent claudication should show lack of response to exercise and pharmacotherapy before revascularization is considered.[5] The only exception is patients with proximal disease location (aortoiliac disease). Those patients could be treated with angioplasty and primary stenting without undergoing exercise therapy and pharmacotherapy.

Box 5 lists the accepted indications for revascularization in patients presenting with intermittent claudication. Box 6 shows factors that increase the risk of limb loss in patients with CLI, and Table 3 lists the clinical categories of acute limb ischemia

Endovascular Interventions

Short stenotic (or occlusive) lesions can generally be successfully treated percutaneously, whereas long lesions usually require surgical treatment. Percutaneous angioplasty carries a lower risk compared with surgical revascularization and can be performed on an outpatient basis. Proposed predictors of favorable long-term outcomes include the locations of treated lesions (better results with the iliac artery compared with femoropopliteal or infrapopliteal arteries); quality of the underlying vessels (better with preserved inflow and distal runoff arteries); patient's comorbid conditions (worse in those who fail to abstain from tobacco, in diabetics, or when the risk factors are poorly controlled); indication for the procedure (claudication better than acute or critical limb ischemia), and immediate postprocedure outcome (return of ABI to normal postintervention value). Although primary stent placement in the iliac arteries appears to improve long-term patency rates, primary stent placement in the superficial femoral artery (SFA) remains controversial. Two recently published studies had contradictory results regarding the use of primary stent in SFA lesions.[84,85] According to the current ACC/AHA guidelines, SFA stent should be reserved for special cases, such as suboptimal angioplasty result, flow-limiting dissection, or acute PTA failure.

Catheter-Directed Thrombolysis

Catheter-directed thrombolytic therapy is an accepted initial treatment strategy for acute limb ischemia.[86-89] It reduces the number of immediate surgical interventions required for acute limb ischemia and therefore markedly reduces perioperative risk. Thrombus resolution allows better visualization of underlying atherosclerotic lesions and offers an opportunity for simultaneous treatment with percutaneous angioplasty. The ACC/AHA guidelines have given catheter-based thrombolysis a grade I recommendation for patients with acute limb ischemia (Rutherford categories I and IIa) (see table 29.4) of less than 14 days' duration and grade IIb for those presenting with a Rutherford category IIb of more than 14 days' duration.[1] Careful patient selection and excluding patients with high bleeding risk are necessary to minimize hemorrhagic complications.

Surgical Procedures

Surgery is advocated for many patients presenting with acute or critical limb ischemia. Occasionally, when disease location is not amenable for endovascular intervention, it is used for patients with lifestyle-limiting claudication. Endarterectomy and bypass grafting are the two most commonly used surgical techniques. Generally, endarterectomy is feasible and offers an excellent success rate when used for proximal arterial segments (aorta, iliac, common femoral, or profunda arteries), and bypass grafting is preferable for distal, long, or diffuse disease. For infrainguinal bypass procedures, autogenous vein grafts have higher patency rates (70%-80% at 5 years) compared with prosthetic grafts.[90,91] Operative complications include myocardial infarction and stroke, wound or graft infection, peripheral embolization, and sexual dysfunction secondary to autonomic nervous system injury. The operative mortality rate ranges from 1% to 3%, and success rates depend on the lesion site and severity, anastomotic site, and status of the outflow system. Use of perioperative beta blockers is indicated because they significantly reduce the risk of cardiovascular complications (including MI and death). With the availability of percutaneous and surgical techniques, the types of revascularization procedures should be individualized depending on the lesion characteristics, the risks for perioperative complications, and patients' preference.

Box 5 Indications for Revascularization in Intermittent Claudication

Before a patient with intermittent claudication is offered the option of any invasive revascularization therapy, endovascular or surgical, the following considerations must be taken into account:

- Predicted or observed lack of adequate response to exercise therapy and claudication pharmacotherapies
- Presence of a severe disability, with the patient being unable to perform normal work or having very serious impairments of other activities important to the patient
- Absence of other disease that would limit exercise even if the claudication was improved (e.g., angina or chronic respiratory disease)
- Anticipated natural history and prognosis of the patient
- Morphology of the lesion, which must be such that the appropriate intervention would have low risk and a high probability of initial and long-term success

The patient desires additional therapy

Adapted from Dormandy JA, Rutherford RB: Management of peripheral arterial disease (PAD). TASC Working Group. TransAtlantic Inter-Society Concensus (TASC). J Vasc Surg 2000;31(Suppl):S1-S296. © 2000, with permission from Elsevier.

Box 6 Factors that Increase Risk of Limb Loss in Patients with Critical Limb Ischemia

Factors that reduce blood flow to the microvascular bed

- Diabetes mellitus
- Severe renal failure
- Severely decreased cardiac output (severe heart failure or shock; is there an ejection fraction here?)
- Vasospastic diseases or concomitant conditions (e.g., Raynaud's phenomenon, prolonged cold exposure)
- Smoking and tobacco use

Factors that increase demand for blood flow to the microvascular bed

- Infection (e.g., cellulitis, osteomyelitis)
- Skin breakdown or traumatic injury

From Hirsch AT, Haskal ZJ, Hertzer NR, et al; American Association for Vascular Surgery; Society for Vascular Surgery; Society for Cardiovascular Angiography and Interventions; Society for Vascular Medicine and Biology; Society of Interventional Radiology; ACC/AHA Task Force on Practice Guidelines Writing Committee to Develop Guidelines for the Management of Patients With Peripheral Arterial Disease; American Association of Cardiovascular and Pulmonary Rehabilitation; National Heart, Lung, and Blood Institute; Society for Vascular Nursing; TransAtlantic Inter-Society Consensus; Vascular Disease Foundation: ACC/AHA 2005 practice guidelines for the management of patients with peripheral arterial disease (lower extremity, renal, mesenteric, and abdominal aortic): A collaborative report from the American Association for Vascular Surgery/Society for Vascular Surgery, Society for Cardiovascular Angiography and Interventions, Society for Vascular Medicine and Biology, Society of Interventional Radiology, and the ACC/AHA Task Force on Practice Guidelines (writing committee to develop guidelines for the management of patients with peripheral arterial disease): Endorsed by the American Association of Cardiovascular and Pulmonary Rehabilitation; National Heart, Lung, and Blood Institute; Society for Vascular Nursing; TransAlantic Inter-Society Consensus; and Vascular Disease Foundation. Circulation 2006;113:e463-e654.

Table 3 Clinical Categories of Acute Limb Ischemia

Category	Description and Prognosis	Sensory Loss	Muscle Weakness	Arterial Doppler Signals	Venous Doppler Signals
Viable	Not immediately threatened	None	None	Audible	Audible
Threatened marginally	Salvageable if promptly treated	Minimal (toes) or none	None	(Often) inaudible	Audible
Threatened immediately	Salvageable with immediate revascularization	More than toes; associated with rest pain	Mild, moderate	(Usually) inaudible	Audible
Irreversible	Major tissue loss or permanent nerve damage	Profound, anesthetic	Profound paralysis (rigor)	Inaudible	Inaudible

Reprinted with permission from Katzen BT: Clinical diagnosis and prognosis of acute limb ischemia. Rev Cardiovasc Med 2002;3(Suppl 2):S2-S6.

CONCLUSION

PAD is a prevalent systemic atherosclerotic disease with associated high cardiovascular morbidity and mortality. Symptomatic PAD often impairs a patient's quality of life, and untreated disease can lead to limb loss. Although PAD can be noninvasively and accurately diagnosed with the ABI, it often remains underdiagnosed and undertreated. Health care providers must make every effort to detect the disease at an early stage, assess associated risk factors, and provide proper long-term care. Aggressive management of atherosclerotic risk factors, a structured exercise program, use of antiplatelet agents, and, when indicated, percutaneous or surgical revascularization are the keys for successful management.

Summary

- PAD is a common but underrecognized cause of morbidity particularly in older adults, those with diabetes, and smokers.
- The risk factors for PAD are similar to the risk factors of atherosclerosis elsewhere; risk factor modification is key to successful management and achieving favorable outcomes.
- Although intermittent claudication is the classic symptom of PAD, the vast majority of those affected are asymptomatic, and PAD is diagnosed by an abnormal ABI value.
- Treatment of leg symptoms includes enrollment in a supervised walking program, use of cilostazol, and, for select patients, percutaneous or surgical revascularization.
- The primary care provider is expected to diagnose and manage most patients with PAD.

Suggested Readings

CAPRIE Steering Committee: A randomised, blinded, trial of clopidogrel versus aspirin in patients at risk of ischaemic events (CAPRIE). Lancet 1996;348:1329-1339.

Norgren L, Hiatt WR, Dormandy JA, et al: Inter-Society Consensus for the Management of Peripheral Arterial Disease (TASC II). Journal of Vascular Surgery, Volume 45, issue 1 – Supplement (January, 2007), p. S5-S67.

Feringa HHH, Bax JJJ, van Waning VH, et al: The long-term prognostic value of the resting and postexercise ankle-brachial index. Arch Intern Med 2006;166:529-535.

Hirsch AT, Criqui MH, Treat-Jacobson D, et al: The PARTNERS program: A national survey of peripheral arterial disease detection, awareness, and treatment. JAMA 2001;286:1317-1324.

Hirsch AT, Haskal ZJ, Hertzer NR, et al: American Association for Vascular Surgery; Society for Vascular Surgery; Society for Cardiovascular Angiography and Interventions; Society for Vascular Medicine and Biology; Society of Interventional Radiology; ACC/AHA Task Force on Practice Guidelines Writing Committee to Develop Guidelines for the Management of Patients With Peripheral Arterial Disease; American Association of Cardiovascular and Pulmonary Rehabilitation; National Heart, Lung, and Blood Institute; Society for Vascular Nursing; TransAtlantic Inter-Society Consensus; Vascular Disease Foundation: ACC/AHA 2005 practice guidelines for the management of patients with peripheral arterial disease (lower extremity, renal, mesenteric, and abdominal aortic): A collaborative report from the American Association for Vascular Surgery/Society for Vascular Surgery, Society for Cardiovascular Angiography and Interventions, Society for Vascular Medicine and Biology, Society of Interventional Radiology, and the ACC/AHA Task Force on Practice Guidelines (writing committee to develop guidelines for the management of patients with peripheral arterial disease): Endorsed by the American Association of Cardiovascular and Pulmonary Rehabilitation; National Heart, Lung, and Blood Institute; Society for Vascular Nursing; TransAlantic Inter-Society Consensus; and Vascular Disease Foundation. Circulation 2006;113:e463-e654.

Deepak L. Bhatt et al. Patients With Prior Myocardial Infarction, Stroke, or Symptomatic Peripheral Arterial Disease in the CHARISMA Trial. J Am Coll Cardiol 2007;49:1982-1988.

Mehler PS, Coll JR, Estacio R, et al: Intensive blood pressure control reduces the risk of cardiovascular events in patients with peripheral arterial disease and type 2 diabetes. Circulation 2003;107:753-756.

Mohler ER 3rd, Hiatt WR, Creager MA: Cholesterol reduction with atorvastatin improves walking distance in patients with peripheral arterial disease. Circulation 2003;108:1481-1486.

Selvin E, Erlinger TP: Prevalence of and risk factors for peripheral arterial disease in the United States. Results from the National Health and Nutrition Examination Survey, 1999–2000. Circulation 2004;110:738-743.

Stewart KJ, Hiatt WR, Regensteiner JG, et al: Exercise training for claudication. N Engl J Med 2002;347:1941-1951.

References

For a complete list of references, log onto www.expertconsult.com.

Venous Thromboembolism

Esther S.H. Kim and John R. Bartholomew

DEFINITION AND CAUSES

Venous thromboembolism (VTE) is a disease that includes both deep vein thrombosis (DVT) and pulmonary embolism (PE). It is a common, lethal disorder that affects hospitalized and nonhospitalized patients, recurs frequently, is often overlooked, and results in long-term complications including chronic thromboembolic pulmonary hypertension (CTPH) and the post-thrombotic syndrome (PTS).

Venous thromboembolism results from a combination of hereditary and acquired risk factors, also known as thrombophilia or hypercoagulable states. In addition, vessel wall damage, venous stasis, and increased activation of clotting factors first described by Rudolf Virchow more than a century ago still remain the fundamental basis for our understanding of thrombosis.

PREVALENCE AND RISK FACTORS

Venous thromboembolism is the third most common cardiovascular illness after acute coronary syndrome and stroke.[1] Although the exact incidence of VTE is unknown, it is believed there are approximately 1 million cases of VTE in the United States each year, many of which represent recurrent disease.[2] Nearly two thirds of all VTE events result from hospitalization, and approximately 300,000 of these patients die.[3] Pulmonary embolism is the third most common cause of hospital-related death and it is the most common preventable cause of hospital-related death.[4,5] Most hospitalized patients have at least one or more risk factors for VTE (Box 1). Long-established and well-known cardiovascular risk factors including hypertension, diabetes mellitus, cigarette smoking, and high cholesterol levels have been linked to acute PE.[6]

PATHOPHYSIOLOGY AND NATURAL HISTORY

Venous thrombi, composed predominately of red blood cells but also platelets and leukocytes all bound together by fibrin, form in sites of vessel damage and areas of stagnant blood flow such as the valve pockets of the deep veins of the calf or thigh. Thrombi either remain in the peripheral veins, where they eventually undergo endogenous fibrinolysis and recanalization, or they embolize to the pulmonary arteries and cause PE.

Deep Venous Thrombosis

The lower extremities are the most common site for DVT, but other affected locations include the upper extremities and the mesenteric and pelvic veins. A proximal lower-extremity DVT (defined as the popliteal vein and above) has an estimated risk of 50% for PE if not treated; approximately 25% of calf vein thrombi propagate (in the absence of treatment) to involve the popliteal vein or higher.

Pulmonary Embolism

Pulmonary emboli commonly result from lower extremity DVTs. These thrombi have the potential to lead to a number of physiologic changes due to their obstruction of the pulmonary arteries. These include increased respiratory rate and hyperventilation, impairment of gas exchange due to impaired perfusion but not ventilation, intrapulmonary shunting leading to hypoxemia, and atelectasis and vasoconstriction resulting from the release of inflammatory mediators (serotonin and thromboxane).

In hemodynamically challenged patients, acutely elevated pulmonary vascular resistance results in decreased right ventricular (RV) output and hypotension. To overcome the obstructing thrombus and maintain pulmonary perfusion, the right ventricle must generate systolic pressures in excess of 50 mmHg and mean pulmonary artery pressures greater than 40 mmHg.[7] The normal right ventricle, however, is unable to generate these pressures, and right heart failure and cardiac collapse ensues. Additionally, elevated RV wall tension can lead to decreased right coronary artery flow and ischemia. Cardiopulmonary collapse from PE is more common in patients with coexisting coronary artery disease or underlying cardiopulmonary disease .[8]

OUTCOMES

Close to 30% of patients who have an acute DVT develop the PTS by year 8 following their initial episode.[9] Most develop signs and symptoms of this condition within 2 years of their acute event, and nearly 25% develop a chronic venous stasis ulcer.

Of the approximately 300,000 Americans who have a fatal PE each year, as many as 15% to 25% present with sudden death or die within 30 days of their diagnosis.[10] The majority of patients die because of a failure in diagnosis rather than inadequate therapy. In fact, the mortality rate for PE without treatment is approximately 30%, whereas it is only 2% to 8% with adequate therapy.[11] In addition, nearly 4% of all PE patients develop CTPH by the second year following their event.[12]

SIGNS AND SYMPTOMS

Deep Venous Thrombosis

Typical symptoms of DVT in the upper and lower extremities include pain or tenderness and swelling. Signs on physical examination include increased warmth, edema, and erythema and the presence of dilated veins (collaterals) on the chest wall or leg. A limb-threatening manifestation of DVT, phlegmasia cerulea dolens, occurs most often in the setting of malignancy, heparin-induced thrombocytopenia (HIT), or other thrombophilic conditions in which the thrombus completely occludes venous outflow, causing massive limb swelling, hypertension in the capillary bed, and eventually ischemia and gangrene if untreated.

Pulmonary Embolism

The most common signs and symptoms of acute PE include dyspnea, tachypnea, and pleuritic chest pain.[13] Other reported findings include apprehension, hemoptysis, cough, syncope, and tachycardia. Fever, gallop heart sounds (S_3 and/or S_4), accentuation of the pulmonary closure sound, rales, and leg erythema or a palpable cord may also be found.

DIAGNOSIS

Deep Venous Thrombosis

Clinical Decision Rules

The clinical examination of DVT is often unreliable; therefore, clinical decision rules (pretest probability scores) based on the patient's signs, symptoms, and risk factors have been developed to stratify

Box 1 Major Risk Factors for Venous Thromboembolism

Hereditary
Factor V Leiden mutation
Prothrombin gene mutation
Protein C or S deficiency
Antithrombin deficiency
Hyperhomocysteinemia
Elevated levels of factor VIII
Dysfibrinogenemia

Acquired
Surgery
Trauma
Medical illness (heart failure, chronic obstructive pulmonary disease)
Immobilization
Pregnancy, oral contraceptives, hormone replacement therapy
Indwelling central venous catheters or pacemakers
Cancer or certain cancer treatments
Antiphospholipid syndrome
Heparin-induced thrombocytopenia
Inflammatory bowel disease
Myeloproliferative disorders
Air travel
Body mass index >30
Previous episode of venous thromboembolism

patients into low, moderate, or high clinical probability.[14,15-18] This approach helps to improve the effectiveness of diagnosing DVT as well as limiting the need for additional testing. Using the clinical decision rule (Table 1), patients in the low pretest probability category have a 96% negative predictive value for DVT (99% if the D dimer is negative as well), and the positive predictive value in patients with a high pretest probability is less than 75%, supporting the need for further diagnostic testing to identify patients with an acute thrombosis.[15-18]

D-Dimer Testing

The sensitivity and negative predictive value of D-dimer assays are high, and their specificity is low. The combination of a low pretest probability or clinical decision rule and a negative D dimer has an extremely high negative predictive value for VTE (approximately 99%).[18] A positive D dimer, however, does not confirm the diagnosis of DVT. False-positive levels are seen in patients with malignancy, trauma, recent surgery, infection, pregnancy, and active bleeding.

Duplex Ultrasonography

Duplex ultrasonography is the imaging procedure of choice for the diagnosis of DVT because it is readily available and is less invasive and less costly than other procedures. It has a sensitivity and specificity of about 95% and 98%, respectively, for detecting DVT in symptomatic patients; however, it is operator dependent and less sensitive in asymptomatic patients and for detecting calf vein thrombi.[19,20] Duplex ultrasonography cannot always distinguish between acute and chronic DVT and may be difficult to perform on obese patients. An inability to compress the vein with the ultrasound transducer is considered diagnostic for DVT. Other findings that are suggestive but not diagnostic include venous distention, absent or decreased spontaneous flow, and abnormal Doppler signals.[21]

Contrast Venography

Contrast venography has been the gold standard test for the diagnosis of DVT. The presence of an intraluminal filling defect is diagnostic, although abrupt cutoffs, nonfilling of the deep venous system, or demonstration of collateral flow may raise suspicion for the presence of DVT. Venography is invasive and requires the use of potentially harmful contrast agents; therefore, it has largely been replaced by noninvasive tests.

Table 1 Pretest probability of Deep Venous Thrombosis (Wells score)[56]

Clinical Feature*	Score
Scoring	
Active cancer (treatment ongoing or within previous 6 months of palliative treatment)	1
Paralysis, paresis, or recent plaster immobilization of the lower extremities	1
Recently bedridden for more than 3 days or major surgery, within 4 weeks	1
Localized tenderness along the distribution of the deep venous system	1
Entire leg swollen	1
Calf swelling by more than 3 cm when compared with the asymtpomatic leg (measured 10cm below tibial tuberosity)	1
Pitting edema (greater in the symptomatic leg)	1
Collateral superficial veins (not varicose)	1
Alternative diagnosis as likely or greater than that of deep-vein thrombosis	–2
Analysis	
High	≥3
Moderate	1 or 2
Low	≤0
Modified Score (adds one point if there is a previously documented DVT	
Likely	≥2
Unlikely	≤1

*In patients with symtpoms in both legs, the more symptomatic leg is used.

Other Diagnostic Tests

Less frequently used tests to detect DVT include magnetic resonance venography imaging (MRV) and computed axial tomography venography.

Pulmonary Embolism

Clinical Decision Rules

Pretest probability scores or clinical decision rules have also been developed to aid in the diagnosis of acute PE.[22] (Table 2). This approach is similar to that employed for DVT; using signs, symptoms, and risk factors to calculate a low, moderate, or high pretest probability score. In a validation study using this approach in combination with a negative D dimer, only 0.5% of patients who were thought unlikely to have a PE later developed nonfatal VTE.[23]

Electrocardiography

The major utility of electrocardiography (ECG) in the diagnosis of PE is to rule out other major diagnoses, such as acute myocardial

Table 2 Clinical Decision Rules (Pre-test Probability for Pulmonary Embolism)[56]

Variable	Points
Clinical signs and symptoms of DVT (minimum of leg swelling and pain with palpation of the deep veins	3.0
Alternative diagnosis less likely than PE	3.0
Heart rate >100 bpm	1.5
Immobilization (>3 days) or surgery in the previous week	1.5
Previous PE or DVT	1.5
Hemoptysis	1.0
Malignancy (receiving treatment or treated in last 6 months or palliative)	1.0

Key: Low probability < 2.0; moderate probability 2.0-6.0; high probability ≥6.0.
DVT, deep venous thrombosis; PE, pulmonary embolism.

infarction (MI). The most specific finding on an ECG is the classic $S_1Q_3T_3$ pattern, but the most common findings consist of nonspecific ST-segment and T-wave changes. Other commonly reported but nonspecific findings include sinus tachycardia, atrial fibrillation, and right bundle-branch block.[24]

Chest Radiography

Chest radiography may also be more helpful in establishing other diagnoses. The most common findings are nonspecific and include pleural effusion, atelectasis, and consolidation.

Arterial Blood Gas Determination

Pulmonary embolism can result in significant hypoxia, and in the Prospective Investigation of Pulmonary Embolism Diagnosis (PIOPED) study, only 26% of patients with angiographically proven PE had a Pao_2 greater than 80 mm Hg.[25] Therefore, a normal Pao_2 cannot rule out PE; however, hypoxia in the absence of cardiopulmonary disease should raise the suspicion for this diagnosis. In patients with cardiopulmonary collapse, a normal Pao_2 suggests an alternative diagnosis. Similarly, an elevated alveolar-arterial gradient is suggestive but not specific for the diagnosis of an acute PE. Therefore if the alveolar-arterial gradient is normal, an acute PE cannot be excluded.[26]

Computed Tomographic Pulmonary Angiography

Because of its wide availability and its ability to directly visualize thrombus, computed tomographic pulmonary angiography (CTPA) imaging has become the standard imaging technique for diagnosing PE. Although initially considered useful only for evaluating central PE and not thought to be the equal to ventilation perfusion ($\dot{V}/\dot{Q}$) scanning, the sensitivity and specificity of newer CTPA scans with multiple slices has increased greatly for diagnosing smaller peripheral or subsegmental PEs. In a recent study by Anderson and colleagues, patients were randomized to undergo PTCA or $\dot{V}/\dot{Q}$ scanning. Their results suggested that CTPA was even more sensitive that $\dot{V}/\dot{Q}$ scans.[27]

CTPA also allows direct imaging of the inferior vena cava and the pelvic and leg veins, as well as identifying other pathologies that can mimic acute PE. The major disadvantages of CTPA are radiation exposure, higher cost, and the possibility of contrast-induced nephrotoxicity. In a meta-analysis of 23 studies involving 4,657 patients with suspicion for PE who had a normal CTPA, only 1.4% developed VTE and 0.51% developed fatal PE by 3 months.[28] These rates are similar to studies of patients with suspected PE who had normal pulmonary angiograms.[29] Computed tomographic pulmonary angiography can also identify right ventricle enlargement (defined as a ratio of right ventricle diameter to left ventricle diameter > 0.9), which has been shown to predict adverse clinical events. This procedure may be an alternative to echocardiography for diagnosing RV enlargement.[30]

Ventilation-Perfusion Scanning

Ventilation-perfusion scanning is now considered a second-line imaging method for the diagnosis of PE. It is helpful in patients who have normal chest radiography or patients who are unable to undergo CTPA (patients with renal insufficiency, contrast allergy, or pregnancy). A normal perfusion scan rules out the diagnosis of a PE, whereas a high-probability scan in the setting of a high clinical suspicion is diagnostic. Unfortunately, nondiagnostic lung scans (intermediate or low probability) are the most common, and in the PIOPED study they occurred in 72% of patients, thereby limiting their usefulness.[31] It must also be noted that in PIOPED, patients with a high or intermediate clinical suspicion for PE but a low-probability scan had a 40% and 16% rate of PE diagnosed by pulmonary angiography, respectively.[31] Hence, it is currently advised that patients with a high or intermediate clinical suspicion for PE but a low-probability $\dot{V}/\dot{Q}$ scan have additional tests to confirm or exclude the diagnosis.

Biomarkers (Troponins and Brain Natriuretic peptide)

Elevated levels of cardiac troponins correlate with echocardiographic findings of RV pressure overload in patients with acute PE and overall mortality. In-hospital complications are higher in these patients compared to those with normal levels.[32] Brain natriuretic peptide (BNP) elevation in the absence of renal dysfunction is also a marker of RV dysfunction in patients with PE and has also been shown to predict adverse outcome in patients with acute PE.[33]

Echocardiography (Transthoracic and Transesophagel)

More than 50% of hemodynamically stable patients with PE do not have evidence of RV dysfunction on transthoracic echocardiography (TTE).[34] Patients with hemodynamic collapse, however, generally suffer severe RV dysfunction, and TTE or transesophageal echocardiography (TEE) can provide rapid bedside assessment in these critically ill patients who are at increased risk for death. Echocardiography findings include RV dilatation, RV hypokinesis, tricuspid regurgitation, septal flattening, paradoxical septal motion, diastolic left ventricular impairment secondary to septal displacement, pulmonary artery hypertension, lack of inspiratory collapse of the inferior vena cava, and occasionally direct visualization of the thrombus. In patients with large PE it has been observed that despite moderate or severe RV free-wall hypokinesis there is relative sparing of the apex. This finding is referred to as *McConnell's sign* and has a specificity of 94% and a positive predictive value of 71% for acute PE.[35] McConnel's sign may be useful in discriminating RV dysfunction resulting from PE versus other causes.

Pulmonary Angiography

Pulmonary angiography remains the reference standard diagnostic test for PE, but it is used infrequently since the advent of CTPA. It is invasive, costly, and associated with nehphrotoxicity due to contrast exposure; however, in experienced centers, associated morbidity and mortality are low. An intraluminal filling defect or an abrupt cutoff of a pulmonary artery is considered diagnostic.

Magnetic Resonance Angiography

Magnetic resonance angiography (MRA) may be an alternative to CTPA for the diagnosis of PE in patients who have contrast allergy or for whom avoidance of radiation exposure is desired. Reports of sensitivity and specificity are varied but compared to CTPA, MRA has been reported to be both less sensitive and less specific and limited by interoberserver variability.[36]

Summary

The American Academy of Family Physicians and the American College of Physicians have published a clinical practice guideline that summarizes current approaches for the diagnosis of venous thromboembolism.[37]

- Clinical prediction rules should be used to estimate the pretest probability of DVT and PE.
- In select patients with a low pretest probability of DVT or PE, a negative high-sensitivity D-dimer indicates a low likelihood of VTE.
- Ultrasound is recommended for patients with intermediate to high pretest probability of DVT in the legs.
- Patients with intermediate or high pretest probability of PE require additional diagnostic imaging studies.

TREATMENT

The main goals of treatment for DVT include prevention of PE, the PTS, and recurrent thrombosis. Once DVT is suspected, anticoagulation should be started immediately unless there is a contraindication.

Anticoagulation

Initial therapy may include heparin (UFH), low-molecular-weight heparin (LMWH), or fondaparinux (Arixtra) followed by an oral anticoagulant (vitamin K antagonist or VKA). LMWH and fondaparinux are renally cleared. The LMWHs can be given in patients with renal insufficiency after dose adjustment; fondaparinux is contraindicated if the creatinine clearance is less than 30 mL/min. Both agents are contraindicated in patients requiring dialysis.

Unfractionated Heparin

Weight-based dosing of UFH (80 U/kg bolus followed by 18 U/kg/hr IV infusion) has been shown to achieve a therapeutic activated partial thromboplastin time (aPTT) more rapidly than fixed-dose regimens. The target aPTT has traditionally been 1.5 to 2.5 times the control aPTT; however, the actual aPTT in seconds varies among laboratories because of the use of different thromboplastin reagents. The American College of Chest Physicians (ACCP) and College of American Pathologists recommend that a therapeutic aPTT range be calibrated for each laboratory by determining the aPTT values that correlate with therapeutic UFH levels of 0.3 to 0.7 IU/mL as determined by factor Xa inhibition.

The aPTT should not be followed in patients with an abnormal baseline aPTT (e.g., in patients with a lupus anticoagulant), in patients who require unusually high doses of UFH such as those with antithrombin deficiency, in select patients with an underlying malignancy, or during pregnancy. In these situations, the anti–factor Xa assay should be used.

Unfractionated heparin can also be administed subcutaneously as an alternative to IV administration, and two dosing nomograms have been recommended. One approach uses an initial IV bolus of 5000 U of UFH followed by a subcutaneous dose of 17,5000 U twice daily.[44] An aPTT is drawn 6 hours after the initiation dose, and subsequent doses are adjusted accordingly to achieve a therapeutic aPTT. Another recently derived nomogram recommends a subcutaneous loading dose of 333 U/kg of UFH followed by fixed doses of 250 U/kg subcutaneously every 12 hours without the need for aPTT monitoring.[38]

Low-Molecular-Weight-Heparin

LMWH is administered as a weight-based subcutaneous injection. Enoxaparin, the most commonly used agent in the United States, is given either as a once-daily injection (1.5 mg/kg/day) or twice per day (1 mg/kg every 12 hr). Two other agents are available, dalteparin and tinzaparin. No monitoring is required except in renal insufficiency or in obese, pediatric, or pregnant patients. If monitoring is required, an anti-Xa level using LMWH as a reference standard should be measured 4 hours after a subcutaneous injection. Therapeutic range is 0.5 to 1.0 IU/mL for the 12 hour regimen and 1.0 IU/mL for the daily dose.

Factor Xa Inhibitors

Fondaparinux is an indirect factor Xa inhibitor that can be used as VTE prophylaxis in medical patients, those undergoing orthopedic procedures (total hip and knee arthroplasty), and those undergoing abdominal surgery. It is also approved as treatment for acute DVT and PE when used in combination with a VKA. Its efficacy and safety in comparison to LMWH for the treatment of acute DVT and in comparison with IV UFH for the treatment of PE has been shown in large randomized, controlled trials.[39,40] Fondaparinux is administered as a once-daily subcutaneous injection of 2.5 mg for DVT prophylaxis and 5 mg, 7.5 mg, or 10 mg based on body weight (<50 kg, 50-100 kg, >100 kg, respectively) for the treatment of DVT or PE. Fondaparinux is contraindicated in patients with severe renal impairment (creatinine clearance <30 mL/min) and bacterial endocarditis.[42] A case of HIT due to fondaparinux, without exposure to UFH or LMWH, has been reported.[42]

Once anticoagulation with UFH, LMWH, or fondaparinux is begun, a VKA may be initiated. An overlap should be continued for a minimum of 5 days and until the international normalized ratio (INR) is within the target range of 2.0 to 3.0 for 24 hours to permit adequate depletion of vitamin K–dependent coagulation factors.[43]

Thrombolytic Therapy

Thrombolytic therapy for DVT may be beneficial in select patients, and although it can be administered systemically, local infusion under catheter guidance is preferred. Both routes carry an increased risk of hemorrhage compared to standard anticoagulation. Although it has been suggested that use of thrombolytics promotes early recanalization and minimizes the incidence of the PTS, their role in the treatment of DVT without a threatened limb is still unclear. The current ACCP guidelines suggest that in selected patients with extensive proximal DVT who are at low risk of bleeding and who otherwise have good functional status and life expectancy of 1 year, catheter-directed thrombolysis may be considered if the expertise and resources are available.[43]

Pulmonary Embolism

Once the diagnosis of PE is suspected, UFH, LMWH, or fondaparinux should be started immediately, unless their use is contraindicated. Anticoagulation with any of these agents should be followed by the addition of a VKA.[44] Risk stratification is felt to be essential for managing acute PE. According to Goldhaber, the clinical examination (including blood pressure, heart rate, and oxygen saturation) biomarkers (troponin, BNP), and echocardiography to assess the right ventricle and PE size should all be used to assist in the acute management of PE.[44] If the patient is normotensive and the right ventricle size and function are normal, standard anticoagulation is advised. If the patient is normotensive, but the right ventricle is abnormal and biomarkers are elevated, treatment is more controversial as noted by the ACCP guidelines. For the patient who is hemodynamically unstable, however, thrombolysis or pulmonary embolectomy should be considered.[44]

Thrombolytic therapy for acute PE remains controversial because there has been no clearly established short-term mortality benefit. Because of favorable outcomes with prompt recognition and anticoagulation for PE, thrombolysis should be reserved for hemodynamically unstable patients with acute PE and low risk of bleeding. An area of ongoing debate is whether there is benefit for thrombolytic therapy in patients who are hemodynamically stable but have echocardiographic evidence of right ventricle dysfunction.

Streptokinase, administered as a 250,000 IU loading dose followed by 100,000 IU/hr for 24 hours and tissue plasminogen activator (rtPA) given as a 100-mg infusion over 2 hours are the current agents approved by the FDA. The ACCP guidelines recommend systemic thrombolytic therapy using an agent with a short infusion time in patients who are hemodynamically unstable. Bleeding remains the most serious complication of thrombolytic therapy. Local administration of these agents via catheter-directed therapy is not recommended due to the risk of hemorrhage at the insertion site.[43] The risk of intracranial bleeding is 1% to 2%.

Pulmonary Embolectomy

According to the ACCP guidelines, pulmonary embolectomy for the initial treatment of PE is reserved for: patients with massive PE (documented angiographically if possible), shock despite heparin and resuscitation efforts, and failure of thrombolytic therapy or a contraindication to its use.[44] To date, there have been no randomized trials evaluating this procedure. Pooled data published by Stein and colleagues report a 20% operative mortality in patients undergoing pulmonary embolectomy from 1985 to 2005.[45]

Other investigational therapies include catheter-based embolectomy procedures that use aspiration, fragmentation, or rheolytic therapy. As of yet, there are currently no guidelines for the use of these therapies and in general they are not advised by the ACCP.[43]

Vena Caval Interruption

Current guidelines recommend against the routine use of inferior vena cava (IVC) filters for the treatment of VTE. Indications for their placement include a contraindication to anticoagulation, complications of anticoagulation, recurrent thromboembolism despite adequate anticoagulant therapy, and patients undergoing pulmonary embolectomy.[44] Relative indications for IVC filters are massive PE, iliocaval DVT, free-floating proximal DVT, cardiac or pulmonary insufficiency, high risk of complications from anticoagulation (frequent falls, ataxia), or poor compliance. Retrievable filters may be considered for situations where anticoagulation is temporarily contraindicated or there is a short duration of PE risk.[47] The consensus guidelines recently published advise that indications for placing a retrievable IVC filter are the same as for permanent devices.[46] IVC filter alone is not effective therapy for DVT, and resumption of anticoagulation as soon as possible after placement is recommended.

Box 2 Risk factors for Recurrence of Venous Thromboembolism

Male gender
Increasing age
Increased body mass index
Neurologic disease (with extremity paresis)
Malignancy
Antiphospholipid syndrome
Idiopathic VTE
Strong family history of VTE
Antithrombin, protein C and S deficiencies
Homozgous for Factor V Leiden
Doubly heterozygous for Factor V Leiden and prothrombin gene mutation
Elevated D dimer following discontinuation of warfarin
Persistent residual DVT
Permanent IVC filter

DVT, deep venous thrombosis; IVC, inferior vena cava; VTE, venous thrombolism.

Direct Thrombin Inhibitors

Three DTIs are currently approved by the FDA for treatment of heparin-induced thrombocytopenia (HIT); however, none have indication for the treatment of VTE. These agents are argatroban (Argatroban), bivalirudin (Angiomax) and lepirudin (Refludan).

Warfarin

Warfarin remains the mainstay of therapy for long-term treatment of VTE. It may be initiated once anticoagulation with UFH, LWMH, or fondaparinux has been started and which should be continued as overlap treatment for a minimum of 5 days and until the INR is at least 2.0 for 24 hours. Recent data suggest that individual variability in response to warfarin dose during initial anticoagulation and time to therapeutic INR may be influenced by genetic variations in the pharmacologic target of warfarin.[47] Physicians are now able to identify whether patients require low, intermediate, or high doses of warfarin, potentially minimizing complications of under- or overdosing (thrombosis or bleeding).

Duration of Treatment

The duration of treatment following the diagnosis of VTE depends on the risk of recurrence. Risk factors for recurrence include idiopathic DVT, underlying hypercoagulable states, and patients with an underlying malignancy. Additional risk factors include placement of a permanent IVC filter, elevated D-dimer levels following discontinuation of warfarin, advanced age, male sex and increased BMI (Box 2). Although the risk of recurrence decreases with longer durations of anticoagulation, clinicians must weigh the risk of bleeding against the risk of new thrombosis.

Current guidelines recommend 3 months of anticoagulation with a VKA targeting an INR of 2 to 3 for patients with a first episode of DVT secondary to a transient cause.[44] Anticoagulation with a VKA for at least 3 months is recommended for patients with a first episode of proximal idiopathic DVT, although consideration should also be given for indefinite anticoagulation (INR 2.0-3.0) in this situation.[43] In patients with unprovoked DVT who prefer less-frequent INR testing after 3 months of conventional intensity VKA therapy (target

INR 2.5), lower-intensity VKA (INR 1.5-1.9) treatment with less-frequent testing is recommended over stopping anticoagulation.[43] Patients who have the antiphospholipid syndrome, who are homozygous for Factor V Leiden, or who are doubly heterozygous for Factor V Leiden and prothrombin gene mutation should be considered for indefinite anticoagulation. Long-term (indefinite) anticoagulation is also recommended in patients with malignancy as long as the cancer remains active and in patients who have unexplained recurrent DVTs.[43]

Compression Stockings

Damage to the venous valves from DVT can lead to venous hypertension and result in the development of the PTS characterized by edema; skin changes, including increased pigmentation and lipodermatosclerosis; pain; and, in severe cases, venous stasis ulceration. Incidence of PTS is drastically reduced with the use of compression stockings. Current ACCP guidelines recommend their use (at a pressure of 30-40 mm Hg) for 2 years following an acute episode of DVT, and the American College of Physicians and American Academy of Family Physicians recommend use for only 1 year.[43,48]

Summary

The American College of Physicians and the American Academy of Family Physicians have published clinical practice guidelines that summarizes current approaches for treating VTE.[49]

- LMWH should be used over UFH if possible for the initial inpatient treatment of DVT; either UFH or LMWH is acceptable for PE.
- Outpatient treatment of DVT with LMWH is safe and cost effective for carefully selected patients.
- Compression stockings should be used to prevent the PTS, beginning within 1 month of diagnosis of a proximal DVT and continued for at least 1 year after diagnosis.
- Both agencies find there is insufficient evidence to make specific recommendations for types of anticoagulation for the treatment of VTE in pregnant patients.
- Anticoagulation should be given for 3 to 6 months for DVT or PE secondary to transient risk factors and for more than 12 months for recurrent VTE. Extended-duration therapy is advisable in patients with an idiopathic VTE.
- LMWH is safe and efficacious for the long-term treatment of VTE in select individuals and may be preferable for cancer patients.

PREVENTION AND SCREENING

Prevention

Approximately two thirds of all VTE events result from hospitalization, yet only one third of all hospitalized patients at risk receive adequate prophylactic treatment.[2] Pulmonary embolism is the most common preventable cause of hospital death in the United States. Without prophylaxis, the incidence of hospital-acquired DVT is 10% to 20% among medical patients and even higher (15%-40%) among surgical patients.[50] Adequate prophylaxis can reduce the incidence of VTE as demonstrated in a meta-analysis involving 19,958 patients. There was a 62% reduction in fatal PE, 57% reduction in fatal and nonfatal PE, and 53% reduction in DVT.[50]

The consequences of VTE if not prevented include symptomatic DVT and PE, fatal PE, the cost of investigating symptomatic patients, the risk and cost of treatment (bleeding), PTS, and CTPH.

Screening

Screening asymptomatic patients for DVT is labor intensive and cost ineffective.[51-54] Thus, prophylaxis in at-risk populations remains the most effective means for preventing complications of VTE.[50]

CONSIDERATIONS IN SPECIAL POPULATIONS

Calf Vein Thrombosis

Anticoagulation is generally indicated for symptomatic calf DVT or when there is propagation into the popliteal vein or more proximally. Typical duration of treatment is 3 months, with a VKA targeting an INR of 2 to 3 for patients with a first episode of symptomatic calf vein DVT secondary to a transient cause.

Monitoring calf vein thrombosis for propagation into the proximal veins with serial ultrasonography (once or twice weekly for 2-3 weeks) without anticoagulation represents an alternative approach to treatment for patients with a contraindication to anticoagulation.

Superficial Venous Thrombosis

Superficial venous thrombosis often occurs as a complication of an intravenous line, but it can occur spontaneously. Anticoagulation is generally not required due to the lower risk of PE unless the thrombosis propagates into the deep venous system or if the event is spontaneous. Guidelines recommend intermediate doses of UFH or LMWH for at least 4 weeks for spontaneous superficial thrombophlebitis.[43]

Deep Venous Thrombosis of the Upper Extremity

Upper-extremity DVT is most often related to central venous catheter placement, pacemaker devices, or intravenous drug abuse. Other, less common causes include thoracic outlet syndrome (also referred to as *effort thrombosis*) and hypercoagulable conditions including malignancy. Patients may be asymptomatic, but more often they complain of arm swelling and pain. Anticoagulation is indicated if there are no contraindications. Thrombolysis should be considered in younger patients with a low risk of bleeding and symptoms of acute onset.[43]

Phlegmasia Cerulea Dolens

Phlegmasia cerulea dolens is a vascular emergency requiring anticoagulation or, in select cases, thrombolysis or surgical or catheter-based thrombectomy. Fasciotomy may also be required to relieve associated compartment syndromes.

Pregnancy and Venous Thromboembolism

Venous thromboembolism is the leading cause of maternal death. The risk of VTE during pregnancy is increased four-fold; this risk is increased five-fold for 6 weeks following delivery. Increased risks for VTE during pregnancy include age older than 35 years, cesarean section, pre-eclampsia, and a history of previous VTE or family history of thrombosis.

Summary

- Venous thromboembolism is the third most common cardiovascular disease after MI and stroke.
- Long-term complications include recurrent VTE, CTPH, and the PTS.
- The recurrence rate for idiopathic VTE approaches 30% after 10 years, the incidence of CTPH is 4% at 2 years, and the rate of PTS is 30% at 8 years.
- D dimer is an excellent test to exclude VTE.
- Duplex ultrasonography is the noninvasive test of choice for the diagnosis of DVT.
- Computed tomographic pulmonary angiography has replaced the ventilation perfusion scan for diagnosing PE.
- Risk stratification is the key to management of patients with VTE.
- Indefinite anticoagulation should be considered for patients with an idiopathic VTE.
- Appropriate prophylaxis remains underused.

References

For a complete list of references, log onto www.expertconsult.com.

Congenital Heart Disease in the Adult

Richard A. Krasuski

DEFINITION

Adults with congenital heart disease (CHD) generally fall into two categories: patients who have been recognized, treated, and followed during their pediatric years and subsequently require follow-up during their adult years; and the de novo, previously unrecognized adults who may or may not be symptomatic at the time of diagnosis. Despite the complexity of this patient population and a well-defined need for subspecialty care, the average adult with CHD is followed primarily by a generalist. It is essential, therefore, that all physicians be familiar with the unique clinical presentations of these patients and have a general understanding of their anatomy and its consequences to facilitate the proper timing of referral for percutaneous, electrophysiologic, and surgical interventions.

PREVALENCE AND RISK FACTORS

CHD in the adult is now more prevalent than ever because of the rapid advances in surgical and medical interventions in the pediatric population. As a result, there are now an estimated 750,000 adults with CHD in the United States,[1] and this figure excludes patients with bicuspid aortic valves, which are present in up to 2% of the population, and mitral valve prolapse. There are a few generalized syndromes in which a toxic exposure during neonatal development has been linked with the development of CHD. Two classic examples are congenital rubella, in which patent ductus arteriosus has been well described, and women who were administered lithium carbonate during their first trimester of pregnancy, which appears to increase the risk of Ebstein's anomaly. Most congenital heart disease, however, appears to be caused by genetic abnormalities, a few of which have been well described, but many of which remain to be elucidated. Evidence to support the importance of genetics in CHD includes the much higher risk in the offspring of CHD patients than the 0.8% general population risk; animal models such as transgenic knockout mice that develop cardiac abnormalities; well-described familial kindreds with lesions such as atrial septal defects; and mendelian patterns of inheritance and the common clinical syndromes such as trisomy 21 (Down syndrome), in which atrioventricular canal–type (primum) septal defects are commonly present, and Noonan's syndrome, in which pulmonic stenosis is often present.[2] In general, routine screening of adults for genetic mutations is not currently advocated for most adults with CHD, even for family planning.

PATHOPHYSIOLOGY

The clinical course of CHD in the adult is most dependent on the anatomic lesions present and the timing and manner of repair. These lesions can be divided into three general categories (by decreasing incidence): simple shunt lesions, obstructive lesions, and complex lesions (acyanotic and cyanotic). The most commonly encountered abnormalities in these categories are described next.

Shunt Lesions

Intracardiac shunts are the most common form of congenital heart lesion and are often diagnosed in otherwise healthy adults. They are associated with increased pulmonary blood flow, which can lead to right heart chamber enlargement and arrhythmias, and with pulmonary hypertension. The surgical correction of many of these lesions has been determined to be safe and efficacious. Percutaneous devices have been increasingly used to close these defects to avoid the morbidity and mortality of surgery. There are three common shunt lesions.

Atrial Septal Defect

The atrial septal defect (ASD) is the most common congenital heart defect encountered in adults, accounting for up to 15% of all adult CHD (Fig. 1). It results from the failure of proper embryologic development of the atrial septum. There are many different types of ASD (Fig. 2), the most common of which is the secundum ASD, in which the defect occurs in the middle of the atrial septum.

The flow of blood across the defect (shunt) is determined by the size of the defect and the compliance of the atria. ASD should be suspected whenever right heart enlargement is present without an alternative explanation. Occasionally, patients present late in life with ASD-related symptoms when the left atrial pressure increases because of a stiff left ventricle and diastolic dysfunction, usually the result of long-standing hypertension or coronary artery disease, resulting in increased shunt.

The larger the left-to-right shunt is in patients with ASD, the greater is the risk for long-term complications, such as atrial fibrillation and pulmonary hypertension. The latter condition affects up to 15% of adults with ASD and, if it remains uncorrected, it can result in Eisenmenger's syndrome (see later). Another condition associated with ASD is stroke, which presumably results from paradoxical embolization—blood clots forming in the extremities and reaching the cerebral circulation by passing through the ASD.

Other, less-common variations of ASD include the sinus venosus ASD, in which there is abnormal fusion of the vena cava (superior or inferior) to the left atrium. This defect is almost always associated with partial anomalous return of the pulmonary veins (right superior or both right pulmonary veins drain into the right atrium). The primum ASD involves the lower portion of the atrial septum and typically affects the ventricular septum as well (the atrioventricular [AV] canal defect). Both AV valves are structurally abnormal, and the mitral valve is typically cleft. The least common form of ASD involves unroofing of the coronary sinus, which results in shunting into the left atrium. At this time, only the secundum ASD has been successfully occluded through percutaneous means.

Ventricular Septal Defect

Ventricular septal defect (VSD) is the most common congenital heart defect seen in children (Fig. 3). Defects can occur at various locations in the septum but most commonly occur in the membranous (Fig. 4) or muscular portions. Small defects often close spontaneously during childhood. One type of defect, the outflow (or supracristal) VSD, can be spontaneously occluded by one of the aortic leaflets prolapsing into it. This can result in the development of significant aortic insufficiency.

Small VSDs are usually asymptomatic, whereas larger defects are more likely to manifest during childhood with heart failure. VSD is the most common cause of Eisenmenger's syndrome.

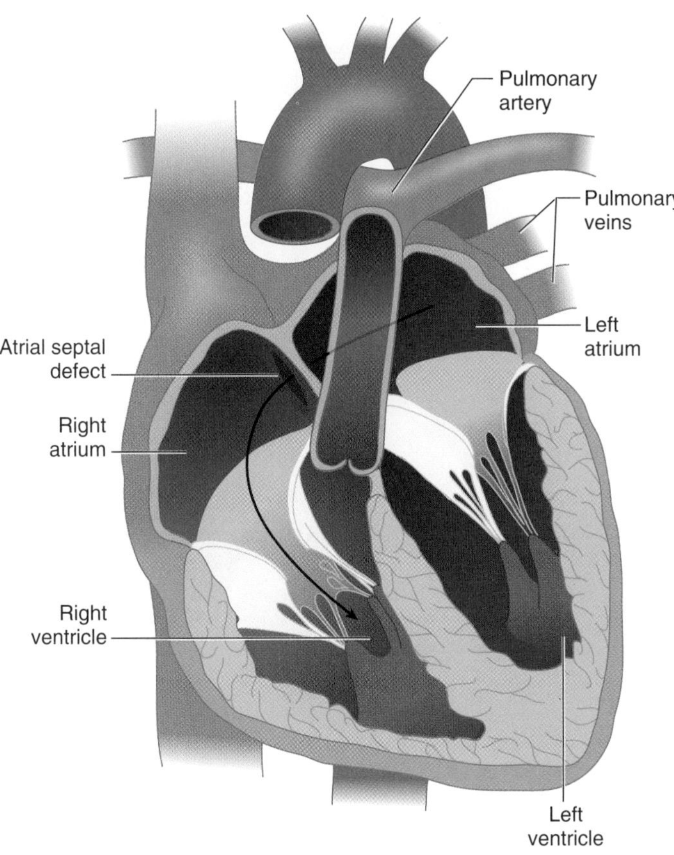

Figure 1 **Atrial septal defect (ASD).** An ASD is the most common congenital heart defect encountered in adults, accounting for up to 15% of all adult congenital heart disease.

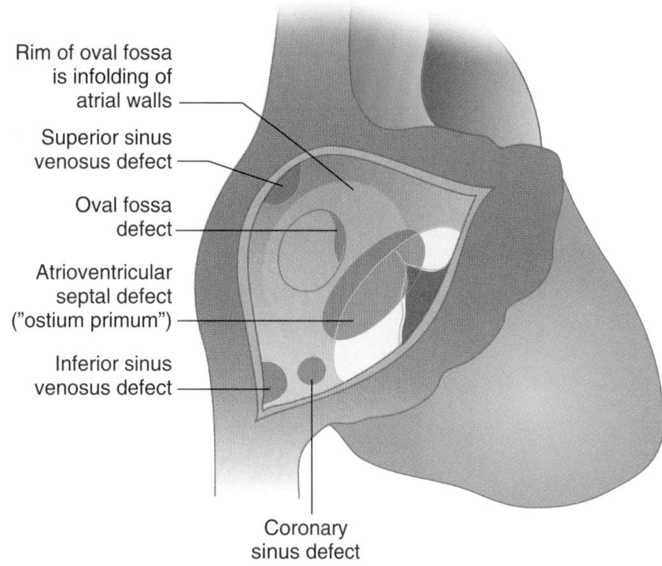

Figure 2 **Types of atrial septal defect.**

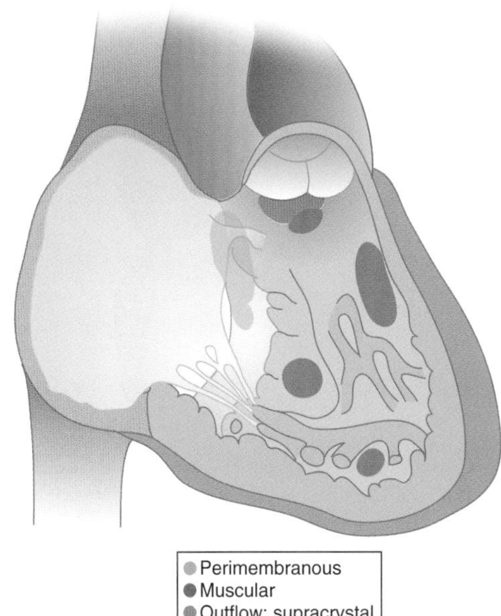

Figure 3 **Types of ventricular septal defect (VSD).** VSD is the most common congenital heart defect seen in children.

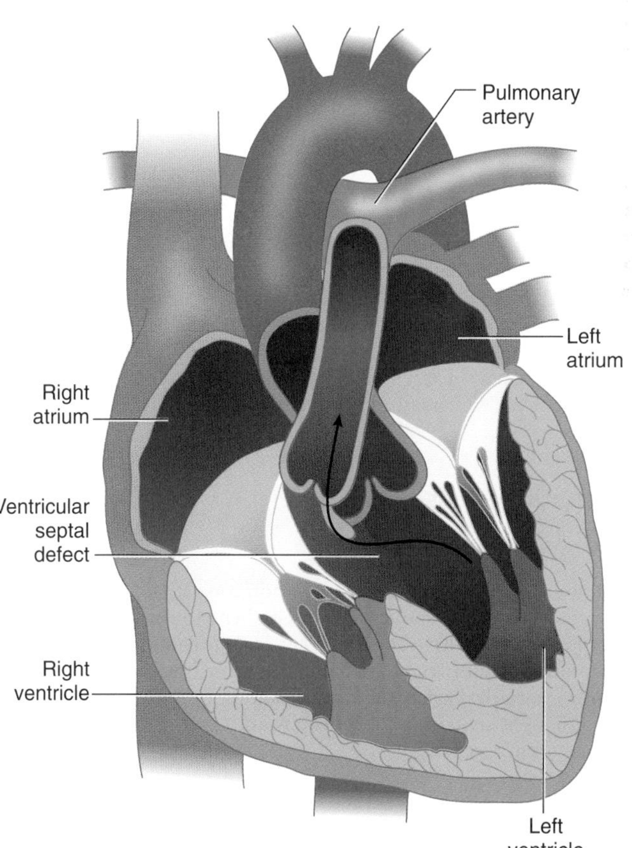

Figure 4 **Membranous ventricular septal defect.** Defects can occur at various locations in the septum, but they most commonly occur in membranous or muscular portions.

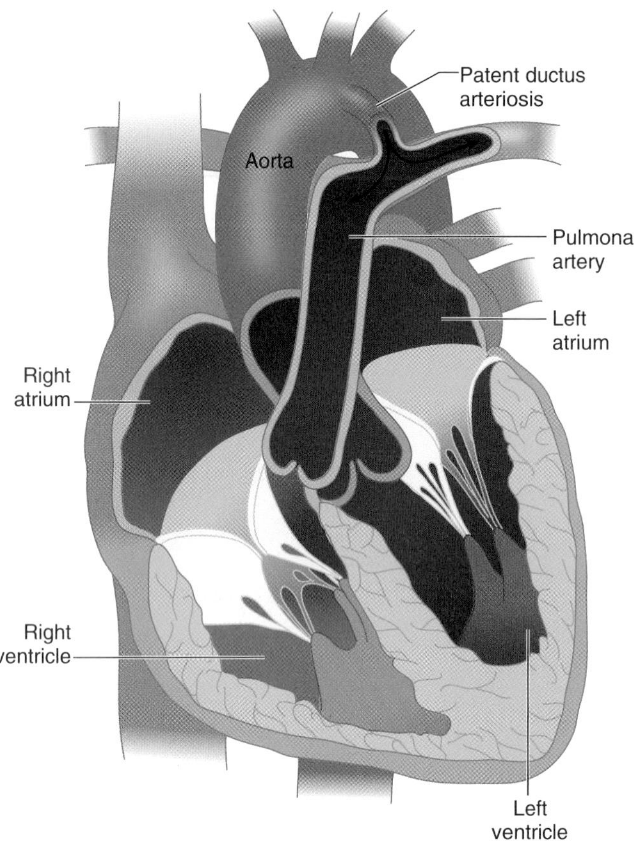

Figure 5 Patent ductus arteriosus. This is the second most common congenital heart defect seen in adults.

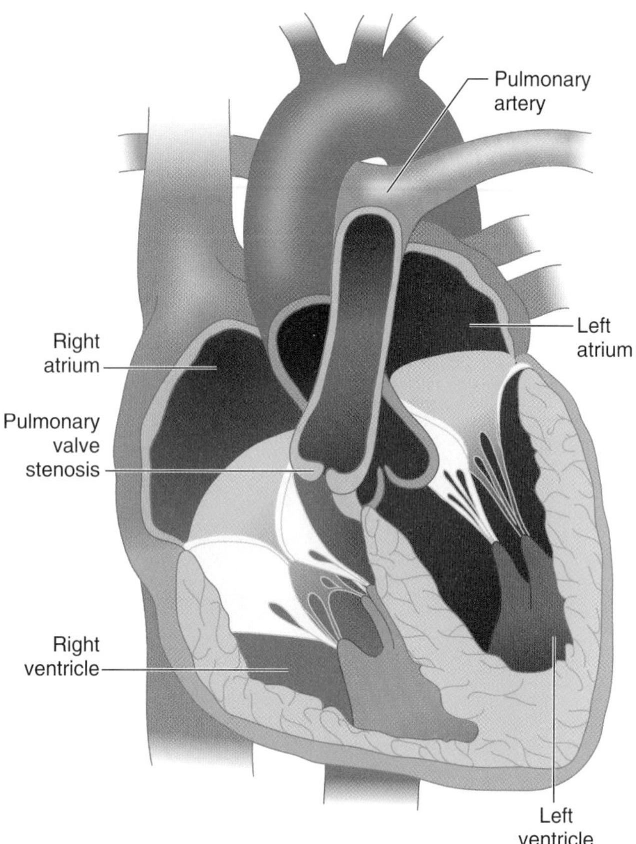

Figure 6 Pulmonary valve stenosis. Excluding mitral valve prolapse and bicuspid aortic valve, this is the most common congenital valve lesion requiring therapy in adults.

Patent Ductus Arteriosus

Patent ductus arteriosus (PDA; Fig. 5) is the second most common congenital heart defect seen in adults (approximately 10%-15% of all CHD in adults). PDA is present as an isolated lesion in most adults, unlike in children, in whom it is often seen with more complex heart defects. The ductus connects the descending aorta at the level of the subclavian artery to the proximal left pulmonary artery. As in VSD, patients with a large uncorrected PDA can develop pulmonary hypertension.

Stenotic Lesions

Pulmonary Stenosis

Pulmonary stenosis is the most common congenital valve lesion that requires therapy in adults (Fig. 6). Gradients across the pulmonary outflow tract usually occur at the valvular level, but it can also involve the infundibulum (right ventricular outflow tract), peripheral pulmonary arteries, or both. Complications of pulmonary stenosis include right ventricular hypertrophy and eventually failure, as well as arrhythmias.

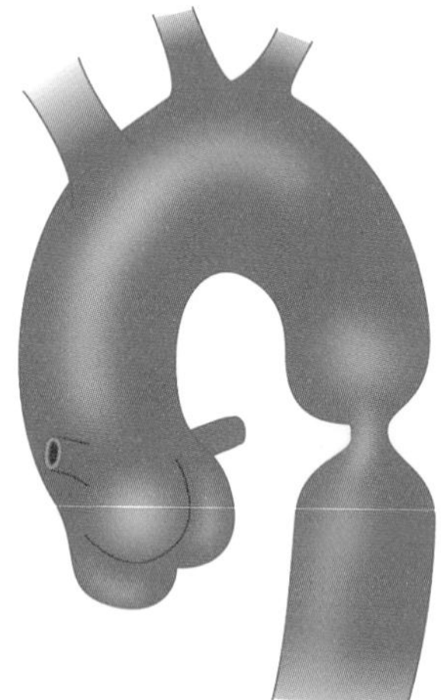

Figure 7 Coarctation of the aorta. This common congenital heart defect accounts for approximately 8% of all congenital defects.

Coarctation of the Aorta

Coarctation of the aorta (CoA) is a common congenital heart defect (Fig. 7) accounting for approximately 8% of all congenital defects. It probably results from extraneous ductal tissue that contracts following birth. Anatomically, it can occur before, at the level of, or after the ductus arteriosus, although adults with previously undiagnosed CoA almost always have postductal lesions. The most common way it is identified in adults is fortuitous discovery during secondary workup for systemic hypertension. Lower extremity and renal hypoperfusion lead to a hyper-renin state that might not abate, even after coarctation repair. In most patients, there is upper extremity hypertension and the development of collateral vessels around the coarctation to the lower extremity.

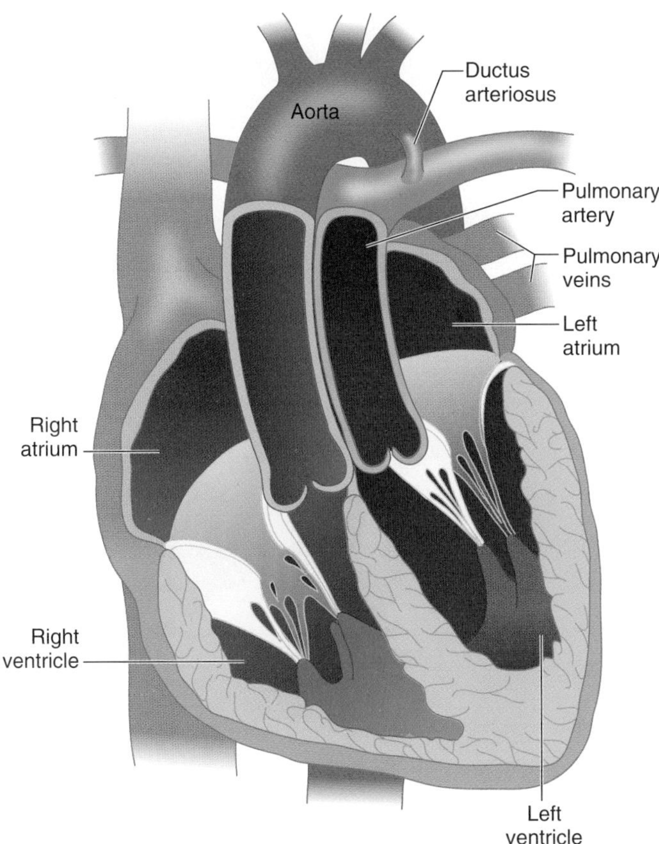

Figure 8 Transposition of the great arteries (TGA). This refers to an abnormality in the developmental separation of the great vessels, which results in the aorta emanating from the venous ventricle and the pulmonary artery coming off the systemic ventricle (ventriculoarterial discordance). In D-TGA, the ventricles are located in their normal anatomic positions (atrioventricular concordance), and in L-TGA, the ventricles are also discordant with the atria.

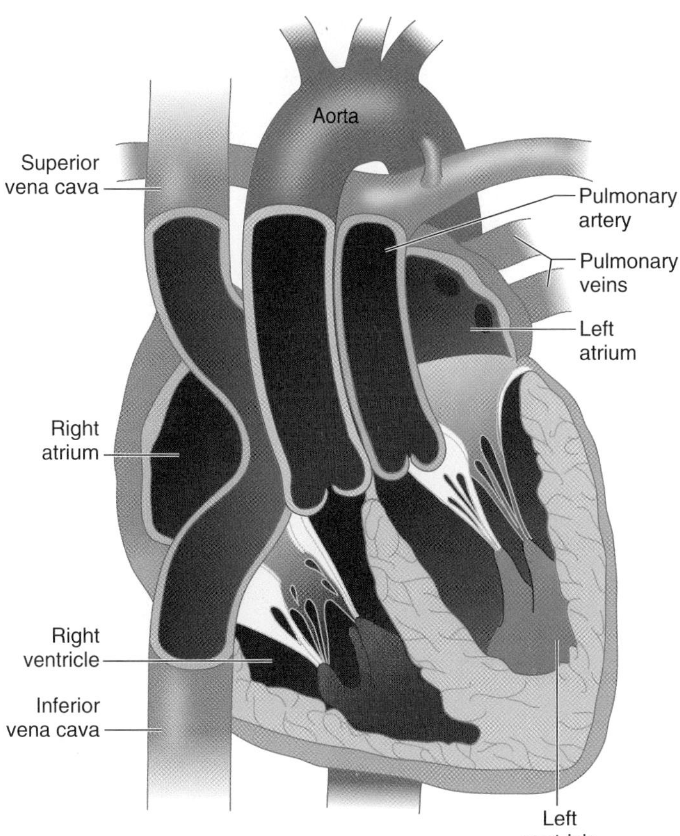

Figure 9 Mustard procedure for dextrotransposition of the great arteries. In this procedure, blood is baffled from the venae cavae to the left atrium and from the pulmonary veins to the right atrium.

Complex Lesions (Acyanotic)

Transposition of the Great Arteries

Transposition of the great arteries (TGA; Fig. 8) refers to an abnormality in the developmental separation of the great vessels, which results in the aorta emanating from the venous ventricle and the pulmonary artery coming off the systemic ventricle (ventriculoarterial discordance). Two varieties are most commonly seen in adults. The first type is dextrotransposition of the great arteries (D-TGA), with "dextro" initially meant to describe the location of the aorta in respect to the pulmonary artery. In this condition, the right ventricle gives rise to the aorta and the left ventricle gives rise to the pulmonary artery, but both atria are appropriately connected to their respective ventricles (AV concordance). This condition is not compatible with life unless there is a naturally occurring shunt (ASD, VSD, or PDA) or surgically created shunt. Often, these patients have undergone repair during childhood with a Senning or Mustard procedure, in which blood is baffled from the venae cavae to the left atrium and from the pulmonary veins to the right atrium (Fig. 9). The primary long-term concern in these patients is that the right ventricle is ill prepared to serve as the systemic ventricle. It can weaken and fail over time (usually when the patient enters the third or fourth decade), and these patients also develop significant systemic AV regurgitation, with the tricuspid valve in the mitral position.

The other type of TGA is the congenitally (naturally) corrected lesion, levotransposition of the great arteries (L-TGA). In this case, the ventricles are also inverted (both AV and ventriculoarterial discordance are present). This variation (see Fig. 8) results in a circulation in which blood flows from vena cava to right atrium to left ventricle to pulmonary artery to pulmonary veins to left atrium to right ventricle to aorta. Again, the problem remains a right ventricle pumping into the systemic circulation. This condition is also associated with about a one in three lifetime prevalence of complete heart block.

Complex Lesions (Cyanotic)

Tetralogy of Fallot

Tetralogy of Fallot (TOF), a conotruncal abnormality, is a constellation of four findings: an aorta that overrides the right ventricular outflow tract; right ventricular outflow obstruction; a large subaortic VSD; and hypertrophy of the right ventricle (Fig. 10). The frequent coexistence of an ASD can make for a pentalogy. Occasionally, patients with unrepaired TOF only present in adulthood because of a remarkable balance between the pulmonic obstruction and the VSD, which limits cyanosis.

Early palliation with a systemic-to-arterial shunt (e.g., Blalock-Taussig), which connects the subclavian and pulmonary arteries (Fig. 11), facilitates growth of the pulmonary arteries and is a precursor to definitive surgical repair in the young child. Definitive repair often involves complete removal of the pulmonic valve (Fig. 12) and therefore results in wide open pulmonic regurgitation. Although the

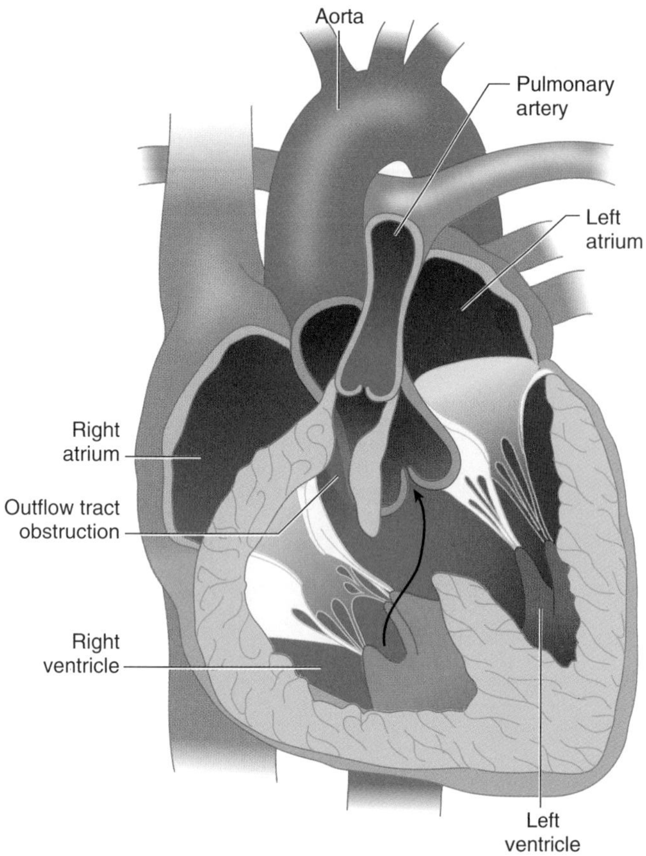

Figure 10 Tetralogy of Fallot. This conotruncal abnormality is the constellation of four findings: an aorta that overrides the right ventricular outflow tract, right ventricular outflow obstruction, a large subaortic ventricular septal defect, and hypertrophy of the right ventricle.

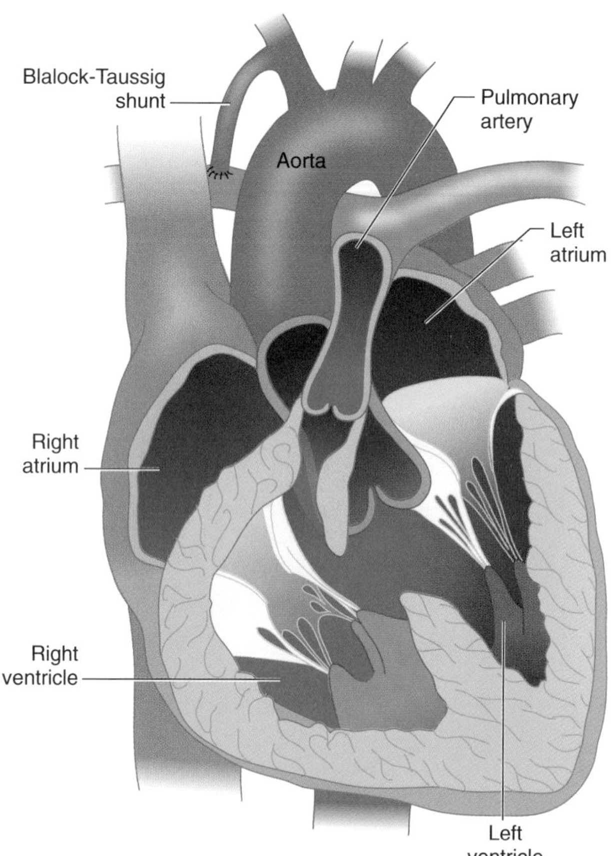

Figure 11 Blalock-Taussig shunt. This connects the subclavian and pulmonary arteries.

repair is tolerated for several years, the right ventricle eventually succumbs to volume overload and progressively increases in size.

Ebstein's Anomaly

Ebstein's anomaly (Fig. 13) is the result of inferior displacement of the tricuspid valve into the right ventricle, which results in atrialization of the right ventricle. As a result, the right ventricle is very small and not infrequently hypocontractile. The posterior and septal leaflets of the tricuspid valve are often small and inadequate, and the anterior leaflet is very large and redundant, resembling a sail. About 25% of Ebstein's anomaly patients have accessory pathways for AV conduction (Wolff-Parkinson-White syndrome), which often are multiple. About 50% of patients also have an ASD or a patent foramen ovale (PFO), and right-to-left shunting through these defects results in cyanosis.

Eisenmenger's Syndrome

Eisenmenger's syndrome (Fig. 14) is a condition in which an intracardiac shunt results in such severe pulmonary hypertension that right-sided pressures eventually exceed systemic pressures and reversal of the intracardiac shunt (becoming right to left) occurs.[3] Oxygen saturation does not improve in patients with this complication when oxygen is administered to them (the telltale sign of a right-to-left shunt). Multiple complications eventually ensue and, until recently, this condition was considered irreversible.

Although patients with Eisenmenger's syndrome have much better long-term survival than comparable patients with idiopathic (primary) pulmonary hypertension, rapid deterioration can be seen during atrial or ventricular arrhythmias or with complications such as pulmonary embolism or infection, or generally with any condition that results in even transient hypotension. Patients with Eisenmenger's syndrome also are at increased risk of developing hemoptysis, which in some cases can be life threatening.

There are also a number of complications that result from longstanding hypoxia, including significant erythrocytosis, elevated red blood cell count. Symptoms of hyperviscosity—changes in mental status, fatigue, and headache—are rare, and phlebotomy should only be performed to relieve these symptoms. Patients with Eisenmenger's syndrome often develop proteinuria and a decreased glomerular filtration rate (GFR). Because of the low GFR and the high turnover of red blood cells, uric acid levels are often elevated and can result in acute renal failure, particularly after administration of contrast dye if the patient is not adequately hydrated.

SIGNS AND SYMPTOMS

The manifestation of CHD varies significantly, according to the type of anatomic defect present. Certain signs and symptoms should prompt an extensive evaluation of adults with CHD, particularly syncope and progression in exertional dyspnea. Simple shunt lesions such as secundum atrial septal defects are often overlooked because the symptoms associated with them, fatigue and breathlessness, can be subtle and nonspecific. Physical examination findings, including a fixed, split, second heart sound (because of loss of differential effects on right- and left-sided filling pressures from a drop in intrathoracic pressure, which normally occur during inspiration) and a pulmonic outflow murmur (the result of increased pulmonary blood volume from shunting) are also commonly missed.

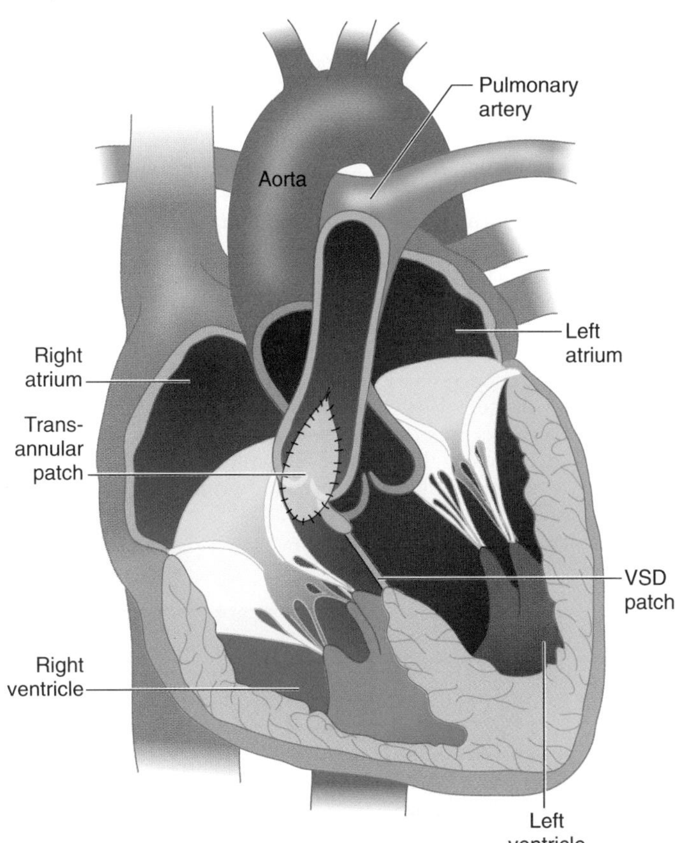

Figure 12 Definitive repair of tetralogy of Fallot. This often results in severe regurgitation of the pulmonic valve.

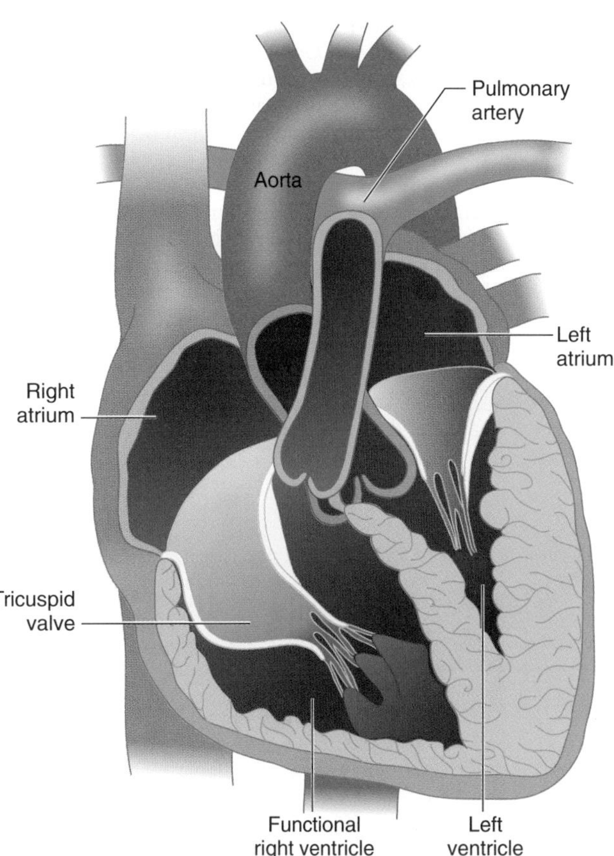

Figure 13 Ebstein's anomaly. This is the result of inferior displacement of the tricuspid valve into the right ventricle, which results in atrialization of the right ventricle.

A small VSD produces a loud systolic murmur and often a palpable thrill at the left sternal border, but patients are generally asymptomatic. Larger defects have softer murmurs, but these are more likely to manifest during childhood with signs and symptoms of congestive heart failure. Patients with PDA have a continuous murmur (systole and diastole) that is often described as a "machinery murmur." This is heard best under the left clavicle and is accompanied by a widened pulse pressure.

Patients with stenotic lesions often remain asymptomatic until significant levels of narrowing develop. In the case of right-sided lesions, fatigue and lower extremity edema develop, whereas in left-sided lesions, shortness of breath predominates, secondary to pulmonary edema. With coarctation of the aorta, patients occasionally complain of leg fatigue during exercise, indicating inadequate lower extremity perfusion caused by the severity of the stenosis and inadequacy of collateral vessels. These patients may also have evidence of a murmur that continues into diastole, as well as a significant brachial-femoral pulse delay.

Patients with L-TGA or surgically repaired D-TGA are typically asymptomatic for many years, until their systemic ventricle begins to fail. Early on, the physical examination can be unremarkable, other than mild systemic AV valve regurgitation (provided no other anatomic defects are present). Once failure ensues, the signs and symptoms are not unlike those of the typical heart failure patient. The acute onset of dizziness or fatigue should prompt a thorough workup to exclude the presence of symptomatic heart block.

In patients with TOF and prior surgical repair, significant pulmonic insufficiency may be present. Because this is low-pressure regurgitation, however, it may be barely audible on examination. In Ebstein's anomaly, on the other hand, the physical examination is usually less subtle. The large anterior leaflet of the tricuspid valve often makes a loud snapping noise described as a "sail sound," which occurs during closure of the valve. It is typically followed by a tricuspid regurgitation murmur, if present. In patients with an accompanying ASD, a fixed, split, second heart sound and pulmonic outflow murmur may also be present. As a result of this interatrial flow communication, right-to-left shunting can occur during physical exertion and lead to cyanosis and reduced exercise tolerance.

The physical examination of a patient with Eisenmenger's syndrome is notable for cyanosis, which typically worsens during exercise, and clubbing. If differential clubbing is present, usually clubbing of the feet and left arm and not the right arm, depending on the location of the PDA, the clinical diagnosis is Eisenmenger's physiology in the context of PDA. Because pulmonary and systemic pressures differ only slightly, a murmur across the shunt lesion is generally not heard in Eisenmenger's syndrome patients.

DIAGNOSIS

An organized approach is especially important in the workup of patients with CHD, and the critical first step is obtaining a complete history. Reviewing the pediatric records, if available, is essential to understand the complexities of the cardiac and vascular anatomy and to define the outcomes of previous diagnostic studies and surgeries. Surgical procedures have changed considerably over the last several decades, and anatomic presumptions based on current practice might not apply.

Early steps in assessing the adult patient with CHD include reviewing the electrocardiogram (ECG) and the chest radiograph. The ECG, by showing tall R waves in the anterior precordial leads with ST-T changes in the opposition direction to the QRS complex, can raise awareness that right ventricular pressure overload is present;

this suggests the presence of pulmonary hypertension or obstruction to right ventricular outflow. ECG might also detect the presence of high-grade heart block, as in the case of corrected transposition; this has an incidence of 1% to 2% per year. In TOF patients who have not yet undergone reoperation for pulmonic insufficiency, a measure of QRS width of more than 180 msec appears to predict a higher risk of sudden death.[4] In the case of atrial septal defect, the ECG can be useful to differentiate between different types (Table 1). The secundum defect often has an incomplete right bundle branch block (RBBB) pattern and a rightward axis, whereas the primum defect has a complete RBBB, a leftward axis, and, occasionally, a first-degree AV block. The ECG of Ebstein's patients shows very tall (Himalayan) P waves, which are a characteristic finding.

The chest radiograph can detect generalized problems, such as increased lung vascularity caused by a shunt lesion (Fig. 15) or the presence of pulmonary vascular congestion in patients with elevated left heart filling pressures. It can also detect specific problems, such as rib notching produced by collateral vessels resulting from an aortic coarctation (Fig. 16).

Echocardiography is widely available and useful in the workup of adults with CHD. Limitations of echocardiography include difficult windows caused by excessive scar tissue from previous surgeries, concomitant lung disease, and obesity. Certain lesions, such as sinus venosus ASD, which are not seen on transthoracic imaging, require transesophageal echocardiography or advanced radiographic imaging to confirm the diagnosis.

The use of computed tomography (CT) or magnetic resonance imaging (MRI) can add substantially to the anatomic description of CHD, especially in patients with unclear great vessel (Fig. 17), pulmonary vascular, or coronary anatomy (Fig. 18). The use of MRI has expanded, with more widely available scanners and simplified scanning protocols. It is important to remember, however, that CT scanning is complicated by the need for intravenous contrast, and MRI is generally not compatible with current implantable cardiac pacemakers and defibrillators.

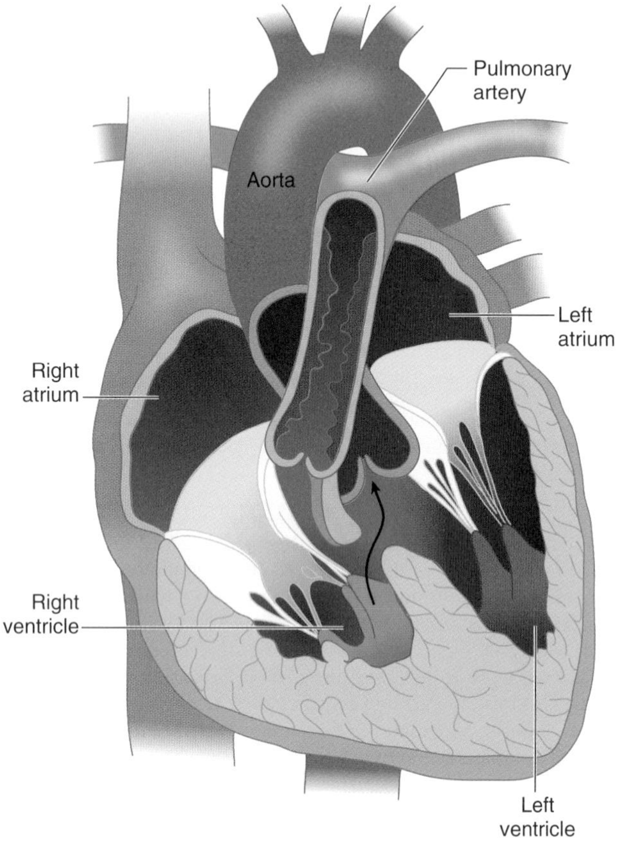

Pulmonary artery

Aorta

Left atrium

Right atrium

Right ventricle

Left ventricle

Figure 14 Eisenmenger's syndrome (ventricular septal defect). This refers to a condition in which an intracardiac shunt results in such severe pulmonary hypertension that right-sided pressures eventually exceed systemic pressures, and the intracardiac shunt is reversed (becoming right to left).

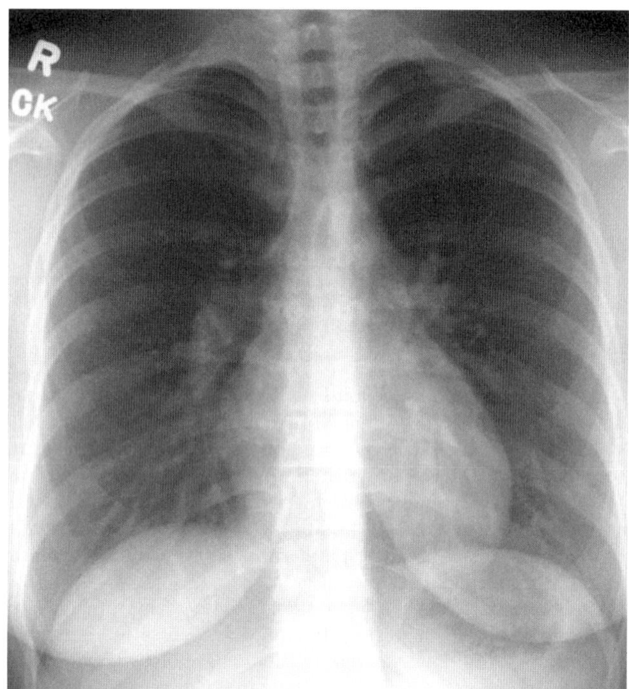

Figure 15 Chest radiograph of a 21-year-old woman with a large secundum atrial septal defect. Prominent pulmonary vascular markings are consistent with increased pulmonary arterial flow because of the shunt lesion. *(Courtesy of Dr. Richard White.)*

Table 1 Unique Features of Atrial Septal Defects

Feature	Secundum ASD	Primum ASD	Sinus Venosus ASD
Anatomic feature	Partial anomalous pulmonary venous return (only ~10%)	Mitral valve involvement; ±?VSD	Partial anomalous pulmonary venous return
Physical examination findings	Fixed split S_2; pulmonic outflow murmur	Same as secundum ASD; murmurs of MR ± VSD	Same as secundum ASD
Electrocardiographic findings	RSR′ pattern; incomplete RBBB; ±right axis	RBBB; left axis; ± 1-degree AV block	Same as secundum ASD; ± leftward-shifted P wave axis (inverted P in lead III)

ASD, atrial septal defect; AV, atrioventricular; MR, mitral regurgitation; RBBB, right bundle branch block; VSD, ventricular septal defect.

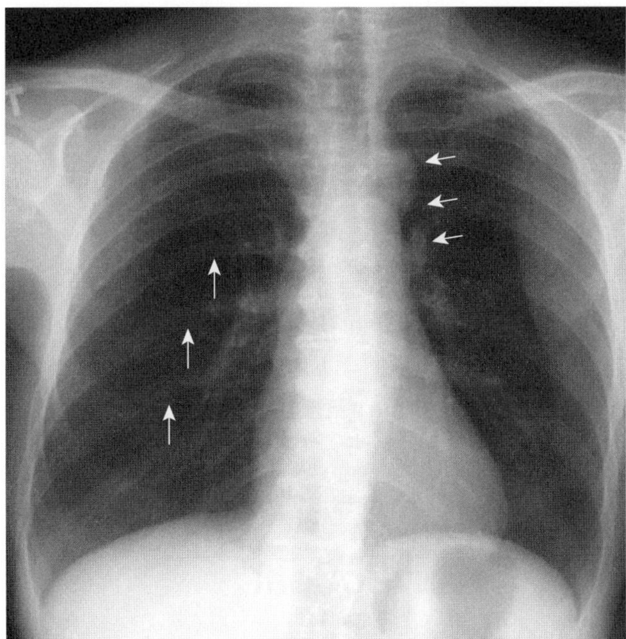

Figure 16 Chest radiograph of a 25-year-old man with unrepaired coarctation of the aorta. The number 3 sign results from the focal narrowing *(short arrows)*. Rib notching *(long arrows)* is seen on the inferior portion of the posterior ribs (ribs 3 to 9) and results from pressure erosion caused by dilated intercostal arteries that serve as collateral blood flow between the internal mammary arteries and the descending aorta. *(Courtesy of Dr. Richard White.)*

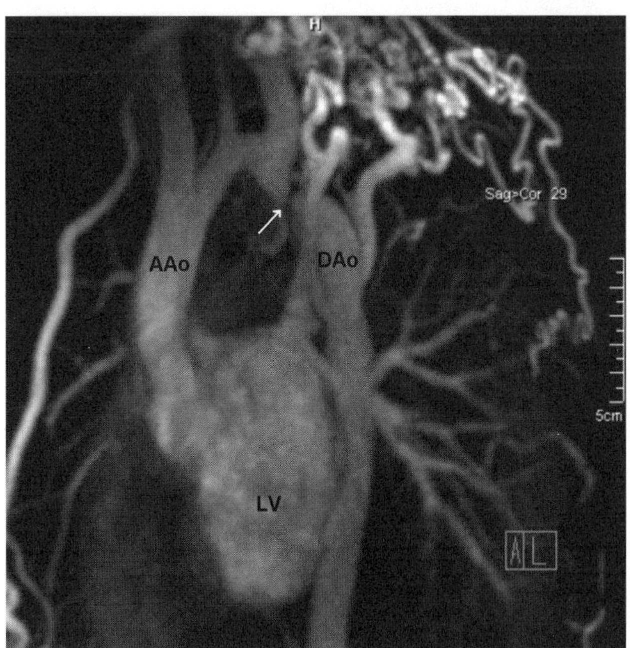

Figure 17 Magnetic resonance angiogram of the heart and great vessels in a young man with unrepaired coarctation of the aorta. There are prominent collateral vessels that drain into the descending aorta below the coarcted segment *(arrow)* and maintain lower extremity perfusion. Aao, ascending aorta; DAo, descending aorta; LV, left ventricle. *(Courtesy of Dr. Janine Arruda.)*

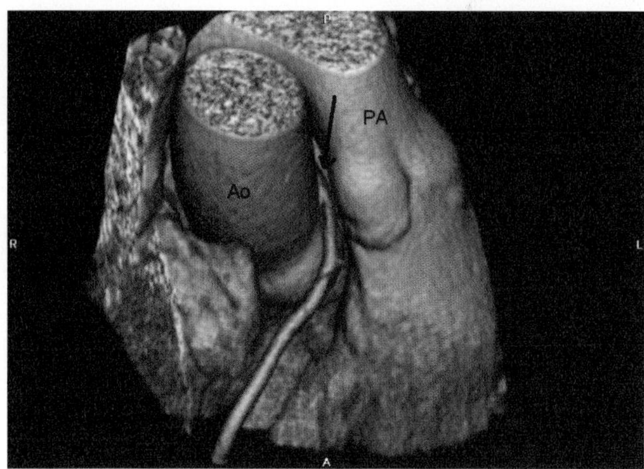

Figure 18 64-slice computer tomography scan of a 52-year-old woman with chest pain and anomalous takeoff of the right coronary artery. The takeoff *(arrow)* comes off the left coronary artery cusp and passes between the aorta (Ao) and the pulmonary artery (PA).

Diagnostic cardiac catheterization, although generally performed later in the diagnostic workup of CHD patients than in the past, remains the gold standard for pressure measurement, cardiac output calculation, and vascular resistance determination. The relative sizes of shunt lesions can be assessed using oximetry, and the hemodynamic consequences of additional blood flow can be assessed. Most importantly, cardiac catheterization affords the opportunity to intervene and palliate or repair anatomic defects or to clarify the suitability of further surgical intervention.[5]

Anatomic shunting can be quantified in the catheterization laboratory by examining the blood oxygen saturations in the respective chambers. The mixed venous (MV) saturation is the saturation of blood returning to the right atrium (RA), with contributions from the inferior vena cava (IVC), superior vena cava (SVC), and coronary sinus (CS). IVC saturation is normally higher than the SVC because of high renal blood flow and less oxygen extraction by the kidneys. The CS saturation is very low, but its volume of contribution is negligible and usually ignored. To normalize the MV saturation, three times the SVC saturation is added to the IVC saturation and the sum divided by 4.

Because so much mixing of blood with differing saturations occurs in the RA, an 11% increase in oxygen step-up (saturation increase from a chamber to its successive chamber) is required to diagnose a shunt lesion between the SVC and the RA. A 7% increase is necessary to detect a shunt between the RA and right ventricle (RV) and a 5% increase is necessary to detect a shunt between the RV and pulmonary artery (PA). A quick and simple measure of the overall size of a left-to-right shunt ratio can be obtained by using the following formula:

$$\text{Size of left-to-right shunt ratio} = (\text{aortic saturation} - \text{MV saturation})/(\text{PV saturation} - \text{PA saturation})$$

The PV saturation can be assumed to be 95% if it is not measured directly.

In general, a significant shunt is present when the shunt ratio is 1.5:1. This simplified definition may not apply to older adults, however. As pulmonary hypertension develops and RV compliance falls, a left-to-right shunt that was 3:1 for 30 years may become lower than 1.5:1 because of the gradual reversing of the shunt. In fact, the left-to-right shunt may totally reverse at some point and result in arterial desaturation (Eisenmenger's syndrome). The significance of a shunt in the adult, therefore, must be examined in the context of other hemodynamic parameters, chamber sizes, and history of the defect over time.

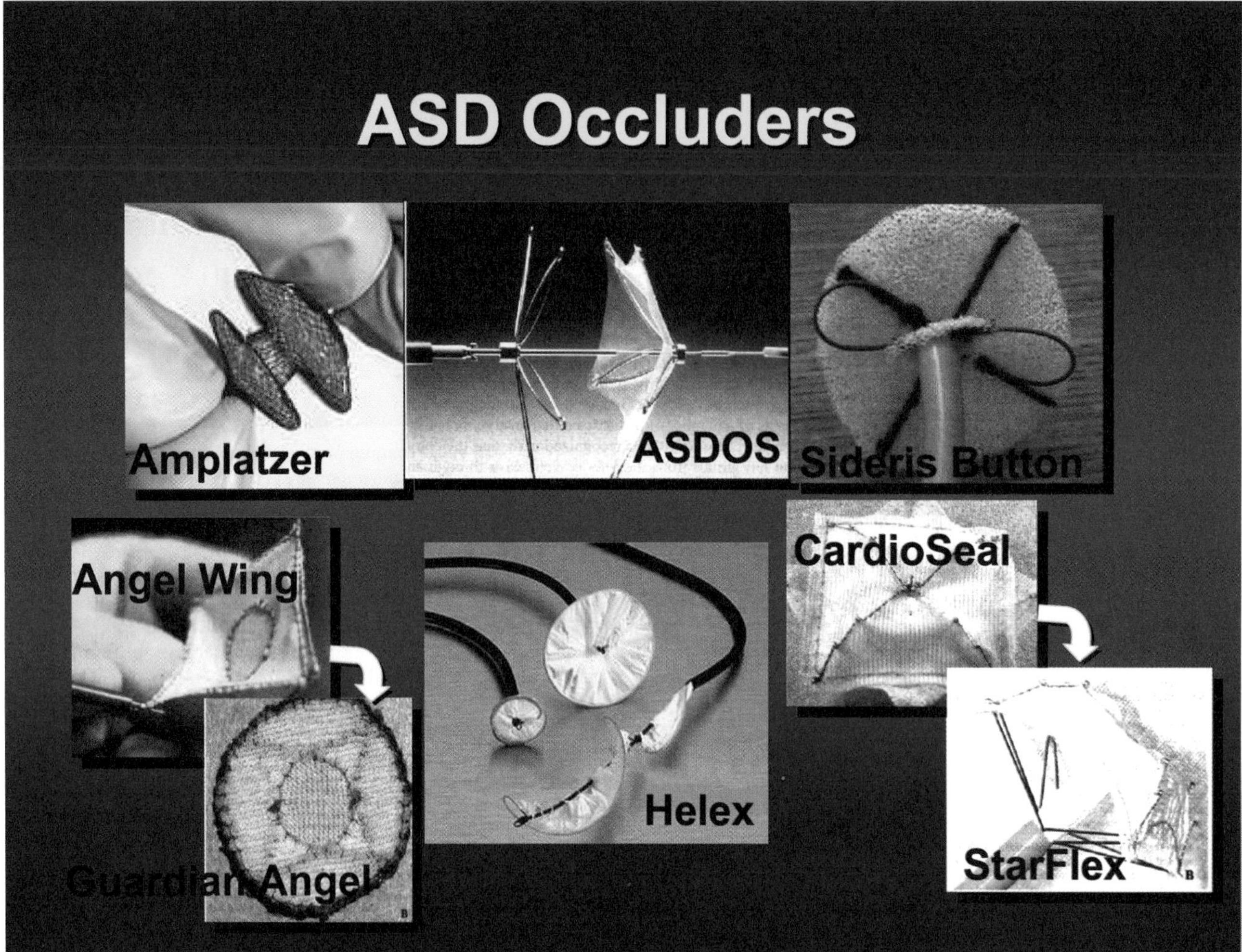

Figure 19 Devices designed to occlude atrial septal defects.

Pulmonary hypertension is a common complication of certain congenital heart diseases and can be secondary to pulmonary venous hypertension from elevated left-sided filling pressures, or it can be the result of systemic-to-pulmonary artery shunting. To help differentiate the cause of pulmonary hypertension, the pulmonary vascular resistance (PVR) can be determined at catheterization:

PVR = (mean PA pressure − mean pulmonary capillary wedge pressure [mm Hg])/(pulmonary blood flow [L/min])

A high resistance (>7 Wood units or a ratio of the pulmonary-to-systemic vascular resistance >0.5 : 1) has been associated with considerably higher perioperative mortality.[6] In addition, assessment of pulmonary vascular reactivity with endothelium-dependent vasodilators, such as inhaled nitric oxide or intravenous adenosine, may provide additional prognostic information in these patients by confirming whether the observed pulmonary hypertension has a vasoconstrictor component.[7]

TREATMENT

Adults with CHD are a unique patient population, particularly those whose CHD has been diagnosed and treated early in life. They are typically accompanied by their parents to office visits, particularly if they have other physical and mental impediments. In some cases, their knowledge and insight into their disorders may be limited and they may depend on their parents to recall their prior history. In other cases, the patient may have an encyclopedic background about the disorder and may know more about state-of-the-art management than the physician. It is always best to obtain as many prior medical records as possible to ensure a clear understanding of the condition and how it has been previously treated.

It is important to recognize that although these patients have been followed by cardiologists, many of them have not been previously instructed about risk factors for atherosclerotic disease. Metabolic syndrome—the constellation of insulin resistance, hypertension, abdominal obesity, and lipid abnormalities—appears at least as prevalent as in the general population; recent studies have shown that many of these patients are in a state of physical conditioning that is on par with that of the heart failure population.[8] In many cases, patients have been instructed to avoid certain activities or have avoided activity because of a fear of possible medical consequences. Generally, exercise should be encouraged and cardiac rehabilitation should be strongly considered.

Patients with metabolic syndrome should be instructed in more heart-healthy diets and encouraged to engage in physical activity. Patients with heart failure should also receive instruction about low-salt diets and how to detect subtle evidence of clinical decompensation before it occurs.

Unlike other areas in cardiovascular medicine, medical therapy in adults with CHD is based on limited clinical data. In general, recommendations are difficult to make and formalized guidelines are not yet available for most of the problems encountered in cyanotic heart disease and for 6 months following most surgical and percutanbous cardiac procedures.

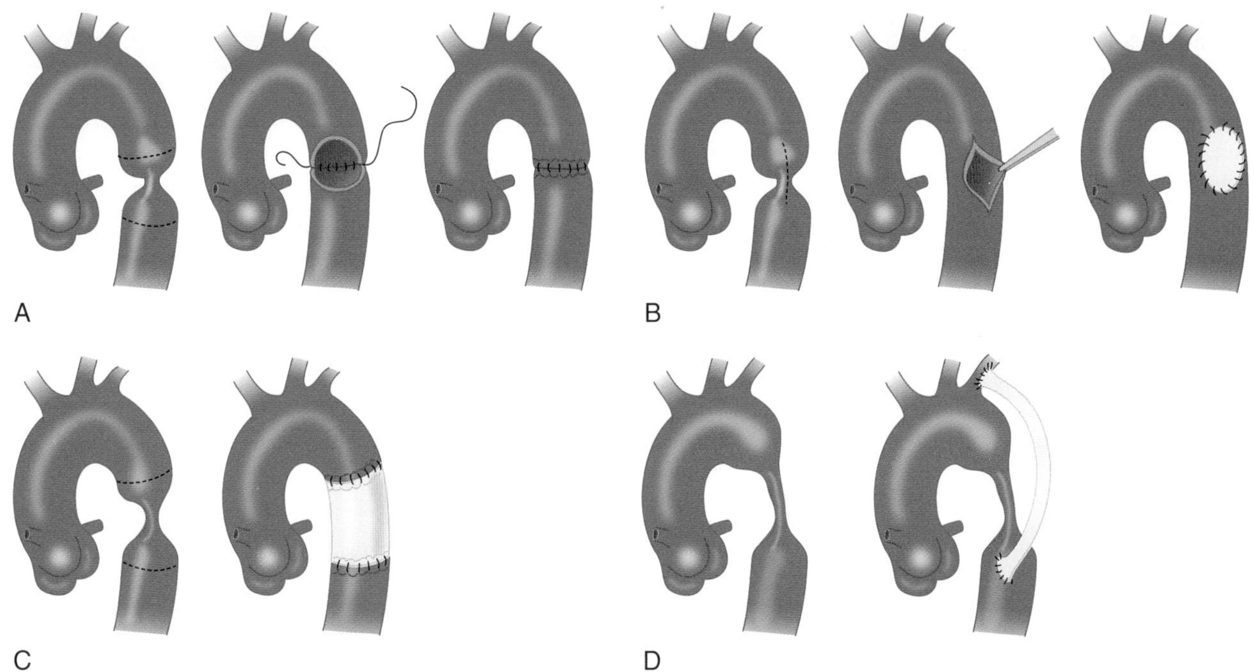

Figure 20 Most commonly used techniques for repairing aortic coarctation. **A,** Resection and end-to-end anastomosis. **B,** Prosthetic patch aortoplasty. **C,** Tube interposition bypass grafting. **D,** Subclavian to aortic bypass.

The adult with CHD and atrial fibrillation should be managed aggressively, because this rhythm can be poorly tolerated. Anticoagulation should be considered in almost all these patients, unless contraindications exist. Certain rhythms, such as atrial flutter, are usually related to scar tissue from previous surgery, and ablation therapy may be curative.[9]

In transposition patients with heart failure and a failing systemic right ventricle, the general approach has been to use commonly accepted heart failure medications: angiotensin-converting enzyme (ACE) inhibitors or angiotensin receptor blockers, beta blockers and spironolactone for possible mortality and heart remodeling benefits, and digoxin and diuretics for symptoms. One must be particularly careful with beta blockers, however, given the risk of precipitating heart block. Whether patients with systemic morphologic right ventricles without heart failure or patients with single ventricles benefit from agents such as ACE inhibitors to prevent heart failure is currently unknown.

For most other conditions, surgical or percutaneous therapy remains the mainstay of management; the details used in selecting therapy follows. Indications to repair an ASD have historically included evidence of right heart volume overload (resulting from the ASD) or the presence of a hemodynamically significant defect (classically a $\dot{Q}_P/\dot{Q}_s$ of 1.5:1). Examples of devices designed to percutaneously close atrial septal defects are illustrated in Figure 19. The timing of closure of an ASD appears important, because repair after the age of 40 years is associated with an increased incidence of arrhythmias (e.g., atrial fibrillation) compared with repair before age 40.[10] Epidemiologic evidence also suggests that long-term survival is worse if ASD is left unrepaired.

Most VSDs encountered in the adult population are small and require little more than observation. However, some experts believe that any PDA should be occluded to prevent endarteritis and to remove any excess flow from the pulmonary circuit, which could result in volume overload over time. PDAs can be ligated surgically or closed percutaneously, using device closure or coils, depending on size.

Careful tracking of the gradient in patients with pulmonic stenosis is critical for decision making. Generally, an intervention is believed to be warranted when the transvalvular gradient exceeds 50 mm Hg (moderate or greater PS), although patients with lesser gradients may benefit if it can be clearly shown that exertional symptoms, typically dyspnea, accompany elevated gradients during provocation. Percutaneous balloon valvuloplasty has proved to be safe and effective in the adult and is the therapy of choice for patients with significant stenosis.

Surgery has previously been the mainstay in the approach to a native CoA, with available options including resection and end-to-end anastomosis, prosthetic patch aortoplasty, interposition (tube bypass) grafting, and subclavian to distal aorta bypass (Fig. 20). Angioplasty and stenting is now considered the procedure of choice in patients with recoarctation following surgery and is experiencing an expanding role in primary treatment.

Surgical repair for systemic AV valve regurgitation in transposition of the great vessels is generally ineffective, and cardiac transplantation is often considered if symptoms of heart failure are severe and refractory. In select medical centers, some success has been achieved in younger patients by using a staged procedure, in which the pulmonic outflow tract is first banded to train the morphologic left ventricle to withstand systemic pressures again. The second step involves removing these bands and performing an arterial switch, with or without takedown of the atrial baffle or the creation of such a baffle.

Surgical repair of pulmonic insufficiency in repaired TOF involves implanting a pulmonic valve bioprosthesis or homograft. This is indicated if progressive decline in exercise tolerance, decrement in right ventricular function, or severe widening of the QRS complex on the ECG can be demonstrated.

Surgery in Ebstein's anomaly involves complex repair of the tricuspid valve in addition to closure of the atrial communication. It should be limited to centers with extensive experience in this area. Indications for surgery include significant cyanosis, severe tricuspid regurgitation and right heart enlargement (often defined as a cardiothoracic ratio >60%), or the development of symptomatic right heart failure.

SPECIAL POPULATIONS

Pregnancy in women with congenital heart disease has important considerations. In most cases, cardiologists with experience in managing congenital disease and specialists in high-risk obstetrics should be consulted early in the process. Usually, it is best for the patient to meet with these physicians before family planning, particularly in cases with a high risk of fetal recurrence. Any medications the prospective mother is taking need to be carefully reviewed to avoid possible teratogenicity. The two groups of women with CHD at highest risk of maternal mortality are those with severe pulmonary hypertension and those with Eisenmenger's syndrome. These patients should be counseled not to become pregnant and, if they do, may need to consider early termination.

Patients with most other lesions can be safely guided through pregnancy, although rates of fetal loss can be significantly higher. Simple shunt lesions are generally well tolerated, but filters should be placed on all IV lines at the time of delivery. Administration of antibiotics at the time of delivery also may be beneficial. Vaginal delivery is generally favored in most women with CHD. However, certain populations, such as those with high-grade obstructive lesions, may benefit from elective cesarean section to avoid prolonged Valsalva maneuvers during labor, which could lead to rapid hemodynamic deterioration.

Summary

- Excluding bicuspid aortic valve and mitral valve prolapse, there are currently over 750,000 adults with CHD.
- Simple shunt lesions (ASD, VSD, and PDA) are the most common forms of CHD and can lead to right heart chamber enlargement, pulmonary hypertension, and arrhythmias.
- Patients with repair of CHD lesions as children still require careful clinical follow-up, and often require further anatomic and electrophysiologic interventions as adults.
- Certain signs and symptoms, particularly syncope and progression in exertional dyspnea, should prompt an extensive workup in adults with CHD.
- Eisenmenger's syndrome occurs when pulmonary pressures exceed systemic pressures in patients with shunt lesions, and results in hypoxia and its sequelae.
- Therapies for CHD are individualized according to the patient's symptoms, underlying lesion(s), and degree of hemodynamic impairment.

Suggested Readings

Blömstrom-Lundqvist C, Scheinman MM, Aliot EM, et al: American College of Cardiology; American Heart Association Task Force on Practice Guidelines; European Society of Cardiology Committee for Practice Guidelines. Writing Committee to Develop Guidelines for the Management of Patients With Supraventricular Arrhythmias: ACC/AHA/ESC guidelines for the management of patients with supraventricular arrhythmias-executive summary: A report of the American College of Cardiology/American Heart Association Task Force on Practice Guidelines and the European Society of Cardiology Committee for Practice Guidelines (Writing Committee to Develop Guidelines for the Management of Patients With Supraventricular Arrhythmias). Circulation 2003;108:1871-1909.

Bush A, Busst CM, Haworth SG, et al: Correlations of lung morphology, pulmonary vascular resistance, and outcome in children with congenital heart disease. Br Heart J 1988;59:480-485.

Diller GP, Dimopoulos K, Okonko D, et al: Exercise intolerance in adult congenital heart disease: comparative severity, correlates, and prognostic implication. Circulation 2005;112:828-835.

Gatzoulis MA, Balaji S, Webber SA, et al: Risk factors for arrhythmia and sudden cardiac death late after repair of tetralogy of Fallot: A multicentre study. Lancet 2000;356:975-981.

Gatzoulis MA, Freeman MA, Siu SC, et al: Atrial arrhythmia after surgical closure of atrial septal defects in adults. N Engl J Med 1999;340:839-846.

Krasuski RA, Bashore TM: The emerging role of percutaneous intervention in adults with congenital heart disease. Rev Cardiovasc Med 2005;6:11-22.

Renforth GL, Wilson DI: Adults with congenital heart disease: A genetic perspective. In Gatzoulis MA, Webb GD, Daubeney PEF (eds): Diagnosis and Management of Adult Congenital Heart Disease. New York, Churchill Livingstone, 2003, pp 19-24.

Warnes CA, Liberthson R, Danielson GK, et al: Task Force 1: The changing profile of congenital heart disease in adult life. J Am Coll Cardiol 2001;37:1170-1175.

Weesner KM: Hemodynamic effects of prostaglandin E1 in patients with congenital heart disease and pulmonary hypertension. Cathet Cardiovasc Diagn 1991;24:10-15.

Wood P: The Eisenmenger's syndrome or pulmonary hypertension with reversed central shunt. Br Med J 1958;46:755-762.

References

For a complete list of references, log onto www.expertconsult.com.

Pregnancy and Heart Disease

Anjli Maroo and Russell Raymond

Cardiac diseases complicate 1% to 4% of pregnancies in women without preexisting cardiac abnormalities. A working knowledge of the normal physiology of pregnancy is often helpful in the management of patients with heart disease. Patients with preexisting cardiac lesions should be counseled in advance about the risk of pregnancy. Women who develop cardiac disorders during pregnancy should be followed closely and counseled about future cardiac risks. Familiarity with the treatment of commonly encountered cardiac diseases during pregnancy is becoming increasingly important for internists and cardiologists as they join the team of obstetricians and anesthesiologists in the care of these complicated patients.

NORMAL PHYSIOLOGIC CHANGES DURING PREGNANCY

Major hemodynamic changes occur during pregnancy, during labor and delivery, and in the postpartum period (Table 1). These changes begin to take place in the first 5 to 8 weeks of gestation and reach their peak late in the second trimester. In patients with preexisting cardiac disease, cardiac decompensation often coincides with this peak.

Blood volume increases 40 to 50% during normal pregnancy. The rise in blood volume is greater than the increase in red blood cell mass, contributing to the fall in hemoglobin concentration, otherwise known as the anemia of pregnancy. Similarly, cardiac output rises 30% to 50% above baseline, peaking by the end of the second trimester and reaching a plateau until delivery. The increase in cardiac output is achieved by three factors: an increase in preload due to greater blood volume, reduced afterload due to a fall in systemic vascular resistance, and a rise in the maternal heart rate by 10 to 15 beats per minute. Stroke volume increases during the first and second trimesters but declines in the third trimester due to compression of the inferior vena cava by the uterus. Blood pressure typically falls about 10 mm Hg below baseline by the end of the second trimester due to reduction in systemic vascular resistance and to addition of new blood vessels in the uterus and placenta.

During labor and delivery, hemodynamic fluctuations can be profound. Each uterine contraction displaces 300 to 500 mL of blood into the general circulation. Stroke volume increases, with a resultant rise in cardiac output by an additional 50% with each contraction. Thus, it is possible for the cardiac output during labor and delivery to be 75% above baseline. Mean arterial pressure also rises, in part due to maternal pain and anxiety. Blood loss during delivery (300-400 mL for a vaginal delivery and 500-800 mL for a cesarian section) can contribute to hemodynamic stress.

The hemodynamic changes during the postpartum state are equally dramatic. Relief of inferior vena caval compression results in an increase in venous return, which in turn augments cardiac output and causes a brisk autodiuresis. The hemodynamic changes return to the prepregnant baseline within 2 to 4 weeks following vaginal delivery and within 4 to 6 weeks after cesarean section.

These marked hemodynamic changes during pregnancy account for the development of several signs and symptoms during normal pregnancy that can mimic signs and symptoms of heart disease. Normal pregnancy is typically associated with fatigue, dyspnea, and decreased exercise capacity. Pregnant women usually have mild peripheral edema and jugular venous distension. Most pregnant women have audible physiologic systolic murmurs created by augmented blood flow. A physiologic third heart sound (S_3), reflecting increased blood volume, can sometimes be auscultated. Signs and symptoms that are abnormal during pregnancy include exertional chest pain, paroxysmal nocturnal dyspnea, orthopnea, sustained atrial or ventricular arrhythmias, pulmonary edema, severe obstructive systolic murmurs, diastolic murmurs, and an S_4 gallop.

Noninvasive testing of the heart may include an electrocardiogram, a chest radiograph, plasma Brain natriuretic peptide (BNP) testing, and an echocardiogram. The electrocardiogram may reveal a leftward shift of the electrical axis, especially during the third trimester when the diaphragm is pushed upward by the uterus. Routine chest radiographs should be avoided, especially in the first trimester. BNP is typically low during normal pregnancy (usually <20 pg/mL); elevations in BNP are a useful guide in managing early cardiac dysfunction and the hypertensive disorders of pregnancy. Echocardiography is an invaluable tool for the diagnosis and evaluation of suspected cardiac disease in the pregnant patient. Normal changes attributable to pregnancy include increased left ventricular mass and dimensions.

ASSESSMENT OF RISK IN PATIENTS WITH PREEXISTING CARDIAC DISEASE

Maternal and Fetal Outcomes

Ideally, women with known preexisting cardiac lesions should discuss the impact of their heart condition on pregnancy well in advance of their pregnancy. They should discuss contraception, the maternal and fetal risks of pregnancy, and the potential long-term maternal morbidity and mortality with their physicians. Combined input from maternal-fetal medicine specialists, the patient's obstetrician, and a cardiologist may be a great asset in managing the pregnancy.

Certain preexisting cardiac conditions carry extremely high maternal risk. Pregnancy in these patients is not advised; it is important for women with these conditions to understand the implications of pregnancy on their health. For example, women with NYHA functional class III and IV heart failure face a mortality rate upwards of 7% and a morbidity rate of more than 30% during pregnancy.

A validated cardiac risk score has been shown to predict a woman's chance of having adverse cardiac complications during pregnancy (Table 2).[1,2] Each risk factor was given a value of one point. The maternal cardiac event rates for 0, 1, and greater than 1 points are 5%, 27%, and 75%, respectively.

Specific Congenital or Acquired Cardiac Lesions

Specific congenital or acquired cardiac lesions can be classified as low, intermediate, or high risk during pregnancy (Box 1).

Low-Risk Lesions

Young women with uncomplicated secundum-type atrial septal defect (ASD) or isolated ventricular septal defect (VSD) usually tolerate pregnancy well. Patent ductus arteriosus (PDA) is not associated with additional maternal risk for cardiac complications if the

Table 1 Normal Hemodynamic Changes During Pregnancy

Hemodynamic Parameter	Change During Normal Pregnancy	Change during labor and delivery	Change during postpartum
Blood volume	↑ 40-50%	↑	↓ (autodiuresis)
Heart rate	↑ 10-15 beats/min	↑	↓
Cardiac output	↑ 30-50 %	↑ additional 50%	↓
Blood pressure	↓ 10 mm Hg	↑	↓
Stroke volume	↑ 1st and 2nd trimester; ↓ 3rd trimester	↑ (300-500 mL per contraction)	↓
Systemic vascular resistance	↓	↑	↓

Table 2 Predictors of Maternal Risk for Cardiac Complications[2]

Criteria	Example	Points*
Prior cardiac events	heart failure, transient ischemic attack, stroke before present pregnancy	1
Prior arrhythmia	symptomatic sustained tachyarrhythmia or bradyarrhythmia requiring treatment	1
NYHA III/IV *or* cyanosis		1
Valvular and outflow tract obstruction	aortic valve area <1.5 cm^2, mitral valve area <2 cm^2, or left ventricular outflow tract peak gradient > 30 mm Hg	1
Myocardial dysfunction	LVEF <40% or restrictive cardiomyopathy or hypertrophic cardiomyopathy	1

*Maternal cardiac event rate for 0,1, and >1 points is 5%, 27%, and 75%, respectively.

LVEF, left ventricular ejection fraction; NYHA, New York Heart Association.

Box 1 Maternal Cardiac Lesions and Risk of Cardiac Complications During Pregnancy

Low Risk

Atrial septal defect
Ventricular septal defect
Patent ductus arteriosus
Asymptomatic aortic stenosis with low mean gradient (<50 mm Hg) and normal LV function (EF >50%)
Aortic regurgitation with normal LV function and NYHA functional class I or II
Mitral valve prolapse (isolated or with mild to moderate mitral regurgitation and normal LV function)
Mitral regurgitation with normal LV function and NYHA class I or II
Mild to moderate mitral stenosis (mitral valve area >1.5 cm^2, mean gradient <5 mm Hg) without severe pulmonary hypertension)
Mild/moderate pulmonary stenosis
Repaired acyanotic congenital heart disease without residual cardiac dysfunction

Intermediate Risk

Large left-to-right shunt
Coarctation of the aorta
Marfan syndrome with a normal aortic root
Moderate to severe mitral stenosis
Mild to moderate aortic stenosis
Severe pulmonary stenosis

High Risk

Eisenmenger's syndrome
Severe pulmonary hypertension
Complex cyanotic heart disease (tetralogy of Fallot, Ebstein's anomaly, truncus arteriosis, transposition of the great arteries, tricuspid atresia)
Marfan syndrome with aortic root or valve involvement
Uncorrected severe aortic stenosis with or without symptoms
Uncorrected severe mitral stenosis with NYHA functional class II-IV symptoms
Aortic and/or mitral valve disease (stenosis or regurgitation) with moderate to severe LV dysfunction (EF <40%)
NYHA class III-IV symptoms associated with any valvular disease or with cardiomyopathy of any etiology
History of prior peripartum cardiomyopathy

EF, ejection fraction; LV, left ventricle; NYHA, New York Heart Association.

shunt is small to moderate and if pulmonary artery pressures are normal. Once these shunts are repaired, the risk during pregnancy is minimal. It is unusual for women with such left-to-right shunts to develop pulmonary hypertension during the childbearing years; however, the presence of pulmonary hypertension with a left-to-right shunt increases the risk of complications during pregnancy substantially.

Chronic mitral regurgitation most commonly is the result of myxomatous degeneration or rheumatic heart disease and usually is well tolerated during pregnancy. However, new-onset atrial fibrillation or severe hypertension can precipitate hemodynamic deterioration. Acute mitral regurgitation (e.g., from rupture of chordae tendineae) can produce flash pulmonary edema and life-threatening cardiac decompensation. Women with severe mitral regurgitation and signs of cardiac decompensation before pregnancy are advised to undergo operative repair before conception. If valve repair is not possible, the decision to undergo valve replacement before conception should be carefully assessed on an individual basis, taking into account the patient's age, clinical status, and plans for future childbearing. Mitral valve prolapse in isolation rarely causes any difficulties during pregnancy.

Aortic regurgitation may be encountered in women with rheumatic heart disease, a congenitally bicuspid or deformed aortic valve, infective endocarditis, or connective tissue disease. Aortic regurgitation generally is well tolerated during pregnancy. Ideally, women with severe aortic regurgitation and signs of cardiac decompensation should undergo operative repair before conception. As with the mitral valve, the decision to undergo valve replacement befoer conception requires careful consideration. Women with bicuspid aortic valves, with or without aortic regurgitation, are at increased risk for aortic dissection and should be followed carefully for signs and symptoms of this complication. Young women who are discovered to have a biscupid aortic valve should be screened for concomitant aortic coarctation.

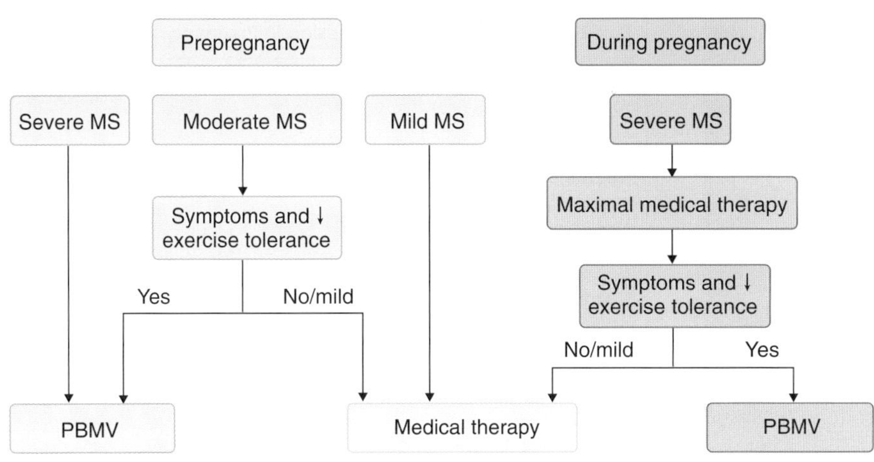

Figure 1 Management strategy for patients with mitral stenosis before and during pregnancy. Algorithm for the management of mitral stenosis in the pregnant patient. MS, mitral stenosis; PBMV, percutaneous balloon mitral valvuloplasty.

Congestive heart failure from either mitral or aortic regurgitation can be treated with digoxin, diuretics, and vasodilators such as hydralazine. Angiotensin-converting enzyme (ACE) inhibitors are teratogenic and therefore contraindicated. Beta blockers are generally safe during pregnancy, although fetal bradycardia and growth retardation have been reported.

Moderate-Risk Lesions

Mitral Stenosis

Mitral stenosis in women of childbearing age is most often rheumatic in origin. Patients with moderate to severe mitral stenosis often experience hemodynamic deterioration during the third trimester or during labor and delivery. The physiologic increase in blood volume and rise in heart rate lead to an elevation of left atrial pressure, resulting in pulmonary edema. Additional displacement of blood volume into the systemic circulation during contractions makes labor particularly hazardous.

The development of atrial fibrillation in the pregnant patient with mitral stenosis can result in rapid decompensation. Digoxin and beta blockers can be used to reduce heart rate, and diuretics can be used to gently reduce the blood volume and left atrial pressure. With atrial fibrillation and hemodynamic deterioration, electrocardioversion can be performed safely. The development of atrial fibrillation increases the risk of stroke, necessitating the initiation of anticoagulation (see “Medication Guidelines During Pregnancy,” later).

Mild mitral stenosis can often be managed with careful medical therapy during pregnancy. In contrast, patients with moderate to severe mitral stenosis should be referred to a cardiologist. Severe mitral stenosis is associated with a high likelihood of maternal complications (including pulmonary edema and arrhythmias) or fetal complications (including premature birth, low birth weight, respiratory distress, and fetal or neonatal death), approaching 80% of pregnancies.[3] These women can require correction via operative repair or replacement or via percutaneous mitral balloon valvotomy before conception. If severe mitral stenosis is discovered during pregnancy, medical therapy with diuretics and digoxin is preferred. If symptoms cannot be controlled with medical therapies, percutaneous valvotomy can be performed in the second or third trimesters to prevent fetal radiation exposure during the first trimester. Treatment options for patients with mitral stenosis are summarized in Figure 1.

Most patients with mitral stenosis can undergo vaginal delivery. However, patients with symptoms of congestive heart failure or moderate-to-severe mitral stenosis may need close hemodynamic monitoring during labor, during delivery, and for several hours into the postpartum period. In these patients, epidural anesthesia is usually better tolerated hemodynamically than general anesthesia during labor and delivery.

Aortic Stenosis

The most common etiology of aortic stenosis in women of childbearing age is a congenitally xxxx bicuspid valve. Mild to moderate aortic stenosis with preserved left ventricular function usually is well tolerated during pregnancy. Severe aortic stenosis (aortic valve area <1.0 cm^2, mean gradient >50 mm Hg), in contrast, is associated with a 10% risk of maternal morbidity (although maternal mortality is rare). Symptoms such as dyspnea, angina pectoris, or syncope usually become apparent late in the second trimester or early in the third trimester. Cardiac surgery is needed in approximately 40% of patients with severe aortic stenosis within 2.5 years of pregnancy.[4]

Women with known severe aortic stenosis should be referred to a cardiologist. Ideally, they should undergo correction of the valvular abnormality before conception. Treatment options include surgical repair, surgical valve replacement, and percutaneous balloon valvotomy. The choice of an appropriate treatment option for severe aortic stenosis before pregnancy is complicated and will likely require multiple discussions. When severe symptomatic aortic stenosis is diagnosed during pregnancy, maximal medical therapy is preferred over any intervention. However, if a patient has refractory symptoms and hemodynamic deterioration despite maximal medical therapy, percutaneous balloon valvotomy may be performed (Fig. 2). Spinal and epidural anesthesia are discouraged during labor and delivery because of their vasodilative effects. As with mitral stenosis, hemodynamic monitoring is recommended during labor and delivery.

High-Risk Lesions

The high-risk conditions listed in Box 1 are associated with increased maternal and fetal mortality. Pregnancy is not advised. If pregnancy should occur, the risk of maternal mortality and morbidity must be assessed on an individual basis. If these risks are extremely high, consideration of medical termination of pregnancy is advised to safeguard the mother’s health. If the pregnancy is continued, these patients are best managed with the assistance of a cardiologist and a maternal-fetal medicine specialist at a center with high-risk obstetrical facilities and a level three neonatal unit.

Prepregnancy Cardiovascular Risk Factors

Since the 1990s, birth rates for older women (ages 25-44 years) have increased. Older women have a higher prevalence of traditional cardiovascular risk factors, such as diabetes and chronic hypertension, and preexisting cardiovascular disease than younger women. The impact of preexisting cardiovascular risk factors on both the mother and the fetus are profound. Traditional risk factors, such as smoking, diabetes, hypertension, hyperlipidemia, and thrombophilia, are associated with increased risks of spontaneous abortion,

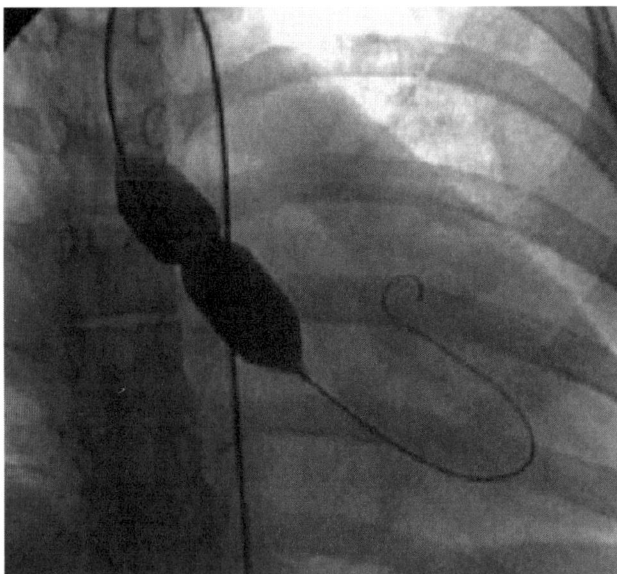

Figure 2 **Percutaneous aortic balloon valvuloplasty.** The valvuloplasty balloon is inserted across the aortic valve over a stiff wire into the left ventricle. The fluid filled balloon is inflated for a few seconds to achieve dilation of the stenotic valve.

maternal placental syndromes (see next section), preterm labor or premature rupture of membranes, and acute arterial or venous thromboses during pregnancy. Furthermore, the presence of such risk factors also predicts future development of coronary artery disease, chronic hypertension, stroke, and peripheral arterial disease in the mother.

Emerging risk factors for future cardiovascular disease in women include maternal obesity and gestational diabetes. Maternal obesity and morbid obesity are associated with increased risks for gestational hypertension, preeclampsia, gestational diabetes, and fetal birth weight of more than 4000 grams.[5] Gestational diabetes can progress to type 2 diabetes. Although the reported incidence of type 2 diabetes in women with gestational diabetes varies widely, the cumulative incidence of type 2 diabetes appears to increase markedly in the first 5 years after pregnancy.[6]

ACQUIRED CARDIOVASCULAR DISORDERS DURING PREGNANCY

Maternal Placental Syndromes

A group of disorders known collectively as *maternal placental syndromes* (MPS) have been associated with increased maternal risk of premature cardiovascular disease. In the CHAMPS (Controlled High-Risk Avonex Multiple Sclerosis Study) study, MPS were defined as the presence of preeclampsia, eclampsia, gestational hypertension, placental abruption, or placental infarction during pregnancy. MPS occurred in 7% of the 1.03 million women who were free from cardiovascular disease before pregnancy. Interestingly, traditional cardiovascular risk factors were more prevalent in women with MPS than in women without MPS. Women with MPS were two times as likely to experience a hospital admission or revascularization procedure for coronary, cerebrovascular, or peripheral vascular disease compared to women without MPS.[7] The growing body of evidence linking cardiovascular risk factors, MPS, and future cardiovascular disease might indicate an underlying abnormal vascular health that predates pregnancy and can manifest as MPS during pregnancy or chronic cardiovascular disease later in life.

Box 2 Drug Therapy of Hypertension in Pregnancy

First Line
Alpha methyldopa (PO)
Labetolol (PO)

Second Line
Hydralazine (PO)
Nifedipine (PO)
Beta blockers (PO)

Contraindicated
Angiotensin-converting enzyme inhibitors (PO)
Angiotensin-receptor blockers (PO)
Aldosterone antagonists (PO)

Avoid
Thiazide diuretics

Severe Hypertensive Urgency or Emergency First Line
Labetolol (IV)
Hydralazine (IV)
Beta blockers (IV)
Nifedipine (PO)

Hypertension in Pregnancy

Hypertension during pregnancy is defined as a systolic pressure ≥140 mm Hg or a diastolic pressure ≥90 mm Hg, or both. Hypertension during pregnancy can be classified into three main categories: chronic hypertension, gestational hypertension, and preeclampsia, with or without preexisting hypertension. In general, hypertensive disorders can complicate 12% to 22% of pregnancies and are a major cause of maternal morbidity and mortality.

Chronic hypertension is defined as blood pressure ≥140/90 mm Hg present before pregnancy, before the 20th week of gestation, or persisting beyond the 42nd postpartum day. Often, women with chronic hypertension must change their medical regimens when they anticipate pregnancy so as to maximize the safety of the growing fetus. Women of childbearing age who take chronic antihypertensive medications should be counseled about the safety of their medications in the event of pregnancy well in advance of a potential pregnancy. Most notably, women who are treated with ACE inhibitors should be made aware of the potential teratogenic effects. Women who become pregnant while taking ACE-inhibitor therapy should discontinue the medication and see their physician for alternative antihypertensive therapies that are safe during pregnancy. Women with chronic hypertension have an increased risk for development of preeclampsia. They should be made aware of the signs and symptoms of preeclampsia and should be instructed in the maintenance of a home blood pressure log. Options for drug therapy during pregnancy are shown in Box 2.

Gestational hypertension is defined as hypertension that develops in the latter part of pregnancy, is not associated with proteinuria or other features of preeclampsia, and resolves by 12 weeks postpartum. This condition is also known as *pregnancy-induced hypertension.* Although it resolves after delivery, women with this condition may be at risk for developing hypertension or cardiovascular disease in the future. They should undergo a physical examination and screening for traditional risk factors for cardiovascular disease annually after their pregnancy.

Preeclampsia, also known as toxemia, occurs in 3% to 8% of pregnancies in the United States. The classic clinical triad involves accelerating hypertension, proteinuria (>300 mg/24 hr), and edema. Symptoms usually begin in the third trimester. BNP can be a useful marker in women with preeclampsia. During normal pregnancy, BNP remains low throughout pregnancy, despite volume overload. In both mild and severe preeclampsia, elevation of BNP can precede other laboratory abnormalities, such as platelet counts and liver function test abnormalities. Although definitive treatment includes delivery of the baby, many women with preeclampsia require treatment with antihypertensive medications before delivery and for some period of time after. Typical antihypertensive medications used to treat preeclampsia include labetolol or hydralazine. Hypertensive urgency due to preeclampsia can be treated with intravenous labetolol or hydralazine. The etiology of preeclampsia is still unclear. Eclampsia is the development of grand mal seizures in a woman with preeclampsia. Both preeclampsia and eclampsia have been linked to future development of cardiovascular disease. As with pregnancy-induced hypertension, women with preeclampsia or eclampsia should undergo a physical examination and screening for traditional risk factors for cardiovascular disease annually after their pregnancy.

Peripartum Cardiomyopathy

Peripartum cardiomyopathy (PPCM) is defined as the development of idiopathic left ventricular systolic dysfunction (demonstrated by echocardiography) in the interval between the last month of pregnancy up to the first 5 months postpartum in women without preexisting cardiac dysfunction. The incidence of PPCM in the United States is estimated to be 1 in 3000 to 1 in 4000 live births. The exact etiology of PPCM is unknown, although viral myocarditis, automimmune phenomena, and specific genetic mutations that ultimately affect the formation of prolactin have been proposed as possible causes.[8]

Although it was believed that women who develop PPCM rarely have symptoms before 36 weeks' gestation, Elkayam and colleagues recently described an earlier presentation, with symptoms occurring as early as the 17th week of gestation.[9] The clinical presentation and outcome of women who developed the early-presentation pregnancy-associated cardiomyopathy was similar to that of women with traditional PPCM. Women with preexisting cardiac dysfunction usually experience cardiac deterioration during the end of the second trimester. Typical signs and symptoms include fatigue, dyspnea on exertion, orthopnea, nonspecific chest pain, peripheral edema, and abdominal discomfort and distension.

Medical therapy for PPCM may be initiated during pregnancy and continue after delivery. Attention to the safety profiles of drug therapies during pregnancy, the postpartum period, and breastfeeding is important. Digoxin, diuretics, and hydralazine may be used safely during pregnancy and while breast-feeding. Beta blockers can improve left ventricular function in patients with cardiomyopathy. Beta blockers are considered safe during pregnancy, although there have been case reports of fetal bradycardia and growth retardation. ACE inhibitors, angiotensin-receptor blockers, and aldosterone antagonists are contraindicated during pregnancy. Most ACE inhibitors can be initiated during the postpartum period, even in women who breast-feed. Anticoagulation can be considered in select patients with severe left ventricular dilatation and dysfunction. As with other etiologies of dilated cardiomyopathy, when conventional medical therapy is not successful, women with PPCM can require intensive intravenous therapy, mechanical assist devices, or even cardiac transplantation. Cardiac transplantation is required in about 4% of women with PPCM.

More than half of women with PPCM completely recover normal heart size and function, usually within 6 months of delivery. Complete recovery is more likely in women with a left ventricular ejection fraction greater than 30% at diagnosis.[9,10] The remainder either experience persistent stable left ventricular dysfunction or continue to experience clinical deterioration. Maternal mortality is approximately 9%. Women with PPCM and persistent left ventricular dysfunction who attempt subsequent pregnancy face a high risk of maternal morbidity and mortality.[10] These women should be counseled against subsequent pregnancies.

Coronary Artery Disease

Acute myocardial infarction (AMI) during pregnancy is rare, occurring in approximately 1 in 35,000 pregnancies. Independent predictors of AMI during pregnancy include chronic hypertension, maternal age, diabetes, and preeclampsia. Most myocardial infarctions occur during the third trimester in women older than 33 years who have had multiple prior pregnancies. Coronary spasm, in situ coronary thrombosis, and coronary dissection occur more often than classic obstructive atherosclerosis. Coronary dissections are thought to result from softening of the media of the artery wall. Coronary dissections in pregnant or postpartum women most commonly affect the left main trunk or the left anterior descending artery. Dissections have been successfully treated medically, with coronary stenting, and with coronary artery bypass graft surgery. Maternal mortality is highest in the antepartum and intrapartum periods. Recent studies have found a 5% to 7% case-fatality rate in women with pregnancy-associated AMI, which might reflect improvements in diagnosis and therapy since the turn of the 21st century.[11]

Medical therapy for AMI must be modified in the pregnant patient. Although thrombolytic agents increase the risk of maternal hemorrhage substantially (8%), their use is permitted in situations where cardiac catheterization facilities are not available. Low-dose aspirin and nitrates are considered safe. Beta blockers are generally safe. Short-term heparin administration has not been associated with increased maternal or fetal adverse effects. ACE inhibitors and statins are contraindicated during pregnancy. Clopidogrel and glycoprotein IIb/IIIa receptor inhibitors have been used safely in individual pregnant patients. Percutaneous coronary intervention with either balloon angioplasty or stenting has been successfully performed in pregnant patients with AMI (using lead shielding to protect the fetus).[12]

Arrhythmias in Pregnancy

Premature atrial or ventricular complexes are the most common arrhythmias during pregnancy. They are not associated with adverse maternal or fetal outcomes per se and do not require antiarrhythmic therapy.

Supraventricular Tachycardia

Supraventricular tachyarrhythmia (SVT) is also common and is often diagnosed with the aid of an event monitor or a Holter monitor. Patients with documented SVT should be instructed on performance of vagal maneuvers. In addition, beta blockers or digoxin, or both, can be useful in controlling the ventricular rate. Adenosine and direct-current cardioversion are both safe during pregnancy and can be used to treat SVT.

Patients with SVT during pregnancy should be observed after delivery. If the frequency of SVT episodes decreases over several months after delivery, the arrhythmia can be managed medically. If SVT continues to occur frequently and with rapid rates, it may be best treated with electrophysiologic ablation.

Atrial fibrillation

De novo atrial fibrillation and atrial flutter are rare during pregnancy. However, women with a history of prepregnancy tachyarrhythmias have a high likelihood of recurrence during pregnancy. Recurrent tachyarrhythmias during pregnancy are associated with an increased risk of adverse fetal complications, including premature birth, low birth weight, respiratory distress syndrome, and death.[13] Rate control of atrial fibrillation and flutter is similar to treatment of SVT. Direct-current cardioversion can be performed safely during any stage of pregnancy. Other arrhythmias should be managed with the assistance of a cardiologist.

Table 3 Cardiovascular Drugs Used During Pregnancy

Drug	Use	Potential Side Effects	Safe During Pregnancy	Safe During Breast-Feeding
Adenosine	Arrhythmia	None reported	Yes	No data
Beta blockers	Hypertension, arrhythmias, MI, ischemia, HCM, hyperthyroidism, mitral stenosis, Marfan syndrome, cardiomyopathy	Fetal bradycardia, low birth weight, hypoglycemia, respiratory depression; prolonged labor	Yes	Yes
Digoxin	Arrhythmia, CHF	Low birth weight, prematurity	Yes	Yes
Diuretics	Hypertension, CHF	Reduced utero-placental perfusion	Yes	Yes
Lidocaine	Arrhythmia, anesthesia	Neonatal CNS depression	Yes	Yes
Low molecular weight heparin	Mechanical valve, hypercoagulable state, DVT, AF, Eisenmenger syndrome	Hemorrhage, unclear effects on maternal bone mineral density	Limited data	Limited data
Nitrates	Hypertension	Fetal distress with maternal hypotension	Yes	No data
Procainamide	Arrhythmia	None reported	Yes	Yes
Unfractionated Heparin	Mechanical valve, hypercoagulable state, DVT, AF, Eisenmenger syndrome	Maternal osteoporosis, hemorrhage, thrombocytopenia, thrombosis,	Yes	Yes
Warfarin	Mechanical valve, hypercoagulable state, DVT, AF, Eisenmenger syndrome	Warfarin embryopathy, fetal CNS abnormalities, hemorrhage	Yes, after the 12th week of gestation	Yes

AF, atrial fibrillation; CHF, congestive heart failure; CNS, central nervous system; DVT, deep vein thrombosis; HCM, hypertrophic cardiomyopathy; MI, myocardial infarction.

Adapted from Elkayam, U. Pregnancy and cardiovascular disease. In: Heart Disease. A Textbook of Cardiovascular Medicine, 6th ed, Braunwald, E, (Ed), WB Saunders, Philadelphia, PA 2001. p. 2184.

Fetal Tachycardia

Fetal tachycardia is a special type of arrhythmia during pregnancy. Fetal tachycardia complicates about 0.5% of all pregnancies and is a significant cause of fetal morbidity and mortality, including fetal congestive heart failure, hydrops fetalis, and fetal demise. Fetal tachycardias include fetal SVT, fetal atrial flutter, and fetal ectopic atrial tachycardia. Fetal echocardiography, using M-mode and pulsed wave Doppler ultrasound, is extremely useful in diagnosing fetal arrhythmias.

Management depends on the fetal condition and gestational age. Therapy includes transplacental therapy, direct fetal therapy, or early delivery and neonatal therapy. Digoxin is the initial drug of choice for transplacental therapy. It can also be delivered via direct fetal injection. Other antiarrhythmic medications that can be used transplacentally include flecainide, sotalol, and amiodraone. It is usually necessary to use higher doses of digoxin and other antiarrhythmic medications in pregnant women due to the increased blood volume and high glomerular filtration rates. These medications require maternal cardiac monitoring during administration.

MEDICATION GUIDELINES DURING PREGNANCY

Cardiovascular Drugs in Pregnancy

Commonly used cardiovascular drug classes and their potential adverse effects during pregnancy are shown in Table 3. For drugs used to treat hypertension, see Box 2.

Antibiotic Prophylaxis

The American Heart Association no longer recommends antibiotic prophylaxis for the preventing bacterial endocarditis during genitourinary procedures, including vaginal delivery and cesarean section, including in high-risk patients.

Anticoagulation

Several conditions require the initiation or the maintenance of anticoagulation during pregnancy, including mechanical valves, certain prothrombotic conditions, prior episode of venous thromboembolism, acute deep venous thrombosis or thromboembolism during pregnancy, antiphospholipid antibody syndrome, and atrial fibrillation. The three most common agents considered for use during pregnancy are unfractionated heparin (UFH), low-molecular-weight heparin (LMWH), and warfarin.

The Seventh American College of Chest Physicians (ACCP) Consensus Conference on Antithrombotic Therapy has recommended three potential strategies for anticoagulation during pregnancy (Fig. 3).[14] In women with venous thromboembolism, LMWH has become the anticoagulant of choice. In women with mechanical heart valves, data are more limited and there has been some concern regarding the efficacy of heparins with respect to preventing valve thrombosis. In these patients, the maternal and fetal risks and benefits must be carefully explained before choosing one of the aforementioned three strategies. When an UFH or LMWH strategy is selected, careful dose monitoring and adjustment is recommended.

Warfarin freely crosses the placental barrier and can harm the fetus. Warfarin is safe during breast-feeding. The incidence of warfarin embryopathy (abnormalities of fetal bone and cartilage formation) has been estimated at 4% to 10%; the risk is highest when warfarin is administered during the sixth through the 12th weeks of gestation. When administered during the second and third trimesters, warfarin has been associated with fetal central nervous system abnormalities. The risk of warfarin embryopathy

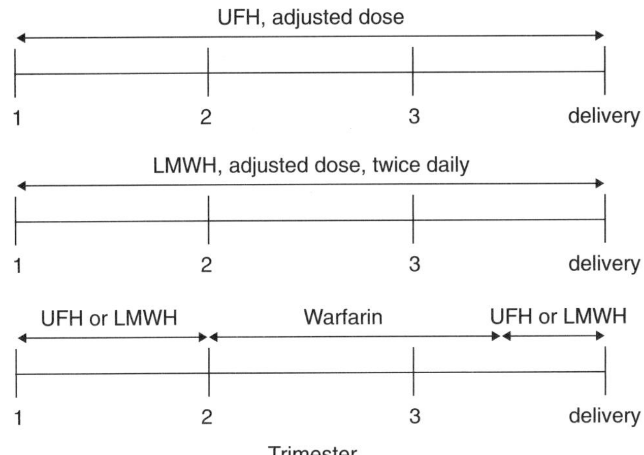

Figure 3 Anticoagulation options during pregnancy. UFH, unfractionated heparin; LMWH, low-molecular-weight heparin.

may be lower in patients who take 5 mg of warfarin or less per day.

Unfractionated heparin (UFH) does not cross the placenta and is considered safer for the fetus. Its use, however, has been associated with maternal osteoporosis; hemorrhage, thrombocytopenia or thrombosis (HITT syndrome); and a high incidence of thromboembolic events with older-generation mechanical valves. UFH may be administered parenterally or subcutaneously throughout pregnancy; when used subcutaneously for anticoagulation of mechanical heart valves, the recommended starting dose is 17,500 to 20,000 units twice daily. The appropriate dose adjustment of UFH is based on an activated partial thromboplastin time (aPTT) of 2.0 to 3.0 times the control level. High doses of UFH are often required to achieve the goal aPTT due to the hypercoagulable state associated with pregnancy. Lower doses of UFH may be appropriate for anticoagulation in situations such as prevention of venous thromboembolism during pregnancy. Parenteral infusions should be stopped 4 hours before cesarean sections. UFH can be reversed with protamine sulfate.

Low molecular weight heparin (LMWH) produces a more predictable anticoagulant response than UFH and is less likely to cause HITT. Its effect on maternal bone mineral density appears to be minimal. LMWH can be administered subcutaneously and dosed to achieve an anti-Xa level of 1.0 to 1.2 U/mL 4 to 6 hours after injection. There are data to support the use of LMWH in pregnant women with deep venous thrombosis, but data on the safety and efficacy of LMWH in pregnant patients with mechanical valve prostheses are limited. Experience with these agents is accruing.

In summary, anticoagulation in the pregnant patient can be difficult because of the risk profile associated with each drug regimen. In planned pregnancies, a careful discussion about the risks and benefits of warfarin, UFH, and LMWH will help the patient and physician choose an anticoagulation strategy. Unplanned pregnancies are often diagnosed partway through the first trimester. It is advisable to stop warfarin when the pregnancy is discovered and to use UFH or LMWH at least until after the 12th week. Dosing regimens for warfarin, UFH, and LMWH may vary by diagnosis; detailed dosing guidelines have been published.[14]

Summary

Heart disease during pregnancy encompasses a wide spectrum of disorders. Basic concepts to keep in mind include:

- Blood volume and cardiac output rise during normal pregnancy, reaching a peak during the late second trimester.
- Preexisting cardiac lesions should be evaluated with respect to the risk they impart during the stress of pregnancy.
- Contraindications to pregnancy include severe pulmonary hypertension or Eisenmenger's syndrome, cardiomyopathy with NYHA class III or IV symptoms, history of peripartum cardiomyopathy, severe uncorrected valvular stenosis, unrepaired cyanotic congenital heart disease, and Marfan syndrome with an abnormal aorta.
- Awareness of major cardiac drug classes that are contraindicated during pregnancy is important for the treatment of hypertension and heart failure during pregnancy.
- Anticoagulation during pregnancy presents unique challenges because of maternal and fetal side effects of warfarin, unfractionated heparin, and LMWH.

Suggested Readings

Bates S, Greer IA, Ginsberg JS, et al: Use of antithrombotic agents during pregnancy. Chest 2004; 126:627S-644S.

Dwyer BK, Taylor L, Fuller A, et al: Percutaneous transluminal angioplasty and stent placement during pregnancy. Obstet Gynecol 2005;106:1162-1164.

Elkayam U, Tummala PP, Rao K, et al: Maternal and fetal outcomes of subsequent pregnancies in women with peripartum cardiomyopathy. N Engl J Med 2001;344:1567.

Hilfiker-Kleiner D, Kaminski K, Podewski E, et al: A Cathepsin-D Cleaved 16 kD form of prolactin mediates postpartum cardiomyopathy. Cell 2007;128:589-600.

James AH, Jamison MG, Biswas MS, et al: Acute myocardial infarction in pregnancy: A United States population-based study. Circulation 2006;113:1564-1571.

Ray JG, Vermeulen MJ, Schull MJ, et al: Cardiovascular health after maternal placental syndromes (CHAMPS): A population-based retrospective cohort study. Lancet 2005;366:1797-1803.

Silversides CK, Harris L, Haberer K, et al: Recurrence rates of arrhythmias during pregnancy in women with previous tachyarrhythmia and impact on fetal and neonatal outcomes. Am J Cardiol 2006;97:1206-1212.

References

For a complete list of references, log onto www.expertconsult.com.

Section 3

DERMATOLOGY

Dermatologic Signs of Systemic Disease

Lisa M. Grandinetti and Kenneth J. Tomecki

COMMON CUTANEOUS DISORDERS

Seborrheic Dermatitis

Seborrheic dermatitis (Fig. 1) is a common chronic, superficial inflammatory disease of the scalp, face (especially the eyebrows and nasolabial folds), ears, and central chest, affecting 2% to 5% of the population. Clinically, the disease is characterized by thin erythematous plaques, often with a fine, greasy scale. Pruritus is common and can be severe.

Recognition of seborrheic dermatitis is important for the primary care physician, because it may be associated with systemic disease, such as Parkinson's disease and human immunodeficiency virus (HIV) infection. Patients who have had a cerebrovascular accident (CVA) can develop seborrheic dermatitis on the scalp in a unilateral distribution, corresponding to the affected hemisphere. The pathophysiology of this phenomenon is not completely understood.

Differential diagnosis includes psoriasis, atopic dermatitis, allergic or irritant contact dermatitis, and dermatophyte (tinea) infections.

Treatment includes medicated shampoos containing zinc pyrithione, selenium sulfide, salicylic acid, coal tar, or ketoconazole in combination with topical corticosteroids. Alternatively, fluconazole 400 mg (one dose) may be effective in combination with a mild topical corticosteroid.

Seborrheic Keratoses

Seborrheic keratoses (Fig. 2), the most common benign cutaneous neoplasms, are warty, age-related hyperkeratotic papules and plaques that appear anywhere on the body, most commonly the trunk. Rarely, seborrheic keratoses indicate an underlying adenocarcinoma of the gastrointestinal tract if they appear suddenly in great numbers (sign of Leser-Trélat).

Differential diagnosis includes verruca vulgaris (warts), epidermal nevus, melanocytic nevi, and melanoma.

No treatment is necessary. If the plaques are pruritic, they can removed by curettage or cryotherapy.

Urticaria

Urticaria (Fig. 3), or hives, is most often caused by medication (commonly penicillin or other antibiotics, sulfa drugs, aspirin) or food (shellfish, nuts, chocolate), and less often by infection. Hives are pruritic, edematous, evanescent wheals that resolve within 24 hours.

Acute urticaria typically lasts less than 6 weeks. Wheals in a fixed location for more than 24 hours suggest the possibility of urticarial vasculitis and warrant a skin biopsy. Chronic idiopathic urticaria for which no trigger can be identified often requires further testing such as serum radioallergosorbent testing (RAST) or skin prick-patch testing.

Differential diagnosis includes erythema multiforme, systemic lupus erythematosus (SLE), bullous pemphigoid, mastocytosis.

Treatment includes elimination of known causes, antihistamines (H_1 and H_2 blockers), oral corticosteroids for acute flares, and, in refractory cases, immunosuppresants such as sulfasalazine and cyclosporine.

Erythema Multiforme

Erythema multiforme (Fig. 4), a cutaneous hypersensitivity reaction, is usually caused by infection (herpes simplex virus or *Mycoplasma pneumoniae*) and less commonly by drug sensitivity (sulfonamides, barbiturates, antibiotics). Division of erythema multiforme into two subsets based on clinical severity has been proposed: erythema multiforme minor and erythema multiforme major or Stevens-Johnson syndrome.[1] Macules, papules, plaques, vesicles, or bullae, often with a targetoid or iris appearance, occur on the skin, often with an acral distribution (extremities). Erythema multiforme can also occur on mucosal surfaces. Prodromal symptoms are uncommon. Erythema multiforme minor is self limited and usually resolves within 2 to 4 weeks.[1]

Differential diagnosis includes urticaria, bullous arthropod reaction, drug eruption, and bullous pemphigoid.

Treatment includes suppressive oral antiviral agents such as acyclovir or valacyclovir, for herpes infection; discontinuation of possible causative medications; and supportive care.

Vitiligo

Vitiligo (Fig. 5) is characterized by a focal or generalized distribution of depigmented macules and patches. The hairs in the vitiliginous areas are usually white. Vitiligo commonly occurs in periorificial areas (mouth, orbits, vagina, anus) or at sites of trauma (hands, elbows, knees). The disorder is often associated with autoimmune thyroid disease, insulin-dependent diabetes mellitus, pernicious anemia, or Addison's disease.

Differential diagnosis includes tinea versicolor, pityriasis alba, postinflammatory hypopigmentation, and hypopigmented mycosis fungoides.

Treatment includes broad-spectrum sunscreens, potent topical corticosteroids, topical calcineurin inhibitors (tacrolimus or pimecrolimus), narrow band ultraviolet (UV) B phototherapy, psoralen with UVA (PUVA) therapy, or total depigmentation for extensive disease.

Erythema Nodosum

Erythema nodosum (Fig. 6), the most common type of panniculitis, is characterized by painful, erythematous nodules on the shins and occasionally elsewhere. Erythema nodosum occurs most commonly in young women, with a peak incidence between 20 and 40 years.[1] In addition to the cutaneous findings, patients can have fever, malaise, arthralgias, or arthritis. Typically the eruption is self limited, lasting an average of 3 to 6 weeks.[1]

The most common cause of erythema nodosum in the pediatric population is streptococcal pharyngitis. Other infectious causes include tuberculosis, gastrointestinal (GI) infections with *Yersinia, Salmonella,* or *Shigella,* and systemic fungal infections. Less common causes include drug sensitivity (sulfonamides, salicylates, iodides, oral contraceptives or hormone replacement therapy), and a variety of systemic diseases, most often inflammatory bowel disease (Crohn's disease more than ulcerative colitis) and sarcoidosis.

Differential diagnosis includes nodular vasculitis and other types of panniculitis.

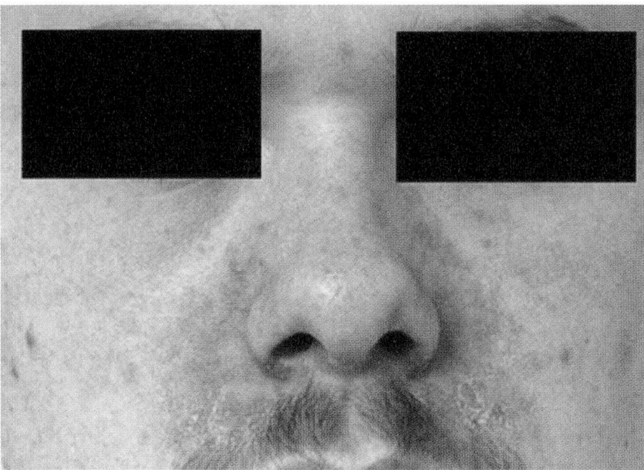

Figure 1 Seborrheic dermatitis along the nasolabial folds in a young man.

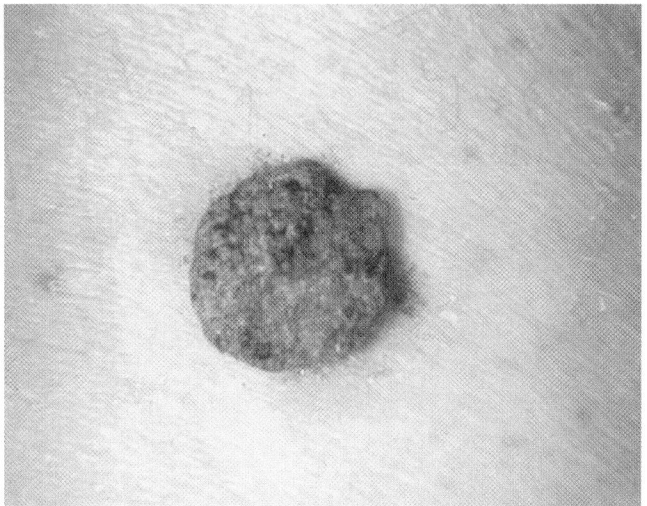

Figure 2 Seborrheic keratosis on the abdomen of an elderly man.

Treatment includes identifying and eliminating known causes, bed rest and elevation of the extremities, aspirin or nonsteroidal anti-inflammatory medications (NSAIDs), colchicine, and supersaturated potassium iodide.

BLISTERING DISEASES

Pemphigus Vulgaris

Pemphigus vulgaris (Fig. 7) is an uncommon chronic and debilitating blistering disease characterized by painful mucosal erosions and flaccid blisters that become erosive. Ninety percent of patients have mucosal disease, and erosions can outnumber intact bullae. Biopsy reveals characteristic suprabasilar acantholysis and intraepidermal bullae formation. Direct immunofluorescence reveals a chicken-wire pattern of deposition of immunoglobulin (Ig) G within the epidermis.

Pemphigus vulgaris can develop at any age, but it most commonly occurs in the fourth to sixth decades of life, usually in people of Mediterranean or Jewish ancestry.[2] Morbidity and mortality are significant, even with treatment.

Differential diagnosis includes bullous pemphigoid, Stevens-Johnson syndrome, and epidermolysis bullosa acquisita.

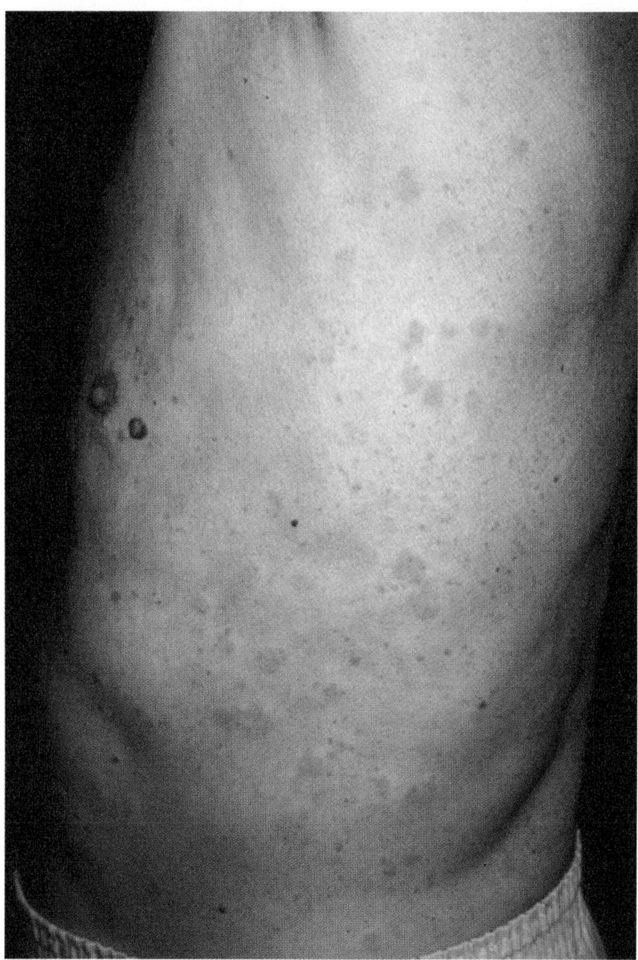

Figure 3 Urticaria on the flank.

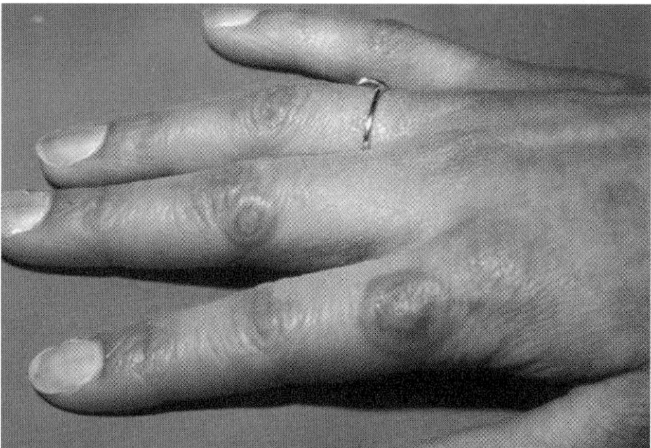

Figure 4 Targetoid plaques on the dorsal surface of the fingers.

Treatment includes good wound care for affected skin, systemic corticosteroids, various steroid-sparing immunosuppressants, rituximab, intravenous immunoglobulin (IVIg), and plasmapheresis.

Bullous Pemphigoid

Bullous pemphigoid (Fig. 8) is the most common bullous disease and is characterized by large, tense subepidermal blisters, which are

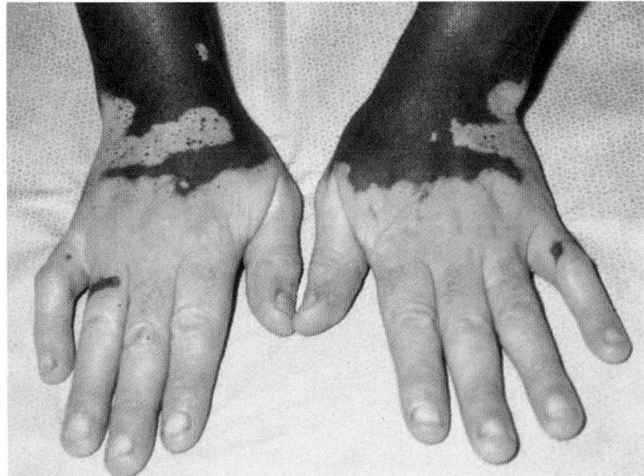

Figure 5 **Vitiligo on the hands.**

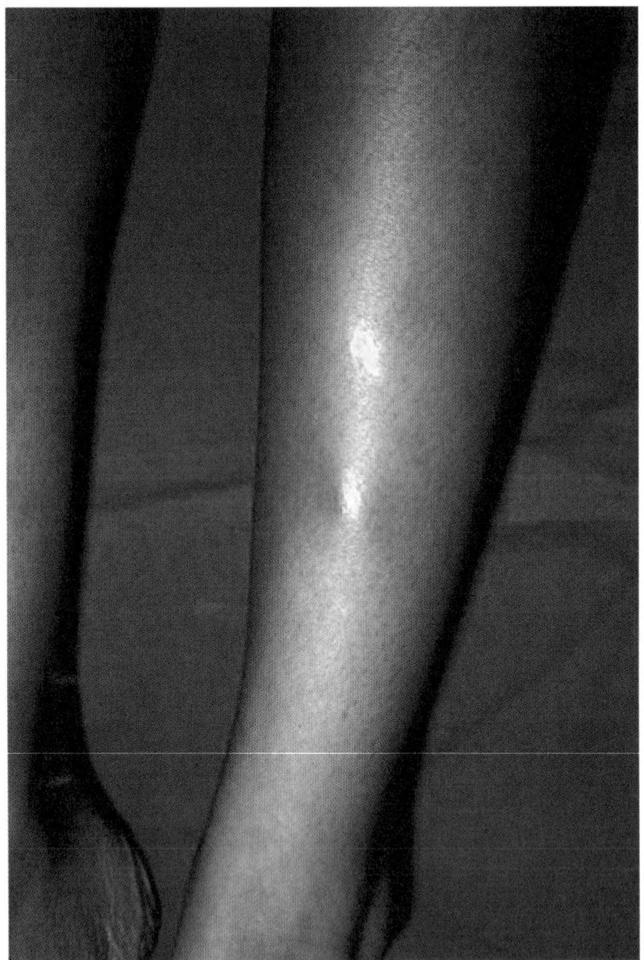

Figure 6 **Erythema nodosum on the leg of a young woman.**

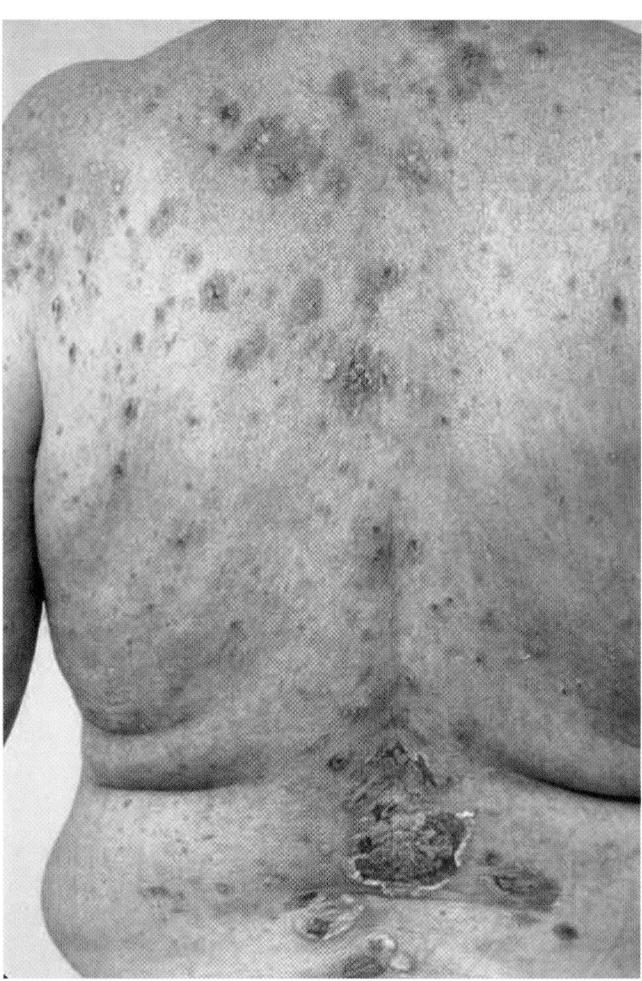

Figure 7 **Eroded bullae on the back of an elderly man with pemphigus vulgaris.**

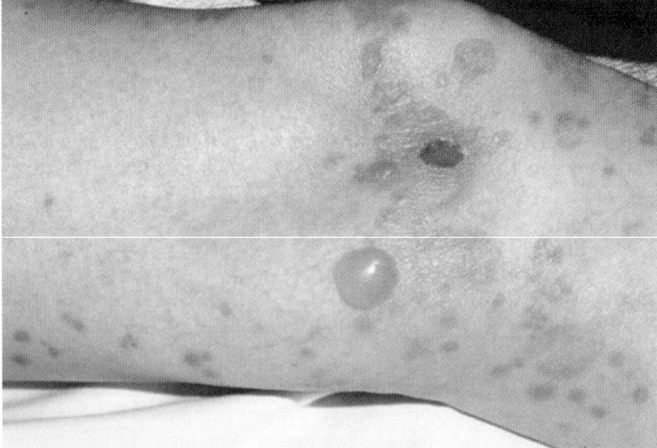

Figure 8 **Intact bullae lateral to the knee in a middle-aged woman with bullous pemphigoid.**

often pruritic. Mucosal disease is rare. Biopsy reveals subepidermal bullae and an infiltrate of eosinophils. Direct immunofluorescence reveals a linear deposition of IgG at the dermal-epidermal junction.

Bullous pemphigoid occurs most commonly in the elderly, with an onset between 65 and 75 years of age. Prognosis is influenced by age and general condition of the patient, not by extent of disease activity.[3] Treatment of older patients in poor health requires caution.

Differential diagnosis includes bullous SLE, epidermolysis bullosa acquisita, cicatricial pemphigoid, and dermatitis herpetiformis.

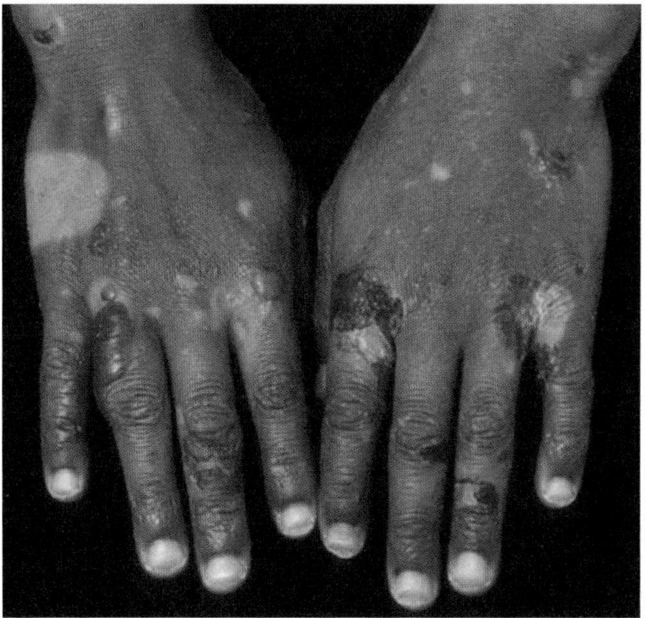

Figure 9 **Bullae and erosions on the hands are characteristic of epidermolysis bullosa acquisita.**

Treatment includes topical and systemic corticosteroids, steroid-sparing immunosuppressants, and tetracycline in combination with niacinamide.

Epidermolysis Bullosa Acquisita

Epidermolysis bullosa acquisita (Fig. 9) is an uncommon bullous disease characterized by skin fragility, milia (small cysts), scarring alopecia, and nail dystrophy. Skin disease typically follows trauma and occurs primarily on the hands, feet, elbows, and knees. Immunofluorescence is similar to bullous pemphigoid, with IgG deposition at the dermal-epidermal junction.

Differential diagnosis includes bullous pemphigoid and bullous SLE.

Treatment includes topical and systemic corticosteroids, steroid-sparing immunosuppressants, colchicine, and plasmapheresis.

INTERNAL MALIGNANCIES

Cutaneous Metastases

Cutaneous metastases (Fig. 10), are uncommon, and the reported prevalence varies from 0.7% to 10% of all patients with cancer.[4] Any malignant neoplasm can metastasize to the skin. Cutaneous metastases from cancers of the lung, large intestine, and kidney are most commonly found in men; cancers of the breast and large intestine are the most likely primary tumors to metastasize to the skin in women.[4] Metastases to the skin are usually flesh-colored to violaceous nodules that appear in close proximity to the primary neoplasm; most common sites are the head (scalp), neck, and trunk.

Differential diagnosis includes pilar or epidermal inclusion cyst, adnexal tumor, neurofibroma, and lipoma.

Treatment depends on the primary neoplasm and overall prognosis.

Paget's Disease

Paget's disease of the breast (Fig. 11) is an uncommon condition characterized by unilateral eczematous plaque of the nipple and

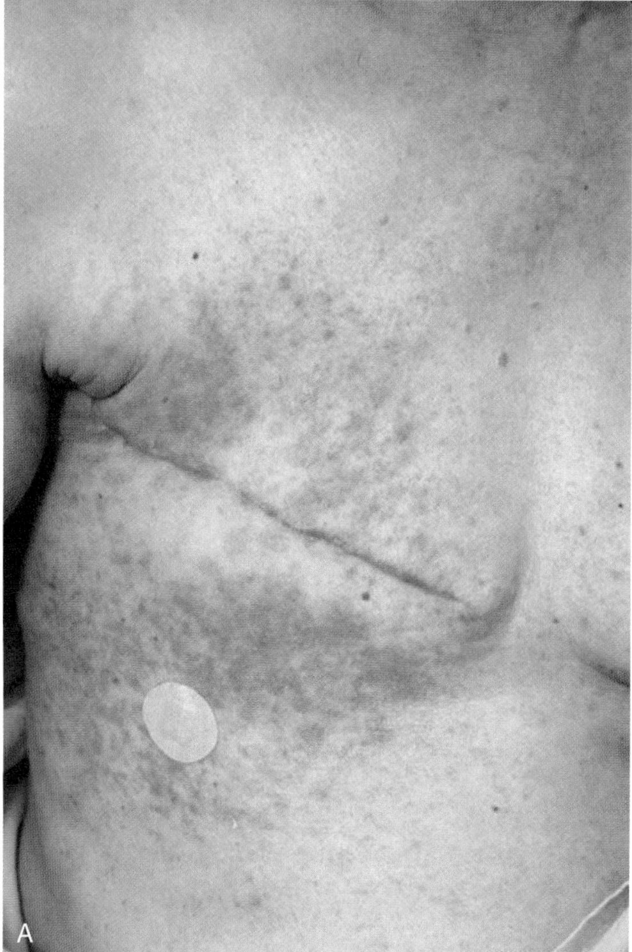

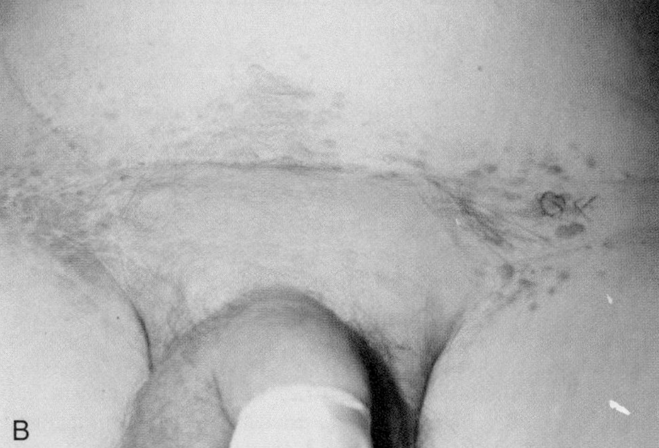

Figure 10 **Cancer. A,** Carcinoma en cuirasse in a woman with metastatic breast cancer. **B,** Metastatic prostate cancer in an elderly man.

areola. The disease is strongly associated with an underlying invasive carcinoma of the affected breast or ductal carcinoma in situ (DCIS).[5]

Extramammary Paget's disease is typically a persistent, eczematous plaque of the anogenital or axillary regions whose morphology and histology strongly resemble Paget's disease of the breast. Extramammary Paget's disease affects older adults and is often associated with an underlying adnexal (apocrine) carcinoma or an underlying cancer of the genitourinary tract or distal gastrointestinal tract.

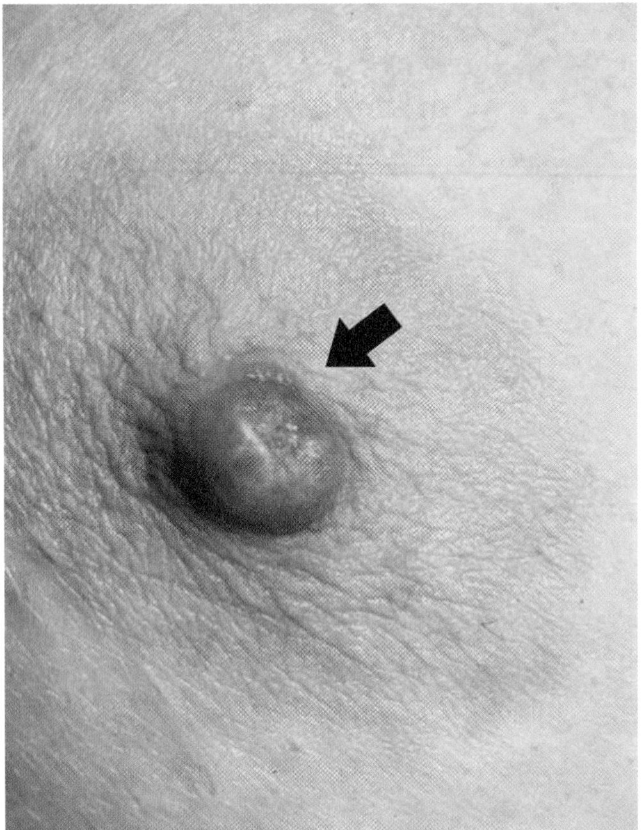

Figure 11 **Paget's disease of the nipple in a middle-aged woman.**

Differential diagnosis includes allergic or irritant contact dermatitis (especially if bilateral), psoriasis, and dermatophyte (tinea) infection.

Treatment includes surgical excision, radiation therapy, and photodynamic therapy. Referral to oncology is recommended.

Acanthosis Nigricans

Acanthosis nigricans (Fig. 12) is characterized by smooth, velvetlike, hyperkeratotic plaques in intertriginous areas (e.g., groin, axillae, neck). Three types of acanthosis nigricans have been recognized.

Type I is associated with malignancy. Occasionally, acanthosis nigricans is a marker of an underlying adenocarcinoma, especially of the gastrointestinal tract (60% gastric). Malignant acanthosis nigricans has a sudden onset and more extensive distribution, including the face, palms, and trunk. Type II is the familial type, with autosomal dominant transmission. It is very rare and appears at birth or soon after. Type II has no malignancy association. Type III acanthosis nigricans is associated with obesity and insulin resistance. Type III is the most commonly occurring type.

Acanthosis nigricans can develop following the use of some medications, such as systemic corticosteroids, nicotinic acid, diethylstilbestrol, and isoniazid (INH).

Differential diagnosis includes confluent and reticulated papillomatosis of Gougerot and Carteaud and Dowling-Degos disease.

Treatment for type I acanthosis nigricans includes identifying and removing the malignant tumor. Treatment for types II and III includes weight loss and treatment of the underlying endocrine disorder, if applicable. Topical treatments including tretinoin, calcipotriol, urea, and salicylic acid may be helpful.

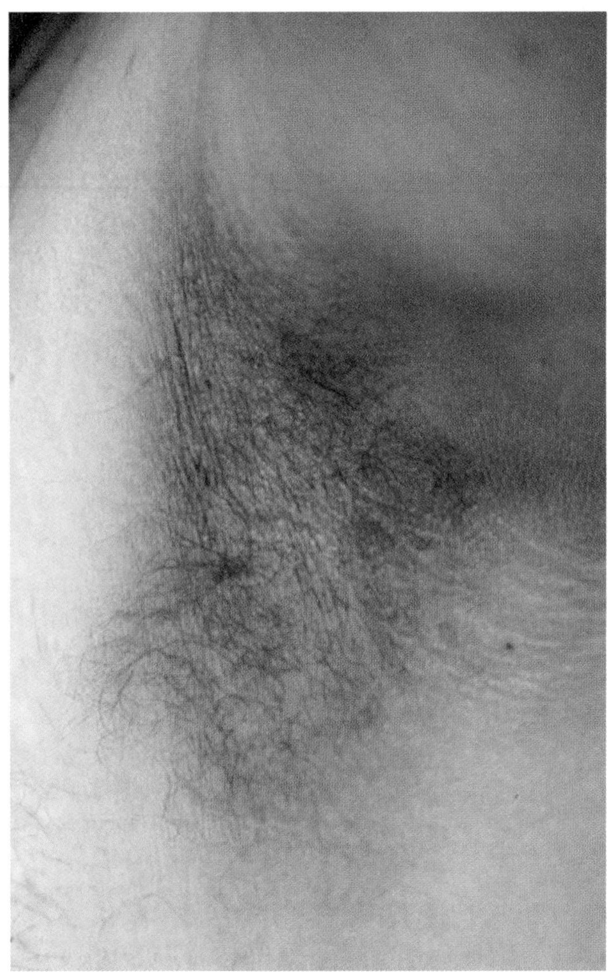

Figure 12 **Acanthosis nigricans in the axilla of an obese man.**

Cowden's Syndrome

Cowden's syndrome, an autosomal dominant cancer syndrome caused by mutations in the tumor suppressor gene *PTEN*, is characterized by multiple tricholemmomas (wartlike growths) around the mouth, nose, and ears; cancer of the breast, endometrium, or thyroid gland; and thyroid disease (adenomas or goiter), mental retardation, and fibrocystic disease of the breast.

Sweet's Syndrome

Sweet's syndrome (Fig. 13), or acute febrile neutrophilic dermatosis, has a strong association with acute myelocytic or myelomonocytic leukemia. Affected patients, usually middle-aged women, have painful erythematous to violaceous plaques on the face, extremities, and trunk. Most have fever, malaise, arthralgias, myalgias, and conjunctivitis.

Sweet's syndrome can occur with inflammatory bowel disease, bowel bypass syndrome, and pregnancy. It occasionally occurs as a reaction to certain medications including all-*trans* retinoic acid and granulocyte colony-stimulating factor.[6]

Differential diagnosis includes erythema multiforme, deep fungal infection, pyoderma gangrenosum, and cutaneous metastases.

Treatment includes systemic corticosteroids, dapsone, and NSAIDs.

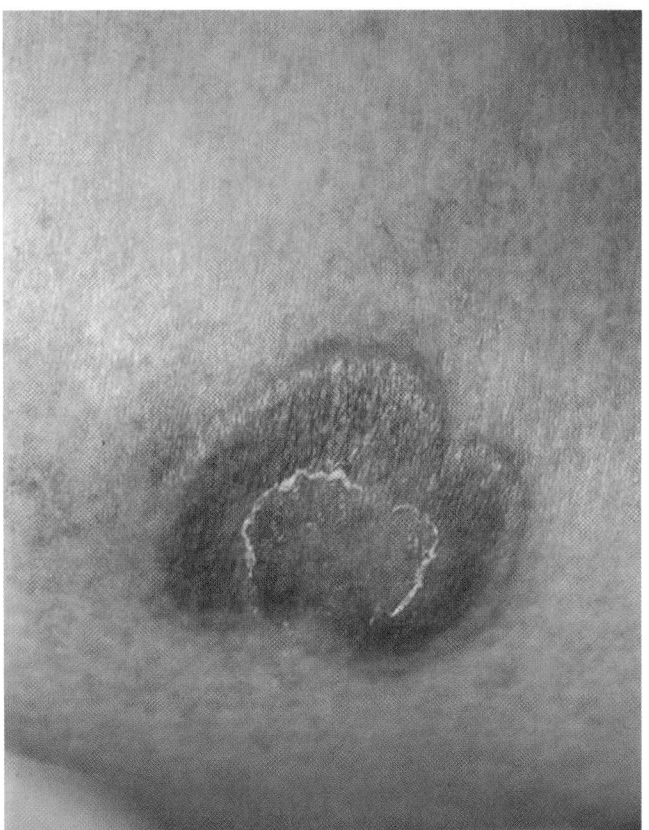

Figure 13 **An erythematous edematous plaque on the arm of a woman with Sweet's syndrome.**

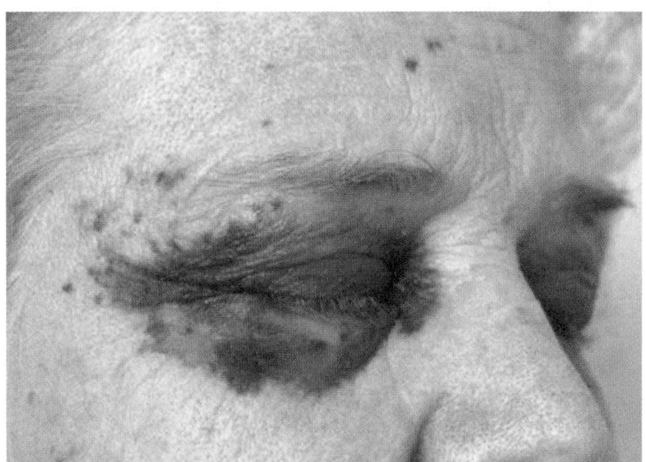

Figure 14 **Pinch purpura in a woman with systemic amyloidosis.**

Amyloidosis

Amyloidosis of the skin may be a sign of multiple myeloma. Affected patients have papules on the eyelids and extremities that become purpuric and ecchymotic due to increased blood vessel fragility secondary to amyloid infiltration of the vessels. The purpura and ecchymosis develop after pressure or rubbing (pinch purpura) (Fig. 14) or may be spontaneous. Many patients have prominent macroglossia. The prognosis for primary systemic amyloidosis is poor.

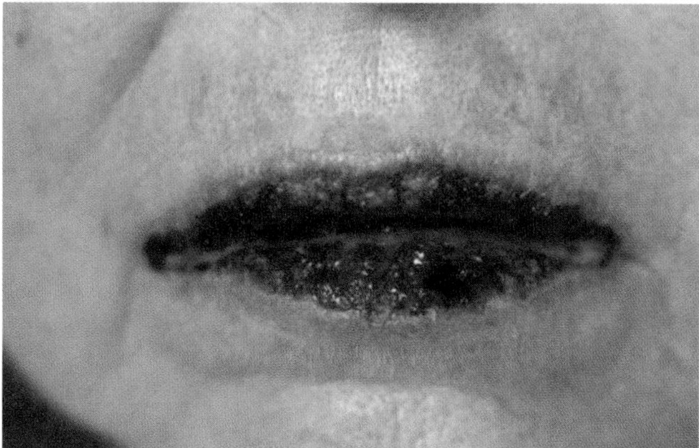

Figure 15 **Severe stomatitis in a woman with paraneoplastic pemphigus.**

Differential diagnosis includes nodular amyloidosis.

Treatment includes systemic chemotherapy and stem cell transplantation.

Paraneoplastic Pemphigus

Paraneoplastic pemphigus (Fig. 15), characterized by intractable stomatitis and blisters on the trunk and extremities, has features of pemphigus and erythema multiforme. Direct immunofluorescence reveals deposition of IgG intercellularly and at the dermal-epidermal junction. Paraneoplastic pemphigus has a strong association with non-Hodgkin's lymphoma, chronic lymphocytic leukemia, and Castleman's disease with or without myasthenia gravis. Severe pulmonary disease (bronchiolitis obliterans) with respiratory failure is often the cause of death in affected patients.[7]

Differential diagnosis includes pemphigus vulgaris, bullous pemphigoid, and erythema multiforme.

Treatment includes treatment of the underlying malignancy, systemic corticosteroids, steroid-sparing immunosuppressants, rituximab, and plasmapheresis.

Erythema Gyratum Repens

Erythema gyratum repens is a rare but very distinctive skin disease characterized by reddened concentric bands in a whorled or woodgrain pattern. Affected patients have severe pruritus and peripheral eosinophilia. Erythema gyratum repens has a strong association with lung cancer; the association with breast, cervical, and gastrointestinal cancers is less strong.

Treatment of the underlying malignancy treats the skin disease.

CARDIOVASCULAR DISEASE

LEOPARD Syndrome

Multiple lentigines occur with LEOPARD syndrome (Fig. 16), an acronym for *l*entigines, *e*lectrocardiographic changes, *o*cular telorism, *p*ulmonary stenosis, *a*bnormal genitalia, *r*etarded growth, and *d*eafness. Inheritance is autosomal dominant, and many cases occur sporadically.

Carney Complex

Carney complex encompasses LAMB syndrome (*l*entigines, *a*trial myxoma, *m*ucocutaneous myxomas, and *b*lue nevi) and NAME syndrome (*n*evi, *a*trial myxoma, *m*yxoid neurofibromas, and *e*phelides), entities known to pediatricians, cardiologists, and dermatologists.

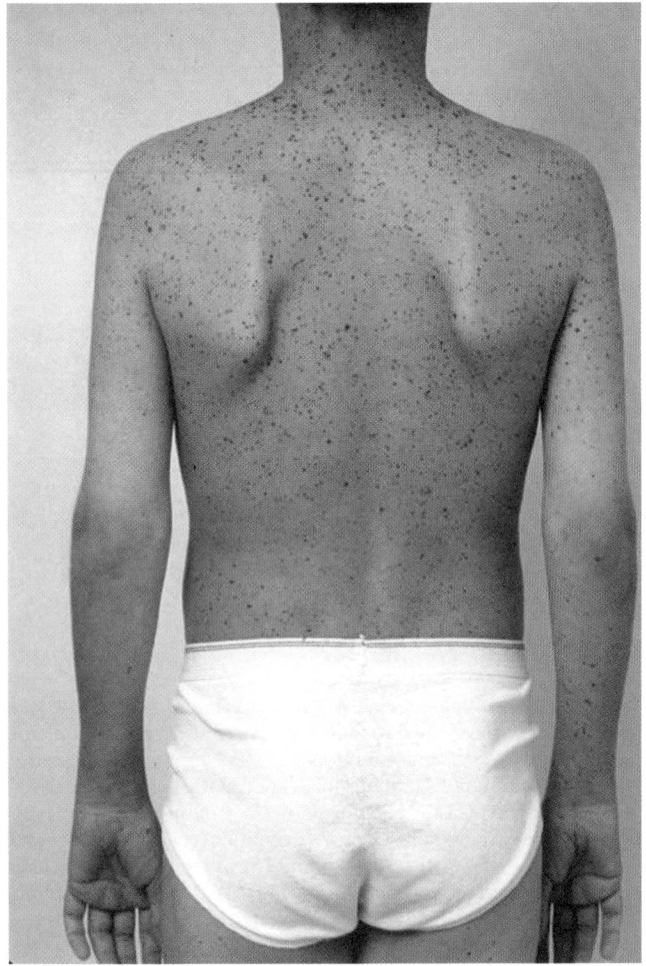

Figure 16 **Multiple lentigines in a boy with LEOPARD syndrome.**

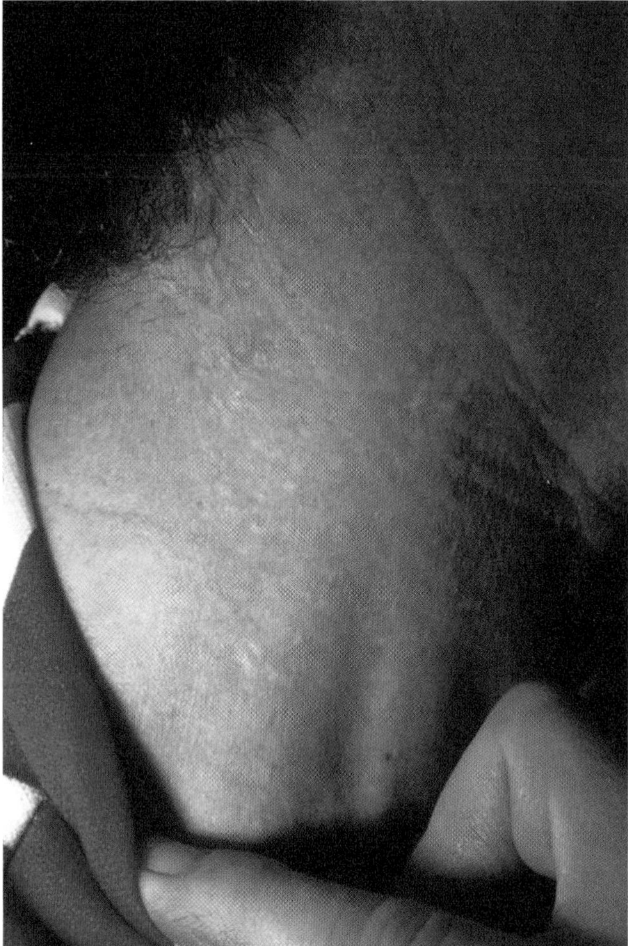

Figure 17 **Yellow papules on the neck of a boy with pseudoxanthoma elasticum.**

Recognition of these syndromes is critical because identification and removal of the associated atrial myxomas may be lifesaving. The inheritance pattern for both syndromes is autosomal dominant.

Pseudoxanthoma Elasticum

Pseudoxanthoma elasticum (Fig. 17) is characterized by yellow papules over redundant skin folds on the neck, abdomen, and groin, giving the skin the appearance of plucked chicken skin. Pseudoxanthoma elasticum represents a defect in elastic fibers, which become brittle and calcified. Skin biopsy reveals swollen, fragmented elastic fibers, and fundoscopic examination reveals angioid streaks in Bruch's membrane. Associated signs of pseudoxanthoma elasticum include hypertension, peripheral vascular and coronary artery disease, retinal and gastrointestinal hemorrhage, and stroke. Disease is transmitted in a sporadic or inherited (autosomal recessive) fashion. Mutations in the gene *ABCC6* on chromosome 16 have been linked to pseudoxanthoma elasticum.

Differential diagnosis includes cutis laxa, Ehlers-Danlos syndrome, and perforating calcific elastosis.

No definitive treatment is available.

Ehlers-Danlos Syndrome

Ehlers-Danlos syndrome is a heterogeneous group of connective tissue disorders characterized by joint hyperextensibility, hypermobility, skin and vessel fragility, and fish-mouth scars. Ehlers-Danlos syndrome is characterized by abnormalities in collagen biosynthesis, which can affect many organ systems.

Eleven types of Ehlers-Danlos syndrome have been identified with varying associated features, including mitral valve prolapse, blue sclerae, vascular aneurysm, aortic dissection, hernias, angina, gastrointestinal bleeding (perforation), and peripheral vascular disease. Genetic testing for specific mutations has demonstrated redundancy and has reduced Ehlers-Danlos syndrome from eleven to seven types. Patients with vascular (type IV) Ehlers-Danlos syndrome are prone to arterial rupture and have the highest mortality.

Differential diagnosis includes cutis laxa.

Treatment includes protecting the skin and treating systemic disease.

PULMONARY DISEASE

Sarcoidosis is a multisystem, granulomatous disease of the lungs, bones, central nervous system, lymph nodes, eyes, and skin. The disease is more common in women and has a higher prevalence in African Americans. Skin disease, affecting 25% to 35% of patients, includes red to purple indurated plaques of the nose (lupus pernio) (Fig. 18), midfacial papules, annular plaques, and plaques or nodules on the trunk and extremities. Sarcoidal disease also has a predilection for scars. Erythema nodosum, an acute, painful panniculitis that usually affects the shins, is the most common nonspecific cutaneous manifestation of sarcoidosis.

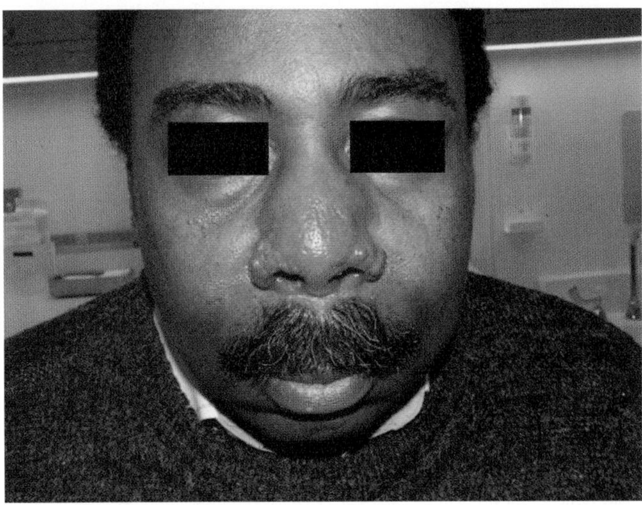

Figure 18 Flesh-colored to erythematous nodules and plaques on the nose of a man with sarcoidosis (lupus pernio).

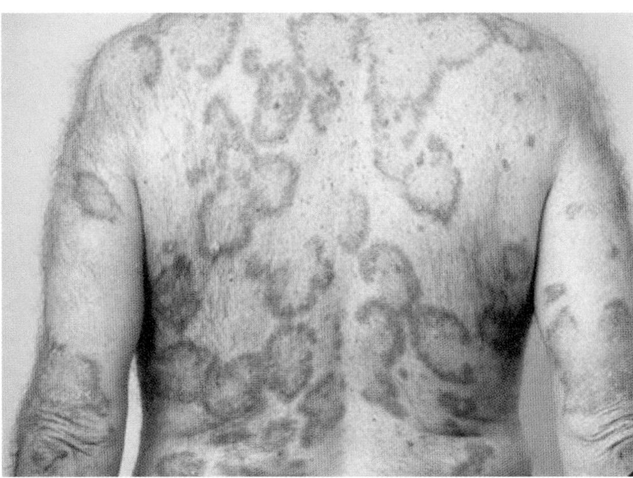

Figure 20 Annular plaques on the back of a man with subacute cutaneous lupus.

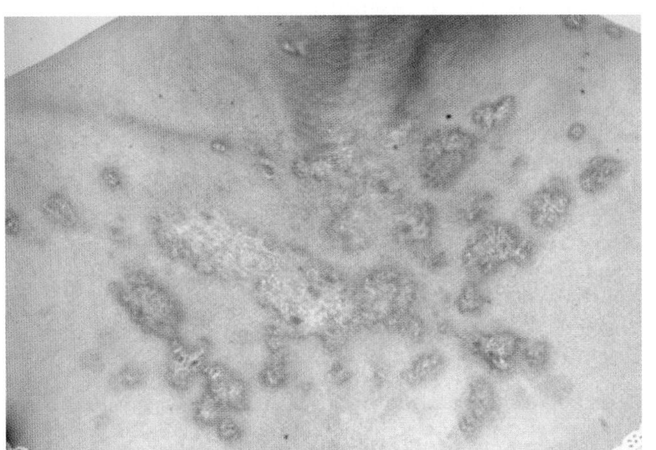

Figure 19 Atrophic red plaques of discoid lupus in a young woman.

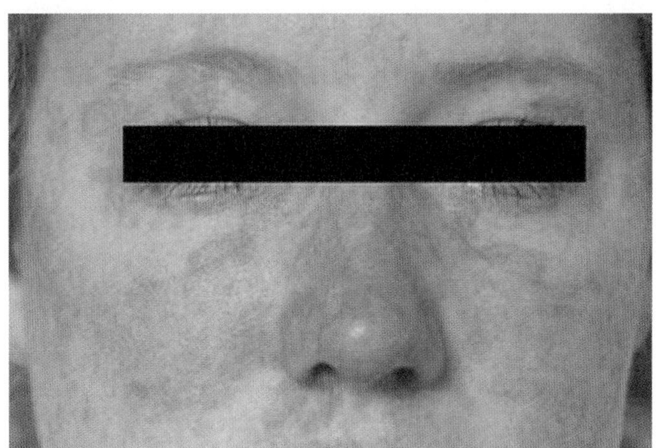

Figure 21 Malar erythema in a young woman with lupus.

Differential diagnosis includes rosacea, trichoepitheliomas, granulomatous syphilis, and granuloma annulare.

Treatment includes systemic corticosteroids, intralesional corticosteroids for localized disease, methotrexate, thalidomide, antimalarials, and tumor necrosis factor-α (TNF-α) inhibitors.

RHEUMATIC DISEASE

Psoriatic Arthritis

Psoriatic arthritis (PsA) affects approximately 5% to 10% of patients with psoriasis. Asymmetric fusiform swelling of the distal interphalangeal joints (sausage digits), in association with oligoarthritis and tenosynovitis can be seen in up to 70% of PsA patients. Other presentations include symmetric polyarticular arthritis (15%), distal interphalangeal joint disease with nail damage (16%), arthritis mutilans with erosion of the phalanges (5%), and ankylosing spondylitis (5%). The arthritis can resemble rheumatoid arthritis. Approximately 50% of affected patients have the HLA-B27 genotype.

Differential diagnosis includes osteoarthritis and rheumatoid arthritis.

Treatment includes TNF-α inhibitors, metrotrexate, NSAIDs, and steroid-sparing immunosuppressants.

Lupus Erythematosus

Lupus erythematosus is an autoimmune photosensitive dermatosis that can be localized or systemic, often with significant overlap. Localized cutaneous (discoid) lupus erythematosus (DLE) (Fig. 19), usually localized to the head or neck, is characterized by atrophic, scarring plaques on sun-exposed areas. Five percent of patients develop SLE.

Subacute cutaneous lupus erythematosus (SCLE) (Fig. 20) is characterized by annular pink to red plaques in a sun-exposed, shawl-like distribution on the chest, back, and arms. Unlike DLE, there is no scarring. Serology is often positive in SCLE-antinuclear antibody (80%) and antibodies to Ro/SSA antigen. SCLE patients account for 10% to 15% of the entire lupus erythematosus population.

The cutaneous manifestations of SLE include malar erythema, photosensitivity, oral ulcers, discoid plaques, bullae, purpura, calcinosis cutis, and alopecia. The butterfly rash (malar erythema) is the most common expression of SLE (Fig. 21).

Differential diagnosis includes dermatomyositis, Sjögren's syndrome, photosensitive drug eruption, acute rheumatic fever, and pellagra.

Treatment includes sun protection; intralesional, topical, and systemic corticosteroids; antimalarials; dapsone; and immunosuppressants.

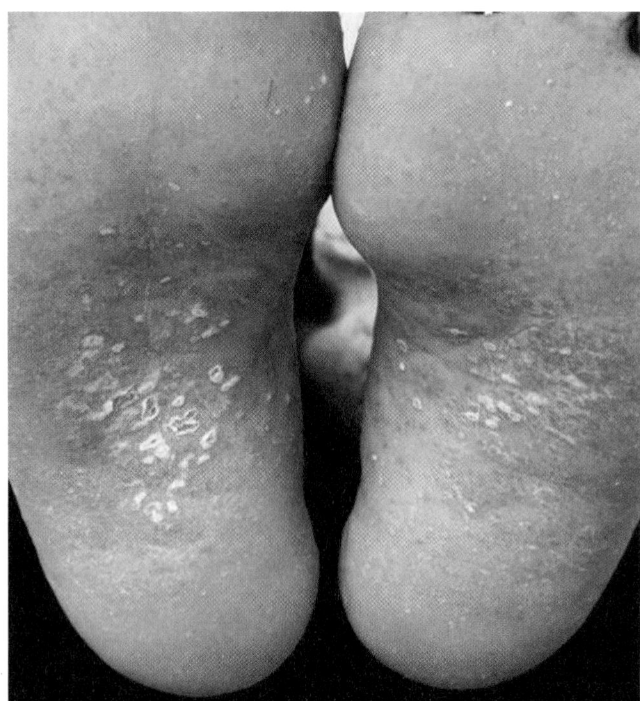

Figure 22 **Pustules and crusted papules on the soles (keratoderma blennorrhagicum) of a young man.**

Scleroderma

Scleroderma is an autoimmune skin disease that can be localized or generalized. The localized form, known as morphea, begins as erythematous patches that evolve into dusky, hypopigmented, indurated plaques with violaceous borders, usually on the trunk. The systemic or generalized forms are subdivided into CREST syndrome (*c*alcinosis, *R*aynaud's phenomenon, *e*sophageal dysmotility, *s*clerodactyly, *t*elangiectasias) and progressive systemic sclerosis. Presence of anticentromere antibodies correlates with CREST syndrome; SCL-70 antibodies correlate with progressive systemic sclerosis. Patients with CREST syndrome have a better prognosis.

Differential diagnosis includes diabetic sclerodema, scleromyxedema, and chronic graft-versus-host disease.

Treatment includes vasodilating drugs, phototherapy (UVA1) for limited disease, methotrexate, and cyclophosphamide.

Reactive Arthritis

Reactive arthritis (Reiter's syndrome with conjunctivitis, urethritis, and diarrhea) (Fig. 22) usually follows a bout of gastroenteritis or urethritis. Implicated organisms include *Campylobacter, Shigella, Salmonella, Ureaplasma,* and *Yersinia* species. Affected patients, usually men, often have vesicles and crusted plaques on the penis (circinate balanitis) and erythematous pustules and papules on the palms and soles (keratoderma blennorrhagicum) that can mimic pustular psoriasis. More than 50% of patients have sacroiliitis, correlating with the presence of HLA-B27 antigen, but few patients have the classic triad of urethritis, conjunctivitis, and arthritis.

Differential diagnosis includes psoriasis, juvenile plantar dermatoses, rheumatoid arthritis, ankylosing spondylitis, and gout.

Treatment includes topical corticosteroids, cyclosporine, or acitretin for refractory disease.

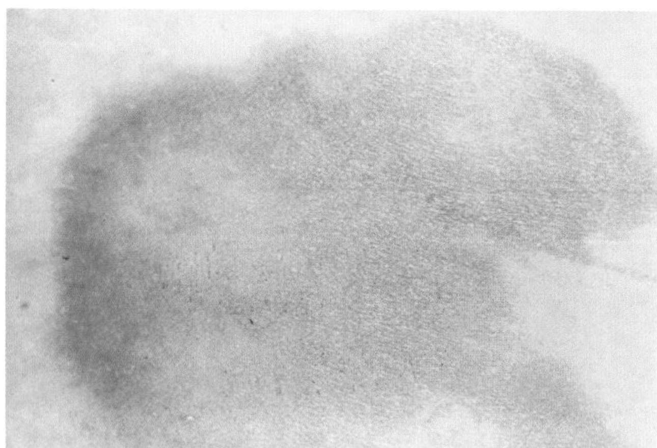

Figure 23 **Annular plaque of erythema chronicum migrans (Lyme disease).**

Erythema Chronicum Migrans

Erythema chronicum migrans, the hallmark of Lyme disease, reflecting early infection with the tick-borne spirochete *Borrelia burgdorferi,* develops as a red macule or papule at the site of the tick bite and gradually enlarges to an annular, reddened plaque (Fig. 23) that surrounds the bite. Affected patients can have fever, arthralgia, and myalgia, and, occasionally, Bell's palsy. Late sequelae include meningoencephalitis, myocarditis, and peripheral neuropathy. Primary endemic areas in the United States are New England, the upper Midwest, and the Pacific Northwest.

Differential diagnosis includes cellulitis, spider bite, erythema multiforme, and erythema annulare centrifugum.

Treatment is doxycycline.

Dermatomyositis

Dermatomyositis, an inflammatory connective tissue disease, is characterized by symmetric proximal muscle weakness (myositis); photosensitivity; papules and plaques on the hands, elbows, and knees (Gottron's papules) (Fig. 24); and periorbital edema with a violaceous hue (heliotrope). Other features include scaly, telangiectatic plaques with atrophy and hypopigmentation (poikiloderma) on the face, neck, trunk, and extremities; malar erythema; and nail abnormalities (periungual telangiectases and cuticular hypertrophy).

Diagnostic criteria include the aforementioned changes plus elevated creatine kinase or aldolase level, positive Jo-1 antibody, and electromyographic changes. In adults, dermatomyositis has a strong association with neoplasm, usually an adenocarcinoma of the breast, gastrointestinal tract, or lung.

Differential diagnosis includes SLE and photosensitive drug eruption.

Treatment includes systemic corticosteroids, methotrexate and other steroid-sparing immunosuppressants, and TNF-α inhibitors.

GASTROINTESTINAL DISEASE

Dermatitis Herpetiformis

Dermatitis herpetiformis (Fig. 25) is a chronic, intensely pruritic blistering disease characterized by symmetric grouped vesicles, papules, and wheals on the elbows, knees, scalp, and buttocks. Biopsy reveals a characteristic neutrophilic infiltrate, and direct immunofluorescence demonstrates deposition of IgA at the dermal-epidermal junction. Most patients have an asymptomatic gluten-sensitive enteropathy or, less commonly, thyroid disease. Approximately 70%

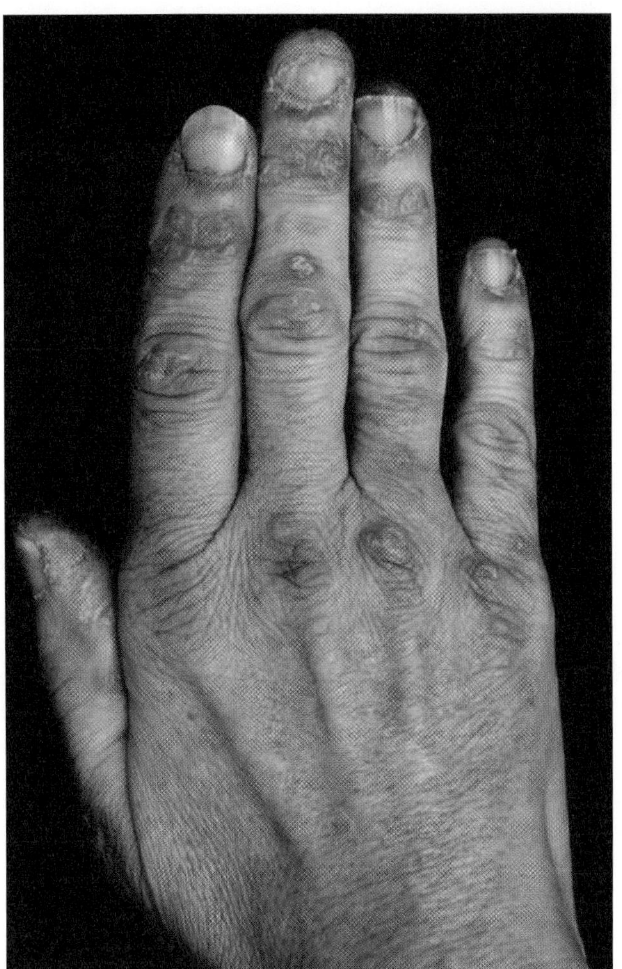

Figure 24 **Gottron's papules on the hands of a woman with dermatomyositis.**

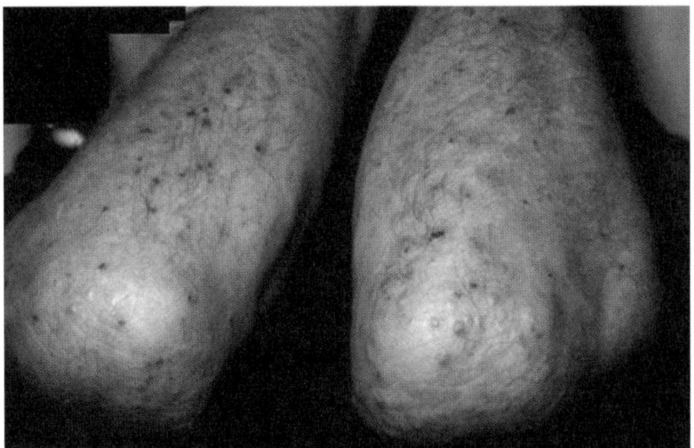

Figure 25 **Pruritic papules on the elbows of a man with dermatitis herpetifomis.**

of patients have circulating IgA antibodies against the smooth muscle cell endomysium (antiendomysial antibodies), which are somewhat peculiar to dermatitis herpetiformis.

Differential diagnosis includes linear IgA dermatosis, bullous pemphigoid, scabies, contact dermatitis, and bullous lupus erythematosus.

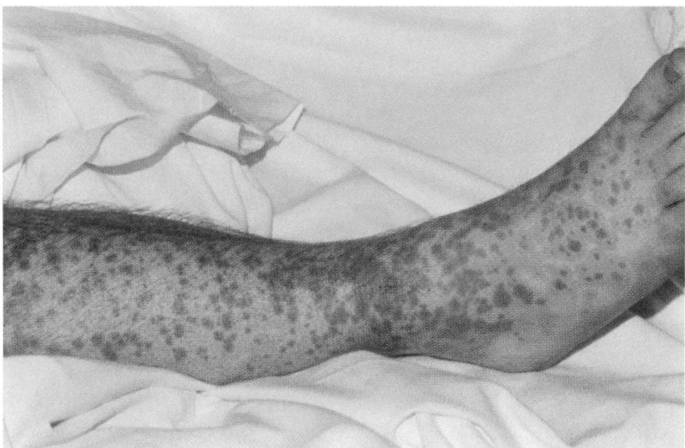

Figure 26 **Leukocytoclastic vasculitis on the leg of a hospitalized patient.**

Treatment includes dapsone, sulfapyridine, and a gluten-free diet.

Acrodermatitis Enteropathica

Acrodermatitis enteropathica is an inherited or acquired condition characterized by pustules, bullae, scaling in an acral and periorificial distribution, and concomitant zinc deficiency. When inherited, acrodermatitis enteropathica results from a mutation in *SLC39A,* which encodes an intestinal zinc transporter.[8] In infants, deficiency can follow breast-feeding, when maternal breast milk contains low levels of zinc. In adults, disease can occur after total parenteral nutrition without adequate zinc supplementation; with alcoholism, other malabsorption states, or inflammatory bowel disease; or as a consequence of bowel surgery. Most patients have diarrhea.

Differential diagnosis includes other nutritional deficiencies, such as niacin or biotin deficiency, and necrolytic migratory erythema.

Treatment is zinc supplementation.

Necrolytic Migratory Erythema

Necrolytic migratory erythema (glucagonoma syndrome) is a rare disease characterized by erythematous, scaly plaques on acral, intertriginous, and periorificial areas, in association with an islet cell tumor of the pancreas. Associated signs include hyperglycemia, diarrhea, weight loss, and atrophic glossitis.

Treatment is rmoval of the tumor.

Hepatitis C Virus–Associated Skin Disorders

Leukocytoclastic vasculitis (cutaneous small vessel vasculitis) (Fig. 26) associated with circulating type II cryoglobulins, usually yields palpable purpura on the lower extremities. Treatment of the hepatitis C infection often leads to resolution of the vasculitis.

Lichen planus (Fig. 27) is characterized by violaceous, flat, polygonal papules, often on the flexor aspects of the wrists, trunk, medial thighs, genitalia, and oral mucosa. Lichen planus also occurs with primary biliary cirrhosis and hepatitis B virus immunization. Oral erosive lichen planus is the most common expression of lichen planus in hepatitis C patients. Treatment includes topical and intralesional corticosteroids, topical immunomodulators, and phototherapy.

Necrolytic acral erythema, characterized by pruritic keratotic plaques on the upper and lower extremities, is a distinctive finding in hepatitis C infection and can resemble a deficiency dermatosis.

Porphyria cutanea tarda is discussed later.

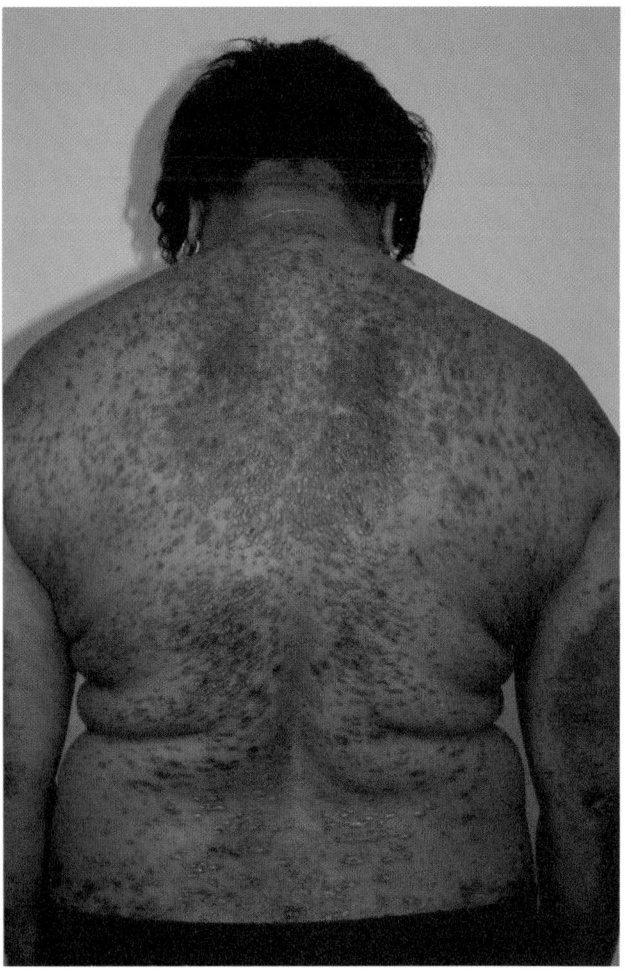

Figure 27 **Generalized lichen planus on the back of a woman.**

Gardner's Syndrome

Gardner's syndrome is an autosomal dominant cancer syndrome characterized by colonic polyposis, osteomas (maxilla, mandible, skull), scoliosis, epidermoid cysts, and soft-tissue tumors (fibromas, desmoids, lipomas). A mutation in the *APC* gene is responsible for Gardener's syndrome. Adenocarcinoma of the colon develops in 60% of patients by the age of 40 years.

Hereditary Hemorrhagic Telangiectasia

Hereditary hemorrhagic telangiectasia (Osler-Weber-Rendu syndrome) is an autosomal dominant disorder characterized by numerous telangiectases on the skin and oral mucosa (Fig. 28). Recurrent epistaxis is the most common presenting manifestation of the syndrome, affecting approximately 85% to 90% of patients. Telangiectases can involve the lungs, liver, brain, eyes, and gastrointestinal tract; hemorrhage can occur at any site. Pulmonary arteriovenous fistulae and central nervous system angiomas can also occur.

Differential diagnosis includes generalized essential telangiectasia.

Treatment includes estrogen therapy or oral contraceptives in postpubertal women, laser cauterization, selective embolization, and supportive care.

Muir-Torre Syndrome

Muir-Torre syndrome is a disorder characterized by one or more sebaceous tumors (adenoma, epithelioma, carcinoma) and one or more internal neoplasms, usually colorectal or genitourinary, rarely lymphoma. This syndrome results from an inactivating germline mutation of the DNA mismatch repair genes, most often *MSH-2*. Treatment is isotretinoin and regular GI and genitourinary evaluation.

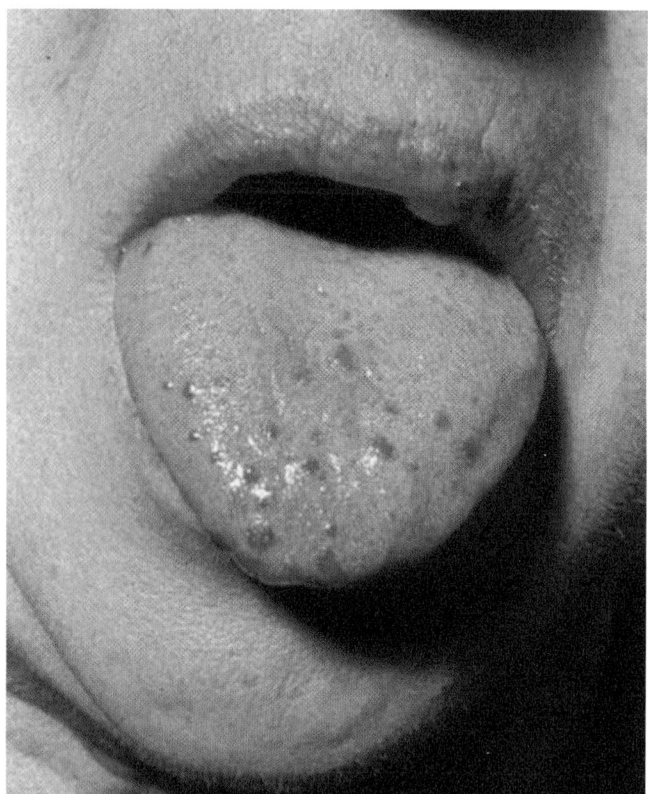

Figure 28 **Telangiectasia on the tongue of a patient with Osler-Weber-Rendu syndrome.**

Peutz-Jeghers Syndrome

Peutz-Jeghers syndrome is an autosomal dominant disease characterized by lentigines on the skin (periorbital region, dorsal surfaces of the fingers and toes) and mucosa (lips, buccal mucosa) and hamartomas of the stomach, small intestine, and colon. The polyps are usually benign with low malignant potential, but patients have a 10 to 18 times greater lifetime risk of cancer, especially GI malignancies.

Differential diagnosis includes LEOPARD syndrome, Carney complex, and Cronkhite-Canada syndrome.

Treatment includes regular and routine endoscopy and symptomatic treatment for hypogeusia and diarrhea.

Pyoderma Gangrenosum

Pyoderma gangrenosum is a neutrophilic dermatosis characterized by painful ulcers with boggy, undermined edges and a border of gray or purple pigmentation (Fig. 29). The ulcers often follow trauma (pathergy) and begin as pustules or nodules that ulcerate and extend centrifugally.[9] All body areas may be involved, but the legs are the most common site. Fifty percent of patients have underlying rheumatoid arthritis or inflammatory bowel disease or, less often, a paraproteinemia, usually an IgA gammopathy.

Differential diagnosis includes infection, vasculitis, spider bite, and factitious disorder.

Treatment includes treatment of underlying disease if applicable, local wound care, systemic and intralesional corticosteroids, cyclosporine, and infliximab.

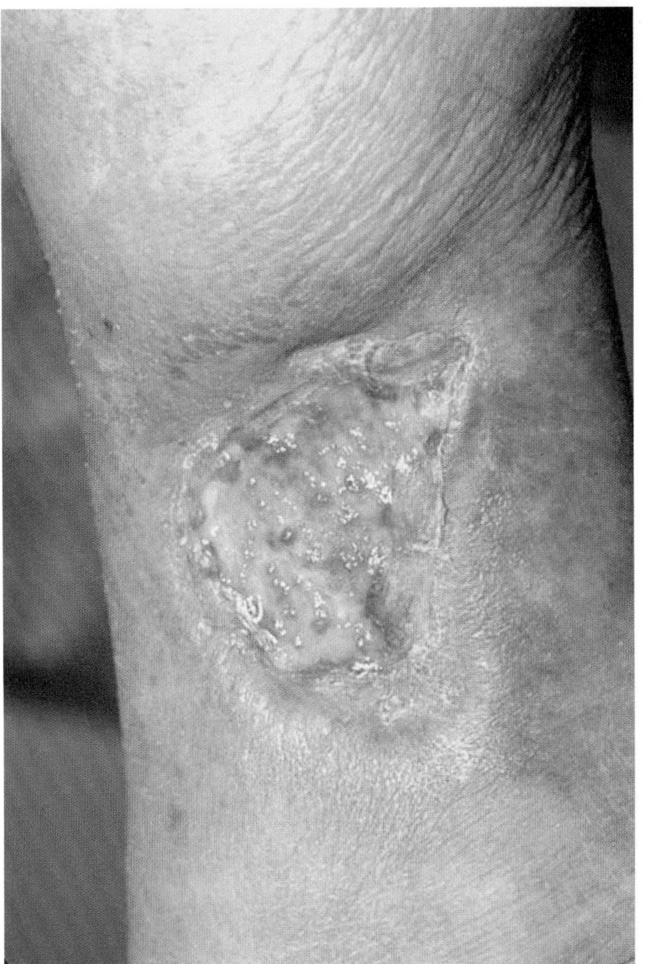

Figure 29 **Ulcer of pyoderma gangrenosum in a man.**

RENAL DISEASE

Nephrogenic Systemic Fibrosis

Nephrogenic systemic fibrosis, also known nephrogenic fibrosing dermopathy, is a recently described disorder that resembles scleroderma. Nephrogenic systemic fibrosis occurs in patients who have end-stage renal disease and are on dialysis and occasionally in patients with acute renal failure or after kidney transplantation. Nephrogenic systemic fibrosis is characterized by thick, indurated plaques on the extremities and the trunk. Disease can be progressive, leading to joint contractures. Autopsies have demonstrated that disease is not limited to the skin; visceral organ and muscle fibrosis has been noted. The cause remains unclear, but the MRI contrast agent gadolinium might have a role in the pathogenesis of this condition.[10]

Differential diagnosis includes scleroderma and scleromyxedema.

Treatment includes immunosuppressive agents, phototherapy, topical steroids, retinoids, and photopheresis, all with little benefit.

Birt-Hogg-Dubé Syndrome

Birt-Hogg-Dubé syndrome is a disorder characterized by multiple fibrofolliculomas and trichodiscomas (skin-colored dermal papules on the face and trunk). Patients have a significantly increased risk of renal oncocytoma and chromophobe renal carcinoma. Spontaneous pneumothorax can occur secondary to rupture of pulmonary cysts. Mutations in the folliculin gene on chromosome 17 are responsible for this syndrome.

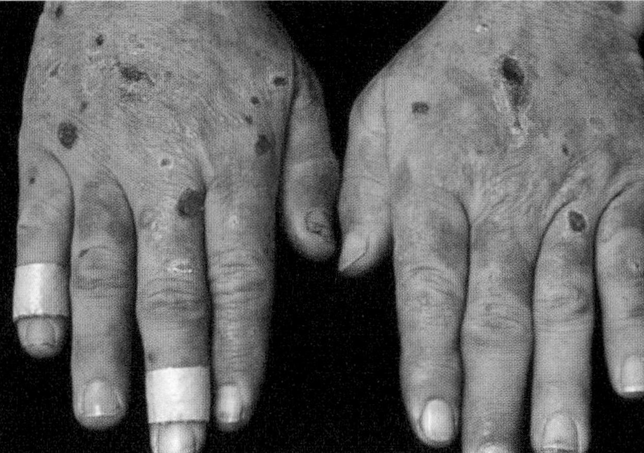

Figure 30 **Eroded blisters on the hands of a man with porphyria cutanea tarda and hepatitis C.**

ENDOCRINE AND METABOLIC DISEASE

Porphyrias

Porphyrias are inherited or acquired disorders of heme biosynthesis and can be erythropoietic, hepatic, or mixed in nature, each associated with a specific enzyme defect in the heme pathway. Porphyria cutanea tarda, the most common porphyria, is a hepatic porphyria with acquired and sporadic forms (Fig. 30). It is caused by a deficiency in uroporphyrinogen decarboxylase, leading to the accumulation of uroporphyrin in the urine and serum.

Precipitating factors include alcohol ingestion, estrogen administration, certain hepatotoxins (dinitrochlorobenzene, carbon tetrachloride), HIV infection, hemochromatosis, and hepatitis C infection. Manifestations of porphyria cutanea tarda include photosensitivity, skin fragility, bullae and erosions on sun-exposed skin (especially dorsal hands), and hypertrichosis. Biopsy reveals a subepidermal bulla with festooning of the dermal papilla. Direct immunofluorescence reveals IgG and C3 at the dermal-epidermal junction and in vessel walls.

Differential diagnosis includes bullous SLE, epidermolysis bullosa acquisita, pseudoporphyria, and variegate porphyria.

Treatment includes phlebotomy and antimalarial drugs.

Pseudoporphyria

Pseudoporphyria mimics porphyria cutanea tarda without an enzyme defect; plasma and urinary porphyrins are normal. Medications (NSAIDs [especially naproxen], furosemide, and tetracycline) are the most common cause of pseudoporphyria. Less common causes are tanning bed use and hemodialysis.

Differential diagnosis is the same as for porphyria cutanea tarda.

Treatment includes removal of the cause.

Diabetes Mellitus-Related Skin Conditions

Approximately 30% to 50% of diabetic patients develop skin disease. Box 1 outlines the most common cutaneous manifestations of diabetes, arranged by frequency of occurrence (most to least frequent).

Summary

- The skin is often a window to systemic disease.
- By recognizing cutaneous manifestations of systemic diseases, the internist can often determine the appropriate diagnosis and therapy or the need for referral to a dermatologist.

SECTION 3 DERMATOLOGY

Box 1 Cutaneous Manifestations of Diabetes Mellitus

Diabetic dermopathy (shin spots)

- Atrophic, hyperpigmented papules and /plaques on the legs
- Very common finding

Diabetic thick skin

- Thickened skin on the hands (dorsum)
- Scleroderma-like changes of the hands with stiffening of the joints
- Scleredema-thickening of the skin on the upper back, posterior neck, and shoulders (uncommon)

Acanthosis nigricans

- Velvety plaques in intertriginous areas (neck, axillae, groin)
- Common with obesity and diabetes

Yellow nails and skin (palms and soles)

- Affects up to 50% of patients

Acquired perforating disorders

- Pruritic hyperkeratotic papules on the legs and trunk
- Histopathologically characterized by the transepidermal elimination of collagen and/or elastin
- Common in patients with diabetes and renal failure

Calciphylaxis

- Painful purpuric plaques with ulceration
- Affected patients often have diabetes and end-stage renal disease with secondary hyperparathyroidism
- Poor prognosis

Necrobiosis lipoidica diabeticorum

- Yellow-orange, atrophic plaques on the legs, especially the shins
- Majority of affected patients have diabetes

Diabetic bullae

- Spontaneous blistering of the hands and feet
- Heals without scarring
- Rare, but distinctive

Suggested Readings

Bystryn JC, Rudolph JL: Pemphigus. Lancet 2005;366(9479):61-73.

Chen CY, Sun LM, Anderson BO: Paget disease of the breast: Changing patterns of incidence, clinical presentation, and treatment in the U.S. Cancer 2006;107(7):1448-1458.

High WA, Ayers RA, Chandler J, et al: Gadolinium is detectable within the tissue of patients with nephrogenic systemic fibrosis. J Am Acad Dermatol 2007;56(1):21-26.

Joly P, Benichou J, Lok C, et al: Prediction of survival for patients with bullous pemphigoid. Arch Dermatol 2005;141:691-698.

Kleyn CE, Lai-Cheong JE, Bell HK: Cutaneous manifestations of internal malignancy. Am J Clin Dermatol 2006; 7(2):71-84.

Kury S, Dreno B, Bezieau S, et al: Identification of SLC39A4, a gene involved in acrodermatitis enteropathica. Nat Genet 2002;31(3):239-240.

Nikolskaia OV, Nousari CH, Anhalt GJ: Paraneoplastic pemphigus in association with Castelman's disease. Br J Dermatol 2003;149(6):1143-1151.

Robson KJ, Piette WW: Cutaneous manifestations of systemic diseases. Med Clin North Am 1998;82(6):1359-1380.

Thompson DF, Montarella KE: Drug-induced Sweet's syndrome. Ann Pharmacother 2007; 41(5):802-811.

Wallach D, Vignon-Pennamen MD: From acute febrile neutrophilic dermatosis to neutrophilic disease: Forty years of clinical research. J Am Acad Dermatol 2006;55(6):1066-1071.

References

For a complete list of references, log onto www.expertconsult.com.

Common Benign Growths

Justin G. Woodhouse and *Kenneth J. Tomecki*

Human skin is subject to a variety of common benign growths, but most never require medical attention. Management (or lack thereof) requires an appreciation of how such growths appear and behave, coupled with the ability to differentiate them from more serious entities. This article provides a selected compilation of the more common benign growths that affect the skin.

SEBORRHEIC KERATOSES

Seborrheic keratoses may be the most common benign tumor of the skin. Typically, they are scaly (hyperkeratotic), brown (hyperpigmented), often somewhat greasy plaques that vary in size and thickness and often appear to be stuck onto the skin surface (Fig. 1). They occur on any surface except the palms, soles, and mucosa. They are common in adults, more so with advanced age, and unusual in children. Their cause is unknown, but a genetic predisposition may be present in some families. The sudden eruption of many, often pruritic seborrheic keratoses on the trunk (Leser-Trélat sign) has been implicated as a cutaneous marker of internal malignancy, commonly gastric adenocarcinoma. Evaluation of such patients should include upper endoscopy and age-appropriate cancer screening.

Therapy is usually not necessary unless plaques are pruritic, irritated or inflamed, or of cosmetic concern. When necessary, cryotherapy (liquid nitrogen) or curettage is usually adequate. If the clinical diagnosis is uncertain, a biopsy is warranted.

DERMATOSIS PAPULOSA NIGRA

Dermatosis papulosa nigra is a condition of hyperpigmented, hyperkeratotic plaques similar to seborrheic keratoses and acrochordons (skin tags), both clinically and histologically. Dermatosis papulosa nigra growths are common and usually are found on the face and neck, with a particular predilection for periorbital skin of darkly pigmented persons (Fig. 2).

Approximately 50% of the black population has these benign growths, and women are more affected than men by a ratio of 2:1.

Therapy is usually not necessary unless the growths become itchy or irritated, although many people desire treatment for cosmetic reasons. Treatment options include scissor excision, curettage, or cryotherapy, all of which can produce hypo- or hyperpigmentation.

SEBACEOUS HYPERPLASIA

Sebaceous hyperplasia is a benign enlargement of sebaceous glands surrounding a follicle characterized by small flesh-colored to yellow papules, often with a central dell, on the face of adults (Fig. 3).

More common in men and in patients with organ transplants, sebaceous hyperplasia lesions are often numerous, and individual papules can resemble basal cell carcinomas (particularly when accompanied by telangiectasias) or even molluscum contagiosum.

Treatment, primarily for cosmesis, includes cryotherapy, curettage, and laser therapy.

EPHILIDES (FRECKLES)

Ephilides are small, discrete, hyperpigmented macules on the sun-exposed skin of fair-complected individuals, usually redheads and blonds.

Ephilides are not growths per se; they represent focal increased melanin in the skin, and they tend to darken in the summer with increased sun exposure and lighten in the winter. When present in large numbers, they indicate excessive sun (photo) damage and an increased risk of sun-induced skin cancer, including melanoma, basal cell carcinoma, and squamous cell carcinoma.

Ephilides are benign and harmless, and treatment is not necessary. Topical bleaching creams, chemical peels, or cryotherapy can lighten ephilides of cosmetic concern.

LENTIGINES (LIVER SPOTS)

Lentigines are hyperpigmented macules or patches that can resemble nevi (moles). Usually pale tan to brown, they typically appear in white adults and increase in number with advancing age (Fig. 4).

Lentigines tend to occur on the sun-exposed skin of the face, neck, upper trunk, forearms, and hands. Unlike ephilides, lentigines are the result of epidermal hyperplasia and of variable proliferation of melanocytes and subsequent melanization. Lentigines are benign, but they occasionally transform into lentigo maligna (superficial melanoma). If change occurs in a lentigo (e.g., rapid growth, change in color or surface contour), a dermatologic evaluation is warranted and a biopsy may be necessary. Many lentigines indicate excessive photodamage and increased risk of sun-induced skin cancer.

Like treatment for ephilides, treatment for lentigines is primarily for cosmetic reasons. Options include cryotherapy, chemical peels, laser therapy, and bleaching creams containing hydroquinone.

NEVUS (MOLE)

Nevi are common benign growths, usually hyperpigmented or skin-colored macules, papules, or small plaques, probably derived from proliferating altered melanocytes (nevus cells). Age, race, and genetic and environmental factors (primarily sun exposure) all contribute to the development of nevi for any particular patient. Nevi can develop anywhere on the body and usually declare themselves by the early adult years. Most nevi are categorized by histologic subtypes: junctional, compound, or intradermal. *Junctional nevi* are hyperpigmented macules composed of nevus cells located in the epidermis (Fig. 5); compound nevi are hyperpigmented papules composed of nevus cells in both the epidermis and dermis; and intradermal nevi are brown to flesh-colored soft papules with nevus cells confined to the dermis (Fig. 6).

The blue nevus is a well-circumscribed, blue-black, dome-shaped papule commonly mistaken for melanoma. Blue nevi are collections of nevus cells, melanocytes, and macrophages containing melanin in the dermis. They are most often found on the dorsal surfaces of the hands and feet (Fig. 7).

Some nevi may be atypical (dysplastic), perhaps portending melanoma. Signs of atypia or perhaps even melanoma include *A*symmetry, irregular *B*order, uneven or multiple *C*olors, and large *D*iameter (>6 mm). These features constitute the ABCDs of melanoma. If such features are present, a dermatologic evaluation is warranted, and a biopsy may be necessary. An excisional biopsy is preferred to allow histologic evaluation of the entire lesion.

Persons who have many atypical moles often have a family history of atypical nevi and might have a family history of melanoma. Such persons have an increased risk of melanoma and deserve a regular dermatologic evaluation in addition to regular self examinations.

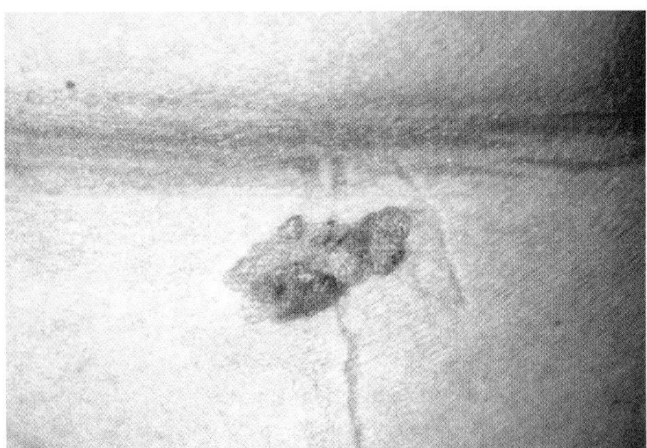

Figure 1 **Seborrheic keratosis.**

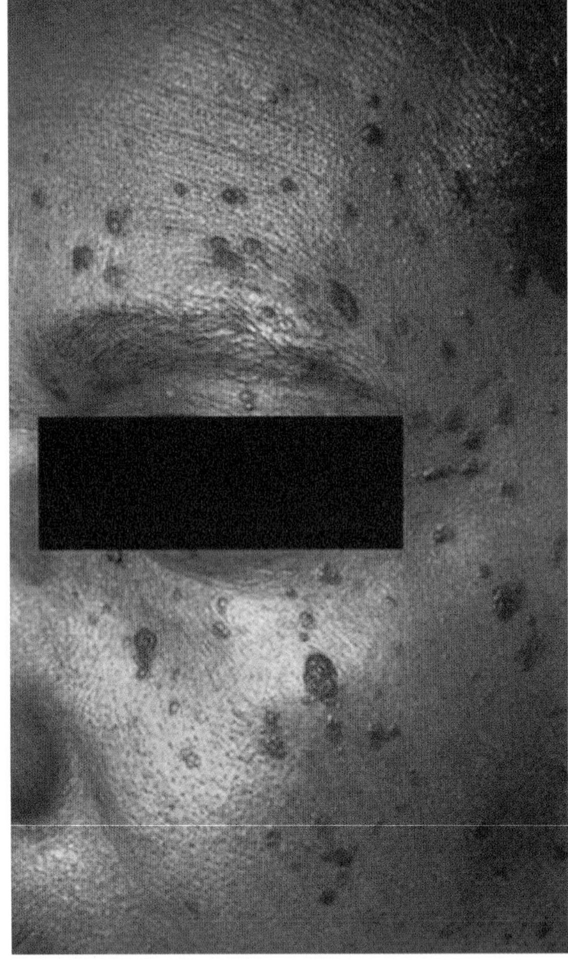

Figure 2 **Dermatosis papulosa nigra.**

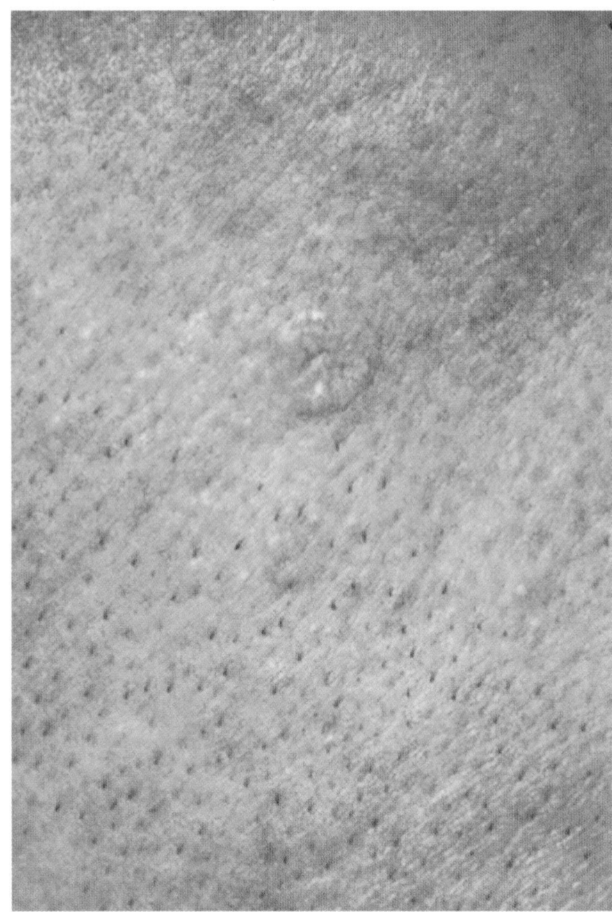

Figure 3 **Sebaceous hyperplasia.**

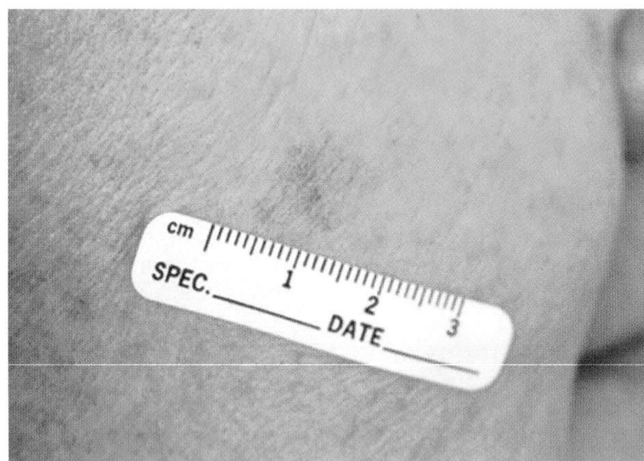

Figure 4 **Solar lentigo.**

CHERRY ANGIOMA

Cherry angiomas are ubiquitous benign vascular growths, usually small red papules or macules, that occur in adults and increase in number with age (Fig. 8).

Angiomas can appear anywhere on the body but tend to be more common on the trunk and proximal extremities. They are invariably asymptomatic but can bleed with trauma. Treatment is not necessary, but laser therapy is the most successful means of destruction for cosmetic purposes.

DERMATOFIBROMA

Dermatofibromas are firm papules or plaques with a dusky red to brown color. They are most commonly found on the extremities (Fig. 9).

With palpation, they often seem to retract, giving the dimple sign. Dermatofibromas are benign tumors of fibroblast and histiocytic origin that can follow trauma. They are usually asymptomatic but occasionally are pruritic or irritated.

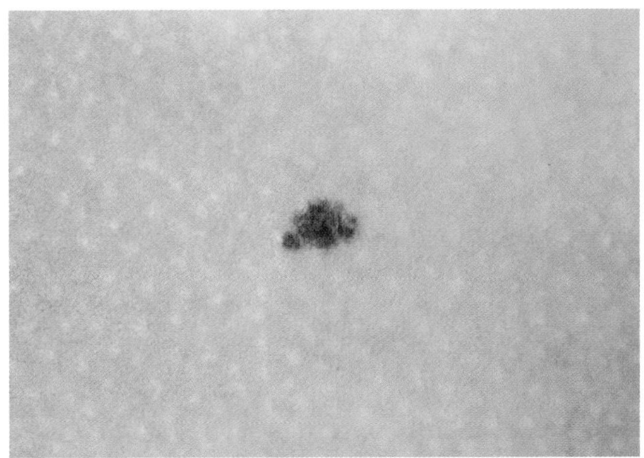

Figure 5 **Junctional nevus.**

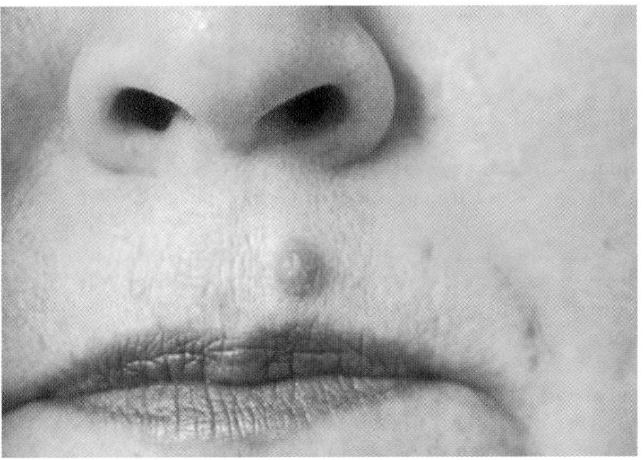

Figure 6 **Intradermal nevus.**

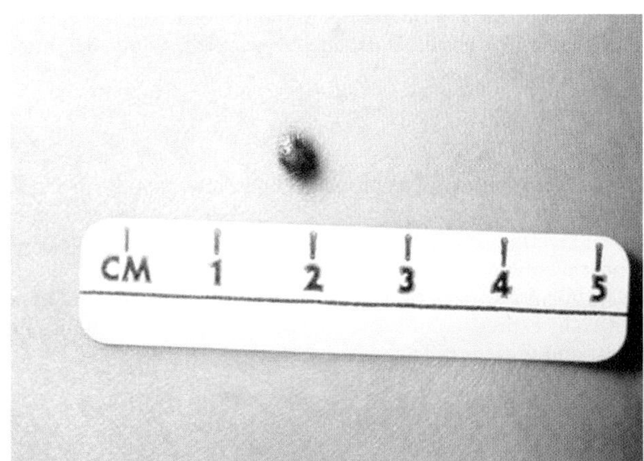

Figure 7 **Blue nevus.**

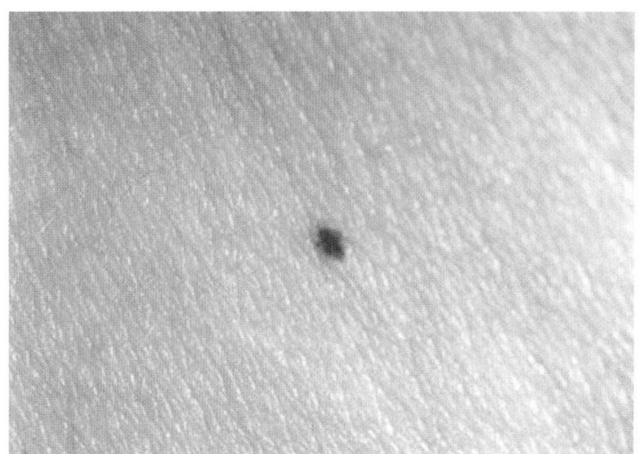

Figure 8 **Cherry angioma.**

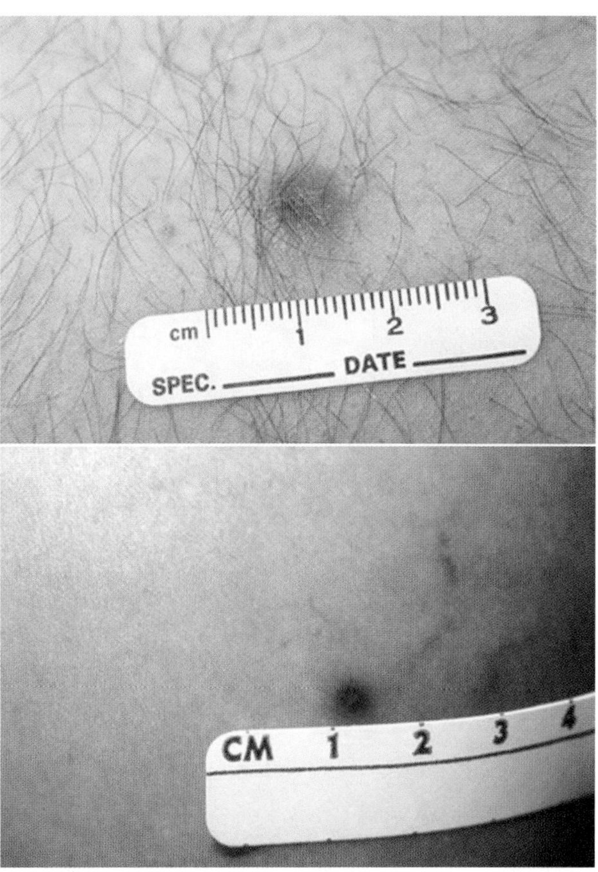

Figure 9 **Dermatofibromas.**

When indicated, therapy involves intralesional corticosteroids or simple excision.

ACROCHORDON (SKIN TAG)

Acrochordons are pedunculated flesh-colored to brown soft papules commonly found in intertriginous areas such as the neck, axillae, and groin (Fig. 10).

Increased numbers of acrochordons tend to occur in obesity and pregnancy. Occasionally, acrochordons twist and strangulate their blood supply, resulting in pain or irritation, or they become irritated from clothing or jewelry.

Treatment with simple snip excision is usually adequate.

LIPOMA

Lipomas are benign, soft, mobile tumors of fat that vary in size from a few millimeters to 10 centimeters or more (Fig. 11).

Lipomas are characterized by slow growth, with eventual stabilization and little tendency to involute. They are usually solitary

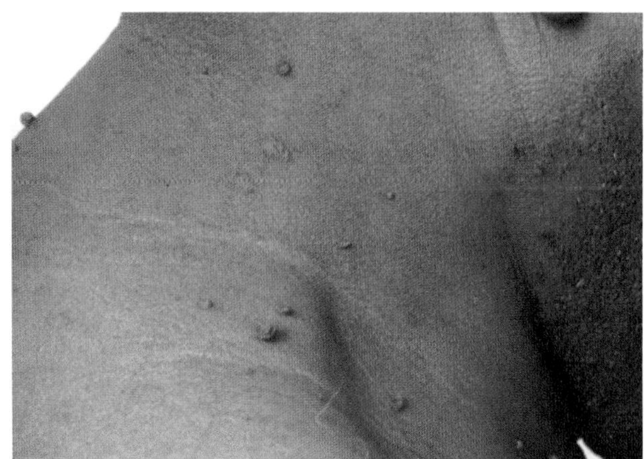

Figure 10 **Acrochordons.**

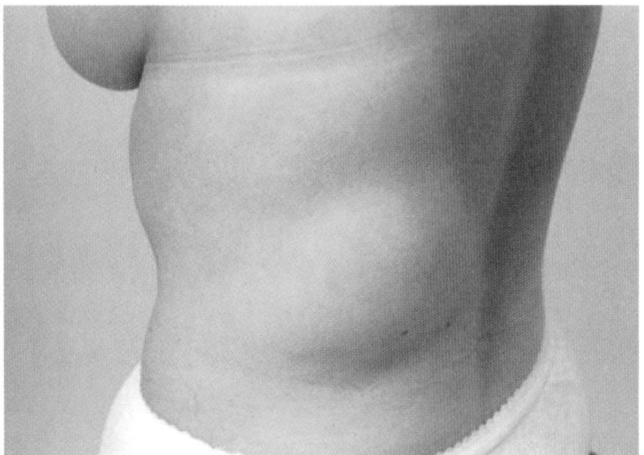

Figure 11 **Lipoma.**

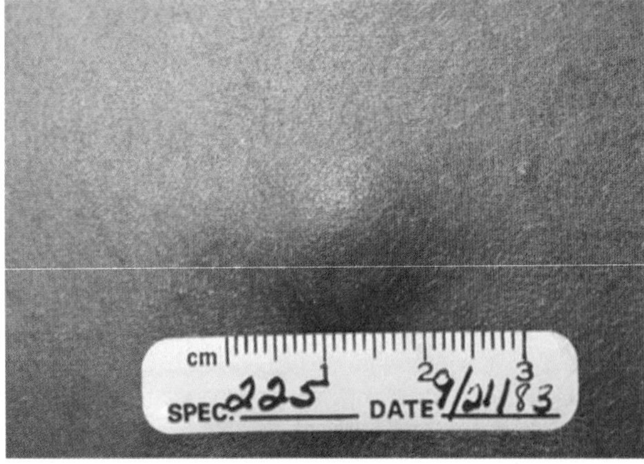

Figure 12 **Epidermal inclusion cyst.**

and asymptomatic but may be painful if they entrap or compress nerves or if they contain thrombosed vessels (a variant termed *angiolipoma*). Some familial syndromes exhibit numerous lipomas, such as Proteus syndrome and Gardener's syndrome. A lipoma overlying the sacrum of an infant can indicate an underlying spinal abnormality, a situation that warrants radiographic evaluation.

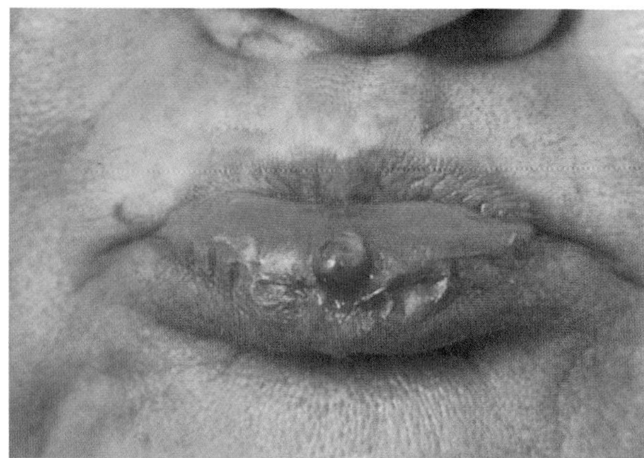

Figure 13 **Pyogenic granuloma.**

Treatment, when desired or necessary, is either excision or liposuction.

EPIDERMAL INCLUSION CYST

Epidermal inclusion cysts (EICs) are flesh-colored, firm nodules with a central punctum, usually found on the face or upper trunk of adults (Fig. 12).

The central punctum is the follicular opening from which the cyst is derived. As the name implies, EICs evolve from fully differentiated squamous epithelium trapped in the dermis with accumulation of keratinaceous debris. "EICs" on the scalp are actually pilar cysts or trichilemmal cysts and can be distinguished histologically. The presence of many EICs is occasionally associated with syndromes that have other dermatologic and internal implications, such as Gardener's syndrome.

Unless the cyst ruptures, EICs do not require therapy. When they do rupture, inflammation and pain occur that warrant treatment with incision and drainage, warm compresses, and often intralesional corticosteroids and even systemic antibiotics for secondary infection. In that scenario, excision is usually recommended after the inflammation subsides.

MILIUM

Milia are asymptomatic small white or yellow papules that occur primarily on the faces of women and newborns. These cystic collections of keratin just under the epidermal surface can also occur with porphyria cutanea tarda and other blistering diseases.

Treatment is usually for cosmetic reasons and consists of incision followed by expression of cystic contents. Topical tretinoin may help to treat and prevent milia in affected persons.

PYOGENIC GRANULOMA

Pyogenic granulomas are solitary, often pedunculated, erythematous papules or small nodules that are often friable and bleed easily with minor trauma. Sites of predilection include the fingers, face, and lips (Fig. 13).

Pyogenic granulomas develop rapidly (over the course of several weeks), and the sudden occurrence can be quite alarming to the patient. They probably represent a reactive neovascularization, potentially in response to injury. Pyogenic granulomas are common in pregnancy; termed *granuloma gravidarum*, they usually arise on the gingival mucosa.

Treatment options include curettage, deep shave excision with fulguration of the base, complete excision, or laser ablation. Recurrence is common, especially after incomplete removal.

Summary

- Most skin growths are benign and harmless, but differentiation from malignancy is essential.
- Certain benign growths can indicate a systemic condition, including hormonal disorders.
- Most benign growths do not require treatment unless they produce symptoms.
- A skin biopsy may be needed to evaluate lesions that have changed or that display characteristics of cutaneous malignancy.

Suggested Readings

Pariser RJ: Benign neoplasms of the skin. Med Clin North Am 1998;82:1285-1307.

Silver SG, Ho VC: Benign epithelial tumors. In Fitzpatrick TB, Freedberg IM, Eisen AZ, et al (eds): Dermatology in General Medicine, 6th ed. New York, McGraw-Hill, 2003, pp 767-785.

Melanoma

Rebecca Tung and *Alison Vidimos*

More than 1 million cases of skin cancer will be diagnosed in the United States this year. About 80% of these new skin cancer cases will be basal cell carcinoma, 16% will be squamous cell carcinoma, and 4% will be melanoma. It has been estimated that regular application of sunscreen with a sun protection factor of 15 or greater for the first 18 years of life would reduce the lifetime incidence of nonmelanoma skin cancers by 78%. Although nonmelanoma skin cancers (basal and squamous cell carcinomas) are the most common types of malignancies in humans, melanoma ranks as the sixth most common cancer.

Although the number of nonmelanoma skin cancers is staggering, they have a better than 95% cure rate if detected and treated early. Mortality is higher with melanoma: An estimated 8110 deaths resulted from melanoma in 2007. Because it has been shown that early detection has led to overall increased survival rates for melanoma patients, it is of utmost importance for all physicians to possess the clinical diagnostic skills necessary to identify early melanoma lesions and then refer patients for further appropriate evaluation and treatment.

DEFINITION

Cutaneous malignant melanoma is a neoplasm arising from the melanocytes that can occur de novo or from a preexisting lesion such as a congenital, acquired, or atypical (dysplastic) nevus. Noncutaneous primary sites of melanocytes also include the mucosal epithelium, retinas, and leptomeninges. Because melanoma is potentially curable with surgical excision of early, thin lesions, prompt detection, diagnosis, and adequate removal of such lesions are of utmost importance. Education of the public with regard to the technique of routine self-examination and proper methods of sun protection can greatly improve the chances for early detection and adequate treatment of melanoma (Box 1). A multidisciplinary approach, including primary care physicians, dermatologists, surgeons, oncologists, immunologists, radiologists, pathologists, and epidemiologists is necessary to optimize detection and treatment of this increasingly common cancer.

PREVALENCE AND RISK FACTORS

Recent U.S. incidence figures estimate that there were about 108,230 new cases of melanoma in 2007: 48,290 in situ (noninvasive) and 59,940 invasive (33,910 men and 26,030 women). At current rates, 1 in 63 Americans will develop an invasive melanoma over a lifetime. One person dies of melanoma every hour. In 2007, about 8110 deaths were attributed to melanoma: 5220 men and 2890 women. Older white men have the highest mortality rates from melanoma. Melanoma is the sixth most common cancer in men and women. Melanoma is the second most common cancer in women ages 20 to 29 in the United States. The incidence of melanoma has increased 690% from 1950 to 2001. Apart from these statistics, if melanoma is detected and treated before it spreads, the 5-year survival rate is 99%.[1,2]

PATHOPHYSIOLOGY

Evidence from epidemiologic studies shows that exposure to solar irradiation is the main cause of cutaneous melanoma in fair-complected persons.[3,4] This causal relation is supported by anatomic differences by sex, migration studies, difference in latitude of residence, and racial differences.

The most common site for melanoma in men is the upper back; in women, the most common sites are the lower legs and upper back.[3] Studies have also shown that persons who immigrated to countries with higher levels of ambient solar radiation have increased rates of melanoma compared with similar people who did not move. Likewise, melanoma incidence and mortality rates in white persons were inversely correlated with distance from the equator. Racial differences also exist with respect to melanoma. The lower rate of melanoma in darkly pigmented persons results from the protective effect of melanin and smaller number of nevi that can serve as precursor lesions for melanoma. The main risk factors for cutaneous melanoma include phenotype (blue eyes, blond or red hair, and fair complexion), cutaneous reaction to sun exposure (freckling, inability to tan, sunburn tendency), history of severe (blistering) sunburns or intense intermittent sun exposures, upper socioeconomic status, family history of melanoma, number and subtypes of nevi (atypical nevi or giant melanocytic nevi), history of prior melanoma, and immunosuppression.[3,5]

Genetic studies have also shown that 50% of familial melanomas and 25% of sporadic melanomas may be due to mutations in the tumor suppressor gene *p16*.[6] Linkage studies have identified chromosome 9p21 as the familial melanoma gene.[6] About 8% to 12% of all melanoma cases are familial melanoma. The familial melanoma syndrome (also known as the dysplastic nevus syndrome) has been defined as melanoma in one or more first- or second-degree relatives; large numbers of melanocytic nevi (often 50 to 100 or more), some of which are atypical and varied in size; and melanocytic nevi demonstrating certain histologic features. The mode of inheritance is most likely polygenic. The cumulative risk of developing cutaneous melanoma among persons with a history of familial melanoma is estimated to be approximately 50% by 50 years of age.[6]

Mutations in the gene *CDKN2A* within the 9p21 region have been demonstrated in familial melanoma kindreds. The *CDKN2A* gene is complex and codes for p16 and p14ARF, which both function to suppress cellular growth. An intact p16 inhibits cyclin-dependent kinases, a critical class of enzymes, whose function is to promote cellular proliferation by inhibiting the retinoblastoma protein. Therefore, an intact p16 is essential to arrest the cell cycle. p14ARF may be important in enhancing the effect of another tumor suppressor, *p53*.[6]

Five stages of tumor progression have been suggested:

1. Benign melanocytic nevi
2. Melanocytic nevi with architectural and cytologic atypia (dysplastic nevi)
3. Primary malignant melanoma, radial growth phase
4. Primary malignant melanoma, vertical growth phase
5. Metastatic malignant melanoma

Each step in tumorigenesis is marked by a new clone of cells with growth advantages over the surrounding tissues.

SIGNS AND SYMPTOMS

Early signs of melanoma include the ABCDEs: *a*symmetry of lesion; *b*order irregularity, bleeding, or crusting; *c*olor change or variegation (some lesions are amelanotic [nonpigmented]); *d*iameter larger than 6 mm or growing lesion; *e*volving (surface changes [raised, bleeding, crusting] or symptomatic [itchiness or tenderness]). About 1% to

Box 1 American Academy of Dermatology Sun Safety Tips

Because overt exposure to ultraviolet light contributes to the formation of skin cancer, dermatologists recommend the following precautions.

Avoid peak sunlight hours—10 A.M. until 4 P.M.—when the sun's rays are the strongest.

Apply a broad-spectrum sunscreen, one that protects against UVA and UVB rays with SPF 15 or higher.

- Sunscreens with the following ingredients provide broad-spectrum protection:
  - Benzophenones (oxybenzone)
  - Cinnamates (octylmethyl cinnamate and cinoxate)
  - Sulisobenzone
  - Salicylates
  - Avobenzone (Parsol 1789), ecamsule (Mexoryl).
- For people with sensitive skin, chemical-free sunblocks containing titanium dioxide or zinc oxide, which also afford broad-spectrum coverage, can be used.

Reapply sunscreen every 2 hours, especially after swimming or heavy perspiration.

Wear protective clothing including a wide-brimmed hat, sunglasses, long-sleeved shirt, and long pants.

Apply lip balm that contains sunscreen with SPF 15 or higher.

Seek shade while outdoors during the day.

Protect children by minimizing sun exposure and regularly applying sunscreen. This is crucial because excessive sun exposure in the first 18 years of life increases a person's chances of developing melanoma. Eighty percent of lifetime sun exposure occurs before age 18 years.

Avoid reflective surfaces such as water, snow, and sand that can reflect up to 85% of the sun's damaging rays.

Avoid tanning beds.

SPF, sun protection factor; UVA, ultraviolet A; UVB, ultraviolet B.

Adapted from Sober AJ, Chuang TY, Duvic M, et al, for the Guidelines/Outcomes Committee. Guidelines of care for primary cutaneous melanoma. J Am Acad Dermatol 2001;45:579-586.

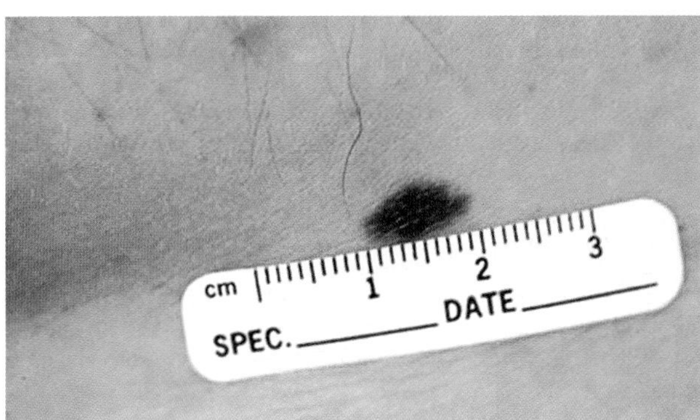

Figure 1 **Atypical nevus on the chest.**

2% of primary melanomas arise from mucous membrane melanocytes. Approximately 5% to 10% of patients present with metastatic disease (usually in the lymph node basin) without an identifiable primary lesion. Less than 2% of patients present with visceral metastases in the absence of an unknown primary lesion.

Precursor Lesions

Acquired dysplastic nevi (Fig. 1) are atypical-appearing melanocytic tumors that are histologically characterized by intraepidermal melanocytic dysplasia. Dysplastic nevi are important because they are potential histogenic precursors of melanoma and markers of increased melanoma risk. Dysplastic nevi are fairly common; in the United States, 1.8% to 4.9% of white adults have dysplastic nevi. Dysplastic nevi start as rather large moles during the first decade of life. Almost 40% of children from families with dysplastic nevi melanoma have dysplastic nevi, and all children in whom melanoma eventually develops have dysplastic nevi. At least 17% of white adults with melanoma outside the familial melanoma setting have one or more dysplastic nevi, illustrating that dysplastic nevi are markers of risk, as well as potential precursors.

Clinically, dysplastic nevi appear by age 20 years as two or more disorderly distributed shades of brown and black. They may be round, oval, or misshapen with an irregular or fuzzy outline. Any site may be affected, even sun-protected sites. The horse-collar area is usually most heavily involved.[7]

Management for patients who have dysplastic nevi, with or without a personal or family history of melanoma, is controversial. Pathologic confirmation of the clinical diagnosis provides a more solid basis for making further management decisions. For people who have one or two suspected dysplastic nevi, excision is reasonable, but periodic examinations should be offered for a lifetime.[7] Prophylactic removal of suspected dysplastic nevi is not feasible for people who have numerous dysplastic nevi. In patients with many dysplastic nevi, excision for hard-to-monitor areas (scalp, perineum, etc.) should be considered, and serial clinical photography of other lesions should be performed to detect new or changing lesions. Persons with dysplastic nevi should also be instructed on how to practice skin self-examination every 4 to 6 weeks at home.

For the removal of dysplastic nevi, lateral margins of about 2 to 3 mm should be taken to ensure complete removal.[7] Dysplastic nevi can remain unchanged, progress to melanoma, or even regress over time. Only a small fraction of dysplastic nevi ever progress to melanoma, even in the familial melanoma setting. It is probable that both environmental and genetic factors play a role in the transition from dysplastic nevus to melanoma. In Greene and colleagues' study of dysplastic nevi-melanoma kindreds, they found the actuarial probability of melanoma developing in persons who have dysplastic nevi in the familial melanoma setting may be as high as 56% from age 20 to 59 years and 100% by age 76 years.[8]

In summary, dysplastic nevi should be considered potential precursor lesions to melanoma and deserve careful surveillance and prompt treatment when required.

A short discussion on congenital nevi (Fig. 2) is presented here because patients often are concerned with the malignant potential of these lesions. A congenital nevus is defined as a melanocytic nevus that is present at birth or appears within the first few months of life. They are classified by size as small (<1.5 cm), medium (1.5-20.0 cm), and large (>20.0 cm). The risk of developing cutaneous melanoma within small- and medium-sized lesions is low but can be 1% over a lifetime. Conversely, large congenital nevi have an increased incidence of melanoma of up to 10% over a lifetime. Approximately 50% of the melanomas that develop within large congenital nevi do so by age 3 to 5 years, and patients have a melanoma risk of approximately 5% during the first 5 years of life.[9] Therefore, smaller congenital nevi can be followed clinically, but early and complete surgical excision of large congenital nevi is usually recommended. If complete removal is not possible, the lesion should be closely observed and any nodules or suspicious changes should be biopsied.

Subtypes

The subtypes of melanoma are distinguished by clinical and pathologic growth patterns: superficial spreading, lentigo maligna, nodular, and acral lentiginous.

Lentigo Maligna and Lentigo Maligna Melanoma

Lentigo maligna (melanoma in situ) (Fig. 3) begins as a tan irregular macule that extends peripherally, with differing shades throughout. It occurs on sun-damaged atrophic skin in elderly persons. Lentigo maligna occurs equally in men and women, usually in the seventh

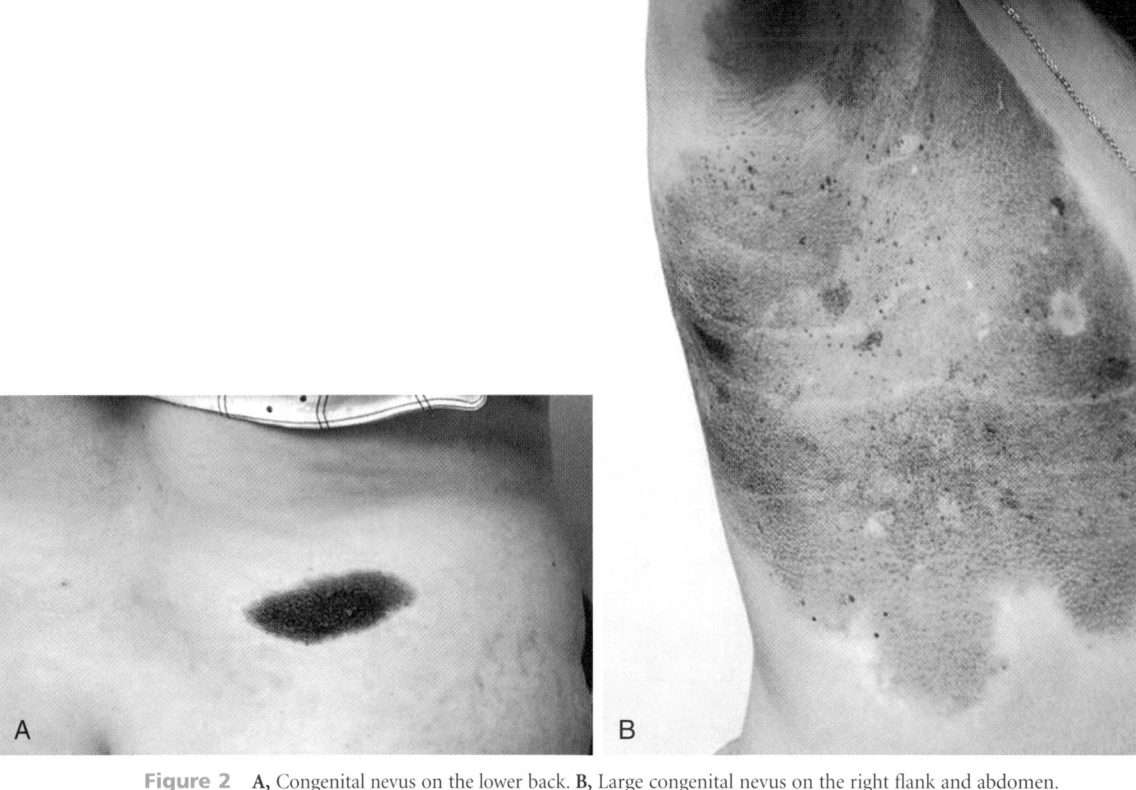

Figure 2 **A,** Congenital nevus on the lower back. **B,** Large congenital nevus on the right flank and abdomen.

and eighth decades of life.[7] The exact percentage of lentigo maligna that progress to invasive lentigo maligna melanoma is unknown, but it is estimated to be less than 30% to 50%. The lesion can grow slowly for 5 to 15 years in the precursor form before invasion.[7] Although lentigo maligna has a prolonged radial growth phase, when invasion occurs, the result can be lethal. Long-term cumulative rather than intermittent sun exposure is believed to confer the greatest risk for developing lentigo maligna.

Lentigo maligna melanoma arises from lentigo maligna, a melanoma in situ (within the epidermis). Lentigo maligna melanoma is the least common subtype of melanoma, accounting for 4% to 15% of all melanoma patients.[7] Lentigo maligna melanoma occurs almost exclusively on the sun-exposed skin of the head and neck; the nose and cheeks are the most common sites.[10] Median age at diagnosis is 65 years. The lesion is usually quite large (3-6 cm or greater), with a variable nodular area from 1 mm to 2 cm in width.[10] Rarely, lentigo maligna and lentigo maligna melanoma are amelanotic.

Superficial Spreading Melanoma

Superficial spreading melanoma (SSM) (Fig. 4) represents approximately 70% of all melanomas and is the most common type of cutaneous melanoma occurring in light-skinned people. It affects adults of all ages, with the peak incidence in the fourth and fifth decades of life. SSM, not uncommonly, can arise in a preexisting melanocytic nevus. The usual history is that of a slowly changing mole over 1 to 5 years.[7] SSM most commonly affects intermittently sun-exposed areas with the greatest nevus density, such as the upper backs of men and women and lower legs of women.

Clinically, SSM starts as a deeply pigmented macule or plaque with intact skin markings. The earliest change in SSM can be a focal area of darkening within a preexisting nevus. Pigment variegation ranges from black and blue-gray to pink or gray-white. Absence of pigmentation within an SSM often represents regression of the melanoma, and the borders are often extremely irregular. The SSM subtype usually manifests with the classic early signs of melanoma (ABCDEs).

Nodular Melanoma

The second most common subtype of melanoma is nodular melanoma (Fig. 5). Nodular melanoma represents 15% of all melanomas. The median age at onset is 53 years. Clinically, nodular melanoma manifests as a uniform blue-black, blue-red, or amelanotic nodule. About 5% of nodular melanomas lack pigment (amelanotic melanoma). The most common sites for nodular melanoma are the trunk, head, and neck. It is more common for nodular melanoma to begin in normal skin rather than in a preexisting lesion. Rapid growth is also a hallmark of nodular melanoma.

Acral Lentiginous Melanoma

Acral lentiginous melanoma (Fig. 6) accounts for 10% of melanomas overall; however, they are the most common types among Japanese, African Americans, Latin Americans, and Native Americans. The median age for occurrence is 65 years, with equal gender distribution. The most common site of melanoma in African Americans is the feet, with 60% of patients having subungual or plantar lesions.[7] Overall, acral lentiginous melanoma can occur on the palms or soles or beneath the nail plate; the sole is the most common site in all races. The average size at diagnosis is 3 cm, which may be related to delayed diagnosis. Clinically, the lesion is characterized by a tan, brown-to-

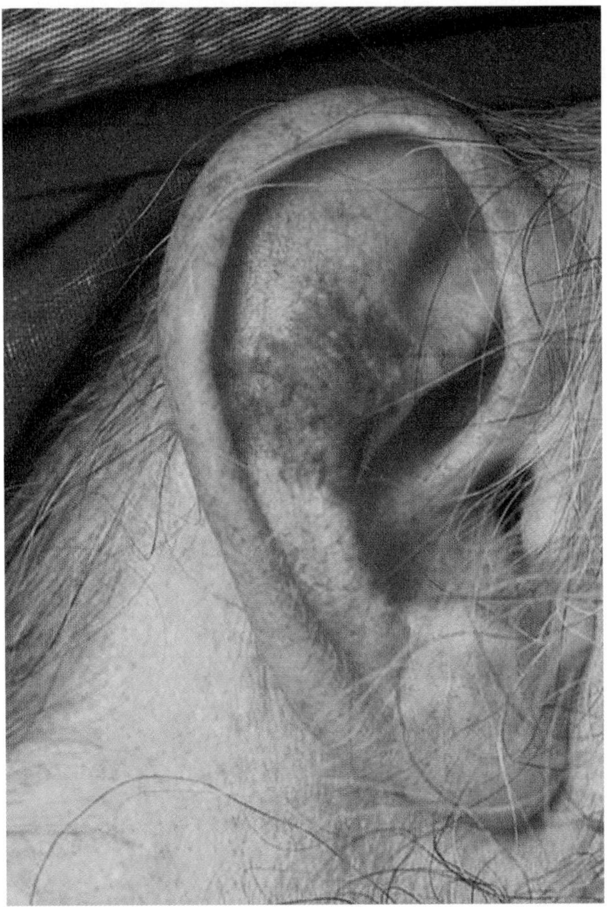

Figure 3 **Lentigo maligna on the right ear.**

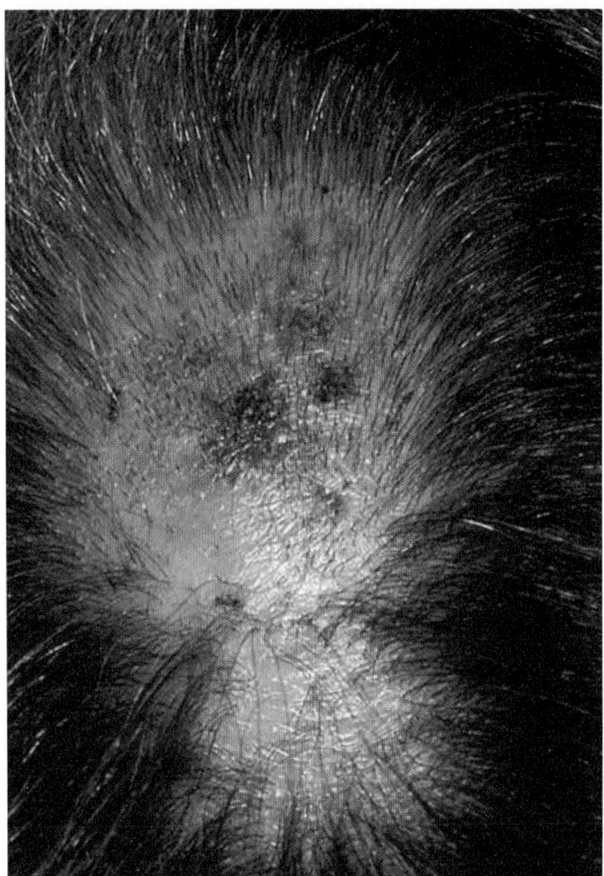

Figure 4 **Superficial spreading melanoma within plaque of lichen planopilaris.**

black, flat macule with color variegation and irregular borders. Unlike lentigo maligna melanoma, development of acral lentiginous melanoma does not seem to be associated with sun exposure.

Subungual melanoma (Fig. 7) is a rare variant of acral lentiginous melanoma. Most subungual melanomas involve the great toe or thumb and generally arise from the nail matrix. Hutchinson's sign is the finding of pigmentation on the posterior nail fold and is associated with advanced subungual melanoma.[7]

Other more uncommon variants of melanoma include melanoma of the mucosa (Fig. 8) and desmoplastic melanoma. When melanoma occurs on the mucosa, it usually develops on the mucosal surfaces of the head and neck (nasal and oral cavities), genital, or anorectal mucosa. Patients can present with bleeding or a mass lesion.

Desmoplastic Melanoma

Desmoplastic melanoma (Fig. 9) is a rare subtype of melanoma that is locally aggressive and has a high rate of local recurrence. It most commonly develops on sun-exposed skin of the head and neck of elderly persons in the sixth or seventh decade of life. Desmoplastic melanoma has a male predominance ratio of approximately 2:1. Approximately one half of desmoplastic melanomas develop in association with a lentigo maligna. Desmoplastic melanoma can manifest clinically as a pigmented macule with or without a nodular component or as a flesh-colored nodule without any surrounding pigmentation. Desmoplastic melanomas often invade perineurally and are, therefore, often symptomatic. Most desmoplastic melanomas are deeply invasive at the time of diagnosis, at least 5 to 6 mm thick. They have a propensity to recur and deeply invade locally.

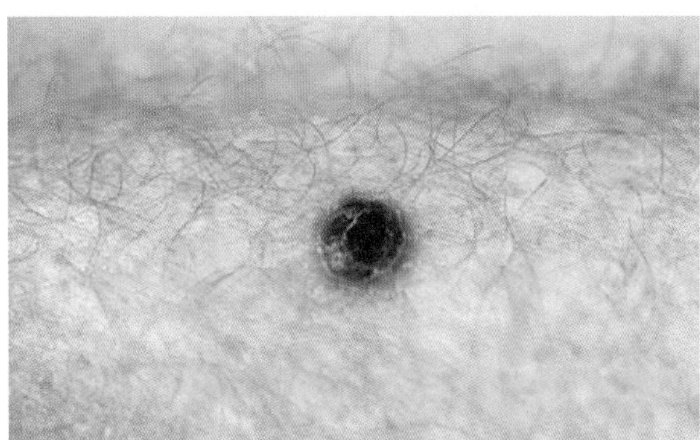

Figure 5 **Nodular melanoma on the forearm.**

DIAGNOSIS

As with nonmelanoma skin cancers, biopsy is indicated for all suspicious pigmented lesions. Surface epiluminescence microscopy (dermatoscopy) and ultrasound are evolving adjunctive noninvasive diagnostic techniques.[4] According to the American Academy of Dermatology (AAD) guidelines, whenever possible the lesion should be excised with narrow margins for diagnostic purposes. An incisional biopsy technique is appropriate when suspicion for melanoma is low, the lesion is large, or it is impractical to perform a complete excision. A repeat biopsy should be performed if the initial biopsy specimen is inadequate for accurate histologic diagnosis or staging. Fine needle aspiration cytology should not be used to assess the primary tumor. Histologic interpretation should be performed by a pathologist experienced in the microscopic diagnosis of pigmented lesions.[4] The differential diagnosis is listed in Box 2.

Determining melanoma stage is important for planning appropriate treatment and assessing prognosis. The American Joint Commission on Cancer (AJCC) has revised the four-stage system, reflecting new findings that the Clark level (level of invasion according to depth of penetration of the dermis) offer little prognostic information for tumors thicker than 1 mm, whereas histologic ulceration consistently worsens prognosis across all tumors depths. There are now a and b (nonulcerated and ulcerated, respectively) categories for each primary tumor level, for a total of eight. A new stage, IIC, has been added, which represents clinically localized melanoma with the worst prognosis (thick, ulcerated primary tumors). The main changes of the revised AJCC staging system include simplified tumor-thickness thresholds from 0.75, 1.5, and 4.0 mm to 1.0, 2.0, and 4.0 mm; reassignment of thick tumors (>4.0 mm) from stage III to stage II; and elimination of the Clark level as a criterion except in tumors 1.0 mm thick. Additional staging criteria include presence or absence of microscopic ulceration, number of nodal metastases, metastatic burden, serum lactate dehydrogenase (LDH) level, and sentinel lymph node status.[11]

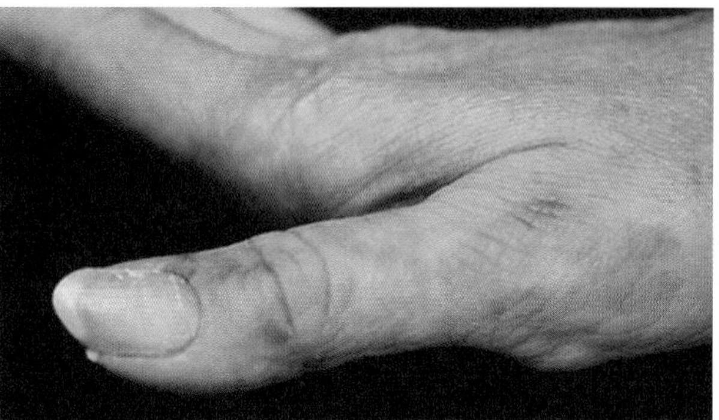

Figure 6 Acral lentiginous melanoma on the right thumb.

Eighty-five percent of melanoma patients have localized disease (stages I and II) on presentation. About 15% of patients have regional nodal disease, and only about 2% of patients have distant metastases at diagnosis. Prognosis for stages I and II melanoma can be affected by many factors. Factors associated with an improved prognosis include younger age, female gender, extremity lesions, and histologically negative nodes. Histologic variables associated with a less-favorable prognosis include increasing tumor thickness, deeper level of invasion, increased mitotic rate, ulceration, diminished lymphoid response, evidence of tumor regression, microscopic satellites, vascular invasion, and non–spindle-cell type tumors.

The presence of regional lymph node metastases imparts an overall 5-year survival rate of 37% and a 10-year survival of 32%.[12]

Box 2 Differential Diagnosis of Melanoma

- Cherry angioma
- Junctional or compound nevi
- Kaposi's sarcoma
- Pigmented basal cell carcinoma
- Pyogenic granuloma
- Seborrheic keratosis

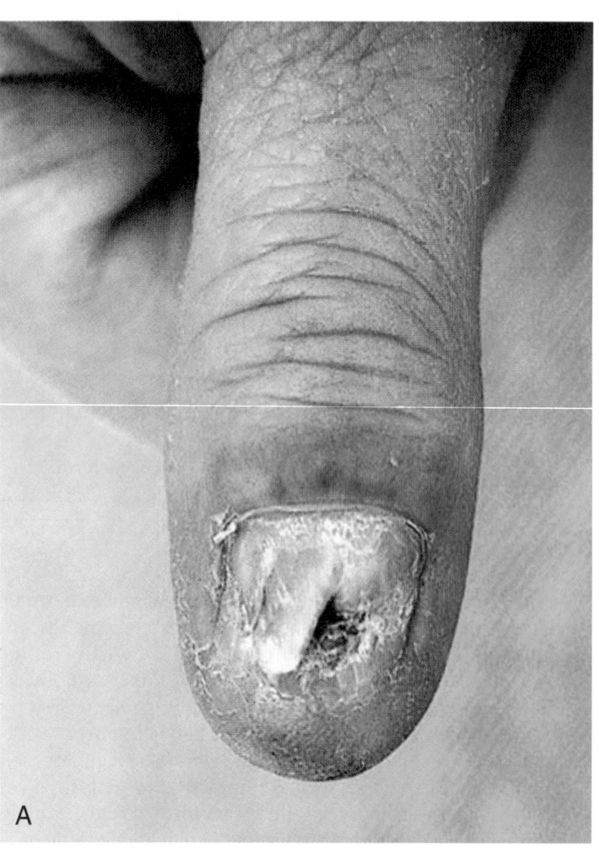

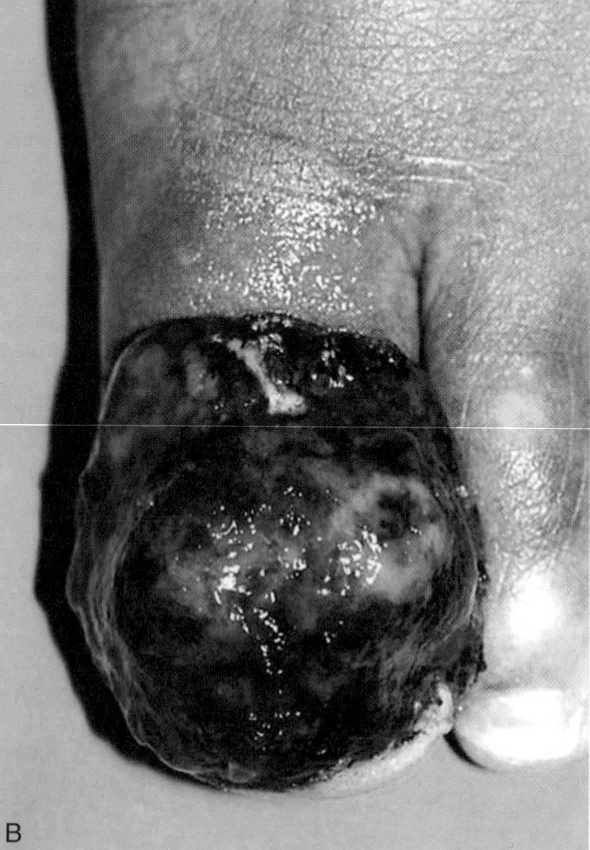

Figure 7 **A,** Subungual melanoma on the right thumbnail. **B,** Melanoma on the left toe.

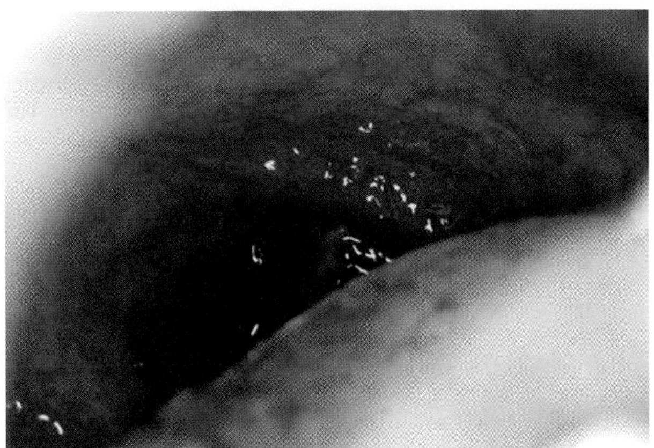

Figure 8 **Tonsillar melanoma.**

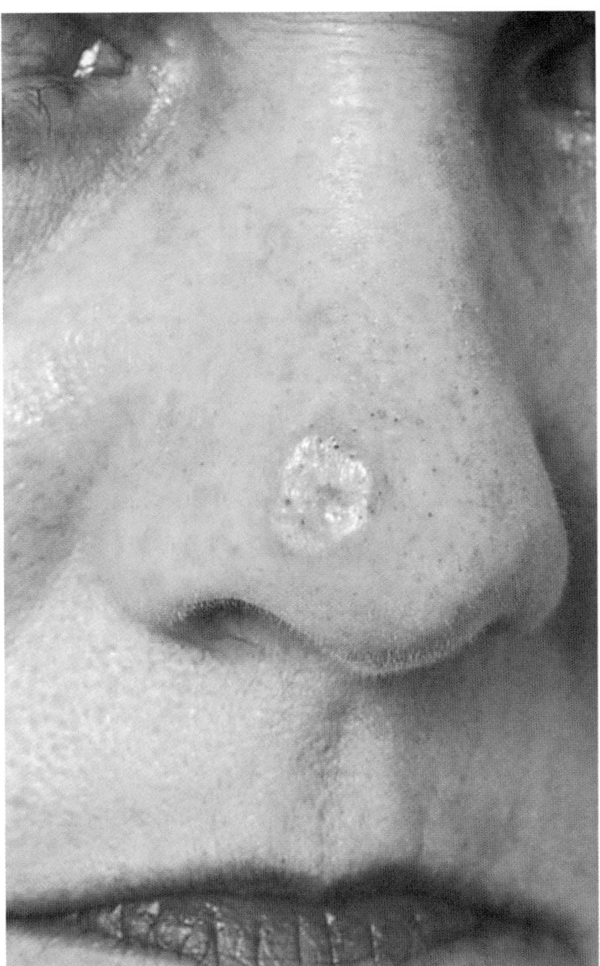

Figure 9 **Desmoplastic melanoma.**

The most important prognostic factor for stage III melanoma is the number of positive lymph nodes. Patients with nodal micrometastases have an improved survival compared with patients with clinically palpable nodes. Patients with melanoma on an extremity and younger age at diagnosis have been shown to have a better prognosis. If there are distant metastases, median survival is about 6 to 9 months.[13] For stage IV patients, the prognostic variables suggesting worse prognosis include increasing number of metastatic sites, visceral location of metastases (lung, liver, brain, bone), absence of resectable metastases, male gender, and shorter duration of remission.[13] Patients with nonvisceral disease (e.g., skin, subcutaneous tissue, lymph nodes) have a better median survival, ranging from 12 to 15 months, and are more likely to respond to chemotherapy.[13]

Summary

- Thickness of lesion
- Presence or absence of ulceration
- Number of lymph nodes involved
- Size of lymph nodes
- Presence or absence of distant metastasis

TREATMENT

According to the AAD's 2001 guidelines, surgical management of primary cutaneous melanoma should focus on obtaining an excision margin based on histologic confirmation of tumor-free margins.[4]

- Melanoma in situ: 0.5-cm margins
- Melanoma with Breslow's thickness <2 mm: 1.0-cm margins
- Melanoma with Breslow's thickness ≥2.0 mm: 2.0-cm margins

In certain circumstances, surgical management needs to be tailored to the individual case. Primary melanomas near a vital structure might require a reduced margin, and aggressive histologic features can suggest a more worrisome tumor and warrant a wider margin. Surgical excision at sites such as the fingers, toes, soles, and ears also need separate surgical considerations.

Mohs' micrographic surgery might prove useful for excision of melanoma, especially lesions located on the head, neck, hands, and feet. However, there are no formal recommendations pending additional studies.[4] Studies suggest that the current recommendation of 0.5-mm margins for lentigo maligna (melanoma in situ) is often insufficient. Mohs' micrographic surgery and margin-controlled excision of lentigo maligna offer lower recurrence rates and allow tissue to be conserved.[14,15] Despite adequate surgical resection of the primary melanoma, approximately 15% to 36% of patients with stages I and II melanoma will have some form of recurrence or metastasis during their clinical course.

Routine laboratory tests and imaging studies are not required for asymptomatic patients with primary cutaneous melanoma 4 mm or less in thickness for initial staging or routine follow-up.[4] Indications for such studies are directed by a thorough medical history and complete physical examination. However, some studies have suggested that a chest x-ray and serum lactate dehydrogenase (LDH) might help detect occult metastases and alter further clinical management.[16,17]

Elective Lymph Node Dissection

Elective lymph node dissection is defined as removing regional lymph nodes that drain the site of the primary melanoma in the absence of any clinical evidence of nodal metastases. Elective lymph node dissection is a much-debated topic in the management of melanoma. Proponents have cited retrospective studies demonstrating improved prognosis for patients with intermediate thickness (1–4 mm) lesions.[18-20] Opponents have cited prospective randomized trials that fail to show a statistically significant difference in survival rates following elective lymph node dissection.[21-23]

Sentinel Lymph Node Biopsy

Sentinel lymph node biopsy, a staging and possibly therapeutic procedure, is the most powerful predictor of melanoma recurrence and survival. Initially, lymphoscintigraphy is used to precisely map the draining nodal basin.[24] The sentinel lymph node biopsy is based on the premise that the first node draining a lymphatic basin (sentinel lymph node) would be expected to predict the absence or presence of melanoma in that area.[24] One percent isosulfan blue (Lymphazurin) dye is injected around the cutaneous lesion to allow intraoperative localization of this sentinel lymph node. Alternately, a radioactive tracer, technetium-99, can be injected at the lesion site. A gamma probe is used to pinpoint the radiolabeled lymph node, which is then removed for histopathologic review. If no melanoma cells are found, no further surgery is done. However, if the node does have melanoma cells, the remainder of the nodes in this area are removed.[24]

Determination of the status of the sentinel lymph node is relevant for several reasons. It has been shown to be an important independent prognostic factor: A positive result predicts high risk of treatment failure. It is a relatively low-risk procedure that can help identify high-risk patients who might benefit from additional therapy, such as selective complete lymphadenectomy or adjuvant interferon alfa-2b. It provides a psychological benefit for the patient whose sentinel lymph node biopsy does not reveal metastases.[2] Because positivity rates for sentinel lymph node biopsy are less than 5% for AJCC T1 melanomas, sentinel lymph node biopsy is considered a low-yield procedure in most thin melanomas. The ideal Breslow criteria for selection of this technique are not yet established.[2]

Adjuvant Treatment with Interferon

In the Eastern Cooperative Oncology Group (ECOG) 1684 study, high-dose interferon alfa-2b was initially reported to improve the survival of patients with melanoma thicker than 4 mm; however, the follow-up trial ECOG 1690 did not show an overall survival benefit. Another major study reported by the Austrian Malignant Melanoma Cooperative Group did show that adjuvant treatment with low-dose interferon alfa-2b decreased the occurrence of metastases and prolonged the disease-free survival in patients with melanoma thicker than 1.5 mm. These studies suggest that the role of interferon in the treatment of melanoma is evolving and needs further study.

Chemotherapy

Systemic chemotherapy is primarily used in patients with advanced stage III (unresectable regional metastases) or stage IV (distant metastases) melanoma. Although most chemotherapy is not that effective, dacarbazine remains the most active drug and is the only FDA-approved chemotherapeutic agent for treating advanced melanoma in the United States.[13] The response rate is in the range of 10% to 20%, and patients with metastases in the skin, subcutaneous tissues, or lymph nodes respond most often. Other combination chemotherapy and biochemotherapy regimens could achieve higher response rates but do not appear to lead to durable remission.[13]

Biologic Treatment

Therapy directed toward modulating or inducing the immune system against melanoma has gathered considerable interest in recent years. Interleukin-2 (IL-2) as a single agent has been used in metastatic melanoma. In one study, 7% of patients had a complete response, which was durable: Patients remained disease-free for up to 8 years after initiation of therapy.[25] Another study also showed positive results in treating patients with their own tumor-infiltrating lymphocytes and IL-2. Monoclonal antibody therapies are still experimental and may be useful in melanoma. Likewise, melanoma vaccines have been developed to stimulate a specific response against melanoma-associated antigens. Vaccines are currently undergoing clinical trials.

Perfusion Chemotherapy

Isolated limb perfusion has been used for melanoma of the extremities. In isolated limb perfusion, the limb is isolated from the systemic circulation with a tourniquet, using arterial and venous cannulation; a chemotherapeutic agent is infused by means of a pump oxygenator, and then the medication is removed from the limb.[26] It has been developed into the most effective method of treatment for local recurrent or in transit metastases of an extremity.[26] Medications used for infusion include melphalan, dacarbazine, cisplatin, carboplatin, thiotepa, and cytokine tumor necrosis factor α.[26]

Radiation

Radiation therapy is used for palliation in certain patients with stage IV disease. Specific indications include brain metastases, pain associated with bone metastases, and superficial skin and subcutaneous metastases.

PROGNOSIS

The prognosis for a patient with stage I or II melanoma is mainly related to tumor thickness[7] (Table 1):

- Melanoma in situ: 100% survival at 5 years and 10 years
- Lesions ≤1 mm: 91%–95% at 5 years; 83%–88% at 10 years
- Lesions 1.01–2 mm: 77%–89% at 5 years; 64%–79% at 10 years
- Lesions 2.01–4 mm: 63%–79% at 5 years; 51%–64% at 10 years
- Lesions >4 mm: 45%–67% at 5 years; 32%–54% at 10 years

If grouped according to stage for localized primary melanoma, the overall survival rate is 80%.[7] For patients with regional lymph node metastases (stage III disease), survival rates were 27% to 69% at 5 years and 18% to 63% at 10 years. Unfortunately, when there is evidence of distant metastases (stage IV disease), the 5-year survival rate is only 9% to 19%, and the 10-year survival rate is 6% to 16% (see Table 1). However, spontaneous regression has been documented in melanoma, even in patients with metastatic disease.[7]

FOLLOW-UP EVALUATION

The goal of regular follow-up evaluation of patients with melanoma is the detection of melanoma recurrence or development of a second primary melanoma. Each visit should include a detailed history and physical examination. For most patients with stage I or II melanoma, it is recommended that follow-up appointments be scheduled initially every 3 months for 2 years, then every 6 months for 3 years, then once yearly thereafter. If the patient has dysplastic nevi, the interval may be continued at every 6 months indefinitely. Photography may be helpful in following multiple clinically atypical nevi. Patients should also be taught and encouraged to practice monthly skin self-examination. Because most experts attribute the rising trend in the overall 5-year melanoma survival rate (some 40% in the 1940s to the current rate of 86%) to improved early detection, it is very important for both physicians and the public to be aware of the early warning signs of melanoma and to get appropriate dermatologic evaluation and treatment as soon as possible.

PREVENTION AND SCREEENING

Primary prevention of melanoma requires reduction of known risk factors in at-risk populations. The most important modifiable behavior for melanoma prevention is reduction of ultraviolet exposure. Education of the public regarding sun protection, risk factors for developing skin cancer, and skin self-examination is essential.[27] The American Academy of Dermatology's skin cancer awareness initiatives such as Melanoma Monday (an annual countrywide event

Table 1 American Joint Committee on Cancer 2002 Revised Melanoma Staging

Histologic Features	TNM Classification	Overall Survival		
		1-yr (%)	5-yr (%)	10-yr (%)
Stage 0				
Intraepithelial or in situ melanoma	Tis N0 M0	—	100	100
Stage I				
A				
≤1 mm without ulceration and Clark level II/III	T1a N0 M0	—	95	88
B				
≤1 mm with ulceration or level IV/V	T1b N0 M0	—	91	83
1.01-2 mm without ulceration	T2a N0 M0	—	89	79
Stage II				
A				
1.01-2 mm with ulceration	T2b N0 M0	—	77	64
2.01–4 mm without ulceration	T3a N0 M0	—	79	64
B				
2.01–4 mm with ulceration	T3b N0 M0	—	63	51
>4 mm without ulceration	T4a N0 M0	—	67	54
C				
>4 mm with ulceration	T4b N0 M0	—	45	32
Stage III				
A				
Single regional nodal micrometastasis, nonulcerated primary	T1-4a N1a M0	—	69	63
2–3 microscopic regional nodes, nonulcerated primary	T1-4a N2a M0	—	63	57
B				
Single regional nodal micrometastasis, ulcerated primary	T1-4b N1a M0	—	53	38
2–3 microscopic regional nodes, ulcerated primary	T1-4b N2a M0	—	50	36
Single regional nodal macrometastasis, nonulcerated primary	T1-4a N1b M0	—	59	48
2–3 macroscopic regional nodes, nonulcerated primary	T1-4a N2b M0	—	46	39
In-transit metastases or satellite lesion(s) *without* metastatic lymph nodes	T1-4a/b N2c M0	—	30–50	
C				
Single microscopic regional node, ulcerated primary	T1-4b N1b M0	—	29	24
2–3 macroscopic regional nodes, ulcerated primary	T1-4b N2b M0	—	24	15
4 or more metastatic nodes, matted nodes/gross extracapsular extension, or in-transit metastases ro satellite(s) *and* metastatic nodes	any T N3 M0	—	27	18
Stage IV				
Distant skin, subcutaneous, or nodal metastases with normal LDH	any T; any N; M1a	59	19	16
Lung metastases with normal LDH	any T; any N; M1b	57	7	3
All other visceral metastases with normal LDH or any distant metastases with increased LDH	any T; any N; M1c	41	9	6

Note: Thickness is defined as the thickness of the lesion using an ocular micrometer to measure the total vertical height of the melanoma from the granular layer to the area of deepest penetration. The Clark level refers to levels of invasion according to depth of penetration of the dermis.

LDH, lactate dehydrogenase; TNM, tumor, node, metastasis.

Adapted with permission from Balch CM, Buzald AC, Soong SJ, et al: Final version of the American Joint Committee on Cancer staging system for cutaneous melanoma. J Clin Oncol 2001;19:3635-3548.

Data from Balch CM, Buzaid AC, Soong SJ, et al: Final version of the American Joint Committee on Cancer staging system for cutaneous melanoma. J Clin Oncol 2001;19:3635-3648.

offering free skin cancer screenings conducted by dermatologists to raise awareness about melanoma and encourage Americans to begin a lifelong habit of regular skin examinations) and Sun Smart programs have been particularly effective in creating positive change in society's approach toward the sun.

Suggested Readings

Ali-Salaam P, Ariyan S: Lymphatic mapping and sentinel lymph node biopsies. Clin Plast Surg 2000;27:421-429.

Bub JL, Berg D, Slee A, Odland PB: Management of lentigo maligna and lentigo maligna melanoma with staged excision: A 5-year follow-up. Arch Dermatol 2004;140:552-558.

Buzzell RA, Zitelli JA: Favorable prognostic factors in recurrent and metastatic melanoma. J Am Acad Dermatol 1996;34:798-803.

Cummins DL, Cummins JM, Pantle H, et al: Cutaneous malignant melanoma. Mayo Clinic Proc 2006;81:500-507.

Klimek VM, Wolchok JD, Chapman PB, et al: Systemic chemotherapy. Clin Plast Surg 2000;27:451-461.

Odom RB, James WD, Berger TG: Melanocytic nevi and neoplasms. In James WD, Berger TG, Elston D (eds): Andrews' Diseases of the Skin, 9th ed. Philadelphia, WB Saunders, 2000, pp 881-889.

Sober AJ, Chuang TY, Duvic M, et al, for the Guidelines/Outcomes Committee: Guidelines of care for primary cutaneous melanoma. J Am Acad Dermatol 2001;45:579-586.

Tsao H, Atkins MB, Sober AJ: Management of cutaneous melanoma. N Engl J Med 2004;351:998-1012.

Tsao H: Update on familial cancer syndromes and the skin. J Am Acad Dermatol 2000;42:939-969.

Wagner JD, Gordon MS, Chuang TY, Coleman JJ 3rd: Current therapy of cutaneous melanoma. Plast Reconstr Surg 2001;105:1774-1799.

References

For a complete list of references, log onto www.expertconsult.com.

Nonmelanoma Skin Cancer

Rebecca Tung and **Allison Vidimos**

More than 1 million cases of skin cancer were diagnosed in the United States in 2007. About 80% of these new skin cancer cases were basal cell carcinoma (BCC), 16% were squamous cell carcinoma, and 4% were melanoma. On a preventive health note, it has been estimated that regular application of sunscreen with a sun protection factor (SPF) of 15 or greater for the first 18 years of life would reduce the lifetime incidence of nonmelanoma skin cancers by 78%. Although nonmelanoma skin cancers (basal and squamous cell carcinomas) are the most common types of malignancies in humans, melanoma ranks as the sixth most common cancer in men and the seventh most common in women. Although the number of nonmelanoma skin cancers is staggering, both basal cell and squamous cell carcinomas have a better than 95% cure rate if detected and treated early.

BASAL CELL CARCINOMA

Definition

BCC is the most common cutaneous malignancy in humans. This tumor is believed to arise from the pluripotential primordial cells in the basal layer of the epidermis and less often from the outer root sheath of the hair follicle or sebaceous gland or other cutaneous appendages.[1] Although BCCs grow slowly and rarely metastasize, they can cause extensive tissue destruction through direct extension, leading to significant patient morbidity if untreated.

Prevalence and Risk Factors

It is estimated that more than 800,000 cases of BCC occurred in the United States in 2007. The annual incidence in Americans is 146 cases per 100,000 people.[2] Although the incidence of BCC increases with advancing age, it is becoming more common in younger adults. An Australian study showed that the incidence of BCC is higher in men, but the incidence in women has been steadily increasing.[3] Factors such as excessive, chronic sun exposure, indoor tanning, fair complexion, prior exposure to ionizing radiation, exposure to chemical cocarcinogens such as arsenic, and genetic determinants are significant risks factors.

Pathophysiology and Natural History

The most common causative factor in the induction of BCC is ultraviolet (UV) light, specifically ultraviolet B (UVB, 290-320 nm). It has been shown that UVB induces characteristic DNA mutations in the skin called pyrimidine dimers. The *p53* tumor suppressor gene is responsible for arresting the cell cycle so that any induced mutations can be repaired by the cell. In BCC, the same UV light-induced pyrimidine dimer mutations have also been found in the *p53* tumor suppressor gene. This mutated *p53* gene is nonfunctional and leads to dysregulation of the cell cycle, with resultant unlimited cell proliferation (cancer).

Although the exact mechanism of BCC propagation is unknown, it is believed that basal cell carcinomas arise when mutations that control cell growth via the hedgehog pathway activate immature pluripotential cells in the epidermis. This most often occurs through inactivation of the tumor suppressor gene *PTC* (patched), located on chromosome 9. Other mutations in *SMO* (smoothened) and *Hh* (hedgehog) have also been seen. *RAS* and *p53* mutations may also play a role in oncogenesis. Additionally, the distinctive biologic behavior of BCC, characterized by local invasiveness but rare metastatic spread, may be related to alterations in certain basement membrane components.[4]

The natural progression of untreated BCC is slow growth with progressive invasion and destruction of adjacent tissues. Metastasis is very rare in BCC, with a relative rate of 0.0028% to 0.1%. When metastasis has occurred, the site of the primary lesion has most often been on the head and neck. The sites of BCC metastasis in order of frequency are the regional lymph nodes, lung, bone, skin, liver, and pleura. The average interval for metastasis is 9 years. Metastatic BCC has a poor prognosis, with a median survival of 8 months. BCC metastasis has usually been observed in men with large neglected ulcerated tumors.

Signs and Symptoms

BCCs are most often found on the head and neck; the nose is the most common site. The typical lesion is a small pearly (waxy) nodule with a central depression and rolled border containing dilated blood vessels. It might have a history of ulceration, crusting, or bleeding. BCC has five clinicopathologic subtypes: nodular-ulcerative, superficial, pigmented, morpheaform (sclerosing), and basosquamous.

Subtypes

Nodular-Ulcerative. The nodular-ulcerative variant (Fig. 1) is the most common type of BCC. It manifests as a small, pearly dome-shaped papule with surface telangiectasias and a typical rolled border. Over time, central ulceration with bleeding or crusting is often seen. Differential diagnosis of this lesion includes sebaceous hyperplasia, squamous cell carcinoma, verruca vulgaris virus, molluscum contagiosum, intradermal nevus, appendageal tumors, amelanotic melanoma, and stasis ulcers (when located on the shins).

Superficial. Superficial BCCs (Fig. 2) are the least aggressive form. They often manifest as several scaly, dry, round-to-oval erythematous plaques with a threadlike raised border on the trunk and extremities. If untreated, superficial BCCs can enlarge to 10 to 15 cm in diameter without ulceration. Differential diagnosis of superficial BCC includes eczema, psoriasis, and Bowen's disease.

Pigmented. Pigmented BCCs (Fig. 3) are seen more often in darker-skinned persons such as Latin Americans and Asians. This subtype has all the characteristics of the nodular-ulcerative variety plus brown or black pigmentation from melanin. A history of arsenic ingestion has been seen with pigmented and superficial BCCs.

Morpheaform (Sclerosing). An indurated yellow to white plaque with an indistinct border and an atrophic surface characterizes morpheaform or sclerosing BCC (Fig. 4). Ulceration and crusting are usually absent. This variety has an aggressive growth pattern, and invasion of muscle, nerve, and bone may be seen. Morpheaform BCC is particularly insidious because of its benign scarlike appearance. Differential diagnosis of morpheaform BCC includes scarring and localized superficial scleroderma (morphea).

Basosquamous. The basosquamous or metatypical variant of BCC is diagnosed on a histologic basis. This tumor possesses features of both BCC and SCC. It is mentioned because it is associated with a higher rate of metastasis.

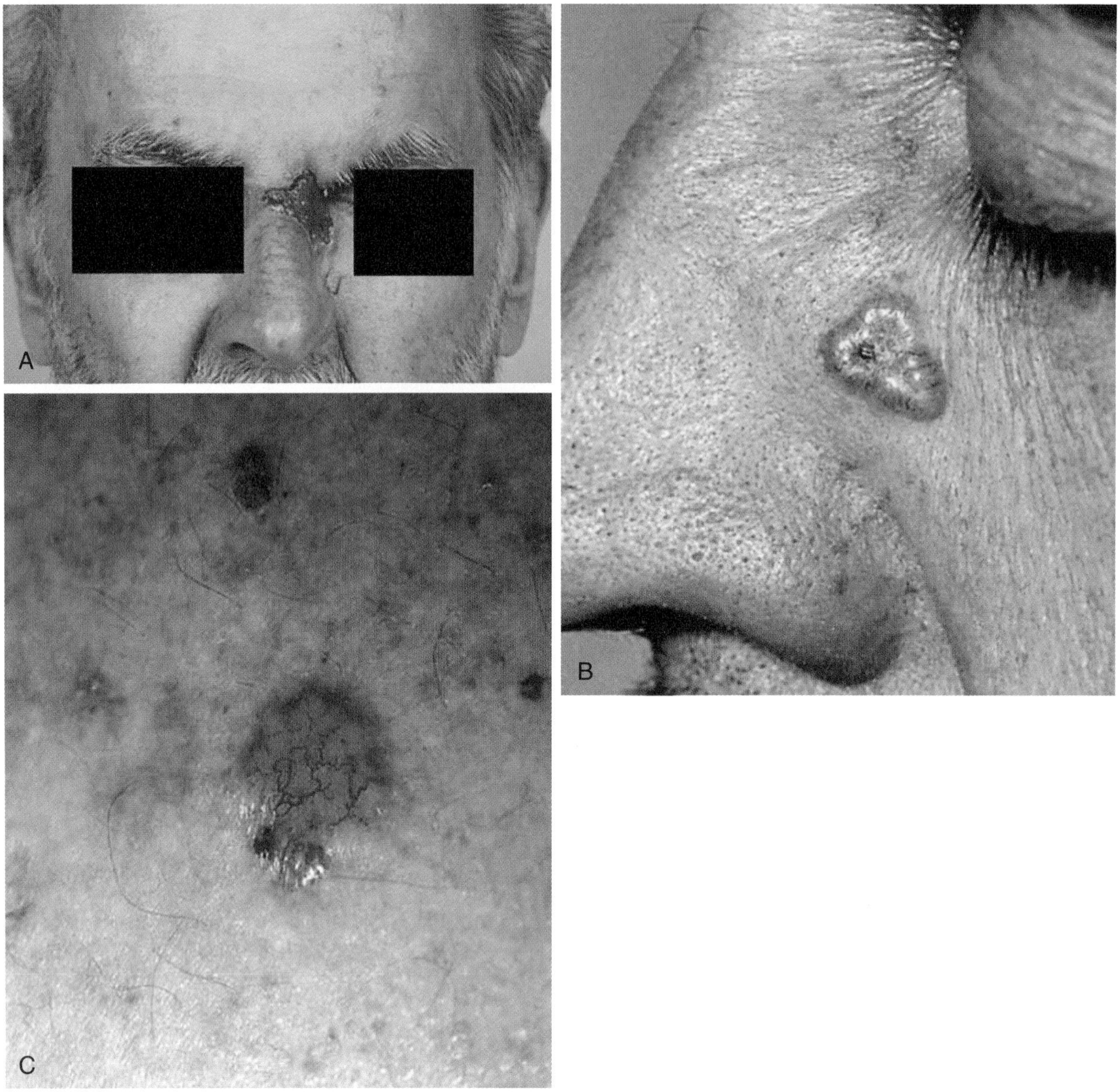

Figure 1 **A,** Noduloulcerative basal cell carcinoma, nasal bridge and medial canthus. **B,** Nodular basal cell carcinoma, left nasofacial sulcus. **C,** Nodular basal cell carcinoma.

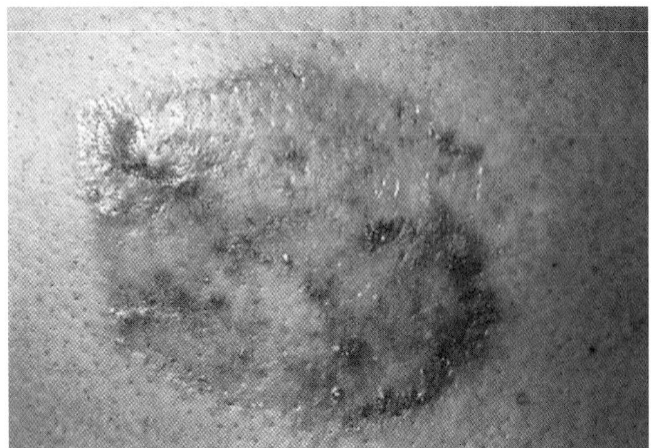

Figure 2 Superficial basal cell carcinoma.

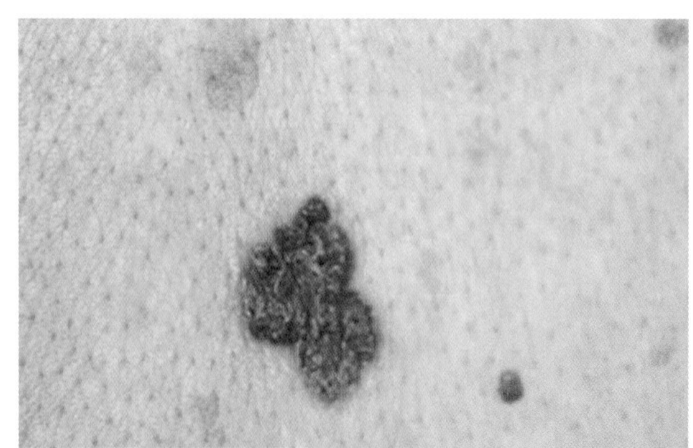

Figure 3 Pigmented basal cell carcinoma, back.

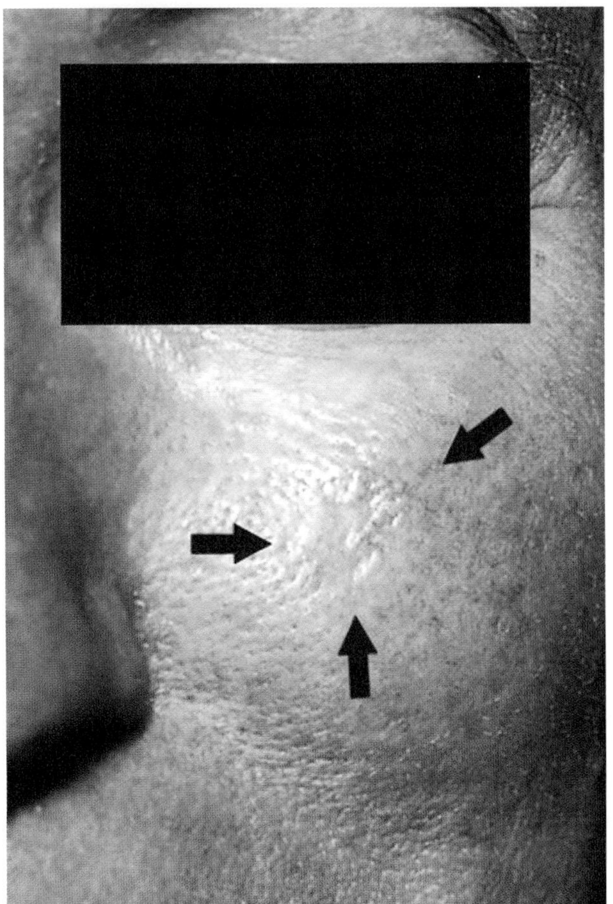

Figure 4 Morpheaform basal cell carcinoma (arrows), left cheek.

Related Syndromes

Two syndromes that have multiple BCCs as a feature include nevoid basal cell carcinoma syndrome (Gorlin's syndrome) and Basex's syndrome. Gorlin's syndrome is characterized by BCCs; odontogenic jaw cysts; pitted depression of the hands and feet; osseous anomalies of the ribs, spine, and skull; and characteristic facies (frontal bossing, hypoplastic maxilla, a broad nasal root, and true ocular hypertelorism).[5] This genetic disorder occurs in an autosomal dominant pattern. There is a mutation of the *PTC* tumor suppressor gene located on chromosome 9.[5] Basex's syndrome is another autosomally dominant inherited disorder. It is characterized by multiple BCCs of the face, follicular atrophoderma of the extremities, localized or generalized hypohidrosis, and hypotrichosis.

Diagnosis

Clinical diagnosis of BCC is confirmed by performing a biopsy of the suspected lesion for histopathologic interpretation. For the majority of BCC subtypes, a shave biopsy suffices. However, when the lesion is believed to be a morpheaform BCC, a deep shave, punch biopsy, or incisional biopsy is recommended to obtain a sufficient tissue sample for correct interpretation.

Treatment

BCC may be effectively treated by a variety of therapeutic modalities. Among the clinical subtypes of BCC, small nodular or superficial BCCs respond to most treatment options; large nodular ulcerative or morpheaform lesions can require more aggressive therapy. No single treatment method is ideal for all lesions. The treating physician should carefully evaluate each BCC on an individual basis and choose the modality that is most appropriate for the lesion's size, site, and histologic type, as well as the patient's age and functional status.[1]

Electrodesiccation and Curettage

According to the American Academy of Dermatology (AAD) Guidelines of Care, electrodesiccation and curettage (ED&C) is best suited for primary lesions, but it may be useful in some recurrent lesions. It is less effective in the cure of recurrent lesions that are in scar tissue.[1] Superficial and nodular BCCs respond especially well to ED&C. It is less effective in the cure of recurrent lesions or in the morpheaform subtype because of indistinct margins. Select low-risk lesions (small, well-defined primary lesions with nonaggressive histology usually in noncritical sites) can achieve 5-year cure rates of up to 97% when treated with ED&C.[6]

Primary nonmorpheaform basal cell carcinomas are more friable than surrounding normal skin and are initially debulked with a curette. The stroma and surrounding dermis are then electrodesiccated. This process is usually repeated two more times. The resulting wound heals with a hypopigmented scar over 2 to 6 weeks. The main disadvantage of this treatment is the absence of histologic margin control. Treatment of facial lesions with this modality is not advocated because of the risk of deep invasion in embryonal fusion planes, the difficulty of adequate curettage in the sebaceous skin of the nose, and poor cosmetic appearance.

Cryosurgery

According to the AAD Guidelines of Care, cryosurgery is useful in treating primary lesions and some recurrent lesions. It is especially useful in certain areas of the body and in patients with multiple lesions.[1] Superficial and small nodular BCCs respond well to liquid nitrogen cryosurgery. Liquid nitrogen (temperature −196° C) produces tissue destruction by reducing the temperature of the skin cancer to tumoricidal levels. It is not indicated for tumors deeper than 3 mm or those with indistinct margins. The main disadvantages include a hypopigmented scar, prolonged healing, pain during the procedure, and risk of recurrence.

Surgical Excision

According to the AAD guidelines, excision is useful in both primary and recurrent tumors. The main goal of any excisional surgery is to remove the tumor entirely. Postoperatively, the surgical margins of the specimen are examined histologically for assessment of adequate tumor removal. The wound defect can be closed primarily with side-to-side closures, flaps, or grafts, or it may be allowed to heal by secondary intention.[1] For small (<20 mm) primary, well-defined BCCs, 3-mm peripheral surgical margins will clear the tumor in 85% of cases, and a 4 to 5 mm margin increases the peripheral clearance rate to approximately 95%.[6] Larger and morpheaform lesions require wider and potentially deeper surgical margins for complete histologic resection. The main disadvantage of surgical excision is incomplete margin control,[6] because the routine vertical sectioning technique (breadloafing and quartering methods of margin checking) only assess 1% of the margin.

Mohs Micrographic Surgery

According to the AAD guidelines, Mohs micrographic surgery (MMS) is particularly efficacious in dealing with recurrent tumors in certain anatomic locations, with tumors that have been present for a long time and have become relatively large, and with certain subtypes including large, nodular, and morpheaform BCCs.[1] MMS consists of the removal of the tumor by scalpel in sequential horizontal layers. Each tissue specimen is mapped, frozen, stained, and microscopically examined. This procedure is especially suited for recurrent lesions and for primary tumors displaying one or more of the risk factors listed in Box 1.[7]

The procedure is predicated on histologically inspecting the entire perimeter and undersurface of the excised specimen to ensure a tumor-free margin. MMS has an extremely high cure rate: 99% for primary BCCs and more than 96% for recurrent lesions. Defects after MMS can be closed immediately, or a delayed repair may be performed in select cases. Repair can be achieved with primary linear closure, adjacent tissue transfer (flap), skin grafting, or healing by second intention.[1]

Box 1 Tumor Features Appropriate for Mohs Micrographic Surgery

Basal Cell Carcinoma

Ill-defined clinical borders

Anatomic sites with a high risk of local recurrence in areas of important tissue conservation:

- Face, including the central one third of the face, nose, nasolabial folds,and periorbital, perioral, and periauricular regions
- Hands
- Feet
- Genitalia

History of incomplete removal

History of prior irradiation therapy

History of recurrence

Large size

Specific histologic patterns including:

- Morpheaform
- Keratinizing
- Metatypical
- Infiltrating
- Contiguous (BCC and SCC)
- Multicentric

Deep tissue or bone involvement

Perineural or perivascular involvement

Rapidly growing or aggressive BCCs

Tumors in immunocompromised patients

Squamous Cell Carcinoma

Size >1 cm

Rapid growth

Ulceration

Growth into deeper tissues

- Subcutaneous fat
- Fascia
- Muscle
- Bone
- Cartilage

Occurrence in a previously inflammatory or degenerative process or scar

Recurrent SCC

Anatomic locations

- Mucous membranes
- Ears
- Temple
- Scalp
- Eyelids
- Other locations

Perineural invasion (may be indicated by pain or paresthesia)

Histologic features

- Undifferentiated histologic pattern
- Depth beyond the subcutaneous fat
- Perineural invasion
- Lymphatic invasion)

Immunocompromised host

Radiation

The AAD guidelines state that radiation is useful for definitive treatment of primary tumors and some recurrent cancers and for palliation of inoperable tumors.[2] This modality is useful for treating elderly patients who are not suitable candidates for surgical procedures. Superficial x-rays are administered in multiple, divided doses over several weeks. In general, 10 treatments are needed. Radiation therapy is contraindicated for morpheaform BCC or recurrent BCC tumors regardless of pathologic subtype.

Evolving Therapies

According to the AAD guidelines, laser surgery is a recognized and evolving therapy that may be used to vaporize superficial and multiple basal cell carcinomas. The laser can also be used in lieu of a scalpel for excisional surgery to provide for improved hemostasis.[1] Other modalities such as retinoids, imiquimod, 5-fluorouracil, immunotherapy (IL-1, IL-2, interferon alfa-2b, and interferon gamma), and photodynamic therapy have been used with varying success. Chemotherapy used in the treatment of metastatic disease may have a role in treating patients with multiple lesions or as adjunctive therapy in patients being treated with radiation.[1]

Outcomes

Five-year recurrence rates after treatment of primary BCC are 1% for MMS, 7.5% for cryotherapy, 7.7% for ED&C, 8.7% for radiation therapy, and 10.1% for surgical excision.[8] The main goal in the treatment of BCC should be complete removal of the malignancy with the highest cure rate and least cosmetic disfigurement or functional impairment.

Prevention and Screening

Monthly self examination and long-term follow-up in patients who have had a BCC are essential because of the possibility of recurrence and because these patients have a much higher propensity to develop new cutaneous malignancies.[1] Studies show that patients who have had one BCC are at significantly higher risk (50%) of developing new primary lesions, which can go undetected by patients.[6] Early detection and appropriate re-treatment of either recurrent BCCs or new primary BCCs can increase the chances of a permanent cure and ultimately can minimize morbidity. Prevention and education are also integral parts of the total care of a patient with BCC.[6] Daily sunscreen application, sun-protective clothing, and sun avoidance during peak hours are essential.

SQUAMOUS CELL CARCINOMA

Definition and Cause

Squamous cell carcinoma (SCC) is a malignant tumor arising from the keratinocytes in the epidermis or its dermal appendages.[9] SCC is the second most common cutaneous malignancy after BCC. Unlike BCC, cutaneous SCC is associated with a greater risk of metastasis.[10] Like BCC, exposure to UV radiation is the most common cause of SCC in fair-complected persons.[10]

Prevalence and Risk Factors

It is estimated that more than 160,000 cases of cutaneous SCC will occur in 2007. The age-adjusted incidence of SCC among whites is 100 to 150 per 100,000 persons per year. The age-specific incidence among persons older than 75 years is approximately 10 times that rate. The most recent data report that the lifetime risk of SCC is 9% to 14% among men and 4% to 9% among women.[5] The incidence of SCC doubles with each 8 to 10 degrees decline in latitude (pro-

Box 2 Risk Factors for Squamous Cell Carcinoma

Photochemotherapy (PUVA) for skin disorders such as psoriasis
Thermal injury to the skin
Exposure to chemical carcinogens

- Arsenic
- Chromates
- Polycyclic aromatic hydrocarbons
- Tars
- Tobacco smoke
- Others

Chronic radiation dermatitis
Human papillomavirus (HPV) infections, especially from HPV types 16, 18, 30, and 33
Previously injured or chronically diseased skin

- Burn sites
- Chronic ulcers
- Scars of various causes
- Sinuses

Genetic determinants
Immunosuppression
Precursor lesions

- Actinic keratosis
- Arsenical keratosis
- Bowen's disease (SCC in situ)
- Erythroplasia of Queyrat (SCC in situ of the penis)
- Radiation-induced keratosis

SCC, squamous cell carcinoma.

ximity to the equator). Since the 1970s, the age-adjusted incidence of SCC has increased by 50% to 200%.[11]

Pathophysiology and Natural History

Although UVB (wavelength 290-320 nm) is mainly responsible, UVA is also important. Any exposure to UV radiation produces mutations in the DNA by forming thymidine dimers in the *p53* tumor-suppressor gene. Mutations in *p53* result in a nonfunctional protein that cannot repair a mutated keratinocyte. This leads to uncontrolled growth and proliferation of these aberrant cells (malignancy).[10] Other factors that have been associated with the development of SCC are listed in Box 2.

Invasive SCC can recur and metastasize. The 5-year recurrence of primary cutaneous lesions is 8%, and the 5-year metastasis rate is 5%.[10] Risk factors for metastasis include size >2 cm, site (lip, ear), immunosuppression, history of prior treatment, and aggressive histologic features (depth >4 mm, poorly differentiated appearance, and perineural invasion).[10] Additional variables that put SCC in the high-risk category include cause (scar, chronic ulcer, sinus tract, radiation dermatitis) and rapid growth pattern.[11]

Signs and Symptoms

Actinic Keratosis

Actinic keratoses are premalignant skin lesions that result from chronic sun exposure and are found chiefly on the face, ears, dorsal hands, and forearms. They are usually multiple, discrete, flat or raised, verrucous or keratotic, pigmented, erythematous or skin-colored. The surface is usually scaly (Fig. 5).

Actinic keratoses are potential precursors to SCC. The annual transformation rate into SCC is 0.24% for each actinic keratosis.[11] However, approximately 5% to 20% of actinic keratoses develop into invasive SCC over 10 to 25 years.[11] The transformation may be heralded by the development of erosion, induration, inflammation, or enlargement.

Options for treatment include cryosurgery, ED&C, topical fluorouracil, photodynamic therapy, dermabrasion, chemical peel, and laser resurfacing. It has been calculated that there is a 10.2% chance of at least one actinic keratosis on a given patient transforming into an SCC within a 10-year period. However, this rate might actually be much higher, especially in immunocompromised patients such as organ transplant recipients.

Bowen's Disease

Well-demarcated erythematous, scaly, slowly enlarging plaques that can occur on any part of the body characterize Bowen's disease or SCC in situ (Fig. 6). When it occurs on the glans penis, it is referred to as *erythroplasia of Queyrat.* The development of ulceration or induration can portend transformation into invasive SCC, which occurs in up to 5% of cases. Bowen's disease affects mostly older white men. Chronic sun damage and arsenicism have been implicated in Bowen's disease. Treatment options include excision, ED&C, photodynamic therapy, imiquimod, cryosurgery, 5-fluorouracil, and MMS.

Keratoacanthoma

This rapidly growing tumor is believed to be a low-grade SCC. Keratoacanthomas usually start out as a 1-mm flesh-colored macule or papule and grow to as large as a 2.5-cm nodule with a keratin-filled crater in only 3 to 8 weeks (Fig. 7). In most cases, solitary keratoacanthomas involute over 2 to 6 months, often healing with scarring. Keratoacanthomas are generally found on sun-exposed areas such as the central face, dorsal hands, arms, and legs, although they can occur anywhere on the body including the mucosa. Although keratoacanthomas might ultimately involute, the duration of regression is unpredictable.

Keratoacanthomas can also mimic invasive SCC with regard to rapid growth pattern and clinical characteristics.[10] Therefore, a method of removal that ensures adequate depth for histopathologic review is important. Options for therapy include observation, surgical excision, ED&C, topical or intralesional 5-fluorouracil, cryosurgery, radiation, and MMS.

Squamous Cell Carcinoma

SCC can occur on the skin or mucous membranes. It generally occurs in middle-aged and elderly adults, and more lesions occur in men. The most common sites affected are the scalp, dorsal hands, ears, lower lip, neck, forearms, and legs. Clinically SCC manifests as an enlarging indurated erythematous papule, nodule, or plaque with scale (Fig. 8). Ulceration and crusting occur later, followed by possible invasion of underlying structures and development of regional lymphadenopathy. On the lower lip, SCC arises on the chronically sun-damaged skin of the vermilion border. Patients usually note the presence of a firm nodule growing either inward or outward with ulceration. Squamous cell carcinomas of the lip metastasize approximately 10% to 15% of the time.

Verrucous Carcinoma

Verrucous carcinoma is a variant of well-differentiated invasive SCC. They manifest as indolent cauliflower-shaped nodules that resemble warts (Fig. 9). They are locally aggressive but are less likely to metastasize.[10] Verrucous carcinoma can occur on the soles, glans penis, scrotum, vulva, scalp, face, back, nail beds, or larynx. The most effective treatment is excision, and MMS is required in some cases.[10]

Diagnosis

As with BCC, a total body examination of the skin is the only screening test available for cutaneous SCC. A physical examination of a patient with SCC should always include a thorough examination of the areas of lymphatic drainage.[9] The clinical presence of lymphade-

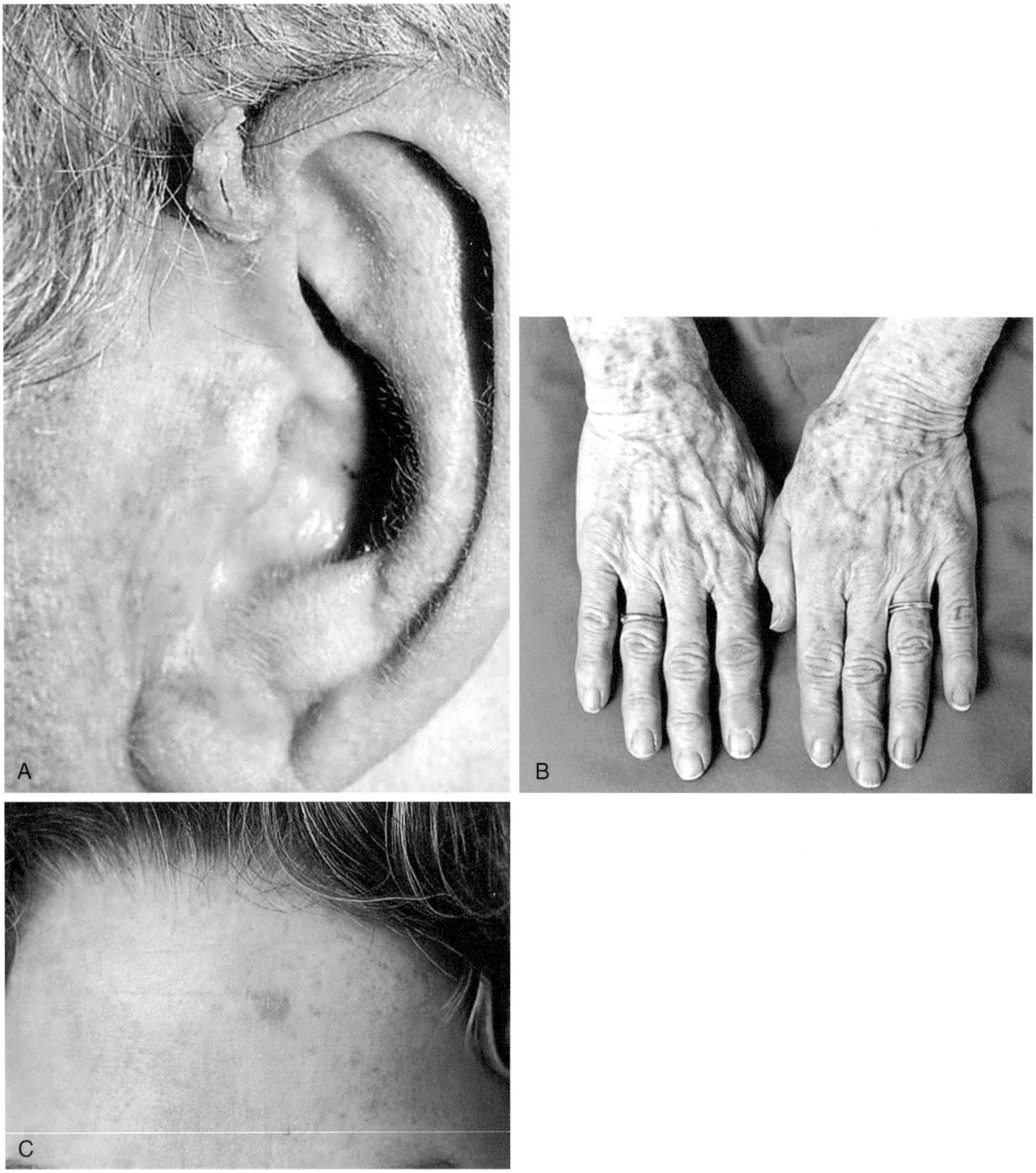

Figure 5 **A,** Actinic keratosis with cutaneous horn, left ear. **B,** Multiple actinic keratoses, dorsal hands. **C,** Actinic keratosis, forehead.

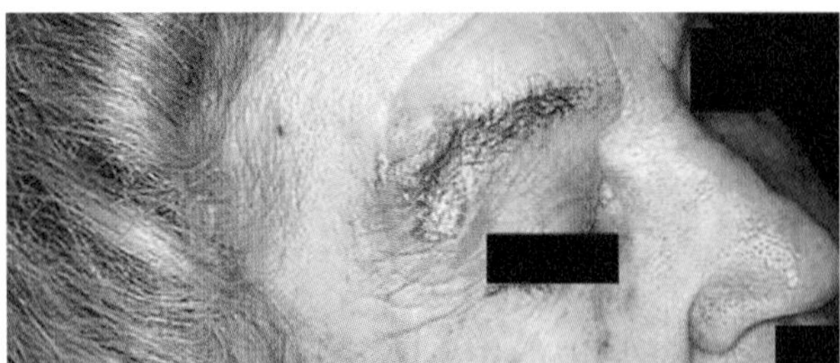

Figure 6 Bowen's disease, right temple.

nopathy necessitates exclusion of metastatic disease. Suspicious cutaneous lesions for SCC should be promptly biopsied. Because even the most astute physicians can make incorrect clinical diagnoses, most biopsies of all suspected nonmelanoma skin cancers should be adequate to allow proper diagnosis and treatment. This sample can be obtained as a shave or punch biopsy. The tissue is then sent for histopathologic review.

Treatment

Fortunately, most SCCs are small, low-risk tumors.[11] A variety of surgical and nonsurgical therapeutic modalities provide effective treatment of SCC.

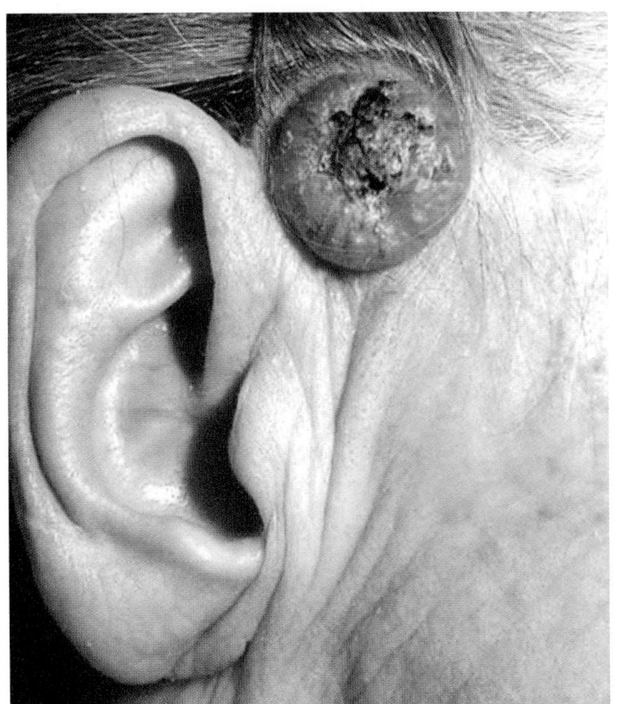

Figure 7 Squamous cell carcinoma, right preauricular skin.

Electrodesiccation and Curettage

According to the AAD guidelines, ED&C may be suitable for small primary lesions on sun-exposed skin. In select patients, curettage used alone or in conjunction with cryosurgery or ionizing radiation is an acceptable treatment method. ED&C is less effective in curing recurrent lesions that have associated scar tissue. Tumors that extend into the subcutaneous tissues histologically or are found to have clinically invaded the subcutaneous fat at the time of treatment are less likely to result in cure when treated with this method.[9]

ED&C is a process used to sequentially scrape the tumor away followed by destruction of an extra margin of normal skin by electrodesiccation performed up to three times to maximize the possibility of complete removal. Five-year cure rates with small primary SCCs treated with ED&C may be as high as 96%.[10] The main drawbacks with ED&C are that there is no tissue available for histologic evaluation to ensure tumor-free resection. ED&C can also have a poor cosmetic outcome. ED&C is not advisable for treating tumors on the face because the tumor can extend along the hair follicles beyond the reach of the curette.

Cryosurgery

This modality uses liquid nitrogen to destroy the tumor by lowering the temperature to tumoricidal levels. According to the AAD guidelines, it is especially useful in patients with bleeding disorders. It is also a good alternative in patients for whom other forms of surgery are contraindicated or who refuse other forms of surgery.[9] During treatment, it is important to include a rim of 3 to 4 mm of normal tissue beyond clinically visible margins of the tumor.

Excision

According to AAD guidelines, this surgical procedure is useful for primary and recurrent tumors. The advantages are that tissue can be assessed microscopically, the wound heals rapidly, and the cosmetic result is good.[9] The wound is closed primarily with side-to-side closure, flaps, or grafts or is allowed to heal by second intention.[9] Chance of clearance is 95% in SCCs that are well differentiated; are smaller than 2 cm; do not occur on the scalp, ears, eyelids, lips, or nose; do not involve the subcutaneous fat; and are removed with a margin of 4 mm around the clinical border of the lesion. For tumors that have a high risk of recurrence and are larger than 2 cm, a 6-mm margin is recommended.[10]

Mohs Micrographic Surgery

According to AAD guidelines, MMS is particularly efficacious in dealing with some recurrent and some primary tumors that display risk factors associated with aggressive biologic behavior (see Box 1).[9] The Mohs procedure offers the highest cure rates for patients with high-risk, primary, or recurrent SCC.

MMS uses horizontal frozen sectioning of the tumor to provide a view of 100% of the peripheral and deep margins of the specimen to ensure tumor-free planes.[10] The 5-year rates of local control for primary SCC at any site, except for the lips and ears, for MMS is 96.9% compared with 92.1% with other forms of treatment.[10] In patients with recurrent SCC, MMS is associated with 5-year cure rates of 90% to 93.3%, compared with a rate of 76.7% for recurrent tumors treated with standard excision.[10] SCCs that have lymph node involvement are additionally treated with radiation and lymph node dissection. This therapy combination offers the 5-year cure rate of 30% to 40%.[10] Cases involving distant metastases may be treated with systemic chemotherapy or other biologic response modifiers.[10]

Laser Surgery

According to AAD guidelines, the CO_2 laser may be used to excise or destroy SCC. The laser excises tissue in a bloodless fashion because the laser seals small blood vessels during the treatment, while also allowing margin control by histopathologic evaluation.[9]

Ionizing Radiation

According to AAD guidelines, this modality is useful for definitive treatment of primary tumors in select patients and some recurrent cancers. It is also used for palliation of inoperable tumors. Radiation is not used for treatment of verrucous carcinoma because some evidence suggests that the metastatic potential may be enhanced.[9]

Evolving Treatments

Photodynamic therapy employs a photoactive compound applied to the SCC lesion followed by photoirradiation. Intralesional interferon and other agents might also prove useful in the future. Oral and topical retinoids are being evaluated for therapeutic and chemoprophylaxis management.[9]

Outcomes

Most patients with primary cutaneous SCC have a very good prognosis.[10] Conversely, those with metastatic disease have a poor long-term prognosis. Patients with regional lymphadenopathy have a less than 20% 10-year survival rate, and patients with distant metastases have a less than 10% 10-year survival rate.[10]

When metastasis does occur, it mainly involves the regional lymph nodes.[10] Distant sites, including the lungs, liver, brain, skin, and bone, are less often affected.[10] Patients with SCC are at risk for developing other malignancies such as cancers of the respiratory organs, buccal cavity, pharynx, small intestines (in men), non-Hodgkin's lymphoma, and leukemia.

The natural course of invasive SCCs in the skin is variable. The incidence of metastases from cutaneous SCC ranges from 1% to 20% in most surveys. In reference to metastatic disease, the metastatic rates result from SCCs arising in scars (37.9%), the lip (13.7%), and the external ear (8.8%). Five-year cure rates after treatment for

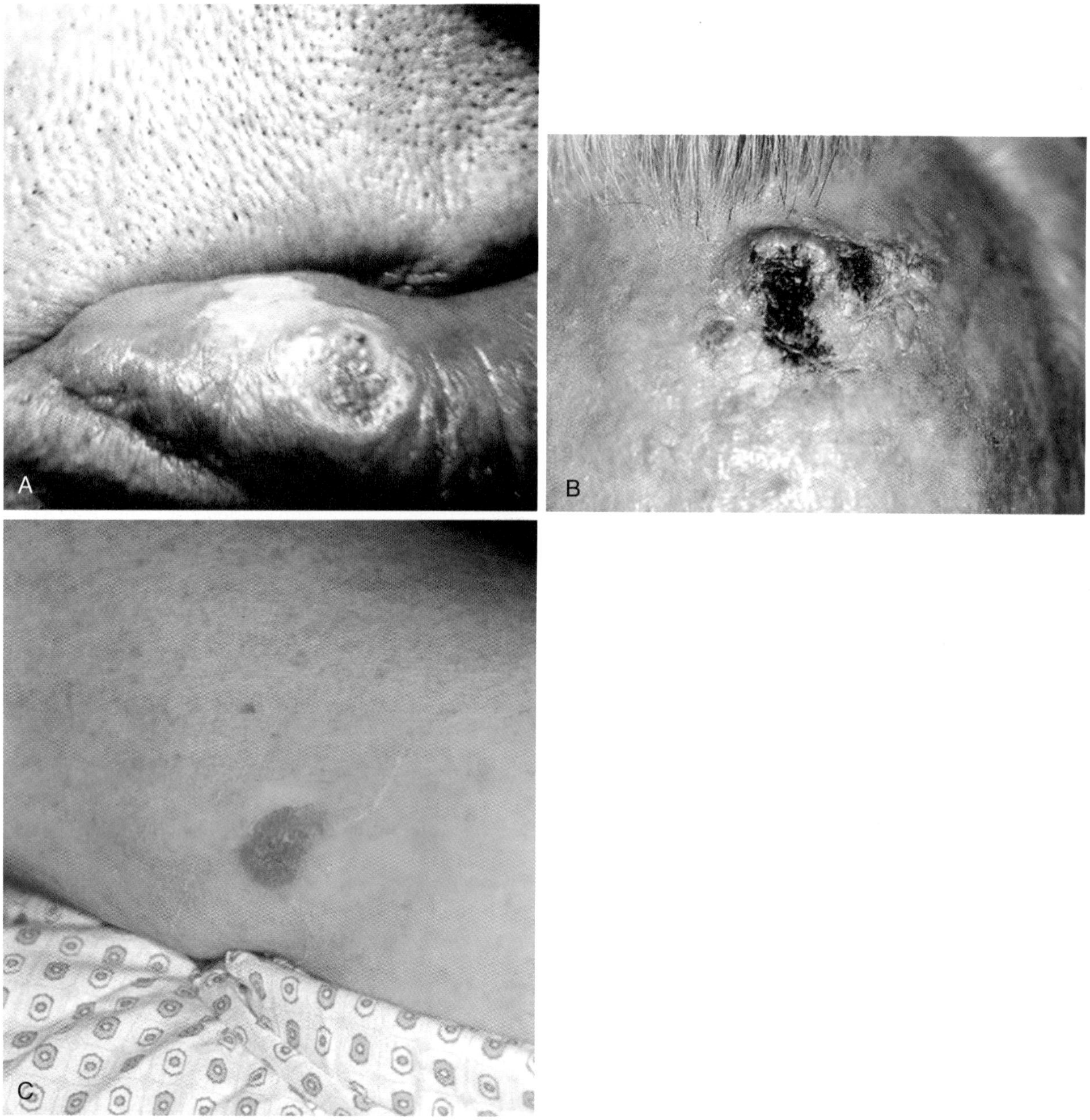

Figure 8 **A,** Squamous cell carcinoma, right side lower lip. **B,** Multiply recurrent squamous cell carcinoma, forehead. **C,** Squamous cell carcinoma, upper arm.

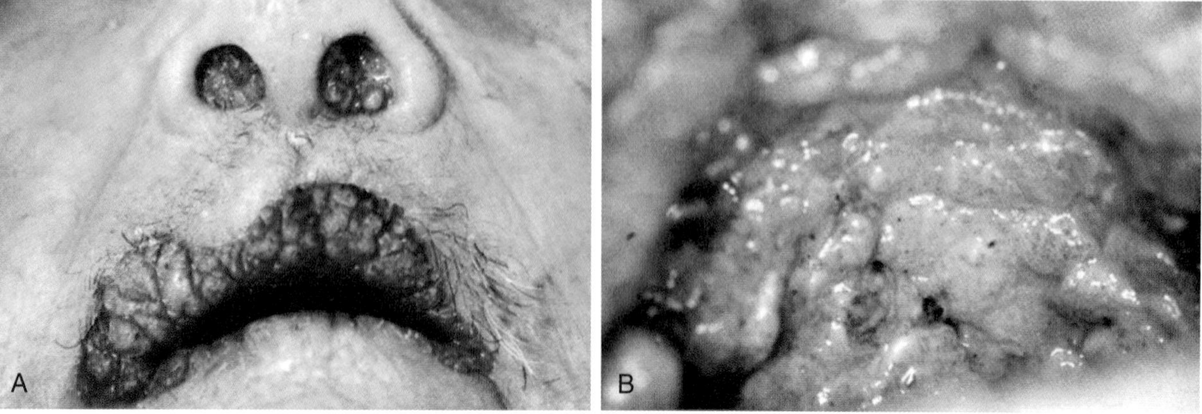

Figure 9 **A,** Verrucous carcinoma, intranasal and intraoral. **B,** Verrucous carcinoma, roof of mouth.

Box 3 American Academy of Dermatology Sun Safety Tips

Because overt exposure to ultraviolet light contributes to the formation of skin cancer, dermatologists recommend the following precautions.

Avoid peak sunlight hours—10 A.M. until 4 P.M.—when the sun's rays are the strongest.

Apply a broad-spectrum sunscreen, one that protects against UVA and UVB rays with SPF 15 or higher.

- Sunscreens with the following ingredients provide broad-spectrum protection:
  - Benzophenones (oxybenzone)
  - Cinnamates (octylmethyl cinnamate and cinoxate)
  - Sulisobenzone
  - Salicylates
  - Avobenzone (Parsol 1789), ecamsule (Mexoryl).
- For people with sensitive skin, chemical-free sunblocks containing titanium dioxide or zinc oxide, which also afford broad-spectrum coverage, can be used.

Reapply sunscreen every 2 hours, especially after swimming or heavy perspiration.

Wear protective clothing including a wide-brimmed hat, sunglasses, long-sleeved shirt, and long pants.

Apply lip balm that contains sunscreen with SPF 15 or higher.

Seek shade while outdoors during the day.

Protect children by minimizing sun exposure and regularly applying sunscreen. This is crucial because excessive sun exposure in the first 18 years of life increases a person's chances of developing melanoma. Eighty percent of lifetime sun exposure occurs before age 18 years.

Avoid reflective surfaces such as water, snow, and sand that can reflect up to 85% of the sun's damaging rays.

Avoid tanning beds.

SPF, sun protection factor; UVA, ultraviolet A; UVB, ultraviolet B.

Adapted from Sober AJ, Chuang TY, Duvic M, et al, for the Guidelines/Outcomes Committee. Guidelines of care for primary cutaneous melanoma. J Am Acad Dermatol 2001;45:579-586.

primary SCC were 96.9% with MMS compared with 92.1% with all other forms of treatment.

Prevention and Screening

As with all skin cancer treatment, therapy should be carefully tailored to the specific lesion and influenced by the medical status of the patient. Because there is a 30% risk of having a second primary SCC within 5 years after therapy for the first malignancy, skin cancer patients should have a total body examination once or twice yearly.[10] Patients with squamous cell carcinoma should also follow sun-safety tips (Box 3).

Considerations in Special Populations

In the United Stated more than 100,000 people have solid organ transplants. Due to their heavy immunosuppressive regimens, they are at risk for developing both internal and cutaneous malignancies. Skin cancer is the most common type of cancer after transplantation. The ratio of BCC to SCC is reversed in this population. These patients should be screened before transplantation to assess their risk of developing skin cancer, and they must be educated regarding safe sun protection measures and skin self examination. Aggressive screening and early treatment of skin cancers are imperative.[12]

Summary

- Basal and squamous cell carcinomas are the most common cancers.
- Sunlight exposure is the primary cause of nonmelanoma skin cancer.
- Most nonmelanoma skin cancers have a high cure rate with early diagnosis and treatment.
- Patients with a history of skin cancer deserve a full skin examination on a regular basis, perhaps every 6 months, coupled with education about ultraviolet sun exposure and the regular use of sunscreen.
- Immunosuppressed patients have a higher incidence of skin cancer, especially squamous cell carcinoma, which can be more aggressive, with appreciable morbidity and mortality.

Suggested Readings

Alam M, Ratner D: Cutaneous squamous cell carcinoma. N Engl J Med 2001:344:975-983.

Berg D, Otley CC: Skin cancer in organ transplant recipients: Epidemiology, pathogenesis, and management. J Amer Acad Dermatol 2002;47:1-17.

Committee on Guidelines of Care, Task Force on Cutaneous Squamous Cell Carcinoma: Guidelines of care for cutaneous squamous cell carcinoma. J Am Acad Dermatol 1993;28:628-631.

Czarnecki D, Meehan C, O'Brien T, et al: The changing face of skin cancer in Australia. Int J Dermatol 1991;30:715-717.

Drake LA, Ceilley RI, Cornelison RL, et al, for the Committee on Guidelines of Care, Task Force on Basal Cell Carcinoma: Guidelines of Care for Basal Cell Carcinoma. J Am Acad Dermatol 1992;26:117-120.

Drake LA, Dinehart SM, Goltz R, et al, for the Guidelines/Outcomes Committee, Task Force on Mohs Micrographic Surgery: Guidelines of care for Mohs micrographic surgery. J Am Acad Dermatol 1995;33:271-278.

Johnson TM, Rowe DE, Nelson BR, Swanson NA: Squamous cell carcinoma of the skin (excluding the lip and oral mucosa). J Am Acad Dermatol 1992;26:467-484.

Korman NJ, Hrabovsky SL: Basal cell carcinomas display extensive abnormalities in the hemidesmosome anchoring fibril complex. Exp Dermatol 1993;2:139-144.

Miller DL, Weinstock MA: Non-melanoma skin cancer in the United States: Incidence. J Am Acad Dermatol 1994;30:774-778.

Rowe DE, Carroll RJ, Day CL: Long-term recurrence rates in previously untreated (primary) basal cell carcinomas: Implications for patient follow-up. J Dermatol Surg Oncol 1989;15:315-328.

Telfer NR, Colver GB, Bowers PW: Guidelines for the management of basal cell carcinoma. Br J Dermatol 1999;141:415-423.

Tsao H: Update on familial cancer syndromes and the skin. J Am Acad Dermatol 2000;42:939-969.

References

For a complete list of references, log onto www.expertconsult.com.

Acne and Rosacea

Jennifer L. Lucas and *Kenneth J. Tomecki*

ACNE

Definition

Acne is a chronic inflammatory disease typically involving the face, neck, upper torso and shoulders and characterized by comedones (blackheads and whiteheads), oily skin, and inflammatory papules, pustules, cysts, or nodules.

Prevalence and Risk Factors

Affecting 40 to 50 million people in the United States, acne is the most common skin condition. It is predominantly a disease of teenagers and affects boys more commonly than girls. Resolution typically occurs by age 25 years. Adult acne occurs less often and is more common in women.[1] Mechanical or frictional forces (frequent washing, headgear, hats) and occlusion (cosmetics, hair products) can aggravate or induce acne. Numerous medications can produce acneiform eruptions (corticosteroids, anabolic steroids, anticonvulsants, lithium, potassium iodide, bromides, and isoniazid). Chloracne, a subtype of acne, occurs after exposure to chlorinated aromatic hydrocarbons.

Pathophysiology and Natural History

Acne is a follicular disease consisting of a comedonal and inflammatory stage. Defective keratinization produces a hyperkeratotic plug that blocks the opening of the pilosebaceous unit, forming a comedo. Seborrhea (increased sebum production) dilates the follicle and leads to subsequent bacterial overgrowth. *Propionibacterium acnes,* a colonizer of the follicle, proliferates, leading to leukocyte invasion and rupture of the follicle. The follicular contents and bacterial metabolites produce an inflammatory response, forming papules and pustules. Androgens, mainly dehydroepiandrosterone sulfate (DHEAS), stimulate sebaceous gland enlargement and secretion, which exacerbate the cycle.[2] Postinflammatory hyperpigmentation and scarring are common residua.

Signs and Symptoms

Acne often begins with open and closed comedones (whiteheads and blackheads) followed by inflammatory papules and pustules on the face, neck, chest, back, and shoulders (Fig. 1). Occasionally cysts and nodules are also present. Most patients have increased sebum production and oily skin.

Acne severity is commonly categorized as[3]:

- Mild: Comedones and some papules or pustules
- Moderate: Several papules, pustules, and comedones with increased truncal involvement
- Moderately severe: Many papules, pustules, and comedones; nodules; and widespread involvement (face, chest, shoulders, and back)
- Severe: Nodules and cysts

Acne conglobata is a severe form of truncal acne characterized by deep inflammatory cysts and nodules, often with interconnecting sinuses and fistulas (Fig. 2). Acne conglobata with systemic involvement, including fever, arthralgias, and leukocytosis, is referred to as acne fulminans.

Inflammatory and traumatized disease often yields hyperpigmentation and scarring, most commonly on the cheeks with an ice-pick or atrophic appearance. These residual changes are usually permanent but become less apparent with time.

Acne can affect a patient's self-esteem, confidence, and sense of well-being. Some patients become depressed.

Diagnosis

Acne is a clinical diagnosis. Evaluation should include inquiry about current and previous treatments, cosmetics, and systemic medications. In female patients, hirsutism, menstrual irregularities, androgenic alopecia, perimenstrual flares, and recalcitrant or late-onset acne should suggest the possibility of androgen excess.

Laboratory tests are usually not necessary. However, signs of androgen excess deserve further evaluation for elevated serum DHEAS and free testosterone.

The differential diagnosis of acne includes rosacea, acneiform drug reactions, folliculitis, gram-negative folliculitis, and pseudofolliculitis (ingrown hairs).

Summary

- Acne is a common, benign disease of the pilosebaceous apparatus.
- Acne is characterized by comedones, papules, and pustules in teenagers and young adults.

Treatment

The American Academy of Dermatology's 2007 guidelines of care for managing acne vulgaris outline a multitiered approach to therapy tailored to the individual patient based on lesion type and severity.[4] Box 1 gives recommended treatment guidelines.

Topical retinoids are a mainstay of treatment, reducing follicular obstruction in comedonal and inflammatory acne. Several formulations are available as creams and gels: tazarotene (Tazorac), tretinoin (Retin-A, Avita, Retin-A Micro), and retinoid-like adapalene (Differin). Nightly application of a thin film of medication is preferred but can lead to dryness and irritation. Implementing the medication three or four times weekly and increasing to nightly as tolerated enhances compliance. If irritation occurs, use should be decreased.

Benzoyl peroxide is an important acne therapy with its bactericidal, anti-inflammatory, and comedolytic properties. It is generally well tolerated and may be the most cost-effective acne treatment. Benzoyl peroxide is available in varying concentrations from 2.5% to 10% and as washes, gels, and cleansing pads. Its use helps to minimize antimicrobial resistance.[5]

Topical antibiotics, such as clindamycin 1% or erythromycin 2%, are helpful in inflammatory disease. However, given the increasing rates of bacterial resistance they should not be used as monotherapy. Combined use with a benzoyl peroxide prevents bacterial resistance, and a benzoyl peroxide or topical retinoid makes them more effective.[3] Other topical agents, such as azelaic acid and products containing salicylic acid, sulfur, or sodium sulfacetamide, have minimal efficacy.

Most patients benefit from combination treatment using two or three agents. For mild to moderate acne, benzoyl peroxide and a topical retinoid with or without a topical antibiotic are often used.

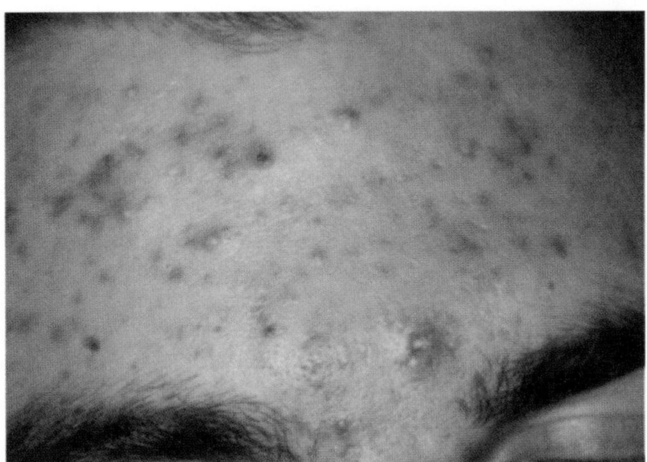

Figure 1 **Acne.** Inflammatory papules and pustules, comedones, and postinflammatory hyperpigmentation.

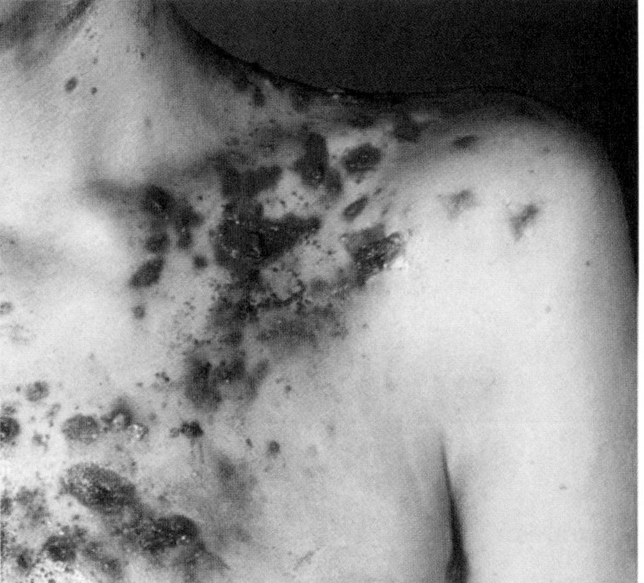

Figure 2 **Acne conglobata.** Nodules and cysts with interconnecting sinus tracts.

Box 1 Acne Treatment

Mild
Topical retinoid nightly as tolerated and/or benzoyl peroxide daily

Moderate to Severe
Topical retinoid *plus* benzoyl peroxide *plus* topical or oral antibiotic

Severe
Dermatology evaluation, isotretinoin
Acne conglobata or fulminans: systemic steroids *plus* isotretinoin

To facilitate treatment and patient compliance, combined formulations are available, such as benzoyl peroxide and clindamycin (Duac, BenzaClin) tretinoin and clindamycin (Ziana) & benzoyl peroxide & adapelene (Epiduo).

For more severe or extensive inflammatory acne, a systemic antibiotic is often warranted in addition to a benzoyl peroxide and/or topical retinoid. Doxycycline 100 to 200 mg/day, minocycline 100 to 200 mg/day, or tetracycline 500 mg to 1 g/day are effective options.[4] Side effects are relatively uncommon, although gastrointestinal distress and vaginal candidiasis are possible. Doxycycline is a photosensitizer, and minocycline can induce pigmentation, dizziness, and a systemic lupus erythematosus (SLE)–like syndrome. These antibiotics should be avoided in children younger than 9 years, because dental or skeletal abnormalities can develop. Typically prescribed for rosaeia, submicrobial doxycycline (Oracea) 40 mg daily has anti-inflammatory properties and minimizes the potential for bacterial resistance. Sustained-release weight based minocycline (Solodyn) has exhibited good efficacy with minimal put Solodyn prior to oracea side effects. Alternatives to tetracycline include trimethoprim-sulfamethoxazole and erythromycin. Maximum improvement should not be expected for at least 3 months, regardless of the antibiotic chosen.[3]

For some women, hormonal therapy with low-progestin oral contraceptives or antiandrogenic agents can enhance treatment. FDA-approved oral contraceptives for acne include those containing norgestimate with ethinyl estradiol (Ortho Tri-Cyclen) and norethindrone acetate with ethinyl estradiol (Estrostep).[4] Drospirenone with ethinyl estradiol (Yasmin, YAZ) has also been used effectively (Author's first choice). Spironolactone (Aldactone), an antihypertensive with antiandrogenic properties, has been effective in some women by decreasing DHEAS.[6]

For severe or extensive disease, isotretinoin (Accutane), a vitamin A derivative, at a dose of 0.5 to 2 mg/kg per day for 20 weeks may be necessary. Potential side effects include skin dryness, bone and muscle pain, ocular dryness, headaches, pseudotumor cerebri, mood instability including depression, hyperlipidema, transaminitis, and teratogenicity. Highly regulated by the FDA, isotretinoin requires enrollment in a national registry, close follow-up including pregnancy testing, and sexual abstinence or two forms of birth control.

Adjunctive therapeutic measures include intralesional corticosteroids for inflammatory cysts and nodules, chemical peels (glycolic and salicylic acids), comedo extraction, photodynamic therapy (PDT), and diode (smooth beam) or pulsed-dye laser therapy. If postinflammatory hyperpigmentation is present the patient should avoid sun exposure and liberally use sunscreen to prevent further darkening.

Acneiform eruptions from the use of occlusive products, mechanical forces, corticosteroid application, or a medication reaction often respond to simply discontinuing the offending agent.

Despite the lack of a cure, acne can be minimized with early and thoughtful treatment, and most patients ultimately do well. Any treatment regimen deserves at least 6 to 8 weeks of consecutive, diligent treatment to assess clinical responsiveness.[3]

Summary

- Benzoyl peroxide or a topical retinoid, or both, are the first-line therapy for mild acne.
- Moderate to severe inflammatory acne often requires a systemic antibiotic.
- Severe and scarring acne might require isotretinoin.

Prevention and Screening

Acne cannot be prevented, but it can be minimized by therapy.

Considerations in Special Populations

Treatment should be minimized or avoided during pregnancy and is often limited to topical or oral erythromycin and azelaic acid. Epileptic and bipolar patients can develop severe acneiform eruptions secondary to their medications.

Table 1 Rosacea

Rosacea Type	Clinical Features	Treatment
Erythematotelangiectatic (vascular rosacea)	Flushing, persistent central face erythema, and telangiectasias	Trigger avoidance, vascular laser, beta blockers, over-the-counter redness relief, green-tinted make-up
Papulopustular	Inflammatory papules and pustules of the central face	Trigger avoidance, sodium sulfacetamide and sulfur agents, metronidazole cream or gel, doxycyclin, minocycline, or tetracycline
Ocular	Blepharitis, ± conjunctival injection	Oral doxycyclin, minocycline, or tetracycline
Phymatous	Soft tissue hypertrophy, rhinophyma (nose)	Ablative laser, dermabrasion, heated scalpel excision, oral antibiotics

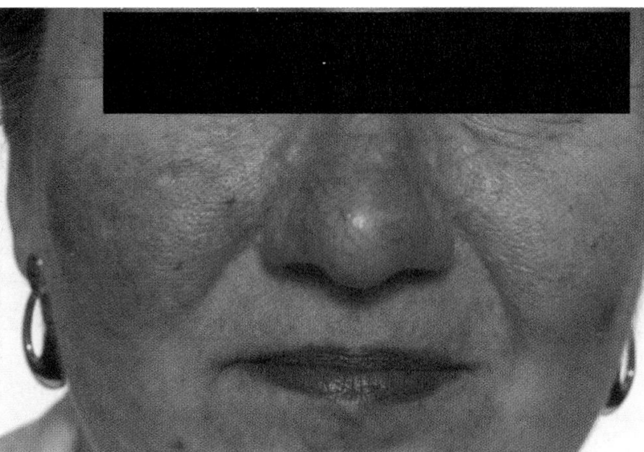

Figure 3 Erythematotelangiectatic rosacea.

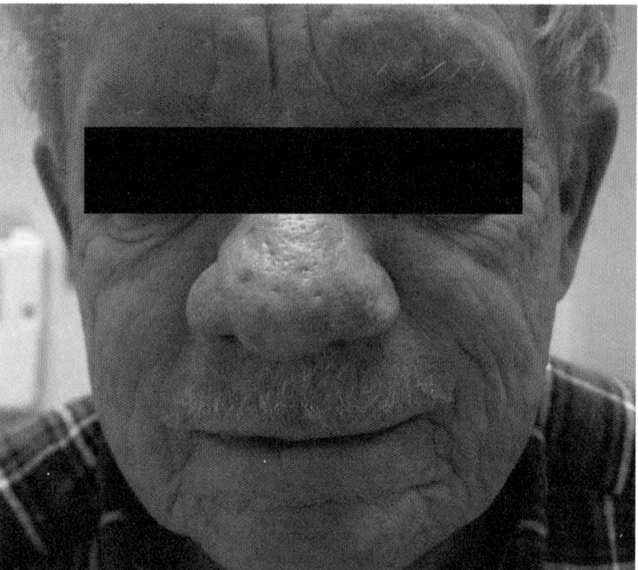

Figure 4 Rhinophyma.

ROSACEA

Definition

Rosacea is a chronic inflammatory disease characterized by easy flushing, persistent erythema on the central face with telangiectasias, and occasional flares of inflammatory papules and pustules.

Prevalence and Risk Factors

Rosacea affects approximately 14 million Americans and primarily occurs in middle-aged, fair-skinned adults of northern European heritage. It has a female predominance, but men more commonly develop phymatous rosacea (rhinophyma).[7]

Besides a genetic predisposition, disease-aggravating factors include spicy foods, alcohol, caffeine, especially hot coffee or tea, exercise, stress, and extremes of temperature.

Pathophysiology and Natural History

The pathophysiology of rosacea remains unclear, although genetic predisposition and vascular reactivity are likely factors involved. Persistent disease often leads to sebaceous hyperplasia and soft tissue hypertrophy (phymatous rosacea).

Signs and Symptoms

Rosacea is a polymorphic disease often divided into four subtypes that commonly overlap (Table 1 and Figs. 3 and 4).[7,8] Unlike acne, seborrhea and comedones do not occur. Ocular rosacea may be subtle, exhibiting only ocular dryness and a foreign body sensation.

Diagnosis

Rosacea is a clinical diagnosis. The patient with rosacea deserves inquiry regarding frequency of flushing, possible triggers, and eye symptoms including dryness, irritation, and redness. Laboratory tests are usually not necessary unless lupus erythematosus, another connective tissue disease, or carcinoid syndrome enters the differential diagnosis. Physiologic flushing can mimic erythematotelangiectatic rosacea and can actually precede rosacea. The differential diagnosis of rosacea includes chronic sun damage, chronic use of topical corticosteroids, seborrheic dermatitis, carcinoid syndrome, mastocytosis, and some connective tissue diseases, such as SLE, dermatomyositis, and mixed connective tissue disease.[8]

Summary

- Rosacea is a polymorphic disease characterized by facial erythema with telangiectasias, papules, and pustules.
- Rosacea is often exacerbated by alcohol, caffeine, spicy foods, exercise, stress, and extremes of temperature.

Treatment

The treatment of rosacea depends on the disease subtype (see Table 1).[9] Erythematotelangiectatic rosacea responds well to vascular laser therapy. Beta-blockers can decrease the frequency and severity of flushing. For inflammatory disease, with papules or pustules, metronidazole 0.75% or 1% gel or cream, sodium sulfacetamide and sulfur agents, and azelaic acid are effective therapies.

Some patients, especially those with moderate to severe papulopustular, phymatous, or ocular disease, should receive oral antibiotics, such as doxycycline 100 to 200 mg/day, minocycline 100 to 200 mg/day, or tetracycline 250 mg to 1 g/day. Submicrobial doses of doxycycline, (Oracea) 40 mg daily, have also shown promising results from the anti-inflammatory properties of the drug while minimizing the potential for antibacterial resistance. For phymatous rosacea, especially rhinophyma, surgical treatment with ablative laser, dermabrasion, or heated scalpel excision can help to restore the normal skin contours.

Summary

- Rosacea therapy is often multifactorial.
- Laser therapy is used for telangeictasias.
- Metronidazole, sodium sulfacetamide and sulfur combinations, azelaic acid, or oral antibiotics are used for the inflammatory papules and pustules.

Prevention and Screening

Rosacea can be minimized by avoiding its known triggers: alcohol, caffeine, and spicy foods. Therapy is directed at the telangiectasias and inflammatory papules and pustules.

Suggested Readings

Crawford GH, Pelle MT, James WD: Rosacea: I. Etiology, pathogenesis, and subtype classification. J Am Acad Dermatol 2004;51(3):327-341.

Degitz K, Placzek M, Borelli C, Plewig G: Pathophysiology of acne. J Dtsch Dermatol Ges 2007;5(4):316-323.

James WD: Clinical practice. Acne. N Engl J Med 2005;325(14):1463-1472.

McDonnell JK, Tomecki KJ: Rosacea: An update. Cleveland Clin J Med 2000;67(8):587-590.

Ozolins M, Eady EA, Avery AJ, et al: Comparison of five antimicrobial regimens for treatment of mild to moderated inflammatory facial acne vulgaris in the community: Randomised controlled trial. Lancet 2004;364:2188-2195.

Pelle MT, Crawford GH, James WD: Rosacea: II. Therapy. J Am Acad Dermatol 2004;51(4):499-512.

Strauss JS, Krowchuk DP, Leyden JJ, et al: Guidelines of care for acne vulgaris management. J Am Acad Dermatol 2007;56(4):651-663.

White GM: Recent findings in the epidemiologic evidence, classification, and subtypes of acne vulgaris. J Am Acad Dermatol 1998;39:S34-S37.

Yemisci A, Gorgulu A, Piskin S: Effects and side-effects of spironolactone therapy in women with acne. J Eur Acad Dermatol Venereol 2005;19(2):163-166.

References

For a complete list of references, log onto www.expertconsult.com.

Psoriasis

Charles Camisa

DEFINITION AND ETIOLOGY

Psoriasis is a common papulosquamous skin disease that may be associated with a seronegative spondyloarthropathy. The etiology of psoriasis is unknown.

PREVALENCE AND RISK FACTORS

Psoriasis affects 2% of the U.S. population, and about 11% of these patients have psoriatic arthritis (PSA). Psoriasis may begin at any age, but the mean age at onset is 30 years. Men and women are affected equally.

U.S. primary care physicians initially see 58% of the estimated 150,000 new cases of psoriasis per year, but dermatologists handle 80% of the 3 million office and hospital visits for psoriasis each year.

The form that psoriasis takes in a patient depends on a combination of genetic influences, environmental factors (e.g., trauma and climate), associated diseases (especially infections), and concomitant medications. Certain drugs, notably lithium, antimalarials, β-adrenergic blockers, interferons, and ethanol (if abused) have been reported to induce psoriasis or aggravate preexisting disease in some patients. Emotional stress may also lead to a flare of psoriasis.

PATHOPHYSIOLOGY

The psoriatic skin lesions are the result of inflammation in the dermis and hyperproliferation with abnormal differentiation of the epidermis. The primary pathologic process is most likely dysregulation of activated T cell interactions with antigen-presenting cells and overproduction of proinflammatory cytokines such as interferon-α and tumor necrosis factor-α (TNF-α). Evidence for this theory derives from the dramatic improvement of severe psoriasis in patients treated with broadly immunosuppressive drugs used in organ transplantation, such as cyclosporine and tacrolimus.

SIGNS AND SYMPTOMS

Although considered a single disease, psoriasis has several morphologic expressions and a full range of severity. *Plaque-type psoriasis*, or psoriasis vulgaris, is the most common form, occurring in about 80% of all psoriasis patients. A typical lesion is a well-demarcated, red-violet plaque surmounted by white silvery scales (Fig. 1).

Symmetry of lesions is the rule, and the face is usually spared. The most commonly involved areas are the elbows, knees, scalp, sacrum, umbilicus, intergluteal cleft, and genitalia. About 70% of patients complain of pruritus, skin pain, or burning, especially when the scalp is involved.

Guttate psoriasis (Fig. 2), named for its small droplet-shaped lesions, accounts for about 18% of all cases. This type is more common among children and young adults and is more likely to involve the face. Patients frequently have a history of upper respiratory tract infection or pharyngitis. Some cases of acute guttate flares following streptococcal throat infection are precipitated by the superantigen exotoxin.

C. *Pustular psoriasis* (Fig. 3) accounts for about 1.7% of cases. It is characterized by sterile pustules, which may be generalized or localized to the palms and soles. There is a female predominance in localized pustular psoriasis, but the incidence is equal in men and women in the generalized type. The average age at onset for pustular psoriasis is 50 years.

The least common form of psoriasis is exfoliative dermatitis or *psoriatic erythroderma* (Fig. 4) accounting for 1% to 2% of all cases. Erythroderma is defined as a scaling pruritic, inflammatory skin eruption that involves almost 100% of the body surface. Erythrodermic psoriasis usually develops gradually or acutely during the course of chronic plaque-type psoriasis, but it may be the first manifestation of psoriasis, even in children. The mean age at onset is about 50 years. Men with the condition outnumber women, and concomitant psoriatic arthropathy is common. The most common precipitating factor is the inappropriate or excessive use of potent topical, oral, and intramuscular corticosteroids. Patients are at risk for *Staphylococcus aureus* septicemia as a result of their compromised skin barrier.

The nails are involved in up to 50% of psoriasis patients; in patients with PSA, the prevalence exceeds 80%. Pitting of the nail plate is the most common manifestation. The pits tend to be large, deep, and randomly dispersed on the nail plate. Small red spots in the lunula or yellow-brown spots (*oil droplet sign*) in the nail bed correspond to lesions of psoriasis there.

PSA affects up to one third of patients with psoriasis. PSA is a destructive arthropathy and enthesopathy with some clinical features in common with rheumatoid arthritis. Arthritis occurs after the onset of the skin eruption in two thirds of cases. The severity of skin and nail involvement does not correlate with the severity of joint disease in patients with PSA. Although the systemic agents used to treat psoriasis are often effective for PSA, the specific management of PSA is beyond the scope of this chapter.

DIAGNOSIS

A clinical diagnosis is usually sufficient for classic skin and nail lesions. The differential diagnosis includes eczema, pityriasis rubra pilaris, drug reactions, tinea corporis, secondary syphilis, and cutaneous T cell lymphoma. Therefore, it may be necessary to perform skin biopsy, potassium hydroxide (KOH) examination of scales, and serologic tests.

THERAPY

Treatments for psoriasis are divided into six levels (Table 1). The choice of treatment depends on the severity of disease and response in the individual patient.

Level 1: Topical Treatments

Emollients (bland lubricants) should be tried first, followed by keratolytic lotions containing salicylic acid or urea. Most patients are treated with both topical corticosteroids and calcipotriene. A new vitamin D analogue calcitriol ointment was approved in 2009. A combination ointment containing calcipotriene and betamethasone for once daily application was introduced in 2006.

Level 2: Phototherapy

Phototherapy is highly effective, clearing 80% to 100% of the skin. However, some maintenance therapy is usually necessary. The disadvantages to this treatment method are that it requires special equipment, two or three office visits a week, and is expensive. Additionally, it carries a short-term risk of sunburn and a theoretical long-term risk of skin cancer. As alternatives, natural sunlight and ultraviolet light (UVA) tanning beds are only mildly therapeutic.

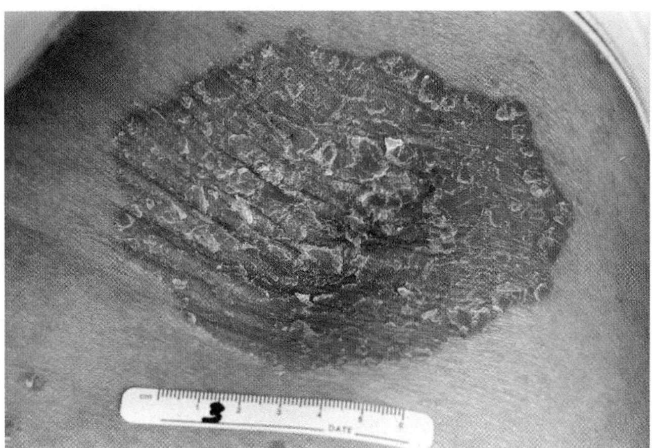

Figure 1 Plaque-type psoriasis. Well-demarcated red plaque with white-to-silvery scales on the surface.

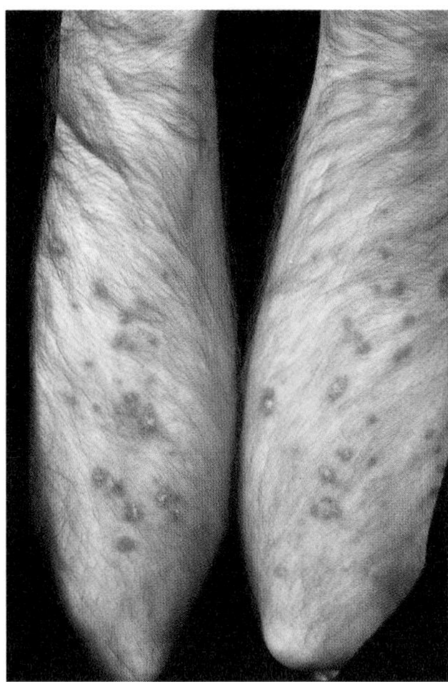

Figure 2 Guttate psoriasis. Widespread small, drop-like, red scaly papules that can coalesce into plaques.

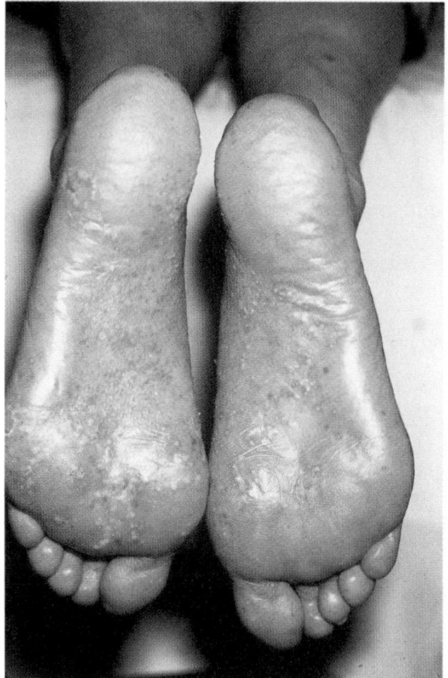

Figure 3 Pustular psoriasis, localized to the soles. Many small sterile pustules on a background of erythema that can coalesce and become hemorrhagic.

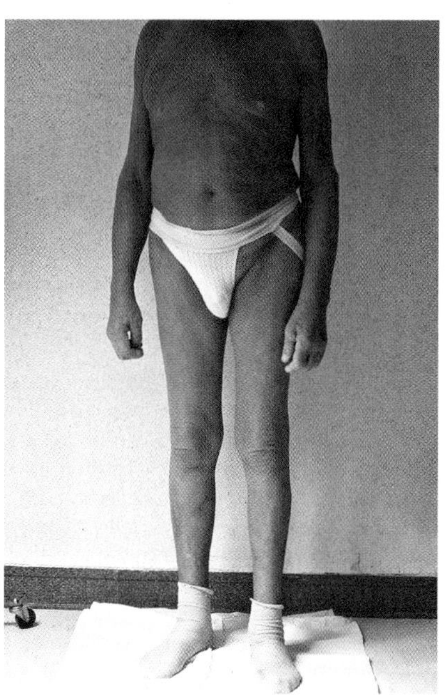

Figure 4 Psoriatic erythroderma or exfoliative dermatitis. Nearly the entire body skin is red. Scaling is less predominant than the plaque type, and a few pustules may form.

Level 3: Systemic Treatments

Systemic treatments are more effective than level 2 treatments, but they are usually more expensive and have greater potential for toxicity. Systemic treatments for psoriasis are generally prescribed after consultation with the dermatologist.

Methotrexate is the antimetabolite most often prescribed by dermatologists for moderate-to-severe psoriasis. Hepatotoxicity is the primary clinical concern when planning long-term methotrexate therapy. Mild transaminase elevations (less than twice the upper limit of normal) are to be expected during therapy, but these levels do not correlate with hepatic fibrosis. The guidelines for monitoring for liver damage differ for rheumatologists and dermatologists. The American College of Rheumatology (ACR) does not recommend liver biopsy during treatment unless 5 of 9 or 6 of 12 liver enzyme levels in a 12-month period are elevated or unless the serum albumin concentration decreases below normal. A 1998 consensus conference of the American Academy of Dermatology recommends liver biopsy at baseline only if the patient has significant risk factors. The initial liver biopsy is done after a 1 g to 1.5 g cumulative dose and is repeated after 3 g and 4 g cumulative doses. A 2009 consensus conference now advocates following ACR guidelines for patients with no risk factors, for liver injury and considering liver biopsy or switching to another treatment after 3.5 to 4 g to total cumulative methotrexate dosage. Folic acid supplementation 1 mg/day is recommended because it mitigates the gastrointestinal effects of methotrexate without reducing efficacy. It also prevents megaloblastic anemia.

Nephrotoxicity and hypertension are the two most serious side effects of cyclosporine therapy. Although it is very effective for severe

Table 1 Treatments for Psoriasis

Level 1	Level 2	Level 3	Level 4*	Level 5*	Level 6
Emollients	Natural sunlight	Acitretin (may be combined with UVB light or with PUVA)	Sulfasalazine	Azathioprine	Alefacept
Keratolytics: salicylic acid, lactic acid, urea	Ultraviolet B (UVB) light	Methotrexate	Hydroxyurea	6-Thioguanine	Efalizumab†
Calcipotriene calcitriol	UVB light and coal tar (Goeckerman regimen)	Cyclosporine	Calcitriol	Mycophenolate mofetil	Etanercept
Anthralin (usually short contact)	UVB light and anthralin (Ingram regimen)		Antibiotics	Tacrolimus	Infliximab
Corticosteroids: topical, hydrocolloid occlusive, intralesional injections	UVB narrowband light (311-313 nm)				Adalimumab
Coal tar	Psoralen and ultraviolet A (UVA) light (PUVA)				Ustekinumab*
Tazarotene	Psoralen, UVA light and UVB light				

*Not approved for psoriasis treatment by the U.S. Food and Drug Administration.
†Withdrawn from U.S. market in 2009.

psoriasis, cyclosporine has been relegated to brief intermittent courses or crisis intervention after the approval of safer biologic immunomodulators (level 6).

Levels 4 and 5: Experimental Treatments

Treatments in levels 4 and 5 are not approved by the U.S. Food and Drug Administration (FDA) for psoriasis. Level 4 treatments are slightly to moderately effective but are less toxic than level 5 treatments. Level 5 treatments are reserved for the most severe and recalcitrant cases, including PSA.

Level 6: Biologic Immunomodulators

Level 6 treatments are the biologic immunomodulators—some of which are currently FDA-approved for psoriasis, PSA, and other indications. The biologics are monoclonal antibodies and fusion proteins that represent a new paradigm for treatment of moderate-to-severe psoriasis. These compounds are designed to antagonize cell-cell interactions, memory-effector T cells, or proinflammatory cytokines.

Alefacept is a fusion protein composed of leukocyte function antigen-3 and human immunoglobulin 1 (IgG1) domains that is administered as a once weekly intramuscular dose of 15 mg for 12 weeks. In double-blind placebo-controlled phase III studies, 21% of patients achieved more than 75% improvement at 14 weeks compared with 5% receiving placebo. Alefacept was the first biologic to receive FDA approval for psoriasis in 2003. Although no serious side effects have been encountered, alefacept is now the least often prescribed biologic because of insufficient therapeutic response rates.

Efalizumab is a humanized monoclonal antibody directed against the CD-11a subunit of leukocyte function antigen-1 (LFA-1) expressed on T cells. By blocking the interaction of LFA-1 and its ligand intercellular adhesion molecule-1, T cell activation and migration into psoriatic plaques are decreased. In phase III trials, efalizumab injected once weekly at 1 mg/kg achieved >75% improvement after 12 weeks in 27% of patients compared with 4% receiving placebo. About 50% of patients maintained more than 75% improvement after 3 years of open-label treatment. Efalizumab was also approved by the FDA for psoriasis in 2003. After three cases of progressive multifocal leukoencephalopathy caused by the JC virus were reported in association with efalizumab therapy for psoriasis, the manufacturer voluntarily withdrew the drug from the U.S. market in June 2009. About 10% of patients experience a flare of their disease either during or after abruptly stopping efalizumab.

Tumor Necrosis Factor Inhibitors

Etanercept is a cloned and engineered fusion protein made of two p75 TNF receptors and the Fc portion of human IgG. It binds and inactivates TNF and prevents its significant proinflammatory effects in the target tissue of skin and joints. Etanercept is a disease modifying antirheumatic drug that is FDA approved for rheumatoid and psoriatic arthritis with and without methotrexate. In the pivotal phase III studies of etanercept in psoriasis, 25 mg administered twice weekly by subcutaneous injection and 50 mg twice weekly gave more than 75% improvement in 34% and 49% of patients, respectively, after 12 weeks compared with 4% receiving placebo. Etanercept was approved for psoriasis by the FDA in 2004 at a starting dose of 50 mg twice weekly for 12 weeks followed by 25 mg twice weekly for maintenance. Slight recrudescence of disease occurred in some patients after the step down in dosage, but the mean percent improvement was stable after 48 weeks. In studies, only wheal-like injection site reactions occurred at higher frequency with etanercept than placebo. Infrequent associations of new onset or aggravation of demyelinating diseases, congestive heart failure, and aplastic anemia have been observed without assigning cause and effect. No baseline or monitoring laboratory tests are required.

Infliximab is a chimeric (human-mouse) monoclonal antibody that binds TNF. It is FDA approved for rheumatoid and psoriatic arthritis and *Crohn's disease* with and without methotrexate. It is delivered by an intravenous infusion over a 2-hour period. Phase II trials of infliximab as monotherapy indicated high efficacy in psoriasis. In phase III trials, 1462 patients were treated with placebo, 3 mg/kg, or 5 mg/kg infliximab infusions given at weeks 0, 2, and 6. The proportion of patients achieving more than 75% improvement in the severity score at 10 weeks was 3%, 71%, and 79%, respectively. Maintenance therapy was continued at 5 mg/kg every 8 weeks, and the response was sustained for 26 weeks. The serious immediate infusion reaction rate is 1%, and about 1% of patients experience delayed hypersensitivity reactions consisting of myalgia, arthralgia, fever, or rash. Neutralizing antibodies are formed in about 20% of patients treated for 1 year, which can result in dose creep, whereby dose escalation or more frequent dosing of infliximab becomes necessary to keep symptoms under control. Concomitant methotrexate administration reduces the development of antichimeric antibodies. Current practice is to repeat infusions of 5 mg/kg every 6 to 8 weeks to maintain response.

Adalimumab is a human anti-TNF monoclonal antibody that blocks the interaction of TNF with the p55 and p75 cell-surface receptors. It is currently approved for rheumatoid and psoriatic arthritis. Phase III studies of patients with both psoriasis and PSA showed that 59% achieved more than 75% improvement in skin disease after 24 weeks at a dosage of 40 mg every other week by subcutaneous injection.

The greatest theoretical risks associated with the biologic immunomodulators discussed here are serious infections, particularly granulomatous, and increased rates of malignancy, particularly the lymphoproliferative diseases. To date, controlled trials and postmarketing surveillance studies have not conclusively demonstrated a higher-than-expected frequency of lymphomas in patients who have been treated the longest with anti-TNF agents; however, the risk for reactivating *tuberculosis* is considered greater for infliximab and adalimumab than with etanercept. Therefore, screening for tuberculosis is required before administering the monoclonal antibodies.

A novel mechanism of action employs monoclonal antibodies directed against the cytokines interleukin 12 and 23 which are postulated to regulate the inflammatory responses in psoriasis. In a phase III double-blind placebo-controlled study of 766 patients, 67% of patients who received ustekinumab by subcutaneous injection at week 0 and week 4 achieved greater than 75% improvement by week 12 compared to 3% of placebo-treated patients. Dosing of ustekinumab every 12 weeks maintained this response in most patients for up to 76 weeks.

Summary

- Psoriasis affects 2% of the U.S. population; about 11% of these patients have psoriatic arthritis.
- There are four clinical variants of psoriasis, but plaque type is the most common (80% of cases).
- Consultation with a dermatologist is recommended if the patient fails to respond to topical therapy (level 1) and natural sunlight or tanning bed exposure.
- Psoriasis is considered moderate to severe if it involves more than 5% of body surface area.
- Phototherapy, systemic, or biologic therapies (levels 2 through 6) are recommended for moderate-to-severe psoriasis.

Suggested Readings

Boenhnke W-H, Prinz J, Gottlieb AB: Biologic therapies for psoriasis. A systematic review. J Rheumatol 2006;33:1-5.

Callen JP, Krueger GG, Lebwohl M, et al: AAD consensus statement on psoriasis therapies. J Am Acad Dermatol 2003;49:897-899.

Helm TN, Camisa C: "Psoralens and photochemotherapy (PUVA)." In Camisa C (ed): Handbook of Psoriasis, ed.2. Blackwell, Oxford, UK, 2004, pp 191-214.

Kalb RE, Strober B, Weinstein G, Lebwohl M: Methotrexate and psoriasis: 2009 National Psoriasis Foundation consensus conference. J Am Acad Dermatol 2009;60:824-837.

Krueger GG, Feldman SR, Camisa C, et al: Two considerations for patients with psoriasis and their clinicians: What defines mild, moderate, and severe psoriasis? What constitutes a clinically significant improvement when treating psoriasis? J Am Acad Dermatol 2000;43:281-285.

Lebwohl M, Ali S: Treatment of psoriasis. Part 1. Topical therapy and phototherapy. J Am Acad Dermatol 2001;45:487-498.

Lebwohl M, Ali S: Treatment of psoriasis. Part 2. Systemic therapies. J Am Acad Dermatol 2001;45:649-661.

Leonardi C, Powers JL, Matheson RT, et al: Etanercept as monotherapy in patients with psoriasis. N Engl J Med 2003;349:2014-2022.

Leonardi CL, Papp KA, Gordon KB, et al: Extended efalizumab therapy improves chronic plaque psoriasis: Results from a randomized phase III trial. J Am Acad Dermatol 2005;52:425-433.

Leonardi CL, Kimball AB, Papp KA, et al: Efficacy and safety of ustekinumab, a human inter-leukin-12/23 monoclonal antibody, in patients with psoriasis: 76-week results from a randomised, double-blind, placebo-controlled trial (PHOENIX1). Lancet 2008 May 17;371(9625):1639-1640.

Mease PJ, Gladman DD, Ritchlin CT, et al: Adalimumab for the treatment of patients with moderately to severely active psoriatic arthritis. Results of a double-blind, randomized, placebo-controlled trial. Arthritis Rheum 2005;52:3279-3289.

Reich K, Nestle FO, Papp K, et al: Infliximab induction and maintenance therapy for moderate-to-severe psoriasis: A phase III, multicentre, double-blind trial. Lancet 2005; 366:1367-1374.

Stern RS: Utilization of outpatient care for psoriasis. J Am Acad Dermatol 1996;35:543-545.

Other Papulosquamous Diseases

Mandi P. Sachdeva and Kenneth J. Tomecki

PITYRIASIS ROSEA

Definition

Pityriasis rosea is an acute self-limited papulosquamous disease that most commonly affects adolescents and young adults during the spring and fall seasons. It affects both genders, with a slight female predominance.

Pathogenesis

The exact cause of pityriasis rosea is unknown, but a viral cause has been suggested. Recent literature has supported an association of pityriasis rosea with human herpesvirus-6 and -7.

Clinical Features

Classic pityriasis rosea initially manifests with a solitary oval, pink to tan, scaly plaque on the neck or trunk, termed the *herald patch* because it heralds the onset of disease. Following the appearance of the herald patch, similar smaller scaly papules and plaques develop on the trunk and proximal extremities in a striking and characteristic Christmas tree or fir tree pattern, with the long axis of the plaques running parallel to the lines of skin cleavage (Fig. 1).

The exanthem of pityriasis rosea typically lasts 6 to 8 weeks, and recurrences are uncommon. Some patients complain of pruritus, but most are asymptomatic. A small percentage of patients experience mild prodromal symptoms including malaise, fever, headache, and arthralgias.

Diagnosis

Diagnosis is usually based on clinical appearance, history, and the self-limited course of disease. Differential diagnosis includes tinea corporis, tinea versicolor, small-plaque parapsoriasis, drug rash, and syphilis. Skin biopsy is usually not necessary except in atypical cases.

Treatment

Pityriasis rosea usually requires no treatment except patient education and reassurance. For symptomatic patients, oral antihistamines a mid-potency topical corticosteroid, or both, may be helpful. Phototherapy with narrow-band ultraviolet B (UVB) and oral antiviral medication have both been anecdotally reported to decrease the duration of disease.

PITYRIASIS RUBRA PILARIS

Definition

Pityriasis rubra pilaris (PRP) is an uncommon papulosquamous skin disease characterized by erythematous papules that coalesce into large, orange-red, scaly plaques with classic islands of sparing. Keratoderma of the palms and soles and nail dystrophy are also common. PRP affects men and women equally with a bimodal age of onset during the first 5 years and then in the fifth decade of life.

Pathogenesis

The exact cause of PRP is not known, but it may be related to abnormal keratinization of the epidermis or abnormal vitamin A metabolism. Associations with autoimmune disease, internal malignancy, infection, minor trauma to the skin, and human immunodeficiency virus have also been suggested.

Clinical Features

Patients with PRP have small, hyperkeratotic, follicular-based red papules that coalesce into large scaly plaques. The plaques have a distinctive orange-red or salmon color with characteristic islands of normal-appearing skin interspersed within (Fig. 2). The most common form of PRP begins on the scalp and spreads caudally in a symmetrical and generalized pattern with a predilection for the sides of the neck, trunk, and extensor surfaces of the extremities. Some patients have an associated waxy keratoderma of the palms and soles and thickened, yellow nails with subungual debri.

Griffith's classification helps to distinguish subtypes of PRP based on age of onset, duration of disease, and type of cutaneous involvement. Type I, classic adult PRP, is the most common form. It is typically self-limited, and skin disease resolves in the majority of patients within 3 years of onset. Type II includes patients with an associated palmoplantar keratoderma and differs from type I in that disease clears in only approximately 20% of patients within 3 years of onset. Types III and IV are juvenile forms of PRP. A sixth type has been proposed to describe patients with HIV infection who develop PRP that is often recalcitrant to therapy.

Diagnosis

The diagnosis of PRP is based on clinical presentation. If necessary, a skin biopsy can be taken to assist in diagnosis, but results are often nonspecific. Classic histopathology reveals epidermal hyperplasia with hyperkeratosis and alternating parakeratosis in a characteristic checkerboard pattern. Hair follicles are dilated and filled with keratin plugs correlating to the follicular-based keratotic papules seen clinically.

The main differential diagnosis is psoriasis, which is characterized by silvery white scale overlying the plaques and a lack of follicular papules.

Treatment

The mainstay of treatment for PRP is systemic retinoid therapy. Acitretin is the most commonly used oral retinoid for PRP. Alternatively, isotretinoin can be used. Both can take 6 to 9 months to achieve full therapeutic effect. Methotrexate, either used alone or in combination with an oral retinoid, is another therapeutic option. When using combination therapy, an increased risk of hepatotoxity must be kept in mind. Topical corticosteroids, vitamin D analogues, and creams containing lactic acid or urea can be useful adjuvant therapies.

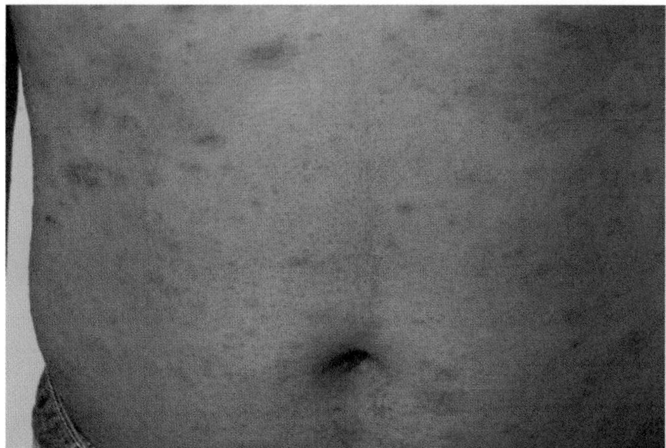

Figure 1 **Pityriasis rosea.**

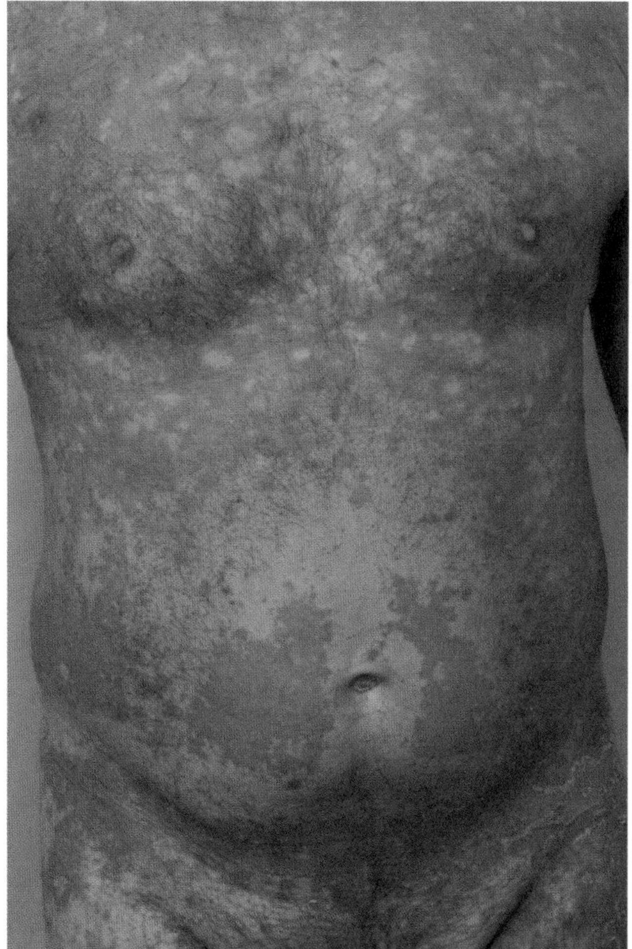

Figure 2 **Pityriasis rubra pilaris.**

PARAPSORIASIS

Definition

Parapsoriasis is a chronic T-cell predominant dermatitis categorized as either large-plaque (LPP) or small-plaque (SPP) disease. Both have similar clinical and histopathologic findings as well an association with cutaneous T-cell lymphoma (CTCL). Middle-aged and elderly adults are most commonly affected without gender or race predilection.

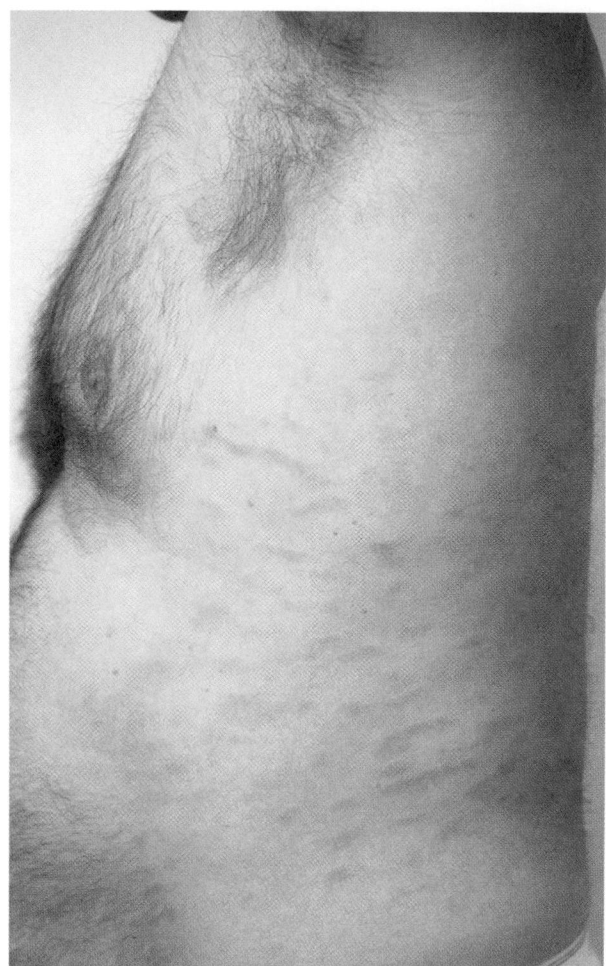

Figure 3 **Small-plaque parapsoriasis.**

Pathogenesis

The etiology of parapsoriasis is unknown. Both LPP and SPP are characterized by superficial lymphocytic infiltrates composed of predominantly $CD4^+$ T cells. T-cell clonality occurs in both LPP and SPP, but it is more common in LPP; therefore, LPP is often considered an intermediate on a spectrum of disease between chronic lymphocytic dermatitis and CTCL.

Clinical Features

Parapsoriasis is characterized by pink to tan plaques with fine, delicate overlying scale that favor sun-protected areas. In SPP, the plaques are small, usually less than 5 cm in diameter, and digitate, with elongated finger-like patches distributed symmetrically on the flanks (Fig. 3). The plaques of LPP are larger than 5 cm and vary in size and shape compared with those of SPP (Fig. 4). LPP plaques may be atrophic, with overlying telangiectasia and varying hyper- and hypopigmentation. Parapsoriasis is usually asymptomatic and tends to run a chronic course.

Diagnosis

Diagnosis is based on clinical and histopathologic findings. Clinically, LPP and SPP are distinguished from each other based on the

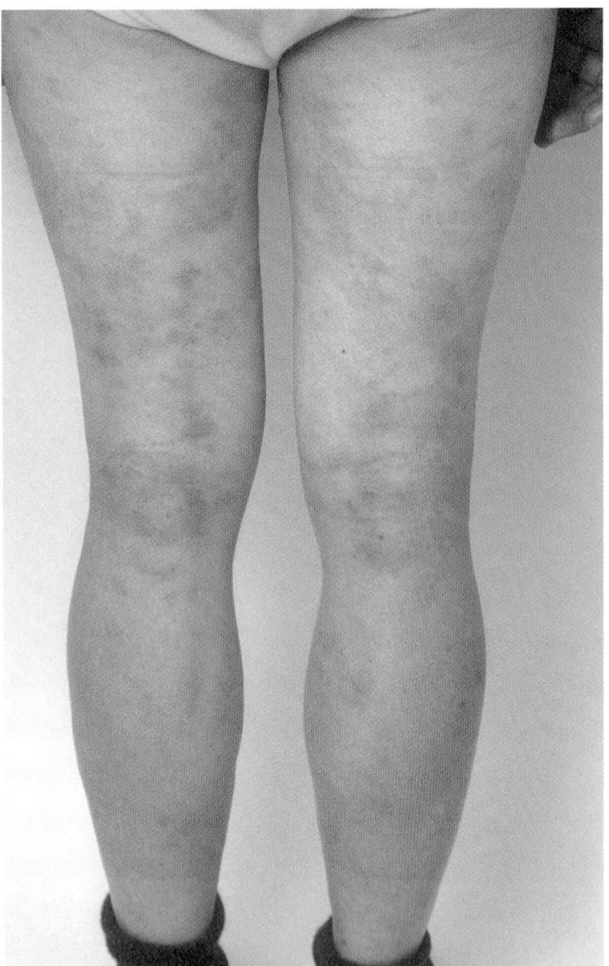

Figure 4 Large-plaque parapsoriasis.

size of the plaques. Both have similar histopathologic findings, with a superficial perivascular lymphocytic infiltrate composed primarily of $CD4^+$ lymphocytes. The epidermis shows focal spongiosis with overlying confluent parakeratosis. Cytologic atypia and epidermotropism are not present.

SPP can resemble pityriasis rosea clinically, but unlike pityriasis rosea, SPP lacks a herald patch and runs a chronic course. Other diseases that may be included in the differential include nummular dermatitis, psoriasis, and secondary syphilis. The most important differential concern for LPP is CTCL of the mycosis fungoides type.

Treatment

Therapy for parapsoriasis is predicated on the use of topical corticosteroids, phototherapy, or both. Parapsoriasis can progress to CTCL, and therefore all patients with parapsoriasis should be evaluated regularly for disease progression.

CUTANEOUS T-CELL LYMPHOMA

Definition

Cutaneous T-cell lymphoma is a broad term that describes a group of heterogeneous skin lymphomas composed of helper T cells. CTCL accounts for 75% to 80% of all skin lymphomas. Different subtypes exist based on clinical presentation, histopathology, immunophenotype, and prognosis. Mycosis fungoides is the most common variant of CTCL and is the one focused on in this chapter.

Mycosis fungoides is a rare disease with approximately 1000 new cases diagnosed per year. It can affect any age group, but it most commonly occurs between the fourth and sixth decades of life. Men are affected almost twice as often as women.

Pathogenesis

The exact cause of mycosis fungoides is unknown, but genetic, environmental, and immunologic factors might all play roles.

Clinical Features

Classically, patients with mycosis fungoides progress from patch to plaque and finally tumor-stage disease over a variable, but usually protracted period. Early patch stage is characterized by thin, well-demarcated, erythematous plaques of varying size with fine scale that have a predilection for the buttocks, trunk, or other sun-protected areas. With progression of disease, plaques gradually enlarge and become thickened, indurated, and reddish-brown, often forming annular, polycyclic, or horseshoe-shaped configurations (Fig. 5). Many patients never progress beyond the plaque stage, but some eventually develop nodules and tumors.

The risk of developing extracutaneous disease correlates with the extent and duration of skin disease. It is most common in patients with skin tumors or erythroderma. Extracutaneous disease is rare in patients with limited patch or plaque stage disease.

Diagnosis

Most patients with mycosis fungoides carry a long history of chronic dermatitis, with past skin biopsies showing nonspecific changes. Any patient with chronic dermatitis that does not respond to standard therapies should be evaluated for CTCL, specifically with repeat skin biopsies to assess the quality of the lymphoid infiltrate in the skin.

The diagnosis of mycosis fungoides can be confirmed with routine histopathology. Early patch disease shows a superficial bandlike and perivascular lymphocytic infiltrate. Atypical lymphocytes and epidermotropism are characteristic features of mycosis fungoides that differentiate it from other benign lymphocytic dermatoses. Immunohistochemical analysis and detection of T cell receptor gene rearrangement by polymerase chain reaction can also assist in making the diagnosis of mycosis fungoides. Further workup should include a complete blood count, peripheral blood smear, flow cytometry of the blood, and a lactic acid dehydrogenase level. Radiographic imaging including chest x-ray or pan-computed tomography may be performed if extracutaneous disease is suspected.

Patch stage mycosis fungoides can mimic several benign dermatoses including eczema, psoriasis, drug reaction, and fungal infection. These can be differentiated and excluded with standard dermatologic examination and histopathology when necessary. Small- and large-plaque parapsoriasis are also in the differential diagnosis of CTCL and can be difficult to differentiate both clinically and histopathologically.

Treatment

Initial treatment depends on the stage of the disease. Patch stage disease is best managed with topical therapies including corticosteroids, retinoids, and possibly topical chemotherapy agents including nitrogen mustard (mechlorethamine) or carmustine. Phototherapy can be effective in the management of early disease, especially if pruritus is present. For plaque stage disease, focal radiotherapy or total skin electron beam radiation can be considered based on extent of disease. Tumor disease requires a combination of chemotherapy, radiotherapy, and phototherapy. Newer immunomodulatory therapies, including targeted cytotoxic fusion proteins and various vaccination strategies, are emerging potential treatments for CTCL.

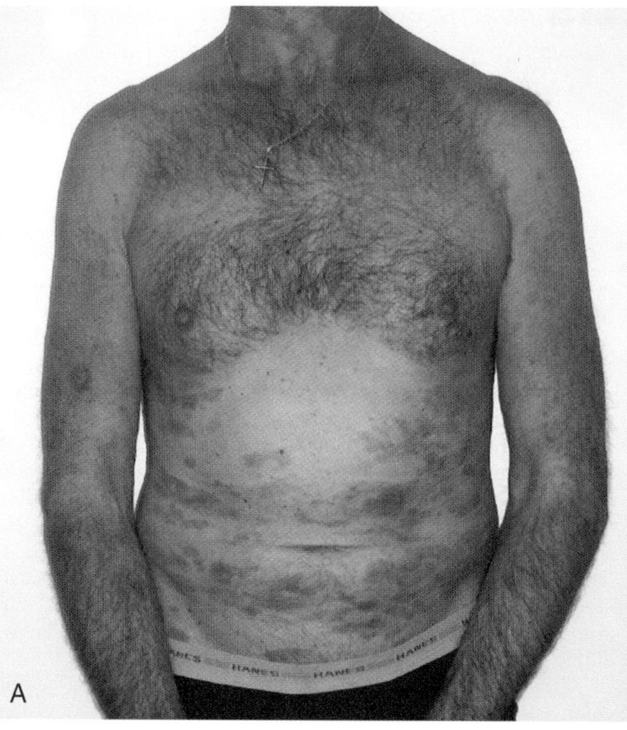

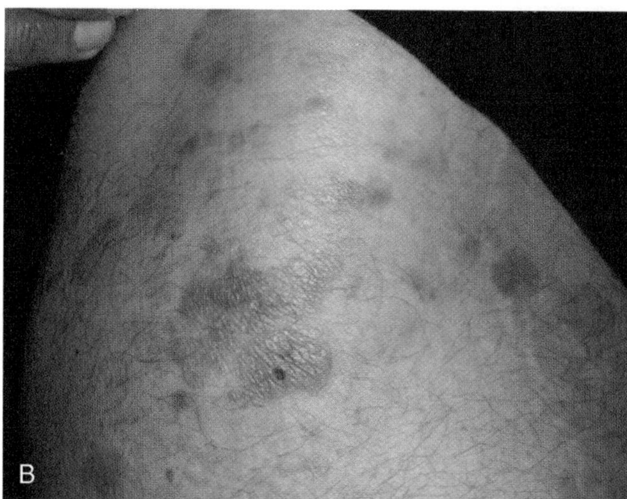

Figure 5 Plaque-stage cutaneous T cell lymphoma.

Summary

- Other papulosquamous diseases that may be encountered by the internist include pityriasis rosea, pityriasis rubra pilaris, parapsoriasis, and cutaneous T-cell lymphoma.
- Pityriasis rosea is a benign, self-limited, likely viral-induced papulosquamous eruption that most commonly occurs in adolescents and young adults.
- Pityriasis rubra pilaris is a rare skin disease that resembles psoriasis clinically and responds well to oral retinoids.
- Parapsoriasis is a lymphocytic dermatitis that is sometimes considered a precursor to cutaneous T-cell lymphoma.
- Cutaneous T-cell lymphoma should be considered in any patient with long-standing dermatitis that has not responded to standard therapies.

Suggested Readings

Albert MR, Mackool BT: Pityriasis rubra pilaris. Int J Dermatol 1999; 38(1):1-11.

Gonzalez LM, Allen R, Janniger CK, Schwartz RA: Pityriasis rosea: An important papulosquamous disorder. Int J Dermatol 2005;44(9):757-764.

Kazakov DV, Burg G, Kempf W: Clinicopathological spectrum of mycosis fungoides. J Eur Acad Dermatol Venereol 2004;18(4):397-415.

Norman RA, Blanco PM: Papulosquamous diseases in the elderly. Dermatol Ther 2003;16(3):231-242.

Slater, DN: The new World Health Organization-European Organization for Research and Treatment of Cancer classification for cutaneous lymphomas: A practical marriage of two giants. Br J Dermatol 2005;153(5):874-880.

Atopic Dermatitis

Melissa Piliang

DEFINITION

Atopic dermatitis (Fig. 1) and hereditary eczema are interchangeable terms for an inflammatory condition of the skin characterized by erythema, pruritus, scaling, lichenification, and papulovesicles. Atopic dermatitis is a distinct condition in persons who are genetically predisposed to developing immunoglobulin (Ig) E-mediated hypersensitivity reactions. It is characterized by the itch-scratch cycle: Affected persons have the sensation of itch, followed by scratching and the subsequent creation of a rash. The classic triad of atopy includes eczema, asthma, and allergies. A wide range of environmental factors, such as contact allergens, stress, food, skin flora, and humidity, play roles in the development and severity of atopic dermatitis.

PREVALENCE

Atopic dermatitis is a common condition affecting approximately 17% of the population,[1] with a slight female preponderance (1.3:1 in children). The incidence has increased twofold to threefold since the 1970s. The basis of this increase in not well understood; however, environmental factors appear to play an important role in disease prevalence.

Some factors associated with an increased risk of atopic dermatitis include small family size, higher socioeconomic and educational levels regardless of ethnicity, movement from rural to urban environment, and increased use of antibiotics (the Western lifestyle). This has led to the hygiene hypothesis, which postulates that infections in early childhood (from less-hygienic practices and older siblings) might prevent atopic dermatitis. This hypothesis is supported by evidence that infections induce type-1 helper T cells (Th1), whereas there is a predominance of type-2 helper T cells (Th2) in atopic dermatitis. Th1 responses antagonize the development of Th2 cells, thereby potentially decreasing the incidence of atopic dermatitis.[2]

PATHOPHYSIOLOGY

Atopic dermatitis is a type I IgE-mediated hypersensitivity reaction, but the exact etiology is unknown. The pathogenesis is multifactorial and involves a complex immunologic cascade, including disruption of the epidermal barrier, IgE dysregulation, defects in the cutaneous cell-mediated immune response, and genetic factors.

The major elements in immune dysregulation are Langerhans' cells, inflammatory dendritic epidermal cells, monocytes, macrophages, lymphocytes, mast cells, and keratinocytes, all of which interact through an intricate cascade of cytokines leading to a predominance of Th2 cells over (Th1 cells).[3] The Th2 cytokines, interleukin (IL)-4, IL-5, IL-10, and IL-13, are increased in the skin, and there is a corresponding decrease in Th1 cytokines, mainly interferon-γ and IL-2.

Patients with atopic dermatitis often have dry, sensitive skin due to changes in the epidermis, which serves as a barrier to the environment by maintaining the water balance of the skin. Essential fatty acids (EFAs), such as linoleic and linolenic acid, are important components of the epidermal barrier. In atopic dermatitis, Δ6-desaturase activity is deficient, which leads to decreased linoleic and linolenic acid metabolites. Loss of EFAs results in increased transepidermal water loss and subsequent xerosis (dryness). The EFAs form the substrate of the inflammatory mediators (prostaglandins and leukotrienes), resulting in a secondary deficiency of prostaglandin E_1 (PGE_1).

Defects in the epidermal barrier also lead to increased susceptibility to atopens (atopic allergens such as house dust mites, grass, or pollen). When such allergens contact atopic skin, they stimulate Th2 lymphocytes to produce cytokines such as IL-4, IL-5, and IL-13, which in turn promote an increase in IgE synthesis.[4] Atopic dermatitis patients often have high levels of IgE antibodies to house dust mites and other allergens. Elimination of these allergens from the environment, an extremely difficult undertaking, can lead to improvement of atopic dermatitis.

Defective cell-mediated immunity leads to increased susceptibility to many bacterial, viral, and fungal infections of the skin. Children with atopic dermatitis are particularly susceptible to severe, widespread herpes simplex virus infection (eczema herpeticum), a systemic and potentially fatal infection affecting primarily areas of active eczema. Widespread infections with human papillomavirus (warts) and molluscum contagiosum are also common in children with atopic dermatitis.

Many factors exacerbate or trigger atopic dermatitis, including colonization with *Staphylococcus aureus,* stress, anxiety, systemic illness, and xerosis. The most common trigger is *S. aureus* colonization. More than 90% of patients with atopic dermatitis have *S. aureus* colonization of lesional skin, and more than 75% have colonization of uninvolved skin.[5] Staphylococci exacerbate atopic dermatitis by two mechanisms: acting as superantigens by stimulating an augmented T cell response, thereby leading to exacerbation of skin disease, and promoting increased production of IgE. IgE has anti–*S. aureus* properties and helps to control colonization and infection in normal persons. In atopic dermatitis patients, the elevated IgE levels contribute to immune dysregulation. Treatment with topical or oral antistaphylococcal antibiotics (or both) decreases the colonization of the skin and often leads to improvement of the dermatitis.

Family studies support a genetic basis for atopic dermatitis. When both parents are atopic, their offspring have a 70% risk for atopic dermatitis,[6] with a higher risk of inheritance if the mother is atopic. The mode of inheritance appears to be complex and likely involves several genes. To date, no specific single gene has been identified as a unique marker for atopic dermatitis or atopy.[7]

SIGNS AND SYMPTOMS

Atopic dermatitis is a chronic disease with periods of remissions and exacerbations. Three age-related stages exist: the infantile stage (up to 2 years old), the childhood stage (from 2 to 12 years), and the adult stage (puberty onward). The manifestations vary with age, even in the same patient. All stages are characterized by xerosis, fissures, pruritus, and lichenification. The main differentiating factor is the area of involvement.

The infantile stage is characterized by very pruritic, red, eczematous plaques on the cheeks and extensor extremities. Secondary impetiginization, with honey-colored crust, is common in infants. Scalp involvement can resemble seborrheic dermatitis. The diaper area is spared.

The childhood stage is primarily a papular dermatitis affecting the flexural areas, especially the antecubital and popliteal fossae, wrists, ankles, and neck. Thickened, lichenified plaques with excoriation (Figs. 2 to 4) are common. In darker-pigmented children, follicular papules may be the only manifestation. Hypopigmentation and hyperpigmentation can occur, which can cause great anxiety in parents. Pityriasis alba, characterized by hypopigmented, scaly patches on the face, is commonly seen. Keratosis pilaris, or spiny hair

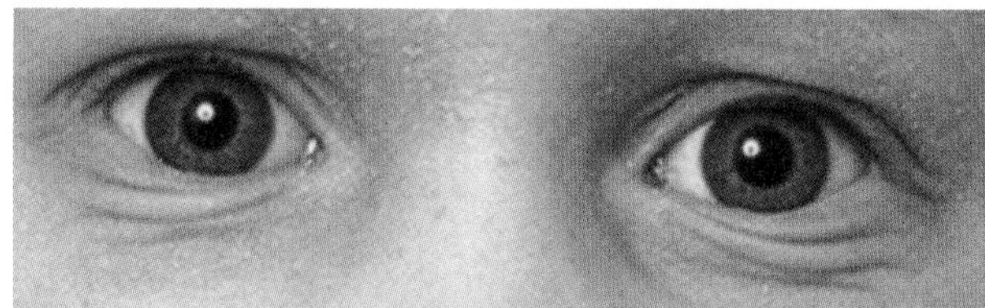

Figure 1 Perioral and periorbital dermatitis with hyperlinearity on the lower eyelid (Dennie-Morgan lines).

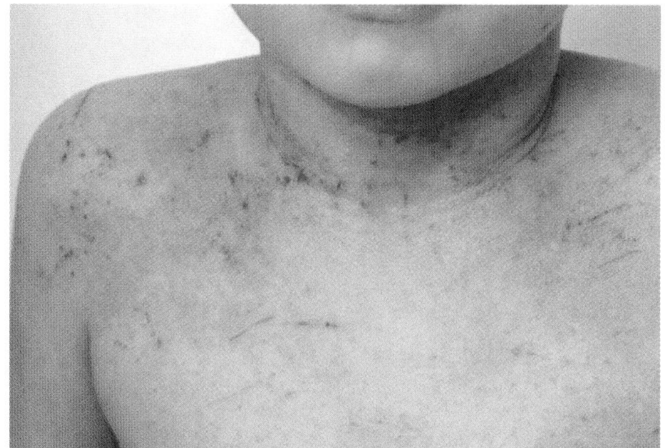

Figure 2 Linear superficial erosions of the neck and upper chest consistent with excoriations.

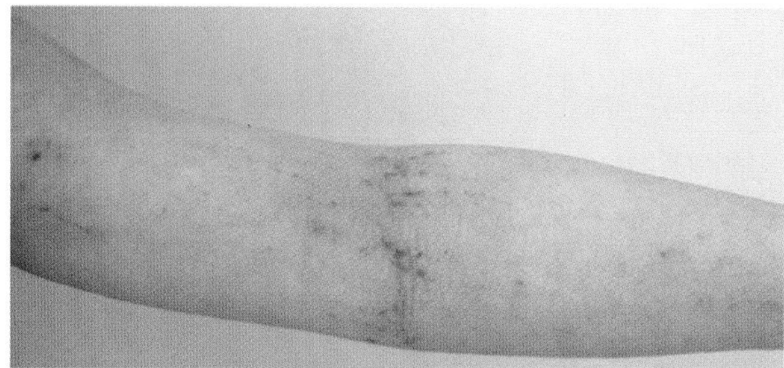

Figure 3 Excoriations and lichenification of the antecubital fossa.

follicles, commonly affect the posterior aspects of the upper arms and the anterior thighs.

The adult stage is unpredictable. Affected patients may have had only a few outbreaks since infancy, or they may have had a chronic, relapsing course. The hand dermatitis is common and may be the only manifestation of adult atopic dermatitis, which can lead to significant disability. Like affected children, adults also commonly have lichenification of the flexures and facial dermatitis.

DIAGNOSIS

The diagnosis of atopic dermatitis depends on a personal and/or family history of atopy coupled with the clinical signs and symptoms described by Hanifin (Box 1).[8] Pruritus and xerosis are key elements; without them, the diagnosis should be questioned.[5]

Atopic dermatitis can resemble other types of dermatitis (seborrheic dermatitis, allergic contact dermatitis, irritant contact dermatitis) and dermatophytosis. It may be a component of rare genetic diseases such as Netherton's syndrome, ichthyoses, and immunodeficiency syndromes (e.g., X-linked agammaglobulinemia, Wiskott-Aldrich syndrome, isolated IgA deficiency, and severe combined immunodeficiency disease). Helpful diagnostic tests include a serum IgE level, serum protein electrophoresis, fungal scraping for potassium hydroxide preparation and culture, and skin biopsy.

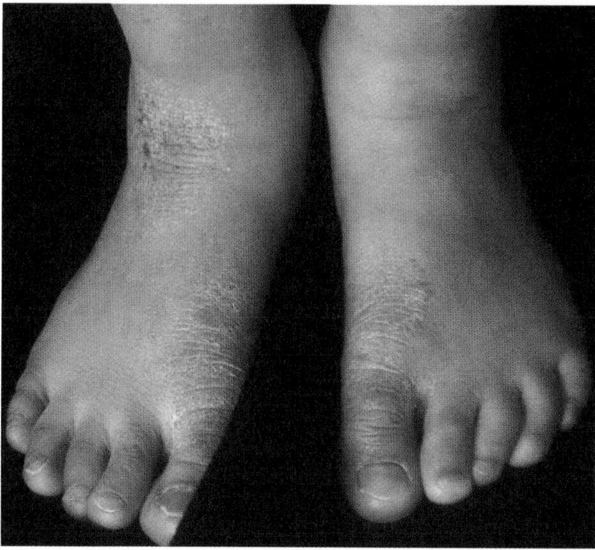

Figure 4 Lichenified, xerotic plaques on the dorsal feet.

Box 1 Hanifin Criteria for Atopic Dermatitis

Major Features (Must Have Three)

Pruritus

Typical morphology and distribution

- Facial and extensor involvement during infancy and childhood
- Flexural lichenification and linearity in adults

Chronic or chronically relapsing dermatitis

Personal or family history of atopy (asthma, allergic rhinoconjunctivitis, atopic dermatitis)

Minor or Less-Specific Features

Cheilitis

Hand or foot dermatitis

Ichthyosis, hyperlinearity, keratosis pilaris

Immunoglobulin E (IgE) reactivity (increased serum IgE, radioallergosorbent, or prick test reactivity)

Periauricular fissures

Perifollicular accentuation (especially in pigmented areas)

Scalp dermatitis (cradle cap)

Susceptibility to cutaneous infections (especially Staphylococcus aureus and herpes simplex virus)

Xerosis

Data from Hanifin JM: Atopic dermatitis in infants and children. Pediatr Clin North Am. 1991;38:763-789.

TREATMENT

Atopic dermatitis tends to be a chronic relapsing disease. The goals of therapy should be to reduce the number and severity of flares and to increase the number of disease-free periods. The mainstay of treatment for atopic dermatitis is hydrating the skin with the regular use of emollients and suppressing cutaneous inflammation with topical corticosteroids. Topical calcineurin inhibitors have become an important adjunctive therapy. For severe disease, especially during acute flares, systemic corticosteroids may be necessary. Secondary infections require treatment with topical or oral antibiotics, or both. Oral antihistamines can help decrease pruritus. In severe, recalcitrant cases, phototherapy or systemic immunosuppressive medications may be necessary.

Most patients with atopic dermatitis require hydration though the liberal use of bland emollients, which serve to hydrate the stratum corneum and maintain the lipid barrier. Sufficient emollients applied liberally several times a day may be enough to significantly reduce the disease activity of atopic dermatitis. Parents of infants and toddlers should apply a bland emollient to the entire body with each diaper change. Older children should apply bland emollients in the morning, after school, and at bedtime. Bathing should be limited to brief, cool showers once daily. Soap, which dries and irritates the skin, should be avoided, but gentle lipid-free cleansers are beneficial.

Corticosteroids suppress lymphocyte activity in the skin, thereby decreasing inflammation. Patients can use a low-potency topical steroid (hydrocortisone or desonide) for day-to-day control of mild disease and a medium-potency steroid (triamcinolone acetonide, fluticasone, or fluocinolone) for more severe flares. Low-potency topical steroids are suitable for infants and for intertriginous and sensitive areas (face, genitals); more potent steroids should be avoided on these sites. Severe, widespread disease can require systemic corticosteroids. Because of the well-known side effects of systemic corticosteroids (e.g., adrenal suppression, osteoporosis, hypertension, diabetes, obesity, striae), their use should be limited to the most severe disease.

Topical calcineurin inhibitors (tacrolimus, pimecrolimus) are effective alternatives to the chronic use of topical corticosteroids. Topical calcineurin inhibitors bind calcineurin and block the activation of T cells by cytokines, thus halting the inflammatory cascade that leads to atopic dermatitis. Topical calcineurin inhibitors are especially suitable for more delicate areas such as the face and genitals because they do not carry the risks of atrophy, telangectasias, and striae associated with the chronic use of steroids. Reports have surfaced suggesting a possible risk of lymphoma associated with high-dose oral pimecrolimus in animal studies,[9] prompting the FDA to put out a black box warning advising against the use of topical calcineurin inhibitors in children younger than 2 years. However, there are no data to support an increased risk of lymphoma with topical treatment in humans.[9] Topical calcineurin inhibitors should be used for a limited time and only on affected skin. They should not be used as a daily moisturizer, first-line therapy, or preventive therapy.

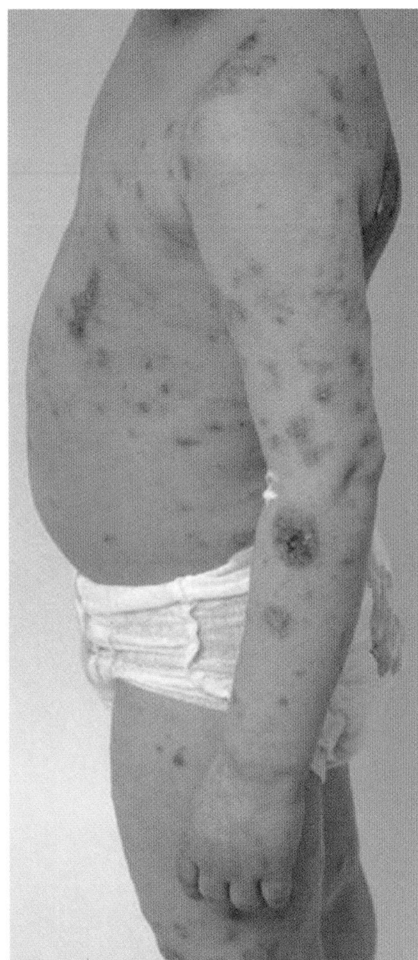

Figure 5 Atopic dermatitis with secondary impetiginization.

The pruritus associated with atopic dermatitis can be severe and often interferes with school, work, and sleep. Despite a lack of objective data to support their use, antihistamines are commonly used to break the itch-scratch-itch cycle.[10] Nonsedating antihistamines such as fexofenadine, cetirizine, loratidine, and desloratidine can help offset daytime itching without somnolence. Sedating antihistamines such as diphenhydramine or hydroxyzine are often helpful for nighttime pruritus.

Patients with atopy have an abnormal tolerance to *S. aureus* colonization of the skin, which can exacerbate the dermatitis. Affected patients should use lipid-free antibacterial cleansers. For open wounds, a topical antibiotic such as mupirocin can help to prevent secondary impetiginization (Figs. 5 and 6). An oral antibiotic with *S. aureus* coverage and good skin penetration, such as ampicillin-clavulanic acid, cephalexin, or azithromycin, is necessary for extensive excoriations and impetigo.

In severe, recalcitrant cases, ultraviolet (UV) light treatments (UVB or psoralen plus UVA [PUVA]) and immunosuppressive medications (e.g., methotrexate, cyclosporine, azathioprine, mycophenolate mofetil) may be helpful.[10] These should be used very cautiously and with close monitoring and should be reserved for the most severe cases.

Allergic contact dermatitis from topical medications, cosmetics, or metals should be considered in patients with recalcitrant disease. Evaluation by an environmental dermatologist and an allergist, including patch, pinprick, and serum radioallergosorbent testing (RAST), may be warranted. Topical medications that are known sensitizers, such as lidocaine, doxepin cream, and diphenhydramine cream, as well as topical antibiotics such as neomycin, should be strictly avoided. Allergic contact dermatitis to topical steroids should

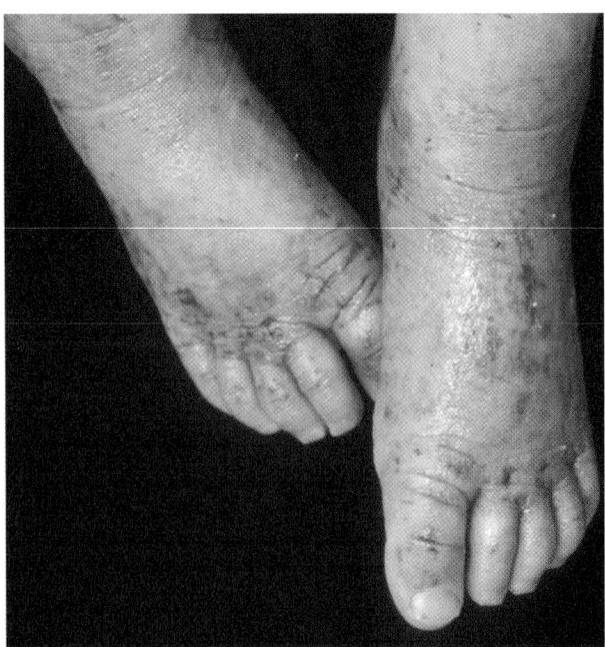

Figure 6 Weeping, lichenified, erythematous plaques with honey-colored crust (atopic dermatitis with secondary impetiginization).

be considered in any patient who fails to improve or worsens with the use of topical steroids.

OUTCOMES

Atopic dermatitis is a chronic disease with intermittent flares and spontaneous remissions. Approximately 40% to 60% of children with atopic dermatitis have the disease in adulthood, usually manifested as hand dermatitis. More than 75% of children with atopic dermatitis also have asthma or allergic rhinitis.

With good skin care, moisturization, and the use of topical corticosteroids or topical calcineurin inhibitors, most patients with atopic dermatitis do well.

Summary

- Atopic dermatitis is a common childhood condition in all races.
- Atopic dermatitis has an increased incidence in industrialized countries.
- It is associated with asthma and airborne allergies (atopic triad).
- First-line treatment consists of applying bland emollients, limiting soap, and decreasing bath temperature.
- Associated pruritus is severe and can interfere with social and scholarly activities.

Suggested Readings

Fonacier L, Spergel J, Charlesworth EN, et al: Report of the Topical Calcineurin Inhibitor Task Force of the American College of Allergy, Asthma and Immunology and the American Academy of Allergy, Asthma and Immunology. J Allergy Clin Immunol 2005;115:1249-1253.

Hanifin JM: Atopic dermatitis in infants and children. Pediatr Clin North Am 1991;38:763-789.

Klein PA, Clark RA: An evidence-based review of the efficacy of antihistamines in relieving pruritus in atopic dermatitis. Arch Dermatol 1999;135:1522-1525.

Kondo H, Ichikawa Y, Imokawa G: Percutaneous sensitization through barrier-disrupted skin elicits a TH2-dominant cytokine response. Eur J Immunol 1998;28:769-779.

Laughter D, Istvan JA, Tofte SJ, Hanifin JM: The prevalence of atopic dermatitis in Oregon school children. J Am Acad Dermatol 2000;43:649-655.

Leung DY, Bieber T: Atopic dermatitis. Lancet 2003;361:151-160.

MacLean JA, Eidelman FJ: The genetics of atopy and atopic eczema. Arch Dermatol 2001;137:1474-1476.

Rudikoff D, Lebwohl M: Atopic dermatitis. Lancet 1998;351:1715-1721.

Ruzicka T: Atopic eczema between rationality and irrationality. Arch Dermatol 1998;134:1462-1469.

Williams HC: Is the prevalence of atopic dermatitis increasing? Clin Exp Dermatol 1992;17:385-691.

References

For a complete list of references, log onto www.expertconsult.com.

Contact Dermatitis and Related Conditions

James S. Taylor and Antoine Amado

DEFINITION

Contact dermatitis is an acute or chronic immunologic (allergic) or nonimmunologic (irritant) inflammation of the skin usually caused by contact with chemicals but occasionally by biologic or physical agents.[1] Of the more than 85,000 chemicals in our environment, many can be irritants and more than 4350 have been identified as contact allergens. The potential for these substances to cause contact dermatitis varies greatly, and the severity of the dermatitis or eczema, the most common clinical expression, ranges from a mild, short-lived condition to a severe, persistent, job-threatening disease.

PREVALENCE AND RISK FACTORS

The prevalence of contact dermatitis in the general U.S. population has been variably estimated between 1.5% and 5.4%. Contact dermatitis is the third most common reason for patients to seek consultation with a dermatologist, accounting for 9.2 million visits in 2004. It also accounts for 95% of all reported occupational skin diseases.[1]

Exogenous and endogenous risk factors are listed in Boxes 1 and 2, respectively. Although genetics, gender, and age can be risk factors, the inherent nature, toxicity, and degree of cutaneous exposure to chemicals are probably more important. A history of atopic dermatitis is linked to an increased susceptibility to irritant dermatitis because of a lower threshold for skin irritation, impaired skin barrier function, and slower healing process.[2] Wet work and chemical exposure are major precipitating factors for the development of irritant contact dermatitis (ICD) in patients with atopic eczema. Although atopic patients downregulate Th1 cells with a decreased propensity to contact sensitization, allergic contact dermatitis (ACD) is often seen in patients with atopic eczema, and nickel sensitization is increased in atopic patients.[3] Other skin conditions with the highest risk of ACD include stasis dermatitis,[1] hand and foot eczemas, and chronic actinic dermatitis.[1]

Irritant Contact Dermatitis

Irritants cause as much as 80% of cases of contact dermatitis. ICD follows exposure to chemical or physical substances capable of direct damage to the skin.[1,2]

There are two major types of ICD. Chronic cumulative (traumiterative, marginal) ICD is the type of contact dermatitis most commonly encountered in clinical practice. Cumulative ICD develops as a result of repeated insults to the skin, where the chemicals involved are often multiple and weak.[3] The most common irritants include soap, detergents, surfactants, organic solvents, and oils (Box 3).[1] Dry skin with a glazed, parched appearance may be the initial sign; erythema, hyperkeratosis, and fissuring can supervene.[3] The second major type is acute ICD, which generally results from a single skin exposure to a strong irritant or caustic chemical (alkalis and acids). Most cases are the result of occupational accidents. Depending on the type of exposure to the irritant, the patient can develop erythema, edema, vesicles, and tissue necrosis.[1]

Allergic Contact Dermatitis

Pathogenesis

ACD is a T cell delayed-type (type IV) hypersensitivity reaction that arises from direct skin exposure to an exogenous allergen. These allergens are low-molecular-weight (<500 Da) lipophilic chemicals called haptens that penetrate the skin and covalently bind to carrier proteins to become fully immunogenic. The new antigen-protein complex is processed by Langerhans cells in the epidermis and then travels to the regional draining lymph nodes and is presented to naïve Th1 cells. There, cytokines such as interleukin 2 and interferon-γ are secreted, leading to clonal proliferation of the newly sensitized memory Th1 cells in the paracortical region of the lymph nodes and are released into the circulation. This is the sensitization phase, which takes 5 to 21 days. On re-exposure to the same antigen, the elicitation phase, the previously sensitized person elicits a clinical dermatitis, usually after 12 to 48 hours.[1,3]

Clinical Features

The clinical features of ACD are often indistinguishable from those of ICD. In the acute stage, erythematous papules, oozing vesicles, and crusted lesions predominate; these can occur anywhere but are best visualized on the palms, sides of the fingers, periungual areas, and soles. Frequently occurring or persistent episodes of acute contact dermatitis often become chronic, with thickening associated with lichenification, scaling, and fissuring. Postinflammatory hyperpigmentation or hypopigmentation can occur. Pruritus is a hallmark of most forms of contact dermatitis.[1] Major causes of ACD are listed in Box 4.

Systemic Contact Dermatitis

Systemic reactivation of ACD, or systemic contact dermatitis (SCD), occurs when persons with contact allergy to a hapten are exposed systemically to the same hapten via the oral, subcutaneous, transcutaneous, intravenous, inhalation, intra-articular, or intravesical route.[1,3,5]

Clinical features of SCD include flare-up of sites of previous dermatitis or of prior positive patch tests and development of dermatitis in previously unaffected areas, such as vesicular hand eczema, flexural dermatitis, nonspecific maculopapular eruptions, vasculitis-like lesions, and the baboon syndrome,[3] which is a well-demarcated eruption on the buttocks, genital area, and inner thighs. Associated systemic symptoms of headache, nausea, vomiting, arthralgias, and diarrhea can accompany the cutaneous findings.

SCD has primarily been caused by medications (e.g., antibiotics, corticosteroids, iodine, alcohol-containing drugs, nonsteroidal anti-inflammatory drugs [NSAIDs], vitamin B, iodine). But metals (nickel, cobalt, chromium, gold, mercury), *Myroxylon pereirae* (balsam of Peru) from spices and flavorings, and certain foods or food additives (e.g., garlic, onion, herbs, quinine tonic water, propylene glycol) are other causes. A relatively high dose of hapten is usually needed. Other variables include route of administration, bioavailability, individual sensitivity to the allergen, and interaction with amino acids and other allergens.

DIAGNOSIS

Diagnostic history and physical examination clues are discussed in the overview of ICD and ACD. The appearance of the lesions often corresponds to whether the patient's dermatitis is acute or chronic at the time of presentation. Most of the diagnostic discussion focuses on ACD, which is easier to diagnose than ICD. A summary of the diagnostic workup is listed in Box 5. The differential diagnosis of contact dermatitis is listed in Box 6.

Box 1 Exogenous Factors Influencing Contact Dermatitis

Body temperature
Cutaneous penetration of chemical
Environment (temperature, humidity)
Mechanical factors (pressure, friction, abrasion)
Properties of the chemical (pH, chemical activity)
Other exposure factors: duration, prior or simultaneous exposures, direct versus airborne

Box 2 Endogenous Factors Influencing Contact Dermatitis

Age
Atopic dermatitis
Individual susceptibility
Lack of hardening
Primary sensitive (hyperirritable) skin
Race
Secondary hyperirritability of the skin (status eczematicus)
Sensitivity to ultraviolet light
Skin permeability

Box 3 Causes of Irritant Contact Dermatitis

Animal products
Cosmetics
Degreasing agents
Detergents
Dusts
Foods
Friction
Low humidity
Metalworking fluids
Solvents
Tear gases
Topical medications
Water and wet work

Box 4 Principal Causes of Allergic Contact Dermatitis*

Bacitracin
Balsam of Peru
Cobalt
Formaldehyde
Fragrance mix
Gold sodium thiosulfate
Neomycin sulfate
Nickel
Quaternium 15
Methyldibromoglutaronitrile/phenoxyethanol

**Top 10 patients list reactions in North America.*

Irritant Contact Dermatitis

No universally accepted test exists for diagnosing ICD, which is often diagnosed by excluding other types of dermatitis including ACD. Because of the clinical similarity of ACD and ICD, it is important that patients believed to have either disorder undergo patch testing, which is positive in the former and negative in the latter.

Allergic Contact Dermatitis

History

Diagnosis of ACD is based on the history; on the appearance, periodicity, and localization of the eruption; and on the clinical course. History is especially important in cases of chronic dermatitis and

Box 5 Diagnostic Workup for Contact Dermatitis

History

Physical history

- Duration
- Site of onset
- Progression
- Symptoms (itching, burning, pain)
- Improvement away from work or hobbies
- Treatment to date including response
- History of any overt contact allergies

Occupational history

- Job description
- Protective clothing used if any
- Other workers affected

Hobbies and part-time jobs
Medical history

- Atopic dermatitis
- Seasonal allergies
- Asthma
- Other dermatologic problems
- Surgery

Family history

- Atopy
- Psoriasis
- Other chronic skin conditions

Examination

Morphology of lesions (erythema, eczema, lichenification, pigmentary changes, urticaria, etc.)
Pattern of involvement
Site(s) of eruption

Diagnostic Tests

Fungal, bacterial, and viral smears and cultures
Patch testing
Potassium hydroxide examination for fungi, glass fibers
Skin biopsies
Tests for contact urticaria and photocontact dermatitis if those diagnoses are suspected

putative occupational contact dermatitis. History alone may be accurate only 50% of the time, on average, ranging from 80% correct for nickel to 50% for moderately common allergens to about 10% for less-common allergens. Even with obvious causes, the specific allergen might not be known, and ACD to other chemicals may be associated.

Skillful history taking is required to differentiate ACD from contact urticaria and ICD, which is especially difficult in chronic cases. Detailed questioning of the patient about all topical medications (over-the-counter and prescription), systemic medications, cosmetics, lotions and creams, occupation, hobbies, travel, and clothing is also important. A past history of ACD to one or more of the major contact allergens, such as nickel, rubber, topical medicaments, cosmetics (fragrances, preservatives, and dyes), or obvious occupational or avocational exposures such as chrome, epoxy, acrylics, gloves, clothing, first aid creams, preservatives, plants, and other chemicals, can point to inadvertent ACD in another unexplained eruption.[1,3-5]

Physical Examination

The distribution of dermatitis is often the single most important clue to the diagnosis of ACD. The area of most intense dermatitis usually corresponds to the site of the most intense contact with the allergen. Exceptions exist, such as nail polish allergy, which typically occurs on ectopic sites, especially the eyelids, face, and neck. In addition to the transfer of allergens to distant sites, volatile airborne chemicals can cause dermatitis on exposed body areas. Regional differences in susceptibility to contact allergens exist. The thinner eyelid and genital

Box 6 Differential Diagnosis of Contact Dermatitis

Other Types of Eczema or Dermatitis
Asteatotic eczema (dry skin)
Atopic dermatitis
Dyshidrotic eczema
Factitial dermatitis
Numular eczema
Photoallergic contact dermatitis
Phototoxicity
Seborrheic dermatitis
Stasis dermatitis with autoeczematization
Sunburn

Other Dermatoses
Psoriasis
Superficial fungal infections
Lupus erythematosus
Parapsoriasis
Cutaneous T-cell lymphoma
Contact urticaria

Infections
Cellulitis
Impetigo
Herpes simplex
Varicella-zoster

skin is more susceptible to ACD and ICD. Scalp hair is often protective, with allergic reactions to hair cosmetics involving the upper face, eyelids, postauricular area, and neck. Other areas have higher or lower exposures to allergens that are not always obvious and that are reflected in unusual distributions of dermatitis. Allergens in lotions and creams which are applied all over the body sometimes produce reaction in skin folds and intertriginous areas, where the chemicals tend to concentrate.

Attempting to recognize ACD on the basis of physical examination alone may be only partially accurate. Linear vesicular streaks are commonly seen in poison ivy, oak, and sumac dermatitis, but contact with other plants can give a similar picture. Contact with liquids can also produce linear vesicles. Failure to examine the entire skin can result in misdiagnosis. Eczema on the trunk and arms might in fact represent autoeczematization from contact or stasis dermatitis of the legs. There are significant regional variations in contact dermatitis, and knowledge of substances that cause dermatitis of specific body sites facilitates the diagnosis (Box 7).

Box 7 Contact Allergen Exposures by Location of Dermatitis[1,2]

Face, Eyelids, and Neck
Airborne allergens
Cosmetics
Hair cosmetics
Hair dyes and shampoos (hairline area)
Jewelry, especially in piercings (eyebrows, nose, lips)
Musical instruments that rest between the neck and shoulder
Nail polish
Perfumes
Photosensitizers
Plants (poison ivy, oak, and sumac)
Topical antibiotics for ears and eyes

Extremities
Coins and keys (buttocks)
Gloves (hands)
Lotions and creams
Plants
Shoes (feet)

Trunk and Flexural Areas
Belt buckle (umbilical area)
Clothing
Lotions and creams
Plants
Rubber elastic band of underwear (bra line and waistline)
Snap of jeans (umbilical area)

Genital Area
Bubble baths
Condoms
Cosmetics
Douches
Fasteners
Plants
Spermicides
Topical medications

Mouth
Dental materials (e.g., amalgams, brackets, acrylics)
Piercings (tongue)
Foods
Flavors
Medications

Data from Cao LY, Taylor JS: V Contact Dermatitis and Related Disorders. 2 Dermatology. ACP Medicine. Dale DC, Federman DD, Eds. BC Decker Inc, Hamilton, ON, September 2008. http://www.acpmedicine.com. (accessed August 6, 2009), and Chew AL, Maibach HI: Occupational issues of irritant contact dermatitis. Int Arch Occup Environ Health 2003;76:339-346.

Patch Testing

If the history and the clinical presentation reveal one or more risk factors for ACD, patch testing is indicated. The patch test is the only useful and reliable method—the gold standard—for diagnosing ACD, and its proper performance and interpretation require considerable experience.[1,6] The patch test aims to reproduce in miniature the clinical eczematous dermatitis by applying allergens under occlusion on intact skin of patients with suspected contact dermatitis. A positive patch test represents an in vivo visualization of the elicitation phase of contact dermatitis. Patch testing for ACD is not meant to reflect an irritant reaction. The patch test is typically better than relying on history alone, trial and error, or in vitro tests.[1,6]

Commercially available individual patch test allergens in a dilute, nonirritating concentration are applied to the upper back for 48 hours. After the patch tests are removed, the sites of the patch tests are evaluated twice, usually after removal at 48 hours and again at 96 hours or beyond. Results at both readings are graded according to intensity of the reaction at the patch test site on a scale of 0 to 3^+.[1] Relevance of positive reactions to present or past episodes of dermatitis is determined by correlating the patch test results with chemicals, products, and processes encountered in the environment.[1]

Patch tests should generally not be applied if the patient's dermatitis is active or involves the back. A screening patch test series is typically applied and supplemented by aimed patch testing with other patch test chemicals based on the patient's history and occupation. Limited screening patch test series diagnose only 20% to 50% of a patient's contact allergens, and additional testing is often indicated to more adequately diagnose ACD.

Skin Biopsy

Histopathology is of limited value in diagnosing contact dermatitis. Findings depend on the stage of the process and the nature of the contactant. Most types of eczema show similar histopathologic changes and cannot be distinguished with certainty.[1]

TREATMENT

Identifying and Avoiding Irritants and Allergens

Identification and elimination of the offending irritant or allergen and protection from further exposure are important in managing contact dermatitis of all causes and types. Patients with ACD must be educated about potential sources of exposure and cross-reacting allergens, and they must be provided with lists of potential products and processes that contain the allergen and a list of nonsensitizing substitutes.[1] Examples of allergen alternatives include topical erythromycin or mupirocin as substitutes for neomycin. Neomycin can cross-react with gentamycin and tobramycin. Bacitratin should generally be avoided in neomycin-sensitive patients because of coreactivity.

Reasons for persistence of ACD include unidentified sources of allergens or irritants at home or at work, exposure to cross-reacting allergens, presence of underlying endogenous (e.g., atopic) eczema, and adverse reactions to therapy.

In the case of hand dermatitis, practical management must include protective measures as well as the use of topical corticosteroids and lubrication. The use of vinyl gloves with cotton liners to avoid the accumulation of moisture that often occurs during activities involving exposure to household or other irritants and foods (e.g., peeling or chopping fruits or vegetables) may be helpful.[7] In the workplace, verify that gloves are safe to use around machinery before recommending their use. Protective devices themselves can introduce new allergic or irritant hazards in the forms of rubber in gloves and solvents in waterless cleansers. Automation of industrial processes can reduce exposure but is the most expensive preventive measure. Barrier creams are generally a last resort and are probably best used in workers with no dermatitis.

Topical Treatment

Once dermatitis develops, use of topical treatment is helpful. *Topical corticosteroids* are the mainstay of ACD therapy; however, their use in ICD is controversial. For mild or moderate localized dermatitis, topical corticosteroids applied twice daily are usually effective within a few days and should be continued for 2 weeks. Lower-potency agents should be applied to the face and intertriginous areas, and higher-potency steroids should be reserved for the extremities and torso. Frequent and prolonged use of topical corticosteroids in fold areas can cause atrophy, telangiectasia, or striae, and their use on the face can also cause steroid rosacea. *Topical calcineurin inhibitors* (e.g., tacrolimus or pimecrolimus) may be used as an alternative to low-potency topical corticosteroids in chronic ICD.[8]

Emollients or occlusive dressings may improve barrier repair in dry, lichenified skin.[1] Traditional petrolatum-based emollients are accessible and inexpensive, and they have been shown to be as effective as an emollient containing skin-related lipids. To relieve pruritus, a lotion of camphor, menthol, and hydrocortisone (Sarnol HC) is soothing, drying, and antipruritic. Pramoxine, a topical anesthetic in a lotion base (Prax) can also relieve pruritus. Phototherapy with bath PUVA (psoralen plus ultraviolet A) therapy may be helpful for chronic contact dermatitis of the palms and soles.

Systemic Treatment

Most cases of contact dermatitis are effectively managed without the use of systemic corticosteroids. Short courses of *systemic corticosteroids* are indicated for patients with severe vesiculobullous eruptions of the hands and feet or the face or with severe disseminated ACD, such as poison ivy, sumac, or oak.[1] Also *systemic drugs* such as cyclosporine may be effective, but they should be prescribed for limited periods by those experienced in their use. When dermatitis is complicated with a secondary infection, systemic antibiotics against *Staphylococcus aureus* and *Staphylococcus pyogenes* are preferred.[1] *Sedating antihistamines* such as diphenhydramine hydrochloride, hydroxyzine hydrochloride, and doxepin hydrochloride may be administered at night for intense itching.[1]

PREVENTION AND SCREENING

Once a contactant has been identified as the causal factor, patients should be educated about avoidance, including everyday practices that can cause or contribute to the contact dermatitis. For ICD, less irritating substances, such as emollients and soap substitutes, should be used rather than soap when washing. Moisturizers are believed to increase hydration or prevent transepidermal water loss, thereby maintaining skin barrier function and reducing the risk of ICD.[2]

In the occupational arena, strategies for preventing contact dermatitis include administrative measures, environmental measures, and personal measures. Administrative measures include worker education and training regarding specific job hazards. Environmental measures include eliminating hazardous materials or finding substitutes for them, isolating and enclosing the work process, providing exhaust ventilation, and observing good housekeeping. Personal measures include applying emollients, adjusting personal cleansing and hygiene routines, and wearing personal protective equipment.[3]

CONSIDERATIONS IN SPECIAL POPULATIONS

Pregnant Women

The safety of patch testing in pregnancy has not been studied. Although the minute amounts of allergens applied during patch testing appear unlikely to be absorbed in sufficient amounts to harm the fetus, most physicians defer such testing in pregnancy. As with all treatments in pregnant women, the benefits of testing should be weighed against any potential risk.[9]

Children

Contact dermatitis has been well documented in children, and nickel and rubber allergies appear to be increasing in this age group. Patch testing with a limited series of allergens is indicated in small children with limited back areas.[10]

Immunosuppressed Patients

Skin hyporeactivity or anergy is not well understood and may be observed in patients taking corticosteroids, immunomodulators, or ultraviolet light therapy and in patients with cancer, sarcoidosis, and viral infections such as human immunodeficiency virus (HIV) and measles.[11]

Summary

- Contact dermatitis is an acute or chronic immunologic (allergic) or nonimmunologic (irritant) inflammation of the skin caused by contact with chemicals or biologic or physical agents.
- Contact dermatitis accounts for 95% of occupational skin diseases, and is one of the most common reasons for consultation in a dermatology office.
- Irritant contact dermatitis accounts for up to 80% of cases and is most often caused by cumulative exposure to marginal irritants such as soap and water.
- Allergic contact dermatitis accounts for 20% or more of cases. Major allergens include urushiol (poison ivy), metals (nickel, chromium, cobalt), rubber accelerators, topical medications (neomycin), and cosmetics (preservatives, fragrances, hair dyes).
- Patch testing is the gold standard for diagnosing allergic contact dermatitis. Negative patch tests favor a diagnosis of irritant contact dermatitis by exclusion.
- Identification and avoidance of the causative agent are the mainstays of treatment.

Suggested Readings

Amado A, Taylor JS: Women's occupational dermatologic issues. Dermatol Clin 2006;24(2):259-269.
Beattie PE, Green C, Lowe G, Lewis-Jones MS: Which children should we patch test? Clin Experimental Dermatol 2006:32:6-11.
Brancaccio RR, Alvarez MS: Contact allergy to food. Dermatol Ther 2004;17:302-313.
Cohen DE, Heidary N: Treatment of irritant and allergic contact dermatitis. Dermatol Ther 2004;17:334-340.
Chew AL, Maibach HI: Occupational issues of irritant contact dermatitis. Int Arch Occup Environ Health 2003;76:339-346.
Frosh PJ, MennéT, Lepoittevin J-P (eds): Contact Dermatitis. 4th edition. Berlin, Springer-Verlag, 2006.
Koehler AM, Maibach, HI: Skin hyporeactivity in relation to patch testing. Contact Dermatitis 2000;42:1-4.
Rietschel RL: Clues to an accurate diagnosis of contact dermatitis. Dermatol Ther 2004;17(3):224-230.
Rietschel RL, Fowler JF, Jr (eds): Fisher's contact dermatitis. Philadelphia, Lippincott Williams & Wilkins, 2001.
Cao LY, Taylor JS: V Contact Dermatitis and Related Disorders. 2 Dermatology. ACP Medicine. Dale DC, Federmann DD, Eds. BC Decker Inc, Hamilton, ON, September 2008. http://www.acpmedicine.com (accessed August 6, 2009).
Hogan D: Skin Allergies. Belsito D, Vinson RP, Callen JP, Gelfand JM, James WD (eds): WebMD Allergies Guide. Available at http://www.webmd.com/allergies/guide/skin-allergies (accessed November 24, 2007).

References

For a complete list of references, log onto www.expertconsult.com.

Hair Disorders

Shannon Harrison, Melissa Piliang, and Wilma Bergfeld*

DEFINITION

Alopecia is the general term for hair loss. Hair loss can occur from the scalp and any hair-bearing part of the body. Hair has great social and cultural importance, and patients with hair loss experience anxiety and concern. The management of hair disorders is complex. This chapter focuses on the common causes of alopecia.

PREVALENCE

Hair loss, a common presenting symptom, affects males and females of all ages. The most common form of hair loss is androgenetic alopecia (pattern hair loss), which increases with age; at least 80% of white men show some degree of thinning by the age of 70 years.[1,2] Androgenetic alopecia occurs with the onset of puberty and in males is dependent on circulating androgens.[3] Female pattern hair loss, (female androgenetic alopecia) also starts after puberty[4] and by 70 years of age, 38% of women have some degree of hair loss.[5] The role of androgens in female-pattern hair loss still remains uncertain.[3,4]

Another common cause of hair loss, telogen effluvium (hair shedding), usually begins within 3 months after a trigger such as childbirth, a new medication, endocrine abnormality, severe illness, a major operation, crash dieting, or nutritional deficiencies.[6] Alopecia areata (patchy hair loss) has a lifetime incidence of 1.7%,[7] commonly occurring in children and adolescents, but it can occur at any age.[6] Trichodystrophies (hair shaft disorders) can cause hair fragility or unruly hair. Trichodystrophies can be acquired, and a history of multiple cosmetic hair treatments, such as perming or coloring, is common. Rarely, they are hereditary conditions.

PATHOPHYSIOLOGY AND NATURAL HISTORY

Most cases of hair loss are due to hair cycle alterations or hair shaft abnormalities. Multiple factors such as diet, chronic illness, endocrine disorders, genetic factors, and medications can play a role in hair loss.[8]

Normal Hair Cycling

Accurate analysis of hair loss is based on knowledge of the hair cycle. Scalp hair grows in a cyclical three-part process. Scalp hairs are all at different stages in the growth cycle and do not grow in a synchronous manner. Anagen is the growing phase, and normally 80% of hair follicles are in anagen at any one time.[8,9] The remaining 10% to 20% are in an involuting phase called *catagen* and a resting phase called *telogen*[8,9] (Fig. 1). Telogen hairs shed in 3 to 5 months, and the scalp normally loses approximately 100 telogen hairs per day.[6] The average rate of scalp hair growth is 0.35 mm a day and can be reduced by age, poor nutrition, and illness.[8,9]

Changes in the hair cycle manifest as hair loss. In androgenetic alopecia, the hair cycle shortens, and hair follicles progressively miniaturize under the influence of androgens.[8,9]

Telogen effluvium results from an abrupt shift of large numbers of anagen hairs to telogen hairs, which shed typically 3 months after a trigger.[6] This recovers usually 6 months after the trigger is removed. Persistent telogen shed over 6 months heralds chronic telogen effluvium, female pattern hair loss, or other metabolic or endocrine states, such as androgen excess or thyroid disorders.[9]

Inflammation of the hair follicle in alopecia areata, an autoimmune condition of the hair follicle, terminates hair growth, causing anagen hair shedding.[6,8] Coin-shaped patches of hair loss are often reversible but tend to recur.[6] Some patients progress to a total loss of scalp hair (alopecia totalis) (Fig. 2) and even all body hair (alopecia universalis).[6]

Hair Structure

Trichodystrophies are usually separate from the hair cycle. Inherited trichodystrophies are rare and associated with hair shaft structural or chemical defects. Acquired trichodystrophies from environmental and cosmetic trauma (hot combing, blow drying and perming) or weathering are more common and can cause fragile, breakable hair.[8]

Hair follicles cycle throughout life, if the bulge region of the hair shaft remains intact.[8] Hair stem cells are located in the bulge in the midportion of the follicles, at the level of the sebaceous glands.[8,10] Inflammation or injury to the bulge can damage the stem cells so hair is unable to regenerate, causing a cicatricial (scarring) alopecia.[8,11] In other conditions, inflammation spares the bulge, leading to a noncicatricial (nonscarring) alopecia, and follicles have regrowth potential.[11] Most types of hair loss can be divided into cicatricial and noncicatricial alopecias.[6] (Box 1)

SIGNS AND SYMPTOMS

Clinical history should include duration of hair loss and pattern of loss (localized or diffuse scalp hair loss and involvement of other hair-bearing areas of the body). A family history of androgenetic alopecia, alopecia areata, autoimmune conditions, and thyroid disorders can be helpful. A history of childbirth, new medication, severe illness, or loss of weight should be sought. Female patients should be asked about acne, irregular menses, and hirsutism.[6] A history regarding hair care habits should be obtained.[6] A history of nail conditions, autoimmune disease, and skin rashes should also be sought.

The clinical appearance of alopecia can be a progressive patterned thinning in androgenetic alopecia (Fig. 3), to a diffuse hair loss without noticeable thinning in telogen effluvium, or discrete circular nonscarring patches of hair loss in alopecia areata. Cicatricial alopecias cause discrete irregular-shaped areas of permanent hair loss with loss of follicular openings.[6] Trichodystrophies result in fragile hairs of irregular length or unruly hair. Infections such as tinea capitis can cause irregular patches of alopecia with associated scale.

History and examination should establish whether the hair is shedding, fragile and breaking, or progressively thinning.[6,8] The way the hair loss occurs is crucial in determining the nature and type of the hair loss.[8] (Table 1)

DIAGNOSIS

In assessing hair disorders, a detailed history and examination are most important. The scalp and all hair-bearing areas of the body should be examined for pattern and degree of hair loss. The scalp should be examined for inflammation and scaling.[6] Scarring should be determined by the presence (noncicatricial) or absence (cicatricial) of hair follicle openings on the scalp. The hair shafts should be assessed for length, diameter, and dystrophy.[6] Nails and skin should

*Dr. Harrison is funded by the Australasian College of Dermatologists and the F.C. Florance Bequest.

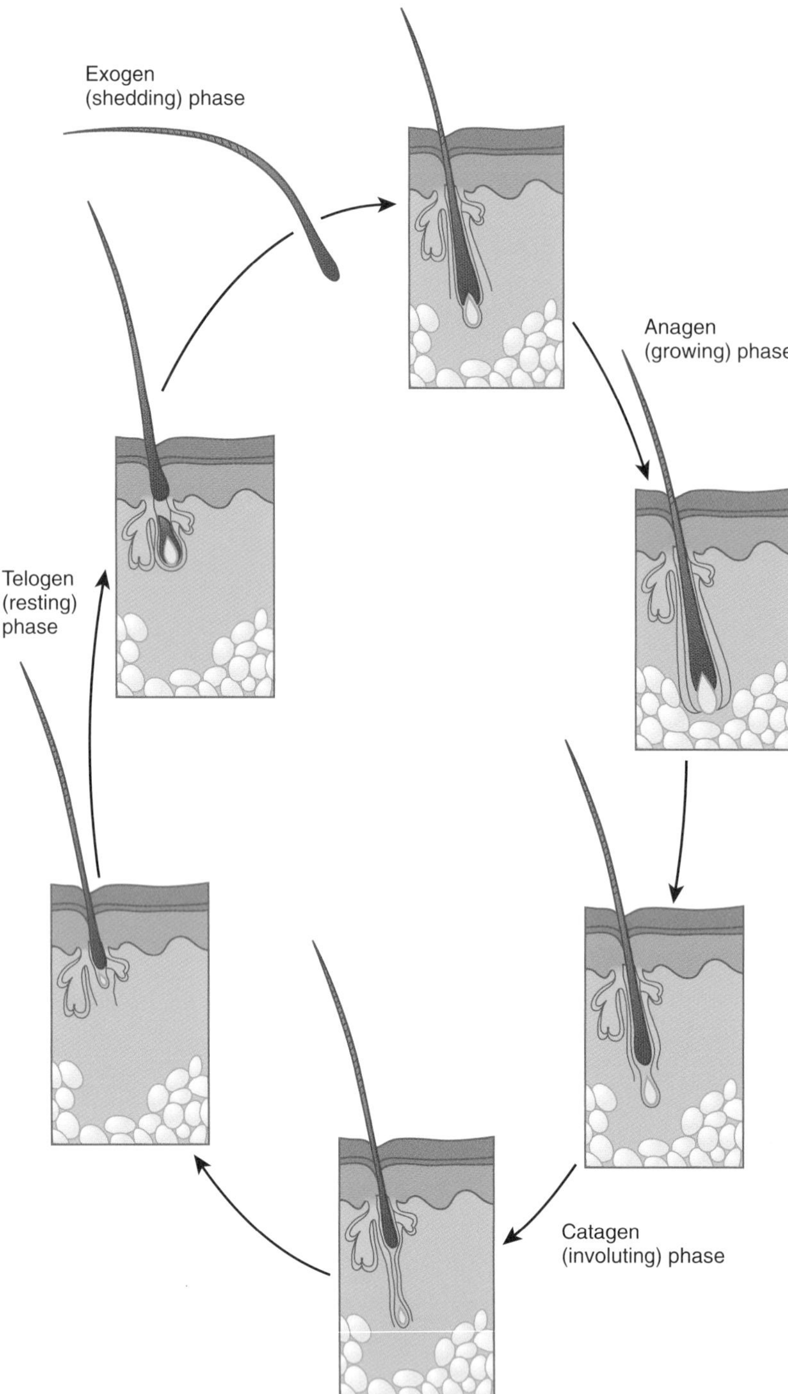

Figure 1. **The hair growth cycle.**

be examined to exclude concomitant skin lesions and nail dystrophy. Inherited trichodystrophies and alopecia areata may be associated with nail dystrophy.[6,8]

Further diagnostic tests such as hair pulls, clippings, and collections (shed hair); light microscopy of hair shafts; scrapings of scalp scales for fungal culture; and a Wood's lamp examination of the scalp can add information to the final diagnosis.[6,8](Table 2)

A scalp biopsy is useful in most cases of hair loss.[6] A 4-mm scalp biopsy is the most helpful. Laboratory workup, such as a complete blood count, ferritin level, androgen panel, and thyroid screening is also helpful[3,6] (see Table 2). Ferritin level should usually be 70 ng/mL to enhance hair growth.[12]

Male androgenetic alopecia is hereditary and has a well-recognized pattern of hair loss; usually no further investigation is required. Female-pattern hair loss tends to occur in women with a family history of baldness.[3] Most women have no clinical or biochemical evidence of hyperandrogenism.[3,6] In women with pattern hair loss associated with acne, hirsutism, and irregular menses (signs of androgen excess), the total and free testosterone level, sex-hormone binding globulin, and dihydroepiandrosterone sulfate (DHEAS) levels should be investigated[3,6] (see Table 2).

Alopecia areata is usually a clinical diagnosis, although a scalp biopsy is occasionally required for diagnosis. Characteristically, an exclamation mark hair (broken off hair narrower closer to the scalp)

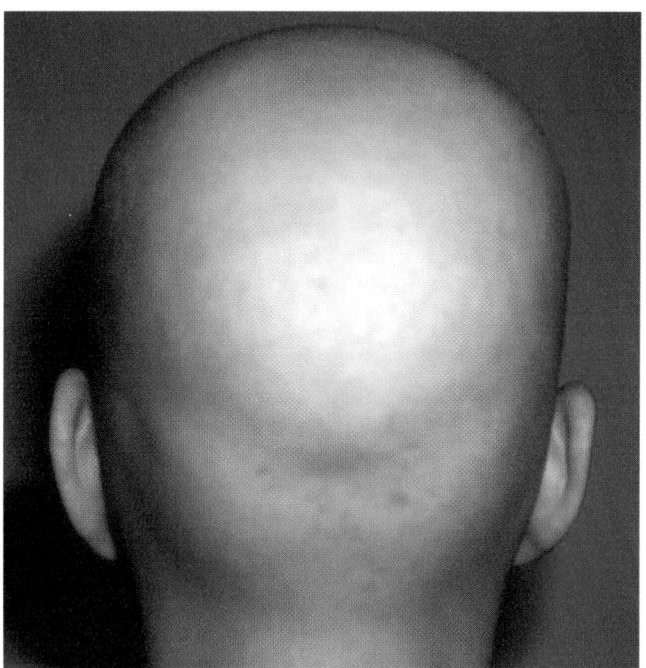

Figure 2. Alopecia totalis.

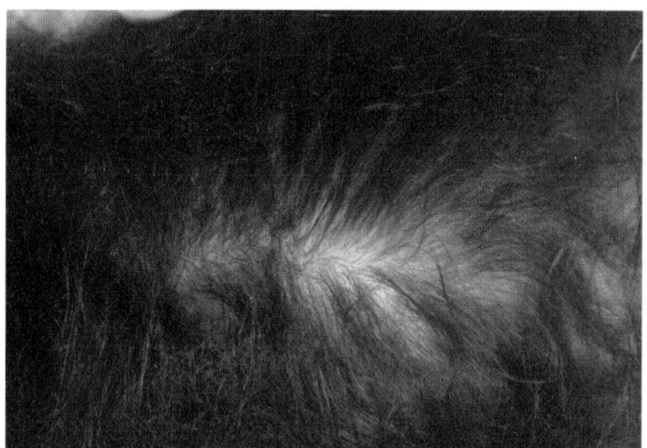

Figure 3. Female pattern hair loss.

Box 1 Types of Hair Loss

Noncicatricial Alopecias
Androgenetic alopecia
Female pattern hair loss
Alopecia areata
Trichodystrophies
Telogen effluvium
Thyroid disease

Cicatricial Alopecias
Lichen planopilaris
Folliculitis (acne) keloidalis
Folliculitis decalvans
Discoid lupus erythematosus
Central centrifugal cicatricial alopecia (CCCA)
Dissecting cellulitis

Table 1 Relationship Between Symptoms and Hair Loss Disorder

Symptom	Hair Disorder
Progressive patterned scalp hair thinning, typically without increased shedding Rarely, associated with diffuse hair loss.	Androgenetic alopecia (pattern hair loss)
Diffuse hair shedding	Telogen effluvium
Hair shedding with patchy irregular shaped areas of scalp hair loss.	Cicatricial alopecia
Hair fragility and breakage Unruly hair Hair that does not grow long	Trichodystrophy
Circular or oval areas of scalp hair loss with shedding ± Involvement of other hair-bearing areas ± Eyelash or eyebrow loss	Alopecia areata
Irregular patch of alopecia with scale and pruritus ±Hair breakage ±Pustules	Infection (tinea capitis)

is seen on the scalp[13] (see Table 2). A hair pull is positive from the margin of the active patch.[13]

Trichorrhexis nodosa, a node-like fragile area in the hair shaft, can be diagnosed from a hair clipping using light microscopy and indicates hair weathering.[8] It can be associated with acquired and inherited trichodystrophies.[8] Certain inherited hair shaft disorders can be recognized by the microscopic hair shaft abnormality. For example, trichorrhexis invaginata or bamboo hair is characteristic of Netherton's syndrome.

In patients with telogen effluvium, hair collections of daily shedding can be diagnostic.[8] Hair pull can be positive. In chronic telogen effluvium, blood workup should be done to exclude disease states, iron deficiency, and thyroid disorders.[6] A scalp biopsy may be needed to differentiate between early female-pattern hair loss and chronic telogen effluvium[3,6] (see Table 2).

Scalp biopsy for accurate diagnosis is required for cicatricial alopecias[6,8] (see Table 2).

For infections of the scalp, such as tinea capitis, hair clipping and microscopy, in addition to culture of the scalp scales, should be performed[6] (see Table 2). A Wood's lamp can be helpful because some fungi—*Microsporum canis* and *Pityrosporum* species—show a green or orange fluorescence, respectively, under Wood's lamp.[6]

TREATMENTS AND OUTCOMES

A range of therapeutic options exist for hair loss. Referral to a dermatologist is often necessary. In all cases, an adequate diet should be maintained and damaging hair care procedures should be avoided.[3]

Androgenetic Alopecia

Male-Pattern Hair Loss

Pharmacological treatment of male androgenetic alopecia includes topical minoxidil 2% or 5% (Rogaine for Women and Rogaine for Men) and selected antiandrogens. Placebo-controlled trials of target hair counts and expert panel review of scalp photographs at 1 year confirm continued use of topical minoxidil helps maintain hair counts and slows further loss.[3,14] With a dropper, 1 mL should be applied twice daily to a dry scalp.[3] Scalp irritation and allergic contact dermatitis have been reported.[3]

Table 2 Diagnosis of Common Types of Hair Loss

Clinical Findings	Investigations
Androgenetic Alopecia	
Thinning of hair in patterned areas of scalp Negative hair-pull test (usually) Exclude other signs of hyperandrogenism	Consider 4-mm scalp punch biopsy and androgen panel in females Nutritional screen to exclude exacerbating factors of hair loss: TSH, T_4, iron and ferritin, zinc, vitamin A, calcium
Alopecia Areata	
Localized coin shaped areas of scalp baldness ± eyebrow, eyelash, and body hair loss Exclamation mark hairs Positive hair-pull test of dystrophic anagen hairs Possible nail changes	Investigate for associated autoimmune disease[13]: TSH, T_4 level, thyroid autoantibodies and vitamin B_{12}
Infective Process (eg., tinea capitis)	
Localized area of alopecia and broken hairs Scalp scale and inflammation ± pustules	Hair clipping and fungal culture Hair shaft light microscopy Scalp scale fungal culture Wood's lamp examination
Telogen effluvium	
Diffuse thinning scalp hair Positive hair pull test of telogen hairs	Identify trigger Hair collection Laboratory investigations (iron level, ferritin level, TSH, T_4) Consider scalp punch biopsy
Trichodystrophy	
Irregular hair breakage and shortening	Hair clipping with light and polarized microscopy of hair shafts Chemical hair analysis if available
Cicatricial Alopecia	
Loss of scalp hair follicular openings Scalp inflammation scale	Scalp 4 mm punch biopsy ANA titer, TSH, thyroid antibodies Bacterial and fungal microscopy and culture.

ANA, antinuclear antibody; T_4, thyroxine; TSH, thyroid-stimulating hormone.

Oral finasteride 1 mg (Propecia), a 5α-reductase inhibitor, competitively blocks the peripheral conversion of testosterone to dihydrotestosterone. Serum and tissue (scalp) dihydrotestosterone concentrations are decreased in men taking finasteride.[3] Studies show that 50% of men aged 18 to 41 years have increased hair growth by 1 year, and 66% of men have increased hair growth by 2 years, compared to 7% and 7% at 1 and 2 years for placebo.[3,15] Reversible sexually related side effects have been reported.[3] A study has shown a decrease in low-grade prostate cancers by 25% in men on finasteride but an increase in high-grade prostate cancers of 6.4% compared to 5.1% of men on placebo.[16]

Neither drug restores all hair lost, and the main aim of treatment is to prevent further hair loss. There are no well-controlled studies combining topical minoxidil and finasteride.[3] Hair pieces, hair transplantation, and scalp reduction can be helpful in selected patients.[8]

Female-Pattern Hair Loss

In female-pattern hair loss, minoxidil 2% and 5% (Rogaine for Women and Rogaine for Men) can also be used; however, only the 2% solution is FDA-approved for women. The 5% solution has been shown to be more effective, but women are more likely to experience facial hypertrichosis.[3,17]

Antiandrogens are also used for female-pattern hair loss. Antiandrogens cause feminization of the male fetus, and therefore all women of child bearing years should be using a reliable form of contraceptive. Small studies show spironolactone in doses of 50 to 200 mg daily has successfully been used as an antiandrogen.[3,18] Hyperkalemia is a risk with spironolactone and potassium levels need to be monitored. Combined oral contraceptives such as 30 μg ethinyl estradiol and 3 mg drosperidone (Yasmin) can be useful with spironolactone in the treatment of female-pattern hair loss. Finasteride appears to be unhelpful in female-pattern hair loss.[3]

Cyproterone acetate 100 mg on days 5 to 15 combined with 50 μg ethinyl estradiol on days 5 to 25 of the menstrual cycle can be effective, but it is not available in the United States.[3,19]

Baseline photographs (typically of the midline scalp part) repeated every 6 to 12 months can be useful to monitor treatment.[6] Hair transplants may be considered in some women with female-pattern hair loss depending on their existing hair density.[3]

Telogen Effluvium

No treatment is usually required for acute telogen effluvium once the initial trigger is corrected or eliminated.[8] The precipitating trigger is usually identified from the history, with attention to events that preceded the effluvium by 6 weeks to 4 months.[8,9] Recognizing the cause is important for preventing relapses and further shedding periods.[6,8] Nutritional deficiencies should be corrected. For a diagnosis of chronic telogen effluvium, a chronic disease state and early female-pattern hair loss must be excluded.[3]

Alopecia Areata

The extent and pattern of hair loss and age of the patient help determine the treatment of alopecia areata.[8] All patients should be informed that alopecia areata can resolve spontaneously over time and no treatment alters the natural history of the disease.[13] However, alopecia areata can be psychologically distressing, and most patients elect treatment. A source of information and support, such as the

National Alopecia Areata Foundation (http://www.naaf.org), is an important part of treatment.

For mild to moderate patchy alopecia areata, potent topical corticosteroids with or without occlusion daily are the favored treatment.[13] Skin atrophy, folliculitis, and adrenal suppression are possible complications.[13] Larger areas or refractory disease can require triamcinolone acetonide suspension (Kenalog, 5-10 mg/mL) injected into involved sites with a 30-gauge needle, providing small amounts of 0.1 mL to each site.[8] Triamcinolone should not exceed a total of 10 to 20 mg per visit every 6 to 8 weeks.[8,13] Complications are pain at injection site and local skin atrophy.[13] If skin atrophy occurs, triamcinolone acetonide 2.5 mg/mL may be used or injections may be discontinued until the skin has recovered.

Extensive or severe disease is better treated with topical agents such as topical minoxidil (Rogaine), anthralin (Dritho-Scalp, Micanol), and topical contact sensitizers such as diphenylcyclopropenone (DPCP).[8] Anthralin cream (0.5%-1.0%) may be applied overnight or as short contact therapy, initially for 5 to 10 minutes, increasing up to 1 hour.[7,13] New hair growth can be noted after 3 to 4 months.[7,13] With DPCP therapy, increasing strengths must be used, and a cosmetically acceptable regrowth can be seen in up to 60% of patients.[7,13] Side effects include irritation, regional lymphadenopathy, and postinflammatory dyspigmentation.[7,13]

Systemic corticosteroids in the treatment of severe alopecia areata is controversial because of the prolonged course required and the potential side effects including cataracts, osteoporosis, and growth retardation.[7,8,13] Cyclosporine in severe alopecia areata is controversial given its side-effect profile and high recurrence rate after cessation of treatment.[7] Some case reports show cyclosporine can be helpful in maintaining hair growth, but treatment must be continued.[7] Thus, the risk-to-benefit ratio is usually not acceptable. The new biological agents have not been helpful in alopecia areata.[20]

Trichodystrophies

Excessive environmental exposure and cosmetic hair care practices cause fragile hair and should be avoided.[8] Management consists of minimizing the handling of the hair and leave-on conditioners and volumizers.[8] Once the injury ceases, the hair typically recovers within a few months in acquired trichodystrophies.[8] Treatment for inherited trichodystrophies depends on the underlying defect, but avoidance of hair-weathering practices is the mainstay of treatment.

Other Causes of Hair Loss

Tinea capitis responds to systemic antifungal treatment.[6]

Cicatricial alopecias encompass a variety of conditions and usually require specialist referral. Only case reports and case series exist for management options. Central centrifugal cicatricial alopecia (CCCA), a condition predominantly of African American women, is treated with avoidance of all hair grooming practices and potent topical corticosteroids.[21]

For folliculitis decalvans, long-term broad-spectrum antistaphylococcal and antineutrophilic antibiotics are needed. Combination rifampicin and fusidic acid with zinc is also useful in some cases.[21]

Isotretinoin is now the first choice in treating dissecting cellulitis of the scalp.[21]

For folliculitis keloidalis, staged intralesional triamcinolone acetonide is helpful in conjunction with oral or topical antibiotics.[21]

For lichen planopilaris and discoid lupus erythematosus, initial treatment starts with a potent topical corticosteroid or intralesional corticosteroid injections.[21] Systemic corticosteroids have also been used short term to gain control of rapid or severe disease.[21] Antimalarials and acitretin may also be needed in the treatment of discoid lupus erythematosus and lichen planopilaris, respectively.[21]

Summary

- Identify and replace reversible nutritional deficiencies to correct contributing causes of hair loss.
- Topical minoxidil or antiandrogens can be used to treat androgenetic alopecia.
- Topical and intralesional corticosteroids are an effective treatment for alopecia areata.
- Removal and correction of the trigger in telogen effluvium usually leads to resolution.
- Avoidance of hair weathering procedures is important with trichodystrophies.
- Identification of the type of cicatricial alopecia is important for correct management.
- Hair pieces, wigs, and hair transplants can be used in some patients.

Suggested Readings

Bergfeld WF, Mulinari-Brenner F: Hair Disorders. Cleveland Clinic: Disease Management Project. Cleveland: Center for Continuing Education, Cleveland Clinic Foundation, 2003.

Birch MP, Messenger AG: Genetic factors predispose to balding and non-balding in men. Eur J Dermatol 2001;11:309-314.

Birch MP, Messenger JF, Messenger AG: Hair density, hair diameter and the prevalence of female patterned hair loss. Br J of Dermatol 2001;144:297-304.

Dombrowski NC, Bergfeld WF: Alopecia areata: What to expect from current treatments. Cleve Cl J Med 2005;72(9):758-768.

Kaufman KD, Olsen EA, Whiting D, et al: Finasteride in the treatment of men with androgenetic alopecia. J Am Acad Dermatol 1998;39:578-589.

Lucky AW, Piacquadio DJ, Ditre CM, et al: A randomized placebo-controlled trial of 5% and 2% topical minoxidil solutions in the treatment of female pattern hair loss. J Am Acad Dermatol 2004;50:541-553.

Olsen EA, Messenger AG, Shapiro J, et al: Evaluation and treatment of male and female pattern hair loss. J Am Acad Dermatol 2005;52:301-311.

Ross EK, Tan E, Shapiro J: Update on primary cicatricial alopecias. J Am Acad Dermatol 2005;53:1-37.

Shapiro J: Hair loss in women. N Eng J Med 2007;357:1620-1630.

Thompson IM, Goodman PJ, Tagen CM, et al: The influence of finasteride on the development of prostate cancer. N Engl J Med 2003;349:213-222.

References

For a complete list of references, log onto www.expertconsult.com.

Nail Disease

Sharon Longshore Thornton and Kenneth J. Tomecki

The primary function of the nail is protection. Nail concerns are common, but the exact prevalence of nail disease is unknown. Nail disease occurs with certain skin diseases (psoriasis, eczema), often follows external trauma, may be an adverse effect of medication, and can occur with certain illnesses. The most common cause of nail disease is infection, usually fungal (onychomycosis) and less often bacterial. In many respects, the nails can indicate or reflect medical illness.

BASIC NAIL ANATOMY

The nail plate is a hard keratinized structure derived from keratinocytes within the nail matrix, which begins proximal to the nail plate and extends to the lunula, the white half-moon-shaped portion often seen through the nail plate. The proximal and distal nail matrices generate the dorsal and ventral nail plate, respectively. The nail bed beneath the nail plate extends from the lunula to the hyponychium, and the hyponychium lies under the free edge of the nail plate. The proximal and lateral nail folds compose the paronychium.

NAIL ABNORMALITIES AND SYSTEMIC DISEASE

Beau's Lines

Beau's lines (Fig. 1) are transverse depressions in the nail plate that often follow local trauma. They can reflect poor nutritional status, febrile illness, or a reaction to medication. Occasionally they occur with eczema, usually atopic or chronic hand eczema. Beau's lines are a temporary cessation in nail growth and tend to appear about 1 month after the inciting event. Beau's lines tend to resolve spontaneously by moving distally.

Onycholysis

Onycholysis (Fig. 2) is the distal separation of the nail plate from the underlying nail bed. Onycholysis often occurs with thyroid disease, either hyperthyroidism or hypothyroidism, and commonly occurs with psoriasis and eczema. It can occur with porphyria cutanea tarda, lichen planus, eczema, and some of the autoimmune blistering diseases. It might also indicate an adverse reaction to medication, for example, tetracycline. Onycholysis may be persistent.

Onychomadesis

Onychomadesis is the proximal separation of the nail plate from the nail bed, which typically results in shedding of the nail. Trauma is the usual cause. Less common causes include poor nutritional status, febrile illness, or drug sensitivity. The inciting event causes complete cessation of nail matrix activity. Loss of the nail might or might not be permanent.

Onychorrhexis

Onychorrhexis (Fig. 3) is the presence of longitudinal striations or ridging of the nails. These striations can simply reflect advanced age, but they do occur in some patients with rheumatoid arthritis, peripheral vascular disease, lichen planus, or Darier's disease. Longitudinal red and white striations invariably occur with Darier's disease, and V-shaped notching or nicking of the free edges of the nails are also common. Onychorrhexis is usually persistent.

Koilonychia

The spoon-shaped, concave nails of koilonychia (Fig. 4) commonly occur with iron-deficiency anemia and Plummer-Vinson syndrome, as a result of thinning and softening of the nail plate. Spoon-shaped nails are a normal physiologic occurrence in children. Koilonychia tends to resolve, either with treatment or with aging (children).

Clubbing

Clubbing (Fig. 5) is an increase in the transverse and longitudinal nail curvature and fibrovascular hyperplasia of the soft tissue proximal to the cuticle. With clubbing, the angle (Lovibond's angle) formed between the dorsal distal phalanx and the nail plate is increased. Clubbing often occurs with cardiopulmonary disease, for example, aortic aneurysm and bronchogenic carcinoma. The change is usually permanent.

Splinter Hemorrhages

Splinter hemorrhages often follow trauma to the nail, but they classically occur in patients with bacterial endocarditis, less so in patients with rheumatoid arthritis, trichinosis, and renal disease, especially those on dialysis. Splinter hemorrhages represent extravasation of blood from the vessels of the nail bed. They can resolve, recur, or persist.

Leukonychia

Leukonychia (Fig. 6) is a white discoloration of the nail secondary to color change in the nail bed. Leukonychia includes Terry's nails, half-and-half nails, and Muehrcke's lines. Terry's nails exhibit almost complete discoloration except for the distal edge; they occur most commonly with cirrhosis and congestive heart failure. The discoloration of half-and-half nails affects the proximal one half of the nail; they occur with chronic renal failure. Muehrcke's lines (Fig. 7) are narrow white transverse lines (usually two); they occur with hypoalbuminemia. Mee's lines resemble Muehrcke's lines, but the lines are thicker and may be single or multiple. Mee's lines occur with arsenic exposure.

Yellow Nail Syndrome

Yellow nail syndrome (Fig. 8) is a permanent cessation of nail growth resulting in hard, thickened, curved, yellow nails, occasionally with onycholysis. Yellow nails occur with lymphedema, chronic bronchitis, or bronchiectasis. Yellow nails tend to be persistent.

Pitting

Pitting (Fig. 9), or small punctate depressions in the nail plate, most commonly occurs with psoriasis, less so with alopecia areata and eczema. The pits represent abnormal keratinization in the nail matrix. In most cases, the treatment of skin disease has little if any effect on the nail disease.

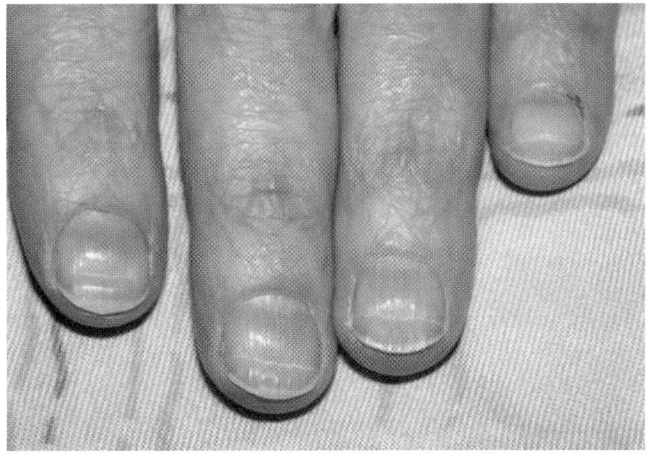

Figure 1 Beau's lines with transverse depressions in the nail plate.

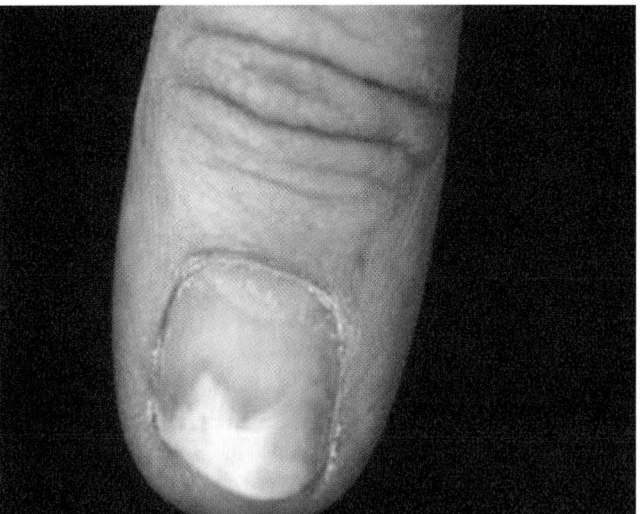

Figure 2 Onycholysis with distal separation of the nail plate from the nail bed.

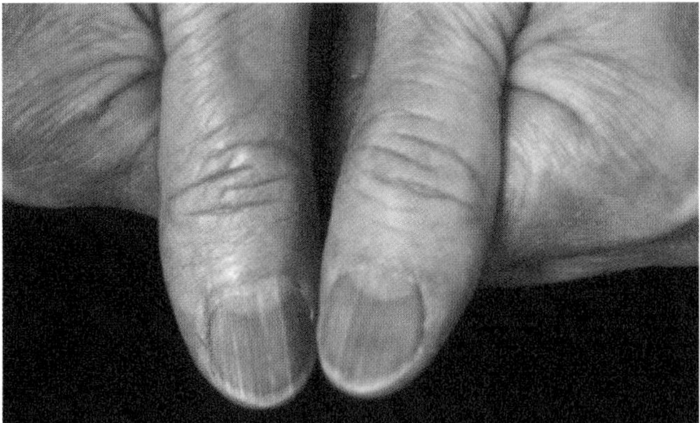

Figure 3 Longitudinal ridging of the nails, or onychorrhexis.

Trachyonychia

Trachyonychia (Figs. 10 and 11), or twenty-nail dystrophy, is a longitudinal ridging and roughness of the nails. Although uncommon, it occurs with psoriasis, lichen planus, alopecia areata, and eczema. Treatment of the skin disease usually has no effect on the ridging and roughness.

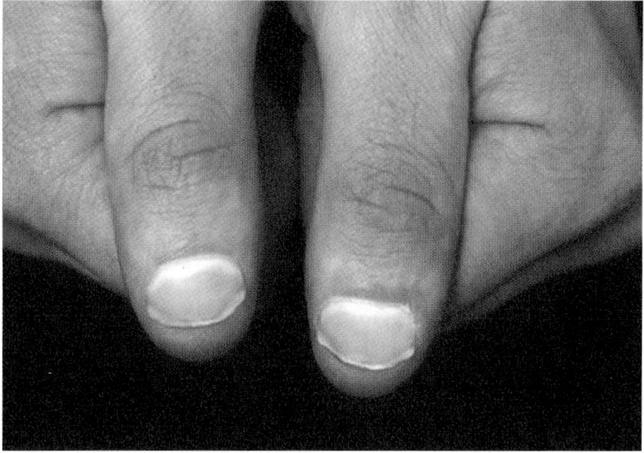

Figure 4 Spoon-shaped nails of koilonychia.

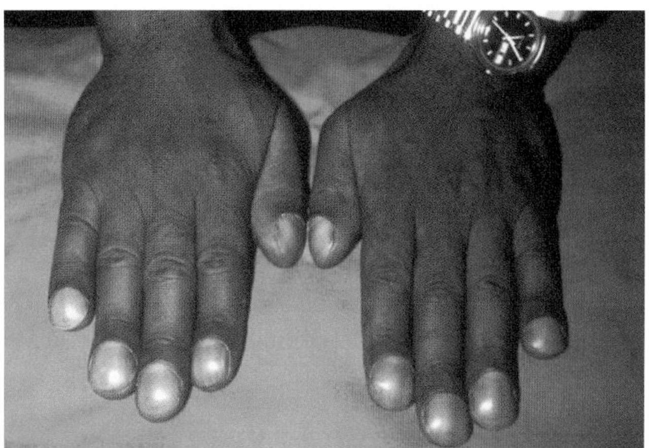

Figure 5 Increased nail curvature results in clubbing of the nails.

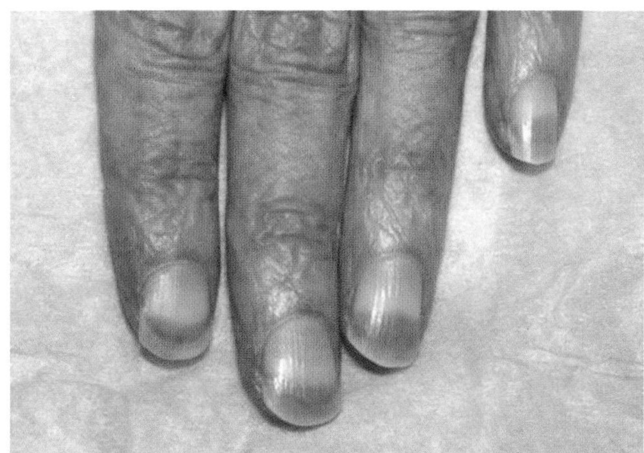

Figure 6 White discoloration of the nails, or leukonychia.

Oil Spots

Oil spots or oil droplets—orange-brown patches seen through the nail plate—are characteristic of psoriasis. Psoriatic nail disease is often associated with psoriatic arthropathy.

Pterygium

Pterygium (Fig. 12) is an adhesion of the proximal nail fold to the proximal nail bed following inflammation that destroys the nail

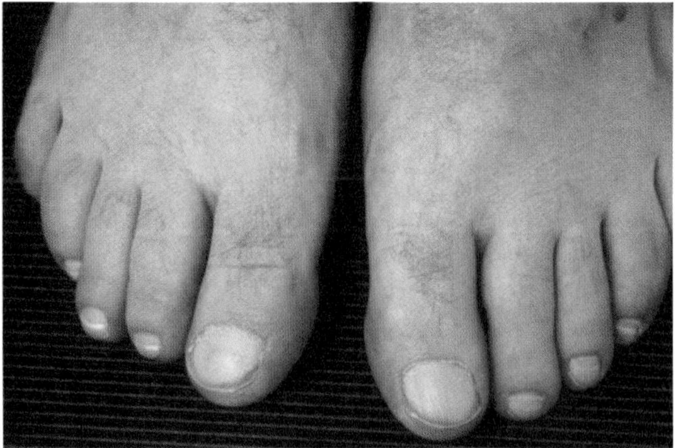

Figure 7 Muehrcke's lines associated with hypoalbuminemia.

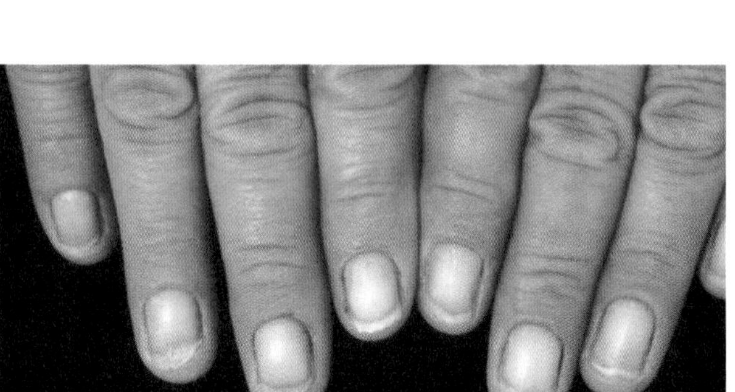

Figure 8 Hard, thick, curved nails of yellow nail syndrome.

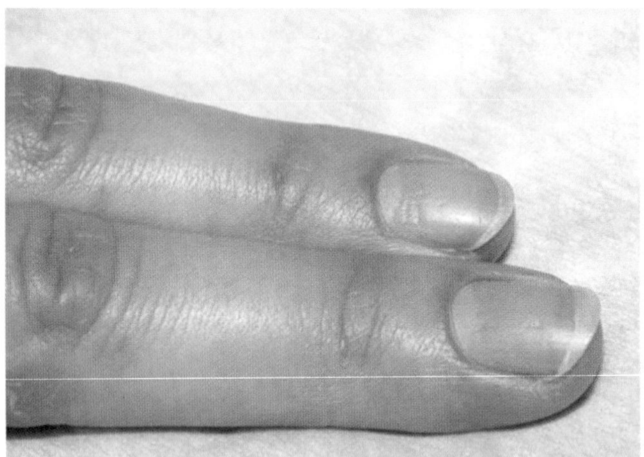

Figure 9 Punctate depressions in the nail plate, or pitting.

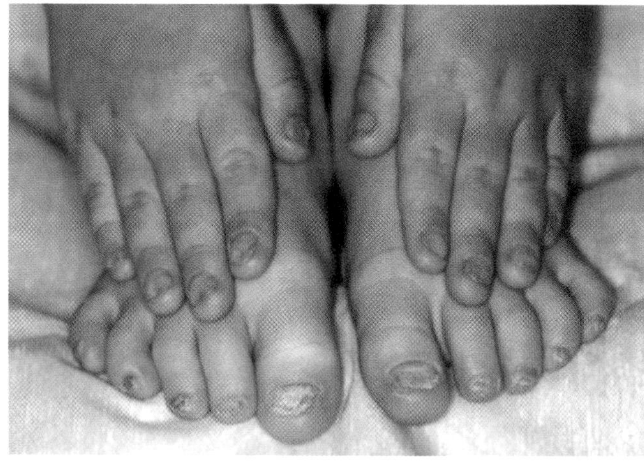

Figure 10 Fingernails and toenails affected by twenty-nail dystrophy.

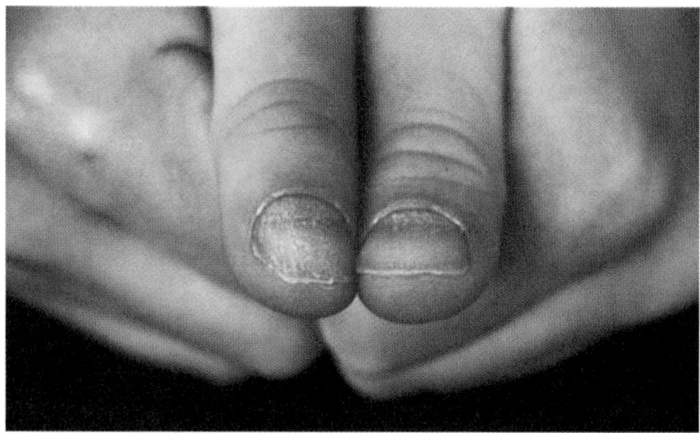

Figure 11 Roughness of the nails of twenty-nail dystrophy.

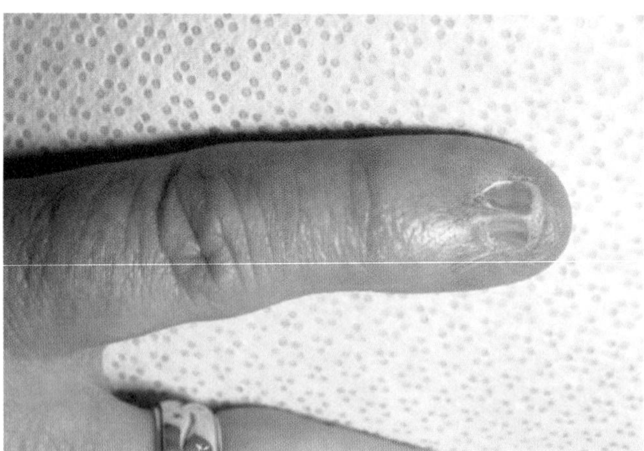

Figure 12 Pterygium with adhesion of the proximal nail fold to the proximal nail bed.

matrix. A scar can form, leading to partial loss of the nail plate. Pterygium occurs almost exclusively with lichen planus.

Pterygium Inversus Unguis

Pterytium inversus unguis, or ventral pterygium, occurs with connective tissue disease, especially progressive systemic scleroderma and systemic lupus erythematosus. Pterygium inversus is an adhesion of the distal nail bed to the ventral nail plate; soft tissue is attached firmly to the underneath side of the nail plate. There is no satisfactory treatment for pterygium.

DRUG-INDUCED NAIL ABNORMALITIES

Many drugs can produce nail disease. Some characteristic abnormalities include those listed in Box 1. If the offending drug is discontinued, the abnormality typically disappears, except for pyogenic granuloma.

Box 1 Systemic Drugs Inducing Nail Changes

Antineoplastic Drugs
Beau's lines
Hyperpigmentation
Leukonychia
Onycholysis
Onychomadesis
Splinter hemorrhages

Arsenic
Mees' lines

Azidothymidine
Melanonychia

Beta Blockers
Beau's lines
Ischemic changes
Thickening and pitting

Chloroquine
Blue-gray to yellow pigmentation

Chlorpromazine
Blue-purple pigmentation

Indinavir
Paronychia
Pyogenic granuloma

Minocycline
Blue-gray pigmentation

Psoralens and PUVA
Photo-onycholysis

Retinoids
Brittleness
Pyogenic granuloma-like growths

Tetracycline
Photo-onycholysis

PUVA, psoralen plus ultraviolet A light.

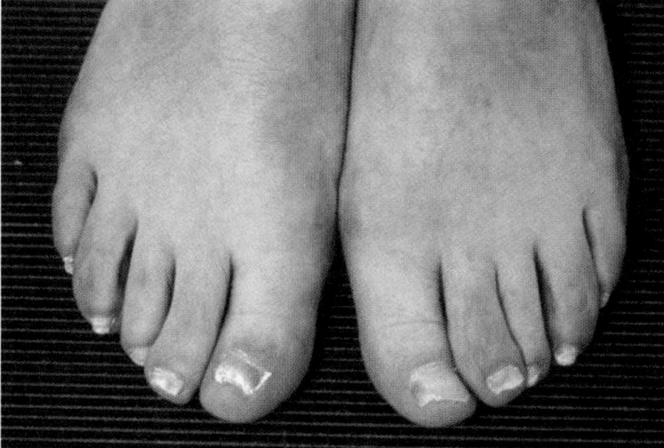

Figure 13 Dystrophic, hyperkeratotic nails affected by onychomycosis.

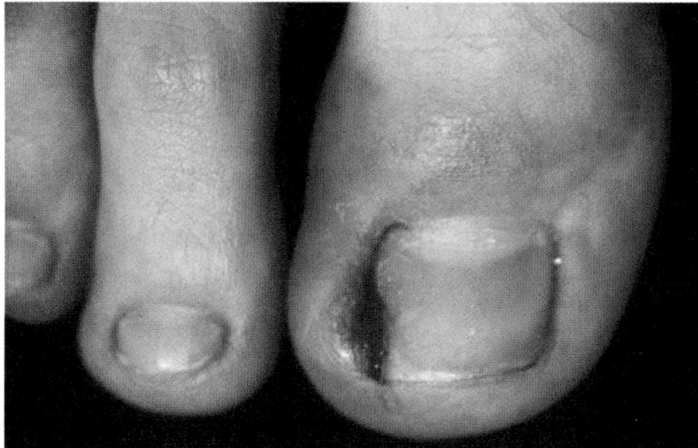

Figure 14 Acute paronychia with inflammation of the lateral and proximal nail folds.

INFECTIONS OF THE NAIL

Onychomycosis

Onychomycosis (Fig. 13), or tinea unguium, is a fungal or yeast infection of the nail, usually caused by *Tinea rubrum, Tinea mentagrophytes,* or *Candida albicans.* Onychomycosis is the most common nail disorder. Predisposing factors for infection include heat, moisture, trauma, diabetes mellitus, and tinea pedis. Affected nails are dystrophic and hyperkeratotic (thickened), often yellow-brown, and sometimes painful. Treatment is warranted for onychomycosis of the fingernails and whenever discomfort occurs. Treatment can be symptomtatic, commonly with the aid of a podiatrist for toenail onychomycosis. If warranted, systemic treatment involves either terbinafine or itraconazole. Success with either agent is less than 50%, and recurrences are common.

Paronychia

Acute paronychia (Fig. 14) is an inflammation of the proximal and lateral nail folds characterized by erythema, edema, and pain. Purulent drainage with compression behind the cuticle can also occur. Trauma is often the initial event, with secondary infection with *Staphylococcus aureus* or *Streptococcus pyogenes.* Treatment usually requires compresses and an oral antistaphylococcal antibiotic.

Chronic paronychia is usually a noninfectious disease that follows irritant or allergic contact dermatitis of the proximal nail fold. The cuticle is invariably absent. Affected persons often trim the cuticles aggressively and meticulously or do wet work with their hands. Secondary infection with *C. albicans* is common. Treatment involves aeration, topical corticosteroids, and perhaps an oral antifungal agent, for example, terbinafine, for secondary infection.

Warts

Warts, or verruca vulgaris, are an infection of the proximal and lateral nail folds caused by human papillomavirus (HPV). HPV types 1, 2, and 4 are primarily responsible for periungual warts. Because of the location, these warts are particularly difficult to treat, especially if they extend subungually. Subungual warts can cause deformity or discoloration of the nail plate. Affected patients are often nail biters.

TUMORS OF THE NAIL

Benign Tumors

Mucous Cyst

A mucous or myxoid cyst (Fig. 15) is a soft nodule at the proximal nail fold, which can intermittently drain viscous fluid; less

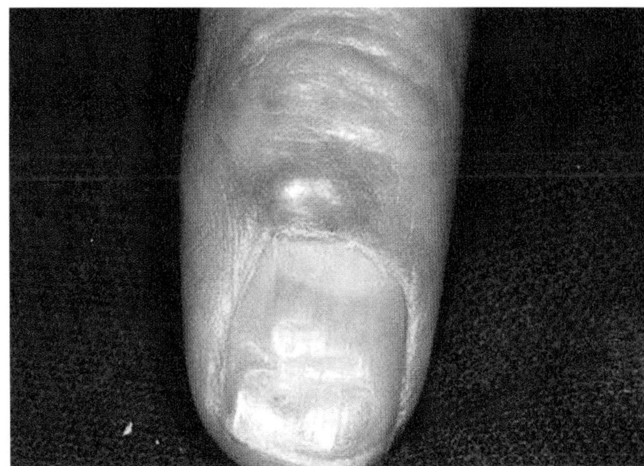

Figure 15 Mucous cyst of the proximal nail fold causing nail dystrophy.

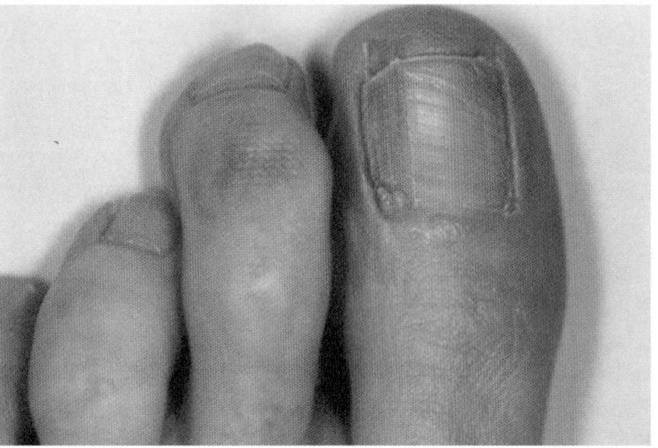

Figure 16 Periungual fibroma causing longitudinal depressions in the nail plate.

commonly, it can occur subungually. The cyst, a collection of degenerative collagen, can cause a longitudinal depression or groove in the nail plate from compression of the nail matrix. Occasionally, it connects to the underlying joint space and is often associated with osteoarthritis of the distal interphalangeal joints. Treatment is excision.

Subungual Exostosis

Subungual exostosis is essentially a hard, painful, subungual tumor, most commonly on the great toe. The exostosis typically occurs with trauma and often causes elevation of the distal nail plate. Exostosis is an outgrowth of normal bone. Treatment is symptomatic, for example, orthotics and analgesics, although surgery may be necessary for some patients.

Periungual Fibromas

Periungual fibromas (Fig. 16), or Koenen's tumors, are flesh-colored to pink papules that originate from the nail bed and cause a longitudinal depression in the nail plate. These fibromas can occur spontaneously, but they are often associated with tuberous sclerosis. Treatment is often unnecessary; however, excision is curative.

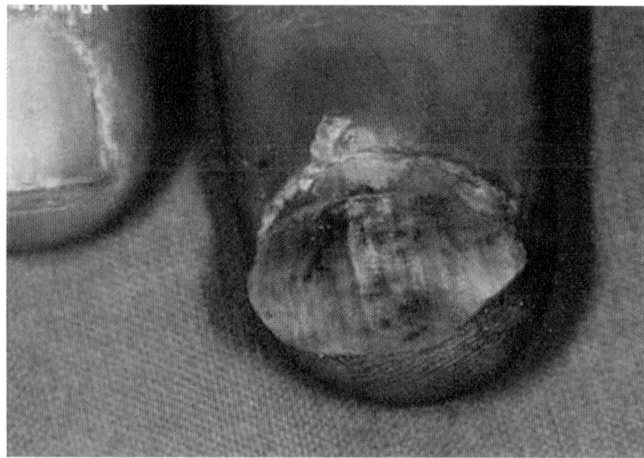

Figure 17 Nail dystrophy secondary to a glomus tumor.

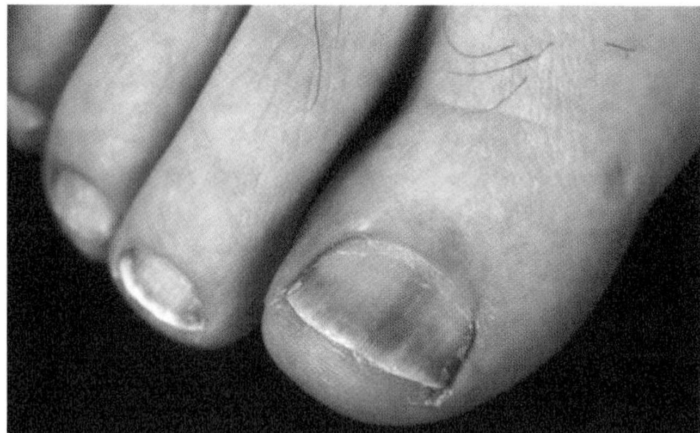

Figure 18 Brown-pigmented longitudinal streak of the nail, or longitudinal melanonychia.

Pyogenic Granuloma

A pyogenic granuloma is a benign vascular tumor that usually develops after trauma and occasionally with pregnancy and some medications (see Box 1). Characterized by rapid growth and a blue-red color, the nodule or tumor bleeds easily with minimal trauma. Surgical excision is the treatment of choice.

Glomus Tumor

The glomus tumor (Fig. 17) is a benign vascular growth arising from glomus cells of the nail bed. The tumor is usually a red-blue macule (patch) within the nail bed visible through the nail plate. Pain or pressure and sensitivity to changes in temperature are common. Treatment, via excision, is often necessary for symptomatic relief.

Malignant Tumors

Longitudinal Melanonychia and Melanoma

Longitudinal melanonychia (Fig. 18), brown-pigmented longitudinal streaks of the nail, may be a normal variant in darker-skinned persons (Fig. 19), or they might actually be nevi. Less commonly, they represent Addison's disease, acanthosis nigricans, Peutz-Jeghers syndrome, trauma, subungual hemorrhage, or fungal infection.

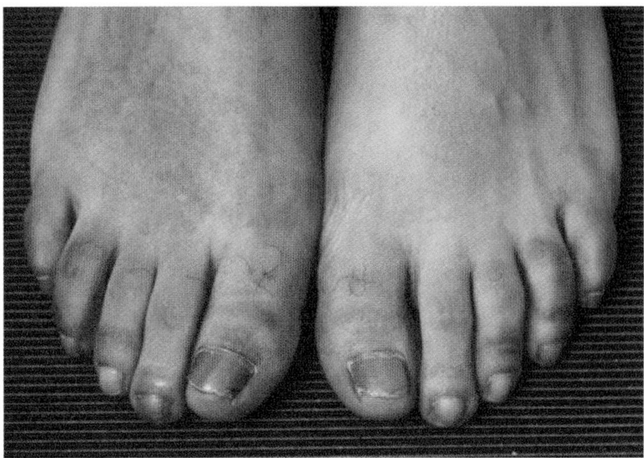

Figure 19 Longitudinal melanonychia as a normal variant in a darker-skinned person.

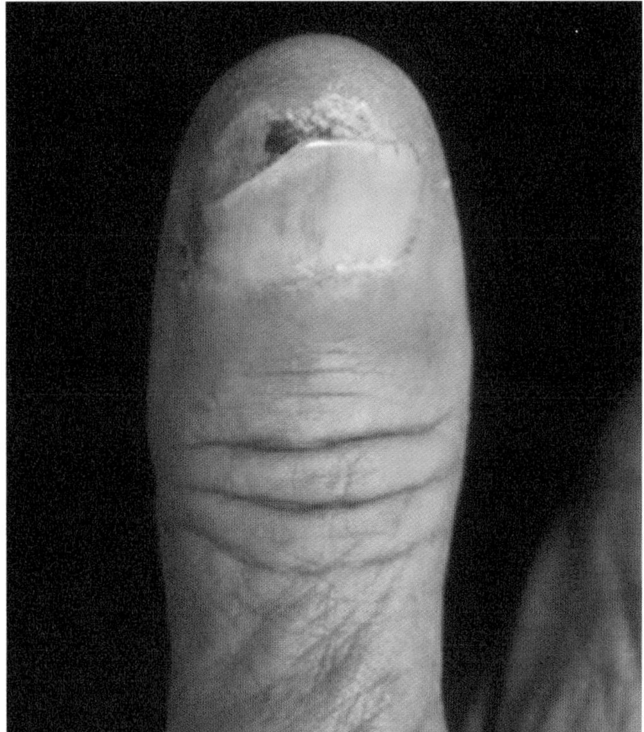

Figure 20 Verrucal plaque of squamous cell carcinoma of the nail unit.

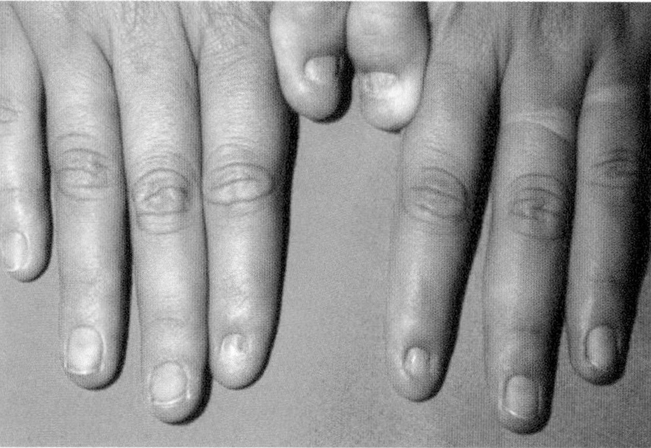

Figure 21 Triangular lunulae of nail-patella syndrome.

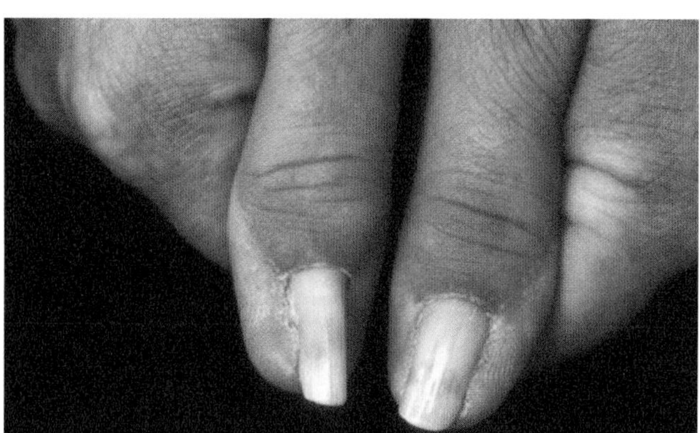

Figure 22 Pincer nails of pachyonychia congenita.

They can also be a sign of underlying melanoma, especially when they occur on the thumb (most common site for melanoma of the nail unit). Black discoloration of the proximal nail fold at the base of the pigmented streak (Hutchinson's sign) is an ominous sign for melanoma. Longitudinal melanonychia in one nail without an obvious explanation warrants a biopsy of the nail matrix. Melanoma of the nail unit has a poor prognosis.

Squamous Cell Carcinoma

Squamous cell carcinoma is the most common malignancy of the nail unit (Fig. 20). Squamous cell carcinoma is usually a verrucal (warty) plaque on the lateral nail fold of the finger and can resemble a wart unresponsive to traditional therapy. Squamous cell carcinoma is associated with HPV-16 infection and with trauma and radiation. Squamous cell carcinoma of the nail unit grows slowly, and metastasis is rare.

GENETIC NAIL ABNORMALITIES

Many genetic disorders have distinctive nail abnormalities. Triangular lunulae are a feature of nail-patella syndrome (Fig. 21), renal disease, and skeletal abnormalities. Pachyonychia congenita, an ectodermal dysplasia, exhibits marked subungual hyperkeratosis and increased transverse curvature of the nails (pincer nails, Fig. 22). Other genetic disorders with nail findings include hidrotic ectodermal dysplasia (thickening, longitudinal striations, absence of nails), dyskeratosis congenita (pterygium, absence of nails), epidermolysis bullosa (absence of nails), and Darier's disease (V-shaped nicking, red-and-white longitudinal striations, onychorrhexis, Fig. 23).

Summary

- An underlying systemic or skin disease may be associated with nail dystrophy.
- In other cases, trauma, medications, or nail unit tumors may be responsible.
- Definitive treatment is often difficult.
- Treatment for infections and tumors is usually straightforward, although many nail disorders simply require observation and reassurance.

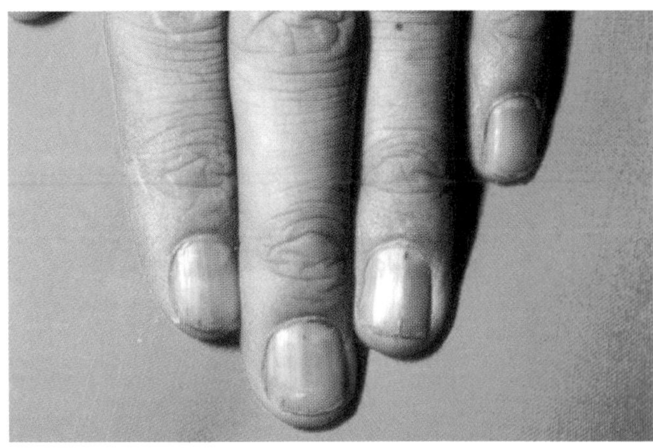

Figure 23 V-shaped nicking and red-and-white longitudinal striations of Darier's disease.

Suggested Readings

Drake LA, Dinehart SM, Farmer EM, et al: Guidelines of care for nail disorders. J Am Acad Dermatol 1996;34:529-533.

Piraccini BM, Tosti A: Treatment of common nail disorders. Derm Clinics 2000;18: 339-348.

Rich P: Nail biopsy: Indications and methods. Dermatol Surg 2001;27:229-234.

Rich P: Nail disorders: Diagnosis and treatment of infectious, inflammatory, and neoplastic nail conditions. Med Clin North Am 1998;82:1171-1183.

Rogers M: Nail manifestations of some important genetic disorders in children. Dermatol Ther 2002;15:111-120.

Spencer JM: Malignant tumors of the nail unit. Dermatol Ther 2002;15:126-130.

Drug Eruptions

Ann R. Kooken and Kenneth J. Tomecki

DEFINITION AND ETIOLOGY

An adverse drug reaction is any unintended or undesirable response to a medication given at an appropriate dose. Predictable adverse drug reactions, including toxicity, side effects, and drug interactions, are dose dependent and related to the pharmacologic actions of the drug. Unpredictable reactions, such as idiosyncratic and allergic reactions, are independent of dose and drug pharmacology.

PREVALENCE AND RISK FACTORS

Cutaneous reactions account for approximately 2% to 3% of all adverse drug reactions. Various patient- and drug-related factors contribute to the risk of adverse drug reactions. Patient factors include age (highest prevalence in the elderly); gender (more common in women); underlying disease (most prevalent in renal or hepatic disease, cystic fibrosis, and human immunodeficiency virus); and genetic differences in metabolizing enzymes. Drug factors include route of administration (more common with topical and intramuscular administration and less so with intravenous or oral administration); duration (more common with chronic or frequent use rather than short-term or intermittent use); dose; and variation in metabolism. Reactions are more common for drugs with low therapeutic indices, high levels of drug–drug interactions, and a tendency to form reactive intermediates or toxins. Even environmental factors can contribute to an adverse reaction. For example, ultraviolet light can alter the immunogenicity of certain medications, and viral infection, such as mononucleosis, can exacerbate the well-documented ampicillin-induced morbilliform reaction.

PATHOPHYSIOLOGY

The mechanisms of drug-induced cutaneous reactions have not yet been clearly defined. Classically, there are four types of allergic reactions: type I, an immediate immunoglobulin E (IgE)-mediated hypersensitivity reaction; type II, a cytotoxic antibody reaction; type III, an immune-complex reaction; and type IV, a delayed hypersensitivity reaction, such as contact dermatitis.

However, most adverse drug reactions are not allergic and include toxicity, drug–drug interactions, and exacerbation of preexisting dermatologic diseases. Nonimmunologic activation of effector pathways, such as direct release of mast cell mediators and activation of complement without antibody formation, are also possible. Drugs also can alter arachidonic acid metabolism, explaining why aspirin and other nonsteroidal anti-inflammatory drugs (NSAIDs) can induce anaphylactic-type reactions without the formation of antibodies.

SIGNS AND SYMPTOMS

Drug reactions can be systemic or organ specific. Systemic reactions are anaphylaxis, vasculitis, serum sickness, and drug fever. Organ-specific reactions commonly affect the skin but can be hematologic, pulmonary, hepatic, or renal. The most common types of adverse cutaneous reactions are exanthems (46%), followed by urticaria (23%), fixed drug eruptions (10%), erythema multiforme (5.4%), and all other forms (less than 5%).

ACUTE CUTANEOUS DRUG INDUCED REACTIONS

Exanthems

These can be maculopapular, morbilliform, or erythematous (Fig. 1). They are often bilateral and symmetrical in distribution and typically begin on the trunk or on pressure areas of bedridden patients. Mucosal involvement varies. Pruritus is usually present. Differentiating between drug-induced and infectious exanthems is often difficult. Drug-induced exanthems usually occur within a week of drug therapy, but they can occur as late as 2 weeks after therapy has ended. They often last 1 to 2 weeks and have a benign course. Any drug can cause an exanthem, but the most common agents are beta-lactam antibiotics, sulfonamides, erythromycin, gentamicin, anticonvulsants, and gold salts.

Urticaria and Angioedema

Urticaria and angioedema are less-common drug reactions, but they can progress to systemic anaphylaxis. Reaction can be immediate or delayed for days. Skin disease ranges from small papules to large annular (urticarial) plaques, often with pruritus. Individual lesions typically last less than 24 hours, but they can reappear. When the drug is discontinued, the lesions resolve rapidly. In angioedema, the mucous membranes are congested; when angioedema is severe, breathing and swallowing may be impaired. Allergic IgE-mediated urticaria and angioedema are often caused by antibiotics, especially penicillin, radiographic contrast media, and anesthetics. In contrast, angiotensin-converting enzyme inhibitors, NSAIDs, opiates, and curare can produce urticaria and angioedema that are not IgE mediated.

Vasculitis

Vasculitis can affect the skin and other organs. Drug-induced cutaneous vasculitis typically begins as erythematous macules and papules on dependent areas (Fig. 2), which become tender and purpuric. Bullae and necrosis can occur. Affected patients often have fever, myalgias, arthralgias, and fatigue. Histologic changes include fibrinoid necrosis of small blood vessels and infiltration of leukocytes with disintegrating nuclei (leukocytoclastic vasculitis). Immunoglobulins within vessel walls suggest that vasculitis is an immune-complex disease, but the exact mechanism is unknown. Common culprits for drug-induced vasculitis include allopurinol, cimetidine, furosemide, penicillins, sulfonamides, hydantoins, and thiazide diuretics.

Fixed Drug Eruption

Fixed drug eruption is an uncommon occurrence characterized by a single or several erythematous, eczematous, or bullous plaques. Pruritus is rare, but burning and discomfort are possible. The face and genitalia are common sites of involvement. By definition, fixed drug reactions recur in the same location with repeated drug administration. The mechanism of action is unknown. Commonly implicated drugs are penicillins, tetracycline, sulfonamides, barbiturates, phenolphthalein, and gold salts. When the reaction resolves, it is often followed by hyperpigmentation.

Erythema Multiforme and Stevens-Johnson Syndrome

Erythema multiforme is a hypersensitivity reaction characterized by macules, papules, and vesicles on the extremities and trunk, which often appear in a targetoid configuration (Fig. 3). Fever usually accompanies the reaction. The most common cause of erythema multiforme is infection, most often herpes simplex virus or mycoplasma, followed by drug sensitivity. Erythema multiforme can evolve to the more serious Stevens-Johnson syndrome, an extensive

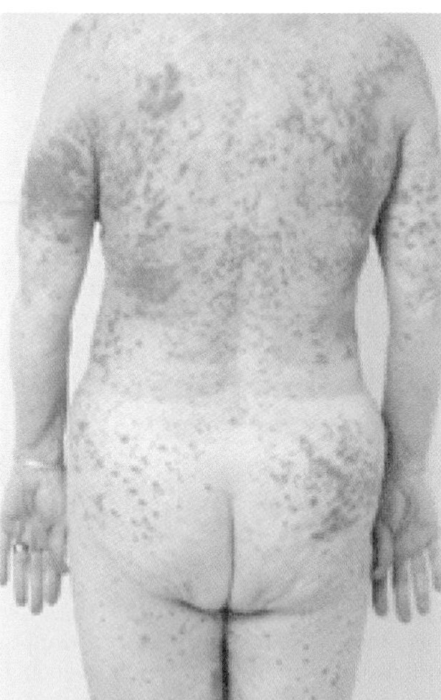

Figure 1 Exanthem. Symmetrical erythematous macules and papules.

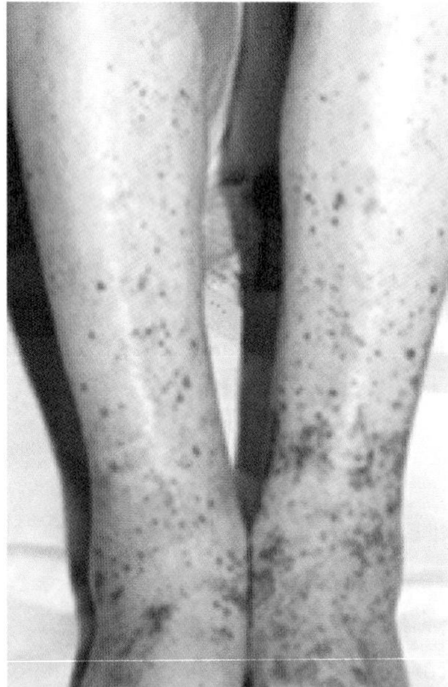

Figure 2 Vasculitis. Purpuric macules and papules.

blistering disease involving two or more mucous membranes. The disease can be life threatening, with 5% mortality. Unlike erythema multiforme, Stevens-Johnson syndrome is usually drug induced. Signs and symptoms generally appear within 1 to 3 weeks of drug initiation. Incriminating drugs for both erythema multiforme and Stevens-Johnson syndrome include sulfonamides; aromatic anticonvulsants, such as phenobarbital, phenytoin, and carbamazepine; penicillins; quinolone; cephalosporins; NSAIDs; and allopurinol.

Toxic Epidermal Necrolysis

Toxic epidermal necrolysis is a severe life-threatening drug reaction that affects the skin and mucous membranes. It is characterized by

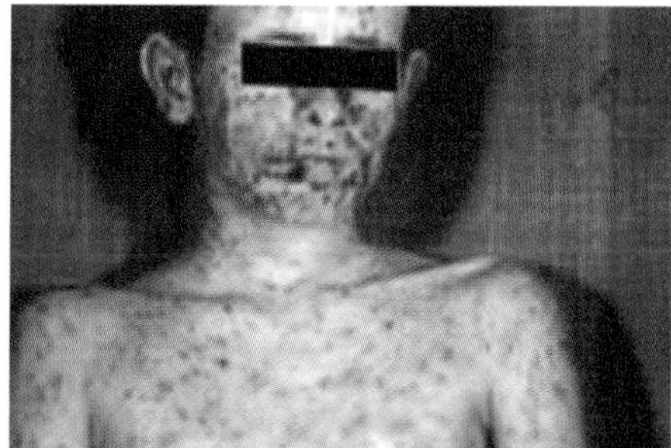

Figure 3 Erythema multiforme. Targetoid macules, papules, and vesicles with involvement of the oral mucosa.

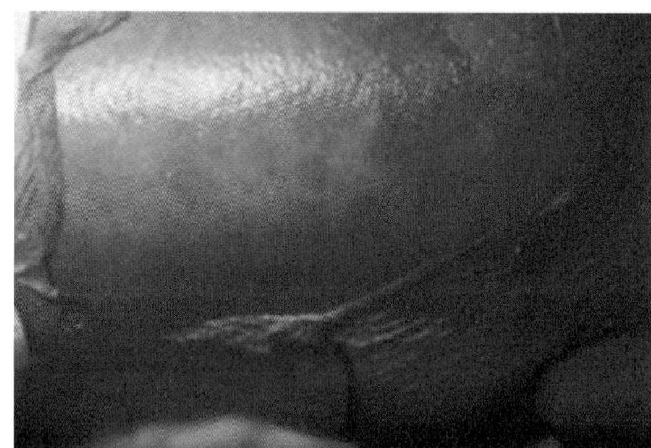

Figure 4 Toxic epidermal necrolysis. Sheet-like epidermal shedding.

confluent bullae and sheet-like epidermal shedding (Fig. 4). Fever and pain are common. Disease spreads quickly (within 2 to 3 days), and mortality can approach 30%. Infection is the leading cause of death. Affected patients experience impaired thermoregulation and electrolyte imbalance. Re-epithelialization occurs with scarring and pigmentation. Some patients have ocular sequelae, such as persistent dryness, photophobia, visual impairment, and even blindness. Histologically, epidermal necrosis occurs, whereas the dermis remains relatively unaffected. The etiologic agents for toxic epidermal necrolysis are the same as those for erythema multiforme and Stevens-Johnson syndrome.

Anticoagulant Skin Necrosis

Warfarin and heparin can induce skin necrosis. Warfarin necrosis occurs in 1 in 10,000 patients. It most commonly affects obese women who develop painful red plaques on the breasts, hips, and buttocks 3 to 5 days after therapy is initiated. Hemorrhagic bullae and necrosis follow and may require surgical débridement. Patients with protein C deficiency are at high risk for such skin necrosis because warfarin depresses this natural anticoagulant and induces a transient hypercoagulable state. Prompt recognition and treatment of warfarin necrosis can minimize fatalities.

Heparin necrosis is typically a localized reaction at injection sites and usually appears as purpuric plaques. Necrosis is triggered by thrombosis via platelet aggregation and the formation of fibrin thrombi. Thrombocytopenia is common, but fibrinogen and fibrin split products are normal. The reaction is probably immune mediated.

Systemic Lupus Erythematosus

Systemic lupus erythematosus most commonly occurs with hydralazine and procainamide but can also occur with isoniazid, chlorpromazine, penicillamine, phenytoin, and sulfasalazine. The syndrome consists of constitutional symptoms (malaise, myalgias, arthralgias), fever, and erythematous plaques on the face. Affected patients have antinuclear antibodies that react only with histones; anti-DNA antibodies remain negative, and complement levels are normal. Other laboratory findings include elevated erythrocyte sedimentation rate, anemia, and leukopenia. Patients who have slow acetyltransferase activity are more likely to develop the syndrome.

Contact Dermatitis

Allergic contact dermatitis is the most common delayed-type hypersensitivity reaction. Skin disease follows topical application of an allergen and is characterized by erythematous, papular, urticarial, or vesicular plaques. Pruritus is common. If chronic, lichenification and thickening of the skin ensue. Sensitization occurs within 5 to 7 days, but the dermatitis recurs within 24 hours with reapplication of the allergen. Cross-reactivity with structurally related substances is possible. Any topical agent can induce contact dermatitis, but most common agents include topical antibiotics (neomycin, bacitracin), benzocaine, paraben, ethylenediamine, formaldehyde, para-aminobenzoic acid (PABA), and topical antihistamines. Although rare, allergic contact dermatitis can develop after application of topical corticosteroids and should be suspected if symptoms worsen during use of these preparations. Patch testing is a diagnostic tool used to identify the sensitizing agent.

Photodermatitis

Photosensitive dermatitis is the interaction between a drug and ultraviolet radiation. The reaction can be phototoxic or photoallergic. Disease begins after exposure to light, usually ultraviolet A (UVA) light. Phototoxic reactions resemble sunburn and are dose related. The drug probably absorbs and concentrates ultraviolet radiation in the skin. Phototoxicity can occur with use of coal tar derivatives, psoralen, chlorpromazine, tetracycline, and doxycycline. Reactions resolve when either ultraviolet radiation or the drug is discontinued. Photoallergic reactions are rare and vary from erythematous and eczematous plaques to bullae on sun-exposed skin. They appear within 1 to 3 weeks of treatment with a drug such as promethazine, PABA, NSAIDs, sulfonamides, griseofulvin, or psoralen. The exact mechanism is unknown, but photodermatitis may be a form of delayed-type hypersensitivity. In contrast to phototoxic reactions, photoallergic reactions can persist after discontinuation of the medication.

Pigmentary Changes

Various drug mechanisms can induce pigmentary changes in the skin. Some drugs, such as oral contraceptives, stimulate melanocytic activity. Others, including phenothiazines and heavy metals such as silver, mercury, and gold, become lodged within the skin and alter pigmentation directly. Antimalarials produce a slate gray or yellow pigmentation, and clofazimine produces a characteristic red color. Tetracycline can permanently stain teeth if taken during early childhood or pregnancy. Minocycline can produce a blue discoloration on mucosa, within scars, and on the shins. Amiodarone produces a characteristic slate blue discoloration in sun-exposed areas.

DIAGNOSIS

Accurate diagnosis of drug eruptions can be challenging. Clinical evaluation should include history and physical examination, with an attempt to distinguish drug eruptions from viral exanthem or preexisting skin disease. Sequence of events can help to differentiate the type of reaction. For example, urticaria and angioedema occur immediately after drug exposure in contrast to most other reactions. Any new dermatitis in a patient without prior skin disease should prompt consideration of drug sensitivity. The diagnosis can be straightforward when a patient who takes few or no medications develops a rash after starting a new drug. The challenge arises when a patient takes many medications, including a few new ones, any one of which can cause an adverse reaction.

To evaluate a patient's drug sensitivity, the clinician needs to be aware of a drug's potential to produce an adverse reaction, especially a drug's dosing frequency and morphology of reactions. Evaluation should begin with a drug history, including identification of all drugs the patient has taken in the recent past. The clinician also needs to understand that adverse reactions can occur as late as 2 weeks after a medication has been discontinued. Knowledge of prior allergies helps to identify any cross-reactivity to current medications. For example, a patient with a penicillin allergy may develop an adverse reaction to other beta-lactam antibiotics. Once the suspected drug (or drugs) has been identified, discontinuation of the drug is warranted. If possible, all suspected drugs should be discontinued.

Several diagnostic tests can help to identify a suspected drug allergy; however, most have limited usefulness because many allergic reactions result from drug metabolites, which cannot be detected. Nonspecific hypersensitivity tests include a blood eosinophil count and measurement of the IgE level. For immediate-type reactions, determining the tryptase level may be helpful, because tryptase is a marker of mast cell degranulation. Immediate-type IgE reactions can be identified through skin testing; however, only a few drugs can be tested this way, with the most common being penicillin, cephalosporin, and latex. Assays to detect drug-specific IgG and IgM antibodies are also available. If medication toxicity is suspected, drug levels are essential.

Skin biopsy can be helpful for identifying a drug eruption. The presence of eosinophils, edema, and inflammation all suggest hypersensitivity. Vasculitis and necrotic changes may suggest erythema multiforme, Stevens-Johnson syndrome, or toxic epidermal necrolysis.

Patch testing is an important tool to evaluate the possibility of allergic contact dermatitis. As a test for reactivity, the application of specific allergens to the patient's skin for 48 to 72 hours may identify an allergen to be avoided. Photopatch testing helps to evaluate photoallergic reactions. The approach is similar to standard patch testing except that the patient is exposed to both the drug and ultraviolet light.

Perhaps the most sensitive and specific diagnostic test for drug eruptions is the rechallenge. Whereas allergic drug reactions by definition should recur, nonallergic reactions may not. In fact, with some adjustments, such as elimination of drug-drug interactions or changing the dose to accommodate impaired metabolism, many drugs can be safely readministered. Drugs suspected to have caused severe reactions should never be taken again.

TREATMENT

Treatment of drug eruptions is generally supportive. Symptomatic treatment primarily is predicated on the discontinuation of the offending agent, if possible. Antihistamines help to relieve pruritus and symptoms of urticaria and angioedema. Topical and systemic corticosteroids can provide additional relief. Topical corticosteroids are most beneficial for eczematous disease, but they provide little benefit in urticaria. Life-threatening reactions such as angioedema and anaphylaxis require prompt treatment with epinephrine, antihistamines, and/or systemic corticosteroids. The treatment of Stevens-Johnson syndrome and toxic epidermal necrolysis includes fluid replacement, pain control, and often antibiotics to prevent secondary infection. The role of systemic corticosteroids, intravenous immunoglobulin, and plasmapheresis in these conditions is controversial. With parenteral vitamin K therapy, warfarin necrosis can be reversed, and systemic anticoagulation can be resumed using heparin. Treatment with monoclonal protein C concentrate is also helpful. Because the mechanisms of heparin and warfarin-induced necrosis are different, treatment with antiplatelet agents or warfarin can be helpful in heparin-induced necrosis.

If a patient requires a medication that previously produced a non–life-threatening drug reaction, premedicating each dose with systemic corticosteroids and antihistamines can significantly reduce the severity of the reaction. This approach is often used for patients who receive radiocontrast media. Desensitization can be considered for patients with an allergy to penicillins, cephalosporins, or sulfonamides.

OUTCOMES

Most drug eruptions are benign, but a small percentage can be extremely dangerous, including angioedema, vasculitis, Stevens-Johnson syndrome, toxic epidermal necrolysis, and anticoagulant necrosis. Therefore, prompt diagnosis and treatment—as well as future avoidance of the medication—are essential to reduce morbidity and mortality. If a medication is necessary, careful monitoring for severe reactions is important. The main caveat is that any medication has the potential to produce an adverse reaction, and any reaction has the potential to be life threatening.

Summary

- Various patient- and drug-related factors contribute to adverse drug reactions.
- The mechanism of many drug reactions is unknown.
- Adverse drug reactions can be systemic or organ specific.
- The clinician needs to be aware of a drug's potential to produce an adverse reaction, especially a drug's frequency and pattern of reactions.
- Adverse reactions can occur as late as 2 weeks after a medication has been discontinued.
- Allergic drug reactions recur, whereas nonallergic reactions might not. With adjustments, such as elimination of drug-drug interactions or changing the dose to accommodate impaired metabolism, many drugs can be safely readministered.
- Treatment of drug eruptions is generally supportive.
- Most drug eruptions are benign, but a small percentage, including angioedema, vasculitis, Stevens-Johnson syndrome, toxic epidermal necrolysis, and anticoagulant necrosis can be life threatening.

Suggested Readings

Anderson JA, Adkinson NF Jr: Allergic reactions to drugs and biologic agents. JAMA 1987;258:2891-2899.

deShazo RD, Kemp SF: Allergic reactions to drugs and biologic agents. JAMA 1997;278:1895-1906.

Gruchalla R: Understanding drug allergies. J Allergy Clin Immunol 2000;105:S637-S644.

Roujeau JC, Stern RS: Severe adverse cutaneous reactions to drugs. N Engl J Med. 1994;331:1272-1285.

VanArsdel PP Jr: Allergy and adverse drug reactions. J Am Acad Dermatol 1982;6:833-845.

Wintroub BU, Stern R: Cutaneous drug reactions: Pathogenesis and clinical classification. J Am Acad Dermatol 1985;13:167-179.

Wolkenstein P, Revuz J: Allergic emergencies encountered by the dermatologist. Severe cutaneous adverse drug reactions. Clin Rev Allergy Immunol 1999;17:497-511.

Yates, AB, deShazo, RD: Allergic and nonallergic drug reactions. South Med J 2003;96(11):1080-1087.

Pruritus

James S. Taylor, Matthew J. Zirwas, and Apra Sood

DEFINITION AND ETIOLOGY

Pruritus or itch is defined as an unpleasant sensation of the skin that provokes the urge to scratch. It is a characteristic feature of many skin diseases and an unusual sign of some systemic diseases.[1,2] Pruritus may be localized or generalized and can occur as an acute or chronic condition. Itching lasting more than 6 weeks is termed *chronic pruritus.*[2] Itching can be intractable and incapacitating, as well as a diagnostic and therapeutic challenge.

PREVALENCE, RISK FACTORS, AND NATURAL HISTORY

Prevalence estimates, risk factors, and natural history exist for only a few specific disorders associated with itching and are mentioned in the discussion of those conditions.

PATHOPHYSIOLOGY

Peripheral Mechanisms

Physical Stimuli and Neural Pathways

Itch can be produced by mechanical (gentle touch, pressure, vibration, and wool), thermal and electrical stimuli such as transcutaneous or direct nerve stimulation. The sensation is received by free nerve endings in the skin and transmitted via unmyelinated C fibers and myelinated Aδ fibers to the central spinothalamic tracts.[1,2] Microneurography studies have demonstrated that itch and pain are transmitted by separate neural pathways.[3,4]

Chemical Mediators

Histamine is one of the most important mediators of itch, although other chemical substances have also been implicated.[3] Some, such as neuropeptides, act by releasing histamine from mast cells, and itching caused by them responds to antihistamines. Others act independently; therefore antihistamines are not effective in some forms of pruritus. Opioids have a central pruritic action and also act peripherally by augmenting histamine itch.

Central Mechanism

Patients with tumors and lesions of the central nervous system have been reported to have intractable pruritus.[1,5-7] Administration of opioids in epidural anesthesia can also lead to pruritus.

Etiology

Itching is associated with dermatologic and systemic causes, and it is important to determine whether there is an associated skin eruption. A characteristic rash usually establishes the diagnosis of a primary dermatologic disorder. Several skin diseases are associated with pruritus; some are listed in Box 1. Itching is an important component of some disorders (atopic eczema, dermatitis herpetiformis, lichen simplex chronicus, and nodular prurigo) and these conditions are rarely diagnosed in its absence. In conditions such as mild urticaria or aquagenic pruritus, the levels of histamine are sufficient for a sensory but not a vascular response, and there may be no skin findings. Bullous pemphigoid can manifest with a prebullous pruritic phase for several months before the characteristic blisters appear.[8] An invisible form of mycosis fungoides can occur as pruritus without a rash and is diagnosed on biopsy.[9]

It is important to establish if pruritus preceded the appearance of a skin eruption. Severe itching leads to scratching that causes secondary skin changes of excoriation, lichenification, dryness, eczematization, and infection. Excessive bathing and contact allergy to topical therapies can lead to dermatitis. These findings should not be interpreted as the primary skin disorder.

Select systemic conditions associated with itching are listed in Box 2. Several are potentially serious, and it can be dangerous to label a case of generalized pruritus "nonspecific eczema" until these conditions are excluded. Pruritus of systemic disease is usually generalized, it may be the only manifesting symptom, and a specific rash is not present. Neurologic and psychiatric conditions associated with chronic pruritus are included in Box 2.

DIAGNOSIS

History

A detailed history is the single most important step toward diagnosing the cause of itching. This should include information on the onset, extent (generalized vs. localized), severity, type of itch, aggravating and alleviating factors, diurnal and seasonal variations, bathing, occupation, hobbies, medication history and allergies, and past medical and surgical history. Inquire about personal or family history of atopy (childhood eczema, allergic rhinitis, asthma), household and other contacts, pets, travel history, sexual history, and history of intravenous drug use (human immunodeficiency virus [HIV] or hepatitis C infection). If the patient has recently undergone surgery, ask if hydroxyethyl cellulose was used as a plasma expander, because this substance can be associated with intense generalized pruritus lasting for up to one year.

Review of Systems

A detailed history is important in chronic pruritus of unknown origin, including general health (fever, chills, weight loss); skin (pigmentation, sweating, asteatosis, plethora, and jaundice); hair (growth, texture, loss); nails (Beau's lines, onycholysis, color changes); eyes (exophthalmos, color changes); and endocrine, hematopoietic, gastrointestinal, genitourinary, neurologic, and mental status.[5-7,10]

Physical Examination

The skin should be examined for evidence of any recognizable disorder. Scratching (causing excoriations) or rubbing (producing papules, nodules, and lichenified plaques) can lead to secondary changes that should not be interpreted as a primary skin disorder but can mimic one. Examination of the upper midback can help in this distinction, because it is relatively inaccessible and unavailable for scratching.

Look for evidence of parasitic infestation, especially scabies and lice. Examination of the skin, hair, and genitalia with surveillance scrapings can identify either disorder. Examination of clothing seams can identify body lice in the unkempt (vagabond's disease).

A complete physical examination to look for other cutaneous signs mentioned in the "Review of Systems" section is essential.

Box 1 Select Dermatologic Disorders Associated with Chronic Pruritus*

Autoimmune
Dermatitis herpetiformis
Dermatomyositis
Pemphigoid
Sjögren's syndrome

Genetic
Darier's disease
Hailey-Hailey disease
Ichthyoses
Sjögren-Larsson syndrome

Infections and Infestations
Arthropod reactions
Dermatophytosis
Folliculitis
Impetigo and other bacterial infections
Insect bites
Pediculosis
Scabies
Viral

Inflammatory
Asteatosis (dry skin), including aging and senile pruritus
Atopic eczema
Contact dermatitis (irritant, allergic)
Drug reactions
"Invisible dermatoses"
Lichen planus
Lichen simplex chronicus
Mastocytosis (urticaria pigmentosa)
Miliaria
Psoriasis
Scars
Urticaria

Neoplastic
Cutaneous T-cell lymphoma or mycosis fungoides (especially Sézary syndrome)
Cutaneous B-cell lymphoma
Leukemia cutis

Pregnancy
Pemphigoid gestationis
Polymorphic eruption of pregnancy
Prurigo gestationis

**Generalized or localized depending on extent of disease*

Adapted from Pujol RM, Gallardo F, Llistosella E, et al: Invisible mycosis fungoides: A diagnostic challenge. J Am Acad Dermatol 2002;47:S167-S171; and Ständer S, Weisshaar E, Mettang T, et al: Clinical Classification of itch: A position paper of the International Forum for the Study of Itch. Acta Derm Venereol 2007:87 291-294.

Box 2 Select Systemic Causes of Chronic Pruritus

Endocrine and Metabolic Diseases
Chronic renal failure
Diabetes mellitus (questionable; may be localized to scalp)
Hyperthyroidism
Hypothyroidism
Liver disease (with or without cholestasis)
Malabsorption
Perimenopausal pruritus

Infectious Diseases
Helminthosis
HIV infection
Parasitosis

Neoplastic and hematological
Hodgkin's disease
Iron deficiency
Leukemia
Non-Hodgkin's lymphoma
Multiple myeloma
Plasmacytoma
Polycythemia rubra vera

Visceral Neoplasms
Carcinoid syndrome
Solid tumors of the cervix, prostate, or colon

Pregnancy
Pruritus gravidarum (with or without cholestasis)

Drugs
Allopurinol
Amiodarone
Angiotensin-converting enzyme inhibitors
Estrogen
Hydrochlorothiazide
Hydroxyethyl cellulose
Opioids
Simvastatin

Other
Neurologic disease

- Abscess
- Infarcts
- Multiple sclerosis
- Nostalgia paresthetica
- Tumors

Psychiatric disease

- Anxiety disorders
- Depression
- Obsessive-compulsive disorder

Adapted from Pujol RM, Gallardo F, Llistosella E, et al: Invisible mycosis fungoides: A diagnostic challenge. J Am Acad Dermatol 2002;47:S167-S171; and Ständer S, Weisshaar E, Mettang T, et al: Clinical Classification of itch: A position paper of the International Forum for the Study of Itch. Acta Derm Venereol 2007:87 291-294.

Pelvic and rectal examination as well as examination of the lymph nodes, liver, and spleen is important.[5-7,10]

Investigations

In some cases, the diagnosis is apparent from the history, physical examination, or bedside studies (such as a scabies preparation). When the diagnosis is not apparent, laboratory studies may be indicated.

In general, the laboratory investigation should be directed by the findings of the history and physical examination. In a patient with no pertinent findings, a reasonable initial screen consists of complete blood count, complete metabolic panel, hepatitis C antibodies, TSH, and chest x-ray. Based on the initial results and the course of the pruritus, further testing may be indicated (Box 3).

Histopathologic examination of the skin lesions may be required. In pruritus without a rash, a biopsy specimen for direct immunofluorescence from normal-appearing skin might show immune deposits in early cases of pemphigoid or findings diagnostic of mycosis fungoides in routine histopathology.

Patients with chronic idiopathic pruritus should be followed with periodic re-evaluation if the symptoms persist, because an underlying disorder can manifest later.[5-7,10]

Box 3 Laboratory Investigations for Generalized Pruritus

Initial Screening Studies
Complete blood count with differential
Blood urea nitrogen, creatinine
Aspartate transaminase, alanine aminotransferase, alkaline phosphatase, bilibrubin
Hepatitis C antibodies
Thyroid-stimulating hormone
Chest x-ray

Other Studies*
Allergy panel

- Histamine
- Mast cell metabolites
- Serotonin
- Total IgE
- Urine 5-HIAA

Antinuclear antibody
Antimitochondrial antibodies
Antitissue transglutaminase antibodies
Calcium and phosphate levels
Erythrocyte sedimentation rate
Fasting glucose, hemoglobin A_{1C}
HIV screen
Pan–computed tomography scan
Prick testing, patch testing
Serum and urine immunofixation
Serum and urine protein electrophoresis
Serum iron and ferritin
Skin biopsy with immunofluorescence
Stool for occult blood, ova, and parasites
Upper and/or lower endoscopy

**To be considered based on history and physical examination, results of initial laboratory screening, and pruritus.*
5-HIAA, 5-hydroxyindoleacetic acid; IgE, immunoglobulin E.
Adapted from Kantor GR, Bernhard J: Investigation of the pruritic patient in daily practice. Semin Dermatol. 1995;14:290-296.

Box 4 Outline for Selected Treatments for Pruritus

Topical
Anesthetics
Antipruritics
Cooling agents
Corticosteroids
Emollients

Systemic
Antihistamines
Corticosteroids
Opioid-receptor antagonist

Phototherapy
Ultraviolet B, broad band or narrow band
Ultraviolet A_1

Miscellaneous
Acupuncture
Capsaicin
Transcutaneous electrical stimulation

Adapted from Hagermark O, Wahlgren C: Treatment of itch. Semin Dermatol 1995;14:320-325.

TREATMENT

General Concepts and Topical and Systemic Treatments

Identifying and treating the underlying cause is the most effective therapy for pruritus. Symptomatic treatment should be prescribed while the primary condition is being treated. Cool compresses and cool baths might help relieve the itch; a cool environment in the home and workplace also helps. Cooling lotions with calamine, pramoxine, or menthol and camphor are helpful (Box 4).

Pruritus due to dry skin, especially in the elderly, responds to generous amounts of emollients such as petrolatum and white paraffin, as well as correcting the temperature and humidity. Patients should avoid frequent and hot baths and excessive use of soap, which further dries the skin. Topical corticosteroids should not be prescribed indiscriminately but should be used only if there are signs of cutaneous inflammation. Topical tacrolimus may be prescribed for limited use in patients with atopic dermatitis. Topical capsaicin may be useful in chronic localized pruritus such as notalgia paresthetica.

H_1-receptor antihistamines are the drugs of choice for urticaria. The newer nonsedating antihistamines are less effective in atopic dermatitis; the older sedating antihistamines might work better. Tricyclic antidepressants such as doxepin have antihistamine activity in addition to central effects and are useful in chronic, severe pruritus. Gabapentin, buspirone, and selective serotonin reuptake inhibitors (SSRIs) may be considered in select patients. Ultraviolet (UV) B phototherapy is very effective in uremic pruritus and may be helpful in patients with prurigo nodularis, atopic dermatitis, HIV infection, and aquagenic pruritus. Opioid-receptor antagonists, such as naloxone, have occasionally been used for intractable pruritus of renal and cholestatic diseases. Other measures that have been tried for chronic pruritus are acupuncture and transcutaneous electrical nerve stimulation (TENS) (see Box 4).

Aggressive treatment of the eczema may be the only way to control the pruritus in patients with atopic dermatitis. Limited use of systemic corticosteroids as well as other systemic immunosuppressives may be needed to treat the eczema.[1,10]

Treatment of Specific Disorders

Chronic Renal Disease

Other than general treatments as mentioned earlier, mild disease might respond to UVB phototherapy and erythropoietin. Second-line treatments include oral activated charcoal, cholestyramine, and the opioid antagonist naltrexone. Third-line therapies include thalidomide and parathyroidectomy.[1,10]

Dialysis can provide some relief but rarely improves itching significantly. Parathyroid hormone levels have been found to be increased and have been implicated as a cause. These patients experience relief of pruritus after parathyroidectomy.[6] Renal transplantation is the definitive treatment.[1,10]

Cholestatic Disease

Ion-exchange resins, such as cholestyramine, probably act by lowering levels of bile salts and other pruritogens. Altered central opioidergic neurotransmission is believed to be a contributing factor,[12] and opioid antagonists such as naloxone and naltrexone have been found useful.[13] Second-line therapies include rifampicin, which has been shown to reduce pruritus in patients with primary biliary cirrhosis,[14] ursodeoxycholic acid, SSRIs, and *S*-adenosylmethionine. Third-line treatment includes UVB phototherapy, extracorporeal albumin dialysis, plasmapheresis, and dronabinol, a cannabinoid.[1,10]

Polycythemia Rubra Vera

Antihistamines are usually ineffective, but psoralen plus ultraviolet A (PUVA) phototherapy has been helpful in some patients. Aspirin has been reported effective, and a trial showed SSRIs to be effective.[1,10]

Summary

- Pruritus or itch is a characteristic feature of many skin diseases and an unusual sign of some systemic diseases.
- The presence of skin changes does not exclude the possibility of an underlying systemic cause of the pruritus.
- The absence of a rash does not automatically mean that the underlying cause of the itching is a systemic disease.
- Dermatologic and internal medicine evaluations, including laboratory tests, skin biopsy, and radiographic studies as dictated by history and physical findings, should be considered for patients with generalized pruritus lasting longer than 6 weeks.
- Identifying and treating the underlying cause are the most effective therapies for pruritus.

Suggested Readings

Alonso-Llamazares J, Rogers RS III, Oursler JR, Calobrisi SD: Bullous pemphigoid presenting as generalized pruritus: Observation in six patients. Int J Dermatol 1998;37:507-514.

Bernhard JD: Pruritus in skin disease. In Bernhard JD: Itch: Mechanisms and Management of Pruritus. New York, McGraw-Hill, 1994, pp 37-67.

Greaves M: Mediators of pruritus. In Bolognia JL, Jorizzo JL, Rapini RP (eds): Dermatology. St Louis, Mosby, 2003, pp 85-94.

Hagermark O, Wahlgren C: Treatment of itch. Semin Dermatol 1995;14:320-325.

Kantor GR, Bernhard J: Investigation of the pruritic patient in daily practice. Semin Dermatol. 1995;14:290-296.

Pujol RM, Gallardo F, Llistosella E, et al: Invisible mycosis fungoides: A diagnostic challenge. J Am Acad Dermatol 2002;47:S167-S171.

Ständer S, Steinhoff M, Schmelz, M, et al: Neurophysiology of pruritus: cutaneous elicitation of itch. Arch Dermatol 2003;139:1463-1470.

Ständer S, Weisshaar E, Mettang T, et al: Clinical Classification of itch: A position paper of the International Forum for the Study of Itch. Acta Derm Venereol 2007:87 291-294.

Ward JR, Bernhard JD: Pruritus. In Lebwohl M, Heymann WR, Berth-Jones J, Coulson I (eds): Treatment of Skin Disease, 2nd ed. St Louis, Mosby Elsevier, 2006, pp 533-537.

Zirwas MJ, Seraly MP: Pruritus of unknown origin: A retrospective study. J Am Acad Dermatol 2001;45:892-896.

References

For a complete list of references, log onto www.expertconsult.com.

Pigmentary Disorders

Apra Sood and Kenneth J. Tomecki

Normal skin color depends on melanin, hemoglobin (oxidized and reduced), and carotenoids. Melanin is the major color determinant and is responsible for variations in skin color. Pigmentary disorders typically indicate an increased amount of melanin, leading to darker color of the skin, called hypermelanosis or hyperpigmentation (Box 1). Decreased or absent pigment makes the skin appear lighter or white, known as hypomelanosis or hypopigmentation (Box 2). The disorders can be genetic or acquired.

DISORDERS OF HYPERMELANOSIS

Melasma (Chloasma)

Definition

Melasma is an acquired hypermelanosis, seen predominantly on sun-exposed areas in women. Most patients are pregnant women in whom the darkening is considered physiologic, although nonpregnant women taking oral contraceptives or estrogens can also develop melasma. Women of all ethnic groups are equally affected, but dark-skinned persons tend to be more affected. Approximately 10% of affected persons are men, thereby suggesting other causes.

Signs and Symptoms

Affected patients have asymptomatic brown patches symmetrically on the upper lips, cheeks, forehead, and chin. Pigmentation tends to be persistent but can fade slowly after pregnancy or after discontinu- discontinuing ating oral contraception.

Diagnosis

The diagnosis is usually straightforward. Biopsy shows increased pigment in the epidermis and dermis.

Treatment

The use of sunscreen (SPF 30 or greater) is essential to minimize further darkening. Bleaching agents with hydroquinone (a hydroxyphenolic compound that inhibits the conversion of dopa to melanin), in concentrations of 2% to 4%, can help to minimize (lighten) the pigmentation. Alternatively, tretinoin cream and α-hydroxy acids can be effective. Mixed topical combinations of hydroquinone, tretinoin, and a fluorinated corticosteroid are particularly effective as short-term treatment. If the pigmentation is deeper (within the dermis), laser therapy combined with topical therapy is often very effective.

Postinflammatory Hyperpigmentation

Any inflammatory condition in the skin (e.g., eczema, psoriasis), especially in dark-skinned patients, can lead to postinflammatory hyperpigmentation, a common late sequela characterized by patches of brown skin. Pigmentation follows the pattern of the initial disease, making the diagnosis straightforward in most patients.

DISORDERS OF HYPOMELANOSIS

Vitiligo

Definition

Vitiligo is an acquired disorder of melanocytes characterized by complete loss of pigment within the skin to yield depigmented macules and patches. The disease usually begins in childhood or early adulthood and is occasionally associated with autoimmune disorders, most often thyroid disease (30% of patients have Graves' disease or hypothyroidism), and less so pernicious anemia, Addison's disease, diabetes mellitus, myasthenia gravis, and alopecia areata. Affected patients can have circulating autoantibodies, including antithyroglobulin, antimicrosomal antibodies, and antiparietal cell antibodies.

Prevalence

Vitiligo affects approximately 1% of the population and both genders equally. Approximately 30% to 40% patients have a family history of vitiligo, and disease has occurred in monozygotic twins.

Signs and Symptoms

Disease usually occurs in childhood or early adulthood. The depigmented patches are sharply delineated, surrounded by normal or darker skin, and are usually symmetrical. A segmental pattern occasionally occurs, usually in children. Vitiligo often follows trauma, with disease common on extensor sites, such as the hands, elbows, and knees. Another pattern is orificial, with depigmented areas surrounding orifices (nares, mouth, vagina, urethra, and anus).

Treatment

Treatment of choice for limited disease is mid- to high-potency topical corticosteroids, although topical calcineurin inhibitors, such as tacrolimus or pimecrolimus, can also be very beneficial. If treatment is successful, repigmentation usually occurs within 3 to 4 months. Narrow-band ultraviolet B and PUVA (topical or systemic psoralens followed by ultraviolet [UV] A exposure) therapy twice weekly is effective treatment for extensive disease. Unresponsive areas can be camouflaged with make-up or self-tanning creams containing dihydroxyacetone. Epidermal grafting can help some patients with stable disease.

Ash Leaf Spots

Oval (ash leaf) hypopigmented macules are the earliest cutaneous sign of tuberous sclerosis. Such light patches can occur at birth or in early infancy; they are often multiple and irregularly scattered on the body. A Wood's light examination highlights the macules and helps to identify them in fair-skinned patients. Other cutaneous signs of tuberous sclerosis include facial angiofibromas (adenoma sebaceum), fibrous plaques on the forehead, periungual fibromas (Koenen's tumors), and connective tissue nevi (shagreen patches).

Box 1 Disorders of Hypermelanosis

Genetic
Café-au-lait macules

- Albright's syndrome
- Neurofibromatosis

Freckles and lentigines; multiple lentigines syndrome
Mongolian spots

Acquired
Deposition

- Metals
  - Silver (argyria)
  - Gold (chrysiasis)
- Tattoos

Endocrine

- Addison's disease
- Melasma (pregnancy, oral contraceptives, estrogens)

Medications

- Chemotherapeutic (busulfan, bleomycin)
- Phenothiazines (chlorpromazine)
- Antibiotics (minocycline)

Nutritional

- Pellagra
- Vitamin B_{12} deficiency

Postinflammatory hyperpigmentation
Systemic diseases

- Hemochromatosis
- Porphyria

Ash leaf spots can resemble nevus depigmentosus, a single, stable, well-circumscribed hypomelanotic macule present at birth.

Idiopathic Guttate Hypomelanosis

Idiopathic guttate hypomelanosis is a common benign acquired disorder characterized by small, well-defined, round white macules on the sun-exposed areas of the legs and forearms. The patches are usually asymptomatic and can resemble vitiligo. Women are more commonly affected. Treatment is not necessary.

Box 2 Disorders of Hypomelanosis

Genetic
Albinism
Nevus depigmentosus
Piebaldism
Tuberous sclerosis (ash leaf macules)
Vitiligo
Acquired
Chemical leukoderma

- Phenolic compounds

Papulosquamous or eczematous

- Pityriasis alba
- Pityriasis versicolor

Miscellaneous
Idiopathic guttate hypomelanosis

Summary

- Melasma is an acquired hypermelanosis seen predominantly on sun-exposed areas in women.
- Any inflammatory condition in the skin (e.g., eczema, psoriasis), especially in dark-skinned patients, can lead to postinflammatory hyperpigmentation.
- Vitiligo is an acquired disorder of melanocytes and is characterized by complete loss of pigment.
- Oval (ash leaf) hypopigmented macules are the earliest cutaneous sign of tuberous sclerosis.
- Idiopathic guttate hypomelanosis is a common acquired benign disorder characterized by small, well-defined, round white macules on the sun-exposed areas of the legs and forearms.

Suggested Readings

Grimes PE: New insights and new therapies in vitiligo. JAMA 2005;293:730-735.

Ortonne J-P, Passeron T: Melanin pigmentary disorders: Treatment update. Dermatol Clin 2005;23:208-226.

Yoshimura K, Sato K, Aiba-Kojima E, et al: Repeated treatment protocols for melasma and acquired dermal melanocytosis. Dermatol Surg 2006;32;365-371.

Blistering Diseases

Brandie Tackett and David Hamrock

Autoimmune mucocutaneous blistering diseases (AMBDs) are a group of conditions that manifest with blisters on the skin or mucous membranes.

BULLOUS PEMPHIGOID

Summary

- Bullous pemphigoid is the most common autoimmune mucocutaneous blistering disease.
- Blisters are subepidermal.
- Oral involvement is rare.

Prevalence

Bullous pemphigoid is the most common AMBD, with an estimated prevalence of 1 in 40,000. It usually manifests in the sixth or seventh decade of life.

Signs and Symptoms

Scattered urticarial papules and plaques on the trunk, arms, and legs are common when the disease first appears. Acral sites such as the palms can be involved. Itching can be intense. With this presentation, the condition is often misdiagnosed as urticaria. Later in the course of the disease, tense vesicles and bullae develop on an urticarial base (Fig. 1). Bullae can reach a size of several centimeters before rupturing. Blisters in the oral cavity are rare, and they usually occur when the cutaneous disease is extensive. Occasionally, bullous pemphigoid can be induced by medications such as furosemide, captopril, and penicillin.

Diagnosis

Skin biopsies for hematoxylin and eosin (H&E) staining and direct immunofluorescence (DIF) are needed to confirm the diagnosis. Histopathologic findings of an early vesicle show a subepidermal vesicle with an inflammatory infiltrate of neutrophils and eosinophils in the upper dermis. Normal skin adjacent to an urticarial plaque is ideal for DIF. Almost all biopsies reveal linear C3 at the basement membrane zone, and 80% of biopsies also show linear immunoglobulin (Ig) G at the basement membrane zone. Biopsies for DIF should be placed in Michel's transport media for processing rather than saline to avoid false-negative results.

Serologic studies for indirect immunofluorescence (IIF) can help to confirm the diagnosis. This should be performed at the same time as the cutaneous biopsies. Circulating IgG antibodies to the basement membrane zone can be detected in approximately 80% of patients with bullous pemphigoid. Diagnosis of bullous pemphigoid is summarized in Box 1.

Treatment

Systemic corticosteroids provide the most rapid and effective control of disease. Initial doses of oral prednisone at 0.5 to 1.0 mg/kg per day, based on ideal body weight, often halts formation of new blisters. The dose of prednisone can be tapered slowly over a period of several months to a maintenance dose between 5 and 10 mg/day. Often, dapsone at a dose of approximately 100 mg/day is started at the same time as prednisone. The addition of dapsone often allows quicker control of disease and thus allows a faster prednisone taper.

When the dose of prednisone cannot be lowered to less than 10 mg/day due to continued blister formation, immunosuppressive agents (ISAs) such as methotrexate, mycophenalate mofetil, azathioprine, or cyclophosphamide may be added. In cases refractory to this conventional immunosuppressive therapy, intravenous immunoglobulin (IVIg) administered monthly has been shown to induce control of disease, and continued use following a defined protocol has led to long-term remissions. Rituximab has been used successfully in refractory cases.

It is essential that frequent bacterial cultures of cutaneous erosions be performed to identify early infections. Erosions become infected quickly, especially when taking immunosuppressive therapy for control of the disease process. Appropriate antibiotics should be initiated promptly. To aid in healing moist cutaneous erosions, topical soaks with aluminum acetate (Domeboro) for 10 minutes, two to four times a day, is very beneficial. Treatment of bullous pemphigoid is summarized in Box 2.

PEMPHIGUS VULGARIS

Summary

- Pemphigus vulgaris begins with jagged intraoral erosions.
- Intraepidermal acantholysis is seen in early vesicles.
- It is more difficult to treat than bullous pemphigoid.

Prevalence

Pemphigus vulgaris is an intraepidermal AMBD that typically manifests in the fifth or sixth decade of life. It is the most common type of pemphigus, accounting for 70% of pemphigus patients. It occurs in both sexes with equal frequency. It can occur in all ethnic groups but is most common in those of Ashkenazi Jewish descent. The prevalence in Jerusalem is 1.6 cases per million.

Signs and Symptoms

Pemphigus vulgaris usually manifests with painful erosions in the oral mucosa. The earliest erosions are often located on the buccal mucosa, adjacent to the lower molars. However, the fixed gingiva , soft palate, and tongue are often affected. These erosions have a characteristic jagged appearance (Fig. 2A). When the disease is limited to the oral cavity, it is often misdiagnosed as candidiasis or herpes.

As the condition progresses, flaccid blisters develop on cutaneous surfaces. These blisters quickly rupture and become crusted erosions. Erythema surrounding the base of a blister is variable. Common sites of involvement are on the scalp, face, chest, upper arms, and back (Fig. 3).

Any mucosal site can be affected. Nasal involvement manifests with bleeding and crusting. The upper one third of the esophagus can be affected, resulting in dysphagia. A hoarse voice is a good indication of vocal cord involvement. Erosions can also occur on the palpebral conjunctiva and the genital and anal mucosa (see Boxes 1 and 2).

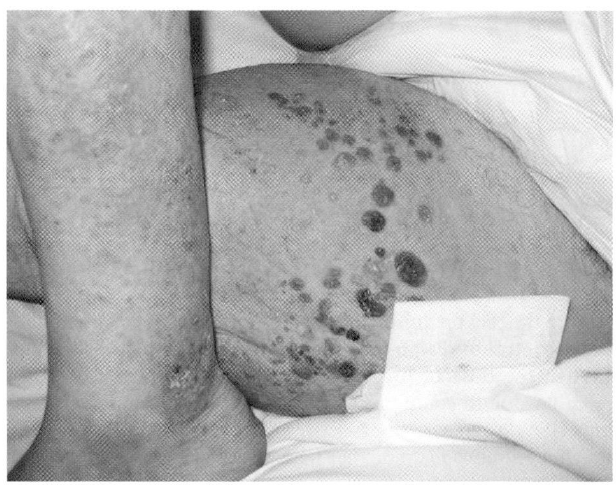

Figure 1 Bullous pemphigoid. Tense bullae on an urticarial base.

Box 46.2-1 Diagnosis of Blistering Diseases

Bullous Pemphigoid
H&E: Subepidermal bullae
DIF: Linear C3 and IgG at basement membrane zone

Pemphigus Vulgaris
H&E: Intraepidermal acantholysis
DIF: Intercellular IgG and C3 in the epidermis

Mucous Membrane Pemphigoid
H&E: Subepidermal bullae
DIF: linear IgG and C3 deposition at the basement membrane zone

Pemphigus Foliaceus
H&E: Superficial epidermal acantholysis
DIF: Intercellular IgG deposition in the stratum corneum

DIF, direct immunofluorescence; H&E, hematoxylin and eosin; Ig, immunoglobulin.

Diagnosis

Oral or cutaneous biopsies for H&E staining and DIF are needed to confirm the diagnosis. Histopathologic findings of an early vesicle show intraepidermal acantholysis, which is a loss of adhesion between keratinocytes. Normal skin adjacent to an early blister is ideal for DIF, which shows intercellular IgG and C3 within the epidermis.

Serologic studies for IIF should be performed at the same time as the biopsies. Circulating intercellular IgG antibodies can be detected in approximately 80% of patients with pemphigus vulgaris. A more sensitive enzyme-linked immunosorbent assay (ELISA) is available for detecting antibodies to desmoglein 3, an intercellular adhesion protein. Diagnosis of pemphigus vulgaris is summarized in Box 1.

Treatment

Pemphigus vulgaris is typically more difficult to treat than bullous pemphigoid. The circulating autoantibody can bind directly to the intercellular proteins that hold keratinocytes together and cause acantholysis. Neither complement fixation nor an inflammatory response is required for blister formation. Thus, medications with anti-inflammatory effects that can benefit patients with bullous pemphigoid are not as effective in patients with pemphigus vulgaris. Suppression of autoantibody formation is important for long-term control of disease.

Systemic corticosteroids provide the most rapid and effective control of disease. Prednisone at a dose of 0.5 to 1.0 mg/kg per day, based on ideal body weight, often halts formation of new blisters.

Box 46.2-2 Treatment of Blistering Diseases

Bullous Pemphigoid
Prednisone and dapsone, taper off prednisone to <10 mg/day
If refractory to prednisone <10 mg/day, add an immunosuppressive agent
If refractory to conventional therapy, try IVIg or rituximab

Pemphigus Vulgaris
Prednisone plus an immunosuppressive agent
IVIg or rituximab in refractory cases

Mucous Membrane Pemphigoid
Topical and intralesional corticosteroids
Dapsone ± prednisone
Prednisone plus an immunosuppressive agent, if unresponsive

Pemphigus Foliaceus
High-potency topical corticosteroids
Hydroxychloroquine
Prednisone plus an immunosuppressive agent
IVIg or rituximab in refractory patients

IVIg, intravenous immunoglobulin.

Often, ISAs such as methotrexate, mycophenolate mofetil, or azathioprine are used together with prednisone at the outset of treatment. The long-term goal is to taper the dose of prednisone slowly over a period of several months to a maintenance dose between 5 and 10 mg/day. Dapsone is not as effective in treating pemphigus vulgaris as it is for bullous pemphigoid. In cases refractory to conventional immunosuppressive therapy, IVIg, administered in monthly cycles following a defined protocol, and rituximab have shown promise in treating patients with refractory disease.

Obtaining frequent bacterial cultures of open cutaneous erosions and topical therapies as discussed for bullous pemphigoid greatly enhances the success of the systemic therapy.

To minimize the formation of new oral blisters, patients should avoid eating foods with jagged edges such as potato chips, toast, and pretzels. A soft toothbrush should be used and care should be taken not to aggressively brush the fixed gingiva. The regular use of a steam inhaler, particularly in months of low humidity, can greatly decrease the amount of nasal crusting and bleeding. Treatment of pemphigus vulgaris is summarized in Box 2.

MUCOUS MEMBRANE PEMPHIGOID

Summary

- Mucous membrane pemphigoid has smooth-bordered intraoral erosions.
- All mucosal sites are potentially affected.
- Blindness can occur.

Prevalence

Mucous membrane pemphigoid (MMP), also termed *cicatricial pemphigoid,* is a subepidermal blistering disease that typically manifests in the sixth or seventh decade of life. The female-to-male ratio is about 2:1.

Signs and Symptoms

MMP differs from bullous pemphigoid in that individual lesions heal with scarring. There are varying manifestations of the disease depending on which protein in the basement membrane is involved in the

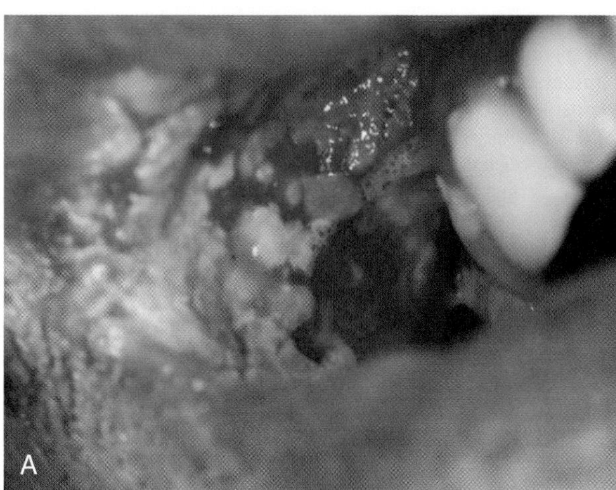

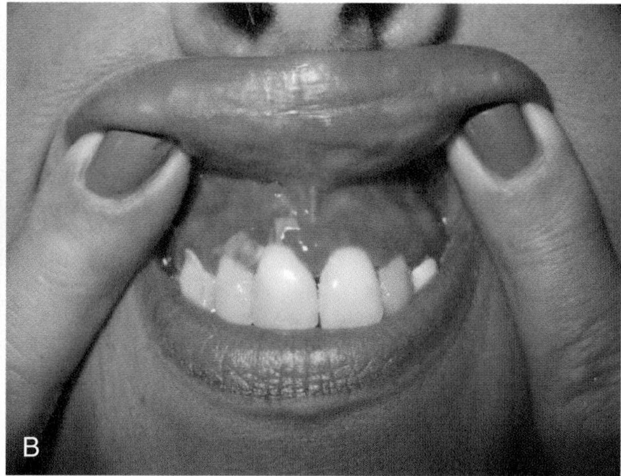

Figure 2 **A,** Jagged oral erosions of pemphigus vulgaris. **B,** Smooth oral erosions of mucous membrane pemphigoid.

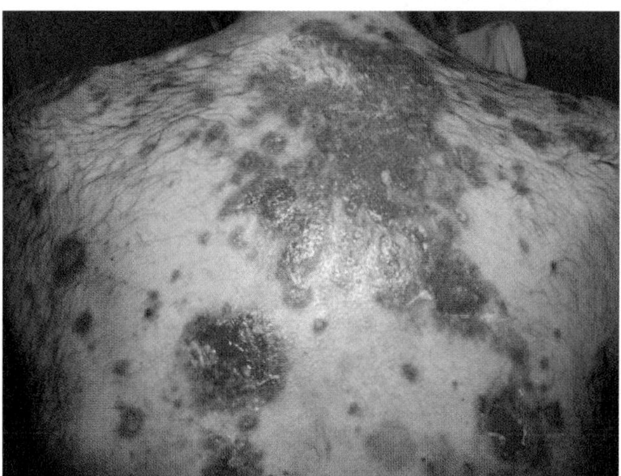

Figure 3 **Pemphigus vulgaris.** Flaccid bullae and erosions.

autoimmune process. A common presentation is that of smooth-bordered erosions in the oral mucosa (see Fig. 2B). Approximately 90% of patients with MMP have oral erosions. If the oral mucosa is the only mucosal site involved, the condition is termed *oral pemphigoid.*

As in pemphigus vulgaris, any mucosal site can be affected. Involvement of the nasal mucosa can lead to strictures. Repeated coughing and a hoarse voice are good indicators of blistering in the pharynx and larynx. Repeated blistering and subsequent scarring in these areas can result in strictures. Involvement of the conjunctiva, which manifests clinically as conjunctivitis and xerosis, results in scarring between the palpebral and bulbar conjunctiva (symblepharon), entropion, and subsequent trichiasis. Progressive scarring can lead to blindness. Ocular cicatricial pemphigoid is a subset of MMP that manifests solely as conjunctival involvement.

Involvement of the genital and anal mucosa is fairly common. Persistent blistering and scarring of the vaginal mucosa can result in stenosis that prohibits screening pelvic examinations. Anal involvement manifests as localized pain and bleeding, which can lead to stenosis if left untreated.

Cutaneous tense blisters similar to those seen in bullous pemphigoid occur in only 20% of patients. Healing occurs with pink, atrophic scarring.

Another type of MMP, termed *antiepiligrin cicatricial pemphigoid,* occurs when antibodies are formed against laminins 5 and 6 in the basement membrane. In this subset, there is an association with solid organ malignancies. The relative risk is approximately sixfold to eightfold, approximately the same as the association with malignancy in patients with dermatomyositis.

Diagnosis

Biopsies for H&E and DIF should be performed to confirm the diagnosis. Histologically, findings are almost identical to bullous pemphigoid. A subepidermal vesicle is seen with an inflammatory infiltrate of neutrophils and eosinophils in the upper dermis. Scarring can be seen in the upper dermis. DIF of perilesional mucosa reveals linear IgG and C3 deposition at the basement membrane zone in 95% of patients. Because there are low amounts of circulating antibodies, IIF testing is not generally helpful. Diagnosis of MMP is summarized in Box 1.

Treatment

Patients with localized oral involvement often respond to topical clobetasol gel or intralesional triamcinolone 5 to 10 mg/mL injected sublesionally every 3 weeks as needed.

Patients with multiple mucosal sites should be treated with systemic therapy such as dapsone or prednisone. If the lesions are unresponsive to this, ISAs in combination with prednisone should be used. Treatment of MMP is summarized in Box 2.

PEMPHIGUS FOLIACEUS

Summary

- Pemphigus foliaceus is a superficial acantholytic autoimmune mucocutaneous blistering disease.
- There is no oral involvement.
- Avoid trauma to the skin.

Prevalence

Pemphigus foliaceus is an AMBD that typically manifests in the sixth or seventh decade of life. Fogo selvagem, the endemic form of pemphigus foliaceus seen in Brazil and other regions of South America, commonly manifests in the third and fourth decades. In western Europe, the incidence of pemphigus foliaceus is 0.5 to 1 case per million population per year. In Brazil, where the endemic form of pemphigus foliaceus is common, the incidence is as high as 50 cases per million population per year.

Signs and Symptoms

Pemphigus foliaceus is characterized by superficial flaccid bullae that easily rupture, leaving erosions. Blisters appear on an erythematous base with associated crusting and scaling. Patients typically present with crusted erosions on the scalp, face, and upper trunk in a seborrheic distribution. In contrast to pemphigus vulgaris, pemphigus foliaceus does not involve the oral mucosa.

Pemphigus foliaceus can be idiopathic or it may be triggered by certain medications such as penicillamine, captopril, or other thiol drugs. Pemphigus foliaceus occurs in up to 7% of patients treated with penicillamine, and it can occur up to 1 year after starting treatment. An arthropod vector carrying an infectious agent can induce fogo selvagem in endemic areas.

Diagnosis

Biopsy of lesional and perilesional skin is needed to confirm the diagnosis. Histopathology shows acantholysis in the superficial layers of the epidermis. DIF reveals intercellular IgG deposition in the superficial epidermis. The antibody is of the IgG4 subclass and directed against desmoglien 1 (dsg-1).

Serum can be tested for IIF and ELISA to detect anti–dsg-1 antibodies. Pemphigus foliaceus can be distinguished from pemphigus vulgaris, because patients with pemphigus foliaceus only have antibodies directed against dsg-1. Diagnosis of pemphigus foliaceus is summarized in Box 1.

Treatment

All patients should be encouraged to avoid sun exposure because it can exacerbate the condition. Any trauma or pressure to the skin commonly produces new lesions.

High-potency topical corticosteroids can be used for mild cases of pemphigus foliaceus. In more-extensive cases, suppression of autoantibody formation with systemic corticosteroids and ISAs is considered conventional therapy. Prednisone at a dose of 0.5 to 1.0 mg/kg per day, based on ideal body weight, often halts formation of new blisters. Hydroxychloroquine 200 mg twice a day has been shown effective in some patients with pemphigus foliaceus. Another effective steroid-sparing regimen is a combination of nicotinamide 1.5 g/day and either tetracycline 2 g/day or minocycline 100 mg/day. In patients with disease refractory to these treatments, IVIg or rituximab may be effective.

Frequent bacterial cultures of open cutaneous erosions should be performed to identify early infections. Appropriate oral antibiotics should be initiated promptly. Treatment of pemphigus foliaceus is summarized in Box 2.

Suggested Readings

Darling MR, Daley T: Blistering mucocutaneous diseases of the oral mucosa—a review: Part 2. Pemphigus vulgaris. J Can Dent Assoc 2006;72(1):63-66.

Eschle-Meniconi ME, Ahmad SR, Foster CS: Mucous membrane pemphigoid: An update. Curr Opin Ophthalmol 2005;16(5):303-307.

McCuin JB, Hanlon T, Mutasim DF: Autoimmune bullous diseases: Diagnosis and management. Dermatol Nurs 2006;18(1):20-25.

Patton T, Korman NJ: Bullous pemphigoid treatment review. Expert Opin Pharmacother 2006;7(17):2403-2411.

Schmidt E, Hunzelmann N, Zillikens D, et al: Rituximab in refractory autoimmune bullous diseases. Clin Exp Dermatol 2006;31(4):503-508.

Stoopler ET, DeRossi SS, Sollecito TP: Mucous membrane pemphigoid. Update for the general practitioner. N Y State Dent J 2003;69(8):28-31.

Walsh SR, Hogg D, Mydlarski PR: Bullous pemphigoid: From bench to bedside. Drugs 2005;65(7):905-926.

Yeh SW, Sami N, Ahmed RA: Treatment of pemphigus vulgaris: Current and emerging options. Am J Clin Dermatol 2005;6(5):327-342.

The Aging Skin

Oren H. Lifshitz and *Kenneth J. Tomecki*

The number and percentage of older persons in industrialized nations continue to increase. In the United States, in 2004, there were more than 36 million people older than 65 years,[1] representing approximately 12% of the population.[1] By 2030, there will be 71 million, or 20% of the population.[1] Skin diseases of the elderly will therefore represent a significant part of general dermatology. This chapter reviews the more common disorders of aging skin, such as actinic (photo) damage, pruritus, eczematous dermatitis, purpura, and venous insufficiency.

BASIC SCIENCE

The structure and the function of skin change with age. In aging skin, the epidermis becomes thinner and loses its undulating rete pattern; the stratum corneum loses its ability to retain water, and cell replacement, barrier function, and wound healing decrease; the dermis becomes thinner and loses its elasticity, partly because of a decrease in the number of fibroblasts; the eccrine sweat glands shrink and secrete less sweat; and Langerhans cells decrease in number, affecting immune responsiveness.[2] All of these changes contribute to many of the skin conditions of the elderly.

DIAGNOSIS, EVALUATION, AND TREATMENT

Intrinsic factors (e.g., genetics) and extrinsic factors (e.g., ultraviolet [UV] exposure) affect the rate at which the skin ages. Excessive UV exposure produces structural changes (photo damage) in all layers of the skin: Collagen and elastic fibers in the dermis become frayed (solar elastosis); elastic tissue loses its integrity and sags or droops, clinically appearing as wrinkles; and connective tissue weakens and predisposes to traumatic solar purpura.

The stigmata of aging skin include wrinkles (rhytides), furrows, sagging, and sunken cheekbones (Fig. 1). Treatment is not necessary, but therapeutic options include topical retinoids (e.g., tretinoin to soften fine wrinkles); chemical peels using salicylic acid or glycolic acid for exfoliation; microdermabrasion; laser therapy (e.g., carbon dioxide for resurfacing); fillers such as botulinum toxin, hyaluronic acid, and collagen, to enhance volume; and plastic surgery.

Photo (sun) damage is the most common and most pervasive change of aging (white) skin, commonly identified as solar lentigines and actinic keratoses (see Fig. 1). Solar lentigines are benign growths—tan or brown macules or patches on sun-exposed areas (head, hands, forearms)—representing epidermal hyperplasia and proliferation of melanocytes. Their presence reflects appreciable sun exposure and can portend an increased risk of sun-induced skin cancer. Treatment is not necessary, except for cosmetic reasons. In contrast, actinic keratoses—rough, reddened, ill-defined plaques on sun-exposed areas—are precancerous growths. Malignant potential is extremely low, but left untreated, approximately 5% to 20% of actinic keratoses deteriorate to invasive squamous cell carcinoma within 10 to 25 years.[3] Actinic keratoses deserve treatment to forestall progression into squamous cell carcinoma. Options include local destruction with either cryotherapy (liquid nitrogen) or curettage and the topical application of 5-fluorouracil (Efudex, Fluoroplex, Carac), imiquimod (Aldara), or diclofenac (Solaraze) for more extensive disease. Obviously, sun avoidance and the use of sunscreens help to minimize photo damage, solar lentigines, and actinic keratoses.

Solar or traumatic purpura (also known as senile purpura) is a common and benign condition of extravasated blood in the dermis characterized by ecchymotic, purpuric patches on the forearms, arms, or legs of older persons. The condition usually follows minor trauma and commonly affects those who take aspirin or other blood thinners (Fig. 2). Treatment is unnecessary and the extravasated blood is eventually reabsorbed.

Seborrheic keratoses are probably the most common benign growths on adult skin. Typically, they are greasy brown hyperkeratotic plaques that appear stuck to the skin surface; they can appear anywhere, except for palms and soles, and tend to congregate on the trunk. Their cause is unknown, but a genetic predisposition might exist in some families. Therapy is usually not necessary unless they are pruritic, irritated, or inflamed. Angiomas are benign vascular growths that commonly occur in adults as red macules and papules on the trunk and proximal extremities. Similar to seborrheic keratoses, therapy for angiomas is usually not necessary unless they are pruritic, irritated, or inflamed. Laser treatment is a successful method of destruction.

Pruritus (itching) is a common condition of advanced age, affecting nearly one half of older adults (older than 60 years) at some time, usually without a rash. Patients with chronic renal or hepatic insufficiency, anemia, thyroid disease, diabetes mellitus, drug allergy, or underlying malignancy might have itch with or without a rash. For patients without a rash, treatment is symptomatic (e.g., lubrication with emollients, and perhaps an antihistamine, coupled with treatment of any underlying problem). For patients with a rash, the treatment is the same, plus treatment of the skin disease (usually a secondary eczema) with topical or systemic corticosteroids.

Dermatitis (eczema) is a common cause of pruritus regardless of age. In older persons the most common cause of dermatitis is xerosis (asteatosis, i.e., dry skin), followed by seborrheic dermatitis, stasis dermatitis, and contact dermatitis. Asteatotic eczema, or winter itch, often affects aging skin, usually as itchy, scaly, cracked, red plaques on the extremities, most commonly the legs. Seasonal changes (e.g., low humidity and cold temperatures) aggravate the disease, which tends to occur more often in winter, especially in northern climates. The mainstay of treatment is dry skin care (minimizing bathing and hot water; avoiding harsh soap; pat drying afterwards) and hydration (liberal and frequent use of emollients, especially after bathing) and topical corticosteroids (e.g., triamcinolone or fluocinolone twice daily as needed) for the eczema.

Seborrheic dermatitis is a common type of eczema characterized by scaly, red plaques on the scalp, face, and central chest. The prevalence and severity are higher in patients with neurologic disease (e.g. Parkinson's disease). Treatment includes shampoo for the scalp, such as those containing zinc pyrithione, selenium sulfide, or ketoconazole, and a mild topical corticosteroid.

Stasis dermatitis, also known as gravitational eczema, affects approximately 7% of older adults, usually the obese.[4] Patients initially experience heaviness and swelling in their feet, which worsens with standing and progresses through the day, followed by the dermatitis—scaly, red, edematous plaques on the feet, ankles, calves, and shins, all as a result of vascular insufficiency or venous hypertension (Fig. 3). Secondary ulceration, cellulitis, and later postinflammatory hyperpigmentation can follow. If venous or stasis ulcers develop, they are typically shallow and irregularly shaped and usually occur just above the medial malleolus. Treatment involves compression, leg elevation, and often débridement, sometimes followed by skin grafting. Aspirin or pentoxifylline is a helpful adjunctive treatment to improve peripheral blood flow, allowing ulcers to heal more rapidly.

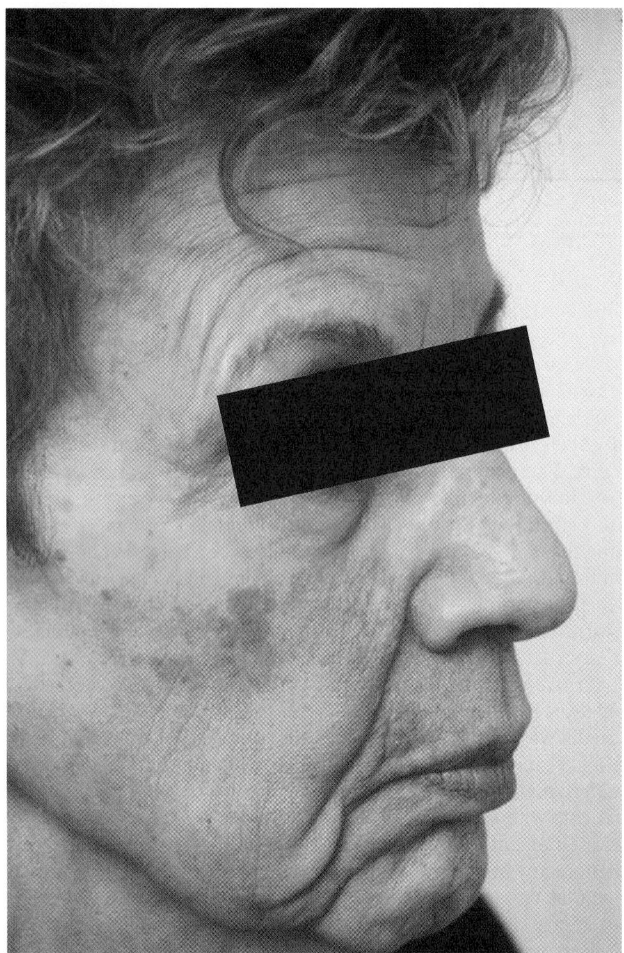

Figure 1 Solar lentigines. Solar lentigines often manifest as brown patches on sun-exposed areas.

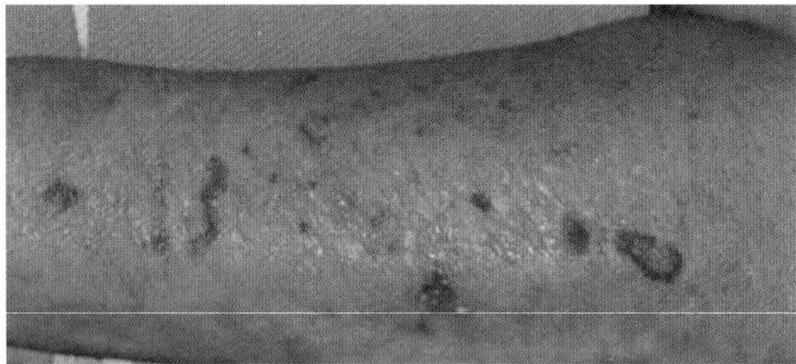

Figure 2 Solar purpura. Solar purpura often manifests as purpuric patches on the forearms.

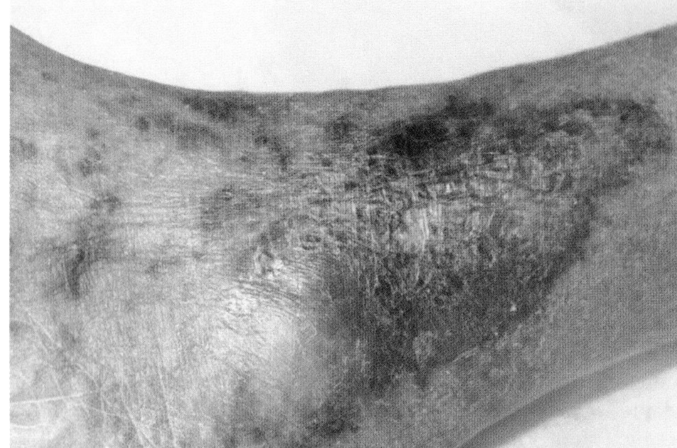

Figure 3 Stasis dermatitis. Stasis dermatitis typically occurs on the lateral aspects of the shins.

Other causes of leg ulcers in the elderly are neuropathy, trauma, neoplasia, infection, panniculitis, and pyoderma gangrenosum. Vascular disease is the most common cause of leg ulcers in the elderly, and venous insufficiency is the most common etiology, accounting for approximately 60% to 70% of all leg ulcers.[5]

Vascular insufficiency can represent venous insufficiency or perhaps even venous thrombosis, valvular incompetence, or arterial insufficiency. Treatment should include weight reduction when warranted, compression stockings to reduce edema, leg elevation as much as possible, and reduction of prolonged standing. Affected areas require regular lubrication with emollients and topical corticosteroids if eczema occurs. Patients with stasis dermatitis and chronic leg ulcers have an increased risk for contact dermatitis, based on the likely use of multiple topical medications. When contact dermatitis is suspected, patch testing can help to resolve the issue and determine the likely allergen; its yield in elderly patients with stasis dermatitis is 60%.[6] Contact dermatitis in older people is often persistent and recalcitrant to standard treatment (i.e., topical and oral corticosteroids as well as antihistamines).

Varicosities (varicose veins) occur commonly with venous insufficiency, characteristically as tortuous vascular channels on calves, thighs, and popliteal fossa. Sclerotherapy or laser treatment can minimize the appearance. Lipodermatosclerosis is an uncommon sequela of chronic venous insufficiency and is characterized by subcutaneous fibrosis with firm, indurated plaques on the legs. Treatment is analogous to the measures outlined for venous insufficiency.

Decubitus ulcers (bed sores, pressure sores or ulcers) can be an unfortunate occurrence in debilitated elderly patients, especially for hospitalized or bedridden patients, where 40% of all nursing care is devoted to skin care and decubital care.[5] Such ulcers follow friction, pressure, or shearing forces over bony prominences, and affect underlying skin, muscle, connective tissue, cartilage, or bone; common sites are the sacrum, ischial tuberosities, and heels. Risk factors include immobility, fecal or urinary incontinence, diabetes, glucocorticoid use, and poor nutrition. Treatment includes surgical débridement if warranted; positional rotation every 2 hours to distribute the compressive forces and to minimize further injury; elevation of the head of the bed to increase upper body pressure; and cleansing the affected area in incontinent patients. All patients need an adequate diet, with vitamin supplementation, and treatment of any underlying conditions. A variety of dressings is available to improve wound or ulcer repair (e.g., transparent films, hydrogels, hydrocolloids, polysaccharides, alginates, foam, and laminates). Selection depends on the state of the ulcer (infected, soupy, or clean), the amount of exudate, ulcer depth, and patient compliance. Absorbent wound dressings (alginates) are useful for moist wounds; films for wounds without drainage; and hydrocolloids for ease of use and expense, which enhance patient compliance.

CONCLUSION

Skin disease in the aging population is common. Evaluation and treatment are usually straightforward, and diagnostic testing is usually not necessary. An understanding of the changing structure and function of aging skin helps to address the disease processes and their treatment.

Summary

- Dermatologic conditions in elderly patients are common. Given the increasing number of elderly patients in the United States, disorders of aging skin are becoming a significant part of general dermatology.
- Common skin conditions in the elderly include: actinic damage, benign and malignant growths, pruritus, eczematous dermatitis, purpura, and vascular insufficiency.
- Intrinsic and extrinsic factors affect the structure and function of the skin and contribute to disorders of aging skin.

Suggested Readings

A Profile of Older Americans. Administration on Aging U.S. Department of Health and Human Services, 2004, pp 1-18.

Beauregard S, Gilchrest BA: A survey of skin problems and skin care regimens in elderly. Arch Dermatol 1987;123:1638-1643.

Lebwohl M: Actinic keratosis: Epidemiology and progression to squamous cell carcinoma. Br J Dermatol 2003;Suppl 66:31-33.

Nedorost ST, Stevens SR: Diagnosis and treatment of allergic skin disorders in the elderly. Drugs Aging 2001;18:827-835.

Thomas DR: Issues and dilemmas in the prevention and treatment of pressure ulcers: A review. J Gerontol 56A:M328, 2001.

Yaar M, Gilchrest BA: Skin aging: Postulated mechanisms and consequent changes in structure and function. Clin Geriatr Med 2001;17:617.

References

For a complete list of references, log onto www.expertconsult.com.

Common Skin Infections

Nathaniel C. Cevasco and Kenneth J. Tomecki

BACTERIAL INFECTIONS

Humans are natural hosts for many bacterial species that colonize the skin as normal flora. *Staphylococcus aureus* and *Streptococcus pyogenes* are infrequent resident flora, but they account for a wide variety of bacterial pyodermas. Predisposing factors to infection include minor trauma, preexisting skin disease, poor hygiene, and, rarely, impaired host immunity.

Impetigo

Definition and Etiology

Impetigo is a superficial skin infection usually caused by *S. aureus* and occasionally by *S. pyogenes*.

Prevalence and Risk Factors

Impetigo affects approximately 1% of children.

Pathophysiology and Natural History

S. aureus produces a number of cellular and extracellular products, including exotoxins and coagulase, that contribute to the pathogenicity of impetigo, especially when coupled with preexisting tissue injury. Impetigo commonly occurs on the face (especially around the nares) or extremities after trauma.

Signs and Symptoms

Two clinical types of impetigo exist: nonbullous and bullous. The nonbullous type is more common and typically occurs on the face and extremities, initially with vesicles or pustules on reddened skin. The vesicles or pustules eventually rupture to leave the characteristic honey-colored (yellow-brown) crust (Fig. 1). Bullous impetigo, almost exclusively caused by *S. aureus*, exhibits flaccid bullae with clear yellow fluid that rupture and leave a golden-yellow crust.

Diagnosis

Diagnosis is by clinical presentation and confirmation by culture.[1]

Treatment

For most patients with impetigo, topical treatment is adequate, either with bacitracin (Polysporin) or mupirocin (Bactroban), applied twice daily for 7 to 10 days. Systemic therapy may be necessary for patients with extensive disease (Table 1).[2,3]

Folliculitis, Furunculosis, and Carbunculosis

Definition and Etiology

Folliculitis is a superficial infection of the hair follicles characterized by erythematous, follicular-based papules and pustules. Furuncles are deeper infections of the hair follicle characterized by inflammatory nodules with pustular drainage, which can coalesce to form larger draining nodules (carbuncles).

Pathophysiology and Natural History

S. aureus is the usual pathogen, although exposure to *Pseudomonas aeruginosa* in hot tubs or swimming pools can lead to folliculitis. In general, folliculitis is a self-limited entity. Occasionally, a pustule enlarges to form a tender, red nodule (furuncle) that becomes painful and fluctuant after several days. Rupture often occurs, with discharge of pus and necrotic material. With rupture, the pain subsides and the redness and edema diminish.

Signs and Symptoms

Folliculitis is generally asymptomatic, but it may be pruritic or even painful. Commonly affected areas are the beard, posterior neck, occipital scalp, and axillae (Fig. 2). Often a continuum of folliculitis, furunculosis (furuncles), arises in hair-bearing areas as tender, erythematous, fluctuant nodules that rupture with purulent discharge (Fig. 3). Carbuncles are larger and deeper inflammatory nodules, often with purulent drainage (Fig. 4), and commonly occur on the nape of the neck, back, or thighs. Carbuncles are often tender and painful and occasionally accompanied by fever and malaise.[1-3]

Diagnosis

Diagnosis is by clinical presentation and confirmation by culture.

Treatment

Topical treatment with clindamycin 1% or erythromycin 2%, applied two or three times a day to affected areas, coupled with an antibacterial wash or soap, is adequate for most patients with folliculitis. Systemic antistaphylococcal antibiotics are usually necessary for furuncles and carbuncles, especially when cellulitis or constitutional symptoms are present.[2] Small furuncles can be treated with warm compresses three or four times a day for 15 to 20 minutes, but larger furuncles and carbuncles often warrant incision and drainage. If methicillin-resistant *S. aureus* (MRSA) is implicated or suspected, vancomycin (1-2 g IV daily in divided doses) is indicated coupled with culture confirmation. Antimicrobial therapy should be continued until inflammation has regressed or altered depending on culture results. Treatment is summarized in Table 2.

Ecthyma

Definition and Etiology

Ecthyma is a cutaneous infection characterized by thickly crusted erosions or ulcerations. Ecthyma is usually a consequence of neglected impetigo and often follows impetigo occluded by footwear or clothing.

Prevalence and Risk Factors

Ecthyma typically occurs in homeless persons and soldiers based in hot and humid climates.

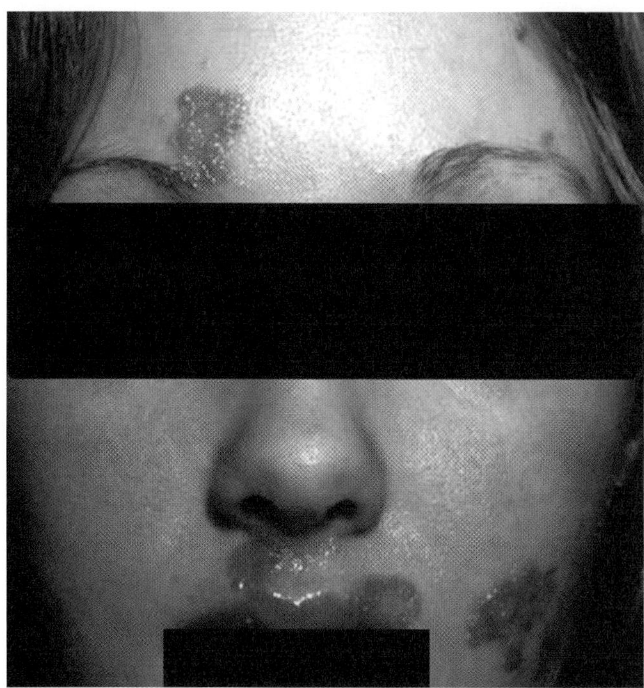

Figure 1 Impetigo.

Table 1 Treatment of Impetigo

Topical	Systemic	Dosing
First-Line Treatment		
Mupirocin bid for 7-10 days	Dicloxacillin	250-500 mg PO qid for 5-7 days
	Amoxicillin plus clavulanic acid; cephalexin	25 mg/kg PO tid; 250-500 mg PO qid for 10 days
	Clavulanic acid	
Second-Line Treatment (Penicillin allergy)		
	Azithromycin	500 mg PO × 1, then 250 my PO daily for 4 days
	Clindamycin	15 mg/kg/day PO tid for 10 days
	Erythromycin	250-500 mg PO qid for 5-7 days

Pathophysiology and Natural History

S. aureus or *S. pyogenes* is the usual pathogen of ecthyma. Untreated staphylococcal or streptococcal impetigo can extend more deeply, penetrating the dermis, producing a shallow crusted ulcer. Ecthyma can evolve from a primary pyoderma, in a pre-existing dermatosis, or at the site of trauma.

Signs and Symptoms

Infection begins with vesicles and bullae that progress to punched-out ulcerations with an adherent crust, which heals with scarring. The most common site of infection is the legs.

Diagnosis

Diagnosis is by clinical presentation and confirmation by culture.[3,4]

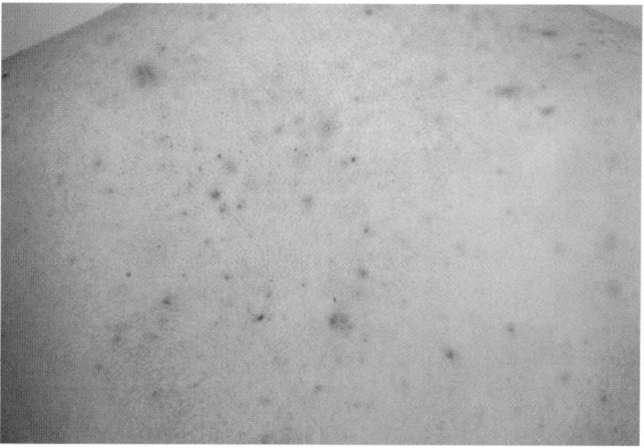

Figure 2 Folliculitis.

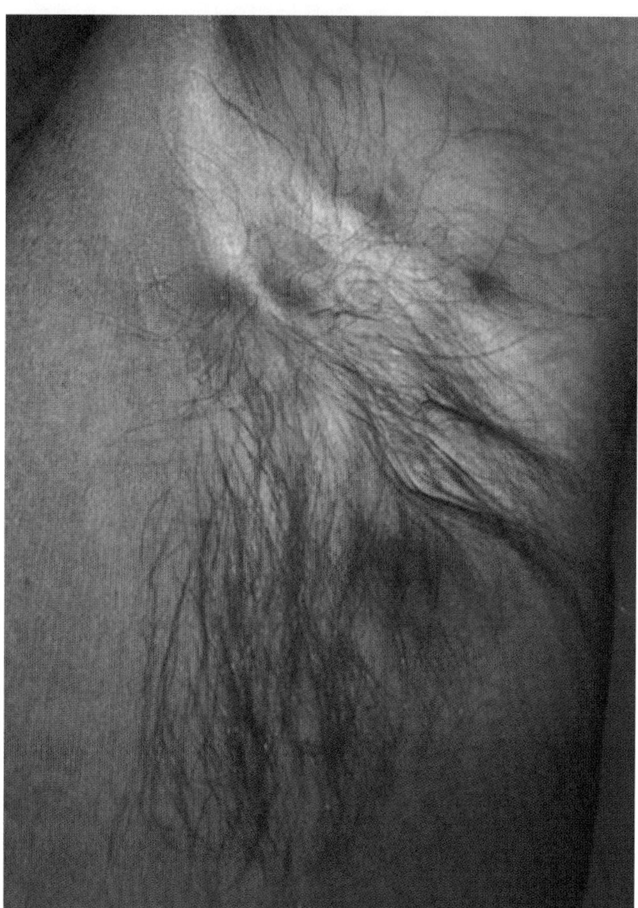

Figure 3 Furuncles.

Treatment

Treatment is summarized in Table 3.[3]

Erysipelas and Cellulitis

Definition and Etiology

Erysipelas is a superficial cutaneous infection of the skin involving dermal lymphatic vessels. Cellulitis is a deeper process that extends to the subcutis.

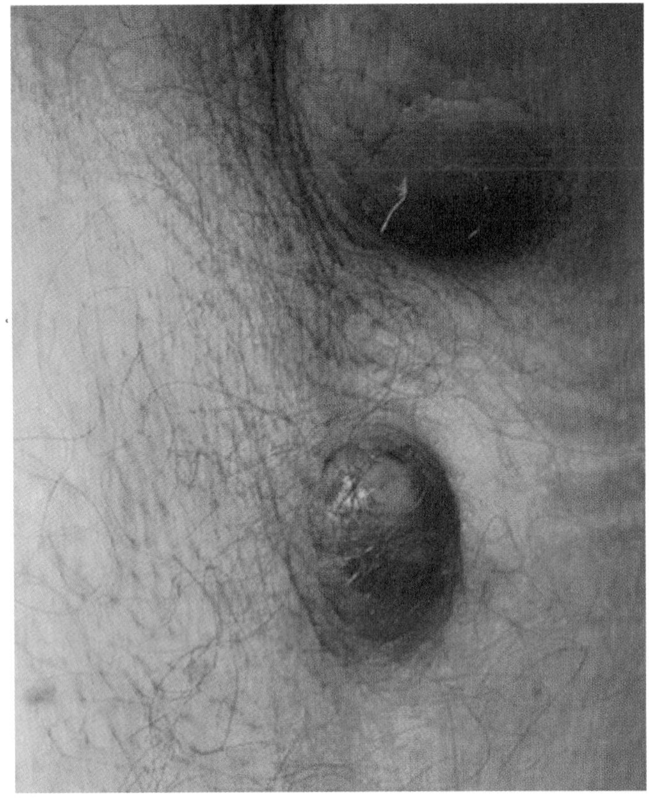

Figure 4 Carbuncles.

Table 2 Treatment of Folliculitis, Furunculosis, and Carbunculosis

Folliculitis	Furunculosis/ Carbunculosis	Dosing
First-Line Treatment		
Topical clindamycin/ erythromycin bid	Incision and drainage	bid
	Dicloxacillin	250-500 mg PO qid for 5-7 days
	Amoxicillin plus calvulanic acid; cephalexin	25 mg/kg PO tid; 250-500 mg PO qid for 10 days
Antibiotic wash (e.g. chlorhexidine) bid	Clavulanic acid;	bid
	Warm compresses	tid
Second-Line Treatment (MRSA)		
Doxycycline (2-8 weeks depending on severity)	Doxycycline	100 mg PO bid (2-8 weeks depending on severity)
	Vancomycin	1-2 g IV daily in divided doses for 7 days

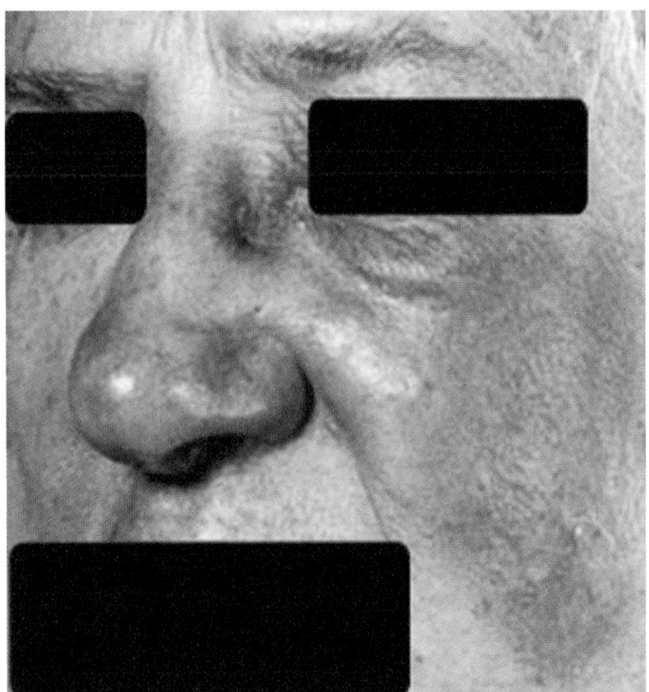

Figure 5 Erysipelas.

Prevalence and Risk Factors

Erysipelas has a predilection for young children and the elderly. Lymphedema, venous stasis, web intertrigo, diabetes mellitus, trauma, alcoholism, and obesity are risk factors in the adult patient.[3,4]

Pathophysiology and Natural History

Group A β-hemolytic streptococcus is the most common pathogen responsible for erysipelas, and *S. aureus* is by far the most common pathogen for cellulitis. *S. pyogenes* produces enzymes that promote infection with systemic manifestations, such as fever and chills, tachycardia, and hypotension. Left untreated, cellulitic skin can become bullous and necrotic, and an abscess or fasciitis, or both, can occur.

Signs and Symptoms

Classically, erysipelas is a tender, well-defined, erythematous, indurated plaque on the face or legs (Fig. 5). Cellulitis is a warm, tender, erythematous, and edematous plaque with ill-defined borders that expands rapidly. Cellulitis is often accompanied by constitutional symptoms, regional lymphadenopathy, and occasionally bacteremia (Fig. 6).[3,4]

Diagnosis

Diagnosis is by clinical presentation and confirmation by culture (if clinically indicated, ie., bullae or abscess formation).

Treatment

Penicillin (250-500 mg, qid × 7-10 days) is the treatment of choice for erysipelas; parenteral therapy may be necessary for extensive or facial disease. An oral antistaphylococcal antibiotic is the treatment of choice for cellulitis; parenteral therapy is warranted for patients with extensive disease or with systemic symptoms as well as for immunocompromised patients. Good hygiene, warm compresses three or four times a day for 15 to 20 minutes, and elevation of the

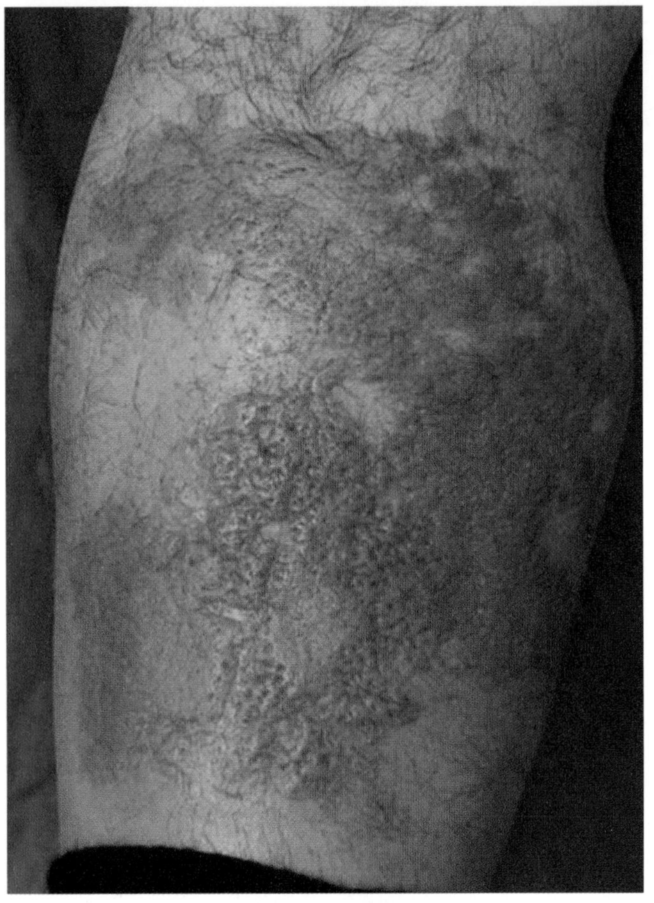

Figure 6 Cellulitis.

Table 3 Treatment of Ecthyma

Topical	Dosing	Systemic	Dosing
First-Line Treatment			
Warm compresses	qid	Dicloxacillin	250-500 mg PO qid for 5-7 days
		Amoxicillin plus clavulanic acid	25 mg/kg PO tid
		Clavulanic acid	
		Cephalexin	40-50 mg/kg/day PO for 10 days
Second-Line Treatment (Penicillin Altergy)			
		Azithromycin	500 mg PO × 1, then 250 mg PO daily for 4 days
		Clindamycin	15 mg/kg/day PO tid for 10 days
		Erythromycin	250-500 mg PO qid for 5-7 days

Table 4 Treatment of Erysipelas and Cellulitis

Erysipelas	Dosing	Cellulitis	Dosing
First-Line Treatment			
Penicillin	500 mg PO qid for 10 days	Dicloxacillin	250-500 mg PO qid for 5-7 days
Dicloxacillin	500 mg PO qid for 5-7 days	Amoxicillin plus clavulanic acid	25 mg/kg PO tid
Warm compresses	tid	Warm compresses	tid
Second-Line Treatment			
***Methicillin-Resistant* Staphylococcus aureus**			
Linezolid	600 mg PO bid for 7-14 days	Linezolid	600 mg PO bid for 7-14 days
Vancomycin	1-2 g IV daily in divided doses for 7 days	Vancomycin	1-2 g IV daily in divided doses for 7 days
Penicillin Allergy			
Clindamycin	15 mg/kg/day PO tid for 10 days	Azithromycin	500 mg PO × 1, then 250 mg PO daily for 4 days
		Clindamycin	15 mg/kg/day PO tid for 10 days
		Erythromycin	250-500 mg PO qid for 5-7 days

affected limb help to expedite healing. Treatment is summarized in Table 4.[3]

Necrotizing Fasciitis

Definition and Etiology

Necrotizing fasciitis is a rare infection of the subcutaneous tissues and fascia that eventually leads to necrosis. Predisposing factors include injuries to soft tissues, such as abdominal surgery, abrasions, surgical incisions, diabetes, alcoholism, cirrhosis, and intravenous drug abuse.[5,6]

Pathophysiology and Natural History

S. pyogenes can be the sole pathogen responsible for necrotizing fasciitis, but most patients have a mixed infection with other aerobes (groups B and C streptococci, MRSA) and anaerobes (*Clostridium* spp).

Signs and Symptoms

Infection begins with warm, tender, reddened skin and inflammation that rapidly extends horizontally and vertically. Necrotizing fasciitis commonly occurs on the extremities, abdomen, or perineum or at operative wounds (Fig. 7). Within 48 to 72 hours, affected skin becomes dusky, and bullae form, followed by necrosis and gangrene, often with crepitus. Without prompt treatment, fever, systemic toxicity, organ failure, and shock can occur, often followed by death. Computed tomography (CT) or magnetic resonance imaging (MRI) can help to delineate the extent of infection. Biopsy for histology, Gram stain, and tissue culture help to identify the causative organism(s).[5,6]

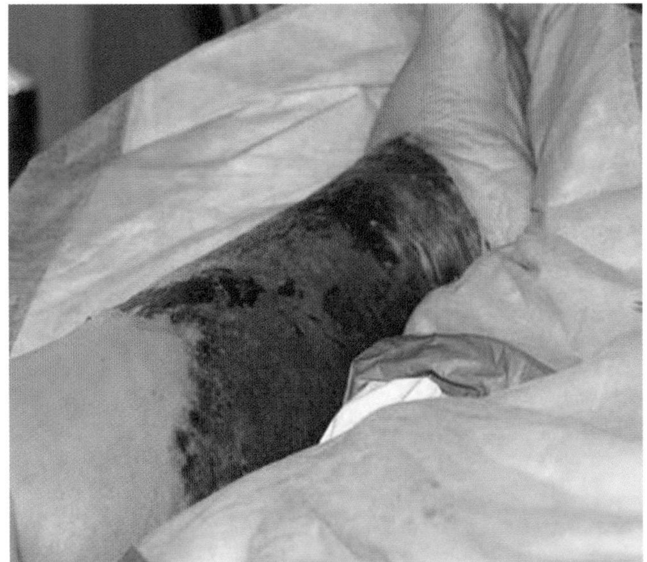

Figure 7 Necrotizing fasciitis.

Diagnosis

Diagnosis is by clinical presentation; CT or MRI; skin biopsy for pathology, Gram stain, and tissue culture; culture of fluid from bullae or fluctuant plaques; and blood cultures.

Treatment

Necrotizing fasciitis is a surgical emergency requiring prompt surgical debridement, fasciotomy, and, occasionally, amputation of the affected extremity to prevent progression to myonecrosis. Treatment with parenteral antibiotics (usually gentamicin and clindamycin) is mandatory. Even with treatment, mortality approaches 70%.

FUNGAL AND YEAST INFECTIONS

Dermatophytosis

Definition and Etiology

Dermatophytosis implies infection with fungi, organisms with high affinity for keratinized tissue, such as the skin, nails, and hair. *Trichophyton rubrum* is the most common dermatophyte worldwide.

Pathophysiology and Natural History

Three fungal genera—*Trichophyton, Microsporum,* and *Epidermophyton*—account for the vast majority of infections. Fungal reservoirs for these organisms include soil, animals, and infected humans.

Signs and Symptoms

Tinea pedis (athlete's foot) is the most common fungal infection in humans in North America and Europe.[4] Affected skin is usually pruritic, with scaling plaques on the soles, extending to the lateral aspects of the feet and interdigital spaces (Fig. 8), often with maceration.

Tinea cruris (jock itch) occurs in the groin and on the upper, inner thighs and buttocks as scaling annular plaques (Fig. 9); disease is more common in men and typically spares the scrotum.

Tinea capitis, or fungal infection of the scalp, is most common in children. It is characterized by scaly, erythematous skin, often with hair loss. Tinea capitis can resemble seborrheic dermatitis. Kerion celsi is an inflammatory form of tinea capitis, characterized by boggy nodules, usually with hair loss and regional lymphadenopathy.

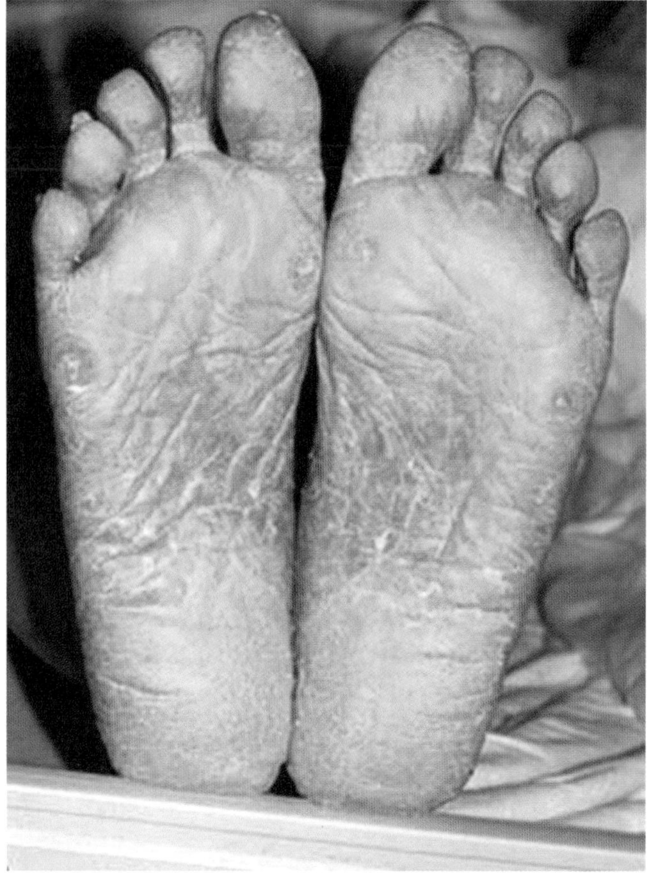

Figure 8 Tinea pedis.

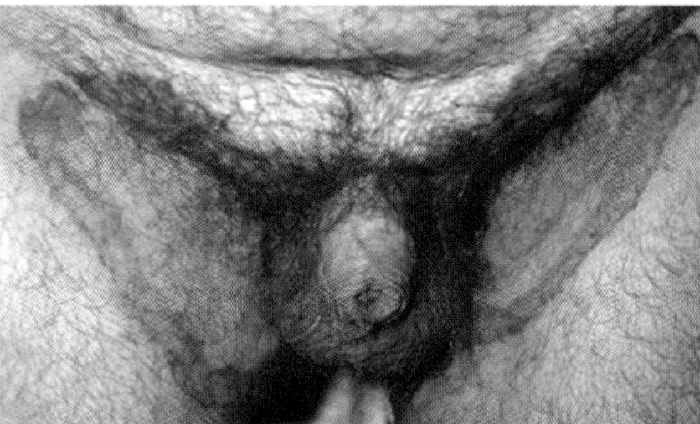

Figure 9 Tinea cruris.

Tinea corporis (body), faciei (face), and manuum (hands) represent infections of different sites, each invariably with annular scaly plaques. Tinea unguium (onychomycosis) is fungal nail disease, characterized by thickened yellow nails and subungual debris (Fig. 10).

Potassium hydroxide preparation or culture help to establish the diagnosis for all forms of fungal infections.[2]

Diagnosis

Diagnosis is by clinical presentation, KOH examination, and fungal culture.

Treatment

For most patients, topical treatment with terbinafine (Lamisil), clotrimazole (Lotrimin, Mycelex), or econazole (Spectazole) cream is

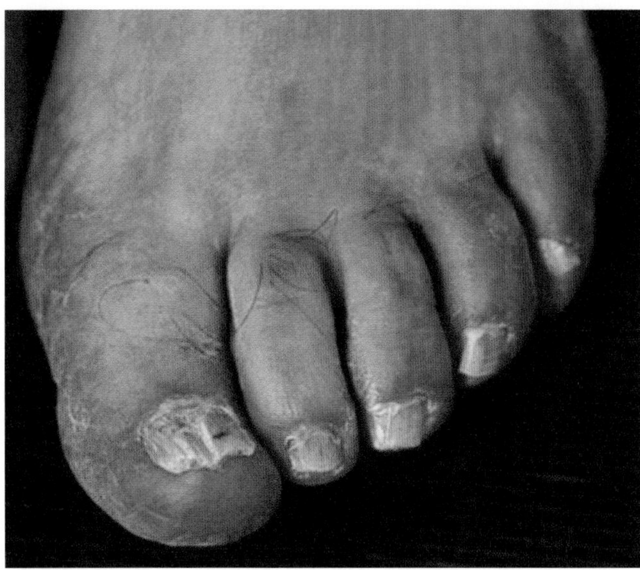

Figure 10 Onychomycosis.

Table 5 Treatment of Dermatophytosis

Limited Disease	Onychomycosis	Tinea Capitis, Extensive Dermatophyte Disease
Terbinafine bid for 4 weeks	Itraconazole 3-5 / kg/day PO for 4-6 weeks	Griseofulvin 20-25 /kg/ day PO for 8 weeks*
Clotrimazole bid for 4 weeks	Terbinafine 3-6 /kg/ day PO for 4-8 weeks	Fluconazole 6 /kg/day PO for 20 days
Econazole bid for 4 weeks		

*Pediatric dose for microsize form.

adequate when applied twice daily for 6 to 8 weeks. For onychomycosis, tinea capitis, and extensive dermatophyte disease, systemic treatment is often necessary: itraconazole (Sporanox) or terbinafine (Lamisil) for nail disease, and griseofulvin or fluconazole for scalp or extensive dermatophyte disease.[7-9] Treatment is summarized in Table 5.

Candidiasis

Definition and Etiology

Candidiasis refers to a diverse group of infections caused by *Candida albicans* or by other members of the genus *Candida*. These organisms typically infect the skin, nails, mucous membranes, and gastrointestinal tract, but they also cause systemic disease.

Prevalence and Risk Factors

Infection is common in immunocompromised patients, diabetics, the elderly, and patients receiving antibiotics.

Pathophysiology and Natural History

Candida albicans accounts for 70% to 80% of all candidal infections. *C. albicans* commonly resides on skin and mucosal surfaces. Alterations in the host environment can lead to its proliferation and subsequent skin disease.

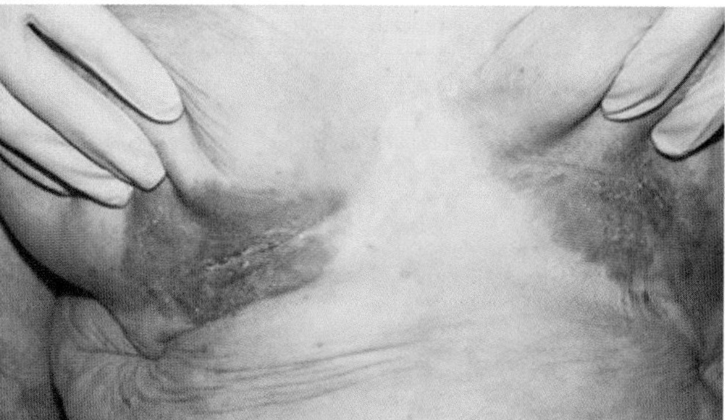

Figure 11 Intertrigo.

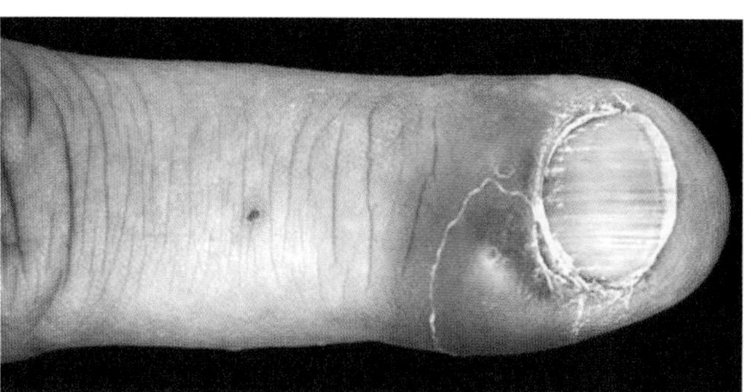

Figure 12 Paronychia.

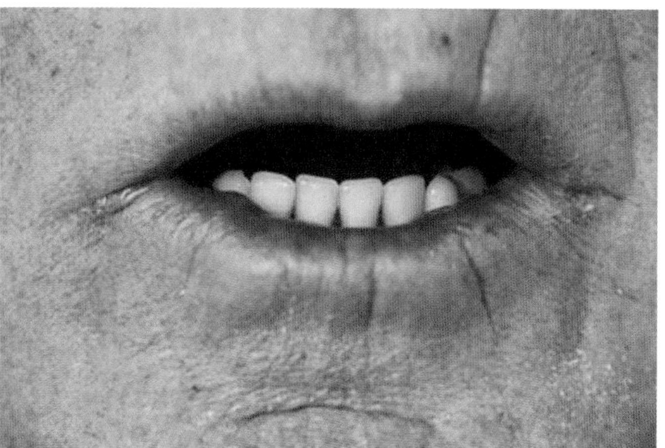

Figure 13 Angular cheilitis.

Signs and Symptoms

Candidal intertrigo is a specific infection of the skin folds (axillae, groin), characterized by reddened plaques, often with satellite pustules (Fig. 11). Thrush is oropharyngeal candidiasis, characterized by white nonadherent plaques on the tongue and buccal mucosa. Paronychia is an acute or chronic infection of the nail characterized by tender, edematous, and erythematous nail folds, often with purulent discharge (Fig. 12); this disease is common in diabetics. Angular cheilitis is the presence of fissures and reddened scaly skin at the corner of the mouth, which often occurs in diabetics and in those who drool or chronically lick their lips (Fig. 13).

Candidal vulvovaginitis is an acute inflammation of the perineum characterized by itchy, reddish, scaly skin and mucosa; creamy discharge; and peripheral pustules. The counterpart in men is balanitis, characterized by shiny reddish plaques on the glans penis, which can

Box 1 Treatment for Candidiasis

Intertrigo or Balanitis
Terbinafine bid for 4 weeks
Clotrimazole bid for 4 weeks
Econazole bid for 4 weeks
Aeration

Paronychia
Terbinafine bid for 2-3 months
Clotrimazole bid for 2-3 months
Econazole bid for 2-3 months
Minimzize wet work

Oral Candidiasis
Nystatin suspension/clotrimazole troches, 5 × daily
Fluconazole 100-200 mg/day PO for 5-10 days
Itraconzazole 100-200 mg/day PO for 5-10 days

Vulvovaginal Candidiasis
Fluconazole 150 mg PO × 1 dose
Aeration

affect the scrotum. Balanitis occurs almost exclusively in uncircumcised men.[2]

Diagnosis

Diagnosis is by clinical presentation, KOH examination, and fungal culture.

Treatment

For candidal intertrigo and balanitis, topical antifungal agents such as clotrimazole, terbinafine, or econazole cream, applied twice daily for 6 to 8 weeks, is usually curative when coupled with aeration and compresses. For thrush, the treatment is nystatin suspension or clotrimazole troches four to six times daily until symptoms resolve. Systemic antifungal drugs, such as fluconazole 100 to 200 mg/day or itraconazole 100 to 200 mg/day, for 5 to 10 days may be necessary for severe or extensive disease. For paronychia, treatment consists of aeration and a topical antifungal agent such as terbinafine, clotrimazole, or econazole for 2 to 3 months; occasionally, oral antistaphylococcal antibiotics are needed, coupled with incision and drainage for secondary bacterial infection. Cheilitis resolves with aeration, application of a topical antifungal agent, and discontinuation of any aggravating factors. A single 150-mg dose of fluconazole, coupled with aeration, is usually effective for vulvovaginitis.[10] Treatment is summarized in Box 1.

Tinea (Pityriasis) Versicolor

Definition and Etiology

Tinea versicolor is a common opportunistic superficial infection of the skin caused by the ubiquitous yeast *Malassezia furfur.*

Prevalence and Risk Factors

Prevalence is high in hot, humid climates. Purported risk factors include oral contraceptive use, heredity, systemic corticosteroid use, Cushing's disease, immunosuppression, hyperhidrosis, and malnutrition.

Pathophysiology and Natural History

M. furfur may filter the rays of the sun and also produces phenolic compounds that inhibit tyrosinase, which can produce hypopigmentation in many patients.

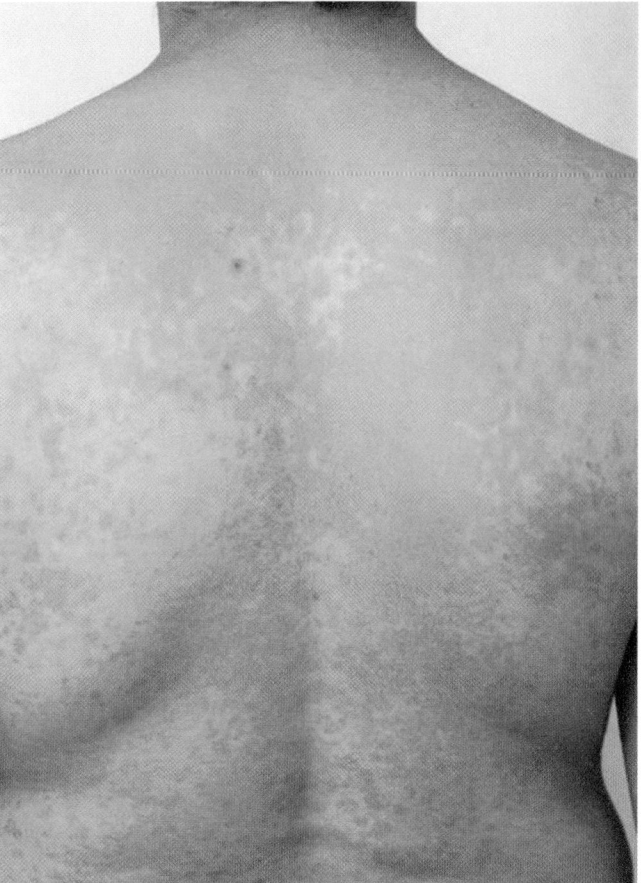

Figure 14 Tinea versicolor.

Signs and Symptoms

Infection produces discrete and confluent, fine scaly, well-demarcated, hypopigmented or hyperpigmented plaques on the chest, back, arms, and neck (Fig. 14). Pruritus is mild or absent.

Diagnosis

Diagnosis is by clinical presentation. Potassium hydroxide preparation exhibits short hyphae and spores with a spaghetti-and-meatballs appearance.

Treatment

Selenium sulfide shampoo (2.5%) or ketoconazole shampoo is the mainstay of treatment, applied to the affected areas and the scalp daily for 3 to 5 days, then once a month thereafter. Alternatively, a variety of topical antifungal agents, including terbinafine, clotrimazole, or econazole cream, applied twice daily for 6 to 8 weeks, constitute adequate treatment, especially for limited disease.[11] Systemic therapy may be necessary for patients with extensive disease or frequent recurrences, or for whom topical agents have failed. Treatment is summarized in Box 2.

VIRAL INFECTIONS

Herpes Simplex

Definition and Etiology

Herpes simplex virus (HSV) infection is a painful, self-limited, often recurrent dermatitis, characterized by small grouped vesicles on an

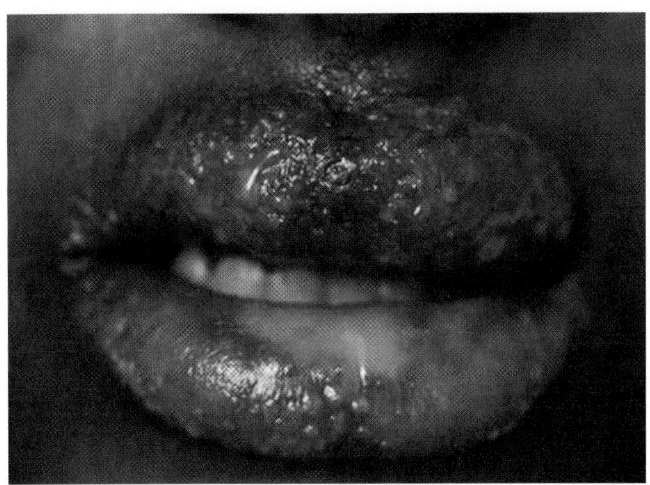

Figure 15 Herpes simplex.

Box 2 Treatment of Tinea (Pityriasis) Versicolor

Mild Disease

Selenium sulfide shampoo for 3-5 days, then once monthly thereafter
Ketoconazole shampoo/cream for 3-5 days, then once monthly thereafter
Econazole cream bid for 6-8 weeks, then once monthly thereafter

Extensiveor Recurrent Disease

Ketoconazole 200 mg PO daily for 7 days
Itraconazole 200-400 mg PO daily for 3-7 days
Fluconazole 400 mg PO × 1

erythematous base. Disease is often mucocutaneous. HSV type 1 is usually associated with orofacial disease, and HSV type 2 is usually associated with genital infection.

Prevalence and Risk Factors

Eighty-five percent of the population has antibody evidence of HSV type 1 infection. HSV type 2 infection is responsible for 20% to 50% of genital ulcerations in sexually active persons.

Pathophysiology and Natural History

Disease follows implantation of the virus via direct contact at mucosal surfaces or on sites of abraded skin. After primary infection, the virus travels to the adjacent dorsal ganglia, where it remains dormant unless it is reactivated by psychological or physical stress, illness, trauma, menses, or sunlight.

Signs and Symptoms

Primary infection occurs most often in children, exhibiting vesicles and erosions on reddened buccal mucosa, the palate, tongue, or lips (acute herpetic gingivostomatitis). It is occasionally associated with fever, malaise, myalgias, and cervical adenopathy (Fig. 15). Herpes labialis (fever blisters or cold sores) appears as grouped vesicles on red denuded skin, usually the vermilion border of the lip; infection represents reactivated HSV. Primary genital infection is an erosive dermatitis on the external genitalia that occurs about 7 to 10 days after exposure; intact vesicles are rare. Recurrent genital disease is common (approximately 40% of affected patients). Prodromal symptoms of pain, burning, or itching can precede herpes labialis and genital herpes infections.

Table 6 Treatment of Herpes Simplex

Indication	Acyclovir	Famciclovir	Valacyclovir
Primary HSV	200 mg PO 5× /day or 400 mg PO tid for 10 days	500 mg PO bid or 250 mg PO tid for 7 days	1 g PO bid for 10 days
Recurrent HSV	400 mg PO tid for 5 days	750 mg PO bid for 1 day	2 g PO bid for 1 day
Suppression	400 mg PO bid	250 mg PO bid	1 g PO or 500 mg PO qd

HSV, herpes simplex virus.

Diagnosis

Viral culture helps to confirm the diagnosis; direct fluorescent antibody (DFA) is a helpful but less-specific test. Serology is helpful only for primary infection. The Tzanck smear can be helpful in the rapid diagnosis of herpesviruses infections, but it is less sensitive than culture and DFA.

Treatment

Acyclovir remains the treatment of choice for HSV infection; newer antivirals, such as famciclovir and valacyclovir, are also effective. For recurrent infection (more than six episodes per year), suppressive treatment is warranted. Primary infection in immunosuppressed patients requires treatment with acyclovir 10 mg/kg every 8 hours for 7 days. Treatment is summarized in Table 6.

Herpes Zoster

Definition and Etiology

Herpes zoster (shingles) is an acute, painful dermatomal dermatitis that affects approximately 10% to 20% of adults, often in the presence of immunosuppression.

Pathophysiology and Natural History

During the course of varicella, the virus travels from the skin and mucosal surfaces to the sensory ganglia, where it lies dormant for a patient's lifetime. Reactivation often follows immunosuppression, emotional stress, trauma, and irradiation or surgical manipulation of the spine, producing a dermatomal dermatitis.

Signs and Symptoms

Herpes zoster is primarily a disease of adults and typically begins with pain and paresthesia in a dermatomal or bandlike pattern followed by grouped vesicles within the dermatome several days later (Fig. 16). Occasionally, fever and malaise occur. The thoracic area accounts for more than half of all reported cases. When zoster involves the tip and side of the nose (cranial nerve V) nasociliary nerve involvement can occur (30%-40%). Most patients with zoster do well with only symptomatic treatment, but postherpetic neuralgia (continued dysthesias and pain after resolution of skin disease) is common in the elderly. Disseminated zoster is uncommon and occurs primarily in immunocompromised patients.

Diagnosis

Diagnosis is by clinical presentation, viral culture, or direct fluorescent antibody.

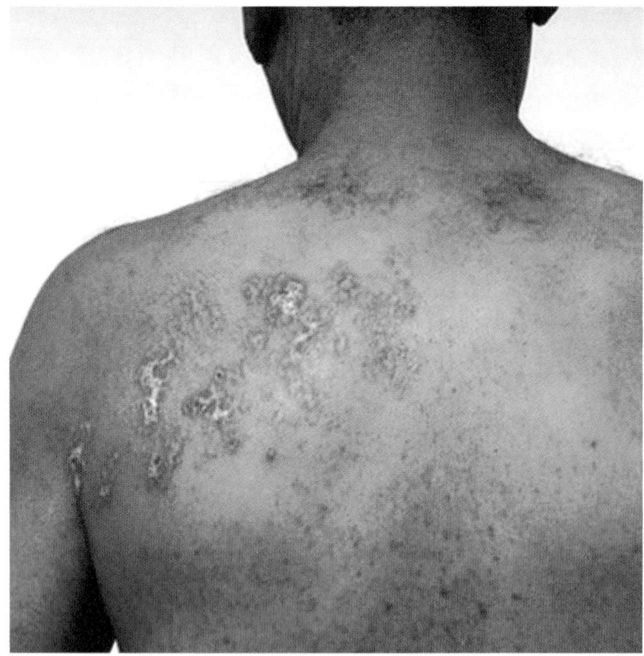

Figure 16 Herpes zoster.

Table 7 Treatment of Herpes Zoster

Indication	Acyclovir	Famciclovir	Valacyclovir
Herpes zoster	800 mg 5×/day for 7-10 days	500 mg tid for 7 days	1 g tid for 7 days
Disseminated zoster	10 mg/kg IV q8hr for 7 days		

Treatment

Zoster deserves treatment, with rest, analgesics, compresses applied to affected areas, and antiviral therapy, if possible, within 24 to 72 hours of disease onset. Disseminated and ophthalmic zoster warrants treatment with acyclovir 10 mg/kg intravenously every 8 hours for 7 days. Treatment is summarized in Table 7.

Warts

Definition and Etiology

Warts are common and benign epithelial growths caused by human papillomavirus (HPV).

Prevalence and Risk Factors

Warts affect approximately 10% of the population. Anogenital warts are a sexually transmitted infection, and partners can transfer the virus with high efficiency. Immunosuppressed patients are at increased risk for developing persistent HPV infection.

Pathophysiology and Natural History

HPV infection follows inoculation of the virus into the epidermis through direct contact, usually facilitated by a break in the skin. Maceration of the skin is an important predisposing factor, as suggested by the increased incidence of plantar warts in swimmers. After inoculation, a wart usually appears within 2 to 9 months. The rough surface of a wart can disrupt adjacent skin and enable inoculation of virus into adjacent sites, leading to the development and spread of new warts.

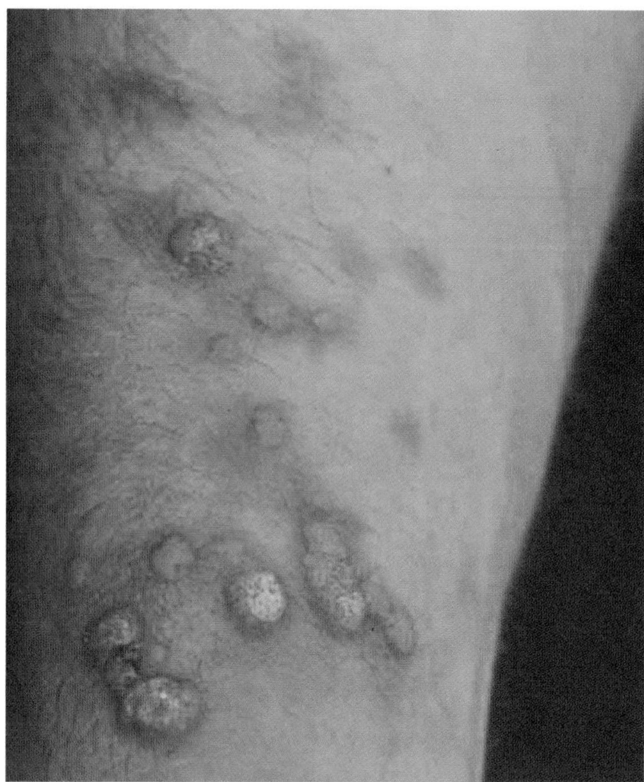

Figure 17 Verruca vulgaris.

Signs and Symptoms

The common wart is the most common type: It is a hyperkeratotic, flesh-colored papule or plaque studded with small black dots (thrombosed capillaries) (Fig. 17). Other types of warts include flat warts (verruca plana), plantar warts, and condyloma acuminatum (venereal warts).

Diagnosis

The clinical appearance alone should suggest the diagnosis. Skin biopsy may be performed, if warranted.

Treatment

Therapy is variable and often challenging. Most modalities are destructive: cryosurgery, electrodesiccation, curettage, and application of various topical products such as trichloroacetic acid, salicylic acid, topical 5-fluorouracil, podophyllin, and canthacur. For stubborn warts, laser therapy or injection with candida antigen may be helpful. The immunomodulator imiquimod cream (Aldara) is a novel topical agent recently approved for treating condyloma acuminatum, and it might help with common warts as well, usually as adjunctive therapy. Sexual partners of patients with condyloma warrant examination, and women require gynecologic examination. Treatment is summarized in Box 3.

Prevention and Screening

For common warts, no approaches have been documented to prevent transmission. For genital warts (condyloma), the risk correlates with the number of sexual partners. A quadrivalent HPV vaccine

Box 3 Treatment of Warts

Destructive Methods
Cryosurgery*
Electrodessication
Curettage
Laser therapy

Chemotherapeutic Agents
Podophyllin
Canthacur
5-fluorouracil

Caustics and Acids
Salicylic acid*
Trichloracetic acid

Immunotherapies
Imiquimod
Candida antigen

**First line therapy*

(Gardasil) has been available since 2006, and this represents the newest approach to preventing genital HPV infection and ultimately cervical cancer in women. The vaccine is safe and 100% effective and is recommended for girls and women ages 9 to 26 years.

Molluscum Contagiosum

Definition and Etiology

Molluscum contagiosum is an infectious viral disease of the skin caused by the poxvirus.

Prevalence and Risk Factors

The prevalence is less than 5% in the United States. Infection is common in children, especially those with atopic dermatitis, sexually active adults, and patients with human immunodeficiency virus (HIV) infection. Transmission can occur via direct skin or mucous membrane contact, or via fomites.

Pathophysiology and Natural History

The disease follows direct contact with the virus, which replicates in the cytoplasm of cells and induces hyperplasia.

Signs and Symptoms

Molluscum are smooth pink, or flesh-colored, dome-shaped, umbilicated papules with a central keratotic plug (Fig. 18). Most patients have many papules, often in intertriginous sites, such as the axillae, popliteal fossae, and groin. They usually resolve spontaneously, but they often persist in immunocompromised patients.

Diagnosis

Diagnosis is by clinical presentation and by skin biopsy, if warranted.

Treatment

Treatment might not be necessary because the disease often resolves spontaneously in children. Treatment is comparable to the modalities outlined for warts; cryosurgery and curettage are perhaps the easiest and most definitive approaches. In children, canthacur, applied topically then washed off 2 to 6 hours later, is well tolerated, and is very effective.

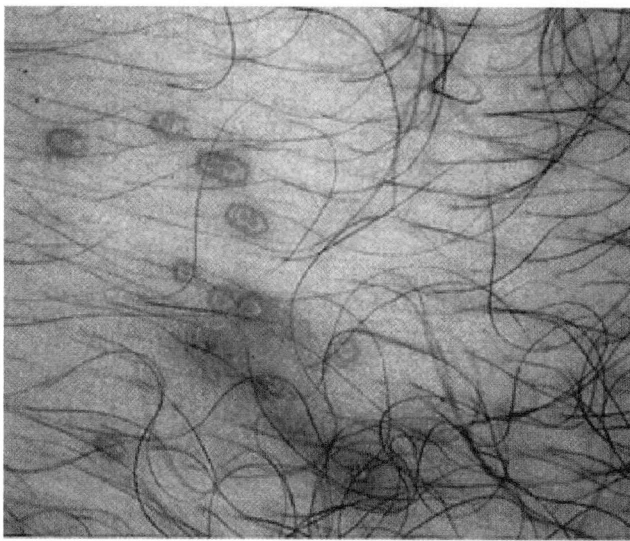

Figure 18 Molluscum contagiosum.

Summary

- Impetigo is a superficial skin infection usually caused by *Staphylococcus aureus* and occasionally by *Streptococcus pyogenes*.
- Folliculitis is a superficial infection of the hair follicles characterized by erythematous, follicular-based papules and pustules.
- Ecthyma is a deep infection of the skin that resembles impetigo. Ecthyma is somewhat common in patients with poor hygiene or malnutrition.
- Erysipelas is a superficial streptococcal infection of the skin.
- Necrotizing fasciitis is a rare infection of the subcutaneous tissues and fascia that eventually leads to necrosis.
- Dermatophytosis implies infection with fungi, organisms with high affinity for keratinized tissue, such as the skin, nails, and hair. *Trichophyton rubrum* is the most common dermatophyte worldwide.
- Cutaneous candidiasis is a yeast infection caused primarily by *Candida albicans*.
- Tinea versicolor is a common superficial infection of the skin caused by the ubiquitous yeast *Malassezia furfur*.
- Herpes simplex virus infection is a painful, self-limited, often recurrent dermatitis, characterized by small grouped vesicles on an erythematous base.
- Herpes zoster (shingles) is an acute, painful dermatomal dermatitis that affects approximately 10% to 20% of adults, often in the presence of immunosuppression.
- Warts are common and benign epithelial growths caused by human papillomavirus.
- Molluscum contagiosum is an infectious viral disease caused by the poxvirus.

Suggested Readings

Bisno AL, Stevens DL: Streptococcal infections of skin and soft tissues. N Engl J Med 1996;334:240-245.
Diven DG: An overview of poxviruses. J Am Acad Dermatol 2001;44:1.
Drake LA, Dinehart SM, Farmer ER, et al: Guidelines of care for superficial mycotic infections of the skin: Onychomycosis. Guidelines/Outcomes Committee. American Academy of Dermatology. J Am Acad Dermatol 1996;34:116-121.
Drake LA, Dinehart SM, Farmer ER, et al: Guidelines of care for superficial mycotic infections of the skin: Tinea corporis, tinea cruris, tinea faciei, tinea manuum, and

tinea pedis. Guidelines/Outcomes Committee. American Academy of Dermatology. J Am Acad Dermatol 1996;34:282-286.
Drake LA, Dinehart SM, Farmer ER, et al: Guidelines of care for superficial mycotic infections of the skin: Pityriasis (tinea) versicolor. Guidelines/Outcomes Committee. American Academy of Dermatology. J Am Acad Dermatol 1996;34:287-289.
Drake LA, Dinehart SM, Farmer ER, et al: Guidelines of care for superficial mycotic infections of the skin: Tinea capitis and tinea barbae. Guidelines/Outcomes Committee. American Academy of Dermatology. J Am Acad Dermatol 1996;34:290-294.
Gnann JW Jr, Whitley RJ: Herpes zoster. N Engl J Med 2002;347:340.
Hay RJ: The management of superficial candidiasis. J Am Acad Dermatol 1999;40(6 Pt 2):S35-S42.
Ko WT, Adal KA, Tomecki KJ: Infectious diseases. Med Clin North Am 1998;82:1001-1031.
Rand S: Overview: The treatment of dermatophytosis. J Am Acad Dermatol 2000;43:S104.
Vinh DC, Embil JM: Rapidly progressive soft tissue infections [Review]. Lancet Infect Dis 2005;5:501.

References

For a complete list of references, log onto www.expertconsult.com.

Bugs, Bites, and Stings

Esteban Faith-Fernandez

SCABIES

Definition and Etiology

Scabies is an ectoparasite infestation caused by the female mite *Sarcoptes scabiei* var. hominis. Norwegian scabies is a more severe infestation found in immunocompromised patients with decreased sensory function and in institutionalized persons.

Prevalence and Risk Factors

The prevalence varies with location, but children and teenagers are most commonly affected. Risk factors include low socioeconomic status, crowded living conditions, and limited access to water.

Pathophysiology and Natural History

Transmission usually occurs by close body contact. Clothing and bedding occasionally act as fomites for transmission. The female mite burrows into the epidermis at a rate of 0.5 to 5 mm/day, lives for 4 to 6 weeks, and produces 2 to 4 eggs daily. An infested patient usually harbors less than 15 mites.

Signs, Symptoms, and Diagnosis

In primary cases, signs and symptoms occur several weeks after infestation. In subsequent episodes, hypersensitivity reactions can develop within a day. Pruritus is usually severe and most prominent at night. Typical skin disease is erythematous papules and vesicles in the interdigital spaces, flexural surface of the wrists and elbows, axillae, areolae, and genitals (Figs. 1 and 2). Face, scalp, and neck are rarely affected except in infants and children. Secondary changes, such as excoriations, eczema, and secondary infection, often follow, especially if disease is persistent.

The burrow—a 1- to 10-mm threadlike plaque—is pathognomonic for scabies, though it is not always easily identified. Reddened nodules can develop on the elbows, anterior axillary folds, penis, and scrotum; these represent a hypersensitivity reaction that can persist for weeks. Itching and the presence of flexural vesicles and burrows should suggest the diagnosis. Identification of the scabies mite, eggs, or fecal pellets from skin scrapings confirms the diagnosis.

Treatment

Permethrin 5% cream (Elimite) is the treatment of choice for uncomplicated scabies in adults, including pregnant women, and in children as young as 1 month. The cream is applied to the trunk and extremities, washed off after 8 to 14 hours, then followed by a second application 7 days later. This routine is approximately 95% successful.

Although it is not yet approved as a treatment for scabies, ivermectin has proved to be very effective. The usual dose is 200 μg/kg as a single dose, then repeated in 10 to 14 days. Its safety has not been proved in pregnancy or in children who weigh less than 15 kg.

Prevention

Close contacts deserve treatment even in the absence of symptoms. Bed linen and clothing should be washed in hot water and dried on high heat, or it may simply be placed in closed plastic bags for 5 to 7 days.

Considerations in Special Populations

Crusted scabies, also known as Norwegian scabies, is a hyperinfestation with thousands of mites that results from the host's inability to mount an immune response to control the infestation. Those at risk are patients with HIV infection, leprosy, hematologic malignancy, graft-versus-host disease, or immunosuppressive therapy; patients with nutritional disorders; and patients with Parkinson's disease, Down's syndrome, and mental retardation.

Crusted scabies, with its hyperkeratotic plaques or nodules, has a predilection for the hands and feet, often resembling psoriasis. Despite the dramatic skin disease and the number of mites, pruritus is usually mild, but lymphadenopathy and eosinophilia can occur.

Crusted scabies is highly infectious, and prompt diagnosis and treatment are essential. Affected patients deserve treatment with permethrin and ivermectin, coupled with vigorous cleaning of clothing and bedding.

Summary

- Scabies is caused by the female mite *Sarcoptes scabiei* var. hominis.
- Diagnosis is based on clinical presentation and demonstration of the mite or eggs (or both) microscopically.
- Permethrin 5% cream is the treatment of choice for uncomplicated scabies, coupled with treatment of close contacts, bed linen, and clothing.
- Crusted scabies is a hyperinfestation in compromised persons unable to mount an appropriate immune response.

PEDICULOSIS

Lice produce three main infestations in humans, depending on the affected body site: pediculosis capitis (head), corporis (body), and pubis (perineum).

Definition and Etiology

Head lice (pediculosis capitis) is caused by the louse *Pediculus humanus* var. capitis; Pediculus humanus var. humanus is responsible for body lice. The crab louse, *Phtirus pubis,* infests the pubic hair and occasionally the eyelashes, beard, and axillae.

Prevalence and Risk Factors

Head lice infestation occurs worldwide, with a reported incidence of 12 million cases per year in the United States. It primarily affects children aged 3 to 11 years. It affects all socioeconomic and ethnic groups, less so African Americans.

Body lice occurs in people living in crowded, often unsanitary conditions, such as homeless persons and refugees.

Pubic lice primarily affects sexually active persons, particularly teenagers and young adults.

Pathophysiology and Natural History

Transmission of all forms of human lice requires close contact. Head lice are transmitted by head-to-head contact; it is transmitted less

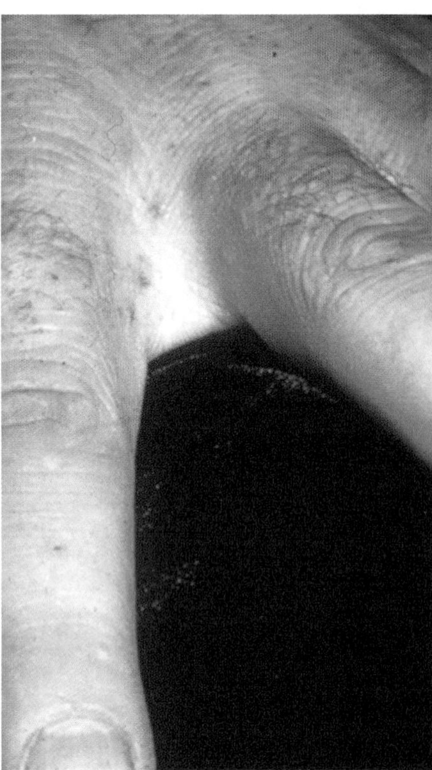

Figure 1 **Scabies.** Erythematous papule-vesicles in web space.

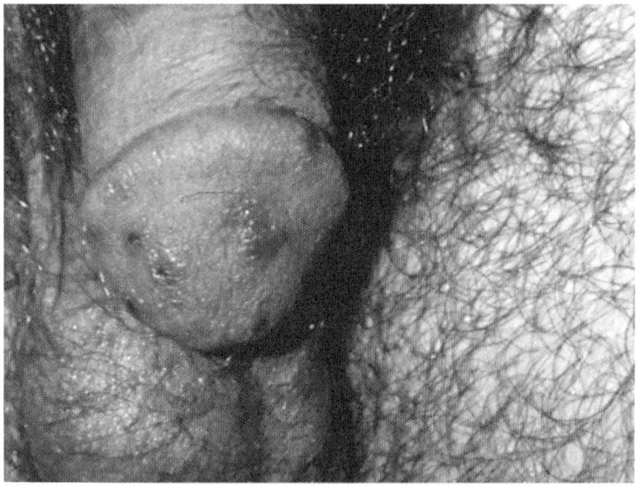

Figure 2 **Scabies.** Erythematous papule-vesicles on penis.

often by fomites. Pubic lice is transmitted by sexual, contact with an infested partner, or less so by contact with the infested person's bed linens, towels, or clothes. Body lice are transmitted by contact with infested persons, who usually live in close, crowded conditions and cannot bathe or change clothes regularly. Head lice and pubic lice or their eggs or nits attach to hairs. body lice live and lay eggs in clothing, not on humans.

Signs, Symptoms, and Diagnosis

Pruritus is the hallmark of all forms of lice. Eczematous changes and secondary infection can follow a patient's scratching. The presence of lice or nits (nodularities on the hair) establishes the diagnosis (Fig. 3). The presence of nits alone can simply indicate past infestation.

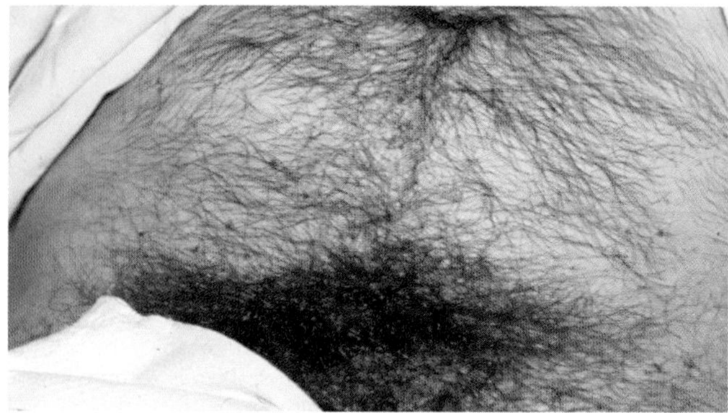

Figure 3 **Pubic lice attached to pubic hair.**

Brushing with a fine-toothed comb can enhance detection of head lice. Pubic lice often produce bluish macules (maculae ceruleae) on the buttocks, upper thighs, and lower abdomen; these macules are thought to be hemosiderin deposition at the site of bites.

Treatment

For head lice, current recommendations include permethrin 1% cream, lindane 1%, or pyrethrins, each applied to a dry scalp for 5 to 10 minutes, followed by rinsing. Malathion 0.5% applied for 8 to 12 hours, then rinsed off can also be used. Each approach should be repeated in 1 week.

For body lice, laundering of clothes and linens coupled with enhanced hygiene is also essential.

For pediculosis pubis, treatment options include permethrin 1% cream applied for 10 minutes or lindane 1% applied for 4-5 minutes or a pyrethrin with piperonyl butoxide applied for 10 minutes, followed by rinsing.

In addition, bedding and clothing should be machine washed and dried with high heat. Close contacts and sexual partners should be treated in similar fashion. Affected patients should be evaluated for other sexually transmitted diseases.

Lindane is not recommended as treatment of infestations in children younger than 2 years and in pregnant women.

Summary

- Head lice (pediculosis capitis) is caused by *Pediculus humanus* var. capitis.
- Body lice (pediculosis corporis) is caused by *Pediculus humanus* var. humanus.
- Pubic lice (pediculosis pubis) is caused by *Pthirus pubis.*
- Pruritus is the hallmark of all lice infesations.
- Pubic lice should raise the possibility of other coexistent sexually transmitted diseases.

BEDBUGS

Definition and Etiology

Bedbugs are blood-sucking insects of the order Cimicidae. The most common species is *Cimex lenticularis.*

Pathophysiology and Natural History

Bedbugs typically feed on sleeping persons, attracted by their body temperature and carbon dioxide production. They tend to live under carpets or floorboards and along the seams of mattresses. They feed

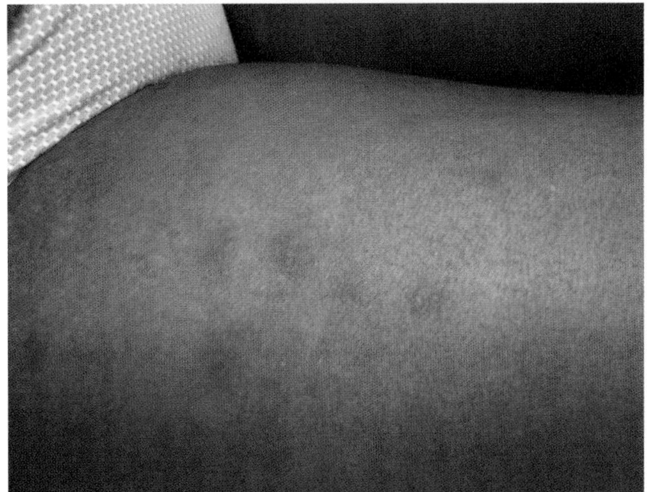

Figure 4 **Bedbug bites.** Nondescript grouped urticarial papules.

infrequently but can live for 1 year. Bedbug resurgence has occurred within the last decade.

Signs, Symptoms, and Diagnosis

Bedbug bites vary from itchy erythematous macules to itchy indurated papules, wheals, vesicles, or bullae, usually on exposed areas of the face, neck, and extremities. They tend to resolve within 2 weeks (Fig. 4). Bites often occur in groups of three, known as the "breakfast, lunch, dinner" pattern. Bedbugs do not transmit diseases.

Treatment

Treatment of patients with bedbug bites is symptomatic, usually nothing more than topical coritocosteroids. Pesticides with dichlorvos, malathion, and pyrethrins are effective in eliminating bedbugs. Prevention of infestation can be achieved with repellents or permethrin-impregnated bed nets.

Summary

- *Cimex lenticularis* is the most common bedbug.
- An itchy nighttime dermatitis, especially grouped papules, should suggest bedbug bites.
- Treatment is symptomatic, such as topical corticosteroids.

FIRE ANTS

Definition and Etiology

Fire ants include the red fire ant *(Solenopsis invicta)* and the black fire ant *(Solenopsis richteri)*. They are well established in the southeastern United States after their importation from South America in the early 20th century. Approximately 30% to 60% of residents in that area are stung every year.

Signs, Symptoms and Diagnosis

Fire ants are aggressive critters, attacking in groups when the anthill is disturbed. The initial bite or sting has a burning sensation followed by an erythematous wheal-and-flare reaction. Within hours, sterile pustules form at the sites of the stings. The pustules are commonly arranged in a rosette or ring pattern, because the ants bite, then pivot and sting in a circular fashion. True anaphylaxis affects 1% of affected persons, usually within hours of the sting.

Treatment

Local reactions deserve symptomatic treatment with compresses, elevation of the affected extremity, and topical corticosteroids. For anaphylactic reactions, immunotherapy with imported fire ant whole body extract has been effective in selected cases.

Summary

- Fire ants *(Solenopsis invicta* and *Solenopsis richteri)* are endemic in the southeastern United States.
- Sterile pustules are the characteristic clinical finding, usually with a burning or stinging sensation.
- Anaphylactic reactions occur in 1% of stung persons.

CUTANEOUS MYIASIS

Definition and Etiology

Cutaneous myiasis, an infestation by larvae of the order Diptera, has three main clinical patterns: furuncular myiasis, wound myiasis, and migratory myiasis. *Dermatobia hominis* (the human bot fly) is the most common agent of cutaneous and furuncular myiasis in North America, usually occurring in travelers from Central and South America, where the fly is common. Though rare, the most common cause of US-acquired furuncular myiasis is the rodent or rabbit bot fly of the genus *Cuterebra*. Wound myiasis is most commonly caused by *Cochliomyia hominivorax*.

Prevalence and Risk Factors

Wound myiasis is the most common type of myiasis in the United States. Risk factors include advanced age, poor social and hygiene conditions, open wounds, psychiatric illness, alcoholism, diabetes, and vascular occlusive disease. Travel to tropical and subtropical areas is the main risk factor for furuncular and migratory myiasis.

Pathophysiology and Natural History

The mode of transmission varies among genera. The adult female bot fly lays eggs on foliage or insects (mosquitoes, flies, ticks), which are then transferred to human skin by direct contact with foliage or biting insects. Once the larva hatches, it burrows into the skin.

Signs, Symptoms, and Diagnosis

Furuncular myiasis exhibits solitary or multiple boil-like nodules on exposed skin, occasionally with drainage (serosanguineous or seropurulent) and surrounding erythema. Patients often have pruritus and local tenderness, and sometimes the larva can be seen protruding from a central pore (Fig. 5). When the nodule is submerged, bubbling occurs if the larva is still alive.

Patients with creeping or migratory myiasis have pruritic, linear, reddened, serpentine plaques, which differ from cutaneous larva migrans in that it extends more slowly. The fly larvae are usually larger in size and survive longer.

In wound myiasis, larvae are readily visualized with varying degrees of tissue destruction. Larvae can invade mucous membranes and body cavities.

Diagnosis of cutaneous myiasis is based on the clinical presentation and presence of the larvae.

Treatment

Removal of the larvae is curative in all cases. The nodule can be occluded by application of a substance (e.g., petrolatum, nail polish,

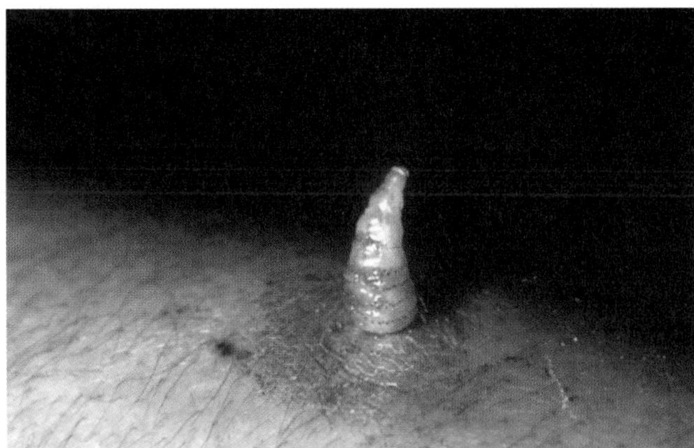

Figure 5 **Furuncular myiasis.**

animal fat, beeswax, paraffin, mineral oil) to asphyxiate the larva and force its exit. The larva can be removed manually or mechanically. Larvicides (topical or oral e.g., ivermectin), mineral turpentine, ethanol spray, and oil of betel leaf kill the larva, which can then be removed.

Summary

- Cutaneous myiasis is an infestation by larvae of the order Diptera.
- There are three types of myiasis: furuncular, wound and migratory or creeping.
- Treatment requires removal of the larva by occlusion, by manual or mechanical means, or with larvicides.

CUTANEOUS LARVA MIGRANS

Definition and Etiology

Cutaneous larva migrans (CLM) is an infestation by a nematode, most often the animal hookworm *(Ancylostoma caninum* or *Ancylostoma braziliense),* less often the human hookworm *(Ancylostoma duodenale* and *Necator americanus).*

CLM occurs most commonly in areas with warm climates such as Africa, Asia, Latin America, and the southeastern United States. It is the most common travel-related skin disease, often occurring in travelers who have visited these areas.

Pathophysiology and Natural History

CLM is a self-limited disease, invariably acquired when the skin has contact with sand or soil contaminated with animal feces. The feet are the most common affected site, and the legs and buttocks are less so. Left untreated, the disease resolves within a few months.

Signs, Symptoms, and Diagnosis

Affected patients have itchy erythematous, serpiginous tracks, usually on the feet, buttocks, or thighs (Fig. 6). The track advances 1 to 2 cm/day.

The history and pattern of skin disease (serpiginous tracks) and its location should suggest the diagnosis.

CLM must be clinically differentiated from migratory myiasis and cutaneous larva currens. Migratory myiasis extends more slowly; the fly larvae are usually larger and survive longer. Cutaneous larva currens is the infestation with the roundworm *Strongyloides stercoralis.* The sign is pruritic, serpiginous, erythematous tracks on the perineal area, buttocks, and thighs, which evolve rapidly at a rate of 5 to 15 cm/hr. This differentiation is important, because cutaneous larva currens may be associated with systemic or disseminated infection with a mortality rate of up to 70% to 90%

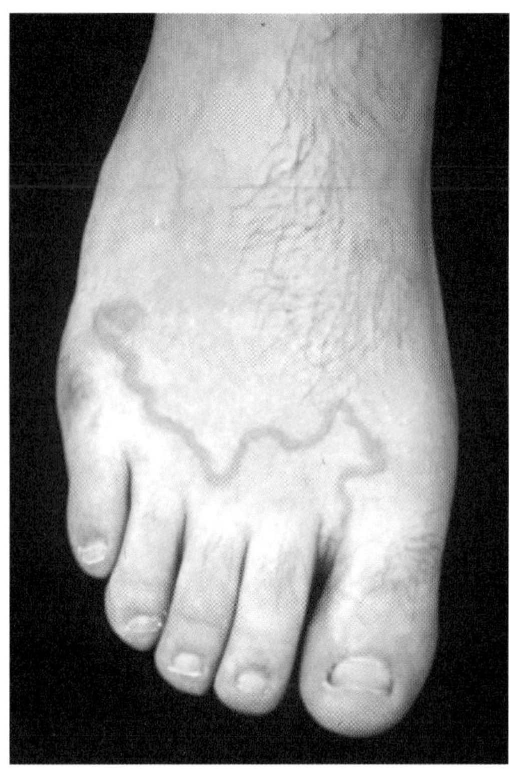

Figure 6 **Cutaneous larva migrans.** Erythematous serpiginous track on foot.

Treatment

Several treatment strategies exist. The most common treatments are thiabendazole cream 2 or 3 times a day for 5 to 10 days, albendazole 400 mg orally daily for 3 to 5 days, and ivermectin as a single dose of 12 mg (200 μg/kg).

Summary

- CLM is the most common travel-related skin disease.
- CLM is caused by a nematode (hookworm).
- Itchy, reddened, serpiginous tracks on the feet or buttocks are characteristic findings.
- Anthelminthics, either topical or oral, are the treatment of choice.

SEABATHER'S ERUPTION

Definition and Etiology

Seabather's eruption, or sea lice, is an acute dermatitis that begins after exposure to seawater containing the thimble jellyfish *Linuche unguiculata.* The eruption is a dermatitis caused by the sting of the jellyfish larvae trapped within a bathing suit.

Prevalence and Risk Factors

Seabather's eruption occurs in the spring and summer, most commonly along the coasts of Florida and in the Caribbean. Children,

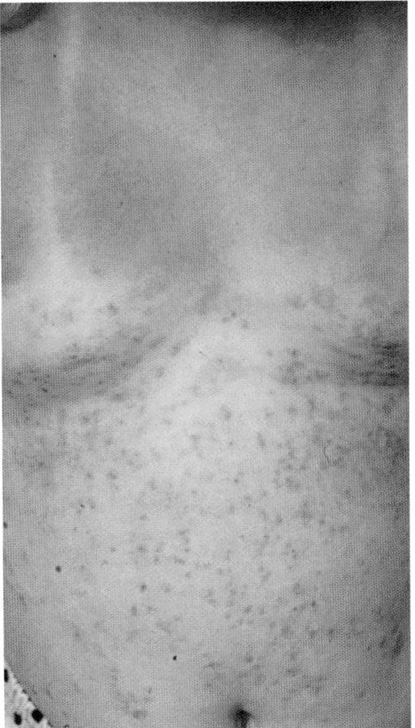

Figure 7 **Seabather's eruption.** Erythematous papules on skin covered by bathing suit.

surfers, and those with a prior occurrence are most commonly affected.

Signs, Symptoms and Diagnosis

Within 24 hours after exposure to infested seawater, erythematous macules, papules, or wheals appear on areas of the body that were covered by the bathing suit) (Fig. 7). The dermatitis results from the firing of the nematocyst after a change in osmotic pressure. Occasionally, systemic symptoms (fever, chills, nausea, headache) occur, particularly in children and adolescents. The dermatitis resolves in 7 to 10 days. The diagnosis is based on the clinical appearance of the dermatitis on covered skin after seawater exposure.

Treatment

Treatment is symptomatic and consists of antihistamines and topical corticosteroids. Severe cases can require systemic corticosteroids. Removal of the bathing suit and showering after seawater exposure is protective.

Summary

- Seabather's eruption is a dermatitis caused by stings of the larval form of the jellyfish *Linuche unguiculata.*
- The dermatitis appears on covered areas after seawater exposure.

SWIMMER'S ITCH

Definition, Etiology and Risk Factors

Swimmer's itch, or cercarial dermatitis, is a pruritic skin disease caused by penetration of cercariae (trematode larvae of the genera Schistosoma and Trichobilharzia). These larvae are common in fresh water (lakes, ponds) and occasionally in salt water.

Cercarial dermatitis is common in children during the summer months after exposure to fresh water, particularly in shallow waters.

Signs, Symptoms and Diagnosis

A few hours after cercarial contact, a pruritic monomorphic dermatitis appears, characterized by erythematous macules and papules on uncovered skin. The larvae die within few hours, and the dermatitis spontaneously resolves in 1 to 2 weeks, even without treatment.

Treatment

Treatment is symptomatic with antihistamines and topical corticosteroids. For severe, generalized disease, systemic glucocorticoids may be necessary.

Summary

- Swimmer's itch (cercarial dermatitis) is caused by invasion of the skin by larvae of trematodes, usually acquired in fresh water.
- Skin disease is essentially a dermatitis on exposed skin after fresh water contact, e.g. swimming.

Suggested Readings

deShazo RD, Butcher BT, Banks WA: Reactions to the stings of the imported fire ant. N Engl J Med 1990;323(7):462-466.

Galiczynski EM Jr, Elston DM: What's eating you? Pubic lice *(Pthirus pubis)*. Cutis 2008;81(2):109-114.

Heukelbach J, Feldmeier H: Epidemiological and clinical characteristics of hookworm-related cutaneous larva migrans. Lancet Infect Dis 2008;8(5):302-309.

Heukelbach J, Feldmeier H: Scabies. Lancet 2006;367(9524):1767-1774.

Jacobson CC, Abel EA: Parasitic infestations. J Am Acad Dermatol 2007;56(6):1026-1043.

Kumar S, Hlady WG, Malecki JM: Risk factors for seabather's eruption: A prospective cohort study. Public Health Rep 1997;112(1):59-62.

Lebwohl M, Clark L, Levitt J: Therapy for head lice based on life cycle, resistance, and safety considerations. Pediatrics 2007;119(5):965-974.

McGraw TA, Turiansky GW: Cutaneous myiasis. J Am Acad Dermatol 2008;58(6):907-926.

Mumcuoglu KY, Barker SC, Burgess IE, et al: International guidelines for effective control of head louse infestations. J Drugs Dermatol 2007;6(4):409-414.

Steen CJ, Carbonaro PA, Schwartz RA: Arthropods in dermatology. J Am Acad Dermatol 2004;50(6):819-842.

Strong M, Johnstone PW: Interventions for treating scabies. Cochrane Database Syst Rev 2007;(3):CD000320.

Ter Poorten MC, Prose NS: The return of the common bedbug. Pediatr Dermatol 2005;22(3):183-187.

Verbrugge LM, Rainey JJ, Reimink RL, Blankespoor HD: Prospective study of swimmer's itch incidence and severity. J Parasitol 2004;90(4):697-704.

Section 4

ENDOCRINOLOGY

Diseases of the Adrenal Gland

Adriana G. Ioachimescu and *Amir H. Hamrahian*

ANATOMY AND PHYSIOLOGY OF THE ADRENAL GLANDS

Each adrenal consists of two functionally distinct endocrine glands: the cortex, derived from mesenchymal cells, and the medulla, derived from neuroectodermal cells. The adrenal cortex consists of three concentric zones: The outer glomerulosa secretes the mineralocorticoid aldosterone, the intermediate fasciculata secretes cortisol, and the inner reticularis secretes androgens. The endocrine cells of the adrenal medulla are the chromaffin cells, which are part of the sympathetic nervous system and produce the catecholamine epinephrine.

ADRENAL INSUFFICIENCY

Etiology

Glucocorticoid insufficiency can be primary, resulting from the direct insult to the adrenal cortex, or secondary, from adrenocorticotropic hormone (ACTH) or corticotropin-releasing hormone (CRH) hyposecretion as a result of pituitary or hypothalamic dysfunctions.

Primary adrenal insufficiency affects glucocorticoid and mineralocorticoid secretion and may be fatal if untreated. Autoimmune destruction of the adrenal glands (Addison's disease) is the most common cause of primary adrenal insufficiency in United States (70%-90%), whereas tuberculosis is now the second most common cause worldwide. Some other causes of primary adrenal insufficiency include bilateral adrenal hemorrhage, drugs (e.g., mitotane, etomidate, ketoconazole) and other infectious diseases (e.g., HIV infection, disseminated histoplasmosis, paracoccidiomycosis). HIV infection may result in both primary and secondary adrenal insufficiencies (AI). Addison's disease may coexist with other autoimmune conditions, such as type 1 diabetes, hypothyroidism, or hypoparathyroidism.

Secondary and tertiary adrenal insufficiencies occur commonly after the discontinuation of glucocorticoids. Less frequently, ACTH deficiency may be caused by pituitary macroadenomas, pituitary surgery or radiation, and parasellar diseases. Megestrol acetate, an appetite stimulator used in some patients with advanced cancer or cachexia related to AIDS may be associated with secondary AI. Tertiary adrenal insufficiency results from the inadequate secretion of CRH. Secondary and tertiary adrenal insufficiencies only affect cortisol secretion, because ACTH has only a minor role in regulation of aldosterone secretion.

Manifestations

All patients with primary adrenal insufficiency complain of fatigue, anorexia, and weight loss. Other clinical and laboratory manifestations of primary adrenal insufficiency are presented in Table 1. Skin hyperpigmentation, initially on the extensor surfaces, palmar creases, and buccal mucosa, results from increased levels of ACTH and other pro-opiomelanocortin–related peptides, including melanocyte-stimulating hormone. Secondary adrenal insufficiency manifests more insidiously with lack of skin hyperpigmentation, salt craving, metabolic acidosis, and hyperkalemia, because mineralocorticoid secretion is intact. Fatigue, hyponatremia, and hypoglycemia are some of the clinical manifestations in secondary adrenal insufficiency.

Evaluation

Evaluating a patient with suspected adrenal insufficiency is a three-step process: establishing the diagnosis, differentiating between primary and secondary adrenal insufficiencies, and looking for the cause of adrenal insufficiency.

Establishing the Diagnosis. Because of circadian secretion of cortisol and overlap among patients with adrenal insufficiency and those with normal adrenal function, determining the random serum cortisol level is only of value during stress (see later, "Adrenal Insufficiency in the Critically Ill Patient"). An algorithm for the evaluation of adrenal function is shown in Figure 1. An early morning (8 AM) plasma cortisol level lower than 3 μg/dL confirms adrenal insufficiency, whereas a value higher than 15 μg/dL makes the diagnosis highly unlikely. Cortisol levels in the range of 3 to 15 μg/dL may be seen in patients with primary, secondary, or tertiary adrenal insufficiency.

These patients should be further evaluated by the cosyntropin (Cortrosyn) stimulation test (CST), which can be performed at any time during the day. The standard-dose CST uses an intravenous or intramuscular injection of 250 μg cosyntropin with plasma cortisol before and 30 and 60 minutes after the injection. A normal response is a plasma cortisol concentration higher than 18 μg/dL at 30 minutes. Most individuals with normal adrenal function achieve much higher cortisol levels at 60 minutes after cosyntropin injection. For this reason, the 18 μg/dL cutoff value should be applied only for the 30-minute cortisol level. The standard-dose CST is excellent for excluding primary adrenal insufficiency. However, patients with mild partial or recent-onset pituitary ACTH or hypothalamic CRH deficiency (e.g., within 2-4 weeks after pituitary surgery) may have a normal response to 250 μg of cosyntropin in the CST, because the adrenal glands have not undergone significant atrophy and will still respond to very high concentrations of ACTH stimulation. The sensitivity of CST to pick up mild adrenal insufficiency improves when using the low-dose CST (1 μg ACTH[1-2] given intravenously); however, this may result in a higher false-positive rate. The lack of a commercially available 1-μg cosyntropin dose may be a potential for error. In most clinical situations, the 30-minute cortisol value during a standard-dose CST has a diagnostic accuracy close to that of a low-dose CST.[1]

The insulin tolerance test (ITT) and metyrapone test are generally used for the evaluation of patients suspected to have secondary adrenal insufficiency. ITT is considered the gold standard test for the evaluation of hypothalamic-pituitary-adrenal (HPA) axis. The ITT is contraindicated in older patients (>65 years) and those with acute illness, seizure disorders, or cardiovascular-cerebrovascular disease. The result of the metyrapone test has been validated compared with the ITT. Metyrapone blocks the final step in cortisol biosynthesis, resulting in a reduction in cortisol secretion, which in turn stimulates ACTH secretion. This leads to higher levels of 11-deoxycortisol, which is the precursor to cortisol.

The CRH stimulation test requires intact pituitary and adrenal glands for a response. The test has not been well validated for the evaluation of adrenal function and its current role in the evaluation of adrenal function is limited to research protocols.

Table 1 Clinical Manifestations of Primary Adrenal Insufficiency

Parameter	Frequency (%)
Symptoms	
Weakness, fatigue	100
Anorexia	100
Nausea	86
Vomiting	75
Constipation	33
Diarrhea	15
Abdominal pain	31
Salt craving	16
Postural dizziness	12
Muscle and joint pain	10
Signs	
Weight loss	100
Hyperpigmentation	90
Vitiligo	15
Hypotension (systolic blood pressure <110 mm Hg)	92
Laboratory Abnormalities	
Hyponatremia	90
Hyperkalemia	64
Hypercalcemia	5
Azotemia	55
Anemia	40
Eosinophilia	17

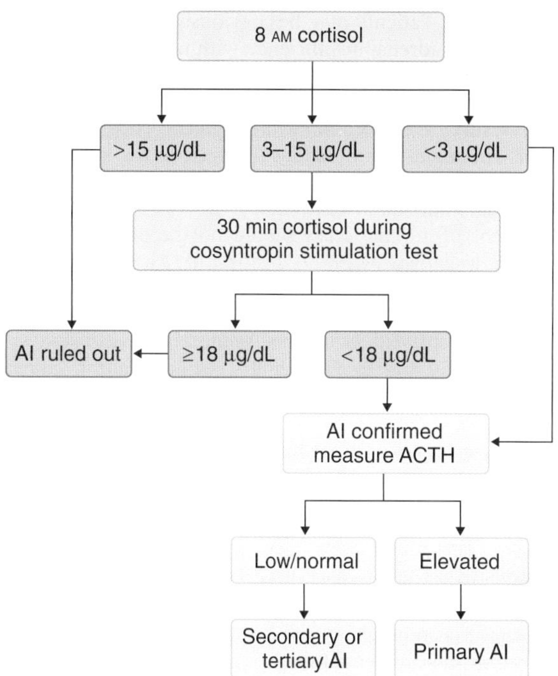

Figure 1 Algorithm for the diagnosis of adrenal insufficiency (AI). The standard cosyntropin stimulation test (CST) may be used as the first-line test for evaluation of adrenal function. The CST may be unreliable in patients with new-onset (<2-4 weeks) secondary or tertiary AI. ACTH, adrenocorticotropic hormone.

Differentiation Between Primary and Secondary Adrenal Insufficiencies. This is done through the measurement of the basal plasma ACTH level. An elevated ACTH level is consistent with primary adrenal insufficiency. A low or normal-range ACTH level, with a low cortisol level, confirms the diagnosis of secondary or tertiary adrenal insufficiency.

Determining the Cause of Adrenal Insufficiency. When the biochemical workup is consistent with primary adrenal insufficiency, computed tomography (CT) scanning of the adrenal glands may help with the differential diagnosis. Enlarged adrenal glands or calcifications suggest an infectious, hemorrhagic, or metastatic cause. In rare circumstances, CT-guided percutaneous fine-needle aspiration of enlarged adrenal glands may help establish the diagnosis. Patients with tuberculous adrenal insufficiency usually have evidence of active systemic disease. When the biochemical work up suggests secondary or tertiary adrenal insufficiency, magnetic resonance imaging (MRI) of the pituitary gland is indicated if glucocorticoid therapy as the cause of the secondary adrenal insufficiency has been ruled out.

Treatment

Patients with Addison's disease require lifelong replacement with glucocorticoids and mineralocorticoids. The minimal dosage to treat symptoms should be used, starting with hydrocortisone, 12.5 to 15 mg in the morning, and 2.5 to 5 mg at noon to mimic the physiologic pattern. Some patients may need another dose of 2.5 to 5 mg hydrocortisone at about 6 PM if fatigue continues later in the day. Patients require fludrocortisone, 0.05 to 0.2 mg, for mineralocorticoid replacement. The dose is adjusted based on clinical status, including the presence or absence of orthostatic hypotension, hypertension, and electrolyte imbalance. Patients may need to double the dose of fludrocortisone or increase salt intake during the summer, when the weather is hot. Patients with secondary or tertiary adrenal insufficiency do not need mineralocorticoid replacement.

During minor illness (e.g., flu or fever >38° C [100.4° F]) the hydrocortisone dose should be doubled for 2 or 3 days. The inability to ingest hydrocortisone tablets warrants parenteral administration. Most patients can be educated to self administer hydrocortisone, 100 mg IM, and reduce the risk of an emergency room visit. Hydrocortisone, 75 mg/day, provides adequate glucocorticoid coverage for outpatient surgery. Parenteral hydrocortisone, 150 to 200 mg/day (in three or four divided doses), is needed for major surgery, with a rapid taper to normal replacement during the recovery. Patients taking more than 100 mg hydrocortisone/day do not need any additional mineralocorticoid replacement. All patients should wear some form of identification indicating their adrenal insufficiency status.

Adrenal Crisis

Acute adrenal insufficiency (adrenal crisis) is a life-threatening emergency, which usually manifests with nausea, vomiting, abdominal pain, and shock. Patients may be previously undiagnosed or have chronic primary adrenal insufficiency, with no or inadequate glucocorticoid replacement. Abdominal tenderness and fever are common findings, and adrenal crisis may manifest as an acute abdomen. In these cases, surgical exploration without glucocorticoid coverage can be lethal. The major hormonal factor precipitating adrenal crisis is mineralocorticoid deficiency. Therefore, adrenal crisis rarely occurs with secondary adrenal insufficiency.

Treatment of adrenal crisis should not be delayed. Diagnostic workup in a patient with no history of AI should include a plasma sample for cortisol and ACTH level determination, immediately followed by an IV bolus of hydrocortisone, 100 mg, and adequate fluid replacement (normal saline). Hydrocortisone should be continued, 50 mg every 8 hours, while awaiting laboratory results.

Adrenal Insufficiency in the Critically Ill Patient

The overall incidence of AI in critically ill patients is less than 10%, but an incidence as high as 50% in a patient with septic shock has been reported. The concept of total adrenal insufficiency has gradually been replaced by relative adrenal insufficiency, which may be fatal in critically ill patients. Hypotension in patients with adrenal insufficiency may mimic hypovolemic or septic shock and should be considered in the differential diagnosis. Serial follow-up of adrenal function in critically patients with clinical features suggestive of AI is recommended.

Intensive care unit (ICU) patients with hemodynamic instability, despite fluid resuscitation (especially in the presence of shock), should be tested for AI. A random serum cortisol level determination and the standard CST are the two commonly used tests for evaluating adrenal function in these patients. However, the cortisol level that reflects an adequate response is uncertain. In critically ill patients with near-normal albumin levels (>2.5 g/dL), a random plasma cortisol level lower than 15 µg/dL, and a maximum cortisol level lower than 20 µg/dL during the CST strongly suggest adrenal insufficiency. In patients with equivocal biochemical results, a trial of 2 or 3 days of stress dosage glucocorticoids is appropriate, as long as it will be discontinued in the absence of any significant hemodynamic improvement. The value of the delta cortisol during the CST (stimulated minus basal cortisol levels) of 9 µg/dL or lower as an indicator of partial AI during septic shock is a matter of debate and does not have strong literature support.

More than 90% of circulating cortisol is bound to cortisol-binding globulin (CBG) and albumin. Free cortisol is biologically active. During severe illness caused by a marked decrease in the CBG level, albumin has a more significant influence on the total concentration of cortisol. Critically ill patients with significant hypoalbuminemia (albumin level >2.5 g/dL) have subnormal serum total cortisol concentrations, but their baseline or cosyntropin-stimulated serum free cortisol level is in the high-normal range or elevated.[3] In patients with hypoalbuminemia, total serum cortisol is a poor indicator of glucocorticoid activity. Studies are needed to establish normative ranges for free cortisol for different levels of stress, including septic shock.[3]

Hydrocortisone, 50 mg IV every 6 to 8 hours is an adequate replacement dose for critically ill patients with suspected adrenal insufficiency. Treatment with this dose should be continued for 2 or 3 days. After hemodynamic improvement, a gradual taper of hydrocortisone, depending on the patient's condition, should be instituted. A subset of patients with septic shock may benefit from physiologic stress dose glucocorticoids. Such therapy has not yet been proven to be effective and safe in all patients with septic shock. Lifelong glucocorticoid replacement therapy should not be sanctioned on the basis of an equivocal biochemical test result in an acutely ill patient. Adrenal function should be re-evaluated after recovery from acute illness.

Box 1 Etiology of Endogenous Cushing's Syndrome

ACTH-Dependent
Cushing's syndrome (67%)
Ectopic ACTH secretion (12%)
Ectopic CRH secretion (<1%)

ACTH-Independent
Adrenal adenoma (10%)
Adrenal carcinoma (8%)
Micro- and macronodular adrenal hyperplasias (1%)

ACTH, adrenocorticotropic hormone; CRH, corticotropin-releasing hormone.

Summary

- Autoimmune destruction of the adrenal glands is the most common cause of primary adrenal insufficiency in the United States.
- Almost all patients with primary adrenal insufficiency present with fatigue, anorexia, and weight loss.
- Primary and secondary adrenal insufficiencies are differentiated through measurement of the plasma ACTH level.
- Acute adrenal insufficiency is a medical emergency that should be treated with IV hydrocortisone and fluids as soon as the diagnosis is suspected.
- Adrenal insufficiency should be suspected in critically ill patients with septic shock or hypotension refractory to intravenous fluids and pressors.

SYNDROMES OF ADRENAL HYPERFUNCTION

Diseases related to adrenal hyperfunction are relatively rare, but they have significant mortality and morbidity if untreated. In the following sections, Cushing's syndrome, primary hyperaldosteronism, pheochromocytoma, and androgen-producing adrenal tumors are reviewed.

Cushing's Syndrome

Definition and Classification

Cushing's syndrome (CS) is composed of symptoms and signs associated with prolonged exposure to inappropriately high levels of plasma glucocorticoids. Exogenous glucocorticoid intake is the most common cause of CS. The endogenous causes are divided into ACTH-dependent and ACTH-independent CS, as shown in Box 1.

Clinical Features

Harvey Cushing initially described the clinical features of CS in the early 20th century, including centripetal obesity, moon face, hirsutism, and plethora; however, such a classic clinical picture is not always present and a high index of suspicion is usually required. Box 2 describes some of the clinical features suggestive of CS. Weight gain is almost always present, except in ectopic ACTH secretion (EAS) caused by malignancy. The striae in CS are red-purple and usually wider than 1 cm. The skin is thin and minimal trauma results in easy bruising. Patients have a plethoric appearance and acne may be present. Proximal myopathy involving the lower limb and shoulder girdle may be present. Moon face and supraclavicular and dorsocervical fat pads (buffalo hump) are nonspecific and accompany obesity from other causes.

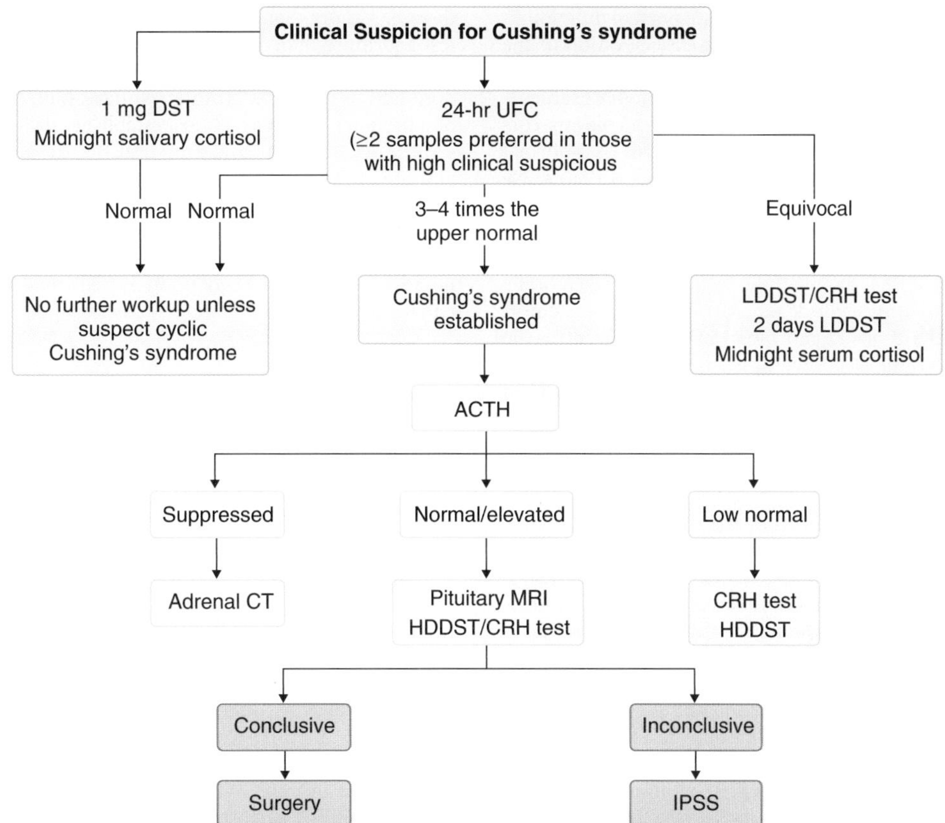

Figure 2 **Algorithm for evaluation of patients suspected of having Cushing's syndrome (CS).** Screening for Cushing's syndrome may be done by a 24-hour urinary free cortisol (UFC) assay, 1-mg dexamethasone suppression test (DST), or midnight salivary cortisol determination. Values of the 24-hour UFC more than three or four times the upper normal for the assay are usually diagnostic for CS, especially once repeated and confirmed. CRH, corticotropin-releasing hormone; HDDST, overnight high-dose (8 mg) dexamethasone suppression test; IPSS, inferior petrosal sinus sampling; LDDST, low-dose dexamethasone suppression test; MRI, magnetic resonance imaging.

Box 2 Clinical Features Suggestive of Cushing's Syndrome

- Central obesity
- Proximal myopathy
- Spontaneous bruising
- Facial plethora
- Wide purplish striae (>1 cm)
- Changes in serial photographs
- Hypokalemia
- Osteoporosis

Women have menstrual irregularity and hirsutism. Men and women exhibit loss of libido. Agitated depression and lethargy are among the most common psychiatric abnormalities seen in CS patients, but paranoia and overt psychosis may occur. Irritability is an early symptom and insomnia is common. CS has profound effects on bone, causing poor linear growth in children and osteoporotic vertebral collapse and pathologic fractures in adults.

Patients with ectopic ACTH syndrome caused by small cell lung carcinoma lack many of the typical clinical features. The rapid course and high levels of ACTH and cortisol often result in hyperpigmentation, myopathy, peripheral edema, glucose intolerance, and hypokalemic alkalosis. Female patients with adrenal carcinomas often present with signs and symptoms of virilization (hirsutism and acne), breast atrophy, deepening of the voice, temporal hair recession, and clitoromegaly caused by hypersecretion of androgens, along with the cortisol.

Pseudo-Cushing's syndrome refers to features of CS combined with some features of hypercortisolism that resolve after resolution of the underlying cause, such as psychiatric disorders (e.g., major depression, anxiety disorder, obsessive-compulsive disorder, anorexia nervosa), morbid obesity, poorly controlled diabetes, and chronic alcoholism.

CS as a result of exogenous administration of glucocorticoids must be excluded. The diagnosis of Cushing's syndrome then involves two steps: demonstration of inappropriate cortisol secretion and localization of its cause.

Establishing the Diagnosis

Screening for CS may be done by a 24-hour urinary free cortisol (UFC) determination, 1-mg dexamethasone suppression test (DST), or midnight salivary cortisol test (Fig. 2). Currently, a 24-hour UFC test (with simultaneous urinary creatinine level measurement) is the most widely used initial screening test but a midnight salivary cortisol determination is becoming a good alternative. An elevated salivary cortisol level in most cases should be confirmed by a 24-hour UFC test before referral to surgery. A normal sleeping pattern is necessary for an accurate salivary cortisol level measurement for the evaluation of CS. Values of UFC above three or four times upper normal for the assay are usually diagnostic for CS, especially when repeated and confirmed. In patients with a glomerular filtration rate lower than 20 mL/min, urinary cortisol excretion is significantly decreased and may thus be normal, despite excessive cortisol production. On the other hand, normal individuals with excess fluid intake (>4 L/day) may have a false elevation of the UFC.

The 1-mg DST is performed by the administration of dexamethasone, 1 mg at 11 PM, followed by measurement of the plasma cortisol level at 8 AM. A cortisol level lower than 1.8 μg/dL is a normal response. It is an excellent test to rule out CS, with less than a 2% false-negative test result; however, because of a high false-positive rate (≤40%), a positive test result needs to be further confirmed by other tests, such as a 24-hour UFC assay.

During the low-dose DST, dexamethasone, 0.5 mg, is taken orally every 6 hours, for a total of eight doses, starting at 6 AM. A cutoff cortisol value of 1.8 μg/dL in the morning (at 7 or 8 AM), after the last dose of dexamethasone at midnight, has been reported to have an excellent sensitivity and specificity of about 98% in the evaluation of patients suspected to have CS. Measurement of the 24-hour UFC during the second day of the low-dose DST is of lesser value, and usually does not add any further to the diagnostic accuracy of the baseline 24-hour UFC test.

The combined DST-CRH stimulation test may be used for differentiating between CS and pseudo-Cushing's syndrome. The test consists of the oral administration of 0.5 mg dexamethasone every 6 hours for eight doses, starting at noon, followed by the IV administration of 100 μg CRH at 8 AM (2 hours after the last dose of dexamethasone). A plasma cortisol level higher than 1.4 μg/dL 15 minutes after the CRH injection strongly suggests CS.

Certain drugs, such as phenytoin, phenobarbitals, and rifampin, increase the clearance rate of dexamethasone, resulting in false-positive results during a DST. In these cases, it may be necessary to measure the plasma dexamethasone level. It is always important to remember the effect of increased levels of CBG on serum cortisol levels during pregnancy or in women taking estrogens. These states do not affect the 24-hour UFC or midnight salivary cortisol levels.

Because of the challenging nature of CS, reaching the proper diagnosis requires a stepwise evaluation, knowledge of the limitations of each test, and avoidance of shortcuts (see Fig. 2). Discrepant or inconclusive test results require re-evaluation of the entire clinical picture and a biochemical workup, because CS is almost always a progressive disease. Another clinical scenario that may be associated with normal screening tests is cyclic CS, which needs to be ruled out by periodic evaluation. Fortunately, true cyclic CS is a rare condition.

Differential Diagnosis: ACTH-Dependent Versus Primary Adrenal Disease

Once Cushing's syndrome is biochemically confirmed, the plasma ACTH level should be measured, preferably in the morning. Normal values typically range between 5 and 50 pg/mL. A suppressed or low ACTH level (<10 pg/mL) is consistent with ACTH-independent CS and should be followed by adrenal CT scanning. ACTH values of 10 to 20 pg/mL may be seen in patients with both adrenal and pituitary causes for CS; these patients should undergo a CRH stimulation test. A flat response of ACTH to CRH during the test suggests an adrenal cause, but a more than 50% increase in the ACTH level during the test is consistent with Cushing's disease. ACTH levels higher than 20 pg/mL suggest ACTH-dependent CS. About 90% of patients with ACTH-dependent CS have a pituitary cause and the rest are ectopic in origin. Pituitary MRI with gadolinium enhancement should be performed. In patients with ACTH-dependent CS, the presence of a pituitary adenoma larger than 6 mm strongly suggests a pituitary origin, but 50% of CS patients do not have any abnormality on MRI.[4] ACTH levels tend to be higher in ectopic CS compared with Cushing's disease, but there is significant overlap.

A combination of the CRH stimulation test and an overnight high-dose DST are used to differentiate ectopic CS from Cushing's disease. A more than 50% increase in the ACTH level after the CRH test and more than an 80% reduction in the morning cortisol level (8-9 AM) after taking 8 mg dexamethasone at 11 PM during a high-dose DST is consistent with a pituitary source, and in the presence of a pituitary adenoma, almost establishes the definitive diagnosis of CS. If the CRH stimulation test and DST results are not concordant and MRI does not show a pituitary adenoma, then inferior petrosal sinus sampling to distinguish ectopic from Cushing's disease is indicated. Localizing tumors that produce ectopic ACTH is accomplished by chest and abdominal CT studies, followed by neck CT if no source is found. An octreotide scan may be of some value in patients with ectopic CS and negative imaging studies.

Treatment

Surgical (trans-sphenoidal) removal of the ACTH-secreting pituitary tumor is the treatment of choice. Experienced neurosurgeons usually achieve 70% to 80% long-term remission rates following surgery. An undetectable cortisol level postoperatively, when the patient is off glucocorticoids, is considered to be an excellent indication of long-term cure.

Cushing's syndrome caused by an adrenal adenoma is usually cured by laparoscopic unilateral adrenalectomy. Adrenal carcinoma is typically an aggressive tumor with a poor prognosis; surgical resection at an early stage, along with lifelong mitotane therapy started soon after surgery, offers the only chance for cure or long-term remission.

Surgical removal of an ectopic ACTH-producing tumor, if possible, results in cure. When the tumor is not resectable, bilateral adrenalectomy is performed to correct hypercortisolemia. Medical therapy with ketoconazole, metyrapone, aminoglutethimide, or mitotane may be considered for patients with a limited life expectancy or for alleviation of hypercortisolemic symptoms before surgery.

National Guidelines

During an international workshop in Italy, in October 2002, a relatively comprehensive consensus statement about the diagnosis and complications of Cushing's syndrome was published.[4] The workshop recommended a low threshold for screening patients for CS, including patients with metabolic syndrome, especially if young and resistant to conventional treatment. The consensus emphasized that if the diagnosis of Cushing's is suspected clinically but initial screening tests are normal, the patient should be re-evaluated at a later date and invasive procedures postponed. A 24-hour UFC assay, overnight 1-mg DST, and midnight salivary cortisol determination were described as first-line screening tests for CS. The workshop briefly discussed the promising results from the midnight salivary cortisol test, which we believe should be part of the diagnostic workup for most patients suspected to have CS, particularly if early disease is suspected.

Evaluation for the plasma circadian rhythm, midnight plasma cortisol level, 2-day low-dose dexamethasone suppression test (LDDST), and combined LDDST-CRH test were described by the workshop as second-line screening tests. In our experiences and in spite of being labor intensive, the combined LDDST-CRH test is of significant value in differentiating CS from pseudo-Cushing's syndrome. The workshop recommended the use of bilateral inferior petrosal sinus sampling (BIPSS) in patients whose clinical, biochemical, or radiologic study results are discordant or equivocal. We usually carry out BIPSS in most of our patients with ACTH-dependent CS who have no clear adenoma on pituitary MRI. After pituitary tumors are treated, lifelong medical follow-up is necessary to detect early recurrence, monitor hormone replacement, and treat any complications related to the tumor.

Summary

- Screening for Cushing's syndrome may be done by a midnight salivary cortisol level assay, 1-mg DST, or 24-hour urinary free cortisol test.
- Certain drugs, such as phenytoin, phenobarbitals and rifampin, increase the clearance rate of dexamethasone, resulting in false-positive results during DSTs.
- Because of the challenging nature of Cushing's syndrome, obtaining a proper diagnosis requires a stepwise evaluation, knowledge of the limitations of each test, and avoidance of shortcuts.
- Once Cushing's syndrome has been biochemically confirmed, the plasma ACTH level should be measured to differentiate between ACTH-dependent and ACTH-independent CS.

Primary Hyperaldosteronism

Prevalence and Etiology

Conn first described primary hyperaldosteronism in 1955 in a patient with an adrenal adenoma. Hyperaldosteronism may be more common than once believed. Some investigators have proposed a prevalence as high as 10% in hypertensive patients.[5] Women in their fourth to sixth decade of life are affected more often than men. A solitary aldosterone-producing adenoma (65%) and bilateral idiopathic hyperplasia (30%) are the most common subtypes of primary aldosteronism. The adenomas are usually benign and smaller than 2 cm in diameter. Idiopathic adrenal hyperplasia may be accompanied by adrenocortical nodules and is associated with lower aldosterone levels and less severe hypertension, compared with adenomas.

Two forms of familial hyperaldosteronism (FH) have been described: FH type I and FH type II. FH type I, or glucocorticoid-remediable hyperaldosteronism (GRH), is an autosomal dominant disease characterized by a chimeric gene between the 11β-hydroxylase and aldosterone synthase, with varying degrees of hyperaldosteronism, which responds to exogenous glucocorticoids. FH type II is an autosomal dominant disorder of both the aldosterone-producing adenoma (APA) and idiopathic hyperaldosteronism (IHA).

Clinical Presentation

The clinical picture varies from asymptomatic to symptoms related to hypertension, hypokalemia, or both. Patients may have headaches, polyuria, nocturia, polydipsia, parasthesias, weakness, and muscle cramps. There are no specific physical findings. The degree of hypertension is usually moderate to severe, and may be refractory to conventional antihypertensive agents. Malignant hypertension and leg edema are rare. The left ventricular hypertrophy is disproportionate to the level of blood pressure and improves after treatment of hyperaldosteronism, even if hypertension persists.

Routine laboratory tests may show slightly high serum sodium levels (143-147 mEq/L), hyperglycemia, hypokalemia, metabolic alkalosis, and hypomagnesemia. Although most patients with hyperaldosteronism are not hypokalemic, a low serum potassium level may be noted, either spontaneously or after thiazide or loop diuretic use. Hypokalemia may be severe and difficult to correct. Its presence reduces the secretion of aldosterone and thus should be corrected before the laboratory evaluation of hyperaldosteronism.

Diagnosis

The workup of a patient for primary hyperaldosteronism involves the following steps: screening tests for primary hyperaldosteronism, establishing the autonomy of aldosterone secretion, and determination of the source of hyperaldosteronism (Fig. 3).

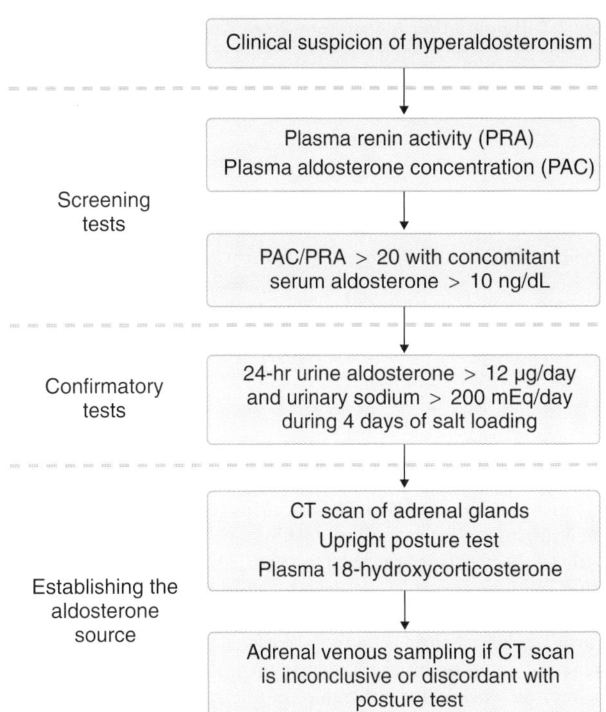

Figure 3 Algorithm for workup of patients with suspected primary hyperaldosteronism. Plasma 18-hydroxycorticosterone level higher than 100 ng/dL is suggestive of an aldosterone-producing adenoma. CT, computed tomography.

The following categories of patients should be tested with priority for primary hyperaldosteronism:

- Hypertensive patients with spontaneous or thiazide-induced hypokalemia
- Hypertensive patients resistant to therapy
- Hypertensive patients with adrenal incidentalomas

Screening Tests

Although hypokalemia in a hypertensive patient is suggestive of hyperaldosteronism, normokalemia does not exclude the diagnosis. Up to 60% of patients with hyperaldosteronism do not have hypokalemia. Adequate sodium intake may be necessary to unmask the hypokalemia. Measurement of the 24-hour urinary potassium level can be useful in assessing the cause of a low potassium level, including surreptitious vomiting or laxative abuse. Inappropriate urinary potassium excretion of more than 30 mEq/24 hours in a patient with hypokalemia suggests primary hyperaldosteronism, especially if plasma renin activity (PRA) is low.

The ratio of the plasma aldosterone concentration (PAC) to PRA (PAC/PRA) is the best screening test for primary hyperaldosteronism. The test can be done while the patient is on antihypertensive medications (except spironolactone and eplerenone), without requiring postural stimulation. Both spironolactone and eplerenone should be discontinued for 6 weeks before biochemical testing and after the potassium level reaches the normal range. A PAC/PRA above 20, with a concomitant PAC above 10 ng/dL, needs to be pursued by confirmatory tests (see Fig. 3). Low or suppressed PRA during therapy with angiotensin-converting enzyme (ACE) inhibitors or angiotensin receptor blockers (ARBs) suggests hyperaldosteronism.

Table 2 Differentiating Aldosterone-Producing Adenoma From Idiopathic Hyperaldosteronism*

Parameter	APA	IHA
HTN, potassium concentration [K⁺]	HTN more severe, higher likelihood of hypokalemia	HTN less severe, less likelihood of hypokalemia
Upright posture test	Decrease or <30% increase of serum aldosterone level	Increase by >30% of serum aldosterone level
18-Hydroxycorticosterone	>100 ng/mL	<100 ng/mL
Computed tomography scan	>1-cm adrenal tumor, with normal contralateral adrenal	No adrenal tumor, bilateral thickening of adrenals
Bilateral adrenal venous sampling	Lateralization	No lateralization

*Clinical, biochemical, and radiologic findings.
APA, aldosterone-producing adenoma; HTN, hypertension; IHA, idiopathic hyperaldosteronism.

Establishing Autonomous Aldosterone Secretion. An elevated PAC/PRA by itself is not diagnostic for hyperaldosteronism and must be confirmed by a 24-hour urinary aldosterone level determined during 4 days of oral salt loading by adding one flat teaspoon of salt to the meals every day. Diuretics, ACE inhibitors, and ARBs should be discontinued for 2 weeks before the tests and potassium needs to be replaced to the normal range. Hypertension may be controlled by calcium channel blockers, beta blockers, or α_1-adrenergic receptor blockers, which do not significantly affect the biochemical workup for hyperaldosteronism. Potassium supplementation is stopped in most patients without any underlying heart disease at the beginning of the salt-loading test. During day 4 of salt loading, a 24-hour urine sample must be collected by the patient for aldosterone, sodium, potassium, and creatinine level testing. A urinary sodium level higher than 200 mEq/24 hours confirms an adequate salt load. An aldosterone level higher than 12 µg/day during salt loading is almost always diagnostic of hyperaldosteronism. Hypokalemia with an inappropriately high urine potassium loss supports the diagnosis. Another supportive measure is correction of hypokalemia with the addition of aldactone at the end of biochemical workup.

IV administration of 2 L of isotonic saline over 4 hours in the recumbent patient is a less favored way to establish the diagnosis. A plasma aldosterone level higher than 10 ng/dL at the end of the infusion supports the diagnosis of primary hyperaldosteronism. The test may entail risk in older patients, those with uncontrolled hypertension, or those with decompensated heart disease.

Establishing the Source of Aldosterone Excess. Because of differences in therapy, distinguishing an aldosterone-producing adenoma APA and idiopathic hyperaldosteronism is important (Table 2). Patients with an APA generally have more severe hypertension, more frequent hypokalemia, higher plasma (>25 ng/dL) and urinary (>30 µg/24 hr) aldosterone levels, and are younger (<50 years). The APA is typically hypodense and smaller than 2 cm on a CT scan of the adrenals. The presence of a solitary adrenal tumor with a normal contralateral adrenal gland is usually consistent with an APA. Determination of plasma aldosterone levels before and 2 hours after an upright posture (with ambulation) and a plasma 18-hydroxycorticosterone level can further help distinguish APA from IHA. Patients with a solitary adrenal tumor, a plasma 18-hydroxycorticosterone level higher than 100 ng/dL, and no significant increase (less than 30%) or a paradoxical decrease in the aldosterone level during a posture test are presumed to have an APA and should be referred for surgery. Patients with an inconclusive adrenal CT scan or discordant results are referred for adrenal venous sampling.

Adrenal venous sampling is technically difficult because the right adrenal vein is small. Adrenal venous sampling is performed during continuous ACTH infusion and relies on demonstration of a gradient for plasma aldosterone in unilateral disease. The cortisol level should be measured to confirm proper catheter placement.

Treatment

The treatment goals are to reduce the morbidity and mortality associated with hypertension, hypokalemia, and cardiovascular damage by normalization of blood pressure and aldosterone levels. Unilateral adrenalectomy, usually by a laparoscopic approach, results in normalization of hypokalemia and improvement in hypertension in all patients. About 50% of patients continue to have a milder hypertension. The blood pressure response to spironolactone before surgery often predicts the blood pressure response to surgery in those with an APA.

Medical treatment is reserved for patients with IHA or those with APAs who are poor surgical candidates. Spironolactone, 50 to 200 mg/day, is the treatment of choice. Side effects include painful gynecomastia, nausea, headaches, impotence, and irregular menstruation. Serum potassium and magnesium levels should be monitored to avoid hyperkalemia and hypomagnesemia. Eplerenone is a steroid-based antimineralocorticoid that blocks the aldosterone receptor selectively and has a better side effect profile. However, spironolactone is the favored initial treatment, because it is more potent and costs less. Alternatively, potassium-sparing diuretics such as amiloride or triamterene may be used, but they lack the mineralocorticoid receptor antagonist benefits.

For the first few weeks after surgery, patients should increase their salt intake to compensate for hypoaldosteronism that may occur because of chronic suppression of the renin-angiotensin system. The use of a mineralocorticoid is usually not necessary.

Summary

- Hypokalemia may not be present in up to 60% of patients with primary hyperaldosteronism.
- The ratio of plasma aldosterone concentration to plasma renin activity (PAC/PRA) is the best screening test for primary hyperaldosteronism.
- Spironolactone and eplerenone should be discontinued for 6 weeks before biochemical testing and potassium needs to be replaced to the normal range.
- Adrenal venous sampling is of value in some patients with primary hyperaldosteronism to differentiate between an aldosterone-producing adenoma and idiopathic hyperaldosteronism

Glucocorticoid-Remediable Hyperaldosteronism

Familial hyperaldosteronism type I, or glucocorticoid-remediable hyperaldosteronism (GRH), is an autosomal dominant disease in which aldosterone is synthesized in the zona fasciculata of the adrenal gland under the control of ACTH.[6] Affected individuals are usually younger than 40 years, exhibit hypertension resistant to standard therapy, and have a family history of primary hyperaldosteronism or a cerebrovascular accident at a young age. Most patients have a normal serum potassium level.

Similar to other causes of primary hyperaldosteronism, the PAC/PRA ratio is higher than 20. A 2-day low-dose DST (0.5 mg dexamethasone orally, every 6 hours) will suppress aldosterone to levels lower than 4 ng/dL. The test is not specific. A very high urinary 18-hydroxycortisol level (>3000 nmol/24 hr) or genetic testing to detect a chimeric gene establishes the diagnosis. Genetic testing for glucocorticoid-remediable aldosteronism (GRA) is available for no charge through the International Registry for Glucocorticoid-Remediable Aldosteronism (available at www.brighamandwomens.org/gra). Affected individuals should have neurovascular screening for cerebral aneurysms. Treatment with glucocorticoids is effective to normalize blood pressure. Eplerenone, spironolactone, amiloride, and triamterene have also been used successfully.

National Guidelines

There are no consensus statements for the evaluation and therapy of patients with hyperaldosteronism. Although some experts have advocated screening all hypertensive patients for hyperaldosteronism, we recommend screening only high-risk patients. The PAC/PRA ratio is widely accepted as the best initial screening test, with some variations in cutoff values because of differences in patient preparation (e.g., diet, medications, position) or assays used.

There is some disagreement about the role of adrenal venous sampling in patients with biochemical proof of hyperaldosteronism. Adrenal venous sampling is selectively used in some centers, whereas some other centers perform the test in almost all patients.[7] In our opinion, if there is a clear adenoma on CT scan on one of the adrenals and the results of the posture test also suggest APA, the patient can be assumed to have the disease and should be referred for surgery. Surgery for APA is more cost-effective than long-term medical therapy.[8]

Pheochromocytoma

Pheochromocytomas (PHEOs) are rare chromaffin cell tumors that may occur at any age. Although their true prevalence is unknown, they occur in about 0.3% of hypertensive patients. If untreated, the disease can have severe consequences, such as myocardial infarction, heart failure, cerebrovascular accident, and death.

Anatomic Considerations and Etiology

Most PHEOs are benign, sporadic, unilateral, and located within the adrenal gland. Extra-adrenal pheochromocytomas (paragangliomas) occur in about 15% of cases in the superior and inferior para-aortic areas, including the Zuckerkandl organ (75%), bladder (10%), thorax (10%), and head, neck, and pelvis (5%). Paragangliomas tend to occur in younger patients (<20 years) and are uncommon in those older than 60 years. They are multifocal in about 15% to 30% of cases. Bilateral adrenal pheochromocytomas (5%-10% of cases) are usually seen as part of familial syndromes. Malignant pheochromocytomas (10% of adrenal cases) have a higher prevalence in ectopic PHEOs and lower prevalence in familial PHEOs. No clinical, imaging, or laboratory criteria absolutely predict malignancy; tumors larger than 5 cm have a greater potential to metastasize. The diagnosis of malignant pheochromocytoma relies on the presence of metastases and not on the histology of the tumor.

About 10% to 15% of PHEOs are hereditary in nature. Familial predisposition to pheochromocytoma is seen in patients with multiple endocrine neoplasia (MEN) types IIA and IIB, von Hippel-Lindau disease, neurofibromatosis type 1, and familial paragangliomas. Genetic screening in patients with apparently sporadic pheochromocytoma is recommended for the following categories of patients: age younger than 20 years, bilateral disease, multiple paragangliomas, or family history of pheochromocytoma or paraganglioma.

Clinical Manifestations

Patients with PHEO may have paroxysmal hypertension (48%) or persistent hypertension (29%), or be normotensive (13%).[9] Wide fluctuations in blood pressure and resistance to antihypertensive medications are typical of those with pheochromocytoma. Norepinephrine-secreting tumors are associated with sustained hypertension and norepinephrine and epinephrine-secreting tumors are associated with labile hypertension. Large cystic PHEOs may not be associated with hypertension because most of the catecholamines are metabolized within the tumor before being released into circulation. Those with a familial form of PHEO are also more likely to be normotensive.

The triad of headaches, palpitations, and diaphoresis suggests the diagnosis of PHEO, but absence of these symptoms does not exclude the disease. Attacks are usually precipitated by emotional stress, exercise, anesthesia, abdominal pressure, or ingestion of tyramine-containing foods. Both pallor and flushing may be seen in patients. Other symptoms include orthostatic hypotension, weight loss, dyspnea, polyuria, polydipsia, visual blurring, focal neurologic symptoms, and change in mental status.

Diagnosis

Testing for PHEO is indicated for any patient with suggestive clinical manifestations. Priority has to be assigned to monitoring patients with the following:[9]

- Episodic symptoms of headaches, tachycardia, and diaphoresis (with or without hypertension)
- Family history of PHEO or familial syndromes that may include PHEO
- Adrenal incidentalomas
- Unexplained paroxysms of tachyarrythmias or bradyarrythmias or hypertension during intubation, induction of anesthesia, parturition, or prolonged and unexplained postoperative hypotension
- Adverse cardiovascular reactions to certain drugs, including anesthetic agents, beta blockers, glucagon, tricyclic antidepressants, histamine, phenothiazine, and tyramine-containing foods
- Spells or attacks during exertion, movements of torso, straining, coitus, or micturition

No single test achieves 100% diagnostic accuracy. Plasma-free metanephrines (total free normetanephrine and metanephrine) have 99% and 97% sensitivity, respectively, for sporadic and familial PHEOs, but there is approximately a 10% to 15% false-positive rate for sporadic PHEO. Clinicians should be familiar with their assay's diagnostic characteristics. In general, a plasma-free metanephrine level more than three or four times the upper normal has 100% specificity for PHEO. Renal failure is only associated with mild increases in plasma-free metanephrine levels. If the plasma-free metanephrine concentration is normal, no other diagnostic test is necessary except in those with small tumors found during workup for familial disease, patients with a history of PHEO or, rarely, patients with a dopamine-producing paraganglioma.

Patients with indeterminate levels of plasma-free metanephrines should have their urinary metanephrine and serum catecholamine levels measured (Fig. 4). Urinary total metanephrine levels higher than 1.8 mg/day are diagnostic for PHEO. Total plasma catecholamine (norepinephrine plus epinephrine) concentration higher than 2000 pg/mL is diagnostic of PHEO, values between 1000 and 2000 pg/mL are highly suggestive of the disease, and values lower than 1000 pg/mL in a patient with severe signs and symptoms at the time of sampling almost always rules out the disease. Urinary vanillylman-

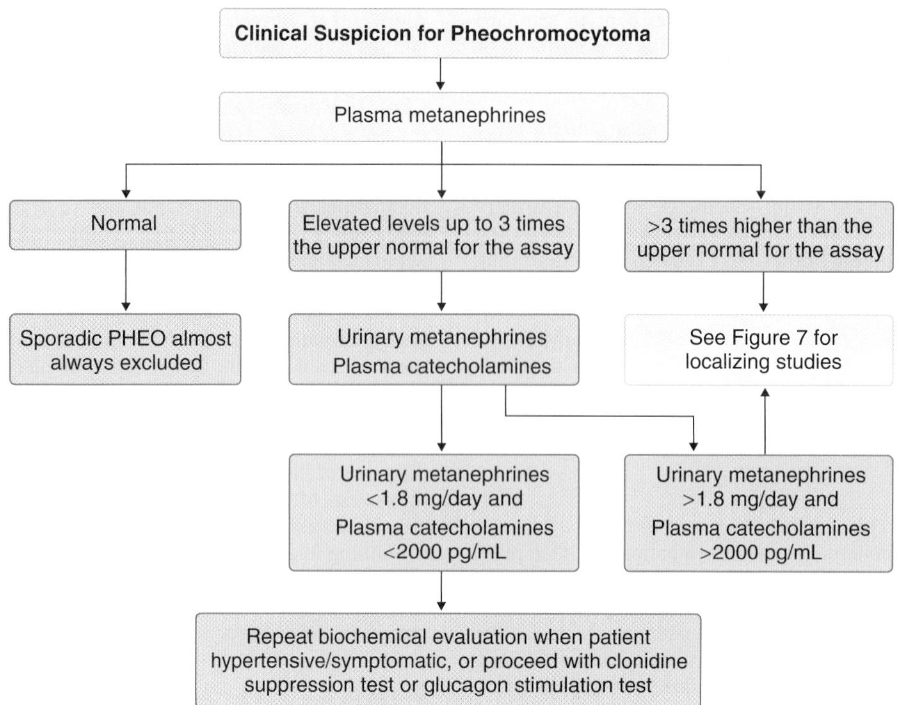

Figure 4 **Algorithm for biochemical evaluation of patients with suspected pheochromocytoma.** A false-positive result caused by drugs needs to be excluded (see Box 3).

delic acid (VMA) measurement has a high false-negative rate (41%) and should not be used for screening purposes, but a positive result has approximately 86% and 99% specificity for sporadic and hereditary PHEOs, respectively.

In patients with nondiagnostic ranges of plasma and urine catecholamine and metanephrine levels, and clinical features suggestive of PHEO, repeating the measurements at the time of symptoms or proceeding with dynamic testing may be used to support or exclude the diagnosis.[10] Clonidine normally suppresses plasma catecholamines, a response that is lost in PHEO. During the clonidine suppression test, clonidine, 0.3 mg, is administered orally and plasma catecholamine and metanephrine levels are measured before and 3 hours after clonidine is administered. Normalization of the plasma metanephrine level or a decrease in the plasma catecholamine levels by at least 50%, into the normal range for the assay, is considered a normal response.

The list of medications and interfering substances varies according to what is measured-plasma or urine catecholamines or their metabolites-and to the specific assay used. Thus, it is usually more practical to try to avoid all of them (Box 3). Patients should abstain from caffeinated beverages and alcohol for 24 hours and medications listed in Box 3 for 3 to 5 days before biochemical evaluation. Selective $alpha_1$ blockers (e.g., doxazosin), calcium channel blockers, and beta blockers such as metoprolol or atenolol can be used for blood pressure control during biochemical evaluation and do not cause any significant false-positive results. Because of the potential for inducing a hypertensive crisis, beta blockers should never be used without simultaneously using alpha blockers.

Box 3 Medications and Stimulants to Avoid Before Measurement of Plasma and Urinary Catecholamines and Metanephrines

Tricyclic antidepressants
Acetaminophen
Phenoxybenzamine
Monoamine oxidase inhibitors
Antipsychotics
Buspirone
Sympathomimetics-ephedrine, pseudoephedrine, amphetamines, albuterol
Stimulants-caffeine, nicotine, theophylline
Miscellanous-levodopa, carbidopa, alcohol, cocaine

Caffeinated beverages and alcohol should preferably be avoided for 24 hours. Medications should be stopped for 3 to 5 days, except labetalol, which needs to be discontinued for 2 weeks (causes analytic interference with some assays).

Imaging Studies

PHEO is diagnosed in about 6.5% of incidentally discovered adrenal tumors. PHEOs are usually larger than 3 cm in diameter and tend to be cystic, with areas of necrosis with increased size. In a patient suspected to have PHEO, CT scanning of the abdomen and pelvis should be performed first, followed by CT of the chest and neck if no tumor is found (Fig. 5). An adrenal tumor with a noncontrast Hounsfield unit (HU) lower than 10 is extremely unlikely to be PHEO. In a review of more than 30 proven PHEO cases at the Cleveland Clinic, all patients had a noncontrast CT scan HU of more than 20.[11]

Chemical shift MRI has a sensitivity of 93% to 100% and specificity of approximately 50% in detecting pheochromocytomas. The low lipid content of PHEO tumors results in a signal intensity decrease from the in-phase to opposed-phase T_1-weighted image. PHEO tumors typically exhibit signal isointensity with the liver, kidneys, and muscle on T_1-weighted images and a characteristically bright, high signal intensity on T_2-weighted images (Fig. 6). We usually prefer CT scanning over MRI as the initial imaging study with a biochemical workup diagnostic for PHEO because of cost and widespread availability.

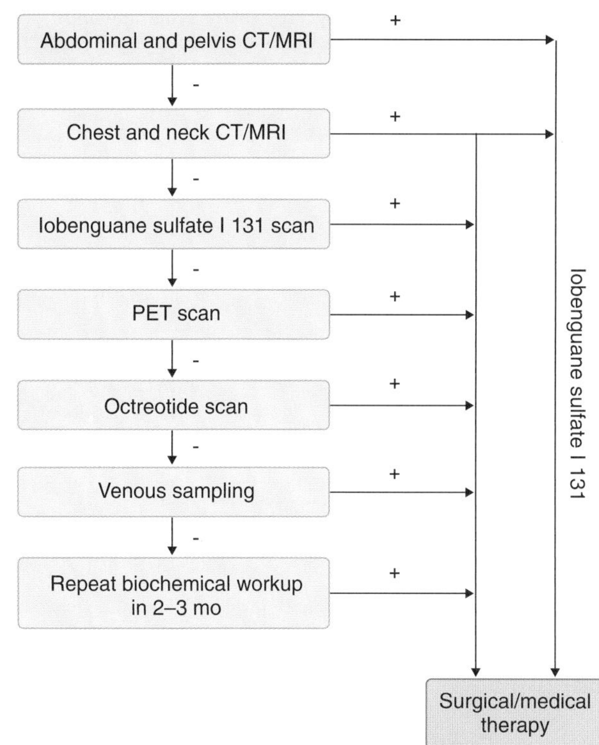

Figure 5 Algorithm for tumor localization in patients with biochemically proven pheochromocytoma (PHEO). Computed tomography (CT) or magnetic resonance imaging (MRI) of the abdomen and pelvis is the initial imaging of the choice. *In patients with positive findings on a CT or MRI scan, an iobenguane sulfate ^{131}I scan may be considered for those with familial PHEO, age younger than 20 years, ectopic PHEO, and tumors larger than 5 cm. PET, positron emission tomography.

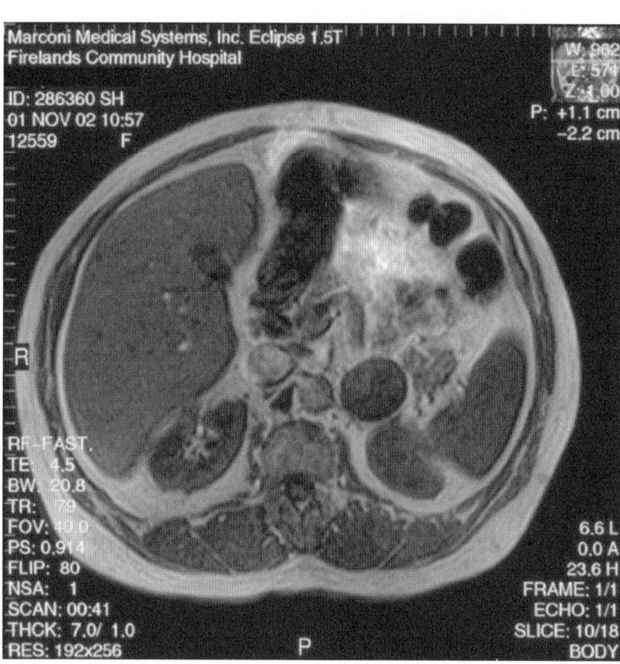

Figure 6 T1- and T2-weighted MRI images of a left adrenal mass in a patient with pheochromocytoma. The adrenal mass shows the characteristic high signal intensity on the T2-weighted image.

Functional imaging using iobenguane sulfate ^{131}I (formerly called meta-iodobenzylguanidine [MIBG]) should be used when multiple or metastatic tumors are suspected, such as in younger patients (<20 years), those with familial pheochromocytoma, tumors larger than 5 cm, or an extra-adrenal tumor, or when CT and MRI fail to localize the tumor despite biochemical evidence supporting the diagnosis of pheochromocytoma (see Fig. 5). The specificity of iobenguane sulfate ^{131}I is very high, 95% to 100%, and the sensitivity is about 85%. Nasal decongestants, some antihypertensives, antidepressants, antipsychotics, and cocaine affect iobenguane sulfate ^{131}I uptake and have to be withheld for 1 to 3 days before the study. Labetolol in particular has been shown to decrease iobenguane sulfate ^{131}I uptake. Uptake of iodine by the thyroid gland should be blocked with potassium iodide (SSKI; five drops three times a day, starting on the day of iobenguane sulfate ^{131}I and 3 days afterward). If the iobenguane sulfate ^{131}I study is negative, fluorodeoxyglucose positron emission tomography (PET) scanning or oxidronate (Octreoscan) may be used with some success for visualization (see Fig. 5).

Treatment

Surgical resection is the treatment of choice for pheochromocytoma. Adequate medical preparation is essential and usually achieved in 10 to 14 days. α_1-Adrenergic receptor blockers (e.g., doxazosin) are first-line therapy, with increasing dosage as tolerated. Beta blockers (e.g., metoprolol, atenolol) are added if tachycardia develops while the patient is adequately hydrated. Beta blockers should be added only after alpha blockade has been instituted to prevent unopposed alpha receptor activation, which may result in hypertensive crisis. Calcium channel blockers (CCBs) can be used for medical preparation or may be added if there is persistent or labile hypertension. The nonspecific α_1-adrenergic blocker phenoxybenzamine has a greater side effect profile and may result in prolonged hypotension after surgery.

Surgery for PHEO has shifted from the open conventional procedure to the laparoscopic approach over the past decade. Patients should have electrocardiography and cardiac echocardiography before surgery, with further cardiac evaluation if any abnormality is detected. It is preferable that patients be admitted to the hospital 1 day before surgery for close observation. In those with orthostatic hypotension, an isotonic saline infusion at a rate of 100 to 200 mL/hr should be started. Close blood pressure monitoring is necessary during surgery. The anesthesia team should be familiar with the care of patients with PHEO during surgery. After surgery, blood pressure and blood glucose levels need to be closely monitored, antihypertensive agents withheld, and normal saline infusion continued. Fluid overload should also be avoided. Antihypertensive agents may be resumed if the patient continues to be hypertensive. Lifelong follow-up is necessary for all patients, with closer follow-up of those with familial, large, extra-adrenal, or bilateral tumors.

Acute hypertensive crises can be treated with IV nitroprusside, nitroglycerin, the short-acting α-adrenergic blocker phentolamine (competitive α_1-adrenergic and weak α_2-adrenergic receptor antagonist), magnesium sulfate, or nicardipine, a calcium channel blocker. Metastatic lesions should also be resected if possible. In patients with aggressive tumors, combination chemotherapy (cyclophosphamide, vincristine, dacarbazine) or iobenguane sulfate ^{131}I-tagged radiotherapy may be considered, but results have not been promising.

National Guidelines

There are no consensus statements for the evaluation and therapy of PHEO patients. Most experts' opinions are based on personal experience in centers with large referral bases. Although there are still disagreements about the best initial screening test for PHEO, serum metanephrine or 24-hour urinary metanephrine level determination appears to be the most favored initial test of choice.

Summary

- The triad of headaches, palpitations, and diaphoresis suggests the diagnosis of pheochromocytoma, but absence of these symptoms do not exclude the disease.
- Beta blockers should not be used in patients with suspected pheochromocytoma until alpha blockade has been instituted.
- Plasma-free metanephrines have 99% and 97% sensitivity for sporadic and familial pheochromocytomas, respectively. However, there is approximately a 10% to 15% false-positive rate for sporadic pheochromocytoma.
- Adequate medical preparation is essential and should be initiated at least 10 to 14 days before surgery.

Adrenal Hyperandrogenism

The adrenal glands are an important source of androgens, especially in children and women. The primary adrenal androgens, dehydroepiandrosterone (DHEA) and dehydroepiandrosterone sulfate (DHEAS sulfate), are under ACTH control and have little intrinsic androgenic activity. However, they are converted to androstenedione and then to testosterone (and estrogen) in both the adrenal gland and peripheral tissues. DHEA and DHEA sulfate are responsible for adrenarche (pubic hair development). Peak levels occur in the third decade of life and decline progressively to 25% of peak levels around the age of 80 years.

Clinical Manifestations

Features of adrenal androgen excess differ with age and gender. In female neonates, androgen excess causes female pseudohermaphroditism (ambiguous genitalia). Male infants exhibit penile enlargement.

In prepubertal children, boys and girls, androgen excess manifests as increased rate of growth in height and skeletal maturation, leading to premature epiphyseal fusion and short adult height. In addition, boys exhibit penile enlargement, hair growth in androgen-dependent areas, deepening of the voice, and other secondary sexual characteristics (isosexual precocious puberty). Girls have hirsutism, acne, and clitoromegaly (heterosexual precocious puberty).

Androgen excess with onset at puberty causes premature skeletal maturation and short adult height in boys. In girls, it manifests as primary or secondary amenorrhea, different degree of virilization, and increased skeletal maturation, resulting in short adult height.

Manifestations of androgen excess with onset at adult age are limited in men. A decrease in size of the testicles, testosterone secretion, and spermatogenesis caused by inhibition of gonadotropin secretion may occur. In women, hirsutism, acne, menstrual irregularities, male pattern baldness, infertility, decreased breast tissue, increased muscle mass, android body habitus, and clitoromegaly may occur, depending on the degree of hyperandrogenism.

Of the various causes of adrenal hyperandrogenism, nonclassic (adult-onset) congenital adrenal hyperplasia (CAH), and androgen-producing adrenal tumors are discussed in this section. Exogenous androgen intake for body building or to increase erythropoiesis may cause acne, hirsutism, and oligomenorrhea or amenorrhea in women and small testes, gynecomastia, and impaired spermatogenesis in men. Hyperprolactinemia may cause an increase in serum DHEAS and androstenedione levels by direct stimulation of the adrenal gland.

Table 3 Differences Between Polycystic Ovary Syndrome and 21-Hydroxylase-Deficient Nonclassic Congenital Adrenal Hyperplasia

Parameter	PCOS	NCAH
Prevalence in reproductive age women	4%-6%	0.1%-0.05%
Prevalence in hyperandrogenic patients	50%-80%	1%-10%
Racial, ethnic distribution	No predilection	Predominantly white or Ashkenazic Jews
Inheritance mechanism	Complex trait	Autosomal recessive
Specific hormonal diagnosis	None	ACTH-stimulated 17-HP >15 ng/mL

ACTH, adrenocorticotropic hormone; 17-HP, 17-hydroxyprogesterone; NCAH, nonclassic congenital adrenal hyperplasia; PCOS, polycystic ovary syndrome.

Nonclassic Congenital Adrenal Hyperplasia

Nonclassic congenital adrenal hyperplasia (NCAH) is an autosomal recessive disorder, with most patients exhibiting a defect in 21-hydoxylase enzyme activity, resulting in decreased cortisol production. The associated increased ACTH secretion stimulates adrenal steroid production upstream of the defective enzyme, resulting in increased androgen secretion. Hyperandrogenic symptoms are usually diagnosed in late puberty and early adulthood. NCAH affects from 1% to 10% of hyperandrogenic women, depending on their ethnic background. It is rare among African Americans. The main differential diagnosis for NCAH is polycystic ovary syndrome (PCOS), which is about 40 to 50 times more common (Table 3).[12] Distinguishing the two only on clinical grounds is difficult, because both can be associated with varying degrees of hyperandrogenism and ovulatory dysfunction. (See elsewhere in this text, "Polycystic Ovary Syndrome," for further discussion.) DHEAS and testosterone levels are not reliable in differentiating the two. The diagnosis of NCAH is established based on a basal or post–250-µg cosyntropin-stimulated level of 17-hydoxyprogesterone higher than 15 ng/mL (45 nmol/L). Morning basal 17-hydroxyprogesterone levels during the follicular phase of the menstrual cycle (shortly after spontaneous or induced vaginal bleeding) lower than 2 ng/mL essentially rules out NCAH. The diagnosis can usually be confirmed by genotyping.

Glucocorticoids, oral contraceptives (OCPs), antiandrogens such as aldactone, or a combination of these medications are used to treat women with NCAH. OCPs and antiandrogens are usually adequate for therapy when fertility is not desired. Glucocorticoid therapy is often necessary when the patient plans to get pregnant. Prednisone, 2.5 mg orally twice daily, is our preferred initial glucocorticoid therapy, with further adjustment depending on androgen levels. Both CAH and NCAH are associated with an increased incidence of adrenal adenomas and testicular adrenal rest tumors.[13] This warrants CT scanning of the adrenal glands and testicular ultrasonography (men) in patients with biochemical confirmation. The consensus statement from the Lawson Wilkins Pediatric Endocrine Society and the European Society for Pediatric Endocrinology about CAH almost exclusively discusses the diagnosis and management of the classic form of the disease. The National Institutes of Health sponsored a clinical staff conference about CAH and NCAH in 1999.[13]

Summary

- Nonclassic congenital adrenal hyperplasia (NCAH) is mostly caused by a defect in the 21-hydroxylase enzyme and manifests as hyperandrogenism in young adolescent and adult women.
- The main differential diagnosis for NCAH is polycystic ovary syndrome, which is about 40 to 50 times more common.
- The diagnosis of NCAH is established in most patients by measurement of the 17-hydroxyprogesterone response to 250 μg of cosyntropin.

Androgen-Secreting Adrenal Tumors

Primary adrenocortical carcinoma may be associated with excess androgen secretion. Production of steroid intermediates and sometimes cortisol may also occur. It is a rare disease, with an incidence of 1 per 600,000 to 1,600,000 and a prevalence of 4 to 12 per 1,000,000. Female patients may exhibit virilization with very high levels of DHEA sulfate (500 μg/dL or higher), testosterone, and urinary 17-ketosteroids. Primary adrenocortical carcinomas are highly malignant, with a poor prognosis. Tumors are usually larger than 6 cm, invade the capsule, metastasize early, and typically recur after surgery. Surgical resection at an early stage, along with lifelong mitotane therapy starting soon after surgery, offers the only chance for cure or long-term remission. Androgen-secreting adrenal adenomas are rare, typically smaller than 4 cm, and are associated mostly with high levels of DHEAS and testosterone. Surgical resection is the therapy of choice.

Adrenal Incidentaloma

Definition and Prevalence

An adrenal incidentaloma is an adrenal mass larger than 1 cm in diameter discovered during radiologic examination done for a reason not related to the adrenal gland. The definition of incidentaloma excludes patients undergoing imaging procedures as part of staging and workup for cancer. Incidental adrenal masses are found in 0.5% to 5% of patients undergoing CT of the abdomen and in up to 9% of postmortem autopsies in unselected populations.

Evaluation

Management decisions are based on the need to address whether the tumor is functional (i.e., producing hormones) or malignant.

Evaluation for Hormonal Hypersecretion. Up to 35% of adrenal incidentalomas may be functional. All patients should undergo hormonal evaluation for Cushing's syndrome and pheochromocytoma, and those with hypertension should also be evaluated for hyperaldosteronism. Isolated excess androgen secretion by adrenal adenomas or carcinomas is rare. Thus, only women with an adrenal mass and physical findings suggestive of hyperandrogenism should have their testosterone and DHEAS levels measured.

Subclinical Cushing's syndrome (SCS) is a relatively recent and poorly described disorder, occurring in about 5% to 24% of patients with adrenal incidentalomas. The prevalence varies greatly, depending on the diagnostic criteria and the screening methods used. Patients do not have the typical signs and symptoms of Cushing's syndrome, but generally have increased frequency of hypertension, glucose intolerance, diabetes, and possibly osteopenia. We support the 2002 NIH consensus panel recommendation of a 1-mg overnight DST as the initial biochemical evaluation of choice. Some experts have recommended two or more of the following abnormal tests of the HPA axis for the diagnosis of SCS: lack of suppression during 1-mg overnight DST, increased urinary free cortisol levels, loss of diurnal cortisol rhythm, low or suppressed ACTH level, and impaired ACTH response to CRH. Development of adrenal insufficiency after surgical removal of the adrenal tumor is the best way to confirm the diagnosis.

Evaluation for Malignancy. Adrenal tumor size has been used to differentiate between benign and malignant adrenal masses. Risk of malignancy increases with adrenal tumor size. Cutoff values ranging from 4 to 6 cm have been proposed by different clinicians for surgical resection of adrenal masses. In spite of a relationship between the risk of malignancy and adrenal tumor size, there is a significant overlap, and even a cutoff value of 2 cm could not achieve a 100% specificity to rule out a malignant adrenal mass.[11]

A noncontrast CT attenuation coefficient (in HU) is the most promising imaging tool to differentiate benign adrenal masses from malignant tumors. Intracytoplasmic fat is often abundant in adrenal adenomas, but rare in adrenal metastases, pheochromocytoma, and adrenocortical carcinomas. Adrenal masses with a noncontrast HU of less than 10 are always benign.[11] The noncontrast HU is superior to adrenal size in differentiating benign from malignant adrenal tumors.

Some studies have reported the value of delayed enhancement washout percentage in attenuation value during CT scanning of the adrenal glands to differentiate lipid-poor adrenal adenomas (noncontrast HU of >10) from nonadenomas. An absolute enhancement washout percentage of less than 60% at 15 minutes postcontrast had 95% to 100% specificity in identifying nonadenomas.[14] This needs to be further validated by studies of large numbers of patients. MRI is another noninvasive method used to differentiate benign and malignant adrenal masses. Its sensitivity and specificity for diagnosis of a benign adrenal mass seem to be close to the noncontrast CT attenuation value.

Algorithm for Evaluation and Treatment of Adrenal Incidentalomas

Our approach to incidentally discovered adrenal masses is shown in Figure 7. We usually do not routinely obtain any follow-up imaging studies in nonfunctional adrenal masses with a noncontrast HU of less than 10. Such patients undergo annual follow-up evaluations for any excess hormone hypersecretion for 5 years and then intermittently afterward. We recommend that all adrenal tumors larger than 6 cm be surgically removed; however, myelolipoma is an exception, with a characteristically low attenuation value on noncontrast CT scan. Adrenal masses smaller than 6 cm with a noncontrast HU of more than 10 need to have their absolute percentage washout calculated at 15 minutes and undergo follow-up imaging studies in 6 to 12 months (see Fig. 7). There is no good evidence supporting continued radiologic surveillance if the follow-up study at 6 to 12 months shows no change in adrenal tumor size.

Fine-needle aspiration of an adrenal mass may be done to rule out metastasis once pheochromocytoma has been ruled out. Adrenal biopsy may not differentiate adrenocortical carcinomas from adenomas. Surgical resection of the adrenal mass is usually considered for patients with functional or malignant adrenal masses. Medical therapy may be acceptable in the case of primary hyperaldosteronism secondary to adrenocortical adenoma or hyperplasia.

National Guidelines

The National Institute of Health (NIH) held a state-of-the-science conference in February 2002, during which the management of adrenal incidentalomas was discussed by a 12-member panel.[15] The panel recommended measuring serum aldosterone levels and plasma renin activity only in patients with hypertension and an overnight

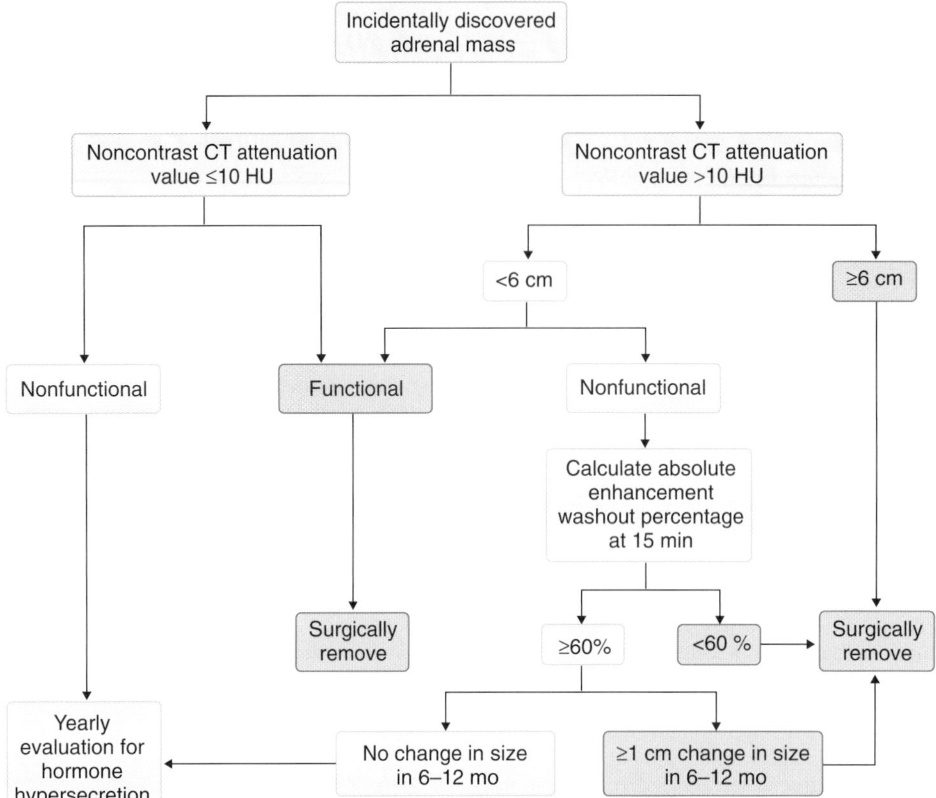

Figure 7 **Algorithm for evaluation of patients with adrenal incidentalomas.** Adrenal tumors with a noncontrast computed tomography (CT) Hounsfield unit (HU) of 10 or less are only followed for hormone hypersecretion. Masses with noncontrast CT HU of more than 10 and larger than 6 cm are surgically resected.

1-mg DST and plasma or urine metanephrine levels for all patients with an adrenal incidentaloma.

The panel recommended a noncontrast CT HU threshold of 10 as a reliable radiologic feature to differentiate benign from malignant adrenal tumors. The panel recommended surgical resection of all adrenal masses larger than 6 cm and a repeat CT scan in 6 to 12 months for those with adrenal incidentalomas that are not surgically removed. The panel concluded that there are no data supporting continued radiologic evaluation if an adrenal mass is stable in size. We usually do not obtain a routine follow-up imaging study in adrenal masses with a noncontrast CT HU of lower than 10, because the risk of developing a primary adrenocortical carcinoma from an adenomatous or hyperplastic adrenal mass is extremely rare.

Summary

- All patients with adrenal incidentaloma should undergo hormonal evaluation for Cushing's syndrome and pheochromocytoma and those with hypertension should also be evaluated for hyperaldosteronism.
- Adrenal masses with a noncontrast CT attenuation coefficient (in HU) of less than 10 are almost always benign.
- Fine-needle aspiration of an adrenal mass may be done to rule out metastasis once pheochromocytoma has been ruled out.

CONSIDERATIONS OF THE PHARMACOLOGIC USE OF GLUCOCORTICOIDS

Pharmacologic doses of synthetic glucocorticoids are used in a wide variety of diseases for their anti-inflammatory and immunosuppressive effects.

Endocrine Problems with Chronic Glucocorticoid Treatment

Two main clinical problems arise with the chronic use of pharmacologic doses of glucocorticoids, iatrogenically induced Cushing's syndrome and adrenal insufficiency on abrupt cessation of therapy. Cushing's syndrome may become clinically apparent within 1 month after onset of treatment. The duration of glucocorticoid therapy, the highest dose, and the total cumulative dose have long been considered important predictors of suppression of the HPA axis. Secondary adrenal insufficiency caused by exogenous steroid intake should be anticipated in any patient who takes more than 30 mg of hydrocortisone (or 7.5 mg prednisone) per day for more than 3 weeks.[16] Excluding depot glucocorticoid injections, therapy for less than 2 weeks rarely results in clinically significant suppression of HPA axis.

Alternate-day therapy and avoidance of nighttime doses are associated with less suppression of the HPA axis. The time to recovery of the HPA axis after discontinuation of glucocorticoid therapy is variable and can be as short as 2 to 5 days or as long as 9 to 12 months.

Inhaled glucocorticoid use for a long duration may result in suppression of the HPA axis. All topical glucocorticoids are absorbed to some extent, depending on the area of the body (intertriginous area absorption higher than forehead and scalp absorption; least absorption is in the forearm). Inflammation of the skin and application of occlusive dressings increase systemic absorption. Case reports have been published, with patients demonstrating a grossly cushingoid appearance after long-term use of steroid-containing topical creams or eye drops.

Recommendations for Glucocorticoid Treatment Withdrawal

There are two important issues that need particular attention when trying to wean a patient from chronic steroid therapy. First, the underlying condition for which the steroid therapy was initiated should always be kept in mind, and any tapering of the dose should be done accordingly. For example, too rapid tapering of glucocorticoid therapy in a patient with asthma may result in exacerbation of the underlying condition. Second, if the underlying disorder for which glucocorticoid therapy was initiated has been resolved, then a rapid tapering of the glucocorticoid dose to about 2 to 3 times the physiologic replacement dose is safe in most patients.

Our approach is to change different glucocorticoid preparations to hydrocortisone, 20 mg in the morning and 10 mg at noon, which after 2 to 4 weeks is changed to 20 mg hydrocortisone once daily in the morning. While on hydrocortisone therapy, patients are advised to double their dose for 2 to 3 days if they develop any acute illness. Patients are then followed at 1- to 2-month intervals, measuring the serum cortisol level during a CST after holding the morning hydrocortisone. A cortisol value higher than 18 μg/dL at 30 minutes during a low-dose (1 μg) or standard-dose (250 μg) CST indicates normal recovery of adrenal function. Those patients with levels between 14 and 18 μg/dL may only take hydrocortisone during acute illness, with re-evaluation of their adrenal axis at 2- to 3-month intervals to ensure full recovery. All patients chronically treated with glucocorticoids should wear medical alert tags and be instructed about supplemental coverage during infection or surgery and the need for parenteral glucocorticoid therapy if unable to tolerate oral medications.

Summary

- Secondary adrenal insufficiency caused by exogenous glucocorticoid intake should be anticipated in any patient who takes more 7.5 mg prednisone/day for longer than 3 weeks.
- Inhaled glucocorticoid use for long periods may result in suppression of the hypothalamic-pituitary-adrenal axis.
- Morning serum cortisol determination and the CST may be used to evaluate the recovery of adrenal function during glucocorticoid taper and withdrawal.

Suggested Readings

Annane D, Sebille V, Charpentier C, et al: Effect of treatment with low doses of hydrocortisone and fludrocortisone on mortality in patients with septic shock. JAMA 2002;288:862-871.

Arnaldi G, Angeli A, Atkinson AB, et al: Diagnosis and complications of Cushing's syndrome: A consensus statement. J Clin Endocrinol Metab 2003;88:5593-5602.

Bravo EL, Tagle R: Pheochromocytoma: State-of-the-art and future prospects. Endocr Rev 2003;24:539-553.

Caoili EM, Korobkin M, Francis IR, et al: Delayed enhanced CT of lipid-poor adrenal adenomas. AJR Am J Roentgenol 2000;175:1411-1415.

Cooper MS, Stewart PM: Corticosteroid insufficiency in acutely ill patients. N Engl J Med 2003;348:727-734.

Gordon RD, Stowasser M, Rutherford JC: Primary aldosteronism: Are we diagnosing and operating on too few patients? World J Surg 2001;25:941-947.

Grumbach MM, Biller BM, Braunstein GD, et al: Management of the clinically inapparent adrenal mass ("incidentaloma"). Ann Intern Med 2003;138:424-429.

Hamrahian AH, Ioachimescu AG, Remer EM, et al: Clinical utility of noncontrast computed tomography attenuation value (Hounsfield units) to differentiate adrenal adenomas/hyperplasias from nonadenomas: Cleveland Clinic experience. J Clin Endocrinol Metab 2005;90:871-877.

Hamrahian AH, Oseni TS, Arafah BM: Measurements of serum free cortisol in critically ill patients. N Engl J Med 2004;350:1629-1638.

Ilias I, Pacak K: Current approaches and recommended algorithm for the diagnostic localization of pheochromocytoma. J Clin Endocrinol Metab 2004;89:479-491.

Mayenknecht J, Diederich S, Bahr V, et al: Comparison of low and high dose corticotropin stimulation tests in patients with pituitary disease. J Clin Endocrinol Metab 1998;83:1558-1562.

McMahon GT, Dluhy RG: Glucocorticoid-remediable aldosteronism. Cardiol Rev 2004;12:44-48.

Merke DP, Bornstein SR, Avila NA, Chrousos GP: NIH conference. Future directions in the study and management of congenital adrenal hyperplasia caused by 21-hydroxylase deficiency. Ann Intern Med 2002;136:320-334.

Moran C, Azziz R: 21-Hydroxylase-deficient nonclassic adrenal hyperplasia: The great pretender. Semin Reprod Med 2003;21:295-300.

Sywak M, Pasieka JL: Long-term follow-up and cost benefit of adrenalectomy in patients with primary hyperaldosteronism. Br J Surg 2002;89:1587-1593.

Young WF Jr: Minireview: Primary aldosteronism-changing concepts in diagnosis and treatment. Endocrinology 2003;144:2208-2213.

References

For a complete list of references, log onto www.expertconsult.com.

Diabetes Mellitus: Disease Management

Byron J. Hoogwerf

Diabetes mellitus (DM) is historically characterized by hyperglycemia. The pathophysiologic processes causing hyperglycemia include insulin deficiency, impaired glucose disposal (insulin resistance), and increased hepatic glucose production. Type 1 diabetes mellitus (T1DM) results from an insulin deficiency state usually caused by immunologic damage to beta cells. Some patients with T1DM also have features of insulin resistance. Type 2 diabetes mellitus (T2DM) results from insulin resistance, often associated with central obesity, increased hepatic glucose production, and a progressive decline in beta cell function that is not immunologically mediated. Secondary forms of diabetes can occur as a result of pancreatectomy (insulin-deficient state), administration of glucocorticoids (glucocorticoid use may simply be unmasking a predisposition for diabetes), hemochromatosis, and rare syndromes such as antibodies to the insulin receptor. Gestational diabetes occurs during pregnancy as a result of production of glucose counterregulatory hormones; it and may be more common in patients genetically predisposed to develop T2DM.

This disease management article is limited to the common forms of diabetes, T1DM and T2DM. Approximately 20 million people in the United States have DM and one third are not aware of their diagnosis.

The processes by which hyperglycemia contributes to the complications of diabetes are not yet established. However, the following are considerations. Hyperglycemia is associated with the glycation of many proteins, including structural proteins. This can result in advanced glycation end products (AGEs), modified protein products that have been associated with many of the complications of diabetes. Glycation of low-density lipoprotein (LDL) makes it more susceptible to oxidation. Lipid oxidation is one of the proposed mechanisms for atherosclerosis. Hyperglycemia increases sorbitol accumulation in tissues and has been invoked as a mechanism for neuropathy and retinopathy. Hyperglycemia increases the concentration of protein kinase C β (PKC β) in the retina, which in turn is associated with increased concentrations of vascular endothelial cell growth factor (VEGF). VEGF contributes to the increased risk for proliferative changes in the eye and to loss of endothelial cell integrity and associated risk for macular edema.

DIAGNOSTIC CRITERIA

The diagnosis of diabetes is based on several findings. The following criteria have been established by the American Diabetes Association (ADA)[1]:

- Fasting glucose level higher than 126 mg/dL on two occasions. This fasting glucose value is consistently associated with the risk for retinopathy. This cut point value will miss a number of patients who have diabetes based on oral glucose tolerance testing results. Observational data suggest that this threshold fasting glucose for diagnosing diabetes may be too high, because patients with impaired glucose tolerance develop retinopathy.
- Random or casual glucose higher than 200 mg/dL, with symptoms of DM. This is a common way to diagnose DM. Many patients do not have obvious symptoms, but that should not alter the fact that a random blood glucose level in this range generally establishes the diagnosis of DM. This criterion is not affected by the time of the last meal.
- Oral glucose tolerance test (OGTT) result after a 75-g oral glucose load, 2-hour value higher than 200 mg/dL. The oral glucose tolerance test is not generally recommended in clinical practice. Such testing requires 3 days of high carbohydrate intake, and tests are not always reproducible.

Hemoglobin A_{1c} (HbA_{1c}) values are too insensitive to be used as a screening test for DM. Elevated values (e.g., higher than 6.2%) are usually associated with a diagnosis of DM, but patients can have DM with values below this range. Thus, elevated HbA_{1c} values are a specific test for the diagnosis of DM, but they are not highly sensitive.

LIFESTYLE TREATMENT

Medical Nutrition Treatment

Guidelines for medical nutrition therapy[2-7] have been established by the ADA and are summarized in Box 1. The primary focus of these guidelines is targeted to outcomes including glycemic control, weight reduction (as appropriate), blood pressure control, and a favorable lipid profile. There is clear evidence that excess saturated fat in the diet has a detrimental effect on lipid profiles, and therefore restriction of saturated fat is recommended. The data supporting absolute restriction of carbohydrates are not robust, so the ADA guidelines allow flexibility in intake of carbohydrates and nonsaturated fat. Separate guidelines have been published about the carbohydrate content and composition of the diet.[8]

The most important variable in prandial glycemic excursion is total carbohydrate intake. Low glycemic index foods consumed alone result in lower prandial glucose excursion than high glycemic index foods. However, in the context of a mixed meal, differences between low and high glycemic index foods are attenuated. The amount[8-10] and source[10,11] of carbohydrates are important determinants of postprandial glucose. The relative effects of each have been recently studied. Brand-Miller and colleagues[12,13] have reported that they analyzed the relative impact of the glycemic index and total carbohydrate content of individual foods on glycemic load—the product of glycemic index and total grams of carbohydrate—using linear regression analysis. Carbohydrate content (total grams) alone explained 68% of the variation in glycemic load, and the glycemic index of the food explained 49%. When total carbohydrate and glycemic index were both included in the regression analysis, the glycemic index accounted for 32% of the variation.

Restriction of alcohol and sodium is generally advised. Supplements are not necessary in patients who are otherwise consuming a well-balanced diet. Many recommendations for weight management propose restriction of calories based on the degree of obesity and propose 30 to 45 minutes of exercise 3 to 5 days a week. Exercise is an important component of any regimen for weight reduction and glycemic control. Other nutritional guidelines for patients with diabetes are generally consistent with the ADA guidelines.[5,14-28]

Exercise

Guidelines for exercise have not always been specific with regard to exact exercise prescriptions, especially regarding aerobic and resistance exercises.[14,29,30] The commonly proposed recommendation that

Box 1 Goals of Medical Nutrition Therapy

For All Persons With Diabetes
- Attain and maintain optimal metabolic outcomes, including the following:
  - Blood glucose levels in the normal range or as close to normal as is safely possible
  - Lipid and lipoprotein profile that reduces risk for macrovascular disease
  - Blood pressure levels that reduce risk for vascular disease
  - Modify nutrient intake and lifestyle as appropriate to prevent and treat obesity, dyslipidemia, cardiovascular disease, hypertension, and nephropathy.
- Improve health through healthy food choices and physical activity.
- Address individual nutritional needs, taking into consideration personal and cultural preferences and lifestyle while respecting the individual's wishes and willingness.

Specific Situations

Children and Adolescents with Type 1 Diabetes
- Provide adequate energy to ensure normal growth and development.
- Integrate insulin regimens into usual eating and physical activity habits.

Children and Adolescents with Type 2 Diabetes
- Facilitate changes in eating and physical activity habits that reduce insulin resistance and improve metabolic status.

Pregnant and Lactating Women
- Provide adequate energy and nutrients needed for optimal outcomes.

Older Adults
- Provide for the nutritional and psychosocial needs of aging adults.

Persons Treated with Insulin or Insulin Secretagogues
- Provide self-management education for treatment (and prevention) of hypoglycemia, acute illnesses, and exercise-related blood glucose problems.

Persons at Risk for Diabetes
- Decrease risk by encouraging physical activity and promoting food choices that facilitate moderate weight loss or at least prevent weight gain.

Adapted from Bantle JP, Wylie-Rosett J, Albright AL, et al: Nutrition recommendations and interventions for diabetes—2006: A position statement of the American Diabetes Association. Diabetes Care 2006;29:2140-2157.

150 minutes of moderate-intensity (or 90 minutes of vigorous) aerobic exercise a week is generally the amount of exercise required to achieve benefits on glycemic control and reduce coronary heart disease (CHD) risk and has been supported by ADA/American Heart Association (AHA) recommendations.[6,7]

Regular exercise is encouraged, but complications of diabetes need to be taken into account. Injury to patients with loss of sensation in their feet is a limitation for weight-bearing exercise. Because of risk of CHD in patients with diabetes, appropriate screening for CHD should be performed before patients engage in any rigorous exercise program.[14,17,29-32] Benefits of exercise include weight control and improved glycemic control, often due to improvement in insulin resistance.

COMPLICATIONS

The complications of diabetes include retinopathy, nephropathy, neuropathy, and increased risk for atherosclerotic vascular disease. Diabetes is the leading cause of blindness in young people and is comparable with macular degeneration as a cause of blindness in older adults. DM is the leading cause of end-stage renal disease requiring dialysis or transplantation. DM is the leading cause of nontraumatic amputations of the lower extremity, a result of peripheral neuropathy and peripheral vascular disease. DM is associated with a twofold to fivefold increased risk for CHD.[33]

Two large trials—the Diabetes Control and Complications Trial (DCCT) and the United Kingdom Prospective Diabetes Study (UKPDS)—have demonstrated clear relation between glucose control and the risks for retinopathy (onset and progression), nephropathy (measured by albuminuria), and neuropathy (clinical and electromyographic measures).[34-38] The relation between the degree of hyperglycemia and CHD risk has also been established.[39,40] Risk begins well below the glycemic threshold for the diagnosis of diabetes.[23,25-28,41,42]

Screening

Patients should be screened for diabetic complications (Table 1).

Diabetic Retinopathy

Dilated eye examinations by ophthalmologists or optometrists should be performed within 5 years of onset in T1DM and at the time of diagnosis in T2DM, because the actual date of onset is

Table 1 Microvascular Complications in Diabetes Mellitus: Screening and Interventions

Complication	Detection	Primary Prevention	Secondary Prevention
Retinopathy	Dilated eye examination (fundus photography) Intravenous fluorescein angiography Optical coherence imaging	Glycemic control BP control Lipid-lowering therapy (?)	Glycemic control BP control Laser therapy Lipid-lowering therapy (?) Corticosteroid injections (?) Anti-VEGF injections (?) PKC β therapy (?)
Nephropathy	Urine micoalbumin	Glycemic control BP control ACEI-ARB therapy (?) Lipid-lowering therapy (?)	Glycemic control BP control ACEI-ARB therapy Lipid-lowering therapy (?)
Neuropathy	Monofilament testing (see Fig. 1)[50]	Daily foot inspection	Proper footwear Podiatry management: foot calluses, ulcers, deformities*

*See elsewhere in this section, "Prevention and Treatment of Leg and Foot Ulcers in Diabetes Mellitus."

ACEI, angiotensin-converting enzyme inhibitor; ARB, angiotensin receptor blocker; BP, blood pressure; PKC β, protein kinase C β; VEGF, vascular endothelial cell growth factor.

unknown in T2DM.[14,29] Follow-up examinations should be performed annually in patients with no or minimal background retinopathy. More frequent follow-up examinations should be performed in patients who have more advanced retinopathy. Handheld ophthalmoscopy in the office may be able to detect diabetic retinopathy but offers limited view of the retina and difficulty detecting diabetic macular edema. Macular edema is a significant cause of vision loss in DM. Macular edema is easier to detect with binocular vision and, in difficult cases, IV fluorescein angiography and confocal microscopy are used. Technology is available for screening with fundus photographs obtained in the physician's office and then read by an experienced reader. However, these methods are not yet sufficiently standardized to use as routine screening tools.

Diabetic Nephropathy

The hallmark of early diabetic nephropathy is albumin excretion. Sensitive assays to detect very low levels of albumin, or microalbuminuria, have been available for many years.[14,29] The simplest screening measure is a spot urine test adjusted for the urine creatinine level. Timed overnight collections and 24-hour collections may also be used. In general, microalbuminuria is defined as more than 30 mg albumin per gram of creatinine (spot urine test) or 30 to 299 mg per 24 hours and more than 300 mg/g creatinine (or 24 hours) as albuminuria. Serum creatinine determinations should be performed at least annually in patients with albuminuria; when estimated glomerular filtration rate (GFR) values are declining, more-specific measures of GFR (most commonly, creatinine clearance) should be used.

Peripheral Neuropathy

Monofilament testing in the office is the easiest way to test for the insensate foot.[43-50] The 5.07-mm monofilament should be applied to the bottoms of the feet (Fig. 1).[50] Any loss of sensation is associated with an increased risk for ulcer formation. Any patient who has had a foot ulcer is at increased risk for further foot ulcers.

Patients should be instructed to look at their feet daily. Patients who have difficulty looking at their feet should have someone else look at their feet, especially if the patient has impaired vision, or should use a mirror, such as a magnifying shaving mirror, if they have trouble seeing the bottoms of their feet (see elsewhere in this section, "Prevention and Treatment of Leg and Foot Ulcers in Diabetes Mellitus").

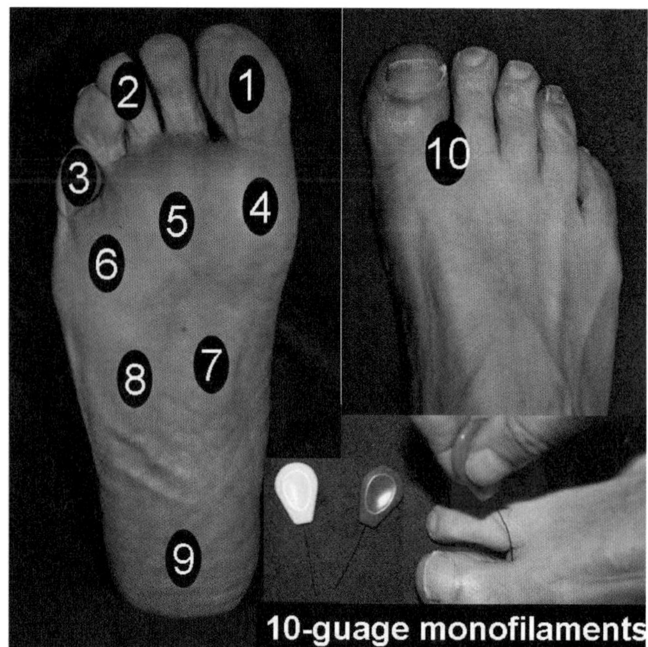

Figure 1 Nylon monofilament test. There is a risk of ulcer formation if the patient is unable to feel the monofilament when it is pressed against the foot with just enough pressure to bend the filament. The patient is asked to say "yes" each time that he or she feels the filament. Failure to feel the filament at 4 of 10 sites is 97% sensitive and 83% specific for identifying the loss of protective sensation. *(From Armstrong DG, Lavery LA: Diabetic foot ulcers: Prevention, diagnosis and classification. Am Fam Physician 1998;57:1325-1328.)*

Coronary Heart Disease

Careful questioning about symptoms of ischemic coronary disease is still one of the most important ways to screen for symptomatic disease. Many patients with diabetes do not have typical exertional chest pain. Consequently, clinicians must ask about reduced exercise tolerance, dyspnea, or exercise-induced nausea.

Various studies have considered the issue of screening for CHD.[14,17,29,51-54] The guidelines and individual recommendations are not entirely concordant. Whereas nearly every group suggests stress tests for patients with symptoms of CHD or electrocardiographic changes suggesting ischemia, recommendations on screening for asymptomatic disease are less consistent. The ADA considers that candidates for a screening cardiac stress test should include those with a history of peripheral or carotid occlusive disease; persons with a sedentary lifestyle, who are older than 55 years, and who plan to begin a vigorous exercise program; and two or more of the risk factors noted earlier.[29] The American Association of Clinical Endocrinologists (AACE) guidelines state:

> *Screening for asymptomatic coronary artery disease is an important consideration in patients with diabetes. An appropriate protocol for such screening has not been adequately tested. Increasing age, gender, cardiovascular risk factors, microalbuminuria, and retinopathy may identify high-risk groups for whom such testing is indicated.*[14]

The AHA consensus group has provided a thoughtful approach to screening for CHD in patients with diabetes. They noted:

> *Screening is defined here as the detection of disease in asymptomatic persons. Because screening tests are intended for widespread application, they should be rapid and inexpensive. In addition, to be useful, the results of testing should lead to a change in management, and the results of testing should improve outcome.*[17]

The American College of Cardiology (ACC)/AHA Guidelines for Exercise Testing give screening by exercise treadmill testing in patients with diabetes a data quality rating of IIb; that is, its usefulness or efficacy is less well established by evidence or opinion.[54] They add that exercise testing "might be useful in people with heightened pretest risk." Most consensus statements and guidelines on diabetes and CHD have suggested that noninvasive cardiac testing be performed in patients with diabetes and one additional criterion: peripheral arterial disease, cerebrovascular disease, rest changes on the electrocardiogram (ECG), or the presence of two or more major coronary vascular disease (CVD) risk factors. According to these guidelines, risk assessment begins with a medical history, including special attention to symptoms of atherosclerotic disease, such as angina, claudication, or erectile dysfunction. Electrocardiographic changes showing left ventricular hypertrophy and ST-T changes suggest increased cardiovascular risk. The ongoing DIAD study, which is designed to determine risk factors associated with clinically silent myocardial disease using stress tests with cardiac imaging, has suggested that the presence of neuropathy may be one of the most important predictors of cardiovascular risk.

It is not yet clear exactly how noninvasive testing changes risk management strategies in diabetes, because DM is already considered a coronary heart disease risk equivalent. Thus, noninvasive testing should be targeted as much as possible to detect patients who might have CHD amenable to surgical intervention. Whereas noninvasive screening in asymptomatic patients might detect disease amenable to percutaneous intervention or coronary artery bypass grafting, the cost-effectiveness and determination of how much such screening affects long-term outcomes are still uncertain.

I believe that careful attention to history of changes in exercise tolerance, atypical symptoms that suggest angina, or suggestive electrocardiographic abnormalities are reasons to consider stress testing. In addition, dyslipidemia, obesity, and hypertension, albuminuria and a family history of CHD may be reasons to consider stress testing in patients who do not have clinical symptoms of CHD. This approach is most consistent with the AACE guidelines and should select patients at highest risk for CHD. In the absence of robust evidence, as noted by the AHA, physicians still need to make decisions about patients who might have silent myocardial disease. Soon, imaging techniques such as computed tomography (CT) angiography will help characterize patients at risk for an acute event, even in the absence of symptoms.

Management of Coronary Heart Disease Risk

Dyslipidemia. Guidelines for the management of dyslipidemia have been published by the National Cholesterol Education Program (NCEP; several expert panels since 1988), AACE, ACP, ADA, ACC, and AHA (Table 2). They are generally consistent in recommending aggressive lipid-lowering management in diabetes, which is considered a coronary risk equivalent.*

Physicians should note that not all patients with diabetes have a 20% risk of a cardiac event over a 10-year period as determined by the UKPDS risk engine,[39] so some discretion may be used with the guidelines. The proposed LDL cholesterol level targets are as follows:

- The LDL cholesterol level is lower than 100 mg/dL for any patient with DM.
- If the LDL cholesterol level is below 100 mg/dL, but triglyceride (and very LDL [VLDL] cholesterol) levels are elevated, then the non–high-density lipoprotein (HDL) cholesterol level should be lower than 130 mg/dL.
- The optional guidelines for patients at very high risk, such as diabetic patients with a prior myocardial infarction (MI), are an LDL cholesterol level lower than 70 mg/dL (and non-HDL cholesterol level lower than 100 mg/dL).
- Patients who have an LDL cholesterol level lower than 100 mg/dL without medication should be treated to achieve a more than 30% reduction in their LDL cholesterol level.

These guidelines were developed based on findings from lipid-lowering trials that included diabetic patients and were confirmed by subsequent trials.

Post hoc analyses of diabetic patients who were included in lipid-lowering trials have supported the notion that diabetic patients have comparable relative reductions (or perhaps greater absolute reductions) in the risk for CHD events than their nondiabetic counterparts. These data have been summarized as part of the ACP guidelines.[20] The ADA and AHA guidelines[6,7,29,55,56] have suggested an LDL cholesterol level target of less than 100 mg/dL for patients with diabetes and an optional target of less than 70 mg/dL for patients with DM who already have CHD; this recommendation is based on several clinical trials including, the HPS, ASCOT-LLA, and CARDS trials.[57-60] The CARDS trial, in 2838 patients with T2DM, showed a 37% reduction in cardiovascular events, with a mean in-trial LDL cholesterol level of approximately 80 mg/dL in the atorvastatin group

Table 2 Goals for Risk Factor Management in Patients With Diabetes

Risk Factor	Goal of Therapy	Recommending Body
Cigarette smoking	Complete cessation	ADA
Blood pressure	<130/85 mm Hg <130/80 mm Hg	JNC VI (NHLBI) ADA
LDL cholesterol level	<100 mg/dL	ATP III (NHLBI), ADA
Triglyceride level 200-499 mg/dL	Non-HDL cholesterol level <130 mg/dL	ATP III (NHLBI)
HDL cholesterol level <40 mg/dL	Raise HDL (no set goal)	ATP III (NHLBI)
Prothrombotic state	Low-dose aspirin therapy (patients with CHD and other risk factors)	ADA
Glucose	Hemoglobin A_{1c} < 7%	ADA
Overweight and obesity (BMI ≥ 25 kg/m^2)		OEI (NHLBI)
Physical inactivity	Exercise prescription depending on patient's status	ADA
Adverse nutrition	See text	ADA, AHA, and NHLBI's ATP III, OEI, and JNC VI

ADA, American Diabetes Association; AHA, American Heart Association; ATP III, National Cholesterol Education Program Adult Treatment Panel III; BMI, body mass index; CHD, coronary heart disease; HDL, high-density lipoprotein; JNC VI, Sixth Report of the Joint National Committee on Prevention, Evaluation, and Treatment of High Blood Pressure; LDL, low-density lipoprotein; NHLBI, National Heart, Lung, and Blood Institute; OEI, Obesity Education Initiative Expert Panel on Identification, Evaluation, and Treatment of Overweight and Obesity in Adults.

Adapted from Grundy SM, Howard B, Smith S Jr, et al: Prevention Conference VI: Diabetes and Cardiovascular Disease: Executive summary: Conference proceeding for health care professionals from a special writing group of the American Heart Association. Circulation 2002;105:2231-2239.

compared with 119 mg/dL in the placebo group. The HPS and CARDS studies have shown favorable effects in diabetic patients whose LDL cholesterol levels were lower than 100 mg/dL. In addition, these guidelines have recommended that in patients with elevated triglyceride levels, and a corresponding increase in VLDL cholesterol levels, that the non-HDL cholesterol value (LDL plus VLDL cholesterol level) be set at 30 mg/dL higher than the LDL target—that is, a non-HDL cholesterol level lower than 130 mg/dL, with an optional target of less than 100 mg/dL.

Since these guidelines were written, two major trials have been reported whose results are less convincing about the benefits of the lower LDL cholesterol level target and the effects of triglyceride level reduction. The ASPEN trial studied 2410 T2DM subjects who were randomized to 10 mg atorvastatin versus placebo.[61] At baseline, LDL cholesterol levels were 113 mg/dL (atorvastatin group) and 114 mg/dL (placebo group). The atorvastatin group had a mean in-treatment LDL cholesterol level of 79 mg/dL, and the placebo group's level was essentially unchanged (LDL cholesterol level, 113 mg/dL). This difference was associated with a 10% reduction in the primary composite end point (*P* was not statistically significant [NSS]) and a 27% reduction in fatal-nonfatal MI (*P* = NSS). Although these results were not as robust as in the similarly designed CARDS study, the authors concluded that the "present data do not detract from the imperative that the majority of diabetic patients, especially those with

*See references 6, 7, 14, 16, 17, 20, 29, 32, 54.

SECTION 4 ENDOCRINOLOGY

existing CHD, are at risk of CHD and deserve LDL cholesterol lowering to the currently recommended targets."[61]

The FIELD trial was designed to assess the effects of fenofibrate (vs. placebo) on cardiovascular disease events in 9795 T2DM subjects.[62,63] The difference in total cardiovascular events was 11% (P = .035) and in MI plus CHD death it was 11% (P = .16). This trial was confounded by very high levels of statin drop-in, especially in the placebo arm. The ACCORD trial results should help clarify the effects of fibrates. In the lipid-lowering arm of this trial, the participants were all provided simvastatin therapy and then randomized to fenofibrate versus placebo. Results should be available by 2010.

Hypertension and Renin-Angiotensin-Aldosterone System Blockade. Blood pressure control has a greater effect on reducing the risk for stroke than the risk for MI. The largest blood pressure trials in diabetic patients have demonstrated favorable effects on reduction in CVD. Current clinical guidelines recommend BP targets of 130/80 (or 130/85) mm Hg.[14,29,64,62,63] Few clinical trials have actually achieved these goals, but there does not appear to be any risk in reaching these targets. Multidrug regimens (often three or more drugs) are usually required. Based on several studies (especially HOPE and the EUROPA study, which demonstrated favorable cardiovascular effects with the ACE inhibitors ramipril and perindopril, respectively, in diabetic cohorts), these agents should be considered part of initial therapy in hypertensive T2DM subjects.[65,66-68] ONTARGET (N = 25,620, 38% with diabetes) compared ramipril to telmisartan and to the combination of both drugs on CVD outcomes. There were no differences among the three arms.[69] The beneficial effects could not be entirely attributed to blood pressure reduction in these trials.

Aspirin. Aspirin (ASA) therapy is recommended for patients with diabetes in the ADA and other guidelines.[29,70] There are few data to suggest benefits for patients without established CHD. Because most patients with T2DM are at increased risk for CHD compared with their nondiabetic counterparts, aspirin use in high-risk patients is prudent. The guidelines originally recommended 81 to 325 mg daily because there are no outcomes data comparing ASA doses. ADA/AHA guidelines now recommend 75 to 162 mg daily.[6,7] The concept of aspirin resistance is evolving, and some patients with diabetes may be aspirin resistant. If this observation is supported by future studies, then doses above 81 mg may be prudent for diabetic patients.

Smoking. All the DM- and CHD-related guidelines recommend smoking cessation.

Glycemic Control. Intervention trials have shown a somewhat modest relation between glycemic control and CHD risk. In the UKPDS trial, a delta HbA_{1c} value of 0.9% was associated with a 14% reduction in the risk for MI (P = .052) in the intention to treat analyses and a 16% reduction for every 1% HbA_{1c} level change as a post hoc observational analysis.[36,38,71] The metformin arm in obese patients in the UKPDS demonstrated a 39% reduction in MI compared with the conventional arm (P = .010).[37] ACCORD (N = 10,251) and ADVANCE (N = 11,140) did not demonstrate beneficial effects of intensive control (HbA_{1c} < 7.0%) on CVD events.[72,73]

In the DCCT/EDIC study, there was no statistically significant reduction in CHD risk at the end of the DCCT—this was expected, because the trial included a population at low risk for CHD at randomization—but a 42% reduction (P = .016) in risk of any cardiac event during the duration of the DCCT/EDIC study, 20 years in subjects randomized early in the trial.[74] Thus, the annualized effect of glycemic control on CHD risk is less than that generally associated with other interventions, especially lipid lowering.

Summary

The watchword of the ADA several years ago was "diabetes is serious." Careful screening for complications, including retinopathy, nephropathy, and neuropathy clearly are associated with opportunities to reduce the risk for disease progression. Aggressive interventions with glycemic control, as well as management of lipids and blood pressure, seem to have favorable effects on many complications of diabetes. Aspirin therapy also reduces the risk for CHD risk in patients with DM. These screening and intervention strategies are supported by robust observational and intervention trial data and, in turn, are endorsed by the various organizations that have written disease management guidelines.

Summary

- Diabetes mellitus is a leading cause of blindness, end-stage renal disease, and nontraumatic lower extremity amputations.
- Diabetes mellitus increases the risk for coronary heart disease by two- to fivefold.
- Glycemic control is associated with a reduced risk for the microvascular and neuropathic complications of diabetes mellitus.
- Treatment of CHD risk factors, especially dyslipidemia, is associated with a reduced risk for CHD.
- Early detection of microvascular and neuropathic complications and implementation of appropriate treatment strategies, such as laser therapy (retinopathy), use of ACE inhibitors and ARBs (nephropathy), and proper footwear (neuropathy), will reduce the risk for adverse outcomes from these complications.

Suggested Readings

Adler AI, Stratton IM, Neil HA, et al: Association of systolic blood pressure with macrovascular and microvascular complications of type 2 diabetes (UKPDS 36): Prospective observational study. BMJ 2000;321:412-419.

American Diabetes Association: Standards of medical care in diabetes-2007. Diabetes Care 2007;30(Suppl 1):S4-S41.

Bantle JP, Wylie-Rosett J, Albright AL, et al: Nutrition recommendations and interventions for diabetes-2006: A position statement of the American Diabetes Association. Diabetes Care 2006;29:2140-2157.

Buse JB, Ginsberg HN, Bakris GL, et al: Primary prevention of cardiovascular diseases in people with diabetes mellitus: A scientific statement from the American Heart Association and the American Diabetes Association. Diabetes Care 2007;30:162-172.

Diabetes Control and Complications Trial Research Group: The relationship of glycemic exposure (HbA_{1c}) to the risk of development and progression of retinopathy in the Diabetes Control and Complications Trial. Diabetes 1995;44:968-983.

Diabetes Control and Complications Trial/Epidemiology of Diabetes Interventions and Complications Research Group: Retinopathy and nephropathy in patients with type 1 diabetes four years after a trial of intensive therapy. N Engl J Med 2000;342:381-389.

Gibbons RJ, Balady GJ, Beasley JW, et al: ACC/AHA guidelines for exercise testing: Executive summary. A report of the American College of Cardiology/American Heart Association Task Force on Practice Guidelines (Committee on Exercise Testing). Circulation 1997;96:345-354.

Grundy SM, Cleeman JI, Merz CN, et al: Implications of recent clinical trials for the National Cholesterol Education Program Adult Treatment Panel III guidelines. Arterioscler Thromb Vasc Biol 2004;24:e149-e161.

Stratton IM, Adler AI, Neil HA, et al: Association of glycaemia with macrovascular and microvascular complications of type 2 diabetes (UKPDS 35): Prospective observational study. BMJ 2000;321:405-412.

Strippoli GF, Craig M, Deeks JJ, et al: Effects of angiotensin-converting enzyme inhibitors and angiotensin II receptor antagonists on mortality and renal outcomes in diabetic nephropathy: Systematic review. BMJ 2004;329:828.

References

For a complete list of reference, log onto www.expertconsult.com.

Microvascular Complications of Diabetes

Robert Zimmerman

DEFINITION

The microvascular complications of diabetes encompass long-term complications of diabetes affecting small blood vessels. These classically have included retinopathy, nephropathy, and neuropathy. *Retinopathy* is divided into two main categories: nonproliferative retinopathy and proliferative retinopathy. *Nonproliferative retinopathy* can be recognized by development of microaneurysms, venous loops, retinal hemorrhages, hard exudates, and soft exudates. *Proliferative retinopathy* is defined as presence of new blood vessels with or without vitreous hemorrhage. Proliferative retinopathy represents a progression of nonproliferative retinopathy.

Diabetic nephropathy is defined as the presence of persistent proteinuria greater than 0.5 g/day. *Overt nephropathy* is characterized by progressive decline in renal function resulting in end-stage renal disease.

Neuropathy is a group of conditions characterized by nerve dysfunction. The condition is classified according to the nerves affected. The classification of neuropathy includes focal, diffuse, sensory, motor and autonomic neuropathy.

PREVALENCE

In patients with type 1 diabetes mellitus (T1DM), 13% have retinopathy at 5 years and 90% have retinopathy after 10 to 15 years. Twenty-five percent of type 1 diabetics develop proliferative retinopathy after 15 years of diabetes.[1] Patients with type 2 diabetes mellitus (T2DM) taking insulin have a 40% prevalence of retinopathy at 5 years, and those taking oral hypoglycemic agents have a 24% prevalence. By 15 to 19 years of diabetes, the rates increase to 84% and 53%, respectively. Proliferative retinopathy develops in 2% of type 2 patients with less than 5 years of diabetes and in 25% with 25 or more years of diabetes.[2] The prevalence of nephropathy in diabetes has not been determined. Thirty percent of patients with type 1 diabetes and 5% to 10% with type 2 diabetes become uremic.[3] The prevalence of neuropathy as defined by loss of ankle jerk reflexes is 7% at 1 year of diabetes, increasing to 50% at 25 years[4] for both T1DM and T2DM.

PATHOPHYSIOLOGY

Microaneurysm formation is the earliest manifestation of diabetic retinopathy. Microaneurysms can form due to release of vasoproliferative factors, weakness in the capillary wall or increased intraluminal pressures. Microaneurysms can lead to increased vascular permeability, which can lead to macular edema and threatens central vision. Obliteration of retinal capillaries can lead to intraretinal microvascular abnormalities (IRMA). As capillary closure becomes extensive, intraretinal hemorrhages develop.

Proliferative retinopathy develops due to ischemia and release of vasoactive substances that stimulate new blood vessel formation as a progression of nonproliferative retinopathy. These vessels erupt through the surface of the retina and grow on the posterior surface of the vitreous. These vessels are very friable and can lead to vitreous hemorrhages. The vitreous can then contract, leading to retinal detachment.

The pathophysiology of neuropathy is complex. Diabetes is associated with dyslipidemia, hyperglycemia, low insulin, and growth factor abnormalities. These abnormalities are associated with glycation of blood vessels and nerves. In addition, autoimmunity can affect nerve structure. Trauma and neuroentrapment can lead to structural nerve damage, including segmental demyelination, axonal atrophy or loss, and progressive demyelination. Several agents, including laminin B2, insulin-like growth factor (IGF) 1 and 2, nerve growth factor (NGF), insulin, and neurotrophin 3 (NT-3) are potential growth factors that might restore nerve function.

Diabetic nephropathy results from increased glomerular capillary flow, which leads to increased extracellular matrix production and endothelial damage. This leads to increased glomerular permeability to macromolecules. Mesangial expansion and interstitial sclerosis ensues, resulting in glomerular sclerosis.

SIGNS AND SYMPTOMS

Symptoms of retinopathy are minimal until advanced disease ensues with loss or blurring of vision. Signs of nonproliferative retinopathy include microaneurysm, venous loops, retinal hemorrhages, hard exudates, and soft exudates. Proliferative retinopathy includes new vessels in the eyes or vitreous hemorrhage.

The earliest sign of nephropathy is hypertension. Development of hypertension often coincides with the development of microalbuminuria. As nephropathy worsens, patients can develop edema, arrhythmias associated with hyperkalemia, and symptoms related to renal failure.

Signs and symptoms of neuropathy depend on the type of neuropathy. Most commonly patients develop symptomatic distal polyneuropathy. Signs include depression or loss of ankle jerks and vibratory sensation, with hyperalgesia and calf pain in some patients. The deficit is in a stocking-and-glove distribution. Wasting of the small muscles of hands and feet can also occur.

Patients may present with focal neuropathies either due to mononeuritis or entrapment syndromes. These produce focal neurologic deficits confined to a single nerve. A rare but severe form of diabetic neuropathy is *diabetic amyotrophy*. It begins with pain followed by severe weakness and spreads from a unilateral distribution to a bilateral one. It resolves spontaneously in 18 to 24 months.

DIAGNOSIS

The diagnosis of nephropathy is initially based on development of *microalbuminuria*. Microalbuminuria is defined as an albumin excretion rate of 20 to 200 µg/min. Because the average daily albumin excretion rate can vary by 40%, it is recommended that three urine collections be made over several weeks before making this diagnosis. Overt nephropathy is defined as an albumin excretion rate greater than 300 mg in 24 hours. This is associated with a linear decline in glomerular filtration rate (GFR) ranging from 0.1 to 2.4 mL/min/month.

Diagnosis of retinopathy is based on finding the diagnostic signs of retinopathy on eye examinations as discussed earlier.

The diagnosis of neuropathy is based on presence of weakness or diminished sensation as described earlier. These findings can be confirmed with nerve conduction studies.

TREATMENT

Prevention is the primary therapy for microvascular complications of diabetes. The main approaches to preventing retinopathy and nephropathy are intensive glycemic control and aggressive control of hypertension. Intensive glycemic control has been the most effective approach to preventing neuropathic complications of diabetes.

Glycemic Control

The Wisconsin Epidemiologic Study[1,2,6-10] demonstrated that in diabetics younger than 30 years and those older than 30 years treated with oral hypoglycemic agents or insulin, baseline hemoglobin A_{1c} (HbA_{1c}) level correlated with the incidence of retinopathy, progression of retinopathy, and progression of proliferative retinopathy.

The Diabetes Control and Complications Trial[11] (DCCT) enrolled 1441 people with type 1 diabetes. Of these, 726 had no retinopathy, had normal albumin excretion, and had had diabetes for less than 5 years. The other 715 had mild-to-moderate background retinopathy with normal albuminuria or microalbuminuria at baseline.

The subjects received intensive therapy or conventional treatment. The intensive treatment was either given with insulin pumps or multiple daily injections (three or more injections per day.) The insulin dosage was guided by self-monitoring of blood glucose three or four times per day. The participants were seen every month.

The conventional group received no more than two shots per day. Urine and blood glucose were monitored up to two times per day. They had clinic visits every 2 or 3 months over an average of 6.5 years. The average HbA_{1c} was 9.1% in the conventional group and 7.2% in the intensively treated group throughout the study. Risk reduction was 70% for clinically important sustained retinopathy, 56% for laser photocoagulation, 60% for sustained microalbuminuria, 54% for clinical grade nephropathy, and 64% for clinical neuropathy. Four years after the close of the DCCT, HbA_{1c} levels in the two groups narrowed to 8.2% in the conventional treatment group and 7.9% in the intensive treatment group. Retinopathic events including proliferative retinopathy, macular edema, and need for laser therapy were 74%, 77%, and 77% lower, respectively, in the intensively treated group. Incidence of microalbuminuria was 53% lower and albuminuria was 86% lower in the intensively treated group.[12]

In the Kumamato trial[13] in 102 patients with T2DM, intensive therapy with multiple daily injections (preprandial, regular, and bedtime intermediate-acting insulin) compared with once or twice daily insulin injections resulted in a decrease in HbA_{1c} from 9.4% to 7.1%. Two-step progression of retinopathy decreased 69%, nephropathy progression decreased 70%, and nerve conduction velocities improved.

The United Kingdom Prospective Diabetes Study (UKPDS)[14,15] evaluated 5102 patients with T2DM. The study maintained an average HbA_{1c} of 7.9% in the conventional treatment group compared to 7% in the intensive treatment group. There was a 27% risk reduction for retinal photocoagulation at 12 years, 33% risk reduction at 12 years for microalbuminuria, and 74% risk reduction for doubling of creatinine at 12 years.

Blood pressure control has been shown to reduce the risk for both retinopathy and nephropathy. The Hypertension and Diabetes Study[16,17] was part of the UKPDS study. The subjects were 1148 patients with T2DM and coexisting hypertension. Tight-control subjects were given a blood pressure goal of lower than 150/85 mm Hg. Most patients were treated with captopril or atenolol. The control group was given a blood pressure goal of lower than 180/105 mm Hg. On average, the tight-control group averaged 144/82 mm Hg and the control group averaged 154/87 mm Hg. The tight-control group had a 35% reduction in retinal photocoagulation ($P < 0.025$), 34% reduction in two-step deterioration of retinopathy, and 47% risk reduction in three-line deterioration in the ETDRS chart ($P < 0.005$) over 7.5 years.

The Euclid (EUrodiab Controlled trial of Lisinopril in Insulin-Dependent Diabetes) study[18] in 354 normotensive type 1 diabetics aged 20 to 59 years demonstrated that lisinopril treatment resulted in a 50% reduction in retinopathy progression, 73% reduction in two-grade retinopathy progression, and an 82% reduction in development of proliferative retinopathy.

Several studies have been performed in T1DM and T2DM patients to assess the effects of blood pressure control on nephropathy. Parving[19] demonstrated that blood pressure control in diabetes with nephropathy decreased the albumin excretion rate by 50% and the rate of decline of GFR from 0.29 to 0.1 mL/min/month. A recent meta-analysis[20] demonstrated that angiotensin-converting enzyme (ACE) inhibitors can delay progression to overt nephropathy by 62% in type 1 diabetics with microalbuminuria. Many also decreased their albumin excretion rate. No studies in T1DM patients show that starting ACE inhibitors when albumin excretion rate is normal delays the development of microalbuminuria.[21-31] In overt nephropathy, Lewis[32] studied 409 type 1 diabetics with protein excretion greater than 500 mg/day and creatinine less than 2.5 mg/dL. Creatinine doubled in 12.1% of the patients receiving captopril and 21.3% in the patients receiving a placebo (a 48% reduction in risk.)

In type 2 diabetic patients with microalbuminuria with or without hypertension, several studies have found that ACE inhibitors delay progression to overt nephropathy, decrease albumin excretion rate, and diminish decline in GFR.[33-40] Only one study has demonstrated that in type 2 diabetics who are normotensive and normoalbuminuric, enalapril attenuates the increase in albumin excretion rate and decreases the likelihood of development of microalbuminuria (a 12.5% risk reduction).[41] Several studies[42-45] using angiotensin II receptor blockers have been published.[36-39] These studies show that in T2DM, there is a slowing of progression of microalbuminuria to overt nephropathy.

Management

Based on these studies, the American Diabetes Association (ADA)[46] recommends a goal preprandial plasma glucose of 70 to 130 mg/dL. The postprandial glucose goal is lower than 180 mg/dL. Normal HbA_{1c} is less than 6%. Goal is less than 7%. The ADA target for blood pressure is less than 130/80. The American Association of Clinical Endocrinology recommends preprandial glucose targets of less than 110 mg/dL, postprandial glucose less than 140 mg/dL, and HbA_{1c} less than 6.5%.[47] They also recommend a blood pressure goal of lower than 130/85. HbA_{1c} measurements are suggested every 3 months. Blood sugar testing in type 1 diabetics or pregnant women with diabetes is suggested at least three times a day. The frequency of glucose monitoring for type 2 diabetics is not known but should be sufficient to facilitate achievement of the glucose goals.

In hypertensive patients with microalbuminuria or albuminuria, ACE inhibitors or angiotensin II receptor blockers should be strongly considered. Patients with T1DM should have an initial dilated and comprehensive eye examination within 3 to 5 years of the onset of diabetes. Patients with T2DM should have an eye examination shortly after diagnosis. Both type 1 and type 2 diabetics should have subsequent eye examinations annually; these should be performed by an ophthalmologist or optometrist knowledgeable and experienced in diagnosing retinopathy.

Once retinopathy is established, the best treatment to prevent blindness in those with proliferative retinopathy is laser photocoagulation.[48-52] The Diabetic Retinopathy Study found that a 50% reduction in severe visual loss could be achieved by treating eyes with neovascularization associated with vitreous hemmorhage or neovascularization on or near the optic disc and eyes with proliferative retinopathy or very severe nonproliferative retinopathy.[48-52] If vitreous hemorrhage occurs and does not resolve, vitrectomy can be performed to restore vision.

Early nephropathy is associated with microalbuminuria, hypertension, and possible elevation in creatinine. First-line therapy is directed toward controlling the hypertension. Generally, ACE inhibitors are agents of first choice. If patients develop a cough, angiotensin receptor blockers have shown similar efficacy at decreasing microalbuminuria, lowering blood pressure, and preventing worsening renal function. Certain calcium channel blockers (cardizem and verapamil) have been shown to decrease microalbuminuria and may be added to these medications if necessary. If creatinine increases above 2 to 3 mg/mL, ACE inhibitors should be avoided because overt renal failure can result. If renal failure develops, treatment with dialysis or kidney transplantation should be considered.

The DCCT found some improvement in neuropathy with intensive diabetes control. If this is not successful, further treatment of neuropathy is centered around pain control. The most common neuropathy is bilateral distal polyneuropathy. Increasing doses of tricyclic antidepressants, neurontin, dilantin, tegretol, and benzodiazepines have been used with varying degrees of success. Gastroparesis is treated with metoclopramide (Reglan).

OUTCOMES

Patients with diabetes should be referred to an endocrinologist if targets for glycemic control cannot be achieved or if patients are experiencing significant hypoglycemia. It is important to refer early to help patients avoid long-term complications of diabetes. Patients who are developing complications of diabetes should be referred to an endocrinolgosit to see if any further treatments are available to improve glycemic control or to treat the complications.

Summary

- Glucose control is strongly associated with development of microvascular complications.
- Hypertension contributes to the development of microvascular complications, too.
- Rates of microvascular complications are similar in type 1 and type 2 diabetes mellitus.
- Once developed, retinopathy, nephropathy, and neuropathy are for the most part irreversible.

References

For a complete list of references, log onto www.expertconsult.com.

Diabetes Mellitus Treatment

Tania Babar and Mario Skugor

After diagnosis of diabetes, the importance of protecting the body from damage caused by hyperglycemia cannot be overstated. In the United States, 57.9% of diabetic patients have one or more diabetes complications, and 14.3% have three or more.[1] Strict glycemic control is the primary method of reducing the development and progression of microvascular complications, such as retinopathy, nephropathy, and neuropathy. Aggressive treatment of dyslipidemia and hypertension decreases macrovascular complications.[2-3,6]

GLYCEMIC CONTROL

There are two primary techniques available for physicians to assess the quality of a patient's glycemic control: self-monitoring of blood glucose (SMBG) and interval measurement of hemoglobin A_{1c} (HbA_{1c}).

Self-Monitoring of Blood Glucose

SMBG is an effective way to evaluate short-term glycemic control. It helps patients and physicians assess the affect of food, medications, stress, and activity on blood glucose levels. The frequency of checking depends on the type of medical therapy, risk for hypoglycemia, and need for short-term adjustment of therapy.

For patients with type 1 diabetes mellitus (T1DM) and insulin-dependent type 2 diabetes (T2DM) patients, clinical trials have demonstrated that SMBG plays a role in effective glycemic control because it helps to refine and adjust insulin doses by monitoring for and preventing asymptomatic hypoglycemia and preprandial and postprandial hyperglycemia.[2,4-5,7] The current American Diabetes Association (ADA) guidelines recommend that T1DM patients self-monitor their glucose at least three times per day. Those who use basal–bolus regimens should self-monitor before each meal and at bedtime (four times daily). Initially some patients require more frequent monitoring, including both preprandial and postprandial readings. Patients with gestational diabetes who are taking insulin should monitor their blood glucose three or more times daily. Patients should be educated on how to use real-time blood glucose values to adjust their food intake and medical therapy.

It is commonly recommended that T2DM patients who use insulin self-monitor their blood glucose levels, but the evidence to support the effectiveness of this practice is inconclusive. Initial studies showed that SMBG in T2DM patients results in reduction in HbA_{1c}, but the inclusion of health-improving behavior such as diet and exercise in many of the analyses made it difficult to assess the degree of contribution of SMBG alone.[2,9] Follow-up studies that attempted to correct for this found there was not a significant improvement in glycemic control after 12 months.[8]

It is important to establish individual goals with patients regarding target blood glucose measurements. The ADA recommends preprandial blood glucose levels in nonpregnant adults to be 70 to 130 mg/dL and less than 180 mg/dL for peak postprandial levels.[10,12] The ADA's goals for gestational diabetes is preprandial blood glucose 95 mg/dL or less and either 1 hour postprandial glucose no more than 140 mg/dL or 2 hours postprandial no more than120 mg/dL. For pregnant women with preexisting T1DM or T2DM, goals are preprandial, bedtime, and overnight glucose levels of 60 to 99 mg/dL and peak postprandial levels between 100 and 129 mg/dL.[12] The American Association of Clinical Endocrinologists (AACE) recommends in nonpregnant adults a fasting blood glucose level lower than 110 mg/dL and a 2-hour postprandial level lower than 140 mg/dL.[11]

Hemoglobin A_{1c}

HbA_{1c} measures nonreversible glycosylation of the hemoglobin molecule, which is directly related to blood glucose concentrations. It reflects a mean of the patient's blood glucose values over a 2- to 3-month period and can be used as a predictor of a patient's risk of microvascular complications.[13] Periodic testing is recommended in all patients with diabetes. The frequency of testing depends on the clinical situation and the patient's treatment regimen. The ADA recommends that patients with stable glycemic control be tested at least twice a year. Quarterly testing is suggested for those with a recent change in therapy or not meeting glycemic goals.[12]

HbA_{1c} testing does have some limitations. HbA_{1c} is influenced by rapid red blood cell turnover and blood loss; therefore, anemia and hemoglobinopathies can result in inaccurate values. Physicians should consider these conditions when there is a discrepancy between HbA_{1c} and SMBG values. Episodes of hypoglycemia and hyperglycemia cannot be determined with HbA_{1c} values alone. Table 1, adapted from the ADA's 2009 Executive Summary on diabetes management, demonstrates that correlation between HbA_{1c} and average blood glucose values.

Traditionally it has been recommended that therapy be adjusted to maintain HbA_{1c} values near or less than 7% in nonpregnant adults. This target has been shown to reduce microvascular complications. For patients with T1DM or T2DM who become pregnant, the goal is less than 6.0%.[12] The AACE recommended an HbA_{1c} of less than 6.5% in nonpregnant adults.[11] The ADA recommends that selected patients, especially those with a long life expectancy and little comorbidity, adopt glycemic targets close to normal, providing the target can be achieved without significant hypoglycemia.[12]

PHARMACOLOGIC TREATMENT

When considering appropriate pharmacologic therapy, a major factor to consider is whether the patient is insulin deficient, insulin resistant, or both. Treatment options can be divided into insulin sensitizers, secretagogues, alpha glucosidase inhibitors, incretins, and insulin. Table 2 summarizes the different noninsulin therapies available.

Insulin Sensitizers

Biguanides (Metformin)

Available since the late 1950s, metformin can trace its roots back to medieval Europe, where biguanides in the form of French lilac were used in diabetes treatment. Its primary mechanism of action is suppression of hepatic glucose output, but it also enhances insulin sensitivity of muscle and fat. It affects primarily fasting glycemia; however, some decreases in postprandial glucose concentrations, especially after the midday meal, can also be seen.

Metformin is well tolerated, with the most common side effect being gastrointestinal complaints, such as diarrhea, nausea, abdominal discomfort, and a metallic taste. All of these improve with time and dose reduction. Metformin causes a small increase in basal and postprandial lactate concentrations in the blood, leading to potential to produce very rare but life-threatening lactic acidosis (<1 in 100,000). It is best to avoid use in patients with hepatic impairment. The use of metformin is contraindicated in patients with a serum creatinine 1.5 mg/dL or higher in male patients or 1.4 mg/dL or higher in female patients.

The major benefits of metformin are that it usually does not lead to hypoglycemia when used as monotherapy. It can lead to weight loss, and it has been shown to decrease plasma triglycerides concentration (10% to 20%).

Dosing is typically twice daily; however, it can be dosed three times daily or once daily (extended release). The typical starting dose is 500 mg daily. The maximum dose is 2550 mg per day. Gradual titration of metformin, starting at 500 mg with breakfast and increasing by 500 mg in weekly intervals until a dose of 1000 mg with breakfast and dinner is reached help to prevent GI side effects.[12,14-18]

Table 1 Correlation between HbA_{1c} and Average Blood Glucose Values

HbA_{1c} (%)	Mean Plasma Glucose (mg/dL)
6	126
7	154
8	183
9	212
10	240
11	269
12	298

HbA_{1c}, glycated hemoglobin.
Data from ADA's 2009 Executive Summary on diabetes management.

Thiazolidinediones

Thiazolidinediones (TZDs) are agonists of peroxisome proliferator-activated receptor gamma (PPARγ) and primarily enhance sensitivity of muscle and fat, and mildly of the liver, to exogenous and endogenous insulin. TZDs lower fasting and postprandial blood glucose levels.

Major side effects include weight gain, with an increase in subcutaneous adiposity, and fluid retention which typically manifests as peripheral edema, but heart failure has been shown to occur on occasion. These agents should be avoided in patients with functional class III or IV heart failure. These effects are mostly seen at higher doses. The PROactive trial (PROspective pioglitAzone Clinical Trial In macroVascular Events) showed that compared with placebo, pioglitazone does not increase cardiovascular risks. TZDs have been shown to have an association with an increased risk of fractures, particularly in women. The TZDs do not cause hypoglycemia when used as monotherapy. Pioglitazone use leads to lowering triglycerides, increasing high-density lipoprotein cholesterol (HDL), and increasing the low-density lipoprotein cholesterol (LDL) particle size.

Dosing is once a day. It takes 2 to 12 weeks for TZDs to become fully effective. For rosiglitazone, starting dose is 4 mg/day and maximum dose is 8 mg/day. For pioglitazone, the starting dose is 7.5 mg/day and the maximum dose is 45 mg/day.[12,14,17-21]

Insulin Secretagogues

Insulin secretagogues stimulate secretion of insulin from the pancreas, thereby decreasing hepatic glucose production and enhancing glucose uptake by muscles and fat.

Sulfonylureas

Sulfonylureas lower fasting and postprandial glucose levels. Main adverse effects include weight gain (about 2 kg upon initiation) and

Table 2 Noninsulin Therapies

Subgroup	Generic Name	Class	Route	Comments
Biguanides	Glucophage (Metformin)	Sensitizer	Oral	Weight loss No hypoglycemia GI upset
Thiazolidinediones	Rosiglitazone (Avandia) Pioglitazone (Actos)	Sensitizer	Oral	Weight gain Peripheral edema
Alpha glucosidase inhibitors	Acarbose (Precose) Miglitol (Glyset)		Oral	GI upset No hypoglycemia
Sulfonylureas	Chlorpropamide (Diabinese) Glimepiride (Amaryl) Glyburide (Glynase) Glipizide (Glucotrol) Tolazamide (Tolinase) Tolbutamide (Orinase)	Secretagogue	Oral	Hypoglycemia Weight gain
Glinides	Nateglinide (Starlix) Repaglinide (Prandin)	Secretagogue	Oral	Weight gain
Exenatide	Byetta	Incretin	Subcutaneous	Weight loss GI upset
Pramlintide	Symlin	Incretin	Subcutaneous	Weight loss GI upset Adjunctive therapy with insulin
Dipeptidyl peptidase-4 inhibitors (DPP-4s)	Sitagliptin (Januvia) Saxagliptin (Onglyza)	Incretin	Oral	No hypoglycemia Nasopharyngitis Weight neutral

GI, gastrointestinal.

hypoglycemia. The hypoglycemia episodes can be significant (leading to need for assistance, coma, or seizure) and are seen more often in the elderly. The benefits include a 25% reduction in microvascular complications with or without insulin found by a UKPDS trial. Dosing is typically once or twice daily. Caution should be used in patients with liver or kidney dysfunction or patients who often skip meals.[12,17-18,20,23]

Glinides

Glinides work in a manner similar to sulfonylureas; however, they have a more-rapid onset of action and a short duration of action, so they are a good option for patients with erratic timing of meals. They have a lower risk of hypoglycemia than sulfonylureas; they have a similar to lower risk of weight gain with initiation of therapy. Caution must be used in patients with liver dysfunction. Dosing is before meals.[12,14,20]

Alpha Glucosidase Inhibitors

Alpha glucosidase inhibitors competitively block the enzyme alpha glucosidase in the brush borders of the small intestine, which delays absorption of carbohydrates (absorbed in the mid and distal portions of the small intestine instead). They primarily target postprandial hyperglycemia without causing hypoglycemia. Gastrointestinal complaints, such as bloating, abdominal cramps, flatulence, and diarrhea are the main side effects. Use should be avoided in patients with severe hepatic or renal impairment. Dosing must be prior to carbohydrate-containing meals.[12,17-18,20,22]

Incretins

Exenatide

Exenatide is a synthetic form of exendin 4, hormone found in the saliva of the Gila monster, that mimics glucagon-like peptide type 1 (GLP-1). GLP-1 is produced in the small intestine and stimulates insulin secretion and inhibits glucagon secretion and hepatic glucose production in a glucose-dependent manner. It also delays gastric emptying and suppresses appetite through central pathways. It primarily decreases postprandial blood glucose levels; however, a moderate reduction in fasting blood glucose levels can also be seen.

Due to its delaying effects on gastric emptying, the major side effect is gastrointestinal complaints such as nausea, vomiting, and diarrhea. Hypoglycemia does not occur when exenatide is used as monotherapy or with metformin, but it does occur when exenatide is combined with a sulfonylurea. Benefits include weight loss up to 2 to 3 kg in the first 6 months and up to 5.5 kg in the first 2 years.

Dosing is twice daily by subcutaneous injection. Start with a dose of 5 μg. If this dose is tolerated, titrate after 1 month to 10 μg.[12,14,20]

Pramlintide

Pramlintide is a synthetic form of amylin, a hormone secreted by beta-cells that acts to suppress glucagon secretion, slow gastric emptying, and suppress appetite through central pathways. It acts primarily on postprandial blood glucose levels.

As with exenatide, the major side effects are gastrointestinal complaints, especially nausea, and hypoglycemia. Benefits of therapy include weight loss of 1-1.5 kg over 6 months and up to 4.5 kg after chronic therapy.

Currently in the United States it is approved only as an adjunctive therapy with insulin, but it can be used both T1DM and T2DM. Patients can see up to a 50% reduction in their insulin requirements with the addition of pramlintide. Starting dose for T2DM is generally 60 μg subcutaneously before meals and for T1DM is 15 μg before each meal. It can be used in patients taking insulin, metformin, or sulfonyureas.[12,14,20]

Dipeptidyl Peptidase 4 Inhibitors

Dipeptidyl peptidase 4 (DPP 4) is a cell membrane protein that rapidly degrades GLP-1 and glucose-dependent insulinotropic polypeptide (GIP). Suppression of DPP 4 leads to higher levels of insulin secretion and suppression of glucagon secretion in a glucose-dependent manner.

DPP 4 inhibitors act primarily on postprandial blood glucose levels, but reductions in fasting glycemia are also seen. It is generally well tolerated, and the most common side effect is headache. An increase in nasopharyngitis has also been seen. Benefits include that it is weight neutral and does not cause hypoglycemia when used as monotherapy or in combination with metformin or TZDs.

Dosing is 100 mg orally once daily with or without meals. Dose reduction in needed in renal impairment. In patients with a creatinine clearance 30 to 50 mL/min, dosing is 50 mg once daily. Those patients with a creatinine clearance less than 30 mL/minute, dosing is 25 mg once daily.[12,14]

Insulin

Insulin is the oldest therapy available for diabetes. It was discovered in 1921, and clinical testing in humans started in 1922.

To this date it remains the most effective method of reducing hyperglycemia. There is no upper limit in dosing for therapeutic effect, so it can be used to bring any HbA_{1c} down to near normal levels. Other benefits of insulin include its effects on reducing triglycerides levels and increasing HDL.

Hypoglycemia is a concern for many, but the actual risk of severe episodes is small. Studies have shown that episodes where the patient required assistance from another due to the hypoglycemia occurred between 1 and 3 per 100,000 patient-years. Weight gain can occur after initiation and is typically about 2 to 4 kg.

Most brands are available in both vial and pen form for delivery. Table 3 summarizes the different formulations of insulin available.[4,11-12,14,17-18,24]

INITIATION AND TITRATION OF THERAPY

There are several different regimens for insulin therapy. These are summarized in Table 4. All patients with T1DM require therapies with insulin products. There are two available regimens: basal–bolus and insulin pump therapy. Patients with T2DM often require insulin, which can be combined with oral hypoglycemic agents. Regimens include basal insulin only, twice-daily premixed insulin, basal–bolus, and insulin pump therapy.

Type I Diabetes

Basal–Bolus

The basal–bolus regimen involves combining a long-acting agent that is used once or twice daily and provides basal insulin needs and a rapid-acting agent for prandial coverage used with meals. When initiating therapy with glargine or detemir as the basal insulin, traditionally 50% of the total daily dose is given as basal insulin and the rest as prandial insulin divided equally before meals. Meal dose of insulin can be fixed, but it is better to determine the dose based on carbohydrate content of the meal. This requires learning carbohydrate counting and knowing the dose of insulin required to cover counted carbohydrates. Help of a diabetic educator is needed for this to be achieved.

Starting daily insulin dose is typically 0.3 U/kg total (divided between long acting and rapid acting) daily. Key to good control is blood glucose self-monitoring by the patient and frequent adjustment of the regimen until control is achieved.[11,14]

Table 3 Forms of Insulin

Insulin (Brand)	Onset	Peak	Effective Duration
Rapid-Acting			
Aspart (NovoLog)	5-15 min	30-90 min	<5 h
Lispro (Humalog)	5-15 min	30-90 min	<5 h
Glulisine (Apidra)	5-15 min	30-90 min	<5 h
Short-acting			
Regular	30-60 min	2-3 h	5-8 h
Intermediate, Basal			
Neutral protamine Hagedorn (NPH)	2-4 h	4-10 h	10-16 h
Long-acting, Basal			
Insulin glargine (Lantus)	2-4 h	No peak	20-24 h
Insulin detemir (Levemir)	3-8 h	No peak	5.7-23.2 h
Premixed			
75% Insulin lispro protamine/25% insulin lispro (Humalog Mix 75/25)	5-15 min	Dual	10-16 h
50% Insulin lispro protamine/50% insulin lispro (Humalog Mix 50/50)	5-15 min	Dual	10-16 h
70% Insulin lispro protamine/30% insulin aspart (Novolog Mix 70/30)	5-15 min	Dual	10-16 h
70% NPH/ 30% regular	30-60 min	Dual	10-16 h

Data from Rodbard HW, Blonde L, Braithwaite SS, et al. American Association of Clinical Endocrinologists medical guidelines for clinical practice for the management of diabetes mellitus. Endocr Pract 2008;14(6):802-803.

Insulin Pump Therapy

The insulin pump allows use of different basal insulin rates in different periods of day and administration of the meal bolus as a single discrete bolus or as an extended bolus (square bolus) over a certain amount of time, which allows a better match between insulin delivery and glucose absorption from the meal in patients with abnormalities of gastric emptying. This use of this therapy is spreading in all diabetic populations and particularly should be considered in the following patients:

- Those unable to achieve target goals with basal–bolus regimens
- Patients with frequent hypoglycemia, dawn phenomenon, or brittle diabetes
- Pregnant patients
- Patients with insulin sensitivity or requiring more intense monitoring due to complications
- Patients who are able to monitor blood glucose several times daily and make insulin dosage adjustments

Type 2 Diabetes

The ADA and the AACE have different algorithms for initiation and maintenance of therapy. No studies are available comparing the efficacy of either method or comparing the two. Each algorithm is summarized in Box 1 and Figure 1. We support the AACE's algorithm (see Box 2), because the ADA's algorithm is significantly influenced by cost of therapy.[12] Figure 2 gives a summary of titration of insulin therapy. Starting daily insulin dose is typically 0.5 U/kg total (divided between long-acting and rapid-acting) daily. Therapy can be combined with oral insulin sensitizers but not secretagogues.

Gestational Diabetes

In patients with gestational diabetes, insulin therapy is indicated when exercise and nutritional therapy are ineffective in controlling prandial and fasting blood glucose levels. Basal therapy alone may be sufficient, but often basal–bolus regimens are required.

Table 4 Regimens for Insulin Therapy

Insulin Regimen	HbA_{1c} (%)	Medication	Pattern	Diet History	Lifestyle	Monitoring
Basal-only	>7.5-10	Oral medications adequately control postprandial glucose excursions	High fasting glucose with minimal glucose rise during the day	Small, regular meals; large meals will result in postprandial hyperglycemia	Reluctance to do MDI; requires oral agents	Fasting
Basal–bolus (MDI)	>7.5	—	Regimen can be matched to any pattern to achieve glycemic control	Regimen can be matched to any diet to achieve glycemic control	Erratic schedule, motivated to achieve tight glycemic control	Frequent blood glucose monitoring (minimum before meals and bedtime)
Once- or Twice-Daily Premixed						
Rapid-acting analogue and intermediate acting	>7.5	Oral agent failure (maximum tolerated dosages, contraindications, cost issues)	Any fasting glucose; glucose rises during the day	Large suppers, small lunches	Consistent daily routine, reluctance to do MDI	Fasting and presupper (if insulin is administered twice daily)
Regular and NPH	>7.5%	Oral agent failure (maximum tolerated dosages, contraindications, cost issues)	Any fasting glucose; glucose rises during the day	Isocaloric meals or larger lunches	Consistent daily routine, reluctance to do MDI	Fasting and presupper (if insulin is administered twice daily)

HbA_{1c}, glycated hemoglobin; MDI, multiple daily injections.

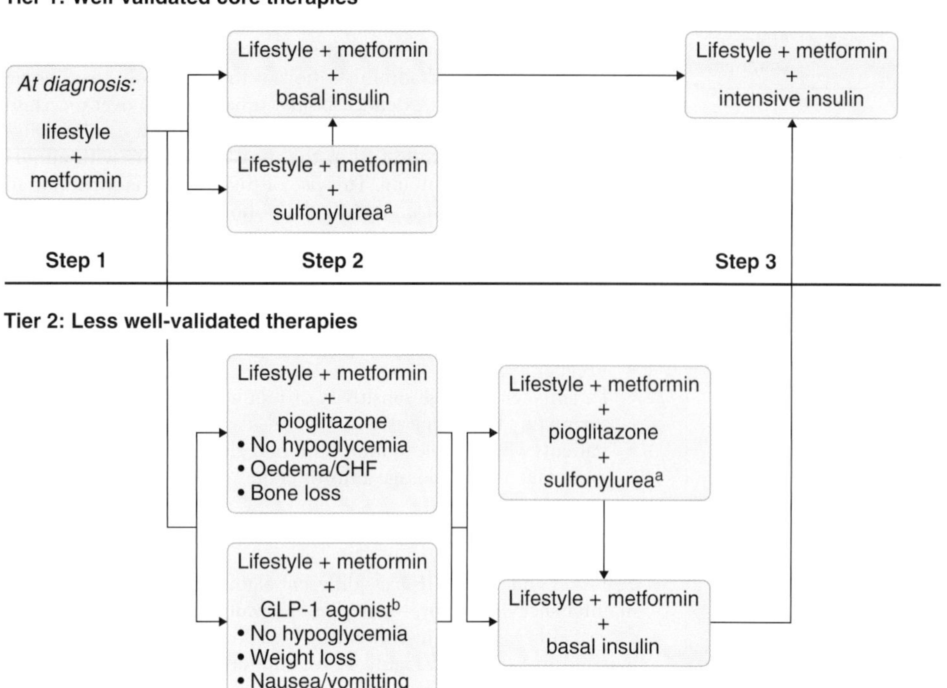

Figure 1 **ADA algorithm for initiation and maintenance of therapy.** *(Adapted from Executive summary: standards of medical care in diabetes—2009. Diabetes Care 2009;32(Suppl 1):S6-S12.)*

Box 1 Examples of Pharmacologic Regimens for Treating Type 2 Diabetes Mellitus*

Patients Naive to Pharmacologic Therapy

Monotherapy

Initiate monotherapy when HbA_{1c} levels are 6% to 7%

Options include:

- Metformin
- Thiazolidinediones
- Secretagogues
- Dipeptidyl-peptidase 4 inhibitors
- α-Glucosidase inhibitors

Monitor and titrate medication for 2 to 3 months

Consider combination therapy if glycemic goals are not met at the end of 2 to 3 months

Combination Therapy

Initiate combination therapy when levels are 7% to 8%

Options include:

- Secretagogue + metformin
- Secretagogue + thiazolidinedione
- Secretagogue + α-glucosidase inhibitor
- Thiazolidinedione + metformin
- Dipeptidyl-peptidase 4 inhibitor + metformin
- Dipeptidyl-peptidase 4 inhibitor + thiazolidinedione
- Secretagogue + metformin + thiazolidinedione
- Fixed-dose (single pill) therapy
  - Thiazolidinedione (pioglitazone) + metformin
  - Thiazolidinedione (rosiglitazone) + metformin
  - Thiazolidinedione (rosiglitazone) + secretagogue (glimepiride)
  - Thiazolidinedione (pioglitazone) + secretagogue (glimepiride)
  - Secretagogue (glyburide) + metformin

Rapid-acting insulin analogues or premixed insulin analogues may be used in special situations

Inhaled insulin may be used as monotherapy or in combination with oral agents and long-acting insulin analogues

All oral medications may be used in combination with insulin; therapy combinations should be selected based on the patient's profiles of self-monitoring of blood glucose

Initiating or Intensifying Therapy

Initiate or intensify combination therapy using options listed above when HbA_{1c} levels are 8% to 10% to address fasting and postprandial levels

Initiate or intensify insulin therapy when HbA_{1c} levels are >10%

Rapid-acting insulin analogue or inhaled insulin with long-acting insulin analogue or NPH

Premixed insulin analogues

Patients Currently Treated Pharmacologically

The therapeutic options for combination therapy listed for patients naive to therapy are appropriate for patients being treated pharmacologically

Exenatide may be combined with oral therapy in patients who have not achieved glycemic goals

Approved exenatide + oral combinations:

- Exenatide + secretagogue (sulfonylurea)
- Exenatide + metformin
- Exenatide + secretagogue (sulfonylurea) + metformin
- Exenatide + thiazolidinedione

Pramlinitide may be used in combination with prandial insulin

Add insulin therapy in patients on maximum combination therapy (oral-oral, oral-exenatide) whose HbA_{1c} levels are 6.5% to 8.5%

Consider initiating basal–bolus insulin therapy for patients with HbA_{1c} levels >8.5%

**The options listed are in no order of preference.*

HbA_{1c}, glycated hemoglobin; NPH, neutral protamine Hagedorn.

Adapted from Rodbard HW, Blonde L, Braithwaite SS, et al: American Association of Clinical Endocrinologists medical guidelines for clinical practice for the management of diabetes mellitus. Endocr Pract 2008;14(6):802-803.

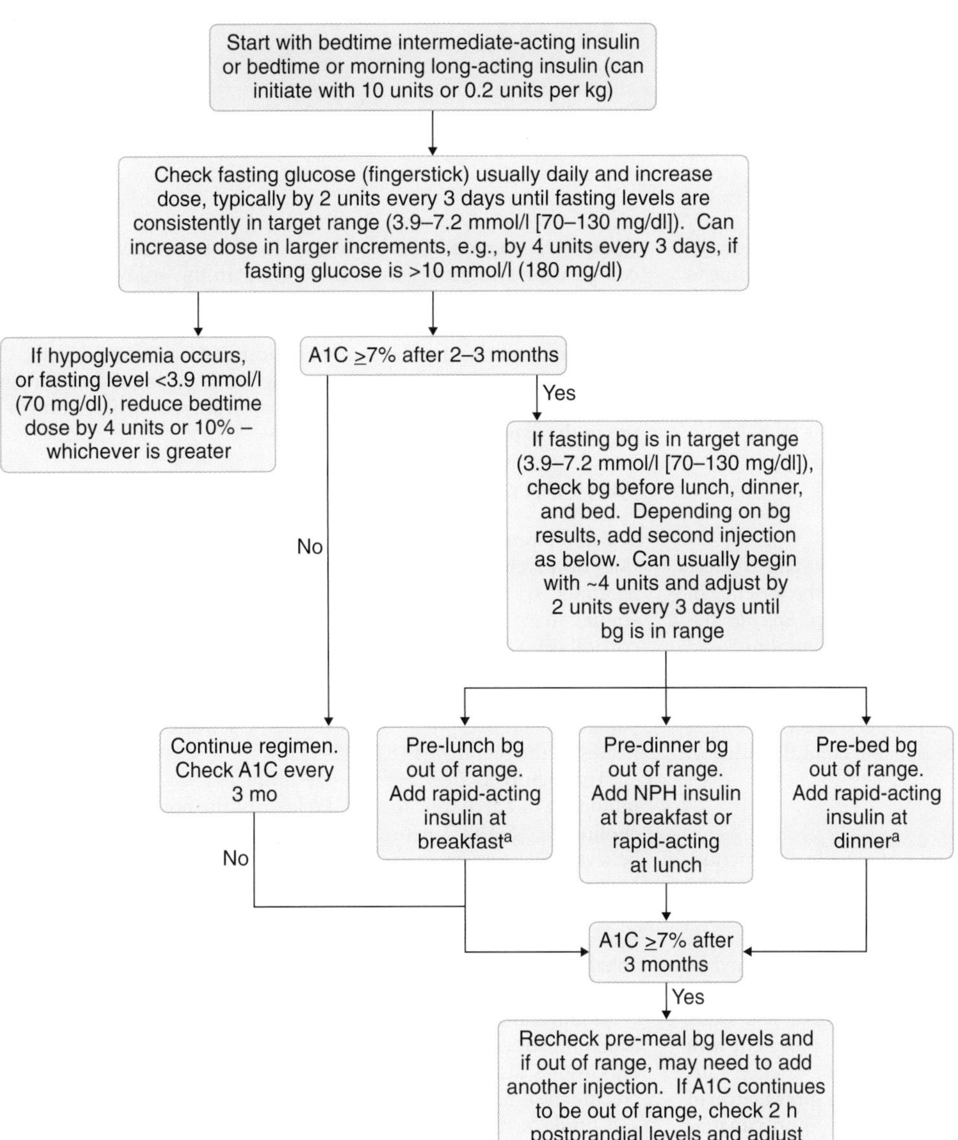

Figure 2 Summary on titration of insulin therapy. *(Adapted from Executive summary: standards of medical care in diabetes—2009. Diabetes Care 2009;32(Suppl 1):S6-S12.)*

SECTION 4 ENDOCRINOLOGY

Summary

- Glycemic control is critical for preventing microvascular complications.
- Type 2 diabetes is progressive disease and requires therapy intensification with time.
- Insulin sensitizers and incretin-based therapy should be used early in the course of the disease.
- Type 1 diabetes must be treated with insulin.
- Multiple daily doses of insulin providing basal, prandial, and supplemental insulin are a mainstay of insulin treatment.

Suggested Readings

Chase HP, Jackson WE, Hoops SL, et al. Glucose control and the renal and retinal complications of insulin-dependent diabetes. JAMA 1989;261: 1155-1160.

Diabetes Control and Complications Trial Research Group: The effect of intensive treatment of diabetes on the development and progression of long-term complications in insulin-dependent diabetes mellitus. N Engl J Med 1993; 329:977-986.

Executive summary: standards of medical care in diabetes—2009. Diabetes Care. 2009;32(Suppl 1):S6-S12.

Fonseca V, Kulkarni K. Management of type 2 diabetes: oral agents, insulin, and injectables. J Am Dietetic Assoc 2008; 108(4):S29-S33.

Nathan DM, Buse JB, Davidson MB, et al. Management of hyperglycemia in type 2 diabetes: A consensus algorithm for the initiation and adjustment of therapy: Update regarding thiazolidinediones. Diabetes Care 2008; 31(1):173-175.

Rodbard HW, Blonde L, Braithwaite SS, et al. American Association of Clinical Endocrinologists medical guidelines for clinical practice for the management of diabetes mellitus. Endocr Pract 2008;14(6):802-803.

Saudek CD, Derr RL, Kalyani RR: Assessing glycemia in diabetes using self-monitoring blood glucose and hemoglobin A_{1c}. JAMA 2006;295(14): 1688-1697.

UK Prospective Diabetes Study (UKPDS) Group: Effect of intensive blood-glucose control with metformin on complications in overweight patients with type 2 diabetes (UKPDS 34): UK Prospective Diabetes Study (UKPDS) Group. Lancet 1998;352:854-865.

References

For a complete list of reference, log onto www.expertconsult.com.

Erectile Dysfunction

Milton Lakin

Since the 1990s, there has been increasing recognition that erectile dysfunction is a common problem. Although many patients come to their general practitioner's or internist's office with erectile dysfunction as a primary complaint, there are still many patients who feel reluctant or embarrassed to discuss this problem. Many physicians also feel uncomfortable discussing and evaluating sexual dysfunction. It is important for us as physicians to feel comfortable discussing and evaluating sexual dysfunction and hopefully to help our patients feel comfortable talking about these issues.

DEFINITION

Erectile dysfunction is the inability to develop and maintain an erection for satisfactory sexual intercourse or activity in the absence of an ejaculatory disorder such as premature ejaculation. *Erectile dysfunction* is the preferred term rather than the more commonly used term, *impotence.* There are no universally agreed on criteria for how consistent the problem has to be and for what duration it needs to be present to fulfill the definition. A period of persistence for longer than 3 months has been suggested as a reasonable clinical guideline.

PREVALENCE

Several studies have looked at the prevalence of erectile dysfunction. The Massachusetts Male Aging Study, conducted from 1987 to 1989 in areas around Boston, was a cross-sectional random sample community-based survey of 1290 men ages 40 to 70 years.[1] Erectile dysfunction was self-reported and the condition was classified as mild, moderate, or complete. The combined prevalence of minimal, moderate, and complete erectile dysfunction was 52%. The study demonstrated that erectile dysfunction is increasingly prevalent with age. At age 40, there is an approximately 40% prevalence rate, increasing to almost 70% in men at age 70. The prevalence of moderate erectile dysfunction increases from 17% to approximately 34%; the prevalence of complete erectile dysfunction increases from 5% to 15% as age increases from 40 to 70 years.

Although age was the variable most strongly associated with erectile dysfunction, following adjustment for age, a higher probability was noted with heart disease, hypertension, diabetes, and associated medications. Cigarette smoking in this study did not correlate with a greater probability of complete erectile dysfunction. However, when it was associated with heart disease and hypertension, a higher probability of erectile dysfunction was noted. The study concluded that erectile dysfunction is a major health concern in light of its high prevalence.

Incidence estimates have been published using data compiled from the Massachusetts Male Aging Study.[2] Incidence data are necessary to assess risk and plan treatment and prevention strategies. The Massachusetts study data have suggested there will be approximately 17,781 new cases of erectile dysfunction in Massachusetts and 617,715 in the United States annually. The national incidence estimate might underestimate the true incidence, because Massachusetts is largely white, so likely the data are underestimated nationally for African Americans, Latin Americans, and other groups.

A larger national study, the National Health and Social Life Survey, looked at sexual function in men and women.[3] This study surveyed 1410 men ages 18 to 59 years, and it also documented an increase in erectile dysfunction with age. Additionally, the study found a decrease in sexual desire with increasing age. The oldest cohort of men (ages 50-59 years) was more than three times as likely to experience erection problems and to report low sexual desire in comparison with men ages 18 to 29 years. In this study, there was a higher prevalence of sexual dysfunction in men who had never married or were divorced. Experience of sexual dysfunction was more likely among men in poor physical and emotional health. It was also concluded that sexual dysfunction is an important public health concern and added that emotional issues are likely to contribute to the experience of these problems.

PATHOPHYSIOLOGY

The development of an erection is a complex event involving integration of psychological, neurologic, endocrine, vascular, and local anatomic systems. Positron emission tomography (PET) scanning studies[4] have suggested that sexual arousal is activated in higher cortical centers, which then stimulate the medial preoptic and paraventricular nuclei of the hypothalamus. These signals ultimately descend through a complex neural network involving the parasympathetic nervous system and eventually activate parasympathetic nerves in the sacral area (S2 to S4).

The neurovascular events that ultimately occur result in the inhibition of adrenergic tone and release of the nonadrenergic, noncholinergic (NANC) neurotransmitter nitric oxide. Nitric oxide is believed to be released from NANC nerves and endothelial cells. Nitric oxide stimulates the guanylate cyclase enzyme system in penile smooth muscle. This results in increased levels of cyclic guanosine monophosphate (GMP) and ultimately in smooth muscle relaxation, enhancement of arterial inflow, and veno-occlusion, producing adequate firmness for sexual activity.

Abnormalities in any of these systems can produce erectile dysfunction. For example, cerebral vascular accidents, multiple sclerosis, Parkinson's disease, and spinal cord injury can result in neurogenic erectile dysfunction. More commonly, vascular disease and diabetes can produce neurovascular abnormalities resulting in erectile dysfunction. Surgery for cancers of the prostate, bladder, and colon can also produce neurovascular abnormalities resulting in erectile dysfunction. Diseases such as Peyronie's disease, in which patches or strands of dense tissue surround the cavernous body of the penis, and traumatic perineal and penile injuries can also interfere with neurovascular and anatomic structures, producing erectile dysfunction.

Hormone deficiency or hypogonadism, whether primary or secondary, can result in erectile dysfunction. Hormone deficiency, however, is less often the cause of erectile dysfunction than is diabetes or vascular disease. How often erectile dysfunction is caused by hormone deficiency remains somewhat controversial, but estimates of approximately 3% to 5% of cases are probably reasonable. Medications and recreational drugs can also produce erectile dysfunction by various poorly understood mechanisms.

SIGNS AND SYMPTOMS

Although erectile dysfunction is a common problem, many patients are reluctant to discuss it. Certainly, some patients who present with issues relating to depression or anxiety disorders actually have a significant problem with erectile dysfunction. Additionally, patients who are poorly compliant with medication prescribed for hypertension may be experiencing significant erectile dysfunction. The best way to elicit whether the problem is present is to ask questions about sexual function as a routine part of the examination.

Some health questionnaires help screen for and evaluate erectile dysfunction[5] and may help in the primary care setting. It is important, however, to recognize that abbreviated questionnaires might not evaluate specific areas of the sexual cycle, such as sexual desire, ejaculation, and orgasm. Nonetheless, they can be useful in helping patients discuss the problem and in signaling the need for an evaluation.

DIAGNOSIS

If it is determined that erectile dysfunction is a problem, a detailed sexual and medical history should be elicited and a physical examination should be done to evaluate the problem. In particular, it is important to evaluate the erectile dysfunction and make sure that the problem is not premature ejaculation, which is also a common sexual dysfunction.[6]

A number of specific questions relating to sexual function help evaluate the complaint of erectile dysfunction. Questions should focus on the following:

- How long has the erectile dysfunction been a problem, and did it start gradually or suddenly?
- How frequent is intercourse currently, and how frequent was it in the past? Is there difficulty with vaginal penetration and/or loss of the erection intravaginally in the absence of premature ejaculation?
- How firm are the erections (use a scale of 1 to 10)? Do erections vary under different circumstances, such as with different partners, oral stimulation, or masturbation?
- Are morning or evening erections present and, if so, what is the quality of these erections?
- Is there any new curve or bend to the penis to suggest Peyronie's disease? If curvature is present, is it painful? What are the location and severity of the curvature?
- Are there any difficulties with sexual desire, arousal, ejaculation, or orgasm (climax)? If there are difficulties, did these difficulties occur with the onset of the erectile dysfunction or are they separate issues?

Once questions related to the specific erectile complaint have been reviewed, additional questions relating to medical and psychosocial factors need to be evaluated. In particular, these include the following: symptoms suggesting the presence of diabetes, peripheral vascular disease, neurologic disease, or chronic liver or kidney disease; a complete list of medications and recreational drugs, including alcohol, and questions about cigarette smoking; previous history of surgery or radiation therapy, particularly procedures related to genitourinary or gastrointestinal malignancy; a history of pelvic genital, perineal, or spinal cord trauma; and the quality of the marital or partner relationship and expectations of both patient and partner.

Following a review of the medical history, the salient features of the physical examination should include the following:

- An assessment of the patient's general health and affect, as well as secondary sexual characteristics, noting in particular gynecomastia and hair loss (axillary or pubic)
- Careful peripheral vascular examination that includes palpation of the lower extremity pulses as well as auscultation for bruits in the abdominal and femoral regions
- Detailed neurologic examination to include gait and postural instability, with blood pressure changes, distal extremity and saddle sensation, and reflexes, including cremasterics and bulbocavernosus
- Careful genital examination, noting testicular size and palpating for Peyronie's plaques
- Rectal examination to assess sphincter tone and evaluate the prostate
- Careful abdominal examination looking for organomegaly masses or other signs of liver or kidney disease
- Cardiopulmonary examination to help evaluate the patient's fitness for future treatment options

Once a complete sexual and medical history has been completed, appropriate laboratory studies can be considered. In the initial evaluation of erectile dysfunction, sophisticated laboratory testing is rarely necessary. Laboratory studies should include hormonal evaluation to exclude a diagnosis of hypogonadism (testosterone and prolactin levels) and testing to screen for diabetes if the patient is not known to be diabetic (hemoglobin A_{1c} or glucose tolerance testing). Most patients usually have had a general survey, but this is certainly appropriate if it has not been done to assess for kidney or liver disease. A lipid panel is also appropriate as a screen for risk factors.

In most cases, a tentative diagnosis can be established with a complete sexual and medical history, physical examination, and limited laboratory testing. In many cases, the diagnosis still remains somewhat ambiguous. However, with the availability of oral medication for treatment of erectile dysfunction that is safe and has minimal or tolerable side effects, additional diagnostic testing is probably unnecessary or can be delayed until a therapeutic trial of oral medication has proved ineffective.

TREATMENT

Oral Treatment

The current nonsurgical treatments are listed in Box 1. Although there are a number of options for nonsurgical treatment, it is clear that oral therapy has revolutionized the treatment approach to patients with erectile dysfunction. As noted, once an initial appropriate evaluation has been performed and a tentative diagnosis is made, a trial of oral therapy is usually the preferred treatment choice for most patients. Currently, there are three oral agents approved for use by the U.S. Food and Drug Administration (FDA). These are sildenafil citrate (Viagra), vardenafil hydrochloride (Levitra), and tadalafil (Cialis).

All three drugs reversibly inhibit the penile-specific phosphodiesterase type 5 (PDE5) and enhance the nitric oxide–cyclic GMP pathways of cavernous smooth muscle relaxation; that is, all three prevent the breakdown of cyclic GMP by PDE5. In several double-blind, placebo-controlled studies of patients with erectile dysfunction of varied causes, all three drugs demonstrated improvement in erectile function, with success rates varying between 70% and 90%, depending on the populations studied.[7-10]

Clinical studies have demonstrated that sildenafil is a durable therapy, with patients able to remain on the medication and use it effectively. Some of these studies have also documented improved quality of life for both patient and partner with use of this medication. Vardenafil and tadalafil were more recently approved by the FDA, so existing clinical studies documenting effectiveness are short term. Hopefully, studies investigating their durability will be forthcoming.

Box 1 Nonsurgical Treatment Options for Erectile Dysfunction

Oral therapy
Withdrawal of offending medication
Hormonal therapy and dopamine agonists
Intracavernous injection therapy
Vacuum constriction devices
Intraurethral therapy
Sex therapy
Transluminal angioplasty, venoablation, or both
Topical agents

The success rate of all three drugs is reduced in some patient groups. For example, success in diabetic patients is probably closer to 50% to 60%, with demonstrated effectiveness for those with type 1 or 2 diabetes. Although patients who have had a radical prostatectomy might respond to any of these drugs, the best response occurs in patients whose procedure was bilateral nerve sparing. In patients whose procedure was bilateral nerve sparing, success rates vary but approach 70% in some series. However, if a single nerve was spared, success is reduced and, if no nerves were spared, results are generally poor, with a success rate of less than 15%.

All three drugs require sexual stimulation to be effective. The usual dose of sildenafil is 50 or 100 mg taken approximately 1 hour before intercourse, on an empty stomach and avoiding a fatty meal. Vardenafil is also taken 1 hour before intercourse, with a usual dose of 10 or 20 mg. Vardenafil may be less affected by food intake, but absorption may be delayed if a high-fat meal is ingested. Tadalafil may be taken 2 hours before intercourse, but its longer half-life (17.5 hours) allows greater flexibility in deciding when it can be taken before initiating intercourse (e.g., 6, 8, or perhaps 12 hours before). Tadalafil may be taken without regard to food intake.

All three drugs are generally well tolerated. Side effects of all three include headache, flushing, dyspepsia, and nasal congestion. Visual abnormalities are encountered with sildenafil, but they are less likely with vardenafil and unlikely with tadalafil. Back pain and myalgia can occur with tadalafil, but are unusual with sildenafil or vardenafil.

All three drugs are contraindicated in patients who use nitroglycerin or nitrate-containing compounds. Combining any of these three drugs with nitroglycerin or nitrates can result in significant hypotension. Vardenafil is contraindicated in patients using doxazosin (Cardura), terazosin (Hytrin), or tamsulosin (Flomax). Tadalafil is contraindicated in patients using doxazosin or terazosin. It may be safely taken with tamsulosin at the 0.4-mg dose. In patients who take 50 mg of sildenafil or higher and use alpha blockers, sildenafil dosing should be avoided for at least 4 hours after the dose of the alpha blocker. In patients who take 25 mg of sildenafil, use of any of the alpha blockers is considered safe. These drugs are often used for the treatment of benign prostatic hypertrophy and, perhaps less often, used for hypertension.

Although some initial concerns were raised about the use of sildenafil and other PDE5 inhibitors in patients with cardiovascular disease, ongoing studies, as well as clinical experience, have suggested that these medications are safe in patients with stable cardiovascular disease who are not using nitroglycerin or nitrate-containing compounds. Guidelines for evaluating cardiac patients before using PDE5 inhibitors have been published.[11,12]

Although vardenafil does not seem to produce significant clinical QT prolongation, it has been suggested that it be avoided in patients who have congenital QT prolongation abnormalities and in patients using class I antiarrhythmic drugs, such as quinidine and procainamide. It is also best to avoid the use of vardenafil with Class III antiarrhythmic drugs, such as amiodarone or sotalol.

Withdrawal of Offending Medications

It is extremely important to take a complete drug history, particularly with regard to antihypertensive medications and drugs used for cardiovascular disease, anxiety, depression, or psychosis in any patient complaining of erectile dysfunction (Box 2). Antihypertensive drugs, such as diuretics and beta blockers, may be associated with erectile dysfunction and perhaps can be discontinued or switched to alternative drugs, such as angiotensin-converting enzyme inhibitors or calcium channel blockers (e.g., diltiazem, nifedipine, amlodipine), which might cause less of a problem. The newer angiotensin II receptor antagonists may also be less problematic, but more long-term data are needed to confirm this.

Of the drugs used for depression, tricyclic antidepressants may be associated with erectile problems and other drugs may be substituted to prevent this complication. Currently available drugs such as bupropion, nefazodone, and trazodone may be helpful in this regard. The selective serotonin reuptake inhibitors (e.g., fluoxetine, sertraline, paroxetine, citalopram) can also cause difficulties with erectile dysfunction, but they might also have other significant sexual side effects, including decreased libido and anorgasmia.

Box 2 Drugs and Drug Classes Reported to Affect Erectile Function*

Antihypertensives
Beta blockers
Clonidine
Methyldopa
Thiazide diuretics

Psychiatric Medications
Antidepressants

- Amitriptyline
- Doxepin

Antipsychotics

- Phenothiazines
- Haloperidol
- Benzisoxazole (Risperidone)

Recreational Drugs
Alcohol
Heroin

Antiandrogens
Estrogen-containing medications
Cimetidine (in very high doses)
Gonadotropin-releasing hormone agonists
Ketoconazole
Spironolactone

Antiarrhythmics
Digoxin
Disopyramide

**This list is by no means comprehensive.*

Clinical experience in switching medication has overall been disappointing, and improvement does not seem to occur often. Nonetheless, it is important to try to discontinue possible offending medications before moving on to more-invasive options. Oral therapy has also basically changed how discontinuing medications may work as well and has improved the approach. For example, a patient might develop erectile dysfunction on a thiazide diuretic. The drug may be withdrawn, but a trial of oral therapy can be initiated during the observation period while the patient is waiting to see whether any spontaneous improvement in erectile function occurs after drug withdrawal. Alternatively, if diuretic therapy is effective, well tolerated, and controlling the blood pressure, oral therapy can be used to deal with the sexual side effects on an ongoing basis, which is often what is done.

If a trial of oral therapy and withdrawal of offending medications prove to be ineffective in restoring erectile function, it is probably appropriate for most primary care practitioners to consider referral to a specialist for additional evaluation and discussion of alternative treatment options. These include intracavernous injection therapy, vacuum constriction devices, intraurethral therapy, and possible surgery.

Vacuum Constriction Devices

As noted, if a trial of oral therapy and withdrawal of offending medications do not restore erectile function, most primary care practitioners will probably consider referral to a specialist for additional evaluation and discussion of alternative treatment options. Some, however, may recommend vacuum constriction devices, and several treatment guidelines have suggested that they represent a first-line treatment modality.[13,14] The concept of using a vacuum constriction device to help facilitate erectile function is almost 75 years old, but it is only within the past 15 years that such devices have become widely used.

The device consists of an acrylic cylinder placed over the penis that uses a lubricant to achieve a good seal between the body and cylinder. An erection is then achieved by creating a vacuum inside the cylinder with a pump connected to the cylinder. Once an erection is achieved, a constriction band is applied to the base of the penis to maintain the erection. The cylinder can then be removed and the patient can engage in intercourse with the constriction band(s) at the base of the penis maintaining the erection. The bands can remain on for approximately 30 minutes and then must be removed. The erection produced by the device differs from a normal erection; it is believed to involve venous occlusion from the constriction band resulting in generalized swelling of the entire penis, with probable preservation of arterial inflow.

A growing body of clinical studies has suggested that these devices are effective and acceptable to a large number of patients with erectile dysfunction of varying causes, including psychogenic erectile failure. Although the initial overall response rate is approximately 80% to 90%, longer-term follow-up studies suggest that satisfaction with this device approaches satisfaction with other modalities, suchas intracavernous injection therapy, which may be in the range of 50% to 60%.

There are relatively few contraindications to the use of this device. Some conditions can predispose to priapism or perhaps bleeding with constriction, such as sickle cell disease, polycythemia, and other blood dyscrasias. Patients on anticoagulation (with warfarin) can safely use vacuum constriction devices but need to accept a higher risk of bleeding (ecchymosis). Good manual dexterity is also needed to use the device; if manual dexterity is impaired, a willing sexual partner can learn to apply the device.

These devices are alternatives for patients who have failed or otherwise are unable to use oral therapy or injection therapy and do not desire surgery. Vacuum constriction devices are considered first-line therapy but in most cases, if oral therapy is effective, patients find that taking a pill is more desirable then using these devices. These devices, however, are useful for patients with marginal cardiac function or cerebral vascular disease who are not good candidates for any other treatment, such as oral therapy or injection therapy.

Complications from the use of a vacuum constriction device are relatively minor. They include the development of petechiae or ecchymosis, numbness or coolness of the penis, trapping of the ejaculate, and pivoting of the penis at the base. Although these complications are troublesome to some patients, they are not significant for most patients. Other complaints regarding the device include its being cumbersome, nonspontaneous and, in some cases, unacceptable to the partner. Despite problems, these devices have become an important nonsurgical option for some patients with erectile dysfunction.

NATIONAL PRACTICE GUIDELINES

The American Urological Association published treatment guidelines for organic erectile dysfunction in 2007.[15] They emphasize, as this chapter does, that yohimbine is not effective for organic erectile dysfunction.

The American Association of Clinical Endocrinologists (AACE) issued clinical practice guidelines in 1998 and then updated them in 2003.[16] This was the first year that oral therapy became available. The basic recommendations in this guideline have been incorporated into this chapter. This guideline mentions trying nonspecific treatment such as yohimbine but, as noted, clinical experience suggests that this drug is generally ineffective for organic erectile dysfunction and probably should be avoided.

The Veterans Health Administration (VHA) guidelines and the process of care model are useful; these incorporate the notion of lifestyle changes and interventions that may be helpful to patients with risk factors for erectile dysfunction.[13,14] However, currently there is limited evidence that these lifestyle interventions are actually beneficial for erectile dysfunction.

An additional interesting observation in the VHA guidelines[14] relates to some patients with spinal cord injury lesions above the T5-T6 level who may be prone to autonomic dysreflexia. This is a life-threatening situation that occasionally requires nitrites for the emergency management of hypertension, which interact adversely with sildenafil, producing severe hypotension. I have not personally seen this, but it is perhaps worth remembering if a physician is evaluating a patient with spinal cord injury for the treatment of erectile dysfunction.

Summary

- Erectile dysfunction, defined as the inability to develop and maintain an erection for satisfactory sexual intercourse, is common in men with diabetes mellitus.
- Associated risk factors include increasing age, dyslipidemia, hypertension, and antihypertensive and psychotropic medications.
- Proper evaluation includes a careful history, physical examination, and evaluation for possible endocrine causes (e.g. low testosterone, high prolactin levels).
- Because erectile dysfunction is caused by a complex set of psychosocial, neurologic, and vascular factors, a specific cause in a patient may remain ambiguous.
- Oral therapy with PDE5 inhibitors is often successful and safe for appropriately selected diabetic patients.
- Vacuum constriction devices provide acceptable alternative therapy for some patients.

Suggested Readings

American Association of Clinical Endocrinologists Male Sexual Dysfunction Task Force: American Association of Clinical Endocrinologists medical guidelines for clinical practice for the evaluation and treatment of male sexual dysfunction: A couple's problem-2003 update. Endocr Pract 2003;9:77-95.

Brock GB, McMahon CG, Chen KK, et al: Efficacy and safety of tadalafil for the treatment of erectile dysfunction: Results of integrated analyses. J Urol 2002;168:1332-1336.

DeBusk R, Drory Y, Goldstein I, et al: Management of sexual dysfunction in patients with cardiovascular disease: Recommendations of the Princeton Consensus Panel. Am J Cardiol 2000;86:175-181.

DeBusk RF, Pepine CJ, Glasser DB, et al: Efficacy and safety of sildenafil citrate in men with erectile dysfunction and stable coronary artery disease. Am J Cardiol 2004;93:147-153.

Feldman HA, Goldstein I, Hatzichristou DG, et al: Impotence and its medical and psychosocial correlates: Results of the Massachusetts Male Aging Study. J Urol 1994;151:54-61.

Goldstein I, Lue TF, Padma-Nathan H, et al: Oral sildenafil and the treatment of erectile dysfunction. N Engl J Med 1998;338:1397-1404.

Goldstein I: Male sexual circuitry. Working Group for the Study of Central Mechanisms in Erectile Dysfunction. Sci Am 2000;283:70-75.

Hellstrom WJ, Gittelman M, Karlin G, et al: Vardenafil for the treatment of men with erectile dysfunction: Efficacy and safety in a randomized double-blind placebo-controlled trial. J Androl 2002;23:763-771.

Johannes CB, Araujo AB, Feldman HA, et al: Incidence of erectile dysfunction in men 40 to 69 years old: Longitudinal results from the Massachusetts Male Aging Study. J Urol 2000;163:460-463.

Lakin M: The evaluation and nonsurgical management of impotence. Semin Nephrol 1994;14:544-550.

Langtry HD, Markham A: Sildenafil: A review of its use in erectile dysfunction. Drugs 1999;57:967-989.

Laumann EO, Paik A, Rosen RC: Sexual dysfunction in the United States: Prevalence and predictors. JAMA 1999;281:537-544.

Montague DK, Barada JH, Belker AM, et al: Clinical guidelines panel on erectile dysfunction: Summary report on the treatment of organic erectile dysfunction. The American Urological Association. J Urol 1996;156:2007-2011.

Pharmacy Benefits Management—Medical Advisory Panel: The Primary Care Management of Erectile Dysfunction (VHA PBM-SHG Publication No. 99-0014). Hines, Ill: Pharmacy Benefits Management Strategic Healthcare Group, Veterans Health Administration, Department of Veterans Affairs, June, 1999.

Process of Care Consensus Panel: The process of care model for evaluation and treatment of erectile dysfunction. Int J Impot Res 1999;11:59-70.

Rosen RC, Cappelleri JC, Smith MD, et al: Development and evaluation of an abridged five-item version of the International Index of Erectile Function (IIEF 5) as a diagnostic tool for erectile dysfunction. Intl J Impot Res 1999;11:319-326.

References

For a complete list of references, log onto www.expertconsult.com.

Flushing

Christian Nasr

DEFINITION

Flushing describes episodic attacks of redness of the skin together with a sensation of warmth or burning of the face, neck and, less frequently, the upper trunk and abdomen. It is the transient nature of the attacks that distinguishes flushing from the persistent erythema of photosensitivity or acute contact reactions. Repeated flushing over a prolonged period can lead to telangiectasia and occasionally to classic rosacea of the face.[1]

Flushing can be an exaggeration of a physiologic process or a manifestation of a serious condition that needs to be identified and treated. A biochemical workup of every case of flushing is neither practical nor cost-effective; in this chapter, we present guidelines that will help determine when a workup is warranted.

PREVALENCE

The prevalence of flushing has not been determined.

PATHOPHYSIOLOGY

Redness of the skin may be caused by an increased amount of saturated hemoglobin, an increase in the diameter or actual number of skin capillaries, or a combination of these factors.[2] Flushing is caused by increased blood flow through the skin, causing warmth and, because of engorgement of the subpapillary venous plexus, redness. The vasodilation of flushing may be caused by a direct action of a circulatory vasodilator substance—for example, histamine—or it may be caused by changes in the neurologic control of the cutaneous vasculature in the affected areas. In the face, neck, and upper trunk, where flushing is most frequent, the neurologic control of vascular tone is predominantly exerted by autonomic vasodilator nerve fibers. These fibers are found in somatic nerves supplying the affected skin, including the trigeminal nerve. Because autonomic nerve fibers also supply eccrine sweat glands, neurally activated flushing is frequently associated with sweating (wet flushing) as opposed to flushing caused by circulating vasodilator mediators, which frequently does not involve sweating (dry flushing). The presence or absence of sweating has therefore been proposed as a clinical guide to the mechanisms of flushing, although in practice this is not always reliable. Examples of wet flushing are physiologic flushing and menopausal flushing. An example of dry flushing is niacin-provoked flushing.[1]

The diameter of the blood vessels of the cheeks is wider than elsewhere, the vessels are nearer to the surface, and there is less tissue thickness obscuring them. This may explain why flushing occurs in that limited distribution.[3] Polycythemia produces the characteristic ruddy complexion, but it may also cause a peculiar coloration termed *erythremia*, which is a combination of redness and cyanosis. The tongue, lips, nose, earlobes, conjunctivae, and fingertips especially demonstrate this coloration. Erythremia results when there is a combination of increased amounts of saturated and desaturated hemoglobin.

In some carcinoid tumors, fibrosis of the right side of the heart may lead to a combination of stenosis and regurgitation at the tricuspid valve, as well as pulmonary stenosis. If cyanosis occurs, the combination of flushing and cyanosis may produce the reddish cyanotic erythremia.[2]

FLUSHING SYNDROMES

Physiologic Flushing

Embarrassment or anger may cause flushing in some individuals in whom the threshold for this response may be low or the reaction itself unusually intense; this is also known as blushing.[1,2] Explanation and reassurance are usually sufficient. If necessary, propranolol or nadolol may be used to alleviate the symptom.[1]

Heat causes flushing in many patients, and overheating can lower the threshold to flushing from other causes, such as menopause.[3] Overheating, such as after exercise or sauna, can cause physiologic flushing because of the effect of the rise in blood temperature on the thermoregulatory center in the anterior hypothalamus. A similar mechanism is responsible for facial flushing caused by hot drinks, which produce a rise in temperature of blood in the oral cavity, in turn leading to an increase in temperature of blood perfusing the hypothalamus. The temperature of hot coffee, rather than its caffeine, causes flushing.

A useful maneuver for patients faced with a brief thermal exposure is to suck on ice chips carried in an insulated cup. This attenuates flushing for the first 20 to 30 minutes.[3]

Menopausal Flushing

About 80% of postmenopausal women experience flushing associated with sweating. A similar syndrome may also occur in men with prostate cancer receiving treatment with gonadotropin-releasing hormone analogues, such as buserelin. About 65% of postmenopausal women have hot flushes for 1 to 5 years, 26% for 6 to 10 years, and 10% for more than 11 years. There is considerable variation in the frequency, intensity, and duration of hot flushes within and among individuals.

A typical hot flush begins with a sensation of warmth in the head and face, followed by facial flushing that may radiate down the neck and to other parts of the body; it is associated with an increase in temperature and pulse rate and followed by a decline in temperature and profuse perspiration over the area of flush distribution. Visible changes occur in about 50% of women. Each hot flush lasts for 1 to 5 minutes.

The primary role of estrogen deficiency has been questioned and a deficit of thermoregulation has been proposed. Rapid estrogen withdrawal rather than a low estrogen level by itself is likely to induce hot flushes.[4] Synchronous with the onset of each hot flush is the release of a pulse of luteinizing hormone; this does not seem to be responsible for the hot flush, because flushing can occur after hypophysectomy. The anterior hypothalamus has estrogen and progesterone receptors, and both hormones can be used effectively to treat hot flushes through binding with their respective hypothalamic receptors. Neurotransmitters that may be involved in the pathogenesis of hot flushes include norepinephrine and other noradrenergic substances. The central noradrenergic system in the hypothalamus triggers the hot flushes via α_2-adrenergic receptors on the noradrenergic neurons. Thus, clonidine, an α_2-adrenergic agonist, effectively alleviates hot flushes through reduction of noradrenergic release.[4]

Pharmacologic menopause with flushing can be induced by various drugs 4-hydroxyandrostenedione, danazol, tamoxifen, clomiphene citrate, and leuprolide. Certain characteristics suggest the diagnosis of climacteric flushing, such as drenching perspiration,

Box 1 Flushing Caused By Drugs

All vasodilators (e.g., nitroglycerin, prostaglandins)
All calcium channel blockers
Nicotinic acid (not nicotinamide)
Morphine and other opiates
Amyl nitrite and butyl nitrite
Cholinergic drugs (e.g., metrifonate, anthelmintic drug)
Bromocriptine used in Parkinson's disease
Thyrotropin-releasing hormone (TRH)
Tamoxifen
Cyproterone acetate
Oral triamcinolone
Cyclosporine
Rifampin
Sildenafil citrate

Adapted from Cutaneous manifestations of disorders of the cardiovascular and pulmonary systems. In Freedberg IM, Eisen AZ, Wolff K, et al (eds): Fitzpatrick's Dermatology in General Medicine, 5th ed, vol 2. New York, McGraw-Hill, 1999, pp 1935-1945.

a prodromal sensation of overheating before the onset of flushing and sweating, and waking episodes at night, with the typical symptoms. Alcohol can enhance a menopausal flush.[5] Veralipride, an antidopaminergic drug, can cause reductions in the frequency and intensity of menopausal flushing in premenopausal women pretreated with goserelin (a gonadotropin-releasing hormone agonist) for endometriosis.[6]

Flushing Caused by Drugs

Other medications that can cause flushing are corticotropin-releasing hormone, doxorubicin, and niacin (Box 1). Flushing is a side effect of sildenafil citrate in 12% of patients.[7] Systemic administration of morphine can cause flushing of the face, neck, and upper shoulders, which is believed to be histamine-mediated.[5] Patients can develop facial flushing, generalized erythema, or both after epidural or intra-articular administration of glucocorticoids. The exact pathophysiology is unclear but could be related to distention of the joint capsule.[8]

Flushing Associated with Alcohol Intake

Asians with certain genotypes show extensive flushing in response to low doses of alcohol. They have been found to have higher plasma levels of acetaldehyde. This abnormality is probably related to a deficiency of an isoenzyme of liver aldehyde dehydrogenase. This population can be detected by using an ethanol patch test, which produces localized erythema. A special type of alcohol flush is also associated with chlorpropamide, the oral antihyperglycemic agent. Even small amounts of alcohol provoke intense flushing within a few minutes of ingestion. This flushing is not associated with sweating but, in some cases, tachycardia, tachypnea, and hypotension may be seen. The flush is mediated by elevated acetaldehyde plasma levels and possibly by the release of prostaglandins. Alcohol ingestion can also trigger flushing in those with carcinoid tumors, mastocytosis, medullary thyroid carcinoma, and certain lymphoid tumors.

Trichloroethylene, a chemical that has been abandoned in recent years because of its carcinogenic potential, can cause flushing. When inhaled following ingestion of alcoholic beverages, a striking cutaneous reaction results, consisting in the sudden appearance of erythema of the face, neck, and shoulders, a reaction that has been termed *degreaser's flush*. Nausea and vomiting can also occur.[5]

Flushing Associated with Food

Eating spicy or sour foods can cause facial flushing. This gustatory flushing is caused by a neural reflex involving autonomic neurons carried by the branches of the trigeminal nerve. The flushing may be unilateral.

The flushing of monosodium glutamate (MSG) is controversial. Oral challenge with MSG has failed to provoke flushing in volunteers with a history of MSG flushing. Patients should be encouraged to look beyond MSG at other dietary agents, such as red pepper, other spices, nitrites and sulfites (additives in many foods), thermally hot foods and beverages, and alcohol.[5] Scombroid fish poisoning (tuna and mackerel) is caused by the ingestion of fish that was left in a warm temperature for hours. In addition to flushing, patients with scombroid fish poisoning experience sweating, vomiting, and diarrhea. These symptoms are caused by intoxication with histamine, which is believed to be generated by histidine decarboxylation by bacteria in spoiled fish.

Carcinoid Syndrome

Carcinoid syndrome describes the manifestations of carcinoid tumors-flushing, bronchoconstriction, gastrointestinal hypermotility, and cardiac disease. Carcinoid tumors are neuroendocrine tumors derived from a primitive stem cell that may differentiate into any of various adult endocrine-secreting cells, producing peptides, hormones, and neurotransmitters. The annual incidence is 1.5 per 100,000 population.[9] The average age of patients is 50 years, and there is no gender predominance.[10]

Carcinoid syndrome occurs in about 10% of patients with these tumors.[10] In 75% of patients, episodes of severe flushing are precipitated by exercise, alcohol, stress, and certain foods (e.g., spices, chocolate, cheese, avocados, plums, walnuts,[1] red sausage, red wine). With time, the flushing may appear without provocation.[9] The character of the flush differs, depending on the site of origin of the tumor (Figs. 1 and 2). Tumors of the foregut (stomach, lung, pancreas) are associated with a bright red geographic flush of a more sustained duration, as well as lacrimation, wheezing, sweating, and a sensation of burning. In ileal tumors, the flush is patchier and more violaceous, intermingled with areas of pallor, and does not last as long. Flushing of either type may be associated with facial edema, which may persist and lead to telangiectasia and even facial rosacea. With extensive disease, pellagra-like skin lesions can also be seen; these result from excessive uptake of tryptophan by the carcinoid tumor, leaving little for the daily niacin requirement. These lesions include hyperkeratosis, xerosis, scaling of the legs, forearms, and trunk, angular cheilitis, and glossitis (Fig. 3). Seventy percent of patients also have watery diarrhea, and 35% develop right-sided endocardial fibrosis, leading to congestive heart failure. Diarrhea and other gastrointestinal manifestations may precede or coexist with the flushing.[5]

Ninety-five percent of all carcinoids are found in the appendix, rectum, or small intestine.[9] The remainder arise outside of the intestinal tract (e.g., in the ovary or testis). In general, the larger the primary tumor, the greater the likelihood of metastasis, which provides prognostic implications.[9] Carcinoids of the appendix and rectum rarely manifest with the carcinoid syndrome. Forty percent to 50% of patients with carcinoids of the small intestine or proximal colon have manifestations of the carcinoid syndrome.[10] Tumors that secrete their hormonal product into the portal venous system do not cause flushing, because the released amines are inactivated by the liver. In contrast, liver metastases may escape hepatic inactivation and deliver their product directly into the systemic circulation, hence causing flushing.[9] Pulmonary or ovarian carcinoids release pharmacologic products directly into the venous circulation, bypassing the portal system, and can therefore cause symptoms without metastasizing to the liver.[1,10]

Pathophysiology

The flushing seen with foregut carcinoids is caused by the release of histamine. Flushing seen with ileal carcinoids cannot be explained solely by the production of serotonin.[1] Serotonin may or may not be

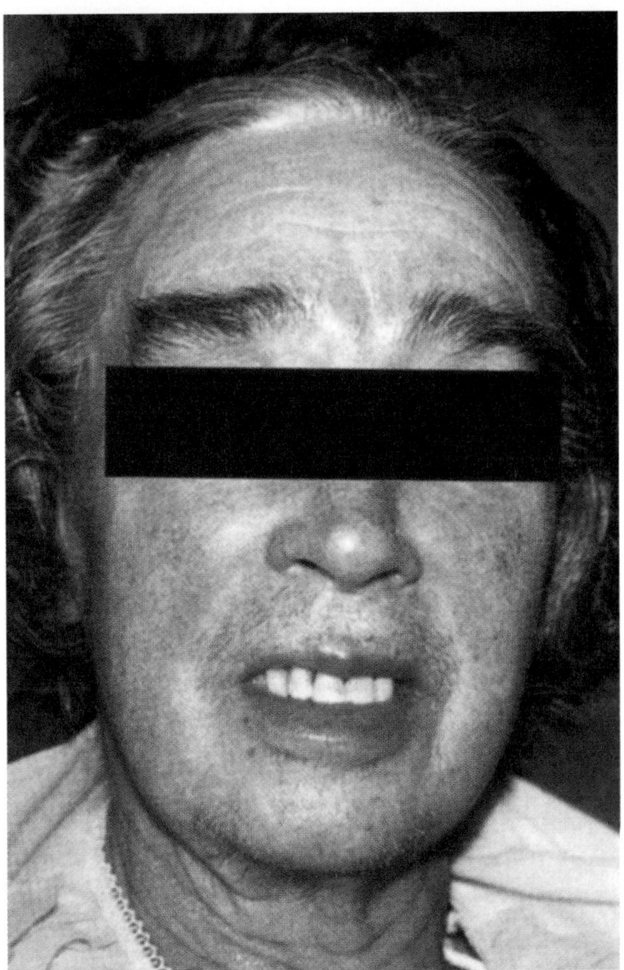

Figure 1 **Flushing of carcinoid syndrome.**

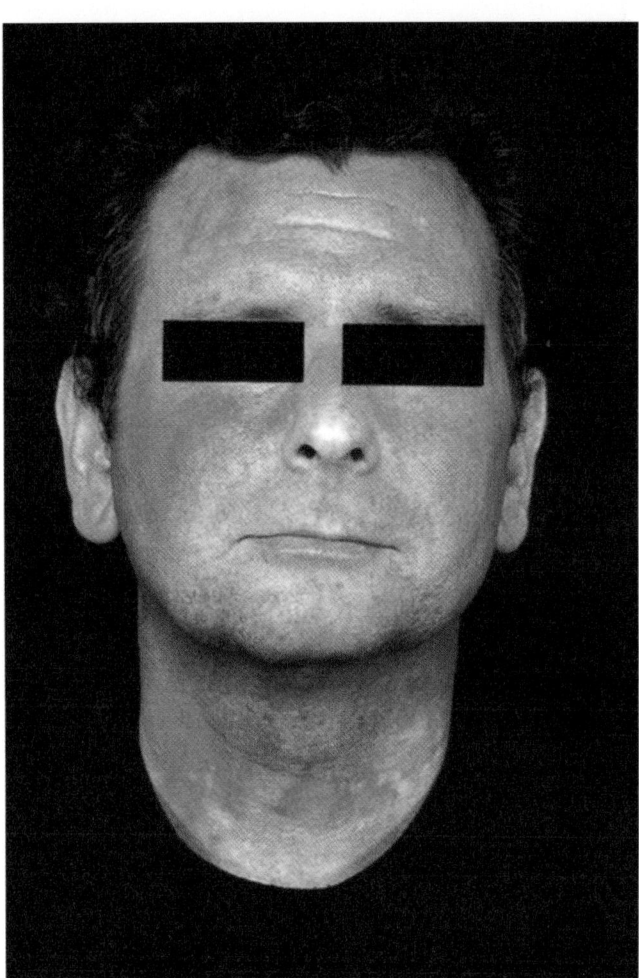

Figure 2 **Histamine-evoked flushing of foregut carcinoid tumor.**

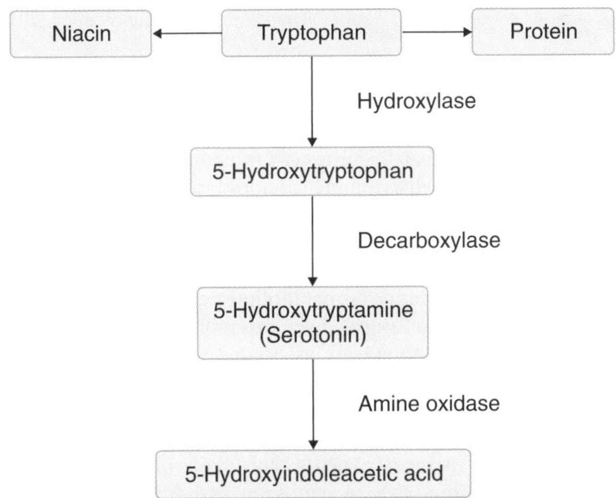

Figure 3 **Pathway for transformation of tryptophan to 5-hydroxytryptamine, niacin, and protein.** *(Adapted from Greaves MW: Mastocytoses. In Champion RH, Burton JL, Burns T, Breathnach S [eds]: Rook/Wilkinson/Ebling Textbook of Dermatology, 6th ed, vol 3. Oxford, England, Blackwell Scientific, 1998, pp 2337-2346.)*

released into the circulation during flushing, and IV infusion of serotonin does not cause flushing. Foregut carcinoids do not generally secrete serotonin but, instead, its precursor, 5-hydroxytryptamine. Screening should therefore seek this product if the other metabolites are not elevated.[9] Other mediators that have been proposed include prostaglandins and tachykinins. Tachykinins are believed to be mediators of the flushing in tumors of the midgut. They exert vasodilation and contraction of various types of smooth muscle. These peptides include substance P, substance K, and neuropeptide K. Urine excretion of histamine is usually increased in patients who have gastric carcinoids (Table 1).[9]

Diagnosis

Clinical diagnosis is not difficult in patients with flushing episodes associated with systemic symptoms (e.g., diarrhea, wheezing, weight loss) and hepatomegaly. It is more difficult in patients who have occasional flushing and no associated symptoms.[1] Only when there is reasonable clinical suspicion should biochemical testing be done, and localization studies must be reserved for those cases proven biochemically.[10] When in doubt, a carcinoid flush can be provoked by alcohol ingestion (4 mL of 45% ethanol) or the infusion of 6 μg noradrenaline, an effect that can be blocked by phentolamine (5-15 mg IV). Calcium gluconate, 10 to 15 mg/kg, administered IV over 4 hours, may produce a flush mimicking a spontaneous attack.[5] Epinephrine reverses flushing in patients with mastocytosis but provokes flushing in patients with the carcinoid syndrome. The procedure should only be performed in a controlled environment. A 1-μg/

Box 2 Factors that Can Precipitate Flushing in the Carcinoid Syndrome

Foods and Beverages
Hot foods or beverages
Spicy foods
Chocolate
Cheeses
Tomatoes
Avocados
Red plums
Walnuts
Eggplant
Alcohol

Other Causes
Emotional stress
Valsalva maneuver
Straining
Vigorous coughing
Sudden direct pressure on a large carcinoid tumor

Adapted from Cutaneous manifestations of disorders of the cardiovascular and pulmonary systems. In Freedberg IM, Eisen AZ, Wolff K, et al (eds): Fitzpatrick's Dermatology in General Medicine, 5th ed, vol 2. New York, McGraw-Hill, 1999, pp 1935-1945.

Table 1 Classification of Carcinoid Tumors According to Site of Primary Tumor

Site	Biochemistry	Clinical Picture
Foregut bronchi, stomach, first part duodenum	5-Hydroxytryptophan, adrenocorticotropin, growth hormone, gastrin, growth hormone releasing hormone	Protracted, purplish or violaceous flush, manifestation of other ectopic hormone secretion
Midgut second part of duodenum, jejunum, ileum, ascending colon	Serotonin, kinins, neuropeptides, prostaglandins	Pink-red flush
Hindgut transverse, descending colon and rectum	None	Only local symptoms

Adapted from Vinik AI: Neuroendocrine tumors of carcinoid variety. In DeGroot LJ (ed): Endocrinology, 3rd ed, vol 3. Philadelphia, WB Saunders, 1995, pp 2803-2812.

Box 3 Factors that Interfere with Determination of Urinary 5-HIAA

Factors that Produce False-Positive ResultsFoods
Avocados
Bananas
Eggplants
Pineapples
Plums
Walnuts

Drugs
Acetaminophen
Acetanilid
Caffeine
Fluorouracil
Guaifenesin
Lugol's (iodine) solution
Melphalan
Mephenesin
Methamphetamine
Methocarbamol
Methysergide maleate
Phenacetin
Phenmetrazine
Reserpine

Factors that Produce False-Negative Results
Drugs
Corticotropin
p-Chlorophenylalanine
Chlorpromazine
Heparin
Imipramine
Isoniazid
Methenamine mandelate
Methyldopa
Monoamine oxidase inhibitors
Phenothiazine
Promethazine
Methenamine mandelate

5-HIAA, 5-hydroxyindoleacetic acid.
Adapted from O'Toole D, Ducreux M, Bommelaer G, et al: Treatment of carcinoid syndrome: A prospective crossover evaluation of lanreotide versus octreotide in terms of efficacy, patient acceptability, and tolerance. Cancer 2000;88:770-776.

mL solution of epinephrine in normal saline is administered by an IV bolus, beginning with an initial dose of 0.05 μg. The dose is doubled at intervals of 10 minutes until flushing appears or until a maximum of 6.4 μg is given. When flushing occurs, it usually begins within 60 seconds after epinephrine administration and dissipates after 3 or 4 minutes.[10]

The diagnosis should be confirmed by determining urinary excretion of 5-hydroxyindoleacetic acid (5-HIAA), the major metabolite of serotonin, which is normally 2 to 10 mg (10-50 μmol)/24 hours.[5] A value of more than 150 μmol/24 hours (30 mg/24 hours) usually confirms the diagnosis, and in carcinoid syndrome it is often above 40 mg/day.[5] This test has a sensitivity of 75% and a specificity of up to 100%. The degree of elevation of 5-HIAA does not always correlate with the severity of flushing.[9] Excretion fluctuates, so that repeat measurements may be necessary. Some patients with carcinoid may lack the metabolic machinery to convert serotonin to 5-HIAA, so they have high blood levels of serotonin but normal urinary 5-HIAA levels.[5] Dietary factors may cause confusion; the patient should therefore receive a diet free of the culprit items (Box 2) for 3 days before the urine collection is made. Although the levels of serotonin in patients with tumors usually far exceed those found after food ingestion, this precaution helps exclude carcinoid in individuals with borderline high 5-HIAA levels.[9] Measuring the blood serotonin level is helpful when the urinary 5-HIAA level is equivocal. Patients with carcinoid syndrome have very high blood levels of serotonin. Measurement of serotonin and its metabolites permits the detection of 84% of neuroendocrine tumors. Even carcinoids that predominantly secrete 5-hydroxytryptophan are associated with increased urinary excretion of 5-HIAA because the released 5-hydroxytryptophan is converted to serotonin in other tissues and is subsequently metabolized to 5-HIAA.[9] Chromogranin A, a peptide cosecreted with serotonin, is elevated in most patients with carcinoid tumors. In the evaluation of flushing with an equivocal 24-hour urinary 5-HIAA level, a normal plasma chromogranin A value suggests nonendocrine causes. This test is sensitive but not specific, and its predictive value in carcinoid is still uncertain.[10] Flushing was associated with a rise in circulating substance P in 80% of patients with gastric carcinoid. Neurokinin A levels are elevated in certain patients (Box 2 and Box 3).[9]

Treatment

Corticosteroids, phenothiazines, and bromocriptine have been effective in the treatment of patients with bronchial carcinoid tumors.

The mechanism of action of these agents is unknown. Cyproheptadine, a serotonin antagonist, may control the flushing. Methysergide can control the diarrhea but has no effect on flushing. Combined administration of histamine types 1 and 2 (H_1 and H_2) receptor antagonists may prevent attacks of flushing in patients with foregut carcinoid tumors that produce histamine.[10] Alpha-interferons may control symptoms of carcinoid syndrome and produce objective biochemical responses (>50% suppression of 5-HIAA) with a median duration of approximately 4 weeks.10 Because catecholamines are known to precipitate attacks, a trial of clonidine is worthwhile. Somatostatin is a potent antagonist of the flushing reaction associated with both gastric and ileal carcinoid tumors but has a short half-life. The somatostatin analogue octreotide has a much longer half-life, making subcutaneous therapy possible. It must be given by subcutaneous injection one to three times/day and should be titrated in increments of 50 μg every 8 hours.[10] Octreotide lowers plasma levels of serotonin and tachykinins and relieves flushing and diarrhea. Amelioration of these manifestations is accompanied by a marked reduction in the urinary excretion of 5-HIAA.[10] Lanreotide, a long-acting analogue of somatostatin administered IM every 14 days, is effective at controlling the flushing of carcinoids.[11,12] A depot form of octreotide (Sandostatin LAR Depot) has been shown to control flushing at a dose of 20 mg IM every month.[13] Flushing may relapse with continued treatment.[9] The patient should receive an adequate niacin supplement (nicotinamide rather than nicotinic acid, because the latter causes flushing) and should avoid foods, agents, and activities that precipitate symptoms.[5]

In some patients, failure of medical treatment may necessitate carrying out hepatic artery embolization. This treatment is based on the dependence of metastatic malignant tissue but not healthy liver parenchyma on an intact hepatic arterial blood supply. Antitumor chemotherapy remains experimental. Alpha-interferon causes symptomatic relief accompanied by lowering of the urinary 5-HIAA level.

Prognosis

Approximately 20% of patients with the carcinoid syndrome undergo a protracted course. In the remainder, deterioration can be rapid. The mean survival is about 8 years, with some surviving up to 20 years. Mean survival is 36 months after the first flushing episode.[9]

Mastocytoses

Causative Factors

Mastocytoses are benign proliferative disorders of the reticuloendothelial system and familial cases have been reported. Mastocytoses are caused by a hyperplastic rather than neoplastic process. They are often self limited, especially in childhood (Box 4). Mast cells contain the enzyme histidine decarboxylase, which enables them to synthesize and store histamine. Other preformed mediators include tryptase, chymase, and carboxypeptidase. Serotonin has not been detected in human mast cells.[14]

Histopathology

There are increased numbers of normal-looking mast cells in the dermis. These cells may be predominantly perivascular or may show a nodular distribution. The epidermis is normal, apart from increased melanization.[14]

Biochemical Markers

Symptoms of mastocytosis are mainly the result of release of products of mast cell activation. Plasma histamine levels are frequently increased in patients with systemic symptoms, and elevated urinary excretion of histamine and its metabolite methyl imidazole acetic acid (MIAA) can also be seen. Plasma tryptase levels can also be elevated. Prostaglandin D_2 (PGD_2) is another product of mast cell activation. Urinary excretion of this substance and its major metabolites can be elevated severalfold in patients with mastocytoses. Urine should be collected within a few hours of an attack.[14]

Box 4 Classification of Mastocytoses

Benign
Cutaneous
Urticaria pigmentosa
Solitary mastocytoma
Diffuse and/or erythrodermic (systemic involvement common; can be fatal)
Telangiectasia macularis eruptiva perstans

Systemic
Myeloproliferative, myelodysplastic
Gastrointestinal
Skeletal

Malignant
Lymphadenopathic with eosinophilia
Mast cell leukemia

Clinical Presentation

Episodic bright red flushing occurs spontaneously or after rubbing the skin or exposure to alcohol or mast cell degranulating agents. Flushing attacks may be accompanied by headache, dyspnea and wheezing, palpitations, abdominal pain, diarrhea, and syncope and may closely resemble the flushing episodes of the carcinoid syndrome, especially the foregut variety, which are also mediated by histamine. Rosacea may develop rarely. PGD_2 might be associated with the symptoms of flushing and diarrhea.[14] The flushing of cutaneous mastocytosis typically lasts more than 30 minutes, unlike the typical carcinoid flush, which lasts less than 10 minutes.[5] In urticaria pigmentosa, the diagnosis is established by demonstrating that gentle rubbing of the lesional skin causes local itching, redness, and whealing (Darier's sign). This reaction is caused by local histamine release. Darier's sign may also be demonstrated in skin without lesions. Confirmation of the diagnosis is obtained by skin biopsy. In patients with systemic symptoms, bone marrow biopsy and liver and spleen scans are usually performed. Bone scans should only be carried out in the presence of localized bone symptoms.[5,14]

Treatment

Treatment of nonlocalized forms of mastocytosis is mainly symptomatic. Patients should avoid known histamine-degranulating agents. Antihistamines remain the preferred treatment for most patients with uncomplicated urticaria pigmentosa. Human skin blood vessels possess H_1 and H_2 receptors, which are involved in both vasodilation and increased vascular permeability evoked by histamine. Thus, combination treatment with an H_1 antihistamine (hydroxyzine 10-20 mg) and H_2 antihistamine (cimetidine 200-500 mg) is logical and sometimes effective at controlling the flushing episodes. Oral administration of the mast cell stabilizing agent disodium cromoglycate has proved effective in some patients. The drug does not decrease urinary excretion of histamine and the histamine metabolite MIAA. Some experts have recommended using this agent only in patients with systemic mastocytosis who suffer from gastrointestinal symptoms. Photochemotherapy has been reported to cause symptomatic relief as well as objective reduction in the population of mast cells and the urinary excretion of MIAA.[14]

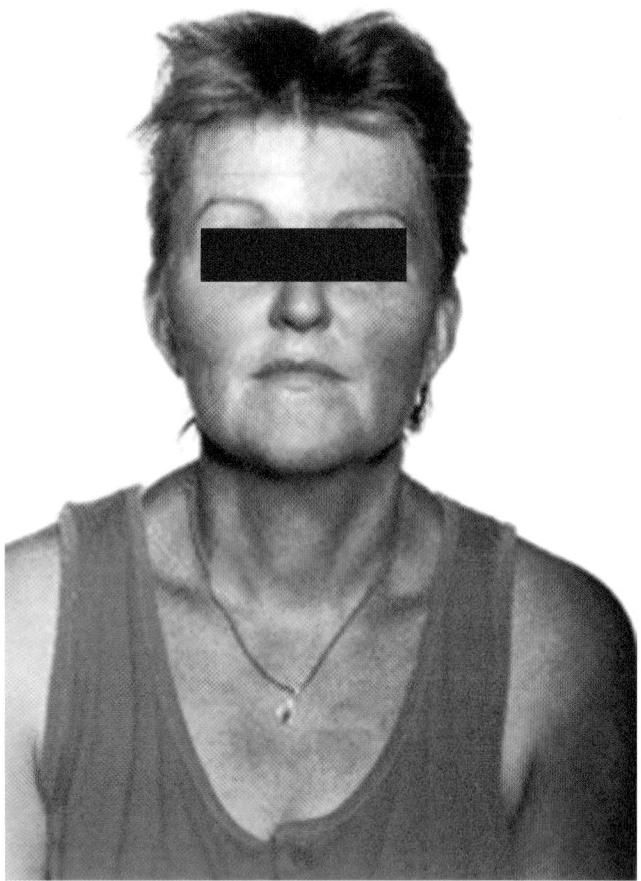

Figure 4 Harlequin syndrome.

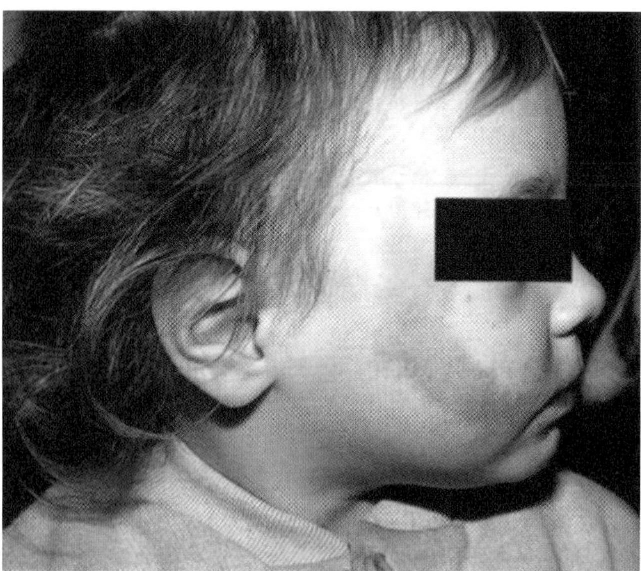

Figure 5 Auriculotemporal nerve syndrome (Frey's syndrome).

Medullary Thyroid Carcinoma

The range of substances secreted by medullary carcinoma of the thyroid is considerable, whether sporadic or familial. Flushing is the most common symptom after diarrhea. Occurring in one third of the patients with diarrhea, there is pronounced episodic flushing, which, as in the carcinoid syndrome, may be induced by alcohol ingestion. Calcitonin gene-related peptide, which is an extremely powerful peripheral vasodilator, is the most likely mediator that causes flushing.[5] The other possible explanation is that calcitonin stimulates prostaglandins, which in turn cause the symptoms.[12]

Harlequin Syndrome

This describes hemifacial flushing and sweating sometimes associated with warmth and anhidrosis of the contralateral arm and leg (Fig. 4). This may be induced by exercise. The suggested cause is a lesion involving preganglionic or postganglionic cervical sympathetic fibers and parasympathetic neurons of the ciliary ganglion.[15] Harlequin syndrome has been described in patients with a contralateral lung cancer invading the spine, Pancoast's syndrome, and Horner's syndrome.[5]

Auriculotemporal Nerve Syndrome (Frey's Syndrome)

This syndrome usually manifests as immediate unilateral or bilateral flushing, sweating in the distribution of the auriculotemporal nerve, or both in response to gustatory or tactile stimuli. In adults, this syndrome is a well-recognized sequela of parotid surgery, trauma, or infection. It occurs rarely in children, most often noted after the introduction of solid food. The flushing is often attributed erroneously to food allergy. It typically begins at 2 to 6 months of age when solid foods, mostly fruit, are introduced. Occurring within a few seconds of eating, it has a peculiar distribution in a triangular area that extends from the tragus of the ear to the midpoint of the cheek. It is not associated with sweating and persists for 20 to 60 minutes. The flushing continues to occur for up to 5 years. In adults, gustatory sweating is the predominant feature of auriculotemporal nerve syndrome; flushing happens less often. One half of pediatric patients with this symptom were delivered with forceps assistance, which possibly causes trauma to the nerve. The likely mechanism is misdirection of parasympathetic fibers along sympathetic pathways during the nerve regeneration that follows trauma. This may account for erythema when eating. The emergence of symptoms several months after the proposed trauma (usually 3-6 months) is probably related to the time required for nerve regeneration, and it is possible that vigorous chewing causes intense stimulation of the parotid gland. Auriculotemporal nerve syndrome is benign in infants and does not tend to worsen. Furthermore, the severity of the flushing tends to diminish with age in most patients. The physician can reassure parents and avoid unnecessary testing and maneuvers (Fig. 5).[16] A similar syndrome can develop after facial herpes zoster.[17]

Flushing with Pseudocarcinoid Syndrome in Secondary Male Hypogonadism

A series of three male patients with secondary hypogonadism has been described, in whom flushing was associated with elevated 24-hour urine 5-HIAA levels. Flushing disappeared, and 5-HIAA levels normalized after starting testosterone enanthate treatment. Male patients with flushing and increased urinary 5-HIAA levels should undergo assessment for hypogonadism after screening for carcinoid tumor.[18]

Treatments that lower the serum testosterone level, such as orchiectomy or luteinizing hormone-releasing hormone analogues, cause hot flushes in more than 50% of men. Lack of regulatory feedback in the hypothalamus from circulating serum testosterone is the presumed mechanism. Most often, hot flushes are only mildly bothersome and can be tolerated without the need for treatment. However, if flushes are particularly annoying or problematic, treatment should be offered. Small doses of diethylstilbestrol are effective in relieving hot flushes but cause gynecomastia. Megestrol acetate, 20 mg twice daily, completely eliminates hot flushes in most men, and the dose can be progressively lowered in some.[19]

Other Diseases Causing Episodic Flushing

Cheung and colleagues[20] have described a family with monoamine oxidase deficiency causing episodes of flushing affecting the face and chest precipitated by emotion or certain foods, followed by diarrhea, headaches, and sometimes palpitations. Blood serotonin levels in this family were elevated secondary to decreased activity of monoamine oxidase. Sertraline hydrochloride controlled the symptoms by depleting platelet serotonin.

Flushing is rare in patients with pheochromocytoma. If flushing occurs at all, it is seen after a paroxysm of hypertension, tachycardia, palpitations, chest pain, severe throbbing headaches, and excessive perspiration. Pallor is typically present during the attack, and mild flushing may occur after the attack as a rebound vasodilation of the facial cutaneous blood vessels.[5] Facial flushing and headache can happen along with sweating of the face, neck, and upper trunk in patients with spinal cord lesions above T6. This may occur as an exaggerated response to bowel or bladder distention.[1] Other causes are certain pancreatic tumors, insulinoma, and POEMS (polyneuropathy, organomegaly, endocrinopathy, monoclonal proteinemia, and skin changes). Transient flushing of the face, chest, or arms has been noted after neurologic deterioration secondary to a rapid increase in intracranial pressure.[21]

Rosacea

Persistent flushing from any cause may eventually lead to rosacea. The lesions of rosacea that initially occur in the central convex areas of the face consist of papules and pustules against a background of erythema, telangiectasia, edema, and eventual permanent induration or thickening of affected skin.[2] Patients with severe flushing caused by mastocytosis can develop rosacea in less than 1 year after the onset of flushing episodes.[5]

EVALUATION OF THE PATIENT WITH A FLUSHING DISORDER

It is important to consider the clinical characteristics of the flushing before embarking on expensive laboratory evaluation.[5] The physician should consider four clinical characteristics in the initial evaluation of a patient with flushing: provocative and palliative factors, morphology, associated features, and temporal characteristics.[2]

Provocative or Palliative Factors. Certain agents that trigger the flush suggest an underlying systemic disease as the cause for the flushing, such as mastocytosis and carcinoid syndrome.

Morphology

- Is there a basic feature that comes and goes?
- Is the redness patchy or confluent?
- What is the color of the flush?
- Is there cyanosis?
- Is the flushing preceded or followed by pallor?[2]

The morphology of the flushing may suggest not only the cause of the flushing but also, in the case of carcinoids, the anatomic origin of the disorder.[5]

Associated Features. Associated features may include respiratory symptoms, gastrointestinal symptoms, headache, urticaria, facial edema, hypertension, hypotension, palpitations, or sweating.

Temporal Characteristics. Temporal characteristics are the frequency of the flushing and the timing of the specific features during each flushing reaction. Important information can be obtained from a 2-week diary in which the patient records qualitative and quantitative aspects of the flushing event and lists exposure to all exogenous agents.[2] When the diagnosis remains obscure after evaluation of the 2-week diary, the patient is given an exclusion diet listing foods high in histamine, foods and drugs that affect urinary 5-HIAA tests, and foods and beverages that cause flushing. If the flushing reactions completely disappear, restoring the excluded items individually can identify the causative agent. If the flushing reactions continue unchanged, then further metabolic workup may be undertaken.[5]

Summary

- It is important to differentiate physiologic flushing from flushing associated with more serious diseases.
- Distinguish wet flushing from dry flushing.
- Look for flush distribution, triggers, reproducibility, and associated symptoms.
- Do not forget to look for drugs that are known to cause flushing.
- Alcohol and certain foods can cause physiologic flushing but may also trigger flushing in carcinoid syndrome.
- The character of the flushing in carcinoid syndrome depends on the location of the tumor.

Suggested Readings

Corbett M, Abernethy DA: Harlequin syndrome. J Neurol Neurosurg Psychiatry 1999;66:544.

Cutaneous manifestations of disorders of the cardiovascular and pulmonary systems. In Freedberg IM, Eisen AZ, Wolff K, et al (eds): Fitzpatrick's Dermatology in General Medicine, 5th ed, vol 2. New York, McGraw-Hill, 1999, pp 1935-1945.

Dawood MY: Menopause. In Copeland LJ (ed): Textbook of Gynecology, 2nd ed. Philadelphia, WB Saunders, 2000, pp 603-629.

Freedberg IM, Eisen AZ, Wolff K, et al (eds): Fitzpatrick's Dermatology in General Medicine, 5th ed., vol. 1 New York, McGraw Hill, 1993, pp 142-1659.

Greaves MW: Flushing and flushing syndromes, rosacea and perioral dermatitis. In Champion RH, Burton JL, Burns T, Breathnach S (eds): Rook/Wilkinson/Ebling Textbook of Dermatology, 6th ed, vol 3. Oxford, England, Blackwell Scientific, 1998, pp 2099-2104.

Greaves MW: Mastocytoses. In Champion RH, Burton JL, Burns T, Breathnach S (eds): Rook/Wilkinson/Ebling Textbook of Dermatology, 6th ed, vol 3. Oxford, England, Blackwell Scientific, 1998, pp 2337-2346.

Larsen PR (ed): Williams Textbook of Endocrinology, 10th ed. Philadelphia, WB Saunders, 2003.

Vinik AI: Neuroendocrine tumors of carcinoid variety. In DeGroot LJ (ed): Endocrinology, 3rd ed, vol 3. Philadelphia, WB Saunders, 1995, pp 2803-2812.

Wilkin J: Flushing and blushing. In Moschella SL, Hurley HJ (eds): Dermatology, 3rd ed, vol 2. Philadelphia, WB Saunders, 1992, pp 2080-2083.

Wilson JD (ed): Williams Textbook of Endocrinology, 9th ed. Philadelphia, WB Saunders, 1998.

References

For a complete list of references, log onto www.expertconsult.com.

Hirsutism

Priya Chinnappa and Adi Mehta

DEFINITION

Hirsutism is defined as a male pattern of hair distribution in a female, with the hair being transformed from fine villous hair to visible, coarse, terminally medullated hair under the influence of androgens.[1] Hirsutism must be distinguished from hypertrichosis and lanugo. Hypertrichosis is the growth of villous hair that is not androgen dependent and that is prominent in sexual and nonsexual areas. Lanugo is very soft, villous, nonpigmented hair that covers the body.

EPIDEMIOLOGY

Overall, the prevalence of hirsutism is unknown but may be as high as 50%. It is said that "even a single hair casts a shadow," so that in cultures in which a lack of hair is a feature of female beauty, minimal hirsutism is considered a disorder, whereas in other cultures, in which some excess hair growth is acceptable, a significant change in the pattern and texture of the hair needs to be present before it is deemed a problem. In a classic British study of 430 normal women, there was no hair seen on the upper back or abdomen, indicating that the presence of hair in these areas is abnormal. In this study, 10% had hair on the chest, 22% had chin hair, and 49% had hair on the upper lip. The distribution of hair was very scanty in all these areas. Hence, the ethnic background, as well as distribution and density of hair growth, determine the degree of hirsutism. The practicing physician must place the patient in the spectrum of individuals in the locality in which he or she practices to be able to assess the severity of hirsutism objectively. In addition, the age at onset, rate of growth and progression, and associated symptoms and signs can determine the severity of the problem.

ETIOLOGY AND PATHOGENESIS

Androgens are a prerequisite for sexual hair development. Hirsutism can arise from increased androgen production or from increased sensitivity of the hair follicles to circulating androgens.

Testosterone is the most important circulating androgen because of its relatively high plasma concentration and greater potency at the target organ level. Circulating testosterone is the sum of the secretion from the ovaries (35%-40%) and adrenals (40%) in response to the tropic hormones—luteinizing hormone (LH) and adrenocorticotropic hormone (ACTH)—respectively. The remaining circulating testosterone is derived from the conversion of androgenic precursors, mainly androstenedione (derived from the ovaries and adrenals) and dehydroepiandrosterone (DHEA; derived almost exclusively from the adrenals).[1-3] Peripheral conversion of androgenic prohormones to testosterone occurs in the liver, skin, and adipose tissue.[1-3] Testosterone is present in the circulation as the free or conjugated form. Almost 98% to 99% of plasma testosterone is bound to steroid hormone-binding globulin (SHBG), to cortisol-binding globulin, or nonspecifically to albumin and other proteins and is biologically inactive. The free portion of testosterone is biologically active. In the hair follicles, testosterone is converted to its biologically active form, dihydrotestosterone, by the enzyme 5α-reductase.[1-3]

Sex hormones work independently in the liver to control SHBG production. Estrogens increase and androgens decrease the production of SHBG. Thus, in hyperandrogenic states, the SHBG level is decreased, thereby allowing even higher free androgen levels. The other major modulator of SHBG is insulin. Insulin decreases the production of SHBG so that in conditions of insulin resistance and compensatory hyperinsulinemia, the SHBG level is decreased.

Pilosebaceous Unit

The pilosebaceous unit (PSU) consists of a pilary component and sebaceous component. Each PSU has the capacity to form either a terminal hair (a dark, pigmented, large medullated hair) as its prominent structure or a sebaceous follicle in which the hair remains villous and the sebaceous gland is more prominent. Androgens play a key role in the development of the PSU. Before the onset of puberty, in androgen-sensitive areas, the hair is villous and sebaceous glands are small. When androgen levels increase during puberty or hyperandrogenic states, PSUs form terminal hairs in sexual areas and increase the size of sebaceous glands in sebaceous areas. Formation of terminal hairs, when excessive, leads to hirsutism; excess secretion from sebaceous glands predisposes to acne.[8]

Mechanism of Action of Androgens

The hair follicle is one of the androgen-sensitive appendages in the skin and is a major site for the formation of testosterone from its precursors. Also, the 5α-reductase enzyme present in the outer root sheath cells converts testosterone to its active metabolite, dihydrotestosterone. The dermal papilla cells are believed to be the target cells releasing the growth factors that act on other cells of the hair follicles.

Sensitivity to Androgens

Development of hirsutism is determined by androgen levels and the sensitivity of the PSU to androgens. Thus, the level of androgens does not always correlate to the degree of hirsutism. Increase in sensitivity is believed to be caused by exaggerated peripheral 5α-reductase activity, androgen receptor polymorphism, or altered androgen metabolism.[2]

Causes of Androgen-Mediated Hirsutism

Polycystic ovary syndrome (PCOS) and idiopathic causes account for 90% of cases of hirsutism.[2-3] The androgen source is a mixture of contributions from the ovaries and adrenal glands. Other conditions can be classified according to the source of excess androgens. Ovarian causes are mainly ovarian tumors and hyperthecosis. Adrenal causes include Cushing's syndrome, androgen-producing tumors, and congenital adrenal hyperplasia (CAH), most commonly resulting from 21-hydroxylase deficiency. Other causes of CAH are 11β-hydroxylase deficiency and 3β-hydroxysteroid dehydrogenase deficiency. Hyperprolactinemia can stimulate adrenal DHEA sulfate (DHEAS) production, thus predisposing to hirsutism.

In patients predisposed to hirsutism, exogenous androgens can cause hirsutism and should not be used. Androgen preparations, mainly estrogen-testosterone combinations, have been approved for treating postmenopausal symptoms, and need to be stopped. Tibolone, a steroid with estrogenic, progestogenic, and androgenic effects, should also be discontinued.[4]

Valproic acid, a commonly used antiepileptic agent, has been associated with PCOS. History of the use of this medication should be specifically determined in the evaluation of women with hirsutism.[5] Although insulin resistance is a feature of PCOS, severe insulin resistance syndromes such as maturity-onset diabetes of the young and lipodystrophies are rarer causes of hirsutism.

Hirsutism can occur in older women, beginning a few years before menopause, and can continue for a few years after menopause. Ovarian estrogen secretion declines rapidly, whereas ovarian androgen production continues for a few years after menopause. Androgen production after menopause is gonadotropin dependent and, when excessive, can lead to hirsutism.[6,7]

SIGNS AND SYMPTOMS

History should include age at onset, rate of progression, virilization, family history, and current medications. Idiopathic hirsutism typically begins at the peripubertal age. Rate of progression is important because hirsutism caused by malignant lesions progresses rapidly. The presence of virilizing signs such as change in voice, male-pattern baldness, clitoromegaly, change in muscle distribution, and increase in libido make the presence of a serious underlying disorder likely. Family history, race, and ethnicity are important determinants of hirsutism; patients of Mediterranean, Middle Eastern, or South Asian descent are more likely to be hirsute without necessarily having significantly elevated androgen levels. Finally, current medications should be evaluated to screen for the use of androgenic steroids.

The amount and distribution of hair are an index of androgen effect. As noted, before puberty, most of the body is covered by fine, nonpigmented, nonmedullated hair called villous hair. In the presence of androgens, these hairs are converted to coarse, pigmented, medullated terminal hairs. Terminal hair on the face, around the areola, and on the abdomen below the level of the umbilicus is present in 10% of "normal" women. Terminal hairs of the upper back, shoulders, sternum, and upper abdomen suggest a more marked androgen effect.

Grading of hirsutism is done using the Ferriman-Gallway scale, which semiquantitatively measures the amount of hair growth; however, it is subject to large observer variability. Examination should include a search for signs of virilization such as male-pattern baldness, decreased voice pitch, increases muscle bulk, and clitoromegaly (length >10 mm or clitoral index [length × width] >35 mm^2). Signs of insulin resistance (e.g., acanthosis nigricans, abdominal obesity), Cushing's syndrome, and ovarian enlargement should be sought during the examination.

DIAGNOSIS

The goals of biochemical assessment are to evaluate the source of hyperandrogenism and to rule out the presence of a malignancy. Some physicians recommend no further evaluation in patients with mild hirsutism and regular ovulatory menses because these women do not have a serious underlying disorder.[1] The major biochemical parameters tested are discussed next.

Testosterone, total and free, should be measured. In most patients with hirsutism, especially that associated with abnormal periods, the testosterone levels are high-normal or just above the upper limit of normal. The free testosterone level is also similarly affected. Values of total testosterone higher than 200 ng/mL suggest an androgen-producing tumor. Because testosterone has a diurnal rhythm and varies with the menstrual cycle, most norms are standardized to early morning blood samples drawn between days 4 and 10 of the cycle. In the absence of cycles, a random early-morning sample usually suffices.

DHEAS should be measured, but marginal elevations of the DHEAS level are common. Elevated values suggest an adrenal source of androgens. Levels higher than 700 μg/dL suggest an androgen-producing adrenal tumor. These patients should undergo further evaluation with computed tomography or magnetic resonance imaging to check for a tumor.

17-Hydroxyprogesterone, a precursor of cortisol, should be measured. To screen for adult-onset CAH, it should be measured between 7 AM and 9 AM in the early follicular phase of the menstrual cycle. Levels lower than 200 ng/dL exclude the disease. Mildly increased levels, from 300 to 1000 ng/dL, require an ACTH stimulation test. Cosyntropin (synthetic ACTH), 250 μg, is administered intravenously, and levels of 17-hydroxyprogesterone are measured before and 1 hour after the injection. Poststimulation values that exceed 1000 ng/dL indicate a positive test result.

Free cortisol in a 24-hour urine sample should be measured in women with signs and symptoms of Cushing's syndrome.

Prolactin levels should be measured because an occasional woman with hirsutism and irregular menses could have hyperprolactinemia caused by hypothalamic disease or a pituitary tumor. Levels are also mildly elevated in up to 20% of patients with PCOS.

Serum follicle-stimulating hormone (FSH) level should be measured if ovarian failure is a consideration, but otherwise it is of minimal help.

Serum LH level should be measured because women with PCOS tend to have higher serum LH levels and a ratio of LH to FSH levels higher than 3. This is believed to be significant by some, but most authorities do not consider this a requirement for the diagnosis of PCOS. Ratios less than 3 do not exclude the diagnosis. Routine measurements of FSH and LH are therefore not needed.

Fasting plasma glucose and lipid profiles are not necessary for the diagnosis of PCOS. However, in patients suspected to have PCOS, insulin resistance, or both, these profiles are helpful to define the presence of metabolic risk, which over the long term can significantly affect a patient's morbidity and mortality.

Ultrasound evaluation of the ovaries, adrenals, or both, may be useful for screening if the symptoms or biochemical levels suggest the presence of a neoplasm. Pelvic sonography findings have been included in the criteria for the diagnosis of PCOS.

TREATMENT

Principles

The underlying cause should be treated. These guidelines refer to the treatment of hirsutism caused by PCOS and idiopathic hirsutism. Hirsutism is a cosmetic and psychological problem, not a life-threatening illness. Therefore, the risks and benefits of treatment have to be weighed.

Before beginning treatment, women should be warned that they might not see improvement in hair growth for 3 to 9 months. Drug treatment affects the growth of new hair follicles, but the half-life of established follicles is up to 6 months, so it takes that much time to see its effect.

Nonpharmacologic Treatment

Because of the significant association of insulin resistance and obesity with PCOS, therapy to reduce insulin resistance is appropriate. Diet, exercise, and weight loss should be prescribed for all women with PCOS. Diet therapy, consisting of decreased total caloric intake and an appropriately mixed high-fiber diet, in addition to a daily exercise program to induce weight loss, have been shown to reduce androgen production. A modest weight loss of 7 to 15 pounds with an appropriate exercise program are all that is needed to relieve menstrual and biochemical abnormalities.[8]

Mechanical hair removal can be achieved by shaving, waxing, or plucking or the use of depilatory creams. These treatments do not compound the problem. Bleaching can mask hair growth. Electrosurgical methods include electrosurgical epilation and laser treatment. Electrosurgical epilation was formerly the only commercially available method of long-term hair removal until the availability of laser treatment, but it is time-consuming, causes discomfort, and requires many treatments. There is a small but definite risk of punctate scarring and postinflammatory skin color changes. Laser treatment was introduced to remove hairs over larger areas effectively, with few complications. There are several different methods, and further studies are needed to determine the ideal treatment.

Pharmacologic Treatment

Antiandrogens

The antiandrogens are effective in the treatment of hirsutism. Their main effect is to inhibit the binding of testosterone and dihydrotestosterone to the androgen receptor.[9] They all share the potential risk of teratogenicity to the developing fetus and should always be used with adequate contraception in women of childbearing age.

Spironolactone is a potent antiandrogen. In addition to binding testosterone and dihydrotestosterone to the androgen receptor, it can inhibit ovarian testosterone synthesis.[9] The starting dose is 50 mg twice daily, which may be increased to a total daily dose of 200 mg/day. It takes at least 6 months for it to be fully effective. Numerous studies have shown its efficacy in the treatment of hirsutism, reducing clinical hirsutism scores by 15% to 40%. Side effects include nausea, fatigue, headaches, mastodynia, and irregular menses. There is a theoretical risk of an increase in serum potassium levels; renal insufficiency can predispose patients to this adverse effect. This drug can interfere with the appropriate sexual maturation of the fetus, especially a male fetus, and we strongly recommend the use of oral contraceptives along with spironolactone. In addition to protecting against pregnancy, and therefore against potential teratogenic effects, the oral contraceptives overcome irregular menses, a side effect of spironolactone. However, spironolactone use as an antiandrogen is not licensed in the United States.

Cyproterone acetate is a potent progestin and moderately potent antiandrogen. Like spironolactone, it inhibits the binding of dihydrotestosterone to the androgen receptor and suppresses gonadotropins. Side effects include nausea, breakthrough bleeding, decreased libido, and depression. It is generally used in combination with ethinyl estradiol. Cyproterone can cause fatal hepatitis and has not been licensed for use in the United States.

Flutamide is another androgen receptor blocker; it is used more commonly for the hormonal treatment of prostate cancer. Flutamide has been shown to be as effective as spironolactone, although some studies have suggested that it is more potent. Dosages of 125 to 500 mg/day are effective for hirsutism. Flutamide is not licensed in the United States for the treatment of hirsutism and, because of the significant risk of hepatoxicity, off-label use for hirsutism is discouraged by the U.S. Food and Drug Administration (FDA).

Cimetidine is a weak antiandrogen and is rarely used in the treatment of hirsutism.

Finasteride is an agent that inhibits 5α-reductase. Its efficacy is similar to that of cyproterone, spironolactone, or flutamide, but it can cause fatal hepatitis and is associated with a significant risk of teratogenicity; hence, it is rarely used. There are reports of a significant synergistic effect when combined with spironolactone.

Eflornithine cream (Vaniqa) is a topical agent that is believed to inhibit hair growth by inhibiting ornithine decarboxylase; this enzyme is modulated by androgens and regulates matrix cell proliferation in the hair follicle and thereby hair growth. The cream is applied to the face twice daily. Gradual improvement is seen in 4 to 6 weeks. Patients should be advised to use mechanical hair removal methods along with this treatment. However, 8 weeks after stopping this agent, hair growth reappears, without change from the pretreatment appearance.[9]

Ovarian Suppression

Estrogen-progesterone combinations act by reducing gonadotropin secretion and thereby reducing ovarian androgen production. They also increase levels of SHBG, resulting in lower levels of free testosterone, and they inhibit adrenal androgen production.[9] Oral contraceptive pills (OCPs) containing progestins that are low in androgenic activity should be used. OCPs that contain norgestrel and levonorgestrel are more androgenic than others and must be avoided. The newer progestins, such as norgestimate, norethindrone, and desogestrel, have a lower androgenic potential and are preferable. We recommend starting with 35 μg of ethinylestradiol and one of the progestins mentioned earlier. If there is no response in biochemical parameters such as testosterone after two or three cycles of treatment, the pill can be changed to one with 50 μg ethinylestradiol. These agents are also effective in controlling hirsutism in the older woman at about the time of menopause.[7]

Yasmin is a newer contraceptive pill that contains 30 μg of estradiol and 3 mg of drospirenone as the progestin and has been shown to have the antiandrogenic action of spironolactone. Yaz is a similar preparation containing a lower dose (20 μg) of estradiol with the same amount of drospirenone. The antiandrogen effect of 3 mg of drospirenone is equivalent to that of 25 mg of spironolactone.

Long-acting gonadotropin-releasing hormone (GnRH) analogues (GnRH agonists) decrease gonadotropin secretion, reducing ovarian stimulation and hence testosterone. Estrogen production is also reduced, so this treatment is usually combined with an OCP containing estrogen and progestin. This therapy is parenteral and expensive, however, and is reserved for women with severe hirsutism who do not respond to a combination of an OCP and antiandrogen. Because GnRH agonist therapy causes a medical menopause, there is a significant risk for premature bone loss; therefore, bone mineral density must be tested and therapies to prevent bone loss may need to be simultaneously started.

Adrenal Suppression

Oral glucocorticoids cause a decrease in androgen levels in most women. We suggest prednisone 2.5 mg or dexamethasone 0.25 mg at bedtime. Side effects at these doses are small. Higher doses are associated with significant side effects, including a cushingoid habitus; weight gain; osteoporosis; glucose, lipid, and blood pressure abnormalities; and possible vascular disease. These drugs have a definite role in the treatment of hirsutism secondary to CAH. In other forms of hirsutism, they are best if combined with antiandrogens and should be reserved for severe cases, where the risk-to-benefit ratio is appropriate.

PCOS is strongly and significantly related to the presence of insulin resistance and its consequent hyperinsulinemia; thus, the use of insulin sensitizers for PCOS has gained wide acceptance. They improve ovulatory function and pregnancy rates in women with PCOS. Thus, metformin is used as a first-line therapy for infertile women with PCOS. Glitazones, because of their direct effect on nuclear receptors and ability to activate numerous gene products, are not often used to induce ovulation because of undetermined potential effects on embryo development. The effect of insulin sensitizers on hirsutism is debated and possibly marginal.[10]

Surgical Treatment

Ovarian wedge resection was a frequently used option in the past. Currently, however, it has little to no usefulness. Laser drilling has been attempted and can restore ovulation but rarely improves hirsutism. All operative procedures carry a significant risk of postoperative adhesions and therefore mechanical infertility. Oophorectomy for perimenopausal or menopausal women with increasing severe hyperandrogenism is sometimes necessary.

CONCLUSIONS

Hirsutism is a distressing condition for most women. Although it is sometimes the harbinger of a more serious metabolic disorder, it often is not associated with significant underlying pathology. The principles of treatment include patience to wait and see the efficacy of treatment and a combination of nonpharmacologic and pharmacologic measures. Combining pharmacologic measures such as OCPs and antiandrogenic therapy yields the best results, making the problem more acceptable to the patient so that over time, she usually can balance the need for treatment with its cosmetic benefits.

Summary

- Hirsutism is common; moderate to severe forms indicate significant other disorders such as insulin resistance and the subsequent risk of cardiovascular disease, tumors, or congenital hormonal disorders.
- Hormonal evaluation, including testosterone, DHEAS, and 17-hydroxyprogesterone measurements, are useful for moderate to severe forms.
- Nonpharmocologic therapies such as diet and exercise are an integral part of therapy.
- Pharmacologic measures need to be maintained long term because the clinical effects lag behind biochemical improvements.
- Antiandrogens with or without suppression of androgen secretion is the most effective treatment.
- Local depilation measures, including electrolysis and lasers, are powerful adjuncts to medical therapy.
- Insulin-sensitizing therapy is efficacious for the restoration of ovulation but has weaker effects on hirsutism.

Suggested Readings

Azziz R, Carmina E, Sawaya ME: Idiopathic hirsutism [review]. Endocr Rev 2000;21: 347-362.

Azziz R, Sanchez LA, Knochenhauer ES, et al: Androgen excess in women: Experience with over 1000 consecutive patients. J Clin Endocrinol Metab 2004;89:453-462.

Barth JH, Jenkins M, Belchetz PE: Ovarian hyperthecosis, diabetes and hirsuties in post-menopausal women. Clin Endocrinol (Oxf). 1997;46:123-128.

Deplewski D, Rosenfield RL: Role of hormones in pilosebaceous unit development [review]. Endocr Rev 2000;21:363-392.

Genton P, Bauer J, Duncan S, et al: On the association between valproate and polycystic ovary syndrome [review]. Epilepsia 2001;42:295-304.

Khorram O: Potential therapeutic effects of prescribed and over-the-counter androgens in women [review]. Clin Obstet Gynecol 2001;44:880-892.

Kiddy DS, Hamilton-Fairley D, Bush A, et al: Improvement in endocrine and ovarian function during dietary treatment of obese women with polycystic ovary syndrome. Clin Endocrinol (Oxf) 1992;36:105-111.

Lindgren R, Gunnarsson C, Jakobsson A, Hammar M: Hypersecretion of ovarian androgens may be gonadotrophin-dependent years after menopause. Maturitas 2000;34:43-46.

Marx TL, Mehta AE: Polycystic ovary syndrome: Pathogenesis and treatment over short and long term [review]. Cleve Clin J Med. 2003;70:31-33, 36-41, 45.

Moghetti P, Toscano V: Treatment of hirsutism and acne in hyperandrogenism. Best practice and research. Clin Endocrinol Metab 2006;20:221-234.

Practice Guidelines

Practice Committee of the American Society for Reproductive Medicine: The evaluation and treatment of androgen excess. Fert Steril 2006;86(Suppl 4):S241-S247.

Practice Committee of the American Society for Reproductive Medicine: Use of insulin-sensitizing agents in the treatment of polycystic ovary syndrome. Fert Steril 2006;86(Suppl 4):S221-S223.References

1. Deplewski D, Rosenfield RL: Role of hormones in pilosebaceous unit development [review]. Endocr Rev 2000;21:363-392.
2. Azziz R, Carmina E, Sawaya ME: Idiopathic hirsutism [review]. Endocr Rev 2000;21:347-362.
3. Azziz R, Sanchez LA, Knochenhauer ES, et al: Androgen excess in women: Experience with over 1000 consecutive patients. J Clin Endocrinol Metab 2004;89:453-462.
4. Khorram O: Potential therapeutic effects of prescribed and over-the-counter androgens in women [review]. Clin Obstet Gynecol 2001;44:880-892.
5. Genton P, Bauer J, Duncan S, et al: On the association between valproate and polycystic ovary syndrome [review]. Epilepsia 2001;42:295-304.
6. Lindgren R, Gunnarsson C, Jakobsson A, Hammar M: Hypersecretion of ovarian androgens may be gonadotrophin-dependent years after menopause. Maturitas 2000;34:43-46.
7. Barth JH, Jenkins M, Belchetz PE: Ovarian hyperthecosis, diabetes and hirsuties in post-menopausal women. Clin Endocrinol (Oxf) 1997;46:123-128.
8. Kiddy DS, Hamilton-Fairley D, Bush A, et al: Improvement in endocrine and ovarian function during dietary treatment of obese women with polycystic ovary syndrome. Clin Endocrinol (Oxf) 1992;36:105-111.
9. Moghetti P, Toscano V: Treatment of hirsutism and acne in hyperandrogenism. Best practice and research. Clin Endocrinol Metab 2006;20:221-234.
10. Marx TL, Mehta AE: Polycystic ovary syndrome: Pathogenesis and treatment over short and long term [review]. Cleve Clin J Med 2003;70:31-33, 36-41, 45.

References

For a complete list of references, log onto www.expertconsult.com.

Hypocalcemia and Hypercalcemia

Mario Skugor

HYPOCALCEMIA

Hypocalcemia can vary from a very mild and asymptomatic biochemical abnormality to severe life-threatening hypocalcemia depending on rapidity of development, duration, and severity. Box 1 summarizes the causes of hypocalcemia.

Hypoparathyroidism is most commonly caused by surgery requiring radical neck resections due to head and neck cancers.[1] The hypoparathyroidism may be transient, permanent, or intermittent (e.g., when needs exceed parathyroid reserve, such as with vitamin D deficiency during winter months). Autoimmune hypoparathyroidism can be an isolated defect or part of the polyglandular autoimmune syndrome type I (with adrenal insufficiency and mucocutaneous candidiasis).[2] Congenital causes of hypocalcemia include activating mutations of *CaSR* and mutations affecting intracellular processing of the pre-pro-parathyroid hormone (pre-pro-PTH) molecule. Finally, some cases of congenital hypoparathyroidism are associated with hypoplasia or aplasia of parathyroid glands (best known is *DiGeorge syndrome*).[3]

Pseudohypoparathyroidism is group of disorders that involve postreceptor resistance to the effects of PTH. The classical variant is known as *Allbright's hereditary osteodystrophy* and is associated with short stature, round facies, short digits, and mental retardation. Hypomagnesemia induces resistance to PTH and also affects PTH production. Severe hypermagnesemia (>6 mg/dL) can lead to hypocalcemia by inhibiting PTH secretion. Deficiency of vitamin D can lead to hypocalcemia when it is associated with decreased dietary calcium intake.

When large amounts of phosphate are released from the intracellular pool (rhabdomyolysis or tumor lysis syndrome), hypocalcemia occurs due to precipitation of calcium in bone and extraskeletal tissues.

In acute pancreatitis, calcium is precipitated as diffuse calcium soaps in the abdominal cavity.

Hungry bone syndrome refers to hypocalcemia after surgical correction of long-lasting severe hyperparathyroidism. Serum calcium is rapidly taken from the circulation and deposited into the bone.

Several medications chelate calcium in the circulation and produce hypocalcemia. These medications include ethylenediaminetetraacetic acid (EDTA), citrate (present in transfusing blood), lactate, and foscarnet. Patients receiving chemotherapy including cisplatin, 5-fluorouracil, and leucovorin develop hypocalcemia mediated through hypomagnesemia. Extensive osteoblastic skeletal metastases, especially from prostate and breast cancer, can also lead to hypocalcemia. Low serum calcium levels seen in patients after surgeries can be mediated by the citrate content of transfused blood or by large fluid administrations and hypoalbuminemia. Patients with sepsis demonstrate hypocalcemia that is usually associated with hypoalbuminemia.

Signs and Symptoms

Chronic moderate hypocalcemia may be completely asymptomatic. Acute hypocalcemia causes increased neuromuscular irritability. The clinical manifestation is tetany, characterized by repetitive neuromuscular discharge after a single stimulus. Tetany is seen in more-severe hypocalcemia (Ca^{2+} <1.1 mmol/L). Milder forms manifest as paresthesias and numbness of the fingertips and perioral area. Twitching of the ipsilateral facial musculature (not only the oral angle) by tapping over cranial nerve VII at the ear is known as *Chvostek's sign. Trousseau's sign* consists of carpal spasm provoked by ischemia (induced by inflation of the blood pressure measuring cuff around the arm) or alkalosis (provoked by hyperventilation for a couple of minutes). Spontaneous muscle cramps are commonly seen in hypocalcemia. Prolonged contraction of the respiratory and laryngeal muscles causes stridorous breathing and can cause cyanosis. Other symptoms and signs are listed in Box 2.

Alkalosis (e.g., induced by hyperventilation), hypokalemia, epinephrine (e.g., due to emotional stress), and hypomagnesemia aggravate symptoms and acidosis decreases symptoms of hypocalcemia (as seen in patients with chronic renal failure who often tolerate marked hypocalcemia).

Diagnostic Evaluation

When diagnosis of hypocalcemia is confirmed (serum calcium <8.2 mg/dL or Ca^{2+} <1.1 mmol/L), attention should turn toward seeking the cause.

History can establish an etiology in patients with post-surgical hypoparathyroidism, chronic renal insufficiency, or phosphate administration. Laboratory evaluation of patients with confirmed hypocalcemia should be guided by history and physical examination. Renal failure, cell lysis syndromes, hypomagnesemia or hypermagnesemia, and acute pancreatitis can be diagnosed or excluded using measurements of serum creatinine, creatine phospokinase (CPK), magnesium, and amylase. In the absence of these conditions, disorders affecting production or action of PTH or vitamin D should be considered. Measurement of intact parathyroid hormone (iPTH), 25(OH) vitamin D, and $1,25(OH)_2$ vitamin D need to be obtained, but the results are often delayed (2-7 days).

The serum phosphate level can be helpful in interpreting causes of hypocalcemia. Low phosphate levels signify either excess PTH activity (secondary hyperparathyroidism) or low dietary phosphate intake. High levels of phosphate in the absence of the tissue breakdown or renal failure signify hypoparathyroidism or pseudohypoparathyroidism.

Interpretation of the iPTH level requires simultaneous determination of serum calcium. A low or even normal iPTH level associated with hypocalcemia is a powerful sign of hypoparathyroidism. Table 1 illustrates iPTH findings in different hypocalcemic disorders.

Measurements of 25(OH) vitamin D (calcifediol) are more informative in most patients with hypocalcemia than measurements of $1,25(OH)_2$ vitamin D (calcitriol), which is dependent on PTH levels. However, calcitriol levels are low despite normal or high calcifediol levels in patients with renal insufficiency, in patients with deficiency of renal 1-α-hydroxylase (vitamin D–dependent rickets type 1), and in patients with hypoparathyroidism. High levels of calcitriol are seen in hereditary vitamin D–resistant rickets (formerly called *vitamin D–resistant rickets type 2*).

Treatment

Patients with acute symptomatic hypocalcemia should be treated promptly with intravenous calcium. Calcium gluconate is preferred over calcium chloride because it causes less tissue necrosis if extravasated. The first 100 to 200 mg of elemental calcium (1-2 g of calcium

Box 1 Causes of Hypocalcemia

Decreased Entry of Calcium into the Circulation

Hypoparathyroidism (absence of PTH hormone secretion)

- Postoperative
- Autoimmune (isolated or part of polyglandular autoimmune syndrome).
- Congenital (mutations of *CaSR*, PTH, and parathyroid aplasia)
- Pseudohypoparathyroidism

Magnesium depletion
Severe hypermagnesemia
Deficiency of vitamin D

Increased Loss of Calcium from Circulation

Hyperphosphatemia

- Renal failure
- Rhabdomyolysis
- Tumor lysis
- Phosphate administration

Acute pancreatitis
Hungry bone syndrome
Chelation

- Citrate
- EDTA
- Lactate
- Foscarnet

Widespread osteoblastic metastases

- Prostate cancer
- Breast cancer

Other Causes

Sepsis
Flouride administration
Surgery
Chemotherapy

- Cisplatin
- 5-flourouracil
- Leucovorin

EDTA, ethylenediaminetetraacetic acid; PTH, parathyroid hormone.

gluconate) should be given over 10 to 20 minutes. Faster administration could result in cardiac dysfunction or even arrest. This should be followed by slow calcium infusion at 0.5 to 1.5 mg/kg/hr. Calcium infusion should be continued until the patient is receiving effective doses of oral calcium and vitamin D. Calcium should be diluted for infusion (in saline or dextrose solution) to avoid vein irritation. The infusion solution should not contain bicarbonate or phosphate because these can form insoluble calcium salts. If bicarbonate or phosphate administration is necessary, separate intravenous lines should be used.

Coexisting hypomagnesemia should be considered in every patient, and it must be corrected if present. Great care should be taken in patients with impaired renal function because they cannot excrete excess magnesium

In patients with severe hyperphosphatemia, treatment is focused on correcting the hyperphosphatemia. Acute hyperphosphatemia usually resolves in patients with intact renal function. Hemodialysis may be necessary in patients who have symptomatic hypocalcemia and hyperphosphatemia, especially if renal function is impaired. Chronic hyperphosphatemia should be managed with a low-phosphate diet and use of phosphate binders with meals.

Chronic hypocalcemia (e.g., hypoparathyroidism) is treated by administration of oral calcium and, if necessary, vitamin D. The serum calcium level should be targeted to about 8.0 mg/dL. Most patients are asymptomatic at this level, and further elevation can lead to hypercalciuria (because of the lack of PTH effect on the renal tubules) and development of nephrocalcinosis, nephrolithiasis, and renal impairment.

Several oral calcium and vitamin D preparations are available (Table 2 and 3). If oral calcium preparations alone are insuficient, vitamin D should be added. The usual initial daily dose is 50,000 IU or 0.25 to 0.5 µg of $1{,}25(OH)_2$ vitamin D. Appropriate doses of calcium and vitamin D are established by gradual titration. When

Box 2 Clinical Manifestations of Hypocalcemia

Neuropsychiatric Symptoms

Seizures (all types)
Dementia (in adults), mental retardation (in children)
Emotional problems (anxiety, depression)
Extrapyramidal symptoms (Parkinsonism is most common)
Calcifications of basal ganglia (in long standing disease)
Papilledema

Increased Neuromuscular Irritability

Chvostek's sign
Trousseau's sign
Paresthesias in circumoral and acral areas (fingers, toes)
Muscle stiffness, myalgias, and spasms

Cardiovascular Symptoms

Prolongation of QT interval
Congestive heart failure
Hypotension

Autonomic Symptoms

Biliary colic
Bronchospasm
Diaphoresis

Other Symptoms

Cataracts
Dry coarse skin, dermatitis, hyperpigmentation and eczema
Steatorrhea
Gastric achlorhydria

Table 1 iPTH Findings In Hypocalcemic Disorders

Disease	iPTH level
Hypoparathyroidism	Mostly reduced, occasionally normal
Pseudohypoparathyroidism	Elevated
Vitamin D abnormalities	Elevated
Hypomagnesemia	Low, normal, or high
Autosomal dominant hypocalcemia	Normal

iPTH, intact parathyroid hormone.

Table 2 Oral Calcium Preparations

Calcium Preparation	Calcium Content	Tablet Weight
Calcium carbonate	250 mg (6.25 mmol)	650 mg
Calcium gluconate	90 mg (2.25 mmol)	1000 mg
Calcium citrate	200 mg (5 mmol)	950 mg
Calcium lactate	60 mg (1.5 mmol)	300 mg

Table 3 Vitamin D Preparations

Vitamin D Preparation (Brand)	Half-Life	Form of Therapy
1,25 Dihdroxycholecalciferol (Rocaltrol, Calcijex)	2-6 hours	Capsule 0.25, 0.5 μg Injection 1 μg/mL, 2 μg/mL Solution 1 μg/ml
25 hydroxycholecalciferol (Calderol [requires activation in the kidneys])	12-22 days	Capsule 20, 50 μg
Ergocalciferol (Vitamin D_2)	Long (month)	Capsule 1.25 mg, 50,000 IU
Calciferol (Drisdol)		Solution 12.5 mg/mL Drops 200 μg/mL, 8000 IU
Cholecalciferol (Vitamin D_3) (Delta-D)	Long (month)	Tablet 400,1000 IU

adequate calcemia is achieved, urinary calcium excretion needs to be measured. If hypercalciuria is detected, a thiazide diuretic may be added to the regimen.

If phosphorus is more than 6.0 mg/dL when calcium is satisfactory, an unabsorbable phosphate binder should be added to the regimen. Once therapeutic goals are achieved, the patient should be monitored every 3 to 6 months for serum calcium and phosphorus levels as well as for urinary calcium excretion.

Special consideration is necessary in treating women who have hypoparathyroidism during pregnancy and nursing. Vitamin D requirements increase gradually during pregnancy and can reach three times pre-pregnancy needs. Supplementation doses of vitamin D should be titrated using frequent serum calcium measurements. After delivery, if there is no plan to nurse, the dose could be decreased to pre-pregnancy level. If the baby will be nursed, the dose of calcitriol should be decreased to one half of the pre-pregnancy dose because endogenous calcitriol production and PTH-related peptide are stimulated by prolactin.

Box 3 Etiology of Hypercalcemia

Primary hyperparathyroidism
Hypercalcemia of malignancy

- Osteolytic hypercalcemia
- Humoral hypercalcemia of malignancy
- Ectopic production of calcitriol (lymphoma)

Hypercalcemia of granulomatous disease
Tertiary hyperparathyroidism
Acute renal failure
Familial hypercalcemic hypocalciuria
Lithium associated hypercalcemia
Vitamin D intoxication
Other causes

- Increased calcium intake
- Pheochromocytoma
- Congenital lactase deficiency
- Hyperthyroidism
- Vitamin A intoxication
- Adrenal insufficiency
- Thiazides
- Milk-alkali syndrome
- Immobilization

HYPERCALCEMIA

Pathophysiology

Hypercalcemia typically manifests as mild chronic calcium elevation. Hypercalcemic emergencies do exist. Hypercalcemia is usually detected as elevation of total plasma calcium or ionized calcium levels. Approximately 50% of calcium is protein bound, and total calcium level varies with protein-binding capacity. This rarely results in pseudohypercalcemia, for example, in patients with hyperalbuminemia secondary to dehydration, and with multiple myeloma. More commonly, lowering of total calcium levels is observed in patients with low levels of binding proteins (hypoalbuminemia). This physiology requires a correction of total plasma calcium for albumin level:

$$\text{Corrected Ca} = \text{total Ca} + 0.8 \times (4.5 - \text{albumin level})$$

where total calcium is in milligrams per deciliter and 4.5 is the average albumin level. Normal calcium levels range from 8.5 to 10.5 mg/dL.

Acidosis decreases the amount of bound calcium, and alkalosis increases it. A small amount of calcium (about 6%) is complexed to anions such are citrate and sulfate. The remainder is ionized calcium that is biologically active.

The most common causes of hypercalcemia (90% of all patients) are primary hyperparathyroidism (HPT) and malignancies (Box 3).

Signs and Symptoms

Symptoms of hypercalcemia (Table 4) are nonspecific, and they are more severe with acute changes than with chronic elevation of calcium level. Symptoms of underlying diseases causing hypercalcemia can dominate the clinical picture.

Normal extracellular calcium concentration is essential for normal neuromuscular function, and neuromuscular dysfunction is major feature of hypercalcemia. Symptoms vary from slight difficulties in concentrating to depression, confusion, and coma. Muscle weakness is common.

Chronic hypercalcemia can lead to nephrolithiasis. Hypercalciuria is a main factor in stone formation, but increased calcitriol production in HPT also plays a role.

Nephrogenic diabetes insipidus caused by downregulation of water channels (aquaporin 2), and tubulointerstitial injury by calcium deposition is seen in about 20% of patients.[4] Renal tubular acidosis and renal insufficiency are rare.

Hypertension associated with hypercalcemia may be caused by renal insufficiency or calcium-mediated vasoconstriction.[5] Hypertension might or might not resolve after correction of hypercalcemia. Cardiac effects consist of short QT interval, which can cause increased sensitivity to digitalis and deposition of calcium in heart valves, myocardium, or coronary arteries.

Constipation, anorexia, nausea, and vomiting are common symptoms, but acute pancreatitis (via activation of trypsinogen in pancreatic parenchyma) and peptic ulcer disease (via stimulation of gastrin secretion) are unusual. Fatigue, musculoskeletal weakness, and pain are common and correlate with levels of serum calcium.

Table 4 Signs and Symptoms of Hypercalcemia

Signs and Symptoms	Associated Conditions
Neuropsychiatric	
Anxiety	Organic brain syndromes
Cognitive dysfunction	
Depression	
Fatigue	
Headache	
Renal	
Nocturia	Nephrogenic diabetes insipidus
Polydipsia	Nephrolithiasis
Polyuria	Renal insufficiency
	Renal tubular acidosis
Cardiovascular	
Short QT interval	Cardiovascular calcifications
Hypertension	
Gastrointestinal	
Abdominal pain	Acute pancreatitis
Anorexia	Peptic ulcer disease
Constipation	
Musculoskeletal	
Aches/pain	Brown tumors
Fractures	Calciphylaxis
Muscle weakness	Chondrocalcinosis
	Osteitis fibrosa cystica
	Osteopenia/osteoporosis
	Pseudogout
Other	
	Hypercalcemic crisis

Primary Hyperparathyroidism

Primary hyperparathyroidism (HPT) occurs at all ages but is most common in the sixth decade of life. The female-to-male ratio is 3:1. In children, HPT it is likely a component of familial syndromes such as the multiple endocrine neoplasia (MEN) syndromes type I or II or familial hyperparathyroidism. The incidence of HPT is approximately 42 per 100,000.

HPT is caused by excessive secretion of parathyroid hormone (PTH) leading to increased bone resorption by osteoclasts, increased intestinal calcium absorption, and increased renal tubular calcium reabsorption. The consequent hypercalcemia is often accompanied by low normal or decreased serum phosphate levels because PTH inhibits proximal tubular phosphate reabsorption.

Most cases of HPT (80%) are discovered accidentally by the use of automated blood sample analyzers. These patients have very few symptoms, and calcium levels are mildly elevated (<12 mg/dL). Patients with HPT can present with any of the clinical manifestations summarized in Box 2, and diagnosis needs to be considered in any patient presenting with kidney stones, bone disease, and hypercalcemic crisis.

Renal calculi are seen in 15% to 20% of patients with HPT, and, about 5% of patients with renal calculi have HPT. Some patients have calcium levels in the upper range of normal. Most calculi are made of calcium oxalate, and the main factor in pathogenesis is hypercalciuria. Although PTH stimulates calcium reabsorption in the distal tubules, the kidney is overwhelmed by the amount of filtered calcium from high serum calcium levels.[6] Patients with increased calcitriol levels are more likely to have hypercalcemia and nephrolithiasis.

The classic bone disease of HPT manifests with brown tumors, osteitis fibrosa cystica, and subperiosteal resorption on the radial aspect of the middle and distal phalanges. These are seen only in severe and long-standing disease, and today they are seen very rarely, usually when disease is caused by parathyroid carcinoma and in secondary or tertiary hyperparathyroidism associated with chronic renal insufficiency.[7] Low bone mineral density is found in some patients with HPT, but it is unclear if this occurs more often than in the normal population. However, there is an increased risk for vertebral fractures in patients with HPT. Several studies found excess mortality in patients with HPT, with most of the excess due to cardiovascular disease.[8]

Hypercalcemic crisis is rare and is characterized by high calcium levels (>15 mg/dL) and severe symptoms, particularly central nervous system (CNS) dysfunction. Abdominal pain, pancreatitis, peptic ulcer disease, nausea, and vomiting are also seen in these patients. The mechanism by which crisis develops is not clear, but dehydration, intercurrent illness and, possibly, infarction of a parathyroid adenoma in some patients all play a role. Treatment consists of rapid correction of hypercalcemia (see later) and surgical parathyroidectomy.

Diagnosis

The diagnosis of HPT requires elevated serum calcium with simultaneous demonstration of PTH levels that are elevated (80%-90% of patients) or inappropriately normal (10%-20% of patients). The PTH should be determined as the intact PTH molecule. Phosphorus may be low but is usually just in the low-normal range. Urinary calcium excretion is measured by 24-hour urine collection; hypercalciuria is defined as calcium excretion of greater than 400 mg/day. Low calcium excretion (<150 mg/day) might signify familial hypocalciuric hypercalcemia, which does not require treatment.

In familial forms of primary hyperparathyroidism, urinary screening for catecholamine overproduction is important before surgical treatment.

Preoperative imaging by the means of ultrasound, ^{99}Tc-sestamibi scintigraphy, or magnetic resonance imaging (MRI) does not improve outcome of treatment but might offer a possibility for a less-invasive surgical approach. Selection of these tests should be left to the surgeon.

Treatment

Removal of the hyperfunctioning parathyroid tissue cures HPT in 96% of patients. Because most patients are asymptomatic and because there is a lack of reliable predictive indices regarding development of HPT-related clinical problems, the following criteria are proposed as indications for parathyroidectomy[9,10]:

- Serum Ca more than 1 mg/dL above the upper limit of normal
- Marked hypercalciuria of more than 400 mg/d
- Creatinine clearance reduced more than 30% compared with age-matched controls
- Reduction in bone mineral density (BMD) of the femoral neck, lumbar spine, or distal radius of more than 2.5 standard deviations below peak bone mass (T score < −2.5)
- Age younger than 50 years
- Patients for whom medical surveillance is not desirable or possible
- Presence of any complications (nephrolithiasis, overt bone disease)
- An episode of hypercalcemic crisis.

Surgical Treatment. Parathyroid surgery remains the single most effective treatment option in HPT. Only about 10% of all patients come to surgery, because most patients have biochemically mild HPT that might not be identified or are managed with conservative measures and surveillance.

Surgery consists of bilateral exploration of the neck to identify all (typically four) parathyroids, assess which are abnormal, and remove only the abnormal glands. The setting of multigland hyperplasia requires subtotal parathyroidectomy or total parathyroidectomy with reimplantation of parathyroid tissue into the sternocleidomastoid or forearm muscles. Newer, minimally invasive methods (smaller incisions under local anesthesia) are currently being evaluated.

Medical Treatment. Patients not treated surgically should maintain good hydration, avoid thiazide diuretics, and stay physically active. Excessive calcium intake can aggravate hypercalcemia, especially in patients with high calcitriol levels, and low calcium intake can stimulate PTH secretion. Bisphosphonates may be used to lower serum calcium in patients with symptomatic hypercalcemia (see the later discussion of treatment of severe hypercalcemia).

Calcimimetics are emerging as safe and effective treatment for hypercalcemia caused by all forms of hyperparathyroidism. These medications stimulate the calcium-sensing receptors on the parathyroid cells and reduce PTH secretion. The effect of medication is quick (days) and is sustained for at least a year.[11]

Familial Forms of Hyperparathyroidism

Up to 10% of cases of primary HPT may be hereditary. The most commonly it is associated with MEN type I. In MEN I, primary HPT is present in about 95% patients by the age of 65 years. Indications for surgical intervention are the same as in sporadic cases. Pancreatic tumors are present in 30% to 80% of patients. Most common are gastrinoma and insulinoma. Pituitary adenomas affect 15% to 50% of patients and are mostly prolactinomas.

MEN type II is dominated by the development of medullary thyroid carcinoma, which affects virtually all patients. Primary HPT occurs in about half of the patients (most are asymptomatic). Pheochromocytoma or adrenal medullary hyperplasia are associated features. Genetic testing (*RET* proto-oncogene) of family members at risk is feasible and desirable because it identifies persons at risk, and timely thyroidectomy is life saving.

Other familial syndromes—HPT–jaw tumor syndrome and familial isolated primary hyperparathyroidism—are rare.

Secondary and Tertiary Hyperparathyroidism

During the prolonged states of secondary HPT, such as are seen in patients with end-stage renal disease and states of vitamin D resistance, the parathyroid glands undergo hypertrophy and eventually develop autonomous PTH secretion, which leads to hypercalcemia and resembles primary HPT. This condition is called *tertiary HPT.* Cure requires surgical intervention to reduce the amount of parathyroid tissue. Suppression of PTH secretion in secondary HPT with calcium, vitamin D analogues, phosphate binders, limited phosphate intake, and, lately, calcimimetic medications prevents or delays development of tertiary HPT.

Other Causes of Hypercalcemia

Familial Hypocalciuric Hypercalcemia

Familial hypocalciuric hypercalcemia is a rare familial condition caused by an inactivating disorder of the calcium-sensing receptor. The disorder is autosomal dominant and decreases the sensitivity of receptors to calcium, requiring higher calcium levels to suppress PTH secretion. Heterozygous patients present with hypercalcemia, hypocalciuria, and mild hypermagnesemia. Fractional excretion of calcium is less than 1% despite hypercalcemia (about 75% of patients excrete <100 mg/day). The PTH level is normal or slightly elevated. These patients are asymptomatic, and treatment is unnecessary. However, familial hypocalciuric hypercalcemia is easily mistaken for primary HPT, and these patients are referred for parathyroidectomy, which cannot correct hypercalcemia. These patients sometime have multiple surgeries.[12]

Humoral Hypercalcemia of Malignancy

Humoral hypercalcemia of malignancy is caused by secretion of PTH-related peptide (PTHrP) and, rarely, excessive production of PTH and calcitriol by tumor.[13] Patients with humoral hypercalcemia of malignancy make up about 80% of all patients with hypercalcemia associated with malignancy. PTHrP causes hypercalcemia via action on PTH receptor and is most commonly seen with squamous carcinomas (e.g., lung, esophagus, cervix, head and neck) and renal, bladder and ovarian cancers.

Therapy for humoral hypercalcemia of malignancy is aimed at reducing the tumor burden, reducing osteoclastic resorption of the bone, and increasing calcium excretion trough.

Most cases of hypercalcemia associated with Hodgkin's disease and about one third of those seen in non-Hodgkin's lymphoma are caused by increased production of calcitriol by the malignant cells. Hypercalcemia usually responds well to treatment with corticosteroids.

Hypercalcemia of Malignancy Associated with Localized Bone Destruction

Multiple myeloma affects the skeleton in almost all patients. In addition, about one third to one half of all malignant tumors spread to bone. Most of the bone metastases are destructive to the bone tissue (osteolytic) and can cause hypercalcemia . Myelomas cause bone destruction by the secretion of cytokines that activate osteoclasts.

Treatment with bisphosphonates improves hypercalcemia but also inhibits bone resorption and thus improves bone fragility. Intravenous pamidronate and zoledronate are effective in practically every patient.

Hypercalcemia Associated with Granulomatous Diseases

Although sarcoidosis is the most common cause, virtually all granulomatous diseases can lead to hypercalcemia (Box 4). With these disorders, the mechanism of hypercalcemia is increased intestinal absorption of calcium induced by elevated calcitriol levels. Calcitriol-mediated increase in bone resorption might have some role, too.

Monocyte-macrophage cells express the identical 1-hydroxylase expressed in the kidneys that converts 25(OH) vitamin D to $1,25(OH)_2$ vitamin D. However, in granulomatous disorders, normal feedback inhibition of the enzyme by PTH is abolished, leading to increased calcitriol production.

Corticosteroid treatment (prednisone 10-30 mg for sarcoidosis and more for lymphoma) decreases production of $1,25(OH)_2$ vitamin D in the macrophages. This in turn results in gradual decrease in serum calcium levels, usually starting after 2 days of treatment and reaching full response in 7 to 10 days. The antimalarial medications chloroquine and hydroxychloroquine may be used, but this treatment should be left to endocrinologists. Bisphosphonates have been used with success in patients not responding to these measures.

Vitamin D Intoxication

Both 25(OH) vitamin D and $1,25(OH)_2$ vitamin D circulate in blood partially bound to vitamin D–binding protein. In the case of ingestion of large amounts of 25(OH) vitamin D or its analogues, calcitriol is displaced from the binding protein, resulting in increased free levels (the total level can be low because calcitriol production is inhibited). Elevated free calcitriol levels, in turn, cause hypercalcemia by increasing intestinal calcium absorption and increased bone resorption. The hypercalcemic episode is usually prolonged and

Box 4 Granulomatous Diseases Associated with Hypercalcemia

Berylliosis
Candidiasis
Crohn's disease
Coccidiomycosis
Histiocytosis X
Histoplasmosis
Hodgkin's lymphoma
Non-Hodgkin's lymphoma
Pneumocystis jiroveci pneumonia
Sarcoidosis
Silicone-induced granulomas
Tuberculosis
Wegener's granulomatosis

often requires therapy with corticosteroids and bisphosphonates in addition to routine nonspecific measures.

In patients who ingest calcitriol, the total calcitriol level in serum is increased, and hypercalcemia is short lived after calcitriol is discontinued because calcitriol has a short half-life. Ensuring adequate hydration is usually enough for fast correction of hypercalcemia.

Thiazide Diuretics

Thiazide diuretics decrease renal calcium excretion by about 50 to 150 mg/day, which can result in hypercalcemia, especially in patients with hyperparathyroidism. Another result is increased bone resorption.

Lithium Therapy

Patients treated with lithium commonly develop mild hypercalcemia. It appears that lithium increases the set point for PTH suppression by calcium. Hypercalcemia usually, but not always, resolves if therapy with lithium is discontinued.

Thyrotoxicosis

Mild hypercalcemia occurs in up to half of patients with thyrotoxicosis. The PTH and $1,25(OH)_2$ vitamin D levels are both low. Increased bone resorption caused by thyroxine (T_4) and triiodothyronine (T_3) is believed to be responsible for hypercalcemia.

Adrenal Insufficiency

Hypercalcemia is usually seen with adrenal insufficiency during adrenal crisis. The simple volume contraction and hemoconcentration are likely responsible. Hypercalcemia usually responds to volume replacement and glucocorticoid replacement.

Immobilization

Immobilization causes hypercalcemia in patients whose underlying bone resorption is elevated. These include children and adolescents, patients with Paget's disease of bone, patients with mild primary and secondary hyperparathyroidism, and patients with mild hypercalcemia of malignancy. Bisphosphonates can decrease hypercalcemia, but resumption of weigh bearing is essential for resolution of hypercalcemia and hypercalciuria.

Milk-Alkali Syndrome

This is a rare condition caused by ingestion of large amounts of calcium together with sodium bicarbonate. Currently it is associated with ingestion of calcium carbonate in over-the-counter antacid preparations and those used to treat and prevent osteoporosis. Features of the syndrome include hypercalcemia, renal failure, and metabolic alkalosis. The exact pathophysiologic mechanism is unknown. The amount of calcium ingested may be as low as 2000 to 3000 mg/day in rare patients, but in the majority of patients it is between 6000 and 15,000 mg/day. Therapy consists of stopping the ingestion of calcium and antacids and promoting rehydration and diuresis. If diuresis is impossible because of renal failure, dialysis against a dialysate with low calcium concentration is very effective. Kidney failure usually recovers in short-lived cases, but it can persist in chronic cases.

Vitamin A Intoxication

Vitamin A in large doses (>50,000 IU/day) sometimes causes hypercalcemia. It appears to be caused by increased osteoclast bone resorption. It is seen in patients taking retinoic acid derivatives for treatment of acne, neuroblastoma, and other malignancies.

Theophylline

Cases of hypercalcemia associated with theophylline are usually seen in asthmatic patients. The theophylline level is usually above the normal therapeutic level. Hypercalcemia resolves when the theophylline level returns to the normal range. The mechanism is unknown.

Treatment of Hypercalcemia

If calcium levels are less than 12 mg/dL and a patient has no symptoms it is unnecessary to treat hypercalcemia. In patients with moderate calcium elevations (12-14 mg/dL) and symptoms consistent with hypercalcemia, aggressive treatment is necessary. In patients with moderate calcium elevations but without symptoms, treatment may consist only of adequate hydration. Patients with calcium levels over 14 mg/dL should be treated aggressively regardless of symptoms. Patients with treatable conditions should be treated more aggressively than those with incurable diseases.

Measures undertaken to treat hypercalcemia are aimed at increasing renal calcium excretion and decreasing intestinal absorption of calcium, slowing bone resorption, removing calcium from circulation, and controlling underlying diseases causing hypercalcemia.

Calcium is passively reabsorbed in the proximal tubule and in the thick ascending limb of the loop of Henle and is actively reabsorbed (via PTH action) in the distal tubule. Excretion of calcium can be achieved by inhibiting sodium resorption in the proximal tubules and loop of Henle. inhibition of sodium resorption is accomplished by volume expansion using an IV normal saline infusion (1-2 L over 1 hour). This results in a marked increase in sodium, calcium, and water delivery to the loop of Henle. Using a loop diuretic (furosemide 20-40 mg IV every 2 hours), it is possible to block transport of sodium in the loop. These actions result in a marked increase in urinary excretion not only of calcium but also of sodium, potassium, chloride, magnesium, and water. It is important to continuously replace water, sodium, potassium, and chloride, and, if this regimen is prolonged (>10 hours), to replace magnesium (15 mg/hour). Urinary flow should exceed 250 mL/hour. Serum calcium level will start decreasing within 2 to 4 hours and approach the normal range in 12 to 24 hours.[14]

Increased calcitriol production in activated macrophages (granulomatous diseases and lymphomas) can be decreased using corticosteroids (10-30 mg/day of prednisone, and more in the cases of lymphomas). If this is ineffective, ketoconazole, chloroquine, and hydroxychloroquine may be used to block calcitriol production.

Intestinal calcium absorption can be partially blocked by ingestion of phosphate-containing drugs, which form insoluble calcium phosphate complexes and prevent absorption. Reducing calcium intake to 400 mg/day or less is also beneficial.

When bone resorption causes hypercalcemia, inhibition of this process with calcitonin and bisphosphonates results in lowering of serum calcium. Calcitonin is given subcutaneously or intramuscularly every 12 hours (4 IU/kg). Its action is rapid (4-6 hours) and calcium is usually lowered by 1-2 mg/dL. However, calcitonin is effective in only 60% to 70% of patients, and most of them develop tachyphylaxis over 48 to 72 hours (most likely due to receptor down-regulation).

Bisphosphonates accumulate in bone and inhibit osteoclast-mediated bone resorption. They very effectively lower serum calcium. Their maximum effect is seen in 2 to 4 days. Duration of effect is usually several weeks and varies among patients and with the type of bisphosphonate. Pamidronate, etidronate, alendronate, and zoledronate are currently available in the United States. Zoledronate appears to have longest-lasting effect (1-1.5 months); it is given in a 15-minute IV infusion (4 mg). Pamidronate is given by IV infusion over 4 to 24 hours. The initial dose is 30 mg if the calcium level is less than 12 mg/dL, 60 mg if the calcium is 12 to 13.5 mg/mL, and 90 mg for calcium above this level. Subsequent doses should not be given more often than every 7 days. Because of the lag in the onset of effect, bisphosphonates should be combined with faster-acting therapeutic modalities such as IV saline infusion and calcitonin injections.

Hemodialysis or peritoneal dialysis with low calcium levels in dialysis fluid is very effective for removing calcium from circulation. These methods are used in patients with renal insufficiency and congestive heart failure in which saline infusion is not feasible.

References

For a complete list of references, log onto www.expertconsult.com.

Prevention and Treatment of Leg and Foot Ulcers in Diabetes Mellitus

Allan Boike, Michael Maier, and Daniel Logan

DEFINITION

An ulcer is defined as a breakdown in the skin that may extend to involve the subcutaneous tissue or even to the level of muscle or bone. These lesions are common, particularly on the lower extremities. Leg and foot ulcers have many causes that may further define their character.

PREVALENCE

The prevalence of leg ulceration is approximately 1% to 2%, and is slightly higher in the older adult population.[1] Venous ulcers are the most common form of leg ulcers, accounting for almost 80% of all lower extremity ulcerations.[2] Peak prevalence is between 60 and 80 years.[3] Approximately one third of patients with chronic venous insufficiency will develop venous ulceration before the age of 40 years.[2] In addition, venous ulcers may have a prolonged duration and are associated with a high rate of recurrence, which contributes to their prevalence.

Ulcerations associated with diabetes are the most common cause of foot ulcers. Most of these ulcers are a direct result of loss of sensation secondary to peripheral neuropathy.

Approximately 15% of persons with diabetes will develop foot ulceration during their lifetime.[4] Most lower extremity amputations in the United States are preceded by a foot ulcer.[5]

Arterial ulcers account for 10% to 20% of lower extremity ulcerations. Other causes of lower extremity ulceration are uncommon. Many ulcers may be of mixed cause, with two or more contributing factors leading to ulceration present in the same patient. We focus on the most common causes of ulceration.

PATHOPHYSIOLOGY

Neurotrophic Ulcers

The development of neurotrophic foot ulcers in patients with diabetes mellitus has several components, including neuropathy, biomechanical pressure, and vascular supply. Peripheral neuropathy is clearly the dominant factor in the pathogenesis of diabetic foot ulcers.

The neuropathy associated with diabetes is a distal symmetrical sensorimotor polyneuropathy. There is a clear correlation between the presence of hyperglycemia and the development of neuropathy. The mechanism by which this occurs, although extensively studied, continues to be investigated. Much attention has been focused on the polyol pathway. This pathway may result in the deposition of sorbitol within peripheral nerves. In addition, oxygen radicals may be produced, which may contribute to nerve damage. Vascular disease of nerve-supplying vessels may contribute to neuropathy. More recently, increased susceptibility to compression in diabetic patients as a contributor to the development of neuropathy has been postulated.[6]

The sensory component of the neuropathy results in a decreased ability to perceive pain from foreign bodies, trauma, or areas of increased pressure on the foot. Loss of sensation accompanied by trauma or increased pressure contributes to skin breakdown, often accompanied by ulcer formation at the site of pressure.

The motor component of neuropathy can lead to atrophy of the intrinsic musculature of the foot, resulting in digital contractures and areas of elevated pressure on the plantar foot. In addition, weakness of the anterior leg musculature may contribute to equinus deformity with lack of adequate dorsiflexion at the ankle joint, leading to elevated plantar pressures in the forefoot.

Autonomic neuropathy may occur, with loss of sympathetic tone and arteriovenous shunting of blood in the foot. Sweat glands may also be affected; the resultant anhidrosis leads to dry, cracked skin and predisposes the skin to breakdown.

There is a well-established association between diabetes and increased risks for the development of atherosclerosis and peripheral arterial disease. This is more likely to occur in smokers. This is not microvascular but macrovascular disease, predominantly of the infragenicular (tibial and peroneal arteries) vessels, with sparing of the vessels in the foot. Ischemia may therefore contribute at least in part to the development or persistence of foot ulcers in diabetic patients.

Venous Ulcers

Venous ulceration is the eventual result of venous hypertension. This has multiple causes, but the most common cause is venous valvular incompetence or insufficiency, which may be congenital or acquired. Failure of the venous or muscle pump or venous obstruction may also contribute to venous hypertension. The end result is transmission of elevated venous pressure from the deep to superficial system of the veins, with local effects leading to ulceration. Although it is accepted that venous hypertension plays a dominant role in the development of ulceration, there are multiple hypotheses attempting to explain the direct cause of ulceration.

The fibrin cuff theory, proposed by Browse and colleagues,[7] has asserted that as a result of increased venous pressure, fibrinogen is leaked from capillaries. This results in the formation of pericapillary fibrin cuffs that serve as a barrier to the diffusion of oxygen and nutrients. This theory has lost favor as the sole cause, because fibrin is probably not as significant a barrier to diffusion as previously believed.

The trapping of white cells to capillary endothelium is another hypothesis. Venous hypertension results in decreased flow in the capillaries, resulting in the accumulation of white cells. These white cells may then release proteolytic enzymes, as well as interfere with tissue oxygenation.[8]

A different trap hypothesis has been proposed. This suggests that venous hypertension causes various macromolecules to leak into the dermis and trap growth factors. These growth factors are then unavailable for repair of damaged tissue.[9]

Arterial Ulcers

Atherosclerosis is the most common cause of peripheral arterial occlusive disease. This predominantly affects the superficial femoral and popliteal vessels, reducing blood flow to the lower extremities. When the ischemia is severe enough, ulceration will develop.

Thromboangiitis obliterans (Buerger's disease) is an inflammatory segmental thrombotic disease of the medium and small vessels of the extremities usually associated with smoking. This is a cause of peripheral arterial disease and ulceration.

Atheroembolism may cause peripheral arterial occlusion when proximal plaques break off and travel distally. This is referred to as cholesterol emboli or blue toe syndrome.

SIGNS AND SYMPTOMS

Venous Ulcers

Patients with venous ulcers may complain of tired, swollen, aching legs. These ulcers may be painful but not as severe as those seen with ischemic ulcers. The legs will typically be edematous, often with hyperpigmentation of the lower legs from chronic venous stasis. The skin around the ulcer is hyperpigmented. These ulcers are usually on or near the malleoli, usually the distal medial leg. The margins of the ulcers are irregular, with a shallow base. Lipodermatosclerosis may be present, a condition of the skin whereby it becomes indurated and fibrotic in a circumferential pattern, resembling an inverted champagne bottle.

Neurotrophic Ulcers

With neuropathy being the underlying cause of ulceration, many patients complain of burning, tingling, or numbness of the feet on presentation. The ulcer is usually on the plantar foot, most commonly under the great toe or first metatarsal head. Because of pressure, it is often surrounded by a rim of hyperkeratotic tissue, which may even cover the ulcer and give the illusion that the ulcer has healed, when it in fact has not. Infected ulcers may be associated with cellulitis, lymphangitis, adenopathy, calor, edema, foul odor, and purulent drainage. Systemic signs such as fever and chills may be related, but are often absent, even in the presence of severe infection. There may be foot deformity or prominent areas of pressure associated with the ulcer.

Arterial Ulcers

Arterial ulcers are almost always painful. Patients may relate intermittent claudication, pain in the extremities or buttocks with activity that is relieved with rest. If occlusion is severe enough, there may be pain even at rest. A familiar complaint is pain in the legs when lying in bed at night that is relieved by dangling the legs off the side of the bed. Physical examination reveals diminished or absent lower extremity pulses, trophic changes in the skin, decreased hair growth, and nails that may be thickened or ridged. The skin may be shiny, smooth, cool, and demonstrate pallor or a reddish-blue discoloration. The ulcers have a predilection for the lateral aspect of the leg, posterior heel, distal aspects of the digits, medial aspect of the first metatarsal head, and lateral aspect of the fifth metatarsal. The ulcer itself will often have a dry, dark base of eschar. Gangrene may be present. The lesions are often punched out, with a well-demarcated border.

DIAGNOSIS

Accurate diagnosis is the foundation of ulcer care. Misdiagnosis may result in mismanagement, with failure to heal, and may even have devastating consequences. For example, venous ulcers are treated with compression. If an ischemic ulcer is mistakenly diagnosed as a venous ulcer and treated with compression, there may be a further progression of ischemia in the affected limb.

Usually, the history and physical examination are the primary means of obtaining the correct diagnosis. The signs and symptoms previously described will allow clinicians to make the correct diagnosis for the most common types of ulcers. Those with an atypical appearance may require further investigation or referral to a specialist. Long-standing ulcers may require biopsy to rule out malignancy.

Diabetics should be tested for neuropathy. Vibratory testing may be performed with a 128-Hz tuning fork on the dorsum of the great toe. Achilles tendon and patellar reflexes should be examined. The response on these tests is diminished with neuropathy. However, the simplest and most effective means of detecting neuropathy is examination with a 10-g monofilament. An inability to detect the monofilament when applied under the metatarsal heads or digits is indicative of neuropathy. A patient with a history of neuropathy who complains of new-onset pain in the extremity should raise concern for a pathologic process, such as infection or Charcot's neuropathic arthropathy.

A proper vascular assessment is critical to the evaluation of the diabetic foot. Vascular examination, including palpation of the dorsalis pedis and posterior tibial pulses, as well as general inspection of the extremities, should be performed. Patients with evidence of ischemia should be further investigated with vascular studies. An excellent tool is the ankle-brachial index (ABI), which is determined by dividing the higher systolic pressure of the anterior tibial or posterior tibial vessels by the highest systolic brachial pressure. Ankle pressure is determined with the assistance of a Doppler probe; a result of 1.0 to 1.1 is normal. Values less than 1.0 are abnormal and reflect decreased perfusion to the lower extremity. Medial calcification of the tibial vessels, which is common in diabetics, may falsely elevate the ankle pressure. Toe pressures in such patients more accurately reflect perfusion. Segmental pressure determination, pulse volume recordings, duplex scanning, transcutaneous oxygen diffusion, contrast angiography, and magnetic resonance angiography are other vascular studies that may assess perfusion.

All ulcers should be assessed for potential infection. Infected ulcers may be limb- and even life threatening. In addition to the signs previously noted, the ulcer base should be inspected. Diabetic foot ulcers should be probed, because they often reveal a tract under the skin that may harbor an abscess. In addition, probing may assess the depth of the ulcer. Grayson and associates[10] have found a positive predictive value of 89% when an ulcer probes to the depth of bone. Leukocytosis may be present, but is often absent in diabetic patients. The erythrocyte sedimentation rate is frequently elevated in infected ulcers, and values higher than 70 mm/hr should heighten suspicion for osteomyelitis. Deep culture of tissue or purulence is helpful in establishing the microbiology of the infection. Superficial swabbing of sinus tracts is unreliable. Bone culture is the definitive method to diagnose osteomyelitis.

When bone infection is suspected, radiographs should be obtained. Films should be inspected for gas in the tissues. Signs of osteomyelitis include periosteal reaction, osteopenia, and cortical erosion. Unfortunately, these signs are delayed because approximately 50% of bone must be destroyed before osteomyelitis is evident radiographically. Bone scanning and magnetic resonance imaging (MRI) are other useful means for establishing the diagnosis of bone infection.

TREATMENT

Venous Ulcers

When speaking of any lower extremity ulceration, the best treatment is prevention. Management of edema should be instituted before the development of ulceration. Mechanical therapy is the gold standard for treatment of venous insufficiency. Elevation of the legs above the level of the heart for 30 minutes three or four times daily may reduce edema and improve the cutaneous microcirculation.[11] Elevation of the legs while sleeping at night also reduces swelling.

Compression stockings are the primary method of edema management, particularly in the active patient. These methods are also the mainstay of treatment once a venous ulcer develops. Compression stocking use in compliant patients increases the ulcer healing rate and reduces the rate of recurrence.[12] Compression therapy is believed to exert its positive effect on venous ulcers by increasing fibrinolysis, reducing venous hypertension, and improving the cutaneous microcirculation. Stockings exerting a pressure of 30 to 40 mm Hg are typically used in the setting of venous ulceration. Multilayered compression bandages are also effective at reducing edema. Compression should generally not be used in the setting of peripheral arterial disease or uncompensated congestive heart failure.

Although compression therapy is the key to venous ulcer treatment, some patients require adjunctive therapy to attain ulcer healing. In addition, some patients have venous ulcers combined with arterial occlusive disease, making excessive compression therapy a hazardous intervention. Pharmacologic therapy is sometimes used in these cases.

Pentoxifylline has been shown to improve venous ulcer healing, with and without compression therapy.[13] A double-blind, randomized, clinical trial of 20 patients treated with enteric-coated aspirin, 300 mg daily, found that the aspirin-treated group had a significantly better reduction in ulcer size.[14]

Diuretics may be used for a short time in cases of severe edema. Venous edema is difficult to mobilize with diuretic therapy, so volume depletion may occur with prolonged use.

Neurotrophic Ulcers

Neuropathy is the gateway to the development of foot ulceration in diabetic patients. Intensive treatment of blood glucose concentration has been shown to delay the onset and slow the progression of peripheral neuropathy.[15] It is therefore critical that patients with or at risk for foot ulceration receive appropriate glucose concentration management from their primary care physician or endocrinologist. Regular screening for the development of neuropathy, intensive podiatric care, and custom footwear may all reduce the risk of foot ulceration.[16] Once ulceration develops, treatment should focus on pressure relief, débridement, and treatment of infection.

Total contact casting is the gold standard for off-loading the diabetic foot. The cast cannot be removed, reducing the risk of patient noncompliance with pressure relief. The cast application is technically demanding and should only be applied with care and expertise. It should not be used in the presence of infection or excessive drainage. Removable cast walkers are commonly used to off-load the diabetic foot in place of the total contact cast. Because the device is removable, the wound may be monitored daily and can be used in the presence of infection. It also allows the patient to remove the device during sleep and bathing. However, because this device is removable, its success is dependent on patient compliance.

Wound débridement removes nonviable tissue that if left in the wound might promote infection. Hyperkeratotic tissue that increases plantar pressures is also removed. Débridement may serve to promote healing by converting a chronic wound to an acute wound. Platelets aggregate in the débrided wound, initiating the inflammatory phase of wound healing.

Management of infection is the most critical aspect of treating the diabetic foot. Infected foot ulcers are commonly limb- or even life threatening. Infections should be treated empirically until test results are available. Cefazolin and beta-lactamase inhibitor agents are effective empirical agents for such infections. Definitive therapy may then be instituted when culture and sensitivity results have been obtained. Incision and drainage should be performed when deep infection or abscess is present. When osteomyelitis is present, antibiotic therapy combined with surgical débridement, with removal of infected bone, is generally necessary.

Arterial Ulcers

In regard to arterial ulcers, a vascular medicine or surgery specialist should be consulted. It should be determined whether the patient is a candidate for a peripheral revascularization procedure. Interventional radiologists also perform less invasive vascular procedures, which may increase peripheral blood flow. Without sufficient tissue oxygenation, these wounds will not heal. Tissue that is infected or gangrenous must be removed, often requiring partial amputation. Vascular consultation is needed to determine the appropriate level of amputation when necessary.

Wound Care

In general, wounds should be kept clean and moist to promote granulation and prevent infection. There is a vast array of wound care products and dressings available that are beyond the scope of this discussion. Clinicians often erroneously rely on a topical therapy alone to heal a wound. It must be stressed that, in most cases, it is adherence to the principles outlined earlier and not what is put on a wound that will lead to a successful result. Wounds resistant to healing, however, may benefit from the many wound care modalities available. Topical growth factors, negative pressure wound therapy, living skin equivalents, and silver-impregnated dressings are among the many adjunctive therapies available for ulcer care, particularly for the specialist.

CONCLUSION

The evaluation and treatment of the most common types of leg and foot ulcers have been discussed. The general principles presented may be used to successfully treat most leg and foot ulcers. However, when presented with a wound that is atypical in presentation or fails to respond to conventional therapy, clinicians should have a low threshold for referral to a specialist.

Summary

- Leg and foot ulcers in diabetic patients have three common underlying causes: venous insufficiency, peripheral neuropathy (neurotrophic ulcers), or peripheral arterial occlusive disease.
- The locations of the ulcers and associated clinical findings, such as edema, callus or decreased pulses, help characterize the predominant cause of an ulcer. However, careful examination of vascular and neuropathic status is important for proper management.
- Management strategies include compression therapy (venous ulcers), unloading treatments (neurotrophic ulcers), and possibly arterial revascularization.
- Infection in an ulcer contributes to the risk for adverse outcomes and can be managed with local and systemic therapy.

National Practice Guidelines

American College of Foot and Ankle Surgeons: http://www.acfas.org/press/backgrounders/Diabetic+Foot+Conditions.htm.

National Guideline Clearinghouse: Clinical guidelines for type 2 diabetes. Prevention and management of foot problems, 2008. Available at http://www.guideline.gov/summary/summary.aspx?doc_id=5062&nbr=3546&string=ulcer.

National Guideline Clearinghouse: Diagnosis and treatment of diabetic foot infections, 2008. Available at http://www.guideline.gov/summary/summary.aspx?doc_id=5888&nbr=3874&string=ulcer.

Suggested Readings

American Diabetes Association: Consensus development conference on diabetic foot wound care. 7-8 April 1999, Boston, MA. Adv Wound Care 1999;12:353-361.

Aszmann OC, Kress KM, Dellon AL: Results of decompression of peripheral nerves in diabetics: A prospective, blinded study. Plast Reconstr Surg 2000;106:816-822.

Browse NL, Burnand KG: The cause of venous ulceration. Lancet 1982;2:243-245.
Gonsalves CF: Venous leg ulcers. Techniques in vascular and interventional radiology 2003;6:132-136.
Grayson ML, Gibbons GW, Balogh K, et al: Probing to bone in infected pedal ulcers. JAMA 1995;27:721-723.
Mayberry JC, Moneta GL, Taylor LM, Porter JM: Fifteen-year results of ambulatory compression therapy for chronic venous ulcers. Surgery 1991;109:575.
Mekkes JR, Loots MAM, Van Der Wal AC, Bos JD: Causes, investigation and treatment of leg ulceration. Br J Dermatol 2003;148:388-401.
Pecoraro RE, Reiber GE, Burgess EM: Pathways to diabetic limb amputation: Basis for prevention. Diabetes Care 1990;13:513-521.
Singh N, Armstrong DG, Lipsky BA: Preventing foot ulcers in patients with diabetes. JAMA 2005;293:217-228.
The Diabetes Control and Complications Trial Research Group: The effect of intensive treatment of diabetes on the development and progression of long-term complications in insulin-dependent diabetes mellitus. N Engl J Med 1993;329:977-986.

References

For a complete list of references, log onto www.expertconsult.com.

Obesity

Stacy Brethauer, Sangeeta Kashyap, and Philip Schauer

DEFINITION AND ETIOLOGY

Obesity has become an important public health problem in industrialized countries throughout the world. The body mass index (BMI = weight [in kg]/height^2 [in m^2]) is the primary measurement used to categorize obese patients (Table 1). Excess body weight (EBW) is defined as the amount of weight present in excess of ideal body weight (IBW), as determined by Metropolitan Life Tables. In 1991, the National Institutes of Health defined morbid obesity as a BMI of 35 kg/m^2 or higher with severe, obesity-related comorbidity or a BMI of 40 kg/m^2 or higher without comorbidity.[1]

The development of obesity involves the interactions between excessive intake, inefficient calorie use, reduced metabolic activity, a reduction in the thermogenic response to meals, and an abnormally high set point for body weight. Genetic, environmental, and psychosocial factors all contribute to this problem.

PREVALENCE AND RISK FACTORS

The prevalence of obesity in the United States has increased from 15% in 1980 to 32% in 2004.[2] The prevalence of extreme obesity (BMI > 40 kg/m^2) is 2.8% in men and 6.9% in women. The prevalence of childhood and adolescent obesity has tripled since 1980 and, currently, 17% of U.S. children and adolescents are overweight. Obesity and morbid obesity affect women and minorities (particularly middle-aged black and Hispanic women) more than white males. However, in almost every age and ethnic group, the prevalence of overweight or obesity exceeds 50%.

Recent studies have also delineated the importance of childhood weight for influencing adulthood weight. Being overweight during older childhood is highly predictive of adult obesity, especially if a parent is also obese. Being overweight during the adolescent years is an even greater predictor of adult obesity. Obesity is now the second leading cause of preventable death after cigarette smoking, despite expenditures of over $45 billion annually on weight loss products.[3]

PATHOPHYSIOLOGY AND NATURAL HISTORY

Adipose tissue is primarily stored in the subcutaneous tissue and abdominal cavity. In general, females are more likely to deposit fat in the peripheral tissues and males tend to deposit fat in the abdominal compartment. As obesity develops, the size and number of fat cells increase. As fat cells grow, they release increasing amounts of cytokines (and lower amounts of adiponectin); these changes have deleterious effects on glucose and lipid metabolism and contribute to the proinflammatory state associated with obesity.

Obesity shortens the life span of those who suffer with it. The mortality rate of an individual with a BMI higher than 40 kg/m^2 is double that of a normal-weight individual.[4] It is estimated that a man in his twenties, with a BMI higher than 45 kg/m^2 has a 22% reduction in life expectancy: 13 years.[5] Most obesity-related deaths result from complications related to diabetes and cardiovascular disease. Worldwide, approximately 2.5 million deaths occur annually because of obesity-related comorbidities.

SIGNS, SYMPTOMS, AND RELATED DISEASES

There are more than 30 comorbid conditions associated with severe obesity. Insulin resistance and diabetes mellitus occur in 15% to 25% of obese patients. Increased abdominal fat raises the intra-abdominal pressure and contributes to gastroesophageal reflux, stress urinary incontinence, venous stasis disease, and abdominal hernia in obese patients. Fatty deposits in the liver can progress to nonalcoholic steatohepatitis (NASH) and ultimately to liver failure. Excess weight causes joint and back stress that can lead to debilitating joint disease. The low-grade inflammatory state associated with morbid obesity has been implicated in the development of vascular and coronary artery disease and the hypercoagulable state seen in these patients. Obese patients have impaired pulmonary function, particularly decreased functional residual capacity, and frequently suffer from asthma, obstructive sleep apnea, and obesity hypoventilation syndrome (pickwickian syndrome). Other comorbidities include hypertension, dyslipidemia, asthma, and sex hormone dysfunction. Obesity is associated with an increased incidence of uterine, breast, ovarian, prostate, and colon cancer and of skin infections, urinary tract infections, migraine headaches, depression, and pseudotumor cerebri.

DIAGNOSIS AND EVALUATION OF COMORBIDITIES

The diagnosis of morbid obesity is established by determining the patient's BMI and the presence of any significant comorbid conditions. A thorough history, physical examination, and focused testing will uncover previously undiagnosed comorbidities in up to two thirds of obese patients.

Visceral, or central, adiposity is more metabolically active than peripheral fat and is associated with type 2 diabetes, dyslipidemia (elevated triglyceride and reduced high-density lipoprotein [HDL] levels), high blood pressure, and increased risk for cardiovascular atherosclerotic disease. The waist-to-hip ratio helps to identify patients with excess visceral adiposity. Women with a waist-to-hip ratio of more than 0.8 and men with a ratio of more than 1.0 are considered to have excess central adiposity that confers risk for developing the metabolic syndrome. The diagnostic criteria for the metabolic syndrome are shown in Table 2.

The pretreatment evaluation performed at the Cleveland Clinic is consistent with published guidelines.[6] Because obese persons are at higher risk for cardiovascular disease, a baseline electrocardiogram should be performed. Cardiology evaluation is carried out when there is evidence of cardiac disease based on clinical symptoms or electrocardiographic findings. Chest radiography and baseline laboratory testing, including a complete blood count, chemistry panel, liver function tests, thyroid function tests, and a lipid profile, should be performed as well.

Obstructive sleep apnea frequently goes unrecognized in this patient population until a thorough history prompts further evaluation. Patients with symptoms of loud snoring, daytime hypersomnolence, or a neck circumference of 43 cm or more should undergo polysomnography and, if positive, be treated with nasal continuous positive airway pressure. Asthma and obesity hypoventilation syndrome (chronic hypoxemia, hypercarbia, pulmonary hypertension, and polycythemia) are also severe pulmonary complications of obesity and should be evaluated by a pulmonologist.

Dietary counseling and psychological testing are required for patients being referred for bariatric surgery.

Table 1 Definitions of Obesity

Category	Body Mass Index (kg/m²)	Over Ideal Body Weight (%)
Underweight	<18.5	
Normal	18.5-24.9	
Overweight	25.0-29.9	
Obesity (class 1)	30-34.9	>20%
Severe obesity (class 2)	35-39.9	>100%
Severe obesity (class 3)	40-49.9	
Superobesity	>50	>250%

Table 2 Adult Treatment Panel III Criteria for the Metabolic Syndrome*

Parameter	Criterion
Central obesity	
Waist circumference in men	>102 cm
Waist circumference in women	>88 cm
Hypertriglyceridemia	≥150 mg/dL
Low high-density lipoprotein cholesterol	
Men	<40 mg/dL
Women	<50 mg/dL
High blood pressure	≥130/≥85 mm Hg
Fasting blood glucose	≥110 mg/dL

*Three or more of these criteria need to be present.

Adapted from National Cholesterol Education Program (NCEP) Expert Panel on Detection, Evaluation, and Treatment of High Blood Cholesterol in Adults (Adult Treatment Panel III): Third Report of the National Cholesterol Education Program (NCEP) Expert Panel on Detection, Evaluation, and Treatment of High Blood Cholesterol in Adults (Adult Treatment Panel III) final report. Circulation 2002;106:3143-3421, with permission.

Summary

- Severe obesity can adversely affect every organ system.
- Detailed evaluation of symptoms can uncover serious comorbidities.
- Diabetes and cardiovascular disease are common in obese patients.
- Central obesity is associated with the presence of the metabolic syndrome.

TREATMENT

Lifestyle Modifications

According to the clinical guidelines published by the American College of Physicians, all patients with a BMI of 30 kg/m² or higher should be counseled intensively on lifestyle and behavioral modifications, such as appropriate diet and exercise.[7,8] An algorithm by the American College of Physicians for medically managing obesity is shown in Figure 1.[8] The patient's goals for weight loss should be individually determined and may encompass other related parameters, such as decreasing blood pressure or fasting blood glucose levels. When establishing realistic weight loss goals, it is important to realize that modest weight loss (10%-15%) of baseline weight is sufficient to result in health benefits.[9,10]

General diet guidelines for achieving and maintaining a healthy weight include eating balanced, nutritious foods to avoid vitamin deficiencies. Avoiding foods high in fat and simple sugars should be emphasized. In addition, eating about 50% to 55% of calories from complex carbohydrates and educating patients regarding portion sizes and caloric content of foods is recommended by several national scientific organizations, such as the American Dietetics Association and American Diabetes Association. Referral to a registered dietitian helps patients initiate and adhere to these dietary guidelines.

Every physician should include an exercise regimen as part of a comprehensive lifestyle modification plan. Moderate exercise has been shown to decrease blood pressure, increase HDL and reduce triglyceride levels, and is predictive of maintenance of weight loss and delaying onset of type 2 diabetes.[11] General exercise recommendations include 20 to 30 minutes of moderate exercise 5 to 7 days a week, and up to 60 minutes a day most days of the week for maintenance of weight and 90 minutes a day for achieving weight loss.

Medical Options

Pharmacologic therapy can be offered to obese patients who have failed to achieve their weight loss goals through lifestyle modification alone or have significant comorbidities. Before initiating therapy, patients must understand the drug's side effects, the lack of long-term safety data, and the temporary nature of the weight loss achieved with medications. Table 3 lists the medications reviewed in the 2005 American College of Physician clinical practice guideline for obesity management.[7]

The choice of agent depends on the side effect profile of each agent and the patient tolerance of those side effects. The amount of extra weight loss attributable to weight loss medications is modest (<5 kg at 1 year). However, even modest weight loss, as seen with medical management, can slow the progression of diabetes and positively influence cardiovascular risk factors There is no evidence that modest weight loss affects mortality.

The optimal duration of treatment with obesity medications has not yet been determined. Data from randomized controlled trials have examined only up to 12 months of therapy; thus, more long-term clinical trials need to be performed. There are no long-term data on whether these drugs decrease morbidity or mortality from obesity-related conditions.

Surgical Options

Indications

Patients with a BMI higher than 35 kg/m² with obesity-related comorbidities and those with a BMI higher than 40 kg/m² with or without comorbidities are eligible for bariatric surgery (Box 1).[1]

Patients must have attempted medical weight loss programs and should be highly motivated to change their lifestyle after surgery. The NIH guidelines of 1991 have recommended age limits between 18 and 60 years. At that time, there was insufficient evidence to make recommendations about surgery for patients at the extremes of age. Although advanced age has been a predictor of increased mortality after bariatric surgery,[12,13] there is some evidence (case series) that supports bariatric surgery in carefully selected adolescents and older patients.

Contraindications

Patients who cannot tolerate general anesthesia because of cardiac, pulmonary, or hepatic insufficiency are not candidates for surgery.

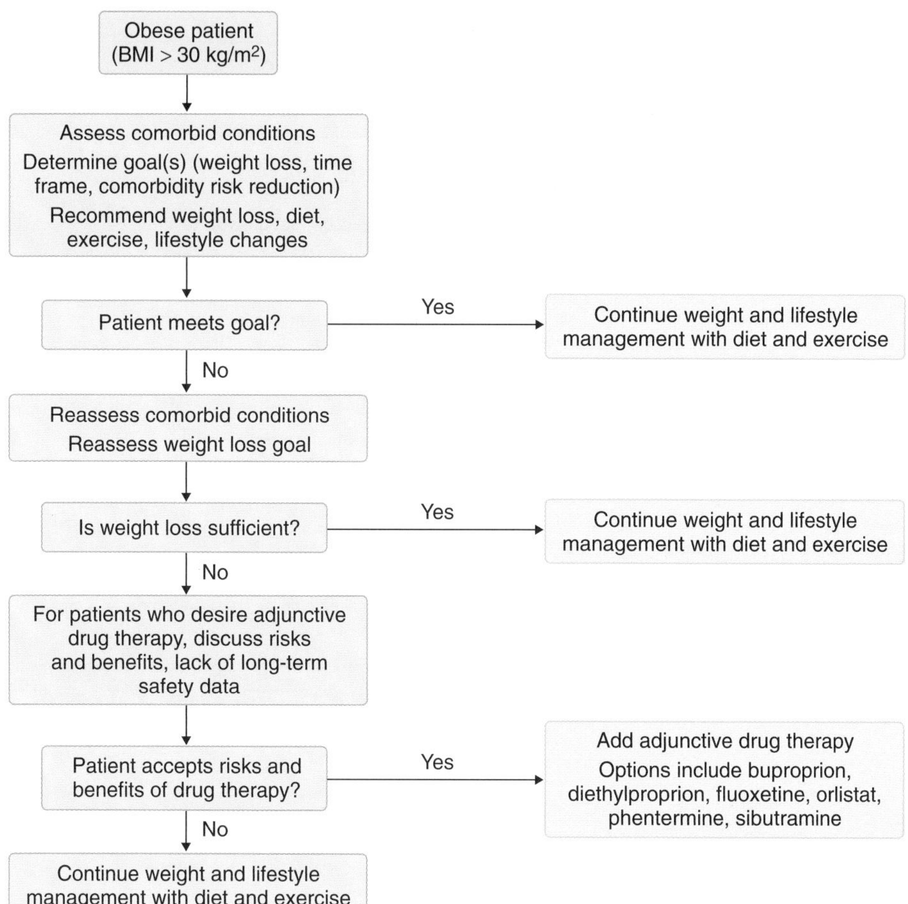

Figure 1 Algorithm for the medical management of obesity. BMI, body mass index. *(With permission from Snow V, Barry P, Fitterman N, et al: Pharmacologic and surgical management of obesity in primary care: A clinical practice guideline from the American College of Physicians. Ann Intern Med 2005;142:525-531.)*

Box 1 Candidates for Bariatric Surgery

- BMI > 40 kg/m^2, or BMI > 35 kg/m^2 with significant obesity-related comorbidities
- Acceptable operative risk
- Documented failure of nonsurgical weight loss programs
- Psychologically stable, with realistic expectations
- Well-informed and motivated patient
- Supportive family and social environment
- Absence of active alcohol or substance abuse
- Absence of uncontrolled psychotic or depressive disorder

Additionally, patients must be able to understand the consequences of the surgery and comply with the extensive preoperative evaluation and postoperative lifestyle changes, diet, vitamin supplementation, and follow-up program. Patients who have ongoing substance abuse issues or unstable psychiatric illness are poor candidates for bariatric surgery.

Follow-up

Bariatric surgery patients require lifetime follow-up.[1] Early postoperative visits focus on complications and the dramatic changes in dietary habits. Later follow-up visits focus on psychological support, nutritional assessment and vitamin supplementation, and adherence to exercise programs. Patients who present with new onset abdominal pain, vomiting, or gastroesophageal reflux months to years after bariatric surgery should be referred to their bariatric surgeon. These symptoms may be secondary to an anastomotic ulcer or stricture or an intermittent bowel obstruction after Roux-en-Y gastric bypass (RYGB). After laparoscopic adjustable gastric banding (LAGB), new onset of gastroesophageal reflux or dysphagia may suggest gastric prolapse through the band. These patients require prompt evaluation and treatment for these conditions.

Procedures

Roux-en-Y Gastric Bypass. RYGB combines a restrictive and a malabsorptive procedure and is the most common bariatric procedure performed in the United States (80%). Most RYGB procedures are now performed laparoscopically, which results in faster recovery and fewer pulmonary and wound complications compared with open surgery. A small, 15- to 30-mL gastric pouch is created to restrict food intake, and a Roux-en-Y anastomosis bypasses the duodenum and proximal jejunum and provides a malabsorptive component. The risks and benefits associated with RYGB are shown in Figure 2. RYGB results in superior weight loss when compared with restrictive procedures with excellent long-term reduction in EWL (50% at 14 years) comorbidity resolution.

Laparoscopic Adjustable Gastric Banding. The LAGB is a restrictive procedure and the device (Lap-Band System, Inamed Health, Santa Barbara, Calif) was approved for use in the United States in 2001 after having excellent results in Europe and Australia. The silicone band, with an inflatable inner collar, is placed around the upper portion of the stomach to create a small gastric pouch. The band is connected to a port that is placed in the subcutaneous tissue of the abdominal wall. The inner diameter of the band can be adjusted by injecting saline through the port.

The adjustable nature of the LAGB is a major advantage that distinguishes it from vertical-banded gastroplasty. Band adjustments are made according to weight loss by injecting or removing saline from a subcutaneous port. Severe complications and mortality rates

Table 3 Medications Used for Weight Loss

Drug	Mechanism of Action	Side Effects
Sibutramine	Appetite suppressant: combined norepinephrine and serotonin reuptake inhibitor	Modest increases in heart rate and blood pressure, nervousness, insomnia
Phentermine	Appetite suppressant: sympathomimetic amine	Cardiovascular, gastrointestinal
Diethylpropion	Appetite suppressant: sympathomimetic amine	Palpitations, tachycardia, insomnia, gastrointestinal
Orlistat	Lipase inhibitor: decreased absorption of fat	Diarrhea, flatulence, bloating, abdominal pain, dyspepsia
Bupropion	Appetite suppressant: mechanism unknown	Paresthesia, insomnia, central nervous system effects
Fluoxetine	Appetite suppressant: selective serotonin reuptake inhibitor	Agitation, nervousness, gastrointestinal
Sertraline	Appetite suppressant: selective serotonin reuptake inhibitor	Agitation, nervousness, gastrointestinal
Topiramate	Mechanism unknown	Paresthesia, changes in taste
Zonisamide	Mechanism unknown	Somnolence, dizziness, nausea

From Snow V, Barry P, Fitterman N. et al: Pharmacologic and surgical management of obesity in primary care: A clinical practice guideline from the American College of Physicians. Ann Intern Med 2005;142:525-531, with permission..

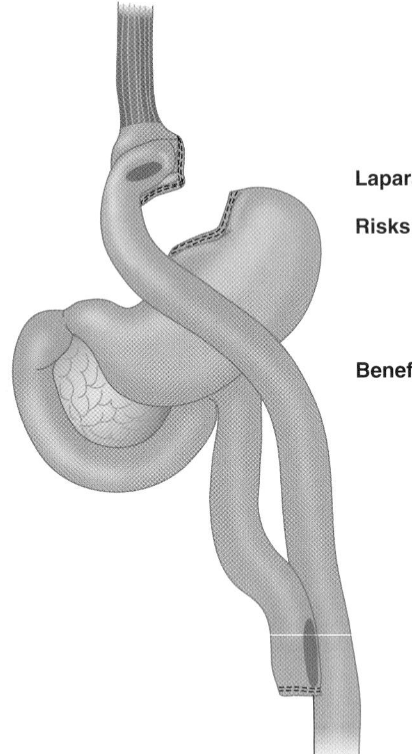

Laparascopic Roux-en-Y Gastric Bypass

Risks:
- 0-5% anastomotic leak rate
- 2-10% anastomotic stricture rate
- 1-5% anastomotic ulcer rate
- 1-5% late bowel obstruction
- 0.5% mortality rate

Benefits:
- 65-80% excess weight loss
- 84% resolution of diabetes
- 97% improvement in hyperlipidemia
- 68% resolution of hypertension
- 78% resolution of sleep apnea

Figure 2 Risks and benefits of Roux-en-Y gastric bypass.

are lower for LAGB than RYGB, but LAGB typically results in less and more gradual weight loss. Common risks and benefits of LAGB are shown in Figure 3.

Vertical Banded Gastroplasty. Vertical banded gastroplasty (VBG) is a restrictive procedure that creates a small gastric pouch with a fixed banded outlet. However, 10-year follow-up data have shown that only 26% to 40% of patients maintain acceptable weight loss (>50% EWL) and one third of patients in these series returned to or exceeded their preoperative weight.[14]

Early complications after VBG are infrequent, but late complications have resulted in a 17% to 30% reoperation rate.[15] Because of the poor long-term weight loss and high late complication rate, VBG has largely been abandoned. Patients with weight regain or severe gastroesophageal reflux disease (GERD) symptoms after VBG should be referred to a bariatric surgeon to discuss revision to RYGB.

Biliopancreatic Diversion. Biliopancreatic diversion is a malabsorptive procedure performed by less than 3% of bariatric surgeons in the United States. This procedure, and a modification called the

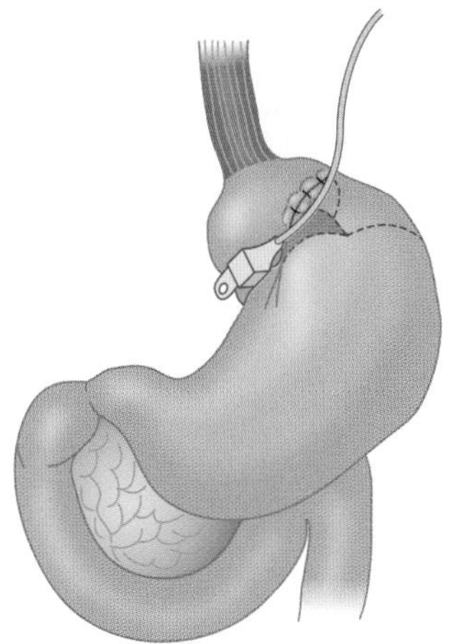

Laparoscopic Adjustable Gastric Banding

Risks:	1% bowel perforation 2-25% slippage/prolapse 0-2% band erosion 1-7% tube or port malfunction 0.1% mortality rate
Benefits:	40-60% excess weight loss 55% resolution of diabetes 60% improvement in hyperlipidemia 45% resolution of hypertension 95% resolution of sleep apnea

Figure 3 **Risks and benefits of laparoscopic adjustable gastric banding.**

duodenal switch, are designed to limit intestinal energy absorption to the length of the distal common channel. Although these procedures offer the best and most durable weight loss results of any bariatric procedure performed today, higher complication rates, nutritional deficiencies, and a higher mortality rate have limited their widespread use.

Summary

- All obese patients (BMI > 30 kg/m^2) should be counseled on lifestyle and behavioral modifications, such as appropriate diet and exercise.
- Pharmacologic therapy can be offered to obese patients who have failed to lose weight with diet and exercise.
- Bariatric surgery should be considered for morbidly obese patients who have failed medical weight loss programs (diet and exercise, with or without pharmacotherapy). Patients with a BMI higher than 40 kg/m^2, or higher than 35 kg/m^2 with obesity-related comorbidities, are candidates for bariatric surgery.

OUTCOMES

In a meta-analysis of sibutramine in patients with a BMI of 25 kg/m^2 or higher, sibutramine was more effective than placebo in promoting weight loss in overweight and obese adults, with an average increased weight loss of 4.5 kg at 1 year compared with placebo.[16,17]

In a meta-analysis of 29 studies of orlistat, the pooled mean weight loss for orlistat-treated patients was 2.59 kg at 6 months and 2.89 kg at 12 months. The average age of patients enrolled was 48 years and the average BMI was 36.7 kg/m^2.[18]

Other agents, such as phentermine, diethylpropion, and fluoxetine, result in a 3.0- to 3.6-kg weight loss after 1 year when used in combination with lifestyle interventions. There is a paucity of data regarding sertraline, bupropion, topiramate, and zonisamide on weight loss outcomes. Therefore, recommendations cannot be made until further studies have been completed.[19]

A randomized controlled trial evaluating use of the Lap-Band for mild to moderate obesity (BMI 30-35 kg/m^2) has demonstrated significantly greater weight loss and comorbidity resolution in the surgical group compared with those enrolled in an aggressive medical weight loss program. After 2 years, EWL was 87% in the surgical group and 21% in the nonsurgical group. Metabolic syndrome resolved in 93% of surgical patients and in 47% of nonsurgical patients. A large, prospective, matched cohort study (Swedish Obese Subjects Study) demonstrated the durability of weight loss and comorbidity reduction 10 years after bariatric surgery.[18] Another large, matched cohort study demonstrated a significant reduction in mortality (89% relative reduction compared with the medical group) 5 years after bariatric surgery.[20] A meta-analysis analyzing 22,094 patients in 136 studies found that for all bariatric procedures, the average excess weight loss was 61.2%. Biliopancreatic diversion or duodenal switch procedures had the highest overall EWL (70%), followed by gastroplasty (68%), gastric bypass (61%), and gastric banding (47%). Overall, diabetes improved or resolved in 86%, hyperlipidemia improved in 70%, hypertension improved or resolved in 78.5%, and obstructive sleep apnea improved or resolved in 83.6% of patients.[21]

The operative mortality rates for restrictive procedures, gastric bypass, and biliopancreatic diversion are 0.1%, 0.5%, and 1.1%, respectively.[21] Mortality after bariatric surgery is primarily the result of pulmonary embolism and anastomotic leak. Early postoperative complications, particularly septic complications, are less common after restrictive procedures such as VBG and LAGB.

Suggested Readings

Arterburn DE, Crane PK, Veenstra DL: The efficacy and safety of sibutramine for weight loss: A systematic review. Arch Intern Med 2004;164:994-1003.

Buchwald H, Avidor Y, Braunwald E, et al: Bariatric surgery: A systematic review and meta-analysis. JAMA 2004;292:1724-1737.

Christou NV, Sampalis JS, Liberman M, et al: Surgery decreases long-term mortality, morbidity, and health care use in morbidly obese patients. Ann Surg 2004;240:416-423.

Consensus Development Conference Panel: NIH conference. Gastrointestinal surgery for severe obesity. Ann Intern Med 1991;115:956-961.

Demaria EJ, Jamal MK: Surgical options for obesity. Gastroenterol Clin North Am 2005;34:127-142.

Flegal KM, Graubard BI, Williamson DF, Gail MH: Excess deaths associated with underweight, overweight, and obesity. JAMA 2005;293:1861-1867.

Flum DR, Salem L, Elrod JA, et al: Early mortality among Medicare beneficiaries undergoing bariatric surgical procedures. JAMA 2005;294:1903-1908.

Fontaine KR, Redden DT, Wang C, et al: Years of life lost due to obesity. JAMA 2003;289:187-193.

Haddock CK, Poston WS, Dill PL, et al: Pharmacotherapy for obesity: A quantitative analysis of four decades of published randomized clinical trials. Int J Obes Relat Metab Disord 2002;26:262-273.

Harris MI, Flegal KM, Cowie CC, et al: Prevalence of diabetes, impaired fasting glucose, and impaired glucose tolerance in U.S. adults. The Third National Health and Nutrition Examination Survey, 1988-1994. Diabetes Care 1998;21:518-524.

Knowler WC, Barrett-Connor E, Fowler SE, et al: Reduction in the incidence of type 2 diabetes with lifestyle intervention or metformin. N Engl J Med 2002;346:393-403.

Livingston EH, Huerta S, Arthur D, et al: Male gender is a predictor of morbidity and age a predictor of mortality for patients undergoing gastric bypass surgery. Ann Surg 2002;236:576-582.

McTigue KM, Harris R, Hemphill B, et al: Screening and interventions for obesity in adults: Summary of the evidence for the U.S. Preventive Services Task Force. Ann Intern Med 2003;139:933-949.

National Cholesterol Education Program (NCEP) Expert Panel on Detection, Evaluation, and Treatment of High Blood Cholesterol in Adults (Adult Treatment Panel III): Third Report of the National Cholesterol Education Program (NCEP) Expert Panel on Detection, Evaluation, and Treatment of High Blood Cholesterol in Adults (Adult Treatment Panel III) final report. Circulation 2002;106:3143-3421.

Ogden CL, Carroll MD, Curtin LR, et al: Prevalence of overweight and obesity in the United States, 1999-2004. JAMA 2006;295:1549-1555.

Pi-Sunyer FX. A review of long-term studies evaluating the efficacy of weight loss in ameliorating disorders associated with obesity. Clin Ther 1996;18:1006-1035.

Ramsey-Stewart G: Vertical banded gastroplasty for morbid obesity: Weight loss at short and long-term follow up. Aust N Z J Surg 1995;65:4-7.

Sauerland S, Angrisani L, Belachew M, et al: Obesity surgery: Evidence-based guidelines of the European Association for Endoscopic Surgery (EAES). Surg Endosc 2005;19:200-221.

Sjostrom L, Lindroos AK, Peltonen M, et al: Lifestyle, diabetes, and cardiovascular risk factors 10 years after bariatric surgery. N Engl J Med 2004;351:2683-2693.

Snow V, Barry P, Fitterman N, et al: Pharmacologic and surgical management of obesity in primary care: A clinical practice guideline from the American College of Physicians. Ann Intern Med 2005;142:525-531.

Wadden TA, Bartlett SJ, Foster GD, et al: Sertraline and relapse prevention training following treatment by very-low-calorie diet: A controlled clinical trial. Obes Res 1995;3:549-557.

Wolf AM, Colditz GA: The cost of obesity: The U.S. perspective. Pharmacoeconomics 1994;5(Suppl 1):34-37.

References

For a complete list of references, log onto www.expertconsult.com.

Male Hypogonadism

Charles Faiman

DEFINITION AND PREVALENCE

Male hypogonadism is defined as the failure of the testes to produce androgen, sperm, or both. Although the disorder is exceedingly common, its exact prevalence is uncertain.

Testosterone production declines with advancing age; 20% of men older than 60 years and 30% to 40% of men older than 80 years have serum testosterone levels that would be subnormal in their younger adult male counterparts. This apparent physiologic decline in circulating androgen levels is compounded in frequency by permanent disorders of the hypothalamic-pituitary-gonadal axis (see later). These include the transient deficiency states associated with acute stressful illnesses, such as surgery and myocardial infarction, and the more chronic deficiency states associated with wasting illnesses, such as cancer and acquired immunodeficiency syndrome.

Male factor infertility is probably responsible for one third of the 10% to 15% of couples who are unable to conceive within 1 year of unprotected intercourse. Most of these male-associated cases result from diminished, absent, or faulty spermatogenesis. In addition to abnormal sperm production, other conditions, including obstructive ductal disease, epididymal hostility, immunologic disorders, and erectile or ejaculatory dysfunction should be considered. Finally, because combined female-male infertility is common, and fertility as well as psychological well-being are ultimate goals, both partners must be assessed from the outset.

PATHOPHYSIOLOGY

The physiologic regulation of the hypothalamic-pituitary-gonadal axis is shown in Figure 1. Circulating testosterone is largely protein-bound—the major protein is sex hormone–binding globulin (SHBG)—with only 2% present as the biologically active or free fraction. Some clinicians believe that the bioavailable fraction, the fraction present in the supernatant after ammonium sulfate precipitation, representing testosterone loosely bound predominantly to serum albumin, is more meaningful. Hepatic SHBG production rises with aging and thyroid hormone excess and declines in hyperinsulinemic states (obesity and type 2 diabetes), so that free testosterone values may not always be concordant with total testosterone values. The biologic effects of testosterone may be mediated directly by testosterone or by its metabolites 5α-dihydrotestosterone or estradiol (Fig. 2).

Male hypogonadism is caused by a primary (hypergonadotropic) testicular disorder or is secondary (hypo- or normogonadotropic) to hypothalamic-pituitary dysfunction, as illustrated in Figure 3. Combined disorders also occur. Examples of the major causes of male hypogonadism are shown in Boxes 1 and 2.

SIGNS AND SYMPTOMS

Birth and Infancy

Persistent failure of the testes to descend may be an early manifestation of testicular dysfunction. In addition, a normally formed but hypotrophic penis may provide a clue to an abnormality of the hypothalamic-pituitary-gonadal axis.

Puberty

Delayed, arrested, or absent testicular growth and secondary sexual characteristic development are hallmarks of pubertal disorders. Skeletal proportions may be abnormal (eunuchoid) with more than a 5-cm difference between span and height and between pubis-floor and pubis-vertex dimensions.

Adulthood

Manifestations in adults are generally more subtle. Perhaps the minor contribution of adrenal androgens (or androgenic precursors) may substitute for testicular deficiency once the target tissues have been fully developed. Moreover, ingrained behavior patterns may be resistant to androgenic hormone deficiency. Certainly, prolactin excess, testosterone deficiency, or both in men may result in impaired libido and erectile dysfunction. The yield of finding hyperprolactinemia or testosterone deficiency, or both, in patients presenting with these symptoms is generally considered to be low, usually less than 5%. However, a large survey of patients with erectile dysfunction presenting to a Veterans Affairs center has suggested that the prevalence of these abnormalities is substantial: 18.7% of patients with low testosterone levels and 4.6% with elevated prolactin levels.[1]

The first manifestation of hypogonadism may be a consequence of a large space-occupying intrasellar or parasellar lesion manifested by headaches, bitemporal hemianopia, or extraocular muscle palsy. Galactorrhea as a manifestation of hyperprolactinemia is rare, but rarely sought. Unexplained osteoporosis or mild anemia sometimes is the clue to an underlying hypogonadal state. Some common clinical conditions associated with male hypogonadism are listed in Box 3. The subject of androgen deficiency and the aging man is dealt with in greater detail later in this chapter.

DIAGNOSIS

Because of the well-known diurnal rhythm of serum testosterone, which appears to be lost with age (>60 years), with values 30% or so higher near 8 AM versus the later day trough, a testosterone value should be determined first thing in the morning. Normal ranges vary among laboratories. Although the usually quoted range for young men is 300 to 1000 ng/dL, the lower limit reported for the Cleveland Clinic is 220 ng/dL. In general, values below 220 to 250 ng/dL are clearly low in most laboratories; values between 250 and 350 ng/dL should be considered borderline low. Because the acute effect of stressful illness may result in a transient lowering of testosterone levels, a confirmatory early morning specimen should be obtained. Measurement of free testosterone levels or bioavailable testosterone levels, determined adequately in select commercial laboratories, may provide additional information (see later, "Pathophysiology"). For example, free testosterone levels may be lower than expected from the total testosterone level as a result of aging and higher than expected in insulin-resistant individuals, such as in obesity. In addition, serum follicle-stimulating hormone (FSH), luteinizing hormone (LH), and prolactin levels should be determined to help delineate the cause of the testosterone-deficient state.

If gonadotropin levels are not elevated, despite clearly subnormal testosterone values, anterior pituitary (thyroid-adrenal) function should be determined by measuring free thyroxine and thyroid-stimulating hormone levels, as well as an early morning cortisol level. A magnetic resonance imaging (MRI) scan of the brain and sella should be considered. An exception to this recommendation is the condition of morbid obesity, in which both total and free testosterone levels are typically low and gonadotropin values not elevated. Hyperprolactinemia, even of a small degree, may also warrant ordering MRI, because interference of hypothalamic-pituitary vascular flow by space-occupying, stalk-compressing lesions will lead to disruption of the tonic inhibitory influence of hypothalamic dopamine, and result in modest hyperprolactinemia (usually 20 to 50 ng/mL range).

A semen analysis should be performed when fertility is in question.

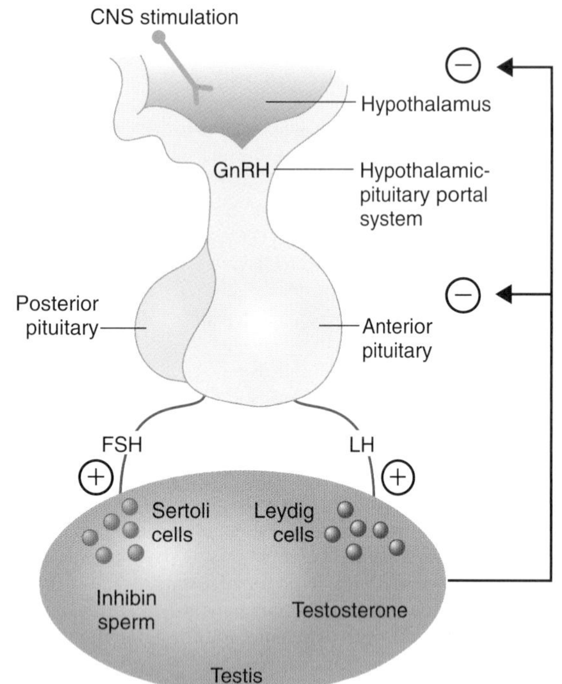

Figure 1 Regulation of testicular function. Note that the single decapeptide gonadotropin-releasing hormone (GnRH) stimulates the release of follicle-stimulating hormone (FSH) and luteinizing hormone (LH). Pulsatile GnRH is required. Chronic exposure downregulates the GnRH receptor and causes impaired FSH and LH release, the mechanism whereby pharmacologic GnRH agonists result in chemical castration. Prolactin excess also results in impaired GnRH pulse generator function and hypogonadotropic hypogonadism. Feedback inhibition of LH secretion is a sex steroid–mediated event, whereas FSH secretion has dual feedback regulation involving inhibition by sex steroids and the Sertoli cell product inhibin. Accordingly, a monotropic elevation of the FSH level (normal LH and testosterone levels) may result from deficient Sertoli cell-spermatogenic function. CNS, central nervous system.

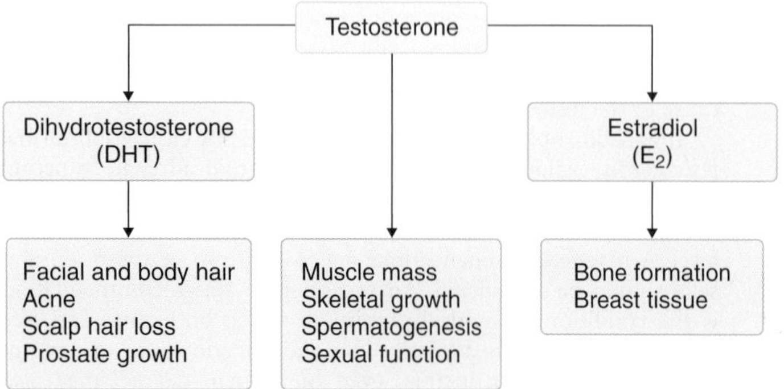

Figure 2 Effects of testosterone and its metabolites in the male (simplified).

TREATMENT

Androgen Replacement Therapy

Androgen replacement therapy is relatively straightforward; see Box 4 for testosterone preparations currently available in the United States. Typically, the depot esters are administered by the deep intramuscular route once every 2 weeks at a dose of 200 mg in adults. A usual dosage for the transdermal or the buccal preparations results

Box 1 Primary (Hypergonadotropic) Hypogonadism: Major Causes

- Genetic: Klinefelter's syndrome
- Congenital: anorchia
- Toxins: alcohol, heavy metals
- Orchitis
- Trauma
- Infarction
- Aging

Box 2 Secondary (Hypogonadotropic) Hypogonadism: Major Causes

- Pubertal delay
- Hypogonadotropism
  - Congenital or acquired
  - Isolated or combined pituitary disease
  - Space-occupying lesions of pituitary, hypothalamus
  - Hyperprolactinemia per se
  - Infiltrative, infectious
  - Suppression
  - Sex steroids
  - Gonadotropin-releasing hormone analogues
- Aging (?)

Box 3 Conditions Associated with Male Hypogonadism

- Aging
- Chronic illness
  - Diabetes
  - Acquired immunodeficiency syndrome (AIDS)
  - Chronic renal failure
  - Rheumatoid arthritis
- Cancer cachexia
- Corticosteroid use

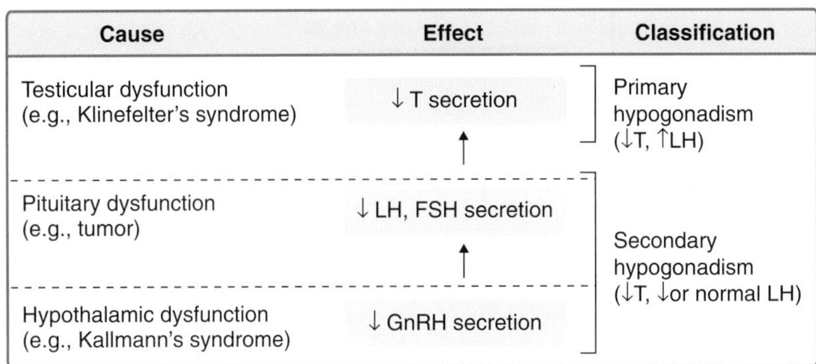

Figure 3 Examples of primary and secondary causes of male hypogonadism. Klinefelter's syndrome results from the 46,XXY karyotypic abnormality present in approximately 1 in 500 male births. The example of Kallmann's syndrome is a rare isolated deficiency of GnRH, resulting in hypogonadotropic hypogonadism associated with olfactory lobe dysgenesis and anosmia. FSH, follicle-stimulating hormone; GnRH, gonadotropin-releasing hormone; LH, luteinizing hormone; T, testosterone.

Table 1 Choice of Testosterone Preparation

	Type of Preparation			
Parameter	**Intramuscular**	**Gel**	**Patch (Genital and Nongenital)**	**Buccal**
Convenience	—	+++	++	?
Stigma	No	No	Yes	No
Physiologic	No	Yes	Yes	Yes
Side effects	Systemic	Local, +	Local, +++	Local, ++
Cost	$	$$$$	$$$	$$$

+, ++, and +++ are semiquantitative assessments of effect.

Box 4 Testosterone Preparations Available in the United States

Depot esters (Depo-Testosterone, Delatestryl)
Genital skin patch (Testoderm)
Nongenital skin patch (Androderm)
Gel (AndroGel, Testim)
Buccal (Striant)

in the systemic absorption of 2.5 to 10 mg daily. If the parenteral route is chosen, patients should and can be taught to self inject. The major disadvantage with the parenteral route is that testosterone levels exhibit a saw-toothed pattern, with high-normal or supranormal levels on days 2 to 4 and low-normal or borderline low trough values before the next injection. Mood, sense of well-being, and libido may vary accordingly in some patients.

Dosages may be adjusted by aiming for midnormal (400-600 ng/dL) testosterone levels after 1 week or at the low end (250-350 ng/dL) just before the next injection is due at 2 weeks. Values are stable within a few days or weeks of the skin patch, gel, or newer buccal preparation. It must be ascertained that the preparation was actually used on the day the sample was drawn; again, a value in the midnormal range (400-600 ng/dL) is the goal. Although comparable testosterone levels are reached by the patch and the gels, skin reactions at the application site are much more common with the patch. Also, the buccal preparation is difficult for patients to get used to. Alkylated oral androgens should be viewed as potentially hepatotoxic and should not be used. Useful criteria for selecting preparations for individual patients are summarized in Table 1.

Monitoring and Screening

In addition to monitoring testosterone levels periodically, prostate screening and measurement of hemoglobin and hematocrit levels must also be performed at intervals when the patient is on therapy.[2]

Prostate Screening

Levels of prostate-specific antigen (PSA) should be checked at 3, 6, and 12 months. If the patient is truly hypogonadal to begin with, expect a significant rise at the 3-month assessment. Thereafter, the usual criteria apply regarding the possible presence of an underlying malignancy (>4 ng/mL, or rate of increase >1.5 ng/mL/2 yr or >2 ng/mL overall). These criteria continue to be revised by our urology colleagues, tending to become more stringent with time. For example, a PSA rise of more than 1 ng/mL/year has been suggested as an early warning guide, and closer surveillance has been recommended, even at rates of 0.7 to 0.9 ng/mL/year.[2] A digital rectal examination should be performed at 3 to 6 months and at 1 year after therapy is initiated. A urologic consultation should be obtained if indicated.

Hemoglobin and Hematocrit Levels

Hemoglobin (Hb) and hematocrit (Hct) levels should be checked periodically. Incremental increases are to be expected, but an Hb level higher than 17.5 g/dL, Hct higher than 55%, or both suggests overtreatment, occasionally abuse. Greater increments tend to occur more frequently with the intramuscular than with the transdermal preparations. If dosage adjustments do not solve the problem, look for another underlying cause.

Contraindications

Physicians should take into consideration a number of clinical situations in which absolute or relative contraindications for the use of testosterone exist (Box 5). It should be noted that no long-term studies in large numbers of patients (neither young or old)

Box 5 Contraindications for Testosterone Replacement

Breast carcinoma (history or presence)
Prostate carcinoma (history or presence)
Severe benign prostatic hyperplasia
Abnormal digital rectal examinations
Elevated levels of prostate-specific antigen
Age (no limit established; possibly older than 80 years)
Psychopathology
Sleep apnea (potential for worsening)
Hypercoagulable states
Polycythemia (hematocrit >51%)

Box 6 Potential Benefits of Testosterone Therapy

Body composition
- Increase in lean body mass
- Decrease in fat mass

Bone
- Increased bone density
- No fracture data available

Mood, well-being
Sexual function
Cognitive function
Muscle strength, physical function

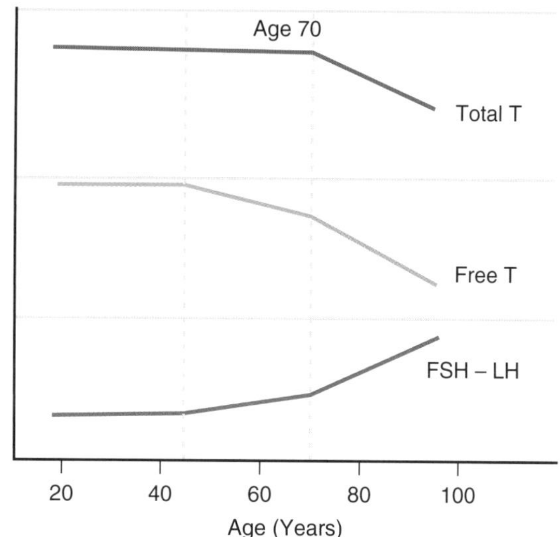

Figure 4 Declining testicular function with age. FSH, follicle-stimulating hormone; LH, luteinizing hormone; T, testosterone.

have been performed, so potential risks and benefits need to be individualized.

OUTCOMES

Benefits

In genuinely hypogonadal men, testosterone administration can be expected to result in improvements in a variety of clinical areas (Box 6). Least predictable are the effects on sexual function, cognitive function, and muscle strength.

Risks

Concerns regarding the use of testosterone have been noted in Box 5 and by Rhoden and Morgentaler.[2] There is no evidence that the incidence of prostate cancer is increased by testosterone replacement. The underlying concern is that it might alter the course of an occult malignancy estimated to be present in more than 50% of men older than 50 years. On the other hand, no one would recommend prophylactic castration to prevent prostate cancer so that, in my view, testosterone replacement in the hypogonadal man should not be avoided. Although there are genuine concerns about worsening of benign prostatic hyperplasia, this may apply only to severe cases with large prostate volumes. Indeed, one study in older men has even suggested improvement in benign prostatic hyperplasia symptoms, although not statistically significant and by an unknown mechanism.[3]

Older Men

The aging man represents a special case and has been the subject of a review.[4] There is a well-known decline in testosterone production with aging in otherwise healthy men. This decline in mean values can be seen in free testosterone levels, beginning in the mid-40s (some clinicians suggest even earlier), as a consequence of increasing SHBG levels, mechanism unknown. Total testosterone levels decline on average beyond 70 years. The diurnal rhythm, seen in younger men, is lost beyond 60 years.[5] Although testicular volume also declines in this age group, spermatogenesis may be well maintained into the 80s or even beyond. Gonadotropin levels tend to rise after 70 years, indicating that the testosterone deficiency is usually primary.[6] Figure 4 schematically presents these hormonal changes with age. Using the criterion of a low testosterone value, and remembering that there is considerable variability in commercially available tests regarding normal young adult ranges, it has been estimated that 7% of 40- to 60-year-olds, 22% of 60- to 80-year-olds, and 36% of 80- to 100-year-olds are hypogonadal.[7]

The ultimate issue as to whether these changes are normal and physiologic or should be considered pathologic, thus demanding therapy, remains unresolved. Indeed, it is a situation analogous to the ongoing dilemma of hormone replacement therapy for postmenopausal women, although in this group the hormonal deficiency state is usually more abrupt and symptomatic.

The scientific basis to help formulate guidelines for dealing with the issue of hormone replacement therapy in men was reviewed in a December 17, 2003, conference by the Institute of Medicine's Committee on Testosterone and Aging (IMCTA).[8] Many of the potential benefits of therapy (see Box 6) have been realized in small, well-controlled studies of older men. Moreover, none of the risks has been proven in a clinical trial. The IMCTA has not recommended a large-scale study to determine whether the risk for prostate cancer would be increased, because the costs of such a study were deemed to be too prohibitive.

In the meantime, practical guidelines for dealing with hypogonadism in older men have been suggested.[9] I have found the recent overview in the Cleveland Clinic Men's Health Advisor newsletter to be useful for patients.[10]

NATIONAL GUIDELINES

The American Association of Clinical Endocrinologists has published 2002 updated guidelines for the evaluation and treatment of hypogonadism in adult male patients.[11] This review, geared particularly for endocrinologists, expands on some of the areas reviewed in this chapter and provides a more detailed look into aspects of male infertility.

The Endocrine Society has published clinical practice guidelines[12] for testosterone replacement therapy. The major recommendations are summarized in Box 7.

Box 7 Endocrine Society Clinical Practice Guidelines for Testosterone Replacement Therapy

Recommend diagnosis of androgen deficiency only in men with consistent symptoms and signs and with unequivocally low serum testosterone levels.

- Measure morning total testosterone level by a reliable assay as an initial test.
- Confirm with repeat total testosterone and free or bioavailable testosterone using accurate assays.

Do not start testosterone therapy in patients with the following:

- Breast or prostate cancer
- Palpable prostate nodule or induration or prostate-specific antigen level >3 ng/mL without urologic evaluation
- Severe lower urinary tract symptoms
- Hematocrit >50% or hyperviscosity (not defined)
- Untreated obstructive sleep apnea
- Severe coronary heart failure (Class III or IV)

Treatment goal and comments (no comments about age or duration limits)

- Aim to achieve testosterone levels in midnormal range.
- Men receiving testosterone therapy should be monitored using a standardized plan.

Adapted from Bhasin S, Cunningham GR, Hayes FJ, et al: Testosterone therapy in adult men with androgen deficiency syndromes: An endocrine society clinical practice guideline. J Clin Endocrinol Metab 2006;91:1995-2010.

Summary

- Male hypogonadism is defined as the failure of the testes to produce androgen, sperm, or both. Although the disorder is exceedingly common, its exact prevalence is uncertain.
- Signs and symptoms vary according to age.
- Diagnosis requires the determination of low testosterone levels. Normal ranges vary among laboratories. Measurement of free testosterone levels or bioavailable testosterone levels (performed adequately in select commercial laboratories) may provide additional information, in addition to serum follicle-stimulating hormone, luteinizing hormone, and prolactin levels. MRI scans of the brain and sella should be considered.
- Androgen replacement therapy is used for the treatment of male hypogonadism. In addition to monitoring testosterone levels periodically, prostate screening by digital rectal examination and prostate specific antigen determinations at periodic intervals when the patient is on therapy should be carried out. Hemoglobin and hematocrit levels should also be checked periodically.

Suggested Readings

American Association of Clinical Endocrinologists: American Association of Clinical Endocrinologists Medical Guidelines for clinical practice for the evaluation and treatment of hypogonadism in adult male patients-2002 update. Endocr Pract 2002;8:440-456.

Bhasin S, Cunningham GR, Hayes FJ, et al: Testosterone therapy in adult men with androgen deficiency syndromes: An endocrine society clinical practice guideline. J Clin Endocrinol Metab 2006;91:1995-2010.

Bodie J, Lewis J, Schow D, Monga M: Laboratory evaluations of erectile dysfunction: An evidence-based approach. J Urol 2003;169:2262-2264.

Bremner WJ, Vitiello MV, Prinz PN: Loss of circadian rhythmicity in blood testosterone levels with aging in normal men. J Clin Endocrinol Metab 1983;56:1278-1281.

Hajjar RR, Kaiser FE, Morley JE: Outcomes of long-term testosterone replacement in older hypogonadal males: A retrospective analysis. J Clin Endocrinol Metab 1997;82:3793-3796.

Lang RS (ed): Testosterone: Anti-aging jump start? Men's Health Advisor 2003;5:1-7.

Liverman CT, Blazer DG (eds): Testosterone and Aging: Clinical Research Directions. National Academies. Washington, DC, National Academies Press, 2004.

Rajfer J: Decreased testosterone in the aging male. Rev Urol 2003;5(Suppl 1):S49-S50.

Rhoden EL, Morgentaler A: Risks of testosterone-replacement therapy and recommendations for monitoring. N Engl J Med 2004;350:482-492.

Snyder PJ: Hypogonadism in elderly men-what to do until the evidence comes. N Engl J Med 2004;350:440-442.

Stearns EL, MacDonnell JA, Kaufman BJ, et al: Declining testicular function with age. Hormonal and clinical correlates. Am J Med 1974;57:761-766.

Vermeulen A, Kaufman JM: Aging of the hypothalamo-pituitary-testicular axis in men. Horm Res 1995;43:25-28.

References

For a complete list of references, log onto www.expertconsult.com.

Osteoporosis

Mario Skugor

DEFINITION

Primary osteoporosis is a metabolic bone disease characterized by low bone mass and microarchitectural deterioration of bone tissue, leading to enhanced bone fragility and increased fracture risk.[1] It also has normal mineral-to-collagen ratio. Primary osteoporosis represents bone mass loss that is unassociated with any other illness and is related to aging and loss of the gonadal function in women and the aging process in men.

Secondary osteoporosis can result from a variety of the chronic conditions that significantly contribute to bone mineral loss, or it can result from the effects of medications and nutritional deficiencies (Box 1).

The World Health Organization (WHO) defines osteoporosis as bone density that is 2.5 standard deviations (SDs) or more below the young adult mean value (T-score <–2.5). Patients with bone density between 1 and 2.5 SDs below average (T-score –1 to –2.5) are said to have osteopenia.[2] Decreased bone density imparts increased risk for bone fracture. Every 1 SD decrease in bone density of the spine increases risk for new vertebral fracture by factor of 2.0 to 2.4.[3]

PREVALENCE

Osteoporosis is the most common metabolic bone disease. About 54% of postmenopausal white women in the United States have osteopenia and 30% have osteoporosis. Men and nonwhite women at risk add 30 million to 54 million affected persons in the United States.

About 2.0 million osteoporotic fractures occur each year in the United States. Approximately one half are vertebral fractures, one quarter are hip fractures, and one quarter are Colles' fractures.[1]

Significant ethnic and geographic differences exist in the prevalence of osteoporosis and osteoporotic fractures. The risk of hip fracture is considerably higher in whites than in blacks. Two factors contribute to this difference: higher peak bone mass (highest bone mass achieved by a person in his or her lifetime) and slower postmenopausal bone loss in African American women.[4] Bone mineral density (BMD) is lower in Asians than in whites. However, when adjusted for body size, most of the difference disappears, suggesting that the lower BMD in Asians is due to their smaller body size.

Decreased BMD and osteoporotic fracture rate increases with age. Wrist fracture incidence starts increasing at about 50 years of age, vertebral fractures in the 60s, and hip fractures in the 70s.

Increased mortality rate associated with hip and vertebral fractures may be the worst consequence, but the loss of independence and lowered quality of life of patients might be the greatest burden of the osteoporosis.[5]

Osteoporosis in men has been recognized as an important health problem. Incidence of hip fracture increases exponentially with age in men as well as in women, although the incidence in men occurs about 5 to 10 years later than in women.[6]

PATHOPHYSIOLOGY

Basic mechanisms responsible for development of osteoporosis are poor bone mass acquisition during growth and development and accelerated bone loss in the period after peak bone mass is achieved. Both processes are modulated by environmental and genetic factors.

About two thirds of the risk for fracture in postmenopausal women is determined by premenopausal peak bone mass.[5] Peak bone mass is higher in blacks than in whites and Asians, and it is higher in men than women.

Approximately half of the bone mass is accumulated during pubertal development.[7] This is associated with the increase in sex hormone levels and is almost completed with closure of the end plates. There is only minimal additional accumulation of the bone minerals during the next 5 to 15 years (skeletal consolidation). Peak bone mass is achieved during the third decade of life.

Studies in twins and mother-daughter pairs suggest that 40% to 80% of the variability in the bone mass is determined by genetic factors. The genes implicated in osteoporosis include those for the estrogen receptor, transforming growth factor-β, and apolipoprotein E and collagen.

Bone loss, in contrast, appears to be mostly determined by environmental factors (nutritional, behavioral, and medications). However, genetic factors also play a role, mostly acting on a person's estrogen status.

Nutritional Factors

Important nutritional factors include dietary calcium intake, Vitamin D status, protein intake, and caloric intake. Phosphorus, vitamins C and K, copper, zinc, and manganese also play a role.

Low calcium intake during childhood increases risk of fracture later in the life[8] and is positively correlated with bone mineral mass at all ages. Supplementation is shown to reduce rate of bone loss and decreases incidence of fractures in calcium deficient elderly persons.

Optimal calcium intake varies among different age groups and is population specific. The typical U.S. diet is rich in sodium and protein, both of which increase urinary calcium excretion, thus increasing dietary requirements.

Vitamin D is essential for bone mineral metabolism through its role in calcium absorption and osteoclast activity. Vitamin D nutritional status is best assessed by measurement of serum 25(OH)-vitamin D levels. Vitamin D levels decrease with increasing age. Supplementation reduces the rate of all fractures in the elderly population.

Protein or caloric malnutrition predisposes to falls and decreases soft tissue cover over bony prominences. Protein intake is the major determinant of outcome after hip fracture, and serum albumin level is the single best predictor of survival in these patients. The body weight history of girls and women with anorexia nervosa is the most important predictor for the development of osteoporosis.

Behavioral Factors

Behavioral factors important in pathogenesis of osteoporosis include physical activity, smoking, and alcohol consumption.

Bone mass is higher in top-level athletes than in nonathletes. This is particularly pronounced in athletes engaging in strength training. The data are hard to interpret because top athletes might have different skeletal and muscular characteristics than the average population even before beginning training. However, mechanical loading is shown to increases bone mass, and with decreasing mechanical load, bone mass is lost. The relationship between load and BMD is curvilinear and much more pronounced at low levels of loads. In completely immobilized patients, bone mass loss may be up to 40% in 1 year. On the other hand, active people who further increase their levels of physical activity may expect only modest gains in BMD.[9]

Box 1 Causes of Secondary Osteoporosis

Chronic Diseases
Anorexia nervosa
Chronic liver disease
Chronic renal insufficiency
Cushing's syndrome
Disseminated carcinomatosis
Ehlers-Danlos syndrome
Hemochromatosis
Homocystinuria
Hypercalciuria
Hyperparathyroidism
Hyperprolactinemia
Hyperthyroidism
Hypophosphatasia
Marfan syndrome
Mastocytosis
Multiple myeloma
Osteogenesis imperfecta
Renal tubular acidosis

Medications
Cyclosporine
Excess thyroid hormones
GnRH agonists
Heparin
Methotrexate
Phenobarbital
Phenothiazines
Phenytoin
Steroids

Conditions Causing Nutritional Deficencies
Alcoholism
Calcium deficiency
Gastric and bowel resections
Malabsorption syndromes
Vitamin D deficiency

Other Causes
Athletic amenorrhea
Pregnancy
Tobacco use

Optimal bone metabolism is the result of hormonal, nutritional, and mechanical harmony, and a deficit in one area is usually impossible to overcome by improvements in others.

Chronic alcohol use has been associated with decreased BMD in the femoral neck and lumbar spine and is commonly listed as a risk factor for osteoporosis. Prevalence of osteoporosis in alcoholics is 28% to 52%.[10] Other nutritional deficiencies associated with chronic alcohol abuse play an important role in development of osteoporosis in alcoholics. Smoking is often associated with alcoholism and is an independent risk factor for low bone mass.[11] Smoking affects peak bone mass development and accelerates bone loss.

Medications

Among several medications (see Box 1), glucocorticoids are the most important cause of bone loss (mostly trabecular). Fractures occur most commonly in vertebrae, ribs, and the ends of the long bones. Bone loss occurs very rapidly and may be as high as 20% during the first year of steroid use. The incidence of osteoporotic fractures in patients taking corticosteroids for more than 6 months is 30% to 50%. The dose of steroid that is detrimental to BMD in most people appears to be more than 7.5 mg of prednisone daily.[12]

Female sex hormones (estrogens) are mandatory for acquisition of the peak bone mass and for maintenance of bone in women and men. Estrogen deficiency is considered a principal cause of postmenopausal osteoporosis.[13] It might play important role in male osteoporosis as well. Risk factors for low BMD are summarized in Box 2.

Box 2 Risk Factors Associated with Development of Osteoporosis

Not Modifiable
Age
Calcium deficient diet
Family history of osteoporosis
Low body weight
Nulliparity
Race (white or Asian)
Use of medications

Modifiable
Estrogen-deficient states
Excessive alcohol intake
Sedentary lifestyle
Smoking

SIGNS AND SYMPTOMS

The clinical expression of osteoporosis is a skeletal fracture. Vertebral fracture is the most common. Many patients (up to two thirds) remain asymptomatic after compressive vertebral fracture, and osteoporosis is diagnosed accidentally on the x-rays taken for other reasons. Incidence of new fracture has been estimated to be 19% in the year after the initial fracture.[14]

Fracture usually occurs during routine daily activities such as bending of the body, coughing, or lifting and is most common in the lumbar spine and the lower thoracic vertebrae. Occurrence of the fracture may be accompanied by acute onset of pain, which might disappear or turn into chronic dull back pain. Multiple fractures can lead to significant height loss and development of thoracic kyphosis (Dowager's hump). Patients notice protuberance of the abdomen, a change in the way clothes fit, and loss of the waist. Restrictive respiratory problems are seen because of diminished volume of the thoracic cage and poor expansion with breathing.

Hip fractures are another common fracture seen in osteoporotic persons and affect about 15% of women and 5% of men older than 80 years. They usually occur after falls or other trauma, but subchondral-insufficiency fractures of the femoral head have been described.

Fractures of the distal radius (Colles' fractures) occur more often in patients with osteoporosis and may be caused by falls on an outstretched hand or after minor trauma.

DIAGNOSIS

History and physical examination are important for identifying secondary causes of osteoporosis and to record behavioral risk factors, use of medications, and presence of signs and symptoms of osteoporotic complications. Use of risk factors as a prescreening device to select patients for further diagnostic procedures is inefficient and fails to identify a substantial portion of patients who have osteoporosis.

Laboratory Evaluation

Laboratory evaluation should be aimed toward diagnosis of secondary osteoporosis. The specific test used depends on the specific clinical situation (Table 1).

Assessment of bone metabolism using markers of bone turnover can yield useful information and guide management decisions in some cases. These tests are noninvasive and can indicate changes in the bone metabolism much faster than measurements of BMD. However, their role in patient management is still being defined. Box 3 lists the tests.

Table 1 Selected Laboratory Tests for Secondary Causes of Osteoporosis

Cause	Appropriate Tests
Hyperparathyroidism	Intact PTH Serum Calcium
Hyperthyroidism	TSH T_4 and FTI T_3
Hypogonadism	Testosterone in men Estradiol in females LH and FSH
Osteomalacia	25-hydroxyvitamin D
Cushing's syndrome	24-hour free urinary cortisol Dexamethasone suppression test
Addison's disease	ACTH stimulation test
Renal disease	Serum creatinine Glomerular filtration
Liver disease	Liver function tests
Malabsorption	24-hour urinary calcium excretion Serum albumin level Serum calcium Serum carotene
Multiple myeloma	Serum protein electrophoresis Urine for Bence Jones proteinuria Serum calcium Intact PTH Erythrocyte sedimentation rate
Hemochromatosis	Serum iron panel
Hyperprolactinemia	Serum prolactin
Acromegaly	Serum IGF-1
Renal tubulopathy	Urinalysis including pH Acid-base studies Urine calcium, phosphorus, amino acid, and glucose
Mastocytosis	Serum tryptase Urine N-methylhistamine Iliac bone biopsy with double tetracycline labeling
Inflammatory and rheumatic diseases	Erythrocyte sedimentation rate ANA Anti DNA antibodies RF

ACTH, adrenocorticotropic hormone; ANA, antinuclear antibody; FSH, follicle-stimulating hormone; FTI, free thyroxine index; IGF, insulin-like growth factor; LH, luteinizng hormone; PTH, parathyroid hormone; RF, rheumatoid factor; T_3, triiodothyronine; T_4, thyroxine; TSH, thyroid-stimulating hormone.

During bone resorption, type I collagen is degraded, and the degradation products are released into circulation and excreted from the body via the kidneys. These degradation products are the most useful bone mineral metabolism markers. Clinical use of the bone metabolism markers determined in the urine has been limited by the need to collect 24-hour urine or to correct results for creatinine levels. Serum markers are free of these problems, but there are marked circadian variations in serum levels, and timing of blood sample collection may be important.

With successful antiresorptive therapy there is a decrease in levels of bone mineral resorption markers within 4 to 6 weeks a decrease in and bone mineral formation markers in 2 to 3 months.[15] These levels remain reduced for the duration of therapy.

Box 3 Biochemical Markers of Bone Metabolism

Serum Markers of Bone Formation

Amino-terminal propeptide of type I collagen
Bone-specific alkaline phosphatase
Carboxy-terminal propeptide of type I collagen
Osteocalcin (bone Gla protein)

Urine Markers of Bone Resorption

Hydroxylysine
Hydroxyproline
C-telopeptide of collagen cross-links
N-telopeptide of collagen cross-links
Total and free deoxypyridinoline
Total and free pyridinoline

Serum Markers of Bone Resorption

Bone sialoprotein
C-telopeptide of collagen cross-links
N-telopeptide of collagen cross-links
Tartarate resistant acid phosphatase

Bone Density Measurements

Although diagnosis of osteoporosis is clinical, BMD must be measured to establish the diagnosis. The American Association of Clinical Endocrinologists lists indications for BMD determination:

- Perimenopausal or postmenopausal women who are willing to accept therapeutic or preventive interventions if osteoporosis diagnosed
- Persons whose x-ray findings suggest osteoporosis
- Persons starting or receiving long-term glucocorticoid therapy if therapeutic or preventive intervention is acceptable
- Persons with asymptomatic primary hyperparathyroidism in whom evidence of bone mineral loss would result in parathyroidectomy.
- Persons treated for osteoporosis as a tool for monitoring response to therapy.

Techniques of measurement include quantitative ultrasound, measuring the speed of sound and attenuation of the ultrasonic beam in the bone. Measurements are limited to peripheral bone (usually the calcaneus) and are very precise (coefficient of variation <1%). Currently, ultrasound results suggesting osteoporosis should be followed by BMD measurement using dual x-ray absorptiometry (DEXA).

DEXA is widely accepted as a standard technique for BMD measurements. Standard measurement consists of imaging the spine in the anteroposterior (AP) projection and imaging the hip area. Spinal measurements in the lateral projection are also possible and may be better for predicting spinal fracture than the AP projection. Approximately 15% of patients have high bone density at one site and low bone density at another, and measurements at multiple sites is desirable. DEXA measures area (apparent) bone density rather than true, volumetric bone density. Density is expressed as bone mineral content per unit of projected bone area (g/cm^2).

Quantitative computed tomography (QCT) is only method able to measure true (volumetric) bone density, expressed as g/cm^3. However, QCT is seldom used due to expense, higher radiation dose, and lower reproducibility than DEXA.

Table 2 Recommended Calcium Intake for Various Population Groups

Recommending Agency	Children	Adolescents	Adults	Elderly
US RDA Ca	800 mg/d	1200 mg/d	800 mg/d	800 mg/d
Consensus development conference Ca	None provided	1200 mg/d	1000 mg/d	1500 mg/d
NIH Consensus Development Conference	800-1200 mg/d	1200-1500 mg/d	1000 mg/d	<65 yr on HRT: 1000 mg All others: 1500 mg/d.

HRT, hormone replacement therapy; NIH, U.S. National Institutes of Health; RDA, U.S. recommended daily allowance.

Table 3 Bisphosphonate Medications

Generic Name	Trade Name
Alendronate	Fosamax
Risedronate	Actonel
Etidronate	Didronel
Tiludronate	Skelid
Pamidronate	Aredia
Ibandronate*	Boniva
Clodronate*	
Zoledronate	Zometa, Reclast

*Not available in the United States.

Preventive Measures

General preventive measures against osteoporosis should be emphasized whenever possible. Adequate dietary calcium intake is one of the mainstays (Table 2). The needs may be met through a diet rich in calcium (e.g., milk, dairy products, calcium-fortified fruit juices) or by use of calcium supplements. Patients with untreated hypercalciuria should not take calcium supplements because of the risk of renal calculi. Vitamin D should be prescribed whenever there is suspicion of inadequate intake and particularly in elderly patients. About 800 IU/day is considered sufficient. Good nutrition with adequate caloric and protein intake should be promoted.

Use of tobacco and excessive alcohol use should be strongly discouraged. Regular exercise is integral for development of the skeleton during growth and development and might slow bone loss in the elderly. In addition, it promotes agility, flexibility, and strength, possibly preventing falls.

Medications

Selective Estrogen-Receptor Modulators

Selective estrogen-receptor modulators (SERMs) are a group of medications that are useful in treating osteoporosis and that may be free of undesirable estrogen effects on reproductive tissues.[16] They consist of tissue-selective receptor agonists raloxifene and tamoxifen, which have both estrogen agonist and antagonist properties. Raloxifene has estrogen-like activity on estrogen receptors in bone and cardiovascular tissue but not in endometrium and breast. Raloxifene preserves bone density, decreases serum total cholesterol level, and inhibits aortic accumulation of cholesterol. It does not cause endometrial or breast tissue hyperplasia.

In clinical trials, raloxifene caused a modest increase in BMD in all tested skeletal sites (2.4% in lumbar spine and 2.0% for whole body) over 2 years. These changes persisted during the third year, and markers of bone turnover were suppressed to the normal premenopausal range in raloxifene-treated women. It appears that the antagonistic effect on breast has a protective effect on the incidence of breast cancer in women treated with raloxifene. There was no increase in endometrial cancer, but an increased incidence of thromboembolic disease is observed. Raloxifene is approved for osteoporosis prevention by the U.S. Food and Drug Administration (FDA).

Bisphosphonates

Bisphosphonates are medications that inhibit bone resorption and have minimal side effects. After administration they attach to bone surfaces. During osteoclast resorption of the bone, bisphosphonates are released and prevent osteoclast activity.[17] Bisphosphonates are widely used for prevention and treatment of osteoporosis, as well as hypercalcemia of malignancy. Table 3 lists the available bisphosphonates.

Alendronate is shown to increase BMD in the spine, femoral neck, and greater trochanter area and to decrease the risk of vertebral fracture at dose of 10 mg/day in postmenopausal women,[18] even if they have already had a vertebral fracture or are older than 75 years. The BMD is maintained in those continuing alendronate, and BMD decreased in those switched to placebo. Alendronate is used for osteoporosis treatment (10 mg/day and 70 mg/week orally) and prevention (5 mg/day or 35 mg/week orally).[19]

Although rare, pill-induced esophagitis and ulcers can occur, and can be severe enough to warrant hospitalization and cause esophageal stricture. Hence, alendronate should not be given to patients with active upper GI disease, and it should be stopped if patients develop any symptoms of esophagitis. Alendronate should be taken on empty stomach with a glass of water (240 mL) while standing or sitting to facilitate passage of the pill from esophagus to stomach. The patient should stay upright for 30 minutes after taking the pill and not eat anything so as to improve absorption of the drug and prevent reflux.

Risedronate is safe and effective in preventing bone loss caused by corticosteroids and in postmenopausal women with normal bone density.[20] The gastrointestinal side effects of risedronate may be less severe than with alendronate as demonstrated by a lower incidence of gastric ulcers (4.1% vs. 13.2%) after 2 weeks of daily therapy. Daily, weekly, and monthly oral dosing is available.

Ibandronate in a daily or monthly oral regimen or by IV every 3 months is also approved for treating postmenopausal osteoporosis.

Pamidronate given by IV infusion is not approved by the FDA but has been used to treat postmenopausal and corticosteroid-induced osteoporosis and to prevent postmenopausal osteoporosis.

Zoledronate is administered once a year as an infusion of 5 mg in 15 minutes. It powerfully increases BMD and reduces fractures. It avoids GI side effects and is well tolerated. Flulike illness is main side effect, and that can be mitigated by administration of acetaminophen or other NSAID before infusion.

The one rare complication common to all bisphosphonates is jaw osteonecrosis. Unfortunately, definition of this disorder is not clear and many patients in whom jaw osteonecrosis is diagnosed had other dental conditions when they were evaluated by experts.

Calcitonin

Calcitonin is used in injection form (SC or IM) and as intranasal spray. Calcitonin injections are shown to increase BMD in the spine and reduce vertebral fracture better than calcium alone. Calcitonin has a significant analgesic effect on bone pain by an unknown mechanism,[21] and it might have potential for reducing the pain of vertebral fracture in the acute setting.

Anabolic Therapy

Recombinant human PTH (hrPTH) is anabolic therapy. Given as a once-daily SC injection in humans, it has demonstrated a marked increase of BMD of the lumbar spine and hip. Vertebral fractures were reduced about 70% and nonvertebral fractures were reduced about 50% in studies.[22] hrPTH is approved for use up to 24 months.

OUTCOMES

Treating and preventing osteoporosis has a goal of preventing fracture. Raloxifene has a demonstrated ability to reduce vertebral fracture risk in postmenopausal women who have osteoporosis regardless of the presence of prevalent vertebral fracture, reducing the risk to 0.45 if there is no prevalent fracture and to 0.70 if prevalent fracture is present. The same study could not demonstrate an effect of therapy on nonvertebral fractures.

Alendronate is quite effective in reducing the incidence of new vertebral fractures in patients with or without prevalent vertebral fracture (48%), as well as hip fractures (51%) and wrist fractures (48%).[23]

Risedronate has been shown to reduce vertebral fractures by 41% and 49% in patients with and without prevalent vertebral fractures, respectively.[24] These studies also demonstrated reduction in nonvertebral fractures by 33% to 39%. Significant reduction in hip fractures has been shown. A significant effect on fracture risk is seen after only 1 year of treatment.

Calcitonin has been shown to modestly reduce the risk of hip fracture if given by injection, in comparison with the patient's taking only calcium (relative risk, 0.69 and 0.75, respectively). It reduces the risk of vertebral fractures if given as nasal spray.[25]

The hrPTH has reduced vertebral fracture between 66% and 69% and has reduced nonvertebral fractures by 53%. Benefit was apparent after 8 months of treatment.[22]

CLINICAL GUIDELINES FOR PRIMARY CARE PHYSICIANS

In light of presented information I propose the following guidelines for testing and treatment of patients with suspected or established osteoporosis.

Recommendations for Average-Risk Patients

A careful history should be taken to assess for risk factors for osteoporosis (see Box 2) and falling in each patient. Patients should be educated about osteoporosis and the importance of prevention and treatment. Instructions for adequate nutrient intake, especially calcium, vitamin D, and protein should be provided. Benefits of engaging in physical regular activities should be emphasized. Patients should be educated about the detrimental effects of alcohol and tobacco abuse. Willingness of the patient to accept preventive measures and medications for osteoporosis should be established.

Recommendations for Patients Perceived to be at Higher Risk

Patients perceived to be at higher risk include those with a history of hip or vertebral fracture in first-degree relative, patients with low body weight (<127 lbs in women), all women ages 20 to 55 years with a history of fracture not caused by significant trauma, patients with history of falling, patients with medical conditions that cause secondary osteoporosis, patients taking medications detrimental to bone health, and women 65 years old or older.

Evaluation

The evaluation should consist of laboratory testing and BMD measurements. Laboratory testing includes serum calcium, phosphorus, 25(OH) vitamin D, alkaline phosphatase, liver enzymes, indices of renal function, total protein and albumin, and 24-hour urinary calcium excretion. Tests aimed at secondary causes of osteoporosis should be performed in patients with clinical suspicion of these conditions (see Table 1). BMD measurement should be performed on the nondominant hip and an AP scan should be made of the spine using DEXA at the facility where it will be possible for patient to have subsequent BMD measurements performed (to ensure use of the same DEXA machine). Patients who are suspected of having osteoporosis based on quantitative ultrasound should have the diagnosis confirmed by DEXA.

Prevention

Based on the results of the evaluation, patients should be advised about preventive measures against osteoporosis and falling, offered treatment, or referred to an osteoporosis specialist.

Preventive measures consist of adequate nutrition (calcium, vitamin D, protein), regular physical exercise, cessation of smoking, and fall prevention (adequate lightning, hand rails, anchored rugs, and adequate shoes). Prevention only, without further intervention, should be implemented by patients with normal BMD at all measured sites (T-score no less than −1), those with BMD T-score between −1 and −2.5 at any site and without risk factors, patients taking medications that may increase propensity to fall, and patients not willing to accept any other form of treatment.

Treatment

Treatments of osteoporosis available to primary care physician include alendronate, risedronate, zoledronate, ibandronate raloxifene, calcitonin, and rhPTH in addition to preventive measures. Candidates for treatment include patients with BMD T-score less than −2.5, patients with BMD T-scores less than −1.5 and presence of one or more risk factors for osteoporosis, patients with demonstrated bone loss despite adequate prevention measures, and patients with low-trauma bone fracture and BMD T-score less than −1.0.

Consultation

Osteoporosis specialist should be consulted for further management of exceptional patients:

- Patients with unusually severe osteoporosis (BMD T-score < −3.0)
- Osteoporosis in young patients, premenopausal women, or men younger than 60 years.
- Patients with fractures despite normal or low normal BMD.
- Patients with transplanted organs.
- Patients with secondary causes of osteoporosis.
- Patients showing no response on treatment (fractures or continuing bone loss while on therapy).
- Patients who cannot tolerate FDA-approved treatment.

Re-evaluation

Patients who are evaluated for osteoporosis should be re-evaluated on a yearly basis to assess their adherence to the recommended prevention and therapeutic measures and to seek new signs or symptoms suggesting osteoporotic complications. These patients should have serial BMD measurements performed on the same DEXA machine.

Patients with unusually high BMD might not need further measurements. Patients with normal BMD may have repeated measurements at 3- to 5-year intervals. Patients who are implementing an osteoporosis prevention program and who ahve borderline BMD (T-score between –1 and –2.5) should have BMD measurements at intervals of 1 to 2 years until BMD is stabilized and then at 2 to 3-year intervals. Patients treated for established osteoporosis should have BMD measurements every year until stable BMD is demonstrated, and then every 2 years after that. However, insurance companies and government regulations might limit the number and frequency of serial BMD measurements.

References

For a complete list of references, log onto www.expertconsult.com.

Pituitary Disorders

Mario Skugor and Amir H. Hamrahian

ANATOMY AND PHYSIOLOGY OF THE PITUITARY GLAND

The pituitary gland weighs about 0.5 to 1 g and is divided into anterior and posterior lobes. It sits in the sella turcica immediately behind and superior to the sphenoid sinus. Cavernous sinuses are located laterally on each side of the sella, inclusive of the internal carotid artery and cranial nerves III, IV, V_1, V_2 and VI (Fig. 1).

Anterior pituitary hormones are regulated by hypothalamic releasing and inhibitory hormones and by negative feedback of the target glandular hormones at the pituitary and hypothalamic levels (Table 1). Among pituitary hormones, only the secretion of prolactin is increased in the absence of hypothalamic influence, because it is mainly under tonic suppression by dopamine, the main inhibitory factor. Antidiuretic hormone (ADH, vasopressin) is produced by the supraoptic and paraventricular nuclei of the hypothalamus and travels in the axons through the pituitary stalk to the posterior pituitary gland.

PITUITARY TUMORS

Definition and Prevalence

Pituitary adenomas arise from adenohypophyseal cells and are almost always benign (Table 2). They are arbitrarily designated as microadenomas (<10 mm) and macroadenomas (≥10 mm). Autopsy studies suggest that up to 20% of normal persons harbor pituitary microadenomas.[1] Pituitary tumors discovered by computed tomography (CT) or magnetic resonance imaging (MRI) examination, in the absence of any symptoms or clinical findings, are referred to as *pituitary incidentalomas.* The prevalence of pituitary incidentalomas found by MRI is about 10%, and the majority are microadenomas.[2]

Pituitary adenomas are rarely associated with parathyroid and neuroendocrine hyperplasia or neoplasia as part of the multiple endocrine neoplasia type I (MEN I) syndrome. Pituitary carcinomas are extremely rare, but metastases from other solid malignancies (mainly breast and lung) can occur.

Signs and Symptoms

Pituitary tumors can manifest with signs and symptoms of pituitary hypofunction, hormone hypersecretion, or mass effect. Impingement on the chiasma by a pituitary tumor results in visual field defects, most commonly bitemporal hemianopia (Fig. 2). Patients with sellar mass pressing on the optic chiasma should have a Humphrey visual field test. Lateral extension of the pituitary mass to the cavernous sinuses can result in diplopia, ptosis, or altered facial sensation. There is no specific headache pattern associated with pituitary tumors and, in some patients, the headache is unrelated to pituitary adenoma.

Diagnosis

MRI is the best method for the visualizing hypothalamic-pituitary anatomy. Once a pituitary adenoma is found, it is necessary to determine the type of adenoma (secretory vs. nonsecretory), pituitary function, and whether there is any visual field defect.

Treatment

The goals for treatment of a pituitary tumor include reduction or complete removal of the tumor, elimination of mass effect, normalization of hormone hypersecretion, and restoration of normal pituitary function. Some patients, especially those with large tumors, require several therapeutic modalities, including medical, surgical, and radiation therapies. The most important factor in pituitary surgery is the availability of an experienced neurosurgeon.

HYPOPITUITARISM

Pituitary adenomas are the most common cause of hypopituitarism, but other causes include parasellar diseases, pituitary surgery, radiation therapy, inflammatory and granulomatous diseases, and head injury. The sequential loss of pituitary hormones secondary to a mass effect is in the following order: growth hormone (GH), luteinizing hormone (LH), follicle-stimulating hormone (FSH), thyroid-stimulating hormone (TSH), adrenocorticotropic hormone (ACTH), and prolactin. Isolated deficiencies of various anterior pituitary hormones can occur. In general, pituitary microadenomas are rarely associated with hypopituitarism. Diabetes insipidus is almost never seen in patients with pituitary adenomas at presentation.

Somatotropin (Growth Hormone) Deficiency

The symptoms of GH deficiency in adults are subtle, consisting of decreased muscle strength and exercise tolerance and reduced sense of well-being (e.g., diminished libido, social isolation). Patients with GH deficiency have increased body fat and decreased lean body mass, and they might have decreased bone mineral density.

Random measurements of GH and gender- and age-adjusted insulin-like growth factor-1 (IGF-1) levels are not reliable to diagnose GH deficiency because GH secretion is pulsatile, and up to 65% of patients with GH deficiency have a normal IGF-1 level. Therefore, GH deficiency is best evaluated by dynamic testing, including the insulin tolerance test or GH-releasing hormone (RH)/arginine test.[3]

Gonadotropin Deficiency

In reproductive-aged women, gonadotropin deficiency causes infertility and oligomenorrhea or amenorrhea. It is often associated with lack of libido, hot flushes, and dyspareunia. In men, hypogonadism is diagnosed less often, because decreased libido and impotence may be considered functions of aging. Hypogonadism is often diagnosed retrospectively in men and postmenopausal women when patients present with mass effect. Osteopenia is a consequence of long-standing hypogonadism and responds to hormone replacement therapy.

Gonadotropin deficiency is diagnosed in the presence of low or normal LH and FSH levels in postmenopausal women, in reproductive-aged women with amenorrhea, or in men with low testosterone levels (<200 ng/dL). Measurement of gonadotropin and estradiol levels in reproductive-aged women with irregular menstruation is usually not informative. The presence of normal menstruation is the best indicator of the integrity of the gonadotropin axis in women of reproductive age.

Testosterone may be replaced by intramuscular injection, transdermal patch, or a gel. Oral testosterone is not recommended because

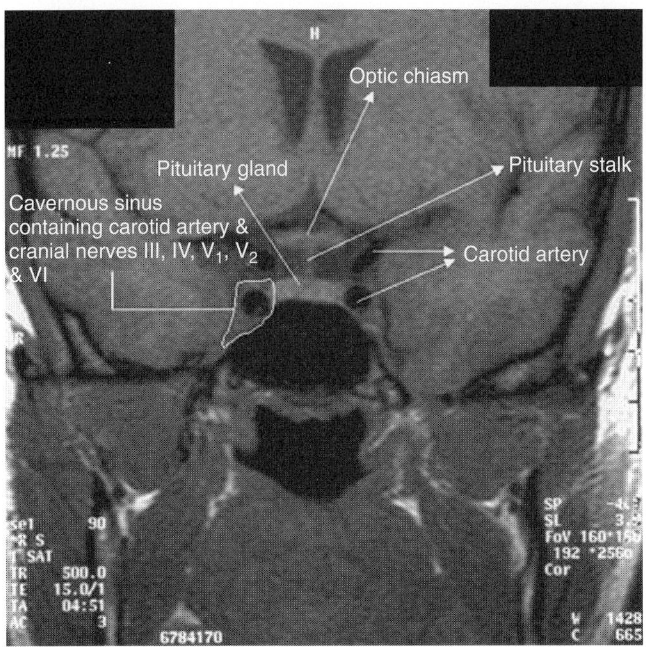

Figure 1 **Magnetic resonance imaging scan of a normal pituitary gland and perisellar structures.**

Table 1 Relationship Among Hypothalamic, Pituitary, and Feedback Hormones and Target Glands

Target Gland	Hypothalamic Regulatory Hormone	Pituitary Hormone	Feedback Hormone
Thyroid gland	TRH	TSH	T_4, T_3
Gonad	LHRH	LH	E_2, T
Gonad	LHRH	FSH	Inhibin, E_2, T
Many organs	GHRH, SMS	GH	IGF-1
Breast	PIF	Prolactin	?
Adrenal	CRH, ADH	ACTH	Cortisol

ACTH, adrenocorticotropic hormone; ADH, antidiuretic hormone; CRH, corticotropin-releasing hormone; E_2, estradiol; GHRH, growth hormone–releasing hormone; IGF-1, insulin-like growth factor 1; LHRH, luteinizing hormone–releasing hormone; PIF, prolactin release inhibitory factor; SMS, somatostatin; T, testosterone; T_3, triiodothyronine; T_4, thyroxine; TRH, thyrotropin-releasing hormone.

of the potential risk for liver toxicity. The serum prostate-specific antigen (PSA) level, hematocrit, and lipid profile should be monitored in men during testosterone replacement therapy. Estrogen replacement is necessary in hypogonadal women of reproductive age to prevent osteoporosis and to treat hot flushes, decreased libido, and vaginal dryness.

Corticotropin Deficiency

Patients with ACTH deficiency maintain their mineralocorticoid secretion because aldosterone is regulated primarily by the renin-angiotensin system and serum potassium concentration. Symptoms usually include chronic malaise, fatigue, anorexia, low-grade fever, and hypoglycemia. Patients might present with hyponatremia, which is secondary to inappropriate ADH secretion.

Table 2 Prevalence of Pituitary Adenomas

Adenoma Type	Prevalence (%)
GH cell adenoma	15
PRL cell adenoma	30
GH and PRL cell adenoma	7
ACTH cell adenoma	10
Gonadotropic cell adenoma	10
Nonfunctioning adenoma	25
TSH cell adenoma	1
Unclassified adenoma	2

ACTH, adrenocorticotropic hormone; GH, growth hormone; PRL, prolactin; TSH, thyroid-stimulating hormone.

An ACTH stimulation test and early morning (8 AM) plasma cortisol level measurement are reasonable initial tests for evaluating the corticotropin axis. An early morning cortisol level lower than 3 µg/dL confirms adrenal insufficiency, and a level higher than 15 µg/dL makes the diagnosis highly unlikely. Cortisol levels in the range of 3 to 15 µg/dL are indeterminate and should be further evaluated by the cosyntropin stimulation test (CST), which can be performed at any time during the day. The standard-dose CST uses an IV or intramuscular injection of 250 µg cosyntropin, and plasma cortisol levels determined before and 30 minutes after the injection. A normal response is a plasma cortisol concentration higher than 18 µg/dL at 30 minutes. Patients with mild partial or recent-onset pituitary ACTH or hypothalamic corticotropin-releasing hormone (CRH) deficiency (e.g., within 2 to 4 weeks after pituitary surgery) may have a normal response to 250 µg CST because the adrenal glands have not undergone sufficient atrophy and still respond to very high concentrations of ACTH stimulation.

The suggested replacement regimen is 15 to 20 mg hydrocortisone/day, usually given in two or three divided doses, with the highest dose given in the morning. Patients should be instructed to carry a medical alert, double their replacement dosage for 2 to 3 days in case of an acute disease, and should be covered by stress doses of hydrocortisone if undergoing surgery.

Thyrotropin Deficiency

The symptoms of thyrotropin (TSH) deficiency are similar to those in patients with primary hypothyroidism, including malaise, fatigue, leg cramps, dry skin, and cold intolerance.

The diagnosis cannot be established only through measurement of TSH because these patients might have a normal TSH level. For this reason, if secondary hypothyroidism is clinically suspected, TSH and free thyroxine (T_4) should be measured together. Usually, patients have a low or normal TSH level along with a low free T_4 level.

Therapy for TSH deficiency is similar to that for primary hypothyroidism. The levothyroxine replacement dose should be adjusted according to the patient's clinical status and free T_4 and free triiodothyronine (T_3) levels, but not TSH. In general, one should try to keep the free T_4 level in the upper normal range while the free T_3 level stays in the normal range. It is important to evaluate the corticotropin axis before initiating levothyroxine replacement, because therapy in those with underlying undiagnosed ACTH deficiency can result in an adrenocortical crisis secondary to an increase in metabolic demand.

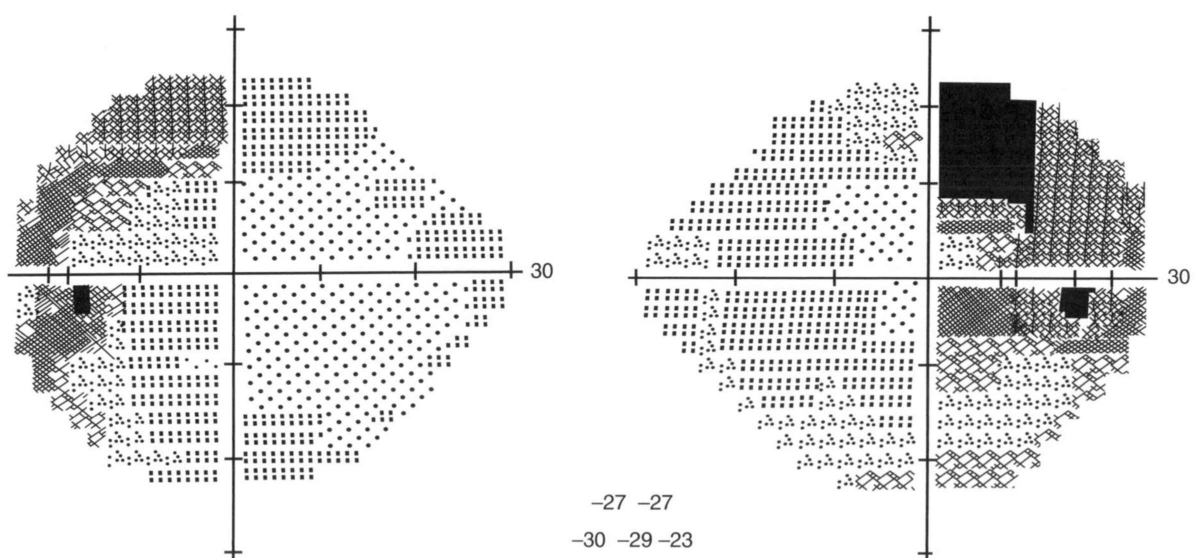

Figure 2 **Bitemporal hemianopsia secondary to a pituitary macroadenoma.**

EXCESS PITUITARY HORMONE SECRETION

Prolactinomas

Prolactinomas are pituitary adenomas that secret prolactin in varying degrees and account for about 30% of all pituitary adenomas. They are seen in all age groups but are more common in women, with a peak incidence during the childbearing years.

Clinical features of prolactinomas may be related to excess prolactin and associated secondary hypogonadism or mass effect. Women of reproductive age mainly present with oligomenorrhea, amenorrhea, galactorrhea, or infertility. Men and postmenopausal women usually come to medical attention because of mass effect, such as headaches and visual field defects. All patients with macroprolactinomas and most patients with microprolactinomas require treatment. Some indications for treatment of patients with microprolactinomas include bothersome galactorrhea, oligomenorrhea or amenorrhea, infertility, and sexual dysfunction.

Hyperprolactinemia can be physiologic or pathologic (Box 1). Pregnancy should always be ruled out. Biochemical analysis to evaluate renal and hepatic function and the TSH determination should be carried out. The drug history is an important part of the initial evaluation, because some medications are associated with hyperprolactinemia and their discontinuation for at least 3 days, if possible, will prevent any further and often expensive workup (Fig. 3). The majority of patients with a serum prolactin level above 100 µg/L have prolactinoma. A serum prolactin level lower than 100 µg/L in the presence of a large pituitary adenoma suggests stalk compression.

Dopamine agonists are the therapy of choice for most patients, and they are effective in decreasing adenoma size and restoring normal prolactin level in most patients. Dopamine agonists usually restore visual field defects to an extent similar to surgery.[4] Therefore, visual field defects associated with prolactinomas are not a neurosurgical emergency. Cabergoline and bromocriptine are potent inhibitors of PRL secretion and often cause tumor shrinkage. Dopamine agonists should be initiated slowly, because side effects often occur at the beginning of treatment. The most common side effects include nausea, headache, dizziness, nasal congestion, and constipation. Bromocriptine is the drug of choice in women planning pregnancy because there is considerable worldwide experience with the drug. Cabergoline is more potent, may be taken only twice a week, and is better tolerated by most patients. Few reports associate high-dose cabergoline with valvular heart disease in patients with Parkinson's disease, but risk seems to be insignificant with the doses used for treatment of prolactinoma.[5-6] Surgery is reserved for patients who are intolerant of or refractory to medical therapy. Radiation therapy may be considered for patients who poorly tolerate dopamine agonists and cannot be cured by surgery.

Box 1 Differential Diagnosis of Hyperprolactinemia

Physiologic considerations
Pregnancy, postpartum, suckling, stress, intercourse, exercise
Pituitary disorders
Prolactinomas, mixed pituitary tumors, pituitary tumors or disorders with stalk effect
Hypothalamic, stalk disorder
Aneurysm, inflammatory or granulomatous disease, tumors such as craniopharyngioma and meningioma, metastasis, trauma, radiotherapy

Drugs
Neuroleptics, metoclopramide, verapamil, methyldopa, reserpine, opiates, cocaine
Tricyclic antidepressants, monoamine oxidase inhibitors, some selective serotonin reuptake inhibitors (SSRIs)
Estrogen, antiandrogens

Systemic Diseases
Hypothyroidism
Chronic renal failure
Cirrhosis

Neurogenic factors
Chest wall disorders
Spinal nerve or cord lesion
Seizures

Ectopic factors
Hypernephroma
Gonadoblastoma
Ovarian teratomas

Idiopathic
Mostly secondary to a small microprolactinoma not identified by magnetic resonance imaging

Acromegaly

Acromegaly is a rare disease caused by a GH-secreting pituitary adenoma in more than 99% of patients. At diagnosis, about 75% of

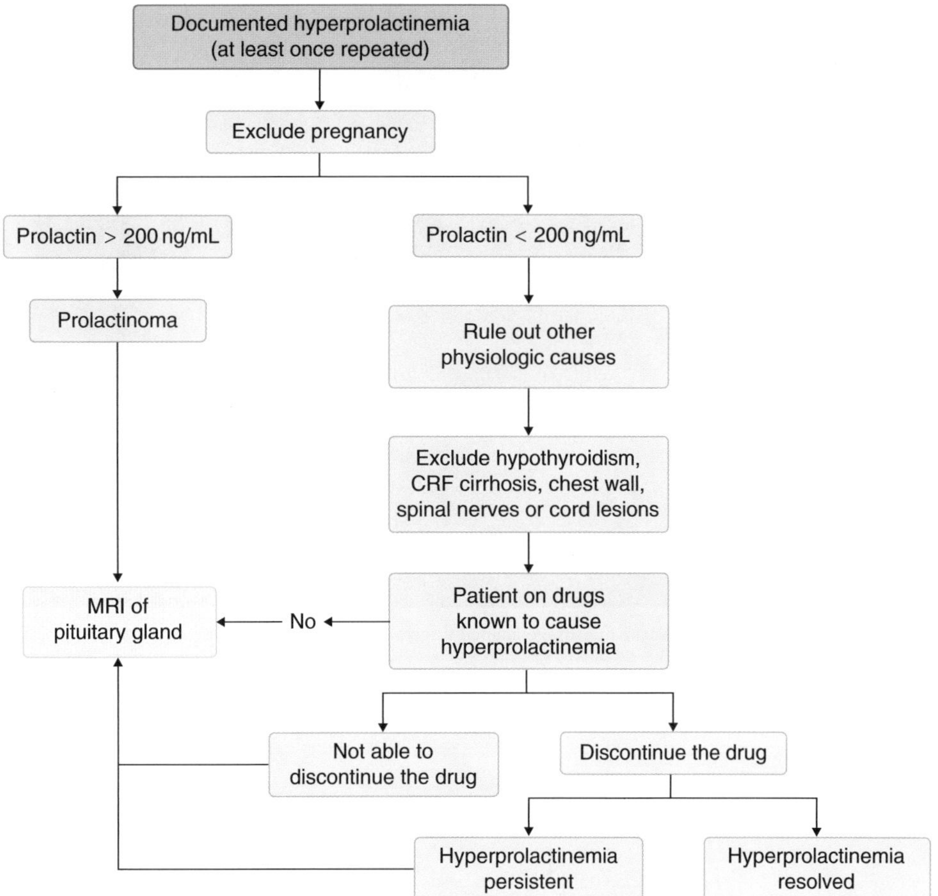

Figure 3 **Algorithm showing diagnostic approach to patients with hyperprolactinemia.** CRF, chronic renal failure; MRI, magnetic resonance imaging.

Box 2 Clinical Features of Patients with Acromegaly

- Acral enlargement
- Arthralgias, neuropathic joints
- Carpal tunnel syndrome
- Coarsening of facial features
- Excessive sweating
- Goiter
- Hypertension, congestive heart failure, arrhythmias
- Impaired glucose tolerance, diabetes mellitus
- Macroglossia
- Malocclusion and tooth gaps
- Pituitary mass effect, including headache and visual field defect
- Pituitary insufficiency
- Sensory and motor peripheral neuropathies
- Snoring, sleep apnea
- Symptoms associated with hyperprolactinemia
- Thick and coarse skin, skin tags

patients have macroadenomas. The mean age at diagnosis is about 45 years. Clinical features of acromegaly may be related to excess GH or IGF-1 or to associated mass effect including hypopituitarism, because most patients present with pituitary macroadenomas (Box 2 and Fig. 4). Excess growth hormone before the fusion of the epiphyseal growth plates results in gigantism. Acromegalic patients probably carry an increased risk of malignancy such as premalignant adenomatous colon polyps and colon cancer, although published data vary greatly in their findings.

Because of the pulsatile nature of GH secretion, random GH levels can overlap in acromegalic patients and normal persons. IGF-1 has a longer plasma half-life than GH and is the best single test for the diagnosing acromegaly (Fig. 5).[7] Acromegaly is associated with increased morbidity and mortality if untreated. The goal of therapy for most patients is to achieve a normal sex- and age-adjusted IGF-1 and GH less than 2 ng/mL.[8]

Surgery is the treatment of choice for most patients presenting with acromegaly even if a cure cannot be achieved. Even a subtotal resection of the tumor will improve the efficacy of subsequent adjuvant therapy. Medical treatment of acromegaly has gained significance since the limitations of radiation and surgical therapy have become evident. Somatostatin analogues inhibit GH secretion mainly by binding to somatostatin receptors and result in normalization of IGF-1 in up to 65% of patients. The most common side effects are gastrointestinal, including diarrhea, abdominal pain, and nausea. Gallbladder sludge and cholelithiasis have been reported in up to 25% of patients on long-term therapy with somatostatin analogues, but most patients were asymptomatic. Dopamine agonists have variable efficacy in patients with acromegaly but may be an attractive first-line therapy, especially in those with cosecretion of prolactin and GH. Pegvisomant has higher affinity to GH receptors than native GH but inhibits its dimerization, which is necessary for the action of GH. It is administered once daily and is usually reserved for patients not responding to other medical therapies. It is very effective, normalizing IGF-1 in up to 95% of patients. The tumor size and liver function need to be monitored during therapy. During therapy with pegvisomant, IGF-1 is used to monitor therapy. Radiotherapy is

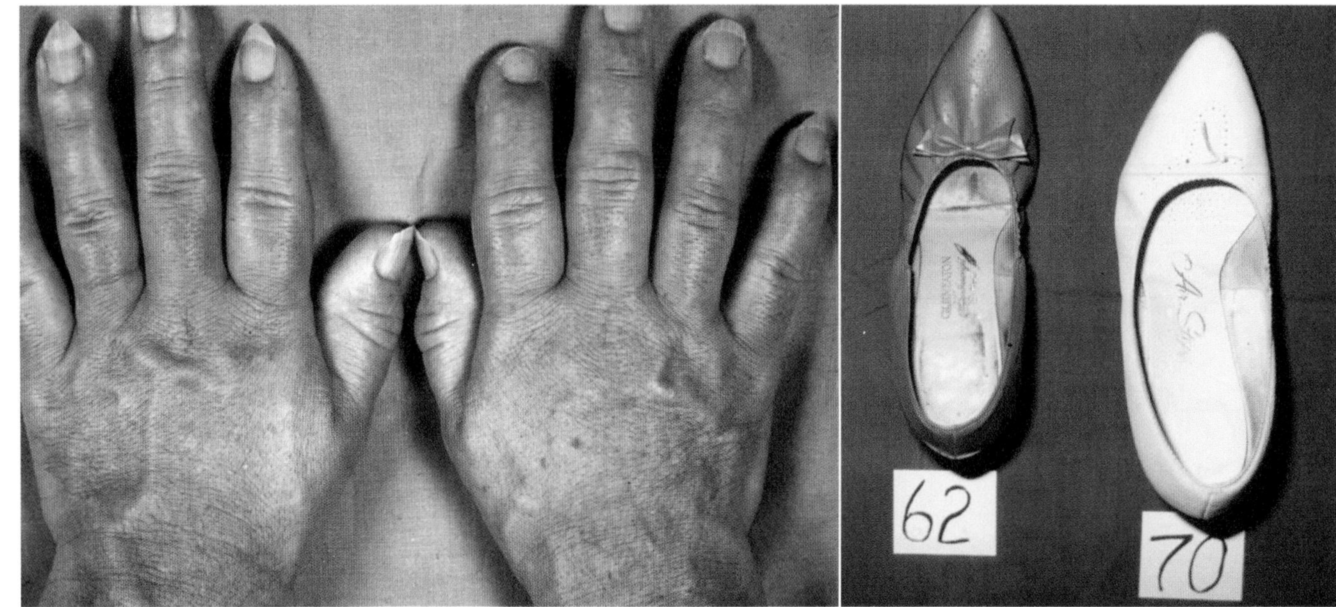

Figure 4 **Hands of an acromegalic patient with sausage-shaped fingers.** Note the change in her shoe size over a period of 8 years.

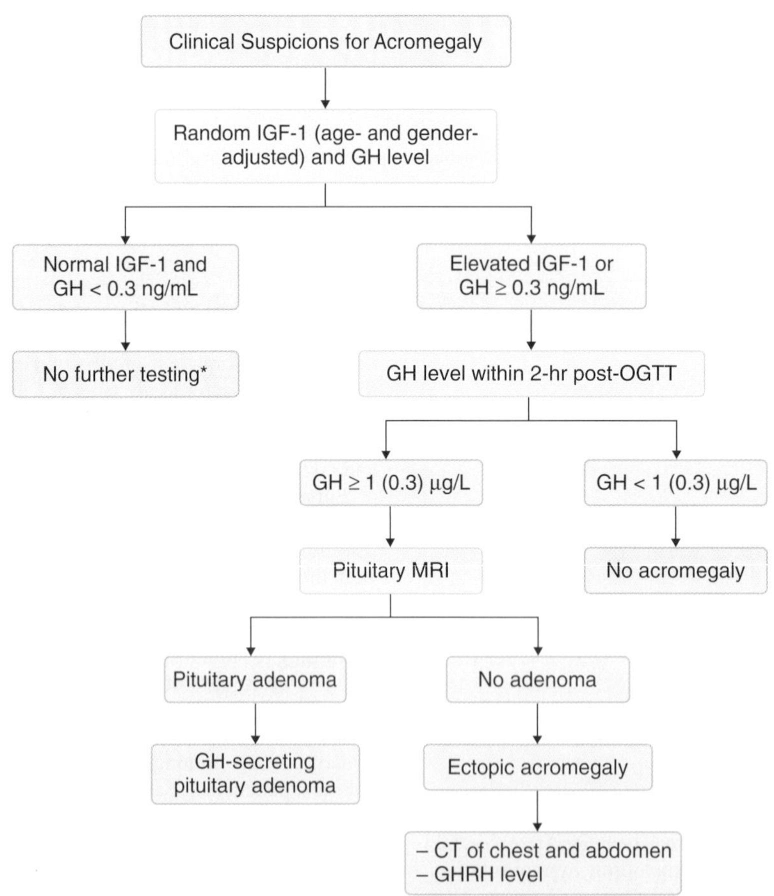

Figure 5 **Diagnostic workup of acromegaly.** CT, computed tomography; GH, growth hormone; GHRH, growth hormone-releasing hormone; IGF-1, insulin-like growth factor-1; OGTT, oral glucose tolerance test.

reserved for patients who cannot be cured by surgery and do not respond to or tolerate medical therapy.

Cushing's Disease

Cushing's syndrome (CS) comprises symptoms and signs associated with prolonged exposure to inappropriately high levels of plasma free glucocorticoids (Box 3). Exogenous glucocorticoid intake is the most common cause of CS. The endogenous causes are divided into ACTH-dependent and ACTH-independent CS (Box 4). In contrast to pale striae that occur postpartum or with weight gain, the striae in CS are usually red-purple, more than 1 cm wide, and located on the abdomen, upper thighs, breasts, and arms (Fig. 6). Increased skin pigmentation is rare and only occurs in the ectopic ACTH syndrome. Supraclavicular and dorsocervical fat pads (buffalo hump) and moon face are nonspecific and are seen in many patients of obesity clinics. Women complain of menstrual irregularity (84%) and hirsutism (especially vellous hypertrichosis of the face), and men and women exhibit loss of libido (≤100%). Psychiatric abnormalities occur in 50% of patients, with agitated depression and lethargy being the most common manifestations. A high clinical suspicion, attention to suggestive clinical features (see Box 3), and an appropriate screening test are the keys to early diagnosis of CS (Fig. 7).[9] Because of the challenging nature of diagnosing CS, it is important to follow a stepwise evaluation, know the limitations of each test, and avoid shortcuts.

Pseudo-Cushing's disease refers to features of CS along with some evidence of hypercortisolism that resolve after resolution of the underlying cause, such as chronic alcoholism, psychiatric disorders (e.g., major depression, anxiety disorder, obsessive-compulsive disorder), anorexia nervosa, morbid obesity, and poorly controlled diabetes. Cyclic CS is characterized by periods of excess alternating with intervals of normal or decreased cortisol production, which occurs in some patients with CS.

Surgical removal of the ACTH-secreting pituitary tumor is the treatment of choice.[10] Availability of an experienced neurosurgeon is crucial, and the long-term remission rate is about 60 to 80% following surgery. A low (<3 μg/dL) or undetectable postoperative cortisol level off glucocorticoids is considered to be a good marker for long-term cure. For those not cured by the surgery, other options include reoperation and radiotherapy. Bilateral adrenalectomy is reserved for those who continue to be hypercortisolemic. Medical therapy for Cushing's syndrome has limited value because of the associated toxicity and gradual decrease in efficacy. Among the available agents, ketoconazole is the most commonly used. During therapy, liver function tests need to be closely monitored.

Box 3 Clinical Features Suggesting Cushing's Syndrome

Central obesity
Unexplained osteoporosis
Proximal myopathy
Wide purplish striae (>1 cm)
Facial plethora
Spontaneous bruising
Hypokalemia
Serial photographs

Box 4 Causes of Endogenous Cushing's Syndrome

ACTH-Dependent Cushing's Syndrome
Cushing's disease (67%)
Ectopic ACTH secretion (12%)
Ectopic CRH secretion (<1%)

ACTH-Independent Cushing's Syndrome
Adrenal adenoma (10%)
Adrenal carcinoma (8%)
Micro- and macronodular adrenal hyperplasia (1%)

ACTH, adrenocorticotropic hormone; CRH, corticotropin-releasing hormone.

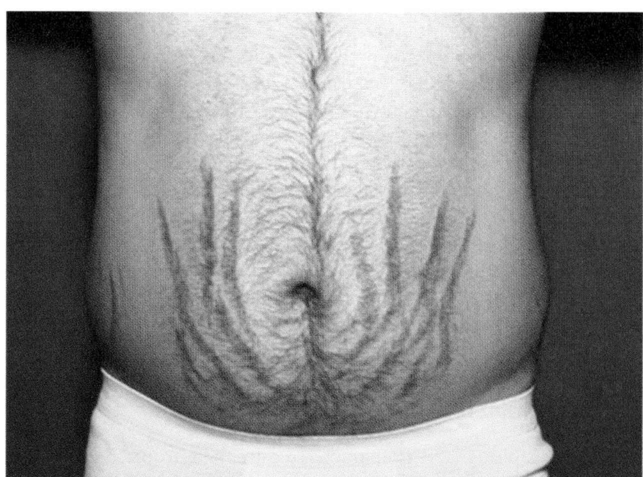

Figure 6 **Red purplish abdominal striae >1 cm in width in a patient with Cushing's syndrome.**

Thyrotropin-Secreting Adenoma

Thyrotropin (TSH)-secreting pituitary adenomas account for less than 1% of all pituitary tumors. The mean age at presentation is about 40 years, with a slight female predominance. Symptoms secondary to hyperthyroidism and goiter are the initial complaints in most patients, followed by pituitary mass effect if the disease remains undiagnosed. The most important biochemical feature is elevation of serum thyroid hormone levels (T_4 and T_3), with an inappropriately normal or elevated TSH level.

In patients with TSH-secreting adenomas, surgery is the primary therapeutic approach. Radiation is generally used for those with residual tumor. Somatostatin analogues are effective in most patients for control of excess TSH production leading to improvement in hyperthyroidism and possibly to a decrease in tumor size.[11] Beta blockers should be initiated in patients with uncontrolled hyperthyroidism, and antithyroid medications may be used only for a short period before surgery (if somatostatin analogues cannot be used) because long-term use can stimulate tumor growth.

NONFUNCTIONAL AND GLYCOPROTEIN-SECRETING PITUITARY ADENOMAS

Nonfunctional and glycoprotein-secreting pituitary tumors account for about 25% to 30% of all pituitary adenomas. Many clinically nonfunctional pituitary adenomas are glycoprotein-producing tumors. They can secrete intact glycoprotein hormones or their alpha and beta subunits. They usually manifest with clinical features related to mass effect, including visual field defect, hypopituitarism, and headache.[12]

Patients with small nonfunctional pituitary adenomas are usually observed; however, the standard treatment for those with mass effect is surgery, mainly through the trans-sphenoidal approach. Radiotherapy is indicated in those with residual pituitary tumor following surgical debulking or in those who are not surgical candidates. The use of high-dose dopamine agonists has been associated with a decrease in tumor size in only about 10% of patients.

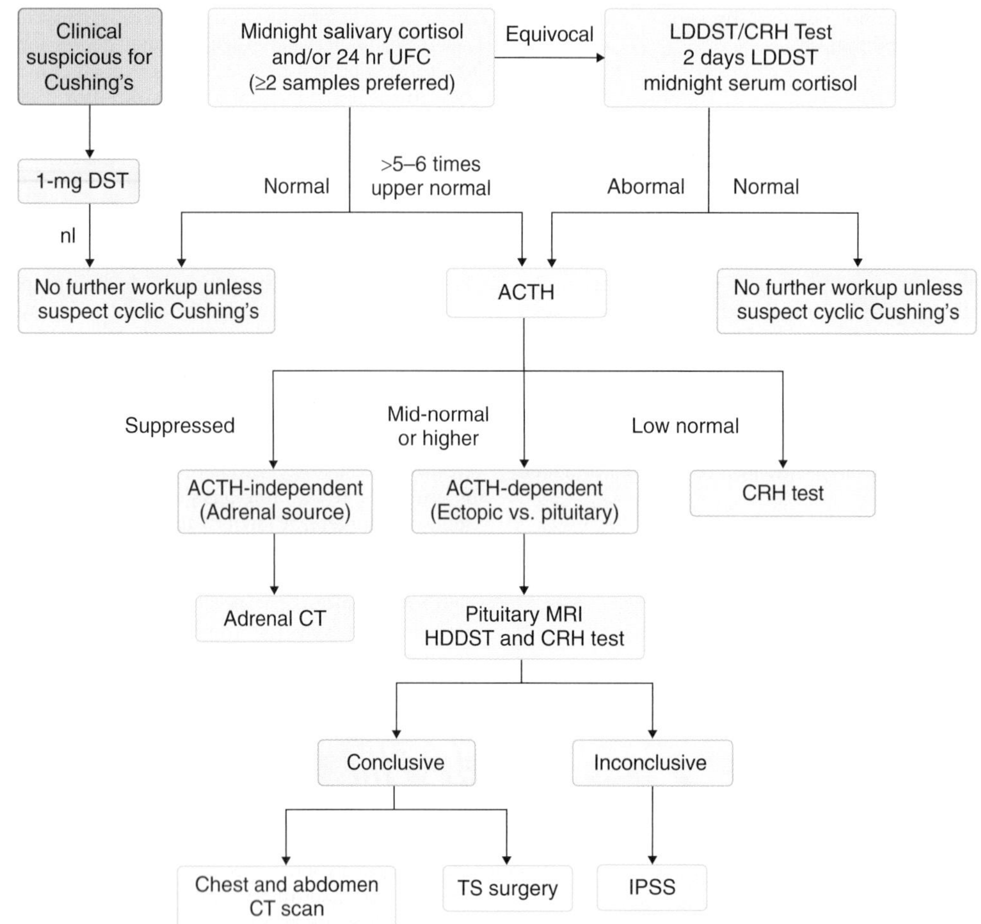

Figure 7 Algorithm showing diagnostic workup for Cushing's syndrome. CRH, corticotropin-releasing hormone; DST, dexamethasone suppression test; HDDST, high-dose dexamethasone suppression test; IPSS, inferior petrosal sinus sampling; LDDST, low-dose dexamethasone suppression test; nl, normal; TS, trans-sphenoidal; UFC, urinary free cortisol.

LYMPHOCYTIC HYPOPHYSITIS

Lymphocytic hypophysitis is a rare inflammatory lesion of the pituitary gland, commonly affecting young women during late pregnancy or in the postpartum period. This disorder probably has autoimmune pathogenesis and is associated with other autoimmune disorders, mainly Hashimoto's thyroiditis and Addison's disease. The clinical manifestations relate to mass effect or hypopituitarism. The corticotropin axis is the most commonly affected axis. The chronologic association with pregnancy or the postpartum period and isolated ACTH deficiency is a diagnostic clue.

Trans-sphenoidal surgery is the therapy of choice for those with pituitary mass effect. It is important to monitor patients with varying degrees of hypopituitarism, because some have partial or full recovery of their pituitary axes.

EMPTY SELLA

The empty sella is defined as a sella that, regardless of its size, is completely or partly filled with cerebrospinal fluid. An empty sella of normal size is a common incidental autopsy finding. An empty sella is called secondary when it is seen after surgery, irradiation, or medical treatment for a pituitary pathology. Most patients have no pituitary dysfunction, but partial or complete pituitary insufficiency has been reported. The discovery of an empty sella needs to be followed by an endocrine evaluation to determine whether there is any associated pituitary dysfunction. Management usually involves reassurance and hormone replacement, if necessary.

PITUITARY APOPLEXY

Pituitary apoplexy is a rare endocrine emergency resulting from hemorrhagic infarction of a preexisting pituitary tumor (Fig. 8). The clinical manifestations are related to rapid expansion of the tumor secondary to hemorrhage, with compression of the pituitary gland and the perisellar structures leading to headache, hypopituitarism, visual field defect, and cranial nerve palsies.[13] Headache is the most prominent symptom in most patients with clinically evident pituitary apoplexy. Once pituitary apoplexy is suspected, stress-dose glucocorticoids (e.g., dexamethasone 4 mg every 8 hours IV) should be initiated and pituitary MRI should be performed. Patients with mass effect benefit from tumor and blood clot debulking, which leads to resolution of visual field defects and improvement of cranial nerve palsies in most patients.

DIABETES INSIPIDUS

Diabetes insipidus (DI) is characterized by the chronic excretion of abnormally large volumes (>50 mL/kg) of dilute urine. The true prevalence of DI is unknown, but it is usually underdiagnosed because the symptoms and signs are benign and many patients ignore

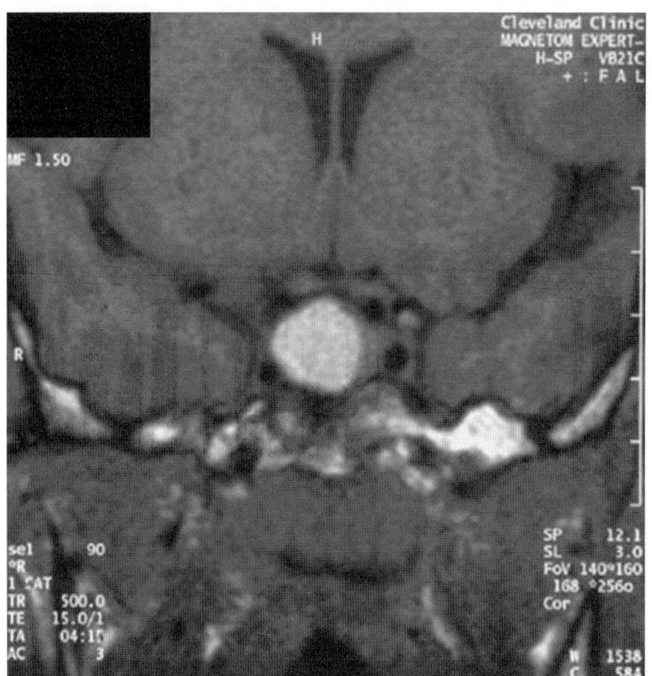

Figure 8 **Pituitary apoplexy with hemorrhage in the pituitary macroadenoma, causing sudden expansion of the tumor.**

them or are unaware of them. There are four major types of DI: central (neurogenic) DI, nephrogenic DI, primary polydipsia, and gestational DI. Central DI is secondary to inadequate ADH secretion that is insufficient to concentrate the urine.

Diabetes insipidus by itself is usually well tolerated and results in few symptoms, including polydipsia and polyuria. Nocturia of a large urine volume is often the primary reason for which patients seek medical attention. In most patients, DI is not associated with any abnormality on the physical examination or routine laboratory evaluation, except a low urine osmolality. Overt disturbances in fluid and electrolytes are uncommon unless other factors interfere with the normal compensatory mechanism of polydipsia, such as loss of consciousness.

Once diabetes mellitus and hypercalcemia have been excluded, patients should have their 24-hour urinary volume measured during ad libitum fluid intake. DI is diagnosed in those with abnormally high urinary output (>50 mL/kg/day), low urinary osmolality (<300 mOsm/kg), and an appropriate creatinine excretion (14-18 mg/kg body weight) as an indicator of an accurate 24-hour urine collection.[14] Measurement of spot urine osmolality is usually unreliable to exclude or diagnose DI, because it may be decreased significantly in an otherwise healthy person who drinks large amounts of water and can be increased to normal by fasting in a patient with partial DI. Patients with DI who are conscious usually have sufficient thirst to maintain a normal serum sodium level in spite of polyuria. Once the diagnosis has been established, the next step is to differentiate the type of DI. A water deprivation test may need to be performed by an experienced endocrinologist to differentiate among types of partial DI.

The therapy of choice for central DI is the administration of the ADH analogue desmopressin (DDAVP). It is available in a subcutaneous form or as an oral or nasal spray. The spray or oral form of desmopressin is usually started at bedtime and is gradually titrated for the desired antidiuretic effect.

Suggested Readings

Arnaldi G, Angeli A, Atkinson AB, et al: Diagnosis and complications of Cushing's syndrome: A consensus statement. J Clin Endocrinol Metab 2003;88:5593-5602.

Bonadonna S, Doga M, Gola M, et al: Diagnosis and treatment of acromegaly and its complications: Consensus guidelines. J Endocrinol Invest 2005;28(Suppl 11): 43-47.

Casanueva FF, Molitch ME, Schlechte JA, et al: Guidelines of the pituitary society for the diagnosis and management of prolactinomas. Clin Endocrinol 2006;65:265-273.

Ezzat S, Asa SL, Couldwell WT, et al: The prevalence of pituitary adenomas: A systematic review. Cancer 2004;101:613-619.

Ezzat S, Serri O, Chik CL, et al: Canadian consensus guidelines for the diagnosis and management of acromegaly. Clin Invest Med 2006;29:29-39.

Findling JW, Raff H: Cushing's syndrome: Important issues in diagnosis and management. J Clin Endocrinol Metab 2006;91:3746-3753.

Fleseriu M, Lee M, Pineyro MM, et al: Giant invasive pituitary prolactinoma with falsely low serum prolactin: The significance of 'hook effect.' J Neurooncol 2006;79:41-43.

Freda PU, Reyes CM, Nuruzzaman AT, et al: Basal and glucose-suppressed GH levels less than 1 microg/L in newly diagnosed acromegaly. Pituitary 2003;6:175-180.

Krikorian A, Aron D: Evaluation and management of pituitary incidentalomas-revisiting an acquaintance. Nat Clin Pract Endocrinol Metab. 2006;2:138-145.

Molitch ME, Clemmons DR, Malozowski S, et al: Evaluation and treatment of adult growth hormone deficiency: An Endocrine Society Clinical Practice Guideline. J Clin Endocrinol Metab 2006;9:1621-1634.

Ness-Abramof R, Ishay A, Harel G, et al: TSH-secreting pituitary adenomas: Follow-up of 11 cases and review of the literature. Pituitary. 2007;10:307-310.

Robertson GL: Diabetes insipidus. Endocrinol Metab Clin North Am 1995;24:549-572.

Schade R, Andersohn F, Suissa S, et al: Dopamine agonists and the risk of cardiac-valve regurgitation. N Engl J Med 2007;356:29-38.

Vance ML: Treatment of patients with a pituitary adenoma: One clinician's experience. Neurosurg Focus 2004;16:E1.

Verrees M, Arafah BM, Selman WR: Pituitary tumor apoplexy: Characteristics, treatment, and outcomes. Neurosurg Focus 2004;16:E6.

References

For a complete list of references, log onto www.expertconsult.com.

Hypothyroidism and Hyperthyroidism

Mario Skugor and Maria Fleseriu

ANATOMY AND PHYSIOLOGY

A normal adult thyroid weighs 10-20 g and receives blood from bilateral superior and inferior thyroid arteries and a small artery called the thyroid ima. The thyroid secretes two hormones. Thyroxine (T_4) makes 90% of hormone production, and triiodothyronine (T_3) produces the other 10%. Peripheral tissues convert T_4 to T_3, and most of T_3 is derived from T_4. Thyroid hormone secretion is regulated by hypothalamo-pituitary-thyroid axis through actions of TRH and TSH.

Thyroid hormones are transported in serum bound to carrier proteins (0.03%-0.04% of T_4 and 0.3%-0.4% of T_3 are free hormone). Thyroid hormone binding globulin (TBG) is the main carrier, accounting for 75% of bound T_4 and all of bound T_3. Thyroxine binding prealbumin and albumin are responsible for the rest.

PHYSIOLOGIC EFFECTS

Most thyroid hormone actions (metabolic and developmental) are mediated via nuclear receptors through gene expression regulation. Thyroid hormone receptors are found in most body tissues. T_3 is biologically much more active than T_4. Thyroid hormones increase the basal metabolic rate by stimulating catabolic and anabolic reactions in metabolism of carbohydrates, fat, and proteins and by stimulating thermogenesis. Thyroid hormone deficiency during embryonic development leads to cretinism and dwarfism (congenital myxedema).

HYPOTHYROIDISM

Definition and Prevalence

Hypothyroidism results from reduced effects of thyroid hormone on tissues. Hypothyroidism is more common in women, has total prevalence of 1% to 2%,[1] and increases with age (~10% adults >65 years). In the U.S. population, prevalence of biochemical hypothyroidism is 4.6%, but clinically evident hypothyroidism is present in 0.3%.[2] Congenital hypothyroidism is among the most common congenital diseases, with an incidence of 1/4000 newborns. Higher risk of hypothyroidism is seen in persons with the conditions listed in Box 1.

Hypothyroidism can be congenital or acquired, subclinical or overt, and, according to the site of abnormality, primary (thyroid level) or secondary (pituitary or hypothalamic). The most common causes (Box 2) are Hashimoto's thyroiditis, postsurgical or postablative hypothyroidism, amiodarone-induced hypothyroidism, and postpartum thyroiditis.

Specific Syndromes

Hashimoto's Thyroiditis

Hashimoto's thyroiditis is an autoimmune disorder directed against thyroid antigens and is the most common cause of hypothyroidism. The incidence is 0.3 to 1.5 per 1000 person-years, and it is 4 to 10 times more common in women than in men. Hashimoto's thyroiditis is more prevalent in areas with a high dietary iodine intake, and smoking increases the risk. Goiter can be seen on presentation, but thyroid atrophy is more common. Hashimoto's thyroiditis is associated with other endocrine diseases in polyglandular autoimmune failure syndrome (Addison's disease, type1 diabetes mellitus, and hypogonadism).

The diagnosis is made by clinical features, elevated TSH, low thyroid hormone, and the presence of anti–thyroid peroxidase antibodies (anti-TPO).

Amiodarone-Induced Hypothyroidism

Excess iodine from amiodarone exerts an acute, transient inhibition of iodide organification, the Wolff-Chaikoff effect, but the normal gland escapes this effect due to adaptation of the iodide transport system. In some persons, the thyroid gland is unable to escape the block, and hypothyroidism ensues. Thyroid function tests should be checked before starting amiodarone therapy, after 3 to 4 months of therapy, and 1 year after discontinuing therapy.

Postpartum Thyroiditis

Postpartum thyroiditis usually manifests with hyperthyroidism (see later) followed by a hypothyroid phase (transient or permanent).

Signs and Symptoms

Symptoms of hypothyroidism depend on pathogenesis, duration, severity, and the age of the patient. Symptoms of mild hypothyroidism are nonspecific: fatigue, cold intolerance, sleepiness, weight gain and muscle aches. These symptoms are also seen with a variety of other conditions; however, such patients should be tested for hypothyroidism. Other symptoms include bradycardia, constipation, menstrual irregularities, dry skin, coarse or brittle hair, edema (especially periorbital), and difficulty with concentration and memory. Laboratory tests might also show elevated cholesterol, prolactin, and creatine phospokinase.

Hypothyroidism is associated with impaired endothelial function, left ventricular diastolic dysfunction, and higher diastolic blood pressure due to increased systemic vascular resistance. These abnormalities are reversible with L-T_4 replacement therapy.[3]

Myxedema coma is the most serious form of hypothyroidism; it is often precipitated by other diseases. Patients have profound hypothermia, bradycardia, and typical skin and facial changes. Mortality is 100% if not treated. Myxedema coma is seen extremely rarely today.

Diagnosis

A TSH level is the best screening test for detecting hypothyroidism. A normal TSH rules out primary hypothyroidism in asymptomatic patients. Abnormal TSH should be followed by determination of thyroid hormone levels.

Overt hypothyroidism is defined as a clinical syndrome of hypothyroidism associated with elevated TSH and decreased serum levels of T_4 or T_3. Subclinical hypothyroidism is defined as a condition without typical symptoms of hypothyroidism, elevated TSH (>5 μU/mL), and normal circulating thyroid hormone.

Box 1 Conditions Indicating Higher Risk for Hypothyroidism

Family or personal history of autoimmune disease
Women in the postpartum period
Personal history of neck or head irradiation
Primary pulmonary hypertension
Genetic syndromes: Turner's and Down syndromes
Patients treated with amiodarone, interferon-alpha, or lithium
Persons over 65 years of age

Box 2 Causes of Hypothyroidism

Primary
Agenesis
Gland destruction

- Surgical removal
- Irradiation (therapeutic radioiodine, external irradiation)
- Autoimmune disease (Hashimoto's, atrophic thyroiditis)
- Idiopathic atrophy
- Infiltrative process

Inhibition of thyroid hormone synthesis and release

- Iodine deficiency
- Excess iodide in susceptible persons
- Drugs: interferon alpha, lithium, amiodarone, aminoglutethimide, thalidomide, sunitinib, sovafenib
- Inherited enzyme defects

Transient

- After surgery or therapeutic radioiodine
- Postpartum
- Thyroiditis

Secondary
Hypothalamic disease
Pituitary disease

- Genetic forms of pituitary hormone deficiencies
- Infiltrative disorders
- Sheehan's syndrome
- Surgery or irradiation
- Trauma
- Tumors

Resistance to thyroid hormone

The measurement of thyroid autoantibodies helps in diagnosing autoimmune process. However, this test should be ordered only if it will influence the decision to treat.

Treatment

Treatment is with thyroid hormone supplementation. Levothyroxine (L-T_4) is acceptable therapy for most patients. The starting dose should be 1.6 µg/kg of body weight. In elderly patients and patients with cardiac disease, we recommend starting at a lower dose (25-50 µg/day) and increase by 25 µg/d until the patient is clinically and biochemically euthyroid. The dose should be adjusted about 6 to 8 weeks after treatment is initiated (unless symptoms of overtreatment occur). Once the patient is euthyroid and TSH is stable, an annual follow-up with TSH measurement should suffice. During pregnancy, more-frequent TSH determination are needed because of increasing needs secondary to an increase in binding protein levels. TSH should be checked 2 months after the start or discontinuation of HRT.

The patient should be advised to take the T_4 preparation 2 to 4 hours before or after meals or using preparations known to impede T_4 absorption: calcium, magnesium, iron, sucralfate, and aluminum hydroxide.

Box 3 Causes of Thyrotoxicosis

Thyroid hormone overproduction

- Graves' disease
- Toxic multinodular goiter
- Toxic adenoma
- Metastatic thyroid carcinoma
- Human chorionic gonadotropin–mediated thyrotoxicosis
- Thyroid-stimulating hormone–mediated thyrotoxicosis, pituitary resistance to T_4 and T_3
- Iodide excess (Jod-Basedow)

Uncontrolled release of preformed thyroid hormones

- Subacute thyroiditis
- Painless thyroiditis
- Postpartum thyroiditis
- Hashimoto's thyroiditis
  Amiodarone induced thyroiditis
  Nonthyroidal excess
  Thyrotoxicosis factitia
  Struma ovarii

If any signs or symptoms suggest adrenal insufficiency, this should be investigated and, if confirmed, glucocorticoids should be given before starting T_4. Failure to do so can precipitate adrenal crisis.

In selected circumstances, T_3 may also be used to treat hypothyroidism. Drawbacks to routine use of T_3 include short half-life, requiring multiple daily doses, and fluctuating symptoms when doses are missed.

Combination therapy using both T_4 and T_3 (dessicated thyroid extract, compounded T_4-T_3 preparation) has been proposed to improve mood and quality of life, but most studies did not show benefit.[4] We do not recommend routine use of combination therapy except in cases where fast improvements in clinical condition are required (profound hypothyroidism).

Myxedema coma requires aggressive treatment with intravenous T_4 (≤500 µg/day), and some authors recommend addition of T_3.[5]

Consultation with an endocrinologist should be sought in hypothyroid patients who are 18 years old or younger, unresponsive to therapy, or pregnant; who have cardiac disease, goiter, nodule, or other structural abnormality of thyroid gland; or who have another coexisting endocrine disease

HYPERTHYROIDISM

Definition and Prevalence

Thyrotoxicosis is a clinical condition resulting from the action of excess thyroid hormone on tissues. The term *hyperthyroidism* is usually reserved for thyrotoxicosis caused by excessive production of thyroid hormone (Boxes 3 and 4). Other forms of thyrotoxicosis include thyrotoxicosis factitia and those associated with different forms of thyroiditis. Overt thyrotoxicosis is defined as the syndrome of hyperthyroidism associated with suppressed TSH and elevated serum levels of T_4 or T_3. Subclinical thyrotoxicosis is devoid of symptoms, but TSH is suppressed although there are normal circulating levels of thyroid hormone.

Prevalence of overt thyrotoxicosis is about 0.5%. However, 1% to 2% of patients have a below-normal TSH level. Low TSH is seen in 3% of the population older than 80 years.[6]

Signs and Symptoms

Thyrotoxic signs and symptoms vary with the level of thyroid hormone excess, age of the patient, and duration of the disease. Some features are characteristic of all types of thyrotoxicosis, and some are related to the specific etiology (e.g., exophthalmos with Graves' disease).

Box 4 Signs and Symptoms of Thyrotoxicosis

Symptoms

Nervousness
Fatigue
Weakness,
Palpitations
Heat intolerance
Excessive sweating
Dyspnea
Diarrhea
Insomnia
Poor concentration
Oligomenorrhea

Signs

Weight loss
Hair loss
Tachycardia
Proximal myopathy
Warm, moist skin
Hyperkinesis
Stare, lid lag, lid retraction, and exophthalmos (with Graves' disease)
Emotional liability
Hyperactive reflexes
Thyroid enlargement (in most cases)

Graves' Disease

Graves' disease is an autoimmune disorder in which autoantibodies bind and stimulate the TSH receptor. It is the most common cause of thyrotoxicosis. Receptor activation stimulates thyrocyte growth and function.

The disease is more common in whites and Asians, and the incidence is lower in African Americans. The female-to-male ratio is 3.5 : 1.[6] It is more common in patients with a family history of thyroid disease, especially Graves' disease.

Graves' disease has some specific features: swelling over the anterior shin (pretibial myxedema), thyroid eye disease (prominence of eyes, lid lag, globe lag, exophthalmos, lid edema, chemosis, and extraocular muscle weakness); and increased pigmentation and vitiligo.

Thyroid ophthalmopathy is present in about 50% of Graves' patients. Smoking is a risk factor. Therapeutic options include local measures to combat inflammation—glucocorticoids, plasmapheresis, and immune suppressants—as well as orbital radiation, decompressive surgery, and thyroid ablation. Treatment should be managed by an endocrinologist and an ophthalmologist specializing in thyroid eye disease.

Toxic Multinodular Goiter

Toxic multinodular goiter (MNG) is defined as the presence of two or more thyroid nodules secreting excess thyroid hormone and causing hyperthyroidism. Hyperthyroidism in an MNG can be potentiated by iodine-containing drugs (e.g., IV contrast dye, amiodarone).

Patients are typically older than those with Graves' disease. The disease has an insidious onset, and patients often have apathetic hyperthyroidism, presenting with weight loss, atrial fibrillation, and depression and few other symptoms. On examination, patients have MNG and, sometimes, compressive symptoms (dysphagia, dyspnea, neck pressure, and Pemberton's sign).

Diagnosis is confirmed by low TSH, high T_4, high T_3, and thyroid scintigraphy demonstrating multiple functioning nodules (hot nodules).

Toxic Adenoma

Toxic thyroid nodules are histologically usually benign. Scintigraphy shows increased RAI uptake in the nodule (hot nodule), with various degrees of suppression of remaining thyroid. Toxic nodules may be solitary or present in MNG.

Thyroiditis

All types of thyroiditis cause inflammation of thyroid tissue and can release preformed hormone from the colloid space, causing thyrotoxicosis, which is transient and followed by recovery or development of hypothyroidism. Approximately half the patients with subacute and postpartum thyroiditis develop permanent hypothyroidism.

In acute and subacute thyroiditis, thyroid tenderness and neck pain are often present. Silent thyroiditis is, by definition, devoid of local symptoms. Thyroiditis reduces iodine uptake in thyroid cells, and scintigraphy shows very little RAI accumulation.

Supportive measures are adequate treatment in most patients (see later).

Postpartum thyroiditis presents as hypo- or hyperthyroidism in women who were euthyroid during pregnancy. The incidence of postpartum thyroiditis ranges from 3% to 16% judging by biochemical studies. Clinically apparent disease is much less common. Postpartum thyroiditis appears 3 to 6 months after delivery. Women may have small goiter or no physical findings. Symptoms and signs can be very subtle. Laboratory tests in thyroiditis show a triphasic presentation: hyperthyroidism 2 to 4 months after delivery, continuing with hypothyroid phase of 4 to 8 months, and then recovery in up to 90% of cases.[7] Women with other autoimmune disease have a three-fold increased risk for postpartum thyroiditis. The recurrence risk in subsequent pregnancies is about 25%.

Iodide-Induced Thyrotoxicosis (Jod-Basedow Phenomenon)

Jod-Basedow phenomenon refers to induction of hyperthyroidism after a large load of iodine is administered to a susceptible patient. Symptoms are usually mild and resolve spontaneously. Most patients have MNG, and hyperthyroidism is not associated with autoimmunity. Thyrotoxicosis after iodide exposure appears also in patients with latent or drug-treated Graves' disease.

Amiodarone-Induced Hyperthyroidism

Amiodarone-induced hyperthyroidism is seen in 3% of patients (10% in iodine-deficient areas)[8] Symptoms may be masked by amiodarone effects on the heart (beta blocking).

Hyperthyroidism may be caused by increased T_4 and T_3 production. It is seen usually in patients with underlying MNG with autonomy that is fed by iodine from amiodarone (type I hyperthyroidism) or by thyroiditis (type II hyperthyroidism). The hyperthyroid phase can last up to several months. Differentiating between the two types may be very difficult, and the two types can coexist.

Diagnosis

A clinical picture of hyperthyroidism, suppressed TSH, and high or high normal T_4 or T_3 (or both) confirms the diagnosis. The typical eye findings (exopthalmos) make a diagnosis of Graves' disease almost certain.

Radioactive Iodine (RAI) uptake and scan differentiates between different causes of hyperthyroidism. Graves' disease has increased uptake and smooth distribution of RAI in the gland. Thyroiditis is characterized by diffusely diminished RAI uptake (this picture also can be seen in patients with high body iodine load and in those with factitious thyrotoxicosis). Toxic adenomas and toxic MNG show areas of increased RAI uptake (hot nodules), with different degrees of suppression of remaining thyroid parenchyma.

The thyroid receptor antibodies (TRABs) are specific for Graves' disease. This test is useful in patients who had recent iodine load or in pregnant women in whom RAI cannot be used. If factitious hyperthyroidism is suspected, serum thyroglobulin is typically undetectable. High iodine load can be confirmed by measurement of urinary Iodine excretion.

Treatment

Untreated hyperthyroidism can lead to hypertension, heart failure, atrial fibrillation, bone mass loss, and thyroid storm. During pregnancy, hyperthyroidism can result in maternal or fetal complications, miscarriage, preterm delivery, placental abruption, fetal or neonatal hyperthyroidism, intrauterine growth retardation, or still birth. Treatment is aimed at reducing the risk of these complications. Treatment consists of supportive measures to relieve effects of thyrotoxicosis and specific measures aimed to specific cause.

In thyrotoxicosis, the catecholamine receptor number is increased, so beta blockers have an important role in blocking catecholamine response. If tolerated, propranolol should be used (usually 40-120 mg in two or three daily doses) because it blocks conversion of T_4 to T_3. Atenolol can also be used (25-50 mg once a day).

In severe thyroiditis, anti-inflammatory agents (NSAIDs, corticosteroids) may be necessary.

Radioiodine Ablation

Graves' disease is usually treated with RAI (^{131}I) administered orally. RAI dosing is based on thyroid size, RAI uptake, and prior use of thionamide agents. In most cases, complete ablation of the thyroid gland is attempted. Permanent hypothyroidism results and requires permanent thyroid hormone replacement. If ablation is unsuccessful, RAI administration should be repeated.

RAI has an essential role in treating toxic adenomas and toxic MNG when surgery is contraindicated. Toxic MNG requires a higher dose of radioiodine, and the risk of permanent hypothyroidism is lower.

The RAI treatment is safe and has few long-term consequences. Side effects include gustatory disturbances, sialoadenitis, hypoparathyroidism, and transient worsening of hyperthyroidism in some patients. Allergy to iodine is not seen, and RAI can be used even in patients sensitive to iodinated contrast agents.

Antithyroid Drugs

Propylthiouracil (PTU) and methimazole are the U.S. Food and Drug Administration (FDA)-approved thionamides. Both antithyroid drugs inhibit thyroid hormone synthesis by interfering with thyroid peroxidase–mediated iodination of thyrosine residues in the thyroid gland. PTU also blocks the conversion of T_4 to T_3. However, methimazole is widely used due to a better side-effect profile (less neutropenia and agranulocytosis) and improved adherence with a simpler schedule (once or twice a day vs. three daily doses). The usual starting doses for methimazole are 20 to 40 mg in one or two daily doses or PTU 300 to 600 mg in three daily doses. [8]

Follow-up is recommended every 4 to 6 weeks, with dose adjustment until euthyroidism is achieved. Maintenance usually requires a lower dose (5-10 mg of methimazole of 100-200 mg of PTU). Antithyroid drugs are used for 12 to 18 months and then discontinued. Relapse typically occurs in the first 3 to 6 months, but it can be as late as 40 years. The risk of relapse is very high with pregnancy. When antithyroid drugs are used in preparation for RAI treatment, they must be stopped several days before RAI, and the dose of RAI needs to be increased, because of the radioprotective effect of antithyroid drugs.

Minor side effects of antithyroid drugs include skin reactions, arthralgias, gastrointestinal effects, and sialadenitis. The most serious side effect is agranulocytosis, which has been reported to occur in 0.3% to 0.6% of cases. A baseline complete blood count is recommended, but further follow-up with differential white cell count in asymptomatic patients is not recommend. All patients should be instructed about this risk and told to stop the drug if signs of infection develop and seek urgent medical care. Other rare side effects include hepatotoxicty, vasculitis, cholestasis, hypoglycemia, and hives.

Surgery

Surgical therapy is a safe and effective for Graves' disease when performed by an experienced thyroid surgeon. Surgery is not first-line therapy, but it is helpful when rapid control of hyperthyroidism is important, in patients with large glands, in children, and in women of childbearing age. Hyperthyroidism should be controlled before surgery with antithyroid drugs, corticosteroids, and elemental iodine to minimize the risk of thyroid storm during the surgery. Surgery is a safe and effective treatment for toxic adenoma (unilateral thyroidectomy) and MNG.

Treatment of Specific Maladies

Amiodarone-Induced Hyperthyroidism. The high iodine content of amiodarone limits the effectiveness of RAI treatment. Discontinuing amiodarone is generally helpful, but many patients cannot stop treatment because of an underlying heart condition. The half-life of amiodarone in the body is about 100 days, and no immediate benefit can be expected from stopping therapy.

Type I Hyperthyroidism. Type I hyperthyroidism should be treated with thionamide drugs (although the response may be slower than in other forms of hyperthyroidism), and high doses may be necessary. If thyrotoxicosis is severe, perchlorate (to enhance iodine clearance from the thyroid gland) and lithium may be used in association with antithyroid drugs to enhance the therapeutic response.

Type II Hyperthyroidism. Type II hyperthyroidism may be treated with corticosteroids (prednisone 30-60 mg once daily). If amiodarone can be discontinued, thionamides and iopanoic acid (not available in the United States) have a potential role. When the mechanism of hyperthyroidism is not known, a combination therapy with corticosteroids and thionamides is started. If hyperthyroidism is impossible to control, surgery is indicated (this is rarely necessary).

Thyroid Storm. Thyroid storm is rare, but mortality is still high. In the past it was seen in hyperthyroid patients poorly prepared for thyroid or other surgery. Today it is seen in patients who have severe thyrotoxicosis and who are noncompliant with medication or who have severe comorbidities. The clinical picture is that of life-threatening thyrotoxicosis. Symptoms include severe tachycardia or atrial fibrillation, fever (even hyperpyrexia), change in mental status (tremulousness, restlessness agitation, delirium, psychosis, lethargy, seizure, coma), pulmonary edema or congestive heart failure, nausea, vomiting, abdominal pain, diarrhea, jaundice, and profuse sweating.

Treatment of thyroid storm usually requires monitoring in the intensive care unit (ICU). Therapy includes high doses intravenous beta blockers (propranolol) to control symptoms of increased adrenergic tone and acetaminophen to control fever (aspirin should not be used because it increases free level of thyroid hormone). Antithyroid drugs (given orally, via nasogastric tube, or rectally) are used to suppress thyroid hormone production and release. Iodinated contrast dyes (currently not available in the United States) are given to inhibit peripheral T_4 to T_3 conversion. Iodine containing solutions block release of thyroid hormone from the thyroid and can be used 1 or 2 hours after antithyroid drugs are given. Corticosteroids reduce T_4 to T_3 conversion and possibly affect the autoimmune process in Graves' disease. Because thyrotoxic patients have an increased thyroid hormone enterohepatic circulation, cholesteramine has a role in treatment.

THYROID FUNCTION IN NONTHYROIDAL ILLNESS

Thyroid hormone alterations seen during nonthyroidal illness (euthyroid sick syndrome) include reduced production of T_3 in the majority of patients due to decreased T_4 conversion (inhibition of 5′-monodeiodinase), decreased serum T_4 (≤50% of patients in the ICU) because of decreased levels of binding proteins and inhibition of thyroid hormone-protein binding, and somewhat inhibited TSH secretion. In severe illness these effects occur sequentially, and early phases of euthyroid sick syndrome have low T_3, followed by reduction in T_4 and then TSH.

In the recovery phase of nonthyroidal illness, TSH can transiently rise abnormally high. Reverse T_3 is usually elevated and can be measured to confirm the diagnosis. The finding of altered thyroid hormone levels in hospitalized patients confirms the participation of these factors in the adaptive response to illness. Thyroid function should not be routinely checked during serious illnesses unless there is a strong suspicion of thyroid disorder.

EFFECTS OF MEDICATIONS ON THYROID FUNCTION TESTS

Dopamine is a potent inhibitor of TSH secretion. Corticosteroids and dobutamine also can decrease TSH levels slightly. Estrogens and selective estrogen-receptor modulators increase TBG production and increase total T_4 level; androgens and nicotinic acid decrease TBG production. High dose-salicylates (aspirin, salasalate) displace T_4 from binding proteins. Phenytoin and carbamazepine can artificially lower measured values of free T_4 and T_3 in standard assays. In patients using these medications, only TSH measurements should be used.

Summary

Screening

- TSH is a sufficient test for screening asymptomatic patients.
- We consider screening for:
  - Women and men older than 35 years every 3 years
  - Women older than 60 years every year
  - Persons with family history of spontaneous hypothyroidism and who are older than 35 years once a year
  - Patients with personal history of another autoimmune disease once a year
  - Routine screening of women planning pregnancy is not recommended
- TSH and thyroid hormone levels (preferably free thyroid hormone) should be ordered in all patients suspected to have thyroid disorder and in pregnant women.

Treatment

- We recommend treatment with T_4 with goal TSH below 3.0.
- If symptoms are still present, it is acceptable to increase T_4 dose to achieve TSH below 2.0.
- We advise against routine treatment of subclinical hyperthyroidism.
- We use antithyroid medications to treat patients with persistent subclinical hyperthyroidism and symptoms that are consistent with hyperthyroidism. If symptoms improve, definite treatment is instituted.[9]
- We treat patients with TSH higher than 5.0 µU/mL if anti-TPO antibodies are positive or if symptoms of hypothyroidism are present. We reassess symptoms in 2 and 6 months and stop treatment if there is no improvement.[9]
- We do not routinely use combination T_4/T_3 therapy or preparations derived from animal thyroid glands. Patients desiring these therapies should be referred to an endocrinologist.

Suggested Readings

American Association of Clinical Endocrinologists: Medical guidelines for clinical practice for the evaluation and treatment of hyperthyroidism and hypothyroidism. Endocrine Practice 2002;8(6):457-469.

Benbassat C, Mechlis-Frish S, Cohen M, Blum I: Amiodarone-induced thyrotoxicosis type 2: A case report and review of the literature. Am J Med Sci 2000;320(4):288-291.

Biondi B, Klein I: Hypothyroidism as a risk factor for cardiovascular disease. Endocrine 2004;24(1):1-13.

Canaris G, Manowitz N, Mayor G, Ridgway E: The Colorado thyroid disease prevalence study. Arch Intern Med 2000;160(4):526-534.

Cooper D: Antithyroid drugs. N Engl J Med 2005;352(9):905-917.

Gharib H, Tuttle RM, Baskin HJ, et al: Subclinical thyroid dysfunction: A joint statement on management from the American Association of Clinical Endocrinologists, the American Thyroid Association, and the Endocrine Society. J Clin Endocrinol Metab 2005;90(1):581-585.

Glinoer D: The regulation of thyroid function during normal pregnancy: Importance of the iodine nutrition status. Best Pract Res Clin Endocrinol Metab 2004;18(2):133-152.

Hollowell J, Staehling N, Flanders W, et al: Serum TSH, T_4, and thyroid antibodies in the United States population (1988 to 1994): National Health and Nutrition Examination Survey (NHANES III). J Clin Endocrinol Metab 2002;87(2):489-499.

Sawka A, Gerstein H, Marriott M, et al: Does a combination regimen of thyroxine (T_4) and 3,5,3′-triiodothyronine improve depressive symptoms better than T_4 alone in patients with hypothyroidism? Results of a double-blind, randomized, controlled trial. J Clin Endocrinol Metab 2003;88(10):4551-4555.

References

For a complete list of references, log onto www.expertconsult.com.

Section 5

GASTROENTEROLOGY

Structural Disorders of the Esophagus

Edgar Achkar

Dysphagia, a common symptom in those with esophageal disorders, can arise from a multitude of underlying causes. Dysphagia, or difficulty swallowing, refers to a sensation of impairment of the normal progression of the bolus from the mouth into the stomach. Dysphagia should be distinguished from odynophagia or pain on swallowing. Recognizing dysphagia and gauging its clinical significance appear simple. There are, however, several important points that may be brought up with the following questions:

- Is the patient truly complaining of dysphagia? In most cases, patients can clearly express symptoms of difficulty in swallowing. Alternative terms, such as *food sticking* or *food moving down slowly into the chest* can assist in identifying those with dysphagia.
- Is the dysphagia for solids, liquids, or both? Mucosal lesions, benign or malignant, that produce a narrowing of the esophageal lumen do not usually interfere with the passage of liquid substances, and dysphagia is limited to solid foods. On the other hand, disorders impairing esophageal peristalsis cause difficulty with both solids and liquids.
- Is the dysphagia intermittent or progressive? Structural lesions of the lower esophagus, such as rings and strictures, produce intermittent obstruction related to the size of the bolus, often with prolonged periods free of symptoms. In motor disorders, on the other hand, dysphagia is insidious and becomes progressively worse.

The proper clinical evaluation of dysphagia requires a detailed history.[1] Several diagnostic techniques are available; their use depends on the manifesting clinical features. The initial test, however, is often a barium swallow or an endoscopic examination. The choice between these two techniques—determining which is more useful and less costly for evaluating dysphagia—has been the subject of debate. In a patient who presents with intermittent solid dysphagia, suggesting a benign obstructing lesion such as a peptic stricture or ring, starting with endoscopy is reasonable, because it allows making the diagnosis and simultaneously treating the lesion by dilation. In cases of dysphagia to both solids and liquids and suspicion of a motor disorder, a barium swallow provides more useful information by evaluating esophageal peristalsis. The guidelines of the American Gastroenterological Association (AGA) have supported the choice of barium swallow in these cases, a recommendation with which most clinicians would agree.[2]

Various known causes of esophageal disorders may be classified into four different groups: disorders caused by mucosal injury, neoplastic disorders, esophageal lumen anomalies, and motor disorders.

DISORDERS CAUSED BY MUCOSAL INJURY

Definition

Mucosal injury is defined as mucosal damage resulting from an intrinsic or extrinsic agent capable of disrupting the integrity of the mucosa, leading to acute inflammation and potentially chronic inflammation, with possible permanent scarring. The most common syndromes of mucosal injuries are gastroesophageal reflux disease (GERD), infectious esophagitis, radiation esophagitis, esophagitis caused by caustic ingestion, pill esophagitis, and eosinophilic esophagitis. GERD disease is discussed in detail elsewhere in this section ("Acid Peptic Disorders").

Prevalence

Although GERD is prevalent, causing symptoms in 20% of the population at least once a week, other causes of mucosal injury are less common.

Infectious esophagitis is rare in normal persons. In an immunocompromised patient, infection occurs today at a lesser rate than in the past because of better diagnostic and therapeutic techniques. *Candida* is the organism most often responsible for causing esophagitis. Radiation esophagitis is reported by some patients during treatment, but long-term lesions occur infrequently.

Caustic ingestions have been reduced dramatically since protection laws have been instituted. It is estimated that 5000 cases per year occur in the United States. The prevalence of pill-induced esophagitis is unknown. An increasing number of cases are reported, but these are few compared with the innumerable pills ingested by the public.

Eosinophilic esophagitis has gained recognition in the last few years either because of rising prevalence or increased awareness. It was originally described in children and young men, but more recent reports have involved all age groups.[3]

Pathophysiology

Almost all mucosal injuries are accompanied by inflammation with varying degrees of severity, including inflammation resulting from erythema, frank ulcers with potential scarring and bleeding, and strictures.

Infectious esophagitis occurs almost always in immunocompromised patients, such as post-transplantation patients or those with cancer or AIDS. Predisposing factors include diabetes, alcoholism, malnutrition, and older age, as well as treatment with corticosteroids. Diseases leading to stasis, such as achalasia, can also predispose to some infections.

Radiation esophagitis occurs with radiation therapy to the chest and mediastinum. It is dependent on the total dose administered and the duration of treatment. Injury by caustic ingestion is most commonly caused by alkali agents producing burns or by acidic agents producing necrosis.

Pill esophagitis was first reported with tetracycline. Doxycline and other tetracyclines account for most cases, but injuries have been reported with other antibiotics, antiviral agents, nonsteroidal anti-inflammatory drugs, potassium preparations, and many other medications.[4] There is some evidence that sustained-release medications are more commonly associated with injury. The lesion occurs most often between the junction of the proximal and midesophagus at the point of impression by the aortic arch or above the esophagogastric junction.

Eosinophilic esophagitis is characterized by intense infiltration of eosinophils in the esophagus. An allergic reaction secondary to prior sensitization to food or an airborne agent is invoked as a potential pathophysiologic mechanism.

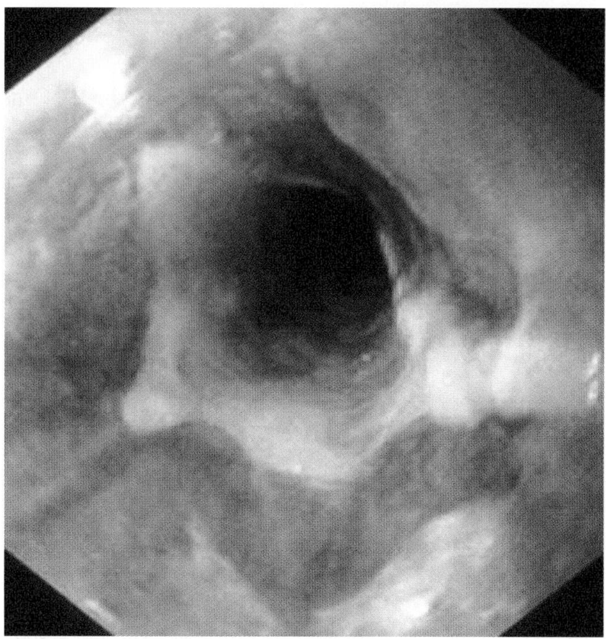

Figure 1 ***Candida esophagitis.*** Endoscopy shows white exudates.

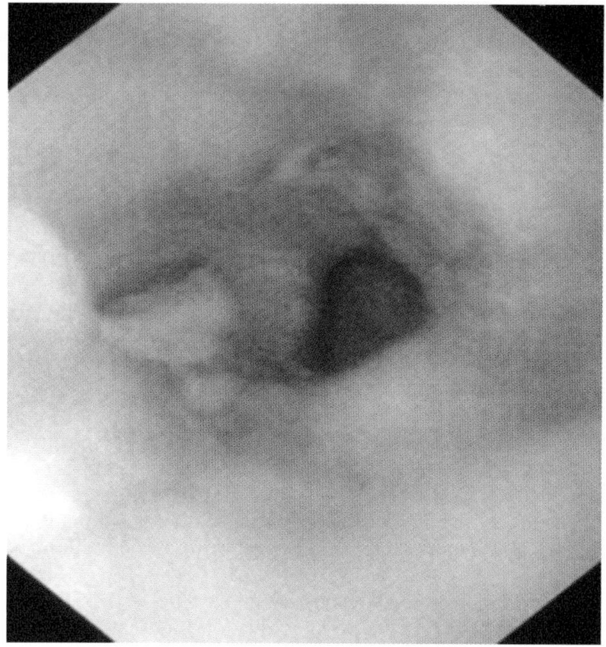

Figure 2 **Esophageal ulcer caused by medication (pill ulcer).** The ulcer is well demarcated and has clear edges.

Signs and Symptoms

Mucosal injury may be asymptomatic or may be manifested by dysphagia, odynophagia, or chest pain. Patients whose nutrition may already be affected by their immunocompromised status and anorexia are further jeopardized by their inability to eat.

Candida esophagitis is often asymptomatic and is discovered at endoscopy. Pill injury is accompanied by sudden onset of severe pain over 1 to 3 days. Pain is aggravated by eating.

Eosinophilic esophagitis is manifested by dysphagia, food impaction, and chest pain. Although the condition is seen at all ages, it should be particularly suspected in young adults with dysphagia or chest pain.

Diagnosis

The diagnosis of mucosal injury is suspected based on the patient's background and is established by a barium swallow but more precisely by endoscopy.[5]

Candida esophagitis shows typical white plaques scattered throughout the esophagus (Fig. 1). Viral infections caused by herpes simplex virus or cytomegalovirus (CMV) reveal focal or disseminated ulcers; the diagnosis is established by biopsy and special stains. About 40% of ulcers seen in patients with AIDS are not caused by a specific infection and are termed *idiopathic ulcers*. They are typically large and deep.

Radiation esophagitis is characterized by erythema and friability during the acute stages and by strictures in the late stages. Caustic ingestion is rare in the adult population and is almost always caused by suicidal attempts. Endoscopy is relatively contraindicated in the acute stages. Pill-induced esophagitis causes a typical discreet ulcer, surrounded by a normal-appearing surrounding mucosa (Fig. 2).

In eosinophilic esophagitis, endoscopy reveals multiple concentric rings or furrows (Fig. 3), but it appears normal in many cases. Barium swallow shows a narrow esophageal lumen. The diagnosis is based on the presence of 15 or more eosinophils per high-power field on esophageal biopsies.

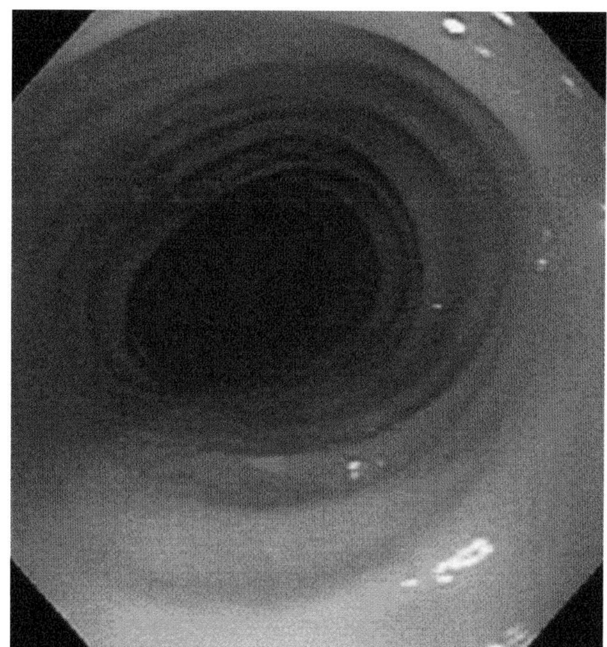

Figure 3 **Eosinophilic esophagitis.** Endoscopy reveals multiple concentric rings or furrows.

Treatment and Outcomes

The treatment of infectious esophagitis depends on isolating the causative agent. In immunocompromised patients, multiple infections can coexist. *Candida* esophagitis is best treated with ketoconazole 200 to 400 mg/day or with fluconazole 100 mg/day for 7 to 14 days. Nystatin in an oral solution may be effective for mild cases and in the absence of immunodeficiency. Viral infections respond somewhat to antiviral agents. Idiopathic ulcers of AIDS are treated with prednisone 40 mg/day, with tapering over 4 weeks by 10 mg/week,[6] or thalidomide 200 to 300 mg/day for 4 weeks. The potential risk of birth defects limits the use of thalidomide.

In pill injury, the offending medication should be withdrawn and antireflux therapy prescribed to prevent exacerbation of the injury. When odynophagia is pronounced, topical anesthetic agents administered orally might help relieve the pain. In most cases, symptoms disappear within a few days, and bleeding and perforation are rare. More importantly, pill injury should be prevented by encouraging patients to drink large amounts of fluid with their pills, to remain upright for 30 minutes after taking the pills, and to avoid pills known to cause frequent injury, particularly in patients who have esophageal strictures or who are bedridden. These preventive measures are very important in older patients, who tend to take multiple medications, particularly at bedtime.[5]

Eosinophilic esophagitis is treated by some with proton pump inhibitors. Periodic dilations are necessary to relieve dysphagia and are effective albeit somewhat riskier than for peptic strictures. Inhaled corticosteroids are used and give temporary relief. Oral steroids have also been used. In children, allergy testing and food elimination are effective. New reports show some benefit from good elimination in adults.

Chronic lesions caused by mucosal injury often lead to strictures. Strictures are managed by periodic dilations and antireflux treatment. In GERD, the use of potent acid-suppressing agents has reduced the frequency with which dilation needs to be performed.

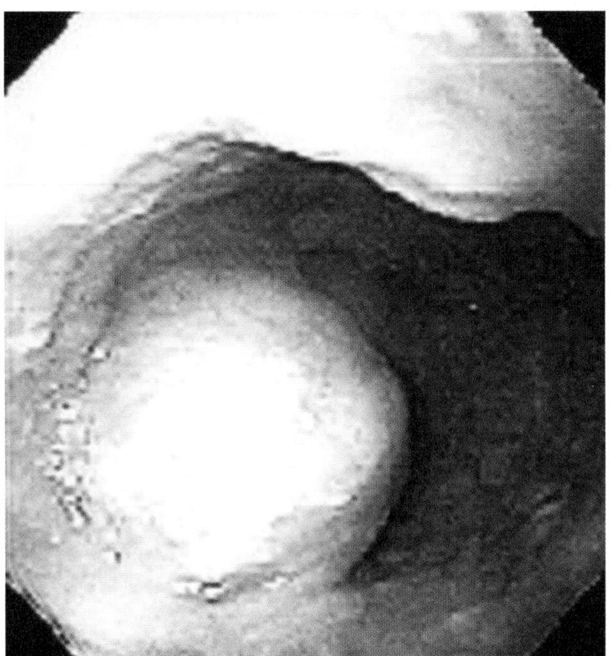

Figure 4 Leiomyoma of the midesophagus. The tumor is covered by normal mucosa.

NEOPLASTIC DISORDERS

Benign Tumors

Benign esophageal tumors are nonmalignant neoplasms arising from the mucosal or muscular layers of the esophagus. Benign tumors of the esophagus are rare. Leiomyoma, the most common, has been described in 5% of autopsy specimens. Benign tumors are classified as mucosal or intramural. *Mucosal tumors* tend to produce a filling defect in the lumen; they include fibrovascular polyps, granular cell tumors, papillomas, and lipomas. *Intramural lesions,* such as leiomyomas and cysts, are more common than mucosal tumors. They produce an extrinsic mass projecting from the wall into the lumen.

Signs and Symptoms

Most benign tumors of the esophagus are asymptomatic and are discovered by chance during an examination done for other reasons. When symptomatic, benign tumors cause mostly dysphagia and, in some cases, chest pain and regurgitation. The most important issue is to differentiate them from malignant tumors.

Diagnosis

A barium swallow often determines if the lesion is intramural or mucosal. Endoscopy is usually helpful in determining the tumor's nature (Fig. 4). Some polyps appear on a long stalk and may be seen flopping into the lumen. Endoscopic examination reveals intramural tumors as smooth protrusions covered by normal mucosa. Cysts appear round and smooth. Mucosal lesions sometimes ulcerate. Endoscopic ultrasound is helpful in distinguishing a leiomyoma from a leiomyosarcoma. Unfortunately, when the tumor is large, the differentiation is more difficult.

Treatment and Outcomes

Small asymptomatic lesions require no treatment. Surgical enucleation is the treatment of choice for symptomatic intramural lesions or when intervention is necessary because malignancy cannot be definitively ruled out. Polyps are treated with local resection.

Malignant Tumors

Definition and Classification

Malignant tumors of the esophagus constitute most esophageal tumors. Different types of tumors have been described, such as squamous cell carcinoma, adenocarcinoma, sarcoma, lymphoma, primary melanoma, and metastatic tumors (e.g., breast, lung, melanoma).

Squamous cell carcinoma and adenocarcinoma represent the largest number of esophageal malignancies.[7] About 13,000 cases per year of esophageal cancer are diagnosed in the United States. Squamous cell carcinoma used to account for most malignancies, but the incidence of adenocarcinoma has been rising steadily and now accounts for about 50% of all tumors. Squamous cell carcinoma arises from the squamous epithelium and is encountered most commonly in the midesophagus. A smaller number of tumors arise in the distal and upper portions of the esophagus.

Environmental factors seem to play an important role in the genesis of squamous cell carcinoma, with wide geographic variations. Other predisposing factors include alcohol use, tobacco use, long history of achalasia, previous ingestion of caustic agents, and genetic factors.

In the United States, squamous cell carcinoma is more common in African Americans. Adenocarcinoma of the esophagus is increasing in frequency and is more commonly seen in white men.

Most tumors arise in the distal one third of the esophagus. Barrett's esophagus is the major predisposing factor for adenocarcinoma of the esophagus. Tylosis, or hyperkeratosis of the palms and soles, is an autosomal dominant disorder strongly associated with gastrointestinal malignancy, particularly squamous cell carcinoma of the esophagus.

Although there are differences between squamous cell carcinoma and adenocarcinoma in epidemiology, location, and patterns of spread, both diseases tend to spread early outside the esophagus, and both share a poor prognosis unless discovered early. Therefore, efforts are undertaken to detect early signs of cancer or precancer. The ACG guidelines recommend screening for Barrett's esophagus

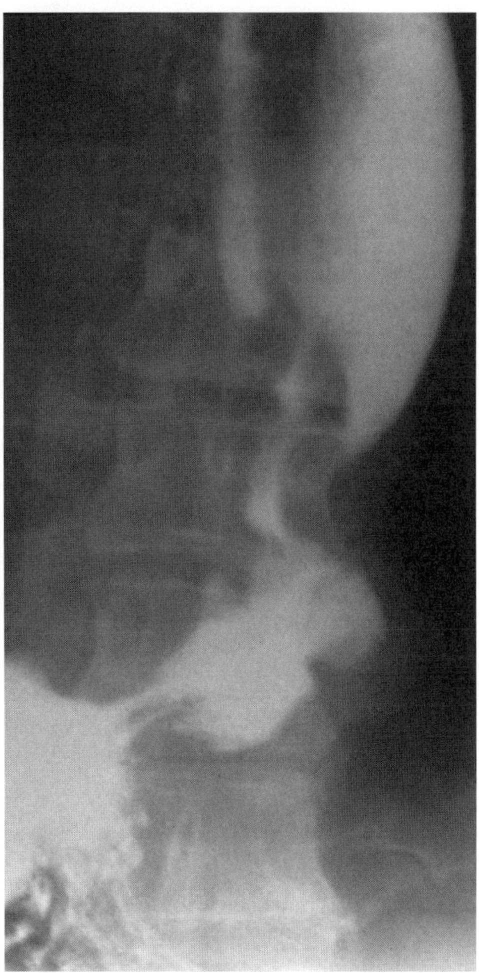

Figure 5 **Carcinoma of the esophagus.** There is a large, irregular filling defect, with proximal dilation.

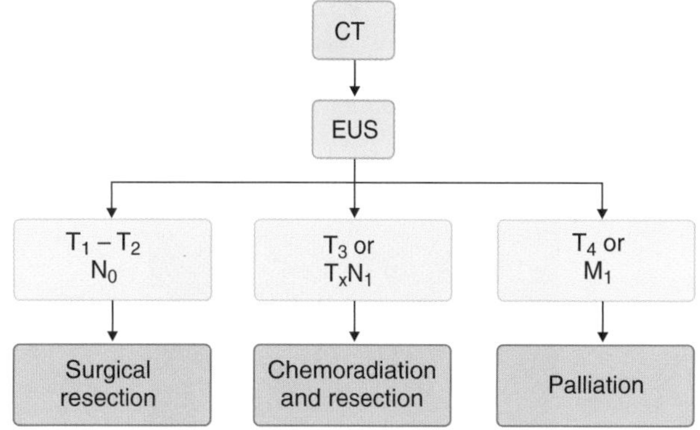

Figure 6 **American Society for Gastrointestinal Endoscopy algorithm for treating esophageal cancer.** CT, computed tomography; EUS, endoscopic ultrasound. *(Adapted from Jacobson BC, Hirota W, Baron TH, et al; Standards of Practice Committee. American Society for Gastrointestinal Endoscopy: The role of endoscopy in the assessment and treatment of esophageal cancer. Gastrointest Endosc 2003;57:817-822.)*

in white men older than 50 years who have long-standing heartburn, although there is no documented impact on mortality from esophageal adenocarcinoma.[8] Screening is not recommended in achalasia.

Signs and Symptoms

The most common clinical manifestation of esophageal tumors is dysphagia, which occurs to solid foods first, then progresses to soft foods and eventually to liquids. Odynophagia is reported in some cases. Chest pain, when present, may be an ominous sign, because it indicates invasion to the mediastinum. Weight loss is common as a result of difficulty swallowing and, in late stages, because of anorexia. Bleeding is rare. The physical examination reveals signs of weight loss. In some cases, supraclavicular nodes may be detected.

Diagnosis

Carcinoma of the esophagus should be suspected in any patient with recent-onset dysphagia, particularly after the age of 50 years. A long history of reflux diseases raises the possibility of carcinoma arising in Barrett's esophagus, especially in white men. The diagnostic modalities used in evaluating malignant neoplasms include barium swallow, endoscopy, computed tomography (CT), endoscopic ultrasound (EUS), and bronchoscopy.

Barium swallow provides an indication of tumor location and size (Fig. 5). Endoscopy determines the size of the esophageal lumen. Biopsy and cytologic brushings establish the tumor's histologic type. The central issue, at that point, is the appropriateness of surgical intervention. The decision to operate is based on tumor staging. Both squamous cell carcinoma and adenocarcinoma are staged according to the TNM system (tumor invasion, lymph nodes, and metastasis). EUS is more sensitive than CT, but a combination of both improves the accuracy of the staging.[9]

The AGA guideline has listed CT scanning as the first staging study and, if no metastases are found, EUS is then recommended.[10]

Treatment and Outcomes

Curative Treatment. When full evaluation reveals a favorable stage and the patient's general condition is not a contraindication to surgery, tumor resection represents the most promising treatment. Surgical resection is indicated when the lesion is considered curable. Combined chemotherapy and radiotherapy, followed by surgery, is offered to patients with local extension. Even in adenocarcinoma, which is less sensitive to chemotherapy and radiotherapy, combined treatment improves prognosis. The best chance of significant survival in esophageal cancer resides in a multidisciplinary approach in institutions possessing good experience in gastroenterology, thoracic surgery, chemotherapy, and radiation oncology. The ASGE guideline[11] has outlined the advantages of and the treatment approach for esophageal cancer with an algorithm (Fig. 6).

Palliative Treatment. When surgery is ruled out because of tumor extension or complications, and in cases of tumor recurrence, several palliative methods are available. Esophageal cancer is often diagnosed at an advanced incurable stage; when patients present with dysphagia, 50% of the lumen may already be occluded. Palliation methods include radiotherapy and the following endoscopic modalities: periodic dilation, esophageal stenting, photodynamic ablation, laser ablation, and endoscopic mucosal resection.

Endoscopic techniques have varying rates of success, and all carry a risk of complications, including perforation, infection, and bleeding, as well as worsening of the initial symptoms. In late stages and in patients whose dysphagia is insurmountable, insertion of a gastrostomy feeding tube is often necessary.

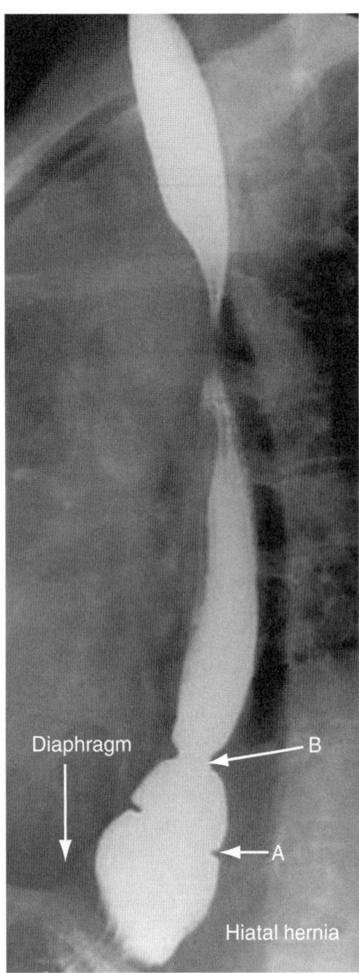

Figure 7 **Esophageal hiatal hernia.** A rings (mucosal rings, also known as Schatzki's rings) and B rings can be seen.

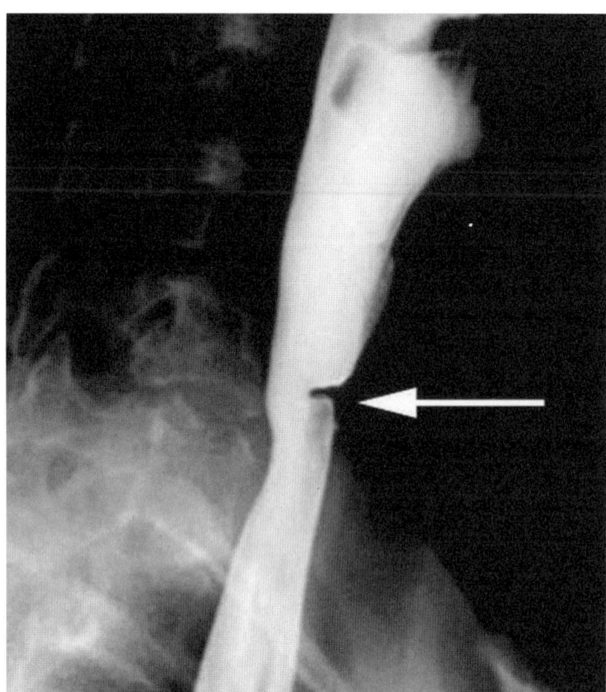

Figure 8 **Esophageal web.** The indentation is anterior *(arrow)*.

ESOPHAGEAL LUMEN ANOMALIES

Rings and Webs

Definition

The definition of webs and rings is confusing because the terms have been used interchangeably. A web is a thin membrane occupying part of the esophageal lumen and is most commonly seen on the anterior aspect of the area just below the cricopharynx. Rings are concentric narrowings of the lumen and are usually seen in the lower esophagus. The B ring, or muscular ring, occurs at the junction of the tubular portion of the esophagus and the most distal part, the vestibule. The ring is often described by radiologists but is rarely symptomatic. The A ring, or mucosal ring, occurs most distally at the esophagogastric junction and usually occurs in association with a hiatal hernia. Also known as Schatzki's ring,[12] it deserves particular attention because it is often symptomatic (Fig. 7).

Prevalence

Both webs and rings are frequently seen during radiologic or endoscopic examination. It is estimated that webs are present in 0.5% to 1% of asymptomatic people. Lower esophageal rings are found in 10% to 15% of barium swallow studies. Currently, it is not known how many are symptomatic.

Pathophysiology

The exact nature of webs is unknown. It is believed that webs result from an anomaly of development in the epithelium of the upper esophagus.

Schatzki's ring consists of esophageal mucosa and submucosa. This ring is almost always associated with a hiatal hernia. Although it is histologically and probably pathogenetically different from esophageal peptic strictures, the association of a lower esophageal ring with gastroesophageal reflux occurs commonly. In addition, distinguishing one from the other endoscopically is sometimes difficult. Therefore, many clinicians manage esophageal rings as they do strictures. The Plummer-Vinson and Paterson-Kelly syndromes refer to the association of webs with iron deficiency anemia and other oropharyngeal abnormalities. These associations are rarely described today, and the terms have largely been abandoned.

Signs and Symptoms

When a cricopharyngeal web or ring causes difficulty, the patient presents with dysphagia. In the case of a web, the dysphagia is oropharyngeal, is associated with solid foods, and is rarely severe. The dysphagia associated with a lower esophageal ring is intermittent, occurring with solid foods (particularly meat), with occasional impaction. It was formerly referred to, in the old literature, as the "steakhouse syndrome."

Diagnosis

Barium x-ray is the most sensitive method to detect webs and rings. Webs should not be confused with the normal impression of the cricopharynx. On x-ray, a web is seen as an indentation on the anterior aspect of the pharynx (Fig. 8). The diagnostic yield for a ring is higher when a solid bolus is given during the test. Endoscopic examination is less sensitive in detecting subtle rings, particularly with the use of the newer thin endoscopes, which may pass through the ring without the endoscopist's seeing the luminal narrowing.

Treatment and Outcomes

Most webs do not require treatment. When they are symptomatic, however, endoscopic dilation is useful but has to be performed with caution by an experienced operator. Lower esophageal rings are treated easily with dilation by bougies or over a guidewire. The response to treatment is generally good in most patients. There is a small risk of perforation. An acid-suppressing agent is usually prescribed.

Diverticula

Definition

An esophageal diverticulum is a sac protruding from the esophageal wall that contains all layers of the esophagus. Esophageal diverticula may be congenital or acquired. The simplest way to classify them is according to anatomy: Zenker's diverticula, midesophageal diverticula, epiphrenic diverticula, and intramural pseudodiverticulosis.

Prevalence

Esophageal diverticula have been described in all age groups but are most commonly seen in adults. They are rare, occurring in less than 1% of upper gastrointestinal x-rays and accounting for less than 5% of dysphagia cases.[13]

Pathophysiology

Zenker's diverticulum, or pharyngoesophageal diverticulum, occurs in a location proximal to the esophagus, above the upper esophageal sphincter. The diverticulum bulges posteriorly and its size increases over time. The most widely accepted mechanism for a Zenker's diverticulum is a functional disturbance of the hypopharynx. The most popular explanation is an incoordination between the pharynx and the cricopharyngeus muscle, termed *cricopharyngeal achalasia*. Most recent evidence, however, has suggested that the diverticulum occurs because of reduced compliance of the upper sphincter, rather than because of incoordination.[14]

Midesophageal diverticula have been classified as traction or pulsion diverticula. This distinction has no practical value. The exact cause of a midesophageal diverticulum is not known, but the condition has been associated with scarring and various esophageal motor abnormalities.

Epiphrenic diverticula are almost always the result of an esophageal motor abnormality, namely an incoordination between the distal esophagus and lower esophageal sphincter.[15]

Esophageal intramural pseudodiverticulosis is characterized by numerous, minute, flasklike outpouchings along the esophageal wall.[16] They can be segmental or generalized and are associated with strictures, carcinoma, candidiasis, and motor abnormalities (Fig. 9).

Signs and Symptoms

Many esophageal diverticula are discovered by chance during radiologic evaluation. In early stages of Zenker's diverticulum, the patient might complain of vague throat irritation and, when the sac becomes large, more severe symptoms develop, particularly dysphagia, regurgitation of food ingested several hours earlier, and gurgling sounds on swallowing. Complications of Zenker's diverticulum, such as bleeding, obstruction, or fistulization, are rare. Midesophageal diverticula are often asymptomatic unless they become so large that food becomes trapped in the pouch. For epiphrenic diverticula, the severity of symptoms depends on the associated motor abnormality. The conditions most commonly associated with such diverticula are achalasia and diffuse spasm.

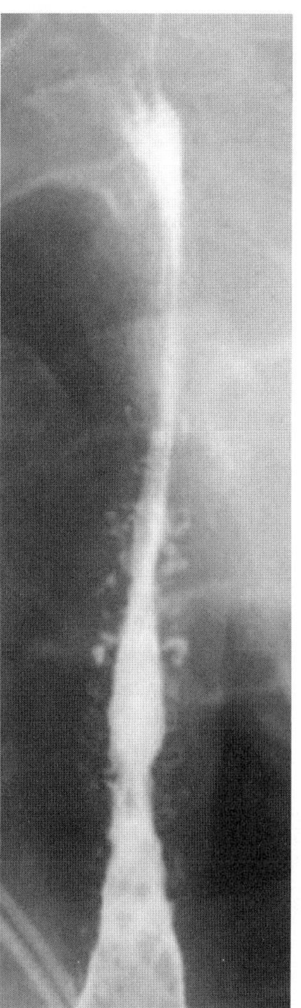

Figure 9 Segmental intramural pseudodiverticulosis.

Diagnosis

A barium esophagram with special attention to the oropharyngeal phase of swallowing is the best diagnostic test for Zenker's diverticulum. The diverticulum is seen to protrude posteriorly and the barium tends to fall into the pouch before progressing into the esophagus (Fig. 10). Endoscopy adds little to the evaluation of Zenker's diverticulum. Manometric testing of upper esophageal function is not clinically useful. Midesophageal (Fig. 11) and epiphrenic diverticula (Fig. 12) are best diagnosed by barium swallow, and an associated motor disorder is usually suspected when these are found.

Treatment and Outcomes

Symptomatic Zenker's diverticula can be treated by surgical excision. Newer treatments are applied endoscopically. A transection is made to create a communication between the diverticulum and the esophagus, allowing the diverticulum to drain into the esophagus. This technique can be carried out with or without the assistance of laser.[17,18] Most surgeons agree that whatever the surgical technique, a myotomy of the cricopharyngeus muscle is necessary to prevent recurrence of the diverticulum. Midesophageal diverticula are treated by surgical excision. For an epiphrenic diverticulum, the goal of therapy should be to treat the underlying motor disorder, with the hope of preventing further enlargement of the diverticulum. In the absence of achalasia, a long esophagomyotomy is recommended, but published results have involved only a small number of patients.

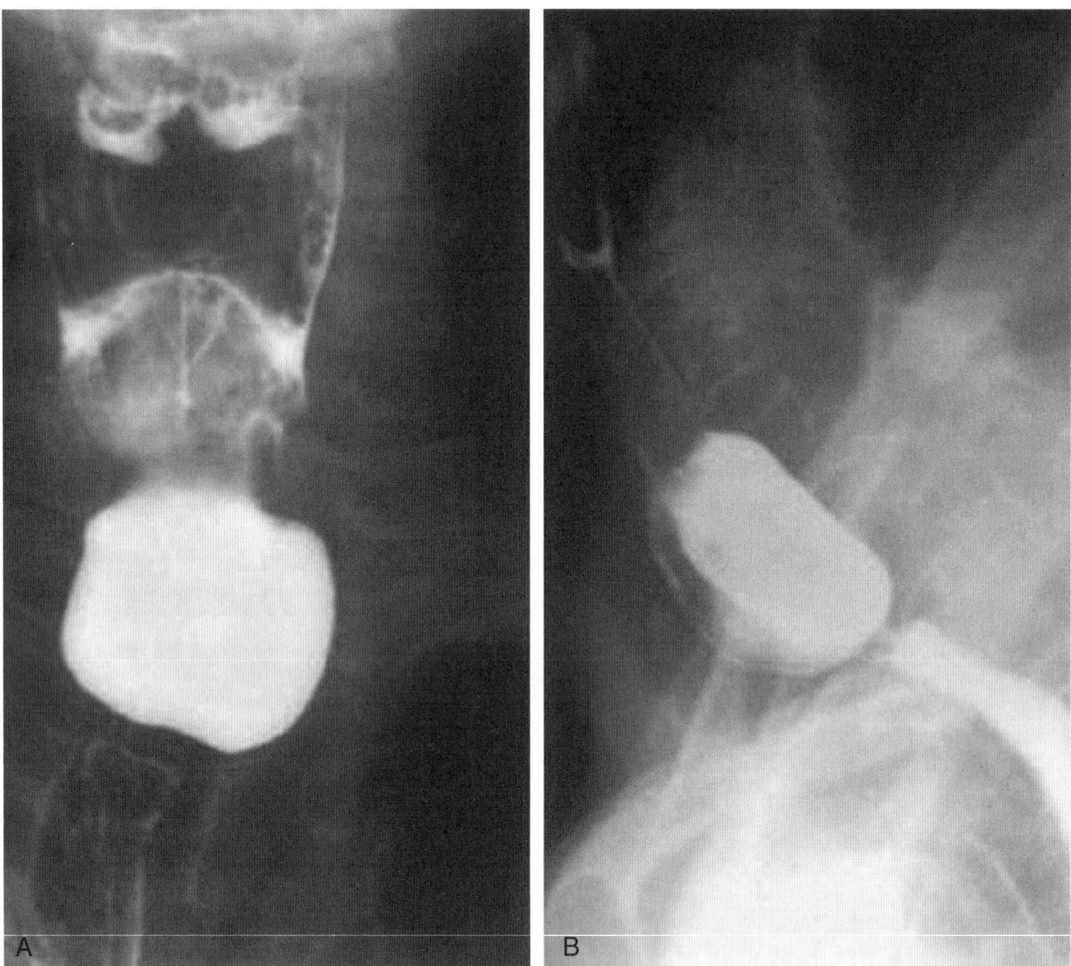

Figure 10 **Zenker's diverticulum.** Anteroposterior (**A**) and lateral (**B**) views show the pouch above the cricopharynx.

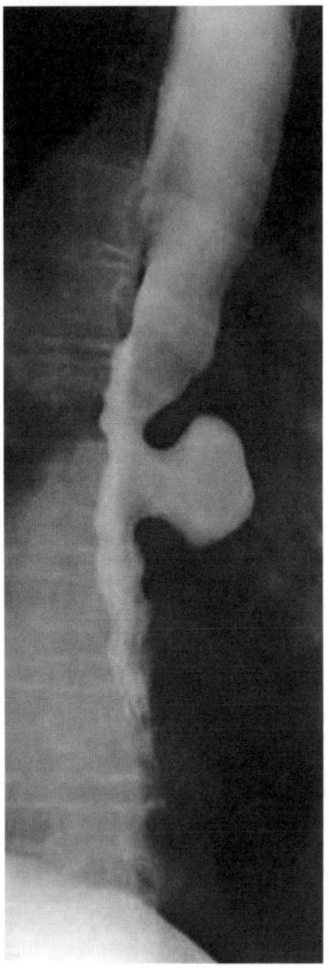

Figure 11 Midesophageal diverticulum.

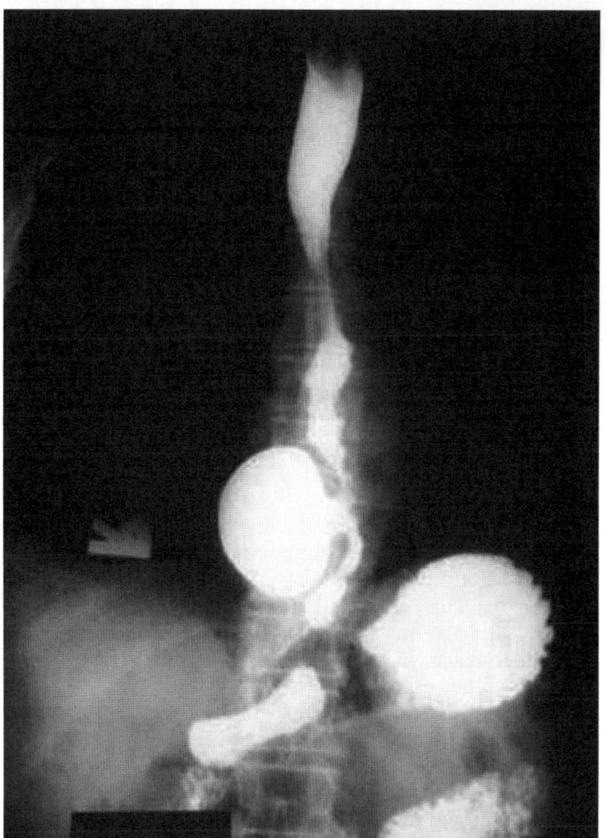

Figure 12 Epiphrenic diverticulum.

Intramural pseudodiverticulosis requires treatment of the underlying infection or obstruction, with dilation in the case of a distinct obstructing area.

Summary

- The most common cause of esophagitis is acid reflux. Other causes include infection, radiation, pills, and eosinophilic esophagitis.
- Eosinophilic esophagitis is a disease of young people, with multiple rings, dysphagia, and, occasionally, history of allergy or asthma.
- *Candida* and other infections tend to occur in immunocompromised patients.
- Cancer of the esophagus tends to spread quickly beyond the esophageal wall.
- Combined chemotherapy and radiation followed by surgery improves survival from esophageal cancer.
- Webs, rings, and diverticula require intervention only if symptomatic.

Suggested Readings

Byrne MF, Jowell PS: Gastrointestinal imaging: Endoscopic ultrasound. Gastroenterology. 2002;122:1631-1648.

Furuta GT, Liacouras CA, Collins MH, et al: Eosinophilic esophagitis in children and Adults: A systematic review and consensus recommendations for diagnosis and treatment. Gastroenterology 2007;133:1342-1363.

Kahrilas PJ, Dodds WF, Dent J, et al: Upper esophageal sphincter function during deglutition. Gastroenterology 1988;95:52-62.

Kikendall JW: Pill-induced injury. In Castell DO, Richter JE (eds): The Esophagus, 4th ed. Philadelphia: Lippincott Williams & Wilkins, 2003, pp 572-584.

Schatzki R: The lower esophageal ring. Long-term follow-up of asymptomatic rings. Am J Roentgenol Radiat Ther Nucl Med 1963;90:805.

Spechler SJ: AGA technical review on treatment of patients with dysphagia caused by benign disorders of the distal esophagus. Gastroenterology 1999;117:233-254.

Spechler SJ: American Gastroenterological Association medical position statement on treatment of patients with dysphagia caused by benign disorders of the distal esophagus. Gastroenterology 1999;117:229-232.

Stoeckli SJ, Schmid S: Endoscopic stapler-assisted diverticuloesophagostomy for Zenker's diverticulum: Patient satisfaction and subjective relief of symptoms. Surgery 2002;131:158-162.

Wang KK, Wongkeesong LM, Buttar NS: American Gastroenterological Associations medical position statement: Role of the gastroenterologist in the management of esophageal carcinoma. Gastroenterology 2005;128:1468-1470.

Zuccaro G Jr: Tumors of the esophagus. In Castell DO, Richter JE (eds): The Esophagus, 4th ed. Philadelphia, Lippincott, Williams, & Wilkins, 2003, pp 275-289.

References

For a complete list of references, log onto www.expertconsult.com.

Motor Disorders of the Esophagus

Edgar Achkar

Dysphagia, a common symptom in those with esophageal disorders, may arise from a multitude of underlying causes. Dysphagia, or difficulty swallowing, refers to a sensation of impairment of the normal progression of the bolus from the mouth into the stomach. Dysphagia should be distinguished from odynophagia or pain on swallowing. Recognizing dysphagia and gauging its clinical significance appears not to difficult. There are, however, several important points that may be brought up by the following questions:

- Is the patient actually complaining of dysphagia? In most cases, patients can clearly express symptoms of difficulty in swallowing. Alternative terms, such as *food sticking* or *food moving down slowly into the chest*, may assist in identifying those with dysphagia.
- Is the dysphagia for solids, liquids, or both? Mucosal lesions, benign or malignant, that produce a narrowing of the esophageal lumen will not usually interfere with the passage of liquid substances, and dysphagia is limited to solid foods. On the other hand, disorders impairing esophageal peristalsis will cause difficulty with both solids and liquids.
- Is the dysphagia intermittent or progressive? Structural lesions of the lower esophagus, such as rings and strictures, produce intermittent obstruction related to the size of the bolus, often with prolonged periods free of symptoms. In motor disorders, on the other hand, dysphagia is insidious and becomes progressively worse.

A proper clinical evaluation of dysphagia requires a detailed history.[1] A number of diagnostic techniques are available and their use depends on the manifesting clinical features. The initial test is often a barium swallow or an endoscopic examination. The choice between these two techniques, as the most useful and least costly for the evaluation of dysphagia, has been the subject of debate. In a patient who presents with intermittent solid dysphagia, suggesting a benign obstructing lesion such as a peptic stricture or ring, starting with endoscopy is reasonable because it allows making the diagnosis and treating the lesion by dilation simultaneously. In cases of dysphagia with solids and liquids and suspicion of a motor disorder, a barium swallow provides more useful information by evaluating esophageal peristalsis. The guidelines of the American Gastroenterological Association (AGA)[2] have supported the choice of barium swallow in these cases, a recommendation with which most clinicians would agree.

Various known causes of esophageal disorders may be classified into four different groups:

1. Disorders caused by mucosal injury
2. Neoplastic disorders
3. Anomalies of esophageal lumen
4. Motor disorders

DEFINITION AND CLASSIFICATION

The term *esophageal motor disorder* or *esophageal motility disorder* is used to describe abnormal esophageal motility patterns found in the process of testing patients with chest pain, dysphagia, or both or in patients being considered for surgical treatment of acid reflux disease. This definition implies the absence of an obstructing lesion of the esophagus. Motility disorders may be caused by an abnormality of the proximal striated muscle portion of the esophagus or of the distal smooth muscle portion. Proximal motor disorders are neurogenic or myogenic in origin, such as disturbances seen after cerebral vascular accidents or in the course of a progressive degenerative muscular disorder. The discussion here will be limited to disorders of the smooth portion of the esophagus, which is responsible for the involuntary phase of swallowing. These diseases may be primary, in which the abnormality is limited to the esophagus, or secondary, in which the esophageal lesion is part of a systemic disorder. Primary disorders include achalasia, diffuse esophageal spasm, nutcracker esophagus, motility changes caused by gastroesophageal reflux disorder (GERD), and nonspecific abnormalities. Secondary disorders include scleroderma, chronic idiopathic intestinal pseudo-obstruction, diabetes, and other systemic disorders.

PRIMARY MOTOR DISORDERS

Prevalence

The exact prevalence of esophageal motor disorders is unknown. In one study, 28% of patients presenting with chest pain were found to have abnormal esophageal motility test results.[1] The annual incidence of achalasia is estimated at 0.4 to 1.2 per 100,000 in the Western world. Diffuse esophageal spasm is found in 2% of patients referred to a motility laboratory. These figures do not reflect the prevalence of any of these disorders in the general population and may indicate that such disorders are generally rare. They are, however, frequent enough to be encountered by every gastroenterologist in his or her practice as well as by general internists who are occasionally faced with these problems.[3]

Pathophysiology

Esophageal motor disorders involve a disturbance of esophageal peristalsis. In the normal state, once the voluntary oropharyngeal phase of swallowing takes place, a well-coordinated peristaltic sequence travels distally toward the lower esophageal sphincter (LES). The orderly succession of contractions from one segment to the next is possible because of a progressively longer latency period to stimulus from one esophageal segment to the next. The LES relaxes almost immediately after relaxation of the upper sphincter, thus providing an open passage in anticipation of the incoming bolus. Both esophageal peristalsis and relaxation of the lower sphincter are mediated by the vagus nerve, but the function is controlled by the intramural plexus of Auerbach.

In achalasia, there is a total loss of peristalsis and the LES relaxes poorly.[4] The disease results from a neurologic deficit in the myenteric plexus. There is a marked decrease in myenteric ganglion cells with marked inflammatory changes.[5] The lower esophageal sphincter dysfunction is caused by the destruction of inhibitory nerve fibers, which normally reduce sphincter tone and control sphincter relaxation. Their absence leads to poor reduction of the sphincter's resting tone. The cause of the disorder is unknown.[6]

In diffuse esophageal spasm, there is intermittent loss of peristalsis, resulting in simultaneous, often repetitive, contractions, but peristalsis is recovered intermittently. LES is usually normal.[7] Severe reflux esophagitis is often accompanied by low LES pressure and decreased distal contraction amplitude. In the nutcracker esophagus, peristalsis is normal but the contraction amplitude is much higher than usual. Duration is also prolonged.[8]

Signs and Symptoms

Dysphagia

The cardinal symptom in esophageal motor disorders is dysphagia. This is most typical of patients with achalasia although, in the early phases, dysphagia may be limited to solids. As the disease progresses, patients avoid meat but continue to report difficulty with leafy vegetables, bread, pastas, and frequently liquids. Symptoms are aggravated by hasty eating or emotional upset. Patients learn to eat slowly and use certain maneuvers, such as arching the back or raising the arms, to ease progression of the food bolus. "Washing foods down" with liquids is often ineffective, and relief is only obtained by belching and regurgitation of undigested food. The process may become so embarrassing that patients avoid eating in public. Patients with motility disorders other than achalasia seem to have less-frequent and less-severe dysphagia.

Chest Pain

When chest pain occurs in a patient with dysphagia and in whom a structural lesion and all causes of esophagitis have been ruled out by x-ray and endoscopy, a motility disorder is suspected. In diffuse esophageal spasm, chest pain varies in frequency, intensity, and location. Patients report some relief with nitroglycerin or calcium channel blockers. In achalasia, chest pain is reported by approximately 50% of patients and is prominent in the early stages of the disease. The pain is retrosternal, may be aggravated by meals, and is occasionally nocturnal. It may be partially relieved by antacids or calcium channel blockers. The pain is significantly less frequent and less severe in older adults than in younger patients.

Recurrent chest pain, in the absence of dysphagia, is a frequent reason for gastroenterologic consultation from internists and cardiologists. Most patients are men, complaining of retrosternal pain, who have had several visits to the emergency department and in whom cardiac disease has been ruled out. The concept of noncardiac chest pain caused by esophageal disease has been exaggerated. The term *esophageal spasm* is often used without any objective evidence; the chest pain has sometimes been attributed to nonspecific motor changes noted on manometry or to the nutcracker esophagus. The most frequent cause of chest pain originating from the esophagus is related to acid reflux. Motor disorders account for less than 30% of cases of chest pain studied in a manometry laboratory.

Heartburn

Heartburn is not characteristic of disturbed esophageal motility. In achalasia, however, patients may complain of retrosternal burning, a symptom caused by food stasis and not by acid reflux. Unfortunately, I have seen many patients treated for a long time for gastroesophageal reflux disease based on the presence of heartburn because no inquiry is made about dysphagia.

Regurgitation

Regurgitation is often seen in patients with achalasia who are unable to facilitate the passage of solid foods by drinking fluids. The food particles are undigested and may be brought up several hours after ingestion.

Weight Loss

Weight loss is rare in esophageal motility disorders. In spite of the struggle associated with eating, weight loss is surprisingly mild or nonexistent in most patients with achalasia. Review of more than 400 of our patients with achalasia seen at the Cleveland Clinic revealed weight loss at the time of presentation in 57% of patients, but it was generally mild. In a few patients, however, weight loss is so prominent that achalasia may be mistaken for anorexia nervosa, particularly in adolescent girls. The issue is complicated by the fact that esophageal motor disorders are common in patients fulfilling the diagnostic criteria for primary anorexia nervosa and because psychiatric symptoms are common in patients with esophageal motor abnormalities. Therefore, in an adolescent girl with weight loss and regurgitation, esophageal motor abnormalities such as achalasia must be ruled out.

Cancer and Achalasia

Achalasia may predispose to squamous cell carcinoma. Indeed, cases of squamous cell carcinoma of the esophagus have been reported in patients with achalasia, perhaps as a result of prolonged stasis, but the review of large series does not indicate a significantly increased risk. Therefore, surveillance endoscopy for cancer screening in achalasia is not recommended (American Society for Gastrointestinal Endoscopy [ASGE] guideline).

Pseudoachalasia is a syndrome simulating achalasia and caused generally by malignant tumors near or at the esophagogastric junction. The clinical, radiologic, and manometric findings are often indistinguishable from those of primary achalasia. Although most cases are seen in older patients with recent-onset dysphagia, the abnormality has been observed in young people.[9] For this reason, all patients with achalasia should undergo endoscopy and any suspicious lesion should be biopsied before definitive treatment is entertained.

Diagnosis

History

The history is of extreme importance in the diagnosis of esophageal motor disorders. As mentioned earlier, patients with motor disorders are often treated for acid reflux or worked up for cardiac disease. In particular, the diagnosis of achalasia is entertained with a high degree of suspicion if a detailed history is obtained.

Physical Examination

The physical examination is usually unremarkable, except in patients who suffer from malnutrition.

Diagnostic Tests

Barium Swallow. When a barium swallow is performed in a patient suspected of esophageal motility disorder, it should be accompanied by a videographic study. A solid bolus such as a barium tablet should always be used. The examiner is able to observe peristaltic abnormalities.

In diffuse esophageal spasm, tertiary contractions produce multiple indentations and pseudodiverticular deformities (Fig. 1). The presence of these changes, however, does not allow the diagnosis of symptomatic spasm without knowledge of associated symptoms. In achalasia, the x-ray reveals a typical smooth tapering of the esophagogastric junction, which has been compared with a bird's beak (Fig. 2). Esophageal peristalsis is abnormal and the passage of both solid and liquid media is delayed. In later stages, the esophagus is dilated and food residue may be present. Large diverticula develop over time and the esophagus becomes tortuous, assuming a sigmoid shape (Fig. 3).

Endoscopy. The upper endoscopic examination is usually normal, unless the motor abnormality is associated with severe reflux disease. The importance of endoscopy in detecting tumors that cause pseudoachalasia has already been mentioned.

Esophageal Manometry. Esophageal manometry is the most specific test for determining the exact nature of the motor abnormality. The test is indicated in cases of dysphagia in which structural lesions have already been ruled out by x-ray or endoscopy. The yield

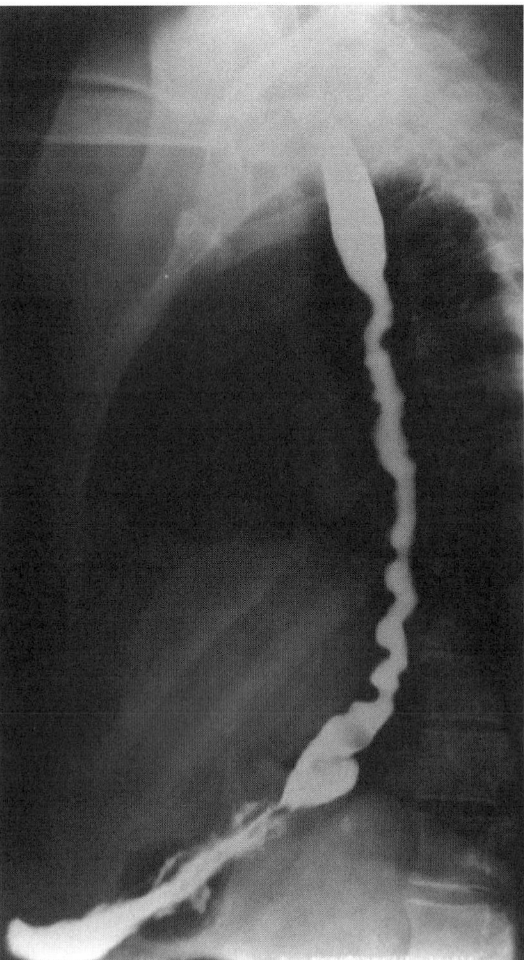

Figure 1 **Diffuse esophageal spasm.** Tertiary contractions.

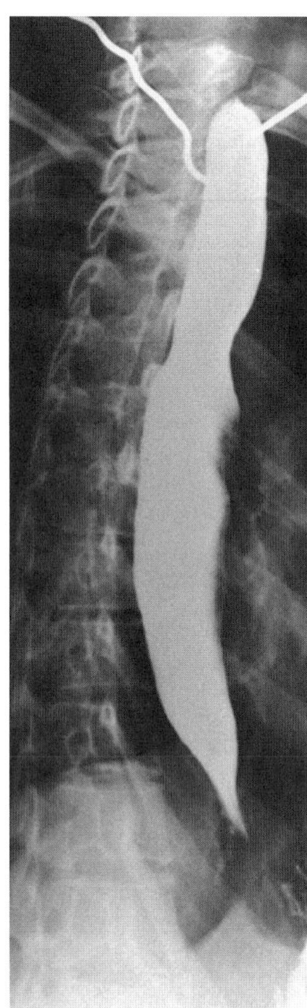

Figure 2 **Achalasia.** Smooth tapering of the gastroesophageal junction (bird's beak).

is very low in patients with noncardiac chest pain without dysphagia. In those cases, prolonged pH monitoring is more useful, because acid reflux causing chest pain is more frequent than disordered peristalsis. AGA guidelines have appropriately outlined the indications for esophageal manometry.[10]

Esophageal manometry is indicated for the following:

- Establishing the diagnosis of achalasia and diffuse spasm
- Detecting motor abnormalities associated with systemic disease if diagnosis or management is affected by the results
- Placing intraluminal devices (pH monitoring)
- Preoperative evaluation of patients considered for antireflux surgery

Esophageal manometry is not indicated for the following:

- As a screening test
- As an initial test for chest pain
- To establish the diagnosis of acid reflux
- To assess the results of antireflux surgery

In normal persons, esophageal motility testing reveals normal progression of the peristaltic wave, with timely relaxation of the lower esophageal sphincter (Fig. 4). In achalasia, LES relaxation is partial and ill-timed and peristalsis is totally absent. In diffuse esophageal spasm, tertiary contractions are seen with alternating normal contractions. The nutcracker esophagus reveals high-amplitude, long-duration contractions. Patients with ineffective motility most often caused by reflux disease show intermittent lack of progression in the distal esophagus and low-amplitude contractions. Other motor abnormalities do not correspond to any clinical syndrome; these are referred to as nonspecific motor changes, a convenient but not clinically relevant category.[11]

Treatment

The treatment of esophageal motor disorders depends on establishing a specific diagnosis. In some patients, numerous investigations do not provide enough information for such a purpose. In those cases, reassurance and advice to eat with caution are generally sufficient. Empirical dilation with bougie dilators is sometimes helpful.

For diffuse esophageal spasm, calcium channel blockers, anticholinergics, and mild sedatives have had varying degrees of success. As already noted, diffuse spasm is a rather rare disorder and symptoms are rarely disabling. A long surgical myotomy is indicated in extremely rare cases in which dysphagia is disabling.

The treatment of achalasia includes several options, although no therapeutic modality can restore muscular activity to the denervated achalasic esophagus. Treatment is therefore limited to reducing the gradient of pressure represented by the lower sphincter. This goal may be accomplished by one of four methods: pharmacologic agents, forceful (pneumatic) dilation, surgical myotomy, or endoscopic injection of botulinum toxin.

Pharmacologic Agents

Long-acting nitrates and calcium channel blockers reduce LES pressure and improve esophageal emptying. However, effective doses can produce

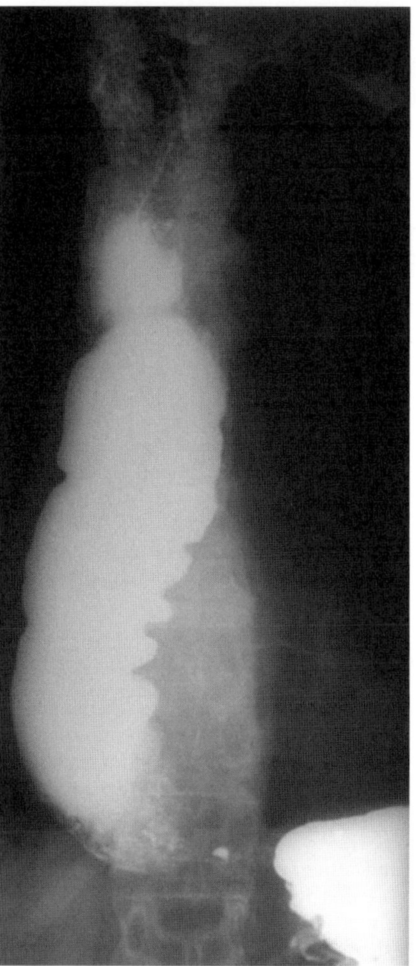

Figure 3 **Advanced achalasia.** The esophagus is dilated and tortuous.

adverse side effects, such as headaches and hypotension, and the drugs tend to become less effective with time. It is recommended that calcium channel blockers be used sublingually to ensure absorption, because delayed passage through the esophagus would retard their effect.

Pneumatic Dilation

Dilation with bougies and small balloons produce brief results. In older and frail patients, periodic bougie dilations offer temporary relief and should not be entirely disregarded. Pneumatic dilation is a forceful disruption of the lower esophageal sphincter using a large balloon capable of achieving high pressures. Most specialists in the United States use the Rigiflex balloon (Fig. 5), which can be passed around a guidewire during endoscopy, is visible under fluoroscopy, and is easy to maneuver. The procedure is carried out with sedation and under fluoroscopy so that the balloon is positioned at the level of the diaphragm. The balloon is inflated until the waist at the gastroesophageal junction disappears. The duration of the distention has varied in different studies, but an inflation time of 30 seconds is reasonable. The patient experiences some chest pain and, on withdrawal of the device, blood streaks are often seen on the balloon. There is a 2% to 6% risk of perforation, which is why a radiologic study is performed immediately after the procedure to rule out perforation; if perforation is present, it requires thoracotomy and surgical repair. The procedure is successful in 65% to 90% of patients. The technique of graded dilation has been advocated by starting with a smaller balloon size of 3 cm and repeating the procedure with larger balloons at later dates. This method is accompanied by a lower initial success rate but seems to reduce the number of complications.

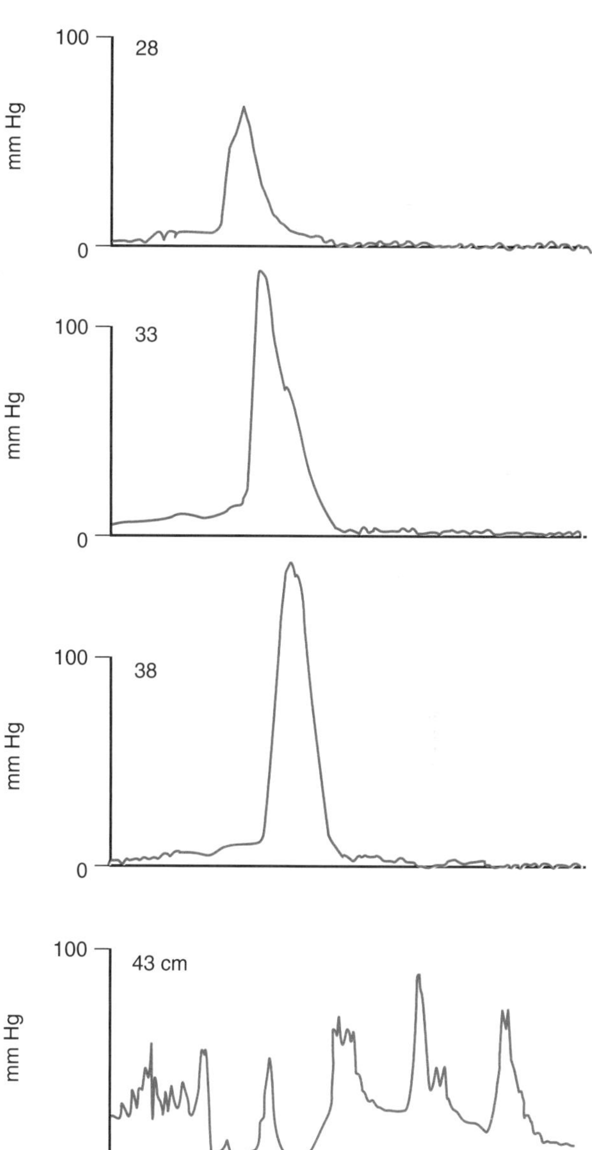

Figure 4 **Normal esophageal motility.** Normal progression of the contraction with relaxation of the lower esophageal sphincter (LES). Recording sites are 5 cm apart (distance from the nares).

Surgical Myotomy

Surgical myotomy, or Heller's myotomy, named for the German surgeon who first performed it in 1914, aims at releasing LES pressure by performing a longitudinal muscular incision that extends above the esophagogastric junction, but not too far distally to avoid acid reflux. There have been few studies comparing pneumatic dilation with Heller's myotomy for the treatment of achalasia.[12,13] Myotomy appears more successful than pneumatic dilation, with success rates of 85% to 95%.

The advent of laparoscopic myotomy, resulting in less morbidity and a shorter hospital stay, has made the procedure much more attractive as an initial treatment option.[14] The choice between pneumatic dilation and surgical myotomy should be made by the patient, with the assistance of his or her physician. The patient should be treated in an institution that offers expertise in both procedures. Failure of pneumatic dilation does not preclude surgical treatment. Some patients have also undergone pneumatic dilation after surgery. The Society for Surgery of the Alimentary Tract (SSAT) has published a guideline on the surgical treatment of achalasia.[15] The recommendations are vague; the required qualifications to perform this type of surgery are based on board certification and eligibility and training and experience.

Botulinum Toxin

Botulinum toxin acts by inhibiting the release of acetylcholine from nerve terminals at the level of the LES.[16] A powder containing 100 U of the toxin is diluted with normal saline and injected during endoscopy in a quadrant fashion at the level of the gastroesophageal junction. Swallowing improves in about 85% of patients, but the effect of the drug wanes with time so that at 6 months, only 50% report improvement. Repeated injections are necessary. The best indication for botulinum toxin is for older patients whose general condition is deemed too risky for pneumatic dilation or surgery, or for patients who refuse both treatment modalities.

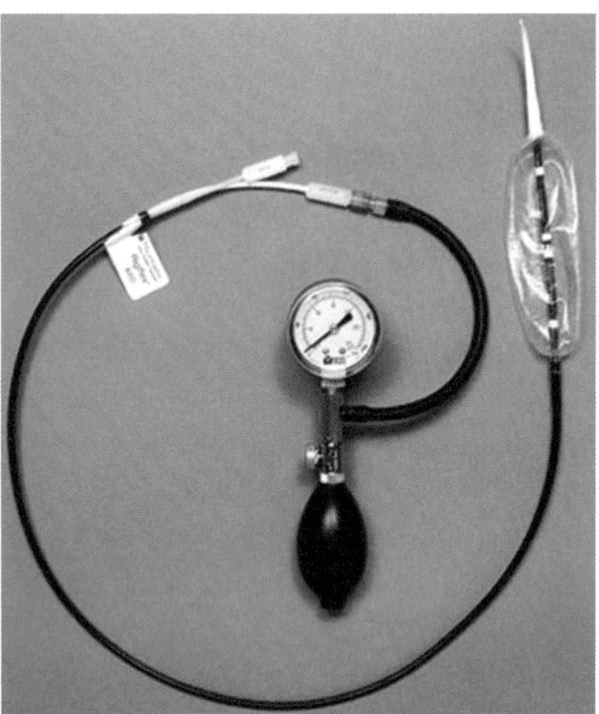

Figure 5 Rigiflex balloon used for pneumatic dilation.

The approach to treatment of patients with achalasia has been summarized in a practice guideline document from the American College of Gastroenterology, which discusses treatment options in great detail and provides a good algorithm for management of achalasia (Fig. 6).[17]

Outcomes

Treatment results and long-term follow-up studies are available only for patients with achalasia. Treatment of achalasia is a lifetime process. Various analyses have been carried out to find predictors of outcome. It appears that younger patients—those 40 years of age or younger—require more aggressive treatment. Young men have generally been shown to have a less favorable response to pneumatic dilation than older men and women.[18]

SECONDARY MOTOR DISORDERS

In those with secondary motor disorders, the esophageal abnormality is secondary to a generalized disorder and other organs in addition to the esophagus are affected. Although esophageal motor changes have been noted in various disorders, the following are the most common: scleroderma, chronic idiopathic pseudo-obstruction, and diabetes.

Diabetes and other systemic diseases produce some changes in esophageal peristalsis but patients are usually asymptomatic. Chronic idiopathic pseudo-obstruction is a diffuse motor disorder of the gastrointestinal tract manifested by recurrent attacks of intestinal obstruction. The study of esophageal function reveals repetitive contractions, segmental loss of peristalsis, and other nonspecific find-

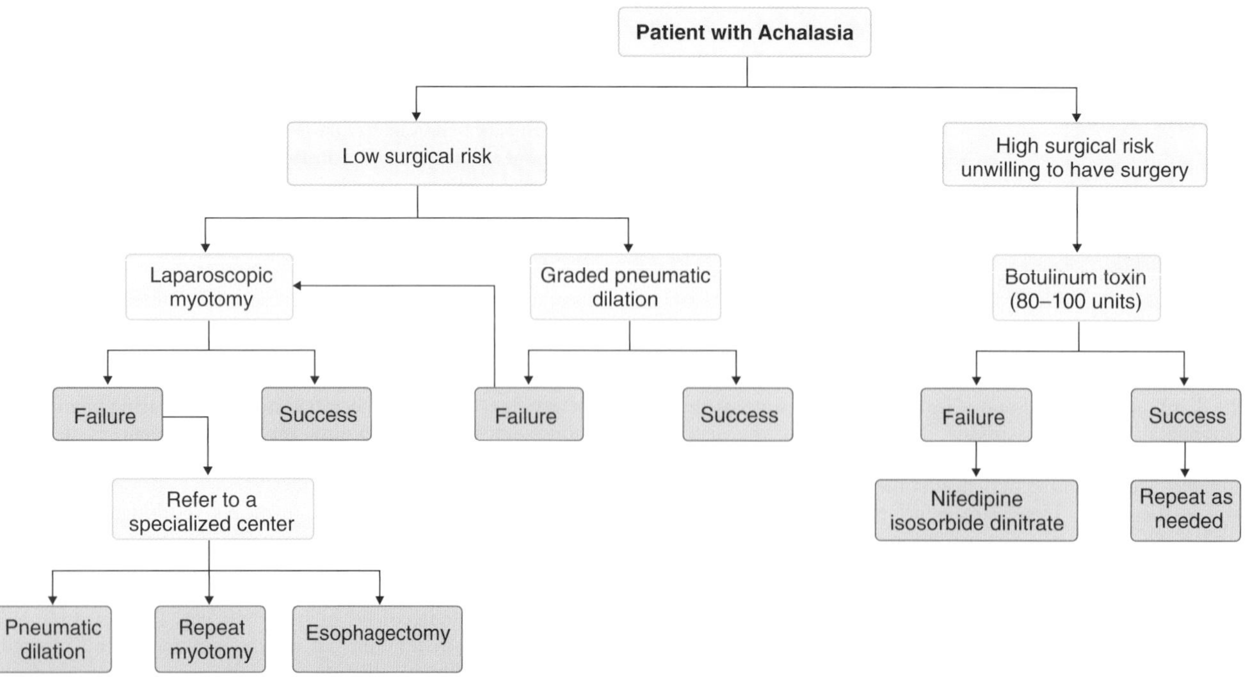

Figure 6 American College of Gastroenterology algorithm for treatment of achalasia. *(Adapted from Vaezi MF, Richter JE: Diagnosis and management of achalasia. American College of Gastroenterology Practice Parameter Committee. Am J Gastroenterol 1999;94:3406-3412.)*

ings. Patients, however, infrequently report esophageal symptoms. An abnormal esophageal manometry test may lead to the diagnosis if the esophagus is affected. A significant motor abnormality is associated most often with progressive systemic cirrhosis or scleroderma.

Scleroderma is a multisystem sclerosing disease affecting most notably the skin, lungs, and esophagus. Of patients with scleroderma, 75% have esophageal involvement but only a fraction have symptoms referring to the esophagus.

Pathogenesis

The esophagus reveals atrophy and sclerosis of the distal smooth muscle with fragmentation of connective tissue. The lower esophageal sphincter is also affected. As a result, normal peristalsis is lost and the lower esophageal sphincter pressure is decreased.

Signs and Symptoms

Patients with scleroderma present with signs of gastroesophageal reflux disease. Dysphagia is not common until a stricture develops. This is probably because the poor peristaltic activity is offset by the reduced lower esophageal sphincter pressure, which enables food to pass through the esophagogastric junction.

Raynaud's phenomenon correlates best with the presence of abnormal esophageal motility, whether skin changes are present or not.

Diagnosis

The barium swallow shows a normal swallowing mechanism in the upper one third of the esophagus but delay in progression of the bolus in the distal part of the esophagus. The lower esophageal sphincter is patent and free reflux is often reported at fluoroscopy. Strictures, may be encountered (Fig. 7). Endoscopy confirms the presence of esophagitis and allows gauging the severity of the inflammation as well as ruling out ulcers and strictures. Esophageal manometry reveals low esophageal sphincter pressure and weak simultaneous contractions in the distal two thirds of the esophagus (Fig. 8). The proximal esophagus may reveal normal contractions, although occasionally the entire esophagus is involved.

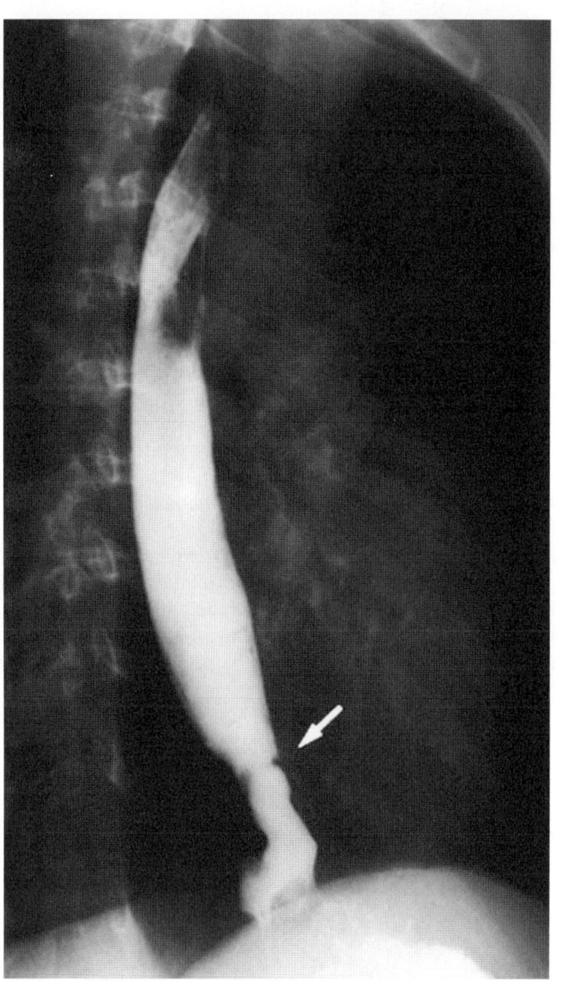

Figure 7 **Scleroderma.** The esophagus is mildly dilated, and a stricture is seen at the gastroesophageal junction proximal to a small bilateral hernia *(arrow).*

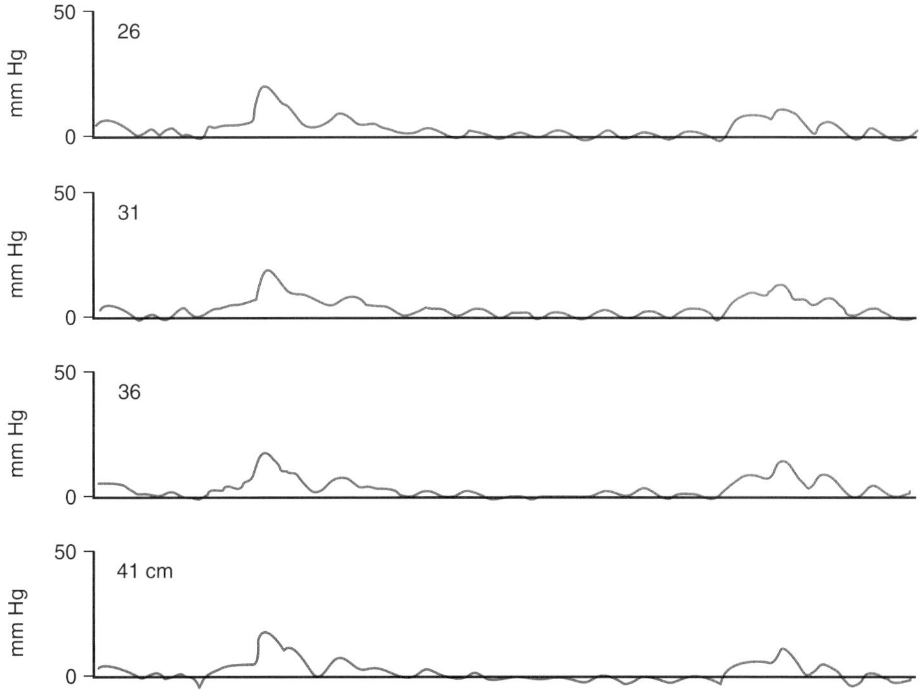

Figure 8 **Scleroderma.** Weak simultaneous contractions occur throughout the esophagus.

Treatment

The treatment of scleroderma is directed to reflux, involving potent acid-suppressing agents and dilation of strictures, when necessary. Strictures tend to be recalcitrant to treatment and frequent dilations are necessary.

Summary

- The differential diagnosis of dysphagia depends primarily on a detailed, carefully obtained history.
- Esophageal motor disorders may be classified as primary (esophagus only involved) or secondary (esophageal abnormality is part of a systemic disease).
- Achalasia is the most common esophageal motor disorder, manifested by dysphagia and chest pain.
- Achalasia may be treated by surgical myotomy or pneumatic dilation. Endoscopic botulinum injection should be reserved for older or high-risk patients.
- In scleroderma, the main clinical issue is acid reflux. Dysphagia does not usually occur until a stricture develops.

Suggested Readings

Achkar E: Achalasia. Gastroenterologist. 1995;3:273-288.

American Gastroenterological Association: An American Gastroenterological Association Medical Position Statement on the clinical use of esophageal manometry. Gastroenterology 1994;107:1865-1884.

Goldblum JR, Whyte RI, Orringer MB, Appelman HD: Achalasia. A morphologic study of 42 resected specimens. Am J Surg Pathol 1994;18:327-337.

Katz PO, Castell JA: Nonachalasia motility disorders. In Castell DO, Richter JE (eds): The Esophagus, 3rd ed. Philadelphia, Lippincott, Williams & Wilkins, 1999, pp 215-234.

Parkman HP, Reynolds JC, Ouyang A, et al: Pneumatic dilitation or esophagomyotomy treatment for idiopathic achalasia: clinical outcomes and cost analysis. Dig Dis Sci 1993;38:75-85.

Pasricha PJ, Ravich WJ, Hendrix TR, et al: Intrasphincteric botulinum toxin for the treatment of achalasia. N Engl J Med. 1995;322:774-778.

Rozman RW Jr, Achkar E: Features distinguishing secondary achalasia from primary achalasia. Am J Gastroenterol 1990;85:1327-1330.

Society for Surgery of the Alimentary Tract: Patient Care Guidelines: Esophageal Achalasia, 2000. Available at http://www.ssat.com/cgi-bin/achalasia.cgi.

Spechler SJ: American Gastroenterological Association medical position statement on treatment of patients with dysphagia caused by benign disorders of the distal esophagus. Gastroenterology 1999;117:229-232.

Vaezi MF, Richter JE: Diagnosis and management of achalasia. American College of Gastroenterology Practice Parameter Committee. Am J Gastroenterol 1999;94:3406-3412.

References

For a complete list of references, log onto www.expertconsult.com.

Acid Peptic Disorders

Mohammed A. Qadeer and Gary W. Falk

Acid peptic disorders include a number of conditions whose pathophysiology is believed to be the result of damage from acid and pepsin activity in the gastric secretions. This chapter focuses on gastroesophageal reflux disease (GERD) and peptic ulcer disease, the two most common and well-defined disease states.

GASTROESOPHAGEAL REFLUX DISEASE

Definition

GERD is defined as chronic symptoms of heartburn, acid regurgitation, or both, or mucosal damage produced by the abnormal reflux of gastric contents into the esophagus.[1] Reflux esophagitis occurs in a subgroup of GERD patients with histopathologically demonstrated characteristic changes in the esophageal mucosa.

Nonerosive reflux disease, also known as endoscopy-negative reflux disease, occurs in patients who have typical GERD symptoms caused by intraesophageal acid but who do not have visible mucosal injury at endoscopy. Functional heartburn is defined as episodic retrosternal burning without evidence of increased esophageal acid exposure or other structural esophageal abnormalities.

Prevalence

GERD is generally considered to be one of the most prevalent conditions affecting the gastrointestinal (GI) tract; however, figures on the precise prevalence and incidence of GERD are based more on estimates than on actual data. A population-based study, using a validated questionnaire, found that 58.7% of the population has heartburn or acid regurgitation at least once during the course of a year and that 19.8% experience symptoms at least once weekly.[2] It is estimated that approximately 50% of patients with typical reflux symptoms have erosive esophagitis (Fig. 1).

Pathophysiology

GERD occurs when the normal antireflux barrier between the stomach and esophagus is impaired, either transiently or permanently. Therefore, defects in the esophagogastric barrier, such as lower esophageal sphincter incompetence, transient lower esophageal sphincter relaxation, and hiatal hernia, are the primary factors involved in the development of GERD. Symptoms develop when the offensive factors in the gastroduodenal contents, such as acid, pepsin, bile acids, and trypsin, overcome several lines of esophageal defense, including esophageal acid clearance and mucosal resistance. As more components of esophageal defense break down, the severity of the reflux increases.

Signs and Symptoms

Classic symptoms of GERD are heartburn, defined as a retrosternal burning discomfort, and acid regurgitation. Symptoms often occur after meals and can increase when a patient is recumbent. Other ancillary symptoms seen in typical reflux are dysphagia, odynophagia, and belching. Atypical GERD symptoms include chest pain, asthma, cough, hoarseness, sore throat, globus, and repetitive throat clearing.

Diagnosis

Although GERD is a common clinical problem, there is no diagnostic gold standard for this disease. Classic symptoms of acid regurgitation and heartburn are specific but not sensitive for the diagnosis of GERD, as determined by abnormal 24-hour pH monitoring. It is reasonable to consider an empirical trial of antisecretory therapy in a patient with classic symptoms of GERD in the absence of alarm signs.[1] Considerable attention has been given to the role of an empirical trial of proton pump inhibitor (PPI) therapy in the diagnosis of GERD. However, recent meta-analyses have shown that successful PPI therapy may be useful in the diagnosis of GERD-related noncardiac chest pain, but it is not very useful in the diagnosis of GERD; the sensitivity and specificity are 0.78 (95% confidence interval [CI], 0.66-0.86) and 0.54 (95% CI, 0.44-0.65), respectively.[3] Endoscopic evaluation should be performed under the following conditions[1]:

- Failure to respond to an empirical course of antisecretory therapy
- Alarm signs suggesting complicated reflux disease (e.g., dysphagia, odynophagia, bleeding, weight loss, anemia)
- Chronic symptoms (>10 years) in a patient at risk for Barrett's esophagus
- Patients requiring chronic antisecretory therapy

Endoscopy is the technique of choice to evaluate the mucosa in patients with symptoms of GERD. Erosions or ulcerations at the squamocolumnar junction, as well as the findings of Barrett's esophagus, are diagnostic of GERD. However, Barrett's epithelium must be confirmed by a biopsy revealing intestinal metaplasia. When mucosal breaks are present, the patient is classified as having erosive esophagitis. The Los Angeles (LA) classification is used to grade the severity of the esophagitis.

Unfortunately, in the absence of mucosal breaks, there is no definitive standard for the diagnosis of GERD. Although ambulatory 24-hour pH monitoring has long been believed to be the most useful for the diagnosis of GERD, this test has limitations that remain underappreciated. Results are normal in 25% of patients with erosive esophagitis and in approximately 33% of patients with nonerosive reflux disease.[4] Nevertheless, 24-hour pH testing is useful to document acid exposure and allows symptoms to be correlated to acid reflux events. Determining how long the pH is lower than 4 (expressed as a percentage of total recording time) is the single most important parameter in these studies. At present, the barium esophagram has no role in the routine evaluation of GERD. This test demonstrates reflux in only 25% to 75% of symptomatic patients and it can yield false-positive results in 20% of normal controls.[5]

Because of the limitations of standard 24-hour pH monitoring, several new diagnostic modalities for GERD are under investigation. These include multichannel intraluminal impedance (MII) and the Bravo pH probe. Impedance uses changes in resistance to alternating current between two metal electrodes to detect the presence of a bolus in the esophageal lumen. When combined with 24-hour pH monitoring, this system allows the detection not only of acid reflux but also of nonacid reflux. The Bravo pH probe is a catheter-free monitoring system in which a pH monitoring probe approximately the size of a medication capsule is placed endoscopically. The pH data are then transmitted to a recording device worn on the patient's waist. In addition to being catheter free, the Bravo system has the advantage of recording 48 hours of pH data. This allows improved evaluation of the relation of symptoms to reflux events.

Treatment and Outcomes

The goals of treatment in GERD are to relieve symptoms, heal esophagitis, prevent recurrence of symptoms, and prevent complications.

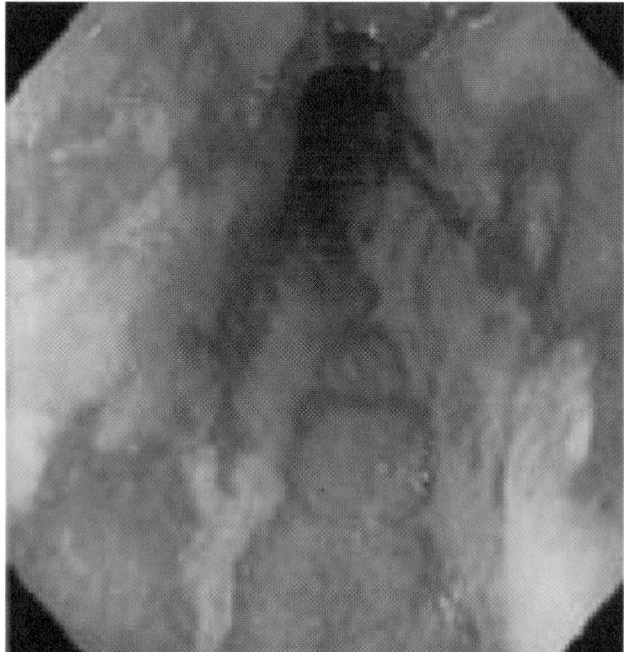

Figure 1 Erosive esophagitis.

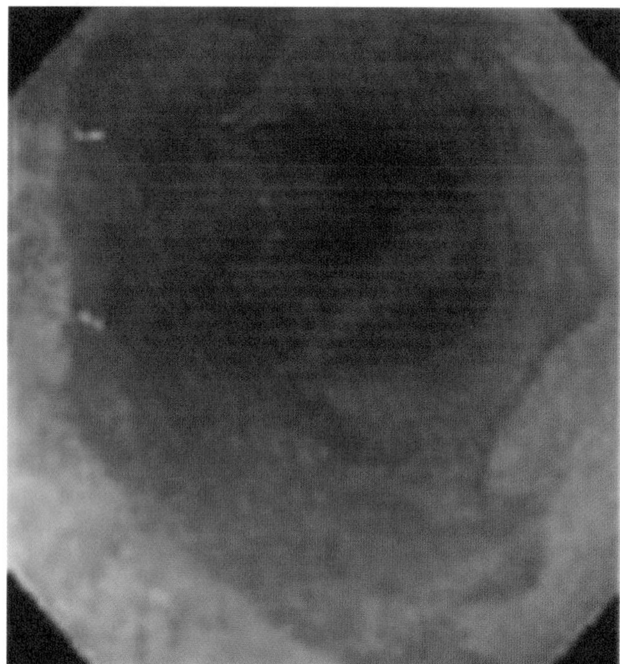

Figure 2 Barrett's esophagus.

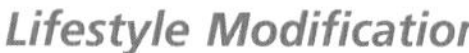

Lifestyle Modification

Various lifestyle modifications are recommended for the treatment of GERD. However, although all these measures make sense physiologically, few data are available in the literature to support them. Lifestyle measures include avoiding precipitating foods (e.g., fatty foods, alcohol, caffeine), avoiding recumbency for 3 hours postprandially, elevating the head of the bed, quitting smoking, and losing weight.[6]

Medication

The cornerstone of GERD therapy is the administration of agents that decrease gastric acid secretion, thereby decreasing esophageal acid exposure.[7] An antacid, which only neutralizes acid that is already secreted, and antirefluxants such as alginates may be used for patient-directed immediate symptom relief, but they are not recommended as chronic therapy. Approximately 20% of patients experience symptom relief with these therapies. Administration of histamine-2 (H_2) receptor antagonists (H_2RAs) in standard divided doses achieves complete symptom relief in approximately 60% of patients and heals esophagitis in about 50%.[7] Doubling the dose does not further improve the response.[8] Over-the-counter H_2RAs are particularly useful when taken before any reflux. The peak potency of antacids and H_2RA is identical, but H_2RAs have a much longer duration of action, up to 10 hours. PPIs are superior to H_2RAs in regard to healing erosive esophagitis and relieving symptoms, with healing rates approaching 90% and symptom relief in 83%.[7]

For most patients, GERD is a chronic relapsing disease with almost universal recurrence of symptoms after treatment withdrawal; thus, it requires maintenance therapy. Long-term therapy with PPIs is again superior to H_2RAs, with remission maintained in 80% compared with 50% of patients, respectively.[9] PPIs should always be given before meals; a single dose may be given in the morning to patients with daytime symptoms and in the evening to those with nighttime symptoms. PPIs are generally well tolerated, with the most common side effects being diarrhea and headache.[10] Observational studies have raised concerns about the possibility of an increased risk of community-acquired pneumonia, *Clostridium difficile* infections, and hip fractures in patients on long-term PPI therapy.[11-13]

Because of their superiority in healing esophagitis and maintaining symptom relief, PPIs are the treatment of choice in patients with frequent reflux symptoms or complications from reflux disease. Dose escalation may be necessary in those rare patients who do not respond to a standard dosing regimen. On the other hand, patients whose GERD is well controlled on PPI therapy may consider step-down therapy to an H_2 receptor blocker.

Surgery

Antireflux surgery, now performed primarily by the laparoscopic approach, remains an option for carefully selected patients with well-documented GERD.[11] The ideal candidate is the patient with typical symptoms who responds completely to antisecretory therapy. Patients in this category who opt for surgery typically have concerns regarding the cost or potential adverse effects associated with long-term PPI therapy. Patients with predominant regurgitation symptoms, which are often nocturnal, are also good candidates. However, because patients refractory to medical therapy are uncommon with the use of high-dose PPI therapy, any consideration of surgery in this group must first document continued evidence of ongoing acid exposure or esophageal damage while PPIs are being used. Evidence indicates that fundoplication works better than low-dose PPIs but in a manner similar to that of high-dose PPIs; however, 10-year follow-up results have indicated that up to 62% of patients initially treated with surgery go back on reflux medications.[1]

Cancer Prevention

Barrett's esophagus (Fig. 2) is a potentially serious complication of chronic GERD. It is present when the normal stratified squamous epithelium of the distal esophagus is replaced by intestinal columnar metaplasia. It is the most significant histologic outcome of long-standing GERD; the odds of developing Barrett's epithelium increase by about sixfold after 10 years of symptoms.[14] It is estimated that 6% to 12% of patients undergoing endoscopy for GERD have Barrett's esophagus.[15] The most dreaded complication of Barrett's epithelium is esophageal adenocarcinoma. However, the incidence rate for developing esophageal carcinoma is still low, approximately 0.5%

Table 1 Barrett's Dysplasia Grade and Surveillance Interval

Documentation	Follow-Up
No Dysplasia	
Two EGDs with biopsy within 1 year	Endoscopy every 3 years
Low-Grade Dysplasia	
Highest grade on repeat EGD with biopsies within 6 months	1 year interval until no dysplasia × 2
Expert pathologist confirmation	
High-Grade Dysplasia	
Mucosal irregularity	ER
Repeat EGD with biopsies to rule out EAC within 3 months	Continued 3-month surveillance or intervention based on results and patient
Expert pathologist confirmation	

EAC, esophageal adenocarcinoma; EGD, esophagogastroduodenoscopy; ER, endoscopic resection.

Wang KK, Sampliner RE: Updated guidelines 2008 for the diagnosis, surveillance and therapy of Barrett's esophagus. Am J Gastroenterol 103(3):788-797.

annually.[16] Unfortunately, symptoms do not predict the development of Barrett's epithelium in patients with chronic GERD. Thus, these patients require not only acid suppression with PPIs to control symptoms but also continued endoscopic surveillance to detect the development of dysplasia and adenocarcinoma.

Surveillance intervals for Barrett's esophagus are based on the presence and degree of dysplasia (Table 1), as outlined in the updated practice guidelines of the American College of Gastroenterology (ACG).[17] Because endoscopic surveillance is cumbersome and imperfect, risk stratification to make surveillance more efficient is desirable. Biomarkers and genomic profiles have promise in this regard.

The role of chemoprevention is also being actively investigated. A systematic review has demonstrated a protective association between any use of aspirin or nonsteroidal anti-inflammatory drugs (NSAIDs) and esophageal cancer (odds ratio, 0.67; 95% CI, 0.51 to 0.87).[18] Use of this class of medications was protective against adenocarcinoma and squamous cell carcinoma, and there was a dose-related effect. The mechanism may be related to the inhibition of cyclooxygenase (COX)-2 enzyme, which is induced in the development of esophageal maligancies.[19] Additionally, studies have demonstrated that administration of a selective COX-2 inhibitor decreases cell growth and increases apoptosis in esophageal adenocarcinoma lines.[20]

PEPTIC ULCER DISEASE

Definition

Peptic ulcers (gastric and duodenal) are defects in the GI mucosa that extend through the muscularis mucosa.

Prevalence

The lifetime prevalence of peptic ulcer disease is approximately 5% to 10%.[21] In *Helicobacter pylori*–positive subjects, the lifetime prevalence is significantly higher, 10% to 20%.[22] In patients with dyspepsia, a positive urea breath test for *H. pylori* was found to be associated with duodenal ulcer in 40% and gastric ulcer in 13% of patients, whereas a negative test result was associated with duodenal and gastric ulcers in only 2% and 3% of patients, respectively.[23]

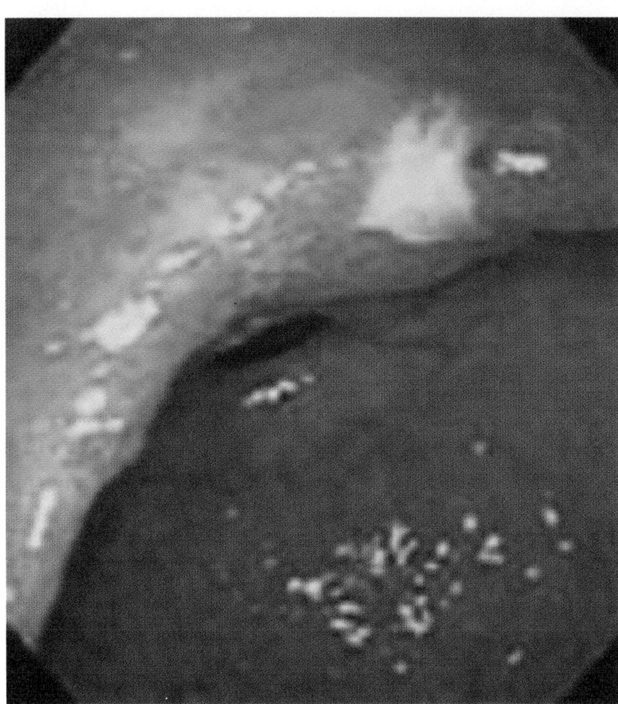

Figure 3 **Gastric ulcer in the antrum.**

Pathophysiology

Peptic ulcer disease is the end result of an imbalance between aggressive and defensive factors in the gastroduodenal mucosa. *H. pylori* infection, NSAIDs, and acid secretory abnormalities are the major factors that disrupt this equilibrium. Although acid peptic injury is necessary for ulcers to form, acid secretion is normal in almost all patients with gastric ulcers (Fig. 3) and increased in only one third of patients with duodenal ulcers. A defect in bicarbonate production and, in turn, acid neutralization in the duodenal bulb is also seen in patients with duodenal ulcer disease. This abnormality resolves with eradication of *H. pylori* infection when it is present. However, a small percentage of ulcers is not related to *H. pylori* infection or NSAID use. These are classified as idiopathic and may be related to defective mucosal defense mechanisms, tobacco use, genetics, rapid gastric emptying, or psychological stress.

Signs and Symptoms

Dyspepsia, the classic symptom of peptic ulcer disease, is defined as pain centered in the upper abdomen or discomfort characterized by fullness, bloating, distention, or nausea.[24] Symptoms may be chronic, recurrent, or new.

Dyspepsia is a common clinical problem that may be seen in 25% to 40% of adults. Only 10% of patients with upper GI symptoms are found to have a gastric or duodenal ulcer.[24] Up to 60% of patients have no definitive diagnosis and are classified as having functional dyspepsia, a condition probably related to visceral hypersensitivity. When ulcers are present, they may be asymptomatic, especially in patients ingesting NSAIDS. Patients might also present with complications of ulcer disease: Hemorrhage can develop in 20%, perforation in 5%, and gastric outlet obstruction in 2%.

Diagnosis

There are several possible diagnostic approaches to the patient with dyspepsia[24]:

- Instituting a short trial of empirical antisecretory therapy (H_2RAs or PPIs) for 4 to 8 weeks
- Conducting noninvasive testing for *H. pylori* infection followed by antibiotic treatment of patients with positive test results (test-and-treat strategy)
- Performing early endoscopy
- Performing endoscopy after failure of acid suppression or test and treating for *H. pylori*

These approaches are outlined in the American Gastroenterological Association's medical position statement on the evaluation of dyspepsia.[24]

Early endoscopic evaluation is indicated for patients older than 55 years with new-onset dyspepsia. It is also indicated for younger patients with alarm features such as unintended weight loss, bleeding, dysphagia, odynophagia, iron-deficiency anemia, persistent vomiting, palpable mass or lymphadenopathy, jaundice, or family history of gastric cancers. If a gastric ulcer is found at endoscopy, multiple biopsies and a brush cytologic examination are required to exclude malignancy. Endoscopy is also indicated for patients whose disease does not respond to empirical therapy. There is no longer any role for barium radiography in the evaluation of dyspepsia because of its poor sensitivity and specificity.

In patients younger than 55 years without alarm features, an initial *H. pylori* test-and-treat strategy is a reasonable approach if the population prevalence of *H. pylori* is higher than 10%. The rationale for this is that *H. pylori* eradication helps in peptic ulcer healing, improves symptoms of nonulcer dyspepsia, and prevents any potential future complications. At the same time, empirically treating dyspepsia patients with antibiotics for only presumed *H. pylori* infection is not supported by any model to date and should not be done. In *H. pylori*–negative patients, an empirical trial of acid suppression for 4 to 8 weeks should be instituted. Empirical PPI therapy as the initial choice is a most cost-effective approach when the *H. pylori* prevalence in a population is lower than 10%. Patients who respond to an *H. pylori* test-and-treat strategy or PPI therapy may be managed without further investigations. Initial concerns about exacerbating GERD symptoms following *H. pylori* eradication have remained unsubstantiated.

H. pylori testing is essential for patients with peptic ulcer disease. A negative test result will focus subsequent diagnostic evaluation on ruling out other causes of peptic ulcer disease. However, an initial negative test result in patients with newly diagnosed peptic ulcer disease should be confirmed by a second test, given the importance of diagnosing *H. pylori* infection. Diagnostic tests for detecting *H. pylori* are subdivided into nonendoscopic and endoscopic techniques. Enzyme-linked immunosorbent assay (ELISA) serologic tests, formerly the cornerstone of *H. pylori* testing, are no longer recommended because of the poor performance characteristics of these tests: a sensitivity rate of 85% and specificity rate of 79%.[25] Furthermore, serologic test results can remain positive for up to 3 years after bacteria are eradicated, which limits the role of such testing in the documentation of response to therapy.

Urea breath tests are more accurate than serologic tests and are now the noninvasive test of choice for diagnosing *H. pylori* infection and documenting successful *H. pylori* eradication after antibiotic therapy. Patients should not receive PPIs for at least 14 days before administration of breath tests to avoid false-negative results. Stool antigen tests are an acceptable alternative to the urea breath test, with a sensitivity rate of 89% to 98% and a specificity of more than 90%.[26] If endoscopy is performed, the diagnosis is made by the rapid urease test or histologic examination of biopsy specimens. Recent treatment with antibiotics or proton pump inhibitors decreases the diagnostic yield of both these biopsy tests.

A subset of patients also requires post-treatment testing to confirm the eradication of *H. pylori* infection. Post-treatment testing is mandatory for patients with complicated peptic ulcer disease, in which there is bleeding, perforation, or obstruction. Such post-treatment testing may also be performed in all patients with newly diagnosed peptic ulcer disease or when persistent infection is a particular concern. Because antibiotic treatment suppresses the organism, even if it is not eradicated, testing to confirm cure should not be done until 4 weeks after completion of therapy.

Treatment and Outcomes

A number of treatment options are available for the healing of peptic ulcers. These include antacids, H_2RAs, and PPIs. Antacids are potentially effective agents for healing ulcers and controlling symptoms; however, because they neutralize only acid that is already secreted, their greatest buffering capacity is active when they are taken 1 hour after eating. From a practical perspective, this inconvenient dosing frequency and the adverse effects of therapy, such as diarrhea, limit the use of antacids to symptom control only.

H_2RAs are better than antacids for ulcer healing. Acid secretion is decreased by competitive and selective inhibition of the H_2 receptor of the parietal cell. The four available H_2RAs are cimetidine, ranitidine, famotidine, and nizatidine. All these compounds act by the same mechanism but have different relative potencies for inhibiting gastric acid secretion. The inhibition of acid secretion results in an increase of the gastric pH and a decrease of pepsin activity. This class of drugs is uniformly safe and well tolerated, although the risk of adverse effects is slightly increased with cimetidine because it interacts with cytochrome P-450, causing increased drug-drug interactions. H_2RAs heal 90% to 95% of duodenal ulcers and 88% of gastric ulcers within 8 weeks. Given as a single full dose at bedtime, each of the available compounds has a comparable efficacy for ulcer healing.

The PPIs are substituted benzimidazoles that bind irreversibly to the H^+,K^+-ATPase (adenosine triphosphatase) enzyme of the gastric parietal cell. This blocks the final step of gastric acid secretion in response to any type of stimulation and results in long-lasting inhibition of gastric acid secretion. For gastric secretory activity to be restored, new enzymes need to be resynthesized, a process that normally takes 2 to 5 days. PPIs are generally well tolerated and effective; they achieve duodenal ulcer healing rates at 4 weeks (90%-100%) typically seen at 8 weeks with H_2RAs. Additionally, PPIs relieve symptoms more rapidly than H_2RAs.[27] Gastric ulcer healing is also more rapid with PPIs, but an 8-week course of therapy is still needed to achieve healing rates higher than 90%.[28] Table 2 outlines the dosing and duration of therapy of agents used to treat peptic ulcer disease. Maintenance antisecretory therapy is rarely needed, except in circumstances such as unsuccessful *H. pylori* eradication or chronic NSAID use.

Eradication of *H. pylori* infection accelerates the rate of duodenal and gastric ulcer healing, approximating the rate obtained with omeprazole at 4 weeks, and essentially cures them. Therefore, eradication should be attempted in all patients with current or past documented peptic ulcer disease and evidence of infection. Recent meta-analyses have confirmed that for duodenal ulcer healing, *H. pylori* eradication therapy is superior to ulcer-healing drugs (relative risk [RR] = 0.66; 95% CI, 0.58-0.76) and no treatment (RR = 0.37; 95% CI, 0.26-0.53).[29] Eradication therapy was also superior to no treatment for preventing recurrent duodenal ulcers (RR = 0.20; 95% CI, 0.15-0.26) and recurrent gastric ulcers (RR = 0.29; 95% CI, 0.20-0.42). However, there was no significant difference between eradication therapy and ulcer-healing drugs for gastric ulcer healing or preventing recurrent gastric and duodenal ulcers. Because eradication therapy is much more cost effective than ulcer-healing drugs and is better tolerated by patients, it should be routinely instituted whenever feasible.

The in vivo activity of antibiotics is variable, so combinations of two antibiotics plus a PPI are used to maximize the chance of eradication. Usually, the efficacy of these regimens is approximately 90%. Current treatments are shown in Box 1.[30] A reasonable approach is to use a metronidazole- or clarithromycin-based triple-therapy

Table 2 Antisecretory Therapy for Peptic Ulcer Disease

	Duodenal Ulcer		Gastric Ulcer	
Agent	Dose (mg)	Duration (wk)	Dose (mg)	Duration (wk)
H_2 Receptor Antagonists				
Cimetidine	800	8	800	8
Ranitidine	300	8	300	8
Famotidine	40	8	40	8
Nizatidine	300	8	300	8
Proton Pump Inhibitors				
Esomeprazole	20	4	40	8
Omeprazole	20	4	40	8
Lansoprazole	15	4	30	8
Rabeprazole	20	4	20	8
Pantoprazole	40	4	40	8

Box 1 Preferred Therapies for *Helicobacter pylori* Infection

Twice-Daily Proton Pump Inhibitor (PPI) or Ranitidine Bismuth Citrate Triple Therapies

PPI or ranitidine bismuth citrate plus two of the following three agents for 10-14 days:
Amoxicillin 1 g bid
Clarithromycin 500 mg bid
Metronidazole 500 mg bid

Quadruple Therapy

PPI bid
Tetracycline 500 mg qid
Metronidazole 500 mg tid or 250 mg qid
Bismuth subsalicylate or subcitrate 525 mg PO qid

Adapted from Graham DY: Therapy of Helicobacter pylori: *Current status and issues. Gastroenterology 2000;118(Suppl 1):S2-S8.*

Box 2 Risk Factors for NSAID-Induced GI Ulceration

Age older than 60 years
Prior history of peptic ulcer disease or GI hemorrhage
Concurrent use of NSAIDs and corticosteroids
Concurrent use of NSAIDs and anticoagulants
High dosage of NSAIDs or use of more than one NSAID

GI, gastrointestinal; NSAID, nonsteroidal anti-inflammatory drugs.

regimen as first-line therapy. If that fails, second-line therapy involves the antimicrobial not used initially, with quadruple therapy reserved as the third-line option. Because resistance to metronidazole is approximately 35% and resistance to clarithromycin is 11% in the United States, using these two agents together in the initial treatment of *H. pylori* is not recommended. Recent reports have documented clarithromycin resistance in up to 24% of patients, believed to be related to a gene mutation *(A2143G)*. Therefore, sequential therapy with four medications (PPI, bismuth, metronidazole, and tetracycline) for 10 to 14 days, rather than typical 1-week therapy, has been suggested in such patients. This regimen successfully eradicated *H. pylori* infection in 85% of patients who live in areas of high metronidazole resistance and in 95% of patients with clarithromycin resistance.

For patients who develop ulcers while ingesting NSAIDs, NSAID therapy should be stopped, if possible, and the patient placed on conventional doses of PPIs. It is important to realize that even low-dose aspirin used for cardiac prophylaxis is a risk factor for bleeding from peptic ulcer disease.[31] Therapy with a nonaspirin antiplatelet agent such as clopidogrel carries a similar risk as low-dose aspirin. In a meta-analysis of aspirin and clopidogrel for peptic ulcer bleeding, it was noted that low-dose aspirin doubles the risk of major GI bleeding compared with placebo, but the absolute increase was only 1.2 in 1000 patients. Aspirin increases major GI bleeding by 1.5-fold compared with clopidogrel. However, switching to clopidogrel is not cost effective compared with adding a PPI to aspirin. In fact, the risk of recurrent peptic ulcer bleeding is significantly higher with clopidogrel compared with aspirin and a PPI.[32] Therefore, patients with aspirin-related peptic ulcer bleeding should not be switched to clopidogrel; instead, a PPI needs to be added to aspirin.

Even though COX-2 inhibitors have a lower incidence of peptic ulcers than nonselective NSAIDs, the combination of a COX-2 inhibitor and low-dose aspirin has the same risk as a nonselective NSAID. Conversely, the combination of a PPI and an NSAID has a similar incidence of peptic ulcers as COX-2 inhibitors. Evidence indicates that the combination of a PPI and COX-2 inhibitor is superior to using COX-2 inhibitors alone for reducing peptic ulcers. However, concerns continue to be raised about cardiovascular adverse events with COX-2 inhibitors and, therefore, these agents should be used judiciously, if at all.

Patients should be tested for *H. pylori* infection and treated if infection is confirmed. For patients who need continued NSAID therapy, the NSAID dosage should be reduced as much as possible. Because prophylactic medications are expensive and NSAID use is common, ulcer prophylaxis should be considered only for high-risk patients. Misoprostol is a prostaglandin E_1 analogue that is effective for the prophylaxis of NSAID-induced ulcers and decreases the incidence of serious GI complications, such as bleeding, perforation, and gastric outlet obstruction. Although misoprostol at a dose of 200 µg three or four times daily is effective for ulcer prevention, adverse events such as diarrhea and abdominal cramps are common and limit its use.[33]

Box 2 lists risk factors based on the guidelines for the treatment and prevention of NSAID-induced ulcers from the American College of Gastroenterology.[32]

Summary

- Gastroesophageal reflux disease is one of the most common GI disorders, affecting about 50% of the U.S. population annually.
- Barrett's esophagus is a serious complication of chronic gastroesophageal reflux and the most important risk factor for the increasing incidence of esophageal adenocarcinoma.
- Barrett's esophagus requires regular surveillance for early detection of dysplasia, which may be aggressively treated with several available therapeutic options.
- Currently, *H. pylori* infection and NSAIDs cause more than 90% of peptic ulcers.
- Successful treatment of *H. pylori* infection significantly decreases the risk of peptic ulcers, MALToma, and possibly gastric cancers.
- PPI therapy has been demonstrated in several trials to reduce the incidence of recurrent peptic ulcer bleeding in patients taking NSAIDs.

National Guidelines

For more information on the diagnosis and treatment of gastroesophageal reflux disease and gastric and duodenal ulcers, please refer to the following guidelines:

American College of Gastroenterology: Guidelines for the Diagnosis and Treatment of Gastroesophageal Reflux Disease, 2005. Available at http://www.acg.gi.org/physicians/guidelines/GERDTreatment.pdf.

American College of Gastroenterology: Guidelines for Dyspepsia, 2005. Available at http://www.acg.gi.org/physicians/ guidelines/dyspepsia.pdf.

American College of Gastroenterology: Guidelines for the Management of *Helicobacter pylori* Infection, 2007. Available at www.acg.gi.org/physicians/guidelines/ManagementofHpylori.pdf.

American College of Gastroenterology: Guidelines for the Treatment and Prevention Of NSAID-Induced Ulcers, 1998. Available at www.acg.gi.org/acg-dev/staging/members/guides/nsaid_ulcer.html.

American College of Gastroenterology: Updated guidelines 2008 for the diagnosis, surveillance and therapy of Barrett's esophagus. Available at www.acg.gi.org/acgdev/staging/ members/guides/barretts.html.

American College of Gastroenterology: Guidelines for the Management of Peptic Ulcer Disease. Available at www.acg.gi.org/acg-dev/staging/members/guides/pudabs.html.

American College of Gastroenterology: Medical Position Statement: Evaluation of Dyspepsia, November 2005. http://www.gastrojournal.org/article/PIIS0016508505018172/fulltext.

American Gastroentological Association: Esophageal Cancer, May 2005. Available at http://www2. us.elsevierhealth.com/inst/serve?action=searchDB&searchDBfor=art&artType=fullfree&id=as0016508505006050&special=hilite&query=[all_fields]esophageal+carcinoma.

Suggested Readings

Chan FK, Ching JY, Hung LC, et al: Clopidogrel versus aspirin and esomeprazole to prevent recurrent ulcer bleeding. N Engl J Med 2005;352:238-244.

DeVault KR, Castell DO: Updated guidelines for the diagnosis and treatment of gastroesophageal reflux disease. The Practice Parameters Committee of the American College of Gastroenterology. Am J Gastroenterol 2005;100:190-200.

Falk G: Barrett's esophagus. Gastroenterology 2002;122:1569-1591.

Ford AC, Delaney BC, Forman D, Moayyedi P: Eradication therapy for peptic ulcer disease in *Helicobacter pylori* positive patients. Cochrane Database Syst Rev 2006;(2):CD003840.

Graham DY: Therapy of *Helicobacter pylori*: Current status and issues. Gastroenterology 2000;118(Suppl 1):S2-S8.

Howden CW, Hunt RH: Guidelines for the management of *Helicobacter pylori* infection. Ad Hoc Committee on Practice Parameters of the American College of Gastroenterology. Am J Gastroenterol 1998;93:2330-2338.

Lanza FL: A guideline for the treatment and prevention of NSAID-induced ulcers. Members of the Ad Hoc Committee on Practice Parameters of the American College of Gastroenterology. Am J Gastroenterol 1998;93:2037-2046.

Numans ME, Lau J, de Wit NJ, et al: Short-term treatment with proton-pump inhibitors as a test for gastroesophageal reflux disease: A meta-analysis of diagnostic test characteristics. Ann Intern Med 2004;140:518-527.

Sampliner RE: Updated guidelines for the diagnosis, surveillance, and therapy of Barrett's esophagus. Am J Gastroenterol 2002;97:1888-1895.

Talley NJ: American Gastroenterological Association: American Gastroenterological Association medical position statement: Evaluation of dyspepsia. Gastroenterology 2005;129:1753-1755.

References

For a complete list of references, log onto www.expertconsult.com.

Celiac Disease and Malabsorptive Disorders

Jamilé Wakim-Fleming

DEFINITION

Celiac disease (CD) is an immune-mediated disorder that develops in genetically susceptible persons when gluten, a major protein found in wheat, barley, and rye is ingested in the diet. Also called nontropical sprue, celiac sprue, or gluten-sensitive enteropathy, CD is primarily an enteropathy characterized by inflammation of the small bowel mucosa and atrophy of the villi, resulting in nutrient malabsorption, wasting, and diarrhea. These symptoms define the classic or typical symptoms of CD (Table 1).

Any organ system may be involved in CD, and patients can develop extraintestinal manifestations—also called atypical manifestations—such as anemia, bone disease, infertility, unfavorable outcomes of pregnancy, lymphoma, and liver disease. The clinical presentation can include a wide range of symptoms, or even lack of symptoms as in silent CD, but patients can have abnormal celiac serology (endomysial [EMA] and tissue transglutaminase [tTG] antibodies) and varying degrees of small bowel involvement on biopsy. A definition of the various forms of CD based on clinical, pathologic and serologic findings is listed in Table 1.

Genetic susceptibility defines persons who possess the gene pair encoding the major histocompatibility complex class II HLA DQ2 or DQ8. These genes are virtually required for CD to occur, and lack of these genes makes CD very unlikely.

PREVALENCE AND EPIDEMIOLOGY

Availability of highly sensitive and specific serologic tests such as endomysial and tissue transglutaminase antibodies (EMA and tTG) has made it possible to assess the true prevalence of CD. Epidemiologic studies using such tests along with small bowel biopsies report a higher prevalence of CD than previously thought. Prevalence in Western Europeans and in the United States is reported to range between 1 in 250 and 1 in 133, and it is higher in relatives of persons with CD, occurring in 1 in 22 first-degree relatives and in 1 in 39 second-degree relatives. It is rarely, if ever, reported in people with pure ethnic backgrounds from Africa, the Caribbean, China, and Japan. Women are affected more commonly than men, but there is no age predilection.

Other than persons who have relatives with CD, persons at increased risk include those with Down syndrome, Turner syndrome, type 1 diabetes mellitus, thyroid disease, lymphocytic colitis, and autoimmune disorders (Box 1).

PATHOPHYSIOLOGY

Celiac disease is a multifactorial and a multisystem disorder involving a genetic predisposition, environmental exposure of the small bowel mucosa to gluten, and an immunologic response to gluten.

Genetic

The majority (>90%) of persons with CD possess the HLA DQ2 haplotype, and 5% to 10% possess the DQ8 haplotype, conferring a negative predictive value greater than 98%. These haplotypes are encoded within the HLA class II region of the major histocompatibility complex on chromosome 6p. However, about 40% of the general population carry these haplotypes without having the disease, which makes their presence necessary but not sufficient for its development. Other non-HLA genes have been proposed, but their role in influencing the disease has not been clearly defined.

Environmental

It was a serendipitous observation that children with CD improved during World War II when cereals used to make bread were scarce, and they relapsed after the war when the supply of these cereals was reinstituted. Risk for developing CD is increased with the introduction of gluten in the diet of infants before the age of 4 months. Grains that activate the disease contain proteins that can form gluten (prolamins: glutenins and gliadins) and include wheat, barley, and rye. Grains that do not activate the disease include rice, corn, sorghum, and millet. Oats contain a very small proportion of prolamins and should be avoided initially.

Immunologic

Exposure of the upper small bowel mucosa to gluten in susceptible persons precipitates an inflammatory reaction characterized by infiltration of the lamina propria and the epithelium with inflammatory cells, which eventually leads to destruction and atrophy of the mucosa.

Ingestion of gluten induces the antigen-precipitating cells, which express HLA DQ2/DQ8, in lamina propria to sensitize T lymphocytes in both lamina propria and in epithelium. Activated T lymphocytes, particularly CD8+ intraepithelial lymphocytes expressing γ/δ receptors, become abundant and their numbers increase about sixfold. These in turn activate B lymphocytes and other lymphocytes to secrete immunoglobulins, cytokines, interferons, tumor necrosis factor, and other inflammatory mediators, notably interleukin (IL)-15, and cause damage to the enterocytes, resulting in villous atrophy. Additionally, tTG, a ubiquitous enzyme that is released by inflammatory and endothelial cells, deamidates glutamine residues in gluten to glutamic acid, which is negatively charged and in turn facilitates further reactivation of more lymphocytes and potentially affects more organ systems in the body.

CLINICAL MANIFESTATIONS

Celiac disease exhibits a spectrum of clinical and pathologic manifestations. Left untreated, CD can progress to involve multiple organ systems with severe complications and nutritional deficiencies.

Symptoms can manifest in infancy and as early as cereals are introduced in the diet. Crampy abdominal pain, steatorrhea, failure to thrive, apathy and irritability, muscle wasting, and hypotonia are described. Any of these symptoms should trigger a diagnostic workup. Catch-up growth is well documented once a gluten free-diet is introduced.

In adults, the clinical symptoms are variable and not specific. The classic symptoms of malabsorption are less and less encountered since testing with serological antibodies has become available, and diagnosis is recognized before the full-blown clinical wasting occurs. On the other hand, atypical presentations are increasingly recognized and becoming more common.

Patients with CD can exhibit weakness, fatigue, and dyspnea as a result of vitamin B_{12}, folate, and iron deficiency; bone fractures,

Table 1 Types of Celiac Disease

Type	Symptoms	Serology	Villous atrophy
Classic CD	Malabsorption	Abnormal	Yes
Atypical CD	Extraintestinal	Abnormal	Yes
Silent CD	None	Abnormal	Yes
Latent CD	None	Abnormal	No villous atrophy
Potential CD	Symptoms	Abnormal	Increase IELs only
Refractory CD symptoms	Abnormal	Villous atrophy but no response to 6 months on gluten-free diet	
Collagenous symptoms	Abnormal	Villous atrophy and failure of therapy	

CD, celiac disease; IEL, intraepithelial lymphocytes.

Box 1 Patients Who Are at Risk for Celiac Disease and Should Be Tested

- Patients with gastrointestinal and classic symptoms: diarrhea, weight loss, abdominal distention, failure to thrive
- Patients with autoimmune diseases, type 1 diabetes, thyroid disorders, Sjögren's syndrome, microscopic colitis, inflammatory bowel disease
- First-degree relatives
- Patients with elevated liver enzymes
- Patients with Down syndrome
- Patients with Williams syndrome
- Patients with iron deficiency anemia
- Patients with osteoporosis
- Patients with delayed puberty
- Infertile patients
- Patients with irritable bowel syndrome

muscular atrophy, and tetany as a result of osteoporosis and osteopenia due to vitamin D and calcium deficiencies; peripheral neuropathy and ataxia as a result of cerebellar and posterior column inflammatory damage; and secondary hyperparathyroidism, edema, petechiae, and dermatitis herpetiformis. Infertility is observed in men and women. Amenorrhea, intrauterine growth retardation, and unfavorable outcomes of pregnancy have been reported. Liver enzyme abnormalities and nonspecific hepatitis have been incidentally recognized in patients with CD, and advanced liver disease and cirrhosis have been reported, with improvement of the liver disease upon withdrawal of gluten from the diet. It is generally accepted that patients with abnormal elevation of liver enzymes should be tested for celiac disease.

Dermatitis herpetiformis may be the clinical presentation of a latent CD. It is characterized by a papulovesicular rash that is intensely pruritic and affects the buttocks and the extensor surfaces of elbows and knees. It is characterized by granular immunoglobulin (Ig)A deposits in the dermo-epidermal junction. Most patients have abnormalities of the intestinal mucosa. Treatment consists of withdrawing gluten from the diet. If skin lesions do not improve, dapsone may be added at 1 to 2 mg /day.

Other manifestations of CD include weight gain and obesity, gastroesophageal reflux disease, irritable bowel syndrome with abdominal pain and constipation, pancreatitis, myocarditis, aphthous ulcers of the oral mucosa, lymphocytic and collagenous colitis, hyposplenism, and asymptomatic IgA nephropathy. There is a slightly higher risk for gastrointestinal malignancies and lymphomas in CD patients than in the general population.

Box 2 Histologic Spectrum of Intestinal Involvement in Celiac Disease

- Marsh 0 or type 0: preinfiltrative or normal
- Marsh I or type 1: infiltrative lesion; increased intraepithelial lymphocytes
- Marsh II or type 2: hyperplastic lesion (type 1 plus crypt hyperplasia)
- Marsh III or type 3: destructive lesion (type 2 plus villous atrophy)
- Marsh IV or type 4: hypoplastic lesion seen in T cell lymphoma

DIAGNOSIS

Once the clinical suspicion in patients at risk factors is raised, the initial step toward a diagnosis is to obtain celiac serology antibody testing. This should be followed by a small bowel biopsy. The patient should be tested while following a gluten-containing diet.

The most sensitive and specific serologic tests are endomysial antibody IgA EMA and tissue transglutaminase antibody IgA tTG. Sensitivities and specificities are higher than 85% and 97%, respectively, for EMA and 90% and 97%, respectively, for tTG. Gliadin antibodies have lower sensitivities and specificities and are not recommended for screening; however, gliadin antibodies may have a role in monitoring adherence to a gluten-free diet.

About 2% to 5% of patients with CD have selective IgA deficiency, in which case serum IgG tTG or IgG EMA testing should be performed.

Pathologic changes on small-bowel biopsy are characterized by a spectrum of abnormalities described by Marsh and known as the Marsh criteria (Box 2). The hallmark of CD is Marsh 3 or villous atrophy; however, this may be patchy or present in other disorders as in hypogammaglobulinemia, acute infectious gastroenteritis, or milk intolerance. Additionally, there is growing evidence that CD may be diagnosed when changes of earlier phase on biopsy such as Marsh 1 or Marsh 2 are seen.

Establishing Diagnosis in the Absence of Typical Symptoms

The wide range of clinical manifestations of the disease coupled with less than Marsh 3 on biopsy makes the diagnosis of CD challenging for the clinician. In these situations, genetic testing or gluten challenge may be necessary for a definite diagnosis. A few scenarios may be encountered in a clinical setting and their proposed diagnostic workups include:

- Positive serology and villous atrophy: Diagnosis established. Patient should be treated.
- Positive serology and normal small bowel mucosa biopsy: Disease is considered latent and biopsy should be repeated after a gluten challenge or a few months later on a normal diet.
- Positive serology and increased intraepithelial lymphocytes: Potential celiac disease; repeat biopsy after a gluten challenge or in a few months on a normal diet, or obtain HLA typing. If any is positive, start a gluten-free diet.
- Normal serology and normal biopsy: Look for other causes of the patient's symptoms.
- Normal serology and villous atrophy: Exclude other causes of villous atrophy, immunodeficiency, IgA deficiency.

Gluten challenge should be done in patients who embarked on a gluten-free diet empirically without serologic or pathologic abnormalities. It can also be done in patients with latent celiac disease and in patients with potential celiac disease. Gluten should be started in small increments beginning with one slice of bread and doubling this amount every 3 days if tolerated until at least 10 g of gluten are ingested daily or the equivalent of 4 slices of bread, after which serologic testing and small bowel biopsy should be repeated and signs and symptoms observed. If tests remain negative, patients should remain on a normal diet.

Screening

Although CD is fairly common, is underdiagnosed, and can lead to serious complications, mass screening is not yet recommended. Screening with EMA and tTG may be warranted in patients with high risk factors, notably first-degree relatives of patients with the disease.

COMPLICATIONS

Patients with refractory disease have persistent symptoms despite 6 months on a gluten-free diet. Glucocorticoids and at times immunosuppressants are indicated to induce remission. Patients often progress to ulcerative jejunitis or malignancy.

Malignancy, including intestinal lymphoma such as enteropathy-associated intestinal lymphoma or enteropathy-associated T-cell lymphoma, is usually not responsive to a gluten-free diet. Other malignancies include various carcinomas along the gastrointestinal tract.

Ulcerative jejunoileitis consists of ulcers and strictures of the small bowel, requiring surgical resections.

Acute celiac crisis is rare and usually occurs when patients undergo rapid and nonincremental gluten challenge. It is characterized by severe diarrhea, electrolyte abnormalities, and metabolic acidosis. Glucocorticoids and volume replacement are often required.

Collagenous sprue defines CD that is refractory to therapy and characterized by the deposition of collagen in subepithelial regions of the small bowel with a thickness greater than 10 mm. Prognosis is very grim.

TREATMENT

Treatment consists of withdrawing gluten from the diet for life. It entails eliminating wheat, barley, and rye. This allows healing of the small bowel mucosa and restitution of nutritional status. Oats may initially be withdrawn in severely symptomatic patients until symptoms begin to resolve.

Lactose-containing products can worsen gastrointestinal symptoms and should be avoided in these situations until restitution of normal mucosa. Deficiencies of vitamins D and B_{12}, folic acid, calcium, and iron and nutritional deficiencies should be replaced as necessary. Prevention of bone loss and pneumococcal vaccination due to hyposplenism are necessary. Complications of CD should be managed appropriately, and increased vigilance in recognizing and managing lymphoma and cancer is important.

Adherence to a gluten-free diet is often difficult because of cost and lack of palatability and because it requires the patient's commitment and perseverance. Therefore, alternative therapies are increasingly in demand, and trials are ongoing to assess for their efficacy. These therapies include gluten-degrading enzymes, modified grains that lack immunogenic compounds, zonulin inhibitors that decrease intestinal permeability, and anti-inflammatory and immunotherapy.

Referral of patients to nutritional counseling for education and for monitoring adherence and response to therapy is essential to safeguard and good outcome. Information on gluten-containing and gluten-free foods is available on various websites along with a wide variety of gluten-free recipes.

Response to the gluten-free diet is assessed by clinical and serologic improvement. There is no clear consensus on whether a repeat small bowel biopsy is necessary. However, repeat biopsy may be indicated in cases where adherence to diet is proved but response to diet is equivocal or lacking.

OTHER MALABSORPTION DISORDERS

The small intestine is the site of absorption of nutrients necessary to maintain life. Several disorders, including CD, affect the intestinal mucosa or the intestinal chyme and can cause malabsorption and wasting. These may be classified into small bowel mucosal diseases and luminal or digestive diseases. Potential etiologies include infectious causes, as in parasitic or bacterial and viral enteritis; iatrogenic causes by means of surgical resection of the small bowel or administration of medications; structural defects, as in strictures causing stasis with bacterial overgrowth; and lack of digestive enzymes in the brush border or the lumen of the gastrointestinal tract (Table 2 and Box 3).

CONCLUSION

CD is a multisystem disorder with a wide range of clinical presentations. Clinicians should have a heightened awareness of these presentations and a low threshold for testing with EMA and tTG antibodies. Education and surveillance of patients on a gluten-free diet are crucial to safeguard adherence to the diet and prevent further complications of the disease.

Other malabsorptive disorders should be included in the differential diagnosis of CD, bearing in mind the similarities in signs and symptoms even pathologic findings on biopsy. Further testing may be required, and a multidisciplinary approach may be necessary for a definite diagnosis.

Box 3 Differential Diagnosis of Celiac Disease

- Pancreatic insufficiency, chronic pancreatitis, cystic fibrosis: lack of pancreatic enzymes
- Zollinger-Ellison syndrome, inactivation of pancreatic enzymes by excess gastric acid secretion
- Gastrectomy, ileal resection, or short gut syndrome
- Cholestatic liver disease and severe chronic liver disease
- Parasitic infestation
- Lymphoma
- Bacterial overgrowth
- Drugs
  - Bile salt binders (decrease micelle formation)
  - Antacids (chelation)
  - Metothrexate (villlus blunting)
  - Sulfasalazine (inhibits folate hydrolase)

Summary

- Celiac disease is an immune-mediated disorder that develops in genetically susceptible persons when gluten is ingested in the diet. Exposure of the upper small bowel mucosa to gluten precipitates an inflammatory reaction characterized by infiltration of the lamina propria and the epithelium with inflammatory cells, which eventually leads to destruction and atrophy of the mucosa.
- Prevalence in Western Europe and in the United States ranges between 1 in 250 and 1 in 133. It is higher in relatives of persons with celiac disease, occurring in 1 in 22 in first-degree relatives and in 1 in 39 in second-degree relatives. It is rarely if ever, reported in people with pure ethnic backgrounds from Africa, the Caribbean, China, and Japan. Women are affected more commonly than men, but there is no age predilection.

Continued

Table 2 Differential Diagnosis of Celiac Disease, Malabsorption due to Mucosal Abnormalities

Disease	Etiology	Diagnosis	Therapy
Tropical sprue	Nonspecific enterotoxigens	Acute enteric infection in visitors of endemic locales	Antibiotics
Whipple disease	*Tropheryma whippelli*	Small bowel biopsy, PAS+ laden macrophages	Antibiotics
Disaccharidase deficiency (lactose intolerance)	Lactase deficiency of villous epithelial cells	Hydrogen breath test	Avoidance of milk products
Abetalipoproteinemia	Autosomal recessive inability to synthesize abetalipoproteins	Absence in plasma of chylomicrons, VLDLs, and LDLs Burr cells on blood smear	
Crohn's disease	Autoimmune disorder of the GI tract	Clinical, endoscopic and histological	5 ASA and immunosuppressants
Eosinophilic gastroenteritis, mastocytosis	Inflammation	Histologic	Steroids
Gastrectomy	Surgical, iatrogenic	Clinical history, B_{12} deficiency	B_{12} supplementation
Short gut syndrome	Surgical, iatrogenic	Clinical history	Nutrient supplementation
Graft versus host disease	Iatrogenic	Clinical history	Withdrawal of offending agents
Giardia	Protozoa	Histologic	antibiotics
AIDS	Infectious agents, AIDS enteropathy	Possibly histologic	Antibiotics, antiretroviral therapy

ASA, acetylsalicylic acid; GI, gastrointestinal; LDL, low-density lipoprotein; PAS, periodic acid–Schiff; VLDL, very-low-density lipoprotein.

SECTION 5 GASTROENTEROLOGY

Summary—cont'd

- Diarrhea and fat malabsorption is most often observed. Often patients present with extraintestinal manifestation of deficiencies caused by prolonged malabsorption, including anemia, bone disease, infertility, unfavorable outcomes of pregnancy, lymphoma, and liver disease.
- The diagnosis should be suspected in any patient with chronic diarrhea, and in those with unexplained deficiency states including iron, folate, and fat-soluble vitamins. The most sensitive and specific serologic tests are endomysial antibody IgA EMA and tissue transglutaminase antibody IgA hTTG. Biopsy of the small intestine plays a confirmatory role.
- Treatment consists of withdrawing gluten from the diet for life. It entails eliminating wheat, barley, and rye. This allows healing of the small bowel mucosa and restitution of nutritional status. Oats may initially be withdrawn in severely symptomatic patients until symptoms begin to resolve.

Suggested Readings

AGA Institute: AGA Institute medical position statement on the diagnosis and management of celiac disease. Gastroenterology 2006;131(6);1977-2002.

Dickey W: Symposium 1; Joint BAPEN and British Society of Gastroenterology Symposium on Coeliac Disease: "Basics and Controversies". Coeliac disease in the twenty-first century. Proc Nutr Soc 2009;3:1-8.

Kaukinen K, Collin P, Mäki M: Latent celiac disease or celiac disease beyond villous atrophy? Gut 2007;56(10):1339-1340.

Kurppa K, Collin P, Viljamaa M, et al: Diagnosing mild enteropathy celiac disease: A randomized, controlled clinical study. Gastroenterology 2009;136(3):816-823.

Marsh MN: Gluten, major histocompatibility complex, and the small intestine. A molecular and immunobiologic approach to the spectrum of gluten sensitivity ("celiac sprue"). Gastroenterology 1992;102(1):330-354.

NIH Consensus Development Conference on Celiac Disease. NIH Consens State Sci Statements. 2004;21(1):1-23.

Qiao SW, Sollid LM, Blumberg RS: Antigen presentation in celiac disease. Curr Opin Immunol 2009;21(1):111-117.

Richey R, Howdle P, Shaw E, Stokes T: Recognition and assessment of celiac disease in children and adults: Summary of NICE guidance. Guideline development group. BMJ 2009;338:b1684.

Sollid LM, Markussen G, Ek J, et al: Evidence of a primary association of celiac disease to a particular HLA DQ γ/δ heterodimer. J Exp Med 1989;169(1):345-350.

Pancreatic Disorders

Tyler Stevens

ACUTE PANCREATITIS

Definitions

Acute pancreatitis (AP) is an inflammatory condition of the pancreas that can extend to extrapancreatic tissues. AP is broadly classified as mild or severe. Mild AP is often referred to as interstitial pancreatitis, based on its radiographic appearance. The pancreatic blood supply is preserved in interstital pancreatitis. Severe AP implies organ failure, local complications, or pancreatic necrosis. There is disruption of the pancreatic blood supply in necrotizing pancreatitis, with resulting ischemia.

Different types of fluid collections develop in the setting of AP. Acute fluid collections occur early in the course of AP in the peripancreatic areas and are not encapsulated by a fibrous wall. Acute pseudocysts are well-developed collections of pancreatic juice encapsulated by a nonepithelialized wall of granulation tissue (Fig. 1). Pseudocysts typically form 4 to 6 weeks after an episode of AP. A pseudocyst that has become infected is a pancreatic abscess. Pancreatic abscesses can also form through encapsulation of areas of infected pancreatic necrosis. The terms *pancreatic phlegmon* and *hemorrhagic pancreatitis* are no longer used in the current American College of Gastroenterology (ACG) guidelines.

When acute pancreatitis occurs on two or more occasions, it is classified as acute recurrent pancreatitis. In some cases, acute recurrent pancreatitis progresses to chronic pancreatitis, characterized by parenchymal fibrosis and loss of exocrine function.

Prevalence

The yearly incidence of AP in the United States is approximately 17 new cases per 100,000 popuation. Acute pancreatitis results in more than 100,000 hospitalizations per year. Eighty percent of cases of AP are mild; the remaining 20% are severe. Approximately 2000 patients per year die from complications related to AP.

Etiology

Gallstones and alcohol are the two most common causes of AP in Western countries, accounting for 80% of cases. Gallstone (biliary) pancreatitis results from transient obstruction of the ampulla of Vater by small stones or crystals (microlithiasis). Clinical features suggesting biliary pancreatitis include preceding biliary colic, the presence of cholelithiasis or biliary dilation on gallbladder ultrasound, and liver function test abnormalities. Biliary pancreatitis typically does not recur after cholecystectomy or endoscopic therapy (biliary sphincterotomy and stone extraction). Alcohol is the second leading cause of AP. Acute recurrent pancreatitis from alcohol often leads to chronic pancreatitis.

Numerous less-common causes have been described (Box 1). Hypertriglyceridemia produces acute pancreatitis if triglyceride levels are above 1000 mg/dL. Markedly elevated triglyceride levels may be encountered in the setting of diabetes, alcoholism, and inherited disorders of lipoprotein metabolism (Fredrickson types I, II, and V). Hypercalcemia produces AP through calcium-mediated activation of trypsinogen and subsequent glandular autodigestion. Hypercalcemia-associated AP can occur in the setting of primary and secondary hyperparathyroidism, malignancy, and metabolic bone disease. Certain medications (e.g., sulfa drugs, 6-mercaptopurine, didanosine, furosemide, and valproate) have also been implicated as causes of acute pancreatitis.

Obstruction of the pancreatic duct can produce acute or chronic pancreatitis. Causes of obstructive AP include ductal adenocarcinoma, ampullary tumors and polyps, neuroendocrine and cystic pancreatic tumors, and intraductal papillary mucinous tumors. Congenital abnormalities such as pancreas divisum and annular pancreas can also result in obstructive AP in adult patients.

Pathophysiology

The pathogenesis of AP has been studied extensively using animal models. Although different etiologies produce distinct inciting events, the final common pathway is premature activation of enzymes. Ordinarily, pancreatic proenzymes become activated on release within the duodenum. Pancreatitis results when activation of pancreatic enzymes occurs early within the acinar cells, producing autodigestion of the pancreas and surrounding tissues. Exposure of trypsinogen to lysosomal enzymes such as cathepsin B has been shown as a mechanism for early trypsin activation.

Signs and Symptoms

Acute pancreatitis manifests with the sudden onset of epigastric pain radiating to the back. The pain may be severe and worsens after meals. Abdominal pain can last for days and is associated with anorexia, nausea, and vomiting. In alcohol-related AP, pain occurs from hours to days after binge drinking. Most patients present to the emergency department. However, occasional patients manage their symptoms at home by minimizing oral intake for a few days.

Physical examination often reveals systemic signs such as fever, tachycardia, and hypotension. Abdominal examination reveals epigastric tenderness, with localized guarding and rebound. Sluggish or absent bowel sounds indicate coexisting ileus. Less-frequent findings signal complications, including Grey Turner's (flank ecchymosis) or Cullen's (umbilical ecchymosis) signs suggesting retroperitoneal hemorrhage, a palpable mass suggesting a pseudocyst, panniculitis suggesting subcutaneous fat necrosis, and dullness to percussion of lung fields suggesting pleural effusion. The differential diagnosis of upper gastrointestinal bleeding in acute pancreatitis includes erosion of a pseudocyst into the splenic artery (hemosuccus pancreaticus) or bleeding from gastric varices that arise secondary to splenic vein thrombosis.

Diagnosis

The diagnosis of AP is supported by an elevation of the serum amylase and lipase levels in excess of three times the upper limit of normal. These enzyme levels are elevated because of leakage from pancreatic acinar cells into the interstitial space and subsequent absorption into the circulation. The amylase level becomes elevated within hours of the development of pain and can remain elevated for 3 to 5 days. The differential diagnosis for hyperamylasemia includes intestinal obstruction, visceral perforation, tubo-ovarian abscess, renal failure, and salivary gland disease. Macroamylasemia is a condition in which amylase is chronically elevated because of its binding to an abnormal serum protein, leading to delayed clearance. Serum lipase has higher specificity for pancreatic disease, but its level may be elevated in other conditions as well. The severity of pancreatitis does not correlate well with the magnitude of elevation of the serum amylase and lipase levels. There is no value in following daily trends of serum amylase and lipase levels because they do not correlate with recovery or prognosis.

Laboratory abnormalities encountered in AP include hyperglycemia, hypocalcemia, leukocytosis, and mild elevations of liver function test results. Elevation of the serum alanine aminotransferase level to greater than 80 U/mL is highly specific and poorly sensitive for biliary pancreatitis. An elevated hematocrit at admission is now recognized as an important marker of severity in AP.

Simple plain films of the chest and abdomen are appropriate for the initial radiographic assessment of AP. An abdominal radiograph is helpful for excluding other causes of acute abdominal pain, such as obstruction and perforation. In AP, the abdominal radiograph is typically normal or might demonstrate ileus. A chest radiograph can detect pulmonary complications of AP such as atelectasis, pleural effusions (most commonly left-sided), or infiltrates suggesting acute respiratory distress syndrome.

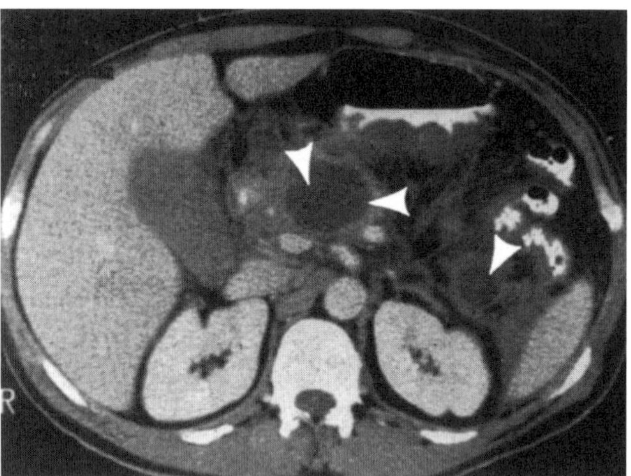

Figure 1 Abdominal computed tomography scan of acute pancreatitis. Pseudocyst formation can be noted *(arrowheads)*.

Box 1 Causes of Acute Pancreatitis

- Gallstones (45%)
- Alcohol (35%)
- Other (10%)
- Medications
- Hypercalcemia
- Hypertriglyceridemia
- Obstruction
- After endoscopic retrograde cholangiopancreatography
- Heredity
- Trauma
- Viral infection
- Vascular ischemia
- Idiopathic (10%)

Although transabdominal ultrasound is poorly reliable for imaging the pancreas itself, it is the best initial radiographic test for the evaluation of mild AP because it detects gallstones as a potential cause, it rules out acute cholecystitis as a differential cause of pain and hyperamylasemia, and it detects biliary dilation, which suggests the need for early endoscopic retrograde cholangiopancreatography (ERCP).

Contrast-enhanced computed tomography (CT) of the abdomen is the preferred test for evaluating severe pancreatitis and detecting complications. CT features in interstitial pancreatitis include homogenous contrast enhancement; diffuse or segmental pancreatic enlargement; irregularity, heterogeneity, and lobularity of the pancreas; and obliteration of the peripancreatic fat planes. CT detects areas of pancreatic necrosis (Fig. 2), which significantly influences subsequent management. The presence of necrosis predicts a substantial increase in mortality compared with interstitial pancreatitis. A CT should not be routinely ordered for all patients with AP; however, the ACG practice guidelines state that "a dynamic contrast-enhanced CT is recommended at some point beyond the first 3 days in *severe* acute pancreatitis (on the basis of a high APACHE score or organ failure) to distinguish interstitial from necrotizing pancreatitis." It is unlikely that intravenous contrast worsens or precipitates pancreatic necrosis, and abdominal CT should generally not be withheld on this basis. A CT may also be considered for those in whom a localized pancreatic complication is suspected (e.g., pseudocyst, splenic vein thrombosis, splenic artery aneurysm). A CT is also appropriate 4 to 6 weeks after resolution of AP to exclude a tumor if the cause of the attack is unclear.

Endoscopic ultrasound (EUS) and magnetic resonance cholangiopancreatography (MRCP) are emerging as potentially valuable tests in the evaluation of AP. Both are helpful in detecting stones in the common bile duct and in directly assessing the pancreatic parenchyma. Magnetic resonance imaging is similar or superior to contrast CT in its ability to stage AP and detect necrosis and complications, and it does not require intravenous contrast.

Treatment

Supportive Care

The primary goals of therapy in AP are meticulous supportive care and prevention of pancreatic necrosis, infection, and organ failure. The primary treatment is pancreatic rest and analgesia. Patients should be given nothing by mouth, and intravenous fluids should be given with careful attention to volume status. The ACG guidelines state, "all patients should receive close supportive care including pain control, fluid resuscitation, and nutritional support." A therapeutic algorithm closely based on the ACG guidelines is shown in (Fig. 3).

The importance of vigorous hydration to optimize outcomes has been increasingly recognized. The ACG guidelines stress, "Patients with evidence of significant third-space losses require aggressive fluid resuscitation." Many patients sequester substantial amounts of fluid into the retroperitoneal space, producing very high fluid require-

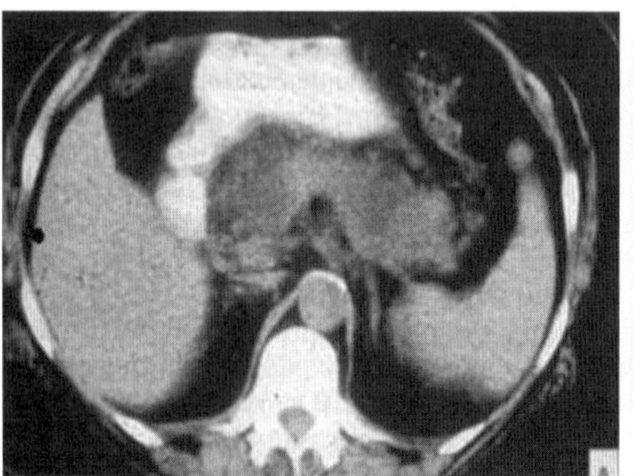

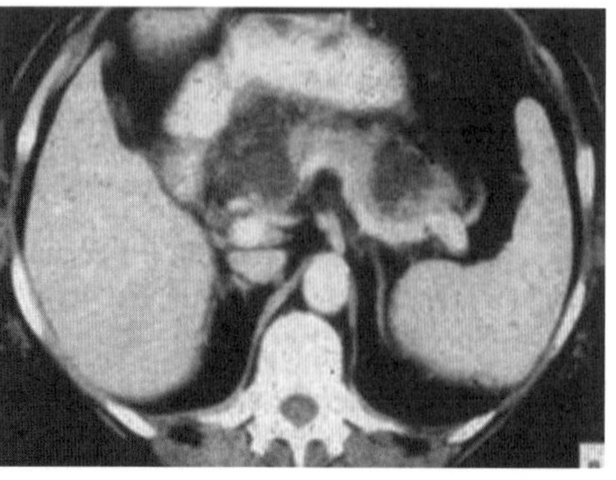

Figure 2 Computed tomography appearance of necrotizing pancreatitis. The image on the *left* is before contrast. The image on the *right* is after contrast. The lack of contrast enhancement of the entire gland suggests areas of necrosis.

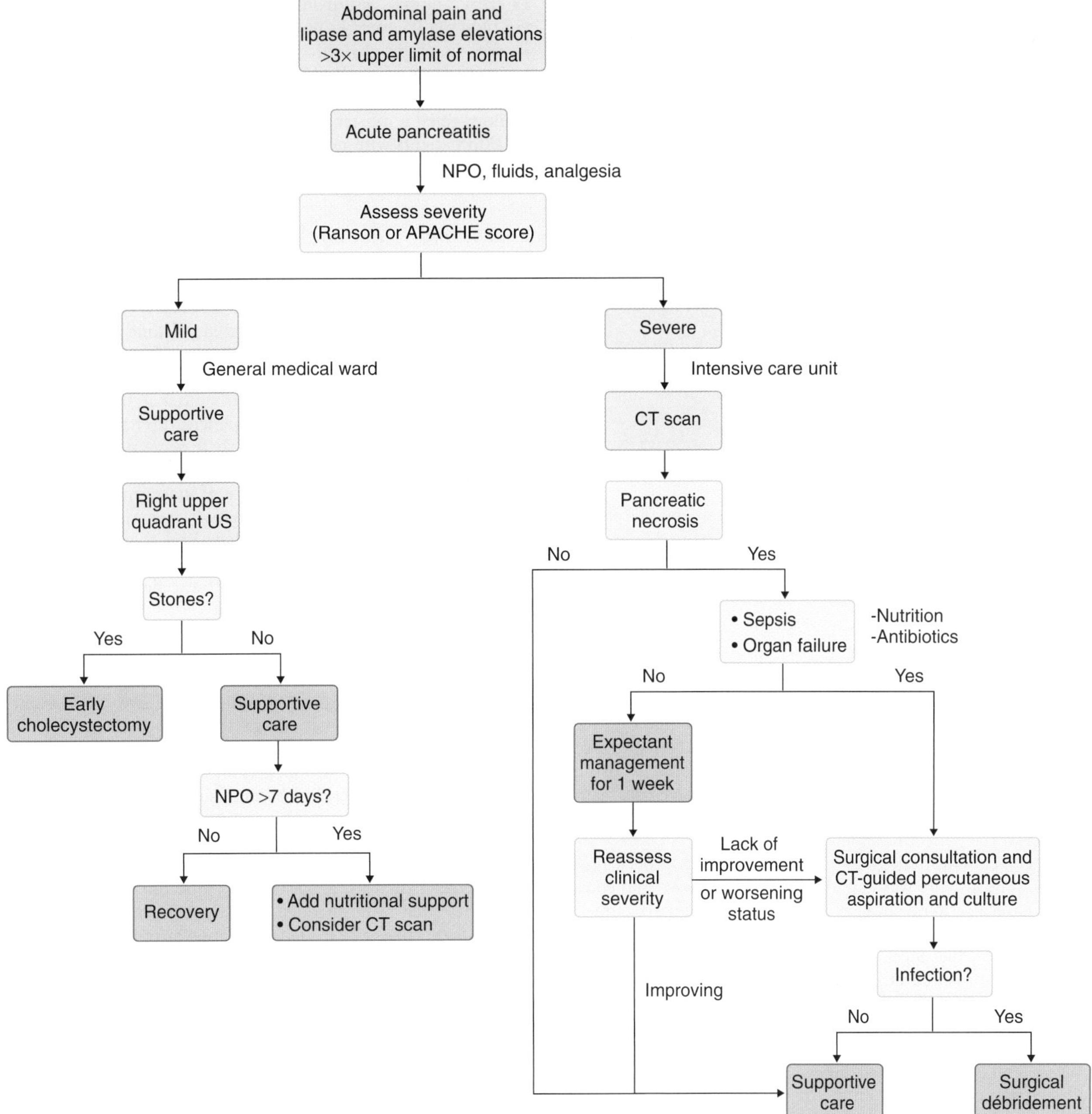

Figure 3 Approach to the management of acute pancreatitis. This algorithm is based on the practice guidelines from the American College of Gastroenterology. CT, computed tomography; US, ultrasound.

ments. Intravascular volume depletion can lead to tachycardia, hypotension, renal failure, hemoconcentration, and generalized circulatory collapse. More than 6 L of fluid sequestration within the first 48 hours is considered a marker of increased severity, according to the Ranson criteria (Box 2). Patients with evidence of hemoconcentration resulting from intravascular water loss appear to be at increased risk for the development of pancreatic necrosis and organ failure. In addition to maintenance fluid requirements, the amount sequestered should be monitored and replaced with isotonic fluids such as normal saline, with a goal of euvolemia and hemodilution. Some patients require as much as 250 to 350 mL/hour, particularly in the early phases of AP. Of course, the aggressiveness of fluid replacement must be tempered in the presence of underlying cardiac or renal disease.

Oral intake should be severely limited initially and then carefully advanced as pain subsides and hunger returns. Carbohydrate-containing foods are best for early refeeding because they do not stimulate the pancreas as much as fat- and protein-containing foods. A nasogastric tube is necessary only in the presence of vomiting or ileus. Intravenous narcotics by injection or by patient-controlled analgesia should be used liberally during the attack and tapered as the diet is advanced to enable prompt bowel recovery.

The ACG guidelines advise nutritional support if NPO status is maintained for longer than 5 to 7 days. All patients with severe AP should receive nutritional support because of the inherently high level of stress and hypercatabolism. Nasojejunal feeding past the ligament of Treitz does not stimulate the pancreas and is preferred over parenteral feeding because of decreased infection complication rates. Studies have shown improved humoral and cellular immunity, decreased systemic inflammatory response, and decreased bacterial translocation for enteral feeding compared with parenteral nutrition.

Box 2 Ranson Criteria for Severity of Acute Pancreatitis

At Admission

Age >55 yr
WBC >16,000/mL
LDH >350 IU/L
AST >250 IU/L
Glucose >200 mg/dL

At 48 Hours

Hematocrit decrease >10%
BUN increase >5 mg/dL
Calcium <8 mg/dL
Pao_2 <60 mm Hg
Base deficit >4 mg/dL
Fluid sequestration >6 L

AST, aspartate aminotransferase; BUN, blood urea nitrogen; LDH, lactate dehydrogenase; Pao_2, partial pressure of arterial carbon dioxide; WBC, white blood cell.

The presence of a severe intestinal ileus or delay in tube placement can limit the use of enteral feeding. Many patients with AP develop gastric and colonic ileus but maintain adequate small bowel motility for enteral feeding.

Assessment of Severity

An important initial step in management is the assessment of severity by clinical and radiographic criteria. Severe AP implies organ failure or pancreatic necrosis and carries a mortality rate of 10%. According to the ACG guidelines, severe pancreatitis is recognized on the basis of early clinical prognostic signs, evidence of organ failure, or local complications. Early recognition of severe pancreatitis improves outcomes by prompting aggressive fluid resuscitation and transfer of the patient to an intensive care unit.

Several clinical and radiographic severity scores have been proposed. The Ranson score was developed for alcoholic AP and comprises five clinical criteria measured at admission and six clinical criteria measured at 48 hours (see Box 2). The criteria measured at admission reflect the local inflammatory effects of pancreatic enzymes; those measured at 48 hours represent the later systemic effects. Three or more Ranson criteria predict a severe course and increased mortality. The APACHE II and III scores (acute physiology, age, chronic health evaluation) are generated from multiple parameters and are considered highly accurate. APACHE scores allow prediction of severity from the day of admission and may be recalculated on a daily basis. Unfortunately, the APACHE score is rarely used in clinical practice because of its time-consuming and cumbersome nature.

In addition to formal scoring systems, patients should be followed closely for other markers of increased severity, including signs of hemodynamic instability or organ failure. Respiratory failure can occur through the development of large pleural effusions or acute respiratory distress syndrome. Rarely, hemorrhage into retroperitoneal tissues results in further hemodynamic compromise. Extra vigilance for these complications will result in more timely and aggressive management and improved patient outcomes.

Preventive Measures

Prevention of Infection. Because superinfection of pancreatic necrosis dramatically increases the mortality rate of AP compared with sterile necrosis, a major goal in management is the prevention of infection. Some randomized trials have suggested a benefit for early initiation of broad-spectrum antibiotics in necrotizing AP. Antibiotics with good pancreatic tissue penetration, such as imipenem (500 mg IV every 8 hours), cefuroxime (1.5 g IV every 8 hours), or ciprofloxacin (400 mg IV every 12 hours) are favored in this setting. Potential drawbacks of prophylactic antibiotics include the development of resistant organisms and fungal infections. Although antibiotics have been shown to decrease infection rates, they have not consistently demonstrated a mortality benefit. The ACG guidelines recommend that "in patients with necrotizing pancreatitis associated with organ failure, it is reasonable to initiate treatment with antibiotics with good spectrum of activity against aerobic and anaerobic bacteria."

Endoscopic Retrograde Cholangiopancreatography. Although the ACG guidelines state that "patients with severe pancreatitis caused by gallstones should undergo urgent ERCP," there has been much recent debate over the benefit of early endoscopic removal of common bile duct stones in suspected gallstone pancreatitis. There is strong evidence to suggest a benefit for ERCP with papillotomy and stone extraction in the setting of stone impaction and cholangitis. However, randomized trials of early ERCP in the management of all patients with suspected gallstone pancreatitis have shown conflicting results. ERCP can further exacerbate acute pancreatitis. Guidelines from the British Society of Gastroenterology advise that "severe gallstone pancreatitis in the presence of increasingly deranged liver function tests and signs of cholangitis (fever, rigors, and positive blood cultures) require an immediate and therapeutic ERCP." If there is only moderate suspicion of retained stones, EUS and MRCP are less risky alternatives to ERCP, with excellent sensitivity for the detection of common bile-duct stones.

Surgery

Surgical management of AP is indicated in two clinical settings: infected pancreatic necrosis and gallstone pancreatitis.

Pancreatic Necrosis. Confirmation of the diagnosis of infected pancreatic necrosis is critical because surgical management is indicated. Clinical and radiographic criteria are not sufficiently reliable for detecting pancreatic infection. Infection is confirmed through ultrasound- or CT-guided aspiration of areas of pancreatic necrosis or suspected pancreatic abscesses. This procedure is safe and reliable, and it has been recommended for all patients with CT criteria for pancreatic necrosis and evidence of sepsis or organ failure.

The ACG guidelines differentiate necrotizing pancreatitis with and without clinical improvement. Patients with evidence of slow clinical improvement may be managed expectantly, without needle aspiration; however, "in the absence of clinical improvement, guided percutaneous aspiration should be performed." This approach is reasonable if the patient is hemodynamically stable and has not developed significant organ failure or a septic syndrome. It is advisable to obtain a surgical consultation before performing this procedure, given the potential need for surgical débridement.

In the setting of infected pancreatic necrosis, resection of all devitalized pancreatic and surrounding tissue is performed. Multiple re-explorations may be required for adequate débridement. Recent studies have suggested that a delayed approach to surgical débridement improves outcomes by allowing time for adequate separation of necrotic and vital areas. In experienced centers, endoscopic transmural necrosectomy is an alternative to surgical débridement for walled off pancreatic necrosis. Cholecystectomy is indicated to prevent recurrence of gallstone pancreatitis. In mild disease, an early cholecystectomy performed during the same hospitalization is favored. In severe gallstone pancreatitis, cholecystectomy may be delayed until clinical improvement or performed at the time of necrectomy.

Idiopathic Acute Pancreatitis. Ten percent of cases of acute pancreatitis are idiopathic acute pancreatitis (IAP). Potential underlying causes of idiopathic pancreatitis include biliary microlithiasis, sphincter of Oddi dysfunction, and undiagnosed genetic defects.

Biliary microlithiasis has been implicated as a common cause of IAP. Recurrent acute episodes of pancreatitis can develop in the absence of gallstones on ultrasound, with or without elevated liver enzyme levels. Repeat ultrasound examinations might eventually reveal biliary sludge or small stones. The finding of cholesterol monohydrate or calcium bilirubinate crystals on microscopic biliary analysis after cholecystokinin stimulation strongly supports the diagnosis of microlithiasis; however, it is not completely sensitive. Laparoscopic cholecystectomy prevents recurrence in patients with IAP and should be considered in all patients with acute recurrent pancreatitis of unclear cause. Endoscopic sphincterotomy or stone dissolution therapy with ursodiol (8-10 mg/kg/day, in two divided doses) are valid options in patients with high surgical risk. Stone dissolution therapy is effective only for noncalcified, cholesterol monohydrate stones smaller than 1 cm in diameter.

ERCP may be helpful in elucidating the cause of IAP. ERCP allows the detection of ampullary tumors, mucinous ductal ectasia, common bile duct stones, pancreas divisum, and pancreatic ductal adenocarcinoma. Biliary manometry allows the diagnosis of sphincter of Oddi dysfunction. ERCP is most strongly indicated for patients who are older than 40 years to rule out neoplasia. MRCP is a safer alternative to ERCP for detecting diseases of the pancreatic duct; however, it is less sensitive for small duct processes, and does not allow inspection of the ampulla or functional assessment of the sphincter of Oddi. EUS is also recognized as a sensitive structural investigation for ampullary, biliary, and pancreatic causes of AP.

There are no published guidelines for the approach to recurrent IAP. Most clinicians do not favor extensive evaluation for the first episode of IAP, because it does not recur in most patients after the first episode; however, CT after resolution is probably reasonable for excluding pancreatic cancer. It is best to tailor the diagnostic approach individually based on patient characteristics. One suggested approach to the patient with idiopathic recurrent acute pancreatitis is demonstrated in Fig. 4.

Outcomes

Mortality rates for hospitalized patients vary from 5% to 10% in most series. In patients with interstitial pancreatitis, mortality is close to zero. Mortality is substantially increased in necrotizing pancreatitis (<1% for interstitial pancreatitis, 10% for sterile necrosis, 30% for infected necrosis).

CHRONIC PANCREATITIS

Definition

Chronic pancreatitis (CP) is defined as a progressive inflammatory disease of the pancreas, characterized by irreversible morphologic changes and gradual fibrotic replacement of the gland. Loss of exocrine and endocrine function results from parenchymal fibrosis. The primary symptoms of CP are abdominal pain and maldigestion. Because of diagnostic and therapeutic challenges, an interdisciplinary management strategy is required.

Epidemiology

The incidence of CP ranges from 1.6 to 23 cases per 100,000 population per year worldwide. Chronic pancreatitis in the United States results in more than 122,000 outpatient visits and more than 56,000 hospitalizations per year.

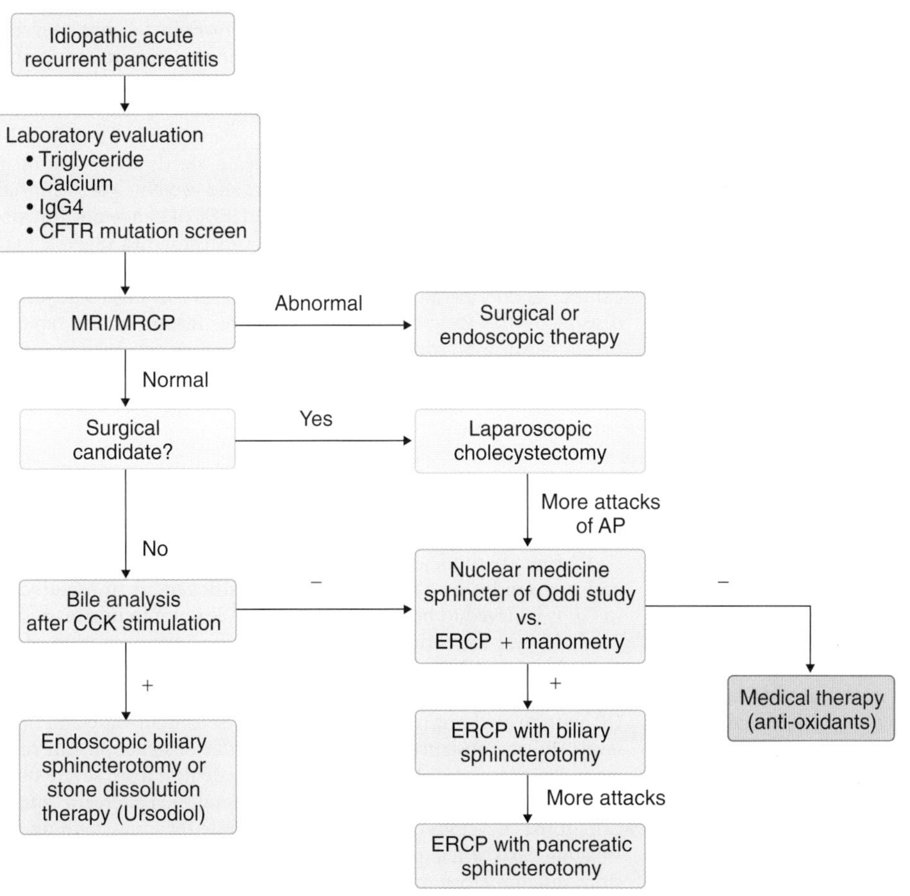

Figure 4 Approach to the management of idiopathic recurrent acute pancreatitis (AP). IgG4, immunoglobulin G4, CCK, cholecystokinin; CFTR, cystic fibrosis transmembrane regulator; ERCP, endoscopic retrograde cholangiopancreatography; MRI, magnetic resonance imaging; MRCP, magnetic resonance cholangiopancreatography.

Pathophysiology

Grossly, the pancreas may be enlarged or atrophic, with or without cysts or calcifications. The ducts may be dilated, irregular, or strictured. Essential pathologic features include irregular and patchy loss of acinar tissue, chronic inflammation, ductal changes, and fibrosis.

Several important pathogenic theories have been developed. The premise of the oxidative stress hypothesis is that reactive by-products of hepatic mixed function oxidase activity damage the pancreas through chronic reflux of bile into the pancreatic duct. The toxic-metabolic theory is that alcohol is directly toxic to the acinar cell through a change in intracellular metabolism. This metabolic effect results in pancreatic lipid accumulation, fatty degeneration, cellular necrosis, and eventual widespread fibrosis. The stone and duct obstruction theory suggests that alcohol increases the lithogenicity of pancreatic juice, leading to stone formation. Chronic contact of the stones with duct epithelial cells produces ulceration and scarring. Eventually, atrophy and fibrosis result from chronic obstruction of the acini. The necrosis-fibrosis theory differs from other theories in that it emphasizes that acute and chronic pancreatitis represents a spectrum of disease. Inflammation from acute pancreatitis leads to scarring and extrinsic compression of the pancreatic ductules. Obstruction results in stasis, atrophy, and stone formation.

A major advance in understanding the underlying cellular mechanisms of pancreatic fibrogenesis is in the primary role of pancreatic stellate cells. Stimulated by alcohol and oxidative stress, activated stellate cells migrate to the periacinar areas to deposit collagen and fibronectin. Stellate cells are also stimulated by specific cytokines, many of which are emitted during the inflammatory phase of acute pancreatitis.

Etiology

Heavy and prolonged alcohol use is the most common cause of CP. In contrast to other causes, alcohol-related CP is associated with more-severe pain, extensive calcification and ductal changes, and more rapid progression to endocrine and exocrine insufficiency. Most patients experience recurrent episodes of acute pancreatitis for several years before CP develops. Interestingly, only a small percentage of alcoholics develop CP, implying the presence of cofactors that amplify the effect of alcohol. A high-fat diet and smoking might also contribute to pancreatic disease in alcoholics. Smoking adversely affects pancreatic bicarbonate and water secretion, induces oxidative stress, and increases the rate of pancreatic calcification.

Tropical pancreatitis is endemic to certain developing regions, such as India, Africa, and South America. Episodic abdominal pain begins in childhood and is followed by rapid progression to endocrine and exocrine insufficiency. Nutritional factors such as dietary toxins (cyanogens in the cassava plant) and micronutrient deficiencies (zinc, copper, and selenium) may be involved in the pathogenesis of tropical pancreatitis.

Causes of obstructive CP include pancreatic adenocarcinoma, neuroendocrine tumors, and intrapapillary mucinous tumors. Autoimmune chronic pancreatitis is a rare but increasingly recognized condition. It is often associated with other autoimmune diseases, such as Sjögren's syndrome and primary sclerosing cholangitis. Laboratory features include an elevated immunoglobulin (Ig)G-4 level. Imaging features include focal or diffuse pancreatic enlargement and a narrowed pancreatic duct. The clinical and radiographic features of the disease improve rapidly with corticosteroid therapy.

Important discoveries have been made in the genetic basis of pancreatic disease. Hereditary pancreatitis is a rare autosomal dominant disease that causes recurrent painful episodes of acute pancreatitis in childhood, leading to CP and pancreatic cancer in adulthood. Hereditary pancreatitis occurs through a mutation of the cationic trypsinogen gene, leading to loss of autoregulation of activated trypsin. Additionally, studies have demonstrated a high prevalence of *CFTR* gene mutations in patients presenting with idiopathic acute and chronic pancreatitis. Although 85% of cystic fibrosis patients have the severe form of cystic fibrosis, with respiratory disease and pancreatic insufficiency, the remaining 15% possess lower sweat chloride levels and might express other phenotypes, including pancreatitis. Most patients who present with pancreatitis as the sole phenotypic feature of cystic fibrosis have one or two mild *CFTR* mutations.

Severe hypercalcemia is known to trigger episodes of acute pancreatitis through trypsin-mediated mechanisms and can progress to CP. Chronic renal failure is associated with an increased prevalence of CP, perhaps related to a direct toxicity of uremia on the pancreas. Hypertriglyceridemia and gallstones rarely cause CP.

Ten percent to 30% of patients with CP possess no identified risk factors. Idiopathic CP has a bimodal age presentation. Early-onset idiopathic CP manifests with severe abdominal pain in childhood, with relatively few structural and functional changes. Late-onset idiopathic CP manifests in late adulthood, often with minimal pain and pronounced exocrine insufficiency.

Signs and Symptoms

Abdominal pain occurs in 50% to 80% of cases and is responsible for most hospitalizations related to this illness. Pancreatic pain is dull or boring in quality and worsens after eating. The pain is located in the epigastric area and often radiates to the back. There may be associated nausea and vomiting with exacerbations of pain. Two patterns of abdominal pain have been described in CP. Type A pain is characterized by short relapsing episodes lasting days to weeks, separated by pain-free intervals. Type B pain implies prolonged, severe, unrelenting pain. Pain exacerbations are not always associated with elevations of serum amylase and lipase levels. Some studies have demonstrated a gradual diminishment of pancreatic pain over years. Proposed clinical predictors of this pancreatic burnout include calcifications, exocrine insufficiency, and endocrine insufficiency. There are several proposed pathogenic mechanisms of abdominal pain in CP, including intraductal hypertension, neural inflammation, neurohormonal changes, concomitant gastroparesis, and elevated cholecystokinin (CCK) levels. Some patients develop nonvisceral (central) pain, often after years of narcotic dependency.

Gradual pancreatic fibrosis produces a steady deterioration in enzyme output, leading to steatorrhea and weight loss. Clinically apparent steatorrhea does not occur until 90% of pancreatic function has been lost. The sudden development of steatorrhea suggests main pancreatic duct obstruction by inflammatory strictures, stones, or cancer. Endocrine insufficiency does not occur until late in the disease course. Pancreatic diabetes requires insulin and is typically brittle because of concomitant glucagon deficiency. Weight loss in CP is multifactorial, related to maldigestion, fear of eating, anorexia, nausea, and vomiting. Severe or rapid weight loss is a red flag for pancreatic cancer.

Complications

Complications of chronic pancreatitis are listed in Table 1.

Chronic pseudocysts are benign cysts formed of pancreatic fluid and surrounded by a fibrous wall. The pathogenesis of pseudocysts in CP is believed to be ductal obstruction, leading to upstream dilation and cyst formation. ERCP might show communication of the cyst with the main pancreatic duct. The typical clinical presentation of a pseudocyst is worsening abdominal pain in the setting of known CP, with or without mild elevation in the serum amylase and lipase levels. Biliary obstruction and gastric outlet obstruction can result from compression of the bile duct and duodenum from severe fibrosis, enlarging pseudocysts, or pancreatic cancer. Pancreatic adenocarcinoma develops in 4% of patients with long-standing CP. Imaging tests often produce uncertainty in differentiating cancer from inflammatory masses.

Pancreatic fistulas, ascites, and pleural effusions arise from a communication of pancreatic pseudocysts with adjacent cavities or from disruption of the pancreatic ducts. The diagnoses of pancreatic ascites and pleural effusions are based on the finding of elevated fluid amylase. Endoscopic stent placement across the pancreatic duct disruption can ameliorate these complications. Splenic vein thrombosis is common and usually asymptomatic; however, recurrent bleeding from secondary gastric varices develops in some patients.

Table 1 Complications of Chronic Pancreatitis

Signs and Symptoms	Treatment
Pseudocysts	
Increased pain	Drainage for large or symptomatic pseudocysts
Vomiting	Endoscopic drainage (transmural or transpapillary)
Mild elevations in amylase and lipase levels	Surgical drainage (cyst gastrostomy or cyst jejunostomy)
Biliary Obstruction	
Jaundice	Drainage of obstructing pseudocyst Endoscopic decompression Surgical decompression
Gastric Outlet Obstruction	
Abdominal pain	Drainage of pseudocyst
Early satiety	Surgical gastrojejunostomy
Nausea and vomiting	
Pancreatic Adenocarcinoma	
Increased pain	Consider surgical resection
Weight loss	Palliation
Pancreatic Ascites	
Increased abdominal girth	Endoscopic stent placement
High-amylase ascites	Total parenteral nutrition
Pleural effusion	
Shortness of breath	Therapeutic thoracentesis
High-amylase pleural fluid	Endoscopic stent placement Total parenteral nutrition
Splenic vein thrombosis	
Bleeding from gastric varices	Splenectomy

Diagnosis

Diagnostic tests for chronic pancreatitis are shown in Table 2.

Advanced CP is most easily diagnosed with a pancreatic-protocol CT scan. The cardinal CT features of CP are pancreatic atrophy, calcifications, and main pancreatic duct dilation. Using these criteria, CT has a sensitivity of 74% to 90% and a specificity of 84% to 100%. Additionally, CT can detect CP complications, including pseudocysts, splenic artery pseudoaneurysm, and biliary obstruction. The finding of pancreatic head enlargement suggests pancreatic cancer or an inflammatory mass.

The diagnosis of early (minimal change) CP is more challenging. ERCP involves the endoscopic injection of contrast into the pancreatic duct via the papilla of Vater for fluoroscopic imaging. ERCP ductal changes are graded from equivocal (class I) to severe (class IV) (Cambridge classification). Although ERCP is considered accurate for early CP, it carries a 5% to 10% risk of acute pancreatitis. The role of ERCP in the diagnosis of chronic pancreatitis has recently decreased because safer and less-invasive techniques are available.

EUS is a minimally invasive test that allows a close sonographic inspection of the head, body, and tail of the pancreas from gastric and duodenal stations. The finding of five or more EUS criteria has been an approximate sensitivity of 75% and specificity of 80% for CP in studies incorporating ERCP as reference standard (Box 3).

MRCP is comparable to CT for detecting major structural abnormalities (atrophy, pseudocysts). Gadolinium-enhanced MRCP can offer improved differentiation of neoplastic and inflammatory masses compared with CT. T_1-weighted images showing parenchymal abnormalities can correlate with early parenchymal fibrosis. Heavily T_2-weighted images produce bright enhancement of fluid-

Box 3 Endoscopic Ultrasound Features of Chronic Pancreatitis

Parenchymal Features
- Hyperechoic foci
- Hyperechoic stranding
- Cysts
- Lobularity

Ductal Features
- Dilation
- Irregularity
- Calculi
- Side branch dilation
- Hyperechoic walls

Table 2 Diagnostic Tests for Chronic Pancreatitis

Test	Sensitivity	Invasiveness, Risk	Cost	Comments
KUB	+	0	+	Reasonable screen Almost 100% specificity
CT	++	0	++	Detects advanced disease
MRI/MRCP	+++	0	+++	Assesses ducts and parenchyma Operator dependence Secretin enhancement may improve sensitivity
EUS	+++	++	+++	Assesses ducts and parenchyma Limited availability
ERCP	++++	+++	+++	Detects early ductal changes
Hormone-stimulated PFT	++++	++	++	Traditional methods not widely available Endoscopic methods in development

CT, computed tomography; ERCP, endoscopic retrograde cholangiopancreatography; EUS, endoscopic ultrasound; MRI/MRCP, magnetic resonance imaging/MR cholangiopancreatography; PFT, pancreatic function test.

filled structures, allowing a noninvasive alternative to ERCP for imaging the pancreatic duct. Secretin-enhanced MRCP allows a functional assessment of the pancreas by visualizing and quantifying duodenal fluid volume after secretin stimulation of the exocrine pancreas. Although EUS and MRCP are now commonly used for diagnosing CP, there are many unanswered questions regarding the true accuracy, interobserver variability, and cost-effectiveness of these tests.

When imaging test results are negative or equivocal, direct, hormone-stimulated pancreatic function tests are helpful to confirm or rule out the presence of mild exocrine insufficiency as a surrogate marker of early CP. Pancreatic function tests involve stimulating the pancreas with intravenous CCK or secretin and then collecting fluid from the duodenum. Pancreatic fluid is analyzed for enzyme and bicarbonate production. Several noninvasive indirect tests of pancreatic function are also available, including fecal fat analysis, fecal chymotrypsin, and fecal elastase assays. These tests are sensitive for moderate and late-stage exocrine insufficiency but lack sensitivity for detecting early disease.

Treatment

Three components are essential to the optimal management of CP: control of pain, improvement of maldigestion, and management of complications.

Control of Abdominal Pain

The management of chronic pancreatic pain is challenging. The AGA has published an evidence-based technical review on the management of pain in CP. In this review, the available medical, endoscopic, and surgical techniques for pain control are critically evaluated in the context of existing literature. The following discussion reflects these guidelines.

Some have advocated supportive therapy for abdominal pain on the premise that fibrosis and scarring ultimately progress to pancreatic burnout and spontaneous relief of pain. Although long-term improvement in pain has been observed in some patients with CP, a significant subset of patients experiences debilitating pain for decades. The AGA technical review has stated that "a strategy of waiting for spontaneous pain relief is not reliable and may be unreasonable advice for the patient with persistent, severe pain." Medical options for pain relief include abstinence from alcohol, analgesics, and pancreatic enzymes. Abstinence from alcohol is critical because continued use can hasten disease progression, aggravate chronic pain, and increase mortality. Non-narcotic analgesics (e.g., nonsteroidal anti-inflammatory drugs, acetaminophen, and tramadol) are the next step in managing painful CP. If pain persists, low doses of mild narcotics may be added. Severe or recalcitrant pain can warrant the use of stronger opiates in selected cases.

Pancreatic enzymes are presumed to improve pain by suppressing CCK release from the duodenum, leading to decreased pancreatic stimulation. The AGA review has critically appraised the literature regarding the controversial use of enzymes for pain. A meta-analysis of six randomized, placebo-controlled trials did not reveal a statistically significant benefit for supplemental pancreatic enzyme therapy for pain relief. However, there was substantial methodological heterogeneity among the included trials. Uncoated preparations might work better by enhancing delivery to the proximal small bowel. Uncoated pancreatic enzymes may be worth trying in all patients because of their safety and minimal side effects. However, the AGA technical review has cautioned that "additional studies are required to establish the effectiveness of this modality of treatment and to define whether certain subsets are more likely to benefit from enzyme therapy."

Interestingly, many patients with CP have nonvisceral pain (central or somatosensory in origin). A differential nerve blockade is helpful in determining whether there is a central or somatosensory component to the pain syndrome. A differential nerve blockade is indicated for any patient with pancreatic pain that does not respond to simple medical therapeutic measures such as non-narcotic analgesics and enzymes. Antidepressants, anticonvulsants (gabapentin), topical therapy, psychiatric counseling, and opioid rehabilitation may be of use for patients with nonvisceral pain. Celiac or sphlanchnic nerve blockade may be used in select patients with visceral pancreatic pain. Limited studies have suggested that a subset of patients obtain significant short-term pain relief from CT-guided celiac plexus blockade. EUS-guided celiac plexus blockade has emerged as an effective and perhaps safer alternative to percutaneous methods.

It is generally accepted that pain in CP can result in part from obstruction of the main pancreatic duct from stones and strictures, leading to increased ductal and parenchymal pressure. Because obstruction contributes to pain, patients with an enlarged, obstructed main pancreatic duct might benefit from endoscopic or surgical duct decompression therapy. Endoscopic techniques include biliary or pancreatic sphincterotomy (or both), removal of pancreatic duct stones, and placement of pancreatic stents.

Several surgical options exist for select patients with visceral pain resulting from CP. In patients with a dilated main pancreatic duct, a side-to-side pancreaticojejunostomy (Puestow procedure) may be performed. Most studies of surgical and endoscopic decompressive therapy in CP have revealed good short-term but poor long-term pain control. The AGA technical review has stated that these procedures are best performed based on "need for long-term narcotic therapy, marked diminution of the quality of life because of intractable pain, or major nutritional consequences of pain."

Pancreatic resection is reserved for patients with disease of the small duct and pain unresponsive to medical therapy. The Whipple procedure and distal pancreatectomy have been used in the past to treat patients with small-duct CP. Newer resection techniques have offered substantial relief of pain related to an inflamed and scarred gland, with preservation of surrounding structures. For example, the Beger procedure involves resection of the inflamed pancreatic head with careful sparing of the duodenum; the Frey procedure adds a longitudinal duct decompression to the pancreatic head resection. The AGA review has cited several potential drawbacks of resection procedures, including paucity of randomized trials; loss of exocrine and endocrine function, including diabetes; technical expertise required for organ-sparing methods; and lack of pain relief in some patients, even after total pancreatectomy. In spite of these drawbacks, resection offers significant relief to a subset of carefully chosen patients, particularly if performed in high-volume centers. Total pancreatectomy with auto–islet cell transplantation (TP/AIT) has been performed at several centers in the United States. TP/AIT involves removing the entire pancreas. The pancreatic explant is enzymatically digested to isolate the insulin-producing islet cells. In a second surgery, the islet cells are infused through the portal vein to engraft within the liver. Case series of TP/AIT suggest that most patients receive substantial relief of pain and have no or minimal insulin requirement.

Improvement of Maldigestion

Pancreatic enzymes are used for the treatment of maldigestion in CP. Exogenous pancreatic enzymes are safe, are well tolerated, and produce few side effects. Pancreatic enzyme preparations differ based on enzyme content, the use of microspheres versus microtablets, and the presence of a coating for delayed release. Lipase is the most important determinant of the effectiveness of individual preparations. A minimum of 30,000 U lipase per meal allows adequate intraluminal digestion of fat and protein in most patients. The dose might need to be titrated to as much as 80,000 U lipase per meal, because not all the lipase may reach the proximal small intestine in active form. Dosing of enzymes is most physiologic if one half the amount is taken at the onset of the meal and the other half is taken

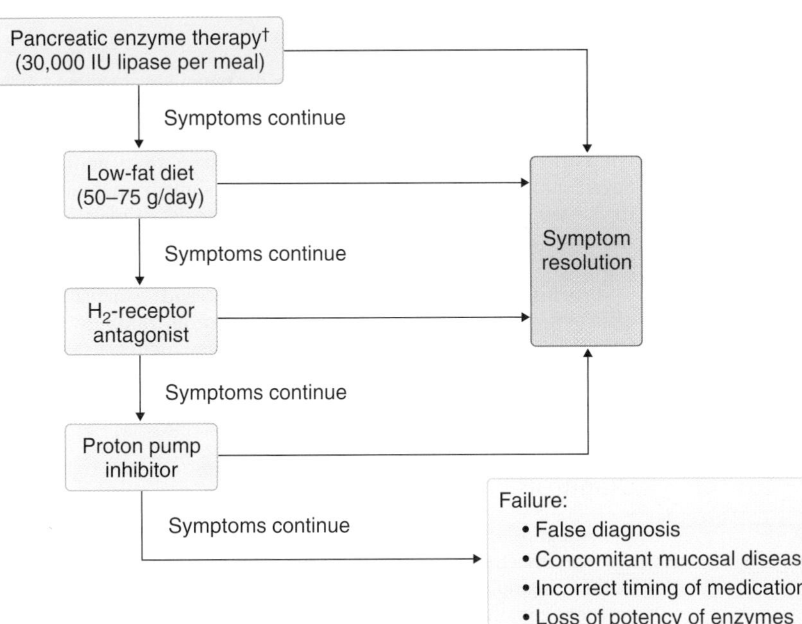

Figure 5 **Approach to the management of pancreatic maldigestion.**

approximately 15 minutes into the meal. Because uncoated preparations are more easily denatured by gastric acid, acid suppression with a proton pump inhibitor (e.g., omeprazole 20 mg once daily) or histamine-receptor antagonist (e.g., famotidine 20 mg twice daily) is required.

Response to enzyme therapy may be monitored through an assessment of symptoms or, more objectively, through 72-hour stool fat quantification. A poor response to pancreatic enzymes can suggest noncompliance, loss of enzyme potency, improper timing of enzymes in relation to meals, or coexisting mucosal disease. A daily proton pump inhibitor may be added for those refractory to therapy because gastric acid can denature exogenous enzymes. A general approach to the treatment of maldigestion in CP is shown in Figure 5.

Management of Complications

Large or symptomatic pseudocysts may be drained endoscopically through transmural or transpapillary approaches. Large pseudocysts may also be drained surgically through cyst gastrostomy. Biliary and gastric outlet obstructions are best managed through surgical decompression. The initial management of the complications of pancreatic duct disruption or fistulas (pancreatic ascites or pleural effusions) includes prolonged pancreatic rest (parenteral nutrition), octreotide, and endoscopic placement of pancreatic duct stents. In some cases, surgical resection may be necessary.

Cleveland Clinic Approach

Because of the significant challenges inherent in the management of this disease, we have developed a multidisciplinary approach similar to the AGA algorithm. Patients first undergo a diagnostic and staging evaluation (Fig. 6). Most patients undergo CT as an initial diagnostic test. Secretin-stimulated endoscopic pancreatic function tests and EUS are used as second-line tests to diagnose early CP in patients in whom initial imaging is negative.

Once the diagnosis of CP has been established, patients with severe pancreatic pain refractory to initial conservative management may be referred for a differential nerve blockade to clarify the origin of their pain syndrome (Fig. 7). Patients with nonvisceral pain are referred for psychotherapy and treatment of chemical dependency. Patients with visceral pain are first given a trial of conservative medical management. If pain persists, patients with large-duct disease

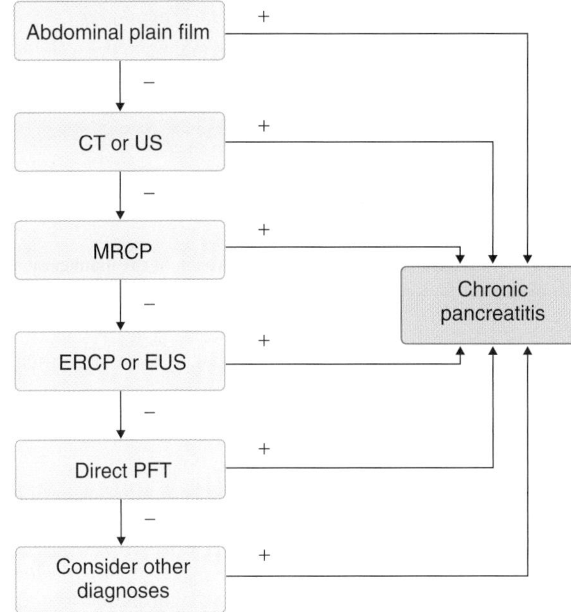

Figure 6 **Approach to the diagnosis of chronic pancreatitis.** CT, computed tomography; ERCP, endoscopic retrograde cholangiopancreatography; EUS, endoscopic ultrasound; MRCP, magnetic resonance cholangiopancreatography; PFT, pancreatic function test; US, ultrasound.

or pseudocysts are referred for surgical management or endoscopic therapy. Patients with small-duct disease (or those with large-duct disease failing duct-decompression measures) are referred for an EUS-guided celiac plexus blockade. Other options for these patients include sphlanchnic radio-frequency ablation, spinal cord stimulation, and total pancreatectomy with auto–islet cell transplantation.

PANCREATIC NEOPLASMS

Pancreatic ductal adenocarcinoma accounts for 90% of cancers of the pancreas. The diagnostic and therapeutic approaches outlined

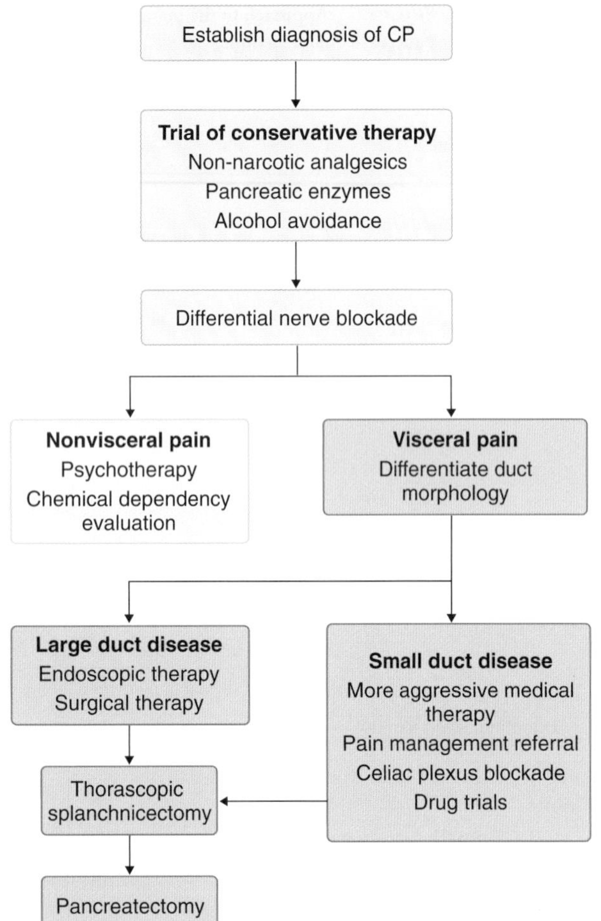

Figure 7 **Cleveland Clinic Foundation approach to the management of pain in chronic pancreatitis (CP).**

here integrate the AGA guidelines for the diagnosis and treatment of pancreatic ductal adenocarcinoma (Fig. 8).

Prevalence

Pancreatic cancer is the fourth and fifth most common cancer in men and women, respectively. It accounts for more than 30,000 new cases and 20,000 cancer-related deaths each year. Most patients are older than 60 years. The male-to-female ratio is 2:1. It has the lowest 5-year survival of any cancer, reflecting late diagnosis and low resection rates.

Risk Factors

The AGA guidelines have recommended smoking cessation for preventing pancreatic cancer. Based on animal experiments, the aromatic amines present in cigarette smoke, meats, and fish oil may be the specific pathogenic factor predisposing to neoplastic transformation. Occupations with a high exposure to amines (e.g., chemistry, hairdressing, rubber work) can confer an increased risk. Certain diseases, including chronic pancreatitis, diabetes mellitus, and hereditary cancer syndromes, predispose toward pancreatic cancer. Patients with hereditary pancreatitis develop acute recurrent pancreatitis in childhood, which usually progresses to chronic pancreatitis and pancreatic cancer in early adulthood. Patients with a significant familial risk (>2 first-degree relatives, multiple second-degree relatives, early onset of pancreatic cancer before age 50 years) might qualify for a surveillance strategy such as yearly endoscopic ultrasound.

Signs and Symptoms

Of pancreatic cancers, 60% develop in the pancreatic head and 40% develop in the body and tail. Symptoms include abdominal pain, anorexia, weight loss, and jaundice. The pain is located in the epigastrium and has a quality characterized as deep and boring. Severe abdominal pain suggests neural plexus involvement, location in the tail, unresectability, and a poor prognosis. Painless jaundice indicates a potentially resectable lesion located in the pancreatic head.

Pruritis and steatorrhea suggest biliary and pancreatic duct obstruction, respectively. Physical examination findings include jaundice, cachexia, a palpable abdominal mass, ascites, left cervical lymphadenopathy (Virchow's node), a palpable gallbladder (Courvoisier's sign), and migratory superficial thrombophlebitis (Trousseau's syndrome).

Diagnosis

The diagnosis and staging of pancreatic cancer is accomplished through imaging tests and pathologic diagnosis (see Fig. 8). The best initial imaging test for diagnosis and staging of pancreatic cancer is contrast-enhanced, dual-phase, helical CT, with thin cuts through the pancreas. CT allows assessment of the primary tumor, local invasiveness, regional lymph node involvement, liver metastases, and peritoneal spread (Fig. 9). The sensitivity of helical CT for detecting pancreatic cancer ranges from 85% to 95%. Dual-phase CT helps determine surgical resectability through assessment of invasion of major vessels. CT can underestimate hepatic and lymph node involvement.

Magnetic resonance imaging (MRI) with gadolinium enhancement compares favorably with CT in the assessment of local tumor extent, relation to vascular structures, lymph node involvement, and distant metastases. MRI can improve differentiation of a pancreatic cancer from chronic pancreatitis and offers simultaneous assessment of the pancreatic and bile ducts by heavily T_2-weighted imaging (MRCP).

Several studies have suggested increased sensitivity of endoscopic ultrasound (EUS) compared with conventional, single-phase CT for detecting and local staging of pancreatic cancer. The greatest advantage of EUS is that it allows fine needle aspiration (FNA) of the tumor to provide a tissue diagnosis. Problems with EUS include operator dependency and lack of widespread availability. The AGA guidelines have suggested that EUS has the greatest role in detecting small tumors missed by CT and in tissue acquisition.

The role of endoscopic retrograde cholangiopancreatography (ERCP) in the diagnosis of pancreatic disease has diminished in recent years as a result of improved noninvasive and less-risky imaging techniques. ERCP is most useful for palliating unresectable tumors that cause biliary obstruction. Diagnostic features on ERCP include an irregular solitary pancreatic duct stenosis more than 1 cm long, an abrupt cutoff of the main pancreatic duct, or an obstruction of both pancreatic and bile ducts (double-duct sign). Importantly, these findings are nonspecific, because they may also be observed in chronic pancreatitis.

Tumor markers are adjunctive tests for diagnosing gastrointestinal cancers. A CA19-9 concentration higher than 70 U/mL has a sensitivity of 70% and specificity of 87% for pancreatic cancer. The CA19-9 level may also be significantly elevated in benign conditions such as choledocholithiasis and cholangitis. In the absence of a mass, elevated levels of CA19-9 and other tumor markers are difficult to interpret.

Biopsy of a pancreatic mass or metastasis may be done percutaneously under CT guidance or by EUS with FNA. Biopsy is indicated in unresectable disease to confirm the diagnosis and aid in decision making regarding chemotherapy and radiation therapy. The use of biopsy in resectable disease is more controversial. Critics have argued that the theoretical risk of peritoneal seeding and procedure compli-

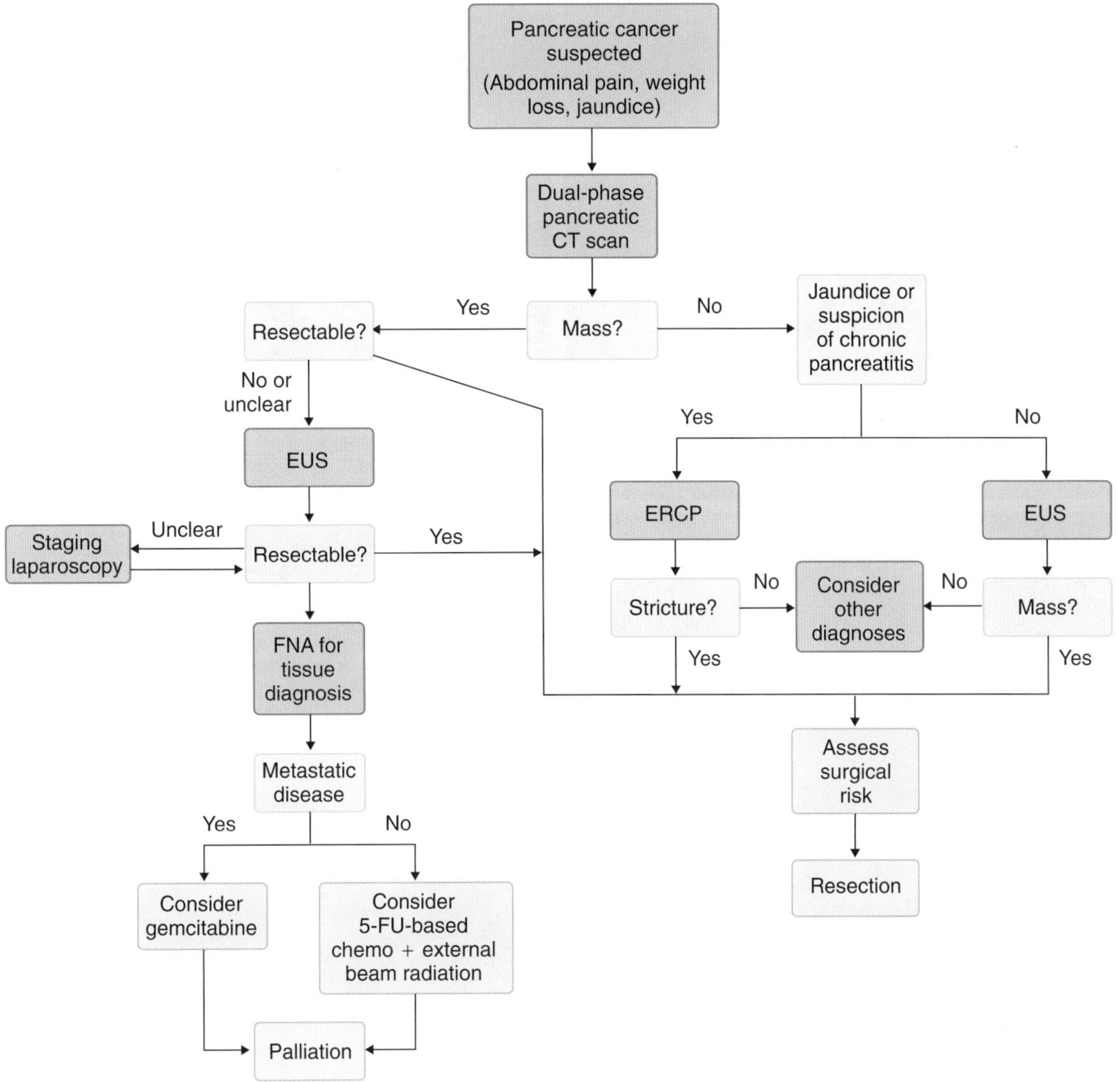

Figure 8 **Approach to the diagnosis and management of pancreatic adenocarcinoma.** CT, computed tomography; EUS, endoscopic ultrasound; ERCP, endoscopic retrograde cholangiopancreatography; FNA, fine needle aspiration; 5-FU, 5-fluorouracil. *(Adapted from DiMagno EP, Reber HA, Tempero MA: AGA technical review on the epidemiology, diagnosis, and treatment of pancreatic ductal adenocarcinoma. American Gastroenterological Association. Gastroenterology 1999;117:1464-1484.)*

cations outweigh the benefit. Proponents of routine biopsy have cited the rare possibility of detecting a chemosensitive tumor (lymphoma) and the desire of many patients to know their diagnosis before major surgery. The AGA guidelines have recommended FNA only for patients with unresectable lesions. However, individual circumstances may dictate otherwise.

All the current imaging tests can underestimate tumor, nodal, and metastatic staging. Staging laparoscopy with or without laparoscopic ultrasound improves accuracy through the detection of small hepatic or peritoneal metastases, widespread sampling of regional lymph nodes, and direct visualization of the primary tumor and its relation to peripancreatic vessels. The AGA guidelines have recommended staging laparoscopy if there is a high likelihood of unresectability that has not been confirmed by imaging tests.

Treatment

The only potentially curative therapy for pancreatic cancer is surgical resection. Pancreatic cancer is resectable if the tumor is confined to the pancreas and does not have encasement of adjacent surrounding major vessels (superior mesenteric artery or vein, portosplenic confluence, celiac trunk, or aorta), does not have extensive peripancreatic lymph node involvement, or does not have distant metastases. Unfortunately, because of late presentation and delay in diagnosis, only 20% of patients present with resectable disease. The long-term prognosis is poor, even among those who undergo resection and have tumor-free margins (5-year survival rate after resection is 10%-25%). Because the only chance of cure is through resection, all patients with potentially resectable lesions by CT criteria should be referred for surgical consultation.

The standard operation for adenocarcinoma in the pancreatic head or uncinate process is pancreaticoduodenectomy, or Whipple procedure. This involves resection of the pancreatic head, duodenum, common bile duct, distal stomach, and gallbladder. Reconstruction involves pancreaticojejunostomy, hepaticojejunostomy, and gastrojejunostomy. Although the perioperative mortality in high-volume centers is less than 2%, several short- and long-term complications can occur, including anastomotic leaks and ulcerations, dumping syndrome, and bile gastritis. The AGA guidelines have stressed the importance of cardiac, pulmonary, and nutritional

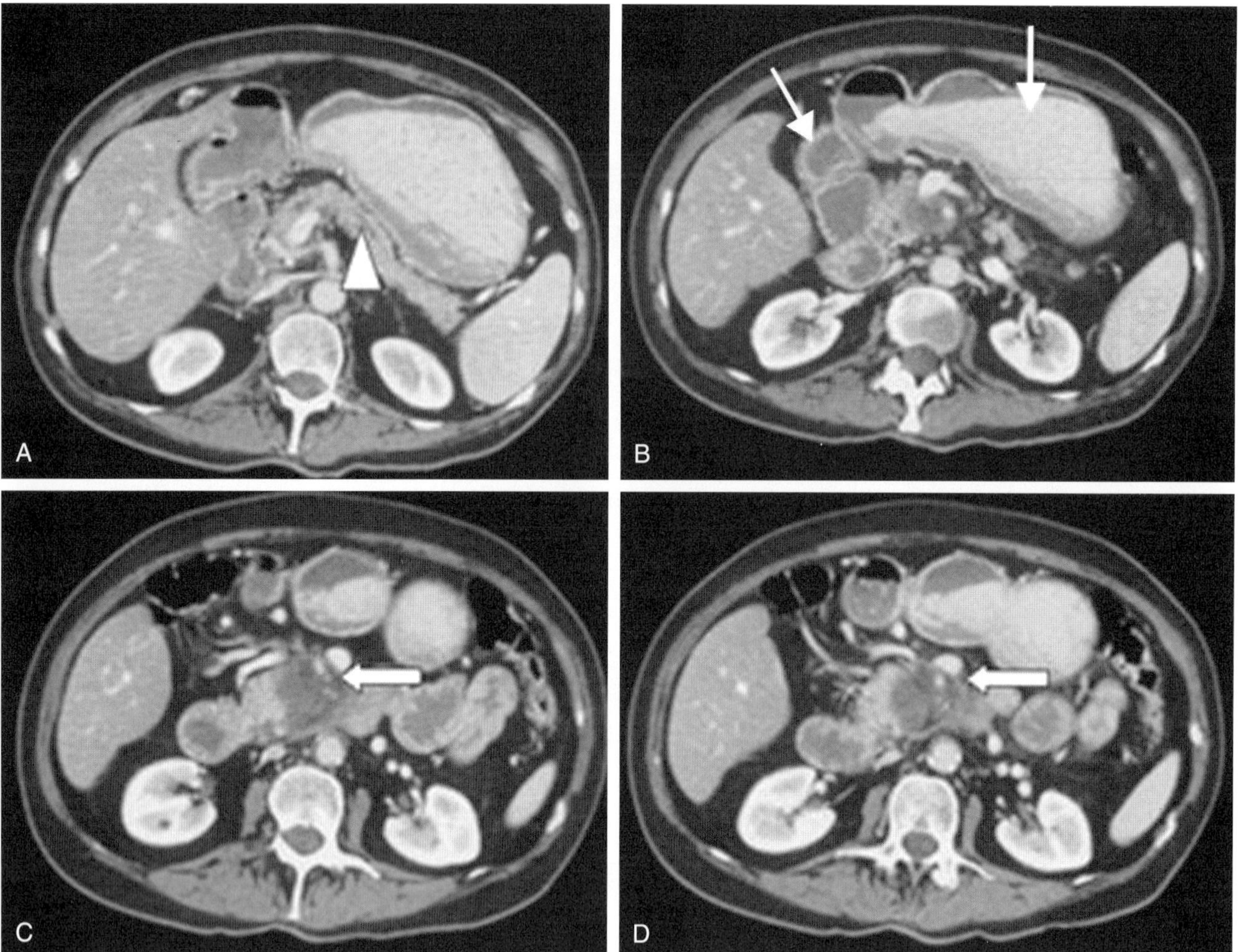

Figure 9 Computed tomography scan showing pancreatic head cancer. A, Upstream pancreatic duct dilation *(arrowhead)*. **B,** Dilation of the stomach and proximal duodenum, suggesting gastric outlet obstruction *(thin arrows)*. This cancer is unresectable on the basis of superior mesenteric artery encasement (**C,** *thick arrow*) and the presence of hepatic metastases (**D,** *thick arrow*).

optimization before pancreatic surgery. Although commonly performed, routine preoperative endoscopic biliary decompression is not beneficial and can actually worsen outcomes. The AGA guidelines have recommended preoperative biliary stenting for jaundiced patients in whom surgery will be delayed for several weeks or in patients with unresectable tumors.

Although chemotherapy and radiotherapy are not curative, they can offer some clinical benefits, including shrinkage of the primary tumor, improvement of symptoms, and prolongation of survival. These modalities have been studied in locally metastatic disease and advanced disease and as surgical adjuvant therapies. The AGA guidelines have stated that "all patients with unresectable locoregional or metastatic pancreatic cancer should be considered for inclusion into investigational trials." Single-agent gemcitabine is often administered in patients with advanced metastatic pancreatic cancer. Studies with gemcitabine have demonstrated a significant clinical response (decreased pain, increased functional status), even in the absence of a measurable tumor response. Patients with locally advanced cancer may be considered for combined 5-fluorouracil-based chemotherapy and external beam radiation, which has been shown to improve median survival compared with radiation therapy alone. The benefits of chemotherapy and radiation as therapies adjuvant to surgical resection have not been proved.

The palliation of symptoms is arguably the most important goal in patients with locally advanced and metastatic disease. Patients with pancreatic cancer may develop debilitating symptoms of pain (neural plexus invasion), jaundice (biliary obstruction), or vomiting (gastric outlet obstruction). Pain can usually be managed with escalating doses of narcotic agents. In spite of their benefits, narcotics can cause constipation and depressed mental status. EUS-guided celiac nerve neurolysis can offer significant pain control and decrease narcotic requirements. Diarrhea and weight loss from maldigestion may be palliated through the use of pancreatic enzymes. Patients with biliary obstruction might require surgical or endoscopic biliary decompression. Gastric outlet obstruction can be managed by surgical gastrojejunostomy or endoscopic stenting. Not all vomiting arises from outlet obstruction. Many patients have impaired gastric motility as a result of the local invasion of nerve fibers.

Types of Tumors

Pancreatic Neuroendocrine Tumors

Neuroendocrine tumors (NETs) are rare tumors (incidence rate, 5 cases per 1 million person-years) that arise from endocrine cells within or near the pancreas. NETs can occur sporadically or as part

Table 3 Pancreatic Neuroendocrine Tumors

Tumor Type	Number (%)*	Secretory Products	Clinical Features	Laboratory Tests	Symptomatic Treatment
Insulinoma	40-60	Insulin	Hypoglycemia; symptoms of catecholamine excess; 90% benign	Insulin level, C-reactive protein; 72-hr inpatient fasting, with monitoring of glucose and insulin levels	Dietary measures; octreotide; diazoxide
Gastrinoma	20-50	Gastrin	Peptic ulcer disease; GERD; secretory diarrhea; most common NET in MEN-I; 60%-90% malignant	Fasting serum gastrin; gastric pH analysis; gastrin provocation testing (calcium or secretin challenge)	Proton pump inhibitor; octreotide
Glucagonoma	Rare	Glucagon	Glucose intolerance; migratory necrolytic erythema; weight loss; anemia; 90% malignant	Serum glucagon	Octreotide; insulin; zinc supplement (rash); TPN (malnutrition)
Somatostatinoma	Rare	Somatostatin	Diabetes; gallstones; secretory diarrhea	Clinical and pathologic diagnoses; increased somatostatin-like immunoreactivity in resected tumor	Octreotide
VIPoma	Rare	Vasoactive intestinal peptide	Cholera-like, secretory diarrhea; hypokalemia; hypochlorhydria	Serum VIP	Octreotide

*Percentage among neuroendocrine tumors.

GERD, gastroesophageal reflux disease; MEN-I, multiple endocrine neoplasia type I; NET, neuroendocrine tumor; TPN, total parenteral nutrition; VIP, vasoactive intestinal polypeptide.

of multiple endocrine neoplasia type 1. Most primary NETs arise within the gastrinoma triangle, composed of the joining of the cystic and common hepatic ducts, second and third portions of the duodenum, and border of the body and tail of the pancreas. Although a subset of NETs is nonfunctional, most secrete hormones that can result in various clinical syndromes (Table 3). Carcinoid tumors are considered NETs but are rarely found in the pancreas. Most NETs are listed in the differential diagnosis for secretory diarrhea, although the yield of testing in this setting is extremely low. Nonfunctional tumors are most often indolent but can demonstrate malignant behavior, including metastases.

When a NET is suspected, imaging tests are used to locate the primary tumor and determine the presence of metastases (Fig. 10). NETs may be difficult to localize. Contrast-enhanced CT and MRI may be used as initial tests; however, they have a low yield for small tumors. EUS is a more sensitive test for detecting small pancreatic neuroendocrine tumors and allows simultaneous FNA for tissue diagnosis. Nuclear imaging after administration of radiolabeled octreotide aids in localizing some neuroendocrine tumors. Insulinomas are not well visualized with octreotide scans because they do not possess high concentrations of somatostatin receptors.

NETs confined to the pancreas should be surgically resected after symptoms of hormonal excess have been treated and controlled (see Box 1). Patients with metastatic disease can be managed medically with octreotide, chemotherapy (streptozocin), or radiographic embolization of the primary tumor and metastases. Debulking of primary and metastatic disease may also be considered for patients with debilitating symptoms related to tumor secretory products.

Pancreatic Cystic Neoplasms

Up to 90% of pancreatic cysts are inflammatory pseudocysts arising from acute or chronic pancreatitis. Cystic neoplasms are reported to account for less than 1% of pancreatic cancers. Generally, they are indolent tumors with varying malignant potential (Table 4). The primary aim of diagnosis is to differentiate benign cysts (e.g., pseudocysts, serous cystadenoma) from malignant cysts (e.g., mucinous cystadenoma, premalignart intraductal papillary mucinous neoplasms [IPMNs]) (Fig. 11). Small (<1 cm), simple, asymptomatic cysts discovered incidentally may be observed using follow-up imaging. A history of past acute pancreatitis or imaging criteria suggesting chronic pancreatitis should increase suspicion of a pseudocyst. In the absence of pancreatitis, radiographic features are poorly reliable in differentiating mucinous from other types of pancreatic cysts. Cystic masses larger than 3 cm and producing symptoms should be resected.

In asymptomatic patients, EUS allows improved characterization of cyst features and also simultaneous aspiration of cyst fluid for chemical analysis. Fluid may be analyzed for cytology, tumor markers (carcinoembyonic antigen [CEA]), and amylase. A positive mucin stain of cyst fluid may also be helpful in ruling in a mucinous cystic neoplasm. The primary diagnostic test for IPMN is ERCP. The ERCP features of IPMN include a gaping papilla, with the extrusion of mucin, and global or segmental main duct or side branch dilation, with papillary projections (Fig. 12).

Mucinous cystic neoplasms and IPMNs should be resected because they have potential for malignant transformation. Resection should also be considered for serous cystademomas that are symptomatic or enlarging.

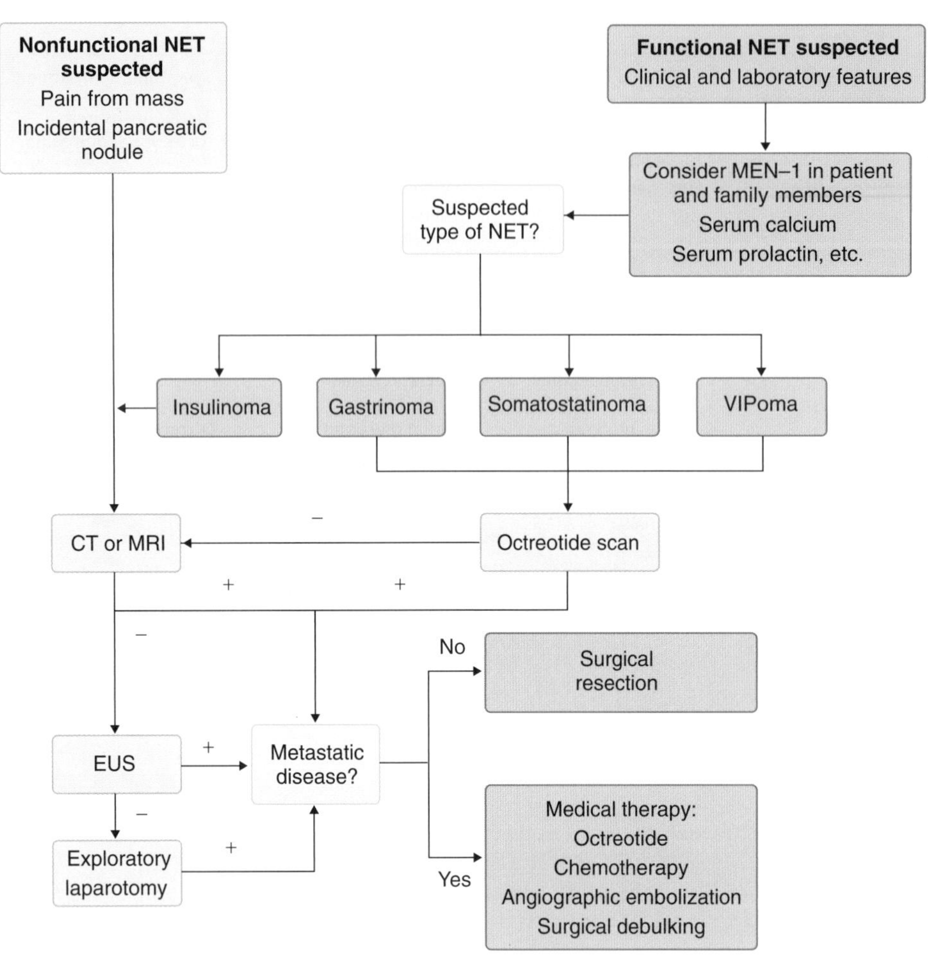

Figure 10 **Approach to the diagnosis and management of pancreatic neuroendocrine tumors (NETs).** CT, computed tomography; MEN-I, multiple endocrine neoplasia type I; MRI, magnetic resonance imaging.

Table 4 Types of Pancreatic Cysts

Type	Demographic	Malignant Potential	Location	Radiographic Features	Cyst Fluid Analysis
Pseudocyst	History of pancreatitis	No	Throughout	Unilocular; thick-walled	↑ amylase level
Serous cystadenoma	Middle-aged women	No	Throughout	Multicystic; calcifications; central scar	↑ Ca19-9 level
Mucinous cystadenoma or cystadenocarcinoma	Middle-aged women	Yes	Body and tail	One or few cysts; thick or irregular walls	Positive mucin stain; ↑CEA level; positive cytology
Intrapapillary mucinous neoplasia	Middle-aged and older men	Yes	Diffuse or localized	Pancreatic duct dilation; papillary projections	
Papillary cystic neoplasm	Rare; young women	Yes; locally aggressive	Body and tail		

CEA, carcinoembryonic antigen.

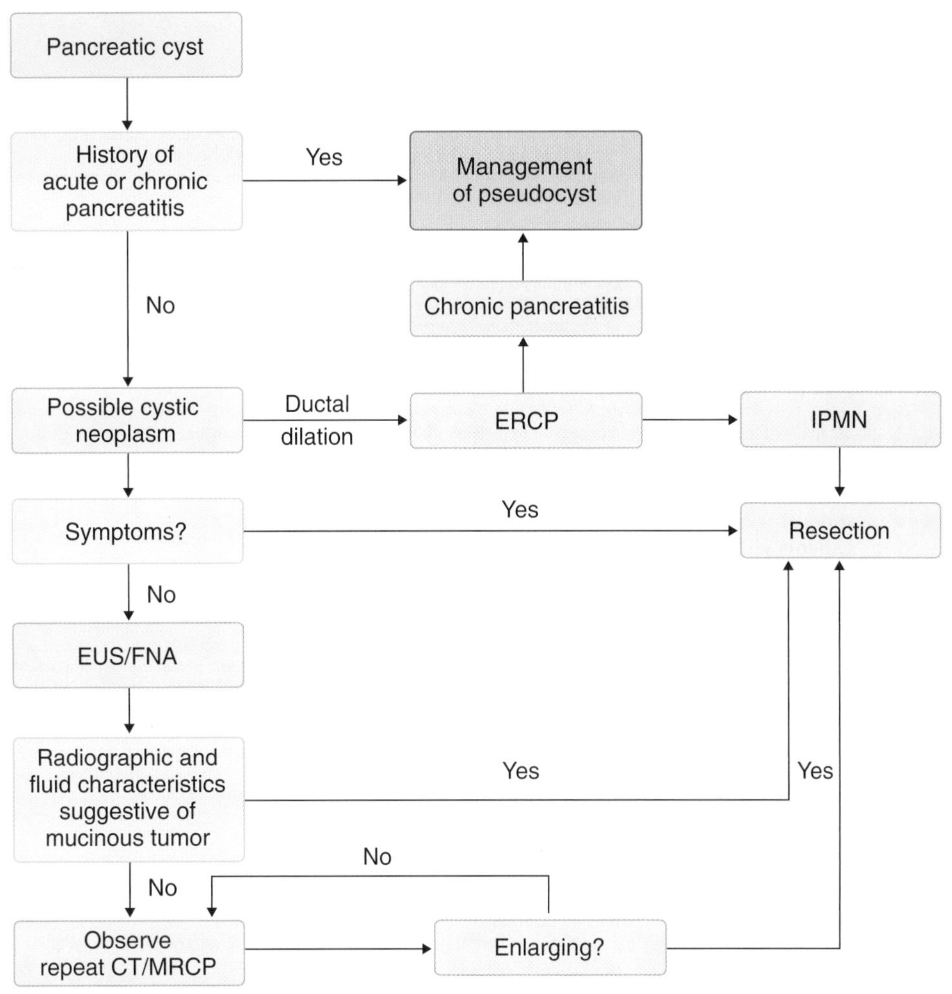

Figure 11 **Approach to the diagnosis and management of pancreatic cysts.** ERCP, endoscopic retrograde cholangiopancreatography; EUS, endoscopic ultrasound; FNA, fine needle aspiration; IPMN, intradutal papillary mucinny neophy.

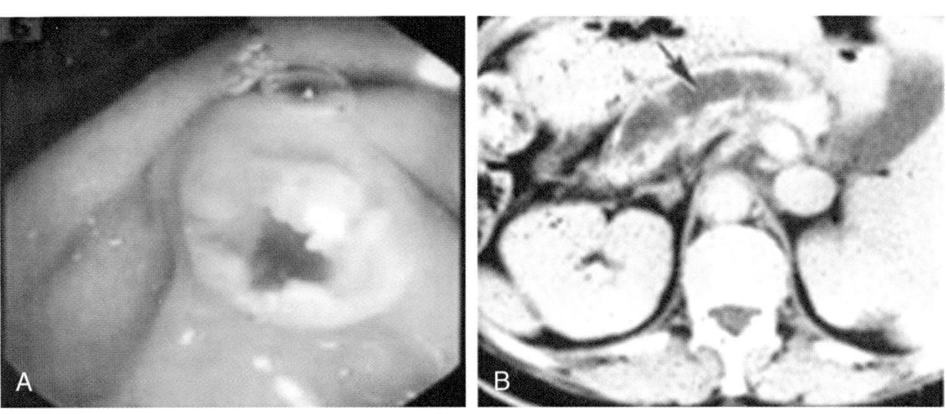

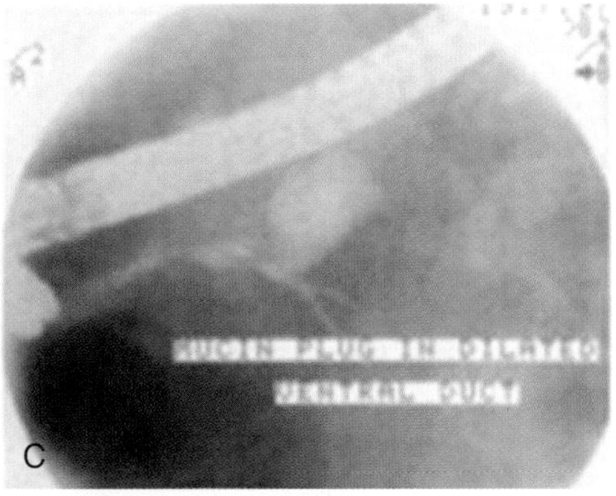

Figure 12 **Endoscopy, computed tomography (CT), and endoscopic retrograde cholangiopancreatography (ERCP) appearance of intradutal papillary mucinny neophy (IPMN).** **A,** Endoscopic image shows a gaping papilla, with extrusion of mucin. **B,** CT scan shows a dilated pancreatic duct, with papillary projections. **C,** ERCP image shows a dilated pancreatic duct, with mucin plugs.

Summary

Acute Pancreatitis

- The management of acute pancreatitis includes meticulous supportive care and aggressive but careful volume resuscitation.
- Assessment of severity is an important initial step in the care of all patients with acute pancreatitis.
- A contrast-enhanced pancreatic CT scan should be considered for patients with severe acute pancreatitis.
- Endoscopic retrograde cholangiopancreatography should be performed in patients with gallstone pancreatitis and signs of ongoing biliary obstruction or cholangitis.
- Nutritional support should be administered to all patients with prolonged NPO status or severe acute pancreatitis.
- Surgical consultation and percutaneous aspiration of pancreatic necrosis should be considered for patients with clinical deterioration or multiorgan system failure.

Chronic Pancreatitis

- Computed tomography scanning detects advanced chronic pancreatitis.
- Endoscopic ultrasound and pancreatic function tests detect early (minimal change) chronic pancreatitis.
- Management strategies for chronic pancreatic pain include analgesics, pancreatic enzyme supplementation, celiac plexus blockade, endoscopic or surgical duct decompression therapy, and total pancreatectomy with auto–islet cell transplantation.

Pancreatic Cancer

- Dual phase contrast-enhanced computed tomography scanning is the initial test of choice in the diagnosis and staging of pancreatic cancer.
- Radical pancreaticoduodenectomy (Whipple procedure) is the treatment of choice for patients with resectable pancreatic cancer.
- Although chemotherapy and radiation therapy have roles in the management of unresectable pancreatic cancer, palliation of symptoms is the primary therapeutic goal.
- EUS-guided fine needle aspiration and fluid analysis aid in differentiating pancreatic cysts with and without malignant potential.

Suggested Readings

American College of Gastroenterology: Practice Guidelines: Acute Pancreatitis, 2006. Available at http://gi.org/physicians/guidelines/AcutePancreatitis.pdf.

Ammann RW, Muellhaupt B: The natural history of pain in alcoholic chronic pancreatitis. Gastroenterology 1999;116:1132-1140.

Axon AT, Classen M, Cotton P, et al: Pancreatography in chronic pancreatitis: International definitions. Gut 1984;25:1107-1112.

Balthazar EJ, Robinson DL, Megibow AJ, Ranson JH: Acute pancreatitis: Value of CT in establishing prognosis. Radiology 1990;174:331-336.

Bradley EL 3rd: A clinically based classification system for acute pancreatitis. Summary of the International Symposium on Acute Pancreatitis, Atlanta, Ga, September 11 through 13, 1992. Arch Surg 1993;128:586-590.

British Society of Gastroenterology: United Kingdom guidelines for the management of acute pancreatitis. Gut 1998;42(Suppl 2):S1-S13.

Brown A, Hughes M, Tenner S, Banks PA: Does pancreatic enzyme supplementation reduce pain in patients with chronic pancreatitis: A meta-analysis. Am J Gastroenterol 1997;92:2032-2035.

DiMagno EP, Reber HA, Tempero MA: AGA technical review on the epidemiology, diagnosis, and treatment of pancreatic ductal adenocarcinoma. American Gastroenterological Association. Gastroenterology 1999;117:1464-1484.

Folsch UR, Nitsche R, Ludtke R, et al: Early ERCP and papillotomy compared with conservative treatment for acute biliary pancreatitis. The German Study Group on Acute Biliary Pancreatitis. N Engl J Med 1997;336:237-242.

Lee SP, Nicholls JF, Park HZ: Biliary sludge as a cause of acute pancreatitis. N Engl J Med 1992;326:589-593.

Lu DS, Reber HA, Krasny RM, et al: Local staging of pancreatic cancer: Criteria for unresectability of major vessels as revealed by pancreatic phase, thin-section helical CT. AJR 1997;168:1439-1443.

Marik PE, Zaloga GP: Meta-analysis of parenteral nutrition versus enteral nutrition in patients with acute pancreatitis. BMJ 2004;328:1407.

National Comprehensive Cancer Network Clinical Practice Guidelines in Oncology: Neuroendocrine tumors, 2007. Available at www.nccn.org/professionals/physician_gls/PDF/neuroendocrine.pdf (accessed March 12, 2009).

Niederau C, Grendell JH: Diagnosis of chronic pancreatitis. Gastroenterology 1985;88:1973-1995.

Powell JJ, Miles R, Siriwardena AK: Antibiotic prophylaxis in the initial management of severe acute pancreatitis. Br J Surg 1998;85:582-587.

Remer EM, Baker ME: Imaging of chronic pancreatitis. Radiol Clin North Am 2002;40:1229-1242.

Sahai AV, Zimmerman M, Aabakken L, et al: Prospective assessment of the ability of endoscopic ultrasound to diagnose, exclude, or establish the severity of chronic pancreatitis found by endoscopic retrograde cholangiopancreatography. Gastrointest Endosc 1998;48:18-25.

Saleh MM, Norregaard P, Jorgensen HL, et al: Preoperative endoscopic stent placement before pancreatoduodenectomy: A meta-analysis of the effect on morbidity and mortality. Gastrointest Endosc 2002;56:529-534.

Scheiman JM: Cystic lesions of the pancreas. Gastroenterology 2005;128:463-469.

Schneider A, Whitcomb DC: Hereditary pancreatitis: A model for inflammatory diseases of the pancreas. Best Pract Res Clin Gastroenterol 2002;16:347-363.

Steer ML: Pathogenesis of acute pancreatitis. Digestion 1997;58:46-49.

Walsh RM, Henderson JM, Vogt DP, et al: Prospective preoperative determination of mucinous pancreatic cystic neoplasms. Surgery 2002; 132: 628-633.

Warshaw AL, Banks PA, Fernandez-Del Castillo C: AGA technical review: Treatment of pain in chronic pancreatitis. Gastroenterology 1998;115:765-776.

Inflammatory Bowel Disease

Bret A. Lashner

DEFINITION

The two main categories of inflammatory bowel disease are ulcerative colitis and Crohn's disease. *Ulcerative colitis* is characterized by recurring episodes of inflammation of the mucosal layer of the large bowel not related to an intestinal infection or nonsteroidal anti-inflammatory drug (NSAID) use. The inflammation involves the rectum and can extend proximally in a continuous fashion. *Ulcerative proctosigmoiditis* refers to inflammation extending into the sigmoid colon. *Left-sided colitis* refers to inflammation extending up to, but not beyond, the splenic flexure. *Pancolitis refers* to disease that extends proximal to the splenic flexure.

Crohn's disease is characterized by recurring episodes of inflammation of any part of the bowel, from the mouth to the anus. This inflammation is transmural and can result in strictures, microperforations, and fistulae. The inflammation is noncontiguous and thus can produce skip lesions throughout the bowel. Histologically, Crohn's disease can have either transmural lymphoid aggregates or non-necrotizing granulomas. Although granulomas strongly suggest Crohn's disease as the diagnosis, they are seen in only 10% of patients with Crohn's disease.

INCIDENCE AND PREVALENCE

The annual incidence of ulcerative colitis and Crohn's disease ranges from 1 to 10 cases per 100,000 people annually depending on the region studied. The peak age-specific incidence occurs near 20 years of age, and a second smaller peak occurs near age 50 years. The prevalence of ulcerative colitis and Crohn's disease ranges from 10 to 70 per 100,000 people, but some North American studies have shown a prevalence as high as 200 per 100,000 people.[1,2] In the United States, males and females are equally affected, but both whites and Ashkenazi Jews are at much higher risk of developing inflammatory bowel disease than the rest of the population.

PATHOPHYSIOLOGY

The causes of ulcerative colitis and Crohn's disease are not known. However, a reasonable hypothesis for the pathogenesis of inflammatory bowel disease can be presented. As yet unidentified antigens, possibly a mycobacterium, paramyxovirus, or components of cigarette smoke, activate resting macrophages to release a wide variety of cytokines.[3] *Cytokines* is a collective term for a group of low-molecular-weight peptides that are active at low concentrations and bind to specific receptors to produce autocrine, paracrine, and endocrine effects. The most abundant cytokine is interleukin-1 (IL-1), which not only causes diarrhea but also acts as a pyrogen. Other cytokines activated in the inflammatory process are IL-6, tumor necrosis factor-α (TNF-α), and the chemokine IL-8. Cytokines cause differentiation of lymphocytes to different types of T cells. Helper T cells, type 1 (Th1), are associated principally with Crohn's disease, whereas Th2 cells are associated principally with ulcerative colitis. These cytokines serve to stimulate the immune system and cause an inflammatory reaction, thus producing tissue damage in the intestinal mucosa.

There is a genetic predisposition for both ulcerative colitis and Crohn's disease. For example, mutations in the *NOD2/CARD15* gene on chromosome 16 are associated with stricturing Crohn's disease of the ileum, and mutations in the IL-23 receptor gene on chromosome 1 are protective for the development of Crohn's disease.

SIGNS AND SYMPTOMS

Ulcerative colitis patients typically present with rectal bleeding, diarrhea, tenesmus (urgent desire to evacuate the bowels but with passage of little stool), and abdominal pain. Patients with fulminant or toxic colitis usually have more than ten bowel movements daily, continuous bleeding, abdominal distention and tenderness, and radiologic evidence of edema and possibly bowel dilation.

Crohn's disease patients typically present with diarrhea, abdominal pain, and weight loss. The abdominal pain usually is insidious, is in the right lower quadrant, occurs soon after eating, and may be associated with a tender inflammatory mass. There may be hematochezia, but bleeding is much less common than in ulcerative colitis patients. Fever, weight loss, stomatitis, perianal fistulae or fissures (or both), arthritis, and erythema nodosum are all commonly seen.

There are many extraintestinal manifestations in inflammatory bowel disease. Approximately 2% of ulcerative colitis patients develop primary sclerosing cholangitis, a cholestatic liver disease diagnosed by the appearance of extrahepatic and intrahepatic strictures on a cholangiogram. Primary sclerosing cholangitis is seen more often in ulcerative colitis than in Crohn's disease patients. Other hepatic manifestations of inflammatory bowel disease include fatty liver, chronic active hepatitis, amyloidosis, and complications from medications used to treat inflammatory bowel disease (e.g., steroids, azathioprine, 6-mercaptopurine [6-MP], sulfasalazine, infliximab).

Erythema nodosum, seen in up to 3% of patients, is characterized by raised tender, erythematous nodules appearing typically on the extremities. Pyoderma gangrenosum, a rare ulcerating necrotic lesion, is seen in both Crohn's disease and ulcerative colitis. Arthritis usually is seronegative, mono- or pauciarticular, and asymmetrical. The large joints are most often affected, and there is no synovial destruction. Ocular manifestations include blurred vision, eye pain, photophobia, and keratitic precipitates. Patients with uveitis often have human leukocyte antigen B27 (HLA-B27), whereas patients with episcleritis and iritis usually do not. Cerebrovascular accidents and other thromboembolic events can result from hypercoagulability secondary to chronic inflammation or to other inherited syndromes, such as the factor V Leiden mutation. Patients are susceptible to nephrolithiasis from calcium oxalate stones.

DIAGNOSIS

The diagnosis of ulcerative colitis or Crohn's disease is established by finding characteristic intestinal ulcerations and excluding alternative diagnoses, such as enteric infections, ischemia, diverticulitis, or NSAID-induced enteropathy. Active disease in ulcerative colitis is characterized by the endoscopic appearance of superficial ulcerations, friability, a distorted mucosal vascular pattern, and exudates (Fig. 1). Patients with severely active disease can have pseudopolyps and deep ulcers and friability that result in spontaneous bleeding. The typical distribution of disease is continuous from the rectum proximally. However, patients with partially treated ulcerative colitis might have discontinuous or patchy involvement.

The ulcerations of Crohn's disease may appear aphthoid, but they could also be deep and serpiginous. Skip areas, a cobblestone appearance, pseudopolyps, and rectal sparing are characteristic findings (Fig. 2). On a small bowel series, Crohn's disease often is manifested

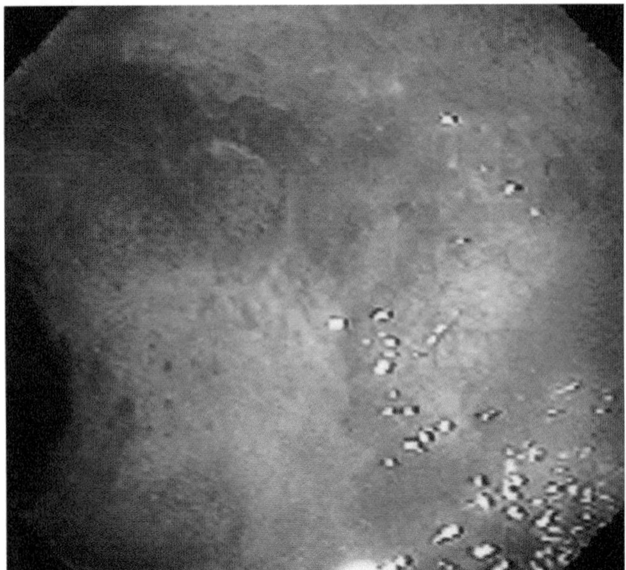

Figure 1 Endoscopic photograph of ulcerative colitis. This is characterized by erythema, submucosal hemorrhage, granularity, and a loss of mucosal vascular pattern.

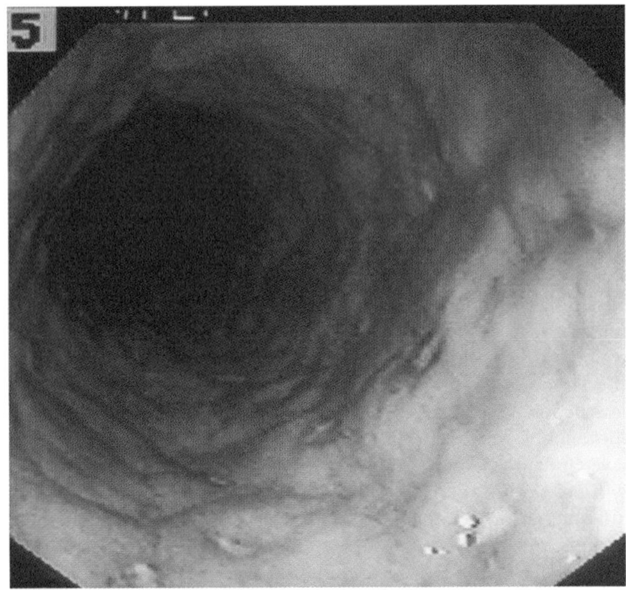

Figure 2 Endoscopic photograph of Crohn's disease of the colon. This is characterized by punched-out ulcerations and a cobblestone appearance.

by separation of bowel loops and a narrowed terminal ileal lumen, the string sign.

Histologic features of ulcerative colitis include disease limited to the mucosa and submucosa, mucin depletion, ulcerations, exudate, and crypt abscesses. In Crohn's disease, non-necrotizing granulomas, transmural lymphoid aggregates, and microscopic skip lesions can be seen. Typical lesions of Crohn's disease also may be seen in the upper gastrointestinal tract. The inflammation is localized in the ileocecal region in 50% of cases, in the small bowel in 25%, in the colon in 20%, and in the upper gastrointestinal tract or perirectum in 5%.

The diagnosis of inflammatory bowel disease can be made only when other reasonable alternatives in the differential diagnosis have been excluded (Box 1). The most common diagnoses that mimic ulcerative colitis are the infectious colitides. It is imperative to check stool for enteric pathogens, including ova and parasites, *Escherichia coli* O157:H7, and *Clostridium difficile.* Infection with *Yersinia enterocolitica* or *Mycobacterium tuberculosis* can cause inflammation in the terminal ileum resembling Crohn's disease. Other important diseases in the differential diagnosis of Crohn's disease include intestinal lymphoma, celiac sprue, radiation enteropathy, and NSAID-induced enteropathy.

Box 1 Principal Alternatives in the Differential Diagnosis of Inflammatory Bowel Disease—Ulcerative Colitis and Crohn's Disease

Ulcerative Colitis

Infectious colitis
Antibiotic-associated colitis
Amyloidosis
Solitary rectal ulcer syndrome
Diarrhea of acquired imuunodeficiency syndrome (AIDS)

Crohn's Disease

Appendicitis
Bacterial overgrowth
Bowel tuberculosis
Small bowel cancer
Nonsteroidal enteropathy
Diverticulitis
Celiac sprue
Lymphoma
Postsurgical adhesions
Behçet's disease
Ischemic colitis
Radiation enteropathy

TREATMENT

Ulcerative Colitis

Management of ulcerative colitis is described in practice guidelines published in 2004. The severity of the ulcerative colitis flare is based on patient symptoms and on the extent of colitis, not on the histologic severity of inflammation.

For patients with mild to moderate distal or left-sided colitis, therapy includes oral or topical agents, or both. Mesalamine (5-aminosalicylic acid [5-ASA]) enemas (Rowasa) are commonly used topical agents and given 4 g daily. They are effective for both active colitis and for maintaining a patient in remission, and they are superior to rectal corticosteroids for distal disease. Steroid enemas are effective in active disease, but they are not useful in maintaining a remission. Mesalamine suppositories (Canasa) are also useful for patients with proctitis. Mesalamine therapy has not failed until a patient has been given maximum doses of the drug or has experienced intolerable side effects. Asacol 2.4 g per day is given for maintenance, up to 4.8 g per day for active disease. Sulfasalazine 2 g per day is given for maintenance, and up to 8 g per day for active disease. Pentasa 2 g per day is given for maintenance, and up to 4 g per day for active disease (Table 1). Colazal 6.75g daily is particularly effective for left-sided colitis. Lialda, and Apriso a once-daily formulations, are effective in inducing remission.

The combination of oral and topical mesalamine is more effective than either alone for active disease. Although sulfasalazine is less expensive than the other 5-ASA agents, it has a high incidence of side effects, such as nausea, vomiting, anorexia, dyspepsia, malaise, and headaches. Some rare idiosyncratic reactions include fever, rash, hepatitis, pancreatitis, pneumonitis, and agranulocytosis. Folate supplementation is recommended, because sulfasalazine can inhibit folate absorption. The other 5-ASA agents can be more expensive but generally are better tolerated.

Table 1 Aminosalicylates and Intestinal Activity

Medication	Dosage (g/day)	Colon Activity		Small Bowel Activity
		Distal	Proximal	
Sulfasalazine	2-8	++	+++	–
Olsalazine (Dipentum)	1-3	++	+++	–
Balsalazide (Colazal)	6.75-12	+++	+++	–
Mesalamine (5-Aminosalicylic Acid)				
Pentasa	2-4	++	++	++
Asacol	2.4-4.8	++	+++	+
Lialda	2.4-4.8	++	++	–
Apriso	1.5	++	++	++
Rowasa enemas	4	+++	–	–
Canasa suppositories	2-4	+	–	–

For patients with mild to moderate pancolitis, first-line therapy involves oral 5-ASA agents. If this therapy is ineffective, oral steroids can be used for active disease, with the usual starting prednisone dose of 40 mg/day. For patients with mild to moderate disease who do not completely respond to or are dependent on oral steroids, immunosuppressives such as 6-MP or azathioprine can be used. These purine analogues act by causing chromosome breaks and blunt the proliferation of rapidly dividing cells, such as lymphocytes. These agents are effective for active disease and for maintaining remission.

Thiopurine methyltransferase (TPMT) activity should be measured before initiating therapy to determine the optimal starting dose. Metabolite levels of 6-MP (6-thioguanine [6-TG] and 6-methylmercaptopurine [6-MMP]) can be measured to determine the optimal therapeutic dose with the minimal risk of toxicity. Measurements of metabolite levels are best done on patients who are not responding but who are taking adequate doses. Metabolite levels can be used to distinguish between those who are nonresponders, those who are not compliant with medication, and those in whom the dose can be safely increased. One shortcoming, however, is that 6-MP and azathioprine usually require 3 to 6 months to become maximally effective. In addition, they have the rare side effects of allergy (e.g., abdominal pain, fever, rash), pancreatitis, and bone marrow suppression.

Infliximab (Remicade), a monoclonal chimeric anti-TNF antibody, has been approved for use in ulcerative colitis and is especially helpful in patients with moderately active disease that does not respond to 5-ASA agents, immunosuppressive medications, or corticosteroids.

For ulcerative colitis patients with severe colitis refractory to maximal oral therapy, admission to the hospital and intravenous steroids are required. The usual dosage of intravenous steroids is 0.5 to 0.75 mg/kg/day of prednisone equivalence. Usual regimens include intravenous hydrocortisone 100 mg every 8 hours or intravenous methylprednisolone 40 mg daily. It is important to rule out toxic megacolon by checking a radiograph of the abdomen, as well as CMV infection with serologic and histologic studies. A colorectal surgery consultation should be obtained, because a significant number of these patients require surgery during their hospitalization. Indications for a colectomy during a colitis flare include massive hemorrhage, perforation, toxic megacolon, or active disease unresponsive to conventional therapy. Surgery is also indicated for patients with persistent moderate disease that is medically refractory or for those with intolerable steroid side effects.

Cyclosporine has been shown to be useful in the treatment of severely active ulcerative colitis as an alternative to colectomy. However, because cyclosporine has many side effects and has not been shown to be effective in maintaining remission over the long term, this medication is not widely used in the treatment of severe ulcerative colitis. Infliximab can induce remission in severely active cases. Maintenance therapy with infliximab and an immunosuppressive agent should be considered in patients whose remission was induced with infliximab.

Crohn's Disease

Therapy for Crohn's disease has been discussed in practice guidelines published in 2009. These guidelines set up a definition for the severity of a Crohn's disease flare. Mild to moderate disease is indicated when patients can tolerate oral intake without dehydration, high fever, abdominal pain, abdominal mass, or obstruction. Moderate to severe disease describes the disorder in patients who have failed to respond to therapy for mild or moderate disease or those with fevers, weight loss, abdominal pain, anemia, or nausea and vomiting without frank obstruction.

Severe to fulminant disease is found in patients with persisting symptoms despite the introduction of steroids on an outpatient basis or those presenting with high fever, persistent vomiting, obstruction, rebound tenderness, cachexia, or an abscess. In addition, it is important to distinguish between differing behaviors of disease: inflammatory, fistulizing, or fibrostenotic.

For Crohn's disease patients with mild to moderate disease, oral mesalamine is only modestly effective and is not approved for use. Sulfasalazine has some potential benefit in the treatment of colonic disease, but it is not useful for isolated small bowel disease. Budesonide is a topically active corticosteroid that, when given orally, is effective in treating mucosal inflammation and is then inactivated through first-pass metabolism. The side-effect profile of budesonide is much better than that of oral corticosteroids. In patients with mildly to moderately active Crohn's disease, budesonide 9 mg daily was found to be significantly better in inducing remission than 4 g daily of a mesalamine preparation. Gastroduodenal Crohn's disease has been shown to improve with oral proton pump inhibitors.

For moderate to severe Crohn's disease, oral steroids are often necessary. Prednisone is dosed as in ulcerative colitis patients at 40 mg per day. It is important to rule out any concomitant infection or abscess before initiating steroid therapy. For patients who are steroid-resistant or who have become steroid-dependent, 6-MP, azathioprine, or methotrexate may be used. These agents have been shown to be safe and effective in Crohn's disease, enabling patients to avoid long-term use of corticosteroids. Infliximab has been shown to be effective for the acute management of both inflammatory and fistulous Crohn's disease. Infliximab also is effective for maintenance therapy of both inflammatory and fistulous Crohn's disease. Infliximab is given as a loading regimen of three doses over 6 weeks and then typically dosed at 5 mg/kg over 2 hours and given every 8 weeks. Adverse side effects include infusion reaction, infections (including tuberculosis and other opportunistic infections), and lymphoma. A skin test (e.g., purified protein derivative or Mantoux test) and a hepatitis B surface antigen test should be performed before initiating infliximab therapy to assess a patient's risk for developing tuberculosis or fulminate hepatic failure from recurrent hepatitis B.

Adalumimub (Humira) is a fully human anti-TNF antibody that is approved for induction and maintenance therapy for Crohn's disease. It is given as a loading dose of 160 mg at week 0 and 80 mg at week 2 and then as a 40-mg subcutaneous injection every 2 weeks. Its effectiveness and toxicities are very similar to infliximab's with the exception of lower antibody formation. Certolizumab (Cimzia) is a pegylated Fab fragment of a humanized anti-TNF antibody. Its effectiveness and toxicity is similar to that of infliximab and adalimumab, and it is given as a monthly subcutaneous injection. Natalizumab (Tysabri), an anti-integrin antibody, is another biologic agent approved for use in Crohn's disease. Its effectiveness appears to be similar to that of other biologic agents, and rate of opportunistic infections may be lower. Natalizumab was associated with a case of progressive multifocal leukoencephalopathy (PML) in a Crohn's disease patient in a clinical trial (as well as sight cases in multiple sclerosis patients), causing its use to be restricted to patients enrolled into a national registry.

For Crohn's disease patients with severe or fulminant disease, hospitalization is advisable. An abdominal computed tomography (CT) scan should be obtained if an abscess is clinically suspected. Stool studies should be done to rule out infection. Once abscess and infection have been excluded, intravenous steroids should be instituted in the same doses as those used for ulcerative colitis. Surgical intervention is indicated with perforation, obstruction, abscess, or fulminant disease unresponsive to medical therapy.

OUTCOMES

Colorectal Cancer

Patients with ulcerative colitis or Crohn's disease have an increased risk of colonic epithelial dysplasia and carcinoma. Ulcerative colitis patients have a colon cancer risk at least three times higher than that in the general population. This risk of colon cancer is higher with both increasing duration and extent of disease, as well as with primary sclerosing cholangitis. Crohn's disease patients with at least 30% of the colon involved with disease might have an increased risk of colorectal dysplasia and cancer.

Entering a patient into a cancer surveillance program is important in both these groups. However, the exact method and timing of surveillance are still matters of much debate. Most guidelines recommend beginning screening colonoscopies after 8 years of disease. Multiple biopsies should be taken at regular intervals throughout the colon; these include polypoid lesions and examination for the premalignant neoplastic lesion of dysplasia. All specimens with any grade of dysplasia should be reviewed by an expert gastrointestinal pathologist to confirm the findings.

It is generally agreed that high-grade dysplasia is an absolute indication for a colectomy, because these patients have a 42% risk for concurrent cancer. Low-grade dysplasia in flat mucosa also is an indication for colectomy, because progression to more advanced neoplasia often occurs.

The frequency with which colonoscopic screenings should be performed varies according to the extent of colitis, duration of disease, and history of primary sclerosing cholangitis. Because the risk of cancer is low throughout the first decade after the diagnosis of ulcerative colitis, surveillance need not be performed more frequently than every 3 years. As the cancer risk increases, the testing interval should shorten. One reasonable approach calls for tests every 3 years for 12 years, then every 2 years for 10 years, and annually thereafter. Patients with primary sclerosing cholangitis have an increased risk of colorectal cancer, so endoscopic surveillance examinations should be performed annually.

Ileal Pouch–Anal Anastomosis

Ulcerative colitis patients who require surgery are often offered an ileal pouch–anal anastomosis. At surgery, a total proctocolectomy is done, the distal small bowel is fashioned into a J-shaped reservoir, and the ileal pouch is stapled to the anal verge. Following surgery, patients usually have four to seven bowel movements daily and occasional or minimal incontinence. Acute pouchitis, the most common complication, occurs in about 25% to 50% of patients within 5 years. Acute pouchitis is usually successfully treated with antibiotics such as metronidazole or ciprofloxacin. Other, less-common complications of the ileal pouch include chronic pouchitis (inadequate response of pouchitis to multiple rounds of antibiotics), irritable pouch syndrome (bowel symptoms without endoscopic inflammation), cuffitis (recrudescence of colitis in the retained rectal cuff), or even unsuspected Crohn's disease. Irritable pouch syndrome often responds to antispasmodics or antidepressants, cuffitis responds to 5-ASA suppositories, chronic pouchitis responds to long-term antibiotics, probiotics, or immunosuppressive therapy, and Crohn's disease of the ileal pouch requires immunosuppressive therapy for treatment.

Summary

- Ulcerative colitis is characterized by mucosal inflammation of the colon, and Crohn's disease is characterized by transmural inflammation involving any part of the gastrointestinal tract.
- The diagnosis of ulcerative colitis or Crohn's disease is based on a constellation of positive endoscopic, radiographic, and histologic findings, with negative stool cultures.
- The differential diagnosis of inflammatory bowel disease includes infectious colitis, celiac sprue, intestinal lymphoma, radiation enteropathy, NSAID use, and ischemic colitis.
- First-line therapy for ulcerative colitis patients includes 5-aminosalicylic agents, and some patients also need corticosteroids, immunosuppressives, and biologic agents.
- First-line therapy for Crohn's disease patients often includes budesonide, and some patients also need other corticosteroids agents, immunosuppressives, antibiotics, and biologic agents.
- Colorectal cancer risk is an important concern for patients with ulcerative colitis or Crohn's colitis.

Suggested Readings

Colombel JF, Sandborn WJ, Rutgeerts P, et al: Adalimumab for maintenance of clinical response and remission in patients with Crohn's disease: The CHARM trial. Gastroenterology 2007;132:52-65.

Dubinsky MC, Lamothe S, Yang H, et al: Pharmacogenomics and metabolite measurement for 6-mercaptopurine therapy in inflammatory bowel disease. Gastroenterology 2000;118:705-713.

Duerr RH, Taylor KD, Brant SR, et al: A genome-wide association study identifies IL23R as an inflammatory bowel disease gene. Science 2006;314:1461-1463.
Fiocchi C: One commensal bacterial molecule—all we need for health? N Engl J Med 2005;353:2078-2080.
Lichtenstein GR, Hanauer SB, Sandborn WJ: Management of Crohn's Disease in Adults. Am J Gastroenterology 2009;104:465-483.
Jarnerot G, Hertervig E, Friis-Liby I, et al: Infliximab as rescue therapy in severe to moderately severe ulcerative colitis: A randomized, placebo-controlled study. Gastroenterology 2005;128:1805-1811.
Kornbluth A, Sachar DB; Practice Parameters Committee of the American College of Gastroenterology: Ulcerative colitis practice guidelines in adults (update): American College of Gastroenterology, Practice Parameters Committee. Am J Gastroenterol 2004;99:1371-1385.
Loftus EV Jr, Silverstein MD, Sandborn WJ, et al: Crohn's disease in Olmsted County, Minnesota, 1940-1993: Incidence, prevalence, and survival. Gastroenterology 1998;114:1161-1168.
Loftus EV Jr, Silverstein MD, Sandborn WJ, et al: Ulcerative colitis in Olmsted County, Minnesota, 1940-1993: Incidence, prevalence, and survival. Gut 2000;46:336-343.
Ogura Y, Bonen DK, Inohara N, et al: A frameshift mutation in *NOD2* is associated with susceptibility to Crohn's disease. Nature 2001;411:603-606.
Ponsioen CI, Tytgat GN: Primary sclerosing cholangitis: A clinical review. Am J Gastroenterol 1998;93:515-523.
Present DN, Rutgeerts P, Targan S, et al: Infliximab for the treatment of fistulas in patients with Crohn's disease. N Engl J Med 1999;340:1398-1405.
Rutgeerts P, Sandborn WJ, Feagan BG, et al: Infliximab for induction and maintenance therapy for ulcerative colitis. N Engl J Med 2005;353:2462-2476.
Sandborn WJ, Feagan BG, Stoinov S, et al: Certolizumab pegol for the treatment of Crohn's disease. N Engl J Med 2007;357:228-238.
Sands BE, Anderson FH, Bernstein CN, et al: Infliximab maintenance therapy for fistulizing Crohn's disease. N Engl J Med 2004;350:876-885.
Schreiber S, Khaliq-Kareemi M, Lawrance IC, et al: Maintenance therapy with certolizumab pegol for Crohn's disease. N Engl J Med 2007;357:239-250.
Shapiro BD, Lashner BA: Cancer biology in ulcerative colitis and potential use in endoscopic surveillance. Gastrointest Endosc Clin N Am 1997;7:453-468.
Shen B, Achkar J-P, Lashner BA, et al: Endoscopic and histologic evaluation together with symptom assessment are required to diagnose pouchitis. Gastroenterology 2001;121:261-267.
Targan SR, Hanauer SB, van Deventer SJ, et al: A short-term study of chimeric monoclonal antibody cA2 to tumor necrosis factor alpha for Crohn's disease. Crohn's Disease cA2 Study Group. N Engl J Med 1997;337:1029-1035.
Targan SR, Feagan BG, Fedorak RN, et al. Natalizumab for the treatment of active Crohn's disease: Results of the ENCORE Trial. Gastroenterology 2007;132:1672-1683.
Thomsen OO, Cortot A, Jewell D, et al: A comparison of budesonide and mesalamine for active Crohn's disease. N Engl J Med 1999;340:370-374.
Ullman T, Croog V, Harpaz N, et al: Progression of flat low-grade dysplasia to advanced neoplasin in patients with ulcerative colitis. Gastroenterology 2003;125:1311-1319.
Van Assche G, D'Haens G, Noman M, et al: Randomized, double-blind comparison of 4 mg/kg versus 2 mg/kg intravenous cyclosporine in severe ulcerative colitis. Gastroenterology 2003;25:1025-1031.

References

For a complete list of references, log onto www.expertconsult.com.

Irritable Bowel Syndrome

Katherine Freeman

Irritable bowel syndrome (IBS) is common in the general population and has a significant medical and socioeconomic impact. Its pathophysiology is still not entirely clear, and the diagnosis and management can be challenging. It is desirable to make a positive diagnosis rather than to rely on a diagnosis of exclusion. A step-by-step approach for management and a realistic goal of therapy is advocated. An effective treatment strategy should address the dominant symptoms, their severity, and psychosocial factors.

DEFINITION

IBS is defined on the basis of the recently modified Rome III criteria as recurrent abdominal pain or discomfort at least 3 days per month in the last 3 months that started at least 6 months before diagnosis, cannot be explained by a structural or biochemical abnormality, and is associated with at least two of the following: improvement with defecation, onset associated with a change in frequency of stool, and onset associated with a change in form (appearance) of stool.[1] Other symptoms that support the diagnosis but are not part of the criteria include abnormal stool frequency (≤3 bowel movements per week or >3 bowel movements per day), abnormal stool form (lumpy/hard or loose/watery), defecation straining, urgency, or feeling of incomplete bowel movement, passing mucus, and bloating. Four possible IBS subtypes include IBS with constipation (IBS-C), IBS with diarrhea (IBS-D), mixed IBS (IBS-M) and un-subtyped IBS depending on the predominant stool pattern.[2]

PREVALENCE

IBS is one of the most commonly diagnosed gastrointestinal (GI) conditions and also one of the most common functional GI disorders seen in clinical practice.[3] Estimates of prevalence vary, largely because of the differences among epidemiologic studies (e.g., the use of different diagnostic criteria, population selection, and data sources). Approximately 10% to 20% of the general adult population has reported symptoms compatible with IBS.[4,5] However, only 15% of those affected actually seek medical attention.[5,6] IBS accounts for 12% of primary care patients and 28% of gastroenterology practice patients (41% of all functional GI disorders).[6] Patients often experience the onset of symptoms as young adults, but the prevalence is similar in older adults. IBS is diagnosed in women more than twice as often as men; however, studies have found the prevalence of pain-related symptoms of IBS to be equal among men and women and the prevalence of symptoms not related to pain, such as constipation, bloating and extra-intestinal manifestations, to be greater among women.[7]

The financial burden of IBS is high, both in direct and indirect costs.[8] IBS has a major impact on the quality of life of those afflicted, affecting social interactions and professional opportunities.[9]

PATHOPHYSIOLOGY

To date, no physiologic mechanism unique to IBS has been identified. Rather, it is currently viewed as a biopsychosocial disorder resulting from an interaction among a number of factors: visceral hyperalgesia, genetic and environmental factors, infection, inflammation, gut motility, and psychological factors[10] Dietary factors, GI dysmotility dysfunction, and the role of gut flora are evolving mechanisms.

Visceral Hypersensitivity

Many studies have shown that in patients with IBS, both awareness and pain caused by balloon distention in the large and small bowel are experienced at significantly lower balloon volumes than those reported by healthy subjects.[11-13] It is not known at which level of pain-signal transmission (starting at the receptor in the gut wall, through the spinal cord to the brain) this increased sensitivity is expressed, but it is selective to visceral stimuli, because patients with IBS have normal or even decreased sensitivity to somatic stimuli.[14,15]

Abnormal Gut Motility

The changes in gut motility observed in IBS are qualitative, with no distinct pattern that can distinguish patients from healthy subjects. Two major changes are observed: Changes in gut transit and increased motility. Enhanced gut transit is seen in some patients with diarrhea-predominant IBS, and decreased gut transit is seen in some patients with constipation-predominant IBS. Increased motility compared with healthy subjects is seen in response to various stimuli, such as psychological stress, meals, and balloon inflation in the gut.[10]

Psychosocial Factors

IBS has long been dismissed as a psychosomatic condition because it has no clear cause or pathophysiology. Psychological stress and emotional events, such as physical or sexual abuse, can result in GI symptoms in healthy subjects, but they affect patients with IBS to a greater degree. The common psychological symptoms associated with IBS are depression, somatization, anxiety, hostility, phobia, and paranoia. Up to 50% of patients with IBS meet criteria for a psychiatric diagnosis as compared with an average of 20% with organic GI disorders and 15% of control subjects.[10] Although there are no psychological or psychiatric disorders specific to IBS, identification of such disorders can help in planning psychological or psychopharmacologic treatment.

Brain-Gut Interaction

The central nervous system (CNS) modulates various functions such as secretion, motility, and blood flow.[16] Signals from the gut, in turn, are involved in regulating reflexes. Perception of events in the gut involves activation of afferent pathways, with information being modulated at different levels, peripheral as well as central.[17] A major advance in our understanding of brain-gut interaction and its alteration in IBS occurred with the introduction of functional magnetic resonance imaging (MRI). This technique allowed assessment of the difference in cortical function in response to gut stimulation between healthy subjects and IBS patients,[18] opening the door for potential pharmacologic and behavioral interventions.

Latent or Potential Celiac Disease

The concept of latent or potential celiac disease has recently been introduced into the pathogenesis of IBS. Abdominal symptoms in the absence of mucosal abnormalities are features of IBS and latent or potential celiac disease.[19] In a study of genetic, serologic, and histologic markers of celiac disease in 102 patients with diarrhea-predominant IBS, 35% of the patients had positive findings for human leukocyte antigen (HLA)-DQ2, 23% had increased intraepithelial lymphocyte counts, and 30% had increased celiac disease–associated antibodies in the duodenal aspirates, including antibodies against gliadin, tissue transglutaminase, β-lactoglobulin, and ovalbumin.[19] Stool frequency and the intestinal immunoglobulin A (IgA) level decreased significantly under a gluten-free diet in a subgroup of IBS patients with positive HLA-DQ2 and positive intestinal celiac disease–associated antibodies when compared with IBS patients without these markers.[19] Celiac disease–associated IgG and HLA-DQ2 expression can identify likely responders to gluten-free diet in patients with IBS-D (diarrhea predominant IBS).[20]

Infection and Inflammation

Clinical, epidemiologic, and physiologic studies have shown that acute, transient GI infection is associated with a syndrome that often meets diagnostic criteria for the diagnosis of IBS. This was observed after documented outbreaks of enteric infections with organisms such as *Campylobacter jejuni* or *Salmonella*.[21,22] IBS and small intestine bacterial overgrowth might share similar symptoms. In a study of 202 patients with IBS, 157 (78%) had small bowel bacterial overgrowth. Intraepithelial lymphocytes, lamina propria CD3 and CD25 cells, neutrophils, and mast cells are increased in patients with IBS.[23]

The exact mechanisms whereby the inflammatory changes cause the symptoms are not clear. The inflammatory response may be associated with activating enterochromaffin cells to produce 5-hydroxytryptamine (5-HT) and CD3 cells to produce cytokines, which in turn leads to enhanced motility, increased intestinal permeability, and lowered visceral sensation thresholds.[24] In one prospective study of postinfectious IBS, it was found that patients whose symptoms remained 3 months after an enteric infection not only had increased mucosal cellularity but also had increased psychosocial distress at the time of the infection. Lowered visceral sensation thresholds and increased motility were present after the infection, regardless of whether or not the symptoms remained.[25] Therefore, in patients with IBS refractory to a gluten-free diet, small bowel bacterial overgrowth may be suspected, and prompt hydrogen breath testing may be warranted.

Fructose and Lactose Intolerance

Common symptoms of dietary fructose and lactose intolerance include bloating, flatulence, pain, and diarrhea which have also been found in patients with unexplained dyspepsia or functional bowel disorders such as IBS. It has been shown that approximately one third of patients with suspected IBS might also have fructose intolerance as identified by a positive fructose breath test. Although there are no data documenting the efficacy of a fructose-restricted diet, a study of 80 suspected IBS patients showed significant relief of symptoms in those who were compliant with a fructose-restricted diet.[26] Patients with IBS have subjectively reported higher incidence of lactose intolerance, but it is hard to tell whether reported symptoms are secondary to lactose intolerance or IBS in the absence of documented lactose malabsorption. A period of avoiding dairy products or requesting a test for lactose malabsorption (or both) may be beneficial in this area.

SIGNS AND SYMPTOMS

Patients with IBS can present with a wide variety of GI and extraintestinal symptoms. However, the symptom complex of chronic abdominal pain and altered bowel habits that cannot be explained by identifiable structural or biochemical abnormalities is the main clinical pattern of IBS.

Chronic abdominal pain in IBS is usually described as a crampy sensation, with varying intensity and periodic exacerbation. The pain is generally located in the lower abdomen, although the location and character of the pain can also vary. Emotional stress and eating can exacerbate the pain, whereas defecation often provides some relief. Progressive pain that awakens the patient from sleep or prevents sleep should prompt a search for causes other than IBS.

Because the range of normal bowel habits is broad, a careful history should include the volume, frequency, and consistency of the patient's stool. Assuming no use of laxatives or antidiarrheals, subtyping of IBS by predominant stool pattern has been divided into the following: IBS with constipation (IBS-C), IBS with diarrhea (IBS-D), mixed IBS (IBS-M) and unsubtyped IBS. The frequency of bowel movements in normal persons is variable, and it range from three times a day to three times a week. Patients with IBS complain of diarrhea, constipation, alternating diarrhea and constipation, or normal bowel habits alternating with diarrhea or constipation reflecting intestinal transit time.[2]

Irritable Bowel Syndrome with Diarrhea

Diarrhea is generally characterized as a condition of at lea[illegible] frequent loose stools of small and moderate volume without ab[illegible]inal comfort in at least 75% of stools[2] or Bristol Stool Form Scale [illegible] (fluffy pieces with ragged edges, a mushy stool or watery, no so[illegible] pieces, entirely liquid). In addition, hard and lumpy stool typically occurs in less than 25% of bowel movements. Bowel movement generally occurs during waking hours, most often in the morning or after meals. Most bowel movements are preceded by urgency and may be followed by a feeling of incomplete evacuation. Pseudodiarrhea—frequency defecation and urgency without solid stools—is not considered diarrhea.[27] Nocturnal diarrhea, bloody stools, dehydration, or weight loss are not features of IBS.

Irritable Bowel Syndrome with Constipation

Constipation can last from days to months, with interludes of diarrhea or normal bowel function. Stools are often hard and may be described as pellet shaped in at least 25% of bowel movements, or Bristol Stool Form Scale 1-2 (separate hard lumps like nuts that are difficult to pass, or sausage shaped but lumpy). In addition, loose (mushy) or watery stools account for less than 25% of bowel movements. Patients might also experience a sense of incomplete evacuation, even when the rectum is empty. This can lead to straining with defecation, prolonged time on the toilet, and inappropriate use of enemas or laxatives.

Mixed Irritable Bowel Syndrome

Mixed IBS is defined as hard or lumpy stool at least 25% of bowel movements and loose or mushy stools at least 25% of bowel movements using Bristol scale 1-2 for constipation and scale 6-7 for diarrhea.

Unsubtyped Irritable Bowel Syndrome

Unsubtyped IBS is defined as insufficient abnormality of stool consistency to meet criteria for IBS-D, IBS-C or IBS-M.

Other Gastrointestinal Symptoms

Upper GI symptoms are not uncommon in patients with IBS. These include symptoms of heartburn, dysphagia, nonulcer dyspepsia, nausea, and noncardiac chest pain.[28] Patients with IBS often complain of abdominal bloating and increased gas production in the form of flatulence or belching.

Extraintestinal Symptoms

Patients with IBS have a high frequency of non-GI symptoms, including rheumatologic symptoms, headache, genitourinary symptoms such as urinary frequency ?d urgency, dyspareunia, sexual dysfunction, and sleep-related di urbances.[29]

ACTIVE DIAGNOSIS

A diagnosis is based o ientifying positive symptoms consistent with IBS and excludi her conditions with similar clinical presentations in a cost-eff manner. In the absence of biologic markers, attempts have be ade to standardize the diagnosis of IBS using symptom-base ria. These include criteria proposed by Manning and colleag 1978[30] and the international workshop criteria, Rome I a with the updated current Rome III criteria.[1] In the criteria anning and associates,[1] the symptoms associated with IBS i relief of pain with bowel movements, looser and more fre ools with onset of pain, passage of mucus, and a sense of i ete evacuation. The current Rome III criteria, described g are a simplification of the Rome II criteria—for example, by stool form as a criterion. A key feature of the Rome III defini- n is the presence of abdominal discomfort or pain.

The diagnostic evaluation of patients with IBS can be challenging. It is generally agreed that the initial diagnosis of IBS can be fulfilled by the following: symptom-based diagnostic criteria are met, such as Rome III; negative results are obtained on physical examination; and a cost-effective, conservative set of screening studies has been performed. It is important to exclude organic causes of symptoms compatible with IBS. However, to avoid unnecessary and costly testing, the diagnosis of IBS should not be made simply by excluding organic disorders. Emphasis should be placed on identifying a symptom complex compatible with IBS and then using prudent, although not exhaustive, testing to make a positive diagnosis. The Rome and Manning criteria provide guidelines to identify patients with suspected IBS.

In 2002, the American Gastroenterological Association (AGA) published an extensive review and position statement[6] regarding pathophysiology, role of psychosocial factors, diagnosis, and treatment of IBS, and in April 2006, the Rome III criteria were again modified to include the IBS bowel habit subgroups that emphasized the use of the stool consistency as outlined in April 2006 *Gastroenterology*. It has been acknowledged that evidence exists for a diagnostic and treatment approach based on the predominant symptom, its severity, and associated psychosocial features, although more studies are needed to understand the mechanism underlying these symptoms and to develop effective treatments (Box 1).

The predominant symptom subtype is helpful for clinicians to determine the type of evaluation. For example, for the constipation-predominant subtype, a therapeutic trial of fiber may be sufficient. If symptoms persist, confirmation of a slow colonic transit test with a whole-gut transit test or evaluation for obstructed defecation (pelvic floor dysfunction) may be indicated. For the diarrhea-predominant subtype, clinical judgment determines the choice of studies. Particularly for loose or watery stools, a lactose-dextrose hydrogen breath test, celiac serology, or small bowel or colon biopsy may be indicated. If results of these tests are negative, a therapeutic trial of loperamide may be ordered. For patients with predominant symptoms of abdominal pain, a plain abdominal x-ray during an acute episode to exclude bowel obstruction and other abdominal pathology is recommended. If the x-ray is negative, a therapeutic trial of an antispasmodic agent may be tried.[6]

Box 1 Stepwise Approach to Irritable Bowel Syndrome

Step 1: Assessment of Symptoms

Use nonjudgmental, open-ended questions that include dietary history and medications.

Identify abdominal pain as the dominant symptom, with altered bowel function.

Consider psychological factors by gently questioning the patient about physical and sexual abuse once the physician–patient relationship has been established.

Identify red flag symptoms such as weight loss, fever, persistent diarrhea, rectal bleeding, anemia, nocturnal symptoms of pain and abnormal bowel habit, new onset of symptoms in patients >50 yr old, and the family history of gastrointestinal (GI) malignancy, inflammatory bowel disease, and celiac disease.

Step 2: Physical Examination

The physical examination findings are generally normal in IBS. The patient may have nonspecific abdominal tenderness.

Identify red flag signs such as anemia, jaundice, organomegaly, and abdominal mass.

Step 3: Laboratory Tests

Complete blood count, chemistry panel, and thyroid function studies help exclude organic diseases.

Stool analysis for ova, parasites, and fecal leukocytes should be done if diarrhea is the predominant symptom.

Because of overlap of clinical presentations of celiac disease and IBS, antigliadin and antiendomysial IgA antibody serologies may be reasonably effective screening tests, given that the sensitivities and positive predictive values range from 90% to 100%. However, in populations in which the prevalence of celiac disease is low, many positive serologic tests will be false-positives.

These tests are indicated for most patients for exclusion and inclusion of diagnosis.

Step 4: Invasive Tests

Invasive tests include flexible sigmoidoscopy and colonoscopy.

Invasive tests are indicated for select patients, in particular:

- Age >50 years with chronic, stable symptoms
- Age >50 years and recent onset
- Persistent diarrhea, rectal bleeding

Routine flexible sigmoidoscopy with biopsy has a low diagnostic yield and is not cost effective, particularly in young patients. It might help reassure an anxious patient or may be performed in an older patient with chronic, stable symptoms.

Colonoscopy is recommended for patients older than 50 years (because of a higher pretest probability of colon cancer), but in younger patients, performing a colonoscopy or sigmoidoscopy is determined by clinical features suggestive of structural disease (e.g., hematochezia, diarrhea, weight loss) and might not be indicated.

In patients with persistent diarrhea, if inflammatory bowel disease or microscopic colitis is suspected, a mucosal biopsy should be taken.

Step 5: Initiate a symptom-oriented treatment program

The treatment goal should be relief of symptoms and addressing the patient's concerns.

Step 6: Follow-up

Assess clinical response in 3 to 6 weeks.

TREATMENT

IBS is a chronic disorder with no specific cause, and there is no cure. The patient's confidence in the physician's diagnosis, explanation, and reassurance are vital therapeutic tools.

General Principles

The treatment strategy is based on the nature and severity of the symptoms, the character and degree of functional impairment, and the presence of psychosocial difficulties affecting the course of the illness. Patients with mild symptoms usually respond to education, reassurance, and simple treatments not requiring prescription medication. Some patients with moderate symptoms have more disability and require pharmacologic therapy directed at altered gut physiology or psychological treatments. A small group of patients with severe and refractory symptoms seen more often at referral centers may benefit from antidepressant therapy and psychological treatment.[6]

The treatment goal should be set on relief of symptoms and addressing the patient's concerns.[31] An important question is why the patient is seeking help at this time. Possible reasons may include recent exacerbating factors (e.g., concurrent medical disorders, new medications, dietary changes), concern about serious illness (e.g., recent family death), environmental stressors (e.g., major loss, abuse history), psychiatric comorbidity (e.g., depression, anxiety), impairment of daily function (e.g., recent inability to work), or a hidden agenda (e.g., disability claims, narcotic requests, laxative abuse, secondary gain). In a subgroup of patients with clear concurrent psychosocial disturbance, specific treatments for the triggering factors are reasonable. An effective treatment strategy should address the dominant symptoms, their severity, and psychosocial factors.

Therapeutic Relationship and Patient Education

As proposed by Drossman,[31] the most important component of treatment is to establish a therapeutic physician-patient relationship coupled with patient education, with the following steps:

1. Obtain the history through a nonjudgmental and patient-centered interview.
2. Conduct a careful examination and cost-efficient investigation.
3. Determine the patient's understanding of the illness and his or her concerns ("What do you think is causing your symptoms?").
4. Provide information regarding proposed mechanisms of IBS, which helps validate the patient's disease experience and sets the basis for therapeutic interventions.
5. Explain to patients that their symptoms of IBS are real and not life-threatening, the disease course is likely to be chronic, the diagnosis, if well established, is not likely to be changed, and that he or she should have a normal life span.
6. Establish realistic expectations with consistent limits ("I appreciate how bad the pain is, but narcotic medication is not indicated"), and involve the patient in treatment decisions ("Let me suggest some treatments for you to consider"). IBS is a condition that can be managed but not cured.

Modification of Diet

A diet history might reveal patterns of symptoms related to dairy or gas-producing foods. Exclusion of foods that increase flatulence (e.g., beans, onions, celery, carrots, raisins, apricots, prunes, Brussels sprouts, wheat germ, pretzels, bagels) should be considered in patients with symptoms of bloating or gas. Underlying visceral hyperalgesia in IBS may explain the exaggerated discomfort experienced with the consumption of gas-producing foods.

An increase in the intake of fiber is generally recommended, through diet or the use of commercial bulking supplements. Although the efficacy of fiber supplements has not been proved, some improvement has been demonstrated in patients with IBS whose primary complaints are abdominal pain and constipation.[32,33]

Many types of fiber supplements are available; some are synthetic, such as polycarbophil or methylcellulose, and others are from natural sources, such as bran or psyllium compounds. All types of fiber can cause increased bloating and gaseousness because of the colonic metabolism of nondigestible fiber.

Because of its safety, a trial of fiber supplementation is advised for patients with IBS, especially those with constipation-predominant symptoms. The amount should be titrated to symptoms.

Psychosocial Treatment

Psychological therapy is initiated when symptoms are severe enough to impair the health-related quality of the patient's life. Mental health referral may also be made for the treatment of associated psychiatric disorders, such as major depression or history of physical and sexual abuse that interferes with adjustment to illness.

Behavioral treatment may be considered for motivated patients who associate symptoms with stressors. Cognitive-behavioral treatment, interpersonal (psychodynamic) therapy, hypnosis, biofeedback, stress management and relaxation training, and family or group therapy can be tried. They help reduce anxiety levels, encourage health-promoting behavior, increase patient responsibility and involvement in the treatment, and improve pain tolerance. Factors that favor a good response to psychotherapy include[34]:

- The patient is motivated.
- The patient has predominant diarrhea or pain.
- IBS is associated with overt psychiatric symptoms.
- Intermittent pain is exacerbated by stress.

Patients with constant abdominal pain do poorly with psychotherapy or hypnotherapy.

Medications

Pharmacologic agents are only adjuvants to the treatment of IBS. The drug chosen depends on the patient's major symptoms; diarrhea-predominant IBS is treated differently from constipation-predominant disease. Common strategies include using dietary fiber for constipation, loperamide or diphenoxylate for diarrhea, and anticholinergic, antispasmodics, tricyclic antidepressants, or selective serotonin reuptake inhibitors (SSRIs) for pain (Table 1).

Chronic use of drugs should be minimized or avoided because of the lifelong nature of the disorder and the lack of convincing therapeutic benefit. The difficulty in demonstrating efficacy may in part be a result of the heterogeneous population with IBS, the lack of disease markers, and high placebo-response rates.[35]

Smooth-Muscle Relaxant Agents

Smooth-muscle relaxants include those directly affecting intestinal smooth muscle relaxation (e.g., mebeverine, pinaverium) and those that act in a similar fashion via anticholinergic pathways (e.g., dicyclomine, hyoscyamine). The rationale for using smooth-muscle relaxants to treat patients with IBS is based on the hypothesis that intestinal dysmotility results in abdominal pain, bloating, and disturbed defecation. Overall, the published trials with smooth-muscle relaxants were generally of short duration and included small numbers of patients. These agents may be beneficial in patients with postprandial abdominal pain, gas, bloating, and fecal urgency.

In a meta-analysis of randomized, controlled trials, 13 of 16 studies of smooth-muscle relaxants have shown these agents to be efficacious in global or symptomatic improvement.[36] The meta-analysis of the effects of smooth-muscle relaxants found them to be helpful, with 4.1 patients needing to be treated for each therapeutic success, although the effects on patient symptoms were relatively modest.[37] In a separate meta-analysis, four smooth-muscle relaxants that directly affect intestinal smooth muscle relaxation—cimetropium, pinaverium, otilonium, and trimebutine—have been consistently shown to be efficacious.[38] However, these smooth-muscle relaxants are currently not approved in the United States.

Common side effects of anticholinergic agents are dry mouth, dizziness, blurred vision, drowsiness, and tachycardia. Because of these side effects and the intermittent nature of pain in IBS, we advise using such agents on an as-needed basis or in anticipation of stressors with known exacerbating effects. Hyoscyamine (Anaspaz, Cystospaz, Levsin, Neoquess) can be given for pain at a dose of 0.125 mg to 0.25 mg sublingually or orally, three or four times daily, or sustained-release tablets, 0.375 mg to 0.75 mg orally every 12 hours. The

Table 1 Select Drug Therapies for Irritable Bowel Syndrome

Pharmacologic Agent	Usual Adult Dosage
Diarrhea-Predominant IBS	
Opioid μ-Receptor Agonists	
Loperamide (Imodium)	2-4 mg, up to qid prn
Diphenoxylate (Lomotil)	5 mg qid prn
Smooth-Muscle Relaxants	
Dicyclomine (Bentyl)	20 mg qid initially, then up to 40 mg qid
Hyoscyamine (Levsin, NuLev, Levbid)	0.125 mg sublingually tid prn or 0.375 mg bid PO
Tricyclic Antidepressants	
Amitriptyline (Elavil, Endep)	10-25 mg bid or 25-50 mg qhs
Desipramine (Norpramin)	50 mg tid
Selective 5-HT$_3$ Receptor Antagonist	
Alosetron (Lotronex)	1 mg qd × 4 wk, may increase to 1 mg bid × 4 wk*
Constipation-Predominant IBS	
Bulking Agents	
Psyllium (Metamucil)	20 g/day, divided, with >250 mL water
Polycarbophil (Konsyl Fiber)	1-6 g/day, divided, with >250 mL water
Methylcellulose (Citrucel)	3-6 g/day, divided, with >250 mL water
Osmotic Laxatives	
Polyethylene glycol (MiraLax)	1 dose (17 g in glass of water) qd or bid
Lactulose (Kristalose, Cephulac, Chronulac, Constulose, Duphalac, Enulose, R O Lactulose)	15-60 mL/day, divided
Sorbitol (Ora-Sweet)	120 mL of 25% solution
Pain	
Smooth-muscle relaxants	
Dicyclomine (Bentyl)	20 mg qid initially, then up to 40 mg qid
Hyoscamine (Levsin, NuLev, Levbid)	0.125 mg sublingually tid prn or 0.375 mg bid PO
Tricyclic Antidepressants	
Amitriptyline (Elavil, Paregoric)	10-25 mg bid or 25-50 mg qhs
Desipramine (Norpramin)	50 mg tid

*Prescribing physicians need to enroll in a special Lotronex Risk Management Program.

typical dose of dicyclomine is 20 mg orally three or four times daily or three or four times daily as needed.

Antidepressants

Antidepressants are purported to be beneficial and are often used in patients with chronic refractory symptoms. These drugs are particularly helpful for patients with comorbid depressive and anxiety disorders. The odds ratio for improvement with antidepressant therapy from the pooled data of seven randomized trials was 4.2 (95% confidence interval [CI], 2.3-7.9), with substantial improvement in severity of pain.[39] A randomized, controlled study has shown that desipramine improves pain in women with IBS who can tolerate the drug.[40] Tricyclic antidepressants and possibly selective serotonin reuptake inhibitors (SSRIs) modulate visceral afferent activity from the GI tract and might improve abdominal pain.[41] Tricyclic antidepressants are helpful in patients with diarrhea-predominant IBS,[42] possibly because of the constipating effect of this class of drugs. Conversely, if SSRIs are to be used, they should be avoided in patients with diarrhea-predominant IBS because diarrhea is a side effect of some of these agents, such as sertraline.

Improvement in neuropathic pain with tricyclic antidepressants occurs at lower doses than those required for treating depression. Thus, low doses should be tried initially and titrated to pain control or tolerance. Because of the delayed onset of action, 3 to 4 weeks of therapy should be attempted before considering treatment insufficient and increasing the dose. The medications often used include amitriptyline (Elavil, Endep) 10 to 25 mg orally every hour at bedtime, and imipramine (Tofranil) 25 to 50 mg orally every hour at bedtime. The initial dose should be adjusted based on tolerance and response.

Although SSRIs are increasingly preferred over tricyclic agents because of their low adverse-effect profile, data on the use of SSRIs in IBS are limited.[36,39] As with tricyclic antidepressants, treatment should start with a once-daily low dose of paroxetine (Paxil) 20 mg orally, fluoxetine (Prozac, Sarafem) 20 mg orally, or sertraline (Zoloft) 100 mg orally.

Antidiarrheal Agents

Loperamide (Imodium, Pepto Diarrhea Control) has been shown to be beneficial in diarrhea-predominant IBS by slowing whole-gut transit and enhancing intestinal water and electrolyte absorption.[43] It does not require a prescription and is the antidiarrheal drug of choice. Diphenoxylate (Logen, Lomanate, Lomotil, Lonox) can be tried next if loperamide is not effective.

Serotonin Receptor Agonists and Antagonists

5-HT serves both as a neurotransmitter and as a paracrine signaling molecule in the bowel.[37] 5-HT is distributed throughout the gut, predominantly within enterochromaffin cells in the mucosal crypts and, to a lesser extent, within the nerve fibers of the myenteric and submucosal plexuses. The concentration of 5-HT in the bowel is substantially greater than that in the brain. It is estimated that 95% of the body's 5-HT is synthesized and stored in the enterochromaffin cells of the gut. Thus, 5-HT has become a primary focus of recent research.

The postprandial plasma level of 5-HT in patients with diarrhea-predominant IBS is significantly higher than that in healthy controls.[44] 5-HT$_3$ antagonists were shown to increase colonic compliance, delay colonic transit, improve stool consistency, and increase thresholds for sensation and discomfort during distention of the rectum.[45] Alosetron produced statistically significant improvements in abdominal pain, stool consistency, frequency, and urgency in women with IBS, although symptoms rapidly returned after cessation of therapy.[46] The U.S. Food and Drug Administration (FDA) first approved alosetron (Lotrinex), a 5-HT$_3$ antagonist, for treating women who have diarrhea-predominant IBS in February 2000. After its introduction, serious and life-threatening cases of ischemic colitis and complications of constipation, including deaths, were reported. The cumulative incidence of ischemic colitis in women receiving alosetron was 0.3% in 6 months. The drug was withdrawn from the market in November 2000 and reintroduced in 2002 with limited approval through the enrollment in the Lotronex Risk Management Program.

Tegaserod (Zelnorm) is an aminoguanidine indole with selective and partial 5-HT_4 receptor agonist activity. 5-HT_4 agonists possess GI stimulatory effects, partially by facilitating enteric cholinergic transmission. In a randomized, double-blind, placebo-controlled study of patients with constipation-predominant IBS, tegaserod significantly improved abdominal pain and bowel function.[47] The medication was approved by the FDA for treating female patients who have constipation-predominant IBS. However, it was removed from the market because of cardiovascular adverse effects.

Lubiprostone (Amitiza, a locally acting type II sodium channel blocker) was the subject of a 4-week double-blind, placebo-controlled multicenter trial in patients with chronic diarrhea. The study showed that stool consistency, straining, consiptation severity, and patient-reported treatment effectiveness were significantly improved with lubiprostone compared with placebo at all weeks of the trial. The most commonly reported adverse event was mild to moderate nausea, which resulted in treatment discontinuation in 5% of treated patients.[48] This agent has been approved since 2006 by the FDA for IBS-C in women and has been shown to have similar efficacy in elderly patients (>65 years).

The cornerstone of IBS therapy is a strong patient-physician relationship that is based on empathy, education, and reassurance. Active dialogue about treatment risk and benefits has been shown to lead to compliance and treatment efficacy as shown by the risk-management program following the reintroduction of Lotronex to the U.S. market for women with severe IBS-D. Patients ultimately engaged in active dialogue about their symptoms with their physicians, leading to better compliance and treatment outcome.[49]

Probiotics and Antibiotics

Probiotics are live microbial organisms provided as food supplements. Preliminary studies in patients with IBS have demonstrated that *Bifidobacterium infantis* reduces inflammatory mediators.[50] Various commercial preparations are available, and studies have shown a potential benefit for such agents in the treatment of IBS.[51] In addition, multispecies probiotics such as *Lactobacillus rhamnosus* GG, *L. rhamnosus* LC705, *Bifidobacterium breve,* and *Propionibacterium freudenreichii* have shown promising results, with decreased symptom severity and decreased serum inflammatory markers when used for greater periods of time (5-6 months).[52] In a double-blind, randomized study of IBS patients, treatment with the antibiotic rifaximin resulted in a greater improvement in symptoms as compared with placebo.[53] Prebiotics, short-chain carbohydrates that allow for changes in the gut composition and activity of gut microflora, and symbiotics (combination of prebiotics and probiotics) will likely be in the future of IBS-C. These studies suggest that manipulation of gut flora may be a promising new modality of treatment for IBS.[52]

OUTCOMES

IBS is a chronic disease with an extremely variable clinical course in the general population. IBS is a safe diagnosis; patients with a diagnosis of IBS seldom turn out to suffer from serious organic disease, and the time-honored clinical strategy of reassuring the patient that the diagnosis is benign, without significant risk of missing an organic disease, is well justified.[54,55]

Summary

- Irritable bowel syndrome (IBS) is common in the general population and has significant medical and socioeconomic impact.
- IBS is defined on the basis of the modified Rome III criteria as recurrent abdominal pain or discomfort at least 3 days per month in the last 3 months that started at least 6 months before diagnosis, cannot be explained by a structural or biochemical abnormality, and is associated with improvement with defecation, onset associated with a change in frequency of stool, and onset associated with a change in form (appearance) of stool.
- IBS pathophysiology is still unclear, and the diagnosis and management are often challenging. Research is inconclusive, but evidence supports a role for visceral hypersensitivity, abnormal gut motility, psychosocial factors, neurotransmitter imbalance, latent or potential celiac disease, infection, and inflammation.
- A diagnosis is based on identifying positive symptoms consistent with IBS and excluding other conditions with similar clinical presentations in a cost-effective manner.
- IBS is a chronic disorder with no specific cause, and there is no cure. The patient's confidence in the physician's diagnosis, explanation, and reassurance are vital therapeutic tools. The treatment goal should be focused on relieving symptoms and addressing the patient's concerns.
- IBS is a safe diagnosis; patients with a diagnosis of IBS seldom turn out to suffer from serious organic disease, and the time-honored clinical strategy of reassuring the patient that the diagnosis is benign, without significant risk of missing an organic disease, is well justified.
- IBS as a multifactorial disease will continue to evolve as pathophysiologic mechanisms become clearer.

Suggested Readings

Camilleri M: Probiotics and irritable bowel syndrome: Rationale, putative mechanisms, and evidence of clinical efficacy. J Clin Gastroenterol 2006;40:264-269.

Drossman DA, Toner BB, Whitehead WE, et al: Cognitive-behavioral therapy versus education and desipramine versus placebo for moderate to severe functional bowel disorders. Gastroenterology 2003;125:664-671.

Drossman DA, Camilleri M, Mayer EA, Whitehead WE: AGA technical review on irritable bowel syndrome. Gastroenterology 2002;123:2108-2131.

Gwee K-A: Irritable bowel syndrome in developing countries–a disorder of civilization or colonization? Neurogastroenterol Motil 2005;17:317-324.

Longstreth GF, Thompson WG, Chey WD, et al: Functional bowel disorders. Gastroenterology 2006;130:1480-1491.

Longstreth GF, Wilson A, Knight K, et al: Irritable bowel syndrome, health care, and costs: A U.S. managed care perspective. Am J Gastroenterol 2003;98:600-607.

Mayer AE: The neurology of stress and gastrointestinal disease. Gut 2000;47:861-869.

Mearin F, Pérez-Oliveras M, Perelló A, et al: Dyspepsia and irritable bowel syndrome after a *Salmonella* gastroenteritis: One-year follow-up cohort study. Gastroenterology 2005;129:98-104.

O'Mahony L, McCarthy J, Kelly P, et al: *Lactobacillus* and *Bifidobacterium* in irritable bowel syndrome: Symptom responses and relationship to cytokine profile. Gastroenterology 2005;128:541-551.

Pimentel M, Park S, Mirocha J: The effect of a nonabsorbable oral antibiotic (rifaximin) on the symptoms of the irritable bowel syndrome: A randomized trial. Ann Intern Med 2006;145:626-628.

Saito WA, Schoefeld P, Locke GRI: The epidemiology of irritable bowel syndrome in North America. Am J Gastroenterol 2002;97:1910-1915.

Whitehead WE, Paulsson O, Jones KR: Systematic review of the comorbidity of irritable bowel syndrome with other disorders: What are the causes and implications? Gastroenterology 2002;122:140-156.

Wilson A, Longstreth GF, Knight K, et al: Quality of life in managed care patients with irritable bowel syndrome. Manage Care Interface 2004;17:24-28.

References

For a complete list of references, log onto www.expertconsult.com.

Acute Diarrhea

David S. Lever and *Edy Soffer*

DEFINITION AND CAUSES

Normal bowel frequency ranges from three times a day to three times a week in the normal population. Increased stooling, with stool consistency less solid than normal, constitutes a satisfactory, if somewhat imprecise, definition of diarrhea. *Acute diarrhea* is defined as a greater number of stools of decreased form from the normal lasting for less than 14 days. If the illness persists for more than 14 days, it is called *persistent*. If the duration of symptoms is longer than 1 month, it is considered *chronic diarrhea*. Most cases of acute diarrhea are self-limited, caused by infectious agents (e.g. viruses, bacteria, parasites), and do not require medication unless the patient is immunocompromised.

PREVALENCE

Worldwide, acute diarrhea constitutes a major cause of morbidity and mortality, especially among the very young, very old, and infirm. It is estimated that each year, U.S. adults experience 99 million episodes of acute diarrhea or gastroenteritis, resulting in about 8 million physician visits and more than 250,000 hospital admissions each year (1.5% of adult hospitalizations) caused by acute diarrhea or gastroenteritis. Most cases are caused by enteric infections. Food- and waterborne outbreaks involving a relatively small subset of population and recurrent bouts of illness in others comprise most cases.

Diarrhea is more prevalent among adults who are exposed to children and non-toilet-trained infants, particularly in a daycare setting. It is also more prevalent in travelers to tropical regions; homosexual males, persons with underlying immunosuppression, and those living in nonhygienic environments, with exposure to contaminated water or foods.

PATHOPHYSIOLOGY

Approximately 8 to 9 L of fluid enter the intestines daily—1 to 2 L represents food and liquid intake, and the rest is from endogenous sources such as salivary, gastric, pancreatic, biliary, and intestinal secretions. Most of the fluid, about 6 to 7 L, is absorbed in the small intestine, and only about 1 to 2 L is presented to the colon. Most of this is absorbed as it passes through the colon, leaving a stool output of about 100 to 200 g/day. Although many organisms simply impair the normal absorptive processes in the small intestine and colon, others, organisms, such as *Vibrio cholerae,* secrete a toxin that causes the colonic mucosa to secrete, rather than absorb, fluid and electrolytes. Voluminous diarrhea may result.

Diarrhea-causing pathogens are usually transmitted through the fecal-oral route. Risk factors for this type of transmission include improper disposal of feces and lack of proper hand washing following defecation and feces contact before handling food. Other risk factors include improper food hygiene, inadequate food refrigeration, food exposure to flies, and consumption of contaminated water. Multiple host factors that determine the level of illness once exposure to infectious agents has occurred include age, personal hygiene, gastric acidity and other barriers, intestinal motility, enteric microflora, immunity, and intestinal receptors.

Viruses (e.g., adenovirus, rotavirus, Norwalk virus) are the most common cause of diarrhea in the United States. *Escherichia coli, Clostridium difficile,* and *Campylobacter, Salmonella,* and *Shigella* spp. are common bacterial causes. *Bacillus cereus, Clostridium perfringens, Staphylococcus aureus, Salmonella* spp., and others cause food poisoning. *Entamoeba histolytica* and *Giardia, Cryptosporidium,* and *Cyclospora* spp. are parasitic or protozoal agents that cause diarrhea.

Acute watery diarrhea is most commonly seen with traveler's diarrhea caused by enterotoxigenic *E. coli* (ETEC), parasite-induced diarrhea from *Giardia* and *Cryptosporidium* spp. and, in cases of food poisoning (ingestion of preformed toxins), from *B. cereus* and *S. aureus.*

Some infectious agents cause mucosal inflammation, which may be mild or severe. Bacteria such as enteroadherent or enteropathogenic *E. coli* and viruses such as rotavirus, Norwalk agent, and HIV can cause minimal to moderate inflammation. Bacteria that destroy enterocytes such as *Shigella,* enteroinvasive *E. coli,* the parasite *E. histolytica,* and bacteria that penetrate the mucosa such as *Salmonella, Campylobacter jejuni,* and *Yersinia enterocolitica* result in moderate to severe inflammation with or without ulceration.

Ingestion of preformed toxin produced by bacteria such as *B. cereus, S. aureus,* and *Clostridium perfringens* can result in acute jejunitis. *Aeromonas, Shigella,* and *Vibrio* spp. (e.g., *V. parahaemolyticus*) produce enterotoxins and also invade the intestinal mucosa. Patients therefore often present with watery diarrhea, followed within hours or days by bloody diarrhea. Bacteria that produce inflammation from cytotoxins include *Clostridium difficile* and hemorrhagic *E. coli* O157:H7.

Exudative diarrhea results from extensive injury of the small bowel or colon mucosa as a result of inflammation or ulceration, leading to a loss of mucus, serum proteins, and blood into the bowel lumen. Increased fecal water and electrolyte excretion results from impaired water and electrolyte absorption by the inflamed intestine rather than from secretion of water and electrolytes into the exudates.

Noninfectious causes of diarrhea include inflammatory bowel disease, irritable bowel syndrome, ischemic bowel disease, partial small bowel obstruction, pelvic abscess in the rectosigmoid area, fecal impaction, and the ingestion of poorly absorbable sugars, such as lactulose and acute alcohol ingestion. Diarrhea is one of the most frequent adverse effects of prescription medications; it is important to note that drug-related diarrhea usually occurs after a new drug is initiated or the dosage increased.

SIGNS AND SYMPTOMS

Clinical features sometimes provide a clue to the cause. Diarrhea caused by small intestine disease is typically high volume, watery, and often associated with malabsorption. Dehydration is frequent. Diarrhea caused by colonic involvement is more often associated with frequent small-volume stools, the presence of blood, and a sensation of urgency.

Important factors in evaluating acute diarrhea include travel history, sources of water (e.g., well water), recent food intake, history of profuse diarrheal episodes, dehydration, fever, hematochezia, nausea, vomiting, and abdominal pain. Important clinical features include abrupt versus gradual onset of symptoms, symptom duration, including bowel movement frequency, stool quantities, dysentery with fever, tenesmus, hematochezia or pus in the stool, signs of volume depletion, including thirst, tachycardia, orthostasis, decreased urine output, skin turgor, and lethargy or confusion, or both.

Patients ingesting toxins or those with toxigenic infection typically have nausea and vomiting as prominent symptoms, along with watery diarrhea, but rarely have a high fever. Vomiting that begins within 6 hours of ingesting a food should suggest food poisoning caused by preformed toxin from bacteria such as *S. aureus* or *B. cereus.* If diarrhea disease begins within 8 to 14 hours of food ingestion, *C. perfringens* should be suspected. When the incubation period is longer than 14 hours and vomiting is also a significant symptom, along with the diarrhea, viral agents should be considered. Parasites that do not invade the intestinal mucosa, such as *Giardia lamblia* and *Cryptosporidium,* usually cause only mild abdominal discomfort. Giardiasis may be associated with mild steatorrhea, gaseousness, and bloating.

Infection with invasive bacteria such as *Campylobacter, Salmonella,* and *Shigella* spp., and organisms that produce cytotoxins, such as *C. difficile* and enterohemorrhagic *E. coli* (serotype O157:H7), often result in abdominal pain, and low-grade fever; occasionally, peritoneal signs may suggest a surgical abdomen. *Yersinia* organisms often infect the terminal ileum and cecum and manifest with right lower quadrant pain and tenderness suggesting acute appendicitis.

Hemolytic-uremic syndrome and thrombotic thrombocytopenic purpura can occur in infections with enterohemorrhagic *E. coli* and *Shigella* organisms, particularly in young children and older adults. *Yersinia* infection and other enteric bacterial infections may be accompanied by Reiter's syndrome (arthritis, urethritis, and conjunctivitis), thyroiditis, pericarditis, or glomerulonephritis. Enteric fever, caused by *Salmonella typhi* or *Salmonella paratyphi,* is a severe systemic illness manifested initially by prolonged high fevers, prostration, confusion, and respiratory symptoms, followed by abdominal tenderness, diarrhea, and rash.

Epidemiologic risk factors should be investigated for certain diarrheal diseases and their spread. They include recent travel to an underdeveloped area, daycare center exposure, consumption of raw meat, eggs, shellfish, and unpasteurized milk products, contact with reptiles or pets with diarrhea, a history of other ill people in a shared dormitory facility, recent antibiotic use, and a history of HIV or medically induced immunosuppression. In cases of homosexual males, in addition to immunosuppression, there are two other disease transmission routes that lead to an increased susceptibility to infectious agents that cause diarrhea. These include an increased rate of fecal-oral transmission of all infectious agents spread by this route, including *Shigella, Salmonella, Campylobacter,* and intestinal protozoa and anal intercourse. Anal intercourse can lead to a direct rectal inoculation, resulting in proctitis associated with rectal pain, tenesmus, and passage of small-volume, bloody, mucous stools.

DIAGNOSIS

History and Physical Examination

Conducting a careful interview can provide valuable clues that will aid in diagnosing and choosing the most appropriate and cost-effective investigation. Acute diarrheas are usually infectious in origin and, for the most part, resolve with or without intervention before a diagnosis is made.

The presence of blood is a useful clue, suggesting infection by invasive organisms, inflammation, ischemia, or neoplasm. Large-volume diarrhea suggests small bowel or proximal colonic disease, whereas small frequent stools associated with urgency suggest left colon or rectal disease. All current and recent medications should be reviewed, specifically new medications, antibiotics, antacids, and alcohol abuse. Nutritional supplements should also be reviewed, including the intake of sugar-free foods (containing nonabsorbable carbohydrates), fat substitutes, milk products, and shellfish, and heavy intake of fruits, fruit juices, or caffeine. Food- or waterborne outbreaks of diarrhea are becoming more common. The history should include place of residence, drinking water (treated city water or well water), rural conditions, with consumption of raw milk, consumption of raw meat or fish, and exposure to farm animals that may spread *Salmonella* or *Brucella* organisms. Sexual history is important, because specific organisms can cause diarrhea in homosexual men and HIV-infected patients.

A medical evaluation of acute diarrhea is not warranted in the previously healthy patient if symptoms are mild, moderate, spontaneously improve within 48 hours, and are not accompanied by fever, chills, severe abdominal pain, or blood in the stool. On the other hand, evaluation is indicated if symptoms are severe or prolonged, the patient appears toxic, there is evidence of colitis (occult or gross blood in the stools, severe abdominal pain or tenderness, and fever), or empirical therapy has failed. Passage of many small-volume stools containing blood and mucus, temperature higher than 38.5° C (101.3° F), passage of more than six unformed stools in 24 hours, or a duration of illness longer than 48 hours, diarrhea with severe abdominal pain in a patient older than 50 years, diarrhea in older adults (>70 years) or in the immunocompromised patient (e.g., those with AIDS, after transplantation, or undergoing cancer chemotherapy) are all indications for a thorough medical and bacteriologic evaluation.

The physical examination in acute diarrhea is helpful in determining the severity of disease and hydration status. A directed physical examination may lead to a more focused evaluation. Vital signs (including temperature and orthostatic evaluation of pulse and blood pressure) and signs of volume depletion (including dry mucous membranes, decreased skin turgor, and confusion) should be carefully evaluated. A careful abdominal examination to evaluate for tenderness and distention and a stool examination to evaluate for grossly bloody stools are warranted. Nonbloody stools should be evaluated for heme positivity.

The history and physical examination can help lead to a diagnosis but, for treatment of some organisms, a specific diagnosis is required, which will lead to more specific therapy and prevention of unneeded interventions. Fecal testing should be performed in patients with a history of diarrhea longer than 1 day who have the following symptoms: fever, bloody stools, systemic illness, recent or remote antibiotic treatment, hospital admission, or signs of dehydration, as described earlier.

Studies in Selected Patients with Acute Diarrhea

In patients with acute diarrhea, the following studies should be carried out:

- Fecal leukocyte determination
- Stool culture for enteric pathogens
- Stool examination for ova and parasites
- Flexible sigmoidoscopy with biopsy

Stool evaluation for fecal leukocytes (or lactoferrin, a by-product of white blood cells) is a useful initial test, because it may support a diagnosis of inflammatory diarrhea. If the test is negative, stool culture may not be necessary, but culture is indicated if the test is positive. However, clinicians should remember that inflammatory diarrhea with a noninfectious cause, such as inflammatory bowel disease, ischemic or radiation-induced colitis, and diverticulitis, can be positive for stool leukocytes.

Indications for stool culture are bloody diarrhea, a toxic-appearing patient (fever, severe abdominal pain), possible epidemic, history of traveler's diarrhea, immunosuppression, or persistent diarrhea. A positive stool culture can be considered to be a true positive. Multiple stool cultures are usually not necessary because bacteria usually shed continuously. The culture medium routinely used can identify *Campylobacter, Salmonella, Shigella,* and *Aeromonas* organisms. Stool cultures are of little value if first performed more than 72 hours after admission. In outbreaks of diarrhea secondary to *Salmonella* and *E. coli,* routine culture is critical for antibiotic resistance testing and serotype subtyping. In patients with bloody diarrhea or hemolytic-uremic syndrome, the stool should be evaluated for *E. coli* O157 by the presence or absence of Shiga toxin. Stool culture for *Vibrio* spp. should be performed for those with diarrhea who have a previous history of shellfish ingestion within three days of onset of the illness. Cultures for *Y. enterocolitica* should be performed for at-risk populations (Asian Americans in California and African American infants) who develop diarrhea in the fall or winter. The rapid enzyme-linked immunoassay (ELISA) for *C. difficile* toxins A and B is most often used for high-risk patients who have taken antibiotics or have hospital-acquired diarrhea that develops three or more days after admission. The evaluation and management of antibiotic-associated diarrhea, including *C. difficile,* are considered elsewhere in this section ("Antibiotic-Associated Diarrhea").

A negative stool culture in a patient with acute diarrhea with fecal leukocytes is helpful for suggesting the acute onset of idiopathic inflammatory bowel disease (e.g., Crohn's disease, mucosal ulcerative colitis). A flexible sigmoidoscopy with biopsy may provide additional support.

Stool testing for ova and parasites should be done if the patient is at risk for parasitic infection. Multiple stool samples should be collected at different times because shedding of parasites may be intermittent.

When organisms are not identified on stool cultures for ova and parasites, a sigmoidoscopy should be performed and biopsies obtained. Mucosal biopsy is helpful in differentiating infectious colitis from inflammatory bowel disease. Further investigations will depend on the results of sigmoidoscopy, severity of diarrhea, immune status of the host, and presence of systemic toxicity. A general algorithm for the evaluation and management of acute diarrhea is shown in Figure 1.

TREATMENT

The principal components of the treatment of acute diarrhea are fluid and electrolyte replacement, dietary modifications, and drug therapy. All recommendations agree with the guidelines on acute infectious diarrhea in adults published by the American College of Gastroenterology.

Rehydration

In most cases of acute diarrhea, fluid and electrolyte replacement are the most important forms of therapy. If patients are otherwise healthy and are not dehydrated, adequate oral intake can be achieved with soft drinks, fruit juice, broth, soup, and salted crackers. In those with excessive fluid losses and dehydration, more aggressive measures such as IV fluids or oral rehydration therapy with isotonic electrolyte solutions containing glucose or starch should be instituted. Oral rehydration therapy is less expensive, often just as effective, and more practical than intravenous fluids. A number of oral rehydration solutions are available, including Pedialyte, Rehydralyte, Ricelyte (Infalyte), Resol, the World Health Organization formula, and the newer reduced osmolarity formula for children. An equally effective homemade mixture is 1/2 tsp salt (3.5 g), 1 tsp baking soda (2.5 g $NaHCO_3$), 8 tsp sugar (40 g), and 8 oz orange juice (1.5 g KCl), diluted to 1 L with water. Fluids should be given at rates of 50 to 200 mL/kg/24 hr, depending on the patient's hydration status. IV fluids (e.g., lactated Ringer's solution) are preferred acutely for patients with severe dehydration and for those who cannot tolerate oral fluids.

Diet

Total food abstinence is unnecessary and not recommended. Foods providing calories are necessary to facilitate renewal of enterocytes. Patients should be encouraged to take frequent feedings of fruit drinks, tea, flat carbonated beverages, and soft, easily digested foods such as bananas, applesauce, rice, potatoes, noodles, crackers, toast, and soups. Dairy products should be avoided, because transient lactase deficiency can be caused by enteric, viral, and bacterial infections. Caffeinated beverages and alcohol, which can enhance intestinal motility and secretions, should be avoided.

Pharmacologic Measures

Antidiarrheal Agents

Antidiarrheal agents can be useful for the amelioration of symptoms. The most effective agents are the opioid derivatives-loperamide, diphenoxylate-atropine, and tincture of opium. These agents inhibit

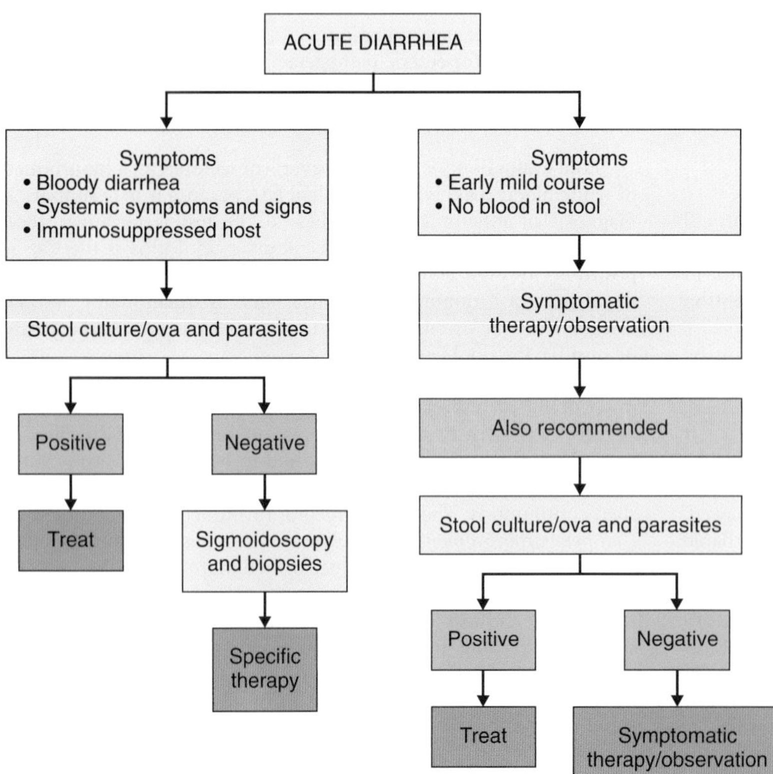

Figure 1 **Algorithm for the evaluation of a patient with acute diarrhea.** *(Adapted from Soffer EE: Diarrhea. In Andreoli TE, Carpenter CCJ, Griggs R, Loscalzo J [eds]: Cecil Essentials of Medicine, 5th ed. Philadelphia, WB Saunders, 2001, pp 316-320.)*

intestinal peristalsis, facilitating intestinal absorption, and have antisecretory properties. Loperamide may reduce the duration of diarrhea in those with traveler's diarrhea and bacillary dysentery. These agents should be avoided in patients with fever, bloody diarrhea, and possible inflammatory diarrhea because they may be associated with prolonged fever in patients with shigellosis, toxic megacolon in patients with *C. difficile* infection, and the hemolytic-uremic syndrome in children with Shiga toxin–producing *E. coli.*

Bismuth subsalicylate, somewhat less effective than loperamide, is effective in relieving symptoms of diarrhea, nausea, and abdominal pain in patients with traveler's diarrhea. Bismuth subsalicylate is contraindicated in HIV-infected patients because it may cause bismuth encephalopathy.

Antimicrobial Treatment

Because most patients have mild, self-limited disease caused by viruses or noninvasive bacteria, routine empirical treatment is not warranted. Empirical treatment is indicated for those patients with suspected invasive bacterial infection, traveler's diarrhea, or immunosuppression. Empirical antibiotic treatment is also appropriate specifically for early *Campylobacter* infections and *C. difficile*–associated diarrhea as well as for the febrile patient with fecal leukocytes and hemoccult-positive stools. Empirical treatment for *Giardia* can be prescribed for those with a 2-week or longer history of diarrhea. Empirical parasitic treatment should be considered for those in the following situations:

- History of diarrhea following travel to Russia, Nepal, or other endemic areas
- Exposure to infants in daycare centers
- Homosexual exposure or exposure to patients with AIDS
- Community waterborne outbreak
- History of bloody diarrhea with a history of few or no white blood cells (WBCs), suggesting amebiasis

OUTCOMES

Diarrhea is one of the most common illnesses in all age groups and is second only to the common cold as a cause of lost days of work or school. It is estimated that there are almost 100 million cases of acute diarrhea per year in U.S. adults. Adults experience an average of more than one bout of diarrhea per year. Most patients with acute diarrhea have a mild and self-limited illness; most treat their illness at home and usually get better without medical intervention. However, diarrhea is responsible for more than 300 deaths per year in North America. Diarrhea and related complications can cause severe illness, especially in high-risk groups, such as patients with severe comorbid conditions, underlying immunosuppression, and advanced age.

Summary

- Acute diarrhea is a common problem worldwide, with high morbidity and mortality in high-risk groups, such as the very young, older adults, and immunocompromised individuals.
- Most cases remit spontaneously and do not need diagnostic studies or specific therapy. Diagnostic studies are warranted for patients with fever or bloody diarrhea, or if the affected individual is immunocompromised.
- Infectious agents are responsible for most cases of acute diarrhea, and may act via numerous mechanisms.
- Prevention of dehydration is the most important therapeutic intervention for the management of individuals with acute diarrhea. Oral hydration is preferred in most cases.
- The use of nonspecific antidiarrheals, especially loperamide, is safe for most cases of acute diarrhea. Caution in use of these agents is urged when there is fever, chills, or bloody diarrhea, or when Clostridia difficile is suspected (diarrhea occurring after antibiotic use).
- Antibiotics such as ciprofloxacin may be used empirically for traveler's diarrhea. Antibiotics may also be used for early *Campylobacter* infection and for suspected or confirmed cases of *C. difficile* infection, as well as for the febrile patient who is positive for fecal leukocytes.

Suggested Readings

Dupont HL: Guidelines on acute infectious diarrhea in adults. The Practice Parameters Committee of the American College of Gastroenterology. Am J Gastroenterol 1997;92:1962-1975.

Fine KD: Diarrhea. In Feldman M, Scharschmidt BF, Sleisenger MH, Fordtran JS (eds): Sleisenger & Fordtran's Gastrointestinal and Liver Disease: Pathophysiology/Diagnosis/Management, 6th ed. Philadelphia, WB Saunders, 1998, pp 128-152.

Gangarosa RE, Glass RI, Lew JF, Boring JR: Hospitalizations involving gastroenteritis in the United States, 1985: The special burden of disease among the elderly. Am J Epidemiol 1992;135:281-290.

Garthright WE, Archer DL, Kvenberg JE: Estimates of incidence and costs of intestinal infectious diseases in the United States. Public Health Rep 1988;103:107-115.

Guerrant RL, Van Gilder T, Steiner TS, et al; Infectious Diseases Society of America: Practice guidelines for the management of infectious diarrhea. Clin Infect Dis 2001;32:331-350.

Musher DM, Musher BL: Contagious acute gastrointestinal infections. N Engl J Med 2004;351:2417-2427.

Scheidler MD, Giannella RA: Practical management of acute diarrhea. Hosp Pract 2001;36:49-56.

Schiller LR: Diarrhea. Med Clin North Am 2000;84:1259-1274.

Sellin JH: Intestinal electrolyte absorption and secretion. In Feldman M, Scharschmidt BF, Sleisenger MH, Fordtran JS (eds): Sleisenger & Fordtran's Gastrointestinal and Liver Disease: Pathophysiology/Diagnosis/Management, 6th ed. Philadelphia, WB Saunders, 1998, pp 1451-1471.

Thielman NM, Guerrant RL: Acute infectious diarrhea. N Engl J Med 2004;350:38-47.

Antibiotic-Associated Diarrhea and *Clostridium difficile*

Ronnie Pimental** and **Anuja Choure

DEFINITION

The first report of antibiotic-associated diarrhea (AAD) was found in the *Bulletin of the Johns Hopkins Hospital* of 1893, where John Finney and Sir William Osler described the case of a young woman who died of a severe case of "diphtheric colitis" shortly after gastric surgery.[1] It was not until the mid-1900s, with the use of preoperative antibiotics, that AAD became a common medical problem.

For years, the cause of the pseudomembranous colitis remained elusive; indeed, the term *staphylococcal enterocolitis* was used, reflecting the belief that the disease was commonly caused by staphylococci. In the 1970s, important clinical observations of clindamycin-associated pseudomembranous colitis and the demonstration of the potent cytopathic effects of *Clostridium difficile*–derived toxin in animal models established the cause and pathogenesis of this condition.[2]

Today, the term *antibiotic-associated diarrhea* refers to a benign, self-limited diarrhea following the use of antimicrobials. Typically, no pathogens are identified and the diarrhea is caused by changes in the composition and function of the intestinal flora. Most patients respond to supportive measures and discontinuation of antibiotics. On the other hand, *C. difficile* diarrhea refers to a wide spectrum of diarrheal illnesses caused by the potent toxins produced by this organism, including cases of severe colitis with or without the presence of pseudomembranes.

PREVALENCE

The occurrence of AAD varies greatly and is influenced by a number of factors, including nosocomial outbreaks, patterns of antimicrobial use, and individual susceptibility. It is estimated that 10% to 15% of all hospitalized patients treated with antibiotics will develop AAD. Most important, twice as many will become asymptomatic carriers. Risk factors include compromised immune status, advanced age, abdominal surgery, comorbidity, types and prolonged use of antibiotics, and the length of hospitalization. For example, infection rates for *C. difficile* are reported to be around 10% after 2 weeks of hospitalization but may reach 50% after 4 or more weeks.[2]

All groups of antibiotics may cause AAD, but those with broad-spectrum coverage-in particular cephalosporins, extended-coverage penicillins, and clindamycin-are the most common culprits.[3] *C. difficile* diarrhea is largely a nosocomial disease and is the most frequent cause of diarrhea in hospitalized patients. Its occurrence in the outpatient setting other than in patients confined to nursing homes is much less common.[2]

Epidemiologic studies have shown that *C. difficile* is often isolated in hospital wards, including the floors, door handles, and furniture, even weeks after patients with AAD have been removed from the area. Less frequently, similar observations have been made among asymptomatic medical personnel and in hospital wards occupied by unaffected patients. Patients readmitted after recent hospitalizations are found to have a high prevalence of *C. difficile* colonization, representing an important source of infection. Because of the sporulating properties of this organism, all these observations have suggested an important role for cross-contamination between patients, contact with environmental surfaces, and transmission via hands of medical personnel.[4] During the past few years, there has been renewed interest in *C. difficile* diarrhea reflecting a form of disease that is more frequent, more severe, and more refractory to standard treatment. These observations are explained by the presence of a new strain of *C. difficile*, designated NAP-1, that produces more toxins A and B in vitro, produces binary toxin that is of uncertain significance, and is resistant to fluoroquinolones.[16]

PATHOGENESIS

The prolonged use of multiple antibiotics, especially broad-spectrum agents with poor intestinal absorption or high biliary excretion, induces a change in the composition and function of the intestinal flora and therefore results in a higher incidence of AAD.[2,5] The degree of alteration will be influenced by the ability of the normal flora to resist colonization and the type of antibiotic used. A decrease in the colonic anaerobic flora interferes with carbohydrate and bile acid metabolism. Osmotic or secretory diarrhea may occur. Overgrowth of opportunistic pathogens takes place as a result of microbiologic and metabolic alterations.

C. difficile, an anaerobic gram-positive rod, accounts for 15% to 20% of all AAD cases. In particular, this organism can be isolated in a great number of AAD cases with evidence of colitis and in all those with pseudomembranes. It is widely present in the environment, may survive for a considerable time, and is transmitted by the fecal-oral route to susceptible individuals. It is considered part of the normal flora of infants and can be isolated in about 5% of healthy adults and in up to one third of asymptomatic or colonized hospitalized patients.

Both *C. difficile* toxins A and B exhibit potent enterotoxic and cytotoxic effects that are responsible for the clinical manifestations. The mechanism of action is by toxin binding on intestinal receptors, leading to disruption of the cellular skeleton and intracellular junctions. Protein synthesis and cell division are inhibited. Important inflammatory mediators attract neutrophils and monocytes, increasing capillary permeability, tissue necrosis, hemorrhage, and edema.

Serum and fecal antibodies to *C. difficile* infection are detected in many infected patients. The host's immune response appears to be critical in the clinical outcome. Elevated levels of serum immunoglobulin G and A (IgG and IgA) and fecal IgA against toxin A have been demonstrated in asymptomatic patients and in those with mild forms of *C. difficile* colitis, in contrast to those with severe illness, showing that antibodies provide a protective function.[6]

Histologically, three different stages in *C. difficile* colitis can be identified. Initially, focal epithelial necrosis, along with fibrin-rich exudates and neutrophils, is present. In the second phase, a marked exudate protruding through an area of mucosal ulceration represents the classic volcano lesion (Fig. 1). The third stage is characterized by diffuse and more severe mucosal ulceration and necrosis, often associated with a pseudomembrane composed of fibrin, leukocytes, and cellular debris.[7]

SIGNS AND SYMPTOMS

The clinical manifestations of AAD may vary from mild diarrhea to fulminant colitis.[8] The severity of *C. difficile* colitis appears to be

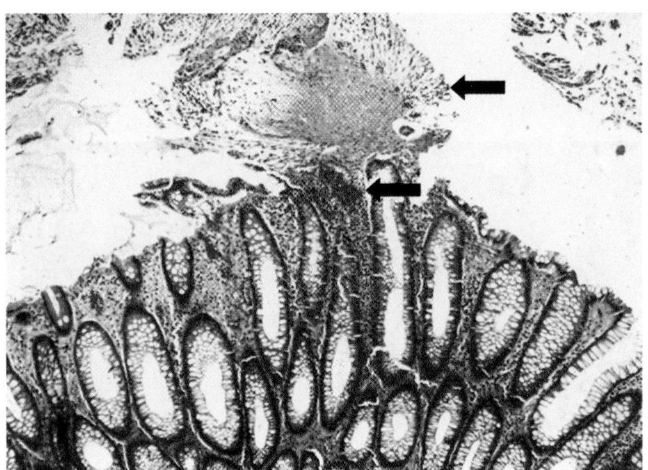

Figure 1 Typical volcano lesion. A marked exudate can be seen protruding through an area of mucosal ulceration (*arrows*). *(Hematoxylin and eosin stain ×105.5) (From Feldman M, Friedman LS, Brandt LJ [eds]: Sleisenger and Fordtran's Gastrointestinal and Liver Diseases, 8th ed. Philadelphia, WB Saunders, 2006.)*

influenced by a myriad of factors, including age, comorbidity, host's immune response, and the use of antiperistaltic agents. Interestingly, bacterial genotype and toxin production appear to play minimal roles.[9] The cardinal symptom of the disease is diarrhea, which commonly develops during treatment but may appear as late as 8 weeks after discontinuation of antibiotics. In most cases of AAD, patients present with loose stools, minimal signs of colitis, and no constitutional symptoms. The diarrhea promptly responds to supportive measures and withdrawal of the antimicrobial agent.[8]

In contrast, typical cases of *C. difficile* infection manifest with a profuse, mucous, foul-smelling diarrhea associated with cramps and tenesmus. Frank bleeding is rare, although fecal occult blood and leukocytes are frequently detected. The abdomen is generally soft, with increased bowel sounds and mild tenderness over the left lower quadrant. Constitutional symptoms are common, and include nausea, vomiting, dehydration, and low-grade fever. Mild leukocytosis is frequently present and may occur even in the absence of diarrhea. An occasional leukemoid reaction has been reported. For colitis limited to the right colon, prominent findings of localized abdominal pain, leukocytosis, and fever can be found in the presence of minimal diarrhea.

In severe cases, toxic megacolon may occur along with the deceiving findings of "improved diarrhea." A dramatic clinical picture of marked colonic distention, peritoneal irritation, fever, and elevated white blood count is commonly found. Hypoalbuminemia, hypovolemia, and ascites are common. A plain abdominal x-ray may show marked colonic distention or thumbprinting, with or without pneumatosis intestinalis. Computed tomography often reveals colonic wall thickening, lumen obliteration, pericolonic fat stranding, and ascites. Surgical intervention is often required, and carries significant morbidity and mortality.[10]

The diagnosis of AAD should be considered in any patient recently treated with antibiotics and presenting with new-onset diarrhea. Exposure up to 8 weeks before onset to any antimicrobial, including antifungal agents, should be considered. Clinical presentation, laboratory data, imaging studies, and endoscopic examinations are all useful. Atypical subtle presentations, especially in ambulatory patients with a remote and brief antibiotic exposure, require high suspicion. Leukocytosis, fecal leukocytes, and fecal occult blood are supportive of the diagnosis but not always present. Imaging studies, including plain radiographic films and computed tomography, are of marginal benefit as diagnostic tools but become helpful in severe cases to identify complications.

The cornerstone of the diagnosis of *C. difficile* colitis is identification of *C. difficile* toxins in the stool. Culture assays are considered to be the gold standard, based on the demonstration of toxin B cytopathic effects on cell culture monolayers. This test carries great specificity and sensitivity, detecting minimal toxin concentrations. Unfortunately, cell culture tests are expensive, time-consuming, and rarely used in clinical practice.

The most preferred diagnostic method in *C. difficile* colitis is the enzyme-linked immunosorbent assay (ELISA), based on toxin detection in the stool. Today, most commercially available methods detect both A and B toxins, obviating the problems of missing certain *C. difficile* strains that produce only toxin B. ELISA is fast, relatively inexpensive, and has excellent specificity; its sensitivity, however, is 75% to 85%. Serial stool determinations on different days are suggested for suspected cases with initial negative results.

The latex agglutination test is based on the detection of the enzyme glutamate dehydrogenase rather than on *C. difficile* toxin. Nontoxigenic strains of *C. difficile*, as well as other colonic organisms, may produce this enzyme. Latex agglutination tests are rarely used today because of their lack of specificity.

Endoscopy is a rapid but invasive and expensive diagnostic test for *C. difficile* colitis. Often, nonspecific findings of colitis such as edema, erythema, and loss of vascular pattern are the only findings. In cases of pseudomembranous colitis, endoscopy is diagnostic, because it may reveal typical raised, yellow nodules over areas of normal mucosa or minimal erythema. In more severe cases, coalescent nodules forming extensive areas of pseudomembranes over a background of inflammation and ulcerations are found (Fig. 2). In most cases, pseudomembranes are distributed throughout the colon and are readily identified within the reach of the sigmoidoscope. In a few cases, the pseudomembranes are confined to the right colon. Endoscopy should be used with caution and reserved for patients with severe colitis of unclear cause in whom a prompt diagnosis is needed.

TREATMENT

The current guidelines from the American College of Gastroenterology (ACG) for the initial management of *C. difficile* colitis are clear and widely accepted (Box 1).[5] In the vast majority of patients AAD is a mild and self- limited illness that responds to the discontinuation of antibiotics, supportive care, and fluid and electrolyte replacement. On the other hand, in cases in which signs and symptoms of colitis develop, the use of effective oral antimicrobial agents against *C. difficile* is often necessary. Although the diagnosis of *C. difficile* colitis should always be established before antimicrobial therapy is implemented, we strongly agree with the current ACG guidelines in that empirical therapy should be initiated in highly suggestive cases of severely ill patients.[11]

Pharmacologic Agents

Many antimicrobials have been used to treat *C. difficile* colitis. Oral vancomycin and metronidazole used for 7 to 10 days are considered the first line of therapy by most clinicians and current guidelines.[11] Multiple studies have reported initial response rates greater than 90% and comparable failure rates of 15% to 20%.[12] Metronidazole at a dosage of 250 mg four times daily is recommended by most clinicians and ACG guidelines as the drug of choice for the initial treatment of *C. difficile* colitis. These recommendations are largely based on efficacy, lower costs, and concerns about the development of vancomycin-resistant strains. Major disadvantages of metronidazole include a less desirable drug profile and contraindications for children and pregnant women.

An albumin level of 2.5 g/L and intensive care unit stay were predictors of failure of metronidazole therapy for *C. difficile*-associated diarrhea. These patients may benefit from oral vancomycin at the outset. Vancomycin at a dosage of 125 mg four times daily,

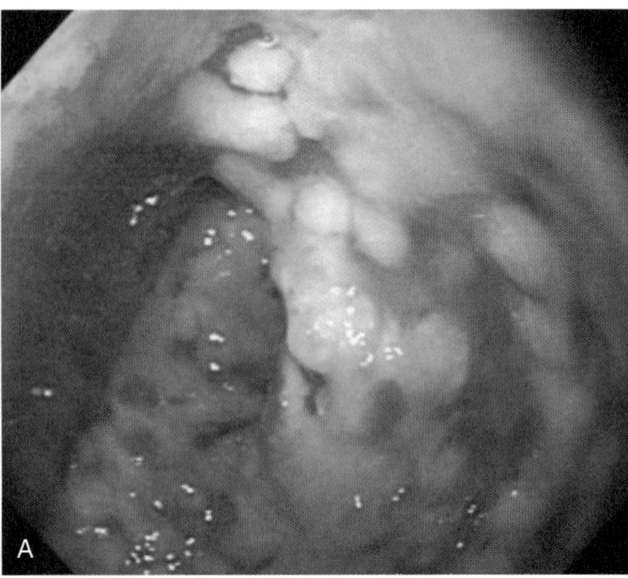

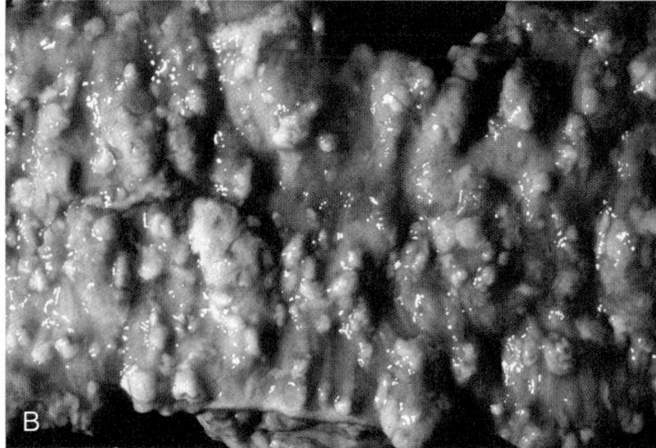

Figure 2 Pseudomembranous colitis. A, Multiple yellow coalescent plaques throughout the colonic mucosa, typical findings for pseudomembranous colitis. **B,** Flat raised lesions that vary in size with intervening hyperemic mucosa. *(From Feldman M, Friedman LS, Brandt LJ [eds]: Sleisenger and Fordtran's Gastrointestinal and Liver Diseases, 8th ed. Philadelphia, WB Saunders, 2006.)*

Box 1 Guidelines for the Treatment of *Clostridium Difficile* Colitis

Discontinue antibiotics.
Initiate supportive therapy. Prophylactic antibiotic therapy should not be given routinely.
Once the diagnosis of *C. difficile* diarrhea is confirmed and specific therapy is indicated, metronidazole given orally is preferred.
If diagnosis is highly likely and the patient is seriously ill, metronidazole may be given empirically before the diagnosis is established.
Vancomycin given orally is reserved for the following conditions:

- The patient has failed therapy with metronidazole.
- The patient's organism is resistant to metronidazole.
- The patient is allergic, cannot tolerate metronidazole, or is being treated with ethanol-containing solutions.
- The patient is either pregnant or a child under 10 years of age.
- The patient is critically ill because of *C. difficile*-associated diarrhea or colitis.
- There is evidence suggesting the diarrhea is caused by *Staphylococcus aureus*.

is safe, well tolerated, and achieves stool levels 20 times the required minimal inhibitory concentration required for the treatment of *C. difficile*. Higher doses of the drug have failed to show significant benefits.[12] Main disadvantages with this agent are cost and the potential development of vancomycin-resistant strains. We concur with the current ACG guideline in considering vancomycin the drug of choice for severely ill patients and for those in whom the use of metronidazole is precluded.

The treatment of patients with severe ileus is challenging and not clearly addressed by the ACG practice guidelines. Most reports have suggested the use of parenteral metronidazole in these patients. In animal studies, intravenous metronidazole has been shown to achieve reasonable concentrations in the intestinal lumen. Unfortunately, most studies are based on small clinical trials with contradictory results.[13] Few anecdotal reports of vancomycin enemas can be found in the literature, but good scientific data are lacking to recommend its use in these patients.

Because of their potential role in binding *C. difficile* toxin, anion exchange resins such as cholestyramine and colestipol were introduced in the management of AAD in an attempt to decrease relapses. These agents, in particular colestipol, have been shown to reduce titers, concentration, and time exposure of the *C. difficile* toxin in the colons of infected patients.[14] Although subsequent binding of vancomycin occurs with cholestyramine, the minimal inhibitory concentration for *C. difficile* is maintained. Other antimicrobial agents, in particular bacitracin and teicoplanin, were used with some success in the past. Today, however, their use is limited to special situations in which metronidazole or vancomycin cannot be used or has failed.[15]

The NAP-1 strain has forced us to take a closer look at the current therapeutic options; therefore, newer drugs have been proposed for the treatment including Nitazonide and Rifaximine both of which achieve high colonic levels and have been used for other indications and others including Ramoplanin a new lipoglycodepsipeptide and Difimicin (OPT-80 and PAR 101), a new macrolide antibiotic with no approved indications. Tolevamer, a nonantibiotic polymer that binds *C. difficile* toxins A and B to neutralize biologic activity had promising results in phase 2 clinical trials but in phase 3 trials, it was shown to be inferior to Metronidazole and Vancomycin for initial therapy although relapse rates were significantly lower again suggesting the limitations of treating AAD with antibiotics.[16]

Probiotics, a group of agents designed to resist colonization and restore normal flora have been tried in AAD. The most promising probiotic agent is *Saccharomyces boulardii*, a live nonpathogenic yeast shown to have some benefit in the treatment of AAD by binding to the glycoprotein receptor site for toxin A at the intestinal brush border. When given prophylactically to patients receiving antibiotics in a prospective, double-blind, controlled study,[17] *S. boulardii* was shown to be safe and beneficial in reducing the incidence of *C. difficile* colitis in comparison with placebo (22% vs. 9.5%). Unfortunately, *S. boulardii* is not commercially available in the United States.[17] Lactobacillus GG, another popular probiotic, has been shown to improve intestinal immunity by increasing IgG and IgA levels at the intestinal mucosal level. Clinical studies have been tried but with limited success.[18]

Surgical Treatment

Surgical treatment of *C. difficile* colitis is rarely needed. It is reserved for patients with toxic megacolon who do not respond to medical therapy and carries a mortality rate close to 40%. Comorbidity and late intervention are largely responsible for the poor outcomes of these patients. Segmental resections are commonly ineffective. Early

Box 2 Oral Regimens for Treating Relapsing *Clostridium Difficile* Colitis

I. Vancomycin Plus Anion Exchange Resin[23]
  1. Vancomycin 125 mg PO qid for 7-10 day
  2. Vancomycin 125 mg PO bid for 5-7 day
     plus
     Colestipol 5 g PO bid for 5-7 day
  3. Vancomycin 125 mg PO qd for 5-7 day
     plus
     Colestipol 5 g PO bid for 5-7 day
  4. Colestipol 5 g PO bid for 14 day

II. Vancomycin Plus Rifampin[20]
  Vancomycin 125 mg PO qid for 7 day
  plus
  Rifampin 600 mg PO bid for 7 day

III. Antibiotic Plus *Saccharomyces*[17]
  Metronidazole 250 mg PO qid for 14 day
  or
  Vancomycin 125 mg PO qid for 14 day
  plus
  Saccharomyces boulardii, 250 mg PO bid, for 4 wk*

**Not commercially available in the United States.*
bid, twice daily; qd,each day; qid, four times daily.

intervention with total colectomy and diversion is the recommended approach.[10]

Relapses

The most difficult problem in the management of *C. difficile*-associated colitis is relapse, reported to occur in 15% to 20% of cases, regardless of the initial treatment used. Relapse appears to be facilitated by the sporulating properties of *C. difficile*. Some conditions identified as potential markers for relapse include previous relapses, chronic renal failure, marked leukocytes, and continued antibiotic use.[19]

For a first relapse, the current guidelines of the ACG recommend treating patients with a second course of metronidazole or vancomycin for a total of 7 to 10 days.[11] Nevertheless, most studies advocate for a longer course of treatment, a total of 2 weeks.

In cases of more than one failure, when the relapse rate could be as high as 65%, a different approach is needed. Confirmation of the diagnosis and avoidance of unnecessary antibiotics is strongly advised. Different agents, regimens, doses, and even unusual forms of therapy, such as fecal enemas, have been tried, with varying success. Limitations in the actual management of repetitive relapses are acknowledged in the ACG practice guidelines.[11] However, most of the recommended regimens available, although reported to be effective, are based on small uncontrolled studies (Box 2).[19,20]

Based on stool clearance by culture, toxin detection, and some limited clinical data, vancomycin appears to be a superior agent for cases of multiple relapse. Probably the most popular approach today is the use of vancomycin in a tapered dose regimen over several weeks or in combination with other agents, including anion-binding resins and rifampin.[20-23] The design of most of these regimens is based on the sporulating properties of *C. difficile*, and combine the antimicrobial action of different agents along with the constipating effects and potential for toxin-binding properties of anion resins. Probiotics such as *S. boulardii* in combination with vancomycin or metronidazole are frequently used in Europe for relapse prevention. When available, this agent may play a more important role in the future management of these patients in other parts of the world. Tolevamer can also be used to prevent relapses.[16] In case of multiple relapses or refractory disease, consider the use of probiotics, immunoglobulin, or steroids. However, in all cases, strict isolation of the patient is essential for controlling the spread of the disease to other patients.

OUTCOMES

Most AAD cases are mild and self limited. Most patients recover completely with supportive measures and antibiotic withdrawal. Relapses are unlikely in this group of patients. In cases of well-established colitis that is probably associated with *C. difficile* infection, specific antimicrobial therapy is needed. Most patients respond to treatment and recover without sequelae, but relapses are common. The rates of recurrence in this group of patients vary but can be as high as 65% after the first recurrence. Antibiotic use in the months to come should be avoided unless strictly necessary.

In general, medical therapy is effective and surgical intervention is rarely necessary. Medical failures, particularly in cases of fulminant colitis, require prompt surgical intervention. These patients tend to be older and suffering from other comorbid conditions. Total colectomy with ileostomy is the recommended approach. Mortality in these patients has been reported to be as high as 40%, in contrast with the minimal mortality in medically treated patients. Preventive strategies are based on the fact that AAD is usually a nosocomial disease. Preventive measures for colonization of hospitalized patients with *C. difficile* are widely recommended and supported, as stated in the ACG guidelines.[11] Avoidance of unnecessary use of antibiotics is of paramount importance. Hospital antibiotic use should be limited and regulated. Medical personnel should be enforced to follow simple enteric precautions and educated about the disease and its epidemiology.

Summary

- Antibiotic-associated diarrhea is the most common cause of diarrhea in hospitalized patients, representing an important source of morbidity, mortality, and cost.
- Although no infectious agent is found in most cases of AAD, *Clostridium difficile* is frequently identified in patients with signs and symptoms of colitis.
- All types of antimicrobial agents have been implicated, leading to a wide range of clinical manifestations, from asymptomatic carrier state to severe pseudomembranous colitis.
- Most cases of AAD respond to supportive measures and withdrawal of antibiotics.
- In patients with severe and persistent symptoms, effective antibiotic therapy is available, but relapses are common.

Suggested Readings

Bartlett JG: New antimicrobial agents for patients with Clostridium difficile infection, Curr Infect Dis Rep. 2009 Jan;11(1):21-28.

Cheng SH, Lu JJ, Young TG, et al: *Clostridium difficile*-associated diseases: Comparison of symptomatic infection versus carriage on the basis of risk factors, toxin production, and genotyping results. Clin Infect Dis 1997;25:157-158.

Fekety R, Kim KH, Brown D, et al: Epidemiology of antibiotic-associated colitis. Isolation of *Clostridium difficile* from the hospital enviroment. Am J Med 1981;70:906-908.

Fekety R: Guidelines for the diagnosis and management of *Clostridium difficile*-associated diarrhea and colitis. American College of Gastroenterology, Practice Parameters Committee. Am J Gastroenterol 1997;92:739-750.

Gorbach SL, Chang TW, Goldin B: Successful treatment of relapsing *Clostridium difficile* colitis with *Lactobacillus* GG. Lancet. 1987;2:1519.

Grundfest-Broniatowski S, Quader M, Alexander F, et al: *Clostridium difficile* colitis in the critically ill. Dis Colon Rectum 1996;39:619-623.

McFarland LV, Mulligan ME, Kwok RYY, Stamm WE: Nosocomial acquisition of *Clostridium difficile* infection. N Engl J Med 1989;320:204-210.

Price AB, Davies DR: Pseudomembranous colitis. J Clin Pathol 1977;30:1-12.

Tedesco FJ: Treatment of recurrent antibiotic-associated pseudomembranous colitis. Am J Gastroenterol 1982;77:220-221.

References

For a complete list of references, log onto www.expertconsult.com.

Colonic Diverticular Disease

H. Nail Aydin and Feza Remzi

Colonic diverticulosis is among the most common diseases in developed Western countries. In the United States, diverticulosis occurs in approximately one third of the population older than age 45 and in up to two thirds of the population older than 85 years,[1,2] and it also affects a significant proportion of younger adults.

DEFINITION AND CAUSES

A diverticulum is a saclike protrusion in the colonic wall that develops as a result of herniation of the mucosa and submucosa through points of weakness in the muscular wall of the colon. The colonic diverticulum is a false or pulsion diverticulum-that is, it does not contain all layers of the colonic wall. Diverticulosis indicates the presence of multiple diverticula and generally implies an absence of symptoms (Fig. 1). Diverticular disease implies any clinical state caused by diverticula, including hemorrhage, inflammation, or their complications. Diverticulitis describes the presence of an inflammatory process associated with diverticula. Its pathogenesis is attributed to genetic and environmental factors (Box 1).

PREVALENCE

The actual prevalence of diverticulosis is difficult to measure because most individuals are asymptomatic. Comparisons of the earliest and most recent autopsies and barium enema studies have indicated that the worldwide prevalence is increasing over time (Box 2).[1,3,4]

Studies so far include barium examinations and necropsy series. These may be misleading for determining the actual prevalence rate, however, mainly because barium studies may overestimate the prevalence of diverticulosis in people who have been referred for gastrointestinal (GI) symptoms, and necropsy series may either overestimate the frequency of diverticula in older age groups or miss the presence of small diverticula in younger populations.[5,6] Whether these findings are the results of increased numbers of older individuals in the population, increased screening, or an actual increase in prevalence is unknown. Younger patients presenting earlier than age 40 years have a prevalence rate of 5% and are more commonly male.[7-9]

PATHOPHYSIOLOGY

Colonic diverticulosis in general is an acquired disease, developing as mucosal and submucosal herniations through the circular muscle layer at vulnerable weak points of the colonic wall. Diverticula are covered only by serosa, and tend to develop at four well-defined points around the circumference of the colon, where the vasa recta penetrate the muscular layer.[10,11] These vessels enter the colonic wall on either side of the mesenteric teniae and on the mesenteric border of the two antimesenteric teniae. Diverticula do not develop in the rectum, presumably because of the coalescence of the teniae with the longitudinal muscle layer that marks the junction between the sigmoid colon and the rectum. In the colon, the presence of anatomic and physiologic changes contributes to the development of diverticula (Box 3). Mycosis, a set of findings consisting of the thickening of the muscular layer, shortening of the teniae, and luminal narrowing, is found in most patients with sigmoid diverticula.

The mechanical features of the colonic wall change with increasing age.[12,13] Combined barostat-manometry studies of the entire colon have demonstrated that compliance is lowest in the sigmoid and descending colon and greatest in the transverse and ascending colon.[13] This difference in mechanical properties between the right and left sides might partly account for the left-sided predominance of diverticulosis.[14]

Structural components of the extracellular matrix of the colonic wall, including collagen, elastin, and proteoglycans, are likely to be important in maintaining the strength and integrity of the colonic wall.[15,16] Changes in these components of the bowel wall, such as damage and breakdown of mature collagen, and consequently its immature synthesis can lead to a change in bowel consistency.[17] These changes may be related to a genetic predisposition such as that seen in Ehlers-Danlos and Marfan's syndromes, which may be responsible for the occurrence of diverticula at an early age, or to the natural course of the aging process itself. In one study, it has been reported that collagen fibrils in the left colon are smaller and more tightly packed than those in the right colon with increasing age, and that this difference is accentuated in diverticular disease.[16]

The thickening of longitudinal and circular muscles in diverticular disease is neither hyperplastic nor hypertropic, but appears to be related to a contractile state. An increase in the number of elastic fibers has been observed only in the longitudinal muscle.[18] It has been suggested that this process is responsible for longitudinal contraction, with subsequent thickening of both muscle layers.[18] All these changes, along with elastin deposition in the teniae coli, lead to an irreversible state of contracture, with substantial bowel shortening, which may result in decreased resistance of the colon wall to persistent intraluminal pressure.[19]

In addition to other predisposing factors, diverticula are believed to develop as a result of elevated intraluminal pressure generated by tonic and rhythmic contractions, resulting in segmentation. If contractions occur relatively close to each other and form an enclosed space, pressure within that intervening segment of colon may exceed 90 mm Hg. However, segmentation on its own separates the colonic lumen into a series of chambers, with each having a different amount of pressure that is closely related to the chamber's diameter. These isolated increases of intraluminal pressure are believed to predispose to herniation through the previously mentioned weak points of the colon.

The fiber content of the diet plays a large role in the pathogenesis of diverticular disease. Fiber has been found to be protective. Most fiber in the human diet is of plant origin and this type of fiber binds water and salt in the colon, leading to bulkier and more voluminous stools. Therefore, fiber decreases the frequency of contractions and prevents an exaggerated form of segmentation.[6,20,21] In addition, dietary fiber influences the content of colonic bacterial flora, forms the main substrate for bacterial carbohydrate fermentation, and produces energy-yielding substrates—short-chain fatty acids—for growth and maintenance of colonic cellular function. Consequently, a fiber-deficient diet increases the chances of intense, more frequent segmentation, thus predisposing to herniation of mucosa by allowing isolated increases of intraluminal pressure.[6,22]

After the development of colonic diverticula, a spectrum of inflammatory changes or bleeding caused by the traumatic injury to penetrating vessels may occur.[20,21] Changes within these vessel walls, such as eccentric intimal thickening and thinning of the media of the vessel facing the bowel lumen, result in segmental weakness of these vessels and render them vulnerable to injury and bleeding.

The term *diverticulitis* represents a spectrum of inflammatory changes that ranges from localized subclinical inflammation to generalized peritonitis, with free perforation (Fig. 2). In turn, this leads to hyperplasia of the lymphoid tissue within the mucosa at the base of the diverticulum, one of the earliest signs of diverticulitis. Inflam-

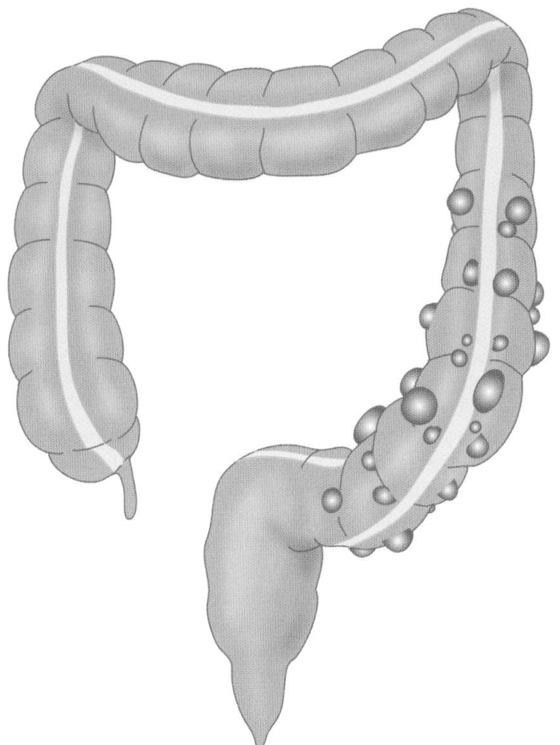

Figure 1 **Colonic diverticulosis.** © 2008 The Cleveland Clinic Foundation.

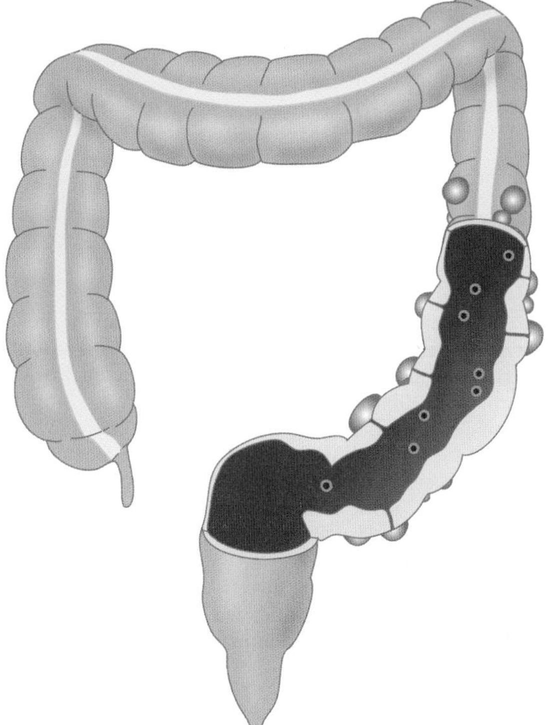

Figure 2 **Colonic diverticulosis: generalized peritonitis, with free perforation.** © 2008 The Cleveland Clinic Foundation.

Box 1 Factors Involved in the Pathogenesis of Colonic Diverticula

Genetic factors
Environmental factors

- Low-fiber diet
- Obesity
- Decreased physical activity
- Corticosteroids
- NSAIDs
- Alcohol
- Caffeine intake
- Cigarette smoking
- Polycystic kidney disease

Epidemiologic factors

- Age
- Geography
- Life style
- Ethnicity

Box 2 Prevalence of Diverticulosis

5% to 10% before age 50
30% after age 50
50% after age 70
66% after age 85

Box 3 Physiologic and Anatomic Colonic Changes in Diverticula Formation

Mycosis
Changes in mechanical features of colonic wall
Changes in structural components of colonic wall
Elevated intraluminal pressure
Segmentation

mation usually begins at the apex of the diverticulum and seldom involves the neck or mucosa proximal to the neck. However, there is active inflammation of the pericolic and mesenteric fat, with peridiverticular abscess formation. These peridiverticular abscesses often involve areas of subserosa and are closely related to the outer aspect of the muscularis propria; they can spread circumferentially and longitudinally and may be responsible for the pathologic picture of diverticular colitis. Longitudinal tracking, especially, may result in fissuring, along with the lymphoid aggregates, which resembles the distinctive feature of colonic colitis in Crohn's disease.[23] This may cause misinterpretation of the pathologic study of the specimen. Therefore, the differential diagnosis of these two conditions in terms of pathologic interpretation of the resected specimen is important. Persistent localized inflammation after diverticular rupture results in a phlegmon, a thickened, firm segment of bowel wall, which ultimately may manifest as acute or subacute large bowel obstruction. If left untreated or treated inadequately, it may result in extensive fibrosis around the affected segment of the colon, giving it a mass appearance indistinguishable macroscopically from that of a neoplasm.

Another pathologic entity that may be encountered during progression of the disease, with recurrent attacks of diverticulitis, is the formation of a localized abscess with chronic inflammation and involvement of other neighboring luminal organs, such as the bladder, small and large bowel loops, uterus, and vagina. Fistulae may develop within this contained area, between involved segment(s) of colon and these organs. Fistulae occur in 2.4% to 20% of cases; 65% of these fistulae are colovesical and 20% are colovaginal fistulae.[24-26]

SIGNS AND SYMPTOMS

Most people with uncomplicated colonic diverticulosis are asymptomatic. A small fraction of these patients may have troublesome symptoms, such as colicky abdominal pain, bloating, flatulence, or altered bowel habit. The symptoms characteristically disappear after

Box 4 Manifestation of Acute Diverticulitis

Acute left lower quadrant pain (93%-100%)
Fever, chills (57%-100%)
Leukocytosis (69%-83%)
Nausea, vomiting
Mass
Constipation
Diarrhea
Urinary symptoms

Box 5 Differential Diagnosis of Acute Diverticulitis

Irritable bowel syndrome
Gastroenteritis
Cholecystitis
Bowel obstruction
Appendicitis
Ischemic colitis
Colorectal cancer
Urologic disorders
Gynecologic disorders

defecation or passage of flatus. On clinical examination, they may have tenderness in the left iliac fossa with no signs or symptoms of peritonitis or systemic illness, and all laboratory values may be within normal limits. The clinical picture of symptomatic uncomplicated diverticulosis often overlaps with that of irritable bowel syndrome (IBS), because these two clinical entities are usually diagnosed after other pathologies are excluded. IBS-type symptoms are independent of the presence or absence of diverticulosis on double-contrast barium enema studies. Bleeding alone can sometimes be the only sign of diverticulosis.[27]

Signs and symptoms of acute diverticulitis may vary from local findings and manifestations to a wide variety of clinical pictures, with signs and symptoms of intra-abdominal sepsis, depending on the stage of disease (Box 4).

Patients with acute uncomplicated diverticulitis classically present with left-sided lower abdominal pain, fever, and leukocytosis.[28] The site of pain often depends on the segment of colon affected. Right-sided symptoms may occur in the presence of right-sided diverticulosis, as well as in redundant sigmoid colon lying on the right side of the abdomen. Patients with left-sided pain may also have right-sided symptoms. Other common manifestations are frequently related to GI disturbances, with alteration in bowel habits, constipation, either alone or alternating with bouts of diarrhea, anorexia, and nausea and vomiting. Urinary symptoms such as dysuria, frequency, and urgency may develop in a minority of patients, probably because of the proximity of the bladder to the inflamed sigmoid colon. In acute presentations, fever is almost always present, but high fever must suggest the possibility of advanced disease and sepsis from generalized peritonitis caused by perforation and spreading of inflammation in the peritoneum.

Abdominal findings reflect the severity and localization of the disease. In cases of diffuse peritonitis, generalized tenderness, involuntary guarding, or decreased or absent bowel sounds are noted. Severe abdominal distention with nausea and vomiting suggests bowel obstruction. The presence of pneumaturia and fecaluria signifies the presence of a colovesical fistula.

Immunocompromised and immunosuppressed patients constitute the most important group needing special attention in diagnosis and treatment. This patient group may lack a normal inflammatory response and present with minimal classic signs and symptoms, which may delay the diagnosis and treatment. This may result in sepsis and death. It is preferable to operate semielectively on these patients during the first episode of their initial hospitalization.

DIAGNOSIS

The initial assessment of patients with suspected acute diverticulitis is comprised of a thorough history and physical examination, including abdominal, rectal, and pelvic examinations. Useful initial examinations may include a complete blood cell count, urinalysis, and flat and upright abdominal radiography. If the clinical picture is clear enough to diagnose diverticulitis, no other tests are indicated.[1] When the diagnosis is in question, other tests such as computed tomography (CT), water-soluble contrast enema, cystography, endoscopy, and ultrasound may be performed. The differential diagnosis of acute diverticulitis should also be considered,[29] not only during examination of the patient but also while ordering the tests (Box 5). In particular, the differential diagnosis of colorectal cancer, as well as the detection of its possible coexistence, is important.[30,31] A barium enema examination should be avoided in acute presentations in patients with suspected acute diverticulitis and localized peritoneal signs because of a possible extravasation of barium into the peritoneal cavity, which can increase the morbidity and mortality related to barium-induced chemical peritonitis.[31] In the emergency setting, water-soluble enemas are safer.

Abdominal ultrasound, with a sensitivity of 84% to 98% and a specificity of 80% to 97%, is a noninvasive screening tool with the potential drawback of the interpretation of the study, which may differ from one examiner to another.[32,33] It is helpful, especially in female patients, to exclude pelvic and gynecologic pathology. CT, with a sensitivity of 69% to 95%, a specificity of 75% to 100%, and a low false-positive rate, is generally superior to contrast studies.[30,34-36] CT with triple contrast—oral, rectal, and IV contrasts—is being used more frequently as the initial imaging study, especially in the acute setting, particularly whenever moderately severe disease or abscess is anticipated. In addition to the identification of complications such as phlegmon, abscess, adjacent organ involvement and distant septic complications, it also is a useful therapeutic tool for percutaneous drainage of intra-abdominal abscesses, providing the opportunity to downstage the intra-abdominal pathology so that it can be treated with a single-stage surgical procedure. The positive predictive value for diverticulitis by CT scanning is 73% for the presence of sigmoid diverticula, 88% for pericolic inflammation, 85% for wall thickness of 7 to 10 mm, and 100% for wall thickness more than 10 mm.[34] Severity staging by CT scanning may allow not only the selection of patients most likely to respond to conservative treatment, but may also predict the risk of failure of medical therapy and of secondary complications after initial conservative treatment. The incidence of subsequent complications is highest in patients with severe disease on initial CT.[37-39] CT is not useful in differentiating cancer from diverticulitis and must be supplemented by contrast enema studies or endoscopy. Although endoscopy is rarely indicated in an acute setting, if required, it should be done with gentle and cautious insufflation and manipulation because of the risk of perforation of an acutely inflamed colon, either by insufflation of air or by the instrument itself. It can be performed more safely after the patient recovers from the acute attack.

TREATMENT

Medical Treatment

Complicated diverticulitis refers to acute diverticulitis accompanied by abscess, fistula, obstruction, or free intra-abdominal perforation. In the absence of complications and systemic signs and symptoms, patients with mild abdominal tenderness may be treated conservatively. Conservative treatment typically includes dietary modification and oral or IV antibiotics. This has been shown to be successful in 70% to 100% of patients.[37,38,40]

Uncomplicated diverticulitis may be managed in the outpatient setting with dietary modification and oral antibiotics for those without fever, excessive vomiting, or marked peritonitis, as long as there is the opportunity for follow-up. If these conditions are not met or the patient fails to improve with outpatient therapy, hospital admission is required.

Antibiotic selection should be based on appropriate coverage for gram-negative rods and anaerobic bacteria.[41] Conservative treatment will resolve acute diverticulitis in 85% of patients, but approximately one third will have a recurrent attack, often within a year.[5,42,43]

After recovery from the first episode, use of fiber prevents recurrence in more than 70% of patients.[44,45] Immunosuppressed or immunocompromised patients are more likely to present with perforation and fail medical treatment.[41,42,46]

Approximately 15% of patients develop pericolonic or intramesenteric abscess.[47,48] Abscesses smaller than 2 cm in diameter may resolve with antibiotic treatment without any further intervention, whereas larger abscesses may require percutaneous drainage. This may prevent an emergency operation and multistaged surgeries involving the creation and closure of stoma.[42,48,49]

After resolution of the initial acute attack, the colon should be thoroughly evaluated with colonoscopy or contrast enema radiography.

Surgical Treatment

Surgical treatment of the disease can be evaluated emergently or electively, based on the stage of the disease and clinical presentation. Emergent sigmoid colectomy is required for patients with the following:

- Diffuse peritonitis
- Failure of conservative treatment
- Persistent sepsis despite percutaneous drainage
- Very low threshold, immunosuppressed, and immunocompromised patients who are likely to fail medical treatment and present with perforation.

Intraoperative surgical options are based on the status of the patient and the severity of intra-abdominal contamination (Hinchey classification; Box 6 and Figs. 3 to 6).[50] The desired surgical option is resection of the diseased segment with primary anastomosis, with or without intraoperative lavage or resection, and anastomosis with a temporary diverting ileostomy (Figs. 7 and 8). In advanced stages of peritonitis, Hartmann's procedure (sigmoid colectomy, end colostomy, and closure of the rectal stump; Fig. 9) is the preferred operation, but it has been shown that the closure operation (Hartmann's reversal) is not only technically challenging, but may be also associated with significant postoperative morbidity and mortality.[51]

The decision for elective colectomy after recovery from acute diverticulitis should be made on a case by case basis. After the first attack, about one third of the patients will have a later, second attack. After the second attack, another one third of patients will have another attack.[40,42] Factors affecting decision making for elective surgery include the following:

- Age
- Medical condition of the patient
- Frequency, persistence, and severity of the attacks
- CT-graded severity of the attack as a predictor of failure of medical treatment and possible risk of secondary complications

Box 6 Hinchey Classification

Stage I: Diverticulitis with confined paracolic abscess
Stage II: Diverticulitis with distant (pelvic, retroperitoneal) abscess
Stage III: Diverticulitis with purulent peritonitis
Stage IV: Diverticulitis with fecal peritonitis

- Inability to exclude carcinoma.
- Conservative treatment of a complicated diverticulitis attack

There is no clear consensus regarding two widely debated points in management. First, the number of attacks of uncomplicated diverticulitis is not necessarily a determinant for appropriateness of surgery, because it has been shown that elective surgery after recovery from uncomplicated episodes might not decrease the likelihood of later emergency surgery or overall mortality.[40,46,52-54] Second, patients younger than 50 years may have a higher cumulative risk for recurrent diverticulitis; however, whether they are at increased risk of complications or recurrent attacks remains debatable.[5,28,40-42,54]

There are several important points regarding surgical technique. From a technical standpoint, the resection should be carried proximally to the compliant bowel and extend distally to the upper rectum. After sigmoid colectomy, an important predictor of recurrence is a colosigmoid rather than colorectal anastomosis. The proximal margin of resection should be in an area of pliable colon without hypertrophy or inflammation. Resection of the diseased colon must be the desired goal, along with removal of the entire thickened colonic segment(s) but not necessarily all the proximal diverticula-bearing colon. Laparoscopic colectomy is appropriate in select patients and has advantages over open laparotomy, including less pain, smaller incisions, and shorter recovery. There is no increase in early and late complications[55,56] and cost and outcome are comparable with those of open resection.[57]

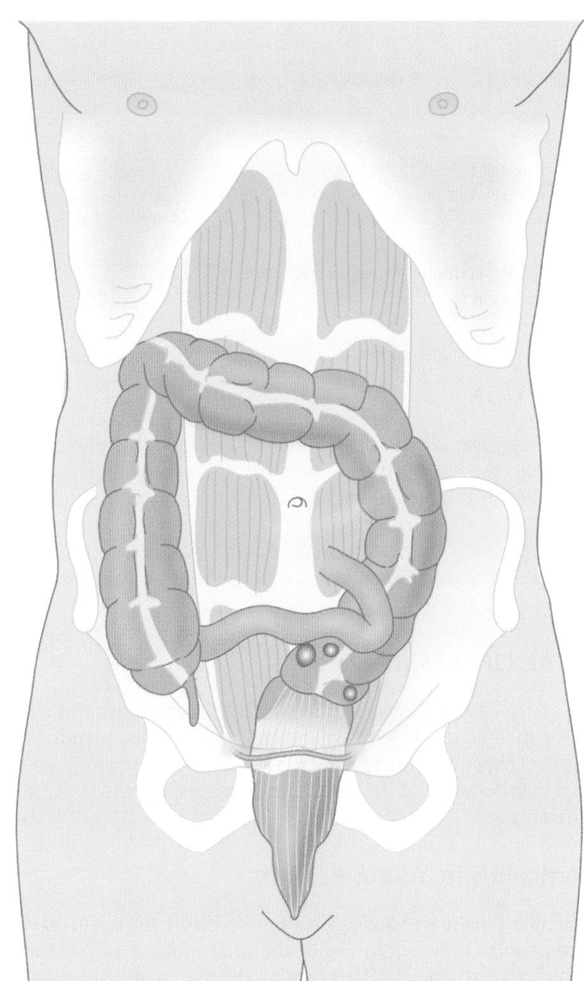

Figure 3 Resection and anastomosis. © 2008 The Cleveland Clinic Foundation.

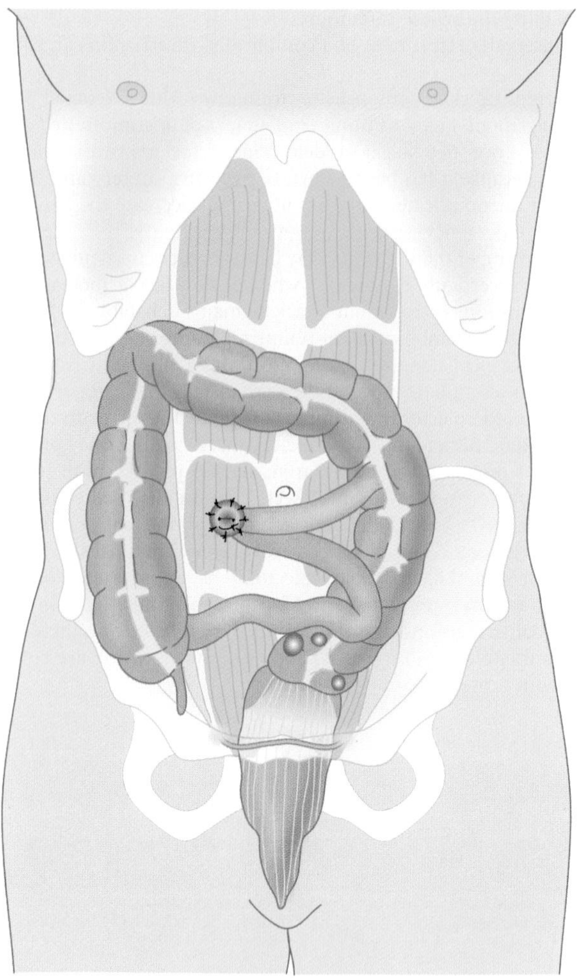

Figure 4 **Resection and proximal diversion.** © 2008 The Cleveland Clinic Foundation.

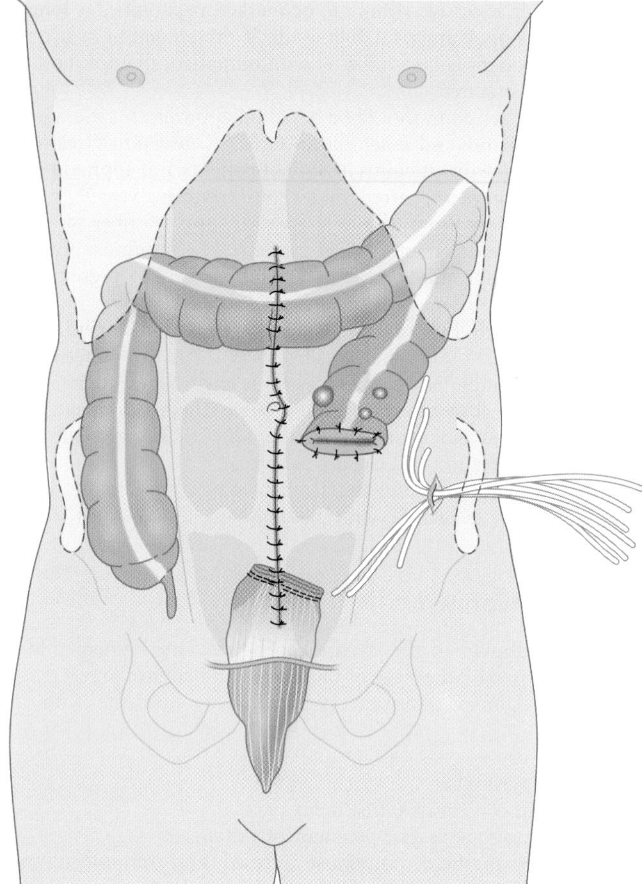

Figure 5 **Resection and colostomy.** © 2008 The Cleveland Clinic Foundation.

PREVENTION

Prevention can be achieved by elimination of the factors involved in the pathogenesis of this disease (see Box 1). Increasing the proportion of fiber in the diet, along with an increase in fluid intake, will help keep more diverticula from forming and also will help keep the existing condition from worsening. Additionally, alteration of lifestyle by weight reduction and exercise can limit the contribution of other causative factors.

SPECIAL CIRCUMSTANCES

There are special circumstances in which the general recommendations for the diagnostic workup and treatment of diverticulitis may not apply. These are closely associated with the presence of factors such as manifestation of the disease, patient's response to the disease, and treatment.

Diverticulitis in Young Patients

Diverticular disease is relatively uncommon before the age of 40 years and constitutes only 2% to 5% of the total number of patients in multiple large studies.[58,59] Diverticular disease in the younger age group occurs more commonly in men, with obesity (84%-96%) being a major risk factor.[60,61] There is ongoing controversy not only about the nature and course of the disease in this younger patient

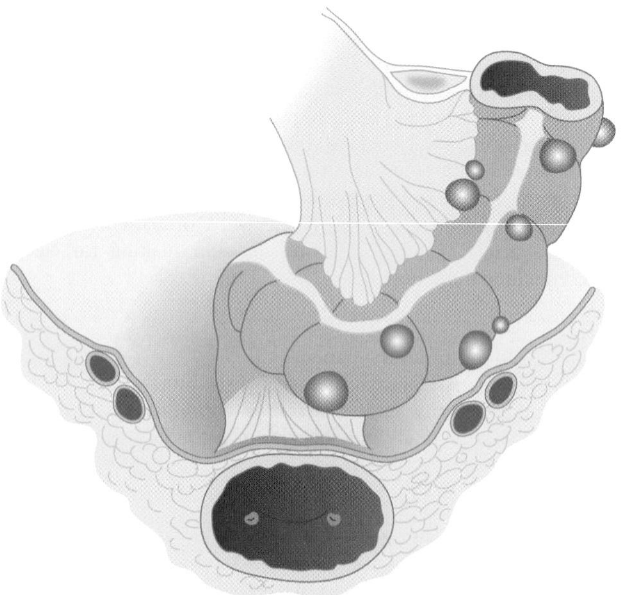

Figure 6 **Hinchey, stage I.** © 2008 The Cleveland Clinic Foundation.

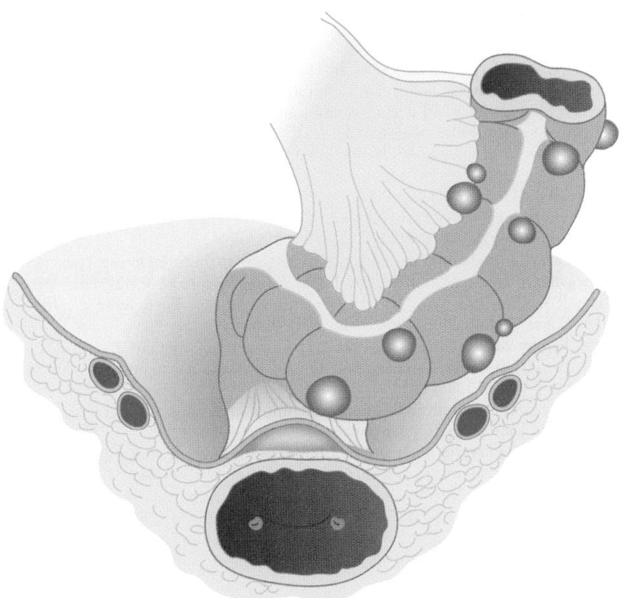

Figure 7 **Hinchey, stage II.** © 2008 The Cleveland Clinic Foundation.

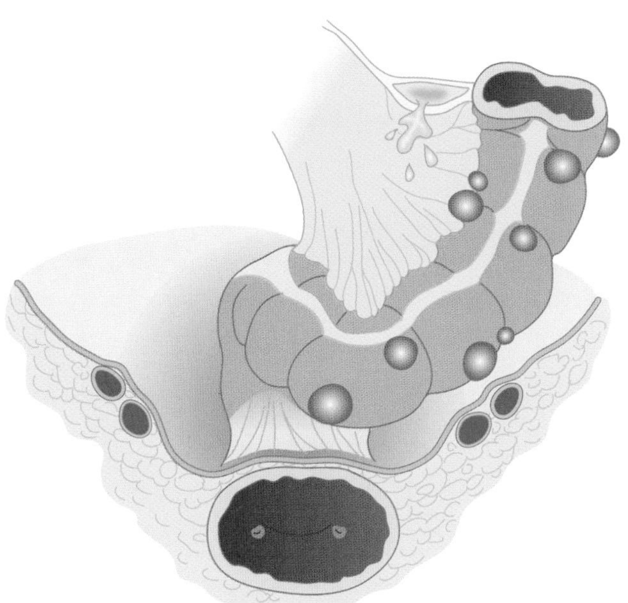

Figure 8 **Hinchey, stage III.** © 2008 The Cleveland Clinic Foundation.

population, but also about the timing of the operation.[62-66] The disease trend in this patient group is toward more recurrence and an increased incidence of poor outcomes, ultimately requiring surgery.[67] This might be related to the fact that younger patients have a longer life expectancy, which increases the possibility and risk of subsequent episodes and related complications. Therefore, surgery may be often regarded as the treatment of choice for younger symptomatic patients.

Diverticulitis in Immunocompromised Patients

Conditions that represent an immunocompromised state include severe infection, steroids, diabetes mellitus, renal failure, malignancy, cirrhosis, and chemotherapy or immunosuppressive therapy. Although the incidence of diverticulitis does not appear to be

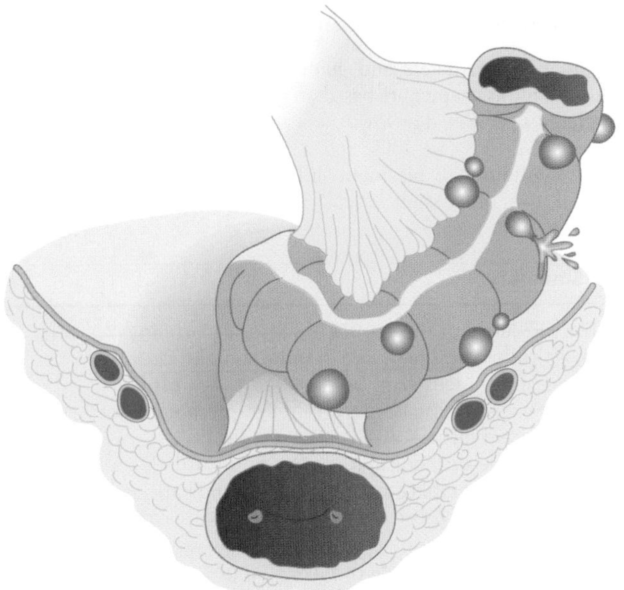

Figure 9 Hinchey, stage IV. © 2008 The Cleveland Clinic Foundation.

increased in this population, the complications and sequelae of the diverticulitis are more severe. This group of patients may lack a normal inflammatory response and present with minimal or subtle signs and symptoms, which may delay the diagnosis and treatment. There is an increased rate of free perforation (43% vs. 14% in immunocompetent patients), increased need for surgery (58% vs. 33%), and increased postoperative mortality (39% vs. 2%).[68,69] Specifically, it is preferable to operate on transplant patients, immunocompromised patients, and patients under immunosuppression semielectively during the first episode of initial hospitalization. Primary resection with proximal diversion is the desired operation and should be attempted, whenever possible.

Recurrent Diverticulitis after Resection

Recurrent diverticulitis after surgical treatment is rare, with the incidence ranging from 1% to 10%. In general, the progression of diverticular disease in the remaining colon is approximately 15%.[70] In such cases, the previous diagnosis and treatment can be questioned and investigated. Important factors to be considered in terms of surgery are the adequacy of resection, meaning the degree of proximal resection and level of distal anastomosis.[69,71] The use of the rectum as the distal margin decreases the rate of recurrence.

Care also must be taken to exclude other components of differential diagnosis, especially irritable bowel syndrome, inflammatory bowel disease, and ischemic colitis.

Right-Sided Diverticulitis

Diverticulosis in Asia is predominantly a right-sided phenomenon. Diverticula of the right colon may be singular or multiple. The diagnosis of right-sided diverticulitis is difficult to differentiate from appendicitis with a similar clinical picture and presentation. An abdominal mass is usually found in 26% to 88% of cases.[72,73] Surgical treatment is reserved for recurrent and complicated episodes if the diagnosis of right-sided diverticulitis has been made with confidence. If extensive inflammation is present or multiple diverticula are found, a right hemicolectomy with primary anastomosis is indicated. In selected cases, a simple diverticulectomy may be done.[74]

PRACTICE PARAMETERS AND GUIDELINES

The practice parameters and guidelines for sigmoid diverticulitis discussed in this chapter are based on guidelines for the treatment of diverticulitis published by the American Society of Colon and Rectal Surgeons (ASCRS) in 2000 and a recent revision, published in 2006.[28,75] Additional pertinent information was retrieved and reviewed from other studies.

Summary

- The incidence of diverticular disease, particularly diverticulitis, has increased in industrialized countries.
- Diverticular disease can be classified as symptomatic uncomplicated disease, recurrent symptomatic disease, and complicated disease.
- Conservative or medical management is usually indicated for acute uncomplicated diverticulitis. Indications for surgery include recurrent attacks and complications of the disease.
- Surgical treatment options have changed considerably over the years, along with the development of new diagnostic tools and surgical approaches.
- Indications and timing for surgery of diverticular disease are determined mainly by the stage of the disease. In addition, individual patient risk factors, along with the course of the disease after conservative or operative therapy, play a significant role in decision making and treatment.
- In this context, the purpose of this chapter has been to review colonic diverticular disease and its treatment.

Suggested Readings

Aydin HN, Remzi FH, Tekkis PP, et al: Hartmann's reversal is associated with high postoperative adverse events. Dis Colon Rectum 2005:48:2117-2126.

Chapman J, Davies M, Wolff B, et al: Complicated diverticulitis: Is it time to rethink the rules? Ann Surg 2005; 242:576-583.

Janes S, Meagher A, Frizelle A: Elective surgery after diverticulitis. Br J Surg 2005; 92; 133-142.

Mueller MH, Glaetzer J, Kasparek MS, et al: Long-term outcome of conservative treatment in patients with diverticulitis of the sigmoid colon. Eur J Gastroenterol Hepatol 2005; 17:649-654.

Patient Care Committee of the Society for Surgery of the Alimentary Tract (SSAT): Surgical treatment of diverticulitis. J Gastrointest Surg 1999; 3:212-213.

Rafferty J, Shellito P, Hyman NH, et al: Practice parameters for sigmoid diverticulitis. Dis Colon Rectum 2006; 49:939-944.

Roberts P, Abel M, Rosen L, et al: Practice parameters for sigmoid diverticulitis. The Standards Task Force American Society of Colon and Rectal Surgeons. Dis Colon Rectum 1995; 38:125-132.

Salem L, Veenstra DL, Sullivan SD, et al: The timing of elective colectomy in diverticulitis: A decision analysis. J Am Coll Surg 2004; 199:904-912.

Thaler K, Baig MK, Berho M, et al: Determinants of recurrence after sigmoid resection for uncomplicated diverticulitis. Dis Colon Rectum 2003; 46:385-388.

Wong WD, Wexner SD, Lowry A, et al: Practice parameters for the treatment of sigmoid diverticulitis-supporting documentation. The Standards Task Force. The American Society of Colon and Rectal Surgeons. Dis Colon Rectum 2000; 43:290-297.

References

For a complete list of references, log onto www.expertconsult.com.

Colorectal Neoplasia

Carol A. Burke and Laura K. Bianchi

Colorectal cancer is one of the few preventable cancers. The removal of precancerous polyps during colonoscopy inhibits their progression to cancer. Widely available screening tests such as the fecal occult blood test (FOBT), sigmoidoscopy, and colonoscopy are associated with a decrease in colorectal cancer mortality. Unfortunately, less than 50% of eligible Americans have undergone screening, and more than 45% of cancers s are diagnosed at a time when the cancer is incurable.

DEFINITION

The colorectum is the portion of the gastrointestinal (GI) tract most commonly affected by tumors. Most colonic tumors are benign epithelial polyps. *Polyp* is an inexact term that indicates a protuberance of tissue into the colonic lumen. There are many histologic types of polyps. The best characterized and most common cancer precursor is the adenomatous polyp. The size, number of adenomas, and degree of villous features predict the future risk of advanced neoplasia, including malignancy in patients who harbor adenomas. An additional precursor to colorectal cancer called a *sessile serrated adenoma* has been identified. Persons who harbor such lesions should be managed similarly to those with adenomas.

This chapter focuses on the most common neoplastic epithelial tumors, including adenomatous polyps and adenocarcinoma of the colon and rectum.

PREVALENCE AND RISK FACTORS

The incidence of colorectal carcinoma has been decreasing an average of 1.5% annually since the mid-1980s. Research has suggested that the decline may be caused by an increased use of screening and polyp removal, which prevents progression from polyp to cancer. Although almost 40% of Americans 50 years and older harbor adenomatous polyps, it is estimated that only 2% of adenomas will progress to cancer.

Adenocarcinoma of the colon and rectum is the third most common cancer and cause of cancer deaths in the United States. Both men and women face a lifetime risk of almost 6% for the development of invasive colorectal cancer (Table 1).[1] It is estimated that approximately 149,000 new cases of colorectal cancer were diagnosed in 2008 and that 50,000 deaths from colorectal cancer will occur. The only known race predilection is in African Americans, who have higher colorectal cancer incidence and mortality rates.

Epidemiologic studies have implicated a number of environmental cofactors in the development of colorectal cancer. They include advanced age, a diet high in red meat, a diet high in fat, smoking, alcohol consumption, and obesity. In approximately 30% of patients with colorectal cancer, risk factors have been identified (Box 1), and the remaining 70% of newly diagnosed colorectal cancers arise in patients without any identifiable risk factors.

PATHOPHYSIOLOGY AND NATURAL HISTORY

Well-established and newly discovered molecular and genetic pathways of colorectal carcinogenesis including chromosomal instability, microsatellite instability, and CpG island methylation (CIMP) have broadened our understanding of the precursors to colorectal cancer.[1] In approximately 80% of cases, colorectal carcinoma arises from an adenomatous polyp. Observational studies have suggested that the adenoma-to-carcinoma sequence takes approximately 10 years. This pathway traditionally was believed to result from multiple acquired genetic alterations in tumor tissue and is called the *chromosomal instability pathway.* The remainder of colorectal cancers arise from alterations in DNA repair genes, which are characterized by extensive instability in simple repeated nucleotide sequences (microsatellites) called *microsatellite instability* or by widespread hypermethylation in gene promoter regions (CIMP).[2] Convincing evidence shows that serrated polyps, in particular sessile serrated adenomas, are the precursor to CIMP cancers. These precursor serrated lesions are usually large and have high levels of CIMP, *BRAF* mutations, and a proximal colon predilection.

A personal history of adenomatous polyps or colorectal cancer increases the risk for metachronous colorectal cancer. First-degree relatives of patients with colorectal cancer have a two- to threefold increased risk for colorectal cancer and adenomatous polyps. A systematic review and meta-analysis has proved that first-degree family members of patients with adenomatous polyps also have an increased risk of colorectal cancer themselves, particularly when the relative's adenoma is diagnosed before age 60 years.[3]

Patients with the highest risk for colorectal cancer are those who have a hereditary colorectal cancer syndrome. The dominantly inherited syndromes include familial adenomatous polyposis (FAP) and Lynch syndrome, which has also been known as hereditary nonpolyposis colorectal cancer (HNPCC). An autosomal recessive colon cancer syndrome has been discovered, *MYH*-associated polyposis (MAP).

FAP is caused by a mutation in the tumor suppressor gene *APC* on the long arm of chromosome 5. Germline mutations in *APC* can be detected in approximately 80% of patients with FAP. The *APC* mutation results in the development of hundreds to thousands of colonic adenomas, usually by the second decade of life. Colon cancer develops in all FAP patients by age 40 years if prophylactic colectomy is not performed. Attenuated FAP is a phenotypically distinct form of colonic polyposis. The number of colonic polyps in these patients usually numbers less than 100, and the age of onset of polyposis and cancer is shifted 1 to 2 decades later. Duodenal adenomas are common in either form of FAP, and periampullary cancer is the second leading cause of cancer death in this population. Gardner's syndrome is a phenotypic variant of FAP. In addition to colonic polyposis, other manifestations may be seen, such as benign soft tissue tumors, osteomas, supernumerary teeth, desmoid tumors, and congenital hypertrophy of the retinal pigment epithelium.

MAP is associated with mutations of the *MYH* gene. Biallelic germline mutations in *MYH* are responsible for 10% of the *APC*-negative cases of FAP and up to 29% of patients with numerous adenomas (>15) during their lifetime. The affected patients usually have fewer than 100 colorectal adenomas and an increased risk of cancer.[4]

Lynch syndrome is caused by genetic alterations in one of the mismatch repair genes. Alterations in these genes prevent adequate repair of DNA, resulting in a change of length of nucleotide bases (MSI) when compared with those of normal tissue. MSI can be investigated in a colon cancer specimen in a molecular pathology laboaratory. If MSI is present, immunohistochemistry (IHC) should be performed to assess for the lack of protein expression from one of the mismatch repair genes. MSI or abnormal IHC can suggest the tumor has developed in a patient with Lynch syndrome. In Lynch syndrome, colorectal cancer occurs in up to 80% of those affected, usually by the age of 50 years, and is often right-sided and associated with unusual pathologic features. Extracolonic cancers, such as

Table 1 Lifetime Probability of Developing Invasive Colorectal Cancer in the United States (%)

Gender	<40 Yr	40-49 Yr	50-59 Yr	60-69 Yr	≥70 Yr
Male	0.08	0.92	1.60	4.78	5.65
Female	0.07	0.72	1.12	4.30	5.23

Adapted from Jemal A, Siegel R, Ward E, et al: Cancer statistics, 2008. CA Cancer J Clin 2008;58;71-96.

Box 1 Risk Factors for Colorectal Cancer

Personal history of adenomas or colorectal cancer
Family history of colorectal adenoma or colorectal cancer
First-degree relative younger than 60 years *or* two first-degree relatives of any age
Inherited colorectal cancer syndromes
Hereditary nonpolyposis colorectal cancer
Familial adenomatous polyposis
MYH-associated polyposis
Ulcerative colitis and Crohn's colitis

Table 2 U.S. Multi-Society Task Force Recommendations for for Average-Risk Colorectal Cancer Screening*

Method	Interval
Stool DNA	Unknown
Fecal occult blood test (FOBT)	Annual
Flexible sigmoidoscopy	Every 5 yrs
CT Colonography	Every 5 yrs
Double Contrast Barium Enema	Every 5 yrs
Colonoscopy	Every 10 yr

*Begin screening at age 50 years.
Adapted from Levin B, Lieberman D, McFarland B, et al.: Screening and surveillance for the early detection of colorectal cancer and adenomatous polyps, 2008: A joint guideline from the American Cancer Society, the US Multi-Society Task Force on Colorectal Cancer and the American College of Radiology 2008;58:130-160.

endometrial, ovarian, small bowel, transitional cell of the ureter or bladder, and gastric cancer, often occur in patients with Lynch syndrome. The risk of endometrial carcinoma has been reported in up to 60% and ovarian carcinoma in up to 20%. Therefore, aggressive gynecologic screening for endometrial and ovarian cancers is recommended in women in Lynch kindreds.

Clinical criteria have been developed to identify families with Lynch syndrome. The strictest criteria include the Amsterdam criteria:

- Three or more relatives with colorectal cancer, with one a first-degree relative of the other two
- At least two successive generations affected
- One cancer diagnosed before age 50 years

Many researchers have found the Amsterdam criteria neither sufficiently sensitive nor specific for use as the sole criterion for determining which families should undergo intensive surveillance or genetic evaluation. The Amsterdam II criteria broadened the original criteria to include other HNPCC-associated cancers, including colorectal cancer or cancer of the endometrium, small bowel, ureter, or renal pelvis.[5]

The revised Bethesda criteria were formulated to identify tumors that should be tested for MSI[6]:

- Colorectal cancer diagnosed before the age of 50 years
- Presence of synchronous or metachronous colorectal or other HNPCC-associated tumors, regardless of age
- Colorectal cancer with MSI diagnosed in a patient younger than 60 years
- Colorectal cancer diagnosed in a patient with one or more first-degree relatives with an HNPCC-related tumor, with one of the cancers being diagnosed before age 50 years
- Colorectal cancer diagnosed in a patient with two or more first- or second-degree relatives with HNPCC-related tumors, regardless of age

The chronic inflammatory colitides, ulcerative colitis and Crohn's disease, are associated with an increased risk of colorectal cancer. The proximal extent of colonic involvement, duration of disease, and activity of disease stratify the level of risk. Risk is highest in patients with pancolitis and is negligible in patients with proctitis. After a decade of disease, the cancer risk increases yearly by 1% to 2%.

SIGNS AND SYMPTOMS

Colon polyps and early colon cancer are often asymptomatic until they are advanced. GI blood loss is the most common sign and can include a positive FOBT result, iron-deficiency anemia, or hematochezia. When tumors are advanced, unexplained anorexia, weight loss, or symptoms from obstruction or local invasion, such as a change in bowel habits, abdominal pain, or obstruction, can occur.

DIAGNOSIS

The diagnosis of colorectal polyps and cancer is most often made during a colonic evaluation performed for GI symptoms, for colorectal cancer screening, or as part of endoscopic surveillance.

Screening

National organizations, including the American Cancer Society, United States Preventive Services Task Force, and U.S. Multi-Society Task Force on Colorectal Cancer, have established guidelines for colorectal cancer screening and surveillance. Various options are recommended for average-risk patients (Table 2).[7] Colonoscopy is recommended by the American College of Gastroenterology as the preferred colorectal cancer screening strategy. The evidence to support colonoscopy has been derived from data showing a decreased incidence of colorectal cancer mortality in subjects who have undergone colonoscopic adenoma removal. Additionally, colonoscopic screening has been shown to have favorable cost effectiveness when compared with other screening strategies. Unfortunately, lesions may be missed on colonoscopy, and up to 5% of patients in whom colorectal cancer is diagnosed had undergone colonoscopy within the previous 3 to 5 years.[8]

Patients with symptoms of colorectal cancer and those with more than a moderate to high risk for colorectal cancer should undergo colonoscopy (Table 3). Surveillance intervals differ based upon risk factors including adenoma characteristics of size, multiplicity, histology, and family history.

Fecal Occult Blood Test

Randomized trials have found that the use of annual guaiac based FOBTs (g-FOBT) has decreased the mortality from colorectal cancer by up to 33%. Traditional guaiac FOBTs take advantage of the peroxidase activity of hemoglobin from bleeding colonic lesions that can be detected in the stool by a color change when it catalyzes the oxida-

Table 3 U.S. Multi-Society Task Force on Colorectal Cancer and American Cancer Society Guidelines for Surveillance of Colorectal Cancer (CRCa) and polyps

Risk Level	Recommendation	Interval
High Risk		
One or two small (<1 cm) tubular adenomas	Colonoscopy	5-10 yr after polyp removal; if normal, resume average-risk screening
More than two adenomas; any adenoma > 1 cm*; any adenoma with villous features or high-grade dysplasia	Colonoscopy	3 yr after complete polyp removal; if normal, repeat every 5 yr
More than 10 adenomas	Colonoscopy	<3 yr-interval based on clinical judgment
Hyperplastic polyposis syndrome	Colonoscopy	<3 yr-interval based on clinical judgment
Personal history of curative intent resection for CRCa	Colonoscopy	1 yr after surgery; if normal, repeat in 3 yr; if normal, repeat every 5 yr
CRC or adenomas in FDR age <60 yr, or two or more FDRs at any age	Colonoscopy	Every 5 yr, beginning at age 40, or 10 yr younger than the youngest cancer in FDR, whichever is earlier
Highest Risk		
Family history of FAP	Refer to specialty center for genetic counseling and consideration of genetic testing Sigmoidoscopy or colonoscopy	At time of diagnosis Every 1-2 yr, beginning at puberty
Family history of HNPCC	Refer to specialty center for genetic counseling and consideration of genetic testing Colonoscopy	At time of diagnosis Every 2 yr, beginning at age 21-25 until age 40, then annually
Inflammatory bowel disease	Refer to specialty center for colonoscopy with biopsies for dysplasia	Every 1-2 yr, beginning 8 yr after start of pancolitis or 12-15 yr after start of left-sided colitis

*If a polyp is removed piecemeal, recommendation is for repeat colonoscopy in 2-6 mo for verification of complete removal.
FAP, familial adenomatous polyposis; FDR, first-degree relative; HNPCC = hereditary nonpolyposis colorectal cancer.
Adapted from Levin B, Lieberman D, McFarland B, et al.: Screening and surveillance for the early detection of colorectal cancer and adenomatous polyps, 2008: A joint guideline from the American Cancer Society, the US Multi-Society Task Force on Colorectal Cancer and the American College of Radiology 2008;58:130-160.

tion of guaiac by a peroxide reagent. A special diet (e.g., a meat-free, high-residue diet without vegetables that have peroxidase activity, such as turnips and horseradish) is recommended for at least 24 hours before three separate stool specimens are collected at least 1 day apart. Unrehydrated test sensitivity is low at approximately 80%, with a specificity of up to 98%.

Immunochemical methods for FOBT (i-FOBT) use antibodies to human globin. The potential advantages of the i-FOBT include automation of test results and a potential increase in compliance, because no dietary restrictions are needed because the antibodies do not cross-react with nonhuman hemoglobin or peroxidases from food sources and the collection method is simpler, requiring only one or two samples. In addition, because globin does not survive passage through the upper GI tract, the test is specific for bleeding in the colon and rectum. A distinct advantage of i-FOBT is that the clinician can determine the fecal hemoglobin threshold to determine test characteristics and the level at which colonoscopy should be performed. When Levi and colleagues set the hemoglobin threshold at a cutoff of greater than 75 ng/mL, they found a sensitivity and specificity for cancer of 94% and 87.5%, respectively. The corresponding accuracy for all clinically advanced neoplasia was 67% and 91.4%, respectively.[9]

Although i-FOBT has not been studied in widespread randomized, controlled screening trials, in case-control studies a reduction of colorectal cancer mortality of up to 80% has been shown.[10-12]

The accuracy of a one-time brush-sample i-FOBT has been studied and shows improved test characteristics compared with g-FOBT. In a study of more than 2500 subjects, i-FOBT was positive significantly more often than g-FOBT in subjects with cancer (87.5% vs. 54.2%) and with significant adenomas (42.6% vs. 23.0%).[13] Beneficial results were also confirmed for a study of nearly 6000 subjects. The sensitivity for detecting cancer was 82% for i-FOBT and 64.3% for g-FOBT. The sensitivity for detecting advanced neoplasia was 41% and 29%, respectively. The specificity of each modality was greater than 98%.[14] The 2008 US PSTF guidelines for CRC screening recommend using an FOBT with a high sensitivity for the detection of colorectal cancer.

Stool DNA Testing

Stool DNA testing takes advantage of the potential for exfoliated neoplastic cells to pass into stool in order to detect mutations from within the molecular pathway that leads from adenoma to carcinoma. The largest study that compared fecal DNA to g-FOBT (Hemoccult II) in a screening population who underwent colonoscopy used a fecal DNA panel consisting of 21 mutations (three in the *Kras* gene, 10 in the *APC* gene, and eight in the *p53* gene), the microsatellite instability marker BAT-26, and a marker of long DNA thought to reflect disordered apoptosis of cancer cells sloughed into the colonic lumen. The fecal DNA panel detected 52% of the cancer cases vs. 13 % of the g-FOBT. The corresponding results for the detection of advanced neoplasia was 18% versus 11 %.[15] The results were disappointing, and the poor accuracy of fecal DNA was thought to be due to problems with technologic aspects of the DNA testing.

A second-generation fecal DNA test, which stabilizes DNA for transport and allows better extraction of DNA from stool, was tested in a small study and showed an increase in sensitivity for cancer to 72.5% and a specificity of 89%.[16] When a methylation marker of the vimentin gene was combined with the DNA integrity (DIA) assay, the performance of those two markers alone had an improved sensitivity of 87.5% and an 82% specificity.

Computed Tomography Colonography

Over the last decade, significant advances have occurred in computed tomography (CT) technology, and there is widespread interest in the use of CT colonography (CTC) for colorectal cancer screening. Many studies have been conducted to determine the accuracy of CTC for detecting colorectal neoplasia. The best accuracy was reported by Pickhardt and colleagues, who found the sensitivity of CTC comparable to colonoscopy for detecting adenomas larger than 6 mm (86%) and 92% for adenomas larger than 10 mm.[17] Poorer results came from Cotton and colleagues, with a sensitivity 32% for lesions larger than 6 mm and 52% for lesions larger than 10 mm. Rockey and colleagues found a sensitivity of 47% for polyps 6 to 9 mm and 53% for polyps larger than 1 cm.[18-19] The exact reasons for the disparity in the results are unknown. The results of the National CT Colonography Trial (ACRIN) of 2531subjects has not been published yet; however, preliminary reports (auntMinnie.com 9/28/2007) found the sensitivity for detecting lesions larger than 5 mm was 65% and for lesions larger than 9mm was 90%. The specificity was approximately 86% for any size.

Advocates of CTC suggest that patient compliance with screening will improve if CTC is an option. The fact that it is less invasive, is not associated with sedation, has little procedure-related risk, and has the potential to assess for lesions outside the colon might make it attractive to patients. However, the detection of insignificant extracolonic lesions might result in unnecessary health care expenditures, and the lifetime radiation-induced risk is a consideration. Other drawbacks include lack of reimbursement for screening by third-party payers, need for bowel preparation, and lack of detection of polyps smaller than 5 mm. Multidisciplinary collaboration between gastroenterologists and radiologists regarding the delivery of care between the radiology and endoscopy suite, interpretation and reporting of intraluminal and extraluminal findings, and proper follow-up of patients with detected lesions are necessary before widespread use of CTC is implemented.

Sigmoidoscopy

Results of several case-control studies have shown a reduction in deaths from colorectal cancer in subjects who have undergone sigmoidoscopic examinations. The reported reduction in mortality varies between 59% and 80%. The best-known study compared the use of rigid sigmoidoscopic screening in 261 patients who died from cancer of the distal colon or rectum with 868 control subjects. Screening reduced the rectosigmoid cancer mortality rate by 60%, and the protective effect of sigmoidoscopy was noted to last for up to 10 years. This reduction in mortality may have resulted from earlier detection of cancer and removal of premalignant polyps.

Sigmoidoscopic screening allows the lower one third of the colorectal mucosa to be visualized directly and diagnostic biopsy to be performed at the time of examination. Sensitivity and specificity are high for detecting polyps and cancer in the segment of the bowel examined. Unfortunately, however, almost 50% of polyps and cancers are beyond the limits of detection of the longest (e.g., 60 cm) flexible sigmoidoscope.

Opinions vary regarding the need for colonoscopy for patients in whom a single small (<1 cm) adenoma is found on flexible sigmoidoscopy. Studies have shown that the prevalence of advanced proximal neoplasms in patients with distal adenomas is up to 9%. Therefore, the use of colonoscopy to detect proximal neoplasia in patients with distal adenomas continues to be recommended.

Barium Enema

Barium enema has the advantage of imaging the entire colon. However, recent evidence has suggested that it is inaccurate for detecting polyps and early cancers and suboptimal for colorectal cancer screening or surveillance. In a prospective study comparing the use of double-contrast barium enema and colonoscopy, barium enema missed 52% of polyps larger than 1 cm.[20] If barium enema is the only option for screening or surveillance, it should be coupled with flexible sigmoidoscopy. The use of flexible sigmoidoscopy allows visualization of the rectosigmoid, which might not be well seen on barium enema because of the overlapping loops of bowel. Lesions detected on barium enema warrant colonoscopic evaluation.

Colonoscopy

Colonoscopy is the gold standard for detecting colonic neoplasms and is the preferred colorectal cancer screening strategy. The incidence rate of colorectal cancer has been shown to be reduced up to 90% in subjects who had polypectomy versus patients in three reference groups, including two cohorts in whom colonic polyps were not removed and one general population registry. Colonoscopy can be completed in more than 95% of examinations with negligible risk. Colonoscopic screening in average-risk patients has been found to be cost effective, and it is similar to cervical or breast cancer screening techniques in cost effectiveness per life-year saved. Medicare has approved the use of screening colonoscopy in average-risk beneficiaries. Unfortunately, not all Americans younger than 65 years have health care benefits that cover the charges for colonoscopy, which could affect patient compliance with screening colonoscopy.

The stage of colorectal cancer is the most important feature predicting curability and survival in colorectal cancer. The depth of tumor invasion and lymph node involvement are the two major components constituting the basis for colorectal cancer tumor staging. The first colorectal cancer staging system was developed in 1932 and is known as the Dukes' classification. Since then, many modifications in the Dukes' scheme have been made. In an effort to minimize confusion over which Dukes' stage is implied and to standardize all organ system cancer staging, the TNM (tumor, nodal status, and presence of metastases) system has been adopted. Stages II and III have been further stratified based on tumor size. In addition, investigators used the surveillance, epidemiology, and end results (SEER) data to calculate 5-year survival rates, and patients with stage IIIA colon cancer were found to have significantly better survival than patients with stage IIB disease.

TREATMENT

The primary treatment of colorectal cancer is surgical resection of the primary tumor and regional lymph nodes. Surgery is curative for most early-stage colorectal tumors. For more advanced stages, surgery and adjuvant therapy are recommended to prevent recurrence and prolong survival.[20-22]

Colon Cancer

Studies have proved the benefit of adjuvant chemotherapy in prolonging disease-free and overall survival in patients with stage III colon cancer compared with patients who received surgery alone.[20] Patients with stage III colon cancer who undergo surgery alone have a 50% risk of relapse; these patients benefit from 5-fluorouracil (5-FU)-based adjuvant therapy, with a 30% reduction in risk of death. Despite this recommendation for postoperative chemotherapy, there is documented underuse of adjuvant therapy in patients with stage III colon cancer.

Use of adjuvant therapy in patients with stage II colon cancer has been actively debated. Currently, the American Society of Clinical Oncologists does not recommend routine use of adjuvant chemotherapy in patients with stage II colon cancer. Certain patient populations, however, may be considered for adjuvant treatment, including patients with inadequately sampled nodes, T4 lesions, perforation, or poorly differentiated histology. Additionally, patients with stage II disease should be encouraged to participate in clinical trials aimed at determining the true benefit, if any, of adjuvant therapy in this patient population.

Rectal Cancer

The major limitation of rectal cancer surgery is the inability to obtain wide margins because of the confined space of the bony pelvis. Adjuvant radiation therapy decreases the rate of local recurrence, whereas the addition of systemic chemotherapy further enhances local control and improves survival. A 1990 NIH Consensus Development Conference recommended that postoperative 5-FU–based chemotherapy combined with irradiation should be the standard clinical practice in stages II and III rectal cancer because of its proven decrease in local recurrence, cancer-related deaths, and overall mortality.[21]

In the last decade, subsequent randomized trials have been challenging that recommendation. The debate is fueled, in part, by refinements in surgical techniques. Total mesorectal excision (TME) is one of the most exciting recent developments in surgical oncology. The sharp dissection follows along the mesorectal fascia, with removal of the rectum and of all tissue invested by the adjacent visceral fascia, including fatty tissue, lymph nodes, and lymphatic vessels. This technique has been associated with a reduction in local recurrence rates from 39% to less than 10%. These low rates have led some investigators to question the routine use of adjuvant radiation therapy. One study has compared the use of TME plus preoperative radiotherapy versus TME alone.[25] Short-term survival was no different in the two groups, but the rate of local recurrence was 2.4% for TME with preoperative radiotherapy versus 8.2% for TME alone.

There is also controversy over the best timing of radiotherapy. Compared with postoperative irradiation, preoperative treatment might have lower toxicity and might increase the chance of preserving the sphincter. The information from all controlled trials reported so far shows that the fraction of local recurrences is reduced to less than 50% when radiotherapy, up to moderately high doses, is given preoperatively. This reduction is smaller with postoperative radiotherapy, even if higher doses are used. Improved survival has been seen in trials using postoperative radiotherapy, but only when combined with chemotherapy. In one trial, a survival benefit was incurred with preoperative radiotherapy versus surgery alone. Randomized trials comparing preoperative and postoperative combined modality therapy are in progress.

Outside of clinical trials, curative-intent surgery combined with radiochemotherapy remains the recommended standard for treatment of stages II and III rectal cancer.

PREVENTION

Epidemiologic studies have found a modest decrease in colorectal cancer in patients using nonsteroidal anti-inflammatory drugs, particularly aspirin. Two randomized, controlled trials have found that aspirin substantially reduces the risk of recurrent and advanced adenomas in high-risk populations.[23,24] Two randomized, placebo-controlled trials have found a moderate reduction in recurrent adenomas with calcium supplementation.[25,26]

A 6-month placebo-controlled trial of a selective cyclooxygenase (COX)-2 inhibitor, celecoxib, in FAP patients resulted in a 28% reduction in polyp size and number.[27] The U.S. Food and Drug Administration has approved the use of celecoxib as an adjunct for managing colorectal adenomas in patients with FAP. The value of COX-2 inhibitors celecoxib and rofecoxib in the sporadic adenoma population has been investigated in three large multicenter studies of patients with a history of colorectal adenoma. The efficacy results of these 3-year trials all demonstrated a significant reduction in the recurrence of both adenomas and advanced adenomas. Unfortunately the studies were stopped prematurely because of adverse cardiovascular events.[28-30]

The increased cardiovascular risk of COX-2 inhibitors appears to outweigh the potential for preventing colorectal neoplasia in patients with sporadic colorectal adenomas.[31] The effectiveness and cost-effectiveness of chemopreventive agents in different risk populations needs to be confirmed before widespread recommendations for their use can be given.

CONCLUSIONS

Colorectal cancer is one of the leading causes of cancer and death from carcinoma in the United States. Increasing awareness regarding the preventable nature of this disease, along with widespread use of screening, should favorably affect the incidence of colorectal cancer. Colorectal cancer screening and polyp removal can save lives, and the most exciting area of future research will be the primary prevention of adenomas and colorectal cancer through chemoprevention.

Summary

- Adenocarcinoma of the colon and rectum is the third most common cancer and cause of cancer deaths in the United States, but studies have suggested that the incidence is declining because of the increased use of screening and polyp removal.
- Colon cancer screening and surveillance strategies must be individualized based on a patient's risk factors, including personal history of adenomas or colorectal cancer, family history of adenomas or colorectal cancer, family history of an inherited colorectal cancer syndrome, and personal history of inflammatory bowel disease.
- The stage of colorectal cancer is the most important feature predicting curability and survival in colorectal cancer.
- Continued investigations of chemopreventive agents are needed to identify a means of primary prevention of adenomas and colorectal cancer.

Suggested Readings

Baron J, Cole B, Sandler R, et al: A randomized trial of aspirin to prevent colorectal adenomas. N Engl J Med 2003;348:891-899.

Benson AB: Adjuvant chemotherapy of stage III colon cancer. Semin Oncol 2005; 32(Suppl 9):S74-S77.

Giardello FM, Brensinger JD, Petersen GM: AGA technical review on hereditary colorectal cancer and genetic testing. Gastroenterology 2001;121:198-213.

Lieberman DA, Weiss DG: One-time screening for colorectal cancer with combined fecal occult-blood testing and examination of the distal colon. N Engl J Med 2001;345: 555-560.

Sieber OM, Lipton L, Crabtree M, et al: Multiple colorectal adenomas, classic adenomatous polyposis, and germ-line mutations in MYH. N Engl J Med 2003;348:791-799.

Bertagnolli MM, Eagle CJ, Zauber AG, et al: Celecoxib for the prevention of sporadic colorectal adenomas. N Engl J Med 2006;355:873-884.

Umar A, Boland C, Terdiman J, et al: Revised Bethesda guidelines for HNPCC and microsatellite instability. J Natl Cancer Inst 2004;96:261-268.

Levin B, Lieberman D, McFarland B, et al: Screening and surveillance for the early detection of colorectal cancer and adenomatous polyps, 2008: A joint guideline from the American Cancer Society, the US Multi-Society Task Force on Colorectal Cancer and the American College of Radiology. CA Cancer J Clin 2008;58:130-160.

References

For a complete list of references, log onto www.expertconsult.com.

Section 6

HEPATOLOGY

Approach to the Patient with Liver Disease: A Guide to Commonly Used Liver Tests

William D. Carey

Laboratory assessment of the patient with suspected or clinically obvious liver disease is context dependent. For example, the acutely ill jaundiced patient with a history of prolonged alcohol ingestion requires a different laboratory assessment than the well patient in whom one or more standard liver test results are discovered to be abnormal during routine testing. Additionally, the sequence of liver tests depends heavily on the question asked. If it is to determine whether this well person whose brother was recently diagnosed with hemochromatosis also has this genetic disease, then a series of tests will be initiated to detect iron overload. If it is to determine whether this spouse has been infected with hepatitis B, then blood tests related to hepatitis B will be required. Thus, algorithms for the evaluation of liver disease need to be considered skeptically.

This chapter is designed to discuss a useful way of thinking about liver tests. It emphasizes limitations of and alternative explanations for isolated abnormalities of common liver test results. Information in this chapter should be combined with discussions of specific liver diseases elsewhere in this section. A final caveat relates to terminology. Tests done in clinical laboratories do not measure any functional capacity of the liver. Hence, the commonly used term *liver function tests* is inaccurate, and the term *liver tests* is used in this chapter. Guidelines on the interpretation and evaluation of abnormal liver test results have been published.[1,2] Useful algorithms are presented that parallel the recommendations in this chapter.

ISOLATED ABNORMALITIES IN LIVER TEST RESULTS

A common clinical scenario is the unanticipated discovery of an abnormal liver test result, obtained when a bundle of tests has been done for other reasons. Most clinical laboratories offer bundled blood tests, which often contain all or most of the following:

- Bilirubin
- Aspartate transaminase (AST, formerly referred to as serum glutamic-oxaloacetic transaminase, SGOT)
- Alanine transaminase (ALT, formerly called serum glutamic-pyruvic transaminase, SGPT)
- γ-Glutamyl-transpeptidase (GGTP)
- Alkaline phosphatase
- Lactate dehydrogenase (LDH)

An isolated elevation of just one test result should raise suspicion that a source other than the liver is the cause. Table 1 indicates nonhepatic sources of elevated values for certain tests commonly considered as liver tests. When several liver test results are simultaneously out of the normal range, consideration of nonhepatic sources becomes irrelevant.

Special note should be made of the GGTP and LDH as liver tests. The GGTP level is too sensitive, frequently elevated when no liver disease is apparent. The only usefulness of the GGTP test is that it confers liver specificity to an elevated alkaline phosphatase level. An isolated elevation of the GGTP level does not need to be further evaluated unless there are additional clinical risk factors for liver disease.[3] The LDH assay is insensitive and nonspecific because LDH is present in tissues throughout the body.

EVALUATION OF LIVER DISEASE BASED ON ENZYME LEVELS

It is customary and useful to categorize liver diseases into three broad categories—hepatocellular, in which primary injury is to the hepatocytes; cholestatic, in which primary injury is to the bile ducts; and infiltrative, in which the liver is invaded or replaced by nonhepatic substances, such as neoplasm or amyloid. Although there is a great deal of overlap in liver test result abnormalities seen in these three categories, particularly in cholestatic and infiltrative disorders, an attempt to characterize an otherwise undifferentiated clinical case as hepatocellular, cholestatic, or infiltrative often makes subsequent evaluation faster and more efficient. The AST, ALT, and alkaline phosphatase tests are most useful to make the distinction between hepatocellular and cholestatic disease.

The normal range for aminotransferase levels in most clinical laboratories is much lower than that for the alkaline phosphatase level. Accordingly, when considering levels of elevations, it is necessary to consider them relative to the respective upper limit of normal for each test compared. Consider a patient with an AST level of 120 IU/mL (normal, ≤40 IU/mL) and an alkaline phosphatase of 130 IU/mL (normal, ≤120 IU/mL). This represents a hepatocellular pattern of liver injury because the AST level is three times the upper limit of normal, whereas the alkaline phosphatase level is only marginally higher than its upper limit of normal.

Serum aminotransferase levels—ALT and AST—are two of the most useful measures of liver cell injury, although the AST is less liver specific than the ALT level. Elevations of the AST level may also be seen in acute muscle injury, cardiac or skeletal muscle. Lesser degrees of ALT level elevation may occasionally be seen in skeletal muscle injury or even after vigorous exercise. Diseases that primarily affect hepatocytes, such as viral hepatitis, will cause disproportionate elevations of the AST and ALT levels compared with the alkaline phosphatase level. The ratio of AST/ALT is of little benefit in sorting out the cause of liver injury except in acute alcoholic hepatitis, in which the ratio is usually greater than 2 *and* the AST level is 400 IU/mL or lower.

Mild elevations of the AST level, less than two times the upper limit of normal, are common. In part, this is explained by how normal values are calculated; normal is defined as the mean of the distribution ± 2 standard deviations (SDs). By this definition, 2.5% of normal persons have values above the normal range.[2] Common causes of mild increases in AST and ALT levels include reduction effect (e.g., status) and fatty liver disease seen most often in those with obesity, diabetes, or elevated blood lipid levels. Fatty liver is also seen in those who drink alcohol.

Serum alkaline phosphatase is comprised of a heterogeneous group of enzymes. Hepatic alkaline phosphatase is most densely represented near the canalicular membrane of the hepatocyte.

Table 1 Nonhepatic Sources of Abnormalities for Select Laboratory Tests

Test	Nonhepatic Source
Bilirubin	Red blood cells (e.g., hemolysis, intra-abdominal bleed, hematoma)
AST	Skeletal muscle, cardiac muscle
LDH	Heart, red blood cells
Alkaline phosphatase	Bone, first-trimester placenta, kidneys, intestines

AST, aspartate transaminase; LDH, lactate dehydrogenase.

Table 2 Category of Liver Disease by Predominant Serum Enzyme Abnormality

	Liver Disease Category		
Test	Hepatocellular	Cholestatic	Infiltrative
AST, ALT higher than alkaline phosphatase level	Typical	—	—
Alkaline phosphatase higher than AST, ALT levels	—	Typical	—
Elevation of alkaline phosphatase with near-normal AST, ALT levels	—	Typical	Typical

ALT, alanine aminotransaminase; AST, aspartate transaminase.

Accordingly, diseases that predominately affect hepatocyte secretion (e.g., obstructive diseases) will be accompanied by elevations of alkaline phosphatase levels. Bile duct obstruction, primary sclerosing cholangitis and primary biliary cirrhosis, are some examples of diseases in which elevated alkaline phosphatase levels are often predominant over transaminase level elevations (Table 2).

It is apparent that infiltrative liver diseases most often result in a pattern of liver test result abnormalities similar to those of cholestatic liver disease. Differentiation often requires imaging studies of the liver. Liver imaging by ultrasound, computed tomography (CT), or magnetic resonance imaging (MRI) most often identifies infiltration of the liver by mass lesions such as tumors. Imaging by cholangiography—endoscopic retrograde cholangiography, transhepatic cholangiography, or magnetic resonance cholangiography—identifies many bile duct lesions that cause cholestatic liver disease. Liver biopsy is often needed to confirm certain infiltrative disorders (e.g., amyloidosis) and microscopic biliary disorders such as primary biliary cirrhosis.

Bilirubin Level Elevations

Bilirubin is produced by the normal breakdown of pigment-containing proteins, especially hemoglobin from senescent red blood cells and myoglobin from muscle breakdown. Bilirubin released from such sources, tightly albumin bound, is delivered to the liver, where it is efficiently extracted and conjugated by hepatic glucuronidation and sulfation. Conjugated bilirubin is rapidly excreted into bile and removed from the body through the gut. Therefore, the amount of conjugated bilirubin present in serum in healthy subjects is trivial (<10% of measured total bilirubin). An elevated level of

Table 3 Bilirubin Fractions Present in Blood and Urine

Fraction	In Serum As	Measured As	Present in Urine
Unconjugated	Albumin-bound	Indirect-reacting bilirubin	Never
Conjugated	Unbound	Direct-reacting bilirubin	Yes, when serum bilirubin level exceeds 3-4 mg/dL

conjugated serum bilirubin implies liver disease. Because only conjugated bilirubin appears in urine, the finding of bilirubinuria also implies liver disease.

Most laboratories report only total bilirubin levels, the sum of the conjugated and unconjugated portions. It is sometimes useful to determine the fraction of total serum bilirubin that is unconjugated versus conjugated, usually referred to as fractionation of bilirubin. The main clinical situation in which this is useful is when all the standard liver test results are normal, except the total bilirubin. Laboratories report the total bilirubin as well as the conjugated and unconjugated portions. To make matters more confusing, the conjugated bilirubin is sometimes referred to as the direct-reacting bilirubin and the unconjugated as the indirect-reacting bilirubin (Table 3).

Normally, 90% or more of measured serum bilirubin is unconjugated (indirect-reacting). When the total bilirubin level is elevated and fractionation shows that the major portion (≥90%) is unconjugated, liver disease is never the explanation. Instead, the clinical suspicion should turn to one of two explanations. If the patient is young and healthy, an inherited decrease in the inability to conjugate bilirubin is likely; it is referred to as Gilbert's syndrome. It causes no symptoms and is associated with no liver disease. Interestingly, fasting and intercurrent illnesses such as influenza often make the level of unconjugated bilirubin even higher in those with Gilbert's syndrome. This syndrome is easily diagnosed when all the standard liver test results are normal, and 90% or more of the total bilirubin is unconjugated. There is no need for an imaging study or liver biopsy in cases of suspected Gilbert's syndrome.

Elevations of the unconjugated bilirubin level, when the conjugated bilirubin level remains normal, may also indicate an increased load of bilirubin caused by hemolysis. Anemia and an elevated reticulocyte count are usually present in such cases (Table 4).

Many mistakenly interpret elevations of direct-reacting bilirubin to indicate that cholestatic (obstructive) liver disease is present. It is apparent from Table 2 that the serum bilirubin level plays no useful role in categorizing a case as hepatocellular, cholestatic, or infiltrative. The bilirubin level may be normal or elevated in each type of disorder. Viral hepatitis A, a prototypic hepatocellular disease, may frequently be associated with bilirubin levels that are high, whereas primary biliary cirrhosis, a prototypic cholestatic disorder, is associated with a normal serum bilirubin level except in later stage disease. Serum bilirubin levels should be disregarded when trying to decide whether the liver test pattern is more suggestive of hepatocellular or cholestatic disease.

DETERMINATION OF SPECIFIC DISORDERS

Acute Alcoholic Hepatitis

Acute alcoholic hepatitis may be mild or life threatening. The pattern of liver test abnormality is hepatocellular. Additionally, the AST level is higher than the ALT level but rarely exceeds 400 IU/mL. The AST is typically in the 100 to 200 IU/mL range, even in severe disease, and

Table 4 Common Causes of Isolated Bilirubin Elevation

Cause	Direct-Reacting Bilirubin	Indirect-Reacting Bilirubin	Associated Features
Liver disease (many types)	Elevated	Elevated or normal	Liver enzyme levels often elevated
Hemolysis	Normal	Elevation represents more than 90% of total bilirubin	Anemia usual; increased reticulocyte count; normal liver enzyme levels (although LDH may be elevated)
Gilbert's syndrome	Normal	Elevation represents more than 90% of total bilirubin (common)	No abnormal liver tests; no anemia; onset in late adolescence; fasting makes bilirubin rise

LDH, lactate dehydrogenase.

Table 5 Hepatitis A Antibody Testing In Different Clinical States

State	Anti-HAV Total (IgG, IgM)	IgM Anti-HAV
Acute hepatitis A	Positive	Positive
Resolved hepatitis A	Positive	Negative
Immunization	Positive	Negative

HAV, hepatitis A virus; IgG, immunoglobulin G; IgM, immunoglobulin M.

the ALT level may be normal, even in severe cases. The degree of bilirubin level increase and prothrombin time elevation are better indicators of severity of disease than the level of enzyme elevation. The important corollary of this observation is that an AST or ALT elevation, or both, of, for example, 800 IU/mL is not likely to be explained by acute alcoholic hepatitis, even in an alcoholic.

Viral Hepatitis

Viral hepatitis most often produces a hepatocellular pattern of injury (AST and ALT level elevations predominate). Persons with no symptoms and normal aminotransferase levels may be infected. In addition, a great deal of confusion is caused by abnormal viral markers, many of which do not indicate active infection but rather immunity. These concepts are more fully developed elsewhere in this section in the chapters on viral hepatitis. A clinical practice guideline on viral hepatitis is also available.[4]

Hepatitis A

Hepatitis A virus (HAV) infection is an acute self-limited disease in most cases, although it may rarely be fatal. Diagnosis is made through the use of antibody tests (anti-HAV). The standard screening tests contain reagents that will test positive for the presence of immunoglobulin M (IgM) anti-HAV or immunoglobulin G (IgG) anti-HAV. This test will therefore be positive with any exposure: acute, remote, or via immunization. Thus, it is not useful to determine whether a patient with acute hepatitis has hepatitis A.

Because IgM anti-HAV is present for only a few months after acute infection, the key to diagnosis of acute hepatitis A is to measure IgM anti-HAV. Selective testing of IgM anti-HAV is required to establish the serologic diagnosis of acute hepatitis A (Table 5).

Hepatitis B

Like hepatitis A, hepatitis B produces hepatocellular enzyme level elevations (AST and ALT predominate). In adults who acquire hepatitis B, the infection almost always clears, but antibodies persist. In a few, the disease does not resolve, but becomes chronic. These patients retain serum markers of viral infection. Many blood tests are available for hepatitis B antigenic determinants and their antibodies. It is best to separate testing appropriate for the acute hepatitis situation from testing for chronic liver disease caused by hepatitis B. Only a few tests need to be considered by the generalist to determine the status of a patient with possible hepatitis B.

Acute Hepatitis B. Within 2 weeks of exposure, but often delayed for weeks or months, hepatitis B surface antigen (HBsAg) emerges. This antigen is present in the blood for a variable period, usually encompassing the time during which the patient is clinically ill and most likely to seek medical attention. For patients with mild symptoms whose testing may be delayed, the HBsAg level may have already declined. In this case, a second chance to make the diagnosis comes from detection of the IgM antibody directed against the hepatitis B core antigen, anti-HBc-IgM (Table 6).

Chronic Hepatitis B. Chronic hepatitis B is characterized by a long-lasting persistence of HBsAg and anti-HBc (IgG). Anti-HBs is absent. An additional antigen-antibody system requires mention, the hepatitis B e antigen (HBeAg) and its antibody (anti-HBe). These tests are only relevant in the individual in whom the HBsAg is chronically positive. In chronic B infection in which HBeAg is also positive, there are usually active viral replication and significant liver injury. In time, HBeAg may be lost, replaced by its antibody, anti-HBe. This transformation is often associated with lower level infection (less viral replication) or HBV DNA, lower AST and ALT values, and less (or no) hepatic inflammation. These concepts and exceptions are discussed more fully elsewhere in this section in the chapters on viral hepatitis. A clinical practice guideline on viral hepatitis B has provided additional information on laboratory testing in various contexts of hepatitis B infection.[5]

Resolved Hepatitis B and Immunization Status. Confusion may arise in the interpretation of hepatitis B tests in a patient who has received hepatitis B immunization or has had previous hepatitis B. When such an individual develops a different type of liver disease, certain test results for hepatitis B will also be positive and interpretation may be difficult. In those immunized, only the antibody directed against the surface antigen (anti-HBs) will be present; in a patient with resolved hepatitis B, anti-HBs and the antibody directed against the hepatitis B core (anti-HBc) will usually be present. In this case, the anti-HBc will be of the IgG class, not IgM.

In acute hepatitis B in which delay in testing has occurred, the HBsAg may be absent. In such cases, the anti-HBc will be positive (but not anti-HBs). In remote (resolved) infection, only IgG anti-HBc is present. In acute infection, IgM anti-HBc will be detected.

Hepatitis C

Because infection with hepatitis C usually produces no symptoms or mild, nonspecific, flulike symptoms, it is not frequently diagnosed during the acute phase. The virus clears spontaneously in only about 15% of those infected. Although generally helpful for the diagnosis of chronic infection, antibody tests are not usually useful for acute

Table 6 Hepatitis B Testing in Different Clinical States

	Basic Tests			Ancillary Tests		
State	**HBsAg**	**Anti-HBc**	**Anti-HBs**	**HBeAg**	**Anti-HBe**	**HBV DNA**
Acute, early	+	+ or –	–	+	–	+
Acute, late	+ or –	+ IgM	–	+	–	+
Resolved	–	+ IgG	+	–	+	–
Chronic carrier	+	+	–	Variable	Variable	–
Chronic with active features	+	+	–	+	–	+
Successful immunization	–	–	+	–	–	–

HBc, hepatitis B core; HBeAg, hepatitis B e antigen; HBs, hepatitis B surface; HBV, hepatitis B virus.

Table 7 Hepatitis C Testing in Different Clinical States

State	Anti-HCV (EIA)	Anti-HCV (RIBA)	HCV RNA (PCR or bDNA)	Genotype
Acute	–	–	+	Types 1-6
Resolved (spontaneous or after treatment)	+	+	–	Undetectable
Chronic	+	+	+	Types 1-6

EIA, enzyme immunoassay; HCV, hepatitis c virus; PCR, polymerase chain reaction; RIBA, radioimmunoblot assay.

hepatitis C virus (HCV) because emergence of the antibody is delayed for several months after infection.

To test for chronic HCV infection, the most commonly used anti-HCV antibody test is an enzyme immunoassay (EIA) or a variant. False-positive results may occur. The radioimmunoblot assay (RIBA) adds specificity to a positive anti-HCV EIA, but is probably of lesser use now that direct measurement of viral products in serum (HCV RNA) is widely available. HCV RNA is usually determined by the polymerase chain reaction (PCR) assay, although a simpler test, HCV RNA by bDNA is still done in some laboratories, but this latter test is not as sensitive as the PCR assay. HCV RNA in serum definitively establishes the presence of HCV infection. Some have wondered whether the initial screening test for HCV should therefore be the HCV RNA rather than an antibody test. Currently, however, because of cost considerations, the initial test for HCV should be an anti-HCV antibody test.

Once the presence of HCV is established, the genotype should be determined. There are six major HCV genotypes (1-6). Genotype has increasing importance for treatment determinations. This is discussed more fully elsewhere in this section ("Hepatitis C") (Table 7).

Iron and Copper Overload Diseases

Diseases characterized by iron overload and copper overload are discussed in detail elsewhere in this section ("Inherited Metabolic Liver Diseases: Hemochromatosis, Wilson's Disease").

Iron Tests

Two paths may be considered to establish a diagnosis of hemochromatosis, genotypic and phenotypic. Diagnosis is most often made by phenotypic expression of disease—that is, by demonstration of excess circulating iron, ferritin, or iron accumulation within organs, especially the liver. Despite the excitement surrounding the genotypic diagnosis of hereditary hemochromatosis, it has been shown that phenotypic demonstration of iron overload is the most cost-efficient strategy.[6] A practice guideline has been published that confirms this approach.[7]

The most useful tests for iron overload in serum are iron, iron-binding capacity, and percentage transferrin saturation. Serum ferritin levels are also useful and easily obtained. Hemochromatosis should be suspected in the following:[8]

- Any adult with liver disease, especially men
- Transferrin saturation higher than 55%
- Ferritin level elevations higher than 200 μg/L in premenopausal women or higher than 300 μg/L in men and postmenopausal women

These thresholds are low; most patients who exceed them will not prove to have iron overload. Many inflammatory conditions, and especially other liver diseases, will result in elevations of ferritin or iron levels, or both, in the absence of total body iron excess.

Limitations of Serum-Based Tests of Iron Overload. Because both iron and ferritin are stored in liver cells, any condition that results in hepatocyte injury and release of intracellular contents into the blood will falsely raise iron, transferrin saturation, and ferritin levels. Therefore, in acute hepatic injury of any source, these tests will falsely suggest iron overload. Acute inflammation outside the liver may also falsely elevate serum-based iron tests. Tests of serum ferritin levels, iron, iron-binding capacity, and percentage saturation determined in the setting of markedly elevated aminotransferase levels (AST and ALT), such as those seen in acute viral hepatitis or massive hepatic necrosis, will be identical to those seen in hemochromatosis. Iron studies cannot be interpreted in the face of major elevations of transaminase levels.

Another limitation of iron studies relates to the time it takes for an individual with genetic hemochromatosis to accumulate excessive iron. In a young patient with this condition, who has not yet had enough time to accumulate iron (especially the premenopausal woman), screening tests for iron overload may be normal, even though the individual is at risk for the subsequent development of iron overload.

Confirmation of suspected iron overload from serum-based tests requires demonstration of an increased hepatic iron level, usually by liver biopsy. The value of the biopsy is twofold: It provides information about the degree of fibrosis or cirrhosis present, which is vital in predicting the risk of subsequent development of hepatoma, and it provides an assessment of iron stores. Because there is an age-dependent increase in hepatic iron in normal individuals, it is necessary to create an index that takes this into account. The hepatic iron index is calculated as follows:

$$\text{Hepatic iron index} = \text{hepatic iron concentration } (\mu\text{mol/g dry weight}) \div \text{patient age (in years)}$$

A hepatic iron index lower than 2.0 is normal; values higher than 2.0 are seen in hemochromatosis.[9] Renewed interest in the assessment of hepatic iron by the evaluation of iron stains of liver biopsy material indicates that this is a satisfactory alternative to quantitative iron determination.[10] Bone marrow iron stores are not adequate to assess total body iron stores; cases of hemochromatosis with absent stainable bone marrow iron have been reported.

Genotypic Diagnosis of Genetic Hemochromatosis. It has been known for years that many cases of hemochromatosis are inherited as an autosomal recessive trait. In many cases, a defective gene, called the *HFE* gene, is implicated. The presence of this inherited gene results in the production of a protein in which a tyrosine amino acid rather than a cysteine amino acid is present at position 282 of the HFE protein. A second missense gene that results in an aspartic acid (instead of histidine) at position 63 of the same protein may increase iron absorption in some patients. The abnormalities are called *C282Y* and *H63D* mutations, respectively.

The patient with hereditary hemochromatosis usually must have two abnormal genes (homozygosity). Most often, two *C282Y* genes are present, but occasionally a compound heterozygote (*C282Y-H63D*) will also have excess iron. Homozygosity for *H63D* does not usually result in excess iron absorption.

The value of genotypic diagnosis is primarily limited to the identification of at-risk family members after an index case has been discovered. *HFE* determination can identify young individuals at risk for iron overload before iron becomes excessive. In Australia, where almost all patients with genetic hemochromatosis demonstrate such genetic abnormalities, gene diagnosis can replace iron testing. However, in most parts of the world, only 60% to 80% of those with hemochromatosis have an *HFE* abnormality. Therefore, *HFE* testing is generally not a suitable screening test for iron overload. Reliance on phenotypic expression (iron overload) is still required.

Copper Tests

Although copper may accumulate to moderate excess in the liver in any chronic cholestatic liver condition, it does not appear to be injurious in these conditions. Wilson's disease is the main disease in which pathologic copper deposition results in serious liver injury, cirrhosis, and death. In Wilson's disease, copper also accumulates in the basal ganglia of the brain, where it produces a wide gamut of neurologic abnormalities. Patients may present with liver disease, brain disease, or both. This disorder is discussed in more detail elsewhere in this section ("Inherited Metabolic Liver Diseases: Wilson's Disease").

Wilson's disease is rare. Untreated, it usually produces death before age 40 years. Therefore, it is most appropriate to consider this potential cause in a child or young adult with otherwise unexplained liver disease. Laboratory diagnosis is most often based on the finding of a low ceruloplasmin level. Because most acute and chronic liver diseases cause the ceruloplasmin level to be elevated, the finding of a low-normal or depressed ceruloplasmin level in a young patient with liver disease is suggestive of Wilson's disease. There are a few exceptions to this. A patient with acute fulminant liver failure of any sort may no longer have a liver capable of ceruloplasmin synthesis, so that patient may have a low serum level. Similarly, the patient with terminal end-stage liver disease may have a falling ceruloplasmin level. Finally, a few individuals have congenital hypoceruloplasminemia without copper accumulation and are healthy.

Autoimmune Liver Diseases: Autoimmune Chronic Hepatitis and Primary Biliary Cirrhosis

The two most common forms of autoimmune liver disease are autoimmune chronic hepatitis and primary biliary cirrhosis. Ninety percent of those with each disorder are women. Autoimmune chronic hepatitis is characterized by very high serum aminotransferase (ALT and AST) levels, whereas primary biliary cirrhosis is associated with predominant elevations of the alkaline phosphatase level, a cholestatic disorder. Each is associated with autoantibodies in the serum. The treatment for each is different, so accurate diagnosis is essential. Table 8 contrasts the laboratory findings of these two autoimmune liver disorders.

Interpretation of autoimmune markers in a patient with liver disease is highly context-dependent. Autoantibodies are common in low titer in a number of acute and chronic liver conditions, such as viral hepatitis. Therefore, the finding of autoantibodies in low titer is not sufficient evidence with which to make a diagnosis of autoimmune chronic hepatitis or primary biliary cirrhosis.

Autoimmune hepatitis should be rapidly recognized by its propensity to occur in women (90%) and to be associated with high

Table 8 Contrasting Features of Two Autoimmune Liver Diseases

Feature	Autoimmune Chronic Hepatitis	Primary Biliary Cirrhosis
AST, ALT	7-10 times upper limit of normal (ULN)	1-3 times ULN
Alkaline phosphatase	1-3 times ULN	2-10 times ULN
Anti-smooth muscle antibody positive	90% (usually high titer)	10%-20% (usually low titer)
Antimitochondrial antibody positive	10%-20% (usually low titer)	90%-100% (usually high titer)
Liver-kidney microsomal antibody positive	Positive in some cases in which smooth muscle antibody is negative (rare in North America)	Negative

ALT, alanine aminotransaminase; AST, aspartate transaminase.

transaminase levels (200 IU/mL or higher). In this disease, elevations of the gamma globulins (especially IgG) are pronounced. A myriad of autoimmune markers may be positive in autoimmune chronic hepatitis, but only a few are measured regularly: smooth muscle antibody, antinuclear factor, and liver-kidney microsomal (LKM) antibody. A liver biopsy is often done to establish the diagnosis of autoimmune chronic hepatitis.

Primary biliary cirrhosis is discussed in detail elsewhere in this section ("Primary Biliary Cirrhosis, Primary Sclerosing Cholangitis, and Other Cholestatic Liver Diseases"). In this condition, serum-based liver tests reveal a predominant elevation of the alkaline phosphatase level. An autoantibody most likely to be present in high titer in primary biliary cirrhosis is the antimitochondrial antibody, but determination of its presence may not be needed in clear-cut cases.[11] An occasional patient may have features of autoimmune chronic hepatitis and primary biliary cirrhosis.

Summary

- Laboratory assessment of the patient with suspected or clinically obvious liver disease is context dependent. It is useful to categorize liver diseases into three broad categories: hepatocellular, cholestatic, and infiltrative.
- Acute alcoholic hepatitis may be mild or life threatening. The pattern of liver test abnormality is hepatocellular. The AST level is higher than the ALT level but rarely exceeds 400 IU/mL, and the ALT level may be normal. The level of bilirubin elevation and prothrombin time elevation are better indicators of severity of disease than the level of enzyme elevation.
- Viral hepatitis most often produces a hepatocellular pattern of injury (AST and ALT elevations predominate). Specific antigens and antibodies establish the diagnosis of viral hepatitis.
- Two paths may be considered to establish a diagnosis of iron-loading disease (hemochromatosis), genotypic and phenotypic. Diagnosis is most often made by the phenotypic expression of disease. Wilson's disease is rare; untreated, it usually produces death before age 40 years. Laboratory diagnosis is usually based on the finding of a low ceruloplasmin level and increased copper levels.
- Autoimmune chronic hepatitis is characterized by very high serum aminotransferase levels and high smooth muscle antibody titer. Primary biliary cirrhosis is mainly associated with alkaline phosphatase level elevations and a high antimitochondrial antibody titer.

Suggested Readings

Adams PC, Valberg LS: Screening blood donors for hemochromatosis: Decision analysis model comparing genotyping to phenotyping. Am J Gastroenterol 1999;94:1593-1600.

American Gastroenterological Association: Medical position statement: Evaluation of liver chemistry tests. Gastroenterology 2002;123:1364-1366.

Bassett ML, Halliday JW, Powell LW: Value of hepatic iron measurements in early hemochromatosis and determination of the critical iron level associated with fibrosis. Hepatology 1986;6:24-29.

Carey WD: How should a patient with an isolated GGT be evaluated? Cleve Clin J Med 2000;67:315-316.

Deugnier YM, Turlin B, Powell LW, et al: Differentiation between heterozygotes and homozygotes in genetic hemochromatosis by means of a histological hepatic iron index: A study of 192 cases. Hepatology 1993;17:30-34.

Green RM, Flamm S: AGA technical review on the evaluation of liver chemistry tests. Gastroenterology 2002;123:1367-1384.

Heathcote EJ: Management of primary biliary cirrhosis. The American Association for the Study of Liver Diseases practice guidelines. Hepatology 2000;31:1005-1013.

Lok AS, McMahon BJ: Chronic hepatitis B. Hepatology 2001;34:1225-1241.

Powell LW, George DK, McDonnell SM, Kowdley KV: Diagnosis of hemochromatosis. Ann Intern Med 1998;129:925-931.

Tavill AS, American Association for the Study of Liver Diseases, American College of Gastroenterology, American Gastroenterological Association: Diagnosis and management of hemochromatosis. Hepatology 2001;33:1321-1328.

Younossi ZM: Viral hepatitis guide for practicing physicians. Cleve Clin J Med 2000;67(Suppl 1):S16-S45.

References

For a complete list of references, log onto www.expertconsult.com.

Gallbladder and Biliary Tract Disease

David S. Barnes

GALLBLADDER DISEASES

Gallbladder diseases considered here include gallstones, tumors, and acute acalculous cholecystitis.

Gallstones and Cholecystitis

Definition and Etiology

Gallbladder stones are an extremely common disorder and are usually asymptomatic. Some patients experience biliary colic, an intermittent and often severe pain in the epigastrium or right upper quadrant, and at times between the scapula because of temporary obstruction of the cystic duct with a gallstone. If the cystic duct obstruction persists, the gallbladder becomes inflamed and the patient develops cholecystitis, an acute inflammation and infection of the gallbladder.

Prevalence and Risk Factors

It is estimated that there are 20.5 million cases of gallbladder disease in the United States, 14.2 million of whom are in women.[1] More than 600,000 cholecystectomies per year are performed in the United States, most of which are for symptomatic gallstone disease. Epidemiologic studies have shown variations in the prevalence of gallstones in different ethnic populations, with particularly high rates in Native Americans. In addition to ethnic background, other risk factors for the development of gallstones include diabetes, rapid weight loss, morbid obesity, cirrhosis, and conditions associated with infrequent gallbladder emptying, such as total parenteral nutrition.

Pathophysiology and Natural History

Most gallstones are composed primarily of cholesterol, with smaller amounts of mucus, calcium bilirubinate, and protein. Pigment stones, a result of hemolysis, are less common and are made primarily of calcium bilirubinate. Symptoms occur with gallstones when the gallbladder contracts, often after a meal, resulting in occlusion of the cystic duct with a stone that produces symptoms, typically pain.

Signs and Symptoms

The vast majority of patients with gallstones are asymptomatic. Symptomatic gallstones typically manifest with right upper quadrant abdominal pain, often accompanied by nausea and vomiting. The pain is often severe, may abate over several hours (biliary colic), or may progress to cholecystitis, with persistent pain and fever. On examination, there is pain to palpation in the right upper quadrant (Murphy's sign).

Diagnosis

The imaging study of choice is a right upper quadrant ultrasound, which, in the presence of cholecystitis, typically shows the presence of gallstones, a thickened gallbladder wall, and pericholecystic fluid. In those patients with symptomatic gallstones and a negative ultrasound examination, endoscopic ultrasound may be helpful.[2] To confirm the suspicion of cholecystitis, a hydroxyiminodiacetic acid (HIDA) scan can be useful. The radionuclide material is concentrated in the liver and excreted into the bile but does not fill the gallbladder because of cystic duct obstruction.

Summary: Acute Cholecystitis

- Right upper quadrant abdominal pain, nausea, and vomiting
- Ultrasound reveals
- Thickened gallbladder wall
- Pericholecystic
- HIDA scan reveals nonvisualized gallbladder

Treatment

The primary treatment for symptomatic gallstone disease is cholecystectomy. Prophylactic cholecystectomy for silent gallstones is not warranted.[3] Most cholecystectomies in the United States are done laparoscopically. A patient with an acute episode that resolves should see a surgeon within a few weeks and elective cholecystectomy should be considered. Patients who have persistent right upper quadrant tenderness and develop fever or an elevated white blood cell count should be seen more urgently.

Common bile duct stones can accompany acute cholecystitis in up to 10% of cases. These stones can be removed endoscopically before or after cholecystectomy, or surgically at the time of laparoscopic or open cholecystectomy.

Most good-risk patients who undergo elective laparoscopic cholecystectomy are sent home within 24 hours. Patients who undergo open cholecystectomy may require hospitalization for several days. It is estimated that 95% of patients experience relief of pain after cholecystectomy. The remaining patients probably had symptoms not related to gallbladder disease before surgery.

Practice guidelines for the treatment of gallstones and gallbladder disease are available from the Society for Surgery of the Alimentary Tract (SSAT). These guidelines (available at http://www.ssat.com/cgi-bin/guidelines.cgi) review the symptoms and diagnosis of gallstone disease and make treatment recommendations regarding surgical consultation and indications for surgery. They review the risks of cholecystectomy, both laparoscopic and open, and the expected outcomes. There are also recommendations for the treatment of common duct stones.

Gallbladder Tumors

Benign and malignant tumors can occur in the gallbladder. Benign tumors consist of papillomas, adenomyomas, or cholesterol polyps. Malignant tumors of the gallbladder are uncommon. The most common malignant tumor of the gallbladder is adenocarcinoma, although squamous cell carcinoma, cystadenocarcinoma, and adenoacanthomas have been reported. Adenocarcinoma of the gallbladder is associated with chronic cholecystitis; exposure to rubber or petroleum products has also been suggested as a cause. It occurs more commonly in women and those older than 50 years.

Patients with small gallbladder tumors may present with symptoms suggesting cholecystitis (e.g., abdominal pain, fever), whereas larger tumors may manifest late with jaundice and an abdominal mass. Computed tomography (CT) or ultrasound scans will reveal a gallbladder mass and, in the case of larger tumors, a mass in the liver and evidence of biliary obstruction. Patients with the incidental finding of gallbladder carcinoma at the time of cholecystectomy have a good prognosis. Otherwise, the 5-year survival rate of patients with gallbladder cancer is only about 5%.

Special mention should be made of the finding on ultrasound of polypoid lesions of the gallbladder, gallbladder polyps. Histologically, there are four types of polypoid lesions, including cholesterol polyps, adenomas, adenomyomatous hyperplasia, and malignant polyps. Although polyp size (larger than 10 mm) and patient age (older than 60 years) are more suggestive of malignancy, no radiologic test can distinguish benign from malignant polyps in the absence of metastatic or invasive cancer.[4] Although there are no firm guidelines, cholecystectomy for patients with polyps larger than 10 mm seems warranted.[4,5] Regular follow-up ultrasound examination for patients with polyps smaller than 10 mm has been suggested, but prospective studies confirming the benefit of such a surveillance program have not been done.[4]

Acute Acalculous Cholecystitis

Acute acalculous cholecystitis is an acute inflammatory disease of the gallbladder not associated with gallstones. About 10% of the 500,000 cholecystectomies performed each year in the United States are for acalculous cholecystitis. The pathogenesis is believed to be an ischemic injury to the gallbladder wall, compounded by chemical injury caused by bile acids. It is often seen in patients hospitalized for trauma or burns who have a superimposed sepsis and are on mechanical ventilation. It is also associated with patients with vascular disease and immunodeficiency.

Clinical manifestations can be similar to those seen with calculous cholecystitis (right upper quadrant pain, fever, and a positive Murphy sign [pain during inspiration associated with palpation of the right upper quadrant]) but are typically subtler in a ventilated patient in the intensive care unit, in whom usual clinical clues are absent. When acalculous cholecystitis is being considered, ultrasound is the diagnostic test of choice and shows a thickened gallbladder wall, pericholecystic fluid, and a sonographic Murphy's sign. Cholecystectomy, open or laparoscopic, is the definitive therapy. In patients who are a prohibitively high surgical risk, an ultrasound-guided percutaneous cholecystostomy tube provides drainage of the gallbladder without surgery. Another nonsurgical approach is transpapillary endoscopic drainage of the gallbladder.[6] The outcome of patients with acalculous cholecystitis depends to a large extent on the underlying illness, but mortality can be as high as 30% when perforation of the gallbladder occurs as a complication.[7]

BILIARY TRACT DISEASES

Choledocholithiasis

Definition and Causes

One of the most common causes of extrahepatic biliary obstruction is choledocholithiasis, with one or more stones in the common bile duct or common hepatic duct causing biliary obstruction.

Prevalence and Risk Factors

Up to 10% of patients with gallstones have common bile duct stones. Common bile duct stones have been discovered days to several years after surgery in as many as 5% of patients who have undergone cholecystectomy.[8] It is believed that the stones represent retained stones or stones that have formed de novo after the operation.

Pathophysiology and Natural History

Stones in the bile duct can cause biliary obstruction and cholestasis. This can lead to infection in the bile duct (bacterial cholangitis), which requires urgent medical therapy. The long-standing presence of stones in the bile duct can lead to secondary biliary cirrhosis. Choledocholithiasis can also lead to gallstone pancreatitis.

Signs and Symptoms

Most patients with choledocholithiasis report upper abdominal pain, although some patients may remain asymptomatic. Because complete obstruction of the bile duct by the stone may be intermittent, patients may report episodic jaundice.

The initial manifestation of choledocholithiasis can also be heralded by an episode of cholangitis. Gallstone pancreatitis manifests with typical features of pancreatitis, including epigastric pain, nausea, and vomiting.

Diagnosis

Several diagnostic tools can be used when evaluating patients suspected of having choledocholithiasis. Ultrasound is the preferred initial screening test because it is usually less expensive than CT or magnetic resonance imaging (MRI), does not use ionizing radiation, and is highly accurate in detecting gallbladder stones and bile duct dilation.[9] MR cholangiography has gained acceptance as a tool for diagnosing choledocholithiasis. Its accuracy in detecting bile duct stones approaches that of endoscopic retrograde cholangiography.[10] Abdominal CT scanning can also be helpful in evaluating patients with obstructive jaundice. It is as accurate as ultrasound in detecting common duct stones and may help localize the level of obstruction in the biliary tree.

Once biliary dilation or the presence of a common duct stone is noted on an imaging study, or biliary obstruction is strongly suspected on clinical grounds despite negative imaging studies, endoscopic retrograde cholangiopancreatography (ERCP) is recommended. ERCP provides a means of visualizing the biliary tree and the opportunity for therapy. Percutaneous transhepatic cholangiography can be a useful alternative when ERCP is not successful, although it is sometimes not successful in the absence of dilated bile ducts. Practice guidelines from the Society for Surgery of the Alimentary Tract for the treatment of gallstone and gallbladder diseases can be found online (www.ssat.com/cgi-bin/chole7.cgi).

Treatment

The goals of therapy for choledocholithiasis are to remove the stones from the biliary tree and to decompress the biliary tree urgently if bacterial cholangitis is present. Stone extraction can be accomplished with ERCP, often preceded by an endoscopic sphincterotomy. In the presence of bacterial cholangitis, when a stone cannot be removed for technical reasons—for example, because of its large size—an endoscopically placed biliary stent can be useful for decompressing the biliary tree. An alternative to ERCP for the treatment of choledocholithiasis is percutaneous transhepatic cholangiography (PTHC). PTHC can be used for emergent drainage of the biliary tree in the presence of cholangitis. Passage of a wire into the duodenum via a percutaneous approach can also help guide an endoscopist when performing an ERCP with stone extraction if ERCP had previously failed because of technical factors.

Cholangiocarcinoma

Definition

Cholangiocarcinoma is an adenocarcinoma of the intrahepatic or extrahepatic bile duct.

Prevalence and Risk Factors

There are 2000 to 3000 new cases per year of cholangiocarcinoma in the United States, accounting for 10% to 15% of all primary hepatobiliary malignancies.[11] It is most common in middle-aged men. Primary sclerosing cholangitis (PSC) is a major risk factor for the development of cholangiocarcinoma. In a large Swedish study, 8% of patients with PSC developed cholangiocarcinoma over a mean follow-up period of 5 years.[12] However, this study might have underestimated the actual incidence of PSC-associated cholangiocarcinoma. Other diseases associated with the development of cholangiocarcinoma include choledochal cysts and infection with liver flukes, including *Opisthorchis* (formerly *Clonorchis*) *sinensis*, *O. felineus*, and *O. viverrini*.

Pathophysiology and Natural History

Cholangiocarcinoma is a malignant transformation of the bile ducts, including the ducts in the intrahepatic, perihilar, or extrahepatic biliary tree. A commonly used classification system for cholangiocarcinoma is based on the anatomic location of the tumor.[13] The natural history is one of progression, with a poor 5-year survival rate, lower than 5%. A tissue diagnosis is often difficult to obtain and, in the absence of obviously metastatic disease or extensive local spread, surgical exploration is the only way to determine resectability.

Signs and Symptoms

Patients typically present with jaundice and pruritus and more generalized symptoms, such as weight loss, anorexia, and fatigue. Cholangiocarcinoma should always be suspected in a previously stable patient with PSC who has a rapid clinical decline.

Diagnosis

Initial diagnostic testing for cholangiocarcinoma is similar to that used for other causes of cholestasis. Laboratory testing typically shows an elevated level of alkaline phosphatase of liver origin, with or without an elevation of the bilirubin level. Ultrasound examination, MRI, or CT scanning may reveal areas of focal biliary dilation. MRI is the optimal imaging study when cholangiocarcinoma is suspected.[14] Direct cholangiography with ERCP or PTHC cholangiography with brush cytology of the biliary tree can be useful for diagnosis, although the sensitivity for detecting malignancy with brush cytology is less than 75%.[15]

Blood testing for cancer antigens, particularly CA19-9, has been shown to be useful in detecting cholangiocarcinoma, as has an index using CA19-9 and carcinoembryonic antigen (CEA).[16-18] Neither method is highly sensitive or specific but can help confirm suspected cholangiocarcinoma.

Treatment

Surgical resection of cholangiocarcinoma has resulted in a 5-year survival rate of 16% to 44%.[19,20] Liver transplantation for cholangiocarcinoma is not offered by most transplantation centers because of a high recurrence rate after transplantation. Some centers have had a more favorable outcome with radiation and chemotherapy followed by liver transplantation in patients with early-stage disease.[21,22] Palliative therapy includes percutaneously or endoscopically placed biliary stenting. Photodynamic therapy has also been used with some success.[23]

Miscellaneous Conditions Causing Biliary Tract Obstruction

Benign Tumors

Although most bile duct tumors are malignant, some benign biliary lesions result in biliary obstruction and cholestasis. These include papillomas, adenomas, and cystadenomas.[24]

Ampullary Tumors

Tumors of the ampulla of Vater can be benign (adenomas) or malignant (ampullary carcinoma). Either can result in biliary obstruction and can be confused with cholangiocarcinoma and pancreatic adenocarcinoma. At presentation, patients are often jaundiced and may have a palpable gallbladder because of bile duct obstruction distal to the cystic duct. Laboratory findings typically show an elevation of alkaline phosphatase and bilirubin levels.

Imaging studies of the biliary tree will often show dilation, suggesting a distal bile duct obstruction. Further investigation with a side-viewing duodenoscope will reveal the presence of the ampullary tumor. Ampullary adenomas, often seen with familial adenomatous polyposis, can be treated with surgical excision of the ampulla.[25,26] Whipple's procedure is the treatment of choice for those with resectable ampullary carcinoma.

The 5-year survival rate is as high as 60% in patients with tumor-free surgical margins.[27] For patients who are not surgical candidates, ERCP with sphincterotomy can provide palliation for what are often slow-growing tumors.

Pancreatic Disorders

Carcinoma of the head of the pancreas can manifest with painless jaundice caused by obstruction of the bile duct as it passes through the head of the pancreas. Weight loss, fatigue, and other constitutional symptoms often accompany the cholestasis. CT scanning or ultrasound typically reveal biliary ductal dilation to the level of the pancreatic head and a pancreatic mass.

Cholestasis can also result from benign pancreatic disorders such as chronic pancreatitis resulting in pancreatic fibrosis leading to common duct narrowing and cholestasis or a pancreatic pseudocyst causing compression of the biliary tree.

Mirizzi's Syndrome

Mirizzi's syndrome is caused by an impacted cystic duct stone, leading to gallbladder distention and subsequent compression of the extrahepatic biliary tree. Occasionally, the gallstone erodes into the common hepatic duct, producing a cholecystocholedochal fistula. The original classification of Mirizzi's syndrome has been expanded to include hepatic duct stenosis caused by a stone at the junction of the cystic and hepatic ducts or as a result of cholecystitis, even in the absence of a obstructing cystic duct stone.[28]

Patients present with jaundice, right upper quadrant, pain and fever. Ultrasound or CT scanning reveals biliary dilation above the cystic duct. ERCP may reveal the obstructing stone, which can occasionally be removed, but the definitive treatment is usually surgical, consisting of cholecystectomy with surgical repair of the bile duct, if necessary.

AIDS Cholangiopathy

Cholestasis can be seen in AIDS as a result of biliary ductal changes seen on a cholangiogram that resemble primary sclerosing cholangitis. The ductal strictures are believed to be caused by infections, including *Cryptosporidium* spp, cytomegalovirus, microsporidian, and *Cyclospora* spp.[29]

Patients present with right upper quadrant pain and laboratory tests suggesting cholestasis. A wide variety of other hepatobiliary abnormalities may also occur in those with HIV infection, including granulomatous liver disease from mycobacteria, fungi, or drugs, bacterial abscesses, neoplasms such as Kaposi's sarcoma or lymphoma, and drug toxicity. Initial evaluation should include ultrasound and ERCP if the ultrasound is abnormal.[30] ERCP should also be carried out despite a normal ultrasound if there is evidence of severe abdominal pain. Endoscopic therapy is useful in certain circumstances. Endoscopic sphincterotomy is useful for those patients with symptoms of papillary stenosis (e.g., abdominal pain, jaundice, cholangitis). Endoscopic stenting of the dominant structure of the biliary may also be helpful.

Parasites

Extrahepatic biliary obstruction has been seen with various parasitic infections, such as *Strongyloides* and *Ascaris* spp, and liver flukes, such as *Opisthorchis sinensis* and *Fasciola hepatica*.

Suggested Readings

Anthony PP: Tumors of the hepatobiliary system. In Fletcher CDM (ed): Diagnostic Histopathology of Tumors. London, Churchill Livingstone, 2000, pp 411-460.

Balfe DM, Ralls PW, Bree RL, et al: Imaging strategies in the initial evaluation of the jaundiced patient. American College of Radiology. ACR Appropriateness Criteria. Radiology 2000;215(Suppl):125-133.

Broomé U, Olsson R, Lööf L, et al: Natural history and prognostic factors in 305 Swedish patients with primary sclerosing cholangitis. Gut 1996;38:610-615.

de Groen PC, Gores GJ, LaRusso NF, et al: Biliary tract cancers. N Engl J Med 1999;341:1368-1378.

Everhart JE, Khare M, Hill M, Maurer KR: Prevalence and ethnic differences in gallbladder disease in the United States. Gastroenterology 1999;117:632-639.

Heimbach JK, Gores GJ, Haddock MG, et al: Liver transplantation for unresectable perihilar cholangiocarcinoma. Semin Liver Dis 2004;24:201-207.

Hermann RE: The spectrum of biliary stone disease. Am J Surg 1989;158:171-173.

Khan SA, Davidson BR, Goldin R, et al: Guidelines for the diagnosis and treatment of cholangiocarcinoma: Consensus document. Gut 2002;51:7-9.

Ransohoff DF, Gracie WA: Prophylactic cholecystectomy or expectant management for silent gallstones. Ann Intern Med 1983;99:199-204.

Torok N, Gores GJ: Cholangiocarcinoma. Semin Gastrointest Dis 2001;12:125-132.

References

For a complete list of references, log onto www.expertconsult.com.

Alcoholic Liver Disease

Kyrsten D. Fairbanks

DEFINITION AND ETIOLOGY

Liver disease related to alcohol consumption fits into one of three categories: fatty liver, alcoholic hepatitis, or cirrhosis (Table 1). Fatty liver, which occurs after acute alcohol ingestion, is generally reversible with abstinence and is not believed to predispose to any chronic form of liver disease if abstinence or moderation is maintained. Alcoholic hepatitis is an acute form of alcohol-induced liver injury that occurs with the consumption of a large quantity of alcohol over a prolonged period of time; it encompasses a spectrum of severity ranging from asymptomatic derangement of biochemistries to fulminant liver failure and death. Cirrhosis involves replacement of the normal hepatic parenchyma with extensive thick bands of fibrous tissue and regenerative nodules, which results in the clinical manifestations of portal hypertension and liver failure.

PREVALENCE AND RISK FACTORS

The prevalence of alcoholic liver disease is influenced by many factors, including genetic factors (e.g., predilection to alcohol abuse, sex) and environmental factors (e.g., availability of alcohol, social acceptability of alcohol use, concomitant hepatotoxic insults), and it is therefore difficult to define. In general, however, the risk of liver disease increases with the quantity and duration of alcohol intake.[1,2] Although necessary, excessive alcohol use is not sufficient to promote alcoholic liver disease. Only one in five heavy drinkers develops alcoholic hepatitis, and one in four develops cirrhosis.[3]

Different alcoholic beverages contain varying quantities of alcohol (Table 2). Although fatty liver is a universal finding among heavy drinkers,[3] up to 40% of those with modest alcohol intake (≤10 g/day) also exhibit fatty changes.[1] Based on an autopsy series of men, a threshold daily alcohol intake of 40 g is necessary to produce pathologic changes of alcoholic hepatitis. Consumption of more than 80 g per day is associated with an increase in the severity of alcoholic hepatitis, but not in the overall prevalence.[1] There is a clear dose-dependent relation between alcohol intake and the incidence of alcoholic cirrhosis. A daily intake of more than 60 g of alcohol in men and 20 g in women significantly increases the risk of cirrhosis. In addition, steady daily drinking, as compared with binge drinking, appears to be more harmful.[3]

PATHOPHYSIOLOGY AND NATURAL HISTORY

The liver and, to a lesser extent, the gastrointestinal tract, are the main sites of alcohol metabolism. Within the liver, there are two main pathways of alcohol metabolism, alcohol dehydrogenase and cytochrome P-450 (CYP) 2E1. Alcohol dehydrogenase is a hepatocyte cytosolic enzyme that converts alcohol to acetaldehyde. Acetaldehyde subsequently is metabolized to acetate via the mitochondrial enzyme acetaldehyde dehydrogenase. CYP 2E1 also converts alcohol to acetaldehyde.[4]

Liver damage occurs through several interrelated pathways. Alcohol dehydrogenase and acetaldehyde dehydrogenase cause the reduction of nicotinamide adenine dinucleotide (NAD) to NADH (reduced form of NAD). The altered ratio of NAD/NADH promotes fatty liver through the inhibition of gluconeogenesis and fatty acid oxidation. CYP 2E1, which is upregulated in chronic alcohol use, generates free radicals through the oxidation of nicotinamide adenine dinucleotide phosphate (NADPH) to NADP.[4] Chronic alcohol exposure also activates hepatic macrophages, which then produce tumor necrosis factor α (TNF-α).[5] TNF-α induces mitochondria to increase the production of reactive oxygen species. This oxidative stress promotes hepatocyte necrosis and apoptosis, which is exaggerated in the alcoholic who is deficient in antioxidants such as glutathione and vitamin E. Free radicals initiate lipid peroxidation, which causes inflammation and fibrosis. Inflammation is also incited by acetaldehyde that, when bound covalently to cellular proteins, forms adducts that are antigenic.[4]

With abstinence, morphologic changes of the fatty liver usually revert to normal. Although the short-term prognosis in patients with alcoholic steatosis is excellent, with longer follow-up it has been found that cirrhosis develops more commonly in alcohol abusers with fatty liver changes than in those with normal liver histology.[6] Morphologic features that predict progression to fibrosis, cirrhosis, or both include severe steatosis, giant mitochondria, and the presence of mixed macrovesicular-microvesicular steatosis.[7]

Historically, the 30-day mortality rate in patients with alcoholic hepatitis ranges from 0% to 50%.[8] Clinical and laboratory features are powerful prognostic indicators for short-term mortality. Hepatic encephalopathy, derangement in renal function, hyperbilirubinemia, and prolonged prothrombin time are seen more often in patients who succumb to their illness than in those who survive.[9] Both the discriminant function[10] and the model for end-stage liver disease (MELD) score[11] can be used to predict short-term mortality in patients with alcoholic hepatitis. The MELD score is calculated based on a patient's prothrombin time, serum creatinine, and bilirubin; a calculator can be found on the United Network for Organ Sharing website.[12] Long-term survival in patients with alcoholic hepatitis who discontinue alcohol is significantly better than in those who continue to drink, although it remains considerably below that of an age-matched population. Three-year survival approaches 90% in abstainers, whereas it is less than 70% in active drinkers.[9]

Cirrhosis has historically been considered an irreversible outcome of severe and prolonged liver damage. However, studies involving patients with liver disease from many distinct causes have shown convincingly that fibrosis and cirrhosis might have a component of reversibility.[13] For patients with decompensated alcoholic cirrhosis who undergo transplantation, survival is comparable to that of patients with other causes of liver disease (approximately a 70% 5-year patient survival rate.)[14]

SIGNS AND SYMPTOMS

Patients with fatty liver typically either are asymptomatic or present with nonspecific symptoms that do not suggest acute liver disease. Supporting features on physical examination include an enlarged and smooth, but rarely tender, liver. In the absence of a superimposed hepatic process, stigmata of chronic liver disease such as spider angiomas, ascites, or asterixis should be absent.

Alcoholic hepatitis is a syndrome with a spectrum of severity, and therefore manifesting symptoms vary. Symptoms may be nonspecific and mild and include anorexia and weight loss, abdominal pain and distention, or nausea and vomiting. Alternatively, more severe and specific symptoms can include encephalopathy and hepatic failure. Physical findings include hepatomegaly, jaundice, ascites, spider angiomas, fever, and encephalopathy.[15]

Table 1 Forms of Alcoholic Liver Disease

Parameter	Fatty Liver	Alcoholic Hepatitis	Cirrhosis
Histologic specificity for alcoholic cause	No	No	No
Prognosis	Excellent	Variable	Guarded
Reversible	Yes	Variable	Generally, no

Table 2 Alcohol Content of Some Common Beverages

Drink	Amount (oz)	Absolute Alcohol (g)
Beer	12	12
Wine	5	12
Liquor (80 proof)	1.5	12

Established alcoholic cirrhosis can manifest with decompensation without a preceding history of fatty liver or alcoholic hepatitis. Alternatively, alcoholic cirrhosis may be diagnosed concurrently with acute alcoholic hepatitis. The symptoms and signs of alcoholic cirrhosis do not help differentiate it from other causes of cirrhosis. Patients may present with jaundice, pruritus, abnormal laboratory findings (e.g., thrombocytopenia, hypoalbuminemia, coagulopathy), or complications of portal hypertension, such as variceal bleeding, ascites, or hepatic encephalopathy.

DIAGNOSIS

Fatty liver is usually diagnosed in the asymptomatic patient who is undergoing evaluation for abnormal liver function tests; typically, aminotransferase levels are less than twice the upper limit of normal. No laboratory test is diagnostic of fatty liver. Characteristic ultrasonographic findings include a hyperechoic liver with or without hepatomegaly. Liver biopsy is rarely needed to diagnose fatty liver in the appropriate clinical setting, but it may be useful in excluding steatohepatitis or fibrosis. Typical histologic findings of fatty liver include fat accumulation in hepatocytes that is often macrovesicular, but it is occasionally microvesicular (Fig. 1). The centrilobular region of the hepatic acinus is most commonly affected. In severe fatty liver, however, fat is distributed throughout the acinus.[16] Fatty liver is not specific to alcohol ingestion; it is associated with obesity, insulin resistance, hyperlipidemia, malnutrition, and various medications. Attribution of fatty liver to alcohol use therefore requires a detailed and accurate patient history.

The diagnosis of alcoholic hepatitis is based on a thorough history, physical examination, and review of laboratory tests. Characteristically, the ratio of aspartate aminotransferase to alanine aminotransferase (AST/ALT) is approximately 2:1, and the absolute aminotransferase level does not exceed 300 U/L unless a superimposed hepatic insult exists, such as acetaminophen toxicity. Other common and nonspecific laboratory abnormalities include anemia and leukocytosis. Liver biopsy is occasionally necessary to secure the diagnosis. The classic histologic features of alcoholic hepatitis include inflammation and necrosis, which are most prominent in the centrilobular region of the hepatic acinus (Fig. 2). Hepatocytes are classically ballooned, which causes compression of the sinusoid and reversible portal hypertension. The inflammatory cell infiltrate, located primarily in the sinusoids and close to necrotic hepatocytes, consists of polymorphonuclear cells and mononuclear cells. In addition to inflammation and necrosis, many patients with alcoholic hepatitis have fatty infiltration and Mallory bodies, which are intracellular perinuclear aggregations of intermediate filaments that are eosinophilic on hematoxylin-eosin staining. Neither fatty infiltration nor Mallory bodies are specific for alcoholic hepatitis or necessary for the diagnosis.[15]

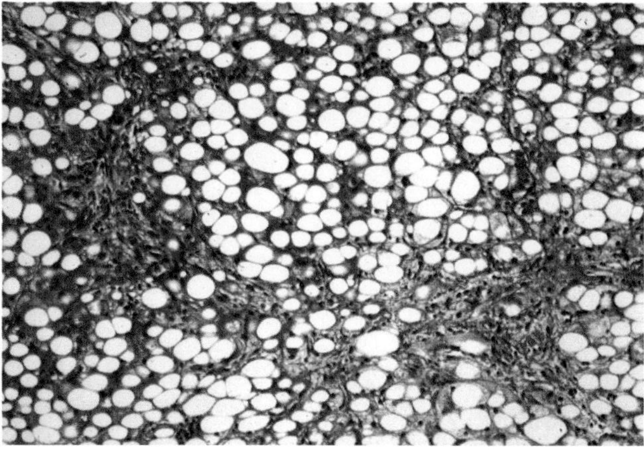

Figure 1 Classic histologic findings in alcoholic liver disease: Alcoholic fatty liver disease. Diffuse macrovesicular steatosis is associated with perisinusoidal fibrosis and lobular necroinflammatory activity (trichrome stain, ×200). *(Courtesy of Dr. Ana Bennett.)*

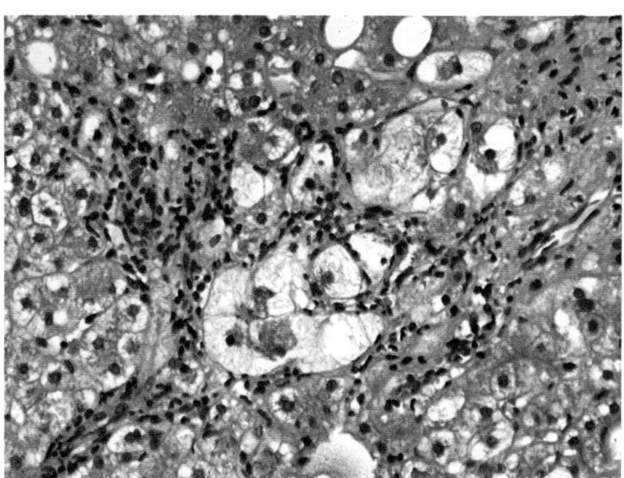

Figure 2 Alcoholic hepatitis: Macrovesicular steatosis associated with hepatocyte ballooning and Mallory bodies. These inclusions are a characteristic but nonspecific feature of alcoholic liver disease (hematoxylin-eosin stain, ×200). *(Courtesy of Dr. Ana Bennett.)*

The diagnosis of alcoholic cirrhosis rests on finding the classic signs and symptoms of end-stage liver disease in a patient with a history of significant alcohol intake. Patients tend to underreport their alcohol consumption, and discussions with family members and close friends might provide a more accurate estimation of alcohol intake. Patients can present with any or all complications of portal hypertension, including ascites, variceal bleeding, and hepatic encephalopathy. The histology of end-stage alcoholic cirrhosis, in the absence of acute alcoholic hepatitis, resembles that of advanced liver disease from many other causes, without any distinct pathologic findings (Fig. 3)[17].

The overall clinical diagnosis of alcoholic liver disease, using a combination of physical findings, laboratory values, and clinical acumen, is very accurate (Box 1). However, liver biopsy can be justified in select cases, especially when the diagnosis is in question. In addition to confirming the diagnosis, liver biopsy is also useful for

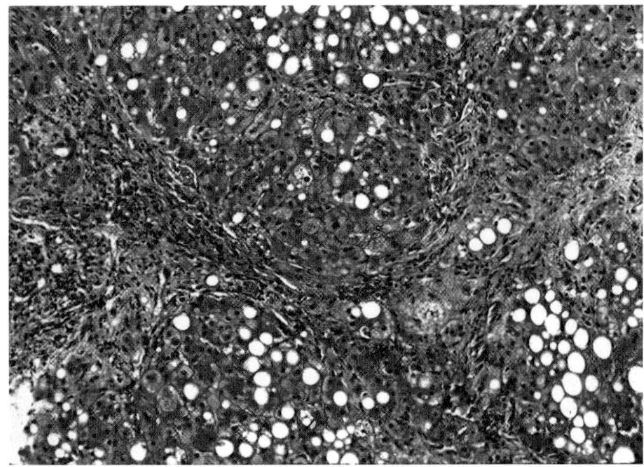

Figure 3 Alcoholic cirrhosis. Fibrous septa act as a bridge between centrilobular regions and portal tracts with the development of cirrhosis (trichrome stain, ×200). *(Courtesy of Dr. Ana Bennett.)*

Box 1 Physical Examination and Laboratory Findings in Alcoholic Liver Disease

Physical Examination

Constitutional: Fever
Skin: Spider angioma
Parotid and lacrimal gland enlargement
Palmer erythema
Jaundice
Decreased body hair
Gynecomastia
Musculoskeletal: Dupuytren's contracture
Clubbing
Muscle wasting
Genitourinary: Testicular atrophy
Abdomen: Hepatomegaly or small shrunken liver
Splenomegaly
Ascites
Hepatic tenderness
Neurologic: Asterixis
Confusion, stupor

Laboratory Findings

Liver synthetic function: Hyperbilirubinemia (usually conjugated)
Prolonged prothrombin time
Hypoalbuminemia
Liver enzyme levels: Aspartate aminotransferase (AST) and alanine aminotransferase (ALT) levels elevated, usually <300 U/L; AST/ALT ratio ~ 2:1
Hematologic: Anemia
Leukocytosis or leukopenia
Thrombocytopenia
Increased serum globulin levels
Metabolic: Elevated blood ammonia level
Hyperglycemia
Respiratory alkalosis
Hypomagnesemia
Hypophosphatemia
Hyponatremia
Hypokalemia

ruling out other unsuspected causes of liver disease, better characterizing the extent of the damage, providing prognosis, and guiding therapeutic decision making. As emphasized in the recent practice guidelines for alcoholic liver disease from the American College of Gastroenterology,[18] liver biopsy is a relatively safe procedure, with morbidity lower than 0.6% and mortality lower than 0.03%.

Summary

- All patients should be screened for alcoholic liver disease.
- Alcoholic liver disease is a heterogeneous disease.
- No physical examination finding or laboratory abnormality is specific for alcoholic liver disease.
- The diagnosis of alcoholic liver disease requires a detailed patient history, with supportive laboratory and imaging studies.
- Liver biopsy may be useful to confirm the diagnosis, rule out other diseases, and prognosticate.

TREATMENT

The foundation of therapy for alcoholic liver disease is abstinence. Patients are often unable to achieve complete and durable alcohol abstinence without assistance, and referral to a chemical dependency team is appropriate. Hospitalization is indicated to expedite a diagnostic evaluation of patients with jaundice, encephalopathy, or ascites of unknown cause. In addition, patients with known alcoholic liver disease who present with renal failure, fever, inadequate oral intake to maintain hydration, or rapidly deteriorating liver function, as demonstrated by progressive encephalopathy or coagulopathy, should be hospitalized.

Nutritional Support

Supportive care for all patients includes adequate nutrition. Almost all patients with alcoholic hepatitis have some degree of malnutrition, but estimating the severity of malnutrition remains a challenge because sensitive and specific clinical or laboratory parameters are lacking. The nutritionist plays a valuable role in assessing the degree of malnutrition and guiding nutritional supplementation in malnourished alcoholic patients. The degree of malnutrition correlates directly with short-term (1-month) and long-term (1-year) mortality. At 1 year from the time of diagnosis of alcoholic hepatitis, patients with mild malnutrition have a 14% mortality rate, compared with a 76% mortality rate in those with severe malnutrition.[19] Attempts to correct protein-calorie malnutrition with supplemental oral or parenteral nutrition, or both, have met with mixed results. In general, enteral nutrition is preferable over parenteral supplementation, and protein should be supplied to provide positive nitrogen balance. Branched-chain amino acids are useful as a supplement to maintain positive nitrogen balance in patients who do not tolerate liberal protein intake because of the development of encephalopathy; however, their expense limits routine use in all alcoholic malnourished patients. Nutritional supplementation is generally associated with an improvement in liver test results, but only rarely with a mortality benefit.[20] Refer to the most recent practice guidelines for a summary of recommendations for daily feeding in patients with alcoholic liver disease[18].

Medical Therapy

The use of corticosteroids as specific therapy for alcoholic hepatitis has received a great deal of interest. The rationale behind their use is the possible role of the immune system in initiating and perpetuating hepatic damage. Three randomized, controlled trials that investigated the use of corticosteroids (prednisolone 40 mg/day, or the equivalent methylprednisolone 28 mg/day, for 28 days) for patients with severe acute alcoholic hepatitis have suggested a significant decrease in short-term (30-day) mortality in patients randomized to prednisolone, but only those with more-severe liver dysfunction, as manifested by hepatic encephalopathy or a markedly abnormal discriminant function.[10,21,22] The discriminant function predicts the risk of early mortality in acute alcoholic hepatitis, and is calculated using the following formula:

$$(4.6 \times [\text{prothrombin time} - \text{control time}]) + \text{serum bilirubin (mg/dL)}$$

with the prothrombin and control times in seconds.

Results from other randomized, controlled trials have been contradictory.[23,24] Several meta-analyses have been conducted in an effort to overcome low statistical power in individual trials.[25-27] Analyses by Mathurin and colleagues[27] and Imperiale and McCullough[25] support the use of corticosteroids in a select group of patients with severe alcoholic hepatitis manifested by a discriminant function of more than 32, hepatic encephalopathy, or both. Christensen and Gluud[26] found no effect of corticosteroids on mortality. Most recent trials of corticosteroids for alcoholic hepatitis have excluded patients with certain coexisting conditions, such as gastrointestinal bleeding, active infection, diabetes, viral hepatitis, or acute pancreatitis, and therefore the applicability of these study findings is limited. Practice guidelines[18] support the use of corticosteroids in patients with severe alcoholic hepatitis in whom the diagnosis is certain.

The most recent practice guidelines[18] did not addressed the use of pentoxifylline in the treatment of alcoholic hepatitis, because studies with pentoxifylline were published after the guidelines. Pentoxifylline is an inhibitor of TNF synthesis. Elevated TNF levels have been associated with higher mortality from alcoholic hepatitis.[28] A randomized, double-blind, controlled trial investigated the effects of treatment with pentoxifylline on short-term survival and progression to the hepatorenal syndrome in patients with severe alcoholic hepatitis.[29] Pentoxifylline-treated patients had a significant decrease in mortality (24% vs. 46%, $P = .037$). The survival advantage was primarily due to a decrease in the development of hepatorenal syndrome in pentoxifylline-treated patients (50% vs. 91.7%, $P = .009$). Although promising, these findings have yet to be validated by independent investigation.

Other therapies that have been investigated in the treatment of alcoholic hepatitis but not found to be beneficial include propylthiouracil,[30] infliximab,[31] insulin and glucagon,[32,33] calcium channel blockers,[34] and antioxidants, such as vitamin E.[35]

General Treatment

Treatment of the patient with alcoholic cirrhosis mirrors the care of patients with any other type of cirrhosis, and includes prevention and management of ascites, spontaneous bacterial peritonitis, variceal bleeding, encephalopathy, malnutrition, and hepatocellular carcinoma. Once advanced cirrhosis has occurred with evidence of decompensation (ascites, spontaneous bacterial peritonitis, hepatic encephalopathy, variceal bleeding), patients should be referred to a transplantation center.

Acute alcoholic hepatitis, no matter how severe, is an absolute contraindication for liver transplantation. For more than a decade, alcoholic cirrhosis has been the second leading indication for liver transplantation in the United States. Most transplantation centers currently require patients with a history of alcohol abuse to have documented abstinence of at least 6 months before undergoing transplantation. This requirement theoretically has a dual advantage of predicting long-term sobriety and allowing recovery of liver function from acute alcoholic hepatitis. This 6-month abstinence rule might not have much prognostic significance in predicting recidivism, however. Alcohol use of any quantity after transplantation for alcohol-related liver disease approaches 50% during the first 5 years, and abuse occurs in up to 15% of patients.[36]

Table 3 summarizes investigated treatments for alcoholic liver disease.

Table 3 Treatments Investigated for Alcoholic Liver Disease

Treatment	Routine Use Recommended	Potential Benefit
Abstinence	Yes	Survival
Nutritional support	Yes	Survival, laboratory
Corticosteroids	Consider if DF ≥32	Survival
Pentoxifylline	Consider (preliminary data)	Survival, less renal failure
Propylthiouracil	No	No
Infliximab	No	No
Colchicine	No	No
Insulin, glucagon	No	No
Calcium channel blocker	No	No
Vitamin E	No	No
Liver transplantation	Consider (for decompensated cirrhosis)	Survival ~ 70% at 5 yr

DF, discriminant function.

Summary

- Abstinence is the cornerstone of treatment of alcoholic liver disease.
- Nutritional deficiencies should be sought and treated aggressively.
- Corticosteroids should be used in patients with a definite diagnosis of severe alcoholic hepatitis, who have a discriminant function of more than 32, hepatic encephalopathy, or both. Corticosteroids have not been evaluated in patients with renal failure, active infection, pancreatitis, or gastrointestinal bleeding.

PREVENTION AND SCREENING

As emphasized in the most recent national practice guidelines,[18] health care providers must be attentive for signs of covert alcohol abuse. Many patients do not openly disclose an accurate history of alcohol use. In addition, no physical examination finding or laboratory abnormality is specific for alcoholic liver disease. All patients should therefore be screened for alcohol abuse or dependency. The CAGE questionnaire (*c*utting down on drinking, *a*nnoyance at others' concerns about drinking, feeling *g*uilty about drinking, using alcohol as an *e*ye opener in the morning) is the preferred screening tool, with two or more positive answers providing a sensitivity of 70% to 96% and a specificity of 91% to 99% for alcohol dependency.[18]

Suggested Readings

Christensen E, Gluud C: Glucocorticoids are ineffective in alcoholic hepatitis: A meta-analysis adjusting for confounding variables. Gut 1995;37:113-118.

Grant BF, Dufour MC, Harford TC: Epidemiology of alcoholic liver disease. Semin Liver Dis 1988;8:12-25.

Imperiale TF, McCullough AJ: Do corticosteroids reduce mortality from alcoholic hepatitis? Ann Intern Med 1990;113:299-307.

Maddrey WC. Alcoholic hepatitis: Clinicopathologic features and therapy. Semin Liver Dis 1998;8:91-102.

Mathurin P, Mendenhall CL, Carithers RL, et al: Corticosteroids improve short-term survival in patients with severe alcoholic hepatitis (AH): Individual data anlysis of the last three randomized placebo controlled double blind trials of corticosteroids in severe AH. J Hepatology 2002;36:480-487.

McCullough AJ, O'Connor JFB: Alcoholic liver disease: Proposed recommendations for the American College of Gastroenterology. Am J Gastroenterol 1998;93:2022-2036.

Savolainen VT, Liesto K, Männikkö A, et al: Alcohol consumption and alcoholic liver disease: Evidence of a threshold level of effects of ethanol. Alcohol Clin Exp Res 1993;17:1112-1117.

Schenker S, Halff GA: Nutritional therapy in alcoholic liver disease. Semin Liver Dis 1993;13:196-209.

Stewart S, Jones D, Day CP: Alcoholic liver disease: New insights into mechanisms and preventative strategies. Trends Mol Med 2001;7:408-413.

United Network for Organ Sharing: Model for End-Stage Liver Disease (MELD) Calculator, 2007. Available at http://www.unos.org/resources/MeldPeldCalculator.asp?index=98 (accessed March 15, 2009).

References

For a complete list of references, log onto www.expertconsult.com.

Inherited Metabolic Liver Diseases

Anthony S. Tavill

There are many inherited metabolic diseases that may have a pathologic impact on the liver. In many cases, the liver component of these diseases is an epiphenomenon of a more generalized systemic disorder. Examples of such epiphenomena are glycogen and lipid storage diseases, in which hepatomegaly is a manifestation of the underlying metabolic defect, although the liver is not necessarily the major target organ. However, there are three genetically determined diseases in which the liver may be the principal target organ, with manifestations of acute, subacute, or chronic disease that can become evident in early or later life. These are hereditary hemochromatosis, a major disorder of iron overload; Wilson disease, a genetic disorder of copper overload; and alpha$_1$-antitrypsin (α_1-AT) deficiency, a disorder in which the normal processing of a liver-produced protein is disturbed within the liver cell.

In some cases, the awareness of these conditions is brought about by suspicion based on a specific clinical syndrome. In other cases, these conditions have to be excluded when faced with nonspecific liver disease abnormalities, such as elevated liver enzyme levels, hepatomegaly, or previously undiagnosed portal hypertension. In the case of hemochromatosis, the approach to early diagnosis has moved one step further, with an awareness that markers of iron overload may be present in the serum long before liver disease has developed. This chapter focuses on discussions of these three conditions.

Certain key concepts are common to all three conditions and need to be emphasized at the outset. First, although the recognition of inherited liver disease is often a process of exclusion of more common causes (e.g., viruses, alcohol, autoimmunity), it is important to emphasize that awareness of the clinical features of these metabolic liver diseases should promote a proactive diagnostic evaluation. Second, inherited metabolic liver disease can manifest in childhood or may be delayed until adult life; in some cases it can regress after childhood or adolescent years, only to reappear later in life. Third, with the advent of molecular diagnostic testing, phenotypic assessment of these conditions may be now complemented in certain cases by genotypic evaluation. Fourth, with the availability of effective treatments, there has been a dramatic impact on the prognosis of metabolic liver diseases in both childhood and adult life, further emphasizing the importance of early diagnosis. Finally, in several conditions (e.g., α_1-AT deficiency, Wilson disease), liver transplantation corrects the primary biochemical abnormality in the liver and effectively cures the disease.

Summary

- Awareness of the clinical features of inherited metabolic liver diseases should promote proactive diagnostic evaluation.
- The clinical features of certain inherited metabolic liver diseases can manifest in childhood, disappear during growth and development, and reappear in adult life.
- Molecular diagnostic testing has made genotypic evaluation available for some diseases to complement phenotypic diagnosis.
- Preemptive treatment may prevent the development of phenotypic complications in some diseases (e.g., hereditary hemochromatosis and Wilson disease), and liver transplantation may be curative in others (e.g., alpha$_1$-antitrypsin deficiency and Wilson disease).

Alpha$_1$-Antitrypsin Deficiency

Anthony S. Tavill and Loutfi S. Aboussouan

DEFINITION

α_1-AT deficiency is a common inherited disorder associated with retention of the liver-produced protein α_1-AT in the liver and low levels of α_1-AT in the serum. In the most severe form of α_1-AT deficiency, the clinical features consist of early-onset emphysema, neonatal hepatitis, chronic hepatitis, cirrhosis, and hepatocellular carcinoma. However, phenotypic expression throughout life is extremely variable. The gene for α_1-AT is located on chromosome 14, and mutations at the protease inhibitor (PI) locus lead to a single amino acid substitution (glutamic acid for lysine 342) that impairs secretion of the mutant gene product, leading to retention of α_1-AT in the hepatocyte and low levels of α_1-AT in the serum. Because the phenotype is expressed by autosomal codominant inheritance, each allele is responsible for 50% of the circulating α_1-AT level. More than 100 allelic variants have been described, only some of which are associated with liver disease. The *Z* allele is the mutation associated with maximum deficiency in α_1-AT.

EPIDEMIOLOGY

The frequency of this pathogenic PI *Z* allele in the U.S. population of European descent is between 0.01 and 0.02, with the homozygous deficiency state affecting 1 in 2000 to 7000 of the population. The major deficiency occurs in the PI *ZZ* phenotypes, with indirect epidemiologic approaches, and more direct population-based screening methods estimating that about 60,000 people in the United States are homozygous for this phenotype. In Scandinavia, the frequency of the *Z* allele is considerably higher, resulting in one PI *ZZ* in 1600 live births. The PI *Z* allele is confined predominantly to whites and is found rarely in African Americans or Asians. There are many other allelic combinations that might have clinical relevance, including the *MZ* heterozygous state and other combinations, such as PI *SZ,* which are also associated with α_1-AT deficiency in the serum.

PATHOPHYSIOLOGY

α_1-AT is the predominant serine PI in the blood, accounting for the α_1 peak on serum protein electrophoresis. α_1-AT functions by inhibition of tissue proteinases that include enzymes such as neutrophil elastase, cathepsin G, and various other proteinases. This is a relatively low-molecular-weight protein, composed of 394 amino acids and several carbohydrate side chains. α_1-AT is also an acute-phase protein, and its synthesis can increase significantly in response to injury or inflammation.

Despite its name, α_1-AT reacts much more readily with neutrophil elastase than with trypsin, in a mutually suicidal interaction that normally maintains an adequate protective screen against the elastolytic burden of neutrophil elastase.

α_1-AT is synthesized within the endoplasmic reticulum of the hepatocyte and undergoes multiple complex foldings and insertions of carbohydrate side chains. Genetic mutations responsible for α_1-AT deficiency can interfere with synthesis, export from the cell, and the ability to function as a proteinase inhibitor.

The *Z* variant results from a single point mutation leading to the substitution of glutamic acid for lysine at position 342. The resultant variant polypeptide is relatively unstable and becomes polymerized within the endoplasmic reticulum, resulting in the periodic acid–Schiff (PAS)-positive globules that can be seen on light microscopy. Only the α_1-AT variants that lead to this type of polymerization are associated with a gain-of-function defect leading to liver cell damage. The rare null variant is not characterized by accumulation of α_1-AT within the hepatocyte and is not associated with liver damage.

Polymerization of mutated antitrypsin prevents its secretion from the hepatocyte, so that only about 15% of the PI *ZZ* antitrypsin is secreted into the plasma. Polymerization and the rare null variant both result in a loss-of-function defect, which increases the risk of developing emphysema.

The most common genetic variant, PI *M,* is present in approximately 95% of the U.S. white population and is regarded as the normal variant associated with normal serum levels of functional α_1-AT. Deficiency alleles, such as PI *Z* and PI *S,* can result in decreased levels of circulating α_1-AT but with completely normal-functioning proteins. The *MM* phenotype is therefore designated as manifesting 100% concentration of circulating α_1-AT. The heterozygous combination *MZ* yields 57.5%, *SZ* 37.5%, and *ZZ* 15% of this normal *MM* value. Approximately 95% of all α_1-AT deficiency states leading to clinical manifestations are made up of PI *ZZ* homozygotes. Certain alleles, such as the *S* allele, either in the homozygous state or associated with the *M* allele, do not appear to be associated with the abnormally polymerized molecules within the endoplasmic reticulum and have not been incriminated in the development of liver or lung disease unless combined with the *Z* allele. The products of these various alleles have distinctive characteristics on isoelectric focusing, which provides a means for the specific identification of the PI types (see later, "Diagnosis").

SIGNS AND SYMPTOMS

The association of α_1-AT deficiency and liver disease in children was first described in 1969 by Dr. Harvey Sharp. Many subsequent clinical studies have observed that liver disease occurrence in α_1-AT deficiency is bimodal, affecting children in neonatal life or early infancy and, less commonly, adults in late middle life. In both these groups, the homozygous form of α_1-AT deficiency is the underlying genetic predeterminant (Box 1).

Box 1 Clinical Manifestations of Alpha$_1$-Antitrypsin Deficiency*

Children
Neonatal or infant hepatitis
Prolonged cholestasis in infancy
Hepatosplenomegaly

Adults
Chronic obstructive pulmonary disease
Chronic hepatitis
Cirrhosis with or without portal hypertension
Hepatocellular carcinoma

**Alpha$_1$-antitrypsin deficiency may also be asymptomatic.*

Children with PI *ZZ* Deficiency of Alpha$_1$-Antitrypsin

Much of the information on the clinical presentation of α_1-AT deficiency in this population has come from Scandinavia. Two thirds of newborns deficient in α_1-AT have abnormal liver enzyme levels, and approximately 10% develop persistent cholestasis during the first year of life. Many of these infants appear to undergo a spontaneous remission, and only about 3% progress to fibrosis or cirrhosis during childhood and teenage years. Nevertheless, careful surveillance has revealed that many of these children have persistently abnormal liver enzyme levels.

Newborns with the most fully expressed form of the disease show evidence of acute neonatal hepatitis, with a predominantly conjugated hyperbilirubinemia. This jaundice can persist for as long as 1 year, with associated evidence of defective growth and the consequences of malabsorption of fat-soluble vitamins. Physical signs also include hepatomegaly and splenomegaly

Adults with PI *ZZ* Deficiency of Alpha$_1$-Antitrypsin

Most adults with PI *ZZ* α_1-AT deficiency are identified by their pulmonary symptoms and show signs and symptoms of chronic obstructive pulmonary disease, with emphysema developing in about 80% to 100% of patients. This condition is often aggravated by cigarette smoking. The emphysema associated with α_1-AT deficiency has distinctive features, including early onset (in the fourth or fifth decade of life), predominant involvement of the lung bases, and panacinar pathology.

The prevalence of associated liver disease has probably been underestimated, but 10% to 40% of these adults might have evidence of cirrhosis. The risk of cirrhosis becomes higher with advancing years, particularly in men. In these cases, a man older than 50 years with evidence of cirrhosis, portal hypertension, or hepatocellular carcinoma and no underlying predisposing cause should evoke suspicion for an underlying metabolic defect such as hemochromatosis or α_1-AT deficiency. The features of the liver disease appear to be rapidly progressive when diagnosed at this stage, with a high likelihood of death within 4 years of the identification of liver disease.

Heterozygous Alpha$_1$-Antitrypsin Deficiency

A number of studies have asserted a role for a single mutant allele in the development of cryptogenic liver disease in adults. Because many of these heterozygous states are associated with intermediate α_1-AT deficiency, it will be necessary to carry out prospective studies to evaluate the pathophysiologic consequences of the heterozygous state. It has been suggested that the presence of a single *Z* allele might act synergistically with other risk factors for liver disease. These associated conditions include chronic viral hepatitis, alcoholic liver disease, and nonalcoholic steatohepatitis.

Box 2 Diagnostic Tests for Alpha$_1$-Antitrypsin Deficiency

Determination of quantitative level of serum alpha$_1$-antitrypsin *and* phenotypic analysis of alpha$_1$-antitrypsin by isoelectric focusing
Gene analysis
Liver biopsy for:

- Light microscopy with evaluation of diastase-resistant, periodic acid–Schiff–positive globules
- Immunochemistry for alpha$_1$-antitrypsin
- Electron microscopy

DIAGNOSIS

α_1-AT deficiency is an example of an inherited metabolic disorder in which the definition of the phenotype also defines the genotype (Box 2). Determination of the α_1-AT serum level by quantitative immunoprecipitation is insufficient evidence for the diagnosis of α_1-AT deficiency. This is because serum levels may be falsely elevated as a result of the particularly robust acute-phase response of this protein. Therefore, determination of the quantitative level of α_1-AT must be combined with phenotypic analysis. This defines the phenotype of the variant PI proteins in the serum and is performed by isoelectric focusing. Patients with the most severe form of deficiency have an allelic variant that migrates to a higher isoelectric point and can be defined as PI *ZZ* phenotypes, and therefore by inference as PI *ZZ* genotypes. Interpretation of the electrophoretic patterns on isoelectric focusing determines the homozygous or heterozygous states, and defines the specific mutant alleles based on their relative position between anode and cathode. Finally, the molecular genetic tools for defining the defect in the nucleotide coding sequence for each of the defective alleles have been developed for population studies but are not currently routinely available in diagnostic laboratories.

Epidemiologic considerations have established a threshold amount of α_1-AT necessary to protect the lung from emphysema. This protective threshold level is 80 mg/dL by radial diffusion, and it is 11 µmol when referenced to functional elastase activity (normal values, 150-350 mg/dL or 20–53 µmol, respectively). In PI *ZZ* individuals, serum α_1-AT levels cluster around a mean value of approximately 6 µmol.

The American Thoracic Society and European Respiratory Society have provided guidelines that recommend testing for α_1-AT deficiency in cases of early-onset emphysema (<45 years); emphysema in the absence of a recognized risk factor; emphysema with prominent basilar hyperlucency; unexplained liver disease; necrotizing panniculitis; antiproteinase 3–positive vasculitis (C-ANCA positive vasculitis); family history of emphysema, bronchiectasis, liver disease, or panniculitis; or bronchiectasis without evident cause.

In patients with manifestations of liver disease, liver biopsy for light microscopy and histochemistry and possibly electron microscopy is valuable for staging liver disease and for identifying the PAS-positive diastase-resistant globules within the hepatocytes. In neonates, the globules may be indistinct and ill developed, but they increase with age. In adult patients, in particular, the globules may be associated with portal and periportal inflammation. Confirmation of the nature of the globules may be provided by immunohistochemical techniques, using immunoperoxidase coupled to α_1-AT antibody. The location of these globules within the endoplasmic reticulum may be confirmed by electron microscopy.

TREATMENT

In advanced and decompensating liver disease, the only available treatment is liver transplantation. α_1-AT deficiency is the most common inherited disorder leading to liver transplantation in children. As in Wilson disease, the outcome of orthotopic liver transplantation is extremely good, and replacement of the liver provides the recipient with the donor's α_1-AT phenotype.

Newer approaches that can have an effect on the secretion of α_1-AT from the hepatocyte can prove helpful, but these are in the experimental stage of development. Although gene therapy might ultimately provide the most hopeful approach for α_1-AT deficiency, it will have to be achieved with the removal of the aberrant mutant gene, which will pose a considerable challenge.

Because α_1-AT deficiency is associated with variable phenotypic expression, it is reasonable to counsel patients with regard to all other possible sources of liver injury, such as alcohol abuse. A similar approach has been adopted for those with lung injury, counseling patients regarding the deleterious effects of smoking.

Augmentation therapy refers to the exogenous infusion of purified pooled human plasma α_1-AT. It can be given on a weekly, biweekly, or monthly basis. Although this has become the mainstay of specific therapy in α_1-AT deficiency with emphysema, the technique offers no significant help in improving the liver injury.

OUTCOMES

The outcomes of treatment, short of liver transplantation, present conflicts of purpose when they are aimed at preventing both liver and lung diseases. This is because the benefits of any approach that increases the serum levels of α_1-AT to protect the lungs do not always offer similar protection to the liver. Only liver transplantation offers an effective cure for the condition by correcting the recipient phenotype and normalizing the circulating levels of α_1-AT.

Summary

- α_1-AT deficiency is an inherited liver disorder caused by disordered α_1-AT secretion by the hepatocyte, with varying phenotypic features.
- The most severe forms are characterized by neonatal hepatitis, chronic hepatitis, cirrhosis, hepatocellular cancer, and early-onset emphysema.
- More than 100 allelic variants of the α_1-AT gene have been described. The *Z* variant is the one associated with the most-severe phenotypic features.
- Diagnosis is confirmed by phenotypic analysis of the variant forms of α_1-AT in the serum and, when there are manifestations of liver disease by a liver biopsy, with immunohistochemical and ultrastructural evaluations.
- Treatment is by liver transplantation for decompensated liver disease and by augmentation therapy for the relief and prevention of symptomatic emphysema.
- Liver transplantation cures the metabolic defect in α_1-AT deficiency.

Suggested Readings

American Thoracic Society/European Respiratory Society Statement: Standards for the diagnosis and management of individuals with alpha-1 antitrypsin deficiency. Am J Respir Crit Care Med 2003;168:818-900.

Berg NO, Eriksson S: Liver disease in adults with alpha-1-antitrypsin deficiency. N Engl J Med 1972;287:1264-1267.

Carrell RW, Lomas DA: Alpha 1-antitrypsin deficiency-a model for conformational diseases. N Engl J Med 2002;346:45-53.

Fairbanks KD, Tavill AS: The liver in alpha 1-antitrypsin deficiency. Amer J Gastroenterol 2008;103:2136-2141.

Perlmutter DH: The cellular basis for liver injury in alpha 1-antitrypsin deficiency. Hepatology 1991;13:172-185.

Perlmutter DH: Clinical manifestations of alpha 1-antitrypsin deficiency. Gastroenterol Clin North Am 1995;24:27-43.

Rosen HR: Liver disease associated with alpha 1-antitrypsin deficiency. In Rosen HR, Martin P (eds): Metabolic Liver Disease: Clinics in Liver Disease, vol 2. Philadelphia, WB Saunders, 1998, pp 175-185.

Sharp HL, Bridges RA, Krivit W, Freier EF: Cirrhosis associated with alpha-1-antitrypsin deficiency: A previously unrecognized inherited disorder. J Lab Clin Med 1969;73:934-939.

Stoller JK, Aboussouan LS: Alpha1-antitrypsin deficiency. Lancet. 2005;365:2225-2236.

Hemochromatosis

Anthony S. Tavill

DEFINITION

Hereditary hemochromatosis (HH) is defined as an inherited disorder of iron metabolism that can lead to progressive parenchymal cellular iron overload in many tissues of the body—in particular in the liver, pancreas, and heart (Box 3). When the degree of iron overloading reaches a critical level, structural and functional damage to these organs can become apparent, and these constitute the phenotypic evidence for HH. The genotypic definition is based on a single missense mutation, the C282Y mutation, of the *HFE* gene on the short arm of chromosome 6, which has a major role in regulating iron metabolism. When this mutation is present in both copies of the gene, homozygous HH is said to be present. Not every person who is homozygous for this mutation develops phenotypic evidence of iron overload. Furthermore, there are other hereditary forms of iron overload based on alternative mutations of the *HFE* gene or mutations of other genes that also play a role in the regulation of iron metabolism (see Box 3).

PREVALENCE

The *HFE* gene and its mutation were first described in 1996. The principal mutation at amino acid position 282 in the protein product of this gene leads to the substitution of tyrosine for cysteine, which has a profound effect on the function of this protein. Retrospective analyses of persons in the United States with phenotypic or familial evidence for homozygous HH have revealed that 83% to 100% were homozygous for the C282Y mutation. Approximately 10% of persons with a clinical condition that is phenotypically similar to HH lack the C282Y mutation. Mutations of other genes not located on chromosome 6 also play a role in iron metabolism and account for the majority of non–*HFE* related HH (see Box 3). In particular, hepcidin synthesized in the liver appears to play a central role in the transport of iron among the enterocyte, macrophage, and the hepatocyte and may be the crucial link in all forms of HH.

It is now evident that HH is the most common identified mendelian genetic disorder in the white population. Although its geographic distribution is worldwide, it is particularly common in persons of Northern European descent, particularly of Nordic or Celtic ancestry. Overall, its prevalence in the white population is approximately 1 in 300, with a higher prevalence of 1 in 150 to 200 in the Anglo-Celtic-Nordic population.

Box 3 Causes of Iron Overload

Hereditary Hemochromatosis
***HFE*-related (Type 1)**
C282Y homozygotes
C282Y : H63D compound heterozygotes
Rare alternative *HFE* mutations

Non-*HFE* related:
Type 2, Juvenile hemochromatosis

- 2A Hemojuvelin (HJV) mutation
- 2B Hepcidin (HAMP) mutation

Type 3, Transferrin receptor 2 (TfR 2)mutation
Type 4, Ferroportin mutation (autosomal dominant)

Secondary Iron Overload
Iron-loading anemias with or without blood transfusion
Chronic liver diseases
Hepatitis B and C
Alcoholic liver disease
Nonalcoholic fatty liver disease
Porphyria cutanea tarda
Miscellaneous causes
Dietary iron overload
African iron overload with or without genetic predisposition
Neonatal iron overload
Aceruloplasminemia
Atransferrinemia

PATHOPHYSIOLOGY

Before mutational analysis was available, it was believed that the homozygous genetic abnormality inevitably led to progressive iron overload. With the availability of genotypic analysis, it is now apparent that the homozygous state for the mutation does not invariably lead to iron overload. In those who do fully express, there appears to be a pathophysiologic predisposition to increased inappropriate absorption of dietary iron, which can lead to the progressive development of life-threatening complications of cirrhosis, hepatocellular cancer, diabetes, and heart disease.

The normal HFE protein is expressed predominantly in the crypt cells of the upper intestine where, in association with the transferrin receptor, it might play a role in sensing the iron status of the body. Evidence has suggested that the mutant HFE protein is unable to provide this sensing, leading to upregulation of the iron transport protein normally expressed on the villous cell.

Although the genetic predisposition to increased iron absorption is present at birth, the disease can take 40 to 50 years or longer to progress to significant organ damage. Therefore, it is useful to think of the evolution of this clinical condition as a series of stages that begins with clinically insignificant iron accumulation based on the genetic abnormality (from 0 to 20 years of age, 0-5 g parenchymal iron storage). Subsequently, this evolves to a stage of iron overload without evident disease (at approximately 20 to 40 years of age, 5-20 g parenchymal iron storage). If left untreated, the condition can progress to the stage of iron overload with organ damage (usually at 40 years of age or older, and with >20 g of parenchymal iron storage).

SIGNS AND SYMPTOMS

In the past 40 years, the percentage of patients with this condition who are symptomatic, with evidence of target organ damage, has been overtaken by a predominance of persons who are asymptomatic, with only laboratory evidence for iron overload. The classic triad of cirrhosis, diabetes mellitus, and skin pigmentation—bronzed diabetes—is now a rare finding.

Even in the absence of early diagnosis based on abnormal serum iron markers, or on abnormal liver function found incidentally or by appropriate family screening, many early symptoms of HH are nonspecific. These consist of weakness, malaise, fatigue, lethargy, and weight loss that might not evoke an awareness, even in the astute clinician, unless appropriate laboratory tests are performed. Development of arthralgias, loss of libido, or impotence also might not arouse the suspicion of HH unless appropriate laboratory tests are performed. These features can antedate the more classic and specific clinical findings associated with involvement of the liver, pancreas, heart, and skin. At this later point, patients may reveal marked hepatomegaly, abnormal liver enzyme levels, skin pigmentation resulting from iron deposition and increased melanin, glucose intolerance, and cardiac signs indicating a dilated cardiomyopathy, with associated cardiac dysrhythmias and congestive heart failure.

As the liver disease progresses, portal hypertension with ascites, splenomegaly, and additional cutaneous features of chronic liver disease become apparent. These features of progressive liver disease are greatly accelerated in the face of coexisting risk factors such as alcohol abuse, hepatitis C, or nonalcoholic steatohepatitis. Features of hypogonadism may be difficult to interpret as specific for iron overload because they are common complications of end-stage liver disease.

DIAGNOSIS

Target Population

Target populations (Box 4, Fig. 1) may be symptomatic individuals with unexplained features of liver disease, diabetes mellitus associated with hepatomegaly and elevated liver enzyme levels, and early-onset atypical arthropathy, cardiac disease, and male sexual dysfunction. Alternatively they may be asymptomatic first-degree relatives or just persons with abnormal serum iron markers during routine testing or unexplained elevation of liver enzyme levels, hepatomegaly, or radiologic features on computed tomography (CT) scanning or magnetic resonance imaging (MRI) that suggest hepatic iron overload.

Box 4 Target Populations for the Diagnosis of Hereditary Hemochromatosis

Patients with clinical manifestations compatible with hereditary hemochromatosis

- Unexplained liver disease, hepatomegaly, or elevated liver enzyme levels
- Type 2 diabetes mellitus with associated liver disease, cardiomyopathy, or early-onset sexual dysfunction
- Early-onset arthropathy, cardiomyopathy, cardiac dysrhythmias. or sexual dysfunction

Patients without clinical manifestations of HH

- First-degree relatives of a patient with identified hereditary hemochromatosis
- Incidental finding of elevated serum iron markers (e.g., iron saturation or serum ferritin)
- Incidental finding of elevated liver enzyme levels or hepatomegaly, or a compatible computed tomography or magnetic resonance imaging scan of the liver

Because it is agreed that clinical HH is the result of iron overload, the diagnosis is based on the documentation of increased iron stores, namely, increased hepatic iron concentrations associated with elevated serum ferritin levels. As serologic iron markers have become more widely available, most patients with HH are now identified while they are still asymptomatic and without evidence of target organ damage. Now, with the availability of mutational analysis, HH may be further defined genotypically in a first-degree relative by the finding of C282Y homozygosity or C282Y-H63D compound heterozygosity. There is evidence to support the cost effectiveness of sequential testing of these target populations by a combination of indirect phenotypic markers of iron overload in the serum followed by mutational analysis to confirm the presence of classic *HFE*-related HH (see Fig. 1).

Diagnostic Algorithm

The diagnostic algorithm (see Fig. 1) from the guidelines adopted by the liver and gastroenterology subspecialty societies proceeds in three steps, beginning with phenotypic evaluation and followed by mutational analysis of persons with confirmed elevated serum iron markers.

The initial step in the diagnostic approach to HH is the fasting transferrin iron saturation (TS). This is the ratio of serum iron to total iron binding capacity, expressed in micrograms per deciliter multiplied by 100. An elevated TS value (>45%) may be the earliest phenotypic manifestation of HH. The presence of an associated elevated serum ferritin level usually indicates increased iron stores.

Serum ferritin is susceptible to nonspecific elevation, particularly in the presence of inflammatory diseases and other causes of liver disease. Nevertheless, a normal serum ferritin level in combination

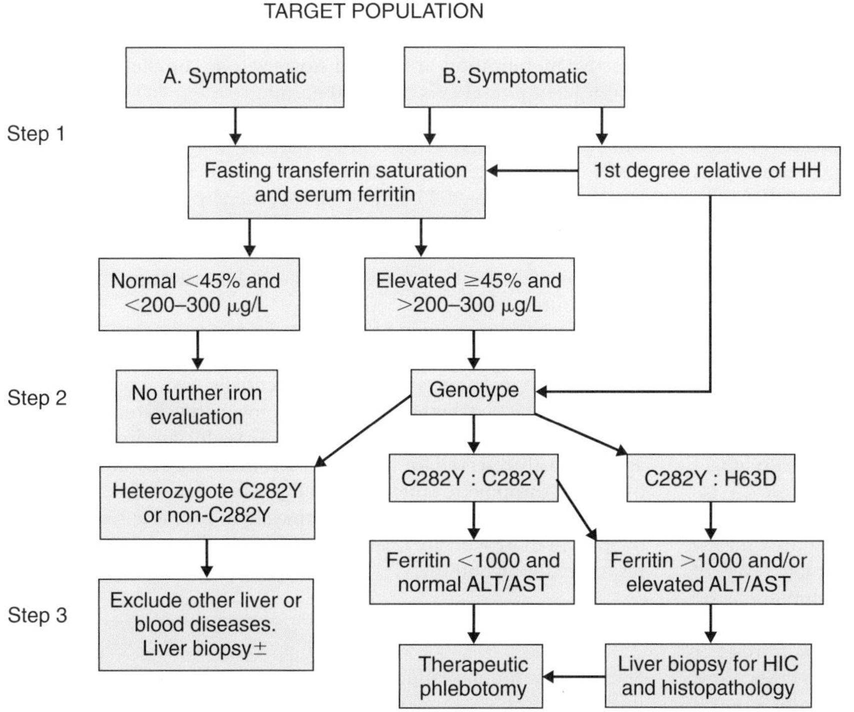

Figure 1 Diagnostic algorithm for investigating patients for hemochromatosis. ALT, alanine aminotransferase; AST, aspartate aminotransferase; HH, hereditary hemochromatosis; HIC, hepatic ion concentration. *(Reproduced with permission from Tavill AS, Adams PC: A diagnostic approach to hemochromatosis. Can J Gastroenterol 2006;20:535-540.)*

with a TS value lower than 45% has a negative predictive value of 97%, and a combination of elevated TS and ferritin has been found in more than 75% of C282Y homozygous males and about 50% of females in population studies. However, it is recognized that values in excess of 45% often include C282Y heterozygotes, and elevated serum ferritin is observed in patients with relatively minor degrees of secondary iron overload (e.g., those with alcoholic liver disease, nonalcoholic steatohepatitis, and chronic hepatitis C, and those who have had surgical portacaval shunts). Finally, the serum ferritin level may have an additional prognostic value: Patients with a ferritin level higher than 1000 ng/mL have a greatly increased likelihood of developing hepatic fibrosis or cirrhosis.

The second stage in the algorithm is genetic mutation analysis for the C282Y and H63D mutations of the *HFE* gene. This step is reserved for persons with a fasting TS value higher than 45% and an elevated serum ferritin level. The presence of *HFE* mutations can now be detected by commercially available polymerase chain reaction testing on samples of whole blood. Persons with serum indicators of iron overload who are found to be homozygotes for the C282Y mutation are candidates for phlebotomy therapy; in those with no risk factors for significant liver injury, therapeutic phlebotomy may be undertaken without need for a liver biopsy. These usually include those with no clinical evidence of liver disease (e.g., increased liver enzyme levels, hepatomegaly) whose serum ferritin level is lower than 1000 ng/mL.

Finally, the current recommendation is to offer mutation analysis to first-degree relatives of known HH patients, regardless of the phenotypic markers of iron overload. In such persons, the presence of homozygosity for the major mutation provides an indication for subsequent regular evaluation of transferrin saturation and serum ferritin levels. Adults who are determined to be homozygous for the major mutation may be offered guidance about the likelihood of the presence of the mutation in their children by appropriate mutation analysis in the spouse. The failure to detect either mutation in the spouse offers reassurance that the children can be only obligate heterozygotes.

The third step of the algorithm provides the option to perform a liver biopsy when there is unexplained elevated liver enzymes or a strong suggestion of fibrosis. Liver biopsy is also recommended for compound heterozygotes with elevated TS and abnormal liver enzyme levels or clinical evidence of liver disease.

The liver is the most easily accessible tissue for accurately assessing the level of iron stores. The degree and cellular distribution of iron stores are assessed using Perls' Prussian blue test, which provides a qualitative assessment of iron stores based on stainable iron. Grade IV staining is defined as deposition of iron in all zones of the acinus. In addition, quantitative iron determination may be made on fresh-frozen or formalin-fixed tissue. A hepatic iron concentration (HIC) of more than 1800 μg/g dry weight (approximately 32 μmol/g) indicates excess iron in the tissue.

Because excessive iron deposition in homozygotes who develop iron overload is usually a lifelong progressive accumulation, the rate of iron accumulation itself may provide powerful evidence of homozygous HH. A rate in excess of 1.9 μmol/g/year is found in most symptomatic HH homozygotes. This rate is defined as the hepatic iron index, which used to be regarded as the gold standard for homozygous HH. It is now recognized that up to 15% of symptomatic homozygotes have a rate of iron accumulation lower than 1.9 μmol/g/year; such a definition, based on the hepatic iron index, is no longer regarded as essential for diagnosis.

In persons with HH who are older than 20 years, the HIC is usually at least three times the upper limit of normal (approximately 5400 μg/g), although it is recognized that spuriously low levels of hepatic iron can occur for various reasons, including voluntary blood donation. The HIC is usually elevated to levels exceeding 14,000 μg/g dry weight in those who have already developed hepatic fibrosis or cirrhosis; they are usually older than 40 years. In certain cases, these manifestations of liver damage occur at a younger age and at lower levels of hepatic iron. In the absence of cofactors such as alcohol or hepatitis, it is rare to see fibrosis or cirrhosis in those younger than 40 years.

It is therefore important to emphasize that the value of liver biopsy is not limited to determination of the HIC. Rather, the documentation of cirrhosis on liver biopsy also has a significant impact on the prognosis in terms of morbidity and mortality in HH patients. Patients who are treated before cirrhosis develops usually have a normal life expectancy.

Box 5 Treatment of Hereditary Hemochromatosis

Initial Treatment

Phlebotomy of one unit of blood (500 mL) once or twice weekly as tolerated

Check hematocrit and hemoglobin before each phlebotomy to assure that they fall no more than 20% below starting value

Check serum ferritin at intervals and stop frequent phlebotomy when it falls below 50 ng/mL

Avoid vitamin C supplements

Maintenance Treatment

One phlebotomy every 2-3 months (approx) to maintain serum ferritin between 25 and 50 ng/mL

Avoid vitamin C supplements

TREATMENT

The treatment of HH is simple and relatively safe. Therapeutic phlebotomy effectively mobilizes and removes iron stores and, when adhered to on a regular basis, maintains them at normal levels (Box 5). Patients should be encouraged to adhere to a regimen of phlebotomy of one unit of blood once or twice weekly as tolerated initially. This removes approximately 250 mg of iron for each unit of blood, depending on the starting hematocrit value. In situations in which total body iron stores exceed 20 to 30 g, this regimen of phlebotomy can take as long as 2 to 3 years to complete. The aim is to reduce iron stores to a level just short of iron deficiency. The hematocrit value should be monitored before each phlebotomy and should be postponed if it falls by more than 20% of its starting value. It is reasonable to check the serum ferritin level after every 10 to 12 phlebotomies. The serum ferritin level may be expected to fall progressively with iron mobilization, and it can be confidently assumed that effective mobilization of the iron stores will be completed when the serum ferritin level falls below 50 ng/mL.

Subsequently, a maintenance schedule may be initiated, and it can be expected that a one-unit phlebotomy may be necessary every 2 to 3 months. The aim of maintenance therapy is to keep the serum ferritin level between 25 and 50 ng/mL, thereby avoiding overt iron deficiency. Currently, phlebotomy is a therapeutic procedure, with a coding recognized by the Centers for Medicare and Medicaid Services (formerly the Health Care Finance Administration) and third-party insurers.

It is important to avoid pharmacologic doses of vitamin C, which can result in accelerated mobilization of iron. This might saturate the circulating transferrin and lead to potentially toxic complications, such as cardiac dysrhythmias and cardiomyopathy. Parenteral deferoxamine (Desferal) or oral deferasirox (Exjade) are iron-chelating agents usually reserved for those with secondary iron overload caused by dyserythropoietic anemia. Finally, many specialists prescribe erythropoietin, which is given systemically to promote red cell production in those who are unable to mount an adequate bone marrow response to phlebotomy.

OUTCOMES

Several longitudinal studies have provided powerful evidence that initiation of phlebotomy therapy before cirrhosis or diabetes develops significantly reduces the morbidity and mortality of HH by attenuating or preventing progressive organ damage. Certain clinical symptoms and signs may be improved by phlebotomy (e.g., fatigue, malaise, skin pigmentation, abdominal pain, level of insulin requirements in diabetics). Other clinical features may be less responsive to iron mobilization (e.g., arthropathy, hypogonadism, established cirrhosis). Primary liver cell cancer accounts for about 30% of all iron-related deaths in HH, with another 20% ascribed to complications of cirrhosis Therefore, prevention of fibrosis and cirrhosis is a paramount aim.

Because the definition of HH is still based initially on phenotypic manifestations, there are no convincing arguments to treat genetically predisposed persons who have no indirect markers of iron overload. This has been used as one of the proposed arguments against any recommendation at present for widespread genetic screening for hereditary hemochromatosis. Nevertheless, evidence points to a majority of genetically predisposed persons—that is, C282Y homozygotes—particularly males exhibiting elevated iron markers. We do not have accurate predictors of how many of these will develop tissue iron overload, and most specialists currently favor prophylactic phlebotomy in these cases.

Because cirrhosis in its fully developed form is very rarely reversible by iron removal, the potential remains for decompensated liver disease in these patients and can provide an indication for considering transplantation. To optimize a favorable outcome, it has been suggested that every endeavor should be made to diagnose HH at an early enough time point to permit adequate removal of excess iron stores before transplantation. Again, iron removal treatment in HH before cirrhosis or diabetes develops can help maintain normal life expectancy, providing a persuasive argument for preventive therapy.

Summary

- Hemochromatosis is defined as iron overload affecting the parenchymal cells of the liver and other organs caused either by inherited or acquired (secondary) disorders.
- Hereditary hemochromatosis (HH) is most commonly caused by homozygous C282Y mutations of the *HFE* gene on the short arm of chromosome 6, leading to excessive absorption of dietary iron by the enterocyte.
- Although the phenotypic features of elevated iron markers in the serum are seen in the majority of persons with the homozygous mutations C282Y, particularly males, the classic findings of cirrhosis and bronzed diabetes occur in a variable minority (5%-10%).
- Diagnosis of hemochromatosis is by phenotypic evaluation of iron overload using indirect serum markers and, ultimately, in select persons, by liver biopsy, and by genotypic evaluation using mutation analysis of the *HFE* gene in blood samples.
- Treatment of HH is by iron removal using phlebotomy in those with confirmed iron overload. Early treatment before evidence of tissue damage prevents cirrhosis, with complicating liver cancer, and diabetes. Removal of iron in secondary forms of iron overload has not been evaluated to date in controlled trials. In iron-loading anemia, early treatment with iron chelators is indicated.

Suggested Readings

Adams P, Brissot P, Powell LW: EASL international consensus conference on haemochromatosis. J Hepatol 2000;33:485-504.

Allen KJ, Gurrin LC, Constantine CC, et al:. Iron-overload-related disease in *HFE* hereditary hemochromatosis. N Engl J Med 2008;358: 221-230.

Bacon BR, Britton RS: Clinical penetrance of hereditary hemochromatosis (editorial). N Engl J Med 2008; 358:291.

Bacon BR, Olynyk JK, Brunt EM, et al: HFE genotype in patients with hemochromatosis and other liver diseases. Ann Intern Med 1999;130:953-962.

Beutler E, Felitti VJ, Koziol JA, et al: Penetrance of 845 G→A (C282Y) *HFE* hereditary haemochromatosis mutation in the USA. Lancet 2002;359:211-218.

Feder JN, Gnirke A, Thomas W, et al: A novel MHC class 1–like gene is mutated in patients with hereditary haemochromatosis. Nat Genet 1996;13:399-408.

Niederau C, Fischer R, Purschel A, et al: Long-term survival in patients with hereditary hemochromatosis. Gastroenterology 1996;110:1107-1119.

Olynyk JK, Cullen DJ, Aquilia S, et al: A population study of the clinical expression of the hemochromatosis gene. N Engl J Med 1999;341:718-724.

Tavill AS; American Association for the Study of Liver Diseases; American College of Gastroenterology; American Gastroenterological Association: Diagnosis and management of hemochromatosis. Hepatology 2001;33:1321-1328.

Tavill AS, Adams PA: A diagnostic approach to hemochromatosis. Can Gastroenterology 2006;20:535-540.

U.S. Preventive Services Task Force: Screening for hemochromatosis: Recommendation statement. Ann. Intern Med 2006;145;204-208.

Whitlock EP, Garlitz BA, Harris EL, et al: Screening for hereditary hemochromatosis: A systematic review for the U.S. Preventive Services Task Force. Ann Intern Med 2006;145:209-223.

Wilson Disease

Anthony S. Tavill

DEFINITION

Wilson disease (WD) is a genetic disorder in which there is excessive accumulation of copper in the liver and brain because of an inherited defect in the biliary excretion of copper. A comprehensive practice guideline has been published by the American Association for the Study of Liver Diseases and represents the state of the art management of Wilson disease. Recommendations in this review are consistent with that guideline.

PREVALENCE

WD is transmitted from generation to generation by autosomal recessive inheritance. Only homozygotes for this disorder who inherit disease-specific mutations of both alleles of the Wilson disease gene may go on to manifest clinical evidence of the condition. Such persons have been described in many different ethnic groups and number about 1 in 30,000 of the worldwide population. As described later, particular mutations are found more frequently in specific populations or ethnic groups, with varying phenotypic expression in some of these mutations. However, it is known that heterozygotes with a mutation of a single allele do not develop disease, although they may show varying degrees of abnormality in serum copper markers.

PATHOPHYSIOLOGY

The transport of copper from the hepatocytes to bile is critical in overall copper homeostasis, because biliary excretion undergoes minimal enterohepatic recirculation. The protein ATP7B is important in the vesicular pathway of hepatic copper transport into bile. The WD gene mutation occurs on chromosome 13, and in homozygous form it leads to the absence or diminished function of the hepatic protein ATP7B, resulting in a decrease in biliary copper excretion and ultimately in accumulation of copper in the liver. Along with this failure of biliary excretion, there is also reduced hepatic incorporation of copper into ceruloplasmin, a process also dependent on ATP7B, leading to a reduced circulating level of serum ceruloplasmin in most patients.

When copper accumulates beyond the normal safe storage capacity of the liver, hepatocellular injury results. Furthermore, when the liver's storage capacity for copper is exceeded or when additional cellular copper is released because of hepatocellular damage, levels of non–ceruloplasmin-bound copper in the circulation are elevated and copper accumulates in a number of extrahepatic sites, in particular the brain. As copper spills over to other organs from the liver, pathologic manifestations become evident in the brain, kidneys, eyes, and joints.

The pathologic evidence for copper accumulation in the liver evolves from early infancy to adult life. The earliest pathologic changes can consist of steatosis and distinctive mitochondrial changes. With progression and without treatment, the liver can show signs indistinguishable from chronic hepatitis and ultimately develops cirrhosis. In some cases, there is fulminant hepatic failure with parenchymal necrosis and collapse of lobular architecture. In the brain, the predominant neuropathologic changes of advanced untreated WD are concentrated in the lenticular nuclei, which have the highest copper levels and with increasing copper accumulation undergo various forms of degeneration. Similarly, abnormalities in the renal tubules and glomeruli, periarticular and articular tissues, and the eyes can all become sites that manifest copper damage.

Box 6 Signs and Symptoms of Wilson Disease

Asymptomatic

Biochemical abnormalities alone

Biochemical abnormalities and Kayser-Fleischer rings

Symptomatic

Hepatic disease

- Chronic active hepatitis
- Cirrhosis
- Fulminant hepatitis

Neurologic disease: features of cerebellar or extrapyramidal disease

- Dystonia
- Dysarthria
- Tremors
- Involuntary choreiform movements

Psychiatric disease, particularly with associated organic neurologic disease

Renal disease

- Aminoaciduria
- Nephrocalcinosis

Arthropathy with osteochondritis dissecans

Opthalmologic manifestations

- Kayser-Fleischer rings
- Sunflower cataracts

Hematologic manifestations

- Hemolysis

SIGNS AND SYMPTOMS

Signs and symptoms of liver, neurologic, and psychiatric disease are the most common clinical manifestations of symptomatic WD (Box 6). In contrast, those found by family screening are often asymptomatic. Failure to diagnose and treat WD results in the development of hepatic insufficiency, ultimately hepatic failure, and, in some patients, neuropsychiatric disease.

The clinical spectrum of liver disease in WD patients varies widely. Overt disease can occur in childhood or may be delayed to adolescence or adulthood. Patients might present with features of chronic liver disease indistinguishable from other forms of chronic active hepatitis or end-stage liver disease. In the latter case, with established cirrhosis, features of portal hypertension such as ascites, edema, or hypersplenism and hepatic encephalopathy may be observed. If WD is left untreated, these patients ultimately progress to hepatic insufficiency, liver failure, and death. Others present acutely with fulminant hepatic failure and associated hemolytic anemia. These are circumstances that are commonly fatal without timely, life-saving liver transplantation.

There are other patients with WD whose first presenting symptoms are neurologic or psychiatric; often they are patients in the third decade of life or even older. Most of these patients with central nervous system disease have occult significant liver disease at the time of presentation. The neurologic disease manifests predominantly as motor abnormalities, with disabling parkinsonian features of dystonia, hypertonia, and rigidity, with tremors and dysarthria. In rarer cases, WD manifests with abnormalities of other organ systems—namely, renal tubular abnormalities, arthropathy, and cardiomyopathy with dysrhythmias.

Ophthalmologic findings include Kayser-Fleischer (KF) rings and sunflower cataracts. KF rings are most marked at the upper and lower poles of the limbus, the junction between the cornea and sclera, and are caused by the granular deposition of elemental copper on the inner surface of the cornea in Descemet's membrane. The rings have a golden brown or greenish appearance on slit-lamp examination. By the time the neurologic changes occur, usually in the third decade of life, KF rings are almost invariably present, although there are exceptions to this rule.

DIAGNOSIS

WD should be considered and excluded in any patient who has unexplained hepatic, neurologic, or psychiatric disease (see Box 6). In particular, it should be considered in children or young adults with atypical extrapyramidal or cerebellar motor dysfunction, neuropsychiatric disease, elevated aminotransferase levels, or other features of acute or subacute liver disease and with unexplained non–immune-mediated hemolysis. In these cases, WD must be considered whether or not there is a family history of liver or neurologic disease. Usually, the diagnosis can be confirmed on the basis of clinical and biochemical evaluations without the need for liver biopsy.

As a practical algorithm, there are three levels of tests used to confirm the diagnosis of Wilson disease (Box 7). Level 1 tests consist of determining the serum ceruloplasmin concentration, total serum copper concentration, and, by derivation, the circulating non–ceruloplasmin-bound copper concentration and 24-hour urine copper excretion, together with slit-lamp examination of the eyes for KF rings. Testing for the serum ceruloplasmin concentration is routinely available in all clinical laboratories; the normal range is 20 to 50 mg/dL. Approximately 95% of homozygous WD patients have values lower than 20 mg/dL. However, approximately 5% of all homozygotes, whether symptomatic or not, and 15% to 50% of WD patients with liver disease, can maintain normal levels of ceruloplasmin. Spuriously normal levels of ceruloplasmin can occur as a result of acute-phase responses based on active inflammation. Conversely, low serum ceruloplasmin concentrations can occur in various hypoproteinemic states and in up to 20% of asymptomatic WD heterozygotes. A rare cause of extremely low ceruloplasmin levels may be hereditary aceruloplasminemia.

Box 7 Diagnostic Tests for Wilson Disease

Level 1 Tests
Low serum ceruloplasmin(<20 mg/dL)
Kayser-Fleischer rings
Raised serum free copper (non–ceruloplasmin-bound) (>25 μg/dL)
24-hour urinary copper (>100 μg/24 hr)

Level 2 Tests
Liver histopathology and stainable copper
Liver copper concentration (>250 μg/g dry weight)

Level 3 Tests
Ultrastructural study of hepatocytes
Mutational gene analysis for Wilson disease
Incorporation of radiocopper in to ceruloplasmin

Adapted from Roberts EA, Schilsky ML. AASLD Practice Guidelines. Diagnosis and Treatment of Wilson Disease: An Update. Hepatology 2008;47:2089–2111.

The total serum copper concentration is made up of ceruloplasmin-bound copper and free copper, bound more loosely to albumin or smaller circulating peptides. The ceruloplasmin and therefore the ceruloplasmin copper levels are typically low in WD and might explain an overall reduction in total serum copper concentration. However, when the free (i.e., non–ceruloplasmin-bound) copper is calculated by subtracting the ceruloplasmin copper from the total serum copper level, it is usually found to be elevated, typically to more than 25 μg/dL in WD. To calculate the free copper level, the ceruloplasmin (in mg/dL) is multiplied by 3; this value is then subtracted from the total serum copper level (in μg/dL). The non–ceruloplasmin-bound copper may be elevated in acute liver failure of any cause, not just WD, and in chronic cholestasis.

Slit-lamp evaluation of the cornea for KF rings should be performed by an experienced ophthalmologist. KF rings are present in almost every patient with neurologic disease, but they may be absent in younger patients with hepatic manifestations only.

The measurement of 24-hour urinary copper excretion usually exceeds 100 μg/24 hours in WD and reflects the increased plasma non–ceruloplasmin-bound copper. Spuriously elevated increases in urinary copper levels can occur in the face of fulminant liver failure and in patients with nephrotic levels of proteinuria. The 24-hour urine samples must be collected in metal-free containers.

In the absence of Kayser-Fleischer rings, level 2 tests are important for the diagnostic confirmation of WD. Liver biopsy for hepatic copper concentrations is an invaluable diagnostic tool. Most homozygotes for WD have levels higher than 250 μg/g dry weight, with normal values rarely exceeding 50 μg/g. Intermediate values may be seen in heterozygotes. A number of hepatic conditions manifesting extreme cholestasis can have elevated hepatic copper concentrations but can usually be diagnosed by other clinical, serologic, or histopathologic criteria. Immunohistochemical staining for copper is relatively insensitive.

Level 3 tests include incorporation of radiocopper into ceruloplasmin and molecular genetic studies to provide evidence for mutations in the *ATP7B* gene. Incorporating isotopes of copper into ceruloplasmin is impractical in most centers.

Currently, molecular genetic studies include haplotype analysis of family members of an affected person with WD gene mutation. Such tests involve evaluation of DNA polymorphisms in the nucleotide regions surrounding the *ATP7B* gene. There have been multiple disease-specific mutations of the WD gene described in probands with the disorder. Even the most common of these mutations account for only 15% to 30% of most WD populations. Newer technologies that use whole-gene sequencing are available on referral to selected genetics laboratories in North America and Europe.

Table 1 Treatment of Wilson Disease*

Drug	Dose and Route of Administration
Penicillamine (Cupramine, Depen)	250 mg PO tid or qid
Trientine (Syprine)	250 mg PO tid or qid
Zinc salts†: sulfate, gluconate, or acetate	50 mg PO tid (as elemental zinc)

*In all therapies, the goal is to reduce serum free copper (non–ceruloplasmin bound) to <10 μg/dL.
†Zinc salts may be substituted as a maintenance therapy after adequate decoppering has been achieved, but they may be the treatment of choice in selected asymptomatic Wilson disease patients.

TREATMENT

Depending on the mode of manifestion of WD, treatment options consist of orally administered pharmacologic agents (Table 1) or transplantation. Liver transplantation should not be regarded as a treatment of last resort, but it may be the only means of timely intervention in patients presenting with acute or subacute liver failure or decompensating end-stage liver disease. Ideally, diagnosis should be early enough for medical therapy to attenuate or abolish symptoms and prevent progression of the disease.

It is generally agreed that patients with symptoms or signs of hepatic insufficiency or chronic active hepatitis with or without neurologic manifestations should be offered chelation therapy with penicillamine or trientine. These drugs are administered orally and remove copper from potentially toxic sites. In contrast, zinc salts serve to block the intestinal absorption of dietary copper. Penicillamine was the first copper chelator to be developed; unfortunately, it has been incriminated as causing some toxic side effects, which leads to discontinuation of the drug in 10% to 15% of patients. Trientine was developed more recently and is considered preferable by many experts as first-line therapy in patients with hepatic or neurologic disease, or both. Zinc salts may be considered as initial therapy for asymptomatic patients or for those intolerant of penicillamine or trientine. With any of these treatments, patients should be evaluated for clinical and biochemical improvements and normalization of markers of copper metabolism, in particular the level of free serum copper and urinary copper output. With stabilization of these clinical and biochemical parameters, patients can be switched to maintenance therapy. This may consist of a reduced dose of penicillamine or trientine or, in some cases, switching from these chelating agents to zinc salts (see Table 1).

Dietary intake of foods rich in copper should be avoided, particularly during the initial phase of treatment. Organ meats, nuts, chocolate, and shellfish should be avoided. These restrictions may be partially lifted during the maintenance phase of treatment.

For WD patients who become pregnant, the doses of penicillamine or trientine should be reduced during the second trimester and the first 2 months of the third trimester, to 500 mg/day maximum, and to 250 mg/day for the month before delivery and for up to 1 month after delivery. A similar approach to reduction in therapy with chelating agents is applied to patients undergoing surgery to allow complete wound healing.

The key to long-term success of pharmacologic treatment for WD is the patient's adherence to treatment. Evaluation of response is based on improvement in the signs of liver or neurologic disease and improvement in biochemical markers of liver function. Further assessment is based on regular periodic monitoring of urinary copper output, slit-lamp examinations, and, most importantly, by reduction in the level of non–ceruloplasmin-bound copper in the serum. With adequate treatment, the non–ceruloplasmin-bound copper level should decrease to 10 μg/dL or less. Inadequate treatment or lack of compliance is usually associated with a level above 25 μg/dL. In the context of chelation therapy, urinary copper excretion initially exceeds 1000 μg/day, and on maintenance treatment it should be between 250 and 500 μg/day. Values lower than this usually suggest nonadherence to treatment. In contrast, on zinc therapy, urinary copper excretion usually falls to less than 150 μg/day. All patients should receive regular monitoring at least annually for serum copper, ceruloplasmin, urinary copper, complete blood count, liver tests, and urinalysis.

Liver transplantation is indicated in the extreme circumstances mentioned when there is evidence of impending liver failure. Transplant recipients develop the normal donor phenotype with regard to markers of copper metabolism and do not require additional pharmacologic therapy for WD, except possibly in the case of residual neurologic symptoms and signs.

OUTCOMES

Even with established cirrhosis or chronic active hepatitis, the prognosis is excellent for patients who adhere fully to pharmacologic therapy. Neurologic or psychiatric symptoms may be slow to recover and might not be completely reversible. However, features of both neurologic disease and hepatic insufficiency usually stabilize on treatment, and only a watch-and-wait approach can be recommended. In cases of liver decompensation, following liver transplantation, the 1-year survival rate is comparable with that for other causes of liver failure. Although neurologic symptoms can improve after liver transplantation, the extent of neurologic involvement itself in the absence of liver failure is not an indication for liver transplantation.

Summary

- Wilson disease (WD) is a genetic disease of the liver that leads to excessive copper storage in the liver, brain, and, to a lesser degree, in other organs, occurring in about 1 in 30,000 persons worldwide.
- Genetic mutation leads to defective hepatic secretion of copper into bile and copper incorporation into ceruloplasmin.
- Clinical features relate to the toxic effects of excessive copper in the liver, brain, corneas, blood, kidneys, and joints and can manifest from childhood to adulthood.
- A diagnostic algorithm has been published using ascending levels of clinical, laboratory, and tissue biochemical testing. Molecular genetic testing is not yet routinely available in the clinic but can be obtained in specialist WD or genetics referral centers.
- Early treatment using zinc to diminish intestinal copper absorption and oral chelators to remove excessive tissue copper have been shown to prevent progression, reverse clinical complications of tissue copper damage, and improve survival in patients with WD.
- Liver transplantation is life-saving in those with complications of irreversible end-stage liver disease and acute liver failure.

Suggested Readings

Brewer GJ, Johnson VD, Dick RD, et al: Treatment of Wilson's disease with zinc. XVII: Treatment during pregnancy. Hepatology 2000;31:364-370.

Petrukhin K, Fischer SG, Pirastu M, et al: Mapping, cloning and genetic characterization of the region containing the Wilson disease gene. Nat Genet 1993;5:338-343.

Roberts EA, Schilsky ML; AASLD Practice Guidelines. Diagnosis and treatment of Wilson disease: An Update. Hepatology 2008;47:2089-2111.

Scheinberg IH, Gitlin D: Deficiency of ceruloplasmin in patients with hepatolenticular degeneration (Wilson's disease). Science 1952;116:484-485.

Schilsky ML, Scheinberg IH, Sternlieb I: Liver transplantation for Wilson's disease: Indications and outcome. Hepatology 1994;19:583-587.

Schilsky ML, Tavill AS: Wilson disease. In Schiff ER, Sorrell M, Maddrey W (eds): Schiff's Diseases of the Liver, 10th ed. Philadelphia, Lippincott Williams & Wilkins, 2007, pp 1023-1040.

Sternlieb I, Scheinberg IH: Prevention of Wilson's disease in asymptomatic patients. N Engl J Med 1968;278:352-359.

Sternlieb I: Wilson's disease and pregnancy [editorial]. Hepatology 2000;31:531-532.

Tanzi RE, Petrukhin K, Chernov I, et al: The Wilson disease gene is a copper-transporting ATPase with homology to the Menkes disease gene. Nat Genet 1993;5:344-350.

Walshe JM: Copper chelation in patients with Wilson's disease: A comparison of penicillamine and triethylene tetramine dihydrochloride. Q J Med 1973;42:441-452.

Chronic Autoimmune Hepatitis

William D. Carey

Chronic autoimmune hepatitis (CAIH) is a serious liver disease that occurs throughout the world. It represents an immunologic attack against hepatocytes, produces a myriad of symptoms, is frequently fatal if untreated, and is often exquisitely sensitive to the effects of corticosteroid therapy. It occurs in all age groups, although it most often emerges in the young. More than 90% of CAIH cases occur in women. A clinical practice guideline is available. The information in this chapter applies to those older than 16 years. Younger patients with suspected CAIH should be referred to a specialist. Although many patients with this condition will be seen by a specialist, all clinicians should be aware of the principles on which therapy is based and of the monitoring needed to ensure optimal patient outcomes.

CAUSES AND PATHOGENESIS

The causes of CAIH are unknown. It behaves as an autoimmune disease, often with multiple organ involvement (e.g., thyroid, joints). It is often associated with major histocompatibility complex (MHC) class II DRB1 alleles, DRB1*0301 and DRB1*0401.

SYMPTOMS

The onset of autoimmune chronic hepatitis most often begins with insidious constitutional symptoms, such as fatigue, joint aches, loss of appetite, and malaise. Oligomenorrhea may be present. In one third of cases, the onset is abrupt and mimics that of acute hepatitis. In the acute presentation, jaundice is frequent but not necessarily present.

DIAGNOSIS

Laboratory test results in most cases are dramatic. Liver function tests reveal a "parenchymal" pattern—that is, levels of aspartate transaminase (AST) and alanine aminotransferase (ALT) predominate over elevations of alkaline phosphatase levels, which may be normal. Classic severe autoimmune hepatitis results in AST and ALT levels at least 7 to 10 times the upper limit of normal (e.g., an ALT level of 300-800 U/L) or higher. The laboratory tests that most characterize CAIH are autoimmune markers. Most characteristic is the smooth muscle antibody (SMA). Although this test is not by itself diagnostic, the combination of very high AST and ALT levels, without other obvious explanations, together with a positive SMA in high titer (>1:80), strongly suggests autoimmune hepatitis and should be considered as such unless proven otherwise. Some patients may have typical features of CAIH but lack autoantibodies. Others, particularly in Europe, may express anti–liver-kidney microsomal (LKM) antibody. Those who lack autoantibodies may respond equally well to treatment.

Although usually straightforward, variations in presentation occasionally create difficulty for the clinician. An international panel of experts has created a robust although unwieldy scoring system that delineates most patients with this disorder (Table 1).

Simpler means will suffice. Evaluation of suspected CAIH should include consideration of the following:

- Liver panel, including AST, ALT: Levels 7 to 10 times the upper limit of normal are expected.
- Exclusion of other causes of liver injury, especially drug-induced hepatitis (e.g., by nitrofurantoins, isoniazid, amoxicillin-clavulanic acid, propylthiouracil, statins) and viral hepatitis A, B, and C. In patients younger than 40 years, measure the ceruloplasmin level. If the value is low or low-normal, consider Wilson's disease and refer the patient to a specialist.
- Quantitative autoantibodies, especially SMA and antinuclear antibody (ANA): Expect a high titer of SMA (e.g., >1:160). Perform second-tier tests, such as for LKM antibody, when SMA and ANA values are negative.
- Quantitative immunoglobulins: Gamma globulin levels are often 150% or more of normal.
- Liver biopsy is optional but often helpful.

Due diligence requires exclusion of other conditions, such as drug-induced hepatitis, viral hepatitis, and Wilson's disease in those younger than 40 years. Although a practice guideline has incorporated the need for liver tissue examination as a diagnostic criterion for CAIH, there is no clear evidence that a liver biopsy is required in all cases. It is helpful but not necessary in the diagnosis of autoimmune hepatitis. Treatment should not be delayed when the findings are otherwise typical. I often delay liver biopsy until after treatment has improved liver synthetic function.

Typical histologic findings include portal inflammation with mononuclear cells, most often lymphocytes. Plasma cells are often highly represented. The inflammation is not limited to the portal area, but spills out into the parenchyma, near the portal tracts. This is currently termed *interface hepatitis* (formerly known as "piecemeal necrosis"). Varying degrees of fibrosis may be present, up to and including cirrhosis.

Many cases are atypical, causing a diagnostic problem. Occasional confusion with other autoimmune liver diseases, especially primary biliary cirrhosis, may occur. Such cases are best referred to a gastroenterologist or hepatologist.

TREATMENT

The mainstay of treatment is corticosteroid therapy, given for months or years. In many cases, lifelong therapy is needed to keep the disease at bay. Prednisone or prednisolone are each effective in this disorder (Table 2). Another agent, azathioprine, is ineffective in the initial control of disease, but permits lower doses of prednisone to be used; this results in lower rates of side effects. For the individual who can tolerate both drugs, combination therapy is preferred. Budesonide used in combination with azathioprime may be an alternative to prednisone. An initial budesonide dose of 3 mg TID, then reduced to 3 mg BID may be as effective as prednisone and be associated with fewer corticosteroid side effects. The cost of this agent for exceeds that of prednisone.

When initiating treatment, moderately high doses of prednisone or prednisolone are used. The patient should be evaluated after 4 to 6 weeks. Expect normal or near-normal enzyme levels.

After 4 to 6 weeks, gradual dose reduction is usually possible. By this time, AST and ALT values should be approaching normal. Con-

Table 1 Diagnostic Scoring in Chronic Autoimmune Hepatitis

Factor	Score
Female gender	+2
Alkaline phosphatase Ratio	
AST or ALT < 1.5	+2
AST or ALT > 3.0	−2
Serum globulin Elevation	
2-fold	+3
1.5-2-fold	+2
1-1.5-fold	+1
SMA, ANA, or LKM Antibody	
>1:80	+3
1:80	+2
1:40	+1
Other positive autoantibodies	+2
AMA positive	−4
Viral Markers	
Positive	−3
Negative	+3
Alcohol intake	
<25 g	+2
>60 g	−2
Liver histology	
Interface hepatitis	+3
Lymphoplasmacytic infiltrate	+1
Piecemeal necrosis	+1
None of the above	−5
Biliary changes	−3
Features of other diseases	−3
Other autoimmune diseases	+2
HLA DR3 or DR4	+1
Response to treatment	
Complete remission	+2
Remission then relapse	+3
Interpretation	**Aggregate Score**
Pretreatment Score	
Definite CAIH	>15
Probable CAIH	10-15
Post-treatment Score	
Definite CAIH	>17
Probable CAIH	12-17

ALT, alanine aminotransferase; ANA, antinuclear antibody; AST, aspartate transaminase; CAIH, chronic autoimmune chronic hepatitis; HLA, human leukocyte antigen; LKM, liver-kidney microsomal; SMA, smooth muscle antibody.

Table 2 Pharmacotherapy for Chronic Autoimmune Hepatitis

Agent	Initial Dosage for Active Disease (mg/day)	Maintenance Dose (mg/day)	Duration of Treatment Before Attempted Withdrawal
Prednisone (or prednisolone) plus azathioprine	30	10	
	50	50	9-12 mo
Prednisone (or prednisolone) monotherapy	60	20	9-12 mo
Azathioprine monotherapy	Not recommended	100 mg/day or ≤2 mg/kg/day (see text)	1 yr*

*More than one unsuccessful attempt to withdraw therapy probably means that the patient is treatment dependent.

tinue treatment for 9 to 12 months before considering withdrawal of treatment.

Azathioprine has also been shown to be effective in the maintenance of remission. After remission with dual-drug therapy has been achieved for 1 year, more than 80% of patients will remain in remission when the prednisone is discontinued and azathioprine is given in a dosage of 2 mg/kg/day. As a matter of practice, I suggest that the dosage of azathioprine used to maintain remission be capped at 100 mg/day to avoid problems of bone marrow suppression that may be seen at higher doses. It is important to monitor liver function and complete blood cell count on a quarterly basis to ensure that neither a breakthrough nor bone marrow toxicity ensues.

Patients receiving azathioprine should be advised that this drug may have an adverse effect on the fetus. When pregnancy can be planned, cessation of azathioprine 3 months ahead of time is advised. In case pregnancy occurs while a woman is on azathioprine, it should be stopped and the dosage of prednisone adjusted upward. Other therapies have been reported in small series of patients. Mycophenolate, ursodiol, and budesonide, have been tried. Patients who are not well controlled with prednisone-prednisolone and azathioprine should be referred to a gastroenterologist or hepatologist for further management.

OUTCOMES

Most patients have resolution of adverse liver test results within a few weeks. Very young patients often respond less favorably. Improvement in liver histology is delayed for many months. Responders treated for 9 to 12 months who have persistently normal enzyme levels have a 40% to 60% likelihood of remaining in remission off therapy. Those who require continuous therapy can often be converted to treatment with azathioprine alone. If a patient is to spend years on corticosteroid therapy, care must be taken to assess for bone loss. Bone densitometry is recommended annually. Those who fail therapy and develop liver failure are often excellent liver transplantation candidates. Even after liver transplantation, prednisone therapy is often required to prevent disease recurrence in the transplanted liver.

Summary

- CAIH is an autoimmune disease that affects primarily women. It may be insidious in onset. It progresses to cirrhosis and death in most patients if untreated.
- CAIH is usually easy to treat. Use of prednisone or prednisolone, generally with adjunctive azathioprine, provides prompt dramatic improvement in most.
- Many patients with CAIH remain dependent on treatment for life.
- Liver transplantation remains an option for those who fail therapy, although vigilance to monitor for disease recurrence after liver transplantation is necessary.

Suggested Readings

Alvarez F, Berg PA, Bianchi FB, et al: International autoimmune hepatitis group report: Review criteria for diagnosis of autoimmune hepatitis. J Hepatol 1999;31:929-938.

Czaja AJ, Freese DK: Diagnosis and treatment of autoimmune hepatitis. Hepatology 2002;36:479-497.

Johnson PJ, McFarlane IG, Williams R: Azathioprine for long-term remission in autoimmune hepatitis. N Engl J Med 1995;333:958-963.

Complications of Cirrhosis: Ascites, Hepatic Encephalopathy, and Variceal Hemorrhage

Karin B. Cesario, Anuja Choure, and William D. Carey

ASCITES

Definition and Etiology

Ascites is defined as the accumulation of fluid in the peritoneal cavity. It is a common clinical finding, with various extraperitoneal and peritoneal causes (Box 1), but it most often results from liver cirrhosis. The development of ascites in a cirrhotic patient generally heralds deterioration in clinical status and portends a poor prognosis.

Prevalence

Ascites is the most common major complication of cirrhosis and is an important landmark in the natural history of chronic liver disease. If observed for 10 years, approximately 60% of patients with cirrhosis develop ascites requiring therapy.

Pathophysiology

Cirrhotic ascites forms as the result of a particular sequence of events. Development of portal hypertension is the first abnormality to occur. As portal hypertension develops, vasodilators are locally released. These vasodilators affect the splanchnic arteries and thereby decrease the effective arterial blood flow and arterial pressures. The precise agent(s) responsible for vasodilation is a subject of wide debate; however, most the recent literature has focused on the likely role of nitric oxide.

Progressive vasodilation leads to the activation of vasoconstrictor and antinatriuretic mechanisms, both in an attempt to restore normal perfusion pressures. Mechanisms involved include the renin-angiotensin system, sympathetic nervous system, and antidiuretic hormone (vasopressin). The ultimate effect is sodium and water retention. In the late stages of cirrhosis, free water accumulation is more pronounced than the sodium retention and leads to a dilutional hyponatremia. This explains why cirrhotic patients with ascites demonstrate urinary sodium retention, increased total body sodium, and dilutional hyponatremia, a challenging concept for many physicians.

Signs and Symptoms

The symptoms of ascites vary from patient to patient and largely depend on the quantity of fluid. If trace ascites is present, the patient may be asymptomatic and fluid can be detected only on physical or radiologic examination. If a large amount of fluid is present, the patient might complain of abdominal fullness, early satiety, abdominal pain, or shortness of breath.

Physical examination findings are equally variable. The accuracy of detecting ascites depends on the amount of fluid present and the body habitus of the patient: ascites may be more technically difficult to diagnose in obese patients. If ascites is present, typical findings include generalized abdominal distention, flank fullness, and shifting dullness. If the physical examination is not definitive, abdominal ultrasonography can be used to confirm the presence or absence of ascites.

Two grading systems for ascites have been used in the literature (Table 1). An older system has graded ascites from 1+ to 4+, depending on the detectability of fluid on physical examination. More recently, a different grading system has been proposed, from grade 1 to grade 3. The validity of this grading system has yet to be established.

Diagnosis

If a noncirrhotic patient develops ascites, diagnostic paracentesis with ascites fluid analysis is an essential part of the medical evaluation. In a patient with well-established cirrhosis, the exact role of a diagnostic paracentesis is less clear. Our opinion is that for a highly functional outpatient with documented cirrhosis, the new development of ascites does not routinely require paracentesis. Cirrhotic patients should, however, undergo paracentesis in the case of unexplained fever, abdominal pain, or encephalopathy or if they are admitted to the hospital for any cause. It is common for hospitalized cirrhotic patients to have infected ascites fluid (spontaneous bacterial peritonitis, SBP) even if no symptoms are present. This is particularly true in the case of a significant gastrointestinal hemorrhage.

Complications from abdominal paracentesis are rare, occurring in less than 1% of cases. A low platelet count or elevated prothrombin time is not considered a contraindication, and prophylactic transfusion of platelets or plasma is almost never indicated. Insertion of the paracentesis needle is most commonly performed in the left or right lower quadrant, but it can also be performed safely in the midline. An abdominal ultrasound can guide the procedure if the fluid is difficult to localize or if initial attempts to obtain fluid are unsuccessful.

Valuable clinical information can often be obtained by gross examination of the ascites fluid (Table 2). Uncomplicated cirrhotic ascites is usually translucent and yellow. If the patient is deeply jaundiced, the fluid might appear brown. Turbidity or cloudiness of the ascites fluid suggests that infection is present and further diagnostic testing should be performed. Pink or bloody fluid is most often caused by mild trauma, with subcutaneous blood contaminating the sample. Bloody ascites is also associated with hepatocellular carcinoma or any malignancy-associated ascites. Milky-appearing fluid usually has an elevated triglyceride concentration. Such fluid, commonly referred to as *chylous ascites,* can be related to thoracic duct injury or obstruction or lymphoma, but it is often related primarily to cirrhosis.

Many ascites fluid tests are currently available, yet the optimal testing strategy has not been well established. Generally, if uncomplicated cirrhotic ascites is suspected, only a total protein and albumin concentration and a cell count with differential are determined (Box 2). Less than 10 mL of fluid is required to perform these basic tests. The albumin concentration is used to confirm the presence of portal hypertension by calculating the serum-to-ascites

Box 1 Common Causes of Ascites

Extraperitoneal Causes
Budd-Chiari syndrome
Chylous ascites
Cirrhosis
Congestive heart failure
Hypoalbuminemia

- Nephrotic syndrome
- Malnutrition
- Protein-losing enteropathy

Myxedema
Pancreatitis

Peritoneal Causes
Endometriosis
Infection

- Tuberculosis
- Bacterial
- Fungal
- Parasitic

Malignancy

- Ovarian cancer
- Pancreatic cancer

Other

Table 1 Grading Systems for Ascites

Grade	Severity	Score
1	Minimal	1+
2	Moderate	2+
3	Severe	3+
4	Tense	4+

Table 2 Gross Appearance of Ascites Fluid

Color	Association
Translucent or yellow	Normal/sterile
Brown	Hyperbilirubinemia (most common) Gallbladder or biliary perforation
Cloudy or turbid	Infection
Pink or blood tinged	Mild trauma at the site
Grossly bloody	Malignancy Abdominal trauma
Milky ("chylous")	Cirrhosis Thoracic duct injury Lymphoma

albumin gradient, or SAAG. The SAAG is determined by subtracting the ascites albumin value from a serum albumin value obtained on the same day:

$$\text{Albumin}_{\text{serum}} - \text{albumin}_{\text{ascites}} = \text{SAAG}$$

The SAAG has been proved in prospective studies to categorize ascites better than any previous criteria. The presence of a gradient higher than 1.1 g/dL indicates that the patient has portal hypertension–related ascites with 97% accuracy. Portal hypertension is usually caused by liver cirrhosis or, less commonly, outflow obstruction from right-sided heart failure or Budd-Chiari syndrome. A SAAG value lower than 1.1 g/dL indicates that the patient does not have portal hypertension–related ascites, and another cause of the ascites should be sought. Determination of the SAAG does not need to be repeated after the initial measurement.

The cell count and differential are used to determine if the patient is likely to have SBP. Patients with an ascites polymorphonuclear (PMN) count greater than 250 cells/mm^3 should receive empiric antibiotics, and additional fluid should be inoculated into blood culture bottles to be sent for culture. The PMN count is calculated by multiplying the white cells/mm^3 by the percentage of neutrophils in the differential. In a bloody sample, which contains a high concentration of red blood cells, the PMN count must be corrected: 1 PMN is subtracted from the absolute PMN count for every 250 red cells/mm^3 in the sample.

Based on clinical judgment, additional testing can be performed on ascites fluid including total protein, lactate dehydrogenase (LDH), glucose, amylase, triglyceride, bilirubin, cytology, or tuberculosis smear and culture. These tests are generally only useful when there is suspicion of a condition other than sterile cirrhotic ascites. Tests that are not routinely helpful include determination of pH, lactate levels, and Gram staining. Results of Gram staining are of particular low yield unless a large concentration of bacteria, such as in the case of a free gut perforation, is suspected.

Box 2 Ascites Fluid Testing

Routine
Cell count with differential
Albumin
Total protein
Culture*

Sometimes Useful
Lactose dehydrogenase level
Glucose
Amylase
Triglyceride
Bilirubin
Cytology
Tuberculosis smear and culture

Rarely Helpful
pH
Lactate
Gram stain

*If infection is suspected and/or corrected polymorphonuclear count is ≥250 cells/mm^3.

Summary

- Cirrhotic patients should undergo diagnostic paracentesis in cases of unexplained fever, abdominal pain, or encephalopathy or when admitted to the hospital for any cause.
- Paracentesis is a safe procedure, with a low risk of serious complication.
- The serum-to-ascites albumin gradient (SAAG) can be calculated to determine whether the patient has portal hypertension–related ascites.
- The ascites fluid cell count and differential are used to determine whether the patient is likely to have spontaneous bacterial peritonitis (SBP).

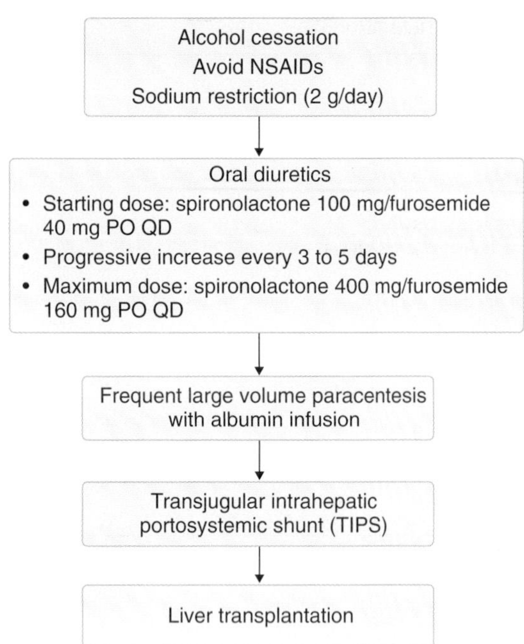

Figure 1 Treatment options for cirrhotic ascites.

Treatment

Successful treatment of cirrhotic ascites is defined as the minimization of intraperitoneal fluid without intravascular volume depletion. Despite a lack of data supporting decreased mortality, minimizing the amount of ascites fluid can decrease infection-related morbidity in the cirrhotic patient. Treatment of ascites can dramatically improve quality of life by decreasing abdominal discomfort or dyspnea, or both. General ascites management in all patients should include minimizing consumption of alcohol, nonsteroidal anti-inflammatory drugs (NSAIDs), and dietary sodium. The use of more-aggressive interventions largely depends on the severity of ascites and includes oral diuretics, therapeutic (or large-volume) paracentesis, transjugular intrahepatic portosystemic shunt (TIPS), and orthotopic liver transplantation (Fig. 1).

Low-Volume Ascites

All patients with cirrhotic ascites should be encouraged to minimize consumption of alcohol. Even if alcohol is not the cause of their liver disease, cessation can lead to decreased fluid and improved response to medical therapies. Patients with ascites should also minimize use of all NSAIDs; these agents inhibit the synthesis of renal prostaglandin and can lead to renal vasoconstriction, decreased diuretic response, and acute renal failure. Finally, ascites patients should be counseled to limit their sodium consumption to no more than 2 g/day. Because fluid passively follows sodium, a salt restriction without a fluid restriction is generally all that is required to decrease the amount of ascites. In patients with minimal fluid, the restriction of alcohol, NSAIDs, and salt may be all that is needed to control ascites formation adequately.

Moderate-Volume Ascites

Patients with moderate fluid overload who do not respond to more conservative measures should be considered for pharmacologic therapy. A rapid reduction of ascites is often accomplished simply with the addition of low-dose oral diuretics in the outpatient setting.

First-line diuretic therapy for cirrhotic ascites is the combined use of spironolactone (Aldactone) and furosemide (Lasix). Beginning dosages are 100 mg of spironolactone and 40 mg of furosemide by mouth daily. If weight loss and natriuresis are inadequate, both drugs can be simultaneously increased after 3 to 5 days to 200 mg of spironolactone and 80 mg of furosemide. To maintain normal electrolyte balance, the use of the 100:40 mg ratio of spironolactone to furosemide is generally recommended. Maximum accepted dosages are 400 and 160 mg/day of spironolactone and furosemide, respectively.

The response to diuretics should be carefully monitored on the basis of changes in body weight, laboratory tests, and clinical assessment. Patients on diuretics should be weighed daily; the rate of weight loss should not exceed 0.5 kg/day in the absence of edema and should not exceed 1 kg/day when edema is present. Serum potassium, blood urea nitrogen (BUN), and creatinine levels should be serially followed. In the event of marked hyponatremia, hyperkalemia or hypokalemia, renal insufficiency, dehydration, or encephalopathy, diuretics should be reduced or discontinued. Routine measurement of the urinary sodium level is not necessary, but it can be helpful to identify noncompliance with dietary sodium restriction. Patients excreting more than 78 mmol of sodium/day (88 mmol dietary intake − 10 mmol nonurinary excretion) detected on a 24-hour urinary collection should be losing fluid weight. If not, they are noncompliant with their diet and should be referred to a dietician. The spot urine sodium-to-potassium ratio might ultimately replace the cumbersome 24-hour collection: A random urine sodium concentration higher than the potassium concentration has been shown to correlate with a 24-hour sodium excretion higher than 78 mmol/day with approximately 90% accuracy. Because of the potentially severe complications associated with diuretic use, patients with ascites should be assessed by a health care provider at least once weekly until they are clinically stable.

Large-Volume Ascites

Large-volume ascites is defined as intraperitoneal fluid in an amount that significantly limits the activities of daily life. With additional fluid retention, the abdomen can become progressively distended and painful. This is commonly referred to as *massive* or *tense ascites.*

Therapeutic (or large-volume) paracentesis is a well-established therapy for large-volume ascites. However, the use of postprocedural colloid, usually albumin, continues to be a controversial issue. Studies have shown that patients who do not receive intravenous albumin after large-volume paracentesis develop significantly more changes in their serum electrolyte, creatinine, and renin levels. The clinical relevance of these findings, however, is not well established. In fact, no study to date has been able to demonstrate decreased morbidity or mortality in patients given no plasma expanders compared with patients given albumin after paracentesis. In view of the high cost of albumin and its uncertain clinical role, more studies certainly need to be conducted. Until these studies are carried out, current practice guidelines state that it is reasonable, although not mandatory, to give albumin for paracenteses greater than 5 L. Although no direct comparisons have been studied, 25% albumin at doses of 5 to 10 g/L of ascites removed is generally used.

To prevent the reaccumulation of ascites fluid, patients with large-volume ascites should be counseled about limiting consumption of alcohol, NSAIDs, and sodium. They should also be placed on an aggressive diuretic regimen. Diuretic-sensitive patients are generally treated with lifestyle modifications and medications, not serial paracentesis.

Refractory Ascites

Refractory ascites occurs in 5% to 10% of cirrhotic ascites patients and portends a poor prognosis. The definition of refractory ascites is (1) lack of response to high-dose diuretics (400 mg of spironolactone and 160 mg of furosemide/day) while remaining compliant with a low-sodium diet or (2) frequent ascites recurrence shortly after therapeutic paracentesis. Patients with recurrent side effects from

Table 3 Child-Pugh Classification*

Clinical or Biochemical Parameter	Points		
	1	2	3
Bilirubin (mg/dL)	<2	2-3	>3
Albumin (g/dL)	>3.5	2.8-3.5	<2.8
Ascites	Absent	Moderate	Tense
Encephalopathy	Absent	Moderate (I or II)	Severe (III or IV)
Prothrombin time			
Seconds prolonged or	<4	4-6	>6
International normalized ratio (INR)	<1.7	1.7-2.3	>2.3

*Child-Pugh score: A = 5-6, B = 7-9, C = 10-15.

diuretic therapy, including symptomatic hyponatremia, hyperkalemia or hypokalemia, renal insufficiency, or hepatic encephalopathy, are also considered to have refractory ascites. Treatment options include large-volume paracentesis with albumin infusion, placement of a TIPS, or liver transplantation. Surgical shunts (e.g., LeVeen or Denver shunt) have essentially been abandoned because controlled trials have shown poor long-term patency, excessive complications, and no survival advantage over medical therapy.

Frequent therapeutic paracentesis with or without albumin infusion is the most widely accepted treatment for patients with refractory ascites (see "Large-Volume Ascites" for controversy and dosing of albumin use). For those who have loculated fluid or are unwilling or unable to receive frequent paracentesis, TIPS placement can also be considered. In the appropriately selected patient, TIPS is highly effective for preventing ascites recurrence by decreasing the activity of sodium-retaining mechanisms and improving renal function. Ongoing studies will determine whether TIPS might also provide a survival benefit.

In the United States, TIPS is most commonly performed under conscious sedation by an interventional radiologist. The portal system is accessed through the jugular vein, and the operator inserts a self-expanding shunt between the portal (high-pressure) and hepatic (low-pressure) veins. The ultimate goal of the procedure is to lower portal pressures to less than 12 mm Hg, the level at which ascites begins to accumulate. Complications are relatively common and include hemorrhage (intrahepatic or intra-abdominal) and stent stenosis or thrombosis. Other important complications include hepatic encephalopathy and decompensation of liver or cardiac function. Therefore, TIPS is generally not recommended for patients with pre-existing encephalopathy, an ejection fraction lower than 55%, or a Child-Pugh Score higher than 12 (Table 3). Additional disadvantages of the procedure are high cost and lack of availability at some medical centers.

Liver transplantation is the ultimate treatment for cirrhosis and cirrhotic ascites. Appropriate timing for referral is debated, but should be considered when a cirrhotic patient first presents with a complication from cirrhosis, such as ascites. Because refractory ascites portends a particularly poor prognosis, immediate referral to an experienced liver transplantation center is recommended.

The 2-year survival rate for a patient with cirrhotic ascites is approximately 50%. Once a patient becomes refractory to routine medical therapy, 50% die within 6 months and 75% within 1 year. Because liver transplantation is associated with 2-year survival rates of almost 85%, it should be considered as an important treatment option in all appropriate patients.

Many with ascites will develop infection, most often without a known precipitating factor (such as diverticulitis, bowel perforation, etc). This is referred to as spontaneous bacterial peritonitis (SBP). SBP should be suspected whenever there is clinical deterioration in a cirrhotic with ascites. Diagnosis rests on ascitic fluid cell count (more than 250 polymorphonuclear cells/mm^3) or a positive ascitic fluid culture. Treatment should be undertaken whenever SBP is suspected. Most often intravenous therapy with a third undertaken whenever SBP is suspected. Most often intravenous therapy with a third generation cephalosporin (e.g., cefotaxime 2 gm every 8 hours) is used. Quinolones may also be effective, including oral agents such as ofloxacin (400 mg twice per day). Intravenous albumin (1.5 gm/kg body weight on day zero and 1.0 gm/kg on day 3 has been shown to improve survival in SBP, particularly in those with renal insufficiency and should be used if the creatinine or BUN are elevated. Antibiotic treatment should be continued for 5 days. The presence of bacteremia does not influence treatment duration. Longer therapy may be warranted in individual cases. Those who survive SBP are at risk for a second bout. Prophylactic antibiotics are recommended, e.g., norfloxacin 400 mg daily, or trimethoprim/sulfamethoxazole (160/800). A clinical practice guideline updated in 2009 suggests a role for SBP prophylaxis even in those who have never had SBP. Primary SBP prophylaxis should be considered in patients with ascites containing <1.5 gm/dl and one or more of the following: serum creatinine >1.2 mg/dl; BUN >25 mg/dl; serum sodium concentration <130 mEq/L, Childs Pugh score >9 together with a bilirubin >3 mg/dl.

Hepatorenal Syndrome

A feared complication of advanced liver disease is hepatorenal syndrome (HRS). In its most virulent form (type I) there is an inexorable worsening of renal function reflecting in rising creatinine and BUN, resulting in death. This syndrome almost always occurs in the setting of ascites. A diagnosis is established when other causes of acute renal insufficiency are excluded, especially hypovolemia due either to diuretic use, infection, or bleeding. HRS is established in a patient with a creatinine of >1.5 mg/dl that does not improve with withdrawal of diuretics, volume expansion with albumin, absence of obstructive or parenchymal renal disease (indicated by ultrasonography, proteinuria), and absence of recent use of nephrotoxic drugs or administration of IV contrast material. Treatment of HRS is frustrating and often unsuccessful. Studies suggest a possible role for use of intravenous albumin (e.g., 25 grams daily) together with octreotide (200 ug sc TID) and midodrine (5 mg TID, titrating to a maximum of 12.5 mg TID). Referral for liver transplantation services should be considered for appropriate patients. A less severe form of HRS (type II) is recognized. In this variant, non-progressive renal impairment without another etiology than cirrhosis is seen.

HEPATIC ENCEPHALOPATHY

Definition and Etiology

Hepatic encephalopathy (HE) is defined as mental or neuromotor dysfunction in a patient with acute or chronic liver disease. Several forms of HE have been described (Box 3). The acute form of HE is often associated with fulminant hepatic failure and can rapidly progress to seizures, coma, and death. In patients with cirrhosis, acute encephalopathy is most commonly associated with a precipitating factor, such as electrolyte disturbance, medications, gastrointestinal hemorrhage, or infection. Recurrent HE can occur with or without a precipitating factor and is usually easily reversible. Persistent HE is rare and is defined as the persistence of neuropsychiatric symptoms despite aggressive medical and dietary therapy. The most common form of HE is not always clinically apparent: A patient with subclinical HE has only mild cognitive deficits or subtle personality changes. Recent evidence demonstrates individuals with even

Box 3 Precipitating Factors in Hepatic Encephalopathy

Anemia
Azotemia, uremia
Constipation
Dehydration
Excessive dietary protein
Gastrointestinal bleeding
Hepatoma
Hypokalemia, metabolic alkalosis
Hypoglycemia
Hypothyroidism
Hypoxia
Infection (e.g., urinary tract, ascites)
Medications (e.g., narcotics, sedatives)
Vascular occlusion

miximal hepatic encephalopathy have impacted driving skills and a high rate of motor vehicle accidents. Specific neuropsychological or neurophysiologic testing may be required to secure the diagnosis in these cases.

Prevalence

HE may be clinically apparent in as many as one third of cirrhotic patients and, if rigorously tested, up to two thirds have some degree of mild or subclinical HE.

Pathophysiology

The exact etiology of how HE develops is largely unknown. The premise of most pathophysiologic theories involves the accumulation of ammonia in the central nervous system, producing alterations of neurotransmission that affect consciousness and behavior. These ammonia toxicity theories have been supported by studies demonstrating increased ammonia levels in patients with both fulminant hepatic failure and chronic liver disease. The lack of strong correlation between serum ammonia levels and stage or degree of encephalopathy has been used in the argument that hyperammonemia might not be the sole factor in HE pathogenesis.

Most ammonia is produced in the intestine by colonic breakdown of nitrogenous compounds and enterocytic catabolism of amino acids. Other sources of ammonia are the kidneys and skeletal muscle. Normally, ammonia is metabolized in the liver and promptly excreted through the kidneys or colon. Formation of glutamine from glutamate, by glutamine synthetase, in the liver and brain is another means of detoxifying ammonia. Impaired liver function, shunting of blood around the liver, and increased muscle wasting all lead to increased serum ammonia levels in cirrhotic patients.

Ammonia interferes with brain function at many sites. Ammonia crosses the blood-brain barrier and directly depresses the central nervous system. There is also evidence that hyperammonemia might facilitate the brain's uptake of tryptophan, a substance with neuroactive metabolites such as serotonin. Excess ammonia can reduce brain adenosine triphosphate (ATP) levels, resulting in impaired cerebral energy. Lastly, the metabolism of ammonia to glutamine in the brain increases the intracellular osmolarity of astrocytes, inducing astrocyte swelling and vasodilation. Increased astrocyte hydration without overt increased intracranial pressure is currently considered a major factor in the development of HE in patients with chronic liver disease.

Toxins other than ammonia have also been implicated in the pathogenesis of HE. Excesses of neurotoxic short-chain fatty acids and mercaptans have received attention in the past. Patients with cirrhosis have also been shown to have decreased branched-chain amino acid (BCAA) to aromatic amino acid (AAA) ratios. It has been postulated that the increased AAA level in the cirrhotic patient's brain might competitively inhibit normal neurotransmitters. Cirrhotic patients with HE have been shown to have greatly increased serum manganese levels. Manganese can deposit directly in the basal ganglia and induce extrapyramidal symptomatology. Manganese can also act synergistically with ammonia to activate peripheral-type benzodiazepine receptors and the gamma-aminobutyric acid (GABA)-ergic neuroinhibitory system.

Table 4 Clinical Characteristics of Various Forms of Hepatic Encephalopathy

Form	Precipitating Factors	Clinical Course	Reversibility
Acute	+	Short*	±*
Recurrent	±	Short	+
Persistent	–	Continuous	–
Subclinical	–	Insidious	–

*May be fatal or irreversible as in fulminant hepatic failure.

Signs and Symptoms

In patients with progressive HE, there is a gradual decrease in level of consciousness, intellectual capacity, and logical behavior, along with the development of specific neurologic deficits. Two staging systems have been described. Numerous studies have used the West Haven criteria of altered mental status in patients with HE (Table 4). Although the Glasgow coma scale has not been rigorously evaluated in this specific patient population, its widespread use in various other disorders of brain function makes it applicable for patients with acute or chronic liver disease (Table 5).

Diagnosis

HE is a diagnosis of exclusion. Similar neuropsychiatric symptoms are seen in various metabolic disorders, toxic ingestions, or intracranial processes (Table 6). In certain patients, brain imaging or electroencephalography (EEG) may be indicated to exclude an intracranial abnormality. Lumbar puncture with cerebrospinal fluid analysis may also be required for patients with unexplained fever, leukocytosis, or symptoms suggesting meningeal irritation. Knowledge of the existence of acute or chronic liver disease, history of HE, or both is often helpful in heightening clinical suspicion and securing the diagnosis.

The most commonly studied laboratory test in HE is the venous ammonia level. Because of inconsistent elevation and lack of correlation with the stage of encephalopathy, determination of ammonia levels is not considered to be a good screening tool. Measurement of serum ammonia can be helpful, for example, when the level is elevated and there is doubt regarding the presence of significant liver disease. The arterial ammonia concentration provides a more accurate assessment of the amount of ammonia at the blood-brain barrier, but it is also of limited clinical use.

Because of implications in diagnosis and treatment, a search for a precipitating factor should be sought in all cirrhotic patients hospitalized for HE (Box 4). Serum determination of the complete blood count, electrolyte levels, and renal function is indicated in almost all cases. Recent use of psychoactive medications, such as narcotics or sedatives, should also be investigated. In a confused patient who cannot give a reliable history, the examination of stool or placement of a nasogastric tube may help in detecting gastrointestinal bleeding. Because infection is a common precipitating factor in HE, the culture of body fluids (urine, blood and ascites, if present) should be routinely performed. Lastly, the consumption of excessive dietary protein and constipation can precipitate HE. This is believed to be the result of an increased nitrogen load in the gastrointestinal tract. Rare precipitants, such as hepatoma or vascular occlusion, need only be investigated if no other factors are believed to be contributing or with clinical suspicion.

Table 5 West Haven Criteria of Altered Mental Status in Hepatic Encephalopathy

Stage	Consciousness	Intellect and Behavior	Neurologic Findings
0	Normal	Normal	Normal examinationImpaired psychomotor testing
1	Mild lack of awareness	Shortened attention span Impaired addition or subtraction	Mild asterixis or tremor
2	Lethargic	Disoriented Inappropriate behavior	Obvious asterixis Slurred speech
3	Somnolent but arousable	Gross disorientation Bizarre behavior	Muscular rigidity and clonus Hyperreflexia
4	Coma	Coma	Decerebrate posturing

Table 6 Glasgow Scale of Level of Consciousness

Best Motor Response (M)	Score	Best Verbal Response (V)	Score	Eyes Open (E)	Score
Obeys verbal orders	6				
Localizes painful stimuli	5	Oriented and conversant	5		
Withdraws from painful stimuli	4	Disoriented and conversant	4	Spontaneously	4
Flexion in response to pain	3	Inappropriate words	3	To command	3
Extension in response to pain	2	Inappropriate sounds	2	To pain	2
No response	1	No response	1	No response	1

M + V + E = 3 to 15. Severe encephalopathy is defined as a score ≤12.

Box 4 Differential Diagnostic Considerations in Hepatic Encephalopathy

Metabolic
Hypo- or hyperglycemia
Hypo- or hypercalcemia
Hypokalemia
Hypoxia
Uremia

Toxic
Alcohol intoxication
Alcohol withdrawal
Carbon monoxide narcosis
Illicit drugs
Medications

Central Nervous System
Bleed or infarction
Abscess, meningitis
Encephalitis
Trauma
Tumor

Summary

- HE is a diagnosis of exclusion.
- Determination of a serum ammonia level can be helpful but is not a good screening tool.
- All cirrhotic patients hospitalized for HE should be evaluated for a precipitating factor.

Treatment

The main objectives in the treatment of HE are fourfold: provide supportive care, correct any precipitating factors, reduce the nitrogen load in the gastrointestinal tract, and assess the need for long-term therapy. Each of these objectives is discussed separately here.

Standard supportive care is required for all hospitalized patients with HE. Patient safety and frequent monitoring of mental status are crucial. This can require additional personnel and, in the case of comatose patients, admission to the intensive care unit, endotracheal intubation, or both. Patients with HE should also avoid prolonged periods of fasting. Although the restriction of dietary protein at the time of acute HE can be part of therapy, protracted nitrogen restriction can lead to malnutrition. Appropriate enteral nutrition, by mouth or nasogastric feeding tube, should be administered as soon as feasible.

A methodical search to identify and treat any precipitating factors is crucial in reversing the signs and symptoms of HE. (See earlier, "Diagnosis," for a more detailed discussion.)

Because the toxins believed to be responsible for HE arise in the gastrointestinal tract, removal of the nitrogenous load is the mainstay of therapy. Various pharmacologic agents may be used, but the nondigestable disaccharide known as lactulose is currently the first-line therapy. After consumption, lactulose passes through the small bowel completely undigested. Once in the colon, lactulose is metabolized by colonic bacteria and the pH is lowered. This acidification of the bowel is believed to underlie the cathartic effect; ammonia can then pass from the blood stream into the colonic lumen to be excreted. As a result, peripheral ammonia levels are reduced.

For acute encephalopathy, lactulose can be administered either orally (by mouth or through a nasogastric tube) or via retention enemas (Table 7). The usual oral dose is 45 mL followed by dosing every hour or two until evacuation occurs. At that point, dosing is

Table 7 Commonly Used Medications for Hepatic Encephalopathy

Drug	Dose (Acute)	Dose (Chronic)	Side Effects
Lactulose			
Oral	45 mL PO q1-2hr	15-45 mL PO q6-12hr	Diarrhea, flatulence, cramps
Enema	300 mL in 1 L of water q4-6hr	Not used chronically	Diarrhea, flatulence, cramps
Antibiotics			
Metronidazole	250 mg PO q8-12hr	250 mg PO q8-12hr	Peripheral neuropathy
Rifaximin	400 mg PO q8hr	400 mg PO q8hr	Rare flatulence, constipation
Neomycin	1000 mg PO q4-8hr	500 mg PO q6-12hr	Rare nephro- and ototoxicity

adjusted to attain two or three soft bowel movements daily. This usually requires 15 to 45 mL every 6 to 12 hours. Lactulose by enema is administered as 300 mL in 1 L of water and should be retained for 1 hour. Because of the difficulty of administration, lactulose by enema is not generally used for chronic therapy. Common side effects include flatulence, bloating, and diarrhea.

For patients who do not tolerate lactulose or have continued symptoms, antibiotics are a second-line alternative for therapy. Antibiotics are believed to reverse HE by its alteration of colonic bacteria. Metronidazole (Flagyl) and neomycin are most commonly used. Metronidazole is generally administered at 250 mg every 8 to 12 hours. Dose and duration of metronidazole should be minimized as much as possible to avoid peripheral neuropathy, a side effect associated with its long-term use. Neomycin is as effective as metronidazole and is administered at 3 to 6 g/day in acute encephalopathy and 1 to 2 g/day when used chronically. Neomycin use should also be limited, if possible, because long-term use can lead to rare ototoxicity, renal failure, or both. If administered chronically to control HE symptoms (with or without lactulose), periodic renal and annual auditory monitoring should be performed.

Rifaximin (Xifaxon®) is a nonabsorbable derivative of rifampin that has been used in Europe for a wide variety of gastrointestinal problems, including HE, for many years. In 2005, the drug received approval from the U.S. Food and Drug Administration (FDA) for HE therapy in the United States. Previous studies have demonstrated that rifaximin at doses of 400 mg every 8 hours is as effective as lactulose and neomycin at improving HE symptoms. Rifaximin has few side effects, making it an appealing alternative to other antibiotics, particularly when prolonged therapy is required.

Several other HE therapies have been investigated, but they are not routinely used. These include zinc, ornithine aspartate, flumazenil, and bromocriptine. In experimental models, zinc supplementation has been shown to decrease ammonia levels. Human studies, however, are conflicting, and zinc is currently only recommended in patients with known zinc deficiency. Some studies using ornithine aspartate have been encouraging, but the drug is not currently available in the United States. Flumazenil may also be helpful, but it is currently only indicated for patients with acute HE and suspected benzodiazepine intake. No oral or long-acting preparations are currently available, which would make flumazenil cumbersome to use long term. Improvements of extrapyramidal symptoms have also been reported when bromocriptine was added to more conventional therapies. Bromocriptine, at 30 mg orally twice daily, can be considered in patients who are refractory to other therapies.

Occasionally, a portosystemic shunt (spontaneous, surgical, or from placement of a TIPS) is believed to be the primary cause of recurrent or chronic HE. In these rare cases, the shunt can be occluded. This is generally accomplished by placement of occlusive coils by an interventional radiologist. This advanced procedure should only be undertaken at experienced medical centers and after all other measures have failed.

Before discharge from the hospital, all cirrhotic patients with HE should be assessed for the need for long-term therapy. Patients should be counseled on avoiding precipitating factors such as constipation and psychoactive medications. Compliance with chronic medications, including lactulose, antibiotics, or both, should be emphasized. They should also be counseled about their higher risk of motor vehicle accidents and advised to curtail driving of appropriate. Appropriate candidates should be referred to a liver transplantation center after the first episode of overt encephalopathy. The ultimate therapy for cirrhosis and HE is orthotopic liver transplantation.

Some forms are reversible, but the development of overt HE overall carries a poor prognosis. Recovery and recurrence rates are variable but, without liver transplantation, the 1-year survival is only 40%. Both acute and chronic HE, once advanced to stage 4 (coma), is associated with an 80% overall mortality rate.

Summary

- The main objectives in the treatment of HE are to provide supportive care, correct any precipitating factors, reduce the nitrogen load in the gastrointestinal tract, and assess the need for long-term therapy.
- Lactulose is generally considered first-line therapy for acute and chronic HE.
- Antibiotics are second-line therapy for HE, but they can have many potential side effects and complications.
- Rifaximin was recently FDA approved for use in HE and appears to have fewer side effects than other antibiotics.
- Development of overt HE is a poor prognostic indicator.

VARICEAL HEMORRHAGE

Definition and Etiology

Varices are dilated submucosal veins, most commonly detected in the distal esophagus or proximal stomach, but they can occur anywhere in the gastrointestinal tract. Varices are associated with portal hypertension of any cause, including cirrhosis. Any cirrhotic patient with varices is placed at risk for variceal hemorrhage, the most lethal complication of cirrhosis. Despite advances in therapy over the last decade, variceal hemorrhage is associated with a mortality of at least 20% at 6 weeks.

Prevalence

Esophageal varices are present in approximately 50% of patients with cirrhosis. Gastric varices are less prevalent, occurring in 5% to 33% of these patients. Variceal hemorrhage occurs at a yearly rate of 5% to 15%. Clinical and endoscopic predictors of a first variceal hemorrhage include advanced Child-Pugh score (see Table 3), continued alcohol use, large varices, and presence of red wale markings.

Pathophysiology

In cirrhosis, portal pressures initially increase as a consequence of resistance to blood flow within the liver. This resistance is due mainly to fibrous tissue and regenerative nodules in the hepatic parenchyma. In addition to this structural resistance, there is intrahepatic vasoconstriction, as well. This is believed to be due to decreased production of endogenous nitric oxide.

Varices are the portosystemic collaterals that form after pre-existing vascular channels are dilated by portal hypertension. Dilation generally is clinically significant once the wedged hepatic venous pressure (WHVP) gradient is elevated above 12 mm Hg (normal, <5 mm Hg). The WHVP is defined as the gradient between the wedged hepatic venous pressure and the free hepatic venous pressure measured by a catheter threaded down through the jugular vein. It is important to remember that varices do not invariably form once the WHVP is above 12 mm Hg, so this pressure gradient is generally considered necessary but not sufficient.

Signs and Symptoms

Nonbleeding varices are generally asymptomatic. Once varices are bleeding, patients classically present with symptoms of an upper gastrointestinal hemorrhage such at hematemesis, passage of black or bloody stools, lightheadedness, or decreased urination. Associated signs of variceal hemorrhage include decompensated liver function manifested as jaundice, hepatic encephalopathy, worsened or new-onset ascites. Physical examination will likely reveal hypotension or shock (in severe cases), pallor and stigmata of chronic liver disease such as spider angiomatas, palmar erythema, gynecomastia, or splenomegaly. A rectal examination should be performed on all patients without obvious bleeding. A black tarry stool on the gloved finger suggests an upper gastrointestinal source, and further workup needs to be pursued. Hemoccult testing is not necessary because clinically significant bleeding should be apparent with visual inspection of the stool alone.

Diagnosis

The gold standard for the diagnosis of varices is esophagogastroduodenoscopy (EGD). It is generally recommended that patients with cirrhosis undergo elective endoscopic screening for varices at the time of diagnosis and periodically thereafter if no or small varices are detected (Fig. 2). If screening EGD reveals appreciable esophageal varices, a size classification should be assigned. Different size classification systems have been used over the years; however, a recent consensus meeting proposed that varices be categorized in only two grades, small and large. An appropriate cut-off was determined to be 5mm; that is, small varices are those less than 5 mm and large varices are those greater than 5 mm.

Another procedure that is currently being studied for screening for varices is esophageal capsule endoscopy. Pilot studies suggest it is safe and well tolerated (and does not require sedation), although its sensitivity and cost effectiveness still needs to be established.

EGD is also the main method for diagnosing variceal hemorrhage. The diagnosis is secured when endoscopic evaluation reveals active bleeding from a varix or clinical evidence of a recent bleed, such as an overlying clot. Esophageal or gastric varices should be indicted as the most likely source of hemorrhage when varices are present and no other potential source of bleeding is found.

Treatment

Practice guidelines have recently been updated regarding the prevention and management of gastroesophageal varices and variceal hemorrhage in cirrhosis. Treatment of varices is best considered in three distinct phases: prevention of the first variceal hemorrhage (primary prophylaxis), control of acute hemorrhage, an prevention of a second hemorrhage in a patient who has already bled (secondary prophylaxis).

Primary Prophylaxis

If a patient has small varices that have never bled and has no risk factors for a first variceal hemorrhage (high Child-Pugh score, continued alcohol use, presence of red wale markings), prophylactic strategies can be considered, although the long-term benefit has never been established. In our practice, primary prophylaxis for bleeding has often been reserved for high-risk patients who have small varices and for all patients with large varices.

The primary pharmacologic strategy for preventing variceal hemorrhage is use of nonselective beta blockers, particularly propranolol and nadolol. These medications reduce portal pressures both by decreasing cardiac output and by producing splanchnic vasoconstriction. Several studies have shown that nonselective beta blockers decrease the risk for first variceal hemorrhage by 40% to 50% when compared to patients taking placebo. A meta-analysis has also showed a statistically significant decrease in overall mortality. Selective beta-blockers, such as atenolol and metoprolol, are less effective and are not currently recommended for primary prophylaxis. Likewise, use of isosorbide mononitrate (alone or with nonselective beta blockers) is not currently recommended.

Propranolol is usually started at a dose of 20 mg twice daily and nadolol at a dose of 40 mg daily. The goal of therapy is to reduce the WHVP by at least 20% or to a gradient of less than 12 mm Hg. However, because WHVP measurement is not widely available, most clinicians aim to titrate the dose of beta blockers to achieve a resting heart rate of 55 beats/min or a reduction of heart rate by 25% from baseline. Unfortunately, beta blockers have some significant side effects, so often the dose is simply adjusted to a maximally tolerated dose. The most common side effects reported are lightheadedness, fatigue, shortness of breath, and impotence in men. Relative contraindications to the use of beta blockers include reactive airways disease, insulin-dependent diabetes (with episodes of hypoglycemia), and peripheral vascular disease.

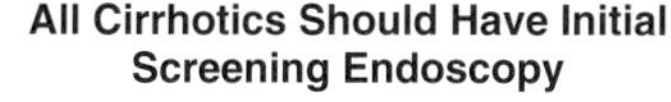
All Cirrhotics Should Have Initial Screening Endoscopy
Child-Pugh ≤ 7
Child-Pugh > 7
No varices at screening
Small varices at screening
Large varices at screening
No or small varices at screening
EGD in 2–3 yr
EGD in 1 yr
Band ligation or beta blocker
EGD in 1 yr

Figure 2 **Endoscopic surveillance for esophageal varices in cirrhosis.**

Patients who meet criteria for primary prophylaxis but who cannot tolerate or have contraindications to beta blocker therapy should be considered for prophylactic endoscopic variceal ligation (EVL). Although studies have been conflicting, a recent consensus panel of experts concluded that both nonselective beta blockers and EVL are effective in preventing first variceal hemorrhage. The decision on whether to treat pharmacologically or via EVL should be based on patient characteristics and preferences, local resources, and expertise.

Acute Variceal Hemorrhage

Cirrhotic patients with suspected acute variceal hemorrhage should be admitted directly to an intensive care unit setting for frequent monitoring and aggressive management (Fig. 3). While still in the emergency department, initial resuscitation can begin by securing large-bore IVs and sending bloodwork to the lab, including a type and crossmatch for blood products. Volume resuscitation should be undertaken promptly but with caution because vigorous resuscitation can actually increase portal pressures to levels higher than baseline, thereby prompting rebleeding. In our practice we usually start the resuscitation with normal saline and switch to blood or albumin (or both), once available, with the goal to maintain hemodynamic stability. Transfusion of fresh frozen plasma and platelets can be considered in patients with a severe coagulopathy or thrombocytopenia. Low threshold should be taken to intubate the patient for airway protection, particularly if the patient is in shock or encephalopathic, because aspiration of blood often occurs.

Antibiotics are routinely administered in cirrhotic patients who are admitted to the hospital with variceal hemorrhage. Several randomized clinical trials were able to show that antibiotics not only decreased the rate of bacterial infection in these patients but also decreased the incidence of early rebleeding and increased overall survival. The optimal antibiotic and duration is unclear, because benefit was detected from many different regimines. In general, oral norfloxacin at doses of 400 mg twice daily for 7 days or IV ciprofloxacin (in patients in whom oral administration is not possible) is the recommended antibiotic. In patients with advanced cirrhosis or at hospitals with a high incidence of quinolone resistance, ceftriaxone at a dose of 1 g IV daily may be preferable.

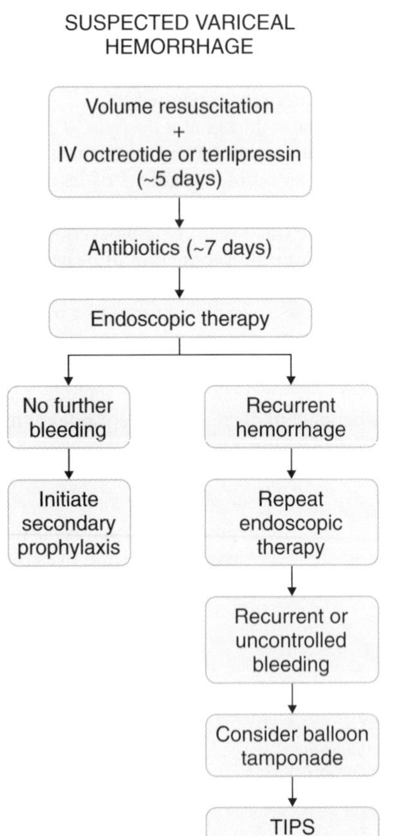

Figure 3 **Mangement of acute variceal hemorrhage.** TIPS, transjugular intrahepatic portosystemic shunt.

Pharmacologic therapy to decrease portal pressures is critically important and should be considered the first-line treatment for acute variceal hemorrhage. It should be initiated as soon as the diagnosis of variceal hemorrhage is suspected and before EGD. The most common pharmacologic agent used in the United States for this purpose is octreotide, a somatostatin analogue that causes splanchnic vasoconstriction. The advantage of octreotide is that it can stop variceal hemorrhage in up to 80% of patients and is nearly devoid of side effects. It has been most widely used as an initial IV bolus of 50 µg followed by 50 µg/hour. This agent should be administered ideally for 5 days, even after bleeding is controlled. Vasopressin (most often used with nitroglycerin) is the most potent splanchnic vasoconstrictor, but it is rarely used for control of variceal hemorrhage due to its multiple vascular side effects including myocardial and mesenteric ischemia and infarction. Terlipressin is a vasopressin analogue that has significantly fewer side effects. It is effective in controlling variceal hemorrhage and reducing mortality. It is administered at an initial dose of 2 mg IV every 4 hours and then titrated down to 1 mg every 4 hours once bleeding is controlled. Terlipressin is currently used extensively in other parts of the world but is not widely available in the United States.

Even though pharmacologic therapy can be effective at controlling suspected variceal hemorrhage, EGD should be performed as soon as possible to confirm the diagnosis and implement endoscopic therapy. Endoscopic therapy is highly effective and can control variceal bleeding in 80% to 90% of patients. Sclerotherapy, widely used in the past, is now nearly obsolete because of improvement in EVL devices and risk of complication. Indeed, recent consensus determined EVL to be the preferred form of endoscopic therapy for acute esophageal variceal bleeding, although sclerotherapy is still recommended in patients in whom EVL is not technically feasible. Gastric varices, which are often not amenable to either EVL or sclerotherapy, may be more difficult to treat. *N*-butyl-2-cyanoacrylate glue injected directly into the varix has been shown to be effective for control of bleeding gastric varices.

Despite endoscopic and pharmacologic therapies, variceal bleeding cannot be controlled or recurs in up to 20% of patients. It is at this time that portal decompressive therapy, either shunt surgery or TIPS, can be considered. As TIPS has become more widely available, this is becoming the preferred decompressive procedure. However, performance of either TIPS or shunt surgery largely depends on local expertise. Because TIPS and surgery are both invasive procedure with a high risk of complication, they are reserved for patients who fail pharmacologic therapy and repeated attempts at endoscopic therapy.

Balloon tamponade applies direct pressure to the ruptured varix and can be highly effective for immediate control of variceal hemorrhage. Unfortunately, recurrent bleeding is common after the balloon is decompressed, and balloon tamponade is associated with potentially fatal complications such necrosis or perforation of the esophagus. Therefore, tamponade should be used only as a rescue procedure and a bridge to more definitive therapy, such as TIPS, in the cases of uncontrolled bleeding.

Secondary Prophylaxis

Patients who survive an episode of acute variceal hemorrhage are at high risk of rebleeding and death. If bleeding is left untreated, the rebleeding rate is nearly 60% within 1 to 2 years, with a mortality rate of 33%. Several studies have demonstrated that combination endoscopic plus pharmacologic therapy is the most effective means of preventing secondary bleeding episodes.

In terms of endoscopic therapies, EVL is the method of choice for secondary prophylaxis. After inital control of the bleeding, EVL should be repeated at 1- to 2-week intervals until varices are completely obliterated. This usually requires 2 to 4 sessions. Once the varices are obliterated, EGD is repeated every 3 to 6-months to evaluate the need for repeat EVL. Complications of EVL include chest pain, dysphagia and ulcers that form at the site of the band ligation, which universally form and can cause significant bleeding. Although not definitively proven to be effective, proton pump inhibition is sometimes used in an attempt to decrease the bleeding risk from these band ulcer sites for 2 weeks after an EVL procedure.

Optimal pharmacologic therapy for secondary prophylaxis appears to be a combination of a nonselective beta blocker and a nitrate. However, this combination has significantly greater side effects compared to beta blockers alone and is overall poorly tolerated. In our clinical practice, most patients end up taking beta blockers alone. Clinical opinion is divided on the need to continue pharmacologic therapy once varices are completely obliterated, but current guidelines suggest that pharmacologic therapy should be continued at the highest tolerated dose indefinitely. TIPS or shunt surgery can be considered in patients who experience recurrent bleeding despite combination pharmacologic and endoscopic therapy.

Most variceal haemorrhages can be controlled with these measures. However, because acute variceal bleeding often precipitates a clinical deterioration and worsening of liver synthetic function, patients who are otherwise transplant candidates should be referred to a liver transplantation center for a liver transplant evaluation after recovery.

Summary

- Cirrhosis sets the stage for risk of GI bleeding once the WHVP rises above 12 mm Hg.
- Primary prophylaxis with either nonselective beta blockers or EVL is warranted in cirrhotic patients with small varices and high-risk features and in all patients with large varices.
- Treatment of acute variceal hemorrhage involves careful volume resuscitation, administration of antibiotics and drugs to reduce portal hypertension and prompt endoscopy therapy.
- Combination of pharmacologic and endoscopy therapy is employed for secondary prevention of variceal hemorrhage.
- TIPS and surgical shunts can be considered in patients in whom recurrent variceal hemorrhage occurs despite maximal pharmacologic and endoscopic therapies.

Suggested Readings

Ascites

Ginès P, Cárdenas A, Arroyo V, Rodés J: Management of cirrhosis and ascites. N Engl J Med 2004;350:1646-1654.

Ginès P, Quintero E, Arroyo V, et al: Compensated cirrhosis: Natural history and prognostic factors. Hepatology 1987;7:122-128.

Ginès P, Tító L, Arroyo V, et al: Randomized study of therapeutic paracentesis with and without intravenous albumin in cirrhosis. Gastroenterology 1988;94:1493-1502.

Moore KP, Wong F, Ginès P, et al: The management of ascites in cirrhosis: Report on the consensus conference of the International Ascites Club. Hepatology 2003;38: 258-266.

Runyon BA: AASLD practice guidelines. Management of adult patients with ascites due to cirrhosis: an update. Hepatology 2009;49:2087-2107.

Runyon BA, Montano AA, Akriviadis EA, et al: The serum-ascites albumin gradient is superior to the exudate-transudate concept in the differential diagnosis of ascites. Ann Intern Med 1992;117:215-220.

Sanyal AJ, Genning C, Reddy KR, et al: The North American Study for the Treatment of Refractory Ascites. Gastroenterology 2003;124:634-641.

Hepatic Encephalopathy

Blei AT, Cordobá J: Practice Parameters Committee of the American College of Gastroenterology: Hepatic encephalopathy practice guidelines. Am J Gastroenterol 2001;96:1968-1976.

Bajaj JS, Saeian K, Schubert CM, et al: Minimal hepatic encephalopathy is associated with motor vehicle crashes. Hepatology 2009;50:1175-1183.

Bustamante J, Rimola A, Ventura PJ, et al: Prognostic significance of hepatic encephalopathy in patients with cirrhosis. J Hepatol 1999;30:890-895.

Cordobá J, Blei AT: Treatment of hepatic encephalopathy. Am J Gastroenterol 1997;92:1429-1439.

Fitz JG: Hepatic encephalopathy, hepatopulmonary syndromes, hepatorenal syndrome, coagulopathy and endocrine complications of liver disease. In Feldman M, Friedman LS, Sleisenger MH (eds): Sleisenger & Fordtran's Gastrointestinal and Liver Disease, 8th ed. Philadelphia, WB Saunders, 2006, pp 1966-1972.

Stahl J: Studies of the blood ammonia in liver disease: Its diagnostic, prognostic, and therapeutic significance. Ann Intern Med 1963;58:1-24.

Variceal Hemorrhage

Garcia-Tsai G, Sanyal AJ, Grace N, Carey WD: Practice Guidelines Committee of American Association for Study of Liver Diseases; Practice Parameters Committee of the American College of Gastroenterology: Prevention and management of gastroesophageal varices and variceal hemorrhage in cirrhosis. Hepatology 2007; 46(3):922-938.

Gotzsche PC, Hrobjartsson A: Somatostatin analogues for acute bleeding oesophageal varices. Cochane Database Syst Rev 2005, CD000193.

Groszmann RJ, Garcia-Tsao G, Bosch J, Grace ND, Burroughs AK, Planas R, et al: for the Portal Hypertension Collaborative Group. Beta-blockers to prevent gastroesophageal varices in patiens with cirrhosis. N Engl J Med 2005;353:2254-2261.

North Italian Endoscopic Club for the Study and Treatment of Esophageal Varices: Prediction of the first variceal hemorrhage in patients with cirrhosis of the liver and esophageal varices. A prospective multicenter study. N Engl J Med 1988;319:983-989.

Sharara AI, Rockey DC: Gastroesophageal variceal hemorrhage. N Engl J Med 2001;345(9):669-681.

Soares-Weiser K, Brezis M, Tur-Kaspa R, Leibovici L: Antibiotic prophylaxis for cirrhotic patients with gastrointestinal bleeding. Cochrane Database Syst Rev. 2002;(2): CD002907.

Nonalcoholic Fatty Liver Disease

Anna Wieckowska and *William D. Carey*

DEFINITION AND CAUSES

Nonalcoholic fatty liver disease (NAFLD) is one of the most common causes of chronic liver disease. It encompasses a spectrum of conditions associated with lipid deposition in hepatocytes. It ranges from steatosis (simple fatty liver), to nonalcoholic steatohepatitis (NASH—fatty changes with inflammation and hepatocellular injury or fibrosis), to advanced fibrosis and cirrhosis (Fig. 1). Studies suggest that although simple fatty liver is a benign condition, NASH can progress to fibrosis and lead to end-stage liver disease. The disease is mostly silent and is often discovered through incidentally elevated liver enzyme levels. It is strongly associated with obesity and insulin resistance and is currently considered by many as the hepatic component of the metabolic syndrome (see later). NASH cirrhosis is now one of the leading indications for liver transplantation in the United States.

Because NAFLD resembles alcoholic liver disease but occurs in people who drink little or no alcohol, excessive daily alcohol consumption must be ruled out before making the diagnosis. Numerous other conditions leading to fatty liver must be excluded by history, physical examination, and appropriate testing (Box 1).

PREVALENCE AND RISK FACTORS

Accurate epidemiologic data are not available because of a lack of population-based studies and reliable noninvasive screening tools. There is disagreement about the methods used to diagnose NASH, and there is no clear consensus on the clinical implications of histologic changes or on the influence of the amount of alcohol ingested. The prevalence of NAFLD is affected by many factors, including genetics (predilection to alcohol abuse, sex) and environment and is therefore difficult to define. In general, however, the risk of liver disease increases with the weight of the patient.

From the available data, NAFLD is estimated to be present in one third of the general population in the United States. The prevalence of NASH is more difficult to determine. It seems to occur in approximately 3% of the population but may be found in more than 25% of obese persons.

The prevalence of overweight persons (body mass index [BMI] ≥25 kg/m^2) in the United States has risen to more than 65%, and obesity (BMI ≥30 kg/m^2) is now present in more than 30% of the adult U.S. population. The increasing prevalence of childhood obesity and NAFLD is equally alarming. Affected persons generally present between the fourth and sixth decades of life and are more often women (50%-80%). However, there are numerous reports of NAFLD in children and nonobese persons. NAFLD has been described in all ethnic groups, with some variation in clinical characteristics.

PATHOPHYSIOLOGY AND NATURAL HISTORY

Pathophysiology

Development of NASH may be the result of two liver insults, a *two-hit process.* With the initial hit, macrovesicular steatosis occurs. Insulin resistance and subsequent hyperinsulinemia seem to lead to alterations in the hepatic pathways of uptake, synthesis, degradation, and secretion of free fatty acids and ultimately to accumulation of lipids in the hepatocytes. These changes seem to make the liver susceptible to a second hit, resulting in an inflammatory response and progression of liver damage. Oxidative stress, mainly caused by mitochondrial dysfunction, and proinflammatory cytokines such as tumor necrosis factor α, are believed to play an important role in the progression of liver damage in NAFLD. Hepatocyte apoptosis, an organized form of cell death, has been identified as a potential key component of the second hit involved in NAFLD progression.

Natural History

Overall, morbidity and mortality have been shown to be significantly higher in NASH patients compared with the general population. Data suggest that the natural history of NAFLD is determined by the severity of the histologic damage. Most patients with NAFLD have pure steatosis without inflammation and are reported to have a benign clinical course. Up to 20% of patients with NASH progress to cirrhosis and its complications. At the time of initial biopsy, as many as one third of NASH patients have advanced hepatic fibrosis, whereas 10% to 15% have well-established cirrhosis. It is now recognized that a large portion of patients with cryptogenic cirrhosis have burned-out NASH: the histologic feature of steatosis or steatohepatitis is replaced by a bland cirrhosis. NASH-associated cirrhosis is an increasing indication for liver transplantation. NASH cirrhosis is also a risk factor for development of hepatocellular carcinoma (HCC). Japanese data suggest that the cumulative rate of HCC at 5 years may be as high as 15%.

Further studies are needed to define the pathogenesis of NAFLD clearly and explain the apparent interindividual variation in the susceptibility to progress to more-advanced liver disease. Genetic factors have been suggested to play an important role in this variation, and several new candidate genes have been proposed.

SIGNS AND SYMPTOMS

Most persons with NAFLD are asymptomatic, and liver disease is often discovered incidentally when laboratory examination shows elevated liver enzyme levels. It is the most common cause of unexplained persistent elevation of liver enzyme levels after hepatitis and other chronic liver diseases have been excluded. The most common symptoms that bring NAFLD to medical attention are malaise, fatigue, and right upper quadrant or diffuse abdominal discomfort. Hepatomegaly may be found on clinical examination. When cirrhosis appears, stigmata of chronic liver disease, such as spider angiomata, ascites, splenomegaly, hard liver border, palmar erythema, or asterixis, can be present. Patients might complain of jaundice or pruritus, or they might present with a complication of portal hypertension (e.g., ascites, variceal bleeding, or encephalopathy). Most patients have associated features of the metabolic syndrome (Table 1): obesity (47%-90%), diabetes mellitus (28%-55%), and variable incidences of hyperlipidemia (4%-92%) and hypertension.

DIAGNOSIS

NAFLD is usually diagnosed during further evaluation for elevated aminotransferase levels found in one of three situations: on routine checkup, when monitoring is performed for possible side effects of drugs (most often cholesterol-lowering medication), or for nonspecific symptoms. NAFLD can also be identified incidentally on

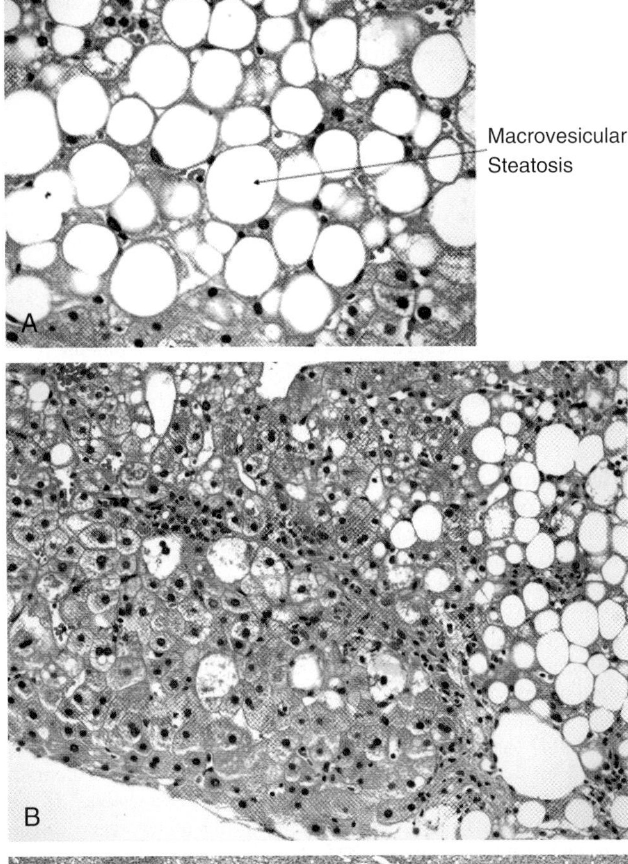

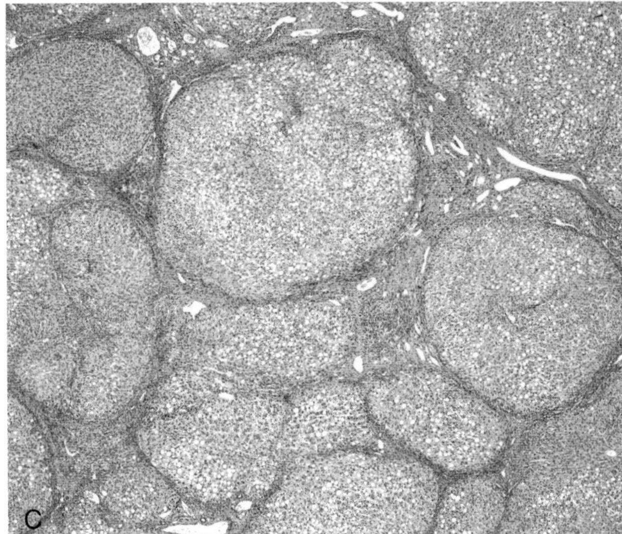

Figure 1 **Spectrum of disease in nonalcoholic fatty liver disease (NAFLD). A,** Nonalcoholic fatty liver (NAFL). **B,** Nonalcoholic steatohepatitis (NASH). **C,** Cirrhosis. *(Courtesy of Dr. Lisa M. Yerian.)*

Box 1 Conditions Associated With Macrovesicular Steatosis

Nonalcoholic fatty liver disease
Alcohol
Drugs

- Estrogens
- Coumadin
- Tamoxifen
- Valproic acid
- Methotrexate
- Isoniazid
- Corticosteroids
- Vitamin A
- Troglitazone
- L-Asparaginase
- Amiodarone
- Perhexiline
- Calcium channel blockers
- Nucleoside analogues

Hepatitis C (genotype 3)
Nutritional factors

- rapid weight loss, total parenteral nutrition

Surgical considerations

- Gastrointestinal surgery for obesity
- Extensive small-bowel resection

Metabolic disorders

- Cystic fibrosis
- Abetalipoproteinemia
- Others

Syndromes associated with obesity and insulin resistance

- lipodystrophies, hypopituitarism, Prader-Willi syndrome

Table 1 Diagnostic Criteria for the Metabolic Syndrome

Parameter*	Value
Impaired glucose tolerance	Fasting blood glucose level ≥110 mg/dL
High blood pressure	≥130/85 mm Hg
Elevated triglyceride levels	>250 mg/dL
Low high-density lipoprotein level	<40 mg/dL for men; <50 mg/dL for women
Abdominal obesity	Waist: >102 cm (40 inches) for men; >88 cm (35 inches) for women

*The metabolic syndrome is diagnosed by the presence of ≥2 of these parameters.

imaging or, less often, on liver biopsy done for other reasons. Some centers screen for NAFLD in high-risk groups that include patients with elements of the metabolic syndrome.

Clinical evaluation includes a careful history and physical examination. It is particularly relevant to inquire about excess alcohol consumption—defined as more than 30 g/day for men and more than 20 g/day for women within the last 5 years; 350 mL (12 oz) of beer, 120 mL (4 oz) of wine, and 45 mL (1.5 oz) of hard liquor each contain 10 g of alcohol—and to define the nonalcoholic nature of the condition. Moreover, it is necessary to exclude the alternative causes of fatty liver (see Box 1). It is most important to include anti–hepatitis C antibody as well as serum ceruloplasmin levels in young patients.

Primary noninvasive evaluation may be used to confirm the diagnosis of fatty liver disease, given the risks and costs of a liver biopsy. Clinical factors and basic laboratory evaluation, particularly in patients aged 45 years and older, or those with obesity, type 2 diabetes mellitus, or an aspartate aminotransferase–to–alanine aminotransferase (AST/ALT) ratio greater than 1, have been shown to be predictors of more-severe histologic disease and may be useful in making a decision regarding when to order a biopsy. Histologic evaluation is the gold standard and should be considered.

Laboratory Evaluation

In a patient with suspected NAFLD or NASH, useful baseline testing should include levels of AST, ALT, total and direct bilirubin, and fasting serum glucose, as well as a lipid panel. Mild to moderate elevation of serum aminotransferase levels is most commonly found (mean range, 100-200 IU/L). Generally, the ratio of AST to ALT is less than 1, but this ratio increases as fibrosis advances. Liver enzyme levels are normal in a large percentage of patients with NAFLD; normal aminotransaminase levels do not exclude the presence of advanced disease. Serum alkaline phosphatase and γ-glutamyl transpeptidase levels may also be mildly abnormal. Given that more than 80% of patients with NAFLD have some components of the metabolic syndrome, serum levels of fasting cholesterol and triglycerides, as well as fasting glucose and insulin, should be determined. Albumin, bilirubin, and platelet levels are usually normal unless the disease has evolved to cirrhosis. Some patients with NAFLD have low titers of autoimmune antibodies (antinuclear and anti–smooth muscle antibody) and an elevation of ferritin. The role of these markers is still unclear.

Imaging

A liver ultrasound examination is useful for confirming steatosis. Fatty infiltration of the liver produces a diffuse increase in echogenicity and vascular blurring (Fig. 2). Unfortunately, ultrasound cannot rule out steatohepatitis or fibrosis, and its sensitivity drops sharply when less than 30% of hepatocytes contain fat droplets. Both computed tomography (CT) and magnetic resonance imaging (MRI) studies, especially the new technique of magnetic resonance spectroscopy, are more sensitive modalities for quantifying steatosis. However, none of these imaging techniques has sufficient sensitivity and specificity for staging the disease and cannot distinguish between simple bland steatosis and NASH with or without fibrosis.

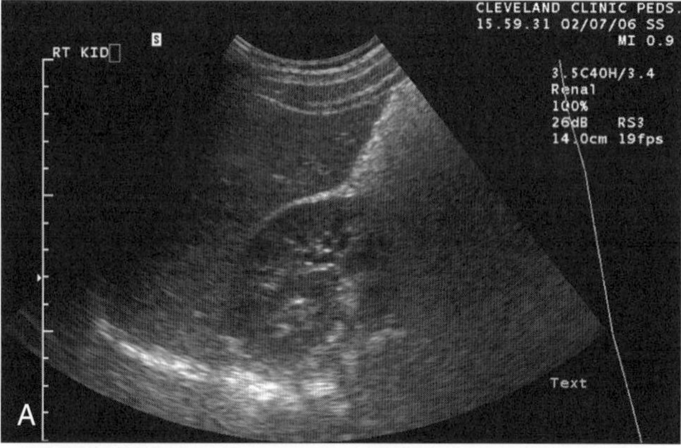

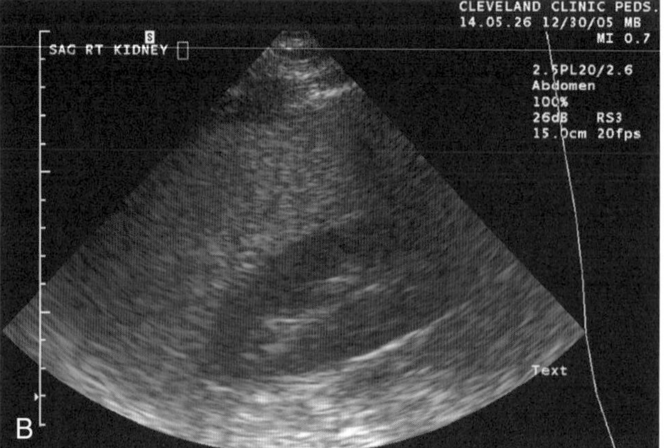

Figure 2 Sonographic features in fatty liver. A, Normal liver: same echogenicity as the kidney. **B,** Fatty liver: increased echogenicity compared with the kidney.

Liver Biopsy

Liver biopsy is of unquestioned value in determining the presence of steatosis, distinguishing steatosis from steatohepatitis, and assessing the degree of fibrosis. Because the diagnostic accuracy of noninvasive diagnostic tools is low, histology is the most reliable means to grade the severity of the disease and thus estimate prognosis. Biopsy is also helpful in ruling out an alternative diagnosis. In addition to establishing the cause and severity of disease, histology permits the monitoring of disease progression and the response to therapy, because aminotransaminase levels can decrease during the course of the disease regardless of whether fibrosis progresses or improves.

NAFLD is histologically indistinguishable from liver damage resulting from alcohol-induced liver injury. The steatosis seen in NAFLD is macrovesicular. In adults, similar histologic findings can be found in a number of conditions (see Box 1). The spectrum of abnormalities varies from simple bland steatosis to NASH, in which steatosis is associated with mixed inflammatory cell infiltration and liver injury. Cell injury is manifested by hepatocyte ballooning and by Mallory hyaline and acidophil bodies.

Despite the advantages of liver biopsy, its overall role in the evaluation of patients with NAFLD is unsettled, in large measure because of its risks and poor patient acceptance. In patients with risk factors for NAFLD (i.e., the metabolic syndrome), 3 to 6 months are often allowed for a trial of weight loss and for possible improvements in imaging studies and biochemical markers of liver disease. In the subset of patients most likely to have NASH or advanced disease (those with older age, higher BMI, type 2 diabetes, AST/ALT ratio = 1, clinical suspicion) and in those with an unclear diagnosis, a liver biopsy should be considered earlier (Fig. 3).

Because of the important limitations of the currently available noninvasive and invasive tests, recent efforts have focused on identifying potential novel noninvasive biomarkers for NASH and assessment of fibrosis.

TREATMENT

The goal of treatment is to improve steatosis and prevent the development of fibrosis, which can lead to cirrhosis and its complications. Because the prognosis of NASH depends on risk factors (e.g., obesity, insulin resistance, type 2 diabetes), these conditions have been the focus of treatment. Treatment proposed for NAFLD has been based on the two-hit hypothesis, the first being fatty liver infiltration (linked to obesity and insulin resistance) and the second being oxidative stress. Patients should avoid alcohol and other hepatotoxins.

Treatment of Obesity

Although no randomized clinical trials exist, weight reduction has been widely studied in adults and has been shown to improve not only the biochemical results but also the histology. Slow, consistent weight loss through diets designed to produce a caloric deficit of 500 to 1000 cal/day is advised. Reduction of dietary carbohydrates, in particular dietary fructose, is the most beneficial and has been found to improve the lipid profile in overweight patients. High- to moderate-intensity exercise (30 minutes, three to five times a week) has also been advocated to reduce the risk of comorbidities associated with obesity. However, more realistically, patients should be encouraged to incorporate moderate activity into everyday life (e.g., climbing stairs, walking instead of driving).

Finally, bariatric surgery is now suggested for patients with a BMI of more than 40 kg/m^2, or for those with a BMI of more than 35 kg/m^2 and obesity-related comorbidities. Resolution in steatosis,

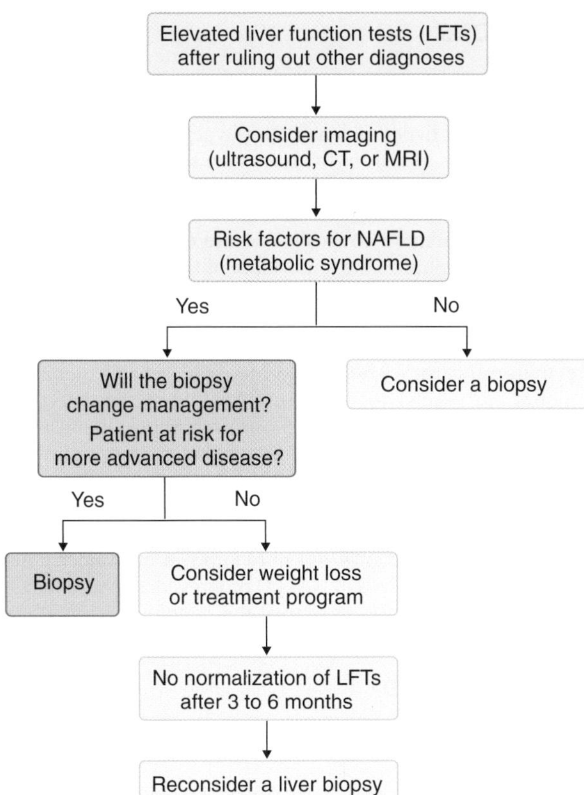

Figure 3 Algorithm for diagnosis in patients with elevated liver enzyme levels. CT, computed tomography; MRI, magnetic resonance imaging.

but not of fibrosis, has been convincingly demonstrated. However, the safety of bariatric surgery in patients with cirrhosis is still under investigation.

Pharmacologic Therapy

Although numerous clinical trials have been undertaken since the last American Gastroenterological Association Technical Review on Nonalcoholic Fatty Liver Disease, there is no consensus on the effectiveness of any therapeutic agent in the treatment of NAFLD. Pharmacologic treatment of obesity in NASH is still experimental. Several drugs have been studied, including sibutramine, a serotonin reuptake inhibitor, and orlistat, producing fat malabsorption, both of which have been shown to improve liver enzyme levels and sonographic signs of fatty liver. A multicentered randomized, controlled of rimonabant, a cannabinoid-1 antagonist, in human NASH is under way.

Insulin-Sensitizing Agents

NASH patients with diabetes are at higher risk of developing more-aggressive disease. Insulin-sensitizing agents have been tested in adults and are of benefit. Studies on metformin have shown discrepant results, but a large randomized trial in children with NASH is under way. Peroxisome proliferator-activated receptor gamma (PPARγ) agonists (thioglitazones) have been shown to improve insulin resistance, surrogate markers of fatty liver, and histology. However, hepatotoxicity has been described with thioglitazones, and a more common side effect is paradoxical weight gain and fat redistribution. Although controversial, increased risk of cardiovascular events and bone loss with the use of rosiglitazone as well as of increased risk of heart failure with pioglitazone have been described.

Box 2 Therapeutic Approaches for Nonalcoholic Fatty Liver Disease

Weight Loss
Caloric restriction, exercise
Sibutramine, orlistat
Weight-reduction surgery

Insulin-Sensitizing Agents
Metformin
Peroxisome proliferator-activated receptor gamma agonists (thiazolidinedione, rosiglitazone, pioglitazone)

Lipid-Lowering Drugs
Fibrates (gemfibrozil)
Fish oil

Antioxidants
N-acetylcysteine
Vitamin E
Betaine

The routine use of these agents in nondiabetic subjects with NAFLD should be discouraged outside of clinical trials.

Lipid-Lowering Agents

The literature concerning lipid-lowering medication and NAFLD is sparse. Reports have demonstrated improvement in transaminase levels with different classes of drugs, but there is a lack of histologic follow-up. Although one of the most common side effect of statins is liver enzyme level elevation, evidence has pointed out that patients with elevated baseline transaminase levels (likely having NAFLD) who receive statin treatment do not have a higher incidence of liver enzyme level elevation or hepatotoxicity than liver disease control subjects who do not receive statins. Moreover, the clinical relevance of the current recommendation that liver biochemistry should be checked before and periodically (usually 12 weeks) after treatment initiation has not been substantiated in the NAFLD population.

Hepatoprotective Therapy

Several therapeutic agents believed to offer hepatocyte protection have been evaluated. Antioxidants have been hypothesized to decrease the oxidative stress and slow the progression of the disease. Several trials in humans with NAFLD have supported an effect of vitamin E on the improvement of transaminase levels and fibrosis. A phase 3 clinical trial is under way. However, a controversial report has shown a mild increase in all-cause mortality in subjects taking vitamin E as a health supplement. Despite small adult studies suggesting a role of ursodeoxycholic acid in the improvement of NASH, a large, randomized, placebo-controlled trial has demonstrated no benefits from ursodeoxycholic acid over placebo on liver biochemistry and histology. Betaine, *N*-acetylcysteine, and pentoxifylline have shown promising effects, but larger trials are needed.

Thus, emerging data from recent trials have suggested that weight loss through lifestyle modifications, as well as several insulin-sensitizing, antioxidant, and hepatoprotective medications, may be of benefit in patients with NAFLD (Box 2). However, many of these interventions need to be evaluated in carefully controlled long-term studies before a treatment recommendation is adopted.

Liver Transplantation

In patients with decompensated NAFLD cirrhosis, liver transplantation should be considered. Coexisting conditions (e.g., morbid obesity, severe complications of diabetes, cardiac disease) and fear of intraoperative and post-transplantation complications, may preclude transplantation candidacy in these patients. A thorough pretransplantation evaluation, as well as better weight and metabolic derangement control, may be necessary. Following transplant, most patients have persistent metabolic syndrome, with long-term implications. Moreover, NAFLD has been shown to recur in the liver allograft, with a possible rapid progression to steatohepatitis and cirrhosis.

PREVENTION AND SCREENING

More than 50 million Americans have been estimated to have the metabolic syndrome, and 80% of them probably have NAFLD. Furthermore, about one third of the U.S. population suffering from type 2 diabetes mellitus has fatty liver. The prevalence of NAFLD in the United States seems to be substantially greater than the 2% prevalence of hepatitis C virus infection and is believed to be increasing. Given such high prevalence, the American Gastroenterological Association Technical Review on Nonalcoholic Fatty Liver Disease, published in 2002, stated that "physicians should actively check for the presence of NAFLD in those who are overweight and/or diabetic." Screening is complicated by the fact that the accuracy of noninvasive diagnostic tools remains poor and, apart from weight loss, there is no clearly established treatment for NAFLD. Basic laboratory evaluation of liver enzyme levels might point to the diagnosis but cannot rule out NAFLD if test results are normal, and imaging techniques have poor sensitivity for low-grade steatosis. Moreover, because these tests do not differentiate simple steatosis from NASH, a liver biopsy must be discussed with the patient if the suspicion of NASH is strong. Therefore, although generalized screening for fatty liver in all at-risk patients may be difficult, it is certainly warranted to look for and actively manage the metabolic syndrome (obesity, diabetes, hyperlipidemia, and hypertension). Prevention of obesity and its complications is now a major public health goal.

Summary

- Nonalcoholic fatty liver disease (NAFLD), a condition associated with obesity and diabetes, is increasingly being recognized in the Western population.
- Simple fatty liver is the most common form of NAFLD and seems to be a benign condition. In contrast, nonalcoholic steatohepatitis can progress to advanced fibrosis and cirrhosis.
- The diagnosis is often made after incidentally finding elevated liver enzyme levels or by clinical suspicion in patients with obesity or diabetes. Laboratory results or imaging examinations can confirm the diagnosis. However, at present, only a liver biopsy can differentiate simple steatosis from NASH.
- There is no clear consensus on the effectiveness of the pharmacologic treatment of NAFLD. Several therapies, including insulin-sensitizing drugs, antioxidant agents, and hepatoprotective medications, have been studied. Lifestyle modifications, particularly weight loss, have been shown to be particularly beneficial.

CONCLUSIONS

NAFLD affects a substantial portion of the general population and is associated with the metabolic syndrome, which includes obesity, insulin resistance, hyperlipidemia, and hypertension. Patients with NAFLD not only suffer from the metabolic sequela of insulin resistance but also have increased overall mortality. Although simple fatty liver seems to be a benign condition, some patients progress to NASH and ultimately to cirrhosis. Because of the consequences of the disease, we emphasize the importance of the detection of NAFLD in high-risk groups, including obese patients, as well as those with evidence of insulin resistance or other components of the metabolic syndrome. Screening and surveillance methods should be applied more uniformly from center to center, and reliable noninvasive techniques are needed to diagnose NAFLD and the detection of progressive liver disease. The diagnosis of NAFLD should prompt management of the metabolic risk factors. Weight loss regimens are believed to be helpful, and numerous drugs have been investigated in small studies. Large randomized clinical trials are necessary to determine the real benefit of these agents. Finally, studies on the pathogenesis of NAFLD may not only improve our understanding of the mechanisms involved in NAFLD progression but also may lead to novel therapeutic strategies to treat this condition.

Suggested Readings

Angulo P: Nonalcoholic fatty liver disease. N Engl J Med 2002;346:1221-1231.

Greenfield V, Cheung O, Sanyal AJ: Recent advances in nonalcholic fatty liver disease. Curr Opin Gastroenterol 2008;24:320-327.

Torres DM, Harrisson SA: Diagnosis and therapy of nonalcoholic steatohepatitis. Gastroenterol 2008;134:1682-1998.

Younossi ZM: Review article: Current management of non-alcoholic fatty liver disease and non-alcoholic steatohepatitis. Aliment Pharmacol Ther 2008;28:2-12.

Ramesh S, Sanyal A: Evaluation and management of non-alcoholic steatohepatitits. J Hepatol 2005;42(Suppl 1):S2-S12.

Sanyal AJ: American Gastroenterological Association: AGA technical review on nonalcoholic fatty liver disease (national guidelines). Gastroenterology 2002;123:1705-1725.

Hepatitis A

Talal Adhami and William D. Carey

DEFINITION AND ETIOLOGY

Hepatitis A virus (HAV) is a cause of acute liver inflammation or hepatitis. It can cause relapsing signs and symptoms but not a chronic infection. The virus is a 27-nm-diameter nonenveloped RNA virus. It belongs to the family Picornaviridae and the genus *Hepatovirus*, and it has characteristics of the enteroviruses.[1] Viral transmission occurs in a fecal-oral fashion. The genome is a positive-strand RNA, 7474 nucleotides long, 7.5 kb in length, that encodes a polyprotein with structural and nonstructural components. Viral replication and assembly occur in the hepatocyte cytoplasm of humans and nonhuman primates, the exclusive natural hosts. The virus is then secreted into the bile and serum.[2]

PREVALENCE

HAV is found throughout the world and is the most common cause of symptomatic acute hepatitis in the United States (annual incidence, 9.1/100,000), occurring largely as sporadic rather than epidemic cases. This figure has been declining since vaccines have become available and given to high-risk persons. The virus is more prevalent in areas with poor sanitary conditions. The most common source of hepatitis A is direct person-to-person exposure and, to a lesser extent, direct fecal contamination of food or water. Consumption of raw or partially cooked shellfish raised in contaminated waterways is an uncommon but possible source of hepatitis A.[3] Vertical transmission from mother to fetus and transmission from blood or blood products have been described on rare occasions. High-risk groups for acquiring HAV infection include travelers to developing nations, children in daycare centers, sewage workers, cleaning personnel, male homosexuals, intravenous drug users, hemophiliacs given plasma products, and persons in institutions. No identifiable source is found in 42% of all cases.[4]

PATHOPHYSIOLOGY

HAV is not directly cytopathic to the hepatocyte. Injury to the liver is secondary to the host's immune response. Replication of HAV occurs exclusively within the cytoplasm of the hepatocyte. Human leukocyte antigen (HLA)-restricted, HAV-specific $CD8^+$ T lymphocytes and natural killer cells mediate hepatocellular damage and destruction of infected hepatocytes. Interferon gamma appears to have a central role in promoting the clearance of infected hepatocytes.[5,6]

SIGNS AND SYMPTOMS

The clinical manifestations of HAV infection are widely variable, depending on the host response. They range from silent infection and spontaneous resolution to fulminant hepatic failure. The incubation period of HAV ranges from 15 to 49 days (mean, 25 days). The prodromal phase is characterized by nonspecific symptoms, such as fatigue, weakness, anorexia, nausea, vomiting, abdominal pain, and, less commonly, fever. Headache, arthralgias, myalgias, rash, or diarrhea can follow. Jaundice begins within 1 to 2 weeks from the onset of the prodrome. It occurs in 70% of adults infected with HAV, with or without pruritus, and in a far smaller proportion of children. Mild hepatomegaly, splenomegaly, and cervical lymphadenopathy are found in 85%, 15%, and 14% of infected patients, respectively.

The host is infective from 14 to 21 days before the onset of jaundice to 7 to 8 days after jaundice has resolved.[7] The host serum and saliva are not nearly as infectious as stool, and urine does not transmit the virus. Anti-HAV antibody (immunoglobulin M [IgM], followed by immunoglobulin G [IgG]) appears shortly before the onset of symptoms and rises to high titers 3 to 4 months after exposure. IgM-specific anti-HAV persists for 4 to 12 months, and IgG-specific anti-HAV persists for life (Fig. 1). Extrahepatic manifestations are uncommon and include a leukocytoclastic vasculitis, glomerulonephritis, arthritis, immune complex disease, toxic epidermal necrolysis, myocarditis, optic neuritis, transverse myelitis, polyneuritis, thrombocytopenia, aplastic anemia, and red cell aplasia.[8]

DIAGNOSIS

Detecting IgM anti-HAV in the serum of a patient with the clinical and biochemical features of acute hepatitis usually confirms the diagnosis of acute hepatitis A.[9] Figure 1 outlines the immune response to HAV infection. HAV antigen can be detected in the stool or body fluids, but there is no commercially available assay. Detecting viral RNA is highly specific but expensive and is rarely used to confirm the diagnosis. Liver biopsy is not indicated. Testing for anti-HAV IgG is not helpful in the diagnosis but is a means of assessing immunity to hepatitis A. When detected in the serum, this IgG remains positive for years.

TREATMENT AND PREVENTION

Acute hepatitis A is usually a self-limited infection. Complete recovery is seen in most patients, and chronic disease does not occur. In rare cases, infection is complicated by fulminant disease, and fatalities occur. Treatment is mainly supportive. Attempts should be made to prevent transmission of the virus within the household and to close contacts. Boiling contaminated water for 20 minutes or exposing the virus to chlorine, formalin, or ultraviolet light reduces the risk of infection.[10]

A safe and effective hepatitis A vaccine is available and is recommended for patients at high risk of acquiring hepatitis A. Patients with chronic liver disease are more likely to develop severe or fulminant liver disease when infected with HAV and should be vaccinated. Hepatitis A vaccine is also recommended for patients with chronic immunodeficiency, those on dialysis, and those on chronic immunosuppressive therapies.

Two formulations of the HAV vaccine are available in the United States; both consist of inactivated hepatitis A antigen purified from cell culture. Havrix is recommended as two injections 6 to 12 months apart in an adult dose of 1440 U of enzyme-linked immunosorbent assay (ELISA; 1.0 mL) and a pediatric dose (ages 2-18 years) of 720 U (0.5 mL). A dose of 360 U administered three times over a 6-month period is an acceptable regimen for children. Travelers to high-risk areas should receive the first dose of vaccine at least 4 weeks before anticipated exposure. Vaqta is recommended for administration as two injections at least 6 months apart in an adult dose of 50 U

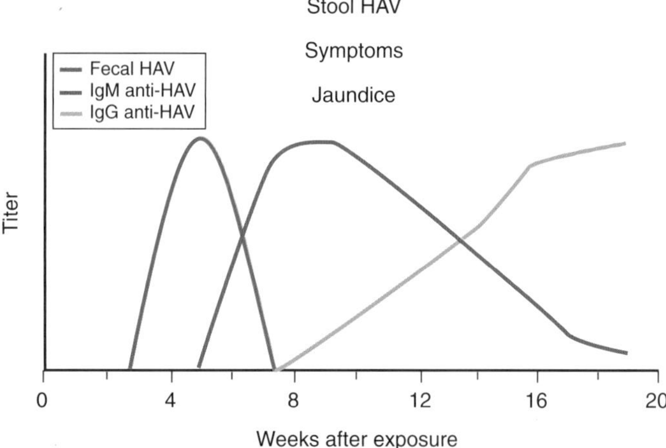

Figure 1 Serology in relation to signs and symptoms. HAV, hepatitis A virus; IgG, immunoglobulin G; IgM, immunoglobulin M.

(1.0 mL) and a pediatric dose (2 to 17 years) of 25 U (0.5 mL). Protection lasts for approximately 15 years.

Hepatitis A vaccines have an excellent safety record, with serious complications in less than 0.1% of recipients. Vaccines used are highly immunogenic, and seroconversion rates after the HAV vaccine is given are higher than 90% but lower in patients with chronic liver disease (possibly as low as 50%). At least 50% of patients who are vaccinated after transplantation have titers below the protective level 2 years after receiving the vaccination. Patients with liver disease should therefore be vaccinated as early in their illness as possible. Follow-up testing for anti-HAV antibody and booster inoculations are not currently recommended. Pooled human immune globulin, 2 mL/kg in adults and 0.02 mL/kg in children, given intramuscularly, is recommended for postexposure prophylaxis.[9]

These recommendations for the prevention of hepatitis A are advocated by the Centers for Disease Control and Prevention (CDC).

OUTCOMES

The course of hepatitis A infection is benign in most of those infected. It is occasionally severe, or fulminant, in adults, particularly in those with chronic liver disease. Jaundice usually resolves in less than 2 weeks, and full recovery usually occurs in 2 months. The illness occasionally persists for several weeks or months, but it never leads to a chronic infection, chronic hepatitis, or cirrhosis. A chronic relapsing hepatitis has been noted to last for as long as 1 year. Hepatitis A can cause a cholestatic hepatitis that usually responds to a short course of prednisolone, 30 mg daily. Pregnancy does not affect the severity or outcome of acute hepatitis A infection. In the rare case of fulminant hepatitis, patients should be evaluated early for possible liver transplantation.[11]

Summary

- Hepatitis A (HAV) is an RNA virus and the most common cause of symptomatic acute hepatitis in the United States. The main mode of transmission is fecal-oral, but consumption of raw shellfish and direct contact with contaminated blood can cause infection.
- HAV causes acute and relapsing hepatitis. It does not cause chronic hepatitis.
- Treatment is usually supportive, and hospitalization may be needed for severe cases. Liver transplantation is recommended in case of fulminant HAV hepatitis.
- There is a safe and effective vaccine to prevent HAV infection. It is recommended for patients at high risk of acquiring hepatitis A and for patients with chronic liver disease.
- Intramuscular human immune globulin is recommended for postexposure prophylaxis.

Suggested Readings

Advisory Committee on Immunization Practices (ACIP): Prevention of hepatitis A through active or passive immunization. MMWR Morb Mortal Wkly Rep 1999;48(RR-12):1-37.

Younossi ZM: Viral hepatitis guide for practicing physicians. Cleve Clin J Med 2000;67(Suppl 1):SI6-SI45.

References

For a complete list of references, log onto www.expertconsult.com.

Hepatitis B

Robert S. O'Shea

EPIDEMIOLOGY

Liver disease related to hepatitis B remains an important public health concern and a major cause of morbidity and mortality. It also presents a common challenging problem for practicing physicians.

Hepatitis B is found throughout the world, but its prevalence varies greatly; it is especially high in Asia, sub-Saharan Africa, and the South Pacific, as well as in specific populations in South America, the Middle East, and the Arctic.[1] Prevalence in the United States varies, based on the population makeup, including the extent of the immigrant population from endemic areas, and on risk factors and behavior, such as the prevalence of intravenous drug use and homosexual practices. Public health agencies estimate that there are about 1.25 million people infected in the United States, but 2 billion people infected worldwide, with approximately 5% of the world's population (or 350 million people) being carriers of chronic hepatitis B.[2] In a typical year, 70,000 Americans become infected with chronic hepatitis B virus (HBV), and approximately 5000 patients with chronic hepatitis B die of complications caused by the disease. Worldwide, chronic hepatitis B is the tenth leading cause of death.

Hepatitis B was first discovered in 1963 by Dr. Baruch Blumberg and colleagues, who identified a protein (the "Australia antigen" that reacted to antibodies from patients with hemophilia and leukemia. The association of this protein with infectious hepatitis was discovered 3 years later by several investigators, and the virus was specifically seen by electron microscopy in 1970.[3]

HBV is a double-stranded hepatotropic DNA virus belonging to the family Hepadnaviridae. The virus infects only humans and some other nonhuman primates. Viral replication takes place predominantly in hepatocytes and, to a lesser extent in the kidneys, pancreas, bone marrow, and spleen. The viral genome is 3.2 kb in length and possesses four partially overlapping open-reading frames that encode various antigens.[4] The intact virion is a spherical double-shelled particle with an envelope of hepatitis B surface antigen (HBsAg), an inner nucleocapsid of core antigen (HBcAg), and an active polymerase enzyme linked to a single molecule of double-stranded HBV DNA. Significant variability of the nucleotide sequence exists, and the virus can be subdivided into eight different genotypes, based on the degree of variation. The clinical importance of these is still uncertain, however.

NATURAL HISTORY

Although HBV can survive outside the body for up to 1 week—and therefore, might be transmitted via indirect contact, such as from open sores—hepatitis B is spread predominantly parenterally, through intimate personal contact, and perinatally. Persons at risk include intravenous drug users, children of mothers with HBV, men who have sex with men, patients on hemodialysis, and those exposed to blood or blood products.

The incubation period of HBV ranges from 45 to 160 days (mean, 100 days). The acute illness is usually mild, particularly in children. In adults, as many as 30% to 50% present with jaundice, and hepatitis may be fulminant in 0.1% to 0.5% of those with acute hepatitis B infection. Symptoms therefore range widely in severity, from asymptomatic subclinical infection to fulminant fatal disease. An insidious onset of nausea, anorexia, malaise, and fatigue, or flulike symptoms, such as pharyngitis, cough, coryza, photophobia, headache, and myalgias, can precede the onset of jaundice. Fever is uncommon, unlike with hepatitis A infection. These symptoms abate with the onset of jaundice, although anorexia, malaise, and weakness can persist. Physical examination features are nonspecific but can include mild enlargement and slight tenderness of the liver, mild splenomegaly, and posterior cervical lymphadenopathy in 15% to 20% of patients. Fulminant disease (acute liver failure) manifests with a change in mental status (encephalopathy) and coagulopathy.[5]

The risk of developing chronic infection, or the carrier state, defined as the persistence of HBsAg in the blood for longer than 6 months, depends on the age and immune function of the patient at the time of initial infection. Ninety percent of infected newborns, 30% of children younger than 5 years, and 10% of adults progress to chronic infection. Of these carriers, 15% to 40% develop hepatitis B-related sequelae in their lifetimes. Patients with chronic infection spontaneously clear surface antigen at a rate of 0.5% per year.[6] Patients with chronic hepatitis B can develop extrahepatic manifestations, including arthralgias, mucocutaneous vasculitis, glomerulonephritis, and polyarteritis nodosa. The glomerulonephritis of hepatitis B occurs more commonly in children than in adults and is usually characterized by the nephrotic syndrome, with little decrease in renal function. Polyarteritis nodosa occurs primarily in adults and is marked by a sudden and severe onset of hypertension, renal disease, and systemic vasculitis with arteritis in the vessels of the kidneys, gallbladder, intestine, or brain. Other rare extrahepatic manifestations are mixed essential cryoglobulinemia, pericarditis, and pancreatitis.

DIAGNOSIS

Viral and immune markers are detectable in blood, and characteristic antigen-antibody patterns evolve over time. The first detectable viral marker is HBsAg, followed by hepatitis B e antigen (HBeAg) and HBV DNA. Titers may be high during the incubation period, but HBV DNA and HBeAg levels begin to fall at the onset of illness and may be undetectable at the time of peak clinical illness.[7] Core antigen does not appear in blood, but antibody to this antigen (anti-HBc) is detectable with the onset of clinical symptoms.

Box 1 Serologic Patterns for Hepatitis B

Immunity

Natural Exposure

HBsAg negative
HBcAb positive (or negative if distant in time)
HBsAb positive

Vaccination

HBcAb negative
HBsAb positive
HBsAg negative

Acute Infection

IgM HBcAb positive
HBsAb negative
HBeAg may be positive or negative, depending on timing
HBsAg positive
HBV DNA-positive (usually)

Chronic Infection

IgG HBcAb positive
HBsAb negative
HBsAg positive
HBV DNA positive (usually)

HBcAb, hepatitis B core antibody; HBsAb, hepatitis B surface antibody; HBeAg, hepatitis B e antigen; HBsAg, hepatitis B surface antigen; HBV, hepatitis B virus; Ig, immunoglobulin.

The IgM fraction is used in an important diagnostic assay for acute hepatitis B infection. Before current molecular assays were available, it was the only marker detectable in the window period, the time between the disappearance of HBsAg and the appearance of anti-HBs. Patients who clear the virus lose HBsAg and develop anti-HBsAb, a long-lasting antibody associated with immunity. The presence of anti-HBsAb and anti-HBcAb (IgG) indicates recovery and immunity in a previously infected person, whereas a successful vaccination response produces antibody only to HBsAg (Box 1).

HBeAg is another viral marker detectable in blood. It correlates with active viral replication and therefore high viral load and infectivity. The antigen is synthesized from a strand of DNA immediately preceding the area that codes for the core antigen.[8] A mutation in this area can occur, preventing the production of the HBeAg. Such viruses are present throughout the world, particularly in Asia and the Mediterranean, and are known as *precore mutants.* The presence of a precore or core mutant, causing HBeAg-negative chronic hepatitis, typically implies disease of longer standing and therefore a higher risk of cirrhosis.

The hepatitis B virus is not cytopathic, and liver injury in chronic hepatitis B is believed to be immunologically mediated. Thus, the severity and course of disease do not correlate well with the level of virus in serum or the amount of antigen expressed in the liver. Antigen-specific cytotoxic T cells are believed to play a role in the cell injury in hepatitis B, but they ultimately account for viral clearance. Specific cytokines produced by cytotoxic and other T cells also have antiviral effects, contributing to viral clearance without cell death. The lack of a vigorous and specific $CD8^+$ cytotoxic T cell and $CD4^+$ helper T cell response can allow chronic infection to develop. Recruitment of nonspecific T cells then results in low-level chronic inflammation and liver damage. Similarly, spontaneous seroconversion from HBeAg to anti-HBeAb during chronic hepatitis B is also immunologically mediated, as is suggested from the transient flare of disease that often immediately precedes clearance of HBeAg.[7]

CLINICAL COURSE

Acute hepatitis B is diagnosed by detecting HBsAg and IgM core antibody, or core antibody alone, in the window period. IgM core

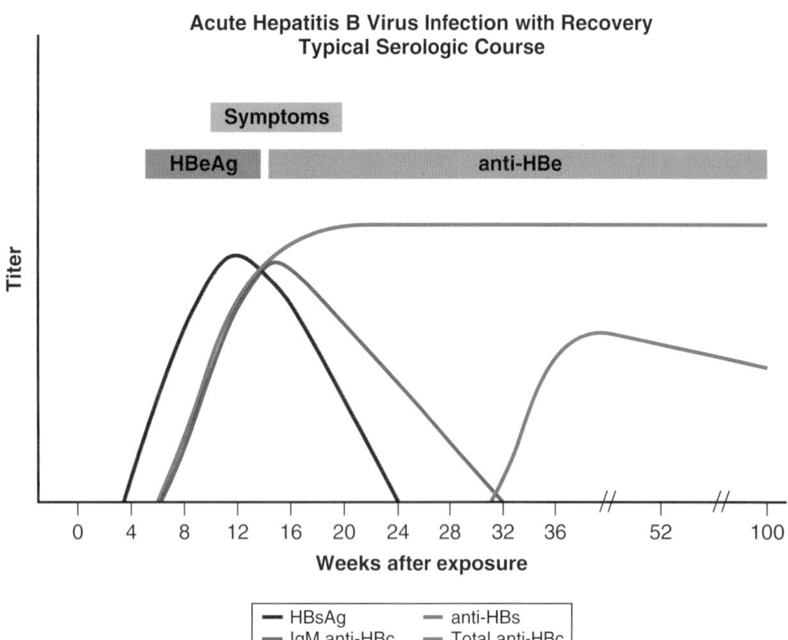

Figure 2 Serologic course of acute hepatitis B.

antibodies are lost within 6 to 12 months of the onset of illness. Biochemically, serum alanine aminotransferase (ALT) and aspartate aminotransferase (AST) levels can increase to between 500 to 5000 U/L and fall after the acute phase of infection. Serum bilirubin levels seldom increase above 10 mg/dL, the alkaline phosphatase level and prothrombin time are usually normal or mildly elevated (e.g., 1 to 3 seconds), and the serum albumin level is normal or minimally depressed. Peripheral blood counts may show mild leukopenia, with or without relative lymphocytosis. Loss of HBsAg and the development of HBsAb signify recovery from the acute infection and the development of immunity (Fig. 2).

Chronic hepatitis B is defined as the persistence of HBsAg in serum for at least 6 months. Patients with chronic infection may be divided into those with evidence of active replication, typically associated with abnormal transaminase levels and higher viral loads, and those in the nonreplicative state, associated with decreased markers of liver inflammation and damage and lower viral loads. Transaminase levels may be normal, or they may be increased anywhere from 1 to 10 times the upper limit of normal. Levels of HBV DNA are usually in the range of 10^5 genome copies/mL, which are readily detectable by hybridization techniques, but the absolute level can fluctuate.

HBeAg in serum reflects active viral replication, and the clinical outcome of infection is correlated with HBeAg status. Conversion to HBeAg-negative and HBeAb-positive status in patients with chronic hepatitis B typically leads to decreased inflammation, with normalizing transaminase levels and decreased levels of HBV DNA in serum: the inactive carrier state. The e antigen marker is also absent in patients with core or precore mutants. Using conventional hybridization assays, HbsAg carriers do not have detectable HBV DNA in serum. Testing for HBV DNA with more sensitive techniques, such as the polymerase chain reaction (PCR) assay, however, usually demonstrates low levels of viral DNA in serum in these carriers (Fig. 3).

The course of chronic hepatitis B is variable. Spontaneous loss of HBeAg occurs at a rate of 8% to 12% per year, associated with a decrease in HBV DNA below levels detected by hybridization techniques. Loss of HBsAg occurs less often (<1%/year). Chronically infected patients without active liver disease or viral replication (inactive carriers) generally have a benign course, with a smaller likelihood of progressing to cirrhosis. Patients who continue to have active viral replication with high levels of HBV DNA and HBeAg in serum have progressive liver injury, and cirrhosis and end-stage liver disease can develop. A transient flare of disease often precedes remission. Loss of HBeAg is not always followed by permanent resolution of disease and disease flares can occur, particularly if a patient is treated with steroids or other immunosuppressive medications. Patients who revert to chronic HBeAg-positive status tend to develop cirrhosis at a substantially increased rate compared with those who remain HBeAg-negative.[9] Patients infected with a core or precore mutant strain, who continue to have high DNA levels and evidence of ongoing hepatic inflammation, tend to have a higher risk of disease progression than patients who are HBeAg-positive.

Chronic HBV infection is associated with a ten-fold increase in the risk of developing hepatocellular carcinoma (HCC). This risk is further magnified in the setting of ongoing inflammation: In patients with both HBsAg and HBeAg, the risk increases to 60-fold compared with the general population.[10] Older men with cirrhosis and those coinfected with hepatitis C are at greatest risk. In regions where HBV is endemic, HCC is the leading cause of cancer-related death. It is therefore recommended that HBV carriers, particularly those at highest risk (men older than 45 years, patients with cirrhosis, and those with a family history of liver cancer) should be screened with ultrasound and alpha-fetoprotein testing for HCC at 6-month intervals.[11]

TREATMENT AND IMMUNIZATION

Effective vaccines for HBV, defined as inducing better than 90% protection against HBV, have been available in the United States since 1982. Hepatitis B vaccine has been described as the first effective anticancer vaccine, and its use has been promoted by the World Health Organization as routine care worldwide since 1997. Early strategies targeted high-risk groups, but they were not successful in materially decreasing incidence rates. Therefore, universal vaccination for HBV has been recommended for infants by the American Academy of Pediatrics since 1991. For patients with a documented exposure, postexposure prophylaxis consists of a single dose of hepatitis B immunoglobulin (HBIg) injected intramuscularly, followed immediately by HBV vaccination. Two recombinant hepatitis B vaccines are available in the United States, Engerix-B. and Recombivax HB. For adults, the recommended regimen is three injections (20 μg of Engerix-B or 10 μg of Recombivax HB) intramuscularly in the

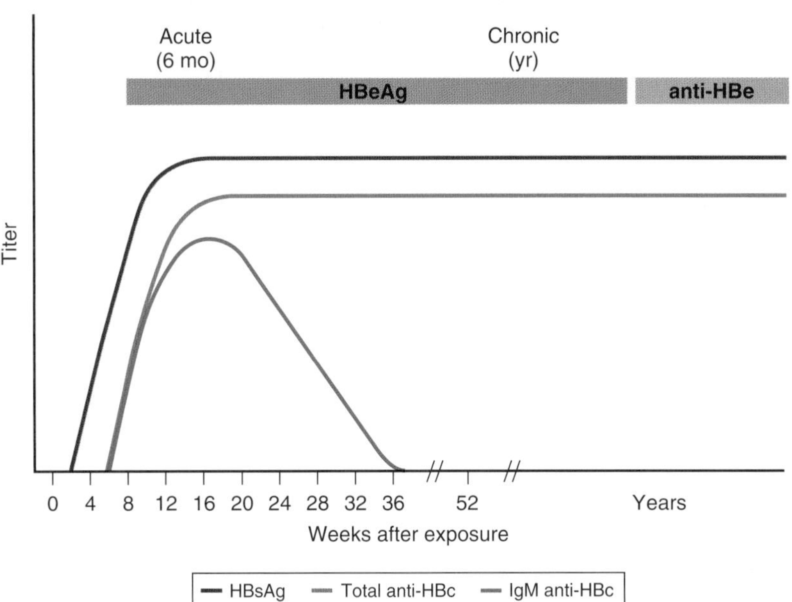

Figure 3 Serologic course of chronic hepatitis B.

deltoid muscle at 0, 1, and 6 months. The seroconversion rate is greater than 90% in adults but may be lower in certain persons, depending on comorbid diseases or genetic factors, as well as in smokers, the obese, older adults, or patients who are immunocompromised. These patients might require higher doses and more injections.

Prevaccination screening for anti-HBs is not recommended except for adult patients who are likely to have been previously exposed, including those in high-risk groups (e.g., injection drug users, male homosexuals). Postvaccination testing for anti-HBs to document seroconversion is not routinely recommended, except for persons who are at risk for lack of response or continued exposure. Booster doses may be appropriate for high-risk patients if titers of anti-HBs fall below what is considered protective (10 IU/mL). The vaccine should be routinely administered to everyone younger than 18 years and to adults at risk of exposure. It should be given to neonates of HBV-infected mothers together with HBIg.[12]

In acute hepatitis B, treatment is supportive. Although several case series have been published, there is no clear evidence that early therapy with antiviral agents for acute hepatitis B decreases the risk of chronicity or speeds recovery. Most patients with acute icteric hepatitis B recover without residual injury or chronic hepatitis. Patients should be followed with repeat testing for HBsAg and ALT levels to determine whether seroconversion and clearance of surface antigen have occurred.[13]

In chronic hepatitis B, therapy is administered to suppress viral replication and prevent progression of liver disease. Although several end points are therefore important, the ability of any medication to prevent liver damage may be related to specific targets, including the prevention of inflammation (leading to decreased liver enzyme levels, a biochemical end point), or the ability of a drug to induce seroconversion (from HBeAg-positive to HBeAg-negative) or a change in fibrosis (i.e., a decrease in scar tissue on repeat liver biopsy). Because the likelihood of developing anti-HBs, and therefore recovery with long-term protection from hepatitis B, is fairly low, measured outcomes of treatment focus on rates of normalization of liver enzyme levels, decreases in viral DNA levels, or seroconversion—that is, from HBeAg-positive to HBeAg-negative, with a positive HBeAb.

In the absence of cirrhosis, therapy is not routinely recommended for patients with normal enzyme levels whether they are chronic inactive carriers or based on their HBeAg status.[14] Therapy is recommended for patients with evidence of active damage to the liver, such as those with abnormal transaminase levels (an ALT level more than twice the upper limit of normal). A liver biopsy before therapy is the gold standard to assess the degree of necroinflammatory activity and fibrosis. Although the data are still evolving, the most recent recommendations of the American Association for the Study of Liver Diseases (AASLD) also include treatment of patients with compensated and decompensated cirrhosis and measurable HBV DNA (>2000 IU/ml) regardless of HBeAg status or degree of elevation of ALT level.[14] This approach is supported by several studies that have shown a decreased rate of development of progressive liver disease or complications in treated patients.

Six agents have been approved by the U.S. Food and Drug Administration (FDA) to treat hepatitis B. Interferon alfa, available since 1992 and injected subcutaneously at a dosage of 5 MU daily, has direct antiviral activity as well as effects on the host immune system. The major side effects of interferon include fatigue, muscle aches, fever, depression, and irritability. Uncommon severe side effects include exacerbation of depression, psychosis, renal and cardiac failure, bacterial infections, and induction of autoimmunity. The FDA approved the use of long-acting interferon (peginterferon alfa-2a, at a dose of 180 µg for 48 weeks) in 2005 for treating patients with chronic hepatitis B; the side-effect profile of peginterferon alfa-2a is very similar to that of shorter-acting interferon. Other treatments available are oral agents and include nucleoside or nucleotide analogues, which interfere with the replication of the hepatitis B virus. The advantages of these medications include a relatively more benign side effect profile compared with interferon; however, the durability of response after treatment might not be as reliable as that of interferon. The first of these was lamivudine, approved by the FDA in 1998. Other medications available for treating HBV include adefovir, approved by the FDA in September 2002, entecavir, approved in March 2005, and telbivudine, approved in October 2006.

Patients who are HBeAg-positive and have evidence of liver disease should be treated. The choice among treatment options is dictated by considerations of the likelihood of response, cost, length of treatment, and side-effect profile, as well as the likelihood of developing resistance. There are some data regarding the likelihood of treatment response in patients treated with interferon, with a higher chance of success in patients with high ALT levels but low HBV DNA levels. Analogously, lamivudine is more likely to be effective in patients with increased ALT levels or inflammation on liver biopsy. Comparable predictors of response for the other antivirals have not been established.

The response rate for these different therapies in this population, defined as seroconversion (from HBeAg-positive to HBeAg-negative, with a positive HBeAb) is variable; published rates are 12% (with adefovir), 16% to 18% with lamivudine, 21% with entecavir, 26% with telbivudine, and 32% to 33% with peginterferon alfa-2a or interferon. Other end points (normalization of liver enzyme levels or improvement in liver histology) are typically seen in 50% to 70% of treated patients. Patients with a beneficial response to interferon therapy often develop a flare of disease, with elevations of serum ALT to levels two to three times the baseline before normalization occurs. Because of the possibility that a flare of liver disease can lead to decompensation, the use of interferon in cirrhotic patients is not recommended. Disease flares, by comparison, are not typically seen in patients treated with lamivudine or adefovir. Preliminary data have suggested that entecavir might also be safe in cirrhotic patients.

Treatment for patients with HBeAg-negative disease is also possible. Several studies have shown efficacy with each of the various approved therapies, in terms of loss of hepatitis B viral DNA or normalization of liver enzyme levels (in approximately 60%-70%). Unfortunately, the response rates are often not sustained, with very high relapse rates after therapy is stopped. As a result, the optimal duration of therapy is not defined in this population.

An important consideration in patients treated with any of the nucleoside or nucleotide analogues is the possibility of emergence of resistant mutants, which increases with increasing duration of treatment. This is particularly true with lamivudine treatment, for which rates of resistance range from 24% at 1 year to 42% by year 2 of continued therapy. Lamivudine resistance is manifested by the reappearance of HBV DNA in serum, most commonly with the YMDD mutant, characterized by an amino acid substitution in the HBV DNA polymerase. The outcomes in these patients are variable, but the emergence of a mutant virus can lead to a serious flare of liver disease. Patients therefore should be monitored for the development of resistance and considered for treatment with another antiviral. Other antivirals are associated with a much lower rate of resistance, but none of them is immune from this possibility. Combination therapy with several agents is likely more effective in preventing the development of resistance, but optimal combinations to improve response rates and clinical outcomes have not yet been defined.

Thus, although the introduction of nucleotide or nucleoside analogues represents a significant advance in the management of chronic hepatitis B, many questions remain regarding optimal dosing, duration, and possible combinations to prevent resistance, increase long-term suppression, or promote eventual clearance. A number of other drugs, including emtricitabine, clevudine, famciclovir, and tenofovir, have also shown some efficacy, often in patients coinfected with HIV, and are therefore being further studied in a number of clinical trials. These emerging therapies, including newer and more potent antiviral agents, coupled with aggressive worldwide vaccination policies, lend promise to the hope that hepatitis B will one day be controlled.

Summary

- Hepatitis B is found throughout the world. Its incidence is especially high in Asia, sub-Saharan Africa, the South Pacific, South America, the Middle East, and the Arctic.
- The most common mode of transmission of hepatitis B worldwide is from mother to infant. Hepatitis B is spread predominantly parenterally, through intimate personal contact, and perinatally.
- Persons at risk include intravenous drug users, children of mothers with HBV, men who have sex with men, patients on hemodialysis, and those exposed to contaminated blood or blood products.
- Most acute infections produce no symptoms. When present, symptoms range widely in severity, from asymptomatic subclinical infection to fulminant fatal disease.
- The risk of developing chronic infection (or the carrier state) depends on the age and immune function of the patient at the time of initial infection.
- Viral and immune markers are detectable in blood, and characteristic antigen-antibody patterns evolve over time. The first detectable viral marker is HBsAg, followed by HBeAg and HBV DNA.
- Effective vaccines for HBV, defined as inducing better than 90% protection against HBV, have been available in the United States since 1982. Hepatitis B vaccine has been described as the first effective anticancer vaccine, and its use has been promoted by the World Health Organization for routine care worldwide since 1997.
- In acute hepatitis B, treatment is supportive. Although several case series have been published, there is no clear evidence that early therapy with antiviral agents for acute hepatitis B decreases the risk of chronicity or speeds recovery. In chronic hepatitis B, therapy is administered to suppress viral replication and prevent progression of liver disease. Many treatment programs have been shown to be effective and have been approved by the FDA and other governmental health agencies around the world.

Suggested Readings

Blumberg BS, Alter HJ, Visnich S: A "new" antigen in leukemia sera. JAMA 1965;191:541-546.

Centers for Disease Control and Prevention: Prevention of perinatal transmission of hepatitis B virus: Prenatal screening of all pregnant women for hepatitis B surface antigen. Recommendations of the Immunization Practices Advisory Committee (ACIP). MMWR Morb Mortal Wkly Rep 1988;37:341-346.

Ganem D, Prince AM: Hepatitis B virus infection-natural history and clinical consequences. N Engl J Med 2004;350:1118-1129.

Hsu YS, Chien RN, Yeh CT, et al: Long-term outcome after spontaneous HBeAg seroconversion in patients with chronic hepatitis B. Hepatology 2002;35:1522-1527.

Keefe EB, Dieterich DT, Han SH, et al: A treatment algorithm for the management of chronic hepatitis B virus infection in the United States. Clin Gastroenterol Hepatol 2004;2:87-106.

Lavanchy D: Hepatitis B virus epidemiology, disease burden, treatment and current and emerging prevention and control measures. J Viral Hepatol 2004;11:97-107.

Liang TJ, Ghany M: Hepatitis B e antigen—the dangerous end game of hepatitis B. N Engl J Med 2002;347:208-210.

Lok AS, McMahon BJ: Chronic hepatitis B. AASLD practice guidelines. Hepatology 2007;45:507-539.

Lok AS, McMahon BJ, Practice Guidelines Committee, American Association for the Study of Liver Diseases (AASLD): Chronic hepatitis B: Update of recommendations. Hepatology 2004;39:857-861.

McMahon BJ, Holck P, Bulkow L, Snowball M: Serologic and clinical outcomes of 1536 Alaska Natives chronically infected with hepatitis B virus. Ann Intern Med 2001;135:759-768.

Nair S, Perrillo RP: Hepatitis B and D. In Zakim D, Boyer TD (eds): Hepatology: A Textbook of Liver Diseases, 4th ed. Philadelphia, WB Saunders, 2003, pp 959-1017.

Seeger C, Mason WS: Hepatitis B virus biology. Microbiol Mol Biol Rev 2000;64:51-68.

World Health Organization: Geographic Prevalence of Hepatitis B, 2004. Available at http://www.who.int/vaccines-surveillance/graphics/htmls/hepbprev.htm (accessed March 9, 2009).

Yang H, Lu SN, Liaw YF, et al: Hepatitis B e antigen and the risk of hepatocelluar carcinoma. N Engl J Med 2002;347:168-174.

References

For a complete list of references, log onto www.expertconsult.com.

Hepatitis C

Robert S. O'Shea

Despite rapid scientific progress in understanding the biology of viral illnesses, viral liver disease remains a common and challenging problem for physicians and their patients. Six viruses, designated hepatitis A, B, C, D, E, and G, primarily target the liver and produce inflammation, or hepatitis, as their primary clinical manifestation. Other viruses, such as Epstein-Barr virus (EBV) and cytomegalovirus (CMV), can cause hepatitis as part of their clinical presentation, but the liver is usually not the primary infected organ. Of the typical hepatitis viruses, chronic infection with hepatitis C remains one of the most important clinical and public health problems. In the Western world, chronic damage from hepatitis C is the primary cause for the end-stage liver disease requiring liver transplantion.

The discovery of the hepatitis C virus (HCV) in 1989 was a major breakthrough. Before that point, it was clear that a major cause of acute hepatitis after a blood transfusion was neither related to hepatitis A nor to hepatitis B—hence the early name for this disease, non-A, non-B hepatitis. After extensive testing of serum from experimentally infected animals, the virus was cloned using molecular biology techniques. It was found to be an RNA virus classified in the Flaviviridae family and genus *Hepacivirus*.[1] It is a double-shelled, enveloped, single-stranded RNA virus, 50 to 60 nm in diameter. HCV replicates in the liver, and it is detectable in serum during acute and chronic infection.

The HCV genome codes for the synthesis of a single large polyprotein of about 3000 amino acids that is then cut by specific enzymes into structural and nonstructural proteins. A schematic of the hepatitis C viral structure is shown in Figure 4, along with the proteins that each section encodes. Based on differences in the amino acid sequence of specific proteins, hepatitis C can be classified into a number of different subtypes, known as *genotypes.* Because of the high error rate in the production of daughter RNA viruses, infected patients typically harbor a heterogeneous group of viruses, with multiple mutations in specific proteins. This variability can be used to divide the HCV infection further in a given patient into subtypes and, beyond that, into specific quasispecies.[2] This has considerable importance in determining the outcome of treatment, although it probably does not affect the natural history of the disease. Although the virus is found throughout the world, the various genotypes of hepatitis C are distributed differently; for example, genotype 4 infection is common in Egypt, but relatively rare in the United States (Fig. 5).

PREVALENCE

Some patients exposed to hepatitis C do not develop chronic infection, perhaps as many as 20%. Similarly, although the remainder develop chronic infection, only a percentage ultimately develop cirrhosis and its complications, usually over a 10- to 20-year time frame.

Because patients who develop a new infection with hepatitis C are usually asymptomatic for many years, the true prevalence is probably underestimated. It is estimated that approximately 170 million people are infected worldwide, equivalent to 3% of the world's population. Based on antibody testing on blood samples from the National Health and Evaluation Nutrition Surveys from 1999 through 2002 in the United States, it was estimated that as many as 4.1 million people were exposed to HCV. Because most patients are unable to clear the infection spontaneously, experts have estimated that between 2.7 and 3.9 million people—or about 1.3% of the U.S. population—have chronic hepatitis C infection.[3]

In the past, a major route of infection was via blood transfusion; after implementing polymerase chain reaction (PCR) assays to screen blood donations, the risk of transfusion-associated HCV fell to less than 1 per 100,000 units transfused. Although the incidence of new infection dropped dramatically, the prevalence of infection (the total population of patients still infected) continues to rise. The most common route of transmission is now believed to be related to intravenous drug use, responsible for perhaps as many as 50% of new infections.

Other potential avenues of infection include having multiple sexual partners, tattooing, body piercing, and sharing straws during intranasal cocaine use, all of which are linked to an increased risk of infection. Maternal-fetal transmission occurs in approximately 10% of cases and is more likely to occur in a mother who is coinfected with HIV. The rate of infection after an HCV-contaminated needlestick injury has ranged from 0% to 10% in various studies. Although possible, viral transmission to a sexual partner in a monogamous relationship is rare, with a less than 5% risk. The Centers for Disease Control and Prevention (CDC) does not advocate any change in sexual practice for partners engaging in a long-term, monogamous, sexual relationship.

Based on epidemiologic studies of transmission and prevalence rates, the CDC recommends screening patients with specific risk factors, including the following:[4]

- Patients who have previously used drugs
- Patients with HIV or hemophilia
- Patients on dialysis in the past, or those who received transplants or transfusions before 1992
- Health care workers after a needle stick injury
- Possibly children of HCV-infected mothers or sexual partners of HCV-infected persons

PATHOPHYSIOLOGY

Although HCV can be found in multiple sites throughout the body, including the liver, peripheral blood mononuclear cells, dendritic

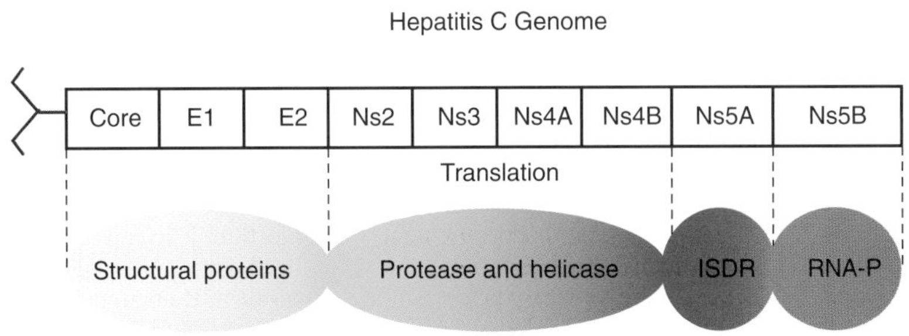

Figure 4 Hepatitis C genome.

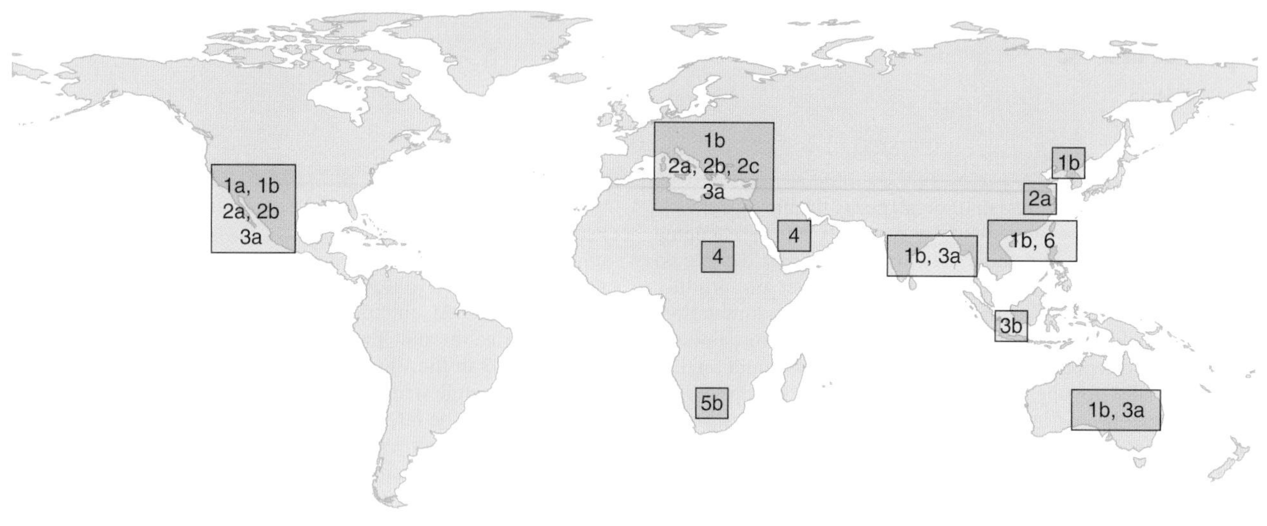

Figure 5 **Geographic distribution of hepatitis C virus genotype.** *(Adapted from Fang JW, Chow V, Lau JY: Virology of hepatitis C virus. Clin Liver Dis 1997;1:493-514.)*

cells, epithelium, and even the central nervous system, HCV replicates in the hepatocytes. However, in the person with a normal immune system, it is not directly hepatotoxic.

Viral replication occurs through an RNA-dependent RNA polymerase process. Lymphocytes recognize infected cells and initiate an immune response to control the virus. Viral clearance is associated with the development and persistence of strong, virus-specific responses by cytotoxic T lymphocytes and helper T cells. Because of the rapid evolution of diverse quasispecies within an infected person, even a brisk B cell (e.g., antibody) response to hepatitis C has been inadequate to clear the infection, because the virus represents a moving target to the immune system. For the same reason, progress in the development of a vaccine to protect patients from an initial infection has been slow.

Damage to the liver parenchyma is mediated by inflammatory cytokines. Persistent inflammatory mediators activate stellate cells in the liver parenchyma, leading to varying degrees of hepatic fibrosis. Why some patients develop progressive fibrosis and eventually cirrhosis, and others do not, is unknown, but some predictors of progression have been identified, including male sex, age at onset of infection, and use of alcohol.

SIGNS AND SYMPTOMS

Acute HCV infection is uncommonly recognized because it is usually accompanied by mild flulike symptoms. Although the vast majority of patients with acute HCV infection are asymptomatic, weight loss, fatigue, muscle or joint pain, irritability, nausea, malaise, anorexia, and jaundice have been reported to occur rarely in the 2- to 26-week incubation period. In chronic symptomatic HCV infection, fatigue is a common complaint, but the degree of fatigue is unrelated to the severity of liver disease. Other complaints can include depression, nausea, anorexia, abdominal discomfort, and difficulty with concentration. Symptoms might first appear only with the onset of more-advanced liver disease. Common extrahepatic manifestations of HCV infection include mixed cryoglobulinemia and porphyria cutanea tarda. Membranoproliferative glomerulonephritis, leukocytoclastic vasculitis, focal lymphocytic sialadenitis, and idiopathic pulmonary fibrosis occur in rare cases and are believed to be secondary to immune-complex deposition in association with intact virus or viral proteins. Many patients have no specific symptoms, and the finding of abnormal hepatic transaminase levels on routine testing often prompts specific testing for hepatitis C.

DIAGNOSIS

Serologic assays for HCV are based on detecting HCV antibodies or HCV RNA. The most commonly used serologic test for detecting antibodies to hepatitis C is ELISA, with a sensitivity and specificity of 95%. Some laboratories automatically confirm a positive ELISA test by a supplemental recombinant immunoblot assay (RIBA) to increase the specificity of the test (e.g., to decrease the number of false positives). In the 15% of infected persons who clear the virus spontaneously, these antibody test results remain positive and thus cannot be used to confirm active infection. This also applies to treated patients who clear the virus, who maintain a positive HCV antibody indefinitely. A very small percentage of patients infected with HCV are unable to mount an immune response to the viral protein and do not produce antibody. These false negatives occur in those with HIV infections, renal failure, or HCV-associated mixed cryoglobulinemia. Confirmation of ongoing infection therefore requires the detection of HCV RNA by PCR using a qualitative or quantitative assay. These assays can detect a viral count as low as 9.6 IU/L. A negative qualitative test result argues strongly against active viral infection. The quantitative HCV RNA test reflects the viral load, which is an important variable to predict the outcome of anti-HCV therapy but not the likelihood of disease progression.[4]

Patients commonly come to medical attention based on elevated alanine aminotransferase (ALT) levels, which are indirect markers of liver cell necrosis. Although ALT measurements have been used to monitor HCV infection and the efficacy of therapy, the recognition that many infected patients have normal ALT levels has limited their usefulness. Furthermore, the normalization of ALT levels with antiviral therapy is not proof of successful virus eradication. Viral quantification has replaced ALT levels, therefore, in monitoring treatment response.

In patients with documented HCV infection, a liver biopsy is often helpful in determining the need for therapy. Although not considered mandatory before initiating treatment, it documents the amount of ongoing destruction (grade) and degree of fibrosis (stage) of disease. Patients with more-advanced fibrosis are at high risk for progressive liver disease and therefore should be considered for therapy. Significant fibrosis may be present in up to 25% of patients with normal transaminase levels. Conversely, patients with minimal fibrosis can choose to forgo immediate therapy, weighing the likelihood of progressive scar tissue development against the side effect profile of current treatment, as well as the likelihood of response.

Viral load and viral genotype help predict the outcome of treatment, because response rates are most strongly linked to these two variables. In addition, they influence the length of therapy: Patients with genotype 1, the most common form in North America, and a high viral load are more resistant to therapy, with response rates of approximately 40%, even after 1 year of combination treatment. By comparison, patients with genotype 2 or 3 may be expected to achieve sustained virologic response rates of almost 80% after 6 months of treatment.[4]

TREATMENT

Treatment outcomes depend on many factors, including whether a patient is being treated for acute or chronic disease. Acute HCV infection is uncommonly diagnosed, because it often manifests with nonspecific flulike symptoms. Available evidence suggests that interferon-based therapy given early in the course of infection decreases the risk of progression to chronic disease.[5] Health care workers, for example, who are accidentally exposed to HCV-infected blood via a needle stick injury, should be followed carefully for evidence of ongoing infection, and if they are unable to clear the infection spontaneously, they should be treated early.

The more common situation facing clinicians is that of patients with chronic hepatitis C, for whom the goal of treatment is elimination of the virus. This is associated with stabilization or even improvements in liver histology and clinical course. Secondary aims are symptom control, improvement in liver function, and prevention of complications of progressive liver disease, including cirrhosis, decompensated liver disease, and hepatocellular carcinoma.

Complete abstinence from alcohol is an extremely important behavioral modification and has been shown to affect the likelihood of progression as well as the efficacy of therapy. The usefulness of other therapies, including dietary supplements, herbs, and unconventional treatments, have not been rigorously studied, and the results are extremely varied.[6] Apart from interferon-based therapy, most interventions have only marginal benefit. Regardless of whether a patient elects to be treated or not, practice guidelines recommend that all patients with hepatitis C and no evidence for immunity be vaccinated for hepatitis A and, if risk factors exist, for hepatitis B as well.

Patients treated with interferon are classified into those who do not respond (i.e., fail to clear HCV from their blood), relapsers (i.e., those who cleared the virus on treatment, but afterward had detectable virus), and those who develop a sustained virologic response (SVR), defined as undetectable virus in the serum 6 months after treatment completion, which correlates well with long-term absence of virus. Although any patient with hepatitis C infection can be considered for therapy, the decision must be individualized, based on the overall risks and benefits of therapy. Patients with chronic HCV infection and evidence of damage, including elevated serum aminotransferase levels, chronic hepatitis on liver biopsy, absence of decompensation, and no contraindications, should be considered for treatment. Specific contraindications include severe concurrent disease, previous solid organ transplantation, autoimmune hepatitis, hyperthyroidism, pregnancy, or uncontrolled depression. Previous contraindications, such as HIV infection or AIDS or otherwise immunocompromised status, are no longer considered obstacles to treatment. Often, HIV-positive patients are coinfected with hepatitis C, because the viruses can share a similar epidemiology. The most recent studies have demonstrated response rates to therapy of 14% to 73% in these patients, depending on genotype, which are somewhat better than those seen with previous treatments. These rates, however, are less than those expected in HIV-negative patients.[7]

Table 1 Sustained Viral Response Rate of Hepatitis C Virus (HCV) with Different Therapeutic Regimens

Interferon	Duration (mo) SSVR	VR Genotype 1 (%)	Genotype 2 or 3 (%)
Interferon plus ribavarin	6	10	20
Pegylated interferon	6-12*	21%	45%
Pegylated interferon plus ribavirin	6-12*	46%	76%
Pegylated interferon plus ribavirin in patients with chronic HCV and low viral load (<2 million copies/mL) 6-12*	56%	81%	

*HCV genotype 2 treated for 12 mo and genotypes 2 and 3 for 6 mo.
SVR, sustained virologic response.

A pretreatment neuropsychiatric assessment should be performed in all patients. If depression, anxiety, or other psychiatric illness is evident by history, a psychiatric consultation should be sought for evaluation, treatment, and follow-up during the interferon treatment period. Psychosis and homicidal or suicidal ideation are strong contraindications to therapy.

Factors predicting a therapeutic response include low pretreatment HCV RNA level, genotype 2 or 3, female sex, low body mass index (BMI), and low hepatic iron load. Patients with advanced liver disease or decompensated cirrhosis are also unlikely to respond and often are unable to tolerate treatment.[4]

Treatment of hepatitis C infection has evolved since the 1990s. It remains based on interferon alfa as an immune modulator. Response rates were modest when it was used as monotherapy (10% in genotype 1 and 30% at best in genotypes 2 and 3). Side effects remain a significant problem and are typically described as flulike symptoms, including fever, arthralgia, headache, depression, injection site inflammation, and bone marrow suppression. The addition of ribavirin, a nucleoside analogue and an inhibitor of viral replication, has improved the SVR rate to approximately 50% (46% in genotype 1 and 76% in genotypes 2 and 3; Table 1). There is some evidence for a dose-response effect, with generally increased response rates in higher doses (usually 1000-1200 mg in divided doses). Ribavirin is cleared by the kidneys and therefore is contraindicated in patients with significant renal dysfunction (a creatinine clearance <50 mL/min). It also has been shown to be teratogenic and is therefore strictly contraindicated in pregnancy. The most common side effect is fatigue in about 15% of patients, resulting partly from hemolytic anemia.

The most recently introduced treatment is pegylated interferon, a form of interferon covalently bound to a large inert polyethylene glycol molecule. The combination serves to prolong the serum half-life by decreasing the excretion rate, thereby increasing the duration of action. Enhanced response rates have been demonstrated for pegylated interferons in combination therapy with ribavirin.[8] If patients are able to complete a full course of treatment at optimal doses (e.g., without dose adjustments for side effects or toxicity), SVR rates may be as high as 88% in genotypes 2 and 3 patients and up to 50% in those with genotype 1 (see Table 1). Side effects, such as injection site reaction and bone marrow suppression, may be more pronounced with different formulations and doses.

Although the usual duration of treatment for patient with genotype 1 is 48 weeks, data from multiple studies have suggested that it is possible to predict the outcome of therapy by 12 weeks of therapy. If a patient fails to clear infection or has at least a 2-log decline in the viral load (measured with the same PCR assay as used at baseline), it is unlikely that the patient will develop a SVR.[9] Studies are ongoing to define new and earlier stopping rules.

Patients on therapy need to be monitored closely for complications or symptoms of the adverse reactions of combination therapy. This should include evaluation for depression, symptoms of irritability, sleep disturbance, and visual disturbances, as well as evidence of hyper- or hypothyroidism. Blood counts should be monitored frequently at the beginning of treatment and at least monthly afterward, if stable. An emerging literature suggests that support of the bone marrow with erythropoietin for anemia and granulating cell-stimulating factor (GCSF) for neutropenia can allow continuation of therapy, even in patients with significantly affected counts. The cost effectiveness of this approach, however, is uncertain.

COMPLICATIONS

Chronic HCV infection is the most common indication for liver transplantation in the United States, and, as complications related to the epidemic continue, a significant impact on the U.S. health care system is expected. It has been estimated that over the next 20 years, the ppercentage of infected patients with cirrhosis will increase from 16% to 32%, and other complications will also increase dramatically, including hepatic decompensation (up 106%), hepatocellular carcinoma (up 81%), and liver-related deaths (up 180%).[10]

CONCLUSIONS

HCV infection typically progresses to chronic infection in more than 60% of patients, and it can lead to cirrhosis in as many as 20% over a 20-year period. Serum aminotransferase levels reflecting hepatocellular injury can fluctuate, as does the viral load.

As the disease evolves, hepatocytes are progressively destroyed and replaced by fibrosis, insidiously leading to the development of bridging fibrosis and ultimately cirrhosis. The course of any individual patient is affected by various factors, such as age at onset of infection, sex, coinfection with other viruses (HAV, HBV or HIV), or other medical conditions, as well as risk behavior, such as alcohol consumption. Interferon-based treatment has a varying success rate in clearing the virus, as noted earlier. Careful selection and monitoring of patients are essential in undertaking therapy. In patients without cirrhosis, hepatitis C–related mortality is only slightly increased. Severe complications usually occur only in those with established cirrhosis. The risk of developing hepatocellular carcinoma (HCC) in chronic HCV patients with cirrhosis is as high as 4% per year. HCV-infected patients with cirrhosis should be screened at intervals with ultrasound and alpha-fetoprotein testing. Some retrospective studies have shown that treatment with interferon is associated with a lower rate of development of HCC, even without an SVR.

Although HCV remains a major global health problem, significant advances in the understanding of its basic biology have allowed significant improvements in treatment since the turn of the 21st century. Treatment, although difficult, has been shown to prolong life, and the pace of discovery in this field gives hope that patients will be able to treated even more effectively in the future.

Summary

- It is estimated that approximately 170 million people are infected worldwide (3% of the world's population). It has been estimated that as many as 4.1 million Americans were exposed to HCV; from 2.7 to 3.9 million people in the United States have chronic hepatitis C infection.
- Chronic HCV infection is the most common indication for liver transplantation in the United States and, as its complications continue, a significant impact on the U.S. health care system is expected. It has been estimated that over the next 20 years, the percentage of infected patients with cirrhosis will increase from 16% to 32% and other complications will also increase dramatically.
- In the past, a major route of infection was via blood transfusion; after implementing the use of polymerase chain reaction (PCR) assays to screen blood donations, the risk of transfusion-associated HCV fell to less than 1/100,000 units transfused. However, the prevalence of infection continues to rise. The most common route of transmission is now believed to be related to intravenous drug use, responsible for perhaps as many as 50% of new infections. Maternal-fetal transmission occurs in approximately 10% of cases.
- Acute HCV infection is uncommonly recognized. Although most patients with acute HCV infection are asymptomatic, fatigue, depression, nausea, anorexia, abdominal discomfort, and difficulty with concentration can occur in chronic symptomatic HCV infection. Common extrahepatic manifestations of HCV infection include mixed cryoglobulinemia and porphyria cutanea tarda. Many patients have no specific symptoms, and the finding of abnormal hepatic transaminase levels on routine testing often prompts specific testing for hepatitis C.
- Serologic assays for HCV are based on detecting HCV antibodies or HCV RNA. Viral load and viral genotype help predict the outcome of treatment, because response rates are most strongly linked to these two variables.
- Treatment of hepatitis C infection is based on interferon alfa administration over many months. Combined with ribavirin, a sustained virologic response rate of approximately 50% (46% in genotype 1 and 76% in genotypes 2 and 3) can be anticipated. Higher response rates may be seen when the patient is younger, thinner, or female and has a low viral load and absence of hepatic fibrosis.

Suggested Readings

Choo QL, Kuo G, Weiner AJ, et al: Isolation of a cDNA clone derived from a blood-borne non-A, non-B viral hepatitis genome. Science 1989;244:359-362.

Chung RT, Andersen J, Volberding P, et al: Peginterferon Alfa-2a plus ribavirin versus interferon alfa-2a plus ribavirin for chronic hepatitis C in HIV-coinfected persons. N Engl J Med 2004;351:451-459.

Davis GL, Albright JE, Cook SF, Rosenberg DM: Projecting future complications of chronic hepatitis C in the United States. Liver Transpl 2003;9:331-338.

Davis GL, Wong JB, McHutchison JG, et al: Early virologic response to treatment with peginterferon alfa-2b plus ribavirin in patients with chronic hepatitis C. Hepatology 2003;38:645-652.

Fried MW, Shiffman ML, Reddy KR, et al: Peginterferon Alfa-2a plus ribavirin for chronic hepatitis C virus infection. N Engl J Med 2002;347:975-982.

Jaeckel E, Cornberg M, Wedemeyer H, et al: German Acute Hepatitis C Therapy Group: Treatment of acute hepatitis C with interferon alfa-2b. N Engl J Med 2001;345:1452-1457.

Kim WR: The burden of hepatitis C in the United States. Hepatology 2002;36(Suppl 1):S30-S34.

Liu J, Manheimer E, Tsutani K, Gluud C: Medicinal herbs for hepatitis C virus infection: A Cochrane hepatobiliary systematic review of randomized trials. Am J Gastroenterol 2003;98:538-544.

Penin F, Dubuisson J, Rey FA, et al: Structural biology of hepatitis C virus. Hepatology 2004;39:5-19.

Strader DB, Wright T, Thomas DL, Seeff LB; American Association for the Study of Liver Diseases: Diagnosis, management, and treatment of hepatitis C. Hepatology 2004;39:1147-1171.

References

For a complete list of references, log onto www.expertconsult.com.

Hepatitis D

Talal Adhami and William D. Carey

VIROLOGY

Hepatitis D or delta virus (HDV) is a defective single-stranded RNA virus requiring the presence of hepatitis B virus (HBV) for its expression and replication. HDV is a 35- to 37-nm spherical particle enveloped by a lipoprotein coat derived from HBsAg. HDV-RNA consists of 1680 nucleotides, and replication is limited to hepatocytes. It is considered to be the smallest RNA genome among the animal viruses.

PREVALENCE

HDV has a worldwide distribution. It is endemic in the developing world, with a high prevalence in South America. HDV infection is limited to patients who have HBV infection and, like hepatitis B, is acquired parenterally. Worldwide, about 5% of HBV carriers are anti-HDV-positive. Delta hepatitis remains a common problem among intravenous drug users.

PATHOPHYSIOLOGY

Patients may be infected with HDV at the same time that they acquire the hepatitis B virus (acute coinfection) or they can acquire the virus after infection with hepatitis B (superinfection). It is still not clear whether the virus is directly cytotoxic or whether an immune-mediated response is responsible for the pathology. An immune response may be the predominant mediator in chronic disease, whereas direct viral cytotoxicity can predominate in acute infection. Necroinflammatory activity is severe, but histologic features are nonspecific for chronic HDV infection.[1]

SIGNS AND SYMPTOMS

Symptoms of HDV infection are nonspecific, and most patients have subclinical illness. Most patients who acquire HDV and HBV simultaneously clear the delta virus, whereas 70% to 90% of those superinfected develop chronic delta infection. Superinfection produces more-severe acute illness than HBV alone and carries a higher risk for fulminant hepatic failure, which occurs in 5% to 20% of cases.[2]

DIAGNOSIS

The diagnosis of delta hepatitis should only be considered if positive HBV infection is present. This is usually reflected by finding a positive serum HBsAg or HBV DNA, or both. Measuring antibodies to delta antigen using ELISA can make the diagnosis. However, it may be positive after viral clearance, especially in case of HBV-HDV coinfection. IgM antibodies are increased when there is liver damage and not just in the acute illness; they apparently disappear when the hepatitis resolves. Presence of HDV antigen in the serum confirms the diagnosis, as does HDV RNA, which is only available in a research setting. Anti-HDV antibody (IgG) can appear in high titers in chronic HDV infection, whereas lower titer may be detected after viral resolution.

TREATMENT

Delta hepatitis can be prevented by vaccination against hepatitis B. At this time, there is no effective vaccine to prevent delta hepatitis in chronic hepatitis B carriers. Delta hepatitis can be treated with high-dose interferon as high as 9 million U three times per week for 1 year. Although as many as 70% of patients clear the virus and normalize liver enzyme levels, almost all patients relapse at some point after therapy. Orthotopic liver transplantation is considered for decompensated patients. Interestingly, patients who have HDV and who receive a liver transplant have a higher chance of graft survival than those who receive a transplant for hepatitis B alone. This phenomenon may be a result of the inhibitory effect of HDV on HBV replication. Hepatitis B immunoglobulin is administered to these patients.

OUTCOMES

Coinfection with HDV and HBV can result in a severe fulminant hepatitis and liver failure or can persist as a chronic infection, resulting in cirrhosis or hepatocellular carcinoma. Chronic infection can persist in an inactive phase, and some patients go into complete remission. The chance of progression to cirrhosis is higher in patients with delta hepatitis than in patients solely infected with hepatitis B, as is the risk for hepatocellular carcinoma. Patients coinfected with human immunodeficiency virus or hepatitis C have a worse outcome.[3,4]

Summary

- Hepatitis D or delta virus (HDV) is a defective single-stranded RNA virus requiring the presence of hepatitis B virus (HBV) for its expression and replication. HDV has a worldwide distribution. It is endemic in the developing world.
- HDV infection is limited to patients who have HBV infection and, like hepatitis B, is acquired parenterally.
- Infection with HDV produces more severe acute illness than HBV alone and carries a higher risk for fulminant hepatic failure, which occurs in 5% to 20% of cases.
- The chance of progression to cirrhosis is higher in patients with delta hepatitis than in patients solely with hepatitis B, as is the risk for hepatocellular carcinoma.
- Delta hepatitis can be prevented by vaccination against hepatitis B.

Suggested Readings

Chu CM, Yeh CT, Liaw YF: Viral superinfection in previously unrecognized chronic carriers of hepatitis B virus with superimposed acute fulminant versus nonfulminant hepatitis. J Clin Microbiol 1999;37:235-237.

Huo TI, Wu JC, Lai CR, et al: Comparison of clinico-pathological features in hepatitis B virus-associated hepatocellular carcinoma with or without hepatitis D virus superinfection. J Hepatol 1996;25:439-444.

Mendez L, Reddy KR, Di Prima RA, et al: Fulminant hepatic failure due to acute hepatitis B and delta co-infection: Probable bloodborne transmission associated with a spring-loaded fingerstick device. Am J Gastroenterol 1991;86:895-897.

Polish LB, Gallagher M, Fields HA, Hadler SC: Delta hepatitis: Molecular biology and clinical and epidemiological features. Clin Microbiol Rev 1993;6:211-229.

References

For a complete list of references, log onto www.expertconsult.com.

Hepatitis E

Talan Adhami and William D. Carey

DEFINITION

Hepatitis E virus (HEV) is a 32-nm nonenveloped single-stranded RNA virus. It belongs to the family Calciviridae and genus *Calcivirus*. It is largely a waterborne epidemic disease (Fig. 6). Increasing evidence has suggested that animals, especially swine, represent an important reservoir for HEV.[1]

PREVALENCE AND RISK FACTORS

HEV is distributed in endemic and epidemic forms in Southeast and Central Asia, the Middle East, Africa, and Mexico (Fig. 7). Seroprevalence studies have indicated that the incidence of hepatitis E is increasing in 8 of 11 countries surveyed. Up to 30% of persons ages 16 to 30 years test positive for anti-E antibodies in most participating countries, except for Spain, Japan, and the United States, where the incidence remains very low.[2] The incidence may be increasing in the United Kingdom.[3] In Nepal, 56% of acute hepatitis is associated with IgM anti–hepatitis E. It is rare in the United States, except in immigrants and travelers returning from endemic regions. Less than 1% of reported cases of acute viral hepatitis in the United States are attributed to hepatitis E. Infection requires ingestion of fecally contaminated water or foods.

PATHOPHYSIOLOGY AND NATURAL HISTORY

HEV replicates in the hepatocytes and is excreted in stool. Transmission is predominantly by the fecal-oral route, usually through contaminated water. Although person-to-person transmission is rare, maternal-neonatal transmission has been documented. Outbreaks occur in conditions of crowding and poor sanitation. A report of hepatitis E among displaced populations in Darfur, Sudan, has indicated an attack rate as high as 3% and a case-fatality rate of 1.7%. Forty-two percent of the deaths occurred in pregnant women.[4]

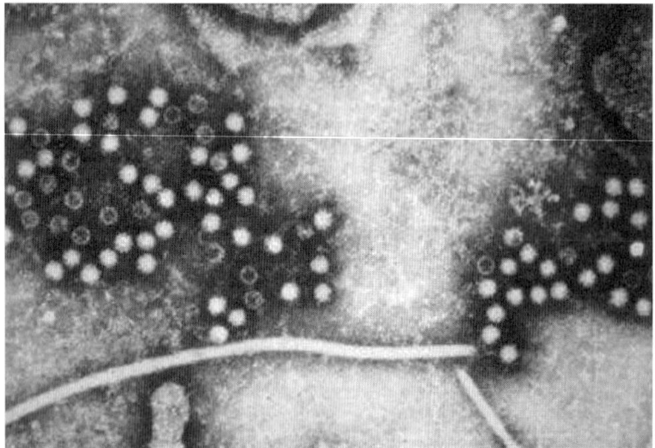

Figure 6 Hepatitis E particles in stool. Hepatitis E virus (HEV), the major causative agent of enterically transmitted non-A, non-B hepatitis worldwide, is a spherical, nonenveloped, single-stranded RNA virus that is approximately 32 to 34 nm in diameter. *(From the Centers for Disease Control: Hepatitis E Virus, 2007. Available at http://www.cdc.gov/ncidod/diseases/hepatitis/slideset/hep_e/slide_1.htm.)*

The incubation period ranges from 15 to 60 days. The virus is detected in stool as early as 1 week before the onset of clinical illness and persists for 1 to 2 weeks afterward, during which stools are highly infectious. Anti-HBE antibody (IgM) appears soon after the onset of the clinical infection, and IgG appears soon after that; IgG remains detectable for as long as 20 months.

Like hepatitis A, HEV is most often a self- limited disease; immunity develops, and no second attacks occur. Hepatitis E occurs, on average, in older persons than those who acquire hepatitis A infection. Severe disease, including fulminant hepatitis and death, occur more often in hepatitis E.[5]

The course of HEV is usually more severe than that seen in other forms of epidemic jaundice. The fatality rate is generally lower than 1%. It is, however, an illness of great concern in pregnant women because it can cause liver failure, with a mortality rate of 20%. Prolonged viremia or fecal shedding are unusual, and chronic infection does not occur.

SIGNS AND SYMPTOMS

HEV causes acute hepatitis. Nonspecific constitutional and gastrointestinal symptoms are similar to those found in other types of viral hepatitis. The onset of symptoms tends to be abrupt, and fever is uncommon. Prodromal symptoms improve or disappear with the onset of jaundice, although anorexia, malaise, and weakness can persist. Without the presence of jaundice, most sporadic episodes are probably misdiagnosed. Nevertheless, in most reported outbreaks, jaundice is present in 90% to 100% of cases, suggesting that HEV may be more likely than hepatitis A, B, or C to produce jaundice.

DIAGNOSIS

In the United States, hepatitis E infection should be considered in patients who present with acute hepatitis and have recently traveled to endemic areas. The disease is often cholestatic, with elevated bilirubin and alkaline phosphatase levels. The presence of anti-HBE antibody (IgM) in the serum confirms the disease and persists for at least 6 weeks after the peak of the illness. IgG antibody peaks soon after that and remains detectable for as long as 20 months. Laboratory diagnosis is based on antibody testing. IgM anti–hepatitis E denotes recent infection, although the IgM can remain positive for more than 1 year. IgM anti–hepatitis E is usually present for years.[6]

TREATMENT AND PREVENTION

Persons traveling to endemic areas should be aware of the virus and avoid water, uncooked food, and contact with contaminated substances. Vaccination and immune globulin are not currently available, but tests have been conducted in human volunteers. Treatment of the acute infection is supportive.

Common sense dictates that societal commitment to good public health, clean water supplies, and personal sanitation will reduce the incidence of HEV, as it has with hepatitis A. However, evidence is meager that such measures have had an impact on HEV infection rates. Passive immunization with gamma globulin is *not* recommended for protection against hepatitis E, in part because gamma globulin produced in countries where the prevalence of HEV is low is expected to have low anti-HEV activity. Even when gamma globulin is produced in high-endemic areas, evidence of benefit of passive immunization is equivocal. No active immunization is currently available.

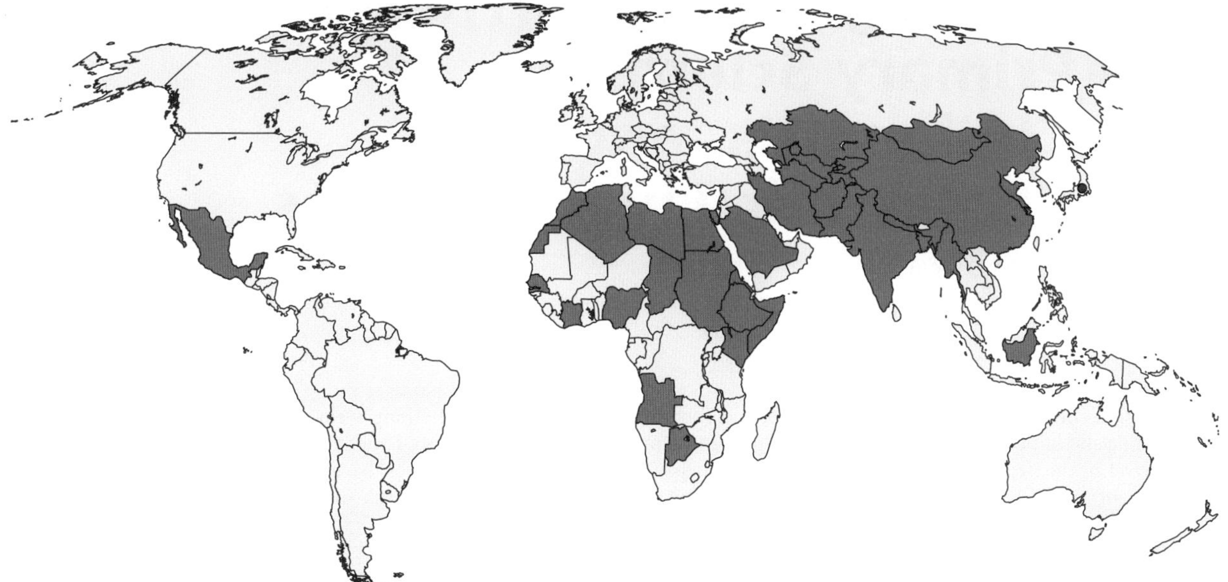

Figure 7 **Geographic distribution of hepatitis E-outbreaks or confirmed infection in more than 25% of cases of sporadic non-ABC hepatitis.** *(From the Centers for Disease Control: Hepatitis E Virus, 2007. Available at http://www.cdc.gov/ncidod/diseases/hepatitis/slideset/hep_e/slide_5.htm.)*

Summary

- Hepatitis E is an RNA virus that infects humans through oral contamination of water. It spreads both from person to person and through animal intermediaries, such as swine.
- Hepatitis E is seen principally in Southeast and Central Asia, the Middle East, and Africa, and in travelers returning from endemic areas.
- Illness caused by hepatitis E might be asymptomatic, but is much more likely to produce jaundice than other forms of acute viral hepatitis. The case-fatality rate is 1.7%, but pregnant women seem especially susceptible to severe disease and a fatal outcome.
- There is no chronic form of hepatitis E. One attack appears to confer immunity.
- Management of acute hepatitis E is similar to that for other forms of acute viral hepatitis. Patients who can maintain hydration and nutrition can be treated at home; those with severe symptomatic disease can require hospitalization. No antiviral agents have yet been shown to affect the course of acute hepatitis E.

Suggested Readings

Abe K, Li TC, Ding X, et al: International collaborative survey on epidemiology of hepatitis E virus in 11 countries. Southeast Asian J Trop Med Public Health 2006;37:90-95.

Chau TN, Lai ST, Tse C, et al: Epidemiology and clinical features of sporadic hepatitis E as compared with hepatitis A. Am J Gastroenterol 2006;101:292-296.

Guthmann JP, Klovstad H, Boccia D, et al: A large outbreak of hepatitis E among a displaced population in Darfur, Sudan, 2004: The role of water treatment methods. Clin Infect Dis 2006;42:1685-16891.

Myint KS, Endy TP, Shrestha MP, et al: Hepatitis E antibody kinetics in Nepalese patients. Trans R Soc Trop Med Hyg 2006;100:938-941.

Sadler GJ, Mells GF, Shah NH, et al: UK acquired hepatitis E-an emerging problem? J Med Virol 2006;78:473-475.

Zheng Y, Ge S, Zhang J, et al: Swine as a principal reservoir of hepatitis E virus that infects humans in eastern China. J Infect Dis 2006;193:1643-1649.

References

For a complete list of references, log onto www.expertconsult.com.

Primary Biliary Cirrhosis, Primary Sclerosing Cholangitis, and Other Cholestatic Liver Diseases

Claudia O. Zein

The term *cholestasis* originally derives from the Greek and literally means "a standing still of bile." This disruption of bile flow can occur on a cellular level in the hepatocyte, at the level of the intrahepatic biliary ductules, or from an extrahepatic mechanical obstruction of the bile ducts. Commonly, bile flow is only partially disrupted, giving rise to anicteric cholestasis, or cholestasis without jaundice. Cholestasis is defined, therefore, both clinically and biochemically, with varying degrees of jaundice, pruritus, and elevated levels of conjugated bilirubin, alkaline phosphatase, γ-glutamyl transpeptidase, 5′-nucleotidase, bile acids, and cholesterol. A conventional categorization of cholestatic liver diseases has divided these factors into intrahepatic and extrahepatic causes (Box 1). This chapter discusses the different types of intrahepatic cholestatic liver disease.

PRIMARY BILIARY CIRRHOSIS

Definition and Etiology

Primary biliary cirrhosis (PBC) is a chronic cholestatic liver disease predominantly affecting middle-aged women. It is hypothesized that PBC begins with loss of immune self tolerance, leading to damage of the biliary epithelial cells of small bile ducts. Ongoing immunologic events perpetuate the biliary epithelial cell destruction via direct cytotoxicity or lymphokine-mediated cell damage, leading to disease progression.

Prevalence and Risk Factors

PBC is most commonly diagnosed after the age of 40 years. Of patients with PBC, 90% are women. The prevalence is higher in northern European population groups and lower in Japan. Disease prevalence estimates have ranged from 40 to 400 cases per 1,000,000 population, with an incidence between 4 and 30 cases per 1,000,000 per year.[1] Recent evidence has suggested that environmental factors, including infectious agents and chemicals, might play a role in inducing PBC in genetically predisposed patients.[2]

Pathophysiology and Natural History

PBC is considered an autoimmune disease, with immune destruction of the interlobular bile ducts resulting in a gradually progressive ductopenia. PBC is generally a progressive disease leading to cirrhosis and death, although there have been reports of prolonged survival, with minimal progression of disease. Patients who are asymptomatic at presentation have a longer survival than those who are symptomatic; however, their survival appears to be shorter than that of an age-matched controlled population. About one third of patients who are asymptomatic at presentation become symptomatic within 5 years. Symptomatic patients have an 8-year survival rate of approximately 50%. Survival models have been developed to predict outcome more precisely and are useful in determining the timing for liver transplantation. If PBC is diagnosed at an early histologic stage and treatment with ursodiol is begun (see later), recent studies have suggested that the long-term survival approaches that of a healthy control population. Patients with more advanced histologic disease at diagnosis, however, have 30% and 50% rates of requiring liver transplantation or death over 10 and 20 years, respectively, despite treatment.[3]

Signs and Symptoms

With the ready availability of automated blood chemistry testing, many cases are diagnosed in an asymptomatic phase. The most common initial symptom is fatigue, which occurs in approximately 70% of patients. Fatigue does not necessarily correlate with the severity of disease, and there is evidence suggesting central nervous system mediation of this symptom. Fatigue severity in PBC has been associated with excessive daytime somnolence, autonomic dysfunction, cognitive impairment, and depression.[4-6] Pruritus is also a common symptom, occurring in 50% to 60% of patients. As the disease progresses, patients can develop symptoms of portal hypertension, such as variceal hemorrhage and ascites. Xanthomata, particularly around the eyes (xanthelasma), are commonly found in patients with PBC. PBC is also associated with metabolic bone disease, resulting in premature osteoporosis.

As the disease progresses, there can be fat-soluble vitamin malabsorption caused by a decrease in the biliary secretion of bile acids. There is an increased frequency of other autoimmune disorders in patients with PBC, including autoimmune thyroid disease, sicca syndrome, CREST syndrome (calcinosis, Raynaud's phenomenon, esophageal dysmotility, and telangiectasia), celiac disease, and inflammatory bowel disease.

Diagnosis

The diagnosis of PBC is based on a combination of findings, including cholestatic liver enzyme levels, positive antimitochondrial antibody (AMA), and characteristic liver biopsy findings. An elevated serum alkaline phosphatase level of liver origin is the most common laboratory finding.

The most characteristic laboratory finding in PBC is the presence of the AMA, generally in a titer of 1:40 or higher. More than 95% of patients with PBC have a positive AMA. A confident diagnosis of PBC may be made in cases with typical clinical presentation of PBC in the setting of a positive AMA (≥1:40), and a cholestatic pattern of liver enzymes with alkaline phosphatase at least 1.5 times the upper limit of normal and AST less than five times the upper limit of normal without the obligation to perform a liver biopsy.[7,8] A liver biopsy should be performed in atypical cases, in cases where an alternative diagnosis is suspected, and to obtain staging information. The liver biopsy findings include portal hepatitis, with granulomatous destruction of bile ducts. The histologic changes are divided into four stages, ranging from stage 1, characterized by portal inflammation and bile duct destruction, through stage 4, characterized by histologic cirrhosis. Overlapping stages can be found in individual patients.

Box 1 Causes of Cholestasis

Intrahepatic Cholestasis
- Primary biliary cirrhosis
- Primary sclerosing cholangitis
- Drugs and toxins
- Sepsis
- Malignancy
- Granulomatous liver disease
- Intrahepatic cholestasis of pregnancy
- Hepatitis (viral and alcoholic)
- Genetic disorders
- Graft-versus-host disease
- Post–liver transplantation

Extrahepatic Biliary Tract Diseases
- Choledocholithiasis
- Bile duct tumors, benign and malignant
- Ampullary tumors, benign and malignant
- Pancreatic carcinoma
- Mirizzi's syndrome
- AIDS cholangiopathy
- Parasites
- Primary sclerosing cholangitis

A subgroup of patients have a positive AMA with normal liver enzyme levels. Most of these patients ultimately develop biochemical evidence of cholestasis and symptomatic disease. Another subgroup, with cholestasis and histology suggesting PBC, are AMA negative (AMA-negative PBC).[9] The natural history of AMA-positive and AMA-negative PBC appears to be similar. A positive AMA, usually in low titer, can be seen in patients with other autoimmune disorders.[10]

Summary

- AMA is positive in 95% of patients.
- Liver biopsy reveals portal hepatitis and granulomatous destruction of bile ducts.
- Biopsies are staged 1 through 4 (cirrhosis).

Treatment

Treatment of PBC is directed at both the underlying disease and its complications. Ursodeoxycholic acid (UDCA) is a dihydroxy bile acid that is hydrophilic and nonhepatotoxic. Several large randomized trials using UDCA have shown biochemical improvement.[11-15] Although controversy exists regarding the effect of UDCA in survival, a survival benefit is demonstrated when only trials with adequate UDCA dosing (13-15 mg/kg/day) and sufficient duration of follow-up are considered. Patients without established cirrhosis at the time of starting UDCA therapy, and those with significant improvement of their alkaline phosphatase with therapy, seem to show the greatest survival benefit. In this regard, the survival of noncirrhotic patients with PBC on UDCA therapy appears similar to that of the general population.[16] Similarly, patients with an adequate biochemical response with UDCA therapy also have survival similar to that of the general population.[17] UDCA is currently the recommended treatment at a dosage of 13 to 15 mg/kg daily, either in divided doses or as a single daily dose.[8]

Other drugs have recently been considered for treatment. Methotrexate in combination with UDCA has been shown not to improve the course of PBC compared with UDCA alone in a large randomized trial.[18] Oral budesonide seems to improve hepatic histology in PBC, but its role in treatment remains undetermined. Liver transplantation is recommended for patients with decompensated liver disease.

The most common symptom of PBC requiring treatment is pruritus. First-line treatment consists of cholestyramine at a dosage of 4 g/day, up to 16 g daily. At least 4 hours should elapse between taking cholestyramine and any other medication. Rifampicin 300 to 600 mg/day is second-line treatment for pruritus in patients who do not respond to cholestyramine. Opioid antagonists such as naltrexone have also been used in treatment-resistant cases, as has plasmapheresis. Unfortunately, there is no therapy proved to be of benefit for fatigue in PBC.

Patients with stage 4 PBC can develop portal hypertension and should be screened for the presence of esophageal varices when PBC is first diagnosed and every 3 years thereafter. If prominent varices are found, consider primary prophylaxis (pharmacologic or endoscopic). Bone mineral density should be assessed at the time of diagnosis and periodically thereafter. If osteoporosis is present, consider treatment with a bisphosphonate.[19] Fat-soluble vitamin deficiency should be considered and screened for in patients with hyperbilirubinemia, and oral replacement may be necessary. The association of thyroid disease with PBC has led to the recommendation of checking the serum thyroid-stimulating hormone level at the time of diagnosis and periodically thereafter. Hypercholesterolemia is commonly seen in PBC, but it has not been demonstrated that this is associated with increased cardiovascular risk. Hypercholesterolemia in these patients should be managed based on each patient's cardiovascular risk profile.

Practice Guidelines

Guidelines on the management of primary biliary cirrhosis have been published and are available online.[8,20] This is a comprehensive review of PBC with discussions of diagnosis, clinical manifestations, associated conditions, and therapy. Recommendations made in the review are judged on the quality of evidence in the medical literature used to formulate each guideline.

Summary

- Treat with ursodeoxycholic acid 13 to 15 mg/kg/day.
- Treat pruritus with a stepwise approach, starting with cholestyramine.
- Screen for esophageal varices, osteoporosis, fat-soluble vitamin deficiency, and hypothyroidism.

PRIMARY SCLEROSING CHOLANGITIS

Definition and Etiology

Primary sclerosing cholangitis (PSC) is a chronic, progressive, cholestatic liver disease resulting from inflammation, fibrosis, and destruction of the intrahepatic and extrahepatic bile ducts. This leads to multiple areas of stricturing in the biliary tree and eventually to cirrhosis.

Prevalence and Risk Factors

The estimated prevalence of PSC is 60 to 80 cases per 1 million population. There is a 2 : 1 male predominance. Approximately 80% of patients with PSC have inflammatory bowel disease, more commonly ulcerative colitis than Crohn's disease.[21]

Pathophysiology and Natural History

The pathophysiology of PSC is unclear, but there is evidence suggesting an autoimmune component to the disease. There is also a genetic predisposition, with an increased prevalence of HLA-B2 and DR3 in patients with PSC. Other proposed causes include chronic portal bacteremia, cytotoxic bile acids, and viral infections. The periductal inflammation leads to progressive multifocal stricturing of the intrahepatic and extrahepatic biliary tree.[21]

PSC is a progressive disease, often leading to biliary cirrhosis within 10 to 15 years. Patients who are asymptomatic at the time of diagnosis fare better than those who are symptomatic, but the disease tends to progress in either case. The average overall survival time is approximately 10 years from the date of diagnosis.

Cholangiocarcinoma is a dreaded complication of PSC, occurring in 4% to 20% of patients; the incidence is even higher in autopsy studies. The development of cholangiocarcinoma is often accompanied by clinical decline but can be difficult to diagnose, even when it is suspected, because of the low sensitivity of biliary brush cytology in this setting. Survival after the diagnosis of cholangiocarcinoma is poor, and cholangiocarcinoma is often considered a contraindication to liver transplantation. Some centers have had favorable outcomes with liver transplantation preceded by radiation and chemotherapy.[22]

Signs and Symptoms

It is common for patients with PSC to be asymptomatic. In one large study, only 56% of patients had one or more symptoms at the time of initial diagnosis.[23] The most common symptom is fatigue, which is nonspecific. Other, less-common symptoms include pruritus, weight loss, and fever. Occasionally, patients present with symptoms of portal hypertension, including the onset of ascites or variceal bleeding, or symptoms of bacterial cholangitis. Physical examination at initial presentation may be normal, although jaundice and hepatosplenomegaly are present in up to 50% of patients.

Diagnosis

The diagnostic test of choice for PSC is cholangiography, typically endoscopic retrograde cholangiography (ERC). Occasionally, percutaneous transhepatic cholangiography is necessary to establish the diagnosis when ERC is unsuccessful. The cholangiogram typically shows multiple strictures of the intrahepatic and extrahepatic biliary tree (Fig. 1). In one large study, 27% of patients had intrahepatic ductal involvement only and 6% had only extrahepatic ductal changes.[23] Magnetic resonance cholangiography (MRC) has also been used in the diagnosis of PSC. When compared with ERC in one study, MRC had a sensitivity of 85% to 88% and a specific of 92% to 97%, with good interobserver agreement.[24] It remains to be seen whether MRC will surpass ERC as the first-line test for the diagnosis of PSC.

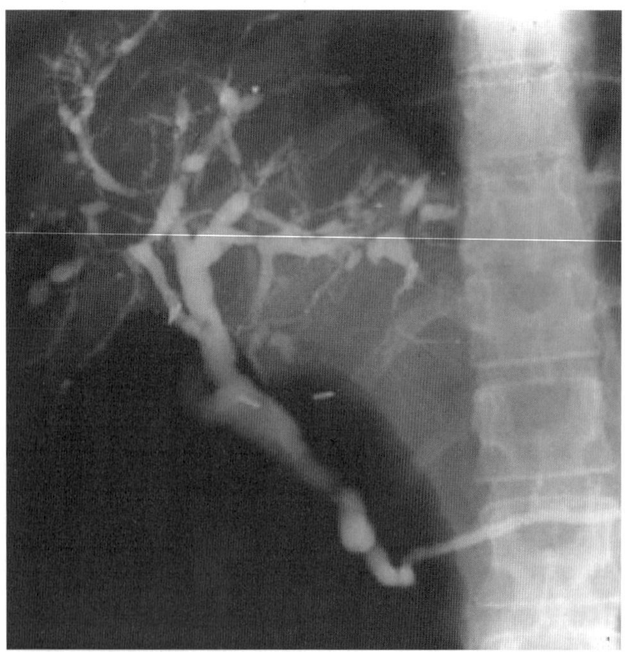

Figure 1 Cholangiogram of primary sclerosing cholangitis (PSC). The areas of stricturing and dilation are typical of PSC.

Liver biopsy is not diagnostic for PSC, but findings often include commonly the absence of intralobular bile ducts (ductopenia), bile duct proliferation, and periductal fibrosis, with an onion-skin fibrosis and nodular fibrous scars. A liver biopsy is often not necessary for the routine diagnosis of PSC.[25] Liver enzyme studies typically show an elevated alkaline phosphatase level of biliary origin, although there is a subgroup of patients with early PSC who present with a normal alkaline phosphatase level.

Summary

- Cholangiography is the diagnostic test of choice.
- Cholangiographic features include areas of stricturing and dilation in the intrahepatic or extrahepatic biliary tree, or both.
- Liver enzyme studies typically show an elevation of the alkaline phosphatase level.

Treatment

"Currently, no medical therapy has been shown to be beneficial in PSC. A 2-year randomized, controlled trial using UDCA at a dose of 12 to 15 mg/kg/d in patients with PSC was associated with improved liver tests, however there was no beneficial effect on survival, liver histology, cholangiographic appearance or symptoms.[26] Subsequently, studies testing higher doses of UDCA (between 17 and 23 mg/kg/d) showed trends towards improved survival but did not reach statistical significance. Recently, a 5-year randomized controlled trial of UCDA at 28 to 30 mg/kg/d demonstrated that high dose UDCA was associated with improved liver tests but did not improve survival and was associated with higher rates of serious adverse events. Based on these results, high dose UDCA (25 to 30 mg/kg/d) cannot be recommended in patients with PSC. Consideration of medical therapy for patients with PSC in the setting of prospective studies is reasonable, but there is not treatment that can be recommended at this time". Medical management of PSC is therefore limited to complications that arise during the course of the disease. Most of these complications and treatments are similar to those listed earlier for the management of PBC.

Up to 20% of patients with PSC develop jaundice, cholangitis, or both, caused by a dominant stricture of the biliary tree, which can be treated with balloon dilation with or without the placement of a biliary stent. This is usually done endoscopically, but it can be done percutaneously. Although there are no established guidelines for surveillance for cholangiocarcinoma in patients with PSC, a high index of suspicion should be maintained.

Liver transplantation is effective for patients who have evidence of end-stage liver disease or who have recurrent bouts of cholangitis that cannot be controlled with dilation of a dominant stricture. Unfortunately, PSC recurs in 15% to 20% of cases, and recurrence is often associated with loss of the graft.

OTHER CONDITIONS ASSOCIATED WITH INTRAHEPATIC CHOLESTASIS

Drug-Induced Cholestasis

Drugs are a common cause of cholestasis. The spectrum of drug-induced liver injury can range from acute reversible cholestasis to chronic cholestasis with loss of bile ducts. In a large study of 1100 cases, acute cholestasis accounted for about 17% of liver-related adverse drug reactions.[30] Drugs can interfere with various stages of bile acid metabolism, including uptake, transport, and secretion at the hepatocyte level.[31]

Drug-induced cholestasis can be categorized into acute and chronic forms (Box 2).[32] The acute forms are subdivided into cholestasis without inflammation (bland cholestasis), cholestasis with inflammation, and cholestasis with bile duct injury. Chronic forms include a vanishing bile duct syndrome and a sclerosing cholangitis-like syndrome.

Drug-induced cholestasis can be accompanied by nausea, anorexia, malaise, and pruritus.[32] Symptoms can occur weeks to months after beginning treatment.

Drugs that cause cholestasis with bile duct injury often are accompanied by additional clinical features, such as fever, rigors, jaundice, and tender hepatomegaly mimicking acute cholangitis. Drugs that result in a vanishing bile duct syndrome can lead to progressive cholestasis, with prolonged jaundice, pruritus, and, occasionally, cirrhosis and liver failure.

The most important tool in the diagnosis of drug-induced cholestasis is a careful medical history, eliciting a history of taking prescribed, over-the-counter, or alternative medications, including herbs. Biliary obstruction should be excluded with an imaging study, ultrasound, or computed tomography (CT) of the biliary tree. The mainstay of treatment is withdrawal of the drug. Management of symptoms associated with cholestasis are similar to those for PBC.

Most cholestatic hepatic injury resolves with withdrawal of the offending medication. A small subgroup of patients develop progressive liver disease, resulting in biliary cirrhosis and liver failure.

Sepsis

Intrahepatic cholestasis is often seen in patients who have sepsis.[33] Circulatory endotoxins associated with sepsis induce cytokine production, including tumor necrosis factor α, interleukin-1, and interleukin 6, which results in impaired bile acid transport. The cholestasis of infection is often seen in severely ill hospitalized patients, often in the intensive care unit (ICU). Other factors can contribute to the cholestasis, including medications and total parenteral nutrition. Calculous or acalculous cholecystitis or biliary obstruction is often a concern in this setting. Ultrasound can be a helpful diagnostic tool in this circumstance. Ultrasound is noninvasive and can be done in the ICU. Therapy for sepsis-induced cholestasis consists of treating the underlying infection. Outcomes usually are dictated more by the patient's underlying disease than by the cholestasis itself.

Malignancy

Primary liver cancer—hepatocellular carcinoma—and metastatic cancer are associated with a liver enzyme pattern suggestive of cholestasis. They are more properly categorized as infiltrative disorders but are discussed here because of their similarity to cholestatic diseases. Hepatocellular carcinoma, once a relatively uncommon tumor, has been increasing in incidence since the 1990s because of its association with hepatitis C–induced cirrhosis. In this setting, the estimated incidence of the development of hepatocellular carcinoma is 1% to 4% per year.[34] Cirrhosis from causes other than hepatitis C, particularly hepatitis B and hemochromatosis, is also associated with the development of hepatocellular carcinoma. Hepatocellular carcinoma is often suspected in patients who have previously stable cirrhosis and who have experienced a precipitous clinical decline without other explanation. The diagnosis is made by abdominal imaging techniques, including ultrasound, CT, and magnetic resonance imaging (MRI).

Therapeutic approaches to hepatocellular carcinoma include surgical resection, liver transplantation, and techniques designed to shrink the tumor, such as alcohol injection or radiofrequency ablation.

Box 2 Drug-Induced Cholestasis

Cholestasis without Hepatitis
Estrogens
Anabolic steroids
Cyclosporine
Tamoxifen
Azathioprine

Cholestasis with Hepatitis
Chlorpromazine
Macrolide antibiotics
Tricyclic antidepressants
Carbamazepine
Amoxicillin-clavulanate
Oxypenicillins
Nonsteroidal anti-inflammatory drugs
Azathioprine

Cholestasis with Bile Duct Injury
Dextropropoxyphene
Flucoxacillin (floxacillin)
Carmustine
Toxins: paraquat, methylenedianiline

Vanishing Bile Duct Syndrome
Chlorpromazine
Flucloxacillin (floxacillin) and other oxypenicillins
Amoxicillin-clavulanic acid
Ampicillin
Amitriptyline
Azathioprine
Barbiturates
Carbamazepine
Chlorothiazide
Cotrimoxazole
Clindamycin
Chlorpromazine
Cimetidine
Cyproheptadine
Dicloxacillin
Erythromycin esters
Estradiol
Flucloxacillin
Glycyrrhiza
Haloperidol
Ibuprofen
Imipramine
Methyltestosterone
Norandrostenolone
D-Penicillamine
Phenytoin
Prochlorperazine
Tetracycline
Terbinafine
Thiabendazole
Tiopronin
Tolbutamide

Sclerosing Cholangitis-like Syndrome
Floxuridine
Intralesional and scolicidal agents

- 2% Formaldehyde
- 20% Hypertonic saline
- Absolute alcohol
- Silver nitrate
- Iodine solution

Data from Chitturi S, Farrell GC: Drug-induced cholestasis. Semin Gastrointest Dis 2001;12:113-124.

SECTION 6 HEPATOLOGY

Metastatic carcinoma can also manifest with cholestasis. The hepatic component is usually found after the diagnosis of carcinoma is made, although it is occasionally the presenting feature. Cholestasis can also occur in patients as a paraneoplastic syndrome in the absence of metastatic disease to the liver. This nonmetastatic cholestasis has been described in non-Hodgkin's lymphoma, prostate cancer, and renal cell carcinoma.[35-38]

Granulomatous Liver Diseases

Granulomatous liver diseases are more accurately classified as infiltrative diseases but are discussed here because the pattern of liver enzyme abnormality resembles that seen with cholestasis. Granuloma formation in the liver occurs in various disorders, including systemic infections from bacteria, viruses, fungi, rickettsia, spirochetes, and parasites; drugs and chemicals; immune-mediated diseases, such as sarcoidosis and primary biliary cirrhosis; and neoplasms, such as Hodgkin's disease (Box 3).[39,40] The list of commonly used drugs that result in hepatic granulomas is extensive; it includes allopurinol, quinidine, sulfonamides, and sulfonylureas. The finding of granulomas on liver biopsy is often expected, for example, in patients with suspected primary biliary cirrhosis who present with cholestasis and a positive mitochondrial antibody or patients with known sarcoidosis who present with cholestasis. On the other hand, when granulomas are found on liver biopsy unexpectedly or as part of an evaluation for a systemic illness, a thorough investigation should be undertaken to look for the underlying cause.

Evaluation should begin with a careful history including, for example, risk factors for HIV, exposure to tuberculosis, or exposure to farm animals, which presents a risk for brucellosis and Q fever.

Because exposure to drugs is a common cause of granulomatous liver disease, a history of medication use is essential. Further diagnostic testing is often necessary to ascertain the cause; this should include chest x-ray; serologic evaluation for fungi, *Brucella, Treponema,* HIV, other viruses, and mitochondrial antibody and angiotensin-converting enzyme levels; tuberculin skin testing; and special stains of the liver biopsy for fungus and acid-fast bacilli (AFB). More-extensive evaluation, such as abdominal or chest CT scanning, may be necessary if lymphoma is suspected.

Treatment of granulomatous liver disease is disease specific. It may be as simple as stopping an offending drug. A trial of corticosteroids in patients with idiopathic granulomatous hepatitis who are symptomatic, with fever, myalgias, and arthralgias, may be helpful. Empirical antituberculous therapy should be considered before instituting corticosteroids.

Box 3 Causes of Hepatic Granulomatous Liver Diseases

Chemicals
Beryllium

Drugs
Allopurinol
Carbamazepine
Chlorpropamide
Hydralazine
Methyldopa
Nitrofurantoin
Phenytoin
Procainamide
Quinidine
Sulfonamides
Sulfonylureas

Infection

Bacteria
Brucellosis
Tularemia
Yersinia
Propionibacterium
Pseudomonas pseudomallei
Spirochetes: *Treponema*
Rickettsia: Q fever

Fungi
Histoplasmosis
Coccidiomycosis
Blastomycosis
Aspergillus
Actinomycosis
Nocardia
Cryptococcus
Candida

Mycobacteria
Tuberculosis
Atypical mycobacteria
Leprosy

Parasites
Ascaris
Toxocara
Schistosoma
Leishmania

Viruses
Epstein-Barr Virus
Cytomegalovirus
HIV

Miscellaneous
Sarcoidosis
Primary biliary cirrhosis
Hodgkin's disease
Non-Hodgkin's lymphoma
Inflammatory bowel disease
Systemic lupus erythematosus
Whipple's disease
Wegener's granulomatosis
Talc in drug abusers

Data from Guckian JC, Perry JE: Granulomatous hepatitis. An analysis of 63 cases and review of the literature. Ann Intern Med 1966;65:1081-1100; Cunningham D, Mills PR, Quigley EM, et al: Hepatic granulomas: Experience over a 10-year period in the West of Scotland. Q J Med 1982;202:162-170.

Intrahepatic Cholestasis of Pregnancy

Intrahepatic cholestasis of pregnancy (ICP) can occur in the second or third trimester. There appears to be a genetic component because it has been reported to occur in family members.[41] It is likely that hyperestrogenemia associated with a pregnancy plays a role.[42] The altered metabolism of progesterone has also been implicated. The hallmark clinical feature of intrahepatic cholestasis of pregnancy is pruritus. Jaundice can occur, and laboratory findings reveal the typical features of cholestasis, including elevated levels of serum bile acids, alkaline phosphatase, and total bilirubin. UDCA has been used in ICP to relieve pruritus, and it appears to be safe for mother and fetus.[43] Symptoms resolve within several days of delivery but can recur during subsequent pregnancies.

Viral and Alcoholic Hepatitis

Occasionally, viral hepatitis manifests with signs and symptoms of cholestasis characterized by jaundice and pruritus. The clinical course can last for several months.[44]

Alcoholic hepatitis generally manifests with features of cholestasis. It is often accompanied by fever, and the clinical presentation can be confused with that of cholangitis. A careful medical history is essential to confirm a history of ethanol abuse or dependency.

Genetic Disorders

Rare syndromes result from mutations of genes responsible for transporting biliary constituents from the space of Disse across the basal lateral (sinusoidal) membrane and across the canalicular membrane into the bile duct. Transporter gene mutations can result in hereditary cholestasis and include such disorders as Byler's disease and benign recurrent intrahepatic cholestasis.[45] Byler's disease is characterized by cholestasis occurring early in life that progresses to cirrhosis and death, usually in early childhood. Benign recurrent intrahepatic cholestasis is characterized by episodic jaundice and pruritus lasting for several weeks to months, with long symptom-free intervals. The disease does not progress to cirrhosis. Multiple family members can be affected. Cystic fibrosis can result in cholestasis caused by gene mutations at the level of the bile duct, resulting in inspissated bile.[46]

Graft-Versus-Host Disease

Graft-versus-host disease (GVHD) can be seen within the first 100 days after bone marrow transplantation (acute GVHD) or after that time (chronic GVHD). It occurs in up to 50% of patients after bone marrow transplantation and is believed to be caused by T cells of the donor marrow reacting against host antigens, resulting in cytokine damage of the affected organ. GVHD can affect the skin, liver, and gastrointestinal tract.

Although hepatic involvement is usually associated with cholestatic liver enzyme levels, other causes of cholestasis are common in this patient population. GVHD often has to be distinguished from viral infections, drug toxicity, and hepatic veno-occlusive disease. Liver biopsy provides the most definitive way to distinguish the various causes of cholestasis in this patient population. Treatment of GVHD consists of prophylactic measures and treatment of active disease. The most common prophylactic regimen is a combination of methotrexate and cyclosporine. Various treatment regimens of acute of GVHD have been used, including corticosteroids, antithymocyte globulin, tacrolimus, and mycophenolate.[47] Chronic GVHD has also been treated with various agents, including prednisone, cyclosporine, thalidomide, psoralen, ultraviolet irradiation, UDCA, tacrolimus, rapamycin, and mycophenolate.[48] Less than 50% of patients treated for GVHD sustain a cure. In general, the more severe the skin, liver, or gut involvement, the less favorable the outcome.

Total Parenteral Nutrition

Total parenteral nutrition (TPN) is associated with liver dysfunction resulting in steatosis, cholestasis, and cirrhosis. Intrahepatic cholestasis can occur after 2 to 3 weeks of TPN therapy and is associated with elevations in serum bilirubin and alkaline phosphatase levels.

Cholestasis usually reverses after TPN is stopped but is of concern if the patient requires long-term TPN. Progressive liver disease, including cirrhosis, may be associated with long-term TPN.[49]

Box 4 Causes of Cholestasis After Liver Transplantation

Infections (bacterial, cytomegalovirus)
Medications (immunosuppressive drugs, antibiotics)
Viral hepatitis B and C
Rejections, acute and chronic
Recurrence of disease (primary biliary cirrhosis, primary sclerosing cholangitis)

Post–Liver Transplantation Cholestasis

Cholestasis is often seen after liver transplantation and is caused by various conditions (Box 4).[50] In the first few months after transplantation, cholestasis is often associated with bacterial infections or viral infections, particularly cytomegalovirus. Medications, both antibiotics and immunosuppressive drugs typically used after transplantation, are also associated with cholestasis. Acute cellular rejection is often heralded by the onset of abnormalities in cholestatic liver enzyme levels. Later after transplantation, other causes of cholestasis are more common, including chronic rejection, fibrosing cholestatic hepatitis resulting from recurrent hepatitis B or C, or a recurrence of the original disease, such as PBC or PSC.

Suggested Readings

Broome U, Olsson R, Loof L: Natural history and prognostic factors in 305 Swedish patients with primary sclerosing cholangitis. Gut 1996;38:610-615.
Chitturi S, Farrell GC: Drug-induced cholestasis. Semin Gastrointest Dis 2001;12: 113-124.
Heathcote JE: Management of primary biliary cirrhosis. The American Association for the Study of Liver Diseases practice guidelines. Hepatology 2000;31:1005-1013.
Heneghan MA, Sylvestre PB: Cholestatic diseases of liver transplantation. Semin Gastrointest Dis 2001;12:133-147.
Kaplan MM, Gershwin ME: Primary biliary cirrhosis. N Engl J Med 2005;353;1261-1274.
Mendes FD, Lindor KD: Primary sclerosing cholangitis. Clin Liver Dis 2004;8:195-211.
Moseley RH: Sepsis and cholestasis. Clin Liver Dis 2004:8:83-94.
Riely CA, Bacq YB: Intrahepatic cholestasis of pregnancy. Clin Liver Dis 2004;8:167-176.
Trauner M, Fickert P, Zollner G: Genetic disorders and molecular mechanisms in cholestatic liver disease-a clinical approach. Semin Gastrointest Dis 2001;12:66-88.

References

For a complete list of references, log onto www.expertconsult.com.

Liver Disease in Pregnancy

Jamilé Wakim-Fleming

DEFINITION AND CAUSES

Liver disease in pregnancy encompasses a spectrum of diseases encountered during gestation and the postpartum period that result in abnormal liver function tests, hepatobiliary dysfunction, or both. It occurs in 3% to 10% of all pregnancies.

Several disorders contribute to liver disease in pregnancy (Box 1). These include diseases induced by the pregnancy such as acute fatty liver of pregnancy (AFLP) and intrahepatic cholestasis of pregnancy (IHCP), diseases that existed before pregnancy that could potentially flare during pregnancy such as autoimmune hepatitis and Wilson's disease, and diseases not related to the pregnancy but that could affect the pregnant woman at any time during gestation such as viral hepatitis.

DIAGNOSIS AND OUTCOMES

The diagnosis of liver disease in pregnancy is challenging and relies on laboratory investigations. Signs and symptoms are often not specific and consist of jaundice, nausea, vomiting, and abdominal pain. The underlying disorder can have a significant effect on morbidity and mortality in both mother and fetus, and a diagnostic workup should be initiated promptly.

The physical examination of a pregnant woman can show skin changes suggesting chronic liver disease, such as palmar erythema and spider angiomas. These changes are the result of hyperesterogenemia of pregnancy and occur in up to 60% of healthy pregnancies.

Alterations of laboratory test results can represent physiologic changes of pregnancy an example of this is a decreased level of serum albumin and increased level of alkaline phosphatase whereas. Elevations of transaminase, bilirubin, and prothrombin time (PT) indicate a pathologic state. The unconjugated hyperbilirubinemia of Gilbert's syndrome is not affected by the pregnancy. Clotting factors are affected by normal pregnancy and favor a hypercoagulable state. Women with inherited thrombophilia, such as factor V Leiden or antithrombin III deficiency, are at increased risk for hepatic vein and portal vein thrombosis during pregnancy.

When diagnostic imaging is needed during the workup of liver test abnormalities in a pregnant woman, ultrasonography becomes the modality of choice because of its safety for the fetus. Magnetic resonance imaging (MRI) may be used as a second line test if additional information is still necessary. Computed tomography (CT) and endoscopic retrograde cholangiopancreatography (ERCP) involve radiation to the fetus and require shielding of the uterus.

Outcome depends on the causative factors. Newly acquired primary herpes simplex hepatitis can cause fulminant liver failure, premature delivery, and stillbirths. On the other hand, pregnancy can induce eclampsia and AFLP with a potential for liver failure and death.

Extreme vigilance in recognizing physical and laboratory abnormalities in pregnancy is a prerequisite for an accurate diagnosis. This could lead to a timely intervention and successful outcome.

PHYSIOLOGIC CHANGES DURING PREGNANCY

Pregnancy induces hemodynamic changes that involve several organ systems throughout gestation, the postpartum period, and lactation. The major physiologic changes in pregnancy (Box 2) include an increase in cardiac output, sodium and water retention, blood volume expansion, and a reduction in systemic vascular resistance and systemic blood pressure. These changes peak in the second trimester and then plateau until the time of delivery. Total blood flow to the liver increases after 28th week driven by the increased flow to the portal vein. Histology of the liver remains essentially normal during pregnancy.

Physiologic changes during pregnancy could be misinterpreted as pathologic. Lack of understanding of these changes can appreciably alter the criteria for diagnosis and therapy and can contribute to the morbidity and mortality associated with the pregnancy.

FACTORS TO CONSIDER DURING PREGNANCY

Safety of Drugs

Treatment of liver disease in pregnancy may involve prompt delivery, supportive management, or drug therapy. The choice of drugs in pregnancy should be based on the U.S. Food and Drug Administration (FDA) classification for drugs and fetal risk (Box 3). Although not all drugs have been tested in pregnant women, the FDA has classified them into five categories based on the level of teratogenicity determined from animal and human studies.

Pregnancy after Liver Transplantation

Women with a liver transplant may increasing in number, and many of them are of reproductive age and attempting pregnancy. Menstrual function, libido, and fertility are usually restored within 6 months after transplantation, and pregnant women can have excellent outcome and deliver healthy babies, especially when pregnancy is planned 2 years after the transplant.

PREEXISTING LIVER DISEASE AND PREGNANCY

The outcome of a pregnancy is greatly affected by the medical condition of the liver before conception. Diagnosis and treatment of a liver disorder before conception will minimize potential exacerbations that could lead to liver failure and fetal loss.

Cirrhosis and Portal Hypertension

The prevalence of cirrhosis in reproductive-age women approximates 0.45 cases per 1000. Etiology of cirrhosis in pregnancy is similar to that in the nonpregnant state and commonly includes alcohol and viral hepatitis C and B. Cirrhosis can affect ovulation and cause infertility. However, women might still become pregnant and should expect a good outcome if their liver function is well compensated (as in noncirrhotic portal hypertension) and if their liver disease is treated before conception and treatment is maintained during pregnancy. Patients with cirrhosis and noncirrhotic portal hypertension are at high risk for premature deliveries. Hepatic decompensation with jaundice, bleeding from esophageal varices, ascites, and fulminant liver failure can occur. In general, diuretics and spironolactone, which are in FDA category D, are not advisable during pregnancy or lactation because of the potential for teratogenicity. Banding of bleeding esophageal varices and octreotide (FDA category B) are safe during pregnancy. Meperidine (Demerol) and midazolam (Versed) are both in FDA category C and safe to use during endoscopy.

Box 1 Physiologic Changes During Pregnancy

Increases
Blood volume, heart rate, and cardiac output rise by 35% to 50%, peak at 32 weeks' gestation; further increase by 20% in twin pregnancies
Alkaline phosphatase levels rise three- to fourfold because of placental production
Clotting factors I, II, V, VII, VIII, X, and XII
Ceruloplasmin level
Transferrin level

Decreases
Gallbladder contractility
Hemoglobin level (because of volume expansion)
Uric acid level
Albumin and total protein levels
Antithrombin III and protein S level
Systemic vascular resistance
Modest decline in blood pressure

No Changes
Liver transaminase levels (aspartate aminotransferase, alanine aminotransferase)
γ-Glutamyl transferase (GGT) level
Bilirubin level
Prothrombin time
Platelet count (or slight decline)

Box 2 Causes of Liver Disease in Pregnancy

Preexisting Liver Disease
Cirrhosis and portal hypertension
Autoimmune hepatitis
Primary biliary cirrhosis, primary sclerosing cholangitis
Wilson's disease
Chronic viral hepatitis B and C

Liver Disease Coincidental with Pregnancy
Budd-Chiari syndrome
Hepatitis

- Viral hepatitis E
- Herpes simplex virus hepatitis
- Acute hepatitis A, B, and C
- Cytomegalovirus hepatitis

Alcohol and pregnancy
Gallstone disease

Liver Disease Unique to Pregnancy
Acute fatty liver of pregnancy
Preeclampsia, eclampsia
HELLP syndrome (*h*emolysis, *e*levated *l*iver enzyme levels, *l*ow *p*latelet count)
Intrahepatic cholestasis of pregnancy
Hyperemesis gravidarum

Box 3 U.S. Food and Drug Administration (FDA) Classification of Drugs and Fetal Risk

Category A: Controlled studies show no risk
Category B: No evidence of risk in humans
Category C: Risk cannot be ruled out
Category D: Positive evidence of risk
Category X: Contraindicated in pregnancy

Autoimmune Hepatitis

Autoimmune hepatitis (see the chapter "Chronic Autoimmune Hepatitis") is a progressive liver disease that predominantly affects women of all ages and can manifest at any time during gestation and the postpartum period.

The disease activity of autoimmune hepatitis is usually attenuated during pregnancy, and dosages of medication can be decreased because of the state of immune tolerance induced by the pregnancy. Nonetheless, flares have occurred in 11% of patients during gestation and up to 25% in the postpartum period. There is an increased risk of prematurity, low-birth-weight infants, and fetal loss. Pregnancy does not contraindicate immunosuppressive therapy. Both prednisone and azathioprine (FDA category D at dosages <100 mg/day) are considered safe during pregnancy and lactation. In one meta-analysis, prednisone given during the first trimester was linked to a marginal risk of oral cleft defect in the newborn.

Primary Biliary Cirrhosis and Primary Sclerosing Cholangitis

Primary biliary cirrhosis and primary sclerosing cholangitis (see the chapter "Primary Biliary Cirrhosis, Primary Sclerosing Cholangitis, and Other Cholestatic Liver Diseases") are autoimmune diseases that can overlap with autoimmune hepatitis. Pregnancy is rare in these conditions and carries a high risk of prematurity, stillbirths, and liver failure.

In patients with primary biliary cirrhosis, pregnancy can induce a new-onset pruritus or worsen a preexisting pruritus. Diagnosis is not different from that in the nonpregnant woman. Ursodeoxycholic acid is considered FDA category B and can be continued safely in pregnancy. However, no large studies have demonstrated its safety during the first trimester and lactation.

Primary sclerosing cholangitis is rarely described in pregnancy; pruritus and abdominal pain seem to be the major symptoms. Alkaline phosphatase and γ-glutamyl transferase levels are elevated. Diagnosis relies on clinical and ultrasound findings. No specific treatment exists for primary sclerosing cholangitis, but ursodeoxycholic acid and stabilization of cirrhosis, when present, have been associated with good outcome.

Wilson's Disease

Wilson's disease (see the chapter "Wilson's Disease") is an inherited autosomal recessive defect of copper transport. Fertility in Wilson's disease is decreased but can improve with therapy. Treatment should be initiated before conception and should not be interrupted during pregnancy, because of the risk of fulminant liver failure. The treatment of choice in pregnancy is zinc sulfate 50 mg three times daily (FDA category C), because of its efficacy and safety for the fetus. Patients who are treated with D-penicillamine (FDA category D) or trientine (FDA category C) before pregnancy require a dose reduction by 25% to 50% of that in the pre-pregnancy state especially during the last trimester, to promote better wound healing if a cesarean section is to be performed.

LIVER DISEASES COINCIDENTAL WITH PREGNANCY

Budd-Chiari Syndrome

Budd-Chiari syndrome is an occlusive syndrome of the hepatic veins that leads to sinusoidal congestion and necrosis of hepatocytes around the central vein. Most cases occur during the postpartum period. Of pregnant women who develop Budd-Chiari syndrome, 25% have an underlying predisposing condition, such as factor V Leiden, antithrombin III, protein C or S deficiency, or the presence of antiphospholipid antibodies. Clinical manifestations include hepatomegaly, ascites, and abdominal pain. On physical examination,

Table 1 Viral Hepatitis in Pregnancy

Virus	Risk of Transmission to Fetus	Signs and Symptoms	Treatment	Outcome
HEV	In utero, 50%	Jaundice, viral syndrome, liver failure	Prevention	Mortality up to 40%
HSV	In utero and during delivery, up to 50%	Increases in bilirubin, transaminase levels, prothrombin time	Acyclovir (often)	Liver failure; mortality up to 40%
HAV	Rare	Viral syndrome or asymptomatic	Supportive	Benign
HBV	High if mother is HBeAg$^+$ and during third trimester	Viral syndrome or asymptomatic	Supportive	Benign
HCV	3.8%	Often asymptomatic	Supportive	Benign
CMV	Up to 30%-40%	Mononucleosis-like	Supportive	High morbidity to child

CMV, cytomegalovirus; HAV, hepatitis A virus; HBeAg, hepatitis B e antigen; HBV, hepatitis B virus; HCV, hepatitis C virus; HEV, hepatitis E virus; HSV, herpes simplex virus.

the liver is palpable and hepatojugular reflux is absent. Doppler ultrasound and MRI are the imaging modalities of choice. Complete anticoagulation throughout pregnancy and the puerperium is required. Liver transplantation is often necessary in the acute phase.

Viral Hepatitis

Acute viral hepatitis (Table 1) is the most common cause of jaundice in pregnancy, with an incidence of approximately 1 to 2 per 1000. The outcome is usually benign, except in viral hepatitis E and herpes simplex virus (HSV) hepatitis.

Viral Hepatitis E

Hepatitis E virus (HEV) is rare in the United States but endemic in Asia and Africa. Acute viral hepatitis E is transmitted via the fecal-oral route and is associated with high morbidity and a maternal mortality rate of 30%. Vertical transmission of HEV to the newborn occurs in 50% of cases if the mother is viremic at the time of delivery. Treatment is supportive, and judicious hand washing prevents contamination. Pregnant women should avoid travelling to high-risk endemic areas, especially during the late stages of pregnancy.

Herpes Simplex Hepatitis

Approximately 2% of women acquire HSV during pregnancy. HSV hepatitis is a rare condition but may be devastating when primary infection occurs in pregnancy because it is associated with a 40% risk for fulminant liver failure and death. Treatment of choice for severe primary HSV infection is intravenous acyclovir (FDA category B).

Recurrent HSV infections usually manifest as genital mucocutaneous lesions. Transmission to the fetus is high (≤50%) when maternal acquisition occurs near the time of delivery. Oral acyclovir 400 mg three times daily for 7 to 10 days should be given. Cesarean section is strongly advisable if lesions are present at delivery.

Acute Viral Hepatitis A

Acute hepatitis A virus (HAV) infection is usually self-limited during pregnancy. Transmission to the newborn can occur when delivery takes place during the incubation period because of viral shedding and contamination during vaginal delivery. Treatment of the mother is supportive. Passive immunoprophylaxis should be given to the newborn.

Viral Hepatitis B

Acute and chronic HBV infections during pregnancy do not seem to affect the course of pregnancy but are associated with an increased risk of transmission to the newborn. The risk of vertical transmission of HBV is minimal if the infection is acquired and resolves in the first trimester. The risk is high, ranging from 60% to 90% if the infection is acquired during the third trimester or if the infected mother is positive for the envelope antigen (eAg) and the viral DNA count is elevated. Therefore, active and passive immunoprophylaxis should be administered to newborns of HBV-infected mothers as recommended by the CDC (Box 4). However, despite these prophylactic measures, failure rates are reported and nucleoside and nucleotide analogues have been used to prevent transmission to newborns of mothers with high HBV viral count. Although this practice appears safe (www.apregistry.com) the use of these agents remains controversial.

Box 4 Centers for Disease Control and Prevention (CDC) Recommendations for Hepatitis B Virus (HBV) Testing and Vaccination During Pregnancy

- All pregnant women should be tested routinely for hepatitis B surface antigen (HBsAg) during the first trimester in each pregnancy, even if they have been previously vaccinated or tested.
- Newborns of pregnant women who test positive for HBsAg should receive HBV vaccine and hepatitis B immunoglobulin during the first 12 hours of life and complete the three-dose HBV vaccine series by 9 to 18 months of age.
- For newborns of mothers not infected with HBV, the first vaccine should start at 1 month of age and the series should be completed by 18 months of age.
- Hepatitis B vaccination is not contraindicated in pregnancy. Limited data indicate no apparent risk for adverse events to developing fetuses when hepatitis B vaccine is administered to pregnant women. Current vaccines contain noninfectious HBsAg and should carry no risk for the fetus.

Viral Hepatitis C

The prevalence of hepatitis C virus (HCV) infection in women of childbearing age in the United States is approximately 1%. Treatment of HCV infection is contraindicated in pregnancy because of the teratogenicity of the drugs used. There is a 3.8% rate of vertical transmission to infants born to mothers who are viremic at the time of delivery. This rate increases to 25% in mothers coinfected with the human immunodeficiency virus (HIV). Breast-feeding should not be discouraged and the indication for cesarean section should be based on obstetrical reasons. The PCR assay is not sensitive for infants younger than 1 month, and the treatment of HCV is contraindicated in children younger than 3 years because of the potential for neurologic damage. Testing for HCV in children should be delayed until age 18 months.

Cytomegalovirus Hepatitis

Infection with cytomegalovirus (CMV) is common and usually inapparent. The overall prevalence in women of childbearing age is 50% to 80%. Acute CMV hepatitis in the pregnant woman can manifest as a mononucleosis-like illness. The risk of transmission to the fetus is high, occurring at a rate of 30% to 40% when the infection is acquired before 22 weeks of gestation. The infection can cause mental retardation and congenital malformations. There is no effective and safe therapy during pregnancy.

Alcohol and Pregnancy

More than 50% of all women of childbearing age have reported alcohol use, and one in eight has reported binge drinking. Many of these women are sexually active and do not take effective measures to prevent pregnancy. Women are more sensitive to the effects of alcohol than men, and ethanol consumption increases the frequency of alcoholic hepatitis, menstrual disturbances, infertility, abortions, and miscarriages. The U.S. Surgeon General and Secretary of Health and Human Services have recommended abstinence from alcohol for women planning pregnancy, at conception, and during pregnancy because a safe level of prenatal alcohol consumption has not been determined. Mothers who consume alcohol during pregnancy can have premature babies, stillbirths, babies with neonatal alcohol withdrawal (characterized by jitteriness, irritability, and poor feeding in the first 12 hours of life), and infants with fetal alcohol syndrome. Fetal alcohol syndrome is a serious congenital malformation diagnosed by the presence of dysmorphic facial features, prenatal and postnatal growth deficits, and central nervous system abnormalities. The prevalence of fetal alcohol syndrome among offspring of moderate to heavy drinkers (1-2 oz/day of absolute alcohol) and chronic alcoholics is 10% to 50%.

Gallstone Disease

Pregnancy and the hyperestrogenemic state promote biliary cholesterol saturation and inhibit the hepatic synthesis of chenodeoxycholic acid, thus favoring lithogenesis. In addition, prepregnancy obesity, low activity level, low serum leptin levels, and a history of gallbladder disease are reported to be strong risk factors for pregnancy-associated gallbladder disease. The risk increases as the pregnancy advances, and by the third trimester approximately 10% of pregnant women may have gallstones, compared with 5% at the beginning of the pregnancy. However, most gallstones regress in the postpartum period.

Symptoms of cholelithiasis are experienced by 8% to 25% of pregnant women and the symptoms recur in 38% during the same gestation, often requiring surgical management. Laparoscopic cholecystectomy for symptomatic cholelithiasis in pregnancy is particularly safe when performed during the second trimester because of the moderate size of the uterus, decreased number of days in the hospital, and reduced rate of labor induction and preterm deliveries.

Choledocholithiasis during pregnancy increases the risks of morbidity and mortality for both mother and fetus because of cholangitis and pancreatitis. Endoscopic retrograde cholangiopancreatography (ERCP) may be needed.

LIVER DISEASES UNIQUE TO PREGNANCY

AFLP, the HELLP syndrome (*h*emolysis, *e*levated *l*iver enzyme levels, *l*ow *p*latelet count), eclampsia, and preeclampsia occur during the third trimester and are associated with increased morbidity and mortality to both the mother and fetus (Table 2). These disorders have been suggested to represent a spectrum of the same pathologic mechanisms, making the differentiation among them challenging. Of patients with AFLP, 50% have preeclampsia, and 20% of patients with severe eclampsia develop the HELLP syndrome. Delivery is the most important step in managing these disorders because it can be lifesaving to mother and child.

Acute Fatty Liver of Pregnancy

AFLP is a rare disorder of the third trimester, affecting less than 0.01% of pregnant women. It is most common in primiparous women older than 30 years and in women with multiple gestations carrying a male fetus. Initial symptoms are nonspecific and include nausea, vomiting, and abdominal pain. These manifestations should prompt vigilant monitoring because progression to jaundice, hypoglycemia, disseminated intravascular coagulation with marked decrease of antithrombin III activity, encephalopathy, and frank liver failure can rapidly ensue.

During pregnancy, levels of free fatty acids (FFAs) increase in maternal blood because of the effects of hormone-sensitive lipase and gestational insulin. Transport of fatty acids into the cell and oxidation of fatty acids by the mitochondrion provide the energy necessary for the growth of the fetus. Defects in the genes encoding for the transport and oxidation pathways of fatty acids are inherited as autosomal recessive traits and are known as *fatty acid oxidation disorders*. These have been shown to be associated with maternal, placental, and fetal complications. During the last trimester, the metabolic demands of the fetus increase, and mothers heterozygous for a fatty acid oxidation disorder and pregnant with an affected fetus can develop AFLP because of their inability to metabolize fatty acids for energy production and fetal growth. Fatty acids then deposit in the liver.

Liver biopsy may be necessary for diagnosis. AFLP is characterized by microvesicular fat deposition in centrilobular hepatocytes. Delivery of the fetus unloads the excess of fatty acid delivery to the liver and leads to rapid recovery without sequelae of chronic liver disease.

The most common disorder of fatty acid oxidation disorder in AFLP is a deficiency of long-chain 3-hydroxylacyl-CoA dehydrogenase (LCHAD). Infants homozygous for LCHAD born to heterozygous mothers suffer from failure to thrive, hepatic failure, cardiomyopathy, microvesicular steatosis, hypoglycemia, and death. Thus, mothers and children born to mothers with AFLP should be screened for the LCHAD gene defect and other disorders of fatty acid oxidation. Treatment of the infant consists of administering formula rich in medium-chain triglycerides. AFLP can recur in subsequent pregnancies, especially in women carrying the LCHAD mutations. However, the overall recurrence rate of AFLP is unclear.

Preeclampsia and Eclampsia

Preeclampsia and eclampsia affect 5% of pregnancies beyond the 22nd week of gestation and are more common in primiparous women with multifetal gestations. Other risk factors include preeclampsia in a previous pregnancy, chronic hypertension, pregestational diabetes, nephropathy, obesity, and antiphospholipid syndrome. Symptoms include hypertension of 140/90 mm Hg or higher and proteinuria higher than 0.3 g in 24 hours. Eclampsia is defined by the additional occurrence of new-onset seizures. Liver test abnormalities are present in 25% of cases. Overlap with the HELLP syndrome occurs in 20% of cases. The underlying mechanism is partly due to abnormal implantation of the placenta, with decreased perfusion, resulting in vasospasm and endothelial injury to various organs, notably the brain, liver, and kidneys. Genetic mechanisms have also been implicated. In a woman with a prior history of eclampsia, the recurrence rate is 20% to 30% for preeclampsia and 2% to 6% for eclampsia.

Liver histology is distinct from that of AFLP. It indicates fibrin deposition in sinusoids, periportal hemorrhage, and liver cell necrosis. Hypertensive crisis, abruptio placentae, and liver failure can occur. Maternal mortality is noted in 1% but can reach 15% of cases in developing countries. Fetal mortality rates range from 5% to 30%. Labetolol (FDA category C) and methyldopa (FDA category B) are the drugs of choice for managing hypertension. Magnesium sulfate (FDA category B) is the drug of choice for preventing and treating

Table 2 Liver Diseases Unique to Pregnancy

Disorder	Gestational Period at Presentation	Prevalence	Symptoms	Specific Laboratory Tests	Outcome	Treatment
HG	First trimester; resolves after 20 wk	<2% primiparous	Nausea and vomiting	AST, ALT <1000 IU/L; ALT >AST; low TSH	Benign for mother and child	IV fluids; thiamine pyridoxine; promethazine; FDA category C
IHCP	Second trimester	<10% multifetal gestations	Pruritus; resolves in postpartum period	AST, ALT <1000 IU/L; GGT normal; bile acid levels high; PT normal; bilirubin <6 mg/dL	Increased gallstones; recurs; risk for fetal distress increases	Ursodiol; delivery when fetal distress is imminent
AFLP	Third trimester; 50% have eclampsia	1/13,000; primiparous, multifetal gestations	Progress quickly to FHF, diabetes insipidus, hypoglycemia	Platelets <100,000/mm^3; AST, ALT >300 IU/L; PT elevated; fibrinogen level low; bilirubin level increased; DIC	Maternal mortality <20%; fetal mortality up to 45%; test for LCHAD	Prompt delivery; liver transplantation
Eclampsia, preeclampsia	Beyond 20 wk; recurs	5% multiparous, multifetal gestations	High blood pressure, proteinuria, edema, seizures, renal failure, pulmonary edema	Uric acid level elevated	Maternal mortality, 1%; prematurity and fetal death, 5%-30%	Beta blocker, methyldopa, magnesium sulfate; early delivery
HELLP syndrome	Beyond 22 wk and after delivery; 20% progress from severe eclampsia	0.5%	Abdominal pain, seizures, renal failure, pulmonary edema, liver hematoma and rupture	Platelets <100,000/mm^3; hemolysis; high LDH level; AST, ALT 70-6000 IU/L; DIC	Hepatic rupture, with 60% maternal mortality; fetal death, 1%-30%	Prompt delivery

AFLP, acute fatty liver of pregnancy; ALT, alanine aminotransferase; AST, aspartate aminotransferase; DIC, disseminated intravascular coagulation; FHF, fulminant hepatic failure; GGT, γ-glutamyl transferase; HELLP syndrome (*h*emolysis, *e*levated *l*iver enzyme levels, *l*ow *p*latelet count).
HG, hyperemesis gravidarum; IHCP, intrahepatic cholestasis of pregnancy; LCHAD, long-chain 3-hydroxylacyl-CoA dehydrogenase; LDH, lactate dehydrogenase; PT, prothrombin time; TSH, thyroid-stimulating hormone.

seizures in preeclamptic and eclamptic women. Early delivery is often required.

HELLP Syndrome

The HELLP syndrome complicates 0.5% of pregnancies and the recurrence rate is high, approaching 20% in severe cases. It is characterized by microangiopathic hemolysis with burr cells and schistocytes on peripheral smear; elevated liver enzyme levels, with aspartate transaminase (AST) exceeding alanine aminotransferase (ALT) levels; and a platelet count lower than 100,000/mm^3.

The HELLP syndrome is more common in multiparous women and can manifest in 30% after delivery. Abdominal pain is the usual symptom, and rapid progression to disseminated intravascular coagulation, renal failure, subcapsular liver hematoma, and hepatic rupture are described. Maternal mortality is about 1% but reaches 60% in cases of hepatic rupture. Perinatal death is variable and can reach 37% when the syndrome occurs at an earlier stage of pregnancy. Immediate delivery is the definitive treatment for HELLP syndrome.

Intrahepatic Cholestasis of Pregnancy

Intrahepatic cholestasis of pregnancy (ICP) occurs in the second half of pregnancy and affects less than 1% of all pregnancies. It is more common in multiparous women with twin gestations. It promptly resolves after delivery and usually recurs in subsequent pregnancies. Generalized pruritus is the main complaint, and jaundice occurs in up to 50% of cases. Bilirubin level remains lower than 6 mg/dL, AST level is increased, and total bile acid levels rise markedly, reaching 20 times normal. The etiology of ICP is unclear but might be due to a genetic mutation in the canalicular transporters of phospholipids.

Pruritus may be intense and distressing to the mother, thus requiring therapy. Ursodeoxycholic acid (FDA category B) is the treatment of choice for reducing pruritus. It also improves biochemical markers without adversely affecting the mother or the baby.

The main risk of ICP is to the fetus. High levels of bile acids have been implicated in premature labor, meconium staining and sudden death. These complications may be prevented with immediate delivery.

Recent data suggest long-term effects of ICP on the mother. Nonalcoholic cirrhosis and gallstone-related complications have been reported.

Hyperemesis Gravidarum

Hyperemesis gravidarum (HG) occurs in less than 2% of pregnancies, starting in the first trimester and resolving by week 20 of gestation. It is characterized by severe nausea and vomiting, with electrolyte disturbances that can require hospitalization. Weight loss exceeds 5% of prepregnancy body weight. HG is more common in primiparous women and may be associated with mild elevation of transaminase levels. The cause of HG is unclear, but predisposing factors might include female gender of the fetus. Rehydration and antiemetics are useful. The outcome for the mother is benign except when severe vomiting causes esophageal rupture, vascular depletion, and renal damage. Adverse infant outcomes such as prematurity and low birth weight are rare and seem to occur because of poor maternal weight gain later in the pregnancy.

CONCLUSIONS

Liver disease in pregnancy can manifest as a benign disease with abnormal elevation of liver enzyme levels and a good outcome, or it can manifest as a serious entity affecting hepatobiliary function and resulting in liver failure and death to the mother and her fetus. There are no clinical markers that predict the course of a pregnancy and the pathophysiologic mechanisms are not always understood, but knowledge and management of the preconception liver disease and efficacious pre-pregnancy and prenatal care are essential. The overall mortality attributed to liver disorders in pregnancy has dramatically decreased in the past few years because of clinicians' understanding of the physiologic changes that occur during pregnancy, their ability to identify and treat preconception liver disorders, and their vigilance in recognizing clinical and laboratory abnormalities in a timely manner. A coordinated team approach that involves the primary care physician, obstetrician, hepatologist, and transplant surgeon is often required to promote good maternal and fetal outcomes.

Summary

- Signs and symptoms of liver disease in pregnancy are not specific, but the underlying disorder can have significant morbidity and mortality effects on the mother and fetus. Early recognition can be lifesaving.
- Acute viral hepatitis is the most common cause of jaundice in pregnancy. The outcome is usually benign. Intervention might not be required except in cases of viral hepatitis E and herpes simplex hepatitis.
- Women with well-compensated cirrhosis and noncirrhotic portal hypertension may become pregnant. Preconception care and management of pregnant women with portal hypertension should be similar to that for nonpregnant women.
- Fertility may be restored after liver transplantation and pregnancy might have a good outcome.
- Vigilance in recognizing liver disorders in pregnancy and early coordinated management among the primary care physician, obstetrician, liver specialist, and transplant surgeon are essential for promoting good maternal and fetal outcomes.

Suggested Readings

ACOG Committee on Practice Bulletins—Obstetrics: ACOG practice bulletin. Diagnosis and management of preeclampsia and eclampsia. Number 33, January 2002. Obstet Gynecol 2002;99:159-167.

Chen MM, Coakley FV, Kaimal A, Laros RK Jr: Guidelines for computed tomography and magnetic resonance imaging use during pregnancy and lactation. Obst Gynecol. 2008 August:112(2 pt 1):333-340.

Chotiyaputta W, Lok AS: Role of antiviral therapy in the prevention of hepatitis B virus infection. J Viral Hepat. 2009 Feb;16(2):91-93.

Czaja AJ, Freese DK: Diagnosis and treatment of autoimmune hepatitis. Hepatology 2002;36:479-497.

Ghany MG, Strader DB, Thomas DL, Seeff LB: Diagnosis, management and treatment of hepatitis C: an update. Hepatology 2009 April;49(4):1335-1374.

Heathcote EJ: Management of primary biliary cirrhosis. The American Association for the Study of Liver Diseases practice guidelines. Hepatology 2000;31:1005-1013.

Mast EE, Hwang LY, Seto DS, et al: Risk factors for perinatal transmission of hepatitis C virus (HCV) and the natural history of HCV infection acquired in infancy. J Infect Dis 2005;192:1880-1889.

Roberts EA, Schilsky ML: Diagnosis and treatment of Wilson disease. Hepatology 2008;47:2089-2111.

Shellock FG, Crues JV: MR procedures: Biologic effects, safety, and patient care. Radiology 2004;232:635-652.

Sibai BM: Diagnosis, prevention, and management of eclampsia. Obstet Gynecol 2005;105:402-410.

Wasley A, Grytdal S, Gallagher K; Centers for Disease Control and Prevention (CDC): Surveillance for acute viral hepatitis—United States 2006. MMWR Surveill Summ 2008;57(2):1-24.

Zapata R, Sandoval L, Palma J, et al: Ursodeoxycholic acid in the treatment of intrahepatic cholestasis of pregnancy. A 12-year experience. Liver Int 2005;25:548-554.

Post–Liver Transplantation Management

Bijan Eghtesad, Charles M. Miller, and John J. Fung

Orthotopic liver transplantation (OLT) replaces the diseased liver with a transplanted allograft liver in the anatomically correct position and has become an increasingly used treatment for end-stage liver disease. Since the first successful OLT, done by Thomas Starzl in 1967, the technique of OLT has been refined to a relatively standardized procedure, but the operation remains a formidable surgical challenge. As such, OLT can be associated with a spectrum of technical and medical complications; the recipient's pretransplantation condition and donor and immunologic factors may all be contributing factors. Preoperative recipient factors such as age older than 60 years, presence of comorbid conditions such as cardiac or pulmonary disease, renal failure, diabetes, and severe malnutrition, and the nature of the liver disease can affect survival. Perioperative factors such as the quality of the donor liver, difficulty of the liver transplantation procedure, development of postoperative infection, and side effects of immunosuppressive agents are important factors influencing outcome.

Patients with end-stage liver disease undergo extensive workups before being listed for liver transplantation. The preoperative condition, nature and severity of the liver disease, and comorbid conditions are assessed during the evaluation process. Patients are presented and discussed in a multidisciplinary committee to be approved for final listing.

The purpose of this chapter is to focus on the perioperative care of OLT patients and delineate potential surgical and medical complications, management of immunosuppressive regimens, and diagnosis and treatment of rejection and other immunologic problems in these patients.

OPERATIVE TECHNIQUE

The technique of OLT has been progressively refined since its introduction in humans in 1963. Several variations are applied selectively, according to the patient's specific situation, transplantation center's routine practice, or both. The traditionally described OLT involves resecting the recipient native liver (hepatectomy) together with the retrohepatic inferior vena cava (IVC), a short anhepatic phase, and implanting a whole deceased donor liver graft with the interposed donor IVC. Restoration of venous continuity during the implantation is achieved by an upper subdiaphragmatic and lower end-to-end donor-to-recipient IVC anastomosis; the donor-to-recipient portal vein and hepatic artery anastomoses are also performed in an end-to-end fashion. The biliary connections involve a primary duct-to-duct technique or the performance of a hepaticojejunostomy.

One modification of the standard procedure is to preserve the retrohepatic IVC in the recipient and restore the venous drainage of the liver allograft by anastomosis of the suprahepatic IVC to a common venous channel. This is made from the confluence of three hepatic veins in the recipient and ligation of the infrahepatic allograft IVC, also referred to as the *piggyback technique.* This technique also allows live donor and segmental liver transplantation, in which venous outflow is connected to the preserved native IVC while the new segment of the liver is revascularized between the corresponding recipient and donor vascular structures, as described for whole-liver transplantation.

Other modifications may be required, depending on the nature of the structures in the recipient. For example, if the portal vein of the recipient is thrombosed, portal vein reconstruction using a conduit from the superior mesenteric vein or portal vein thrombectomy may be required. Similarly, if the hepatic artery is unsuitable for revascularization of the transplanted liver, an arterial conduit from the aorta may be required.

POSTOPERATIVE CARE

General Intensive Care Unit Measures

Immediately following OLT, these patients are returned to the surgical intensive care unit (ICU). In the ICU, they are maintained on a ventilator until fully conscious and able to breathe on their own while being able to protect their airway. During the ICU stay, there is a need for close attention to management of fluid and electrolytes, which could be significantly abnormal as a result of the prolonged operation and massive fluid shifts.

Immunosuppressive agents, based on specific protocols and on the patient's renal function, are started early after OLT. Doses are adjusted according to blood levels and functional status of the transplanted liver and renal function. Most patients with an uncomplicated postoperative course and good liver function remain in the ICU for 1 or 2 days before being transferred to an inpatient transplantation unit.

Transfer to an Inpatient Transplantation Unit

Following transfer to a designated transplantation inpatient unit, the patient should be closely followed by the surgical and medical team, as well as by pharmacists, nutritionists, and physical therapists. Fluid and electrolyte status and kidney and liver function need to be monitored at least daily. Dosages of immunosuppressive agents are adjusted according to blood levels and organ function during this period. The pattern of liver function test (LFT) results are monitored for early signs of dysfunction, which can require further study or intervention. Any major alteration in liver function should initiate a series of studies, which may include Doppler ultrasound to evaluate vascular patency of the new liver, bile duct studies (e.g., T-tube cholangiography, endoscopic retrograde cholangiopancreatography [ERCP], percutaneous transhepatic cholangiography) to evaluate any abnormality of the biliary system (e.g., stricture, bile leak, obstruction), and liver biopsy to rule out rejection. Necessary treatments are initiated based on these findings. Usually, in an uneventful recovery, the patient is discharged within 10 to 14 days after OLT and followed as an outpatient.

During the transition to an outpatient setting, the patient meets with the post-OLT coordinator and goes through extensive teaching regarding his or her medications and immunosuppressive agents and their potential side effects. The patient receives instructions about the schedule for blood work and follow-up clinic visits. The patient receives a book containing after-discharge instructions, including when and how to notify the transplantation program if he or she feels that there is something wrong, such as abnormal pain, fever, diarrhea, and headaches. The recipient is also instructed about physical activities, diet, and general health maintenance, such as vaccinations, avoidance of sun, and cancer screening.

Discharge Instructions

Medications and Prophylactic Measures

The maintenance medications after discharge include immunosuppressive agents, prophylactic medications for prevention of opportunistic infections, such as for *Pneumocystis jiroveci* infection (trimethoprim-sulfamethoxazole, or in case of sulfa allergy, dapsone or pentamidine), herpetic infections (acyclovir), *Candida* esophagitis (nystatin [Mycostatin]), as well as other prophylactic medications, such as acid-reducing agents (proton pump inhibitors, histamine-2 blockers). In addition to these agents, the patient might also require antihypertensive medications, insulin or oral hypoglycemic agents, or mild analgesics. In addition, certain patients require additional medications depending on their original disease; for example, patients who received a transplant for hepatitis B require anti–hepatitis B treatment (hepatitis B immunoglobulin, antivirals), and patients who received a transplant for Budd-Chiari syndrome might require anticoagulation. It is also emphasized that patients call the transplantation program with any new medication started for them by other physicians for assessing compatibility with their immunosuppressive agents.

Blood Work Instructions

Laboratory studies are usually done biweekly for the first 2 weeks, weekly for the next 8 weeks, every other week for 2 months, and then once monthly if laboratory test results are stable. Blood work can be done at the patient's local laboratory. In any case, a prescription listing the needed blood tests and instructions for mailing blood samples for immunosuppression monitoring will be given to the patient. Outpatient laboratory work is reviewed by the post-transplantation coordinator in conjunction with the transplantation surgeon or physician.

Short-Term and Long-Term Problems During Follow-Up

Fever

Fever higher than 101° F or associated with chills should be taken seriously in immunosuppressed patients. The spectrum of potential infectious organisms is large in the immunosuppressed population and might also point to anatomic complications after OLT. In addition, fever could be the primary sign of rejection. The fever workup includes cultures, blood and radiologic diagnostic tests and, if needed, endoscopies and biopsies. Patients might need to be hospitalized and kept on broad-spectrum antibiotics or antiviral agents until results are available. Identifying the cause of the fever allows targeted appropriate treatment.

Increased Liver Function Test Results

Any dramatic or persistent increase in the results of LFTs mandates a series of diagnostic tests to evaluate for possible causes, such as rejection, ischemic insult to the liver (hepatic artery problems), biliary complications, infections (viral hepatitis, bacterial sepsis), or drug toxicities or hypersensitivities. A thorough workup, including blood tests, computed tomography (CT) scanning and ultrasound of the abdomen, radiologic studies of the biliary system, viral studies, and liver biopsy, may be indicated for appropriate therapeutic response.

Immunosuppression

The nature of immunosuppressive agent use in OLT in the United States has been reported by the Scientific Registry of Transplant Recipients, which analyzed data from the United Network for Organ Sharing database. The use of calcineurin inhibitors (CNIs) was reported in 97% of patients discharged from the hospital after OLT in the United States in 2004. Corticosteroid use was reported in more than 80%, mycophenolate mofetil (MMF) in nearly 54%, and azathioprine (AZA) in approximately 4% of patients at discharge. Sirolimus (SRL) use was noted in nearly 5% of OLT patients at discharge. Induction antibody use was noted in 21%, with most antibody use being anti-interleukin-2 receptor (IL-2r) antibodies and the remainder being antithymocyte globulin. It is clear that the overwhelming majority of programs view the use of CNIs as essential to the success of OLT, in both early and later phases after OLT.

Primary Immunosuppressants

CNIs—tacrolimus (TAC) and cyclosporine (CsA)—remain the cornerstone of immunosuppressive therapy; tacrolimus is used in 90% of primary OLT recipients at the time of discharge. Administration of one of these agents at therapeutic doses is the key to preventing rejection of the liver allograft.

Calcineurin Inhibitors. CsA and TAC are CNIs by virtue of their shared property of binding to their specific immunophilin, which leads to inhibition of calcineurin activity. The routine application of CNIs to OLT has dramatically reduced rejection, morbidity associated with treatment of rejection and graft loss, and death caused by rejection. The dosage of CsA or TAC is based on blood levels and is tailored based on time after OLT, presence or absence of renal dysfunction, or other side effects. The usual acceptable trough levels early after OLT are 8 to 12 ng/mL for TAC and 200 to 300 ng/mL for CsA. The side effects of TAC and CsA overlap and include nephrotoxicity, neurotoxicity, diabetogenicity, increased susceptibility to opportunistic infections, and certain de novo malignancies.

Because CNIs are metabolized in the liver by the cytochrome P-450 system, it is important to recognize when other drugs are being used that can increase blood levels of CNIs by inhibiting or competing for this system. Agents such as fluconazole, erythromycin, diltiazem, verapamil, and protease inhibitors are well recognized as causing increased CNI levels, which can result in increased CNI toxicities. Other drugs that enhance cytochrome P-450 activities, such as barbiturates, phenytoin, rifampin, and carbamazepine, can lead to reduction of CNI blood levels; if left untreated, this can lead to insufficient immunosuppression and resultant rejection. Thus, it is important to readjust CNI dosages when these medications are started or discontinued in transplant patients.

Corticosteroids. The most commonly used non-CNI immunosuppressive agents in OLT are corticosteroids. Corticosteroids have been shown to decrease transplant rejection when combined with other immunosuppressive agents. Whereas most post-transplantation protocols rapidly lower the dosage of corticosteroids to a minimum, some protocols also discontinue them shortly after OLT. These practices recognize that acute and chronic dosing of corticosteroids are associated with side effects that include hypertension, hyperglycemia, delayed wound healing, osteoporosis, glaucoma, suppressed growth, hyperlipidemia, increased risk of gastrointestinal ulceration, risk of fungal infections, and suppression of the pituitary-adrenal axis. Thus, attempts to reduce or eliminate corticosteroid use have encouraged the use of other non-CNI immunosuppressive agents with CNI maintenance therapy.

Adjunctive Agents

Adjunctive medications are usually prescribed in addition to a CNI and include the antiproliferative agents MMF, AZA, and SRL. In addition, induction antibody can help decrease the incidence of early rejection.

Mycophenolate Mofetil. Before the availability of MMF, AZA was used as an adjuvant immunosuppressive agent but was associated with significant myelosuppression and hepatotoxicity and was not useful in treating acute cellular rejection (ACR). MMF acts by a similar mechanism as AZA but is more selective, has fewer myelotoxic and hepatotoxic side effects, and appears to be a more effective immunosuppressive agent. When MMF is used in combination with TAC and steroids, the dose of TAC required is usually lowered. This can improve renal dysfunction that results from higher levels of CNI. MMF, as monotherapy after CNI withdrawal, should be used cautiously, because abrupt transition to MMF monotherapy has been associated with an unacceptably high incidence of ACR, severe ductopenic rejection requiring retransplantation, and severe steroid-resistant ACR. Although MMF is not suitable for all OLT candidates, it does have a role as a CNI-sparing agent, particularly in patients with renal dysfunction and neurotoxicity. It can be safely added to the current immunosuppressive regimen without increasing infectious complications.

Sirolimus. SRL is a macrolide antibiotic structurally related to TAC. It binds to the immunophilin FKBP12, but it does not inhibit cytokine gene transcription in T cells. Rather, SRL blocks signals transduced from various growth factor receptors to the nucleus by acting on phosphatidyl inositol kinases, known as mammalian targets of rapamycin. The pivotal prospective controlled trials in kidney transplantation that led to U.S. Food and Drug Administration (FDA) approval in 1999 delineated the efficacy and side effects of SRL, which included leukopenia, thrombocytopenia, elevated serum cholesterol levels, anemia, gastrointestinal disturbances, lymphocele, wound disruptions and infections, oral ulcerations, and elevated triglyceride levels. An increased incidence of pneumonitis and aseptic pneumonia has been reported, which in most cases is reversible with SRL discontinuation; however, it can be fatal.

Because of some reported cases of early vascular thrombosis after OLT, the FDA has not approved the drug to be used in liver transplantation, especially in the early period after OLT. A combination of SRL and low-dose CNIs has been used to protect renal function after OLT. Because of the antiproliferative activities of SRL, it is being tested for preventing recurrence of hepatocellular carcinoma after OLT.

Antibody Induction. Antibody induction therapy has been limited to the perioperative period as a means to reduce early exposure to CNIs or to obviate the need for large doses of perioperative corticosteroids. Antibody therapy can be depleting, receptor-modulating, or both. With the use of depleting antibody preparations, a phenomenon known as a first-dose effect can occur, related to the intravascular release of cytokines by lymphocytes. The symptoms, including fever, chills, tachycardia, gastrointestinal disturbances, bronchospasm, and fluctuations in blood pressure, can be blocked by pretreatment with corticosteroids, diphenhydramine hydrochloride, and acetaminophen.

More common antibodies used in liver transplantation are IL-2r blockers (daclizumab or basiliximab), antilymphocyte globulins (rabbit thymoglobulin), monoclonal anti–T cell antibodies (muromonab-CD3 or OKT-3), or anti-CD52 monoclonal antibody (alemtuzumab). Each of these antibodies has its own place in induction therapy or treatment of rejection.

COMPLICATIONS AND OUTCOMES

The postoperative course in OLT patients ranges from straightforward to extremely complicated, and the outcome depends on the status of the recipient, donor organ, and technical issues in the operation. Complications after liver transplantation can have a significant impact on outcomes and costs of the procedure. Timely diagnosis of alterations in the normal postoperative course is the critical factor to minimize morbidity and mortality and to improve outcomes.

Primary Nonfunction

Primary nonfunction is characterized by post-transplantation encephalopathy, coagulopathy, minimal bile output, and progressive renal and multisystem failure, with increasing serum lactate and rapidly rising liver enzyme levels and histologic evidence of hepatocyte necrosis in the absence of any vascular compromise. With improved donor selection and management, operative techniques, reducing cold ischemia times, and newer preservative solutions, the risk of primary nonfunction has decreased but remains between 4% and 6% following OLT. Patients with initial dysfunction, also known as primary graft dysfunction, might recover with support, but those who progress to show evidence of extrahepatic complications, such as hemodynamic instability, renal failure, or other organ system dysfunction, can require urgent retransplantation.

Hepatic Artery Stenosis and Thrombosis

Angiographic evidence of more than a 50% reduction in the caliber of the hepatic artery lumen is defined as hepatic artery stenosis. When there is no arterial flow, the hepatic artery is thrombosed, which occurs in about 3% to 4% of the cases after liver transplantation. Usually, hepatic artery pathology is detected by ultrasonography, with the presence of a low resistive index, lower than 0.5, often with an increase in focal peak velocity as the first clue of stenosis. Lack of arterial flow, however, should raise suspicion for thrombosis. Clinically, these patients might show no symptoms (most often with stenosis), but generally there is an increase in abnormal LFT results, or fever and infection caused by infarcts in the liver after the hepatic artery is thrombosed. Hepatic artery stenosis can be treated by surgical intervention, especially soon after liver transplantation, whereas percutaneous angioplasty is generally reserved for stenosis occurring several weeks after the transplantation procedure, with more than a 90% success rate.

Complete hepatic artery thrombosis (HAT) usually occurs in the very early stages after liver transplantation, but it can occur many months after the procedure. Because the liver depends on the hepatic artery for most of its oxygenated blood, HAT can lead to acute massive hepatocyte necrosis, formation of a central biloma secondary to intrahepatic duct necrosis, multiple biliary structures, or intermittent bacteremia. Occasionally, rarely in adults and more often in children, HAT can be asymptomatic. The factors that determine whether a liver fails or survives with complete HAT is unknown, but the presence of collateral circulation (e.g., from the phrenic artery via vascularized adhesions to the liver) is usually associated with a more benign course after HAT. Angiography is the gold standard for diagnosis. In cases of early documentation of the problem (i.e., within 24-48 hours), urgent revascularization can result in arterial patency. However, a significant number of patients treated in this manner still require retransplantation because of biliary complications, persistent biliary sepsis, and intra-abdominal infection.

Portal Vein Stenosis and Thrombosis

Portal vein stricture can manifest shortly after liver transplantation because of the increased production of ascites and liver allograft dysfunction. The incidence of portal vein complications is less than 2% of OLT cases. Ultrasonography and CT angiography are usually diagnostic, whereas superior mesenteric artery angiography with late films is the confirmatory test. Treatment is by surgical intervention in early post-transplantation and by percutaneous transhepatic dilation or stenting of the stricture later after liver transplantation. If left untreated, it can progress to complete thrombosis of the vein or severe graft dysfunction and hemodynamic instability secondary to massive ascites.

Hepatic Outflow Obstruction

Complications associated with vena cava stenosis include a 2.5% to 6% incidence of venous outflow obstruction (iatrogenic Budd-Chiari syndrome), caused by rotation of the liver graft or anastomotic stricture. Stenosis of the suprahepatic cava anastomosis can manifest with hepatic outflow obstruction in the form of liver allograft dysfunction, ascites formation, and impairment of renal function. The problem carries a high risk for morbidity and mortality. Treatment is generally radiologic, using stents to treat the stenosis, but the success rate is between 50% and 60%. In some cases, retransplantation may be necessary.

Biliary Complications

Biliary complications continue to be the most common technical complication after liver transplantation, with an overall incidence of 15% to 20%. These complications range from early anastomotic leak to late stricture and obstruction in the extrahepatic or intrahepatic biliary system. The associated mortality rate with biliary complications is about 10%, which is mainly because of the delay in diagnosis or misdiagnosis of the problem, resulting in secondary infectious complications and graft dysfunction.

The biochemical abnormalities of elevated bilirubin and canalicular enzyme levels (e.g., alkaline phosphatase, γ-glutamyl transferase) associated with biliary complications are not specific; these indicators of biliary obstruction are also seen in ischemic graft injury, rejection, recurrent hepatitis C virus (HCV) infection, and sepsis. Imaging modalities such as ultrasonography to detect biliary dilation and radioisotope studies to evaluate anastomotic or cut surface leaks are considered relatively insensitive. The gold standard for evaluating biliary pathology is cholangiography (transhepatic or endoscopic) which helps make an accurate diagnosis. In addition, endoscopically or radiographically detected strictures, leaks, or obstruction can be treated at the time of diagnosis, often with biliary stenting. In fact, biliary leaks that occur after removal of the T-tube are preferentially treated by endoscopic biliary stent placement.

The most common biliary complication is biliary stenosis. This is the result of imperfect anastomotic technique or ischemia of the bile duct, which appears as a stenotic area in the common bile duct, at or slightly proximal to the biliary anastomosis, with proximal biliary dilation. Recurrent bouts of cholangitis or persistent abnormal LFT results can indicate an obstruction to bile outflow. In these cases, endoscopic or percutaneous balloon dilation of the bile duct stricture and stenting have been successful. In cases with no response, revision of the choledochojejunostomy or conversion of duct-to-duct anastomosis to choledochojejunostomy with a Roux-en-Y loop is the treatment of choice. A number of intrahepatic strictures of the biliary tree can be indistinguishable from simple anastomotic strictures at a clinical level and must be evaluated by cholangiography. The etiology and pathophysiology of these intrahepatic strictures have not been clearly elucidated. Often, the strictures seem to be associated with a hepatic artery thrombosis or stenosis, and ischemia of the biliary tree is probably the cause, especially in livers used from non–heart-beating donors. Preservation damage of the allograft can result in multiple intrahepatic biliary strictures, with or without biliary sludge and casts. In some patients, who originally received transplants for primary sclerosing cholangitis, recurrence of the disease seems a possibility. Although some patients with multiple intrahepatic strictures eventually need retransplant, others can live for years with minimal difficulties, especially if they receive chronic antibiotic prophylaxis.

Bleeding

Poor graft function, coagulopathy, imperfect hemostasis, or slippage of a tie can result in postoperative bleeding that requires re-exploration. Postoperative bleeding is reported in 7% to 15% of patients and requires re-exploration in approximately 50% of them. Even if easily controlled, postoperative bleeding leads to increased cost, morbidity, and mortality.

Ascites and Fluid Retention

A possible problem after OLT is fluid retention and the formation of ascites. This is especially more significant in malnourished patients and patients with preexisting ascites and edema. After ruling out the possibilities of renal dysfunction or vascular problems with the liver, these patients should be managed with diuretics and fluid management. Most patients start mobilizing the extra fluid a week after OLT and then can be treated with diuretic therapy if their kidneys are functioning. Nutritional support and careful management of fluid and electrolyte balance, in addition to diuretic therapy, are essential for treatment.

Infection

Infection is one of the leading causes of morbidity and mortality in liver transplant recipients. More than two thirds of liver transplant recipients have an infection in the first year after transplantation, and infection is the leading cause of death in these patients. In addition, the release of cytokines during the infection can have other indirect and negative effects, including allograft injury, opportunistic superinfection, and malignancy. The risk of infection in liver transplant recipients is determined by the intensity of exposure to infectious agents (hospital or community sources) and the overall immunosuppression level. This net state of immunosuppression is influenced by dose, duration, sequence, and choice of immunosuppressive medications; underlying immune deficiencies; presence of neutropenia or lymphopenia; mucocutaneous barrier integrity: presence of necrotic tissue, ischemia, or fluid collection; metabolic conditions such as diabetes mellitus; and activity of immunomodulating viruses.

After OLT, there are three periods during which infections with specific organisms are likely to occur. The patient's susceptibility to infection at these times is strongly influenced by surgical factors, level of immunosuppression and environmental exposure, and doses, duration, and types of prophylaxis. During the first period, the first month immediately after transplantation, most infections are related to technical or surgical issues and complications. Exposure to infectious agents through prolonged hospitalization before transplantation or during postoperative care can also result in infection. Bacterial and candidal wound infections, urinary tract infections, catheter-related infections, bacterial pneumonias, and *Clostridium difficile* colitis predominate during this period; the causative organisms are similar to those for hospital-acquired infections common in other surgical patients. Although its incidence has markedly diminished with prophylaxis, reactivated human herpesvirus (herpes simplex virus) infection can occur in this time frame.

The next period is the second through sixth month after transplantation. During this time, infections from opportunistic organisms predominate as a result of cumulative immunosuppression. Viral infections, predominantly cytomegalovirus, and fungal infections, such as those caused by *Aspergillus*, *Cryptococcus*, *Histoplasma*, and *Coccidioides* species, can occur. Other herpesviruses, such as varicella-zoster virus, and de novo or recurrent hepatitis B and C viruses can cause infections in this period. Some rare bacterial infections caused by *Nocardia* and *Listeria* species, and *Mycobacterium tuberculosis* infection can also occur.

Approximately 7 to 12 months after transplantation, and beyond, most recipients can develop infections such as influenza, urinary tract infections, and community-acquired pneumonias, similar to those acquired by patients who have not received transplants. Reactivation of human herpesvirus 3 can manifest as herpes zoster, and, although it is uncommon, cytomegalovirus infections can occur. Sinister opportunistic fungal infections can occur as a result of cumulatively high levels of immunosuppression, poor graft function, or heavy environmental exposure.

Three notable scenarios can enhance patient susceptibility to opportunistic infections: acute organ rejection necessitating increased immunosuppression therapy; retransplantation, which restarts the immunosuppression and infection time line; and chronic viral infections, such as human immunodeficiency virus or hepatitis B or C.

Rejection

Acute rejection is an ongoing risk in any solid organ transplant, although it is somewhat less of a risk in OLT compared with more immunogenic organs, such as the kidney. Improvements in immunosuppressive therapy have reduced rejection rates and improved graft survival, but acute (cellular) rejection still develops in 25% to 50% of OLT patients treated with CNI-based immunosuppression. Chronic (ductopenic) rejection is somewhat less frequent and is declining; it occurs in approximately 4% of adult OLT patients. The incidence of rejection varies by type of immunosuppressive agent used and by the patient population.

Increases in bilirubin or liver enzyme levels, or both, after OLT in a stable patient may be the first sign of rejection. Histologic evaluation of the liver allograft (liver biopsy) is essential for making the diagnosis of rejection. Based on the presence and then the severity of rejection, the patient receives additional treatments, which could range from an increase in the baseline immunosuppressive regimen to the administration of steroid boluses and the addition of other drugs to the maintenance therapy, or the administration of antilymphocyte antibodies in case of resistance to the primary line of therapy.

Early acute rejection does not generally affect patient or graft outcomes for patients not infected with hepatitis C virus (HCV), except that multiple acute rejection episodes might be a risk factor for chronic rejection. Many patients with focal or mild histologic signs of rejection on protocol biopsy maintain steady graft function, even without treatment, and many centers no longer treat acute rejection aggressively, particularly in the setting of hepatitis C. Studies have shown a higher relative risk of death for HCV-infected patients with rejection versus that for non–HCV-infected patients with rejection (2.9 vs. 0.5, respectively). Therefore, rejection is to be avoided in HCV-infected patients at all times. Late acute rejection, defined as histologically confirmed acute cellular rejection occurring months after transplantation, can result from a precipitous or marked reduction in immunosuppressive agents or with nonadherence to medication.

Chronic rejection is characterized by the destruction of the portal bile ducts or biliary epithelial atrophy, a decreased number of hepatic arterioles in the portal tract, or obliterative arteriopathy. Chronic rejection was once a major cause of liver graft failure; with the newer immunosuppressive agent tacrolimus, the risk of chronic rejection is markedly reduced when used de novo after OLT. This can even successfully reverse chronic rejection, especially in its early stages (also known as *rescue therapy*) when the maintenance immunosuppression does not include tacrolimus.

Electrolyte Imbalances and Other Metabolic Abnormalities

Almost any metabolic imbalance can occur after OLT. This is not surprising, considering the magnitude of the physiologic stress of surgery, fluid shifts, multitude of pharmacologic agents administered, and multisystem complications. The most common imbalances, however, are hypokalemia, hyperkalemia, hyperglycemia, and hypomagnesemia.

Hypokalemia can occur as a side effect of potassium-wasting diuretic therapy, intracellular fluid shifts secondary to metabolic alkalosis, hypothermia, insulin therapy, and corticosteroid therapy. Rarely, if the serum potassium level is monitored regularly and supplementation given when indicated, hypokalemia from any cause is significant enough to produce physical signs.

Hyperkalemia is more often seen after transplantation, beginning 1 to 2 weeks after OLT. It is caused by renal tubular acidosis secondary to CNI use. It is easily manageable with a dietary regimen. Rarely, patients need to be placed on mineralocorticoids or potassium-chelating agents.

The main cause of hyperglycemia in liver transplant patients is preexisting diabetes mellitus. Other important causes are corticosteroids and CNIs. Drug-induced hyperglycemia is usually transient and improves after discontinuation of steroids and reduction in dosage of CNIs. Less than 5% of these patients require long-term treatment.

Hypomagnesemia is another phenomenon after OLT. Many patients are hypomagnesemic from malnutrition before transplantation, and the condition is exacerbated during the postoperative period. The exact nature of this problem is not completely understood. However, contributing postoperative factors are believed to include diuretic therapy and the renal effects of CNIs. Routine monitoring of the serum magnesium level and supplementation with IV or oral magnesium may be indicated.

Patients after transplantation and immunosuppression are prone to develop osteoporosis and other metabolic bone abnormalities. These patients should be monitored regularly by bone densitometry and other metabolic tests and receive appropriate replacement therapies with oral calcium and bisphosphonates.

Renal Dysfunction

Renal dysfunction (acute or chronic) occurs in 17% to 95% of patients after OLT. The wide range of incidence reported could result from the wide disparity in the criteria used to define renal failure and differences in the duration of follow-up. The most common causative factors include acute tubular necrosis secondary to ischemic or toxic insult to the kidneys, preexisting hepatorenal syndrome (HRS) or renal insufficiency, diabetes mellitus, drug-induced interstitial nephritis, and CNI nephrotoxicity. Dialysis requirements in the pre- or post-transplantation period, hepatitis C infection, and age have also been variably shown to be associated with an increased risk for the development of chronic kidney disease.

CNIs are generally considered to be the main cause of post-transplantation nephropathy in liver transplant patients, estimated to be responsible for 70% of progressive end-stage renal failure after OLT. In the presence of renal dysfunction after OLT, as the first line of therapy, these agents are withdrawn from the immunosuppressive regimen or the dose is reduced to minimize their nephrotoxic effect. Many recent immunosuppressive protocols contain fewer CNIs and instead have more of other agents, such as MMF or SRL, as the baseline immunosuppressant. Many patients with end-stage liver disease can have preexisting renal problems, and in the post-OLT period, CNIs should not be considered as the main cause of renal dysfunction. Careful assessment of patients and the cause of their renal dysfunction (possibly performing a renal biopsy) is helpful for decision making and for assessing the recoverability of kidney in order to offer appropriate treatment to these patients. In patients in whom significant and prolonged renal dysfunction occurs before OLT, combined liver and kidney transplantation should be considered.

Neurologic Complications

Natients occasionally experience various neurologic problems after OLT. These are more common in adults than in children. Most neurologic complications are related to the degree of pretransplantation encephalopathy caused by hepatic encephalopathy or electrolyte disturbances, in particular hyponatremia, as well as the idiosyncratic central nervous system effects of metabolic abnormalities caused by immunosuppressive agents, most notably the CNIs. These drugs can produce a wide clinical spectrum of signs and symptoms, from mild tremor and acute confusion to status epilepticus. CNI-related neurotoxicity occurs in approximately 25% of liver transplant recipients. These could be dose-related and include impaired mentation or confusion, psychosis, dysphasia, mutism, cortical blindness, extrapyramidal syndromes, quadriplegia, encephalopathy, seizures, and coma. Treatment includes reducing or completely discontinuing the suspected offending agent. In some cases of suspected CNI toxicity, substitution of one CNI by another is all that is needed. It is also important to identify other drugs on the patient's list that might increase immunosuppressive levels and thereby trigger neurotoxicity.

Malignancy

Solid organ graft survival rates have improved remarkably since the 1990s because of improved immunosuppression, innovative technical procedures, and assiduous post-transplantation monitoring. However, recipient mortality caused by de novo post-transplantation malignancies remains a serious impediment to long-term survival. The increasing prevalence of post-transplantation malignancies has been evidenced by data collected by transplant registries in the United States, Europe, Australia, and New Zealand, as well as a large single-center analysis. In liver transplantation, estimates of cancers approach 15% by 10 years after OLT, with the rate for solid organ tumors being markedly higher in adults than in children and in patients with risk factors, such as colon cancer in OLT patients with ulcerative colitis and aerodigestive cancers in smokers.

Various factors have been proposed to explain the increased cancer risk in transplant recipients. Among the earliest was the concept of impaired immune surveillance resulting from systemic immunosuppression. Long-term antigenic stimulation and environmental influences, such as UV irradiation, genetic predisposition, uremia preceding transplantation, donor-and-host interactions, and mutagenic activity of immunosuppressive agents, have also been implicated as potential causative factors. Many of the cancers with a significantly increased incidence are considered to be associated with viral infections, such as skin cancers, possibly from human papillomavirus (HPV), Kaposi's sarcoma, cervical cancer (from HPV), and lymphomas. As might be expected, post-transplantation malignancies are associated with higher mortality rates, and many of the deaths occur in patients with a fully functioning allograft.

Post-transplantation lymphoproliferative disorders (PTLDs) are a heterogeneous group of hyperplasias and lymphomas that are serious post-transplantation complications for all organ recipients. Most cases of PTLD are believed to arise from Epstein-Barr virus (EBV)-infected B cells. The clinical signs and symptoms of PTLD are diverse and are similar to those seen during primary EBV infection, such as fever, sweats, malaise, and lymphadenopathy. The incidence of PTLD varies with the transplanted organ, with the highest prevalence in the small bowel (approximately 20%) and a lower prevalence in other solid organs (1% to 10%). However, despite identification of EBV as the causative factor in 90% of patients with PTLD, the immunosuppressive drugs used to prevent graft rejection are largely responsible for the deficient immune response to EBV infection or reactivation. In contrast to solid organ cancers after OLT, the preponderant risk is in the pediatric population.

In any case, it is critical that the local physician and transplantation team search diligently for de novo cancers in OLT patients and, most importantly, educate patients about reducing the risk of cancers by routine use of sunscreens, early testing, and vaccinations.

Disease Recurrence

Hepatitis B

A total of 5% to 10% of patients undergoing OLT have HBV-associated chronic or fulminant liver disease. Long-term survival depends on preventing allograft reinfection or slowing disease progression in those who have recurrent disease. In the absence of prophylactic measures, the risk of HBV reinfection after OLT is approximately 80%; it is related mainly to the level of HBV replication at the time of transplantation. Recurrent infection in the graft can lead to graft failure, retransplantation, or death, and in the past this was the most common cause of reduced patient and graft survival.

Significant improvements in patient and graft survival in HBV liver transplant recipients have been made during the past 15 years. The first major therapeutic advance was the use of long-term hepatitis B immune globulin (HBIG) to prevent reinfection. The second major advance came with the availability of highly effective and well-tolerated antiviral agents against HBV, such as lamivudine, adefovir dipivoxil, and more recently, entecavir and tenafovir, which improved the outcomes of patients with decompensated cirrhosis awaiting transplantation as well as transplant recipients who had recurrent HBV disease. Finally, with the use of HBIG in combination with antivirals, the risk of reinfection has been reduced to 10% or lower during the first 2 years following transplantation. As a result of these therapies, the outcomes of patients with acute and chronic HBV-related liver disease undergoing liver transplantation are now similar to or better than those of patients undergoing transplantation for non-HBV indications. Because of the increase in development of resistance to lamivudine, the American Association for the Study of Liver Diseases has recommended entecavir for preventing disease recurrence after OLT.

Hepatitis C

Post-transplantation recurrence of HCV infection is a universal phenomenon, with a highly variable natural history. The histologic progression of chronic hepatitis C is more aggressive and is associated with lower patient and graft survival when compared with that of non-HCV liver recipients. Approximately 40% of the liver recipients develop hepatic decompensation in 1 year, and 10% to 25% develop cirrhosis within 5 years after transplantation. Factors associated with recurrence include donor and recipient age, recipient gender and race, presence of genotype 1, level of viremia at the time of transplantation, the use of strong antilymphocyte induction therapy, and high doses of corticosteroids. No single factor has been uniformly shown to be the strongest predictor of outcome.

Results of antiviral therapy in recurrent HCV after OLT have also not been totally convincing. A number of reports have shown no response to histologic improvement. Unfortunately, there are no standard time courses for treatment, dosages, and modes of follow-up. It seems that only prolonged treatment and histologic follow-up can evaluate whether progression of fibrosis is halted following post-OLT treatment for recurrent HCV infection. The current sustained virologic response after a combination of pegylated interferon and ribavirin in the OLT population is approximately 10% to 25%. Recently, trials with protease inhibitors, alone or in combination with interferon and ribavirin, have shown promising results. Most centers, including our program, start antiviral therapy with interferon and ribavirin in the presence of stage II or III fibrosis in the liver allograft or signs of aggressive recurrence of HCV. During the treatment course, monitoring of platelets, white cell count, hemoglobin, and renal function, in addition to LFTs, is essential. Abnormalities in these tests mandate the dose adjustment of growth factors, such as filgastrim (Neupogen) and epoetin alfa (Epogen). Biochemical, histologic, and virologic responses are followed by LFTs, liver biopsy, and quantitative measurement of HCV RNA.

Cholestatic Diseases

There is approximately a 10% to 20% long-term risk of recurrence for cholestatic liver disorders, such as primary sclerosing cholangitis and primary biliary cirrhosis. Recurrence can occur within months after OLT but generally it takes years for the recurrence to occur. It can mimic rejection or bile duct complications. Diagnosis is made by appropriate histologic, biochemical, and radiologic tests. The impact of recurrent cholestatic disease is minimal in terms of patient and graft survival, with rates of retransplantation in primary biliary cirrhosis lower than 2% and, for primary sclerosing cholangitis, approximately 15% at 10 years.

GRAFT AND PATIENT SURVIVAL

With improvements in immunosuppressive agents and increased knowledge about the care of post-OLT patients since the 1990s, 1- and 2-year patient survival rates have increased from 76% and 72% to 86% and 84% respectively, with a 5-year survival of 72%. During the same period, with increased understanding of organ donor management and better preservation solutions, graft survival at 1 year has increased from 72% to 82% and the 5-year survival has increased to 67%.

CONCLUSIONS

Liver transplantation has progressed to become an acceptable means for treating end-stage liver disease, with excellent long-term outcomes. This was not achievable without multidisciplinary teamwork among transplantation center teams and outside primary physicians and caregivers. Increased understanding of the care of these highly complicated patients and effective communication among team members has benefited these patients, with consequently better long-term functional recovery.

Summary

- Liver transplantation has progressed to become an acceptable means for the treatment of end-stage liver disease, with excellent long-term outcomes. Survival outcomes have dramatically improved over the years; the longest living patient has survived more than 35 years after liver transplantation.
- Orthotopic liver transplantation involves the resection of the recipient native liver followed by the implantation of a whole or partial liver graft from a deceased or living donor.
- Immunosuppressive agents are the mainstay of rejection prevention in liver transplantation. To prevent their long-term toxicity, the patient must adhere to the prescribed regimen and compliance with close follow-up for medication adjustments.
- Complications (e.g., infection, rejection, disease recurrence) are common after liver transplantation and, if untreated, can lead to graft failure and increased morbidity and mortality. Close follow-up of the patients by the transplantation team is essential for prevention, early diagnosis, and treatment of these issues.
- Liver failure secondary to viral hepatitis (especially hepatitis B and C) is a common indication for liver transplantation. Hepatitis B recurrence is manageable with new antiviral drugs. Hepatitis C recurrence is universal, with a highly variable natural history and potentially lower patient and graft survival.
- New treatments for the prevention of recurrent diseases and rejection are being tested and are likely to improve long-term outcomes.

Suggested Readings

Almusa O, Federle MP: Abdominal imaging and intervention in liver transplantation. Liver Transpl 2006;12:184-193.

Amesur NB, Zajko AB: Interventional radiology in liver transplantation. Liver Transpl 2006;12:330-351.

Charlton M: Recurrence of hepatitis C infection: Where are we now? Liver Transpl 2005;11:S57-S62.

Davis JE, Moss DJ: Treatment options for post-transplant lymphoproliferative disorder and other Epstein-Barr virus-associated malignancies. Tissue Antigens 2004;63:285-292.

De la Mora-Levy JG, Baron TH: Endoscopic management of liver transplant patients. Liver Transpl 2005;11:1007-1021.

Lok ASF, McMahon BJ: AASLD practice guideline. Chronic hepatitis B. Hepatology 2007;45:507-539.

Ojo AO, Held PJ, Port FK: Chronic renal failure after transplantation of nonrenal organ. N Engl J Med 2003;349:931-940.

Post DJ, Douglas DD, Mulligan DC: Immunosuppression in liver transplantation. Liver Transpl 2005;11:1307-1314.

Starzl TE, von Kaulla KN, Hermann G, et al: Homotransplantation of the liver in humans. Surg Gynecol Obstet 1963;117:659-676.

Terrault N, Roche B, Samuel D: Management of the hepatitis B virus in the liver transplantation setting: A European and an American perspective. Liver Transpl 2005;11:716-732.

Tzakis AG, Gordon RD, Shaw BW Jr, et al: Clinical presentation of hepatic artery thrombosis after liver transplantation in the cyclosporin era. Transplantation 1985;40:667-671.

Section 7

HEMATOLOGY AND ONCOLOGY

Anemia

Bernard J. Silver

DEFINITION

Generally defined, anemia is present when the hemoglobin concentration is below a normal value based on the reference population. The mean normal value of hemoglobin is dependent on age, gender, race, and altitude. According to WHO criteria, the lower limit of normal in adults is 13 g/dL in men and 12 g/dL in women. The blood hemoglobin concentration is believed to reflect more accurately the total red cell mass or status of the erythron (erythroid precursors of the marrow and circulating mature red cells) compared with the hematocrit. A drop in the hemoglobin level is observed in older men that may be the result of reduced androgen levels. This assumption does not, however, obviate the need for evaluation, especially if the patient is known to have had normal values in the recent past; the detection of a slight decrease in the hemoglobin level is often a signal of underlying disease, such as myelodysplastic syndrome. Other features that should prompt investigation include microcytic or macrocytic indices, elevated reticulocyte count (signifying hemolysis), and leukocyte or platelet abnormalities.

PREVALENCE

It's been estimated that 3.4 million Americans have anemia. Approximately 20% to 30% of hospitalized patients have some degree of anemia, with the highest percentage being found in intensive care units. The most common causes of anemia seen in general practice are illustrated in Figure 1.

PATHOPHYSIOLOGY

Anemia can also be defined physiologically by the degree of impairment of tissue oxygenation. Oxygen supply to tissues is controlled by a well-balanced mechanism that depends on the relative rate of oxygen supply and demand. Tissue oxygen delivery is dependent on the hemoglobin concentration, oxygen saturation and oxygen affinity, the degree and rate of change in blood volume, and the capacity for the cardiovascular and pulmonary systems to compensate. These, in turn, determine the clinical manifestations of anemia, on which the decision to transfuse should ultimately be based. Tissue oxygen delivery is also the major controlling factor of erythropoiesis through the synthesis and release of erythropoietin (EPO) by the proximal tubular cells or the peritubular interstitial cells in the kidney. EPO synthesis is governed by the activation of hypoxia inducible factor-1 (HIF-1), which controls the metabolic responses of multiple gene products to hypoxia. HIF-1 binds and activates the hypoxia-responsive transcriptional enhancer in the erythropoietin gene regulatory region that upregulates EPO expression. EPO stimulates erythroid precursor cells (CFU-E [colony-forming units—erythroid]), leading to increased proliferation and shortening of their maturation time. The marrow responds to increased EPO maximally in 4 to 7 days if enough iron is available. Erythropoiesis can be increased by as much as a factor of 8. Typical of an endocrine loop feedback mechanism, there is an inverse relation between the hemoglobin and EPO levels measured in the blood (Fig. 2). Although this relation holds true in simple iron deficiency, it is somewhat distorted in the anemia associated with inflammation or chronic disease, in which there may be a blunted EPO response. This has made prediction of the hemoglobin response to treatment with exogenous EPO unpredictable, except in limited circumstances (see later).

SIGNS AND SYMPTOMS

The clinical manifestations of anemia depend on the individual's ability to compensate for a loss in oxygen-carrying capacity. The more abrupt the onset of the anemia, the more dramatic the presentation. A sudden loss of more one third of a patient's blood volume, for example, usually results in hypotension, respiratory distress, and acute mental status change, even in a young, previously healthy patient. With the more typical chronic development of anemia, the clinical changes are subtler and depend on the patient's age and comorbid conditions. The most familiar of these changes is an increase in cardiac output causing symptoms of palpitations and tachycardia, breathlessness, especially on exertion, and dizziness or lightheadedness. The patient may also complain of noise in the ears. This is not true tinnitus, but rather a roaring sound caused by accelerated blood flow through the ear. Some patients develop a feeling of profound generalized fatigue that can be accompanied by a loss of mental acuity, resulting in reduced ability to perform simple tasks such as reading a newspaper. These chronic symptoms are made worse by underlying coronary artery disease, congestive heart failure, and intrinsic pulmonary or cerebrovascular disease.

DIAGNOSIS

The evaluation of anemia can be a complex and difficult endeavor that may not yield a definitive diagnosis, even after exhaustive testing, including a bone marrow biopsy. Often, anemia exists in a milieu of chronic organ dysfunction or medical conditions that cloud the diagnosis because of their effect on erythropoiesis or red cell survival. These conditions may also create discrepancies in laboratory results, leading to further obfuscation in the differential diagnosis. Even bone marrow findings can be so subtle as to be nondefinitive, and only after long-term follow-up does the diagnosis become apparent in retrospect.

These difficulties arise in two of the most common types of anemia, iron deficiency anemia and the anemia of chronic disease. This review will emphasize the pathogenesis and diagnosis of these two types of anemias, how they are differentiated from each other, and how erythropoietin is used therapeutically in select patients to avoid or lessen the requirement for transfusion.

Once anemia has been identified, classification of the physiologic mechanism is the most useful first step (Box 1). This kinetic classification is a useful first approach for any type of cytopenia. In this schema, red blood cells are being lost (blood loss), destroyed (hemolysis), or underproduced. The last category is further divided into hypoproliferative and ineffective erythropoiesis. Three patterns of erythropoiesis are identified based on the reticulocyte count, appearance of the bone marrow, and tests for hemolysis, such as the indirect bilirubin assay (Table 1). More than one mechanism can exist, or one category can evolve from another. The last example is best illustrated by iron deficiency anemia, caused first by blood loss and then by underproduction of red cells caused by lack of sufficient iron. Although the mechanism of anemia may be considered in kinetic terms, the mean corpuscular volume (MCV), measured directly by automated cell counters, is used to classify and diagnose the anemia further and guide the rest of the laboratory workup.

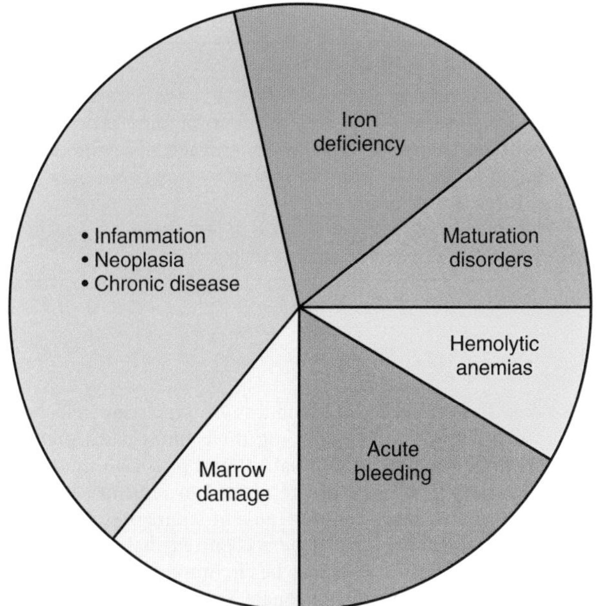

Figure 1 Relative frequencies of anemia seen in clinical practice. *(Adapted from Hillman RS, Finch, CA [eds]: Red Cell Manual, 7th ed. Philadelphia, FA Davis, 1996, pp 67-129.)*

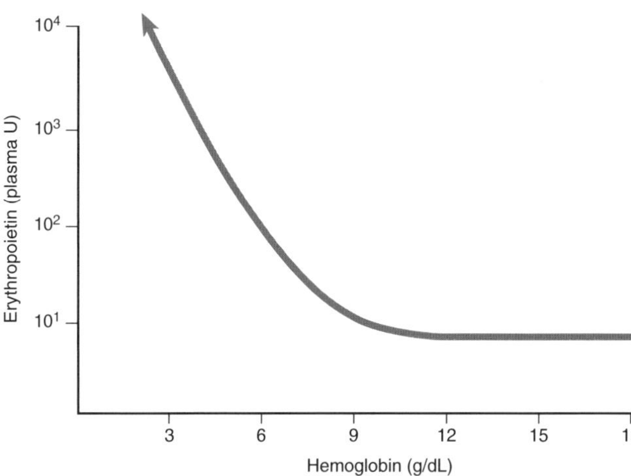

Figure 2 Inverse relation between erythropoietin levels and degree of anemia. *(Adapted from Hillman RS, Finch, CA [eds]: Red Cell Manual, 7th ed. Philadelphia, FA Davis, 1996, pp 1-38.)*

Box 1 Kinetic Classification of Anemia

Red blood cell loss (bleeding)
Red blood cell destruction (hemolysis)
Extracorpuscular hemolytic disease
Antibodies
Infection (e.g., malaria)
Splenic sequestration and destruction
Associated diseases (e.g., collagen-vascular, lymphoproliferative, immunodeficiency)
Drugs, chemicals, physical agents
Red cell trauma (e.g., microangiopathic hemolytic anemia)
Intracorpuscular hemolytic disease, hereditary
Disorders of glycolysis
Faulty synthesis or maintenance of reduced glutathione (e.g., glucose-6-phosphate dehydrogenase [G6PD] deficiency)
Hemoglobinopathies
Red cell membrane abnormalities
Erythropoietic porphyria
Intracorpuscular hemolytic disease, acquired
Paroxysmal nocturnal hemoglobinuria
Lead poisoning
Red blood cell underproduction
Nutritional deficiencies-iron, vitamin B_{12}, folic acid, pyridoxine
Bone marrow aplasia or hypoplasia
Pure red cell aplasia
Bone marrow infiltration
Myelodysplasia
Leukemia, lymphoma
Multiple myeloma
Carcinoma
Myelofibrosis
Endocrinopathy (e.g., thyroid, adrenal, pituitary hypofunction)
Chronic renal disease
Chronic inflammatory disease
Cirrhosis

Adapted from Wintrobe MM, Lukens JN, Lee GR: The approach to the patient with anemia. In Lee G, Bithell T, Foerster J et al (eds): Wintrobe's Clinical Hematology, 9th ed. Philadelphia, Lea & Febiger, 1993, pp 715-744.

Table 1 Patterns of Abnormal Erythropoiesis

Disorder	Reticulocytes	Marrow Erythropoiesis	Bilirubin
Hemolytic anemia	↑(appropriate for Hb)	Erythroid hyperplasia	↑
Hypoproliferative anemia	Inappropriately low for Hb	Erythroid hypoplasia	↓
Ineffective erythropoiesis	Inappropriately low for Hb	Erythroid hyperplasia	↑

Hb, hemoglobin.
Adapted from Hillman, RS, Finch, CA (eds): Red Cell Manual, 7th ed. (1996). Philadelphia, FA. Davis, 1996, pp 1-38.

TYPES OF ANEMIA

Iron Deficiency Anemia

Iron is an essential nutrient found mostly in heme proteins (e.g., hemoglobin, myoglobin), but also in a host of enzymes of intermediary metabolism. About two thirds of the body's iron are incorporated into the hemoglobin of the erythron. The distribution of iron between the erythron, the plasma, and reticuloendothelial storage sites (e.g., hepatocytes, macrophages) is a tightly controlled process; both iron deficiency and iron overload are serious disorders. There has been a rapid increase in our understanding of the regulation of iron distribution. More than 15 newly identified proteins have been described in recent years. These proteins regulate the absorption of iron from the gastrointestinal (GI) tract, transport to the erythron, and storage of iron in reticuloendothelial cells.

Iron deficiency is one of the most common causes of anemia in the United States and worldwide. The three stages of iron deficiency are iron depletion (reduced stores), early iron deficiency anemia (depleted stores, normal MCV, and red cell morphology), and advanced iron deficiency anemia. Bleeding is the most common cause, typically GI bleeding or menstruation, although other causes of blood loss (e.g., pulmonary, urinary, and even factitious) occasionally present themselves (Box 2).[1] A rare cause of iron deficiency is paroxysmal nocturnal hemoglobinuria. Although dietary lack of iron alone is rarely a cause of iron deficiency, it does contribute to the loss of iron brought about by otherwise minor bleeding, such as with normal menstruation. Iron malabsorption is rarely the cause of iron deficiency. Malabsorption of iron may result from achlorhydria

Box 2 Causes of Iron Deficiency

Increased Loss

Gastrointestinal blood loss: epistaxis, varices, gastritis, ulcer, tumor, Meckel's diverticulum, parasitosis

Milk-induced enteropathy of early childhood: vascular malformations, inflammatory bowel disease, diverticulosis

Inadequate Absorption

Poor bioavailability

- Antacid therapy or high gastric pH
- Excess dietary bran, tannin, phytates, or starch
- Competition from other metals (e.g., copper, lead)

Loss or dysfunction of absorptive enterocytes

- Bowel resection
- Celiac disease
- Inflammatory bowel disease
- Intrinsic enterocyte defects

Other blood loss

- Trauma
- Excessive phlebotomy
- Large vascular malformations
- Chronic infection

Pulmonary blood loss

- Pulmonary hemosiderosis
- Infection

Menorrhagia

Cancer

Genitourinary blood loss

Hemorrhoids

Data from Andrews N: Disorders of iron metabolism. N Engl J Med 1999;341:1986-1995.

(e.g., that seen in vitamin B_{12} deficiency), gastric bypass surgery, and celiac disease. Gastric resection alone would not be expected to cause iron deficiency unless the upper duodenum, the major site of iron absorption, was also removed or bypassed. About 50% of patients who have undergone a subtotal gastric resection will have impaired food iron absorption, but will still absorb exogenous iron. Inflammatory bowel disease involving the upper jejunum and duodenum may also cause malabsorption of iron. It has been estimated that approximately two thirds of patients with iron deficiency anemia have GI lesions that can be detected by endoscopy, and 10% to 15% have a GI malignancy.

The clinical manifestations of iron deficiency consist of those related to anemia, but there also appear to be effects on the central nervous system causing neuromuscular abnormalities and cognitive defects, especially in children. Pica occurs in children and adults. Effects on epithelial tissues, such as the nails (koilonychia), oropharyngeal mucosa (glossitis, angular stomatitis, and mucosal webs [Plummer-Vinson syndrome]), are rarely seen today because of earlier diagnosis and treatment.

The pure case of iron deficiency anemia is straightforward to diagnose.[2] By the time red cell production is slowed and microcytic anemia occurs, iron stores are depleted, as determined by a low serum ferritin level, the major iron storage protein. The familiar laboratory tests of determination of the serum iron level, total iron-binding capacity (TIBC; transferrin), transferrin saturation, and ferritin level accurately reflect body iron stores, and obviate the need for a bone marrow biopsy in most cases. Although an MCV lower than 80 fL and a serum ferritin lower than 20 ng/mL are traditionally used to diagnose iron deficiency anemia, an MCV of 95 fL or a serum ferritin lower than 45 ng/mL were found to be predictive of iron deficiency secondary to serious GI lesions in one prospective study.

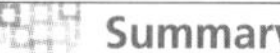

Summary

Diagnosis of Iron Deficiency

- Use all four laboratory parameters to make an accurate diagnosis—serum iron level, total iron-binding capacity, percentage transferrin saturation, and serum ferritin level.
- Bleeding is the most common cause.
- Search for GI malignancy.
- Malabsorption is rarely the cause unless there is a specific defect in the duodenum or upper jejunum.

Treatment

After searching for a source of blood loss, iron replacement is begun, starting with ferrous sulfate, 325 mg three times daily, preferably taken 1 hour before meals. Both patient and physician must realize that several months of therapy are needed to replenish body iron stores. Although the most frequent cause of failure of iron therapy is patient noncompliance, it must be recognized that many patients cannot tolerate oral iron. This may be circumvented by switching to other iron salts (e.g., ferrous gluconate, ferrous fumarate) or to an iron-polysaccharide complex (Nu-IronPlus®) that may produce fewer side effects. Patients may tolerate delayed-release products better, but iron absorption could be impaired because of bypass of the major iron absorption sites in the upper jejunum and duodenum. Some patients tolerate oral iron yet do not respond to therapy. This could result from defects in the iron transport abnormalities in the intestinal epithelium as well as from the more common causes of malabsorption. These patients may benefit from parenteral iron replacement, with iron dextran, sodium ferric gluconate (Ferrlecit®), or iron sucrose (Venofer®). Test doses of iron dextran should be given first because anaphylactic reactions could occur.

Summary

Treatment of Iron Deficiency

- Use ferrous sulfate for iron replacement; if not well tolerated, try other iron salts (e.g., ferrous gluconate, ferrous fumarate) or polysaccharide iron complex.
- Proton pump inhibitors can interfere with iron absorption; add vitamin C.
- IV iron replacement should be done sparingly and only if malabsorption is present.

Chronic Disease Anemia

Chronic disease anemia (CDA), or the anemia of inflammation, is a mild to moderate anemia accompanying infectious, inflammatory, or neoplastic disease that is characterized by abundant reticuloendothelial iron unavailable to bone marrow erythroid precursors.[3] Iron-deficient erythropoiesis results from this defect in iron recycling, triggered by cytokines (e.g., tumor necrosis factor α [TNF-α, interleukin-1 or interleukin-6 [IL-1, IL-6]) that lower the serum iron level and affect macrophage iron storage so as to prohibit iron uptake. Hepcidin is a major regulator of iron absorption and iron efflux from macrophages. Studies have indicated that it may play a major role in the pathogenesis of CDA in that hepcidin decreases iron absorption in the small intestine and inhibits iron release from macrophages. It is also inducible by IL-1 and IL-6 and has been found to cause hypoferremia and anemia. Other mechanisms in CDA that limit erythropoiesis include inappropriately low EPO secretion and diminished EPO responsiveness. This same pattern of iron diversion and altered response to EPO can be seen in acutely ill patients in the intensive care unit with multiorgan dysfunction or sepsis. Although typically found in inflammatory conditions or malignancy, CDA is also associated with noninflammatory disorders, such as congestive heart failure, COPD, alcoholic liver disease, and chronic kidney disease. In diabetics, for example, the EPO response to anemia is blunted, even in those patients without renal insufficiency.[4] In anemic COPD patients, moderately elevated erythropoietin levels have been described, suggesting relative EPO resistance. Anemia develops 1 to 2 months after the onset of illness, does not progress, and parallels the severity of the underlying condition. Iron therapy is ineffective because of limited iron absorption and trapping of iron in macrophage storage sites.

The diagnosis of CDA can be difficult, especially if it coexists with iron deficiency. Other contributing causes of anemia should be ruled out, including blood loss, malnutrition, folate or vitamin B_{12} deficiency, and hemolysis. Myelodysplastic syndrome frequently masquerades as CDA until it progresses, and the threshold for performing a bone marrow biopsy should be low, particularly for those in older age groups or in the absence of an obvious chronic disease. Laboratory findings of CDA include a mild to moderate anemia with normocytic or slightly microcytic indices, reduced serum iron and TIBC (transferrin) levels, and increased ferritin level, reflecting the increase in iron stores (Table 2). Although the serum ferritin level is useful when there is no accompanying inflammation, it is influenced by acute phase responses. The soluble transferrin receptor (TFR) is present in human plasma and its concentration is determined by marrow erythroid activity and iron status. Its synthesis is induced by iron deprivation, so in iron-deficient states the level of TFR rises. The TFR concentration is not increased with infection or inflammation, providing a way of differentiating iron deficiency from CDA. Patients who have a combination of iron deficiency and an infectious, inflammatory, or malignant disorder can be more accurately diagnosed by using a combination of the ferritin and TFR concentrations to derive the TFR-ferritin index. This index is the TFR concentration divided by the log of the ferritin concentration (see Table 2).

Treatment

Whereas CDA will improve with recovery from the chronic disorder, this is usually not possible, although the anemia will wax and wane with the activity of an associated inflammatory process, and may resolve altogether with successful treatment of an underlying infection. Because the anemia is relatively mild and the time course for its development is prolonged, allowing adequate compensatory mechanisms to come into play, patients are usually asymptomatic from the anemia itself and do not require treatment. Patients with compromised cardiac function and other chronic diseases, however, may have more exaggerated anemia-related symptoms. Transfusions result in immediate correction of anemia, and may be useful in differentiating anemic symptoms from those of the underlying disease process. Chronic blood replacement, however, is not recommended because of the potential complications of iron overload, alloimmunization, delayed and immediate transfusion reactions, and potential viral transmission.

Table 2 Iron Values in Chronic Disease Versus Iron Deficiency Anemia

Parameter	Chronic Disease Anemia	Iron Deficiency
Iron level	↓ to N	↓
Transferrin level	↓ to N	↑
Transferrin saturation	↓ to N	↓
Ferritin level	N to ↑	↓
TFR level	N	↑
TFR/log ferritin	Low (<1)	High (>4)

TFR, transferrin receptor.

The major objectives for the use of recombinant human erythropoietin (rHuEPO) therapy are to reduce transfusion requirements and to improve quality of life. Initiation of therapy should be based on the same rationale as one would use in deciding whether a transfusion is indicated—that is, whether or not the patient has clinical signs and symptoms of anemia that would be resolved or lessened by an increase in oxygen delivery. The three approved erythropoietic agents approved for use in the United States are epoetin alfa (Epogen, Procrit) and darbopoetin alfa (Aranesp). The latter is a recombinant erythropoietin that has been modified to increase the plasma half-life. It yields an equivalent erythropoietic response but requires less frequent dosing. Guidelines have been developed for the treatment of the anemia of cancer and for anemia of chronic kidney disease (CKD).[5,6] Erythropoietin therapy has been successful in patients with other types of chronic disease anemia, especially rheumatoid arthritis, in whom improvements in disease activity as well as anemia have been reported.[7]

In patients with cancer, CKD, and chronic inflammatory diseases, erythropoietin levels may be inappropriately low for the degree of anemia, suggesting that measuring EPO levels would be useful in predicting responses to therapy. In myelodysplastic syndromes, for example, an EPO level higher than 200 mU/L predicted a lack of response. Those with a level lower than 100 mU/L are said to be most likely to respond. This was substantiated in patients with advanced cancer, but only when an initial response (within 2 weeks) to rHuEPO was also observed. For other malignancies, and in most other chronic diseases, there is insufficient evidence to show that measuring serum EPO levels alone is clinically useful for predicting treatment responses, and current guidelines do not recommend it because it is unlikely to guide clinical decision making.

In the anemia related to cancer chemotherapy, evidence from clinical trials has supported the use of rHuEPO at a dosage of 150 U/kg subcutaneously three times weekly.[8] Once-weekly dosing, however, has become common practice, at a starting dosage of 40,000 U/week. If there is no response after 4 weeks, the dose can be titrated upward to 60,000 U/week. Randomized, placebo-controlled studies have demonstrated that rHuEPO therapy improves anemia, reduces transfusion requirements, and improves quality-of-life scores in cancer patients.

In general, erythropoietin therapy is safe and, in many cases, results in the resolution of anemic symptoms, allowing responding patients to avoid the detrimental effects of chronic red cell transfusions. An uncommon complication is the development of neutralizing antierythropoietin antibodies and pure red cell aplasia. Most of these cases have been described in Europe in patients treated with either the Eprex brand of epoetin alfa or, to a lesser extent, epoetin beta (NeoRecormon), agents not in use in the United States. Clinicians should also be aware, however, of recent U.S. Food and Drug Administration (FDA) warnings regarding the increased risk of venous thrombosis, stroke, and myocardial infarction in orthopedic, renal failure, and cancer patients treated with rHuEPO. A possible detrimental effect on survival has been noted in patients with head and neck cancers. Further revisions of guidelines for the use of these agents are likely to be forthcoming. Treating physicians are advised to follow the hemoglobin level closely when starting therapy and adjust the dose of erythropoietin to maintain the lowest level required to avoid transfusion.

Iron requirements are increased during rHuEPO therapy. If there is no increase in the hemoglobin level or a patient stops responding during therapy, iron deficiency should be excluded, because it will limit the erythropoietic response. Recommendations for iron replacement, however, are variable, and there is some debate as to the optimal route, dose, and indication for initiating iron supplements in patients receiving rHuEPO. In end-stage renal disease, oral iron supplements have been largely abandoned and replaced by newer generation IV preparations; these are believed to be superior in achieving more rapid repletion of iron stores in patients known to have increased iron losses and possibly poor iron absorption.[9] Rapid responses to rHuEPO and IV iron are observed. However, there are contrasting results among the few published randomized trials. In predialysis patients, for example, a randomized comparison in rHuEPO-treated patients between oral ferrous sulfate and IV iron sucrose showed no differences in hemoglobin response or required rHuEPO doses. Opposite results were seen in chemotherapy-induced anemia. One randomized controlled study has suggested that patients treated with IV iron have a higher hematopoietic response rate to rHuEPO than those given oral iron.[10] Iron dextran preparations have a low but significant incidence of serious adverse effects, including anaphylactic reactions. Newer nondextran iron preparations, such as ferric sodium gluconate (Ferrlecit) and iron sucrose (Venofer), are associated with a lower incidence of immediate toxicities. In these and other patient populations, there is concern that IV nontransferrin bound iron may have long-term effects through the production of excess free radicals, exacerbation of atherosclerosis, and risk of infection. The potential for iron toxicity and iron overload with IV iron supplementation, as well as its role in rHuEPO-treated patients, remain to be determined.

Suggested Readings

Andrews NC: Disorders of iron metabolism. N Engl J Med 1999;341:1986-1995.

Auerbach M, Ballard H, Trout JR, et al: Intravenous iron optimizes the response to recombinant human erythropoietin in cancer patients with chemotherapy-related anemia: A multicenter, open-label, randomized trial. J Clin Oncol 2004;22:1301-1307.

Ioannou GN, Spector J, Scott K, et al: Prospective evaluation of a clinical guideline for the diagnosis and management of iron deficiency anemia. Am J Med 2002;113:281-287.

National Comprehensive Cancer Network: Clinical Practice Guidelines in Oncology, vol 1, 2005. Available at: http://www.nccn.org/professionals/physician_gls/PDF/anemia.pdf.

National Kidney Foundation: IV. NKF-K/DOQI Clinical Practice Guidelines for Anemia of Chronic Kidney Disease: Update 2000. Am J Kidney Dis 2001;37(Suppl 1):S182-S238.

Stoves J, Inglis H, Newstead CG: A randomized study of oral vs intravenous iron supplementation in patients with progressive renal insufficiency treated with erythropoietin. Nephrol Dial Transplant 2001;16:967-974.

Thomas MC, Cooper ME, Tsalamandris C, et al: Anemia with impaired erythropoietin response in diabetic patients. Arch Intern Med 2005;165:466-469.

Weiss G, Goodnough LT: Anemia of chronic disease. N Engl J Med 2005;352:1011-1023.

Wilson A, Yu HT, Goodnough LT, Nissenson AR: Prevalence and outcomes of anemia in rheumatoid arthritis: A systematic review of the literature. Am J Med 2004;116(Suppl 7A):50S-57S.

Witzig TE, Silberstein PT, Loprinzi CL, et al: Phase III, randomized, double-blind study of epoetin alpha compared with placebo in anemic patients receiving chemotherapy. J Clin Oncol 2005;23:2606-2617.

References

For a complete list of references, log onto www.expertconsult.com.

Disorders of Platelet Function and Number

Rachid Baz and Tarek Mekhail

THROMBOCYTOPENIAS

Thrombocytopenia is defined as a platelet count of less than 150,000/mm^3. With normal platelet function, thrombocytopenia is rarely the cause of bleeding unless the count is less than 50,000/mm^3. Thrombocytopenia should always be confirmed by examination of a peripheral smear. It can be caused by decreased platelet production, increased destruction, sequestration, or a combination of these causes.

Etiologic Factors

Platelet Underproduction

The hallmark of platelet underproduction is decreased marrow megakaryocytes or, when available, a decreased peripheral blood reticulated platelet count.[2] Common causes include infections (including HIV), drugs (usually chemotherapeutic agents or alcohol, but other medications in rare cases), radiotherapy, vitamin deficiency (e.g., folate, vitamin B_{12}), or marrow infiltration by tumor, storage diseases, or marrow failure syndromes (e.g., aplastic anemia). In addition, the myelodysplastic syndromes are a commonly overlooked group of disorders associated with thrombocytopenia in older adults.

Management involves treatment of the underlying condition and supportive platelet transfusions if needed. Two first-generation recombinant thrombopoietin (TPO) agents have been evaluated in clinical trials (recombinant human thrombopoietin [rhuTPO] and pegylated recombinant human megakaryocyte growth and development factor [PEG-rhuMGDF]).[3] Both rhuTPO and PEG-rhuMGDF have shown the ability to increase platelet count, reduce the duration of thrombocytopenia, and result in a decrease in platelet transfusion for patients receiving dose-intense chemotherapy for ovarian cancer.[3] However, when PEG-rhuMGDF was administered to platelet donors, it resulted in the development of antibodies that cross-reacted with endogenous TPO and caused severe thrombocytopenia. This led to the discontinuation of investigations using these two products.

Second-generation TPO mimetics (AMG531 [Romiplostin] and SB497115 [eltrombopag]) have undergone evaluation in patients with immune thrombocytopenic purpura, and romiplostin has been approved by the U.S. Food and Drug Administration (FDA) for treating immune thrombocytopenic purpura (ITP). Romiplostin is a recombinant peptibody that is given subcutaneously once weekly. Eltrombopag is an oral daily hydrazone organic compound. Both agents activate the TPO receptor without structural homology to native TPO. These agents are discussed in more detail in the ITP section (later).

Platelet Sequestration

Hypersplenism from a variety of causes, including liver disease or malignancy, can result in platelet sequestration (Box 1). Mild to moderate thrombocytopenia is caused by platelet sequestration when there is an associated mild reduction in neutrophil count and hemoglobin and with minimal impairment of hematopoiesis on bone marrow examination. If physical examination fails to detect splenomegaly, evaluation with ultrasonography or radionuclide imaging is recommended to document splenomegaly.

Management includes treating the underlying condition and transfusing platelets as needed. Cytopenias secondary to hypersplenism are often not sufficiently severe to warrant treatment in the form of total or partial splenectomy, partial splenic embolization, or transjugular intrahepatic portosystemic shunting for congestive splenomegaly.[4]

Increased Platelet Destruction

The hallmark of increased platelet destruction is increased marrow megakaryocytes or, when available, high reticulated platelet count. Platelet destruction results from various immune and nonimmune conditions, including immune thrombocytopenic purpura (ITP), thrombotic microangiopathies, post-transfusion purpura (PTP), heparin-induced thrombocytopenia (HIT), and disseminated intravascular coagulation (DIC).

Immune Thrombocytopenic Purpura

Prevalence

The incidence of ITP in a Danish study was 100 cases per 1 million person-years, with 50% of cases occurring in the pediatric age group. It can be of adult or childhood onset. Adult onset is more likely to be chronic and insidious. Adult-onset ITP is more common in women than men (female-to-male ratio of 1.7 : 1), whereas childhood onset has equal sex distribution.[5]

ITP is subdivided into chronic or acute; acute ITP is 6 months or less in duration.[5]

Etiology

ITP can be primary or secondary. Causes of secondary ITP include systemic lupus erythematosus, antiphospholipid antibody syndrome, immunoglobulin A (IgA) deficiency, common variable hypogammaglobulinemia, lymphoproliferative disorders (e.g., chronic lymphocytic leukemia, lymphomas), viral (e.g., HIV, hepatitis C), or drug-induced.

Many drugs have been linked to thrombocytopenia, but those known to be associated with immune thrombocytopenia are heparin and quinidine. Patients with drug-induced ITP usually present within 1 to 2 weeks from the initiation of the offending drug with petechiae and a platelet count of less than 20,000/mm^3. Recovery usually occurs 5 to 7 days after discontinuation of the offending agent, but it is occasionally more prolonged.

Here we focus on primary ITP. The guidelines are derived from recommendations of the consensus guideline of the American Society of Hematology.[6]

Pathophysiology

The pathophysiology of primary ITP involves the formation of antiplatelet antibodies, often directed at platelet glycoproteins IIb/IIIA, IIb/IX, Ia/IIa, and V, or multiple platelet antigens. A relative impaired platelet production in response to platelet destruction is thought to contribute to the pathophysiology of ITP as evidenced by the clinical success of TPO-mimetic agents.

Box 1 Causes of Splenomegaly

Cirrhosis
Heart failure
Portal or hepatic venous thrombosis
Malignancies and hematologic disorders

- Lymphoma
- Acute and chronic leukemias
- Myeloproliferative disorders
- Metastatic solid tumors
- Hemolytic anemias

Infection

- Epstein-Barr virus
- Cytomegalovirus
- *Salmonella*
- *Brucella*
- Tuberculosis
- Malaria
- *Toxoplasma*
- Leishmania

Infiltrative disease

- Gaucher's disease
- Amyloidosis
- Glycogen storage diseases

Miscellaneous disorders

- Sarcoidosis
- Systemic lupus erythematosus
- Felty's syndrome

Clinical Features

On history and physical examination, the absence of systemic symptoms is helpful in ruling out secondary causes. Evidence of platelet-type (mucosal) bleeding should be noted, and the absence of splenomegaly supports the diagnosis. Bleeding is often less pronounced than in cases of decreased production with similar platelet counts.

Diagnosis

The complete blood cell (CBC) count should be unremarkable except for thrombocytopenia or easy-to-account-for anemia. The peripheral smear must confirm thrombocytopenia, and large immature platelets are often noted. A bone marrow biopsy or aspirate is required in patients older than 60 years, with presence of atypical features (e.g., fatigue, fever, joint pain, macrocytosis, neutropenia), or before splenectomy in the patient whose diagnosis is not definitive. Testing for antiplatelet antibodies is generally not recommended. A negative test result does not rule out the diagnosis.

Treatment

First Presentation. In the asymptomatic patient with a platelet count of less than 30,000/mm^3 or in the symptomatic patient with a platelet count between 30,000 and 50,000/mm^3, treatment with steroids such as prednisone 1 to 1.5 mg/kg/day has an expected response rate of 50% to 75%.[5,6] A response is usually seen after days of treatment. Experts differ on the length of time needed before labeling the patient unresponsive to steroids and changing therapy. Accordingly, a trial of 1 to 3 weeks of a corticosteroid is considered an adequate therapeutic trial.

Intravenous immunoglobulin (IVIg) 1 g/kg/day for 2 to 3 days is used to treat major bleeding, platelet counts of less than 5,000/mm^3 despite 3 days of steroids, or extensive and progressive purpura.[6] It is also the initial agent in patients with platelet counts of less than 50,000/mm^3 with life-threatening bleeding. The response rate for IVIg is 80%.[6] Disadvantages include cost, the low rate of long-term response, and risks of anaphylaxis (especially in patients with IgA deficiency), renal failure, or pulmonary failure.

Rh_o(D) immune globulin (RhoGAM) for Rh-positive patients, 75 µg/kg, is as effective as but less toxic than steroids. Significant adverse effects of this treatment include a hemolytic anemia that rarely results in more than a 2-g/dL drop in the hemoglobin level. It is, however, more expensive than prednisone and affords a similar long-term remission (5%-30%).[6]

Splenectomy should be considered after 3 to 6 months if the patient continues to require 10 to 20 mg/day of prednisone to keep the platelet count higher than 30,000/mm^3 or within 6 weeks of diagnosis in the patient with a platelet count of less than 10,000/mm^3 despite treatment. Laparoscopic splenectomy is increasingly used in high-volume centers and helps decrease the duration of hospitalization. Pneumococcal, meningococcal, and *Haemophilus* vaccination is indicated before splenectomy.

Urgent treatment for ITP patients with neurologic deficits or internal bleeding, or for emergency surgery, includes methylprednisolone 30 mg/kg/day for 2 to 3 days, for a maximum of 1 g/day, and/or IVIg 1 g/kg/day for 2 to 3 days, combined with platelet transfusions. Vincristine, antifibrinolytic therapy, recombinant factor VIIa, or continuous platelet transfusions should also be considered.

Relapsed ITP. Treatment is indicated only for those with a platelet count of less than 30,000/mm^3. Splenectomy (with a 66% response rate) is indicated in patients who relapse and do not respond to treatment with steroids, IVIg, or Rh_o(D) immune globulin. Rh_o(D) immune globulin is traditionally less effective in patients with ITP refractory to treatment.[6]

Rituximab, a monoclonal antibody to CD20, has been used in patients with ITP with varying success. Disadvantages include cost, infusion reactions, and lack on of long-term safety data. The role of rituximab therapy in ITP patients remains to be defined. It is currently being evaluated in the newly diagnosed and relapsed refractory patient.

TPO mimetics have been shown to increase platelet counts in patients with refractory ITP. In a phase I/II study of romiplostin, most patients who received the study drug at doses higher than 1 µg/kg weekly subcutaneously for 1 to 6 weeks achieved a platelet count greater than 50,000/mm^3. Two randomized, placebo-controlled studies in patients with prior splenectomy and patients without splenectomy were recently reported. Romiplostin, the only FDA-approved drug at the time of this publication, was administered for 24 weeks and adjusted to maintain platelet counts of 50,000 to 200,000/mm^3. The overall response rates were 78% in patients with prior splenectomy and 87% in patients without prior splenectomy. Bleeding events were decreased among responders. No patients developed neutralizing antibodies to TPO, and the most common reported event was mild to moderate headache. Reticulin fibrosis in the bone marrow of treated patients was of uncertain significance, but early data suggest it is reversible.

A randomized, placebo-controlled phase II study of eltrombopag administered orally at doses of 30, 50 and 75 mg has also been performed. At the higher two dose levels, a dose-dependent increase in platelet count was noted. A subsequent phase III study randomized 114 adults with ITP to eltrombopag or placebo. Eltrombopag was given at 50 mg daily and could be increased to 75 mg. Platelet responses (platelet count >50,000/mm^3) were noted in 59% and 16% on the eltrombopag and placebo arms, respectively. Clinically significant bleeding was also reduced in patients receiving eltrombopag. Adverse events were not different from placebo-treated patients, and the most commonly reported adverse event was headache.

Thrombotic Microangiopathies and Thrombotic Thrombocytopenic Purpura

Diagnosis

A pentad of signs is classically described to establish a diagnosis of TTP: thrombocytopenia (platelet counts usually <20,000/mm^3), microangiopathic hemolytic anemia, fever, renal dysfunction, and neurologic signs. A clinical triad of thrombocytopenia, red blood cell fragments (schistocytosis), and an increased lactate dehydrogenase (LDH) level is enough to suggest the diagnosis.[7] Examination of the peripheral blood smear in patients with thrombocytopenia of unclear cause is imperative to exclude this diagnosis (Fig. 1). If severe renal failure is a prominent feature of the syndrome, the hemolytic-uremic syndrome may be a more likely diagnosis. Although ADAMTS13 (a zinc-containing metalloprotease enzyme that cleaves von Willebrand factor [vWF]) levels can be measured, the diagnosis of TTP is a clinical one and results are often not available at the time of diagnosis.

Pathophysiology

Thrombotic microangiopathies are characterized by destructive thrombocytopenia, erythrocyte fragmentation, and tissue ischemia and necrosis, as evidenced by increased LDH levels. In nonacquired TTP, systemic clumping of platelets is caused by unusually large amounts of vWF, often caused by a deficiency of the metalloproteinase ADAMTS13 that cleaves vWF into smaller, less-thrombogenic multimers.[7]

Etiology of Thrombotic Thrombocytopenic Purpura

TTP can be familial or acquired. Familial TTP manifests in infancy or childhood and often remits and relapses. Acquired TTP manifests in adults or older children and often occurs as a single acute episode.

Drug-induced TTP often occurs weeks after exposure to the implicated drug. Medications commonly associated with this diagnosis include ticlopidine, mitomycin C, cyclosporine, tacrolimus, quinine, and, less commonly, clopidogrel. Whole-body irradiation and organ transplantation also can result in a clinical syndrome similar to that of TTP.[7]

Treatment

The treatment of childhood TTP (often related to ADAMTS13 deficiency) involves the transfusion of platelet-poor fresh-frozen plasma (FFP), FFP treated with organic solvent, or cryoprecipitate-poor plasma (cryosupernatant) every 3 weeks. The treatment of adults or older children with acquired TTP is by daily plasma exchange until platelet counts and LDH levels normalize.[7] Patients not responding to these modalities might require the addition of steroids, consideration of splenectomy, or administration of vincristine. More recently, rituximab has been used in patients with refractory TTP, with varying efficacy. Platelets should not be transfused unless a life-threatening hemorrhage or intracranial bleed is present.

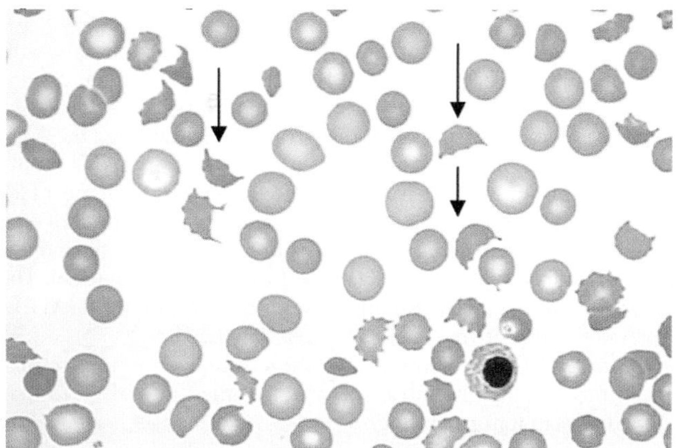

Figure 1 Peripheral blood smear of a patient with microangiopathic hemolytic anemia. Schistocytes *(arrows)* are also noted in patients with severe burns, dysfunctional prosthetic valves, and disseminated intravascular coagulation.

Post-Transfusion Purpura

Diagnosis

PTP is a transfusion reaction characterized by severe thrombocytopenia lasting days to weeks after transfusion of platelet-containing products. Human platelet antigen 1a (HPA-1a) is required to confirm the diagnosis.

Pathophysiology

Patients become sensitized to platelet antigen, most commonly HPA-1a, from prior transfusion of platelet-containing products or from pregnancy. This explains the much higher incidence among women. HPA-1a is also the platelet antigen most commonly involved in the pathophysiology of neonatal alloimmune purpura, thrombocytopenia that occurs in the neonatal period in the offspring of patients with PTP.[8]

Treatment

The treatment of choice is IVIg 400 mg/kg/day for 5 days or 1 g/kg/day for 2 days for severe thrombocytopenia. Further transfusions should be washed or HPA-1a–negative.[8]

Heparin-Induced Thrombocytopenia

Definition

HIT can be of two types. Type I HIT occurs in about 10% of patients receiving heparin, usually within 2 days of heparin initiation, and platelet counts return to normal despite continued heparin exposure. As opposed to type II HIT, thrombocytopenia is mild (usually >100,000/mm^3). It is nonimmune in origin and has no clinical consequences. The incidence of type II HIT varies from 0.3% to 3% in patients who have received more than 4 days of heparin, most commonly unfractionated heparin, and has no relation to the heparin dose. It rarely occurs beyond 2 weeks of exposure.

The remainder of this discussion focuses on type II HIT, because type I HIT is of no clinical consequence.

Pathophysiology

The pathophysiology involves antibody formation against the heparin-platelet factor 4 complex, with resultant thrombosis. Thrombosis is usually venous, in the form of deep venous thrombosis or pulmonary embolism), but it can be arterial as well, in the form of myocardial infarction or stroke.[10]

Clinical Presentation

HIT is rare with platelet counts of less than 20,000/mm^3; the average platelet count nadir is approximately 60,000/mm^3.[10] HIT has an earlier onset with re-exposure to heparin. A high index of suspicion is required, and HIT should be considered in hospitalized patients with nosocomial thrombocytopenia. In addition, thrombosis is often associated with HIT and is usually asymptomatic.[10]

Diagnosis

The diagnosis is clinical, despite the availability of adjunctive laboratory tests. These include the serotonin release assay, which is expensive and not widely available but has high sensitivity and specificity and still remains the gold standard; the heparin-induced platelet aggregation test (HIPA), with a low sensitivity but high specificity; and the platelet-factor IV assays, highly sensitive but with a 10% to 20% clinical discordance with other tests.[10] These adjunctive tests are often used in combination.

Prevention

Because they have been associated with lower rates of HIT (2.2% vs. 7.8% with unfractionated heparin), the use of low-molecular-weight heparin is believed to result in a decreased incidence of HIT. Prophylaxis with fondaparinux can also result in a lower incidence of HIT.

Treatment

Treatment involves discontinuation of all heparins, including IV line flushes and avoidance of warfarin until the platelet count normalizes. This approach carries a 30-day risk of thrombosis (de novo deep venous thrombosis) of 53%.

There are three strategies to decrease the high risk of thrombosis. One is anticoagulation with danaparoid, a heparinoid with a long half-life and 10% cross-reactivity with heparin, which requires monitoring of factor Xa activity.[9] Lepirudin, a renally cleared recombinant hirudin, can be used at a bolus dose of 0.1 to 0.4 mg/kg followed by an infusion of 0.1 to 0.15 mg/kg/hour for a goal activated partial thromboplastin time (aPTT) of 1.5 to 2.5 times normal.[9] Argatroban, a direct thrombin inhibitor metabolized in the liver, can be used in patients with renal failure at a dosage of 2 μg/kg/min, for a goal aPTT of 1.5 to 3 times normal. It has a short half-life—the anticoagulant effect wears off after 3 hours with normal hepatic function—and prolongs both the prothrombin time (PT) and the aPTT in a dose-dependent fashion. In patients with hepatic insufficiency, the dose should be decreased to 0.5 μg/kg/min.[9] Caution must be exercised with the use of argatroban, danaparoid, and lepirudin, because their effects cannot be reversed.

Disseminated Intravascular Coagulation

DIC is a systemic process that results in thrombosis or hemorrhage, or both. Often, one presentation predominates, and patients might have signs of bleeding or thrombosis.[11] It is estimated to occur in 1% of hospitalized patients.

Pathophysiology

DIC represents a massive activation of the coagulation cascade that results in excessive production of thrombin, systemic intravascular fibrin deposition, and consumption of clotting factors and platelets. The initiating factor is the release of tissue factor caused by various mechanisms, including extensive endothelial injury and the monocyte response to endotoxin or various cytokines.

DIC can be acute, decompensated when the generation of clotting factor cannot keep up with the excessive consumption, or chronic, compensated when the clotting factors are generated at the same rate as they are consumed. Acute DIC occurs secondary to various insults (Box 2) and its pathogenesis involves the massive generation of thrombin and consumption of coagulation factors.

Box 2 Common Causes of Disseminated Intravascular Coagulation

Obstetric complications

- Abruptio placentae
- Septic abortion
- Intrauterine fetal death

Infections

- Viral
- Bacterial
- Rickettsial
- Fungal
- Protozoal

Malignancy

- Acute leukemias
- Solid organ malignancies

Intravascular hemolysis

- Transfusion reactions
- Drug-induced hemolysis
- Paroxysmal nocturnal hemoglobinuria

Vascular malformation and aneurysms
Massive tissue injury (includes trauma)
Hypoxia and hypoperfusion

- Pulmonary embolism
- Myocardial infarction,
- Hypothermia
- Others

Miscellaneous factors

- Snake bite
- Head trauma
- Anaphylaxis
- Heat stroke
- Graft-versus-host disease
- Acute pancreatitis
- Status epilepticus
- Acute iron toxicity

Clinical Features

Acute DIC manifests with bleeding and oozing from multiple sites—catheter access or mucosal surfaces—often in a critically ill patient with multisystem organ failure. Chronic DIC is most often associated with malignancy, usually solid tumors, and results from continuous slow exposure of blood to small amounts of tissue factor without overwhelming the compensatory mechanisms that regenerate depleted factors. It most often manifests clinically with thrombosis rather than hemorrhage.

Diagnosis

The diagnosis of acute DIC relies on history and clinical setting, with particular attention to trauma, sepsis, malignancy, pregnancy, and miscarriages; moderate to severe thrombocytopenia; evidence of microangiopathic hemolysis on the peripheral smear (e.g., the presence of schistocytes); and suggestive laboratory test results. Clinically significant DIC is unlikely in the presence of normal fibrin degradation products (FDPs) or D dimers.[11] Prolonged PT and aPTT can also be noted, as well as decreased fibrinogen levels; fibrinogen, however, is an acute-phase reactant and may be falsely normal. The thrombin time (TT) is prolonged, and antithrombin III (ATIII), protein C, and protein S levels are often depressed.

Chronic DIC can manifest with more subtle laboratory results; smear microangiopathy and an elevated D-dimer (or FDP) level may be the only laboratory finding.

Treatment

Acute DIC in the setting of sepsis, trauma, or burns carries 40% to 80% mortality. Increasing age and severity of multiorgan failure represent worse prognostic factors.

Treatment is largely supportive, with platelet or FFP transfusions, or both, in bleeding patients and in those at high risk for bleeding. Cryoprecipitate transfusion in patients with a fibrinogen level lower than 100 mg/dL is often considered, although its benefit is difficult to demonstrate.

Heparin was not shown to be beneficial in acute DIC in controlled trials, and its role is limited to the treatment of DIC associated with the retained products of gestation or with giant hemangiomas.[11] Heparin has been used with varying efficacy in patients with DIC and disseminated malignancy.[11]

Emerging but not yet validated treatment for DIC includes protein C concentrates for patients with homozygous protein C deficiency, antithrombin, and activated protein C, which has demonstrated survival benefit in severe sepsis.

QUALITATIVE PLATELET DISORDERS

Qualitative platelet disorders are suggested by a prolonged bleeding time (abnormal platelet function screen) or clinical evidence of bleeding in the setting of a normal platelet count and coagulation studies. They are most commonly acquired, but they can be inherited. A new platelet function test, PFA-100 (Dade-Behring, Deerfield, Ill), has a 96% sensitivity for detecting von Willebrand disease (vWD) and aspirin-induced platelet defects.[13] It is often used as a screening test for platelet dysfunction but has not been shown to correlate with clinical bleeding. Platelet aggregation studies remain the gold standard diagnostic tests.

Drug-Induced Platelet Dysfunction

The most common drug responsible for platelet dysfunction is aspirin, which irreversibly inhibits cyclooxygenase for 5 to 7 days—hence, the need to hold aspirin for 5 to 7 days before elective surgery. Other common drugs include clopidogrel, ticlopidine, and glycoprotein IIb/IIIa inhibitors. Nonsteroidal anti-inflammatory drugs (NSAIDs) inhibit cyclooxygenase reversibly. Ethanol use and aspirin therapy have synergistic effects. Box 3 lists drugs associated with platelet dysfunction. Treatment includes discontinuation of the offending drug and platelet transfusion in the setting of clinically significant bleeding.

Box 3 Common Drugs Causing Platelet Dysfunction

Interfering with Platelet Membrane
Amitriptyline
Imipramine
Chlorpromazine
Cocaine
Lidocaine
Isoproterenol
Propranolol
Penicillin
Ampicillin
Cephalothin
Promethazine
Diphenhydramine
Carbenicillin

Inhibition of Prostaglandin Pathways
Aspirin
Nonsteroidal anti-inflammatory drugs
Furosemide
Verapamil
Hydralazine
Cyclosporine
Hydrocortisone

Inhibition of Platelet Phosphodiesterase
Caffeine
Dipyridamole
Aminophylline
Theophylline
Vinblastine
Vincristine
Colchicine
Papaverine

Unknown Mechanism of Action
Acetazolamide
Ethacrynic acid
Hydroxychloroquine
Nitroprusside
Cyproheptadine
Nitroglycerin
Famotidine
Cimetidine

Uremia

Uremia imparts a predisposition to bleeding that is incompletely understood. Treatment involves correction of anemia, institution of hemodialysis, and the use of desmopressin[14] (DDAVP; its use is discussed later, "Treatment of von Willebrand Disease"). Platelet transfusions do not correct the coagulopathy because the transfused platelets assume the dysfunction of the uremic platelets.

Liver Disease

Whether acute or chronic, hepatic disease is associated with platelet dysfunction that is multifactorial in origin. Increased FDP levels from activation of the fibrinolytic pathway compromise platelet function and impair release of platelet factor III from platelets because of cirrhosis or manifestations of hepatic dysfunction.

Acquired von Willebrand Disease

Acquired vWD is often described in patients with autoimmune disorders, valvular heart disease, lymphoproliferative disorders, or monoclonal gammopathies. It can also be drug induced (e.g., by dextran or valproic acid). The pathophysiology varies, from adherence of vWF to tumor cells to vWF degradation by proteolytic enzymes. Treatment involves therapy for the underlying disorder, in addition to considering a desmopressin trial, intermediate-purity factor VIII concentrates, high-dose IVIg, or recombinant factor VIIa, depending on availability and urgency.

Paraneoplastic Platelet Dysfunction

Platelet dysfunction has also been associated with plasma cell dyscrasias and is believed to be related to coating of the platelet membrane by monoclonal proteins. Myelodysplastic and myeloproliferative syndromes can result in platelet dysfunction (e.g., through an acquired glycoprotein IIb/IIIa deficiency). The bleeding time is often prolonged but does not correlate with the bleeding tendency.

Other disorders associated with platelet dysfunction include cardiopulmonary bypass or valvular defects, autoimmune disorders (e.g., systemic lupus erythematosus, rheumatoid arthritis, scleroderma), and severe iron or folate deficiency.

Inherited Platelet Disorders: Von Willebrand Disease

Inherited platelet disorders include the common vWD and the less common Glanzmann thrombasthenia and Bernard-Soulier disease. The latter two are beyond the scope of this text.

Prevalence

vWD is the most common inherited bleeding disorder. It affects about 1% of the population, although only a fraction of these persons come to medical attention, often because of the paucity of symptoms in the absence of significant hemostatic challenge but also because of failure to recognize abnormal bleeding. Laboratory testing for mild disease is often difficult to interpret, making its definitive incidence difficult to determine.

Pathophysiology and Types

vWD is subdivided into three types, based on clinical and laboratory features (Table 1).[12]

Type 1 accounts for approximately 70% of patients, has an autosomal dominant inheritance, and represents a mild quantitative deficiency of vWF. Bleeding can be mild to moderately severe. Many patients have not been found to have a detectable mutation in the vWF gene.

Type 2 is further subdivided into types 2A, 2B, 2M, and 2N. Type 2A accounts for about 15% of patients. It is transmitted in an autosomal dominant pattern and involves a deficiency of the high-molecular-weight multimers of vWF.[1] Patients present with moderate to severe bleeding. Type 2B accounts for approximately 5% of patients. It is inherited in an autosomal dominant pattern and involves a gain-of-function mutation that results from increased binding of vWF to platelet glycoprotein 1B and resultant decreased circulating vWF. The hallmark of type 2B vWD is an enhanced aggregation of the patient's platelets in the presence of ristocetin.[1] Patients with type 2B often have mild thrombocytopenia. Bleeding is moderate to severe. Type 2M is a rare autosomal dominant disorder characterized by reduced binding of vWF to platelet glycoprotein 1B.[1] Type 2N is a rare autosomal recessive disorder characterized by decreased binding of vWF to factor VIII, resulting in low factor VIII levels and bleeding patterns similar to those seen in the hemophilias.[1]

Type 3 is a rare autosomal recessive subtype, characterized by a marked decrease in vWF. It can result from different genetic defects in compound heterozygotes.

Treatment

Treatment of vWD involves replacing factor, and this can be difficult to monitor because of the lack of laboratory tests that correlate with bleeding. Hence, commonly monitored parameters include clinical bleeding, factor VIII levels, and ristocetin cofactor levels.

Table 1 Laboratory Diagnosis of von Willebrand Disease by Type

	Type of Von Willebrand Disease					
Diagnostic Test	**1**	**2A**	**2B**	**2M**	**2N**	**3**
Von Willebrand factor (vWF) antigen	↓	↓ or N	↓	↓ or N	N	↓↓↓
Ristocetin cofactor activity	↓	↓↓	↓↓	↓	N	↓↓↓
Factor VIII activity	↓↓	↓ or N	↓ or N	↓ or N	↓↓	↓↓↓
High-molecular-weight vWF multimers	N	↓↓	↓	N	N	↓↓↓
Ristocetin-induced platelet aggregation	↓ or N	↓		↓	N	↓↓↓

N, normal; ↓, mildly decreased; ↓↓, moderately decreased; ↓↓↓, markedly decreased; , increased.

Desmopressin.

Desmopressin promotes the release of vWF from endothelial cells. It is effective for patients with type 1 disease, but it has a varying effect for patients with type 2A disease. It is relatively contraindicated in patients with type 2B disease. It may also be helpful for patients with type 2M or 2N vWD, but it is not helpful for patients with type 3 disease.

Desmopressin can be given intravenously or subcutaneously at 0.2 μg/kg (maximum dose, 20 μg), with a response noted as early as 30 minutes later and lasting 6 to 12 hours. The dose may be repeated in 12 hours and then daily. The intranasal preparation is given at a dose of 150 μg for patients weighing less than 50 kg and 300 μg for those weighing more than 50 kg. A trial infusion is needed to assess the efficacy of treatment and adequacy of prophylactic use. Adverse effects include facial flushing, headaches, hyponatremia with continuous use, and a potential for thrombotic events.

Factor VIII Concentrates.

Intermediate-purity factor VIII concentrates are used for patients who do not benefit from desmopressin and for those with serious bleeding or before major surgery. Intermediate-purity factor VIII concentrate is used to maintain factor VIII levels between 50% and 100% for 3 to 10 days. A dose of 20 to 30 IU/kg is typically used twice daily. Overzealous treatment results in high factor VIII levels, which is believed to increase the risk of thrombosis.

Aminocaproic Acid and Tranexamic Acid.

Aminocaproic acid 50 mg/kg four times daily and tranexamic acid 25 mg/kg three times daily have been used for mild bleeding episodes and for dental procedures. They carry a risk of thrombotic events, which is especially pronounced in older patients and with long-term use.

Topical Treatment.

Topical treatment for oral or nasal bleeding with Gelfoam or Surgicel soaked with thrombin has been used successfully. Topical therapy plays an important role in prophylaxis and treatment after dental procedures.

Recombinant Factor VIIa.

Recombinant factor VIIa has been used successfully in patients with type 3 vWD with alloantibodies. In

Summary

- Thrombocytopenias are generally caused by one or a combination of the following: decreased production of platelets (bone marrow disorders), increased destruction of platelets (immune or mechanical), and splenic sequestration.
- ITP is often an idiopathic immune thrombocytopenia. Treatment includes corticosteroids, antibody therapy (IVIg or $Rh_o(D)$ immune globulin), rituximab, and splenectomy. Thrombopoietic agents are likely useful therapeutic options for refractory patients.
- TTP is characterized by otherwise unexplained thrombocytopenia, microangiopathic hemolytic anemia, and end-organ damage. Treatment involves urgent plasma exchange with or without adjunctive therapies, including corticosteroids, immunosuppressive agents, and rituximab.
- Drugs such as aspirin and clopidogrel are common causes of platelet dysfunction. Other causes include uremia, liver disease, and von Willebrand disease, congenital or acquired.
- Von Willebrand disease is the most common inherited bleeding disorder and mild forms are likely underdiagnosed. Treatment involves factor replacement before anticipated invasive procedures or surgery or after significant trauma. Desmopressin and local therapies are often effective for patients with milder forms.

addition, its use should be considered in patients with life-threatening bleeding in whom other measures have failed. Disadvantages include its high cost and the increased risk of thrombotic events, which are more pronounced in older adults.

Suggested Readings

Cines DB, Blanchette VS: Immune thrombocytopenic purpura. N Engl J Med 2002;346:995-1008.

Feinstein DI: Diagnosis and management of disseminated intravascular coagulation: The role of heparin therapy. Blood 1982;60:284-287.

George JN, Woolf SH, Raskob GE, et al: Idiopathic thrombocytopenic purpura: A practice guideline developed by explicit methods for the American Society of Hematology. Blood 1996;88:3-40.

Kottke-Marchant K: Laboratory diagnosis of hemorrhagic and thrombotic disorders. Hematol Oncol Clin North Am 1994;8:809-853.

Kurata Y, Hayashi S, Kiyoi T, et al: Diagnostic value of tests for reticulated platelets, plasma glycocalicin, and thrombopoietin levels for discriminating between hyperdestructive and hypoplastic thrombocytopenia. Am J Clin Pathol 2001;115:656-664.

Kuter DJ, Begley CG: Recombinant human thrombopoietin: Basic biology and evaluation of clinical studies. Blood 2002;100:3457-3469.

Mammen EF, Comp PC, Gosselin R, et al: PFA-100 system: A new method for assessment of platelet dysfunction. Semin Thromb Hemost 1998;24:195-202.

Mannucci PM: Treatment of von Willebrand disease. Thromb Haemost 2001;86:149-153.

McCrae KR, Herman JH: Posttransfusion purpura: Two unusual cases and a literature review. Am J Hematol 1996;52:205-211.

Moake JL: Thrombotic microangiopathies. N Engl J Med 2002;347:589-600.

Mozes MF, Spigos DG, Pollak R, et al: Partial splenic embolization, an alternative to splenectomy—results of a prospective, randomized study. Surgery 1984;96:694-702.

Warkentin TE, Chong BH, Greinacher A: Heparin-induced thrombocytopenia: Towards consensus. Thromb Haemost 1998;79:1-7.

Warkentin TE: Current agents for the treatment of patients with heparin-induced thrombocytopenia. Curr Opin Pulm Med 2002;8:405-412.

Weigert AL, Schafer AI: Uremic bleeding: pathogenesis and therapy. Am J Med Sci 1998;316:94-104.

References

For a complete list of references, log onto www.expertconsult.com.

Bleeding Disorders

Rachid Baz and *Tarek Mekhail*

EVALUATION

The accurate diagnosis and treatment of patients with bleeding require some basic understanding of the pathophysiology of hemostasis. The process is divided into primary and secondary components. Primary hemostasis is the formation of a platelet plug at the site of injury and occurs within seconds of injury. Secondary hemostasis involves the coagulation system and results in fibrin formation. It requires several minutes to complete. The fibrin strands strengthen the hemostatic platelet plug. This process is particularly important in bleeding originating from large vessels and in preventing recurrent bleeding hours or days after the initial injury (Fig. 1).

Bleeding disorders can thus be categorized into three groups: disorders of platelet function or number, disorders of clotting factors, and a combination of these. Platelet disorders are discussed elsewhere in this section ("Disorders of Platelet Function and Number"). A focused history, physical examination, and screening laboratory tests are of paramount importance in directing the evaluation in a time-saving and cost-effective manner.

HISTORY AND PHYSICAL EXAMINATION

The evaluation of the bleeding patient should be focused primarily on whether and how the patient is bleeding.

Determine if the patient is bleeding. Surrogate markers of bleeding (e.g., a declining hemoglobin level) are often subject to misinterpretation. Hence, deciding whether the patient is bleeding should not be based solely on a declining hemoglobin level or sudden hypotension. Hemolysis or hemodilution represent other causes of a decrease in the hemoglobin level.

If bleeding is suspected, identify the site and severity, duration of bleeding, and clinical setting. Mucocutaneous bleeding suggests a platelet disorder. It manifests as petechiae, ecchymoses, epistaxis, and genitourinary and gastrointestinal bleeding. Bleeding into potential spaces (joints, fascial planes, and retroperitoneum) suggests a coagulation factor deficiency. In hospitalized patients, bleeding from multiple sites can be seen with disseminated intravascular coagulation (DIC) or thrombotic thrombocytopenic purpura (TTP).

A complete history should include a past medical history; a history of human immunodeficiency virus (HIV) infection, liver or kidney disease, or malabsorption is often associated with bleeding. A medication history should be obtained, with particular attention to anticoagulants, nonsteroidal anti-inflammatory drugs (NSAIDs), oral contraceptives, antibiotics, ethanol, and dietary vitamins K and C. The response to past hemostatic challenges, such as trauma, tooth extraction, pregnancy, surgery, sports, and menstruation, should be determined. A family history of bleeding disorders may be helpful for assessing pathologic bleeding.

Acute massive mucocutaneous bleeding in a patient previously without symptoms should suggest immune thrombocytopenic purpura (ITP). Massive bruising and oozing from multiple sites in otherwise asymptomatic patients might suggest accidental warfarin ingestion or acquired factor VIII inhibitors (particularly in older patients). Postoperative bleeding at a surgical site is usually related to a local surgical problem. Spontaneous or excessive posttraumatic (immediate or delayed) bleeding can indicate a localized pathologic process or a disorder of the hemostatic process.

The physical examination should focus on identifying signs of bleeding (e.g., petechiae, mucosal bleeding, soft tissue bleeding, ecchymoses) as well as signs of systemic disease.

DIAGNOSTIC LABORATORY TESTING

Initial laboratory investigations should include a complete blood count (CBC), prothrombin time (PT), activated partial thromboplastin time (aPTT), and peripheral smear. A preoperative screen for a patient with a negative history and examination should include a CBC, PT, and aPTT only. The following is a brief description of tests available for the evaluation of hemorrhagic disorders.

In the platelet count, always verify thrombocytopenia by reviewing a peripheral smear. For example, platelet clumping with ethylenediaminetetraacetic acid (EDTA) does not represent true thrombocytopenia, and an accurate platelet count can be obtained by using citrated, or heparinized tubes.

The aPTT represents the time for clot formation after adding calcium, phospholipids, and kaolin to citrated blood. It is prolonged by heparin, direct thrombin inhibitors, a deficiency of or inhibitor for factors in the intrinsic and common pathways (e.g., factors II, V, VIII, IX, X, XI, and XII) as well as lupus anticoagulant, vitamin K deficiency, or severe liver disease.

The PT represents the time for clot formation after the addition of thromboplastin (tissue factor) and calcium to citrated blood. It is prolonged with deficiencies of factors II, V, VII, and X or fibrinogen; liver disease; vitamin K deficiency; and warfarin use. The international sensitivity index is a measure of thromboplastin sensitivity. Table 1 illustrates causes of a prolonged PT, aPTT, or both.

The thrombin time (TT) is the time to clot formation after the addition of thrombin to citrated blood. The TT is prolonged by heparin, direct thrombin inhibitors, fibrin degradation products (FDPs), paraproteins, and fibrinogen deficiency (qualitative and quantitative). Protamine is added to neutralize the heparin so the TT can be interpreted without heparin interference. This assay has been used to establish the presence of adequate fibrinogen but is not being used as widely now.

Reptilase time measures the time to clot formation after the addition of reptilase, a thrombin-like snake enzyme, to citrated blood. Unlike the TT, it is not affected by heparin. It can be useful to determine whether heparin is the cause of the prolonged TT.

The 1 : 1 mixing study is done when the PT or aPTT is prolonged. The patient's plasma is mixed with normal plasma, and the test is repeated. If the mixing of normal plasma corrects the abnormal result (PT or aPTT), a factor deficiency is suggested; otherwise, an inhibitor is suspected. Similarly, an incubated mixing study is done 1 hour (and occasionally 2 hours) after mixing of the patient's plasma with normal plasma. It is used to differentiate a lupus anticoagulant from clotting factor inhibitors; the latter usually results in immediate-acting inhibitors, whereas the former results in delayed inhibitors).

The urea clot solubility test relies on the ability of urea to dissolve unstable clots, which are formed in the absence of factor XIII. Normal clots are not dissolved by urea or monochloroacetic acid, unlike clots in patients with factor XIII deficiency.

Fibrin degradation products are fragments resulting from the action of plasmin on fibrin or fibrinogen and reflect high fibrinolysis states (such as DIC) when their levels are elevated.

D dimers are FDPs that can be measured specifically by enzyme-linked immunosorbent assay (ELISA). Their level is usually higher in DIC and in thrombotic conditions, such as deep venous thrombosis and pulmonary embolisms. Their elevation in the absence of symptoms does not imply the presence of these disorders.

Platelet function screening is performed on the PFA-100, which is a platelet function analyzer that is slowly supplanting the bleeding

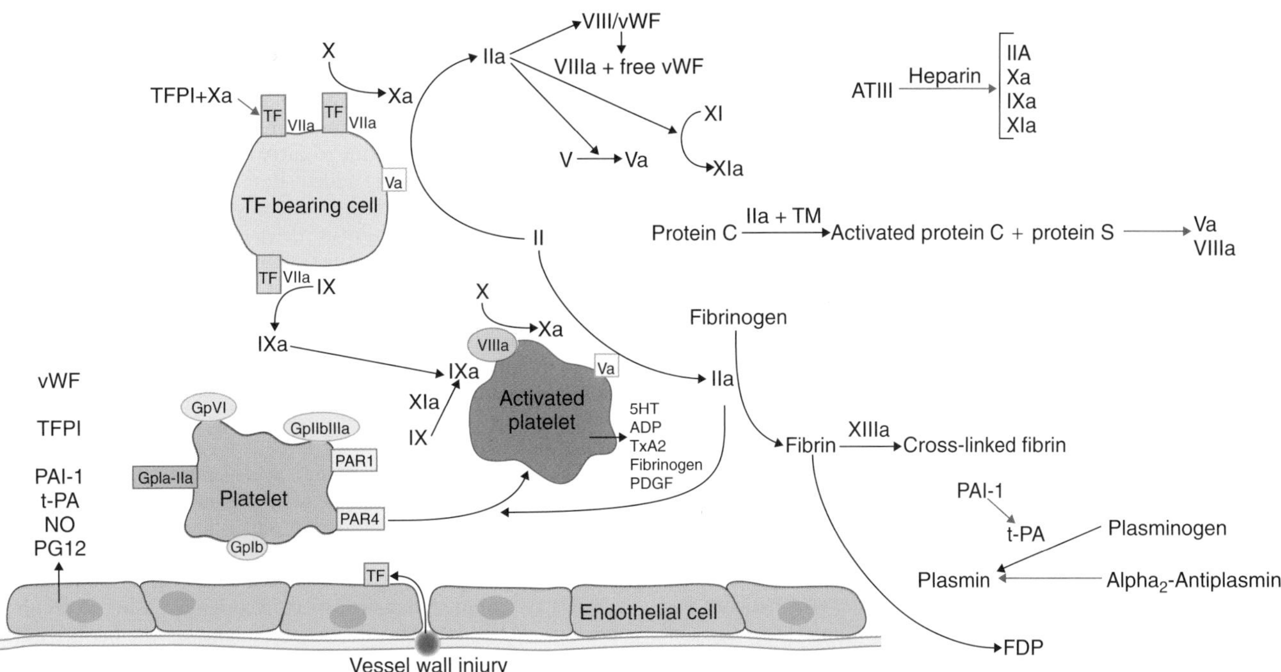

Figure 1 Overview of hemostasis. Vessel wall injury leads to expression of tissue factor (TF) on endothelial cells. TF complexes with factor VIIa to activate factors X and Xa in the presence of factor V, which leads to the activation of thrombin (IIa). Thrombin activates factors VIII, XI, and V fibrinogen to fibrin, as well as activating platelets to degranulate. This extrinsic pathway is turned off by tissue factor pathway inhibitor (TFPI), produced from endothelial cells. The intrinsic pathway-activated factor XIa activates factor IX, which in the presence of factor VIIIa activates factor X, resulting in the thrombin burst. Fibrin complexing with thrombin and factor XIII generates factor XIIIa, which cross-links fibrin strands. The fibrinolytic pathway plasminogen is converted to plasmin by tissue plasminogen activator (t-PA). Plasminogen activator inhibitor-1 (PAI-1) is produced by endothelial factor VIII. Antithrombin III (ATIII), a circulating plasma protease inhibitor, inhibits factors II, X, IX, and XI (its inhibition is further accentuated by binding to heparin). ADP, adenosine diphosphate; GpIa-IIa, glycoprotein Ia/IIa (binds collagen; deficiency causes mild bleeding diathesis); GpIb, glycoprotein Ib (binds vWF; deficiency causes Glanzmann's thrombasthenia); GpVI, glycoprotein VI (binds collagen; deficiency causes a severe bleeding diathesis); 5HT, serotonin; NO, nitric oxide; PAR1 and 4, protease-activated receptors 1 and 4 (thrombin receptors); PDGF, platelet-derived growth factor; PGI_2, prostaglandin I_2; TxA2, thromboxane A2; vWF, von Willebrand factor; *red arrows*, inhibition; *black arrows*, stimulation.

Table 1 Causes of Prolonged Prothrombin Time (PT) and Activated Partial Thromboplastin Time (aPTT)

Prolonged PT	Prolonged aPTT	Prolonged PT and aPTT
Inherited		
Factor VII deficiency	vWF, factor VIII, IX, XI, or XII deficiency	Prothrombin, fibrinogen, factor V, X or combined factor deficiency
Acquired		
Vitamin K deficiency	Heparin use	Liver disease
Liver disease	Inhibitor of vWF, factors VIII, IX, XI or XII	DIC
Warfarin use	Antiphospholipid antibodies	Supratherapeutic heparin or warfarin
Factor VII inhibitor		Combined heparin or warfarin use Inhibitor of prothrombin, fibrinogen, factor V or X Direct thrombin inhibitor

time in the clinical arena. It tests the ability of platelets to aggregate into two cartridges (collagen–adenosine diphosphate [ADP] and collagen-epinephrine). It has a reported sensitivity of approximately 95% and specificity of approximately 89% in detecting platelet dysfunction, and a 98% positive predictive value in detecting aspirin-induced platelet defects.

Platelet aggregation studies remain the gold standard in detecting platelet function defects. In these tests, platelet aggregation is tested in response to various agents: ADP, epinephrine, collagen, arachidonic acid, and ristocetin. Platelets of patients with Glanzmann thrombasthenia (dysfunctional or deficient glycoprotein IIb/IIIa complex in platelets) only aggregate with ristocetin, whereas platelets of patients with Bernard-Soulier syndrome (absent or decreased glycoprotein Ib complex on platelets) have no aggregation with ristocetin, reduced aggregation with collagen, and normal aggregation with ADP, arachidonic acid, and epinephrine.

von Willebrand factor (vWF) screening includes tests of platelet function. It has a low negative predictive value and can require repeat testing. It includes the vWF antigen (vWF:Ag)-immunoassay for circulating vWF, and vWF activity (vWF:RCo), which measures the functional ability of a patient's vWF to agglutinate platelets in the presence of ristocetin. Factor VIII:C activity is a functional assay for factor VIII that is measured by mixing normal plasma with factor VIII-deficient plasma. Levels of vWF:Ag and vWF:RCo may be elevated during pregnancy, oral contraceptive use, and liver disease. They are decreased by hypothyroidism and type O blood.

DISORDERS OF COAGULATION

Deficiencies or inhibitors of clotting factors, whether acquired or inherited, can result in bleeding disorders. Figure 1 illustrates the current understanding of the coagulation cascade. This section provides an overview of the hemophilias and of the less-common coagulation factor deficiencies and inhibitors.

Hemophilias

Inheritance and Incidence

Hemophilias are most commonly X-linked recessive diseases characterized by deficiency of factor VIII (hemophilia A) or factor IX (hemophilia B, or Christmas disease). The incidence is 1 per 5000 live births for hemophilia A and 1 per 30,000 live births for hemophilia B. In 30% of patients, hemophilia is the result of a de novo mutation, and no family history can be elicited. Males are most commonly affected; however, symptomatic females have been documented, and the proposed mechanisms include X chromosome inactivation or deletion, or the presence of a true homozygous offspring of an affected father and a carrier mother. Coinheritance of the factor V Leiden mutation occurs in about 5% of patients and results in a decreased bleeding tendency.[1] The clinical severity correlates well with factor levels, and they are clinically classified as mild (>5% of normal factor activity), moderate (1%-5% factor activity), and severe (<1% factor activity).

Clinical Features

The most common bleeding sites are joints (80% of bleeding), muscles, and the gastrointestinal mucosa. Ankles are the most commonly affected joints in children, whereas knees and elbows are more often involved in adults. Quadriceps and iliopsoas bleeding are the most common sites of muscle hematomas. Abdominal wall bleeding and gastrointestinal mucosal bleeding can occur. In most children, the hemophilia is already known at the time of first bleeding because of previous screening for a positive family history. In severe disease, bleeding occurs in the first 2 years of life; this contrasts with patients with milder disease, whose hemophilia can go undiagnosed for years. Late complications include hemarthroses and joint destruction, blood-borne infectious complications, and development of clotting factor inhibitors.

Diagnosis

The diagnosis is suggested by an elevated aPTT level in a male patient with a positive family history. This is tyically followed by a 1 : 1 mixing study with normal plasma, which corrects the aPTT level. Hemophilia B patients might have a normal aPTT. Factors VIII and IX levels are decreased in hemophilias A and B, respectively. A two-stage assay is recommended. It is more technically demanding but it is also more accurate, especially in patients with a mutation near the A domain of factor VIII, which makes the mutant factor less stable. Carrier detection often relies on DNA-based methodology rather than finding 50% factor activity. Genetic testing can identify patients at risk for inhibitor development; patients with a missense mutation or small deletion are less likely to develop inhibitors than patients with nonsense mutations or large deletions.

Treatment

Prevention. Prevention includes avoidance of contact sports, good oral hygiene, careful immunization techniques, timely replacement therapy after trauma, and treatment of acute bleeding episodes. Primary prophylactic therapy has been shown to reduce the incidence of arthropathy. However, considerable controversy surrounding factor use remains, especially with regard to the age at onset when this therapy is initiated and the expense.

Factor Replacement. Choices for replacing factor include recombinant versus plasma-derived factor VIII. Plasma-derived concentrates vary in purity and undergo viral inactivation procedures. First-generation recombinant products (Bioclate, Helixate FS, Kogenate, Recombinate) have demonstrated efficacy in clinical trials; however, they continue to carry a theoretic risk of viral transmission because of the added human albumin necessary for factor stabilization.[5] Second-generation recombinant products (Kogenate FS and B-domain deleted recombinant factor VIII [BDDrFVIII]) do not require albumin stabilization. Factor IX replacement has traditionally been with prothrombin complex concentrates (PCCs) that contain factors II, VII, and X, as well as IX, and were associated with thrombotic risk. Newer plasma-derived factor IX concentrates are effective, and they undergo viral inactivation. Recombinant factor IX concentrates are also effective and have no added albumin, hence eliminating a theoretic risk of viral infection.

The choice of replacement therapy depends on availability, safety, and cost, with the knowledge that plasma-derived products are becoming safer and recombinant products are less available and two or three times more costly. For patients with HIV infection, the use of recombinant products has been associated with a slower decline in CD4 cell count, and many experts recommend using recombinant products in that setting. However, it is unknown whether this advantage translates into improved clinical outcome. There is a suggestion that using recombinant products can result in a higher likelihood of inhibitor formation, which would be a theoretical benefit to the use of human products.

The desired factor level depends on the site and severity of bleeding: 30% to 40% factor activity is required for early joint or muscle bleeding, 50% factor activity is required for dental surgery or more-severe muscle bleeding, and 80% to 100% factor activity is required for life-threatening or serious bleeding (intracranial, intra-abdominal, or orthopedic surgery). Because the half-life of factor VIII is about 12 hours and that of factor IX 16 hours, factor levels should be checked every 12 hours and 16 hours, respectively.

The following formula is used to calculate the required dosage of factor VIII replacement:

$$\text{Dose (units)} = (\text{desired factor level} - \text{baseline factor level}) \times (\text{patient weight [kg]}/2)$$

For example, if a 60-kg patient with 1% factor level needs to undergo dental surgery, which requires correction to 50% of factor VIII level, 1500 units of factor VIII must be administered initially. This is usually followed by maintenance dosing (every 12 hours for factor VIII–deficient patients) at one half the initial dose. For patients with factor IX deficiency, the initial dose is calculated using the following formula:

$$\text{Dose (units)} = (\text{desired factor level} - \text{baseline factor level}) \times \text{patient weight (kg)} \times 1.2$$

The maintenance dose is usually equal to one half the initial dose and is given daily. Monitoring through factor levels is usually recommended after major trauma, bleeding, or surgery.

Desmopressin. Desmopressin (DDAVP) is the treatment of choice in patients with mild hemophilia A and mild to moderate bleeding, but it has no role in hemophilia B. The use of desmopressin is described for the treatment of von Willebrand disease (vWD) elsewhere in this section ("Disorders of Platelet Function and Number").

Antifibrinolytic Therapy. Antifibrinolytic therapy (in the form of tranexamic acid or ε-aminocaproic acid) is useful in controlling oral cavity bleeding and menorrhagia. For details on dosing, see elsewhere in this section for its use in patients with vWD ("Disorders of Platelet Function and Number").

Recombinant Factor VIIa. Hemophilia patients with high titers of inhibitors respond to recombinant factor VIIa. Although the recommended dosage schedule is 90 µg/kg every 2 hours until hemostasis is achieved, lower doses may be effective. Patients with lower titers of inhibitors might respond to higher doses of factor VIII replacement or factor VIII bypassing products.

Treatment of Long-Term Complications. Treatment of the long-term complications of hemophilia requires a multidisciplinary approach. Chronic hemarthroses may be managed with short-term prophylaxis and, at times, requires synovectomy, which can use arthroscopy or radioactive phosphorus. Experimental treatments with gene-targeted therapies are undergoing testing.

Coagulopathy of Liver Dysfunction

Most clotting factors are synthesized by the liver (except for von Willebrand factor, vWF, and tissue plasminogen activator), and the liver reticuloendothelial system is responsible for metabolizing most clotting factors. The characteristics of the coagulopathy of liver disease are presented in Table 2. Treatment involves correction of vitamin K deficiency, when present, and the judicious use of fresh-frozen plasma (FFP).

Rare Factor Deficiencies

Factor XI Deficiency

Factor XI deficiency is inherited as an autosomal trait. The incidence in the general population is estimated to be 1 in 1 million, but about 10% of Ashkenazi Jews are heterozygous. The bleeding tendency does not correlate with factor levels, and bleeding is worse from areas with high intrinsic fibrinolytic activity, such as the oral cavity or genitourinary tract. The propensity to bleed also seems to be increased in patients with a nonsense mutation compared with patients with a missense mutation. Treatment involves the use of FFP to achieve a factor XI level of 30% to 45% (despite the lack of clear consensus on the target factor XI activity). Factor XI concentrates are available in Europe and have the advantage of undergoing viral inactivation and having a smaller volume. However, they have been associated with DIC and increased thrombogenicity.

Factor X Deficiency

Factor X deficiency is a rare (1/1,000,000) autosomal recessive deficiency characterized by asymptomatic heterozygotes and by homozygotes with bleeding symptoms that correlate with factor activity. It can be acquired in association with amyloidosis, acute respiratory infections, and leukemias. The most common bleeding complications are hematomas, hemarthrosis, epistaxis, and menorrhagia. Treatment involves replacement with 10 to 15 mL/kg of PCCs, which contain a variable concentration of factor X, to a target of 15% to 20% factor X activity.

Factor VII Deficiency

Factor VII deficiency is a rare (1/500,000) autosomal recessive deficiency that exhibits little correlation between bleeding risk and factor activity. In general, less than 1% activity produces severe bleeding similar to that seen in the hemophilias, and more than 5% activity produces mild bleeding that is often localized to mucous membranes. Treatment involves the use of recombinant factor VIIa at a dose of 22 to 26 µg/kg (in contrast to a dose of 90 µg/kg in patients with hemophilia and inhibitors) to normalize the prothrombin time.

Factor V Deficiency

Factor V deficiency is a rare (1/1,000,000) autosomal recessive deficiency in which patients can manifest platelet-type bleeding (easy bruising, epistaxis, and oral bleeding). Patient can have an increased risk of thrombosis. Treatment involves replacement with FFP—an initial dose of 20 mL/kg followed by 5 mL/kg every 12 hours, with monitoring of factor V levels and bleeding—for a goal of 25% factor activity. Platelet transfusion may be required in severe bleeding, because platelets account for 20% of the total pool of factor V.

Factor II Deficiency

Factor II deficiency (prothrombin deficiency) is a rare (1/2,000,000) autosomal recessive disorder associated with mucosal and deep tissue bleeding. Treatment involves the use of PCCs, which contain varying concentrations of prothrombin. Factor survival analyses, measuring

Table 2 Coagulopathy of Liver Dysfunction

Test	Mild Hepatocellular Injury	Severe Hepatocellular Injury	Cirrhosis	Vitamin K Deficiency
PT	↑ N	↑	↑	↑
PTT	↑ N	↑	↑	↑
Factor VII	↓N	↓	↓	↓
Factors II, IX, and X	N	↓	↓	↓
D dimers	N	↑	↑	N
FSPs	N	↑	↑	N
Platelets	N	↓	↓	N
ATIII	N	N	↓	N
TT	N	↑	↑	N
Factor VIII	N	↓	↓	N

ATIII, antithrombin III; FSPs, fibrin split products; N, normal; PT, prothrombin time; PTT, partial thromboplastin time; TT, thrombin time; ↑, increased; ↓, decreased.

the effect of varying amounts of PCCs, are required to ensure proper dosing.

Congenital Afibrinogenemia

Congenital afibrinogenemia is a rare (1/1,000,000) autosomal recessive bleeding disorder characterized by the absence of fibrinogen. A high rate of consanguinity is noted, and carriers often have decreased fibrinogen levels. Early symptoms include umbilical stump bleeding; bleeding later in life can be life-threatening and involve any organ system. Patients with hypofibrinogenemia have mild bleeding only. Low levels of fibrinogen are more commonly seen in clinical practice in liver disease or DIC, or after the use of thrombolytics. Treatment involves replacement with cryoprecipitate—250 mg fibrinogen per 5- to 7-kg loading dose followed by a daily infusion of 250 mg/15 kg—to a target fibrinogen level of of 80 mg/L.1

Factor XIII Deficiency

Factor XIII deficiency is a rare (1/1,000,000) autosomal recessive disorder. Acquired factor XIII deficiency has been noted in patients with Henoch-Schönlein purpura, erosive gastritis, and leukemia. Bleeding occurs early in life, with umbilical stump bleeding. Later in life, bleeding occurs in skin, muscles, and the oral cavity, and it is often delayed after a hemostatic challenge.[11] Intracerebral bleeding occurs in 30% of patients and is a major cause of mortality. Hemarthroses are rare, and female patients have recurrent abortions if they do not receive replacement therapy. Diagnosis is by noting clot solubility in both 5 M urea and 1% monochloroacetic acid, and testing factor XIII activity. Treatment involves using factor XIII concentrates. Some experts have recommended primary prophylaxis with factor XIII concentrates, 1000 units every 6 weeks, or every 3 weeks in pregnant patients. FFP can be used when these concentrates are not available; FFP contains varying concentrations of factor XIII.

COAGULATION FACTOR INHIBITORS

Definition and Characterization

Coagulation factor inhibitors are antibodies that neutralize a specific clotting factor's function. They are called *alloantibodies* when they occur in patients with inherited factor deficiency, and they are called *autoantibodies* when they arise in patients without an inherited factor deficiency. The most commonly inhibited factor in clinical practice is factor VIII. The management of inhibitors of other clotting factors follows the same general guidelines and is not discussed here.

Incidence and Causes

Autoantibodies to factor VIII are characteristically oligoclonal non–complement-fixing immunoglobulin (Ig) G. Patients with lymphoproliferative disorders or multiple myeloma might have IgM or IgA antibodies. The incidence of factor VIII inhibitors is 0.2 to 1 in 1,000,000 person-years, with a higher incidence in older age groups. There is an equal sex distribution.

Associated conditions include connective tissue disorders (e.g., rheumatoid arthritis, systemic lupus erythematosus, myasthenia gravis, temporal arteritis, and pemphigus), drugs (e.g., penicillins, sulfa, interferon alfa), malignancy (e.g., lymphoproliferative disorders, graft-versus-host disease, prostate, renal, lung, or colon cancer), pregnancy (usually within 3 months of an uncomplicated first pregnancy and delivery), and idiopathic causes, especially in older adults.

Clinical Presentation

Soft tissue bleeding, gross hematuria, and postsurgical hemorrhage can occur; however, fatal bleeds take place in 15% of patients. Hemarthroses are rare. Laboratory tests are notable for a prolonged aPTT, which is not corrected by a 1:1 mixing study with normal plasma. Quantification of inhibitor titers is done with a Bethesda inhibitor assay; 1 Bethesda unit (BU) is the amount of antibody in the patient's plasma that permits detection of 50% residual factor activity when mixed with normal plasma.

Treatment

The treatment of factor VIII inhibitor is often directed at the cause, when known. For drug-induced inhibitors, discontinuing the drug responsible results in recovery within several months; most postpartum inhibitors resolve within 2 to 3 months after delivery.

For symptomatic patients, the treatment is aimed at managing the bleed and reducing the antibody titer. The latter involves immunosuppression with steroids, cyclophosphamide or azathioprine, biologic response modifiers (desmopressin), intravenous immunoglobulin (IVIg), or plasmapheresis. Prednisone 1 mg/kg/day for 3 to 6 weeks is the treatment of choice and results in about a 30% response rate. For patients who do not respond to steroids, cyclophosphamide 2 mg/kg/day for 6 weeks results in an added 30% response rate. Azathioprine has also been used as an immune suppressant. IVIg 0.4 g/kg/day for 5 days results in a 25% to 30% response rate. It is used for patients with contraindications to immune suppression.

Plasmapheresis can lower high-titer antibodies. It can be combined with a staphylococcal protein A column, which attaches to the Fc portion of the antibody, and results in a 50% to 90% decrease in circulating antibodies. Disadvantages include cost, difficulty of performing it in unstable patients, the need for central venous access, and the potential for circulatory collapse with the use of staphylococcal protein A.

The management of the bleeding patient includes replacing factor to overwhelm the antibody for low-titer antibody (<5 BU/mL) or using porcine factor VIII, activated thrombin complexes, or recombinant factor VIIa for patients with high-titer antibodies, because these patients would not respond to factor replacement in the form of factor VIII concentrates, FFP, or cryoprecipitate.

Summary

- A focused history and physical examination, as well as routine laboratory tests (including a complete blood count, prothrombin time, and activated partial thromboplastin time) are paramount in the diagnosis of suspected bleeding disorders.
- Hemophilia A, the most common inherited X-linked recessive disorder, is characterized by deficiency of factor VIII, which can be mild, moderate, or severe. Treatment includes prophylactic factor replacement before anticipated invasive procedures or surgery and after trauma.
- Other factor deficiencies are generally less common, and treatment guidelines similar to those for hemophilia therapy generally apply.
- Acquired inhibitors of clotting factors often cause severe bleeding in older patients without a prior history of bleeding diathesis. Treatment involves corticosteroids and immunosuppressive therapy.

Suggested Readings

Blanchette VS, Sparling C, Turner C: Inherited bleeding disorders. Baillieres Clin Haematol 1991;4:291-332.

Board PG, Losowsky MS, Miloszewski KJ: Factor XIII: Inherited and acquired deficiency. Blood Rev 1993;7:229-242.

Bolton-Maggs PH: Factor XI deficiency and its management. Haemophilia 2000;6(Suppl 1):100-109.

Bray GL, Gomperts ED, Courter S, et al: A multicenter study of recombinant factor VIII (recombinate): Safety, efficacy, and inhibitor risk in previously untreated patients with hemophilia A. The Recombinant Study Group. Blood 1994;83:2428-2435.

Kitchens CS: Approach to the bleeding patient. Hematol Oncol Clin North Am 1992;6:983-989.

Kottke-Marchant K: Laboratory diagnosis of hemorrhagic and thrombotic disorders. Hematol Oncol Clin North Am 1994;8:809-853.

Lee DH, Walker IR, Teitel J, et al: Effect of the factor V Leiden mutation on the clinical expression of severe hemophilia A. Thromb Haemost 2000;83:387-391.

Mammen EF: Coagulation abnormalities in liver disease. Hematol Oncol Clin North Am 1992;6:1247-1257.

Mannucci PM, Tuddenham EG: The hemophilias-from royal genes to gene therapy. N Engl J Med 2001;344:1773-1779.

Shapiro A: Inhibitor treatment: State of the art. Semin Hematol 2001;38:26-34.

White GC 2nd, Rosendaal F, Aledort LM, et al: Factor V, factor IXS: Definitions in hemophilia. Recommendation of the scientific subcommittee on factor VIII and factor IX of the scientific and standardization committee of the International Society on Thrombosis and Haemostasis. Thromb Haemost 2001;85:560.

Hypercoagulable States

Steven Deitcher

DEFINITION

The concept of a state of hypercoagulability dates back to 1854, when German pathologist Rudolph Virchow postulated that thrombosis resulted from, and in turn precipitated, three interrelated factors[1]: decreased blood flow (venous stasis), inflammation of or near the blood vessels (vascular endothelial injury), and intrinsic alterations in the nature of the blood itself. These "blood changes" alluded to in Virchow's triad have become what are now known as hypercoagulable states, or thrombophilias.

Hypercoagulable states can be defined as a group of inherited or acquired conditions associated with a predisposition to venous thrombosis (including upper and lower extremity deep venous thrombosis with or without pulmonary embolism, cerebral venous thrombosis, and intra-abdominal venous thrombosis), arterial thrombosis (including myocardial infarction, stroke, acute limb ischemia, and splanchnic ischemia), or both. Venous thromboembolic disease is the most common clinical manifestation resulting from hypercoagulable states. Although most inherited conditions appear to increase only the risk of venous thromboembolic events (VTEs), some of the acquired conditions have been associated with both VTEs and arterial thrombosis. These include cancer, myeloproliferative syndromes, antiphospholipid antibodies (APAs), hyperhomocysteinemia, and heparin-induced thrombocytopenia.

Most hypercoagulable states alter the blood itself, whereas others affect the vasculature directly. Although patients with hypercoagulable states are at greater risk for developing a thrombotic event than those without such disorders, not all persons with a well-defined hypercoagulable state will develop an overt thrombosis and not all persons with thrombosis have an identifiable hypercoagulable state. In fact, in 2003, testing for an inherited hypercoagulable state was likely to uncover an abnormality in more than 60% of patients presenting with idiopathic (i.e., spontaneous or unprovoked) VTEs (Fig. 1).[2] Although the remaining 30% to 40% would have unremarkable test results, this does not imply a true absence of a hypercoagulable state. Some of these individuals may have an acquired condition such as cancer or APA, and others may have a disorder or defect that has not yet been discovered or characterized. This can be illustrated by the fact that before 1993—before the discoveries of factor V Leiden and the prothrombin G20210A mutation—an inherited predisposition to hypercoagulability was identified in only 15% to 20% of patients presenting with idiopathic VTEs.[2]

This chapter will focus on the most common hypercoagulable states and their association with VTEs. Readers are referred to reports on the association between hypercoagulable states and arterial thrombosis.[3,4] Specific derangements that will be reviewed in this chapter include activated protein C resistance, factor V Leiden, prothrombin G20210A mutation, deficiencies of natural anticoagulants (antithrombin, protein C, and protein S), APAs, and hyperhomocysteinemia. Although it is beyond the scope of this chapter to review the association between cancer and thrombosis or to discuss issues pertaining to cancer screening following VTEs, malignant diseases are likely the most common acquired hypercoagulable state. At a minimum, appropriate age- and gender-specific cancer screening must be considered after VTEs, particularly in older individuals and in young patients with idiopathic VTEs but without laboratory evidence for a hypercoagulable state. Guidelines for the early detection of cancer have been updated by the American Cancer Society.[5]

ETIOLOGY

Hypercoagulable states can be inherited, acquired, or both. Activated protein C (APC) resistance secondary to factor V Leiden, prothrombin G20210A mutation, and deficiencies of natural anticoagulants are examples of inherited conditions, whereas APAs are an acquired set of disorders. Hyperhomocysteinemia can be precipitated by both genetic defects and acquired medical conditions, including vitamin deficiency states.

Factor V Leiden, or factor V G1691A, is a single-point mutation in the gene that codes for coagulation factor V.[2] It involves a G (guanine)-to-A (adenine) substitution at nucleotide 1691 (G1691A) in exon 10, which predicts the replacement of arginine at amino acid residue 506 by glutamine (Arg506Gln).[6] The mutation, transmitted through autosomal dominant inheritance, renders factor V resistant to inactivation by APC (a natural anticoagulant protein). Factor V Leiden accounts for 92% of cases of APC resistance (APC-R), with the remaining 8% of cases resulting from pregnancy, oral contraceptive use, cancer, select APA, and other factor V point mutations. Therefore, the terms *factor V Leiden* and *APC-R* should not be considered synonymous; in fact, APC-R is an independent risk factor for VTEs, even in the absence of factor V Leiden. It is estimated that the mutation arose in a single white ancestor some 21,000 to 34,000 years ago, well after the evolutionary separation of non-Africans from Africans (approximately 100,000 years ago) and of Caucasoid (white non-Africans) from Mongoloid (Asians) subpopulations (approximately 60,000 years ago).[7]

Prothrombin G20210A is a single-point mutation (G-to-A substitution at nucleotide 20210) in the 3′ untranslated region of the prothrombin (coagulation factor II) gene.[2] This autosomal dominant mutation appears to result in elevated concentrations of plasma prothrombin. Like factor V Leiden, the prothrombin G20210A mutation arose in a single common white founder, and probably also occurred after the evolutionary divergences of subpopulations.[8]

Over 100 different mutations have been detected in the genes that code for each of the natural anticoagulant proteins (protein C, protein S, and antithrombin), resulting in quantitative (type I) or qualitative (type II) deficiencies.[9] Both antithrombin and protein S deficiencies have an autosomal dominant pattern of inheritance.[10,11] Protein C deficiency was believed to be inherited in an autosomal dominant pattern, with incomplete penetrance. Studies have suggested that protein C deficiency is an autosomal recessive disorder and that coinheritance of another defect, particularly factor V Leiden, results in a high degree of penetrance that appears as dominant inheritance in double-heterozygous carriers.[12,13]

APAs consist of two major subgroups, the lupus anticoagulants and the anticardiolipin antibodies. Lupus anticoagulants are detected by their ability to prolong phospholipid-dependent coagulation tests in vitro (e.g., activated partial thromboplastin time and dilute Russell viper venom time). Anticardiolipin antibodies are detected by the enzyme-linked immunosorbent assay (ELISA).[14] APAs that occur in association with autoimmune disorders, such as systemic lupus erythematosus, Sjögren's syndrome, rheumatoid arthritis, and mixed connective tissue disease, as well as in the setting of cancer, are considered secondary;[15] APAs detected in those without any obvious underlying autoimmune or malignant diseases are called primary. APAs have also been reported in conjunction with idiopathic autoimmune hemolytic anemia, malaria, syphilis, Q fever, infections by mycobacteria, *Pneumocystis jiroveci*, cytomegalovirus, and after exposure to drugs such as neuroleptics, quinidine, and procainamide.[14,16]

The metabolism of the amino acid homocysteine consists of a vitamin B_6-dependent trans-sulfuration pathway involving the enzyme cystathionine β-synthase (CBS) and a folate- and vitamin B_{12}–dependent remethylation pathway involving the enzymes methylenetetrahydrofolate reductase (MTHFR) and methionine synthase (Fig. 2).[17,18] Inherited severe hyperhomocysteinemia (plasma level >100 μmol/L), as seen in classic homocystinuria, may result from homozygous MTHFR or CBS deficiencies and, more rarely, from inherited errors of cobalamin (vitamin B_{12}) metabolism.[19] Inherited mild to moderate hyperhomocysteinemia (plasma level 15-100 μmol/L) may result from heterozygous MTHFR and CBS deficiencies, but most commonly results from the C677T gene polymorphism, which is the most common mutation in the gene that codes for the MTHFR enzyme.[18,19] This single-point mutation (C677T) in the coding region for the MTHFR binding site (exon 4) is autosomal recessive, leads to the substitution of a valine for an alanine, and results in a thermolabile variant of the MTHFR (tlMTHFR).[18] Acquired hyperhomocysteinemia in the absence of any mutation or polymorphism may be caused by folate deficiency, vitamins B_6 and B_{12} deficiencies, renal failure, diabetes mellitus, hypothyroidism, carcinoma, pernicious anemia, inflammatory bowel disease, and methotrexate, theophylline, or phenytoin therapy.[17,18]

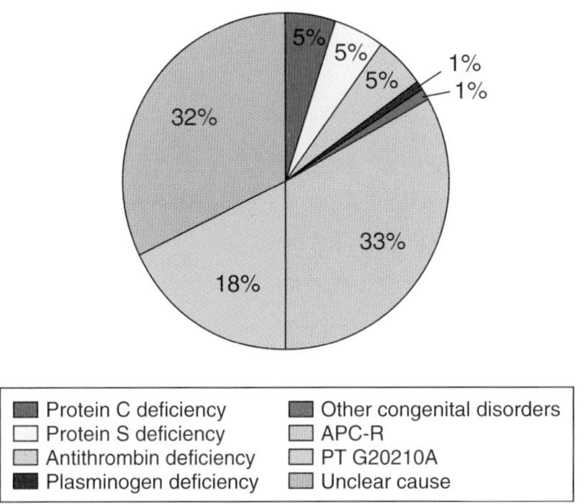

Figure 1 Results of testing for congenital hypercoagulable states projected for patients with idiopathic deep venous thrombosis in 2003. APC-R, activated protein C resistance; PT G20210A, prothrombin G20210A mutation.

Individuals who are heterozygous for the tlMTHFR variant have normal plasma homocysteine levels, whereas homozygous carriers may have mild to moderate fasting hyperhomocysteinemia in the setting of concomitant folate deficiency.[17,19] However, homozygosity for the tlMTHFR in the absence of hyperhomocysteinemia does not appear to be associated with an increased risk of VTEs, and most patients with hyperhomocysteinemia do not have the tlMTHFR polymorphism.[19] Excess homocysteine in the plasma is the risk factor and is the target of therapeutic intervention, not the C677T mutation.

PREVALENCE

The prevalence of hypercoagulable states depends on the ethnicity and clinical history of the studied population. Prevalence is lowest in the general population, greater in individuals with a single VTE, and highest in those with recurrent VTEs or who are from known thrombophilic families (Table 1).[20]

APC-R caused by factor V Leiden is the most common inherited predisposition to hypercoagulability in white populations of northern European background.[2] Factor V Leiden follows a geographic and ethnic distribution; it occurs most frequently in northern and western Europe (the highest prevalence of 15% has been reported in Sweden), but high prevalences are also found in Cyprus (13%), Turkey (9%), and the Middle East (5.4%).[21] The mutation is also found in whites from eastern Europe and South America (prevalences of 2%-4%), but is rare in the Asian and African continents as well as in ethnic groups of Asian descent, such as the Inuit Eskimos, Native Americans, Australian aboriginals, and Polynesians.[21] In the United States, factor V Leiden is most commonly seen in whites (6%), with lower prevalences in Latin Americans (2.2%), African Americans and Native Americans (1.2%), and Asian Americans (0.45%).[22]

The prothrombin G20210A mutation is the second most common inherited predisposition to hypercoagulability, occurring more frequently in whites of southern European background. In fact, the 3%

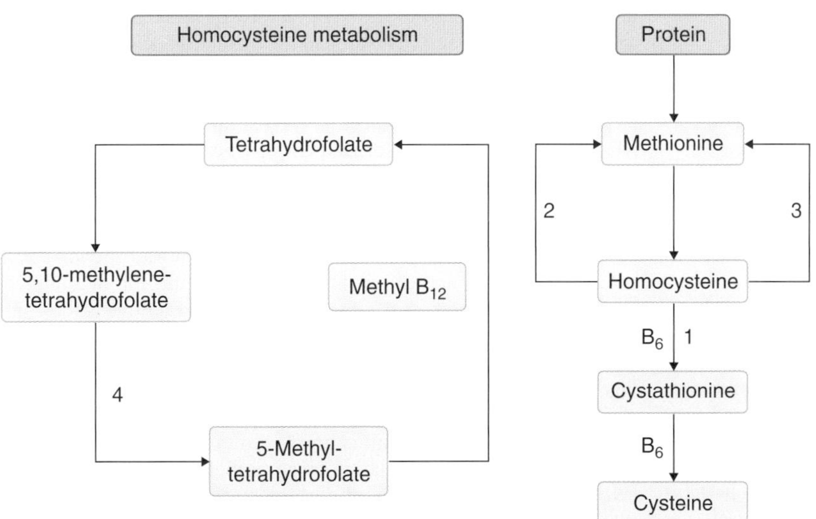

Figure 2 Homocysteine metabolism.

Table 1 Prevalence of Major Hypercoagulable States in Different Patient Populations

Hypercoagulable State	General Population (%)	Patients with Single VTE (%)	Thrombophilic Families (%)
Factor V Leiden	3-7	20	50
Prothrombin G20210A	1-3	6	18
Antithrombin deficiency	0.02	1	4-8
Protein C deficiency	0.2-0.4	3	6-8
Protein S deficiency	N/A	1-2	3-13
Hyperhomocysteinemia	5-10	10-25	N/A
Antiphospholipid antibodies	0-7	5-15	N/A

N/A, not readily available or unknown; VTE, venous thromboembolic event.
Data from Rosendaal FR: Risk factors for venous thrombosis: prevalence, risk, and interaction. Semin Hematol 1997;34:171-187.

prevalence in southern Europe is almost twice the prevalence observed in northern Europe.[23] Similar to factor V Leiden, the prothrombin G20210A mutation is also found in the Middle East and Indian regions, but is virtually absent in individuals of African and eastern Asian backgrounds.[23] These distributions provide support to the estimate that both mutations (factor V Leiden and prothrombin G20210A) originated relatively recently in the European founding population, after the evolutionary divergences of subpopulations.

The deficiencies of natural anticoagulants are rare in the general population and, combined, are found in less than 15% of all individuals with a single VTE (see Table 1 and Fig. 1). The prevalence of APA (an acquired set of disorders) is significantly higher in patients with autoimmune disorders than in healthy individuals from the general population. In patients with systemic lupus erythematosus, the reported average prevalences for lupus anticoagulants and anticardiolipin antibodies are 34% and 44%, respectively.[15]

PATHOPHYSIOLOGY

Appreciation of the mechanisms whereby hypercoagulable states lead to pathologic thrombosis requires an understanding of normal hemostasis, which comprises two equally important processes, primary hemostasis and secondary hemostasis. Although described as separate events, both primary and secondary hemostases occur concurrently at a site of vascular injury.

Primary hemostasis consists of three events that lead to the formation of a platelet plug—namely, platelet adhesion, platelet activation, and platelet aggregation. Platelets adhere to the vascular subendothelium by attaching to subendothelial von Willebrand factor molecules exposed at a site of vascular injury. Once adherent, platelets are activated by a number of agonists, including thrombin, collagen, epinephrine, and thromboxane A_2, and are stimulated to release their alpha and dense granule contents, which further promote platelet recruitment, activation, and aggregation. After additional platelets are recruited, they are linked by fibrinogen through the surface glycoprotein IIb/IIIa receptors to form the platelet plug.

Secondary hemostasis consists of a series of sequential reactions, a coagulation cascade, in which inactive protease zymogens are converted to active serine proteases, ultimately resulting in the production of thrombin and covalently cross-linked fibrin (Fig. 3). In response to vascular injury, the in vivo coagulation cascade is triggered by the exposure of tissue factor. Tissue factor not only

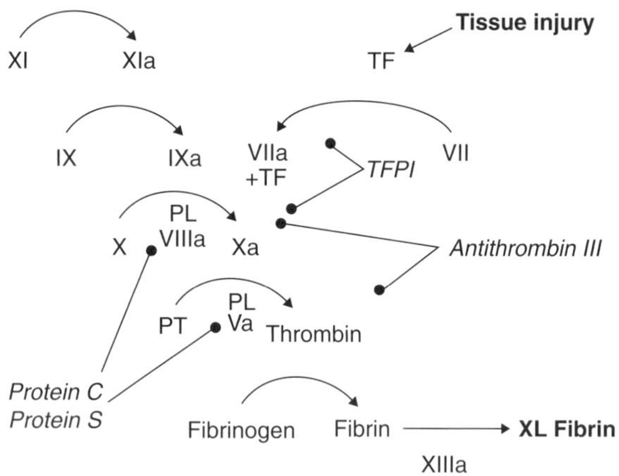

Figure 3 Coagulation cascade. PT, prothrombin time; TF, tissue factor; TFPI, tissue factor pathway inhibitor; XL, cross-linked.

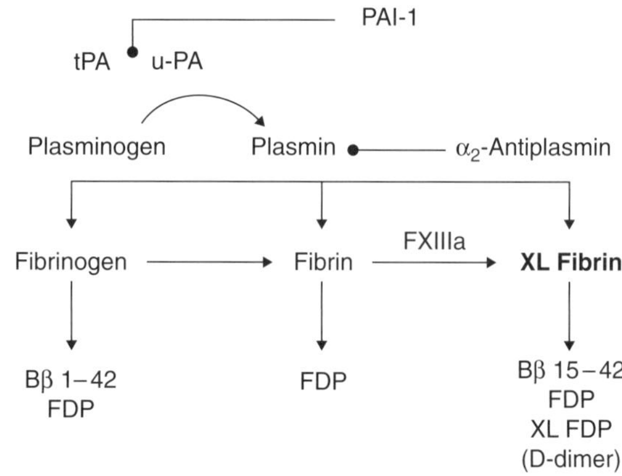

Figure 4 Fibrinolytic pathways. PAI-1, plasminogen activator inhibitor-1; tPA, tissue plasminogen activator; u-PA, urokinase plasminogen activator; FDP, fibrinogen degradation products; XL, cross-linked.

complexes with trace amounts of activated factor VII, present in the circulation of normal individuals, but also activates factor VII to factor VIIa. The complex formed by factor VIIa and tissue factor then activates factors IX and X, leading to the formation of small amounts of thrombin. However, this pathway is rapidly downregulated by tissue factor pathway inhibitor. Nevertheless, potent positive feedback by thrombin itself results in the activation of factor XI to factor XIa, which can activate factor IX, hence perpetuating the production of thrombin and, subsequently, of a fibrin clot. Thrombin also promotes ongoing thrombosis by activation of factors VIII, V, and XIII. Factor VIIIa functions as a cofactor during the activation of factor X to Xa, catalyzed by factor IXa. Factor Va functions as a cofactor during the activation of prothrombin to thrombin, catalyzed by factor Xa. The end result of these sequential reactions is the conversion of fibrinogen to fibrin monomers. Factor XIIIa cross-links fibrin to promote the development of a stabilized platelet plug (see Fig. 3).

The natural anticoagulants function to confine thrombus formation to the site of vascular injury and to limit thrombus size. Whereas it promotes ongoing coagulation by a number of positive feedbacks, thrombin also provides an important negative feedback to limit thrombus formation by binding to thrombomodulin on endothelial cells. The thrombin-thrombomodulin complex then converts protein C to APC. Antithrombin and protein C are the major natural anticoagulants, and protein S serves as a vital cofactor for APC-mediated inactivation of factors Va and VIIIa (see Fig. 3).

Vascular endothelial disruption triggers not only coagulation reactions but also the fibrinolytic pathways (Fig. 4). Physiologic fibrinolysis is initiated by endothelial cell-derived tissue plasminogen activator (tPA)-mediated conversion of plasminogen to plasmin. Plasmin can degrade fibrinogen and fibrin, thus limiting the size of a thrombus and helping to clear a thrombus once the vascular injury has been repaired. The fibrinolytic pathways are regulated by the inhibitory proteins α_2-antiplasmin and plasminogen activator inhibitor-1.

Therefore, the human hemostatic system can be defined as consisting of multiple independent yet integrally related cellular and protein components; these function to maintain blood fluidity under normal conditions and to promote localized, temporary thrombus formation at sites of vascular injury (Fig. 5). The six major components of this hemostatic system are vascular endothelium, platelets, plasma coagulation proteins or "factors," natural anticoagulant proteins, fibrinolytic proteins, and antifibrinolytic proteins. In the presence of an intact endothelium, there is no clot formation taking place inside the blood vessels, even though a low, basal, physiologic level of coagulation factor activation is occurring continuously. This highly regulated hemostatic system maintains a delicate balance between a prohemorrhagic and prothrombotic state, which is maintained by the concomitant actions of platelets, coagulation factors, and fibrinolytic inhibitors (on one side of the hemostatic scale), and of natural anticoagulants and fibrinolytic proteins (on the other side of the scale), as shown in Figure 6. Marked thrombocytosis, accentuated platelet aggregation, increased activity levels of coagulation factors, and excess plasma levels of fibrinolytic inhibitors may lead to pathologic thrombosis. Similarly, quantitative or qualitative deficiencies of a natural anticoagulant coagulation factor resistance to inactivation by a natural anticoagulant (in the specific case of factor V Leiden), and a deficiency of a fibrinolytic protein, may all be associated with a state of hypercoagulability. Thus, it is not surprising that a multitude of potential hypercoagulable states have been described (Box 1).

The factor V Leiden mutation renders factors V and Va partially but not completely resistant to inactivation by APC.[2,6] APC inactivates factor Va in an orderly and sequential series of cleavages, first at Arg506 and then at Arg306 and Arg679.[6] This partial resistance is explained by the fact that cleavage of factor Va by APC at Arg306 continues to occur, although at a slower rate. In fact, factor V Arg-506Gln (factor V Leiden) is inactivated 10 times slower than normal factor Va.[24] This provides a pathophysiologic explanation for why factor V Leiden, although common, is a relatively weak risk factor for VTEs. Because factor Va functions as a cofactor in the conversion of prothrombin to thrombin, the mutation results in greater amounts

Box 1 Established or Potential Hypercoagulable States

- Activated protein C resistance
- Alpha-macroglobulin deficiency
- Anticardiolipin antibodies
- Antithrombin deficiency
- Dysfibrinogenemia
- Factor V Leiden
- Factor V deficiency, excess
- Factor VII excess
- Factor VIII excess
- Factor XI excess
- Heparin cofactor II deficiency
- Hyperhomocysteinemia
- Hyperfibrinogenemia
- Lupus anticoagulants
- PAI-1 excess
- Plasminogen deficiency
- Protein C deficiency
- Protein S deficiency
- Prothrombin G20210A
- tPA deficiency
- TFPI deficiency
- Thrombomodulin deficiency

PAI-1, plasminogen activator inhibitor-1; TFPI, tissue factor pathway inhibitor; tPA, tissue plasminogen activator.

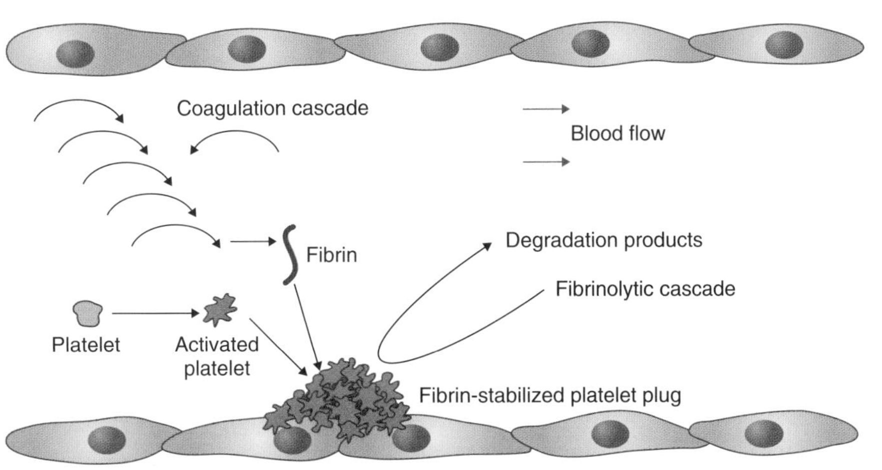

Figure 5 Normal hemostasis.

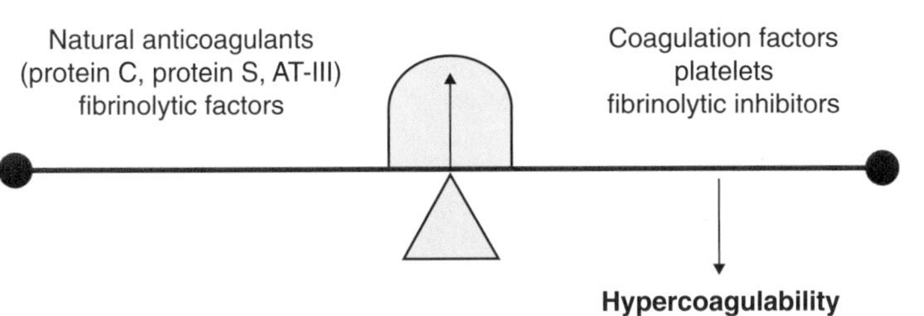

Figure 6 Hemostatic balance. AT-III, antithrombin III.

of factor Va available for coagulation reactions, shifting the hemostatic balance toward more thrombin generation.[2,9]

By unknown mechanisms, the prothrombin G20210A mutation results in elevated concentrations of plasma prothrombin, which is the immediate precursor of thrombin. The tendency to hypercoagulability is believed to be derived from the greater availability of prothrombin for conversion to thrombin.[2]

Antithrombin is the primary inhibitor of thrombin and the other serine proteases, factors XIIa, XIa, Xa, and IXa. Deficiency of antithrombin leads to enhanced thrombin formation. Complete deficiency of antithrombin likely leads to unfettered thrombin formation and hypercoagulability to degrees that are fatal in utero. Protein C, in its activated form (APC), controls the formation of thrombin in the presence of its cofactor, free protein S. Thus, in the setting of protein C or protein S deficiency, thrombin formation is also enhanced, leading to hypercoagulability.[9] Type I deficiencies of natural anticoagulants are characterized by low antigen and activity (functional) levels of the deficient natural anticoagulant, whereas type II defects are characterized by normal (total) antigen levels but low activity, dysfunctional molecules.[6,10,11] Under normal conditions, protein S exists in plasma in two forms, bound to C4b-binding protein (60% of total) and free (40% of total). Because only free protein S has cofactor activity, a type III protein S has been described, consisting of low activity and free antigen levels but with a normal total antigen level.[6,11] This type III protein S deficiency may result from excess C4b-binding protein or free protein S inhibitory and clearing antibodies.[25] The exact mechanisms whereby APAs cause thrombosis are unknown. Some proposed mechanisms include the following: acquired APC-R: stimulation of platelet adhesion, activation, and aggregation; upregulation of the tissue factor pathway; enhanced expression of cell adhesion molecules; and reduction of the free protein S level by inducing protein S binding to C4b-binding protein.[14,16] One mechanism described for APA-associated fetal loss involves the presence of trophoblast-reactive antibodies that disrupt the annexin V shield on trophoblast cell membranes, thus enhancing thromboxane A_2 production and leading to placental insufficiency.[14]

The pathophysiology of thrombosis in hyperhomocysteinemia is also unclear. Proposed mechanisms include direct endothelial injury, increased tissue factor activity, inhibition of protein C activation, increased platelet activation and aggregation, suppression of thrombomodulin expression, and impaired fibrinolysis by inhibition of tPA binding to its endothelial cell receptor.[17,18]

SIGNS AND SYMPTOMS

There are no specific signs or symptoms associated with hypercoagulable states. The finding of livedo reticularis on examination of the skin has been frequently associated with the presence of APA, but a true causality has not been established. The most common clinical manifestation of an underlying hypercoagulable state is lower extremity deep venous thrombosis, with or without pulmonary embolism. Because the clinical signs and symptoms associated with deep venous thrombosis and pulmonary embolism are insensitive and nonspecific, objective diagnostic confirmation by the use of an imaging method, such as contrast venography and duplex ultrasound, is mandatory. Other less common or unusual clinical presentations of venous thrombosis appear to occur more commonly, but not exclusively, in certain hypercoagulable states, as depicted in Table 2.

The risk of a first VTE varies, depending on the hypercoagulable state being considered (Table 3).[2,14,19,20] This risk is usually expressed as relative risk. Although the relative risk is useful in comparing the VTE rates between a patient population with a given disorder and normal controls, the absolute risk is the best measure to assess the importance of a given risk factor for an individual patient.[2] This is particularly important, considering the fact that the baseline risk of thrombosis for women and men increases exponentially with age.[20]

Table 2 Unusual Venous Thrombotic Presentations of Certain Hypercoagulable States

VTE Presentation	Hypercoagulable Condition
Cerebral venous thrombosis	Prothrombin G20210A, antiphospholipid antibodies, antithrombin deficiency, essential thrombocythemia, paroxysmal nocturnal hemoglobinuria
Cerebral venous thrombosis in women using oral contraceptive pills	Prothrombin G20210A
Inferior vena cava, renal venous, mesenteric venous, portal and hepatic venous thromboses	Antiphospholipid antibodies, cancer, antithrombin deficiency, myeloproliferative syndromes, paroxysmal nocturnal hemoglobinuria
Migratory superficial thrombophlebitis (Trousseau's syndrome)	Cancer (particularly adenocarcinoma of the gastrointestinal tract)
Recurrent superficial thrombophlebitis	Factor V Leiden, polycythemia vera, deficiencies of natural anticoagulants
Warfarin skin necrosis	Protein C and protein S deficiencies
Neonatal purpura fulminans	Homozygous protein C and protein S deficiencies
Unexplained fetal loss (three or more first-trimester miscarriages or one second- or third-trimester unexplained death of a morphologically normal fetus)	Antiphospholipid antibodies

VTE, venous thromboembolic event.

DIAGNOSIS

Laboratory testing for hypercoagulable states can uncover an inherited abnormality in more than 60% of patients presenting with a first VTE (see Fig. 1). However, testing is costly, it rarely influences acute VTE management, and its results are frequently misinterpreted, which may lead to a non–evidence-based use of antithrombotic drugs and inappropriate justification of lifelong therapy. More important, a focus exclusively on hypercoagulable state testing may undermine the performance of age- and gender-specific cancer screening in patients with idiopathic VTEs. In the absence of validated guidelines, testing for hypercoagulable states should be performed only in select patients, and only if the results will significantly affect management.

Who Should Be Tested?

Select testing should be considered mainly in the following circumstances:

- Idiopathic (i.e., spontaneous) VTE
- VTE at young age (<45 years)
- Recurrent VTE
- VTE in unusual sites (see Table 2)
- VTE in the setting of a strong family history of VTE
- Recurrent pregnancy loss (more than three consecutive first-trimester pregnancy losses without an intercurrent term pregnancy)

Table 3 Relative Risks of a First VTE in Select Hypercoagulable States

Hypercoagulable State	Relative Risk of Lifetime Single VTE
Factor V Leiden	2-10
Prothrombin G20210A	2-6
Factor V Leiden and prothrombin G20210A ("double heterozygous")	20.0
Protein C deficiency	6.5-31*
Protein S deficiency	2-36*
Antithrombin deficiency	5-40*
Hyperhomocysteinemia	2-4
Lupus anticoagulant	11
Anticardiolipin antibodies	3.2

*Relative risks are highly variable, depending on whether they were derived from population- or family-based studies. Differences in risk can be explained in part by greater difficulty in obtaining reliable population-based estimates because of the overall low prevalence of these disorders. It is also possible that event rates were overestimated in early familial studies.
VTE, venous thromboembolic event.
Data from Deitcher SR, Caiola E, Jaffer A: Demystifying two common genetic predispositions to venous thrombosis. Cleve Clin J Med 2000;67:825-826, 829, 833-836; Levine JS, Branch DW, Rauch J: The antiphospholipid syndrome. N Engl J Med 2002;346:752-763; De Stefano V, Casorelli I, Rossi E, et al: Interaction between hyperhomocysteinemia and inherited thrombophilic factors in venous thromboembolism. Semin Thromb Hemost 2000;26:305-311; Rosendaal FR: Risk factors for venous thrombosis: prevalence, risk, and interaction. Semin Hematol 1997;34:171-187.

Testing should be strongly considered for patients who present with two or more of these criteria. It may also be considered for select asymptomatic individuals, particularly female relatives of patients with known inherited hypercoagulability, provided that the results will affect their decision to begin oral contraceptive pill (OCP) use or hormone replacement therapy (HRT).

Why Should a Patient Be Tested?

Testing should be performed if the results will affect management by guiding the following:

- Duration of anticoagulation therapy
- Choice of anticoagulant agent
- Intensity of anticoagulation therapy
- Therapeutic monitoring strategies
- Family screening
- Family planning
- Choice of concomitant medications

The issue of OCP use and HRT in the setting of an inherited hypercoagulable state remains a matter of intense debate. Both groups of medications are associated with a two- to sixfold increased relative risk of a VTE in women without hypercoagulable states.[26] Based on data from the Leiden Thrombophilia Study,[27] the risk of a VTE is increased sevenfold in heterozygous carriers of factor V Leiden. The relative risk of VTEs is increased exponentially in women taking an OCP who are carriers of factor V Leiden (35-fold) and prothrombin G 20210A (16-fold).[28,29] The VTE risk appears even higher in women homozygous for factor V Leiden, and an absolute risk of VTEs of 4% per year has been reported in women who are taking an OCP and carry a natural anticoagulant deficiency.[30,31] OCP

Table 4 Interaction of Factor V Leiden and Oral Contraceptive Pill (OCP) Use and Relative Risk of Venous Thromboembolic Disease

Parameter	Relative Risk	Absolute Risk*
Noncarrier women	1	0.8/10,000
Noncarrier women on OCP	4	3.2/10,000
Factor V Leiden heterozygosity	7	5.7/10,000
Factor V Leiden heterozygous woman on OCP	35	28.5/10,000

*Estimated number of cases of VTE/10,000 persons/year.[28]
VTE, venous thromboembolic event.

users who carry the prothrombin G20210A mutation also have a 150-fold increased risk of cerebral venous thrombosis.[32]

It is not currently recommended that all asymptomatic women be screened before initiation of such therapies, mainly because it is not cost effective.[33] It is clear, however, that the combination of factor V Leiden with OCP use leads to an exponential increase in the relative risk of VTEs, even though the absolute risk still remains fairly low (Table 4). Thus, in asymptomatic women with a family history of VTEs, select testing may be considered if the results of testing will affect a woman's decision to proceed with OCP use. It is generally recommended that OCP use be avoided in the setting of objectively and properly confirmed antithrombin, protein C, and protein S deficiency states because of the high annual rates of VTEs reported in this group of women.[31,33] However, current evidence does not allow that such a firm recommendation be made regarding OCP use in a woman with factor V Leiden or even prothrombin G20210A mutation heterozygosity. This is because OCPs remain the most effective form of prescribed contraception, and the increased risk of VTEs associated with the presence of factor V Leiden or prothrombin G20210A heterozygosity needs to be balanced against the possibility of unwanted pregnancy, with its attendant 9- to 15-fold increased risk of VTEs in this same population.[34]

The relative risk of VTEs is also further increased (by 15-fold) in women on HRT who are heterozygous for factor V Leiden. The epidemiologic importance of this increased risk lies in the fact that women on HRT belong to an older group than those on OCP, with a baseline risk of VTEs between 1 in 100 to 1000 persons (instead of 1/10,000 persons)/year.[26] Thus, it is likely that the impact of a 15-fold increased risk of VTEs is more significant in women within this age group, and it is possible that the benefits of HRT may not outweigh the risk of VTEs.

What Tests Should Be Performed?

Testing for hypercoagulable states is best performed in stages. Highest yielding assays (screening tests) should be performed first and, if positive, should be followed by appropriate confirmatory tests (Table 5). If screening test results are negative and sufficient suspicion exists, less common disorders can be tested for. Specific testing for factor V Leiden is not necessary if the test result for APC-R is negative. Prothrombin G20210A mutation detection by the polymerase chain reaction assay is preferred over prothrombin activity level quantification because the latter does not sufficiently differentiate carriers from noncarriers of the mutation.[2] Activity assays for antithrombin, protein C, and protein S are initially preferred, because they will be abnormal in both type I (quantitative) and type II (qualitative) deficiencies.[35] If activity assay results are normal, there is no benefit to pursuing antigenic testing. Factor VIII activity testing should also be considered, especially in patients suspected of having protein S deficiency. Both factor VIII activity higher than 250% and APC-R can interfere with some available protein S activity assays.[36]

Table 5 Recommended Laboratory Evaluations for Suspected Underlying Hypercoagulable State

Screening Test	Confirmatory Test
Activated protein C resistance	Factor V Leiden PCR
Prothrombin G20210A mutation testing by PCR	Antigenic assays for antithrombin, protein C, and/or protein S levels
Antithrombin, protein C, and protein S activity (functional) levels	Confirmatory tests for lupus anticoagulants*
Factor VIII activity level	
Screening tests for lupus anticoagulants (sensitive aPTT, aPTT mixing studies, dilute Russell viper venom time)	
Anticardiolipin antibody testing by ELISA	
Fasting total plasma homocysteine level	

*Include at least one of the following: platelet neutralization procedure, hexagonal phase phospholipids, Textarin/Ecarin ratio, platelet vesicles, DVV Confirm assay.[37]

aPTT, activated partial thromboplastin time; ELISA, enzyme-linked immunosorbent assay; PCR, polymerase chain reaction; VTE, venous thromboembolic event.

The International Society on Thrombosis and Haemostasis Guidelines for APA testing have suggested that two distinct lupus anticoagulant assays be carried out, in addition to anticardiolipin antibody testing by ELISA.[37] If either the clot end point lupus anticoagulant assay result (either the activated partial thromboplastin time [aPTT] or the dilute Russell viper venom time [dRVVT]) is abnormal, the assay should be repeated with a phospholipid or platelet neutralization step to increase its specificity. I do not recommend genotyping for the tlMTHFR polymorphism because hyperhomocysteinemia from any cause is the risk factor for thrombosis, not the presence of the tlMTHFR polymorphism.[19] Total plasma homocysteine should be determined in a fasting state.[17,19]

When Should Tests Be Performed?

Ideally, testing should be performed in the outpatient setting at least 4 to 6 weeks after any acute thrombotic event. This is because acute illness states, including VTEs, can cause elevations of a number of acute phase reactants, including factor VIII, C4b-binding protein, fibrinogen, and IgM anticardiolipin antibodies, all of which may interfere with testing and often lead to false-positive diagnoses. Unfractionated and low-molecular-weight heparins can interfere with antithrombin activity and with lupus anticoagulant assays, and warfarin predictably lowers proteins C and S activity levels.[35] Low activity levels of natural anticoagulants also occur as a result of liver disease, because protein C, protein S, and antithrombin are all synthesized in the liver.[10,11,35] Antithrombin activity level may be reduced in nephrotic syndrome and active colitis, and protein S activity may also be reduced in the setting of HIV infection.

TREATMENT

There are no specific therapies to reverse most hypercoagulable states. Recombinant factor concentrates of antithrombin and APC exist and may be useful in select situations beyond the scope of this review. Gene transfer to correct a particular genetic defect is theoretically feasible but likely cost prohibitive at this time. Attempts to eliminate APA by plasmapheresis or immunosuppressive therapy have not been very successful.

Hyperhomocysteinemia is treatable, and plasma homocysteine levels can be lowered in many individuals by folic acid or other B-complex vitamin supplementation.[3] It is not known whether normalization of plasma homocysteine levels reverses the hypercoagulability completely.

Initiation of oral anticoagulation for primary VTE prophylaxis in asymptomatic carriers of any hypercoagulable state has not been advised, mainly because the annual absolute risk of idiopathic VTE is low or not high enough to be favorably balanced against the annual risk of oral anticoagulation-related major and fatal hemorrhage.[38] However, because most VTEs (50%-70%) in patients with a predisposition to hypercoagulability occur following a situational risk factor, such as major or orthopedic surgery, aggressive VTE prophylaxis should be prescribed to asymptomatic carriers of hypercoagulable states during high-risk situations.[2,38]

The presence of a hypercoagulable state should not affect acute VTE treatment (i.e., initial anticoagulation with intravenous unfractionated heparin or subcutaneous low-molecular-weight heparin followed by oral anticoagulation with warfarin) in most patients, except for those with a lupus anticoagulant. Because these antibodies can prolong the activated partial thromboplastin time, monitoring of unfractionated heparin therapy in this scenario should be performed by heparin assay (protamine titration or anti–factor Xa activity assay). If such assays are not immediately available, the use of weight-based, subcutaneous, low-molecular-weight heparin should be considered instead of unfractionated heparin, because the former compounds do not require monitoring. Moreover, 26.8% to 53% of all patients with a lupus anticoagulant have an abnormal, prolonged, baseline prothrombin time, and in many of these patients the international normalized ratio is not an adequate tool for monitoring warfarin therapy. In this situation, monitoring by chromogenic factor X activity assay is recommended.[39]

Many physicians justify hypercoagulable state testing because, if an abnormality is found, prescription of long-term oral anticoagulation is believed to be more appropriate than the recommended 3- to 6-month course. However, it must be emphasized that there currently are no data from prospective, randomized, controlled trials specifically designed to address the optimal duration of anticoagulation therapy in patients with specific hypercoagulable states. Thus, any decisions regarding the ideal duration of therapy must take into account the estimates of VTE recurrence for a given disorder, the nature of the index VTE, and the risk of bleeding associated with prolonged oral anticoagulation. The Sixth American College of Chest Physicians (ACCP) Guidelines to Antithrombotic Therapy do not recommend continuation of anticoagulation therapy beyond 3 to 6 months after a situational VTE in patients with heterozygous factor V Leiden or the prothrombin G20210A mutation, and suggest that such therapy should last "1 year to lifetime" only in individuals with active cancer, persistently elevated anticardiolipin antibodies, and antithrombin deficiency.[40]

Based on available data, it is also reasonable to consider long-term anticoagulation therapy for patients with conditions known to be associated with increased rates of VTE recurrence. These include patients with documented, persistent lupus anticoagulants, homozygous factor V Leiden, and perhaps patients with a deficiency of protein C or protein S, or with double heterozygosity for factor V Leiden and the prothrombin G20210A mutation. However, the simple fact that a condition increases the risk of VTE recurrence should not be viewed as a mandatory indication for long-term or lifelong therapy. This is because most recurrent VTEs tend to occur within the first 1 to 3 years following the index VTE, with the annual rate of recurrence declining thereafter. Conversely, the risk of oral anticoagulation-related major bleeding increases with aging. Therefore, the balance between the benefits of long-term oral anticoagulation in preventing recurrent VTEs and the bleeding risk associated with this therapy, particularly of major and fatal hemorrhage, are likely to evolve over time, with risks outweighing benefits as the patients age.

OUTCOMES

The outcomes of patients with hypercoagulable states are dependent on the rates of VTE recurrence associated with the different disorders. There currently are no data to suggest reduced survival in patients who carry an inherited predisposition to hypercoagulability.

Summary

- More than 60% of patients with an unprovoked venous thromboembolism have an underlying inherited hypercoagulable abnormality.
- Select testing for an inherited hypercoagulable abnormality should be considered in VTE at a young age (<45 years); recurrent VTE, VTE in unusual sites, VTE in the setting of a strong family history of VTE, or recurrent pregnancy loss (more than three consecutive first-trimester pregnancy losses without an intercurrent term pregnancy).
- Testing for hypercoagulable states should be performed in stages, starting with highest yield assays, such as the APC-R, prothrombin G20210A mutation detection by polymerase chain reaction, and activity assays for antithrombin, protein C, and protein S.
- Prevalence of hypercoagulable states follow the following order: factor V Leiden mutation > prothrombin G20210A mutation > antithrombin deficiency ~ protein C deficiency ~ protein S deficiency
- There currently are no data to suggest reduced survival in patients who carry an inherited predisposition to hypercoagulability.

Suggested Readings

Aiach M, Borgel D, Gaussem P, et al: Protein C and protein S deficiencies. Semin Hematol 1997;34:205-216.

Kearon C, Crowther M, Hirsh J: Management of patients with hereditary hypercoagulable disorders. Annu Rev Med 2000;51:169-185.

Kitchens CS: Concept of hypercoagulability: A review of its development, clinical application, and recent progress. Semin Thromb Hemost 1985;11:293-315.

Koeleman BPC, Reitsma PH, Allaart CF, Bertina RM: Activated protein C resistance as an additional risk factor for thrombosis in protein C–deficient families. Blood 1994;84:1031-1035.

Levine JS, Branch DW, Rauch J: The antiphospholipid syndrome. N Engl J Med 2002;346:752-763.

Rosendaal FR: Risk factors for venous thrombosis: prevalence, risk, and interaction. Semin Hematol. 1997;34:171-187.

Seligsohn U, Lubetsky A: Genetic susceptibility to venous thrombosis. N Engl J Med 2001;344:1222-1231.

Smith RA, Cokkinides V, Eyre HJ: American Cancer Society guidelines for the early detection of cancer, 2003. CA Cancer J Clin 2003;53:27-43.

Van Cott M, Laposata M: Laboratory evaluation of hypercoagulable states. Hematol Oncol Clin North Am 1998;12:1141-1166.

Vandenbroucke JP, Rosing J, Bloemenkamp KWM, et al: Oral contraceptives and the risk of venous thrombosis. N Engl J Med 2001;344:1527-1535.

References

For a complete list of references, log onto www.expertconsult.com.

Use of Hematopoietic Growth Factors

Alan Lichtin

Over the past 15 years, a new class of drugs has become available to boost marrow function, the hematopoietic growth factors (HGFs). These growth factors are a major triumph for recombinant technology. Available HGFs are erythropoietin (EPO) to increase red blood cell (RBC) production, granulocyte colony-stimulating factor (G-CSF) and granulocyte-macrophage colony-stimulating factor (GM-CSF) to increase granulocyte production, and interleukin-11 (IL-11) to increase platelet numbers. Other HGFs in clinical trials for which published data exist are stem cell factor, macrophage CSF (M-CSF), IL-3, and thrombopoietin. Because they are costly and may have side effects, careful patient selection is necessary for their use, and only after a search for correctable causes for the cytopenia has been undertaken. All patients on chemotherapy whose blood count drops may, however, become eligible for the use of HGFs. Appropriate use for these agents is discussed in this chapter.

National guidelines for G-CSF and GM-CSF have been published by the American Society of Clinical Oncology (ASCO)[1,2] and a joint American Society of Hematology (ASH)-ASCO guideline has been published for the use of EPO.[3,4]

DEFINITION

HGFs are chemicals, generally cytokines and interleukins, that interact with developing immature marrow cells and lead to greater numbers of red cells, white cells, or platelets, or combinations of these. The locations of the genes responsible for the HGFs are known: chromosome 7 for EPO; the long arm of chromosome 5 for GM-CSF, IL-3, M-CSF, and the M-CSF receptor; and chromosome 17 for G-CSF.

PATHOPHYSIOLOGY

Hypoxia stimulates EPO production by the peritubular cells of the kidney. T lymphocytes, endothelial cells, fibroblasts, and monocytes-macrophages are the sources of the other HGFs. Various stimuli lead to increased levels of these growth factors—for example, endotoxin causes monocytes to release G-CSF and GM-CSF. Tumor necrosis factor α and IL-1, both formed and released by activated monocytes, stimulate endothelial cells and fibroblasts to produce greater amounts of GM-CSF and G-CSF.[5]

These cytokines interact with specific receptors on target cells. EPO binds to EPO receptors on committed RBC precursors; GM-CSF and IL-3 bind to receptors on early granulocyte precursors; and G-CSF binds to receptors on slightly more mature, committed granulocyte precursors.[5]

HGFs also have a role in potentiating the effects of mature cells. GM-CSF and G-CSF increase the functionality of granulocytes, such as in killing microbes and tumor cells. GM-CSF inhibits neutrophil migration; G-CSF does not.[5]

Two different forms of thrombopoietin are in clinical trials, a native molecule and a pegylated truncated form. Both are potent stimulators of thrombopoiesis and increase platelet numbers quickly after chemotherapy. However, this HGF seems to stimulate the production of neutralizing antibodies, sometimes leading to an immune, thrombocytopenic, purpura-like state and even to an immune panhypoplasia.[6] Use of EPO has also been associated with the development of neutralizing antibodies, leading to pure red cell aplasia.[7]

SIGNS AND SYMPTOMS

HGFs owe their success to their alleviation of cytopenia. Renal failure patients on dialysis were universally anemic before the advent of commercial EPO and required transfusions. The signs and symptoms of anemia (e.g., tiredness, dizziness, feeling cold, "I can hardly move my legs") are improved with an increase in the hemoglobin (Hb) level.

The growth of quality-of-life research has been an epiphenomenon of the commercialization of EPOs. For a patient undergoing chemotherapy, measuring the fatigue that led to the inability to juggle a grandchild on his or her lap became the focus of scientific investigation. Measuring tools, such as the Functional Assessment of Cancer—Anemia (FACT-An) and the Linear Analogue Self-Assessment—Anemia (LASA), appeared in the literature of oncology.[3] Other issues included the following:

- Should EPO begin simultaneously with chemotherapy?
- Should EPO be given once the falling Hb level reaches 13, 12, 11, 10, or 9 g/dL?
- Should a patient's Hb level be allowed to rise with EPO to 12, 13, or 14 g/dL?
- Should iron replacement be administered, and if so, should it be IV or oral? (The role of iron in maintaining an EPO response has been studied less intensely.)

The practicing physician still does not know. For EPO, dosing three times weekly versus once-weekly dosing has never been compared directly, but once-weekly dosing has become a standard of care because it is easier.

A major dose-limiting side effect of chemotherapy is febrile neutropenia. The degree of neutropenia will depend on several factors, including previous radiation the patient may have received, the dose intensity of chemotherapy treatments, and any multiple comorbidities. Fever is usually the first clinical symptom of infection. A patient on chemotherapy who presents with an absolute neutrophil count lower than 500/μL and is febrile (>38° C) is usually admitted to the hospital for at least 2 days of IV antibiotics, until it is certain that initial blood cultures are negative. The prophylactic use of G-CSF or GM-CSF is more beneficial than using these HGFs at the point of febrile neutropenia.

Chemotherapy can also lead to severe thrombocytopenia and increased bleeding risk. For leukemia patients, it was once believed that platelet transfusions should begin when the platelet count reaches 20,000/μL.[8] Then, over the years, trials demonstrated that in the absence of ongoing disseminated intravascular coagulation or fever, the platelet transfusion trigger could drop to 10,000/μL. The outpatient management of these patients in my institution usually involves frequent visits to receive platelet transfusions. IL-11 has not achieved the same success as EPO or G-CSF for the treatment of their respective cytopenias.

DIAGNOSIS

The results of the complete blood cell count, differential, and platelet count indicate anemia, neutropenia, or thrombocytopenia; however, the proper workup in patients is important, even for those on chemotherapy. Not every patient on chemotherapy becomes anemic because of the chemotherapeutic effect on marrow only, and the treating physician should not automatically prescribe exogenous erythropoietin. The following often should be checked: stool guaiac status, to ensure that gastrointestinal bleeding is not starting; peripheral smear, searching for the development of schistocytes, as might be seen in disseminated intravascular coagulation; Coombs' testing, especially for lymphoma or chronic lymphocytic leukemia (CLL) patients, to ensure that immune hemolysis is not starting; nutrient status (i.e., iron, vitamin B_{12}, and folate levels), to maintain normal levels as much as possible. In EPO-treated patients, replacing iron will often improve the EPO response.

TREATMENT

When the decision has been made to treat with an HGF, the ASCO guidelines for GM-CSF or G-CSF[2] and the ASH/ASCO guidelines for EPO[3,4] can be used. For chemotherapy-associated anemia, the ASH-ASCO guideline includes recommendations. Evidence in the medical literature was closely analyzed and, for chemotherapy-associated anemia, as the falling Hb level approaches 10 g/dL, initiating EPO prevents transfusions (approximately five patients must be treated to prevent one transfusion) and raises the Hb level.[3,4] Usually, EPO is given as 150 U/kg three times weekly or 40,000 U once weekly. The newer form of EPO, darbepoetin alfa (Aranesp), is given once every 2 weeks, 2.25 μg/kg.

GM-CSF and G-CSF have reduced the incidence of febrile neutropenia by approximately 50% in three major randomized studies in adults in whom the incidence of febrile neutropenia was predicted to be greater than 40% in the control group. As for whether to initiate CSFs in afebrile versus febrile neutropenia patients, the 2000 guideline stated that "current evidence supports the recommendation that CSFs should not be routinely used for patients with neutropenia who are afebrile." and that "the collective results [of the eight trials] provide strong and consistent support for the recommendation that CSFs should not be routinely used as adjunct therapy for the treatment of uncomplicated fever and neutropenia."[2] The eight trials have consistently shown a decrease in the duration of neutropenia when the neutropenia level is less than 500/μL, but clinical benefit has not consistently accompanied the decreased duration.

A special comment should be made about the treatment of anemia and neutropenia in patients with myelodysplastic syndrome (MDS). One randomized controlled trial has compared EPO with placebo in low-risk MDS patients.[9] Low-risk MDS is defined as refractory anemia only, not refractory anemia with ringed sideroblasts or refractory anemia with excess blasts. In this trial, EPO was beneficial in raising the hemoglobin levels of myelodysplastic patients. Also, EPO is more likely to be useful in nontransfused anemic patients as opposed to those who have already begun transfusions. The dosage of EPO in this trial was 150 U/kg three times weekly for 4 weeks, with the option of increasing to 300 U/kg three times weekly after 1 month if there is no response. The ASCO guidelines recommend using G-CSF or GM-CSF to increase the absolute neutrophil count of neutropenic patients with MDS, but no data in the medical literature support the routine, long-term, continuous use of G-CSF or GM-CSF in this setting.

G-CSF and GM-CSF have a special role in the setting of bone marrow transplantation (BMT). First, these cytokines may be given to normal donors to enhance the circulating pool of peripheral blood progenitor cells (PBPCs). Studies have indicated that recipients engraft just as quickly with the use of cytokine-primed PBPCs as they do with bone marrow.[10] Also, the duration of neutropenia for those undergoing autologous and allogeneic BMT is shortened by the use of G-CSF or GM-CSF. EPO has little or no use in the setting of BMT in reducing the need for red blood cell transfusion.

In leukemic patients, CSFs have been used to prime patients, theoretically lining up blasts in the same cell phase so that chemotherapy will be more effective. The best the guideline can state is, "Use of CSFs as primers for chemotherapy might enhance response rates and disease-free survival." In leukemic patients, CSFs do not reverse the severe neutropenia but may shorten its duration.

SIDE EFFECTS

Side effects with EPO are generally well tolerated. Diarrhea and fluid retention may occur. Hypertension may also occur, especially in patients with renal failure and underlying hypertension, who develop a good response with a rise in the hematocrit level. Seizures have been reported. A case of reversible EPO-dependent transformation of MDS to an acute monoblastic leukemia has been reported.[11]

G-CSF is better tolerated than GM-CSF, which usually has greater risks of fever, skin rash, and pericardial effusions. G-CSF has been associated with bone pain and spleen enlargement, and even rupture of the spleen. Other more unusual side effects of G-CSF include pyogenic infections, leukocytoclastic vasculitis, interstitial pneumonitis, acute gouty arthritis, Sweet's syndrome, stroke, acute iritis, and anaphylaxis.[12]

Thrombopoietin has been associated with the development of neutralizing antibodies to native thrombopoietin. Cases of immune thrombocytopenia have been documented.[13]

OUTCOMES

In the ASCO 2000 updated CSF guidelines, each individual guideline is followed by a section called "Clinical Outcomes," which are helpful and insightful commentaries. For example, it was noted that "by design, primary prophylaxis results in unnecessary treatment of at least 50% of patients who should not have experienced febrile neutropenia on standard chemotherapy regimens" and that "the optimal timing and duration of CSF administration are still under investigation."[2]

Summary

- Available hematopoietic growth factors include erythropoietin to increase red blood cell production, granulocyte colony-stimulating factor and granulocyte-macrophage colony-stimulating factor to increase granulocyte production, and interleukin-11 to increase platelet numbers.
- HGFs are used primarily in the setting of renal failure, chemotherapy-induced cytopenias, and bone marrow failure syndromes.
- Colony-stimulating factors should not be used routinely as adjunct therapy for the treatment of uncomplicated fever and neutropenia. Trials have consistently shown a decrease in the duration of neutropenia when the neutropenia level is less than 500/μL, but clinical benefit has not consistently accompanied the decreased duration.

Suggested Readings

Basser RL, O'Flaherty E, Green M, et al: Development of pancytopenia with neutralizing antibodies to thrombopoietin after multicycle chemotherapy supported by megakaryocyte growth and development factor. Blood 2002;99:2599-2602.

Bolwell B: The use of G-CSF and GM-CSF in bone marrow transplantation. Cleve Clin J Med. 1993;60:291-302.

Casadevall N, Nataf J, Viron B, et al: Pure red-cell aplasia and antierythropoietin antibodies in patients treated with recombinant erythropoietin. N Engl J Med 2002;346:469-475.

Groopman JE, Molina JM, Scadden DT: Hematopoietic growth factors. Biology and clinical applications. N Engl J Med 1989;321:1449-1459.

Italian Cooperative Study Group for rHuEPO in Myelodysplastic Syndromes: A randomized double-blind placebo-controlled study with subcutaneous recombinant human erythropoietin in patients with low-risk myelodysplastic syndromes. Br J Haematol 1998;103:1070-1074.

Li J, Yang C, Xia Y, et al: Thrombocytopenia caused by the development of antibodies to thrombopoietin. Blood 2001;98:3241-3248.

Ozer H, Armitage JO, Bennett CL, et al; American Society of Clinical Oncology: 2000 update of recommendations for the use of hematopoietic colony-stimulating factors: Evidence-based, clinical practice guidelines. American Society of Clinical Oncology Growth Factors Expert Panel. J Clin Oncol 2000;18:3558-3585.

Rebulla P, Finazzi G, Maragnoni F, et al: The threshold for prophylactic platelet transfusion in adults with acute myeloid leukemia. N Engl J Med 1997;337:1870-1875.

Rizzo JD, Lichtin AE, Woolf SH, et al: Use of epoetin in patients with cancer: Evidence-based clinical practice guidelines of the American Society of Clinical Oncology and the American Society of Hematology. Blood 2002;100:2303-2320.

Rizzo JD, Lichtin AE, Woolf SH, et al: Use of epoetin in patients with cancer: Evidence-based clinical practice guidelines of the American Society of Clinical Oncology and the American Society of Hematology. J Clin Oncol 2002;20:4083-4107.

References

For a complete list of references, log onto www.expertconsult.com.

Acute Myelogenous Leukemia

Suzanne R. Fanning, Mikkael A. Sekeres, and Karl Theil

DEFINITION

Acute myelogenous leukemia (AML), also known as acute nonlymphocytic leukemia, represents a group of clonal hematopoietic stem cell disorders in which both failure to differentiate and overproliferation into the stem cell compartment result in the accumulation of myeloblasts. It is the most common leukemia in adults.

EPIDEMIOLOGY

There are a number of risk factors for the development of AML.

Genetic Predisposition

Chromosomal instability in several autosomal dominant conditions can lead to AML, including Fanconi's anemia, ataxia-telangiectasia, neurofibromatosis, and Bloom's syndrome. Germline mutations in the *AML-1* gene are known to be associated with an increased risk of the development of AML. Additionally, congenital immunodeficiency disorders. including infantile X-linked agammaglobulinemia and Down syndrome, have also been associated with an increased incidence of AML.

Environmental Exposure

Ionizing radiation and organic solvents such as benzene and other petroleum products have been associated with a higher risk of developing AML. Both *ras* mutations and polymorphisms resulting in the inactivation of nicotinamide adenine dinucleotide phosphate, reduced (NADPH)-quinone oxidoreductase have been found in patients with these exposures.

Prior Therapy

Therapy-related AML typically develops after alkylating agent-induced damage at a median of 5 to 7 years after therapy for the primary malignancy. It is usually associated with an antecedent myelodysplastic disorder. DNA topoisomerase II agents may also produce gene rearrangements leading to AML, with a short latency period of 12 to 18 months following treatment.

Prior Bone Marrow Disorders

Secondary AML can develop in patients with various hematologic disorders, such as aplastic anemia and severe congenital neutropenia. Other inherited hematologic conditions have also been implicated, such as Bloom's syndrome and Fanconi's anemia. Myelodysplastic and myeloproliferative syndromes, present for at least 3 months, can also progress to AML.

Age

The incidence of AML increases with age. In the United States, the median age of patients with AML is 68 years. The age-adjusted population incidence is 17.6 per 100,000 for people older than 65 years, compared with 1.8 per 100,000 for those younger than 65 years. Similarly, chromosomal abnormalities occur with greater frequency among this older population of patients.

PATHOPHYSIOLOGY

Hematopoiesis in normal cells involves the differentiation of a stem cell into myelocytes, lymphocytes, and megakaryocytes. In AML, this process of cell differentiation is interrupted in those cells committed to the myeloid lineage. Some reports have supported the concept of a single transformed hematopoietic stem cell, whereas others have contended that transformation can occur at any point from stem cell to lineage-committed progenitor cell. This transformation can occur either as a de novo event or associated with previous therapy.

Several molecular and genetic lesions have been identified in AML, leading to advances in defining its pathogenesis. The most familiar of these is the t(15;17) translocation, resulting in AML with abnormal promyelocytes, known as acute promyelocytic leukemia (APL). Translocation of these chromosomes results in the fusion of the retinoic acid receptor gene alpha on chromosome 15, with the *PML* gene on chromosome 17, giving rise to a fusion product that prevents differentiation to mature granulocytes. This block in differentiation can be overcome with all-*trans* retinoic acid (ATRA), a vitamin A derivative. The DNA-binding subunit core-binding factor β (CBFβ) produces a transcription factor that regulates numerous hematopoietic-specific genes. The genetic translocations t(8;21), inv(16), and t(16;16) have all been associated with this transcription factor. AML patients with these genetic disorders have a better prognosis. Six percent to 8% of patients with AML have structural alterations of 11q23, leading to the *MLL* rearrangement. The *MLL* gene rearrangement, also known as mixed lineage leukemia, may lead to AML composed of both myeloid and lymphoid cells. The *MLL* gene rearrangement portends a worse outcome in patients with AML.

SIGNS AND SYMPTOMS

AML often manifests with the clinical sequelae attributable to pancytopenia. The deficient production of red cells can lead to patient complaints of weakness, fatigue, or dyspnea on exertion. Pallor is a common finding on physical examination. Infection can result from insufficient numbers of white cells or impaired white blood cell function. Collections of leukemic cells, seen in leukemia cutis, granulocytic sarcomas, or chloromas, can also occur. These collections represent extramedullary sites of disease and often involve cutaneous and visceral tissues. In some cases, hyperleukocytosis can lead to ocular or cerebral dysfunction. Low numbers of platelets can lead to petechiae, gingival bleeding, ecchymosis, epistaxis, or menorrhagia. APL is a distinct entity of AML that often manifests with hemorrhagic complications, including disseminated intravascular coagulation. Palpable lymphadenopathy and hepatosplenomegaly are rare findings in AML. It is typical for patients to complain of flulike symptoms for 4 to 6 weeks before the diagnosis.

In some patients, the diagnosis of AML can constitute a medical emergency, making prompt referral to a medical hematologist or oncologist a requisite. Hyperleukocytosis, leukostasis, or both can cause impairment of blood flow, most often resulting in central nervous system or pulmonary symptoms. Rapid lowering of the white blood cell count can be achieved with the institution of chemotherapy, leukapheresis, or low-dose radiation. Central nervous system leukemia, although less common in AML, can manifest with patient complaints of headache, lethargy, or cranial nerve signs. For these patients, intrathecal chemotherapy or cranial radiation are treatment options. Additionally, metabolic abnormalities, including tumor lysis syndrome, can occur spontaneously because of high tumor burden or as a result of cytotoxic chemotherapy.

DIAGNOSIS

The diagnosis of AML requires the identification of greater than 20% leukemic blasts in the bone marrow (see later). Further analysis then must separate AML from acute lymphoblastic leukemia by showing evidence for commitment to the myeloid lineage. Immunohistochemical staining for myeloperoxidase is the best method for determining which cells are committed to the myeloid lineage (Fig. 1). The leukemic clone giving rise to AML can occur at any point in the differentiation of the myeloid cell, creating heterogeneity among patients. Flow cytometry and cytogenetics are then used to differentiate the various AML subtypes.

The subtypes of AML were previously described as M0 through M7 by the French-American-British (FAB) system. In 1997, however, the World Health Organization (WHO) reclassified AML into four categories (Box 1) in an attempt to predict the prognosis and biologic properties of AML subcategories more accurately and enhance the clinical relevance of the system. This new classification reflected those entities with similar biologic and clinical features. It also takes into account the morphologic, genetic, and immunophenotypic features of the disease entities. The four categories include AML with recurrent genetic abnormalities, AML with multilineage dysplasia, therapy-related AML and myelodysplastic syndromes, and AML not otherwise categorized, which roughly correlates with the FAB classification (Figs. 2 and 3). The WHO classification system differs from the FAB system in that the previous blast cell threshold of 30% for the diagnosis of AML has been reduced to 20%, and patients with recurring cytogenetic abnormalities are now classified as having AML regardless of blast percentage.

The British Medical Research Council (MRC) AML 10 trial and a Cancer and Leukemia Group B (CALGB) trial found that patients could then be categorized prognostically based on their pretreatment cytogenetics. Patients could be separated into three categories based on response to induction treatment, relapse risk, and overall survival: favorable, intermediate, and adverse cytogenetic groups. Typically, patients with favorable-risk cytogenetics have abnormalities of the

Box 1 WHO Classification of Acute Myelogenous Leukemia

Acute myeloid leukemia with recurrent genetic abnormalities

- Acute myeloid leukemia with t(8;21)(q22;q22), (AML1/ETO)
- Acute myeloid leukemia with abnormal bone marrow eosinophils and inv(16)(p13q22) or t(16;16)(p13;q22), (CBFβ/MYH11)
- Acute promyelocytic leukemia with t(15;17)(q22;q12), (PML/RARa) and variants
- Acute myeloid leukemia with 11q23 (MLL) abnormalities

Acute myeloid leukemia with multilineage dysplasia

- Following MDS or MDS/MPD
- Without antecedent MDS or MDS/MPD, but with dysplasia in at least 50% of cells in two or more myeloid lineages

Acute myeloid leukemia and myelodysplastic syndromes, therapy-related

- Alkylating agent, radiation-related type
- Topoisomerase II inhibitor-related type (some may be lymphoid)
- Others

Acute myeloid leukemia, not otherwise categorized; classify as:

- Acute myeloid leukemia, minimally differentiated
- Acute myeloid leukemia without maturation
- Acute myeloid leukemia with maturation
- Acute myelomonocytic leukemia
- Acute monoblastic, acute monocytic leukemia
- Acute erythroid leukemia (erythroid-myeloid and pure erythroleukemia)
- Acute megakaryoblastic leukemia
- Acute basophilic leukemia
- Acute panmyelosis with myelofibrosis
- Myeloid sarcoma

AML1, acute myelogenous leukemia 1; CBFb, core-binding factor b; ETO, eight twenty-one; MDS, myelodysplastic syndromes; MYH11, myosin heavy chain, type 11; MLL, mixed lineage leukemia; MPD, myeloproliferative disease; PML, promyelocytic leukemia; RARa, retinoic acid receptor.

Adapted from Vardiman JW, Harris NL, Brunning RD: The World Health Organization (WHO) classification of the myeloid neoplasms. Blood 2002;100:2292-2302.

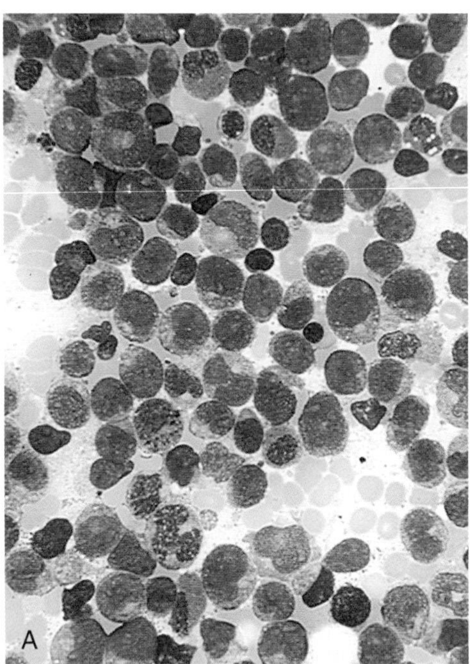

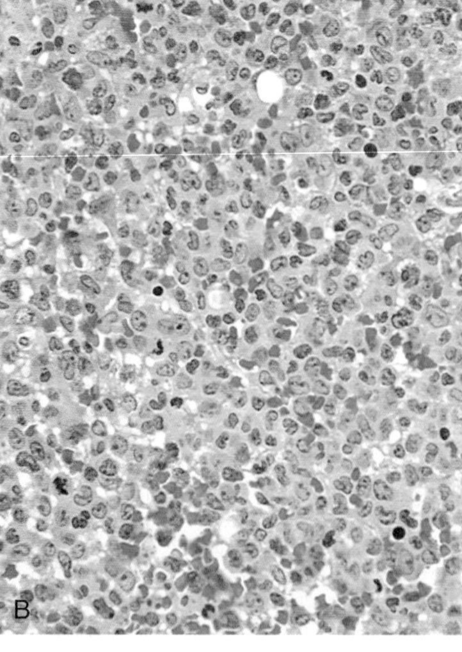

Figure 1 Immunohistochemical diagnosis of acute myelogenous leukemia. A, Bone marrow aspirate shows increased blasts from a patient with acute myeloid leukemia with inv(16) (Wright-Giemsa stain, ×50). **B,** Bone marrow biopsy from the same patient shows 100% cellularity with sheets of blasts (hematoxylin-eosin stain, ×40).

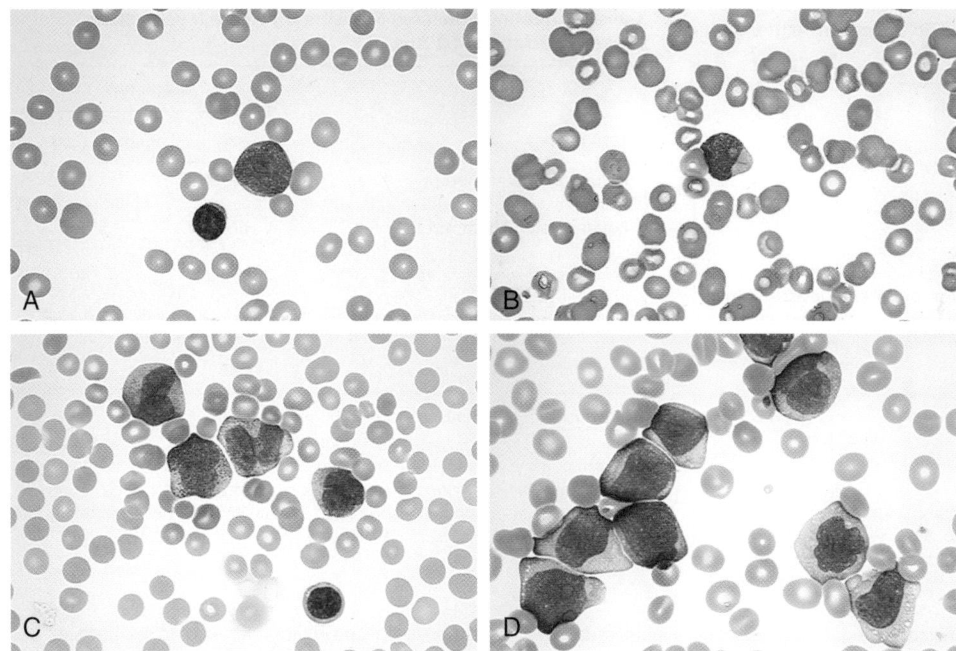

Figure 2 Blast morphology can provide clues about the type of acute myeloid leukemia, but definitive subclassification requires correlation with cytochemistry, flow cytometry, and cytogenetics. **A,** Typical myeloid blast morphology not otherwise diagnostic is shown. The blast is larger than a normal lymphocyte and has less condensed chromatin, scant cytoplasm, and a prominent nucleolus. **B,** Myeloid blasts may contain cytoplasmic Auer rods. **C,** Blasts in acute myeloid leukemia with t(15;17) are larger, have more abundant cytoplasm containing fine azurophil granules, and have characteristic bilobed, folded nuclei. **D,** Blasts in acute monoblastic leukemia have moderate amounts of agranular cytoplasm and may contain cytoplasmic vacuoles (A-D, Wright-Giemsa stains, ×100.)

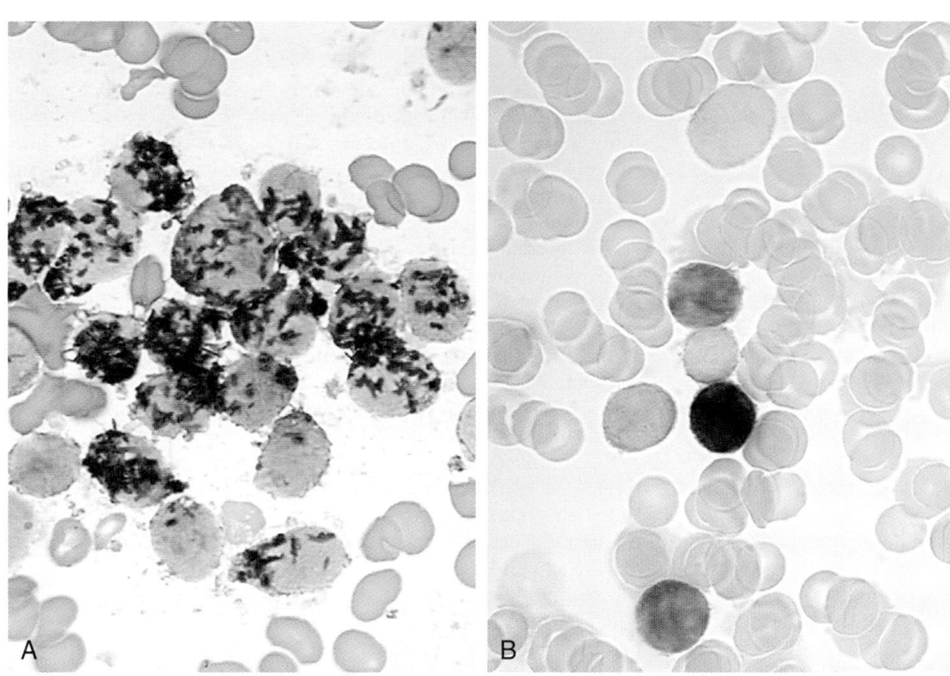

Figure 3 **Cytochemical stains are useful for the subclassification of acute myeloid leukemia.** **A,** Myeloperoxidase stain is positive in blasts and appears as blue-black cytoplasmic granularity. **B,** Nonspecific esterase stain (α-naphthylbutyrate) is useful for the identification of monocytic differentiation and is positive in some (red-brown cytoplasmic staining), but not all, blasts in this case of acute myelomonocytic leukemia.

AML1-CBFβ DNA subunit. This subunit is composed of two proteins, AML1 (also known as core-binding factor 2α, CBF2α) which heterodimerizes with another protein, CBFβ, to form a transcription factor necessary for normal hematopoiesis. Adverse cytogenetics include complex (three or more) abnormalities, deletion of 5q, abnormal 3q, and deletion of chromosome 7. Thus, it is crucial to test for cytogenetics and, when applicable, to use fluorescence in situ hybridization (FISH), because these may help dictate therapy. More recently, gene expression profiling has been shown to improve the molecular classification and prediction of outcome in patients with AML.

Box 2 presents the laboratory and imaging studies needed to diagnose and ultimately treat patients with AML accurately. Baseline evaluation involves routine blood work, including a complete blood count with differential, complete metabolic profile, and coagulation studies. A bone marrow biopsy should be evaluated by cytochemistry, immunophenotyping, flow cytometry, and cytogenetics; this is necessary for determining diagnosis and prognosis. Additional studies, including chest radiography and echocardiography are needed to determine a patient's ability to undergo chemotherapy. A lumbar puncture may be needed if central nervous system (CNS) symptoms are identified. Human leukocyte antigen (HLA) typing and viral serologies are needed if bone marrow transplantation is necessary.

TREATMENT

Therapy for AML includes remission induction followed by postremission chemotherapy for most patients. For some, this is

Box 2 Routine Testing for Diagnosis and Treatment of Acute Myelogenous Leukemia

Complete blood cell count with differential
Determination of the following:

- Blood urea nitrogen, creatinine, electrolyte, uric acid, and blood glucose levels
- Aminotransferases, alkaline phosphatase, bilirubin, lactate dehydrogenase levels
- Calcium, phosphorus levels

Partial thromboplastin time, activated partial thromboplastin time, fibrinogen, D dimer
Bone marrow biopsy with cytochemistry, immunophenotyping, flow cytometry, cytogenetics
Chest radiography
Electrocardiography
Two-dimensional echocardiography in patients with history and/or symptoms of heart-related issues
Lumbar puncture in symptomatic patients
Human leukocyte antigen typing of patient and siblings
Herpes simplex and cytomegalovirus serology

Table 1 Treatment-Related Statistics for Acute Myelogenous Leukemia Stratified by Age

	Age (yr)	
Parameter	**<60**	**≥60**
Induction chemotherapy	7 + 3	7 + 3
Postremission chemotherapy	HiDAC	5 or 5 + 2
Complete response rates (%)	65-85	40-55
Treatment-related mortality (%)	5-10	20-30
5-year disease-free survival (%)	30	5-10

HiDAC, high-dose cytarabine (1000-3000 mg/m^2 IV over 1-3 hr every 12 hr for 6 to 12 doses); 7 + 3, 7 days of cytarabine at 100 mg/m^2 + 3 days of an anthracycline or anthracenedione (most commonly idarubicin, 12 mg/m^2, mitoxantrone, 12 mg/m^2, or daunorubicin, 45 mg/m^2); 5 or 5 + 2, 5 days of cytarabine at 100 mg/m^2 alone or combined with 2 days of an anthracycline or anthracenedione.

followed by hematopoietic stem cell transplantation (see later). Treatment recommendations for AML vary, taking into account patient age, cytogenetics, and prognostic factors. The recommendations are often divided into those for patients younger than 60 and those 60 years and older (Table 1).

The goal of induction chemotherapy is to reduce the number of leukemic cells as well as return proper function to the bone marrow. The 7 + 3 regimen of cytarabine (100 mg/m^2 for 7 days plus an anthracycline or anthracenedione [most often daunorubicin, 45-60 mg/m^2, but other options include idarubicin or mitoxantrone] for 3 days) is the most common induction regimen for both age groups.

A recent study by the Eastern Cooperative Oncology Group has evaluated patients treated with granulocyte-monocyte colony-stimulating factor for priming of the bone marrow before induction chemotherapy. This study revealed a statistically significant difference in complete response rates for patients in whom induction therapy was not delayed for priming. This reinforces the need to refer patients to a hematologist or oncologist as soon as possible for prompt initiation of induction chemotherapy.

Postremission chemotherapy then aims to eradicate any residual disease in an attempt at cure. Postremission chemotherapy includes high-dose cytarabine (ara-c; HiDAC) for patients younger than 60 years, whereas a 5 or 5 + 2 regimen of cytarabine plus an anthracycline or anthracenedione is preferred for patients older than 60 years. HiDAC has proven to be efficacious for young patients with good or intermediate prognosis. In patients younger than 60 years, HiDAC yields a 4-year disease-free survival rate of 44%, with relatively few relapses, but carries with it a 5% treatment-related mortality. In contrast, HiDAC failed to improve the outcome of patients older than 60 years. HiDAC has shown particular efficacy for patients with CBF DNA subunit abnormalities. The HiDAC regimen is 1000 to 3000 mg/m^2 IV over 1 to 3 hours every 12 hours for 6 to 12 doses.

Allogeneic or autologous bone marrow transplantation is an additional option for postremission therapy in adults with AML. For some patients younger than 60 years and for whom an HLA-matched sibling or matched unrelated donor is available, allogeneic stem cell transplantation should follow induction chemotherapy. This procedure is not without risk; it has an associated 20% to 25% treatment-related mortality rate. For patients without a compatible donor or for whom age precludes such treatment, additional chemotherapy or autologous stem cell transplantation are options.

Two novel therapies, arsenic trioxide and gemtuzumab ozogamicin, have recently been approved by the U.S. Food and Drug Administration (FDA) for use in refractory AML. Gemtuzumab ozogamicin, an anti-CD33 immunotoxin conjugate, was shown to have a 30% response rate (complete response plus partial response) in older AML patients in first relapse, with their first remission having lasted 6 months or longer. Studies are ongoing to determine whether initial chemotherapy plus gemtuzumab ozogamicin has a role in previously untreated patients. Arsenic trioxide, which targets intracellular mitochondria, has shown good success in the treatment of relapsed or refractory APL. Single-agent studies with arsenic trioxide in other subtypes of AML have not proven to be as encouraging. In older patients, however, use of arsenic trioxide in combination with ascorbic acid may be a viable treatment option for patients not able to endure intensive chemotherapy.

Farnesyltransferase inhibitors are an emerging class of signal transduction inhibitors. The theorized mechanism of action involves inhibition of several cell-signaling processes. Such inhibition then leads to decreased proliferation of malignant cells. Although not yet approved by the FDA, early studies have demonstrated a 10% to 20% complete response rate among patients with a poor prognosis. Therapy is generally well tolerated. Common side effects include fatigue, nausea, vomiting, and skin rash.

Recommendations for hematopoietic stem cell transplantation (HSCT) in AML rely heavily on risk-stratified cytogenetics (Box 3). In patients with good-risk cytogenetics, induction followed by postremission chemotherapy has shown response rates similar to those of HSCT, with lower treatment-related mortality. There is minimal role for autologous HSCT for those patients who relapse. For those with intermediate-risk cytogenetics, age is often a determining factor, because the risk of treatment-related mortality increases with age. For these patients, treatment options include allogeneic transplantation for those with sibling donors, autologous HSCT, and postremission chemotherapy. For those with poor-risk cytogenetics, allogeneic transplantation with a sibling or matched unrelated donor can be anticipated immediately following induction chemotherapy.

The treatment of APL differs from the recommendations for AML. Instead, ATRA, which promotes differentiation of leukemic promyelocytes into mature cells, has been shown to improve disease-free survival and overall survival compared with chemotherapy alone. ATRA, along with an anthracycline and cytarabine, is currently the standard of care for patients with APL.

OUTCOMES

Over the past few decades, success in the treatment of AML has improved only modestly for patients younger than 60 years. In 1966, the median survival of adult patients with AML was 40 days. Today,

Box 3 Cytogenetic Risk Stratification for Overall Survival

Good Risk
t(8;21)
inv(16)
del(9q)

Intermediate Risk
Normal karyotype
−Y
del(5q)
loss of 7q
t(9;11)
+11
del(11q)
abn(12p)
+13
del(20q)
+21

Poor Risk
Complex karyotype
inv(3)
t(6;9)
t(6;11)
−7
+8
t(11;19)(q23;p13.1)

Data from Byrd J, Mrozek K, Dodge RK, et al: Pretreatment cytogenetic abnormalities are predictive of induction success, cumulative incidence of relapse, and overall survival in adult patients with de novo acute myeloid leukemia: Results from Cancer and Leukemia Group B (CALGB 8461). Blood 2002;100:4325-4336.

AML patients younger than 60 years have complete response rates of 70% to 80% after induction chemotherapy. Overall survival, however, remains at only about 50% for those who go into a complete remission, or 30% overall. In 1998, the MRC AML 10 trial found that patients could be separated into three prognostic groups—favorable, intermediate, and adverse—defined by pretreatment cytogenetics. Overall survival at 5 years was found to be 65%, 41%, and 14%, respectively. If a patient undergoes an allogeneic HSCT while in first remission, the complete response rate ranges from 45% to 65%, although patient selection influences these numbers. In relapsed AML, complete response after allogeneic HSCT is 35% or lower. The prognosis for older patients remains poor, however. In the MRC AML 8 trial, the remission rate was 70% for patients younger than 50 years, 52% for those 60 to 69 years old, but only 26% for those older than 70 years. One theory for such disparity is that neutropenia after chemotherapy lasts longer and is less well tolerated in older adults than in younger patients. Another possible answer is the finding that hematopoietic cells of older patients are derived from a leukemic clone at diagnosis, in contrast to normal stem cells in younger counterparts. The use of granulocyte-monocyte colony-stimulating factors reduces the period of neutropenia and the duration of hospitalization by approximately 2 days; unfortunately, this has not translated into improved overall survival or a decrease in infectious complications. Therefore, their use is not indicated.

Summary

- Acute myelogenous leukemia (AML) represents a group of clonal hematopoietic stem-cell disorders.
- The incidence of AML increases with age.
- A diagnosis of AML requires 20% or more leukemic myeloid blasts.
- Pretreatment cytogenetics are useful in determining prognosis and appropriate treatment.

Suggested Readings

Byrd J, Mrozek K, Dodge RK, et al: Pretreatment cytogenetic abnormalities are predictive of induction success, cumulative incidence of relapse, and overall survival in adult patients with de novo acute myeloid leukemia: Results from Cancer and Leukemia Group B (CALGB 8461). Blood 2002;100:4325-4336.

Byrd JC, Ruppert AS, Mrozek K, et al: Repetitive cycles of high-dose cytarabine benefit patients with acute myeloid leukemia and inv(16)(p13q22) or t(16;16)(p13;q22): Results from CALGB 8461. J Clin Oncol 2004;22:1087-1094.

Grigg AP, Szer J, Beresford J, et al: Factors affecting the outcome of allogeneic bone marrow transplantation for adult patients with refractory or relapsed acute leukaemia. Br J Haematol 1999;107:409-418.

Grimwade D, Walker H, Oliver F, et al: The importance of diagnostic cytogenetics on outcome in AML: Analysis of 1,612 patients entered into the MRC AML 10 trial. Blood 1998;92:2322-2333.

Levine EG, Bloomfield CD: Leukemias and myelodysplastic syndromes secondary to drug, radiation, and environmental exposure. Semin Oncol 1992;19:47-84.

Mayer RJ, Davis RB, Schiffer CA, et al: Intensive postremission chemotherapy in adults with acute myeloid leukemia. Cancer and Leukemia Group B. N Engl J Med 1994;331:896-903.

Rees JK, Gray RG, Swirsky D, Hayhoe FG: Principal results of the Medical Research Council's 8th acute myeloid leukaemia trial. Lancet 1986;2:1236-1241.

Rowe JM, Neuberg D, Friedenberg W, et al: A phase 3 study of three induction regimens and of priming with GM-CSF in older adults with acute myeloid leukemia: A trial by the Eastern Cooperative Oncology Group. Blood 2004;103:479-485.

Stone RM, Berg DT, George SL, et al: Granulocyte-macrophage colony-stimulating factor after initial chemotherapy for elderly patients with primary acute myelogenous leukemia. Cancer and Leukemia Group B. N Engl J Med 1995;332:1671-1677.

Tallman MS, Andersen JW, Schiffer CA, et al: All-trans-retinoic acid in acute promyelocytic leukemia. N Engl J Med 1997;337:1021-1028.

Vardiman JW, Harris NL, Brunning RD: The World Health Organization (WHO) classification of the myeloid neoplasms. Blood 2002;100:2292-2302.

The Myelodysplastic Syndromes

Mikkael A. Sekeres

DEFINITION

Historically, disorders in the myelodysplastic syndrome (MDS) group have been referred to as oligoblastic leukemia, refractory anemia, smoldering acute leukemia, or preleukemia. They represent a collection of heterogeneous hematopoietic disorders derived from an abnormal multipotent progenitor cell, characterized by a hyperproliferative bone marrow, dysplasia of the cellular elements, and ineffective hematopoiesis. MDS can be indolent or aggressive, depending on the subclassification (see later).

PREVALENCE AND RISK FACTORS

MDS is a disease of older adults, with more than 80% of patients older than 60 years. The precise incidence of new diagnoses has been difficult to define in the setting of changing classification systems and difficulty in establishing the diagnosis. In general, MDS affects between 12,000 and 20,000 people in the United States each year, or 22 to 45 per 100,000 people older than 70 years. The population prevalence is estimated to be between 30,000 and 40,000 people in the United States, with most of them having indolent (early) MDS, generally defined as fewer than 5% myeloblasts in the bone marrow. These numbers make it as prevalent as other common hematologic malignancies of older adults, such as multiple myeloma and chronic lymphocytic leukemia.

Risk factors for developing MDS include the following:

- Age: Population studies in England have found that the crude incidence increases from 0.5 per 100,000 people younger than 50 years to 89 per 100,000 people older than 80 years.
- Genetic predisposition: Familial syndromes have been reported but are rare.
- Environmental exposure: This includes particularly benzene and possibly other industrial solvents.
- Prior therapy, including radiation treatment, alkylating agents (e.g., chlorambucil, cyclophosphamide, melphalan), and other chemotherapy agents (on a case report level).

For alkylating agents, the risk of developing a secondary MDS or acute myelogenous leukemia (AML) starts with the end of therapy and peaks at 4 years, with a plateau at 10 years.

PATHOPHYSIOLOGY AND NATURAL HISTORY

In MDS, the hematopoietic stem cells that define the disease are clonally derived. Generally, MDS can be divided into two major subtypes—indolent (or early) MDS, in which pro-apoptotic forces predominate, and aggressive (or advanced) MDS, in which proproliferative factors are more common. In indolent MDS, inhibitory cytokines, including tumor necrosis factor α (TNF-α), interleukin-6 (IL-6), transforming growth factor-β (TGF-β), and Fas ligand promote apoptosis. As genetic lesions accumulate, indolent MDS becomes proliferative MDS and eventually AML. This occurs as oncogenes are activated and tumor suppressor genes are inactivated. In the proliferative categories, *ras*, *FMS*, and *p53* mutations are more common than inhibitory cytokines, and are believed to facilitate the transformation to AML. In general, bone marrow stem cells in MDS are less responsive to and produce fewer hematopoietic growth factors, including IL-3, IL-6, granulocyte colony-stimulating factor (G-CSF), and granulocyte-macrophage colony-stimulating factor (GM-CSF). Peripheral blood cytopenias result from this process. Thus, there is the paradox of having a hypercellular bone marrow in patients requiring blood transfusions.

Cytogenetic abnormalities are found in 40% to 70% of primary and 80% to 90% of secondary MDS patients. Typically, trisomy 8 and monosomy 5 or 7 will be present. Findings of these abnormalities in patients with frank AML indicate probable evolution (which may be subclinical) from an antecedent MDS, which confers a worse prognosis. Therapy-related MDS can be associated with these same abnormalities in addition to translocations or rearrangements involving 11q23 or 21q22. Favorable abnormalities include 5q−, 20q−, Y−, or normal cytogenetics, whereas unfavorable abnormalities are found with complex cytogenetics (three or more cytogenetic abnormalities) or chromosome 7 abnormalities.

Deficiencies in hematopoiesis lead to cytopenias, which may be severe. Not surprisingly, morbidity and mortality result from anemia, bleeding, and infection, along with transformation to AML, which occurs in approximately one third of patients.

SIGNS AND SYMPTOMS

Recognition of this entity has increased over the past decade, and should be suspected in older adults with anemia, thrombocytopenia, leukopenia, or a combination of these abnormalities. MDS often manifests as a refractory cytopenia in an older adult who may be entirely asymptomatic. A macrocytic or normocytic anemia is found in almost all MDS patients, and frequently is accompanied by thrombocytopenia, leukopenia, or both. Typical symptoms reflect underlying cytopenias—patients with anemia frequently complain of fatigue, shortness of breath, loss of appetite, and even exacerbation of underlying cardiac symptoms; patients with thrombocytopenia may have spontaneous bruising, the appearance of petechiae (particularly in dependent areas, such as the shins, or in areas exposed to minor trauma, such as skin under elastic waistbands), or bleeding of mucosal surfaces (including the gums when brushing teeth); and patients with leukopenia may have recurrent infections, particularly of the skin, mucosal surfaces (especially the oral and rectal mucosa), and lungs.

MDS can be associated with paraneoplastic syndromes related to autoimmune processes. These may be dermatologic (e.g., psoriasis, or Sweet's syndrome), rheumatologic (e.g., vasculitis), hematologic (e.g., hemolytic anemia or Glanzmann's disease [an acquired glycoprotein IIB/IIIA inhibition resulting in abnormal platelet function]), or endocrinologic (e.g., hypothyroidism, diabetes insipidus). In addition, a subset of MDS, chronic myelomonocytic leukemia, which actually represents an overlap syndrome with myeloproliferative disorders, may cause splenomegaly and subsequent complaints of left upper quadrant abdominal pain and early satiety. Cytokine release (see earlier, "Pathophysiology and Natural History") may result in constitutional symptoms, such as anorexia, weight loss, and even low-grade fevers.

DIAGNOSIS

MDS is diagnosed through a combination of abnormal findings in the peripheral blood and bone marrow. Morphologic abnormalities should be present in at least 10% of cells in a given lineage. In the peripheral blood, erythrocytes may be macrocytic, nucleated, or stippled, whereas neutrophils may be hyposegmented, hypogranular, or bilobed, with chromatin condensation (pseudo–Pelger-Huët cells). In the bone marrow, erythrocyte precursors may have megaloblastoid changes, contain ringed sideroblasts, or include Howell-Jolly bodies. Myeloid maturation may be stunted, and megakaryocytes can be dysplastic.

Subtypes of MDS are defined using one of two classification systems. The French-American-British (FAB) system has been used widely since 1982 and is useful in predicting rates of survival and transformation to AML (Table 1). In the FAB system, MDS is divided into refractory anemia, refractory anemia with ringed sideroblasts, refractory anemia with excess blasts, refractory anemia with excess blasts in transformation, and chronic myelomonocytic leukemia, an "overlap syndrome" that can include features of a myelodysplastic syndrome, myeloproliferative disorder, or both.

In 1999, the World Health Organization (WHO) published its classification of hematopoietic and lymphoid neoplasms, and in 2002 published a clarification and rationale for differences between the FAB and WHO classifications (Table 2). The most important difference was the lowering of the blast threshold for the diagnosis of AML, from 30% to 20% blasts in the blood or bone marrow. Chronic myelomonocytic leukemia (CMML) was also formally separated from the myelodysplastic syndromes, and a cytogenetically defined MDS subgroup, the 5q− syndrome—which confers a good prognosis, is associated with normal or elevated platelet counts, and is found in 5% to 13% of patients—was identified. The WHO system, which does not differ substantially from the FAB classification, is gaining wider acceptance in clinical practice and in the literature.

A differential diagnosis includes the following:

- Anemia from other causes, such as vitamin deficiencies, iron deficiency from an inadequate diet or blood loss, another cancer with bone marrow involvement, rheumatologic disorders, or medication effect
- Thrombocytopenia resulting from idiopathic thrombocytopenic purpura (ITP), thrombotic thrombocytopenic purpura (TTP), or medication effect
- Leukopenia from other causes, such as infections (from human immunodeficiency virus (HIV), hepatitis, or parvovirus), rheumatologic disorders, or medication effect

If MDS is suspected, a bone marrow biopsy and aspirate should be performed. The diagnosis is made based on cell morphology, immunohistochemistry and, in the case of more advanced subtypes of MDS, flow cytometry. Obtaining a bone marrow aspirate sample for cytogenetics is crucial, because abnormalities may help in establishing the diagnosis and in risk stratification (see later).

Other laboratory tests that should be obtained to narrow the differential diagnosis include vitamin B_{12}, folate, and iron studies, including a ferritin level, serum erythropoietin level determination, certain rheumatologic studies (including antinuclear antibody or rheumatoid factor assay in certain patients), or monitoring for infectious causes, including HIV and hepatitis serologies. Although not specific, determination of the erythrocyte sedimentation rate and lactate dehydrogenase level can establish the presence of an acute process or rapid cell turnover.

Summary

- MDS can be classified into five or eight subtypes, depending on the system (FAB or WHO) used. In general, MDS is indolent (early) or proliferative (advanced).
- In patients with cytopenias, rule out vitamin or iron deficiencies, rheumatologic, or infectious causes.
- Obtain a bone marrow biopsy and aspirate. Always carry out cytogenetic testing on the aspirate.

TREATMENT

Options for the treatment of MDS range from supportive care, which includes blood product transfusions and the use of growth factors, to intensive therapy with allogeneic hematopoietic stem cell transplantation.

Patients with more indolent forms of MDS, without excess myeloblasts. who may be dependent on blood product transfusions, may derive some benefit from the use of growth factors. Often, recombinant human erythropoietin (epoetin alfa [EPO, Procrit, Epogen]) is used initially as a single agent, in escalating doses. G-CSF, filgrastim, GM-CSF, or sargramostim may be combined with epoetin alfa, and may result in higher response rates. Typical response rates, across a number of studies, are in the 15% to 40% range. Growth factor agents tend to be more effective in low-risk MDS patients with lower serum erythropoietin levels, less than 500 U/L, who do not already require frequent blood transfusions (defined as less than 2 units packed red blood cells per month). Darbepoetin alfa (Aranesp) has recently been used for the treatment of patients with MDS, although few clinical trials have supported its use.

In patients who are transfusion dependent, or who are unlikely to respond to growth factors, non–growth factor therapy, such as chemotherapy, may be initiated. Less intensive (midrange) therapeutic options for patients with indolent MDS include the use of

Table 1 French-American-British (FAB) Myelodysplastic Syndrome (MDS) Classification System

MDS Subtype	Peripheral Blasts (%)	Bone Marrow Blasts (%)	AML Transformation	Median Survival (mo)	MDS Diagnoses (%)
Refractory anemia (RA)	≤1	<5	10-20	30-65	10-40
Refractory anemia with ringed sideroblasts (RARS)	≤1	<5	10-35	34-83	10-35
Refractory anemia with excess blasts (RAEB)	<5	5-20	>50	8-18	25-30
Refractory anemia with excess blasts in transformation (RAEB-T)	≥5	21-29	60-100	4-11	10-30
Chronic myelomonocytic leukemia (CMML)	<5	≤20	>40	15-32	10-20

AML, acute myelogenous leukemia.

Table 2 World Health Organization Myelodysplastic Syndrome Classification and Criteria

MDS Subtype	Blood Findings	Bone Marrow Findings
Refractory anemia (RA)	Anemia	Erythroid dysplasia *only*
No or rare blasts		<5% blasts, <15% ringed sideroblasts
Refractory anemia with ringed sideroblasts (RARS)	Anemia	Erythroid dysplasia *only*
	No blasts	>15% ringed sideroblasts, <5% blasts
Refractory cytopenia with multilineage dysplasia (RCMD)	Cytopenias (bi- or pancytopenia)	Dysplasia in ≥10% of cells in 2 or more myeloid cell lines
	No or rare blasts	<5% blasts in marrow
	No Auer rods	No Auer rods
	<1 × 10^9/L monocytes	<15% ringed sideroblasts
Refractory cytopenia with multilineage dysplasia and ringed sideroblasts (RCMD-RS)	Cytopenias (bi- or pancytopenia)	Dysplasia in ≥10% of cells in 2 or more myeloid cell lines
	No or rare blasts	≥15% ringed sideroblasts
	No Auer rods	<5% blasts
	<1 × 10^9/L monocytes	No Auer rods
Refractory anemia with excess blasts-1 (RAEB-1)	Cytopenias	Unilineage or multilineage dysplasia
	<5% blasts	5% to 9% blasts
	No Auer rods	No Auer rods
	<1 × 10^9/L monocytes	
Refractory anemia with excess blasts-2 (RAEB-2)	Cytopenias	Unilineage or multilineage dysplasia
	<5% to 19% blasts	10%-19% blasts
	Auer rods ±<1 × 10^9/L monocytes	Auer rods ±<1 × 10^9/L monocytes
Myelodysplastic syndrome, unclassified (MDS-U)	Cytopenias	Unilineage dysplasia in granulocytes or megakaryocytes
	No or rare blasts	<5% blasts
	No Auer rods	No Auer rods
MDS associated with isolated del(5q)	Anemia	Normal to increased megakarocytes with hypolobated nuclei
	<5% blasts	<5% blasts
	Platelets normal or increased	No Auer rods
		Isolated del(5q)

MDS, myelodysplastic syndrome.
Data from Vardiman JW, Harris NL, Brunning RD: The World Health Organization (WHO) classification of the myeloid neoplasms. Blood 2002;100:2292-2302.

thalidomide (Thalomid), lenalidomide (Revlimid), arsenic trioxide (Trisenox), or immunosuppressive therapy. Thalidomide, whose effects may be mediated through the inhibition of TNF-α, TGF-β and a decrease in microvessel density, appears to be more effective in patients without excess myeloblasts, in whom the response rate—defined as hematologic improvement, improvement in blood product transfusion requirements, or both—may be as high as 19%. Many patients are intolerant of the medication's side effects, which include gastrointestinal toxicity, particularly constipation, somnolence, and neurotoxicity. A thalidomide derivative, lenalidomide, has been investigated in two large phase II trials in patients with the 5q− syndrome and in patients with non-5q− early MDS. Response rates, defined as transfusion independence, in patients with the 5q− abnormality are approximately two thirds, with 44% of patient attaining a cytogenetic remission. In patients with early MDS who lack the 5q− abnormality, the transfusion independence response rate is lower, approximately 25%. Lenalidomide has been approved by the U.S. Food and Drug Administration (FDA) for use in transfusion-dependent patients with early MDS who have the 5q− abnormality.

Arsenic trioxide works through both prodifferentiation and proapoptotic mechanisms and, as a single agent, can yield response rates—defined as improvement in hematologic parameters—of 25% to 30%. This drug can also be used in patients with advanced MDS. Immunosuppressive therapy (which includes the use of antithymocyte globulin (ATG, Atgam) and cyclosporine A (Neoral, Sandimmune)) takes advantage of the immune-mediated aspects of MDS and may be effective in the subset of patients with hypoplastic MDS, MDS that resembles aplastic anemia, with a hypocellular bone marrow. Improved hematologic counts and transfusion independence may be achieved in up to 33% of appropriately treated patients.

For patients with advanced MDS, two drugs approved for use in MDS by the FDA deserve mention, 5-azacitidine (azacitidine; 5-AZA, Vidaza), and decitabine (Dacogen). These hypomethylating agents induce hematopoietic progenitor cell differentiation. In a recent phase III trial, responses occurred in 60% of patients treated with 5-azacitidine compared with 5% of patients receiving supportive care, including 23% complete or partial remissions. Median survival, transformation to AML, and even quality of life were better for patients receiving 5-azacitidine than for those receiving supportive care. Decitabine has been investigated in a multicenter phase III study, in which responses were achieved in 30% of patients, with a complete and partial remission rate in 17%.

Allogeneic hematopoietic stem cell transplantation (HSCT), the only potentially curative approach to MDS, is a realistic option for only about 5% to 10% of patients because MDS is usually diagnosed in patients in their seventh or eighth decade of life. Conditioning regimens typically consist of busulfan (Myleran) and cyclophosphamide (Cytoxan), and long-term (often 2-year) disease-free survival approaches 40%, although studies have often included younger MDS patients (with a median age between 30 and 45 years) in earlier stages of MDS. Treatment-related mortality may be as high as 40% to 50%. Newer approaches take advantage of nonmyeloablative ("mini") conditioning regimens in an effort to reduce treatment-related mortality and to include older patients with MDS. This type of transplantation is still considered experimental, but can be offered to patients up to 70 years of age who otherwise are in good health. Allogeneic HSCT should be considered as up-front therapy in patients with advanced subtypes of MDS, but can be delayed in patients with early MDS.

Summary

- Determine whether the patient has early or advanced MDS.
- For early MDS, growth factors may be initiated once patients are almost or completely transfusion-dependent.
- Once growth factors fail, or in patients less likely to respond to growth factors, non-growth factor approaches lead to responses in 15% to 66% of patients.
- For advanced MDS, HSCT or therapy with hypomethylating agents should be initiated immediately.

OUTCOMES

One of the most widely used prognostic systems for MDS patients is the International Prognostic Scoring System (IPSS; Tables 3 and 4). The IPSS separates patients into four distinct subgroups based solely on the percentage of bone marrow blasts, cytogenetics, and the number of cytopenias. Patients with fewer bone marrow blasts and cytopenias and with better cytogenetic profiles (normal, 5q−, 20q−, Y−) have a prolonged median survival, whereas those with more blasts and cytopenias and worse cytogenetic profiles (complex, or with abnormalities of chromosome 7) have a shorter survival.

Table 3 Myelodysplastic Syndrome International Prognostic Scoring System

Parameter	Score				
Prognostic variable	0	0.5	1.0	1.5	2.0
Bone marrow blasts (%)	<5	5-10		11-20	21-30
Cytogenetics	Good	Intermediate	Poor		
Cytopenias	0/1	2/3			

Adapted from Greenberg P, Cox C, LeBeau MM, et al: International scoring system for evaluating prognosis in myelodysplastic syndromes. Blood 1997;89:2079-2088.

Table 4 Myelodysplastic Syndrome Prognosis

Score	IPSS Subgroup	Median Survival (yr)
0	Low	5.7
0.5-1.0	Intermediate 1	3.5
1.5-2.0	Intermediate 2	1.2
>2.5	High	0.4

IPSS, International Prognostic Scoring System.
Adapted from Greenberg P, Cox1 C, LeBeau MM, et al: International scoring system for evaluating prognosis in myelodysplastic syndromes. Blood 1997;89:2079-2088.

Suggested Readings

Aul C, Gattermann N, Schneider W: Age-related incidence and other epidemiological aspects of myelodysplastic syndromes. Br J Haematol 1992;82:358-367.

Allampallam K, Shetty V, Mundle S, et al: Biological significance of proliferation, apoptosis, cytokines, and monocyte/macrophage cells in bone marrow biopsies of 145 patients with myelodysplastic syndrome. Int J Hematol 2002;75:289-297.

Bennett JM, Catovsky D, Daniel MT, et al: Proposals for the classification of the myelodysplastic syndromes. Br J Haematol 1982;51:189-199.

Fenaux P, Morel P, Lai JL: Cytogenetics of myelodysplastic syndromes. Semin Hematol 1996;33:127-138.

Greenberg P, Cox C, LeBeau MM, et al: International scoring system for evaluating prognosis in myelodysplastic syndromes. Blood 1997;89:2079-2088.

Kernan NA, Bartsch G, Ash RC, et al: Analysis of 462 transplantations from unrelated donors facilitated by the National Marrow Donor Program. N Engl J Med 1993;328:593-602.

List A, Kurtin S, Rose D, et al: Efficacy of lenalidomide in myelodysplastic syndromes. N Engl J Med 2005;352:549-557.

Molldrem JJ, Caples M, Mavroudis D, et al: Antithymocyte globulin for patients with myelodysplastic syndrome. Br J Haematol 1997;99:699-705.

Negrin RS, Stein R, Doherty K, et al: Maintenance treatment of the anemia of myelodysplastic syndromes with recombinant human granulocyte colony-stimulating factor and erythropoietin: Evidence for in vivo synergy. Blood 1996;87:4076-4081.

Silverman LR, Demakos EP, Peterson BL, et al: Randomized controlled trial of azacitidine in patients with the myelodysplastic syndrome: A study of the cancer and leukemia group B. J Clin Oncol 2002;20:2429-2440.

Vardiman JW, Harris NL, Brunning RD: The World Health Organization (WHO) classification of the myeloid neoplasms. Blood 2002;100:2292-2302.

Chronic Leukemias

Ronald M. Sobecks** and **Karl Theil

DEFINITION

The chronic leukemias are a group of malignancies involving the hematopoietic system. Chronic myelogenous leukemia (CML) is a myeloproliferative disease that arises from a clonal process involving an early progenitor hematopoietic stem cell. It also is associated with the Philadelphia (Ph) chromosome, *bcr/abl* fusion gene, or both. Chronic myelomonocytic leukemia (CMML) has recently been reclassified by the World Health Organization as a myelodysplastic-myeloproliferative disease. It originates from a clonal hematopoietic stem cell disorder in which there are dysplastic features in at least one myeloid lineage, less than 20% blasts in the blood and bone marrow, a persistent monocytosis, and no evidence of Ph chromosome or the *bcr/abl* fusion gene. Chronic neutrophilic leukemia (CNL) is a rare myeloproliferative disorder characterized by a sustained, mature neutrophilic leukocytosis. There is no monocytosis, eosinophilia, or basophilia and no associated Ph or *bcr/abl* fusion gene. Chronic eosinophilic leukemia (CEL) is another myeloproliferative disease similar to hypereosinophilic syndrome but that is characterized by a clonal proliferation of eosinophilic precursors with increased blasts. Chronic lymphocytic leukemia (CLL) is a clonal expansion of small, round, and mature-appearing lymphocytes. Hairy cell leukemia (HCL) is a malignancy of small B lymphoid cells that display surface cytoplasmic "hairy" projections.

INCIDENCE

The incidence of CML is approximately 1 per 100,000 population per year. In 2006, it was estimated that there would be 4500 new cases, with 600 estimated deaths. Most CML cases are identified in the fifth and sixth decades of life, and there is a higher incidence in males. The actual incidence of CMML is difficult to determine because patients were previously included in other diagnostic categories, such as CML and myelodysplastic syndrome. However, it has been estimated to occur annually in 3 per 100,000 individuals older than 60 years. The median age at diagnosis is 65 to 75 years, and there has been a higher incidence in men. CNL is rare, with only 33 case reports being identified that appeared to have met the diagnostic criteria. The mean age at diagnosis is 62.5 years, and there is a 2:1 male-to-female ratio. CEL is also rare, but the actual incidence is unknown, because patients with the disease have often been categorized with those having hypereosinophilic syndrome. The incidence is highest in the fourth decade of life, and the disease more commonly affects men. CLL is the most common form of leukemia in Western countries and is more prevalent with increasing age. Most patients are older than 50 years, and there is a 2:1 male-to-female ratio. For patients older than 70 years, the incidence is more than 20 per 100,000 population. In 2006, it was estimated that there would be approximately 10,000 new cases of CLL, with approximately 4,700 estimated deaths. HCL accounts for about 2% of all leukemias, with an estimated 600 new cases in the United States annually. The median age at diagnosis is 55 years, and there is a 5:1 male-to-female ratio.

PATHOPHYSIOLOGY AND NATURAL HISTORY

In chronic leukemias, there is an accumulation of malignant hematopoietic cells in the bone marrow that ultimately may lead to bone marrow failure states. Cytopenias may result in hemorrhage, infection, and organ compromise (e.g., congestive heart failure from severe anemia).

CML is characterized by a balanced reciprocal translocation between the long arms of chromosomes 9 and 22 [t(9;22)(q34;q11.2)] that occurs in about 90% to 95% of cases. This translocation results in the juxtaposition of the *c-abl* proto-oncogene from chromosome 9 with a portion of the *bcr* gene located on chromosome 22, thereby producing a novel *bcr/abl* fusion gene. The gene product results in an 8.5-kb mRNA transcript that generates a 210-kd bcr/abl fusion protein having abnormal tyrosine kinase activity. Through phosphorylation, this enzyme may activate different signal transduction pathways that may result in increased proliferation and decreased apoptosis (programmed cell death) of hematopoietic cells.

CML is also characterized by three phases that occur during the course of the disease. Initially, there is a chronic phase that may last approximately 2 to 5 years, during which time the disease is often indolent. With progression of the disease, there is an accelerated phase that lasts 6 to 18 months and ultimately blast crisis develops, which appears similar to that of an aggressive acute leukemia, with a survival of only about 3 to 6 months. The exact molecular mechanism by which CML transforms to more advanced stages of the disease is unknown. However, it is possible that a series of genetic changes is responsible, which would be supported by the finding of additional chromosomal abnormalities that can develop during disease acceleration, known as clonal evolution.

CMML is suspected to originate from an abnormal hematopoietic stem cell. This disease arises because of dysregulation of myeloid proliferation, maturation, and cell survival. It may result in dysplastic hematopoiesis and cytopenias as well as organ compromise from leukemic infiltration. Abnormalities in the Ras signaling pathway may also be involved in this process. In addition, a single recurrent somatic activating mutation (JAK2V617F) in the Janus kinase 2 (JAK2) tyrosine kinase has been noted in 8% to 13% of cases.

CNL may arise from a granulocyte-committed progenitor. Cytogenetic and molecular studies have demonstrated the clonal nature of the disease; however, most reports have found that patients have normal cytogenetics. Patients eventually develop either progressive neutrophilia or blastic transformation. Somatic mutation in the JH2 autoinhibitory domain of the JAK2 tyrosine kinase has only infrequently been observed in CNL.

CEL may arise from a multipotent, pluripotent, or eosinophil-committed progenitor cell. The disease is also characterized by a chronic phase that may progress to blast crisis. Organ damage may result from leukemic tissue infiltration as well as from eosinophilic cytokine and enzyme release (e.g., major basic protein, eosinophil cationic protein). An interstitial deletion resulting in the FIP1L1-PDGFRα fusion protein, with constitutive tyrosine kinase activity, has been identified in hematopoietic cells of these patients.

In CLL, there is an accumulation of neoplastic lymphocytes, without the increased proliferation that results from abnormalities in apoptosis. The *bcl-2* proto-oncogene produces the bcl-2 protein that inhibits apoptotic cell death. This protein is overexpressed in most cases of CLL. The neoplastic cells, in turn, have prolonged survival, which allows them to increase in the peripheral blood, bone marrow, and other lymphoid tissues. Patients subsequently may develop cytopenias as a result of progressive bone marrow involvement or autoimmune abnormalities. This, as well as hypogammaglobulinemia and T cell dysfunction, may allow bacterial, fungal, and viral infections to occur. CLL may also transform to large cell lymphoma (Richter's syndrome) or prolymphocytic leukemia.

Although the cause of CLL is unknown, chromosomal abnormalities are present in approximately 80% of cases. Most common are deletions of chromosomes 13q14 and 11q22-23, as well as trisomy 12. More recent investigation has suggested that the predominant alterations in the neoplastic cell's genome involve transcriptional and post-transcriptional deregulations of a novel class of genes known as micro-RNAs (miRNAs). In particular, for B cell CLL, the miRNA genes *miR-15a* and *miR-16-1*, located at 13q14.3, are often deleted, downregulated, or both. These miRNAs allow induction of apoptosis by negatively regulating bcl-2. In addition, normal B cells may be distinguished from B cell CLL by miRNA expression profiles, which have also been associated with other prognostic factors in CLL.

HCL has been postulated to originate from a peripheral B cell, but the stage of its development after leaving the germinal center has not been delineated. The leukemia cells release tumor necrosis factor, which may inhibit hematopoiesis and result in cytopenias. More recently, gene expression profiling has demonstrated a distinct homogeneous pattern that differs from those of other B cell non-Hodgkin's lymphomas. These analyses have suggested that HCL cells may be derived from memory B cells. In comparison with memory cells, HCL cells have demonstrated a notable conservation in proliferation, apoptosis, and DNA metabolism programs while having altered gene expression that might affect cell adhesion and response to chemokines. HCL also expresses CD25 (interleukin-2 [IL-2] receptor), which may contribute to the proliferation of the disease.

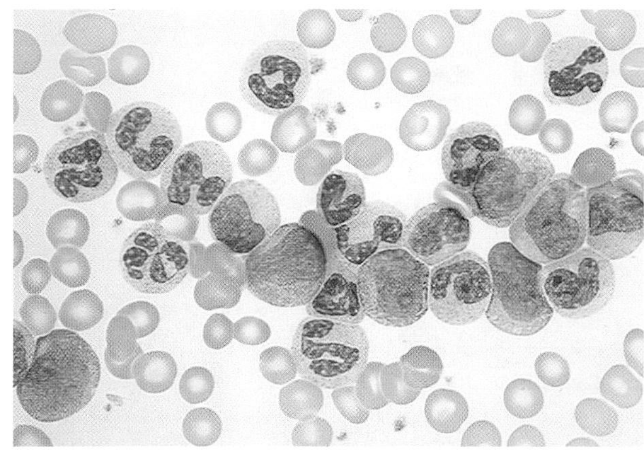

Figure 1 Chronic phase of chronic myelogenous leukemia. The peripheral blood smear is characterized by an elevated white blood cell count showing a left shift in granulocyte maturation, with increased myelocytes. Eosinophilia and basophilia are characteristic (Wright-Giemsa stain, ×100).

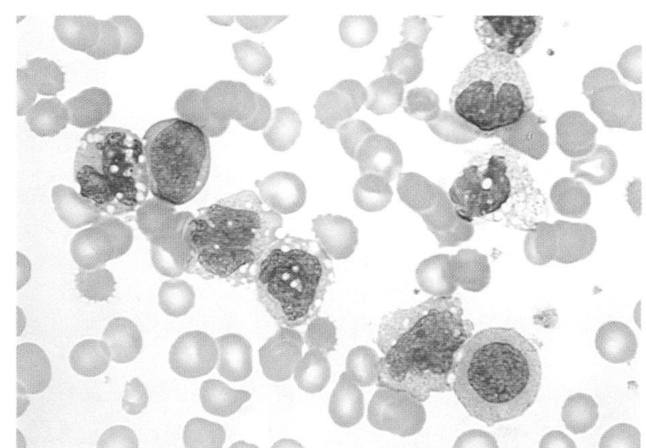

Figure 2 Chronic myelomonocytic leukemia. The peripheral blood smear demonstrates absolute monocytosis (1×10^9/L) as one of the defining criteria. Circulating blasts may also be present (Wright-Giemsa stain, ×100).

SIGNS AND SYMPTOMS

Many patients with chronic leukemias are asymptomatic and their disease is only identified by finding an abnormality during routine laboratory testing. These patients may develop constitutional symptoms such as fatigue, anorexia, weight loss, sweats, and fever. With progressive bone marrow involvement and the development of cytopenias, various infections can occur, as well as hemorrhage, anemia-related symptoms (e.g., dyspnea, lightheadedness, and fatigue), and easy bruising, with petechiae and purpura.

Hepatosplenomegaly and lymphadenopathy may be present and result in a sensation of abdominal fullness, along with discomfort and early satiety. Although lymphadenopathy is uncommon in chronic phase CML, it may develop in more advanced stages of the disease. Some patients with chronic leukemia may present with hyperleukocytosis that can result in marked splenomegaly. In patients with CML, priapism may also develop.

In CEL, other symptoms related to organ infiltration can occur. Cardiac involvement is the most common, with possible necrosis, endomyocardial fibrosis, congestive heart failure, valvular regurgitation, mural thrombosis, and thromboembolic events. In addition, neurologic (e.g., cognitive dysfunction, peripheral neuropathy), pulmonary (e.g., cough), cutaneous (e.g., angioedema, papules, nodules, urticaria), gastrointestinal, ocular, rheumatologic, and renal involvement may develop.

DIAGNOSIS

The initial evaluation of chronic leukemias should include an analysis of the bone marrow, peripheral blood, or both, with morphologic review by an experienced hematopathologist, immunophenotyping, chromosomal analysis, and appropriate molecular studies. In certain cases, a similar pathologic evaluation may be performed on an excised lymph node, spleen, or other tissue biopsy specimen (e.g., endomyocardial biopsy for CEL).

The diagnosis of CML may be established on morphologic review and by demonstrating the presence of the Ph chromosome [t(9;22)] or the *bcr/abl* fusion gene. In chronic phase CML, the peripheral blood shows a neutrophilic leukocytosis, with a left shift revealing immature granulocytic forms. Other findings include a blast count of less than 10%, basophilia, eosinophilia, thrombocytosis, and anemia. The bone marrow findings include myeloid hyperplasia with immature forms, less than 10% blasts, and no dysplasia; mild to moderate myelofibrosis may be present. Fig. 1 illustrates some morphologic findings in chronic phase CML. Figures 2 to 4 demonstrate the characteristic morphology of CMML, CNL, and CEL.

The National Cancer Institute–sponsored Working Group revised guidelines for CLL diagnosis require an absolute lymphocytosis with more than 5×10^9/L mature-appearing lymphocytes and less than 55% atypical cells or prolymphocytes. The bone marrow should demonstrate more than 30% lymphocytic involvement of all nucleated cells. However, a bone marrow analysis is not necessary to establish the diagnosis because of the routine use of peripheral blood flow cytometric analysis for immunophenotyping. Phenotypic features consistent with B cell CLL include most lymphocytes expressing B cell markers (CD19, CD20, and CD23) with CD5 but without other pan-T cell markers; monoclonality of B cells with either kappa or lambda light chain restriction; and low-density surface immunoglobulin. Morphologic findings of CLL are shown in Figure 5.

HCL may be diagnosed on finding hairy cells on morphologic review of the peripheral blood (Fig. 6). The cells are medium-sized lymphoid cells with abundant cytoplasm that extends circumferentially as "hairy" projections. The cells are tartrate-resistant and acid phosphatase-positive, and immunophenotyping demonstrates the expression of CD19, CD20, CD22, CD25, CD11c, and CD103.

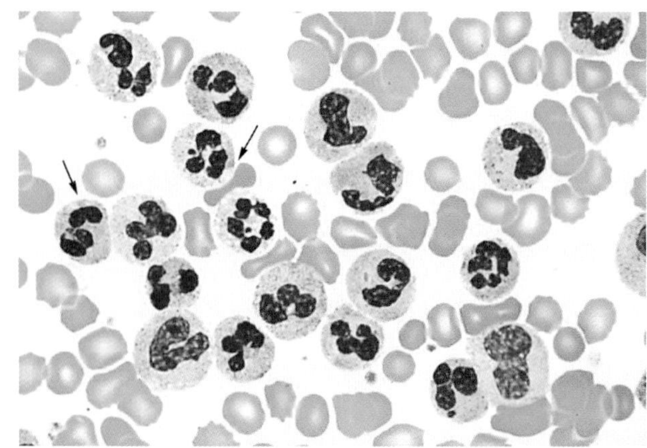

Figure 3 Chronic neutrophilic leukemia. The peripheral blood smear shows an absolute neutrophilia without the significant left shift, vacuolization, or toxic granulation usually associated with a reactive process. Döhle bodies (*arrows*) are often present in the cytoplasm of neutrophils (Wright-Giemsa stain, ×100).

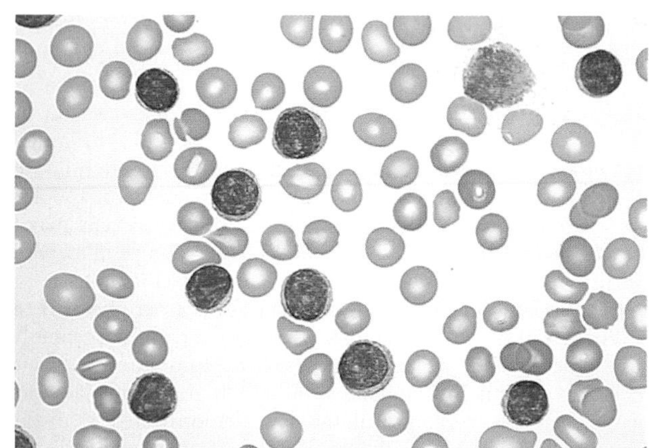

Figure 5 Chronic lymphocytic leukemia. The peripheral blood smear shows an absolute lymphocytosis of small "mature" lymphocytes with clumped, smudgy chromatin and scant cytoplasm. Smudge cells (*near top right*) are a common finding (Wright-Giemsa stain, ×100).

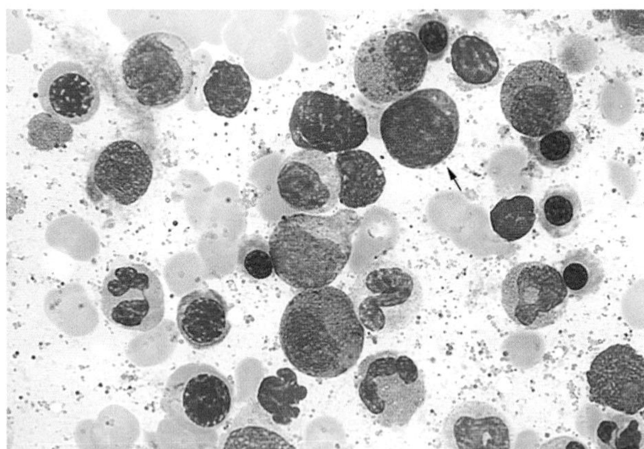

Figure 4 Hypereosinophilic syndrome—chronic eosinophilic leukemia. This bone marrow aspirate smear from a patient with hypereosinophilic syndrome demonstrates marked eosinophilia with mainly mature features. An increase in blasts (*arrow*) should prompt consideration of a neoplastic process. Numerous eosinophil granules from degranulated cells result in a "dirty" background in this illustration (Wright-Giemsa stain, ×100).

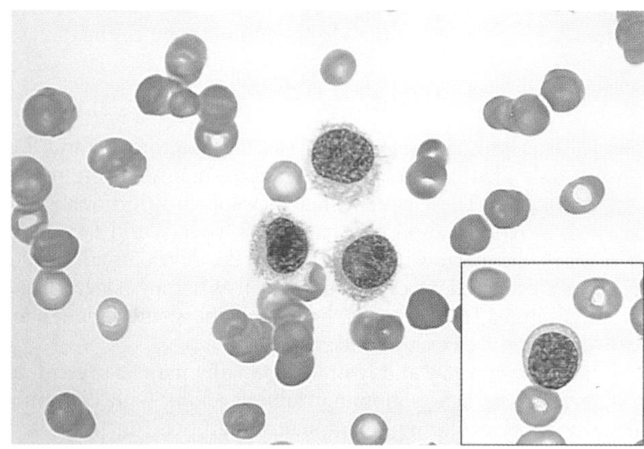

Figure 6 Hairy cell leukemia. Classic hairy cells (*center*) demonstrate cytoplasmic projections. *Inset,* In comparison with a normal lymphocyte, the hairy cells are larger, have slightly less condensed chromatin, and often contain small nucleoli (Wright-Giemsa stain, ×100).

Summary

- Diagnostic criteria for accelerated and blast phase CML, CMML, CNL, and CEL are shown in Boxes 1 to 4, respectively.
- A diagnosis of CLL requires an absolute lymphocytosis with more than 5×10^9/L mature-appearing lymphocytes (with less than 55% atypical cells or prolymphocytes); the diagnosis may be established by peripheral blood flow cytometric analysis, which identifies characteristic immunophenotypic markers.
- HCL may be diagnosed on finding hairy cells on morphologic review of the peripheral blood that are tartrate-resistant and acid phosphatase-positive and have characteristic immunophenotypic markers by flow cytometric analysis.

Box 1 Diagnostic Criteria for Accelerated and Blast Phase Chronic Myelogenous Leukemias

Accelerated Phase*

Blasts composing 10%-19% of peripheral blood WBCs, nucleated bone marrow cells, or both
≥20% peripheral blood basophils
Persistent thrombocytopenia (<100×10^9/L) unrelated to treatment
Persistent thrombocytosis (>1000×10^9/L) unresponsive to treatment
Increasing splenomegaly or leukocytosis unresponsive to treatment
Cytogenetic evidence of clonal evolution

Blast Phase*

Blasts composing ≥20% of peripheral blood WBCs, nucleated bone marrow cells, or both
Extramedullary blast proliferation
Large foci or clusters of blasts in the bone marrow biopsy

**Requires one or more of the criteria listed.*
WBC, white blood cell.
Adapted with permission from Vardiman JW, Pierre R, Thiele J, et al: Chronic myelogenous leukemia. In Jaffe ES, Harris NL, Stein H, Vardiman JW (eds): World Health Organization Classification of Tumours. Pathology and Genetics. Tumours of Haematopoietic and Lymphoid Tissues. Lyon, France, IARC Press, 2001, pp 17-31, 47-52.

Box 2 Diagnostic Criteria for Chronic Myelomonocytic Leukemia

- Persistent monocytosis (>1 × 10^9/L) in the peripheral blood
- No Philadelphia chromosome or *bcr/abl* fusion gene
- <20% blasts and promonocytes in the peripheral blood and bone marrow
- One myeloid lineage or more, with dysplasia:

If there is no dysplasia, the diagnosis of CMML can still be made:

- If the other requirements are satisfied *and* the marrow cells contain an acquired, clonal cytogenetic abnormality.

  or

- If there is persistent monocytosis for 3 months *and* all other causes of monocytosis have been excluded.

Adapted with permission from Vardiman JW, Pierre R, Bain B, et al: Chronic myelomonocytic leukemia. In Jaffe ES, Harris NL, Stein H, Vardiman JW (eds): World Health Organization Classification of Tumours. Pathology and Genetics. Tumours of Haematopoietic and Lymphoid Tissues. Lyon, France, IARC Press, 2001, pp 17-31, 47-52.

Box 3 Diagnostic Criteria for Chronic Neutrophilic Leukemia

Peripheral blood leukocytosis ≥25 × 10^9/L

- Segmented neutrophils and bands >80% of leukocytes
- Immature granulocytes <10% of leukocytes
- Myeloblasts <1% of leukocytes

Hypercellular bone marrow

- Increased number and percentage of neutrophilic granulocytes
- Nucleated marrow cells, with <5% myeloblasts
- Normal neutrophilic maturation pattern

Hepatosplenomegaly
No Philadelphia chromosome or *bcr/abl* fusion gene
No other cause for neutrophilia

- No infectious or inflammatory process
- No evidence of another myeloproliferative disease
- No evidence of a myelodysplastic or myelodysplatic, myeloproliferative disease
- No evidence of a tumor or, if present, myeloid cells must show clonality

Adapted with permission from Imbert M, Bain B, Pierre R, et al: Chronic neutrophilic leukemia. In Jaffe ES, Harris NL, Stein H, Vardiman JW (eds): World Health Organization Classification of Tumours. Pathology and Genetics. Tumours of Haematopoietic and Lymphoid Tissues. Lyon, France, IARC Press, 2001, pp 17-31, 47-52.

TREATMENT

The goals of therapy for an individual patient with chronic leukemia should be determined before formulating a treatment plan. These goals range from cure to improved survival and quality of life to disease palliation and comfort measures.

The principal goal in treating CML is to eliminate the clone of cells that have the Ph chromosome or *bcr/abl* fusion gene. Hydroxyurea has been a standard therapy for chronic phase disease, and it can achieve hematologic remissions as well as decrease splenomegaly. However, this form of therapy does not result in cytogenetic remissions. Subsequently, in the early 1980s, therapy with interferon alfa was demonstrated not only to achieve hematologic remissions in most patients, but also to result in cytogenetic remissions in up to 35% of patients. These patients also had a survival advantage over those treated with hydroxyurea. However, intolerable symptoms from interferon, such as a flulike syndrome, anorexia, and depression, have prevented continuation of this agent in some patients. Subsequently, a specific *bcr/abl* tyrosine kinase inhibitor, imatinib (STI571; Gleevec), was developed. This agent has demonstrated substantial hematologic and major cytogenetic responses in patients with chronic phase CML who were refractory to interferon alfa as well as in patients with accelerated phase CML or blast crisis. A randomized clinical trial of imatinib versus interferon and low-dose cytarabine in patients with newly diagnosed chronic phase CML has revealed imatinib to be vastly superior for achievement of complete hematologic, major cytogenetic, and complete cytogenetic responses, as well as for progression-free survival.

Box 4 Diagnostic Criteria for Chronic Eosinophilic Leukemia

Persistent eosinophilia >1.5 × 10^9/L in blood, increased bone marrow eosinophils
>5% but <19% myeloblasts in bone marrow or >2% in peripheral blood
Clonality of myeloid cells
No reactive eosinophilia caused by allergy, parasitic, infectious, pulmonary, or collagen vascular disease
No reactive eosinophilia caused by other malignancies:

- T cell lymphomas
- Acute lymphoblastic leukemia, lymphoma
- Other myeloproliferative diseases
- Acute myeloid leukemia, including inv(16), t(16;16)
- Mastocytosis
- Chronic myelogenous leukemia
- Myelodysplastic syndrome
- Hodgkin's lymphoma

No T cell population, with abnormal cytokine production and aberrant phenotype

Adapted with permission from Bain B, Pierre R, Imbert M, et al: Chronic eosinophilic leukemia. In Jaffe ES, Harris NL, Stein H, Vardiman JW (eds): World Health Organization Classification of Tumours. Pathology and Genetics. Tumours of Haematopoietic and Lymphoid Tissues. Lyon, France, IARC Press, 2001, pp 17-31, 47-52.

More recently, the novel tyrosine kinase inhibitors dasatinib (BMS-354825; Sprycel) and nilotinib (Tasigna; AMN107), have been shown to induce hematologic and cytogenetic responses in patients with CML or Ph+ ALL who cannot tolerate or are resistant to imatinib. Clinical trials combining STI571 with other agents are currently in progress. Allogeneic hematopoietic stem cell transplantation is a standard therapy for CML, with curative potential. However, this therapy is limited to younger patients with human leukocyte antigen (HLA)-matched donors, and there are significant transplant-related morbidity and mortality risks with this approach. Nonmyeloablative or reduced intensity conditioning, allogeneic, hematopoietic stem cell transplantation has recently been investigated. This has expanded the potential for transplantation to older patients and those not medically suitable for a myeloablative transplant. Autologous hematopoietic stem cell transplantation has been performed for chronic phase CML patients, with substantially fewer transplantation-related mortality risks than with an allogeneic approach. However, most of these patients develop recurrent disease because of the lack of a graft-versus-leukemia effect that may be achieved after allogeneic transplantation. Further evidence of a graft-versus-leukemia effect in the allogeneic setting comes from the observation that durable remissions can be achieved with donor leukocyte infusions in patients who relapse after allogeneic transplantation. The National Comprehensive Cancer Center (NCCN) clinical practice guidelines for CML can be reviewed at online at www.nccn.org/professionals/physician_gls/PDF/cml.pdf.

CMML has previously been classified with and treated as a myelodysplastic syndrome. Therapeutic approaches have included best supportive care measures, such as antibiotics and blood product transfusion support. Other treatment modalities have consisted of growth factors (e.g., granulocyte colony-stimulating factor, granulocyte-macrophage colony-stimulating factor, erythropoietin), amifostine, immunosuppressive therapy (e.g., antithymocyte globulin, cyclosporine), hypomethylating agents (e.g., azacytidine, decitabine), low-intensity chemotherapy (e.g., hydroxyurea), high-intensity chemotherapy (e.g., topotecan), and allogeneic hematopoietic stem cell transplantation.

Therapy for CNL and CEL has included agents such as hydroxyurea, busulfan, 6-thioguanine, and interferon. Although these agents have been able to control the disease burden and reduce splenomegaly, they have not been curative. Imatinib has been demonstrated to be effective in CEL. However, allogeneic hematopoietic stem cell transplantation may potentially cure some patients who are appropriate candidates for this aggressive approach.

Often, patients with CLL require no initial treatment. Therapy is indicated for patients who develop systemic symptoms (e.g., extreme fatigue, fevers, night sweats, weight loss), worsening anemia or thrombocytopenia from progressive bone marrow involvement or an autoimmune cause that is not responsive to corticosteroids; massive or progressive splenomegaly or lymphadenopathy, or a rapid lymphocyte doubling time (<6 months). Therapeutic agents have included chlorambucil, with or without corticosteroids, cyclophosphamide-vincristine-prednisone (CVP), and purine analogues (e.g., fludarabine, cladribine). When compared with chlorambucil, fludarabine has demonstrated an improved disease-free survival but no improvement in overall survival. Rituximab and alemtuzumab, monoclonal antibodies directed against CD20 and CD52, respectively, have demonstrated significant single-agent activity in CLL and are currently being evaluated in combination trials with other agents. For select patients, both autologous and allogeneic hematopoietic stem cell transplantation may also be considered, including nonmyeloablative approaches with reduced intensity conditioning regimens. The National Comprehensive Cancer Center (NCCN) clinical practice guidelines for CLL can be reviewed at www.nccn.org/professionals/physician_gls/PDF/nhl.pdf.

Therapy for HCL previously had been indicated for patients who developed severe infections or cytopenias, as well as for patients with symptomatic splenomegaly. Initial therapeutic approaches consisted of splenectomy and, later, interferon alfa. Subsequently, pentostatin and cladribine were found to be highly effective, with most patients achieving durable long-term remissions. Therefore, treatment with these agents is often administered earlier, before patients become symptomatic. More recently, rituximab and the anti-CD22 recombinant immunotoxin BL22 have also been found to be effective therapy for relapsed or refractory HCL.

Summary

- Although different treatments exist for CML, most patients are now initially managed with imatinib. Allogeneic hematopoietic stem cell transplantation remains a potentially curative treatment approach for suitable patients who do not respond to imatinib and who have HLA-matched donors.
- CMML, CNL, and CEL may be managed with various cytotoxic therapies. However, allogeneic hematopoietic stem cell transplantation may potentially cure some patients who are appropriate candidates.
- Patients with CLL who require treatment may be managed with chemotherapy (e.g., chlorambucil, fludarabine), monoclonal antibodies (e.g., rituximab, alemtuzumab), clinical trials, or hematopoietic stem cell transplantation.
- HCL may be effectively treated initially with a purine analogue (e.g., cladribine, pentostatin), whereas relapsed and refractory disease may be managed well with rituximab or the anti-CD22 recombinant immunotoxin BL22.

OUTCOMES

Patients with chronic phase CML usually have a longer survival than those with a more advanced phase of the disease. However, prognostic systems have been proposed to help predict outcomes more effectively. Initially, before the use of interferon, Sokal and colleagues had found age, spleen size, platelet count, and percentage of myeloblasts to be independent prognostic factors. With the use of a Cox model, patients were then categorized into high-, intermediate-, or low-risk groups, with median survivals of 34, 44, and 57 months, respectively. The Hasford system was developed for patients previously treated with interferon; it was found that the percentage of basophils and eosinophils were other prognostic factors in addition to those from the Sokal scoring system. Respective median survivals for the high-, intermediate-, and low-risk groups were 42, 65, and 98 months, respectively. The Gratwohl risk assessment system was developed for patients before allogeneic stem cell transplantation. Risk factors included stage of the disease, histocompatibility, age, interval from diagnosis to transplant, and donor and recipient gender. Five-year survivals incrementally increased from 18% to 72%, whereas transplantation-related mortality incrementally decreased from 73% to 20% for high-risk to low-risk score patients, respectively. More recently, it has been demonstrated by quantitative real-time polymerase chain reaction assay that those patients on imatinib who achieve a 3-log reduction in bcr-abl transcript levels by 12 months of therapy have a negligible risk of disease progression during the subsequent 12 months.

For CMML, median survivals have often ranged from 20 to 40 months. This disease had been included in the International Prognostic Scoring System for myelodysplastic syndromes. Independent risk factors identified were the percentage of bone marrow blasts, cytogenetic abnormalities, and number of cytopenias. After generating a risk score based on the number of these factors that were present, patients were categorized into low-, first intermediate-, second intermediate-, or high-risk groups, with median survivals of 5.7, 3.5, 1.2, and 0.4 years, respectively.

CNL is a slowly progressive disease, with survivals reported from 6 months to 20 years. Death may occur as a result of progressive refractory neutrophilia or from transformation to acute leukemia. CEL may also have a variable survival, ranging from months to longer than 20 years. The findings of marked splenomegaly, increasing blasts, dysplasia in other myeloid lineages, and severe visceral disease are poor prognostic factors.

Although CLL is considered an indolent disease, standard therapeutic approaches have not been curative. The Rai clinical staging system groups patients into five stages: (0) lymphocytosis only, (1) lymphadenopathy, (2) hepatosplenomegaly, (3) anemia, and (4) thrombocytopenia. Median survivals were 12+, 8.5, 6, 1.5, and 1.5 years, respectively. Other unfavorable prognostic factors include a rapid lymphocyte doubling time (<12 months) and CD38 expression. Genomic aberrations, mutated *IgVH* genes (and its surrogate marker ZAP-70 expression), as well as serum B_2 microglobulin and thymidine kinase, also provide additional prognostic information.

Untreated HCL patients have a median survival of approximately 5 years. However, therapy with cladribine or pentostatin has achieved 10-year overall survival rates of 80% to 90%.

Suggested Readings

Caligaris-Cappio F: Biology of chronic lymphocytic leukemia. Rev Clin Exp Hematol 2000;4:5-21.

Cheson BD, Bennett JM, Grever M, et al: National Cancer Institute-sponsored Working Group guidelines for chronic lymphocytic leukemia: Revised guidelines for diagnosis and treatment. Blood 1996;87:4990-4997.

Greenberg P, Cox C, LeBeau MM, et al: International scoring system for evaluating prognosis in myelodysplastic syndromes. Blood 1997;89:2079-2088.

Harris NL, et al: Mature B-cell neoplasms. In Jaffe ES, Harris NL, Stein H, Vardiman JW (eds): World Health Organization Classification of Tumours. Pathology and Genetics. Tumours of Haematopoietic and Lymphoid Tissues. Lyon, France, IARC Press, 2001, pp 127-130, 138-141.

Jelinek J, Oki Y, Gharibyan V, et al: JAK2 mutation 1849G > T is rare in acute leukemias but can be found in CMML, Philadelphia chromosome-negative CML, and megakaryocytic leukemia. Blood 2005;106:3370-3373.

Jemal A, Siegel R, Ward E, et al: Cancer statistics, 2006. CA Cancer J Clin 2006;56:106-130.

Oliver JW, Deol I, Morgan DL, Tonk VS: Chronic eosinophilic leukemia and hypereosinophilic syndromes. Proposal for classification, literature review, and report of a case with a unique chromosomal abnormality. Cancer Genet Cytogenet 1998;107:111-117.

Reilly JT: Chronic neutrophilic leukaemia: A distinct clinical entity? Br J Haematol 2002;116:10-18.

Sokal JE, Cox EB, Baccarani M, et al: Prognostic discrimination in "good-risk" chronic granulocytic leukemia. Blood 1984;63:789-799.

Vardiman JW, Pierre R, Bain B, et al: Chronic myelomonocytic leukemia. In Jaffe ES, Harris NL, Stein H, Vardiman JW (eds): World Health Organization Classification of Tumours. Pathology and Genetics. Tumours of Haematopoietic and Lymphoid Tissues. Lyon, France, IARC Press, 2001, pp 17-31, 47-52.

Chronic Myeloproliferative Disorders

Anjali Advani and Karl Theil

Chronic myeloproliferative disorders (MPDs) are characterized by the clonal proliferation of one or more hematopoietic cell lineages, predominantly in the bone marrow, but sometimes in the liver and spleen.[1] Traditionally, the chronic myeloproliferative disorders have included polycythemia vera (PV), chronic idiopathic myelofibrosis (CIMF), essential thrombocythemia (ET), chronic myelogenous leukemia (CML), and chronic myelomonocytic leukemia (CMML).[1] The World Health Organization (WHO) has reclassified CMML from the myelodysplastic syndrome (MDS) group into a new group of MDS/MPDs because its clinical and pathologic features overlap those of traditional MDS disorders and MPDs.[2] Revisions to the WHO classification of PV, CIMF, and ET are anticipated, and reflect a new understanding of the role of Janus kinase 2 (*JAK2*) mutation as a molecular marker of myeloid neoplasia.[3] This chapter reviews the definition, prevalence, pathophysiology, signs and symptoms, diagnosis, treatment, and outcomes of each of these clinical entities. CML is discussed elsewhere in this section ("Chronic Leukemias").

POLYCYTHEMIA VERA

Definition and Etiology

PV is a clonal disorder characterized by the overproduction of mature red blood cells in the bone marrow.[1] Myeloid and megakaryocytic elements are also often increased. No obvious cause exists.[4] Genetic and environmental factors have been implicated in rare cases. Familial PV has been associated with mutation of the erythropoietin receptor.[5] An increased number of cases has been reported in survivors of the atomic bomb explosion in Hiroshima during World War II.

Epidemiology

The disorder typically occurs in the sixth or seventh decade of life. The prevalence of the disease is approximately 5 per million population; it occurs more commonly in men and in men and women of East European Jewish ancestry.[1,4]

Pathophysiology

The primary defect involves a pluripotent stem cell capable of differentiating into red blood cells, granulocytes, and platelets.[4] Clonality has been demonstrated through glucose-6-phosphate dehydrogenase (G6PD) studies as well as restriction fragment length polymorphism of the active X chromosome.[5] Erythroid precursors in PV are exquisitely sensitive to erythropoietin, which leads to increased red blood cell production. Precursors in PV are also more responsive to cytokines such as interleukin-3 (IL-3), granulocyte-macrophage colony-stimulating factor, and steel factor. Myeloid and megakaryocytic elements are often increased in the bone marrow (Fig. 1). More than 60% of patients have endogenous megakaryocyte colony unit formation.

Increased red blood cell production in PV leads to an increased red cell mass and increased blood viscosity. This in turn can lead to arterial or venous thrombosis, bleeding, or both.[1] The hematocrit is directly proportional to the number of thrombotic events.[4] Investigators have demonstrated a reduction in cerebral blood flow in patients with hematocrits between 53% and 62%.[5] An increased platelet count can also contribute to bleeding and thrombosis. Although platelet aggregation abnormalities exist in most patients, these abnormalities do not appear to correlate with the risk of bleeding or thrombosis. Increased production and breakdown of blood cells can lead to hyperuricemia and hypermetabolism.

Signs and Symptoms

Patients may be asymptomatic at the time of diagnosis and have only isolated splenomegaly, erythrocytosis, or thrombocytosis.[5] However, most patients develop symptoms as the hematocrit, platelet count, or both increase. An elevated white blood cell (WBC) count is found in 50% to 60% of patients. Symptoms of hyperviscosity associated with an elevated hematocrit include headache, blurred vision, and plethora.[1]

Thrombosis in small blood vessels can lead to cyanosis, erythromelalgia (painful vessel dilation in the extremities), ulceration, or gangrene in the fingers or toes. Thrombosis in larger vessels can lead to myocardial infarction, deep venous thrombosis, transient ischemic attacks, and stroke. A cerebrovascular event precedes the diagnosis in 35% of patients with PV.[4] Unusual sites of thromboses also tend to be seen more frequently in PV—splenic, hepatic, portal, and mesenteric.

Of patients with Budd-Chiari syndrome (hepatic–inferior vena cava obstruction), 10% have coexisting PV. Abnormalities in platelet function lead to epistaxis, bruising, and gastrointestinal and gingival bleeding in 2% to 10% of patients. Severe bleeding episodes are unusual. Hypermetabolism caused by increased blood cell turnover can lead to hyperuricemia, gout, stomach ulcers, weight loss, and kidney stones. Pruritis is especially common after a warm bath or shower. As the disease progresses, many patients develop abdominal pain secondary to hepatomegaly, splenomegaly, or both.

Diagnosis

PV should be suspected in men with a hematocrit higher than 50% and in women with a hematocrit higher than 45%.[5] Confirmation of an elevated hematocrit involves measuring a red blood cell mass[1] using direct tagging of red blood cells with chromium 51, a test unfortunately not widely available. These studies might not be needed in men with hematocrits higher than 60% or in women with hematocrits higher than 55%.

Secondary causes of polycythemia also need to be ruled out: hypoxia caused by heart or lung disease or smoking and cysts or tumors in the liver, kidneys, or brain, all of which can secrete erythropoietin. Serum erythropoietin levels should be low to normal in patients with PV but high in patients with secondary polycythemia, although there may be some overlap. Molecular testing for the *JAK2* V617 or other functionally similar mutation plays a central role in the diagnosis of PV as a way of separating neoplastic from reactive myeloid proliferations.

The initial diagnostic criteria defined by the PVSG (Polycythemia Vera Study Group) have undergone changes over the last several years. The current diagnostic criteria have been published by WHO.[6] A diagnosis of PV is met if a patient has the first two A criteria together with any other A criterion or two B criteria. New proposed

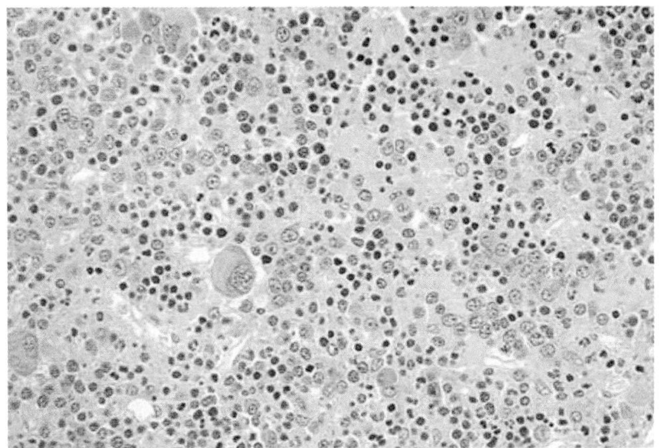

Figure 1 Bone marrow biopsy. The bone marrow in polycythemia vera is hypercellular as a result of an increase in myeloid, erythroid, and megakaryocytic elements. (Hematoxylin-eosin stain, ×40.)

revised WHO criteria for polycythemia vera include major and minor criteria, and diagnosis will require the presence of both major criteria and 1 minor criterion or the presence of the first major criterion together with 2 minor criteria.[3]

A Criteria

Elevated red cell mass more than 25% above mean normal predicted value, or hemoglobin higher than 18.5 g/dL in men or 16.5 g/dL in women, or higher than the 99th percentile of method-specific reference range for age, sex, and altitude of residence

No cause of secondary erythrocytosis, including:

- Absence of familial erythrocytosis
- No elevation of erythropoietin caused by:
  - Hypoxia (arterial Po_2 <92%)
  - High oxygen affinity hemoglobin
  - Truncated erythropoietin receptor
  - Inappropriate erythropoietin production by tumor

Splenomegaly

Clonal genetic abnormality other than the Philadelphia chromosome or *BCR/ABL1* fusion gene in marrow cells

Endogenous erythroid colony formation in vitro

B Criteria

Thrombocytosis higher than 400 × 10^9/ L

Leukocytosis higher than 12 × 10^9/ L

Bone marrow biopsy showing panmyelosis with prominent erythroid and megakaryocyte proliferation

Low serum erythropoietin levels

Major Criteria

Hemoglobin greater than 18.5 g/dL in men, 16.5 g/dL in women or other evidence of increased red cell volume

- Hemoglobin or hematocrit greater than the 99th percentile of method-specific reference range for age, sex, altitude of residence or hemoglobin greater than 17 g/dL in men, 15 g/dL in women if associated with a documented and sustained increase of at least 2 g/dL from a patient's baseline value that cannot be attributed to correction of iron deficiency, or
- Elevated red cell mass greater than 25% above mean normal predicted value

Presence of *JAK2* V617F or other functionally similar mutation such as *JAK2* exon 12 mutation

Minor Criteria

Bone marrow biopsy showing hypercellularity for age with trilineage growth (panmyelosis) with prominent erythroid, granulocytic, and megakaryocytic proliferation

Serum erythropoietin level below the reference range for normal

Endogenous erythroid colony formation in vitro

Treatment

Treatment of PV focuses on decreasing the hemoglobin level, thereby reducing plasma viscosity and its attendant complications. Therapeutic options include phlebotomy, radioactive phosphorus (^{32}P), and myelosuppressive agents. The goal of therapy is a hematocrit of 45% on the basis of cerebral blood flow studies.[4] Several clinical trials have tried to address the optimal treatment of PV.

Treatment for PV should be risk-adapted.[6] Patients at high risk for thrombosis include patients older than 60 years and those with a prior history of thrombosis. Low-risk patients include those who are younger than 60 years with no history of thrombosis, a platelet count below 1500 × 10^9/L, and the absence of cardiovascular risk factors (e.g., smoking, hypertension, congestive heart failure). In the PSVG-01 study, thrombotic events were increased in the phlebotomy arm, particularly in patients with a history of thrombosis, advanced age, or high phlebotomy requirement.[4] Therefore, high-risk patients should be treated with phlebotomy plus hydroxyurea or interferon. Hydroxyurea is typically used as first-line therapy. However, interferon should be used in women of childbearing age and in patients who cannot tolerate hydroxyurea. Low-risk or intermediate-risk patients may be treated with phlebotomy alone.

In the PVSG-01 study, there was an increased risk of leukemia in the ^{32}P and chlorambucil arms (two or three times that seen in the phlebotomy arm).[4] Because of the increased leukemogenicity associated with chlorambucil, hydroxyurea, which inhibits ribonucleotide reductase, is now the most widely used myelosuppressive agent. Side effects of hydroxyurea include myelosuppression, macrocytosis, leg ulcers, increased creatinine level, and jaundice.[5] A recent large study has demonstrated no increased incidence of leukemia in PV patients treated with hydroxyurea.[6] For older high-risk patients, ^{32}P can be used to help with issues of compliance and convenience, especially if the patient's life expectancy is less than 10 years.

Myelosuppressive agents should also be used for symptomatic splenomegaly, pruritis intractable to antihistamines, or patients with poor venous access.[4] Interferon-alfa may also be used in the place of hydroxyurea for myelosuppression, particularly in younger patients and n patients with intractable pruritus. Side effects of interferon include flulike syndromes, fevers, neuritis, and fatigue.[5] Patients with PV who are undergoing surgery are at extremely high risk of developing postoperative complications if their erythrocytosis is not controlled before surgery.

Patients with PV and no drug contraindications or evidence of acquired von Willebrand syndrome should be treated with low-dose aspirin.[6] One study has demonstrated an antithrombotic benefit for low-dose aspirin (100 mg/day) in patients already receiving treatment for PV.[6] Patients with erythromelalgia also experience a rapid relief of their symptoms after low-dose aspirin.[4]

Outcomes

The median survival is more than 10 years with treatment. The major causes of death in untreated patients are thrombosis and hemorrhage.[1] Less than 10% of patients develop acute myelogenous leukemia.[1] Fifteen percent of patients develop postpolycythemic myelofibrosis (MF) at an average interval of 10 years from diagnosis.[4] Once they develop MF, most patients die within 3 years.[4] MF often transforms to acute myelogenous leukemia.

CHRONIC IDIOPATHIC MYELOFIBROSIS

Definition and Causes

Other common names for CIMF include agnogenic myeloid metaplasia and primary myelofibrosis.[1,7] In CIMF, a clonal hematopoietic stem cell expansion in the bone marrow is accompanied by a reactive nonclonal fibroblastic proliferation and marrow fibrosis. As the bone marrow becomes fibrotic and normal hematopoiesis can no longer occur, extramedullary hematopoiesis (myeloid metaplasia) occurs in the liver and spleen.[8] The cause is unknown.

Epidemiology

The prevalence of CIMF is 2 per 1,000,000 population.[1] The risk of developing CIMF is increased by exposure to benzene or radiation. It typically occurs in whites, and the median age at diagnosis is 67 years.[5] Men and women are affected equally. As noted earlier, patients with PV and other myeloproliferative disorders can develop secondary MF late in the course of their disease.[4]

Pathophysiology

Clonal studies have demonstrated a stem cell origin.[8] The clonal proliferation of hematopoietic stem cells is believed to produce growth factors (platelet-derived growth factor, transforming growth factor-β, epidermal growth factor, and basic fibroblastic growth factor) that lead to fibrosis of the bone marrow.[1,5] Initially, the bone marrow is hypercellular, but normal hematopoiesis is diminished as the bone marrow becomes fibrotic and patients become pancytopenic (Fig. 2).[1] Because of this, the extramedullary hematopoiesis occurring in the liver and spleen causes these organs to enlarge.

Signs and Symptoms

Many symptoms are attributable to the pancytopenia associated with myelofibrosis. Pancytopenia occurs as a result of decreased hematopoiesis and splenic sequestration. Most patients are anemic and feel short of breath and fatigued. Thrombocytopenia and neutropenia can lead to hemorrhage and infection, respectively.

Other constitutional symptoms include anorexia, weight loss, and night sweats.[1] The WBC and platelet counts might increase initially but typically decrease as the disease progresses. The blood film displays a characteristic leukoerythroblastic picture (teardrop poikilocytosis, nucleated red blood cells, and immature myeloid elements) caused by crowding out of normal hematopoietic elements by fibrosis in the bone marrow (Fig. 3).[5]

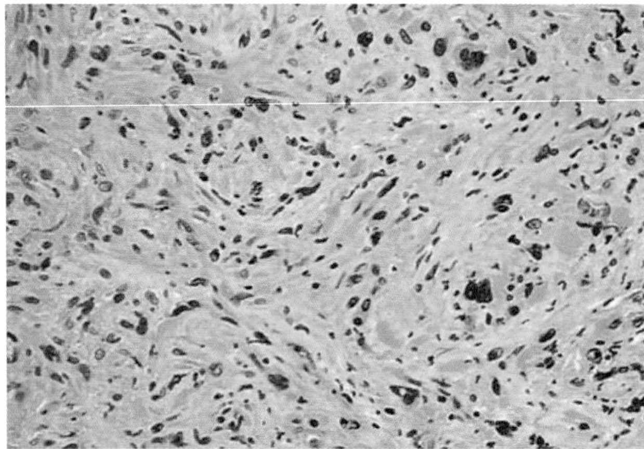

Figure 2 Bone marrow biopsy. The fibrotic stage of chronic idiopathic myelofibrosis is marked by extensive replacement of the normal marrow stroma by fibrous tissue. In this example from an advanced case, several atypical megakaryocytes with hyperchromatic and hyposegmented nuclei are shown, surrounded by pink fibrous tissue. (Hematoxylin-eosin stain, ×40.)

Patients might complain of abdominal discomfort and decreased appetite because of splenic and hepatic enlargement resulting from extramedullary hematopoiesis.[1] Portal hypertension and jaundice can occur as a result of increased hepatic blood flow.[5] Rarely, extramedullary hematopoiesis can occur at other sites, such as the skin, lungs, bladder, genitourinary tract, gastrointestinal tract, and central nervous system. Severe bone pain typically heralds a poor prognosis and often represents a conversion of CIMF to acute leukemia.

Diagnosis

The blood film demonstrates a characteristic leukoerythroblastic picture.[5] Attempts to perform a bone marrow aspirate and biopsy are often complicated by a dry tap.[1] Special stains of the bone marrow biopsy demonstrate increased fibrosis. Stains that contain silver can be used to identify reticulin, the glycoprotein coating of stromal cell strands that appears as black fibers.[8] Trichrome stains identify mature collagen as bluish-green fibers, depending on the stain used (Fig. 4).

The bone marrow biopsy is typically hypercellular, and increased numbers of abnormal megakaryocytes with a tendency to form loose to tight clusters are often present.[1,5] Thirty percent to 75% of patients have cytogenetic abnormalities at the time of diagnosis, with the most common abnormalities being del(13q), del(20q), and partial trisomy 1q. Molecular analysis can reveal a *JAK2* V617F or *MPL* W515L/K in as many as 50% of patients. Secondary causes of marrow fibrosis (e.g., metastatic breast cancer, lymphoma, lung cancer, infection, autoimmune disorders), as well as other hematologic disorders (e.g., hairy cell leukemia, CML), need to be excluded. In addition, acute panmyelosis with myelofibrosis and acute megakaryoblastic leukemia need to be ruled out. These entities also manifest with pancytopenia and marrow fibrosis, but patients typically have no splenomegaly, minimal or absent teardrop poikilocytosis, and increased numbers of blasts.

Proposed revised WHO criteria for CIMF have been published[3] and emphasize the role of assessing megakaryocyte morphology in bone marrow biopsies and excluding secondary causes for marrow fibrosis when establishing a diagnosis.

Treatment

There are no available treatments to reverse the process of idiopathic myelofibrosis short of bone marrow transplantation.[1] Because of their older median age at diagnosis, most patients are not suitable bone marrow transplant candidates. One transplant study has demonstrated a 47% overall survival at 5 years, with regression of fibrosis in 40% of patients.[8] Future studies might clarify the role of nonmyeloablative transplants in CIMF and possibly extend this option to an older patient population. The role and benefit of using chemotherapeutic agents early in the disease to reverse the fibrosis are highly controversial, and randomized clinical trials are needed to address this issue.[5] Most care is directed toward symptomatic management with transfusions (red blood cells, platelets) and growth factors (erythropoietin for anemia, granulocyte-colony stimulating factor for neutropenia). Because of the frequency of red blood cell transfusions, patients can require iron chelation therapy to decrease the risk of iron overload. Androgens (danazol) and, occasionally, low-dose steroids (e.g., prednisone) may also be helpful in managing the anemia associated with ineffective erythropoiesis.

Thalidomide has antiangiogenic, immunomodulatory, and anti-inflammatory properties, and it has been evaluated in the treatment of myelofibrosis. A pooled analysis of small phase 2 studies published between 2000 and 2002 has demonstrated a response (increase in hemoglobin, or reduction or elimination of blood transfusion require-

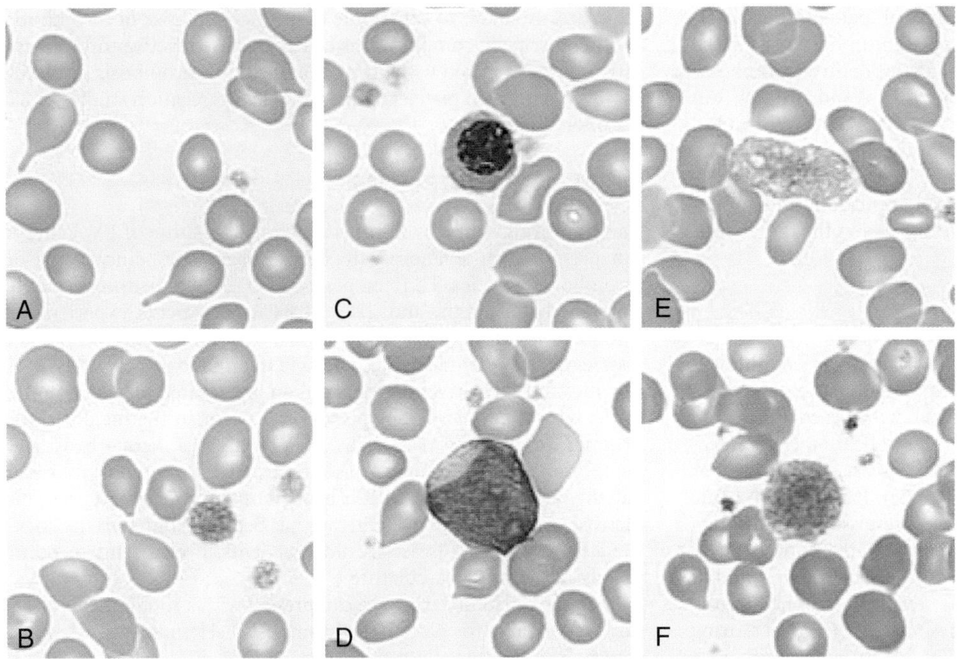

Figure 3 Peripheral blood abnormalities in the fibrotic stage of chronic idiopathic myelofibrosis. These can include teardrop-shaped erythrocytes **(A, B)**, circulating nucleated erythroid precursors **(C)**, occasional blasts **(D)**, and abnormal giant platelets **(E, F)**. (Wright-Giemsa stain, ×100.)

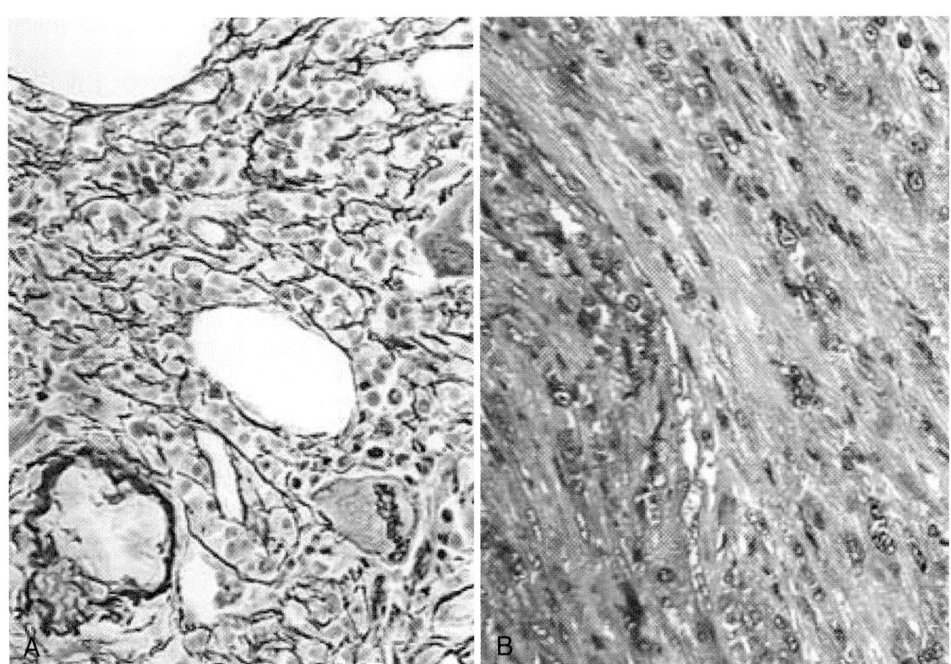

Figure 4 Bone marrow biopsy. **A,** Marrow fibrosis in chronic idiopathic myelofibrosis first appears as increased stromal reticulin; this meshwork of dark fibers can be highlighted using a reticulin stain. **B,** More mature collagenous stromal fibrosis occurs later in the course of the disease, as seen by the blue fibers made visible with a Masson trichrome stain. (A, B, ×40.)

ments) in 29% of patients with moderate or severe anemia receiving thalidomide at a dosage of 200 to 800 mg/day.[9] However, a large number of patients stopped thalidomide secondary to side effects. More recent studies have combined low-dose thalidomide with prednisone, leading to a better-tolerated and possibly more effective regimen.

The immunomodulatory agent lenalidomide (Revlimid) has also been evaluated in two separate, but similarly designed phase 2 studies.[10] Overall response rates were 22% for improvement of anemia, 33% for reduction of splenomegaly, and 50% for improvement of thrombocytopenia.[10] A subset of patients had an impressive improvement in their anemia or resolution of bone marrow abnormalities (fibrosis, angiogenesis), or both.[10] Treatment with hypomethylating agents is currently under investigation.

Splenomegaly can require treatment with myelosuppressive agents, splenectomy, or palliative radiation.[1] Splenic irradiation is typically associated with transient responses and should be considered for patients too ill for splenectomy or chemotherapy.[5] Splenectomy may be considered for symptomatic splenomegaly. In a series of 223 patients at the Mayo Clinic, patients experienced durable remissions in constitutional symptoms (67%), transfusion-dependent anemia (23%), portal hypertension (50%), and severe thrombocytopenia (0%) after splenectomy.[11] The operative mortality rate was 9% and the morbidity rate was 31%, including postoperative thrombotic complications. Sixteen percent of patients developed hepatomegaly, and 22% of patients developed thrombocytosis, which was associated with an increased risk of perioperative thrombosis. Blastic transformation was 16.3% in this series, and the risk was increased in patients with splenomegaly and preoperative thrombocytopenia, suggesting that presplenectomy thrombocytopenia may be a surrogate marker of advanced disease.

In the future, the clinical development of antifibrotic and antiangiogenesis therapies might play an important role in the therapeutic armamentarium.[8]

Outcomes

Patients asymptomatic at the time of diagnosis can have an indolent clinical course for several years. However, among the myeloproliferative disorders, CIMF has the worst prognosis, with a median survival of 3.5 to 5.5 years.[8] The most common causes of death include infection, cardiovascular disease, cerebrovascular disease, hemorrhage or thrombosis, and acute leukemia (10% to 25%). Patients with acute leukemia arising from CIMF rarely achieve a remission from induction chemotherapy.[5] Scoring symptoms have been developed to help determine prognosis for individual patients more definitively and to help identify younger patients who might benefit from bone marrow transplantation. Hoffman and colleagues[5] have defined a scoring system based on hemoglobin (<10 g/dL) and WBC count (either $<4 \times 10^9$/L or $>30 \times 10^9$/L). Patients with none, one, or two of the preceding factors had a median survival of 93, 26, and 13 months, respectively. Bone marrow transplantation might cure a subset of patients, but longer follow-up is needed.

ESSENTIAL THROMBOCYTHEMIA

Definition and Etiology

ET[5] is characterized by a sustained clonal proliferation of megakaryocytes in the bone marrow, with a peripheral blood platelet count greater than 600×10^9/L. Proposed revised criteria suggest lowering the platelet threshold to greater than 450×10^9/L.[3] Causes of reactive thrombocytosis must be excluded. The underlying cause is unknown.[1]

Epidemiology

The incidence of the disease (2.38/100,000 population per year in Olmsted County, Minn) is the lowest among the chronic myeloproliferative disorders.[1,5] There may be a higher prevalence in younger women. ET occurs equally in men and women, and the average age at diagnosis is 50 to 60 years.

Pathophysiology

The proliferation of megakaryocytes is primarily caused by clonal stem cells, as confirmed by enzyme and genetic analysis.[12] Megakaryocyte progenitor cells in ET are hypersensitive to the action of several cytokines, including IL-3 and IL-6, and possibly thrombopoietin.[5,12] This leads to increased platelet production. There is controversy regarding spontaneous megakaryocyte formation in ET. Thrombopoietin and its associated receptor pathways do not appear to be involved in the development of ET.

Increased platelet counts in ET are associated with increased thrombotic and hemorrhagic complications. Decreasing platelet counts in ET (to $<600 \times 10^9$/L) can decrease thrombotic complications (see later).[13] High platelet counts ($>1000 \times 10^9$/L) are associated with acquired von Willebrand disease resulting from the adsorption of von Willebrand multimers onto platelet membranes.[5] A reduction in the platelet count is associated with correction of the defect and cessation of bleeding. Qualitative abnormalities in the platelets themselves are also likely to contribute to the increased risk of thrombotic and hemorrhagic complications in ET, because reactive thrombocytosis is not associated with an increased risk of thrombosis or bleeding, even with high platelet counts. Platelet aggregation studies in ET are often abnormal.

SIGNS AND SYMPTOMS

The clinical signs and symptoms are similar to those of PV. Patients can present with splenomegaly, hepatomegaly, or hemorrhagic or thrombotic episodes. Thirteen percent to 37% of patients experience a hemorrhagic event, and 22% to 84% of patients experience a thromboembolic event. Constitutional symptoms, such as weight loss, fever, and pruritis, can also occur. Other patients may be asymptomatic, and their diagnosis is based on an elevated platelet count.

As with PV, thrombotic episodes can occur in the major vessels or microvasculature (see earlier, "Polycythemia Vera: Signs and Symptoms").[5] Thrombotic episodes occur more often in older patients and in patients with a history of thrombotic events. This increase in thrombotic risk with age has been attributed to the coexistence of vascular disease in older patients. Events tend to occur mainly in the microvasculature.

Women of childbearing age can present with a spontaneous abortion secondary to placental thrombosis.[5] Hemorrhage is most common in the gastrointestinal tract.

Diagnosis

The first step should be examination of the peripheral blood film (Fig. 5).[5] Automated hematology analyzers can erroneously count platelet-sized particles that are red or white cell fragments as platelets (pseudothrombocytosis).

To diagnose ET, causes of reactive thrombocytosis as well as clonal thrombocytosis secondary to another myeloproliferative disorder (e.g., CML) must be excluded. Causes of reactive thrombocytosis can include inflammatory states, infection, malignant disease, trauma, blood loss, and the postsplenectomy state.[5]

In one series of 280 patients with thrombocytosis at a university hospital, 82% of cases were reactive thrombocytosis.[5] Some of these patients have platelet counts greater than 1000×10^9/L, so the degree of thrombocytosis is not always helpful in making a diagnosis. Reactive thrombocytosis is associated with elevated levels of IL-6 or C-reactive protein in 81% of patients, which can help distin-

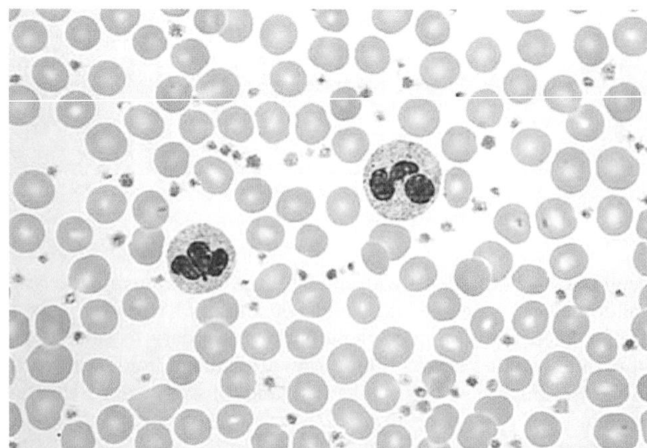

Figure 5 Platelet count in essential thrombocythemia is increased. This is shown in this peripheral blood smear from a patient with platelet count >2,000,000/μL. Although some variation in platelet size is present, the platelets are not otherwise atypical. (Wright-Giemsa stain, ×100.)

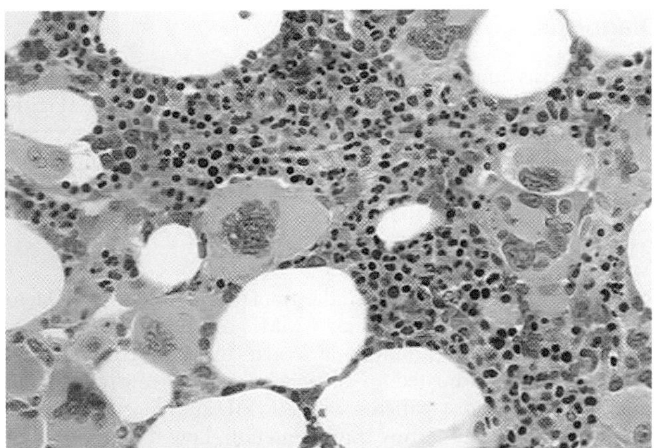

Figure 6 Bone marrow biopsy. Megakaryocytes in essential thrombocythemia not only are increased in size and number but also have deeply lobulated and hyperlobated nuclei and tend to form small clusters. (Hematoxylin-eosin stain, ×40.)

guish it from ET.[12] Patients with uncomplicated thrombocytosis secondary to a myeloproliferative disorder typically have undetectable IL-6 levels.[8]

A bone marrow aspirate and biopsy with cytogenetics (and reverse transcriptase polymerase chain reaction [RT-PCR] for *BCR/ABL1* fusion) can be helpful in excluding CML, which is *BCR/ABL1* positive. Two thirds of patients with ET have bone marrow with marked megakaryocytic hyperplasia, morphologically bizarre megakaryocytes with nuclear pleomorphism, and clustering of megakaryocytes (Fig. 6).[5] Increased myeloid and erythroid precursors, abnormal cytogenetics, minimal reticulin fibrosis, and spontaneous megakaryocyte colony formation may also be present. These features are not typically present in the bone marrow of patients with reactive thrombocytosis. Identifying a *JAK2* V617F mutation can be useful in excluding a reactive thrombocytosis. Additional clinical features that suggest ET rather than reactive thrombocytosis include a chronically elevated platelet count, splenomegaly, and history of thrombosis or hemorrhage. Red cell mass and plasma volume studies may be needed to differentiate ET from PV. Finding significant dyserythropoiesis or dysgranulopoiesis should prompt consideration of MDS rather than ET.

Treatment

A randomized study[13] has demonstrated that hydroxyurea decreases the risk of thrombosis in high-risk patients who have ET from 24% to less than 4% ($P = 0.003$), compared with no treatment, when the platelet count is decreased to less than 600 × 10^9/L. In addition, maintaining a platelet count less than 400 × 10^9/L may be associated with a further reduction in thrombosis, although these data have not been confirmed in a randomized trial.[12] The risk stratification for thrombotic events in ET and PV is the same. Patients older than 60 years or with a history of thrombotic events are considered to be at high risk. Patients with cardiovascular risk factors or extreme thrombocytosis (platelet counts >1500 × 10^9/L) are considered to be at intermediate risk.

In low-risk patients, thrombotic events are too infrequent to justify long-term drug therapy, although the use of low-dose aspirin is optional.[12] Controversy exists regarding the treatment of intermediate-risk patients.

In addition to hydroxyurea, anagrelide can also control thrombocytosis in most patients.[12] The drug works by interfering with megakaryocyte maturation. However, no randomized study has demonstrated that the drug actually decreases the risk of thrombotic events. Therefore, it should be used in patients with ET who do not tolerate hydroxyurea or in younger patients who will need long-term therapy. The main side effects include headaches, palpitations, and, rarely, a nonischemic cardiomyopathy. These effects are secondary to the drug's vasodilative inotropic actions; therefore, it should be used cautiously in patients with cardiac disease.[13] Anagrelide can also decrease the hematocrit (but not the WBC count). A randomized study (the P1 study), has demonstrated that hydroxyurea should be considered first-line treatment for patients with high-risk ET.[14] In this study, 809 patients were randomized to receive low-dose aspirin plus either anagrelide or hydroxyurea. The primary composite end point was the actuarial risk of arterial thrombosis, venous thrombosis, serious hemorrhage, or death from hemorrhagic or thrombotic causes. After a median follow-up of 39 months, patients in the anagrelide arm were more likely than those in the hydroxyurea arm to have reached the primary end point (odds ratio, 1.57; $P = 0.03$).

Interferon-alfa is another option for patients, but its use in ET is limited primarily to high-risk women of childbearing age.[12] There are no specific recommendations for ET during pregnancy. Although 45% of these women have spontaneous abortions, abortions cannot be predicted by the course of disease, platelet count, or specific treatment. Agents such as ^{32}P or busulfan are rarely used in ET but can be used in patients whose life expectancy is shorter than 10 years. Low-dose aspirin can decrease the thrombotic risk in ET, but randomized studies are still pending.

Patients with life-threatening hemorrhagic or thrombotic events should be treated with plateletpheresis in combination with myelosuppressive therapy.[12] Patients with a platelet count greater than 1500 × 10^9/L and acquired von Willebrand disease should be treated with platelet-reduction therapy and should avoid aspirin.[5] These patients also might require treatment with factor VIII concentrates that also contain von Willebrand factor (VWF) and desmopressin in the setting of a bleeding episode. Finally, patients undergoing surgery have an increased risk of thrombotic and bleeding episodes and should have their platelet counts normalized before surgery.

Outcomes

Prognosis is highly dependent on the age and history of thrombosis, because thrombosis can be life-threatening for some patients.[12] One series has demonstrated that most patients with ET die from thrombotic complications.[5] The 10-year survival rate is 64% to 80% for patients with ET. Less than 10% of patients with ET convert to acute leukemia, and 5% of patients develop myelofibrosis.

CHRONIC MYELOMONOCYTIC LEUKEMIA

Definition

Based on the WHO diagnostic criteria for CMML, patients must have a persistent peripheral blood monocytosis exceeding 1 × 10^9/L (Fig. 7), no Philadelphia chromosome or *BCR/ABL1* fusion gene, less than 20% blasts in the blood or bone marrow, and dysplasia in one or more myeloid lineages. If myelodysplasia is absent or minimal, the diagnosis of CMML may still be made if the other requirements are met and an acquired clonal cytogenetic abnormality is present, or if the monocytosis has been persistent for at least 3 months and all other causes of monocytosis have been excluded.[15]

Epidemiology

The disease typically occurs in older patients.[15]

Pathophysiology

CMML was initially characterized as a myelodysplastic syndrome because of the associated dysplasia and cytopenia observed in some

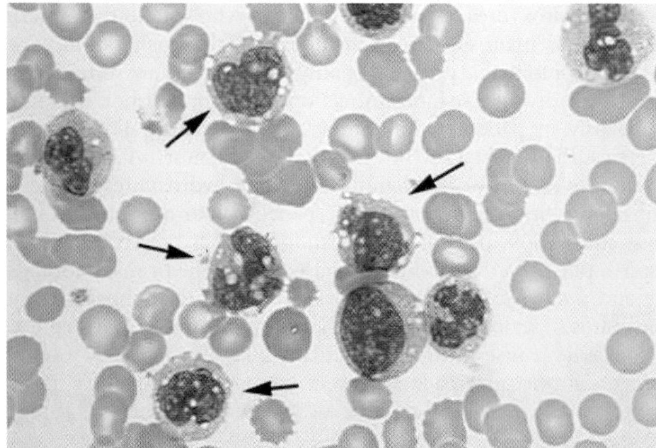

Figure 7 **Persistent peripheral blood monocytosis (*arrows*) >1 × 10^9/L.** This is a hallmark of chronic myelomonocytic leukemia. The degrees of leukocytosis, monocytosis, and dysplasia are variable; in this example, dysplastic hypogranular neutrophils are present. (Wright-Giemsa stain, ×100.)

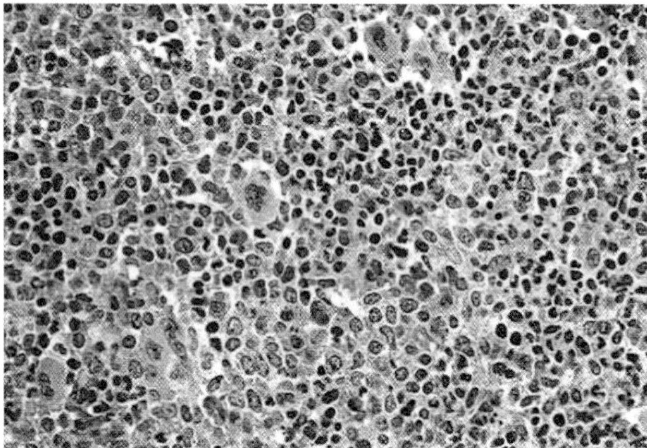

Figure 8 **Bone marrow biopsy.** The bone marrow in chronic myelomonocytic leukemia is typically hypercellular, with an increase in monocytes with folded nuclei and delicate chromatin. The marrow monocytosis may be more readily appreciated in aspirate smears stained with α-naphthylbutyrate esterase (nonspecific esterase). (Hematoxylin-eosin stain, ×40.)

patients; however, some patients display myeloproliferative features (increased myelopoiesis).[5] High peripheral monocyte counts are often associated with pericardial, pleural, synovial, and ascitic effusions, as well as hepatomegaly and splenomegaly secondary to tissue infiltration by monocytes.

Signs and Symptoms

Patients with the dysplastic or proliferative form of CMML may have shortness of breath, fatigue, bleeding or bruising, or they might have infections as the blood counts decrease secondary to splenic sequestration, dysplasia, crowding out of normal hematopoietic cells by myeloproliferation, or a combination of these factors. As noted earlier, patients with the myeloproliferative form can develop splenomegaly, hepatomegaly, skin lesions, and effusions and can present with abdominal pain or swelling, shortness of breath, or joint swelling.[16]

Diagnosis

The diagnosis requires evaluation of peripheral blood monocyte counts, in addition to bone marrow aspirate and biopsy (Fig. 8). Cytogenetics as well as molecular methods including fluorescence in situ hybridization (FISH) or RT-PCR for *BCR/ABL1* fusion should be performed to rule out CML.

Treatment

Supportive care for CMML includes transfusions and growth factor therapy. The active treatment of CMML has been disappointing. Younger patients with a human leukocyte antigen (HLA)–identical sibling should be evaluated for allogeneic bone marrow transplantation.[16] However, most patients with CMML are older and are not candidates for bone marrow transplantation. Low-dose chemotherapy (cytosine arabinoside) has low response rates, and intensive chemotherapy has been less active than in MDS.[16] Hydroxyurea may be used for patients with splenomegaly or high leukocyte counts; however, the responses are often partial, and blood counts can decrease during treatment. Investigators have examined other agents such as etoposide (VP-16). In a randomized trial, hydroxyurea yielded higher response rates and better survival than etoposide in patients with advanced CMML.[16] Other agents, such as topotecan, a topoisomerase I inhibitor, have also been studied. However, their long-term impact, and the result of combining them with other agents, is unknown. Hypomethylating agents and farnesyltransferase inhibitors have also been evaluated.

A subset of patients who have CMML with eosinophilia have a t(5;12)(q33;p13) translocation, encoding a *TEL/PDGFRβ* fusion protein. This group of patients might benefit from treatment with imatinib, which inhibits PDGFR as well as the BCR/ABL1 kinase.

Outcomes

The prognosis in CMML is highly dependent on the number of blasts in the bone marrow.[5] The life expectancy can vary from several months to several years. A study of 213 patients with CMML was used to define a prognostic scoring system.[15] In a multivariate analysis, hemoglobin lower than 12 g/dL, the presence of circulating immature myeloid cells, an absolute lymphocyte count higher than 2.5 × 10^9/L, and 10% or more marrow blasts were associated with a shorter survival.[15] Based on the number of adverse factors (0 to 4), four subgroups of patients could be defined (low, intermediate 1, intermediate 2, and high risk), with respective median survivals of 24, 15, 8, and 5 months. This scoring system has subsequently been validated in a separate set of patients.

JAK2 AND MYELOPROLIFERATIVE DISORDERS

Janus kinase 2 is a tyrosine kinase. Constitutive activation of tyrosine kinases can lead to uncontrolled cell growth. Recently, the V617F mutation in *JAK2* was found in a significant proportion of myeloproliferative disorders (60%-90% of PV and 50%-60% of ET and CIMF).[17] Other *JAK2* mutations have now been identified (i.e., exon 12). The presence of this mutation is determined by PCR assays and may be helpful in differentiating a myeloproliferative disorder from a reactive cause for elevated counts. *JAK2* allele burden might also be important in identifying high-risk patients with PV or ET (i.e. those at risk for requiring treatment with chemotherapy or those at risk for developing major cardiovascular complications).[18] Incorporation of this information may lead to a risk-adapted treatment approach in the future. Clinical trials with small molecule inhibitors of *JAK2* are currently enrolling patients, and these drugs will likely become an important part of the therapeutic armamentarium.

Summary

- The myeloproliferative disorders include polycythemia vera, chronic idiopathic myelofibrosis, essential thrombocythemia, and chronic myelogenous leukemia. Chronic myelomonocytic leukemia has features that overlap traditional myelodysplastic and myeloproliferative disorders.
- Myeloproliferative disorders are characterized by the clonal proliferation of one or more hematopoietic cell lineages.
- Review of the peripheral blood film and a bone marrow aspirate or biopsy is needed to make a definitive diagnosis.
- Reverse transcriptase polymerase chain reaction (RT-PCR) or fluorescence in-situ hybridization (FISH) for the *BCR/ABL1*gene fusion should be performed to rule out chronic myelogenous leukemia.
- Janus kinase 2, a tyrosine kinase, is mutated in a significant proportion of myeloproliferative disorders, and may represent a therapeutic target.

Suggested Readings

Barosi G, Hoffman R: Idiopathic myelofibrosis. Semin Hematol 2005;42:248-258.

Bilgrami S, Greenberg BR: Polycythemia rubra vera. Semin Oncol 1995;22:307-326.

Cortelazzo S, Finazzi G, Ruggeri M, et al: Hydroxyurea for patients with essential thrombocythemia and a high risk of thrombosis. N Engl J Med 1995;332:1132-1136.

De Keersmaecker K, Cools J: Chronic myeloproliferative disorders: A tyrosine kinase tale. Leukemia 2006;20:200-205.

Harrison CN, Campbell PJ, Buck G, et al: Hydroxyurea compared with anagrelide in high-risk essential thrombocythemia. N Engl J Med 2005;353:33-45.

Hoffman R, Benz EJ Jr, Shattil SJ, et al: Hematology: Basic Principles and Practice, 3rd ed. New York: Churchill Livingstone, 2000, pp 1106-1155, 1172-1205.

Onida F, Kantarjian HM, Smith TL, et al: Prognostic factors and scoring systems in chronic myelomonocytic leukemia: A retrospective analysis of 213 patients. Blood 2002;99:840-849.

Talarico LD: Myeloproliferative disorders: A practical review. Patient Care 1998;30:37-57.

Tefferi A: Myelofibrosis with myeloid metaplasia. N Engl J Med 2000;342:1255-1265.

Tefferi A, Mesa RA, Nagorney DM, et al: Splenectomy in myelofibrosis with myeloid metaplasia: A single-institution experience with 223 patients. Blood 2000;95:2226-2233.

Tefferi A, Solberg LA, Silverstein MN: A clinical update in polycythemia vera and essential thrombocythemia. Am J Med 2000;109:141-149.

Tefferi A, Spivak JL: Polycythemia vera: Scientific advances and current practice. Semin Hematol 2005;42:206-220.

Wattel E, Guerci A, Hecquet B, et al: A randomized trial of hydroxyurea versus VP16 in adult chronic myelomonocytic leukemia. Blood 1996;88:2480-2487.

Yavorkovsky LL, Cook P: Classifying chronic myelomonocytic leukemia. J Clin Oncol 2001;19:3790-3792.

References

For a complete list of references, log onto www.expertconsult.com.

Multiple Myeloma

Rachid Baz and Brian Bolwell

DEFINITION

Plasma cell disorders are a heterogeneous group of diseases characterized by a clonal population of B cells (plasma cells) that produce a monoclonal protein (M protein, or paraprotein). The clinical manifestations of these disorders result from the uncontrolled and progressive proliferation of a plasma cell clone, the effect of normal bone marrow replacement, and the overproduction of monoclonal proteins. Multiple myeloma is a plasma cell dyscrasia characterized by destructive lytic bone lesions, a plasma cell infiltrate in the bone marrow, and a monoclonal protein in the serum or urine.[1]

INCIDENCE AND RISK FACTORS

Multiple myeloma was diagnosed in an estimated 19,900 patients in 2008, and about 10,700 patients died of the disease in the same year. Multiple myeloma is a cancer of older adults, with a median age at diagnosis of approximately 65 years. Men and African Americans have twice the incidence of multiple myeloma as women and whites, respectively. Specific genetic disorders and environmental exposures have not been clearly linked to the risk of multiple myeloma, with the possible exception of exposure to ionizing radiation.

PATHOPHYSIOLOGY AND NATURAL HISTORY

Multiple myeloma is a neoplasm of malignant plasma cells phenotypically expressing CD38, CD56, and CD138. In addition, approximately 20% of malignant plasma cells express CD20. Overproduction of interleukin-6 (IL-6), an autocrine and paracrine plasma cell growth factor, is believed to be central to the pathogenesis of multiple myeloma. Alterations in other cytokines and signaling molecules such as tumor necrosis factor α (TNF-α), interleukin 1 (IL-1), vascular endothelial growth factor (VEGF), transforming growth factor β (TGF-β), and receptor activator of NF-κB (RANK) play key roles in the pathogenesis of multiple myeloma (Fig. 1). The interactions between malignant plasma cells and bone marrow stromal cells and osteoclasts are central to the pathogenesis and development of bone lesions and stimulation of bone marrow angiogenesis (Fig. 2).

A number of cytogenetic abnormalities in the malignant plasma cell clone have been described. These include deletions of chromosome 13 (in about 30% of patients), chromosome 17 deletions, and translocations involving the immunoglobulin heavy chain. As a general rule, cytogenetic abnormalities presage an adverse outcome.

The natural history of multiple myeloma is one of progressive bone destruction, refractory cytopenias, and end-organ damage in the form of renal and cardiac dysfunction. Deficits in the humoral immune system, long-term corticosteroid therapy, and progressive leukopenia from bone marrow replacement place patients at increased risk for frequent infectious complications, usually with encapsulated microorganisms.

SIGNS AND SYMPTOMS

The clinical manifestations of multiple myeloma can be divided into three categories: plasma cell growth in bone marrow and skeletal disease, immunologic abnormalities, and effects of abnormal paraprotein.

Plasma Cell Growth in Bone Marrow and Skeletal Disease

The most common manifesting symptom of multiple myeloma is bone pain, usually involving the spine or chest. Although most back pain often results from bone marrow replacement, discrete lytic lesions, or vertebral compression fractures, spinal cord compression must always be considered and ruled out, especially when back pain is not well explained by routine x-rays. Diffuse osteoporosis is often noted radiographically. Characteristic lesions of multiple myeloma are lytic lesions (rounded, punched-out areas of bone) found most commonly in vertebral bodies, the skull, ribs, humerus, and femur (Fig. 3). Lytic lesions are not usually located in the distal extremities. Bone scans might not accurately reflect the destruction seen on plain radiographic films. Accordingly, skeletal surveys are used in the initial evaluation and follow-up of patients with multiple myeloma. Hypercalcemia in patients with multiple myeloma is secondary to bone turnover and is treated with bisphosphonate therapy, which is also useful for treating pain from lytic lesions and in skeleton-related events and may have an antimyeloma effect.[2]

Anemia is present in most patients at diagnosis and during follow-up. Anemia in multiple myeloma is multifactorial and is secondary to bone marrow replacement by malignant plasma cells, chronic inflammation, relative erythropoietin deficiency, and vitamin deficiency. Recombinant human erythropoietin may be effective for the treatment of anemia in multiple myeloma.[3] Mild neutropenia and mild thrombocytopenia are common, but severe cytopenias are uncommon at diagnosis. Plasma cell leukemia, a condition in which plasma cells account for more than 20% of peripheral leukocytes, is typically a terminal stage of multiple myeloma and is associated with short survival.

Immunologic Abnormalities

Commonly, patients exhibit a reciprocal decrease in normal immunoglobulin values in the presence of an elevated M protein level. Patients with myeloma often suffer from repeated infections, similar to those seen in patients with reduced levels of immunoglobulins. Long-term corticosteroid use and use of chemotherapeutic agents also predispose patients to infectious complications. Intravenous immunoglobulins have been used as prophylaxis for patients with repeated severe infections.

Effects of Abnormal Paraprotein

Increased serum viscosity is occasionally noted in patients with multiple myeloma. It is more commonly noted in patients with heavy chain immunoglobulin A. Hyperviscosity is more commonly noted in patients with Waldenström's macroglobulinemia. High viscosity interferes with efficient blood circulation in the brain, kidneys, and extremities. Symptoms of hyperviscosity include headache, dizziness, vertigo, and severe ischemia.

Although peripheral neuropathy secondary to antibodies to myelin-associated glycoprotein (MAG) is occasionally noted in patients with multiple myeloma, it is more often the result of therapeutic agents (e.g., thalidomide, bortezomib, vincristine). Antibodies to factor X are occasionally present in patients with multiple myeloma and result in abnormal bleeding. Abnormal platelet aggregation and

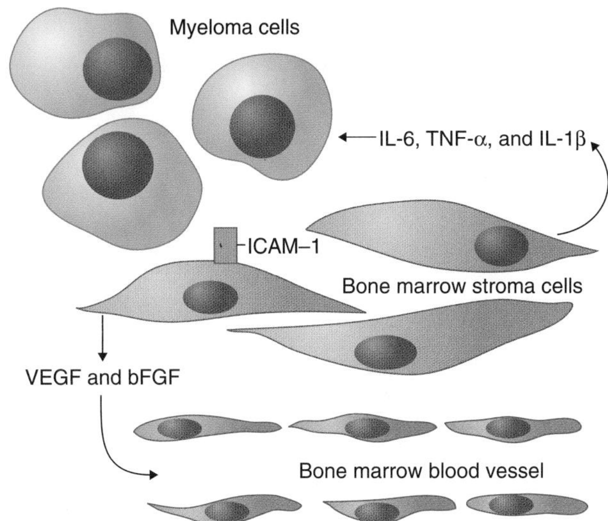

Figure 1 Role of bone marrow stromal cells in the pathogenesis of multiple myeloma. The interaction of malignant plasma cell and bone marrow stromal cells results in the generation of angiogenic cytokines (VEGF and bFGF) and paracrine myeloma growth factors (IL-6, TNF-α, and IL-1β). bFGF, basic fibroblast growth factor; IL-6, interleukin-6; TNF-α, tumor necrosis factor α; VEGF, vascular endothelial growth factor.

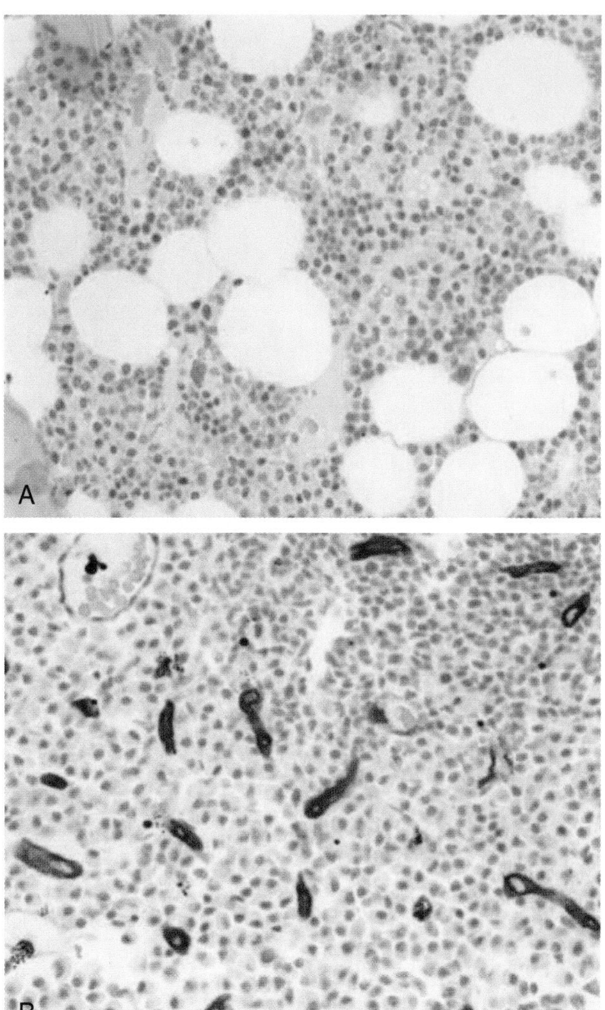

Figure 2 Bone marrow angiogenesis in multiple myeloma. A, Normal bone marrow (CD34 stain). **B,** Bone marrow from a patient with multiple myeloma. New blood vessel formation is noted (CD34 stain). *(Courtesy of Dr. Mohamad Hussein.)*

function are often noted on laboratory testing and can result in clinical bruising.

Renal dysfunction can have many causes in patients with multiple myeloma and is present in about 50% of patients at diagnosis. Hypercalcemia, concomitant medications (e.g., nonsteroidal anti-inflammatory drugs [NSAIDs], intravenous contrast agents, aminoglycoside antibiotics), and intravascular volume depletion are all possible causes. In addition, cast nephropathy (myeloma kidney), amyloidosis, and light chain deposition should be considered when immediately reversible causes are excluded. Therapy directed at the malignant plasma cell clone often treats the myeloma kidney as well. The role of plasma exchange remains controversial, despite a recent trial that showed no advantage for this approach. Proteinuria is present in 90% of patients with multiple myeloma, and abnormal light chains (Bence Jones protein) are found in 80% of patients.

DIAGNOSIS

Multiple myeloma should be suspected in older adults presenting with back pain, constitutional symptoms (sweats, weight loss), and elevated total protein levels. In addition, unexplained renal dysfunction, anemia, or pathologic fracture should prompt evaluation for this diagnosis.

Diagnostic criteria for multiple myeloma from the International Myeloma Workshop rely on a combination of criteria (Table 1).[4] Evidence of end-organ damage (hypercalcemia, renal insufficiency, anemia, lytic bone lesions) is required for the diagnosis of symptomatic multiple myeloma. These criteria diverge from historical diagnostic criteria, which relied on the monoclonal protein concentration and the amount of bone marrow plasma cell infiltrate. These changes stem from the observation that 40% of patients with multiple myeloma have a serum M protein level lower than 30 g/L. Similarly, 5% of patients with multiple myeloma have less than 10% bone marrow plasmacytosis. The difficulty of the present diagnostic system rests in determining whether end-organ dysfunction is related to the monoclonal gammopathy. Often, this requires the exclusion of other causes of end-organ damage.

The differential diagnosis of a patient with a monoclonal protein includes monoclonal gammopathy of undetermined significance (MGUS), amyloidosis, light chain deposition disease, solitary plasmacytomas of bone or extramedullary plasmacytoma, Waldenström's macroglobulinemia, lymphoproliferative disorders (e.g., chronic lymphocytic leukemia), and rheumatologic autoimmune conditions. In addition, patients with metastatic carcinoma occasionally have a monoclonal gammopathy. The metastatic carcinoma is often well characterized when the monoclonal protein is identified, and a search for a metastatic carcinoma usually is not recommended.

STAGING

The staging evaluation of patients with multiple myeloma should include diagnostic tests as well as prognostic tests. Box 1 details the recommended staging work-up of patients with multiple myeloma. The Durie and Salmon staging system for multiple myeloma dates back to 1975 and, although still widely used, is cumbersome in clinical practice (Table 2).[1] The Southwest Oncology Group has proposed a different staging system for multiple myeloma that relies only on serum β_2-microglobulin and serum albumin levels (Table 3).[5] In addition, the latter staging system affords excellent prognostication.

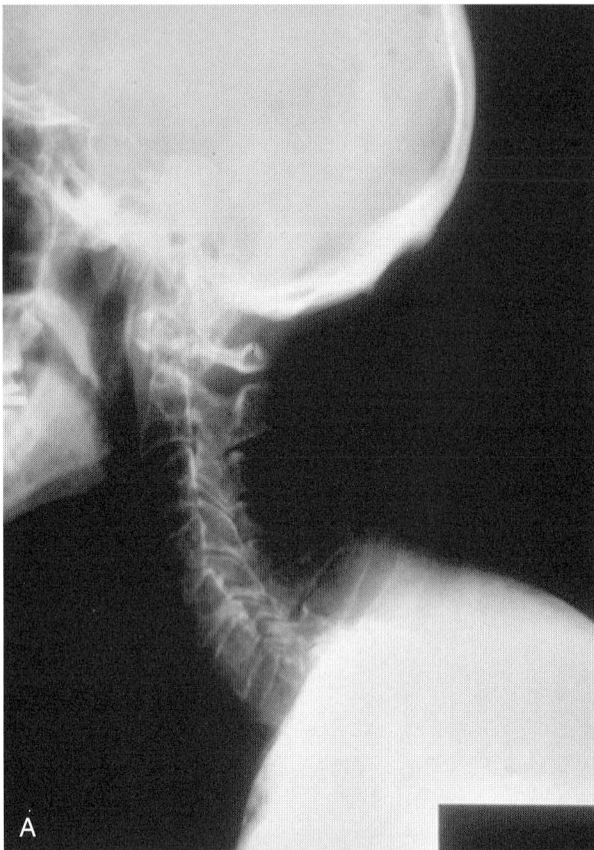

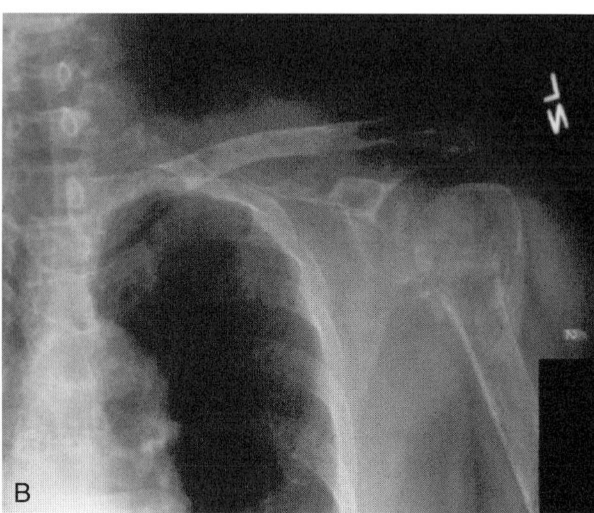

Figure 3 **Lytic skeletal lesions in patients with multiple myeloma. A,** Skull of a patient with multiple myeloma demonstrating lytic lesions. **B,** Proximal humerus of a patient with multiple myeloma displaying multiple lytic lesions. *(Courtesy of Dr. Mohamad Hussein.)*

Table 1 Differential Diagnosis and Diagnostic Criteria for Multiple Myeloma and Monoclonal Gammopathy of Undetermined Significance (MGUS)*

MGUS	Asymptomatic Multiple Myeloma	Symptomatic Multiple Myeloma
Serum M protein <30 g/L	Serum M protein ≥30 g/L	M protein in the serum or urine
Clonal† bone marrow plasmacytosis <10%	Clonal bone marrow plasmacytosis ≥10%	Clonal bone marrow plasmacytosis or plasmacytoma
No other B cell lymphoproliferative disorder	No related organ and tissue impairment	Related organ and tissue impairment
No related organ and tissue impairment		

*Related organ and tissue impairment:

1. Hypercalcemia: serum calcium >2.75 mmol/L
2. Renal dysfunction: serum creatinine >173 mmol/L
3. Anemia: hemoglobin 2 g/dL below lower limit of normal
4. Lytic bone lesions (CT and MRI may be used to identify suspicious findings on plain films)
5. Symptomatic hyperviscosity
6. Amyloidosis
7. Recurrent bacterial infections (more than two episodes in 1 year)

Adapted from International Myeloma Working Group: Criteria for the classification of monoclonal gammopathies, multiple myeloma and related disorders: A report of the International Myeloma Working Group. Br J Haematol 2003;121:749-757.

Box 1 Diagnostic Workup of Patients With Multiple Myeloma*

Routine Laboratory Tests

Complete blood count and differential, peripheral blood smear
Complete metabolic panel (includes calcium, albumin, and creatinine)
Coagulation testing
Serum vitamin B_{12}, folate, and ferritin

Myeloma-Specific Testing:†

Serum protein electrophoresis, monoclonal protein analysis, and immunofixation
24-Hour urine collection for protein, urine protein electrophoresis, and immunofixation
Serum β_2-microglobulin, C-reactive protein, and lactate dehydrogenase
Bone marrow aspirate and biopsy, flow cytometry, and cytogenetics

Imaging Studies

Skeletal bone survey (includes plain films of spine, pelvis, skull, humeri, and femurs)‡
Bone mineral densitometry by DEXA scan at baseline

**Dental evaluation at baseline should be considered in patients with poor dentition.*
†Consideration for serum free light chain assays when available.
‡Consideration for magnetic resonance imaging of spine in patients with back pain unexplained by plain films.
DEXA, dual-energy x-ray absorptiometry.

Table 2 Durie and Salmon Staging System for Multiple Myeloma*

Stage	Criteria
I	All the following: 1. Hemoglobin >10 g/dL 2. Serum calcium value normal (≤12 mg/dL) 3. On radiograph, normal bone structure or solitary bone plasmacytoma only 4. Low M component production rates a. IgG <5 g/dL b. IgA <3 g/dL c. Urine light chain M component on electrophoresis < 4 g/24 h
II	Fitting neither stage I nor stage III
III	One or more of the following: 1. Hemoglobin <8.5 g/dL 2. Serum calcium >12 mg/dL 3. Advanced lytic bone lesions 4. High M component production rates a. IgG >7 g/dL b. IgA >5 g/dL c. Urine light chain M component on electrophoresis >12 g/24 h

*Designations A and B are based on serum creatinine levels (A, serum creatinine <2.0 mg/dL; B, serum creatinine ≥2.0 mg/dL).
IgA, immunoglobulin A; IgG, immunoglobulin G.
Adapted from Durie BG, Salmon SE: A clinical staging system for multiple myeloma: Correlation of measured myeloma cell mass with presenting clinical features, response to treatment, and survival. Cancer 1975;36:842-854.

Table 3 Southwest Oncology Group (SWOG) Staging of Multiple Myeloma and Anticipated Survival per Stage

β_2-Microglobulin (mg/L)	Albumin (g/dL)	SWOG Stage	No. of Patients (%)	Median Survival (mo)
<2.5	Any	I	14	55
≥2.5 and <5.5	Any	II	43	40
≥5.5	≥3.0	III	32	24
≥5.5	<3.0	IV	11	16

Adapted from Jacobson JL, Hussein MA, Barlogie B, et al: A new staging system for multiple myeloma patients based on the Southwest Oncology Group (SWOG) experience. Br J Haematol 2003;122:441-450.

TREATMENT

General Considerations and Supportive Care

Patients with multiple myeloma occasionally have associated complications that require immediate attention, including hypercalcemia, renal failure, and spinal cord compression. These complications should be promptly identified and managed before instituting systemic therapy. Alternatively, patients with asymptomatic (smoldering) multiple myeloma may be followed without specific therapy until clear evidence of progression is noted. Ambulation and hydration should be maintained throughout the initial therapy. Avoidance of potentially nephrotoxic drugs (e.g., NSAIDs, aminoglycosides, IV contrast agent) is important for renal health.

Supportive care has also significantly evolved in the past few decades. Vertebroplasty and kyphoplasty have resulted in major improvement in regard to diminishing the pain of compression fractures.[6] The use of bisphosphonates (pamidronate or zoledronic acid) is recommended for almost all myeloma patients with lytic lesions or significant osteoporosis and normal renal function. Bisphosphonate therapy has been shown to decrease the incidence of skeletal-related problems.[2] In addition, bisphosphonate therapy has analgesic properties for pain related to lytic lesions and possibly antineoplastic properties, and it is effective treatment for hypercalcemia in multiple myeloma patients. Immediate adverse effects of bisphosphonate therapy include flu-like symptoms associated with the first infusion and renal dysfunction, which is in part related to the infusion rate. Long-term use of bisphosphonate therapy has been associated with osteonecrosis of the jaw. Baseline dental evaluation and prompt evaluation of jaw symptoms is recommended for patients receiving these agents. Radiation therapy for painful lytic lesions produces effective palliation of pain. Larger radiation fields are probably best avoided early in the course of the disease because they can impair bone marrow reserve and preclude subsequent therapies.

Granulocyte and erythropoietic growth factors are effective for the neutropenia and anemia of chemotherapy, respectively. In addition, recombinant human erythropoietin is effective for treating anemia associated with relative erythropoietin deficiency.[3] It has been shown to decrease transfusion requirements and possibly improve quality of life.

Patients with multiple myeloma are at increased risk for infectious complications. The use of intravenous immunoglobulin should be considered in the patient with decreased immunoglobulin levels and repeated bacterial infections. A dose of 0.4 g/kg is recommended on a monthly to trimonthly basis.

Patients with plasma cell dyscrasias, and specifically multiple myeloma, have an increased risk of venous thromboembolic events. Immunomodulatory drug therapy (thalidomide and lenalidomide) has also been associated with increased risk of thromboembolic events. Accordingly, particular attention to early mobilization and prophylaxis of thromboembolic events should be considered for patients undergoing surgical procedures or receiving immunomodulatory therapy. For the latter purpose, we recommend low-dose daily aspirin (81 mg) until completion of therapy. Alternative therapies include low-molecular-weight heparins or therapeutic anticoagulation with warfarin.

Response Criteria

A number of response criteria have been used to assess the efficacy of therapy for multiple myeloma. Box 2 describes the response criteria from the International Myeloma Working Group (IMWG)[7]

Treatment for Newly Diagnosed Multiple Myeloma

Induction Treatment

Although conventional therapy cannot cure multiple myeloma, it can effect a temporary remission. The past decade has witnessed the addition of a number of exciting novel therapeutic agents for relapsed and newly diagnosed myeloma. Because of recent advances, a standard first-line therapy has yet to be defined. Accordingly, the choice of first-line therapy is often guided by patient comorbidities and preferences as well as disease characteristics. Enrollment in a clinical trial must be a consideration at all stages of therapy.

The combination of melphalan and prednisone historically has been used in this setting. It produces responses in approximately 50% of patients and a progression-free survival of approximately 15 months. A meta-analysis comparing combination chemotherapy with melphalan and prednisone has shown no statistically significant difference in survival, despite a higher response rate with more-aggressive combination chemotherapy. Despite this finding, the combination of melphalan and prednisone was abandoned as induction therapy, because long-term therapy with alkylating agents compromises the ability to collect stem cells for high-dose therapy and stem

Box 2 Response Criteria From the International Myeloma Working Group (IMWG)

Complete Remission (CR)
The absence of bone marrow or blood findings of multiple myeloma. This includes disappearance of all evidence of serum and urine M-components on electrophoresis as well as by immunofixation studies for 6 weeks. Soft tissue plasmacytoma must have disappeared.

Stringent Complete remission (CRs)
In addition to meeting criteria for a CR, patients with a CRs must have a normal free light chain ratio, absence of clonal cells in the bone marrow by immunohistochemistry and/or immunofluorescence (ratio of kappa to lambda plasma cells between 0.5 and 4.)

Very Good Partial Response (VGPR)
Detectable serum and urine M component on immunofixation but not on electrophoresis or 90% or greater reduction in serum M protein with less than 100 mg/24 h of urinary M protein.

Partial Remission (PR)
A greater than 50% reduction in the serum paraprotein, and if present, a greater than 90% reduction in the urine M protein excretion. Patients must also have a decrease by 50% in the size of soft tissue plasmacytoma. If serum and urine M protein are not measurable, a 50% or greater decreased in the difference of the involved and uninvolved free light chain.

Minimal Remission (MR)
A 25% to 49% reduction in serum paraprotein and a 50% to 89% reduction in urine light chain excretion for 6 weeks. A 25% to 49% reduction in the size of soft tissue plasmacytoma must be demonstrated.

Plateau Phase (P)
A stable serum and urine paraprotein (within 25%) maintained for at least 3 months.

Adapted from Durie BG, Harousseau JL, Miguel JS, et al. International uniform response criteria for multiple myeloma. Leukemia 2006; 20: 1467-1473.

cell transplantation. Accordingly, dexamethasone-based chemotherapy is often used for induction, because it is believed to be safe for stem cell collection. The VAD regimen (infusional vincristine and doxorubicin combined with dexamethasone) results in a response rate of about 70% and does not compromise stem cell collection. Modifications of the VAD regimen have yielded the DVD regimen (pegylated liposomal doxorubicin, vincristine, and dexamethasone), which is given in an outpatient setting and results in a similar response rate.[8]

More recently, thalidomide, lenalidomide and bortezomib have been used in different combinations with corticosteroids and chemotherapy in the initial therapy of myeloma patients.[8-10] Thalidomide, an oral immunomodulatory drug, is efficacious for patients with relapsed and refractory multiple myeloma. It has been combined with dexamethasone, and a recent clinical trial noted a higher response rate (70%) with that combination when compared with dexamethasone alone (50%).[11] However, the thalidomide-dexamethasone combination also results in a higher rate of adverse events, notably neuropathy, somnolence, and deep venous thrombosis. Although survival data are not mature, a survival benefit from the combination was not observed. The increased response rate in that setting must be weighed against increased side effects of the combination; treatment decisions must be individualized.

Lenalidomide has also been used in combination with dexamethasone as induction therapy for newly diagnosed multiple myeloma. Although it has not been formally compared to thalidomide induction, response rates of approximately 85% to 90% are noted. In addition, severe peripheral neuropathy as is sometimes noted with thalidomide has not been seen with this agent. More recently, a decreased dose of dexamethasone in combination with lenalidomide in newly diagnosed myeloma was demonstrated to be superior to a higher dose of dexamethasone in terms of survival but not response rates.

Similarly, the bortezomib and dexamethasone combination has resulted in a superior response rate than VAD chemotherapy, as has the bortezomib and melphalan-prednisone combination when compared to melphalan and prednisone. Although the response rates are exciting, survival data for these new combinations remains immature .

In summary, the optimal first-line therapy remains undefined but likely involves a combination of a novel agent (lenalidomide, thalidomide, or bortezomib) and corticosteroids. A more intensive approach is likely to result in a higher response rate, but this may be offset by a greater likelihood of significant toxicity, and treatment should be individualized.

High-Dose Therapy and Autologous Peripheral Blood Stem Cell Transplantation

Autologous stem cell transplantation generally consists of a collection of the patient's peripheral blood progenitor cells following stimulation by granulocyte colony-stimulating factor (G-CSF), with or without chemotherapy. The patient is then given high-dose chemotherapy (usually melphalan, 200 mg/m^2) as the high-dose preparative regimen of choice. High-dose chemotherapy followed by autologous peripheral blood stem cell transplantation has been demonstrated to result in complete response rates of 40% to 50% as well as 5 years' event-free survival of 28%.[12-15] In addition, a few randomized clinical trials have noted a prolonged overall survival with this approach.

The more recent U.S. intergroup study (S9321) did not show a benefit of high-dose therapy (using melphalan and total body irradiation) when compared with standard therapy.[14] Possible explanations for this finding include the inferiority of total body irradiation as a preparative regimen in multiple myeloma (when compared with high-dose melphalan), and the more intensive standard chemotherapy arm in this study, which consisted of VBMCP therapy (vincristine, carmustine, melphalan, cyclophosphamide, and prednisone in 5-week cycles) for 1 year. Patients randomized to standard therapy in this study had similar response rates as patients who received high-dose therapy, thus implying that a response achieved with either therapy has similar prognostic implications. The combinations of novel therapies in patients with newly diagnosed myeloma often result in high responses rates, similar to those achieved with high-dose therapy.

Accordingly, the precise role of high-dose therapy in the era of novel agents with high response rates remains to be determined. In vitro purging of peripheral stem cells has not been demonstrated to result in superior outcomes and is not routinely recommended. Alternatively, in vivo purging of stem cells by induction chemotherapy before stem cell collection is believed to be beneficial.

Tandem Autologous Stem Cell Transplantation

The success of high-dose therapy followed by peripheral blood stem cell transplantation has prompted French investigators to evaluate tandem autologous stem cell transplantation. The landmark study included 399 patients with newly diagnosed multiple myeloma who underwent three or four cycles of VAD chemotherapy. Patients were subsequently randomized to receive a single autologous stem cell transplant with melphalan 140 mg/m^2 and total body irradiation or a tandem autologous stem cell transplant; the first transplant consisted of melphalan 140 mg/m^2 alone, and the second consisted of melphalan 140 mg/m^2 with total body irradiation.[13] A complete response was observed in 42% of patients with a single transplant compared with 50% in the tandem transplant group. The 7-year event-free survival was 10% versus 20% (P = 0.03), favoring the tandem transplants. In addition, the 7-year overall survival was 21%

versus 42% ($P = 0.01$), also favoring the tandem transplants.[13] Treatment-related deaths were 4% versus 6% ($P = 0.4$), favoring the single transplant.

A planned subgroup analysis has suggested that patients with suboptimal responses who have not achieved a good partial response are more likely to benefit from the second transplant. Two other tandem transplant clinical trials have not demonstrated a survival benefit over a single transplant, and a smaller trial demonstrated superiority of thalidomide maintenance after a single transplant to a tandem-transplant approach. Therefore, tandem transplantation cannot be routinely recommended outside the setting of a clinical trial.

Allogeneic Stem Cell Transplantation

Despite single and tandem high-dose therapy, patients with multiple myeloma relapse. Some investigators have noted prolonged disease-free survival for patients who underwent allogeneic transplantation. A graft–versus–multiple myeloma effect is believed to confer benefits to this approach. Accordingly, the U.S. intergroup (S9321) study included an arm that evaluated allogeneic stem cell transplantation in multiple myeloma. In this study, after three or four cycles of induction therapy with VAD, 36 patients received an allogeneic transplant. The preparative regimen consisted of melphalan 140 mg/m^2 and total body irradiation. The treatment-related mortality rate was 39% and the overall mortality 53%; this arm was stopped early on the recommendation of the data safety monitoring board.[14] However, at 7 years of follow-up, 22% of patients were disease free. Nonmyeloablative allogeneic transplantation has reduced the transplant-related mortality and was reported to result in a survival benefit in a small clinical trial. Confirmatory trials are ongoing.[14] In view of the high transplantation-related mortality, allogeneic transplantation should be considered for young patients in the context of a clinical trial.

Maintenance Treatment

Maintenance therapy following response after first-line therapy has been studied. A number of randomized clinical trials and a meta-analysis have shown a modest benefit to interferon alfa-2b maintenance therapy. Because of significant adverse events from interferon therapy, negative impact on quality of life, and only a modest benefit, this approach has been largely abandoned. Corticosteroid maintenance therapy (prednisone 50 mg every other day) was shown to increase survival in one randomized study, and pulsed dexamethasone maintenance therapy has been used by others, with promising results.[16] More recently, preliminary results of a randomized clinical trial conducted by the Intergroupe Français du Myelome (IFM) have suggested a role for thalidomide maintenance therapy.

Treatment for the Relapsed or Refractory Patient

Despite effective first-line therapy, all patients with multiple myeloma experience a progression of their disease. A number of principles are inherent to the treatment of patients with relapsed or refractory multiple myeloma. In the event of progression after 12 months of completion of therapy, the use of the same therapy is likely to produce responses. Alternatively, a shorter time to progression or refractoriness to therapy implies a change in treatment. Table 4 lists commonly used therapeutic regimens, and Box 3 describes common adverse events of novel agents used for the management of multiple myeloma.

Other combinations of active agents have been reported to result in higher response rates but not in clearly improved outcomes. Clinical trial enrollment should be particularly emphasized in this setting. Novel agents, such as histone deacetylase inhibitors, mammalian target of rapamycin (MTOR) inhibitors, RANK-L antibodies, and other immunomodulatory drugs (e.g., CC-4047 [Actimid]) are currently the subjects of ongoing investigations.

Table 4 Chemotherapeutic Regimens for Multiple Myeloma

Regimen	Dosage and Frequency	Cycle Length
Melphalan	9 mg/m^2 PO, day 1-4	4-6 weeks
Prednisone	100 mg PO, day 1-4	
Dexamethasone	40 mg PO, day 1-4, 9-12, 17-20	28 days
Doxorubicin (Doxil)	40 mg/m^2 IVP, day 1	28 days
Vincristine	2 mg IVP, day 1	
Dexamethasone	40 mg PO, day 1-4	
Thalidomide*	200 mg PO, qhs	
Dexamethasone	40 mg PO, day 1-4, 9-12, 17-20	28 days
Cyclophosphamide	1000 mg/m^2 IV, day 1	21 days
Prednisone	100 mg PO, day 1-5	
Bortezomib	1.3 mg/m^2 IVP, day 1, 4, 8, 11	21 days
Lenalidomide	25 mg PO, day 1-21	28 days
Dexamethasone	40 mg PO, day 1-4, 9-12, 17-20	

IVPB, intravenous piggyback; IVP, intravenous push (injection); qhs, at bedtime.
*Thalidomide and lenalidomide at standard doses have been combined with the following regimens: melphalan and prednisone, dexamethasone, and DVd. Thalidomide and lenalidomide are rarely used as single agents.

Box 3 Notable Adverse Effects of Novel Agents Used for Multiple Myeloma Treatment

Thalidomide
Sedation
Rash
Constipation
Peripheral neuropathy*
Teratogenicity
Bradycardia
Peripheral edema
Tremors
Thromboembolic events†

Lenalidomide plus Bortezomib
Muscle cramps and arthralgia
Myelosuppression
Peripheral edema
Thromboembolic events
Hypothyroidism
Rash
Constipation or diarrhea
Potential birth defects
Thrombocytopenia
Nausea and diarrhea
Rash
Peripheral neuropathy‡

**Peripheral neuropathy from thalidomide is related to the cumulative dose.*
†Thromboembolic events in patients with leprosy are not increased with thalidomide. The rate of thromboembolic events in patients with multiple myeloma receiving concurrent dexamethasone or anthracycline chemotherapy and thalidomide is about 15% and 30%, respectively.
‡Peripheral neuropathy from bortezomib is not dose dependent.

PROGNOSIS

Clinical, laboratory, and cytogenetic prognosticators have been identified. Adverse clinical prognosticators include advanced age, decreased performance status, and the presence of extramedullary plasmacytomas. Adverse laboratory prognostic variables in multiple myeloma include high serum β_2-microglobulin, high serum lactate dehydrogenase, low serum albumin, and high creatinine and C-reactive protein levels. In addition, high plasma cell labeling index is believed to indicate a poor outcome, but this test is not routinely performed in all laboratories. Plasmablastic morphology has been associated with worse outcomes. Cytogenetic abnormalities by metaphase cytogenetics are identified in approximately 50% of multiple myeloma patients. The most common abnormalities include deletion of chromosomes 13 and 17, as well as immunoglobulin heavy chain rearrangement with the cyclin *D1* and *FGFR3* genes. Most cytogenetic abnormalities are associated with adverse outcomes in multiple myeloma.[17]

Summary

- In addition to multiple myeloma, plasma cell dyscrasias include monoclonal gammopathy of undetermined significance, smoldering myeloma, primary systemic amyloidosis, and Waldenström's macroglobulinemia.
- Multiple myeloma is a plasma cell neoplasm characterized by a monoclonal gammopathy, bone marrow plasmacytosis, and end-organ damage.
- Cytogenetic determinations of bone marrow aspirates and serum β_2-microglobulin and albumin are important prognostic tools.
- Multidisciplinary treatment includes systemic therapy—chemotherapy, corticosteroids, and immunomodulatory agents—and the prevention and treatment of skeletal, renal, and infectious complications.

Suggested Readings

Attal M, Harousseau JL, Stoppa AM, et al: A prospective, randomized trial of autologous bone marrow transplantation and chemotherapy in multiple myeloma. Intergroupe Français du Myelome. N Engl J Med 1996;335:91-97.

Attal M, Harousseau JL, Facon T, et al: Single versus double autologous stem-cell transplantation for multiple myeloma. N Engl J Med 2003;349:2495-2502.

Barlogie B, Kyle RA, Anderson KC, et al: Standard chemotherapy compared with high-Dose chemoradiotherapy for multiple myeloma: Final results of Phase III U.S. Intergroup Trial S9321 10.1200/JCO.2005.04.5807. J Clin Oncol 2006;24:929-936.

Berenson JR, Crowley JJ, Grogan TM, et al: Maintenance therapy with alternate-day prednisone improves survival in multiple myeloma patients. Blood 2002;99:3163-3168.

Bergsagel PL, Kuehl WM: Molecular pathogenesis and a consequent classification of multiple myeloma. J Clin Oncol 2005;23:6333-6338.

Durie BG, Harousseau JL, Miguel JS, et al. International uniform response criteria for multiple myeloma. Leukemia 2006;20:1467-1473.

Cavo M, Terragna C, Renzulli M, et al: Poor outcome with front-line autologous transplantation in t(4;14) multiple myeloma: Low complete remission rate and short duration of remission. J Clin Oncol 2006;24:e4-e5.

Child JA, Morgan GJ, Davies FE, et al: High-dose chemotherapy with hematopoietic stem-cell rescue for multiple myeloma. N Engl J Med 2003;348:1875-1883.

Dhodapkar MV, Hussein MA, Rasmussen E, et al: Clinical efficacy of high-dose dexamethasone with maintenance dexamethasone/alpha interferon in patients with primary systemic amyloidosis: Results of United States Intergroup Trial Southwest Oncology Group (SWOG) S9628. Blood 2004;104:3520-3526.

Dudeney S, Lieberman IH, Reinhardt MK, Hussein M: Kyphoplasty in the treatment of osteolytic vertebral compression fractures as a result of multiple myeloma. J Clin Oncol 2002;20:2382-2387.

Durie BG, Salmon SE: A clinical staging system for multiple myeloma. Correlation of measured myeloma cell mass with presenting clinical features, response to treatment, and survival. Cancer 1975;36:842-854.

International Myeloma Working Group: Criteria for the classification of monoclonal gammopathies, multiple myeloma and related disorders: A report of the International Myeloma Working Group. Br J Haematol 2003;121:749-757.

Jacobson JL, Hussein MA, Barlogie B, et al: A new staging system for multiple myeloma patients based on the Southwest Oncology Group (SWOG) experience. Br J Haematol 2003;122:441-450.

Jagannath S, Barlogie B, Berenson J, et al: A phase 2 study of two doses of bortezomib in relapsed or refractory myeloma. Br J Haematol 2004;127:165-172.

Osterborg A, Brandberg Y, Molostova V, et al: Randomized, double-blind, placebo-controlled trial of recombinant human erythropoietin, epoetin beta, in hematologic malignancies. J Clin Oncol 2002;20:2486-2494.

Rajkumar SV, Hayman SR, Lacy MQ, et al: Combination therapy with lenalidomide plus dexamethasone (Rev/Dex) for newly diagnosed myeloma. Blood 2005;106:4050-4053.

Rajkumar SV, Blood E, Vesole D, et al: Phase III clinical trial of thalidomide plus dexamethasone compared with dexamethasone alone in newly diagnosed multiple myeloma: A clinical trial coordinated by the Eastern Cooperative Oncology Group. J Clin Oncol 2006;24:431-436.

Richardson PG, Sonneveld P, Schuster MW, et al: Bortezomib or high-dose dexamethasone for relapsed multiple myeloma. N Engl J Med 2005;352:2487-2498.

Rifkin RM, Gregory SA, Mohrbacher A, Hussein MA: Pegylated liposomal doxorubicin, vincristine, and dexamethasone provide significant reduction in toxicity compared with doxorubicin, vincristine, and dexamethasone in patients with newly diagnosed multiple myeloma: A Phase III multicenter randomized trial. Cancer 2006;106:848-858.

Rosen LS, Gordon D, Kaminski M, et al: Zoledronic acid versus pamidronate in the treatment of skeletal metastases in patients with breast cancer or osteolytic lesions of multiple myeloma: A phase III, double-blind, comparative trial. Cancer J 2001;7:377-387.

References

For a complete list of references, log onto www.expertconsult.com.

Non-Hodgkin's and Hodgkin's Lymphoma

Stephen Smith

DEFINITION AND ETIOLOGY

Non-Hodgkin's lymphoma (NHL) and Hodgkin's lymphoma (HL) are neoplasms arising from cells of the lymphoid lineage. T and B cells originate in the bone marrow, migrate to the thymus or peripheral lymphoid tissues respectively, and develop into highly specialized mediators of the adaptive immune response. The means for generating and maintaining this mobile, interactive, and highly plastic repertoire of cells are complex and prone to error. Lymphoid cells are at various times susceptible to genetic errors, direct viral infection, chronic stimulation by antigen, and effects of generalized host immunodeficiency—four dynamic factors involved in lymphomagenesis. However, it has proved difficult to identify consistent etiologic factors in families or populations. The heterogeneity of lymphomas, reflecting the complexity of the human immune system, implies that a number of genetic and acquired risk factors interact in their pathogenesis.

Lymphomas are divided into two major groups, NHL and HL, based on a range of pathologic and clinical features. The incorporation of genetic and immunologic characteristics into lymphoma diagnosis is a recent advancement, proposed by the 1994 Revised European-American Classification of Lymphoid Neoplasms (known as the REAL classification).[1] Dividing lymphomas into B cell neoplasms, T cell neoplasms, and Hodgkin's disease, the REAL classification was validated and shown to be clinically relevant by subsequent studies. It also served as the basis for the ensuing World Health Organization (WHO) classification of lymphoid neoplasms. The many WHO subtypes of NHL are made more manageable via grouping into indolent, aggressive, or highly aggressive categories based on their natural history (Box 1). HL encompasses two main categories: classic HL (with four further subgroups) and nodular lymphocyte-predominant HL. Classic HL includes nodular-sclerosis, mixed-cellularity, lymphocyte-rich, and lymphocyte-depleted subgroups. The WHO classification, though complex and continually evolving, establishes a common language for researchers and clinicians and is key to collaborative research aimed at curing lymphoma.

PREVALENCE AND RISK FACTORS

According to the National Cancer Institute and Centers for Disease Control and Prevention (CDC) SEER database, lymphoma was diagnosed in about 74,340 people in the United States in 2008, giving an age-adjusted incidence rate of 22.2 per 100,000 per year.[2] In general, NHL is increasing in incidence (especially diffuse large B cell lymphoma), though mortality among those affected with NHL has decreased. HL is much less common than NHL, accounting for about one tenth of all lymphoma cases; its annual incidence is 2.8 per 100,000. The prevalence of lymphomas tends to be much higher than their incidence, given their natural history and availability of effective therapies. For example, the U.S. prevalence of HL was 156,000 (patients with HL or a history of HL) as of January 1, 2005.

As noted, risk factors for the development of lymphoma are not fully understood. Environmental associations with pesticides, agricultural chemicals, and hair dyes have been inconsistently identified. On the other hand, known risk factors for lymphoma include systemic immunosuppression due to inherited conditions, HIV infection, or medications.

PATHOPHYSIOLOGY AND NATURAL HISTORY

The natural history of a given NHL is reflected in its conceptual grouping (e.g. indolent, aggressive, highly aggressive), although heterogeneity even within specific subtypes is observed. This heterogeneity is due to the broad spectrum of genetic changes, cell-signaling aberrations, and features of the tumor microenvironment that can affect the behavior of an individual lymphoma.

Although some population studies have found a higher risk of lymphoma in first-degree relatives of probands, defining the exact inherited genetic lesions has proved difficult.[3] In contrast, genetic abnormalities acquired during early lymphocyte development have been clearly implicated in lymphomagenesis. These include chromosomal translocations and the accidental mutation of bystander genes during immunoglobulin gene remodeling, a complex process providing lymphocytes the diversity needed for effective host defense. Expression of the virus's genetic program by cell machinery (as occurs in chronic Epstein-Barr virus infection) contributes to the pathogenesis of HLs and lymphoproliferative disorders in immunosuppressed patients following organ transplant.

Infection by nonviral microbes can also lead to lymphoma, but not by direct infection of lymphocytes. Instead, chronic infection with organisms such as *Helicobacter pylori* is thought to lead to ongoing antigenic stimulation in lymphoid tissues, creating an environment ripe for selection of a malignant clone. Such stimulation can also follow immune attack on self-antigens, possibly explaining the link between some lymphomas and autoimmune conditions such as rheumatoid arthritis and systemic lupus erythematosis.

Inborn or acquired immunodeficiency is associated with a higher risk of lymphoma. The interaction among these etiologic factors, and in particular the cellular interactions among immune and tumor cells (in the tumor microenvironment), are important topics of research in lymphoma pathogenesis and therapy.

Non-Hodgkin's Lymphoma

Indolent Lymphomas

Follicular lymphoma (FL) and chronic lymphocytic leukemia/ small lymphocytic lymphoma (CLL/SLL) are the most common indolent lymphomas. Survival from diagnosis of indolent lymphoma is generally measured in years. However, although radiation therapy can cure early-stage indolent lymphomas, advanced-stage forms have classically been considered incurable. Despite initial chemosensitivity, such patients tend to face a continual pattern of relapse and treatment-related morbidity until death. Data from Stanford University published in 1984 showed that some asymptomatic patients with advanced follicular lymphoma had no decrement in survival following an initial watch-and-wait approach.[4] Data from the same group have also shown a rate of spontaneous remission in up to 20% of patients with FL.

Based on these factors and the lack of curative therapy, treatment for follicular lymphoma was historically delayed until emergence of disease-related symptoms or organ compromise, and median survival was 8 to 10 years from diagnosis. However, newer treatment approaches using monoclonal antibodies with initial chemotherapy, and autologous stem cell transplantation for patients in relapse, may be prolonging survival and altering the natural history of follicular lymphoma. This has given rise to therapeutic optimism and prompted some to initiate treatment in some groups of patients with newly diagnosed lymphoma who may have been managed expectantly in the past.

In follicular lymphoma, the classic genetic lesion is the translocation between chromosomes 14 and 18 t(14;18), seen in the majority of cases (≥70%). As is typical for lymphomas, this translocation juxtaposes a regulatory sequence next to a normal, intact gene involved in cellular processes. (This contrasts with most leukemias, in which translocations—such as translocation 9;22 in chronic myelogenous leukemia—create a unique fusion gene and protein bearing unique oncogenic properties). Translocation 14;18 places the *BCL2* gene on chromosome 18 under the control of a key regulatory region (the immunoglobulin heavy chain [IgH] enhancer sequence) on chromosome 14. This results in the overexpression of *BCL2,* a protein that renders cells resistant to programmed cell death (apoptosis). Affected cells are, in a sense, excessively durable: They defy the usual checks and balances controlling B lymphocyte growth, and they persist in the lymph node to face chronic antigenic stimulation and ongoing mutagenesis processes that can eventually bring about a malignant clone.

The fact that this translocation exists in a large fraction of healthy adults is evidence that further mutagenic events are crucial for lymphomagenesis. Other notable lesions in indolent lymphomas include t(11;14) in mantle cell lymphoma (causing increased cyclin D expression, and thus cell cycle progression), the deletion of chromosome 13q14 in CLL/SLL (a region containing suppressive micro-RNA that normally silences *BCL2*)[5] and the t(11;18) in extranodal marginal zone lymphomas (producing a true fusion gene that also affects apoptosis) (Table 1). It should be noted that mantle cell lymphoma can behave in an indolent or aggressive manner, and current studies favor high-intensity induction chemotherapy for patients requiring treatment in an effort to improve poor outcomes.

Box 1 Simplified World Health Organization Classification of Non-Hodgkin's Lymphoma by Clinical Behavior

Indolent

B Cell

Follicular lymphoma (grades I and II)
Chronic lymphocytic leukemia/ small lymphocytic lymphoma
Marginal zone: extranodal, mucosa-associated lymphoid tissue (MALT), nodal, splenic
Plasma cell myeloma
Plasmacytoma
Hairy cell leukemia

T Cell

Mycosis fungoides
Sézary syndrome

Aggressive

B Cell

Diffuse large B cell lymphoma and variants
Follicular lymphoma (grade III)
Mantle cell*

T Cell

Peripheral T cell
Anaplastic large cell

Highly Aggressive

Burkitt's lymphoma
Precursor B/T lymphoblastic

**Mantle cell lymphoma may also behave in an indolent fashion.*

Aggressive and Highly Aggressive lymphomas

Survival of patients with aggressive lymphomas is measured in months without treatment, and patients with untreated highly aggressive lymphomas can face even shorter survival (weeks). On the other hand, the curability of a number of these patients is well known, and survival rates are improving for many subtypes with modern treatment regimens. Given their tendency for rapid progression and the availability of effective chemotherapy, aggressive and highly aggressive lymphomas are treated immediately upon diagnosis and at times require urgent hospitalization and tumor lysis precautions.

Diffuse large B cell lymphoma (DLBCL) is the most common subtype of aggressive lymphoma. About half of all patients with DLBCL achieve long-term disease-free survival after initial therapy, and relapses after more than 5 years are uncommon. Genetic errors involving BCL6 (a transcription factor), BCL2 (an antiapoptotic protein) and FAS (CD95, a TNF-family receptor), are often linked to the development and behavior of DLBCL.[6] However, individual lesions fail to explain the pathologic and clinical heterogeneity of DLBCL. To investigate this variability, investigators have applied molecular tools including gene expression profiling to DLBCL tumor samples, which examines tumor mRNA expression patterns. In one study, this approach identified three groups of patients whose gene-expression patterns suggested a distinct cell of origin of their tumor.[7] These groups had significantly different prognoses, and the gene-expression technique provided prognostic information surpassing that gained using the clinically based International Prognostic Index

Table 1 Genetic Pathophysiology of Selected Indolent NHL Subtypes

Disease	Abnormality	Pathophysiology	Significance
Follicular lymphoma	t14:18	BCL2 juxtaposed with IgH regulatory sequence, increasing BCL2 expression	Increased BCL2 expression confers resistance to apoptosis Early step in malignant transformation
Chronic lymphocytic leukemia/ small lymphocytic lymphoma	Deletion 13q14	Causes loss of suppressive micro-RNA elements	Loss of negative regulation of BCL2 confers resistance to apoptosis Seen in a favorable prognosis subset
Mantle cell lymphoma	t11:14	Cyclin D1 juxtaposed with IgH regulatory sequence, increasing cyclin D1 expression	Increased Cyclin D1 expression alters cell cycle control, associated with a high mitotic index Seen in >70% of cases of MCL
Extranodal marginal zone lymphoma	t11:18	Fuses an apoptosis-inhibitor gene with a novel gene	Alters signals controlling apoptosis in these cells

IgH, immunoglobulin heavy chain.

(IPI, discussed later). However, the challenges for expression profiling are to isolate true driver mutations in lymphomagenesis and to prove them valuable in guiding clinical decisions (such as selection of initial therapy) via prospective trials.

Aggressive T cell lymphomas are rarer and less well understood than their B cell counterparts, and they generally have a poorer outcome. Only about one in three patients with advanced-stage nodal T cell lymphomas survives this diagnosis at 5 years. An exception is the group of ALK-positive (anaplastic lymphoma kinase–staining) T cell anaplastic large cell lymphomas, which occur in younger patients and have a more favorable prognosis. These lymphomas usually have a translocation between chromosomes 2 and 5, causing markedly increased ALK expression and altered intracellular signaling involved in disease pathogenesis.

Highly aggressive lymphomas, typified by adult Burkitt's lymphoma and adult B and T cell lymphoblastic leukemia or lymphomas, can require immediate hospitalization and are some of the fastest-growing malignancies known. These diseases are in general highly sensitive to combination chemotherapy, and high cure rates (surpassing 60% in the highest-risk patients) are possible. In contrast to the heterogeneity of DLBCL, the highly aggressive Burkitt lymphoma is defined by the deregulation of a single transcription factor, the myc protein. Myc deregulation is observed in more than 90% of cases to be due to a translocation between chromosome 8 (containing the c-myc gene) and one of various partner chromosomes, most commonly chromosome 14. This results in widespread deregulation of genes involved in cell proliferation.

Hodgkin's Lymphoma

The pathophysiology of HL, which occurs most commonly in adolescents and young adults, has been even more challenging to elucidate. In contrast to follicular or Burkitt's lymphoma, HL lacks the presence of a unifying genetic lesion. The origin of the characteristic Reed-Sternberg cell—long debated—has been traced to a precursor B cell using molecular studies. Such cells account for less than 1% of the lymph node cellularity, and although they originate from a B cell, they downregulate the normal B cell genetic program and do not display typical surface markers. The presence of this unusual cell in the appropriate inflammatory background forms the basis for HL diagnosis. Although EBV is commonly found in Reed-Sternberg cells, and infectious mononucleosis increases the relative risk of developing HL, its role in lymphomagenesis is incompletely understood.

The natural history of HL resembles that of an aggressive lymphoma, and the disease is uniformly fatal over months if untreated. The disease has a predilection for manifesting with mediastinal disease and spreading in an orderly fashion via contiguous lymph node groups. Nodular lymphocyte–predominant HL is characterized by lymphohistiocytic variants of the Reed-Sternberg cell (known as L&H cells, or popcorn cells for their microscopic appearance). This uncommon Hodgkin's variant tends to manifest as localized disease without involvement of bone marrow or spleen and without B symptoms; overall, it has a more indolent clinical course.

SIGNS AND SYMPTOMS

Signs and symptoms of lymphoma may be local or paraneoplastic in nature. Local tumor growth can cause palpable masses, compression of adjacent structures, lymphatic obstruction and extravascular fluid accumulation (ascites), or infiltration and disruption of normal organs. Tumors secreting a paraprotein (plasma cell myeloma, lymphoplasmacytic lymphoma, some other varieties) can cause increased serum viscosity and related symptoms, especially with immunoglobulin (Ig)M and IgA classes. Lymphomas can also manifest a broad range of paraneoplastic effects such as B symptoms, impaired immunity, autoimmune phenomena, thrombophilia, or metabolic and endocrine disturbances.

NHL and HL both commonly manifest with painless enlargement of superficial lymph nodes, with HL usually involving supradiaphragmatic sites. Organomegaly may be present due to liver or spleen involvement, sometimes palpable on physical examination or implied by symptoms such as abdominal discomfort or early satiety. Infiltration of bone marrow can result in anemia or thrombocytopenia. Involvement of nonlymphoid tissues (extranodal involvement) is more commonly seen in more-aggressive lymphomas, as is risk of CNS involvement, which is greatest in highly aggressive forms. Indolent NHL, on the other hand, is often diagnosed on an incidental basis—for example, after lymph node sampling performed during an unrelated surgery, or because an imaging study performed for a different illness leads to detection and biopsy of an enlarged lymph node. In the majority of cases, the detection of indolent lymphomas is preceded by a variable but long period of undetected, slow growth. For this reason, bone marrow involvement at diagnosis in indolent lymphoma is common.

Constitutional symptoms can result in activation of the coagulation system, causing thrombosis, or can result in impaired immunity, leading to recurrent infection. The presence or absence of B symptoms, related to a cytokine release, is considered part of the staging system for lymphomas (Table 2). B symptoms are defined as fevers higher than 38° C, drenching sweats (especially at night), or unexplained weight loss of more than 10% of body weight in the preceding 6 months.

DIAGNOSIS

Laboratory Tests

Routine laboratory studies are used to assess disease-related complications and suitability for therapy. These include a complete blood count with differential and review of the peripheral blood smear (on which circulating lymphoma cells may be observed). A comprehensive metabolic assessment and tests of kidney and liver function are indicated; these can inform the clinician of mass effects or metabolic consequences such as hypercalcemia or tumor lysis syndrome (which can occur before therapy in aggressive subtypes). Lactate dehydrogenase, immunofixation of urine, and serum, monoclonal protein quantification, urinalysis, erythrocyte sedimentation rate (in HL), β_2 microglobulin in plasma cell disorders, and HIV serology in patients with risk factors are also indicated.

Table 2 Ann Arbor Staging System for Lymphoma

Stage	Description
I	Single lymph node region (I) or extranodal site (IE)
II	Two or more nodal regions, same side of the diaphragm (II) or nodal disease plus localized extranodal extension (IIE)
III	Nodal involvement on both sides of the diaphragm (III) with extranodal involvement (IIIE) or splenic involvement (IIIS)
IV	Involvement of one or more extranodal tissues or organs
Further designations:	A: no symptoms B: with B symptoms (fever >38° C, sweats, weight loss >10% in prior 6 months) E: extranodal X: bulky disease

SECTION 7 HEMATOLOGY AND ONCOLOGY

Imaging

Computed tomography (CT) is the best-studied and most universal imaging tool for staging, restaging after treatment, and surveillance. MRI is indicated in some cases when noncontrast CT is deemed inadequate for patients with renal insufficiency or contrast allergy. Positron-emission tomography (PET) is being increasingly used, although its sensitivity and specificity (as well as positive predictive value) vary substantially by NHL subtype and timing of test performance. In general, aggressive lymphomas are more PET-avid than are indolent NHLs. Prospective trials incorporating PET at various time points (e.g., during initial staging, early PET during therapy, in restaging after treatment, or in post-treatment surveillance) and for specific lymphoma subtypes are needed to define its proper role in diagnosis and treatment.

Diagnostic Procedures

Tissue biopsy of affected nodes or tissues is required, but fine needle aspiration is inadequate. A core needle biopsy or an excisional biopsy is needed for accurate diagnosis, to determine the lymphoma growth pattern and content of the surrounding tissue. This also helps provide adequate tissue for specialized studies such as immunohistochemistry, fluorescence in-situ hybridization (FISH), or polymerase chain reaction (PCR). Flow cytometry of the peripheral blood can, in the appropriate clinical context, provide adequate diagnostic material. Bone marrow aspirate and biopsy is generally required, with few exceptions (such as early-stage HL without B symptoms). Lumbar puncture for evaluation of CNS involvement is indicated in patients at higher risk for central involvement (those with >2 extranodal s ites involved, or bone marrow involvement by aggressive lymphoma) or patients who have symptoms or signs suggesting meningeal involvement.

Staging

Staging is performed according to the Ann Arbor staging system (see Table 2). Early-stage disease (stage I or II) involves lymph nodes on one side of the diaphragm, and advanced stages involve nodal sites on both sides of the diaphragm (stage III) and/or extranodal sites (including bone marrow, stage IV). CLL/SLL is staged based on the Rai or Benet staging systems, which emphasize sites of spleen involvement and cytopenias but not localization of involved lymph nodes.

Summary

- Excisional or core needle biopsy is needed to assess nodal architecture. Fine needle aspiration alone is inadequate.
- Contrast-enhanced CT imaging of the chest, abdomen, and pelvis is the standard imaging study for patients with normal renal function.
- PET imaging test characteristics vary among lymphoma subtypes, and PET requires further study before it can be used routinely in decisions regarding diagnosis, staging, or treatment.
- Clinical stage is determined by history and physical examination, imaging studies, and bone marrow biopsy based on the Ann Arbor staging system.

TREATMENT

The expected clinical behavior of a lymphoma (whether indolent, aggressive, or highly aggressive) is useful in planning management (Table 3). However, given the great variability even among disease subtypes, additional clinical and pathologic prognostic information is needed. The presence of disease-related symptoms and patient comorbidities can also affect the selection and timing of treatment. The effectiveness of treatments are measured by several criteria. One is their response rate in a given disease (determined by degree of tumor shrinkage by CT criteria as either partial or complete response; PET scanning is being used for this purpose as well in clinical trials), and other is the progression-free survival of subjects treated with a drug (defined as the duration a patient is living with a disease that does not get worse). Effectiveness is measured especially by the overall survival: the percentage of patients alive at a given time (often 5 years) after therapy.

Chemotherapy's adverse effects have been mitigated by improvements in supportive care, including medications for nausea and growth factors to stimulate production of red blood cells and neutrophils, but adverse effects are still significant and vary by drug. Fatigue and cytopenias leading to potentially serious infections are seen with many drugs. Some notable adverse effects of lymphoma drugs include neuropathy (due to vincristine), cardiotoxicity (doxorubicin), hyperglycemia (prednisone), and T cell immunosuppression with viral (cytomegalovirus) reactivation (nucleoside analogues including fludarabine). Given these and other toxicities, a thoughtful assessment of the individual patient before treatment is key to maximizing its benefit.

Table 3 Management of Lymphoma*

Category	Indolent Non-Hodgkin's Lymphoma	Aggressive Non-Hodgkin's Lymphoma	Hodgkin's Lymphoma
Early stage	Radiation alone may be curative in FL and some other forms	short-course chemotherapy (CHOP) + radiation for some patients Chemotherapy (CHOP) with rituximab	Short-course chemotherapy (ABVD) + radiation for most pts
Advanced Stage	Observation Chemotherapy + rituximab for B cell subtypes Rituximab alone	Chemotherapy (CHOP) with rituximab for B cell subtypes for 6-8 cycles CHOP-based regimen or clinical trial for T cell lymphomas	Chemotherapy with ABVD for 6-8 cycles, then radiation to persistent bulky masses
Relapsed	Different chemotherapy or monoclonal antibody therapy Clinical trial Autologous transplant	Autologous transplant for eligible chemosensitive patients Clinical trial Chemotherapy	Autologous transplant for eligible chemosensitive patients Clinical trial Chemotherapy

*Management may vary substantially based on individual patient/disease characteristics.
ABVD, doxorubicin [Adriamcyin], bleomycin, vinblastine, and dacarbazine; CHOP, cyclophosphamide, hydroxydaunorubicin, vincristine (Oncovin), and prednisone.

Indolent Non-Hodgkin's Lymphoma

In general, NHL is sensitive to a number of chemotherapeutic agents, as well as newer antibody-based treatments, some molecularly targeted small-molecule therapies in development, and radiation. Early-stage indolent lymphoma may be cured with radiotherapy alone, a standard approach for several subtypes. However, only a small fraction of patients with indolent NHL present with stage I or II disease.

Advanced-stage indolent NHL may be managed in a number of ways, often involving the monoclonal antibody rituximab. Binding to the pan–B cell marker CD20, rituximab induces immune-mediated and pro-apoptotic mechanisms resulting in tumor cell death. It was first approved in the late 1990s for treating relapsed FL, and it is likely responsible in part for the improvement in survival observed in FL patients since then.[6] It is safely combined with chemotherapy in many common intravenous regimens, including the rituximab, cyclophosphamide, vincristine, and prednisone (R-CVP) combination for FL and the fludarabine, cyclophosphamide, and rituximab (FCR) combination for CLL/SLL. The addition of the anthracycline doxorubicin to R-CVP (known as RCHOP: H stands for hydroxydaunorubicin; O stands for Oncovin, vincristine's trade name) resulted in a progression-free survival approaching seven years in one study,[8] but no consensus exists regarding its use in the initial treatment of patients with FL.

Chlorambucil, an oral alkylating agent, has been used extensively in a number of indolent NHL subtypes and affords a favorable toxicity profile and relative ease of administration.

Rituximab, when given alone in four weekly doses, produces response rates well over 50% in the initial treatment of FL and is well tolerated; its major adverse effects relate to reactions (fever, chills) during infusion. Extended or maintenance rituximab after initial treatment with the drug prolongs progression-free survival in FL, but its benefit in terms of overall survival, or beyond that achieved with retreatment at progression, is to be determined.

Radioimmunoconjugates, which link radionuclides to monoclonal antibodies, deliver a combined antilymphoma effect (antibody plus radiation-induced cell killing) and have shown high response rates in treating relapsed (60% response rate) and untreated (95% response rate) follicular lymphoma.[9] Although approved for relapsed and refractory FL, the optimal treatment in this setting is unclear due to the paucity of randomized data showing an overall survival benefit using one therapy instead of another.

Autologous stem cell transplantation (high-dose chemotherapy followed by reinfusion of the patient's own early hematopoetic progenitor cells) also suffers from a lack of randomized, prospective studies, especially in the era of rituximab, to inform decision making in this setting of relapsed indolent lymphoma. Allogeneic stem cell transplantation using an HLA-matched donor has been used with variable success, limited by high upfront treatment-related mortality and complications of graft-versus-host disease. Use of a reduced-intensity initial (conditioning) chemotherapy regimen could make stem cell transplantation less toxic while enabling a purported graft-versus-tumor effect of the donor's immune system to take hold. However, this intensive approach is relevant to few patients and is best performed in the context of a clinical trial when feasible.

In general, given the lack of demonstrable survival benefit for one treatment over another in relapsed FL and the increasingly rapid pace of drug development in the field, involvement in clinical trials of new therapies is an important option for patients.

Aggressive and Highly Aggressive Non-Hodgkin's Lymphoma

In DLBCL, treatment is based on disease stage and other factors, and chemotherapy is invariably involved. Initiation of treatment is required soon after diagnosis, and tumor lysis precautions may be indicated. The International Prognostic Index (IPI) is a well-studied and reliable method to estimate prognosis in DLBCL. The IPI has been revised to account for improvements in prognosis seen with widespread use of rituximab (R-IPI, Table 4).

All but some of the earliest-stage cases of DLBCL are treated initially with RCHOP chemotherapy given every 21 days for six to eight cycles. (For some early-stage patients, a strategy involving

Table 4 Revised International Prognostic Index for DLBCL R-CHOP chemotherapy

Risk Factors (1 point each)			
Age >60 years			
Lactate dehydrogenase			
Eastern Cooperative Oncology Group (ECOG) performance status 2-4			
Stage III or IV			
More than one extranodal site of disease			
Score	**Risk Group**	**4-Year PFS**	**4-Year OS**
0	Very Good	94%	94%
1-2	Good	80%	79%
3-5	Poor	53%	55%

OS, overall survival; PFS, progression-free survival.
DLBCL, diffuse large B cell lymphoma;
R-CHOP, rituximab, cyclophosphamide, hydroxydaunorubicin, vincristine (Oncovin), and prednisone
Sehn LH, Berry B, Chhanabhi M, et al: The revised International Prognostic Index (R-IPI) is a better predictor of outcome than the standard IPI for patients with diffuse large B-cell lymphoma treated with R-CHOP. British Columbia Cancer Center. Blood 2007;109:1857-1861.

abbreviated chemotherapy followed by local radiation may be adequate.) This standard is based on several studies showing that CHOP given in this manner is just as effective as more intensive chemotherapy regimens[10] and that the addition of rituximab to three-weekly CHOP improves overall survival.[11] The superiority of eight versus six cycles has not been established. Alterations in the schedule of administration, and the addition of other drugs, are strategies under investigation for patients with high-risk DLBCL subtypes, as defined by the IPI or pathologic features. Burkitt's and lymphoblastic lymphomas are treated initially with more-intense regimens, and treatment-related complications and hospitalizations are common. A 60% cure rate may be achieved even in the worse-prognosis subgroup of Burkitt's lymphoma patients. In these patients, and in some patients with DLBCL (such as patients with large cell involvement of the bone marrow, or more than two extranodal sites involved), prophylactic chemotherapy given into the CSF (intrathecally) via lumbar puncture is used in an effort to reduce the risk of highly morbid CNS relapse.

For patients with DLBCL who relapse but remain sensitive to chemotherapy, an approach using high-dose chemotherapy followed by autologous stem cell transplantation has been proved superior to salvage chemotherapy alone in a landmark prospective, randomized study.[12] However, up to half of patients with relapsed DLBCL do not display further sensitivity to chemotherapy. For these patients, or for patients otherwise ineligible for autologous transplantation, the prognosis tends to be poor (10% long-term disease-free survival), and clinical trials of new drugs are an important option.

Mantle cell lymphoma contrasts with DLBCL in that its survival curve, given by plotting fraction of patients surviving against time, tends to show a continual downward slope in most studies, with a median survival of 2 to 4 years. (This contrasts with DLBCL's survival curve, which decreases quickly but then plateaus, evidence for cure of some patients). This has prompted investigation of more-intense upfront chemotherapy regimens (such as HyperCVAD, modified CHOP alternating with cytarabine and methotrexate), which tend to have more toxicity but higher initial remission rates, and regimens incorporating novel agents (radioimmunoconjugates, proteasome inhibitors).

Peripheral T cell lymphoma (PTCL) has historically been treated with CHOP-based regimens in the initial setting, though only one in three patients achieves long-term survival with this approach. The rarity of T cell lymphomas and their diversity has made conducting prospective, well-powered therapeutic trials difficult. Modifications of CHOP or altogether new regimens (involving gemcitabine or novel targeted agents, for example) are being tested in some cooperative clinical trials in the United States. Patients with relapsed PTCL also tend to fare more poorly than those with relapsed DLBCL in most series, including after autologous transplant, making clinical trials of new therapies an important option in this setting as well.

Hodgkin's Lymphoma

In contrast to the early 20th century, in which most patients succumbed to HL, about 85% of patients with HL are now cured. In testament to therapeutic successes, the focus of clinical research has shifted toward curing highest-risk groups and preventing late therapy-related complications in patients who are cured.

Early-stage HL is generally treated with four cycles of chemotherapy using ABVD (doxorubicin [Adriamcyin], bleomycin, vinblastine, and dacarbazine) followed by radiation therapy. The long-term risks of radiation (including cardiac disease and the risk of secondary, in-field solid tumors) may be lower with modern techniques, because substantial radiation-related morbidity and mortality has been seen with extensive exposures to the chest.

Advanced-stage HL is usually treated with six to eight cycles of ABVD, followed by radiation to residual bulky masses. Some international variation in practice exists, with application of more-intensive chemotherapy regimens to stage III/IV patients with high-risk disease in some countries. Increased toxicity (ranging from treatment-related infertility to mortality) is seen with more-intensive regimens, and how best to apply increased intensity therapy is a point of debate. The use of PET scanning early during treatment is being investigated in a risk-adapted approach, because early PET negativity (after two cycles of chemotherapy) is associated with much better outcomes than a positive PET scan at that time. The latter group of patients is the focus of a number of prospective studies testing whether an early change in treatment (to a new or more intensive regimen) may be of benefit.

New and Emerging Therapies

The impact of rituximab on the treatment of NHL, arguably much greater than was expected during development of the drug, is likely to foreshadow an era of rapid development of antilymphoma drugs with new modes of action and attenuated toxicity. An improved understanding of disease biology is providing a range of rational targets. In addition to improvements of monoclonal antibodies (by enhancing the mechanisms of immune killing, linking to radiation or other anti-lymphoma drugs), new compounds designed with specific pathophysiologic features are under development. Some target restoration of apoptosis, for example, in tumors demonstrating BCL2 dependence for survival. Others target the effect of deregulated transcription factors such as BCL6 in subtypes of DLBCL. Others block key signaling pathways (such as temsirolimus, which blocks the AKT/mTOR pathway) involved in protein translation and cell growth.

The proteasome, which degrades ubiquitinated intracellular proteins, is the target of bortezomib, a drug approved for relapsed mantle cell lymphoma. This drug is thought to induce apoptosis via a massive disruption in cells' disposal of proteins, affecting tumor cells more than normal ones.

Immunomodulation of the lymphoma microenvironment is an area of intense investigation. Thalidomide and lenalidomide, thought to act in part by this mechanism, are approved for the treatment of multiple myeloma, and early reports show activity in B cell malignancies as well.

Histone deacetylase inhibitors, which open chromatin structure to restore normal transcription of a number of genes suspected to be silenced in tumor cells, have shown promise in relapsed cutaneous T cell lymphoma (for which one such agent is approved) and in early studies in HL.

CONCLUSION

In summary, recognition of the heterogeneity of NHL and HL in their natural history, pathophysiology, and response to treatment is key. The WHO classification system has provided a common language for managing and studying lymphomas. Lymphomas can manifest with local or paraneoplastic effects, and HL and NHL are staged relatively similarly. PET scanning offers promise in some lymphomas, although its clinical value and role remains to be defined by ongoing prospective trials. The success of passive immunotherapy using rituximab for NHL has changed outcomes for indolent and aggressive subtypes of NHL alike. Future therapeutic efforts will exploit newly understood aspects of lymphogenesis and will explore unique maintenance or long-term treatment strategies with drugs that can be tolerated on a chronic basis. Cure of lymphoma may be tantamount to elimination with initial induction therapy, suppression using established, chronically administered, well-tolerated therapies, or both.

Suggested Readings

Abramson JS, Shipp MA: Advances in the biology and therapy of diffuse large B-cell lymphoma: Moving toward a molecularly targeted approach. Blood 2005;106(4):1164-1174.

Coiffier B, Lepage E, Briere J, et al: CHOP chemotherapy plus rituximab compared with CHOP alone in elderly patients with diffuse large-B-cell lymphoma. N Engl J Med. 2002;346(4):235-242.

Rizvi MA, Evens AM, Tallman MS, et al: T-cell non-Hodgkin lymphoma. Blood 2006;107:1255-1264.

Rosenwald A, Wright G, Chan WC, et al: The use of molecular profiling to predict survival after chemotherapy for diffuse large-B-cell lymphoma. N Engl J Med 2002;346(25):1937-1947.

Seam P, Juweid ME, Cheson BD: The role of FDG-PET scans in patients with lymphoma. Blood 2007;110: 3507-3516.

References

For a complete list of references, log onto www.expertconsult.com.

Prostate Cancer

Robert Dreicer and Jorge Garcia

DEFINITION

Prostate cancer has evolved from a relatively common but infrequently discussed neoplasm to a major clinical entity with significant public health and economic ramifications. The widespread application of prostate-specific antigen (PSA) into clinical practice in the late 1980s has had a paradigm-shifting impact on the management of prostate cancer. Among the most visible consequences of PSA-based screening is the substantial increase in the percentage of patients who are believed to have clinically localized disease. This, in turn, has translated into a significant increase in the number of patients undergoing curative-intent surgery and radiotherapy. Additional prostate cancer subsets have been created, including patients with PSA-only evidence of disease following curative-intent therapy, termed *biochemical failure,* and patients with rising PSA levels following androgen-deprivation therapy, termed *castrate progressive prostate cancer, biochemically defined.*

EPIDEMIOLOGY

It is estimated that in 2009 approximately 192,280 men in the United States will be given a new diagnosis of prostate cancer. Although the vast majority present with early disease, more than 27,000 men are destined to die from advanced disease yearly. Prostate cancer is the most common malignancy in U.S. men (excluding nonmelanoma skin cancer), and it is the second most common cause of cancer death, after lung cancer, in American men. Worldwide, prostate cancer ranks third in cancer incidence and sixth in cancer mortality in men.

There is, however, a significant disparity in incidence and mortality rates among world regions, with a very low incidence in China and Japan in contrast to the United States and parts of western Europe. This wide variability in incidence is likely multifactorial, with varying effects of genetic predisposition, diet, environmental factors, and the increased frequency of prostate biopsies performed in asymptomatic men undergoing screening with PSA.

Prostate cancer is also a disease of the older adults, as has been demonstrated in various autopsy series showing 70% to 80% of men older than 80 years with some evidence of latent disease. It is this observation that has complicated the prostate cancer screening debate, with critics questioning the ability of screening to discriminate between clinically relevant disease and latent disease that is not destined to cause symptoms or affect survival.

RISK FACTORS

The causes of prostate cancer remain poorly understood. The main predictors of prostate cancer risk are age, race or ethnicity, and family history. The incidence of prostate cancer in U.S. men increases significantly above age 50 years. African American men have a higher incidence of prostate cancer–related death than European American and Latin American men. Prostate cancer can be sporadic, hereditary, or familial; the familial type is defined by a clustering of prostate cancer cases within members of a family. Men with an affected first-degree relative (i.e., father or brother) have a two-fold increase in their risk of developing prostate cancer. Similarly, early age of onset in any family member also increases the risk. In families with two or three affected first-degree relatives, the risk of developing prostate cancer increases 5- to 11-fold.[1]

There are numerous purported molecular, genetic, environmental, and dietary factors, with varying degrees of supporting evidence. Studies have provided compelling data to support the role of elevated serum testosterone and insulin-like growth factor-1 levels as significant risk factors. Many candidate dietary components have been proposed to influence human prostatic carcinogenesis, including animal fat, calories, fruits and vegetables, antioxidants, and various micronutrients, but the specific role of dietary agents in promoting or preventing prostate cancer remains controversial. Also controversial are the data from recent observational studies that have hypothesized statins and nonsteroidal anti-inflammatory drugs (NSAIDs) as agents capable of decreasing the risk of developing any malignancy, including prostate cancer.

PATHOPHYSIOLOGY

The pathophysiology of prostate cancer is poorly understood and, for many years, was an underrepresented area of investigation, in contrast to work in other solid tumors. Over the past decade, there has been a significant increase in prostate cancer research, with a concomitant increase in funding for basic investigation. Among the challenges faced by investigators attempting to understand early steps in the carcinogenic pathway is the lack of a reliable animal model of prostate cancer.

Although prostate cancer typically manifests in men older than 65 years, a growing body of evidence suggests that prostatic carcinogenesis is initiated much earlier. Prostatic intraepithelial neoplasia (PIN) is the histologic entity widely considered to be the most likely precursor of invasive prostate cancer. Although not all patients with high-grade PIN (HGPIN) progress to develop invasive disease, PIN is characterized by cellular proliferation within pre-existing ducts and glands, with cytologic changes that mimic those of cancer.[1] PIN is associated with progressive abnormalities of phenotype and genotype that are intermediate between normal prostatic epithelium and cancer. The recognition of the strong association of HGPIN and cancer has led many investigators to propose its use as an intermediate marker in chemoprevention studies.

Prostate cancer progression has also been related to a number of genetic abnormalities that affect the androgen receptor (AR) and other molecules that are involved in cell survival and apoptosis. In fact, over the past decade, recognition of a hereditary form of prostate cancer has prompted a vigorous research effort into the molecular genetics of prostate cancer, with various research teams performing linkage studies leading to the identification of several chromosomal loci that may be the source of prostate cancer susceptibility genes. At least six prostate cancer susceptibility loci have been identified to date, with increasing evidence that there is no single major gene accounting for a large portion of susceptibility to the disease. The fraction of prostate cancer cases caused by mutations in these genes is estimated to be 5% to 10%, and the hereditary form of the disease is diagnosed, on average, approximately 7 years earlier than the sporadic form of the disease. Despite of the heterogeneity of this tumor and the lack of appropriate model systems of prostate cancer progression, these studies are beginning to provide important insights into the pathogenesis of this neoplasm.

SIGNS AND SYMPTOMS

The clinical manifestations of prostate cancer result from the effects of local growth of the tumor, the spread to regional lymph nodes via the lymphatics, and the hematogenous dissemination to distant metastatic sites.

Although most patients with early-stage prostate cancer are asymptomatic, locally advanced disease can lead to obstructive or irritative voiding symptoms that result from local tumor growth into the urethra or bladder neck, extension into the trigone of the bladder, or both.

Prostate cancer most often spreads to bone, commonly leading to bone pain. A small but important subset of patients develop spinal cord impingement from the epidural spread of disease, resulting in pain and neurologic compromise that, depending on the location of the spinal lesion, could include the irreversible loss of bowel and bladder function and the ability to walk. Other common sites of metastatic spread include lymph nodes, with some patients presenting with progressive lymphedema, renal insufficiency, or both as a consequence of obstruction of pelvic lymphatics and ureteral outlet obstruction.

DIAGNOSIS

With the introduction of PSA into clinical practice in the late 1980s and the subsequent influential recommendations of the American Urological Society and the American Cancer Society, prostate cancer screening (PSA plus digital rectal examination [DRE]) has become widely used in the United States. Prostate cancer screening remains controversial, as evidenced by the wide array of screening recommendations (Box 1), because there is no prospective evidence demonstrating a decrease in prostate cancer-specific mortality.[2]

Several prospective screening trials are ongoing in the United States and worldwide. Among the largest are the European Randomized Screening for Prostate Cancer (ERSPC) trial, with more than 160,000 men, and the Prostate, Lung, Colorectal, and Ovarian Cancer Screening Trial (PLCO), sponsored by the National Cancer Institute, which completed enrolment of more than 154,000 participants, including 75,000 men, in the summer of 2001. It is hoped that the results of these trials will provide more definitive guidance to patients and clinicians about the impact of screening. Until more definitive data are available, many major medical societies have recommended a careful discussion with individual patients, before screening, regarding the potential risks and benefits. Patients with significant comorbid conditions and those with life expectancies of less than 10 years are much less likely to benefit from therapeutic intervention and therefore should not be considered for screening. Alternatively, patients at potentially high risk, such as African Americans and those with one or more affected first-degree relatives, might be appropriate candidates for screening at an earlier age, 40 to 50 years.

Over the last decade, the penetration of PSA-based screening has caused a stage migration, with an increasing percentage of patients with normal rectal examination findings receiving a diagnosis on the basis of an elevated PSA level (clinical stage T1c in the tumor, node, metastasis [TNM] staging classification). There has also been a concomitant dramatic decrease in the number of patients who present initially with evidence of metastatic disease.

Following a biopsy-proven diagnosis of prostate cancer, patients are clinically staged using the TNM system (Table 1) based on the extent of local tumor on rectal examination and the presence or absence of metastatic disease. In the last several years, a series of outcomes-based nomograms have been developed to improve the clinician's ability to predict the patient's pathologic stage (http://urology.jhu.edu/prostate/partintables.php) and his response to therapy (http://www.mskcc.org/mskcc/html/10088.cfm). These nomograms use clinically available parameters such as PSA, Gleason scores obtained from prostate biopsies or surgery, and other known prognostic factors, such as prostate capsule penetration, margin status, involvement of the seminal vesicles, and node status.

Box 1 Summary of Current Prostate Cancer Guidelines From Selected Organizations

American College of Physicians—American Society of Internal Medicine
Physicians should describe potential benefits and known harms of screening, diagnosis, and treatment, listen to the patient's concerns, and then individualize the decision to screen.

American Cancer Society and American Urological Association
Physicians should offer annual DRE and PSA screening, beginning at age 50 years, to men who have at least a 10-year life expectancy and to younger men at high risk.

Canadian Task Force on Preventive Health Care and U.S. Preventive Services Task Force
DRE and PSA tests are not recommended for the general population.

American Academy of Family Physicians
No published standards or guidelines are available for low-risk patients.

American Medical Association
Physicians should provide information regarding the risks and potential benefits of prostate screening.

DRE, digital rectal examination; PSA, prostate-specific antigen.

TREATMENT AND OUTCOMES

Chemoprevention

Features such as a high prevalence rate, a long latency period, and identifiable risk factors have made prostate cancer a desirable tumor to test different chemopreventive strategies.

Several studies have evaluated different agents thought to be capable of reducing the risk of prostate cancer. Although agents such as retinoids and toremifene have failed to show statistical benefits in this setting, finasteride, an inhibitor of 5α-reductase (5-AR) widely used to treat symptoms related to benign prostatic hyperplasia, appears to reduce the risk for developing prostate cancer. A large randomized trial with more than 18,000 participants comparing finasteride with placebo in men with a normal DRE and normal serum PSA values but with an elevated risk for prostate cancer (aged 55 or older, African American ethnicity, or a first-degree relative having prostate cancer) demonstrated a 25% decrease in the incidence of prostate cancer over a 7-year period for men taking finasteride. Despite this result, the controversy about a possible increase in the incidence of high-grade tumors (Gleason scores >7) initially dampened enthusiasm for the use of this agent as a chemopreventive strategy. Subsequent explanations for these findings suggest a diagnostic bias due to the effect of finasteride on prostate size. In fact,

Table 1 TNM Clinical Stages of Prostate Cancer

Stage	Features
T1a	Nonpalpable, with %5% of tissue with cancer, low grade (diagnosed by transurethral resection of the prostate)
T1b	Nonpalpable, with >5% of tissue with cancer, high grade (diagnosed by transurethral resection of the prostate), or both
T1c	Nonpalpable, but prostate-specific antigen level elevated
T2a	Palpable, one half of one lobe or less
T2b	Palpable, more than one half of one lobe, not both lobes
T2c	Palpable, involves both lobes
T3a	Palpable, unilateral capsular penetration

TNM, tumor, node, metastasis.

when prostate size was included in the analysis, the risk for high-grade tumors disappeared.

Currently, an international multicenter double-blind, placebo-controlled chemoprevention trial is evaluating dutasteride, a more potent 5-AR dual inhibitor. Other, smaller studies also continue to evaluate minimally toxic compounds such as vitamins, minerals, and micronutrients as potential chemopreventive agents in prostate cancer.

Localized Prostate Cancer

For appropriately selected patients with clinically organ-confined prostate cancer, potential curative options include radical prostatectomy (RP) and radiation therapy (external-beam radiation therapy [EBRT], brachytherapy, or both). Other options include active surveillance, androgen-deprivation therapy (ADT), and cryotherapy. The optimal treatment for localized prostate cancer remains undefined, in part because of the absence of prospective randomized clinical trials comparing outcomes of surgery and radiotherapy. To date, only one randomized phase III trial has directly compared RP and watchful waiting in men with clinically localized disease. This study demonstrated a significant improvement in disease-specific survival as well as overall survival in men undergoing surgery.

Other factors that complicate our understanding of the impact of these therapies include the stage migration resulting from screening and the long natural history of localized prostate cancer. Using biochemical relapse (BCR)—PSA recurrence following radical prostatectomy (PSA >0.2) or the nadir PSA value + 2ng/mL in patients receiving radiotherapy—as an intermediate end point and after adjustment for stage and grade of tumors, outcomes with EBRT and radical prostatectomy at 8 years' follow-up are equivalent.[3] Among the challenges in identifying the most beneficial therapy for localized disease is the relatively rapid evolution of radiotherapy techniques over time.

Over the last 5 to 10 years, there has been increasing evidence of a dose-response relationship for prostate cancer, leading to an increase in conventional radiotherapy dosages for localized disease from the upper 60-Gy range to current doses of 72 to 78 Gy. This increase in dosage has been made possible by technologic improvements in radiotherapy delivery systems using three-dimensional conformal radiation theray (3D-CRT) (computer-guided dosing techniques that attempt to minimize radiation dosage outside the target field), such as intensity-modulated radiotherapy.

Evidence from contemporary prospective, randomized clinical trials has also demonstrated that for selected patients, such as those with locally advanced disease (large tumor size, high Gleason grade, and high PSA levels), a disease-free survival, time to the development of progressive disease, and overall survival benefit is gained when patients are treated with ADT. The addition of ADT has been prospectively studied in several settings, including neoadjuvant, concurrent, and adjuvant for periods often persisting for 6 to 36 months.

Prostate brachytherapy with ^{125}I or ^{103}Pd, which involves placing radioactive, rice-sized pellets directly into the prostate gland, has increasingly been used in the management of appropriately selected patients opting for radiotherapy. Compared with external beam radiotherapy, it has some important patient advantages, including a single outpatient treatment versus the typical 7-week course of external beam treatment. Some patients undergo brachytherapy followed by supplemental external beam radiotherapy. Whether the addition of supplemental external beam therapy improves outcomes and can justify increases in patient toxicity and cost remains controversial.

Given the lack of definitive evidence of the optimal therapy for localized prostate cancer, an important consideration for patients and the physicians helping guide their decision is the potential side effects of radiotherapy and surgery (Table 2). The major side effects of therapy for localized prostate cancer affect urinary, bowel, and sexual function. Recent evidence has suggested that for patients undergoing radical prostatectomy, urologists with high-volume prostatectomy practices may have better patient outcomes.[4] Although, historically, reports of these side effects in the literature were typically those reported to the treating physicians in retrospective reviews, there has been a large effort by numerous investigators using "modern" quality-of-life assessment tools to quantitate more precisely the impact of local therapies on long-term quality of life.[5] These assessments should be used by patients and physicians to help guide treatment decisions.

Table 2 Common Side Effects of Standard Treatment Modalities for Localized Prostate Cancer

Treatment Modality	Impotence	Urinary Function	Rectal Injury
Brachytherapy	Variable	Acute bladder irritation, common; incontinence, rare	—
External beam radiotherapy	Common	Acute cystitis, common; late cystitis, infrequent	Acute diarrhea, common; rectal bleeding, infrequent; rectal perforation, rare
Radical prostatectomy	Variable	Incontinence (variable)	—

Cryotherapy is another modality of local treatment for prostate cancer that initially had been abandoned because of its high rate of complications. Recently this modality of treatment has regained momentum as new and improved instruments and techniques have allowed reductions in toxicities and and possibly greater efficacy. Currently, cryotherapy remains experimental in the United States.

Metastatic Prostate Cancer

Hormonal therapy—androgen ablation—has for more than 60 years been the primary initial treatment of patients with metastatic prostate cancer. Androgen ablation options for patients with advanced prostate cancer include bilateral orchiectomy, luteinizing hormone–releasing hormone (LHRH) analogues and antagonists, and combined androgen blockade, a combination of either an orchiectomy or LHRH analogue plus an antiandrogen. Although orchiectomy remains the historical gold standard, LHRH therapy is equivalent therapeutically, and patients are increasingly opting for medical therapy, in part because of the psychological implications of surgical castration. Orchiectomy remains an important option for patients presenting with spinal cord compression or diffuse, painful bone metastases, because it leads to the rapid achievement of castrate levels of testosterone (hours) compared with the 14 to 21 days required for LHRH analogues.

In human males, 5% to 10% of circulating testosterone originates from the conversion of adrenal steroid precursors. Nonsteroidal antiandrogens act at the level of the androgen receptor to inhibit the stimulatory effects of testosterone. The use of an antiandrogen, in addition to LHRH or orchiectomy, is referred to as *combined androgen blockade.* The role of combined androgen blockade remains controversial, with meta-analysis evidence of only a modest improvement in survival, with some added toxicity and significant expense.[6] Approximately 10% of patients started on LHRH therapy have an initial testosterone flare, so patients at risk—such as those with known bone or nodal metastases or at risk for urinary outlet problems—should be started concomitantly on an antiandrogen (e.g., bicalutamide, flutamide) for 2 to 3 weeks to minimize this possibility.

Unfortunately, the vast majority of patients with metastatic prostate cancer have evidence of disease progression on hormonal therapy (median response duration to hormonal therapy, 24-36 months). Patients with advanced prostate cancer typically have progressive bone pain, cancer cachexia, and fatigue. Significant anemia is common, although transfusion dependency is rare. Some patients with primarily nodal involvement develop significant lymphedema or ureteral obstruction. Spinal cord compression is relatively common, and a high index of suspicion must be maintained for patients presenting with back pain, even in the absence of neurologic findings. In prostate cancer patients with suspected spinal cord compression (without cervical spine symptoms, clinical findings, or plain film evidence of bone destruction), magnetic resonance imaging (MRI) of the thoracic and lumbosacral spine, with and without gadolinium, should be performed. Given the high incidence of involvement of both the lumbar and thoracic spines, failure to image both areas can compromise radiotherapy if untreated lesions become symptomatic and are detected later.

Historically, management of advanced disease consisted of second-line hormonal therapies and palliative radiotherapy. Palliative radiotherapy remains an important component of patient management. There has been evidence, similar to findings for breast cancer and multiple myeloma, that bisphosphonate therapy with zoledronic acid can decrease skeletal progression rates and complications in patients with androgen-independent metastatic bone disease.[7] Chemotherapy has the potential to provide meaningful palliation for select patients, with improvement in pain and other disease-related symptoms. Two important phase III studies have evaluated docetaxel-based therapies in patients with advanced prostate cancer and demonstrated, for the first time, the ability to improve the survival of patients with advanced disease, albeit modestly.[8] New drugs in development are targeting the androgen receptor directly with androgen-receptor antagonists and by inhibition of androgenic steroid synthesis.

Although recent progress has been made and new agents are on the horizon, advanced prostate cancer remains an incurable disease. Vigorous efforts to manage pain and other disease-related symptoms through the appropriate use of opiods and palliative radiotherapy are essential for the optimal management of patients with progressive disease.

Summary

- Prostate cancer is the most commonly diagnosed neoplasm (excluding nonmelanoma skin cancer) and is the second most common cause of cancer death, after lung cancer, in American men.
- Prostate cancer screening with PSA testing and a digital rectal examination is widely performed, but data supporting an impact on survival are not yet available.
- Chemotherapy for advanced prostate cancer can palliate the disease and modestly improve survival.

Suggested Readings

American College of Physicians: Screening for prostate cancer. Ann Intern Med 1997;126:480-484.

Bianco FJ Jr, Riedel ER, Begg CB, et al: Variations among high-volume surgeons in the rate of complications after radical prostatectomy: Further evidence that technique matters. J Urol 2005;173:2099-2103.

Bostwick DG: High-grade prostatic intraepithelial neoplasia: The most likely precursor of prostate cancer. Cancer 1995;75:1823-1836.

Goodman PJ, Thompson IM, Tangen CM, et al: The Prostate Cancer Prevention Trial: Design, biases and interpretation of study results. J Urol 2006;175:2234-2242.

Harlan LC, Potosky A, Gilliland FD, et al: Factors associated with initial therapy for clinically localized prostate cancer: Prostate Cancer Outcomes Study. J Natl Cancer Inst 2001;93:1864-1871.

Kupelian PA, Elshaikh M, Reddy CA, et al: Comparison of the efficacy of local therapies for localized prostate cancer in the PSA era: A large single-institution experience with radical prostatectomy and external beam radiotherapy. J Clin Oncol 2002;20:3376-3385.

Prostate Cancer Trialists' Collaborative Group: Maximum androgen blockade in advanced prostate cancer: An overview of the randomised trials. Lancet 2000;355:1491-1498.

Saad F, Gleason DM, Murray R, et al: A randomized, placebo-controlled trial of zoledronic acid in patients with hormone-refractory metastatic prostate carcinoma. J Natl Cancer Inst 2002:94:1458-1468.

Tannock I, de Wit R, Berry W, et al: Docetaxel plus prednisone or mitoxantrone plus prednisone for advanced prostate cancer. N Engl J Med 2004:351:1502-1512.

References

For a complete list of references, log onto www.expertconsult.com.

Treatment of Colorectal Cancer

Richard Kim

MANAGEMENT

The primary treatment of early colorectal cancer is surgical resection of the primary tumor and regional lymph nodes. Surgery is curative in early stage tumors but, in more advanced stages, adjuvant therapy is recommended to prevent recurrence and improve survival. Stage IV disease will require systemic chemotherapy.

Stages I to III Colon Cancer

Primary treatment of stages I to III colon cancer is surgical resection of the primary tumor and regional lymph nodes. Adequate lymph node sampling is important, because the number of nodes examined significantly correlates with 5-year relapse-free and overall survival. At least 12 nodes should be examined to determine nodal status accurately.[1]

After surgical resection, adjuvant chemotherapy should be considered in patients with stage II or III disease to reduce the risk of disease recurrence, either as local or distant metastasis. There is no role for adjuvant chemotherapy in stage I disease.

Use of adjuvant therapy in patients with stage II colon cancer is actively debated. Many trials done to address the benefit of chemotherapy in a population consisting entirely or predominantly of stage II disease have been negative, or shown only a modest benefit in terms of disease-free survival (DFS) but not overall survival (OS). The American Society of Clinical Oncology (ASCO) recommends against routine administration of fluorouracil (5-FU)-based chemotherapy for patients with resected stage II colon cancer. However, they have suggested that adjuvant therapy be considered for medically fit patients who have inadequately sampled lymph nodes (fewer than 12 in the surgical specimen), T4 lesions, perforation, or poorly differentiated histology, despite the lack of direct data from randomized controlled trials to support the practice.[2]

Multiple studies have proven the benefit of adjuvant chemotherapy in patients with stage III disease. Adjuvant chemotherapy is associated with an approximately 30% reduction in the risk of disease recurrence, and a 22% to 32% reduction in mortality.[3] The extent of benefit relates to tumor grade, invasion, and nodal involvement. The choice of chemotherapy in stage III is FOLFOX (oxaliplatin plus infusional 5-FU and leucovorin) regimen based on the MOSAIC trial.[4] In this trial, 2246 patients with completely resected stage II or III colon cancer were randomized to a 6-month course of FOLFOX regimen or infusional 5-FU-leucovorin (LV). After a median follow-up of 38 months, 3-year DFS (the primary end point) was significantly higher with FOLFOX (78% vs. 73%; hazard ratio [HR], 0.77). Patients who have contraindications to oxaliplatin (e.g., preexisting neuropathy), 6 to 8 months of LV modulated 5-FU is an acceptable option. Recently, capecitabine (oral fluoropyrimidine) has been approved by the FDA for adjuvant therapy in stage III colon cancer based on the X-ACT study.[5] In this study, capecitabine was at least as effective as 5-FU-LV, and there was some suggestion of superiority in terms of 3-year DFS (64.2% vs. 60.6%; $P = .05$) and OS (81.3% vs. 77.6%; $P = .07$). Currently, there are active trials looking at the impact of molecular factors (e.g., 18q deletion, thymidylate synthetase [TS] overexpression, p53 mutations, microsatellite instability, gene expression profile) on prognosis and the response to adjuvant chemotherapy in patients with stage II or III colorectal cancer.

Stage IV Colorectal Cancer

When diagnosed as advanced metastatic disease, colorectal cancer (CRC) is traditionally associated with a poor prognosis, with 5-year survival rates in the range of 5% to 8%. The actual survival rate has remained unchanged over the past 35 to 40 years. However, during the past 5 years, significant advances have been made in chemotherapy treatment options, such that improvements in 2-year survival rates are now being reported—median survival rates of 21 to 24 months in patients with metastatic disease.

Chemotherapy has been the mainstay approach for patients with advanced colorectal cancer.[6] For nearly 40 years, 5-FU was the only active anticancer agent available to treat advanced colorectal cancer in the first-line setting. In general, response rates to 5-FU in patients with advanced disease are low, in the range of 10% to 15%. To improve the clinical efficacy of 5-FU, the addition of certain biomodulating agents such as the reduced folate LV, a change in the schedule of administration of 5-FU from bolus to continuous infusion, or both have been actively investigated.[7]

Progress in the past five years has been made possible with the introduction of three cytotoxic agents—capecitabine, irinotecan, and oxaliplatin—and with the approval of two biologic agents, bevacizumab and cetuximab. During this time period, the median survival of patients with advanced metastatic disease has gone from 10 to 12 months to almost 24 months.

In the United States, the combination of irinotecan with bolus 5-FU-LV (IFL regimen) was approved for the initial therapy of metastatic CRC based on a randomized phase III study, which resulted in improved clinical efficacy in terms of higher response rate and greater overall and progression-free survival when compared with 5-FU-LV monotherapy.[8] However, as a result of the increased incidence of diarrhea, dehydration, and myelosuppression, the IFL regimen is rarely used today. Instead, FOLFOX has now become the treatment of choice for most oncologists based on the Intergroup trial N9741.[9] This pivotal study showed that FOLFOX had significantly greater clinical efficacy than IFL in terms of response rate (45% vs. 31%; $P = .002$), time to tumor progression (8.7 vs. 6.9 months; $P = .0001$), and median overall survival (19.5 vs. 14.8 months; $P = .0001$).

Capecitabine is a rationally designed oral fluoropyrimidine carbamate that is absorbed intact through the intestinal wall and then converted to 5-FU in three sequential enzymatic reactions. Studies have shown similar efficacy of capecitabine compared with infusional 5-FU and leucovorin.[10] Capecitabine has been approved by the U.S. Food and Drug Administration (FDA) for first-line treatment of metastatic CRC in the setting of irinotecan- and oxaliplatin-intolerant patients. There have been studies designed to determine whether capecitabine can be substituted for infusional 5-FU in combination with irinotecan and oxaliplatin.[11]

Bevacizumab is a recombinant humanized monoclonal antibody that targets all forms of vascular endothelial growth factor A (VEGF-A). Bevacizumab was granted FDA approval in February 2004 as a first-line treatment for metastatic colorectal cancer in combination with any IV fluoropyrimidine-containing regimen based on a phase III trial.[12] The trial has shown that patients with colorectal cancer who received bevacizumab plus standard chemotherapy with the bolus weekly IFL regimen had longer progression-free survival (10.6 vs. 6.2 months; $P < .00001$) and improved median overall survival (20.3 vs. 15.6 months; $P = .00003$) compared with those receiving IFL chemotherapy plus placebo. Today, the greatest use of bevacizumab has been in combination with FOLFOX-based regimens because of the poor toxicity profile of the IFL regimen.

Cetuximab is a chimeric monoclonal antibody directed against the external cell surface of the epidermal growth factor receptor (EGFR). EGFR is a member of the erb-B family of growth factor receptors, and is overexpressed in up to 85% of colorectal tumors. Moreover, its expression has been correlated with metastatic disease and poor prognosis. Currently, cetuximab is approved, in combination with irinotecan, for the treatment of metastatic CRC in patients refractory to irinotecan, and for use as a single agent in the treatment of recurrent metastatic CRC in patients intolerant of irinotecan-based chemotherapy.[13]

Rectal Cancer

Surgical resection is the cornerstone of curative treatment in rectal cancer. Usually, tumors in the upper and middle rectum can be managed with low anterior resection (LAR), coloanal anastomosis, and preservation of the anal sphincter. Distal rectal cancer will require abdominoperineal resection (APR) and entails a permanent colostomy, which maybe burdensome to patients. Total mesorectal excision (TME) has been used in conjunction with APR and LAR and has been associated with decreased local recurrence. TME is a surgical technique that involves sharp dissection along the mesorectal fascia, with removal of the rectum and all tissue invested by the adjacent visceral fascia, including fatty tissue, lymph nodes, and lymphatic vessels.

The use of perioperative chemoradiation therapy (CRT) for rectal cancer continues to evolve. A 1990 NIH Consensus Development Conference recommended that postoperative 5-FU-based chemotherapy combined with irradiation should be standard clinical practice for stages II and III rectal cancer because of its proven decreases in local recurrence, cancer-related deaths, and overall mortality.[14] The success of combined modality treatment in the postoperative setting has led to its use for the preoperative treatment of rectal cancer. Neoadjuvant CRT has many advantages, including tumor downstaging and a higher rate of sphincter preservation.

The German Rectal Cancer Study Group has completed a large, prospective, randomized trial that compared preoperative with postoperative chemoradiation.[15] In this pivotal study, 823 patients with clinically staged T3 to T4 or node-positive rectal cancer were randomized to the same chemoradiotherapy (50.4 Gy in 28 daily fractions to the tumor and pelvic lymph nodes concurrent with infusional 5-FU) regimen administered preoperatively or postoperatively. It was concluded that although there is no difference in overall survival between the two groups, there is a significant reduction in the local recurrence rate (6% vs. 13%; $P = .006$) and treatment toxicity in the preoperative group (27% vs. 40%; $P = .001$). Based on this trial, neoadjuvant CRT should be considered standard treatment for patients with stage II or III rectal cancer. Surgical resection is generally deferred until 6 to 8 weeks following completion of therapy to allow maximal tumor response and to allow patients to recover from the chemoradiation.

No trials have conclusively demonstrated the benefits of postoperative chemotherapy for patients who have already received neoadjuvant CRT. However, preliminary data from EORTC trial 22921 has suggested that there may be improvement in outcomes for patients receiving postoperative adjuvant 5-FU–based chemotherapy.[16] Guidelines from the NCCN (National Comprehensive Cancer Network, www.nccn.org) recommend that all patients receive 5-FU–containing chemotherapy, even if they have a pathologic complete remission (pCR) to neoadjuvant CRT.

Summary

- No adjuvant treatment is recommended for stage I colon cancer.
- Adjuvant therapy is recommended for stage III and high-risk stage II colon cancer patients.
- Treatment for stage IV colon cancer is generally palliative. There are many new cytotoxic chemotherapy and targeted agents available for treating metastatic colon cancer, such as 5-FU, oxaliplatin, irinotecan, cetuximab, and bevacizumab.

Suggested Readings

Andre T, Boni C, Mounedji-Boudiaf L, et al: Oxaliplatin, fluorouracil, and leucovorin as adjuvant treatment for colon cancer. N Engl J Med 2004;350:2343-2351.

Benson AB, 3rd, Schrag D, Somerfield MR, et al: American Society of Clinical Oncology recommendations on adjuvant chemotherapy for stage II colon cancer. J Clin Oncol 2004;22:3408-3419.

Bosset JF, Calais G, Mineur L, et al: Enhanced tumorocidal effect of chemotherapy with preoperative radiotherapy for rectal cancer: Preliminary results-EORTC 22921. J Clin Oncol 2005;23:5620-5627.

Cunningham D, Humblet Y, Siena S, et al: Cetuximab monotherapy and cetuximab plus irinotecan in irinotecan-refractory metastatic colorectal cancer. N Engl J Med 2004;351:337-345.

Goldberg RM, Sargent DJ, Morton RF, et al: A randomized controlled trial of fluorouracil plus leucovorin, irinotecan, and oxaliplatin combinations in patients with previously untreated metastatic colorectal cancer. J Clin Oncol 2004;22:23-30.

Hoff PM, Ansari R, Batist G, et al: Comparison of oral capecitabine versus intravenous fluorouracil plus leucovorin as first-line treatment in 605 patients with metastatic colorectal cancer: Results of a randomized phase III study. J Clin Oncol 2001;19:2282-2292.

Hurwitz H, Fehrenbacher L, Novotny W, et al: Bevacizumab plus irinotecan, fluorouracil, and leucovorin for metastatic colorectal cancer. N Engl J Med 2004;350:2335-2342.

Saltz LB, Cox JV, Blanke C, et al: Irinotecan plus fluorouracil and leucovorin for metastatic colorectal cancer. Irinotecan Study Group. N Engl J Med 2000;343:905-914.

Sauer R, Becker H, Hohenberger W, et al: Preoperative versus postoperative chemoradiotherapy for rectal cancer. N Engl J Med 2004;351:1731-1740.

Twelves C, Wong A, Nowacki MP, et al: Capecitabine as adjuvant treatment for stage III colon cancer. N Engl J Med 2005;352:2696-2704.

References

For a complete list of references, log onto www.expertconsult.com.

Esophageal Cancer

Ahmed Absi, David J. Adelstein, and Thomas Rice

DEFINITION

Esophageal cancer has long been considered one of the deadliest malignancies, and considerable controversy has surrounded its management. The most common histologic types are squamous cell carcinoma (SCC) and adenocarcinoma (AC), which together constitute more than 90% of esophageal malignancies. Rarely, melanoma, sarcoma, small cell carcinoma, or lymphoma may arise in the esophagus. Although SCC is more evenly distributed throughout the length of the esophagus, AC is predominantly a disease of the distal esophagus and gastroesophageal junction, and is rarely found in the cervical esophagus.

PREVALENCE AND RISK FACTORS

Cancers arising from the esophagus and gastroesophageal junction are relatively uncommon in the United States; there were approximately 14,520 new cases and 13,570 deaths in 2005. Worldwide, however, esophageal cancer is the eighth most common malignancy and the sixth most common cause of cancer-related death. The epidemiology of esophageal cancer changed dramatically during the latter half of the 20th century. Although 40 years ago SCC accounted for more than 90% of all esophageal tumors in the United States, diagnoses of esophageal AC have significantly increased and now represent 80% of cases. However, SCC remains the most common worldwide. The mean age at diagnosis is 67 years, and men are affected more frequently than women, particularly among patients with AC.

There are considerable geographic and racial variations in the incidence of this cancer, which is mostly explained by varying exposure to risk factors, although genetic susceptibility may play a partial role. Many of the causative and risk factors for AC and SCC have been well established (Box 1).

PATHOPHYSIOLOGY AND NATURAL HISTORY

Smoking and heavy alcohol intake are important risk factors for the development of SCC. Smoking has a synergistic effect with heavy alcohol consumption, and heavy exposure to both increases the risk of SCC by a factor of more than 100. This is further complicated by the increased risk of other aerodigestive tract cancers in a person who smokes and drinks alcohol.

Dietary and environmental factors, and certain esophageal disorders (e.g., achalasia, diverticuli) that cause chronic irritation and inflammation of the esophageal mucosa may also increase the incidence of SCC. Plummer-Vinson syndrome—the triad of dysphagia, iron deficiency anemia, and esophageal webs—has been associated with this cancer, although it is becoming increasingly rare in the developed world as overall nutrition improves. There are few genetic factors that have been identified as being important in the development of esophageal SCC. One exception is tylosis, a rare autosomal dominant syndrome associated with hyperkeratosis of the palms and soles and a high rate of esophageal SCC. Infectious agents have also been implicated in the pathogenesis of esophageal SCC. Human papillomavirus has received the most attention. It is believed that the infection results in loss of function of the tumor suppressor genes *p53* and *Rb*. The importance of this mechanism is not well established.

The risk factors for AC of the esophagus are different. Chronic gastroesophageal reflux is the most important, with severe, long-standing reflux symptoms increasing the risk of cancer by a factor of 40. Chronic gastroesophageal reflux disease is associated with Barrett's metaplasia (Barrett's esophagus), a condition in which an abnormal columnar epithelium replaces the stratified squamous epithelium that normally lines the distal esophagus. Most esophageal ACs are believed to arise from Barrett's esophagus. Although this mucosal change appears to be a favorable adaptation to chronic reflux—columnar epithelium appears to be more resistant to reflux-induced injury than the native squamous cells—this specialized intestinal metaplasia may become dysplastic and ultimately malignant, with genetic alterations that activate proto-oncogenes, disable tumor suppressor genes, or both. Factors that increase the risk for gastroesophageal reflux, such as obesity or medications that lower the lower esophageal sphincter tone, may result in an increased risk for esophageal AC.

An infectious etiology for this disease has not been identified and, unlike AC of the gastric cardia, the role of *Helicobacter pylori* colonization is unknown. The genetic and molecular changes underlying the development of esophageal AC also remain poorly understood, although allelic losses at chromosomes 4q, 5q, 9p, 9q, and 18q and abnormalities of *p53, Rb, cyclin D1,* and *c-myc* have been implicated.

The esophagus itself has several unique properties that distinguish the behavior of cancer in this organ from those of other gastrointestinal malignancies. In contrast to the rest of the gastrointestinal tract, the esophagus has no serosa, thus reducing the resistance against local spread of invasive cancer cells. Furthermore, the esophagus has an extensive network of lymphatics, allowing for early regional tumor advancement (Fig. 1). The end result is local spread and invasion into surrounding tissue, with early metastatic disease developing in most patients.

SIGNS AND SYMPTOMS

The clinical presentation of patients with esophageal cancer can be attributed to the direct effects of the local tumor, regional or distant complications of the disease, or paraneoplastic syndromes (Box 2). AC and SCC have similar clinical manifestations, which reflect the extent of local esophageal involvement. Dysphagia, the most common manifesting symptom, usually develops in response to dense solid food, and progresses gradually to interfere with the intake of softer foods and, finally, liquids. This can sometimes be accompanied by vomiting or regurgitation of saliva or food uncontaminated by gastric secretions, particularly in patients with advanced local disease. Pain is frequent and can occur in the absence of dysphagia. It can be related to swallowing itself (odynophagia) or to the local extension of the tumor into adjacent structures, such as the pleura, mediastinum, or vertebral bodies. Weight loss is common and correlates with dysphagia, dietary changes, and tumor-related anorexia. Weight loss is noted in more than 70% of patients and, if present, carries a worse prognosis. Other manifesting signs and symptoms reflect complications from disease spread, such as cough or fever from a respiratory tract fistula, upper or lower gastrointestinal bleeding, hoarseness from recurrent laryngeal nerve involvement, and hiccups from phrenic nerve involvement.

Symptoms related to distant metastasis in the lungs, bone, liver, and central nervous system, particularly in the case of AC, can also be found at the initial clinical presentation. Hypercalcemia is the most common paraneoplastic syndrome. In the absence of bone metastases, it is most common in patients with SCC and is believed to be caused by the production of a parathyroid hormone–related

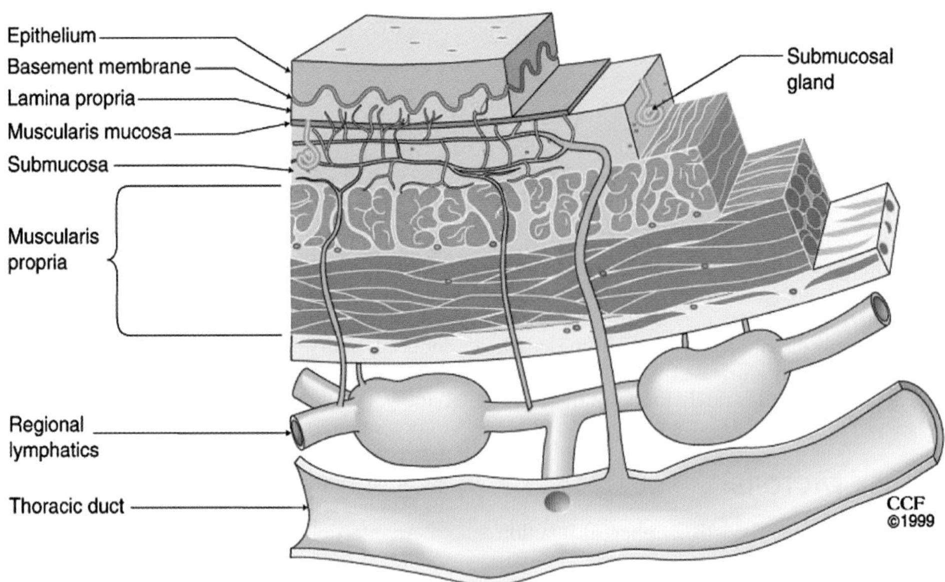

Figure 1 **Anatomic and histologic properties of the esophagus.** The esophagus has no serosa and has an extensive network of lymphatics, thus reducing the resistance against local spread of invasive cancer cells and allowing early regional tumor advancement.

Box 1 Causative and Risk Factors for Adenocarcinoma and Squamous Cell Carcinoma

Adenocarcinoma
Barrett's esophagus
Gastroesophageal reflux disease (GERD)
Obesity (by increasing the risk of GERD)

Squamous Cell Carcinoma
Smoking
Alcohol
Dietary and environmental factors that cause chronic irritation and inflammation of the esophageal mucosa
Predisposing underlying conditions, such as tylosis, achalasia, esophageal diverticula and webs, Plummer-Vinson syndrome, and human papillomavirus (HPV) infection

Box 2 Manifesting Symptoms of Esophageal Cancer

Symptoms Caused by Local Tumor Effects
Dysphagia
Cough and regurgitation
Odynophagia
Weight loss
Upper gastrointestinal bleeding

Symptoms Related to Invasion of Surrounding Structures
Respiratory fistula
Hoarseness from recurrent laryngeal nerve invasion
Hiccups from phrenic nerve invasion
Pain caused by local spread

Symptoms Related to Distant Disease
Metastatic disease to the lungs, liver, and central nervous system
Hypercalcemia

protein. The physical examination is often unremarkable, but should be directed toward finding evidence of metastatic disease, including supraclavicular lymphadenopathy, hepatosplenomegaly, and pleural effusion.

DIAGNOSIS

Dysphagia is an alarming symptom, and mandates the need for an immediate evaluation to define its exact cause and initiate appropriate therapy. Dysphagia in older adults should not be attributed to normal aging. Aging alone causes mild esophageal motility abnormalities, but these are rarely symptomatic. Evaluation of dysphagia starts with a barium swallow examination or an upper endoscopy. Endoscopy will allow the direct visualization of any tumor mass and histologic confirmation with a biopsy or brush cytology. Combining these techniques yields an overall diagnostic accuracy of 98%.

After establishing a diagnosis of esophageal cancer, adequate staging is required, because staging is the most important step in choosing appropriate therapy. More than 50% of patients have unresectable or metastatic disease at the time of presentation. For the others, survival is closely related to the stage of the disease.

The staging evaluation allows patients to be assigned a clinical stage according to the American Joint Committee on Cancer tumor-node-metastasis (TNM) classification (Box 3; Fig. 2). Informed recommendations about therapy and appropriate information regarding prognosis depends on this clinical staging, an assessment that can, however, only approximate the true disease stage

The pathologic extent of disease (pTNM) cannot truly be determined without an esophagectomy, and survival is closely linked to this pathologic stage (Fig. 3). The ability of the clinical (cTNM) stage to predict the pTNM accurately has improved with the development of more modern staging modalities.

Optimal clinical staging for this disease should include at least computed tomography (CT) scanning of the chest and abdomen, endoscopic ultrasonography and, if appropriate, a positron emission tomography (PET) scan. The importance of CT stems from its ability

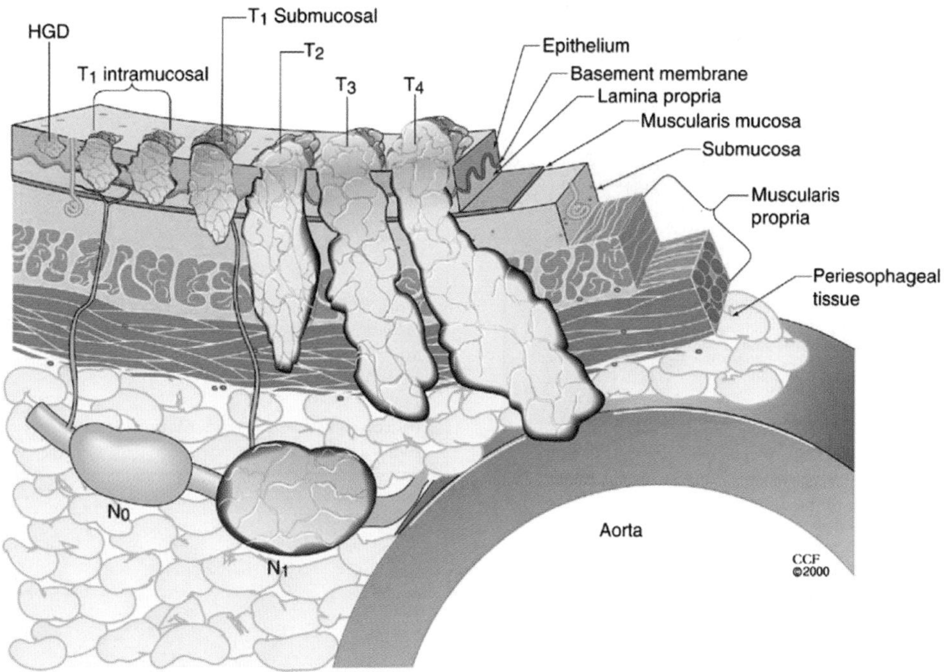

Figure 2 **Tumor-node-metastasis (TNM) staging of esophageal cancer.** Staging of esophageal cancer depends on the pathologic extent of the primary tumor (T), regional lymph nodes (N), and distant metastases.

Box 3 American Joint Commission on Cancer (AJCC) Staging for Esophageal Cancer

TNM Definitions

Primary Tumor (T)

TX: Primary tumor cannot be assessed
T0: No evidence of primary tumor
Tis: Carcinoma in situ
T1: Tumor invades lamina propria (T1a) or submucosa (T1b)
T2: Tumor invades muscularis propria
T3: Tumor invades adventitia
T4: Tumor invades adjacent structures

Regional Lymph Nodes (N)

NX: Regional lymph nodes cannot be assessed
N0: No regional lymph node metastasis
N1: Regional lymph node metastasis
N1a: One to three nodes involved
N1b: Four to seven nodes involved
N1c: More than seven nodes involved

Distant Metastasis (M)

MX: Distant metastasis cannot be assessed
M0: No distant metastasis
M1: Distant metastasis

- Tumors of the lower thoracic esophagus:
  M1a: Metastases in celiac lymph nodes
  M1b: Other distant metastases
- Tumors of the midthoracic esophagus:
  M1a: Not applicable
  M1b: Nonregional lymph nodes and/or other distant metastases
- Tumors of the upper thoracic esophagus:
  M1a: Metastases in cervical nodes
  M1b: Other distant metastases

AJCC Stage Groupings

Stage 0
  Tis, N0, M0
Stage I
  T1, N0, M0
Stage IIA
  T2, N0, M0
  T3, N0, M0
Stage IIB
  T1, N1, M0
  T2, N1, M0
Stage III
  T3, N1, M0
  T4, any N, M0
Stage IV
  Any T, any N, M1
Stage IVA
  Any T, any N, M1a
Stage IVB
  Any T, any N, M1b

to assess the presence of metastatic disease (Table 1) and the extent of direct invasion of local structures, such as the aorta or major airways, any of which will preclude surgical intervention. The technique should use both oral and intravenous contrast media and should include cuts from the thoracic inlet down to the midabdomen. It must be noted, however, that CT is not very accurate in assessing the histologic depth of the tumor (T), nor is it sensitive in assigning lymph node status (N). In fact, the overall accuracy of CT in nodal detection is less than 60%.[1]

PET scanning with 18-fluorodeoxyglucose has been recently incorporated into the staging evaluation of esophageal cancer. This noninvasive test is more sensitive than CT for detecting distant

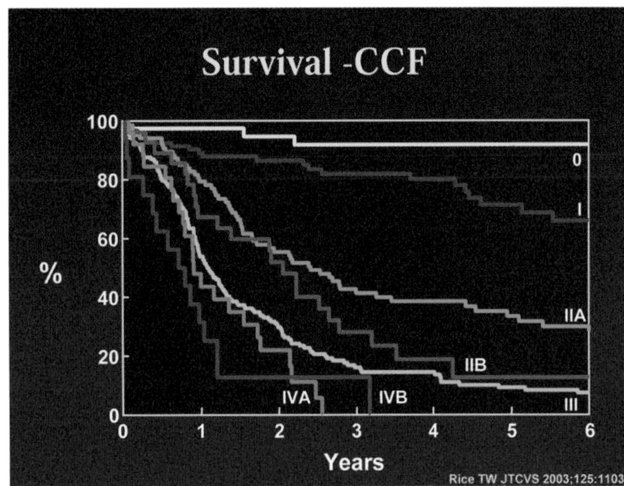

Figure 3 Survival of esophageal cancer. The data are from patients treated at the Cleveland Clinic with surgical resection. Survival is totally dependent on the pathologic stage of the disease.

Table 1 Clinical Usefulness and Accuracy of Modalities Used in Staging of Esophageal Cancer

Modality	Clinical Utility	Overall Accuracy (%)
Computed tomography (chest, abdomen)	Invasion of local structures (airways, aorta)	≥90%
	Metastatic disease	≥90%
Endoscopy	Local tumor (T) staging (operator dependent)	80%-90%
Ultrasonography (with or without fine-needle aspiration of lymph nodes)	Local nodal (N) staging (operator dependent)	70%-90%
Positron emission tomography	Metastatic disease	≥90%

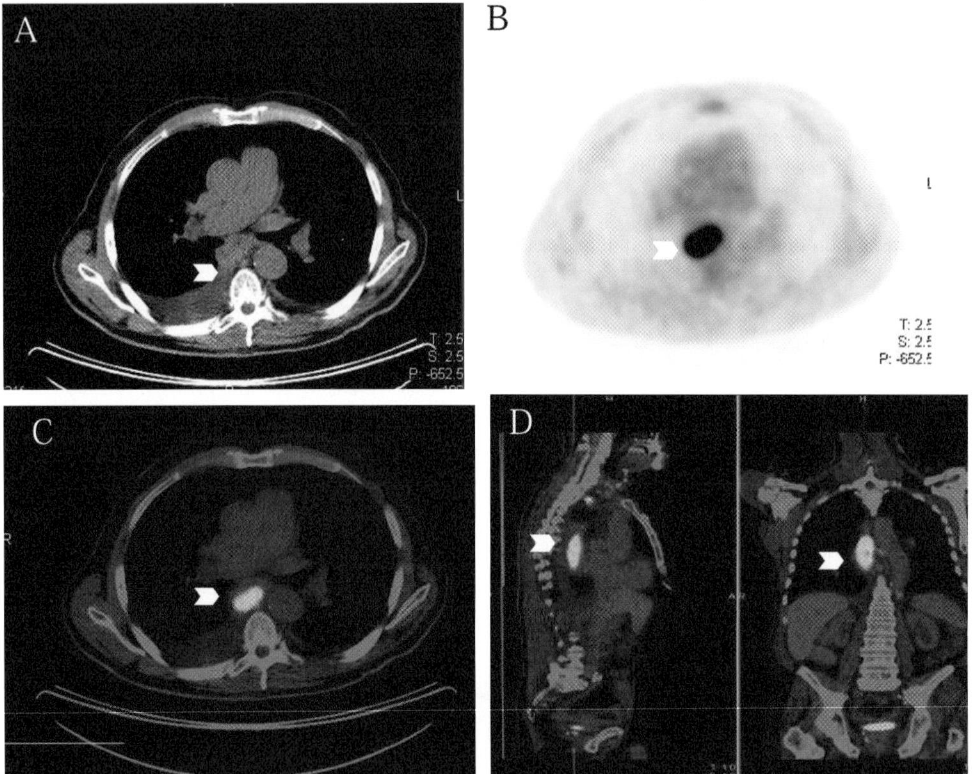

Figure 4 Computed tomography (CT) scan and positron emission tomography (PET) images of a 71-year-old man who presented with abdominal discomfort. A, Chest CT scan showing abnormal esophageal thickening extending from the midesophagus to the distal esophagus. Esophagogastroduodenoscopy showed involvement with a moderately well differentiated esophageal adenocarcinoma extending from 25 to 35 cm of the esophagus. **B** and **C,** PET scan (**B**) and combined PET-CT scans (**C**) show abnormal uptake in that area. **D,** Coronal PET images show extent of the cancer. *(Courtesy of Dr. Bohdan Bybel, Department of Radiology, Cleveland Clinic.)*

metastases. Recent studies have suggested that PET scanning can detect metastatic disease in 15% of patients who were believed, on the basis of conventional diagnostic techniques, to have localized esophageal cancer.[2] The superimposition of CT and PET scans is even more sensitive in identifying patients with occult metastases (Fig. 4).

Endoscopic ultrasonography has proven very useful in assessing the local depth of the tumor (T), lymph node involvement (N) and, with increased clinical experience, involvement of nonregional (M1a) lymph nodes. The overall accuracy of endoscopic ultrasonography in tumor depth assignment is about 80% and improves with more advanced stages of disease. With stringent criteria, the accuracy of

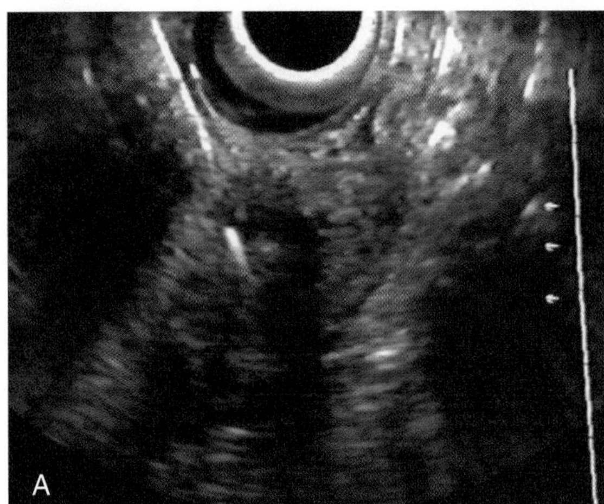

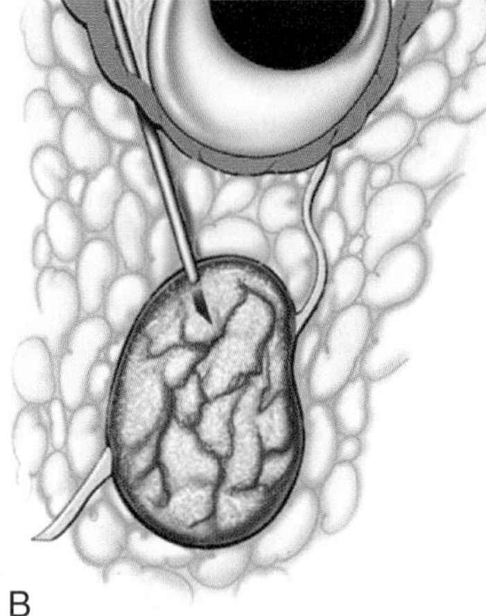

Figure 5 **Endoscopic ultrasonography (EUS). A,** EUS can assess enlarged lymph nodes surrounding the esophageal cancer. Using certain criteria and combining them with fine-needle aspiration of suspicious lymph nodes **(B),** the accuracy can reach almost 95%. This is highly dependent on operator experience.

detecting lymph node involvement approaches almost 75%. This accuracy can be improved further by endoscopic fine-needle aspiration of suspicious lymph nodes, which allows pathologic confirmation of involvement (Fig. 5).[3]

After the clinical disease stage is established, it also becomes important to assess the cardiopulmonary fitness and medical suitability of patients before surgical resection can be undertaken.

TREATMENT

Historically, esophageal cancer has carried a dismal prognosis. This has been attributed to the late presentation of patients with this disease and the technical difficulty of an adequate surgical resection in the presence of advanced local and regional involvement. Furthermore, high-dose definitive radiation therapy, as an alternative to surgical resection, is challenging because of the anatomic location of the esophagus. Any radiation therapy portal encompassing the esophagus will also include other vital structures, such as major blood vessels, major airways, the heart, and lungs. Although modern radiation techniques have fewer adverse side effects, toxicity is still common with the radiation doses required. The frequent medical comorbidities and high incidence of second malignancies in these patients also affect the overall treatment success. Two historical reviews of the outcomes after esophageal cancer treatment, published in 1980, have demonstrated this clearly.[4,5] The overall 5-year survival rate was 4% after surgical resection, with an unacceptable surgical mortality rate of almost 30%. The overall 5-year survival rate was only 6% after radiation therapy.

Surgical results have improved significantly over recent years, however. Multiple surgical series from major medical centers now report that patients undergoing surgery alone have median survival rates between 13 and 19 months, 2-year survival rates between 35% and 42%, and 5-year survival rates of 15% to 24%.[6] Although these numbers are certainly more promising, they can hardly be characterized as a medical success story, especially when we keep in mind that much of this improvement is the result of better clinical staging and better patient selection.

The goal of oncologic surgery for this disease is the resection of the primary tumor and draining lymph nodes. Given the propensity for submucosal skip lesions in the esophagus, this usually requires a subtotal esophagectomy, using a transthoracic or transhiatal approach. The transhiatal approach requires a laparotomy, blunt dissection of the thoracic esophagus, and esophagogastric anastomosis in the neck. This approach saves the patient the cardiopulmonary complications of a thoracotomy, but no prospective clinical trials have demonstrated superiority of this procedure over a thoracoabdominal approach.[7] In patients with tumors of the gastroesophageal junction and significant gastric involvement, a total gastrectomy and Roux-en-Y esophagojejunostomy may be required.

Radiation therapy has been used in the past as a single-modality approach with curative intent. However, except for those with very early-stage disease, radiation has had little impact on long-term survival.[8] For more-advanced disease, single-modality radiation therapy should, in general, be considered a palliative intervention in patients whose underlying medical comorbidities preclude surgical resection or aggressive multimodality treatment.

Multimodality treatment approaches have evolved over recent years in response to the frequent locoregional and distant recurrences identified after surgery or radiation therapy alone. Several different combinations and sequences of treatment modalities have been tried, with mixed results.

Chemotherapy has been given preoperatively, postoperatively, or both. A cisplatin-based regimen is often used. Preoperative chemotherapy has been studied in several randomized clinical trials that compared surgery alone with chemotherapy followed by surgery. These studies have demonstrated that induction chemotherapy can produce up to a 50% clinical response rate but less than a 10% pathologic complete response rate and that the 2-year survival rate after subsequent surgery is approximately 35%. However, the results of these studies have been mixed, and no clear survival advantage has been identified with the induction regimens.[9]

More intensive multimodality approaches have attempted to exploit the radiosensitizing properties of chemotherapy by using concurrent cisplatin-based chemotherapy and radiation as definitive treatment or as a preoperative adjuvant. In 1992, Herskovic and colleagues[8] reported a phase III prospective randomized trial that compared chemotherapy given concurrently with radiation with radiation therapy alone. Surgery was not a planned part of disease management in this trial. A clear survival benefit for the combined approach was identified, with a 5-year survival rate of 25% compared with radiation therapy alone, which produced no long-term survivors.[8] How this approach can be integrated with surgery has remained unclear, however.

Three small phase 3 trials have randomized patients to surgery alone or to preoperative concurrent chemoradiation followed by surgery. Unfortunately, the results have been conflicting, with no consistent survival advantage identified for one approach or another. It is of note, however, that 25% to 30% of patients treated in this fashion achieved a pathologically complete response after concurrent chemoradiation therapy. For obvious reasons, this trimodality approach produces considerable toxicity, with some series reporting treatment-related mortality in excess of 12%.[10] Currently, in many major referral centers in the United States, trimodality therapy is used for suitable patients who have at least T3 lesions, any nodal involvement with esophageal cancer, or both.

Patients with metastatic disease are treated with palliative intent. Palliation should first be directed toward relief of dysphagia and esophageal obstruction. This can be achieved in several ways, including palliative radiation, endoscopic dilation, endoscopic stenting, endoscopic laser therapy, or other light-based therapy (e.g., photodynamic therapy).[11] Palliative chemotherapy has only a limited role in this setting and only a marginal impact on survival. Current efforts are directed toward developing targeted therapies that may prove more active in esophageal cancer.

PREVENTION AND SCREENING

More recently, there has been an effort to discover early, asymptomatic, esophageal adenocarcinoma by screening patients with Barrett's esophagus. The identification of high-grade dysplasia (i.e., carcinoma in situ) is considered to be an indication for esophagectomy, because occult invasive cancer is frequently identified at the time of resection, and because invasive cancer will develop in almost 50% of patients with high-grade dysplasia who do not undergo esophageal resection.[10]

Summary

- Squamous cell carcinoma and adenocarcinoma are distinct malignancies of the esophagus, with different risk factors and different natural histories.
- The epidemiology of esophageal cancer in North America has changed dramatically in recent years with adenocarcinoma now being found in most cases.
- Dysphagia is an alarming symptom that merits careful evaluation for the possibility of esophageal cancer.
- Patients with locoregionally advanced but nonmetastatic disease may be cured with multimodality treatment approaches that often include chemotherapy.
- Although patients with metastatic disease cannot be cured, aggressive symptomatic palliation is appropriate.

Suggested Readings

Adler DG, Baron TH: Endoscopic palliation of malignant dysphagia. Mayo Clin Proc 2001;76:731-738.

Earlam R, Cunha-Melo JR: Oesophageal squamous cell carcinoma: I. A critical review of surgery. Br J Surg 1980;67:381-390.

Earlam R, Cunha-Melo JR: Oesophogeal squamous cell carcinoma: II. A critical view of radiotherapy. Br J Surg 1980;67:457-461.

Fiorica F, Di Bona D, Schepis F, et al: Preoperative chemoradiotherapy for oesophageal cancer: a systematic review and meta-analysis. Gut 2004;53:925-930.

Flamen P, Lerut A, Van Cutsem E, et al: Utility of positron emission tomography for the staging of patients with potentially operable esophageal carcinoma. J Clin Oncol 2000;18:3202-3210.

Greenberg J, Durkin M, Van Drunen M, Aranha GV: Computed tomography or endoscopic ultrasonography in preoperative staging of gastric and esophageal tumors. Surgery 1994;116:696-701.

Herskovic A, Martz K, al-Sarraf M, et al: Combined chemotherapy and radiotherapy compared with radiotherapy alone in patients with cancer of the esophagus. N Engl J Med 1992;326:1593-1598.

Hulscher JB, van Sandick JW, de Boer AG, et al: Extended transthoracic resection compared with limited transhiatal resection for adenocarcinoma of the esophagus. N Engl J Med 2002;347:1662-1669.

Kelsen DP, Ginsberg R, Pajak TF, et al: Chemotherapy followed by surgery compared with surgery alone for localized esophageal cancer. N Engl J Med 1998;339:1979-1984.

Rice TW, Adelstein DJ, Zuccaro G, et al: Advances in the treatment of esophageal carcinoma. Gastroenterologist 1997;5:278-294.

Rice TW, Boyce GA, Sivak MV: Esophageal ultrasound and the preoperative staging of carcinoma of the esophagus. J Thorac Cardiovasc Surg 1991;101:536-543.

References

For a complete list of references, log onto www.expertconsult.com.

Hepatocellular Carcinoma

Federico Aucejo and William D. Carey

DEFINITION

Many cancers develop in or spread to the human liver (Table 1). This chapter deals solely with hepatocellular cancer (HCC). (Fig. 1)

PREVALENCE

HCC is one of the most prevalent cancers in the world (Table 2). It is predominantly a high-risk cancer in less-developed areas of the world. Although the incidence remains relatively low in the United States, unlike many major cancers, the incidence of HCC has doubled in the past 20 years. Throughout the world, men are 2 to 3.5 times as likely as women to develop HCC. Hepatitis B or C is a major association. Aflatoxin exposure in Africa and Asia, oral contraceptive use in Europe and the United States, and alcohol use throughout the world are associated with increased risk. Tobacco use in some but not all studies has also been found to be a risk factor.

Migrants from high endemic areas bring with them a higher risk of HCC compared to those in the host country. The relative risk of HCC in a Chinese immigrant to North America is 3.3 to 11 times higher than in a person born in North America. Similarly, a West African immigrant to England or Wales carries a 32-fold increased risk of HCC compared to a native-born person. This transferable risk is largely associated with the high prevalence of chronic hepatitis B, most often acquired at birth or in early childhood, seen in high incidence in Africa and Asia.

PATHOPHYSIOLOGY

Pathogenesis of HCC is incompletely understood. Much evidence supports the notion that DNA damage occurs, resulting in deregulation of DNA methylation, chromosomal instability, proto-oncogene activation, and tumor suppressor gene inactivation. RAS signaling pathways are observed to be activated, and this serves to activate cell proliferation.

HCC most often occurs in the setting of chronic liver disease, and many cases, particularly in economically developed countries, are found in patients with cirrhosis. Prominent risk factors for HCC include chronic viral hepatitis B or C and alcohol-related liver disease. Cirrhosis of any cause increases the risk of HCC. An emerging threat, therefore, comes from the obesity epidemic, which predisposes to nonalcoholic liver disease and cirrhosis.

In less-developed countries, particularly in tropical and subtropical climates, aflatoxin exposure is a promoter of HCC. Aflatoxins are mycotoxins produced by fungi of the genus *Aspergillus,* which are commonly present in soil and as contaminants of improperly stored nuts, cereals, and other produce. Other risk factors for HCC include inherited disorders such as tyroinemia and hemochromatosis.

Precursor manifestations of HCC may be the development of dysplastic nodules. Until recently, the risk of subsequent HCC in patients in whom dysplasia was reported on liver biopsy was controversial. A recent study reports an odds ratio of 3.2 for subsequent HCC in those with dyslasia (95% confidence interval [CI], 1.7-6.2).[1]

SIGNS AND SYMPTOMS

Small HCC produces no symptoms. Discovery of HCC when symptoms are present provides little value to the patient. Systemic symptoms of cancer such as anorexia, unintended weight loss, and local symptoms such as right upper quadrant pain almost guarantee the disease is untreatable. Often HCC manifests in the cirrhotic patient as worsening of cirrhotic decompensation, such as worsening ascites, hepatic encephalopathy, or gastrointestinal bleeding. Given the lack of effective therapies for advanced or recurrent HCC, early diagnosis is the goal because it allows patients to undergo treatment with good long-term survival (70% at 5 years). Unfortunately, despite earlier detection of HCC, only 20% to 30% of patients are candidates for either surgical or locoregional therapies.

DIAGNOSIS

Imaging study and biopsy are the most useful diagnostic tools. Serum tumor markers are occasionally quite useful. Additional details are discussed later. Discovery of small HCCs is possible through application of screening programs for those at high risk.

In high-risk areas such as Hong Kong, discovery of HCC in adults with HBV (only 11% of whom had clinical cirrhosis) was nearly 7% after 5 years of screening.[2] Multivariate analysis showed that cirrhosis and genotype C HBV was most often associated with the development of HCC. Translation of such yields from high-risk to lower-risk geographic regions must be done with caution. Hepatologists agree on the value of screening, even though rigorous scientific evidence in support of such as a cost-effective lifesaving measure is lacking. Limited cost-to-benefit analyses using modeling methodologies suggest screening is reasonable. Using a standard threshold of utility of less than $50,000 per quality-adjusted life-year (QALY), costs for HCC screening range from $26,000 to $55,000.[3]

A recent practice guideline identifies those who are most likely to benefit from screening (Box 1).[4] Evidence suggests that screening for HCC is inconsistently performed in the United States. Data from Medicare recipients suggests that among more than 3900 patients with HCC, screening had been performed on 25%, and of these, the alpha fetoprotein (AFP) alone was used most often. Patients with known hepatitis B, hepatitis C, or cirrhosis and those who were younger or female were most likely to have been screened. Patients who had been seen by a gastroenterologist were 60% more likely to have received a screening test. These data, if confirmed, suggest that knowledge about screening recommendations has been ineffectively disseminated, particularly to the general medical community.[5]

SCREENING

The mainstay of screening for HCC is liver imaging. Many modalities exist (radioisotope, ultrasound, CT, MRI, PET scanning). Considering sensitivity, cost, and repeated exposure to ionizing radiation, ultrasonography is currently the preferred screening imaging test. Optimal frequency of screening in at-risk populations is not defined by data from randomized, controlled trials. Experts recommend a frequency of no less often than yearly; some suggest intervals of every month.

Nodules are often described in cirrhotic patients without cancer. Most small nodules represent regenerative nodules, some hemangiomas, and other benign growths. Nodules smaller than 1 cm should be followed up with ultrasound at intervals of between 3 and 6 months; if after 2 years the lesion is stable, reversion to routine screening is recommended. When a lesion is 1 to 2 cm in size, further evaluation with either CT or MRI should be considered.

Serum-based tests are quite disappointing as a sole screening tool. AFP is the most commonly used serum marker. The upper limit of normal is typically 10 ng/mL. Values over 200 require further study,

Table 1 Liver Cancers

Disease	Relative Risk	Risk Factors
Primary Cancers of the Liver		
Hepatocellular	Common	Cirrhosis, chronic viral hepatitis, iron overload, aflatoxin exposure
Cholangiocarcinoma	Common	Primary sclerosing cholangitis, liver fluke infection, biliary stone disease, choledochal cyst; possibly hepatitis B and C
Hepatoblastoma	Uncommon	Childhood (<age 4 years)
Fibrolamelllar	Rare	Unknown
Angiosarcoma	Rare	Thorotrast; polyvinyl chloride exposure
Metastatic Cancer to Liver		
Lung	Common	
Colon	Common	
Breast	Common	
Pancreas	Common	
Gastric	Common	
Lymphoma	Common	
Melanoma	Late stage	
Prostate	Late stage	
Ovarian	Late Stage	
Others		

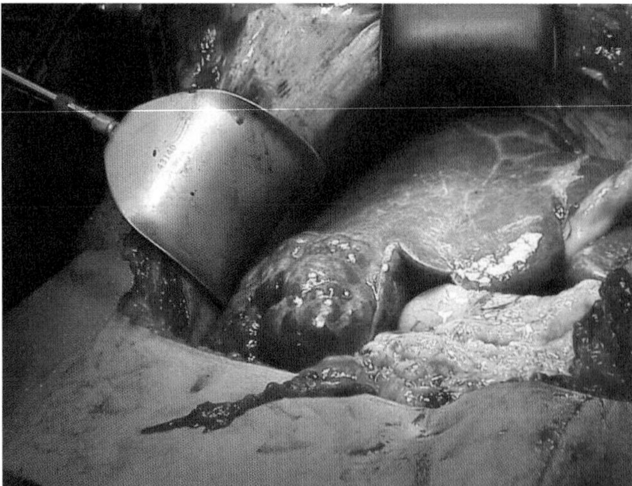

Figure 1 Operating room demonstration of a noncirrhotic liver with a large hepatocellular carcinoma involving the right lobe *(arrow)*. *(Courtesy of Pierre Gholam, MD, University Hospital, Cleveland, Ohio.)*

Table 2 Worldwide Incidence and Mortality of Hepatocellular Cancer

Location	Incidence	Mortality
Worldwide	564,000	548,000
More-developed countries	107,000	106,000
Less-developed countries	457,000	442,000
North America	13,000	12,000

Source: World Health Organization, 2001. Cited in Parkin DM, Bray F, Ferlay J, and Pisani P. CA Cancer J Clin 2005;55:74-108.

Box 1 Surveillance for Hepatocellular Carcinoma

Hepatitis B carriers who meet one or more of the following criteria:

- Asian men 40 years or older
- Asian women 50 years or older
- Cirrhosis
- Family history of HCC
- Africans older than 20 years
- High HBV viral load
- Current or past severe inflammatory liver disease

Non–hepatitis B cirrhosis due to:

- Hepatitis C
- Alcohol
- Primary biliary cirrhosis
- α_1-Antitrypsin deficiency
- Nonalcoholic steatohepatitis
- Autoimmune hepatitis
- Iron overload

Bruix J, Sherman M: Management of hepatocellular carcinoma. Hepatology 2005;42:1208-1236.

and values over 400 in a adult are almost certainly caused by HCC. In most cases of HCC, the AFP levels are normal or only slightly elevated. In addition, patients with chronic viral hepatitis B or C often have AFP levels of up to 100 without evidence of identifiable HCC. The sensitivity and specificity of AFP in detecting measurable HCC is low. Specificity is very high when the AFP value is greater than 400 ng/mL.

Some circulating AFP is in a glycosolated form. Measurement of glycosolated AFP as a percentage of total AFP has been reported to add specificity to AFP. Anotherr protein, DCP (des-γ-carboxy prothrombin, also known as PIVKA-II) might also serve as a serum marker for HCC. The clinical utility of adding these tests to an HCC screening program has not yet been clearly demonstrated.

TREATMENT

In patients with chronic liver disease and portal hypertension, the most effective treatment for HCC confined to the liver in the absence of major vascular invasion is liver transplantation. However, due to organ donor shortage, this approach to HCC has been limited. As a result, surgical resection and locoregional therapies such as radiofrequency ablation (RFA) and transarterial chemoembolization (TACE) have been used to treat and prevent tumor progression in selected cases.

A whole new body of knowledge is being developed regarding HCC biology. Biological tumor features that allow prediction of recurrence or response to treatment permit better patient and treatment selections. New developing molecular targeted therapies will serve as part of the neoadjuvant and adjuvant options to achieve a more comprehensive approach to this complex disease.

Liver Transplantation

Liver transplantation is the treatment of choice for HCC in patients with decompensated cirrhosis, achieving 75% recurrence-free survival at 5 years in the absence of lymphovascular invasion.[6-9]

The early experience with liver transplantation for HCC was discouraging because only patients with extensive tumors were considered to undergo this therapy. However, patients undergoing liver transplantation for other indications who were found to have incidental HCC exhibited promising survival rates. Subsequently, in 1996 Mazzaferro introduced the Milan criteria—a single tumor of 5 cm or up to 3 tumors of 3 cm in size—and showed an 83% recurrence-free survival and 75% actuarial survival at 4 years for patients undergoing liver transplantation meeting these criteria.[10] Currently, patients with HCC meeting the Milan criteria are being given priority for cadaveric donor liver transplantation. As a result, a rising number of patients with cirrhosis and early HCC undergo liver transplantation, accounting for a third of the total liver transplant operations.

In 2001, Yao introduced the University of California at San Francisco (UCSF) criteria showing that patients with a single lesion of 6.5 cm or up to 3 lesions with none larger than 4.5 cm and a total tumor burden less than 8 cm exhibited patient survival of 90% and 75.2% at 1 and 5 years, respectively.[11] Patients with tumors beyond these criteria had 50% 1-year survival. Based on these observations, priority for receiving a donor liver can be obtained for those with tumor burden meeting these criteria. Living donor liver transplantation (LDLT) is an alternative source of liver grafts that has been used to treat patients with end-stage liver disease and HCC.

Locoregional therapies such as RFA and TACE have been implemented to control tumor progression and prevent patient drop-out from the waiting transplant list. The role of these therapies, however, has turned out to be more cost effective in patients with expected waiting time longer than 6 months.

Tumor recurrence rates after liver transplantation in patients within Milan and UCSF criteria ranges between 10% and 15%. Vascular invasion and poor tumor differentiation have been identified as the main risk factors for HCC recurrence. Particularly in the absence of vascular invasion, it seems that the number and size of tumors should not affect patient survival. Vascular invasion is a consequence of aggressive tumor biology. Unfortunately, pretransplant indicators of microvascular invasion remain undiscovered.

Several tumor biological factors such as DNA aneuploidy, high tumor cell proliferation index, high telomerase activity, and mutation of the *p53* gene have been associated with increased risk of postoperative HCC recurrence. However, the prognostic impact of these factors remains uncertain due to a limited number of studies and conflicting data.

There has been growing interest in the study of gene expression profile in relation to prognosis of HCC patients. The copy DNA microarray is a modern technology that allows analysis of thousands of genes simultaneously using gene chips. Several studies have identified gene expression profiles predictive of the recurrence or prognosis of HCC patients.

In a study from the University of Pittsburgh, Marsh and colleagues found that patients with low HCC rates of mutation in critical tumor suppressor genes had lower tumor recurrence rate after liver transplantation, even in the presence of microvascular invasion. Larger studies are needed to confirm these associations, but given the absence of serum markers that can predict tumor behavior, pretransplant HCC biopsy might become a routine practice to assess HCC biology.

Hepatic Resection

Liver resection for HCC is the treatment of choice in noncirrhotic patients. However, unfortunately this option is feasible in only 5% of the cases in Western countries and in 40% of the cases in Asia. Surgical resection is primarily indicated for patients with unifocal HCC not associated with underlying chronic liver dysfunction or for early-stage disease with well-compensated cirrhosis. Determination of tumor extension and liver function are the cornerstone steps to define tumor respectability.

Although noncirrhotic patients tolerate major resections with low morbidity, patients with advanced cirrhosis and portal hypertension are at risk of developing hepatic failure, bleeding, ascites and infection.

Clinical features such as Child A cirrhosis along with platelet count of 100,000/mm^3 and hepatic vein pressure gradient less than 10 mm Hg have been associated with good tolerance to resection, with 5-year survival rate of 70%. However, because of underlying chronic disease in most cases, between 60% and 100% of patients develop HCC recurrence after resection and require additional treatment such as re-resection, ablation, or liver transplantation.

Improvement in surgical technique and patient selection made the perioperative mortality for hepatic resection drop from 10% to 30% to less than 1%. With good surgical technique, blood transfusion during surgical resection may be required in less than 10% of patients. The overall morbidity is between 20% and 50% (pleural effusion, perihepatic abscess, ileus, bile leak, wound infection, deep vein thrombosis, urinary tract infection), and its reduction depends on implementing parenchyma-sparing resections and decreased intraoperative blood loss.

In a large study with case matching by tumor stage and degree of cirrhosis and liver dysfunction, overall 5-year survival rates were similar for patients with HCC treated by liver transplantation or resection, but transplantation provided a clear advantage over resection in terms of recurrence-free survival at 5 years (54% vs 14%, $P < 0.0001$). Long-term outcomes support the use of primary resection in patients with Child A cirrhosis with small unifocal tumors. Multifocal tumors are associated with higher risk of recurrence after resection and are best approached by primary liver transplantation.

Locoregional Therapies

Patients with nonresectable HCC have exhibited survival benefit when treated with radiofrequency ablation (RFA) and transarterial chemoembolization (TACE). Recent studies demonstrated that RFA and TACE had similar efficacy compared to surgery when used to treat small tumors. Refined technique and improvements in technology will continue to expand the indications of these modalities for unresectable HCC, patients waiting for liver transplantation, in need of tumor downstaging, or needing control of progression. The potential combination options of such therapies with resection, or systemic antineoplastic agents such as sorafenib and others, are expected to improve patient outcome, although time is needed to draw this conclusion.

Radiofrequency Ablation

By generating temperatures higher than 60° C with alternating current (±500 kHz) between a radiofrequency probe and grounding pads on the patient's lower extremities, tumor coagulative necrosis is induced when inserting the probe into the tumor substance.

The efficacy of RFA depends on appropriate technical use and size of tumor. Lesions of 3 cm can be effectively treated, achieving complete tumor necrosis in 80% to 90% of cases. However, for lesions of 5 cm, complete tumor necrosis is unlikely, and tumor recurrence is expected in more than 50% of cases.

Tumor location is another important factor to determine treatment efficacy and safety. Lesions adjacent to large vessels might have a worse treatment response due to the thermal protection provided by the contiguous blood flow. Lesions located near the liver hilum should be avoided due to the risk of vascular and bile duct injuries.

Peripheral lesions should also be avoided due to the risk of needle tract tumor dissemination. Overall, the morbidity risk associated with RFA is about 5% to 10%, which includes injury to adjacent anatomic structures, liver failure, hemorrhage, abscess formation, intercostal nerve injury, tumor lysis syndrome, and pneumothorax. The mortality risk has been reported as less than 1%. To reduce the morbidity risk, laparoscopic RFA is a suitable approach when indicated.

Patient survival with unresectable HCC treated with RFA has been reported as 75% to 92% at 1 year, 37% to 59% at 3 years, and 28% at 5 years. In the case of resectable small tumors, RFA has been associated with similar survival rates when compared with resection in selected cases.[12]

Due to technologic improvement and potential association with other locoregional therapies such as TACE, RFA will continue to be a promising tool to approach HCC.

Transarterial Chemoembolization

Selective HCC arterial catheterization followed by the sequential infusion of chemotherapy and embolization particles are the principles of TACE.

Several studies established the efficacy of TACE in treating unresectable HCC. A randomized, controlled trial showed that the 1, 2, and 3-year survival rates were 57%, 31%, and 26% in the treatment group versus 32%, 11%, and 3% in the control group ($P = 0.002$). In a systematic review of randomized trials for unresectable HCC, TACE was shown to improve patient 2-year survival compared to control groups ($P = 0.017$). In addition, a meta-analysis concluded that TACE reduced the 2-year mortality rate compared with control groups ($P = 0.015$).[13]

The role of TACE as a bridging therapy to transplantation has been reported, and conflicting data were observed. The efficacy of TACE in controlling tumor progression and down-staging in patients in the waiting list is accepted, but no conclusive survival benefit has been identified. The current consensus opinion recognizes the benefit of TACE in liver transplant candidates with waiting time longer than 6 months.

The risks associated with TACE for unresectable HCC include death (5%-10% in Child C cirrhotic patients), liver failure (5%-10% in Child C patients), upper gastrointestinal bleeding, abscess formation (30%-80% when the sphincter of Oddi is compromised), encephalopathy, nontarget embolization, tumor lysis syndrome, pulmonary embolism, and acute renal failure. The postchemoembolization syndrome is the most common side effect of TACE. Patients develop abdominal pain, nausea, and fever, which are self-limited in most cases and well controlled with hydration and with pain and antinausea medications.

TACE can be safely used in the absence of portal vein thrombosis and severe liver dysfunction.

Combined Transarterial Chemoembolization and Radiofrequency Ablation

Recent studies have reported improved patient survival when TACE and RFA were implemented in a combined approach to treat HCC larger than 3 cm compared with either RFA or TACE alone. In a randomized, controlled trial including 291 patients with HCC larger than 3 cm, the 1-, 3-, and 5-year survival rates for lesions of 5 cm were superior for TACE followed by RFA over either treatment alone. Further experience is needed to confirm these observations.[14]

Yttrium-90 Microspheres

Selective transarterial radiotherapy able to deliver up to 150 Gy of beta-emitting radiation has been introduced to treat unresectable HCC showing encouraging tumor response. Approximately 50% of patients experience 50% tumor reduction, with a median time to maximum response of 120 days.

Yttrium-90 microspheres (TheraSphere) have been used as a bridge to transplantation to control tumor progression and for downstaging. Also, the capability of this technique to induce tumor burden shrinkage allowed subsequent treatments with surgical resection and RFA.

An important advantage of this technique is that because hepatic artery occlusion is not induced, patients with portal vein thrombosis can be treated safely and in several courses.

Larger clinical experience is needed to provide information regarding the survival benefit of this modality combined with other treatment options such as surgical resection, RFA, TACE, and sorafenib.

Systemic Chemotherapy

There is no evidence that systemic chemotherapy improves overall survival in any subset of HCC patients. The most commonly used agent has been doxorubicin, as a single agent or in combination with other drugs. In all cases, the survival benefit was on the order of weeks. Main drawbacks of conventional cytotoxic chemotherapy have been side effects poorly tolerated in patients with chronic liver dysfunction, as well as HCC intrinsic chemoresistence and advanced stages of HCC at the time of presentation.

Molecular-Targeted Therapies

Several molecular targets, including oncogenes, oncoproteins, and cellular receptors have been identified as key elements in carcinogenic pathways. Many therapeutic agents designed to tackle these targets are currently under evaluation through several clinical trials. In the near future valuable information regarding the efficacy of these new agents will be available, and their potential role as neoadjuvant or adjuvant actors in combination with locoregional therapies or liver transplantation will have to be determined.

Sorafenib (Nexavar), an oral multikinase inhibitor that inhibits Raf serine/threonine kinases and receptor tyrosine kinases, has been approved by the U.S. Food and Drug Administration (FDA) to treat patients with Child A cirrhosis and unresectable HCC.

In an international phase III study, patients with unresectable HCC treated with sorafenib survived 10.7 months versus 7.9 months in the placebo group ($P < 0.001$). Time to cancer progression was also significantly longer in the treatment group: 5.5 versus 2.8 months.

Current trials are evaluating the efficacy of sorafenib and other oral antiangiogenic agents as neoadjuvant and adjuvant therapies to locoregional approaches such as RFA, TACE, yttrium-90 microspheres, and surgical resection. Studies are needed to assess the efficacy of these agents to prevent HCC recurrence after liver transplantation, but interactions with immunosuppression drugs are a matter of concern and safety administration in that scenario is to be determined.

PREVENTION

The most effective strategies to reduce HCC disease burden is to eliminate the precursor disease states. Immunization against hepatitis B has resulted in a sharp decline in HCC. Treatment of chronic hepatitis B and C have similarly been shown to decrease HCC. Effective public health measures related to environmental toxins and control of aflatoxin in food supplies reduce HCC rates. Reduction of high-risk behavior resulting in cirrhosis can also be expected to reduce HCC.

Summary

- HCC is one of the most prevalent cancers in the world. It is predominantly a hig- risk cancer in underdeveloped portions of the world. Although the incidence remains relatively low in the United States, unlike many major cancers, the incidence of HCC has doubled in the in the past 20 years.
- Small HCC produces no symptoms. Discovery of HCC when symptoms are present has little value for the patient. Surveillance by imaging studies and alpha feotprotein provides the best opportunity to discover small, treatable lesions. Those at high risk, especially those with cirrhosis, should be screened twice a year.
- In patients with chronic liver disease and portal hypertension, the most effective treatment for HCC confined to the liver in the absence of major vascular invasion is liver transplantation. Surgical resection and locoregional therapies such as RFA and TACE have been used to treat and prevent tumor progression in selected cases, including patients awaiting liver transplantation.
- Sorafenib (Nexavar), an oral multikinase inhibitor that inhibits Raf serine/threonine kinases and receptor tyrosine kinases, has been approved by the FDA to treat patients with Child A cirrhosis and unresectable HCC. This costly medicine extends life expectancy by a nearly 3 months.
- The most effective strategy to reduce HCC disease burden is to eliminate the precursor disease states. Immunization against hepatitis B and treatment of chronic hepatitis B and C decrease HCC. Effective public health measures related to environmental toxins and control of aflatoxin reduce HCC rates. Reduction of high-risk behavior resulting in cirrhosis may also be expected to reduce HCC.

Suggested Readings

Bruix J, Sherman M: Management of hepatocellular carcinoma. Hepatology 2005;42:1208-1236.

Cheng BQ, Jia CQ, Liu CT, et al: Chemoembolization combined with radiofrequency ablation for patients with hepatocellular carcinoma larger than 3 cm. JAMA 2008;299:1670-1677.

Davila JA, Morgan R, Di, XL, et al: Utilization of screening for hepatocellular carcinoman in the United States. Gastroenterology 2008;134(suppl):A-769.

Georgiades Ch S, Hong K, Geschwind JF: Radiofrequency ablation and chemoembolization for hepatocellular carcinoma. Cancer J 2008;14:117-122.

Ibrahim SM, Lewandowski RJ, Sato KT, et al: Radioembolization for the treatment of unresectable hepatocellular carcinoma: a clinical review. World J Gastroenterol 2008;14:1664-1669.

Kulik LM, Atassi B, Van Holsbeeck L, et al: Yttrium-90 microspheres (TheraSphere) treatment of unresectable hepatocellular carcinoma: Downstaging to resection, RFA and bridge to transplantation. J Surg Oncol 2006;94:572-586.

Llovet JM, Bruix J: Systematic review of randomized trials for unresectable hepatocellular carcinoma: Chemoembolization improves survival. Hepatology 2003;37:429-442.

Mazzaferro V, Chun YS, Poon RT, et al: Liver transplantation for hepatocellular carcinoma. Ann Surg Oncol 2008;15:1001-1007.

Zhu AX: Development of sorafenib and other molecularly targeted agents in hepatocellular carcinoma. Cancer 2008;15:250-259.

References

For a complete list of references, log onto www.expertconsult.com.

Head and Neck Cancer

Cristina P. Rodriguez and David J. Adelstein

DEFINITION AND ETIOLOGY

This chapter reviews squamous cell carcinomas of the head and neck. These are the malignancies arising from the mucosal lining of the oral cavity, oropharynx, nasopharynx, hypopharynx, and larynx. Although there are also a diverse group of tumors that arise from other structures of the head and neck, including the salivary glands, sinuses, thyroid and skin, these primary cancers do not share a similar natural history and should be considered separately.

PREVALENCE AND RISK FACTORS

In 2008 in the United States head and neck cancer was diagnosed in an estimated 35,000 persons, accounting for 3% of all new malignancies. Worldwide, approximately 500,000 new cases are diagnosed annually. Males are at higher risk for developing this disease. In the United States, there are significant racial and socioeconomic disparities in disease incidence. In particular, African Americans have a higher incidence, more-advanced disease at presentation, and greater mortality when compared to whites. Tobacco and alcohol are the most strongly implicated etiologic agents. Occupational exposures to inhaled organic dusts, gases, and asbestos in the construction and mining industries are additional risk factors.

Primary cancers of the nasopharynx are distinct among head and neck cancers in etiology and in racial and geographic distribution. This cancer is endemic to southern China, Southeast Asia and northern Africa, and its association with tobacco and alcohol is weak. Its pathogenesis is thought to involve exposure to unrelated carcinogens, such as nitrosamines from consumption of salted fish in endemic areas. However, there is increasing evidence supporting the oncogenic role of viruses infecting the upper aerodigestive tract. A very strong association between Epstein-Barr virus (EBV) infection and endemic nasopharyngeal cancer has been established. Malignant cells harbor clonal EBV DNA, and antibody titers to EBV are directly related to tumor bulk, stage at presentation, and risk of recurrence.

Since the 1980s, an overall decline in diagnoses of new head and neck cancers has been observed and attributed to public health efforts against tobacco use. The exception to this is oropharyngeal squamous cell carcinoma, which has risen in incidence in the same time frame and has appeared in a younger, nonsmoking population. High-risk human papillomavirus (HPV) subtypes have been identified in a significant fraction of these tumors, including HPV 16, 18, 31, and 33. Greater numbers of sexual partners, early age of first sexual intercourse, and high-risk sexual behavior are emerging as risk factors for HPV-related disease independent of tobacco and alcohol abuse.

PATHOLOGY AND NATURAL HISTORY

Malignant transformation of the involved epithelium is a culmination of constant exposure to carcinogens and an accumulation of genetic alterations. Molecular aberrations have been identified in premalignant lesions of the oral mucosa, which increase in number as lesions progress toward malignancy. Loss of heterozygosity at 9p21 is thought to be an early event, identified in hyperplastic lesions. Mutations in the tumor-suppressor genes *p53* and *Rb* are common in tobacco-related premalignant and malignant lesions. Most HPV-related oropharyngeal head and neck cancers carry wild-type *Rb* and *p53*. Evidence now supports the role of the viral oncoproteins E6 and E7 in the development of malignancy through inactivation of *p53* and *Rb* gene products.

Head and neck squamous cell carcinomas are classified as well, moderately well, or poorly differentiated according to the degree by which their histologic appearance deviates from the normal squamous epithelium. Poorly differentiated carcinomas have little evidence of keratinization, have a more-aggressive clinical behavior, and carry a poorer prognosis. The World Health Organization (WHO) classifies nasopharyngeal carcinomas using a similar principle. Undifferentiated tumors (WHO III) are almost always of the endemic variety and EBV DNA positive. This type is often characterized by a dense lymphocytic infiltrate, hence the term *lymphoepithelioma* previously used to refer to this subtype. The differentiated tumors are divided into keratinizing (WHO I) and nonkeratinizing (WHO II) types. These are less commonly EBV positive and are more prevalent in nonendemic regions.

Head and neck cancer spreads from the primary sites to the draining lymph nodes followed, only late in its natural history, by hematogenous dissemination. Among the different subsites, nasopharyngeal cancer has a more aggressive clinical course and carries the highest risk of systemic involvement at presentation. TNM (tumor, node, metastasis) staging using the 2002 AJCC system correlates with survival outcomes. Approximately 30% of patients present with stage I or II disease, considered early-stage resectable disease. These patients have small primary site lesions and no lymph node disease (T1-2, N0). Another 60% have stage III to IVB cancers, characterized by advanced primary site tumors (T3-4), early or by advanced nodal spread (N1-3) but no with distant hematogenous metastases. Although these cancers are locoregionally advanced, and sometimes unresectable, they are still curable in a significant percentage of patients. Metastatic disease (stage IVC) at presentation is uncommon and incurable. Less than 10% of patients have disseminated disease when it is newly diagnosed.

The association of head and neck cancers with tobacco and alcohol has several implications and has led to the concept of *field cancerization,* wherein the entire exposed aerodigestive tract epithelium is at risk for developing malignancy. Synchronous and metachronous primary cancers of the head and neck and of the lung and esophagus are common. Patients with a prior history of head and neck cancer have a 5% to 7% annual risk of developing a second primary cancer. In addition, tobacco-related cardiac, pulmonary, and vascular comorbidities are significant issues influencing management and mortality.

SIGNS AND SYMPTOMS

The presenting symptoms of head and neck cancer can relate to local effects of the primary tumor, regional spread, metastatic disease, or paraneoplastic phenomena.

Symptoms resulting from local disease vary according to the primary tumor site. Oral cavity, oropharynx, or hypopharynx tumors can result in painful oral mucosal tumors or ulcerations, dysphagia, or odynophagia. Cancers arising from the larynx often cause hoarseness or voice changes. Nasopharyngeal cancer usually arises in the fossae of Rosenmüller, adjacent to the eustachian tube orifices and the base of the skull. Epistaxis, recurrent middle ear effusions, or cranial nerve palsies are common presenting symptoms.

A painless enlarged cervical lymph node may be the only presenting symptom. HPV-related oropharyngeal lesions have been associated with cystic lymph node involvement. The location of lymph node involvement may be helpful in identifying the primary site. Nasopharyngeal primaries are the most common subtype to involve the posterior cervical lymph node chain. The palatine tonsils, nasopharynx, and supraglottis are embedded in a rich lymphatic plexus that drains to both sides of the neck, and these cancers often involve the anterior upper cervical lymph nodes (levels II and III). Oral cavity lesions often spread to the submental and submandibular nodes.

Metastatic head and neck cancer most often involves the lung. Bone and liver involvement is much less common. The squamous cell histology of this disease is also associated with certain paraneoplastic phenomena. These can become evident in advanced disease stages, most commonly hypercalcemia resulting from elaboration of a parathyroid hormone–like peptide. Nasopharyngeal cancer has been associated with leukemoid reactions and paraneoplastic motor neuropathies.

DIAGNOSIS

The diagnosis is often arrived at by a biopsy from the primary site. Evaluation must include a thorough examination of the upper aerodigestive tract, usually under anesthesia, to identify synchronous primary lesions, carefully delineate the extent of the primary tumor, and palpate for cervical lymph nodes. The positron emission tomography (PET) scan, when combined with computed tomography (CT) imaging, may be useful in detecting occult lymph node involvement and metastatic disease.

In the situation where a cervical lymph node is positive without an apparent primary site, a meticulous examination under anesthesia might reveal the primary tumor. If a primary site is not evident by visual inspection or palpation, random biopsies of the nasopharynx, base of tongue, hypopharynx, and an ipsilateral tonsillectomy are often performed. These areas are the most common occult primary sites.

TREATMENT

The treatment of head and neck cancer requires a multispecialty approach coordinated among surgeons, radiation oncologists, and medical oncologists. Surgery and radiation are the only definitive treatment modalities for both early and locally advanced disease. Adequate oncologic surgical resection, wherein the tumor is completely removed with uninvolved resection margins, is often challenging in the head and neck and can involve sacrificing critical structures including the larynx, eye, or mandible. Radiation, when used as definitive therapy, circumvents this difficulty, but it results in significant acute and late toxicity. Chemotherapy alone is not a curative therapeutic modality, but it has been shown to improve outcomes when used in conjunction with radiation for locally advanced disease.

Early Stage Disease

Single-modality surgery or radiation are options for curative-intent treatment in early stage head and neck cancers. Cure rates using either intervention for stage I disease often exceed 90%, but this decreases to approximately 70% for stage II disease. The choice between surgery or radiation is influenced by the location of the primary site, side-effect profile, comorbidity, and institutional experience. Oral cavity lesions of the mobile tongue or floor of mouth, for example, are amenable to surgical resection and reconstruction with acceptable cosmetic and functional results. Radiation therapy, on the other hand, produces a long-term risk of xerostomia and mandibular osteonecrosis. More-limited surgical techniques have been developed and have produced excellent oncologic and functional outcomes in appropriately selected patients with limited primary tumors. The partial laryngectomy and the endoscopic laser resections for T1 or T2 glottic tumors are good examples.

The decision to treat clinically uninvolved cervical lymph nodes with either surgery or radiation is controversial. The rates of occult lymph node metastases in node-negative T1 and T2 tumors varies according to the location of the primary tumor and ranges between 6% and 46%. The estimated risk of occult neck node involvement is used to guide this decision. Early glottic primary tumors have a low rate of occult lymph node involvement due to the paucity of lymphatics in the vocal cords, making it a subsite ideal for local treatment alone. In contrast, at least 20% of clinically N0 supraglottic cancers and a majority of nasopharyngeal primaries have occult lymph node metastases. Treatment of the neck is considered standard for these subsites. Promising reports have emerged about the role of sentinel cervical lymph node biopsy, a procedure under continued investigation.

Locoregionally Advanced Disease

For patients with locoregionally advanced stage III to IV lesions, the historical results with surgery and postoperative radiation have been suboptimal, with reported cure rates ranging from 10% to 50% and with locoregional failure predominating. Early chemotherapy experience using drugs such as methotrexate, 5-fluorouracil, and the platins (cisplatin and carboplatin) suggested significant antitumor efficacy. Response rates as high as 90%, with complete responses in up to 30% of patients, were reported in patients with previously untreated tumors, suggesting that chemotherapy might have a role in the definitive management of this disease. The landmark Veterans Administration Laryngeal Cancer Study Group (VALCSG) trial, reported in 1991, randomized patients with locally advanced larynx cancer to standard treatment with a laryngectomy followed by radiation or to induction chemotherapy using cisplatin and 5-fluorouracil followed by radiation in chemotherapy responders. Survival proved equivalent in both arms, and 64% of patients randomized to induction chemotherapy arm did not require laryngectomy.

The second-generation larynx preservation trial, Radiation Therapy Oncology Group (RTOG) 91-11, sought to determine whether chemotherapy worked in conjunction with radiation to effect organ preservation or if it merely selected patients with better-prognosis disease for nonoperative management. Patients with locally advanced laryngeal cancer were randomized to radiation alone, induction chemotherapy followed by radiation (as in the VALCSG trial), and chemotherapy with single-agent cisplatin given concurrently with radiation. Overall survival was similar in all three groups, and distant metastases were significantly reduced in patients receiving chemotherapy. Organ preservation and locoregional control rates were superior in the concurrent chemotherapy and radiation arm. Disease-free survival and laryngectomy-free survival were improved in the induction and concurrent chemotherapy arms when compared to radiation alone, and no differences in these outcomes were noted between the two chemotherapy-containing arms.

Similar results emerged from a cooperative group study of 295 patients with unresectable stage III and IV head and neck cancer randomized among three arms: radiation alone, radiation with concurrent cisplatin, and split-course radiation concurrent with cisplatin and 5-fluorouracil. Overall and disease-free survival were improved in the radiation and concurrent cisplatin arm, establishing this treatment regimen as the standard of care for locally advanced unresectable head and neck cancer.

The success of concurrent chemotherapy and radiation has also been demonstrated in nasopharyngeal cancer, a disease subsite rarely amenable to surgical resection. The Intergroup 00-99 study randomized 147 patients with locally advanced nasopharyngeal cancer (both endemic and nonendemic), to radiation alone, or to radiation concurrent with cisplatin chemotherapy followed by three cycles of adjuvant chemotherapy with cisplatin and 5-flurururacil. A significant overall survival advantage was noted in the experimental arm, leading to the study's early termination and the adoption of this regimen as the treatment standard for locally advanced nasopharyngeal carcinoma in the United States. The benefit of adding adjuvant chemotherapy has been questioned by many in the Asian oncology community, who have demonstrated similar survival outcomes in patients with endemic nasopharyngeal cancer treated with concurrent chemoradiotherapy alone without additional chemotherapy.

Although concurrent chemoradiotherapy approaches significantly improved survival endpoints, the toxicity resulting from this treatment is quite significant. In the RTOG 91-11 trial, Grade 3 and 4 toxicity was experienced by 77% of the patients on the concurrent treatment arm, compared to 47% of those treated with radiation alone. Twenty-three percent of the concurrently treated patients continued to experience difficulty in swallowing 1 year after treatment was completed. Given the significant comorbidity found in the population affected by this disease, concurrent chemotherapy and radiation might not be feasible for all, underscoring the need to tailor treatment options to the individual patient.

Head and neck cancers often overexpress the epidermal growth factor receptor (EGFr). Cetuximab is a monoclonal antibody that competitively inhibits ligand binding to the EGFr receptor. In a randomized trial of 424 stage III and IV head and neck cancer patients comparing radiation alone to radiation with concurrent cetuximab, a significant difference in overall survival and locoregional control favoring the cetuximab and radiation arm was observed. The subgroup that seemed to benefit most from this treatment were patients with oropharyngeal primary tumors. More importantly, the only toxicity found to be significantly worse in the cetuximab and radiation arm was an acneiform rash.

The detrimental impact of smoking among patients with this disease extends beyond its role as an etiologic agent. Continued smoking during treatment has been associated with adverse treatment outcomes. A study of 115 patients undergoing radiation or radiation with chemotherapy for head and neck cancer found inferior complete response and 2-year overall survival rates in patients who reported that they continued smoking during treatment. This has been attributed to various factors, including nicotine-drug interactions, which might diminish the efficacy of chemotherapy; hypoxemia leading to reduced radiation-induced formation of free radicals; and patient comorbidity, which might limit the patient's ability to complete radiation therapy.

With the improvement in locoregional control and survival from the adoption of concurrent chemotherapy and radiation for locally advanced disease, the pattern of disease failure appears to have changed, and distant metastasis is now emerging as the most common reason for failure. The use of induction chemotherapy before concurrent chemoradiation to decrease the rate of distant metastasis is now under active study.

Metastatic Disease

No curative options exist for metastatic head and neck cancer. Median survival ranges from 5 to 9 months. In patients with distant metastasis, the goal of therapy is palliation of symptoms. A multitude of chemotherapeutic agents and targeted treatments have produced responses. These increase with the use of combination chemotherapy but at the cost of incremental toxicity. Randomized data suggesting the superiority of a particular regimen are scarce. EGFr inhibitors, when used alone, result in response rates of up to 10%, with disease stability in almost half of the patients treated. A study has compared cisplatin and 5-fluorouracil to the same regimen with cetuximab in 442 patients with metastatic disease or locally advanced disease not amenable to local therapy. A modest but significant overall survival advantage was noted in the chemotherapy and cetuximab group, which had a median survival of 10 months, compared to 7 months in the chemotherapy alone group.

Summary

Early-Stage Disease (Stage I-II)

- Surgery or radiation alone results in cure for the majority of patients.
- The choice of treatment modality should be made according to tumor characteristics, patient comorbidity, toxicity profile, and institutional experience.
- Locally Advanced Disease (Stage II-IVA and B).
- Surgery or radiation alone is often unsuccessful.
- Concurrent chemotherapy and radiation improves locoregional control, overall survival. and the risk of distant metastasis. It also can allow organ preservation in larynx and other head and neck cancer subtypes.

Metastatic Disease (Stage IVC)

- Palliation of symptoms is the primary goal of care.
- Chemotherapy combinations result in higher response rates with incremental toxicity.

Suggested Readings

Adelstein DJ, Li Y, Adams GL, et al: An intergroup phase III comparison of standard radiation therapy and two schedules of concurrent chemoradiotherapy in patients with unresectable squamous cell head and neck cancer. J Clin Oncol 2003;21:92-98.

American Society of Clinical Oncology; Pfister DG, Laurie SA, Weinstein GS, et al: American Society of Clinical Oncology clinical practice guideline for the use of larynx-preservation strategies in the treatment of laryngeal cancer. J Clin Oncol 2006;24:3693-3704.

Bonner JA, Harari PM, Giralt J, et al: Radiotherapy plus cetuximab for squamous-cell carcinoma of the head and neck. N Engl J Med 2006;354:567-578.

Browman GP, Wong G, Hodson I, et al: Influence of cigarette smoking on the efficacy of radiation therapy in head and neck cancer. N Engl J Med 1993;328:159-163.

Department of Veterans Affairs Laryngeal Cancer Study Group: Induction chemotherapy plus radiation compared with surgery plus radiation in patients with advanced laryngeal cancer. N Engl J Med 1991;324:1685-1690.

D'Souza G, Kreimer AR, Viscidi R, et al: Case-control study of human papillomavirus and oropharyngeal cancer. N Engl J Med 2007;356:1944-1956.

Forastiere AA, Goepfert H, Maor M, et al: Concurrent chemotherapy and radiotherapy for organ preservation in advanced laryngeal cancer. N Engl J Med 2003;349:2091-2098.

Brain Tumors: Meningiomas and Gliomas

Glen H.J. Stevens

Primary brain tumors are tumors that arise from brain tissue itself as compared with metastatic tumors, whereby tumor cells travel to the brain from a distant site. This chapter deals specifically with primary brain tumors of adults, using the subcategories of benign tumors—meningiomas, realizing that a small subset can be malignant—and malignant gliomas (oligodendrogliomas and astrocytomas).

DEFINITION

Benign Tumors

In 1922, Cushing coined the term *meningioma* to describe tumors originating from the meninges.[1] The World Health Organization (WHO) has now subdivided meningiomas into three separate categories defined as benign (I), atypical (II), and anaplastic or malignant (III) (Table 1).[2]

Malignant Tumors

Oligodendrogliomas are composed of diffusely infiltrating cells resembling oligodendrocytes with aggressive growth potential. WHO has stratified oligodendrogliomas as well-differentiated tumors (II) and anaplastic oligodendrogliomas (III).[2]

Astrocytic neoplasms are characterized by varying degrees of brain infiltration and aggressive growth potential. WHO has stratified astrocytomas as diffuse astrocytoma (II), anaplastic astrocytoma (III), and glioblastoma multiforme (IV).[2] For our purposes here, grade I tumors actually represent a separate tumor genotype and phenotype and are not discussed.

PREVALENCE

The Cancer Brain Tumor Registry of the United States (CBTRUS) was formed in 1992 through the American Brain Tumor Association as a resource for epidemiologic data on primary brain tumors (http://www.cbtrus.org). There are currently eleven state registries involved in data collection. Primary brain tumors represent only 2% of all cancers, with 35,000 new cases diagnosed each year in the United States. Meningiomas occur at a rate of 7.8 per 100,000 per year, but only 25% are believed to be symptomatic, with the others being found incidentally.[3] The male-to-female ratio is 1 : 1.8, and the incidence increases with age, peaking at age 85 years.

According to CBTRUS, the incidence of oligodendrogliomas, including anaplastic oligodendrogliomas, is approximately 0.3 per 100,000 persons. Depending on the study, these tumors account for 4% to 15% of intracranial gliomas.

The most commonly diagnosed primary brain tumor of adults is glioblastoma multiforme (grade IV). The incidence is two to three cases per 100,000 population per year. An estimated 13,000 deaths in 2000 were attributed to primary malignant brain tumors (PMBTs). Approximately 19,500 cases were expected to be diagnosed in 2000. Diffuse astrocytomas (WHO II) represent 10% to 15% of astrocytic brain tumors and have an incidence of 1.4 cases per 1 million population per year.

PATHOPHYSIOLOGY

Only about 5% of primary brain tumors have known hereditary factors. Specifically, the Li-Fraumeni syndrome, *p53* defects, neurofibromatosis 1 (NF1) and 2 (NF2), tuberous sclerosis, von Hippel-Lindau disease, Turcot's syndrome, and familial polyposis increase the risk of brain tumors. The polymerase chain reaction (PCR) assay and direct sequencing analysis can be used to diagnose von Hippel-Lindau disease.

For meningiomas, the strongest genetic link has been associated with NF2, with an almost 50% incidence. Sporadic meningiomas have been linked to chromosome 22 in the region of the NF2 gene.[4] Meningiomas are known to express estrogen and progesterone receptors, with the former being more common. A high incidence of somatostatin receptors has also been found. The significance of these findings is uncertain but has led to diagnostic tests (e.g., octreotide single-photon emission computed tomography [SPECT], using the somatostatin receptors) and treatment strategies (antiprogesterone; mifepristone [RU-486]). Radiation is the only definite cause. Studies have shown that children receiving as little as 10 Gy for tinea capitis have increased risk for meningiomas, with tumor development taking at least 20 years from exposure.[5,6] Head injury is often cited as a causative factor, but a prospective study of 3000 patients with head injuries found no increased incidence.[7]

Viral infections, specifically the JC virus, has been implicated in oligodendrogliomas, but the data are inconclusive. The incidence of PMBTs (specifically astrocytomas) is increased in children with acute lymphocytic leukemia who have had prior brain radiotherapy. There have been reports[8] of low-grade astrocytoma development in patients with inherited multiple enchondromatosis type I. Even though many of the molecular alterations involved in the progression of low-grade astrocytomas to higher grade tumors (glioblastoma multiforme) are known, the underlying causative factors are not well understood (Fig. 1).

SIGNS AND SYMPTOMS

For meningiomas, the clinical symptoms are usually dependent on the anatomic site involved, but many are found incidentally. Most meningiomas are slow growing and cause signs and symptoms by compression of nearby structures. The three most common symptoms are headaches, mental status changes, and paresis, and the most common signs are paresis, normal examinations, and memory impairment.[9] For PMBTs, the most common signs and symptoms are seizures and headache. The lower-grade glial tumors have a more indolent course that may persist over years, whereas the most aggressive tumors (e.g., anaplastic oligodendrogliomas, anaplastic astrocytomas, glioblastoma multiforme) may have a rapid onset of neurologic decline. Patients may, however, present with signs and symptoms of increased intracranial pressure, including nausea, vomiting, headache, and confusion.

DIAGNOSIS

As with most disease processes, the medical history is the most important initial step in the process of brain tumor diagnosis. Because many meningiomas are found incidentally, imaging studies are important. A physical examination usually follows the medical history. Computed tomography (CT) is probably used most often as the initial imaging study, but magnetic resonance imaging (MRI) is considered to be the gold standard when done with and without gadolinium contrast. On MRI, meningiomas are typically isodense, dura-based masses that often show homogeneous enhancement (Fig. 2).

Table 1 World Health Organization (WHO) Classification for Meningiomas

WHO Classification	Description
I	Meningiomas, with low risk of recurrence and/or low risk of aggressive growth
II	Atypical meningiomas, with increased mitotic activity or three or more of the following features: increased cellularity, small cells with high nucleus-to-cytoplasm ratio, prominent nucleoli, uninterrupted patternless or sheetlike growth, and foci of spontaneous or geographic necrosis
III	Anaplastic (malignant) meningiomas: exhibit frank histologic features of malignancy far in excess of the abnormalities present in atypical meningiomas

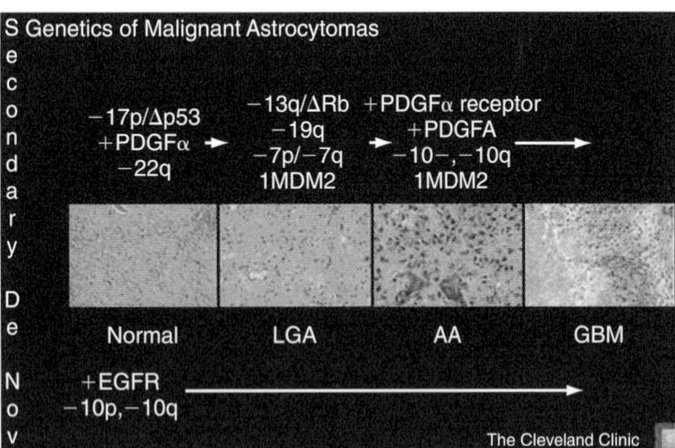

Figure 1 Glioblastoma multiforme development pathway. AA, anaplastic astrocytoma; EGFR, epidermal growth factor receptor; GBM, glioblastoma multiforme; LGA, low-grade astrocytoma; PDGFα, platelet-derived growth factor α. *(Adapted from the Cleveland Clinic).*

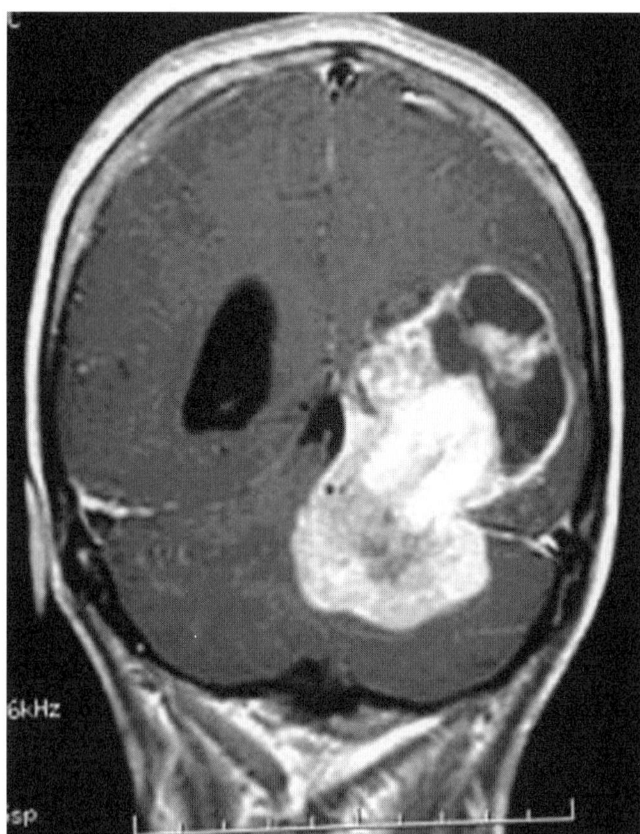

Figure 2 Coronal T1-weighted magnetic resonance imaging scan with gadolinium contrast. Shown is a meningioma crossing the tentorium on the *left*.

Meningiomas

Meningiomas typically appear as extra-axial lesions, and the presence of a dural tail aids in the diagnosis. CT can help evaluate bone involvement and the presence of calcifications, which can be seen in 30% of benign meningiomas but are rare in malignant meningiomas. Although benign tumors can have associated edema, it is much more common in malignant meningiomas. Other noninvasive imaging tests include octreotide SPECT scans, which measure somatostatin levels in meningiomas. Magnetic resonance venograms can help in determining venous sinus patency. Although noninvasive tests are helpful, the definitive diagnostic test is still histologic tissue evaluation after a surgical biopsy or larger resection. Most institutions now use the WHO histologic grading criteria. Grading of tumors is based on cell origin and biologic behavior (see Table 1). Figure 2 demonstrates a very large meningioma that crosses both sides of the tentorium on the left. This tumor was surgically resected in a staged procedure. A typical histologic appearance of a meningioma is shown in Figure 3.

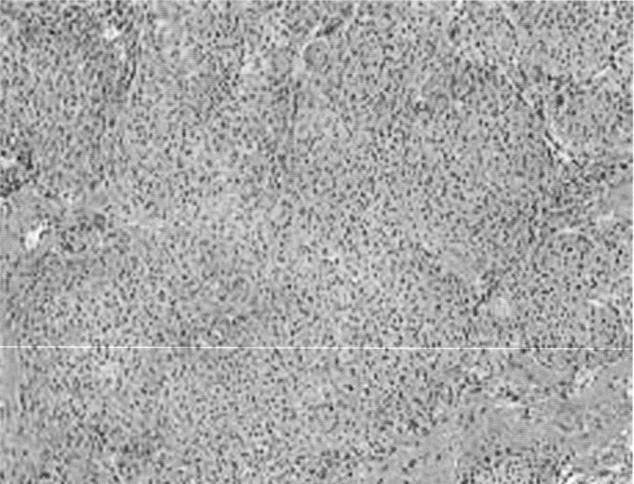

Figure 3 Meningioma with calcified psammoma bodies (hematoxylin-eosin stain, × 50).

Primary Malignant Brain Tumors

As with meningiomas, MRI with and without contrast is the test of choice for PMBTs. Oligodendrogliomas are more likely to demonstrate calcifications on CT than astrocytomas. With MRI scans, PMBTs are typically hypointense on T_1-weighted images and hyperintense on T_2-weighted and fluid-attenuated inversion recovery (FLAIR) images. The higher-grade lesions (WHO III and IV) are more likely to demonstrate enhancement (anaplastic oligodendrogliomas, anaplastic astrocytomas, glioblastoma multiforme), although ring enhancement is less common in anaplastic oligodendrogliomas and usually is associated with a worse prognosis.[10] Glioblastoma multiforme often has ring enhancement around a central area of necrosis (Fig. 4). Tumor-associated cysts are more common with the astrocytomas. The higher-grade lesions also tend to exhibit more peritumoral edema. Newer technologies such as magnetic resonance spectroscopy can help in the differential diagnosis of intracranial lesions. Gliomas tend to demonstrate decreased *N*-acetyl aspartate, increased choline, and decreased creatine levels. A lactate peak is common in higher grade tumors.[11] The diagnosis is ultimately made histologically after surgical biopsy or resection. Figure 5 shows a hematoxylin-eosin slide from an oligodendroglioma, and Figure 6 represents a glioblastoma multiforme at low power. As we increase our understanding of the molecular genetics of tumors, this technology will play an increasing role in tumor diagnosis (see later, "Advances").

TREATMENT

Pharmacologic Treatment

Initial therapy is symptom based and usually involves the use of steroids and anticonvulsant medication. I generally prefer dexamethasone (Decadron) as the steroid of choice. For all tumors other than lymphomas, steroids are used secondary to their antiedema function.

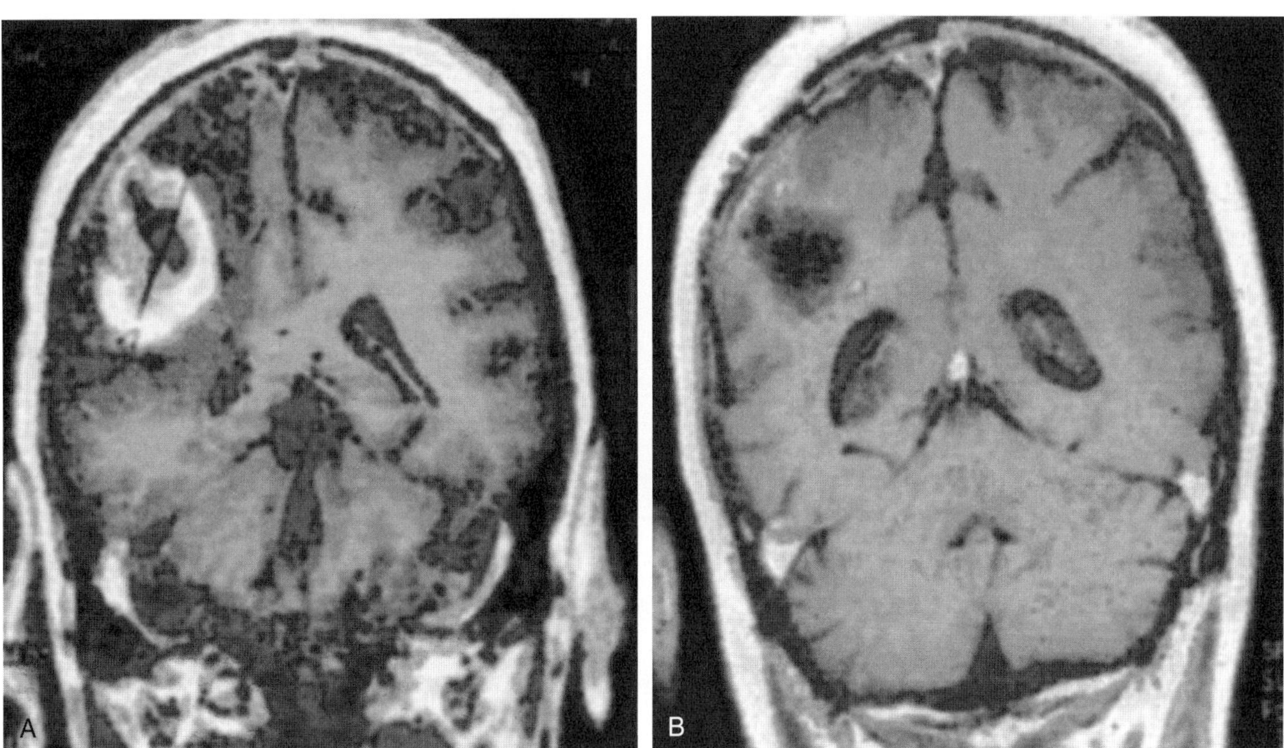

Figure 4 **Malignant glioma (gliobastoma multiforme) in the right frontal lobe.** Coronal T_1-weighted magnetic resonance imaging scan with gadolinium before **(A)** and after **(B)** surgery.

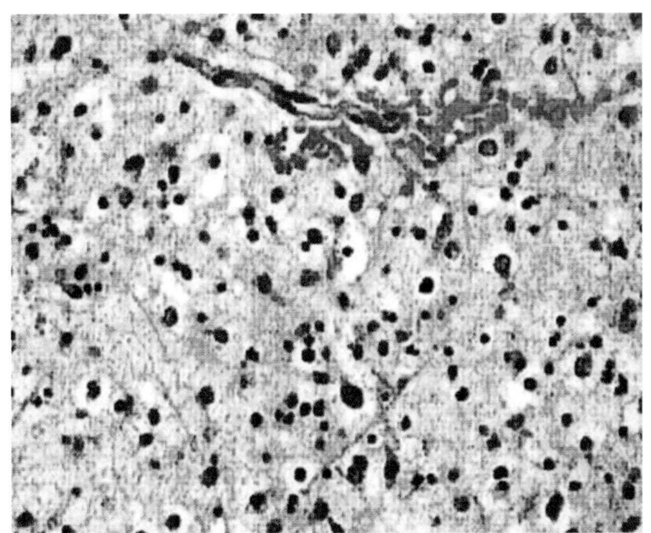

Figure 5 Oligodendroglioma showing the classic fried egg appearance (hematoxylin-eosin stain).

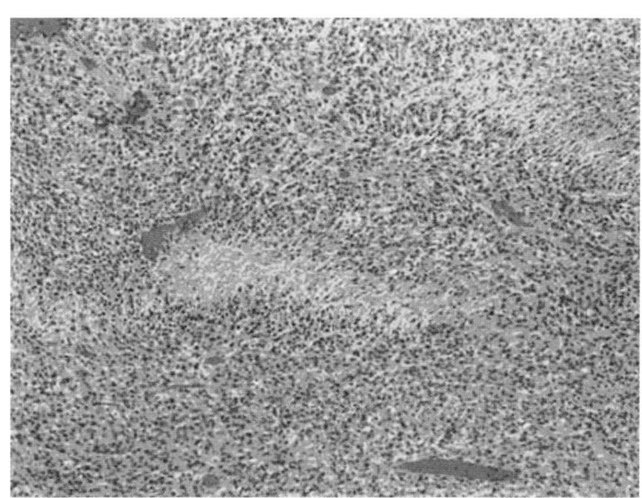

Figure 6 **Low-power slide of gliobastoma multiforme.** Shown is classic pseudopalisading necrosis (hematoxylin-eosin stain).

Side effects can be significant, and all patients should be treated with a histamine 2 (H_2) receptor blocker. The dose of steroids should be tailored for each patient and assessed on a regular basis. I tend to avoid late-night dosing if possible, because it can lead to sleep disturbances and behavioral problems. The typical dexamethasone dosage used by most physicians preoperatively is 4 mg, PO or IV, every 6 hours, and the dose is tapered postoperatively. Patients need to be followed closely during the tapering period. Antiepileptic drug practice has historically depended on the neurosurgeon's preference, and most patients are started on prophylactic anticonvulsants. The American Academy of Neurology issued a position statement in May 2000[12] that recommended not using prophylactic anticonvulsants in patients who have newly diagnosed brain tumors and who have never had a seizure. If patients need to be maintained on an antiepileptic drug, I attempt to convert them to a medication that will not affect the liver's cytochrome P-450 system (Table 2), because this could affect chemotherapeutic drug levels if both drugs are metabolized in the liver.

Surgery, Radiation, and Chemotherapy

Most patients will undergo a surgical procedure for diagnostic and treatment purposes. For patients with meningioma or PMBT, location usually defines the surgical risk. For meningiomas, if the tumor is located in proximity to a venous sinus, a magnetic resonance venogram is generally used and, if the sinus is patent, it usually represents a higher surgical risk. Surgeons may elect to complete cerebral angiography and have the patient undergo tumor embolization before surgical resection to decrease bleeding complications. Postsurgical treatments include observation, usually for WHO I and II meningiomas that undergo a gross total resection; focused external beam radiation for symptomatic tumors that cannot be resected, recurrent tumors, or highly aggressive tumors; chemotherapy (the Southwest Oncology Group currently has an ongoing hydroxyurea study for benign meningiomas); or hormone modulation, because many meningiomas express estrogen or progesterone receptors, or both. However, antihormonal therapy (anti-estrogen tamoxifen or the antiprogestin agent mifepristone) has not been shown to be effective in clinical trials.[13] Interferon alfa-2b has been used with some success for higher-grade meningiomas.[14]

For all grades of glial tumors, surgical resection is often recommended; however, by the very nature of their invasiveness, they cannot be cured surgically. A glioblastoma multiforme before and after surgical resection (see Fig. 4) demonstrates what is referred to as a "gross total resection." Depending on the tumor histology, grade, and patient's functional level (Karnofsky performance status [KPS], Table 3[15]), patients are usually treated after surgery (biopsy or resection) with external beam radiotherapy or chemotherapy. Radiation therapy typically is administered over a 6-week period with limited-field exposure (i.e., not the whole brain). Patients receive approximately 6000 cGy in 30 fractions (200 cGy per fraction). Oligodendrogliomas are usually more chemosensitive than astrocytomas, and hence radiotherapy is often delayed for these tumors.[10] Historically, oligodendrogliomas and anaplastic astrocytomas have been treated with procarbazine-lomustine-vincristine (PCV) chemotherapy, and glioblastoma multiforme has been treated with carmustine (BCNU). The U.S. Food and Drug Administration (FDA) has approved the use of temozolomide (Temodar) for recurrent anaplastic astrocytomas; however, it is clinically being used for tumors of all grades, including meningiomas. The last several years have seen an increase in phases I and II clinical trials. Through our involvement in New Approaches to Brain Tumor Therapy (NABTT), a National Cancer Institute–sponsored consortium of 11 institutions, new and innovative treatments are being developed.

OUTCOMES

Meningiomas

The overall prognosis for meningiomas is good and, as expected, somewhat depends on tumor histopathology. Because many menin-

Table 2 Anticonvulsants

Generic Name	Trade Name
Antiepileptic Drugs that Cause Modest or no Induction of Hepatic Metabolic Enzymes	
Gabapentin	Neurontin
Lamotrigine	Lamictal
Valproic acid	Depakene, Depakote
Felbamate	Felbatol
Levetiracetam	Keppra
Tiagabine	Gabitril
Topiramate	Topamax
Zonisamide	Zonegran
Antiepileptic Drugs That Induce Hepatic Metabolic Enzymes	
Phenytoin	Dilantin
Carbamazepine	Tegretol
Phenobarbital	Phenobarbital
Primidone	Mysoline
Oxcarbazepine	Trileptal

Table 3 Karnofsky Performance Status

Score	Description
100	Normal; no complaints, no evidence of disease
90	Able to carry on normal activity; minor symptoms
80	Normal activity with effort; some symptoms
70	Cares for self; unable to carry on normal activities
60	Requires occasional assistance; cares for most needs
50	Requires considerable assistance and frequent care
40	Disabled; requires special care and assistance
30	Severely disabled; hospitalized but death not imminent
20	Very sick; active supportive care needed
10	Moribund; fatal processes are progressing rapidly
0	Dead

Data from Karnofsky D, Abelman W, Craver L, Burchenal J: The use of nitrogen mustards in the palliative treatment of carcinoma. Cancer 1948;1:634-656.

giomas are found incidentally, observation may be reasonable for many patients. Radhakrishnan and colleagues[3] followed 57 asymptomatic meningiomas for 32 months. None of the patients became symptomatic. A subset of 10 patients showed growth rates of 0.24 cm/year; however, 35 patients showed no growth during an average 29-month follow-up. In a single series of 1799 meningiomas from 1582 patients followed for an average of 13 years after resection, the nonrecurrence rate was 93% of WHO I tumors, 65% of WHO II, and 27.3% of WHO III.[16] Other studies have shown higher recurrence rates after surgery alone.[17] For patients undergoing subtotal resection and radiation therapy, the 5-year progression-free survival for WHO grades I and II was 98% and, for WHO III, slightly less than 50%.[18]

Stereotactic radiosurgery is now being used more commonly, but long-term follow-up data are limited. Lunsford[19] has shown 4-year control rates of 92% for benign meningiomas treated with stereotactic radiosurgery. The roles of hydroxyurea, temozolomide, tamoxifen, mifepristone, and interferon alfa-2b remain to be determined. Several of these are being used in clinical trials but as of now play no real role in initial management and are used when no other treatment options exist.

Gliomas

Outcome for gliomas is based on tumor pathology or grade. For oligodendrogliomas, I retrospectively reviewed the last 96 oligodendrogliomas histologically analyzed at our institution. Prognosis was correlated best with chromosome 1p deletion, not age or tumor pathology grade (also see later, "Advances").[20] Cairncross and associates[10] have shown a median survival time of at least 10 years in anaplastic oligodendrogliomas with a combined 1p-19q deletion. The Radiation Therapy Oncology Group (RTOG) has completed a phase III study evaluating the long-term outcomes of low-grade gliomas (astrocytomas, oligodendrogliomas, and mixed oligoastrocytomas). The study (RTOG 98-02) stratified patients into an observation arm (age <40 years and gross total resection of tumor) and treatment arm (age >40 years plus biopsy or subtotal tumor resection, or both) that randomized patients to external beam radiation alone or external beam radiation followed by PCV chemotherapy. The study closed June 2002, with the results pending at this time.

For higher-grade astrocytic tumors, the RTOG has reviewed 1578 anaplastic astrocytoma-glioblastoma multiforme patients entered in three trials from 1974 to 1989 and performed recursive partition analysis (RPA).[21] Twenty-six pretreatment characteristics and six treatment-related variables were analyzed. Based on this analysis, six classes were developed (Table 4). It will be important in future studies that patient outcomes for new treatments are stratified based on RPA.

ADVANCES

The major advances in brain tumor understanding and treatment over the past 5 years have come from our understanding of oligodendrogliomas, which have specific molecular genetic alterations that distinguish them from astrocytomas. Allelic loss of chromosomes 1p

Table 4 Recursive Partition Analysis

Age (yr)	KPS	Description	Median Survival (mo)	2-yr Survival (%)
Class I				
<50	—	Anaplastic astrocytoma, normal mental status	58.6	76
Class II				
≥50	70-100	Anaplastic astrocytoma, symptom duration >3 mo	37.4	68
Class III				
<50	—	Anaplastic astrocytoma, abnormal mental status	17.9	35
<50	90-100	GBM		
Class IV				
<50	<90	—	11.1	15
≥50	70-100	Anaplastic astrocytoma, symptoms %3 mo		
≤50	70-100	GBM, partial or complete removal, and working neurologic function		
Class V				
≥50	70-100	GBM, partial or complete resection, nonworking neurologic function	8.9	6
≥50	70-100	GBM, biopsy, radiation dose >5440 cGy		
≥50	<70	Normal mental status		
Class VI				
≥50	<70	Abnormal mental status, radiation dose ≤5440 cGy	4.6	4

GBM, glioblastoma multiforme; KPS, Karnofsky performance status (see Table 3).

Data from Reifenberger J, Reifenberger G, Liu L, et al: Molecular genetic analysis of oligodendroglial tumors shows preferential allelic deletions on 19q and 1p. Am J Pathol 1994;145:1175-1190.

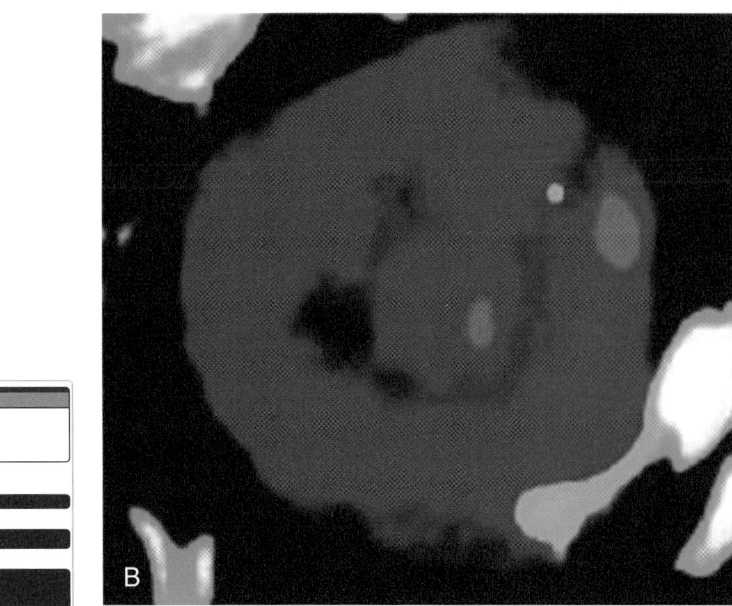

Figure 7 Evaluating the integrity of chromosome 1p using fluorescence in situ hybridization (FISH). Allele for long arm is shown in *red*; allele for short arm is shown in *green*.

and 19q is a molecular signature of oligodendrogliomas and occurs in 50% to 70% of WHO II and III oligodendrogliomas.[22] Molecular testing of brain tumors helps determine their treatment. The loss of heterozygosity (LOH) of chromosome 1p and 19q are predictive of chemosensitivity for oligodendrogliomas, regardless of tumor histology, KPS score, or age.[20] Figure 7 shows how chromosomal LOH is determined in the molecular laboratory. The integrity of chromosome 1p and 19q can be evaluated by fluorescence in situ hybridization (FISH) and the polymerase chain reaction assay.

Cairncross and colleagues[10] were the first to show this relation. They initially looked at 39 patients with anaplastic oligodendrogliomas and correlated chromosome 1p status with treatment effect. They found that allelic loss of chromosome 1p is a significant predictor of chemosensitivity and that combined loss of 1p and 19q shows a significant association with chemosensitivity and recurrence-free survival. These conditions were strongly associated with longer overall survival, and tests for these disorders are now done routinely on all my glioma patients.

The molecular story for malignant gliomas is much more complicated (see Fig. 1). The presence of an epidermal growth factor receptor (EGFR) likely indicates a primary (de novo) glioblastoma multiforme, whereas its absence suggests a secondary glioblastoma multiforme. Mutations of *p53*, on the other hand, are seen most commonly in secondary glioblastoma multiforme and EGFR and *p53* mutations are not found together. Treatments are currently being developed to target these receptors. At my institution, an EGFR antagonist erlotinib (Tarceva, OSI-774) trial has been initiated.

Thus, although mortality statistics for most primary brain tumors have not changed significantly over the past 10 years, morbidity and our understanding of the molecular basis for tumor development have changed. New strategies aimed at targeted sites on tumors are now being developed. We look forward to the challenge.

Summary

- Primary brain tumors represent only 2% of all cancers, with 35,000 new cases diagnosed each year in the United States. Meningiomas occur at a rate of 7.8 per 100,000 per year, but only 25% are believed to be symptomatic, with the others being found incidentally. The most commonly diagnosed primary brain tumor in adults is the glioblastoma multiforme.
- Only about 5% of primary brain tumors have known hereditary factors.
- For meningiomas, the three most common symptoms are headaches, mental status changes, and paresis, and the most common signs are paresis, normal examinations, and memory impairment. For primary malignant brain tumors, the most common signs and symptoms are seizures and headache.
- Computed tomography is probably used most often as the initial imaging study, but magnetic resonance imaging is considered to be the gold standard when done with and without gadolinium contrast.
- Initial therapy is symptom based and usually involves the use of steroids and anticonvulsant medication.

Suggested Readings

Annegers JF, Laws ER Jr, Kurland LT, Grabow JD: Head trauma and subsequent brain tumors. Neurosurgery 1979;4:203-206.

Curran WJ Jr, Scott CB, Horton J, et al: Recursive partition analysis of prognostic factors in three radiation therapy oncology group malignant glioma trials. J Natl Cancer Ins. 1993;85:704-710.

Glantz MJ, Cole BF, Forsyth PA, et al: Practice parameter: Anticonvulsant prophylaxis in patients with newly diagnosed brain tumors. Report of the Quality Standards Subcommittee of the American Academy of Neurology. Neurology 2000;54:1886-1893.

Jaasketainen J: Seemingly complete removal of histologically benign intracranial meningioma: Late recurrence rate and factors predicting recurrence in 637 patients. A multivariable analysis. Surg Neurol 1986;26:461-469.

Kleihues P, Cavenee WB (eds): World Health Organization Classification of Tumors: Pathology and Genetics: Tumors of the Nervous System. Lyon, France, IARC Press, 2000.

Lunsford LD: Contemporary management of meningiomas: Radiation therapy as an adjuvant and radiosurgery as an alternative to surgical removal? J Neurosurg 1994;80:187-190.

Mack EE, Wilson CB: Meningiomas induced by high-dose cranial irradiation. J Neurosurg 1993;79:28-31.

Maier H, Ofner D, Hittmair A, et al: Classical, atypical, and anaplastic meningioma: Three histopathological subtypes of clinical relevance. J Neurosurg 1992;77:616-623.

Radhakrishnan K, Mokri B, Parisi JE, et al: The trends in incidence of primary brain tumors in the population of Rochester, Minnesota. Ann Neurol 1995;37:67-73.

Rohringer M, Sutherland GR, Louw DF, Sima AA: Incidence and clinicopathological features of meningioma. J Neurosurg 1989;71:665-672.

References

For a complete list of references, log onto www.expertconsult.com.

Oncologic Emergencies

Mikkael A. Sekeres

DEFINITION AND ETIOLOGY

Oncologic emergencies, as the term implies, are complications resulting from a cancer itself, a paraneoplastic syndrome, or from treatment of the cancer, that require immediate attention and reversal, if possible. Inpatient treatment is a must, and often these conditions require intervention in an intensive care setting.

TYPES

Examples of oncologic emergencies include tumor lysis syndrome and other metabolic abnormalities, disseminated intravascular coagulopathy (DIC), hyperleukocytosis and leukostasis, fever in the setting of neutropenia, and spinal cord compression from a tumor mass.

Tumor Lysis Syndrome

Tumor lysis syndrome (TLS) is defined by a constellation of metabolic abnormalities seen in tumors with rapid cell turnover, in which the lysis of malignant cells causes release of their contents into the systemic circulation at a rate that exceeds the elimination capacity of the kidneys. TLS occurs most frequently in the acute leukemias, particularly T cell acute lymphoblastic leukemia (ALL), and in highly aggressive lymphomas, such as Burkitt's lymphoma. Risk factors that predispose to TLS include a large tumor burden with rapid cell turnover, elevated lactate dehydrogenase (LDH) level, preexisting hyperuricemia, sensitivity of tumors to chemotherapy, and abnormal baseline renal function.[1]

The sine qua non of TLS includes characteristic metabolic abnormalities, such as hyperuricemia, hyperkalemia (or, rarely, hypokalemia), hyperphosphatemia, hypocalcemia, and an elevated LDH level.

Identifying patients at risk and instituting appropriate prophylactic measures are essential. Electrolyte levels should be monitored frequently and adequate urinary output maintained in anticipation of and during TLS. Aggressive hydration should be initiated, along with urinary alkalinization and specific treatment of individual metabolic abnormalities. This includes measures that prevent uric acid formation and precipitation, and augment uric acid metabolism to allantoin. Allopurinol, which inhibits xanthine oxidase, is administered at a dosage of 300 mg/day to prevent uric acid synthesis from purines released as a result of cell lysis. Urine alkalinization is accomplished with sodium bicarbonate infusions to a target urinary pH of 7.0 or higher to prevent uric acid deposition in the renal tubules. Recombinant urate oxidase (rasburicase) has been recently approved for the treatment of hyperuricemia in pediatric patients with acute leukemia. Although it is extremely effective in reducing serum uric acid to low levels within a few hours of administration, it is reserved for severe cases that have failed traditional prophylactic methods and in which the probability of acute renal failure is very high, for cost reasons, and because it has not been shown to affect outcome.[2]

Disseminated Intravascular Coagulopathy

DIC can be a disorder of excessive bleeding or involving thromboembolic events. It is characterized by excess thrombin generation, usually triggered by an underlying condition, such as cancer or sepsis. DIC can accompany any type of leukemia and is most commonly observed in patients with acute promyelocytic leukemia (APL).[3] The development of DIC in leukemia may be caused by several mechanisms, including release of procoagulant factors, fibrinolytic substances, and inflammatory cytokines, and mechanically via the interaction of the leukemia cell with the vascular endothelium, macrophages, and platelets. Induction chemotherapy itself may transiently worsen the coagulopathy of APL. DIC may also be a sequela of gram-negative septic shock in 30% to 50% of cases; gram-negative shock, in turn, can occur in the setting of the immunosuppression associated with leukemia, its treatment, or both. L-Asparaginase, an agent commonly used as part of induction regimens for ALL, can cause DIC as a drug-related adverse event, frequently leading to a significant drop in fibrinogen levels. This form of DIC is more often associated with episodes of thrombosis rather than bleeding.

Supportive care and treatment of the underlying cause are the cornerstones of therapy of DIC. In patients with DIC in the setting of APL, the risk of bleeding is significantly decreased by institution of differentiation therapy with all-*trans* retinoic acid (ATRA), cytotoxic chemotherapy, and blood product support with platelets and cryoprecipitate.[4] Differentiation is also known to alter the clinical course of the coagulopathy of APL. Aggressive supportive care measures including platelet transfusions, clotting factor and cryoprecipitate replacement, and urgent initiation of definitive therapy; these are the key elements for management of this otherwise potentially fatal condition.

Hyperleukocytosis and Leukostasis

Approximately 5% to 30% of adult patients with acute leukemia will present with a high leukocyte count, usually higher than 100,000/mm^3. This leukocytosis can cause leukostasis, or sludging of the microcirculation with leukemic blasts. This phenomenon occurs more frequently in acute myelogenous leukemia (AML), in which the myeloid blast is larger and has impaired deformability characteristics as compared with a mature granulocyte. Leukemic blasts can also form microaggregates and white bland thrombi in small vessels, leading to impairment in flow, local hypoxemia (exacerbated by the high metabolic activity of the dividing malignant cells), and resultant direct endothelial damage and bleeding. The pulmonary and cerebral vascular beds are the most clinically relevant targets of leukostasis, although the coronary circulation can also be affected. Cerebral involvement can range from subtle confusion and somnolence to frank intracerebral bleeding and coma. Early pulmonary involvement is signaled by mild dyspnea and respiratory alkalosis. Typical chest x-ray findings include diffuse interstitial or alveolar infiltrates, but can be normal in early stages.[5]

The management of hyperleukocytosis and leukostasis is centered on cytoreduction and maximizing vascular flow through supportive measures. In patients with AML, hydroxyurea should be started, 1 to 3 g orally every 6 hours, in combination with emergent leukapheresis for patients presenting with white blood cell (WBC) counts higher than 100,000/mm^3 or signs or symptoms indicative of leukostasis. In ALL, the threshold to initiate leukapheresis is higher, usually higher than 200,000/mm^3, and patients may be treated with vincristine, steroids, or both. The replacement of fresh-frozen plasma that occurs in conjunction with leukapheresis may improve the coagulopathy that may be present in these patients, thereby reducing the risk of hemorrhage. However, leukapheresis has never been shown convincingly to reduce the risk of developing leukostasis or to reduce early mortality.[6] The most definitive therapy for this condition, naturally, involves urgent institution of induction chemotherapy.

Fever and Neutropenia

Patients with malignancies, and particularly those with acute leukemias, in which the cancer involves the immune system directly, often have neutropenia associated with their disease (commonly defined as an absolute neutrophil count lower than 500/mm^3) or with the immunosuppressive chemotherapy used to treat their disease. In particular, they are susceptible to infections with gram-negative organisms, staphylococci, and fungi. The most common sites of infection include the oropharynx, lungs, perirectum, and skin, particularly at IV catheter sites. Broad-spectrum antibiotics should be instituted immediately in the settings of fever and neutropenia to prevent these infections from becoming life threatening.[7] Antibiotics, which must include adequate coverage for *Pseudomonas aeruginosa* and other gram-negative organisms, should be continued until the absolute neutrophil count is higher than 500/mm^3. Antifungal therapy should be instituted if fever persists despite initial broad-spectrum antibiotics, usually 48 to 72 hours after failure of other antibiotics. Although the use of hematopoietic growth factors may reduce the length of hospital stay, they do not improve survival.[8]

Spinal Cord Compression

Compression of the spinal cord from a rapidly growing mass can result in neurologic compromise. Patients will often present with symptoms of back pain and neurologic complaints specific to the dermatome affected by the mass. In patients with cord compression in the lumbosacral area, this can include incontinence of the bowel or bladder or urinary retention, or leg pain or numbness. Without rapid reversal, these neurologic sequelae will become permanent. Malignant causes include liquid tumors, particularly aggressive lymphomas or multiple myeloma, and solid tumors, particularly those with a predilection for bone metastases, such as prostate, lung, or breast cancer. If at all possible, it is imperative first to establish a diagnosis of cancer in a patient previously undiagnosed who presents with cord compression; this can be accomplished through surgical decompression with a biopsy of the culprit lesion. In patients with known cancer diagnoses, nonsurgical interventions can also be used. These include treatment with high-dose steroids and local radiation therapy.

Summary

- Oncologic emergencies include tumor lysis syndrome and other metabolic abnormalities, disseminated intravascular coagulopathy, hyperleukocytosis and leukostasis, fever in the setting of neutropenia, and spinal cord compression from a tumor mass.
- Immediate institution of aggressive supportive measures is warranted, followed quickly by definitive treatment of the underlying malignancy.
- Monitoring electrolyte levels, complete blood cell counts, vital signs, and measures of coagulation are crucial for detecting these abnormalities and quickly initiating appropriate therapy.

Suggested Readings

Barbui T, Falanga A: Disseminated intravascular coagulation in acute leukemia. Semin Thromb Hemost 2001;27:593-604.

Jeha S: Tumor lysis syndrome. Semin Hematol 2001;38(Suppl 10):4-8.

Lichtman MA, Heal J, Rowe JM: Hyperleukocytic leukaemia: Rheological and clinical features and management. Baillieres Clin Haematol 1987;1:725-746.

Pizzo PA: Fever in immunocompromised patients. N Engl J Med 1999;341:893-900.

Porcu P, Danielson CF, Orazi A, et al: Therapeutic leukapheresis in hyperleucocytic leukaemias: Lack of correlation between degree of cytoreduction and early mortality rate. Br J Haematol 1997;98:433-436.

Pui CH, Mahmoud HH, Wiley JM, et al: Recombinant urate oxidase for the prophylaxis or treatment of hyperuricemia in patients with leukemia or lymphoma. J Clin Oncol 2001;19:697-704.

Stone RM, Berg DT, George SL, et al: Granulocyte-macrophage colony-stimulating factor after initial chemotherapy for elderly patients with primary acute myelogenous leukemia. Cancer and Leukemia Group B. N Engl J Med 1995;332:1671-1677.

Tallman MS, Kwaan HC: Reassessing the hemostatic disorder associated with acute promyelocytic leukemia. Blood 1992;79:543-553.

References

For a complete list of references, log onto www.expertconsult.com.

Cancer Pain

Mellar Davis

Cancer occurs in 1.2 million people in the United States each year and nearly one half of cancer patients die as a result of their cancer. Despite all advances in prevention, early detection, and newer treatments, including biologics and target-specific agents, cancer remains one of the most feared, debilitating, and lethal diseases. Cancer is the second leading cause of mortality in the United States.[1] Pain is experienced in more than 50% of these patients, and most of them have pain so severe that it interferes with their normal daily activities.[2,3] Less than half get adequate pain relief. The incidence of pain in advanced cancer is 80%, and 90% of patients with osseous metastases have pain.[4]

There is limited knowledge of the basic neurobiological mechanisms that generate cancer pain. However, empirical strategies for treating cancer pain have been validated and found to be highly successful for relieving pain.[5,6] Guidelines for managing cancer pain, although widely published, have not been universally applied, and as a result, there is considerable variation in the treatment of pain.[7]

DEFINITION

Pain is an unpleasant sensory or emotional experience associated with actual or potential tissue damage or described in terms of such damage.[8] Pain is a state of discomfort (sensory) and distress (affective). Pain corresponds poorly to the degree of tissue destruction, and pain intensity is not proportional to the type or extent of tissue damage. Classic pain categories are chronic and acute, nociceptive and neuropathic, and, within the nociceptive classification, somatic and visceral.[2]

The experience of pain is complex. Pain is modulated at several different central nervous system levels (Fig. 1): the dorsal horn of the spinal cord; the descending tracts through the bulbospinal pathways from the periaqueductal gray and rostral ventral medulla; and the cingulate cortex, within the amygdala, medial thalamus, and limbic cortex.[9] Pain is also influenced by past experience and cognitive function.[10] Psychological factors rarely initiate pain, but they greatly influence intensity.

There is a general tendency to separate malignant from nonmalignant pain and to view cancer pain within a biomedical model and noncancer pain within a biopsychosocial model. However, there is no difference anatomically or physiologically, by biochemical substrate, or through mechanisms of nociception that might be used to justify separating the two.[11] Pain for the cancer patient is a subjective experience, because nociceptive stimuli capable of eliciting pain are modified by genetics, past history, mood, expectation, and culture, just as they are for those with nonmalignant pain.

PREVALENCE AND PAIN INTERFERENCE

The prevalence of cancer pain directly correlates with the stage of disease. Patients with breast and prostate cancers, both of which have a propensity to spread to bone, more often experience pain than patients with uterine and cervical cancers.[12] Pain as an initial manifesting symptom occurs in 20% to 40% of patients. Severe pain (i.e., >5 on a numeric scale 0 being no pain and 10 severe pain) occurs in 20% to 35% of the cancer population and significantly impairs activities of daily living (ADLs). The impact of pain for a given severity varies, depending on the perceived cause of pain. Patients who believe that the pain is a result of their cancer have more pain interference with ADLs for the same degree of pain severity as patients who believe that their pain has a benign cause.[13] Interference with enjoyment of life is greatest when pain is caused by cancer, intermediate when caused by unknown factors, and least when regarded as being caused by treatment.[12]

Despite the direct association of pain prevalence with stage, pain corresponds poorly to the observed tumor burden. For example, only a minority of radiographically apparent metastases to bone are painful. Interestingly, high-dose single-fraction radiation produces rapid analgesia, usually within days, at lower than tumorcidal doses and more rapidly than those projected for tumor response. This indicates that radiation therapy significantly alters the reactive "inflammatory soup around a metastasis" as a means of analgesia, independent of antitumor activity.

Most pain experienced by patients is a result of their underlying cancers: 20% are from treatment sequelae, and less than 10% are the result of comorbidities. This is not the case for the pediatric cancer population, in whom a greater percentage of pain is the result of treatment, and also for those who have undergone bone marrow transplantation, for whom significant stomatitis is a major cause. One third have one pain, one third have two separate pain syndromes, and one third have three or more distinct pains.[13] The most common cause of cancer pain is bone metastases. One third of patients have neuropathic pain, either alone or combined with nociceptive pain. Common causes of pain are listed in Box 1. Pain generally changes little in severity in the last 4 to 6 weeks of life.

PATHOPHYSIOLOGY

Nociceptors are primary sensory neurons activated by stimuli from tissue damage. They are high-threshold receptors that remain silent until significantly stimulated.[14] These nociceptors are polymodal; that is, are capable of responding to physical and chemical stimuli. Various mediators can depolarize these nociceptors (Box 2).

Afferents arise from small- and medium-diameter cell bodies within dorsal root ganglia and trigeminal ganglia and have either unmyelinated (C fibers) or thinly myelinated (Aδ fibers) axons. Interneurons within laminae I and II of the dorsal horn amplify or dampen neurotransmission. Afferent axons terminate on lamina I or II within the dorsal horn, and second-order neurons extend processes to the contralateral spinothalamic tract through the ventral lateral thalamus terminating in the cerebral cortex (see Fig. 1). Sensory fibers associated with affective responses also ascend in the contralateral dorsolateral spinal cord to the medial thalamus or brainstem and then to the cingulate cortex and limbic lobe. Spinothalamics extend axons into the medulla and hypothalamus. Downward modulation occurs through the periaqueductal gray (PAG) and rostral ventral medulla (RVM) with axons that transverse the dorsal lateral funiculus. These modulate pain directly by connections to secondary afferent neurons in the dorsal horn or via connections with interneurons in laminae I and II (see Fig. 1).

Somatic pain is experienced as a fast (Aδ fiber) localizing pain or a slow (C fiber) noxious sensation. Visceral pain is unique because there are no fast or slow components and it is poorly localized compared with somatic pain: ascending second-order neurons cross and ascend in the dorsal lamina fasciculus rather than by lateral spinothalamic.

Peicpheral sensitization results from nerve endings exposed to products of tissue damage and inflammation. Nociceptors also contribute to persistent pathologic pain, in the setting of nerve injury. Central sensitization results from neuroplasticity and lowers nociceptor thresholds. Central sensitization, when nerves are damaged

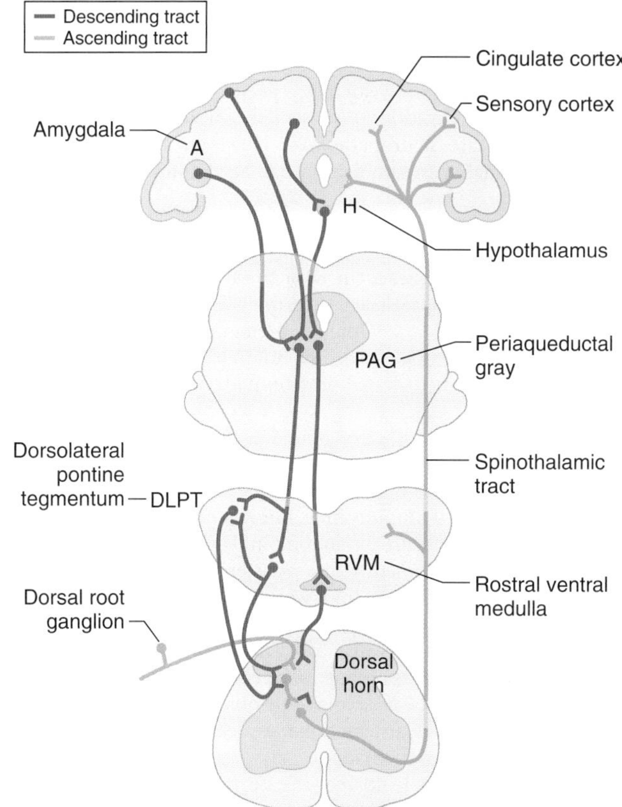

Figure 1 **Pain is modulated at several different central nervous system levels.** *(Adapted from Fields HL, Basbaum AI: Central nervous system mechanisms of pain modulation. In Wall PD, Melzack R [eds]: Textbook of Pain. Edinburgh, Churchill Livingstone, 1999, pp 309-329.)*

Box 1 Common Causes of Pain

Bone metastases
Visceral metastases
Immobility
Neuropathic pain
Soft tissue
Constipation
Esophagitis
Lymphedema
Muscle cramps
Chronic postoperative scar

Adapted from Twycross R, Harcourt J, Bergl S: A survey of pain in patients with advanced cancer. J Pain Symptom Manage 1996;12:273-282.

Box 2 Mediators Capable of Depolarizing Nociceptors

Bradykinin
Heat
Lipids (prostaglandin)
Nerve growth factor
Pressure
Protons
Serotonin

and continuously fire, occur from central algesic receptors, such as *N*-methyl-D-aspartate (NMDA) receptors, and nerve sprouting from lamina IV into laminae I and II, which previously were occupied by secondary sensory neurons. The gate-control theory involves facilitating and inhibitory interneurons, modulated through multiple descending pathways. Whether the gate is opened or closed influences pain intensity according to inhibitory influences from the PAG and RVM on spinal cord interneurons.[15] Central modulation of pain severity by the PAG and RVM is mediated by monoamine neurotransmitters (e.g., serotonin, norephinephrine) and endogenous opioids (e.g., enkephalin, dynorphin). Interneurons release gamma-amino butyric acid (GABA), analgesic amino acids (glycine), algesic amino acids (aspartate, glutamate), and prostaglandins to modulate pain (Fig. 2). Experimental studies have demonstrated that pain generated by bone cancer, inflammation, or neuropathy produces a unique set of sensations and neurochemical changes within the dorsal horn.[16]

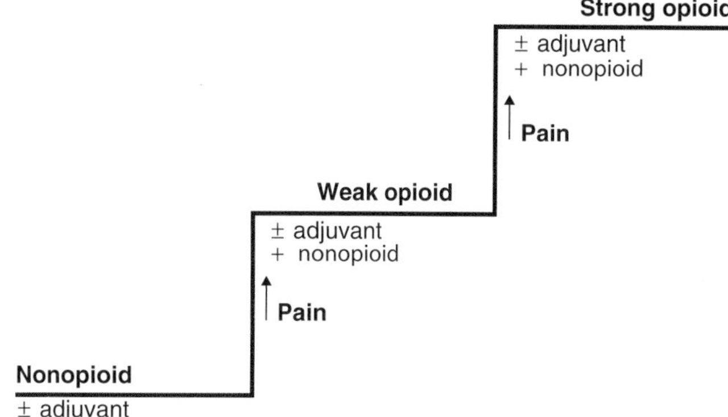

Figure 2 **WHO analgesic ladder.** *(Adapted from Ventafridda V, Stjernsward J: Pain control and the World Health Organization analgesic ladder. JAMA 1996;275:835-836.)*

Cognition and memory play a large role in the experience of pain.[10] Fear and depression reduce pain thresholds and produce anatomic changes that accentuate pain. Long-term neuroanatomic changes have been discovered in amygdala and hippocampus, sites that affect pain memory. These changes involve calcium-calmodulin–dependent protein kinases.[17]

SIGNS AND SYMPTOMS

Pain intensity is pivotal to therapeutic decision making (see Fig. 2). The temporal pattern quality and location of pain suggest its pathophysiology and dictate analgesic dosing strategy.

Somatic pain is well localized, sharp, aching, throbbing, or pressure-like in quality. Visceral pain, on the other hand, is gnawing, crampy, diffuse, and not well localized. Colic occurs with the obstruction of a hollow viscus and with achy, sharp, or throbbing pain, from internal organ capsule invasion or mesenteric infiltration.[2,18]

Neuropathic pain is often associated with allodynia, hyperpathia, or dysesthesia, in an area of neurologic deficit. Pain usually courses in the distribution of the motor, sensory, or autonomic nerve, except when pain is funicular. Funicular pain occurs with impending spinal cord compression. Neuropathic pain is associated with spontaneous, transient breakthrough pain, which is lancinating in quality. Pain might involve injury to a single nerve or to the cervical, brachial, celiac, lumbar, or sacral plexus. Pain may be generated from spinal cord damage and is experienced first as radicular pain, then as ascending levels of sensory loss.[2] Centrally mediated pain may be sympathetic, as in causalgia, or deafferentational, as seen with phantom limb pain.

Cancer pain may be acute and associated with generalized sympathetic hyperactivity, resulting in diaphoresis, hypertension, and tachycardia. Tolerance to sympathetic hyperactivity develops quickly as pain becomes chronic. Overt pain behaviors such as grimacing, moaning, and splinting, as well as sympathetic hyperactivity, are often not present with chronic pain.[19] Acute pain occurring on a background of chronic pain is usually associated with complications related to the cancer or its treatment. Unrelieved chronic pain produces depression, anxiety, anorexia, asthenia, and insomnia. The combination of pain quality, location, and radiation is used to classify pain into recognized cancer pain syndromes.[2,20]

Breakthrough pain is episodic pain that is usually a transient worsening of chronic stable background pain. Few patients have only intermittent pain; most patients have continuous pain, and most patients with chronic pain also have transient worsening of their pain. Incident pain may be voluntary or involuntary but is most often with activity, weight-bearing, cough, or bowel movement and is usually predictable and somatic in origin. Spontaneous lightning is characteristic of neuropathic pain. End-of-dose failure (i.e., pain that occurs before the next dose of analgesia) is caused by undertreatment of chronic pain.

DIAGNOSIS

Accurate assessment is the major step necessary for good pain management. Pain severity can be assessed by unidimensional pain scales, such as the visual analogue, numerical, or category scales.[2,20] Pain-relief scales have the advantage of gauging patient-reported benefits to treatment but do not correlate with unidimensional scales; they tend to be more therapeutically optimistic than unidimensional scales. Patients might have pain relief but still have severe pain that interferes with ADLs.[2,21] Comprehensive multidimensional scales are more burdensome for patients to complete, but they can evaluate the affective component of pain and pain interference with activities. Several general quality-of-life scales include pain-intensity or pain-relief scales. Examples are the QLQ-C30 of the European Organization for Research of Cancer and the Functional Assessment of Cancer Therapy (FACT) Scale.[22]

Adequate assessment requires a thorough history and physical examination before radiographic studies or physiologic testing. Bypassing a good history and physical for radiographs may be misleading, because there is no simple one-to-one correspondence between the report of pain and the presence of underlying pathology.[2,20] The location, radiation, quality, and intensity of pain, along with the palliative and worsening factors associated with pain, often maps the pain source and provide clues to a possible cause. The date of onset, associated symptoms, and pain trajectory measures disease course and prognosis indirectly and crudely. Past trials of therapy, including over-the-counter medications and home remedies, should be recorded. Crescendo or altered pain patterns, in addition to the usual chronic pain, indicate cancer progression or recurrence until proven otherwise. For example, crescendo pain along the course of post-thoracotomy pain indicates recurrence of lung cancer.

Physical examination is centered to the area of pain but should not be misguided by radiating patterns of pains. For example, shoulder pain may be referred from hepatic metastases or splenomegaly. Anatomic examination is followed by maneuvers to elicit or ameliorate pain. Bone metastases are common, and spinal cord compression from epidural tumor extension is most feared by physicians. Hence, a neurologic examination, manual muscle testing, percussion tenderness and joint mobility, and inspection for muscle symmetry are important parts of the physical examination.

Radiographic studies are guided by the history and physical examination as well as the stage of disease, patient performance status, therapeutic options, and goals of care. Terminally ill patients, or those for whom little is gained by defining radiographic pathology, should be treated with palliative measures and not be subjected to painful, unnecessary testing. Plain radiographs of painful areas are still valuable sources of information. Before examination, pain should be treated so that patients are comfortable and able to complete their radiographic procedures. Magnetic resonance imaging (MRI) scanning of the spine and brain and computed tomography (CT) scanning of the chest and abdomen should be completed; these provide the greatest amount of information. Ultrasonographic examination for pericardial effusions and biliary and urinary tract obstructions is easily accomplished, portable, and without radiation exposure. Electrophysiologic studies can separate mononeuropathies or entrapment neuropathies from plexopathies and ulnar or peroneal entrapment syndromes from brachial and lumbar plexopathies, respectively. Conduction velocities, specific latencies, amplitudes, duration, and configurations of sensory and motor evoked potentials identify and locate neuropathology. However, electrophysiologic studies are normal, with significantly damaged nonmyelinated fibers.

TREATMENT

Cancer pain can be relieved in 80% to 90% of patients using an opioid-based analgesic regimen[23] and the WHO analgesic ladder[24] as guidelines (see Fig. 2).[25-27] Opioids, preferably oral, are used with around-the-clock dosing, according to the analgesic ladder, with individualized treatment based on pain patterns and with attention to details.[27]

Morphine should be the first opioid of choice. Alternatively, oxycodone, hydromorphone, or fentanyl may be used initially depending on patient tolerances and clinical context. Efficacy of these other opioids is not better than morphine, but it is not inferior. There may be fewer side effects with oxycodone and fentanyl. Low doses of morphine can be combined with a nonsteroidal anti-inflammatory drug (NSAID) as a substitute for a weak opioid in the second step of the analgesic ladder (see Fig. 2). Avoid codeine, which has excessive side effects, meperidine because of its neuroactive metabolites, and mixed agonist-antagonists because of a ceiling effect. Use oxycodone, fentanyl, and methadone as second-line opioids for patients intolerant to morphine. Drug interactions are least with morphine and more problematic with methadone.

Use around-the-clock normal-release morphine every 4 hours or sustained-release morphine every 12 hours for continuous pain. Reasonable initial doses of morphine in opioid-naive individuals are 5 mg of normal release every 4 hours or 15 mg of sustained release every 12 hours. Rescue doses of normal-release morphine should be provided for breakthrough or incident pain. Doses are based on pain severity; dosing patterns are according to the pain pattern and diurnal variations in pain severity. Alternate routes of administration, such as sublingual, rectal, subcutaneous, IV, or spinal, need to be identified, particularly in dying patients or those unable to take oral medications (Box 3). Analgesic response is quantified by degree and duration of response; dose adjustments are made based on both. Most patients require rescue opioid doses for breakthrough pain. A dose that is 10% to 20% of the total daily opioid dose is a reasonable starting rescue dose, which is repeated every 1 to 2 hours if necessary. Rescue doses need to be titrated to response if the underlying chronic pain is under control. Individualized dosing needs to take into account age, perhaps sex, and renal, liver, and cognitive function.

Alternative opioids may be chosen with organ failure. Methadone and fentanyl are relatively safe, with few dose adjustments necessary for renal failure, whereas morphine is one of the safest opioids for cirrhosis. Oxycodone pharmacokinetics are significantly altered by hepatic and renal failure. Identify dose-limiting side effects and those at risk for respiratory failure, and titrate doses slowly in this group of patients.

An opioid switch is necessary for opioid toxicity, particularly with neurotoxicity (e.g., myoclonus, hallucinations, and confusion) and poorly controlled pain. Adjuvant analgesics and simultaneous opioid reduction (opioid sparing) can accomplish the same (Table 1). Anticipate constipation, and use laxatives such as docusate and bisacodyl, senna, or osmotic laxatives proactively. It is important to be aware of pain syndromes that are relatively opioid-resistant which require the early use of adjuvants, such as antiseizure medications or tricyclic antidepressants, as in the case of neuropathic pain. Interventions such as surgery, radiation, or kyphoplasty may be required for optimal analgesia for some patients with bone metastases. Tables 2 and 3 delineate equianalgesic dosing, opioid rotation, and opioid conversion.[24]

Box 3 Routes of Medication Administration

Oral
Hydromorphone
Methadone
Morphine
Oxycodone

Rectal
Hydromorphone
Morphine
Oxycodone

Sublingual
Fentanyl
Methadone

Spinal
Fentanyl
Hydromorphone
Methadone
Morphine

Intravenous
Fentanyl
Hydromorphone
Methadone
Morphine

Transdermal
Fentanyl

Table 1 Adjuvant Analgesics

Drug	Initial Dose	Maximum Dose
Acetaminophen	500 mg qid	4000 mg/day
Naprosyn	250 mg bid	500 mg tid
Dexamethasone	8 mg bid	Unknown
Nortriptyline	10 mg qhs	100-150 mg qd
Desipramine	10 mg qhs	100-150 mg qd
Valproic acid	250 mg qhs	30-60 mg/kg/day
Gabapentin	300 mg qhs	3600 mg/day

Table 2 Analgesic Equivalents Compared With Morphine

Drug	Potency Ratio	Duration of Action
Tramadol	1:5	2-4 hr
Oxycodone	1:1.5	3-4 hr
Hydromorphone	5	4-5 hr
Fentanyl (transdermal)	100	72 hr
Methadone	4 (<90 mg morphine/day)	8 hr
	8 (90-300 mg morphine/day)	
	12 (>300 mg morphine/day)	

Table 3 Equianalgesic Doses and Conversions

Drug	Oral	Subcutaneous/IV	Rectal
Fentanyl	—	25 μg = 1 mg morphine (parenteral)	—
Hydromorphone	6 mg	2-3 mg	6 mg
Methadone	Linear to total daily morphine	½ oral	1:1 oral to rectal
Morphine	30 mg	10 mg	30 mg

Table 4 Morphine Side Effects and Treatment

Type	Initial Action	Alternative
Gastric stasis, nausea	Metoclopramide 10 mg ½ hr before meals and at bedtime Prochlorperazine 10 mg q6hr	Opioid switch
Sedation	Reduce morphine dose if no pain	Methylphenidate 5 mg q AM and 5 mg at noon Morphine dose reduction plus addition of adjuvant
Cognitive failure	Reduction of morphine dose Deletion of psychosomatic adjuvants	Opioid switch
Myoclonus	Morphine dose reduction	Opioid switch Addition of clonazepam, valproic acid, or gabapentin
Pruritus	Oral antihistaminic	Opioid switch

Opioid side effects are relatively common. There are several ways of managing the more common dose-limiting symptoms (Table 4). The most feared side effect is respiratory depression, which fortunately is uncommon.[24,25] Respiratory compromise, when accompanied by tachypnea or anxiety, is not primarily caused by opioids. Tolerance to respiratory depression occurs quickly. However, care must be taken in those who are frail or opioid-naïve, who have comorbid conditions that predispose to respiratory failure such as chronic obstructive lung disease, or who are given sedative medications. Respiratory depression from opioids is nearly always associated with sedation and miosis. Naloxone is given only if sedation is accompanied by bradypnea and only in doses that reverse respiratory depression and not analgesia, if possible. A 0.4-mg vial of naloxone is diluted in 10 mL of saline; a 1-mL aliquot is given every 1 minute and titrated to the level of consciousness. Patients on sustained-release opioids or methadone might require a continuous infusion of naloxone at the dose that reversed respiratory depression, because the half-life of naloxone is 30 minutes.

Some patients fail to achieve adequate analgesia despite dose escalation because of dose-limiting side effects. Options in these circumstances include the following[24,25,28]:

- Opioid switch, because there is no cross-tolerance between various potent opioids
- Opioid conversion to parenteral or spinal routes
- Opioid sparing with the addition of an adjuvant analgesic
- Neuroblockade, neuroablation, or invasive neurostimulation
- Kyphoplasty, radiation, surgery

Adjuvant analgesics are chosen based on pathophysiology (Fig. 3). The term *adjuvant analgesic* describes a drug that has a primary indication other than pain but has analgesic properties with certain types of pain. Nonsteroidal anti-inflammatory drugs and acetaminophen are not adjuvants, whereas the antiseizure drug gabapentin is an adjuvant analgesic in the case of neuropathic pain. Additional non-pain–related benefits can influence the choice, because several symptoms may be treated by one medication (e.g., corticosteroids for bone pain, nausea, and headaches from cerebral metastases). A dramatic reduction of pain can occur with adjuvant analgesics, precipitating opioid toxicity, and therefore close observation is necessary when adjuvants are initiated. In general, adjuvant analgesics reduce pain and opioid consumption by 30%. Adjuvant analgesics may be started before opioids (e.g., tricyclic antidepressants, valproic acid, or gabapentin for neuropathic pain), depending on the clinical situation and severity of pain. Most adjuvants improve the therapeutic index of opioids but, unlike opioids, have a ceiling effect. Permanent end-organ damage can occur with certain adjuvant medications, unlike opioids. Adjuvants are less flexible and versatile than opioids. The serum level may be helpful in guiding titration, which is not the case with opioids.

Analgesics for somatic pain include NSAIDs. A preferred NSAID is naproxen, because of its twice-daily dosing schedule and low cost. Acetaminophen is an alternative for those with a history of gastrointestinal bleeding or renal dysfunction, but it should be limited to 4 g daily because of the risk of liver toxicity. Corticosteroids can improve multiple symptoms as well as produce a general sense of well-being, but have accumulative side effects that need to be minimized. Doses are reduced to the lowest effective once maximum response has been achieved. Cyclooxygenase-2 (COX-2) selective NSAIDs have a reduced risk of gastrointestinal toxicity and bleeding, but they might not have the analgesia of nonselective COX inhibitors.[29] Pamidronate and calcitonin reduce bone pain, as does a single-fraction radiation therapy.

Neuropathic pain might respond to opioids alone, but it often requires adjuvant analgesics. If pain is limited to a particular area (e.g., a mononeuropathy), a lidocaine 5% patch can be applied for 12 to 24 hours to the affected area without systemic absorption and systemic side effects. The secondary tricyclic antidepressants desipramine and nortriptyline are preferred over the tertiary tricyclics, amitriptyline and imipramine, because of reduced anticholinergic side effects. Of the antiseizure medications, gabapentin, pregabalin, and valproic acid has fewer drug interactions than classic antiseizure medications. Gabapentin has the fewest drug interactions and greatest evidence for benefit, but it is extremely sensitive to renal function and less versatile. Mexiletine is a third-line adjuvant. Electrocardiograms need to be reviewed before starting mexiletine, and some physicians evaluate the therapeutic response to parenteral lidocaine before considering mexiletine. Ketamine, in low doses parenterally or orally, blocks NMDA receptors and can reduce pain without psychotomimetic side effects. Oral doses of 25 mg every 6 hours are reasonable starting doses. Methadone, because of its NMDA receptor blockade, can act the same as ketamine and is also the least expensive of the opioids. Levorphanol has the same receptor-binding profile as methadone but fewer drug interactions.

Celiac plexus blocks are particularly effective for locally extensive pancreatic cancer. Kyphoplasty and vertebroplasty reduce pain associated with unstable vertebral compression fractures. Nonpharmacologic therapies, such as guided imagery, relaxation techniques, hypnosis, and biofeedback, complement pharmacotherapy. Treating depression and delirium with phenothiazines, antidepressants, or atypical antipsychotics, which lower pain thresholds, will reduce pain without the need for opioid titration and might allow opioid dose reduction.

OUTCOMES

Relief of pain is generally measured by unidimensional or pain relief scales. Ancillary outcomes include improved activities, relief of insomnia, and improved appetite, even if pain severity is relatively stable. Patient satisfaction with treatment, in addition to pain relief, reflects the relationship of the patient and the physician. With pseudoaddiction, once pain is relieved, there is a resolution of overt pain behavior. It is generally more difficult to see an improvement in overall quality of life because this is influenced to a significant degree by the burden of multiple symptoms.

CONCLUSION

Pain is one of the most feared symptoms associated with advanced cancer, but it also can be effectively managed in the great majority of patients. Pain assessment is rate-limiting to effective treatment. Numerous opioids are available, but morphine remains the drug of choice. Adjuvant analgesics improve pain control and prevent or ameliorate opioid toxicity by allowing opioid dose reduction. Finally, nonpharmacotherapeutic modalities, as well as treatment of depression and delirium, are important for the overall management of advanced cancer pain.

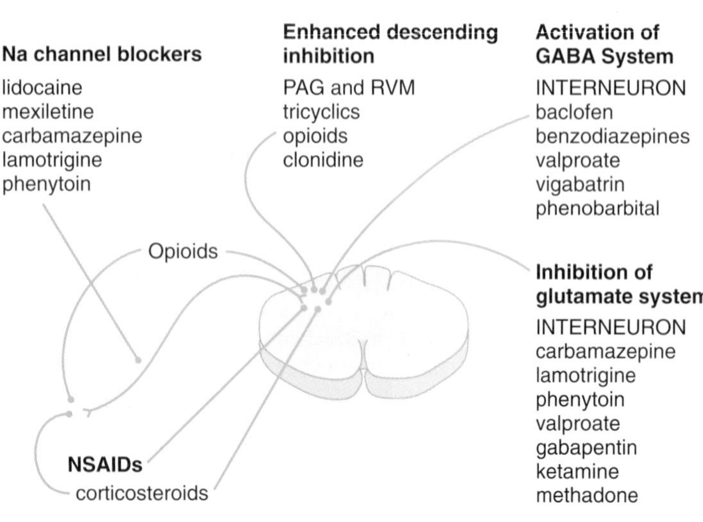

Figure 3 Adjuvant analgesics are chosen based on pathophysiology. *(Adapted from Twycross R: Opioids. In Wall PD, Melzack R [eds]: Textbook of Pain. Edinburgh, Churchill Livingstone, 1999, pp 1187-1214.)*

Summary

- Classic pain categories are chronic and acute, nociceptive and neuropathic, and, within the nociceptive classification, somatic and visceral.
- The temporal pattern quality and location of pain suggest its pathophysiology. Somatic pain is well localized, sharp, aching, throbbing, or pressure-like. Visceral pain is gnawing, crampy, diffuse, and not well localized.
- Overt pain behavior, such as grimacing, moaning, and splinting, as well as sympathetic hyperactivity, are often not present with chronic pain and are derived from personality characteristics.
- The location, radiation quality, and intensity of pain, along with palliative and worsening factors associated with pain, often locate the pain source and provide clues to possible causes.
- Cancer pain can be relieved in 80% to 90% of patients using an opioid-based analgesic regimen and the WHO analgesic ladder as guidelines.

Suggested Readings

Cherny NL: Cancer pain: Principles of assessment and syndromes. In Berger A, Portenoy R, Weissman D (eds): Principles and Practice of Supportive Oncology. Philadelphia: Lippincott-Raven, 1998, pp 3–42.
Dahl JL: Effective pain management in terminal care. Clin Geriatr Med 1996;12:279-300.
Davis M, Walsh D: Cancer pain syndromes. Eur J Pall Care 2000;7:206-209.
DeConno F, Caraceni A, Gamba A, Marianai L, et al: Pain measurement in cancer patients: A comparison of six methods. Pain 1994;57:161-166.
Guay DR: Adjunctive agents in the management of chronic pain. Phamacotherapy 2001;21:1070-1081.
Jemal A, Siegel R, Ward E, et al: Cancer Statistics, 2008. CA Cancer J Clin 2008;58:71-96.
Portenoy RK, Lesage P: Management of cancer pain. Lancet 1999;353:1695-1700.
Turk DC, Monarch ES, Williams AD: Cancer patients in pain: Considerations for assessing the whole person. Hematol Oncol Clin North Am 2002;16:511-525.
Turk DC, Okifuji A: Assessment of patients' reporting of pain: An integrated perspective. Lancet 1999;353:1784-1788.
Ventafridda V, Stjernsward J: Pain control and the World Health Organization analgesic ladder. JAMA 1996;275:835-836.
Walsh D: Pharmacological management of cancer pain. Semin Oncol 2000;27:45-63.
Pharo, GH, Zhou L: Pharmacologic management of cancer pain. J Am Osteopath Assoc 2005;105(11 Suppl 5):S21-S28.
Zech, DF, Grond S, Lynch J, et al: Validation of World Health Organization Guidelines for cancer pain relief: A 10-year prospective study. Pain 1995;63(1):65-76.

References

For a complete list of references, log onto www.expertconsult.com.

Palliative Medicine

Mellar Davis

DEFINITION AND BACKGROUND

Palliative care has been defined by Cairns[1] as follows:

> *Palliative care is an area of health care that specifically addresses the needs of patients who have illnesses that are causing their health to deteriorate progressively, and often rapidly, towards death. The aim of palliative care is the relief of symptoms, the maintenance of the best possible quality of life for the patient within the limitations of their illness, and support for family before and after the death of the patient. Patients and their families are usually introduced to palliative care when it becomes apparent that attempts at cure are no longer possible or are inappropriate. However, from the time of diagnosis of a potentially life-threatening illness or from the time of suspicion of such an illness, patients and their families may face emotional and existential issues that are commonly addressed as part of palliative care.*

Cairns further noted that "Palliative medicine is the medical component of palliative care. Practitioners of palliative medicine employ their knowledge of the pathophysiology of medical management of advanced disease as their particular contribution to the work undertaken by a multidisciplinary palliative care team."[1] The National Comprehensive Cancer Network Clinical Practice Guidelines in Oncology state that "the goals of palliative care are to prevent and relieve suffering and to support the best possible quality of life for patients and their families, regardless of the stage of disease or the need for other therapies. Palliative care can be delivered concurrently with life-prolonging (disease-modifying) care or as the main focus of care." Palliative care is not "end-of-life" care in this regard.[2]

An estimated 12% of patients who are hospitalized for acute illness have advancing chronic illness and are appropriate candidates for palliative care, but only 30% of these patients will be referred to palliative services. Discharges are inaccurately assessed in 27% of these chronically ill patients, resulting in frequent readmissions or excessively long hospital stays. Ongoing continuity of care is provided for only 17% of chronically ill patients.[3] The Study to Understand Prognoses and Preferences for Outcomes and Risks of Treatment (SUPPORT) found that half of patients dying within the hospital suffer from uncontrolled pain and that decisions regarding care are inappropriately timed.[4]

Palliative medicine arose in response to the care of this group of patients. In the past, they were generally managed in an environment with an inappropriately high degree of technology for their stage of disease and with overly optimistic expectations that glossed over the severity of their illness and prognosis. They also may have been in a subspecialty environment that did not provide continuity and that was driven by a disease-centred rather than a patient-centred philosophy.[5] Palliative care is a movement dedicated to making the health care system responsive to quality-of-life concerns so as to avoid the false dichotomy of either cure or care. Palliative care should be intrinsic to the care for all patients.[6]

PATIENT POPULATION AND CHARACTERISTICS

In a population of 1 million, it has been estimated that there will be 2800 cancer deaths annually; in this group, 2400 will have pain and 1300 will have dyspnea.[7] These patients will experience a mean of 11 to 13 different symptoms[8] and, in this group, there will be 6900 deaths caused by nonmalignant disease.[7]

The dying trajectory of patients with nonmalignant disease is distinctly different from that of cancer patients. Functional impairment occurs 1 year before death in 13.9% of cancer patients and increases to 22% to 63% of patients within the last 5 months of life. Greater disability occurs in terminally ill patients with a nonmalignant disease than in cancer patients 1 year before death; 35% of patients with nonmalignant disease are functionally impaired, but most exhibit a more gradual loss of functional activity than cancer patients. Malignancy produces a more precipitous and predictable trajectory of health impairment, whereas nonmalignant illness produces a gradual decline, punctuated by episodic abrupt deterioration, with partial recovery.[9] However, symptom burden can be as high in terminally ill patients with nonmalignant disease as in cancer patients.

ETHICAL FRAMEWORK FOR PALLIATIVE CARE

The lack of integration between the cure and care models of health care delivery forces patients to choose either aggressive medical care to modify the disease process or symptom management. Individual treatment options are limited not by free choice but by policies that force patients to choose between curative or palliative approaches to their disease.[10] Untreated pain and other symptoms associated with illness compromise or destroy patient autonomy.[11] Physicians can protect patients from harm and promote their welfare by palliating pain. The disparity in the provision of palliative care across the health care system violates the ethical concept of distributional justice. Palliative services are unavailable to a large segment of the population who suffer symptomatically and whose lives are disrupted by their disease because they choose disease-modifying or curative therapy. This system provides only comprehensive palliative care within the context of less than 6 months' survival and requires patients to forgo access to acute care and disease-modifying therapy encouraging the hastening of death.

APPROPRIATE REFERRAL

Patients need to have access to palliative care long before the terminal phase of their illness.[12] It is inappropriate to consider a palliative medicine referral only at the point at which all other alternatives have been exhausted, when the patient is highly symptomatic, or when he or she is in social disarray and family life crisis. The United Kingdom's policy framework for commissioning cancer services states that "Palliative care is required for many patients early in the course of their disease, sometimes from the time of diagnosis. It should not be associated with terminal care. The palliative care team should be integrated in a seamless way with all cancer treatment services to provide the best possible quality of life for patients and their families."[13] Similar recommendations can be made for nonmalignant illnesses. The term *end-of-life care*, popularized in 1994, is an inadequate description of palliative services.[14]

PALLIATIVE MEDICINE SERVICES

Clinical palliative care can be made available at three distinct levels. *Primary palliative care* refers to basic skills and competencies required of all physicians and health care workers.[15] These skills are germane to any clinical practice. *Secondary palliative care* refers to specialist clinicians and organizations that provide consultation and specialty care. *Tertiary palliative care* refers to academic centers where specialist knowledge about complex (complicated) problems is practiced, researched, and taught.

PALLIATIVE MEDICINE SKILLS

Palliative medicine incorporates seven major skills: communication, decision making, management of disease-related complications, symptom control, psychosocial and spiritual care, care of the dying, and coordination of care or continuity. These skills are not unique to palliative medicine, but they reflect good medical practice.

Communication

Good communication between the clinician and patient reduces psychological distress, encourages better compliance, instils realistic expectations, and fosters patient satisfaction with care. Communication is particularly important at critical points in the patient's illness, including when breaking bad news, at points of transition in the disease course, when truth telling, and when explaining treatment options so that informed choice and autonomy are possible.[16,17] Communication also requires listening and being present.[18] Delivering bad news requires compassion, suitable physical location, time, and presence of appropriate family members. Physicians need to find out how much the patient knows, what he or she wishes to know, and the way he or she would like to be told information before proceeding.[19] Some patients want information communicated directly, whereas others—usually older or perhaps more dependent patients—want family members informed, deferring autonomy and decision making to them. Information needs to be given in a digestible form and repeated. Physicians need to respond to patients' feelings with empathy. Advance planning care, continuity, and clinical guidance support the patient throughout this process.[19]

Despite the palliative care team's efforts, communication between the palliative care team and the patient is a moderate to severe problem in 20% of cases, and communication between the patient and family members is a moderate to severe problem in 30% to 40% of cases.[17] Respiratory and digestive system malignancies are particularly associated with greater difficulties in communication between patients and families. Earlier referral to palliative care teams can reduce communication problems. Poor communication is associated with greater spiritual needs, poor care planning, and poor patient and family insight. Good communication greatly facilitates the ability to care for patients at home.

Decision Making

When a plan of care that is congruent with disease course is absent, chaos usually reigns. Medical management often is inappropriate for the stage of illness, and medical costs increase as tests and technology become substitutes for wise decision making. Decision making should take into account patient values and beliefs regarding the illness trajectory and should weigh the use of technology against expected benefits and risks. Fragmentation of care in a subspecialty environment can delay transitioning because of an overly optimistic or incomplete understanding of the prognosis, whereas palliative care could better serve the patient's interests. Two of the most important questions physicians need to ask themselves are "What is the plan of care?" and "What are the goals of therapy?"

Treatment of Complications and Symptoms

Palliative medicine defines disease as whatever is experienced by the patient. Physicians grossly underestimate symptoms in most patients with multiple symptoms.[18,20] Patients volunteer an average of two or three symptoms; this figure almost quadruples with a formal review of systems.[8] In a 1000-patient study of advanced cancer patients, the ten most commonly elicited symptoms were pain, easy fatigability, weakness, anorexia, weight loss, lack of energy, dry mouth, constipation, dysphagia, and early satiety. These symptoms were found in more than 50% of patients surveyed. All symptoms were clinically disabling and all contributed to poor quality of life. Gender and age differences in symptom prevalence also exist; for example, nausea and vomiting are more commonly experienced by women, and dysphagia is more common in men. The young experience sleep disturbances, depression, anxiety, and vomiting and have headaches more often than older adults. Symptom clusters and severity change with disease progression. Poor prognostic symptoms are anorexia, dysphagia, hallucinations, weight loss, early satiety, and dyspnea.[21]

Health-related quality-of-life tools can help determine the most prevalent symptoms and measure the detriment that these symptoms have on quality of life.[22] The extent of investigations for symptoms depends on an appropriate patient-centered plan of care, available treatment options, and course of the illness. Prescribing for symptoms has been described in detail in the literature. Principles of good prescribing include the following:

- Using one drug for several symptoms
- Choosing medications with the fewest drug interactions
- Using medications with reduced side effects
- Choosing drugs with multiple routes of administration

Drug efficacy, drug costs, and therapeutic index (dose toxicity to dose response) are other important considerations.

A number of books have been published on the management of symptoms.[23-25]

Psychosocial and Spiritual Care

The family is the primary support for patients with life-threatening illnesses. Patient and family education, counseling, and assessment of family dynamics are particularly important when transitioning patients to palliative care. A social worker is invaluable in this regard. Psychosocial care involves assessing the gaps in communication and understanding between the palliative care team and family as well as evaluating family dynamics, which may be dysfunctional; this is evidenced by disruptive behavior, ambivalence, or discord.[26] Disposition to home requires that the family keep the patient comfortable (maintain symptom control) and safe (maintain a physically and emotionally supportive environment) and maintain the patient's dignity (hygiene). Patient and family evaluation, education, and counselling are effectively done through a family meeting. Critical functioning of the patient and family depend on four common factors: problem solving, adjustment coping, performance status of the patient and caregivers, and communication.[27]

In the hospital environment, a centralized unit fosters multidisciplinary care. In addition to the physical duties of nursing, nurses assess patients' fears and anxieties, provide the palliative care team with insight into family dynamics, act as advocates for family needs, educate, and provide consolation when death occurs. Palliative nurses train families about the special requirements for disposition, such as ostomy care and orthotics aids, review the home medication schedule, and educate families about the signs and symptoms of dying.[26]

A threat to life carries with it a challenge to meaning. A spiritual crisis can manifest itself in somatization and poor symptom control as the patient struggles with a profound sense of meaninglessness and hopelessness.[28] Definitions of spirituality have evolved within certain hospice organizations to mean predominantly a search for meaning, at least in the English-speaking world. Spirituality has been separated from organized religion and traditional orthodox spirituality, which include a relationship with God; this has been replaced by the present wider definition.[29] Fully developed, it is a secularized version of the Christian Reformation; the "priesthood of all the believers" is seen as involving all in palliative care and, as a result, spiritual care is to be done by all.[29]

Such developments in the definition of spirituality have been molded by a recent disenchantment with religious institutions and a strong emphasis on individualism and autonomy, which are fostered by enlightenment principles and humanism. Many, however, hold to

Box 1 Psychological and Biologic Markers of the Imminently Dying

Cognitive failure
Restlessness
Dyspnea
Pain
Anorexia
Bed-bound state
Retained upper respiratory tract secretions (death rattle)
Inability to swallow
Withdrawal hallucinations
Cheyne-Stokes respiration
Reduced blood pressures and pulse pressure
Reduced urinary output
Mottled skin
Incontinence

Adapted from Lichter I, Hunt E: The last 48 hours of life. J Palliat Care 1990;6:7-15.

traditional orthodox spirituality, which will require the attention of a chaplaincy. Traditional orthodoxy uses believing and belonging (ritual and sacrament within community) to bestow hope and continuity. Western society has become a multifaith society, which requires consulting religious leaders of various faiths. The clinician should be aware of the divergent definitions of spirituality and be informed by the patient about his or her particular beliefs (i.e., spirituality as meaning or spirituality in a traditional theistic sense).[30]

Psychological and biological markers of the imminently dying include cognitive failure, restlessness, dyspnea, pain, anorexia, bed-bound state, retained upper respiratory tract secretions (death rattle), inability to swallow, withdrawal, hallucinations, Cheyne-Stokes respiration, reduced blood and pulse pressures, reduced urinary output, mottled skin, and incontinence.[31] However, not all patients present with these signs and symptoms. Additionally, the signs and symptoms of dying are often mistaken for drug side effects, and physicians or families might discontinue medications, which only worsens the situation (Box 1).

Dying patients need symptom relief, the presence of a significant other, physical expressions of affection and caring, and truth telling.[32] Active management is required for pain, dyspnea, nausea, vomiting, myoclonus, and death rattle. Three or four types of medication are generally used; these include opioids for pain and dyspnea; chlorpromazine for dyspnea, delirium, anxiety, and nausea; antimuscarinics (e.g., glycopyrrolate, hyoscyamine, hyoscine hydrobromide) for secretions; and benzodiazepines for myoclonus or seizure. Medications require versatility (multiple routes of administration) because many patients are unable to take medications by mouth near the end of life.[32]

Coordination of Care

Patients can get lost among the various subspecialties involved in multidisciplinary comprehensive oncologic care. Identification with a single physician-nurse dyad improves patient satisfaction, avoids conflicting or overlapping prescribing, and allows a smooth transition to non-antitumor palliative care when appropriate. These goals can be accomplished only by avoiding an either-or approach to palliative care and oncology and by discounting palliative medicine as end-of-life care. Provision for a number of entrance points into palliative-care programs, including inpatient consulting services, outpatient services, and hospice services, is important for timely referral. The availability of such services allows the palliative care team to follow the patient throughout the course of illness wherever the patient may be in an institution or at home. Patients should not be managed by limited palliative services, which is particularly true if services are limited to consultation only.[33] A 24-hour on-call system is part of continuity of care.

PALLIATIVE OUTCOMES

Outcomes to palliative care should be satisfactory control of pain and symptoms, reduction in patient and family distress, an acceptable sense of control, relief of the caregiver's burden, strengthened relationships, optimized quality-of-life as defined by the patient, and personal growth and enhanced meaning.[2]

Summary

- The aim of palliative care is the relief of symptoms, maintenance of the best possible quality of life for the patient within the limitations of the illness, and support for the family before and after the death of the patient.
- An estimated 12% of patients who are hospitalized for acute illness have advancing chronic illness and are appropriate candidates for palliative care, but only 30% are referred to palliative services.
- Palliative medicine incorporates seven major skills: communication, decision making, management of disease-related complications, symptom control, psychosocial and spiritual care, care of the dying, and coordination of care or continuity.

Suggested Readings

American Academy of Pain Medicine: Quality Care at the End of Life: A position statement from the American Academy of Pain Medicine, 1998. Available at http://www.painmed.org/productpub/statements/endoflifestmt.html (accessed March 12, 2009).

American Pain Society: Principles of Analgesic Use in the Treatment of Acute and Cancer Pain (4th ed) Available for order at http://www.ampainsoc.org/pub/principles.htm (accessed March 12, 2009).

Beider S: An ethical argument for integrated palliative care. The Heart Touch Project. Evid Based Complement Alternat Med 2005;2(2):227-231.

Buckman R: How to Break Bad News: A Guide for Health Care Professionals. Baltimore: Johns Hopkins University Press, 1992.

Davis M, Frandsen J, Dickerson D, Ripamonti C: Prescribing for the actively dying patient: Principles and practice. J Termin Oncol 2002;1:19-32.

Edmonds P, Karlsen S, Addington-Hall J: Palliative care needs of hospital inpatients. Palliat Med 2000;14:227-228.

Higgenson I: Palliative and terminal care: Health care needs assessment. In Stevens A, Raftery R (eds): The Epidemiologically Based Needs Assessment Reviews, series 2. New York: Radcliffe Medical Press, 1997.

Higginson IJ, Constantini M: Communication in end-of-life cancer care: A comparison of team assessments in three European countries. J Clin Oncol 2002;20:3674-3682.

Homsi J, Walsh D, Nelson KA, et al: The impact of a palliative medicine consultation service in medical oncology. Support Care Cancer 2002;10:337-342.

Hoyer T: Hospice and future of end-of-life care: Approaches and funding ideas. J Palliat Med 2002;5:259-262.

Lisson E: Ethical issues in pain management. Semin Oncol Nurs 1989;5:114-119.

National Comprehensive Cancer Network: NCCN Clinical Practice Guidelines in Oncology V.I. 2008. Available at http://www.nccn.org (accessed March 12, 2009).

Powazki RD, Palcisco C, Richardson M, Stagno SJ: Psychosocial care in advanced cancer. Semin Oncol 2000;27:101-108.

SUPPORT Principal Investigators: A controlled trial to improve care for seriously ill hospitalized patients. The study to understand prognoses and preferences for outcomes and risks of treatments (SUPPORT). JAMA 1995;274(20):1591-1598.

Teno JM, Weitzen S, Fennell ML, Mor V: Dying trajectory in the last year of life: Does cancer trajectory fit other diseases? J Palliat Med 2001;4:457-464.

von Gunten CF: Secondary and tertiary palliative care in US hospitals. JAMA 2002;287(7):875-881.

Walter T: Spirituality in palliative care: Opportunity or burden? Palliat Med 2002;16:133-139.

Woodruff R: Palliative Medicine: Symptomatic and Supportive Care for Patients with Advanced Cancer and AIDS, 3rd ed. New York: Oxford University Press, 1999.

Adams N: Worldwide Palliative Care Alliance. "Access to pain relief: an essential human right. A report for World Hospice and Palliative Care Day 2007. Help the Hospices for the worldwide Palliative Care Alliance. J Pain Palliat Care Pharmacother 2008;22(2):101-129.

References

For a complete list of references, log onto www.expertconsult.com.

Section 8

INFECTIOUS DISEASE

Travel Medicine for the Primary Care Physician

Steven D. Mawhorter

International tourism and business travel is a growing industry. The World Tourism Organization has estimated that there were 675 million international travelers in 1999, roughly a 50% increase compared with the prior decade.[1] Although most international travel is in developed countries, more than 10 million persons from the United States and Canada travel to developing countries each year.[1] Many destinations lack pure water systems and disease control programs. Travel to these countries requires specific preparation to avoid illness, and general health advice should be sought before international travel. Physicians are often called on to prepare their patients for travel and to treat them afterward. A primary care provider might serve this role, but the constantly changing and highly specialized information makes a dedicated travel medicine expert more likely to be able to handle the individual needs of varied travelers and their unique itineraries. A study by the Centers for Disease Control and Prevention[2] has found that primary care physicians and even the embassy staff of foreign countries could not completely prepare their patients. Consulting an international travel medicine expert before travel reduces the risk of illness associated with travel sevenfold.

This chapter focuses on aiding the primary physician to partner with travel medicine experts. It emphasizes areas of travel medicine that are commonly encountered and therefore most practical for primary care physicians to address.

DEFINITION

A functional definition of the goals of travel medicine is to:

- Counsel patients about how to avoid risky behavior and exposure to infectious agents or disease vectors (pretravel counseling).
- Immunize against illness when it is difficult to limit exposure.
- Use preventive or symptom-triggered medications when immunization vaccines are not available.

There are new consensus guidelines on travel-related health issues in the United States from the Infectious Diseases Society of America. In addition, the Canadian Health System (Health Canada) has published its own set of guidelines on topics related to travel medicine. It should be noted that, like any guidelines, these represent only a starting point for care, which must be individualized for each person coming for travel advice. Moreover, it must be realized that because medicine availability varies among countries, some recommendations may not fit with available resources in the reader's home country. Specifically, there is no oral cholera vaccine available in the United States.

The Centers for Disease Control and Prevention (CDC) has revised its travel notice definitions and uses more common terminology. The four-tiered system is designed to help travelers and health care professionals assess risk in the ever-changing landscape of international travel. The CDC travel section (http://wwwn.cdc.gov/travel/) provides recognized expertise from a U.S. perspective, especially in the *Yellow Book* section.

PREVALENCE

Fifty percent to 75% of travelers to the tropics and subtropics report minor medical complaints, many of which are preventable. This high incidence emphasizes the importance of pretravel counseling. Overall, up to 10% of travelers alter their planned activities because of illness, mostly traveler's diarrhea, 5% become ill enough to require medical attention abroad, and 2% are too ill to be able to immediately return to work after their return.[4]

Fatal illness while traveling is extremely rare. Although 1 in 100,000 Swiss travelers to developing countries has died while traveling, compared with 0.3 in 100,000 travelers to North America, both mortality rates were lower than for those who did not travel.[5] Such statistics reflect the general good health of most travelers.

PRETRAVEL COUNSELING FOR ALL TRAVELERS

Pretravel counseling should be sought before international travel begins. The following health issues and priorities have been outlined.[1,3] The traveler should first be advised about required immunizations based on international regulations. In addition, many other immunizations are recommended to reduce the impact of destination-specific health risks. Second, issues of malaria risk, prevention, and chemoprophylaxis should be reviewed. Third, general health advice should include the following:

- Food and beverage precautions
- Insect bite avoidance
- Accident and injury prevention
- Risk-behavior management—drug use, casual sex, personal safety, high-altitude adjustment

These reflect the most prominent health-related issues associated with international travel, especially travel to lesser developed countries. Tailoring the advice to the individual traveler is important and usually requires the expertise of the travel medicine specialist.

The importance of sunscreen and insect repellent should be stressed. It is good to reinforce food and water precautions, including brushing the teeth with purified or bottled water and avoiding ice in drinks.

Jet Lag

Jet lag is a common unavoidable condition, without any specific therapy. Over the years, many remedies have been sought, but no magic bullet has been found. Adequate hydration and avoidance of excess alcohol are two of the most useful tips.[6] Melatonin is involved in the circadian cycles in many animals, leading to considerable interest in its potential role for treating jet lag. Studies of melatonin in travelers have shown small and inconsistent reductions in jet lag symptoms.[7,8] The safety of melatonin has not been established, although it is widely available in health food stores. Some evidence supports exposure to outdoor sunlight at the travel destination, which may speed acclimatization.[7,8] Important events and meetings are best scheduled at least 48 hours after arrival, if possible.

Electronic Resources

Patients with access to the Internet can review helpful information about medical preparation for foreign travel from several sources (see later, "Resources for Travelers: Electronic Resources"). One of the most notable is the CDC travel information section. The World Health Organization also posts information related to international travel health concerns. A particular advantage of these sources is that they allow the patient to review information related to specific travel plans, which will generate focused questions for review during pre-travel counseling. For practical travel information, including passport and visa questions, as well as U.S. State Department travel advisory information, their website is an excellent resource.

Immunization

More than one dozen vaccines are available for diseases with a high prevalence in developing countries (Box 1). Some are the familiar vaccines recommended for all Americans and others are for diseases mostly found in the developing world or in specific travel destinations. The vaccines that a traveler needs depend on the itinerary and the patient's current immunization status. Primary care physicians should make sure that travelers are up to date in their routine immunizations before going abroad; however, immunizations for rare and travel-related diseases are best left to experts in travel medicine.

Vaccines for Primary Care Administration

Adults who have not completed their primary vaccination series need to complete them for full protection.[9] Updated general vaccine information, as recommended by the Advisory Committee on Immunization Practices (ACIP) can be found at the National Immunization home page on the CDC website (http://www.cdc.gov/vaccines/). Vaccine-based immunity to tetanus, diphtheria, pertussis, polio, and other entities wanes over time, and these diseases are more prevalent abroad; booster vaccination is recommended. Pregnant or immunocompromised travelers should seek specific advice from a travel medicine specialist. Some guidelines regarding vaccines for pregnant travelers can be found at http://www.cdc.gov/vaccines/pubs/preg-guide.htm.

Box 1 Immunizations for Travelers

Routine Vaccinations

Inactivated

Diphtheria-tetanus (Td vaccine for persons ≥7)*
Hepatitis A*
Influenza†
Pneumococcal†
Poliomyelitis (inactivated)*
Hepatitis B†

Live Attenuated

Measles-mumps-rubella†

Travel-Specific Vaccines

Inactivated

Anthrax‡
Japanese encephalitis‡
Meningococcus*
Plague‡
Rabies‡
Typhoid (Vi antigen)†
Diphtheria-tetanus (Td vaccine for persons 7 years of age and older)*
Hepatitis A*
Influenza†
Pneumococcus†
Poliomyelitis (inactivated)*
Hepatitis B†

Live Attenuated

Measles-mumps-rubella†
Typhoid (Ty21a)†
Yellow fever*

**Frequently recommended.*
†Occasionally recommended.
‡Rarely recommended.

Tetanus-Diphtheria. After the initial series, boosters should be given every 10 years. Many of the now-independent former Soviet states have experienced diphtheria outbreaks, which can be life-threatening but are vaccine preventable. A newer formulation of tetanus vaccine now includes both diphtheria and an acellular pertussis component (Tdap). This is the current recommendation of the ACIP when booster doses are needed.

Influenza Vaccine. Influenza vaccine should be given every fall to those older than 65 years or younger people with chronic disease. Of note, the peak influenza incidence in the Southern Hemisphere is during their winter season, June through August.

Pneumococcal Vaccine. Pneumococcal vaccine should be given to all persons older than 65 years.

Polio Vaccine. A single booster of inactivated poliovirus vaccine provides lifelong protection in adults who have received the primary series. The exceedingly rare reports of wild-type polio in the Western Hemisphere make the vaccine optional for travel there. Polio is a viral disease transmitted by oral contamination. Rare outbreaks in Africa and Asia are reinforcing the recommendation for adult travelers to receive a booster before travel to certain destinations.

Measles Vaccine. For travelers born after 1957, a second measles booster, if not previously given, should be considered, given the high prevalence of measles in the developing world. As recent as 2006, mumps outbreaks in the United States and measles (rubeola) in Germany indicate, even travel to developed countries may pose certain vaccine-preventable risks. Two doses of vaccine at least 28 days apart are considered protective for measles, mumps, and rubella (MMR).

Hepatitis A Vaccine. Hepatitis A vaccine is highly recommended for almost all international travelers. Hepatitis A is prevalent and is spread through contaminated food and water. This inactivated virus vaccine achieves 80% to 98% immunity within 15 days after one intramuscular dose.[10] A booster dose at 6 months provides prolonged immunity for up to 10 years or longer. Minimal arm soreness at the site of injection and self-limited headaches are occasionally reported. Safety and efficacy have been shown in patients as young as 1 year of age. Good data support the efficacy of the vaccine, even when given immediately before travel, obviating the need for immune globulin.[11] A combination hepatitis A and B vaccine (Twinrix) produces higher titers to each agent compared with univalent vaccine (see elsewhere in this text, "Hepatitis A").

Hepatitis B Vaccine. Hepatitis B vaccine was recently added to the routine vaccine schedule for children. However, unvaccinated adults typically receive this vaccine only when they expect high-risk exposure to blood or body fluids. The schedule, three shots over 6 months, does not make this vaccine "travel friendly." Travelers planning extended travel to developing countries, or traveling to adopt a child from an endemic area, may benefit from vaccination. Accelerated protocols to achieve protective immunity within four weeks exist using combination hepatitis A and B vaccine.[12] A booster at twelve months was performed in the study participants.

Vaccinations by Travel Medicine Specialists. Some travelers to high-risk areas need vaccinations against meningococcus, yellow fever, and typhoid. These three are generally well-tolerated vaccines. Uncommon diseases such as anthrax, rabies, plague, and Japanese encephalitis are also preventable with immunizations. However, because of the rarity of these diseases and the fairly significant local side effects of their vaccines, these vaccines should only be used for travelers at especially high risk.[9] Knowing when to give these vaccines requires the expertise of a travel health specialist.

Meningococcal vaccination is recommenced for the "meningitis belt" of sub-Saharan Africa and other focal areas, depending on disease prevalence. Physicians must review travel health advisories frequently to stay abreast of this critical information. Because of crowded conditions and extensive international mingling, this vaccine is required for all pilgrims on the Hajj and Umrah to Mecca.

Yellow fever occurs throughout most of urban and rural South America and Africa. The live attenuated vaccine is highly effective, but can only be given at a state-approved center. Although direct travel to a nonendemic area requires no vaccinations, some countries require proof of vaccination before entry if the traveler's itinerary includes any areas of possible yellow fever exposure.[9] Hence, most travelers to South America and Africa need to go to a travel clinic that can give yellow fever vaccine.

The recommendation for typhoid vaccination is itinerary-specific. The original inactivated vaccine had a high incidence of bothersome reactions. Currently, an oral live attenuated typhoid vaccine (*Salmonella typhi* Ty21a) and an improved, inactivated, injectable typhoid vaccine (Vi antigen) are available. Special instructions are needed for the oral vaccine, including avoiding coadministration of antibiotics.

General Issues Related to Travel Vaccination

Coadministration. Multiple vaccinations are often recommended for travel to developing countries. This raises important practical issues about vaccine coadministration. Inactivated vaccines can be given on the same day without altering their immunogenicity,[9] although local reactions such as arm soreness may be greater when this is done. Studies have revealed that diphtheria, pertussis, and tetanus, inactivated poliomyelitis vaccine (or oral poliovirus vaccine), *Hemophilus influenzae* type b, measles, mumps, and rubella, and hepatitis B vaccine may all be given on the same day, with consistent efficacy.

In theory, live virus vaccines may impair the immune responses of each other, and it is suggested that they be given more than 30 days apart. The live attenuated yellow fever and oral poliovirus vaccines are not affected by coadministration.

Immunoglobulin. If it is necessary to give immunoglobulin for passive antibody protection, inactivated vaccines may be given at the same time with no impact on their efficacy. MMR vaccine is best given at least 14 days after immunoglobulin, and 6 months after whole blood or red blood cell transfusion.

Adverse Reactions. The most typical adverse reaction is arm soreness. It is often helpful for the traveler to take acetaminophen regularly for 2 to 3 days after vaccine administration to diminish local arm soreness. The most common adverse allergic vaccine reaction is an egg protein allergy. Because influenza vaccine is developed in embryonic chicken eggs, as is the yellow fever vaccine (see later), caution must be exercised. Also, measles and mumps vaccines are developed in chicken embryo cell cultures. In general, if patients can eat eggs and egg products without reaction, they can receive the vaccines without reaction. Protocols exist to enable vaccination of patients with significant allergy.[13]

Rare patients are allergic to the vaccine antigen, animal proteins, antibiotics, preservatives, or stabilizers used in vaccine preparations. No currently recommended vaccines contain penicillin or penicillin derivatives. MMR vaccine contains trace amounts of neomycin. However, almost all those with neomycin "allergy" actually show a delayed-type hypersensitivity contact dermatitis rather than a systemic allergic response.[9] This reaction is not a contraindication to receiving the vaccine.

Rare anaphylactic reactions to diphtheria and tetanus vaccines have been reported. Skin testing to tetanus toxoid is available to determine whether a patient truly has this sensitivity.

SPECIFIC CONDITIONS

The six leading health problems of travelers are listed in Box 2. Motor vehicle accidents are the leading cause of morbidity and mortality in travelers. Traveler's diarrhea and hepatitis A are examples of common food- and water-borne illnesses. Malaria is a vector-borne illness, and gonorrhea is a sexually transmitted disease. Although routes of acquisition vary, most of these disorders are preventable.

Motor Vehicle Accidents

Motor vehicle accidents remain the leading cause of accidents and mortality around the world for travelers. Hence, the most life-affecting advice we give is to buckle up and drive defensively. When renting a car overseas, travelers should specifically request one with seat belts; they are not standard equipment in all countries. Moreover, taking safety precautions while driving limits the risk of a significant accident with trauma that may require a blood transfusion in a setting in which the blood supply is not necessarily safe.

Traveler's Diarrhea

Traveler's diarrhea is a clinical entity defined as three or more loose or watery stools within 24 hours, associated with one or more additional constitutional symptoms, including crampy abdominal pain, nausea, or both.[6] Most cases are acute, watery, and self limited, without dysenteric or chronic symptoms. Causes of watery diarrhea include bacteria (>80% of cases), viruses, and parasites. Enterotoxigenic *Escherichia coli* is the leading bacterial pathogen (Box 3). Other causes vary by geographic location and time of year. Chronic diarrhea is usually nonbloody, without fever, but extends over a few weeks (Box 4). Dysentery or bloody diarrhea accounts for up to 15% of cases of traveler's diarrhea. Bloody stools indicate a more invasive process, referred to as dysentery, which has an overlapping but slightly different list of causative organisms. Fever more often accompanies dysentery.

Box 2 Leading Health Problems of International Travelers*

Motor vehicle accidents
Diarrhea
Malaria
Upper respiratory tract infection
Hepatitis A
Gonorrhea

**Listed in order of frequency.*

Box 3 Pathogens Associated With Acute Diarrhea in Travelers

Watery Diarrhea
Enterotoxigenic *Escherichia coli*
Salmonella species
Shigella species
Campylobacter species
Vibrio spp., including *V. cholera*
Noroviruses

Dysentery
Shigella species
Salmonella species
Campylobacter species
E. *coli* O157:H7
Entamoeba histolytica

Avoiding Foodborne and Water-borne Illnesses

Some precautions can make eating overseas much safer. Travelers should be counseled to adhere to the following recommendations:

- Choose foods that are thoroughly and recently cooked, not reheated.
- Wash all fruits and vegetable with clean water before slicing them, to avoid carrying bacteria into the otherwise clean inside layers. Raw fruits and vegetables peeled by travelers are usually safe.
- When dining out, where one has less control over food preparation, avoid raw meat, fish, and vegetables, especially salads. Street vendor food is risky unless properly prepared in front of you. Caution must even be exercised regarding airline food prepared in lesser developed countries.
- Avoid drinking tap water; even hotel tap water used for brushing teeth can be a source of infection. Ice should be considered contaminated, including ice cubes on flights that originate in developing countries. Commercially prepared bottled or canned beverages are usually safe alternatives to water.
- Purify drinking water by boiling it, treating it with halogens (chlorine or iodine), or filtering it when reliably clean water is not available. Water brought just to a boil before cooling is generally as safe as water boiled for several minutes.[6] Compared with boiling, halogen treatment is less likely to remove parasites. Because halogens are most effective in clear water, cloudy water should first be allowed to settle until clear. Filters are somewhat expensive, but effective. The combination of halogen treatment and filtering is almost as good as boiling.

Box 4 Causes of Chronic Diarrhea in Travelers

Pathogens

- *Giardia lamblia*
- *Entamoeba histolytica*
- *Cryptosporidium*
- *Cyclospora*
- *Schistosoma mansoni*
- *Schistosoma japonicum*

Malabsorption
Tropical sprue

In summary, regarding food and water precautions, the CDC has developed a simple rule of thumb: "Boil it, cook it, peel it, or forget it."

Prophylaxis

Prophylactic antibiotic use is generally discouraged.[14] Widespread medication use increases the likelihood of side effects, including photosensitivity, vaginal and superficial fungal infections, and severe drug reactions, such as Stevens-Johnson syndrome. It is a nuisance to take a medication every day for a condition that may not develop. Prophylactic medication use may also lead to a false sense of security, resulting in decreased compliance with the more important and effective general recommendations for food and water precautions. Finally, antibiotic resistance is a growing problem, with well-documented examples among diarrheal pathogens. Prophylactic antibiotic use is more likely to induce resistance than the occasional treatment regimens outlined below.

Diagnosis

The diagnosis is clinical. The categorization of routine traveler's diarrhea versus dysentery versus chronic diarrhea has been noted earlier.

Treatment

Dehydration is the major health risk. Oral rehydration solutions containing both carbohydrates or sugar and salt are optimum as fluid replacement. Patients can prepare their own inexpensive solutions, using simple and available ingredients (Fig. 1). The cereal-based formula provides four times as many calories as the glucose-based recipe, and may help decrease the stool volume and duration of diarrhea.[6] Ricelyte, a fully prepared cereal-based oral rehydration solution, can be purchased over the counter.

The principle behind oral rehydration is that glucose facilitates water absorption, and sodium absorption is coupled with glucose absorption. Too much sugar inhibits water absorption and can actually cause water loss via osmotic diarrhea. An ideal glucose concentration for water absorption is about 2.5%. Many drinks, such as

How to Use Oral Rehydration Solutions

If you have more than 3 to 4 episodes of diarrhea per day, you may be in danger of becoming dehydrated. In this situation, you should seek medical attention, or take the medication your physician has already provided to stop the diarrhea. In addition, you should replenish your body fluids by drinking an oral rehydration solution, which you can buy ready-made or prepare yourself.

Cereal-Based Recipe (preferred)

1 to 2 cups rice cereal for infants (e.g., Gerber)
4 cups clean water (boiled or chemically purified)
1/2 teaspoon table salt

Mix salt and water in a clean container. Gradually stir in rice cereal.

Glucose-Based Recipe (use if rice cereal is not available)

4 1/2 cups clean water (boiled or chemically purified)
1/4 teaspoon salt substitute that contains potassium
1/2 teaspoon baking soda
1/2 teaspoon table salt (increase to 1 teaspoon table salt if the salt substitute and baking soda are not available)
2 to 3 tablespoons glucose (table sugar, honey, or corn syrup)

Mix all the ingredients together in a clean container.

With either recipe you may need to drink up to 3 to 6 quarts over 2 to 4 hours to counteract dehydration. Be sure to drink 8 to 12 ounces after each watery stool. If you are nauseated, begin with 1-ounce sips every 5 to 10 minutes, and increase the amount as tolerated.

Figure 1 **How to use oral rehydration solutions.** *(Adapted from Rose SR: International Travel Health Guide, 13th ed. Northampton, Mass, Travel Medicine, 2002.)*

apple juice, cola, sports drinks, and flavored gelatin contain about 6% glucose. These drinks can be diluted by adding approximately 1.5 volumes of water. It is important to dilute with clean (bottled, boiled, or chemically treated) or sterile water to avoid an increased infectious burden or secondary infection.

Untreated, traveler's diarrhea (TD) usually remits spontaneously in 3 to 5 days. Antibiotics often diminish the symptoms of traveler's diarrhea to approximately 1 day, and the addition of loperamide (Imodium) may further reduce the duration of symptoms to less than 1 day.[14] However, loperamide therapy should be avoided if the diarrhea is bloody or fever is present (dysentery). These symptoms should also be used as indicators to seek local medical attention, because they may indicate a more serious medical condition. Symptom-initiated antibiotic treatment is usually effective when taken for 1 to 5 days.[6]

Several options for pharmacologic therapy include bismuth subsalicylate, ciprofloxacin, azithromycin, furazolidone (Furoxone), and rifaximin (Xifaxan). Although bismuth subsalicylate can be effective as prophylaxis and treatment, the large doses required make it impractical. It also binds to antibiotics and limits their effectiveness. The quinolones are rapidly effective for the common causes of traveler's diarrhea. Furazolidone is not as rapidly effective as the quinolones, but can be given to children and has anti-*Giardia* activity (when given for 7-10 days) not seen with the other antibiotics. More recent data make azithromycin an attractive option for children and quinolone-allergic adults.[15] Rifaximin is a newly approved nonabsorbable antibiotic. It is indicated for persons older than 12 years with TD caused by noninvasive strains of *E. coli*. The narrow spectrum of rifaximin and recent availability of generic ciprofloxacin continue to make quinolones my preference for episodic self treatment of TD in adults. Emergence of quinolone-resistant diarrheal pathogens, especially in South Asia, reinforces the need for updated expertise and itinerary-specific recommendations.

Recommendations

I currently recommend ciprofloxacin, twice daily for 3 days, as symptom-initiated treatment for traveler's diarrhea in adults.[6,14] Some newer quinolones such as levofloxacin (Levaquin) may induce more photosensitivity, making them less attractive for travelers. Azithromycin (Zithromax) is a current alternative for children or for those unable to tolerate quinolones, although not U.S. Food and Drug Administration (FDA)-approved for this indication (Table 1).

Table 1 Recommended Medications for Acute Traveler's Diarrhea

Medication	Age Group	Dosage*
Ciprofloxacin (Cipro)	Adults	500 mg twice daily
Ofloxacin (Floxin)	Adults	400 mg twice daily
Azithromycin (Zithromax)	Adults	500 mg once daily
	Children >6 mo	10 mg/kg once daily (max 500 mg/day)
Furazolidone (Furoxone)	Adults	100 mg four times daily
	5-17 yr	25-50 mg four times daily
	1-4 yr	15-25 mg four times daily
	1 mo-1 yr	7-15 mg four times daily

*All medications are recommended for 3 days for this indication (range 1 to 5 days).
Furazolidone duration is 7 to 10 days when treating *Giardia lamblia*.

Chronic Diarrhea

Rarely, travelers experience chronic diarrhea, often with weight loss and malabsorption.[16] Because the pathogens responsible are often not self limited and not sensitive to quinolone antibiotics (see Box 4), further medical care is necessary. These patients typically present to their primary care physician after returning home. Physicians should identify the causative agent and give pathogen-specific therapy in this situation. Dysentery is a serious medical condition. Again, it is important to make a specific diagnosis. Dysentery should be managed under the direct supervision of a physician.

Malaria

This review of travel medicine will not review classic malaria disease issues, but rather will focus on its prevention in international travelers. Each year, more than 7 million Americans travel to countries in which malaria is common.[6] There are 1000 to 1500 reported cases (underreporting is common) of malaria each year, with the greatest number (≤83%) coming after travel to East Africa.[6] Most mosquitoes that transmit malaria are found in rural areas, in contrast to those that transmit yellow fever. Therefore, travel to major urban areas usually does not pose a risk for malaria, but even short trips to rural areas may place travelers at risk.

Avoiding mosquitoes is the first objective. Travelers should use insect repellents and mosquito nets and consider staying indoors in the evening, which is the peak biting time for malaria-carrying mosquitoes. Soaking bed netting and clothing in permethrin can significantly reduce mosquito bites. Permethrin is colorless and odorless and remains active even after laundering. Diethyltoluamide (DEET) is one of the most widely recommended repellents. The product should contain 30% to 50% diethyltoluamide. Products with higher concentrations (≤100% diethyltoluamide) are not necessary and could, rarely, cause serious side effects, especially in young children. Microencapsulated preparations are still effective with the least systemic absorption. A new repellent, picaridin, has efficacy similar to diethyltoluamide when compared on a percentage active ingredient basis. Note that dark clothing, cologne, and perfume attract mosquitoes. Early enthusiasm for Skin-So-Soft, a moisturizing bath oil, has not been borne out as an effective insect repellent.

Given the potential severity of malaria, additional measures are prudent, including prophylaxis.

Prophylactic Drugs

No effective vaccines against malaria are currently available, but prophylactic medications dramatically reduce the risk. To select these medications, physicians need current data on the resistance patterns and relative risk of malaria in the country of destination, and knowledge of side effects and contraindications. The complexity of these considerations mandates referral to a traveler's clinic. Drug resistance and specific travel plans are major reasons to choose one medication over another.

Chloroquine (Aralen) is the oldest, safest, and best tolerated of the available medications. It is safe throughout pregnancy (although pregnant women should avoid malaria-infested areas, if at all possible). Unfortunately, chloroquine-resistant strains of malaria are increasing, nearly all of them in *Plasmodium falciparum*, the most deadly of the parasites that cause malaria. Consequently, the areas of the world where chloroquine is still useful are continually shrinking and now include only Central America, the Caribbean, and limited parts of the Middle East and China.

Mefloquine (Lariam) is an alternative drug in areas of chloroquine resistance. Mefloquine can have unpleasant side effects of dizziness, anxiety, insomnia, and nightmares, which have been much publicized in recent travel literature.[17] However, a similar incidence of central nervous system reactions was noted among Peace Corps volunteers who took chloroquine.[18] Mefloquine reactions are more common in young adults than in older adults and children, and are potentiated by alcohol. The drug should be avoided in patients with a history of seizures or psychiatric disorders. Fairly extensive worldwide use has documented relatively safe use in the second and third trimesters of pregnancy. Because mefloquine works against the blood stage of malaria, which may take up to 4 weeks to appear after a bite, mefloquine must be continued for 4 weeks after leaving a malarial area.

Doxycycline (Vibramycin) is an alternative for patients traveling to areas with chloroquine resistance who are unable or unwilling to take mefloquine.[6,9] However, it must be taken every day, compared with once a week for mefloquine, making it less convenient. Like mefloquine, doxycycline must be taken for 4 weeks after travel. In addition, doxycycline causes a higher incidence of photosensitization reactions, which can be particularly troublesome in sunny tropical countries. It also causes a slightly higher incidence of vaginal yeast infections. On the other hand, it may prevent traveler's diarrhea. Of note, doxycycline is contraindicated throughout pregnancy and for children younger than 8 years.

Combined atovaquone-proguanil (Malarone) is the newest antimalarial drug on the market and is an alternative to mefloquine and doxycycline. It is active against chloroquine-resistant malarial organisms. Daily dosing ensures that a therapeutic level is reached quickly. If an extended trip has a very short segment with malaria exposure, it enables focused preventive treatment starting 1 or 2 days before entering the area. Because it works in the liver, it needs to be taken for only 1 week after leaving a malarial area. It should not be used as prophylaxis during pregnancy or in patients with renal failure.

To ensure the best effect, and because this drug can cause gastrointestinal upset, it should be taken with food or a milk-type drink or dairy product (e.g., milk, milkshake, yogurt), according to the package insert. It is crucial to recall that all such dairy products need to be pasteurized to be safe.

Signs and Symptoms

The onset of malaria can resemble a viral infection, with a fever persisting for several days and possibly weeks. The classic picture consists of shaking chills, with a very high fever and profuse sweating. The patient may also experience joint pain, nausea, vomiting, loss of energy, and headaches. After the acute malarial attack has passed, the disease may become chronic with occasional relapses if the infection is caused by a form with a relapsing liver stage (*Plasmodium vivax* or *P. malariae*, but not *P. falciparum*). An attack is sometimes difficult to recognize in infants and small children with no symptoms other than loss of appetite, extreme fatigue, and agitation. If a parent believes that he or she or their child is suffering an attack of malaria, expert medical assistance should be sought.

It is also important to note that the initial symptoms of malaria may occur up to 1 year after exposure. with or without preventive measures. Thus, it is necessary to emphasize the importance of patients reminding their doctor that they have traveled to an area with malaria when they are evaluated for a fever.

Upper Respiratory Tract Infections

Upper respiratory infections (URIs) are common throughout the world. Traveling brings a large number of people in contact with each other, probably accounting for the perception of increased respiratory illness when traveling. Although air is recirculated on commercial airliners, it is highly filtered, making it unlikely for a traveler to acquire a respiratory infection from another passenger. The few documented cases of severe respiratory infection acquired on airplanes are from people sitting in close proximity to the index patient on long flights.[19] It is often wise to bring a favorite over-the-counter URI medication because selection and availability are unpredictable when traveling.

Severe acute respiratory syndrome (SARS) is an emerging infectious disease caused by a variant of coronavirus, a common cold virus.[20] Its clinical manifestations are highly consistent with those of upper respiratory viral infections, including fever, cough, shortness of breath, and a short incubation period, typically less then 10 days. Unfortunately, SARS appears to have a much higher mortality rate, making it especially concerning. Proper attention to routine public health measures, such as hand washing and general hygiene can significantly minimize risk of infection. The additional use of face masks, especially National Institute for Occupational Safety and Health (NIOSH)-certified N95 fitted masks, can further reduce exposure when contact with a potentially infectious person is more likely. Regular surgical masks may provide some measure of protection, but the exact amount is uncertain. The 2004 SARS epidemic has abated, but it had a chilling affect on international travel during that time. In many ways, this changing nature of human health and its impact on our global world only reinforce the benefit of consultation with specialized international traveler's health clinics before trips abroad. Itinerary review and updates on the latest information help maximize the likelihood of a healthy, productive, and enjoyable travel experience.

Influenza has been an occasional problem at some travel destinations, or rarely on some cruise lines. The issue is usually seasonal, but international travel can alter the usual timing of its occurrence. Older and immunocompromised travelers might consider adding prescription, oral, anti-influenza medication to take in case of exposure, which can be discussed with their travel health advisor. The recent concern regarding avian influenza, or "bird flu," deserves mention. It is a rare disease contracted by those living in close contact with birds, chickens, and ducks. Average international travelers are at limited risk of disease. Precautions to take include avoiding close contact with live birds, eating only fully cooked poultry products, and paying attention to hand hygiene. Helpful information can be found at www.travel.state.gov/travel/tips/health/health_1181.html. Avian influenza pandemic concerns have prompted global efforts to institute pandemic preparedness measures. Information on the U.S. government's overall response is available at www.pandemicflu.gov.

Sexually Transmitted Diseases

With gonorrhea among the top five diseases of international travelers and with HIV infection on the rise,[21] physicians should counsel their patients about the risks and available prophylactic measures for sexually transmitted diseases. However, not all patients will follow this advice. A survey of more than 3000 Swiss travelers to developing counties found that 87% complied with recommended malaria chemoprophylaxis but, remarkably, 50% of the same travelers engaged in casual sex abroad, usually with a partner from the host country.[22] Of the sexual encounters, 38% were unprotected, even though the travelers shared similar knowledge about the risks of HIV virus and other sexually transmitted diseases compared with malaria. Of note, those who engaged in high-risk sexual practices were not the same group who were noncompliant with malaria protective measures.

PATIENTS WITH MEDICAL CONDITIONS

If a patient with a preexisting medical condition is planning an international trip, the physician should ask about the destination and type of trip to decide whether special considerations are necessary. Examples include high-altitude destinations and adventure travel. In addition, some patients, such as those with diabetes, need special diets.[6] Travelers with disabilities have special needs, and more resources are now available to facilitate enjoyable travel. (See later, "Resources for Travelers," which includes helpful references for travelers with disabilities and special medical needs, including the location of dialysis centers.) I strongly encourage independent research to ensure that patients with disabilities plan ahead for their unique needs.

In general, patients with medical conditions should:

- Keep their medications in their original containers to avoid customs delays.
- Take along an epinephrine injection kit if they have severe allergies to foods or insect stings, unless this is otherwise contraindicated.
- Consider taking a copy of their electrocardiogram, a recent medical summary, and the telephone number of their primary care physician in case a treating physician abroad needs to contact them. A list of English-speaking physicians around the world is available from the International Association for Medical Assistance to Travelers, 417 Center Street, Lewiston, NY 14092, 716-754-4883).
- Investigate exactly what their insurance policies cover during travel overseas:
  - Medicare, for example, does not cover medical expenses outside the United States.
  - Supplemental insurance is usually available and is wise to consider.
  - Most pretravel medical evaluations and vaccinations are not covered by medical insurance plans. However, updating patients on routine immunizations, which further protect them overseas, may be covered.

Special Considerations for Coronary Artery Bypass Surgery Patients

Of note, a growing number of international travelers have previously undergone coronary artery bypass grafting (CABG). A survey of 10,000 post-CABG patients has found that 40% had traveled recently to a domestic or foreign location.[23] There was a very low incidence of myocardial infarction or hospitalization during the trip. The only identified health concern was that older post-CABG patients had slightly more shortness of breath when they traveled to Mexico and South America compared with other destinations, probably because of the higher altitudes of many destinations in Central and South America.[22]

CONCLUSION

The goal of travel medicine is to allow the patient to enjoy a long-awaited vacation or work productively when on an important business trip. The needs of travelers to developing countries are unique. To ensure a safe and enjoyable trip, special pretravel counseling and immunizations are usually necessary. Primary care physicians are often the first to be contacted about plans for international travel. Therefore, they can initiate care and select those needing referral to a travel medicine clinic. Understanding the background issues related to the international traveler will facilitate patient care and the referral process. Bon voyage!

Summary

- Basic precautions with food and drinking water are necessary in developing countries. Most cases of traveler's diarrhea respond to a short course of quinolone antibiotics and oral fluid replacement.
- Travelers to countries where malaria is endemic should work to avoid contact with mosquitoes and should take chloroquine, mefloquine, chloroguanide (Malarone), or doxycycline prophylactically. Unfortunately, chloroquine resistance is increasing.
- With gonorrhea among the top five diseases in international travelers and with HIV infection on the rise, physicians should counsel their patients about the risks and prophylactic measures available for sexually transmitted diseases.
- Primary care physicians should make sure that travelers are up to date in their routine immunizations before going abroad; however, immunizations for rare and travel-related diseases are best left to experts in travel medicine. Almost all travelers should be vaccinated against hepatitis A.
- The single most important health advice to travelers is to wear seat belts. When renting a car, travelers should specifically request one with seat belts, not standard equipment in all countries.

Suggested Readings

Centers for Disease Control and Prevention: Travel Notice Definitions, 2004. Available at http://wwwn.cdc.gov/travel/notices.aspx#TravelNoticeDefinitions (accessed March 9, 2009).

Centers for Disease Control and Prevention. Health Information for International Travel, 2008 (The Yellow Book). Philadelphia, Elsevier, 2007.

DuPont HL, Capsuto EG: Persistent diarrhea in travelers. Clin Infect Dis 1996;22:124-128.

Franco E, Giambi C, Ialacci R, Maurici M: Prevention of hepatitis A by vaccination. Expert Opin Biol Ther 2003;3:965-974.

Hill DR, Ericsson CD, Pearson RD, et al: The Practice of Travel Medicine: Guidelines by the Infectious Diseases Society of America. Clin Infec Dis 2006; 43:1499-1539. Available at www.journals.uchicago.edu/doi/pdf/10.1086/508782 (accessed March 9, 2009).

Keystone JS, Dismukes R, Sawyer L, Kozarsky PE: Inadequacies in health recommendations provided for international travelers by North American travel health advisors. J Travel Med 1994;1:72-78.

Mardh PA: What is travel medicine? Content, current position, tools, and tasks. J Travel Med 2002;9:34-47.

Paulson E: Travel statement on jet lag. Can Med Assoc J 1996;155:61-66.

Peiris JS, Yuen KY, Osterhaus AD, Stöhr K: Current concepts: The severe acute respiratory syndrome. N Engl J Med 2003;349:2431-2441.

Pickering L (ed): 2000 Redbook: Report of the Committee on Infectious Diseases. American Academy of Pediatrics, 2000.

Public Health Agency of Canada: Travel health: Know before you go! Available at www.phac-aspc.gc.ca/tmp-pmv/index-eng.php (accessed March 9, 2009).

Steffen R: The epidemiologic basis for the practice of travel medicine. In Lobel HO, Steffen R, Kozarsky PE (eds): Travel Medicine 2. Proceedings of the Second Conference on International Travel Medicine. Atlanta, International Society of Travel Medicine, 1992, pp 11-14.

Yates J: Traveler's diarrhea. Am Fam Physician 2005;71:2095-2100.

Resources for Travelers

Books About Travel Medicine and Personal Safety

Centers for Disease Control and Prevention: Health Information for International Travel, 2008 (The Yellow Book). Philadelphia, Elsevier, 2007.

Dawood R (ed): Travelers' Health: How to Stay Healthy Abroad. New York, Random House, 2002.

Jong EC, McMullen R (eds): The Travel and Tropical Medicine Manual, 3rd ed. Philadelphia, WB Saunders, 2003.

Keystone JS, Kozarsky PE, Freedman DO, et al (eds): Travel Medicine. New York, Mosby, 2004.

Rose SR, Keystone JS: 2006 International Travel Health Guide, 13th ed. New York, Mosby, 2006.

Savage PV: The Safe Travel Book. New York, Lexington Books, 1993.

Scotti AJ: Executive Safety and International Terrorism: A Guide for Travellers. Englewood Cliffs, NJ, Prentice-Hall, 1986.

Worring RW, Hibbard WS, Schroeder S: Travel Safely at Home and Abroad: Don't Be a Target! Helena, Mont, Uniquest Publications, 1996.

Electronic Resources

Centers for Disease Control and Prevention: Travel definitions. Available at http://wwwn.cdc.gov/travel (accessed March 9, 2009); 877-FYI-TRIP; Fax, 888-232-3299.

U.S. Department of State: http://www.travel.state.gov; Overseas Citizens Services, 888-407-4747; from overseas, 202 501 4444.

World Health Organization: http://www.who.int/topics/travel/en.

Newsletters and Periodicals

Consumer Reports Travel Letter, Consumers Union, 101 Truman Ave, Yonkers, NY 10703; 914-378-2000 or 800-234-1645.

Diabetic Traveler Newsletter, Box 8223 RW, Stamford, Conn 06905; 203-327-5832.

Kidney Dialysis Abroad

International Directory of Dialysis Centers. Creative Age Publications, 7628 Densmore Avenue, Van Nuys, Calif 91406; 800-442-5667 or 818-782-7328.

Dialysis Centers Around the World: http://www.globaldialysis.com.

Disability Travel Sites

General access information for the disabled: http://www.access-able.com.

Travel for hearing-impaired people: http://www.sath.org/index.php?sec=768&id=2213.

United Kingdom-based broad listing of information for disabled travelers: http://www.direct.gov.uk/DisabledPeople/fs/en.

U.S. Government Architectural and Transportation Barriers Compliance Board (Access-Board) produces and distributes a variety of publications for travelers with disabilities: http://www.access-board.gov (information can also be obtained via telephone, 800-872-2253 [voice] or 800-993-2822 [TTY]).

Wheelchair travel-oriented website: http://www.disabilitytravel.com.

Wilderness Medicine

Auerbach PS (ed): Wilderness Medicine, 5th ed. St. Louis, Mosby, 2007.

Auerbach PS, Donner H, Weiss E (eds): Field Guide to Wilderness Medicine, 2nd ed. St. Louis, Mosby, 2003.

Houston CS: Going Higher: The Story of Man and Altitude. Boston, Little, Brown, 1987.

Kennedy B: Caring for Children in the Outdoors. Oakland, Calif, Adventure Medical Kits, 1994.

References

For a complete list of references, log onto www.expertconsult.com.

The Microbiology Laboratory and the Internist

Anthony K. Leung and Gary W. Procop

GENERAL PRINCIPLES

Clinical laboratories play a vital part in health care in the United States. Traditionally, clinical laboratories are comprised of the following sections: blood banking, chemistry, hematology, and microbiology. In a university or academic setting, these laboratories are usually under the department of clinical pathology, with the supervision of a board-certified pathologist or microbiologist. Many independent commercial laboratories are now available to provide timely and reliable services to clinicians and hospitals when such services are not locally available. With the advent of molecular and genomic medicine, newer divisions and subspecialties have been created within the arena of clinical pathology. For example, some larger academic and research institutions have divisions that specialize in incorporating molecular methods into their practice.

The primary role of a microbiology laboratory in patient care is to aid clinicians in identifying causative agents of various infectious diseases and help determine the antimicrobial susceptibility profiles, when appropriate.[1] The information provided by the microbiology laboratory enables the clinicians to initiate or modify therapy, which will have a direct impact on patient outcome. The role of the laboratory begins when patient specimens are received in the laboratory; the laboratory should process and handle the specimens appropriately and in a timely fashion—that is, in a manner that ensures that the integrity of the specimen will not be compromised. Depending on the type of specimens and tests requested, the specimens will be worked up accordingly by performing different testing procedures, and accurate and reproducible results will be generated. Clinicians will then use the information obtained to make clinical decisions and initiate treatment options best suited for that particular patient. To facilitate the process, it is of the utmost importance that clear communication exists between the clinician placing the order and the laboratory professionals performing the tests. This communication is critical because it facilitates efficient use of laboratory resources, as well as improving turnaround time for test results.

Ideally, the microbiology laboratory should be under the supervision of a physician or laboratory scientist with expertise in both infectious diseases and microbiology. The insight provided by such a laboratory-based professional helps ensure that quality and clinically relevant information will be provided to health care providers in a timely manner. The microbiology laboratory should be in compliance with the rules and regulations established by the College of American Pathologists (CAP), Clinical Laboratory Improvement Amendments (CLIA) and the Joint Commission (formerly called the Joint Commission on Accreditation of Healthcare Organizations). An accredited microbiology laboratory should be routinely inspected by the CAP or the Joint Commission, to ensure that all standardized laboratory methods and procedures are being followed. Many safety aspects of operating a laboratory will also be evaluated during such an inspection.

CLIA-88 was passed in Congress in 1988 and the final regulations were published in 1992. The purpose of this legislation was to establish that all laboratories that perform clinical testing should provide timely, reliable, and accurate results to clinicians and patients, regardless of where the test was performed. This act has defined that laboratory tests fall under three categories—waived complexity, moderate complexity, and high complexity. Tests that require moderate and high complexity must be performed in a certified laboratory by trained medical technologists. Some of the tests currently available in the marketplace are CLIA waived, which means that testing can be performed outside a laboratory setting. Some examples of these include home pregnancy tests, which may be purchased directly by the consumer (i.e., sold over the counter) and rapid HIV-1 and HIV-2 antibody tests, which can be performed in an outpatient clinic or emergency room.

Medical technologists are an integral part of a microbiology laboratory. These technologists usually possess a baccalaureate degree and have received additional training in accredited medical technology programs in hospitals, colleges, or universities. On completion of this training, they must take the certifying examination offered by the American Society of Clinical Pathologists (ASCP). Only after they have achieved the appropriate certification can the technologist start working in an accredited laboratory. Some technologists choose to be a generalist, meaning that they can rotate to different sections of the laboratory, such as chemistry and microbiology, and perform different assays; conversely, they may elect to specialize in one particular area to gain further experience and expertise.

Communication between the microbiology laboratory and clinicians remains the most important aspect of patient care. The role of the laboratory is to provide advice and guidance to clinicians to optimize specimen collection. Therefore, the laboratory should provide easy access of such information to clinicians and also clearly state the rejection criteria for various tests. With the advent of communication tools such as the Internet, critical clinical information can be provided to clinicians efficiently and in a timely fashion.

It is also prudent to remember that the role of the microbiology laboratory is to identify the causative agent from various specimens, which in turn aids the clinicians to make or confirm a diagnosis, or both. However, it should also be emphasized that the laboratory is providing *clinically* relevant and useful information. Otherwise, if the information is misleading or inaccurate, inappropriate therapy may be prescribed to the patient. This would increase health care costs and expose patients to unwarranted treatment; unnecessary and overused antimicrobial therapy is an important cause of the emergence of antimicrobial resistance.

The following example illustrates this point. A patient with a chronic indwelling catheter for total parenteral nutrition (TPN) administration is admitted to the hospital for general malaise and tiredness. However, no fever is reported. The patient is seen in the emergency department and a single sample of blood is drawn from the catheter for culture while the patient is en route to being admitted to the hospital. Three days later, that single sample indicates growth and a preliminary Gram stain reveals gram-positive cocci in clusters. The diagnosis of catheter-related infection is made and vancomycin therapy is initiated. Subsequently, the isolate from the blood culture is identified as a coagulase-negative *Staphylococcus* and the clinician requests to have antimicrobial susceptibility testing performed on that isolate. Clinically, the patient is doing better after hydration, and repeated blood culture fails to demonstrate any evidence of catheter infection. The positive predictive value of a single sample for blood culture in this setting for a true infection is low; this isolate likely represents a contaminant, given that the isolated organism is a coagulase-negative *Staphylococcus* species. By providing the requested susceptibility, one assumes that the clinician has determined that this isolate is the cause of an infection and that the patient should be treated with an antimicrobial agent. However, in this scenario, no therapy is warranted and the patient improved after proper hydration and adjustment to the TPN formulation and discharged home. In such a case, vancomycin could have been discontinued on speciation of the blood isolate and antimicrobial susceptibility testing was unnecessary; both added to the health care costs, but also implied that the isolate was associated with a bloodstream infection. The usefulness of and issues regarding blood culture will be discussed in more detail.

SPECIMEN REQUIREMENTS

Regardless of the specimen type, it is important for the laboratory to receive an adequate amount of specimen for testing. Unfortunately, it is not uncommon for the laboratory to receive a single swab with requests for viral, aerobic and anaerobic bacterial, fungal, and mycobacterial cultures. The yield of a culture is directly proportional to the amount of specimen initially inoculated onto the primary recover medium. Therefore, to obtain optimal results, a sufficient amount of specimen should be submitted. For example, when submitting an aspirate of an abscess, the clinician should submit more than a few drops of fluid or a swab for culture. Insufficient quantity of specimen will affect the yield of final culture and produce false-negative culture results. The quantity issue is particularly significant if the suspected pathogen is a mycobacterium or filamentous fungus, for which swabs are unacceptable and usually a larger quantity of tissue, fluid, or aspirate is needed.

When the clinician submits specimens to the laboratory for testing, all relevant information, such as the date and time of collection, type of specimen, and brief clinical scenario should be provided on the requisition form. The information is helpful for the laboratory to determine which growth medium to use to optimize growth. In certain cases in which a particularly virulent organism is suspected, the form should clearly indicate this to alert the laboratory technologist to handle the specimens with special safety measures and precautions, such as using a biologic safety cabinet. For example, this should be done if *Brucella* or *Francisella* is suspected clinically, because Petri plates from wound and blood cultures are usually handled on the bench, rather than in a biologic safety cabinet. For some diseases, such as tularemia, caused by *Francisella tularensis*), serologic tests may be the preferred method of diagnosis rather than culture, given the highly contagious nature of this organism and the fastidious growth requirements in vitro. In addition, lymph nodes can be submitted for histopathologic examination, although at times it is difficult to separate tularemia from other granulomatous diseases such as tuberculosis and cat-scratch disease. Serology usually is the preferred method for diagnosing tularemia.

In addition to the issue of quantity, when submitting a specimen, it should be of a quality acceptable for testing. The microbiology laboratory should therefore clarify which types of specimens are acceptable for microbiologic testing. These rejection criteria should be written and be readily available to those collecting the specimens, as well as to the technicians responsible for their processing. A poor-quality specimen is of no use to anyone and may yield unreliable results that could potentially affect patient care. Poor-quality specimens may produce false-negative results, because true pathogens may be overgrown by normal flora, and false-positive results; also, a commensal potential pathogen may be mistaken for the true causative agent of disease.

Blood

Blood culture is the cornerstone of diagnosing many infectious diseases, and is of particular importance for determining the causative agent of endocarditis and other endovascular infections.[2] Different methods and commercial systems are now available for detecting microorganisms. Generally, the blood culture system uses a broth-based medium that supports the growth of aerobic and anaerobic bacteria, depending on the bottle type used, and also some fungi, predominantly yeasts.

A major reason for failing to detect microorganisms in the bloodstream is an inadequate sampling of blood volume. When the recommended blood volume is inoculated (10 mL/bottle for an adult) into the blood culture bottles, most of the bacteremic or fungemic episodes can be recovered from two or three sets of blood cultures.[2] The number of bottles used per draw and the number of draws per blood culture order can be confusing. A single blood culture order consists of two blood culture draws from different anatomic sites, preferably not through an IV catheter. Each of these draws, in turn, consists of filling two blood culture bottles with 10 mL of blood each; usually one aerobic and one anaerobic bottle comprise a blood culture set. It should be emphasized that the recommended volume of 20 to 30 mL is for *each* set of blood cultures, and that at least two sets are used for each blood culture order (i.e., four bottles total).

Further discussion is warranted regarding how many sets of blood cultures should be drawn to detect bacteremia, fungemia, or both in septic patients. A single set of blood cultures is inappropriate for detecting such septic episodes. Some of these are characterized by intermittent bacteremia, and a single set would not be sensitive enough to isolate the causative agent consistently. The clinical objective is to send enough blood to evaluate for microorganisms adequately, without sending so many sets as to produce iatrogenic anemia, which is a real risk in hospitalized patients undergoing numerous blood draws for various tests.

There is little controversy when highly pathogenic microorganisms such as *Staphylococcus aureus* or *Pseudomonas aeruginosa* are isolated from the bloodstream. However, a single set of blood cultures with coagulase-negative staphylococci, *Corynebacterium*, or other gram-positive bacteria consistent with skin flora could represent blood culture contaminants or a true infection (i.e., the positive predictive value of a single blood culture draw is low). In other words, it is difficult to determine the clinical significance of such blood culture findings, because these organisms are part of the normal human skin flora. Clarity may come from assessing the clinical findings in such patients. For example, the patient may have clear evidence of infection associated with an indwelling catheter site. In such a case, clinicians should have a high index of suspicion of an active case of infection, even if it is a single set of blood cultures. It would then be necessary to combine the clinical findings with other laboratory findings (e.g., an elevated neutrophil count) to help interpret the findings of the single blood culture set that turned positive with a common skin commensal.

It is recommended that what would truly be helpful here is an additional blood culture set. Drawing two blood cultures from different sites not only increases the volume sampled, but also helps diagnose infections caused by common skin commensals. The likelihood of a true infection being caused by one of these organisms is increased if more than one blood culture set is positive for the same type of organism—for example, two of two blood culture sets are all found to contain coagulase-negative staphylococci. This is especially true for patients with catheters; the isolation of coagulase-negative staphylococci could be a clue to a catheter-related infection, because its course is usually indolent. Thus, a good rule of thumb is that two or three sets of blood cultures with adequate blood volume should be used and can detect most cases of bacteremia and fungemia.

Prolonged incubation of blood cultures for the detection of fastidious or slow-growing bacteria is controversial. This was a common practice before the use of highly sensitive automated blood culture systems. The concept is to provide more time for the more fastidious organisms to grow, thereby increasing the chances of recovery. This was classically used to detect the HACEK organisms (*Haemophilus aphrophilus*, *Actinobacillus actinomycetemcomitans*, *Cardiobacterium hominis*, *Eikenella corrodens*, and *Kingella kingae*), which were well-described causes of "culture-negative" endocarditis. However, the newer blood culture system technology and improvements in blood culture media have resulted in recovery rates for these organisms that are almost as good as those for more common pyogenic bacteria, such as *Staphylococcus aureus*.[3] Nevertheless, some will still extend incubation or perform terminal subcultures if a fastidious pathogen is a suspected cause of endocarditis. In our experience, we have seen culture and biopsy-proven cases of *Propionibacterium acnes* endocarditis that grew only after extended incubation.

This matter is controversial because it is also well known that the longer a blood culture is incubated, the higher the likelihood that the organisms that grow will be a contaminant, particularly if it is part of the normal skin microbiota. The issue is that even small numbers of contaminating bacteria such as diphtheroids and coagulase-negative staphylococci will grow in the nutrient-rich environment of the blood culture bottle and, given enough time (i.e., extended incubation) will yield positive results. In such cases, these contaminants might be treated as true pathogens, thus exposing patients to unnecessary antibiotics and potentially increasing the length of hospital stay.

Sputum and Other Respiratory Tract Specimens

Diagnosing lower respiratory tract infections and pneumonia remains complicated and requires a combination of clinical and laboratory findings for optimal diagnosis. Expectorated sputum, even with its own limitations, remains the most common and easiest specimen to obtain for diagnosis. However, when a sputum sample is submitted to the microbiology laboratory for routine bacterial culture and stain, clinicians should be familiar with some of the issues regarding this type of specimen.[4] The specimen is first smeared onto a glass slide and Gram staining is performed as a screen. A high-quality purulent sputum specimen should contain many neutrophils and only relatively few epithelial cells. If many epithelial cells are seen—specifically if more than 25 epithelial cells are seen per low-power field—the specimen is contaminated with upper oropharyngeal flora (i.e., saliva) and may not even be from the lower respiratory tract. In such a case, even if microorganisms are seen on Gram staining, it cannot be ascertained whether the organism in question is a pathogen or simply part of the normal upper respiratory tract flora.

It is important to remember that many organisms in the upper respiratory tract (e.g., *Streptococcus pneumoniae*) are also causes of pneumonia. Thus, the positive predictive value of Gram staining and the culture is low for predicting the cause of pneumonia if the sputum specimen is contaminated (i.e., not representative of the lower respiratory tract). Therefore, sputum specimens contaminated with upper respiratory tract contents, as indicated by the presence of excessive squamous epithelial cells, should be rejected and another specimen should be obtained if clinically indicated. It is often helpful to use a respiratory therapist to obtain an induced sputum specimen using hypertonic saline.

If the diagnosis cannot otherwise be confirmed, it may be necessary to perform a bronchoalveolar lavage (BAL) for better assessment of the lower respiratory tract. BAL lavage fluid is the best specimen for diagnosing lower tract infections. This type of specimen is obtained by performing a bronchoscopy, a procedure that requires a physician's time, partial anesthesia, and some degree of risk. When properly done, the chance of contamination by upper respiratory flora is minimized. In addition to sampling the lower respiratory tract for culture and cytologic testing, this procedure affords tissue sampling—transbronchial biopsy—if indicated. More recently, mini-BAL aspirates from endotracheal or tracheostomy tubes have been submitted instead of BAL for patients on mechanical ventilation. These specimens are easier to obtain than those obtained by traditional BAL and are often used as a surrogate specimen to diagnose lower respiratory tract infections, especially ventilator-associated pneumonia (VAP). Although helpful, it should be emphasized that VAP is difficult to diagnose by respiratory culture alone.[5] These specimens, like sputa, may be contaminated with upper respiratory tract flora and therefore have similar limitations. The specificity of diagnosing VAP may be increased by combining several findings, such as respiratory culture, fever, new infiltrate, and leukocytosis. Unfortunately, many specimens obtained from tracheal aspirates contain a mixture of both gram-positive and gram-negative bacteria. The positive predictive value for such specimens is also low and the presence of these organisms might or might not be associated with lower respiratory tract infections. Thus, interpreting culture results is difficult; historical and clinical information should also be included to help determine the presence or absence of infections.

Finally, it is prudent to remember that Gram staining is only a screening tool to aid clinicians in diagnosis. The classic causes of atypical pneumonia, *Mycoplasma pneumoniae*, *Chlamydia pneumoniae*, and *Legionella* species, do not stain (*M. pneumoniae* and *C. pneumoniae*) or do not stain well (*Legionella*) with Gram staining. The diagnosis of infections by these agents uses other methodologies such as serology testing, antigen detection, polymerase chain reaction (PCR) assay, or a combination of these. An astute clinician should have a high index of suspicion for pneumonia if the history, physical examination, and radiograph are suggestive of such an infection, even if the Gram staining result is nondiagnostic or negative for microorganisms, and appropriate empirical antimicrobial treatment should be given.

Stool

Patients with diarrheal illness could have a spectrum of clinical presentations, ranging from mild, self-limited, loose stools, with minimal to moderate abdominal discomfort, to severe abdominal pain, with or without bloody stool. Many bacterial, viral, and parasitic organisms are capable of causing gastrointestinal (GI) infections. It is beyond the scope of this chapter to cover this exhaustive list and many excellent texts and references are available to discuss these pathogens more fully. However, some key concepts should be emphasized to help the clinician obtain maximal laboratory data to make an accurate diagnosis and treat patients appropriately. The laboratory, at the same time, is challenged to perform cost-effective and efficient assays while helping clinicians achieve their diagnostic goals.

Diarrheal illness generally can be divided anatomically into those that predominantly affect the small intestine and those that affect the large intestine. Pathogens that affect the small intestine usually cause a malabsorptive type of symptoms, with loose watery stools. Some classic examples include *Giardia lamblia* and *Cryptosporidium parvum* infections. Infections that affect the large intestine usually manifest with diarrhea caused by colitis that may be bloody; these patients may be toxic or even develop septic shock if the infection is severe enough. Some large intestinal pathogens include *Salmonella*, *Shigella*, *Campylobacter*, and *Clostridium difficile*.

To investigate patients with diarrhea in a hospital setting, a former practice (no longer supported) was to order stool culture and ova and parasite testing (three times) as an initial investigation. However, studies have suggested that there is low predictive value to these tests for patients admitted to the hospital for longer than 3 days, unless the clinical history, epidemiology, and examination suggest an infectious origin.[6] Therefore, stool cultures for typical enteric bacterial pathogens and examinations for parasitic causes of diarrhea should be limited to outpatients with diarrhea, patients with diarrhea on admission, or those who develop it within the first few days of admission. Thereafter, the likelihood of diarrhea being caused by these agents is extremely remote.

It is important to note that most cases of diarrhea develop because of noninfectious causes, and may be medication related. *C. difficile* nonetheless deserves special attention for hospitalized patients. It has been shown that *C. difficile*–associated pseudomembranous enterocolitis is the main cause of hospital-acquired diarrhea, and clinicians should maintain a high index of suspicion for this disease under the appropriate clinical circumstances. Patients with leukocytosis, fever, loose watery stools, and abdominal pain should undergo further investigation and *C. difficile* should be ruled out. The absence of these signs, however, does not specifically diagnose or exclude this disease;

the diagnosis is confirmed by testing the stool, usually for toxins produced by this organism. Ideally, the stool should be loose and free-flowing.

The definitive diagnosis of *C. difficile* infection is made by the detection of the toxins—namely, toxins A and B in the stools of patients suspected of having this disease. The toxins can be detected by enzyme-linked immunoassay (EIA) but, traditionally, the tissue culture method is used for the detection of toxin B. With this method, a cytopathic effect (CPE) is produced that may be blocked using antitoxin. In many laboratories, combined toxins A and B EIAs have replaced tissue culture, generally because they have a more rapid turnaround time and are less labor- and resource-intensive. However, it should be noted that EIA has a sensitivity of only 75% to 85% and a strong clinical suspicion should be entertained, even if there is a negative *C. difficile* toxin EIA result.

Recently, it has been suggested that in addition to toxins A and B detected by EIA, there is also a binary toxin-producing strain of *C. difficile*.[7] Strains of *C. difficile* that produce this toxin usually produce a more fulminant and severe colitis in infected patients. Moreover, strains of *C. difficile* that possess this toxin are also hyperproducers of toxin A or B, or both. Because it is a hyperproducer of toxin, this newly recognized "epidemic" strain of *C. difficile* will be readily detected by commonly used assays, but its specific type will not be detected.

A question that arises is in regard to how many *C. difficile* tests should be ordered to confirm the diagnosis. It has become common practice among house officers to order "*C. difficile* times three" to rule out such infection. This practice was extrapolated from a study by Manabe and colleagues.[8] They found that the sensitivity of EIA is 72% with the first specimen, 84% with the second, and 93% with the third. However, the number of patients required to have three specimens submitted to confirm the diagnosis was small. Moreover, it was found that the negative predictive value with the first stool was 97%. Increasing the number of stool specimens will not increase the sensitivity of detecting *C. difficile* toxin that was not detected in the first two specimens. Therefore, the routine practice of sending stool for *C. difficile* three times should be discouraged. Each *C. difficile* order should be made uniquely by an astute physician who is considering the clinical and laboratory findings, and the inherent limitations of each.

Wound, Wound Drainage, and Cerebrospinal Fluid

Management of wound culture presents some difficult challenges to the microbiology laboratory. Many issues need to be addressed in regard to these types of cultures:

- What is the appropriate method to collect specimens?
- Do swabs have any roles in bacterial cultures?
- What is the clinical significance of cultures that contain mixed flora?
- Should wound drainage (e.g., Jackson-Pratt drain) be cultured routinely to rule out active infections?

These are some questions that should be carefully considered before submitting specimens to the laboratory.

The most effective way to treat an abscess or infected fluid collection is to drain the abscess in conjunction with antimicrobial therapy. Rarely, an abscess can be cured just by medical treatment. Occasionally, fluid to be collected is located in a deep structure in which percutaneous or even surgical drainage is deemed too risky for the patient. In such cases, prolonged antimicrobial therapy is the only viable option and these cases should be followed closely to assess clinical response. In some other cases, a radical surgical procedure might be the best option for managing chronic infection. For example, patients with chronic empyema who have undergone multiple surgical procedures for decortication may be best managed using a Clagett open-window thoracostomy for drainage.

When obtaining specimens from a wound, it is advisable to submit the aspirated fluid in a syringe after removing the needle to help ensure the survival of anaerobic bacteria; an anaerobic transport vial is another alternative. A wound swab is not an appropriate method to collect specimens to assess for anaerobes. Quantity is always an important issue, because the more material one submits, the higher the chance of recovering the causative agent of disease. That is, swabs only hold a limited amount of fluid and anaerobic bacteria may die in transit; the submission of fluid is a superior technique. When submitting a piece of tissue, it should be placed in a sterile container and transported to the laboratory as soon as possible. removing potentially infected tissue and then swabbing it is inappropriate and will yield suboptimal results. The label should clearly contain the name and identification number for the patient and include the type of specimen, source, and a brief clinical description. The requisition, paper or electronic, must denote the microbiologic studies to be performed. This allows for timely, efficient, and accurate processing of specimens.

As noted, swabs generally are the least desirable way to collect a specimen for a wound culture. Organisms isolated from a wound culture obtained by swabbing the wound surface reflect the colonization of that wound (i.e., these do not reflect the organism that may be causing a deeper infection). This is particularly true for a chronic wound, which usually harbors multiple organisms, such as *Pseudomonas aeruginosa*, *Enterococcus* species, and *Staphylococcus aureus*, all of which could be true pathogens in another (deeper) location. In such a case, it is impossible to predict whether the isolated organisms are true pathogens or simply superficial colonizers; that is, there is a poor positive predictive value for a poor wound culture. In this era of health care cost containment one has to ask, "Why then even do it?" To determine the cause of a wound infection definitively, it first needs to be determined clinically whether a wound is thought to be infected. Thereafter, a surgical approach is desired in which the superficial material is débrided and a biopsy of the wound base is submitted for culture. Some clinicians have used screening criteria, which examines the proportion of squamous epithelial cells and neutrophils, to determine the usefulness of subsequent culture. Such approaches may be helpful, particularly in settings in which a high percentage of wound cultures simply reflect superficial colonization.

It has become common practice in many institutions to submit fluid from a surgical drain for culture, even if there is no evidence of infection. It is thought—again, this is not supported—that this is a surrogate marker to diagnose occult infections. However, this practice has been shown to have almost no clinical value for the above-mentioned purposes. Moreover, it may mislead clinicians and result in the institution of inappropriate therapy. Everts and colleagues[9] have shown that there is poor correlation between fluids obtained from a drainage catheter versus those directly aspirated from the collection. Moreover, this group has shown that radiologic studies such as computed tomography (CT) or magnetic resonance imaging (MRI) are the best modalities for diagnosing deep tissue infections.

The appropriate assessment of cerebrospinal fluid (CSF) is absolutely crucial in managing patients with suspected cases of meningitis or encephalitis. The basic tenet for collecting CSF is similar to that for other specimens, but particular attention should be given to the aseptic technique used during collection. Before performing a lumbar puncture, the skin should be thoroughly cleansed with iodophor or chlorhexidine. The patient should preferably be lying in a recumbent position; occasionally, for obese patients it might be easier to obtain the fluid by asking the patient to sit upright and hunch forward to better accentuate the L4-L5 interspace. However, in such a position, the opening pressure cannot be accurately measured. In certain central nervous system infections, an assessment of the initial opening pressure is absolutely crucial for managing the patient. For example, a patient with *Cryptococcus neoformans* meningitis may have an elevated intracranial pressure (ICP), with few or subtle clinical signs and symptoms. Knowing the patient's baseline ICP will assist clinicians and neurosurgeons regarding the performance of shunting, if necessary.

The quantity of CSF is especially crucial and as much fluid as possible should be obtained, because multiple tests are usually ordered and some tests, such as CSF for cytology, require a large amount of sample. For certain pathogens, such as fungi and mycobacterial species, the microbial recovery is directly proportional to the volume of sample used to inoculate the cultures. Therefore, at least 10 to 20 mL of CSF should be submitted to the laboratory for testing. The clinical findings should dictate the type of testing to be performed.

Viral Cultures

Viral diseases are caused by a heterogeneous mixture of viruses and, depending on each virus's unique pathogenesis, the clinician needs to submit the appropriate specimen for testing. Many methodologies can be used for diagnosing viral diseases, such as serologic (antibody and antigen testing), viral culture, and molecular methods, such as the PCR assay and related techniques. Diagnostic virology will not be discussed in detail here; this section will focus specifically on viral cultures.

Molecular methods such as PCR have gained popularity and acceptance in recent years. This methodology is indispensable, especially in the field of clinical virology, One major drawback is the cost of running a molecular assay. Typically, tests using molecular methods are more expensive than conventional viral cultures. Consequently, viral cultures are still being used in many laboratories, especially small hospitals and laboratories in which the volume of testing might be low, and cost containment is important.

When submitting specimens for viral cultures, the principles of aseptic technique, volume, and timely submission of the specimens still apply. However, it should be noted that the specimens are usually stored in a viral transport medium (e.g., M4 medium) to keep the viruses viable. Moreover, submitting specimens with swabs made from calcium alginate can affect the recovery of herpes simplex and varicella zoster virus.[10] If the specimens cannot be processed in a timely fashion, the general rule for keeping the virus viable is to refrigerate the specimens. The clinician should check with the laboratory regarding the specific types of virus collection, transport media, and storage options before obtaining specimens.

CONCLUSION

The clinician and the microbiology laboratory work synergistically to provide optimal care to patients. Open communication between them enables proper collection of specimens and allows appropriate testing to be done. This enables cost-effective and efficient reporting of microbiologic results, which in turn enables the clinician to treat the patient effectively and in a timely fashion. The clinician should also supply adequate clinical information to the laboratory to facilitate proper specimen processing and testing.

Summary

- The clinical microbiology laboratory is an integral part of managing patients with various infectious diseases.
- Clinicians and laboratory personnel should maintain frequent communication so that accurate and clinically relevant test results are available in a timely manner.
- Clinicians should be aware of the limitations and understand the concepts of sensitivity, specificity, and positive or negative predictive value of different microbiology-related assays.
- When submitting specimens to the clinical microbiology laboratory, clinicians should recognize the importance of the quality and quantity of specimens required for that specific assay.

Suggested Readings

American Thoracic Society; Infectious Diseases Society of America: Guidelines for the management of adults with hospital-acquired, ventilator-associated, and healthcare-associated pneumonia. Am J Respir Crit Care Med 2005;171:388-416.

Carroll KC: Laboratory diagnosis of lower respiratory tract infections: Controversy and conundrums. J Clin Microbiol 2002;40:3115-3120.

Everts RJ, Heneghan JP, Adholla PO, Reller LB: Validity of cultures of fluid collected through drainage catheters versus those obtained by direct aspiration. J Clin Microbiol 2001;39:66-68.

Manabe YC, Vinetz JM, Moore RD, et al: *Clostridium difficile* colitis: An efficient clinical approach to diagnosis. Ann Intern Med 1995;123:835-840.

McDonald LC, Killgore GE, Thompson A, et al: An epidemic, toxin gene-variant strain of *Clostridium difficile*. N Engl J Med 2005;353:2433-2441.

Mead PB: Proper methods of culturing herpes simplex virus. J Reprod Med 1986;31:390-394.

Peterson LR, Hamilton JD, Baron EJ, et al: Role of clinical microbiology laboratories in the management and control of infectious diseases and the delivery of health care. Clin Infect Dis 2001;32:605-611.

Washington JA II: Blood cultures: Principles and techniques. Mayo Clin Proc 1975;50:91-98.

Weinstein MP: Emerging data indicating that extended incubation of blood cultures has little clinical value. Clin Infect Dis 2005;41:1681-1682.

Yannelli B, Gurevich I, Schoch PE, Cunha BA: Yield of stool cultures, ova and parasite tests, and *Clostridium difficile* determinations in nosocomial diarrheas. Am J Infect Control 1988;16:246-249.

References

For a complete list of references, log onto www.expertconsult.com.

Community-Acquired Pneumonia

Steven Schmitt

DEFINITION

Pneumonia is an infection of the lung parenchyma. *Community-acquired pneumonia* refers to pneumonia acquired outside of hospitals or extended-care facilities. *Nursing home–acquired pneumonia* refers to infection acquired in an extended-care facility. *Nosocomial pneumonia* and *hospital-acquired pneumonia* describe infections acquired in the hospital setting. The signs and symptoms of acute pneumonia develop over hours to days, whereas the clinical presentation of chronic pneumonia often evolves over weeks to months.

PREVALENCE

Despite a broad armamentarium of antimicrobials available to treat the disease, pneumonia remains the seventh leading cause of death in the United States.[1] In 2003, the age-adjusted death rate caused by influenza and pneumonia was 20.3 per 100,000 persons.[1] Estimates of the incidence of community-acquired pneumonia range from 4 million to 5 million cases per year, with about 25% requiring hospitalization.[2] Nosocomial pneumonia is estimated to occur in 250,000 persons per year, representing about 15% to 18% of all nosocomial infections.[3,4]

MICROBIOLOGY

Streptococcus pneumoniae remains the most commonly identified pathogen in community-acquired pneumonia (Fig. 1). Other pathogens have been reported to cause pneumonia in the community, and their order of importance depends on the location and population studied (Table 1). These include long-recognized pathogens such as *Haemophilus influenzae*, *Mycoplasma pneumoniae*, and influenza A, along with newer pathogens such as *Legionella* species and *Chlamydophilia pneumoniae*. Other common causes in the immunocompetent patient include *Moraxella catarrhalis*, *Mycobacterium tuberculosis*, and aspiration pneumonia. The causative agent of community-acquired pneumonia remains unidentified in 30% to 50% of cases.[5]

Previously seen mainly in extended-care facilities and acute-care hospitals, strains of methicillin-resistant *Staphylococcus aureus* (MRSA) have emerged as prevalent pathogens in community settings.[6] Necrotizing pneumonia is a characteristically severe manifestation of these virulent strains.

A new human pathogen, severe acute respiratory syndrome (SARS)-associated coronavirus, emerged and spread worldwide in the winter of 2002 to 2003. No cases have been identified since 2004. Data regarding this virus and its associated syndrome, SARS,[7] can be found on the SARS page of the website of the Centers for Disease Control and Prevention (CDC), available at http://www.cdc.gov/ncidod/sars.

Influenza continues to be a prevalent seasonal disease in the United States, causing considerable morbidity, loss of productivity, and mortality. A strain of H5N1 influenza has spread rapidly through avian flocks in Asia and Europe. Cases of transmission from birds to humans with severe disease have led to international concern about a possible avian influenza pandemic. Readers are encouraged to check the CDC influenza page, available at http://www.cdc.gov/flu/avian/index.htm, for updated prevention and treatment guidelines, as well as the latest epidemiologic information. Other viral causes of respiratory tract infections include parainfluenza virus, adenovirus, human metapneumovirus, herpes zoster virus (HSV), varicella-zoster virus (VZV), and measles.

Many pathogens listed as potential agents of bioterrorism are spread by the respiratory route. Among the most likely candidates are *Bacillus anthracis*, *Francisella tularensis*, and *Yersinia pestis*. A more extensive discussion of the agents of bioterrorism can be found elsewhere in this section ("Biologic Weapons and the Primary Care Clinician").

Nursing home–acquired pneumonias are often caused by community-acquired pathogens. However, there is an increased influence of pathogens seen with relatively low frequency in the community, such as *S. aureus* and gram-negative organisms.

PATHOPHYSIOLOGY

Six mechanisms have been identified in the pathogenesis of pneumonia in immunocompetent adults (Table 2). Inhalation of infectious particles is probably the most important pathogenetic mechanism in the development of community-acquired pneumonia, with particular importance of pneumonia caused by *Legionella* species and *M. tuberculosis*.

The aspiration of oropharyngeal or gastric contents is the most prevalent pathogenetic mechanism in nosocomial pneumonia, with several contributing factors. Swallowing and epiglottic closure may be impaired by neuromuscular disease, stroke, states of altered consciousness, or seizures. Endotracheal and nasogastric tubes interfere with these anatomic defenses and provide a direct route of entry for pathogens. Impaired lower esophageal sphincter function and nasogastric and gastrostomy tubes increase the risk of aspiration of gastric contents. Fortunately, aspiration rarely leads to overt bacterial pneumonia.

Direct inoculation rarely occurs as a result of surgery or bronchoscopy but may play a role in the development of pneumonia in patients supported with mechanical ventilation. Hematogenous deposition of bacteria in the lungs is also uncommon but is responsible for some cases of pneumonia caused by *S. aureus*, *Pseudomonas aeruginosa*, and *Escherichia coli*. The direct extension of infection to the lung from contiguous areas, such as the pleural or subdiaphragmatic spaces, is rare.

Reactivation of pathogens can take place in the setting of deficits of cell-mediated immunity. Pathogens such as *Pneumocystis jiroveci*, *Mycobacterium tuberculosis*, and cytomegalovirus can remain latent for many years after exposure, with flares of active disease occurring in the presence of immune compromise. Reactivation tuberculosis occasionally occurs in immunocompetent hosts.

Once bacteria reach the tracheobronchial tree, defects in local pulmonary defenses can make infection more likely. The cough reflex can be impaired by stroke, neuromuscular disease, sedatives, or poor nutrition. Mucociliary transport is depressed with the aging process, tobacco smoking, dehydration, morphine, atropine, prior infection with influenza virus, and chronic bronchitis. Anatomic changes such as emphysema, bronchiectasis, and obstructive mass lesions prevent the clearance of microbes. Inflammatory cells drawn to infected areas of the pulmonary tree release proteolytic enzymes, altering the bronchial epithelium and ciliary clearance mechanisms and stimulating the production of excess mucus. Community-acquired MRSA strains contain Panton-Valentine leukocidin, a toxin that creates holes in neutrophil cell membranes, releasing chemotactic and inflammatory factors.[7]

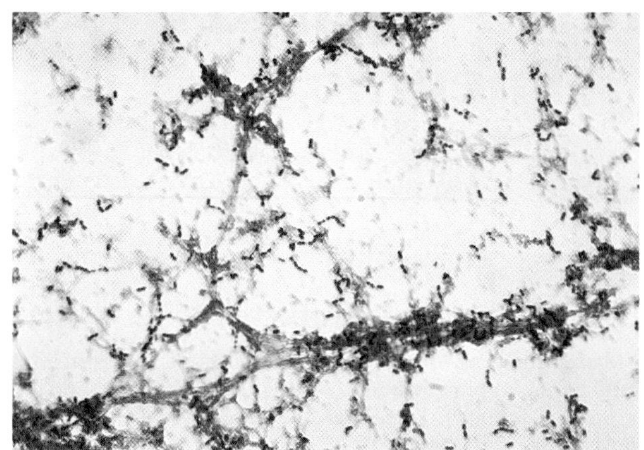

Figure 1 **Streptococcus pneumoniae in blood culture.** Shown are lancet-shaped gram-positive cocci in pairs and chains. *(Courtesy of Dr. Mike Miller, Centers for Disease Control and Prevention.)*

Table 1 Identified Pathogens in Community-Acquired Pneumonia

Pathogen	Cases (%)
Streptococcus pneumoniae	20-60
Haemophilus influenzae	3-10
Staphylococcus aureus	3-5
Gram-negative bacilli	3-10
Legionella species	2-8
Mycoplasma pneumoniae	1-6
Chlamydia pneumoniae	4-6
Viruses	2-15
Aspiration	6-10
Others	3-5

Adapted from Mandell LA, Bartlett JG, Dowell SF, et al: Update of practice guidelines for the management of community-acquired pneumonia in immunocompetent adults. Clin Infect Dis 2003;37:1405-1433.

A blunted cellular and humoral immune response can also increase the risk of pneumonia. For example, granulocyte chemotaxis is reduced with aging, diabetes mellitus, malnutrition, hypothermia, hypophosphatemia, and corticosteroids. Granulocytopenia may be caused by cytotoxic chemotherapy. Alveolar macrophages are rendered dysfunctional by corticosteroids, cytokines, viral illnesses, and malnutrition. Diminished antibody production or function can accompany hematologic malignancies such as multiple myeloma or chronic lymphocytic leukemia.

HISTORY AND PHYSICAL EXAMINATION

Because the clinical syndromes characterizing pneumonic infections caused by various agents often overlap one another and because interobserver variability regarding physical findings of pneumonia is high, the diagnosis of pneumonia can be challenging. A diligent history (Table 3) and physical examination can help narrow the differential diagnosis. In general, typical bacterial pathogens such as *S. pneumoniae, H. influenzae*, and the enteric gram-negative organisms usually manifest acutely with high fever, chills, tachypnea, tachycardia, and productive cough. Examination findings are localized to a specific lung zone and can include rales, rhonchi, bronchial breath sounds, dullness, increased fremitus, and egophony. In contrast, atypical pathogens such as *Mycoplasma, Chlamydophilia*, and viruses can manifest in a subacute fashion with fever, nonproductive cough, constitutional symptoms, and absent or diffuse findings on lung examination. Rapid progression of disease to respiratory failure can be seen in severe pneumococcal or *Legionella* pneumonia. Influenza may be complicated by bacterial pneumonia caused by *S. aureus* or *S. pneumoniae*.

Table 2 Pathogenetic Mechanisms in Pneumonia

Mechanism	Frequency
Inhalation of infectious particles	Common
Aspiration of oropharyngeal or gastric contents	Common
Hematogenous deposition	Uncommon
Invasion from infection in contiguous structures	Rare
Direct inoculation	Less common
Reactivation	More common in immunocompromised hosts

SARS manifests with high fever and myalgia for 3 to 7 days, followed by a nonproductive cough and progressive hypoxemia, with progression to mechanical ventilation in 20% of cases. This can be distinguished from other viral infections by the higher fever and lack of conjunctivitis, sneezing, rhinorrhea, and pharyngitis. Inhalation anthrax can manifest with flulike symptoms of myalgia, fatigue, and fever before rapidly progressing to respiratory distress, mediastinitis, meningitis, sepsis, and death.

The age of the patient can play an important role in disease presentation. Older patients often have humoral and cellular immunodeficiencies as a result of underlying diseases, immunosuppressive medications, and the aging process. They are more commonly institutionalized with anatomic problems that inhibit the pulmonary clearance of pathogens. The presentation is often more subtle than in younger adults, with more-advanced disease and sepsis, despite minimal fever and sputum production.

Extrapulmonary physical findings can provide clues to the diagnosis. Poor dentition and foul-smelling sputum can indicate the presence of a lung abscess with an anaerobic component. Bullous myringitis can accompany infection with *M. pneumoniae*. An absent gag reflex or altered sensorium raises the question of aspiration. Encephalitis can complicate pneumonia caused by *M. pneumoniae* or *Legionella pneumophila*. Cutaneous manifestations of infection can include erythema multiforme *(M. pneumoniae)*, erythema nodosum *(C. pneumoniae* and *M. tuberculosis)*, or ecthyma gangrenosum (*P. aeruginosa*).

DIAGNOSTIC AND TREATMENT CONSIDERATIONS

The composition of the diagnostic workup for pneumonia has been the subject of some disagreement among experts (see later, "National Guidelines"), but a well-chosen evaluation can support a diagnosis of pneumonia and identify a pathogen.

Radiography

A cornerstone of diagnosis is the chest x-ray, which is recommended for diagnosis in every circumstance and usually reveals an infiltrate (Fig. 2) at presentation. However, this finding may be absent in the

Table 3 Microbiologic Differential Diagnosis of Pneumonia: Historical Features

History	Associated Organisms
Alcoholism	*Streptococcus pneumoniae*, oral anaerobes, *Mycobacterium tuberculosis*
Chronic obstructive lung disease (COPD)	*S. pneumoniae, Haemophilus influenzae, Moraxella catarrhalis, Legionella* spp.
Exposure to bat or bird droppings, construction sites, caves	*Histoplasma capsulatum*
Exposure to birds	*Chlamydia psittaci*
Exposure to rabbits	*Francisella tularensis*
HIV infection	"Typical" bacterial pathogens, *M. tuberculosis, Pneumocystis jiroveci,* cytomegalovirus, *Cryptococcus* spp., *Histoplasma* spp., *Coccidioides* spp.
Travel to desert, southwest United States	*Coccidioides* spp., Hantavirus (Sin Nombre virus)
Farm exposure	*Coxiella burnetii* (animals), *Aspergillus* spp. (barns, hay)
Postinfluenza	*S. pneumoniae, S. aureus, Streptococcus pyogenes, H. influenzae*
Aspiration	Mixed aerobic, anaerobic
Marijuana smoking	*Aspergillus* spp.
Anatomic abnormality of lung parenchyma, e.g., bronchiectasis, cystic fibrosis	*Pseudomonas aeruginosa, Burkholderia cepacia, S. aureus*
Injection drug use	*S. aureus*, anaerobes, *M. tuberculosis*, and *S. pneumoniae*
Obstruction of large airway	Anaerobes, *S. pneumoniae, H. influenzae, S. aureus*
Incarceration	*M. tuberculosis*
Neutropenia	*Aspergillus* spp., Zygomycetes
Asplenia	*S. pneumoniae, H. influenzae*

Adapted from Mandell LA, Bartlett JG, Dowell SF, et al: Update of practice guidelines for the management of community-acquired pneumonia in immunocompetent adults. Clin Infect Dis 2003;37:1405-1433.

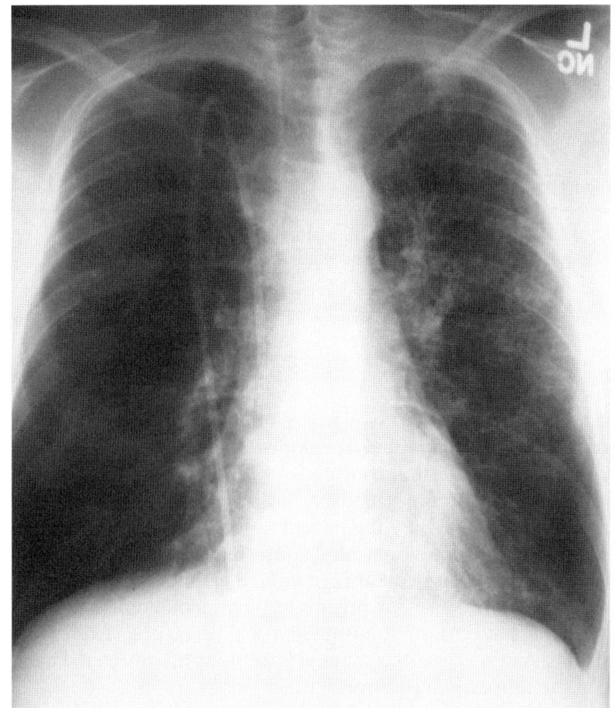

Figure 2 **Radiograph of pulmonary infiltrates in influenza pneumonia.**

dehydrated patient. Also, the radiographic manifestations of chronic diseases such as congestive heart failure, chronic obstructive pulmonary disease (COPD), and malignancy can obscure the infiltrate of pneumonia.

Although radiographic patterns are usually nonspecific, they can suggest a microbiologic differential diagnosis (Table 4).

Initial Management: Risk Stratification and Treatment Setting

When community-acquired pneumonia is strongly suspected on the basis of history, physical examination, and chest radiography, the next critical management decision is whether the patient requires hospital admission. Health care budgetary constraints have given rise to a number of studies addressing the need for hospitalization in community-acquired pneumonia. A study by the Patient Outcome Research Team (PORT) investigators has validated a risk scale, now called the pneumonia severity index (PSI), for mortality in community-acquired pneumonia. Point values are assigned to patient characteristics, comorbid illness, physical examination, and basic laboratory findings (Table 5).[8] Patients younger than 50 years without comorbid illness or significant vital sign abnormalities (risk class I) were found to have a low risk for mortality. The authors suggested that such patients might be eligible for outpatient antibiotic therapy without extensive laboratory evaluation.

All others were evaluated with the laboratory tests listed in Table 5 and assigned to risk classes by point totals (Table 6). Those in

Table 4 Radiographic Patterns of Common Etiologic Agents

Chest Radiographic Pattern	Pathogen
Focal; large pleural effusion	Usually bacteria
Cavitary	Bacterial abscess, fungi, acid-fast bacilli, *Nocardia*
Miliary	Acid-fast bacilli, fungi
Rapid progression/multifocal	*Legionella* spp., *Pneumococcus, Staphylococcus*
Interstitial	Viruses, *Pneumocystis jiroveci, Mycoplasma, Chlamydia psittaci*
Mediastinal widening without infiltrate	Inhalation anthrax

classes I and II are considered excellent candidates for outpatient oral therapy, assuming no hemodynamic instability, no chronic oxygen dependence, immunocompetence, and the ability to ingest, absorb, and adhere to an oral regimen. Patients in risk class III may be considered for outpatient or brief inpatient therapy, depending on clinical judgment. Patients in risk classes IV and V are recommended for hospital admission. Ultimately, each decision to admit must be individualized.

A slightly less complex scheme is the CRB-65. In this algorithm, patients are felt better served by hospitalization if they they meet more than of the following criteria: confusion, respiratory rate greater than 30 breaths per minute, blood pressure less than 90 mm Hg systolic or 60 mm Hg diastolic, or age older than 65 years.[9]

Table 5 Pneumonia Severity Index: Point Assignments in Community-Acquired Pneumonia

Risk Factor	Point Value
Age	
Men	Age (in yr)
Women	Age (in yr) −10
Nursing home resident	+10
Comorbid Illnesses	
Neoplastic disease	+30
Liver disease	+20
Kidney disease	+10
Cerebrovascular disease	+10
Congestive heart failure	+10
Physical Findings	
Altered mentation	+20
Tachypnea (>30 breaths/min)	+20
Systolic hypotension (<90 mm Hg)	+20
Body temperature (<35° or >40° C)	+15
Heart rate >125 beats/min	+10
Laboratory and Radiographic Findings	
Blood pH (arterial) <7.35	+30
Hypoxemia (arterial Pa_{O_2}<60 mm Hg or O_2 saturation <90%)	+10
Serum urea nitrogen (BUN) >30 mg/dL	+20
Na <130 mEq/L	+20
Blood sugar >250 mg/dL	+10
Anemia (hematocrit <30%)	+10
Pleural effusion	10

Adapted from Kolleff MH, Micek ST: Methicillin-resistant *Staphylococcus aureus*—a new community-acquired pathogen? Curr Opin Infect Dis 2006;19:161-168.

Diagnostic Testing

When the patient is not severely ill (ie outpatient treatment or not severely ill in the inpatient setting) and has few risk factors , the consensus guidelines of the Infectious Diseases Society of America (IDSA) and American Thoracic Society (ATS)[10] suggest empirical therapy without extensive laboratory evaluation (Box 1). When identification of a pathogen might change therapy, further studies are indicated (see Box 1). The value of such studies is not uniformly agreed on (see later, "National Guidelines"). However, pathogen identification has important implications for the breadth of therapeutic antibiotic spectrum, development of resistance, and epidemiology.

A Gram-stained sputum specimen can help focus empirical therapy. Unfortunately, sputum is often difficult to obtain from older patients because of a weak cough, obtundation, and dehydration. Nebulized saline treatments might help mobilize secretions. Nasotracheal suctioning can sample the lower respiratory tract directly but risks oropharyngeal contamination. A sputum specimen reflects lower respiratory secretions when more than 25 white blood cells (WBCs) and fewer than 10 epithelial cells are seen in a low-powered microscopic field.[11] Empirical therapy based on a predominant organism in such a specimen is likely to contain appropriate coverage.[12]

Other stains, such as the acid-fast stain for mycobacteria, modified acid-fast stain for *Nocardia*, or toluidine blue and Gomori's methenamine silver stains should be used when directed by the history or clinical presentation. Direct fluorescent antibody (DFA) staining of sputum, bronchoalveolar lavage fluid, or pleural fluid can help identify *Legionella* species. Similarly, DFA testing of nasopharyngeal specimens provides rapid diagnosis of influenza types A and B, as well as other common respiratory viruses such as respiratory syncytial virus, adenovirus, and parainfluenza virus. In an outbreak setting, DFA and other rapid techniques can assist in decision making for therapy and infection control.

The sputum culture remains a controversial tool but is useful to help tailor therapy when the patient is severely ill, has a history of structural lung disease or alcohol abuse, has pleural effusion, or has evidence of pneumococcal or *Legionella* infection. Culture is particularly helpful for identifying organisms of epidemiologic significance, either for patterns of transmission or resistance. Expectorated morning sputum specimens should be sent for mycobacterial culture when the history is suggestive.

Blood cultures can also shed light on a pathogen, and samples should be drawn in severely ill or immunocompromised patients (see

Table 6 Pneumonia Severity Index: Risk of 30-Day Mortality By Point Total

Risk Class	Point Score	Mortality (%)
I	No points assigned	0.1
II	<70	0.6
III	71-90	2.8
IV	91-130	8.2
V	>130	29.2

Adapted from Kolleff MH, Micek ST: Methicillin-resistant *Staphylococcus aureus*—a new community-acquired pathogen? Curr Opin Infect Dis 2006;19:161-168.

Box 1 Diagnostic Testing for Community-Acquired Pneumonia

All patients with suspected pneumonia

- Chest radiography
- Complete blood count
- Complete metabolic profile
- Blood gases or pulse oximetry

Severely ill or immunocompromised patients, patients with anatomic lung disease

- Sputum Gram stain and culture
- Blood cultures: two sets before antibiotics
- *Legionella* serology, urinary antigen, direct fluorescent antibody testing
- Pneumococcal urinary antigen testing

Inpatients with appropriate history or physical findings

- HIV serology
- *Mycoplasma* serology
- *Chlamydia* serology
- Fungal serology
- SARS-associated coronavirus serology or PCR
- Stains or cultures for fungi, mycobacteria, *Pneumocystis jiroveci*

- Analysis or cultures of pleural or cerebrospinal fluid
- Nasopharyngeal swab for viral direct fluorescent antibody or other rapid technique
- Tuberculin skin testing

Deteriorating patient without definitive diagnosis of cause

- Bronchoscopy (bronchoalveolar lavage, protected catheter, transbronchial biopsy)
- Thoracoscopic or open-lung biopsy
- Radiographically guided transthoracic aspirate
- *Legionella*, *Chlamydia*, *Mycoplasma* serology
- Fungal serology
- Evaluation for congestive heart failure, pulmonary embolus, neoplasm, connective tissue disease

PCR, polymerase chain reaction; PORT, Patient Outcome Research Team; SARS, severe acute respiratory syndrome.

Adapted Mandell LA, Wunderink RG, Anzueto A, et al; Infectious Diseases Society of America; American Thoracic Society. Infectious Diseases Society of America/American Thoracic Society consensus guidelines on the management of community-acquired pneumonia in adults. Clin Infect Dis 2007;44 Suppl 2:S27-S72.

later, "Outcomes"). Pleural or cerebrospinal fluid should be sampled when infections in these spaces are suspected.

When these procedures fail to yield a microbiologic diagnosis and when the patient does not respond to empirical antibiotic therapy, more-invasive diagnostic techniques may be indicated. Fiberoptic bronchoscopy allows the use of several techniques for the diagnosis of pneumonia. Bronchoalveolar lavage with saline can obtain deep respiratory specimens for the gamut of stains and cultures mentioned earlier. Transbronchial biopsy of lung parenchyma can reveal alveolar or interstitial pneumonitis, viral inclusion bodies, and fungal or mycobacterial elements. The protected brush catheter is used to distinguish quantitatively between tracheobronchial colonizers and pneumonic pathogens.

A more substantial amount of lung tissue may be obtained for culture and histologic examination by thoracoscopic or open lung biopsy. Because these procedures can carry considerable morbidity, they are usually reserved for the deteriorating patient with a pneumonia that defies diagnosis by less-invasive techniques.

Serologic Testing

Often relegated to retrospective or epidemiologic interest because of delays in testing or reporting, serologic testing for such pathogens as *Legionella* species, *Mycoplasma* species, and *C. pneumoniae* should include sera drawn in the acute and convalescent phases for comparison. A fourfold increase in the immunoglobulin G (IgG) titer suggests recent infection with these organisms. An IgM microimmunofluorescence titer of more than 1:16 is considered diagnostic of *C. pneumoniae* infection. Infection with SARS-associated coronavirus is most often diagnosed by antibody testing and polymerase chain reaction (PCR) testing.

A sensitive enzyme immunoassay has been developed for the detection of *L. pneumophila* type 1 antigen in urine. Because the antigen persists for up to 1 year after infection, it is difficult to differentiate between past and current infections when using this assay.

A urinary assay is also available for detecting *S. pneumoniae* cell wall polysaccharide. This assay may offer some advantage for the rapid diagnosis of pneumococcal pneumonia in culture-proven or unknown cases, but assay specificity is an ongoing question.

Molecular Techniques

Powerful molecular techniques are now being applied to the early diagnosis of pneumonia. DNA probes have been used to detect *Legionella* species, *M. pneumoniae*, and *M. tuberculosis* in sputum. These probes have excellent sensitivity and specificity but can yield false-positive results. The PCR assay has been used for the early detection of various pathogens that are difficult or slow to culture from sputum specimens, including atypical bacteria, viruses (e.g., influenza), and mycobacteria. Given the large percentage of pneumonia cases for which no microbial cause is identified, it is likely that molecular tools will eventually be applied to the identification and antimicrobial susceptibility testing of almost all causative agents of pneumonia.

Summary

- The patient's history can help narrow the microbial differential diagnosis.
- The chest radiograph is the cornerstone of diagnosis.
- The sputum Gram stain and culture are controversial, but they are still useful for targeting antimicrobial therapy when the patient is severely ill or immunocompromised.
- Serologic testing is slow and therefore often not useful for real-time diagnosis.
- Molecular methods are playing an increasing role in identifying difficult-to-culture pathogens.
- The pneumonia severity index uses history, examination, chest radiograph, and initial laboratory test results to identify low-risk patients for outpatient treatment.

ANTIMICROBIAL TREATMENT

Community-Acquired Pneumonia

Antibiotic therapy for community-acquired pneumonia should always be selected with patient characteristics, place of acquisition, and severity of disease in mind. With concerns about antimicrobial overuse, health care costs, and bacterial resistance increasing, many experts believe that therapy should always follow confirmation of the diagnosis of pneumonia and should always be accompanied by a diligent effort to identify a causative agent (see later, "National Guidelines"). When a specific pathogen is identified, pathogen-specific therapy can be used (Table 7).

When a pathogen is yet to be identified, empirical therapy is instituted. A number of expert panels have recommended empirical pneumonia therapy, most prominently IDSA and ATS (Table 8).

Aspiration Pneumonia

Clindamycin is preferred over penicillin for the treatment of community-acquired aspiration pneumonia because of its superiority for treating oral anaerobes such as *Bacteroides melaninogenicus*. Amoxicillin-clavulanic acid also provides excellent coverage in this setting. When large-volume aspiration is documented in the hospital, a beta-lactam–beta-lactamase inhibitor combination or the combination of clindamycin and an antipseudomonal agent should be used.

Other Considerations

Anthrax

Suspected or proven inhalation anthrax should be treated with ciprofloxacin or doxycycline and two other agents (see Table 7). Clinical experience has suggested that rifampin may be an important agent in empirical regimens.[13]

Duration of Therapy

Although few data specifically address the duration of therapy, many cases of pneumonia are adequately treated with 10 to 14 days of antibiotics. Longer courses may be required for certain organisms that cause tissue necrosis, (e.g., *Legionella* spp., *S. aureus, Pseudomonas aeruginosa*), organisms that live intracellularly (e.g., *C. pneumoniae*), or comorbidities that compromise local (COPD) or systemic (hematologic malignancy) immunity.

Table 7 Pathogen-Specific Therapy for Community-Acquired Pneumonia in Adults

Organism	Primary Therapy
Streptococcus pneumoniae, penicillin-susceptible	Penicillin G; amoxicillin
S. pneumoniae, penicillin-resistant	Cefotaxime, ceftriaxone, fluoroquinolone, vancomycin, others, based on susceptibility studies
Haemophilus influenzae	Second- or third-generation cephalosporin, doxycycline, beta-lactam or beta-lactamase inhibitor, azithromycin, TMP-SMX
Moraxella catarrhalis	Second- or third-generation cephalosporin, TMP-SMX macrolide, beta-lactam or beta-lactamase inhibitor
Legionella spp.	Macrolide, tetracycline, fluoroquinolone alone
Mycoplasma pneumoniae	Doxycycline, macrolide
Chlamydia pneumoniae	Doxycycline, macrolide
Anaerobes	Beta-lactam or beta-lactamase inhibitor, clindamycin
Enteric gram-negative bacilli	Third-generation cephalosporin ± aminoglycoside; carbapenem
Pseudomonas aeruginosa	Aminoglycoside + ticarcillin, piperacillin, mezlocillin, ceftazidime, cefepime, aztreonam, or carbapenem
Staphylococcus aureus, methicillin-susceptible	Nafcillin or oxacillin
S. aureus, methicillin-resistant	Vancomycin or linezolid
Bacillus anthracis	Ciprofloxacin or doxycycline + two of the following: rifampin, vancomycin, penicillin, ampicillin, chloramphenicol, imipenem, clindamycin, clarithromycin
Influenza A, within 48 hr of symptom onset or immunocompromised host	Amantidine, rimantadine, oseltamivir, zanamivir
Influenza B, within 48 hr of symptom onset or immunocompromised host	Oseltamivir, zanamivir

*For community-acquired methicillin-resistant *S. aureus*, some clinicians add agents that inhibit toxin production, such as clindamycin, when susceptibility patterns allow.

TMP-SMX, trimethoprim-sulfamethoxazole.

Adapted from Mandell LA, Wunderink RG, Anzueto A, et al; Infectious Diseases Society of America; American Thoracic Society: Infectious Diseases Society of America/American Thoracic Society consensus guidelines on the management of community-acquired pneumonia in adults. Clin Infect Dis 2007;44 Suppl 2:S27-S72.

Table 8 Empirical Antimicrobial Therapy for Community-Acquired Pneumonia In Immunocompetent Adults

Patient, Setting	Common Pathogens	Empirical Therapy
Outpatients		
<60 yr No comorbid diseases	*Streptococcus pneumoniae* *Mycoplasma pneumoniae* *Chlamydia pneumoniae* *Haemophilus influenzae* Viruses	Macrolide or doxycycline
>65 yr or with comorbid disease or antibiotic therapy within last 3 mo	*S. pneumoniae* (drug-resistant) *M. pneumoniae* *C. pneumoniae* *H. influenzae* Viruses Gram-negative bacilli† *S. aureus*†	Macrolide or doxycycline fluoroquinolone* Beta-lactam¶ and macrolide
Inpatients		
Not severely ill	*S. pneumoniae* *H. influenzae* Polymicrobial Anaerobes *S. aureus* *C. pneumoniae* Viruses	Macrolide and cefotaxime or ceftriaxone, or beta-lactam or beta-lactamase inhibitor¶; fluoroquinolone‡ alone
Severely ill	*S. pneumoniae*§ *Legionella* spp. Gram-negative bacilli *M. pneumoniae* Viruses *S. aureus*	Azithromycin, or fluoroquinolone‡ and cefotaxime, ceftriaxone, or beta-lactam or beta-lactamase inhibitor¶ If *P. aeruginosa* possible—IV macrolide or fluoroquinolone and aminoglycoside IV, or antipseudomonal quinolone and antipseudomonal beta-lactam If MRSA possible, add vancomycin or linezolid

*In the outpatient setting, many authorities prefer to reserve fluoroquinolones (levofloxacin, gatifloxacin, moxifloxacin, gemifloxacin) for patients with comorbid diseases or risk factors.
†In most cases, patients with pneumonias caused by these organisms should be hospitalized.
‡Levofloxacin, gatifloxacin, moxifloxacin.
§Critically ill patients in areas with significant rates of high-level pneumococcal resistance and a suggestive sputum Gram stain should receive vancomycin or a newer quinolone pending microbiologic diagnosis.
¶Piperacillin-tazobactam or ampicillin-sulbactam.
¶Cefpodoxime, cefuroxime, high-dose amoxicillin, amoxicillin-clavulanate, or parenteral ceftriaxone followed by oral cefpodoxime.
**Cefotaxime, ceftriaxone, ampicillin-sulbactam, or high-dose ampicillin.
Adapted from Mandell LA, Wunderink RG, Anzueto A, et al; Infectious Diseases Society of America; American Thoracic Society. Infectious Diseases Society of America/American Thoracic Society consensus guidelines on the management of community-acquired pneumonia in adults. Clin Infect Dis 2007;44 Suppl 2:S27-S72.

Oral and Switch Therapies

The use of oral or switch therapies offers potential reductions in duration of stay, antibiotic administration costs, complications of venous access, and disruption of families and careers. Many antibiotics are well absorbed from the gastrointestinal tract, suggesting the possibility of effective fully oral treatment. Because well-controlled, risk-stratified data comparing oral and intravenous therapies are few, appropriate patient populations and treatment settings for full-course oral therapy have yet to be fully defined. Better data exist for the use of IV to oral switch therapies for the stable patient who has good gastrointestinal and swallowing function and adequate social support.[14]

Failure to Respond to Initial Therapy

Worsening of clinical status despite adequate antibiotic therapy should trigger a reassessment of the original clinical impression. First, the diagnosis of infection must be questioned. Entities such as cancers, pulmonary edema, pulmonary embolus, pulmonary hemorrhage, connective tissue diseases, or drug toxicity can mimic the clinical and radiographic appearance of pneumonia. Organisms with inherent (e.g., fungi, mycobacterial, *P. jiroveci*) or acquired (*Pseudomonas aeruginosa*) resistance to drugs commonly used in pneumonia therapy must also be considered. A secondary infection, such as postinfluenza staphylococcal pneumonia, might prove resistant to initial therapy. The patient might fail to respond for reasons of poor adherence, poor drug absorption, or drug interaction. Finally, immunodeficiency (e.g., HIV, hematologic malignancy) or anatomic derangement (e.g., COPD, bronchiectasis, neoplasm) can alter the clinical course of pneumonia and treatment.

Discharge Criteria

Criteria for hospital discharge in community-acquired pneumonia are based on common sense. Candidates for discharge should have no more than one of the following poor prognostic indicators: temperature higher than 37.8° C, pulse higher than 100 beats/min, respiratory rate higher than 24/min, systolic blood pressure lower than 90 mm Hg, oxygen saturation lower than 90%, and inability to maintain oral intake.

Summary

- Antibiotic therapy for community-acquired pneumonia should always be selected with patient characteristics, place of acquisition, severity of disease, and local resistance patterns in mind.
- Antimicrobial therapy should be narrowed whenever a pathogen is identified.
- Most pneumonias, with some exceptions, can be cured with 10 to 14 days of antibiotic therapy.
- Switching to oral therapy is possible and desirable once the patient stabilizes.
- Failure to respond to initial therapy should raise questions of diagnosis, treatment adherence, and antimicrobial resistance.

PREVENTION

Immunization against influenza and increasingly resistant pneumococci can play a critical role in preventing pneumonia, particularly in immunocompromised and older adults. The influenza vaccine is formulated and administered annually. The Centers for Disease Control and Prevention (CDC) recommends that vaccines be offered to persons older than 50 years, residents of extended-care facilities, and patients who have chronic heart and lung disorders, chronic metabolic diseases (including diabetes mellitus), renal dysfunction, hemoglobinopathies, or immunosuppression.[15]

The pneumococcal vaccine has been shown to be 60% to 70% effective in immunocompetent patients. Side effects are rarely serious and consist of local pain and erythema, which occur in up to 50% of recipients. The CDC recommends that vaccines be offered to all persons 65 years of age or older, those at increased risk for illness and death from pneumococcal disease because of chronic illness, those with functional or anatomic asplenia, and immunocompromised persons.[16] Patients who are immunosuppressed by chronic disease or treatment might not have sustained titers of protective antibody and should be considered for revaccination after 6 years.

Residual immunity against *Bordetella pertussis* wanes over time, leading to transmission from older adults to other adults and infants. Because secondary bacterial pneumonia occurs in a significant number of cases of pertussis, the ACIP (Advisory Committee on Immunization Practices) has recommended that the tetanus-diphtheria-acellular pertussis (Tdap) vaccine replace the tetanus-diphtheria (Td) vaccine in the adult immunization schedule.[17]

The emergence of SARS, with significant spread in hospitals, forced an extensive reassessment of respiratory infection control in many institutions. Measures to prevent the spread of SARS-associated coronavirus include close attention to cough hygiene, hand hygiene, contact precautions, and respiratory droplet precautions.

NATIONAL GUIDELINES

A number of expert bodies have developed guidelines for the diagnosis and management of community-acquired pneumonia. The most often cited are the guidelines of IDSA and ATS.[2] Thoughtful and comprehensive, these guidelines provide recommendations for the evaluation and treatment of the patient with community-acquired pneumonia driven by data, when available. Recommendations are classified by strength of supporting data; recommendations formed on the basis of opinion rather than data are identified. There is support for the use of the PSI and CRB scoring systems for risk stratification.

Treatment recommendationsare closely aligned with prior guidelines from the individual organizations. Compromise has been reached between the two organizations regarding the diagnostic evaluation of community-acquired pneumonia. Concerns of drug resistance and epidemiologic tracking have been noted, as have been concerns about lack of sensitivity and specificity in microbiologic testing. The resulting recommendations minimize testing for uncomplicated cases of pneumonia, allowing more extensive testing for sicker patients.

Guidelines for the home care of pneumonia have been published. These seek to ensure the administration of well-tolerated antimicrobial therapy and ongoing professional evaluation.[18]

When new respiratory pathogens emerge or major flares of well-known respiratory diseases occur, information develops quickly and guidelines are altered on a real-time basis. In such situations, the websites of the CDC, World Health Organization, IDSA, and state and local health departments often contain updated authoritative information and guidelines to assist the practitioner.

OUTCOMES AND PERFORMANCE MEASURES

Pneumonia-related outcomes have been measured in several areas. In the area of microbiology, Metlay and colleagues have noted that patients with pneumococci not susceptible to penicillin are more likely to develop suppurative complications than patients infected with susceptible isolates.[19] Overall, pneumococcal pneumonia has been shown by Fine and associates to carry a mortality rate of 12%.[20] This level of mortality is exceeded only by *Legionella* species among community-acquired pathogens. Several pathogens more associated with long-term care facilities, including *P. aeruginosa* (61%) and *S. aureus* (32%), carry substantially higher mortality.

Samples for blood cultures drawn within 24 hours of hospital admission have been associated with improvement in 30-day mortality.[21] Antibiotic therapy initiated within 4 hours of hospital admission has been shown to improve mortality and length of hospital stay in all pneumonia patients.[5,22] Adherence to the IDSA guidelines for antimicrobial therapy improves mortality in patients with community-acquired pneumonia in intensive care units.[23]

With regard to site of care, the PORT data have suggested a less than 1% risk of 30-day mortality for pneumonia sufferers falling into risk classes I and II of the pneumonia severity index, suggesting the possibility of outpatient care for this group. A home hospital model of care with daily home physician visits can reduce the duration of acute care and overall treatment costs in older patients.[24] IV-to-oral switch therapy has been shown to yield no significant reduction in outcome when the switch is instituted after clinical stability.[12]

The Centers for Medicare and Medicaid Services are moving forward with pay-for-performance measures, including certain parts of the IDSA/ATS practice guidelines, as a means of promoting hospital quality. Among the measures adopted are assessment of oxygenation, screening for pneumococcal vaccination, blood cultures before first antibiotic dose, assessment for smoking cessation, antibiotics within 4 to 6 hours of arrival at the hospital, and correct choice of antibiotics.

Suggested Readings

American Thoracic Society: Guidelines for the initial management of adults with community-acquired pneumonia: Diagnosis, assessment of severity, and initial antimicrobial therapy. Am J Resp Crit Care Med 2001;163:1730-1754.

Cassiere HA, Fein AM: Duration and route of antibiotic therapy in patients hospitalized with community-acquired pneumonia: Switch and step-down therapy. Semin Resp Infect 1998;13:36-42.

Centers for Disease Control and Prevention: Prevention and control of influenza: Recommendations of the Advisory Committee on Immunization Practices (ACIP). MMWR Morb Mortal Wkly Rep 2005;54(RR-08):1-40.

Centers for Disease Control and Prevention: Prevention of pneumococcal disease: Recommendations of the Advisory Committee on Immunization Practices (ACIP). MMWR Morb Mortal Wkly Rep 1997;46(RR-08):1-24.

Centers for Disease Control and Prevention: Update: Investigation of bioterrorism-related anthrax and interim guidelines for exposure management and antimicrobial therapy, October 2001. MMWR Morb Mortal Wkly Rep 2001;50:909-919.

Fine MJ, Auble TE, Yealy DM, et al: A prediction rule to identify low-risk patients with community-acquired pneumonia. N Engl J Med 1997;336:243-250.

Fine MJ, Smith MA, Carson CA, et al: Prognosis and outcomes of patients with community-acquired pneumonia. A meta-analysis. JAMA 1996;274:134-141.

Houck PM, Bratzler DW, Nsa W, et al: Timing of antibiotic administration and outcomes for Medicare patients hospitalized with pneumonia. Arch Intern Med 2004;164:637-644.

Mandell LA, Bartlett JG, Dowell SF, et al: Update of practice guidelines for the management of community-acquired pneumonia in immunocompetent adults. Clin Infect Dis 2003;37:1405-1433.

Mandell LA, Wunderink RG, Anzueto A, et al; Infectious Diseases Society of America; American Thoracic Society: Infectious Diseases Society of America/American Thoracic Society consensus guidelines on the management of community-acquired pneumonia in adults. Clin Infect Dis 2007;44 Suppl 2:S27-S72.

Peiris JS, Yuen KY, Osterhaus AD, Stohr K: The severe acute respiratory syndrome. N Engl J Med 2003;349:2431-2441.

References

For a complete list of references, log onto www.expertconsult.com.

Infective Endocarditis

Thomas F. Keys

DEFINITION

Infective endocarditis, an infection of the endocardium that usually involves the valves and adjacent structures, is caused by a wide variety of bacteria and fungi. The disease is known to infectious disease clinicians, but it might not be recognized by a busy general internist who is unlikely to encounter more than several cases a year.

PREVALENCE AND RISK FACTORS

The incidence of infective endocarditis in a general population has been estimated at between 2 and 6 cases per 100,000 person-years, but it is clearly higher in patients with underlying valvular heart diseases and those with intravenous drug abuse (IVDA). Furthermore, invasive procedures performed in our technically robust health care system may cause bloodstream infections and result in endocarditis.

Although historically rheumatic valvulitis was considered a frequent predisposing factor for endocarditis, times have changed. Mitral valve prolapse, aortic sclerosis, and bicuspid aortic valvular heart disease are now more frequent causes. In addition, prosthetic valvular heart disease accounts for about one third of all cases of endocarditis, and occurs in 1% to 3% of patients after valvular heart surgery.

Pacemaker endocarditis, another complication of advancing technology, is caused by microorganisms that usually migrate across a broken skin barrier from an eroding battery pack or generator pocket wound. Early cases are frequently caused by *Staphylococcus aureus* and late cases are caused by *Staphylococcus epidermidis*. Over time, intravascular pacemaker leads encapsulate deeply in the right ventricle, making explantation tedious and difficult.

One study has demonstrated a high frequency of *S. aureus* endocarditis secondary to preventable sources.[3] Of 59 cases reported from Duke University, 23 were caused by intravascular catheters and 14 by infected surgical wounds. Approximately 25% of vascular catheter-associated bacteremias caused by *S. aureus* may result in endocarditis.

A significant risk factor for endocarditis is IVDA. Patients who use injection drugs tend to be younger and may be coinfected with human immunodeficiency virus (HIV). Cases of IVDA-associated endocarditis usually respond quickly to antibiotic therapy, but recurrence is common.[1]

PATHOPHYSIOLOGY

Although uncertain, it is believed that cardiac valves and other endocardial surfaces become infected after exposure to microemboli from bacteria or fungi circulating in the bloodstream. Dextran-producing bacteria, such as *Streptococcus mutans*, have a virulence factor that promotes adherence to endovascular surfaces. Coagulase-negative staphylococci may produce a biofilm on prosthetic surfaces, which also promotes adherence. Beta-hemolytic streptococci and enteric gram-negative bacteria lack recognized adherence factors, and appear less likely to cause endocarditis. Endocardial surfaces previously damaged from valvular heart disease, endocarditis, surgery, or pacemaker wires provide a favorable environment for thrombus formation. Over time, microorganisms proliferate in the thrombus, resulting in a classic vegetation. Microorganisms are released into the circulation, usually on a continuous basis, which often results in interesting findings.

SIGNS AND SYMPTOMS

The disease often begins as a flulike illness with a dry cough, body aches, and fatigue, which follows a subacute or chronic course. Low-grade fevers, night sweats, and weight loss are cardinal manifestations (Table 1). Surprisingly, most patients, especially younger ones, do not seek medical advice until fatigue or fever becomes unbearable or they suffer a major complication, such as an embolic event or heart failure. Patients who have had heart surgery in the recent past usually seek medical advice earlier because of their heightened awareness of post-operative complications.

A careful physical examination may disclose skin or mucosal lesions in about 50% of cases (Fig. 1). These include subconjunctival and soft palate petechiae, hemorrhages within the nail beds (splinter hemorrhages), painful subcutaneous nodules on the palms or soles (Osler's nodes), and generalized rashes. Patients may also present with painful embolic lesions on the fingers or toes, which may be visible.

Almost always, a regurgitant heart murmur is heard, usually in the mitral or aortic valve position. New or changing murmurs in patients with preexisting murmurs are noted in about 30% of cases. A widening of the pulse pressure may be a sign of aortic valve dehiscence, an indication for urgent surgical intervention. Similarly, bradycardia progressing to complete heart block can be caused by a septal abscess, which also requires open surgical débridement and drainage.

Splenomegaly, reported in about 20% of cases, is more likely in patients who have been ill for months rather than days or weeks.

DIAGNOSIS

Diagnostic clues noted by Sir William Osler in 1908 included remittent fever with a valvular heart lesion, embolic findings, skin lesions, and progressive cardiac changes, and these are pertinent today. However, in Osler's time, the diagnosis was confirmed at autopsy, because few, if any, patients survived. Without pathologic evidence, clinical findings are not specific for the diagnosis. Fortunately, with the use of modern blood culture techniques, the diagnosis can usually be confirmed in the microbiology laboratory. A majority of patients with confirmed bacterial endocarditis have positive blood cultures within a 2-day period, provided that they had not recently been on antibiotics. Therefore, it is not necessary to continuously collect blood cultures beyond this point. Three sets should suffice. Recovery of organisms is enhanced with the BACTEC system (Becton Dickinson, Sparks, Md) for gram-negative bacilli and yeasts.

In 1981, Von Reyn and associates published an important article that laid out strict criteria for the diagnosis of endocarditis.[11] A positive valve culture or histology was defined as definite endocarditis. Major criteria for probable endocarditis were persistent bacteremia with a new regurgitant heart murmur or valvular heart disease with vasculitis or negative or intermittent bacteremia with fever and a new regurgitant heart murmur with vasculitis. Further refinements in the diagnosis have occurred with the use of echocardiography. Transesophageal echocardiography is preferred over the transthoracic approach because it usually provides superior imaging for detecting vegetations and abscesses.

Durack and associates[2] at Duke University have subsequently found that an echocardiogram clearly showing vegetations or abscesses of the endocardium is a major criterion, as is positive serology for *Coxiella burnetii* (Box 1).

Table 1 Clinical Findings in Infective Endocarditis Patients*

Symptoms	NVE (%) (*n* = 60)	PVE (%) (*n* = 30)
Fever	75	87
Weight loss	52	20
Skin lesions	51	47
New murmur	33	33
Splenomegaly	20	20

*90 patients.
NVE, native valve endocarditis; PVE, prosthetic valve endocarditis.
Adapted from Keys TF: Infective endocarditis: A continuing challenge. J Crit Illness 1987;2:19-32.

Box 1 Duke Criteria for Diagnosis of Infective Endocarditis

Two major criteria

- Typical organism
- Persistent bacteremia
- Positive serology for *Coxiella brunetii*
- Positive echocardiographic results for vegetations, abscess, or valve

Positive culture or histology of a vegetation or intracardiac abscess dehiscence

Five minor criteria

- Valvular heart disease
- History of IV drug abuse
- Fever higher than 38° C
- Vasculitis, skin lesions
- suggestive echocardiographic results (but not definitive)
- Single positive blood culture

One major and three minor criteria

Adapted from Baddour LM, Wilson WR, Bayer AS, et al: Infective endocarditis: Diagnosis, antimicrobial therapy and management of complications: A statement from the committee on rheumatic fever, endocarditis and Kawasaki disease. Circulation 2005;111:e394-e434.

TREATMENT

Medical Treatment

Streptococci, especially *Streptococcus viridans*, have historically been responsible for the largest percentage of cases of native valve endocarditis (Table 2). However, in more recent series, *S. aureus* may be as common, or even more common. Certain *viridans* streptococci, such as *Streptococcus mitis*, may be nutritionally variant and require active vitamin B_6 and thio compounds for growth. Such variants account for 10% of cases, and tend to be less susceptible to penicillin. Enterococci are responsible for up to 10% of cases; some strains may be not only resistant to penicillin, but to vancomycin and aminoglycosides.

Occasional cases caused by beta-hemolytic streptococci are reported; they often manifest with major embolic events. Rarely, *Streptococcus pneumoniae* may cause endocarditis. Such a case might manifest with the Osler triad of pneumonia, meningitis, and endocarditis. Often associated with alcohol abuse, mortality is extremely high.

S. aureus, in addition to causing endocarditis, may result in a severe sepsis syndrome, with a fulminating coagulopathy. Metastatic foci of infection spread to the brain, lungs, liver, and kidneys, sequelae that result in a high mortality rate. The organism is also a cause of early-onset prosthetic valve endocarditis (PVE), but is not as common as *Staphylococcus epidermidis* (Table 3). This form of endocarditis, occurring within 1 year after surgery, is usually the result of intraoperative contamination by skin bacteria. Currently, infections from vascular catheters and surgical wounds are more frequent sources of infection. *Staphylococcus epidermidis*, the usual cause of early-onset PVE, is almost always resistant to methicillin or oxacillin. *Staphylococcus lugdunensis* is also coagulase-negative, but behaves more like *S. aureus* clinically. Death is almost certain unless infected valves are removed.

The HACEK group of gram-negative bacteria may cause endocarditis. These fastidious microorganisms include *Haemophilus*, *Actinobacillus*, *Cardiobacterium*, *Eikenella*, and *Kingella* species. Patients can be ill for months and may present with a painful embolic lesion to an extremity.

Most cases of fungal endocarditis occur in patients who are receiving prolonged antibiotics or parenteral nutrition through central vascular catheters. Such patients may also be immunocompromised. The most common organism responsible is *Candida albicans*, followed by *Candida parapsilosis*. Endocarditis caused by *Histoplasma capsulatum* or *Aspergillus* spp. is rare.

Finally, unusual cases of endocarditis should be considered when standard microbiologic techniques fail to provide a diagnosis. Q fever endocarditis caused by *Coxiella burnetii* is an example. Patients may not have fever, but they frequently have underlying valvular heart disease and are on immunosuppressive therapy. Vegetations are rarely detected on the echocardiogram. Although routine blood cultures are negative, an alerted microbiology laboratory may recover the organism from buffy coat cultures. Serologic studies are reasonably specific. *Bartonella henselae* may also cause endocarditis, and diagnosis here is also difficult. Infections are seen in the homeless and alcoholic populations. Blood cultures are negative, but again serology may be helpful. Identification by polymerase chain reaction (PCR) assay on resected valve tissue has been reported, but this test is not readily available in most clinical laboratories.

Antimicrobial Selection Guidelines

The penicillins, often in combination with gentamicin, remain the cornerstones of therapy for endocarditis caused by penicillin-susceptible streptococci (Table 4).[4] For penicillin-allergic patients, vancomycin is substituted. IV ceftriaxone (Rocephin), given once daily for 4 weeks, is another option, and even a 2-week course in combination with gentamicin has proven successful. However, short-term therapy is not indicated for patients who have PVE, major embolic complications, or symptoms for longer than 2 months. Furthermore, in this study, 24% of patients required urgent valvular heart surgery within 1 to 5 weeks after beginning treatment. Therefore, careful follow-up is essential, especially for patients who leave the hospital to complete antibiotic therapy at home.

For relatively penicillin-insensitive streptococci (minimal inhibitory concentration >0.1-0.5 μg/mL), the penicillin dosage is higher and duration of therapy is 2 weeks (Table 5).[4] Gentamicin is given for the first 2 weeks; treatment for endocarditis caused by enterococci is longer; both penicillin and gentamicin are given for 6 weeks (Table 6). Patients who are penicillin-allergic, should receive vancomycin, provided the isolate is susceptible. For vancomycin-resistant enterococci (VRE), anecdotal success has been reported using streptogramin quinupristin-dalfopristin (Synercid) either alone or in combination with doxycycline and rifampin. A newer antimicrobial agent, linezolid (Zyvox), has in vitro activity against VRE, and has been reported successful in the treatment of a small series of cases. Daptomycin may also be a promising antibiotic for VRE endocarditis, but has not yet been field tested.

The preferred treatment for native valve endocarditis (NVE) caused by methicillin-susceptible staphylococci is oxacillin or cefazolin for 4 to 6 weeks. If the organism is methicillin-resistant, vancomycin is used. Gentamicin may be added for the first 3 to 5 days. This will shorten the duration of the bacteremia; however, if continued longer, it does not improve the cure rate and may cause renal toxicity.

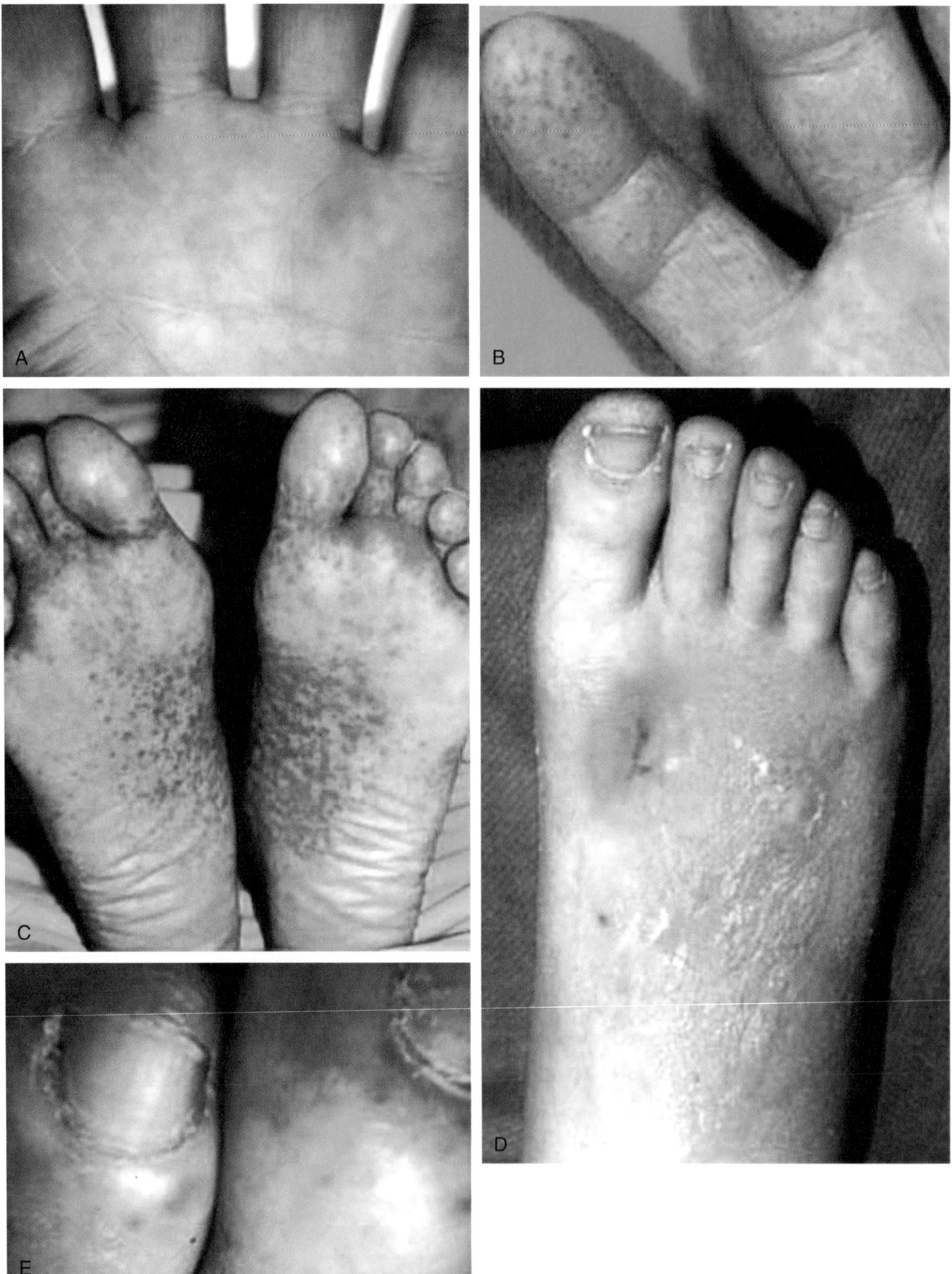

Figure 1 Vascular skin lesions associated with infective endocarditis. **A,** Raised red nodule on palm *(Pseudomonas aeruginosa)*. **B,** Fine raised rash on palms and fingers *(Actinobacillus actinomycetemcomitans)*. **C,** Petechial rash on soles *(Viridans streptococci)*. **D,** Embolic lesion on dorsum of foot *(Acinetobacter calcoaceticus)*. **E,** Flea-bitten rash on toes *(Enterococcus faecalis)*. *(From Keys TF: Infective endocarditis: Prevention, diagnosis, treatment, referral. Cleve Clin J Med 2000;67:353-360.)*

Table 2 Native Valve Endocarditis Microbiology

Organism	Cases (%)
Streptococcus viridans	30-40
Enterococcus spp.	5-18
Other streptococci	15-25
Staphylococcus aureus	10-27
Coagulase-negative staphylococci	1-3
Gram-negative bacilli	2-13
Fungi	2-4
Other	<5
Culture-negative	<5-14

Adapted from Fowler VG, Scheld WM, Bayer AS: Endocarditis and intravascular infections. In Mandell GL, Bennett JE, Dolin R (eds): Principles and Practice of Infectious Diseases, 6th ed. Philadelphia, Churchill Livingstone, 2005, pp 975-1022.

Table 3 Early-Onset Prosthetic Valve Endocarditis*

Organism	Cases (%)
Staphylococcus epidermidis	40 (52)
Staphylococcus aureus	9 (12)
Enterococci	6 (8)
Gram-negative bacilli	4 (5)
Fungi	11 (14)
Others	7 (9)
Total	77 (100)

*Within 12 months of surgery.

Adapted from Gordon SM, Serkey JM, Longworth DL, et al: Early-onset prosthetic valve endocarditis 1992-1997. Ann Thorac Surg 2000;69: 1388-1392.

Table 4 Treatment of Endocarditis Caused by Penicillin-Sensitive Streptococci*

Antibiotic	Dosage Regimen	Duration (wk)
Penicillin G	12-18 MU IV q24hr	4
Ceftiaxone	2 g IV q24hr	4
Ceftriaxone *plus* gentamicin	2 g IV q24hr 1 mg/kg IV q8hr	2
Vancomycin	1 g IV q12hr	4

*Assumes normal renal function.

MU, million units.

Adapted from Baddour LM, Wilson WR, Bayer AS, et al: Infective endocarditis: Diagnosis, antimicrobial therapy and management of complications: A statement from the committee on rheumatic fever, endocarditis and Kawasaki disease. Circulation 2005;111:e394-e434.

Table 5 Treatment of Endocarditis Caused by Penicillin-Insensitive Streptococci*

Antibiotic	Dosage Regimen	Duration (wk)[†]
Penicillin G *or* ceftriaxone *plus* gentamicin	4 MU IV q4hr	4-6
	2 g IV q24hr	4-6
	1 mg/kg IV/IM q8hr	2
Vancomycin	1 g IV q12hr	4-6

*Assumes normal renal function; minimum inhibitory concentration > 0.12-0.5 μg/mL.

[†]Duration-6 wk for prosthetic valve endocarditis.

MU, million units.

Adapted from Baddour LM, Wilson WR, Bayer AS, et al: Infective endocarditis: Diagnosis, antimicrobial therapy and management of complications: A statement from the committee on rheumatic fever, endocarditis and Kawasaki disease. Circulation 2005;111:e394-e434.

Table 6 Treatment of Endocarditis Caused by Enterococci

Isolate	Dosage Regimen	Duration (wk)
Penicillin-Susceptible		
All organisms	Ampicillin 2 g IV q4hr + gentamicin* I mg/kg IV q8hr *or* vancomycin 1 g IV q12hr	4-6
Penicillin-Resistant		
Beta-lactamase[†]	Ampicillin-sulbactam 3 g IV q6hr + gentamicin* I mg/kg IV q8hr	6
Intrinsically resistant	Vancomycin 1 g IV q12hr + gentamicin* 1 mg/kg q8hr	6
Penicillin- and Vancomycin-Resistant		
Enterococcus faecium	Linezolid 600 mg IV or PO q12hr *or* quinupristin-dalfopristin 7 mg/kg q8hr	≥8
Enterococcus faecalis	Imipenem-celastatin 500 mg 7 mg/kg q6hr + ampicillin, 2 g IV q4hr *or* ceftriaxone 2 g IV q24hr + ampicillin 2 g IV q4hr	≥8

*Substitute streptomycin, 7 mg/kg q12hr, if patient is gentamicin-resistant.

[†]Use only when patients cannot tolerate ampicillin (or penicillin).

Adapted from Baddour LM, Wilson WR, Bayer AS, et al: Infective endocarditis: Diagnosis, antimicrobial therapy and management of complications: A statement from the committee on rheumatic fever, endocarditis and Kawasaki disease. Circulation 2005;111:e394-e434.

Antibiotic therapy for staphylococcal PVE must be more aggressive because of the greater likelihood of treatment failure or relapse (Table 7). When the isolate is methicillin-susceptible, oxacillin plus rifampin is given for 6 weeks and gentamicin for the first 2 weeks. When the isolate is methicillin-resistant, vancomycin is substituted for oxacillin.

Endocarditis caused by *S. aureus* associated with IVDA is generally more responsive to short-course antibiotic therapy. In one study, a cure rate of 89% was reported after a 2-week course of IV cloxacillin (not available in the United States).

The preferred treatment for the HACEK group of bacterial endocarditis is ceftriaxone for 4 weeks. Other options are ampicillin-sulbactam or ciprofloxacin (Table 8). Patients with late-onset PVE

Table 7 Treatment of Prosthetic Valve Endocarditis Caused by Staphylococci*

Isolate	Antibiotic	Dosage Regimen	Duration (wk)
MSSA or MSSE	Oxacillin + gentamicin + rifampin	2 g IV q4hr	≥6
		1 mg/kg IVor IM q8hr	2
		300 mg PO q8hr	≥6
MRSA or MRSE	Vancomycin + gentamicin + rifampin	1 g IV q12hr	≥6
		1 mg/kg IV/IM q8hr	2
		300 mg PO q8hr	≥6

*Doses assume normal renal function.

MRSA, *methicillin-resistant Staphylococcus aureus*; MRSE, methicillin-resistant *Staphylococcus epidermidis*; MSSA, methicillin-sensitive *S. aureus*; MSSE, methicillin-sensitive *S. epidermidis*.

Adapted from Baddour LM, Wilson WR, Bayer AS, et al: Infective endocarditis: Diagnosis, antimicrobial therapy and management of complications: A statement from the committee on rheumatic fever, endocarditis and Kawasaki disease. Circulation 2005;111:e394-e434.

Table 8 Treatment of Endocarditis Caused by HACEK Microorganisms*

Antibiotic	Dosage Regimen	Duration (wk)
Ceftriaxone	2 g IV q24hr	4
Ampicillin-sulbactam	3 g IV q6hr	4
Ciprofloxacin	400 mg IV q12hr	4

*Doses assume normal renal function.

HACEK, *Haempohilus, Actinobacillus, Cardiobacterium, Eikenella,* and *Kingella* species of bacteremia.

Adapted from Baddour LM, Wilson WR, Bayer AS, et al: Infective endocarditis: Diagnosis, antimicrobial therapy and management of complications: A statement from the committee on rheumatic fever, endocarditis and Kawasaki disease. Circulation 2005;111:e394-e434.

Table 9 Neurologic Complications in Native Valve Endocarditis (NVE) and Prosthetic Valve Endocarditis (PVE)

Complication	NVE (%)	PVE (%)
Stroke	15	21
Encephalopathy	9	8
Retinal emboli	3	3
Headache	4	3
Mycotic aneurysm	3	—
Abscess	1	2
Menigitis	1	2
Seizures	1	—
Total	37	39

Adapted from Selgado AV, Furlan AJ, Keys TF: Neurologic complications of endocarditis. Neurology 1989;39:173-178.

may be cured medically without requiring valve surgery, provided that only the valve cusps or leaflets are involved.

Fungal endocarditis has a poor prognosis. In a series of prosthetic valve endocarditis reported from the Cleveland Clinic, a 67% survival rate was reported.[12] Survivors not only required aggressive surgery and IV amphotericin B (Fungizone), but received lifelong suppression with an oral antifungal afterward.

From 10% to 20% percent of patients with clinically suspected endocarditis will have negative blood cultures. An empirical trial of ampicillin-sulbactam plus gentamicin for NVE or vancomycin plus ciprofloxacin and gentamicin for PVE should be considered. Although staphylococci or streptococci may not be recovered from blood cultures, they may be seen on smears or recovered from vegetations taken at surgery. About 50% of patients with negative blood cultures will respond to empirical therapy. If not, further investigation is warranted, and unusual microorganisms or noninfectious causes of endocarditis should be considered.

Surgical Treatment

Death from infective endocarditis is usually caused by congestive heart failure, often accompanied by valve dysfunction. In the last 25 years, aggressive surgery has been the most important advance in therapy. Surgery during acute infection does not increase mortality; in fact, restoration of a failing pump improves function and outcome. Valve failure causing moderate to severe congestive heart failure (New York Heart Association Class III or IV) is a strong indication for urgent surgery. An endocardial abscess, which can involve the aortic root, valve ring, or ventricular septum, is another indication for urgent intervention. Other conditions favoring surgery include vegetations larger than 1 cm in diameter, a major embolic event, and failure or relapse of medical therapy.

Even though surgery may not be required during hospitalization, it may be needed later on because of progressive valve damage from healed endocarditis. In one study, 47% of patients eventually required surgery, usually within 2 years after completing medical therapy.[13]

OUTCOMES

Persistent Fever

Persistent fever during the treatment of endocarditis is worrisome. Annular or ring abscesses may cause this and are strong indications for surgery. Other causes of fever include myocarditis, pulmonary and systemic emboli, and intravascular catheter site infections. Drug fevers without other manifestations, such as rash and renal findings, are unusual, but must also be considered.

Neurologic Complications

Neurologic complications from endocarditis are common and can present difficult and sometimes vexing management dilemmas (Table 9). Leading causes are stroke, encephalopathy, and retinal emboli. Brain abscesses and mycotic aneurysms are relatively infrequent. As a general rule, anticoagulation should be avoided because of the increased risk of intracranial bleeding. One may elect to continue anticoagulation in patients with mechanical heart valves, but dosing should be in the low therapeutic range to minimize the risk of bleeding. Fortunately, most mycotic aneurysms do not require surgery, and usually resolve after appropriate antimicrobial therapy.

Survival

In the preantibiotic era, survival after infective endocarditis was unlikely. With effective antimicrobial therapy and surgical intervention, the outcome is no longer bleak. However, despite striking advances in management, mortality remains around 20%. In part, this is because more patients are living longer with prosthetic heart valves and have more comorbidity, and IV drug abuse continues to be a problem. The most frequent cause of death is congestive heart

Table 10 Dental and Cardiac Risk Factors for Infective Endocarditis

Risk Factor	Cases (*n* = 273)	Controls (*n* = 273)
Dental prophylaxis	24	23
Extractions	6	0
Gingival surgery	1	0
History of endocarditis	17	1
Cardiac valvular surgery	37	2
Mitral valve prolapse	52	6

Adapted from Strom BL, Abrutyn E, Berlin JA, et al: Dental and cardiac risk factors for infective endocarditis. Ann Intern Med 1998;129:761-769.

failure, less frequently followed by major embolic events and ruptured mycotic aneurysms. Death is usually not caused by uncontrolled infection. In the past, early-onset PVE mortality was as high as 90% because surgeons were reluctant to reoperate on patients with active infection. Now, with surgical expertise and perioperative support, mortality has been reduced to approximately 25%.

PREVENTION

There is a continued debate about the need for and adequacy of antibiotic prophylaxis to prevent infective endocarditis. In 1986, Bayliss and colleagues[8] reported a presumed dental portal of entry in less than 20% of well-studied cases. Further controversy arose after a case-control study was reported in 1996 from the greater Philadelphia area (Table 10).[9] Patients with well-defined endocarditis were matched with controls for age, gender, and neighborhood. Information was collected through structured telephone interviews and review of outside medical and dental records. Cases of endocarditis were no more likely than controls to have had dental procedures, except for extractions. Cardiac risk factors were more common in these patients, including mitral valve prolapse, congenital heart disease, rheumatic valvular heart disease, previous cardiac surgery, history of infective endocarditis, and a known heart murmur. In an accompanying editorial, the author suggested that only patients with prosthetic valvular heart disease or a history of endocarditis undergoing dental extractions or gingival surgery would benefit from antibiotic prophylaxis.

Box 2 Patients at Highest Risk for Adverse Outcomes from Endocarditis

Prosthetic cardiac valve disease
Previous infective endocarditis
Congenital heart disease (CHD)

- Unrepaired cyanotic CHD
- Completely repaired CHD with prosthetic materials for 6 mo, allowing endothelium formation
- Incompletely repaired CHD with residual defects at prosthetic patches or devices

Cardiac transplantation with valvular defects

Adapted from Wilson W, Taubert KA, Gewitz M, et al; American Heart Association Rheumatic Fever, Endocarditis, and Kawasaki Disease Committee; American Heart Association Council on Cardiovascular Disease in the Young; American Heart Association Council on Clinical Cardiology; American Heart Association Council on Cardiovascular Surgery and Anesthesia; Quality of Care and Outcomes Research Interdisciplinary Working Group: Prevention of infective endocarditis: Guidelines from the American Heart Association: A guideline from the American Heart Association Rheumatic Fever, Endocarditis, and Kawasaki Disease Committee, Council on Cardiovascular Disease in the Young, and the Council on Clinical Cardiology, Council on Cardiovascular Surgery and Anesthesia, and the Quality of Care and Outcomes Research Interdisciplinary Working Group. Circulation 2007;115:1690-1695.

Box 3 Invasive Procedures for Prophylaxis in High-Risk Patients

Any procedure that involves the gingival tissues or periapical region of a tooth or that perforates the oral mucosa
Cystoscopy or other genitourinary tract manipulation in which the urinary tract is infected with *Enterococcus* spp.
Drainage of established infections such as empyema, abscesses, or phlegmons in which *S. aureus*, streptococci, or enterococci are likely or proven pathogens

Adapted from Wilson W, Taubert KA, Gewitz M, et al; American Heart Association Rheumatic Fever, Endocarditis, and Kawasaki Disease Committee; American Heart Association Council on Cardiovascular Disease in the Young; American Heart Association Council on Clinical Cardiology; American Heart Association Council on Cardiovascular Surgery and Anesthesia; Quality of Care and Outcomes Research Interdisciplinary Working Group: Prevention of infective endocarditis: Guidelines from the American Heart Association: A guideline from the American Heart Association Rheumatic Fever, Endocarditis, and Kawasaki Disease Committee, Council on Cardiovascular Disease in the Young, and the Council on Clinical Cardiology, Council on Cardiovascular Surgery and Anesthesia, and the Quality of Care and Outcomes Research Interdisciplinary Working Group. Circulation 2007;115:1690-1695.

Prophylaxis Guidelines

Although the risk of side effects clearly outweighs the benefit in patients at low risk for endocarditis, prophylaxis remains an accepted practice in higher risk patients. Guidelines, published periodically by the American Heart Association, were substantially updated in 2007.[10] After an exhaustive literature search and personal reflections on their own experiences, the expert panel concluded that many of the earlier recommendations had not been based on sound evidence-based studies. They now recommend that prophylaxis should only be given to patients who have the highest risk of complications of endocarditis (Box 2).

Furthermore, the list of procedures for endocarditis prophylaxis has been considerably shortened—for example, only for dental work involving gingival tissue and the periapical regions of the teeth, or for perforations of the oral mucosa (Box 3). Other invasive procedures that might warrant prophylaxis include diagnostic studies or drainage of infected spaces where streptococci, enterococci. or *S. aureus* are proven or likely pathogens.

For recommended dental procedures, the recommended first-line regimen remains amoxicillin, 2 g PO, or ampicillin 2 g IM or IV, 30 to 60 minutes before the procedure (Table 11). The same regimen should apply for patients undergoing cystoscopy or other genitourinary manipulations who have enterococcal bacteriuria.

However, for high-risk patients undergoing diagnostic studies or procedures such as drainage of empyema, abscesses, or phlegmons in which *S. aureus* may be present, prophylaxis should be broadened with a penicillinase-resistant penicillin (oxacillin or nafcillin) or first-generation cephalosporin(cefazolin). Vancomycin should be substituted if the pathogen is suspected or proven resistant to oxacillin or methicillin (methicillin-resistant *S. aureus* [MRSA]).

For patients undergoing cardiac valve surgery, IV preoperative prophylaxis with a first- or second-generation cephalosporin is recommended. This should be given within 30 minutes before opening the skin. If the operation is longer than 4 hours, a second dose can be given intraoperatively before skin closure. Prophylaxis should not be continued longer than 24 hours after surgery. For the penicillin-allergic patient or in hospitals in which there is a high prevalence of MRSA or methicillin-resistant or *S. epidermidis*, vancomycin should be considered.

Table 11 Prophylactic Regimens for Dental Procedures in Adults

Situation	Agent	Dosage Regimen*
Oral	Amoxicillin	2 g
Unable to take oral	Ampicillin *or* ceftriaxone	2 g IM or IV 1 g IM or IV
Penicillin allergy, oral	Cephalexin, *or* clindamycin, *or* azithromycin	2 g 600 mg 500 mg
Unable to take oral	Cefazolin, *or* ceftriaxone, *or* clindamycin	1 g IM or IV 1 g IM or IV 600 mg IM or IV

*30-60 min before procedure.

Adapted from Wilson W, Taubert KA, Gewitz M, et al; American Heart Association Rheumatic Fever, Endocarditis, and Kawasaki Disease Committee; American Heart Association Council on Cardiovascular Disease in the Young; American Heart Association Council on Clinical Cardiology; American Heart Association Council on Cardiovascular Surgery and Anesthesia; Quality of Care and Outcomes Research Interdisciplinary Working Group: Prevention of infective endocarditis: Guidelines from the American Heart Association: A guideline from the American Heart Association Rheumatic Fever, Endocarditis, and Kawasaki Disease Committee, Council on Cardiovascular Disease in the Young, and the Council on Clinical Cardiology, Council on Cardiovascular Surgery and Anesthesia, and the Quality of Care and Outcomes Research Interdisciplinary Working Group. Circulation 2007:115:1690-1695.

Summary

- *Staphylococcus aureus* is probably more common now than *Streptococcus viridans* as the cause of native valve endocarditis.
- A widening pulse pressure and bradycardia are ominous signs that may require early surgical intervention.
- Transesophageal echocardiography is superior to transthoracic imaging for detecting vegetations and abscesses.
- Neurologic complications are frequent but usually do not cause death.
- Antibiotic prophylaxis for invasive dental procedures remains recommended, but only for patients at high risk of complications from endocarditis.

Suggested Readings

Andrews MM, Von Reyn CF: Patient selection criteria and management guidelines for outpatient parenteral antibiotic therapy for native valve infective endocarditis. Clin Infect Dis 2001:32:203-209.

Baddour LM, Wilson WR, Bayer AS, et al: Infective endocarditis: Diagnosis, antimicrobial therapy and management of complications: A statement from the committee on rheumatic fever, endocarditis and Kawasaki disease. Circulation 2005;111:e394-e434.

Bayliss R, Clarke C, Oakley CM, et al: Incidence, mortality and prevention of infective endocarditis. J Royal Coll Physicians Lond 1986;20:15-20.

Durack DT, Lukes AS, Bright KD, et al: New criteria for diagnosis of infective endocarditis. Utilization of specific echocardiographic findings. Am J Med 1994;96:200-209.

Fowler VG, Sanders LL, Kong LK, et al: Infective endocarditis due to *Staphylococcus aureus*. Clin Infect Dis 1994;28:106-114.

Melgar GR, Nasser RM, Gordon SM, et al: Fungal prosthetic valve endocarditis in 16 patients. An 11-year experience in a tertiary care hospital. Medicine 1997;76:94-103.

Miro JM, Angueva I, Cabell CH, et al: *Staphylococcua aureus native* valve endocarditis: Report of 566 episodes from the international collaboration on endocarditis merged database. Clin Infect Dis 2005;41:507-514.

Mylonakis E, Calderwood SB: Infective endocarditis in adults. N Engl J Med 2001;345:1318-1330.

Olaison L, Pettersson G: Current best practices and guidelines indications for surgical intervention in infective endocarditis. Infect Dis Clin North Am 2002;16:453-475.

Strom BL, Abrutyn E, Berlin JA, et al: Dental and cardiac risk factors for infective endocarditis. Ann Intern Med 1998;129:761-769.

Tornos MP, Permanyer-Miralda G, Olona M, et al: Long-term complications of native valve endocarditis in non-addicts: A 15-year follow-up study. Ann Intern Med 1992;117:567-572.

Von Reyn CF, Levy BS, Arbeit RD, et al: Infective endocarditis: an analysis based on strict case definitions. Ann Intern Med 1981;94:505-518.

Wilson W, Taubert KA, Gewitz M, et al; American Heart Association Rheumatic Fever, Endocarditis, and Kawasaki Disease Committee; American Heart Association Council on Cardiovascular Disease in the Young; American Heart Association Council on Clinical Cardiology; American Heart Association Council on Cardiovascular Surgery and Anesthesia; Quality of Care and Outcomes Research Interdisciplinary Working Group: Prevention of infective endocarditis: Guidelines from the American Heart Association: A guideline from the American Heart Association Rheumatic Fever, Endocarditis, and Kawasaki Disease Committee, Council on Cardiovascular Disease in the Young, and the Council on Clinical Cardiology, Council on Cardiovascular Surgery and Anesthesia, and the Quality of Care and Outcomes Research Interdisciplinary Working Group. Circulation 2007;115:1690-1695.

References

For a complete list of references, log onto www.expertconsult.com.

Infectious Disease Emergencies

Nabin K. Shrestha

Infectious disease emergencies are conditions that have potential for significant harm to the patient if not recognized and treated promptly, and for which timely and appropriate intervention may significantly improve outcomes. The following is a discussion of important infectious disease emergencies.

ACUTE BACTERIAL MENINGITIS

Definition, Etiology, and Incidence

Bacterial meningitis is an inflammation of the meninges caused by bacteria. Acute meningitis is characterized by the development of meningeal signs over the course of a few hours to a few days. The important causes of bacterial meningitis are outlined in Box 1.

A passive survey conducted in the United States between 1978 and 1981 revealed an annual incidence rate for bacterial meningitis of 3.0 cases per 100,000 population.[1] During this period, bacterial meningitis was predominantly a disease of children, the most common offending pathogen being *Haemophilus influenzae.* The introduction of routine immunization of children against *H. influenzae* type B in the late 1980s dramatically reduced the incidence of infection with this microorganism. A consequence was a decrease in the overall incidence of bacterial meningitis and particularly in meningitis caused by *H. influenzae*, so that bacterial meningitis is now a disease predominantly of adults.[2]

Pathophysiology

The initial event is usually nasopharyngeal colonization with a pathogenic microorganism.[3] This is followed by mucosal invasion, bacteremia, and meningeal invasion.[4] A marked inflammatory response occurs in the subarachnoid space, but this response is inadequate to control the infection. This inflammatory response results in increased permeability of the blood-brain barrier. This is responsible for the increased cerebrospinal fluid (CSF) protein content seen in patients with meningitis. Progression of meningitis leads to the development of cerebral edema, resulting in increased CSF pressure. Inflammation of blood vessels traversing the subarachnoid space may lead to their thrombosis. This can result in ischemia and infarction of the underlying brain.

Clinical Presentation

Patients with acute bacterial meningitis usually present with headache, neck stiffness, fever, projectile vomiting, and photophobia. In more advanced disease, there is progressive clouding of consciousness. On examination, neck rigidity may be seen and Kernig's and Brudzinski's signs may be elicited. Cranial nerve palsies or focal neurologic signs may be seen in a minority of patients. The presence of petechial skin lesions should raise suspicion for meningococcemia.

Diagnosis

The differential diagnosis includes viral and tuberculous meningitis, viral meningoencephalitis, subarachnoid hemorrhage, and primary amebic meningoencephalitis. Differentiation from viral meningitis on clinical grounds is usually difficult, and requires laboratory testing. Where tuberculosis is prevalent, it must be recognized that tuberculous meningitis can sometimes manifest acutely and could be mistaken for bacterial meningitis. Viral meningoencephalitis may manifest somewhat similarly with headache and fever, but patients would usually have more profound alteration in the sensorium early in the illness and neck stiffness may not be prominent. The most prominent symptom of subarachnoid hemorrhage is a severe headache with a rapid onset. Primary amebic meningoencephalitis is a rare condition with a presentation similar to that of acute bacterial meningitis, but cultures are negative and amebae can be detected in the CSF by careful microscopic examination. There is usually a recent history of swimming in a warm freshwater lake or pond.

The most important diagnostic test is a lumbar puncture, which should always be performed in all patients with suspected acute meningitis. Imaging tests do not help in making the diagnosis or identifying the cause of bacterial meningitis. It is not necessary to obtain a computed tomography (CT) scan before performing a lumbar puncture unless there are focal neurologic deficits.[5] The CSF should be sent for cell count, protein and glucose levels, and Gram staining and culture. Typical CSF findings in acute bacterial meningitis are an elevated opening pressure, increased CSF white blood cell (WBC) count (100-10,000 cells/μL), usually with a predominance of neutrophils, increased CSF protein level (>50 mg/dL) and decreased CSF glucose level (<40% of simultaneously measured serum glucose level).[6] Gram staining may reveal the presence of microorganisms and, if so detected, would be helpful for guiding therapy. In viral meningitis, the CSF WBC count is elevated, but the cells are usually predominantly lymphocytes, and the CSF glucose level may be normal or marginally decreased. The best way to confirm a diagnosis of viral meningitis is by specific polymerase chain reaction (PCR) testing, if available.

Treatment

The management of bacterial meningitis includes appropriate antibiotic therapy and adjunctive corticosteroids.[7,8] Ideally, the lumbar puncture should be done before the administration of antibiotics. However, if there is a delay in performing the lumbar puncture for any reason, antibiotic administration should not be delayed. A lumbar puncture should be performed as soon as possible, even if antibiotics have already been administered; the possibility of being able to make a definite causative diagnosis, and its value in guiding subsequent therapy and managing possible complications, are fully worth the effort. Empirical antibiotics should be selected based on the expected pathogens. The patient's age, presence or absence of risk factors such as middle ear or sinus disease, or recent neurosurgery provide clues about the cause and pathogenesis.

It is recommended that patients be started on adjunctive dexamethasone 10 mg IV every 6 hours for 4 days with the first dose of antibiotics, because this has been shown to improve outcomes in bacterial meningitis.[7] Antibiotic selection and dosing should also take into consideration the ability to cross the blood-brain barrier and achieve an effective concentration in the CSF. In adults, initial empirical treatment should provide adequate therapy for *Streptococcus pneumoniae* and *Neisseria meningitidis.* Increasing resistance of *S. pneumoniae* to beta-lactam antibiotics (including ceftriaxone) has prompted recommendations to initiate empirical antibiotic therapy with a regimen consisting of vancomycin and ceftriaxone.[6] If *Listeria monocytogenes* is a possibility (e.g., in older adults, pregnant women,

Box 1 Important Causes of Bacterial Meningitis*

In Adults
Streptococcus pneumoniae
Neisseria meningitidis
Listeria monocytogenes

In Children
Streptococcus pneumoniae
Neisseria meningitidis
Haemophilus influenzae
Streptococcus agalactiae (in neonates)
Escherichia coli (in neonates)

After Neurosurgery
Staphylococcus aureus
Pseudomonas aeruginosa
Enteric gram-negative bacteria

*Mycobacterium tuberculosis *is also a bacterium and can cause meningitis, but it is usually discussed separately as tuberculous meningitis.*

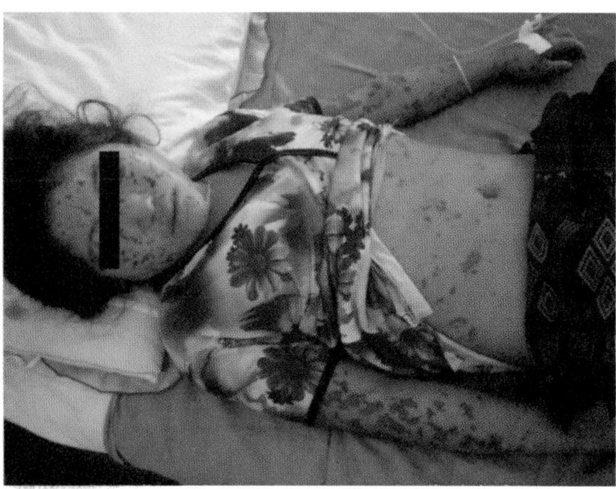

Figure 1 Classic rash of patient with meningococcemia.

and those with cellular immune deficits), ampicillin should be added. If *Pseudomonas aeruginosa* is a possibility, as after neurosurgical procedures, ceftazidime should be used instead of ceftriaxone. Antibiotic therapy should be adjusted once the causative microorganism has been identified. Duration of therapy for bacterial meningitis has not been adequately defined. For meningococcal meningitis, 7 days of therapy is considered adequate. *S. pneumoniae* should be treated for 10 to 14 days. *L. monocytogenes* should be treated for at least 21 days.[9]

Summary

- The differential diagnosis of acute bacterial meningitis includes viral meningitis and meningoencephalitis, tuberculous meningitis, primary amebic meningoencephalitis, and subarachnoid hemorrhage.
- Lumbar puncture should be performed as soon as possible.
- Dexamethasone plus empirical antibiotics should be started without delay.
- Antibiotics should be adjusted subsequently, based on culture and susceptibility data.

ACUTE MENINGOCOCCEMIA

Definition, Etiology, and Incidence

Acute meningococcemia is a disseminated infection caused by *Neisseria meningitidis*, with high mortality rates in those with fulminant disease. Meningococcal infection occurs in an endemic pattern, with periodic epidemics. There are substantial cyclic variations in disease incidence. In the United States, epidemics account for less than 5% of the reported cases. The incidence of meningococcal disease in the United States peaked at 1.7 cases per 100,000 population in 1997.[10]

Pathophysiology

The pathogenesis of meningococcal infection begins with nasopharyngeal colonization. About 10% of the population has asymptomatic nasopharyngeal carriage of *N. meningitidis* during nonepidemic periods. A small proportion of carriers go on to develop invasive meningococcal disease. People who develop invasive disease generally do so soon after acquisition of carriage.[11] Factors that facilitate invasive disease include agent factors such as virulence and transmissibility and host factors.

Deficiencies of the late components of the complement pathway place individuals at markedly increased risk of developing meningococcal infections.[12] These patients have recurrent episodes of meningococcal infection. Genetic variants of mannose-binding lectin (MBL), a plasma opsonin that initiates the MBL pathway of complement activation, may also predispose to increased susceptibility to meningococcal infections.[13]

Clinical Presentation

Meningococcal infection may manifest in different forms: bacteremia without sepsis, meningitis (with or without meningococcemia), acute meningococcemia (with or without meningitis), a meningoencephalitic picture, or chronic meningococcemia. The most fulminant form is acute meningococcemia, in which death may ensue within hours of the onset of symptoms.

The most common manifestation of acute meningococcemia is fever with rash. The rash usually begins as a petechial rash, initially with a few discrete lesions 1 to 2 mm in diameter, which often progress and coalesce to form larger ecchymotic lesions (Fig. 1). If there is associated meningitis, meningeal signs and symptoms may also be present.

The shock state is a dominant feature in patients with acute meningococcemia, and is often accompanied by disseminated intravascular coagulation (DIC). Meningococcemia can lead to complications such as massive adrenal hemorrhage, DIC, arthritis, heart problems such as pericarditis and myocarditis, neurologic problems such as deafness and peripheral neuropathy, and peripheral gangrene.[14] In epidemic settings in third-world countries, case-fatality rates as high as 70% have been recorded. In endemic settings in industrialized countries, the mortality rate is approximately 8%, but could be as high as 19%.

Meningococcemia does not always manifest in a fulminant manner. An unusual manifestation of meningococcal infection is chronic meningococcemia, which manifests with low-grade fever, rash, and arthritis. This manifestation is identical to that of chronic gonococcemia.

Diagnosis

When patients present with an acute febrile illness with the characteristic ecchymotic rash, the diagnosis is not difficult to make. Early infection could be missed if a careful physical examination is not carried out in a patient with an acute febrile illness. Definitive diagnosis requires isolation of the microorganism from a normally sterile site. Samples for blood cultures should always be obtained before the administration of antibiotics, if possible. Antibiotic therapy rapidly sterilizes the blood and CSF in patients with meningococcal infection.[15,16] CSF cultures are often positive for microorganisms, even in patients who do not have clinical evidence of meningitis,[17] and should always be examined when meningococcemia is suspected. Microorganisms may also be identified in the biopsy of petechial skin lesions.

Treatment

The treatment of acute meningococcemia involves appropriate antibiotic therapy, along with supportive therapy for shock, heart failure, DIC, and other complications. Early antibiotic therapy has been conclusively shown to improve outcomes in patients with meningococcal disease.[18] The recommended treatment for severe meningococcal infection is a third-generation cephalosporin with good CSF penetration. Ceftriaxone, 1 g every 12 hours, is the most commonly used treatment.[19] Cefotaxime and ceftazidime should be equally efficacious alternatives. Patients allergic to cephalosporins may be treated with chloramphenicol, 100 mg/kg, in four divided doses, up to a total dosage of 4 g/day.[20] High doses of penicillin G should also usually be adequate; however, small numbers of resistant *N. meningitidis* have been reported, and penicillin G should therefore not ordinarily be the first choice of antibiotic in the absence of susceptibility data. The shock state is a dominant part of the clinical picture of meningococcemia and supportive management is important. The use of steroids for meningococcemia is controversial, and a recommendation for its routine use for treatment of this condition cannot be made.

Prophylaxis

Household contacts are at significantly higher risk of infection.[21] Chemoprophylaxis is recommended for household contacts, daycare center staff and clients, and anyone exposed to the patient's oral secretions. For health care workers, this would include persons who intubated the patient and who provided suction to clear secretions. Effective prophylactic treatments include a single 1-g dose of ceftriaxone intravenously or intramuscularly, a single 500-mg dose of ciprofloxacin, a single 500-mg dose of azithromycin, and 600 mg of rifampin every 12 hours for 2 days.[18]

Summary

- The classic presentation of meningococcemia is fever and rash.
- Prompt antibiotic therapy can be lifesaving.
- Shock is a dominant clinical finding and supportive management is important.
- Close contacts should receive chemoprophylaxis.

CRANIAL SUBDURAL EMPYEMA

Definition, Etiology, and Incidence

Subdural empyema is a condition in which there is collection of pus in the region between the dura and the arachnoid. The most common causes of subdural empyema are aerobic and anaerobic streptococci (especially the *S. milleri* group), *Staphylococcus aureus* and, to a lesser extent, aerobic gram-negative bacilli.[22,23] Studies have found anaerobic infections in varying proportions of infections, with high proportion of patients having anaerobic microorganisms recovered in some studies with careful culturing.[24] This raises the possibility that these infections are usually polymicrobial, with anaerobic microorganisms usually present. Subdural empyemas account for 15% to 20% of all localized intracranial infections.[23]

Pathophysiology

Cranial subdural empyema is usually a complication of infection of the paranasal sinuses.[23] Less commonly, it results from spread from the middle ear.[25] It may also occur as a complication of trauma or neurosurgery. Infection spreads intracranially through the emissary veins that communicate between the veins draining the facial structures and intracranial venous channels. In a small proportion of cases, subdural empyema may occur by metastatic spread, usually from a pulmonary infection, for an unexplained reason.

Clinical Presentation

Patients with this condition usually present acutely, with headache and vomiting. Most patients have an altered mental status at presentation and the level of consciousness deteriorates rapidly. Patients may have neurologic deficits and complications such as local cerebritis, cerebral abscesses, and septic dural venous thromboses may occur.

Diagnosis

The diagnosis should be considered in any patient who presents with features suggestive of meningitis and a focal neurologic deficit or rapid deterioration in the level of consciousness. If recognized, lumbar puncture should not be performed because of the risk of cerebral herniation.[23] CSF findings would be nonspecific, with an elevated opening pressure, neutrophilic pleocytosis, and elevated protein level. Gram staining and culture of CSF are usually negative. The diagnostic procedure of choice is magnetic resonance imaging (MRI). If not available, CT scanning with contrast should be done. CT is inferior to MRI in detecting empyemas at the base of the brain and in the posterior fossa.

Treatment

Effective treatment for cranial subdural empyema requires a combined surgical and medical approach. Empirical antibiotic therapy should be broad spectrum and include coverage for gram-positive pyogenic bacteria and anaerobes. Vancomycin is a reasonable choice for empirical antibiotic therapy. Cultures obtained at the time of surgery will help tailor antibiotic therapy. The goal of surgery is complete evacuation of the purulent collection, which may be accomplished by craniotomy or through burr holes, depending on the circumstances of the case. It is important to evacuate the collection completely, and a craniotomy or multiple surgical procedures may be necessary to accomplish this. Up to 50% of patients who are treated with burr hole drainage require reoperation, compared with 20% of those treated with craniotomy.[26] The duration of antibiotic therapy is usually 3 to 4 weeks after adequate drainage. If there is associated osteomyelitis of the skull, treatment should be extended to approximately 6 weeks.

Summary

- MRI or CT scanning should be performed promptly when cranial subdural empyema is suspected.
- Treatment requires a combined medical and surgical approach.
- Empirical broad-spectrum antibiotic therapy should be started promptly.
- Cultures obtained at the time of surgery will help tailor antibiotic therapy.
- Multiple operations may be necessary.

NECROTIZING SOFT TISSUE INFECTIONS

Definition, Etiology, and Incidence

This term encompasses several specific clinical entities characterized by disease processes that produce necrosis of subcutaneous tissue, muscle, or both that progress rapidly and require a combined emergent surgical and medical approach for optimum outcomes. These entities include necrotizing fasciitis, streptococcal necrotizing myositis, clostridial myonecrosis (gas gangrene), and nonclostridial crepitant myositis.

Type I necrotizing fasciitis is a mixed infection caused by an anaerobic bacterium (usually *Bacteroides* or *Propionibacterium*) in association with a facultative anaerobic microorganism, such as a streptococcus or a member of the *Enterobacteriaceae*. Type II necrotizing fasciitis, hemolytic streptococcal gangrene, is caused by group A streptococci. Other microorganisms may be present in the mix. Community-associated methicillin-resistant *S. aureus* (CA-MRSA) has recently been described as a cause of necrotizing fasciitis.[27]

Clostridial myonecrosis, also commonly known as gas gangrene, and streptococcal necrotizing myositis, as their names imply, are caused by *Clostridium* spp. and by group A streptococci, respectively. The latter can rarely be caused by groups B, C, or G streptococci.

Nonclostridial crepitant myositis encompasses several clinical entities that may result from mixed infection caused by anaerobic streptococci, along with the following: group A streptococci or *S. aureus* (anaerobic streptococcal myonecrosis); a mixture of anaerobic and facultatively anaerobic microorganisms (synergistic nonclostridial anaerobic myonecrosis, or Meleney's bacterial synergistic gangrene); *Proteus* spp., *Bacteroides* spp., and anaerobic streptococci in devitalized limbs (infected vascular gangrene); *Vibrio vulnificus*; and *Aeromonas hydrophila*.

As a group, these illnesses are uncommon but not rare, and prompt recognition and appropriate management will significantly affect outcomes.

Pathophysiology

Necrotizing fasciitis usually begins with the introduction of the offending microorganism to the subcutaneous structures, usually as a result of minor trauma. Gas gangrene occurs in situations in which muscle injury is compounded by wound contamination with soil or other foreign material harboring spores of a tissue-invasive *Clostridium*, such as *C. perfringens*, *C. novyi*, and *C. septicum*. Such injuries include war injuries, compound fractures, and septic abortion. Most cases of streptococcal myositis appear to begin spontaneously. The different forms of nonclostridial myonecrosis usually begin with the introduction of the offending microorganisms at the time of usually minor trauma. *Aeromonas hydrophila* myonecrosis occurs as a result of inoculation of the microorganism at the time of penetrating injury in a freshwater setting or in association with fish or other aquatic animals. In all these conditions, there is rapid progression of disease, often with gas formation in the muscles and subcutaneous tissues, and in many cases associated with the development of gangrene.

Diabetes mellitus is the most important risk factor for the development of necrotizing soft tissue infections.[28] Other risk factors include alcoholism, corticosteroid use, and parenteral drug use.

Clinical Presentation

Necrotizing fasciitis is usually an acute process, with severe infection of the superficial and deep fascia. It most commonly occurs in the extremities. The affected area becomes erythematous, swollen, warm, and painful. It typically progresses rapidly, with the skin becoming darker, and over a few days bullae and skin breakdown develop. In the polymicrobial form, crepitations may be felt subcutaneously, indicating the presence of gas. Development of anesthesia over an erythematous area may precede development of skin breakdown and may serve as a warning sign that the disease process is more serious than cellulitis. Pain out of proportion to the skin changes also may be an indicator of a more serious infection. On palpation, the affected area has a woody hard feel. Increasing tissue edema may lead to the development of compartment syndrome.

Necrotizing myositis or myonecrosis may occur without overt findings on the skin surface. The predominant symptom is intense muscle pain, usually accompanied by fever. Patients usually appear more ill than would be expected from the physical findings. Gas gangrene and other syndromes of necrotizing myositis caused by anaerobic microorganisms will also have crepitations because of the presence of subcutaneous gas.

At initial presentation, it may not be possible to make a clinical distinction between necrotizing fasciitis and necrotizing myositis. Indeed, both processes may occur simultaneously, especially with streptococcal infection. Lack of involvement of the overlying skin does not exclude the presence of an underlying necrotizing process.

Streptococcal necrotizing soft tissue infections are usually associated with the toxic shock syndrome. This is discussed separately (see later). Acute vascular compromise from trauma or embolic occlusion leads to tissue infarction and may progress to infected vascular gangrene if the appropriate microorganisms gain access to the devitalized tissues.

Diagnosis

Clinical suspicion is important if an early diagnosis of a necrotizing soft tissue infection is to be made. A clue to the presence of a deep necrotizing process is the presence of tenderness clearly beyond the areas of apparent involvement in the skin. Leukocytosis is common. The creatine kinase (CK) level is usually elevated, but may be normal in cases of necrotizing fasciitis with minimal muscle involvement. Ultrasonography, CT scanning, or MRI will usually reveal muscle swelling and fluid in muscle compartments, but may not be apparent early in necrotizing fasciitis. Histopathologic examination will reveal the presence of sheets of neutrophils in fascial planes. Gram staining of tissue exudates will reveal the presence of microorganisms.

Treatment

It is not always obvious whether a skin or soft tissue infection is a necrotizing infection. When considered a possibility, aggressive management is important. It is not always possible to predict the causative microorganism from the clinical features accurately. A prudent approach would be to treat with antibiotics that are effective against group A streptococci, *S. aureus*, enteric gram-negative bacteria, and anaerobic microorganisms. The antibiotics of choice for initial empirical therapy are clindamycin plus ampicillin-sulbactam plus ciprofloxacin.[29] If there is reason to suspect MRSA infection, vancomycin may be added. Antibiotic therapy should be modified when culture and susceptibility data become available. A lack of response to a reasonable trial of antibiotics should prompt emergent surgical intervention. Prompt and aggressive fasciotomy and débridement of devitalized tissue are necessary to gain control of the infection. Early surgical intervention reduces mortality.[28] If infection is advanced, amputation may be necessary, and lifesaving.

Summary

- A high index of suspicion will facilitate the early diagnosis of necrotizing soft tissue infections.
- Skin surface findings may be minimal.
- Prompt and aggressive surgical débridement is the most important aspect of treatment.
- Empirical antibiotic therapy should consist of clindamycin plus ampicillin-sulbactam plus ciprofloxacin.
- Antibiotical therapy should be modified once culture data become available.

TOXIC SHOCK SYNDROME

Definition, Etiology, and Incidence

Toxic shock syndrome (TSS) is a severe toxin-mediated bacterial disease characterized by shock resulting from an excess of inflammatory cytokines. Two important syndromes, staphylococcal TSS and streptococcal TSS, are recognized, caused by *S. aureus* and *Streptococcus pyogenes*, respectively. Both are uncommon diseases. The incidence of streptococcal TSS in the United States is 3.5 per 100,000 population per year. Staphylococcal TSS has an overall incidence of about 1 per 100,000, with menstrual TSS about twice as common as nonmenstrual TSS.[30] At the peak of the epidemic of menstrual TSS, before the recognition of the association between the use of certain tampons and TSS, the incidence of menstrual TSS was as high as 10 per 100,000 population per year, and accounted for over 90% of all cases of staphylococcal TSS.

Pathophysiology

Toxic shock syndrome is a toxin-mediated disease.[31] Several exotoxins of *S. aureus* and *S. pyogenes* are capable of stimulating excessive T cell responses, and are thus known as superantigens. These toxins include toxic shock syndrome toxin 1 (TSST-1) and staphylococcal exotoxins A, B, and C (SEA, SEB, SEC) of *S. aureus*, and streptococcal pyrogenic exotoxins A, B, and C (SPEA, SPEB, SPEC) of *S. pyogenes*. These toxins are capable of binding both major histocompatibiliy complex (MHC) class II molecules of antigen-presenting cells and the V_β region of T cell receptors, leading to broad-range induction of T cell proliferation. The resulting excessive production of inflammatory cytokines (interleukin-1 and -6 [IL-1, IL-6], tumor necrosis factors α and β [TNF-α, TNF-β], interferon gamma [IFN-γ]) leads to increased capillary permeability resulting in tissue damage to various organs and shock.

Staphylococcal TSS is commonly associated with menstruation (menstrual TSS).[32] The pathophysiology of menstrual TSS includes a high local protein level and relatively high local pH (caused by the presence of blood and blood products), high partial pressure of carbon dioxide (caused by higher than atmospheric Pco_2 in blood), and high Po_2 (introduced by high-absorbency tampons).[31] In such an environment, the production of TSST-1 by colonizing *S. aureus* is stimulated. Nonmenstrual TSS is caused by *S. aureus* infection at any site in the body, including surgical wounds, the lungs, peritoneal dialysis catheters, and skin and mucosal infections. The illness is mediated by TSST-1 or SEA or SEB produced by the microorganisms at the site of infection.

Clinical Presentation

Toxic shock syndrome manifests as a multisystem illness, with shock being a prominent feature. Clinical features include high fever, hypotension, tachycardia, tachypnea, anasarca, and a morbilliform rash. Many patients also have myalgias and gastrointestinal symptoms, such as vomiting, abdominal pain, and diarrhea. Patients may develop confusion. The disease progresses rapidly and, especially with streptococcal TSS, can lead to death within 24 to 48 hours. Menstrual TSS starts within 2 days of the beginning or end of menses in women using high-absorbency tampons.[32] In many patients with nonmenstrual TSS, the site of infection may show minimal inflammation and may not be readily apparent.

Streptococcal TSS is generally a more serious condition.[33] In this condition, the site of infection with *S. pyogenes* may be obvious. It is usually a necrotizing soft tissue infection, but streptococcal TSS has been described in patients with pneumonia, meningitis, septic arthritis, peritonitis, and other deep infections.[33] Patients are usually very ill and may develop the adult respiratory distress syndrome or DIC. The mortality of adequately treated staphylococcal TSS is about 5%. The mortality of streptococcal TSS is about 50%.

Diagnosis

The diagnostic criteria for TSS are outlined in Boxes 2 and 3.[34,35] In streptococcal TSS, streptococci can usually be detected in culture at the affected site or in blood culture. In staphylococcal TSS, it is rare to detect staphylococci, except if vaginal cultures are obtained from patients with menstruation-associated TSS. Prompt diagnosis requires recognition of the constellation of symptoms and signs, with confirmation by additional laboratory testing to look for abnormalities that indicate damage to the organ systems expected to be involved by the process. CT or MRI helps in defining the presence of deep soft tissue infection in patients with streptococcal TSS. Gas is not produced, but the diagnosis should not be excluded if imaging findings do not appear impressive when clinical features are suggestive of the disease.

Box 2 Diagnostic Criteria for Staphylococcal Toxic Shock Syndrome*

Fever: Temperature ≥102° F (38.9° C)
Rash: Diffuse macular erythroderma
Overt or orthostatic hypotension
Multisystem involvement (three or more of the following):

- Gastrointestinal: Vomiting or diarrhea at the onset of illness
- Muscular: Severe myalgias or creatine kinase level at least twice the upper limit of normal
- Mucous membranes: Vaginal, oropharyngeal, or conjunctival hyperemia
- Renal: Blood urea nitrogen or creatinine level at least twice the upper limit of normal *or* urinary sediment with pyuria (≥5 leukocytes er high-power field) in the absence of urinary tract infection
- Hepatic: Total bilirubin, aspartate transaminase, or alanine aminotransaminase level at least twice the upper limit of normal
- Hematologic: Platelet count ≤100,000/μL
- Central nervous system: Disorientation or alteration in consciousness without focal neurologic signs when fever and hypotension are absent

Negative results on the following tests, if performed:

- Blood, throat, or cerebrospinal cultures (blood cultures may be positive for *Staphylococcus aureus*)
- Rise in antibody titer to Rocky Mountain spotted fever, leptospirosis, or rubeola

Desquamation 1-2 wk after onset of illness, particularly over palms and soles

**All six criteria have to be satisfied to make a definite diagnosis. Fulfillment of the first five criteria makes a probable diagnosis.*

Box 3 Diagnostic Criteria for Streptococcal Toxic Shock Syndrome*

Isolation of *Streptococcus pyogenes*
Hypotension
Two or more of the following:

- Renal impairment: Creatinine level ≥2.0 mg/dL or ≥ twice the upper limit of normal for age
- Thrombocytopenia (platelet count ≤100,000/μL) or disseminated intravascular coagulation
- Liver involvement: Aspartate transaminase, alanine aminotransaminase, or total bilirubin level ≥ twice the upper limit of normal
- Adult respiratory distress syndrome
- Generalized macular erythrodermic rash that may desquamate
- Necrotizing soft tissue infection

**All three criteria have to be met. If* S. pyogenes *is isolated from a normally sterile site, the diagnosis is a definite diagnosis. If isolated from a nonsterile site, the diagnosis is a probable diagnosis.*

Treatment

Management of TSS includes eradication of the focus of infection as well as supportive care, which includes fluid resuscitation and vasopressors, as necessary.[36] Large volumes of crystalloids may be necessary because of the loss of intravascular volume caused by capillary leak. Circulating bacterial hemolysins may lead to moderate to severe anemia, necessitating blood transfusions. When the focus of infection is identified in staphylococcal TSS, it is important to drain abscesses and treat with appropriate antibiotics. In women with hyperabsorbent tampons, the tampons should be removed. Patients with streptococcal TSS do better with combinations of clindamycin and cell wall active agents compared with cell wall active agents alone.[37] Because clindamycin is not affected by bacterial inoculum or stage of growth, and because it inhibits synthesis of bacterial toxin, there are theoretical reasons why it would also be useful for the treatment of staphylococcal TSS. Thus, in both staphylococcal and streptococcal toxic shock syndrome, clindamycin should also be added initially. Staphylococcal TSS should also initially be treated with vancomycin. Antibiotic therapy can be modified once susceptibility data become available. MRSA infections should be treated with vancomycin; MSSA infections should be treated with oxacillin. Penicillin-susceptible *S. aureus* should be treated with penicillin G. Treatment of streptococcal TSS usually includes aggressive surgical débridement, with antibiotic therapy and supportive care. The antibiotic of choice is penicillin G.

Summary

- The toxic shock syndromes are toxin-mediated diseases of *S. aureus* and *S. pyogenes*.
- The site of infection may not be readily apparent, especially in staphylococcal TSS.
- Streptococcal TSS is often associated with necrotizing soft tissue infections.
- Surgical débridement of the focus of infection may be necessary.
- Early antibiotic therapy should include clindamycin in addition to cell wall active agents.

NEUTROPENIC FEVER

Definition, Etiology, and Incidence

Fever in a neutropenic patient is defined as a single temperature higher than 101.3° F (38.3° C) or a sustained temperature higher than 100.4° (38°) for longer than 1 hour.[38] Neutropenia is usually defined as an absolute neutrophil count (ANC) lower than 500 cells µL or less than 1000 cells/µL. with a predicted nadir of less than 500 cells/µL.[38] More than 50% of neutropenic patients who develop a fever have an obvious or occult infection. The risk of invasive infection increases with the degree of neutropenia. At least 20% of patients with an absolute neutrophil count below 100 cells/µL will develop bacteremia.

Pathophysiology and Natural History

Neutrophils and macrophages represent the cellular arm of innate immunity. Neutrophils are recruited to the site of infection, where their role is to ingest the offending microorganisms. Patients with neutropenia have decreased neutrophil numbers, and their inflammatory responses are blunted. These patients may therefore have skin and skin structure infections, with minimal erythema or induration, urinary tract infection without pyuria, and pulmonary infection without chest radiographic infiltrates. The most likely sources of bacterial invasion in such patients are the skin, because of the breaching of skin integrity by invasive vascular catheters, and the gastrointestinal tract, because of mucosal damage from chemotherapeutic agents. The most common bacterial pathogens causing fever in patients with neutropenia are listed in Box 4.

Box 4 Most Common Bacterial Causes of Infection in Patients with Neutropenic Fever

Gram-Positive Bacteria
Staphylococcus spp.
Streptococcus spp.
Enterococcus faecalis or *faecium*
Corynebacterium spp.

Gram-Negative Bacteria
Escherichia coli
Klebsiella spp.
Pseudomonas aeruginosa

Adapted from Hughes WT, Armstrong D, Bodey GP, et al: 2002 guidelines for the use of antimicrobial agents in neutropenic patients with cancer. Clin Infect Dis 2002;34:730-751.

Clinical Presentation

Patients may present with little other than fever. The clinical presentation may appear to be relatively mild, especially to the inexperienced observer. Furthermore, many patients with chemotherapy-induced neutropenia may be on corticosteroids, which may actually mask fever. In neutropenic patients on corticosteroids, hypothermia, hypotension, or other unexplained acute clinical deterioration should be considered as a fever equivalent.

Diagnosis

A careful physical examination should be carried out to identify any possible sources of infection. Two or three sets of blood cultures, urinalysis and urine culture and, if the patient has productive cough, sputum Gram staining and culture should be performed. Chest radiographs should be obtained and there should be a low threshold for obtaining a CT scan of the chest, because the latter is significantly more sensitive for detecting pulmonary processes. Other investigations should be carried out if there are any localizing symptoms or signs. Meningitis is uncommon and lumbar puncture need not be done routinely in all patients.

Treatment

For patients with neutropenic fever, empirical therapy should provide adequate coverage against enteric gram-negative bacteria and *P. aeruginosa*. If *S. aureus* infection is considered a possibility, as in patients with indwelling vascular catheters, vancomycin should also be given until culture data become available. For patients with catheter-related infections, it is usually necessary to remove the catheter unless the microorganism is a coagulase-negative staphylococcus and there is no evidence of tunnel infection or catheter-associated deep venous thrombophlebitis.[39]

Several antibiotic regimens are effective for the empirical treatment of neutropenic fever, but no specific regimen is recommended for all patients. Criteria have been defined to identify those patients considered to be at low risk for progression to severe illness.[40] Patients deemed to be at low risk may be treated with oral ciprofloxacin plus oral amoxicillin-clavulanate. Patients deemed to be at high risk, which would include all patients with an ANC of less than 100 cells/µL, a duration of neutropenia exceeding 7 days, peak temperature 102.2° F (39° C) or higher, active malignancy, lack of early evidence of marrow recovery, and any obvious focus of infection, should receive IV antibiotics.

The decision for these patients will be whether to use vancomycin. Unless such patients can be reasonably excluded from having a serious gram-positive infection, these patients should all receive vancomycin in addition to antibiotics to cover gram-negative bacteria. Regimens for the coverage of gram-negative bacteria must include coverage for *P. aeruginosa*. Effective monotherapy regimens for gram-negative bacteria include imipenem-cilastatin, meropenem, cefepime, and ceftazidime. Effective combination regimens for the empirical treatment of gram-negative bacteria include an aminoglycoside (e.g., gentamicin, tobramycin, amikacin) with an antipseudomonal penicillin (e.g., piperacillin-tazobactam, ticarcillin-clavulanate), an antipseudomonal cephalosporin (e.g., ceftazidime, cefepime), or a carbapenem (e.g., imipenem, meropenem).[38]

Antibiotic therapy should be modified if cultures identify a causative microorganism. If *S. aureus* or another gram-positive bacterium requiring vancomycin is not identified by day 3, vancomycin may be stopped. If there is worsening after 3 days, a change in the antibiotic regimen should be considered. If the fever persists after 5 days, empirical antifungal therapy should be initiated.

The duration of therapy must be based on the clinical response and clinical status of the patient. It is clear that neutropenic patients are a heterogeneous group. Patients who have undergone allogeneic stem cell transplantation, graft-versus-host disease, severe mucosal erosive disease, extensive prior antibiotic treatment, or prolonged hospitalization are at higher risk of subsequent infectious complications.[41] Patients who are neutropenic for less than 7 to 10 days are at low risk of infectious complications. If the fever resolves in 3 to 5 days, antibiotics may be stopped 2 days after the resolution of fever if the ANC is 500 cells/μL or higher for at least 48 hours, or 5 to 7 days after the resolution of fever in low-risk patients if the ANC is 500 cells/μL or lower, but should be continued for at least 2 weeks in high-risk patients with an ANC <500 cells/μL or lower. If the fever persists beyond 5 days, but there is no obvious identified infection, antibiotics may be stopped 4 to 5 days after the ANC recovers above 500 cells/μL, but should be continued for at least 2 weeks if the ANC remains below 500 cells/μL.

Summary

- Neutropenic fever is defined as temperature higher than 101.3° F (38.3° C), or higher than 100.4° F (38° C) for more than 1 hour in a neutropenic patient (actual or predicted ANC of less than 500 cells/μL).
- Signs of inflammation may be minimal.
- There is potential for progression to death within hours.
- Empirical broad-spectrum antibiotic therapy should be instituted immediately and adjusted later.

SEPSIS IN PRIOR SPLENECTOMY OR FUNCTIONAL HYPOSPLENISM PATIENTS

Definition, Etiology, and Incidence

The importance of sepsis in these patients is the potential for progression from a healthy state to death within 24 hours when infected with certain microorganisms. This situation is not common but, when it does occur, the mortality rate is high. It is much more likely to occur at younger ages, with infection rates of 15.7% in infants, 10.4% in children younger than 5 years, 4.4% in children younger than 16, and 0.9% in adults.[42] The lifetime risk of postsplenectomy sepsis has been estimated to be approximately 5%.[43] The risk of infection persists throughout life, but the risk is highest in the first 2 years after splenectomy.[42]

The microorganisms that cause deadly infections in patients with prior splenectomy or functional hyposplenism are *S. pneumoniae, H. influenzae, N. meningitidis, Capnocytophaga canimorsus*, and *Babesia microti* or *B. divergens*. The most common responsible microorganism is *S. pneumoniae*, accounting for 50% to 90% of cases.[42,44]

Pathophysiology

The innate immune system provides immediate protection against invasion by microorganisms. The adaptive immune system provides a more vigorous, targeted, and durable immune response by producing specific antibodies. However, the antigenic priming process for this response takes time, and makes this mechanism protective in subsequent infections, not in initial infections. B-1a B cells are a subset of B lymphocytes that produce antibodies without prior specific exposure.[45,46] These are natural antibodies of the immunoglobulin M (IgM) isotype that target polysaccharides of bacteria.[47] Thus, they are part of the innate immune system and are responsible for the early inhibition of encapsulated bacteria. Splenectomy results in a marked reduction in the number of B-1a B cells.[48] This reduction seriously compromises the ability of the body to mount an early response to infection with encapsulated microorganisms such as *S. pneumoniae, H. influenzae*, and *N. meningitidis*.

The spleen is also responsible for the clearance of erythrocytes with abnormal inclusions from the circulation. Such abnormal inclusions include intraerythrocytic parasites such as *Babesia* species. Most cases of infection with *Babesia* have occurred in splenectomized individuals.[49] The removal of erythrocytes infected with malarial parasites is also affected by splenectomy, but whether this increases the severity of disease is unclear.

Clinical Presentation

The initial presentation, if patients present early, may be no different from a febrile illness in an otherwise healthy patient. Typical symptoms are fever, chills, sore throat, vomiting or diarrhea, and diffuse muscle aches. In young children, meningitis is common. Rapid progression within hours is the usual course. Shock, seizures, and DIC often accompany the clinical deterioration. Purpura fulminans and extremity gangrene can occur. With modern treatment, the mortality rate for postsplenectomy sepsis is in the range of 50% to 70%.[42,44]

Diagnosis

In the setting of prior splenectomy or functional hyposplenism, any febrile illness must raise suspicion for postsplenectomy sepsis. Two to three sets of samples for blood cultures should be obtained. Other investigations should be performed if there are any localizing symptoms or signs. In children, the CSF should be examined. The degree of bacteremia is usually several orders of magnitude greater than in patients with a functional spleen, and blood cultures usually turn positive within 12 to 24 hours. Because of the degree of bacteremia, Gram staining of the buffy coat often reveals the presence of bacteria. Bacteria may even be seen on a peripheral blood smear, which will also show the presence of *Babesia*. Thus, a peripheral smear should always be examined in any patient with postsplenectomy sepsis.

Treatment

The most important aspect of management of postsplenectomy sepsis is to recognize the condition and the potential for its occurrence in any patient with a prior splenectomy presenting with a febrile illness. Antibiotics should be started immediately. Antibiotic therapy should not be withheld if blood cultures cannot be tested immediately. Empirical antibiotic therapy should consist of vancomycin and ceftriaxone. This empirical regimen will adequately treat all the pathogens definitely associated with postsplenectomy sepsis, except *Babesia*. Vancomycin may be stopped if resistance pneumococci are not isolated. The treatment for *Babesia* is quinine plus clindamycin in those rare cases in which it is the causative agent.

Prophylaxis

All patients should receive the 23-covalent bond, unconjugated, capsular pneumococcal polysaccharide vaccine (PPV23) at least 2 weeks before elective splenectomy.[50] If the splenectomy is an emergent procedure, the vaccine should still be given as soon as possible. Revaccination once after 5 years is also recommended.[51] Although there are fewer data on the protective efficacy of the *H. influenzae* type B (Hib) vaccine and meningococcal vaccine, both should be administered as soon as possible, preferably before splenectomy.

Children are often given prophylactic penicillin V for the first few years after splenectomy, which may provide some protection. This approach is not recommended for adults because of the uncertainty of the magnitude of protection offered and the potential for selection of resistant microorganisms.

Summary

- Postsplenectomy sepsis can progress from a healthy state to death within 24 hours.
- The most important responsible microorganisms are *S. pneumoniae* and *H. influenzae*.
- The degree of bacteremia is very high, and bacteria may be seen in the buffy coat or on a peripheral smear.
- Vancomycin plus ceftriaxone will provide adequate antibiotic coverage in most cases.

PLASMODIUM FALCIPARUM MALARIA

Definition, Etiology, and Incidence

Malaria in humans is caused by five species of *Plasmodium*: *P. falciparum*, *P. vivax*, *P. malariae*, *P. knowlesi*, and *P. ovale*. Malaria should always be considered a possibility in any person presenting with fever who has recently been in a malaria-endemic region, even if malaria prophylaxis was taken. Malaria occurs in most of the tropical and subtropical regions of south and southeast Asia, sub-Saharan Africa, and South America. *P. falciparum* malaria is far more dangerous than the non–*P. falciparum* malarias. There are more than 500 million cases of malaria yearly, mostly in sub-Saharan Africa, and millions of deaths.[52] The vast majority of the deaths from malaria are caused by *P. falciparum*. *P. knowlesi* is a newly recognized human malarial parasite and is capable of causing severe malaria. The following discussion focuses on *P. falciparum* malaria, the most important cause of malaria worldwide.

Pathophysiology

The life cycle of *Plasmodium* involves an asexual stage in a mosquito belonging to the genus *Anopheles* and its sexual stage in humans. Humans are infected by the bite of an infected mosquito. In humans, the infective sporozoites initially invade the liver, develop into merozoites in the liver cells, and are released into the bloodstream after several days.[53] *P. vivax* and *P. ovale*, in addition to undergoing immediate development in the liver, are also capable of remaining in liver cells as latent infections for several months to years; the latent forms are known as hypnozoites. These hypnozoites perpetuate what is known as the exoerythrocytic cycle, its importance being that effective treatment for these infections must include medications active against the liver stage of the parasite.

This cycle is not seen with *P. falciparum*. The merozoites released from the liver cells invade red blood cells, where they develop into trophozoites that mature into schizonts, which then divide into several merozoites. The merozoites are in turn released by lysis of the infected cells; the process takes 48 hours in the case of *P. falciparum*. Lysis of infected cells occurs in a coordinated fashion every 24 hours, with two batches undergoing lysis on alternate days. It is at this time that the patient experiences chills and rigors. The released merozoites are capable of infecting other red blood cells, thus perpetuating illness. Some schizonts mature into male or female gametocytes. For transmission of malaria to occur, gametocytes have to be ingested by an appropriate mosquito.[54] Fertilization occurs in the lumen of the mosquito stomach; the resulting zygote penetrates the wall of the stomach and develops into an ookinete on the outer surface of the stomach wall. When the ookinete matures, it develops into an oocyst that multiplies and ruptures to release many sporozoites into the body cavity of the mosquito. The sporozoites then find their way to the mosquito's salivary glands, where they are poised to be transmitted to another human host at the time of the mosquito's next blood meal.

The most important aspect of the pathogenesis of disease caused by *P. falciparum* is the ability of the parasite to sequester in the deep microvasculature. *P. falciparum* erythrocyte membrane protein 1 (PfEMP-1) is a molecule expressed on the surface of infected erythrocytes. This molecule is capable of adhering to various host cell surface ligands, including CD36 on endothelium, monocytes, and platelets and intercellular adhesion molecule-1 (ICAM-1) on endothelial surfaces.[55] Furthermore, PfEMP-1 also mediates rosetting of host erythrocytes.[56] This combination of endothelial binding and rosette formation leads to massive sequestration of parasitized erythrocytes in the cerebral, renal, hepatic, and other microcirculations, leading to the complications of *P. falciparum* malaria.

Clinical Presentation

The most important symptom of malaria is fever. Classic descriptions of malaria include the occurrence of paroxysms that begin with chills and rigors, followed by high fever and then by profuse sweating and defervescence, with the entire paroxysm lasting a few hours. These symptoms classically occurred every 24 hours in patients with *P. falciparum* malaria. Nowadays, paroxysms may not be very prominent, and patients may even have continuous fever. Headache is common, and may be seen even in the absence of cerebral malaria.

P. falciparum malaria is far more likely to lead to complications than the non–*P. falciparum* malarias. The most important complications of *P. falciparum* malaria are severe anemia, hypoglycemia, cerebral malaria, acute renal failure, acute respiratory distress syndrome, acute hepatocellular failure, and DIC.

Several clinical features indicate specific end-organ damage in *P. falciparum* malaria; these include headache, seizures, and loss of consciousness (with cerebral malaria), decreased urine output or blood in urine (blackwater fever), deep jaundice (algid malaria), bleeding from multiple sites (caused by DIC), and respiratory failure (caused by acute respiratory distress syndrome).

Diagnosis

The most important diagnostic and most practical test is the Wright's- or Giemsa-stained peripheral blood smear (thick and thin), which should be examined immediately if malaria is considered a likely diagnosis. These tests can be performed in any laboratory but the limitation in nonendemic areas may be the nonavailability of personnel with experience in reading the slides. The most likely finding in patients with *P. falciparum* malaria is the finding of ring-shaped trophozoites within red blood cells (Fig. 2). Antigen-based tests and serologic tests also exist for the diagnosis of malaria. Although these tests do not require much expertise to read, they are unlikely to be available in areas that are nonendemic for the disease.

Treatment

All patients with *P. falciparum* malaria should be hospitalized, at least for the first 48 hours after initiation of treatment, regardless of how well they may appear at presentation. Patients with severe malaria may require ICU admission. The effectiveness of different antimalarials depends on the geographic area in which the infection was acquired. Treatment regimens effective against *P. falciparum* are outlined in Table 1. The most commonly used drugs are quinine or artemisinin derivatives, which should be effective for almost all cases of malaria in most regions. In many endemic regions, there is significant resistance to pyrimethamine-sulfadoxine, and this drug should be used with caution; if used, patients should be closely monitored for response. The Centers for Disease Control and Prevention (CDC) has published guidelines for the treatment of malaria in the United States (available at http://www.cdc.gov/malaria/pdf/clinicalguidance.pdf).

All patients should be closely monitored for the possibility of hypoglycemia, which occurs as a result of the infection itself and as an adverse effect of antimalarials, and is very common. Patients unable to eat should receive glucose-containing fluids as a continuous infusion. Patients treated with quinine should be monitored for findings suggestive of cinchonism, indicated by tinnitus and hearing loss which, if detected, should prompt dose reduction or change in therapy.

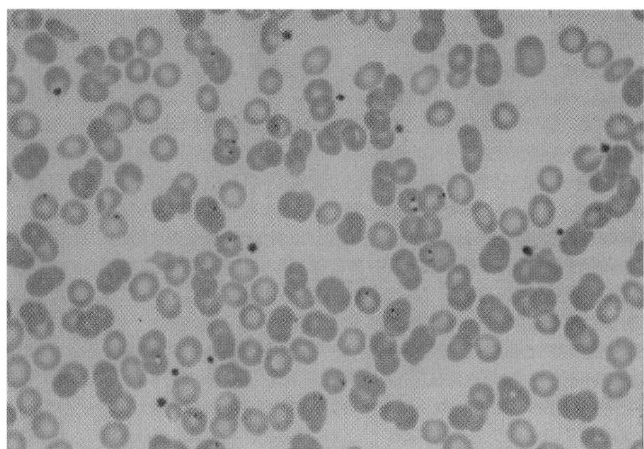

Figure 2 Peripheral blood smear showing numerous ring-shaped trophozoites of Plasmodium falciparum. *(Leishman stain, 1000× magnification).*

Summary

- Most deaths from malaria are caused by *P. falciparum*.
- *P. falciparum* causes sequestration of erythrocytes in the deep microvasculature, resulting in most of the complications from this infection.
- *P. falciparum* must be considered in the differential diagnosis of any patient with fever who has recently been in a malaria-endemic area.
- The diagnostic test of choice is the peripheral blood smear.
- Quinine and artemisinin derivatives are the most commonly used treatments.

CHOLERA

Definition, Etiology, and Incidence

Cholera is a diarrheal disease caused by *Vibrio cholerae*. The disease is widely distributed in Asia, Africa, and South America. It occurs as an endemic form and has the potential to cause pandemics periodically. Of the more than 200 serogroups of *V. cholerae*, only two—O1 and O139—cause clinical cholera. In 2005, the number of reported cases of cholera was 131,943, with 2,272 deaths from 52 countries.[57]

Pathophysiology

The natural reservoir of *V. cholerae* is water, and the predominant mode of spread is contamination of drinking water supplies. The bacterium can survive in a free-living state in water when conditions are favorable and reaches the host's intestinal tract through contaminated food or water. Persons with decreased gastric acidity because of disease or medications have a greater likelihood of becoming infected. Bacteria that survive the gastric environment and gain access to the small intestine cause disease by secreting an enterotoxin that stimulates secretion of fluid and electrolytes into the lumen by the cells lining the small intestine.[58] Excessive secretion leads to dehydration, and the dehydration resulting from cholera is the most severe of any infectious disease. The bacterium does not invade the wall of the small intestine.

Clinical Presentation

Cholera manifests with an abrupt onset of watery diarrhea, soon followed by dehydration. Stools are thin and white, referred to as rice

Table 1 Regimens Effective for Treatment of *P. falciparum* Malaria

Pharmacologic Agent(s)	Dosage Regimen
Quinine + doxycycline	Quinine 10 mg/kg PO or IV q8hr for 7 days *plus* doxycycline 100 mg PO q8hr for 7 days
Atovaquone-chloroguanide	Four adult tablets (each) daily for 3 days (each adult tablet contains 250 mg atovaquone and 100 mg chloroguanide)
Artemether-lumefantrine (Coartem)	Four tablets initially, followed by four tablets 8 hr later, followed by four tablets twice daily on days 2 and 3 (each fixed-dose tablet contains 20 mg artemether and 120 mg lumefantrine)
Pyrimethamine-sulfadoxine	Two or three tablets PO once (each fixed-dose tablet contains 25 mg pyrimethamine and 500 mg sulfadoxine)
Artesunate + mefloquine	Artesunate 4 mg/kg PO daily for 3 days *plus* mefloquine 1250-mg single dose *or* 750 mg followed by 500 mg after 12 hr *or* Artesunate 2.4 mg/kg IV, first dose, followed by 1.2 mg/kg after 12 hr, followed by 1.2 mg/kg q24h × 3 days *plus* mefloquine 1250-mg single dose or 750 mg followed by 500 mg after 12 hr
Artemether + mefloquine	Artemether 3.2 mg/kg IM, first dose followed by 1.6 mg/kg after 12 hr, followed by 1.2 mg/kg q24hr × 3 days *plus* mefloquine 1250-mg single dose or 750 mg followed by 500 mg after 12 hr

water stools. Vomiting is also common, and usually follows diarrhea. The severity of diarrhea and dehydration is variable, and it is important to realize that dehydration from cholera could be so severe that previously healthy people could die of dehydration within hours of the onset of symptoms. In a much smaller proportion of patients, the presentation is abdominal distention rather than diarrhea because of accumulation of fluid within the intestinal lumen, a presentation known as cholera sicca. The most important complication is prerenal acute renal failure, and an incidence rate of 10.6 per 1000 was recognized in an outbreak in Peru in 1991.[59]

Diagnosis

It is not difficult to diagnose a patient with cholera. Patients present with diarrhea, with surprising degrees of dehydration considering the short duration of the illness. For routine clinical care, microbiologic diagnosis cannot be made in a timely manner and is unnecessary.

Treatment

The mainstay of therapy is adequate fluid resuscitation. Patients with mild dehydration can be treated with oral rehydration. Patients with severe dehydration or those with moderate dehydration and unable to tolerate oral rehydration need IV rehydration. Rehydration should be provided in two phases, a rapid rehydration phase lasting 2 to 4 hours and a maintenance phase lasting the duration of the diarrhea. When possible, electrolytes should be monitored and abnormalities corrected. Since 1978, the World Health Organization oral rehydration solution (WHO ORS) has been recommended as the oral rehydration fluid for the management of diarrheal illnesses, including cholera.[60] For IV rehydration, normal saline or Ringer's lactate solution may be used. It must be noted that these fluids have low potassium content, and supplemental potassium may be required. Antibiotics have been shown to reduce the duration of diarrhea and volume of stools;[61] however, their use is of secondary importance in comparison with rehydration. A single 100-mg dose of doxycycline has been shown to be adequate treatment.[62] Alternative agents are trimethoprim-sulfamethoxazole, furazolidone or erythromycin for 3 days, or a single dose of azithromycin, all of which can also be used in pregnant women and children. Practical guidelines for the management of cholera have been published.[63]

The WHO ORS solution is hyperosmolar relative to plasma and concern has been raised that this solution may induce the development of an osmotically driven increase in stool output and hypernatremia.[64] Indeed, the use of this solution does not reduce stool volume or duration of diarrhea.[65] In recent years, the use of reduced osmolarity ORS in areas endemic for cholera has gained favor,[66] and this solution appears to be more effective than standard ORS.[67] Regardless of the nature of the rehydration solution used, the principle of cholera treatment remains adequate rehydration.

Summary

- Cholera is a diarrheal disease transmitted by contaminated drinking water.
- It causes the most severe form of diarrhea caused by any infectious agent.
- Rehydration with repletion of electrolytes is the mainstay of therapy.
- Antibiotic therapy is of secondary importance.

Suggested Readings

Holdsworth RJ, Irving AD, Cuschieri A: Postsplenectomy sepsis and its mortality rate: Actual versus perceived risks. Br J Surg 1991;78:1031-1038.
Hughes WT, Armstrong D, Bodey GP, et al: 2002 guidelines for the use of antimicrobial agents in neutropenic patients with cancer. Clin Infect Dis 2002;34:730-751.
Nathoo N, Nadvi SS, van Dellen JR, Gouws E: Intracranial subdural empyemas in the era of computed tomography: A review of 699 cases. Neurosurgery 1999;44:529-535.
Salzman MB, Rubin LG: Meningococcemia. Infect Dis Clin North Am 1996;10:709-725.
Seas C, DuPont HL, Valdez LM, Gotuzzo E: Practical guidelines for the treatment of cholera. Drugs 1996;51(6):966-973.
Stevens DL, Bisno AL, Chambers HF, et al: Practice guidelines for the diagnosis and management of skin and soft-tissue infections. Clin Infect Dis 2005;41:1373-1406.
Stevens DL: The toxic shock syndromes. Infect Dis Clin North Am 1996;10:727-746.
Tunkel AR, Hartman BJ, Kaplan SL, et al: Practice guidelines for the management of bacterial meningitis. Clin Infect Dis 2004;39:1267-1284.
Tunkel AR, Scheld WM: Pathogenesis and pathophysiology of bacterial meningitis. Clin Microbiol Rev 1993;6:118-136.
Wong CH, Chang HC, Pasupathy S, et al: Necrotizing fasciitis: Clinical presentation, microbiology, and determinants of mortality. J Bone Joint Surg Am 2003;85A:1454-1460.

References

For a complete list of references, log onto www.expertconsult.com.

Upper Respiratory Tract Infections

Sherif B. Mossad

DEFINITION AND CAUSES

Upper respiratory tract infection (URI) is a nonspecific term used to describe acute infections involving the nose, paranasal sinuses, pharynx, larynx, trachea, and bronchi. The prototype is the illness known as the common cold, which is discussed here, in addition to pharyngitis, sinusitis, and tracheobronchitis. Influenza is a systemic illness that involves the upper respiratory tract and should be differentiated from other URIs.

Viruses cause most URIs, with rhinovirus, parainfluenza virus, coronavirus, adenovirus, respiratory syncytial virus, coxsackievirus, and influenza virus accounting for most cases.[1] Human metapneumovirus is a newly discovered agent causing URIs. Group A beta-hemolytic streptococci (GABHS) cause 5% to 10% of cases of pharyngitis in adults.[2] Other less common causes of bacterial pharyngitis include group C beta-hemolytic streptococci, *Corynebacterium diphtheriae, Neisseria gonorrhoeae, Arcanobacterium haemolyticum, Chlamydia pneumoniae, Mycoplasma pneumoniae*, and herpes simplex virus. *Streptococcus pneumoniae, Haemophilus influenzae*, and *Moraxella catarrhalis* are the most common organisms that cause the bacterial superinfection of viral acute sinusitis.[3] Less than 10% of cases of acute tracheobronchitis are caused by *Bordetella pertussis, B. parapertussis, M. pneumoniae*, or *C. pneumoniae*.[4]

PREVALENCE AND RISK FACTORS

Most URIs occur more frequently during the cold winter months, because of overcrowding. Adults develop an average of two to four colds annually. Antigenic variation of hundreds of respiratory viruses result in repeated circulation in the community. A coryza syndrome is by far the most common cause of physician visits in the United States.[1] Acute pharyngitis accounts for 1% to 2% of all visits to outpatient and emergency departments, resulting in 7 million annual visits by adults alone.[1] Acute bacterial sinusitis develops in 0.5% to 2% of cases of viral URIs.[3] Approximately 20 million cases of acute sinusitis occur annually in the United States. About 12 million cases of acute tracheobronchitis are diagnosed annually, accounting for one third of patients presenting with acute cough.[4] The estimated economic impact of non–influenza-related URIs is $40 billion annually.[1]

Influenza epidemics occur every year between November and March in the Northern Hemisphere. Approximately two thirds of those infected with influenza virus exhibit clinical illness, 25 million seek health care, 100,000 to 200,000 require hospitalization, and 40,000 to 60,000 die each year as a result of related complications.[5] The average cost of each influenza epidemic is $12 million, including the direct cost of medical care and indirect cost resulting from lost work days. Pandemics in the 20th century claimed the lives of more than 21 million people. A widespread H5N1 pandemic in birds is ongoing, with threats of a human pandemic. It is projected that such a pandemic would cost the United States $70 to $160 billion.[6]

PATHOPHYSIOLOGY AND NATURAL HISTORY

Transmission of organisms causing URIs occurs by aerosol, droplet, or direct hand-to-hand contact with infected secretions, with subsequent passage to the nares or eyes.[7] Thus, transmission occurs more commonly in crowded conditions. Direct invasion of the respiratory epithelium results in symptoms corresponding to the area(s) involved.

Sinusitis and acute bronchitis are frequently preceded by a common cold. Sinonasal allergies, anatomic abnormalities such as a deviated nasal septum, sinus ostial blockade caused by mucosal edema, immunodeficiency disorders such as hypogammaglobulinemia and human immunodeficiency virus infection, and cocaine abuse predispose to the development of acute sinusitis.[3]

Most influenza epidemics in the 20th century were caused by the influenza A virus, but a few were caused by the influenza B virus. Most epidemics are believed to spread from schoolchildren to their families. Annual influenza epidemics result from the transmission of a mutated influenza virus for which most humans do not have immunity (antigenic drift). Pandemics, on the other hand, occur when a totally new influenza virus is transmitted to humans from other species, most commonly swine and birds (antigenic shift). People older than 65 years and those with comorbidities are at higher risk than healthy people for hospitalization and death because of exacerbation of their underlying medical conditions as a result of influenza.

SIGNS AND SYMPTOMS

Significant overlap exists in the clinical manifestations of the different forms of URIs. Onset of symptoms occurs 1 to 3 days after exposure to the infectious agent. Nasal congestion, sneezing, and sore throat are the hallmarks of the common cold. A predictive index score for the diagnosis of picornavirus infections has been developed, but is not of practical use.[8] Conjunctivitis is characteristically seen with adenovirus infections. Sudden onset of sore throat, fever, absence of cough, and exposure to a person with known streptococcal pharyngitis in the preceding 2 weeks suggest the diagnosis of GABHS-related pharyngitis.[9] Patients with acute sinusitis experience symptoms for more than 1 to 2 weeks after a common cold, including unilateral facial pain, maxillary toothache, headache, and excessive purulent nasal discharge.[10,11] Acute tracheobronchitis is an illness characterized by cough, with or without sputum production, or wheezing, lasting 1 to 3 weeks.[4] Pertussis in adults with waning immunity caused by previous illness or immunization may not manifest with the typical whooping cough seen in children with primary infection. Influenza is a sudden illness characterized by high fever, severe headache, myalgia, and dry cough, followed by significant fatigue and malaise.[12] The constellation of these symptoms during influenza epidemics is 70% to 80% sensitive for making the diagnosis. Older patients with influenza may also present with confusion and somnolence. The presence of sneezing among adults older than 60 years reduces the likelihood of influenza.[12]

On physical examination, patients with common colds may have a low-grade fever, nasal vocal tone, macerated skin over the nostrils, and inflamed nasal mucosa.[8] Patients with GABHS-related pharyngitis may have pharyngeal erythema and exudate, palatal petechiae (doughnut lesions), tender anterior cervical lymphadenopathy, and occasionally a scarlatiniform rash.[9] Pharyngeal or palatal vesicles and ulcers (herpangina) should suggest enteroviral or herpetic pharyngitis. Pharyngeal exudates occur most commonly with GABHS-related pharyngitis, but can also be seen with infectious mononucleosis caused by Epstein-Barr virus, acute retroviral syndrome, candidal infections, and diphtheria. Swelling, redness, and tenderness overlying the affected sinuses and abnormal transillumination are specific for, but not commonly seen, in patients with acute sinusitis.[10]

Generalized lymphadenopathy associated with sore throat, fever, and rash should raise the possibility of a systemic viral infection, such as Epstein-Barr virus, cytomegalovirus, or human immunodeficiency virus. Patients with acute tracheobronchitis may also have audible respiratory wheezes. Patients with influenza appear toxic and may have pulmonary rhonchi and diffuse muscle tenderness.

DIAGNOSIS

Laboratory Tests

Because viruses cause most URIs, the diagnostic role of laboratory investigations and radiologic studies is limited. Viral culture, rapid antigen detection, or polymerase chain reaction (PCR) assay of influenza virus on a nasopharyngeal swab is indicated in patients for whom specific antiviral therapy is recommended. Similar tests are also available for adenovirus, respiratory syncytial virus, and parainfluenza virus. Experience with the use of reverse-transcriptase PCR for the diagnosis of enterovirus and rhinovirus infections is growing, but it is not currently available for daily clinical care.[13] Serologic tests for viruses that can cause a mononucleosis-type illness should be considered in the appropriate clinical setting. Influenza serologies only have epidemiologic value and should not be used for clinical care. A pharyngeal swab for rapid antigen detection of GABHS is 90% sensitive and 95% specific in adults.[14,15] Increased antistreptolysin O titer is not helpful during the acute illness, and is usually detected several days later. Cultures obtained by paranasal sinus puncture should be reserved only for severely ill patients with acute sinusitis and intracranial or orbital complications. In patients with acute bronchitis, a normal C-reactive protein level can reasonably exclude pneumonia, but may be elevated with several other infectious and noninfectious conditions.

Imaging Studies

A lateral neck radiograph should be taken in a patient with stridor to assess the airways. However, this should not deviate attention from close monitoring for patency of the airways if epiglottitis is clinically suspected. Chest radiography should be reserved for patients with acute tracheobronchitis who have other comorbid conditions, those with abnormal vital signs or signs of consolidation on chest examination, or those with persistent symptoms for longer than 3 weeks. Plain radiography has been largely replaced by computed tomography (CT) in the evaluation of sinusitis, particularly in preparation for corrective surgery.[16] Complete opacification and air-fluid level are the most specific findings for acute sinusitis. However, a large proportion of patients with the common cold have radiologic abnormalities on CT. Imaging is recommended for patients who do not respond to treatment with antibiotics and decongestants, but is not advised for the diagnosis of uncomplicated sinusitis. Mastoiditis and other intracranial complications of URIs should be evaluated by CT or magnetic resonance imaging.

Procedural Considerations

Only those experienced in endotracheal intubation should perform laryngoscopic examination of patients with suspected epiglottitis. Paranasal sinus endoscopy is not indicated for patients with uncomplicated acute sinusitis, and endoscopic cultures obtained from the middle meatus should be interpreted with caution because of potential contamination with nasal secretions.

Differential Diagnosis

Prodromal symptoms of viruses that cause systemic syndromes, such as measles and chickenpox, can mimic the common cold. Allergic rhinitis is characterized by itchy eyes and excessive lacrimation; it is often seasonally exacerbated or related to certain allergen exposure, which differentiates it from URIs. Sore throat could be a presenting symptom of acute thyroiditis, Ludwig's angina, and gastroesophageal reflux disease, all of which should be differentiated from pharyngitis. Drug-induced mucositis can cause a noninfectious form of pharyngitis. Wegener's granulomatosis should be considered when sinusitis does not respond to usual therapy. The most important step in the evaluation of someone with acute tracheobronchitis is to exclude pneumonia. If a cough lasts more than 3 weeks, postnasal drip, asthma, and gastroesophageal reflux disease are the most likely considerations.

Summary

- Most URIs are viral in origin. Diagnosis is mainly based on clinical manifestations.
- Adults with clinical findings suggestive of GABHS pharyngitis should have a pharyngeal rapid streptococcal antigen detection test before considering antimicrobial therapy.
- Sinus puncture and sinus CT are not recommended for the diagnosis of uncomplicated sinusitis.
- If pneumonia is unlikely on clinical grounds, chest radiography is not recommended for patients with acute tracheobronchitis.
- A nasopharyngeal swab for influenza rapid antigen detection test or PCR is recommended before considering antiviral treatment for patients and antiviral chemoprophylaxis for their household contacts.

TREATMENT

Lifestyle Modifications

Rest is generally recommended for patients with URIs, mainly to allow patients to cope with their illness. There is no evidence that complete bedrest shortens the duration of illness. Voice rest is important for patients with hoarseness.

Medical Options

Symptomatic treatment for URIs should be directed to maximize relief of the most prominent symptom(s). Increased fluid intake is generally recommended in an attempt to thin respiratory secretions; however, caution about the development of hyponatremia should be considered in certain patients. Hundreds of over-the-counter (OTC) medications are available in various combinations, but none of these agents has proved to be a magic bullet.[17] Americans spend more than $2 billion on OTC medications each year.

A meta-analysis of the literature has shown that nasal symptoms improve after treatment with α-adrenergic agonists such as oxymetazoline HCl, anticholinergic (parasympatholytic) agents such as ipratropium bromide, and first-generation antihistamines such as chlorpheniramine maleate. Only the first dose of decongestants has been proved to be effective, and repeated use may result in a rebound phenomenon—rhinitis medicamentosa—after discontinuation. The sedating effect of first-generation antihistamines can be hazardous in people driving cars or operating heavy machinery, but the effect may be desirable in patients who have difficulty falling asleep at night as a result of their symptoms.

The role of antitussives and expectorants in the treatment of URIs remains controversial. Nonsteroidal anti-inflammatory drugs (NSAIDs) are useful for relieving fever, headache, and malaise, but these agents may be associated with gastrointestinal irritation. In addition, two cyclooxygenase 2 (COX-2) selective NSAIDS, rofecoxib and valdecoxib, have been withdrawn from the market because of increased cardiovascular risks. Warm saline gargles and steam inhalation are inexpensive and relatively safe measures that provide temporary relief of throat symptoms. Camphor and menthol also have been used in various concentrations for temporary relief of various URI symptoms. Mast cell stabilizers such as cromolyn sodium are widely used in preventing asthma attacks, but their role in treating URIs remains unknown. Topical nasal steroids such as fluticasone propionate improve the clinical success rates of patients with chronic or recurrent sinusitis who present with acute exacerbations.[18] Systemic steroids should not be used for the treatment of URIs.

After several decades of debate and numerous studies, the role of vitamin C for the treatment of URIs remains controversial. It appears that large doses of vitamin C are necessary to achieve its beneficial effect as an antioxidant in activated leukocytes. However, doses in excess of 4 g/day have been associated with diarrhea. The average benefit in studies using 2 to 4 g/day of vitamin C has been a decrement of about half a day (15%) in the duration of illness.[19]

Similarly, the role of zinc salts remains controversial, and the specific mechanism of action is unknown. Duration of illness was reduced by about 1 day in studies that showed benefit.[20,21] The ionic bioavailability of zinc salts is an important factor in producing a beneficial effect.[22] Bad taste occurs in up to 80% of patients receiving zinc lozenges, and nausea in about 20%. The long-term effects of cumulative doses of zinc are unknown, and altered lipid metabolism and copper deficiency are potential concerns. An intranasal formulation of zinc gel appears to have the same beneficial effect as oral zinc lozenges, with significantly fewer side effects. If considered, zinc lozenges or intranasal zinc gel should be started within 24 to 48 hours of the onset of cold symptoms.

The therapeutic effectiveness of echinacea in the treatment of URIs has not been established because of the heterogeneous nature of the preparations evaluated in published studies.[23-25] Reports of echinacea-related anaphylaxis in patients with atopy raise the concern of using it in such a common illness. Other traditional medicines, such as troxerutin,[26] *Andrographis paniculata*,[27] and elderberry syrup[28] have been shown in small studies to shorten the duration and decrease the severity of URIs. Because herbal agents are neither patentable nor regulated by the U.S. Food and Drug Administration (FDA), dosages and formulations are not standardized.

Although viruses cause most URIs, antibiotics continue to be inappropriately widely prescribed for these illnesses.[29] Unnecessary adverse effects of antibiotics and the development of antimicrobial resistance can be reduced by judicious use of these drugs.[30] Health care providers should educate their patients about the self-limited nature of most URIs and the hazards of inappropriate use of antibiotics for the individual and the community.

Antibiotics have no role in the management of the common cold or any mild URI.[31] However, almost 75% of adults with URIs are prescribed antibiotics by their physicians.[32] This results in 41 million antibiotic prescriptions per year in the United States, accounting for more than 20% of all antibiotic prescriptions to adults. In addition, 68% of those receiving antibiotics are given nonrecommended, more expensive, broad-spectrum agents, a trend that has been increasing over time.[29] Unnecessary antibiotic prescriptions for treatment of URIs cost approximately $700 million per year. Several symptoms predictive of physicians' behavior to prescribe antibiotics for URIs actually have poor predictive value with respect to the efficacy of antibiotics. These include cough productive of yellow sputum, sore throat, fever, and colored nasal discharge. About 75% of patients with URIs who seek medical attention expect to receive antibiotics, particularly if they have sinus pain. However, studies have shown that patient satisfaction with an office visit is independent of a patient's initial belief about antibiotics and whether antibiotics were prescribed.[33] Satisfaction is more closely related to whether health care providers addressed patients' concerns. Providing patients with written information, in addition to verbal advice about the lack of evidence to support the use of antibiotics, has been found to be valuable.[34] Another approach might involve giving the patient a prescription for an antibiotic, with instructions to fill it only after 3 days if symptoms fail to improve.[35]

Patients with clinical and epidemiologic features consistent with GABHS-related pharyngitis should be started on antimicrobial therapy pending microbiologic confirmation.[2] Oral penicillin or erythromycin (in penicillin-allergic persons), given for 10 days, remains the preferred agent. Fortunately, no resistance to penicillin has been reported so far in GABHS-related pharyngitis patients.

Patients with only mild symptoms of acute sinusitis improve with topical nasal steroids and decongestants. Oral amoxicillin, trimethoprim-sulfamethoxazole, or doxycycline, given for 3 to 10 days, are the recommended first-line antibiotics for the treatment of moderate to severe acute sinusitis.[2,36] The incidence of penicillin-resistant *S. pneumoniae* and beta-lactamase–producing organisms causing acute sinusitis has been steadily increasing in the community. However, larger doses of amoxicillin, up to 3 g daily, or a combination of amoxicillin and clavulanate remain effective in most cases caused by resistant organisms.[3,10,11,36] Alternative agents include cefpodoxime, cefuroxime, and cefdinir. Factors predisposing patients to have antibiotic-resistant organisms include recent antibiotic use and exposure to children who attend daycare centers. Second-line, broad-spectrum, and more expensive agents, including the newer macrolides clarithromycin and azithromycin, and the "respiratory" fluoroquinolones—levofloxacin, gatifloxacin, and moxifloxacin—are no more effective than amoxicillin.[37] These agents should be reserved for use in individuals who are allergic or intolerant to first-line agents, those who do not respond to first-line agents within 3 days, or for confirmed microbiologic resistance. This approach would help contain ever-increasing health care costs and, most importantly, curtail the emergence of drug-resistant organisms as a result of selection pressure.

Treating acute tracheobronchitis with antibiotics is not recommended, because most cases are viral and thus resolve spontaneously.[4,38] In adults with persistent cough who report exposure to a patient with confirmed or suspected pertussis, erythromycin or trimethoprim-sulfamethoxazole should be administered for 14 days. This decreases contagion from bacterial shedding, but it is not expected to improve resolution of symptoms, unless started within 10 days of the onset of illness. Selective β-agonist bronchodilators offer symptomatic relief for cough.

Four agents are currently available for the treatment of influenza. Mild and nonfebrile influenza-like illness should not be treated with antiviral agents. The adamantanes, amantadine and rimantadine, are M2 ion channel blockers that are only active against influenza A and are associated with a high incidence of gastrointestinal and neuropsychiatric side effects, as well as development of viral resistance. The neuraminidase inhibitors (NAIs), oseltamivir and zanamivir, are active against both influenza A and B and have fewer side effects and less propensity to induce viral resistance than the adamantanes, but are considerably more expensive. In January 2006, a report of resistance to the adamantanes in 92% of circulating influenza isolates resulted in a national recommendation to use only NAI until this resistance pattern is reversed, hopefully in the coming years. Anti-influenza agents should be started within 1 to 2 days of onset of illness and continued for 5 days for maximum benefit.

Several antiviral agents with activity against rhinovirus or other viruses that cause URIs have been studied. Interferon is a powerful antiviral drug approved for the treatment of hepatitis B and C virus infections. It has no role in the treatment of viral URIs at this time. Other investigational agents such as pleconaril, a viral capsid inhibitor,[39] and tremacamra, a soluble intercellular adhesion molecule,[40] have shown some promise.

Surgical Options

Patients with suppurative complications of URIs, such as peritonsillar abscess, or mastoiditis, and those with sinusitis refractory to medical treatment should be referred to an ear, nose, and throat surgeon.

Summary

- Symptomatic treatment is the mainstay of treatment for most URIs.
- Vitamin C and zinc remain controversial.
- Antibiotics should be avoided in patients with a common cold or acute bronchitis, but should be prescribed to patients with GABHS pharyngitis and moderate or severe sinusitis. Narrow-spectrum agents such as amoxicillin should be the first-line agents.
- Patients with moderate or severe influenza, and all patients with underlying medical conditions who develop influenza, should be treated with an NAI or an adamantane when the resistance pattern is reversed.

Treatment Outcomes

Most URIs resolve spontaneously in 3 to 10 days with symptomatic therapy alone. In patients with GABHS pharyngitis, moderate or severe sinusitis, and moderate or severe influenza, antimicrobial therapy generally results in symptom relief, and resolution of illness 1 to 2 days sooner than if symptomatic measures alone are used. In addition, prompt initiation of antibiotics in patients with GABHS pharyngitis decreases contagion and may prevent development of suppurative complications, such as peritonsillar abscess. Concerns about preventing immunologic complications, such as rheumatic fever and glomerulonephritis, are more applicable to the developing world. The benefits of anti-influenza drugs are more pronounced in patients presenting with more severe illness. Studies using NAIs have also shown a reduction in the incidence of complications from influenza in the frail older population and in patients with underlying medical conditions, such as chronic obstructive pulmonary disease or cardiomyopathy. However, there are no data on their efficacy in treating influenza pneumonia or their use in severely immunocompromised patients, such as transplant recipients.

PREVENTION AND SCREENING

Frequent hand washing remains the most important preventive measure for most URIs. Simple measures, such as covering the mouth and nose while sneezing, can decrease the risk of transmission of infectious agents. No study has ever shown that prophylactic antibiotics can prevent the development of bacterial superinfection of viral URIs. Aqueous iodine can prevent viral transmission when applied to the hands of patients with viral URIs, but it is cosmetically unacceptable and may be associated with systemic toxicity if ingested. One study has shown that antibacterial home cleaning and hand washing products do not decrease the incidence of URIs.[41] Antimicrobial treatment of the sexual partner can prevent reinfection in cases of gonococcal and herpetic pharyngitis.

Vitamin C is not recommended for prevention of URIs in the general community. However, in marathon runners, skiers, or soldiers, who are exposed to significant cold or physical stress, prophylactic vitamin C may reduce the incidence of colds by 50% and shorten the duration of colds by 8% in adults (approximately 0.6 day).[19]

Multivitamin and mineral supplements, particularly vitamin E, have no effects on the incidence and severity of URIs in well-nourished noninstitutionalized older individuals,[42,43] but they decrease the incidence of common colds in older nursing home residents,[44] as well as infectious illnesses and work-related absenteeism in diabetic community-dwelling adults.[45] These findings are ascribed to micronutrient deficiency.

The trivalent inactivated intramuscular influenza vaccine—the flu shot—is one of the few cost-saving interventions in medicine today. It results in a 30% to 50% reduction of respiratory illnesses, physician visits, and sick leave in vaccinated healthy adults, as well as a reduction in hospitalization related to acute worsening of chronic obstructive pulmonary disease or congestive heart failure, and death from any cause among vaccinated older persons.[46] Vaccination is recommended for almost 50% of the U.S. population, including children aged 6 to 23 months, adults 50 years and older, patients with chronic medical conditions that predispose for the development of influenza-related complications and their household members, residents of extended-care facilities, and health care providers. Influenza vaccine is provided from early fall through early spring and is well tolerated by patients. Local side effects, such as mild redness and soreness at the site of injection, occur in 10% to 40% of patients. Systemic reactions, such as fever, malaise, and myalgia, may develop in about 10% of patients, especially those without prior exposure to the influenza virus antigens in the vaccine.

Contrary to widespread belief among patients, the inactivated influenza vaccine cannot cause influenza. This must be explained to skeptics, emphasizing that the gains of vaccination clearly outweigh its potential risks, and that respiratory illnesses caused by other infectious organisms are not prevented by the vaccine. The only absolute contraindication to the vaccine is severe egg allergy. Patients with mild URIs can still receive the vaccine. Unfortunately, only about 65% of people in the United States who should be vaccinated are getting the vaccine, but the rate of vaccination has been steadily climbing over the past several years. Problems with shortage may hamper vaccination efforts. Automatic reminders and scheduling routine office visits for those at risk during the early fall are some measures that can be used to increase the rate of vaccination. Inpatient computerized standing orders for vaccination, directed at nurses, are actually more effective than computerized reminders to physicians.[47] The live-attenuated, cold-adapted, intranasal influenza vaccine is as effective as the inactivated vaccine, and may be more appealing for those who would like to avoid an injection.[48] However, it is only approved for healthy persons aged 5 to 49 years. In addition, because shedding of live attenuated virus occurs for about 1 week after receiving this vaccine, health care providers and household contacts of severely immunocompromised patients should only receive the inactivated vaccine to avoid the theoretical risk of virus transmission causing disease.

Fortunately, almost all URIs in children caused by *H. influenzae* type B have been eliminated by the widespread use of the *H. influenzae* type B vaccine, but cases of nontypable *H. influenzae* continue to occur in adults. The greatest impact of using the 23-valent pneumococcal polysaccharide vaccine has been on preventing bacteremic pneumonia and meningitis in older adults.[49] Studies have also shown a reduction in invasive pneumococcal disease in adults since the introduction of the pediatric conjugated pneumococcal vaccine as a result of herd immunity.[50] An oral live attenuated adenovirus vaccine is available but is restricted for military use.

Chemoprophylaxis with anti-influenza drugs should be reserved for influenza outbreaks occurring before or despite influenza vaccination, or for immunocompromised patients exposed to a person with proven influenza. Chemoprophylaxis should not be considered as a substitute for vaccination. The cost of a 10-day course for post-exposure prophylaxis or a 6-week course for seasonal outbreaks is much more expensive than the vaccine.

CONSIDERATIONS IN SPECIAL POPULATIONS

Patients who are immunocompromised because of disease or medications are at higher risk for complications caused by URIs. Special attention should be paid to prevention of these infections, if possible, and to treat early to limit morbidity.

Practice Guidelines

Anon JB, Jacobs MR, Poole MD, et al: Sinus and Allergy Health Partnership: Antimicrobial treatment guidelines for acute bacterial rhinosinusitis. Otolaryngol Head Neck Surg 2004;130(Suppl 1):1-45.

Bison AL, Gerber MA, Gwaltney JM Jr, et al: Practice guidelines for the diagnosis and management of group A streptococcal pharyngitis. Clin Infect Dis 2002;35:113-125.
Centers for Disease Control and Prevention: Prevention and control of influenza. Recommendations of the advisory committee on immunization practices (ACIP). MMWR Morb Mort Wkly Rep 2007;56:1-54.
Gonzales R, Bartlett JG, Besser RE, et al: Principles of appropriate antibiotic use for treatment of uncomplicated acute bronchitis: Background. Ann Intern Med 2001;134:521-529.
Institute for Clinical Systems Improvement: Health Care Guideline: Diagnosis and Treatment of Respiratory Illness in Children and Adults, 2008. Available at http://www.icsi.org/guidelines_and_more/respiratory_illness_in_children_and_adults_guideline_13116.html.

Suggested Readings

Aagaard E, Gonzales R: Management of acute bronchitis in healthy adults. Infect Dis Clin North Am 2004;18:919-937.
Arroll B, Kenealy T: Antibiotics for the common cold and acute purulent rhinitis. Cochrane Database Syst Rev 1998;(4):CD000247.
Avenell A, Campbell MK, Cook JA, et al: Effect of multivitamin and multimineral supplements on morbidity from infections in older people (MAVIS trial): Pragmatic, randomised, double blind, placebo controlled trial. BMJ 2005;331:324-329.
Call SA, Vollenweider MA, Hornung CA, et al: Does this patient have influenza? JAMA 2005;293:987-997.
Cooper RJ, Hoffman JR, Bartlett JG, et al: Principles of appropriate antibiotic use for acute pharyngitis in adults: background. Ann Intern Med 2001;134:509-517.
Gonzales R, Malone DC, Maselli JH, Sande MA: Excessive antibiotic use for acute respiratory infections in the United States. Clin Infect Dis 2001;33:757-762.
Musher DM: How contagious are common respiratory tract pathogens? N Engl J Med 2003;348:1256-1266.
Nichol KL, Nordin J, Mullooly J, et al: Influenza vaccination and reduction of hospitalizations for cardiac disease and stroke among the elderly. N Engl J Med 2003;348:1322-1332.
Poole MD, Portugal LG: Treatment of rhinosinusitis in the outpatient setting. Am J Med 2005;118:45S–50S.
Smith MB, Feldman W: Over-the-counter cold medications. A critical review of clinical trials between 1950 and 1991. JAMA 1993;269:2258-2263.

References

For a complete list of references, log onto www.expertconsult.com.

Sepsis

Steven P. LaRosa

DEFINITION

The term systemic inflammatory response syndrome (SIRS) was coined in 1992 by a panel composed of members of the American College of Chest Physicians and Society of Critical Care Medicine. They convened to develop consensus definitions of critical illness for the purposes of clinical trial design.

SIRS describes the host response to a critical illness of infectious or noninfectious cause, such as burns, trauma, and pancreatitis. More specific definitions are as follows:

- Sepsis is SIRS resulting from a presumed or known site of infection.
- Severe sepsis is sepsis with an acute associated organ failure.
- Septic shock, a subset of severe sepsis, is defined as a persistently low mean arterial blood pressure despite adequate fluid resuscitation.
- Refractory septic shock is a persistently low mean arterial blood pressure despite vasopressor therapy and adequate fluid resuscitation.[1]

SIRS can be readily diagnosed at the bedside by the presence of at least two of the following four signs: body temperature alterations (hyperthermia or hypothermia), tachycardia, tachypnea, and changes in white blood cell count (leukocytosis or leukopenia).

PREVALENCE AND INCIDENCE

Sepsis is the leading cause of death in noncoronary intensive care units (ICUs) and the 10th leading cause of death in the United States overall. The incidence of severe sepsis in the United States is between 650,000 and 750,000 cases.[2,3] More than 70% of these patients have underlying comorbidities and more than 60% of these cases occur in those aged 65 years and older. When patients with human immunodeficiency virus are excluded, the incidence of sepsis in men and women is similar. A greater number of sepsis cases are caused by infection with gram-positive organisms than gram-negative organisms, and fungal infections now account for 6% of cases.

After adjusting for population size, the annualized incidence of sepsis is increasing by 8%. The incidence of severe sepsis is increasing greatest in older adults and the nonwhite population. The rise in the number of cases is believed to be caused by the increased use of invasive procedures and immunosuppressive drugs, chemotherapy, transplantation, and prosthetic implants and devices, as well as the increasing problem of antimicrobial resistance.

PATHOPHYSIOLOGY

Inflammatory Cascade

Severe sepsis can occur as a result of infection at any body site, including the lungs, abdomen, skin or soft tissue, or urinary tract and as a result of a primary blood stream infection, such as in meningococcemia. Bacteria are the pathogens most commonly associated with the development of sepsis, although fungi, viruses, and parasites can cause sepsis. The pathophysiology of sepsis can be initiated by the outer membrane component of gram-negative organisms (e.g., lipopolysaccharide [LPS], lipid A, endotoxin) or gram-positive organisms (e.g., lipoteichoic acid, peptidoglycan), as well as fungal, viral, and parasitic components (Fig. 1). Signaling by these mediators occurs via a family of transmembrane receptors known as Toll-like receptors. Within the monocyte, nuclear factor-κB (NF-κB), is activated, which leads to the production of proinflammatory cytokines, tumor necrosis factor α (TNF-α), and interleukin 1 (IL-1). TNF-α and IL-1 lead to the production of toxic downstream mediators, including prostaglandins, leukotrienes, platelet-activating factor, and phospholipase A2. These mediators damage the endothelial lining, leading to increased capillary leakage.[4] Furthermore, these cytokines lead to the production of adhesion molecules on endothelial cells and neutrophils. Neutrophilic endothelial interaction leads to further endothelial injury through the release of the neutrophil components. Finally, activated neutrophils release nitric oxide, a potent vasodilator that leads to septic shock.

Link Between Inflammation and Coagulation

IL-1 and TNF-α also have direct effects on the endothelial surface. As a result of these inflammatory cytokines, tissue factor, the first step in the extrinsic pathway of coagulation, is expressed on the surfaces of the endothelium and of monocytes. Tissue factor leads to the production of thrombin, which itself is a proinflammatory substance. Thrombin results in fibrin clots in the microvasculature, a sequela most easily recognized in meningococcal septic shock with purpura fulminans. Fibrinolysis is also impaired during the septic process. IL-1 and TNF-α lead to the production of plasminogen activator inhibitor-1, a potent inhibitor of fibrinolysis.[5]

Proinflammatory cytokines also disrupt the body's naturally occurring modulators of coagulation and inflammation, activated protein C (APC) and antithrombin. Protein C circulates as an inactive zymogen but, in the presence of thrombin and the endothelial surface-bound protein thrombomodulin, is converted to the enzyme-activated protein C. Studies have shown that proinflammatory cytokines can shear thrombomodulin from the endothelial surface as well as lead to downregulation of this molecule, thus preventing the activation of protein C.[6] APC and its cofactor protein S turn off thrombin production by cleaving factors Va and VIIIa. APC also restores fibrinolytic potential by inhibiting plasminogen activator inhibitor-1.[7,8] In vitro studies have revealed that APC has direct anti-inflammatory properties, including inhibiting the production of proinflammatory cytokines by LPS-stimulated monocytes, inhibiting leukocyte adhesion and rolling, and inhibiting neutrophil accumulation.[9-11]

Antithrombin is the second naturally occurring endothelial regulator affected during sepsis. Antithrombin inhibits thrombin production at multiple steps in the coagulation cascade as well as by binding and inhibiting thrombin directly.[12] Antithrombin, when bound to endothelial cell surface glycosaminoglycans (GAGs), leads to the production of the anti-inflammatory molecule prostacyclin (prostaglandin I_2 [PGI_2]).[13] Evidence exists that neutrophil elastase cleaves GAGs off the surface of the endothelial lining, thus limiting the anti-inflammatory properties of antithrombin.[14]

Immunoparalysis

CD4 lymphocytes play a key role in the inflammatory response seen in sepsis. Early in the sepsis process, these cells assume a TH1 phenotype, where they produce large amounts of the proinflammatory mediators, including interferon gamma, TNF-α, and IL-2. CD4 lymphocytes may evolve over time to a Th2 phenotype, whereby the CD4

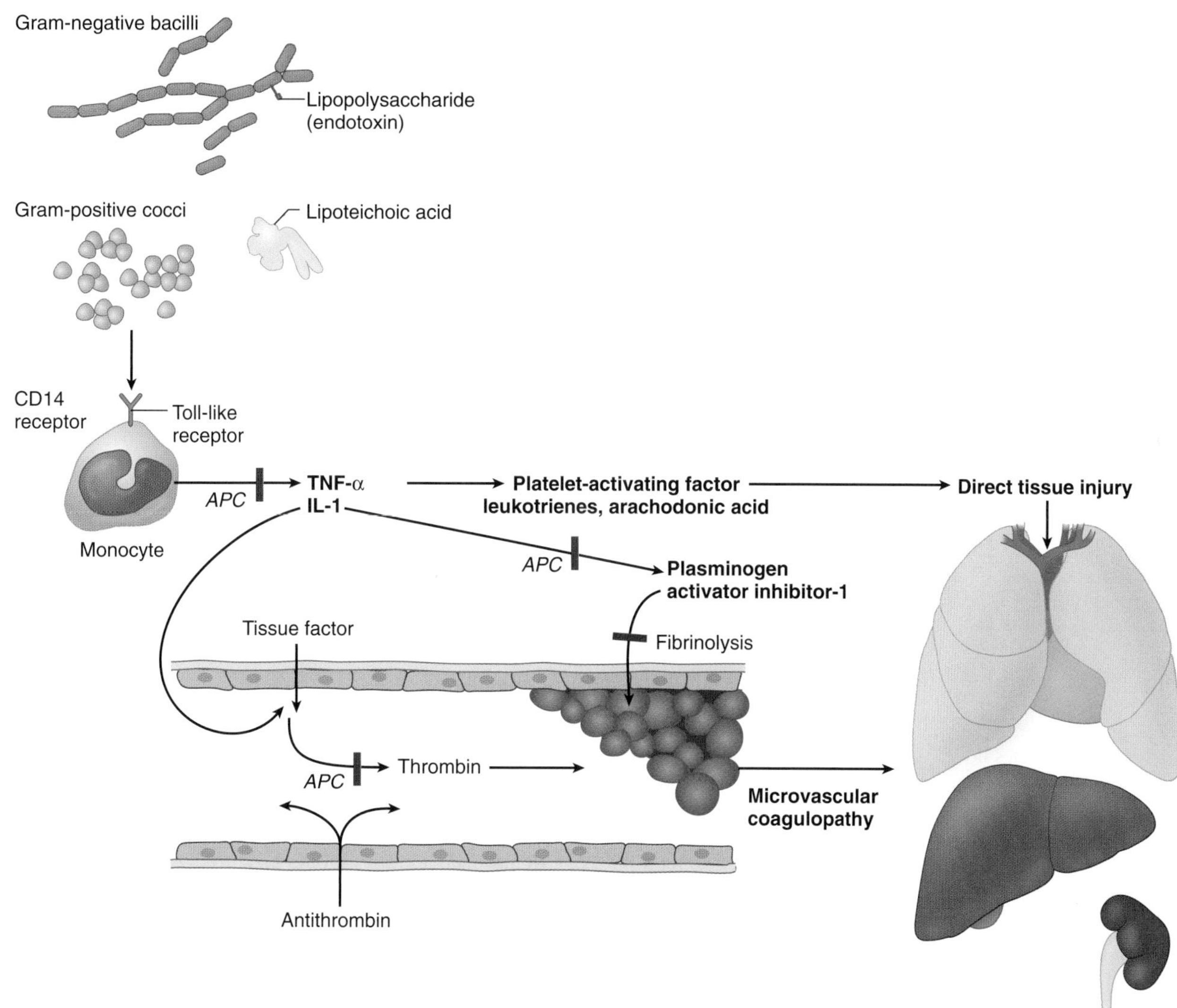

Figure 1 Sepsis leads to organ failure and death via a cascade of inflammation and coagulation. Activated protein C (APC) blocks the cascade at several points. A formulation of recombinant human APC has been approved for treating sepsis. IL-1, interleukin 1; TNF-α, tumor necrosis factor α. © 2002 The Cleveland Clinic Foundation.

lymphocytes produce anti-inflammatory cytokines, including IL-10, IL-4, and IL-13. This is often driven by the release of stress hormones, such as catecholamines and corticosteroids. These cytokines dampen the immune response and can lead to the deactivation of monocytes. Additionally, TNF released early can cause apoptosis of lymphocytes in the gut, leading to further immunosuppression.[15]

Severe Sepsis: The Final Common Pathway

As a result of the vicious cycle of inflammation and coagulation, cardiovascular insufficiency and multiple organ failure occur, and often lead to death. Cardiovascular insufficiency can occur at the level of the myocardium as a result of the myocardial depressant effects of TNF or at the level of the vessel, caused by vasodilation and capillary leak.[16]

SIGNS AND SYMPTOMS

Clinical signs that may lead the physician to consider sepsis in the differential diagnosis include fever or hypothermia, unexplained tachycardia, unexplained tachypnea, signs of peripheral vasodilation, unexplained shock, and unexplained mental status changes. Hemodynamic measurements that suggest septic shock are an increased cardiac output, with a low systemic vascular resistance. Abnormalities of the complete blood count (CBC), laboratory test results, clotting factors, and acute-phase reactants might indicate sepsis (Table 1).

Conditions other than sepsis can produce a systemic inflammatory response and organ dysfunction. Noninfectious illnesses that should be considered in the differential diagnosis include tissue injury caused by trauma, hematoma, venous thrombosis, myocardial or pulmonary infarcts, transplant rejection, pancreatitis, hyperthyroidism, addisonian crisis, drug or blood product reaction, malignancies, and central nervous system hemorrhages.[17]

DIAGNOSIS

The diagnosis of severe sepsis requires the presence of a presumed or known site of infection, evidence of a systemic inflammatory response, and an acute sepsis-associated organ dysfunction. Following is a description of the specific diagnostic criteria used in past clinical trials to define patients with severe sepsis.

Table 1 Laboratory Indicators of Sepsis

Laboratory Test	Findings	Comments
White blood cell count	Leukocytosis or leukopenia	Endotoxemia may cause early leukopenia
Platelet count	Thrombocytosis or thrombocytopenia	High value early may be seen as acute-phase response; low platelet counts seen in overt DIC
Coagulation cascade	Protein C deficiency; antithrombin deficiency; elevated D-dimer level; prolonged PT and PTT	Abnormalities can be observed before onset of organ failure and without frank bleeding.
Creatinine level	Elevated from baseline	Doubling-indicates acute renal injury
Lactic acid level	Lactic acid > 4 mmol/L (36 mg/dL)	Indicates tissue hypoxia
Liver enzyme levels	Elevated alkaline phosphatase, AST, ALT, bilirubin levels	Indicates acute hepatocellular injury caused by hypoperfusion
Serum phosphate level	Hypophosphatemia	Inversely correlated with proinflammatory cytokine levels
C-reactive protein (CRP) level	Elevated	Acute-phase response
Procalcitonin level	Elevated	Differentiates infectious SIRS from noninfectious SIRS

ALT, alanine aminotransferase; AST, aspartate transaminase; DIC, disseminated intravascular coagulation; PT, prothrombin time; PTT, partial thromboplastin time; SIRS, systemic inflammatory response syndrome.

- A presumed or known site of infection is indicated by one of the following:
  - Purulent sputum or respiratory sample, or chest radiograph with new infiltrates not explained by a noninfectious process
  - Spillage of bowel contents noted during an operation
  - Radiographic or physical examination evidence of an infected collection
  - White blood cells in a normally sterile body fluid
  - Positive blood culture
  - Evidence of infected mechanical hardware by physical or radiographic examination
- Evidence of a systemic inflammatory response is indicated by at least two of the following:
  - Fever or hypothermia: core body temperature 38° C or higher or 36° C or lower
  - Tachypnea: 20 breaths/min or more, or need for mechanical ventilation for an acute process
  - Tachycardia: heart rate 90 beats/min or more, unless the patient has a preexisting tachycardia
  - White blood cell count:12,000 cells/mm^3 or higher, 4,000 cells/mm^3 or less, or more than 10% bands on differential
- A sepsis-induced organ failure is indicated by one of the following criteria:
  - Cardiovascular dysfunction: mean arterial pressure 60 mm Hg or lower, the need for vasopressors to maintain this blood pressure in the presence of adequate intravascular volume (central venous pressure >8 mm Hg or pulmonary artery occlusion pressure >12 mm Hg), or after an adequate fluid challenge has been given
  - Respiratory organ failure: an arterial oxygen pressure-to-fraction of inspired oxygen ratio of less than 250 in the absence of pneumonia or less than 200 in the presence of pneumonia
  - Renal dysfunction: urine output less than 0.5 mL/kg/hr for 2 hours in the presence of adequate intravascular volume or after an adequate fluid challenge or doubling of the serum creatinine level
  - Hematologic dysfunction: thrombocytopenia with less than 80,000 platelets/mm^3, or 50% decrease from baseline during the acute illness
  - Unexplained metabolic acidosis: pH lower than 7.30 and plasma lactate level higher than 1.5 times the upper limit of normal for the laboratory

Summary

- The diagnosis of severe sepsis includes the presence of a systemic inflammatory response and an end-organ failure in the setting of infection.
- The inflammatory and coagulopathic responses to infection cause the end-organ failure seen in sepsis.
- Noninfectious causes should be considered in the differential diagnosis of SIRS.
- The physical examination and radiographic tests should focus on three major sites of sepsis: lungs, abdomen, and urinary tract.
- Elevated lactic acid levels and coagulation abnormalities are early laboratory indicators of sepsis.

TREATMENT

Practice Guidelines

Eleven societies involved in the care of the critically ill collaborated to produce guidelines for the care of patients with severe sepsis, published in 2004.[18] However, the individual treatment guidelines have not been universally agreed on. Additionally, new clinical trial data have been reported since these guidelines were initially published.

Appropriate Antimicrobial Treatment

Many clinical studies have demonstrated a twofold increase in mortality caused by sepsis when inappropriate antimicrobial therapy is given. More recent animal and human studies have demonstrated an incremental but statistically significant increase in mortality with each hour delay in the administration of appropriate antibiotic therapy from the onset of septic shock.[19] When the clinician encounters a patient with severe sepsis, the site of infection and causative organism(s) often are unknown. Empirical antibiotics must be given in these cases. Appropriate empirical antimicrobial therapy must be guided by the knowledge of the most common sites of infection and the most common infecting organisms. A clinical trial of patients

Table 2 Empirical Antimicrobial Therapy for Major Sites of Sepsis

Site of Infection	Microorganisms	Therapeutic Choices
Community-acquired pneumonia	*Streptococcus pneumoniae, Haemophilus influenzae, Legionella pneumophila, Mycoplasma pneumoniae*	Third-generation cephalosporin with macrolide or respiratory quinolone
Early hospital-acquired pneumonia (<5 days)	*S. pneumoniae, H. influenzae, L. pneumophila, M.* pneumonia; nonresistant gram-negative rods	Ceftriaxone, respiratory quinolone or ampicillin-sulbactam, or ertapenem
Late hospital-acquired pneumonia	*Pseudomonas aeruginosa, Klebsiella* spp., *Acinetobacter* spp., methicillin-resistant *Staphylococcus aureus*	Antipseudomonal cephalosporin or carbapenem, or antipseudomonal beta-lactam or beta-lactamase inhibitor, *plus* linezolid or vancomycin
Intra-abdominal infections	Enteric gram-negative rods and anaerobes	Third-generation cephalosporin with metronidazole, or beta-lactam or beta-lactamase inhibitor, or carbapenem or moxifloxacin
Urinary tract infections	Gram-negative rods; *Enterococcus* spp.	Extended-spectrum beta-lactam or aztreonam, with or without an aminoglycoside; ampicillin or vancomycin if *Enterococcus* is present

with severe sepsis has revealed that the lungs are the most common sites of infection, followed by the abdomen and urinary tract.[20] In terms of pathogen type, gram-positive organisms cause sepsis slightly more often than gram-negative organisms; fungal organisms account for approximately 6% of cases.[3] The most common gram-positive organisms are *Staphylococcus aureus* and *Streptococcus pneumoniae,* and the most common gram-negative organisms are *Escherichia coli, Klebsiella* spp., *Pseudomonas* spp., and *Enterobacter* spp.[20] Samples for blood cultures should be taken from a percutaneous site and from any intravascular catheters. Samples for Gram staining and culture should be taken from suspected sites of infection. Table 2 indicates appropriate empirical antibiotic choices by site of infection.

Empirical antifungal therapy should be given to patients at high risk for fungemia. High-risk patients include those who have had prior colonization with *Candida* at two or more sites, those being treated with more than two different antibiotics, those who have taken antibiotics for more than 14 days, those who have had prior placement of a Hickman catheter, and those who have undergone prior hemodialysis.[21]

Source Control of Infection

Adequate source control of infection is as important as appropriate antimicrobial therapy in the treatment of a patient with severe sepsis. Source control of infection includes removal of infected foreign bodies, such as urinary catheters, intravascular catheters, peritoneal dialysis cannulas, prosthetic joints, vascular grafts, and mechanical valves. Incision and drainage of cutaneous abscesses as well as open or percutaneous drainage of intra-abdominal abscesses also fall under the principle of adequate source control of infection.[22] Furthermore, one specific clinical scenario requires specific mention. For patients with necrotizing fasciitis, mortality and extent of tissue loss are directly related to the rapidity of surgical intervention.

Optimizing Tissue Oxygenation

Optimizing the delivery of oxygen to critical organs is an urgent priority in the treatment of severe sepsis. The inability to meet tissue oxygen demand can be determined at the time of a patient's presentation to the emergency department by the presence of lactic acidosis (serum lactic acid level >4 mmol/L or 36 mg/dL). In this setting, the use of early goal-directed therapy (EGDT) to achieve a central venous oxygen saturation of 70% or higher has been shown to reduce mortality as well as hospital resources. EGDT is accomplished by first placing a central venous catheter to monitor the central venous oxygen saturation. Crystalloid boluses of 500 mL are given every 30 minutes to reach a central venous pressure (CVP) of 8 to 12 mm Hg. If the mean arterial pressure (MAP) is still below 65 mm Hg, vasopressor agents are added. If after these maneuvers the central venous oxygen saturation remains below 70%, red blood cells are transfused to reach a hematocrit of 30%. If the target is still not reached, dobutamine is then administered.[23]

Fluid Resuscitation

The best type of fluid replacement and optimal volume of resuscitation in the setting of severe sepsis have been heavily debated but studies have provided guidance to the clinician. One trial comparing 4% albumin with normal saline for fluid resuscitation found no difference in mortality at 28 days.[24] A 2004 meta-analysis similarly found no mortality advantage with the use of colloids compared with the use of crystalloids.[25] The trial of EGDT revealed that patients in the treatment arm received far greater volumes of fluid in the first 6 hours of resuscitation than those in the control arm. In a large study of European ICUs, patients with a positive fluid balance at 72 hours had a poor outcome.[26] In a clinical trial of patients with acute lung injury, the use of a conservative fluid strategy targeting a CVP lower than 4 mm Hg and a pulmonary artery occlusion pressure (PAOP) lower than 8 mm Hg was associated with a fewer number of ICU and ventilators days.[27] The preponderance of data would suggest that aggressive fluid management be done in the acute phase of sepsis, followed by a more conservative phase in the following few days.

Vasopressor Treatment

Dopamine and norepinephrine are the first-line agents for the treatment of sepsis shock. Dopamine increases cardiac index and systemic vascular resistance, whereas norepinephrine is a potent vasoconstrictor with few cardiac effects. A clinical trial comparing dopamine and norepinephrine in fluid-resuscitated patients with septic shock demonstrated a greater reversal of hypotension and lower mortality with the use of norepinephrine.[28] Norepinephrine also has the added advantage of causing fewer tachyarrhythmias than dopamine and does not suppress the hypothalamic-pituitary axis. Second-line agents for the treatment of septic shock include epinephrine, phenylephrine, and vasopressin. The use of epinephrine and phenylephrine is hampered by both drugs' negative effects on splanchnic blood flow.[29] Vasopressin has become the agent of choice in cases of septic shock refractory to dopamine, norepinephrine, or both. Studies have demonstrated that vasopressin increases blood pressure and allows dopamine and norepinephrine drips to be weaned.[30]

Low-Dose Corticosteroid Treatment for Septic Shock

Corticosteroids have long been considered to be of potential use in the treatment of severe sepsis because of their anti-inflammatory properties and beneficial effects on vascular tone. Clinical trials of high-dose, short-course corticosteroids have not demonstrated benefits in mortality in patients with severe sepsis; however, trials of long-course, low-dose corticosteroids (<200 mg/day of hydrocortisone for ≥5 days) have demonstrated a shorter time to shock reversal and improved mortality compared with placebo.[31] The largest of these trials, performed by Annane and colleagues,[32] has shown an improved survival time with the use of hydrocortisone, 50 mg every 6 hours, and with fludrocortisone, 50 µg/day for 5 days, in patients with refractory septic shock no longer than 8 hours in duration who did not respond with a 9-µg/dL rise in the cortisol level 1 hour following adrenocorticotropic hormone (ACTH) stimulation. This trial has suggested a treatment benefit with corticosteroids only in patients with adrenal insufficiency or adrenal resistance caused by sepsis. A meta-analysis, however, did not reveal that treatment benefit is related to ACTH test results.[33] A study by Hamrahian and colleagues[34] of free cortisol levels in this population revealed a low incidence of adrenal insufficiency. A larger trial (CORTICUS) in a less severely ill population with septic shock than the Annane trial did not reveal a mortality benefit with low-dose, long-course corticosteroids but suggested a shorter time to shock reversal. A higher incidence of hyperglycemia and superinfections was observed in the corticosteroid-treated arm.[35] Current clinical evidence would suggest treating only patients with shock refractory to vasopressors with low-dose, long-course corticosteroid therapy. Results of an ACTH test are not necessary to determine which patients should be treated.

Recombinant Human Activated Protein C

Activated protein C is a molecule with anti-inflammatory, antithrombotic, and profibrinolytic properties. In a large placebo-controlled, randomized, clinical trial in patients with severe sepsis, recombinant human activated protein C (rhAPC), 24 µg/kg/hour for 96 hours, was associated with a 6% absolute reduction in 28-day all-cause mortality compared with placebo.[20] The treatment benefit was confined to patients with greatest disease severity, as indicated by a baseline APACHE II score higher than 25 or those with two or more organ failures at baseline.[36] Retrospective analyses would suggest that patients with severe sepsis caused by community- acquired pneumonia and those with overt DIC may be the most ideal target populations for this agent.

The main adverse event associated with rhAPC is bleeding. Bleeding tends to occur in patients with severe thrombocytopenia and in those with a known disruption of blood vessels or ulcerative gastrointestinal lesions. RhAPC is not approved for children or surgical patients with sepsis and a single organ failure. Children with purpura fulminans, a profound state of protein C deficiency caused by infection with Neisseria meningitidis or Streptococcus pneumoniae, should be considered for treatment with rhAPC given the high mortality rate and amputation rates associated with this syndrome.

Glycemic Control

Tight control of the blood glucose level during sepsis might be expected to decrease the rate of infectious complications and improve outcomes in patients with sepsis. In a clinical trial conducted in a surgical ICU predominantly in patients following cardiac surgery, maintaining the blood glucose level below 110 mg/dL was associated with improved survival, fewer blood stream infections, shorter ICU stays, and fewer episodes of acute renal failure compared with a group in whom the glucose level was maintained between 180 and 200 mg/dL.[37] A second study completed in the medical ICU showed a mortality benefit with tighter glycemic control only in patients with stays in the ICU of 3 days or longer.[38] A threshold glucose level of 145 mg/dL was associated with improved mortality in a prospective observational study.[39] A German trial (VISEP) was stopped when mortality was not improved in the tight glycemic control arm and more hypoglycemic events were observed.[35] Current data suggest targeting a blood glucose level of no lower than 150 mg/dL in a critically ill patient.

Ventilator Treatment for Acute Respiratory Distress

Thanks to the efforts of organized networks of acute respiratory distress syndrome (ARDS) investigators in the United States and elsewhere, much has been learned about the appropriate ventilator management of patients with ARDS caused by sepsis. A randomized clinical trial has demonstrated lower mortality and an increase in the number of days off the ventilator when a lower (6 mL/kg) tidal volume strategy is used compared with a standard (12 mL/kg) tidal volume strategy.[40] A second study using the lower tidal volume strategy examined the optimal amount of PEEP (positive end-expiratory pressure) that should be administered to patients with ARDS. This study found that low levels of PEEP (<14 cm H_2O) produced similar outcomes as high PEEP (>14 cm H_2O).[41] A clinical trial of nitric oxide indicated that this agent is capable of transient improvements in oxygenation without an improvement in mortality or number of ventilator days.[42] Similar findings were observed with prone position ventilation.[43] However, neither nitric oxide use nor prone position ventilation can be recommended routinely for all patients with sepsis and ARDS based on randomized studies.

Blood Transfusions

Blood transfusions in the critically ill have the potential to increase oxygen-carrying capacity but also entail an increased risk of nosocomial infection. In the EGDT protocol, transfusing red blood cells to achieve a hematocrit of 30% was used as part of the strategy to reach a central venous oxygen saturation of 70% during the first 6 hours of hospital stay. A study by Hebert and colleagues[44] in critically ill patients demonstrated that maintaining hemoglobin between 7 and 9 mg/dL and transfusing only when the hemoglobin drops below 7 mg/dL is not associated with a worse outcome than maintaining the hemoglobin above 10 g/dL. The data would suggest early use of transfusions in the acute setting of sepsis, followed by a conservative strategy once tissue oxygen demands have been reached.

Additional Treatment Components

Three additional components in the care of severe sepsis patients include ensuring adequate nutrition, providing deep venous thrombosis prophylaxis, and providing gastric ulcer prophylaxis.[18] Adequate nutrition is best accomplished enterically to avoid catheter-related blood stream infections, maintain gut mucosa integrity, and prevent the theoretical possibility of translocation of bacteria across the intestinal wall. A mortality benefit with enteral feeds containing omega-3 fatty acids compared with standard enteral feeds was observed in a small clinical trial of patients with severe sepsis.[45] A morbidity benefit was observed with this same formula in patients with ARDS.[46] Deep venous thrombosis prevention can be accomplished with the use of subcutaneous heparin or continuous use of pneumatic compression stockings. Gastric ulcer prophylaxis may be accomplished with sucralfate, an H2 receptor antagonist, or a proton pump inhibitor.

Summary

- Antibiotic therapy should be administered within 1 hour of the acute presentation of sepsis.
- Patients with lactic acidosis should be placed on an early goal-directed therapy protocol.
- A low tidal volume ventilator strategy and a conservative fluid strategy should be used in patients with established acute lung injury.
- Recombinant human activated protein C use should be considered in the setting of an APACHE II score higher than 25 or the presence of two or more organ failures.
- Low-dose corticosteroid therapy should be considered for patients with septic shock refractory to fluid resuscitation and vasopressors (MAP <60 mm Hg).

OUTCOMES

Although the incidence of severe sepsis is increasing, mortality rates continue to decrease. In a recent study in a sepsis cohort, the mortality rate was 24.4%.47 Age was found to be an independent risk factor for death with a mortality rate of 27.7% in those older than 65 years versus 17.7% in those younger than 65 years of age. An increasing number of older survivors of sepsis require skilled nursing facilities following discharge from the hospital.[47]

PREVENTION

Because pneumonia is the most common infection leading to sepsis, efforts to decrease the incidence of this infection would lead to the most rapid reduction in new sepsis cases. Every effort should be made to vaccinate susceptible individuals against influenza, H. influenzae, and S. pneumoniae. Additionally, asplenic patients should receive vaccination against N. meningitidis as should college students living in dormitories. The incidence of intravascular catheter-related blood stream infections can be diminished by strict procedures to ensure sterile insertion, as well as the use of chlorhexidine dressings at the exit site. Cases of ventilator-associated pneumonia can be decreased by maintaining ventilator patients semirecumbent at a 45-degree angle.

Suggested Readings

Acute Respiratory Distress Syndrome Network: Ventilation with lower tidal volumes as compared with traditional tidal volumes for acute lung injury and the acute respiratory distress syndrome. N Engl J Med 2000;342:1301-1308.

Bernard GR, Vincent JL, Laterre PF, et al: Efficacy and safety of recombinant human activated protein C for severe sepsis. N Engl J Med 2001;344:699-709.

Bone RC, Balk RA, Cerra FB, et al: Definitions for sepsis and organ failure and guidelines for the use of innovative therapies in sepsis. The ACCP/SCCM Consensus Conference Committee. American College of Chest Physicians/Society of Critical Care Medicine. Chest 1992;101:1644-1655.

Dellinger RP, Carlet JM, Masur H, et al: Surviving sepsis: Campaign guidelines for management of severe sepsis and septic shock. Crit Care Med 2004;32:858-873.

Finney S, Zekveld S, Alia, A, et al: Glucose control and mortality in critically ill patients. JAMA 2003;290:2041-2047.

Kumar A, Roberts D, Wood KE, et al: Duration of hypotension prior to antimicrobial administration is the critical determinant of survival in human septic shock. Crit Care Med 2006; 34:1589-1596.

LaRosa SP: Sepsis: menu of new approaches replaces one therapy for all. Cleve Clin J Med 2002;69:65-73.

Martin C, Papazian L, Perrin G, et al: Norepinephrine or dopamine for the treatment of hyperdynamic septic shock? Chest 1993;103:1826-1831.

Martin GS, Mannino DM, Eaton S, et al: The epidemiology of sepsis in the United States from 1979 through 2000. N Engl J Med 2003;348:1546-1554.

Minneci PC, Deans KJ, Banks SM et al: Meta-analysis: The effect of steroids on survival and shock during sepsis depends on the dose. Ann Intern Med 2004;141:47-56.

Rivers E, Nguyen B, Havstad S, et al: Early goal-directed therapy in the treatment of severe sepsis and septic shock. N Engl J Med 2001;345:1368-1377.

Roberts I, Alderson P, Bunn F, et al: Colloids versus crystalloids for fluid resuscitation in critically ill patients. Cochrane Database Syst Rev 2004;(4):CD000567.

References

For a complete list of references, log onto www.expertconsult.com.

Acute and Chronic Bacterial Cystitis

Joseph B. Abdelmalak** and **Jeannette M. Potts

Urinary tract infections (UTIs) are the most common nosocomial infections. They account for more than 7 million physician visits and over 1 million hospital admissions in the United States each year.[1,2] They are the most common bacterial infection in older adults and the most frequent source of bacteremia.[3,4] UTIs are second in seriousness only to respiratory infections.

DEFINITION

The term *uncomplicated urinary tract infection* refers to the invasion of a structurally and functionally normal urinary tract by a nonresident infectious organism. Complicated UTI refers to the occurrence of infection in most men and in patients with an abnormal structural or functional urinary tract, or both (Box 1).

PREVALENCE AND RISK FACTORS

In 1995, the estimate for the United States put the direct cost of community-acquired UTIs at $659 million and indirect costs, through lost productivity, at $936 million.[5-8] The UTI incidence ratio in middle-aged women to men is 30 : 1; however, during later decades of life, the ratio of infection in women to men with bacteriuria progressively decreases.[9] Women are especially susceptible to cystitis for reasons that are poorly understood. One factor may be that a woman's urethra is short, allowing bacteria quick access to the bladder. Also, a woman's urethral opening is near sources of bacteria from the anus and vagina. For many women, sexual intercourse seems to trigger an infection, although the reasons for this linkage are unclear.[10] Estimates have suggested that about one third of women will have at least one episode of UTI requiring antibiotic therapy by the time they are 24 years old, and over a lifetime 50% will have had at least one UTI.[5-7] Hormonally induced changes in the vaginal flora associated with menopause are responsible for its higher prevalence in older women.[11]

PATHOGENESIS

The infection spreads to the urinary tract through an ascending route of fecal flora, from the fecal reservoir through the urethra into the bladder, particularly in patients with intermittent or indwelling catheters; hematogenous dissemination, secondary to *Staphylococcus aureus* bacteremia; or by direct extension from adjacent organs via the lymphatic system, as in the case of retroperitoneal abscesses or severe bowel obstruction. In women, colonization of the mucosa of the vaginal introitus is an essential step in the pathogenesis of UTIs.

Some people are more likely to get UTIs than others because of host factors or urothelial mucosal adherence to the mucopolysaccharide lining.[12] Any abnormality of the urinary tract that interferes with the drainage of urine (e.g., kidney stones or an enlarged prostate) sets the stage for an infection, as well as foreign bodies in the bladder, such as catheters and tubes (see Box 1). Diabetes and other immunocompromised patients are at higher risk for a UTI and its complications. Sexual intercourse[10] and women's use of a diaphragm[13] have also been linked to an increased risk of cystitis. Pregnancy does not increase the risk of cystitis; however, it increases the risk of pyelonephritis if UTI occurs.

URINARY PATHOGENS

Escherichia coli is the most common infecting organism in patients with uncomplicated UTIs.[14] It causes 85% of community-acquired infections and approximately 50% of nosocomial infections. Other gram-negative microorganisms causing UTIs include *Proteus, Klebsiella, Citrobacter, Enterobacter,* and *Pseudomonas* spp. Gram-positive pathogens such as *Enterococcus fecalis, Staphylococcus saprophyticus,* and group B streptococci can also infect the urinary tract. Anaerobic microorganisms are frequently encountered in suppurative infections of the genitourinary tract (e.g., periurethral abscess, Fournier's gangrene).

SIGNS AND SYMPTOMS

Cystitis may be asymptomatic. However, some patients report incontinence, a general lack of well-being, or both.[15] Cystitis clinically manifests as irritative voiding symptoms that include frequency, dysuria, urgency, suprapubic or lower abdominal pain, and incontinence. In men, urinary retention should be ruled out, because it is frequently associated with cystitis and possible prostatitis. The manifestations of UTIs in older adults may include confusion, lethargy, anorexia, and incontinence.

DIAGNOSIS

Physical examination, including a pelvic examination, should be carried out in women with lower urinary tract symptoms to exclude gynecologic, neurologic, or colorectal disorders. Physicians should also maintain a high index of suspicion for underlying sexually transmitted disease (STD). Up to 50% of women presenting to an emergency department for symptoms of cystitis were found to have positive STD cultures.[16]

Urine samples are collected for urinalysis in a sterile container through urethral catheterization, especially in women, or by midstream voided urine after the genital area is washed to avoid contamination. The sample is then tested for bacteriuria, pyuria, and hematuria. Indirect dipstick tests are informative but less sensitive than microscopic examination of the urine. About one third of the women who have acute symptoms of cystitis have sterile urine or some other cause for the symptom.[17] Many diseases of the urinary tract produce significant pyuria without bacteriuria, including staghorn calculi, tuberculosis, and infections caused by *Chlamydia* and *Mycoplasma* spp. Microscopic hematuria is found in 40% to 60% of cystitis patients.[18] Associated gross hematuria should be evaluated further by imaging studies. Cystoscopy is indicated for those patients older than 50 years or who have other risk factors for concomitant diseases, such as nephrolithiasis or transitional cell carcinoma (e.g., smoking).

Whereas empirical therapies are acceptable for uncomplicated cystitis (Box 2), culture and sensitivity testing should be performed in all other cases. It should be noted that a large percentage of women with cystitis have been found to have STDs. Additional cultures for *Neisseria gonorrhea, Chlamydia, Mycoplasma hominis,* and *Ureaplasma ureolyticus* should be considered for women with recurrent lower urinary tract symptoms.

Box 1 Functional and Structural Abnormalities of the Genitourinary Tract

Functional Abnormalities
Vesicoureteral reflux
Neurogenic bladder
Obstruction

Congenital Abnormalities
Pelvic-ureteric obstruction
Ureteric and urethral strictures
Urolithiasis
Bladder diverticuli
Tumors

Foreign Bodies
Indwelling catheters

Other
Diabetes mellitus
Renal failure
Urinary diversions
Urinary instrumentation

Box 2 Urinary Tract Infection (UTI) in Adults

Uncomplicated
Acute cystitis in women
Acute pyelonephritis in young healthy women

Complicated
Acute cystitis in men
Acute prostatitis
Chronic prostatitis
Acute pyelonephritis in men
UTI with pregnancy
UTI with gross hematuria
UTI associated with nephrolithiasis
UTI associated with neurogenic bladder
UTI in diabetic or immunocompromised patient
Recurrent UTI (>3 episodes per year)

Radiologic studies are unnecessary for the routine evaluation of patients with cystitis; however, they may be indicated to find the cause of complicated cases, in which UTIs are associated with urinary calculi, ureteral strictures, ureteral reflux, urinary tract tumors, and urinary tract diversions. The following studies may be useful:

- Plain radiography of the abdomen for the detection of radiopaque calculi or abnormal renal contour
- Intravenous pyelography for radiographic images of the bladder, kidneys, and ureters. An opaque dye visible on radiographic film is injected into the vein and a series of radiographs are taken. The films demonstrate the contour of the collecting system, which may reveal filling defects or obstruction.
- Voiding cystourethrography to evaluate neurogenic bladder and urethral diverticulum and to exclude or define the extent of vesicoureteral reflux
- Renal ultrasonography, through interpretation of echogenic patterns generated by sound waves, can detect the presence of hydronephrosis, tumors, pyonephrosis, calculi, or abscesses.
- Computed tomography (CT), a more sensitive means of defining renal parenchyma, especially when used with intravenous contrast material. CT urograms have replaced intravenous pyelograms in the evaluation of the urinary tract and kidneys, particularly in the workup of hematuria. Spiral CT scanning without contrast is the most sensitive means of detecting calculi within the urinary collecting system and is the standard of care for the evaluation of acute flank pain.

Box 3 Factors Influencing Selection of Antimicrobial Agents for Treating Urinary Tract Infections

Patient Factors
History of drug allergy
Medical history (e.g., renal impairment, liver impairment)
Presence of urologic abnormalities

Drug Factors
Safety profile
Spectrum of activity
Route of administration
Costs

Type of Organism
Results of Gram staining
Results of special culture and sensitivity testing

- Magnetic resonance imaging may be indicated for patients who require further evaluation for renal neoplasm, in whom IV contrast is contraindicated. It may also be necessary as the most sensitive modality for the detection of urethral diverticulum.
- The urethra and bladder can be inspected quickly and safely by the use of cystoscopy with a local anesthetic in an office setting.

TREATMENT

Cystitis

For the general management of cystitis, the patient is advised to drink plenty of water, which helps cleanse the urinary tract of bacteria. Cranberry juice and vitamin C (ascorbic acid) supplements inhibit the growth of some bacteria by acidifying the urine. Avoiding coffee, alcohol, and spicy foods is also useful. A heating pad and pain relief medication are helpful for pain management.

Cystitis is treated with antibacterial drugs. The choice of drug and length of treatment depend on several factors (Box 3). The sensitivity test is especially useful for selecting the most effective drug.

Acute Cystitis

Patients who have symptoms of frequency, urgency, pyuria on microscopic examination, and no known functional or anatomic abnormality of the genitourinary tract may be presumed to have acute uncomplicated cystitis. Empirical therapy with a 3-day regimen of trimethoprim-sulfamethoxazole (TMP-SMX) or a fluoroquinolone without pretreatment culture and sensitivity testing is usually effective. Alternative regimens such as a fluoroquinolone, an oral third-generation cephalosporin, or nitrofurantoin (7-day regimen) may have a better result. Generally, for most female patients, a 3-day course seems warranted, because this demonstrates similar efficacy when compared with 7-day therapy, and with lower side effects and cost.[19] Single-dose therapy usually results in lower rates of cure and more frequent recurrences.

Recurrent Cystitis

The most common cause of recurrent UTI in women is reinfection that may occur with varying intervals and different causative organisms. Reinfection in women does not require extensive urologic evaluation. Recurrent episodes of uncomplicated cystitis can be managed by several strategies. Behavioral therapy includes increasing fluid intake, urinating as soon as the need is felt, as well as immediately after intercourse, and changing the method of contraception (for users of a diaphragm or spermicide), because spermicidal jelly contains nonoxynol 9, which decreases vaginal lactobacillus colonization and increases bacterial adherence. Long-term antimicrobial prophylaxis,[20] postcoital prophylaxes with a single-dose antibiotic,[21] or short-course (1- or 2-day) antibiotics for each symptomatic episode is recommended. For postmenopausal women, the use of vaginal estrogen cream may prove an effective preventive measure.[11] Patients with bacterial persistence should be evaluated thoroughly to exclude potential structural or functional abnormalities.

Prostatitis

Prostate infections are more challenging to cure because of the altered microenvironment of the inflamed tissue, which may affect antibiotic efficacy. Therefore, men with acute bacterial prostatitis often need long-term treatment (≥30 days) with a carefully selected antibiotic. Severely ill patients need hospitalization and parenteral antimicrobial agents, such as an aminoglycoside-penicillin combination, until culture and susceptibility results provide guidance for alternative, specific antibiotic regimens. In men with urinary retention, a urethral or suprapubic catheter is necessary. Suprapubic catheterization is preferable to decrease the risk of prostatic abscesses. Mild and moderate cases respond well to fluoroquinolones or TMP-SMX, both of which have a cure rate of 60% to 90%.[22] Chronic bacterial prostatitis may manifest as episodes of recurrent bacteriuria with the same organism between asymptomatic periods. Episodic treatment may be prescribed using the agents mentioned and, in select patients, may be self administered as needed. Daily suppressive therapy should be considered in men with frequent cystitis if other causes are excluded, and the culpable organism is localized to the prostate, using the Meares-Stamey technique.[23]

DIFFERENTIAL DIAGNOSIS

When evaluating patients with LUTS, it is important to consider gynecologic and colorectal diagnoses as well. STDs in either gender may manifest as lower urinary tract symptoms (LUTS), with or without fever. Female patients, especially those presenting with severe symptoms and pain, should be screened for pregnancy, because complications such as ectopic pregnancy or abortion should be ruled out. Chronic appendicitis and sigmoid diverticulitis may be confused with an UTI. We have encountered several patients referred for evaluation of persistent or recurrent UTI or prostatitis, in whom diverticulitis (and, even rarer, chronic appendicitis) was proven to be the cause of their symptoms.

Sexually Transmitted Diseases

Special cultures are needed to diagnose these infections. Antibiotic therapy should be prescribed accordingly. Longer treatment with tetracycline, doxycycline, or any drug appropriate for the treatment of *Mycoplasma hominis* and *Ureaplasma urealyticum* is recommended.[24] The patient's sexual partner must be treated simultaneously.

CONSIDERATIONS IN SPECIAL POPULATIONS

Catheter-Related Infections

Catheterization for longer than 2 weeks is usually associated with bacteriuria. Prophylactic antimicrobial therapy for cystitis during short-term, indwelling, urethral catheterization is not recommended. Symptomatic UTIs in older adults should be treated. Careful consideration should be given to antimicrobial choice and meticulous monitoring of drug levels in this patient population, because the older patient is more susceptible to harmful side effects of many antimicrobial agents. Short-term antimicrobial therapy (5-7 days) is indicated only for symptomatic episodes. In patients requiring long-term urinary catheterization, suprapubic catheter placement should be considered. In men, suprapubic catheterization is associated with decreased risk of meatal erosion or prostatitis. In the short term, suprapubic catheterization may be associated with a decreased risk of bacteriuria or UTI. Unfortunately, this difference is not associated with long-term catheterization.[25]

Funguria is a common finding in catheterized patients. Whereas most patients are asymptomatic, interventions should include change in catheter, elimination of unnecessary antimicrobials, and glycemic control. Although amphotericin B may be used for bladder irrigations, it is less effective and more expensive than oral fluconazole therapy, although the latter is a concern in patients with hepatic vulnerability.

Removal of an indwelling catheter should be prompt; whenever possible, intermittent self catheterization should be used for patients with transient or long-term urinary retention.

Asymptomatic Bacteriuria

Bacteriuria denotes the presence of bacteria in the urine, which may be symptomatic or asymptomatic. Treatment of asymptomatic bacteriuria is indicated for pregnant women and those requiring urologic surgery.[26] Preoperative treatment reduces postoperative complications, including bacteremia.[27]

Cystitis and Pregnancy

Although the prevalence of bacteriuria identified by screening is no higher in pregnant than nonpregnant women, the presence of asymptomatic bacteriuria in a pregnant woman should be treated promptly.[28] The gravid uterus causes physiologic alterations that increase the risk of pyelonephritis. Pyelonephritis has been associated with infant prematurity, low birth weight, perinatal mortality, and high blood pressure.[29] The recommended regimen is 7-day treatment with ampicillin or nitrofurantoin.

Urinary Tract Infection and Renal Failure

When creatinine clearance is significantly impaired, antibiotic dosage should be decreased since the renal blood flow is decreased and the perfusion of antimicrobial agents into the renal tissue and urine is impaired. Ampicillin, TMP-SMX, and fluoroquinolones are all effective for the treatment of UTIs in uremic patients.[30,31] Nitrofurantoin and tetracyclines are contraindicated for the treatment of UTIs in uremic patients.

PROPHYLAXIS

Antimicrobial prophylaxis is recommended to ensure the sterility of urine for those who appear susceptible to developing infections. These include immunocompromised patients, patients with heart disease, people with a prosthetic heart valve, and patients who are scheduled for a procedure such as cystoscopy. Oral or vaginal estrogen administered prophylactically to postmenopausal women also reduces the incidence of cystitis.[26,31]

Summary

- UTI is one of the most common health problems affecting people of all ages. It is the most common nosocomial bacterial infection in older adults. Women are especially prone to UTIs for reasons that are poorly understood.
- Although prostatitis syndrome accounts for 25% of male office visits for genitourinary tract infections, only 5% are attributed to a bacterial cause.
- Acute cystitis or pyelonephritis in adult patients should be considered uncomplicated if there are no known functional or anatomic abnormalities of the genitourinary tract. Most of these infections are caused by *Escherichia coli*.

- Acute uncomplicated cystitis can be effectively treated with a 3-day course of TMP-SMX, but alternative regimens such as a fluoroquinolone, an oral third-generation cephalosporin, or nitrofurantoin (7-day regimen) may have a better result. For acute uncomplicated pyelonephritis, a 10- to 14-day regimen is recommended.
- Sexually transmitted diseases, including those caused by *Chlamydia, Mycoplasma hominis,* and *Ureaplasma urealyticum*, should be considered potential culprits in sexually active patients.
- Complicated UTIs require thorough evaluation and correction of the underlying abnormality to provide a cure and prevent recurrence.

Suggested Readings

Foxman B: Epidemiology of urinary tract infections: Incidence, morbidity and economic costs. Am J Med 2002;113(Suppl. 1A): 5S-13S.

Michota F: Indwelling Urinary Catheters: Infection and Complications. In Potts J (ed): Genitourinary Pain and Inflammation: Diagnosis and Management. Totowa, NJ, Humana Press, 2008.

Parsons CL, Schmidt JD: Control of recurrent lower urinary tract infection in the post-menopausal woman. J Urol 1982;128:1224-1226.

Potts JM, Ward AM, Rackley RR: Association of chronic urinary symptoms in women and *Urea plasm*a urealyticum. Urology 2000;55:486-489.

Raz R, Stamm WE: A controlled trial of intravaginal estriol in postmenopausal women with recurrent urinary tract infections. N Engl J Med 1993;329:753-756.

Ronald A: The etiology of urinary tract infection: Traditional and emerging pathogens. Am J Med 2002;113:14S-19S.

Schaeffer AJ, Rajan N, Cao Q, et al: Host pathogenesis in urinary tract infections. Int J Antimicrob Agents 2001;17:245-251.

Stapleton A, Latham RH, Johnson C, Stamm WE: Postcoital antimicrobial prophylaxis for recurrent urinary tract infection. A randomized, double-blind, placebo-controlled trial. JAMA 1990;264:703-706.

References

For a complete list of references, log onto www.expertconsult.com.

Foodborne Disease

Alan Taege

Foodborne disease is a pervasive problem caused by consumption of contaminated food and drink. More than 200 pathogens are associated with foodborne disease. An estimated 76 million cases occur annually (one in every four Americans), resulting in 300,000 hospitalizations and 5,000 deaths.[1] Fewer cases are documented because of underreporting. International travel and food importation have further expanded the problem. The onset of foodborne disease is generally acute, with resolution of an uncomplicated illness in 72 hours for most episodes. Proper food handling and preparation, personal hygiene, and improved methods of decontamination of consumer products could significantly reduce the extent of morbidity and mortality of this common problem.

Foodborne illness is tracked in the United States through a system called FoodNet, a joint effort of the U.S. Food and Drug Administration (FDA) and the U.S. Department of Agriculture (USDA). Data are collected annually from ten different monitoring sites throughout the country (representing 15% of the population) and compiled by the Centers for Disease Control and Prevention (CDC). Only documented cases are used for reporting. The target organisms include *Campylobacter* spp., *Salmonella* spp., *Shigella* spp., *Listeria* spp., Shiga toxin-producing *Escherichia coli* O157:H7 (STEC O157), non-O157 STEC, *Vibrio* spp., *Yersinia* spp., *Cryptosporidium* spp., and *Cyclospora* spp. The hemolytic-uremic syndrome (HUS) is also tracked.

EPIDEMIOLOGY

Foodborne disease can be caused by bacteria, parasites, toxins, and viruses (Box 1). Despite efforts to investigate foodborne disease, less than 50% of all outbreak causes are identified, usually because of limited diagnostic capabilities. Viruses are likely the most common cause of foodborne disease but are seldom investigated and confirmed because of the short duration and self-limited nature of the illness. In addition, the inherent difficulty of laboratory investigation and subsequent cost of viral studies lead to a lack of clinician investigation and therefore overall underreporting. Bacteria are the most common documented cause.

Cultural and demographic factors, as well as increased mobility, have resulted in major epidemiologic shifts in foodborne disease during recent decades.[2] Previous outbreaks of foodborne disease were smaller and limited in scope, more often originated in the home, and were associated with *Staphylococcus* or *Clostridium* spp. Family picnics or dinners and home-canned foods were the typical sources for the outbreaks. Today, many more people dine outside the home and travel more extensively. As a result, more than 80% of foodborne disease cases occur from exposures outside the home.

Technology has provided the means for mass production and distribution of food. Therefore, foodborne disease often occurs on a massive scale, whereby hundreds or thousands are exposed and may become ill. Mobility and travel have resulted in exposure to foods abroad, where regulation of food safety and food products for sale may vary. When traveling, the axiom "boil it, peel it, cook it, or forget it" remains true in many areas of the world. Travelers bringing home unique foods as gifts may unwittingly expose family members and friends to unexpected illness. International ships discharging their bilge in ports are another possible means of disseminating pathogens.

Food importation has steadily increased to meet the demand for seasonal and nonseasonal foods. Conditions of production and harvest may be unsupervised or uncontrolled, with resultant importation of contaminated foods. Raw manure is frequently used as fertilizer, causing contamination of fresh produce. If improperly cleaned, the fertilized produce may cause illness when consumed.

Unique ethnic food preferences and preparation have been associated with several food-related illnesses. One example is the African American tradition of eating chitterlings (cooked swine intestines) during the Christmas holiday season.[3] This food has been associated with an outbreak of *Yersinia enterocolitica* infection in infants.[4] Fresh cheese made from unpasteurized milk has been associated with episodes of listeriosis in Hispanic neighborhoods.

Foodborne disease is more likely to affect the extremes of age as well as immunocompromised patients and pregnant women. These groups suffer higher incidence, morbidity, and mortality.[5,6] The effect of foodborne disease may extend beyond the immediate illness. This has been shown by a Danish study, which demonstrated a greater than threefold risk of dying in the year after contracting a foodborne illness.[7]

Most foodborne disease has a short duration of illness and a self-limited course. Others may cause a more protracted illness, such as *Cryptosporidium* and *Cyclospora*. However, some foodborne diseases are associated with long-term chronic sequelae (Box 2). *Salmonella, Shigella, Yersinia*, and *Campylobacter* spp. are linked to reactive arthritis; *Campylobacter* has also been associated with the Guillain-Barré syndrome, and STEC O157:H7 has been linked to renal failure.[8]

The most commonly identified pathogens are *Campylobacter* spp., *Salmonella* spp., *Shigella* spp., and STEC O157:H7. These organisms have evolved and now have greater cold, heat, and acid tolerance, as well as resistance to multiple antibiotics. Increased drug resistance has been associated with prolonged illness and a greater risk of hospitalization.[9]

Almost any food can be a source of foodborne disease. Some foods are more commonly associated with particular organisms (Box 3). *Salmonella* has traditionally been associated with poultry and eggs, *Campylobacter* with chicken and unpasteurized milk, and STEC O157:H7 with ground beef. An outbreak of STEC O157:H7 was associated with steak that had been needle-tenderized, thereby exposing the center of the meat to surface organisms. When the steak was not thoroughly cooked to an adequate internal temperature, the microorganisms survived and illness occurred after consumption.

Water may be the vector of illness when contaminated with viruses, bacteria, parasites, or chemicals. Crowding, poor sanitation, disruption of water supplies, and natural disasters are closely linked to waterborne illness. Viruses are the most common cause of waterborne illness and include rotaviruses, enteric adenovirus, astrovirus, caliciviruses and hepatitis A virus. Outbreaks of gastroenteritis aboard cruise ships in recent years were a result of noroviruses. *Salmonella* spp., *Shigella* spp., *E. coli*, and *Vibrio* spp. are the predominant bacterial pathogens involved. *Cryptosporidium* spp. and *Giardia lamblia* are the parasitic pathogens most commonly encountered in water-borne illness. Immunocompromised hosts, particularly organ transplant recipients and HIV-infected patients, should exercise extra precaution in situations of potential waterborne illness.

Incubation periods of foodborne disease may offer clues to the cause. Four time frames may be envisioned: very brief, short, intermediate, and long durations of incubation. The very brief category (<8 hours) is generally caused by preformed toxins, which may be found in staphylococcal or bacillus-contaminated food. Short incubation periods (24-48 hours) are more typical of viral causes. Intermediate incubation periods (1-5 days) correlate with many bacterial pathogens. The long-duration incubation group (>5 days) approximates the time course of parasitic infections. These time frames are crude groupings and areas of overlap exist between them. In addi-

Box 1 Common Causes of Foodborne Disease

Bacteria
Salmonella spp.
Campylobacter jejuni
Shigella spp.
STEC O157:H7
Listeria monocytognes
Vibrio spp.
Yersinia spp.

Parasites
Cryptosporidium spp.
Cyclospora spp.
Trichinella spiralis
Giardia lamblia
Toxoplasma caris
Entamoeba histolytica

Toxins
Enterotoxins
Staphylococcus aureus
Clostridium perfringens
Bacillus cereus

Botulinum toxin
Clostridium botulinum

Fish toxins
Scombrotoxin
Ciguatera toxin
Paralytic shellfish toxin

Mushrooms
Amatoxin
Phallotoxin

Miscellaneous
Niacin
Monosodium glutamate

Viruses
Norwalk
Hepatitis A

Box 2 Sequelae of Foodborne Illness

Reactive Arthritis
Campylobacter
Salmonella
Shigella

Hemolytic-Uremic Syndrome, Renal Failure
STEC O157:H7
Shigella

Neurologic Effects
Listeria
Botulinum toxin
Campylobacter
STEC O157:H7

tion, the inoculum of organisms ingested may influence the incubation period and the rapidity of onset of illness—for example, a large inoculum may cause a shortened time to onset of illness.

Bloody diarrhea or a febrile illness is often associated with invasive organisms. The more common microorganisms associated with bloody diarrhea and fever are listed in Box 4.

Box 3 Pathogens and Food Associations

Campylobacter: chicken, unpasteurized milk and dairy products, water
Salmonella: eggs, poultry, fruits, vegetables, meats
Shigella: fruits, vegetables
Escherichia coli O157:H7: hamburger, salami, alfalfa sprouts, unpasteurized milk and dairy products and juice
Clostridium botulinum: home-canned foods
Cryptosporidium: water
Cyclospora: raspberries
Listeria monocytogenes: delicatessen meats, soft cheeses, unpasteurized milk and dairy products, vegetables
Vibrio vulnificus: shellfish
Yersinia enterocolitica: raw pork, unpasteurized milk and dairy products, water

Box 4 Clinical Manifestations

Bloody Diarrhea
- *Campylobacter*
- *Salmonella*
- *Shigella*
- *Escherichia coli* O157:H7
- *Yersinia*

Fever
- *Salmonella*
- *Campylobacter*
- *Shigella*
- *Listeria*
- *Vibrio*
- *Yersinia*

DIAGNOSIS

Diagnosis is accomplished through a careful history, physical examination, and laboratory evaluation. The history should include questioning about the suspected time of exposure, recent travel, the food and drink consumed, other people who may have been present and eaten similar foods, and the specific symptoms involved (e.g., nausea, vomiting, diarrhea with or without visible blood, cramping, gas, fever, neurologic symptoms, alteration of mental status). Dietary history may include intake during the last 2 to 3 weeks. The physical examination should focus on vital signs, including orthostatic measurements, skin turgor, mental status, abdominal findings, and stool testing for blood. Fresh stool samples for culture and analysis (<6 hours old) provide the highest yield. The clinician must be knowledgeable of the laboratory's assay procedures to facilitate proper sample testing. Specific culture requests for suspected organisms may be necessary, as well as microscopic examination of stool samples for parasites. Three samples on different days will generally provide adequate diagnostic results. Special circumstances may dictate the need to perform special assays for toxins (e.g., botulinum toxin) on gastric aspirates or stool samples. Blood cultures are often useful, particularly if *Salmonella* or *Listeria* is suspected or when evaluation involves high-risk groups and immunocompromised hosts.

DESCRIPTION AND TREATMENT

Most foodborne disease is self limited and requires only supportive care. The very young, older adults, immunocompromised patients, and pregnant women may benefit from antibiotic treatment for certain bacterial or parasitic infections. Drug-resistant pathogens require knowledge of regional, national, and international patterns of resistance to allow appropriate empirical selection of therapy.

Specific Bacteria

Salmonella

The most recent FoodNet data list nontyphoidal *Salmonella* as the most commonly identified bacterial cause of foodborne disease.[10] It is estimated that 1,400,000 cases occur annually. Fever, abdominal cramps, and diarrhea (occasionally bloody in a minority of cases) are the usual manifesting symptoms after 8 to 48 hours of incubation. Although generally self limited, *Salmonella* infection may cause sepsis and localized infections, such as septic arthritis and infection of endovascular prosthetic devices, such as grafts. The most common serotypes are *Salmonella typhimurium* and *S. enteritidis*.

Eggs remain a common source because of vertical transovarial transmission within an infected poultry flock. Poultry itself has become a significant source of *Salmonella* infection. Fruits, vegetables, meats, and ice cream are other reported food associations.

Populations at greatest risk are infants, older adults, and the immunocompromised, but also those with inflammatory bowel disease, hemoglobinopathies, and endovascular prosthetic devices. Patients older than 60 years have the highest rate of hospitalization and highest case-fatality rate.[11] Antibiotic treatment should be considered for these high-risk groups because bacteremia may occur in 2% to 14% of cases. Unfortunately, increasing resistance to the usual antibiotics (cephalosporins, aminoglycosides, and fluoroquinolones) has made therapy more challenging.

Campylobacter

Campylobacter is the second most common identified organism in foodborne disease. Over one million cases are estimated to occur annually. After a 2- to 5-day incubation period, acute dysentery ensues. Nearly two thirds of patients will have fever, and one half will have bloody diarrhea. Illness may last 1 week and then resolve spontaneously. Immunocompromised patients may experience life-threatening sepsis and therefore should receive aggressive therapy.

Age-related biphasic peaks of *Campylobacter* infection occur in infancy and early adulthood. Young men are more often affected because of poor food handling knowledge. Almost all human illness is caused by one species, *Campylobacter jejuni*. Poultry is the overwhelming source. Additional food sources include raw milk, water, and ice cream. When treatment is deemed necessary, a macrolide is preferred or a fluoroquinolone antibiotic can be used, but once again increasing drug resistance may present a therapeutic challenge. Macrolide resistance remains less than 5% but quinolone resistance may be as high as 20%. Regions of southeast Asia have strains of *Campylobacter* that are resistant to both macrolide and quinolone antibiotics. Antibiotic-resistant strains are associated with more invasive disease and increased mortality.[12] Guillain-Barré syndrome may be an unusual delayed sequela of infection with *Campylobacter*.

Shigella

Although less common than *Salmonella* or *Campylobacter*, *Shigella* is a significant cause of foodborne disease. Shigella is responsible for 10% to 20% of cases of bacterial foodborne illness each year in the United States. After 2 to 4 days of incubation, it produces an invasive dysentery syndrome that often includes fever and bloody diarrhea. Shiga toxins are frequently elaborated. Duration is typically 5 to 7 days. Fruits, vegetables, and shellfish are common food associations. Third-generation cephalosporins and fluoroquinolones are the antibiotics of choice; however, drug resistance may be encountered. Long-term sequelae include reactive arthritis and HUS.

STEC O157:H7

STEC O157:H7 infection was initially associated with ground beef. Multiple other food associations have been recognized, such as unpasteurized apple cider, milk and dairy products, juices, and lettuce. In addition, STEC O157:H7 has been associated with nonfoodborne illness after contact with cattle and swimming in contaminated lakes. Crump and colleagues[13] have described an outbreak among a group after they visited a dairy farm.

An estimated 60,000 to 70,000 cases occur annually, resulting in approximately 2000 hospitalizations and 60 to 70 deaths. The average incubation period is 4 to 8 days. Symptoms include abdominal cramps with bloody diarrhea but little or no fever. The diarrhea usually resolves within 1 week. Antibiotics appear to play no role in treatment, because the illness is the result of a Shiga toxin produced by the organism. Five to 10 days after the diarrheal illness, HUS develops. It is more common in the young (<5 years old) and older adults. Manifestations of HUS may include hemolytic anemia, thrombocytopenia, and acute renal failure. Neurologic sequelae (e.g., seizures or stroke) may be additional late complications.

Listeria

Listeriosis is caused by *Listeria monocytogenes*. It is a much less common cause of foodborne disease, with approximately 2500 cases annually. However, it has the highest hospitalization and mortality rates of all foodborne diseases, with approximately 500 deaths each year. It strikes more often at the extremes of age, attacking the young and older adults, as well as those who are immunocompromised, causing a more severe illness in this population. Pregnant women are also at increased risk of infection. Manifestations appear to vary by host-related factors. Older adults and immunocompromised patients often present with sepsis and meningitis, whereas immunocompetent patients develop febrile gastroenteritis. Pregnant women may experience a flulike illness, but granulomatosis infantisepticum may afflict the fetus, resulting in bacteremia, meningitis, or both in the newborn infant.

Data from the CDC have suggested that Latin Americans may have a higher incidence of listeriosis. Latin American women of childbearing age and their infants have an 11-fold increased risk of infection.[14] The reason for this finding is unclear and remains under investigation.

Listeriosis has been associated with delicatessen meats, hot dogs, soft cheeses, and unpasteurized milk and dairy products. Queso fresco, an ethnic homemade soft cheese produced from unpasteurized milk, has been associated with listeriosis in the Hispanic population.

Illness follows a 1- to 2-day incubation period. Clinical symptoms include fever, gastrointestinal upset, and subsequent diarrhea. When treatment is needed, ampicillin appears to be the most effective antibiotic.

Vibrio

Vibrio foodborne disease tends to be seasonal, with a peak incidence in late summer and early autumn. Consumption of raw seafood from the southern United States coast is the most common food association. *V. parahaemolyticus* and *V. vulnificus* are the most frequent species isolated. They are halophilic and cold-tolerant organisms, which allow *Vibrio* to survive in conditions that may normally retard or prevent food contamination.

A clinical syndrome of watery diarrhea, abdominal cramping, nausea, vomiting, and fever occurs 1 to 4 days after ingestion. The illness is usually self limited, with resolution in about 3 days. Persons with liver disease may develop a severe sepsis syndrome, bullous cellulitis, or both, with 50% mortality. *Vibrio* cellulitis and wound infections are occupational risks for fishermen and oyster shuckers. Appropriate antibiotic treatment includes tetracycline or ceftriaxone.

Yersinia

Yersiniosis is an uncommon cause of foodborne disease in the United States. It has been associated with the consumption of raw pork, unpasteurized milk and dairy products, and contaminated water. The preparation, handling, or consumption of chitterlings (see earlier) has been associated with *Yersinia* infections. Young African American children are disproportionately affected by this holiday food tradition.

The incubation period is 4 to 7 days and is followed by fever, abdominal pain, and bloody diarrhea. The abdominal pain may mimic that of appendicitis. Additional manifestations include carditis, joint pain, and sepsis. Although most cases resolve spontaneously, severe cases may require therapy with doxycycline, a fluoroquinolone, aminoglycoside, or trimethoprim-sulfamethoxazole.

Parasites

Parasites are an uncommon form of foodborne illness. The most frequent causes include *Cryptosporidium* spp. and *Giardia lamblia*, which have been associated with contaminated water. Additional foodborne diseases include cyclosporiasis, trichinosis, toxoplasmosis, and amebiasis. Cyclosporiasis has been previously linked to imported raspberries. Trichinosis was traditionally linked to pork but can be contracted through other sources, such as inadequately cooked wild game. Toxoplasmosis has been most often associated with undercooked meat and amebiasis is associated with contaminated water.

Cryptosporidiosis may be difficult to treat. Response has been noted with nitazoxanide, paromomycin, or azithromycin. Metronidazole is the usual treatment for giardiasis. Prolonged treatment with trimethoprim-sulfamethoxazole may be necessary to cure cyclosporiasis.

Toxins

Foodborne disease caused by toxins may have a variety of presentations that include gastrointestinal symptoms, neurologic manifestations, or both. Preformed heat-stable enterotoxins associated with *Staphylococcus aureus* and *Bacillus cereus* have an acute onset of nausea, vomiting, and diarrhea within 1 to 6 hours of ingestion. Fever is not a common component of this self-limited syndrome. Symptoms resolve rapidly, often within 12 hours.

Clostridium perfringens has a slower onset of illness, occurring approximately 12 hours after ingestion, because the heat-labile enterotoxin is produced in vivo after consumption of contaminated food. Cramping and diarrhea are the major manifestations, with resolution of symptoms in about 24 hours.

Botulinus toxin is considered the most potent lethal substance known. It is produced by *Clostridium botulinum*. Illness occurs 18 to 36 hours after ingestion of the source food. Home-canned foods have been the traditional sources. The onset of illness is heralded by nausea, vomiting, and diarrhea, followed by constipation. A descending paralysis then occurs. Antitoxins are available but only prevent further progression of paralysis because they neutralize circulating toxin and have no effect on bound toxin. Foodborne botulism carries a 5% to 10% mortality rate. If the individual survives, many months may be required before recovery.

The onset of paresthesias within minutes to a few hours of food ingestion should alert the clinician to the possibility of niacin, monosodium glutamate, fish, or shellfish poisoning. Marine bacteria present on the surface of some fish produce inhibitors of histamine degradation, resulting in high levels of histamine. When they are consumed, scombroid poisoning (histamine fish poisoning) may occur. The fish most often associated with scombroid poisoning are tuna, mackerel, skipjack, bonito, and mahi-mahi. The syndrome resembles a histamine reaction, with flushing, headache, nausea, vomiting, cramping, and burning in the mouth and throat. Poisoning by ciguatera fish such as grouper and snapper produces nausea, vomiting, and diarrhea as well as paresthesias of the lips, tongue, and throat. Shellfish poisoning causes a similar syndrome except that muscle weakness, paralysis, or amnesia may occur in severe cases. The neurologic manifestations resolve in hours to a few days.

Mushroom poisoning can produce various clinical syndromes. Depending on the toxin involved, symptoms may range from parasympathetic hyperactivity to hallucinations or hepatic and renal failure, in the case of amatoxins or phallotoxins. Onset is rapid, within 2 hours of ingestion, and resolution of symptoms occurs in approximately 24 hours. Organ failure may follow after an additional 1 to 2 days. Without emergent liver transplantation, acute hepatic failure rapidly leads to death.

Viruses

Hepatitis A and Norwalk virus are the two most commonly identified viral sources of foodborne disease. Many additional cases of foodborne disease occur as a result of unidentified viruses. Hepatitis A is often associated with shellfish and infected food handlers. In addition, green onions were determined to be the source of a widespread outbreak in a restaurant chain in 2003.[15]

The high morbidity and overall relatively low mortality of foodborne disease could be significantly reduced. Proper knowledge of food handling, storage, and preservation could have a significant impact on the occurrence of this common problem. Improved conditions in mass production and processing of foods have produced tangible results. New methods of sterilization, such as irradiation, represent avenues of future progress.

Additional information on foodborne illness can be found on the CDC website.[16] This site reviews many of the common syndromes in an educational case scenario format. Several useful tables list causative agents, incubation periods, and major manifestations.

Summary

- Viruses and bacteria are responsible for the vast majority of foodborne diseases.
- The time course of onset from ingestion to illness can be useful in establishing the cause.
- Certain food groups are associated with particular pathogens.
- Supportive care is sufficient for most cases but antibiotics may be lifesaving in others.
- Proper food handling, preparation, and hand hygiene can prevent most foodborne illnesses.

Suggested Readings

Altekruse S, Swerdlow D: The changing epidemiology of foodborne disease. Am J Med Sci 1996;311:23-29.

Bottone EJ: *Yersinia enterocolitica*: The charisma continues. Clin Microbiol Rev 1997;10:257-276.

Buzby JC: Older adults at risk of complications from microbial foodborne illness. Food Rev 2002;25:30-35.

Centers for Disease Control and Prevention (CDC): Diagnosis and management of foodborne illness: A primer for physicians. MMWR Morb Mortal Wkly Rep 2001;50(RR-02):1-69.

Centers for Disease Control and Prevention (CDC): Hepatitis A outbreak associated with green onions at a restaurant—Monaca, Pennsylvania, 2003. MMWR Morb Mortal Wkly Rep 2003;52:1155-1157.

Centers for Disease Control and Prevention (CDC): Preliminary FoodNet data on the incidence of infection with pathogens transmitted commonly through food—10 sites, United States 2002. MMWR Morb Mortal Wkly Rep 2003;52:340-343.

Charles L, Molbak K, Hedler J, et al: Decline in Major Bacterial Foodborne Illnesses in the United States: FoodNet, 1996-2001. Chicago, Infectious Disease Society of America, 2002.

Crump JA, Sulka AC, Langer AJ, et al: An outbreak of *E. coli* O157:H7 infections among visitors to a dairy farm. N Engl J Med 2002;8:555-560.

Helms M, Simonsen J, Olsen K, Molbak K: Adverse health events associated with antimicrobial drug resistance in *Campylobacter* species: A registry-based cohort study. J Infect Dis 2005;191:1050-1055.

Helms M, Vastrup P, Gerner-Smidt P, Molbak K: Short- and long-term mortality associated with food-borne bacterial gastrointestinal infections: Registry-based study. BMJ 2003;326:357-361.

Jones F: From pig to pacifier: Chitterling-associated yersiniosis outbreak among black infants. Emerg Infect Dis 2003;9:1007-1009.

Kennedy M, Villar R, Vugia D, et al: Hospitalizations and deaths due to *Salmonella* infections, FoodNet, 1996-1999. Clin Infect Dis 2004;38(Suppl 3):S142-S148.
Lay J, Varma J, Marcus R, et al; EIP FoodNet Working Group: Higher incidence of *Listeria* infections among Hispanics: FoodNet, 1996-2000. Presented at the International Conference on Emerging Infectious Diseases, Atlanta, March 2002.
Mead PS, Slutsker L, Dietz V, et al: Food-related illness and death in the United States. Emerg Infect Dis 1999;5:607-625.
Tam CC, Rodrigues LC, O'Brien SJ: Guillain-Barré syndrome associated with *C. jejuni* infection in England. Clin Infect Dis 2003;37:307-310.
Varma J, Mølbak K, Rossiter S, et al: Antimicrobial resistance in *Salmonella* is associated with increased hospitalization; NARMS 1996-2000. Presented at the International Conference on Emerging Infectious Diseases, Atlanta, March 2002.

References

For a complete list of references, log onto www.expertconsult.com.

Brain Abscess

Carlos M. Isada

Brain abscess is defined as purulence and inflammation in one or more localized regions within the brain parenchyma. It is one of several forms of severe intracranial infection, with other examples including subdural empyema and intracranial epidural abscess. Brain abscesses are uncommon but are life-threatening. Optimal assessment of the likely pathogenesis of the lesion and causative pathogens is essential for a favorable outcome. With the advent of routine neuroimaging and less invasive neurosurgical techniques, the mortality rate of brain abscesses has fallen, but an understanding of the complexities of this infection is crucial for management.

EPIDEMIOLOGY

There are approximately 1500 to 2000 cases of brain abscess diagnosed in the United States annually, with an estimated 1 in 10,000 being hospitalized for a brain abscess. The infection tends to occur in young men, although infection can occur in all age groups; the male-to-female ratio varies between 2:1 and 3:1. In some series, children account for up to 25% of cases.

There have been several trends in the epidemiology of brain abscess over recent decades. One trend is that there appears to be a trend toward a decreasing incidence of brain abscess. In a population-based study of residents of Olmstead County, Minnesota, the incidence rate was 1.3 per 100,000 patient-years from 1935 to 1944 compared with 0.9 per 100,000 patient-years from 1965 to 1981.[1] In this series, brain abscess rates were highest in children and in adults older than 60 years. Another epidemiologic trend has been the decrease in the incidence of brain abscesses as a complication of otitis media, which has been attributed to the early use of antimicrobial agents for respiratory infections. A third epidemiologic trend is the increasing number of brain abscesses occurring in immunocompromised hosts. These patients are at a higher risk of opportunistic fungal and parasitic infections of the central nervous system (CNS). Most case series still report that most brain abscesses are caused by common bacteria, but the trend for more unusual pathogens as the cause in the immunocompromised patient is likely to increase in the future. Finally, there has been a marked decrease in mortality rate associated with brain abscess. For a number of decades, the mortality associated with brain abscess remained constant, in the 40% to 50% range in the pre-antibiotic era, and did not improve substantially for a number of years during the post-antibiotic era. Antibiotics alone did not appear to be the key factor to improve survival, and neurosurgical drainage had been described since the late 1800s.[2]

However, after the mid-1970s, the case-fatality rate improved, with several case series reporting mortality rates below 20%. This improvement has been attributed to the routine use of brain computed tomography (CT) scanning for initial diagnosis and follow-up of brain abscesses. In one series, the mortality rate from brain abscess from 1970 to 1974, before routine CT scanning, was 36%, but fell to 0% for brain abscesses managed from 1974 to 1977, after routine CT scanning.[3] This improved mortality rate was attributed to multiple factors. including earlier diagnosis, fewer cases with multiple abscesses, more accurate localization of abscesses, greater incidence of total abscess removal, and rapid detection of postoperative complications.

Brain abscesses tend to occur in immunocompetent patients in the general population, with most being polymicrobial with aerobic and anaerobic bacteria. The major predisposing factors in this group include contiguous focus of infection, such as from paranasal sinusitis; hematogenous spread from an extracranial site of infection, such as infective endocarditis or lung abscess; recent neurosurgical procedure; and penetrating head trauma. Brain abscess from a contiguous focus of infection accounts for about 50% of total cases. The epidemiology varies with the location of the primary focus; for example, with sinusitis, older children and young adults are most commonly affected but, with otogenic brain abscesses, young children and older adults are usually involved. There may be a trend away from this particular risk factor, with one study of 100 brain abscesses reporting only 21% associated with ear infections or paranasal sinusitis.[4] In this European series, postneurosurgical cases accounted for 28% of cases. The widespread and early use of antibiotics for otitis and sinusitis has been cited as one reason for this possible shift in epidemiology.

An important risk factor for the development of a brain abscess is an acute or chronic immunosuppressed state, particularly patients who are solid organ transplant recipients, bone marrow transplant recipients, or persons with the acquired immunodeficiency syndrome (AIDS). From epidemiologic and clinical perspectives, brain abscesses that develop in these groups should be considered separately from healthy persons with brain abscesses from traditional risk factors. In persons with AIDS, *Toxoplasma* encephalitis has been the most common focal brain disorder. The annual incidence in the 1980s through the early 1990s was about 0.7 per 100 person-years. Risk factors for CNS toxoplasmosis included low CD4+ cell counts, prior opportunistic infections, injection drug use, and lack of prophylaxis. The annual incidence of toxoplasmosis fell between 1992 and 1996, likely because of the routine use of prophylactic regimens. A further decrease in the annual incidence was seen after the introduction of highly active antiretroviral therapy (HAART) in the mid-1990s. However, in a report from Italy, *Toxoplasma* encephalitis remained a highly prevalent disorder, even during the late HAART era.[5]

In transplant recipients, opportunistic mold or yeast infections predominate and can originate from primary infection or from reactivation of latent infection. In a large retrospective study from Pittsburgh, brain abscesses occurred in 0.61% of solid organ transplant recipients.[6] There appeared to be two distinct populations of patients. The first population consisted of acutely immunosuppressed transplant recipients at risk for a number of fungal infections, including fungal brain abscesses (mainly *Candida* and *Aspergillus* spp.). The lung was the primary site of fungal dissemination for most of these patients. Important factors in this high-risk group included antirejection therapy, need for retransplantation, recent bacteremia or viremia, and multiorgan failure. The second population was made up of transplant recipients who were generally healthy and developed a brain abscess long after transplantation. These late-presentation abscesses were usually of nonfungal origin, including nocardiosis and toxoplasmosis.

Fungal brain abscesses have also been reported in hematopoietic stem cell transplant recipients, despite the routine use of antifungal prophylaxis. At the Fred Hutchinson Cancer Research Center in Seattle, brain abscesses were diagnosed in 58 patients undergoing marrow transplantation between 1984 and 1992.[7] Fungi were isolated in 92% of cases, with *Aspergillus* spp. being the most common isolate, followed by *Candida* spp. Concomitant pulmonary aspergillosis was common. Risk factors for *Candida* brain abscess were prior candidemia and prolonged neutropenia. The incidence of brain abscess in bone marrow transplant recipients overall has been estimated at 1 in 49 persons.

PATHOGENESIS

In a substantial number of cases, the cause of brain abscess is unknown. The percentage of cases of brain abscess in which no primary focus of infection can be identified ranges from 10% to over 60%, although in recent case series the rates of idiopathic brain abscess are in the lower range (≤15%). Direct spread of infection from a site contiguous to the CNS remains the most common route of infection in most case series, comprising about 50% of brain abscess cases. Historically, the common primary sites have been sinusitis, otitis, and dental abscesses. Brain abscess has been described as a complication of infection involving any of the paranasal sinuses, with brain abscesses located mainly in the frontal lobe (frontal and ethmoidal sinusitis), temporal lobe (sphenoid sinusitis), or both, depending on the sinuses involved. Sphenoid sinusitis is particularly problematic, because it carries a higher rate of CNS complications compared with the other paranasal sinuses; it can spread to several contiguous areas, including the temporal lobe, pituitary, cavernous sinus, and sometimes the frontal lobe.

When there is spread of infection from the mastoids or middle ear to the CNS, the cerebellum temporal lobes, or both, are most often involved.[8] The most common predisposing condition is chronic otitis media. Several case series have reported involvement of the cerebellum four times more frequently than temporal lobes,[9] but others have not.[10] Cholesteatoma is seen in 40% to 100% of cases.[8,11] Direct spread from a dental source can account for up to 10% of brain abscesses, although this varies considerably in case series and is highest in developing countries. Dental infection or dental procedures, or both, can also cause brain abscess via a hematogenous route, rather than by direct extension. Brain abscess from direct spread from a dental abscess, often a molar, usually involves the frontal lobe.

Several mechanisms have been proposed to explain the spread from a contiguous focus of infection to the brain: extension from the primary focus to the adjacent bone and then to the brain (e.g., frontal sinusitis complicated by osteomyelitis of the posterior wall of the sinus); spread of local infection to the brain via emissary veins of the skull—bacteria or fungi in the sinuses can spread retrograde from the vasculature of the sinus mucosa, through the extensive valveless network of veins and venous sinuses, and into the cerebral venous system; spread via lymphatics; spread via the internal auditory canal or cochlear structures (for otitis media); and deep inoculation into the brain, such as with neurosurgery.

It should be noted that brain abscess rarely results from meningitis. The finding of a possible brain abscess on neuroimaging should not automatically prompt a lumbar puncture to rule out meningitis, because meningitis is a rare cause of brain abscess. This is particularly true in adults, for whom large series of community-acquired bacterial meningitis have reported no cases of secondary brain abscess. One exception is meningitis caused by *Listeria monocytogenes*, in which small abscesses in the brainstem (rhomboencephalitis) have occasionally been described. In the newborn, some forms of gram-negative meningitis are often complicated by brain abscess; about 70% of neonates with *Citrobacter diversus* meningitis will develop secondary brain abscesses. Conversely, a brain abscess can occasionally rupture into a cerebral ventricle, leading to sudden deterioration and a meningitis-like picture. This is a rare event, with about 140 cases reported in the literature, but with a lethality rate of more than 80%.[12]

Hematogenous spread of infection from a distant source to the CNS represents the second most commonly identified mechanism. This route of infection accounts for about 25% of brain abscesses. However, it should be noted that the vast majority of bacteremic events do not result in brain abscess or any other CNS infections. When bacteremia does result in brain abscess, there is usually an additional predisposing factor. Historically, pulmonary infections were the most common conditions associated with hematogenous brain abscess. The most common pulmonary conditions are lung abscess, empyema, and bronchiectasis. Pulmonary venous malformation is another underlying condition associated with a relatively high rate of brain abscess. Patients with Osler-Weber-Rendu disease, hereditary hemorrhagic telangiectasia, are known to be at higher risk of brain abscess,[13] presumably because bacteremia may result in small infected emboli that travel through the pulmonary arteriovenous malformations and enter the arterial circulation of the brain directly, without first being filtered by the pulmonary vasculature. Cyanotic congenital heart disease is also considered a traditional risk factor for brain abscess because of the increased risk of spread of a blood-borne pathogen to the brain.

Less commonly, brain abscess has also been reported with concomitant liver abscess. Most of these reported cases represent underlying pyogenic liver abscess, with hematogenous spread to the brain. One emerging trend is simultaneous liver and brain abscesses caused by *Klebsiella pneumoniae* in diabetics. This particular association has been described in several series from Taiwan, in which *K. pneumoniae* liver abscess was found to be a leading cause of community-acquired brain abscess.[14,15] Brain abscess has also been described with other gastrointestinal conditions and procedures, such as following sclerosis of esophageal varices. It has also been described as a complication of tongue piercing.[16]

PATHOPHYSIOLOGY

Experimental studies of brain abscesses have led to a four-stage model of disease development.[17-20] Direct inoculation of bacteria into brain parenchyma results in focal inflammation and edema. This has been termed the first stage, or early cerebritis stage, and develops in the first 1 to 3 days after inoculation. Typically, there is neutrophil accumulation, edema, and some tissue necrosis. Astrocytes and microglia are activated early on, and this activation persists afterward. The area of cerebritis expands and a necrotic center develops, termed *late cerebritis*, on days 4 to 9. Macrophages and lymphocytes predominate in the infiltrate. The third stage is characterized by the development of a capsule that is vascularized and ring enhancing on CT scan, days 10 to 14, the early capsule stage. In the fourth stage, the host immune response causes the capsule to wall off, and there is destruction of some surrounding healthy brain tissue in an attempt to sequester the infection. This model can vary considerably based on factors such as the size of the bacterial inoculum, microorganism, immune state of the host, and antimicrobial agent. This model was derived primarily from experimental rodent studies but seems to correlate well with human disease. In both animal modeling and human disease, the key requirements for the formation of a pyogenic brain abscess are a focus of necrotic or ischemic brain tissue, combined with a virulent microorganism.

Animal studies examining the neuroimmunology of brain abscess have shown that the local immune response may contribute to parenchymal brain destruction.[19] In animal and human brain abscess studies, the area of inflammatory response and tissue destruction often appears significantly larger than the more localized area of the initial bacterial infection. In a *Staphylococcus aureus* brain abscess model, bacteria are recognized by Toll-like receptor 2, which leads to activation of astrocytes and microglia, which in turn results in production of proinflammatory cytokines.[20] Cytokine release causes disruption of the blood-brain barrier, with subsequent entry of large molecules into brain parenchyma, such as immunoglobulin G (IgG) and albumin. Adhesion molecules are expressed, such as the intracellular adhesion molecule (ICAM), which facilitate entry of neutrophils, T cells, and macrophages from the circulation into the growing abscess. These immune cells are activated by bacteria and cytokines, leading to a repetitive cycle of inflammation.

Microbiology in the Immunocompetent Host

The pathogens involved in pyogenic brain abscess often can be predicted by the predisposing condition, host immune status, and mode of acquisition. When the predisposing condition is a contiguous focus of infection, such as paranasal sinusitis, otitis media, or dental abscess infection, it is usually polymicrobial (>50%-60% of cases), particularly if culture specimens from the brain abscess are submitted optimally on anaerobic media. The usual pathogens reflect the oral and upper respiratory flora, in which anaerobes are an important component of the normal flora: aerobic and anaerobic streptococci, *Fusobacterium* spp., and anaerobic gram-negative bacilli (e.g., *Bacteroides, Prevotella*). The paranasal sinuses can also be colonized and/or infected with other bacteria, such as *S. aureus* and *Enterobacter* spp., but this is less common than the normal flora.

Following neurosurgery or head trauma, such as a gunshot wound, the likely pathogens for brain abscess are *S. aureus*, coagulase-negative staphylococci, *Pseudomonas aeruginosa, Enterobacter* spp., and some streptococci. *Clostridium* spp. can be seen following contaminated penetrating head trauma.

The spectrum of organisms varies somewhat when the associated condition is a chronic pulmonary infection, such as lung abscess, bronchiectasis, or chronic empyema. Common organisms are *Fusobacterium* spp., anaerobic gram-negative bacilli such as *Bacteroides* spp. (not *B. fragilis*), various aerobic and anaerobic streptococci, and some *Actinomyces* and *Nocardia* spp. For brain abscesses occurring in the setting of bacterial endocarditis or congenital heart disease, the most common organisms are *viridans* streptococci, including the *Streptococcus milleri* group (*S. constellatus, S. anginosus, S. intermedius*, which have a marked tendency for abscess formation), *S. aureus, Haemophilus* spp., and occasionally enterococci.

- Miscellaneous causes of brain abscess in the normal host include the following:
- The endemic mycoses: *Histoplasma capsulatum, Blastomyces dermatitidis, Coccidioides immitis*. The main site of infection for these pathogens is pulmonary, but infection can disseminate to the CNS.
- Protozoa, such as *Entamoeba histolytica, Schistosoma, Paragonimus*.
- Helminths, especially *Taenia solium*, the cause of neurocysticercosis.

The frequency of these causes of brain abscess varies considerably depending on geography, but usually accounts for only a small percentage of cases in most series, including developing countries. *Streptococcus pneumoniae* is the most common cause of community-acquired bacterial meningitis, but is a rare cause of brain abscess.[21]

Microbiology in the Immunocompromised Host

In persons with AIDS, brain abscesses are more likely to be from opportunistic infections, although bacterial brain abscesses have been reported in a small percentage of cases. Common pathogens in AIDS-related brain abscess include *Toxoplasma gondii, Listeria monocytogenes*, and *Cryptococcus neoformans. Toxoplasma* encephalitis is the most common cause of a focal intracranial lesion in AIDS, even in the current era of HAART. In one study from Italy, toxoplasmosis remained the most prevalent cause of HIV-related neurologic disorders.[5] However, the differential diagnosis of one or more focal cerebral lesions in a person with AIDS is wide. The most common causes are *T. gondii* (about 50%), but this is followed by CNS lymphoma (about 20%-30%).

Other pathogens account for the remainder. *Rhodococcus equi*, an intracellular gram-positive coccobacillus, is a known but rare cause of brain abscess in those with AIDS.[22] This zoonotic infection typically causes a chronic cavitary or nodular pulmonary infection and brain abscess has been reported, usually in the setting of a current or prior *Rhodococcus* pulmonary infection. *Mycobacterium tuberculosis* is recognized as a cause of brain abscesses in AIDS patients,[23,24] and has been reported as an isolated ring-enhancing lesion or multiple lesions in the setting of widely disseminated mycobacterial infection. Tuberculosis can infect the CNS in a number of ways, including tubercular meningitis, tuberculous encephalopathy, tuberculous arteritis, tuberculoma, and tuberculous abscess. A true tuberculous abscess is a rare manifestation of CNS tuberculosis, even in countries in which tuberculosis is common. Other causes of focal mass lesions in AIDS include *C. neoformans, H. capsulatum, A. fumigatus*, and others.

In solid organ transplant recipients, the major organisms of concern are fungal (*Aspergillus, Mucorales, Candida, Cryptococcus*) and *Nocardia* spp. Occasionally, other opportunistic infections may be seen, such as *Toxoplasma gondii*,[25-29] as well as polymicrobial bacterial brain abscess. In the neutropenic patient, opportunistic mold infection is the most common cause of brain abscess, particularly *Aspergillus* and *Mucorales* spp. Additional pathogens are *Pseudomonas aeruginosa* and *Enterobacter* spp.

In general, the clinical and radiographic appearances of brain abscess in the immunocompromised host are nonspecific. Microbiologic confirmation from brain tissue is necessary to establish a causative diagnosis in the vast majority of cases.

CLINICAL MANIFESTATIONS

The clinical presentation depends on a number of factors, including the host's immune status, specific pathogen involved, contiguous sites of infection or distant foci of infection, size of the abscess, and location of the lesions. The most common symptom is a headache (about 70% of cases), although the headache tends to be nonspecific and not always localizing. In general, the headaches are dull and subacute or chronic in nature, and not sudden and severe. One exception to this is rupture of a preexisting brain abscess into an adjacent ventricle, which manifests with an acute illness more suggestive of meningitis. Patients may also present with symptoms of increased intracranial pressure such as nausea, vomiting, and advancing lethargy. The classic triad of fever, headache, and altered mental status is unfortunately not reliable and is present in 50% or fewer cases. It is important to note that fever is absent in over 50% of patients with brain abscess at the time of the initial presentation. This is also true for persons with AIDS with CNS toxoplasmosis; fever is not reliably present. Similarly, focal neurologic deficits such as hemiparesis and aphasia are absent in 50% of patients with bacterial brain abscess. Papilledema is also an insensitive sign, being absent in about 75% of cases on presentation. Other clinical manifestations include generalized seizures and neck stiffness if the abscess is close to the meninges.

Certain focal neurologic abnormalities may provide a clue to the location of a space-occupying lesion. A sizable abscess in the frontal lobe may lead to hemiparesis and motor speech deficits. A lesion in the temporal lobe may lead to an ipsilateral headache, aphasia, and possibly a visual field defect. Lesions in the cerebellum may cause ataxia, dysmetria, and nystagmus. However, these relationships are not dependable and, as previously noted, patients with brain abscesses often have no localizing signs on presentation. Thus, the bedside diagnosis of a brain abscess can be challenging, with a number of patients presenting without fever or focal deficits.

DIAGNOSIS

Laboratory Studies

Routine laboratory studies are not helpful for the diagnosis of brain abscess. Leukocytosis may be absent; in some series about 40% of patients have a normal peripheral white blood cell count. Acute-phase reactants are moderately helpful but nonspecific. The C-reactive protein level is elevated in almost all patients, but the sedimentation rate can be only moderately elevated and sometimes is normal. Samples for blood cultures should be obtained in all suspected cases; although the yield is low, a positive result can be extremely valuable.

In immunocompromised patients, several tests may be useful. The tuberculin skin test is an often overlooked screening test that should be administered to an immunosuppressed patient with a brain or lung lesion. The limitations of the tuberculin skin test are false-negative reactions caused by cutaneous anergy from chronic steroids, other medications, and often the primary infection itself. The *Toxoplasma* IgG level is of some potential use in assessing the AIDS patient with afocal CNS lesions. The seroprevalence rate of a positive *Toxoplasma* IgG level is high in the general population, with considerable geographic and international variations, and a positive serum level in isolation is not diagnostic of active toxoplasmosis. The *Toxoplasma* IgG serum level is used to support a presumptive diagnosis of toxoplasmosis when there are also compatible clinical and radiographic features in an individual case. A negative serum *Toxoplasma* IgG level is suggestive of diagnoses other than *Toxoplasma* encephalitis, but does not rule out this diagnosis completely. AIDS patients with a negative serum toxoplasmosis IgG level in the setting of *Toxoplasma* encephalitis have been reported. A negative serum IgG test result may place the diagnosis of toxoplasmosis lower in the differential diagnostic considerations but does not exclude the diagnosis entirely.

Lumbar puncture is often contraindicated in persons with suspected brain abscess. Cerebrospinal fluid (CSF) results, when reported in the literature, have shown nonspecific abnormalities in most cases, usually with mild elevations of the CSF protein level, and varying numbers of CSF leukocytes. The yield of a pathogen from CSF examination with suspected brain abscess is low, less than 10%. There may be an occasional patient in whom the abscesses are small on CT or magnetic resonance imaging (MRI), the lesions exert minimal mass effect, the third and fourth ventricles are open, and there are no other signs of cerebral edema In these cases, lumbar puncture is sometimes considered mainly to obtain CSF for cytologic and flow cytometry studies (to rule out metastases), cryptococcal antigen detection, and polymerase chain reaction (PCR) assay for *T. gondii*. However, this should be undertaken with great caution. Given the risks of brain herniation in the setting of elevated intracranial pressure, and the low yield of diagnostic tests, lumbar puncture should be avoided in the vast majority of cases.

Most patients with a brain abscess will undergo some type of CT-guided aspiration or open evacuation of the abscess. Operative specimens should be routinely submitted for Gram staining, routine culture, and anaerobe culture. Purulent fluid should usually be submitted in a sterile container, in addition to the use of standard Culturette swabs, because the microbiologic yield of larger tissue samples and fluids is significantly higher than the yield of the small specimen submitted for swab cultures. In addition, some microbiology laboratories do not accept specimens submitted on a swab culture for certain organisms, especially acid-fast bacillus (AFB). Because of the important role of anaerobes in brain abscesses, special effort should also be made to optimize recovery of anaerobes. The local microbiology laboratory should be consulted beforehand regarding the preferred specimen collection technique for anaerobes, which generally requires inoculation of specimens directly into anaerobic bottles or rapid transport of a specimen from the operating room to the laboratory using appropriate transport systems. Other stains and cultures include acid-fast staining with mycobacterial culture, fungal stains and cultures, *Nocardia* stain and culture, and culture for *Rhodococcus equi*. Samples for these special stains and cultures should be obtained routinely when the patient is immunocompromised, but should be strongly considered in some immunocompetent patients as well.

PCR molecular testing is available through many reference laboratories for various pathogens from CSF and tissue specimens, particularly *Mycobacterium tuberculosis* and *T. gondii*. It should be emphasized that a number of molecular tests that are potentially useful for the diagnosis of meningitis in the AIDS patient or transplant recipient are not useful for the diagnosis of brain abscess in these patients. For example, cytomegalovirus and varicella zoster virus are known causes of meningoencephalitis in AIDS patients, but do not cause brain abscesses. In patients from whom CSF or tissue may have been obtained to diagnose *Toxoplasma* brain abscesses, several PCR-based tests have been developed, with some commercially available assays able to detect as few as 100 copies of DNA per mL (or down to three oocysts). Commercially available PCR tests for *M. tuberculosis* have a lower limit of detection of 400 cells/mL in CSF and tissue. Many tertiary centers have developed in-house PCR detection systems for these and other unusual organisms. Standardization of the numerous PCR assays reported in the literature, and also the many variations of PCR assays in local laboratories, may have had only in-house validation. Many lack rigorous standardization and validation for multiple specimens, and thus the false-negative and false-positive results for a number of these tests remain unclear. Generally, the decision to order multiple PCR assays on blood, CSF, and brain tissue should be done judiciously, avoiding a shotgun approach when ordering molecular diagnostics, even for an immunocompromised host.

Specimens should also be submitted routinely for cytopathologic and histopathologic testing for special organism stains and also to rule out malignancy. Touch preparations from tissue specimens may be useful for detecting *T. gondii* rapidly. Special stains should be used for pathology specimens, including silver stains for fungi, AFB stains for mycobacteria, and mucicarmine stain for *Cryptococcus neoformans* in select cases. Tissue biopsy will also be useful in diagnosing the rare case of parasitic brain abscess other than *T. gondii*, such as those caused by *Entamoeba histolytica* (extraintestinal amebiasis).

Neuroimaging

Because of the difficulties in clinical diagnosis of brain abscess, neuroimaging is essential.[30-37] In general, radiographic abnormalities depend on the particular stage of the brain abscess. One of the uses of neuroimaging is to estimate the age of the brain abscess. A lesion in the early or late cerebritis stage may be managed somewhat differently compared with a mature, walled-off abscess (see later, "Treatment"). CT scanning with contrast during stage 1 (early cerebritis) may show only edema—an area of hypodensity—which may or may not enhance with contrast. If done very early in the course of infection, a contrast-enhanced CT may be normal. During later stages, there is the development of a space-occupying lesion with a hypodense center and later a ring-enhancing rim, which is often surrounded by a large area of edema. Occasionally, ring enhancement can be seen with late cerebritis; delayed administration of contrast that fills in the central hypodensity is suggestive that the lesion is still in the cerebritis stage. Although contrast-enhanced CT scanning is considered sensitive for the detection of brain abscesses, it is not specific. Brain abscesses tend to have smooth thin-walled capsules, whereas tumors tend to have more irregular capsules. There are additional characteristics of brain tumors, but some overlap exists with brain abscesses. It is important to note that brain abscesses and brain tumors may have an identical appearance on the CT scan.

MR imaging is more sensitive than CT, and MRI can usually detect infection in the early cerebritis stage. The MRI scan in focal cerebritis usually shows an area of hypointensity on T_1- and T_2-weighted imaging. The characteristic appearance of a mature brain abscess on MRI is a focal lesion with low intensity on a T_1-weighted image, with a smoothly marginated capsule that enhances with IV gadolinium (Fig. 1). On T_2-weighted images, the central abscess is hyperintense and the surrounding capsule is hypointense. There is extensive surrounding edema in most cases. The finding of a capsule that is hypointense on a T_2-weighted image and mildly hyperintense on a T_1-weighted image is suggestive of an abscess capsule.

The finding of multiple cerebral abscesses conforming to a vascular distribution is suggestive of a central embolic source. Brain abscesses from a hematogenous source, such as infective endocarditis, tend to be multiple and distribute widely in the middle cerebral artery. Multiple cerebral lesions are present in about 50% of cases of hematogenously acquired brain abscess.[38] However, a single brain abscess can also be seen with endocarditis.

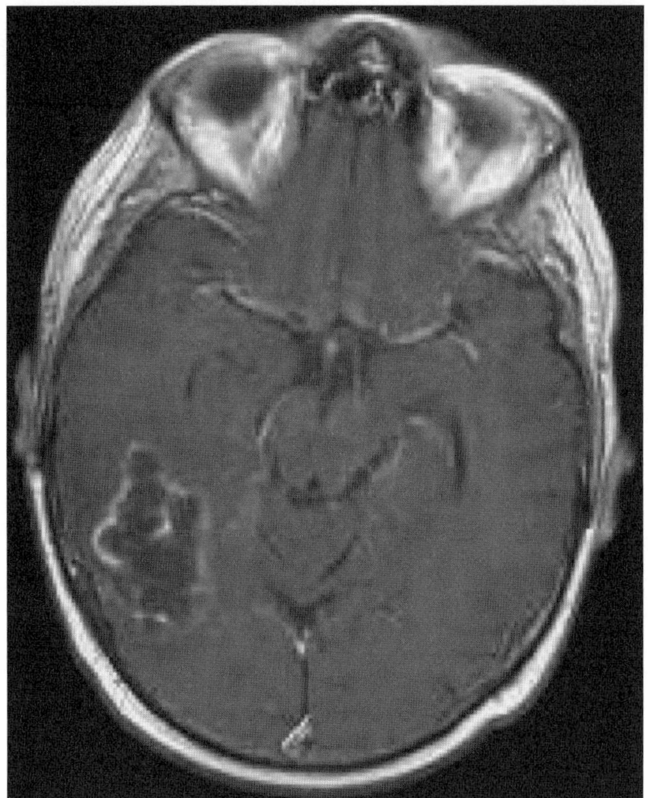

Figure 1 **T_1-weighted MR image of temporal lobe abscess, with gadolinium enhancement.**

In immunocompromised persons, it is not possible to distinguish a bacterial brain abscess from an opportunistic CNS infection on the basis of conventional MR imaging alone. With *Toxoplasma* encephalitis, MRI typically shows multiple, small, ring-enhancing lesions. Any region of the brain may be involved, but the basal ganglia is the most common site. There is frequently some degree of local edema and mass effect as well, which are helpful in distinguishing *Toxoplasma* encephalitis from other brain lesions in AIDS, which lack mass effect (e.g., progressive multifocal leukoencephalopathy, cytomegalovirus encephalitis). CNS lymphoma in AIDS patients also manifests with a ring-enhancing lesion, but tends to be solitary rather than multiple, although multifocal CNS lymphoma does occur. Given the difficulty in distinguishing toxoplasmosis from CNS lymphoma, a number of additional radiographic techniques have been studied, including thallium single-photon emission computed tomography (SPECT) and positron emission tomography. These tests can be useful adjunctive studies in difficult cases.

For transplant recipients, diffusion-weighted imaging in fungal brain abscesses has been reported in one small study of six patients with proven fungal (*Aspergillus*) cerebral abscesses.[39] Conventional MR imaging showed typical ring-enhancing lesions indistinguishable from pyogenic brain abscesses. Most of the patients had restricted diffusion in the center of the abscess, similar to prior reports of diffusion-weighted imaging (DWI) in bacterial brain abscesses. The DWI hyperintensity (restriction) was attributed to cellular infiltration and proteinaceous fluid in the abscess. There were several additional patients who presented with *Aspergillus* and *Rhizopus* cerebritis; these individuals had a fulminant course and expired rapidly. Conventional MRI showed large, nonenhancing cerebral lesions, which did not show ring enhancement. On DWI, the lesions showed a more heterogeneous pattern with some areas of decreased and increased diffusion. Pathology demonstrated cerebritis rather than a purulent abscess. In transplant patients presenting with neurologic changes and ring-enhancing brain lesions, a fungal cause should be high in the differential diagnosis; conventional MRI and DWI abnormalities appear to be similar to those of bacterial brain abscesses.

TREATMENT

The optimal treatment of brain abscess is complex and requires a coordinated approach among multiple teams. There are no large, randomized, clinical trials comparing different antimicrobial regimens or different neurosurgical approaches, but large retrospective series have demonstrated dramatic improvement in survival using a combination of surgical drainage and a prolonged course of IV antibiotics. In most patients, particularly those with abscesses larger than 2.5 cm, stereotactic aspiration or open brain biopsy with evacuation should be strongly considered for microbiologic diagnosis, given the wide range of possible pathogens and the prolonged course of IV antibiotics required. One approach has been to treat neurologically stable patients with early infections in the cerebritis stage with IV antibiotics alone, with aspiration attempted when the infection later appears more encapsulated and liquefied, to maximize the yield of an aspiration procedure. Alternatively, an area of focal cerebritis without a frank abscess may still be aspirated using a stereotactically guided needle procedure through a burr hole, but the volume of fluid and tissue may be small. Large abscesses (>2.5 cm) should generally be aspirated, drained, or completely excised.

For patients with multiple abscesses of varying sizes, one approach would be to aspirate and/or evacuate large collections, and treat smaller abscesses medically. Serial CT scans need to be obtained afterward to assess the stability of the remaining abscesses, because repeat aspirations may be necessary. Patients with multiple small (<2 cm) abscesses may respond to medical therapy alone, particularly if the lesions are smaller than 1 cm, but these patients also need serial neuroimaging. Medical treatment is usually attempted when abscesses are also in deep locations, such as the brainstem. However, a medical approach carries a significant risk of selection of incorrect antibiotics. This is particularly problematic for the immunocompromised patient, in whom the spectrum of pathogens is even more unpredictable. The diagnostic algorithm is somewhat different for immunocompromised patients with suspected cerebral toxoplasmosis (see later).

Immunocompetent Host

In general, the antibiotics used for the treatment of brain abscess should have the following characteristics: favorable brain or CSF drug levels, or both, even in the absence of inflamed meninges; bactericidal activity; minimal side effects over many weeks of treatment; good penetration and activity in the abscess fluid; and good in vitro activity against the most common pathogens, based on the most likely pathogenesis of the infection.

Penicillin G has excellent activity against most aerobic and anaerobic streptococci found in brain abscesses associated with paranasal sinusitis, otitis media, mastoiditis, and dental abscesses. Penicillin G also penetrates relatively well into the CSF and brain tissue, and maintains activity in abscess fluid. Most isolates of *Prevotella*, *Fusobacterium*, and *Porphyromonas* species are susceptible to penicillin G, but there are some resistant clinical strains. Penicillin G is also not reliably active against most anaerobic gram-negative bacilli. Thus, penicillin G is not used by itself for the initial empirical coverage of brain abscesses, and is usually used in combination with a second agent with broader anaerobic coverage, such as metronidazole.

Third-generation cephalosporins, such as ceftriaxone, also achieve effective levels in various compartments of the CNS and are highly active against aerobic streptococci and most gram-negative bacilli, but lack anaerobic activity and generally need to be used in combination with an agent such as metronidazole, because many brain abscesses include anaerobes. Metronidazole has many favorable characteristics for the treatment of brain abscess. It is reliably active against gram-positive and gram-negative anaerobes, retains activity in abscess cavities, and crosses the blood-brain barrier, even when the meninges are not inflamed. Metronidazole has no activity against aerobes, including aerobic streptococci, and thus needs to be used in combination with other agents. The beta lactam–beta-lactamase inhibitor drugs (e.g., ampicillin-sulbactam, ticarcillin-clavulanate, piperacillin-tazobactam) are effective against most organisms that cause contiguous and hematogenous brain abscess. These agents cross the blood-brain barrier and can be used as monotherapy in many cases.

For the treatment of *S. aureus*, antistaphylococcal penicillins such as oxacillin are the drugs of choice for susceptible isolates. The semisynthetic penicillins are rapidly bactericidal for *S. aureus* and penetrate into the CNS, although not as well as penicillin G. However, many hospital-associated isolates of *S. aureus* are methicillin-resistant and antimicrobial susceptibility tests are not available for several days after brain tissue is submitted for culture. The most experience in treating methicillin-resistant *S. aureus* (MRSA) brain abscesses is with vancomycin, which is also active against aerobic and anaerobic streptococci and *Clostridia* spp. The penetration of vancomycin into the CNS is limited with noninflamed meninges. Ceftriaxone has the best activity against *S. aureus* compared with other third-generation cephalosporins. However, its role in the treatment of life-threatening *S. aureus* infections is not clear, and agents with better in vitro activity and clinical use are available.

The carbapenems (e.g., imipenem, meropenem, ertapenem) have the advantage of excellent anaerobic coverage, along with activity against aerobic streptococci and *Enterobacter* spp. Imipenem has good penetration into CSF and brain pus. Anecdotal reports have suggested that imipenem may be effective for bacterial brain abscess, but concerns have been raised regarding seizures induced by the carbapenems, particularly imipenem. In one series of 15 patients, imipenem was used successfully to treat brain abscesses from various gram-positive and gram-negative organisms, with one seizure.[40] In addition, imipenem has been used for the treatment of *Nocardia* brain abscesses without undue reports of seizures. Carbapenems do not appear contraindicated in the setting of brain abscess, but their use should be weighed against the small seizure risk and the risks and benefits of alternative regimens. Quinolones (e.g., ciprofloxacin, levofloxacin) penetrate well into the CNS but experience with this class of antibiotics in CNS infections is still limited. Ciprofloxacin has unreliable activity against a number of gram-positive infections, including *S. pneumoniae* and other streptococcal spp. In general, the quinolones should be reserved for special cases, such as for those with multiple drug allergies.

The decision to treat empirically with antibiotics before a stereotactic or open brain biopsy is not always straightforward and can depend on a number of factors, such as the severity of the illness, presence of mass effect or impending herniation, timing of surgery, and comorbid medical conditions. Administration of empirical antibiotics for several days before a brain biopsy probably does decrease the yield of pathogens in culture, but the exact impact is not known. In practice, a number of patients will receive empirical antibiotics before microbiologic culture, and every effort should be made to submit cultures on appropriate media, including anaerobic cultures at the time of surgery.

For the empirical treatment of brain abscess associated with paranasal sinusitis, otitis, or mastoiditis, one preferred regimen is a third-generation cephalosporin (e.g., ceftriaxone, ceftizoxime) combined with IV metronidazole.[41-45] This regimen covers the common pathogens in this setting but has no activity against MRSA and suboptimal activity against methicillin-susceptible *S. aureus*. However, *S. aureus* is not a pathogen associated with otitis media and dental abscesses, and remains relatively uncommon with brain abscess secondary to paranasal sinusitis. The addition of antistaphylococcal therapy in this setting is optional but may be considered in patients at higher risk for *S. aureus* sinusitis, such as those with recent endoscopic sinus surgery, chronic sinusitis, and recent nasal packing.

Brain abscesses from dental infections or dental procedures can be treated with IV penicillin in combination with metronidazole. Aerobic gram-negative bacilli are not important causes of odontogenic infection and do not require empirical coverage with a third-generation cephalosporin.

S. aureus is a major pathogen when brain abscess is associated with trauma or neurosurgical procedures, and must be covered empirically in this situation. Gram-negative bacilli, including *Pseudomonas aeruginosa*, are also common nosocomial pathogens in neurosurgical infections and should be treated pending culture results. A common empirical regimen in this setting would be vancomycin, or an antistaphylococcal penicillin, in combination with an antipseudomonal third- or fourth-generation cephalosporin, such as ceftazidime or cefepime. Brain abscess associated with lung abscess or bronchiectasis can be empirically treated with a third-generation cephalosporin in combination with metronidazole or with IV penicillin G in combination with metronidazole.

When brain abscess is associated with congenital heart disease, a third-generation cephalosporin covers the usual associated pathogens, *Streptococcus* and *Haemophilus* spp. This regimen does not cover enterococci, which is an occasional pathogen in this setting; IV ampicillin may be added to the third-generation cephalosporin in some cases pending microbiologic information. The empirical treatment of brain abscess associated with endocarditis usually is determined by the treatment of the underlying endocarditis, and depends on whether the patient has native valve or prosthetic valve endocarditis. Empirical regimens include the following: for native valve endocarditis, IV ampicillin and gentamicin; and for prosthetic valve endocarditis, IV vancomycin and gentamicin, with or without rifampin.

The length of therapy for the treatment of bacterial brain abscesses in all these scenarios has not been formally studied. Large series have generally reported good outcomes with prolonged courses of IV antibiotics for 4 to 6 weeks, or longer. One group described cures using an early switch to oral antibiotic therapy in a small number of patients who had refused IV antibiotics.[46]

Immunocompromised Patient

Aspergillus fumigatus brain abscess usually occurs in the setting of disseminated *Aspergillus*, in which there is often evidence of pulmonary and other organ involvement. CNS aspergillosis is often rapidly fatal, even with surgical intervention. Several clinicians have reported a good clinical response to voriconazole for fungal brain abscesses,[47-50] but there have been no comparative trials to date between voriconazole and amphotericin. Animal modeling has shown that voriconazole has high penetration into brain tissue and CSF, with steady-state drug levels in the CNS twice those of plasma levels, and limited human data have suggested favorable pharmacokinetics.[51] Various regimens have been described at a case report level for successful salvage therapy for CNS, including amphotericin B and voriconazole, voriconazole and caspofungin, intrathecal amphotericin administered via an Ommaya reservoir, and others. Overall, the data are sparse and do not permit a specific recommendation for salvage therapy, although a number of options exist.

Toxoplasma encephalitis in AIDS patients is generally treated empirically when there is a compatible presentation (advanced AIDS, positive *Toxoplasma* IgG serum, lack of prophylaxis, multiple ring-enhancing basal ganglia lesions). The regimens of choice are sulfadiazine 6 to 8 g orally, in four divided doses, plus pyrimethamine, 200-mg loading dose orally, followed by 75 mg/day. An alternative regimen is clindamycin, 600 to 1200 mg IV, four times daily (or oral equivalent) with pyrimethamine. Because of the rapid radiographic improvement when *Toxoplasma* encephalitis is treated correctly, serial CT scans should demonstrate improvement within several weeks.

Summary

- Brain abscesses are uncommon but potentially lethal infections of the central nervous system. This infection can occur in various settings, including previously healthy patients, immunocompromised hosts, and after neurosurgical procedures.
- There have been several changes in the epidemiology of this infection, with fewer cases caused by odontogenic or otic causes, and more cases related to opportunistic infections in those who are immunocompromised.
- In otherwise healthy persons, brain abscesses are usually polymicrobial in nature, with both aerobes and anaerobes predominantly.
- In immunocompromised individuals, such as persons with AIDS, neutropenic patients, or organ transplant recipients, the causative organisms are numerous, and range from more uncommon bacteria such as *Nocardia* spp., to fungal organisms such as *Aspergillus* spp., and to parasitic infections such as *Toxoplasma gondii*.
- The diagnosis of brain abscess is difficult to make on clinical grounds alone, and neuroimaging studies are essential.
- The mortality associated with brain abscesses has decreased significantly with a combined medical-surgical approach, particularly for brain lesions larger than 2.5 cm.
- The selection of antimicrobial agents should be directed by microbiologic culture results whenever possible, particularly in immunocompromised patients, in whom there is a wide range of pathogens. Optimal management requires coordinated efforts by a team that includes general internists, neurosurgeons, infectious disease specialists, and others.

Suggested Readings

Antinori A, Larussa D, Cingolani A, et al; Italian Registry Investigative NeuroAIDS: Prevalence, associated factors, and prognostic determinants of AIDS-related *Toxoplasma* encephalitis in the era of advanced highly active antiretroviral therapy. Clin Infect Dis 2004;39:1681-1691.

Calfee DP, Wispelwey B: Brain abscess. Semin Neurol 2000;20:353-360.

Canale DJ: William Macewen and the treatment of brain abscesses: Revisited after one hundred years. J Neurosurg 1996;84:133-142.

Falcone S, Post MJ: Encephalitis, cerebritis, and brain abscess: Pathophysiology and imaging findings. Neuroimaging Clin North Am 2000;10:333-353.

Hagensee ME, Bauwens JE, Kjos B, Bowden RA: Brain abscess following marrow transplantation: Experience at the Fred Hutchinson Cancer Research Center, 1984-1992. Clin Infect Dis 1994;19:402-408.

Heilpern KL, Lorber B: Focal intracranial infections. Infect Dis Clin North Am 1996;10:879-898.

Kielian T: Immunopathogenesis of brain abscess. J Neuroinflammation 2004;1:16.

Mathisen GE, Johnson JP: Brain abscess: State-of-the-art clinical article. Clin Infect Dis 1997;25:763-781.

Osenbach RK, Loftus CM: Diagnosis and management of brain abscess. Neurosurg Clin North Am 1992;3:403-420.

Sennaroglu L, Sozeri B: Otogenic brain abscess: Review of 41 cases. Otolaryngol Head Neck Surg 2000;123:751-755.

References

For a complete list of references, log onto www.expertconsult.com.

Biologic Weapons and the Primary Care Clinician

Thomas Tallman, Steven Gordon, and Thomas P. Noeller

DEFINITION

Recent events have highlighted the need for clinicians to educate themselves and prepare for the threat of biologic terrorism. For many years, these attacks seemed unlikely, but no longer. The events of September 11, 2001, the cases of anthrax caused by letters sent in the mail, and increasing intelligence revealing the existence of biologic agents available to governments and terrorist organizations have awakened health care providers to the need for preparatory measures. Bioterrorism is the intentional use of a pathogen or biologic product to cause harm to humans and other living organisms, influence the conduct of government, or intimidate or coerce a civilian population.

Weapons of mass destruction include nuclear, biologic, and chemical weapons. Biologic weapons disseminate pathogenic microbes or biologic toxins to cause illness or death in human, animal, or plant populations. Potential living biologic warfare agents include bacteria, viruses, rickettsia, and fungi. Why use biologic agents as weapons? They are relatively easy to produce, can disseminate great distances from a target, result in effects ranging from incapacitation to death, and can be difficult to detect, and the threats alone can result in panic.

The ideal biologic weapon is one that can be quickly and easily disseminated to a large population, is highly contagious, causes high rates of morbidity and mortality, requires vast resources to combat, and causes mass panic, confusion, or social disruption. Bioterrorism release types include overt and covert release.

Government agencies, health departments, and the Centers for Disease Control and Prevention (CDC) have identified the most likely agents to be used in a biologic attack (Box 1) and have plans in place to address such attacks.[1] These plans emphasize the important role of frontline medical providers in recognizing and reporting suspected biologic and chemical attacks.

The United States had an offensive biologic weapons program in place from 1943 to 1969 that included lethal agents such as anthrax and botulinum toxins, incapacitating agents such as Brucella suis and Venezuelan equine encephalitis (VEE) virus, and anticrop agents such as wheat stem rust and rice blast. Today, 17 countries are suspected of including or developing biologic agents in their offensive weapons programs. Almost all these countries are signatories to the 1972 Biological Weapons Convention, yet they continued to maintain offensive programs.

PATHOPHYSIOLOGY

Anthrax

Bacillus anthracis is an aerobic, gram-positive, spore-forming, nonmotile bacterium. Spores form when environmental nutrients are exhausted, and they can exist for decades. When exposed to the appropriate nutrient-rich environment, the spores germinate and can potentially cause disease.

Anthrax in nature is a zoonosis; humans become infected through contact or ingestion of contaminated animals or animal products. It is not transmitted via person-to-person contact, so no special isolation of suspected or proven cases is necessary.

Anthrax may cause an acute infectious disease in humans of three types: inhalational, cutaneous, and gastrointestinal. Cutaneous anthrax is the most commonly encountered form, typically following exposure to anthrax-infected animals (Fig. 1). Anthrax spores can enter wounds or broken skin, a route suspected in some of the recent cases of intentional anthrax exposure. Gastrointestinal anthrax is rare, but can follow ingestion of undercooked contaminated meat. Inhalational anthrax, although rare, is the most lethal.

Until the recent bioterrorist events, only 18 cases had been reported in the United States in the last century. As of December 5, 2001, 11 additional cases of inhalational anthrax and 11 cases of confirmed and suspected cutaneous anthrax have been identified as a result of an apparent intentional release into the postal system.[2] The most recent case of anthrax in the United States occurred in a man in New York, in 2006, who had made a drum from infected animal skins.

Once inhaled, spores are transported via lymphatics to mediastinal lymph nodes, where germination can occur up to 60 days or more after exposure. The disease progresses rapidly once germination occurs because replicating bacteria elaborate toxins that lead to hemorrhage, edema, and necrosis. The anthrax genome contains two plasmids, one of which codes for toxin-making genes. In Sverdlovsk, hemorrhagic thoracic lymphadenitis and hemorrhagic mediastinitis occurred in all patients, and hemorrhagic meningitis occurred in 50% of cases.[3]

Smallpox

Once one of the deadliest diseases known to humankind, with a mortality rate of 30%, smallpox is the only human disease that has been successfully eradicated, with the last natural case occurring in 1977. Immunization ceased in 1980 based on recommendations from the World Health Organization.[4] Routine immunizations in the United States ceased in 1972. There is now a large U.S. population that would be very susceptible to this disease.

Caused by variola virus, smallpox is potentially the most devastating of the bioterrorism agents because it has a high infectivity rate, a fatality rate of up to 30%, and a high person-to-person transmission rate. Like anthrax, smallpox can be easily disseminated in aerosol form. Infection occurs after deposition of the virus particles on upper respiratory mucous membranes.

Plague

Plague is well known in history, having caused several pandemics and millions of deaths. Several countries, including the United States, have experimented with plague as a biologic weapon, using flea vectors in World War II and, more recently, an aerosolized form of the causative organism, *Yersinia pestis*. The organism has a high potential to be used as a bioterrorism (BT) weapon, because it is endemic in many animals worldwide, is easy to grow and disseminate, has a high fatality rate, and can be spread from person to person.

Y. pestis is classically transmitted through the bites of infected fleas, resulting in several forms of the disease, including bubonic, pneumonic, and primary septicemia plague. Bubonic plague is historically the most common manifestation, characterized by markedly tender and swollen lymph nodes, or buboes, resulting from local lymphangitic spread of the organism. Necrosis of the involved nodes is followed by endotoxemia, leading to cardiovascular and neurologic collapse.[5]

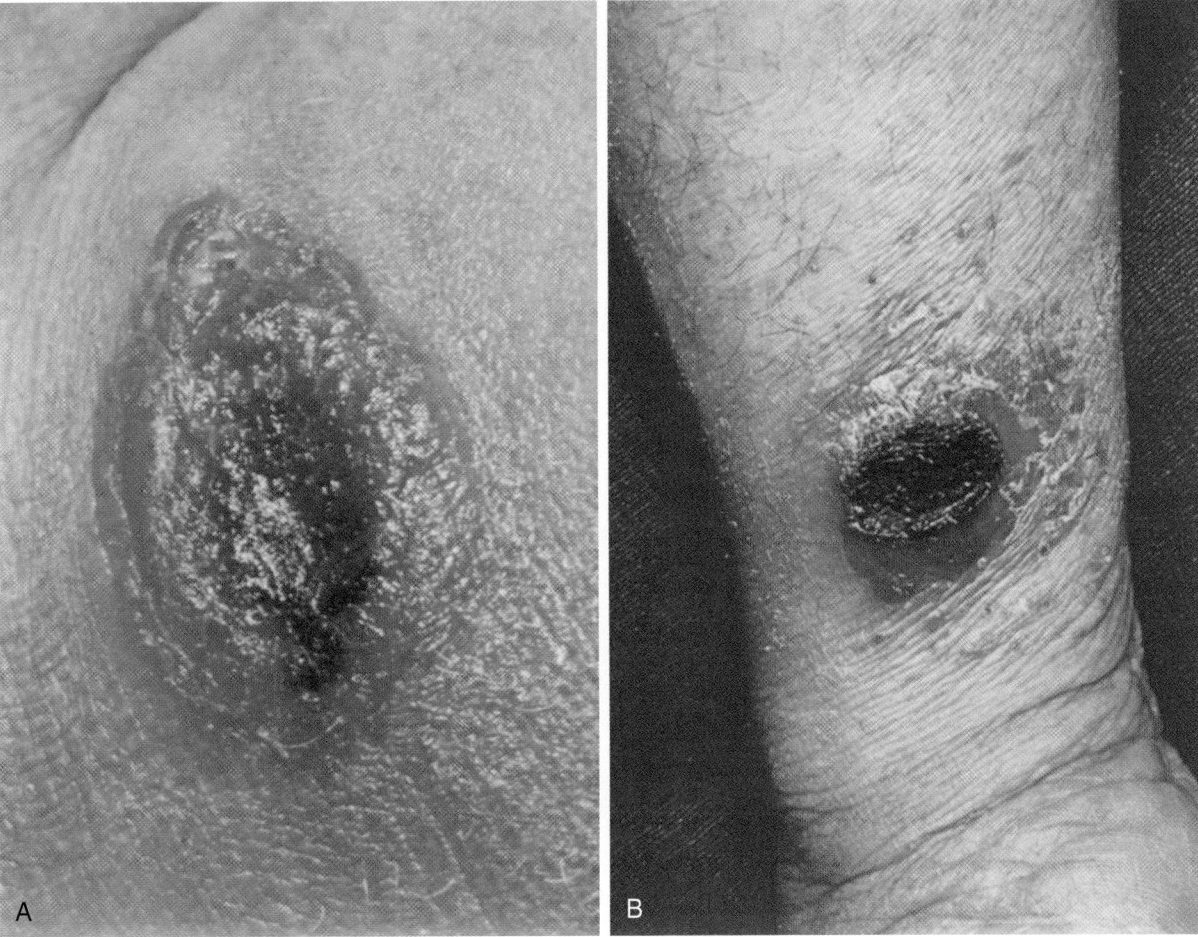

Figure 1 Characteristic black eschar with surrounding erythema and edema. This usually develops 2 to 4 days after incubation. The black scab falls off in 1 to 2 weeks.

Box 1 Most Likely Bioterrorism Agents

Bacillus anthracis (anthrax)
Variola major (smallpox)
Yersinia pestis (plague)
Clostridium botulinum toxin
Francisella tularensis (tularemia)
Viral hemmorhagic fever viruses

Adapted from Centers for Disease Control and Prevention: Biological and chemical terrorism: Strategic plan for preparedness and response. Recommendations of the CDC Strategic Planning Workgroup. MMWR Morb Mortal Wkly Rep 2000;49(RR-40):1-14.

As a biologic weapon, plague would most likely manifest as the primary pneumonic form of the disease resulting from an aerosolized attack. Pneumonic plague is usually a secondary result of bubonic or primary septicemia plague. Primary pneumonic plague is rare in the United States (endemic in parts of the southwest), so such a case should raise the suspicion of a biologic attack.

Botulinum Toxin

As the most potent poison known, *Clostridium botulinum* toxin has been well documented as a biologic weapon, producing paralysis in its victims. Botulinum toxin is a zinc endopeptidase that irreversibly blocks fusion of acetylcholine-containing vesicles with the terminal membrane of the motor neuron, resulting in flaccid paralysis. Natural botulism occurs in three common forms, foodborne, wound, and intestinal.[6] All forms result from toxin absorption through mucosal surfaces or wounds, because botulinum toxin cannot penetrate intact skin. A botulinum toxin attack could take the form of a focused aerosol release in a populated area, or it could be released into a food source.

Tularemia

Francisella tularensis, one of the most infectious pathogenic bacteria known, is the causative organism for tularemia. It is a nonmotile, aerobic, gram-negative, non–spore-forming coccobacillus that can survive for weeks at low temperatures in water, soil, hay, and decaying animal carcasses. Human infection can result from inoculation or inhalation of as few as 10 organisms.[7] Sporadic human cases occur following spread by ticks or biting flies, and occasionally from direct contact with infected animals. Although mortality from tularemia is relatively low and human-to-human transmission is not known to occur, its high infectivity rate and ease of dissemination, coupled with its ability to inflict significant morbidity, make it a candidate for use as a biologic weapon.

Tularemia can assume many clinical forms, depending on the route of exposure. An aerosol release, the most likely route of bioterrorism exposure, would likely result in predominantly pulmonary disease, manifesting in hemorrhagic bronchial inflammation and progressing to pleuropneumonitis. Hilar lymphadenopathy is a common finding. Biologic attack with this agent would most likely occur via aerosolized bacteria, resulting in tularemia with or without pneumonia.

Viral Hemorrhagic Fevers

Four main classes of viruses cause viral hemorrhagic fever (VHF): arenaviruses (Argentine, Bolivian, and Venezuelan hemorrhagic fevers, and Lassa fever), Filovirus (Ebola and Marburg), bunyaviruses (Hantavirus, Congo-Crimean hemorrhagic fever, Rift Valley fever), and flaviviruses (dengue and yellow fever). All are zoonotic RNA (ribonucleic acid) viruses that cause infection naturally in humans by contact with infected animals, most often rodents or arthropods, or through bites or contact with contaminated meat or carcasses. Human-to-human transmission can occur through direct contact with infected fluids and even through contaminated objects.[8] A BT attack most likely would occur from an aerosolized virus. Case-fatality rates range from 0.5% for Omsk hemorrhagic fever to 90% for Ebola.

CLINICAL PRESENTATIONS, SYNDROMES, AND DIFFERENTIAL DIAGNOSES

Table 1[9] summarizes clinical presentations, syndromes, and differential diagnoses of select agents of bioterrorism.

Anthrax

Cutaneous anthrax manifests as a "malignant" ulcer that initially occurs as a painless pruritic papule on the hands or face. The classic coal-appearing black eschar usually evolves over 3 to 7 days.

The clinical diagnosis of inhalational anthrax requires a high degree of suspicion. It generally manifests as a two-stage illness.[10] First, a flulike syndrome begins with nonspecific symptoms of fever, dyspnea, cough, headache, vomiting, rigors, generalized weakness, and abdominal and chest pain. This stage can last from a few hours to a few days.

The second fulminant stage can follow immediately or after a brief period of improvement. The second stage tends to develop abruptly, with fever, dyspnea, diaphoresis, and shock. Stridor can result from upper airway obstruction caused by mediastinal lymphadenopathy and hemorrhage. Chest radiography may demonstrate pulmonary infiltrates, pleural effusions, and a widened mediastinum. The development of hemorrhagic meningitis may be heralded by meningismus, delirium, and obtundation. Death occurs rapidly, and the mortality rate may approach 50%.

Smallpox

Early features of smallpox, which generally begin 12 to 14 days after exposure, include malaise, fever, rigors, vomiting, myalgias, delirium, and rash. Over the next few days, the patient develops mucous membrane lesions and a rash, which progresses from macules to papules to pustules.

Smallpox can be easily confused with varicella (chickenpox), but there are differences. The pustules in smallpox tend to be round, tense, deep, dermal lesions that are all in the same stage of development; in contrast, the pustules of varicella tend to be in various stages of development. In addition, varicella lesions tend to predominate on the trunk, whereas smallpox lesions tend to occur more commonly on the face and extremities, including the palms and soles. Death, which may occur in up to 30% of infected persons, occurs

Table 1 Clinical Presentations, Syndromes, and Differential Diagnoses of Select Bioterrorism Agents

If Patient Has:	Consider:	In Addition to:
Few days of nonspecific flulike symptoms, with nausea, emesis, cough ± chest discomfort, without coryza or rhinorrhea → abrupt onset of respiratory distress ± shock ± mental status changes, with chest x-ray abnormalities (wide mediastinum, infiltrates, pleural effusions)	Inhalational anthrax	Bacterial mediastinitis, tularemia, ruptured aortic aneurysm, SVC syndrome, histoplasmosis, coccidioidomycosis, Q fever, psittacosis, Legionnaires' disease, influenza, sarcoidosis
Pruritic, painless papule → vesicle(s) → ulcer → edematous black eschar ± massive edema and regional adenopathy, ± fever, evolving over 3-7 days	Cutaneous anthrax	Recluse spider bite, atypical Lyme disease, staphylococcal lesion, orf, glanders, tularemia, rat bite fever, ecthyma gangrenosum, plague, rickettsialpox, atypical mycobacteria, diphtheria
Cough, fever, dyspnea, hemoptysis, lung consolidation ± shock	Pneumonic plague	Severe bacterial or viral pneumonia, inhalational anthrax, pulmonary infarct, pulmonary hemorrhage
Sepsis, disseminated intravascular coagulopathy, purpura, acral gangrene	Primary septicemic plague	Meningococcemia; gram-negative, streptococcal, pneumococcal, or staphylococcal bacteremia with shock; overwhelming postsplenectomy sepsis, acute leukemia
Synchronous, progressive papular → vesicular → pustular rash on face, extremities, trunk → generalization ± hemorrhagic component, with systemic toxicity	Smallpox	Atypical varicella, drug eruption, Stevens-Johnson syndrome, atypical measles, secondary syphilis, erythema multiforme, meningococcemia, monkeypox (with African travel history)
Acute febrile illness with pleuropneumonitis, bronchiolitis ± hilar lymphadenopathy, variable progression to respiratory failure	Inhalational tularemia	Inhalational anthrax, influenza, mycoplasma pneumonia, Legionnaires' disease, Q fever, plague
Acute onset of afebrile, symmetrical, descending flaccid paralysis that begins in bulbar muscles, dilated pupils, dry mucous membranes, with normal mental status and absence of sensory changes	Botulism	Brainstem cerebrovascular accident, polio, myasthenia gravis, Guillain-Barré syndrome, tick paralysis, chemical intoxication

SVC, superior vena cava.
Adapted from the Infectious Disease Society of America website. Available at http://www.idsociety.org/WorkArea/showcontent.aspx?id=4284.

from the systemic inflammatory response and cardiovascular collapse.[11,12]

Plague

The onset of plague symptoms follows exposure by 2 to 4 days. Plague is characterized by fever, cough, and dyspnea and may include prominent gastrointestinal symptoms, such as abdominal pain, nausea, vomiting, and diarrhea. The cough may be productive of watery, bloody, or purulent sputum.

Although both inhalational anthrax and pneumonic plague initially have a similar presentation, a productive cough, especially hemoptysis, preferentially suggests plague. Radiographic findings also differ. Plague results in a pneumonic process, whereas anthrax produces a prominent mediastinum in addition to pulmonary infiltrates and pleural effusions.

Botulinum Toxin

Botulism is characterized by descending, symmetrical, flaccid muscle paralysis that first manifests in the bulbar muscles. Regardless of type of exposure to the toxin, acute bilateral cranial neuropathies will occur. Cranial nerve palsies result in diplopia, dysphagia, dysarthria, and ptosis. Other symptoms can include blurred vision, dry mouth, and mydriasis. Fever and sensory complaints or findings are absent. Hypotonia, paralysis of respiratory muscles, and loss of the gag reflex may result in the need for mechanical ventilation. Although the degree of hypotonia can make the patient appear obtunded, the sensorium is preserved, so the clinician must understand that the patient is aware of his or her surroundings.

Tularemia

Naturally occurring forms of tularemia include ulceroglandular, glandular, oculoglandular, oropharyngeal, pneumonic, typhoidal, and septic. Aerosol release of tularemia in a populated area would result in a cluster of people with an acute onset of fever, rigors, headache, coryza, cough, and respiratory distress. Without antibiotic treatment, mortality can reach 30% to 60% for the pulmonic forms, but this drops to 2% with appropriate recognition and antibiotic therapy.

Viral Hemorrhagic Fevers

The syndromes caused by each of the VHF viruses are slightly different, but those that cause the most severe disease have certain characteristics in common. Initially, the clinical syndrome may mimic that of any other viral illness, with fever, generalized malaise, myalgias, dizziness, weakness, and fatigue. Following this nonspecific prodrome, patients may display dermal ecchymosis and bleed from the mouth, eyes, ears, and even internal organs, with predictable presentations and sequelae. Death rarely results directly from blood loss. Rather, end-stage disease is manifest by shock, central nervous system disturbances such as delirium, coma, and seizures, and multisystem organ failure.

DIAGNOSIS

Anthrax

In a previously healthy patient, an overwhelming febrile illness with a widened mediastinum on chest radiography should alert the clinician to the possibility of inhalational anthrax.

Definitive testing can be arranged through local and state health departments or the U.S. Army Medical Research Institute of Infectious Diseases. Rapid diagnostic tests such as the enzyme-linked immunosorbent assay (ELISA) or polymerase chain reaction (PCR) assay are generally available only at reference laboratories. Standard blood cultures and serologic tests are likely the most useful diagnostic tests, but the clinician should alert the laboratory to the possibility of anthrax when the culture is sent. Direct Gram staining of the blood may demonstrate the organism: gram-positive bacilli with bamboo rod appearance. Sputum culture and Gram staining are unlikely to be useful because the disease may not involve a pneumonic process. Postmortem examinations revealing hemorrhagic mediastinitis or hemorrhagic mediastinal lymphadenitis and hemorrhagic meningitis are essentially pathognomonic of inhalational anthrax.[13] Nasal swabs are ineffective for ruling out anthrax and should not be used as a clinical test.

Smallpox

Smallpox virus is shed from the oropharynx and from skin lesions until they are completely healed. The preliminary diagnosis may be made by electron microscopy. Diagnostic confirmation is done through virus isolation, ELISA, and PCR assay from skin scrapings and oropharyngeal swabs in a facility equipped to manage this organism. Once an outbreak has occurred, diagnosis can be made on clinical grounds. The main diagnostic tool for smallpox is the history and physical examination. Public health authorities must be notified based on clinical suspicion alone, without waiting for diagnostic test results.

Plague

Confirmatory tests for plague are generally available only through health departments, which should be notified immediately if plague is strongly suspected. Cultures of blood, sputum, or lymph node aspirate would be useful.[14] The laboratory needs to be notified of the suspicion of plague, because special culturing techniques may be needed. Gram staining may show characteristic safety pin bipolar staining. Chest x-rays reveal patchy infiltrates.

Botulinum Toxin

Botulism is diagnosed clinically. Specialized laboratory testing may take days to confirm the diagnosis, although electromyography may aid in the differential diagnosis. Possible misdiagnoses include Guillain-Barré syndrome, myasthenia gravis, Lambert-Eaton syndrome, tick paralysis, and stroke. Suspected cases of botulism should be reported immediately to local health authorities to expedite epidemiologic investigation, provision of antitoxin when indicated, and prevention of further cases. The CDC is available 24 hours a day to consult with state authorities, facilitate provision of antitoxin when indicated, and provide botulism information.

The CDC emergency operations center can be reached at 770-488-7100 to request equine antitoxin release or consultation about suspected adult botulism cases. The California Infant Botulism Treatment and Prevention Program can be reached at 510-231-7600 for consultation on suspected infant botulism cases.

Tularemia

Diagnosis of tularemia is suspected on clinical grounds when a cluster of patients presents with acute pneumonia, pleuritis, and hilar lymphadenopathy. Routine microbiologic procedures may miss the organism for days or weeks. When tularemia is suspected, direct immunohistochemical or fluorescent antibody stains of fluids or tissue specimens may yield the diagnosis. Growth in culture is the definitive means of diagnosis, but ELISA, PCR assay, and other methods are available in select reference laboratories.[10] Laboratory personnel should be notified promptly whenever tularemia is suspected, because special safety precautions and diagnostic procedures are required.

Viral Hemorrhagic Fevers

Diagnosis of viral hemorrhagic fevers is suspected on clinical grounds, but confirmatory testing with ELISA, PCR assay, and virus isolation is available. Immunoglobulin M and immunoglobulin G titers can also be measured in specialized laboratories. Public health authorities should be notified promptly, even before the diagnosis is confirmed.

TREATMENT AND OUTCOMES

Anthrax

The following information on anthrax therapy and outcomes comes largely from CDC reports and guidelines.[15,16] Antibiotic prophylaxis is indicated based on exposure to known or suspected anthrax spores, not on laboratory testing. Nasal swabs are to be used for epidemiologic but not diagnostic purposes because they can rule in but not rule out exposure.

In suspected cases of active disease, early antibiotic treatment is essential; the clinician should not delay treatment while waiting for disease confirmation. On the basis of past experience and susceptibility testing of recently isolated anthrax strains, the CDC has published antimicrobial recommendations (Table 2). For postexposure prophylaxis, ciprofloxacin or doxycycline is recommended and should be continued for 60 days. Evidence has shown that recently identified strains possess penicillinase and cephalosporinase activity. Concern for a beta-lactamase induction event in the presence of large numbers of organisms has prompted the recommendation that beta-lactams not be used for treatment of active disease.

For treatment of active disease, ciprofloxacin or doxycycline is recommended, given IV for inhalational anthrax and orally for the cutaneous form. This applies even to children and pregnant women, in whom these antibiotics have been generally contraindicated, given the relative risks and benefits.[15-17]

Table 2 Centers for Disease Control and Prevention Recommendations for Antimicrobial Therapy Against Anthrax

Adults	Children
Postexposure Prophylaxis	
Ciprofloxacin, 500 mg PO bid	Ciprofloxacin 10-15 mg/kg PO bid*
or	*or*
Doxycycline, 100 mg PO bid	Doxycycline
	>8 yr and >45 kg, 100 mg PO bid
	>8 yr and ≤45 kg, 2.2 mg/kg PO bid
	>8 yr and ≤45 kg, 2.2 mg/kg PO bid
Cutaneous Anthrax	
Ciprofloxacin, 500 mg PO bid	Ciprofloxacin, 10-15 mg/kg PO bid*
or	*or*
Doxycycline 100 mg PO bid	Doxycycline
	>8 yr and >45 kg, 100 mg PO bid
	>8 yr and ≤45 kg, 2.2 mg/kg PO bid
Inhalation Anthrax	
Ciprofloxacin 400 mg IV bid	Ciprofloxacin, 10-15 mg/kg IV bid*
or	*or*
Doxycycline, 100 mg IV bid	Doxycycline
plus (for either drug)	>8 yr and >45 kg, 100 mg IV bid
One or two additional antibiotics (e.g., rifampin, vancomycin, penicillin, ampicillin, chloramphenicol, imipenem, clindamycin, clarithromycin)	>8 yr and ≤45 kg, 2.2 mg/kg IV bid ≤8 yr, 2.2 mg/kg IV bid *plus* (for either drug) One or two additional antibiotics

*Ciprofloxacin dose in children not to exceed 1 g/day.

Data from Centers for Disease Control and Prevention: Update: Investigation of anthrax associated with intentional exposure and interim public health guidelines, October 2001. MMWR 2001;50:889-893; and Centers for Disease Control and Prevention: Update: Investigation of bioterrorism-related anthrax and interim guidelines for exposure management and antimicrobial therapy, October 2001. MMWR 2001;50:909-919.

The anthrax strains from the postal attack have demonstrated susceptibility to rifampin, clindamycin, vancomycin, and chloramphenicol, although clinical experience with these antibiotics is limited. Erythromycin, azithromycin, trimethoprim-sulfamethoxazole, and cephalosporins should not be used for the treatment of anthrax. The CDC suggests combination therapy with two or more antibiotics until susceptibility testing is performed. IV antibiotics can be switched to oral equivalents when clinically appropriate and continued for 60 days.

If a patient goes to an emergency department or physician's office after being exposed to a suspicious substance, the clinician should isolate the patient and substance while notifying the local health department. Biohazard precautions should be maintained to seal the substance and the patient's clothes in a plastic container, ensuring that the powder is not aerosolized. If the emergency department has decontamination facilities, the patient should shower before entering the clinical care area. The local health department will assist in testing the substance and instituting appropriate infection control measures.

An inactivated acellular vaccine has been used by the U.S. military for several years. The government is stockpiling vaccines against anthrax (75 million doses) and research is under way for an improved anthrax vaccine.

Smallpox

Patients with suspected smallpox should be quarantined, and appropriate respiratory isolation precautions should be taken. Any person known to have been exposed to the virus may be placed in respiratory isolation and observed for signs of the disease until after the standard incubation period, although doing so is considered controversial.

If possible, patients with smallpox should be treated in facilities separate from the usual hospital setting in an effort to minimize the spread of the disease. Even a single case of smallpox would be considered a significant international health event.

There is no specific treatment for smallpox, although cidofovir is effective in vitro.[11] Smallpox vaccine (vaccinia) can be obtained through the CDC, and approximately 35,000 civilian first responders have received booster vaccinations. The federal supply of smallpox vaccine has increased to more than 300 million full doses from an initial stockpile of about 15 million doses. Research is under way to develop a more effective smallpox vaccine for use in immunocompromised persons. Routine vaccination in the United States stopped in 1972, and it is unlikely that people immunized before this time would still have protective immunity.[12] Vaccination up to 4 days after exposure may prevent or attenuate the illness.[13] Vaccinia immune globulin should be given to patients with severe cutaneous reactions to the vaccine and to those with contraindications to vaccination. Secondary bacterial infections are rare, and antibiotic treatment would only be warranted as specific rather than empirical therapy.

Plague

Treatment recommendations for pneumonic plague resulting from a biologic weapons attack are based on limited scientific evidence. The plague vaccine was discontinued in 1999 and is no longer available.

The antibiotic most often recommended and used for the treatment of plague is streptomycin sulfate. Because the availability of streptomycin is now limited, gentamicin is recommended as an alternative.[14] In a large-scale attack, when hospital supplies of IV drugs might be limited, doxycycline is recommended as an alternative for patients suitable for oral therapy. Fluoroquinolones have not been adequately studied in controlled human trials, but have demonstrated clinical efficacy comparable with that of doxycycline in the treatment of pneumonic plague in animal models.[19-21]

Postexposure prophylaxis in the form of IV antibiotics should be given to anyone in an area of a plague outbreak who has a fever. Tachypnea would be considered a sufficient indication in infants. Persons without symptoms who are in close contact with infected patients should receive oral antibiotic prophylaxis with doxycycline for 7 days.[22]

Person-to-person transmission of plague can occur via respiratory droplets, prompting the recommendation that infected patients and asymptomatic close contacts of an infected patient, whether confirmed or suspected, observe strict respiratory isolation precautions until after 48 hours of adequate antibiotic treatment or prophylaxis. Environmental decontamination of plague is not necessary because the organism is sensitive to environmental conditions and is only infective for up to 1 hour after aerosolization.[23]

Botulism

Early recognition of botulism, treatment in an intensive care unit, provision of mechanical ventilation when indicated, and rapid administration of antitoxin (optimally within 12 hours of presentation) are the cornerstones of treatment. An antitoxin available through the CDC and health departments is a trivalent compound active against the three most common types of botulinum toxin. The U.S. Army has an investigational heptavalent antitoxin that may be available during an outbreak. Antitoxin should be given to patients with neurologic signs of botulism at the time of diagnosis unless the patient is already improving.[6] As with any antitoxin, rare adverse reactions may occur, including anaphylaxis and serum sickness. A small test dose should be given before administering the full dose, and appropriate supportive resources should be immediately available.

With improvements in supportive and critical care in the past few decades, mortality from botulism has declined from 25% in the 1950s to 6% in the 1990s.[24] Because botulinum toxin binding is irreversible, patients may remain in critical care units on mechanical ventilation for months while motor neuron fibers regenerate.

Botulism is not transmissible through person-to-person contact, so isolation is unnecessary. Based on risk versus benefit, antitoxin prophylaxis is not recommended for people without symptoms who may have been exposed to the toxin; however, they should remain under close supervision and be treated promptly should symptoms occur. In case of an outbreak, health agencies would work to identify the source of the toxin and perform decontamination procedures, which may be necessary because it could take days for the toxin to degrade naturally.[25]

Tularemia

In addition to supportive care, including appropriate respiratory support and fluid management, antibiotics can significantly decrease the severity of disease and overall mortality. Streptomycin is considered the drug of choice but, because of its limited availability, other aminoglycosides and fluoroquinolones are first-line drugs for the management of tularemia. Alternate choices are doxycycline or chloramphenicol (14-21 days) or ciprofloxacin (10 days).[10]

Viral Hemorrhagic Fevers

Treatment for VHF is mostly supportive. Ribavirin and passive antibody therapy have proved effective in some arenavirus and bunyavirus infections,[9] but no specific therapy has proved useful for *Filovirus* or *Flavivirus* infections. Vaccines are available for yellow fever virus, Rift Valley fever virus, and some of the arenaviruses.[9]

NATIONAL GUIDELINES

Biologic defense is a layered defense system, consisting of accurate threat intelligence, physical countermeasures (e.g., detection, personal protection, decontamination procedures), medical countermeasures (e.g., vaccines, oral chemoprophylaxis, diagnostics, therapeutics), and education and training. Although it is not known whether or when a biologic or chemical attack will take place, clinicians can improve the medical community's readiness for such a situation by disseminating reliable information to others. In the event of a bioterrorism threat, the CDC should be contacted (telephone 1-800-CDC-INFO, or e-mail cdcinfo@cdc.gov). Many resources provide information on chemical and biologic terrorism; however, only reliable sources be contacted because, unfortunately, times like these spawn a few who seek to spread fear and panic through misinformation. For more information, refer to the CDC website at www.cdc.gov, the World Health Organization at www.who.int, and the U.S. Army Medical Research Institute of Infectious Diseases at www.usamriid.army.mil.

Summary

- Biologic warfare and terrorism are real threats and mass casualties could result.
- The U.S. public health system and primary health care providers must be prepared to address various biologic agents, including pathogens that are rarely seen in the United States.
- High-priority agents include organisms that pose a risk to national security because they can be easily disseminated and transmitted from person to person, result in high mortality, might cause public panic and social disruption, and require special action for public health preparedness.
- Such high-priority or category A agents include anthrax, smallpox, plague, botulinum toxin, tularemia, and viral hemorrhagic fevers.
- Medical defenses are available against several threat agents.
- Work needs to be done in many areas before it can be said that we are adequately prepared to respond to an actual biologic weapon attack.

Suggested Readings

Abramova FA, Grinberg LM, Yampolskaya OV, Walker DH: Pathology of inhalation anthrax in 42 cases from the Sverdlovsk outbreak of 1979. Proc Natl Acad Sci USA 1993;90:2291-2294.

Brachman PS: Inhalation anthrax. Ann NY Acad Sci 1980;353:83-93.

Centers for Disease Control and Prevention: Biological and chemical terrorism: Strategic plan for preparedness and response. Recommendations of the CDC Strategic Planning Workgroup. MMWR Morb Mortal Wkly Rep 2000;49(RR–40):1-14.

Dennis DT, Inglesby TV, Henderson DA, et al: Tularemia as a biological weapon: Medical and public health management. JAMA 2001;285:2763-2773.

Franz DR, Jahrling PB, Friedlander AM, et al: Clinical recognition and management of patients exposed to biological warfare agents. JAMA 1997;278:399-411.

Inglesby TV, Dennis DT, Henderson DA, et al: Plague as a biological weapon: Medical and public health management. JAMA 2000;283:2281-2290.

Inglesby TV, Henderson DA, Bartlett JG, et al: Anthrax as a biological weapon: Medical and public health management. JAMA 1999;281:1735-1745.

References

For a complete list of references, log onto www.expertconsult.com.

Sexually Transmitted Diseases

Rabin K. Shrestha and Kristin Englund

The term *sexually transmitted diseases* (STDs) refers to many diseases and the number keeps expanding with the discovery of newer pathogens (e.g., HIV) or a new route of acquisition of a known pathogen (e.g., hepatitis C). The terminology can be confusing as well. Historically, the term *venereal disease* was used for the class of diseases known to be transmitted by sexual intercourse. Other terminology includes sexually transmitted infections, because some infections may be asymptomatic and not cause disease, sexually transmissible diseases and infections, because some diseases such as hepatitis C may be transmitted predominantly by a nonsexual route, and reproductive tract infections, because the sexual transmission of some diseases such as bacterial vaginosis are still debated. In this chapter, STD is used to encompass all these diseases. Although there is a vast number of STDs, only a few important ones that are classically associated with sexual transmission will be discussed. HIV infection is not discussed in this chapter.

STDs have complex social, political, and public health implications, in addition to their medical significance. Even with the introduction of effective treatments such as penicillin for syphilis more than 60 years ago, syphilis continues to remain an important disease. In fact, the rate of syphilis in men who have sex with men (MSM) is on the rise in some areas in the United States. STDs remain among the most common infectious diseases in developed and developing countries. The fact that diseases for which there are effective therapies that can be prevented by changing behavior are still rampant illustrates the complex nature of these diseases and the enormous challenges faced by the medical and public health communities in dealing with them.

The STDs discussed in this chapter can be categorized into two main categories: diseases characterized by genital ulcers and those characterized by genital discharge.

SEXUALLY TRANSMITTED DISEASES WITH ULCERS

Herpes simplex virus (HSV) infections, syphilis, and chancroid account for almost all the STDs characterized by genital ulcers in the United States. More than one may be present in a patient who presents with genital ulcers and each of these diseases has been associated with an increased risk of HIV infection. A diagnosis based only on the patient's medical history and examination is often inaccurate and laboratory confirmation should be sought. Often, the clinician must treat the patient before laboratory results are available. In this case, the clinician should treat based on the clinical presentation or epidemiologic circumstances. Even after a complete diagnostic evaluation, at least 25% of patients who have genital ulcers have no laboratory-confirmed diagnosis. Noninfectious causes of genital ulcers, including Crohn's disease, Behçet's disease, and traumatic ulcers, should be considered.

Herpes Simplex Virus Infections

Genital HSV infection prevalence has markedly increased over the past two decades. About 50 million persons in the United States have genital HSV infection based on seroprevalence studies and most of them remain undiagnosed. Most infections are transmitted by those who are asymptomatic. Two serotypes, HSV-1 and HSV-2 have been identified, and both have been implicated as the pathogen in genital HSV infection. Although genital HSV infections are usually caused by HSV-2, up to 50% of first episodes of genital herpes are caused by HSV-1. However, recurrences are much less frequent for HSV-1; thus, distinction of the serotypes influences prognosis and counseling. HSV-2 infections are almost always sexually acquired, whereas HSV-1 infections may be caused by anogenital or orolabial infections.

Laboratory diagnosis of HSV infections consists of virologic and serologic tests. Viral culture is the preferred test for patients with mucocutaneous lesions. However, the sensitivity is low and declines rapidly as lesions begin to heal. Antigen detection by direct fluorescent antibody (DFA) and polymerase chain reaction (PCR) assays to detect viral DNA are other methods. The PCR assay is not widely available and has not been well studied for genital lesions but is the preferred method of diagnosis in spinal fluid specimens. Type-specific serologic tests are useful for the diagnosis of patients who are asymptomatic or for whom virologic test results are negative. Cytologic detection of cellular changes from lesions (using the Tzanck test) is insensitive and nonspecific and should not be relied on for diagnosis.

The clinical manifestations of first-episode genital HSV infections differ greatly from recurrent episodes and will be discussed separately.

First-Episode Genital Herpes Infection

Primary genital HSV infection is one in which the patient has not had prior infection by any HSV serotype. Patients with primary infection are more likely to have a symptomatic and more severe infection.

First-episode infections often are associated with prolonged systemic and local symptoms. Systemic symptoms include fever, headache, malaise, and myalgias. These appear in the first 3 to 4 days after the onset of lesions and gradually recede over the next 3 to 4 days. Local symptoms are characterized by papules or vesicular lesions that coalesce to form painful ulcers and can also include itching, urethral discharge, dysuria, vaginal discharge, and painful inguinal adenopathy. Cervicitis manifesting with ulcerative lesions in the exocervix and purulent or bloody vaginal discharge may be present. Local symptoms often last 3 weeks and peak at about the end of the first week. Pharyngitis and proctitis can also occur, depending on the site of inoculation of the virus. Complications of first-episode genital HSV infection include aseptic meningitis (usually with HSV-2), urinary retention (because of autonomic dysfunction), transverse myelitis, and extragenital lesions, usually on the buttocks and caused by autoinoculation, disseminated infection with both cutaneous or visceral involvement and pelvic inflammatory disease. Women may also be superinfected by yeast vaginitis during the course of the illness.

Most patients with primary genital herpes should receive antiviral therapy because they may have mild symptoms early but could develop severe disease later. The recommended therapy is acyclovir, 200 mg five times daily or 400 mg three times daily, or famciclovir, 250 mg three times daily, or valacyclovir, 1 g twice daily. The recommended duration of therapy is 7 to 10 days.

Recurrent Genital Herpes

Almost all persons infected with HSV-2 have the infection reactivated in the genital region. About 60% of episodes are preceded by prodromal symptoms, such as a mild tingling sensation or shooting pains in the buttocks or hips. The lesions tend to be more severe in women. As with the primary episode, the lesions are classically described as painful vesicles that ulcerate and later crust, without leaving a scar. However, compared with the primary episode, the lesions are less painful, heal faster, and are not associated with systemic symptoms. Also, the lesions may not be typical, and all genital ulcers should be evaluated for HSV. The frequency of recurrences decreases over time.

The strategy for managing recurrent episodes consists of episodic treatment to ameliorate or shorten the duration of illness or suppressive treatment to reduce the frequency of recurrences. Recommended regimens for episodic treatment include acyclovir, 400 mg three times daily or 800 mg twice daily, famciclovir, 125 mg twice daily, or valacyclovir, 500 mg twice daily or 1 g daily. The recommended duration of therapy is 5 days, except for valacyclovir, 500 mg twice daily, which has been shown to be as effective with 3-day therapy as 5-day therapy. Treatment should be started within 1 day of onset of lesions; hence, the patient should be provided with a prescription for of the relevant drug(s) so that therapy can be self-initiated when symptoms arise.

Suppressive treatment has been shown to reduce the frequency of genital herpes by 70% to 80% in patients who have more than six recurrent episodes per year. Recommendations for suppressive therapy include acyclovir, 400 mg twice daily, famciclovir, 250 mg twice daily, or valacyclovir, 1 g daily. Because the frequency of recurrences decreases over time, continuation of suppressive therapy should be reassessed periodically.

Other Considerations

Severe Disease. In patients with severe disease or with disseminated infection such as meningitis, IV acyclovir should be given. The recommended regimen is acyclovir, 5 to 10 mg/kg body weight every 8 hours for 2 to 7 days, or until clinical improvement is observed, followed by oral therapy for a total of 10 days.

Herpes Simplex Virus in Pregnancy. The risk of neonatal herpes in an infant born to a mother who has primary HSV infection is 30% to 50% and is less than 1% in mothers with a history of recurrent herpes or those who acquire herpes in the first half of pregnancy. Prevention of neonatal herpes depends both on preventing the acquisition of HSV during late pregnancy and avoiding exposure of the infant to herpetic lesions during delivery. It is recommended that mothers with a history of recurrent genital HSV infection who have prodromal symptoms or herpetic lesions on examination undergo cesarean section to lessen the chance of neonatal herpes infection.

Herpes Simplex Virus in HIV infection. HSV infection increases the risk of HIV infection. In addition, HIV patients may have more severe and prolonged episodes of recurrent herpes. The recommendations for episodic and suppressive therapy differ from those for immunocompetent patients. Recommended therapy for episodic treatment is oral therapy for 5 to 10 days with acyclovir, 400 mg three times daily or 200 mg five times daily, famciclovir, 500 mg twice daily, or valacyclovir, 1 g twice daily. Recommended therapy for suppressive therapy is oral therapy as follows: acyclovir, 400 to 800 mg two or three times daily, famciclovir, 500 mg twice daily, or valacyclovir, 500 mg twice daily.

Counseling Discordant Couples. Transmission of HSV from the patient to a seronegative partner can occur during asymptomatic shedding. Hence, discordant couples should be advised to abstain from sexual activity when active lesions are present and encouraged to use condoms consistently at other times. However, condoms do not fully prevent transmission because there can be asymptomatic shedding from areas such as the perineum, which are not protected by condoms.

Syphilis

Syphilis is a systemic disease caused by the spirochete *Treponema pallidum*. The natural history of syphilis consists of different stages with distinctive clinical stages: primary, secondary, latent, and tertiary syphilis. Neurosyphilis, often considered part of tertiary syphilis, can occur with any of the different stages and requires special attention because of its therapeutic implications. Syphilis and its complications were common in medical practice in the earlier part of the 20th century. After the introduction of penicillin and public health efforts to control the disease, its prevalence has declined. Advanced stages of syphilis are now rare and clinicians are often unfamiliar with its various manifestations. However, outbreaks have occurred in several groups and, in the presence of HIV infection, may manifest different signs and symptoms. Thus, there is renewed interest in this disease.

Because it has not been possible to grow the organisms in vitro, definitive diagnosis depends on visualizing the organisms by dark field microscopy or DFA tests of lesion exudates or tissue. A presumptive diagnosis can be made based on two types of serologic tests: nontreponemal tests (e.g., Venereal Diseases Research Laboratory [VDRL]) and rapid plasma reagin [RPR]); and treponemal tests, such as fluorescent treponemal antibody adsorption (FTA-ABS) and *T. pallidum* particle agglutination (TP-PA) assays. Nontreponemal test titers correlate with disease activity and therefore should be quantitative. Treatment can be considered effective if follow-up titers at 6 months have fallen at least fourfold. They usually become negative after treatment. If the titer has dropped at least fourfold, but remains positive, the patient is considered serofast (usually in the 1:2 to 1:4 range). Sequential tests in individual patients should be performed using the same test because the two tests (VDRL and RPR) cannot be compared. Patients who have positive treponemal test results generally remain positive for the rest of their lives.

The incubation period of syphilis is 10 to 90 days (average, 2 weeks). Clinical manifestations depend on the stage of the disease, which are discussed here.

Primary Syphilis

The lesion of primary syphilis starts as a painless papule at the site of inoculation, which subsequently develops into an ulcer (chancre). The chancre is a painless, slightly elongated ulcer 1 to 2 cm across, with a clean base and an indurated margin. Moderate painless, bilateral, inguinal lymphadenopathy is usually present. Lesions are usually solitary and can be missed if they are not in visible regions because of their painless nature. Untreated, they spontaneously heal in 3 to 6 weeks. Treatment is with benzathine penicillin, 2.4 million units IM, in a single dose.

Secondary Syphilis

Secondary syphilis develops 4 to 10 weeks after the initial appearance of primary lesions. It starts as an evanescent macular rash followed in a few days by a symmetrical papular eruption involving the entire trunk and extremities. Characteristically, it involves the palms and soles. The papules are reddish brown and generally scaly, and may be mistaken for psoriasis. Other manifestations could be a patchy alopecia (moth-eaten alopecia), mucosal lesions (painless aphthous ulcers or gray plaques), condyloma latum (raised, moist whitish lesions in warm moist areas such as the axilla or groin region), and lymphadenopathy. It is a systemic disease with possible symptoms of low-grade fever, sore throat, headache, malaise, and weight loss. The lesions of primary and secondary syphilis are highly infectious. Treatment, as for primary syphilis, is benzathine penicillin, 2.4 million units IM in a single dose.

Latent Syphilis

If secondary syphilis is untreated, there is a spontaneous resolution of symptoms in 3 to 12 weeks. The patient then enters into the latent phase, during which the patient is asymptomatic but has serologic evidence of ongoing infection. During the first year of latent syphilis, the patient may have relapses of secondary syphilis. This phase is early latent syphilis. After the first year, during the late latent phase, it is highly unlikely that the patient will have any recurrences of secondary syphilis. Often, the duration of infection cannot be determined to classify the infection as early or late.

These patients, with latent syphilis of unknown duration, should be treated as if they had late latent syphilis. Recommended treatment for early latent syphilis is benzathine penicillin, 2.4 million units IM in a single dose. The recommended treatment for late latent syphilis is benzathine penicillin, 2.4 million units IM given weekly for 3 weeks consecutively.

Tertiary Syphilis

About one third of patients with late latent disease go on to develop tertiary syphilis if left untreated. This includes gummatous disease (benign late syphilis), cardiovascular syphilis, and neurosyphilis.

Gummatous disease, now uncommon, can manifest as recurrent nodular lesions in the skin that ulcerate and heal leaving an atrophic scar. In addition to the skin, skeletal and upper respiratory tract areas are the more common sites involved.

Cardiovascular syphilis consists mainly of an aortitis of the ascending aorta. The aortic valve and coronary ostia may also be involved. Gummatous disease and cardiovascular syphilis are treated with benzathine penicillin, 2.4 million units IM given weekly for 3 weeks consecutively.

Neurosyphilis is classically described as a part of tertiary syphilis. There may be several forms with overlap, among them; these forms include asymptomatic, meningeal, meningovascular, parenchymatous (general paresis and tabes dorsalis), and gummatous disease. Asymptomatic syphilis is manifest by cerebrospinal fluid (CSF) findings suggestive of meningitis. Usually, there is a CSF pleocytosis, predominantly lymphocytic, with more than 5 cells/mm^3. The protein level is elevated and there may be decreased glucose levels. The VDRL test result is positive in most cases; this is specific but not very sensitive. The FTA-ABS test result on the CSF is sensitive but not specific and may be used to exclude a diagnosis of central nervous system (CNS) syphilis when the CSF VDRL test result is negative. Syphilitic meningitis manifests as cranial nerve palsies and hearing loss caused by basilar meningitis. There may also be signs of uveitis. Meningovascular syphilis can result in cerebrovascular accidents.

The recommended treatment regimen for neurosyphilis is aqueous penicillin G, 18 to 24 million units daily, given as 3 to 4 million units IV every 4 hours or as a continuous infusion for 10 to 14 days. Alternatively, procaine penicillin, 2.4 million units IM once daily, plus probenecid, 500 mg PO four times daily, may be given, both for 10 to 14 days. A CSF examination should be repeated every 6 months until the cell count is normal. If the cell count has not decreased after 6 months or the CSF is not normal after 2 years, retreatment should be considered.

Other Considerations

Jarisch-Herxheimer Reaction. After treatment for primary or secondary syphilis patients may have a febrile reaction because of the release of treponemal constituents. It starts 4 to 6 hours after treatment, subsides in 24 hours, and is characterized by fever, chills, headache, arthralgias, and a transient increase in prominence of the lesions. Patients should be managed with an anti-inflammatory agent such as ibuprofen.

Penicillin Allergy. For patients with primary or secondary syphilis or early latent syphilis, other options include doxycycline, 100 mg PO twice daily for 14 days, or tetracycline, 500 mg PO four times daily for 14 days. Ceftriaxone, 1 g IM or IV daily for 8 to 10 days, is another option. Some reports have suggested that azithromycin, 2 g PO as a single dose is effective. However, other reports have suggested that there may be substantial resistance to azithromycin, based on molecular studies, so caution should be used with this approach. For patients with late latent syphilis, doxycycline or tetracycline may be used for 28 days. For patients with neurosyphilis, ceftriaxone, 2 g IV or IM for 10 to 14 days, may be used. Pregnant women who are allergic to penicillin should be desensitized and treated with penicillin.

Follow-up. Because any therapy could fail, follow-up is extremely important. In patients without HIV, 6-month and 1- and 2-year follow-ups are recommended. Patients who have continued signs and symptoms or a fourfold increase in titer during follow-up are considered to be therapeutic failures. Also, if patients do not achieve a fourfold decrease in nontreponemal titers in 6 months, they are considered therapeutic failures. In this case, the patient should be checked for HIV and neurosyphilis. For therapeutic failures, the patient should receive three weekly doses of benzathine penicillin.

Syphilis in HIV-Infected Persons. Patients with HIV infection have an increased risk of developing neurosyphilis, even if they are not severely immunocompromised, and the disease may progress more rapidly. In addition, they may have higher rates of treatment failure. Some specialists have recommended treatment for primary syphilis, secondary syphilis, and early latent syphilis in HIV-infected patients with 2.4 million units of benzathine penicillin every week for 3 weeks. In addition, many specialists would do a CSF examination to rule out neurosyphilis before starting treatment. Follow-up is recommended at 3-month intervals in HIV-infected patients for the first year of follow-up.

Syphilis in Pregnancy. Infants born to mothers at any stage of syphilis are at risk of becoming infected with congenital syphilis. The mode of transmission is transplacental. The risk, however, decreases with later stages of disease. Syphilis during pregnancy is associated with increased risk of miscarriage. All pregnant women should be screened serologically for syphilis at their first prenatal visit. Treatment should consist of the penicillin regimen appropriate for the stage of syphilis. Penicillin-allergic patients should be desensitized and treated with penicillin.

Chancroid

Chancroid is an ulcerative disease caused by *Haemophilus ducreyi*. The U.S. incidence of chancroid has declined since 1987, with less than 100 cases per year reported to the Centers for Disease Control and Prevention (CDC). It usually occurs in discrete outbreaks, although it is endemic in some U.S. regions. About 10% of persons in the United States who acquire chancroid are coinfected with *T. pallidum* or HSV.

Clinically, it manifests as a tender erythematous papule that may develop at the site of inoculation after 4 to 7 days. This then progresses to form a pustule that may rupture after 2 to 3 more days to form painful shallow ulcers. These ulcers typically have a granulomatous base, with purulent exudates and overhanging margins. Painful tender lymphadenopathy is seen in up to 50% of cases and is usually unilateral; this may become fluctuant and drain spontaneously unless aspirated or drained by incision.

Chancroid ulcers take several weeks or months to resolve in the absence of effective therapy. As with other ulcerative diseases, chancroid is a cofactor in the transmission of HIV.

The definitive microbiologic diagnosis of chancroid is challenging, so chancroid is usually diagnosed clinically. A special medium is required to isolate *H. ducreyi* in culture, and is not widely available. Even using this medium, the sensitivity is less than 80%. Several commercial laboratories offer DNA amplification assays for *H. ducreyi* but these are not widely available. For treatment purposes, a probable diagnosis can be made if the following criteria are met: the patient has one or more painful genital ulcers; the patient has no evidence of *T. pallidum* infection by dark field examination of ulcer exudates or by serologic testing for syphilis performed at least 7 days after the onset of ulcers; the clinical presentation, appearance of genital ulcers and, if present, regional lymphadenopathy are typical of chancroid; and a test for HSV performed on the ulcer exudates is negative. It must be remembered that such a definition excludes coinfections.

Treatment

Recommended regimens are as follows:

- Azithromycin, 1 g PO single dose, *or*
- Ceftriaxone, 250 mg IM single dose, *or*
- Ciprofloxacin, 500 mg PO twice daily for 3 days, *or*
- Erythromycin base, 500 mg PO three times daily for 7 days

Patients with HIV and uncircumcised men do not respond well to therapy, compared to those who are HIV negative and circumcised. These patients should be carefully followed. Some specialists recommend using the erythromycin 7-day regimen for HIV-positive patients. Patients should be tested for HIV when chancroid is diagnosed. Patients who test negative for HIV and syphilis when chancroid is diagnosed should be retested again for these diseases after 3 months.

Patients should be re-examined within 3 to 7 days; they should have symptomatic improvement within 3 days and objective improvement within 7 days after therapy is initiated. If no clinical improvement is apparent, consideration should be given to the possibility of an incorrect diagnosis, coinfection with another STD such as HSV or syphilis, HIV coinfection, noncompliance, or resistance of the organism. Complete healing of the ulcer may take longer than 2 weeks. Resolution of fluctuant lymphadenopathy is slower than ulcers. These buboes should be drained to provide symptomatic relief to the patient and avoid spontaneous rupture. Sexual partners of patients with chancroid should be treated regardless of symptoms if they have had sexual contact with the patient within 10 days preceding the patient's onset of symptoms.

Lymphogranuloma Venereum

Lymphogranuloma venereum (LGV) is caused by the L1, L2, and L3 serovars of *Chlamydia trachomatis*. These serovars are more invasive than other *C. trachomatis* serovars. The disease is rare in the United States and other industrialized nations but is endemic in Africa, southeast Asia, Central and South America, and the Caribbean islands.

The clinical manifestations of LGV can be divided into three stages. After an incubation period of 3 to 30 days at the site of inoculation, the patient may develop a painless papule that may ulcerate (primary stage). The lesion is self limited and often may go unnoticed. After several weeks of the primary lesion, the patients may have involvement of the inguinal lymph nodes or the anus and rectum (secondary stage). Inguinal lymph nodes are usually involved in men. The lymphadenopathy is typically unilateral, tender, and firm. It may manifest on both sides of the inguinal ligament, which forms a groove, called the groove sign. Stellate abscesses that are present in the lymph nodes coalesce and form discharging sinuses. Many patients present with systemic complaints such as fever, myalgias, and headache.

Anorectal involvement manifests as an acute hemorrhagic proctitis. Patients present with rectal pain and bleeding and often with pronounced systemic complains. A recent outbreak in the Netherlands in MSM highlights the importance of awareness of this manifestation of LGV.

In untreated LGV, fibrosis caused by chronic inflammation is present (tertiary stage). Fibrosis can lead to lymphatic obstruction and elephantiasis of the genitalia in either gender. Rectal involvement may cause strictures and fistulas. These conditions are more common in women and can lead to widespread destruction of the genitalia, a condition known as *esthiomene* (from the Greek, "eating away").

Diagnosis may be made by serologic testing or detection of the organism. Because the disease is invasive, antibody titers to *Chlamydia* are high. Laboratory criteria consistent with a diagnosis of LGV include a complement fixation titer for *Chlamydia* of 1:64 or higher, or a microimmunofluorescence test for *C. trachomatis* titer of 1:128 or higher. *C. trachomatis* may also be identified in buboes by tissue culture or by DFA staining on a bubo or ulcer smear. A PCR diagnostic assay has been described.

Treatment

Treatment cures infection and prevents ongoing tissue scarring. The recommended regimen is doxycycline, 100 mg PO twice daily for 21 days. An alternative regimen is erythromycin base, 500 mg PO four times daily for 21 days. Some specialists believe that azithromycin, 1 g PO once weekly for 3 weeks is effective, but clinical data are lacking.

Patients should be followed until signs and symptoms have resolved. Sexual partners of the patient within the last 60 days should be evaluated. In the absence of symptoms, sexual partners should be treated with azithromycin, 1 g PO as a single dose, or doxycycline, 100 mg PO twice daily for 7 days.

Granuloma Inguinale (Donovanosis)

Granuloma inguinale is caused by the bacterium *Calymmatobacterium granulomatis*, which has been seldom isolated on culture. The disease is rare in the United States but endemic in Papua, New Guinea, parts of South Africa and India, Brazil, and among aborigines in Australia. In addition to sexual transmission, the disease may also be transmitted during birth and to children, probably when sitting on the laps of infected persons.

The incubation period is uncertain, with estimates ranging from 1 to 360 days. Experimental lesions in humans appear after 50 days of inoculation. The lesions of donovanosis start as a firm papule that ulcerates. Lymphadenopathy is typically absent. Classically, four types of lesions are described: ulcerogranulomatous (nontender beefy red lesions that bleed easily on touch); hypertrophic or verrucous ulcer, with irregular margins; necrotic, foul-smelling deep ulcers causing tissue destruction; and sclerotic or cicatricial lesions, with fibrous or scar tissue. Lesions generally occur in the genital areas or inguinal region. Lesions may also occur in the cervix or upper genital tract of women. Occasionally, lesions may appear in the oral cavity or pharynx. Rarely, disseminated infection is present, which may involve the bone and liver, and is usually associated with pregnancy and cervical infection.

Diagnosis requires visualization of dark-staining Donovan bodies on tissue crush section or biopsy. Other methods of preparation of the specimen have been described. One technique is to firmly roll a cotton-tipped swab across the surface of the lesion after removing debris from the surface of the wound. The swab is then rolled over a glass slide and stained by a rapid Giemsa method. If multiple samples for different tests are taken at the same time, the sample for Donovan bodies should be taken first so that enough cells are obtained.

The treatment regimen recommended by the CDC is as follows:

- Doxycycline, 100 mg PO twice daily for at least 3 weeks, *or*
- Alternative regimens include the following:
- Ciprofloxacin, 750 mg twice daily for at least 3 weeks, *or*
- Erythromycin, base 500 mg PO twice daily for at least 3 weeks, *or*
- Azithromycin, 1 g PO once/week for at least 3 weeks
- Trimethoprim-sulfamethoxazole, one double-strength tablet PO twice daily for at least 3 weeks

Three weeks of the above-recommended therapy is generally sufficient, although the addition of an aminoglycoside such as gentamicin, 1 mg/kg IV every 8 hours, to these regimens may be considered if improvement is not evident in the first few days of therapy.

Despite optimal therapy, relapse can occur after 6 to 18 months. Persons who have had sexual contact with the patient within 60 days before onset of the patient's symptoms should be examined and offered therapy, although the value of treating asymptomatic contacts has not been established.

SEXUALLY TRANSMITTED DISEASES WITH GENITAL DISCHARGE

Pelvic Inflammatory Disease

Pelvic inflammatory disease (PID) is the term used to describe any single infection or combination of infections of the upper female genital tract such as endometritis, salpingitis, tubo-ovarian abscess and pelvic peritonitis. In the United States alone, approximately 1,200,000 women and girls acquire PID annually; of these, 100,000 are likely to become infertile as a result of the infection, and more than 150 will die as a result of PID or its complications. Even mild to moderate or asymptomatic disease could result in long-term morbidity, such as infertility, ectopic pregnancy, and chronic pelvic pain.

PID is caused by various organisms. The sexually transmitted organisms *C. trachomatis* and *Neisseria gonorrhoeae* are believed to be important in the pathogenesis. Gonococcus infection generally causes a more acute illness, whereas that caused by *Chlamydia* tends to be mild or subtle. Other organisms generally found in the vaginal flora have also been implicated: namely anaerobes, facultative gram-negative organisms, and streptococci. In addition, cytomegalovirus, *Mycoplasma hominis*, and *Ureaplasma urealyticum* may be causative agents. Immunologic mechanisms seem to be important, especially in *Chlamydia* infection, in which recurrent episodes tend to be more severe than the first. Risk factors for PID include younger age (teenagers), STDs (*Chlamydia*, gonococcus, and bacterial vaginosis), intrauterine contraceptive devices, and douching. Oral contraceptives have been associated with a decreased severity of PID caused by *Chlamydia*, probably by modifying the immune response of the body.

The diagnosis of PID is difficult and a combination of signs, symptoms, and tests may be used. The clinical diagnosis of PID has a positive predictive value of 65% to 90% compared with that for laparoscopy. Some cases are asymptomatic and many cases go undiagnosed because of mild or nonspecific symptoms. In addition, a delay in initiating treatment has been shown to increase the risk of long-term gynecologic complications. It is therefore recommended that health care providers have a low threshold for the diagnosis of PID and that empirical therapy be initiated promptly. The minimum criteria in women at risk of STDs for the diagnosis of PID, when no other cause of illness can be identified, include uterine or adnexal tenderness and cervical motion tenderness.

Additional criteria used to increase diagnostic specificity, especially in low-risk women, include the following:

- Oral temperature higher than 101° F (38.3° C)
- Abnormal vaginal or uterine mucopurulent discharge
- Presence of white blood cells on saline microscopy of vaginal secretions
- Elevated erythrocyte sedimentation rate
- Elevated C-reactive protein level
- Laboratory documentation of cervical infection with *N. gonorrhoeae* or *C. trachomatis*

If the cervical discharge appears normal and no white cells are seen on a vaginal wet preparation, the diagnosis of PID is unlikely and alternative causes of pain should be considered. More specific criteria for the diagnosis of PID include an endometrial biopsy showing endometritis, transvaginal ultrasound or magnetic resonance imaging showing a fluid-filled salpinx (or salpinges), or laparoscopic findings consistent with PID.

PID may occasionally manifest more acutely with peritonitis and frank vaginal discharge. Acute complications of PID include periappendicitis and perihepatitis (Fitz-Hugh–Curtis syndrome).

Treatment

In the past, many specialists recommended that all patients with PID be hospitalized so that bed rest and parenteral antibiotics could be initiated. However, outpatient therapy is being increasingly used, based on the important PEACH trial data. This randomized clinical trial (*P*ID *e*valuation *a*nd *c*linical *h*ealth [PEACH]) compared short- and long-term outcomes of parenteral (cefoxitin-doxycycline) with oral (cefoxitin-probenecid or ceftriaxone plus doxycycline) for mild to moderate symptomatic PID in several U.S. centers showed no difference in short-term and long-term outcomes.

The treatment regimen generally consists of antibiotics that will be effective against *N. gonorrhoeae*, *C. trachomatis*, anaerobes, facultative gram-negative bacilli, and streptococci.

Recommended Parenteral Treatment. Parenteral treatment regimens include the following:

- Cefoxitin, 2 g IV every 6 hours (or cefotetan, 2 g IV every 12 hours) plus doxycycline, 100 mg PO or IV every 12 hours. IV therapy is continued for 24 hours after clinical improvement. The patient can then take oral doxycycline to complete 14 days of therapy. If the patient has a tubo-ovarian abscess, metronidazole or clindamycin may be added for better anaerobic coverage.
- Clindamycin, 900 mg IV every 8 hours, plus gentamicin, 2-mg/kg IV loading dose followed by 1.5 mg/kg every 8 hours (single daily dosing may be substituted). Parenteral therapy can be discontinued after 24 hours of clinical improvement and the patient can be switched to oral therapy with clindamycin, 450 mg PO four times daily, or doxycycline, 100 mg PO twice daily, to complete 14 days of therapy.

Alternative, less-preferred regimens include the following:

- Ofloxacin, 400 mg IV every 12 hours (or levofloxacin, 500 mg IV every 24 hours), with or without metronidazole
- Ampicillin-sulbactam, 3 g IV every 6 hours, plus doxycycline, 100 mg PO or IV every 12 hours

These regimens can be switched to oral therapy when clinical improvement is apparent.

ORAL AND INTRAMUSCULAR TREATMENTS

Oral or intramuscular treatments can be given to patients who do not appear very ill, are not pregnant, do not have a tubo-ovarian abscess, can tolerate oral therapy, and for whom surgical emergencies such as appendicitis is unlikely. Patients who do not improve despite 72 hours of oral therapy should be admitted for parenteral therapy.

The recommended oral and IM regimens are as follows:

- Ofloxacin, 400 mg PO once daily (or levofloxacin, 500 mg PO once daily), with or without metronidazole, 500 mg PO twice daily, administered for 14 days
- Ceftriaxone, 250 mg IM single dose, or cefoxitin, 2 g IM single dose, and probenecid, 1 g PO administered concurrently or another third-generation cephalosporin administered parenterally, plus doxycycline, 100 mg PO twice daily (with or without metronidazole, 500 mg PO twice daily), administered for 14 days.

Follow-up is necessary, especially for oral therapy. Clinical improvement should be apparent in 72 hours. Some specialists have recommend rescreening for *N. gonorrhoeae* and *C. trachomatis* 4 to 6 weeks after completion of therapy. Male sexual partners of women with PID should be treated empirically, even if they are asymptomatic, with a regimen that covers both *N. gonorrhoeae* and *C. trachomatis* to prevent reinfection.

Bacterial Vaginosis

Bacterial vaginosis (BV) is a clinical syndrome resulting from the replacement of normal hydrogen peroxide–producing *Lactobacillus* in the vagina with high concentrations of anaerobic bacteria, *Gardnerella vaginalis*, and *Mycoplasma hominis*. It does not appear to be a sexually transmitted disease, although it has been associated with having multiple sex partners. However, it is the most common cause of vaginal discharge or malodor and is commonly encountered in the context of STDs. This syndrome will be summarized here.

The clinical diagnosis of BV requires three of the following four symptoms or signs: a homogeneous, white, noninflammatory discharge that smoothly coats the vaginal walls; the presence of clue cells on microscopic examination (clue cells are squamous epithelial cells covered with many vaginal bacteria, giving the cells a stippled appearance); a vaginal fluid pH higher than 4.5; and a fishy odor of vaginal discharge before or after the addition of 10% KOH (positive whiff test).

A diagnosis can also be made based on Gram staining criteria. Scoring for the absence of large gram-positive rods (*Lactobacillus*), and the presence of small gram-negative or variable rods (*Gardnerella*) and curved gram-negative rods (*Mobiluncus*) provides evidence for BV. Commercially available tests such as Affirm VP III (Becton-Dickinson, Sparks, Md), FemExam test card (Cooper Surgical, Shelton, Conn), and QuickVue Advance (Quidel, San Diego, Calif) can also be used.

Treatment

BV has been associated with endometritis, PID, and vaginal cuff cellulitis after invasive procedures. It has also been associated with postabortion PID. Thus, treatment of BV is aimed at relieving symptoms as well as preventing complications after invasive procedures.

Recommended regimens are as follows:

- Metronidazole, 500 mg PO twice daily for 7 days, *or*
- Metronidazole 0.75% cream, one full applicator (5 g) intravaginally once daily for 5 days, *or*
- Clindamycin 2% cream, one full applicator (5 g) intravaginally at bedtime for 7 days

Alternative regimens are less efficacious and include the following:

- Clindamycin, 300 mg PO twice daily for 7 days, *or*
- Clindamycin ovules, 100 g intravaginally, once at bedtime for 3 days

BV occurring during pregnancy has been associated with adverse pregnancy outcomes, including preterm labor, premature rupture of membranes, chorioamnionitis, preterm birth, postpartum endometritis, and postcesarean wound infection. All symptomatic pregnant women should be tested and treated for BV. It is also recommended that all asymptomatic pregnant women at high risk for preterm delivery (i.e., those who have previously delivered a preterm infant) be screened for BV during their first antenatal visit and be treated if positive. Currently, there is no recommendation to do the same for mothers at low risk. Intravaginal therapy is not recommended for pregnant patients.

The regimens recommended for pregnant women are the following:

- Metronidazole, 500 mg PO twice daily for 7 days, *or*
- Metronidazole, 250 mg PO three times daily for 7 days, *or*
- Clindamycin, 300 mg PO twice daily for 7 days

No teratogenic of mutagenic effects of metronidazole have been demonstrated despite concerns about this possibility.

Follow-up visits are unnecessary if symptoms resolve, except in pregnant women who have been treated for asymptomatic BV, for whom a 1-month follow-up is recommended. There has been no benefit shown in treating sexual partners of patients with BV.

Trichomoniasis

Trichomoniasis is caused by the protozoan *Trichomonas vaginalis*. An estimated 3 million American women contract trichomoniasis each year. They usually have a diffuse, malodorous, sometimes frothy, yellow-green discharge with vulvar pruritis, but some women may have no symptoms. On colposcopy, a strawberry cervix may be seen. In men, trichomoniasis may be asymptomatic or may manifest as a nongonococcal urethritis.

Diagnosis of vaginal trichomoniasis is by microscopic examination of a wet mount, which is 60% to 70% sensitive. It is important to obtain a fresh specimen because the organism is identified by its motility and hence must be viable when it arrives in the laboratory. Culture is a more sensitive method.

Recommended treatment for trichomoniasis is metronidazole, 2 g PO in a single dose. Alternatively, metronidazole, 500 mg twice daily for 7 days, is recommended.

Certain strains of *Trichomonas* have diminished susceptibility to metronidazole and respond to higher doses of metronidazole. In case of treatment failure with either regimen, patients should be retreated with metronidazole, 500 mg twice daily for 7 days. If this fails, patients should be treated with 2 g daily for 3 to 5 days. Tinidazole in a single dose of 2 g has recently been approved for treatment of trichomoniasis.

Sexual partners of patients should be treated to avoid reinfection. Pregnant patients with trichomoniasis should be treated if symptomatic with metronidazole, 2 g PO. Although trichomoniasis has been associated with adverse pregnancy outcomes such as premature rupture of membranes, preterm delivery, and low neonatal birth weight, data have not indicated that treating asymptomatic patients reduces this risk.

Gonococcal Infections

In the United States, nearly 340,000 new cases of gonococcal were reported to the CDC in 2005. Although gonococcal infection is a notifiable disease in the United States, it is estimated that about 50% of these infections go unreported. *N. gonorrhoeae*, the causative agent of gonorrhea, is a gram-negative diplococcus. In clinical specimens, a smear is considered positive for gonorrhea when gram-negative diplococci with typical morphology are identified in or closely associated with polymorphonuclear leukocytes. A smear is considered equivocal if the organisms are not cell-associated or intracellular organisms do not have the typical morphology.

Gonococcal infections have a wide variety of clinical manifestations and can manifest as asymptomatic or symptomatic local infections in men and women. It may also manifest as a complicated local infection with systemic dissemination.

Local infections may manifest as urethritis, proctitis, pharyngitis, or cervicitis. Acute anterior urethritis is the most common manifestation in men. Most men are symptomatic after infection. It manifest after an incubation period of 1 to 14 days, usually 2 to 5 days, with purulent discharge and dysuria. Varying degrees of meatal erythema and edema accompany the infection. Untreated, the infection tends to resolve in most patients. Local complications include epididymitis, prostatitis, and seminal vesiculitis. Periurethral abscess, urethral stricture, and fistulas are rare in the era of antibiotic therapy.

Urogenital infection in women has a nonspecific presentation and includes increased vaginal discharge, dysuria, intermenstrual bleeding, and menorrhagia. Many patients have purulent to mucopurulent cervicitis on examination. Purulent exudates may occasionally be expressed from the urethra, periurethral glands, or Bartholin's gland (duct).

Rectal infection is common in women with gonococcal cervicitis and infection is probably from perineal contamination of infected cervical secretions. It is usually asymptomatic. Rectal infection in MSM is caused by direct inoculation. Symptoms range from minimal anal pruritis, mucopurulent discharge, or scant rectal bleeding to overt proctitis, with severe rectal pain and tenesmus.

Orogenital sexual contact can result in pharyngeal infection. Most of these cases are asymptomatic but may occasionally cause acute pharyngitis or tonsillitis associated with cervical lymphadenopathy. Pharyngeal infection may also be a source of gonococcal urethritis in MSM. Rarely, adults may present with conjunctivitis from autoinoculation.

Systemic Complications

Disseminated gonococcal infection (DGI) is the most common systemic complication of acute gonorrhea. DGI manifests with fever accompanied by joint pain and skin lesions: arthritis-dermatitis syndrome. Joint pain is polyarticular in more than 50% of cases, but monoarticular arthritis in a young, sexually active person should have gonococcus (GC) in the differential. Joint pain may be caused by arthralgias or tenosynovitis or possible by frank arthritis with effusion. Joints involved are usually the wrists, metacarpophalangeal joints, ankles, or knees but any joint may be involved. The classic skin lesion is a necrotic pustule on an erythematous base. The skin lesions, however, may manifest as macules, papules, pustules, petechiae, bullae, or ecchymoses. They generally occur in the distal extremities and are sparse. Diagnosis is made by demonstrating the presence of the organism from clinical specimens. The likelihood of recovery of the organism is best from mucosal surfaces (e.g., urethra, pharynx, rectum) when this syndrome is suspected. Other systemic complications are rare and include endocarditis and meningitis.

Diagnosis

Culture and Gram staining of urethral, rectal, or pharyngeal swabs have been the methods traditionally used for diagnosis. A Gram stain showing intracellular diplococci resembling gonococci is highly specific and sensitive in the presence of urethral discharge. However, Gram staining is not sensitive for screening asymptomatic patients. Newer tests include nonamplification tests such as DNA probes or amplification tests such as PCR assay and transcription-mediated amplification. These tests are highly sensitive and specific and can also be used to screen patients for *N. gonorrhoeae* and *Chlamydia* from urine samples. However, they should not be used to test for *N. gonorrhoeae* in pharyngeal or rectal specimens because of the presence of commensal *Neisseria*, which can yield a false-positive result.

Treatment

N. gonorrhoeae was initially sensitive to penicillin, but the 1970s saw the emergence of plasmid-mediated resistance to penicillin (penicillinase-producing *N. gonorrhoeae* [PPNG]). Also, the emergence of chromosomally mediated resistant *N. gonorrhoeae* (CMRNG), resistant to penicillin as well as tetracycline, emerged in the 1970s. In 2003, 16.4% of isolates were penicillin resistant, tetracycline resistant, or both. Quinolones have been increasingly used for oral therapy, but recently there have been reports of strains of increasing quinolone-resistant *N. gonorrhoeae* (QRNG) from different states, especially in MSM. It was recommended that patients who acquired gonorrhea in Asia, the Pacific Islands, Hawaii, or California not be treated with a quinolone because of a high prevalence of resistance in these areas. With the emergence of resistance in MSM, it is now recommended that quinolones not be used for the treatment of MSM with gonorrhea.

Patients infected with *N. gonorrhoeae* are frequently coinfected with *C. trachomatis*. This has led to the recommendation that patients with gonococcal infection be routinely treated with a regimen effective for *Chlamydia* as well. Routine dual therapy without testing for *Chlamydia* is cost-effective for patients in whom coinfection occurs more than 10% to 30% of the time.

Recommended treatment regimens for uncomplicated gonococcal infections of the cervix, urethra, and rectum are as follows:

- Ceftriaxone, 125 mg IM single dose, *or*
- Cefixime, 400 mg PO single dose, *or*
- Ciprofloxacin, 500 mg PO single dose, *or*
- Ofloxacin, 400 mg PO single dose, *or*
- Levofloxacin, 250 mg PO single dose

In addition, treatment for *C. trachomatis* with azithromycin 1 g PO in a single dose, or doxycycline 100 mg PO twice daily for 7 days, may be initiated. Note that cefixime is currently not available in the United States after its manufacturer discontinued making the medication.

Alternative regimens include the following:

- Spectinomycin, 2 g IM single dose, or
- Other single-dose third-generation cephalosporins: ceftizoxime, 500 mg IM, cefoxitin, 2 g IM plus 1 g probenecid, cefotaxime, 500 mg IM
- Other single-dose quinolones: gatifloxacin, 400 mg PO, norfloxacin, 800 mg PO, or lomefloxacin, 400 mg PO
- Azithromycin, 2 g PO single dose, has been shown to be effective but may have high rates of gastrointestinal intolerance.

Uncomplicated gonococcal infections of the pharynx are more difficult to eradicate. The following is recommended:

- Ceftriaxone, 125 mg IM single dose, *or*
- Ciprofloxacin, 500 mg PO single dose

In addition, treatment for *C. trachomatis* with azithromycin, 1 g PO in a single dose, or doxycycline, 100 mg PO twice daily for 7 days, may be initiated.

Other Considerations

Persons who have persistent symptoms should be evaluated by culture and for antimicrobial susceptibility. Persistent symptoms may be caused by untreated coinfection with *Chlamydia* or other infections, such as trichomoniasis.

Patient should abstain from sexual activity for 7 days after therapy is started. All sex partners within 60 days before onset of symptoms or diagnosis should be treated. If the last sexual encounter was more than 60 days before the onset of symptoms or diagnosis, the patient's most recent sex partner should be treated. Pregnant women should be treated with a cephalosporin or spectinomycin; avoid quinolone.

For complicated infections, higher doses of antibiotics are recommended:

- Gonococcal conjunctivitis: ceftriaxone, 1 g IM, single dose
- Disseminated gonococcal infection: ceftriaxone, 1 g IV or IM every 24 hours. Alternative treatment regimens for DGI include the following:
  - Equivalent third-generation cephalosporin, *or*
  - Ciprofloxacin, 400 mg IV every 12 hours (or equivalent quinolone), *or*
  - Spectinomycin, 2 g IM every 12 hours, until 24 to 48 hours of clinical improvement

Therapy can then be completed with oral cefixime, 400 mg twice daily, ciprofloxacin 500 mg twice daily, levofloxacin 500 mg daily, or ofloxacin, 400 mg twice daily, to complete at least 1 week of antimicrobial therapy.

- Gonococcal meningitis or endocarditis, ceftriaxone, 1 to 2 g IV every 12 hours. Therapy is continued for 10 to 14 days for meningitis and at least 4 weeks for endocarditis.

Chlamydia Infection

C. trachomatis infection of the genital tract, a reportable disease in the United States, has been increasing in prevalence probably to the result of an actual increase in prevalence and also increased screening and more sensitive tests. In 2004, there were approximately 930,000 cases reported to the CDC. Underreporting is a major problem because most patients are asymptomatic.

An estimated 2,800,000 Americans are infected each year. Genital infections caused by *Chlamydia* are similar to those of *N. gonorrhoeae* in that similar syndromes develop: urethritis, epididymitis, cervicitis, PID, and proctitis. However, the symptoms tend to be less abrupt in onset and tend to be milder or asymptomatic. The incubation period for chlamydial infection is 1 to 3 weeks, longer than that of gonococcus. Some syndromes are discussed here.

Symptoms of urethritis include dysuria and a mild to moderate whitish to clear urethral discharge. Because coinfection with gonococcus is common, patients may present after being treated for gonococcal urethritis with a persistent discharge, although milder. Urethritis may be asymptomatic, although even these patients will exhibit signs of ongoing inflammation manifested by the presence of urethral leukocytes.

In male patients, chlamydial infection has also been implicated as a common pathogen in epididymitis in sexually active young men. Non-LGV serotypes of *Chlamydia* may cause proctitis. This organism has also been associated with nonbacterial prostatitis and Reiter's syndrome: urethritis, conjunctivitis, arthritis, and skin lesions.

In female patients, chlamydia is frequently isolated from the cervix. Infection is often silent and symptoms such as discharge, if present, are nonspecific. Findings on examination suggestive of chlamydial infection include easily induced endocervical bleeding, mucopurulent endocervical discharge, and edema within an area of ectopy. Mucopurulent discharge from the cervix may have other causes, such as gonococcal cervicitis, endometritis, or PID.

In addition to cervicitis, female patients may also have an acute urethritis, bartholinitis, and PID caused by *Chlamydia*. Fitz-Hugh–Curtis syndrome, perihepatitis as a result of PID, although once considered to be a complication of only gonococcal infection, has been shown to be more often associated with *Chlamydia*.

Diagnosis

The preferred methods of diagnostic testing are molecular. Both DNA probes and amplification assays are available, with the latter being more sensitive. Amplification assays include PCR assay and transcription-mediated amplification. Using these assays may be inhibited in clinical specimens, sometimes yielding a false-negative result. The ligase chain reaction, another amplification assay that was once widely used, is no longer available. Other diagnostic methods include culture, antigen tests (e.g., DFA), enzyme immunoassay (EIA), and serologic assays. Culture needs special precautions during collection and cell culture systems may not be available in many centers. Antigen assays are not very sensitive and serologic assays are difficult to interpret because of the high prevalence of infection in the population and largely asymptomatic infection in women.

Empirical therapy is started in symptomatic patients and often in contacts. However, where possible, a confirmatory test should be done because it helps in tracing contacts and controlling the epidemic.

Treatment

Recommended regimens include the following:

- Azithromycin, 1 g PO single dose, *or*
- Doxycycline, 100 mg PO twice daily for 7 days

Alternative regimens include the following:

- Erythromycin base, 500 mg PO four times daily for 7 days, *or*
- Erythromycin ethylsuccinate, 800 mg four times daily for 7 days, *or*
- Ofloxacin 300, mg twice daily for 7 days, *or*
- Levofloxacin, 500 mg PO daily for 7 days

It is recommended that a test for cure be done at 3 weeks for pregnant women when amplification tests are used. This is not recommended in others unless there is a suspicion of noncompliance. However, because of a high rate of reinfection caused by *C. trachomatis* in patients who have received therapy, and because a second infection confers a higher risk for PID, health care providers should consider rescreening all female patients who have received treatment 3 to 4 months after completion of therapy.

Patients should abstain from sexual activity for 7 days after therapy is started. All sex partners within 60 days before the onset of symptoms or diagnosis should be treated. If the last sexual encounter was more than 60 days before the onset of symptoms or diagnosis, the patient's most recent sex partner should be treated.

In pregnancy, doxycycline and quinolones are contraindicated. Thus, the recommended regimens are as follows:

- Azithromycin, 1 g PO in a single dose, *or*
- Amoxicillin, 500 mg three times daily for 7 days

Alternative regimens during pregnancy are erythromycin base or erythromycin ethylsuccinate for 7 days or 14 days, depending on the dose.

Chlamydial infections and gonococcal infections are frequent in women but often asymptomatic. Even asymptomatic infections can have serious long-term consequences, mainly infertility and ectopic pregnancy. Hence, it is recommended that all sexually active adolescent women and women aged 20 to 25 years be screened for chlamydial infection annually, even if they are asymptomatic. Older women with risk factors (e.g., new sexual partner and those with multiple sexual partners) should also be screened annually.

Urethritis

Urethritis is a syndrome characterized by urethral discharge of mucopurulent or purulent material and sometimes by dysuria or urethral pruritis. Infected patients may also be asymptomatic. It is a syndrome mainly found in men. The principal bacterial pathogens implicated are *N. gonorrhoeae* and *C. trachomatis*. Gonococcal urethritis is diagnosed if intracellular gram-negative diplococci with characteristic morphology are identified on urethral smears.

Otherwise, it is classified as nongonococcal urethritis (NGU). *C. trachomatis* is a frequent cause (15%-55%) of NGU. The cause of most cases of nonchlamydial NGU is unknown. *Ureaplasma urealyticum* and *Mycoplasma hominis* have been implicated in some studies. However, detection of these organisms is often difficult and specific diagnostic tests for these organisms are not indicated. *T. vaginalis* and HSV sometimes cause NGU, and diagnosis should be pursued if these infections are suspected (e.g., nonresponse to therapy or history of exposure).

Diagnosis

A diagnosis of urethritis is made if any of the following are present:

- Mucopurulent or purulent discharge
- Gram staining of urethral discharge demonstrating more than 5 white blood cells (WBCs)/oil immersion field

This is the preferred method for rapid diagnostic testing because it is highly sensitive and specific for documenting urethritis as well as the presence or absence of gonococcal infection.

- Positive leukocyte esterase test on first-void urine or microscopic examination of first-void urine demonstrating 10 WBCs or more per high-power field

If none of these conditions is met, treatment should be deferred and the patient should be tested for *N. gonorrhoeae* and *C. trachomatis* and followed closely if results are negative. Empirical treatment of symptoms without documentation is recommended only for patients at high risk for infection and who are unlikely to return for follow-up. Such patients should be treated for both gonorrhea and chlamydia. Their partners should be also evaluated and treated.

Treatment

Treatment for gonococcal urethritis has been discussed earlier (see "Gonococcal Infections"). For NGU, treatment should begin as soon as possible after diagnosis. Recommended regimens, aimed at treating mainly *C. trachomatis* (but also effective against *Mycoplasma* and *Ureaplasma*), include the following:

- Azithromycin, 1 g PO in a single dose (this regimen has the advantage of compliance and directly observed therapy), *or*
- Doxycycline, 100 mg PO twice daily for 7 days

Alternative regimens include the following:

- Erythromycin base, 500 mg PO four times daily for 7 days, *or*
- Erythromycin ethylsuccinate, 800 mg PO four times daily for 7 days, *or*
- Ofloxacin, 300 mg PO twice daily for 7 days, *or*
- Levofloxacin, 500 mg PO once daily for 7 days

Patients should be instructed to abstain from sexual intercourse for 7 days after therapy is initiated. They should be retested if symptoms persist or recur after completion of therapy. All sex partners within the last 60 days should be evaluated.

For patients with objective signs of recurrent or persistent urethritis, patients should be evaluated for noncompliance or reexposure to an untreated sex partner. After this has been excluded, patients should have a culture of an intraurethral swab as well as a first-void urine specimen tested for *T. vaginalis*. Also, some cases of recurrent urethritis may be caused by tetracycline-resistant *U. urealyticum*. Thus, the recommended regimen for these patients is metronidazole, 2 g PO in a single dose, plus erythromycin base, 500 mg PO four times daily, or erythromycin ethylsuccinate, 800 mg PO four times daily for 7 days.

Mucopurulent Cervicitis

Mucopurulent cervicitis (MPC) is characterized by purulent or mucopurulent endocervical exudate visible in the endocervical canal or in an endocervical swab specimen. It is often asymptomatic, but some patients may have an abnormal vaginal discharge or vaginal bleeding after intercourse. MPC can be caused by *N. gonorrhoeae* or *C. trachomatis*, but in most cases neither organism is isolated. This may be the result of nonmicrobiologic causes (e.g., inflammation of the zone of ectopy).

Patients with MPC should be tested for *N. gonorrhoeae* and *C. trachomatis* using sensitive and specific tests and therapy should be based on these results. Empirical therapy may be given for patients in whom the likelihood of infection is high and who are unlikely to return for follow-up. In patients with MPC, signs of PID should be sought because this may manifest as MPC.

Human Papilloma Virus

Human papilloma virus (HPV) infections of the genital tract can be asymptomatic or can manifest as genital warts or as intraepithelial neoplasia or carcinoma of the vulva, cervix, penis, or anus. About 1% of the sexually active population in the United States has genital warts. There are more than 100 different types of HPV. Types 6 and 11 are the most common types associated with genital warts. Intraepithelial neoplasia is most commonly associated with types 16, 18, 31, 32, and 34 (also called high-risk types). Types 6 and 11 also cause respiratory papillomatosis in infants and children and it is believed that transmission occurs perinatally.

Genital Warts

These commonly manifest as flesh-colored, painless, cauliflower-like lesions (condyloma acuminata), but may also manifest as smooth, dome-shaped papules (papular warts), flat crusty papules resembling seborrheic keratosis (keratotic warts), or macular or slightly raised flat-topped papules. They occur on the penis, scrotum, perianal area, vulva, or perineum. Less often, they may appear on the crural folds, thighs, or pubic area. They may also appear on the vaginal wall, on the cervix, or in the anus. Occasionally, patients report itching, burning, pain, or bleeding. Perianal warts may appear, even in the absence of anal intercourse. Application of 5% acetic acid to genital warts turns the lesion a whitish color, a property sometimes used to differentiate a wart from other lesions.

Genital warts may resolve spontaneously, grow in size or number, or remain the same. Warts that have been present for less than 1 year respond better to therapy. Treatment of genital warts reduces viral DNA and probably reduces infectivity. Response to therapy is variable and recurrences can occur, usually in the first 3 months after therapy. Therapy is usually undertaken to remove aesthetically unpleasant lesions.

Treatment for External Genital Warts. Therapy can be divided into patient-applied or provider-administered therapy. The choice of therapy depends on the patient and provider. Generally, if there is no significant improvement after three provider-administered therapies, or if warts have not completely cleared after six treatments, the treatment modality should be changed. Hypo- or hyperpigmentation or scars can occur at sites of treatment.

Patient-Applied Treatment. Podofilox, 0.5% solution, should be applied with a cotton swab, and podofilox gel should be applied with a finger to visible warts twice daily for 3 days, followed by 4 days of no therapy. This cycle should be repeated for up to four cycles as necessary. No more than 0.5 mL/day should be applied and the total wart area treated should not exceed 10 cm^2.

The patient should apply imiquimod 5% cream once daily at bedtime three times a week for up to 16 weeks. The treatment area should be washed with soap and water 6 to 10 hours after the application.

Provider-Administered Treatment. A small amount of podophyllin resin, 10% to 25%, in a compounded tincture of benzoin, should be applied to each wart and allowed to dry. Because systemic absorption can lead to complications such as bone marrow suppression and neuropathy, less than 0.5 mL of the resin should be applied to a wart area smaller than 10 cm^2 per session. Some experts recommend washing off the area 1 to 4 hours after application to reduce local irritation. The treatment can be repeated weekly if necessary.

A small amount of trichloroacetic acid (TCA) or bicholoroacetic acid (BCA), 80% to 90%, should be applied only to the warts and allowed to dry so that a white frosting develops. Excess acid can be removed by applying powdered talc, sodium bicarbonate (baking soda), or liquid soap to the area. The treatment may be repeated weekly if necessary. Some centers apply a repellent such as petroleum jelly (Vaseline) to the skin area surrounding the warts before applying podophyllin or TCA to prevent application to unaffected areas.

Cryotherapy using liquid nitrogen or cryoprobe and surgical removal by excision, curettage, or electrosurgery are other recommended modalities. Alternative modalities include intralesional interferon and laser surgery.

Treatment for Other Genital Warts. For vaginal warts, recommended treatment includes cryotherapy or TCA or BCA. Urethral meatus warts can be treated with cryotherapy or podophyllin resin. Anal warts can be treated with cryotherapy, TCA or BCA, or surgical excision. For cervical warts, squamous intraepithelial lesions should be excluded from treatment.

Cervical Cancer Screening

It is believed that cervical intraepithelial neoplasia is an early lesion in the continuum of changes leading to cervical cancer after HPV infection. This concept has remained the principle behind cervical cancer screening using the Papanicolaou (Pap) test, which has helped reduce the incidence of cervical cancer in developed countries. Cervical cancer can occur in young, sexually active women as well as in older women, and it is important to ensure that all women presenting with STDs be screened for cervical cancer using the Pap test. It is recommended that women who are sexually active be screened every year for cervical cancer, but can be screened less frequently if three consecutive Pap tests show no abnormality. A thin-preparation medium is widely available in developed countries that allows for Pap smear and HPV testing to be performed on the same sample.

Results are reported as the presence or absence of a low- or high-risk HPV type. High-risk HPV types (16, 18, 31, 32, 34) predict those women who are at greater risk of progressing to high-grade SIL or cervical cancer. Patients with atypical squamous cells of undetermined significance (ASCUS) or low-grade SIL who also have high-risk HPV types as determined by the Pap smear should be referred for colposcopy.

Other Considerations

No evidence exists to suggest that the presence of genital warts (low-risk HPV types) or their treatment is associated with the development of cervical cancer. Thus, HPV typing of patients with genital warts is not recommended, nor is colposcopy or increased frequency of Pap smear recommended.

Genital warts can proliferate and become friable during pregnancy and many experts advocate their removal during pregnancy. Imiquimod, podofilox, or podophyllin should not be used during pregnancy. Although HPV types 6 and 11, which can also cause genital warts, cause respiratory papillomatosis, their transmission is not well understood. Cesarean section is not recommended as a preventive measure in patients with genital warts. A Pap smear is recommended during pregnancy.

The use of latex condoms has been associated with a lower rate of cervical cancer, an HPV-associated disease. However, they are not effective in preventing the transmission of genital warts, because condoms cannot cover all the affected skin.

In June 2006, the U.S. Food and Drug Administration approved a quadrivalent vaccine for HPV. Two low-risk types that cause most genital warts, HPV 6 and 8, are targeted, as well as the two high-risk types that cause 70% of U.S. cervical cancer cases, HPV types 16 and 18. The vaccine is most effective when given before the initiation of sexual intercourse, so recommendations are for girls and young women between the ages of 9 and 26. Approval will eventually be sought for boys and young men because they can develop genital warts and penile or anal cancer from HPV as well. The vaccine is generally well tolerated and is given as a series of three vaccines at 0, 1, and 6 months. Several states have already recommended making HPV vaccination mandatory for middle school–aged girls.

Summary

- STDs are still a major cause of morbidity in the United States and worldwide.
- Pelvic inflammatory disease can lead to devastating long-term sequelae, even when symptoms are mild. If PID is suspected, it should be treated.
- *Neisseria gonorrhoeae* is becoming more quinolone resistant. Thus, quinolone should not be used as first-line treatment for the MSM population, and all other populations should be carefully monitored, because recommendations may change.
- HPV vaccine is available for use in girls and young women aged 9 to 26 years. It is highly effective in preventing genital warts and, most importantly, in preventing cervical cancer.

Suggested Readings

Centers for Disease Control and Prevention, Workowski KA, Berman SM: Sexually transmitted diseases treatment guidelines, 2006. MMWR Morb Mortal Weekly Rep 2006;55(RR-11):1-94.

Centers for Disease Control and Prevention: Quadrivalent human papillomavirus vaccine: Recommendations of the Advisory Committee on Immunization Practices (ACIP). MMWR Morb Mortal Weekly Rep 2007;56(RR-2):1-24.

Holmes KK, Mardh PA, Sparling PF, et al (eds): Sexually Transmitted Diseases, 3rd ed. San Francisco, McGraw-Hill, 1999.

Ness RB, Soper DE, Holley RL, et al: Effectiveness of inpatient and outpatient treatment strategies for women with pelvic inflammatory disease: Results from the Pelvic Inflammatory Disease Evaluation and Clinical Health (PEACH) Randomized Trial. Am J Obstet Gynecol 2002;186:929-937.

Tuberculosis

Octavian C. Ioachimescu and J. Walton Tomford

Man must want to achieve more than he is able to achieve. … If we do not reach for the impossible, we shall never reach far enough to discover the possible. Our wishes should be boundless.

DR. GERHARD DOMAGK *(1947 Nobel Prize in medicine for the discovery of the first antimicrobial drug)*

Over the last century, tuberculosis (TB) has killed more than 100 million people and this has continued relatively unchanged over the last 50 years, despite the development of effective antituberculous drugs. This chapter summarizes the current status of the epidemiology, pathogenesis, diagnosis, treatment, and control of pulmonary tuberculosis. We have excluded nontuberculous mycobacterial disorders and the various forms of extrapulmonary disease, except pleural TB.

HISTORICAL OVERVIEW

- Egyptian mummies with severe skeletal deformities suggest that TB has existed since antiquity (Pott's disease).
- After the plague devastated Europe during the Middle Ages, TB (the "white plague") began to take its heavy toll.
- TB affected famous kings and political figures (e.g., King Edward VI, King Louis VIII of France, John Calvin, Cardinal Richelieu, Napoleon II).
- TB, also called writer's or artist's disease, killed, among others, Nicolo Paganini, Robert Louis Stevenson, Franz Kafka, George Orwell, all five Brontë sisters, Thomas Mann, Albert Camus, and Igor Stravinsky.
- The Nobel Prize for Medicine for TB-related work was given to the following:
- Dr. Robert Koch (Fig. 1) for the discovery of TB bacillus (1905)
- Dr. Gerhard Domagk for the discovery of the first antibacterial drug (Prontosil); also pioneered anti-TB drug development (1947)
- Dr. Selman Waksman for the development of streptomycin as an anti-TB drug (1952)
- In 1993, the World Health Organization (WHO) declared TB a global emergency, the only disease ever so designated. In 2003, WHO reported a continued TB pandemic.

PREVALENCE AND RISK FACTORS

Tuberculosis Worldwide

About one third of the world's population is infected with *Mycobacterium tuberculosis*. Among the communicable diseases, TB is the second leading cause of death worldwide after HIV-AIDS, killing nearly two million people each year. Approximately 13% of TB patients have coexistent HIV infection. There were an estimated eight million to nine million new cases of TB in 2000, but fewer than one half were actually reported. Most cases (5 million to 6 million) occur in those aged 15 to 49 years, with significant socioeconomic impact. More than 50% of TB cases occur in the largest Asian countries (India, China, Indonesia, Bangladesh, Philippines, and Pakistan). Sub-Saharan Africa has the highest incidence rate (approximately 300/100,000 population/year). Even though TB has declined steadily in western Europe and North America, the global TB burden appears on the rise, especially in the former Soviet Union, Eastern Europe, and Africa. HIV infection accounts for much of the recent increase in the global TB incidence.

Tuberculosis in the United States

In the 1900s, TB was one of the leading causes of death in the United States. Here, the most important risk factors for the development of TB are immigration from or travel to an endemic area, close contact with a TB patient, exposure to untreated cases in crowded living facilities, advanced age, residing in an inner city, and host immunodeficiency. Although the TB incidence was already decreasing in the first half of the 20th century because of better nutrition and housing conditions, the introduction of effective chemotherapy produced a steep decline in mortality and an accelerated drop in incidence, reaching an average of a 5.5% decline per year of TB case rates between 1953 and 1983. Between 1985 and 1992, however, the incidence of TB unexpectedly increased by about 20%. The responsible factors were increased immigration from high-prevalence countries, the emergence of the HIV-AIDS epidemic, an increased number of medically underserved persons (e.g., homeless, drug abusers, low-income persons), emergence of drug-resistant TB cases and, most importantly, deterioration of the public health infrastructure for the control of TB.

In 2005, a total of 14,093 TB cases (4.8 cases/100,000 population) was reported in the United States, representing a 3.8% decline in the rate from 2004. These findings indicated that although the 2005 TB rate was the lowest recorded since national reporting began in 1953, the decline has slowed from an average of 7.1% per year (1993-2000) to an average of 3.8% per year (2001-2005). In 2005, the TB rate in foreign-born persons in the United States was 8.7 times that of U.S.-born persons. Hispanics, African Americans, and Asians had TB rates 7.3, 8.3, and 19.6 times higher than whites, respectively. Moreover, the number of multidrug-resistant (MDR) TB cases in the United States increased by 13.3%, with 128 cases of MDRTB in 2004, the most recent year for which complete drug-susceptibility data are available. Effective TB control and prevention in the United States require adequate resources, sustained collaborative measures with other countries to reduce the incidence of TB worldwide, and interventions targeted to populations with the highest TB rates.[1]

ETIOLOGY

Tuberculosis is caused by a group of five closely related species, which form the *Mycobacterium tuberculosis* complex: *M. tuberculosis, M. bovis, M. africanum, M. microti*, and *M. canettii. M. tuberculosis* (Koch's bacillus) is responsible for the vast majority of TB cases in the United States. The main defining characteristic of the genus *Mycobacterium* is the property called acid-fastness, which is the ability to withstand decolorization with an acid-alcohol mixture after staining with carbolfuchsin or auramine-rhodamine. Mycobacteria are primarily intracellular pathogens, have slow growth rates, are obligate aerobes, and produce a granulomatous reaction in normal hosts. In cultures, *M. tuberculosis* does not produce significant amounts of pigment, has a buff-colored, smooth surface appearance, and biochemically produces niacin. These characteristics are useful in differentiating *M. tuberculosis* from nontuberculous mycobacteria. One characteristic but not distinctive morphologic property of *M. tuberculosis* is the tendency to form cords, or dense clusters of bacilli, aligned in parallel (Fig. 2). The biochemical background of cording is called cord factor (a trehalose dimycolate), and its contribution to bacterial virulence is still unclear.

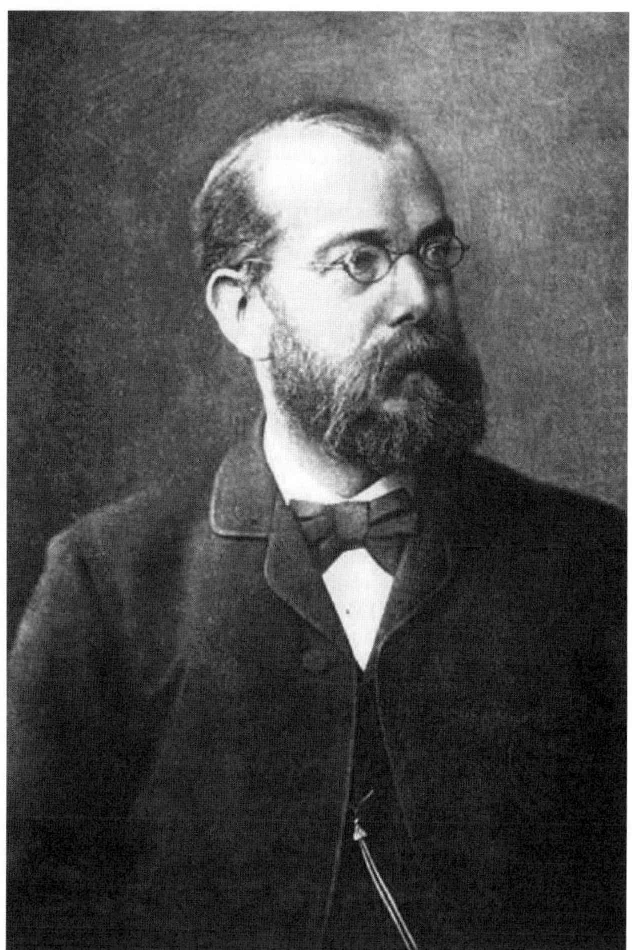

Figure 1 **Robert Koch, 1843-1910.** *(Reproduced with permission from the College of Physicians of Philadelphia).*

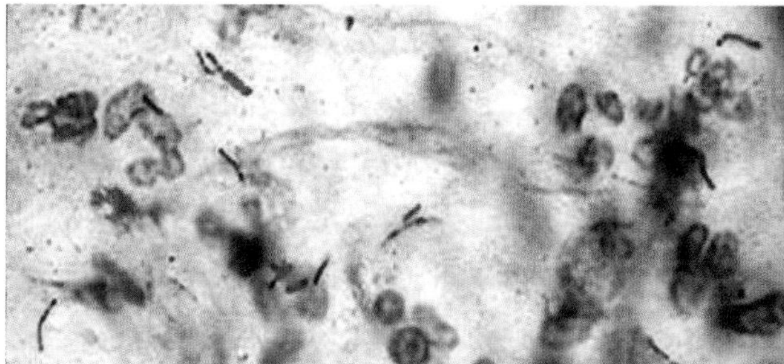

Figure 2 **Ziehl-Neelsen stain of a sputum specimen showing acid-fast bacilli in cords (red; × 1000).**

PATHOPHYSIOLOGY AND NATURAL HISTORY

TB transmission occurs almost exclusively from human to human; a prerequisite is having contact with a source case. More than 80% of new TB cases result from exposure to sputum smear-positive cases, although smear-negative, culture-positive cases can be responsible for up to 17% of new cases. Tuberculosis is spread by airborne droplet nuclei, which are 1- to 5-μm particles containing 1 to 400 bacilli each. They are expelled in the air by, for example, coughing, sneezing, singing, laughing, or talking, and remain suspended in the air for many hours. They can be inhaled and subsequently entrapped in the distal airways and alveoli. There, bacilli are ingested by local macrophages, multiply within the cells and, within 2 weeks, are transported through the lymphatics to establish secondary sites (lymphohematogenous spread). The development of an immune response, heralded by a delayed-type hypersensitivity reaction over the next 4 weeks, leads to granuloma formation, with a subsequent decrease in the number of bacilli. Some of them remain viable, or dormant, for many years. This stage is called latent TB infection (LTBI), which is generally an asymptomatic, radiologically undetected process in humans. Sometimes, a primary complex (Ghon complex) can be seen radiographically, mostly in the lower and middle lobes, and comprises the primary lesion, hilar lymphadenopathy, with or without a lymphangitic track. Later, the primary lesion tends to become calcified and can be identified on chest radiographs for decades. Most commonly, a positive tuberculin test result remains the only proof of LTBI, and therefore does not signify active disease.

Under certain conditions of immature or disregulated immunity, alveolar macrophages and the subsequent biologic cascade could fail in limiting the mycobacterial proliferation, leading to primary progressive tuberculosis; this is seen mostly in children younger than 5 years or in HIV-positive or profoundly immunosuppressed individuals. Factors known to influence this unfavorable course are patient's age, nutritional status, host immunity, and bacterial infective load.

Once infected with *M. tuberculosis*, 3% to 5% of immunocompetent persons develop active disease (i.e., secondary progressive tuberculosis) within 2 years and an additional 3% to 5% later on during their lifetime. Overall, there is a lifetime risk of re-activation of 10%, with one half occurring during the first 2 years after infection—hence, the necessity to treat all tuberculin skin test converters. The lifetime re-activation rate is approximately 20% for most persons with purified protein derivative (PPD) induration of more than 10 mm and either HIV infection or evidence of old, healed tuberculosis; it is between 10% and 20% for recent PPD skin test converters, adults younger than 35 years with an induration of more than 15 mm or on therapy with infliximab (a tumor necrosis factor α [TNF-α] receptor blocker), and children younger than 5 years and a skin induration of more than 10 mm.

Studies performed in New York City and San Francisco using DNA fingerprinting have indicated that recent transmission (exogenous reinfection), especially among HIV patients, could account for up to 40% of new TB cases. This is significantly different from older studies, which have shown that approximately 90% of new TB cases are the result of endogenous re-activation.

After inhalation, the pathogenic bacilli start to replicate slowly and continuously and lead to the development of a cellular immunity in about 4 to 6 weeks. T lymphocytes and local (pulmonary and lymphatic node) macrophages represent key players in limiting further spread of bacilli in the host. This can be seen at the pathologic level, where the bacilli are in the center of necrotizing (caseating) and non-necrotizing (noncaseating) granulomas, surrounded by lymphocytes and macrophages. The infected macrophages release interleukins 12 and 18 (IL-12 and IL-18), which stimulate CD4-positive T lymphocytes to secrete IFN-γ (interferon gamma), which in turn activate the macrophage phagocytosis of *M. tuberculosis* and the release of TNF-α. TNF-α has an important role in granuloma formation and the control of infection.

Genetic defects are illustrated by different polymorphisms of the *NRAMP-1* gene (natural resistance-associated macrophage protein-1); vitamin D receptors, and interleukin-1 have also been shown to be involved in TB pathogenesis. It can be difficult to differentiate between genetic predisposition and overwhelming bacteriologic load, as often seen in countries with a high prevalence of TB.

HIV coinfection is the greatest risk factor for progression to active disease in adults. The relation between HIV and TB has augmented the deadly potential of each disease. Other risk factors include diabetes mellitus, renal failure, coexistent malignancies, malnutrition, silicosis, immunosuppressive therapies (including steroids and anti-TNF drugs), and TNF-α receptor, IFN-γ receptor, or IL-12 β_1 receptor defects.

DIAGNOSIS

Signs and Symptoms

A high index of suspicion is needed in countries with a high prevalence of infection or in patients with immunosuppression, although bacteriologic confirmation is required whenever possible. Persistent cough for more than 2 to 4 weeks should raise the possibility of pulmonary TB. Other common associated symptoms are hemoptysis, dyspnea, malaise, weight loss, night sweats, and chest pain. The symptoms are less pronounced in children, and any exposure to an active TB patient or a positive tuberculin test should raise more concerns about this disease. Box 1 shows the Centers for Disease Control and Prevention (CDC) recommendations for the clinical and laboratory criteria of TB diagnosis.

Laboratory Tests

One inexpensive and rapid diagnostic test is the sputum smear, done by Ziehl-Neelsen (ZN) carbolfuchsin, Kinyoun carbolfuchsin, or fluorochrome staining methods. ZN stain identifies 50% to 80% of culture-positive TB cases and is a useful diagnostic and epidemiologic tool, because smear-positive TB patients are more infectious than smear-negative patients and have a higher fatality rate. Nevertheless, smear-negative cases may account for up to 20% of *M. tuberculosis* transmission. In countries with a high prevalence of TB, a positive smear signifies TB in 95% of ases. The lower limit of detection of ZN staining is 5×10^3 organisms/mL, whereas rhodamine-auramine fluorochrome staining tends to be more sensitive. In children, *M. tuberculosis* can be recovered from gastric aspirates, with yields varying from 30% to 50% in older children to 70% in infants for three consecutive specimens. The role of induced sputum or bronchoscopy in diagnosing TB is well established in patients unable to provide good-quality sputum specimens.

Culture media most often used for diagnosis include the following:

- Solid culture medium: egg-based Löwenstein-Jensen, or agar-based Middlebrook 7H10 or 7H11 (growth can take up to 6 weeks)
- Liquid culture medium (growth in 1-3 weeks)

The speciation can be done with biochemical tests or DNA probes. The direct specimen polymerase chain reaction assay is rapid (1-2 days), although it can lead to false-positive results and has been disappointing in its practicality.

Box 1 Centers for Disease Control and Prevention (CDC) Case Definition of Tuberculosis

Laboratory Criteria

Isolation of *M. tuberculosis* from a clinical specimen *or* (when culture not obtained)

Demonstration of acid-fast bacilli in a clinical specimen

Clinical Elements (All of these are needed when not confirmed by laboratory test results.)

A positive skin tuberculin test

Signs and symptoms compatible with tuberculosis or an abnormal chest radiograph

Treatment with two or more antituberculous drugs

A complete diagnostic evaluation with exclusion of other, alternative diagnoses

Imaging Studies

Radiographic findings suggesting TB include upper lobe infiltrates, cavitary lesions, and hilar or paratracheal lymphadenopathy. In many patients with primary progressive disease and in HIV patients, radiographic findings can be subtle and include lower lobe opacities, a miliary pattern, or both. In a study done on HIV-infected pulmonary TB patients, 8% of cases had normal chest radiographs.

TREATMENT

Lifestyle Modifications

These include good nutrition, which is of paramount importance, and physical activity, which is strongly encouraged.

Treatment Options

- Drug treatment is an individual and public health measure.
- Regimens must contain multiple drugs to which organisms are susceptible, given for a sufficient period of time.
- Adherence to the drug regimen is critical for success. Directly observed therapy (DOT) is cost effective for patients at high risk for nonadherence, and should be used in all cases.
- Chemotherapy can be successful only within a health system infrastructure that addresses the clinical and social management of patients and their contacts.
- Surgery is indicated for TB abscesses or loculated foci of infection that are unresponsive to medical therapy.

Practice Guidelines

- Use the major antituberculous drugs, isoniazid (INH) and rifampin (RIF) throughout the course, unless there is a resistant organism to one of them.
- Use pyrazinamide (PZA) for the first 2 months. Studies have shown that 6 months of INH and RIF with 2 initial months of PZA are as effective as 9 months of INH and RIF alone, but leads to a higher sputum conversion rate and a smaller chance of secondary resistance.
- If PZA cannot be used in the first 2 months, a reasonable alternative is INH and RIF administered for 9 months.
- Use ethambutol (ETB) or streptomycin (SM) as a fourth drug until susceptibilities are known if the patient comes from a community with a higher than 4% chance of drug resistance (currently, in 41 of 50 states), has undergone prior therapy, or has possible exposure to a drug-resistant case.
- Once susceptibilities are known and *M. tuberculosis* is susceptible to INH, RIF and PZA, ETB, and SM can be discontinued.
- If cultures are positive after 2 months of therapy, triple-drug therapy continuation is recommended; the treatment should be continued for about 4 months after the cultures become negative.
- The 7 day/week regimens are interchangeable with 5 day/week regimens for the same duration of therapy if *M. tuberculosis* is susceptible to the respective drugs.
- Corticosteroids have been shown to be of benefit in preventing cardiac constriction from TB pericarditis, decreasing neurologic sequelae in TB meningitis, and (possibly) preventing bronchial stenosis in cases of diffuse endobronchial TB. Once there is absolute assurance that the chemotherapeutic regimen is effective, some have advocated the use of low-dose steroids in the initial phase, especially in malnourished patients, although supporting data are lacking.
- Pregnant women with active TB need to be treated with INH and RIF, which are safe during pregnancy. PZA, although recommended by many, has not been thoroughly studied in pregnancy and should be used at the discretion of the treating physician.

ETM has not been recommended, and SM is definitely harmful during the pregnancy.

- Pulmonology or infectious disease consultations, or both, are recommended for guiding expertise in the management of pulmonary TB.
- Public Health Department notification and assistance are essential for the management of TB, and the institution of DOT.

Treatment Regimens

When discussing treatment regimens for TB, the nomenclature used needs to be defined. The expression $nHRZS(E)_m$ refers to n months of isoniazid, H, rifampin, R, pyrazinamide, Z, and streptomycin, S (or ethambutol, E), for *m* days a week. The first term represents the initial phase and the second term respresents the continuation phase.

For culture-positive pulmonary tuberculosis caused by drug-susceptible organisms, there are four acceptable regimens[2]:

- $2HRZE(S)_7 + 4HR_7$ *(preferred)*
- $0.5HRZE(S)_7 + 1.5HRZS(E)_2 + 4HR_2$
- $2HRSZ(E)_3 + 4HR_3$
  or
- $2HRE_7 + 7HR_7$

For smear-negative, culture-negative TB cases (clinical TB), a 4-month HR regimen ($4HR_7$ or $4HR_2$) is acceptable. The doses used in TB regimens are shown in Table 1.

Drug Resistance Considerations

Antituberculous drug resistance has been increasing worldwide. Treatment of resistant TB, especially MDRTB, is frequently unsuccessful, requiring the use of more toxic, expensive drugs, surgery, or both. Thus, emphasis should be on strategies developed to avoid the emergence of drug resistance. Primary resistance occurs in patients with active TB who have never received antituberculous drugs. Secondary (or acquired) resistance is the occurrence of resistance after a mutant's selection or facilitation in the presence of various antituberculous drugs. A cavitary TB lesion may contain up to 10^9 bacilli in a perfect, culture-type, aerobic environment. *M. tuberculosis* has low rates of spontaneous chromosomal mutations, in the range of $1:10^6$ for INH, $1:10^8$ for RIF and approximately $1:10^{14}$ for both agents. These rates are clinically insignificant, unless suboptimal time intervals or doses of anti-TB drugs facilitate the resistant subpopulation's growth.

MDRTB is defined as the presence of at least 1% of *Mycobacterium* strains in a bacterial population or culture that are resistant to at least INH and RIF. The practices associated with the occurrence of MDRTB include failure to predict, identify, or adequately address nonadherence to therapy, use of an inadequate initial regimen, use of INH monotherapy when the patient actually has active disease (not LTBI), and the addition of a single drug to a failing regimen. The most important demographic clues for drug resistance are being a resident of a large urban, coastal, or border community area (in the United States), or from areas with high MDRTB rates (outside the United States, such as Russia), or being HIV-infected (probably reflecting a higher proportion of disease resulting from recent transmission). The most important historical clues are prior therapy for TB, and, less so, cavitary lesions. MDRTB is treated with four drugs, as in the usual therapeutic regimens, plus at least an additional two drugs to which the patient's infective organism is believed to be susceptible. Patients with culture-confirmed MDRTB should be treated with at least three drugs to which the organism is susceptible for at least 12 months after the sputum conversion. Most experts recommend 18 to 24 months of therapy. INH-resistant cases can be treated with RIF, PZA, and ETB for 6 to 9 months, and patients with RIF-resistant TB are treated with INH, PZA, and ETB for 9 to 12 months after sputum cultures become negative. Consultation with a TB expert and the public health department's assistance are mandatory when managing an MDRTB case.

DISEASE CONTROL

Infection control efforts to stem TB outbreaks among inpatients and health care staff are essential, because they represent the proximal contacts for any TB source in that particular setting. Although most patients do not ultimately need hospitalization (e.g., an isolated TB pleurisy), patients suspected of having active TB are kept in isolation until they are no longer infectious, until TB is ruled out, or three negative sputum specimens are obtained. Isolation rooms should have negative-pressure ventilation, with at least six air exchanges per hour. Health care workers who come in contact with these patients should wear N95 masks or powered air-purifying respirators (PAPRs) to avoid inhaling infectious particles while in the room with the patient. The isolation can be discontinued after 10 to 14 days of therapy if the patient responds to therapy. Patients can be removed from isolation and discharged home if they are returning to their previous residence, where the health department has identified no individuals at risk (children younger than 2 years, immunocompromised patients) and the other possibly exposed individuals are being evaluated for LTBI. Outpatient medications should be given using DOT to ensure adherence to treatment. The recent decline in the United States is largely the result of the implementation and use of DOT, which has been shown to improve therapy completion rates and to prevent the emergence of acquired resistance and MDRTB.[3-5]

Table 1 First-Line Tuberculosis Drugs

Drug	Side Effects	Dosage Regimen (mg/kg)	
		Daily	Two or Three Times/wk
Isoniazid	Hepatitis, peripheral neuropathy, lupus-like syndrome, drug interactions	5 (max, 300 mg)	15 (max, 900 mg)
Rifampin	Drug interactions, orange discoloration of body fluids, gastrointestinal upset, hepatitis, fever, hypersensitivity, acute renal failure, hemolytic anemia	10 (max, 600 mg)	10 (max, 600 mg)
Pyrazinamide	Hyperuricemia, gouty arthritis, rarely hepatitis	15-30 (max, 2 g)	50-70 (max, 4 g)
Ethambutol	Optic neuritis, exfoliative rash	15-25	25-30
Streptomycin	Cochleo- and vestibulotoxicity, nephrotoxicity	15	25-30
Amikacin	Cochleo- and vestibulotoxicity, nephrotoxicity	7.5-10	

SPECIAL CONSIDERATIONS

Latent Tuberculosis Infection

The intradermal administration of tuberculin has been used as a diagnostic test for TB infection since the early 1900s, and the standardized purified protein derivative (PPD-S) since 1939. The diagnosis of TB infection relies on determining the size of the delayed-type hypersensitivity reaction to an injection of 0.1 mL of 5 tuberculin units (TU) after 48 to 72 hours (Mantoux test). The tine test has no role in the evaluation of an individual patient.

Although the PPD is still the best available way to diagnose TB infection, it is not a perfect test because of the following:

- It has low sensitivity in immunosuppressed patients (e.g., HIV-infected patients; the threshold for positivity is 5 mm for these patients), or in the preimmune initial phase of infection.
- It has cross-reactivity with bacille Calmette-Guérin (BCG) vaccine and environmental mycobacteria (low specificity). The larger the induration, the greater is the likelihood that the reaction represents a *M. tuberculosis* infection versus environmental mycobacterial sensitization or reaction from prior BCG vaccination.
- It usually needs a follow-up visit in 48 to 72 hours for reading the results, although e-mail, digital pictures, and other means in this era of telemedicine have become available and are widely used.
- The reading is subjective and requires expertise (low interrater variability).
- There is a booster effect. It is known that delayed-type hypersensitivity reactions from a prior mycobacterial infection or BCG vaccination may wane over time. Although subsequent skin reactions could be still negative for a particular individual, the stimulus of the first test may boost or increase the size of the second test results, generally by less than 5 mm, administered 1 week to 1 year later, suggesting a false conversion. When PPD skin testing is repeated periodically, as in employee health or institutional screening programs, an initial two-step approach can reduce the likelihood that a boosted reaction will be interpreted as a sign of recent infection. If the first PPD skin test is negative, a second 5-TU test should be performed 1 to 3 weeks later; a positive second reaction would indicate boosting of a previous infection or BCG vaccination. The major problem with a booster effect is LTBI overdiagnosis (false-positive result for infection).

The American Thoracic Society (ATS) and the Centers for Disease Control and Prevention (CDC) statement on LTBI[6] has established the thresholds of PPD indurations for different settings and hosts (Box 2). An increase in induration of more than 10 mm within a 2-year period indicates conversion, irrespective of age. In patients at low risk for TB infection, PPD skin testing is not recommended. The ATS-CDC has specifically recommended LTBI screening to be used only for high-risk patients, the concept of targeted LTBI screening. The old term, *INH prophylaxis*, applied to the treatment of LTBI should be abandoned.

Similar to the principle of the Mantoux reaction, a whole-blood IFN-γ release assay (IGRA) evaluates cell-mediated immunity to tuberculin. Although it seems to be less sensitive and less specific, it can differentiate between infection and prior BCG vaccination. An enzyme-linked immunosorbent spot (ELISPOT) assay has been developed that is relatively sensitive and specific for detecting LTBI by targeting early-secreted antigenic target (ESAT-6), which is expressed only by *M. tuberculosis*, and not by other *Mycobacterium* spp. or by BCG. In May 2005, an in vitro test, QuantiFERON-TB Gold (QFT-G, Cellestis Limited, Carnegie, Victoria, Australia), received approval from the U.S. Food and Drug Administration (FDA) as an aid for diagnosing *M. tuberculosis* infection. The test detects the IFN-γ released in fresh heparinized whole blood from sensitized persons when it is incubated with a mixture of synthetic peptides representing two proteins from *M. tuberculosis*, ESAT-6 and culture filtrate protein-10 (CFP-10). These antigens have greater specificity than PPD as the TB antigen. In direct comparisons, the sensitivity of QFT-G was statistically similar to that of the tuberculin skin test (TST) for detecting infection in persons with untreated culture-confirmed TB.

In July 2005, the CDC,[7] after reviewing existing data, recommended that the QFT-G can be used in all cases in which the TST is currently recommended, including contact investigations, evaluation of recent immigrants, and sequential testing surveillance programs for infection control (e.g., those for health care workers). The report provided specific cautions for interpreting negative QFT-G results in persons from select populations. Although approved by the FDA, the cost-effectiveness and practicality of the molecular methods discussed are still unclear.

The recommended approach in LTBI is given in Box 3. The ATS-CDC guidelines[6] for LTBI treatment recommend isoniazid

Box 2 Threshold for Purified Protein Derivative (PPD) Skin Reaction Positivity by Host or Setting

Reaction >5 mm

HIV-positive individuals
Recent contacts of tuberculosis (TB) cases
Fibrotic changes on chest radiograph suggesting old TB
Patients with organ transplants and other immunosuppressed patients (receiving equivalent of >15 mg/day prednisone for 1 mo or longer, or anti-TNF drugs)*

Reaction >10 mm

Recent immigrants (within last 5 yr) from endemic countries
Injection drug users
Residents and employees of certain high-risk congregate settings (e.g., prisons, jails, nursing homes, other long-term facilities, residential facilities for AIDS patients, homeless shelters)
Microbiology laboratory personnel
Patients with certain clinical conditions that place them at risk (e.g., silicosis, diabetes mellitus, chronic renal failure, leukemia, lymphoma, other malignancies [e.g., carcinomas of the head and lung], weight loss of >10% of ideal body weight, gastrectomy, and jejunoileal bypass
Children younger than 4 yr

Reaction >15 mm

Persons with no risk factors for TB

Data adapted from British Thoracic Society Standards of Care Committee: BTS recommendations for assessing risk and for managing Mycobacterium tuberculosis infection and disease in patients due to start anti-TNF-alpha treatment. Thorax 2005;60:800-805.

Box 3 Approach to the Patient with Latent Tuberculosis Infection (LTBI)

Clinical evaluation: cough, chest pain, hemoptysis, fever, chills, night sweats, anorexia, weight loss, fatigue
Past medical history-TB treatment or exposure
Social history: demographic factors increasing the risk of acquiring TB or resistant strains
HIV status; voluntary testing and counseling should be offered routinely
Chest radiographs (posteroanterior and lateral)
Sputum (three specimens) for patients with symptoms (even if chest radiograph is normal) or patients with radiologic abnormalities (images compatible with old fibrotic changes)
Perform baseline laboratory testing for HIV-infected patients, pregnant and postpartum women, those with liver disease, those who use alcohol regurlaly
Those without clinical, radiologic, or microbiologic evidence of active disease: LTBI therapy (those with abnormal liver function tests at baseline require continuous monitoring)

(INH), 5 mg/kg daily to a maximum of 300 mg, or 15 mg/kg twice weekly to a maximum of 900 mg. The duration of therapy recommended is 9 months for all patients (including children); if this cannot be accomplished, 6 months is acceptable. This represents a change in previous recommendations of 6 months of therapy for adults and 12 months for HIV-positive patients, which was based on studies showing that a 9-month course is superior to a 6-month course and almost as effective as 12 months of therapy. Following concerns about decreased rates of adherence to this length of therapy, studies have shown that RIF in doses of 10 mg/kg/day, up to a total of 600 mg for 4 months, or RIF (alternatively, rifabutin, with less interactions with other drugs) with PZA) daily for 2 months in HIV-infected individuals is an effective alternative to INH for 9 months. However, as a result of reports of severe hepatic injury following RIF-PZA combination administration in HIV-negative patients, the ATS-CDC has revised its recommendations, endorsed by the Infectious Diseases Society of America (IDSA), which state that this combination should no longer be offered to persons with LTBI.[8] The tuberculin skin testing is safe during pregnancy.

Bacillus Calmette-Guérin Vaccination

BCG, an attenuated strain of *M. bovis*, was first used as a vaccine in the 1920s. It has become the most widely used vaccine in the world, despite questions regarding its variable efficacy (0%-80%) in preventing TB in adults. Although less than ideal, studies have consistently shown its effectiveness in reducing fatal or severe forms of TB in infants and young children—miliary TB or meningitis. Most countries give only one BCG vaccine, at birth) Only 50% of vaccinated infants ever become PPD-positive, but by 1 to 2 years of age, only 20% are reactors. Of note, there are multiple BCG variants worldwide, with different results and varying rates of PPD conversion, which has greatly confounded their use. The chance of developing a postvaccination positive PPD test increases with the age of the BCG recipient, whereas repeated vaccinations have much higher rates of long-term conversion or booster effects on PPD rechallenge. In BCG recipients, the reactions to PPD are generally smaller than 10 mm, although reactions up to 18 mm have been reported.

In the United States, it is generally accepted that a positive tuberculin reaction in an adult indicates a true infection with *M. tuberculosis*, especially if that individual is a close contact of a TB case, from a high-prevalence area, or at high risk of exposure. BCG's lower efficacy in preventing TB compared with INH, as part of LTBI treatment, and interference with tuberculin skin testing has limited its use in the United States.

Tuberculous Pleural Effusion

Tuberculous Pleurisy

Tuberculous pleurisy is the most common form of extrapulmonary TB; it occurs in 10% of PPD converters. It develops when a subpleural TB focus ruptures into the pleural space and elicits a significant immune response. This can happen after the primary phase (up to 6 months after exposure) or during the secondary phase (endogenous reactivation). Clinically, it often manifests with cough, pleuritic chest pain, dyspnea, low-grade fever, and other nonspecific constitutional symptoms. The PPD skin test is generally positive in 90% of cases. Radiographically, it is generally unilateral, small to moderate in size, more frequent on the right side, and sometimes associated with parenchymal disease (ipsilateral infiltrates).

The pleural fluid is serous or serosanguineous (rarely hemorrhagic), exudative, with high protein concentrations (>5 g/dL), low pH (<7.30), moderately depressed glucose levels (<60 mg/dL), and usually lymphocytic (typically >90% cells). Acid-fast bacilli can be isolated in pleural fluid sediment in less than 5% of cases and, in cultures, in up to 70% of cases. Pleural biopsy specimens can increase the diagnostic yield to 20% of the cases, on microscopy, and to 80% of the cases, in cultures. Closed pleural biopsy, with pleural fluid analysis and sputum examination, yield the diagnosis of pleural TB in more than 80% of cases, whereas video-assisted surgical biopsy has an even higher diagnostic yield. The sputum can be positive for TB from 4% in isolated TB pleurisy to 50% of cases in those with extensive parenchymal infiltrates. A pleural fluid adenosine deaminase (ADA) level higher than 60 U/L may support the diagnosis if rheumatoid arthritis or empyema is unlikely, although this test is not routinely recommended.

Even if the pleurisy is not treated, the clinical course is toward spontaneous resolution, with minimal pleural scarring. However, the reactivation rate is higher for cases with coexistent parenchymal foci, more than 65% of cases at 5 years. Pleural TB is treated with a 4- to $6HR_2$ regimen. Steroids may hasten the pleural fluid resorption and resolution of clinical symptom resolution, although they do not seem to prevent scar formation.

Tuberculous Empyema

Less common than TB pleurisy, tuberculous empyema represents a chronic active infection of the pleural space. Its incidence was higher historically in patients who had undergone therapeutic pneumothorax, oleothorax, Lucite ball plombage, or pneumonectomy. It can run its course for decades, with a surprising paucity of clinical symptoms. On the chest computed tomography (CT) scan, the pleural peel is thickened, calcified, and sometimes loculated; the pleural mass may be accompanied by an extrapleural mass, which is diagnostic of empyema necessitans. The pleural fluid is generally thick, purulent in appearance, and positive on microscopic examination for acid-fast bacilli and occasionally other aerobic and anaerobic bacteria, indicating the presence of a bronchopleural fistula. In general, therapy is surgical, with a wide range of possible interventions, from parietal decortication to thoracoplasty, with or without omentopexy or myoplasty. Medical therapy is mandatory in an attempt to sterilize all residual TB foci.

Tuberculosis and HIV Infection[9]

It is estimated that 33% to 50% of the 20 million individuals infected with HIV worldwide are coinfected with *M. tuberculosis*. In many TB clinics, more than 10% of patients are HIV-seropositive. The AIDS case definition was modified in 1987 to include any form of extrapulmonary TB in an HIV-positive patient. Most cases represent the re-activation of old TB, occurring earlier than other opportunistic infections, because of the virulence of *M. tuberculosis*. There is also a significantly higher fraction of HIV-infected subjects who develop primary progressive TB, especially at the AIDS stage.

There is no evidence that HIV coinfection makes the patient more likely to transmit the disease, although AIDS patients are more predisposed to develop the progressive disease and can be more difficult to diagnose. The mean CD4 count at TB presentation is 200 to 300 cells/mm^3, which is earlier than other opportunistic infections. With a CD4 count higher than 300 cells/mm^3, the clinical presentation is similar to that of those who are HIV-negative—that is, isolated pulmonary disease, with focal apical infiltrates, occasionally with cavitation. As immunosuppression worsens, the incidence of diffuse pulmonary disease without cavitation, miliary TB, and extrapulmonary TB increases, up to 70% of AIDS patients.

Patients with HIV infection have a similar response to anti-TB medications as that of HIV-negative patients. However, drug interactions are important issues. Many of the highly active antiretroviral therapy (HAART) drugs interfere with rifampin's metabolism, which is a potent inducer of the cytochrome P-450 enzyme system. Consequently, the levels of anti-HIV drugs could be suboptimal. Rifabutin, a RIF-derivative, has equivalent efficacy and less effect on hepatic enzymes and therefore is preferred for most HIV-positive patients. Clinical deterioration may occur in patients with active TB started on HAART—for example, worsening infiltrates, severe hypoxemia to full-blown acute respiratory distress syndrome, necrotizing lymphadenitis, enlarging brain tuberculomas, miliary TB, or severe systemic toxicity. This is called immune reconstitution syndrome and is believed to be caused by re-arming of the cellular immune system during the first weeks of HAART. A possible preventive measure is initiating anti-TB treatment 2 weeks before stating HAART.

CONCLUSIONS

Tuberculosis is probably one of the greatest killers of all time, over the centuries taking more than 1 billion lives and up to 2 million people every year (i.e., one life every 15 seconds, as opposed to a life lost in an accident every 50 seconds). Every year, TB infects up to 100 million people worldwide, and up to 8 million develop active disease. If the tuberculosis is not treated, every source case infects, on average, 10 to 15 other persons each year. TB can be considered a social disease, disrupting families emotionally, educationally, and economically. Furthermore, only about 20% of worldwide TB cases are detected and treated successfully.

DOT strategy implemented by the World Heath Organization (WHO) is probably one of the most cost-effective of all health interventions. Achievement of global targets of 70% detection and 85% cure rates would reduce incidence and mortality by 10%. The United States and several other low-incidence countries have embarked on plans to eliminate tuberculosis completely. Important elements in an elimination strategy would be to identify and treat effectively LTBI persons at risk of developing active disease, and to ensure provision of inexpensive and efficacious drugs to countries that cannot afford them. However, even though a constellation of drugs, molecular tools, and public health strategies are on the horizon, newer diagnostic tools, a better vaccine, and novel therapeutic agents are urgently needed to fight this condition more effectively.

Summary

About one third of the world's population is infected with *Mycobacterium tuberculosis*. Once infected with *M. tuberculosis*, 3% to 5% of immunocompetent individuals will develop active disease.

- Among communicable diseases, tuberculosis is the second leading cause of death worldwide.
- Tuberculosis is caused by the *Mycobacterium tuberculosis* complex: *M. tuberculosis, M. bovis, M. africanum, M. microti*, and *M. canettii*.
- TB transmission occurs almost exclusively from human to human, most commonly via airborne droplet nuclei.
- Persistent cough, hemoptysis, dyspnea, malaise, weight loss, night sweats, and chest pain are the common symptoms of tuberculosis.
- Standard anti-TB therapeutic regimens have to be administered after notification of the local public health department, preferably under DOT (directly observed therapy).
- DOT strategy, which is implemented and enforced by the World Heath Organization, is probably one of the most cost effective of all health interventions.

Suggested Readings

American Thoracic Society; Centers for Disease Control and Prevention; Infectious Diseases Society of America: American Thoracic Society/Centers for Disease Control and Prevention/Infectious Diseases Society of America: Controlling tuberculosis in the United States. Am J Respir Crit Care Med 2005;172:1169-1227.

Blumberg HM, Burman WJ, Chaisson RE, et al: American Thoracic Society, Centers for Disease Control and Prevention and the Infectious Diseases Society: American Thoracic Society/Centers for Disease Control and Prevention/Infectious Diseases Society of America: Treatment of tuberculosis. Am J Respir Crit Care Med 2003;167:603-662.

British Thoracic Society Standards of Care Committee: BTS recommendations for assessing risk and for managing Mycobacterium tuberculosis infection and disease in patients due to start anti-TNF-alpha treatment. Thorax 2005;60:800-805.

Centers for Disease Control and Prevention (CDC); American Thoracic Society: Update: Adverse event data and revised American Thoracic Society/CDC recommendations against the use of rifampin and pyrazinamide for treatment of latent tuberculosis infection—United States, 2003. MMWR Morb Mortal Wkly Rep 2003;52:735-739.

Diagnostic Standards and Classification of Tuberculosis in Adults and Children. This official statement of the American Thoracic Society and the Centers for Disease Control and Prevention was adopted by the ATS Board of Directors, July 1999. This statement was endorsed by the Council of the Infectious Disease Society of America, September 1999. Am J Respir Crit Care Med 2000;161:1376-1395.

Jensen PA, Lambert LA, Iademarco MF, Ridzon R: Guidelines for preventing the transmission of Mycobacterium tuberculosis in health-care settings, 2005. MMWR Recomm Rep 2005;54:1-141.

Mazurek GH, Jereb J, Lobue P, et al: Guidelines for using the QuantiFERON-TB Gold test for detecting Mycobacterium tuberculosis infection, United States. MMWR Recomm Rep 2005;54:49-55.

Mofenson LM, Oleske J, Serchuck L, et al: National Institutes of Health; Infectious Diseases Society of America: Treating opportunistic infections among HIV-exposed and infected children: Recommendations from CDC, the National Institutes of Health, and the Infectious Diseases Society of America. MMWR Recomm Rep 2004;53(RR-14):1-92.

Targeted tuberculin testing and treatment of latent tuberculosis infection. This official statement of the American Thoracic Society was adopted by the ATS Board of Directors, July 1999. This is a Joint Statement of the American Thoracic Society (ATS) and the Centers for Disease Control and Prevention (CDC). This statement was endorsed by the Council of the Infectious Diseases Society of America. (IDSA), September 1999, and the sections of this statement. Am J Respir Crit Care Med 2000;161:S221-S247.

Taylor Z, Nolan CM, Blumberg HM; American Thoracic Society; Centers for Disease Control and Prevention; Infectious Diseases Society of America: Controlling tuberculosis in the United States. Recommendations from the American Thoracic Society, CDC, and the Infectious Diseases Society of America. MMWR Morb Mortal Wkly Rep 2005;54(RR-12):1-81.

References

For a complete list of references, log onto www.expertconsult.com.

Nontuberculous Mycobacterial Disorders

Octavian C. Ioachimescu and J. Walton Tomford

TAXONOMY

Mycobacteria other than *Mycobacterium leprae*, *M. tuberculosis*, and *M. bovis* were identified from human sources as early as 1885, but it was not until almost 65 years later that human infection was attributed to these organisms. Between the early 1950s and 1980s, there was increasing awareness of the spectrum of disease caused by the nontuberculous mycobacteria (NTM), although the number of cases was small. In the 1980s, in the early days of HIV infection, it was recognized that *M. avium* complex and *M. kansasii* organisms commonly caused disseminated infections in patients who were severely immunocompromised. Currently, the epidemiology and clinical features of the NTM diseases are dominated by their occurrence in patients with HIV infection and, more recently, in patients on tumor necrosis factor α (TNF-α) pathway blockers. However, disease caused by this group of organisms continues to occur in persons without detectable systemic immune dysfunction (e.g., recipients of prosthetic knees, fish tank granuloma, hot tub lung).

The genus *Mycobacterium* is composed of more than 100 species characterized by complex lipid-rich cell walls, which confer the acid-fast staining property. Mycobacterial species were classically differentiated using cultural and biochemical properties, but genetic differences are now used for this purpose, especially 16S ribosomal RNA sequence differences. The published mycobacterial species and subspecies, which number 139 (as of January 2008), are included in the List of Prokaryotic Names with Standing in Nomenclature. The genus *Mycobacterium* contains two obligate pathogens, the *M. tuberculosis* complex and *M. leprae*. The *M. tuberculosis* complex contains several related mycobacteria (i.e., *M. bovis*—including bacillus Calmette-Guérin [BCG], *M. africanum*, *M. microti*, and *M. cannetti*), which on DNA analysis are all variants of *M. tuberculosis*. The other species live freely in the environment (water and soil) and are thus often termed *environmental mycobacteria* or *nontuberculous mycobacteria;* we prefer the latter term.

NTM have been called in the past "atypical" mycobacterial species or mycobacteria other than tuberculosis (MOTT). These microbes share many common properties, such as acid fastness and the ability to cause pulmonary and extrapulmonary granulomatous disorders. As a group, they comprise diverse organisms with dissimilarities in their cultural characteristics and pathogenicity to humans compared with *M. tuberculosis* (MTB). There are many organisms in this group capable of causing human infections. Infections caused by *M. avium-intracellulare* (MAI) complex became common in patients with severe HIV infection—in patients with low CD4 lymphocyte counts—or in AIDS, for which it is a disease-defining condition. NTM cause significant lung disease in individuals with structural abnormalities (e.g., patients with bronchiectasis and chronic obstructive pulmonary disease with *M. kansasii* infection) and in those with immunodeficiency syndromes (e.g., *M. avium* infection in HIV-AIDS patients).

CLASSIFICATION

NTM classifications have generally not been helpful to the clinician. The most widely used classification in the past, the Runyon system, was based on microbiologic characteristics of the organisms, such as growth rate in cultures and colony pigment formation in the presence or absence of light. Familiarity with the Runyon system remains useful for presumptive laboratory identification of possible NTM pathogens; however, positive identification of NTM species is now largely based on biochemical and molecular biology techniques. Classification of NTMs based on the organ system of primary involvement (e.g., lungs, lymph nodes, disseminated, skin, and soft tissue) is more useful to the clinician and will be used hereafter (Table 1). Based on culture characteristics, NTM are subclassified into the following main groups: the slow, intermediate, and rapid growers, with varying nutritional requirements.

Slow-Growing Mycobacteria

The slow-growing group includes species of mycobacteria that require usually more than 14 days of incubation for mature growth; some may require nutritional supplementation of routine mycobacterial media. The most common clinically important species found in this group include the *M. avium* complex (*M. avium* and *M. intracellulare*), *M. kansasii*, *M. xenopi*, *M. simiae*, *M. szulgai*, *M. scrofulaceum*, *M. malmoense*, *M. terrae-nonchromogenicum* complex, *M. haemophilum*, and *M. genavense*. These organisms grow best at 35° to 37° C, with the exception of *M. haemophilum*, which has a preference for lower temperatures (28° to 30° C) and the presence of iron, and *M. xenopi*, which grows optimally at 42° C. Newer isolated slow-growing species include *M. celatum*, *M. interjectum*, *M. confluentis*, *M. triplex*, *M. lentiflavum*, *M. branderi*, *M. conspicuum*, *M. cookii*, and *M. asiaticum*.

Intermediate-Growing Mycobacteria

The intermediate-growing group includes *M. marinum* and *M. gordonae*. These organisms are usually pigmented and require 7 to 10 days of incubation for mature growth. *M. marinum* has an optimal growth temperature of 30° C, whereas *M. gordonae* prefers 35° C. *M. gordonae* is seldom if ever pathogenic, except in severely immunocompromised hosts.

Rapid-Growing Mycobacteria

The rapid-growing group of organisms includes nonpigmented and pigmented species that produce mature growth on agar plates, usually within 7 to 10 days. Nonpigmented pathogenic species are mostly grouped within the *M. fortuitum* complex, which includes the *M. fortuitum* group (*M. fortuitum*, *M. peregrinum*, and *M. fortuitum* third biovariant complex) and the *M. chelonae-abscessus* group (*M. chelonae*, formerly *M. chelonae* subspecies *chelonae*, *M. abscessus*, formerly *M. chelonae* subspecies *abscessus*, and *M. mucogenicum*, formerly *M. chelonae*-like organism). *M. smegmatis* may be pigmented or nonpigmented.

Pigmented, rapid-growing species are difficult to identify by traditional laboratory methods. Rapid-growing pigmented species occasionally isolated in clinical disease include *M. phlei*, *M. aurum*, *M. flavescens*, *M. neoaurum*, *M. vaccae*, and the thermophilic species *M. thermoresistible*.

EPIDEMIOLOGY

In the United States, the number of significant NTM isolates continues to increase, in parallel with a recent increase in the number of immunocompetent patients with NTM disease (primarily lung disease) and a slow decline of tuberculosis (TB). Factors that may be contributing to this increase include the following:

Table 1 Major Clinical Syndromes Associated with Nontuberculous Mycobacteria Infections

Syndrome	Common Causes	Less-Common Causes
Pulmonary disease (especially in adults)	*Mycobacterium avium-intracellulare, M. kansasii, M. abscessus*	Uncommon: *M. fortuitum, M. malmoense, M. szulgai, M. scrofulaceum, M. smegmatis, M. simiae, M. xenopi* Rare: *M. celatum, M. asiaticum, M. shimodei*
Cervical and lymphadenitis (especially children)	*M. avium, M. intracellulare*	*M. scrofulaceum, M. malmoense, M. abscessus, M. fortuitum*
Skin and soft tissue disease	*M. fortuitum, M. chelonae, M. abscessus, M. marinum*	*M. haemophilum, M. kansasi, M. smegmatis, M. ulcerans*
Skeletal (bones, joints, tendons) disease	*M. marinum, M. avium* complex, *M. kansasii, M. fortuitum* group, *M. abscessus, M. chelonae*	*M. haemophilum, M. scrofulaceum, M. smegmatis, M. terrae-nonchromogenicum* complex
Catheter-related infections	*M. fortuitum, M. abscessus, M. chelonae*	*M. mucogenicum*
Disseminated infection	HIV-seropositive host: *M. avium, M. kansasii*	*M. haemophilum, M. genavense, M. xenopi, M. marinum, M. simiae, M. intracellulare, M. scrofulaceum, M. fortuitum*
	HIV-seronegative host: *M. abscessus, M. chelonae*	*M. marinum, M. kansasii, M. haemophilum, M. fortuitum*

- An increased number of clinical specimens submitted for acid-fast bacilli (AFB) stains and cultures
- Improved laboratory techniques, which have made identification and isolation of NTM more rapid and accurate
- Higher recognition of NTM disease, especially in chronic pulmonary disease and in immunocompetent patients (e.g., older women with MAI disease)

Evidence is mounting to show that the environment is the major source of human NTM infection. NTM are ubiquitous in the environment and have been isolated from water (most cases), soil, dust, domestic and wild animals, milk, and food. DNA fingerprinting techniques—restriction fragment length polymorphism analysis by pulsed field gel electrophoresis and major polymorphic tandem repeat probe sequence analysis—have been useful for epidemiologic investigation (e.g., point source epidemics). These techniques also may provide clues to pathophysiologic differences among NTM species. For example, there appears to be great genetic variability among MAI isolates from different patients and sometimes even from the same patient. In contrast, clinical *M. kansasii* isolates generally have similar genotypes, suggesting that most clinical isolates are clonal. This clonal nature of most clinical isolates of *M. kansasii* would seem unusual for environmental species such as MAI, and suggests that their colonization of environmental sites of human disease acquisition (e.g., municipal water supplies) is fairly recent and involves only select genotypes.

Unlike TB, disease caused by NTM is rarely if ever transmitted from patient to patient. Infection is acquired from the environment; pulmonary disease is probably caused by the inhalation of aerosols of water containing the mycobacteria. The incidence of disease caused by NTM is somewhat independent of that of TB, but is determined by the number, distribution, and species of NTM in the environment and the susceptibility of the human population. In regions where TB is common, only a small minority of cases of pulmonary mycobacterial disease will be caused by NTM. By contrast, in regions where TB is rare, such as rural areas of western Europe and the United States, a much higher proportion of pulmonary mycobacterial disease is caused by NTM. There are geographic variations in distribution of the species of NTM: whereas the MAI complex occurs worldwide, others, such as *M. xenopi* and *M. malmoense*, are restricted to certain regions. *M. xenopi* is the second most common NTM causative organism in Canada and the United Kingdom, and *M. malmoense* is the second most common NTM disease in Sweden and other northern European countries. *M. ulcerans* infections occur mostly in Australia and tropical countries. Although MAI disease has a worldwide distribution, disseminated MAI is rarely seen in people from central Africa who have AIDS, even though MAI can be recovered from that environment. One possible explanation is that those who have AIDS in Africa may die from infection with more aggressive pathogens such as *M. tuberculosis* before their immunosuppression becomes severe enough to develop disseminated MAI. In addition, the distribution of species varies with time, possibly as a result of environmental changes.

Immune reactions elicited by exposure to NTM have been postulated as a cause of the wide geographic variation in the protective efficacy of BCG. One possible explanation is that repeated contact with NTM leads to protective immunity equivalent to that conferred by BCG; in this case, BCG vaccination would not add any protective effect. Another explanation is that the immune response in TB is qualitatively different, eliciting protective immunity or a delayed hypersensitivity reaction, with possible disease progression. The switch between the two responses is determined by helper T cell 1 (Th1) versus helper T cell 2 (Th2) T lymphocyte selection in the immune response. A predominant Th1 response facilitates protective immunity, whereas a superimposed Th2 response seems to be associated with tissue necrosis. When given neonatally, BCG confers protection against TB inducing a Th1 response, but later in life it boosts or fails to downregulate an environmentally determined harmful Th2 component and therefore fails to protect from—and may even predispose to—active TB. A third hypothesis, supported by mouse models, is that environmental sensitization to *M. avium* (but not *M. fortuitum* and *M. chelonae*) prevents the multiplication of BCG in tissues, which is essential for the development of protective immunity. These hypotheses are not mutually exclusive.

VIRULENCE AND PATHOGENICITY

Many questions surround the determinants of virulence of *M. tuberculosis* and *M. leprae*, and even less is known about the virulence of NTM. A mouse model has revealed three patterns of pathogenicity. After intravenous inoculation in immunocompetent mice, most tested species were found to replicate progressively in the liver and spleen; some replicated in these organs in interferon gamma (IFN-γ)-deficient mice, but not in immunocompetent mice (e.g., *M. heidelbergense* and *M. intermedium*). Others were eliminated in both types of mice (e.g., *M. confluentis* and *M. lentiflavum*). The relevance of these findings to human disease remains to be established, but they suggest that IFN-γ is not a crucial determinant of protection in all forms of mycobacterial disease. For the clinician, it is important to emphasize that NTM disease can occur in immunocompetent hosts.

There are few data on the relative virulence of NTM in humans. Although some species such as MAI and *M. kansasii* are recognized as pathogens, others such as *M. gordonae* are often isolated as non-pathogenic contaminants of the respiratory tract but only occasionally as causes of overt disease. In the presence of immunosuppression, all NTM must be regarded as potential pathogens, but some species are particularly associated with disease. For unknown reasons, HIV-positive patients are particularly prone to develop disease caused by certain genetic variants of MAI.

CLINICAL SYNDROMES

Five major clinical syndromes have been described that are attributable to NTM (see Table 1): pulmonary disease; lymphadenitis; skin, soft tissue, and skeletal infections; catheter-related bloodstream infections; and disseminated disease, especially in persons with AIDS or severely immunocompromised hosts (e.g., individuals on high-dose corticosteroids). There is limited documentation (if any) of person-to-person transmission of NTM. Nosocomial infections and outbreaks caused by inadequate disinfection or sterilization of medical devices or environmental contamination of medications or medical devices have been described.

Pulmonary Disease

Pulmonary disease caused by NTM may occur as a component of disseminated infection, but often the disease affects only the lungs (Table 2). Four main categories of pulmonary disease can be nosologically identified. First, the disease occurs in middle-aged or older patients, usually men with a history of lung disease. Second, the disease occurs in otherwise apparently healthy persons, although some may have minor and covert immune defects. Third, the disease occurs in children with more severe immune defects or predisposing pulmonary disease, notably cystic fibrosis or severe fungal infection (e.g., invasive or semi-invasive *Aspergillus* disease). Fourth, the disease occurs in very immunosuppressed patients, of which HIV infection is the prevalent cause worldwide. Also, it is important to emphasize that patients with NTM diseases do not need to be isolated because of the noncontagiousness of these conditions.

Patients with Predisposing Lung Disease

Most patients are men with a history of smoking, bronchiectasis, chronic obstructive lung disease, rheumatoid lung, healed TB, or exposure to industrial dusts as a result of mining, sandblasting, or welding. Risk factors have been evaluated in South African gold miners with pulmonary mycobacterial disease. In this study,[1] 51 patients with disease caused by NTM and 425 with TB were similar with regard to age, education, home region, and smoking habits. Those with disease caused by NTM were more likely to have been previously treated for TB, worked longer underground, or have evidence of silicosis. Patients with disease caused by NTM were less likely to be HIV-positive (35.3%) than those with TB (48.8%), although the difference was not statistically significant. Pulmonary disease caused by *M. kansasii* is particularly associated with underlying lung damage such as pneumoconiosis or silicosis, which leads to slowly progressive and insidious disease in miners and other workers. This species has been recognized since 1977 as the most common cause of NTM pulmonary disease in South African gold miners. The disease occurs in both HIV-positive and HIV-negative patients, and most have had radiologic evidence of silicosis. Disease caused by *M. kansasii* in HIV-positive gold miners differs from that occurring in HIV-positive patients without the risks associated with mining. Thus, in miners, the disease occurs much earlier in the course of HIV infection, with $CD4^+$ T cell counts being significantly higher, and clinically it more closely resembles the disease in HIV-negative patients. It has been noted that assessment of the clinical significance of sputum isolates of *M. kansasii* in this group of patients by American Thoracic Society guidelines[2] is not straightforward.

Old TB lesions may be colonized or infected by NTM. In one study in Japan, 75% of mycobacteria isolated from sputum more than 1 year after completion of therapy for TB were NTM. The presence of such mycobacteria could lead to a false diagnosis of recurrence of TB. In some cases, disease caused by *M. xenopi* has been superimposed on aspergillomas in old cavities; this disease has a generally poor prognosis and response to therapy.

Immunocompetent Hosts

A number of cases, mostly caused by MAI complex, have been reported in older people, principally nonsmoking women with no other evidence of lung disease except for the associated bronchiectasis. It has been postulated that such disease in women is associated with the practice of coughing quietly and covertly, thereby suppressing the clearance of sputum. The disease has accordingly been termed *Lady Windermere syndrome* after the fastidious aristocrat in Oscar Wilde's play, "Lady Windermere's Fan."[3] We prefer not to use "Lady Windermere syndrome," mainly because the term is not

Table 2 Clinical Settings for Nontuberculous Mycobacteria Lung Disease

Radiographic Disease	Setting	Usual Pathogen	Rare Pathogen
Upper lobe cavitary	Male smokers, often abusing alcohol, usually in their early 50s	*M. avium* complex, *M. kansasii*	
RML, lingular nodular bronchiectasis	Female nonsmokers, usually older than 60 yr	*M. avium* complex, *M. abscessus*	*M. kansasii*
Localized alveolar, cavitary disease	Prior granulomatous disease (usually tuberculosis) with bronchiectasis	*M. abscessus*, *M. avium* complex	
Not well established	Adolescents with cystic fibrosis	*M. avium* complex, *M. abscessus*	
Reticulonodular or alveolar lower lobe disease	Achalasia, chronic vomiting secondary to GI disease, exogenous lipoid pneumonia (mineral oil aspiration, etc.)	*M. fortuitum*	*M. abscessus*, *M. avium* complex, *M. smegmatis*
Reticulonodular disease	HIV-positive hosts, patients with preexisting bronchiectasis, others	*M. avium* complex	

GI, gastrointestinal; HIV, human immunodeficiency virus; RML, right middle lobe.

comprehensive and does not illustrate the full spectrum of the disease. If the disorder continues undetected for years, cavities develop in the lungs and respiratory failure may ensue; however, the natural history of this disorder is unpredictable. The causative organisms include MAI and *M. kansasii* and, less frequently, *M. xenopi*, *M. scrofulaceum*, *M. szulgai*, *M. malmoense*, *M. simiae*, *M. celatum*, and *M. chelonae*. A similar but less common form of pulmonary disease caused by NTM has also been reported in apparently immunocompetent men.

A bizarre characteristic of 10 previously healthy patients with diffuse pulmonary disease caused by NTM (*M. avium* in 9 of the 10 cases) was that they all bathed in hot tubs. Although this serious condition was termed *hot tub lung*, further studies are required to confirm whether the use of such tubs is an important predisposing factor.[4] Although the patients described appeared clinically and immunologically normal, it is possible that they had minor immune defects. On detailed investigation, some patients with pulmonary disease caused by NTM have been found to have such defects, although it is not clear whether these were a cause or consequence of the disease.

Children

Although rare in childhood, a few cases caused by MAI, *M. chelonae*, and *M. fortuitum* have been reported in children with cystic fibrosis. Children with deteriorating lung function should be screened for NTM because therapy can, in some cases, halt the deterioration. Familial susceptibility to NTM disease, but not to *M. tuberculosis*, can be linked to different mutations in four genes. These mutations result in eight different clinical syndromes, all characterized by impaired cell-mediated immune responses mediated by IFN-γ. Because these syndromes vary in severity and require different therapeutic strategies, identification of the underlying genetic defect is important.

Immunosuppressed Hosts

Mycobacteria, both *M. tuberculosis* and NTM, are common causes of lung disease in HIV-positive patients. In general, the isolation of NTM, and most notably of MAI complex, from the respiratory tract of an HIV-positive person is more likely to be clinically significant than from an HIV-negative person. Cough is a common complaint irrespective of HIV status, but HIV-positive patients are more likely to have fever. Abnormal chest radiographs are common, with HIV-positive patients being more likely to have diffuse abnormalities. In one study, a specific diagnosis was made in 20 of 25 HIV-positive patients with cavitating lung lesions.[8] Bacteria, often more than one species, were the cause in 17 patients. Mycobacteria were isolated in 8 patients. Mediastinal or hilar lymphadenopathy and additional ill-defined, noncavitating, nodular opacities were seen more frequently in patients with mycobacterial pathogens.

Localized Cutaneous, Soft Tissue, and Bone Infections

Skin and Subcutaneous Diseases

Postinoculation lesions usually affect skin or subcutaneous tissues following a traumatic inoculation. This can take the form of swimming pool (or fish tank) granuloma or Buruli ulcer, the latter mainly outside the United States. Although all species of NTM have been incriminated in cutaneous NTM disease, *M. marinum* and rapid-growing mycobacteria most often cause localized skin infections. *M. marinum* causes an infection historically recognized as swimming pool or fish tank granuloma. Most infections occur 2 to 3 weeks after contact with contaminated fresh or salty water from one of these sources. The lesions are most often small violet papules on the hands and arms that may progress to shallow crusty ulcerations and scar formation. Lesions are usually singular. However, multiple ascending lesions resembling sporotrichosis (sporotrichoid disease) can occasionally occur; in our experience, the antifungal-resistant sporotrichosis is the most common presentation. Most patients are clinically healthy with a previous local hand injury that became infected while cleaning a fish tank, or patients may sustain scratches or puncture wounds from saltwater fish, shrimp, or fins contaminated with *M. marinum*. Diagnosis is made from culture and histologic examination of biopsy material, along with a compatible history of exposure. There is no treatment of choice for *M. marinum*; traditionally, the regimen has been a combination of rifampin and ethambutol or monotherapy with doxycycline, minocycline, clarithromycin, or trimethoprim-sulfamethoxazole, given for a minimum of 3 months. Clarithromycin has been used increasingly because of good clinical efficacy and minimal side effects, although published experience is limited. Because *M. marinum* grows better at lower temperatures, local heat can produce amelioration.

The rapid-growing species *M. abscessus*, *M. fortuitum*, and *M. chelonae* are probably the most common NTM involved in cases of community-acquired infections of skin and soft tissue. Localized traumatic injury, such as puncture wounds from stepping on a nail, and open lacerations or fractures are the usual scenarios. An outbreak in California was associated with contamination of a post–leg shaving solution, causing mycobacterial abscesses of the lower extremities.[5] Occasionally, these infections may involve slow-growing species, including *M. avium* complex, *M. kansasii*, and *M. terrae-nonchromogenicum* complex.

Sporadic cases of nosocomial skin and soft tissue disease have also been described as possible point source outbreaks. These cases include infections of long-term IV or peritoneal catheters, postinjection abscesses, surgical wound infections such as those after cardiac bypass surgery, and augmentation mammaplasty. In ophthalmology, rapid-growing species may cause keratitis and corneal ulceration after surgery, as well as infection after local accidental trauma. Clustered outbreaks or pseudo-outbreaks of mycobacterial skin, soft tissue, or bone infections have been described and usually result from contaminated fluids such as ice made from tap water, water, injectable medicines, and topical skin solutions. Most of these outbreaks have involved the rapid-growing species *M. fortuitum* and *M. abscessus*. The reservoir for these outbreaks has generally been municipal or distilled (hospital) water supplies. These and other species such as *M. avium* complex and *M. xenopi* are incredibly resistant, can endure temperatures of 45° C and higher (MAI complex and *M. xenopi*), and may resist the activity of commonly used disinfectants.

Diagnosis of all types of skin and soft tissue infections is made by culture of specific NTM from drainage material or tissue biopsy (swabs are useless). Treatment may include amikacin, cefoxitin, ciprofloxacin, clarithromycin, doxycycline, sulfonamides, and imipenem for the *M. fortuitum* group, whereas only amikacin, cefoxitin, imipenem, and clarithromycin or only amikacin, imipenem, tobramycin, and clarithromycin have activity against *M. abscessus* and *M. chelonae*, respectively. Clarithromycin is generally the first drug of choice for localized disease caused by *M. fortuitum*, *M. chelonae*, and *M. abscessus*, although its use in combination with at least one other drug is preferred. The duration of therapy is usually 4 to 6 months. Antituberculous agents have no efficacy against any of the rapidly growing mycobacteria other than ethambutol for *M. smegmatis*. Treatment of slow-growing species is similar to that for chronic lung disease, except that the duration of therapy may only be 6 to 12 months.

Two unusual species causing skin and soft tissue infections in select situations are *M. ulcerans* and *M. haemophilum*. *M. ulcerans* is not endemic in the United States, but is endemic in areas of Australia and tropical locations, where it is commonly known as the Buruli ulcer. This infection progresses from an itchy nodule, most often on the extremities, to a necrotic lesion that may result in severe deformity. Treatment success is common in early disease with excisional surgery, rifampin, sulfonamides, and clofazimine but, for advanced ulcerative disease, therapeutic response has generally been poor. Surgical débridement and skin grafting then become the usual therapeutic measures of choice. Studies have suggested that clarithromycin is highly active in vitro.

The second unusual species, *M. haemophilum*, causes cutaneous infections, primarily of the extremities, in immunosuppressed patients, especially in the setting of organ transplantation, long-term high-dose steroid use, or HIV. A review by Saubolle and coworkers has cited more than 50 cases of *M. haemophilum*, with almost 80% of them involving skin and soft tissue infections. Careful attention to culture technique is essential because this species requires heme or iron to grow in culture. Therapy for this species usually includes clarithromycin and rifampin or rifabutin.

Skeletal Disease: Bone, Tendon, Ligament, and Joint Diseases

Both rapid-growing and slow-growing species of NTM have been implicated in chronic granulomatous infections involving tendon sheaths, bursae, bones, and joints after direct inoculation of the pathogen through accidental trauma, surgical incisions, puncture wounds, or injections. Most patients have no underlying immune suppression, but those at high risk for pathogens such as *M. chelonae* and *M. haemophilum* are patients who are immunosuppressed. MAI complex and *M. marinum* have been described as causing tenosynovitis of the hand, although the rapid-growing mycobacteria, *M. kansasii*, and *M. terrae* complex (especially *M. nonchromogenicum*) have also been associated with a chronic type of disease. Osteomyelitis of the sternum caused by *M. fortuitum* and *M. abscessus* has also been found in clustered outbreaks and sporadic cases after cardiac surgery. Additionally, *M. haemophilum* has a tendency to involve bones and joints, usually with concurrent draining skin lesions and bacteremia.

Management of mycobacterial bone and soft tissue infections often requires surgical débridement for both diagnosis and therapy, especially for the closed spaces of the hand and the wrist and for patients with infected bones, such as fractured long bones or the sternum after cardiac surgery. Drug therapy for the specific pathogen is also essential.

Lymphadenitis

Lymphadenitis usually affects the cervical lymph nodes in otherwise healthy children younger than 5 years. Lymphadenitis in older persons usually indicates HIV infection or some other form of immunosuppression. Many mycobacterial species are involved. Since the early 1980s, 80% of cases of culture-positive NTM lymphadenitis in children in the United States have been caused by *M. avium* complex.[6] The remainder of cases in Australia and the United States are caused by *M. scrofulaceum*, and only about 10% of cases have been caused by *M. tuberculosis* (this should serve as a reminder about this condition). Rarely, other species are recovered, including rapid-growing mycobacteria, *M. kansasii*, and *M. haemophilum*. This last species has a special growth requirement for hemin or iron and may present some diagnostic difficulties if iron- or hemin-supplemented media and lower temperatures (incubation at 28°-30° C) are not used. A surprising number of specimens are AFB smear-positive and culture-negative, so a presumptive diagnosis is often based on typical caseating granulomas and a negative culture for *M. tuberculosis* in the common clinical setting. Skin testing with purified protein derivative–Battey (PPD-B), an antigen prepared from *M. avium* complex, has been shown to be useful, but the antigen is unavailable except for use in experimental protocols.

Treatment of NTM cervical lymphadenitis is still evolving. Routine biopsy or incision and drainage should be avoided because these procedures often result in the formation of fistulas and chronic drainage. Fine-needle aspiration with cytology and culture has been used increasingly, with apparently few associated problems. The treatment of choice is excision of the involved nodes by an experienced surgeon. Chemotherapy seems to be of little benefit. The potential role of chemotherapy without surgery or as a supplement to surgery in complicated or recurrent disease is being considered with increasing frequency. Clarithromycin combined with ethambutol or rifabutin is the usual suggested regimen (Box 1). However, the established treatment of routine NTM cervical lymphadenitis remains surgical excision, without chemotherapy.

Box 1 Guidelines for Diagnosing NTM Pulmonary Disease

- Clinical and radiologic features indicative of mycobacterial disease
- AFB smear-positive and/or moderate/heavy growth of NTM on culture in two clinical specimens (e.g., sputum or BAL)
- Absence of other pathogens/conditions (e.g., tuberculosis, aspergillosis)
- Underlying host conditions (e.g., alcoholism, immunosuppressive conditions, chronic lung disease, cystic fibrosis, lung cancer)
- Failure of clearance of the NTM in sputum within 2 weeks of initiation of antimycobacterial therapy
- When sputum evaluation in cavitary or noncavitary disease is negative:
- Transbronchial or open lung biopsy has histopathologic features of mycobacterial disease and grows NTM on culture
- Transbronchial or open lung biopsy does not grow the organism but has histopathologic features of mycobacterial disease and other reasonable causes for granulomatous disease have been excluded

AFB, acid-fast bacilli; BAL, bronchial lavage; NTM, nontuberculous mycobacteria.

Catheter-Related Infections

Currently, catheter-related infections are the most common nosocomial NTM infections encountered. They are usually seen with long-term central IV catheters, but they may also occur with peritoneal or shunt catheters. The usual pathogens are rapid-growing mycobacteria. These infections may be manifested as fever, local catheter site drainage, or bacteremia or occasionally as lung infiltrates or granulomatous hepatitis. The usual treatment is catheter removal combined with pus drainage and appropriate antibiotics for 6 to 12 weeks.

Disseminated Diseases

Localized nonpulmonary lesions in the kidneys, bones, joints, and central nervous system have been described, but are exceedingly rare. Most diseases in this category are multifocal, especially to the skin, or widely disseminated. Such diseases are almost always associated with some form of congenital or acquired immune defect, including post-transplantation immunosuppressive therapy. Most cases at present occur in patients with AIDS, and most are caused by MAI.

In the setting of advanced HIV infection, most disseminated NTM disease is caused by *M. avium*. However, other NTM, including *M. kansasii*, *M. genavense*, *M. intracellulare*, *M. haemophilum*, *M. simiae*, *M. celatum*, *M. malmoense*, *M. marinum*, and rapid-growing mycobacteria, have also been cited. In the absence of HIV infection, cases of disseminated MAI complex are rare. Disseminated infections by other NTM species in non-AIDS patients, such as organ transplant recipients or patients receiving chronic steroids, have occurred in all age groups, almost exclusively in immunosuppressed patients. The most commonly reported physical findings in disseminated *M. avium* infection include fever, weight loss, skin lesions, and enlargement of organs of the reticuloendothelial system. Although anemia often occurs with a hematocrit lower than 25%, and one third of patients with disseminated *M. avium* infection have elevated alkaline phosphatase levels, laboratory studies and chest radiographs are not usually conclusive in establishing the diagnosis of disseminated NTM disease. The usual method of diagnosis is mycobacterial blood cultures in patients with AIDS or, in other patients, by skin biopsy. The diagnosis of disseminated *M. avium* is rare in HIV-infected patients with more than 100 $CD4^+$ lymphocytes. Also, patients with hairy cell leukemia seem to be particularly susceptible to MAI infections.[7]

Disseminated *M. kansasii* is the second most frequent cause of disseminated NTM disease. Pulmonary and cutaneous manifestations have occurred in patients with chronic lymphocytic leukemia, after organ transplantation, and in those infected by HIV. One study has reported five patients with disseminated *M. kansasii* infection, including three patients with pulmonary and extrapulmonary involvement and two patients with exclusive extrapulmonary involvement. All patients had $CD4^+$ lymphocyte counts less than 200 cells/μL. The most common clinical manifestation was pulmonary disease with thin-walled cavitary lesions.

The incidence of disseminated *M. avium* infection can be reduced by the use of prophylactic antimicrobials. Rifabutin, 300 mg daily, clarithromycin, 500 mg twice daily, and azithromycin, 1200 mg weekly either alone or in combination with rifabutin, have all been shown in controlled trials to be effective as prophylactic agents for the prevention of *M. avium*–disseminated disease and are recommended in patients with a $CD4^+$ cell count lower than 75 cells/μL, even when levels improve with HIV therapy.

The diagnosis of central nervous system involvement by NTM is difficult, and therefore it is extremely important to suspect the diagnosis on the basis of the clinical setting. Nontuberculous mycobacteria are rarely found on routine AFB smear analysis of cerebrospinal fluid (CSF), so a positive AFB culture is usually required to make the diagnosis. The CSF in NTM disease usually shows an elevated white blood cell count with a neutrophilic or lymphocytic predominance. CSF protein and glucose levels may vary widely, from within normal limits to far outside the normal range.

DIAGNOSIS

Because there are no typical clinical features of NTM disease, diagnosis depends on having a high index of suspicion. Signs and symptoms of NTM pulmonary disease are variable and nonspecific and include chronic cough, sputum production, and fatigue. Malaise, dyspnea, fever, hemoptysis, and weight loss can also occur, usually with advanced disease, but are less common than with tuberculosis.

Although some differences in radiologic features between TB and diseases caused by NTM-and even between different species of NTM-have been described, there is so much overlap in these features that a radiologic determination of the cause is not possible in the individual patient (see Table 2). A radiologic feature noted in some cases was described as a cluster of homogeneous shadows 1 cm across, surrounding a translucent zone, with line shadows radiating from each lesion. Some patients, notably nonsmokers with no other evidence of lung disease, tend to have nodular lesions localized to the middle lobe or the lingula. When MAI causes chest disease in immunocompetent individuals, there are three categories of chest radiograph patterns seen in clinical practice.

The most common appearance is similar to that of apical postprimary TB, with or without cavities. It is not possible to differentiate this disease from TB, although the cavities have been described as being thinner and smaller. Somewhat common are patchy nodular opacities in any zone of the lung, which on computed tomography (CT) scanning are shown to be associated with local bronchiectasis. Least common is the isolated pulmonary nodule. Mediastinal lymphadenopathy and pleural effusion are also rare, especially in MAI infections. Bizarre and rapidly changing radiologic appearances are seen in patients with AIDS and other immunosuppressive disorders. Chest radiographs may appear normal in up to one third of AIDS patients with NTM pulmonary disease. As with TB, diffuse appearances and lymph node enlargement are more common than in immunocompetent persons and cavitation is less common.

Nontuberculous mycobacterial disease is characterized histopathologically by the presence of caseating and noncaseating granulomatous inflammation, epithelial histiocytes, and occasional giant cells. NTM infection cannot be differentiated definitively histopathologically from tuberculosis. Poorly formed granulomas with histiocytic reactions are more commonly reported in immunodeficient patients, especially those who have AIDS, but they can be seen in immunocompetent patients because not all NTM stimulate granuloma formation equally well. Dimorphic granuloma or the absence of caseating necrosis does not rule out TB nor is this specific for NTM disease, because immune status can modulate the pathologic response.

Definitive diagnosis is made by mycobacteriologic examination, preferably from tissue or aspirated specimens. All mycobacteria are acid-fast and the fluorochrome method (auramine stain) is preferred for microscopic recognition of NTM in clinical samples, although it is important to remember that using only fluorochrome stains, several mycobacterial species can be missed. The appearance of NTM by microscopy is sometimes indistinguishable from that of *M. tuberculosis*, and therefore confirmation of the presence of NTM still requires cultures. Cultures should be inoculated onto one or more solid media (e.g., Löwenstein-Jensen or Middlebrook 7H10 or 7H11) and into a liquid medium as well, given the more rapid recovery of all mycobacteria in broth systems such as the BACTEC system. All skin or soft tissue samples should be incubated at 95° F (35° C) and at 82.4° to 89.6° F (28° to 32° C), because a number of pathogens that infect these tissues, including *M. haemophilum* and *M. marinum*, may grow much better at lower temperatures.

As a consequence of the demand for more rapid diagnosis of *M. tuberculosis*, identification of NTM increasingly focuses on the use of rapid diagnostic systems: high-performance liquid chromatography, which assesses the patterns of long-chain fatty acids (mycolic acids) found in different NTM species, and genetic methods, such as polymerase chain reaction–restriction fragment length polymorphism analysis of a 439-base pair fragment of the 65-kD heat shock protein gene and genetic probes. Commercial genetic probes for mycobacterial RNA are currently available for the identification of *M. tuberculosis* complex, *M. avium*, *M. intracellulare*, *M. gordonae*, and *M. kansasii*. For some of the newer species, such as *M. genavense*, *M. cookii*, and *M. triplex*, high-performance liquid chromatography, 16S ribosomal DNA sequencing, or both are important or essential to make a species identification. Traditional biochemical testing to determine carbohydrate uptake and other standard mycobacterial tests such as arylsulfatase, nitrate reduction, and iron uptake provide alternative, although slower, methods for identification of slow-growing and rapid-growing NTM. For epidemiologic studies, standard biochemical and susceptibility tests have been useful in initial strain comparison for most outbreaks involving NTM, although the latter are rare. Molecular methods such as Southern hybridization with repetitive elements, arbitrarily primed polymerase chain reaction, and pulsed-field gel electrophoresis (DNA fingerprinting) of NTM are now the standard for definitive strain comparison of NTM outbreaks.

Most clinical and public health laboratories now use one or more rapid diagnostic methods for mycobacterial species identification, including high-performance liquid chromatography and commercial DNA probes, which are available for identifying isolates of *M. tuberculosis*, *M. gordonae*, *M. kansasii*, *M. avium*, and *M. intracellulare*. These probes are highly sensitive and specific and can provide species identification using a culture directly from the broth medium.

Various skin test reagents have been prepared from various species of NTM, including purified protein derivative (PPD-A) from *M. avium* and PPD-B from *M. intracellulare*; however, they are not specific, lack standardization and are not clinically useful in the diagnosis of NTM disease. The use of NTM skin test reagents is currently confined to epidemiologic studies and is not available at this time for clinical use in the United States.

One major problem in the diagnosis of pulmonary disease caused by NTM is to establish the clinical significance of these organisms isolated from sputum and other pulmonary specimens by culture or detected by nucleic acid-based techniques. There are no absolute criteria for distinguishing true pulmonary disease caused by NTM from contamination or colonization, but the American Thoracic Society and the British Thoracic Society have issued similar guidelines for reaching a diagnosis, which may be summarized as follows (Boxes 1 and 2):

- Compatible chest radiograph or CT appearance, including infiltrates, multiple nodules, multifocal bronchial disease, and cavities

Box 2 Proposed Diagnostic Criteria for Nontuberculous Mycobacterial Pulmonary Disease

- Compatible clinical presentation based on symptoms, radiographic findings (chest radiograph or high-resolution CT scan) and exclusion of other diagnoses
- Collection of at least three sputum and/or bronchial washing specimens
- One culture-positive sputum or bronchial washing that is heavily (≥2+) smear-positive or heavily (≥2+) culture-positive

  or

- One culture-positive sputum or bronchial washing associated with multiple smear-positive specimens

  or

- Multiple positive cultures (≥3) over 1 year, regardless of smear positivity

For unusual radiographic presentation or nondiagnostic sputum analysis, lung biopsy (bronchoscopy with transbronchial biopsy) demonstrating granulomatous inflammation or culture positive for NTM is required.

In questionable cases, expert consultation is required.

- Compatible clinical symptoms
- Exclusion of other causes of the symptoms and radiologic signs, including TB
- Three sputum specimens positive on culture within a 12-month period or two culture-positive specimens if they are also positive for acid-fast bacilli on microscopic examination
- Heavy growth on culture and AFB seen on microscopic examination of one specimen of bronchial washings
- Isolation of mycobacteria from a sterile site, including lung tissue obtained by transbronchial biopsy or open lung biopsy

It should, however, be noted that these diagnostic criteria were developed principally with respect to disease caused by the common pathogens for MAI, such as *M. kansasii*, and *M. abscessus*. Further clinical experience is required to evaluate the relevance of these criteria to the less frequent, and possibly less pathogenic, NTM. Additionally, as outlined below, these criteria are of limited value in determining the significance of isolates of NTM from certain high-risk groups, such as miners with silicosis.

Bronchial washing of segments draining areas with nodular opacities on a CT scan is useful in the differentiation of causative from casual isolates of MAI and for making a diagnosis when sputum is negative on culture or the patient is incapable of producing sputum. In addition, bronchial washing is more likely to aid in the diagnosis than transbronchial biopsy, even though the latter reveals characteristic granuloma formation.

The presence of an obvious cause of immunosuppression, such as HIV infection, does not per se indicate that an isolated NTM is causing the disease. In a study based on the clinical, bacteriologic, and radiographic diagnostic criteria advocated by the American Thoracic Society, MAI isolates were only considered clinically significant in 7 of 46 HIV-positive patients and 1 of 34 HIV-negative patients.[8] The diagnostic problems are further illustrated by a study in a Dutch TB center where NTM were isolated from 27 patients (25 HIV-negative and 2 HIV-positive patients) but were only considered to be pathogenic in 14 patients. The detection of NTM led to unnecessary or inappropriate treatment (including treatment for TB) in 17 of the patients, and a diagnosis of malignant disease was delayed in 2 patients.

Special Considerations

M. avium-intracellulare Complex Infection

MAI complex is the most common cause of NTM lung disease. In most U.S. patients, MAI lung disease is caused by *M. intracellulare*; in other geographic areas, *M. avium* infection is equally common. Lung disease caused by MAI has traditionally been diagnosed in middle-aged or older white men, usually with a history of cigarette smoking and underlying lung disease, such as chronic obstructive pulmonary disease (COPD), previous tuberculosis, pneumoconiosis, or bronchiectasis. Most of these patients have cavitary changes on chest imaging. This form of disease can be aggressive and causes extensive lung destruction. In our experience, these patients should also be screened for *Nocardia* or *Aspergillus* coinfections.

It is now clear that MAI lung disease has a more heterogeneous clinical presentation, in particular in older female nonsmokers who have no known underlying lung disease.[9] These patients present radiographically with midlung and lower lung field disease characterized by a combination of discrete, small (<5 mm) pulmonary nodules and accompanying bronchiectasis, abnormalities that are especially apparent with high-resolution CT scanning of the chest. Because this form of disease is radiographically atypical for mycobacterial disease, diagnosis may be delayed, even in patients who have persistent cough and progressive radiographic abnormalities. Disease progression is usually indolent; however, this form of MAI lung disease can be associated with significant morbidity and mortality.

It has also become apparent that patients with noncavitary MAI lung disease who are infected by one MAI genotype can be reinfected by another MAI genotype (i.e., polyclonal infections are possible). These patients would previously have been considered treatment failures, but in fact they are actually reinfected by new MAI strains. This phenomenon complicates the evaluation of a patient who has successfully completed therapy but has sputum that again becomes culture-positive for MAI.

M. kansasii Infection

M. kansasii produces pulmonary disease that most closely parallels clinical disease caused by *M. tuberculosis*. Patients with *M. kansasii* lung disease are characteristically older men from urban environments who are cigarette smokers with one or more underlying pulmonary diseases, including COPD, previous TB, bronchiectasis, or pneumoconiosis.[10] The radiographic findings are similar to those of re-activated pulmonary TB, with an upper lobe predilection and cavitation in approximately 90% of patients. Some patients with noncavitary disease, similar to those with MAI lung disease, have also been identified with *M. kansasii* disease. Once isolated, *M. kansasii* should not be considered a colonizer; a pulmonology or infectious disease consultation should be obtained in this setting.

M. abscessus Infection

Patients who have *M. abscessus* lung disease are typically older nonsmoking females with no known underlying or predisposing lung disease.[11] This disease clinically and radiographically most closely resembles noncavitary (nodular bronchiectatic) pulmonary MAI disease. *M. abscessus* and MAI are occasionally isolated concurrently or consecutively in some patients.

TREATMENT

Treatment of NTM infections is not as simple or dependent on in vitro drug susceptibilities as the treatment of TB; some familiarity with the treatment details for each NTM is necessary.[2] Because of the duration of therapy required and the potential toxicity of the medications, not all patients with NTM lung disease will benefit from therapy. For some patients, the treatment is in essence worse than the disease. Older patients who have few symptoms and minimal or slowly progressive disease, or have severe comorbid conditions and limited life expectancy, may not benefit from drug therapy directed at some NTM pathogens, especially MAI. These patients should be selected to receive treatment only after careful evaluation.

Treatment recommendations for NTM diseases in immunocompetent and immunocompromised hosts will probably continue to evolve as new agents with activity against NTM are introduced. The introduction of agents such as clarithromycin, azithromycin, and rifabutin has dramatically improved the treatment outcomes for some NTM infections. The treatment of NTM infections is complicated by the observation that response to therapy for some NTM infections does not correlate with in vitro drug susceptibilities, especially to antituberculous drugs. For example, clinical response to multidrug antimycobacterial regimens for *M. kansasii* correlates only with in vitro susceptibility to rifampin (rifampicin). Response of MAI disease to antimycobacterial drug regimens in the past frequently had no correlation with in vitro drug susceptibilities. In contrast, there is a strong correlation between successful treatment of NTM infections, including MAI infection, with clarithromycin and azithromycin and the in vitro macrolide susceptibility of the specific NTM. Patients with pulmonary or disseminated MAI infection resistant to macrolides will not respond favorably to macrolide-containing regimens.[12,13] Macrolide monotherapy for disseminated or pulmonary MAI disease is associated with a genetic mutation conferring resistance to macrolides and should therefore be avoided.[14]

Recommendations for treating NTM pulmonary disease are given in Table 3. Patients undergoing therapy for NTM pulmonary disease require frequent follow-ups to evaluate symptomatic and objective response to therapy and medication toxicity, and to collect specimens for AFB analysis.

Serial sputum AFB analysis is the most important element of disease monitoring. The sputum analysis is a critical measure of medication efficacy and may provide evidence for treatment failure, which may be caused by the emergence of selective drug resistance, disease relapse or reinfection. Additionally, the duration of therapy for some patients is determined by how long their sputum is AFB-culture negative while on therapy. Patients who have NTM lung disease should not be placed on therapy for extended periods without repeated sputum AFB evaluation. Although periodic chest radiographs are also helpful, the chest radiograph is likely to improve only slowly.

Drug treatment is not successful for all patients with NTM lung disease. Surgical resection of limited disease remains an important option, although surgical morbidity and mortality dictate that the surgical approach should be undertaken only by surgeons experienced with mycobacterial disease and after careful preoperative selection.[15,16] Other approaches, such as cytokine therapy (especially IFN-γ), are promising but remain investigational. Unfortunately, since clarithromycin and azithromycin have become available, there have been few new drugs introduced with activity against NTM. Linezolid, a new oxazolidinone, has in vitro activity against some NTM species, including *M. abscessus*, *M. chelonae*, and MAI, but this is not consistent or predictable for all isolates. Linezolid, currently an expensive drug, is also associated with frequent and severe side effects, such as anemia, peripheral neuropathy, and optic neuritis. Clearly, better antimycobacterial agents for the treatment of NTM infections are needed.

Recommendations for treating disseminated NTM disease in AIDS patients are listed in Table 4. Treatment of disseminated MAI,

Table 3 Treatment Recommendations for Select Nontuberculous Mycobacteria Causing Lung and Disseminated Disease

NTM	Suggested Drug Regimen	Duration of Therapy	Comments
MAI	Clarithromycin, 1 g *or* azithromycin, 600 mg MWF *plus* rifabutin, 300 mg *or* rifampin, 600 mg MWF *plus* ethambutol, 25 mg/kg MWF	12 mo of sputum AFB culture negativity for pulmonary disease, or lifetime therapy for disseminated disease, unless immune status restored	Clarithromycin or azithromycin-not as monotherapy; surgical resection if limited pulmonary disease; streptomycin for 2-3 mo, 500-1000 mg IM MWF *or* amikacin, 400 mg IV daily for severe disease; rifampin contraindicated with protease inhibitors (consider rifabutin 150 mg/day with indinavir)
M. kansasii (rifampin susceptible in vitro)	Rifampin, 600 mg/day *plus* INH, 300 mg/day *plus* ethambutol, 25 mg/kg/day for 2 mo and then 15 mg/kg/day	18 mo and 12 mo of sputum AFB culture negativity for pulmonary disease or lifetime therapy for disseminated disease unless immune status restored	Add streptomycin, 500-1000 mg im MWF *or* clarithromycin, 1 g/day initially (2-3 mo) for advanced disease; treatment success with this regimen dependent on in vitro rifampin susceptibility; PZA not effective
M. kansasii (rifampin resistant in vitro or patient on protease inhibitor)	Clarithromycin, 0.5 g q12 h *plus* ethambutol, 25 mg/kg/day for 2 mo and then 15 mg/kg/day *plus* INH, 900 mg/day (B6 50 mg/day) *plus* sulfamethoxazole, 1.0 g PO q8 h *plus* streptomycin, 500-1000 mg IM MWF (initial 2-3 mo)	12 mo of sputum AFB culture negativity for pulmonary disease or lifetime therapy for disseminated disease, unless immune status restored	In vitro rifampin resistance occurs as consequence of treatment failure (noncompliance) for rifampin-susceptible *M. kansasii* lung disease; rifabutin, 150 mg/day can be used with indinavir (see text for other options in AIDS patients)
M. abscessus	Clarithromycin, 1 g/day *or* azithromycin, 500 mg MWF ± cefoxitin, imipenem, amikacin	12 mo of sputum AFB culture negativity	No drug regimen of proven efficacy; surgical resection of limited pulmonary disease most effective therapy; first-line antituberculosis drugs not useful
M. fortuitum	Two agents, including ofloxacin, 800 mg/day *or* ciprofloxacin, 1500 mg/day, doxycycline 100 mg q12 h, sulfamethoxazole, 1 g q8 h, clarithromycin, 0.5 g q12 h	6 mo	Therapy based on in vitro antibiotic susceptibility; only 50% of *M. fortuitum* isolates susceptible to clarithromycin; for severe disease, amikacin, 400 mg/day IV *or* cefoxitin, 12 g/day IV, until favorable clinical response; first-line antituberculosis drugs not useful
M. chelonae	Clarithromycin, 1 g/day	6 mo	Macrolide monotherapy effective

Other NTM respiratory pathogens that likely would respond to macrolide-containing regimens: *M. xenopi*, *M. malmoense*, *M. simiae*, *M. szulgai*.
Other disseminated NTM pathogens that likely would respond to macrolide-containing regimens: *M. gordonae*, *M. haemophilum*, *M. genavense*.
AFB, acid-fast bacilli; INH, isoniazid; PZA, pyrazinamide; MWF, Monday, Wednesday, and Friday; NTM, nontuberculous mycobacteria.

as well as other NTM pathogens such as *M. kansasii*, results in clinical and bacteriologic improvements as well as increased survival. Treatment of these infections has been complicated by the introduction of protease inhibitors (PIs) and non-nucleoside reverse transcriptase inhibitors (NNRTIs) for the treatment of HIV infection, which interact with rifamycins. There are several options for treating disseminated NTM disease for patients who are also undergoing therapy for HIV infection. One strategy is the use of three nucleoside reverse transcriptase inhibitors (NRTIs) as initial therapy for HIV disease, which would allow the use of rifampin in a multidrug regimen for disseminated NTM infection. Efavirenz, with appropriate dosage adjustment (800 mg/day if used with rifampin), can also be added to a multidrug HIV treatment regimen that contains NRTIs, and the patient could still receive a rifampin-containing regimen for NTM disease. For patients receiving the PIs indinavir, nelfinavir, and amprenavir or the NNRTIs nevirapine and evafirenz, rifabutin could be used instead of rifampin in the NTM treatment regimen. A strategy for boosting PI levels by giving ritonavir has been developed, which might also allow concomitant administration of rifampin with the PIs, but dose adjustments are still required. Clearly, the treatment of NTM disease in HIV-infected patients can be complicated. Inappropriate combinations of drugs may result in treatment failure of one or both infections as well as significant drug-related toxicity. Physicians who do not routinely treat HIV-infected patients or are not familiar with the drugs involved should seek expert consultation for the management of these patients. Effective regimens for prophylaxis against disseminated MAI are outlined in Table 4. The successful treatment of NTM central nervous system (CNS) diseases is difficult because of the relative antibiotic resistance of the organisms, the poor CNS penetration of important agents, such as clarithromycin, and the usually far advanced underlying disease of the host. One useful adjunctive therapeutic strategy would be to taper corticosteroids or lower the level of immunosuppression, if feasible.

Treatment of skin and soft tissue infections caused by *M. fortuitum*, *M. abscessus*, or *M. chelonae* unrelated to disseminated disease involves regimens similar to those recommended for pulmonary or disseminated disease (Table 5).[17,18] Surgical débridement is

Table 4 Prophylactic Agents Against Disseminated *Mycobacterium avium-intracellulare* (MAI) Complex Lung Disease in AIDS Patients

Regimen	Dosage	Comments
Rifabutin	300 mg/day	Rifamycin (rifampin) resistance can emerge with rifabutin monotherapy in patients with occult active tuberculosis; not compatible with some protease inhibitors
Clarithromycin	1 g/day	Well tolerated; clarithromycin resistance will emerge if monotherapy used for active disseminated MAI infection
Azithromycin	1.2 g/wk	Well tolerated; macrolide (clarithromycin) resistance will emerge if monotherapy used for active disseminated MAI infection
Azithromycin plus rifabutin	1.2 g/wk plus 300 mg/day	Very effective prophylaxis regimen; high incidence of rifabutin toxicity

Table 5 Frequently Used Treatment Regimens for Common Nontuberculous Mycobacteria

Pathogen	Disease	Drug	Daily Adult Dosage	Duration of Therapy
M. avium complex	Pulmonary	Clarithromycin *plus*	500 mg bid	Until culture-negative for 12 mo
		Ethambutol *plus*	15 mg/kg	
		Rifampin *or*	600 mg	
		Rifabutin	150-300 mg	
	Disseminated, HIV-positive	Clarithromycin *plus*	500 mg bid	For life (?)
		Ethambutol *plus*	15 mg/kg	
		Rifabutin (?)	300 mg	
	Lymphadenitis, children	Surgical excision		
		Clarithromycin (?) *plus*		
		Rifabutin (?) *or*		
		Ethambutol		
M. kansasii	Pulmonary			
	United States	Isoniazid *plus*	300 mg	18 mo, culture-negative for at least 12 mo
		Rifampin *plus*	600 mg	
		Ethambutol	15 mg/kg	
	United Kingdom	Rifampin *plus*	600 mg	9-12 mo
		Ethambutol	15 mg/kg	
	Disseminated	Same as pulmonary		
	HIV-positive	Same as pulmonary (United States) but replace rifampin with rifabutin *or* clarithromycin	150 mg 500 mg bid	Same as pulmonary (United States)
M. abscessus	Pulmonary	Amikacin IV *plus*	15 mg/kg (see text)	2 wk (designed to improve, not cure)
		Cefoxitin IV *plus*	12 g/day	6 mo
		Clarithromycin	500 mg bid	6 mo
	Cutaneous localized	Clarithromycin	500 mg bid	
	Disseminated or extensive cutaneous	Same three drugs as above		
M. marinum	Cutaneous	Clarithromycin *or*	500 mg bid	3-mo minimum for all regimens
		Minocycline *or*	100 mg bid	
		Rifampin *plus*	600 mg	
		Ethambutol	15 mg/kg	

SECTION 8 INFECTIOUS DISEASE

important for extensive or poorly responsive disease. As a rule, *M. marinum* seems to be the exception among NTM in the sense that it does not develop resistance to monotherapy and it is easier to treat.

Several regimens administered for 3 months are effecti ve for the treatment of *M. marinum* infection, including clarithromycin, 500 mg twice daily; doxycycline, 100 mg twice daily; trimethoprim-sulfamethoxazole (co-trimoxazole), 160/800 mg twice daily; and rifampin, 600 mg/day, plus ethambutol, 15 mg/kg/day.

Surgical débridement may be necessary for extensive disease. Complete surgical excision is the standard treatment for NTM lymphadenitis and is usually curative.[17,19] Antimycobacterial therapy is seldom necessary, except for those patients who are immunocompromised. Regimens that contain the newer macrolides are effective for eradicating disease in patients who are unable to have surgery or who undergo incomplete excision of MAI lymphadenitis.[20]

Summary

- Although less important than tuberculosis, nontuberculous mycobacterial disorders represent a significant morbidity, especially in HIV-infected patients.
- The latest advances in diagnosis and treatment have made the nontuberculous mycobacterial diseases considerably more amenable to diagnosis, treatment, and even cure.

Suggested Readings

Ahn CH, Lowell JR, Onstad GD, et al: A demographic study of disease due to *Mycobacterium kansasii* or *M. intracellulare-avium* in Texas. Chest 1979;75:120-125.

Bennett C, Vardiman J, Golomb H: Disseminated atypical mycobacterial infection in patients with hairy cell leukemia. Am J Med 1986;80:891-896.

Berger C, Pfyffer GE, Nadal D: Treatment of nontuberculous mycobacterial lymphadenitis with clarithromycin plus rifabutin. J Pediatr 1996;128:383-386.

Chaisson RE, Benson CA, Dube MP, et al: Clarithromycin therapy for bacteremic *Mycobacterium avium* complex disease. A randomized, double-blind, dose-ranging study in patients with AIDS. AIDS Clinical Trials Group Protocol 157 Study Team. Ann Intern Med 1994;121:905-911.

Diagnosis and treatment of disease caused by nontuberculous mycobacteria. This official statement of the American Thoracic Society was approved by the Board of Directors, March 1997. Medical Section of the American Lung Association. Am J Respir Crit Care Med 1997;156(2 Pt 2):S1-S25.

Griffith DE, Girard WM, Wallace RJ Jr: Clinical features of pulmonary disease caused by rapidly growing mycobacteria. An analysis of 154 patients. Am Rev Respir Dis 1993;147:1271-1278.

Khoor A, Leslie KO, Tazelaar HD, et al: Diffuse pulmonary disease caused by nontuberculous mycobacteria in immunocompetent people (hot tub lung). Am J Clin Pathol 2001;115:755-762.

Lai KK, Stottmeier KD, Sherman IH, McCabe WR: Mycobacterial cervical lymphadenopathy. Relation of etiologic agents to age. JAMA 1984;251:1286-1288.

Meier A, Heifets L, Wallace RJ Jr, et al: Molecular mechanisms of clarithromycin resistance in *Mycobacterium avium:* Observation of multiple 23S rDNA mutations in a clonal population. J Infect Dis 1996;174:354-360.

Parrot RG, Grosset JH: Post-surgical outcome of 57 patients with *Mycobacterium xenopi* pulmonary infection. Tubercle 1988;69:47-55.

Pomerantz M, Brown JM: Surgery in the treatment of multidrug-resistant tuberculosis. Clin Chest Med 1997;18:123-130.

Prince DS, Peterson DD, Steiner RM, et al: Infection with *Mycobacterium avium* complex in patients without predisposing conditions. N Engl J Med 1989;321:863-868.

Raju B, Schluger NW: Significance of respiratory isolates of *Mycobacterium avium* complex in HIV-positive and HIV-negative patients. Int J Infect Dis 2000;4:134-139.

Reich JM, Johnson RE: *Mycobacterium avium* complex pulmonary disease presenting as an isolated lingular or middle lobe pattern. The Lady Windermere syndrome. Chest 1992;101:1605-1609.

Saubolle MA, Kiehn TE, White MH, et al: *Mycobacterium haemophilum:* Microbiology and expanding clinical and geographic spectra of disease in humans. Clin Microbiol Rev 1996;9:435-437.

Schaad UB, Votteler TP, McCracken GH Jr, Nelson JD: Management of atypical mycobacterial lymphadenitis in childhood: A review based on 380 cases. J Pediatr 1979;95:356-360.

Sonnenberg P, Murray J, Glynn JR, et al: Risk factors for pulmonary disease due to culture-positive M. tuberculosis or nontuberculous mycobacteria in South African gold miners. Eur Respir J 2000;15:291-296.

Wallace RJ Jr: The clinical presentation, diagnosis, and therapy of cutaneous and pulmonary infections due to the rapidly growing mycobacteria, M. fortuitum and M. chelonae. Clin Chest Med 1989;10:419-429.

Wallace RJ Jr, Brown BA, Griffith DE, et al: Initial clarithromycin monotherapy for *Mycobacterium avium-intracellulare* complex lung disease. Am J Respir Crit Care Med 1994;149:1335-1341.

Wallace RJ Jr, Tanner D, Brennan PJ, Brown BA: Clinical trial of clarithromycin for cutaneous (disseminated) infection due to *Mycobacterium chelonae.* Ann Intern Med 1993;119:482-486.

Winthrop KL, Abrams M, Yakrus M, et al: An outbreak of mycobacterial furunculosis associated with foot baths at a nail salon. N Engl J Med 2002;346:1366-1371.

References

For a complete list of references, log onto www.expertconsult.com.

HIV for the Primary Care Physician

Wendy S. Armstrong and *Marisa Tungsiripat*

DEFINITION AND CAUSES

Human immunodeficiency virus (HIV) is a retrovirus that infects primarily CD4$^+$ T helper cells. Depletion of these cells causes progressive immunologic decline. When CD4$^+$ T cell counts fall below 200 cells/mm^3 or opportunistic infections occur, an infected patient is described as having the acquired immunodeficiency syndrome (AIDS).

PREVALENCE AND RISK FACTORS

At the end of 2005, an estimated 1,200,000 million persons in the United States were living with HIV, AIDS, or both, with approximately 25% of those unaware of their HIV infection.[1] According to surveillance data at the end of 2004 obtained from the 35 areas that use name-based reporting, 73% of cases were in males. Almost 50% of infected persons were black non-Hispanic, despite representing only 14% of the U.S. population, 37% were white non-Hispanic, and almost 18% were Hispanic. Among infected men, 60% identified their risk behavior as men having sex with men (MSM), 19% reported a history of injection drug use (IDU), 7% admitted to both MSM and IDU, and 13% reported heterosexual contact as their route of HIV exposure. Of HIV-infected women, 71% identified heterosexual sex as their HIV exposure, and 27% had IDU as a risk factor. Once a predominant mode of transmission, receipt of blood products accounted for less than 2% of cases of HIV/AIDS.[2]

The magnitude of the global HIV/AIDS epidemic vastly exceeds that in the United States. As of the end of 2005, more than 38,600,000 people were estimated to be living with HIV/AIDS. In 2005, 4,100,000 people were newly infected with HIV and 2,800,00 deaths were estimated to have occurred from AIDS. Almost 75% of those with the disease are living in sub-Saharan Africa, where access to antiretroviral therapy is limited.[1]

PATHOPHYSIOLOGY AND NATURAL HISTORY

HIV infection was first described in 1981 when an epidemic of *Pneumocystis jiroveci* (formerly identified as *Pneumocystis carinii*) pneumonia (PCP) was noted in homosexual men.[3] In 1984, HIV was identified as the causative agent of AIDS. Subsequently, two genetic types of HIV were identified. The predominant type worldwide is HIV type 1 (HIV-1). HIV-1 is further subdivided into subtypes (also called clades), designated A through K (collectively referred to as group M), N, and O. More than 98% of HIV-1 infections in the United States are caused by subtype B. HIV type 2 (HIV-2) is found in West Africa, particularly Guinea-Bissau, Gambia, and Senegal, as well as in France, Portugal, Angola, and Mozambique. Disease caused by HIV-2 appears to be less readily transmissible and results in slower disease progression than that caused by HIV-1.[4]

The HIV viruses belong to the lentivirus subfamily of the RNA retroviruses. Like most retroviruses, the HIV genome consists of three structural genes, *gag*, *pol*, and *env*. The *gag* gene codes for viral capsid proteins, *env* for viral envelope proteins, and *pol* for proteins responsible for viral replication, including the RNA-dependent DNA polymerase known as reverse transcriptase. In addition, several other regulatory genes are present, including *nef*, *rev*, and *tat*.

Most commonly, transmission of the virus occurs after a breach in the integument or mucous membranes. HIV infection occurs when the envelope subunit gp120 binds the human CD4$^+$ T cell receptor found primarily on lymphocytes and monocyte-derived macrophages. In addition, binding also requires the presence on the host cell of the chemokine receptor CCR5 or CXCR4. The viral envelope then fuses with the host cell, allowing release of the viral core into the host cell. Viral DNA is synthesized by reverse transcriptase and incorporated into the host genome by the protein integrase. Once the viral gene products are transcribed and assembled, the HIV protease mediates packaging of new virions for release into serum to propagate the infection.[5]

Over time, infected persons have a progressive loss of CD4$^+$ lymphocytes, although in the early stages of infection, this is not associated with increased immunosuppression. The rate of CD4 cell loss is variable and depends on viral and host factors. On average, infected persons lose 40 to 80 CD4 cells/mm^3/year.[6] A subset of patients progress rapidly; however, 5% of infected persons, known as *long-term nonprogressors*, will have little or no progression of clinical disease or decline in CD4$^+$ counts over 10 years, even without antiretroviral therapy.[7]

Transmission of the virus occurs through exposure to infected body fluids, including blood, semen, and vaginal fluid. The most common modes of transmission are sexual contact (male-male or heterosexual sex), parenteral exposure to blood and blood products, and vertical transmission during pregnancy. The magnitude of risk depends on the exposure and degree of viremia of the source. For example, the risk of HIV transmission from a known HIV-positive source from receptive anal intercourse is 0.1% to 0.3%, whereas receptive vaginal intercourse carries a risk per episode of 0.08% to 0.2%. A percutaneous exposure from a needlestick injury or IDU results in transmission 0.3% or 0.67% of the time, respectively.[8] The risk of vertical transmission from mother to fetus without any preventive therapy is approximately 25%.[9] The efficiency of transmission increases with greater degrees of viremia in the source patient and the presence of concurrent sexually transmitted diseases.

SIGNS AND SYMPTOMS

Acute HIV Infection

In an estimated 40% to 90% of individuals, HIV seroconversion is associated with a clinical syndrome known as acute or primary HIV infection, or the acute retroviral syndrome. In one prospective study, among those with symptoms at the time of seroconversion, 95% sought medical care. Nevertheless, acute HIV infection is rarely diagnosed, partly because the symptoms are protean. The onset of illness is between 2 and 6 weeks after viral transmission and is believed to correlate with peak viremia, often in excess of 1 million viral copies/mL. Fever (mean, 38.9° C), rash, lymphadenopathy, and nonexudative pharyngitis are each present in at least 70% of individuals (Table 1). Most often, the rash is reminiscent of a viral exanthem with erythematous maculopapular lesions on the face and trunk, although many types of lesions have been described. Headache with or without cerebrospinal fluid pleocytosis, myalgias, and gastrointestinal symptoms are also common. Although present in only 5% to 20% of patients, oral or genital ulcers can be an important diagnostic clue. Laboratory abnormalities, specifically leukopenia, thrombocytopenia, and elevated transaminase levels, are not uncommon. Opportunistic infections such as mucocutaneous candidiasis and PCP may

Table 1 Acute HIV Infection: Frequency of Associated Signs and Symptoms

Sign or Symptom	Frequency (%)
Fever	96
Headache	32
Lymphadenopathy	74
Nausea and vomiting	27
Pharyngitis	70
Hepatosplenomegaly	14
Rash	70
Weight loss	13
Myalgia or arthralgia	54
Thrush	12
Diarrhea	32
Neurologic symptoms	12
Oral or genital ulcers	5-20

Adapted from Department of Health and Human Services Panel on Antiretroviral Guidelines for Adults and Adolescents: Guidelines for the Use of Antiretroviral Agents in HIV-1 Infected Adults and Adolescents, December 1, 2007. Available at http://www.aidsinfo.nih.gov/contentfiles/AdultandAdolescentGL.pdf.

manifest during acute HIV infection as a result of transient but dramatic $CD4^+$ cell count depletion caused by the high level of viremia.

The symptoms of acute HIV infection are self limited and most likely correlate with viremia. After reaching high levels, the viral load declines to a steady state or set point, and the $CD4^+$ count recovers. HIV-1–specific cytotoxic T lymphocytes are present in high titer and appear to play an important role in controlling viral replication. The magnitude of the viral set point and the severity of initial symptoms predict disease progression. Recognition of this syndrome has obvious implications for public health. Whether early antiretroviral treatment changes an individual's disease course remains unclear.[10] Diagnosis is discussed below.

Chronic HIV Infection

Various historical details, findings on physical examination, and laboratory abnormalities should prompt testing to identify persons with established HIV infection. As expected, these findings are more prominent in patients with more advanced disease. Often, the initial diagnosis of HIV infection is made when the patient develops an AIDS indicator condition (Box 1).[11] However, the astute clinician can often detect signs and symptoms of HIV infection earlier in the course of disease, allowing access to appropriate therapy and prophylaxis before significant illness develops.

A history of certain illnesses can also be suggestive of HIV infection. Infections such as active tuberculosis, recurrent community-acquired pneumonia, esophageal candidiasis, and either multidermatomal herpes zoster or zoster in younger adults should lead to HIV testing. Neoplastic diseases such as B cell lymphoma, severe anal or cervical dysplasia, or invasive carcinoma and Kaposi's sarcoma are indications for HIV testing, as is idiopathic dilated cardiomyopathy. The evaluation of fever of unknown origin or unexplained weight loss should always include an HIV test, even in older patients without identified risk factors.

Box 1 Indicator Conditions in the 1993 AIDS Surveillance Case Definition

Candidiasis of the esophagus, bronchi, trachea, or lungs
Cervical cancer, invasive
Coccidioidomycosis, extrapulmonary
Cryptococcosis, extrapulmonary
Cryptosporidosis, chronic intestinal (>1 mo duration)
Cytomegalovirus disease of any organ other than the liver, spleen, nodes
Encephalopathy, HIV-related
Herpes simplex with mucocutaneous ulcer >1 mo duration, or bronchitis, pneumonitis, or esophagitis
Histoplasmosis, extrapulmonary
Isosporiasis, chronic intestinal (>1 mo duration)
Kaposi's sarcoma
Lymphoma, Burkitt's, immunoblastic, or primary central nervous system (CNS) involvement
Mycobacterium avium complex or *M. kansasii*, extrapulmonary
M. tuberculosis, any site
Pneumocystis jiroveci pneumonia
Pneumonia, recurrent bacterial (two or more episodes in 1 yr)
Progressive multifocal leukoencephalopathy
Salmonella septicemia, recurrent
Toxoplasmosis, CNS
Wasting syndrome caused by HIV

Adapted from Centers for Disease Control and Prevention: 1993 revised classification system for HIV infection and expanded surveillance case definition for AIDS among adolescents and adults. MMWR Morb Mortal Wkly Rep 1992;41(RR-17):1-19.

Various findings on physical examination may suggest coexisting HIV infection. Examination of the skin can be particularly revealing. Seborrheic dermatitis or molluscum contagiosum are common in early disease, as is psoriasis. Oral candidiasis and oral hairy leukoplakia can be seen, typically with $CD4^+$ counts less than 500 cells/mm^3. Generalized lymphadenopathy is common. Recurrent or severe lesions of herpes simplex virus may be indicative of underlying HIV infection. Neurologic findings such as unexplained peripheral neuropathy or dementia are suggestive.

On laboratory evaluation, idiopathic thrombocytopenia, unexplained anemia, neutropenia, and/or leukopenia are frequent early clues to underlying HIV infection. An elevated total protein level or globulin fraction is also suggestive.

DIAGNOSIS

Since the recognition that HIV is the agent causing AIDS, many tests have been developed to aid in establishing the diagnosis of HIV infection and evaluating the stage of infection. However, only a few have application today for routine use.

Serologic Tests

The principal tests for the diagnosis of HIV-1 infection are the HIV enzyme-linked immunosorbent assay (ELISA) and the confirmatory Western blot test. Both detect host antibodies to the HIV virus. ELISA is the initial screening test and has a sensitivity and specificity greater than 99%. A false-negative ELISA result occurs most commonly when the test is performed in a newly infected patient before an antibody response has developed (the window period). Most patients have a positive ELISA finding 10 to 14 days after infection, although seroconversion may be delayed in some. False-negative results occur rarely in patients with late-stage disease and in those with subtype N or O HIV-1 infection. False-positive results occur in various settings, including patients with autoimmune diseases, multiparity, and liver disease, as well as recipients of multiple transfusions, hemodialysis, and vaccinations.[12] An isolated positive ELISA finding should never be considered evidence of HIV infection, and clinicians should counsel patients accordingly.

The confirmatory study for a persistently positive ELISA finding is the Western blot test, which detects antibodies to specific HIV proteins. A positive study is defined as one in which bands are present in two of the following three proteins: the envelope proteins gp41 and gp120/160 and the viral capsid protein p24. A negative Western blot test result has no positive bands, but a study with any positive bands that do not meet the above criteria is considered indeterminate. Of patients with persistently positive ELISA results, 4% to 20% have indeterminate Western blot test findings. Indeterminate findings may occur during the window period between infection and seroconversion. Alternatively, other conditions such as autoimmune disease can lead to an indeterminate study. Western blot tests have a reported specificity of 97.8%; therefore, false-positive results can occur. Patients with both false-positive ELISA and false-positive Western blot test results are rare (6 to 7 in 1,000,000 tests).[12]

The diagnosis of HIV-2 infection requires an ELISA finding that will detect HIV-2 antibodies, followed by an HIV-2–specific Western blot test. Many currently available HIV ELISAs will detect antibodies to HIV-1 or HIV-2; however, HIV-2–specific ELISAs are also available.

Newer diagnostic tests using ELISA or immunofluorescence technology are now available for use in specific circumstances. Most popular are the rapid testing systems, which allow the assay to be run in 5 to 20 minutes. Currently available U.S. Food and Drug Administration (FDA)-approved kits are OraQuick Advance Rapid HIV-1/2 Antibody Test (OraSure Technologies, Bethlehem, Penn), Uni-Gold Recombigen (Trinity Biotech, Wicklow, Ireland), Reveal G2 (MedMira Inc, Halifax, Nova Scotia), and Multispot HIV-1/HIV-2 (BioRad Laboratories, Hercules, Calif). Although these tests are particularly beneficial in the delivery room, emergency room, and after occupational exposures, the availability of Clinical Laboratories Improvement Act-waived testing (OraQuick and Uni-Gold) allows these assays to be run in the community, expanding access to testing. The FDA is currently considering whether to allow rapid test kits to be sold over the counter to the public. In addition, home tests are available that allow patients to collect a blood sample after a finger stick, which is then sent anonymously for testing (Home Access Express Test, Home Access Health, Hoffman Estates, Ill). Body fluids other than blood can also be tested. Both the OraQuick rapid test and the OraSure HIV-1 Oral Specimen Collection Device (OraSure Technologies, Bethlehem, Penn) allow for testing of oral mucosal transudate, the Calypte kit (Calypte, Alameda, Calif) tests for HIV antibodies in urine and most recently, vaginal secretion testing kits (Wellcozyme HIV 1&2, Gracelisa Murex Diagnostics, Danforth, United Kingdom) are available. Of all these test kits, only the OraSure HIV-1 Oral Specimen Collection Device can confirm a positive test with a Western blot test using the same sample; all other methods, including all rapid test kits, require confirmation with standard Western blot testing. Some kits can detect HIV-1 and HIV-2 infection, some can distinguish between the two viruses, and others can detect only samples positive for HIV-1 antibodies. It is important to understand the test characteristics and a patient's risk of HIV-2 infection, highest among immigrants from West Africa or exposure to an individual at risk, before drawing conclusions based on test results.

As with all diagnostic tests, the positive predictive value depends on the rate of disease in the population being screened. In low-prevalence populations, the likelihood that a positive ELISA result represents a false-positive result may exceed the likelihood of the test's indicating true HIV infection.

Quantitative HIV Testing

Quantitative plasma HIV RNA (viral load) testing is most commonly used to measure response to antiviral therapy or to predict disease progression. Several methods of measuring viral load are commercially available, including viral RNA quantification by the polymerase chain reaction (PCR), branched-chain DNA assays, and nucleic acid sequence–based amplification. At present, the RNA PCR assay is most commonly used, but it should not be used for the diagnosis of HIV infection unless acute HIV infection is a consideration. HIV-infected individuals can have undetectable viral loads in the absence of antiviral therapy, and the false-positive rate approaches 3%. When the clinician is concerned about acute HIV infection with a symptomatic patient and ELISA–Western blot test findings are negative or indeterminate, viral load testing can be helpful. With initial viremia, before the development of an immunologic response to the virus, the viral load is extremely high, often higher than 100,000 copies/mL. Low viral loads (<15,000 copies/mL) with negative serologic studies may represent a false-positive RNA PCR result and should be repeated.[12] Qualitative measurements of proviral DNA can also be useful for the detection of viremia before seroconversion.

Measurement of p24 antigenemia has also been used to detect HIV infection before seroconversion. On average, however, HIV DNA or RNA can be detected 2 to 3 days earlier than the p24 antigen. As a result, viral load testing has become the preferred method for the diagnosis of acute HIV infection. Studies of p24 antigen can be useful to help clarify confusing serologic or quantitative viral load results.

In summary, serologic testing is the gold standard for diagnosing HIV infection and should be performed on all patients in whom HIV infection is suspected. Viral load testing has no role in the diagnosis of established HIV infection. When suspicion of acute HIV infection is present, viral load testing can be performed, in addition to serologic studies. Negative serologic studies in the setting of a strongly positive viral load (more than 15,000 copies/mL) suggest acute HIV infection. These patients should be urgently referred to an HIV specialist; however, seroconversion must also be documented in the ensuing weeks to months. Indeterminate Western blot findings can present challenging management issues. At a minimum, the study should be repeated 6 months after the initial result to clarify whether the indeterminate findings were the result of ongoing seroconversion.

TREATMENT

Appropriate treatment of the HIV-infected patient requires much more than consideration of antiretroviral therapy. The initial evaluation of an HIV-infected patient should include a careful medical and social history, a medication history, including alternative and herbal supplements, and a thorough physical examination. The clinician should explore the patient's knowledge of HIV, understanding of the course of disease, emotional well-being, and presence or absence of support systems. A discussion of safer sex practices and contraception is vital. Notification of sex partners should be discussed. Identification of a durable power of attorney and discussion of advanced directives are valuable early in the course of the disease.

Several baseline laboratory studies aid in establishing a treatment plan for the patient, choosing agents for antiretroviral therapy, and guiding prophylaxis (Box 2). HIV infection should be staged with a $CD4^+$ count and HIV viral load measurement. Current guidelines suggest performing HIV resistance testing (HIV genotype) in all newly diagnosed patients, because acquisition of resistant virus is becoming more commonplace (6% to 16%).[13] Recommended studies also include a complete blood cell count with differential and platelet counts, determination of electrolyte, blood urea nitrogen (BUN), creatinine, transaminase, and alkaline phosphatase levels, rapid plasma reagin or VDRL testing to assess for syphilis, *Toxoplasma gondii* IgG serology to assess past exposure, hepatitis B and C serologies, and determination of the glucose-6-phosphate dehydrogenase (G6PD) level. Many clinicians favor cytomegalovirus immunoglobulin G (IgG) and hepatitis A IgG serologies as well. A purified protein

Box 2 Initial Laboratory Evaluation of the HIV-Infected Patient

Complete blood count, including differential and platelets
Determination of levels of electrolytes, blood urea nitrogen, creatinine, transaminases, alkaline phosphate, glucose-6-phosphate dehydrogenase
Rapid plasma reagin (RPR) or VDRL testing
Toxoplasma gondii immunoglobulin G (IgG) determination
Hepatitis B and C serologies
$CD4^+$ count
Quantitative HIV RNA level
HIV genotype
Purified protein derivative (PPD) test
Consider determination of cytomegalovirus IgG, hepatitis A IgG levels, baseline chest x-ray

derivative (PPD) test must be performed if not done in the past year, and exposure to any individuals with active tuberculosis must be assessed. An anergy panel is not necessary. Women should have a Pap smear performed every 6 months until two consecutive smears are negative, and then annually. Women with abnormal Pap smears should be referred for colposcopy. Some authorities recommend that a baseline chest radiograph be obtained for patients.

Annual ophthalmologic and dental visits are recommended. Consultation with a nutritionist experienced in HIV care and a social worker are beneficial.

Preventive Treatment

Preventive care is essential to treating the HIV-infected patient. Some infections can be minimized by avoiding uncooked and undercooked foods such as seafood, eggs, and meats, abstaining from drinking lake and river water, avoiding contact with cat litter boxes and animals with diarrhea, and institution of careful hand washing. The patient's vaccination history should be carefully reviewed. All patients should receive the pneumococcal vaccine, updated every 3 to 6 years. The influenza vaccine is recommended, as is hepatitis B vaccination if the patient is seronegative. Although hepatitis A vaccination is indicated if the patient has existing hepatitis B or C, most clinicians favor vaccinating all seronegative individuals. Tetanus boosters are indicated every 10 years. At present, live vaccines are not recommended for patients with advanced disease. The safety of these vaccines (e.g., varicella, measles-mumps-rubella, and yellow fever) early in disease is unknown and should be considered on an individual basis. The inactivated vaccines for typhoid (Typhim Vi capsular polysaccharide vaccine, ViCPS) and polio should be administered when required rather than live vaccines.[14]

Patients with advanced HIV disease require prophylaxis to prevent opportunistic infections. With a $CD4^+$ count less than 200 cells/mm^3 (or CD4 percentage lower than 14), prophylaxis against PCP should be initiated promptly, because the incidence of disease approaches 20% per year in these patients in the absence of prophylaxis. The first-line agent is trimethoprim-sulfamethoxazole (TMP-SMX), one double-strength tablet daily. Dapsone, 100 mg/day, is recommended for patients who are TMP-SMX–intolerant and not G6PD-deficient. When the $CD4^+$ count falls below 100 cells/mm^3, patients with positive *T. gondii* IgG serologies require prophylaxis to prevent reactivation. Daily TMP-SMX is again the drug of choice. Patients receiving dapsone require the addition of pyrimethamine. Although *Mycobacterium avium* complex (MAC) prophylaxis is recommended at CD4 counts below 50 cells/mm^3, initiation is never emergent, and active MAC disease should be ruled out before starting prophylaxis if the patient has any suggestive symptoms. The most common regimen is azithromycin, 1200 mg/week. More detailed information can be obtained from the U.S. Public Health Service and Infectious Disease Society of America guidelines for the prevention of opportunistic infections.[14]

Highly Active Antiretroviral Therapy

In the past decade, selection of highly active antiretroviral therapy (HAART) has become increasingly complex. A single regimen is no longer appropriate for all patients, even as initial therapy. Furthermore, textbook chapters often become obsolete almost as soon as they are printed as new classes and agents become available and recommendations for use change. Appropriate individualized selection of HAART should be left to an HIV specialist.

The ideal time to start HAART therapy remains unclear. Recent guidelines suggest initiating HAART later than previously recommended because of the emerging problems of drug resistance and medication side effects, coupled with uncertain benefit. Although the decision to start HAART must be individualized in every case, current guidelines recommend starting antiretroviral therapy for patients with $CD4^+$ cell counts lower than 200 cell/ mm^3 or patients with AIDS-defining illnesses, regardless of $CD4^+$ cell count. Therapy should be offered to patients with CD4 counts below 350 cells/mm^3. Most clinicians defer therapy at $CD4^+$ cell counts above 350 cells/mm^3 but may consider therapy if the viral load exceeds 100,000 copies/mL.[13]

Current therapy should almost always include a minimum of three agents and often more, selected from among four presently licensed drug classes: nucleoside nucleotide reverse transcriptase inhibitors (NRTIs), non-nucleoside reverse transcriptase inhibitors (NNRTIs), protease inhibitors (PIs), and entry (fusion) inhibitors. Agents in other classes, such as chemokine receptor antagonists, integrase inhibitors, and maturation inhibitors are in development.

Recommended first-line regimens consist of a backbone of therapy with two NRTI agents and either an NNRTI or one or two PIs. Currently, PIs are most commonly prescribed in a boosted formulation, which means that low-dose ritonavir is added to an active PI, not for antiviral activity but as an inhibitor of the hepatic metabolism of the active agent. This increases the levels of the active drug, improving its potency and often allowing longer dosing intervals. An added benefit is that boosted PIs have a higher barrier to resistance, improving regimen durability when compared with nonboosted PI regimens. The Department of Health and Human Services (DHHS) has designated one NNRTI-containing antiretroviral regimen and three PI-containing regimens as preferred regimens for patients without prior therapy or primary resistance. These are as follows: efavirenz (or lopinavir-ritonavir) twice daily, or fosamprenavir plus ritonavir twice daily (or atazanavir plus ritonavir) plus zidovudine-lamivudine or tenofovir-emtricitabine.[13] Several alternative regimens are also available and final selection must include consideration of many additional factors, including comorbidities, other prescribed or over-the-counter medications, lifestyle, and family history.

Once HAART is initiated, the most critical and modifiable factor affecting success is patient adherence. Only 45% of patients taking 90% to 95% of their prescribed doses of antiretroviral medications will achieve viral suppression (<400 copies/mL) compared with 78% in those taking more than 95% of their doses.[15] Incomplete viral suppression leads to the development of drug resistance. Adherence to the antiviral regimen should be addressed at every visit with every physician in a detailed fashion, and the importance of careful adherence should be stressed. Once-daily dosing of many treatment regimens is now possible and changes in pill formulations have allowed more potent regimens to be prescribed with fewer total pills. Both pill burden and dosing frequency have been shown to correlate with adherence.

Side effects of the currently available antiretroviral agents are considerable, and the general practitioner should be aware of them (Table 2). Those that are the most common and potentially serious include cytopenias with zidovudine, pancreatitis with didanosine, peripheral neuropathy with didanosine and stavudine, hypersensitivity, including rash, fever, and risk of death with abacavir, Fanconi's syndrome with tenofovir, rash with all NNRTIs, hepatitis with nevirapine, nephrolithiasis with indinavir, unconjugated hyperbilirubi-

Table 2 Select Common Adverse Events (AEs) Caused by Antiretroviral Agents

Agent	AEs Unique to Agent	AEs Common Across Class
Nucleoside and Nucleotide Reverse Transcriptase Inhibitors		
Zidovudine (AZT, ZDV)	Anemia, neutropenia, myopathy	Lactic acidosis with hepatic steatosis (higher incidence with d4T) Lipodystrophy*
Didanosine (ddI)	Peripheral neuropathy, pancreatitis	
Zalcitabine (ddC)	Peripheral neuropathy	
Stavudine (d4T)	Peripheral neuropathy	
Lamivudine (3TC)		
Abacavir	Hypersensitivity syndrome	
Tenofovir	Fanconi's syndrome	
Non-nucleoside Reverse Transcriptase Inhibitors		
Nevirapine	Hepatitis	Rash
Delavirdine		
Efavirenz	CNS symptoms	
Protease Inhibitors		
Indinavir	Nephrolithiasis, unconjugated hyperbilirubinemia	Fat maldistribution,* GI intolerance, hyperglycemia, lipid abnormalities
Ritonavir		
Nelfinavir		
Saquinavir		
Fosamprenavir		
Lopinavir-ritonavir		
Atazanavir	Unconjugated hyperbilirubinemia	
Tipranavir		
Darunavir		
Entry Inhibitors		
Enfuvirtide	Injection site reactions	

*The role of various antiretroviral agents in the development of lipodystrophy is not fully understood.
CNS, central nervous system; GI, gastrointestinal.
Adapted from Department of Health and Human Services Panel on Antiretroviral Guidelines for Adults and Adolescents: Guidelines for the Use of Antiretroviral Agents in HIV-1 Infected Adults and Adolescents, December 1, 2007. Available at http://www.aidsinfo.nih.gov/contentfiles/AdultandAdolescentGL.pdf.

nemia with indinavir or atazanavir, and gastrointestinal toxicity, including diarrhea and nausea, with all protease inhibitors.

More recently appreciated are the metabolic abnormalities that can occur in patients taking HAART. Hyperglycemia, hypercholesterolemia, and hypertriglyceridemia should be carefully monitored and treated (with attention to interactions between the protease inhibitors and many 3-hydroxy-3-methylglutaryl coenzyme A [HMG-CoA] reductase inhibitors). Additionally, studies have suggested an association between antiretroviral therapy use and increased relative risk of cardiovascular end points, such as myocardial infarction.[16] Fat distribution abnormalities (e.g., lipodystrophy, fat accumulation) are frequently noted, including wasting of the limbs and face as well as enlargement of the dorsocervical fat pad and central obesity, with increased visceral adipose tissue. An increased risk of osteopenia and avascular joint necrosis has been noted. Mitochondrial dysfunction with potentially fatal lactic acidosis is well described.

In addition, significant drug interactions can occur between antiretroviral agents and commonly prescribed drugs that can lead to drug toxicities or reduction in levels of the drug or the antiretroviral agent, rendering them ineffective. For a complete listing of adverse effects, toxicities, and medication interactions, refer to the DHHS Antiretroviral Guidelines.[13]

OUTCOMES

The advent of HAART has improved mortality for HIV-infected patients who have access to these medications. In the United States, deaths caused by AIDS declined sharply in 1996 and 1997, when protease inhibitors were first introduced. Death rates decreased from 29.4 per 100 person-years in 1995 to 8.8 per 100 person-years by 1997 in a cohort of adults with advanced HIV infection.[17] Other studies in a pediatric population have mirrored these results.[18] Morbidity has declined as well, as measured by the incidence of opportunistic infections.[17] Between 1994 and 1997, the incidence of PCP, MAC disease, and cytomegalovirus retinitis combined decreased by 83% (21.9 to 3.7 per 100 person-years). A study using a computer simulation of HIV disease has estimated that a total of 2,100,000 years of life have been saved by prophylactic therapy and antiretroviral therapy between 1989 and 2003. The per-person survival gain attributed to HAART for HIV infection is estimated to be 180 months, nine times that of coronary artery bypass surgery.[19] Current efforts are focused on improving ease of use and decreasing toxicity of HAART in hopes of enhancing the quality of life in those infected with HIV.

PREVENTION AND SCREENING

Physicians must conduct a thorough, nonjudgmental assessment of risk factors for HIV infection. Persons at increased risk for HIV infection include those with a history of IDU, sexually transmitted diseases, including human papillomavirus, hemophilia, and receipt of blood products between 1977 and 1985. Men who have had sex with men, sex workers, and heterosexual persons with more than one partner since their last HIV test are also considered to be at high risk, as are the sexual partners of high-risk or HIV-infected persons. Mental illness and incarceration may serve as markers for high-risk behavior, as does a history of hepatitis B or C infection. Persons who consider themselves at risk should receive testing, even if risk behaviors are not disclosed. Past efforts have focused on testing individuals perceived to be at increased risk for HIV infection. The Centers for Disease Control and Prevention (CDC) has now recommended that all persons aged 13 to 64 be screened for HIV infection at least once, and that this should be done unless the patient declines testing (opt-out testing).[20] Individuals at high risk should be screened more regularly and all pregnant women should be screened for HIV unless they choose to opt out of testing. The availability of reliable, CLIA-waived rapid tests (see earlier, "Diagnosis") increases the feasibility of this approach.

CONSIDERATIONS IN SPECIAL POPULATIONS

Pregnant Women

Treatment of pregnant women poses special considerations. Antiretroviral therapy in pregnancy has been shown to decrease the risk of transmission to the child dramatically. Therapy with zidovudine in the third trimester, followed by IV infusion of zidovudine in labor and administration to the infant for the first 4 weeks of life, have been shown to lead to a 66% reduction in the risk of transmission of HIV to the infant.[9] Currently, combination antiretroviral therapy during pregnancy is recommended. Delivery by cesarean section further reduces that risk, from approximately 8% to 2%. When the maternal viral load is reduced to less than 1000 copies/mL with HAART therapy, however, the likelihood of transmission to the fetus is less than 1%, whether the child is delivered vaginally or by cesarean section. Although counseling regarding the risks of antiretroviral medications to the fetus is necessary, the transmission benefits of antiretroviral therapy generally outweigh the risks of teratogenicity. Efavirenz is a pregnancy category D agent and should be avoided.[21]

Postexposure Prophylaxis

Health care workers are at risk for contracting HIV infection through exposure to infectious body substances. Blood, cerebrospinal fluid, semen, and vaginal, peritoneal, synovial, pleural, and amniotic fluids, as well as tissue samples, can all transmit the HIV virus, although nonbloody urine, saliva, tears, sweat, and vomitus do not. Percutaneous exposures (needlesticks) carry a risk of transmission of 0.3%, whereas mucus membrane exposures (e.g., a splash) transmit less virus and are less likely to lead to seroconversion (0.01% of the time). The risk of a percutaneous exposure is increased when blood is visible on the device causing the injury, when the device was in the source patient's artery or vein, when the injury is deep, or when the source patient died within 60 days of the event. Retrospective data, animal data, and mother-to-child transmission data all suggest that immediate antiretroviral therapy after an exposure reduces the risk of HIV seroconversion in the exposed individual. Currently, administration of a basic (two-drug) or expanded (three or more drug) antiretroviral regimen is recommended, based on the severity of the exposure and degree of viremia in the source patient. Most commonly, zidovudine-lamivudine or tenofovir-emtricitabine are prescribed, with the addition of lopinavir-ritonavir or efavirenz if an expanded regimen is favored. The specific regimen may be altered if the source patient has known resistant virus. The postexposure regimen should be continued for 4 weeks if no toxicities occur and the first dose should be administered as soon as possible. Follow-up testing is recommended at 6 weeks, 3 months, and 6 months.[8]

Summary

- Acute HIV infection is associated with fever, rash, lymphadenopathy, and nonexudative pharyngitis. Up to 70% of seroconverters are symptomatic but are rarely diagnosed. The appropriate tests to establish the diagnosis are an HIV screening antibody test and HIV RNA by PCR assay.
- More than 250,000 individuals in the United States are HIV infected but unaware of their diagnosis. Current CDC guidelines recommend screening all individuals ages 13 to 64 years at least once in their lifetime and annually for higher risk behavior. Consent for testing should be obtained using opt-out approaches.
- Antiretroviral therapy is recommended for patients with a $CD4^+$ T cell count of less than 350 cells/mm^3.
- Currently recommended initial antiretroviral regimens include at least thee and sometimes four different medications to suppress the virus successfully. Combination antiretroviral therapy should also be administered to HIV-positive pregnant women, which can reduce the risk of transmission of HIV to the fetus to less than 1%.
- Long-term complications of antiretroviral therapy are increasingly recognized. These include hyperlipidemia, insulin resistance, accelerated bone loss, increased cardiovascular disease, lipoatrophy, and fat accumulation.

Suggested Readings

Cao Y, Qin L, Zhang L, et al: Virologic and immunologic characterization of long-term survivors of human immunodeficiency virus type 1 infection. N Engl J Med 1995;332:201-208.

Centers for Disease Control and Prevention: 1993 revised classification system for HIV infection and expanded surveillance case definition for AIDS among adolescents and adults. MMWR Morb Mortal Wkly Rep 1992;41(RR-17):1-19.

Kahn JO, Walker BD: Acute human immunodeficiency virus type 1 infection. N Engl J Med 1998;339:33-39.

Mellors JW, Muñoz A, Giorgi JV, et al: Plasma viral load and $CD4^+$ lymphocytes as prognostic markers of HIV-1 infection. Ann Intern Med 1997;126:946-954.

Mylonakis E, Paliou M, Lally M, et al: Laboratory testing for infection with the human immunodeficiency virus: Established and novel approaches. Am J Med 2000;109:568-576.

Palella FJ Jr, Delaney KM, Moorman AC, et al: Declining morbidity and mortality among patients with advanced human immunodeficiency virus infection. HIV Outpatient Study Investigators. N Engl J Med 1998;338:853.

Paterson DL, Swindells S, Mohr J, et al: Adherence to protease inhibitor therapy and outcomes in patients with HIV infection. Ann Intern Med 2000;133:21-30.

References

For a complete list of references, log onto www.expertconsult.com.

Hospital-Acquired, Health Care–Associated, and Ventilator-Associated Pneumonia

Justin L. Ranes, Steven Gordon, and *Alejandro C. Arroliga*

In 2005, the American Thoracic Society and Infectious Disease Society of America published an evidenced-based guideline for the management of hospital-acquired pneumonia (HAP), ventilator-associated pneumonia (VAP), and health care–associated pneumonia (HCAP).[1] This chapter provides basic information for the clinician and reviews guidelines for the management of HCAP. The key summary principles are summarized here.

Summary

- HCAP is included in the spectrum of HAP and VAP, and patients with HCAP need therapy for multidrug resistant (MDR) pathogens.
- Early, appropriate, broad-spectrum antimicrobial therapy should be prescribed at adequate doses for all patients with suspected HCAP.
- A lower respiratory tract culture should be collected on all patients before antimicrobial therapy, but collection should not delay initiation of empirical therapy in critically ill patients.
- An empirical therapy regimen should not include antimicrobial agents that the patient has recently received.
- De-escalation of antibiotics (changing to narrow spectrum or oral therapy) should be considered once the results of cultures and the patient's clinical response are known.

DEFINITIONS

HAP is defined as pneumonia that occurs 48 hours or more after admission and that was not incubating at the time of admission. VAP refers to pneumonia that occurs more than 48 hours after endotracheal intubation. HCAP includes patients with pneumonia who are hospitalized in an acute care hospital for more than 2 days within 90 days of the pneumonia; those who resided in a long-term care facility (e.g., nursing home); those who received recent parenteral antimicrobial therapy, chemotherapy, or wound care within 30 days of pneumonia; or those who received treatment in a hospital or hemodialysis clinic. For practical purposes, most principles for HCAP, VAP, and HAP overlap.

EPIDEMIOLOGY

HAP is the second most common nosocomial infection in the United States. There are 300,000 cases of HAP annually, and it carries an associated mortality rate of 30% to 70%.[2] It is difficult to determine the fraction of patients with HAP whose mortality is directly attributable to their pneumonia (the attributable mortality), but this rate is estimated to be between 27% and 50%.[2,3] This means that of the patients who develop HAP, it will be the proximate cause of death in 25% to 50% of them, and the remaining 50% to 75% will develop HAP but die from some other cause. HAP lengthens the hospital stay by 7 to 9 days and is associated with a higher cost of medical care.

General risk factors for developing HAP include age older than 70 years, serious comorbidities, malnutrition, impaired consciousness, prolonged hospitalization, and chronic obstructive pulmonary diseases.[2]

HAP is the most common infection occurring in patients requiring care in an intensive care unit (ICU) and accounts for almost 25% of all nosocomial infections in ICU patients, with incidence rates ranging from 6% up to 52%.[3] This increased incidence is because patients located in an ICU often require mechanical ventilation, and mechanically ventilated patients are 6 to 21 times more likely to develop HAP than nonventilated patients. Mechanical ventilation is associated with high rates of HAP because the endotracheal tube bypasses upper respiratory tract defenses, allows for pooling of oropharyngeal secretions, prevents effective cough, and can be a nidus for infection.[2] The development of HAP in mechanically ventilated patients portends a poor prognosis, with a rate of mortality 2 to 10 times higher for this group than for mechanically ventilated patients without HAP.

The timing of HCAP is an important epidemiologic variable and risk factor for pathogens and outcomes in patients with VAP and HAP. Early-onset pneumonia (within 96 hours) usually is associated with a better prognosis and fewer MDR pathogens than late-onset (5 days or more) VAP and HAP.[1]

PATHOGENESIS

HAP, VAP, and HCAP are likely to occur when a sufficiently large number of organisms are delivered to the lower respiratory tract so that host defenses are overwhelmed (e.g., by aspiration or contaminated respiratory therapy equipment), when host defenses are impaired (e.g., by immunodeficiency or steroids), or if particularly virulent organisms are involved.[2] Gram-negative bacteria (GNB) account for 55% to 85% of HAP infections, and gram-positive cocci account for 20% to 30%.[4] GNB rarely causes community-acquired pneumonia, but hospitalized patients are exposed to organisms that nonhospitalized patients are not exposed to, and many factors directly related to hospitalization make patients more likely to develop and less able to fight infection.

Microaspiration of contaminated oropharyngeal secretions seems to be the most important of these factors, because it is the most common cause of HAP.[2] Microaspiration is a common event, even in nonhospitalized patients, occurring in as many as 50% of normal sleeping subjects and 70% of patients subject to some degree of sedation or depressed consciousness. Microaspiration in a hospitalized patient is more serious and more likely to cause infection because the oropharyngeal secretions aspirated are likely to contain organisms that are not present under normal circumstances but that frequently cause HAP. The oropharynx of hospitalized patients becomes colonized by GNB in as many as 35% of moderately ill and 73% of critically ill patients, often within the first 4 days of admission. With the introduction of these new pathogenic organisms into the oropharynx, the previously benign event of microaspiration now becomes a mechanism whereby virulent organisms are introduced into the lower respiratory tract and cause pneumonia.

CAUSES

HAP, VAP, and HCAP are caused by a spectrum of bacterial pathogens, may be polymicrobial and rarely due to viral and fungal pathogens (unless immunocompromised patients; e.g., bone marrow transplants). Common pathogens include aerobic gram-negative bacilli (e.g., *Pseudomonas aeruginosa*, *Klebsiella pneumoniae*, *Escherichia coli*) as well as gram-positive organisms such as *Staphylococcus aureus*.

Rates of HAP caused by MDR pathogens have been increasing and affect empirical therapy. A discussion of the mechanisms of resistance for specific bacterial pathogens is beyond the scope of this chapter but includes the following:

- Methicillin-resistant *S. aureus* (MRSA)
- MDR *Pseudomonas aeruginosa* (with resistance to carbapenems, fluoroquinolones, and antipseudomonal penicillins and cephalosporinases)
- Extended-spectrum beta-lactamase (ESBL) producing *Enterobacter*, *E. coli*, and *K. pneumoniae*
- *Acinetobacter* species, *Stenotrophomonas* (*Pseudomonas*) *maltophilia*, and *Burkholderia cepacia*, all of which have increasing resistance to commonly used antimicrobials

Summary

Risk Factors for Multidrug-Resistant Pathogens[1]

- Antimicrobial therapy was initiated within the preceding 90 days.
- Onset of pneumonia occurred after 4 days of hospitalization.
- Known MDR pathogens are circulating in the community or hospital.
- Immunosuppressive disease is present or immunosuppressive therapy has been initiated.

DIAGNOSIS

Testing for and diagnosing HAP are difficult, because there are no reliable tools to determine whether the patient has pneumonia as the explanation for the clinical signs and symptoms seen at the bedside and no reliable method for determining the causative pathogen when pneumonia is present.[6] The diagnosis is initially made on clinical grounds by the finding of a new infiltrate on chest radiograph, fever, purulent sputum, or other signs of clinical deterioration. Unfortunately, this clinical method was shown to be specific for HAP in only 27 of 84 patients in a series reported by Fagon and colleagues,[7] because other conditions, such as congestive heart failure, pulmonary embolism, atelectasis, acute respiratory distress syndrome (ARDS), pulmonary hemorrhage, or drug reactions, may mimic pneumonia, particularly in critically ill patients.[1] Lack of specificity in the clinical diagnosis gives rise to the need for more reliable diagnostic tools so that fewer patients will be treated with antibiotics for noninfectious causes. Although there are many different testing modalities that can be used, all have their limitations and none is sufficiently sensitive and specific to be considered a gold standard test.[3]

Blood cultures have diagnostic and prognostic values but their reported sensitivity is only 8% to 20%, and their role is therefore limited. Similarly, examination of expectorated sputum is neither sensitive nor specific and should not be routinely used.[1] The most useful noninvasive test is the examination of tracheobronchial aspirates (TBAs). This method has a high degree of sensitivity, as demonstrated in a study in which the offending organism was recovered from tracheal secretions in 29 of 31 patients.[4] The weakness of this test is its inability to differentiate between the organism responsible for causing the pneumonia and harmless colonizers. Because of this limitation, the use of TBA lies in its negative predictive value and its ability to exclude the presence of resistant organisms, thus narrowing antibiotic coverage.

Invasive bronchoscopic techniques are able to take samples directly from the lower respiratory tract without contamination from upper airway or oral secretions and would seem to provide an advance in identifying the responsible pathogen.[8] Surprisingly, when bronchoscopic techniques such as bronchoalveolar lavage (BAL) or the use of protected specimen brushes (PSBs) have been compared with less invasive methods, they do not appear to differ significantly in terms of sensitivity, specificity or, more importantly, patient morbidity and mortality.[9] There is currently a lack of consensus on the role of invasive diagnostic testing for HAP, and it is the subject of ongoing debate.

One study regarding this issue compared the results of bronchoscopically obtained PSBs with those of TBAs in 76 mechanically ventilated patients who were already receiving empirical antibiotic therapy.[9] In this study, more patients who received bronchoscopy with PSB had a change in their antibiotic regimen, but there were no significant differences in length of stay, days requiring mechanical ventilation, or mortality between the two groups. This study concluded that outcome is "not influenced by techniques used for microbial investigation."

Another study compared the use of invasive testing, such as PSBs and BAL, with the use of noninvasive TBAs in 413 patients.[10] This study showed an initial decrease in mortality, antibiotic use, and organ dysfunction at 14 days in patients in whom invasive techniques were used, but at a 28-day analysis the difference in mortality could not be similarly demonstrated. These and other studies have led many clinicians to the conclusion that noninvasive and invasive tools achieve similar diagnostic performance and therefore the use of invasive techniques cannot be justified in every patient with HAP.[8] Others argue that if invasive testing is done within the first 12 hours after diagnosis and before antibiotics are administered, the improvement in diagnostic yield may be sufficient to merit its use.[3]

A review of this issue by Ewig and Torres[8] has stated that invasive and noninvasive techniques do not differ significantly, both are less sensitive than specific, and the false-negative rate for these tests ranges from 30% to 40% and the false-positive rate from 20% to 30%. The review also stated that invasive diagnostic testing should not be performed early in the course of HAP, and the best way to make adjustments to the empirical antibiotic regimen is by the use of TBAs rather than invasive techniques. Furthermore, they stated that because of the poor sensitivity associated with invasive methods, empirical coverage should not be stopped on the basis of negative diagnostic testing alone, and that the potential role for invasive diagnostic evaluation lies in cases of nonresponse to initial treatment.

TREATMENT

After HAP is diagnosed, it is imperative that antimicrobial therapy begin promptly, because delays in the administration of antibiotics have been associated with worse outcomes.[3] One study in support of this concept has reported a mortality rate of 30% in patients who receive early appropriate therapy compared with a rate of 91% in patients who do not.[11] The initial selection of an antimicrobial agent is almost always made on an empirical basis and is based on factors such as severity of infection, patient-specific risk factors, and total number of days in hospital before onset.

Pneumonia is defined as severe if there is need for admission to an ICU, radiographic evidence of rapid progression, need for mechanical ventilation or high levels of inspired oxygen, or evidence of sepsis. Regardless of severity, the initial empirical treatment regimens for HAP or VAP in patients with no known risk factors for MDR pathogens, and who have early-onset pneumonia (within 5 days of hospitalization) should include coverage for a group of core organisms that includes antibiotic-sensitive, aerobic, enteric, gram-negative bacilli (*Enterobacter* spp., *E. coli*, *Klebsiella* spp., *Proteus* spp., and *Serratia marcescens*) community pathogens such as *Haemophilus influenzae* and *Streptococcus pneumoniae*, as well as methicillin-sensitive *S. aureus*. Recommended antibiotics would include ceftriaxone or a quinolone (e.g., ciprofloxacin or levofloxacin) or ampicillin-sulbactam or eratpenem.[1] Although it is acceptable to use a fluoroquinolone in the empirical regimen of patients with penicillin allergies, one study evaluated the use of penicillin skin testing in these patients.[12] It was found that most patients with a history of penicillin allergy can safely be treated with penicillin antibiotics, so penicillin skin testing may be a means whereby the use of fluoroquinolones can be decreased.

Regardless of the severity of infection, the initial empirical treatment regimens for HAP or VAP in patients at risk for infection with MDR pathogens should be targeted with agents known to be effective against these organisms. This would include patients with late-onset disease (within 4 days of hospitalization), other risk factors (e.g., prior use of broad-spectrum antibiotics), or both. The potential pathogens include *P. aeruginosa*, *K. pneumoniae* (ESBL strains), *Acinetobacter* spp., and MRSA. Empirical combination antimicrobial therapy should include an antipseudomonal cephalosporin (e.g., ceftazidime), antipseudomonal carbapenem (e.g., imipenem), or beta-lactam-beta-lactamase inhibitor (e.g., piperacillin-tazobactam), plus an antipseudomonal fluoroquinolone (e.g., ciprofloxacin) or aminoglycoside (e.g. tobramycin) plus vancomycin or linezolid (for MRSA). If *Legionella* is suspected, then this combination should also have a macrolide (e.g., azithromycin) added if a fluoroquinolone that has *Legionella* activity is not already part of the regimen[1] (Table 1).

Duration of Treatment

There is no consensus regarding the duration of antibiotic treatment for all patients with HAP, although if the initial clinical suspicion was low, antibiotics may be safely discontinued after 72 hours if the clinical picture has not changed significantly.[13] Recommendations from the American Thoracic Society have suggested that the duration of treatment should be guided by severity, time to clinical response, and the pathogenic organism[1]; however, a panel of experts has suggested that "the main factor for deciding the duration of therapy should be the time to clinical response and not the pathogen involved"[3] and that patients should be treated for at least 72 hours after a clinical response is achieved.

Clinical response to antimicrobial therapy is not likely in the first 48 to 72 hours, so the empirical antibiotic regimen should not be changed during this time unless as directed by the results of microbiologic investigation.[1] In patients who fail to respond after this initial period, recommendations are that antibiotic coverage should be broadened, noninfectious causes considered, and invasive diagnostic testing performed. Appropriate diagnostic testing may include bronchoscopy with PSBs and BAL, radiographic tests to evaluate for the possibility of pleural effusions or abscesses that limit response, and computed tomography (CT) scanning of the sinuses to evaluate for sinusitis, because this may be a cause of persistent symptoms. After excluding all other causes in the nonresponding patient, it may be advisable to perform open lung biopsy for diagnostic purposes, even though this technique has not been shown to improve outcomes.[2]

Table 1 Antibiotics for Empirical Therapy of Hospital-Acquired Pneumonia* in Patients at Risk for Multidrug-Resistant Pathogens

Antibiotic	Adult Dosage†
Antipseudomonal Cephalosporin	
Cefepime	1-2 g q8-12hr
Ceftazidime	2 g q8hr
Carbepenems	
Imipenem	500 mg q6hr or 1 g q8hr
Meropenem	1 g q8hr
Beta-Lactam–Beta-Lactamase inhibitor	
Piperacillin-tazobactam	4.5 g q6hr
Aminoglycosides	
Gentamicin	7 mg/kg/day
Tobramycin	7 mg/kg/day
Amikacin	20 mg/kg/day
Antipseudomonal Quinolones	
Levofloxacin	750 mg/day
Ciprofloxacin	400 mg q8hr
Vancomycin	15 mg/kg q12hr
Linezolid	600 mg q12hr

*Including ventilator-associated and health care–associated pneumonia.
†Dosages are based on normal renal and hepatic function. Trough levels for gentamicin and tobramycin should be less than 1 mg/mL, and for amikacin they should be less than 4-5 mg/mL. Trough levels for vancomycin should be 15-20 mg/mL.
Adapted from Niederman MS, Craven DE, Bonten MJ, et al: Guidelines for the management of adults with hospital-acquired, ventilator-associated, and healthcare-associated pneumonia. Am J Respir Crit Care Med 2005;171:388-416.

Summary[1]

Recommendations for Assessing Response to Treatment

- Modifications of empirical therapy should be based on results of microbiology testing in conjunction with clinical parameters.
- Clinical improvement of HCAP usually takes 2 to 3 days and therefore therapy should not be changed during this period unless there is a rapid clinical decline.
- Narrowing therapy to the most focused regimen possible on the basis of culture data (de-escalation of antimicrobials) should be considered for the responding patient.
- The nonresponding patient should be evaluated for possible MDR pathogens, extrapulmonary sites of infection, complications of pneumonia and its therapy, and mimics of pneumonia. Testing should be directed to whichever of these causes is likely after physical examination of the patient.

PREVENTION

Prevention is important because even when appropriate diagnostic and therapeutic procedures are used, HAP is associated with a high rate of mortality. Prevention strategies should focus on general measures for infection control, measures directed at specific patient risk factors, and measures to limit the use of antibiotics in an attempt to decrease the prevalence of resistant organisms.

Although most clinicians think that strategies for prevention are important, it must be noted that few techniques have been shown in well-designed experimental or epidemiologic studies to be of definite value, so most specific recommendations for the prevention of HAP are made on the basis of expert opinion rather than hard data. The Centers for Disease Control and Prevention has published a set of 74 recommendations for preventing bacterial nosocomial pneumonia[14]; only 15 of these recommendations were "strongly supported by well-designed experimental or epidemiologic studies" and 14 of those 15 recommendations dealt with general issues such as surveillance, education, hand washing, sterilization, proper use of gloves, value of vaccination, and sanitation. The recommendation that prophylactic antibiotics not be routinely administered was the only specific recommendation supported by well-designed studies; all other specific recommendations, such as prevention of aspiration and prevention of colonization, were based on less-stringent evidence or on expert opinions.

General measures for infection control such as proper hand washing, use of gloves, and measures to reduce contamination from respiratory therapy equipment are important factors in preventing HAP. Although the benefits of these practices are universally recognized, they are often not performed, as evidenced by an observational study performed in an ICU setting where only 10% of health care workers washed their hands before having direct patient contact and only 32% washed their hands after patient contact.[15] Compliance with these general measures has repeatedly been shown to correlate with favorable outcomes, and stricter adherence to these guidelines is needed.

Patient-specific measures should be considered and, if other circumstances allow, followed for every hospitalized patient. Efforts should be made to reduce immunosuppression, reduce sedation, avoid transportation of patients out of the ICU, and provide adequate nutrition, because these measures have been shown to reduce the incidence of HAP. It has been shown that pneumonia is more common in patients with sinusitis.[2] Because the presence of nasally placed tubes is associated with sinusitis, it is recommended that endotracheal or gastric tubes be placed orally if possible.

Another intervention with proven benefit for mechanically ventilated patients is the use of subglottic secretion drainage, a method whereby oropharyngeal secretions are continuously suctioned in an effort to prevent pooling and thus aspiration.[1] Finally, body positioning seems to have an impact on the development of HAP. This has been evidenced by a study[16] that was stopped early after an interim analysis found a significant difference in the development of HAP between patients in a supine position and patients in a semirecumbent position, probably because of the protective effects of the semirecumbent position against aspiration of refluxed gastric contents.

Other techniques, such as administration of prophylactic antibiotics or nonabsorbable antibiotics for the purpose of gastrointestinal decontamination, have been attempted in the past, with varying degrees of reported success. More recent literature has suggested that these methods should not be used because they have not consistently been shown to influence mortality or length of stay, and the use of antibiotics in this manner may lead to the development of resistant organisms.[3] On the other hand, the results regarding the role of histamine blockers in the development of HAP are conflicting, but their use should not be specifically avoided in patients for this reason.[1]

The notion that antibiotics select out resistant or virulent organisms, or both, has been suggested in a study that found that in mechanically ventilated patients who had previously received antibiotics, 65% of pneumonias were caused by *Acinetobacter* or *Pseudomonas*, but in antibiotic-naïve patients, only 19% of infections were caused by these pathogens.[17] In another study, 11 of 14 patients who had previously received ceftazidime developed HAP caused by resistant strains of *Acinetobacter* but only 11 of 29 control patients developed similar infections.[15] These observations have resulted in efforts to decrease the use of antibiotics, which in turn decreases the incidence of antibiotic-resistant pathogens and potentially improves patient outcomes.[18,19]

Suggested Readings

Drakulovic MB, Torres A, Bauer TT, et al: Supine body position as a risk factor for nosocomial pneumonia in mechanically ventilated patients: a randomised trial. Lancet 1999;354:1851-1858.

Fagon JY, Chastre J, Domart Y, et al: Nosocomial pneumonia in patients receiving continuous mechanical ventilation. Prospective analysis of 52 episodes with use of a protected specimen brush and quantitative culture techniques. Am Rev Respir Dis 1989;139:877-884.

Kollef MH: Current concepts: The prevention of ventilator-associated pneumonia. N Engl J Med 1999;340:627-634.

Niederman MS, Craven DE, Bonten MJ, et al: Guidelines for the management of adults with hospital-acquired, ventilator-associated, and healthcare-associated pneumonia. Am J Respir Crit Care Med 2005;171:388-416.

Ruiz M, Torres A, Ewig S, et al: Noninvasive versus invasive microbial investigation in ventilator-associated pneumonia: evaluation of outcome. Am J Respir Crit Care Med 2000;162:119-125.

Singh N, Rogers P, Atwood CW, et al: Short-course empiric antibiotic therapy for patients with pulmonary infiltrates in the intensive care unit. A proposed solution for indiscriminate antibiotic prescription. Am J Respir Crit Care Med 2000;162:505-511.

Weber DJ, Raasch R, Rutala WA: Nosocomial infections in the ICU: The growing importance of antibiotic-resistant pathogens. Chest 1999;115:34S-41S.

Yates RR: New intervention strategies for reducing antibiotic resistance. Chest 1999;115:24S-27S.

References

For a complete list of references, log onto www.expertconsult.com.

Tick-Related Infections

Alan Taege

Ticks are the vectors of at least 10 clinically significant zoonotic illnesses in the United States (Box 1). These illnesses may be caused by bacterial, viral, or parasitic pathogens, some of which may occur simultaneously during the bite of a single tick. Humans are often an accidental host to these increasingly recognized conditions by virtue of our intrusion into the natural habitat of the ticks and their reservoirs, the white-footed mouse and whitetail deer. Geographically distinct areas exist for most of the vectors, reservoirs, and diseases; however, recreational travel into these regions may result in illness for nonresidents. Continued encroachment into forested and uncultivated areas will likely lead to a further increase in the incidence of tick-related infections. Many of these infections may be contracted in urban or semirural areas as well. Therefore, they should not be viewed as occurring only in remote or rural regions.

The common arthropod vectors are listed in Table 1. Each has the potential to carry more than one pathogen. The illnesses they cause often have a nonspecific manifestation that requires astute physician recognition. A careful history and physical examination, with particular attention to travel and recreational activities, may be lifesaving. Early recognition, diagnosis, and treatment result in fewer complications and less morbidity and death. Seroconversion is often delayed; therefore, empirical therapy is frequently necessary. A dated but useful overview of these infections has been given by Spach and colleagues.[1]

LYME DISEASE

Lyme disease is currently the most common vector-borne disease in the United States. It was described in Lyme, Connecticut, in the 1970s and also exists in Europe with a different clinical presentation. Although rarely fatal and seldom a serious illness, Lyme disease has been widely publicized, frequently overdramatized, and sometimes linked to unproven conditions. *Borrelia burgdorferi*, a gram-negative spirochete, is the causative organism. *Ixodes scapularis* ticks in the eastern and midwestern regions of the United States and *I. pacificus* in the northern Pacific areas carry this bacterium. The white-footed mouse is the natural reservoir. Although Lyme disease has been reported in nearly every state, it is considered endemic to the northeast coastal, mid-Atlantic, upper Midwest, northern California, and Pacific northwest regions (Fig. 1), with seasonal peaks of infection occurring in May through August.

Ixodes tick attachment for 48 to 72 hours is generally required for infection.[2] After an incubation period of 7 to 10 days (range, 3-30 days), the illness may evolve through three stages. Other than erythema migrans (EM), the characteristic rash of Lyme disease, symptoms of Lyme disease are nonspecific. Stage 1, or early localized disease, is characterized by EM in approximately 90% of cases. EM is a rapidly expanding erythematous macule varying in size from 5 to 70 cm. It is generally solid, especially in the early period, but may show central clearing or a target-like appearance (Fig. 2). EM may resolve without therapy; it is usually asymptomatic but may be associated with fever, malaise, arthralgia, myalgia, or headache. Occasionally, the lesion may be pruritic. A history of a tick bite or exposure and the development of EM are diagnostic for Lyme disease.

Stage 2, early disseminated disease, may occur if stage 1 was not treated. It may manifest as multiple EM lesions (generally smaller) 3 to 5 weeks after the bite. Cranial nerve palsies (especially cranial nerve VII, or Bell's, palsy), meningitis, or carditis (variable atrioventricular block) may also occur.

Stage 3, late disease, may evolve if stage 2 was not treated. Monoarticular or oligoarticular arthritis is the most common manifestation of stage 3. The knee is the most commonly involved joint. It is likely an autoimmune arthritis, which does not respond well to antibiotic therapy. Encephalitis, encephalopathy, and polyneuropathy may be late-stage sequelae, but are uncommon.

Diagnosis is best accomplished by recognition of EM and the compatible history in stage 1 or 2. Culture of the organism, most often from an EM lesion, is the standard of diagnosis but is technically slow and difficult.[3] Serology detects antibodies but does not establish the diagnosis by itself because other spirochetes (e.g., syphilis, relapsing fever, oral spirochetes) as well as varicella, cytomegalovirus, Epstein-Barr virus, and parvovirus may cause false-positive test results. In addition, rheumatoid arthritis and systemic lupus may cause erroneous serologic results. Serology is best performed as a two-step process using an enzyme-linked immunosorbent assay (ELISA; high sensitivity) as the first step, followed by a Western blot test for confirmation (high specificity). Immunoglobulin M (IgM) antibodies may be detected in only 20% to 30% of cases during the first 2 weeks; however, 70% to 80% of cases develop IgM antibodies by 1 month. IgG antibodies will be present by 6 to 8 weeks. Early antibiotic therapy may delay, blunt, or block the antibody response, making the clinical diagnosis even more important.

Therapy is well established and defined (Table 2). There appears to be no indication for prolonged therapy. Shorter courses may be as effective as the current recommendations. Stage 1 is treated with oral antibiotics for 14 to 21 days with doxycycline, amoxicillin, or cefuroxime. Stage 2 disease may be treated with the same regimens as for stage 1 unless meningitis or severe carditis occurs, in which case ceftriaxone, 100 mg/kg/day (maximum, 2 g/day) for 14 to 28 days, is recommended. Stage 3 arthritis may be treated with oral doxycycline or amoxicillin for 14 to 21 days. If it recurs, therapy with ceftriaxone would be used for 14 to 28 days. Late-stage neurologic disease is also treated with ceftriaxone.[4]

Human Lyme disease vaccine is no longer available in the United States (it is available in Europe), but animal vaccine is still used. Also, Lyme vaccine results in reactive ELISA (but negative Western blot) results.

ROCKY MOUNTAIN SPOTTED FEVER

Rocky Mountain spotted fever (RMSF) is caused by the obligate intracellular, pleomorphic, gram-negative rod *Rickettsia rickettsii*. Although it is considered the most common rickettsial disease in the United States, its declining incidence (Fig. 3) may yield this position to ehrlichiosis. RMSF occurs in the south Atlantic coastal, south central, and western regions, being most concentrated in North and South Carolina, Tennessee, and Oklahoma. The tick vectors are *Dermacentor variabilis* in the East and *D. andersoni* in the West.

Infection can occur year-round but is most commonly encountered from April through September. Most cases occur in children with exposures to dogs and wooded areas. Tick attachment of 6 to 10 hours is required for transmission, followed by an incubation period of 5 to 7 days (range, 2-14 days) until infection is manifest. Only 60% to 70% of patients recall a tick bite.

The classic triad of fever, rash, and headache occurs in a minority of cases, particularly early in the course. The vasculitic rash, which often begins on the wrists and ankles and then spreads centrally (Fig. 4), is uncommon during the first 3 days of illness; however, 10% of patients may not develop a rash. When it occurs, it may first have a maculopapular appearance, which progresses to a petechial rash. Abdominal symptoms of nausea, vomiting, and diarrhea may be present in one third of cases.[5] Myalgia, arthralgia, and confusion may also be parts of the clinical picture.

Early diagnosis may be difficult because of the nonspecific nature of the symptoms. Because of overlapping symptoms and geographic distribution, RMSF may be confused with ehrlichiosis. Fortunately, both may be treated with doxycycline. Serologic diagnosis is delayed and therefore seldom useful in the acute situation. Antibodies measured by indirect immunofluorescence have a 90% sensitivity but do not become positive until 10 to 14 days into the course.[6] Direct immunofluorescence of a skin biopsy from the rash may prove useful early in the course of the illness. General laboratory tests have a limited role, although a finding of thrombocytopenia may be helpful. Ehrlichiosis is more likely to be associated with leukopenia and ele-

Box 1 Tick-Related Infections

- Lyme disease
- Ehrlichiosis
- Granulocytic
- Monocytic
- Rocky Mountain spotted fever
- Babesiosis
- Tularemia
- Relapsing fever
- Tick paralysis
- Q fever
- Colorado tick fever
- Tick encephalitis
- Southern tick rash

Table 1 Tick Vectors

Vector	U.S. Location
Ixodes scapularis	East, Northeast, Midwest
Ixodes pacificus	West, Northwest
Dermacentor variabilis (dog tick)	East, Midwest
Dermacentor andersoni (wood tick)	West
Amblyoma americanum (Lone Star Tick)	South, Central

Table 2 Treatment of Lyme Disease

Stage	Features	Dosage Regimen	Duration of Therapy (days)
1	Erythema migrans	Doxycycline, 100 mg PO bid; amoxicillin, 500 mg PO tid; cefuroxime 500 mg PO bid	14-21 14-21 14-21
2	Severe carditis, meningitis	Doxycycline, 100 mg PO bid	14-21
		Amoxicillin, 500 mg PO tid	14-21
		Cefuroxime, 500 mg PO bid	14-21
		Ceftriaxone, 100 mg/kg/day (max, 2 g/day)	14-28
		Ceftriaxone, 100 mg/kg/day (max, 2 g/day)	14-28
3	Arthritis, recurrent arthritis, neurologic disease	Doxycycline, amoxicillin, or cefuroxime PO, as above	14-21
		Ceftriaxone, as above	14-28
		Ceftriaxone, as above	14-28

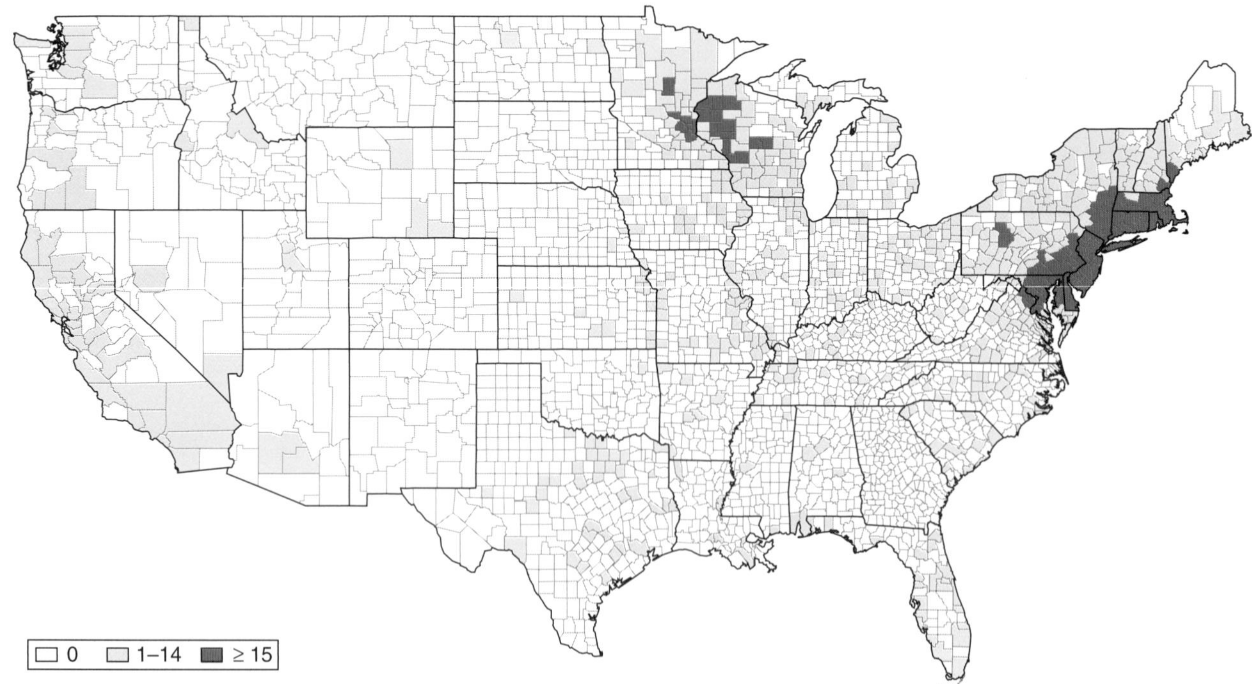

Figure 1 **Lyme disease, reported cases by county, United States, 2000.** The total number of cases from these counties (marked in green) represented 90% of all cases reported in 2000. *(From the Centers for Disease Control and Prevention.)*

vated liver enzyme levels, whereas RMSF is more likely to be associated with thrombocytopenia.

Recommended treatment is doxycycline, 100 mg twice daily for 5 to 7 days, or for 2 days after defervescence occurs.[7] Many believe that doxycycline may be used to treat children, because this short course has a low risk for staining teeth. Chloramphenicol may be the best therapy during pregnancy.

Adverse prognostic factors include age older than 40 years, male gender, thrombocytopenia, hyponatremia, renal insufficiency, neurologic symptoms, delayed diagnosis, and lack of initial treatment with doxycycline.

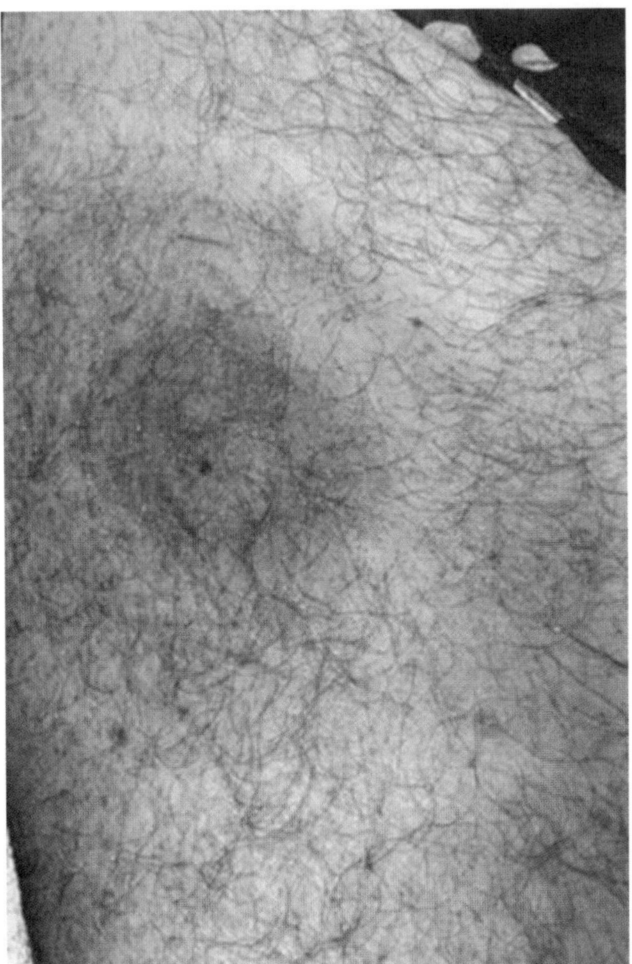

Figure 2 **Erythema migrans (EM).** This is the characteristic rash of Lyme disease.

EHRLICHIOSIS

Ehrlichiosis is a rather recently recognized rickettsial infection. This pleomorphic gram-negative rod infects white blood cells (WBCs). Two geographically distinct but clinically similar diseases exist and are named for the WBCs they inhabit: human monocytic ehrlichiosis (HME) and human granulocytic ehrlichiosis (HGE) (Table 3). *Ehrlichia chaffeensis* is responsible for HME, and *Anaplasma phagocytophila* and *E. ewingii* are associated with HGE. Clumps of organisms, morulae, may be found in the cytoplasm of the WBCs (Fig. 5).

HME occurs in the mid-Atlantic, southeast, and south central regions, and in California, most often from April through September (Fig. 6). The largest numbers of cases have been encountered in Missouri, Oklahoma, Arkansas, and North Carolina.

Transmission occurs after 24 to 48 hours of attachment by *Amblyomma americanum* (the Lone Star tick) followed by a 7- to 10-day incubation period. The illness may be mild or progress to multiorgan system failure and death. The onset is abrupt, with fever, chills, myalgia, arthralgia, and headache. Rash may occur in as many as 40% of HME cases but is uncommon early in the illness. It manifests as a macular or maculopapular exanthem, which may become petechial. In contrast to RMSF, the rash generally starts centrally and moves peripherally. Secondary opportunistic infections may occur and may be the result of an immunosuppressive phenomenon. A 2% to 3% mortality rate has been noted. HME may be a more severe infection than HGE and is particularly severe in immunocompromised patients.[8]

HGE occurs in southern New England, the mid-Atlantic coastal and upper Midwest regions, and northern California (Fig. 7). The tick vectors are *Ixodes scapularis* in the east and *I. pacificus* in the west. The white-footed mouse is the reservoir for HGE and HME. Both tick vectors may also infect whitetail deer, coyotes, and rats.

HGE occurs most often in the summer months after a 1- to 2-week incubation. The symptoms are similar to those of HME, although rash is less common (2%-5%), and HGE may be less severe.

Laboratory evaluation may reveal leukopenia, thrombocytopenia, and elevated transaminase levels in both forms. Serologic diagnosis by immunofluorescent assay is delayed because antibodies are

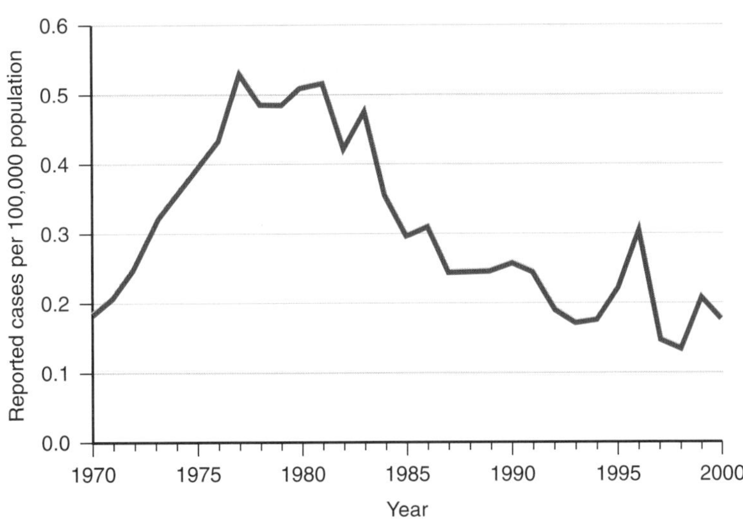

Figure 3 **Rocky Mountain spotted fever, reported cases/100,000 population in the United States by year, 1970 to 2000.** *(From the Centers for Disease Control and Prevention.)*

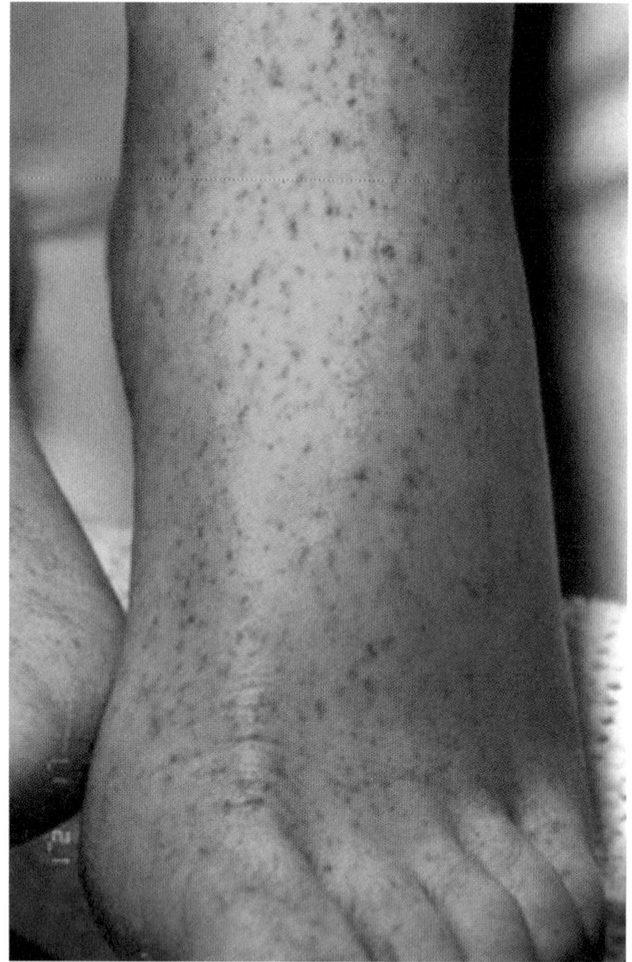

Figure 4 **Vasculitic rash.** This rash often begins on the wrists and ankles and then spreads centrally.

Table 3 Ehrlichiosis

Human Monocytic Ehrlichiosis	Human Granulocytic Ehrlichiosis
Ehrlichia chaffeensis	*Anaplasma phagocytophila* *Ehrlichia ewingii*
Amblyoma americanum	*Ixodes scapularis* *Ixodes pacificus*
Midwest, South	East, Midwest, West

seldom present in the first week. A fourfold rise from acute to convalescent sera or titers of 1:256 for HME or 1:80 for HGE is considered diagnostic. The polymerase chain reaction assay may be useful in the first week, and has a sensitivity rate of 67% to 87% and a specificity of approximately 100%.[9] Morulae may be found in peripheral blood smears in about 50% of cases of HGE and 7% to 17% of HME cases, although a trained microscopist and careful search are necessary. Morulae may also be found in bone marrow aspirates.

Doxycycline, 100 mg twice daily for 14 days, is the treatment of choice. Shorter courses may be as effective. The organisms appear to be resistant to chloramphenicol. Quinolones may be used for second-line therapy.

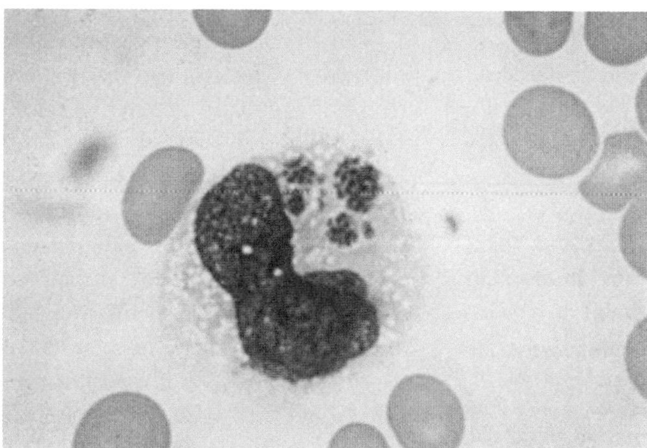

Figure 5 **Clumps of organisms (morulae) may be found in the cytoplasm of the white blood cells.**

BABESIOSIS

Babesiosis is a protozoan, parasitic, malaria-like infection of red blood cells that results in hemolysis. The causative organisms are *Babesia microti* in the northeast United States, *B. divergins* in California, and an unnamed *Babesia* spp. in Washington (WA-1) and Missouri (MO-1). It may be transmitted by tick bites or, rarely, through blood transfusions. It is not a reportable disease; therefore, the incidence and number of infections are unknown. The vectors and reservoirs are the same as those for ehrlichiosis and Lyme disease, resulting in occasional cases of coinfection.

Infection occurs in the summer months. The Northeast, Midwest, and upper Pacific regions harbor the most cases (Maryland, Virginia, Georgia, Wisconsin, California, and Washington). Disease occurs in all age groups but is more severe in those older than 50 years, splenectomized individuals, and immunocompromised patients. After a 1- to 6-week incubation, infection may result in subclinical, mild, or fulminant disease. Mortality may be 5% to 10%.[10] Symptoms include fever, chills, drenching sweats, headache, nausea, and abdominal pain. Mild hepatosplenomegaly may be found on examination.

Diagnosis is made by a compatible clinical picture and laboratory findings of hemolytic anemia, thrombocytopenia, and elevated transaminase levels. Thick and thin blood smears may show the parasite in the ring form (Fig. 8) or its characteristic tetrad, which resembles a Maltese cross. Serologic testing with an immunofluorescence assay may help confirm the diagnosis. The polymerase chain reaction assay is also available and may be a useful diagnostic modality.

Treatment with clindamycin, 600 mg four times daily, and quinine, 650 mg three times daily, is the standard therapy, although atovaquone, 750 mg twice daily, and azithromycin, 500 to 600 mg followed by 250 to 600 mg daily for 7 to 10 days, may be better tolerated and as effective. Exchange transfusions may be helpful in severe cases.

TULAREMIA

Tularemia is caused by *Francisella tularensis*, a gram-negative coccobacillus that is virulent and highly infectious. Tick (*Dermacentor* and *Amblyomma*), deer fly, or mosquito bites, or contact with or consumption of poorly cooked infected meat (rabbit) may result in infection. Accidental aerosolization may cause outbreaks as well.[11] Most cases occur in geographic regions similar to those for RMSF, but they also reach Texas and Utah. The largest number of infections is concentrated in Missouri, Oklahoma, Arkansas, and Tennessee; however, the incidence is declining.[12] Six clinical syndromes exist

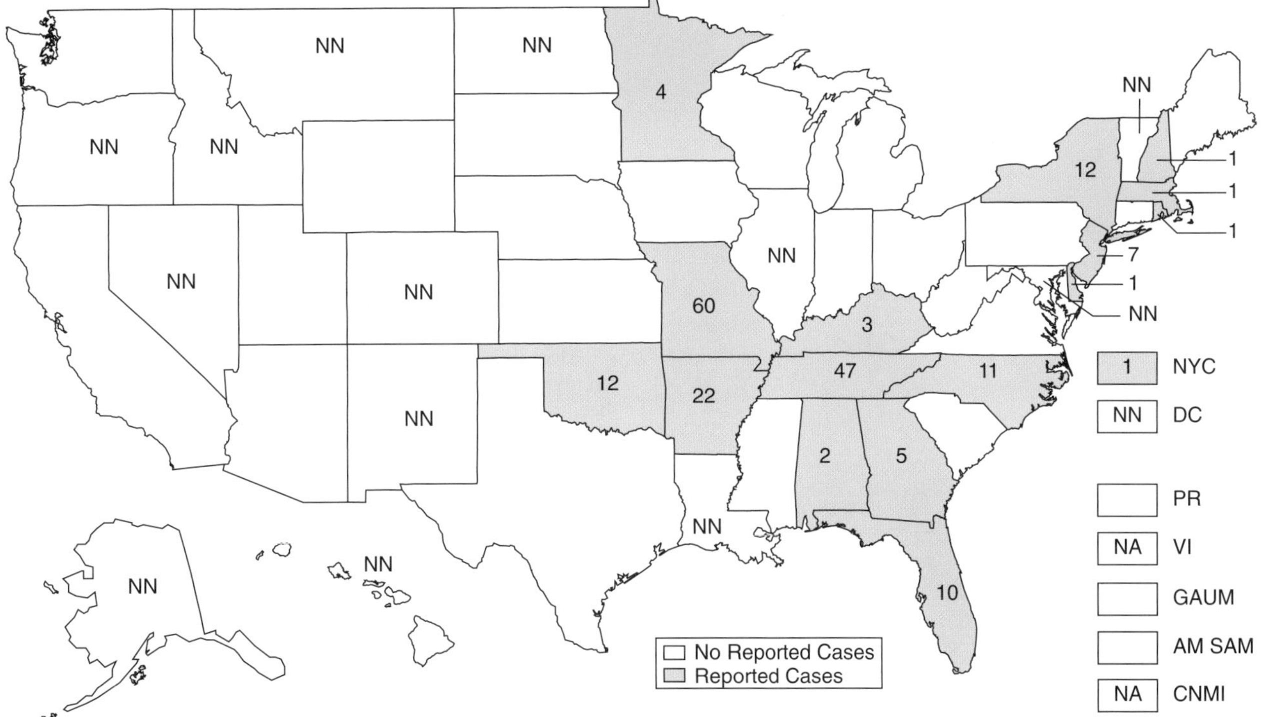

Figure 6 Human monocytic ehrlichiosis, number of reported cases in the United States and U.S. territories, 2000. AM SAMOA, American Samoa; CNMI, Commonwealth of the Northern Mariana Islands; DC, District of Columbia; NYC, New York City; PR, Puerto Rico; VI, Virgin Islands. *(From the Centers for Disease Control and Prevention.)*

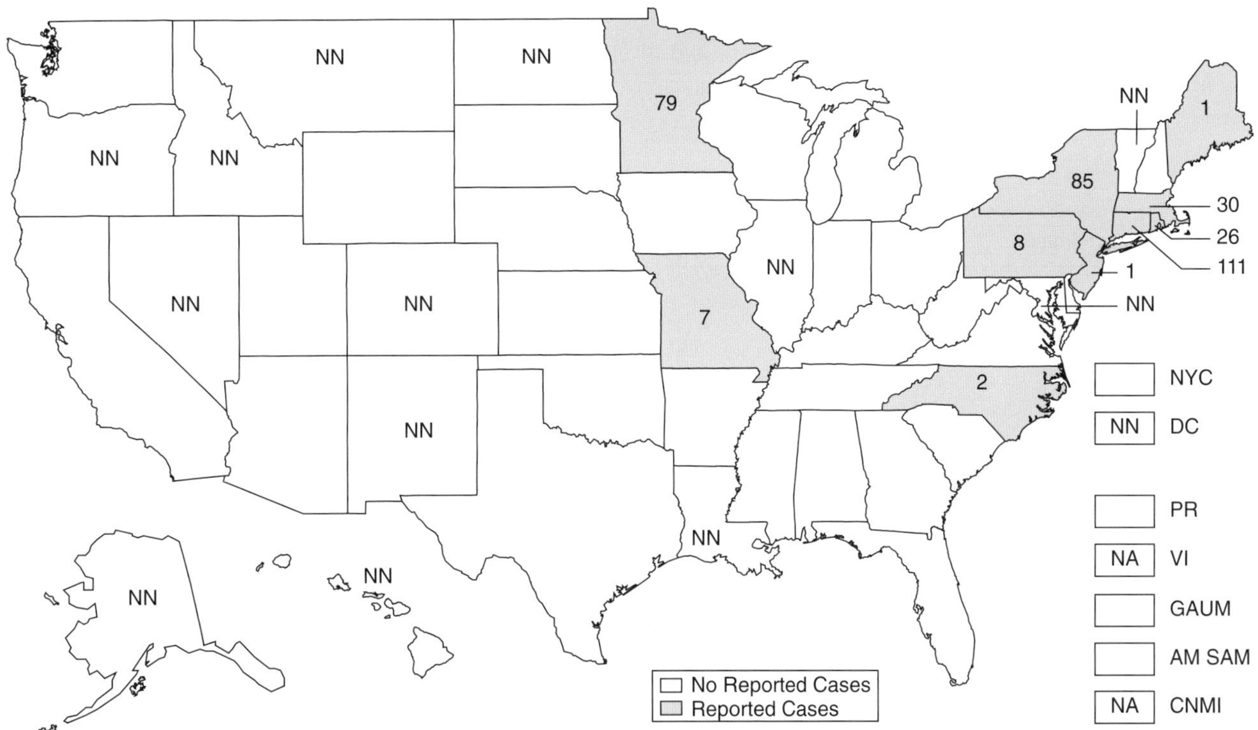

Figure 7 Human granulocytic ehrlichiosis, number of reported cases in the United States and U.S. territories, 2000. AM SAMOA, American Samoa; CNMI, Commonwealth of the Northern Mariana Islands; DC, District of Columbia; NYC, New York City; PR, Puerto Rico; VI, Virgin Islands. *(From the Centers for Disease Control and Prevention.)*

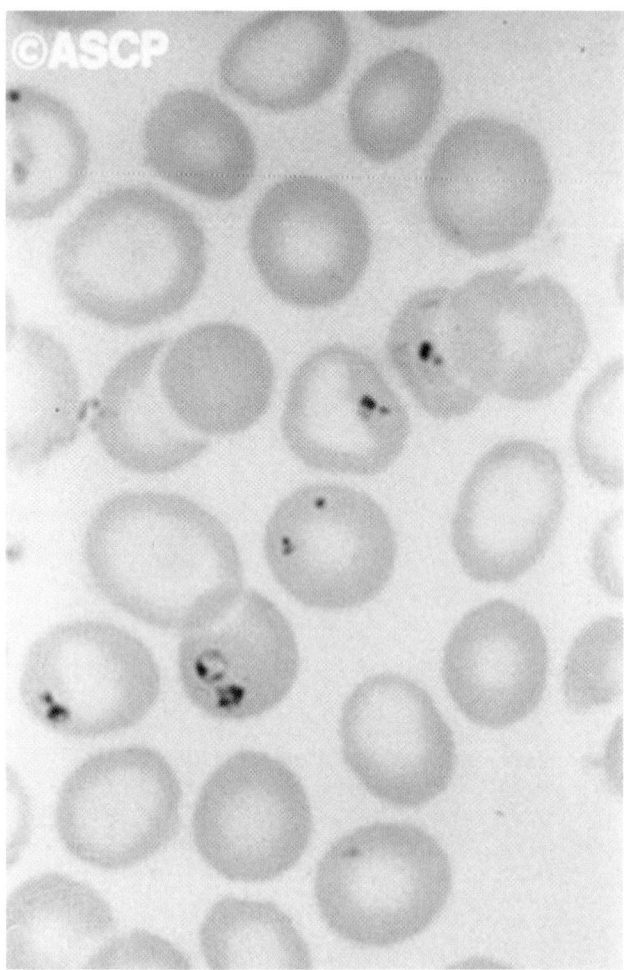

Figure 8 **Thick and thin blood smears may show the parasite in the ring form.**

Box 2 Tularemia Syndromes
Ulceroglandular Glandular Oculoglandular Oropharyngeal Typhoidal Pneumonic

(Box 2), corresponding to the portal of entry or the clinical manifestation. Ulceroglandular tularemia is the most common type. An incubation period of 2 to 14 days leads to a clinically variable illness, depending on the form that develops.

The organism can be cultured from blood, body fluids, and tissues but requires special media (cysteine-enriched). Laboratory personnel should be notified, because it is highly contagious and represents a laboratory hazard. Serodiagnosis may be obtained through agglutination tests. Elevated liver enzyme levels occur in about 50% of cases.

The standard of treatment is streptomycin, but because of difficulties in procurement, gentamicin has been substituted. Tetracyclines and quinolones may also be effective but usually require longer courses of therapy. Mortality may occur in 2% to 4% of cases.

MISCELLANEOUS INFECTIONS

Q Fever

Coxiella burnetti, the causative agent of Q fever, is another gram-negative intracellular organism. Its nonspecific manifestation of fever and headache may be associated with various clinical syndromes, most commonly pneumonia, hepatitis, and endocarditis. Based on serology, however, most patients appear to have an asymptomatic illness. Although Q fever has been associated with ticks, acquisition usually occurs by inhalation of the organism during exposure to infected animals, such as cattle, sheep, or goats, although many other animals have been known to be sources.

Most infections are self-limited. Pneumonia frequently resembles an atypical pneumonic picture. Multiple round infiltrates have also been described. Hepatitis is usually anicteric. Endocarditis occurs in the setting of previous valvular disease in which the patient is frequently immunocompromised.

Doxycycline or a tetracycline derivative remains the mainstay of therapy. Quinolones and rifampin also have therapeutic efficacy. A brief course of a tetracycline suffices for acute disease, when not self limited. The chronic form of Q fever may require months or years of treatment.

Relapsing Fever

Relapsing fever is another tick-borne disease caused by the spirochete *Borrelia hermsii* or *B. duttonii* occurring in the southwest United States. After approximately 7 days of incubation, a 3- to 6-day illness characterized by fever, headache, and rash will be followed by an asymptomatic week, and then a recurring cyclic illness. The organism can be demonstrated on thick and thin blood smears. Treatment with doxycycline or ceftriaxone is effective. A Jarisch-Herxheimer reaction may occur during treatment.

Colorado Tick Fever

Colorado tick fever is a viral illness caused by the Coltivirus, which is transmitted by *Dermacentor andersoni* tick bites in the Rocky Mountains, California, and Pacific Northwest. Clinical manifestations include high fever, chills, headache, and myalgia. Serologic diagnosis is available. No specific treatment is known; therefore, supportive and symptomatic care is administered.

Tick Paralysis

Tick paralysis is caused by a neurotoxin elaborated by female *Dermacentor*, *Amblyomma*, and *Ixodes* ticks after prolonged attachment for 2 to 7 days. It is most common in young children, especially girls in the northwest and Rocky Mountain areas. It manifests as a rapidly progressive Guillain-Barré–like syndrome, with ascending motor paralysis and sparing of sensation and the sensorium.[13] It can be fatal unless the tick is located and removed. Thereafter, rapid improvement ensues.

Tick Encephalitis

The arbovirus that causes tick encephalitis belongs to the Flaviviridae family, is endemic in Russia and Eastern and Central Europe, but is rare in the United States.[14] It is transmitted by *Ixodes* ticks. After 1 to 2 weeks of incubation, a biphasic illness may occur, characterized by fever, headache, and myalgia. After a 2- to 4-week asymptomatic period, aseptic meningitis or meningoencephalitis may occur. No specific therapy is available; therefore, supportive care is rendered.

Southern Tick Rash. Southern tick rash is an incompletely characterized illness probably transmitted by *Amblyomma americanum*, infecting the individual with a *Borrelia* species that causes an erythema migrans–like rash. It responds to the same treatment as Lyme disease.

Summary

- Ticks are not insects but arthropods (eight legs, two parts to the body).
- The most common tick-borne illness in the United States is Lyme disease, and erythema migrans (expanding target-like rash) is characteristic.
- A high index of suspicion is required because tick-borne illnesses often have a nonspecific presentation.
- Empirical therapy is often necessary for the treatment of tick-borne illness, usually with doxycycline.

Suggested Readings

Bunikis J, Barbour AG: Laboratory testing for suspected Lyme disease. Med Clin North Am 2002;86:311-340.
Choi E: Tularemia and Q fever. Med Clin North Am 2002;86:393-416.
Des Vignes F, Piesman J, Heffernan R, et al: Effect of tick removal on transmission of Borrelia burgdorferi and Ehrlichia phagocytophila by Ixodes scapularis nymphs. J Infect Dis 2001;183:773-778.
Dumpis U, Crook D, Oksi J: Tick-borne encephalitis. Clin Infect Dis 1999;28:882-890.
Feldman KA, Enscore RE, Lathrop SL, et al: An outbreak of primary pneumonic tularemia on Martha's Vineyard. N Engl J Med 2001;345:1601-1606.
Felz MW, Smith CD, Swift TR: A six-year-old girl with tick paralysis. N Engl J Med 2000;342:90-94, 127-129.
Holman RC, Paddock CD, Curns AT, et al: Analysis of risk factors for fatal Rocky Mountain spotted fever: evidence for superiority of tetracyclines for therapy. J Infect Dis 2001;184:1437-1444.
Krause P: Babesiosis. Med Clin North Am 2002;86:361-373.
Olano J, Walker DH: Human ehrlichiosis. Med Clin North Am 2002;86:375-392.
Safdar N, Love RB, Maki DG: Severe Ehrlichia chaffeensis infection in a lung transplant recipient: A review of ehrlichiosis in the immunocompromised patient. Emerg Infect Dis 2002;8:320-323.
Sexton DJ, Kaye KS: Rocky Mountain spotted fever. Med Clin North Am 2002;86:351-360.
Shapiro ED, Gerber MA: Lyme disease. Clin Infect Dis 2000;31:533-542.
Spach DH, Liles WC, Campbell GL, et al: Tick-borne diseases in the United States. N Engl J Med 1993;329:936-947.
Zaidi S, Singer C: Gastrointestinal and hepatic manifestations of tickborne diseases in the United States. Clin Infect Dis 2002;34:1206-1212.

References

For a complete list of references, log onto www.expertconsult.com.

Clostridium difficile

Thomas G. Fraser and James F. Swiencicki

DEFINITION AND CAUSES

Clostridium difficile is an obligate anaerobic, spore-producing, gram-positive rod that was first described in 1935. Its link with pseudomembranous colitis and *Clostridium difficile*–associated diarrhea (CDAD) was established in 1978.[1,2] It is the implicated pathogen in 20% to 30% of patients with antibiotic-associated diarrhea, 50% to 75% of those with antibiotic-associated colitis, and more than 90% of those with antibiotic-associated pseudomembranous colitis.[3] CDAD is an important hospital-acquired infection associated with an increase in length of hospital stay and cost and substantial morbidity and mortality.[4,5]

INCIDENCE AND PREVALENCE

Prevalence rates of *C. difficile* depend on the patient population, antibiotic prescribing patterns, endemic strains, and criteria used to define antibiotic-associated diarrhea.[2,6] The estimated prevalence of *C. difficile* colonization varies from 7% to 11% in hospitalized patients, 5% to 7% in residents of long-term care facilities, and generally less than 2% in ambulatory adults.[2] Carriage rates are higher in hospitalized patients who have received antibiotics. The reported incidence of *C. difficile* colitis among hospitalized inpatients ranges from 1 to 10 cases per 1000 discharges and it has been shown that these rates may vary over time in a given institution.[6] These numbers likely increase in direct proportion to hospital length of stay. The incidence of CDAD is increasing.[7]

PATHOPHYSIOLOGY AND NATURAL HISTORY

The current understanding of the natural history of *C. difficile* infection can be conceptualized as a three-step process.[8] As outlined in Figure 1, the first step is alteration of the normal gut flora, usually as a result of administration of an antibiotic. Clindamycin was the first antibiotic to be associated with pseudomembranous colitis, identified as a precipitant before the establishment of *C. difficile* as the causal pathogen.[9] Since that initial observation, almost all antimicrobials have been associated with CDAD including the cephalosporins and the penicillins.[2] Recently, attention has focused on a growing link between the widespread use of fluoroquinolones and CDAD.[10] Chemotherapeutic agents, particularly those with antimicrobial properties, have also been associated with the development of CDAD.

The second step is acquisition of a toxigenic strain of *C. difficile*. It is primarily a nosocomially acquired pathogen and its spores can be found in the hospital environment, with the chance of contamination being highest for those in closest proximity to symptomatic patients.[11] Most disease transmission is caused by transient carriage on health care workers' hands. The direct effect of the environment on transmission is difficult to assess, although studies have shown that the more contaminated the environment, the more likely health care workers' hands are contaminated.[12]

Once a patient has acquired *C. difficile*, he or she will develop clinical disease or will remain asymptomatically colonized, the final step in the process. Although the exact incubation time for CDAD is unknown, the time from acquisition to disease is relatively short, perhaps no longer than 7 days.[13] Whether a patient will develop CDAD once exposed to the pathogen has been shown to correlate with the ability to mount a humoral immune response.[14] Further clinical risk factors for the development of acute disease have also been identified (Box 1).

The pathogenicity of *C. difficile* is because it is a spore-forming toxigenic organism. The spore form of the organism is resistant to gastric acid and can therefore readily pass through the stomach to the intestine, where it changes to a vegetative life cycle.[2] As this occurs, the organism releases two potent exotoxins, toxin A (a 308-kd enterotoxin) and toxin B (a 269-kd cytotoxin).[6] These toxins not only open tight junctions between the cells of the intestine that result in increased vascular permeability and hemorrhage, but they also induce the production of tumor necrosis factor α and proinflammatory interleukins that cause a large inflammatory response and ultimately formation of pseudomembranes. Toxin A was previously believed to play a more important role in the development of diarrhea because animal models demonstrated more extensive tissue damage and fluid accumulation in the intestine compared with toxin B, which appeared to cause its effects only after the intestinal walls were damaged by toxin A. However, toxin A is not essential for virulence because virulent strains of *C. difficile* that are toxin A–negative but toxin B–positive have been described.

The genes that encode toxins A, *tcd*A, and B, *tcd*B, are found on the pathogenicity locus in *C. difficile*. These genes are situated in close proximity on this locus and are transcribed in the same direction.[36] Three other genes, *tcd*C, *tcd*D, and *tcd*E, are also located on the pathogenicity locus and are believed to play a role in regulation of toxin production.[36] The *tcd*C gene lies downstream of *tcd*A and is transcribed in the opposite direction from *tcd*A and *tcd*B. It functions as a negative regulator of toxin production. The *tcd*D gene is found upstream from *tcd*B and is believed to be a major positive regulator of toxins A and B production. The *tcd*E gene lies between *tcd*A and *tcd*B and is believed to facilitate the release of toxins A and B through permeabilization of the *C. difficile* cell wall.

Recently, there has been the emergence of a new epidemic strain of *C. difficile* responsible for increases in the incidence and severity of disease.[15] This strain is characterized by the deletion of *tcd*C and the hyperproduction of toxins A and B. It is also characterized by the production of binary toxin, as well as a more resistant antimicrobial susceptibility pattern. The significance of binary toxin production is still being investigated.

SIGNS AND SYMPTOMS

C. difficile infection manifests as a spectrum of disease, including asymptomatic carriage, simple antibiotic-associated diarrhea, pseudomembranous colitis, and fulminant colitis with toxic megacolon.[16] Symptoms include watery, nonbloody diarrhea accompanied by lower abdominal pain and cramping (20%-33%), fever (30%-50%), and leukocytosis (50%-60%).[6] Nausea, malaise, anorexia, hypoalbuminemia, and occult colonic bleeding may also be present. Fulminant colitis is characterized by a toxic appearance, fever, diffuse abdominal pain, and distention. These patients may develop toxic megacolon and paralytic ileus, with little or no diarrhea, which ultimately can result in colonic perforation and peritonitis with substantial mortality.[2] The incidence of severe disease has increased recently.

Extracolonic manifestations of *C. difficile* infection have been described. They are rare and include bacteremia, splenic abscess, osteomyelitis, reactive arthritis: Reiter's syndrome, tenosynovitis, pleural effusion, empyema, and infections of prosthetic devices.[17]

Recurrent diarrhea can occur in up to 40% of patients with CDAD.[2] Re-infection accounts for almost 50% of these cases, which suggests continued exposure to a *C. difficile* endemic environment as well as persistence of risk factors for disease in affected patients.

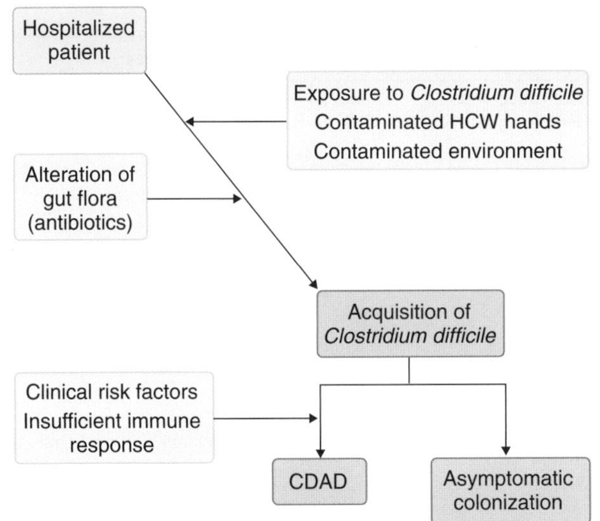

Figure 1 Pathophysiology and natural history of *Clostridium difficile*–associated diarrhea (CDAD). HCW, health care worker.

Box 1 Risk Factors for the Development of *Clostridium difficile*–Associated Diarrhea (CDAD)

Age
Severity of illness
Antacid therapy
Cathartics
Stool softeners
Gastrointestinal surgery
Enteral feeds
Nasogastric or oral gastric tubes

Adapted from Poutanen SM, Simor AE: Clostridium difficile*–associated diarrhea in adults. CMAJ 2004;171:51-58; and Thielman NM, Wilson KH: Antibiotic-associated colitis. In Mandell GL, Bennett JE, Dolin R (eds): Principles and Practice of Infectious Diseases, 6th ed, vol 1. Philadelphia: Elsevier, 2005, pp 1249-1262.*

Commonly, patients have received another course of antibiotics that predisposes to the second episode. The intraluminal presence of *C. difficile* spores likely contributes to recurrence of symptoms in those with true relapses. Most relapses will occur within 1 month of the end of therapy. Relapse caused by antibiotic resistance is not common. One recurrence is a risk factor for a subsequent episode.

The differential diagnosis of CDAD depends on the severity of the clinical presentation. Considerations in those with symptoms limited to diarrhea or mild colitis should include antibiotic-associated diarrhea, food-borne illness caused by enteric pathogens, and viral gastroenteritis. In those presenting with more severe disease, particularly with ileus or abdominal distention, colitis, diverticulitis, and other causes of a surgical abdomen must be considered ischemic.

DIAGNOSIS

CDAD should be considered in any currently or recently hospitalized patient treated with antibiotics who develops diarrhea. This holds for residents of long-term care facilities or rehabilitation centers. Community-acquired CDAD does occur but the vast majority of patients will have had recent exposure in a traditional health care setting.

Table 1 outlines the tests used for the diagnosis of *C. difficile*. No single best testing algorithm has been established for the diagnosis of CDAD, but some broad comments can be made. Typically, a single unformed stool specimen is sufficient to detect *C. difficile* toxins; however, repeat testing may be required.[2,6] Multiple specimens on the same day are seldom useful. Patients successfully treated can still shed toxin in their stool and therefore testing cure specimens should not be done because the results can be misleading.

The tissue culture cytotoxin assay, which detects toxin B from stool filtrate, is considered the gold standard because of its high sensitivity and specificity.[2] The disadvantages are its need for 24 to 48 hours for completion, as well as requiring tissue culture capability.

The most common test used to establish a diagnosis of *C. difficile* is an enzyme-linked immunosorbent assay (ELISA) for toxin A or toxins A and B.[18] The ELISA test is less technically demanding as compared with the cytotoxin assay. Although not as sensitive as the gold standard, the test performs well and has been widely adopted by clinical microbiology laboratories. Repeated testing may improve its sensitivity, although one specimen should usually be sufficient for diagnosis.[6]

Although inexpensive and easy to perform, a latex agglutination test for glutamate dehydrogenase, or common antigen, which is an enzyme-produced in *Clostridium* spp. as well as other bacteria, is not recommended for use in *C. difficile* diagnosis. This is because of its low poor sensitivity and specificity compared with other available testing strategies.[6]

Stool culture for *C. difficile* is rarely performed in clinical microbiology laboratories because of inconvenience compared with other marketed tests. Culture is very sensitive but not specific, because it will not distinguish between toxigenic and nontoxigenic strains.[6] This question can be answered if a toxin assay is added as a second step in the test. The benefits of stool culture include the ability to perform epidemiologic investigations and strain typing of isolates.

The polymerase chain reaction (PCR) assay for *C. difficile* toxins is currently a research method that shows promise as a more sensitive and specific test as compared with ELISA, with results similar to those of cytotoxin assays.[2] Its use in the clinical setting may be limited because of its cost compared with ELISA.[16]

Endoscopy should be considered when a rapid diagnosis is required, the patient has an ileus and stool is unable to be obtained, and other colonic diseases are being considered, such as inflammatory bowel disease.[6] Sigmoidoscopy or colonoscopy is required to visualize the colonic mucosa to establish the diagnosis of pseudomembranous colitis. Pseudomembranes are 2- to 10-mm raised yellow plaques that may have areas of normal mucosa or may coalesce to form larger plaques. Flexible sigmoidoscopy can miss up to 10% of cases of pseudomembranous colitis. If pseudomembranes are not visualized on endoscopy, then the findings of *C. difficile* colitis may be nonspecific and biopsies should be taken. Endoscopy should be used judiciously in patients with fulminant colitis given the incumbent risk of perforation.[2]

Findings of a thickened, edematous bowel wall (thumbprinting) may be seen on abdominal plain radiographs as well as on computed tomography (CT) scans in patients with pseudomembranous colitis.[2,16] Imaging studies are adjunctive but not diagnostic, can demonstrate the extent of colon involvement, and can assist in evaluating for other diagnoses in the differential.

Summary

- Consider CDAD infection in any patient with nosocomial diarrhea or diarrhea following recent antibiotic administration.
- A single unformed stool specimen is usually adequate for *C. difficile* testing.
- Most clinical laboratories use ELISA tests for *C. difficile* toxins because of their cost, convenience, and sensitivity.
- Endoscopy is required to establish the diagnosis of pseudomembranous colitis or when stool samples are unable to be obtained secondary to ileus.

Table 1 Tests Used for the Diagnosis of *Clostridium difficile*–Associated Diarrhea[2,6,16,19]

Test	Sensitivity (%)	Specificity (%)	Advantages	Disadvantages
Cytotoxin assay	80-90	99-100	Standard highly sensitive and specific; considered as gold standard	Takes 24-48 hr to complete; requires tissue culture facility; cost; detects only toxin B
ELISA toxin test	65-85	95-100	Fast (2-6 hr), easy to perform, high specificity	Not as sensitive as cytotoxin assay
Stool culture	90-100	98-100	Allows strain typing in epidemics	Takes 2-5 days to complete; labor intensive; not specific for toxin-producing bacteria
Latex agglutination assay for glutamate dehydrogenase	58-68	80-96	Fast, inexpensive, easy to perform	Poor sensitivity and specificity needed to establish diagnosis; requires confirmatory test
PCR assay toxin gene detection	92-97	100	Excellent sensitivity and specificity compared with cytotoxin assay	Research test only; no commercial assays available
Endoscopy	51	~100	Diagnostic of pseudomembranous colitis; can be used without need to collect stool sample	Cost; invasive test; risk of perforation

ELISA, enzyme-linked immunosorbent assay; PCR, polymerase chain reaction.

Data from Poutanen SM, Simor AE: *Clostridium difficile*–associated diarrhea in adults. CMAJ 2004;171:51-58; Thielman NM, Wilson KH: Antibiotic-associated colitis. In Mandell GL, Bennett JE, Dolin R (eds): Principles and Practice of Infectious Diseases, 6th ed, vol 1. Philadelphia: Elsevier, 2005, pp 1249-1262; Hurley BW, Nguyen CC: The spectrum of pseudomembranous enterocolitis and antibiotic-associated diarrhea. Arch Int Med 2002;162:2177-2184; and Gerding DN, Johnson S, Peterson LR, et al: *Clostridium difficile*–associated diarrhea and colitis. Infect Control Hosp Epidemiol 1995;16:459-477.

TREATMENT

The most important aspect of management of CDAD is rapid recognition of the disease and discontinuation of the inciting agent.[2] Historically, as many as 50% of patients will respond to stopping the precipitating antibiotic. Medical therapy for CDAD is necessary in moderate to severe disease and surgery may be necessary for severe disease. Adequate hydration and electrolyte replenishment should accompany medical and surgical therapy. Antiperistaltics should be avoided because these can exacerbate toxin-mediated damage to the mucosa.

Medical Options

Oral metronidazole, 500 mg three times daily, or vancomycin, 125 to 250 mg four times daily for 10 to 14 days is considered first-line therapy for *C. difficile*–associated dirarrhea.[19] Both agents have been found to have similar efficacy in prospective randomized control trials.[20,21] Metronidazole is the preferred first-line therapy because of its lower cost and concerns that oral vancomycin selects for vancomycin-resistant *Enterococcus*.[16,19] Oral vancomycin should be reserved for those patients with intolerance to metronidazole, those who fail to respond to metronidazole, or those who have more severe disease. Recently, there have been concerns that metronidazole is inferior to vancomycin. This observational data are noteworthy but as of yet there is no evidence that metronidazole should be abandoned for this disease.[22-24] The epidemic strain that has been recently identified reminds us of the potentially severe consequences of this disease and the need for careful clinical attention. If a patient on metronidazole deteriorates, a change to vancomycin is likely warranted. It usually takes 3 or 4 days for a patient to begin to improve with appropriate therapy. To date, there has been no documentation of metronidazole or vancomycin resistance to *C. difficile*.

In patients who are unable to tolerate oral medications or who have severe ileus, IV metronidazole in combination with intracolonic vancomycin via nasogastric tube is appropriate.[26] In addition, vancomycin enemas have been used for the patient with severe disease and ileus (Box 2). Timely surgical and infectious disease consultations are critical for these complicated patients. IV vancomycin is not efficacious in *C. difficile* infection because the drug is not excreted in the colon.[2,16]

Box 2 Management of *Clostridium difficile*–Associated Diarrhea (CDAD)

Metronidazole, 500 mg PO tid for 10 days (preferred)
Vancomycin, 125-250 mg PO qid for 10 days if metronidazole-intolerant or if patient fails to respond to metronidazole
For moderate to severe disease,* vancomycin should be used
CDAD with ileus or critical illness
Surgical and infectious disease consultation
Vancomycin orally or via nasogastric tube, 500 mg q6h
Metronidazole, 500 mg q6h IV
Vancomycin enema, 500 mg q6h

**White blood cell count > 20,000/mm^3, acute renal failure, abdominal distention, hemodynamic instability.*

Adapted from Olson MM, Shanholtzer CJ, Lee JT, et al: Ten years of prospective Clostridium difficile*–associated disease surveillance and treatment at the Minneapolis VA Medical Center 1982-1991. Infect Control Hosp Epidemiol 1994;15:371-381; and from Apisarnthanarak A, Razavi B, Mundy LM: Adjunctive intracolonic vancomycin for severe* Clostridium difficile *colitis: Case series and review of the literature. Clin Infect Dis 2002;35:690-696.*

CDAD can recur after treatment with metronidazole or vancomycin.[19] A first relapse should be treated with the same antimicrobial used in the initial regimen.[16] Multiple relapses have been treated with various medical regimens, including pulsed and tapered metronidazole and vancomycin, combinations with rifampin, colestipol, or cholestyramine.[16,19,25,27,28] Small case series have shown IV immunoglobulin to be helpful in both recurrent and severe disease.[29] Studies using adjunctive probiotics such as *Saccharomyces boulardii* and *Lactobacillus* GG have had mixed results.[30] The lack of standardization of probiotic preparations makes endorsement of these approaches difficult. There are also reports of severe consequences of this adjunctive therapy.[31] Finally, attempts to reconstitute the protective flora with fecal infusions via nasogastric tube or rectally have been reported to have great success.[32,33]

Newer agents in the treatment of *C. difficile* are currently in development. These include not only antimicrobials but also toxin-neutralizing agents and vaccines.

Surgical Options

Early surgical consultation should be considered for severe CDAD, especially if toxic megacolon is present, because operative intervention can be lifesaving.[6] Various surgical procedures have been described, including diversion of fecal stream by ileostomy, decompressive colostomy, or subtotal colectomy, the procedure of choice with toxic megacolon. Cases requiring surgery carry high mortality rates, ranging from 30% to over 50%.

Summary

- Oral metronidazole remains the preferred initial agent in the treatment of *C. difficile*–associated diarrhea.
- Oral vancomycin should be considered if the patient fails to respond to metronidazole or has severe disease.
- The severely ill patient with CDAD requires a multidisciplinary approach, and surgery may be lifesaving.
- The first relapse should be treated with the same antimicrobial used for the initial therapy.
- Recurrent infection can be difficult to manage and includes various treatment strategies.

PREVENTION

Box 3 reviews practice guidelines for the prevention of CDAD. The proper use of antibiotics is essential for prevention. Institutional antimicrobial restriction of agents associated with an increased risk of *C. difficile* (e.g., clindamycin, cephalosporins) can be effective in controlling outbreaks.[34,35]

The Centers for Disease Control and Prevention has recommended measures to prevent the nosocomial transmission of *C. difficile*. These can be found at http://www.cdc.gov/ncidod/dhqp/id_CdiffFAQ_HCP.html.

Institution of these measures requires an ongoing surveillance program to identify patients with CDAD. Patients should be placed in a private room, if possible, particularly if they have fecal incontinence. If private rooms are not available, cohorting of affected patients is acceptable. Hands should be washed with soap and water or alcohol hand rub after contact with infected patients. In outbreak settings, the preferential use of soap and water should be considered, because alcohol rubs may not be as effective in removing spores from the hands. Gloves should be worn when entering the room of a patient with CDAD. Gowns should be worn for significant patient contact. Equipment should be dedicated whenever possible. Meticulous cleaning of all environmental surfaces must be ensured and, if ongoing cross-transmission occurs, a hypochlorite-based solution is recommended.

Box 3 Practice Guidelines for the Prevention of *Clostridium difficile*–Associated Diarrhea

Limit use of antimicrobial agents.
Wash hands between contact with all patients.
Use private rooms with enteric precautions for patient with *C. difficile*–associated diarrhea.
Wear gloves when contacting patients with *C. difficile* or their environment.
Disinfect objects contaminated with *C. difficile* with sodium hypochlorite, alkaline glutaraldehyde, or ethylene oxide.

Adapted from Hurley BW, Nguyen CC: The spectrum of pseudomembranous enterocolitis and antibiotic-associated diarrhea. Arch Int Med 2002;162:2177-2184.

Suggested Readings

Gerding DN, Johnson S, Peterson LR, et al: *Clostridium difficile*–associated diarrhea and colitis. Infect Control Hosp Epidemiol 1995;16:459-477.

Johnson S, Gerding GN: *Clostridium difficile*–associated diarrhea. Clin Infect Dis 1998;26:1027-1036.

McDonald LC, Killgore GE, Thompson A, et al: An epidemic, toxin gene–variant strain of *Clostridium difficile*. N Engl J Med 2005;353:2433-2441.

McFarland LV, Mulligan ME, Kwok RYY, Stamm WE: Nosocomial acquisition of *Clostridium difficile* infection. N Engl J Med 1989;320:204-210.

McFarland LV, Surawicz CM, Stamm WE: Risk factors for *Clostridium difficile* carriage and *C. difficile*–associated diarrhea in a cohort of hospitalized patients. J Infect Dis 1990;162:678-684.

Muto CA, Pokrywka M, Shutt K, et al: A large outbfeak of *Clostridium difficile*–associated disease with an unexpected proportion of deaths and colectomies at a teaching hospital following increased fluoroquinolone use. Infect Control Hosp Epidemiol 2005;26:273-280.

Poutanen SM, Simor AE: *Clostridium difficile*–associated diarrhea in adults. CMAJ 2004;171:51-58.

Shim JK, Johnson S, Samore MH, et al: Primary symptomless colonization by *Clostridium difficile* and decreased risk of subsequent diarrhea. Lancet 1998;351:633-636.

Thielman NM, Wilson KH: Antibiotic-associated colitis. In Mandell GL, Bennett JE, Dolin R (eds): Principles and Practice of Infectious Diseases, 6th ed, vol 1. Philadelphia: Elsevier, 2005, pp 1249-1262.

References

For a complete list of references, log onto www.expertconsult.com.

Adult Immunization

Robin Avery

Morbidity and mortality from vaccine-preventable diseases remain substantial, particularly in adults. In the United States, between 50,000 and 90,000 adult deaths per year are caused by pneumococcal disease, influenza, and hepatitis B, whereas 300 to 500 deaths in children are caused by vaccine-preventable diseases.[1] Research on the reasons for vaccine underuse, and strategies to increase levels of vaccination coverage in the adult population, are areas of active endeavor.[2-6]

Several national organizations and other groups have provided detailed guides to immunization in adults, regarding both specific vaccines and proposed comprehensive vaccination schedules.[1,5-31] The Centers for Disease Control and Prevention (CDC) Advisory Committee on Immunization Practices (ACIP) is the source of many monographs containing definitive recommendations for immunization in general,[6,14,24] vaccine adverse effects,[17] safety and efficacy of specific vaccines,[16,18-20,22-23,25,26] and vaccination in immunocompromised persons[15,27,28] and in health care workers.[21] The American Academy of Pediatrics,[12,24] the American Public Health Association,[13] the Infectious Diseases Society of America,[9,10] the American College of Physicians—American Society of Internal Medicine,[9,11] the American Medical Association,[24] and the American Association of Family Physicians[24] have all participated in the formulation of guidelines for immunization. The Institute of Medicine (IOM) has convened a panel of experts to review specific vaccine safety issues,[29] and the National Coalition for Adult Immunization[30] has been formed for the purpose of increasing vaccination coverage and meeting national Healthy People goals.[31] The U.S. Preventive Services Task Force has included immunizations among the recommendations for general preventive measures.[6] Detailed recommendations for adult immunization have also been issued by the Mayo Vaccine Research Group.[1] The March 2001 issue of *Infectious Disease Clinics of North America* was devoted to "Vaccine Recommendations: Challenges and Controversies." This compendium of reviews by experts is highly recommended for additional in-depth reading on these topics.[7,8,32,33]

In 1994, the National Vaccine Advisory Committee (NVAC) reported on the status of adult vaccination in the United States and cited missed opportunities to vaccinate adults during health care visits.[5] The American College of Physicians Task Force on Adult Immunization and the Infectious Diseases Society of America (IDSA) recommended linking an assessment of vaccination status with other preventive measures at age 50 years.[9] This approach has been endorsed by the ACIP of the CDC, which recommends that all primary care physicians schedule a prevention visit at age 50 years,[34] at which time the patient's vaccination status can be reviewed, tetanus-diphtheria toxoid vaccine can be updated, and it can be determined whether the patient has an indication for the pneumococcal vaccine,[22] initiation of annual influenza vaccination, or both. The preventive visit at age 50 is all the more important because new recommendations from the CDC include influenza vaccination annually, beginning at age 50.[23]

In 1991, the U.S. Public Health Service introduced national goals for health promotion and disease prevention under the heading of Healthy People 2000.[31] At the start of this campaign, in the 50- to 64-year-old age group, only 9% and 15% of persons with cardiac or pulmonary high-risk conditions, respectively, had ever received pneumococcal vaccination, and only 21% and 28%, respectively, had received influenza vaccine the previous year,[34] although vaccination levels were higher in the over-65 age group.[34] The Healthy People 2000 national goals included an increase to 60% vaccination levels for these vaccines. Although many states met this objective with regard to influenza vaccination, pneumococcal vaccine coverage lagged considerably behind. The recently released Healthy People 2010 goals include achievement of 90% pneumococcal vaccination coverage in older adults and high-risk younger individuals.[32]

Current ACIP recommendations for adult immunization, endorsed by the IDSA and many of the above organizations, are summarized in Table 1.

SPECIFIC VACCINES

Pneumococcal Vaccine

The complex issues surrounding pneumococcal vaccination have been well summarized by Poland.[32] The pneumococcus bacteria is responsible for 500,000 cases of pneumonia, 50,000 cases of sepsis, 3,000 cases of meningitis, 40,000 deaths, and 7 million cases of otitis media annually in the United States. Unfortunately, pneumococcal vaccination is severely underused. The 23-valent pneumococcal polysaccharide vaccine, licensed in 1980, contains the serotypes responsible for 85% to 90% of invasive pneumococcal disease in adults, including the six pneumococcal serotypes, which are most frequently drug resistant.[32] The reported efficacy of the pneumococcal polysaccharide vaccine has ranged from 55% to 80% and varies between different risk groups, but its benefits in preventing invasive disease are significant despite less than 100% efficacy.[32] A 7-valent conjugated pneumococcal vaccine was licensed in 2000 and has been recommended for young children, for whom it is more immunogenic than the standard vaccine, but data in adults are limited.[32]

Current ACIP recommendations[22] (see Table 1) state that the pneumococcal vaccine should be administered to all adults age 65 years or older; individuals ages 2 to 64 years with chronic cardiovascular or pulmonary disease, diabetes, alcoholism, chronic liver disease, cerebrospinal fluid (CSF) leaks, functional or anatomic asplenia, who are immunocompromised, and those in high-risk environments, including residents of nursing homes or long-term care facilities, Alaskan natives, and Native American populations (who have high rates of pneumococcal disease). Reimmunization is recommended after 5 years, in patients older than 65, if the patient is immunocompromised, has chronic renal failure or nephrotic syndrome, has had organ or bone marrow transplantation, or had the first dose before age 65. Patients ages 10 to 65 years with splenic dysfunction or who are immunocompromised should receive reimmunization after 5 years.[22]

One report has highlighted the fact that smoking is a major risk factor for pneumococcal disease.[35] Given that approximately one third of adults smoke, and other risk factors are common in the age 50 to 64 group, some experts have anticipated that recommendations for universal pneumococcal vaccination may be extended to the age 50 to 64 group in the future, analogous with influenza vaccination.[32] As with influenza vaccine, strategies such as standing orders at hospital discharge and in long-term care facilities have the potential to increase pneumococcal vaccination levels significantly.[6]

Tetanus-Diphtheria Toxoid and Tetanus-Diphtheria-Acellular Pertussis Vaccine

Tetanus and diphtheria are rare diseases in the United States today. However, there has been a recent widespread outbreak of diphtheria

Table 1 Recommendations for Immunizations in Adults

Vaccine	Recommendations
Measles-mumps-rubella (MMR)*,†	Two doses for persons born after 1956 who are at high risk of exposure; one dose for persons born after 1956 who are at low risk of exposure.
Tetanus-diphtheria* and tetanus-reduced diphtheria-acellular pertussis (Tdap)[19]	Tetanus-diphtheria primary series consisting of first dose, second dose after 1 mo, and third dose 6-12 mo later, followed by a booster every 10 yr or once at age 50 yr; substitute Tdap for Td booster for adults ages 19-64; health care workers or those in close contact with infants should receive Tdap even if Td received within 10 yr
Influenza‡,§	Annual vaccination (see text)
Pneumococcal‡,¶	One vaccination, with possible revaccination after 6 yr or more (see text)
Hepatitis B∥,**	First dose, followed by second dose 1-2 mo later, third dose 5 mo later
Varicella∥,†† and zoster vaccine[38]	Varicella vaccine for seronegative, nonimmunocompromised adults-first dose, followed by second dose 1-2 mo later Zoster vaccine for nonimmunocompromised adults age 60 yr and older-single dose
Hepatitis A∥,‡‡	First dose, followed by second dose 6-12 mo later
Human papillomavirus vaccine	Three doses for girls ages 11-12 yr, with catch-up vaccination for girls and women ages 13-26 yr

*For all adults lacking immunity.

†Adults born in or before 1956 are considered naturally immune; adults born after 1956 should receive one dose of MMR vaccine; some adults, such as college students, persons working in health care facilities, and international travelers, may need two doses.

‡For all adults 65 yr of age and older and for persons with chronic illnesses (all adults 50 yr of age and older, as per updated recommendations for influenza).

§Includes other persons at high risk, such as those with chronic cardiopulmonary disease, chronic metabolic diseases (including diabetes mellitus), chronic renal dysfunction, hemoglobinopathies, and immunosuppression, as well as residents of long-term care facilities, providers of home health care or health care to high-risk persons, and others who wish to avoid influenza.

¶Includes younger individuals with high-risk conditions such as cardiopulmonary disease, diabetes, alcoholism, chronic liver disease, chronic renal failure, or cerebrospinal fluid leaks or immunocompromise because of conditions such as splenic dysfunction or asplenia, Hodgkin's disease, lymphoma, multiple myeloma, nephrotic syndrome, and organ transplantation. Revaccination should be considered for persons at highest risk who have received the 14-valent vaccine or the 23-valent vaccine 6 years or more previously.

∥For all adults in high-risk groups.

**Includes those who are exposed to blood and blood products during their work (e.g., health care workers), clients and staff of institutions for the developmentally disabled, hemodialysis patients, sexually active homosexual or bisexual males, injection drug users, recipients of certain blood products such as factor VIII and IX concentrates, household and sexual contacts of hepatitis B virus (HBV) carriers, sexually active heterosexual individuals with multiple partners or a recent episode of a sexually transmitted disease, inmates of long-term correctional facilities, individuals from high-risk populations (e.g., Pacific Islanders, Alaskan natives, and first-generation immigrants and/or refugees from countries where HBV infection is of high or intermediate endemicity), and international travelers planning prolonged visits to areas with high rates of hepatitis B infection.

††Includes susceptible persons who may be at increased risk of exposure or who have close contact with persons at high risk for serious complications from varicella infection, including health care workers, susceptible family contacts of immunocompromised individuals, teachers of young children, daycare workers, residents and staff in institutional settings, college students, inmates and staff of correctional institutions, military personnel, nonpregnant women of childbearing age, and international travelers.

‡‡Includes persons traveling to or working in countries with high rates of hepatitis A virus (HAV) infection, persons who live in communities with high rates of HAV infection (e.g., Native Americans, Alaskan natives, and Pacific Islanders), homosexual and bisexual males, injection drug users, persons with chronic liver disease, and food handlers (optional.)

Used with permission from Gershon AA, Gardner P, Peter G, et al: Quality standards for immunization. Clin Infect Dis 1997;25:782-786. Copyrighted 1997, University of Chicago.

in the states of the former Soviet Union, prompting concerns about the possibility of transmission to other populations with waning immunity, such as older adults in the United States. The tetanus-diphtheria toxoid vaccine (Td) is composed of bacterial toxins rendered inactive by chemical treatment. It is safe and efficacious and is currently recommended to be administered as a booster every 10 years, or earlier if a tetanus-prone wound occurs.[19] Some experts have questioned the need for a booster every 10 years, instead recommending a single booster dose at midlife for persons who previously received a full primary immunization series.[7] For individuals not previously immunized, a three-dose primary series should be administered (see Table 1).

In recognition of the underreported burden of pertussis in adults, a new vaccine—tetanus toxoid, reduced diphtheria toxoid, and acellular pertussis vaccine (Tdap)—was licensed in 2005 in the United States for those ages 11 to 64 years. In 2006, the ACIP recommended that adults ages 19 to 64 should receive a single dose of Tdap in place of a Td booster if their last dose of Td was 10 years previously or earlier. Tdap can also be given even if the Td dose was more recent if protection against pertussis is desired. This is particularly important for health care workers and those expected to have close contact with an infant younger than 12 months.[19]

Meningococcal Vaccine

Meningococcal vaccine is a polysaccharide vaccine that covers serogroups A, C, Y, and W-135, but not B. This vaccine is not required for all adults. Recent recommendations from the American College Health Association and the ACIP[20] have encouraged physicians to inform incoming college freshmen about the vaccine. The risk for meningococcal disease is higher among college freshmen than in other college students.

Arguments for and against routinely vaccinating college-bound freshmen have been summarized by Gordon[36]; these include the devastating nature of the illness, safety and efficacy of the vaccine, higher risk among college freshmen, experience with vaccination of military recruits, and the fact that the serogroup distribution in the United States is moving toward those serotypes covered by the vaccine. Arguments against routine vaccination of freshmen include the cost of the vaccine ($54-$88/person) for 2 million incoming freshmen and 500,000 freshmen already living in dormitories, the lack of protection against serogroup B, decline of antibody levels over 2 to 3 years, and only 5% of all cases occurring in college students.[36] At present, counseling and offering the vaccine to interested incoming and current freshmen are recommended, but administration of the vaccine is not required.[20]

Influenza Vaccine

There are fewer cost-effective, efficacious medical interventions subject to more mythology than the influenza vaccine. Barriers to immunization include patient concerns about potential adverse effects or induction of illness, or both. Sadly, these concerns are reinforced by some clinicians. In actuality, the trivalent influenza vaccine is extremely safe and effective. It is an inactivated vaccine, not a live vaccine, and therefore cannot transmit infection. Since the swine flu vaccine of 1976, no vaccine preparations have been associated with a significantly increased risk of Guillain-Barré syndrome.[33] The trivalent influenza vaccine is composed of two strains of influenza A and one strain of influenza B, which are the strains predicted to be circulating during the upcoming influenza season. Because these strains vary from year to year, annual immunization is recommended. Allergic hypersensitivity to egg proteins is a contraindication.

Influenza accounts for approximately 20,000 deaths and 200,000 hospitalizations each year, and is also responsible for many days of work lost and many visits to health care providers.[33] About 10% of adults develop influenza each year.[33] The burden of illness is most significant in older adults, in whom mortality can result from postinfluenza bacterial pneumonia and exacerbations of cardiopulmonary conditions.[33] The efficacy of influenza vaccine has been estimated to be 70% to 90% in healthy persons[23] and, although lower in older adults, it still has significant benefit in the prevention of overall mortality.[23] Although past recommendations focused on those 65 years of age and older, and younger individuals with chronic medical conditions, the most recent ACIP recommendations target persons 50 years of age and older, because it has been noted that age-based recommendations result in higher immunization rates than risk-based recommendations. Immunization continues to be recommended for persons younger than 50 years who are residents of nursing homes or other chronic care facilities or who have chronic cardiac or pulmonary conditions or chronic metabolic disease, including diabetes, renal dysfunction, hemoglobinopathies, or immunosuppression. In addition, women who will be in the second or third trimester of pregnancy during the influenza season, and children and adolescents receiving long-term aspirin who are at risk for Reye's syndrome, are among those for whom vaccination is recommended.[23]

A live, attenuated, trivalent intranasal vaccine for influenza has also been licensed for healthy individuals ages 5 to 49 years. This vaccine is not recommended for those who are immunocompromised.

Strategies for increasing immunization rates are of paramount importance[6] (see later). The importance of immunization of health care workers cannot be overemphasized. Immunosuppressed patients such as transplant recipients may not develop adequate antibody titers after immunization, and are at risk for nosocomial transmission of influenza when hospitalized during the influenza season, as well as for community-acquired infection. Therefore, immunization of health care workers and family members can be an effective means of augmenting the protection of immunocompromised patients.

Varicella Vaccine and Zoster Vaccine

The varicella vaccine is a live, attenuated vaccine that provides long-lasting immunity. Although most adults are seropositive from prior infection, seronegative adults are susceptible to varicella primary infection, which is often more severe in adults than in healthy children. Current recommendations are to immunize susceptible adults (not immunocompromised adults), with priority given to those at increased risk of exposure or those who could expose persons at risk for serious complications of varicella. These groups include seronegative health care workers, family members of immunocompromised patients, teachers and child care workers, residents and staff of long-term care facilities or prisons, college students, military personnel, nonpregnant women of childbearing age, adolescents and adults in households with children, and international travelers.[10,16] Because the varicella vaccine is a live vaccine, it is not administered to immunocompromised patients. Although the fraction of those vaccinated who develop a rash after vaccination could theoretically transmit the vaccine strain of the virus to household contacts, such transmission is considered to be unlikely and the disease would most likely be mild. In addition, the risk of exposing an immunocompromised family member to actual varicella is much more serious, so administration of the varicella vaccine to seronegative household contacts of immunocompromised patients is encouraged rather than contraindicated.[12]

Postexposure prophylaxis with varicella-zoster immune globulin (VZIg) is not recommended routinely for all susceptible adults exposed to varicella, but is indicated for immunocompromised or pregnant seronegative patients. VZIg should be given within 96 hours for maximum effectiveness.[13,16] Some clinicians also administer antiviral therapy to exposed seronegative immunocompromised patients.

Herpes zoster (shingles) is caused by re-activation of the varicella virus. In addition to the pain of the acute zoster episode, post-herpetic neuralgia is a major cause of chronic pain, particularly in older adults. A live attenuated vaccine for shingles prevention has been licensed on the basis of a placebo-controlled trial of over 38,000 adults, in whom zoster vaccine was associated with a reduction in zoster from 11.1 to 5.4 cases per 1000 person-years.[37] The ACIP has provisionally recommended a single dose of zoster vaccine for administration to adults 60 years of age and older, whether or not they have had a prior zoster episode.[38] The vaccine is contraindicated for immunocompromised and pregnant patients, and those on immunosuppressive medications or with active tuberculosis.

Measles-Mumps-Rubella Vaccine

The measles-mumps-rubella (MMR) vaccine is a live vaccine that prevents potentially serious diseases, including congenital rubella syndrome. A measles outbreak between 1989 and 1991 in under-vaccinated inner city residents was a reminder that these diseases remain a threat and reinforced the need to maintain high immunization levels in the general population. Persons born before 1956 are considered to have natural immunity to these infections. Traditionally, a single dose of MMR vaccine was given, but more recent childhood recommendations are for two doses, one at 12 to 15 months and the second at 4 to 6 years or 11 to 12 years, because immunity can wane after a single dose. For adults born after 1956 who are not immune, a single dose of MMR should be administered, but high-risk groups such as college students, health care workers, and international travelers should receive two doses.[10] Because MMR is a live vaccine, it is not generally administered to immunocompromised patients, with the exception of HIV patients with early disease[27] and stable bone marrow transplant (BMT) recipients 2 years or more after transplantation without graft-versus-host disease.[28]

Hepatitis A Vaccine

There are currently two formulations of hepatitis A vaccine, which are inactivated, safe, and immunogenic. Administration of a two-dose series is recommended for adults in high-risk groups, which include international travelers, residents of communities with high rates of infection (Native Americans, Alaskan natives, and Pacific Islanders), homosexual and bisexual men, injection drug users, persons with chronic liver disease, and food handlers.[10] Persons with chronic liver disease appear to be particularly susceptible to fulminant disease when they develop hepatitis A infection and should be high-priority candidates for vaccination.[39]

Hepatitis B Vaccine

Two formulations of recombinant hepatitis B vaccine are available in the United States. Recently, the ACIP released a comprehensive strategy to prevent transmission of hepatitis B virus (HBV) in the United States.[26] A strategy of vaccinating high-risk groups was devised originally, but current recommendations are for universal infant vaccination and catch-up vaccination of nonimmune older children and adolescents. For adults, high-risk groups should be the top priority for vaccination, with a three-dose series. These groups include health care workers and others who may be exposed to blood and blood products, residents and staff of long-term care facilities or prisons, homosexual or bisexual men or heterosexuals with multiple partners, injection drug users, recipients of clotting factor concentrates, household or sexual contacts of HBV carriers, and persons from high-risk populations (Pacific Islanders, Alaskan natives, and immigrants from countries of high endemicity).[10] International travelers planning lengthy stays in endemic areas should be vaccinated.

Human Papillomavirus Vaccine

Human papillomavirus (HPV) is the cause of anogenital warts and is associated with cervical cancer in women and other anogenital cancers in men and women. It has been estimated that 6,200,000 new cases of HPV infection occur every year in the United States.[40]

The HPV vaccine was recently licensed for girls and young women ages 9 to 26 years, with recommended immunization at age 11 to 12 years using a three-dose series, and catch-up vaccination for girls and women 13 to 26 years who have not yet received it. The ideal time to vaccinate is before the onset of sexual activity, but women who have been infected with one type of HPV may benefit from prevention of infection with the other types included in the vaccine. The components are antigenic materials related to HPV types 6, 11, 16, and 18. Types 6 and 11 are responsible for 90% of anogenital warts, whereas types 16 and 18 are associated with cervical cancer. The vaccine is not live and can be given to immunocompromised patients, although its efficacy in those who are immunocompromised is unknown.

POTENTIAL AGENTS OF BIOTERRORISM: ANTHRAX, SMALLPOX, AND PLAGUE

With the events of the past few years, attention has been focused on the possibility of deliberately induced larger outbreaks of infectious diseases. Vaccines exist for some of the pathogens mentioned as possible agents of bioterrorism, including anthrax, smallpox, and plague (*Yersinia pestis*). The Working Group on Civilian Biodefense has published recommendations for the management of anthrax[41] and smallpox[42] as public health threats, and updated information on all topics related to bioterrorism can be found on the CDC website.[43] The anthrax vaccine is a cell-free inactivated vaccine given in a six-dose series, and is currently available in the United States only for military personnel or certain high-risk persons, such as laboratory workers working directly with *Bacillus anthracis*.[13] Currently, efforts to manufacture much larger numbers of doses of vaccine are underway. The safety of the vaccine remains a controversial issue. The CDC website[43] has up-to-date information on the indications for and safety of anthrax vaccine.

Smallpox was the first disease for which vaccination was found to be effective. It now has been certified as eradicated, with the last naturally acquired case in the world having occurred in 1977. However, the specter of smallpox has again been raised with the threat of bioterrorism. The current vaccine for smallpox is derived from vaccinia virus, which is a live attenuated viral vaccine, of which supplies are currently limited and not available for the general public.[13] During the era when smallpox vaccination was universal, adverse reactions to the vaccine were not uncommon, including neurologic effects, and inadvertent vaccination of immunocompromised patients sometimes resulted in severe progressive or disseminated vaccinia infection.[44] Current efforts are focused on dramatically increasing the production of smallpox vaccine and the development of measures to render the vaccine safer.

An inactivated whole cell bacterial vaccine is available for the prevention of bubonic plague, but may not be effective against pneumonic plague.[13] It is currently recommended only for persons at high risk, such as laboratory workers working with the organism.

OTHER VACCINES

Bacillus Calmette-Guérin (BCG) vaccination is not routinely recommended in the United States for the prevention of tuberculosis, although it is administered to children in many other countries in which the prevalence of tuberculosis is higher. BCG is a live attenuated vaccine that should *not* be administered to immunocompromised persons, including those with HIV. The efficacy of BCG vaccine for prevention in adults has varied in different studies, and currently is recommended in the United States only for the following: infants and children who live where the likelihood of TB transmission is high; and health care workers highly likely to be exposed to multidrug-resistant TB (MDR-TB) in settings where other TB prevention measures have failed. If the incidence of MDR-TB rises, these indications could be expanded in future.[25]

There are currently three rabies vaccines licensed in the United States; the human diploid cell vaccine (HDCV) is most commonly used. It is indicated for pre- and postexposure prophylaxis in conjunction with rabies immune globulin (RIg). Persons at high risk because of potential occupational exposure or travel are candidates for pre-exposure prophylaxis.[13]

Vaccines for international travel are discussed in more detail elsewhere in this section ("Travel Medicine for the Primary Care Physician").

STRATEGIES FOR INCREASING ADULT VACCINATION RATES

Given the morbidity and mortality of vaccine-preventable diseases in adults, and the documented underuse of safe and cost-effective vaccines, it is appropriate that significant attention has been drawn to strategies to increase vaccination rates.[1-6,30-34] Many organizations involved in the development of guidelines for immunization have published or endorsed such measures. Standing orders at hospital discharge or in long-term care facilities have the potential to increase opportunities for vaccination. Within the context of individual clinical practices, patient reminder or recall systems have been found to be effective. More educational materials for clinicians and patients and other interventions are actively promoted by organizations such as the National Coalition for Adult Immunization; details can be found on their website.[30]

CONCLUSION

Adult immunizations are extremely important. Guidelines for immunization standards from national organizations should be implemented and the preventive visit at age 50 should be used to update vaccination status. Interventions such as standing orders at hospital discharge and in long-term care facilities should be pursued. Educational efforts to reduce barriers to vaccination for clinicians and patients should be actively pursued. Changing guidelines for vaccination can be found in the recommendations of the Advisory Committee on Immunization Practice, which are frequently updated. Further information and recommendations for vaccines against agents of bioterrorism will undoubtedly be forthcoming.

Summary

- Vaccine-preventable diseases remain significant causes of morbidity and mortality in the United States.
- There is widespread undervaccination, even of high-risk individuals.
- Recent additions to the list of recommended vaccinations for particular groups of adults include the tetanus-reduced diphtheria-acellular pertussis vaccine, zoster (shingles) vaccine, and human papillomavirus vaccine.
- Physicians and patients should familiarize themselves with currently recommended vaccinations and should use the primary care visit, particularly at age 50, for reassessment of immunization status and administration of needed vaccines.

Suggested Readings

Centers for Disease Control and Prevention: A comprehensive immunization strategy to eliminate transmission of hepatitis B virus infection in the United States. Recommendations of the Advisory Committee on Immunization Practices ACIP): Part II: Immunization of Adults. MMWR Morb Mortal Wkly Rep 2006;55(RR-16):1-25.

Centers for Disease Control and Prevention: Preventing tetanus, diphtheria, and pertussis among adults: Use of tetanus toxoid, reduced diphtheria toxoid and acellular pertussis vaccine recommendations of the Advisory Committee on Immunization Practices and (ACIP), and recommendation of ACIP, supported by the Healthcare Infection Control Practices Advisory Committee (HICPAC), for use of Tdap among health care personnel. MMWR Recomm Rep 2006;55(RR-17):1-37.

Centers for Disease Control and Prevention: Prevention and control of influenza: Recommendations of the Advisory Committee on Immunization Practices (ACIP). MMWR Morb Mortal Wkly Rep 2006;55(RR-10):1-42.

Centers for Disease Control and Prevention: Prevention and control of meningococcal disease: Recommendations of the Advisory Committee on Immunization Practices (ACIP). MMWR Morb Mortal Wkly Rep 2005;54(RR-07):1-21.

Centers for Disease Control and Prevention: Prevention of hepatitis A through active or passive immunization-recommendations of the Advisory Committee on Immunization Practices (ACIP). MMWR Morb Mortal Wkly Rep 2006;55(RR-07):1-23.

Centers for Disease Control and Prevention: Prevention of pneumococcal disease: Recommendations of the Advisory Committee on Immunization Practices (ACIP). MMWR Morb Mortal Wkly Rep 1997;46(RR-8):1-24.

Centers for Disease Control and Prevention: Prevention of varicella: Updated recommendations of the Advisory Committee on Immunization Practices (ACIP). MMWR Morb Mortal Wkly Rep 1999;48(RR-06):1-5.

Centers for Disease Control and Prevention: Quadrivalent human papillomavirus vaccine. Recommendations of the Advisory Committee on Immunization Practices (ACIP). MMWR Morb Mortal Wkly Rep 2007;56(RR-02):1-24.

Gardner P, Eickhoff T, Poland GA, et al: Adult immunizations. Ann Intern Med 1996;124:35-40.

Gordon SM: Should all college-bound freshmen receive meningococcal vaccine? Cleve Clin J Med 2001;68:9-10.

References

For a complete list of references, log onto www.expertconsult.com.

Adolescent Immunization

Camille Sabella

The success of the immunization program in the United States is exemplified by the fact that all vaccine-preventable diseases have been reduced by at least 95% as compared with baseline pre-vaccine morbidity. This success has been the result of the effectiveness of vaccination programs aimed at infants and children. It has become clear, however, that childhood vaccination alone does not provide sufficient protection against all vaccine-preventable diseases. Although adolescent immunizations have been recommended since 1996, an estimated 35 million adolescents in this country still lack one or more recommended vaccinations, leaving them at risk for vaccine-preventable diseases such as measles, mumps, tetanus, hepatitis B, and varicella.

Vaccine coverage in adolescents is inadequate because in general they have less contact with physicians than younger children, many lack access to health care, and opportunities to vaccinate are missed by the provider. In addition, because adolescence is a time for exploration and experimentation, adolescents engage in high-risk activities that increase their risk for various infectious diseases, such as hepatitis B and human papillomavirus (HPV).

Two important infections (*Neisseria meningitidis* and pertussis), for which effective vaccination now is available, are especially prevalent in the adolescent years, making the adolescent age group the ideal target age for prevention. In addition, a safe and effective vaccine against HPV will soon be available and will be recommended for the adolescent age group. Similarly, a vaccine against herpes simplex type 2 is currently being evaluated and, if proven safe and effective, will likely be targeted to protect adolescents.

Recommendations regarding childhood and adolescent immunization schedules are developed collaboratively by the Advisory Committee on Immunization Practices (ACIP) of the Public Health Service, the American Academy of Pediatrics Committee on Infectious Diseases (the Red Book Committee), and the American Academy of Family Practice. A continuously updated version of the harmonized schedule is available at http://www.cdc.gov/vaccines/recs/schedules/default.htm. This chapter will review the most recent immunization recommendations for adolescents.

RECOMMENDED IMMUNIZATIONS

With the exception of conjugate meningococcal vaccine (MCV4) and the adolescent preparation of tetanus and diphtheria toxoids and acellular pertussis vaccine (Tdap), which are primarily recommended for adolescents, the adolescent years serve as a time that warrants special effort to administer those vaccines not previously administered (catch-up vaccination).

Hepatitis B

Hepatitis B vaccines in the United States are produced by recombinant DNA technology and are highly effective and safe. The strategy for prevention of hepatitis B relies on the universal vaccination of neonates and infants, so that the immunization series is complete by 18 months of age. Despite the fact that adolescents are at higher risk of infection, this strategy was chosen because neonates and infants are more likely to receive medical care. Since implementation of this strategy in 1992, the incidence of hepatitis B has dropped markedly. Nevertheless, adolescents who were born before universal immunization or who have not received the three-dose hepatitis B series remain at risk, especially those who have one or more risk factors for hepatitis B infection (Box 1). Thus, routine immunization of adolescents who previously have not been immunized is recommended. A three-dose series is recommended; there is no need to restart the series for those who received one or two doses in the past. Because immune memory remains intact for 15 years or longer, a booster dose is not recommended for adolescents who have completed the three-dose series.

Measles-Mumps-Rubella (MMR)

Of children immunized with measles-mumps-rubella (MMR) vaccine at 12 to 15 months of age, 95% to 98% develop protective and durable, probably lifelong, antibodies against measles, mumps, and rubella. A second dose is recommended to protect the approximately 5% of vaccine recipients who do not respond to the first dose, and is usually given between 3 and 6 years of age. This second dose does not serve as a booster dose; rather, it is recommended to protect against primary vaccine failure, ensuring high levels of protection and thus preventing outbreaks of infection. More than 99% of patients who receive two doses of MMR vaccine separated by at least 1 month, with the first dose administered on or after the first birthday, develop immunity to measles. Thus, the status of immunization against measles, mumps, and rubella should be addressed in every adolescent to ensure that they have received two doses of MMR vaccine.

Measles and mumps both occur in highly immunized populations. In recent years, periodic outbreaks of measles among high school and college students and, more recently, an outbreak of mumps in the Midwestern United States, have served to underscore the importance of ensuring that all adolescents have received two doses of this vaccine.[1] Although postnatal rubella is a mild disease characterized by low-grade fever, generalized lymphadenopathy, and a discrete maculopapular rash, congenital rubella syndrome is a devastating disease, characterized by a high rate of congenital anomalies and long-term neurodevelopmental problems. Thus, emphasis must be placed on ensuring that postpubertal patients are immunized against rubella. This entails immunizing postpubertal women who do not have documentation of rubella immunity unless they are known to be pregnant, assessing postpubertal women for rubella susceptibility during health care encounters, and routine prenatal screening for rubella immunity.

Because MMR is a live virus vaccine, it should not be given to pregnant women or to those who have altered immunity. Adverse effects of vaccination occurring mostly in susceptible children include rash, fever, and lymphadenopathy. Adverse reactions seen more commonly among postpubertal female vaccinees include arthralgias (25%) and transient arthritis (10%) following vaccination.

Varicella

Varicella vaccine was introduced in 1995 and is recommended for all children between 12 and 18 months of age. Children who are not vaccinated early in life may be vaccinated at any time, but preferably before their 13th birthday. This is because before the age of 13 years, only one dose of vaccine is needed, whereas two doses of vaccine are recommended for adolescents 13 years of age and older and adults. In addition, vaccination before age 13 years is strongly advisable, because varicella in adolescents and adults is associated with a higher risk of serious illness and complications.

Thus, susceptible children up to 13 years of age should receive one dose of vaccine, whereas susceptible adolescents 13 years of age and older should receive two doses 4 to 8 weeks apart. Individuals

Box 1 Adolescents at High Risk for Hepatitis B Infection

Those who engage in injection drug use
Sexually active heterosexuals with more than one partner during previous 6 months or who have had a sexually transmitted disease
Men who have sex with men
Household contacts and sexual partners of people with chronic hepatitis B infection
Those at occupational risk of exposure to blood or blood-contaminated body fluid
Those undergoing hemodialysis
Members of household with adoptees who are chronic carriers of hepatitis B
Inmates of juvenile detention and other correctional facilities
Adolescents with bleeding disorders who receive clotting factor concentrates
Those who are long-term international travelers to areas where hepatitis B infection is endemic

who have a reliable history of varicella can be assumed to be immune and do not need to be immunized. Although it may be cost-effective to perform serologic testing of adolescents and adults and only vaccinate those who are seronegative, the American Academy of Pediatrics recommends that adolescents who lack a reliable history of varicella should be considered susceptible and immunized without serologic testing. This recommendation takes into account that the vaccine is well tolerated, even in immune persons, and that universal immunization of this age group is easier to implement than serologic testing and tracking of seronegative patients.

Since the introduction of the varicella vaccine and the implementation of universal immunization for all children, the incidence of varicella and its related complications and hospitalizations has dramatically declined.[2] Because less virus is now circulating in the community, nonvaccinated children and adolescents are less likely to become infected and will be susceptible into their adult years. Because it is possible that many adolescents today were not vaccinated since the vaccine was introduced in 1995, it is especially important to target this age group to ensure that they are immune or have been vaccinated.

Because varicella vaccine is a live attenuated vaccine, it should not be administered routinely to adolescents with altered immunity, including T lymphocyte immunodeficiency and those receiving corticosteroid therapy (≥20 mg/day of prednisone), or during pregnancy.

Hepatitis A

Hepatitis A vaccine is indicated for adolescents who are at increased risk of acquiring hepatitis A or at increased risk of severe disease from hepatitis A infection. This includes adolescents who travel internationally to areas where hepatitis A is endemic, male adolescents who have sex with men, those who use illegal drugs, and those with clotting factor disorders. In addition, adolescents with chronic liver disease should be vaccinated because they are at increased risk of fulminant infection if they become infected.

Hepatitis A vaccine has been shown to be safe and has a protective efficacy of more than 95%. Adolescents can be immunized at any age and should receive a two-dose schedule of the pediatric-adolescent formulation, with the booster dose given at least 6 months after the first dose. An adult formulation is available for those 19 years of age and older.

Influenza

Annual influenza vaccination, administered during the autumn, is recommended for adolescents with risk-factors for severe infection (Box 2). Adolescents who have contact with high-risk persons, including children younger than 5 years, should also be immunized.

Box 2 High-Risk Conditions for Severe Influenza Infection

Asthma and other chronic pulmonary diseases
Hemodynamically significant cardiac disease
Immunosuppressive disorders or therapy
Hemoglobinopathies
Diseases requiring long-term salicylate therapy, such as Kawasaki disease or rheumatoid arthritis
Chronic renal dysfunction
Chronic metabolic disorders such as diabetes mellitus

Immunization is also recommended for pregnant adolescents, which benefits the unborn infant by the transmission of transplacentally acquired antibody. Finally, influenza vaccination should be considered for adolescents whose close contact with others facilitates rapid transmission, which may result in disruption of routine activities (e.g., those who reside in dormitories or are members of athletic teams).

One dose of inactivated influenza virus vaccine, given annually in the autumn, is recommended for adolescents at risk for severe influenza infection. A cold-adapted, trivalent, live attenuated influenza vaccine administered intranasally is also available but should be given only to healthy, nonpregnant patients 5 to 49 years of age who do not have contact with severely immunocompromised persons.

Meningococcal Disease

Although the annual incidence of invasive meningococcal disease in the United States is relatively low (0.5-1.1/100,000 population), case-fatality rates approach 10% to 14% and sequelae such as neurologic disabilities, limb or digit amputation, and skin scarring in survivors are significant. Invasive meningococcal disease can manifest as meningococcemia, with relatively high mortality and morbidity rates, or as meningitis, with a lower mortality rate but a significant risk of hearing loss and long-term neurologic sequelae. Because of the success of conjugate vaccines against *Haemophilus influenzae* type b and *Streptococcus pneumoniae*, *Neisseria meningitidis* has become the leading cause of bacterial meningitis in children.

The incidence of invasive meningococcal disease in pediatric patients has two peaks. The highest incidence is in infants younger than 12 months. A second peak occurs between 15 and 18 years of age (Fig. 1).[3] The overall rate of invasive disease among adolescents 11 to 19 years of age is 1.2 per 100,000, which is higher than that for the general population, but the case-fatality rate in adolescents is 20%, the highest of any age group. This is likely because adolescents 15 years of age or older are more likely to develop meningococcemia without meningitis and to have shock at presentation.

In the United States, most cases of invasive meningococcal disease (98%) are sporadic, but the frequency of localized outbreaks, especially in schools, has been increasing over the past decade. Serogroups B, C, and Y are the major causes of meningococcal disease in this country, with each responsible for approximately one third of cases. However, the proportion of these serogroups causing disease at different age groups differs. Whereas serogroup B accounts for over 50% of cases of meningococcal diseases in infants, it accounts for less than 25% of cases in adolescents 11 to 18 years of age. Thus, serogroups A, C, Y, and W-135, for which a licensed and available vaccine exists, are responsible for 75% of cases of invasive meningococcal disease in the adolescent age group. The incidence of invasive meningococcal disease caused by these vaccine-preventable serotypes begins to increase substantially at 15 years and peaks at 18 years of age (see Fig. 1).

U.S. surveillance data from the 1998-1999 school year have revealed the incidence of meningococcal disease in college students. Although the incidence of meningococcal disease is lower in all college students than in nonstudents, the rate of disease in freshmen students living in dormitories is significantly higher than in any other subgroup of 18- to 23-year-olds (Table 1).[4]

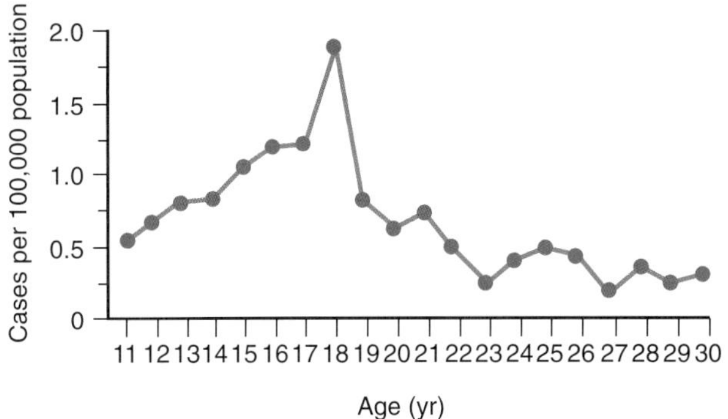

Figure 1 **Rates of meningococcal disease in 11- to 30-year-olds in the United States, 1991-2002.** *(Data from Centers for Disease Control: Active bacterial core surveillance. MMWR Morb Mortal Wkly Rep 2005;54(RR-07);1-21.)*

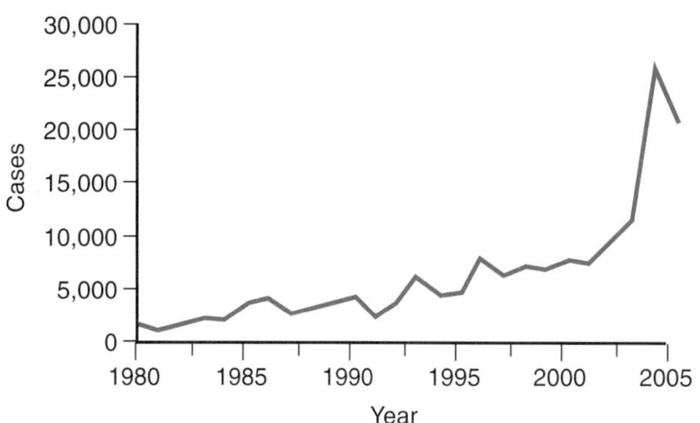

Figure 2 **Pertussis, United States, 1980-2005.** *(Data from Centers for Disease Control and Prevention: Epidemiology and prevention of vaccine-preventable diseases. U.S. Department of Health and Human Services, January 2006.)*

Table 1 Rates of Meningococcal Disease in U.S. College Students, September 1998-August 1999

Population	Rate/100,000
18- to 23-yr-old	1.4
18- to 23-yr-old, nonstudents	1.4
All college students	0.6
Undergraduates	0.7
Freshmen	1.9
Dormitory residents	2.3
Freshmen living in dormitories	5.1

Data from Bruce MG, Rosenstein NE, Capparelle JM, et al: Risk factors for meningococcal disease in college students. JAMA 2001;286:688-693.

Two vaccines are currently licensed for the prevention of meningococcal disease. Meningococcal polysaccharide vaccine (MPSV4) was licensed in 1981 for use in persons 2 years of age and older. This vaccine has never been recommended for routine use, but rather for those individuals who are at increased risk for meningococcal disease. MCV4 was licensed in 2005 for use in persons 11 to 55 years of age. Both vaccines provide protection against serogroups A, C, Y, and W-135. A vaccine that protects against serogroup B meningococcus has not yet been developed. The effects of conjugating the polysaccharide to a protein carrier allows induction of a T cell-dependent response, which in turn results in an improved primary response to the polysaccharide as well as a strong booster response on re-exposure. In addition, experience with previous conjugate vaccines has revealed that the use of these vaccines results in reduction of nasopharyngeal carriage of the organism, thus protecting nonimmunized individuals through a herd immunity effect. It is also expected that the conjugate vaccine will provide longer lasting immunity. Therefore, the conjugate vaccine offers advantages over the polysaccharide vaccine and is preferred for those aged 11 to 55 years.

Given the epidemiology of meningococcal disease in adolescents, and the availability of a safe and effective conjugate meningococcal vaccine, adolescents should be routinely immunized with MCV4. The vaccine should be administered routinely at the 11- to 12-year preadolescent visit. Those who have not been previously vaccinated with MCV4 should be immunized at high school entry or 15 years of age, whichever comes first. Other adolescents at increased risk for meningococcal disease should also be routinely immunized. This includes college freshmen living in dormitories; patients with a terminal complement deficiency, anatomic or functional asplenia; and person who travel to or reside in countries in which *N. meningitidis* is hyperendemic or epidemic. For adolescents previously immunized with MPSV4, re-immunization with MCV4 should be considered 3 to 5 years after receiving MPSV4 if they remain at risk for meningococcal disease.

Prelicensure safety studies have shown that MCV4 has rates of systemic and local adverse reactions similar to MPSV4. Since the licensure of MCV4, eight cases of Guillain-Barré syndrome (GBS) occurring within 6 weeks after vaccination have been reported, raising suspicion of a possible association between the vaccine and GBS. However, investigation by the Centers for Disease Control and Prevention to date indicate that even with these reported cases, the incidence of GBS remains similar to the expected incidence. Thus, a causal relation between MCV4 and GBS cannot be proved or disproved at this time, and close monitoring is ongoing. The CDC continues to recommend the use of MCV4 for those for whom the vaccine is indicated.[5]

Pertussis

Before the availability of whole-cell pertussis vaccines in the late 1940s, pertussis was a major cause of morbidity and mortality in the United States, accounting for almost 300,000 cases and 10,000 deaths annually. Following introduction of an effective vaccine, a dramatic decrease in cases ensued and, by the early 1970s, the incidence had declined by 99% as compared with that in the prevaccine era, with a record low number of 1010 cases reported in 1976. Since the early 1980s, however, the incidence of pertussis in this country has steadily increased (Fig. 2).[6] Although the disease is endemic, epidemic peaks occur every 3 to 5 years, and several large outbreaks in North America have been reported in the past several years. These outbreaks have occurred in highly immunized populations and in infants who had not completed their primary immunization series.

Over the past several decades, the age distribution of pertussis has changed dramatically. In the prevaccine era, the peak incidence of disease occurred in children ages 1 to 5 years. With widespread vaccination, and by the late 1980s, infants younger than 1 year had the highest age-specific incidence, which declined with increasing age. Since the early 1990s, however, there has been a dramatic increase in reported cases in children ages 10 years and older. Data from the National Notifiable Diseases Surveillance System between 2001 and 2003 have revealed that children ages 10 to 19 years comprised 33% of all reported cases, whereas 23% of cases occurred in persons 20 years and older.[7] During the same time period, infants younger than 1 year accounted for 23% of all cases. Infants younger than 1 year of age, however, continue to have the highest average annual incidence (55.2/100,000 population), as compared with 7.7 per 100,000 for persons ages 10 to 19 years and 1.1 per 100,000 for adults. The overall number of cases of pertussis, however, is likely underestimated, because the infection is often underdiagnosed in adolescents and adults.

Although chronic carriage of the organism does not occur, it is clear that subclinical or mild illness commonly occurs in fully or partially immunized, as well as naturally immune, persons. This occurs because immunity wanes within 3 to 5 years of vaccination or natural infection and is often undetectable at 12 years. Thus, neither vaccination nor natural disease provides long-lasting immunity, and U.S. adults do not have adequate protection against pertussis. Importantly, adults and adolescents with pertussis serve as important reservoirs for infection and are often the index cases for younger infants and children. An example of this occurred during an outbreak of pertussis in Chicago in 1993, during which mothers served as an important source of pertussis for their infants.

Many studies have proven that pertussis is a common cause of prolonged cough in adolescents and adults, accounting for 12% to 32% of cases of cough lasting 2 weeks or longer. A prospective U.S. population-based study with active surveillance has revealed that 13% of study participants between the ages of 10 and 49 years who presented to their community clinic with an acute paroxysmal cough or a persistent cough illness longer than 2 weeks' duration have evidence of an acute pertussis infection. A Canadian study,[8] the largest prospective study examining the rates of pertussis disease in adolescents and adults, has demonstrated that 20% of 442 adolescents and adults with cough illness lasting 7 to 56 days had pertussis.

Universal immunization with pertussis vaccines for children younger than 7 years is recommended by the American Academy of Pediatrics and is the mainstay of prevention. Vaccination of all children starting in infancy has resulted in more than a 97% decrease in the incidence of pertussis in the United States as compared with the prevaccine era. The currently available acellular vaccines, which are purified subunit vaccines combined with diphtheria and tetanus toxoids (DTaP), have been shown to be 75% to 90% effective and are well tolerated.

Despite the successes of universal immunization, there continues to be a steady increase in reported cases of pertussis in this country, with resultant significant morbidity and mortality. This appears to occur because of waning immunity after vaccination and natural infection, underdiagnosis of mild disease, and infants who have not completed their primary immunization series, who remain susceptible to infection.

Because of the role that adolescents and adults play in the transmission of pertussis, much interest has been generated in studies evaluating the efficacy and safety of pertussis vaccination in these age groups. Traditionally, pertussis vaccine have not been recommended for persons 7 year of age and older, relating to past concerns about the safety of the previously used whole-cell vaccines in this age group. However, with the advent of the less reactogenic acellular vaccines over the last decade, there has been great interest in studying these vaccines in adolescents and adults. Adverse reactions to these vaccines in adolescents and adults have been mild, with local swelling and redness as the most commonly reported events. A National Institutes of Health–sponsored prospective multicenter trial,[9] in which 2781 healthy subjects ages 15 to 65 years were randomized to receive acellular pertussis vaccine or hepatitis A vaccine, found that the acellular pertussis vaccine is safe, immunogenic, and effective in preventing clinical pertussis.

Given the immunogenicity and safety of these vaccines in adolescents and adults, adolescents ages 11 to 18 years should receive acellular pertussis vaccine combined with tetanus and reduced diphtheria toxoid, Tdap (Box 3).[6]

Box 3 Recommendations for the Use of Tetanus and Diphtheria Toxoids and Acellular Pertussis (Tdap) Vaccines in Adolescents

Single dose of Tdap instead of tetanus and diphtheria toxoids (Td) vaccine is recommended for booster immunization for adolescents 11-18 years of age.

Preferred age for Tdap immunization is 11-12 years.

Adolescents 11-18 yr of age who have received Td but not Tdap are encouraged to receive a single dose of Tdap. An interval of at least 5 years between Td and Tdap is suggested, but intervals shorter than 5 years are acceptable, particularly in settings of increased risk of acquiring pertussis, having complicated disease, or transmitting infection to vulnerable contacts.

Administer Tdap and conjugate meningococcal vaccine (MCV4) during the same visit if both vaccines are indicated.

FUTURE VACCINES

Human Papillomavirus

HPV infection is the cause of anogenital warts and most cancers of the anogenital tract. It is estimated that over 6 million new infections occur every year in the United States, and that 20 million persons are infected. Epidemiologic data have shown that the highest rate of HPV infection occurs in adolescents and young adults, placing women at risk of developing cervical cancer later in life.[10] HPV types 16 and 18 are responsible for approximately 70% of cases of cervical cancers and types 6 and 11 are responsible for more than 90% of anogenital warts. Two prophylactic HPV-type specific vaccines have been developed that appear to be efficacious and well-tolerated-a quadrivalent vaccine targeting high-risk cervical cancer types 16 and 18, as well as the genital wart-associated types 6 and 11, and a bivalent vaccine targeting high-risk cervical cancer types 16 and 18. A vaccine against HPV infection represents the second vaccine aimed at preventing cancer (after hepatitis B) and would likely have an enormous public health impact. Because most women acquire HPV soon after becoming sexually active, these vaccines are targeted at preadolescent or adolescent girls before the onset of sexual activity. Recommendations regarding the clinical use of HPV vaccines are forthcoming.

Herpes Simplex Type 2

Twenty percent to 30% of persons in the United States are infected with herpes simplex virus type 2 (HSV-2) and most are asymptomatic. Although persons with symptomatic HSV-2 infection can suffer significant morbidity, asymptomatic persons infected with HSV-2 can transmit the virus. The most feared complication of HSV-2 infection is neonatal infection, which most commonly occurs from an infected maternal genital tract at the time of delivery and is associated with high rates of mortality and morbidity. Clinical trials are under way to evaluate a candidate HSV-2 glycoprotein vaccine. If such a vaccine is found to be safe and effective, the adolescent and preadolescent age groups would likely be targeted for prevention.

Summary

- The adolescent years serve as a time that warrants special effort to administer routinely recommended vaccines not previously administered, such as hepatitis B, hepatitis A, varicella, and measles-mumps-rubella vaccines.
- Given the increased incidence and case-fatality rate of meningococcal disease in the adolescent age group, adolescents should be routinely immunized with conjugate meningococcal vaccine.
- Pertussis is common among adults and adolescents; these individuals serve as important reservoirs for infection and are often the index cases for younger infants and children.
- Adolescents ages 11 to 18 years should be routinely vaccinated with acellular pertussis vaccine combined with tetanus and reduced diphtheria toxoid (Tdap).

Suggested Readings

Bruce MG, Rosenstein NE, Capparelle JM, et al: Risk factors for meningococcal disease in college students. JAMA 2001;286:688-693.

Centers for Disease Control and Prevention: Notice to readers: Update recommendations of the advisory committee on immunization practices (ACIP) for the control and elimination of mumps. MMWR Morb Mortal Wkly Rep 2006;55:629-630.

Centers for Disease Control and Prevention: Pertussis, 2001-2003. MMWR Morb Mortal Wkly Rep 2005;54:1283-1286.

Centers for Disease Control and Prevention: Preventing tetanus, diphtheria, and pertussis among adolescents: Use of tetanus toxoid, reduced diphtheria toxoid and acellular pertussis vaccines. MMWR Morb Mortal Wkly Rep 2006:55(RR-03):1-34.

Centers for Disease Control and Prevention: Prevention and control of meningococcal disease. MMWR Morb Mortal Wkly Rep 2005;54(RR-07):1-21.

Centers for Disease Control and Prevention: Update: Guillain-Barré syndrome among recipients of Menactra meningococcal conjugate vaccine-United States, October 2005-February 2006. MMWR Morb Mortal Wkly Rep 2006:55:364-366.

Kulasingam SL, Hughes JP, Kiviat NB, et al: Evaluation of human papillomavirus testing in primary screening for cervical abnormalities: Comparison of sensitivity, specificity, and frequency of referral. JAMA 2002;288:1749-1757.

Senzilet LD, Halperin SA, Spika JS, et al: Pertussis is a frequent cause of prolonged cough illness in adults and adolescents. Clin Infect Dis 2001;32:1691-1697.

Strebel P, Nordin J, Edwards K, et al: Population-based incidence of pertussis among adolescents and adults, Minnesota, 1995-1996. J Infect Dis 2001;183:1353-1359.

Ward JI, Cherry JD, Chang SJ, et al: Efficacy of an acellular pertussis vaccine among adolescents and adults. N Engl J Med 2005;353:1555-1563.

Zhou F, Harpaz R, Jumaan AO, et al: Impact of varicella vaccination on health care utilization. JAMA 2005;294:797-802.

References

For a complete list of references, log onto www.expertconsult.com.

Mycoses

Alice Kim

DEFINITION AND CAUSES

The incidence of superficial and deep fungal infections has increased in the era of increasing immunosuppression due to underlying disease states such as HIV/AIDS in addition to immunomodulatory therapy for the prevention of rejection in solid organ and hematopoietic cell transplantation. The spectrum of fungal infections ranges from localized skin and soft tissue infections to fungemia with disseminated disease to almost any organ system.

Mycoses can be further defined into fungi that are yeasts or molds. The terms *yeast form* and *yeastlike* describe fungi that reproduce by budding. Yeasts include the *Candida* spp., *Cryptococcus* spp., and *Pneumocystis jiroveci*. *Candida* species grow by forming pseudohyphae. The pathogenic species of *Candida* include *C. albicans*, *C. krusei*, *C. parapsilosis*, *C. tropicalis*, *C. lusitaniae*, *C. glabrata* (*Torulopsis glabrata*), *C. guilliermondii*, *C. pseudotropicalis*, and *C. dubliniensis*.

Molds are filamentous fungi composed of hyphae. Molds include *Aspergillus* spp. and the agents of mucormycosis. *Aspergillus fumigatus* is the most pathogenic of the molds and the most common of that species to cause invasive disease. Other species of aspergillus include *A. flavus*, *A. terreus*, and *A. niger*. These pathogens grow as molds in the environment and as hyphal forms in tissue.

The dimorphic fungi are capable of producing both hyphal and yeastlike forms depending on temperature. They typically grow as yeasts at body temperature and as molds at room temperature. The dimorphic fungi include the agents of histoplasmosis, blastomycosis, sporotrichosis, coccidiomycosis, paracoccidioidomycosis, and chromoblastomycosis.

A definitive review of mycoses is beyond the scope of this chapter. Therefore, this discussion will be limited to and focus on the more common fungal infections caused by *Candida*, *Aspergillus*, and the endemic fungi, histoplasmosis, blastomycosis, and coccidiomycosis.

PREVALENCE AND RISK FACTORS

Fungi are ubiquitous in nature and are found in the air, soil, and decaying matter. The scope of fungal infections can manifest from asymptomatic colonization to invasive disease. *Candida* spp. are commensals of human mucocutaneous surfaces and of the gastrointestinal, respiratory, and female genital tracts. Colonization with *Aspergillus* appears most commonly in the respiratory tracts of those with underlying chronic pulmonary disease. Colonization does not occur with coccidioidomycosis and blastomycoses.

The major risk factor for invasive, disseminated fungal disease is an immunocompromised state. This includes patients with HIV/AIDS, who are neutropenic from an underlying hematologic malignancy or from cytotoxic therapy, as well as patients treated with prolonged corticosteroids.

The most common human pathogenic fungi are the *Candida* species. *Candida* is now recognized as the fourth most common organism recovered from blood culture isolates in the United States,[1] accounting for 8% to 10% of all nosocomial bloodstream infections. Invasive candidiasis is associated with an attributable mortality rate of up to 49%.[2,3] *C. albicans* is the most commonly recovered species, followed by *C. glabrata*, *C. tropicalis*, and *C. parapsilosis*. The risk factors that have been identified for invasive candidal infections include intensive care unit stay, presence of indwelling vascular catheters, treatment with broad-spectrum antibiotics, colonization with *Candida*, renal failure, and having undergone abdominal, gastrointestinal, or cardiac surgical procedures.

Aspergillus is the most common invasive mold. Invasive aspergillosis has become the major cause of morbidity and mortality in immunocompromised patients, with mortality rates as high as 88%. Almost two thirds (61%) of patients with invasive aspergillosis have an underlying hematologic disease, or have undergone bone marrow transplantation (BMT). Risk factors for the development of invasive aspergillosis include prolonged or repeated episodes of profound neutropenia, solid organ or hematopoietic stem cell transplantation, grade III or IV graft-versus-host disease, and steroid therapy.

The endemic mycoses have specific geographic distributions. *Histoplasma capsulatum* is endemic in the midwestern and southeastern United States, notably highly prevalent in the Ohio and Mississippi River valleys. *Blastomyces dermatitidis* is endemic in southeastern and south central states that border the Mississippi and Ohio Rivers, the midwestern states, and Canadian provinces bordering the Great Lakes and the St. Lawrence River. Most cases of blastomycosis are reported in Mississippi, Arkansas, Kentucky, Tennessee, and Wisconsin. In the United States, the endemic regions for *Coccidioides immitis* and *C. posadasii*, the agents of coccidiomycoses, include southern Arizona, central and southern California, southern New Mexico, and west Texas.

Residence in or travel to these endemic areas is a risk factor. Sporadic and epidemic cases of the endemic mycoses have been associated with disruption and exposure to infected soil. Histoplasmosis has a strong association with bird and bat guano and persons at high risk include spelunkers who explore caves where bats reside. Persons at highest risk for exposure to and infection by histoplasmosis and coccidioidomycosis also include workers in agriculture, outdoor construction, and excavation. Blastomycosis is isolated from soil containing decayed vegetation or decomposed wood.

PATHOPHYSIOLOGY AND NATURAL HISTORY

Mycoses that are pathogenic to humans are rarely transmissible from person to person and are usually acquired via inhalation or ingestion of spores and, in some cases, direct inoculation. Severity of illness is dependent on the intensity of exposure and the immune status of the patient. Inhalation allows initial infection in the lungs, which can result in subsequent dissemination to other body sites. Most acute infections go unrecognized with asymptomatic or mild illness.

Intact human defense mechanisms are needed to prevent and contain fungal disease. The cell-mediated arm of the immune system is important in producing granulomatous inflammation and in cytokine and chemokine production for the recruitment of macrophages and neutrophils. The hallmark of tissue response is the development of caseating or noncaseating granulomas. Granulomas consist of an admixture of mononuclear phagocytes and lymphocytes, principally T cells. The function of the granuloma is to contain fungal growth.

SIGNS AND SYMPTOMS

Candidiasis

Candidal infection manifests as superficial mucocutaneous disease to invasive disease with dissemination. Oral candidiasis (thrush) and esophageal candidiasis are characterized by white patches (pseudomembranes) on the tongue or mucosal surfaces, which can be removed by scraping. Vulvovaginitis is seen in the settings of oral contraceptive use, diabetes mellitus, pregnancy, and antibiotic therapy; it manifests with vaginal discharge and vulvar edema and pruritis. Chronic mucocutaneous candidiasis (CMC) is associated with failure of T cells to respond to candidal antigen stimulation, resulting in onset in childhood of persistent candidal infections of the mucous membranes, nails, hair, and skin. There is an association of CMC with the autoimmune polyendocrinopathy-candidiasis-ectodermal dystrophy (APECED) syndrome.

Candiduria is common and usually asymptomatic. Most cases represent colonization of the bladder, perineum, or indwelling urinary catheter. However, it can represent upper and lower urinary tract involvement or candidemia, and this should be considered in patients with recurrent or relapsing infection. Risk factors for candiduria include increased age, female gender, antibiotic use, urinary drainage devices, prior surgical procedures, and diabetes mellitus. Of note, discontinuation of urinary catheter use alone results in eradication of candiduria in almost 40% of patients.[4]

Candidal pneumonia exists in two forms, primary pneumonia from an aspiration event and pulmonary lesions from hematogenous dissemination. More common, however, is benign colonization of the airways or contamination by oropharyngeal material. Therefore, identifying yeast forms from cultured sputum or endotracheal aspirates is unreliable and definitive diagnosis requires histopathologic evidence of fungal invasion of pulmonary tissue.

Invasive candidiasis manifests as candidemia, infective endocarditis, joint and bone infection, and endophthalmitis. Clinical signs of disseminated disease may include skin lesions described as painless, erythematous, pustular to macronodular lesions. Notable features of candidal infective endocarditis are larger vegetations and the propensity of embolization to major vessels. Candidal endophthalmitis occurs from hematogenous seeding in as many as 28% of patients. It is manifested by symptoms of blurry vision, floaters, and pain. Prompt recognition and diagnosis are necessary, because permanent blindness may ensue. Hepatosplenic or chronic disseminated candidiasis is a distinct entity in patients with hematologic malignancies in the setting of recovering neutropenia. Patients classically present with persistent fever, right upper quadrant pain, nausea, and vomiting.

Candidal brain abscess and meningitis occur in the setting of disseminated infection, local trauma or surgery, or ventricular shunt. Symptoms are similar to those of bacterial meningitis. A notable frequent complication is hydrocephalus.

Aspergillosis

The clinical spectrum of aspergillosis ranges from allergic reaction and colonization to invasive disease. The three main diseases caused by *Aspergillus* species include allergic bronchopulmonary aspergillosis (ABPA), invasive aspergillosis, and aspergilloma.

Allergic bronchopulmonary aspergillosis (ABPA) is diagnosed by the following criteria[5]: asthma; central bronchiectasis on chest computed tomography (CT) scan; immediate cutaneous reactivity to *Aspergillus* species; total serum immunoglobulin E (IgE) concentration higher than 417 IU/ml; elevated serum IgE and/or IgG antibody to *A. fumigatus*; fleeting infiltrates on the chest radiograph; serum precipitating antibodies to *A. fumigatus*; and peripheral blood eosinophilia. The usual course of disease is one of remissions and exacerbations, which can eventually lead to pulmonary fibrosis.

Invasive disease occurs most commonly in the lungs and sinuses. Invasive pulmonary aspergillosis (IPA) occurs in the setting of profound neutropenia. Patients present with fever, progressive dry cough, dyspnea, fever, and pleuritic chest pain, as well as hemoptysis. In IPA, vascular invasion and pulmonary infarction are classic and can lead to fatal pulmonary hemorrhage. Distinctive radiographic findings include pleura-based, wedge-shaped densities or cavitary lesions on chest radiographs. On CT scan early IPA has a halo sign, which is an area of low attenuation surrounding a nodular lesion, representing edema or bleeding surrounding an ischemic area. Later in the course of disease, the classic air crescent sign is seen near the periphery of a lung nodule, caused by contraction of infarcted tissue and signifying cavitation of the nodular lesions. This finding is seen in association with neutrophil recovery.

Cerebral aspergillosis is the second most common site of invasive disease. It occurs in the setting of sinonasal disease causing acute or chronic indolent invasion in the immunocompromised host and presents with epistaxis and naso-orbital pain.

Chronic invasive pulmonary aspergillosis manifests as an aspergilloma or fungus ball. An aspergilloma is a solid mass of hyphae growing in a previously existing pulmonary cavity or ectatic bronchus and typically develops in patients with chronic lung disease. Patients present with hemoptysis and chest radiograph findings of an apical solid, rounded mass within a spherical or ovoid cavity, and positive *Aspergillus*-specific serum precipitins.

Histoplasmosis, Blastomycosis, and Coccidiomycosis

Histoplasmosis can manifest as asymptomatic infection to progressive pulmonary and disseminated disease. Pulmonary histoplasmosis can be subdivided into acute, subacute, and chronic forms. Acute disease manifests with diffuse interstitial or reticulonodular infiltrates associated with fever, sweats, and weight loss. The subacute form occurs over weeks to months and is characterized by hilar or mediastinal lymphadenopathy and focal or patchy infiltrates. Chronic pulmonary disease may show calcifications and consolidation with upper lobe thin- or thick-walled cavitary lesions. A histoplasmoma is a mass lesion that resembles a fibroma and, on chest radiograph, has either a central core of calcium or rings of calcium, which are useful to exclude malignancy.

Five percent to 10% of patients with histoplasmosis suffer from acute pericarditis and other rheumatologic syndromes. Rheumatologic manifestations of arthralgias, erythema nodosum, and erythema multiforme may be present in cases of acute pulmonary histoplasmosis, and can also be seen in cases of coccidiomycosis.

Mediastinal lympadenopathy is common in acute and subacute cases. A late complication that may develop is fibrosing mediastinitis. This can lead to subsequent impingement of mediastinal structures, with a progressive fatal course.

In disseminated histoplasmosis, patients present with fever, sweats, weight loss, fatigue, and respiratory symptoms. Physical findings include hepatosplenomegaly (in almost all patients), lymphadenopathy of the cervical chain, oropharyngeal ulcer (tongue, buccal mucosa, larynx, gums, and lips), and cutaneous lesions (maculopapular eruption, petechiae, or ecchymosis). Central nervous system involvement occurs in 5% to 20% of cases of acute disseminated histoplasmosis, presenting as chronic meningitis—usually lymphocytic—or focal brain lesions. Disseminated disease can be self limited or progressive. Laboratory findings include bone marrow suppression and elevated alkaline phosphatase and lactic acid dehydrogenase levels.

Blastomycosis can manifest as nonspecific febrile illness to acute or chronic pulmonary disease mimicking community-acquired pneumonia and malignancy, and ultimately to disseminated disease involving cutaneous, genitourinary, and bony lesions. Pulmonary infection can have alveolar or reticulonodular infiltrates or mass lesion. Cutaneous blastomycosis is reported in 40% to 80% of cases and is the marker for multiorgan involvement. Skin or naso-oropharyngeal mucosal lesions may be seen. Superficial skin lesions can be verrucous or ulcerative and deep lesions can be noted as subcutaneous nodules or cold abscesses. Skeletal blastomycosis most commonly involves the long bones, vertebrae, and ribs and is typically a well-circumscribed osteolytic lesion manifesting as a soft tissue abscess, chronic draining sinus, or septic arthritis. Ten percent to 30% of cases in men with blastomycosis have involvement of the genitourinary tract, primarily of the prostate and epididymis.

Primary coccidioidomycosis manifests with pulmonary involvement and in most cases is asymptomatic. Symptomatic coccidioidomycosis usually presents with fever, cough, and chest pain and may mimic community-acquired pneumonia. Laboratory findings include an increased erythrocyte sedimentation rate and peripheral eosinophilia. Chest radiographs may show infiltrates, nodules, or peripheral, solitary thin-walled cavities and parapneumonic effusion. More than 95% of patients recover spontaneously from the acute illness. Chronic pulmonary disease occurs in 5% of those with symptomatic primary pulmonary infection. This results in nodular lesions that may cavitate and subsequently rupture, causing pneumothorax or hemorrhage and then may become secondarily infected. Disseminated disease can occur locally with pleural or pericardial invasion or hematogenously to involve any organ of the body, most commonly the lungs, skin and soft tissue, bones, joints, and meninges. Central nervous system involvement manifests as meningitis and obstructive or communicating hydrocephalus. More severe and disseminated disease is seen in immunosuppressed women in the third trimester of pregnancy, and in those of Filipino and African American descent.

DIAGNOSIS

A prompt and accurate diagnosis of fungal infections is the key to affecting mortality. A comprehensive history, including a detailed travel history, and physical examination are needed for initial evaluation.

Chest x-ray and CT scanning of the chest, abdomen, and brain are useful in finding characteristic features of disease. Isolation of the organism with histopathology or culture is the gold standard to confirm fungal infections; however, this can be time consuming and delay prompt diagnosis. Therefore, various laboratory tests have been developed that may provide early clues to the diagnosis.

Preliminary identification of a fungal infection by direct microscopy can be done using several different stains of clinical specimens:

- Fungal specific stains include the Gomori methenamine-silver (GMS), periodic acid–Schiff reagent (PAS), and calcofour white. GMS stains target the fungal cell wall in all fungi, whereas PAS will identify the polysaccharide component in the cell wall in viable fungi. Calcofour will stain all fungi white or green under the fluorescent microscope.
- Routine Gram staining is useful only for *Candida* and stains gram positive.

A rapid presumptive diagnosis of *C. albicans* can be done using the germ tube test. This involves placing the organism in serum and observing germ tube formation, which are small projections from the cell surface that reflect initiation of hyphal growth.

Currently used automated blood culture methods have improved the isolation of fungal organisms, but blood culture isolation of fungi may be negative, even in disseminated fungal disease. The most common fungi recovered from blood cultures include *Candida* spp. and *Histoplasma* spp. Blood cultures and bone marrow are usually positive in up to 50% of disseminated histoplasmosis cases.

Tissue culture technique can take weeks for definitive results and most fungi require special fungal media for growth. Histopathologic diagnosis can yield faster presumptive diagnosis, as well as help distinguish between truly invasive tissue disease versus contamination or colonization. Distinctive histopathologic characteristics include the following:

- *Candida* spp.: oval, budding yeast with hyphae and pseudohyphae; microabscesses
- *Aspergillus* spp.: septate, acute-angle branching, nonpigmented hyphae
- *Histoplasma*: small ovoid, intracellular yeast forms with narrow-based budding, granulomas
- *Blastomyces dermatitidis*: large, thick-walled budding yeast with broad-based budding, daughter cell, often as large as mother cell before detachment
- *Coccidiomycosis immitis*: thick-walled spherules with endospores

The laboratory should be alerted and notified of a presumptive diagnosis of coccidiomycosis because of the potential of secondary infection when plates are examined.

Other diagnostic tests include serologic studies with antigen and antibody assays. Important limitations include lack of antibody response due to the immunocompromised state of the patient and cross-reactions resulting in false positivity.

Galactomannan is an immunoassay for the diagnosis of invasive *Aspergillus* infections. Galactomannan is a polysaccharide specific to *Aspergillus* that is detectable in serum, urine, cerebrospinal (CSF), and bronchoalveloar lavage (BAL) specimens by enzyme immunoassay (EIA), enzyme-linked immunosorbent assay (ELISA), and immunoblot testing. These assays have reported positive predictive values of 54% and negative predictive values of 95% in bone marrow transplant recipients.[6] There have been conflicting and varying results and further studies need to be performed to test the validity of these assays. No antigen tests are currently approved for use in the United States.

Histoplasma antigen detection of fungal cell elements in urine, serum, and CSF by ELISA has proven to be important in the diagnosis, monitoring, and prognosis of acute disseminated histoplasmosis. The sensitivity of *Histoplasma* antigen is higher in urine (92%) than in serum (60%-80%). Antigen concentrations in both urine and serum decline with effective treatment. Therefore, failure of the antigen concentration to fall during therapy may suggest treatment failure or relapse and should prompt further investigation.

Serologic testing is the most frequent means of diagnosing primary coccidioidal infections. Early infection can be detected by tube precipitin antibodies as IgM and by complement-fixing antibodies as IgG. A titer of 1:16 or higher has been associated with extrathoracic dissemination and is especially important in the diagnosis of coccidioidal meningitis because CSF cultures are usually negative. More recently, ELISA for coccidioidal IgG and IgM antibodies has been used with 100% sensitivity and 99% specificity and positive predictive value (PPV) of 82% and negative predictive value (NPV) of 100%.[7]

Other nonculture diagnostic techniques include molecular techniques using nucleic acid (DNA and RNA) probes via polymerase chain reaction (PCR) technology and fluorescent in situ hybridization (FISH). PCR modalities allow rapid and definitive identification and are promising, but to date lack sufficient validity and standardization to be used clinically.

Summary

- The spectrum of fungal infection can range from asymptomatic infection to disseminated disease.
- The major risk factor for invasive fungal disease is immunosuppression.
- Diagnosis requires a thorough history, including travel history, and physical examination.
- A rapid presumptive diagnosis can be made by the use of staining, histopathologic characteristics, and serologic testing results.

TREATMENT

Early diagnosis, efforts to improve immune function, and prompt administration of appropriate antifungal therapy are key to favorable outcomes.

A detailed review of the available antifungal agents and guidelines for treatment are beyond the scope of this chapter; therefore, a brief overview is presented here. Referral to medication package inserts, the Infectious Diseases Society of America practice guidelines, and management of cases in consultation with an infectious disease specialist are strongly recommended.

Classes of Antifungal Agents

Four classes of antifungal agents are approved for the treatment of fungal infections.

Polyenes

Amphotericin B deoxycholate (Fungizone) is the mainstay of antifungal therapy, with the broadest spectrum of activity. It is rapidly fungicidal by binding to ergosterol on the fungal cell membrane, causing disruption of the membrane and ultimately cell death. The few pathogens that are resistant to amphotericin include *Candida lusitaniae* and *C. guilliermondii*, *A. terreus*, and *Fusarium*, *Rhizopus*, *Mucor*, and *Scedosporium* spp.

Limiting factors in the use of amphotericin are associated toxicities, most importantly nephrotoxicity (elevation of serum creatinine level, hypokalemia, hypomagnesemia, and renal tubular acidosis), and infusion-related adverse affects, such as fever, chills, rigors, and hypotension. Amphotericin B–associated nephrotoxicity can be ameliorated or prevented by maintaining intravascular volume by with 500 to 1000 mL of normal saline before infusion and also by avoiding concurrent potentially nephrotoxic agents, such as radiocontrast dyes, nonsteroidal anti-inflammatory drugs, aminoglycoside antibiotics, and immunosuppressive agents, such as cyclosporine and tacrolimus. Infusion-related symptoms can be minimized by premedication with acetaminophen, diphenhydramine, and meperidine. Importantly, most patients develop tolerance over time to the acute infusion-related toxicities.

Lipid formulations (liposomal amphotericin B [L-AmB; AmBisome]) and amphotericin B lipid complex [ABLC, Abelcet]) and amphotericin B colloidal dispersion (ABCD; Amphotec) have a reduced toxicity profile but are more expensive. All are indicated for patients with systemic mycoses who are intolerant of or refractory to conventional amphotericin B, defined as follows: development of renal dysfunction (serum creatinine level higher than 2.5 mg/dL) during antifungal therapy; severe or persistent adverse events, despite premedication or comedication regimens; and disease progression after a 50-g total dose of amphotericin B. A triad of infusional toxicity has been characterized with the liposomal preparation, manifested as pulmonary toxicity (chest pain, dyspnea, hypoxia), abdominal, flank, or leg pain, or flushing and urticaria.

Dosages are as follows:

- Amphotericin B 0.1 to 1.5 mg/kg/day
- Liposomal amphotericin B 1 to 5 mg/kg/day
- ABLC and ABCD 3 to 5 mg/kg/day

Pyrimidines

The only approved drug in this class is flucytosine (5-fluorocytosine). It is a pyrimidine analogue that inhibits DNA and protein synthesis. Its limited spectrum of activity includes *Candida* spp., *Cryptococcus neoformans*, and some molds. Significant potential for toxic effects such as rash, nausea, vomiting, diarrhea, liver dysfunction, and bone marrow suppression limits its use. Because of emergence of resistance, it is used primarily in combination with amphotericin B as therapy for select life-threatening and disseminated fungal infections. Its dosage regimen is 50 to 150 mg/kg/day, divided into four doses.

Azoles

Azoles also target the fungal cell membrane by inhibiting ergosterol synthesis through inhibition of cytochrome P-450–dependent 14a-lanosterol demethylation. The agents available are fluconazole (Diflucan), itraconazole (Sporanox), and ketoconazole (Nizoral). The second-generation azoles voriconazole (Vfend) and posaconazole (Noxafil) are synthetic triazole derivatives of fluconazole.

In general, azoles demonstrate fungistatic activity against *Candida* spp., but they have varying potency against endemic fungi such as *C. immitis*, *B. dermatitidis*, and *H. capsulatum*. Itraconazole, voriconazole, and posaconazole have increased spectrum of activity against molds such as *Aspergillus*.

Fluconazole, itraconazole, and voriconazole are available in oral and IV formulations. Itraconazole has unreliable oral absorption and requires an acidic gastric environment for the capsules and an empty stomach for the solution for optimal absorption. Both fluconazole and voriconazole achieve good CSF levels as well.

The azoles overall as a class are well tolerated. Side effects include gastrointestinal (GI) upset and elevated liver enzyme levels. Therefore, it is recommended to monitor liver functions every 2 to 4 weeks and to discontinue the medication if elevations of more than five times the normal are noted. The most common adverse effect with voriconazole is a transient and reversible visual disturbance in 30% of cases. This is manifested as bright spots and wavy lines, altered color discrimination, blurred vision, and photophobia; it usually appears during the first week of therapy and abates in most patients on continued therapy.

Both itraconazole and voriconazole are limited because of significant drug-drug interactions with other drugs metabolized by cytochrome P-450. Refer to Table 1 and medication package insert for details. IV intraconazole and IV voriconazole are contraindicated in patents with renal insufficiency (creatinine clearance <50 mL/min) because of concerns of accumulation of the cyclodextrin component in these formulations.

Recommended dosages are as follows:

- Fluconazole 100 to 400 mg/day
- Ketoconazole 200 to 400 mg/day
- Itraconazole 200 to 400 mg/day
- Voriconazole: PO 200 mg every 12 hours; IV 6 mg/kg every 12 hours on first day, then 4 mg/kg/day
- Posaconazole 600 to 800 mg/day (in two to four divided doses)

Echinocandins

The echinocandins are the newest class of antifungal agents. This class targets cell wall synthesis by inhibiting β-1,3-D-glucan synthase, resulting in selective inhibition of glucan synthesis. The agents in this class include caspofungin (Cancidas), micafungin (Mycamine), and anidulafungin (Eraxis). All are administered intravenously.

The echinocandins have fungicidal activity against most *Candida* species, including azole-resistant strains, and have been shown to be as efficacious as amphotericin and fluconazole in cases of candidemia or invasive candidiasis. The echinocandins are fungistatic against *Aspergillus* spp. Caspofungin is currently U.S. Food and Drug Administration (FDA)-approved for the treatment of invasive aspergillosis as a salvage or secondary agent in patients with an initial response to voriconazole or amphotericin B, or in combination therapy with these agents. The echinocandins have no activity against the endemic mycoses.

The side effect profile of the echinocandins is relatively safe. The most common adverse reactions include headache, nausea, vomiting, flushing and infusion-related pruritis, erythema, and pain. Approximately 10% of patients will have elevations of liver enzyme levels.

Caspofungin distributes well into tissues but has little penetration into the brain and CSF. It does not inhibit or induce cytochrome P-450 (CYP450) but inducers of CYP450, such as rifampin, phenytoin, and carbamazepine reduce serum concentrations of caspofungin so that a higher daily dosage is needed. It is not recommended to be given with cyclosporine because it can result in an increased

Table 1 Antifungal Agents

Drug	Route of Administration	Dosage	Side Effects	Comments
Polyenes				
Amphotericin B (Fungizone)	IV	0.5-1.0 mg/kg/day	Infusion-related: fever, chills, rigors, hypotension; thrombophlebitis, azotemia, renal tubular acidosis (RTA), K^+, Mg^{2+}, HCO_3, wasting	Toxicities ameliorated or prevented by normal saline; avoid concurrent nephrotoxic agents, premedication with acetaminophen, diphenhydramine, meperidine
Lipid Formulations				
liposomal amphotericin B (AmBisome); amphotericin B lipid complex (ABLC, Abelcet); amphotericin B colloidal dispersion (ABCD, Amphotec)	IV	Liposomal amphotericin B, 1-5 mg/kg/day; ABLC and ABCD, 3-5 mg/kg/day	Infusion-related: chest pain, dyspnea, hypoxia, flushing, urticaria	
Pyrimidine				
Flucytosine	PO	50-150 mg/kg/day, qid	Rash, gastrointestinal (GI) upset, bone marrow suppression	Used primarily in combination therapy
Azoles				
Fluconazole (Diflucan)	PO, IV	100-800 mg/day	GI upset, elevated liver function tests (LFTs); drug-drug interactions: contraindicated with cisapride	Monitor liver enzyme levels, renal function
Ketoconazole (Nizoral)	PO, topical	200-400 mg/day	Significant drug-drug interactions: contraindicated with cisapride, midazolam, triazolam, ergot alkaloids, lovastatin, simvastatin, pimozide; hepatoxicity	Monitor liver enzyme levels
Itraconazole (Sporanox)	PO (capsule, 100 mg; solution, 100 mg/10 mL), IV	100-400 mg/day	Significant drug-drug interactions: contraindicated with cisapride, dofetilide, ergot derivatives, levomethadyl, lovastatin, midazolam, pimozide, quinidine, simvastatin, triazolam; rash; elevated LFTs; congestive heart failure	Bioavailability of capsule increased with food in acidic gastric environment: coadminister with cola beverage and avoid use with H_2 blockers; bioavailability of suspension increased with empty stomach; monitor liver enzyme levels; avoid in patients with active liver disease; avoid IV formulation in renal insufficiency
Voriconazole (Vfend)	PO, IV	200 mg q12h; loading, 6 mg/kg q12h bid; maintenance, 4 mg/kg q12h	Significant drug-drug interactions: contraindicated with cisapride, pimozide, quinidine, long-acting barbiturates, carbamazepine, efavirenz, ergot alkaloids, rifampin, rifabutin, ritonavir, sirolimus; reversible photopsia in ~30%; rash; elevated LFTs	Bioavailability of PO form increased when given 1 hr before or after meal, decreased with fatty foods; dose adjustment for liver dysfunction; avoid IV formulation in renal insufficiency
Posaconazole (Noxafil)	PO	600-800 mg/day (two to four divided doses)	Drug-drug interactions: contraindicated with cisapride, pimozide, quinidine, ergot alkaloids; GI upset; rash	Requires high-fat meals for absorption; monitor liver enzyme levels
Echinocandins				
Caspofungin (Cancidas)	IV	Loading, 70 mg × one dose; maintenance, 50 mg/day	Histamine-like infusion reaction; elevated LFTs; thrombophlebitis	Monitor liver enzyme levels; dose adjustment in liver dysfunction
Micafungin (Mycamine)	IV	150 mg daily	Thrombophlebitis; elevated LFTs; leukopenia	Monitor liver enzyme levels
Anidulafungin (Eraxis)	IV	Loading, 100-200 mg × one dose; maintenance, 50-100 mg/day	Histamine-like infusion reaction; elevated LFTs	Monitor liver enzyme levels

Adapted from Cisneros Herreros JM, Cordero Matia E: Therapeutic armamentarium against systemic fungal infections. Clin Microbiol Infect 2006;12(Suppl 7):53-64; Dimukes WE: Introduction to antifungal drugs. Clin Infect Dis 2000;30:653-657; Kauffman CA: Clinical efficacy of new antifungal agents. Curr Opin Microbiol. 2006;9:483-488; Vazquez JA, Sobel JD: Anidulafungin: A novel echinocandin. Clin Infect Dis 2006;43:215-222; and Wong-Beringer A, Kriengkauykiat J: Systemic antifungal therapy: New options, new challenges. Pharmacotherapy 2003;23:1441-1462.

serum concentration of caspofungin and transient elevations of serum transaminase levels.

Recommended dosages are as follows:

- Caspofungin: 70-mg load, then 50 mg/day
- Anidulafungin: initial dose of 100 to 200 mg, followed by 50 to 100 mg/day
- Micafungin: 150 mg/day

Combination Antifungal Therapy

Combination therapy for invasive mold infections with different classes of antifungal drugs has shown to be promising according to their different mechanisms of action. For example, triazoles and echinocandins or echinocandins with amphotericin B have been used for the treatment of invasive aspergillosis (IA). However, further well-designed, randomized trials need to be done to establish their usefulness. The routine use of antifungal combinations as primary therapy is currently not recommended.

Guidelines for Treatment

Candidiasis

- Susceptibility patterns of note: *C. lusitaniae* isolates are often resistant to amphotericin B. *C. guilliermondii* and *C. parapsilosis* may be less susceptible to echinocandins. *C. glabrata* and *C. krusei* are less susceptible to azoles.
- Esophageal candidiasis: fluconazole is used as primary therapy. Refractory cases can be treated with voriconazole, caspofungin, or intraconazole solution or amphotericin B formulations.
- Invasive candidal infections: amphotericin B preparations or caspofungin can be used for critically ill patients, given the increasing incidence of fluconazole-resistant non–*C. albicans* strains. Once the candidal isolate and susceptibility are known, the triazoles, fluconazole, itraconazole, and voriconazole (for salvage therapy) can be used.
- Other interventions: removal of indwelling catheters, ophthalmology examination to rule out endophthalmitis.

Aspergillosis

- Susceptibility patterns of note: itraconazole, voriconazole, and posaconazole have fungicidal activity against *Aspergillus* spp. Echinocandins are fungistatic against *Aspergillus* spp.
- APBA: the use of corticosteroids (prednisone 10 mg/day) is indicated for patients with increasing IgE levels, new or worsening infiltrate on chest radiograph, or worsening spirometry, with gradual dose reduction dependent on individual response. Itraconazole (200 mg twice daily) may be useful as a corticosteroid sparing agent.
- Invasive aspergillosis (IA): voriconazole has become the drug of choice for IA based on a large randomized trial that showed higher response rates and significantly improved survival rates in patients receiving voriconazole versus amphotericin B.[8] Amphotericin B preparations (amphotericin B, 1 to 1.5 mg/kg/day or 5 mg/kg/day of lipid formulations of amphotericin, up to 400 mg/day) should be used in life-threatening cases. Itraconazole can be used as a second-line agent and for those with non–life-threatening infection. Caspofungin is the only echinocandin FDA-approved for salvage therapy in IA. Posaconazole is also an alternative for salvage therapy for those refractory or intolerant of previous therapy.[9] The length of therapy is unknown; it should be dependent on the patient's response to therapy based on resolution of clinical and radiographic abnormalities and improvement of the patient's underlying condition or immune status.
- Aspergilloma: surgical removal is definitive therapy but is associated with high morbidity and mortality; it is usually reserved for those with life-threatening hemoptysis, the immunocompromised, and those with increasing *Aspergillum*-specific IgG titers. Bronchial artery embolization should be considered as a temporizing procedure until more definitive therapy can be done. Additional therapies that need further study and validation include radiation, intracavitary or endobronchial instillation of amphotericin B, and systemic antifungals (itraconazole).

Endemic Mycoses (Histoplasmosis, Blastomycosis, Coccidioidomycosis)

- Susceptibility patterns of note: voriconazole and posaconazole have in vitro activity but no trials have been done. The echinocandins are not active in vitro and should not be used.

Histoplasmosis

- Asymptomatic patients do not require treatment.
- Acute pulmonary histoplasmosis: Amphotericin B should be used for severe cases and itraconazole can be used for milder cases. The optimal duration has not been determined but should be at least 3 months if there is no evidence of disseminated disease.
- Subacute pulmonary histoplasmosis: Most cases do not require treatment, however, it should be considered in immunosuppressed patients or those with underlying lung disease with 6 to 12 weeks of therapy.
- Chronic pulmonary histoplasmosis: This entity becomes progressive without therapy, so severe cases should be treated with amphotericin B. Milder cases can be treated with itraconazole. Duration of therapy should be continued for at least 1 year because of the high relapse rate (10%-25%), until radiographic abnormalities stabilize.
- Mediastinal lympadenopathy: For patients who do not show spontaneous improvement after 1 month of illness, a trial of itraconazole for 3 to 6 months can be used if there is response to therapy.
- Mediastinal fibrosis: There is no role for or effect of antifungal therapy or anti-inflammatory medications. Stents or surgery can be considered but this is high risk.
- Progressive disseminated histoplasmosis: This can be treated with liposomal amphotericin B (3-5 mg/kg/day), changing to intraconazole (200 mg three times daily × 3 days and then twice daily) if there is initial response. Therapy should be continued for at least 6 to 12 months, and until clinical findings and antigen levels resolve.
- Central nervous system involvement: Treat with liposomal amphotericin B (105-175 mg/kg over the total course), followed by itraconazole or posaconazole for at least 1 year of therapy.

Coccidioidomycosis

- Uncomplicated: No treatment is required but close monitoring should be done every 3 to 6 months for up to 2 years with serologic testing, because a rise in antibody titers may be associated with progressive disease.
- Acute, diffuse pneumonia: Treat with amphotericin B for 3 to 6 months and then consider oral azole for at least 1 year.
- Chronic cavitary pneumonia: If asymptomatic, only close monitoring is needed, with consideration of resection if there are complications, enlargement, or persistence of the lesion after 2 years. If there is symptomatic disease, treat with fluconazole or itraconazole for at least 1 year. Voriconazole and posaconazole are other options for therapy. Surgical resection may need to be considered for refractory lesions.
- Disseminated coccidioidomycosis: Treat with fluconazole (400 or 800 mg/day) or intraconazole (200 mg twice daily) or amphotericin B for 6 to 12 months followed by close observation for years, given the risk of relapse in more than one third of cases.

- Central nervous system, meningitis: Treat with fluconazole (800 mg/day) or itraconazole (400-600 mg/day). Consider intrathecal amphotericin (0.01-1.5 mg) for those who do not respond to azoles. Azole therapy is continued for life. Other measures include ventriculoperitoneal (VP) shunting in cases with obstructive hydrocephalus.

Blastomycosis

- Uncomplicated/immunocompetent: Close monitoring is needed.
- Pulmonary (mild to moderate disease): Treat with itraconazole (200-400 mg/day) or ketoconazole (400-800 mg/day) or fluconazole (400-800 mg/day).
- All immunocompromised patients and those with progressive pulmonary and disseminated disease should be treated, because spontaneous resolution is uncommon and untreated cases are associated with mortality rates as high as 60%. Treatment options include amphotericin B (0.7-1.0 mg/kg/dose, with 1.5- to 2.5-g total dosage) for life-threatening infections, which can be changed to itraconazole (200-400 mg/day) if stabilized. Those patients with less severe infection can be treated with ketoconazole (400 mg/day, increased to maximum 800 mg/day for those who do not respond), itraconazole, or fluconazole. Treatment duration is at least 6 months.
- CNS infection: Treat with amphotericin B, with the total dosage at least 2 g.

Summary

- Amphotericin B should be the first-line agent in life-threatening fungal infections.
- There are significant drug-drug interactions with azoles that need close review when using this class of antifungals.
- Voriconazole is now considered the drug of choice for invasive aspergillosis.
- The echinocandins are well tolerated and are treatment options for infections with *Candida* and *Aspergillus* spp.
- Consultation with an infectious disease specialist is recommended.

PREVENTION AND SCREENING

Local measures including hygienic means to decrease colonization, careful attention to intravascular catheter use and care, judicious use of antibiotics, and strict infection control measures, can decrease the risk of fungal infections. High-risk patients should avoid environmental exposure or wear approved respiratory devices during recreation or if working at construction sites where soil or building disruption may cause high numbers of yeasts to be aerosolized.

For pathogenic molds, the use of high-efficiency particulate air (HEPA) filters, frequent air exchanges, and positive pressure ventilation are recommended to limit nosocomial exposure.

CONSIDERATIONS IN SPECIAL POPULATIONS

Amphotericin B is the tratment of choice for pregnant women. Echinocandins and azoles (fluconazole and itraconazole) are designated category C (risk to fetus cannot be ruled out) and voriconazole as category D (positive evidence of human fetal risk).

Suggested Readings

Alexander BD, Pfaller MA: Contemporary tools for the diagnosis and management of invasive mycoses. Clin Infect Dis 2006;43:S15-S27.

Chapman SW, Bradsher RW, Campbell GD, et al: Practice guidelines for the management of patients with blastomycosis. Clin Infect Dis 2000;30:679-683.

Dimukes WE: Introduction to antifungal drugs. Clin Infect Dis 2000;30:653-657.

Galgiani JN, Ampel NM, Catanzaro A, et al: Practice guidelines for the treatment of coccidioidomycosis. Clin Infect Dis 2000;30:658-661.

Kauffman CA: Clinical efficacy of new antifungal agents. Curr Opin Microbiol 2006;9:483-488.

Kauffman CA: Endemic mycoses: Blastomycosis, histoplasmosis, and sporotrichosis. Infect Dis Clin North Am 2006;20:645-662.

Pappas PG, Rex JH, Sobel JD, et al: Guidelines for treatment of candidiasis. Clin Infect Dis 2004;38:161-189.

Stevens DA, Kan VL, Judson MA, et al: Practice guidelines for diseases caused by *Aspergillus*. Clin Infect Dis 2000;30:696-709.

Wheat J, Sarosi G, McKinsey D, et al: Practice guidelines for the management of patients with histoplasmosis. Clin Infect Dis 2000;30:688-695.

References

For a complete list of references, log onto www.expertconsult.com.

Section 9

NEPHROLOGY

Kidney Function Assessment by Creatinine-Based Estimation Equations

Martin E. Lascano and Emilio D. Poggio

Chronic kidney disease (CKD) has been recognized as a common health care problem, and therefore the National Kidney Foundation (NKF) has published the Kidney Disease Outcomes Quality Initiative (KDOQI) Practice Guidelines for the early detection, evaluation, diagnosis, and treatment of this condition (http://www.kidney.org/professionals/kdoqi/guidelines.cfm). As recommended by this initiative, the degree of kidney dysfunction, as assessed by the estimation of the glomerular filtration rate (GFR), is essential for the diagnosis, classification, and staging of CKD; see elsewhere in this section ("Chronic Kidney Disease"). Among the various alternatives available for the assessment of GFR, the NKF, and the National Kidney Disease Education Program (NKDEP) recommend that renal function be estimated by creatinine-based GFR estimation equations, and these are the focus of this chapter.

EVALUATION OF GLOMERULAR FILTRATION RATE

Among the many physiologic roles of the renal system, GFR is considered the best indicator of overall kidney function and therefore its assessment has become an important clinical tool in the daily care of patients. GFR cannot be measured directly, but instead it can be assessed by the renal clearance of filtration markers.[1] The total kidney GFR is the sum of the filtration rates of all single functional nephrons—that is, it is determined by the total number of functional nephrons. Because of its highly dynamic and adaptive nature, despite initial structural damage to the renal parenchyma (i.e., reduction in functional nephron number), an individual's total GFR may not proportionally decrease because of the compensatory features of the remaining renal units, enabling the kidneys to maintain kidney function temporarily despite the loss of functional tissue. Moreover, the GFR may also be affected in the absence of parenchymal renal disease because of hemodynamic, pharmacologic factors, or both. The clinical assessment of GFR can aid the clinician in measuring the degree of renal dysfunction, progression of established kidney disease, or both; however, it is not informative in the determination of the cause of kidney disease, making it imperative to interpret the GFR in the context of the clinical setting.

The GFR can be determined from the renal clearance of a marker that achieves stable plasma concentration, is inert, and is freely filtered by the glomeruli but not reabsorbed, secreted, or metabolized.[1,2] Such an ideal endogenous marker does not exist. Serum creatinine, one of the clinically useful analytes (others are serum urea and, more recently, serum cystatin C), has long been used by clinicians as a marker of renal function. However, it is important to emphasize that often the isolated use of serum creatinine concentration may not reflect the actual degree of kidney function of a particular subject. This is because multiple factors affect the concentration of serum creatinine (Table 1) and that the inverse relation between serum creatinine and GFR is nonlinear, particularly when patients have near-normal renal function (Fig. 1). An alternative to this approach is the measurement of creatinine clearance. This determination does not require highly trained personnel or expensive assays and can be performed by standard laboratories. However, this approach is limited by the difficulties in obtaining accurate urine collections and its potential misinterpretation because of the large biologic variability of creatinine metabolism in various clinical settings, including the unpredictable level of creatinine secretion at different levels of GFR. This method, however, is widely available and familiar to the health care community. On the other hand, more exact methods of GFR measurement, such as the clearance of exogenous markers such as inulin or renally excreted isotopes, are expensive and usually not readily available. More novel serum measurements of analytes, such as cystatin C, are under investigation and are not yet fully validated in all clinical settings; therefore, this approach remains a research tool at present.

Rapid estimation of GFR by using creatinine-based mathematical equations is an attractive alternative to the clinician. These models rely on the inverse relation of serum creatinine with GFR, along with adjustment factors for measurable determinants of serum creatinine concentration (e.g., age, sex, body size, race).

CREATININE-BASED ESTIMATION EQUATIONS

Numerous kidney function estimation equations, used to estimate creatinine clearance or GFR, have been published over the past few decades. However, the most commonly used formulas, the Cockcroft-Gault formula and the modification of diet in renal disease (MDRD) study equation, have been recommended by the KDOQI practice guidelines to be used for the estimation of GFR. These equations rely heavily on the reciprocal relation between serum creatinine and GFR but also incorporate demographic and anthropometric variables to complement the GFR estimation derived from the use of serum creatinine alone. It is important to emphasize that these mathematical models will reflect the clinical setting used to originate them.[3]

Cockcroft-Gault Formula

The Cockcroft-Gault formula was developed in 1976 with data from 249 men, primarily in an inpatient setting, with a wide range of renal function.[4] It uses age, the inverse of serum creatinine, and lean body weight to estimate creatinine clearance in milliliters per minute (Box 1); it was not originally intended to be adjusted for body surface area (BSA). The inclusion of the weight factor is intended to adjust for muscle mass, a determinant of serum creatinine concentration. This implies that in clinical situations in which a change in weight is not the result of a similar change in muscle mass (e.g., edematous states, pregnancy, third spacing, overweight, obesity), the weight factor will adversely affect the performance of this formula. Because the original mathematical model was derived from data obtained predominantly in a male population, an arbitrary adjustment for female sex by a factor of 0.85 was incorporated. This equation has become popular because of its simple mathematical formulation and bedside applicability. It is important to note that this formula estimates creatinine clearance; this is known to overestimate GFR because of tubular secretion of creatinine, which is not adjustable.

Modification of Diet in Renal Disease Formula

The MDRD equation was developed in 1999 using data from 1628 patients with established chronic kidney disease.[5] Whereas the

Table 1 Factors Affecting Serum Creatinine Concentration

Factor	Effect on Serum Creatinine Level	Comment
Demographics		
Aging	Decreased	Caused by decline in muscle mass
Female sex	Decreased	Reduced muscle mass
Ethnicity*		
African American	Increased	Higher average muscle mass in African Americans
Hispanic	Decreased	
Asian	Decreased	
Body Habitus		
Muscular	Increased	Increased muscle mass
Muscle wasting, amputation, malnutrition	Decreased	Reduced muscle mass ± decreased protein intake
Obesity	No change	No change in muscle mass
Diet		
Vegetarian	Decreased	Decrease in creatinine generation
Ingestion of cooked meats	Increased	Transient increase in creatinine generation
Medications, Endogenous Substances		
Cimetidine, trimethoprim, probenecid, potassium-sparing diuretics	Increased	Reduced creatinine tubular secretion
Ketoacids, ascorbic acid, glucose, some cephalosporins	Increased	Interference with alkaline picrate assay (Jaffé reaction) for creatinine
Bilirubin, hemoglobin	Decreased	Interference with alkaline picrate assay (Jaffé reaction) for creatinine
Flucytosine, praline, hemoglobin	Increased	Interference with enzymatic assays for creatinine
Metamizole, methyldopa, ethamsylate	Decreased	Interference with enzymatic assays for creatinine

*Whites used as reference group.

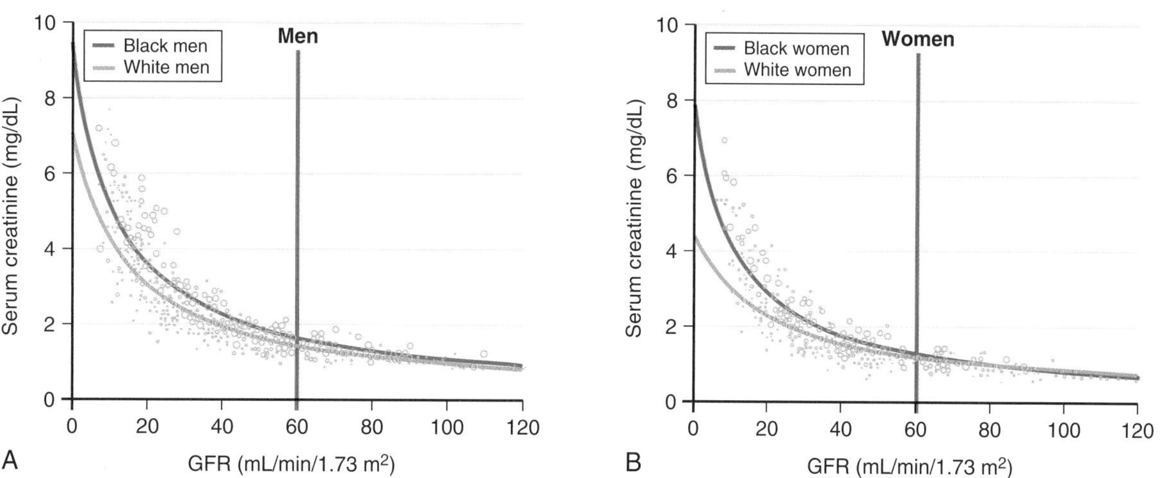

Figure 1 Relation between serum creatinine levels and measured glomerular filtration rate (GFR) by 125I-iothalamate GFR among black and white men (A) and women (B). Note how a significant decrease in GFR can occur, despite normal or near-normal serum creatinine values. *(From Levey AS, Bosch JP, Lewis JP, et al: A more accurate method to estimate glomerular filtration rate from serum creatinine: a new prediction equation. Ann Intern Med 1999;130:461-470.)*

Box 1 Creatinine-based Glomerular Filtration Rate (GFR) Estimation Equations

Cockcroft-Gault formula = ([140 − age] × weight)/(72 × SCr)*
Abbreviated MDRD equation = 186 × ($SCr^{-1.154}$) × ($age^{-0.203}$)†
Re-expressed MDRD equation‡ = 175 × ($SCr^{-1.154}$) × ($age^{-0.203}$)†

Note: *Weight in kilograms, age in years.*
**Multiply by 0.85 if female; expressed in mL/min.*
†*Multiply by 0.742 if female, by 1.212 if African American; expressed in mL/min/1.73 m^2.*
‡*To be used with assays that have been calibrated to be traceable to an isotope dilution mass spectrometry (IDMS) reference method (gold standard), as specified by the National Institute of Standards and Technology (NIST).*
MDRD, modification of diet in renal disease; SCr, serum creatinine level, expressed in mg/dL.

Cockcroft-Gault formula estimates creatinine clearance, the set of equations developed from the data derived from the MDRD study are aimed at estimating GFR as measured by ^{125}I-iothalamate urinary clearance, the reference method used by this study. The base population for these equations was outpatients with established CKD. Various MDRD equations have been published; however, the most widely used equation by the health care community is the abbreviated (four-variable) MDRD equation, which has been reformulated to be used with a standardized serum creatinine assay (see Box 1). It uses age, the inverse of serum creatinine, gender, and race (African American versus non–African American). In contrast to the Cockcroft-Gault formula, this model accounts for the biologic relation of creatinine metabolism observed in African Americans, but there is no adjustment for other ethnicities. This equation directly relates the accounted variables (e.g., serum creatinine, age, gender, race) to GFR adjusted for BSA—that is, the determinants of body size are prepackaged in the equation and thus additional adjustment is not required. A relative limitation of this equation is the need for a calculator. The NKF and the NKEDP now recommend using this equation, rather than the Cockcroft-Gault formula, to estimate kidney function.

Serum Creatinine Assay Calibration

Serum creatinine measurements are susceptible to calibration bias. This refers to a systematic absolute difference in measured serum creatinine concentrations throughout the whole range of creatinine values among laboratories because of variations in the assay calibration. This issue is critical in the application of estimation equations, especially at the normal levels of serum creatinine values.[2,3,6] Data derived from the College of American Pathologists have suggested that there is a bias of up to 0.37 mg/dL in measured serum creatinine levels among U.S. laboratories. The importance of this difference is exemplified by the fact that a serum creatinine level of 0.8 mg/dL in one laboratory could represent a value of 1.2 mg/dL in a different one, with both falling within the "normal" range. Assuming that this sample belongs to a 60-year-old white woman, the estimated GFR could range from 78 to 49 mL/min/1.73 m^2, clearly indicating the possibility of decreased kidney function.

To generalize the applicability of creatinine-based estimation equations among clinical laboratories, reference materials must be standardized, traceable to a gold standard from the National Institute of Standards and Technology (NIST). Clinical laboratories are expected to recalibrate their serum creatinine assays in the near future. The MDRD formula was re-expressed in 2005 to be used with serum creatinine measurements from clinical laboratories that have recalibrated their assays traceable to a standardized assay. This yields a value approximately 5% lower when compared with the measurements obtained by the original MDRD laboratory (see Box 1). Otherwise, until the transition to the recalibrated serum creatinine assay has been completed, the conventional abbreviated MDRD equation should be used.

CLINICAL APPLICABILITY OF CREATININE-BASED ESTIMATION EQUATIONS

One of the main limitations of the currently available GFR estimation equations is the lack of universality across the multiple clinical situations encountered by the clinician. However, growing evidence has suggested that the overall performance of the abbreviated MDRD equation is superior to the GFR estimates obtained by use of the Cockcroft-Gault formula, partially because the latter method estimates creatinine clearance and not GFR. Recognition of the limitations of these estimation equations is essential to using the information obtained from them properly.[3] In general, the applicability of the MDRD equation is clinically satisfactory in settings that resemble the original population and methods used to develop the model, with expected poor performance in settings that deviate from the original. None of the available equations is applicable in cases of acute kidney injury, mostly because the serum creatinine level itself is not predictive of the acute changes in GFR.

Subjects with Established Chronic Kidney Disease

Several studies have reported on the performance of the Cockcroft-Gault and MDRD formulas in estimating GFR in subjects with established CKD and different levels of kidney function. Direct comparison between studies is challenging because of different methodologies used but, in general, both formulas perform better at lower GFR values (e.g., estimated GFR from 15 to 60 mL/min/1.73 m^2), with the MDRD equation providing a lower bias (absolute or relative difference between estimated and measured GFR) and higher accuracy (percentage of estimated GFR within 30% of measured GFR) than the Cockcroft-Gault formula.[7,8] Their performance is compromised as the level of GFR increases because of the caveats presented earlier (Fig. 2). Nevertheless, the abbreviated conventional MDRD equation performs better than the Cockcroft-Gault formula in subjects with known CKD, including those with diabetic nephropathy, and it is considered a reliable method to estimate GFR in this particular setting.

Subjects with Normal-Range Glomerular Filtration Rate

One particular area of interest is the validity of GFR estimation equations in subjects with or without CKD but with normal ranges of renal function. Several studies have reported on the performance of these equations in potential kidney donors (considered healthy) or in subjects with known or at high risk for CKD but with normal GFR levels. The two largest studies that analyzed the performance of estimation equations in healthy subjects have reported underestimation of GFR, which can vary anywhere from 5% to 29%, depending on methodologic issues related to the study.[7,8] Results obtained from subjects with CKD or at risk for CKD (e.g., subjects with type 1diabetes mellitus, but no established CKD) but with a normal GFR range have provided results similar to those obtained from the healthy population. In this particular setting, current estimation equations are not precise and accurate enough to provide exact estimates of GFR, and can potentially misclassify patients as having a low GFR because of the trend for underestimation of renal function—hence, the importance of interpreting the obtained data in the context of the subject's clinical situation. For example, in the absence of risk factors for CKD such as hypertension or diabetes, absence of evidence of parenchymal renal disease (e.g., abnormal urine analysis results), and a single measurement of the serum creatinine level, an estimated GFR in the range of 60 mL/min/1.73 m^2 should be viewed as a possible laboratory error. Because of this limitation of creatinine-based GFR estimation models, the NKEDP has recommended reporting specific values only if the estimated GFR is lower than

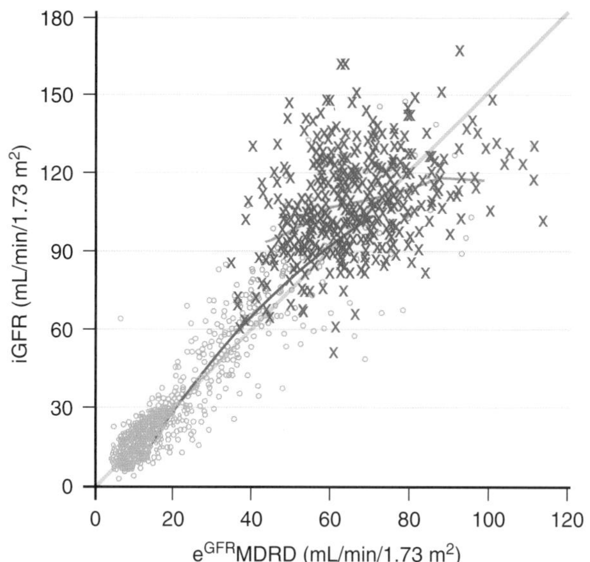

Figure 2 Relation between estimated (by the four-variable modification of diet in renal disease [MDRD] equation) and measured glomerular filtration rate (GFR) in subjects with chronic kidney disease and in potential kidney donors. In the case of subjects with kidney disease, changes in estimated GFR tracks well with similar changes in measured GFR by 125I-iothalamate clearances, whereas this is not true for subjects without kidney disease. *(From Poggio ED, Hall PM: Estimation of glomerular filtration rate by creatinine-based formulas: Any room for improvement? NephSAP 2006;5:131-140.)*

60 mL/min/1.73 m^2; for higher values, "estimated GFR higher than 60 mL/min/1.73 m^2" should be reported instead.

Subjects of Different Races and Ethnic Origins

The current MDRD equation incorporates African American race as a factor to account for the different creatinine metabolism in this population; hence, good performance is expected when applied to an African American population. A deficit of the current MDRD equation is the lack for adjustment, if needed, for Hispanic origin of the target subject. The Hispanic population is the fastest growing minority group in the United States, and is one of the largest populations in certain areas of the country. It is likely that biologic variations of creatinine metabolism, as well as different cultural and social habits (e.g., different diets), affect serum creatinine levels, thus requiring an adjustment. Correction factors may also be needed for other ethnic populations, such as Asians.

Renal Transplant Recipients

Various factors in kidney transplant patients may affect the metabolism of creatinine that will then translate into varying performance of estimation equations. Nevertheless, different estimation equations, including the Cockcroft-Gault and the MDRD formulas, have been used by different investigators for this purpose, along with the Nankivell equation, which was derived from mostly white renal transplant recipients who underwent ^{99}Tc-diethylenetriaminepentaacetic acid (DTPA) clearances.[3] Several studies using different methodologies have compared the performance of these equations, with varying results. In one study, the MDRD formula was found to be superior to the Nankivell and Cockcroft-Gault formulas in an American population that included African American subjects and used the same GFR analytical reference method as the MDRD study. In contrast, other authors have reported better performance of the Nankivell formula over the MDRD equation in a Canadian population, in which GFR was measured by clearance of ^{99}Tc-DTPA, the same method used to develop the Nankivell formula. In this study, serum cystatin C-based estimation equations were clearly superior to all creatinine-based models.

Other Considerations

Because of the steady aging of the population and the increase in illness severity of hospitalized patients, estimation of renal function is often needed for drug dosing or patient care in these settings. In older adults, the strength of the association between age and GFR may be overestimated by the Cockcroft-Gault formula; however, this varies among studies. It is not clear whether any of these formulas apply to older adults, but they are currently the best available alternative to assess kidney function quickly. In sick hospitalized patients, both the MDRD and the Cockcroft-Gault formulas significantly overestimate GFR and their poor performance is not clinically acceptable.[9] By introducing other variables that may adjust for severity of illness, performance of the six-variable MDRD equation, which includes corrections for albumin and blood urea nitrogen levels, is partially improved, suggesting that future models should incorporate multiple surrogate markers of GFR to improve the estimation.

Summary

- Estimation of glomerular filtration rate (GFR) to assess kidney function facilitates the detection, evaluation, and management of kidney disease.
- Estimation equation results should be interpreted in the context of the clinical setting being applied.
- An important aspect of creatinine-based GFR estimation equations is the recognition and acknowledgment of their limitations in each clinical setting.
- The applicability of these estimation equations is satisfactory in settings that resemble the original population and methods used to develop the model, such as patients with established chronic kidney disease, and are an invaluable tool for the assessment of patients with kidney disease.

Suggested Readings

Cockcroft DW, Gault MH: Prediction of creatinine clearance from serum creatinine. Nephron 1976;16:31-41.

Coresh J, Astor BC, McQuillan G, et al: Calibration and random variation of the serum creatinine assay as critical elements of using equations to estimate glomerular filtration rate. Am J Kidney Dis 2002;39:920-929.

Levey AS, Bosch JP, Lewis JB, et al: A more accurate method to estimate glomerular filtration rate from serum creatinine: A new prediction equation. Modification of Diet in Renal Disease Study Group. Ann Intern Med 1999;130:461-470.

Stevens LA, Coresh J, Greene T, Levey AS: Assessing kidney function—measured and estimated glomerular filtration rate. N Engl J Med 2006;354:2473-2483.

Stevens LA, Levey AS: Measurement of kidney function. Med Clin North Am 2005;89:457-473.

Poggio ED, Hall PM: Estimation of glomerular filtration rate by creatinine-based formulas: Any room for improvement? NephSAP 2006;5:131-140.

Poggio ED, Nef PC, Wang X, et al: Performance of the Cockcroft-Gault and modification of diet in renal disease equations in estimating GFR in ill hospitalized patients. Am J Kidney Dis 2005;46:242-252.

Poggio ED, Wang X, Greene T, et al: Performance of the modification of diet in renal disease and Cockcroft-Gault equations in the estimation of GFR in health and in chronic kidney disease. J Am Soc Nephrol 2005;16:459-466.

Rule AD, Larson TS, Bergstralh EJ, et al: Using serum creatinine to estimate glomerular filtration rate: Accuracy in good health and in chronic kidney disease. Ann Intern Med 2004;141:929-937.

References

For a complete list of references, log onto www.expertconsult.com.

Hyponatremia and Hypernatremia

Benjamin J. Freda and Saul Nurko

PHYSIOLOGY OF WATER AND BODY FLUIDS

Disorders of sodium concentration result from a perturbation in water balance. Water is the most abundant body fluid. In lean individuals, water accounts for 60% of total body weight, with approximately two thirds residing intracellularly and one third in the extracellular space. Of the water in the extracellular space, approximately 75% is in the interstitium and 25% in the intravascular space. Because fat contains less water than lean muscle, water accounts for a lower percentage of total body weight in women, older adults, and obese persons. Additionally, water can move between these compartments, resulting in changes in plasma sodium concentration. Water movement between body fluid compartments is regulated by the effective osmolality of the solutes within each compartment. Sodium is the main determinant of plasma osmolality, and water moves toward body compartments with higher osmolality and away from those with lower osmolality.

Plasma water is regulated by an interaction between sensory organs (e.g., carotid body and hypothalamus), antidiuretic hormone (ADH or vasopressin), and the kidney. Although the gastrointestinal tract, skin, and bronchial tree are capable of sodium and water loss, the kidney is the only organ able to conserve or excrete sodium and water under tight regulatory control.

Alterations in arterial blood pressure and plasma osmolality are the main physiologic signals regulating ADH secretion. As plasma water decreases, increases in plasma sodium concentration and osmolality are sensed by nuclei in the hypothalamus, with a resultant increase in production of ADH by the supraoptic and paraventricular nuclei. ADH acts to increase renal free water reabsorption in the collecting tubule to restore plasma water, resulting in a correction of plasma sodium concentration back toward the normal range. The antidiuretic effect of ADH is mediated by binding to the vasopressin type 2 (V_2) receptor in the basolateral membrane of the collecting tubule. Binding of ADH leads to an increase in intracellular cyclic adenosine monophosphate (cAMP) and ultimately to the insertion of a water channel (aquaporin 2) into the luminal membrane and an increase in the aquaporin 2 mRNA level. Alternatively, as plasma water increases, plasma sodium concentration, osmolality, and ADH secretion decrease and the collecting tubule becomes impermeable to water, resulting in excretion of free water and restoration of the plasma sodium concentration.

Decreased arterial blood pressure can also act as a potent stimulus to ADH secretion, probably mediated by angiotensin II and neural inputs, even in the presence of hypo-osmolality. Decreased arterial pressure is sensed via baroreceptors in the aorta and carotid arteries. This can occur acutely during hypovolemia (e.g., blood loss) or chronically in disorders associated with decreased arterial perfusion (effective arterial blood volume), such as cirrhosis and heart failure.[1]

Disorders of water metabolism result from loss or gain of plasma water, often caused by or in association with altered conservation or release of water by the kidneys. Most of these disorders are caused by dysfunctional release or renal response to ADH.

Summary

- Hyponatremia and hypernatremia result mainly from disorders of water metabolism.
- Water metabolism is tightly regulated by hypothalamic osmoreceptors, ADH release, and an adequate renal response to ADH.
- Most disorders of water metabolism are caused by dysfunctional release or renal response to ADH.

HYPONATREMIA

Definition and Etiology

Hyponatremia is defined as a serum sodium concentration lower than 136 mmol/L.[2] It can result from a particular laboratory technique or from improper blood collection, excessively high water intake, or, most commonly, an inability of the kidneys to excrete free water (see later, "Pathophysiology and Natural History").[3]

Prevalence and Risk Factors

Hyponatremia is one of the most common electrolyte abnormalities. Indeed, approximately 15% of hospitalized patients have a plasma sodium concentration lower than 134 mmol/L. Patients with underlying severe dysfunction of the heart, liver, or kidneys are at greatest risk of developing hyponatremia. In addition, older women being treated with thiazide diuretics and premenstrual girls and women in the postoperative period, if given hypotonic fluids, are at higher risk for developing hyponatremia. Acute hyponatremia has also been reported in marathon runners and in those who ingest 3,4-methylenedioxymethylamphetamine (ecstasy).

Pathophysiology and Natural History

Hyponatremia can result from improper collection of a blood sample from a vein that is being infused with hypotonic medications. Additionally, if older techniques (e.g., flame photometry using whole plasma) for sodium measurement are being used, high levels of protein or triglyceride in the sample can cause the sodium concentration to be falsely low (pseudohyponatremia).[4] Hyperglycemia can also cause hyponatremia, via osmotically induced water movement from cells into the blood (translocational hyponatremia), resulting in a relative decrease in serum sodium concentration in the absence of hypo-osmolality. The sodium concentration should be increased by approximately 1.6 to 2 mmol/L for each 100-mg/dL increase in glucose concentration above 100 mg/dL.[4]

Excess water intake is a rare cause of hyponatremia. In persons with preserved renal function, any extra water intake above obligatory water loss is usually excreted in a dilute urine, hyponatremia does not develop. However, in psychogenic polydipsia, ingesting

Box 1 Drugs Associated With Increased Antidiuretic Hormone Release or Action

Amiodarone
Bromocriptine
Ciprofloxacin
Cisplatin
Desmopressin
Methylenedioxymethamphetamine (Ecstasy)
Oxytocin
Prostaglandin inhibitors
Phenothiazines
Tricyclics
Serotonin-reuptake inhibitors
Opiate derivatives
Chlorpropamide
Clofibrate
Carbamazepine
Cyclophosphamide
Vinblastine
Vincristine

Box 2 Causes of Hyponatremia Based on Extracellular Fluid Volume Status

Hypovolemia
Gastrointestinal solute loss (diarrhea, emesis)
Third-spacing (ileus, pancreatitis)
Diuretic use
Addison's disease
Salt-wasting nephritis

Euvolemic
Syndrome of inappropriate antidiuretic hormone (SIADH)
Diuretic use
Glucocorticoid deficiency
Hypothyroidism
Beer drinker's potomania, psychogenic polydipsia
Reset osmostat

Hypervolemia with Decreased Effective Circulating Blood Volume
Decompensated heart failure
Advanced liver cirrhosis
Renal failure with or without nephrosis

large volumes (>15-20 L/day) of water can result in hyponatremia, despite preserved renal function and diluting ability.

However, most cases of hyponatremia are caused by decreased renal excretion of water, secondary to persistent action of ADH or the use of medications that interfere with urinary dilution (e.g., thiazide diuretics and nonsteroidal anti-inflammatory drugs [NSAIDs]). Most of these clinical disorders (e.g., congestive heart failure, nephrotic syndrome, cirrhosis) share a reduction in effective arterial blood volume, resulting in persistent ADH activity despite hypo-osmolar plasma. In addition, acute or chronic renal failure results in reduced functional nephron mass, decreased glomerular filtration rate, and therefore decreased capacity for water excretion.

The drugs most commonly associated with the development of hyponatremia are thiazide diuretics and NSAIDs. The mechanism of diuretic-induced hyponatremia is complex and includes interference with urinary dilution by the thick ascending loop of Henle and the distal convoluted tubule, as well as volume contraction–induced increase in ADH secretion. Hyponatremia occurs almost exclusively with thiazide diuretics because of preservation in medullary osmolality and urine-concentrating ability. NSAIDs can lead to hyponatremia via a decrease in prostaglandin-mediated suppression of ADH. Many other drugs can be associated with hyponatremia via the augmentation of ADH release or action (Box 1).

Hyponatremia can also be seen in hypovolemic disorders where solute and water losses (e.g., diarrhea) result in hemodynamically mediated ADH release. Importantly, hyponatremia results only if these losses are replaced with a source of free water (e.g., hypotonic fluids).

Other, less-common causes of hyponatremia include a reset osmostat, adrenal insufficiency, hypothyroidism, low dietary solute intake, beer drinker's potomania, and salt-wasting nephropathy. Although the mechanisms of hyponatremia associated with adrenal or thyroid dysfunction are complex and not entirely clear, replacement of the deficient hormone usually leads to resolution of the hyponatremia, barring any other concomitant cause.

Signs and Symptoms

Most symptoms of hyponatremia are caused by cerebral edema from transcellular shifts of plasma water into cells of the central nervous system (CNS). Symptoms and signs usually do not manifest until the sodium concentration is lower than 125 mmol/L. These can include nausea, emesis, headache, seizures, lethargy, development of focal neurologic deficits, respiratory depression, and coma. Serious neurologic changes such as seizure and coma are usually not seen until the sodium concentration is lower than 110 to 115 mmol/L. Patients with rapidly developing severe hyponatremia (<120 mmol/L over 24-48 hours) are at highest risk for developing serious, life-threatening CNS disturbances.

Diagnosis

After sampling error, hyperglycemia, and pseudohyponatremia have been ruled out, the diagnosis of hyponatremia begins with careful examination of the patient's extracellular fluid (ECF) volume status (Box 2). Patients are classified as hypovolemic, euvolemic, or hypervolemic according to features of the history (e.g., emesis, diarrhea) and physical examination findings (e.g., flat or distended neck veins, dry or moist skin or mucosa, heart rate, blood pressure, orthostatic vital signs, presence of edema or ascites).

Patients with edema or ascites are, by definition, hypervolemic. Patients with hypotension, flat neck veins, dry mucosa, and no edema are hypovolemic. Other patients may be euvolemic or might have clinically undetectable forms of hypovolemia. Additional testing using determination of spot urine sodium, blood urea nitrogen (BUN), and serum uric acid levels and response to isotonic intravenous fluids may be helpful in this patient subgroup.

The presence of low urinary spot sodium (<10 mmol/L), normal or elevated serum uric acid, and elevated BUN levels suggest hypovolemia, whereas levels of urinary spot sodium higher than 10 to 20 mmol/L, low serum uric acid, and normal BUN imply that the ECF volume is not decreased. Additionally, the response of the serum sodium concentration to volume replacement may be helpful. In patients with hypovolemia, the serum sodium level should increase following administration of 1 to 2 L of normal saline. In patients with euvolemia, the serum sodium level will decrease further (e.g., syndrome of inappropriate antidiuretic hormone, SIADH) as water is reclaimed by the nephron, or the level will remain unchanged.

Urine osmolality is inappropriately high (>100 mOsm/kg)) in almost every patient with hyponatremia. It should be checked to confirm inappropriate urinary dilution, but it does not help delineate the cause of hyponatremia, except in patients found to have dilute urine (psychogenic polydipsia and reset osmostat).[3] Plasma osmolality (P_{osm}) is almost always low (<270 mOsm/kg) in patients with hyponatremia, because serum sodium is the major determinant of P_{osm}. If measured P_{osm} is more than 10 mOsm/kg higher than calculated osmolality ([2Na + BUN/2.8] + [glucose/18]), there is an effective osmole in the plasma other than sodium or glucose (e.g., mannitol, glycine, or sorbitol), or high levels of plasma protein or lipid causing pseudohyponatremia.

In euvolemic patients, or those with clinical suspicion of endocrine disorders, measures of thyroid function (thyroid-stimulating hormone [TSH] and free thyroid hormone level determination) and adrenal function (cosyntropin [Cortrosyn] stimulation test) can be assessed. Euvolemic patients with normal thyroid, adrenal, and renal function might have SIADH. This syndrome is associated with various drugs (see Box 1) and clinical disorders including pulmonary infections, ectopic production by certain cancers (particularly small cell lung carcinoma), various CNS disorders, and pain.

Treatment

Appropriate treatment of any patient with truly hypo-osmolar hyponatremia, regardless of its cause or the patient's ECF volume status, begins with a thorough clinical assessment that aims to answer the following questions[5]:

- Is the patient having any signs or symptoms of cerebral edema?
- What is the time frame for the development of the hyponatremia?
- Does the patient have risk factors for developing neurologic complications from hyponatremia or its treatment?

Hyponatremia is considered to be of acute onset if it develops in less than 48 hours. Patients who develop hyponatremia acutely almost always do so during hospitalization, and often during the postoperative period. Chronic hyponatremia is defined as that developing over a time course longer than 48 hours. In patients for whom the time frame is unknown, it should be assumed that they developed hyponatremia chronically. Alternatively, an imaging study assessing for cerebral edema can be performed.

The distinction between acute and chronic hyponatremia is made to alert the clinician to the clinical consequences associated with the timing of the cerebral response to hyponatremia. As water enters the brain cells during acute hyponatremia, there is a loss of intracellular sodium and potassium in an attempt to prevent further water entry. Over the next several days, additional osmolytes are lost from the brain (e.g., inositol). If hyponatremia is corrected too rapidly, regardless of the method of correction, excess water can be lost from the cells, resulting in cellular dehydration and central pontine myelinosis (CPM).[2] CPM is characterized by demyelination of neurons and the development of neurologic dysfunction, including seizures, dysphagia, dysarthria, paresis, and even death. Thus, the patient with chronic hyponatremia is at greater risk of developing CPM if the hyponatremia is corrected too rapidly.

All patients with symptomatic hyponatremia should be treated with hypertonic (3%) saline at 1 to 2 mEq/L/hour along with intravenous furosemide if there is evidence of hypervolemia.[5] The saline is used to increase free water excretion via interference with urinary-concentrating ability and to avoid worsening of hypervolemia from the intravenous sodium load. The serum sodium level should be followed closely and should not be corrected to normal with hypertonic saline. The goal of hypertonic saline is to bring sodium up to a safer level—usually approximately 125 mEq/L—while ameliorating neurologic signs and symptoms.[6]

Although the exact rate of correction is a matter of debate, acute hyponatremia should not be corrected by more than 2 mEq/L/hour. Chronic hyponatremia or hyponatremia of unknown duration should be corrected by no more than 0.5 mEq/L/hour or no more than 10 to 12 mEq/day. If the patient with chronic hyponatremia presents with severe symptoms, a more rapid initial rate of correction, 1 to 2 mEq/L/hour over the first few hours, is advisable to ameliorate neurologic morbidity. However, the sodium level should not be raised more than 12 mEq/L during the first day of treatment.

The clinician should be aware that the risk of hyponatremia-induced cerebral edema is increased in certain patient groups and characteristics, including hypoxemia, older women on thiazide diuretics, postoperative menstruating girls and women, children, and patients with psychogenic polydipsia.[5] Additionally, patients at higher risk for developing CPM include alcoholics, older women on thiazide diuretics, burn victims, and patients with malnutrition or severe concomitant potassium depletion.[5] Patients at higher risk for CPM should be monitored closely and undergo slower rates of correction.

Patients with asymptomatic chronic hyponatremia do not need immediate correction. The clinician should focus on determining the cause of the hyponatremia (see earlier, "Diagnosis") and assessing the ECF volume status. The ECF volume status directs the initial therapeutic approach.

Hypovolemia

In patients with hypovolemia, volume should be restored with normal saline to reduce the nonosmotic stimulus to ADH secretion.

Hypervolemia

Patients with clinical evidence of hypervolemia should undergo sodium and water restriction. Furosemide should be used to control volume and promote free water excretion. If possible, the underlying illness should be treated (e.g., angiotensin-converting enzyme [ACE] inhibitor for heart failure). This is often difficult, because hyponatremia is usually a manifestation of severe underlying disease (e.g., severe decompensated heart failure or cirrhosis). Data from clinical trials indicate that V_2 receptor antagonists (e.g., tolvaptan) promote solute-free water loss and thus may be effective therapies for hypervolemic hyponatremia.[7]

Euvolemia

In patients who are euvolemic, there are three methods to raise the serum sodium level: fluid restriction, increased solute intake (salt tablets or oral urea) plus furosemide to increase obligate water excretion, and pharmacologic inhibition of ADH action with lithium, V_2 receptor antagonists, or demeclocycline. Pharmacologic inhibition of ADH is generally reserved for patients who are unresponsive to or cannot tolerate fluid restriction or increased solute intake plus furosemide. Lithium use has declined secondary to the frequent development of adverse effects. Demeclocycline is usually started at a dose of 300 mg twice daily and the dosage titrated to up to 1200 mg/day in divided doses. Vasopressin antagonists have been reported to be efficacious in treating the hyponatremia associated with SIADH.[7]

Vasopressin Receptor Antagonists

Pharmacologic antagonists of the V_2 receptor exert their aquaretic effect via a decrease in transcription and insertion of aquaporin-2 channels into the apical collecting duct membrane, resulting in decreased water permeability even in the presence of circulating vasopressin. Vasopressin action (agonism) occurs via interactions with various receptor subtypes including V_{1a} (vasoconstriction, platelet aggregation, ionotropic stimulation, myocardial protein synthesis), V_{1b} (ACTH secretion) and V_2 (water reabsorption, von Willebrand factor and factor VIII release).

Conivaptan is a combined V_{1a}/V_2 antagonist that has been FDA approved for the treatment of euvolemic and hypervolemic hyponatremia.[8] As a result of concerns regarding drug interactions due to its inhibition of the cytochrome P-450 (CYP) 3A4 system, use of conivaptan has been limited to the hospital setting using the intravenous formulation for up to 4 days. Dosing recommendations are for an initial 20-mg infusion over 30 minutes, followed by daily continuous infusions of 20 to 40 mg/day. Dosing adjustments in renal and hepatic impairment have not been well defined. Conivaptan should not be used in patients with hypovolemic hyponatremia due to concerns with V_{1a} blockade causing hypotension or V_2

blockade producing water excretion and a worsening of the volume-depleted state. Further studies are needed in patients with cirrhosis, because V_{1a} antagonism may be expected to cause a decrease in systemic blood pressure or even a worsening of portal hypertension via splanchnic vasodilation. Alternatively, patients with heart failure and hyponatremia theoretically might benefit from V_{1a} antagonism-induced vasodilatation, but further studies are needed to clarify this issue.

Tolvaptan is an oral selective V_2 receptor antagonist that is effective at raising serum sodium in patients with hypervolemic and euvolemic hyponatremia. Data indicate that this agent might improve symptoms and result in enhanced weight loss in patients with decompensated heart failure.[9] However, long-term end points including mortality and rehospitalization rate were not significantly improved.

Although there have been some cases of excessive increase in serum sodium during therapy with vasopressin antagonists, available data suggest that these agents are safe, with no reported case of CPM in any of the clinical trials. An increase in thirst has been described in some of these studies, highlighting the need to continue with water restriction and careful monitoring of serum sodium levels when these agents are made available for use in clinical practice. No data are available regarding the use of vasopressin antagonists in the treatment of hyponatremia in the presence of severe neurologic symptoms. Hypertonic saline should be considered the treatment of choice in this population.

Summary

- Determine the patient's volume status.
- Classify rate of development of hyponatremia: acute versus chronic.
- Determine the proper rate of correction: Acute hyponatremia must be corrected rapidly but not faster than 2 mEq/L/hr; chronic hyponatremia must be corrected slowly, 0.5 mEq/L/hr.

HYPERNATREMIA

Definition and Causes

Hypernatremia is defined as a serum sodium concentration greater than 145 mmol/L.[10] It is most commonly caused by the loss of water via the skin, urine, or gastrointestinal (GI) tract. In all cases, loss of access to water or impaired thirst sensation is required to maintain the hypernatremic state (see later, "Pathophysiology and Natural History").

Prevalence and Risk Factors

Hypernatremia can develop in outpatient and inpatient settings. When it develops in the outpatient setting, it is most commonly seen in patients at the extremes of age. In the hospital, hypernatremia develops across a more general age distribution. In both settings, patients at highest risk are those who depend on others to adequately assess and provide water intake, such as breast-feeding infants, older nursing home residents, and the critically ill. Although estimates in large populations are not available, one observational study has suggested that approximately 1% of hospitalized patients have a serum sodium level higher than 150 mmol/L.[11]

Pathophysiology and Natural History

An increase in serum sodium concentration is almost always a reflection of water loss rather than sodium gain. Water loss results in the development of plasma hyperosmolality; via hypothalamic sensors, this acts as a stimulant to thirst and production of ADH. Ultimately, free water is ingested and reclaimed via the kidneys, and sodium concentration and osmolality are restored to normal. Thus, the maintenance of hypernatremia requires diminished thirst sensation or decreased access to water. Even in states of impaired ADH release or reduced ADH function at the level of the kidneys (e.g., central or nephrogenic diabetes insipidus), hypernatremia is avoided if thirst is intact and access to free water is maintained in adequate amounts to compensate for renal losses.

Hypernatremia is not always associated with pure water loss. It can be associated with concomitant loss of sodium via hypotonic fluids (e.g., diarrheal fluid) or the addition of hypertonic fluids (e.g., excessive sodium from parenteral nutrition or sodium bicarbonate infusion).

Hypernatremia causes a loss of intracellular water into the ECF space and can be associated with cellular shrinkage. In the CNS, this can be catastrophic, with ensuing cell death or rupture of blood vessels. To protect against cell shrinkage, electrolytes enter into the ICF, usually in the first few hours. When hypernatremia persists beyond 2 or 3 days, the cells begin to generate intracellular osmolytes to maintain intracellular fluid (ICF) osmolarity further and avoid water loss into the ECF.

Signs and Symptoms

Most signs and symptoms relate to the underlying illness that is driving water loss (e.g., diarrhea, nausea, emesis, insensible loss from fever) and the condition causing decreased intake of water (e.g., delirium, dementia). Hypernatremia should cause an increase in thirst in the absence of altered sensorium or a new neurologic lesion involving the hypothalamus. The presence of polyuria (>3 L urine/day) should be noted, because this indicates renal loss of water via a solute diuresis (e.g., mannitol, urea, glucose) or pure water diuresis (e.g., diabetes insipidus). As noted, hypernatremia causes cellular dehydration, leading to a myriad of findings, including muscle cramps, seizures, headache, intracranial hemorrhage, lethargy, coma, and death. Patients might also have signs and symptoms of volume depletion if sodium has been lost along with water (e.g., hypotonic losses with diarrhea).

Diagnosis

Figure 1 illustrates important causes of hypernatremia correlating with the bedside determination of the ECF volume status. Patients with euvolemia usually have had a pure water loss. Patients with evidence of reduced ECF volume and hypernatremia have predominantly developed a water loss; however, they have also had some loss of sodium from the ECF to account for the clinical signs of hypovolemia.

Accurate diagnosis requires that the clinician uncover the source of water loss or sodium gain. A careful assessment of the patient's volume status, access to water, ongoing water losses, and renal response to water loss are also important (see Fig. 1). Additionally, if impaired thirst is present, the clinician should inquire into possible causes, such as delirium (e.g., from any cause) or the development of a new lesion in the CNS (e.g., stroke).

Whereas the cause of hypernatremia is usually apparent (e.g., diarrhea), the urine osmolality may be useful in clarifying the cause in patients without obvious GI or insensible water losses. During hypernatremia caused by extrarenal water losses, the renal response should be to generate a hypertonic urine with an osmolality of 700 to 800 mOsm/kg.

If the urine osmolality (U_{osm}) is lower than 300 mOsm/kg, then water loss is occurring via the kidneys, secondary to decreased hypothalamic release of ADH (central diabetes insipidus) or impaired sensation in the cortical collecting tubule (nephrogenic diabetes insipidus). In central diabetes insipidus, provision of ADH results in

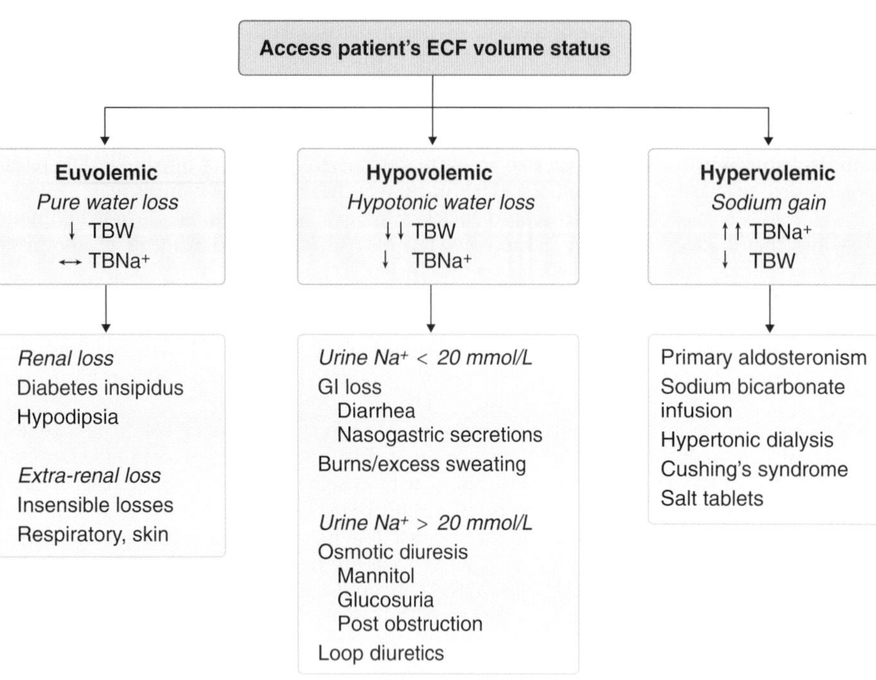

Figure 1 Important causes of hypernatremia correlating with the bedside determination of the ECF volume status. ECF, extracellular fluid; GI, gastrointestinal; $TBNa^+$, total body sodium; TBW, total body water.

an increase in U_{osm}, whereas in nephrogenic diabetes insipidus, it results in little to no increase in U_{osm}.

If U_{osm} is between 300 and 800 mOsm/kg, patients might have partial forms of nephrogenic or central diabetes insipidus or an osmotic diuresis from urea or glucose. In patients believed to have diabetes insipidus, a water deprivation test can be performed to assess the integrity of pituitary release and renal response to ADH.[12]

Treatment

The management of hypernatremia involves the following principles:

- Replacement of the water deficit
- Correction of the underlying cause of water loss

Importantly, if hypovolemia is present, plasma volume should be restored with isotonic saline or colloid *before* the correction of the water deficit. Correction of the underlying cause of the water losses can include withdrawal of loop diuretics or mannitol, treatment of diarrhea with antimotility agents or antibiotics, provision of ADH to correct central diabetes insipidus, or use of pharmacologic agents to treat nephrogenic diabetes insipidus (see later).

Correction of the water loss requires an assessment of the current water deficit and ongoing rate of water losses. The following equation can be used to estimate the water deficit:

$$\text{Water deficit} = \text{TBW} \times \left(1 - \text{current}\left[\text{Na}^+\right]/140\right)$$

where TBW (total body weight) = 0.6 × weight (in kg) for male patients, or 0.5 × weight (in kg) for female and obese patients. The factor of multiplication may be closer to 0.4 in critically ill cachectic patients.

The rate of correction is controversial, but most experts recommend that in the absence of symptoms of hypernatremia, the serum sodium level should be corrected by no more than 0.5 mEq/L/hour. To avoid the development of cerebral edema, the water deficit should not be replaced too quickly. Severely symptomatic patients require a more rapid correction to ameliorate symptoms. Once symptoms have abated, the pace of water provision is decreased to allow a rate of correction of 0.5 mEq/L/hour. The actual rate of fluid replacement needs to account for ongoing fluid losses (e.g., GI and insensible).

It must be remembered that this is only an estimate. The serum sodium level and neurologic function should be monitored frequently to ensure the proper rate of correction.

In patients with central diabetes insipidus, ADH must be provided exogenously via intranasal or oral desmopressin (DDAVP). In more acute cases, with large water losses, ADH can be replaced with subcutaneous aqueous vasopressin. In the absence of a reversible cause (e.g., hypercalcemia, hypokalemia), patients with nephrogenic diabetes insipidus are generally treated chronically with a low-sodium, low-protein diet along with a thiazide diuretic. The diuretic and low-sodium diet act to create a mild volume depletion and therefore result in a reduction in urine output. A decrease in protein intake results in a decrease in obligate renal solute excretion and therefore a decrease in water excretion and urine flow.

In patients with hypervolemic hypernatremia, sources of hypertonic fluids containing excess sodium (e.g., parenteral nutrition, sodium bicarbonate) should be eliminated. In addition, a loop diuretic is administered to promote sodium loss and correct hypervolemia. Dialysis may be required if there is concomitant renal failure.

Summary

- Calculate the water deficit.
- Replace isotonic losses if the patient is hypovolemic.
- Replace water deficit plus ongoing fluid losses.
- The rate of correction should be approximately 0.5 mEq/L/hr to avoid cerebral edema.

Suggested Readings

Adrogue HJ, Madias NE: Hypernatremia. N Engl J Med 2000;342:1493-1499.

Adrogue HJ, Madias NE: Hyponatremia. N Engl J Med 2000;342:1581-1589.

Freda BJ, Davidson MB, Hall PM: Evaluation of hyponatremia: A little physiology goes a long way. Cleve Clin J Med 2004;71:639-650.

Gross P, Reimann D, Neidel J, et al: The treatment of severe hyponatremia. Kidney Int Suppl 1998;64:S6-S11.

Lauriat SM, Berl T: The hyponatremic patient: Practical focus on therapy. J Am Soc Nephrol 1997;8:1599-1607.

Oster JR, Singer I: Hyponatremia, hyposmolality, and hypotonicity: Tables and fables. Arch Intern Med 1999;159:333-336.

Palevsky PM, Bhagrath R, Greenberg A: Hypernatremia in hospitalized patients. Ann Intern Med 1996;124:197-203.

Pham PC, Pham PM, Pham PT: Vasopressin excess and hyponatremia. Am J Kidney Dis 2006;47:727-737.

Sands JM, Bichet DG: Nephrogenic diabetes insipidus. Ann Intern Med 2006;144:186-194.

Schrier RW: Body fluid volume regulation in health and disease: A unifying hypothesis. Ann Intern Med 1990;113:155-159.

References

For a complete list of references, log onto www.expertconsult.com.

Hypokalemia and Hyperkalemia

Boon Wee Teo and Saul Nurko

PHYSIOLOGY OF POTASSIUM HANDLING

Potassium (K^+) is the most abundant cation in the body. About 90% of total body potassium is intracellular and 10% is in extracellular fluid, of which less than 1% is composed of plasma. The ratio of intracellular to extracellular potassium determines neuromuscular and cardiovascular excitability, which is why serum potassium is normally regulated within a narrow range of 3.5 to 5.0 mmol/L. Dietary K^+ intake is highly variable, ranging from as low as 40 mmol/day to more than 100 mmol/day.[1,2] Homeostasis is maintained by two systems. One regulates K^+ excretion, or external balance through the kidneys and intestines, and the second regulates K^+ shifts, or internal balance between intracellular and extracellular fluid compartments. Internal balance is mainly mediated by insulin and catecholamines.

Cellular Shifts

Ingested K^+ is absorbed rapidly and enters the portal circulation, where it stimulates insulin secretion. Insulin increases Na^+,K^+-ATPase activity and facilitates potassium entry into cells, thereby averting hyperkalemia. β_2-Adrenergic stimulation also promotes entry of K^+ into cells through increased cyclic adenosine monophosphate (cAMP) activation of Na^+,K^+-ATPase.

Renal Handling

An increase in extracellular potassium concentration also stimulates aldosterone secretion (via angiotensin II), and aldosterone increases K^+ excretion. In the steady state, K^+ excretion matches intake, and approximately 90% is excreted by the kidneys and 10% in the stool. Renal K^+ excretion is mediated by aldosterone and sodium (Na^+) delivery (glomerular filtration rate [GFR]) in principal cells of the collecting ducts.[3] K^+ is freely filtered by the glomerulus, and almost all the filtered K^+ is reabsorbed in the proximal tubule and loop of Henle (Fig. 1). This absorption in the proximal part of the nephron passively follows that of Na^+ and water, whereas reabsorption in the thick ascending limb of the loop of Henle is mediated by the $Na^+,K^+,2Cl^-$ carrier (NKCC2) in the luminal membrane. K^+ is secreted by the connecting segment, the principal cells (see Fig. 1) in the cortical and outer medullary collecting tubule, and the papillary (or inner medullary) collecting duct via luminal potassium channels (ROMK). Secretion in these segments varies according to physiologic requirements, and is responsible for most of the urinary potassium excretion. Secretion in the distal segments is also balanced by K^+ reabsorption through the intercalated cells (see Fig. 1) in the cortical and outer medullary collecting tubules. This process is mediated by an active H^+,K^+-ATPase pump in the luminal membrane and results in both proton secretion and K^+ reabsorption. The kidneys are better at increasing K^+ excretion than decreasing excretion. As a result, K^+ depletion and hypokalemia can occur from inadequate intake. Hyperkalemia usually occurs when renal excretion is impaired (GFR <20 mL/min).

Summary

- Potassium homeostasis is maintained by the balance of potassium excretion and potassium cellular shifts.
- Potassium excretion is tightly regulated by the kidneys.
- Potassium cellular shifts are principally mediated by hormones.

HYPOKALEMIA

Definition

Hypokalemia is defined as a serum potassium concentration below 3.5 mmol/L. Hypokalemia can be further arbitrarily graded by severity.

Relative severity is defined as:

$$3.5 < [K^+] < 4.0 \text{ mmol/L}$$

This applies to certain high-risk patient populations with cardiac disease, such as ischemic or scarred myocardium, left ventricular hypertrophy, congestive heart failure, or myocardial infarction).

Moderate severity is defined as:

$$2.5 < [K^+] < 3.5 \text{ mmol/L}$$

Severe hypokalemia is defined as:

$$[K^+] < 2.5 \text{ mmol/L}$$

Prevalence

Hypokalemia is found in about 20% of hospitalized patients, but it occurs in less than 1% of otherwise healthy adults.

Pathophysiology

Hypokalemia can result from transcellular shifts (from extracellular into intracellular spaces), or when potassium losses are increased; these losses can be from renal or nonrenal causes (Box 1). Transcellular shifts can occur in pathologic conditions associated with a catecholamine surge, such as chest pain syndromes, or mediated by acid-base disturbances. Loop or thiazide diuretic use, aldosteronism, or other renal diseases (e.g., postobstructive diuresis, cortical necrosis) can cause excessive renal potassium losses. The renal and nonrenal causes of K^+ loss can be determined by laboratory tests (Fig. 2).

Clinical Effects

Normal individuals with hypokalemia are usually asymptomatic. Manifestations of hypokalemia include generalized muscle weakness, ileus, and cardiac arrhythmias. In patients with ischemic or scarred myocardium, left ventricular hypertrophy, congestive heart failure,

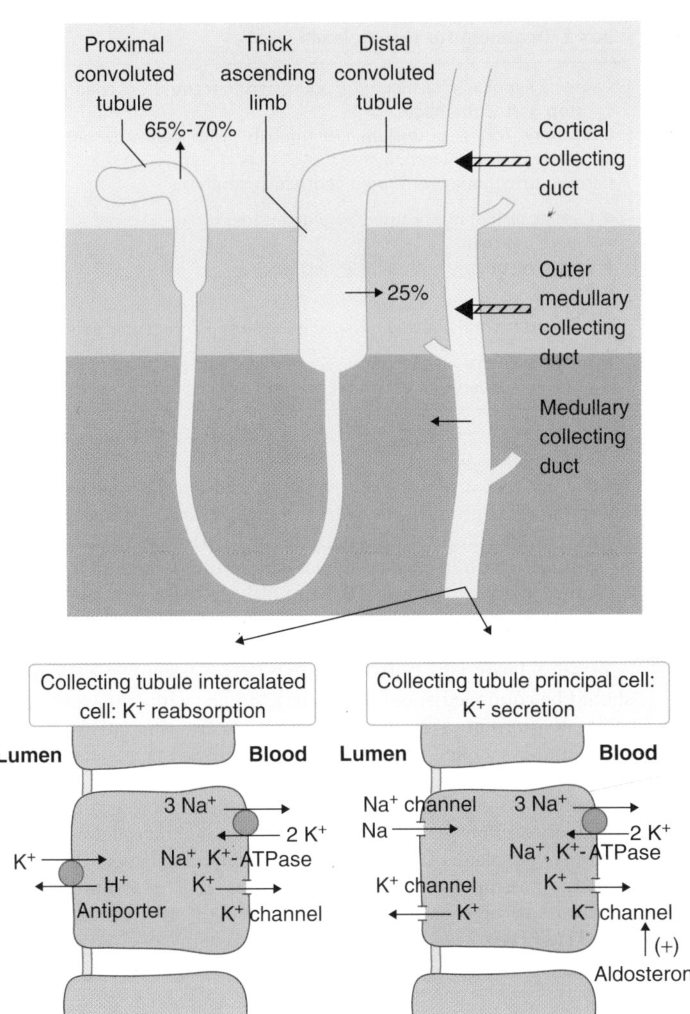

Figure 1 **Renal handling of potassium.** Almost all of the filtered K is reabsorbed in the proximal tubule and the loop of Henle. *Black arrows* represent percent of potassium reabsorbed at proximal tubule (thick ascending limb and medullary). *Dashed arrows* represent sites of potassium secretion in the cortical collecting duct (CCD) and medullary collecting duct.

or myocardial infarction, hypokalemia is associated with an increased incidence of ventricular ectopy, ventricular tachycardia, and ventricular fibrillation. In those patients with heart disease at risk for serious ventricular tachyarrhythmias, even relative hypokalemia ($[K^+]$ = 3.5 to 4.0 mmol/L) may require potassium supplementation to prevent development of overt hypokalemia. More severe hypokalemia (<2.5 mmol/L) can cause myopathy that can progress to rhabdomyolysis, and ascending paralysis with respiratory arrest (<2.0 mmol/L; see Box 1).

Diagnostic Workup

When hypokalemia is reported, the initial step is to ascertain whether it is associated with clinical symptoms or arrhythmias that would require prompt intervention. In the absence of compelling indications for immediate therapy, a careful history and physical examination should be performed. Important clinical clues such as medication, vomiting, and hypertension should be specifically sought. Factitious or spurious hypokalemia, which can occur in patients with leukemia or elevated white cell counts because K^+ is taken up by these metabolically active cells in the test tube, should be ruled out. If true hypokalemia is present, then determine whether it was caused by a transcellular shift or a decrease in total body potassium. Hypokalemia from transcellular shift is managed by treating the underlying condition or removing the offending agent. Decreased total body K^+ require further diagnostic workup. Urine potassium, chloride, creatinine, and serum aldosterone levels are determined to distinguish the causes of extrarenal and renal losses of K^+ so that the primary condition can be treated, in addition to replacement therapy (see Fig. 2).

Urine Potassium, Fractional Excretion, and Transtubular Potassium Gradient

The spot urine potassium concentration, fractional excretion of potassium (FE_K), and transtubular potassium gradient (TTKG) can be used to help differentiate between renal and nonrenal causes of hypokalemia and hyperkalemia.[4-7] The spot urine K^+ level is helpful for determining renal and nonrenal causes of hypokalemia; a urinary potassium (U_K) level higher than 20 mmol/L is suggestive of renal causes and a U_K level lower than 20 mmol/L suggestive of nonrenal causes. Accuracy is improved with a 24-hour urine collection for K^+ because K^+ secretion and water reabsorption affect K^+ excretion.[7,8]

When serum and urine creatinine levels are known, FE_K can be calculated.[4,5] FE_K is the percentage of filtered potassium that appears in the urine; it represents the K^+ clearance (Cl_K) corrected for the GFR, as determined by creatinine clearance (Cl_{Cr}): Cl_K/Cl_{Cr}. Because clearance for any substance is UV/P, where U is the concentration of that substance in urine, V is the volume per unit time, and P is the plasma concentration, then:

$$FE_K = (U_K V/P_K)/(U_{Cr} V/P_{Cr}) \times 100\%$$

Or, to simplify, because V cancels out,

$$FE_K = (U_K/P_K)/(U_{Cr}/P_{Cr}) \times 100\%$$

Box 1 Causes of Hypokalemia

Increased Excretion

Nonrenal losses (urine $K^+ < 20$ mmol/L)

- Diarrhea, laxative abuse
- Vomiting

Renal losses (urine K^+ >?20 mmol/L)

- Loop diuretics (furosemide, bumetanide, torsemide): block chloride-coupled sodium reabsorption in the loop of Henle
- Thiazide diuretics (hydrochlorothiazide): block distal tubule chloride-coupled sodium reabsorption
- Osmotic diuresis (uncontrolled diabetes)

Hypokalemia with hypertension

- Mineralocorticoid excess
- Primary hyperaldosteronism
- Glucocorticoid-remediable aldosteronism: renovascular hypertension, renin-secreting tumor, Liddle syndrome
- Apparent mineralocorticoid excess: 11β-hydroxysteroid dehydrogenase deficiency (genetic, drug induced [chewing tobacco, licorice], congenital adrenal hyperplasia)

Hypokalemia with normal blood pressure

- Bartter's syndrome
- Gitelman's syndrome
- Magnesium depletion (*cis*-platinum, alcoholism)
- Renal tubular acidosis (types 1 and 2)

Transcellular Shifts

Drugs-insulin administration

β-Adrenergic agonists (bronchodilators, decongestants, tocolytic agents)-theophylline, caffeine

Acute catecholamine surge from stress (e.g., acute myocardial infarction)

Delirium tremens

Thyrotoxic hypokalemic paralysis

Familial hypokalemic periodic paralysis

Barium poisoning-metabolic alkalosis

In a person with normal renal function and average potassium intake, FE_K is approximately 10%. Hypokalemic patients with a lower FE_K would suggest extrarenal loss of K^+, whereas hypokalemia from renal losses would be associated with an elevated FE_K.

The TTKG estimates the potassium gradient between the urine and blood in the distal nephron.[6,7] It is calculated as

$$TTKG = (U_K/P_K)/(U_{Osm}/P_{Osm})$$

where U_{Osm} and P_{Osm} are the urine and plasma osmolalities, respectively. The numerator is an estimate of the luminal potassium concentration, and the osmolality ratio is used to correct for the increase in U_K caused by water extraction. In normal individuals under normal conditions, the TTKG is about 6 to 8. Hypokalemia associated with a high TTKG (>10) suggests excessive renal potassium loss, whereas a low TTKG (<2) would suggest nonrenal losses. A value of 5 to 7 suggests aldosterone deficiency or resistance. In hyperkalemic patients, a value greater than 10 suggests normal aldosterone action and an extrarenal cause of hyperkalemia.

The usefulness of the FE_K and TTKG is limited by their variability with diet and chronic kidney disease. These indices increase and decrease with dietary K^+ accordingly. Moreover, in patients with chronic kidney disease (lower GFR), adaptive responses increase K^+ excretion, with resultant increases in FE_K and TTKG. Therefore, the normal values will vary, making the interpretation of significance difficult.

Treatment

Intravenous potassium administration is rarely indicated because of the risk of hyperkalemia, except for cardiac arrhythmias (rapid ventricular response), severe myopathy, and paralysis (usually $[K^+]$ lower than 2.0 mmol/L, or with familial periodic paralysis). Continuous cardiac monitoring is preferred, with no more than 20 mmol/hr administered, and reassessment of the serum potassium level after 60 mmol is given. For every 0.3-mmol/L decrease in serum potassium concentration, the total body potassium deficit is approximately 100 mmol/L. Patients with relative hypokalemia (e.g., congestive heart failure [CHF] patients on diuretics or digoxin), should be counseled about adequate K^+ intake with fruits and vegetables to prevent overt hypokalemia. Because almost all dietary potassium is coupled with phosphate, hypokalemia associated with chloride depletion (e.g., diuretic use, vomiting, nasogastric drainage) can only be effectively corrected with potassium chloride administration. Concomitant hypomagnesemia has to be corrected as well to correct hypokalemia fully. Magnesium depletion reduces the intracellular potassium concentration and causes renal potassium wasting; it appears to be caused by an impairment of cell membrane Na^+, K^+-ATPase (Box 2).

Box 2 Treatment for Hypokalemia

Cause of hypokalemia should be addressed (remove drug, change diet, stop gastric drainage).

Indications for IV potassium (20 mmol/hr with cardiac monitoring, reassess after 60 mmol):

Cardiac arrhythmias with rapid ventricular response

- Cardiac arrhythmias caused by digoxin toxicity
- Severe diarrhea
- Severe myopathy with muscle necrosis
- Paralysis

Indications for oral potassium chloride (20-80 mmol/day in divided doses):

- All other situations except for renal tubular acidosis: replace with oral potassium bicarbonate, citrate, acetate, or gluconate.

Summary

Management of Hypokalemia

- Ascertain whether it is associated with clinical manifestations, such as arrythmias, which require immediate treatment.
- Even relative hypokalemia can be of consequence in high-risk patients.
- A careful history and a physical examination should be done, especially looking for evidence of catecholamine surge, hypertension, vomiting or diarrhea, and medication use.

HYPERKALEMIA

Definition

Hyperkalemia is defined as a serum potassium concentration higher than 5.0 mmol/L, and severe hyperkalemia is defined as a serum potassium concentration higher than 6.5 mmol/L. An elevated potassium level occurs when potassium homeostasis is disrupted. Pseudohyperkalemia can occur with thrombocytosis, hemolysis, and extremely high white cell counts. In these cases, lysis of the cells in the test tube releases potassium into the serum and increases potassium concentrations. Repeated fist clenching with a tourniquet can also release K^+ from muscle cells and increase potassium concentrations factitiously.

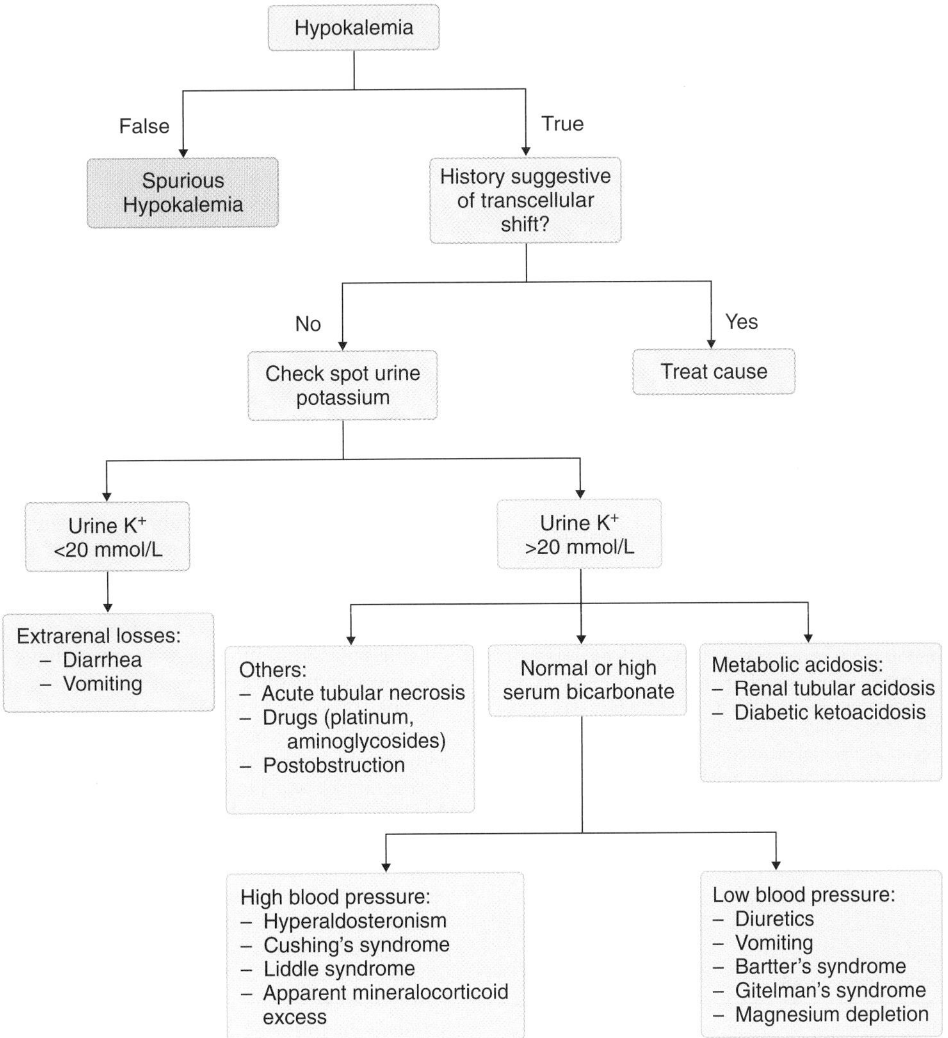

Figure 2 **Hypokalemia-diagnostic algorithm.**

Prevalence

The reported incidence of hyperkalemia is from 1.1% to 10% of all hospitalized patients. Mortality data caused by hyperkalemia are unavailable for the general population but accounted for 1.9% of patients with end-stage renal disease in the United States in 1993.

Pathophysiology

More than 80% of hyperkalemic episodes are caused by impaired potassium excretion from renal insufficiency.[1] Usually, another event that prevents or overcomes the renal adaptation precipitates the hyperkalemia. Supplemental potassium chloride administration is commonly the second event and this added potassium can be from exogenous (e.g., diet, salt substitutes) or endogenous sources (e.g., tumor lysis, gastrointestinal bleed, rhabdomyolysis). Impaired K^+ excretion or impaired potassium entry into cells accounts for all other causes of hyperkalemia. Drugs such as potassium-sparing diuretics (e.g., spironolactone, triamterene), or drugs that block aldosterone production or receptors (e.g., eplerenone, angiotensin-converting enzyme [ACE] inhibitors, nonsteroidal anti-inflammatory drugs [NSAIDs], heparin) impair the excretion of K^+. Potassium entry into cells is impaired with insulin deficiency, hypertonicity, or drugs (e.g., beta blockers, digoxin; Box 3).

Clinical Effects

Patients with hyperkalemia are usually asymptomatic, although some patients may present with generalized muscle weakness, and cardiac conduction may be impaired. The earliest electrocardiographic changes are tenting of T waves, followed by widening of the QRS complex, atrioventricular conduction block, ventricular fibrillation, and then asystole. The serum potassium concentrations are poorly correlated to the electrocardiographic and conduction abnormalities. However, the toxic effects of hyperkalemia are enhanced by hypocalcemia, hyponatremia, and acidemia.[9]

Diagnostic Workup

The initial step with reported hyperkalemia is to ascertain whether it is associated with clinical symptoms or arrhythmias that would require prompt intervention. If no compelling indication for immediate therapy exists, a careful history and physical examination should be performed, with particular emphasis on medication, diet, and chronic kidney disease. Spurious hyperkalemia should be excluded. This can occur with hemolysis in vitro, fist clenching during blood draw, leukocytosis (>50,000/mm^3), or severe thrombocytosis (>1,000,000/mm^3). A plasma K^+ determination, instead of serum determination, is sometimes necessary in addition, spurious hyperkalemia will not be associated with abnormalities on the electrocardiogram (ECG). If hyperkalemia is indeed present, then determine whether it occurred with a transcellular shift or reduction in potassium excretion, or in the setting of preserved renal function.

Box 3 Causes of Hyperkalemia

Spurious

- Thrombocytosis (>1,000,000/mm^3)
- Leukocytosis (>50,000/mm^3)
- Hemolysis
- Repeated fist clenching with tourniquet in place

Impaired potassium excretion

- Renal insufficiency or failure
- Mineralocorticoid deficiency
- Addison's disease
- Hyporenin hypoaldosteronism (type 4 renal tubular acidosis)
- Hereditary enzyme deficiencies

Pseudohypoaldosteronism
Drugs

- Block sodium channel in distal nephron-trimethoprim, pentamidine, potassium-sparing diuretics (amiloride, triamterene)
- Block aldosterone production: ACE inhibitors, angiotensin receptor blockers, NSAIDs, and COX-2 inhibitors, heparin, tacrolimus
- Block aldosterone receptors: spironolactone, eplerenone
- Block Na^+,K^+-ATPase activity in the distal nephron: cyclosporine

Impaired transcellular shift-insulin deficiency
Hypertonicity (uncontrolled diabetes): familial hyperkalemic periodic paralysis

- Drugs-beta blockers, digoxin (at toxic levels), succinylcholine, arginine, lysine

Excessive potassium load
Massive tissue breakdown (rhabdomyolysis, burns, trauma)

ACE, angiotensin-converting enzyme; COX-2, Cyclooxygenase-2; NSAID, nonsteroidal anti-inflammatory drug.

Hyperkalemia from transcellular shift occurs with insulin deficiency, hypertonicity (e.g., uncontrolled diabetes), massive tissue breakdown (e.g., rhabdomyolysis, burns, trauma), or familial hyperkalemic periodic paralysis. Impaired renal function (usually, estimated GFR from stable serum creatinine level <20 mL/min) can cause hyperkalemia. In the setting of preserved renal function (GFR >20 mL/min), serum aldosterone, renin, and cortisol levels can distinguish other causes (Fig. 3).

The urine potassium concentration, FE_K, and TTKG can also be used to help distinguish between renal and nonrenal causes of hyperkalemia. Renal causes will be associated with a low TTKG (see earlier, "Urine Potassium, Fractional Excretion, and Transtubular Potassium Gradient").

Treatment

We believe that therapy should be initiated regardless of the cause of hyperkalemia when potassium levels are higher than 6.5 mmol/L or if there are conduction abnormalities on the ECG. Intravenous calcium is required for rapid reversal of conduction abnormalities that are present. An exception to this is hyperkalemia caused by digoxin toxicity because acute hypercalcemia can potentiate the toxic effects of digoxin. Acute therapy is also directed at rapidly moving potassium into cells with intravenous dextrose and insulin. This moves potassium into cells within 10 to 20 minutes and lowers the potassium level by 0.5 to 1.0 mmol/L, with the effect lasting for about 2 to 3 hours. Longer term therapy for hyperkalemia without conduction abnormalities should be directed toward minimizing intake and increasing excretion of potassium. Medications that affect potassium homeostasis should be stopped, if possible. Although there are no prospective studies on inpatient versus outpatient management of hyperkalemia, it would seem intuitive that patients with hyperkalemia associated with abnormalities on the ECG, or rapid increases in or large changes from baseline potassium concentrations, should be admitted for therapy under continuous cardiac monitoring.[9] Patients with less severe hyperkalemia (lower than 6.0 mmol/L) and without cardiac conduction abnormalities can probably be safely managed in an outpatient setting (Table 1).

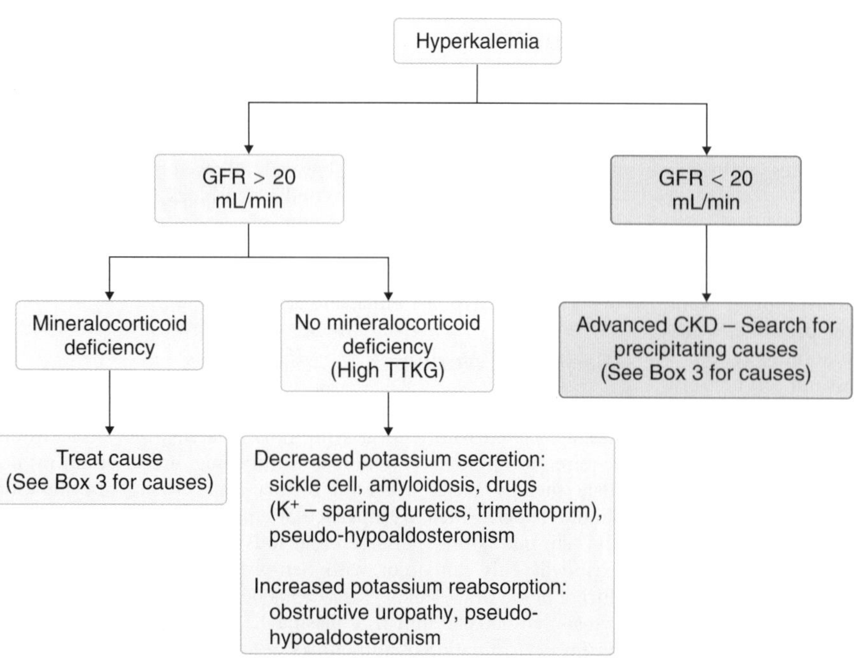

Figure 3 Hyperkalemia. CKD, chronic kidney disease; GFR, glomerular filtration rate; TTKG, transtubular potassium gradient.

Table 1 Treatment for Hyperkalemia

Clinical Situation	Treatment	Response Time	Duration of Effect
Emergency Treatment			
Electrocardiographic abnormalities	IV calcium gluconate or chloride (10 mL of 10% solution)	Immediate	15-30 min
$[K^+]$> 6.5 mmol/L or rising	IV Glucose (50 mL of 50%) + IV regular insulin, 10 U	10-20 min	2-3 hr
	Albuterol (10-20 mg) by inhaler over 10 min	20-30 min	2-3 hr
	IV sodium bicarbonate (only if metabolic acidosis)	Delayed	
	Kayexalate (sodium polystyrene), 15-30 g, with sorbitol	4-6 hr (PO); 1 hr (as retention enema)	
	Loop diuretic (IV)	1 hr	
	Hemodialysis	15-30 min	
Long-Term Treatment			
	Dietary potassium restriction, 2-3 g/day		
	Discontinue supplemental potassium (salt substitutes)		
	Discontinue drugs that interfere with potassium homeostasis		
	Augment potassium excretion with loop diuretics, thiazide diuretics, fludrocortisone, if hypoaldosteronism present		
	Chronic Kayexalate therapy		

Summary

Treatment of Hyperkalemia

- Ascertain whether it is associated with clinical symptoms, such as changes on the ECG, which require immediate attention.
- Rule out spurious elevation, hemolysis, difficult blood draw, or abnormal blood count.
- Careful history and physical examination should be done, looking specifically for chronic kidney disease, medications, dietary, or clinical situations associated with transcellular shifts, such as hyperglycemia.

Suggested Readings

Batlle DC, Arruda JA, Kurtzman NA: Hyperkalemic distal renal tubular acidosis associated with obstructive uropathy. N Engl J Med 1981;304:373-380.

Charytan D, Goldfarb DS: Indications for hospitalization of patients with hyperkalemia. Arch Intern Med 2000;160:1605-1611.

Cohn JN, Kowey PR, Whelton PK, Prisant LM: New guidelines for potassium replacement in clinical practice: A contemporary review by the National Council on Potassium in Clinical Practice. Arch Intern Med 2000;160:2429-2436.

Elisaf M, Siamopoulos KC: Fractional excretion of potassium in normal subjects and in patients with hypokalaemia. Postgrad Med J 1995;71:211-212.

Ethier JH, Kamel KS, Magner PO, et al: The transtubular potassium concentration in patients with hypokalemia and hyperkalemia. Am J Kidney Dis 1990;15:309-315.

Gennari FJ: Disorders of potassium homeostasis. Hypokalemia and hyperkalemia. Crit Care Clin 2002;18:273-288.

Gennari FJ, Segal AS: Hyperkalemia: An adaptive response in chronic renal insufficiency. Kidney Int 2002;62:1-9.

Kamel KS, Ethier JH, Richardson RM, et al: Urine electrolytes and osmolality: When and how to use them. Am J Nephrol 1990;10:89-102.

West ML, Marsden PA, Richardson RM, Zettle RM, Halperin ML: New clinical approach to evaluate disorders of potassium excretion. Miner Electrolyte Metab 1986;12:234-238.

References

For a complete list of references, log onto www.expertconsult.com.

Diabetic Nephropathy

Saud Butt, Phillip Hall, and Saul Nurko

DEFINITION AND CAUSES

Diabetic nephropathy (DN) is typically defined by macroalbuminuria—that is, a urinary albumin excretion of more than 300 mg in a 24-hour collection—or macroalbuminuria and abnormal renal function as represented by an abnormality in serum creatinine, calculated creatinine clearance, or glomerular filtration rate (GFR). Clinically, diabetic nephropathy is characterized by a progressive increase in proteinuria and decline in GFR, hypertension, and a high risk of cardiovascular morbidity and mortality.

PREVALENCE AND RISK FACTORS

Diabetes has become the primary cause of end-stage renal disease (ESRD) in the United States, and the incidence of type 2 diabetes mellitus continues to grow in the United States and worldwide. Approximately 44% of new patients entering dialysis in the United States are diabetics. Early diagnosis of diabetes and early intervention are critical in preventing the normal progression to renal failure seen in many type 1 and a significant percentage of type 2 diabetics.

In the United States, approximately 20.8 million people, or 7.0% of the population, are estimated to have diabetes, with a growing incidence. Roughly one third of this population, 6.2 million, is estimated to be undiagnosed with type 2 diabetes. The prevalence of diabetes is higher in certain racial and ethnic groups, affecting approximately 13% of African Americans, 9.5% of Hispanics, and 15% of Native Americans, primarily with type 2 diabetes.[1,2] Approximately 20% to 30% of all diabetics will develop evidence of nephropathy, although a higher percentage of type 1 patients progress to ESRD.

PATHOPHYSIOLOGY AND NATURAL HISTORY

The common progression from microalbuminuria to overt nephropathy has led many to consider microalbuminuria to define early or incipient nephropathy. Renal disease is suspected to be secondary to diabetes in the clinical setting of long-standing diabetes. This is supported by the history of diabetic retinopathy, particularly in type 1 diabetics, in whom there is a strong correlation. The natural history of diabetic nephropathy is a process that progresses gradually over years.

Early diabetes is heralded by glomerular hyperfiltration and an increase in GFR. This is believed to be related to increased cell growth and expansion in the kidneys, possibly mediated by hyperglycemia itself. Microalbuminuria typically occurs after 5 years in type 1 diabetes. Overt nephropathy, with urinary protein excretion higher than 300 mg/day, often develops after 10 to 15 years. ESRD develops in 50% of type 1 diabetics, with overt nephropathy within 10 years.

Type 2 diabetes has a more variable course. Patients often present at diagnosis with microalbuminuria because of delays in diagnosis and other factors affecting protein excretion. Fewer patients with microalbuminuria progress to advanced renal disease. Without intervention, approximately 30% progress to overt nephropathy and, after 20 years of nephropathy, approximately 20% develop ESRD. Because of the high prevalence of type 2 compared with type 1 diabetes, however, most diabetics on dialysis are type 2 diabetics.

Long-standing hyperglycemia is known to be a significant risk factor for the development of diabetic nephropathy. Hyperglycemia may directly result in mesangial expansion and injury by an increase in the mesangial cell glucose concentration. The glomerular mesangium expands initially by cell proliferation and then by cell hypertrophy. Increased mesangial stretch and pressure can stimulate this expansion, as can high glucose levels. Transforming growth factor β (TGF-β) is particularly important in the mediation of expansion and later fibrosis via the stimulation of collagen and fibronectin. Glucose can also bind reversibly and eventually irreversibly to proteins in the kidneys and circulation to form advanced glycosylation end products (AGEs). AGEs can form complex cross-links over years of hyperglycemia and can contribute to renal damage by stimulation of growth and fibrotic factors via receptors for AGEs. In addition, mediators of proliferation and expansion, including platelet-derived growth factor, TGF-β, and vascular endothelial growth factor (VEGF) that are elevated in diabetic nephropathy can contribute to further renal and microvascular complications.

Proteinuria, a marker and potential contributor to renal injury, accompanies diabetic nephropathy. Increased glomerular permeability will allow plasma proteins to escape into the urine. Some of these proteins will be taken up by the proximal tubular cells, which can initiate an inflammatory response that contributes to interstitial scarring eventually leading to fibrosis. Tubulointerstitial fibrosis is seen in advanced stages of diabetic nephropathy and is a better predictor of renal failure than glomerular sclerosis. Hyperglycemia, angiotensin II, TGF-β, and likely proteinuria itself all play roles in stimulating this fibrosis. There is an epithelial-mesenchymal transition that takes place in the tubules, with proximal tubular cell conversion to fibroblast-like cells. These cells can then migrate into the interstitium and produce collagen and fibronectin.

In diabetic nephropathy, the activation of the local renin-angiotensin system occurs in the proximal tubular epithelial cells, mesangial cells, and podocytes. Angiotensin II (ATII) itself contributes to the progression of diabetic nephropathy. ATII is stimulated in diabetes despite the high-volume state typically seen with the disease, and the intrarenal level of ATII is typically high, even in the face of lower systemic concentrations. ATII preferentially constricts the efferent arteriole in the glomerulus, leading to higher glomerular capillary pressures. In addition to its hemodynamic effects, ATII also stimulates renal growth and fibrosis through ATII type 1 receptors, which secondarily upregulate TGF-β and other growth factors.

Control of hypertension has clearly shown to be an important and powerful intervention in decreasing the progression of diabetic nephropathy. In diabetics who have disordered autoregulation at the level of the kidney, systemic hypertension can contribute to endothelial injury. Human studies of type 2 diabetics have shown that blood pressure lowering, regardless of the agent used, retards the onset and progression of diabetic nephropathy. In animal studies, the degree and severity of the diabetic nephropathy were strongly linked to systemic blood pressure.

The fact that most types 1 and 2 diabetics do not develop diabetic nephropathy (DN) suggests that other factors may be involved. Genetic factors clearly play a role in the predisposition to diabetic nephropathy in family members who have DN, and linkage to specific areas on the human genome is evolving. The theory of a reduction in nephron number at birth indicates that individuals born with a reduced number of glomeruli may be predisposed to subsequent renal injury and progressive nephropathy. This has been shown in animal studies in which the mother was exposed to hyperglycemia at the time of pregnancy. If this linkage is true in humans, that would have important implications concerning the role of maternal factors in the eventual development of kidney disease.[3]

SIGNS AND SYMPTOMS

Early signs and symptoms of kidney disease in patients with diabetes are typically unusual. However, a vast array of signs and symptoms listed below may manifest when kidney disease has progressed:[4]

- Albumin or protein in the urine
- High blood pressure
- Ankle and leg swelling, leg cramps
- Going to the bathroom more often at night
- High levels of blood urea nitrogen (BUN) and serum creatinine
- Less need for insulin or antidiabetic medications
- Morning sickness, nausea, and vomiting
- Weakness, paleness, and anemia
- Itching

The differential diagnosis of diabetic nephropathy is vast, but it includes the following in a patient with known diabetes mellitus:

- Primary or secondary glomerular disease
- Nephrosclerosis
- Renovascular hypertension
- Renal artery stenosis
- Renal vein thrombosis
- Multiple myeloma
- Cholesterol embolization
- Chronic obstruction
- Interstitial nephritis
- Amyloidosis

DIAGNOSIS

Laboratory Tests

In screening for diabetic nephropathy, we recommend early testing for glucose intolerance and diabetes to identify patients who are at risk for developing microalbuminuria, particularly if they have other risks for type 2 diabetes, such as hypertension, lipid abnormalities, or central obesity. As noted, approximately one third of type 2 diabetics are believed to be undiagnosed. Once the diagnosis of diabetes has been made, we routinely check urinary protein levels only to guide therapy and prognosis.

It is not uncommon to find microalbuminuria or macroalbuminuria in a type 2 diabetic at or soon after the initial diagnosis of diabetes. This may be because the patient has had undiagnosed diabetes for many years, or it may relate to the contributions of hypertension or other processes that may cause proteinuria independently of diabetes, such as small-vessel atherosclerosis. Microalbuminuria is now recognized as an independent cardiac risk factor, even in the absence of diabetes. Screening for microalbuminuria in nondiabetics may have important implications for cardiac risk, and should lead to instituting some of the same therapies as those used for diabetic nephropathy (Table 1).

Imaging Studies

A renal ultrasound is typically obtained to observe for kidney size. In the early stages of diabetic nephropathy, kidney size may be enlarged from hyperfiltration. With progressive kidney disease from diabetes, the kidneys diminish in size from glomerulosclerosis. In addition, a renal ultrasound can assess for hyperechogenicity that suggests chronic kidney disease and can assist in ruling out obstruction.

Diagnostic Procedures

Frequently, the question is raised as to whether proteinuria is from diabetes or from a primary renal disease. Suspicion may arise in patients with significant proteinuria without a long history of diabetes or without other signs of end-organ damage, such as retinopathy or neuropathy. Although the presence of retinopathy supports a diabetic source of proteinuria, the lack of diabetic retinopathy does not rule out diabetic nephropathy, particularly in type 2 diabetics.

Patients with diabetes can develop nephrotic-range proteinuria (higher than 3.5 g/24 hr), but typically only after long-standing diabetes. A bland urine sediment supports the diagnosis of diabetes, although it is not uncommon to have some microscopic hematuria with advanced diabetic nephropathy. The presentation of an acute nephrotic syndrome, rapidly rising urinary protein level, or rapidly declining GFR should lead to consideration of renal biopsy. The finding of red cell or white cell casts in the urine should also suggest a biopsy. Renal biopsy findings consistent with diabetic nephropathy in the early stages are mesangial expansion and glomerular basement membrane thickening. Eventual progression of diabetic nephropathy can lead to nodular glomerulosclerosis, also referred to as Kimmelstiel-Wilson disease.

Often, a patient will present without available history and may be frankly nephrotic in the face of long-standing diabetes. In cases of uncertainty such as this, it is not wrong to consider a renal biopsy, because the finding of a primary glomerular disease could potentially change the course of management.

Staging

See Table 2.

Table 1 Methods of Measuring Urinary Protein and Ranges of Abnormal Excretion

Method	Normal Value	Abnormal Values	
		Microalbuminuria	Macroalbuminuria
24-hour urine collection	<150 mg/day	150-300 mg/day	>300 mg/day
Spot protein-to-creatinine ratio (mg/mg)*	Estimate 1 g creatinine excretion/1.73 m^2 (ratio of 0.15 = 150 mg protein/24 hr/1.73 m^2) *Or* estimate per 20 mg/kg creatinine excretion for men, 15 mg/kg for women	Ratio: 0.18-0.36 for 60-kg male, 0.135-0.27 for 60-kg female	Ratio: >0.36 for 60-kg male, >0.27 for 60-kg female
Albumin-to-creatinine ratio (µg/mg)†	<30 µg/mg	30-300 µg/mg	>300 µg/mg

*Good for screening; does not correlate well with 24-hr urinary protein at higher (nephrotic) levels of proteinuria.
†Good for screening; does not account for patient weight or muscle mass; some recommend ratio of 17-249 µg/mg for women and 25-354 µg/mg for men to define microalbuminuria.

Table 2 Stages of Chronic Kidney Disease

Stage	Description	GFR (mL/min)
1	Kidney damage with normal or raised GFR	≥90
2	Kidney damage with mild decrease in GFR	60-89
3	Moderate decrease in GFR	30-59
4	Severe decrease in GFR	15-29
5	Kidney Failure	<15

GFR, glomerular filtration rate.
From National Kidney Foundation: GFR, 2008. Available at http://www.kidney.org/professionals/KLS/gfr.cfm#20.

Summary

- In the United States, approximately 20.8 million people, or 7.0% of the population, are estimated to have diabetes.
- Progressive renal disease in diabetes is a multifactorial process that begins initially via a process of glomerular hyperfiltration and increased glomerular filtration rate.
- Diabetic nephropathy is typically defined by macroalbuminuria or macroalbuminuria and abnormal renal function as represented by an abnormality in serum creatinine, calculated creatinine clearance, or glomerular filtration rate.
- Microalbuminuria is now recognized as an independent cardiac risk factor, even in the absence of diabetes.
- Findings of diabetic nephropathy on kidney biopsy include mesangial expansion, glomerular basement membrane thickening, glomerulosclerosis, or a combination of these.

TREATMENT

Lifestyle Modification

One keystone in the prevention and management of diabetic nephropathy is tight glycemic control. In the Diabetes Control and Complications Trial, type 1 diabetics were randomized to intensive or conventional insulin treatments and followed for an average of 6.5 years.[5] Average hemoglobin A_{1c} (HbA_{1c}) values were 7.2% versus 9.2%. There was a 39% risk reduction in the development of microalbuminuria and a 54% reduction in the development of macroalbuminuria in the intensive treatment group.

In the UK Prospective Diabetes Study (UKPDS), 3867 patients with newly diagnosed type 2 diabetes were randomized to oral or insulin therapy versus dietary control and followed for 11 years.[6] The difference in HbA_{1c} was 7.0% versus 7.9%. After 9 years, there was a significant risk reduction in the intensive group, with a relative risk of 0.76 for the development of microalbuminuria.

The complete correction of hyperglycemia with pancreatic transplantation in type 1 diabetics has led to a dramatic resolution in glomerular and tubular expansion and fibrosis over time.[7] With a drop in HbA_{1c} from an average of 8.7% to 5.5% in eight transplanted patients, there was a significant reduction in basement membrane thickening and mesangial expansion on repeat biopsies over time. Even glomerular sclerosis appeared to resolve, showing that renal fibrosis may be reversible, although it took 10 years after transplantation to see these significant changes.

Medical Options

Control of blood pressure is the other keystone in prevention and treatment. Blood pressure control is critical in slowing the natural history of diabetic nephropathy in types 1 and 2 diabetics. Parving and colleagues studied 12 type 1 diabetics and treated hypertension before angiotensin inhibitors were available.[8] Using metoprolol, hydralazine, and diuretics, patients with macroalbuminuria and declining GFR were treated to reduce mean arterial pressure from 120 to lower than 105 mm Hg. An initial decline in GFR was noted in most patients immediately after blood pressure lowering. However, a 2-year subsequent follow-up showed a slowing in the rate of reduction of GFR from an average of 0.91 to 0.39 mL/min/month, with significant preservation of GFR above that expected from pretreatment measurements. The initial drop in GFR illustrated a functional or hemodynamic effect of antihypertensive treatment, which does not lead to permanent renal damage but rather to renal preservation. One review has recommended maintaining antihypertensive therapy in renal disease, even if therapy causes some hemodynamic drop in GFR, provided there is a stabilization in the creatinine level, with an increase of less than 30% of baseline.[9]

The UKPDS studied 1148 hypertensive patients who had recently been diagnosed with type 2 diabetes.[10] Patients were assigned to tight blood pressure control, achieving a mean level of 144/82 mm Hg, or less tight control, with a mean pressure of 154/81 mm Hg. After a median follow-up of 8.4 years, there was significant reduction in risk of death related to diabetes, stroke, and microvascular disease in the tight control group. There was no difference in outcomes within the tight control group in patients assigned to atenolol or captopril, although captopril was given only twice daily at 25 to 50 mg/dose.

The importance of blood pressure control, no matter what agent is used, cannot be emphasized enough in diabetes, both for slowing progression of nephropathy and for preventing cardiovascular morbidity and mortality. Currently, the recommendation from the most recent Joint National Committee guidelines is that blood pressure in diabetics be reduced to lower than 130/80 mm Hg.[11] Some studies of hypertension treatment in diabetics have shown benefit with lowering blood pressure even further. For example, in the Hypertension Optimal Treatment trial, diabetics with a target diastolic pressure of 80 mm Hg had 50% of the cardiovascular events seen in patients with a target of 90 mm Hg.[12]

Furthermore, the Modification of Diet in Renal Disease Study has found value in further reduction in a diverse group of patients with renal disease and proteinuria.[13] In patients with 24-hour urinary protein of more than 1 g, a blood pressure level at or below 125/75 mm Hg was shown to slow the decline in GFR. Based on these data, we recommend a target blood pressure of 130/80 mm Hg or lower in all diabetics, with a further goal of 125 to 130/75 to 80 mm Hg in diabetics with macroalbuminuria (Table 3). These blood pressure goals may seem difficult to accomplish in some patients but, in clinical trials, preset goals have been consistently achieved. It is important for clinicians and patients to be aware early on that three or more agents may be required to achieve the blood pressure goal, and that these agents will likely be needed long term.

It is important to emphasize that diuretics are extremely beneficial adjuncts for blood pressure control and are often missing in patients who are not close to meeting blood pressure goals. Diuretics are first-line agents for many hypertensives, and we routinely add a diuretic as a second-line agent after angiotensin blockade in diabetics. Thiazide diuretics work well, even at low dosages for patients with normal renal function. For example, just 12.5 to 25 mg/day of hydrochlorothiazide is often effective. When the GFR is below 60 mL/min, we often institute loop diuretics for a better natriuretic effect. Short-acting loop diuretics such as furosemide work better when given at least twice daily to avoid rebound sodium retention.

Specific use of agents that block the renin-angiotensin system appears to be particularly beneficial in the prevention or slowing of progression of diabetic nephropathy. ATII can increase glomerular capillary pressure by preferentially constricting the renal efferent arteriole. ATII also stimulates renal cell growth and fibrosis, independently of hemodynamic effects. Even with blood pressure at goal and without microalbuminuria, we consider initiation of low dosages

Table 3 Blood Pressure Goals and Recommended Agents

Patient	Goal Blood Pressure (mm Hg)	Recommended Blood Pressure Agents
Type 1 diabetic	≤130/80	ACEI; ARB if ACEI not tolerated; diuretic as second-line agent
Type 2 diabetic	≤130/80	ARB; ACEI as alternative; diuretic as second-line agent
Diabetic with macroalbuminuria	≤130/80	Angiotensin blockade in conjunction with diuretic; beta blocker or calcium channel blocker as third-line agent
Diabetic with congestive heart failure	≤130/80	ACEI remains a first-line agent, followed by beta blocker
Diabetic with coronary artery disease	≤130/80	Beta blocker is first-line agent, followed by ACEI; diuretic as third-line agent

ACEI, angiotensin-converting enzyme inhibitor; ARB, angiotensin II receptor blocker.

of angiotensin-blocking agents, with titration up as tolerated. Other antihypertensives may not offer this antiproliferative effect and may cause adverse hemodynamic effects. For example, the calcium channel blockers, in particular the dihydropyridines, cause afferent dilation and thus may increase glomerular capillary pressure. Dihydropyridines may best be reserved as third- or fourth-line agents in patients with diabetes, only after angiotensin blockade and diuretics have already been instituted.

The benefits of angiotensin-converting enzyme inhibitors (ACEIs) have been shown by the Collaborative Study Group using captopril compared with placebo in 409 patients with type 1 diabetes and macroalbuminuria.[14] Patients with a creatinine level higher than 1.5 mg/dL had a significant reduction in risk of doubling serum creatinine and of the composite of death, dialysis, or transplantation when treated with captopril, even after controlling for changes in blood pressure.

A substudy of the Heart Outcomes Prevention Evaluation (HOPE) looked at 3577 patients ages 55 years or older with diabetes and randomized to ramipril, 10 mg/day, or placebo.[15] All patients had at least one other cardiac risk factor in addition to diabetes, including lipid abnormalities, hypertension, microalbuminuria, and current smoking. Patients with dipstick-positive proteinuria and overt nephropathy were excluded, as were patients with congestive heart failure. The ramipril group had a reduction in blood pressure of 2.5 mm Hg systolic and 1 mm Hg diastolic. When corrected for blood pressure, there were significant reductions in risk of stroke and cardiovascular morbidity and mortality. There was also a relative risk reduction of 24% in the progression to diabetic nephropathy in all patients, although this was not controlled for the minor change in blood pressure. In subgroup analysis, the diabetics who had significant benefit were those who already had coronary disease or microalbuminuria.

Angiotensin receptor blockers (ARBs) have also shown renal protection in type 2 diabetics. Two studies of the prevention of progression in patients with microalbuminuria have been published.[16,17] Both irbesartan and valsartan were shown to lower albumin excretion and prevent development of diabetic nephropathy, even when controlling for changes in blood pressure. The effects of irbesartan appeared to be dosage dependent, with greater protection at 300 mg/day versus 150 mg/day. The study using valsartan did not stratify for dosage, and the average dosage was 122 mg/day. Two trials of ARBs in patients with overt diabetic nephropathy have also shown a decline in rate of progression of disease.[18,19] Both studies have shown a slowing in the rate of progression to doubling of creatinine or to ESRD using irbesartan titrated to 300 mg/day or losartan at an average dosage of 85.5 mg/day. The benefit in both studies was impressive, although more importantly the treatment only decreased the rate of progression of disease but did not halt it. The average patient had a delay in progression to ESRD of about 2 years.

Angiotensin blockade should be started early and may have its greatest benefit in prevention or reversal of early kidney disease. The benefits of angiotensin blockade have been shown in both trials of irbesartan and valsartan in type 2 diabetics with microalbuminuria in which a significant percentage of treated patients had albumin excretion reduction into the normal range. Administration of irbesartan, 300 mg/day, led to a 34% incidence of normalization of protein excretion compared with 21% in the placebo group. Similarly, valsartan treatment led to an approximately 30% normalization compared with 14.5% in the placebo group. Early treatment is important to prevent and possibly even reverse diabetic nephropathy.

The combination of an ACEI and an ARB in diabetic nephropathy has been studied in several small randomized trials.[20] The largest analysis, the Candesartan and Lisinopril Microalbuminuria (CALM) study, involved lisinopril, 20 mg/day, and candesartan, 16 mg/day, given individually and then in combination in patients with type 2 diabetes, hypertension, and microalbuminuria. Any patient with a diastolic blood pressure lower than 80 mm Hg was not eligible to receive the combination, thus excluding 25% of the original participants. In the remaining patients receiving the combination, there was a further lowering in blood pressure and in urinary protein excretion compared with either agent alone, and the treatment was well tolerated.

We recommend attempting to maximize angiotensin blockade as much as patients will tolerate, especially given the dosage-related benefits shown in some studies. The benefit of using an ACEI-ARB combination over a higher dosage of a single agent alone appears to provide a greater reduction in protein excretion, although long-term studies are needed to prove the efficacy of the ACEI-ARB combination. If the maximal dosage of one agent has been achieved, it may be reasonable to introduce the second agent. Some clinicians have recommended adding an ARB to an ACEI once a moderate dosage of the ACEI is achieved. There may be ATII formation independent of ACE, and blocking the receptor should block this ATII activity. Angiotensin blockade may reach a threshold above which further benefit will not be gained, and animal studies at supramaximal dosages of ACEIs and ARBs have shown incomplete blockage of TGF-β. However, many patients are underdosed and could gain more benefit from maximal therapy.

At this point, it is difficult to recommend one type of renin-angiotensin blockade over another for initial treatment in diabetics. There are ample data supporting ACEIs for type 1 diabetics. Based on data from the HOPE trial, it would seem acceptable also to choose an ACEI in type 2 diabetics with coronary artery disease, although beta blockers remain first-line agents. Similarly, in patients with congestive heart failure, ARBs may be used in patients who are intolerant of ACEIs, but ACEIs remain first-line agents. Patients with type 2 diabetes and microalbuminuria or overt nephropathy but no known cardiac disease should probably receive an ARB as first-line treatment based on data reviewed earlier (Table 3).

It is important to treat with angiotensin blockade, even in patients with baseline renal insufficiency. Patients with a high serum creatinine level are still candidates for angiotensin blockade, although they need close follow-up, with cautious titration. As noted, GFR often drops somewhat at the initiation of therapy, and close monitoring of renal function should take place within 1 or 2 weeks of starting medication. Provided there is a bump of no more than 30% in the serum creatinine level, and it remains stable, therapy may be continued.[9]

ACEIs and ARBs are generally both well tolerated. However, attempting to institute and titrate either agent must be done while monitoring for side effects, such as symptomatically low blood pressure or hyperkalemia. Patients should be monitored for hyperkalemia and an increase in creatinine level within 1 week of starting or changing the dosage of either agent, and should be counseled on limiting potassium in the diet. Diuretics such as thiazides or loop diuretics are often useful and necessary adjunctive treatments for blood pressure control, and can have the added benefit of offsetting a rise in serum potassium level. The side effect of cough secondary to bradykinin accumulation with an ACEI may necessitate conversion to an ARB.

Rarely, severe, life-threatening angioedema can occur with ACEIs or ARBs. This side effect has been reported even months or years after starting an ACEI. The incidence of angioedema appears to be less frequent with ARBs. In a patient with a history of ACEI-induced angioedema, an ARB may be started cautiously at a low dosage if there is a strong indication, such as diabetes and microalbuminuria, but should probably be held if there is no abnormal urinary albumin excretion.[21] ACEIs and ARBs are also both contraindicated in pregnancy, and should be used with caution in women of childbearing potential.

There are other classes of agents for diabetic nephropathy that may show hope for the future. Aldosterone receptor antagonists decrease proteinuria further in patients with diabetes on ACEIs.[22] Eplerenone, a new aldosterone blocking agent, has been approved by the U.S. Food and Drug Administration. It is similar to spironolactone but lacks the sex steroid side effects, such as impotence and gynecomastia. In a small randomized study of type 2 diabetics already treated with an ACEI, eplerenone caused a significant reduction in urinary albumin excretion.[23] One side effect noted in the study that needs to be monitored is hyperkalemia, which may be increased with this combination. Further long-term studies will be needed to decipher the benefit of this combination.

3-Hydroxy-3-methylglutaryl coenzyme A (HMG-CoA) reductase inhibitors, or statins, are also being studied. There are already recommendations for tight lipid control in diabetics because of the high cardiac risk in these patients. Statins may have additional unique benefits, independent of lipid lowering. In animal models of diabetic nephropathy, statin treatment was found to block intracellular signaling and decreases the mRNA expression of TGF-β.[24]

Agents that directly inhibit or degrade TGF-β or inhibit AGEs have shown success in animals and are being developed for clinical human trials. One such agent, known as ALT-711, breaks cross-links in AGE complexes. It has been shown to improve vascular endothelial function in diabetes and may have promise for diabetic nephropathy.[25]

Dietary Changes

A common question from patients and primary care providers is whether the reduction of dietary protein is beneficial in diabetic nephropathy. Many animal studies of glomerulopathies have shown reduction in decline in renal function by restricting dietary protein. The data in humans remain inconclusive, however. We currently counsel patients to avoid protein supplements such as protein shakes or powders, but do not otherwise restrict protein from the diet. Others recommend a restriction of 0.8 g/kg/day in patients with overt nephropathy, or even 0.6 g/kg/day in the presence of a falling GFR.

It is important to maintain a low-sodium diet in diabetic nephropathy. Many diabetics with renal disease are salt-sensitive and minimizing salt intake can help in reaching blood pressure goals, with secondary benefits of decreased stroke risk, regression of left ventricular hypertrophy, and reduction in proteinuria. We advocate a low-sodium diet of 2.3 g or lower (5.8 g of NaCl) or 100 mEq/day in patients with diabetes and hypertension or any degree of proteinuria.

Avoidance of Nephrotoxins

It is important to avoid nephrotoxic agents, if possible, in patients with diabetic nephropathy. Nonsteroidal anti-inflammatory drugs (NSAIDs) can cause a significant drop in GFR in patients with diabetic nephropathy, particularly when used with angiotensin-blocking agents. Daily low-dosage aspirin is safe in diabetics, and the cardiac benefits greatly outweigh any risk. However, aspirin at higher dosages and other NSAIDs should be avoided if possible. Cyclooxygenase 2 (COX-2) inhibitors are similar to other NSAIDs in their potential for renal toxicity.

Radiocontrast media are also particularly nephrotoxic for diabetics. Even with a normal serum creatinine level, patients with diabetes and proteinuria should be volume-loaded 12 hours before and after exposure to contrast, if possible. Diuretics should be temporarily discontinued, and hyperglycemia should be controlled. Other agents such as dopamine-like agonists and acetylcysteine may help prevent contrast nephropathy in diabetics but require further study.

Nephrology Referral

Referral to a nephrologist should be considered if the GFR is steadily declining or is already below 60 to 70 mL/min. Challenges in blood pressure control, hyperkalemia, or rising creatinine level on angiotensin blockade may also prompt a referral. We consider it appropriate to refer a patient in any situation in which the primary physician feels that he or she needs additional input or assistance with the management of diabetic nephropathy.

Surgical Options

Surgical care in diabetic nephropathy typically entails complications that can arise from peripheral vascular disease or diabetic foot ulcers. Surgical issues also arise in the context of the creation of a native or artificial access in preparation for dialysis. Lastly, transplantation options may be pursued in the form of kidney or pancreas transplantation, or both, in select individuals.

Practice Guidelines

The American Diabetes Association Standards of Medical Care in Diabetes has published treatment practice guidelines.[26] These are available at http://care.diabetesjournals.org.

Summary

- One keystone in the prevention and management of diabetic nephropathy is tight glycemic control.
- Joint National Committee guidelines recommend that blood pressure in diabetics be reduced to less than 130/80 mm Hg.
- Specific use of agents that block the renin-angiotensin system appears to be particularly beneficial for the prevention or slowing of progression of diabetic nephropathy. Current recommendations are the use of an ACE inhibitor in type 1 diabetes and an angiotensin receptor blocker in type 2 diabetes.

PREVENTION AND SCREENING

Practice Guidelines

The American Diabetes Association Standards of Medical Care in Diabetes has published prevention and screening practice guidelines.[26] These are available at http://care.diabetesjournals.org.

CONSIDERATIONS IN SPECIAL POPULATIONS

Special attention should be given to women of reproductive age who become pregnant and who are taking ACEIs or ARBs. Pregnancy in a patient with diabetic nephropathy does not seem to accelerate functional loss, however this issue is controversial. A more increased range of proteinuria and hypertension may occur after midgestation.

Suggested Readings

American Diabetes Association: Standards of medical care in diabetes-2007. Diabetes Care 2007;30:S4-S41.

Brenner BM, Cooper ME, de Zeeuw D, et al; RENAAL Study Investigators: Effects of losartan on renal and cardiovascular outcomes in patients with type 2 diabetes and nephropathy. N Engl J Med 2001;345:861-869.

Hall P: Prevention of progression in diabetic nephropathy. Diabetes Spectrum 2006; 19:18-24.

Hansson L, Zanchetti A, Carruthers SG, et al: Effects of intensive blood-pressure lowering and low-dose aspirin in patients with hypertension: Principal results of the Hypertension Optimal Treatment (HOT) randomised trial. Lancet 1998;351: 1755-1762.

Heart Outcomes Prevention Evaluation Study Investigators: Effects of ramipril on cardiovascular and microvascular outcomes in people with diabetes mellitus: Results of the HOPE study and MICRO-HOPE substudy. Lancet 2000;355:253-259.

Lewis EJ, Hunsicker LG, Bain RP, Rohde RD: The effect of angiotensin-converting-enzyme inhibition on diabetic nephropathy. The Collaborative Study Group. N Engl J Med 1993;329:1456-1462.

Lewis EJ, Hunsicker LG, Clarke WR, et al; Collaborative Study Group: Renoprotective effect of the angiotensin-receptor antagonist irbesartan in patients with nephropathy due to type 2 diabetes. N Engl J Med 2001;345:851-860.

Peterson JC, Adler S, Burkart JM, et al: Blood-pressure control, proteinuria, and the progression of renal disease: The Modification of Diet in Renal Disease Study. Ann Intern Med 1995;123:754-762.

UK Prospective Diabetes Study Group: Intensive blood-glucose control with sulphonylureas or insulin compared with conventional treatment and risk of complications in patients with type 2 diabetes. Lancet 1998;352:837-853.

UK Prospective Diabetes Study Group: Tight blood pressure control and risk of macrovascular and microvascular complications in type 2 diabetes: UKPDS 38. BMJ 1998;317:703-713.

References

For a complete list of references, log onto www.expertconsult.com.

Primary Glomerular Diseases

Brian R. Stephany

Primary glomerular diseases include a group of disorders characterized by pathologic alterations in normal glomerular structure and function, independent of systemic disease processes. This distinction is important because the clinical presentation and pathologic findings of glomerulopathies secondary to systemic diseases may mirror primary glomerular disorders, yet the correct diagnosis of the underlying systemic disease may significantly alter the treatment of the patient. Furthermore, an understanding of the typical clinical signs of patients with primary glomerular disorders (e.g., proteinuria, hematuria, hypertension, decline in glomerular filtration rate [GFR], edema, and abnormal urine sediments) is essential. From this, the clinician can classify the clinical presentation of the patient, which is the first step to defining the exact disease accurately (Table 1). However, it should be noted that the same primary glomerular disease as diagnosed on pathologic grounds may manifest differently in patients, from the benign to the severe (Box 1). This likely reflects our poor understanding of their underlying pathophysiology and how a particular disease may actually represent a spectrum of disorders that pathologically may be similar but phenotypically manifest as a wide spectrum.

MINIMAL CHANGE DISEASE

Pathologic Definition

Minimal change disease (MCD), historically referred to as nil disease, is characterized by an absence of glomerular pathology by light microscopy or immunofluorescence. There may be extraglomerular findings by light microscopy, including intratubular lipid and protein resorption droplets—hence the alternate name, lipoid nephrosis—and focal proximal tubular epithelial flattening. However, although not specific to MCD, the classic finding of MCD is effacement of visceral epithelial cell foot processes seen using electron microscopy.

Prevalence and Risk Factors

MCD is the most common primary glomerular disease in children, accounting for 70% to 90% of cases of nephrotic syndrome for those younger than 10 years, with the incidence peaking between ages 2 and 4 years.[1] The prevalence declines with age, whereby it is responsible for only 10% to 20% of cases of nephrotic syndrome in adults. There appears to be a higher predominance in Asia compared with the United States and Europe, although no strong gender predominance exists.[2]

Pathophysiology and Natural History

The underlying mechanism(s) leading to MCD is unknown. Some studies have implicated upregulation of various cytokine activities, including interleukin-2, during disease activity. It has been postulated that this may induce glomerular permeability factor(s) that interfere with normal function of the charge-selective barrier to filtration of serum proteins.[3] As with all primary glomerular disorders, when approaching a patient with a new diagnosis of MCD, it is important to exclude secondary causes. Most notable on this list is the use of medications that have a strong association with MCD, including nonsteroidal anti-inflammatory drugs and certain antibiotics, including rifampin. Additionally, although rare, lymphoid malignancies such as Hodgkin's disease and leukemia may manifest along with nephrotic syndrome from MCD.

Signs and Symptoms

Patients with MCD typically present with findings consistent with the nephrotic syndrome (see Table 1). Although not specific to primary glomerular disorders, the abrupt onset and generalized distribution of edema are typically what lead the patient to medical attention and should indicate that the clinician consider a primary kidney disorder as the causative factor. More common in children, visceral effusions (pleural, peritoneal, and pericardial) may also accompany the peripheral edema. Children are typically normotensive, but elevated blood pressures may be present in adults. Finally, patients may also present with syndromes resulting from the biologic complications of the nephrotic syndrome that are not necessarily specific to MCD. Venous and, much less commonly, arterial, thromboses may occur, caused by several factors that lead to thrombophilia, including loss of normal anticoagulants in the urine (e.g., antithrombin III, plasminogen) and excessive hepatic production of procoagulants (e.g., fibrinogen, factors II, V, VII, VIII, X, and XIII).[4] Additionally, loss of immunoglobulins in the urine may predispose patients to infections of various types.

Diagnosis

Albuminuria detectable by urine dipstick is the most common laboratory finding in patients with MCD. When quantified by a 24-hour urine collection or spot urine protein-to-creatinine concentration ratio, the degree of proteinuria may be severe. Microscopic hematuria is not the norm, but may occur in up to 25% of patients, and macroscopic hematuria is decidedly rare. Active urine sediment changes (e.g., dysmorphic RBCs and RBC casts) should not be present in patients with MCD. However, lipiduria in the forms of free fat, oval fat bodies, and lipid casts may be present on urine microscopy. Hypoalbuminemia correlates with the severity of the degree of proteinuria, and in children can be severely depressed to lower than 1 g/dL. As a result, the hypoalbuminemia and total serum calcium levels are low, but the corrected calcium and ionized calcium levels are usually normal.

Renal function, as evidenced by serum creatinine level, is typically normal, especially in children. However, some patients with MCD also present in acute renal failure, with an elevated serum creatinine level.[5] Risk factors for this include age older than 45 years, the coexistence of hypertension, and heavier degrees of proteinuria. Pathologically, these patients exhibit concomitant acute tubular necrosis on their biopsy specimens. Clinically, successful treatment of the nephrotic syndrome invariably is associated with resolution of the acute renal failure.[5]

An increase in total and low-density lipoprotein (LDL) cholesterol levels is often seen, as is hypertriglyceridemia. If the hyperlipidemia is severe enough, pseudohyponatremia may be present.

Although the circulating red blood cell mass remains normal in the absence of renal failure, given that plasma volume is often decreased in patients with MCD and the nephrotic syndrome, elevations of the hematocrit and hemoconcentration can be observed. Erythrocyte sedimentation rate is often elevated because of hyperfibrinogenemia, but complement levels are normal.

Table 1 Common Clinical Syndromes of Primary Glomerular Diseases

Symptom	Nephrotic Syndrome	Acute Glomerulonephritis	Rapidly Progressive Glomerulonephritis	Asymptomatic Hematuria and/or Proteinuria
Proteinuria	>3.5 g/1.73 m^2/per day*	May be in nephrotic range	May be in nephrotic range	No or non-nephrotic range
Hematuria	Variable and usually monomorphic if present	Micro- or macroscopic with RBC casts and dysmorphic RBCs	Micro- or macroscopic with RBC casts and dysmorphic RBCs	Micro- or macroscopic (may be dysmorphic with RBC casts)
Blood pressure	Normo- or hypertension	Hypertension	Hypertension	Normotension
GFR	Variable decline, depending on diagnosis	Rapid decline (days to weeks)	Progressive decline (weeks to months)	Decline uncommon

*In children, >40 mg/m^2/hr; often accompanied by edema, hypoalbuminemia, hyperlipidemia, with or without lipiduria.
GFR, glomerular filtration rate; RBC, red blood cell.

Box 1 Classification of Primary Glomerular Disease Based on Clinical Syndrome

Nephrotic Syndrome
Minimal change disease
Membranous glomerular nephropathy
Focal segmental glomerulosclerosis
Membranoproliferative glomerulonephritis*
C1q nephropathy†
Fibrillary glomerulonephritis†

Acute Glomerulonephritis
Membranoproliferative glomerulonephritis
IgA nephropathy

Rapidly Progressive Glomerulonephritis
Antiglomerular basement membrane disease
Immune complex crescentic glomerulonephritis
Pauci-immune crescentic glomerulonephritis
Membranoproliferative glomerulonephritis
IgA nephropathy
Membranous glomerular nephropathy (rare)

Asymptomatic Hematuria and/or Proteinuria
IgA nephropathy
Membranoproliferative glomerulonephritis

**Usually with active sediment; e.g., red blood cell casts, dysmorphic red blood cells), unlike other causes of nephrotic syndrome.*
†Extremely rare disorders.

Diagnostic Procedures

Given the predominance of MCD as the leading cause of nephrotic syndrome in children younger than 10 years, many clinicians will treat empirically in this age group, resorting to a kidney biopsy only in cases of treatment failure. In older age groups, however, given that the causes of nephrotic syndrome by primary glomerular disorders are varied, a kidney biopsy for older children and adults is indicated.

Summary

- MCD is the most common cause of primary glomerular disease in children.
- The typical presentation is the nephrotic syndrome.
- Renal failure is uncommon, except in older adults.

Treatment

After the diagnosis of MCD is made, therapy should concentrate on management of the biologic consequences of the nephrotic syndrome (e.g., edema, proteinuria, hypertension if present, and hyperlipidemia), as well as on induction of remission with immunosuppressive agents. Regarding the former, escalating doses of loop diuretics given at least twice daily, with or without concomitant thiazide-type diuretics, may be necessary to maintain euvolemia. Additionally, the use of angiotensin-converting enzyme (ACE) inhibitors and/or angiotensin receptor blockers (ARBs) reduce proteinuria to some degree; these are the agents of choice if concomitant hypertension is present. Controlling blood pressure to lower than 130/80 mm Hg is advocated for any patient with kidney disorders.[6,7] Use of antihyperlipidemic agents, including 3-hydroxy-3-methylglutaryl coenzyme A (HMG-CoA) reductase inhibitors are recommended, although often not sufficient to reach the treatment goals in patients with kidney disease[8] if the degree of proteinuria remains severe.

Beyond this symptomatic treatment, induction of remission using immunosuppressive agents is indicated for all patients with MCD if not contraindicated. In select patient populations, up to 90% of children and 80% of adults enter complete remission (i.e., absence of dipstick proteinuria) after 2 and 4 months, respectively, of therapy with prednisone. Typical dosing regimens include daily prednisone (1 mg/kg/day for adults, 60 mg/m^2/day for children, maximum 80 mg/day), generally using alternate-day dosing soon after remission or sometimes from onset of therapy, with tapering doses for a total course of 2 to 6 months.[9,10] Relapses of MCD after steroid withdrawal or during steroid wean (steroid dependence) are common, especially in children. If frequent relapses occur, or in cases of steroid dependence, alternate therapies using cytotoxic agents (usually cyclophosphamide) are indicated as steroid-sparing agents. Steroid-resistant patients may respond to therapy with cyclosporine, but often relapse with withdrawal of that agent.

Summary

- Nonimmunosuppressive management includes diuretics, ACE inhibitors, ARBs, and statins.
- Patients are exquisitely steroid sensitive, with a high remission rate.
- Relapses and steroid dependence are common and may require cytotoxics; steroid resistance is rare and may be treated with cyclosporine.

Prognosis

MCD in general carries with it a good renal prognosis and ESRD is extremely rare. However, management of complications of the nephrotic syndrome (e.g., edema, infections, thrombophilia) and complications of the immunotherapy, most notably those related to corticosteroids, may prove challenging to the clinician and affect the morbidity of the patient.

FOCAL SEGMENTAL GLOMERULOSCLEROSIS

Pathologic Definition

Focal segmental glomerulosclerosis (FSGS) defines a characteristic pathologic pattern of glomerular injury and is not necessarily a distinct disease. The hallmark of kidney biopsy is an increased degree of scarring seen on light microscopy of some but not all of the glomeruli present (focal) that involves some but not all portions of the affected glomeruli (segmental). There are five distinct pathologic variants of FSGS. The importance of distinguishing these variants involves their different natural histories and responses to therapy. Apart from this, other nonspecific pathologic manifestations include low-level staining for immunoglobulin M (IgM) or C3 in sclerosed portions of the mesangium and fusion of epithelial foot processes in sclerosed and nonsclerosed portions of affected glomeruli. This pattern of injury can be seen as a manifestation of chronic injury induced by many different kidney disorders, and thus is regarded as secondary FSGS. For example, kidney biopsy specimens of patients with chronic vesicoureteral reflux may show FSGS-like patterns of injury. Conversely, patients with an appropriate clinical presentation (see later) lacking other identifiable kidney disorders who exhibit this pathologic pattern are correctly regarded as having idiopathic or primary FSGS. Such differentiation between primary and secondary FSGS may prove difficult at times, but is crucial when it comes to accurate treatment and prognosis.

Prevalence and Risk Factors

Primary FSGS is one of the two most common causes of idiopathic glomerular disease in adults, accounting for up to 25% to 35% of cases of nephrotic syndrome in all adults.[11] There is a two to four times higher prevalence of the disease in African Americans compared with whites. It is the most common primary glomerular disorder to cause ESRD in the United States, accounting for approximately 2.3% of the ESRD population.[12]

Pathophysiology and Natural History

Similar to MCD, primary FSGS is believed to occur as a result of a T-cell disorder resulting in the production of a circulating permeability factor, the identification of which has proven elusive, but may be a cytokine or lymphokine. This permeability factor is believed to lead to glomerular injury and proteinuria, hyperfiltration, and scarring. A small fraction of primary FSGS cases result from an inherited disorder of structural parts of the glomerular basement membrane or podocyte that results in altered glomerular function; these are not caused by a circulating factor. Secondary FSGS is known to occur in the setting of many different renal disorders, which can be classified based on the following: those leading to reduced nephron mass and/or glomerular hyperfiltration (e.g., aplasia or dysplasia, vesicoureteral reflux, morbid obesity); inflammatory renal disorders causing glomerular epithelial cell injury and subsequent scarring (e.g., lupus, focal proliferative glomerulonephropathy, vasculitis); infectious (e.g., HIV-associated FSGS); and toxins (e.g., heroin nephropathy).

Signs and Symptoms

As with MCD, the hallmark of FSGS is the presence of proteinuria, which can vary in severity from only 1 to 2 g/day to more than 10 g/day. Unlike MCD, at presentation, patients with FSGS are more prone to have concomitant microscopic hematuria (up to 50% of the time), hypertension (33% of the time), and a depressed glomerular filtration rate leading to elevated serum creatinine levels (33% of the time). Typically, patients with heavy proteinuria present clinically with signs and symptoms of the nephrotic syndrome (see earlier). As with MCD, serum complement levels are normal.

Diagnosis

The laboratory findings in FSGS are similar to those of MCD, with the exception of a higher likelihood of patients presenting with significant azotemia. Red blood cell (RBC) casts or dysmorphic RBCs are not characteristic of FSGS; their presence should point the clinician to disorders that can manifest with the nephritic syndrome. As with MCD, a kidney biopsy is usually necessary to establish the diagnosis.

Summary

- FSGS is the most common cause of primary glomerular disease in African American adults.
- It typically manifest with the nephrotic syndrome.
- Patients are likely to present with an elevated creatinine level.
- It is the most common primary glomerular disease leading to ESRD.

Treatment

Similar to MCD, the treatment of FSGS involves conservative measures (e.g., edema control with diuretics, hypertension management, treatment of hyperlipidemia, ACEs and/or ARBs) and those that target the proposed immune basis of the disorder specifically. The former (see earlier, MCD section), is indicated for all patients with FSGS, primary or secondary, regardless of the degree of proteinuria or azotemia. The latter is reserved for those patients with primary FSGS with nephrotic-range proteinuria and the absence of advanced azotemia. The options for immunosuppressive therapy include steroids alone (prednisone, 1 mg/kg daily or 2 mg/kg every other day) or, if comorbid conditions preclude the safe use of high-dose steroids, calcineurin inhibitors such as cyclosporine, 3 to 4 mg/kg/day in divided doses, with or without low-dose steroids. Use of calcineurin inhibitors should be avoided in patients with estimated GFRs lower than 40 mL/min/1.73 m^2 because of the concern for nephrotoxicity associated with their prolonged use.

The success of therapy is measured by the nephrotic patient's response in terms of proteinuria reduction: complete remission (CR), lower than 200 mg/day; partial remission (PR), 200 to 3500 mg/day; partial responder (PR), more than 50% reduction in proteinuria from baseline but still >3500 mg/day; and nonresponder (NR), less than 50% reduction in proteinuria and still >3500 mg/day. The success of therapy should not be determined for at least 4 months after initiation of therapy because of the well-described occurrence of fairly late treatment responses that may be missed if therapy is abandoned too soon after initiation. Duration of therapy should continue for 6 to 12 months after the onset of remission, with tapering prednisone doses. Patients who fail to reach a CR or PR with an adequate steroid trial are termed *steroid-resistant* and deserve a trial of a calcineurin inhibitor, if not contraindicated. Those who reach a CR or PR, but then subsequently develop recurrent nephrotic-range proteinuria during or shortly after steroid weaning, are termed *steroid-dependent* and may be tried on cytotoxic agents, such as cyclophosphamide, or other novel agents, such as mycophenolate mofetil or sirolimus. On average, approximately 40% to 80% of patients will achieve CR or PR with therapy, although the chance of relapse is high after cessation of cyclosporine (approximately 75%).

Summary

- Prednisone therapy is used at 1 mg/kg/day for at least 4 months.
- Monitor degree of proteinuria to determine therapeutic success.
- Calcineurin inhibitors are useful for those intolerant of high-dose steroids but without advanced azotemia.

Prognosis

As noted, primary FSGS is the most common cause of any primary glomerular disease leading to ESRD. Determining a patient's risk of this and pace of progression of azotemia is dependent on factors determined at clinical presentation (e.g., severity of proteinuria, degree of azotemia, pathologic variant, degree of interstitial disease on biopsy) and during therapy (e.g., CR vs. PR vs. NR). Regarding the former, subnephrotic patients with a normal serum creatinine level at baseline have the slowest rate of progression to kidney failure (i.e., 80% survival-free of ESRD at 10 years) compared with heavily nephrotic patients with more than 10 g/day (i.e., almost all ESRD by 3 years).[13,14] Regarding the latter, those achieving CR or PR have a superior renal survival compared with nonresponders: less than 15% ESRD at 5 years versus 50% ESRD at 6 months, respectively.[15]

MEMBRANOUS GLOMERULAR NEPHROPATHY

Pathologic Definition

Membranous glomerular nephropathy (MGN) is a kidney disorder defined by characteristic microscopic and immunofluorescence findings. On light microscopy, there is diffuse thickening of glomerular capillary walls without associated hypercellularity. On immunofluorescence, there is diffuse granular staining of the glomerular capillary loops: typically, for IgG more than IgA or IgM, as well as C3. On electron microscopy, the pathologic hallmark confirming MGN is electron-dense deposits in the subepithelial region of the glomerular basement membrane. These deposits correspond to the immunoglobulins seen on immunofluorescence. Occasionally, these deposits are large enough that they can be seen with special stains on light microscopy directly, or may induce adjacent changes of glomerular basement membrane material, leading to a spike appearance on either side of the deposit.

Prevalence and Risk Factors

Similar to FSGS, MGN is one of the most common primary glomerular diseases to cause nephrotic syndrome, accounting for 33% of cases,[11] with a predominance in men older than 40. And, similar to FSGS, MGN can result as part of a multisystem disease process such as lupus or chronic hepatitis B, or as a paraneoplastic manifestation of extrarenal carcinomas, appropriately called secondary MGN. Although primary MGN can occur in children, it is typically found in adults, with a peak incidence in the fourth or fifth decade of life.

Pathophysiology and Natural History

The cause of immunoglobulin deposition in the subepithelial location of the glomerular basement membranes in MGN, and its subsequent damage and altered structure, function, or both, are not completely known. It is believed that antigen-antibody complexes form in situ in the subepithelial space, possibly as a result of a freely circulating antibody recognizing and binding to a resident antigen within the glomerulus. Whatever the antigen stimulus may be, when the complex is formed, it is believed that complement activation occurs that produces toxic substances (e.g., the C5b-9 membrane attack complex); these directly induce damage to nearby cells and lead to the pathologic changes seen on biopsy and to the clinical manifestation of proteinuria or azotemia, or both. In the absence of other causes, which can accelerate the rate of loss of renal function (e.g., superimposed drug-induced acute interstitial nephritis, bilateral renal vein thrombosis), chronic kidney disease progression in MGN patients is slow in those who remain free of remission, with progression rates to ESRD averaging 30% to 40% at 10 to 15 years.[16] Clinical factors associated with an increased risk of this include age older than 50 years, male gender, proteinuria higher than 8 g/day, an elevated creatinine level at presentation, and higher scores of tubulointerstitial damage seen on biopsy. However, there is a well-documented occurrence of spontaneous remission of proteinuria in those with MGN who initially presented as nephrotic, ranging in up to 50% of cases, if followed untreated long enough: at least 5 years.[17]

Signs and Symptoms

Although patients with MGN may present with asymptomatic proteinuria, most present with signs and symptoms typical of the nephrotic syndrome. Up to 50% of patients may have some degree of hypertension at the onset of the disease. Rarely, patients will present with symptoms attributable to the hypercoagulability that may accompany nephrotic syndrome, most notably lower extremity venous thrombi causing pain or renal vein thrombosis with flank pain. Renal function is usually preserved at presentation unless MGN has gone undiagnosed for many years. Although only 3.5 g of proteinuria/day is sufficient to be regarded as in the nephrotic range, patients with MGN commonly have massive proteinuria, exceeding 10 to 20 g/day. Microscopic hematuria is seen in up to 50% of cases, although as with FSGS, RBC casts or dysmorphic RBCs should not be present. Although known as an immune complex disease, serum complement levels of C3 and C4 are normal.

Diagnosis

Adults presenting with the nephrotic syndrome and a relatively normal serum creatinine level are likely to have MGN in the absence of signs or symptoms suggestive of a systemic disease process. As noted, a kidney biopsy is necessary to delineate the pathology from the other disorders mentioned. However, given that MGN may be the presenting manifestation of a yet undiagnosed systemic disease, combined with the clinical importance of diagnosing such diseases early, all adults diagnosed with MGN on biopsy deserve a dedicated evaluation of secondary causes. This includes a remote hepatitis panel, VDRL, serologic markers of autoimmune disorders (e.g., lupus or mixed connective tissue disease), and age-appropriate cancer screening.

Summary

- MGN is one of the two most common primary glomerular diseases to cause nephrotic syndrome in adults.
- Severe proteinuria of more than 10 g/day and relatively normal serum creatinine level at presentation are not uncommon.
- Normal C3 and C4 levels are present, despite immune complex deposition seen pathologically on biopsy specimens.

Treatment

Given the relatively benign course in remission-free patients, together with a moderate chance of spontaneous remission without specific therapy, much controversy exists regarding the appropriate intensity of treatment for MGN. All patients deserve the conservative treatment of blood pressure control to lower than 130/80 mm Hg, ACE or ARB use, or both, and treatment of lipid disorders. Regarding the use of immunosuppressive therapy, however, scrutiny must be given to the risk of such treatment versus a potential benefit over the long term. This risk-to-benefit ratio only favors intense treatment for those patients who have a high likelihood of faster progression of kidney disease, which may be predicted by the presence of additive clinical risk factors present at diagnosis (see earlier). For those patients deemed high risk and in need of dedicated immunotherapy, treatment options include steroid-only regimens (e.g., prednisone at a dose of 2 mg/kg on alternate days for at least 8 weeks), alkylating agent-based regimens (e.g., 6 months of alternating steroids and cyclophosphamide),[18] and cyclosporine-based regimens (e.g., 6 months of twice-daily cyclosporine, targeting a trough level of 150 µg/L, plus low-dose prednisone).[19] Remission (complete or partial) rates vary among the treatment protocols, from 20% to 40% for steroid alone to almost 67% for alkylating agent or cyclosporine-based regimens, although the latter is complicated by a significantly higher relapse rate.

Summary

- **Immunosuppressive therapy is controversial, given the relatively benign course and moderate chance of spontaneous remission.**
- **Immunosuppressive therapy is reserved only for those at highest risk for faster progression to ESRD.**
- **Steroid-only, alkylating agent–based, or cyclosporine-based regimens are all used, with varying degrees of success.**

Prognosis

As noted, the prognosis of MGN is diverse and varied, based on pertinent clinical factors at presentation and the occurrence of remission, whether it is spontaneous or induced by specific immunotherapy. In general, those patients free of remission typically have a slow progressive loss of renal function, leading to ESRD. A pertinent caveat of MGN is the higher degree of hypercoagulability with the nephrotic syndrome compared with other primary glomerular disorders. Although any venous thrombosis event appears to be more likely in patients with MGN compared with other primary glomerular diseases, a significant consideration that may significantly affect renal and patient survival is the development of renal vein thrombosis, which may occur in approximately 15% of cases.

IMMUNOGLOBULIN A NEPHROPATHY

Pathologic Definition

The hallmark of IgA nephropathy (IGAN) is the presence of IgA deposits, predominantly in the mesangium, on biopsy specimens. Other immunoglobulins may also be present to a lesser degree, such as IgG or IgM. On light microscopy, pathologic findings may vary, from completely lacking to a severe diffuse proliferative glomerulonephritis, depending on the severity of clinical presentation. Typically, mesangioproliferative and focal proliferative findings are evident. The most severe cases will show diffuse proliferation as well as more than 50% of glomeruli with cellular crescents. Electron microscopic findings include electron-dense deposits in an expanded sclerotic mesangium.

Prevalence and Risk Factors

IGAN is believed to be the most common primary glomerular disease worldwide, but its incidence is likely underestimated by a bias against doing a biopsy in patients with a relatively benign presentation and clinical course. This is seen by the discrepancy in prevalence rates in Asia (>40% of biopsy specimens), where patients are more likely to receive a kidney biopsy with any urine sediment alterations as opposed to North America, where biopsies are typically reserved for patients with heavier degrees of proteinuria accompanying hematuria.[20] Although seen at all ages, it is predominant in the second and third decades of life, with a male predominance.

Pathophysiology and Natural History

Although not exactly known, it is believed that IGAN represents abnormal polyclonal IgA production as part of mucosal host defense, specifically a post-translational glycosylation defect of that protein. This abnormal glycosylation impairs the normal clearance from the bloodstream of the circulating IgA molecules, as well as predisposing their deposition within the kidneys. Given the inability of IgA molecules to fix complement once it is deposited, the mechanism of renal injury is poorly understood. In the absence of a severe presentation of IGAN, with heavy proteinuria and azotemia, most patients have a favorable renal course. Most will have one or a few intermittent episodes of IGAN that spontaneously resolve, without long-term effects on renal function. Indeed, only 1% to 2% of patients will develop ESRD as a result of IGAN. However, with extended follow-up of higher risk patients, especially those with persistent microscopic hematuria and heavier proteinuria, up to 20% to 30% will develop ESRD two decades after diagnosis.[21]

Signs and Symptoms

Patients with IGAN present on a wide spectrum, from asymptomatic microscopic hematuria to rapidly progressive renal failure, with heavy degrees of proteinuria. Knowing how IgA production is related to a mucosal host defense mechanism, it has been found that many patients present with abnormal urine findings soon after a current or recently resolved upper respiratory tract infection.

The most common presentation (40%-50% of cases) of IGAN is a single or sparsely recurrent episodes of gross hematuria at the time of or soon after a respiratory infection; this occurs more in children than in adults. Patients may also complain of dysuria and be mistakenly diagnosed with a urinary tract infection or with fevers and myalgias, and deemed to have a nonspecific viral syndrome. Such patients typically present with normal renal function and dysmorphic RBC, or RBC casts may be present.

The next most common presentation of IGAN (40% of cases), and the most predominant in adults, is asymptomatic microscopic hematuria with dysmorphia or RBC casts, with or without concomitant proteinuria or intermittent gross hematuria. Renal function is typically normal at baseline, although it may worsen slowly over time.

The final 20% of patients with IGAN present with hematuria and the nephrotic syndrome or, rarely, with the nephritic syndrome and rapidly progressive renal failure because of a crescentic glomerulonephritis.

Diagnosis

Given the appropriate clinical scenario—new hematuria in the setting of an upper respiratory tract infection with no significant proteinuria and normal renal function—many clinicians would opt for expectant management and reserve kidney biopsy for those with persistent abnormal urine findings, significant proteinuria (>500 mg/day), or an abnormal serum creatinine level. Serum IgA levels may be modestly elevated, although this usually is not helpful in the diagnosis. As expected, serum complement levels are normal.

Summary

- IGAN is the most common primary glomerular disorder worldwide.
- It involves the temporal relation of hematuria to an upper respiratory tract infection.
- Intermittent macroscopic hematuria, without proteinuria, and persistent microscopic hematuria, with or without proteinuria, are the most common presentations.

Treatment

Treatment of IGAN nephropathy is dictated by the clinical presentation of the patient and, if obtained, the pathologic changes seen. Those patients with isolated or recurrent gross hematuria following a respiratory tract infection, without alteration in renal function or significant proteinuria, may be observed without specific treatment. Similarly, patients with isolated microscopic hematuria, or with minimal proteinuria and favorable pathologic changes on biopsy, may be observed without specific treatment. In patients with significant proteinuria or azotemia, treatment with ACEs or ARBs is warranted, with blood pressure targeted at lower than 130/80 mm Hg. One study used ACEs plus ARBs, with favorable results on long-term renal function compared with either agent alone.[22] Controversy exists about whether treatment with fish oil in such patients is beneficial but, because of apparently little toxicity with their use, this is reasonable to try in patients at risk for progressive disease. Immunosuppressive therapy should be reserved for patients with the most severe clinical presentation or biopsy findings, or both. Patients with nephrotic syndrome may be tried on steroid-only regimens, such as prednisone, 2 mg/kg every other day for 3 months, tapered off over 3 months. For the most severe cases of rapidly progressive crescentic glomerulonephritis, a combined regimen of oral or intravenous cyclophosphamide along with steroids should be used for 3 months, followed by a prolonged steroid taper.

Summary

- Treatment is dictated by clinical presentation and biopsy findings.
- Moderate-risk patients should receive ACE inhibitors or ARBs, or both, statins, and possibly fish oil therapy.
- Severe cases are treated with steroids, with or without cyclophosphamide.

Prognosis

Generally, the long-term renal prognosis of IGAN is favorable. The most common clinical and most benign course is isolated events of macroscopic hematuria without proteinuria and normal renal function. These patients do well over time, without significant renal events. Patients with persistent urine abnormalities, especially those with higher degrees of proteinuria, are at risk for progression of renal disease over time, although the pace may be significantly slowed by the treatment regimens discussed. The worst prognosis is limited to those with crescentic glomerulonephritis, as would be expected.

MEMBRANOPROLIFERATIVE GLOMERULONEPHRITIS

Pathologic Definition

Biopsy specimens from patients with membranoproliferative glomerulonephritis (MPGN) are characterized by global capillary wall thickening and glomerular hypercellularity. The increased cellular content occurs because of proliferation of resident glomerular cells, as well as infiltrating mononuclear cells and neutrophils. Often seen, but not necessarily specific to MPGN, is double contouring or splitting of the glomerular capillary basement membranes. A subset of patients with MPGN may exhibit cellular crescents within Bowman's space. Immunofluorescence studies demonstrate diffuse granular or bandlike intense staining of capillary loops and mesangium with C3, and to a lesser extent IgG and IgM. MPGN pathognomonic changes on electron microscopy are subendothelial and mesangial electron-dense deposits; the former are found in an expanded subendothelial region of the glomerular basement membrane formed by projections of mesangial cytoplasm. Some subepithelial deposits may also been seen, but they are not as prominent as in cases of MGN. A subset of MPGN cases (type II MPGN) have a different hallmark electron microscopic finding than the discrete subendothelial deposits (type I MPGN). In the former, a bandlike, almost continuous, ribbon of the electron-dense material is found in the subendothelial space.

Prevalence and Risk Factors

MPGN is a rare primary glomerular disorder and appears to be decreasing in frequency. A possible reason for this is correction of what used to be known as primary MPGN, but actually was a renal manifestation of hepatitis C virus infection and mixed essential cryoglobulinemia. Such cases are now correctly defined as secondary MPGN. Primary MPGN is a disease mostly found in children, with more than 75% of cases diagnosed between ages 8 and 16 years.[23] It accounts for approximately 10% of biopsy specimens of primary glomerular disorders.

Pathophysiology and Natural History

Similar to MGN, MPGN is classified as an immune complex disease and the presumptive pathophysiologic mechanism is the inappropriate production of antibodies recognizing a nephritogenic antigen. Unlike MGN, in which it is believed that antigen is inherent in the glomerular structure itself, MPGN is believed to occur as a result of deposition of circulating antigen-antibody complexes. These traverse the large pores found between glomerular endothelial cells and deposit between them and the glomerular basement membrane. Complement activation results from the deposition of these antigen-antibody complexes and results in a cascade of proinflammatory signals that stimulate local cell proliferation and recruitment of circulating immune cells, which augments the inflammatory reaction. This ongoing inflammation is believed to be the major reason for the ensuing renal damage.

Signs and Symptoms

Patients with MPGN may present with different clinical syndromes. Approximately 50% exhibit signs and symptoms typical of the nephrotic syndrome, whereas 25% of patients only present with asymptomatic hematuria and proteinuria. The remaining 25% present more severely, with the acute nephritic syndrome. Although 50% of all patients may have some degree of azotemia at presentation, those exhibiting a nephritic as opposed to a nephrotic picture tend to have more depressed renal function at baseline, which declines rapidly.

Diagnosis

As with all glomerular diseases, one must be cognizant of systemic processes in which MPGN may be a common renal manifestation. These include autoimmune diseases such as lupus, viral infections such as hepatitis C or B, and chronic bacterial infections such as endocarditis or chronic abscesses. Rarely, MPGN may represent a paraneoplastic manifestation of solid or liquid malignancies. Correct identification of a systemic disease leading to MPGN is critical because treatment of the underlying disorder, and not the renal lesion itself, is appropriate. Beyond the typical findings of the nephrotic or nephritic syndrome, few other symptoms may aid the clinician in distinguishing primary MPGN from other primary glomerular disorders. However, the urine sediment becomes a valuable tool in this setting. Unlike the other primary glomerular diseases that cause nephrotic syndrome, patients with MPGN exhibit an active sediment, defined by hematuria with associated dysmorphic RBCs (e.g., acanthocytes) as well as RBC casts. Additionally, because the inflammatory reaction induced by the deposition of the immune complexes is in the subendothelial space and directly in contact with circulating complement, which they can fix and activate, hypocomplementemia is characteristic of all types of MPGN. C3 and C4 levels are more equally depressed in type I MPGN because of activation of the classic complement pathway as opposed to type II MPGN, in which C3 levels are lower than C4 because of preferential activation of the alternative complement pathway.

Summary

- MPGN is more prevalent in children and young adults.
- The clinical presentation may be nephrotic syndrome, nephritic syndrome, or asymptomatic hematuria and proteinuria.
- An active urine sediment and hypocomplementemia in the absence of systemic diseases are useful clinical clues.

Treatment

Patients with MPGN follow the rule of thirds. That is, approximately one third will have a spontaneous remission, one third will have persistent manifestations that intermittently wax and wane, and one third will have a progressive decline to ESRD. Factors that may predict the latter include heavier degrees of proteinuria or the nephrotic syndrome, or both, hypertension, advanced azotemia at baseline, and a nephritic presentation, especially with crescents on biopsy. After excluding important secondary causes of MPGN, most notably hepatitis C infection, immunosuppressive therapy should be tried for these patients, in addition to conservative management. Most data on treatment have come from pediatric studies,[24] but a potential adult regimen includes prednisone, 2 mg/kg every other day for 3 to 12 months, depending on the rate of response. If a significant response is seen, with a decline in proteinuria, stabilization of serum creatinine level, and improvement in activity of the urine sediment, the steroids may be tapered to 20 mg every other day and maintained for another few years. Other therapies, in addition to steroids, such as antiplatelet agents (e.g., aspirin, dipyridamole), with or without cytotoxic agents, have not convincingly proven to be of benefit.

Summary

- Restrict immunosuppressive patients to those at highest risk for progression-heavier proteinuria, nephritic syndrome, elevated creatinine level at baseline, and crescents on biopsy.
- It is crucial to exclude secondary causes, most notably hepatitis C, before initiating immunosuppressive therapy.
- Prednisone, 2 mg/kg every other day for many months, tapered to 20 mg every other day for several years, may be given.

Prognosis

Given the rule of thirds, the renal prognosis of patients with MPGN depends exactly on presentation. Those with asymptomatic hematuria and non-nephrotic proteinuria have a relatively benign course, whereas those with more severe presentations who fail to remit spontaneously or with therapy will progress to ESRD faster. On average, progression to ESRD 10 years after diagnosis will occur in is 35% to 60% of patients with MPGN.[25,26]

SPECIAL CASES OF CRESCENTIC GLOMERULONEPHRITIS

Pathologic Definition

As discussed for MPGN and IGAN, there are some severe forms of primary glomerular diseases that manifest clinically, with rapid deterioration of renal function associated with diffuse cellular crescents on biopsy. However, there are other forms of primary crescentic glomerular diseases pathologically distinct from those discussed that also lead to rapidly progressive glomerulonephritis (RPGN). Anti–glomerular basement membrane (anti-GBM) disease refers to cases of RPGN characterized by linear staining, as opposed to granular patterns (as in MPGN or IGAN) of IgG along the glomerular basement membranes, almost always in the presence of cellular crescents and fibrinoid necrosis, but usually in the absence of significant hypercellularity. Although most cases of anti-GBM disease occur as part of a systemic process involving other systems—most notably the lungs in the form of Goodpasture's syndrome, with pulmonary hemorrhage—idiopathic anti-GBM disease can occur as a renal-limited disorder.

Pauci-immune antineutrophil cytoplasmic antibody (ANCA)-associated crescentic glomerulonephritis is characterized by a necrotizing, hypercellular, crescentic, glomerular lesion similar to that in anti-GBM disease that lacks any significant immunoglobulin staining in a granular or linear pattern. Again, although usually occurring with multisystem small-vessel ANCA-associated vasculitis syndromes (e.g., Wegener's granulomatosis, Churg-Strauss syndrome), patients can present with a renal-limited pauci-immune glomerulonephritis. Rarely, there are some forms of crescentic glomerulonephritis with granular immunoglobulin staining similar to but not completely classifiable as other lesions, such as IGAN or MPGN, and are thus known as idiopathic immune complex glomerulonephritis.

Prevalence and Risk Factors

Anti-GBM disease is rare, accounting for less than 20% of all cases of crescentic glomerulonephritis,[27] and has a bimodal distribution, the first in the second to third decade of life and the second in the sixth and seventh decades. Pauci-immune ANCA-associated crescentic glomerulonephritis, renal-limited or as part of a systemic vasculitis syndrome, is the most common cause of RPGN in older adults, with a predominance in whites observed.[28]

Pathophysiology and Natural History

Although many antigens have been described to which the IgG of anti-GBM disease binds, 90% of the time they are directed toward a mutated α_3 chain of type IV collagen, which is a predominant component of the GBM. It is believed that once bound, these IgG molecules stimulate a T lymphocyte-dependent inflammatory reaction that leads to the pathologic and clinical findings observed, including crescent formation and rapid deterioration of renal function. In cases of pauci-immune glomerulonephritis, because of the absence of immunoglobulin deposition, it is believed that the ANCAs directly stimulate a neutrophilic inflammatory process and subsequent damage. If left untreated, both syndromes will lead to complete loss of renal function over a short period of time, in weeks to months).[29]

Signs and Symptoms

Patients with crescentic glomerulonephritis syndromes in the absence of systemic processes present with the nephritic syndrome with varying degrees of proteinuria, hematuria with dysmorphic RBCs and RBC casts, hypertension, and some degree of azotemia at the time of diagnosis. Patients may also exhibit concomitant or subsequent extrarenal signs and symptoms if the anti-GBM disease is present as part of Goodpasture's syndrome (e.g., hemoptysis or frank pulmonary hemorrhage, respiratory failure), or if the pauci-immune glomerulonephritis is part of systemic small-vessel vasculitis syndromes (e.g., recurrent sinusitis, hemoptysis, abdominal pain, arthralgias, mononeuropathies).

Diagnosis

Although pathologic determination is necessary to classify the exact glomerular syndrome, patients exhibiting the nephritic syndrome should also undergo a serologic workup, including determination of complement levels, which are normal in anti-GBM or pauci-immune cases but are usually depressed in cases of idiopathic immune complex glomerulonephritis. Additionally, the presence of circulating anti-glomerular basement antibodies or ANCAs (e.g., c-ANCA against proteinase-3 antibodies or p-ANCA against myeloperoxidase) should be investigated. However, because significant time may elapse before the results of these assays are available, combined with the rapid deterioration of renal function if appropriate therapy is delayed, the clinician should not delay pursuing a renal biopsy if clinical suspicion is high.

Summary

- These rare disorders can manifest with the nephritic syndrome as a renal-limited process or as part of a multisystem disease.
- Although serologic markers are specific, the delay in obtaining the results of such assays should not postpone a kidney biopsy for a definitive diagnosis if clinical suspicion is high.
- Immunofluorescence staining is necessary to differentiate between specific causes, which affect the correct treatment modality to be used.

Treatment

Once the specific type of crescentic glomerulonephritis is determined by kidney biopsy, appropriate treatment should be instituted immediately to preserve renal function and optimize patient survival. Anti-GBM disease treatment includes daily or alternate-day plasmapheresis for 2 to 3 weeks and immunosuppressive therapy with steroids and a cytotoxic agent, such as cyclophosphamide. The goal of the former is to remove the pathologic circulating anti-GBM antibody and the latter is to decrease its production. A typical daily regimen is 1 mg/kg of prednisone plus 2 mg/kg of oral cyclophosphamide. The duration of cyclophosphamide therapy is usually 3 months, with a slow taper of the prednisone over a 6- to 9-month period after cessation of the cytotoxic agent.[30]

In general, all patients with anti-GBM should be treated, but some caveats do exist. In patients requiring dialysis, the chance of renal recovery is sufficiently low that the potential toxicity outweighs the chance of success and should be avoided.[30] A possible exception to this involves patients with crescentic glomerulonephritis who have circulating anti-GBM antibodies and ANCAs. In such cases, cytotoxic therapy may lead to a late renal recovery, despite early dialysis requirements, and so its use should at least be contemplated.[31] Similarly, those patients who present with pulmonary hemorrhage should undergo treatment regardless of their renal status because patient, and not just renal, survival takes precedence in this situation.

Optimal treatment for pauci-immune ANCA-associated crescentic glomerulonephritis is different than that for anti-GBM disease. In this case, plasmapheresis has not shown to add any advantage to a combination of cytotoxic and steroid therapies unless the patient also has hemoptysis or anti-GBM antibody present. Initial steroid dosing should be more aggressive in the form of pulse intravenous high doses, such as methylprednisolone, 1000 mg daily for 3 consecutive days, followed by oral prednisone at a dosage of 1 mg/kg daily. Cytotoxic therapy should accompany this steroid therapy, typically either 2 mg/kg of oral cyclophosphamide daily, or monthly intravenous pulse cyclophosphamide. Typical duration of therapy is 6 to 12 months, depending on how quickly the patient has entered remission. Patients who need dialysis should still be treated unless contraindicated, because the chance for renal recovery is higher than with anti-GBM disease, although adjusting down the dose of cyclophosphamide is necessary.

Summary

- Early institution of plasmapheresis and cytotoxic therapy is essential in anti-GBM disease, because there is a small chance of renal recovery when progression to dialysis dependence has occurred.
- Steroid dosing should be more aggressive in patients with pauci-immune crescentic glomerulonephritis and cytotoxic therapy should be used, even for patients requiring dialysis, unless otherwise contraindicated.

Prognosis

The renal and patient prognoses of untreated crescentic glomerulonephritis are dismal and bely the aggressiveness of treatment. In general, with early intervention, patient response to therapy is good, with renal and patient survival approaching 70% and 90%, respectively. Relapses can occur and, when present, adversely affect overall outcome. As expected, success of treatment and prognosis is highly dependent on the degree of renal dysfunction at the time of diagnosis.

Suggested Readings

Cattran DC, Appel GB, Hebert LA, et al: Cyclosporine in patients with steroid-resistant membranous nephropathy: A randomized trial. Kidney Int 2001;59:1484-1490.

Couser WG: Rapidly progressive glomerulonephritis: Classification, pathogenetic mechanisms, and therapy. Am J Kidney Dis 1988;11:449-464.

Haas M, Meehan SM, Karrison TG, et al: Changing etiologies of unexplained adult nephrotic syndrome: A comparison of renal biopsy findings from 1976-1979 and 1995-1997. Am J Kidney Dis 1997;30:621-631.

Hogan SL, Muller KE, Jennette JC, et al: A review of therapeutic studies of idiopathic membranous glomerulopathy. Am J Kidney Dis 1995;25:862-875.

Jennette J, Mandal A: The nephrotic syndrome. In: Mandal A, Jennette J (eds): Diagnosis and Management of Renal Disease and Hypertension. Durham, NC, Carolina Academic Press, 1994, pp 235-272.

Kitiyakara C, Eggers P, Kopp JB: Twenty-one-year trend in ESRD because of focal segmental glomerulosclerosis in the United States. Am J Kidney Dis 2004;44: 815-825.

Korbet SM: Primary focal segmental glomerulosclerosis. J Am Soc Nephrol 1998;9:1333-1340.

Nakao N, Yoshimura A, Morita H, et al: Combination treatment of angiotensin-II receptor blocker and angiotensin-converting-enzyme inhibitor in non-diabetic renal disease (COOPERATE): A randomised controlled trial. Lancet 2003;361:117-124.

National Heart, Lung and Blood Institute: Seventh Report of the Joint National Committee on Prevention, Detection, Evaluation, and Treatment of High Blood Pressure (JNC 7), 2003. Available at www.nhlbi.nih.gov/guidelines/hypertension.

Nolasco F, Cameron JS, Heywood EF, et al: Adult-onset minimal change nephrotic syndrome: A long-term follow-up. Kidney Int 1986;29:1215-1223.

West CD: Childhood membranoproliferative glomerulonephritis: An approach to management. Kidney Int 1986;29:1077-1093.

References

For a complete list of references, log onto www.expertconsult.com.

Hematuria

Richard Fatica and Adele Fowler

Blood in the urine can originate at any point along the urinary tract and both gross and microscopic hematuria may represent serious underlying disease. Gross hematuria is often alarming and will prompt the patient to seek medical attention. Similarly, the office practitioner may be faced with the incidental finding of asymptomatic microscopic hematuria. Patient characteristics and the clinical presentation will help guide the clinician in the proper evaluation and diagnosis.

DEFINITION

Hematuria is defined as the abnormal presence of red blood cells (RBCs) in the urine and is commonly divided into gross and microscopic hematuria. Gross, or visible, hematuria can result from as little as 1 mL of blood in 1 L of urine, and therefore the color does not reflect the degree of blood loss. Also, numerous other substances can induce such a color change (see later, "Signs and Symptoms"). When true gross hematuria exists, the literature universally supports a full evaluation.[1]

Microscopic hematuria is often found incidentally during office evaluation of urinary tract infection symptoms or during routine health screening. Approximately one million RBCs pass into the urine daily, which corresponds to 1 to 3 RBCs/high-power (HPF) field in centrifuged urine sediment examined microscopically.[2] Although much controversy exists, the American Urological Association (AUA) defines microscopic hematuria as 3 RBCs/high-power field on microscopic examination of the centrifuged urine specimen in two of three freshly voided, clean catch, midstream urine samples.[3] Confirmation on repeat testing takes into account the intermittent nature of hematuria found in some diseases.

PREVALENCE

The reported prevalence of asymptomatic hematuria in adults varies widely. Population-based studies have shown prevalence rates of less than 1% to as high as 16%. This range is attributed to differences in patient demographics, amount of follow-up, definition and diagnostic technique, and the number of screening tests per patient.[1] Patients at high risk for urologic disease, such as older men, have a higher prevalence of hematuria.[4]

PATHOPHYSIOLOGY

The pathophysiology of hematuria depends on the anatomic site in the urinary tract from which blood loss occurs. A distinction has conventionally been drawn between glomerular and extraglomerular bleeding, separating nephrologic and urologic disease.

Blood originating from the nephron is termed *glomerular* or *nephronal hematuria.*[5] RBCs can enter the urinary space from the glomerulus or, rarely, from the renal tubule. Disruption of the filtration barrier in the glomerulus may result from inherited or acquired abnormalities in the structure and integrity of the glomerular capillary wall. These RBCs can be trapped in Tamm-Horsfall mucoprotein and will be manifest in the urine by RBC casts. Finding casts in the urine represents significant disease at the glomerular level. However, in disease of the nephron, casts can be absent and isolated RBCs may be the only finding. The presence of proteinuria helps support a glomerular source of blood loss.

Hematuria without proteinuria or casts is termed isolated hematuria. Although a few glomerular diseases may produce isolated hematuria, this finding is more consistent with extraglomerular bleeding. Anything that disrupts the uroepithelium, such as irritation, inflammation, or invasion, can result in normal-appearing RBCs in the urine. Such insults may include malignancy, renal stones, trauma, infection, and medications. Also, nonglomerular renal causes of blood loss, such as tumors of the kidney, renal cysts, infarction, and arteriovenous malformations, can cause blood loss into the urinary space. Clues to the specific causes of hematuria are discussed in the next section.

Summary

- Microscopic and macroscopic hematuria may represent serious underlying disease.
- Gross hematuria needs full evaluation.
- Microhematuria needs confirmation as it can be intermittent.
- Hematuria can be divided into glomerular and extraglomerular (nephrologic and urologic) diseases.
- The presence of proteinuria and red cell casts suggests glomerular involvement.
- The presence of clots suggests urologic involvement.

SIGNS AND SYMPTOMS

The history, physical examination, and review of systems can provide important clues to the nature of the underlying disease, narrow the differential diagnosis, and separate glomerular from extraglomerular bleeding in the patient who presents with hematuria. One of the most important considerations is age, because childhood causes of hematuria may differ greatly from those in the adult. For example, hypercalciuria is a common cause of hematuria in children but is rare in adults.[2] In older adults, even transient hematuria carries an appreciable risk of cancer and should be strongly considered for further evaluation.[1]

A family history of renal failure and cerebral aneurysms suggests polycystic kidney disease. Hearing loss and renal failure in male members of a family are seen in Alport's disease. A family history without these symptoms may suggest thin basement membrane disease. A tendency to form kidney stones may run in families.

Many ingested substances can cause color change in the urine that can be mistaken for blood, and careful dietary and medication histories may elucidate a cause that can spare costly medical evaluations (Box 1).[6] Recent strenuous exercise can produce transient hematuria by traumatic and nontraumatic mechanisms.[7] Increased glomerular permeability may result from ischemic damage to the nephron as blood is shunted to exercising muscle or from an increased perfusion pressure secondary to efferent arteriolar vasoconstriction.

Constitutional symptoms such as fever, arthritis, and rash may suggest a glomerulonephritis associated with a connective tissue disease such as systemic lupus erythematosus. Hematuria or cola-colored urine following an upper respiratory illness is seen in immunoglobulin A (IgA) nephritis. Henoch-Schönlein purpura (HSP), the systemic variant of IgA nephritis, is commonly associated with palpable purpura of the skin and gastrointestinal manifestations. Absence of constitutional symptoms does not rule out a glomerulonephritis, however, because many primary renal diseases may manifest with only hematuria or proteinuria (or both).

Box 1 Substances that Can Cause Red Pigmenturia

Endogenous Sources
Bilirubin
Myoglobin
Hemoglobin
Porphyrins

Foods
Rhubarb
Blackberries
Blueberries
Paprika
Beets
Fava beans
Artificial food colorings

Drugs
Rifampin
Nitrofurantoin
Sulfonamides
Metronidazole
Phenytoin
Prochlorperazine
Phenolphthalein
Quinine
Chloroquine
Phenazopyridine
Levodopa
Methyldopa
Adriamycin
Desferoxamine

Data from Sokolosky MC: Hematuria. Emerg Med Clin North Am 2001;19:621-632.

A careful history of pain symptoms should be conducted. Suprapubic tenderness accompanied by dysuria, urgency, or hesitancy is found in cystitis. Prostatitis and urethritis also result in symptoms with urination. Severe pain in the flank, with radiation into the groin, is seen in ureteral distention or irritation by stones, clots, or other debris, such as that found in papillary necrosis. The rare loin pain–hematuria syndrome can have a similar pain pattern. Renal capsular distention from inflammation (pyelonephritis) or hematoma (trauma) can result in costovertebral angle tenderness. Bleeding or infection in a renal cyst can also result in costovertebral angle tenderness.

The characteristics of the hematuria can often help distinguish the cause and location of bleeding. A glomerular source of bleeding usually results in persistent microscopic hematuria, with or without periods of gross hematuria. In renal sources of hematuria, the blood is equally dispersed throughout the urine stream and does not clot.[6] If clots are present, it is important to ascertain where in the urine stream they occur. Hematuria or clots at the beginning of the urine stream, initial hematuria, is a symptom of a urethral cause. Terminal hematuria, occurring at the end of the urine stream, may occur with a prostatic, bladder, or trigonal cause of hematuria.[6]

Important physical examination findings in the patient with hematuria may include fever and hypertension. The examination should include a search for signs of the above-mentioned systemic illnesses, such as rash and joint tenderness. Complete abdominal and back examinations should be performed to evaluate for tenderness or masses. In men, a complete genitourinary examination, including the prostate, is important to look for any visible urethral lesion or evidence of prostatitis. A pelvic examination should be done in women to exclude the possibility of contamination of urine by vaginal bleeding.

DIAGNOSIS

Before any imaging studies, the urinalysis can provide a great deal of information. Many urine specimens are first tested by dipstick. The dipstick urinalysis records a reaction between hydrogen peroxide and Chromagen that is catalyzed by hemoglobin. This reaction results in a green color change of the Chromagen that is visible on the dipstick.[3] The sensitivity of the dipstick to detect hematuria at a concentration of more than 3 RBCs/HPF is more than 90%.[6]

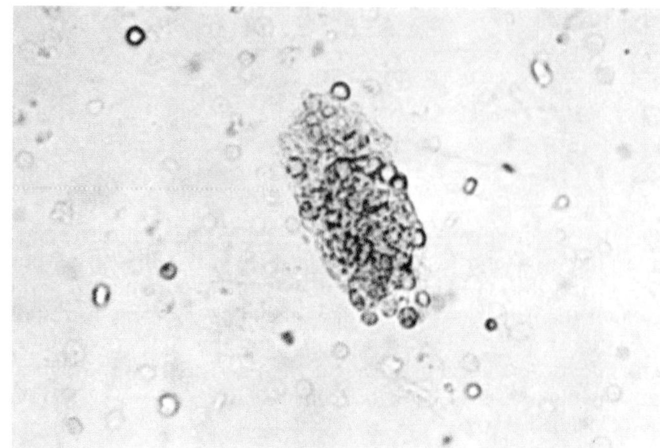

Figure 1 Red blood cell cast (400×).

However, many factors can result in false-positive and false-negative results. A false-negative can result from vitamin C ingestion, urine pH lower than 5.1, or a dipstick that has had prolonged exposure to air before testing.[1,3] A false-positive result may be seen by contamination of the urine with menstrual blood, myoglobinuria, and bacterial peroxidases. For these reasons, all positive dipstick results and all negative results with a high index of suspicion should undergo microscopy. Samples sent for microscopy should be evaluated within 1 hour, because casts will begin to disintegrate and RBCs may lyse. Cellular elements may be preserved a few more hours by refrigeration of the sample.[6]

On microscopy, dysmorphic red cells and RBC casts are consistent with a glomerular source of bleeding. These findings, especially in conjunction with significant proteinuria, should lead to an evaluation for glomerular disease. These patients do not need evaluation for urologic disease.[8,9] RBCs from a nonglomerular source more closely resemble peripheral blood on microscopy, with isomorphic RBCs and absence of casts.[6]

Another helpful practice in locating the source of bleeding is the three-tube test. Three consecutive samples of the urine stream are collected: the first few milliliters, midstream, and the last few milliliters. Similar to that described for the location of clots in the urine stream, hematuria primarily in the first sample is consistent with a urethral source, whereas hematuria primarily at the end of the urine stream is more likely a lesion at the bladder trigone. Equivalent hematuria in all three samples is seen in renal, ureteral, and diffuse bladder lesions.[8]

As mentioned, the presence of proteinuria, typically higher than 500 to 1000 mg/day along with hematuria, is highly suggestive of a renal parenchymal disease. Abnormal RBC morphology (e.g., dysmorphic RBCs) and the presence of RBC casts are almost pathognomonic for parenchymal disease. Dysmorphic RBCs have irregular membrane blebs or shapes, often with reduction in the hemoglobin level. The presence of more than 80% dysmorphic cells in a sample is highly suggestive of a glomerular source, whereas the presence of less than 20% dysmorphic cells is associated with a urologic source.[10] Dysmorphic RBCs may be better appreciated under phase contrast microscopy.

RBCs that escape through the glomerular filter may be trapped in Tamm-Horsfall mucoprotein excreted by the distal tubule and appear in the urine as a RBC cast (Fig. 1). Primary renal diseases such as membranoproliferative glomerulonephritis (MPGN), acute glomerulonephritis such as poststreptococcal glomerulonephritis (PSGN), and rapidly progressive glomerulonephritis (RPGN) may all have RBC casts in the urine. The presence of RBC casts in the urine should initiate a prompt nephrologic referral for further diagnosis and treatment.

Hematuria may be seen in various other renal parenchymal disorders without glomerulonephritis, such as acute allergic interstitial nephritis, chronic interstitial nephritis, papillary necrosis, or pyelonephritis. The RBCs in these disorders are more commonly free RBCs, not associated in casts, and may not be the predominant abnormal finding on the urinalysis.

TREATMENT

Any evidence of renal parenchymal disease should prompt a referral to a nephrologist for consideration of a kidney biopsy and treatment. Many renal diseases are slowly progressive and much therapy may be performed in the general practitioner's office.

If the clinical picture is suspicious for nephrolithiasis, various imaging studies can be helpful in making a definitive diagnosis. A plain film x-ray of the abdomen and pelvis has the advantages of being quick and noninvasive. However, it is not particularly sensitive and many stones can be missed, including calcium-containing stones smaller than 2 mm and stones that are radiolucent (e.g., uric acid, xanthine, triamterene). Bony pelvic structures and overlying bowel contents can also obscure stones.

A long-standing gold standard in the diagnosis of kidney stones is intravenous pyelography (IVP), which can detect both anatomic abnormalities and ureteral obstruction as a result of stones. It is also relatively inexpensive and safe in the patient with normal renal function, except for the obvious risks associated with IV contrast. Many institutions have replaced the IVP with helical computed tomography (CT). It is reported to have 97% sensitivity and 96% specificity in identifying ureteral stones.[11,12] It also has the advantage of finding other disease that is being mistaken for renal colic. Another option is ultrasound, which can evaluate for stones by direct visualization of the stone or by the finding of unilateral hydronephrosis. It is less sensitive than IVP or CT but safe in patients with renal insufficiency.

Kidney stones smaller than 4 mm are likely to pass spontaneously, whereas those larger than 7 mm have a low likelihood of passing spontaneously.[13] Any symptoms such as pain, fever, or obstruction with hydroureter should prompt a referral to a urologist for possible stone extraction. Recurrent stone formers should undergo metabolic testing to prevent or reduce the frequency of development of subsequent stones.

The difficult decision for the general practitioner is the extent of evaluation needed for the patient with no symptoms and no evidence of renal parenchymal disease, stones, or infection. Numerous studies[4,14,15] have been done to determine the significance of asymptomatic microscopic hematuria and its likelihood of predicting significant urologic disease. Most of the studies have been done in referral-based populations made up of patients referred to urologists for evaluation of asymptomatic microscopic hematuria. These studies tend to find a higher incidence of significant urologic disease and malignancy than studies in non–referral-based populations because those believed to be at higher risk are more likely referred for further evaluation. Mariani and associates[14] have found the incidence of life-threatening disease to increase with age, especially after age 50 years, and to be higher in men than women in a group of 1000 patients referred for urologic evaluation of hematuria. Mohr and colleagues[15] have investigated the prevalence of urologic disease in 286 patients with asymptomatic hematuria from 2697 patients sampled. The percentage of asymptomatic hematuria was relatively constant across age groups, at 13%; however, the presence of serious urologic disease, such as renal neoplasia and cancer of the prostate, increased with advancing age. There were no women with serious urologic disease younger than 75 years, regardless of the degree of hematuria. There was no disease discovered in 63% of men younger than 55 years with hematuria. It was concluded that the positive predictive value of asymptomatic hematuria is low, and that the patient age could be used as a guide to determine whether further workup is needed.[15]

Box 2 Risk Factors for Significant Disease in Patients With Microscopic Hematuria

- Smoking history
- Occupational exposure to chemicals or dyes (e.g., benzenes, aromatic amines)
- Age older than 40 years
- History of urologic disorder or disease
- History of irritative voiding symptoms
- History of urinary tract infection
- Analgesic abuse
- History of pelvic irradiation

Adapted from Grossfeld GD, Wolf JS, Litwin MS, et al: Evaluation of asymptomatic microscopic hematuria in adults: The American Urological Association best practice policy recommendations. Urology 2001;57:599-610.

In their review of published studies of referral- and non–referral-based patients with asymptomatic microscopic hematuria, Grossfeld and Carroll[1] have described the incidence of urologic malignancy as ranging from 0% to 26%. This wide range likely reflects the different populations studied in terms of age, gender, and whether it was a referral-based population.

The current AUA best practice policy recommendations are based on presence of risk factors for significant urologic disease (Box 2).[16] Low-risk patients should undergo urine cytology examination or cystoscopy, along with upper tract imaging (CT or IVP). Patients with suspicious findings on cytology should then be referred for cystoscopy. Patients with significant risk factors should undergo a complete evaluation including upper tract imaging, urine cytology, and cystoscopy (Fig. 2).

All patients with an initial negative evaluation should have follow-up, especially those in higher risk groups. This should include repeat urinalysis, urine cytology, and blood pressure, as outlined in Figure 2.

OUTCOMES

Hematuria will continue to be a common problem in the outpatient setting and therefore the primary care physician will frequently be faced with the initial workup. Infection accounts for 25% of all cases[15] and stones account for another 20%.[2] Despite workup, a urologic cause of hematuria is not discovered in approximately 10% of patients.[6] The incidence of urologic malignancy increases with advancing age, and even low-grade hematuria in high-risk patients should prompt an evaluation.

Summary

- Forty-five percent of cases are attributed to infection and nephrolithiasis.
- Evidence of renal parenchymal disease should prompt nephrology referral.
- The frequency of significant urologic disease found in patients without renal parenchymal disease, infection, or stones increases with age, with a predominance in men.
- Most patients with an initial negative workup should have follow-up, specially if in a high-risk population.

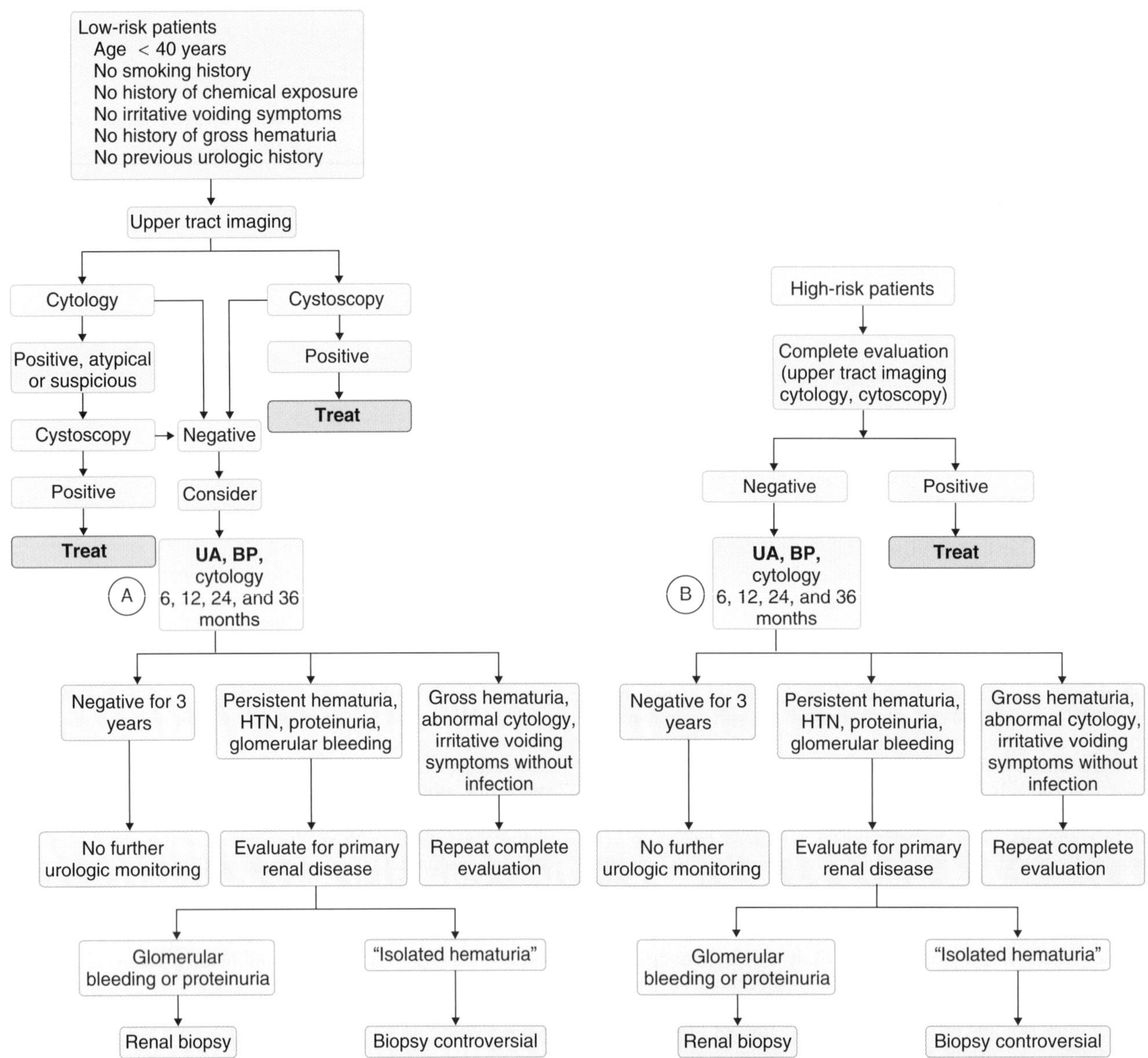

Figure 2 **Urologic evaluation of asymptomatic hematuria.** **A**, Low-risk patients. **B**, High-risk patients. BP, blood pressure; HTN, hypertension; UA, urinalysis. *(Adapted from Grossfeld GD, Wolf JS, Litwin MS, et al: Evaluation of asymptomatic microscopic hematuria in adults: The American Urological Association best practice policy recommendations. Urology 2001;57:599-610.)*

Suggested Readings

Froom P, Ribak J, Benbassat J: Significance of microhaematuria in young adults. Br Med J 1984;288:20-22.

Grossfeld GD, Carroll PR: Evaluation of asymptomatic microscopic hematuria. Urol Clin North Am 1998;25:661-676.

Grossfeld GD, Wolf JS Jr, Litwan MS, et al: Asymptomatic microscopic hematuria in adults: Summary of the AUA best practice policy recommendations. Am Fam Physician 2001;63:1145-1154.

Grossfeld GD, Wolf JS, Litwin MS, et al: Evaluation of asymptomatic microscopic hematuria in adults: The American Urological Association best practice policy recommendations. Urology 2001; 57:599-610.

Handrigan MT, Thompson I, Foster M: Diagnostic procedures for the urogenital system. Emerg Med Clin North Am 2001;19:745-761.

Mariani AJ, Mariani MC, Macchioni C, et al: The significance of adult hematuria: 1,000 hematuria evaluations including a risk-benefit and cost-effectiveness analysis. J Urol 1989;141:350-355.

Mohr DN, Offord KP, Owen RA, et al: Asymptomatic microhematuria and urologic disease. A population-based study. JAMA 1986;256:224-229.

Pollock C, Liu PL, Gyory AZ, et al: Dysmorphism of urinary RBCs-value in diagnosis. Kidney Int 1989;36:1045-1049.

Sokolosky MC: Hematuria. Emerg Med Clin North Am 2001;19:621-632.

Thaller TR, Wang L: Evaluation of asymptomatic microscopic hematuria in adults. Am Fam Physician 1999;60:1143-1152.

References

For a complete list of references, log onto www.expertconsult.com.

Acute Kidney Injury

Sevag Demirjian and Joseph Nally

DEFINITION

Acute renal failure (ARF) is characterized by azotmeia that progresses over several hours or days, with or without oliguria. Recently, the term *acute kidney injury* (AKI) has been popularized to increase awareness of milder degrees of renal impairment and to better describe the underlying pathobiology. Azotemia, on the other hand, signifies the accumulation of nitrogenous waste (urea) and other solutes.

A consensus classification for acute renal failure has been proposed by the the Acute Dialysis Quality Initiative (ADQI) group to standardize the definition and severity categories of AKI. The entry criteria for RIFLE (*r*isk of renal dysfunction, *i*njury to the kidney, *f*ailure of kidney function, *l*oss of kidney function, and *e*nd-stage kidney disease) are based on changes in serum creatinine or urine output (Table 1).[1]

PREVALENCE

Acute renal failure is common, with a reported incidence of 2% to 5% of all patients admitted to general medical-surgical hospitals. Up to 50% of patients who develop ARF die; survivors face marked increases in morbidity and prolonged hospitalization. The high incidence and substantial morbidity and mortality of ARF demand a logical approach to its prevention and early diagnosis, prompt recognition, and management of its complications.

PATHOPHYSIOLOGY

Once ARF is discovered, it is important to determine the cause—prerenal, postrenal, or intrinsic—because the initial evaluation and management are tailored to the particular cause (Fig. 1).

Prerenal Acute Renal Failure

Prerenal ARF, caused by underperfusion of an otherwise normal kidney, accounted for 21% of cases of ARF in a multicenter study in Madrid.[2] The hallmark of prerenal failure is that it is quickly reversible with appropriate therapy. Thus, it can be thought of as "a good kidney looking at a bad world."

Prerenal kidney failure can be a result of volume depletion from renal or extrarenal losses, fluid sequestration in liver failure or other edematous states, or inadequate perfusion pressure caused by heart failure. The urinalysis is bland and the urinary sodium level is low, but urine osmolality is high.

Treatment is imperative, because continued renal hypoperfusion can progress to intrinsic renal failure. Renal perfusion and volume status must be optimized by giving isotonic fluids. Underlying diseases such as heart failure should be treated.

Postrenal Acute Renal Failure

Postrenal ARF, caused by obstruction of the urinary tract, accounted for 10% of cases in the Madrid study.[2] Urinary tract obstructions may be within the urinary tract (e.g., blood clots, stones, sloughed papillae, fungus balls), or extrinsic (e.g., tumors, retroperitoneal fibrosis, even inadvertent ligation).

Renal ultrasonography, when used to detect obstructions, has a sensitivity and specificity of 90% to 95%. Unfortunately, it is also highly operator-dependent, so it should be performed by a highly experienced radiologist. Ultrasonography can yield false-negative results if the obstruction is caused by retroperitoneal fibrosis or certain malignancies that encase the entire system. It might also fail to detect an obstruction in extremely volume-depleted patients who do not have enough fluid buildup to reveal the obstruction.

Treatment should focus on removing the obstruction. Techniques vary with the type of obstruction.

Intrinsic Acute Renal Failure

Once prerenal and postrenal causes are ruled out, intrinsic renal failure is likely. Intrinsic ARF, caused by disease of the renal parenchyma, accounted for 69% of cases in the Madrid study.[2] Acute tubular necrosis (ATN), the most common type of intrinsic ARF, accounted for 45% of all cases of ARF. Most of the following discussion is therefore focused on ATN; other types of intrinsic ARF have been reviewed in detail in studies by Glassock and colleagues.[3]

ATN is most often caused by renal hypoperfusion and renal ischemia. Other causes include various endogenous nephrotoxic substances (e.g., myoglobin and hemoglobin after trauma; cellular products in tumor lysis syndrome; crystals of uric acid, calcium, or oxalate) and a host of exogenous substances (Box 1). If a patient develops ATN while receiving medications, each medication must be reviewed for the possibility of nephrotoxicity.

In oliguric ATN, renal plasma flow declines, but the glomerular filtration rate declines even more. This dichotomy suggests that constriction of the afferent arterioles contributes to the pathophysiologic process. Ischemic injury to epithelial cells can lead to tubular back leak, which allows filtrate back into the bloodstream, and tubular obstruction.

The distribution of tubular necrosis in the kidneys is patchy, and the degree of necrosis does not correlate with the level of renal dysfunction. This is because the medulla of the kidneys, containing the thick ascending limbs of Henle, is less well vascularized and perfused than the cortex and therefore is disproportionately affected by ischemia. The ischemic insult in this region is worsened by reperfusion injury. Persistent vasoconstriction and congestion from white cells and cell debris lead to ongoing hypoxia and necrosis.

Summary

- Acute renal failure is common in hospitalized patients.
- Early recognition is important but still elusive.
- Acute renal failure results in substantial morbidity and mortality.
- Intrinsic acute renal failure is the most common cause; acute tubular necrosis is the most common intrinsic acute renal failure.

SPECIAL RISK GROUPS

Bone marrow transplant recipients are at increased risk of ARF and have a poor prognosis. Perioperative ATN can result from tumor lysis, sepsis, and nephrotoxins, including antibiotics and contrast agents. If ARF develops 10 to 16 days after transplantation, the most likely immediate cause is hepatic veno-occlusive disease that mimics acute hepatorenal syndrome. ARF developing 4 to 12 months after bone marrow transplantation may be caused by hemolytic uremic syndrome, perhaps related to cyclosporine or radiation therapy.

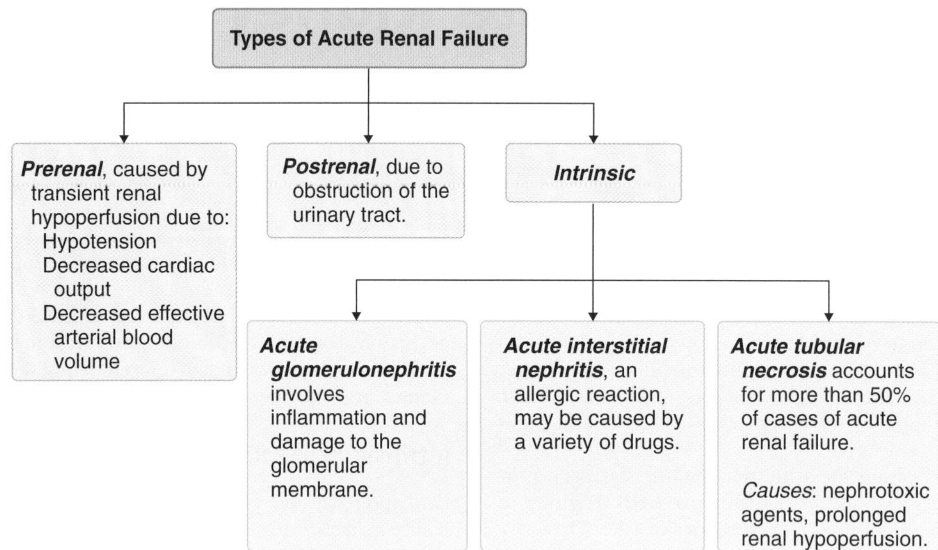

Figure 1 Types of acute renal failure.

Table 1 RIFLE Criteria

Category	GFR Criteria	Urine Output Criteria
Risk	Increased creatinine ×1.5 GFR decrease >25%	UO < 0.5 mL/kg/h × 6 hr
Injury	Increased creatinine ×2 GFR decrease >50%	UO < 0.5 mL/kg/h × 12 hr
Failure	Increase creatinine ×3 GFR decrease >75%	UO < 0.3 mL/kg/h × 24 hr Anuria × 12 hr
Loss	Persistent ARF = complete loss of kidney function >4 weeks	
ESKD	End-stage kidney disease (>3 months)	

ARF, acute renal failure; GFR, glomerular filtration rate; RIFLE, *r*isk of renal dysfunction, *i*njury to the kidney, *f*ailure of kidney function, *l*oss of kidney function, and *e*nd-stage kidney disease; UO, urine output;

HIV patients are also at risk of ARF not only from the usual nephrotoxic insults but also from potential nephrotoxicity of protease inhibitors. Other agents with similar risks include acyclovir and foscarnet.

DIAGNOSIS

The diagnosis of AKI traditionally has been based on functional parameters; an increase in serum creatinine is most commonly used as surrogate for impaired glomerular filtration rate (GFR). However, estimation of GFR with creatinine in the setting of AKI is inaccurate due to lag time to steady state, as well as other changing determinants of serum creatinine such as volume and nutrition. In addition, significant renal impairment can occur with only subtle variation in serum creatinine due to renal reserve or increased secretion (or both).

There is great interest in biomarkers of kidney injury that are elevated with ischemia and within hours of the event. NGAL (neutrophil gelatinase-associated lipocalin) and KIM-1 (kidney injury molecule-) are two of a dozen biomarkers that showed promising preliminary results but need further validation.[4]

A patient with ARF requires a complete evaluation by the physician (Box 2). The medical history should be reviewed for possible nephrotoxic insults, such as exposure to contrast materials, medications, or hypotension. The physical examination should focus on volume status. It is also prudent to screen for signs of systemic diseases that might affect kidney function, such as lupus erythematosus or Wegener's granulomatosis. Renal ultrasonography should be performed to screen for urinary tract obstruction.

In addition, urine studies need to be performed, such as urinalysis and measurement of urine volume. Urine chemistry studies may provide additional information. Anuria is a clue that ARF has one of three causes: urinary tract obstruction, a severe type of ATN called *cortical necrosis,* or a blood vessel blockage by a clot or another obstruction. Urinalysis, especially examination of the sediment, is fundamental to the evaluation (see Box 2). Low fractional excretion of sodium in a patient with acute oliguria is a classic sign of prerenal failure, and it is also associated with hepatorenal syndrome and acute glomerulonephritis. However, some types of ATN also have low sodium excretion, specifically postcontrast ATN, rhabdomyolysis, and multisystem organ failure.

TREATMENT

Treatment for intrinsic ARF is largely supportive, including adjusting medications, providing appropriate nutrition, and correcting volume status, hyperkalemia, and acidosis. The leading indications for dialysis are volume overload and hyperkalemia.

Cessation of Nephrotoxic Medications

With any patient with ARF, prescription and nonprescription medications should be reviewed immediately so that any potentially nephrotoxic drugs can be stopped. In addition to contrast media, other nephrotoxic agents include aminoglycosides and amphotericin (see Box 1). Outside the hospital, the main nephrotoxic agents are nonsteroidal anti-inflammatory drugs (NSAIDs). Patients can also be put at risk by angiotensin-converting enzyme (ACE) inhibitors, cisplatin, ifosfamide, and even Chinese herbal remedies.

Treatment of Endogenous Nephrotoxic Insults

If endogenous nephrotoxicity is diagnosed early enough, it can often be reversed with urinary alkalinization, which can prevent kidney failure and the need for dialysis. For example, pigment nephropathy from myoglobin, hemoglobin, or methemoglobin can be treated with urinary alkalinization. These types of nephrotoxicity often result

Box 1 Drugs and Other Exogenous Causes of Acute Renal Failure

Analgesics

- Nonsteroidal anti-inflammatory drugs (NSAIDs)

Anesthetics

- Enflurane
- Methoxyflurane

Angiotensin-Converting Enzyme Inhibitors
Antimicrobials

- Acyclovir
- Aminoglycosides
- Amphotericin B
- Bacitracin
- Cephalosporins
- Foscarnet
- Leflunomide
- Pentamidine
- Polymyxin, colistin
- Sulfonamide, cotrimoxazole
- Tetracyclines
- Vancomycin

Antiulcer agents

- Cimetidine
- Milk-alkali (in excess)

Recreational drugs

- Amphetamines
- Heroin
- Others

Bacterial toxins
Chinese herbs
Dextrans
Contrast media

- Bunamiodyl
- Diatrizoate
- Iopanoic acid
- Iothalamate
- Diuretics
- Mercurials
- Ticrynafen

Chemotherapy agents and immunosuppressants

- 5-Azacitidine
- Carboplatin
- Cisplatin
- Cyclosporine A and tacrolimus
- D-Penicillamine
- Ifosfamide
- Interferon alfa or gamma 1B
- Methotrexate
- Mitomycin
- Nitrosourea
- Plicamycin
- Recombinant interleukin 2

HIV protease inhibitors

- Indinavir
- Ritonavir

EDTA
ε-Aminocaproic acid
Heavy metals
Industrial chemicals
Organic solvents
Pesticides
Radiation
Silicone
Snake or insect venom

Adapted from Nally JV Jr: Acute renal failure. In Stoller JK, Michota, Mandell BF (eds): The Cleveland Clinic Intensive Review of Internal Medicine, 4th ed. Philadelphia, Lippincott, Williams & Wilkins, 2005, pp 577-584.

Box 2 Evaluation of Patients With Acute Renal Failure

1. Review records, perform history and physical examination
   Findings that suggest prerenal causes:
   - Volume depletion
   - Congestive heart failure
   - Severe liver disease or other edematous states

   Findings that suggest postrenal causes:
   - Palpable bladder or hydronephrotic kidneys
   - Enlarged prostate
   - Abnormal pelvic examination
   - Large residual bladder urine volume
   - History of renal calculi, perform ultrasound to screen for urinary tract obstruction)

   Findings that suggest intrinsic renal disease:
   - Exposure to nephrotoxic drugs or hypotensive
   - Recent radiographic procedures with contrast
2. Examine the urine sediment
   - If no abnormalities: suspect prerenal or postrenal azotemia
   - If eosinophils: suspect acute interstitial nephritis
   - If red blood cell casts: suspect glomerulonephritis or vasculitis
   - If renal tubular epithelial cells and muddy brown casts: suspect acute tubular necrosis
3. Calculate urinary indices
   Findings that suggest prerenal azotemia or glomerulonephritis:
   - Urinary sodium concentration <20 mEq/L
   - Urine : plasma creatinine ratio >30
   - Renal failure index <1

     Renal failure index = (urinary sodium concentration × plasma creatinine concentration)/ urinary creatinine concentration
   - Urine osmolality >500 mOsm/kg

   Findings that suggest acute tubular necrosis or postrenal azotemia:
   - Urinary sodium concentration >40 mEq/L
   - Urine:plasma creatinine ratio <20
   - Renal failure index >1
   - Urine osmolality <400 mOsm/kg

from tumor-specific or plasma cell dyscrasias (e.g., myeloma kidney).[3]

Increasing Urine Output

Acute renal failure patients who make urine tend to have lower morbidity and mortality rates. They are at less risk of hypervolemia, there is room for bicarbonate and nutrition, and there is less likelihood of hyperkalemia. This suggests that increasing urine output should be attempted. Unfortunately, much of the literature on this subject is dated, the studies were poorly designed, and a beneficial effect on mortality is not clear.

Mannitol should be avoided in patients with established ARF because it is an osmotic agent that can induce hypervolemia.[5] To increase urine output, hydrate the patient with saline and then start a loop diuretic.

Dopamine in renal doses should probably be used sparingly, if at all, because data on its effectiveness and safety are scant. In normal subjects, dopamine increases renal blood flow by approximately 40% and the glomerular filtration rate by approximately 10%, resulting in increases in salt and water excretion. It is not clear whether these increases are caused by a direct effect on the kidneys or are the result of cardiac effects. Little information is available about how to apply these results to patients with ARF. Data are not available for routine clinical use, so a trial of dopamine should be for no longer than 24 to 48 hours, followed by a taper.[5]

New Directions for Treatment

In cells that recover from an ischemic insult, growth factors play a role in recovery. This phenomenon has led to research with epidermal growth factor, insulin-like growth factor, and hepatocyte-type growth factor as therapy for ischemic ATN. Other researchers are investigating endothelium receptor blockers to address the ongoing vasoconstriction, and antiadhesion molecule antibodies to prevent vessel congestion by leukocytes.

Summary

- Treatment is largely supportive.
- Stop nephrotoxic medications and manage endogenous nephrotoxic insults.
- Leading indications for dialysis are volume overload and hyperkalemia.

OUTCOMES

The mortality rate in severe ARF is almost 50%, depending on the type of ARF and comorbidities of the patient. In the Madrid study, patients with ATN had a mortality rate of 60%, whereas those with prerenal or postrenal disease had a 35% mortality rate.[2]

Most deaths are not caused by the ARF itself but rather by the underlying disease or complications. In the Madrid data, 60% of deaths were caused by the primary disease and the remaining 40% were caused by cardiopulmonary failure or infection.[2]

ARF is not merely a marker of illness. In a follow-up report[7] of 16,000 patients who were studied by computed tomography with contrast, 183 developed ARF. The mortality rate among those with ARF was 34%, compared with only 7% in a matched cohort from the similarly exposed group.

About 50% of people who survive ATN recover renal function completely and another 40% have an incomplete recovery. Only approximately 5% to 10% require maintenance hemodialysis.

PREVENTION

Because few measures exist to treat ARF actively, clinicians should try to prevent it. Issues to consider are correcting volume status, avoiding exposure to nephrotoxins, and preparing for high-risk procedures, such as using contrast agents (Box 3).

Box 3 Measures to Prevent Acute Renal Failure in Hospitalized Patients

- Prevent hypotension, and correct it rapidly when it does occur.
- Evaluate renal function before any surgery.
- Avoid prescribing nephrotoxic drugs.
- Correct volume deficits or electrolyte imbalances, especially before surgery.
- Replace traditional contrast agents with nonionic contrast, and use contrast sparingly.
- Treat infection quickly.
- Treat oliguria quickly.

Preventing Contrast Nephropathy

The incidence of contrast nephropathy can be reduced by adequately hydrating patients before the procedure, replacing traditional agents with nonionic contrast, and limiting the quantity of any contrast agent used.[5]

Using nonionic contrast agents can cut the overall risk of contrast nephropathy by 50%, from about 6% to 3%. In the study by Rudnick and colleagues, risk factors for contrast nephropathy were baseline chronic kidney disease (serum creatinine level higher than 1.5 mg/dL) and diabetes; the use of nonionic contrast agents reduced the incidence in the highest risk patients who had both risk factors from 24% to 12%.

The most effective strategy to hydrate patients is to give IV normal saline, 1 mL/kg/hour, before the procedure. No benefit is gained by adding mannitol or a loop diuretic. Pretreating with acetylcysteine can reduce the rise of creatinine levels slightly but might have minor clinical impact. One report has suggested a benefit of IV sodium bicarbonate hydration before contrast exposure.[6]

Suggested Readings

Bellomo R, Ronco C, Kellum JA, Mehta RL, Palevsky P. Acute renal failure—definition, outcome measures, animal models, fluid therapy and information technology needs: the Second International Consensus Conference of the Acute Dialysis Quality Initiative (ADQI) Group. Crit Care 2004;8(4):R204-12.

Glassock RJ MS, Massry SG, Humes, HD: Diagnosis, clinical presentation and management. In Glassock RJ, Massry SG (eds): Massry and Glassock's Textbook in Nephrology, 4th ed. Baltimore, Lippincott Williams & Wilkins 2001, pp 956-977.

Liano F, Junco E, Pascual J, Madero R, Verde E. The spectrum of acute renal failure in the intensive care unit compared with that seen in other settings. The Madrid Acute Renal Failure Study Group. Kidney Int Suppl 1998;66:S16-S24.

Merten GJ, Burgess WP, Gray LV, Holleman JH, Roush TS, Kowalchuk GJ, et al. Prevention of Contrast-Induced Nephropathy With Sodium Bicarbonate: A Randomized Controlled Trial. JAMA 2004;291(19):2328-2334.

Rudnick MR, Goldfarb S, Wexler L, Ludbrook PA, Murphy MJ, Halpern EF, et al. Nephrotoxicity of ionic and nonionic contrast media in 1196 patients: a randomized trial. The Iohexol Cooperative Study. Kidney Int 1995;47(1):254-261.

Thurman JM, Parikh CR. Peeking into the black box: New biomarkers for acute kidney injury. Kidney Int 2008;73(4):379.

References

For a complete list of references, log onto www.expertconsult.com.

Chronic Kidney Disease

Martin E. Lascano, Martin J. Schreiber, and Saul Nurko

Chronic kidney disease (CKD) is an important source of long-term morbidity and mortality. It has been estimated that CKD affects more than 20 million people in the United States. Given that most patients are asymptomatic until the disease has significantly progressed, they remain unaware of the condition. Thus, it is essential to have clinical practice guidelines aimed at early detection, evaluation, diagnosis, and treatment of this condition. This chapter reviews the medical management of patients with CKD, emphasizing measures aimed at slowing disease progression and treatment of its common complications. Methods used for estimating the level of renal function are presented elsewhere in this section ("Kidney Function Assessment: Creatinine-Based Estimation Equations").

DEFINITION AND STAGING

CKD is an irreversible, progressive reduction in renal function. The National Kidney Foundation's Kidney Disease Outcomes Quality Initiative (K/DOQI) guidelines define CKD as sustained kidney damage indicated by the presence of structural or functional abnormalities (e.g., microalbuminuria/proteinuria, hematuria, histologic or imaging abnormalities), and/or reduced glomerular filtration rate (GFR) to less than 60 mL/min/1.73 m^2 for at least 3 months. Based on GFR estimation, the National Kidney Foundation has classified CKD into five stages (Table 1).[1]

In addition to GFR estimation, the evaluation of all patients with suspected or confirmed CKD should include a urinalysis, with testing for proteinuria. In addition to being a marker of kidney damage, proteinuria is a strong predictor of increased risk of cardiovascular morbidity and mortality in patients with or without CKD. To quantify the level of proteinuria, rather than using a 24-hour urine collection, the determination of the protein-to-creatinine or albumin-to-creatinine ratio in a random urine specimen is recommended. Urinary ratios are also useful for monitoring changes in the degree of proteinuria in CKD patients.

EVALUATION AND TREATMENT

Once the presence of CKD and the disease stage have been established, the K/DOQI recommends following a stage-specific clinical action plan (see Table 1). During stages 1 and 2, the focus should be on treating comorbid conditions, addressing reduction of cardiovascular risk factors. and instituting measures to slow the progression of kidney disease. During these early stages, aggressive blood pressure control is the mainstay of therapy. In stage 3, in addition to continuing with the measures described, the focus shifts to evaluating and treating complications of CKD, such as anemia and the effects of abnormal mineral metabolism on bone and overall health. By stage 4, preparations for renal replacement therapy (dialysis, transplantation, or both) should begin. When stage 5 is reached, or when symptoms of the uremic syndrome ensue, renal replacement therapy is started.

SLOWING DISEASE PROGRESSION

Given the progressive nature of most forms of CKD, with a continued decrease in the GFR over time, it is important to address factors known to contribute to loss of renal function. Primary renoprotective strategies for limiting the progression of CKD are presented in Table 2.

Hypertension

The progression of CKD is strongly linked to hypertension control. A number of studies have shown that for diabetic and nondiabetic kidney disease, elevated blood pressure is associated with a faster decline in GFR. The Modification of Diet in Renal Disease (MDRD) study has shown that control of hypertension is even more important in patients with proteinuria higher than 1 g/day, because lowering blood pressure to a target of 125/75 mm Hg in these patients achieves a greater decrease in the rate of decline of GFR than in patients with less proteinuria.[2] For patients with proteinuria higher than 3 g/day, the impact of blood pressure lowering was even greater. The MDRD study also showed that hypertensive African Americans have faster progression of CKD compared with their white counterparts. However, reduction of blood pressure to lower than 125/75 mm Hg reduced the rate of decline by 50% in this group.

The Ramipril Efficacy in Nephropathy (REIN) trial followed nondiabetic renal disease patients with proteinuria higher than 1 g/day. It demonstrated that patients being treated with an angiotensin-converting enzyme (ACE) inhibitor have more effective preservation of renal function at similar levels of blood pressure reduction. This effect was most profound in those patients with the highest levels of baseline proteinuria.

In the African American study of kidney disease (AASK), metoprolol, amlodipine, and ramipril were compared as first-line drugs in patients with nondiabetic nephropathy. Blood pressure control was similar among the three groups. However, only in the patients treated with ramipril were there significant reductions in rates of renal disease progression and in composite end points (22%-38% reduction in renal function, need for dialysis, or death).

These combined results support the hypothesis that reduction in systemic hypertension slows or prevents progression of proteinuric and nonproteinuric renal disease. Studies have shown that even treating isolated systolic hypertension in older patients slows the progression of CKD.

Most classes of antihypertensive medication can be used to treat patients with CKD because many of these trials required additional drugs to achieve their goals. However, it has also been shown that at similar degrees of blood pressure control, ACE inhibitors are more protective, particularly in proteinuric disease. In patients who cannot tolerate ACE inhibitors, an angiotensin receptor blocker (ARB) may reasonably be prescribed. In spite of these observations, the therapeutic goal of reducing the blood pressure to target, regardless of agent used, should not be sacrificed.

It is worth noting that CKD may alter some of the pharmacologic characteristics of multiple medications, including the antihypertensive medications. However, specific pharmacologic information is beyond the scope of this chapter.

Proteinuria

Microalbuminuria and proteinuria are well-recognized prognostic factors for the development and progression of CKD. The MDRD study has shown that severe proteinuria (>3 g/day) is associated with a higher rate of decline in GFR. Other studies have shown that this holds true for the glomerular and nonglomerular forms of CKD. Interventions aimed at reducing proteinuria, including ACE inhibition and dietary modifications, have been shown to predict outcomes better in diabetic and nondiabetic CKD patients. Proposed

Table 1 Stages of Chronic Kidney Disease and Clinical Action Plans

Stage	Description	GFR (mL/min/1.73 m^2) Action	Plan
1	Kidney damage with normal or elevated GFR	≥90	Diagnosis, treatment of underlying condition and comorbidities, cardiovascular disease risk reduction
2	Kidney damage with mildly decreased GFR	60-89	Estimating progression
3	Moderately decreased GFR	30-59	Evaluating and treating complications
4	Severely decreased GFR	15-29	Preparation for renal replacement therapy
5	Kidney failure (ESRD)	<15 (or dialysis, transplantation)	Replacement therapy (dialysis or transplantation)

ESRD, end-stage renal disease; GFR, glomerular filtration rate.
Adapted from the National Kidney Foundation: K/DOQI Clinical practice guidelines for chronic kidney disease: Evaluation, classification, and stratification. Am J Kidney Dis 2002;39:S1-S266.

Table 2 Renoprotective Strategies for Slowing Progression of Chronic Kidney Disease

Parameter	Goal	Intervention
Blood pressure control (mm Hg)	<130/80 if proteinuria <1 g/day; <125/75 if proteinuria >1 g/day	ACE inhibitors, ARBs, sodium, restriction, diuretics
Reduction in proteinuria	<0.5 g/day	ACE inhibitors, ARBs
Glycemic control	$HgbA_{1c}$< 7%	Dietary counseling, oral hypoglycemic agents, insulin
Dietary protein restriction	0.6-0.8 g/kg/day	Dietary counseling
Lipid lowering	LDL <100 mg/dL	Dietary counseling, statins
Lifestyle modifications	Smoking cessation, achieving ideal body weight, regularly exercising	Counseling, exercise program

ACE, angiotensin-converting enzyme; ARB, angiotensin receptor blocker; LDL, low-density lipoprotein.

mechanisms for the effects of proteinuria include initiation and progression of tubulointerstitial fibrosis and inflammation through toxicity from filtered compounds (e.g., transferrin-iron, albumin-bound fatty acids, inflammatory cytokines).

Dietary Protein Restriction

Extensive studies of chronic renal failure in animal models have shown that reduced dietary protein is associated with a reduction in glomerular hyperfiltration and slows the progression of renal disease. Although animal models of disease and treatment do not always apply to humans, a number of human studies in nondiabetic and diabetic renal disease have tested whether dietary protein restriction ameliorates the rate of progression of disease. The MDRD study was the largest controlled multicenter trial to compare usual protein intake (1 g/kg/day) with low (0.6 g/kg/day) and very low (0.28 g/kg/day) protein intake in nondiabetic patients.[2] Although the primary outcome was inconclusive, several subanalyses have suggested that a prescribed dietary protein intake of 0.6 g/kg/day as compared with 1 g/kg/day reduces the rate of progression by about 28%, the same benefit seen in achieving the low blood pressure goal. A meta-analysis of five of the best studies of both diabetic and nondiabetic renal disease has suggested that a small reduction in rate of progression occurs with dietary protein restriction. In an analysis of the MDRD data, Locatelli and Del Vecchio have found that adherence to a low (0.6 g/kg/day) versus a usual (1 g/kg/d) protein diet for 9 years would delay the need for renal replacement therapy by approximately 1 year.[3] The difficulty of achieving consistent dietary protein restriction, however, makes the application of this intervention unwieldy and prone to failure, especially in diabetic patients. Compliance in the MDRD was successful but required intensive regular interaction by dietitians.

Summary

Clinically proven strategies to slow the progression of nondiabetic renal disease include the following:

- Blood pressure reduction to lower than 130/80 mm Hg, especially in patients with proteinuric renal disease (<125/75 mm Hg if proteinuria is >1 g/day). Most antihypertensive medications can be used but ACE inhibitor therapy is recommended.
- Dietary protein restriction (0.6-0.8 g/kg/day) is reasonable for patients who are willing to follow dietary restrictions.
- Proteinuria reduction, by blocking the renin-angiotensin-aldosterone system, should be initiated.

COMPLICATIONS

As GFR declines, a wide range of disorders develop, including fluid and electrolyte imbalances, such as volume overload, hyperkalemia, metabolic acidosis, and hyperphosphatemia[4]; hormonal imbalances leading to anemia and secondary hyperparathyroidism, which accompanies bone disease (renal osteodystrophy); and systemic dysfunction that develops in the uremic syndrome, such as neuropathy, anorexia, nausea, vomiting, fatigue, and malnutrition.

Given these considerations, every patient with CKD should undergo evaluation by a nutritionist. Box 1 shows typical dietary recommendations for CKD patients; specific recommendations should be modified based on the needs of the individual patient.[5,6]

Sodium and Water Imbalance

Sodium and intravascular volume balance are usually well maintained until the GFR falls below 15 mL/min/1.73 m^2. This is caused by an increase in the fractional excretion of salt and water by the remaining nephrons. However, the ability to respond to rapid infusions of sodium with volume expansion will be reduced, even in patients with CKD stages 3 and 4, making them prone to fluid overload. The optimal level of daily salt intake varies from patient to

Box 1 Typical Dietary Recommendations for Chronic Kidney Disease Patients

Protein: 0.6-0.8 g/kg/day
Sodium: <2 g/day (<6 g/day of salt)
Potassium: 40-70 mEq/day
Phosphate: 600-800 mg/day
Calcium: 1400-1600 mg/day (not to exceed 2000 mg/day)
Free water (in excess of urine output): 1-1.5 L/day

patient. Less than 6 g/day of sodium chloride (<2 g/day of sodium) is the typical initial recommendation. Adjustments need to be made depending on the patient's volume status, aiming to achieve normotension and only trace pedal edema. Patients with a GFR below 20 mL/min/1.73 m^2 in whom, despite sodium restriction, edema ensues, respond well to diuretic therapy, usually a loop diuretic. Given that the ability to concentrate or dilute the urine maximally becomes progressively impaired as GFR declines, patients with stage 4 or 5 CKD tend to be isosthenuric. Therefore, these patients are at risk for developing hypo- or hypernatremia caused by positive or negative water balance, respectively. Free water intake should be approximately equal to urine output plus an additional 1 to 1.5 L/day to account for insensible losses.

Potassium Imbalance

Renal potassium excretion is preserved at near-normal levels in patients with CKD as long as both the renin-angiotensin-aldosterone system (RAAS) and distal nephron flow are maintained. Therefore, hyperkalemia generally develops in oliguric patients with a GFR lower than 10 mL/min/1.73 m^2 or in those who experience an additional alteration in potassium metabolism because of increased intake or from certain medications (e.g., ACE inhibitors, ARBs, nonsteroidal anti-inflammatory drugs). See elsewhere in this section for further information ("Hypokalemia and Hyperkalemia").

Dietary restriction is the mainstay of management of chronic hyperkalemia in these patients (40-70 mEq/day). If it persists, the next step is the addition of a loop diuretic (more so if hypertension or volume overload is an issue) to promote kaliuresis by increasing sodium delivery to the distal nephron. If acidosis is present, sodium bicarbonate is helpful by increasing distal nephron sodium delivery, inducing kaliuresis, and promoting intracellular potassium shift. An additional alternative is the use of potassium-binding resins such as sodium polystyrene sulfonate (Kayexalate) combined with sorbitol to avoid constipation, at smaller doses than those typically used for the treatment of acute hyperkalemia, given daily or every other day.

Metabolic Acidosis

The kidneys' ability to regenerate bicarbonate consumed in buffering the daily net acid production diminishes as nephron mass decreases. This occurs because of reduced production of ammonia, decreased filtration of titratable acids (e.g., sulfates, phosphates, urates, hippurates), decreased proximal tubular bicarbonate reabsorption, and decreased renal tubular hydrogen ion secretion. The resultant metabolic acidosis is initially of the nonanion gap type but, as GFR declines, the anion gap widens—because of retained titratable acids—with the serum bicarbonate concentration tending to stabilize between 12 and 20 mEq/L. Buffering of excess hydrogen ions occurs in bone, contributing to the development of renal osteodystrophy (see later). Additionally, chronic acidosis leads to muscle protein breakdown and reduced albumin synthesis.

The goal of therapy is to maintain the serum bicarbonate concentration at or above 22 mEq/L to avoid the deleterious effects of acidosis on bone histology and protein catabolism. The first-line agent is sodium bicarbonate, 0.5 to 1 mEq/kg/day; a typical starting dosage is 650 mg three times daily. Sodium citrate, generally better tolerated than bicarbonate, should be restricted to patients who are not taking aluminum-containing phosphate binders because it enhances intestinal aluminum absorption.

Renal Osteodystrophy and Calcium and Phosphorus Imbalance

As functional nephron mass declines, the fractional excretion of phosphate drops, leading to an increase in the serum phosphate level. This is accompanied by a reciprocal decrease in serum calcium concentration. These events lead to an increase in parathyroid hormone (PTH) release; this has a phosphaturic effect, resulting in the return of phosphate and calcium to normal levels. As GFR continues to decline, this cycle maintains serum calcium and phosphate concentrations within the normal ranges, at the expense of rising PTH levels. When further renal mass is lost and GFR drops below 30 mL/min/1.73 m^2, despite the compensatory hyperphosphaturia, hyperphosphatemia becomes sustained.[7]

Parallel to this, as nephron mass decreases, the 1α-hydroxylation in the kidney of 25-hydroxyvitamin D [25-(OH)D] declines, leading to lower serum levels of 1,25-dihydroxyvitamin D [1,25-(OH_2)D]. This lack of 1,25-(OH_2)D contributes to the development of hypocalcemia, given its role of enhancing calcium absorption in the gut and enhancing PTH-mediated calcium release from bone. The combination of all these factors contributes to the development of secondary hyperparathyroidism and renal osteodystrophy.

The primary goals in the management of these abnormalities are maintaining phosphate levels within target range (2.7-4.6 mg/dL for CKD stages 3 and 4; 3.5 to 5.5 mg/dL for CKD stage 5 or end-stage renal disease, ESRD) and the calcium-phosphorus product at lower than 55 mg^2/dL^2.[8] Treatment should begin with dietary phosphorus restriction to approximately 800 mg/day. In addition to dietary restriction, patients with a GFR of lower than 30 mL/min/1.73 m^2 will generally need oral phosphate binders given with meals to decrease gut absorption of phosphate. These are available as calcium-containing or non–calcium-containing binders. The decision as to which class of binder to use initially is based on the starting phosphate level and the calcium-phosphorus product. When the serum phosphate level is higher than 7 mg/dL or the calcium-phosphorus product is higher than 63 mg^2/dL^2, the initial choice should be a non–calcium-containing binder.

Calcium-containing binders are available as calcium carbonate or calcium acetate (PhosLo); the latter is suggested as a more efficient binder. Calcium citrate is avoided in CKD patients because it markedly increases intestinal aluminum absorption. Because of the risk of vascular calcification, the aim is to maintain the total elemental calcium intake (including both dietary calcium intake and calcium-based phosphate binders) under 2000 mg/day. Among non–calcium-containing binders, current available options include sevelamer (Renagel), a cationic polymer that binds phosphate through ion exchange, and lanthanum carbonate (Fosrenol), a rare earth element. Aluminum hydroxide is an effective phosphate binder but can lead to osteomalacia and neurologic complications and should be limited to short-term use only.

Vitamin D or vitamin D analogues should be given to treat secondary hyperparathyroidism. The CKD stage-specific target levels of intact PTH are shown in Box 2. Once the PTH level is established, the next step is assessment of 25-(OH)D levels and replacement with vitamin D_2 (ergocalciferol) if levels are lower than 30 ng/mL. If the intact PTH level is elevated and the serum 25-(OH)D level is higher than 30 ng/mL, treatment with an active form of vitamin D is indicated. Available options are calcitriol, alfacalcidol, or doxercalciferol. During vitamin D therapy, serum calcium and phosphorus levels need to be monitored closely to prevent hypercalcemia and hyperphosphatemia, aiming for levels lower than 10.2 mg/dL and lower than 4.6 mg/dL, respectively. Calcimimetics are agents that increase the sensitivity of the calcium-sensing receptor in the parathyroid gland to calcium. The only available medication in this category is

Box 2 Target Parathyroid Hormone Ranges for Chronic Kidney Disease Patients

Stage 3: 35-70 pg/mL
Stage 4: 70-110 pg/mL
Stage 5: 150-300 pg/mL

cinacalcet (Sensipar), which can be used if elevated serum phosphorus or calcium levels limit the use of vitamin D analogues.

Anemia

Anemia is almost a universal finding in patients with stages 3 to 5 CKD, and its presence should be sought for when the estimated GFR is lower than 60 mL/min/1.73 m^2. The anemia of CKD is typically normochromic and normocytic and is caused primarily by a decrease in erythropoietin production relative to the degree of anemia. This relative erythropoietin deficiency renders erythropoietin levels not useful for the evaluation of this population, which should begin when the hemoglobin level is lower than 12 g/dL in women and lower than 13.5 g/dL in men.

Before the initiation of erythropoietin replacement, nonrenal causes of anemia need to be excluded. The workup typically includes determination of red blood cell indices, absolute reticulocyte count, serum iron level, total iron binding capacity, percentage transferrin saturation, serum ferritin level, and white blood cell count and differential, platelet count, and testing for occult blood in the stool. Depending on clinical suspicion, laboratory findings, or both, a more extensive workup may be indicated, including serum vitamin B_{12} levels, intact PTH level, serum or urine protein electrophoresis, hemolysis panel, and possibly referral to a hematologist. If no alternative cause for the anemia is found, therapy with erythropoietin-stimulating agents (ESAs) is initiated usually at a nephrologist's office. The potential proven benefits of ESA therapy are reduction in the need for transfusions and of anemia-induced symptoms, with enhanced quality of life. Many observational studies have suggested that treating anemia with ESA improves overall and cardiovascular mortality in CKD. However, there are no randomized trials at present to confirm these observational findings.

There are currently two ESAs available in the United States, epoetin alfa and darbepoetin alfa. Both products are equally effective and mainly differ in their half-lives, so their interval dosing varies.

The target hemoglobin level for both predialysis CKD and end-stage renal disease (ESRD) patients should be 11 to 12 g/dL. Targeting hemoglobin to levels higher than 12 g/dL has been associated with adverse cardiovascular outcomes. The most common cause for suboptimal response to ESA therapy is iron deficiency. ESA-stimulated erythropoiesis is iron restrictive and requires the presence of adequate iron stores. Current K/DOQI guidelines suggest administering iron to maintain the transferrin saturation at or greater than 20%, and serum ferritin level higher than 100 ng/mL.[9] This is typically achieved by oral iron supplementation, with a daily dosage of approximately 200 mg of elemental iron (ferrous sulfate, 325 mg three times daily). Oral iron absorption is best when given without food, typically in between meals. However, this form of therapy is not always well tolerated because of gastrointestinal side effects. Intravenous iron is typically reserved for patients already on dialysis, although it may be used in predialysis CKD patients not achieving targeted iron parameters. In addition to iron deficiency, other causes of poor response to ESA therapy include the presence of an underlying inflammatory state, uremia, hyperparathyroidism, and malignancy.

REFERRAL TO A NEPHROLOGIST

CKD carries a significant burden of morbidity and mortality. Care of patients with CKD requires a multifaceted approach, with focus on close monitoring of GFR and aggressive institution of measures aimed at slowing progression of the disease. Addressing the comorbidities that accompany CKD (e.g., hypertension, diabetes, hyperlipidemia) should occur early in the course of the disease (stages 1 to 3 CKD). These initial measures are best instituted by the primary care provider, with assistance from the nephrologist, if needed, for developing a clinical action plan. As the disease progresses, the roles of the nephrologist widen, including determining the cause of CKD, initiating disease-specific therapies to treat or further slow down progression, diagnosing and treating CKD-related complications and, in the advanced stages, preparing the patient for renal replacement therapy.

The strongest evidence for the importance of referral to a nephrologist is for patients with CKD stages 4 and 5 (GFR <30 mL/min/1.73 m^2). Late referral (less than 3 months before initiation of renal replacement therapy) is associated with an increased mortality rate after starting dialysis. At this point, patients are better served by comanagement between the primary care provider and nephrologist. During this phase, special attention should be given to patient education regarding renal replacement therapy (e.g., hemodialysis, peritoneal dialysis, transplantation), and timely creation of vascular access for those opting for hemodialysis. For those who qualify for kidney transplantation, donor evaluation for preemptive transplantation should begin.

Summary

- Early detection, evaluation, and diagnosis of chronic kidney disease allow for the timely initiation of measures aimed at slowing disease progression.
- Classification of CKD into stages 1 to 5 facilitates patient care through the application of stage-specific clinical action plans.
- During early CKD stages, aggressive blood pressure control is the mainstay of therapy and has a proven effect in limiting the progression of disease.
- The progressive loss of renal function is accompanied by a wide range of adaptive and maladaptive processes as the body attempts to maintain homeostasis resulting in a complex medical clinical picture, with its main manifestations in the cardiovascular, neurologic, hematologic, musculoskeletal, and immunologic systems.
- Given the complexities involved in the care of CKD patients, referral to a nephrologist for evaluation and comanagement is recommended.

Suggested Readings

Ikizler TA: Nutrition and kidney disease. In Greenberg A (ed): Primer on Kidney Diseases. Philadelphia, Elsevier Saunders, 2005, pp 495-501.

KDOQI; National Kidney Foundation: Clinical practice guidelines and clinical practice recommendations for anemia in chronic kidney disease. Am J Kidney Dis 2006; 47(Suppl 3):S11-S145.

K/DOQI; National Kidney Foundation: Clinical practice guidelines for nutrition in chronic renal failure. Am J Kidney Dis 2000;35(Suppl 2):S1-S140.

Klahr S, Levey AS, Beck GJ, et al: The effects of dietary protein restriction and blood-pressure control on the progression of chronic renal disease. Modification of Diet in Renal Disease Study Group. N Engl J Med 1994;330:877-884.

Locatelli F, Del Vecchio L: How long can dialysis be postponed by low-protein diet and ACE inhibitors? Nephrol Dial Transplant 1999;14:1360-1365.

Martin KJ, Gonzalez EA: Metabolic bone disease in chronic kidney disease. J Am Soc Nephrol 2007;18:875-885.

National Kidney Foundation: K/DOQI Clinical practice guidelines for bone metabolism and disease in chronic kidney disease. Am J Kidney Dis 2003;42:S1-S201.

National Kidney Foundation: K/DOQI Clinical practice guidelines for chronic kidney disease: Evaluation, classification, and stratification. Am J Kidney Dis 2002;39:S1-S266.

Wallia R, Greenberg AS, Piraino B, et al: Serum electrolyte patterns in end-stage renal disease. Am J Kidney Dis 1986;8:98-104.

References

For a complete list of references, log onto www.expertconsult.com.

Immunosuppression for Renal Transplant Patients and Common Medical Problems in Renal Transplantation

Naim Issa and William E. Braun

Renal transplantation is the best treatment for most patients with end-stage renal disease and is associated with significant improvements in quality of life and survival of patients with successful kidney grafts. Because patient and graft survival rates 1 year after transplantation are currently higher than 90% for living and deceased donor kidney recipients, there will be large numbers of successful recipients requiring long-term care in the context of chronic immunosuppression. Primary care physicians and internists are becoming increasingly involved in the care of these patients and will need basic information about immunosuppression and the medical management of these patients.

OVERVIEW OF IMMUNOSUPPRESSION FOR RENAL TRANSPLANTATION

Calcineurin inhibitors (CNIs), including cyclosporine (CSA) (Neoral, Gengraf, or the earliest form, Sandimmune) and tacrolimus (TAC; Prograf) have been the cornerstones of an immunosuppressive regimen, which usually includes two or more additional agents, such as glucocorticoids, a purine antagonist (mycophenolic acid [CellCept] or azathioprine [Imuran]). Sirolimus (SRL; Rapamune) has been used as a substitute for CNIs. The choice of agents is often protocol driven but is usually adapted to each recipient's risk profile. High-risk recipients treated with more intensive immunosuppression include those with increased levels of preformed antibody (panel-reactive antibody [PRA] >20%-50%), repeat transplantation after early immunologic loss of a previous graft, and African Americans. High-risk recipients typically receive induction therapy consisting of monoclonal or polyclonal antibodies administered intravenously beginning in the perioperative period. The mechanisms of action of these and other immunosuppressants have recently been reviewed.[1,2]

Agents for Induction Treatment

Polyclonal IgG antibodies are derived from horse (Atgam) or rabbit (Thymoglobulin) sera after injecting the animals with human lymphocytes or human thymocytes, respectively. They target several T cell surface epitopes (CD2, CD3, CD4, and CD25) and, in the case of Thymoglobulin, induce long-term depletion of T lymphocytes. Thymoglobulin's major early side effect is the cytokine release syndrome: fever, chills, myalgias, and shortness of breath. Late side effects include prolonged (up to years) depletion of T lymphocytes, thereby increasing the potential risk of opportunistic infections, post-transplantation lymphoproliferative disorder (PTLD), and possibly autoimmune disease.

Daclizumab (Zenapax) and basiliximab (Simulect) are monoclonal antibodies modified to be humanized or chimeric antibodies that bind to the alpha chain of the interleukin-2 receptor (IL-2R) on T cells and thereby impair lymphocyte proliferation. They typically have minimal side effects and do not increase the recipient's susceptibility to infection or malignancy. Alemtuzumab (Campath), originally approved for the treatment of chronic lymphocytic leukemia, is a humanized murine monoclonal antibody directed against the surface protein CD52 expressed on T and B lymphocytes, monocytes, and macrophages. It can cause prolonged T lymphocyte depletion, with risks for opportunistic infection, PTLD, and possibly autoimmune disease.

Maintenance Immunosuppression

Basic maintenance immunosuppression for many years consisted of three types of drugs in combination: glucocorticosteroid (GC) (prednisone), a purine antagonist (azathioprine or mycophenolate mofetil) and a CNI (CSA) or TAC. Because of numerous potential glucocorticoid (GC) toxicities (Box 1) and CNI toxicities (Table 1), many new regimens have been developed that incorporate rapid GC elimination, or CNI dose reduction or elimination. Rapid GC withdrawal within the first few days after transplantation is usually achieved with antibody induction. Late withdrawal of GC has a high risk of rejection.[3] CNI withdrawal has been attempted by conversion to less nephrotoxic SRL. Alternatively, careful dose reduction can be successfully achieved in select patients.[4] Combined use of a CNI and SRL has the potential for severe nephrotoxicity.

Glucocorticoids

GCs are used for both induction and maintenance immunosuppression. Their immunosuppressant actions are mediated through a number of pathways, mainly directed toward redistribution of lymphocytes and macrophages to the lymphoid tissue and inhibition of the production of cytokines (e.g., IL-1, IL-2, IL-6), tumor necrosis factor α (TNF-α), and interferon gamma (IFN-γ). Prednisone dosage is gradually decreased after transplantation to 5 to 7.5 mg daily unless the patient has been on a rapid GC withdrawal protocol.

Calcineurin Inhibitors

CNIs include CSA and TAC; each functions as a base immunosuppressant agent around which additional agents are added to construct the complete immunosuppressant regimen. Initiation of CSA in the post-transplantation period usually requires signs of renal recovery because of potential nephrotoxicity. The usual starting dosage is about 5 to 6 mg/kg/day, divided into two doses. Many CSA formulations are now available. The original formulation (Sandimmune) has been largely replaced by the newer CSA formulations (Neoral) or modified CSA (e.g., Gengraf, Eon, other generics) that exhibit better absorption and bioavailability. These CSA preparations should not be casually substituted for each other because of increased risk of rejection or toxicity. The interval for monitoring CSA blood levels remains controversial. Monitoring trough levels

Box 1 Important Glucocorticoid Side Effects

Increased susceptibility to infection
Replication of hepatitis B and C viruses
Weight gain (increased appetite)
Cushingoid appearance
Easy bruising, striae, acne
Poor wound healing
Sodium retention
Hypertension
Hypercholesterolemia
Accelerated atherosclerosis
Fatal ventricular arrhythmias (rapid bolus)
Osteoporosis
Avascular necrosis
Arthralgia with rapidly decreasing dose
Myopathy
Diabetes mellitus
Hyperosmotic nonketotic coma
Behavioral changes, psychosis
Posterior subcapsular cataracts
Pancreatitis
Peptic ulcer

Table 1 Important Calcineurin Inhibitor Side Effects

Side Effect	Cyclosporine	vs.	FK506
Nephrotoxicity	++		+
Hypertension	++		+
Hypercholesterolemia	++		+
Gingival hyperplasia	++		?
Hyperglycemia	+		++
Tremor, neuropathy, convulsion	+		++
Susceptibility to malignancy	++		+
Susceptibility to viral infection	+		+
Hypomagnesemia	+		+
Hyperkalemia	++		+
Hyperuricemia	++		+
Hepatotoxicity (cholestatic)	+		+
Nausea, vomiting, diarrhea	+		+
Anaphylaxis	+		+

+, frequency.

Box 2 Calcineurin Inhibitors and Other Drug Interactions*,†

Medications that Increase Calcineurin Levels

Calcium Channel Blockers
Verapamil
Diltiazem
Amlodipine
Nicardipine

Antibiotics
Erythromycin
Clarithromycin
Doxycycline

Antifungal Agents
Ketoconazole
Fluconazole
Itraconazole
Metronidazole

Food
Grapefruit
Grapefruit juice

Protease Inhibitors
Saquinavir
Indinavir
Nelfinavir
Ritonavir

Immunosuppressant
Sirolimus

Medications that Decrease Calcineurin Levels

Anticonvulsants
Barbiturates
Phenytoin
Carbamazepine

Antibiotics
Nafcillin
IV trimethoprim
Cephalosporins
Terbinafine (Lamisil)

Antituberculosis Drugs
Rifampin
Rifabutin

Herbal Preparation
St. John's wort

Other Drugs
Ticlopidine
Octreotide

**The safest procedure is to specifically check any drug added to or eliminated from those taken by a transplant recipient to determine its effect on calcineurin levels. The drugs listed here are only a partial list.*

†Calcineurins can significantly increase the levels, effects, and toxicity of other drugs, notably many statins[7] and sirolimus. Careful dosing and monitoring are necessary.

(C0) is the appropriate way to monitor Sandimmune, but the newer formulations may be better monitored with levels determined 2 hours after the dose is taken (C2). The approximate CSA level is determined by the type of CSA being used, the assay method, the time after transplant, and the clinical status of the patient.[5]

TAC is a macrolide antibiotic somewhat more potent than CSA and has side effects that are distinct from and overlap with those of CSA (see Table 1). TAC has high bioavailability and thus its trough levels correlate with dose. The maintenance dosage is usually approximately 0.1 mg/kg/day divided into two doses, with target trough levels of 5 to 15 ng/mL in the initial 12 months after transplantation and 5 to 10 ng/mL beyond 12 months. Both CSA and TAC are metabolized by the hepatic enzyme system cytochrome P-450 3A4 (CYP 3A4), which is responsible for the metabolism of numerous drugs (Box 2). Consequently, for these drugs and those described later, it is worthwhile to consider the treatment approaches shown in Table 2.

Purine Antagonists

Purine antagonists include azathioprine and mycophenolate mofetil. Azathioprine is a prodrug converted in the body via a nonenzymatic

Table 2 Important Drug Interactions in Renal Transplantation

Transplant Drug	Second Drug	Mechanism	Effect	Strategy
Azathioprine	Allopurinol	Xanthine oxidase inhibition	Increased azathioprine effects	Dose reduction or substitute mycophenolate mofetil (CellCept)
CSA *or* TAC *or* SRL	Azoles, most CCBs, erythromycin, statins	P4503A4	Increased levels of CSA, TAC, SRL, statin	Dose reduction or substitute nifedipine; substitute azithromycin; use ezetimibe (Zetia)
SRL	CSA *or* TAC	P4503A4	Increased nephrotoxicity; increased CSA and TAC levels	Dose reduction or avoid

CCB, calcium channel blockers; CSA, cyclosporine; SRL, sirolimus; TAC, tacrolimus.

reaction to 6-mercaptopurine, a purine analogue that acts as an antimetabolite and blocks the synthesis of nucleotides, thereby inhibiting T and B cell proliferation.[1] Its major side effects are leukopenia and possible myelosuppression, increased susceptibility to infection, increased susceptibility to cancer, particularly PTLD and skin cancer, hepatotoxicity, and alopecia. The usual dosage varies from 1 to 2 mg/kg/day. The concomitant use of azathioprine with allopurinol, a xanthine oxidase inhibitor used to lower serum uric acid levels, typically in patients with gout, increases the risk of side effects and requires dose adjustments (see Table 2). Mycophenolate mofetil has largely replaced azathioprine.

Mycophenolate mofetil (MMF) is converted to mycophenolic acid, which inhibits inosine 5′-monophosphate dehydrogenase, a rate-limiting enzyme in the de novo synthesis of guanine nucleotides, thereby inhibiting DNA synthesis for replication of T and B cells.[1] The usual dose is 1 to 2 g/day in two divided doses. Its major side effects are diarrhea, leukopenia, anemia, and tissue-invasive cytomegalovirus (CMV) disease. Often, diarrhea can be avoided by dosing three times daily rather than twice daily using the same total daily dose.

Mammalian Target of Rapamycin Inhibitors

The immunosuppressants SRL (Rapamune) and everolimus bind to the same immunophilin (FKBP12) as TAC and modulate the intracellular protein mammalian target of rapamycin (mTOR), resulting in cell cycle arrest in the G1-S phase.[1] The maintenance dosage is usually 2 to 5 mg/day, with target trough levels of 5 to 15 ng/mL. SRL has a very long half-life (approximately 65 hours), so that trough level monitoring should be done 5 to 7 days after initiating the medication. It should be noted that although mTOR inhibitors and reduced doses of TAC or CSA may be used together, they can be more nephrotoxic and have inferior graft survival. Initially, mTOR inhibitors alone were not believed to be nephrotoxic. However, SRL may prolong acute tubular necrosis and cause proteinuria, certain glomerulopathies, and thrombotic microangiopathy. SRL, as well as CSA and TAC, also can cause renal magnesium wasting and potentially significant hypomagnesemia. Other side effects, typically dose-related, include hypercholesterolemia, hypertriglyceridemia, edema, hypertension, anemia, thrombocytopenia, leukopenia, interstitial pneumonitis, delayed wound healing, skin rash, mouth ulcers, and myalgia. More frequent acute rejections and inferior allograft survival have been reported with SRL than with CNI.

Approach to Allograft Dysfunction

The frequency of outpatient visits at the transplantation center is generally determined by the individual post-transplantation course of each recipient. Follow-up is focused on monitoring the recipient for acute rejection—an otherwise unexplained rise in serum creatinine level of 20% to 25% and varying clinical signs of decreased urine output, weight gain, edema—and cardiovascular disease, malignancy, infectious complications, usually pulmonary or urinary tract, delayed technical complications (e.g., renal artery stenosis, lymphocele, obstruction), worsening hypertension, new-onset or poorly controlled diabetes mellitus, hyperlipidemia, excessive weight gain, fluid retention and CHF, excessive diuresis and volume contraction, and immunosuppressant management for appropriate blood levels and toxicities. Concurrent management with the primary care physician or local nephrologists may vary among centers but will usually be a joint effort, with continuing contact with the transplantation center's nephrologists.

The advent of new and more potent immunosuppressive agents has reduced the frequency of acute rejection but has introduced other complications of renal transplantation. The differential diagnosis of an acute rise in serum creatinine level of more than 20% to 25% is similar to that for acute renal failure (prerenal, renal arterial, renal parenchymal, postrenal), with special emphasis on the time interval from transplantation, and awareness that the CNI immunosuppressants being used can themselves be nephrotoxic (Fig. 1). Major considerations are acute rejection, CNI nephrotoxicity, uncontrolled hypertension, recurrence of the original kidney disease, infections, and prerenal causes, such as volume depletion (e.g., through gastrointestinal losses, excessive diuretics, uncontrolled hyperglycemia) or hemodynamic alterations (e.g., often caused by combinations of medications, including angiotensin-converting enzyme [ACE] inhibitors, angiotensin-receptor blockers [ARBs], nonsteroidal anti-inflammatory drugs [NSAIDs], and CNIs even with mild volume depletion), and congestive heart failure. Although the frequencies of obstruction and transplantation artery stenosis are low, these need to be evaluated promptly with graft ultrasound or other techniques, because their treatment would usually require a transplantation surgeon or interventional radiologist.

Historical clues to allograft dysfunction include changes in weight and urine output, conditions leading to and symptoms of volume depletion, fever, chills, pain over the allograft, significantly higher or lower blood pressures, failure to adhere to the prescribed immunosuppressant medications, and the addition of a new medication, such as a diuretic, NSAID, ACE inhibitor or ARB, nephrotoxin, or a CYP 3A4 enzyme inhibitor that can increase or a medication that can decrease CNI levels (see Box 2). The physical examination should focus on volume status with orthostatic hypotension, significantly higher or lower blood pressures, allograft tenderness or bruit, swelling in the allograft area, diminished femoral pulses, particularly on the side of the allograft kidney, and evidence of congestive heart failure or infection. Laboratory studies should include a complete metabolic panel, serum phosphorus magnesium and uric acid, complete blood count (CBC) with differential, immunosuppressant blood levels, urinalysis, urine culture, and other studies based on the patient's presentation. An imaging study, including a graft ultrasound to detect evidence of obstruction and evaluate graft arterial and venous blood flow, should be performed promptly. A renal allograft biopsy is essential for determining the full extent of acute rejection.

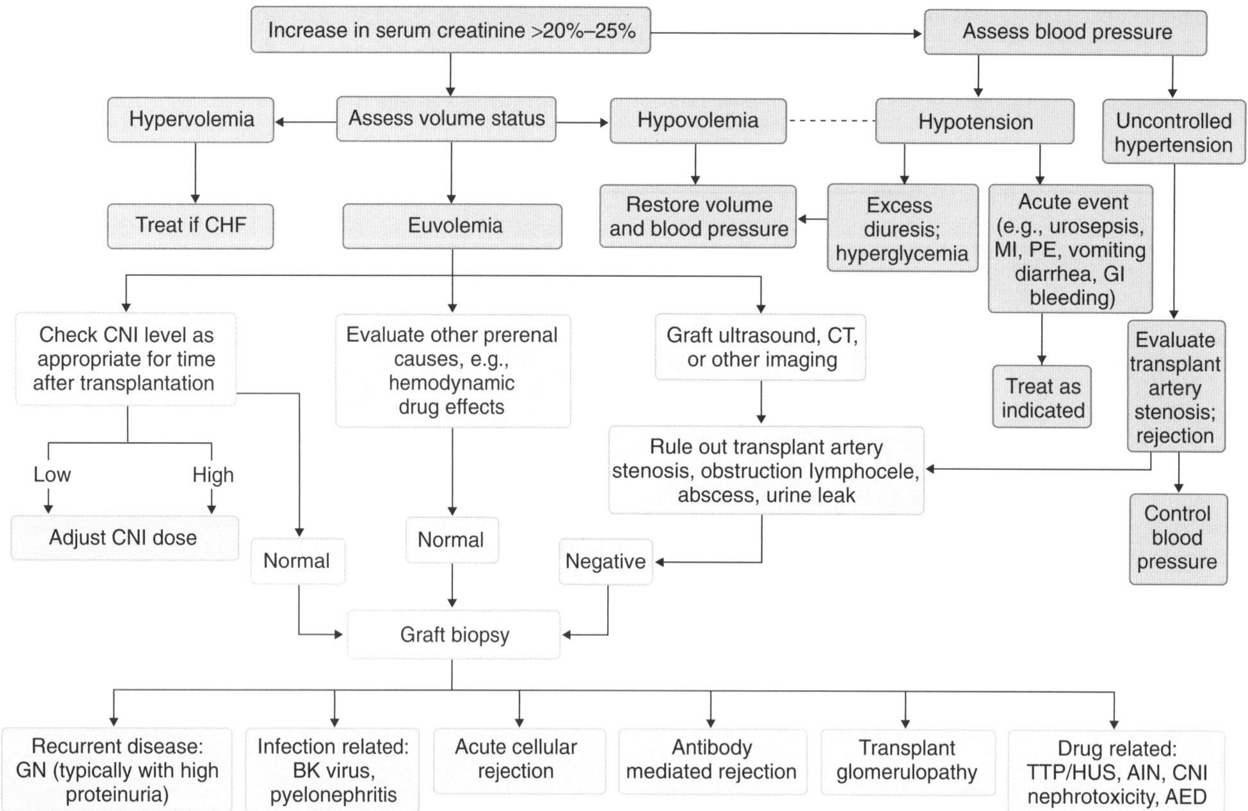

Figure 1 Evaluation of acute rise of serum creatinine level in the renal transplant patient. AED, atheroembolic disease; AIN, acute interstitial nephritis; CHF, congestive heart failure; CNI, calcineurin inhibitor; TTP/HUS, thrombotic thrombocytopenic purpura-hemolytic-uremic syndrome.

Rejection

Acute cellular rejection (ACR) is the most common type of rejection. With current immunosuppression regimens, clinical symptoms including allograft pain, fever, and oliguria, are uncommon. Typically, ACR occurs between 1 and 3 months after transplantation and less commonly after 6 months. Mild ACR (tubulitis) may be successfully reversed with corticosteroids alone, whereas moderate or severe ACR with endotheliitis may require the use of anti–T cell antibodies. Humoral or antibody-mediated rejection (AMR) caused by post-transplantation development of antidonor antibodies is a more serious form of rejection that usually requires plasmaphereses and intravenous immunoglobulin (IVIg) in addition to increased immunosuppression. Acute CNI nephrotoxicity may manifest as the hemolytic-uremic syndrome (HUS) manifested by thrombocytopenia, anemia, elevated lactic dehydrogenase (LDH) levels, and a peripheral blood smear with schistocytes. The definitive diagnosis is made by renal allograft biopsy. Recurrent renal disease in kidney transplant recipients accounts for less than 5% of all graft losses, but some diseases have a higher risk of recurrence, such as focal segmental glomerulosclerosis, immunoglobulin A (IgA) nephropathy, HUS, and membranoproliferative glomerulonephritis. Diabetic nephropathy can recur in renal allografts and has a more rapid onset than that seen in native kidneys, but it still is an uncommon cause of graft loss. Graft pyelonephritis can occur at any time after transplantation, with a clinical presentation ranging from asymptomatic pyuria to severe allograft pain and tenderness, fever, and leukocytosis; graft function usually returns to its baseline with appropriate antibiotics and volume repletion. Acute interstitial nephritis can also be encountered at any time after transplantation and usually responds to removal of the offending agent. BK virus nephropathy has become a more significant problem with the use of more potent immunosuppressant protocols. Full evaluation of BK infection and possible nephropathy should be done in a transplantation center, because treatment involves reduction in immunosuppressants and selection of additional therapy, as well as transplant biopsy with special studies. Similarly, acute rejection and recurrent disease should be managed in the transplantation center with biopsy of the transplanted kidney.

Late allograft dysfunction is usually a slow and progressive process resulting from chronic allograft injury. Biopsies of these kidneys show varying degrees of glomerulosclerosis, vascular damage, tubular atrophy, and interstitial fibrosis caused by both immunologic and nonimmunologic factors.

MEDICAL TREATMENT OF THE RENAL TRANSPLANT RECIPIENT

Medical complications create the most common cause of graft loss, namely, death of the recipient with a functioning graft. The primary causes of recipient death are cardiovascular disease (CVD), infection, and malignancy.[6-8]

Cardiovascular Disease

CVD remains the leading cause of death in kidney transplant recipients. Cardiovascular risk factors, often existing before transplantation, include hypertension, hyperlipidemia, diabetes mellitus, ischemic heart disease, peripheral vascular disease, long duration on dialysis, obesity, physical inactivity, older age, smoking, and male gender.[7,9] Cardiovascular risk reduction includes tight control of blood pressure (to <130/80 mm Hg), hypercholesterolemia (low-density lipoprotein cholesterol [LDL-C] level <100 mg/dL), and diabetes mellitus, if present; smoking cessation, physical activity, and weight control or reduction are also important. Evidence of carotid or peripheral arterial occlusive vascular disease should be checked at least annually on physical examination and followed with duplex ultrasound and pulse volume recordings, respectively. Stress testing is often needed for asymptomatic individuals who are also at high risk but may not experience chest pain because their underlying disease, diabetes mellitus with its neuropathy, can blunt symptoms of angina pectoris.

Hyperlipidemia

Approximately 60% of renal transplant recipients develop hyperlipidemia by 1 month after initiation of immunosuppressive therapy. SRL, CSA, and corticosteroids are major factors contributing to hyperlipidemia, in addition to other more usual factors (e.g., obesity, genetic predisposition, hypothyroidism, diabetes mellitus, nephrotic-range proteinuria, and allograft dysfunction). Recommendations include maintaining total cholesterol level lower than 200 mg/dL, LDL-C level lower than 100 mg/dL, and triglyceride levels lower than 150 mg/dL. First-line therapy should include both a low-fat diet and 3-hydroxy-3-methylglutaryl coenzyme A (HMG-CoA) reductase inhibitor (statin). There is an increased risk of myopathy or rhabdomyolysis because of the pharmacokinetic interaction of statins with CSA, TAC, and SRL. It has been recommended that the maximum dose of statins be reduced in patients receiving either CSA or TAC. Consequently, creatine kinase (CK) enzyme and alanine aminotransferase (ALT) levels should be monitored regularly. If diet and statin treatment fail to control the hypercholesterolemia, other treatment measures include switching from SRL or CSA to TAC, and adding ezetimibe (Zetia).

Hypertension

Hypertension is present in about 90% of kidney transplant recipients. It is well known that increasing levels of hypertension contributed to progressive graft loss. The basis of post-transplantation hypertension is often multifactorial and includes one or a combination of several factors, such as continued renin output from native kidneys, immunosuppressants (CNI, GC), graft renal artery stenosis, chronic allograft injury, liberal sodium intake, excess weight, hyperaldosteronism, and genetic factors. The Seventh Joint National Committee (JNC 7) has recognized the greater risk of hypertension in kidney transplant recipients and recommends a blood pressure goal of 130/80 mm Hg or lower. First-line therapy consists of lifestyle modification. Each class of antihypertensives has advantages and risks in a particular patient. ACE inhibitors and ARBs may be useful to help preserve renal function, particularly in diabetics, but generally should not be used when transplantation renal artery stenosis is present. Other potential side effects include angioedema, cough, hyperkalemia, anemia, and hemodynamic effects that cause a rise in the serum creatinine level. Diuretics may cause hypovolemia, leading to a rise in the serum creatinine level, hypokalemia, hypomagnesemia, and hyperuricemia. Blood levels of CNIs may be increased by some calcium channel blockers (e.g., verapamil, diltiazem, amlodipine), so appropriate monitoring of blood levels is advised with initiation of these calcium channel blockers (see Box 2 and Table 2).

New-Onset Diabetes Mellitus

The cumulative incidence of post-transplantation new-onset diabetes mellitus (NODM) at 12 and 36 months after transplantation has been reported to be approximately 16% and 24%, respectively,[10] but the true incidence is difficult to assess because of the absence of a uniform definition of NODM. Risk factors for NODM are age older than 50 years, obesity, African American and Hispanic ethnicities, family history of DM, hepatitis C, and use of CSA, TAC, and GC. The use of MMF, azathioprine, statins, and ACE inhibitors does not increase the risk for developing NODM. Initial therapy focuses on diabetes education, diet, exercise, and weight reduction. Selection of medications should take into consideration drugs affected by impaired renal function and interaction with immunosuppressants. Because of the surge in new drugs for diabetes treatment, NODM often requires management by an endocrinologist. Modification of the immunosuppressive regimen, if necessary, should be done with the aid of a transplantation nephrologist. GC tapering or discontinuation should be avoided or done with extreme caution because of the high risk of acute rejection.

Calcium and Phosphorus Disorders

Calcium and phosphorus disorders are common after transplantation. Hypophosphatemia may be seen even in the early post-transplantation period and may be caused by residual secondary hyperparathyroidism and impaired proximal tubular phosphate reabsorption because of GC use, and is usually asymptomatic. The phosphorus level should be kept between 2.5 and 4.5 mg/dL, with phosphorus supplementation. Hypercalcemia is most often caused by persistent hyperparathyroidism but may resolve with a longer period of good graft function. However, in some cases of hyperparathyroidism, hypercalcemia may persist, and treatment with the calcium-sensing drug cinacalcet should be considered. Subtotal parathyroidectomy may be needed. Other causes of hypercalcemia should also be evaluated, particularly excessive vitamin D and calcium intake, hyperthyroidism, and malignancies such as lymphomas and multiple myeloma.

Hyperkalemia and Hypomagnesemia

Hyperkalemia can be associated with the use of ACE inhibitors and ARBs, beta blockers, CNI, type IV renal tubular acidosis (RTA), and significant renal failure, especially with high-potassium diets. Hyperkalemia requires treatment that begins with the treatment of any drug or diet cause and, according to the degree of elevation, the use of diuretics, exchange resin, or even dialysis, if extreme.

Hypomagnesemia is commonly the result of the magnesuric effect of SRL and CNI, and may be associated with tremors. Magnesium supplementation should be started when the serum magnesium level falls below the lower level of the reporting laboratory, or kept within the upper normal range if the patient has tremors not due to other causes.

Musculoskeletal Disorders

Osteoporosis

Female and male kidney recipients lose up to 8% of their bone mass during the first 18 months after transplantation. An assessment of kidney transplant recipients at a mean of 6 years after transplantation has shown that bone loss, in the form of osteopenia or osteoporosis, affects 88% of recipients. Corticosteroid use is a major factor in bone loss, along with persistent hyperparathyroidism. Hypothyroidism and hypogonadism are other possible factors that need to be evaluated and treated if indicated.

Guidelines from the American Society of Transplantation recommend a baseline dual-energy x-ray absorptiometry (DEXA) scan at the time of transplantation, at 6 months after transplantation in all patients, and then annually in patients with abnormal results. Prevention and treatment of osteoporosis include appropriate daily elemental calcium (1200 mg/day) and vitamin D (800 U/day) intake, along with daily exercising and avoidance of smoking, caffeine, and alcohol use. The use of bisphosphonates will often depend on the level of renal function. The emerging regimen of GC avoidance may be promising for limiting osteoporosis, whereas GC withdrawal creates a significant risk of rejection.

Gout

Gout occurs in 10% to 20% of kidney recipients at any time after transplantation. Hyperuricemia occurs in a larger number of CNI-treated recipients, primarily those receiving CSA, because of decreased glomerular filtration of uric acid. In addition to the typical site of acute gout in the first metatarsophalangeal joint, post-transplantation gout may occur in the upper extremities and larger joints (e.g., wrists, shoulders, elbows, knees, hips). Acute attacks may be treated with low-dose colchicine or oral GCs. NSAIDs should be avoided.

Allopurinol should be avoided in patients who are taking azathioprine or used in a reduced dosage with lower dose azathioprine because of the high risk of interaction leading to severe myelosuppression, hepatotoxicity, or other adverse effects (see Table 2). Conversion from azathioprine to MMF avoids the problem and usually permits doses closer to those for nontransplantation patients. However, both colchicine and allopurinol can have serious side effects in patients with reduced renal function, and careful consideration must be given to monitoring or even avoiding their use. Major adverse effects of colchicine include diarrhea, myopathy, nausea, vomiting, myelosuppression, teratogenicity, hepatocellular toxicity, and seizures.

Infection

Immunosuppression creates a greater risk of infection, especially in the current era, because many potent immunosuppressants and antibody induction therapies are now used in broad combinations. The spectrum of infections in a renal transplant patient varies over time. In the first few months after transplantation, infections are usually caused by common bacterial and fungal infections associated with the surgical wound, vascular catheters and ureteral stents, organisms transmitted with the donor organ, nosocomial urinary tract infections (UTIs) and pneumonias, and *Clostridium difficile*–associated diarrhea. Infections beyond 4 months often include opportunistic pathogens because of the cumulative effects of intensive immunosuppressive therapy after transplantation. The important pathogens include viruses (CMV, Epstein-Barr virus [EBV], BK polyoma), fungi (*Aspergillus, Cryptococcus*), bacteria (*Listeria monocytogenes*), and other organisms (*Pneumocystis jiroveci, Nocardia*). Beyond 6 months, community-acquired bacterial and viral infections, recurrent urinary tract infections, opportunistic infections, parvovirus B19, and persistent hepatitis B or C virus (HBV, HCV) infections can develop.

Cytomegalovirus Infection

CMV infections represent one of the most common and serious infections in renal transplant recipients. Before prophylaxis programs were used, these infections occurred 1 to 6 months after transplantation, with a peak at approximately 6 weeks. Most transplantation programs now use at least 3 months of prophylactic antiviral therapy. However, experience has shown that CMV may occur within a few weeks after cessation of antiviral prophylaxis. The risk of CMV infection is highest in CMV antibody-negative recipients with CMV antibody-positive donors (CMV D^+/R^-). CMV prophylaxis programs in CMV D^+/R^- pairs may use oral valacyclovir or valganciclovir for 6 months or longer after transplantation.

The clinical presentation ranges from a subtle flulike syndrome to life-threatening pneumonia. It can be tissue invasive and affects the gastrointestinal tract, liver, retinas, central nervous system (CNS), and myocardium. The primary diagnostic test is quantitative CMV DNA determined by the polymerase chain reaction (PCR) assay. CMV infection is usually treated with intravenous ganciclovir for 2 to 4 weeks and reduction of immunosuppression (especially MMF).

Polyoma BK Nephropathy

Polyoma BK virus is a more recently recognized viral infection that can affect the renal allograft early and late after transplantation. Its detection and treatment are best managed in a transplantation center. It is a ubiquitous virus that remains in a latent state in up to 90% of the general population. About 30% to 60% of kidney transplant recipients develop BK viruria after transplantation, and 10% to 20% develop BK viremia. Among those who develop BK viremia, 5% to 10% develop BK nephropathy; of these, approximately 70% lose the allograft and the remainder exhibit some kidney dysfunction. BK infection may be associated with ureteral stenosis and possible obstruction, tubulointerstitial nephritis, and a progressive rise in the serum creatinine level, with ultimate allograft failure. BK infection must be evaluated in any episode of renal dysfunction and prospectively evaluated approximately every 3 to 6 months in the first year after transplantation.

Quantitative measurements of BK virus in the blood can strongly suggest BK nephropathy, but a graft biopsy with in situ hybridization or immunohistochemical techniques is required for a definitive diagnosis. Because there is no proven drug treatment for BK nephropathy, current therapy relies on careful reduction of immunosuppression (with the unavoidable risk of rejection) and options to use intravenous gamma globulin (IVIg) and/or low-dose cidofovir.

Pneumocystis jiroveci Prophylaxis

Prophylaxis of *P. jiroveci* pneumonia for recipients not allergic to sulfa includes single-strength trimethoprim-sulfamethoxazole for at least 1 year or indefinitely, depending on the perceived susceptibility of the transplant recipient and transplantation center practice. For sulfa-allergic patients, prophylaxis is achieved with oral dapsone or monthly inhaled pentamidine for up to 1 year.

Vaccinations

Vaccinations should be administered before transplantation. There are no data regarding timing of vaccines after transplantation. Live or attenuated virus vaccines are contraindicated after transplantation; these include measles-mumps-rubella (MMR), varicella, live oral poliomyelitis (Sabin), oral typhoid, bacillus Calmette-Guérin (BCG), smallpox, yellow fever, and the new varicella zoster virus vaccine. Permitted vaccines include influenza, inactivated injectable poliomyelitis (Salk), pneumococcal (Pneumovax), tetanus, and polysaccharide typhoid vaccines.

Malignancy

The 10-year prevalence of post-transplantation malignancy in the United States is reported to be as high as 30%. There is a twofold increase in common cancers (e.g., lung, colon, stomach, esophagus, pancreas, prostate, breast, and ovary), fivefold increase in melanoma, leukemia, hepatobiliary, cervical, and vulvovaginal cancers, a 15-fold increase in kidney cancer, and a 20-fold increase in Kaposi's sarcoma, non-Hodgkin's lymphoma, and nonmelanoma skin cancers.[11] In addition to the roles of immunosuppression and oncogenic viruses, clinical contributors to the risk of cancer include increasing age, cigarette smoking, and sun exposure.

Skin cancers—squamous cell carcinoma more often than basal cell carcinoma—remain the most common cancers in kidney recipients and are more aggressive than in the general population. The interval between transplantation and diagnosis is age dependent, 8 years for recipients 40 to 60 years of age, and 3 years for those older than 60 years. A dermatologist should be part of the long-term transplant care team for prompt evaluation of suspicious lesions and full skin examinations annually.

PTLD represents a spectrum of tumors, most often in the form of non-Hodgkin's lymphoma (NHL). The incidence of NHL peaks in the first year after transplantation and is associated with EBV virus infection in more than 90% of the cases. It differs from that in the general population by its extranodal, CNS, and allograft involvement. Therapy involves major reduction or complete elimination of nonglucocorticoid immunosuppressants and, in some cases, chemotherapy, surgical excision, and radiotherapy. It may be aggressive and respond poorly to therapy, especially if there is CNS involvement.

Summary

- Maintenance immunosuppression for renal transplantation typically consists of three types of drugs in combination: a glucocorticosteroid, purine antagonist (azathioprine or mycophenolate mofetil), and calcineurin inhibitor (cyclosporine or tacrolimus).
- The most common combination of oral immunosuppressants for renal transplantation currently is prednisone, tacrolimus, and mycophenolate mofetil.
- Any acute rise in the serum creatinine level to more than 20% to 25% in a kidney transplant recipient warrants careful investigation.
- Typically, acute rejection (cellular or antibody mediated) occurs most frequently within the first 6 months after transplantation.
- Cardiovascular disease is the leading cause of death among kidney transplant recipients because of the high prevalence of cardiovascular risk factors before and after transplantation, including hypertension, hyperlipidemia, renal dysfunction, and diabetes mellitus.
- The spectrum of infections in a renal transplant patient varies over time: primarily bacterial and viral infections in the first few months, viral, fungal, and opportunistic pathogens beyond 4 months, and community-acquired bacterial infections at any time.
- The 10-year prevalence of post-transplantation malignancy in the United States is reported to be as high as 30%.

Suggested Readings

Ahsan N, Hricik D, Matas A, et al: Prednisone withdrawal in kidney transplant recipients on cyclosporine and mycophenolate mofetil—a prospective randomized study. Steroid Withdrawal Study Group. Transplantation 1999;68:1865-1874.

Braun WE: Cardiovascular and other non-infectious complications after renal transplantation in adults. In Brady HR, Wilcox CS (eds): Therapy in Nephrology and Hypertension: Companion to Brenner and Rector's The Kidney, 3rd ed. Philadelphia: Saunders, 2008.

Braun WE: The medical management of the renal transplant recipients. In Johnson RJ (ed): Comprehensive Clinical Nephrology, Mosby 2nd ed. St. Louis, Mosby, 2003, pp 1105-1123.

Chobanian AV, Bakris GL, Black HR, et al: The seventh report of the joint national committee on prevention, detection, evaluation, and treatment of high blood pressure: The JNC 7 Report. JAMA 2003;289:2560-2571.

Danovitch GM: Immunosuppressive medications and protocols for kidney transplantation. In Danovitch GM (ed): Handbook of Kidney Transplantation, 4th ed. Philadelphia, Lippincott Williams & Wilkins, 4th ed. 2004, pp 72-134.

Fellstrom B: Risk factors for and management of post-transplantation cardiovascular disease. BioDrugs. 2001;15:261-278.

Gaston RS: Current and evolving immunosuppressive regimens in kidney transplantation. Am J Kidney Dis 2006;47(Suppl 2):S3-S21.

Halloran PF: Immunosuppressive drugs for kidney transplantation. N Engl J Med 2004;351:2715-2729.

Kasiske BL, Snyder JJ, Gilbertson D, Matas AJ: Diabetes mellitus after kidney transplantation in the United States. Am J Transplant 2003;3:178-185.

Kasiske BL, Snyder JJ, Gilbertson DT, et al: Cancer after kidney transplantation in the United States. Am J Transplant 2004;4:905-913.

Norman DJ, Turka LA (eds): Primer on Transplantation, 2nd ed. Mt. Laurel, NJ, American Society of Transplantation, 2001, pp 452-485.

Pascual M, Curtis J, Delmonico FL, et al: A prospective, randomized clinical trial of cyclosporine reduction in stable patients greater than 12 months after renal transplantation. Transplantation 2003:15;75:1501-1505.

References

For a complete list of references, log onto www.expertconsult.com.

Nephrolithiasis

Phillip Hall

DEFINITION

The formation of crystal aggregates in the urinary tract results in kidney stones, the clinical condition referred to as nephrolithiasis. Kidney stones might produce no symptoms or may be associated with one or several of the following: flank pain, gross or microscopic hematuria, obstruction of one or both kidneys, and urinary infections. The stones are usually formed by one of four substances: calcium, uric acid, magnesium ammonium phosphates (or struvite), or cystine.[1] Occasionally, calcium salts and uric acid are present in the same stone. Some rare types of kidney stones include xanthine and triamterene stones, which are seen in patients taking xanthine oxidase inhibitors and triamterene-containing diuretics, respectively. Indinavir stones have been reported in HIV-positive patients treated with this retroviral therapy.[2] In this chapter, I discuss the prevalence, pathophysiology, clinical presentation, and treatment of each of the four major types of stones.

Among American adults, the prevalence of nephrolithiasis is 1 in 1000, with men being almost twice as likely as women to have stones. Among the pediatric population, kidney stones are much less common, but the exact prevalence is unknown.

GENERAL PATHOPHYSIOLOGY

Kidney stones result from the growth of crystals into stones.[3] Crystals form in urine that is supersaturated with particular salts such as calcium oxalate, sodium urate, magnesium ammonium phosphate, or cystine. There is a maximum to the amount of a compound that can be kept in stable solution, which is defined by its solubility or equilibrium concentration product. Supersaturation results when the amount of a compound in solution exceeds the solubility; at that point, there is a process that begins to remove this excess by crystal formation. This can be manipulated in two ways: by changing the amount or concentration of compound available for crystallization or by changing the solubility of the compound. An example of the former is reducing the quantity of calcium or cystine in the urine of a patient with hypercalciuric or cystinuric stone disease, or reducing the concentration of the calcium or cystine by high fluid intake (dilution of the urine). An example of the latter is increasing the solubility by increasing the urinary pH in patients with uric acid or cystine stone disease or by increasing the urinary excretion of naturally occurring inhibitors of crystal formation, such as citrate.

Summary

- Nephrolithiasis has a prevalence of 1 in 1000 U.S. adults and is more common in men.
- Substances found in stones are calcium, uric acid, magnesium ammonium phosphate (struvite), and cystine.
- Stone formation occurs because of urine supersaturation with salts containing these substances.
- Helical computed tomography without contrast is the imaging procedure of choice for initial radiographic investigation.
- Stone analysis is usually necessary to determine the stone's chemical components.
- Most patients present with episodes of flank pain, usually severe and in waves. Often, there is hematuria.

CALCIUM STONE DISEASE

Prevalence

Calcium stone disease is the most common form of nephrolithiasis and represents about 70% of all cases of stone-forming disease. It occurs most often in the third to fifth decades of life and more often in men than women.

Pathophysiology

In 60% to 70% of patients, hypercalciuria is present (defined by 24-hour urinary calcium excretion of >300 mg in males, >250 mg in females, or >4 mg/kg in males or females). In less than 5%, the hypercalciuria may be associated with hyperparathyroidism or sarcoidosis, with or without hypercalcemia. More often, the hypercalciuria occurs with a normal serum calcium level and in the absence of any systemic diseases; this is called *idiopathic hypercalciuria.*[4]

Most patients with idiopathic hypercalciuria exhibit excessive gastrointestinal absorption of calcium (absorptive hypercalciuria). In many such cases, the 1,25-hydroxyvitamin D level is slightly elevated and the serum phosphorus level is slightly low, but parathyroid hormone (PTH) levels are normal. The mechanisms for these derangements are not known. These patients also have inappropriately high levels of urinary calcium excretion, even when on a calcium-restricted diet, which is why a calcium-restricted diet is not advised for these patients.

A minority of hypercalciuric patients have a renal leak of calcium (renal hypercalciuria). These patients have fasting hypercalciuria and slightly elevated levels of PTH and 1,25-hydroxyvitamin D. In these patients, thiazide diuretics reduce urinary calcium excretion, correct the secondary hyperparathyroidism, and return vitamin D levels to normal.

In both forms of hypercalciuria, the degree of hypercalciuria is worsened by high dietary sodium intake, high animal protein intake, and loop diuretics; it is reduced by distally acting thiazide diuretics and amiloride, as well as dietary restriction of sodium and protein. Several studies have shown that a higher dietary calcium intake has been associated with fewer calcium stone events in men and women.[5,6] A study of 120 Italian hypercalciuric calcium oxalate stone patients has demonstrated that a diet with normal calcium, low sodium, and low animal protein resulted in reduced incidence of calcium stones compared with those on a low-calcium diet.[7] In this study, both diets were associated with a reduction in urinary calcium level; however, urinary oxalate excretion rose in the low-calcium diet group and fell in the high-calcium diet group. The reduction in urinary oxalate excretion in persons on a normal calcium diet was attributed to the intestinal binding of dietary oxalate by dietary calcium, thus decreasing the amount of free oxalate available for absorption. Although both groups had reduced calcium oxalate saturation of their urine, the normal-calcium diet group had a more significant reduction. Compared with the patients on a low-calcium diet, the patients on the normal calcium, low-sodium, low-protein diet had a 50% reduction in stone risk at 5 years.

In some calcium stone patients, the mechanism for the increased rate of calcium oxalate stones is the presence of hyperoxaluria.[8] The hyperoxaluria is usually secondary to high dietary oxalate intake caused by ingestion of foods or liquids containing large quantities of oxalate. Some of these foods and liquids include baked beans, collard greens, green beans, rhubarb, tea, cocoa, peanut butter, and vegetable soup. In other cases, the hyperoxaluria occurs in the setting of gastrointestinal malabsorption, seen in patients with inflammatory bowel disease. When patients malabsorb fat, dietary calcium binds to the fat rather than to dietary oxalate, which is the norm. This results in a larger amount of unbound intestinal oxalate that passes into the colon, from which it is absorbed. In patients with ileostomies (colon excluded), this enhanced oxalate absorption does not occur. A rare cause of hyperoxaluria is the inherited condition known as primary hyperoxaluria.[9] In this condition, the hepatic enzyme that converts glyoxylate to glycine is deficient. As a result, there is increased production of oxalate from glyoxylate.

Other risk factors for calcium stones include chronic low urine output, hyperuricosuria, and low urine citrate, which occurs most often in patients with inflammatory bowel disease, chronic metabolic acidosis, and renal tubular acidosis (RTA). Renal stones occur in the distal form of RTA, are often composed of calcium phosphate, manifest as multiple stones on radiography (nephrocalcinosis), and occur in the presence of a persistently alkaline urine (pH >5.5) despite metabolic acidosis.

Signs and Symptoms

Patients often present with episodes of flank pain that radiates to the anterior abdomen or even to the genitalia. The pain is typically severe and comes in waves. Often, there is microscopic or gross hematuria. Calcium oxalate crystals may be seen with urine microscopy, but this finding is not diagnostic because calcium oxalate crystals may be seen in the urine of non–stone-forming patients. In some patients, the renal stones are completely asymptomatic or produce painless hematuria.

Diagnosis

Stone analysis is the best method for diagnosing calcium oxalate or calcium phosphate stones. Calcium-containing stones are radiopaque on routine radiography but show up as bright objects on computed helical tomography without contrast. Ultrasonography detects all types of renal stones if the stone is larger than 3 mm and the ultrasound procedure is technically satisfactory.

At present, helical computed tomography without contrast is the procedure of choice for the initial radiographic investigation. All types of stones located anywhere in the kidneys, ureters, or bladder are demonstrated with this technology. In a patient with azotemia, there is no risk from contrast administration. The anatomic status of the urinary tract will be clarified, and other possible nonstone causes for the patient's symptoms or signs may be identified.[10]

Of the conditions associated with calcium stones, only pyelotubular ectasia—medullary sponge kidney—is better demonstrated by intravenous urography.

Treatment and Outcome

In recurrent hypercalciuric stone patients, treatment should consist of high fluid intake, dietary sodium restriction, and thiazide diuretics. Thiazide diuretics (not loop diuretics) reduce urinary calcium excretion by inducing extracellular volume depletion, which in turn causes increased renal sodium and calcium reabsorption, and by directly increasing distal calcium reabsorption. An additional benefit of thiazide diuretics is that their chronic use is associated with preservation of bone mineral density.[11]

Dietary calcium restriction is not advised because of the potential for negative calcium balance and because a low-calcium diet increases the gastrointestinal absorption of oxalate and increased oxaluria. This increase in urinary oxalate can significantly raise the supersaturation of the urine for calcium oxalate, which in turn increases the stone formation rate. In hypercalcemic hypercalciuric stone-forming patients, the cause of the hypercalcemia should be sought and corrected. Correcting the metabolic acidosis in RTA and inflammatory bowel disease increases the urinary citrate excretion, an inhibitor of crystallization, and lessens the urinary calcium excretion.

Summary

- Calcium stones are the type found in 70% of patients with stones.
- Risk factors include hypercalciuria, low urine output, hyperuricosuria, low urine citrate level, and hyperoxaluria (usually secondary to high dietary intake).
- Most patients (60%-70%) have hypercalciuria. A minority have associated hypercalcemia.
- Idiopathic hypercalciuria is associated with excessive gastrointestinal calcium absorption (mechanism unknown), even on low-calcium diets.
- Hypercalciuria is aggravated by high dietary sodium intake.
- Therapy should include high fluid intake, dietary sodium restriction, and thiazide diuretics.

URIC ACID STONE DISEASE

Prevalence

Uric acid stone disease is found in about 5% to 10% of stone patients.[12] It is more common in patients with chronic diarrheal disorders and in those with hyperuricosuria. Most uric acid stone patients do not have gout. About 30% to 40% of patients have hyperuricosuria. Uric acid stones may also be partially composed of calcium oxalate, and some patients have both uric acid and calcium oxalate stones. In a study by Sakhaee and colleagues,[13] about 30% of normouricosuric stone patients have diabetes and another 23% have abnormal glucose tolerance.

Pathophysiology

Uric acid stones occur especially in patients with a very low urine pH (<5.0) and in those with hyperuricosuria. In some patients, this very low urine pH is caused by a defect in renal ammonia secretion that results in less buffering of secreted hydrogen ions and lower urine pH. Sakhaee and associates[13] have suggested that the very low urine pH is in some way related to the insulin resistance.

Uric acid is rather insoluble (15 mg/dL) in urine at a pH of 5.0, but becomes significantly more soluble in urine at a pH of 7.0 (150 mg/dL). Any combination of low urine pH, concentrated urine (as seen in chronic diarrheal states), and increased urinary uric acid excretion (as seen in patients with gout, chronic probenecid therapy, or high purine intake) increases the risk for uric acid stone disease. Rare congenital disorders of purine metabolism, such as Lesch-Nyhan syndrome, are associated with uric acid stones, hyperuricosuria, and hyperuricemia.

Urate stones are radiolucent and can be visualized by ultrasonography and noncontrast helical computed tomography. If the uric acid is mixed with calcium oxalate, the stone will be radiopaque.

Signs and Symptoms

Patients often present with episodes of flank pain that radiates to the anterior abdomen or even to the genitalia, as in calcium stone disease. The pain is frequently severe and comes in waves. Often there is microscopic or gross hematuria.

Diagnosis

Uric acid stone disease should be suspected in any patient with typical symptoms of renal colic in whom plain radiographs do not show a calcified stone. Urate crystals may be present in the urine, but they occur in patients without stones as well. The urine pH is usually lower than 5.5. Stone analysis provides a definitive diagnosis.

Treatment and Outcome

Because the solubility of uric acid is greatly increased when the urine pH is raised, treatment should consist of alkalinization of urine to a pH higher than 6.5 with potassium citrate solution, 30 to 90 mEq/day in divided doses, and hydration. This treatment has been shown to reduce uric acid stones by 90%. Such treatment, given to a patient with small stones in the kidneys, can also result in dissolution of the stones. When hyperuricosuria is also present, allopurinol may be used to reduce the serum uric acid level and thus reduce the renal excretion of uric acid. Restriction of animal protein is also recommended for patients with hyperuricosuria. Alkalinization of the urine with sodium bicarbonate or sodium citrate is not recommended because the sodium salts will increase calcium excretion, which increases the tendency to form calcium oxalate stones.

Summary

- Uric acid stones represent 5% to 10% of stone cases.
- Risk factors include chronic diarrhea and hyperuricosuria.
- Some patients have both uric acid and calcium oxalate stones.
- Uric acid stones occur in patients with a very low urine pH (<5.0), which reduces uric acid solubility.
- Therapy should include alkalinization of the urine pH to higher than 6.5 with potassium citrate. Uricosuric patients can benefit from allopurinol.

STRUVITE STONE DISEASE

Prevalence

Infection stones, also known as struvite or magnesium ammonium phosphate stones, occur in about 10% to 12% of patients, more often in women. They occur more often also in patients with spinal cord injury, neurogenic bladder, vesicoureteral reflux, chronic indwelling Foley catheters, and recurrent urinary infections, and in those with chronic obstruction of the upper urinary tract.

Pathophysiology

Struvite stones occur only in the presence of urine persistently infected with urease-producing bacteria that split urea and cause persistently alkaline urine.[14] Urea-splitting bacteria include *Proteus* (most commonly), *Pseudomonas*, *Klebsiella*, *Escherichia coli*, and some *Staphylococcus* species. Struvite stones are often branched (staghorn-shaped) and large. Because the stones contain ammonium, they have a tendency to adhere to the uroepithelium, which tends to accelerate the growth of these stones in a very short time. Treatment requires eradication of infection with antibiotics and the removal of the bacteria-laden stones by some interventional technique.

Signs and Symptoms

These stones can cause the typical symptoms of renal colic, but often they are discovered during the course of investigating a patient with recurrent urinary infections or in a patient with asymptomatic bacteriuria. Because these stones can grow to significant size, they are often found in the renal pelvis and infundibula of the kidneys.

Diagnosis

The diagnosis of struvite stones is suspected by finding large or branched stones in the kidneys of a patient with persistently infected urine. Stone analysis confirms the diagnosis.

Treatment and Outcome

Treatment must eradicate the urinary infection. Because the stones themselves are often infected with bacteria, the urinary infection cannot be eradicated without also removing the stones. Thus, surgical removal of the stones accompanied by appropriate antibiotic therapy is necessary. Acetohydroxamic acid is a urease inhibitor and has been used to prevent recurrence. Its effectiveness depends on its presence in the urine; hence, it has limited effectiveness in patients with azotemia. The use of this drug is further compromised because it has potentially serious side effects that include gastrointestinal upset, neurologic deficits, and thrombophlebitis.[15]

Summary

- Magnesium ammonium phosphate stones represent 10% to 12% of stone cases.
- Risk factors include female sex, spinal cord injury, history of obstructive uropathy, and recurrent urinary tract infections.
- They occur only in the presence of persistently infected urine with urease-producing bacteria.
- They are often discovered during a workup for recurrent urinary tract infections.
- Treatment should include eradication of the infection and often requires removal of the stone by some interventional technique.

CYSTINE STONE DISEASE

Prevalence

Cystine stone disease occurs in less than 1% of all adult stone patients and in about 6% to 8% of children with nephrolithiasis.[16]

Pathophysiology

Cystine stone disease occurs in persons who have inherited an autosomal recessive gastrointestinal and renal tubular transport disorder of four amino acids: cystine, ornithine, arginine, and lysine. Of these, cystine is the most insoluble in normally acid urine and thus precipitates into stones.

Signs and Symptoms

The patient presents with symptoms of nephrolithiasis, often at a younger age than a person with calcium stone disease. The stones are radiopaque (ground-glass appearance) and amber. Family history is often helpful (i.e., siblings might have the disorder).

Diagnosis

Normal urine contains less than 20 to 30 mg/day (<100 mg/g creatinine) of cystine. Urinary cystine excretion of more than 250 mg/g creatinine in adults is clearly abnormal and is the usual amount found in patients with cystinuria. The examination of a concentrated acidic urine specimen often reveals the presence of the cystine crystals, which are transparent and hexagonal. Cystine can be detected qualitatively by adding sodium nitroprusside to the urine and observing a purple-red color. Stone analysis is diagnostic.

Treatment and Outcome

Treatment is directed at reducing urinary cystine concentration in the urine or increasing urinary cystine solubility in the urine. The concentration of cystine in the urine is significantly helped by high fluid intake. There is a modest reduction of cystine excretion by reducing methionine in the diet by restricting red meat, fish, poultry, dairy products, and sodium. Alkalinization of the urine with potassium citrate to a pH of 6.5 to 7 is recommended. Sodium bicarbonate may be used for alkalinization, but the high sodium load increases cystine excretion. However, hydration and alkalinization alone are often ineffective at inhibiting recurrent stones.

Cystine is made up of two cysteine molecules connected by a disulfide bond. Thiol derivatives are chelating agents. They contain sulfhydryl groups that can bind with the cysteine molecules, reduce the formation of cystine, and render it more soluble. Therefore, these agents can also help dissolve cystine stones and prevent their formation. D-Penicillamine and α-mercaptopropionyl glycine are examples of such thiol-chelating agents. α-Mercaptopropionyl glycine is slightly more effective and produces fewer side effects. Captopril, which also has sulfhydryl groups, has been used in limited studies with success.[17]

Summary

- Cystine stones occur in patients with an inherited disorder of tubular and intestinal transport of cystine, ornithines, arginine, and lysine.
- Cystine is poorly soluble at normal urine pH.
- Onset of clinical stone events is in the teens and early adulthood
- Therapy requires alkalinization of urine to a pH higher than 7.0, high fluid intake, and using cysteine-binding drugs such as penicillamine or captopril.

Suggested Readings

Asplin JR: Hyperoxaluric calcium nephrolithiasis. Endocrinol Metab Clin North Am 2002;31:927-949.
Borghi L, Schianchi T, Meschi T, et al: Comparison of two diets for the prevention of recurrent stones in idiopathic hypercalciuria. N Engl J Med 2002;346:77-84.
Coe FL, Evan A, Worcester E: Kidney stone disease. J Clin Invest 2005;115:2598-2608.
Curhan GC, Willett WC, Rimm EB, Stampfer MJ: A prospective study of dietary calcium and other nutrients and the risk of symptomatic kidney stones. N Engl J Med 1993;328:833-838.
Curhan GC, Willett WC, Speizer FE, et al: Comparison of dietary calcium with supplemental calcium and other nutrients as factors affecting the risk for kidney stones in women. Ann Intern Med 1997;126:497-504.
Griffith DP: Struvite stones. Kidney Int 1978;13:372-382.
Katz DS, Scheer M, Lumerman JH, et al: Alternative or additional diagnoses on unenhanced helical computed tomography for suspected renal colic: Experience with 1000 consecutive examinations. Urology 2000;56:53-57.
Kok DJ: Clinical implications of physicochemistry of stone formation. Endocrinol Metab Clin North Am 2002;31:855-867.
Kopp JB, Miller KD, Mican JA, et al: Crystalluria and urinary tract abnormalities associated with indinavir. Ann Intern Med 1997;127:119-125.
Moe OW, Abate N, Sakhaee K: Pathophysiology of uric acid nephrolithiasis. Endocrinol Metab Clin North Am 2002;31:895-914.

References

For a complete list of references, log onto www.expertconsult.com.

Hypertension

Mohammed A. Rafey

DEFINITION AND ETIOLOGY

Normal or optimal blood pressure (BP) is defined as the level above which minimal vascular damage occurs. The Joint National Committee 7 (JNC 7) defines normal BP as a systolic BP less than 120 mm Hg and diastolic BP less than 80 mm Hg.[1] There is a continuous, consistent, and independent relationship between elevated BP and risk of cardiovascular events. This was clearly demonstrated in a meta-analysis that evaluated mortality due to vascular events in a million participants that included 61 observational trials. Results from this study demonstrated that a BP level of less than 115/75 mm Hg appears to better define optimal BP.[2]

PREVALENCE AND RISK FACTORS

An estimated 75 million Americans have hypertension, and blood pressure is well controlled to their goal BP level in fewer than one in three.[3] The highest prevalence of hypertension is noted in African Americans. Blood pressure control rate is recognised to be suboptimal or even lower in those who have serious comorbid conditions like chronic kidney disease. In a survey of patients with chronic kidney disease, BP control was found to be a dismal 13.2%.[4] On a global level, hypertension is a greater problem, with 13.5% of all deaths attributed to BP-related diseases. A majority of those who carry this disease burden belong to lower economic strata.[5]

The prevalence of hypertension increases progressively with age. Results from the Framingham study demonstrate that in middle-aged and elderly persons, the residual lifetime risk of developing hypertension is 90%.[6] Hypertension is primary or idiopathic 95% of the time when there is no identifiable risk factor and is of secondary etiologies like renovascular disease, primary aldosteronism, and others in 5% patients.

PATHOPHYSIOLOGY AND NATURAL HISTORY

The role of altered salt excretion by the kidney as a central mechanism in the development of hypertension was proposed by Dr Arthur C. Guyton.[7] According to Guyton's hypothesis, there is impaired excretion of sodium ions by tubular epithelial cells of the kidney. To maintain salt and water hemostasis, the body adapts a pressure-natriuresis approach that ultimately leads to elevation in BP. Animal studies and studies evaluating mendelian forms of syndromes that manifest as hypertension and hypotension, such as Bartter's syndrome and Liddle's syndrome, have provided insight into the pathophysiology of hypertension.[8] These data confirm that the basic problem in conditions leading to alteration in BP lies in the genetic alteration of sodium transport in renal epithelial cells. Several factors including aging, sympathetic overactivity, toxins, and a low nephron number have been proposed as factors that could ultimately damage the renal tubules and alter epithelial cells, resulting in defective sodium excretion.

In addition, several new conditions that can cause hypertension have been identified. The metabolic syndrome, with insulin resistance and elevation in insulin levels, leads to increased sympathetic activity and hypertension. In patients with obstructive sleep apnea, activation of the sympathetic and renin angiotensin systems has been defined as a possible mechanism for elevation in BP.

DIAGNOSIS

A detailed history and physical examination is essential for identifiying risk factors and stratifying patients to target those who need more-aggressive therapy to achieve goal BP. The history should include details of dietary salt intake and should explore lifestyle patterns and social and psychosocial stressors that could potentially affect BP levels. Ophthalmologic assessment and funduscopic examination is a simple technique to identify severity of disease and target organ damage by grading retinal changes.

Office Blood Pressure Measurement

Careful measurement of BP should be an integral part of any physical examination in a physician's office. Because BP inaccuracies are common in clinical practice, the following guidelines[9] should be followed when measuring a patient's BP. The patient should be seated comfortably with the back supported and the upper arm bared without constrictive clothing. The legs should not be crossed. The arm should be supported at heart level, and the bladder of the cuff should encircle at least 80% of the arm circumference. The mercury column should be deflated at 2 to 3 mm/sec, and the first and last audible sounds should be taken as systolic and diastolic pressure. The column should be read to the nearest 2 mm Hg. Neither the patient nor the observer should talk during the measurement.

Ambulatory Blood Pressure Monitoring

In addition to office BP measurements, 24-hour ambulatory BP monitoring and home BP monitoring are now acceptable methods for evaluating BP more comprehensively on an individual basis. Study data further advocate measurement of arterial stiffness parameters and central BP. In the Conduit Artery Function Evaluation (Café) substudy of the Anglo-Scandinavian Cardiac Outcomes Trial (ASCOT), which recruited 2073 patients, radial artery applanation tonometry and pulse-wave analysis was used to derive central aortic pressures and hemodynamic indexes on study visits for up to 4 years. In this trial, greater lowering of central BP appeared to improve cardiovascular outcomes, although peripheral BP reduction was similar in all groups.[10-11] Guidelines of the European Society of Hypertension have incorporated measurement of these vascular parameters at those centers where it is available.

Ambulatory blood pressure monitoring is indicated to rule out white-coat hypertension, to uncover apparent drug resistance (office resistance), to better define resistant hypertension, to identify hypotensive symptoms while the patient is being treated with antihypertensives, to monitor episodic hypertension, and to identify autonomic dysfunction states.

Patterns of Blood Pressure

Based on 24-hour ambulatory BP monitoring and office BP readings, four patterns of BP have been described (Fig. 1).

In *sustained hypertension*, BP measurements taken in the office and at home are elevated. Studies done in patients with sustained hypertension for more than 40 years have consistently demonstrated

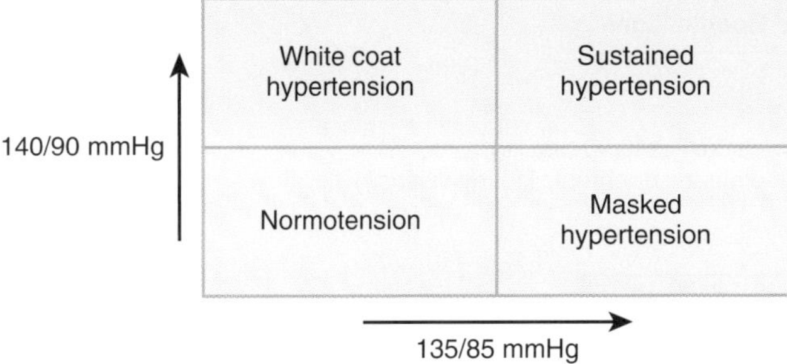

Figure 1 Patterns of blood pressure. Normotension, sustained hypertension, white coat hypertension, and masked hypertension.

that this condition is closely related to target organ damage and worse cardiac and renal events.

Masked hypertension is defined as normal office BP and elevated home BP.[12] Its prevalence ranges from 8% in the general population to as much as 20% in hypertensive patients receiving treatment. Although there are no outcome trials available in patients with masked hypertension, the fact that elevated ambulatory BP is closely related to cardiovascular events implies that its risk profile is similar to that of sustained hypertension. In fact, these patients might have a worse outcome because they are not easily identified and do not receive adequate therapy.

Patients with *white coat hypertension* have an elevated office BP and normal home BPs. Its prevalence has been reported to be 12% to 18 % the general population. Initially it was thought to be a benign condition, because prospective trials evaluating white coat hypertension have shown less target-organ damage (increased left ventricular mass, carotid media intimal thickness) than that with sustained hypertension. Clinical studies evaluating cardiovascular outcomes have consistently demonstrated a lower morbidity with white coat hypertension, supporting a more benign course. Based on these studies, it has been hypothesized that white coat hypertension represents an intermediate risk state between normotension and sustained hypertension. One study that followed white coat hypertension patients demonstrated a significantly elevated risk of stroke in these patients after 6 years of follow-up, emphasizing the importance of long-term follow-up in these patients.[13]

Normally, there is a diurnal variation in BP, with a 10% to 20% decrease in systolic BP during sleep, which is described as the *normal dipping pattern.* Abnormalities in the normal nocturnal dipping pattern of BP have been associated with worse cardiovascular outcomes, even in subjects who are normotensive.[14] A 24 hour ambulatory BP measurement remains the only technique to assess the dipping status of patients. *Nocturnal hypertension* defines a pattern of BP where BP measured during sleep is higher than that measured when the patient is awake. In the African American Study of Kidney Disease and Hypertension (AASK), an abnormal dipping pattern was detected in 80 % of patients and nocturnal hypertension was found in 40%.[15] All of these patients with an abnormal dipping pattern and nocturnal hypertension had hypertension that was apparently well controlled based on office BP readings.

Home Blood Pressure Monitoring

Several prospective trials have demonstrated that home BP is a better predictor of cardiovascular morbidity and mortality than office BP measurements. Based on these data, the first home BP monitoring guidelines endorsed by national societies, including the American Heart Association (AHA) and American Society of Hypertension (ASH), among others, have been published.[16]

These home BP measurement guidelines recommend that a validated device be used to measure BP at home. BP measurements using such validated devices should be taken before an office visit, with at least two morning and two evening readings every day for 1 week (but discarding the readings of the first day), which gives a total of 12 BP readings with which clinical decisions can be made.

Box 1 Baseline Blood Tests Recommended by JNC 7

Routine tests

- Electrocardiogram
- Urinalysis
- Blood glucose, and hematocrit
- Serum potassium, creatinine, or the corresponding estimated glomerular filtration rate, and calcium
- Lipid profile, after 9- to 12-hour fast, that includes high-density and low-density lipoprotein cholesterol, and triglycerides

Optional test

- Measurement of urinary albumin excretion or albumin/creatinine ratio

More extensive testing for identifiable causes is not generally indicated unless blood ressure control is not achieved

Table 1 Tests and Their Clues to the Etiology in Those with Resistant or Secondary Hypertension

Laboratory Test	Possible Clinical Implication	Change in Management
Abnormal urinalysis	Renal disease	Lower blood pressure goal
Low serum potassium	Primary aldosteronism Cushing's syndrome	Further evaluation for secondary hypertension
Serum creatinine concentration	Renal disease and renovascular disease	Further evaluation and more aggressive therapy
Hematocrit	Polycythemia	Further evaluation
Electrocardiogram	Left ventricular hypertrophy	More aggressive therapy
Fasting lipid profile	Elevated risk for cardiovascular events	Aggressive lifestyle modifications

Laboratory Tests

Baseline blood tests are recommended by JNC 7 to identify those at risk for future events (Box 1). In addition, these tests can provide clues to the etiology in those with resistant or secondary hypertension (Table 1).

Summary

- Proper technique of BP measurement should be an integral part in evaluation and management of hypertension.
- Patterns of BP based on ambulatory BP monitoring play an important role in altering therapy and outcomes.
- Laboratory examination helps in stratifying patients who will need more extensive evaluation and aggressive therapy.

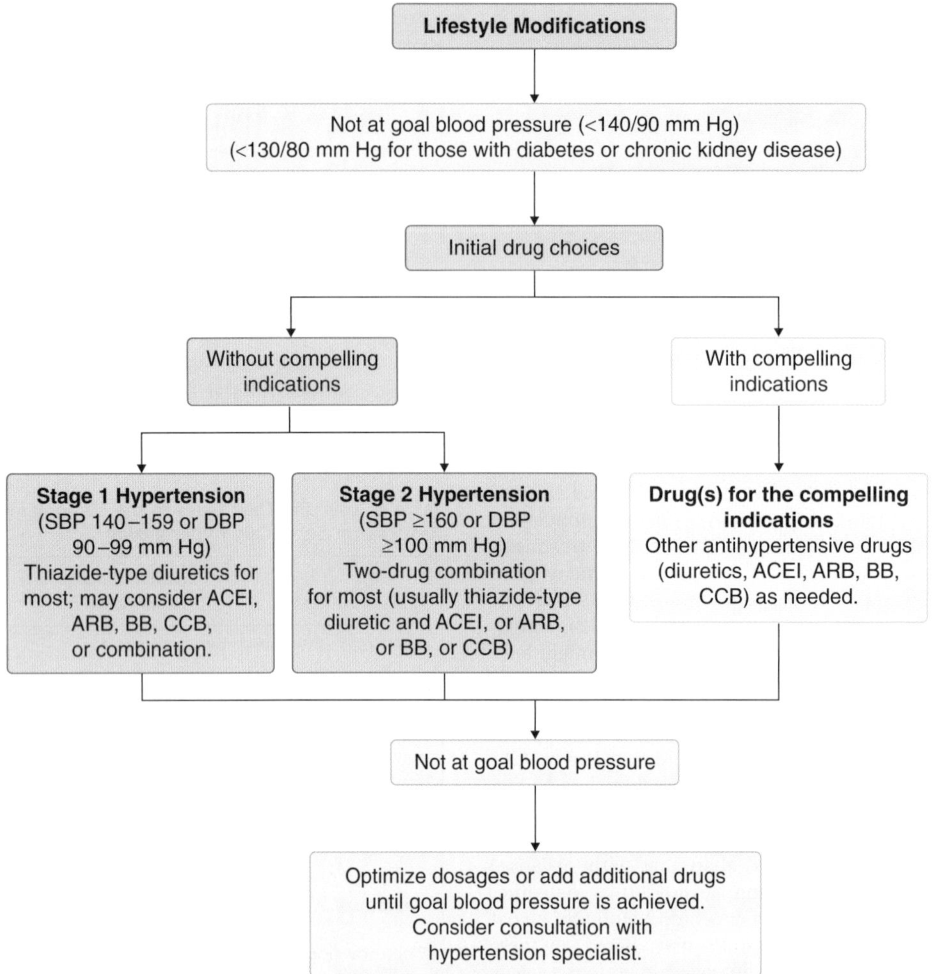

Figure 2 Algorithm for the treatment of hypertension. ACEI, angiotensin-converting enzyme inhibitor; ARB, angiotensin receptor blocker; BB, beta blocker; CCB, calcium channel blocker; DBP, diastolic blood pressure; SBP, systolic blood pressure.

TREATMENT

Current JNC 7 guidelines are still largely based on threshold levels of BP. In addition, JNC 7 guidelines do recognize and incorporate the importance of increased cardiovascular risk across a broad spectrum of BP values, as well as a high lifetime risk of developing hypertension (Fig. 2). The new JNC 8 guidelines are expected to be released in 2009. The European Society of Hypertension (ESH) and European Society of Cardiology (ESC) 2009 guidelines have embraced the concept of global cardiovascular risk in recommending that patients should be classified not only in relation to grades of hypertension but also in terms of their total cardiovascular risk, which represents cumulative risk from the coexistence of multiple risk factors and target organ damage.[17] These guidelines stress that the threshold for hypertension and subsequent drug therapy should remain flexible and should be a function of each patient's individual and total cardiovascular risk.

It is clearly recognized that an increasing BP level is associated with a greater risk of heart attack, stroke, and kidney disease. In fact, for persons aged 40 to 70 years, each increment of 20 mm Hg in systolic BP or 10 mm Hg in diastolic BP actually doubles the risk of cardiovascular disease across the entire range of BP, from 115/75 to 185/115 mm Hg. In an effort to highlight this relationship between elevated BP and cardiovascular disease, a revised classification of hypertension has been provided by JNC 7 (Table 2). Blood pressures below 120/80 mm Hg are now considered normal, whereas the previous categories of normal and high-normal BP have been combined into the new classification of prehypertension (systolic BP 120-139 mm Hg, and diastolic BP 80-89 mm Hg).

Table 2 Classification of Blood Pressure (BP)

Classification	Systolic BP (mm Hg)	Diastolic BP (mm Hg)
Normal	<120	*And* <80
Prehypertension	120-139	*Or* 80-89
Stage 1 hypertension	140-159	*Or* 90-99
Stage 2 hypertension	>160	*Or* >100

BP, blood pressure.
Data from http://www.nhlbi.nih.gov/guidelines/hypertension/index.htm (accessed March 12, 2009).

Based on JNC 7, patients with sustained hypertension are further divided into stage 1 hypertension (systolic BP 140-159 or diastolic BP 90-99 mm Hg), stage 2 hypertension (systolic BP =160 or diastolic BP =100 mm Hg), and those with compelling indications that include diabetes, cardiovascular disease, and renal disease.

Lifestyle Modification

Educating patients regarding the importance of nonpharmacologic interventions for effective BP control is an important component of reducing cardiovascular risk in the general population. This is particularly true for the prehypertensive and hypertensive patient. However, aggressive efforts are needed to ensure optimal adherence to recommendations.

Lifestyle modifications include limiting alcohol intake, increasing physical activity, and reducing sodium intake to less than 6 g of sodium chloride daily. Results from the long-term follow-up of the Trials of Hypertension Prevention (TOHP) study demonstrated that patients who were randomized to a low-salt diet (sodium <1800 mg/24 hr) had a 25% risk reduction in cardiovascular events.[18]

Weight reduction of as little as 10 to 12 pounds in the obese hypertensive patient can have a considerable impact on elevated BP. Appropriate nutritional counselling can encourage a diet with reduced total fat and cholesterol intake, in addition to providing an adequate daily intake of potassium, calcium, and magnesium. The dietary approaches to stop hypertension (DASH) trial has provided substantial data that a diet rich in fruits, nuts, vegetables and low-fat dairy products and with an emphasis on fish and chicken rather than red meat lowered BP even without weight reduction and was particularly effective in those who also restricted sodium chloride intake.[19] Dietary recommendations must be made on an individualized basis and should be well supported with continued educational and counselling efforts.

Cigarette smoking is a recognized accelerator of cardiovascular disease. Smoking cessation should therefore be strongly encouraged for all patients, and education, counselling, and medication should be provided as needed.

Table 3 lists lifestyle modifications for which evidence-based data are available to support BP reductions. The effects of implementing these modifications are both dose dependent and time dependent and could be greater for some patients. Also, a combination of two or more lifestyle modifications can achieve even better results. Lifestyle modifications not only reduce BP but also enhance the efficacy of antihypertensive drugs and decrease cardiovascular risk.

Medical Treatment

Prehypertension

An estimated 70 million Americans have prehypertension. The Framingham study demonstrates that if their prehypertension is left untreated, these patients go on to develop hypertension. Current recommendations center around nonpharmacological interventions, which include lifestyle modifications like weight reduction, increased physical activity, and reduced dietary salt intake. Antihypertensive therapy is not indicated in those with prehypertension at this time.

The Trial of Preventing Hypertension (TROPHY) was conducted to explore whether temporary treatment of prehypertension patients with an antihypertensive agent would reduce their future risk of developing hypertension.[20] Patients were randomized in a double-blind manner to treatment with candesartan (16 mg daily; $n = 391$) or matching placebo ($n = 381$) for a 2-year period, after which all patients were treated with placebo for an additional 2 years. At the 4-year follow-up, hypertension was noted to have developed less often in the group initially randomized to candesartan (53.2% vs 63.0%, relative risk [RR], 0.84; $P = 0.007$). The overall relative risk of hypertension in candesartan group was decreased (RR, 0.58; $P < 0.001$).

Stage 1 and Stage 2 Hypertetension

Based on Antihypertensive and Lipid Lowering to Reduce Heart Attack Trial (ALLHAT) data, JNC 7 recommends diuretics as first-line therapy for the management of stage 1 hypertension and a combination of two drugs as an initial therapy in those with stage 2 hypertension, one of which should preferably be a diuretic.[21]

The ALLHAT trial was designed to compare antihypertensive therapy using an ACE inhibitor, a dihydropyridine calcium antagonist, and an α-adrenergic blocker with treatment with an oral diuretic, chlorthalidone, as the standard of therapy. The α-adrenergic blocker arm of this study was discontinued early in the trial because it was observed that patients receiving an α-adrenergic blocker as monotherapy demonstrated twice the risk of congestive heart failure when compared with those treated with an oral diuretic. The diuretic, calcium antagonist, and angiotensin-converting enzyme (ACE) inhibitor groups were continued to an average follow-up of 4.9 years, at which time no differences were noted among groups with regard to the primary outcome (fatal coronary disease or nonfatal myocardial infarction) or all-cause mortality. However, compared with the diuretic (chlorthalidone) group, the calcium antagonist (amlodipine) group had a significantly higher cumulative incidence of heart failure, and the ACE inhibitor (lisinopril) group

Table 3 Lifestyle Modifications to Manage Hypertension*†

Modification	Recommendation	Approximate SBP Reduction Range
Weight reduction	Maintain normal body weight (body mass index, 18.4-24.9 kg/m^2)	5-20 mm Hg; 10-kg weight loss
Adopt DASH eating plan	Consume diet rich in fruits, vegetables, low-fat dairy products, with reduced content of saturated and total fats	8-14 mm Hg
Dietary sodium reduction	Reduce dietary sodium intake to no more than 100 mmol/day (2.4 g sodium or 6 g sodium chloride)	2-8 mm Hg
Physical activity	Engage in regular aerobic physical activity (e.g., brisk walking) at least 30 min/day, most days of the week	4-9 mm Hg
Moderation of alcohol consumption	Most men: limit consumption to no more than two drinks/day‡ Most women and those who weigh less than normal: no more than one drink/day	2-4 mm Hg

*For overall cardiovascular risk reduction, stop smoking.

†The effects of implementing these modifications are dose- and time-dependent and could be more effective for some patients.

‡1 oz or 30 mL ethanol: 12 oz beer, 5 oz wine, 1.5 oz of 80-proof whiskey.

DASH, Dietary Approaches to Stop Hypertension; SBP, systolic blood pressure.

Data from Chobanian AV, Bakris GL, Black HR, et al; Joint National Committee on Prevention, Detection, Evaluation, and Treatment of High Blood Pressure; National Heart, Lung, and Blood Institute; National High Blood Pressure Education Program Coordinating Committee: Seventh report of the Joint National Committee on Prevention, Detection, Evaluation, and Treatment of High Blood Pressure. Hypertension 2003;42(6):1206-1252. Available at http://www.nhlbi.nih.gov/guidelines/hypertension/index.htm (accessed March 12, 2009).

Table 4 Classification and Management of Blood Pressure for Adults

BP Classification	SBP,* mm Hg	DBP,* mm Hg	Lifestyle Modifications	Initial Drug Therapy: With Compelling Indications	Initial Drug Therapy: Without Compelling Indications
Normal	<120	And <80	Encourage		
Prehypertension	120-139	*Or* 80-89	Yes	No antihypertensive drug indicated	Drug(s) for compelling indications†
Stage 1 Hypertension	140-159	*Or* 90-99	Yes	Thiazide-type diuretics for most. May consider ACEI, ARB, BB, CCB, or combination	Drug(s) for the compelling indications.‡ Other antihypertensive drugs (diuretics, ACEI, ARB, BB, CCB) as needed
Stage 2 Hypertension	>160	*Or* >100	Yes	Two-drug combination for most† (usually thiazide-type diuretic and ACEI or ARB or BB or CCB)	

*Treatment determined by highest blood pressure category.
†Initial combined therapy should be used cautiously in those at risk for orthostatic hypotension.
‡Treat patients with chronic kidney disease or diabetes to blood pressure goal <130/80 mm Hg.
ACEI, angiotensin-converting enzyme inhibitor; ARB, angiotensin receptor blocker; BB, beta blocker; CCB, calcium channel blocker; DBP, diastolic blood pressure, SBP, systolic blood pressure.
Data from Chobanian AV, Bakris GL, Black HR, et al; Joint National Committee on Prevention, Detection, Evaluation, and Treatment of High Blood Pressure; National Heart, Lung, and Blood Institute; National High Blood Pressure Education Program Coordinating Committee: Seventh report of the Joint National Committee on Prevention, Detection, Evaluation, and Treatment of High Blood Pressure. Hypertension 2003;42(6):1206-1252. Available at http://www.nhlbi.nih.gov/guidelines/hypertension/index.htm (accessed March 12, 2009).

had significantly higher incidences of heart failure, stroke, and angina pectoris.

Trial-design issues subsequently generated significant debate regarding the ALLHAT results, particularly the magnitude of the differences noted. Nevertheless, it was concluded from this trial that diuretic therapy is as effective as a calcium channel blocker or an ACE inhibitor from the standpoint of the primary outcome of the trial, and diuretic therapy is superior for select subgroup analyses. A critical look at the trial design suggests a more prudent conclusion that diuretics should be part of all antihypertensive regimens unless they are clearly contraindicated.

In addition, there was also a concern that diuretics might worsen glucose tolerance and insulin resistance. Recent data demonstrates that the higher incidence of diabetes mellitus related to thiazides does not appear to be responsible for the increase in risk for coronary heart disease.[22]

In addition to thiazide diuretics, JNC 7 guidelines also recommend ACE inhibitors, angiotensin receptor blockers (ARBs), beta blockers, and calcium channel blockers as first-line therapy for hypertension. Since the publication of JNC 7 guidelines, studies have shown that beta-blocker therapy might not be effective and in fact might increase the risk of stroke.[23,11] In the newer guidelines published by various national societies, beta blockers have been removed as first-line therapy and are recommended only with a compelling indication in those with cardiac disease.

Based on evidence of improved outcomes, JNC 7 has recommended several medications for compelling indications (Tables 4 and 5). These include beta blockers and aldosterone antagonists in those with cardiac disease, ACE inhibitors and ARBs in those with chronic kidney disease, and diuretics and calcium channel blockers in those with isolated systolic hypertension. A combination of ACE inhibitors and diuretics instead of ACE inhibitors alone is recommended for preventing recurrence of stroke based on findings of Perindopril Protection Against Recurrent Stroke Study (PROGRESS), which showed a 42% stroke reduction in those treated with this combination of therapy.[24]

Further complexity in instituting an antihypertensive combination regimen was introduced by results of the ASCOT, study which showed that a calcium channel blocker and ACE inhibitor combination had a better outcome when compared to a beta blocker and diuretic combination regimen. A better outcome was shown to occur even though there was a similar BP reduction in both treatment arms.

A lower BP goal appears to be a clear winner in most antihypertensive trials to reduce cardiovascular and renal outcomes. Experts in hypertension, however, continue to be perplexed by the fact that certain classes of medications appear to have a more beneficial effect than others. In the Café study, a further reduction of central systolic BP in calcium channel blockers and ACE inhibitors arm appeared to better explain the beneficial outcomes with this combination therapy in the main ASCOT study.[11]

Summary

- Classification of hypertension is based on BP levels as well as comorbidities like heart disease, diabetes, and renal disease.
- Lifestyle intervention should be recommended for patients with prehypertension and all stages of hypertension.
- Compelling indications mandate therapy with specific medications.

CONCLUSIONS

The ultimate public health goal of antihypertensive therapy is to reduce the morbidity and mortality from cardiovascular and renal events. It is well established that lowering BP reduces cardiovascular risk. Numerous clinical trials have also made it clear that treating to achieve lower BP goals can be associated with further risk reduction. A report using data from the National Health and Nutrition Examination Survey (NHANES) Epidemiologic Follow-up Study has estimated the absolute benefit associated with a 12-mm Hg reduction in systolic BP over 10 years. For the patient with stage 1 hypertension (systolic BP 140-159 mm Hg and/or diastolic BP 90-99 mm Hg) and additional cardiovascular risk factors, one death would be prevented for every 11 patients treated. In the presence of cardiovascular disease

Table 5 Clinical Trial and Guideline Basis for Compelling Indications for Individual Drug Classes

Compelling Indication*	Recommended Drugs						Clinical Trial Basis[†]
	Diuretic	BB	ACEI	ARB	CCB	Aldo ANT	
Heart failure	✓	✓	✓	✓		✓	ACC/AHA heart failure guideline, MERIT-HF, COPERNICUS, CIBIS, SOLVD, AIRE, TRACE, ValHEFT, RALES
Postmyocardial infarction		✓	✓			✓	ACC/AHA post-MI guideline, BHAT, SAVE, Capricorn, EPHESUS
High coronary disease risk	✓	✓	✓		✓		ALLHAT, HOPE, ANBP2, LIFE, CONVINCE
Diabetes	✓	✓	✓	✓	✓		NKF-ADA guideline, UKPDS, ALLHAT
Chronic kidney disease			✓	✓			NKF guideline, captopril trial, RENAAL, IDNT, REIN, AASK
Recurrent stroke prevention	✓		✓				PROGRESS

*Compelling indications for antihypertensive drugs are based on benefits from outcome studies or existing clinical guidelines; the compelling indication is managed in parallel with the BP.

[†]Conditions for which clinical trials have demonstrated benefit of specific classes of antihypertensive drugs.

ACEI, angiotensin-converting enzyme inhibitor; Aldo ANT, aldosterone antagonist; ARB, angiotensin receptor blocker; BB, beta blocker; CCB, calcium channel blocker.

Data from Chobanian AV, Bakris GL, Black HR, et al; Joint National Committee on Prevention, Detection, Evaluation, and Treatment of High Blood Pressure; National Heart, Lung, and Blood Institute; National High Blood Pressure Education Program Coordinating Committee: Seventh report of the Joint National Committee on Prevention, Detection, Evaluation, and Treatment of High Blood Pressure. Hypertension 2003;42(6):1206-1252. Available at http://www.nhlbi.nih.gov/guidelines/hypertension/index.htm (accessed March 12, 2009).

with target organ damage, only nine patients would require BP reduction to prevent a death. Because most persons with hypertension, particularly those older than 50 years, reach their diastolic BP goal once systolic BP is at goal, the primary focus in hypertension therapy should be on achieving the systolic BP goal. Evidence exists that treating systolic BP and diastolic BP to a target below 140/90 mm Hg is associated with reduction in cardiovascular disease complications. Data now support treatment to a BP goal below 130/80 mm Hg in patients with hypertension, diabetes mellitus, or renal disease.

Hypertension is an important modifiable risk factor. Although a majority of patients with hypertension remain asymptomatic, a careful early evaluation identifies those with or at risk for target organ damage for left ventricular hypertrophy and microalbuminuria, which portend serious future cardiovascular and renal events. Early identification of these patients and achieving BP goals could potentially reverse early end-organ damage and improve outcomes in these patients. The effective management of hypertension is therefore an important primary health care objective in managing cardiovascular and renal disease.

The disappointing control rates of hypertension can be significantly improved if both health care providers and patients can be encouraged to embrace lower target BPs as suggested by recent results from clinical trials. The majority of patients with uncontrolled hypertension are older adults with isolated stage 1 or 2 systolic hypertension, most of whom have access to and regular visits with their health care providers.

References

For a complete list of references, log onto www.expertconsult.com.

General Medical Care of Patients on Dialysis

Robert Heyka

DEFINITION AND ETIOLOGY

Among patients with end-stage renal disease (ESRD) who require dialysis support, the age at onset, survival rates, and complexity of comorbidities are increasing. Patients with ESRD usually start dialysis with problems that require general medical care in addition to their dialytic care. Patients may choose to continue to see their primary care physician or may request that their nephrologist also assume that aspect of their care. Sometimes the choice is made for the patient by a physician familiar with the management of the patient's problems or contractual insurance demands.

A survey of nephrologists found that nearly two thirds of respondents stated they provided most of the primary care to at least some of their dialysis patients. Additional medical care was most commonly delivered in the dialysis units. However, few nephrologists had written policies for primary care, and 75% did not follow clinical practice guidelines, were not familiar with guidelines, or had not read them but were aware of their existence. Thus, primary care physicians can still play an important role in the general medical care of patients with ESRD.

How can the care of ESRD patients be approached to ensure that a renal-related problem best managed by the nephrologist remains the province of the attending nephrologist while the primary care specialist provides the general medical care? Boxes 1 and 2 provide a framework for this division of patient care. Individual circumstances that take into consideration the skills and knowledge sets of the attending physicians are also of paramount importance.

What medical problems and practices can be altered to improve the outcome of ESRD patients? In addition to the processes related to the dialysis procedure itself, management of comorbid conditions and attention to preventive care can have a significant impact on patient morbidity and mortality and, in many instances, are better provided by a primary care physicians. However, approaches to the general medical care of an ESRD patient more often reflect the age- and gender-appropriate medical care that a patient should receive while taking into consideration the increased comorbidities and mortality associated with ESRD rather than medical care appropriate for a patient who was not on dialysis.

PREVALENCE AND RISK FACTORS

The two major causes of ESRD in the United States are diabetes mellitus and hypertension. As with most patients with end organ failure, ESRD patients often have a slowly declining course marked by periods of life-threatening events or complications. Any approach to general care must address both realities. Most patients starting dialysis have already experienced comorbid events relating to these two entities. There is also a high prevalence of prior cardiovascular disease, which approaches 80% in prospective studies. The care of these patients can reflect a primary or secondary strategy to prevent new or additional morbidity and mortality. As a manifestation of patient comorbidities, many patients die in the first year of dialysis, and 46% of those deaths occur in the first 4 months, primarily from cardiovascular disease, infection, liver disease, and withdrawal of treatment. One-year survival on dialysis is associated with several risk factors including lack of pre-ESRD care, positive HIV status, diabetic status, and low serum calcium levels.

LABORATORY TESTS

Altered serum concentrations of commonly measured enzymes due to impaired renal excretion or decreased synthesis can affect the interpretation of some common laboratory tests. Historically, values for aminotransferases tend to be lower with ESRD. The exact cause is not known but might relate to lower pyridoxine levels due to impaired synthetic pathways. Although most reports are from the 1970s, a marginally elevated value still may be clinically significant.

Alkaline phosphatase can be of hepatobiliary, placental, or bone origin. Most elevations with ESRD are a manifestation of renal osteodystrophy, specifically high bone turnover disorder (osteitis fibrosa and cystica). Verification of source using a serum gammaglutamyl transpeptidase or alkaline phosphatase iosenzyme assay can settle the issue.

Lipase and amylase tend to be elevated due to impaired renal excretion of these fairly large enzymes. Increases of three to five times normal are seen in true pancreatitis, and lesser degrees might reflect the patient's ESRD status rather than the etiology of abdominal pain.

Both serum troponin and creatine kinase (CK) levels are affected in ESRD. Troponins, especially troponin T (cTnT), are commonly elevated in asymptomatic patients, and many studies have associated elevated cTnT with survival in these patients. Troponins are also useful for acute coronary syndromes, although false-positive elevations in cTnT can occur. Total CK can be elevated in asymptomatic ESRD patients, but the use of the MB fraction provides good evidence of acute cardiac injury.

IMAGING

There are no data suggesting that ESRD patients need additional dialytic support after receiving iodinated contrast. Given the low osmotic load of current contrast agents, the risk of causing pulmonary edema is negligible. However, gadolinium used with magnetic resonance imaging (MRI) or magnetic resonance angiography (MRA) procedures should be avoided because it is highly toxic and can lead to nephrogenic fibrosing dermopathy.

Summary

- The numbers of patients living with ESRD is growing, and they commonly have associated general medical problems.
- The major causes of death are cardiovascular disease, infections, and malignancies
- Patients may choose to continue with their primary care giver or their nephrologist for general medical problems.
- Some common laboratory tests are affected by ESRD. Diagnostic procedures, especially MRI with gadolinium, are potentially harmful.

TREATMENT

Lifestyle Modifications

As outlined in Box 2 the recommendations for lifestyle changes are the same as in the general population, especially initiatives for

Box 1 Medical Problems Usually Managed in the Dialysis Unit

Dialysis support
Control of hypervolemia and hypertension
Treatment of anemia with EPO
Replenishment and maintenance of iron stores
Control of renal bone disease (osteodystrophy), including dietary counseling, medications and treatment of vitamin D deficiency
Vaccinations, including hepatitis B, influenza, pneumococcal , tetanus
Tuberculosis testing
Vascular access for dialysis
Perioperative management
Social work support

smoking cessation. Dietary restrictions unique to ESRD patients can make it more difficult for patients to achieve dietary changes, but the effort should still be made.

Medical Treatment

Cancer Screening

Estimated days of life saved by cancer screening is a function of life expectancy and lifetime risk of developing a cancer that will cause significant morbidity or death. This depends on the prevalence of the disease in the ESRD population, the sensitivity and specificity of the screening test used, the efficacy (and potential toxicity) of any interventions should the disease be present, and the overall survival with or without the disease. A financial evaluation of cancer screening in ESRD patients found the least efficient and cost-effective screening in female or white patients 50 to 70 years of age.

Cancer remains an uncommon cause of death in the ESRD population. This is in part due to the high risk for cardiovascular disease and infections. A report of international cancer registries found that certain malignancies are more common in patients with ESRD than in the general population. Cancer of the kidney, liver, bladder, cervix, thyroid, or tongue; Hodgkin's lymphoma; and multiple myeloma were more prevalent, with the highest relative risk at a younger age and decreasing risk with aging. The incidence of lung, breast, colon, rectal, and prostate cancers are not increased. This pattern is the same as that seen after renal transplantation.

Uncertainty remains about the cost-to-benefit ratio of screening ESRD patients for malignancy given their higher mortality rates. Some argue that the benefits of screening disappear in patients who are diabetic, European American, or older than 65 years. However, each patient must be approached on an individual basis with consideration given to age, sex, comorbidities, transplant waiting-list status, ethnicity, and family and personal history. For example, targeted screening of mammography to women who have an expected survival of at least 5 years would greatly decrease the cost of screening but not affect the survival of patients who died.

Vaccination

Routine vaccination for hepatitis B, influenza, diphtheria, tetanus, and pneumococcal infection are recommended for all patients with ESRD. Vaccination done earlier in the course of chronic kidney disease seems to be more effective and is encouraged. The Centers for Disease Control and Prevention (CDC) provide regular updates on vaccination practices and recommendations with ESRD; these are available at their website (http://www.cdc.gov/vaccines/). The schedule for hepatitis B vaccination is different, and the use of or exposure to live influenza vaccine must be avoided. A large percentage of patients have evidence of exposure to hepatitis C, but screening is not routine.

Box 2 Common Medical Problems in ESRD Patients that May Be Managed by Primary Care or Subspecialist Physicians

Diabetic Care
Control of serum glucose and hemoglobin A_{1c}
Foot screening and care
Eye screening and care

Dermatologic Care
Pruritus
Xerosis
Prurigo nodularis
Infections
Calcific uremic arteriolopathy (calciphylaxis)

Dental Care
Poor oral hygiene
Xerostomia
Loss of tooth integrity with bone disease
Oral biofilm control
Gingivitis
Periodontal disease
Mucositis
Antibiotic prophylaxis

Gastrointestinal Care
Gastritis
Duodenitis
Ateriovenous malformations
Hepatitis B and C infections

Bone Abnormalities
Osteoporosis
Carpal tunnel syndrome
Frozen shoulder
Pseudogout
Hip and spine fractures
Amyloidosis

Geriatrics
Depression evaluation
Dementia evaluation
Frailty
Risk for falls

Sleep Disorders
Obstructive sleep apnea
Restless leg syndrome
Poor sleep hygiene

Neurologic Disorders
Seizures
Neuropathy
Gait abnormalities

General Health Care Screening
Age- and sex-appropriate cancer screening
Cardiovascular screening and treatment of cardiovascular disease
Vision and hearing evaluation
Sexual dysfunction
Smoking cessation
Accident prevention
Exercise
Alcohol intake
Safety evaluation at home
Risk for falling

Monitoring of Medication Use
Coumadin
Antiepileptic drugs
Lipid-lowering agents

Advanced Care Planning
Advance directives
Power of attorney for medical affairs
End of life care
Hospice
Withdrawal of treatment

Cardiac Disease

Because cardiac disease remains the cause of death in more than 40% of patients, its evaluation and treatment remain vitally important in ESRD. However, few randomized, prospective studies are available to guide patient care. Screening with stress testing and echocardiograms is recommended. Among patients undergoing evaluation for renal transplantation, the test most often performed is a treadmill or dobutamine stress echocardiogram. We usually order this test for our other ESRD patients as well.

Numerous risk factors have been promulgated to be etiologic in ESRD patients, but at a minimum, traditional risk factors should be assessed and treated. Medication use as necessary for hypertension or dyslipidemia follows standard practice, although no data from randomized, controlled trials are available regarding the use of statins.

If intervention is necessary, coronary artery bypass grafting has been considered the treatment of choice. Newer data on the use of stents, which had been found inferior in the past, is in the state of re-evaluation.

PRACTICE GUIDELINES

The National Kidney Foundation has several evidence-based clinical practice guidelines available to assist in the care of patients with ESRD. These include the Kidney Disease Quality Improvement Initiative (KDOQI) and Kidney Disease Improving Global Outcomes (KDIGO). The American Heart Association also has a variety of policy statements and guidelines.

Summary

- General guidelines for primary care apply to ESRD patients in most instances.
- Cancer screening should be appropriate for age and comorbidity and targeted to malignancies seen in transplant patients.
- Cardiac disease is the major cause of death in ESRD patients but no randomized, controlled trials have been done to clarify best practices.
- Cardiac serum markers and diagnostic tests have a high level of false-positive results in ESRD patients and require care in interpretation.

Suggested Readings

Bradbury BD, Fissell RB, Albert JM, et al: Predictors of early mortality among incident US hemodialysis patients in the Dialysis Outcomes and Practice Patterns Study (DOPPS). Clin J Am Soc Nephrol 2007;2:89-99.

Excerpts From the United States Renal Data System 2008 Annual Data Report Atlas of Chronic Kidney Disease & End-Stage Renal Disease in the United States. Am J Kidney Dis 2009;531(Suppl), S1-S374.

Holley JL: Screening, diagnosis, and treatment of cancer in long-term dialysis patients. Clin J Am Soc Nephrol 2007;2:604-610.

Ifudu O: Care of patients undergoing hemodialysis. N Engl J Med 1998;339:1054-1062.

Janus N, Vacher LV, Karie S, et al: Vaccination and chronic kidney disease. Nephrol Dial Transplant 2008;23: 800-807.

McCullough PA: Coronary artery disease. Clin J Am Soc Nephrol 2007;2:611-616.

Walter LC, Lindquist K, O'Hare AM, Johansen KL: Targeting screening mammography according to life expectancy among women undergoing dialysis. Arch Intern Med 2006;166:1203-1208.

Section 10

NEUROLOGY

Stroke

Asma M. Moheet and *Irene Katzan*

DEFINITION AND ETIOLOGY

A stroke is defined as an acute loss of neurological function due to an abnormal perfusion of brain tissue. Most strokes are ischemic (87%) in nature and commonly result from an arterial obstruction by a thrombus or embolus. Hemorrhagic strokes (13%) are caused by rupture or leak of a blood vessel either within the primary brain tissue or subarachnoid space. This chapter provides a clinical approach to the evaluation and management of stroke, with a focus on ischemic stroke.

PREVALENCE AND RISK FACTORS

Because stroke is the leading cause of morbidity and the third-leading cause of death in the United States today, optimal reduction of risk factors is paramount in preventing and managing stroke. Modifiable and nonmodifiable stroke risk factors are listed in Table 1. In 2005, the prevalence of stroke in noninstitutionalized adults was 5.8 million in the United States alone. Based on American Stroke Association data, the estimated direct and indirect cost of stroke for 2008 was $65.5 billion, with an estimated lifetime cost of $140,000 per patient.

PATHOPHYSIOLOGY AND NATURAL HISTORY

Ischemic Stroke

Based on prior clinical trials, a subclassification scheme of five categories of ischemic stroke has become widely accepted. These categories are based on etiology and are as follows: large-artery atherosclerosis, embolism, small-vessel disease, stroke of other determined etiology, and stroke of undetermined etiology.

Large-Artery Atherosclerosis

High-grade stenosis or occlusion of the major intra- and extracranial arteries, which include the internal carotid artery, the vertebral artery, the basilar artery, and other major branches of the circle of Willis, occur due to deposition of plaque and often leads to a flow-dependent state of perfusion. With interruption of flow due to acute plaque rupture or a prolonged low-flow state due to relative hypotension, a loss of adequate cerebral perfusion results in ischemia and focal neurologic deficit.

Embolism

Turbulent or stagnant flow states in the heart can result in formation of thrombi. These thrombi can dislodge and occlude blood vessels in the intracranial circulation farther downstream. The most common cause of cardioembolic stroke is atrial fibrillation. Other causes include severe left ventricular dysfunction resulting in a low ejection fraction, paradoxical embolus from the venous system due to a shunt through a septal defect such as an aneurysm or patent foramen ovale, or vessel-to-vessel atheroembolism due to atherosclerotic disease in the vertebral arteries, carotid arteries, and aortic arch.

Small-Vessel Disease

Changes in the arterial vasculature of small perforating arteries can result in narrowing of the vessel lumen and eventual occlusion. Chronic hypertension is one state that leads to vessel damage secondary to lipohyalinosis and endothelial damage. Hyperlipidemia, smoking, and diabetes also lead to changes in the vessel wall that result in decreased compliance and intraluminal stenosis. These changes often result in lacunar infarcts, which are small infarcts defined by their size (<15 mm^3) and are typically located in deep structures such as the internal capsule, basal ganglia, thalamus, and brainstem.

Stroke of Other Determined Etiology

The majority of ischemic strokes are classified in one of the previous categories. Rarely, other causes must be investigated, particularly in patients who are young and have no risk factors for stroke. Among these causes are coagulopathies, vasculopathies, genetic disorders, and metabolic disorders.

Stroke of Undetermined Etiology

In a significant number of cases (≤40%), no clear explanation can be found for an ischemic stroke despite an extensive diagnostic evaluation. These strokes are classified as strokes of undetermined etiology, or cryptogenic strokes. This is a diagnosis of exclusion, however, and should only be made once a thorough search for both common and uncommon causes of stroke has been completed.

Intracerebral Hemorrhage

Intracerebral hemorrhage occurs when a blood vessel within the brain parenchyma ruptures and causes accumulation of blood within the brain tissue. Weakening of the blood vessel wall is often a result of chronic uncontrolled hypertension or a problem intrinsic to the blood vessel such as amyloid angiopathy or other vascular malformation. In hypertension, microaneurysms in perforating vessels, known as Charcot-Bouchard aneurysms, can rupture and cause bleeding. The thalamus, basal ganglia, pons, and cerebellum are the most common sites for these hypertensive bleeds. Lobar hemorrhages more commonly result from amyloid angiopathy, which is typically seen in older patients. This should be suspected when there is evidence of prior areas of hemorrhage manifested as hemosiderin deposits on magnetic resonance imaging (MRI). Other causes of intracerebral hemorrhage include the use of anticoagulants, thrombolytics, and antiplatelet agents, particularly when levels are supratherapeutic. They may also be caused by an underlying primary or metastatic brain tumor, especially when there are focal areas of necrosis and hemorrhage within the tumor bed.

Subarachnoid Hemorrhage

Subarachnoid hemorrhage is most commonly due to trauma and typically occurs adjacent to areas of bony prominence, such as the temporal poles and the frontal poles. Subarachnoid hemorrhage can also result from rupture of a cerebral aneurysm. Aneurysms are usually located at vulnerable branch points in the circle of Willis and occur due to weakening of the vessel wall. The most common sites of aneurysm formation and rupture are in the distribution of the anterior communicating artery and the posterior communicating artery. Uncontrolled chronic hypertension, smoking, and a family history of aneurysms are risk factors for formation and rupture of aneurysms. In 10% to 20% of cases of spontaneous, nontraumatic subarachnoid hemorrhage, no cause is found despite serial angiography. The prognosis for these patients is typically benign.

SIGNS AND SYMPTOMS

An acute stroke is signified by a sudden onset of focal neurologic deficit and is variable depending on the area of tissue ischemia. Localization can often be made by the pattern of clinical findings. Common stroke syndromes are listed in Table 2 according to vascular distribution. Although headache might accompany an ischemic stroke, an acute and severe headache that is maximal at onset more commonly represents a subarachnoid or intraparenchymal hemorrhage, especially if this is followed by somnolence or decreased mental status. Seizures can also occur at the onset of ischemic or hemorrhagic strokes.

Motor symptoms consist of facial droop, hemiparesis, or isolated weakness of the arm or leg. Dizziness, slurred speech, problems with coordination, or difficulty with gait and balance may also be reported and may be due to involvement of cerebellar fibers. Sensory symptoms include numbness or altered sensation, with tingling paresthesias of one side of the body or face, or both. Vision loss in one eye or both eyes as in a homonymous hemianopsia can also occur.

Patients with an acute stroke might also present with confusion or are sometimes perceived as being confused when there is an expressive or receptive aphasia or a visuospatial neglect phenomenon.

One of the most urgent and potentially devastating stroke syndromes is thrombosis of the basilar artery, which can manifest with acute quadriparesis, loss of consciousness, and respiratory failure.

Table 1 Cerebrovascular Disease Risk Factors

Disease	Modifiable	Not Modifiable
Ischemic stroke	Hypertension Diabetes Atrial fibrillation Smoking Hyperlipidemia Carotid stenosis	Age >55 Male gender Black race Family history of stroke Personal history of stroke
Intraparenchymal hemorrhage	Hypertension Amyloid angiopathy Anticoagulant use Thrombolytic use	Vascular malformation Neoplasm Trauma Acute ischemic stroke
Subarachnoid hemorrhage		Aneurysm Family history of aneurysm or connective tissue disease Other vascular malformation Trauma

DIAGNOSIS

The first step in correctly identifying a stroke is a rapid, thorough neurologic assessment consisting of a focused history and neurologic examination. A differential diagnosis is listed in Box 1. It is of utmost importance to establish a time of symptom onset when eliciting the history from the patient or witnesses. If the patient woke with symptoms, onset is determined at the time the patient was last seen normal, which for many would be when they went to bed the night before.

Vital signs should be assessed frequently, with particular attention to blood pressure and heart rate. It is also necessary to obtain a blood glucose level immediately because both hypo- and hyperglycemia can manifest clinically with acute neurologic deficits, mimicking a stroke.

Regarding the physical examination, a variety of tools in the form of validated scales are available for evaluation of the patient at presentation. The NIH Stroke Scale is a widely accepted and useful tool that is recommended in the acute phase for the purpose of quickly

Table 2 Overview of Selected Stroke Syndromes

Vascular Territory	Area Affected	Signs and Symptoms
Anterior cerebral artery	Frontal pole and mesial frontal lobe	Contralateral: leg > face and arm weakness Frontal signs such as abulia
Middle cerebral artery	Posterior frontal, temporal, parietal lobes	Contralateral: face and arm > leg weakness, sensory loss to all modalities, visual field cut, visual-spatial neglect Ipsilateral: gaze preference Dominant hemisphere affected: aphasia, alexia, agraphia, acalculia
Posterior cerebral artery	Occipital lobe	Contralateral: homonymous hemianopia With thalamic involvement: Sensory loss to all modalities or pain
Anterior inferior cerebellar artery	Lateral pontine syndrome	Contralateral: hemiparesis and hemisensory loss of pain and temperature Ipsilateral: ataxia
Posterior inferior cerbellar artery	Lateral medulla (Wallenberg syndrome)	Contralateral: hemibody pain and temperature loss Ipsilateral: facial pain, hemifacial pain and temperature loss, ataxia, nystagmus, nausea/vomiting, vertigo, Horner's syndrome, dysphagia Hiccups
Basilar artery	Pons (locked-in syndrome)	Bilateral: progressive quadriplegia, facial weakness Lateral gaze weakness with sparing of vertical gaze
Vertebral artery	Medial medulla	Contralateral: hemibody weakness, loss of vibration and proprioception Ipsilateral: tongue weakness and/or atrophy
Vertebral artery	Lateral medulla	Wallenberg syndrome

Box 1 Differential Diagnosis of Stroke

Complex or atypical migraine
Conversion disorder
Electrolyte disturbance
Hypoglycemia or hyperglycemia
Intracranial neoplasm
Meningitis, encephalitis, or systemic infection
Multiple sclerosis exacerbation
Seizure
Subdural hemorrhage

identifying focal neurologic deficits and their severity (Class I, Level B recommendation).

Laboratory Tests

In patients presenting with sudden onset of focal neurologic deficit, baseline laboratory testing should be performed. This consists of point-of-care blood glucose testing, basic metabolic panel, complete blood count, cardiac enzymes, and coagulation studies (Class I, Level B recommendation). A 12-lead electrocardiogram (ECG) should be performed in all stroke patients (Class I, Level B recommendation). If subarachnoid hemorrhage is suspected, cerebrospinal fluid should be obtained and sent for differential red blood cell counts in serial tubes.

Once the patient is stabilized, further testing such as lipid panel and hemoglobin A_{1C} studies should be sent to assist in identifying risk factors. If no clear etiology is identified, further laboratory testing to assess for a hypercoagulable state, genetic or metabolic disturbance, or inflammatory conditions should be performed.

Imaging

With advances in technology, imaging has become integral in the evaluation and management of acute stroke patients. In all patients who present to the hospital with a suspected stroke, the first imaging study should be an emergent noncontrast computed tomography (CT) scan of the brain to assess for intracranial hemorrhage. CT angiography with and without perfusion studies rapidly provides visualization of blood flow and is used in the acute setting at some tertiary stroke centers to identify the location of vascular occlusion and assess for salvageable brain tissue (Class I, Level A recommendation). However, because the study uses contrast, renal function should ideally be known and documented before proceeding. Cerebral angiography may also be undertaken emergently, particularly in cases when vascular intervention is being considered.

In the last several years, MRI has emerged as an invaluable tool in the care of stroke patients. A specialized MRI sequence that measures the diffusion of water, known as diffusion-weighted imaging (DWI), allows visualization of acute strokes that range in age from a few hours to 1 week. This is especially helpful in stroke patients who present within 24 to 48 hours of symptom onset because an acute ischemic lesion can often be missed on a routine CT scan early on. MR angiography is also a useful method for evaluating intra- and extracranial vasculature, although the degree of stenosis in diseased vessels is often overestimated by this technique. Other studies that assess cerebral blood flow include carotid ultrasound and transcranial Doppler ultrasonagraphy (TCD), which are noninvasive tests that use pulsatility indices and mean flow velocities to evaluate the vasculature.

Other Diagnostic Tests

All patients with ischemic stroke should have a transthoracic echocardiogram (TTE) to assess for a cardioembolic source, which includes left ventricular or valvular dysfunction, intracardiac thrombus, and patent foramen ovale. In patients who are strongly suspected to have a cardioembolic stroke despite a negative TTE, further testing with transesophageal echocardiogram or TCD with breath-holding should be performed as these studies increase the detection of an intra-cardiac shunt. Duplex ultrasonography of the legs should also be considered in patients in whom a paradoxical embolus is suspected.

Box 2 Exclusion Criteria for Treatment of Acute Ischemic Stroke with rtPA

Onset of symptoms >3 hours
CT with acute hemorrhage or hypodensity involving >1/3 of the hemisphere
Systolic blood pressure >185 mm Hg and diastolic blood pressure >110 mm Hg
Evidence of active bleeding or acute trauma on exam
Anticoagulant therapy with INR >1.7 (or elevated PTT if receiving heparin)
Platelet count <100,000 mm^3
Blood glucose <50 mg/dL
Seizure at symptom onset
History of prior intracranial hemorrhage, neoplasm, or vascular malformation
Head trauma or stroke in past 3 months
Myocardial infarction in past 3 months
Gastrointestinal or urinary tract hemorrhage in past 3 weeks
Major surgery in past 14 days
Arterial puncture at a noncompressible site in past 7 days
Rapid, spontaneous improvement of neurologic signs
Symptoms suggesting subarachnoid hemorrhage
Mild neurologic deficit

CT, computed tomography; INR, international normalized ratio; PTT, partial thromboplastin time; rtPA, recombinant tissue plasminogen activator.

TREATMENT

Acute Management and Interventions

The first step in the appropriate management of acute stroke is early identification at symptom onset. Early notification of emergency medical services (EMS) with use of stroke-identification algorithms, management in the field with stroke protocols, and emergent transport to the nearest center capable of treating acute stroke is recommended (Class I, Level B evidence). Airway, breathing, and circulation should be stabilized, with airway support and ventilatory assistance in the appropriate patients (Class I, Level C evidence). Initial laboratory testing and CT brain scan should be performed as detailed earlier.

In patients who present with stroke symptoms within 3 hours of onset and have no evidence of hemorrhage or infarct size greater than one third of the middle cerebral artery territory on CT brain, treatment with IV recombinant tissue plasminogen activator (rtPA) is recommended at a dose of 0.9 mg/kg (maximum dose, 90 mg) over 1 hour, with the first 10% given as a bolus over 1 minute (Class I, Level A evidence). Studies have demonstrated that 31% to 50% of patients treated with rtPA experienced improved recovery at 3 months as compared to 20% to 38% of patients in the placebo arm. However, strict adherence to national guidelines in the administration of rtPA and postlysis management is critical, given the 6% risk of intracranial hemorrhage. Box 2 lists conditions excluding patients from t-PA therapy.

In selected patients who are not candidates for IV rtPA therapy, intra-arterial thrombolysis by a qualified neuro-interventionalist may be considered in stroke patients who present within 6 hours of onset (Class I, Level B recommendation). However, the availability of intra-arterial thrombolysis should not preclude the administration of IV rtPA in eligible patients (Class III, Level C evidence). Endovascular intervention, including angioplasty and disruption or removal of the clot, is another option available at some specialized stroke centers.

Although used previously, urgent anticoagulation in acute ischemic stroke is not recommended and should not be used to replace IV rtPA therapy in eligible patients (Class III, Level A evidence). Oral aspirin therapy at a dose of 325 mg daily is recommended 24 to 48 hours after stroke onset in most patients (Class I, Level A evidence), but it should not be given within 24 hours following rtPA therapy (Class III, Level A and B).

In patients who are eligible for rtPA, treatment of arterial hypertension is recommended (Class I, Level C evidence) with a goal blood pressure of less than 185/110 mm Hg before rTPA is administered. Close post-lysis monitoring, with antihypertensive treatment given according to the rtPA protocol, is also crucial to prevent hemorrhage (Class I, Level B evidence). In patients who are not candidates for rtPA, blood pressure management in the acute setting is still controversial, but the consensus is that antihypertensive medications should be withheld unless systolic blood pressure is higher than 220 or diastolic blood pressure is higher than 120 (Class I, Level C evidence). After 24 hours, initiation of antihypertensive agents is considered relatively safe for patients with pre-existing hypertension.

Hypoxemia should be treated with supplemental oxygen, and fever should be treated with antipyretic agents (Class I, Level C evidence). Euglycemia should be targeted, because persistent hyperglycemia has been associated with poor outcomes (Class IIa, Level C evidence).

Patients should be admitted to specialized stroke care units incorporating rehabilitation when possible (Class I, Level A evidence). Close monitoring during the first 72 to 96 hours of acute ischemic stroke is important to assess for signs of hemorrhagic transformation or brain edema (Class I, Level B evidence). Decompressive surgery in the setting of malignant edema may be life-saving, but the morbidity is unknown in the setting of major cerebral hemispheric infarctions (Class IIa, Level B evidence).

Treatment of concomitant medical illnesses, pneumonia, and urinary tract infections is recommended (Class I, Level B and C evidence). Screening swallow evaluations should be performed to assess the patient's risk for aspiration pneumonia (Class I, Level B evidence). Subcutaneous anticoagulation or sequential compression devices should be instituted to prevent formation of deep venous thrombosis, especially in patients with decreased mobility (Class I, Level A evidence). Additional early and late complications are listed in Box 3.

Box 3 Early and Late Complications of Stroke

Early Complications (within 7 days)

Cerebral edema and herniation (within 72 hr)
Expansion of the infarct/recurrent infarction
Hemorrhagic transformation of the infracted area
Seizure
Aspiration pneumonitis
Gastrointestinal ulcers and/or bleeding
Deep vein thrombosis and thromboembolism
Myocardial infarction

Late Complications (>7 days later)

Recurrent stroke
Seizure
Aspiration pneumonitis
Deep vein thrombosis and thromboembolism
Persistent cognitive or language dysfunction
Persistent loss of mobility
Spasticity

Primary Prevention

In 2006, the American Heart Association and American Stroke Association issued a guideline for the primary prevention of ischemic stroke, which is summarized here.

- Each patient should undergo formal assessment of his or her stroke risk (Class I, Level A evidence).
- Those with coronary artery disease, heart failure, or symptomatic peripheral arterial disease are 1.73 times more likely to have a first stroke as compared to those without these conditions. Antiplatelet therapy is recommended in these patients.
- Hypertension has been well documented to increase the risk of stroke, and current recommendations are to perform screening for hypertension at least every 2 years in adults (Class I, Level A evidence). Diet and lifestyle should be modified and pharmacologic treatment should be prescribed according to the JNC 7 recommendations. Currently, guidelines emphasize individualization of therapy, with the overall goal being blood pressure reduction to at least less than 140/90 mm Hg.
- In patients with diabetes, stricter blood pressure control to less than 130/80 mm HG with use of angiotensin-converting enzyme (ACE) inhibitors or angiotensin receptor blockers (ARBs) is recommended (Class I, Level A evidence). In these patients, a statin to lower the risk of first stroke is also recommended (Class I, Level A evidence). Tight glycemic control is encouraged to reduce microvascular complications, but evidence showing a reduction in stroke risk is lacking.
- In patients with dyslipidemia, recommendations state that those with known coronary disease and high-risk hypertensive patients be treated with lifestyle measures and a statin, even in the presence of a normal LDL (Class I, Level A evidence). In patients with atrial fibrillation, warfarin therapy with a target international normalized ratio (INR) of 2.0 to 3.0 is recommended in those without contraindications to oral anticoagulants (Class I, Level of A evidence).
- Smoking doubles the risk of ischemic stroke and doubles or quadruples the risk of hemorrhagic stroke. Smoking cessation is recommended (Class I, Level B evidence) and the use of counseling, nicotine replacement, and oral medications should be considered (Class IIa, Level B evidence).
- Currently, aspirin therapy is not recommended for primary stroke prevention in men (Class III, Level A evidence), but it may be helpful in primary stroke prevention among women older than 65 years who have well-controlled hypertension (Class IIa, Level B evidence).
- Carotid endarterectomy is recommended for patients with symptomatic high-grade carotid artery stenosis because surgery was shown to be beneficial in significantly reducing stroke risk (9%) at 2 years versus medical therapy with aspirin alone (26%). In patients with asymptomatic carotid artery stenosis, screening for other treatable causes of stroke with aggressive control of all risk factors is recommended (Class I, Level C evidence). Aspirin therapy is recommended in the absence of contraindications (Class I, Level of B evidence). Prophylactic carotid endarterectomy is recommended in selected patients with high-grade asymptomatic carotid stenosis; endarterectomy should be performed by surgeons with less than 3% morbidity and mortality postoperative complication rates (Class I, Level of A evidence). Carotid artery angioplasty and stenting may be considered in asymptomatic patients who are at high surgical risk for endarterectomy (Class IIb, Level B evidence).

Secondary Prevention

Following a stroke, lifestyle changes should be made, with particular attention to reducing risk factors for stroke as outlined earlier. In patients with atrial fibrillation, warfarin therapy is recommended for preventing recurrent stroke in the absence of contraindications. In patients with a history of noncardioembolic ischemic stroke, antiplatelet therapy is recommended. Aspirin, clopidogrel, and dipyridamole in combination with low-dose aspirin have all been shown to be beneficial in reducing the risk of recurrent stroke in multiple clinical trials. The most recently published study, the PRoFESS trial from 2008, directly compared clopidogrel alone and dipyridamole in combination with low-dose aspirin for preventing recurrent stroke. Although the results did not meet the predefined statistical criteria for noninferiority, there was no statistically significant difference between the groups in the primary outcome of recurrent stroke. However, there was an increase in the rate of intracranial hemorrhage with the dipyridamole and aspirin arm, which was not seen in prior studies evaluating this combination. Currently there is no clear uniform recommendation of one agent over another, and therapy must be tailored to individual patients based on availability, cost, and side-effect profile.

Considerations in Special Populations

In patients with known medical conditions that increase the risk of stroke, such as sickle cell disease, vasculitis, or cardiomyopathy, the approach to stroke prevention should be a coordinated effort among the patient, the primary care physician, and involved specialists. Often, it is important to aggressively manage the underlying disease state. The risk of ischemic stroke or intracerebral hemorrhage is 2.4 times greater during pregnancy and the first 6 weeks following delivery. Focal neurologic signs in this population merits prompt evaluation by a neurologist. Other special considerations include children or young adults with stroke and patients in whom no clear etiology of stroke is determined. Further workup may include referral to a geneticist for evaluation of potential genetic or metabolic causes of stroke in these populations.

OUTCOMES

During the hospitalization for an acute stroke, intensive speech, physical, and occupational therapy should be initiated as soon as the patient is stable enough to participate. Most functional recovery occurs within the first 3 months. After this, further recovery is possible, but it is generally limited. The 1-year mortality in first-time stroke sufferers is 14% to 24% in persons aged 40 to 69 years, and the 1-year mortality increases to 22% to 27% in patients aged 70 years and older. Following a first stroke, the mean survival for persons aged 60 to 79 years ranges from 5.4 to 7.4 years. After age 80 years, the mean survival decreases to 1.8 years for men and 3.1 years for women.

Temporary stroke symptoms due to ischemia that last less than 24 hours are typically referred to as a *transient ischemic attack* (TIA). After a TIA, the 90-day risk of stroke is 3% to 17.3%, and the risk is highest within the first 30 days. Within a year of a TIA, up to 25% of patients die.

Summary

- A stroke is defined as a sudden focal loss of neurologic function due to decreased perfusion of brain tissue.
- In patients who present with stroke symptoms, a rapid, focused neurologic history and physical examination should be performed, making every attempt to establish a specific time of onset because this helps to guide further therapy.
- Patients presenting within a 3-hour time window of symptom onset should receive IV rtPA at a dose of 0.9 mg/kg (maximum dose 90 mg) after a CT brain excludes the presence of an intracranial hemorrhage and there are no other contraindications to therapy. The dose is administered over 60 minutes, with 10% of the total dose being given initially as a bolus.
- The remaining hospital course is focused on evaluating potential etiologies of stroke, preventing early complications, and performing intensive rehabilitation.
- Anticoagulation should be considered for patients with a history of cardioembolic stroke, and antiplatelet therapy should be considered for ischemic strokes of noncardiac etiology.
- Optimization of stroke risk factor reduction is critical in both primary and secondary prevention.

The recommendations on early management of adults with ischemic stroke and prevention are based on guidelines from the American Heart Association and American Stroke Association. Data regarding clinical trials in ischemic stroke are available at www.strokecenter.org.

Suggested Readings

Adams HP Jr, del Zoppo G, Alberts MJ, et al: Guidelines for the Early Management of Adults With Ischemic Stroke: A Guideline From the American Heart Association/American Stroke Association Stroke Council, Clinical Cardiology Council, Cardiovascular Radiology and Intervention Council, and theAtherosclerotic Peripheral Vascular Disease and Quality of CareOutcomes in Research Interdisciplinary Working Groups. Stroke 2007;38:1655-1711.

American Heart Association: Heart Disease and Stroke Statistics—2008 Update. Dallas: American Heart Association, 2008.

Goldstein LB, Adams R, Alberts MJ, et al: Primary Prevention of Ischemic Stroke: A Guideline From the American Heart Association/American Stroke Association Stroke Council: Cosponsored by the Atherosclerotic Peripheral Vascular Disease Interdisciplinary Working Group; Cardiovascular Nursing Council; Clinical Cardiology Council; Nutrition, Physical Activity, and Metabolism Council; and the Quality of Care and Outcomes Research, Interdisciplinary Working Group. Stroke 2006;37:1583.

National Institute of Neurological Disorders and Stroke rt-PA Stroke Study Group: Tissue plasminogen activator for acute ischemic stroke. N Engl J Med 1995; 333(24):1581-1587.

North American Symptomatic Carotid Endarterectomy Trial Collaborators: Beneficial effect of carotid endarterectomy in symptomatic patients with high-grade carotid stenosis. N Engl J Med 1991;325:445-453.

Sacco RL, Diener HC, Yusuf S, et al, and the PRoFESS Study Group: Aspirin and extended-release dipyridamole versus clopidogrel for recurrent stroke. N Engl J Med 2008;359:1238-1251.

References

For a complete list of references, log onto www.expertconsult.com.

Epilepsy

Dileep R. Nair

DEFINITION

Seizures result from paroxysmal and excessive electrical neuronal discharges in the brain that cause a variety of clinical manifestations. The term *epilepsy* is usually restricted to those cases with a tendency for recurrent seizures. The identification of a seizure as a symptom and not a disease diagnosis is an important distinction. Seizures are the clinical manifestation of epilepsy; the challenge is to identify the disease that explains the symptom. Often the underlying disease is epilepsy, but at other times it may be a nonepileptic disorder that causes symptoms that resemble an epileptic seizure.

The term *epilepsy* encompasses a group of syndromes that vary in its associated pathology and seizure types. The diagnosis of the epileptic syndrome is one of the primary objectives undertaken when managing a patient with seizures.

PREVALENCE

Epilepsy can manifest itself at any age; however, the incidence and prevalence are highest in the very young and the elderly. Depending on age at manifestation, the causes for epilepsy can differ widely. In the United States, there are approximately 1.6 million people who have epilepsy (roughly 0.6% of the population). Epilepsy has a lifetime prevalence of 3%—that is, 7.2 million persons will become affected by this disorder.[1] Almost 10% of the population will experience at least one epileptic seizure in 80 years of life.

PATHOPHYSIOLOGY

Two sets of changes can determine the epileptogenic properties of neuronal tissues. Abnormal neuronal excitability is believed to occur as a result of disruption of the depolarization and repolarization mechanisms of the cell (this is termed the *excitability of neuronal tissue*). Aberrant neuronal networks that develop abnormal synchronization of a group of neurons can result in the development and propagation of an epileptic seizure (this is termed the *synchronization of neuronal tissue*).[2]

A hyperexcitability of neurons that results in random firing of cells, by itself, may not lead to propagation of an epileptic seizure. Indeed, both normal and abnormal patterns of behavior require a certain degree of synchronization of firing in a population of neurons. Epileptic seizures originate in a setting of both altered excitability and altered synchronization of neurons. The excitability of individual neurons is affected by

- Cell membrane properties and the microenvironment of the neuron
- Intracellular processes
- Structural features of neuronal elements
- Interneuronal connections

The *membrane properties* and *microenvironment of neurons*, which maintain potential differences of electrical charge, are determined by selective ion permeability and ionic pumps. Excitatory neurotransmitters usually act by opening Na^+ or Ca^{2+} channels, whereas inhibitory neurotransmitters usually open K^+ or Cl^- channels. The mechanism of action of certain anticonvulsant medications is by Na^+ or Ca^{2+} channel blockade, which likely prevents repetitive neuronal firing. Extracellular ionic concentrations also can contribute to neuronal excitability; for example, an increase in extracellular K^+ concentrations (such as in rapid neuronal firing or dysfunction of glia, which are mainly responsible for K^+ reuptake) causes membrane depolarization.

Various *intracellular processes* are controlled by genetic information. Neuronal excitability can be preprogrammed by DNA-controlled effects on cell structure, energy metabolism, receptor functions, transmitter release, and ionic channels. The mechanisms that induce these changes, either phasic or long term, appear to be linked to ionic currents, especially Ca^{2+} influx. Intracellular Ca^{2+} mediates changes in membrane proteins to initiate transmitter release and ion channel opening; it also activates enzymes to allow neurons to cover or uncover receptor sites that alter neuronal sensitivity. Various plastic or persistent changes in excitability can result by influencing the expression of genetic information through Ca^{2+} influx. This may occur by selectively inducing genes to synthesize a protein for a specific reason. One example is the induction of the *c-fos* gene to produce c-fos protein in neurons involved in an epileptic seizure by the administration of pentylenetetrazol. The exact effects of this coupling are not known, but it provides a means to study the effects of neuronal excitation on cell growth and differentiation as a model for epilepsy, learning, and memory.[3]

In regard to the *structural features of neuronal elements* in relation to epilepsy, the two primary regions of the brain that are involved in epilepsy are the cerebral neocortex and the hippocampus. In the neocortex, excitatory synapses are made primarily on the dendritic spines and shaft. The release of neurotransmitters at these sites gives rise to excitatory postsynaptic potentials. The inhibitory synapses are more prominent on the soma or proximal dendrites, and give rise to inhibitory postsynaptic potentials. The placement of these synapses effectively prevents distal excitatory events from reaching the axon hillock. Alterations of neuronal morphology, either spontaneously or as a response to injury, could enhance excitability with either an actual increase in the number of excitatory synapses or a decrease in the number of inhibitory synapses. Such alterations could consist of reduced dendritic branching with excitatory synapses placed closer to the axon hillock, or loss of spines, allowing more excitatory synapses to occur directly on the shaft. Lesions in the neuronal cell body or tracts lead to degeneration of the axon terminal and a new terminal may sprout to make contact with the vacated postsynaptic membrane. This may in turn lead to an increase in the excitatory potential of the neuron.[4] Ca^{2+} currents that occur predominantly at the dendrites causing a high-amplitude prolonged depolarization that can evoke a rapid train of Na^+ action potentials (burst-firing of Na^+), which is followed by a prolonged after-hyperpolarization. These discharges are believed to contribute to the paroxysmal depolarization shifts and after-hyperpolarization in experimental epileptic foci.[5]

Neurons are influenced by synaptic and nonsynaptic *interconnections*. Neurochemical transmission between neurons involves a number of steps that can be selectively altered to affect neuronal excitability. These steps result in the release of neurotransmitters into the synaptic cleft and the postsynaptic membrane, resulting in excitatory or inhibitory postsynaptic potentials via Ca^{2+} and other second messengers. The transmitters are deactivated by enzymes, by reuptake into axon terminals, or by uptake by glia. The primary excitatory neurotransmitters in the central nervous system are the amino acids glutamate and aspartate. The primary inhibitory neurotransmitters in the central nervous system are gamma-aminobutyric acid (GABA) and glycine. Neurotransmitters and neuromodulators exert their effects by acting on receptors. Specific properties of receptors have been identified on the basis of the effects of certain agonist and antagonist agents, some of which are anticonvulsant drugs. $GABA_A$ receptor drugs, which activate Cl^-, appear to be more effective as anticonvulsants than $GABA_B$ receptor agents, which activate K^+. The $GABA_A$ receptor is of primary importance in absence epilepsy due to its role in the synchronization and desynchronization of thalamocortical pathways. The oscillatory and burst-firing of these circuits is attributed to neurons in the reticular nucleus of the thalamus and leads to synchronization and desynchronization of the electroencephalogram (EEG). Alterations of this mechanism produce absence seizures. Kainic acid, quisqualic acid, and *N*-methyl-D-aspartate (NMDA) are excitatory amino acid analogues used to define the classes of receptors responsive to glutamate and aspartate. NMDA antagonists are one potential mechanism for some of the anticonvulsants.

Two hypotheses are associated with cortical dysplasia, which is a frequent cause of medically intractable focal epilepsy. The first hypothesis suggests that epileptogenesis results from a change in the synaptic properties of interneurons. The second hypothesis suggests abnormal intrinsic properties in the neurons, such as a mutation in the ion channel.

SIGNS AND SYMPTOMS

The diversity of symptoms that can result from an epileptic seizure arises from the differing brain regions that gives rise to the particular features of an individual seizure. The determination of seizure types can often help in the identification of the epileptic syndrome (Table 1). In spite of the technologic advances that have contributed to the understanding and treatment of epilepsy, the initiation and selection of treatment rely on the observed details of the seizure phenomenology. In this regard, obtaining an accurate seizure history from the patient as well as from observers who have witnessed the patient's seizures is extremely important.

There have been many attempts at a classification system for epileptic seizures. The most widely used classification system is the one developed by the International League Against Epilepsy (ILAE), which is an electroclinical classification system (Table 2).[6] This classification assumes that there is a one-to-one correlation between the phenomenology of the actual seizures and electrical abnormalities on the EEG seen with the seizure. This, however, is not always the case and these exceptions highlight the main weakness of the ILAE classification.

There is an active effort to improve the ILAE classification. One such classification system is already in use in many centers that perform evaluations for epilepsy surgery.[7] The advantage of such a semiologic classification is that it does not rely on knowledge of the electrical abnormalities in a patient, which are frequently unavailable. The classification of seizures can be either vague or more specific with this type of classification, depending on the accuracy of the information available.

Table 1 Features of Primary Generalized and Partial Epilepsies

Epilepsy	Primary Generalized Epilepsy	Focal or Partial
Seizure Features		
Auras	Not present	Present
Prodrome	Occasionally present	Occasionally present
Starting with LOC	Present	Present
Starting with automatisms	Not usually present	Present
Prolonged postictal confusion without generalization	Not usually present	Present
Generalized tonic-clonic seizure	Present	Present
True versive head movements	Not present	Present
Focal motor clonic or tonic seizures	Not usually present	Present
Risk Factors for Epilepsy		
Family history of seizures	May be present	Not usually present
History of CNS infections, significant head trauma, febrile seizures, CNS tumors, CNS vascular malformation	Not usually present	May be present
Examination Findings		
Neurologic examination	Usually normal	May be abnormal
Neuroimaging Findings		
Brain MRI	Usually normal	May be abnormal
EEG Findings		
Generalized epileptiform activity	Present	Not present
Focal epileptiform activity	Not present	Present

CNS, central nervous system; EEG, encephalogram; LOC, loss of consciousness; MRI, magnetic resonance imaging.

Data from Commission on Classification and Terminology of the International League Against Epilepsy. Proposal for revised clinical and electroencephalographic classification of epileptic seizures. Epilepsia 1981;22:489-501.

DIAGNOSIS

The initial evaluation in patients who present with spells or seizures is to determine whether these episodes are epileptic in nature. A false diagnosis can have severe repercussions for the patient, including the expense of medications as well as their potential adverse effects. Other hazards include the loss of driving privileges, loss of income, and the expense of unnecessary visits to the emergency department. Disorders that can be confused with epilepsy include migraine, syncope, transient ischemic attacks, nonepileptic events (pseudoseizures), movement disorders, Menière's disease, and rage attacks. In pediatric patients, the differential also includes breath-holding spells, pallid infantile syncope, tics, night terrors, somnambulism, and long QT syndrome.[8]

As soon as epileptic seizures are diagnosed, the next step is to determine the epileptic syndrome and then the seizure type. This is helpful for choosing medications as well as for evaluating a patient for surgical treatment. The epileptic syndrome is determined based on the history, physical examination, EEG findings, and neuroimaging studies. Epileptic syndromes can be divided primarily into two types: generalized epilepsies and focal (or partial) epilepsies. The primary distinction is that the generalized epilepsies have generalized epileptiform abnormalities on EEG, whereas focal epilepsies have focal abnormalities on EEG. Table 1 shows some of the differentiating points between these two types of epilepsies.

The patients with focal epilepsies are candidates for epilepsy surgery if their seizures are intractable to medications. Wilder Penfield in 1956 established the concept of the epileptogenic anatomic lesion and the epileptogenic physiologic lesion.[9] The physiologic epileptic lesion was the part of the brain that demonstrated abnormalities on EEG that appeared to extend beyond the anatomic boundaries of the identified pathology responsible for the epilepsy. These areas are not always contiguous.

Table 2 International League Against Epilepsy Classification of Epileptic Seizures

Seizure Types	Features
Partial Seizures	*EEG findings suggest focal onset
Simple Partial Seizures	Consciousness not impaired
With motor symptoms	
Focal motor	
Focal motor march (Jacksonian)	
Versive	
Postural	
Phonatory	Vocalization arrest of speech
With somatosensory or special sensory symptoms	Simple hallucinations
Somatosensory	
Visual	
Auditory	
Olfactory	
Gustatory	
Vertiginous	
With autonomic symptoms or signs	Epigastric sensations, pallor, sweating, flushing, piloerection, pupillary dilation
With psychic symptoms	Disturbance of higher cortical function
Complex partial seizures	Consciousness impaired
Absence Seizures	
Typical absence	Regular and symmetrical 3-Hz †SWC on EEG
Atypical absence	Irregular slow SWC on EEG
Myoclonic Seizures	Polyspike or slow SWC on EEG
Clonic Seizures	Fast activity or slow SWC on EEG
Tonic Seizures	Low-voltage fast EEG
Tonic-Clonic Seizures	Rhythm of less than 10 Hz on EEG
Atonic Seizures	Poly SWC or low-voltage fast

*EEG, encephalogram.
†SWC, spike-wave complex.
Data from Commission on Classification and Terminology of the International League Against Epilepsy. Proposal for revised clinical and electroencephalographic classification of epileptic seizures. Epilepsia 1981;22:489-501.

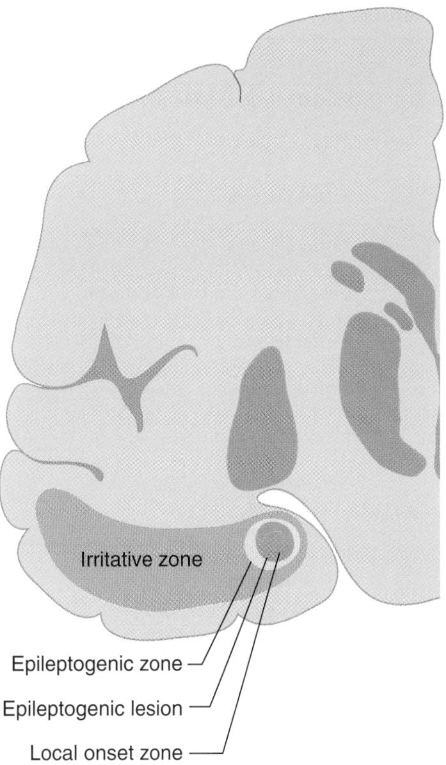

Figure 1 For epilepsy surgery to be successful, the various defined areas usually need to converge in one particular region.

There are further subdivisions that one can use to differentiate regions associated with epileptogenicity. For example, the epileptogenic lesion may be mesial temporal sclerosis, which may have a surrounding large region of interictal epileptiform activity (abnormal EEG activity not associated with a clinical seizure) described as the irritative zone. The area representing the detected ictal onset (the EEG findings *during* an epileptic seizure) is referred to as the *ictal-onset zone.* The area which, when removed by surgery and results in rendering the patient seizure free, is referred to as the *epileptogenic zone.* The epileptogenic zone can be inferred only retrospectively after surgery. For epilepsy surgery to be successful, the various defined areas usually need to converge in one particular region (Fig. 1).[10]

The EEG helps to confirm the diagnosis of epilepsy and provides information regarding the epileptic syndrome and, in focal epilepsies, the location of the seizure focus. However, the EEG records cerebral activity only during the time of recording, and so its information is only a snapshot in time—it cannot confirm the diagnosis of epilepsy in all patients with epilepsy. Certain activation procedures such as sleep deprivation, photic stimulation, and hyperventilation can improve the detection of epileptiform activity as can obtaining more prolonged EEG recordings. In some cases, when the diagnosis is uncertain, video EEG monitoring can help clarify the epileptic syndrome or identify nonepileptic events. In about 10% of patients with epilepsy, multiple EEG studies could show no abnormalities.[8]

Neuroimaging, especially with magnetic resonance imaging, is likely to show abnormalities in patients with focal epilepsy. These include vascular abnormalities such as strokes, arteriovenous malformations, cavernous angiomas, brain tumors, mesial temporal sclerosis, cortical dysplasia, and encephalomalacias.

TREATMENT

The first-line treatment of epilepsy is administration of an antiepileptic drug (AED). The selection of an appropriate AED is based on

Table 3 Characteristics of Various Antiepileptic Drugs (AEDs)

AED	Efficacy	Comments
Carbamazepine	Partial seizures, generalized seizures	Cytochrome P-450 (autoinducer); active metabolite
Ethosuximide	Absence seizures	No cytochrome P-450 induction or inhibition; can induce SLE-like syndrome
Gabapentin	Partial seizures	Minimal drug control; renal clearance of unmetabolized form
Lacosamide	Partial seizures	Minimal drug interactions
Lamotrigine	Generalized and partial seizures	Induced by phenytoin, carbamazepine; inhibited by valproate
Levetiracetam	Partial seizures	Minimal drug control; renal metabolism
Oxcarbazepine	Partial seizures	Prodrug of monohydroxy-carbamazepine
Phenobarbital	Generalized and partial seizures	Cytochrome P-450 inducer; excessive sedative effects
Phenytoin	Generalized and partial seizures	Cytochrome P-450 inducer
Pregabalin	Partial seizures	Minimal drug interactions
Tiagabine	Partial seizures	High protein binding; no enzyme induction or inhibition; may precipitate spike-wave stupor
Topiramate	Generalized and partial seizures	May increase phenytoin levels; no AED enzyme induction; alters efficacy of birth control medication
Valproate	Generalized and partial seizures	Cytochrome P-450 inhibitor; active metabolites
Zonisamide	Partial seizures	Minimal drug interactions

AEDs, antiepileptic drugs; SLE, systemic lupus erythematosus.

Data from Commission on Classification and Terminology of the International League Against Epilepsy. Proposal for revised clinical and electroencephalographic classification of epileptic seizures. Epilepsia 1981;22:489-501.

diagnosis of the epileptic syndrome of the patient (Table 3). First-line therapy for patients with focal seizures includes phenytoin, carbamazepine, and valproate. Drugs for adjunctive therapy for focal seizures include levetiracetam, topiramate, zonisamide, lamotrigine, gabapentin, oxcarbazepine, phenobarbital, and tiagabine. Drugs used in generalized seizures include valproate, lamotrigine, phenytoin, phenobarbital, and ethosuximide, which is specific for absence seizures.

These drugs have initial starting doses, and subsequent titration is based on response to medication and side-effect profile (Table 4). In patients who do not respond to medication, epilepsy surgery is a potential mode of treatment that can offer up to a 70% to 90% chance of seizure freedom (defined as no seizures or auras only, on medication) in some patients. Other novel modes of therapy include the vagal nerve stimulator (VNS), which is usually reserved for those patients with intractable epilepsy who are not surgical candidates. The VNS usually is as effective as a typical AED and usually does not provide a seizure-free state. Its mechanism of action is not known. The benefits of the VNS as opposed to AEDs is that it does not have the neurotoxicities associated with AEDs. Some adverse effects of the VNS include coughing, hoarse voice, bradycardia, and exacerbation of sleep apnea.

OUTCOMES

Seizures are well controlled with a single anticonvulsant in most patients with epilepsy. However, approximately 20% of patients with primary generalized epilepsy and 35% of patients with focal epilepsy have medically intractable seizures.[11,12] If seizures are not controlled with the initial dose of a first-line AED and there is no evidence of toxicity, the dose of the drug should be systematically increased. If the seizures are still not under control, a second first-line drug should be tried as monotherapy. If a second monotherapy trial fails, some experts may attempt a combination of two anticonvulsants. The practice of rational polytherapy is the use of two AEDs with differing modes of action, and that do not lead to worsening of adverse effects for the patient. After the third or fourth AED has been tried at appropriate levels and the patient still has seizures, the likelihood of finding an AED that will render that patient seizure free drops to as low as 5%. These patients who are recalcitrant to medical therapy should be referred to an epilepsy surgery center to determine if they are candidates for surgery.

In those patients who become seizure free with medications, withdrawal of the AED can be considered after a seizure-free interval has been maintained for 2 years. The risk of recurrent seizures after discontinuation is 25% in those patients without risk factors and 50% in those patients with risk factors (e.g., structural lesion, abnormal EEGs, or history of intractable epilepsy). The decision to stop medications should be individualized, and discontinuation should be done gradually, such as by decreasing the daily dose by 25% every 2 or 4 weeks.[13]

Summary

- Epilepsy is a disorder that gives rise to seizures of various pathologies and etiologies—an abnormal, synchronized electrical discharge within the brain causes the seizure.
- Seizures are currently based on an electroclinical classification; however, in addition to history, EEG recordings, imaging studies (such as MRI) may help in the diagnosis of epilepsy.
- Epilepsy surgery may be helpful the treatment of medically refractory focal epilepsy and should be considered once it has been established that medications have failed.

Table 4 Characteristics of Various Antiepileptic Drugs (AEDs)

AED	Typical Adult Starting Dose (mg/day)	Titration	Some Common Side Effects
Carbamazepine	400	200 mg/day at 1-wk intervals	Neurocognitive effects, rash, nausea, vomiting, hyponatremia
Ethosuximide	250-500	250 mg/day at 1-wk intervals	Neurocognitive effects, anorexia, nausea, vomiting, weight loss, diarrhea, abdominal pain, headache, mood changes, rash, hirsutism, and gingival hyperplasia
Gabapentin	300-900	300 mg/day at 24-hr intervals	Neurocognitive effects, weight gain, mood changes, dry mouth, periorbital edema, myalgias
Lacosamide	100	100 mg/day at 1-wk intervals	Neurocognitive, nausea, vomiting, cardiac conduction abnormalities
Lamotrigine	25-50	50 mg/day at 2-wk intervals	Neurocognitive effects, headache, rash, mood changes, nausea, vomiting
Levetiracetam	500-1000	1000 mg/day at 2-wk intervals	Neurocognitive effects, mood changes, behavior changes, anesthesia
Oxcarbazepine	600	600 mg/day at 1-wk intervals	Neurocognitive effects, rash, nausea, vomiting, hyponatremia
Phenobarbital	30-90	30 mg/day at 4-wk intervals	Neurocognitive effects, mood changes, nausea, vomiting, rash, porphyria exacerbation, physical dependence
Phenytoin	300	100 mg/day at 4-wk intervals	Neurocognitive effects, hirsutism, gingival hyperplasia, nausea, vomiting, coarse facies, headache, lymphadenopathy, osteomalacia
Pregabalin	150	150 mg/day at 1-wk intervals	Neurocognitive effects, weight gain, peripheral edema
Tiagabine	4	4-8 mg/day at 1-wk intervals	Neurocognitive effects, mood changes, asthenia, nausea, vomiting
Topiramate	25-50	25-50 mg/day at 1-wk intervals	Neurocognitive effects, language problems, psychomotor slowing, mood changes, paresthesia, weight loss, renal stones
Valproate	250-500	250 mg/day at 1-wk intervals	Neurocognitive effects, weight gain, nausea, vomiting, headache, hair loss, menstrual irregularities
Zonisamide	50-100	100 mg/day at 2-wk intervals	Neurocognitive effects, mood changes, insomnia

Neurocognitive side effects include dizziness, drowsiness, unsteadiness, blurred vision, ataxia, tremor, nystagmus, impaired memory, and fatigue.

Data from Commission on Classification and Terminology of the International League Against Epilepsy. Proposal for revised clinical and electroencephalographic classification of epileptic seizures. Epilepsia 1981;22:489-501.

Suggested Readings

Browne TR, Holmes GL: Epilepsy [comments]. N Engl J Med 2001;344:1145-1151.

Cascino GD: Intractable partial epilepsy: Evaluation and treatment. Mayo Clin Proc. 1990;65:1578-1586.

Commission on Classification and Terminology of the International League Against Epilepsy. Proposal for revised clinical and electroencephalographic classification of epileptic seizures. Epilepsia 1981;22:489-501.

Dinner DS, Lüders HO, Klem G: Chronic electrocorticography: Cleveland Clinic experience. Electroencephalogr Clin Neurophysiol 1998;48(suppl):58-69.

Engel J, Jr: Seizures and Epilepsy: Philadelphia, FA Davis, 1989.

Hauser WA, Hesdorffer DC: Epilepsy: Frequency, Causes and Consequences. New York, Demos, 1990.

Lüders H, Acharya J, Baumgartner C, et al: Semiological seizure classification. Epilepsia 1998;39:1006-1013.

Matsumoto H, Ajmone-Marsan C: Cortical cellular phenomena in experimental epilepsy: Interictal manifestations. Exp Neurol 1964;9:286-304.

Messenheimer JA, Harris EW, Steward O: Sprouting fibers gain access to circuitry transsynaptically altered by kindling. Exp Neurol. 1979;64:469-481.

Morgan JI, Cohen DR, Hempstead JL, Curran T: Mapping patterns of c-fos expression in the central nervous system after seizure. Science. 1987;237:192-197.

Penfield W: Epileptic lesions. Acta Neurol Psychiatry Belg 1956;2:75-88.

Reutens DC, Berkovic SF: Idiopathic generalized epilepsy of adolescence: Are the syndromes clinically distinct? Neurology 1995;45:1469-1476.

Spencer SS, Spencer DD, Williamson PD, Mattson RH: Ictal effects of anticonvulsant medication withdrawal in epileptic patients. Epilepsia 1981;22:297-307.

References

For a complete list of references, log onto www.expertconsult.com.

Multiple Sclerosis

Robert J. Fox

Multiple sclerosis (MS) is a chronic inflammatory disorder of the central nervous system (CNS). It usually affects people beginning in their 20s or 30s and is one of the most common causes of nontraumatic disability among young and middle-aged people. MS-related health care costs are estimated to be more than $10 billion annually in the United States. Symptoms of MS are extremely variable and often subtle, so diagnosis and management have been greatly enhanced by the development of magnetic resonance imaging (MRI). Because therapies that slow the progression of the disease are now available, early diagnosis and treatment are important in limiting the impact of this potentially devastating disease.

DEFINITION

As outlined in Figure 1, there are several different forms of MS. Because these classifications were based on clinical characteristics, they are empirical and do not reflect specific biologic pathophysiology. Nonetheless, they provide an organized framework for diagnosis and long-term management. Relapsing-remitting MS (RRMS) is the most common form of the disease, wherein symptoms appear for several days to weeks, after which they usually resolve spontaneously. After tissue damage accumulates over many years, patients typically enter the secondary progressive stage of MS (SPMS), in which preexisting neurologic deficits gradually worsen over time. Relapses can be seen during the early stages of SPMS, but they become uncommon as the disease progresses. About 15% of patients have gradually worsening manifestations from the onset without clinical relapses, which defines primary progressive MS (PPMS). Patients with PPMS tend to be older, have fewer abnormalities on brain MRI, and generally respond less effectively to standard MS therapies.[1] Progressive relapsing MS is defined as gradual neurologic worsening from the onset with subsequent superimposed relapses. Progressive relapsing MS (and possibly a portion of PPMS) is suspected to represent secondary progressive MS, in which the initial relapses were unrecognized, forgotten, or clinically silent.

Neuromyelitis optica (NMO), or Devic's disease, is an uncommon variant of MS.[2] NMO manifests as recurrent optic neuritis and longitudinally extensive transverse myelitis (extending over three or more vertebral segments). A relatively specific antibody, named NMO antibody, has been identified and recognizes the aquaporin-4 water channel in astrocyte foot processes located adjacent to capillary walls.[3,4] Recognition of the NMO antibody suggests the pathogenic role of autoantibodies in this form of MS, which has therapeutic implications.

PREVALENCE

MS affects more than 350,000 people in the United States and 2.5 million worldwide. In the United States, prevalence estimates are approximately 90 per 100,000 population. MS symptoms can start anywhere between 10 and 80 years of age, but they usually begin between 20 and 40 years, with a mean age of 32 years. Women outnumber men by a ratio of almost 2 to 1, although in PPMS the ratio is closer to equal. MS affects whites more than blacks, although blacks appear to become disabled earlier, suggesting more destructive tissue injury in blacks. The prevalence of MS varies by location, and it generally increases the farther one travels from the equator in either hemisphere. It remains unclear whether this altered incidence represents an environmental influence, genetic difference, or variable surveillance.

PATHOPHYSIOLOGY

Initially in the disease course, MS involves recurrent bouts of CNS inflammation that result in damage to both the myelin sheath surrounding axons and to the axons themselves. Histologic examination reveals foci of severe demyelination, decreased axonal and oligodendrocyte numbers, and gliotic scarring. The exact cause of inflammation remains unclear, but an autoimmune response directed against CNS antigens is suspected. Recent pathologic studies suggest that different patients might have different etiologies for inflammation: Some patients appear to have T cell–mediated or T cell–plus-antibody–mediated autoimmune responses, whereas others have a primary disorder within the myelin-producing oligodendrocyte cells.[5] This latter mechanism is reminiscent of virus- or toxin-induced demyelination rather than autoimmunity in this subset of patients. Further research is needed to understand how these different pathologic subtypes affect prognosis and response to treatments. Currently, brain biopsy is the only method to determine pathologic subtype, but studies are under way to find blood, cerebrospinal fluid (CSF), or MRI markers.

In the past, inflammation was believed to involve only demyelination, but pathologic studies have found significant axonal pathology as well. In active MS lesions, observed transected axons were an average of more than 11,000/mm^3, whereas control brain tissue had less than 1/mm^3.[6] Clearly, axonal injury is significant in the early stages of disease.

Later in the disease course, gradual progression of disability is observed. However, there is little active inflammation during this period, so this clinical progression probably involves significant degenerative changes. Nonetheless, oligodendrocyte progenitor cells capable of remyelinating axons have been observed, even in white matter plaques from patients with chronic MS (Fig. 2).[7] This observation suggests that the potential for remyelination persists even very late in the disease course, which is an encouraging indicator for possible therapeutic targets at this late stage of disease.

Current concepts of the pathophysiology of MS are illustrated in Figure 3. On average, patients have clinical relapses every 1 to 2 years during the relapsing-remitting phase of the disease. Serial MRI studies have shown that lesions develop up to 10 to 20 times more frequently than clinical relapses. Thus, although relapsing-remitting MS appears to have clinically active and quiescent periods, inflammatory lesions are developing and evolving almost continuously. A current hypothesis states that overt progression of disability (secondary progressive MS) occurs when ongoing irreversible tissue injury exceeds a critical threshold beyond which the nervous system can no longer compensate. It is believed that at this point the disease has become essentially a degenerative process, with neurologic deterioration independent of ongoing inflammation.

An important implication of this hypothesis is that the accumulation of irreversible tissue damage limits the potential for benefit from disease-modifying immunomodulatory therapy as the disease progresses and becomes a degenerative process. To be maximally effective, disease-modifying immunomodulatory therapy should be started early in the relapsing-remitting phase and before permanent disability develops.

SIGNS AND SYMPTOMS

Because MS can affect any area of the brain, optic nerve, or spinal cord, MS can cause almost any neurologic symptom. Typical relapses

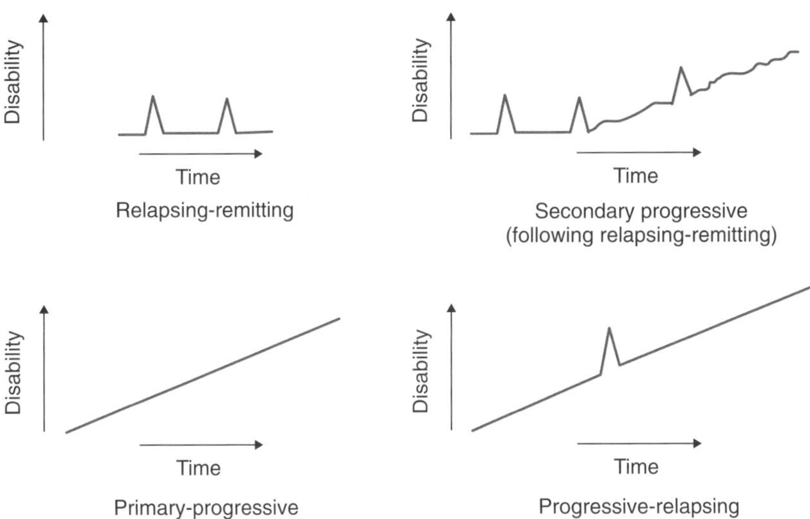

Figure 1 Illustration of different clinical courses of MS. *(Adapted from Lublin FD, Reingold SC. Defining the clinical course of multiple sclerosis: results of an international survey. Neurology 1996;46:907-911.)*

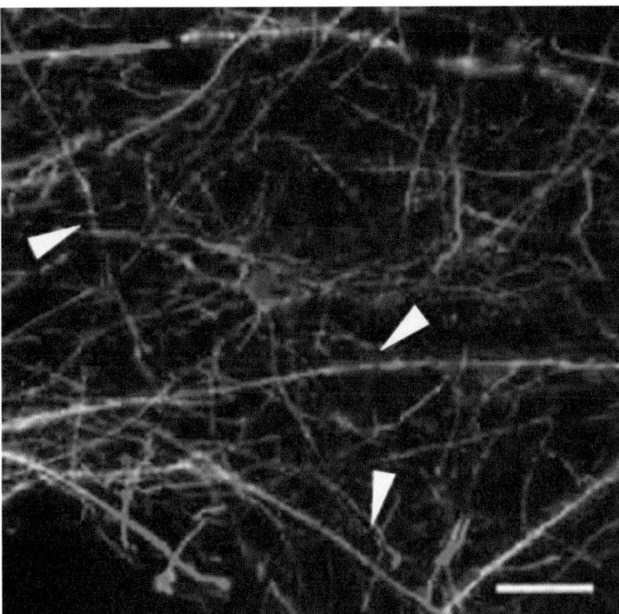

Figure 2 Remyelinating oligodendrocyte in a demyelinated region of brain from a patient with chronic MS. There are straight, healthy-appearing axons *(green)* and an oligodendrocyte *(red)* extending processes *(arrowheads)* to myelin internodes. *(Adapted from Chang A, Tourtellotte WW, Rudick R, Trapp BD: Premyelinating oligodendrocytes in chronic lesions of multiple sclerosis. N Engl J Med 2002;346:165-173.)*

of MS involve episodes of numbness, weakness, or dyscoordination affecting an arm, a leg, or both. Disease localized to the spinal cord can cause sensory or motor changes involving one side of the body or below a certain spinal cord level (i.e., hemiparesis or paraparesis). Brainstem involvement can manifest as diplopia, altered sensation in the face, or ataxia. Inflammation of the optic nerve (optic neuritis) usually manifests as blurry vision with painful eye movements.

Of all the lesions in MS, cerebral lesions are most common, but they cause the fewest symptoms. Very large cerebral lesions can manifest with weakness or numbness and rarely cause aphasia or other cortical dysfunction. Most cerebral lesions are not in eloquent regions and so are clinically silent and identified only by brain MRI. Lhermitte's sign is a nonspecific sign, whereby flexion of the neck causes an electric shock–like shooting sensation extending into the arms or down the back. Lhermitte's sign is believed to arise from partially demyelinated tissue, whereby mechanical stimulation leads to axonal activation.

Other common symptoms of MS include bladder and bowel dysfunction, decreased memory, fatigue, and affective disorders such as depression. Although these symptoms are not uncommon at the diagnosis of MS, they are also nonspecific and can be seen in a multitude of disorders.

DIAGNOSIS

There are no pathognomonic clinical, laboratory, or imaging findings in MS. The diagnosis ultimately is a clinical decision based on weighing the factors that support the diagnosis against those that fail to support it or point to the possibility of an alternative diagnosis.

The Schumacher criteria from 1965 capture the essence of the diagnosis of MS: CNS lesions disseminated in space and time, and the elimination of alternative diagnoses.[8] These criteria render MS a diagnosis of exclusion, which continues today. However, the Schumacher criteria also required that the patient's age be between 10 and 50 years and required the finding of objective abnormalities on examination, both of which are now outdated. However, the main concepts captured by these criteria remain relevant today.

Criteria from the Revised International Panel on MS Diagnosis, also called the Revised McDonald Criteria, is the latest attempt to clearly define diagnostic criteria for MS.[9] Diagnostic classifications are reduced to definite MS and possible MS (Boxes 1 and 2). Advantages to the Revised International Panel criteria include the capability of making a definitive diagnosis of MS either after a monosymptomatic presentation or in the context of a primary progressive course. As the boxes illustrate, the diagnostic classification scheme and MRI criteria remain complicated and tedious, and this complexity limits their use in everyday practice. Furthermore, the specificity of these criteria is relatively low, emphasizing the importance of clinical judgment in excluding other diagnoses. Finally, studies have observed that standard MS disease-modifying medications can benefit patients who do not yet fulfill these diagnostic criteria.

TREATMENT

Initial treatment of MS usually starts during the acute relapse. Several studies have found that treatment with corticosteroids can shorten the length of relapse and might even improve long-term outcome.[10,11] A typical regimen is 500 to 1000 mg of intravenous methylprednisolone followed by a tapering dose of oral prednisone over several

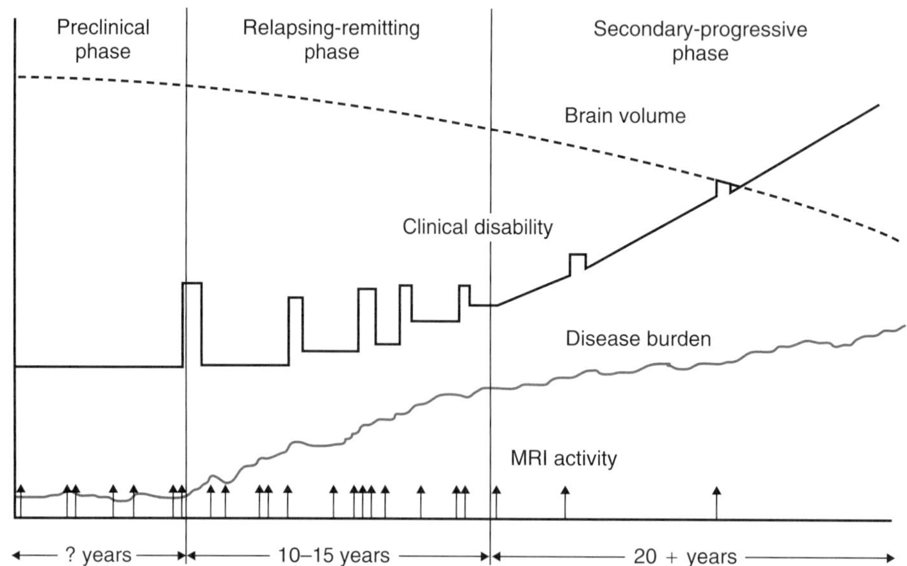

Figure 3 Typical clinical and magnetic resonance imaging (MRI) course of multiple sclerosis. MRI activity *(vertical arrows)* indicates an inflammatory process as measured on brain MRI by gadolinium enhancement or new T2 hyperintense brain lesions. MRI activity typically is more frequent than clinical relapses (*spikes* in clinical disability), which indicates that more disease activity is taking place than is clinically apparent. Loss of brain volume and increase in disease burden (total volume of lesions), both measured on MRI, indicate permanent tissue damage, which is present early in the disease and gradually progresses over time. *(Adapted from Fox RJ, Cohen JA: Multiple sclerosis: the importance of early recognition and treatment. Cleve Clin J Med 2001;68:175-171.)*

weeks. The standard protocol at the Mellen Center, Cleveland Clinic Foundation, is 1000 mg of intravenous methylprednisolone daily for three days, followed by a 12-day prednisone taper (60 mg daily, decreasing every 4 days by 20 mg). Evaluation of a relapse should include a search for precipitating factors such as bladder infection.

After the acute relapse is treated, consideration should turn to disease-modifying therapy. Current therapies target the immune dysfunction in MS and resultant neural tissue damage with the goal of preventing or at least reducing the long-term risk of clinically significant disability. Four first-line therapies are currently available in the United States: interferon (IFN) β-1a (Avonex, weekly intramuscular injection), IFNβ-1a (Rebif, three times-weekly subcutaneous injection), IFNβ-1b (Betaseron, alternate-day subcutaneous injection), and glatiramer acetate (Copaxone, daily subcutaneous injection). The IFN medications are recombinant products with an amino-acid sequence that is identical or nearly identical to that of human IFNβ-1. Glatiramer acetate is a random polypeptide based on the amino-acid sequence of a myelin protein. All of these medications appear to modulate the immune response in MS, although glatiramer acetate and interferon medications probably work through different mechanisms.

In randomized, placebo-controlled trials, all of these medications were shown to decrease the rate of clinical relapses by about 30%, decrease the severity of the relapses, and have beneficial effects on measures of disease activity on MRI.[12-15] Based on these studies, The Medical Advisory Board of the National Multiple Sclerosis Society has recommended that treatment with MS disease-modifying agents should be initiated as soon as possible following a definite diagnosis of MS and determination of a relapsing course. Furthermore, the Board recommends that "therapy is to be continued indefinitely, unless there is clear lack of benefit, intolerable side effects, new data that reveal other reasons for cessation or better therapy is available." If a patient chooses not to start treatment, routine clinical visits and interval brain MRI evaluations are strongly encouraged to monitor for active disease.

The International Panel Criteria for diagnosis of MS aimed to be specific, and as a result, they have limited sensitivity for making the correct diagnosis at very early points in the disease. Several treatment trials have involved patients with a single inflammatory event who were at increased risk of developing MS, and these trials found that interferon medications are beneficial at this very early stage of disease.[16,17] The benefits were observed despite MS not having been formally diagnosed in these subjects. Accordingly, a report from a Consensus Panel of the Consortium of Multiple Sclerosis Centers emphasizes that the new diagnostic criteria should be used for diagnosis only and not to make treatment decisions. Treatment decisions should be made based on the judgment of a clinician experienced in the diagnosis and treatment of MS.

The optimal initial treatment for relapsing MS remains controversial. Several head-to-head studies comparing interferon to glatiramer acetate found their efficacy to be similar on both clinical and imaging outcomes. Studies evaluating different doses and frequencies of interferon found greater short-term efficacy with high-dose, high-frequency interferon, which is balanced by increased adverse effects and greater incidence of neutralizing antibodies. Neutralizing antibodies significantly reduce the long-term efficacy of these medications, which is important when therapy is expected to continue for many years.[18-20] Each of these treatments (interferons and glatiramer acetate) offers different advantages and disadvantages. All four medications are appropriate first-line therapies in relapsing-remitting MS and have rather similar efficacies. Perhaps the most important decision is determining when to initiate treatment. Currently, early treatment is recommended because it offers the greatest chance of preventing or delaying tissue injury and long-term disability.

It is important to note that all of these first-line, disease-modifying medications have limitations. All are given by injection, and all are expensive, costing between $25,472 and $26,832 per year. The most important limitation of these agents is their partial effectiveness. A substantial percentage of patients treated with each of these medications continue to have evidence of clinical disease as measured by clinical relapse, progression of disability, or new T2 lesions (i.e., lesions seen on T2-weighted images) on brain MRI. Monitoring patients clinically and with surveillance MRIs during treatment is important to detect nonresponders and to modify therapy accordingly.

Natalizumab (Tysabri) is the most recent MS therapy, first approved by the U.S. Food and Drug Administration (FDA) in November 2004. Natalizumab is a monoclonal antibody targeting the

Box 1 International Panel Criteria (McDonald Criteria) for the Diagnosis of Multiple Sclerosis

Additional data needed for a diagnosis of multiple sclerosis for a given clinical presentation (in descending order of objective clinical evidence).

Two or More Attacks

Objective Clinical Evidence of Two or More Lesions

None*

Objective Clinical Evidence of One Lesion

Dissemination in space demonstrated by:

- MRI† *or*
- Two or more MRI lesions consistent with MS plus positive CSF‡ *or*
- Await further clinical attack implicating a different site

One Attack

Objective Clinical Evidence of Two or More lesions

Dissemination in time demonstrated by:

- MRI† *or*
- Second clinical attack

Objective Clinical Evidence of One lesion (Clinically Isolated Syndrome)

Dissemination in space demonstrated by:

- Two or more MRI lesions consistent with MS plus positive CSF‡

and

Dissemination in time demonstrated by:

- MRI† *or*
- Second clinical attack

Insidious Neurologic Progression Suggesting MS

One year of disease progression and dissemination in space, demonstrated by two of the following:

- ≥9 T2 lesions in brain, or four to eight T2 lesions in brain with positive visual-evoked potentials *or*
- ≥2 T2 focal lesions in spinal cord
- Positive CSF‡

**Brain MRI is recommended to help exclude other etiologies.*

†MRI criteria for dissemination in space or time are described in Box 2.

‡Positive CSF defined as oligoclonal bands different from those in serum or raised immunoglobulinG index.

CSF, cerebrospinal fluid; MRI, magnetic resonance imaging; MS, multiple sclerosis.

Adapted from Polman CH, Reingold SC, Edan G, et al: Diagnostic Criteria for Multiple Sclerosis: 2005 Revisions to the "McDonald Criteria." Ann Neurol 2005;58:840-846.

Box 2 MRI Criteria for Brain Abnormality: Space and Time Dissemination

MRI Lesions Disseminated in Space

At least three of the following criteria must be met:

- One gadolinium-enhancing lesion or nine T2-hyperintense lesions in the brain or spine
- At least one infratentorial or spine lesion
- At least one juxtacortical lesion
- At least three periventricular lesions

MRI Lesions Disseminated in Time

At least one criterion must be met:

- Gadolinium-enhancing lesion ≥3 mo after initial presentation, but in a different location from the initial event.
- New T2 lesion, compared with a reference MRI done ≥30 days after onset of initial event

Adapted from Polman CH, Reingold SC, Edan G, et al: Diagnostic Criteria for Multiple Sclerosis: 2005 Revisions to the "McDonald Criteria." Ann Neurol 2005;58:840-846.

cellular adhesion molecule α_4 intregin and is administered by intravenous infusion every 4 weeks. Adhesion molecules play an important role in attracting circulating leukocytes to leave the bloodstream and enter the brain parenchyma to cause inflammation. With blockade of α_4 integrin, fewer inflammatory cells are allowed to enter the brain, and CNS inflammation is thus blunted. α_4 integrin blockade within brain tissue can also lead to other beneficial immunologic effects, including anergy from lack of costimulation and apoptosis. Results from phase III clinical trials showed that natalizumab reduces clinical relapses by 55% to 67% and new brain lesions by 92%,[21,22] although it is currently unclear whether the drug enters the central nervous system or exerts its effect entirely from the periphery.

Natalizumab is relatively well tolerated. Mild headache, fatigue, anxiety, menstrual irregularities, peripheral edema, and routine infections (upper respiratory infection, pharyngitis) are occasionally observed. Infusion-related hypersensitivity reactions (hives, pruritus, and rarely anaphylactoid) were observed in 2% to 4% of patients and are believed to represent immune-mediated hypersensitivity reactions. Patients who demonstrate an infusion hypersensitivity reaction should discontinue natalizumab immediately and not be re-treated.

Three cases of progressive multifocal leukoencephalopathy (PML) have been reported in patients treated with natalizumab.[23] PML is a serious viral infection of the brain, arising from the ubiquitous JC virus carried by more than 85% of all adults. During periods of severe immune deficiency (i.e., acquired immunodeficiency syndrome [AIDS], solid organ transplantation, and cancer), the JC virus can enter the brain and cause a severe lytic infection. There are no known treatments for JC virus infection of the CNS, although prompt restitution of the aberrant immune system has helped some patients in the setting of AIDS. Plasmapheresis can accelerate removal of natalizumab and desaturation of α_4 integrin, although its efficacy in treating natalizumab-related PML remains unknown.

Because of the serious complication of PML, natalizumab is not currently a first-line therapy for MS. Natalizumab is reserved generally for patients who respond suboptimally or who are unable to tolerate the standard MS therapies described earlier. Discussions with potential natalizumab recipients should review the risks and potential benefits of natalizumab. A decision to initiate therapy should be made only after a full appreciation of the risks involved. Monitoring for PML is currently limited to clinical surveillance, although ongoing studies are examining biomarkers that might indicate PML reactivation. Monitoring includes a screening questionnaire administered before each monthly infusion of natalizumab, at least semiannual evaluations by the prescribing clinician, and urgent brain MRI or cerebrospinal fluid testing (or both) for patients with suspected or possible PML.

Mitoxantrone (Novantrone) is a chemotherapy medication with demonstrated efficacy in very active relapsing and progressive MS.[24] FDA labeling recommends intravenous infusion every 3 months, although a monthly induction course is sometimes used in patients with very active disease. Infusion side effects include nausea and alopecia. Long-term toxicities include cardiac injury and lymphoproliferative disorders, such as leukemia. Cardiac toxicity is cumulative over time, which limits its use to approximately 2 years. Cardiac monitoring with a transthoracic echocardiogram prior to each mitoxantrone infusion is recommended. The safety concerns of mitoxantrone limit its use to patients with persistently active MS despite standard injection therapy. As with natalizumab, the potential risks and benefits of mitoxantrone need to be weighed carefully and discussed in detail with the patient.

Cyclophosphamide, methotrexate, azathioprine and cyclosporine all have been studied in small- to medium-sized trials. An evaluation by the Therapeutics and Technology Assessment Subcommittee of the American Academy of Neurology and MS Council for Clinical Practice Guidelines has made recommendations regarding these therapies.[25] Methotrexate, azathioprine, and cyclosporine were each found to be possibly effective (Type C recommendation) in altering the course of disease, but cyclosporine was found to have an unacceptable risk-to-benefit ratio. In their review, pulse cyclophosphamide treatment was found to not alter the course of MS (Type B recommendation), although a more recent clinical trial observed reduced relapses and MRI lesions in patients treated with cyclophosphamide.[26]

It is important to note that current therapies are preventive, not restorative. As the disease progresses, response to therapy typically declines. The key to successful treatment of MS is to slow the inflammatory process early in the disease. It is likely that the accumulation of irreversible tissue damage limits the potential for benefit from disease-modifying immunomodulatory therapy as the disease progresses. The therapeutic nihilism of the past should be replaced by aggressive treatment and monitoring, with a careful balancing of risks with potential benefits.

Treatment of SPMS is more difficult. Although interferon medications were found in some trials to prevent progression of disability in SPMS, the effect was modest. It appears worthwhile to use interferons during this stage if there are persistent clinical relapses and side effects are tolerated, but caution regarding reasonable clinical expectations is appropriate. There are no treatments with demonstrated clinical efficacy in primary progressive multiple sclerosis, although anecdotal evidence suggests that intermittent pulses of intravenous methylprednisolone can help slow the progression of clinical disability in some patients. Intermittent pulses of intravenous methylprednisolone also may be helpful in SPMS.

In addition to neurologic disability, MS can produce a variety of other symptoms that can interfere with daily activities. Identification and treatment of these symptoms should be considered throughout the disease course. Specific recommendations for management of fatigue and urinary dysfunction have been outlined by the Multiple Sclerosis Council for Clinical Practice Guidelines. Aggressive evaluation and treatment for these and other symptoms of MS can improve quality of life significantly and are an important component of long-term management of patients with MS.

OUTCOMES

MS is a heterogeneous disease with a variable clinical course. Patients can progress rapidly over several months to death, or they might have a few relapses and then remain clinically stable for many decades. Although there is significant variability between patients, average time from disease onset to difficulty with walking is 8 years; walking with a cane is 15 years; and wheelchair-bound is 30 years. These observational studies were performed before the use of disease-modifying therapies, so these estimates may be different in patients receiving treatment.

It is difficult to predict which patients will progress and which will remain relatively stable over time. Although there are clearly patients in whom the disease remains benign, it is difficult to predict which patients eventually will follow this course. There are several prognostic factors of later outcome. Older age at onset, initial symptoms involving cerebellar, spinal, or pyramidal systems, and higher initial clinical activity (e.g., high attack frequency and increased disability progression in the first 5 years) are all unfavorable prognostic factors. Initial symptoms of optic neuritis or sensory dysfunction are favorable prognostic factors. Prognostic radiologic measures include brain and spinal cord atrophy and gadolinium-enhancing lesions. MRI measures are also useful tools when evaluating the effects of MS therapies.[27]

Pregnancy appears to decrease the incidence of relapses, but there is a rebound in relapse frequency after delivery.[28] The effect of vaccines on MS has been studied very carefully in the past several years, and there appears to be no adverse effect of vaccines on the course of disease.[29] Vaccines can be given safely in MS and should be administered if clinically indicated.

Summary

- MS is a chronic inflammatory disorder affecting the brain, optic nerve, and spinal cord.
- Because symptoms of MS can involve almost any neurologic function, the diagnostic evaluation should include a thorough history, neurologic examination, MRI, and, sometimes, cerebrospinal fluid analysis.
- Many therapies are available to decrease the clinical episodes of inflammation, slow progression of disability, and ameliorate the symptoms from previous injury.
- Early diagnosis and treatment are of key importance, because effective treatment is difficult after the patient has progressed into the later stages of MS.

Suggested Readings

Chang A, Tourtellotte WW, Rudick R, Trapp BD: Premyelinating oligodendrocytes in chronic lesions of multiple sclerosis. N Engl J Med 2002;346(3):165-173.

Confavreux C, Hutchinson M, Hours MM, et al: Rate of pregnancy-related relapse in multiple sclerosis. N Engl J Med 1998;339:285-291.

Francis GS, Rice GP, Alsop JC: Interferon beta-1a in MS: Results following development of neutralizing antibodies in PRISMS. Neurology 2005;65(1):48-55.

Lennon VA, Wingerchuk DM, Kryzer TJ, et al: A serum autoantibody marker of neuromyelitis optica: Distinction from multiple sclerosis. Lancet 2004;364(9451):2106-2112.

Lucchinetti C, Brèuck W, Parisi J, et al: Heterogeneity of multiple sclerosis lesions: Implications for the pathogenesis of demyelination. Ann Neurol 2000;47(6):707-717.

Polman CH, O'Connor PW, Havrdova E, et al: A randomized, placebo-controlled trial of natalizumab for relapsing multiple sclerosis. N Engl J Med 2006;354(9):899-910.

Polman CH, Reingold SC, Edan G, et al: Diagnostic Criteria for Multiple Sclerosis: 2005 Revisions to the "McDonald Criteria." Ann Neurol 2005;58:840-846.

Trapp BD, Peterson J, Ransohoff RM, et al: Axonal transection in the lesions of multiple sclerosis. N Engl J Med 1998;338:278-285.

Wingerchuk DM, Lennon VA, Pittock SJ, et al: Revised diagnostic criteria for neuromyelitis optica. Neurology 2006;66(10):1485-1489.

Yousry TA, Major EO, Ryschkewitsch C, et al: Evaluation of patients treated with natalizumab for progressive multifocal leukoencephalopathy. N Engl J Med 2006;354(9):924-933.

References

For a complete list of references, log onto www.expertconsult.com.

Alzheimer's Disease

Jinny Tavee and Patrick Sweeney

DEFINITION

Originally described by Alois Alzheimer in 1907, Alzheimer's disease (AD) has emerged as the most common type of dementia in the elderly today.[1] Although the definitive diagnosis of AD requires histologic confirmation, in the absence of a readily discernible cause, the clinician may establish the diagnosis antemortem, with a fair degree of certainty, based on the clinical findings of a gradually progressive cognitive decline that results in the loss of memory, language skills, activities of daily living, and executive function.

As the aging population continues to grow at a vigorous pace, it becomes increasingly important to recognize the clinical spectrum of AD because of the possible benefit of medical intervention and its tremendous impact on society. The cost of caring for patients with AD in the United States has been estimated to be $100 billion annually and climbing.[2] In recent years, research studies have made major advances in our understanding of the histopathogenesis, genetic risk factors, and treatment options for this devastating neurodegenerative disease.

PREVALENCE

Epidemiology

In 1996, AD was clinically diagnosed in approximately 4 million people in the United States; this figure is expected to triple in the next 50 years.[3] Women are more affected than men at a ratio of almost 2:1, partly because of the larger population of women who are older than 70 years; however, the prevalence is still higher in women even after statistical correction for longevity.[4] Age is another important risk factor. At the age of 60 years, the risk of developing AD is estimated to be 1%, doubling every 5 years to reach 30% to 50% by the age of 85.[5] Other reported risk factors include lower levels of intelligence and education (defined as primary education only), small head size, and a family history of the disease.[6] A meta-analysis of head injury as a risk factor for Alzheimer's disease also demonstrated a definite association in men.[7]

Genetics

Genetic risk factors are clearly involved in the pathogenesis of AD. In particular, the gene for apolipoprotein E (ApoE) on chromosome 19 has gained much recent attention. ApoE is a protein modulator of phospholipid transport that might have a role in synaptic remodeling.[8] ApoE has three common alleles, ApoE ε2, ε3, and ε4, which are expressed in varying amounts in the normal person. It is the ApoE ε4 genotype that is associated with the risk of AD. Postulated mechanisms include amyloid deposition and abnormal tau phosphorylation, a major component of neurofibrillary tangles. Unlike the chromosomal mutations that are responsible for early-onset AD, the presence of ApoE in itself does not cause AD nor does it guarantee that the carrier will develop any clinical manifestations. Therefore, at this time it should not be used as a screening tool for normal patients who are concerned about developing the disease.

PATHOPHYSIOLOGY

The classic neuropathologic findings in AD include amyloid plaques, neurofibrillary tangles, and synaptic and neuronal cell death. Granulovacuolar degeneration in the hippocampus and amyloid deposition in blood vessels might also be seen on tissue examination, but they are not required for the diagnosis (Figs. 1 to 3).

Amyloid Plaques

Although amyloid plaques or senile plaques may be classified further according to their composition, all contain forms of β-amyloid protein (Aβ). Aβ is a 39- to 42-amino acid peptide that is formed by the proteolytic cleavage of β-amyloid precursor protein (APP) and is found in extracellular deposits throughout the central nervous system (CNS).[9] Aβ is believed to interfere with neuronal activity because of its stimulatory effect on production of free radicals, resulting in oxidative stress and neuronal cell death.[6]

Neurofibrillary Tangles

Neurofibrillary tangles are paired helical filaments composed of tau protein, which in normal cells is essential for axonal growth and development. However, when hyperphosphorylated, the tau protein forms tangles that are deposited within neurons located in the hippocampus and medial temporal lobe, the parietotemporal region, and the frontal association cortices, leading to cell death.

Neuron and Synapse Loss

Areas of neuronal cell death and synapse loss are found throughout a distribution pattern similar to that of the neurofibrillary tangles, but they greatly affect neurotransmitter pathways. The death of cholinergic neurons in the basalis nucleus of Meynert leads to a deficit in acetylcholine (Ach), a major transmitter believed to be involved with memory. In addition, loss of serotoninergic neurons in the median raphe and adrenergic neurons in the locus ceruleus lead to deficits in serotonin and norepinephrine, respectively.

Chromosomal Mutations

Genetic mutations in chromosomes 21, 14, and 1 have been shown to cause familial early-onset AD. Inherited in an autosomal-dominant pattern, the chromosomal mutations account for less than 5% of all cases and result in the overproduction and deposition of Aβ.[10] Chromosome 21, which codes for APP, was first evaluated for an association with AD when Down syndrome patients with the trisomy 21 aberration were observed to develop dementia in the fourth decade. Mutations in presenilin 1 (PS-1) on chromosome 14 and presenilin 2 (PS-2) on chromosome 1 also cause AD and are responsible for the majority of familial early-onset cases.

Inflammation

The exact role of inflammation in the pathogenesis of AD is still controversial. Although some studies have been able to demonstrate the presence of activated microglia (a marker of the brain's immune response) in patients with probable AD, a number of prospective clinical trials evaluating the use of drugs targeting various aspects of the immune system such as prednisone, hydroxychloroquine, and selective COX-2 inhibitors have been able to demonstrate only marginal benefits at best.[11]

Although some studies have suggested a neuroprotective role for nonsteroidal anti-inflammatory drugs, a recent large study of 351 patients revealed that these medications did not slow progression and

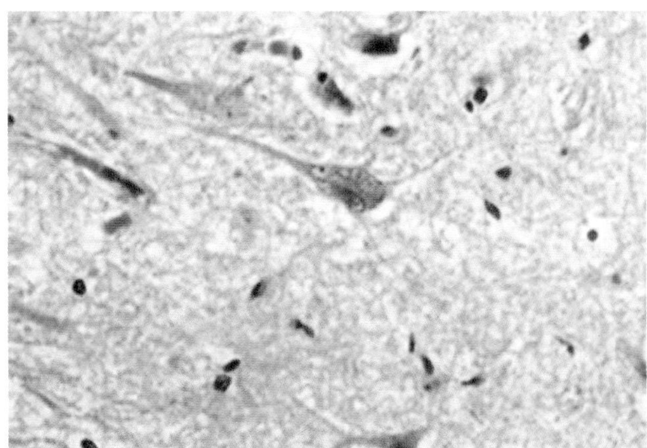

Figure 1 **Neurofibrillary tangles are seen in the cytoplasm of affected neurons as demonstrated in the center of this slide (Bodian method).**

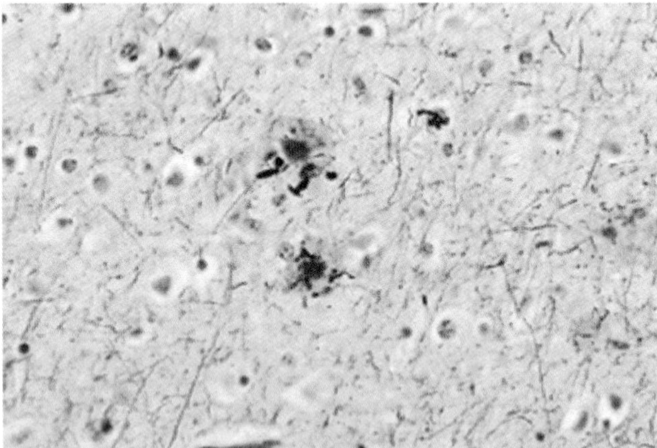

Figure 2 **Extracellular deposits of senile plaques are shown (Bielschowsky's method).**

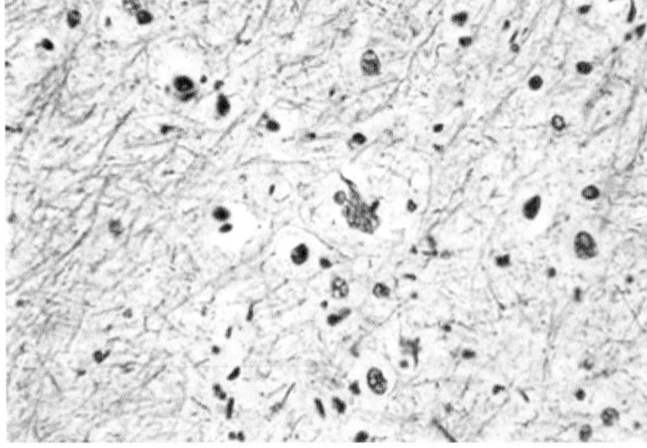

Figure 3 **Granulovacuolar degeneration.** This condition is manifested here as cytoplasmic clearing with granular deposits (hematoxylin-eosin stain).

cognitive decline in established mild-to-moderate Alzheimer's disease.[12,13]

SIGNS AND SYMPTOMS

AD is a progressive dementia with memory loss as the major clinical manifestation. Although short-term memory impairment is often the manifesting symptom, remote memory loss also appears to be affected over time. Another important feature of AD is the disturbance of language. Initially, AD patients might search for words when naming objects or while engaged in a simple conversation. But with progression of the disease, the language difficulties evolve into an inability to communicate as the patient struggles with a markedly limited vocabulary, nominal aphasia, and defects in verbal comprehension.

Other cortical signs and symptoms such as apraxia, acalculia, and visuospatial dysfunction may become apparent over the course of the disease. With the development of apraxia, patients lose the ability to carry out such simple tasks as combing their hair or turning on a water faucet. Acalculia may become evident when the patient is no longer able to maintain a checkbook or household accounts. Visuospatial abnormalities can be seen as patients become disoriented with their body position in space.

Behavioral problems emerge throughout the various stages of the disease. Mood disturbances such as depression, anxiety, or apathy may be present early on in AD, whereas delusions, hallucinations, and psychosis can be prominent in later stages. In addition, aggression and inappropriate sexual behavior can be particularly problematic for the caregiver.

In advanced stages of AD, patients might exhibit extrapyramidal signs such as tremor and gait disturbance, frontal lobe release phenomena, urinary incontinence, and myoclonus. Seizures can also be seen in some patients with late-stage disease. Patients with end-stage AD almost invariably enter a vegetative state when all cognitive activity ceases.

DIAGNOSIS

Clinical Diagnosis

In 1984, the National Institute of Neurological and Communicative Disorders and Stroke and the Alzheimer's Disease and Related Diseases Association (NINCDS-ADRDA) established diagnostic criteria designed for research purposes and clinical definition.[14] Now recommended by the American Academy of Neurology (AAN) for the diagnosis of AD, this classification is divided into definite, probable, and possible AD.[15] (See the AAN national guidelines for the diagnosis and management of Alzheimer's disease, the contents of which are summarized in the following paragraphs.)

In addition to histopathologic confirmation, definite AD requires the clinical finding of dementia as determined by the Mini-Mental State Examination (MMSE) or other standardized neuropsychological testing; the examination must demonstrate deficits in two or more areas of cognition, with progressive memory loss in the absence of delirium.

Probable AD is the clinical determination of dementia as just described and is supported by the findings of impaired activities of daily living, loss of specific cognitive functions such as language and motor skills, and a family history.[14] Other clinical findings that support the diagnosis in patients with advanced AD are myoclonus, gait disorder, and increased muscle tone. Possible AD is considered when there is variation in the onset, presentation, or clinical course of the dementia and when a second brain disease or systemic disorder is present. Clinical factors that make the diagnosis of AD unlikely include sudden onset and focal neurologic findings such as hemiparesis and visual field deficits. Clinically, both the NINCDS-ADRDA criteria and the Diagnostic and Statistical Manual of Mental Disorders IIIR definition of dementia of the Alzheimer type (DAT) may be used to diagnose AD with 90% accuracy.[15]

Differential Diagnosis

The differential diagnosis for AD is extensive and includes a multitude of neurodegenerative diseases that are associated with the development of dementia including Pick's disease, Lewy body disease, and other diseases such as vascular dementia and Creutzfeldt-Jakob disease. Most of these entities can be differentiated from AD by the clinical history and a careful examination. Potentially treatable diseases that can mimic the dementia caused by AD include depression, thyroid disease, vitamin B_{12} deficiency, normal pressure hydrocephalus, and neurosyphilis, all of which should be effectively ruled out in the evaluation of AD.

Imaging Studies

In advanced cases of AD, computed tomography (CT) and magnetic resonance imaging (MRI) demonstrate diffuse cortical atrophy with disproportionate volume loss in the medial temporal lobe structures. However, only mild atrophy and normal age-related changes may be present early on in the disease. Therefore, the use of imaging studies in the diagnostic workup of AD is mainly to exclude structural lesions such as subdural hemorrhage and brain tumors. Functional imaging studies used in clinical research include positron emission tomography (PET) and single-photon emission computed tomography (SPECT) scans, which demonstrate hypometabolism and hypoperfusion, respectively, in the temporal-parietal regions bilaterally. Amyloid burden imaging compounds are under development (Pittsburgh Compound B).

Box 1 Drug Therapy for Alzheimer's Disease

Acetylcholinesterase Inhibitors

Donepezil

- 5 mg once daily, can increase to 10 mg daily after 4-6 wk

Rivastigmine tartrate

- Pill: 1.5 mg bid initially, then titrate by 1.5 mg bid every 2 wk up to 12 mg daily
- Patch: 4.6 and 9.5 mg patch size daily

Galantamine*

- 4 mg bid initially, then titrate by 4 mg bid every 4 wk up to 24 mg daily

Galantamine ER

- 8 mg daily, the titrate by 8 mg/d every 4 wk up to 24 mg daily

NMDA Receptor Antagonists

Memantine (Namenda)

- 10 mg bid

**Renal and hepatic dose adjustments are required.*
NMDA, N-methyl-d-aspartate.

Laboratory Studies

Routine chemistry panels, blood counts, metabolic panels (e.g., TSH) spinal fluid analyses, and inflammatory markers are all within normal limits in patients with AD. Electroencephalographic (EEG) recordings are usually normal or show diffuse slowing in later stages of the disease.

TREATMENT

Management of Cognition

The major issues in treating AD are the improvement of memory and cognition and the delay of disease progression. At present there are no proven medications that cure or slow progression in Alzheimer's disease. Temporary improvements in cognition and behavior can be seen with the two existing drug classes of cholinesterase inhibitors and *N*-methyl-D-aspartate (NMDA) receptor antagonists.

The three cholinesterase inhibitors as well as the NMDA receptor antagonist memantine are listed in Box 1. The new patch formulation of rivastigmine (Exelon) allows the convenience of once-daily administration, with a marked decrease in the common gastrointestinal (GI) side effects seen with the cholinesterase inhibitors. Efficacy appears to be similar among the cholinesterase inhibitors. The only reported differences are the dosing schedule and side-effect profile of each individual drug.

The second drug class widely used in the treatment of Alzheimer's disease recognizes the increasing role of glutamate overstimulation of NMDA receptors on the surface of neurons. It is believed that this results in long-term excessive calcium influx into the neuron through the NMDA surface channel. By inhibiting this excessive influx, some improvements in cognition and behavior have been demonstrated in severe Alzheimer's disease.

An evidence review of the effectiveness of these drugs in the treatment of dementia concluded that "they can result in statistically significant but clinically marginal improvements in the measures of cognition and global assessment of dementia."[16]

Management of Noncognitive Symptoms

Depression is common in patients with AD and can require pharmacologic treatment. Serotonin reuptake inhibitors are relatively well tolerated by patients and are preferred over tricyclic antidepressants, which often exacerbate the cognitive impairment as a result of their anticholinergic properties. Behavioral disturbances such as psychosis and agitation require an investigation for a correctable underlying cause—such as a urinary tract infection—before a neuroleptic agent should be considered. If there is no external etiology, then establishing a quiet, controlled, and familiar environment for the patient can help to decrease confusion and disorientation.

Behavioral disturbances in AD may also be treated pharmacologically with both traditional and atypical neuroleptics. Although haloperidol can be effective, the atypical antipsychotics, which include risperidone, quetiapine, and olanzapine, may be better tolerated than traditional agents. There is not enough evidence to support the use of benzodiazepines, lithium, and anticonvulsants for the treatment of psychosis in patients with AD.[17]

Special care units within long-term care facilities are another consideration; some studies have shown a reduced need for antipsychotics and physical restraints as well as a decrease in behavioral disturbances in AD patients who reside there.[17] Psychosocial intervention for the caregiver is also an integral part of managing patients with AD. Education, support groups, and respite care services are should be suggested to family members and friends who provide the primary care for AD patients.[18]

The Future

A number of novel approaches are being studied in the hope that one or more might prevent or even reverse the accumulation of the toxic substance β-amyloid discussed earlier. These include the development of vaccines to remove or prevent amyloid accumulation and the manipulation of enzyme systems referred to as secretases. Unfortunately, the Ginkgo Evaluation of Memory (GEM) study showed that *Gingko biloba* extract, when taken by normal patients older than 85 years, failed to alter the risk of progression from normal to Clinical Dementia Rating (CDR) stage 0.5 and had no beneficial effect in preserving memory function.[19]

OUTCOMES

With the number of AD patients expected to grow exponentially over the next few decades, further studies are needed to elucidate our understanding of the disease, its risk factors, and potential treatments. This is critical not only for those at risk who can be identified in the preclinical state for early intervention but also for the patients and their caregivers whose lives are forever changed by the tragedy of this disease.

Summary

- Worldwide estimates of dementia prevalence increase from 24 million today to 81 million in 2040.
- Increasing age is the most powerful nonmodifiable risk factor.
- Potentially treatable causes of cognitive decline need to be excluded before establishing the diagnosis of AD.
- Current drug therapy offers mild benefit.

Suggested Readings

Aisen PS, Schafer KA, Grundman M, et al: Effects of rofecoxib or naproxen vs. placebo on Alzheimer's disease progression. JAMA 2003;289:2819-2826.

Alzheimer A: Über eine eigenartige Erkangkung der Hirnrinde. Allgemeine Zeitschr Psychisch-Gerichtliche Medizin 1907;64:146-148. (English translation: Arch Neurol 1967;21:109-110.)

Bird TD: Clinical genetics of familial Alzheimer's disease. In Terry RD, Katzman R, Bick KL (eds): Alzheimer Disease. New York: Raven, 1994, pp 65-74.

Canadian Study of Health and Aging Working Group. Canadian study of health and aging: Study methods and prevalence of dementia. Can Med Assoc J 1994;150:899-913.

Cummings JL, Vinters HV, Cole GM, Khachaturian ZS: Alzheimer's disease: Etiologies, pathophysiology, cognitive reserve, and treatment opportunities. Neurology 1998;51(S1):S2-S17.

Dodge H, Zitzleberg T, Oken B, Howieson D, Kaye J. A randomized placebo-controlled trial of ginkgo biloba for the prevention of cognitive decline. Neurology 2008;70:1809-1817.

Doody RS, Stevens JC, Beck C, et al: Practice parameter: Management of dementia (an evidence-based review). Report of the Quality Standards Subcommittee of the American Academy of Neurology. Neurology 2001;56:1154-1166.

Ernst R, Hay J: The US economic and social costs of Alzheimer's disease revisited. Am J Public Health 1994;84:1261-1264.

Fleminger S, Oliver DL, Lovestone S, et al: Head injury as a risk factor for Alzheimer's disease: The evidence ten years on. J Neurol Neurosurg Psychiatry 2003;74:857-862.

Geldmacher DS: Whitehouse PJ. Differential diagnosis of Alzheimer's disease. Neurology 1997;48(S6):S2-S9.

Graves AB, Kukull WA: The Epidemiology of Dementia. In Morris JC (ed): Handbook of Dementing Illneses. New York: Marcel Dekker, 1994, pp 23-69.

Haley WE: The family's caregiver role in Alzheimer's disease. Neurology 1997;48(S6):S25-S29.

Jones RW: Inflammation and Alzheimer's disease. Lancet 2001;358:436-437.

Knopman DS, DeKosky ST, Cummings JL, et al: Practice parameter: Diagnosis of dementia (an evidence-based review). Report of the Quality Standards Subcommittee of the American Academy of Neurology. Neurology 2001;56:1143-1153.

McKhann G, Drachman DD, Folstein M, et al: Clinical diagnosis of Alzheimer's disease: Report of the NINCDS-ADRDA Work Group under the auspices of the Department of Health and Human Services Task Force on Alzheimer's Disease. Neurology 1984;34:939-944.

Poirer J: Apolipoprotein E in animal models of CNS injury and in Alzheimer's disease. Trends Neurosci 1994;17:525-530.

Raina P, Santaguida P, Ismaila A, et al. Effectiveness of cholinesterase inhibitors and memantine for treating dementia: evidence review for a clinical practice guideline. Ann Intern Med 2008;148:379-397.

Sano M, Ernesto C, Thomas RG, et al: A controlled trial of selegiline, α tocopherol, or both as treatment for Alzheimer's disease. N Eng J Med 1997;336:1216-1222.

Swartz RH, Black SE, St. George-Hyslop P: Apolipoprotein E and Alzheimer's disease: A genetic, molecular, and neuroimaging review. Can J Neurol Sci 1999;26:77-88.

Veld BA, Ruitenberg A, Hofman A, et al: Nonsteroidal antiinflammatory drugs and the risk of Alzheimer's disease. N Engl J Med 2001;345:1515-1521.

References

For a complete list of references, log onto www.expertconsult.com.

Peripheral Neuropathy

Robert W. Shields, Jr.

DEFINITION AND ETIOLOGY

Peripheral neuropathy, in the broadest sense, refers to a range of clinical syndromes affecting a variety of peripheral nerve cells and fibers, including motor, sensory, and autonomic fibers (Box 1). Most peripheral neuropathies affect all fiber types to some extent. However, a single fiber type may be predominantly or exclusively affected in some disorders. For example, in small-fiber neuropathy (SFN) (Table 1), small-caliber, unmyelinated, or only thinly myelinated autonomic fibers and somatic sensory fibers that subserve pain and thermal receptors are predominantly involved.[1] Thus, patients with SFN present primarily with pain and autonomic dysfunction. Peripheral neuropathies are also defined by the pattern of nerve-fiber involvement. For example, some disorders involve single individual peripheral nerves—*mononeuropathies*—and some involve numerous individual peripheral nerves, the *mononeuritis multiplex syndrome.* In addition, peripheral nerve disorders can involve the brachial plexus, lumbosacral plexus, or a single root, resulting in signs and symptoms in one limb.

Most generalized disorders conform to a polyneuropathy syndrome, which usually implies both sensory and motor fiber involvement in a relatively symmetrical fashion and typically with a distal-to-proximal gradient of involvement. These disorders are termed *generalized sensorimotor polyneuropathies,* and they represent the most common form of peripheral neuropathy. This review focuses primarily on this form of peripheral neuropathy.

The peripheral nervous system can be involved in a wide range of medical disorders with various pathophysiologies (see Box 1). It may be affected by numerous toxins, drugs (Table 2), and industrial agents (Table 3) and by a variety of chronic infections, including human immunodeficiency virus (HIV). A number of apparently immune-mediated disorders result in peripheral neuropathies, including Guillain-Barré syndrome (GBS), chronic inflammatory demyelinating polyradiculoneuropathy (CIDP), and multifocal motor neuropathy with conduction block syndrome (MMNCB). A host of hereditary polyneuropathies can cause a wide range of peripheral neuropathy syndromes (Box 2).

This diverse array of possible etiologies can make the diagnosis of peripheral neuropathies challenging. Nevertheless, the diagnosis can be facilitated with a systematic approach that classifies the peripheral neuropathy on the basis of clinical features, taking into account the type of peripheral nerve fiber that may be involved (i.e., sensory, motor, or autonomic), the distribution or pattern of peripheral nerve fiber involvement (generalized and symmetrical versus asymmetrical and multifocal), and the mode of evolution (acute, subacute, or chronic).

PREVALENCE AND RISK FACTORS

Peripheral nerve disorders are relatively common conditions that affect 2.4% of the population.[2] However, the prevalence increases to 8.0% with advancing age.

The most common generalized polyneuropathy is diabetic sensorimotor polyneuropathy, which may be present in as many as 66% of type 1 diabetes patients and in nearly 59% of type 2 diabetes patients.[3] Even higher prevalence rates have been reported depending on the criteria used to diagnose polyneuropathy. Considering that the prevalence rate of diabetes is approximately 1.3%, this common complication of diabetes could affect nearly 1% of the general population.

The most common genetic sensorimotor polyneuropathy is Charcot-Marie-Tooth disease type 1a, which has a prevalence of approximately 30 per 100,000 population. Carpal tunnel syndrome, caused by chronic entrapment of the median nerve in the carpal tunnel, is the most common mononeuropathy, with a prevalence estimated to be between 3% and 5% of adults.

PATHOPHYSIOLOGY AND NATURAL HISTORY

Despite the diverse array of medical disorders that cause peripheral neuropathies, peripheral nerves exhibit only a few distinct pathologic reactions to an insult or disease: wallerian degeneration, axonal degeneration, and segmental demyelination. The specific mechanisms by which the various disorders affecting peripheral nerves induce these pathologic changes are largely unknown.

In wallerian degeneration, the axon degenerates distal to a focal lesion that interrupts the continuity of the axon. This reaction often occurs in focal mononeuropathies that result from trauma or nerve infarction.

Axonal degeneration, sometimes referred to as the dying-back phenomenon, results in axonal degeneration at the most distal extent of the axon. Axonal degenerative polyneuropathies are usually symmetrical, and as the disorder progresses, the axons typically degenerate in a distal-to-proximal gradient. Axonal degeneration is the most common type of pathologic reaction in generalized polyneuropathies, and it is often attributed to a metabolic cause.

Segmental demyelination refers to focal degeneration of the myelin sheath with sparing of the axon. This reaction can be seen in focal mononeuropathies and in generalized sensorimotor or predominantly motor neuropathies. Acquired segmental demyelinating polyneuropathies are often immune-mediated or inflammatory in origin. However, segmental demyelination can also occur in some hereditary polyneuropathies.

In peripheral nerve disorders that are characterized by either wallerian degeneration or axonal degeneration, prognosis is less favorable because the axon must regenerate and reinnervate muscle, the sensory organ, blood vessels, and other structures before clinical recovery is noted. Recovery may be more rapid with segmental demyelination because remyelination is accomplished more quickly, thereby re-establishing normal conductivity of the axon and return of function.

SYMPTOMS AND SIGNS

A host of symptoms and signs that reflect sensory, motor, and autonomic nerve fiber dysfunction are typical of peripheral neuropathies, and some combinations of symptoms and signs may be recognized as specific syndromes of peripheral nerve disease. Sensory symptoms include sensory loss, often described by patients as a sense of numbness or a "Novocain-like" feeling. In most generalized polyneuropathies, these symptoms begin in the most distal extent of the longest sensory fibers (i.e., those that subserve sensation in the toes and feet). The pathologic changes in most of these polyneuropathies are those of a distal-to-proximal axonal degeneration that have been referred to as *distal axonopathies* or *dying-back neuropathies.* Similar

Box 1 Peripheral Neuropathy Syndromes

Acute-Subacute Generalized Polyneuropathies

Sensorimotor
Acute motor and sensory axonal neuropathy syndrome
Alcohol or nutritional deficiencies
Toxins (metals)

Motor More than Sensory
Acute motor axonal neuropathy syndrome
Diphtheria
Guillain-Barré syndrome
Porphyria
Toxins (dapsone, vincristine)

Sensory
Human immunodeficiency virus
Paraneoplastic/autoimmune (anti-Hu-associated)
Toxins (cisplatin)
Vitamin B_6 toxicity

Chronic Generalized Symmetrical Polyneuropathies

Sensorimotor
Alcohol or nutritional deficiencies
Connective tissue diseases
Diabetes
Dysproteinemias
Uremia

Motor More than Sensory
Chronic inflammatory demyelinating polyradiculoneuropathy
Dysproteinemias
Hypothyroidism
Toxins (amiodarone, cytosine arabinoside, metals, tacrolimus)

Sensory
Paraneoplastic or autoimmune (anti-Hu-associated)
Sjögren's syndrome
Vitamin B_6 toxicity
Vitamin E deficiency

Inherited Generalized Symmetrical Sensory and Motor Polyneuropathies
Charcot-Marie-Tooth disease types 1, 2, 3, and X
Familial amyloidosis
Hereditary predisposition to pressure palsies (focal and symmetrical)

Asymmetrical Generalized Sensory and Motor Polyneuropathies
Diabetes
Lyme disease
Sarcoidosis
Vasculitis

Mononeuropathies
Compression and entrapment neuropathies
Diabetes
Vasculitis

symptoms may be seen in hereditary or acquired demyelinating polyneuropathies.

Sensory Symptoms

Typically, all sensory modalities are affected to some extent, including light touch, pain, thermal sensation, vibratory sense, and joint position sense. As the disease progresses, sensory loss ascends the lower extremities, typically in a symmetrical fashion. When the sensory loss is at or above the level of the knee, the axons supplying the distal fingertips begin to be involved, and the length-dependent process then begins in the upper extremities. In addition to sensory

Table 1 Drugs that Can Induce Polyneuropathies

Drug	Clinical Features of Polyneuropathy
Antibiotic	
Chloramphenicol	Sensory, optic neuropathy
Chloroquine	Sensory
Dapsone	Motor
Didanosine	Sensory
Ethambutol	Sensorimotor
Ethionamide	Sensory
Isoniazid	Sensory (vitamin B_6 deficiency)
Metronidazole	Sensory
Nitrofurantoin	Sensorimotor
Savudine	Sensory
Suramin	Suramin
Sensorimotor	
Zalcitabine	Sensory
Chemotherapeutic	
Cisplatin	Sensorimotor, ototoxicity
Cytarabine	Sensory
Docetaxel	Sensorimotor
Paclitaxel	Sensorimotor
Procarbazine	Sensorimotor
Vinblastine	Sensorimotor
Vincristine	Sensorimotor
Cardiovascular	
Amiodarone	Sensorimotor, ototoxicity
Captopril	Sensorimotor
Enalapril	Sensorimotor
Flecainide	Sensory
Hydralazine	Sensory (vitamin B_6 deficiency)
Perhexiline	Sensorimotor
Rheumatologic	
Allopurinol	Sensorimotor
Colchicine	Sensory
Gold	Sensorimotor
Indomethacin	Sensorimotor
Miscellaneous	
Disulfiram	Sensory
Interferon alfa	Sensorimotor
Lithium	Sensorimotor
Lovastatin	Sensorimotor
Phenytoin	Sensorimotor
Pyridoxine	Sensory
Simvastatin	Sensorimotor
Thalidomide	Sensorimotor

Table 2 Environmental and Industrial Toxins That Cause Polyneuropathy

Toxin	Clinical Features of the Polyneuropathy
Acrylamide	Sensorimotor, ataxia
Allyl chloride	Sensory
Arsenic	Sensorimotor
Carbon disulfide	Sensorimotor
Ethylene oxide	Sensorimotor, ataxia
Hexacarbons	Sensorimotor
Lead	Sensorimotor, motor > sensory
Mercury	Sensorimotor, motor > sensory
Organophosphorus esters	Sensorimotor, autonomic (cholinergic)
Thallium	Sensorimotor
Trichloroethylene	Cranial neuropathies

Box 2 Small-Fiber Neuropathies

Diabetes mellitus
Alcohol or nutritional deficiency
Amyloidosis (familial and primary)
Drugs or toxins

- Cisplatin
- Disulfiram
- Isoniazid
- Metals (gold, arsenic, thallium)
- Metronidazole

Primary biliary cirrhosis
Hypothyroidism
Heredofamilial

- Hereditary sensory and autonomic neuropathy types I, III, and IV
- Fabry's disease
- Tangier disease
- Dominantly inherited burning foot neuropathy
- Sjögren's syndrome

Human immunodeficiency virus
Hyperlipidemia
Monoclonal gammopathy of uncertain significance
Idiopathic neuropathies

Table 3 Heredofamilial Polyneuropathies

Disorder	Inheritance	Clinical	Pathology
CMT type 1	AD	Common, childhood onset, S/M	D
CMT type 2	AD	Rare, later onset than type 1, EM	A
CMT type 3 (Dejerine-Sottas disease) AD	Rare, infantile onset, severe S/M, D		
CMT, X-linked	XR	Second-most common, S/M, earlier onset, more severe D	D
HNPP	AD	Variable onset, compression neuropathies, S/M	D
Familial amyloidosis	AD	Variable onset, autonomic and S/M	A
Refsum's disease	AR	Variable onset, ataxia, retinitis pigmentosa	D
Tangier disease	AR	Very rare, variable onset, splenomegaly, orange tonsils	A
Fabry's disease	XR	Childhood onset, SFN	A

AD, autosomal dominant; AR, autosomal recessive; A, axon loss; CMT, Charcot-Marie-Tooth disease; D, demyelinating; HNPP, hereditary neuropathy with liability to pressure palsies; S/M, sensorimotor; SFN, small-fiber neuropathy; XR, X-linked recessive.

loss, patients often complain of paresthesias and dysesthesias, often characterized by a sense of numbness, tingling, prickling, and pins-and-needles sensations. They might also complain of intense band-like sensations and feelings of pressure.

The sensory examination often discloses a distal-to-proximal loss of the various sensory modalities. In certain polyneuropathies, pain predominates in the clinical picture, and the sensory examination tends to disclose deficits predominantly of pain and thermal sensation, conforming to an SFN. On occasion, when significant proprioceptive deafferentation occurs, patients are found to have altered joint position sense that can manifest as an ataxia or tremor of the affected limbs and an imbalance of gait and station.

Pain is a serious symptom for many patients. It may be described as a dull aching sensation, an intense burning sensation or, occasionally, as intermittent lancinating pulses of pain. On occasion, patients notice that their skin is hypersensitive to tactile stimulation such as from the touch of bed sheets or clothing or from standing on their feet. Some patients note an exaggerated painful sensation resulting from any stimulus to the affected area, a form of pain termed *allodynia*.

Weakness

Impairment of motor function typically produces weakness in a distal-to-proximal gradient consistent with a length-dependent axonal degeneration. As with sensory loss, weakness begins in the toes, and as the polyneuropathy progresses, it ascends up the distal lower extremities to the level of the knees, at which time motor involvement in the hands may be observed. Similar patterns of weakness may be seen in demyelinating polyneuropathies. However, in the acquired segmental demyelinating polyneuropathies such as CIDP and related disorders, proximal muscle weakness resulting from root involvement may be observed outside the proximal-to-distal gradient of the dying-back mechanism. This pattern of involvement is termed a *polyradiculoneuropathy*.

Axonal degenerative polyneuropathies tend to produce weakness along with muscle atrophy, but atrophy is much less conspicuous in segmental demyelinating polyneuropathies because in these disorders the axon remains in continuity with the muscle, preventing denervation atrophy. The most common symptom in polyneuropathy is weakness in dorsiflexion of the feet at the ankles. This can result in a partial or complete foot drop that typically causes the feet to slap while walking and predisposes the patient to stumble and fall when the toes catch on an uneven surface.

Tendon reflexes are usually depressed or absent in a distal-to-proximal pattern of involvement, with the lower extremities affected more than the upper extremities. An exception to this is in SFN, in which the large-caliber sensory afferent fibers from muscle spindles are relatively preserved and the tendon reflexes might remain intact.

Autonomic Symptoms

In some polyneuropathies, typically in SFN, autonomic fibers are also affected. In these disorders, a variety of autonomic symptoms may be present, although certainly the most dramatic and incapacitating is orthostatic hypotension, which causes postural light-headedness, syncope, or both. However, orthostatic hypotension typically occurs only with advanced autonomic involvement.

Earlier in the course of autonomic neuropathy, patients might notice reduced or absent sweating (i.e., anhidrosis) often in a distal-to-proximal gradient. Some patients complain of excessive sweating confined to the head and neck region. This is most often secondary to anhidrosis in the limbs and thorax and reflects compensatory hyperhidrosis in the restricted areas that maintain normal sweating.

Other autonomic symptoms include dryness of the eyes and mouth and gastrointestinal dysmotility, often manifested by alternating constipation and diarrhea or by early satiety from gastroparesis. In addition, patients may have urinary bladder dysfunction caused by an atonic bladder, which results in overflow incontinence. In men, erectile dysfunction can represent an early autonomic symptom, reflecting parasympathetic autonomic nervous system involvement.

Other Symptoms and Signs

Various limb deformities and trophic changes may be observed in chronic polyneuropathies. Pes cavus, characterized by high arches and hammer toes and the clawfoot deformity, are typical foot deformities in hereditary polyneuropathies with childhood onset. These deformities are a result of progressive weakness and atrophy of intrinsic foot muscles. A similar claw-like deformity may be observed in the hand.

Autonomic involvement of a limb may, at times, cause the affected area to appear warm, red, and swollen and at other times pale and cold because of abnormal regulation of small vessels as a result of autonomic denervation. Various trophic changes can occur including tight, shiny skin.

In patients who have had severe sensory loss in the limbs, the affected areas may be subject to incidental traumas, including burns, pressure sores, and other injuries that are not perceived by the patient. In these patients, repeated injuries and traumas can result in chronic infections, sometimes leading to osteomyelitis.

In peripheral nerve disorders that are focal and asymmetrical, sensory and motor—and occasionally autonomic—symptoms and signs may conform to a specific peripheral nerve distribution. For example, in carpal tunnel syndrome, patients might complain of intermittent numbness and tingling in the median nerve distribution in the hand or, as the entrapment progresses, atrophy and weakness of the thenar muscle group. In the mononeuritis multiplex syndrome, multiple individual peripheral nerves may be affected, and the sensory, motor, and autonomic symptoms and signs will be distributed in a multifocal pattern conforming to numerous individual peripheral nerve lesions. On occasion, some peripheral nerve disorders cause generalized sensory and motor fiber involvement with asymmetrical and focal features (see Box 1).

DIAGNOSIS

Diagnosis begins by recognizing typical symptoms of peripheral nerve disease and identifying the pattern of peripheral nerve involvement. For example, if the symptoms are highly restricted and focal, they might conform to the distribution of an individual peripheral nerve or, possibly, to an individual root. More-diffuse involvement of an entire limb might be caused by involvement of the brachial or lumbosacral plexus. Alternatively, if generalized symptoms are distributed in an asymmetrical and focal fashion, they may be consistent with a mononeuritis multiplex picture or possibly a polyradiculoneuropathy or polyradiculopathy syndrome. Most often, peripheral neuropathies produce symptoms that are generalized and relatively symmetrical, conforming to a distal-to-proximal gradient typical of a distal axonopathy.

History and Physical Examination

As soon as their distribution is recognized, the symptoms should be analyzed to determine which fiber types appear to be involved (i.e., sensory, motor, autonomic). In addition, the temporal profile of the disorder (i.e., chronic, subacute, acute) is noted. The neurologic examination is then helpful in confirming signs of sensory, motor, or autonomic dysfunction and in documenting the pattern and fiber type involved. These clinical features, which can be derived solely from the history and physical examination, are valuable for characterizing the nature of the peripheral nerve syndrome, which is essential in constructing a differential diagnosis (see Box 1 and Table 3).

Electrodiagnostic Studies

Another important component to the evaluation of peripheral nerve disease is electrodiagnostic studies, primarily nerve conduction studies and the needle electrode examination. Electrodiagnostic testing can document the presence of peripheral nerve disease, define the distribution and pattern of various sensory and motor fibers, and characterize the underlying pathologic processes (i.e., wallerian degeneration, axonal degeneration, segmental demyelination, or some mixture of these pathologic reactions). Characterizing the electrodiagnostic features, particularly whether the process is axonal or demyelinating, adds additional information.[4]

Medical Studies

Other special studies include lumbar puncture for cerebrospinal fluid analysis, which may be useful in diagnosing inflammatory or infectious causes of polyneuropathy, in evaluating acquired demyelinating polyneuropathies such as those in GBS and CIDP, and in a variety of immune-mediated polyneuropathies.

Nerve biopsy, typically sural nerve biopsy, is most often recommended in patients with asymmetrical or focal polyneuropathies in whom a diagnosis of vasculitis is being considered. In addition, biopsies may be used to assist in the diagnosis of some inflammatory, infectious, and metabolic polyneuropathies. Nerve biopsy can help to establish the pathologic basis of the polyneuropathy when electrodiagnostic studies cannot conclusively distinguish an axonal from an acquired segmental demyelinating disorder.

Special autonomic studies, particularly those that measure cardiovascular autonomic reflexes (including heart rate response to deep breathing, heart rate and blood pressure responses to the Valsalva maneuver, and heart rate and blood pressure responses to head-up-tilt) may also be valuable in documenting autonomic cardiovascular involvement. Various tests of sudomotor function including the sympathetic skin response, quantitative sudomotor axon reflex test, and thermoregulatory sweat testing can provide valuable information regarding the extent and distribution of sudomotor impairment in polyneuropathy.

Skin biopsy to measure epidermal nerve fiber density is also a helpful test for the diagnosis of SFN. Quantitative sensory testing is a technique that allows precise measurement of sensory perception thresholds of various fiber types, which can also be helpful in assessing peripheral neuropathy, especially SFN, in which the electrodiagnostic studies are often normal.

Laboratory Studies

By recognizing the peripheral nerve syndrome and appreciating the potential differential diagnosis, one may systematically perform appropriate medical tests to explore the various possible causes. The most common peripheral nerve syndrome is the generalized sensorimotor polyneuropathy with electrodiagnostic features of a distal axonopathy. For this disorder, it is usually appropriate to pursue a history of toxin exposure (see Tables 2 and 3) and alcoholism with nutritional deficiency. It is also reasonable to perform routine laboratory screening studies including a complete blood cell count; erythrocyte sedimentation rate; a blood chemistry panel encompassing hepatic function, renal function, and electrolytes; thyroid function studies; and vitamin B_{12} level.

It is important to screen patients for diabetes mellitus. In the past, a fasting blood sugar or hemoglobin A_{1c}, or both, was often performed, but recent reports suggest that impaired glucose tolerance detected on a glucose tolerance test might provide more meaningful information regarding diabetes as a potential cause for polyneuropathy.[5]

Screening the serum and urine with protein electrophoresis with immunofixation is also important in assessing patients with generalized polyneuropathy. In one series, the only laboratory tests that were helpful in establishing a precise cause for the polyneuropathy were vitamin B_{12}, serum protein electrophoresis with immunofixation, and serum glucose.[6] Additional laboratory and radiographic studies may be considered pending the specific clinical features, and may include chest radiograph, skeletal bone survey, antinuclear antibodies, rheumatoid factor, and angiotensin-converting enzyme level.

In patients with an aggressive, evolving polyneuropathy or a specific paraneoplastic syndrome, additional testing for an occult malignancy is often performed, usually in conjunction with autoantibodies, especially anti-Hu. A variety of autoantibodies have been associated with different polyneuropathy syndromes. The most useful of these include anti-GM_1 antibodies in the setting of MMNCB, anti-Hu antibodies in the context of a sensory neuronopathy, and anti-myelin-associated glycoprotein antibodies in acquired demyelinating polyneuropathy with predominately sensory features and with a distal pattern of involvement.[7,8] Most of the other antibodies are much less specific, and their roles in the mechanism of the polyneuropathies are less certain. Thus, the precise value of performing panels of antibody tests is unclear at this time.[9]

Lumbar puncture is often reserved for patients with possible immune-mediated polyneuropathies, particularly those with demyelinating features on electrodiagnostic testing. However, CSF studies are also often assessed in cryptogenic axonal degeneration polyneuropathies and in patients with possible infectious or inflammatory disorders.

Additional Tests

In patients with electrodiagnostic features suggesting acquired segmental demyelination, a variety of tests are indicated to assess for CIDP and related disorders (Box 3), including serum and urine for protein electrophoresis with immunofixation, skeletal bone survey for myeloma or osteosclerotic myeloma, and HIV testing in patients at risk.

In patients with SFN, various hereditary diseases must also be considered if the more common acquired disorders are not present (see Table 1). In the asymmetrical polyneuropathies, particularly those of acute or subacute evolution, the differential diagnosis includes various connective tissue disorders associated with vasculitis. Appropriate laboratory studies must be obtained to investigate these disorders.

The acute polyneuropathies are a special category that includes GBS, although variants and other less-common causes must also be considered. The inherited polyneuropathies are, of course, identified by a typical chronic course, often with onset in childhood and a family history of similar illness. Some of the hereditary polyneuropathies, in particular Charcot-Marie-Tooth disease, may be confirmed with genetic tests performed on blood.

Box 3 Autonomic Neuropathies and Polyneuropathies with Prominent Autonomic Features

Acute

Acute pandysautonomia (paraneoplastic and idiopathic)
Botulism
Guillain-Barré syndrome
Porphyria
Toxins (vincristine, amiodarone, cisplatin, organic solvents, metals)

Chronic

Amyloidosis
Chronic pandysautonomia (paraneoplastic and idiopathic)
Diabetes
Riley-Day syndrome

Despite comprehensive testing and assessments, an etiologic diagnosis is not determined in nearly 25% of patients with polyneuropathy.[10] In this group, particularly those with chronic sensorimotor polyneuropathies, careful assessment of first-degree relatives may be helpful in identifying an unrecognized familial disorder. In addition, in patients with idiopathic polyneuropathy, judicious reassessment of their laboratory investigations should be performed periodically, particularly if symptoms and signs progress.

TREATMENT

Medical Treatment

Specific therapies for polyneuropathy are based on the precise etiologic diagnosis. In disorders attributed to underlying medical conditions, management is focused on the medical disorder. For example, optimizing glycemic control in diabetic polyneuropathy often stabilizes or improves the polyneuropathy.

In patients with idiopathic immune-mediated polyneuropathies, including GBS, CIDP, and MMNCB, specific immune-modulating therapies are often recommended.[8,11] For GBS, intravenous gamma globulin (IVIg), typically administered at a dosage of 400 mg/kg daily for 5 consecutive days, is initiated early in the patient's course. Alternatively, plasmapheresis may also be instituted as initial therapy.

Treatment of CIDP may begin with corticosteroid therapy. However, chronic IVIg or plasmapheresis, or both, are usually effective and obviate the need for long-term steroid therapy. Alternative therapies including azathioprine, cyclophosphamide, cyclosporine, mycophenolate mofetil, methotrexate, and rituximab have also been used in patients who have not responded to initial standard therapies.

Toxic polyneuropathies are managed by discontinuing the offending drug or removing the industrial toxin from the patient's environment.

Management of hereditary polyneuropathies includes education of the affected family members regarding the nature and genetic features of the disorder and judicious screening of family members at risk.

Supportive Therapy

For all patients, and particularly for those without a specific or treatable cause, therapy focuses on supportive measures. This may include the use of various physical therapy and occupational therapy modalities including bracing and aids to ambulation. An ankle-foot orthosis may be effective in improving ambulation in a patient with foot drop. In patients with severe sensory loss in the feet and lower extremities, careful daily foot inspection for signs of trauma and

Table 4 Drug Therapy for Neuropathic Pain

Drug	Daily Dosage, Range	Comments
Antidepressants		
Amitriptyline	10-150 mg	Sedation, anticholinergic side effects, weight gain, arrhythmia
Nortriptyline	10-150 mg	Similar to amitriptyline but less sedating
Imipramine	10-300 mg	Similar to amitriptyline but less sedating
Desipramine	10-300 mg	Similar to amitriptyline but least sedating
Duloxetine	60-120 mg	Nausea, dry mouth, constipation
Venlafaxine XR	37.5-225 mg	Asthenia, nausea, sweating, ejaculatory dysfunction
Antiepileptics		
Gabapentin	300-3600 mg	Sedation, dizziness
Pregabalin	150-300 mg	Sedation, dizziness
Carbamazepine	200-1200 mg	Sedation, dizziness, nausea, bone marrow suppression
Oxycarbazepine	600-2400 mg	Fatigue, nausea, dizziness, leukopenia
Lamotrigine	50-500 mg	Serious rash, dizziness, nausea, sedation
Topiramate	25-400 mg	Sedation, weight loss, nephrolithiasis, myopia, angle closure glaucoma
Miscellaneous		
Mexiletine	150-750 mg	Dyspepsia, dizziness, tremor, arrhythmia
Tramadol	50-400 mg	Dizziness, nausea, constipation, seizures
Capsaicin 0.075%	Topical tid-qid	Burning, erythema

infection are essential to prevent serious infections and other complications.

Pain Management

In patients who have associated pain, particularly patients with SFN, specific neuropathic pain management is instituted. Neuropathic pain typically does not respond to simple analgesics, and its potential chronicity precludes narcotic therapy as a first choice. Typically, patients with SFN and other painful polyneuropathies respond to drugs known to be effective for neuropathic pain, including tricyclic antidepressants and a variety of antiepileptic drugs and membrane stabilizers (Table 4).[1,6,12]

The choice for each patient must be individualized, taking into account potential side effects and drug interactions, among other factors. For patients requiring sedation because of disturbed sleep from the pain, a sedating tricyclic drug taken at bedtime, such as amitriptyline, is a good choice. However, the anticholinergic side effects of the tricyclic antidepressants make them a poor choice in patients with prominent dysautonomia because they are likely to worsen gastrointestinal dysmotility and bladder dysfunction.

Because most of these drugs can potentially cause sedation, it is customary to begin therapy with small doses and gradually escalate as needed and tolerated. However, it is important to increase a drug to a reasonable dosage before determining its clinical efficacy. Drugs with little efficacy despite high doses should be tapered and discontinued before starting an alternative drug. Alternatively, drugs that provide some relief but are not controlling the pain adequately may be maintained in some circumstances, and another drug may be added to the regimen.

OUTCOMES

Peripheral neuropathies are common disorders associated with a wide range of medical conditions and immune-mediated mechanisms. With a systematic approach to the evaluation of these disorders, approximately 75% of patients have a specific etiologic diagnosis. Despite comprehensive evaluations, the peripheral nerve disorder must be regarded as cryptogenic or idiopathic in nearly 25% of patients. In most patients with a peripheral neuropathy related to a medical disorder or immune-mediated mechanism, specific therapies directed at the underlying mechanism are usually effective in controlling the peripheral neuropathy. Despite these therapies, the symptoms and signs of the peripheral neuropathy remain a chronic problem in most patients. Even in the absence of a specific treatable cause, the symptoms of polyneuropathy can be treated with a variety of supportive measures including medications for neuropathic pain, physical therapy modalities, and orthotic devices. Fortunately, for most of these patients, the peripheral nerve disorder does not result in serious disability.

Summary

- Peripheral neuropathy encompasses a wide spectrum of clinical disorders affecting sensory, motor, and autonomic peripheral nerve fibers.
- Generalized peripheral neuropathy often manifests with symptoms and signs of sensory and motor deficits distributed symmetrically in a distal-to-proximal gradient, with the lower extremities more affected than the upper extremities.
- The diagnosis of peripheral neuropathy depends on the recognition of the symptoms and signs of peripheral nerve dysfunction. Electromyography can be helpful in confirming the diagnosis and in defining the nature and extent of the peripheral neuropathy.
- The etiologic diagnosis of peripheral neuropathy can be challenging and depends on a careful and methodologic assessment for underlying medical conditions that can cause peripheral neuropathy, as well as other causes including hereditary, toxic, and primary autoimmune peripheral nerve disorders.
- Management of the peripheral neuropathy is directed first at the specific cause if it is treatable and second at the alleviation of symptoms, including managing neuropathic pain and bracing and physical therapy for weakness.

Suggested Readings

Donofrio PD, Albers JW: Polyneuropathy: Classification by nerve conduction studies and electromyography. AAEM Minimonograph #34. Muscle Nerve 1990;13:889-903.
England JD, Asbury AK: Peripheral neuropathy. Lancet 2004;363:2151-2161.
Lacomis D: Small-fiber neuropathy. Muscle Nerve 2002;26:173-188.

Lindenbaum Y, Kissel JT, Mendell JR: Treatment approaches for Guillain-Barré syndrome and chronic inflammatory demyelinating polyradiculoneuropathy. Neurol Clin 2001;19:187-204.

Mauermann ML, Burns TM: The evaluation of chronic axonal polyneuropathies. Semin Neurol 2008;28:133-151.

Pourmand R: Evaluating patients with suspected peripheral neuropathy: Do the right thing, not everything. Muscle Nerve 2002;26:288-290.

Saperstein DS: Chronic acquired demyelinating polyneuropathies. Semin Neurol 2008;28:168-184.

Sindrup SH, Jensen TS: Pharmacologic treatment of pain in polyneuropathy. Neurology 2000;55:915-920.

Singleton JR, Smith AG, Bromberg MB: Painful sensory polyneuropathy associated with impaired glucose tolerance. Muscle Nerve 2001;24:1225-1228.

Wolfe GI, Barohn RJ: Cryptogenic sensory and sensorimotor polyneuropathies. Semin Neurol 1998;18:105-111.

References

For a complete list of references, log onto www.expertconsult.com.

Myopathy

Preetha Muthusamy and Jinny Tavee

DEFINITION

Myopathy refers to a clinical disorder of the skeletal muscles. Abnormalities of muscle cell structure and metabolism lead to various patterns of weakness and dysfunction. In some cases, the pathology extends to involve cardiac muscle fibers, resulting in a hypertrophic or dilated cardiomyopathy.

PATHOPHYSIOLOGY

Disruption of the structural integrity and metabolic processes of muscle cells can result from genetic abnormalities, toxins, inflammation, infection, and hormonal and electrolyte imbalances.

CLASSIFICATION

Myopathies may be divided into two main categories: inherited and acquired. The temporal course, the pattern of muscle weakness, and the absence or presence of a family history of myopathy help distinguish between the two types. An early age of onset with a relatively longer duration of disease suggests an inherited myopathy, and a sudden or subacute presentation at a later age is more consistent with an acquired myopathy. Inherited myopathies can be further subclassified as muscular dystrophies, congenital myopathies, mitochondrial myopathies, and metabolic myopathies. Acquired myopathies can be subclassified as inflammatory myopathies, toxic myopathies, and myopathies associated with systemic conditions. The more commonly seen inherited and acquired myopathies are listed in Box 1.

CLINICAL FEATURES

Myopathies are characterized by motor symptoms in the absence of any sensory involvement. Most myopathies manifest with weakness involving the proximal muscles. Commonly, pelvic girdle muscles are involved before and much more severely than shoulder girdle muscles. Some myopathies are associated with atypical distributions of weakness, such as inclusion body myositis, an inflammatory myopathy seen typically in older men that manifests with weakness in the finger flexors and quadriceps. Table 1 gives the distribution patterns of specific muscle disorders.

Cramps, myalgias, and exertional fatigue are other common presenting symptoms. Many patients complain of difficulty rising from a chair, climbing stairs, changing a light bulb, or washing and combing their hair. In metabolic myopathies associated with rhabdomyolysis (defined as creatine kinase elevation 10 times the normal value), patients may report tea-colored or dark urine, especially after intense exercise. Rhabdomyolysis may also be seen with infectious etiologies, alcohol, and toxic exposures.

On physical examination, many myopathy patients, especially those with acquired myopathies, demonstrate symmetrical muscle weakness in a proximal to distal gradient. Sensation is intact, and deep tendon reflexes are preserved unless there is severe weakness. In the muscular dystrophies, which tend to manifest in childhood or adolescence, dyspnea, cardiac abnormalities, contractures, scapular winging, calf hypertrophy, and skeletal deformities may be present in addition to slowly progressive weakness. Respiratory compromise is a common feature of critical illness myopathy, amyloid myopathy, interstitial lung disease associated with dermatomyositis, acid maltase deficiency, and, very rarely, a subtype of limb girdle muscular dystrophy (LGMD 2I). Myopathies with other extramuscular manifestations are listed in Table 1. Some patients actually have a normal examination, such as those with metabolic myopathies, in which symptoms are transiently present only after physical exertion.

DIAGNOSIS

The clinical history is essential in identifying the presence of a myopathy and narrowing down the differential diagnosis. In particular, the patient should be questioned about medication and recreational drug history (especially alcohol), chemical exposures, exercise intolerance, childhood development, and family history of muscle disease or developmental motor delay.

Laboratory Testing

Serologic testing, which can indicate muscle damage, includes elevations in creatine phosphokinase (CPK), aldolase, lactate dehydrogenase (LDH), and liver function enzymes. A screening panel of laboratory tests may also be obtained to rule out more common causes of myopathy, which are listed in Box 2. In cases suspected to be a primary inflammatory myopathy, specific autoantibodies can be considered to determine the prognosis and rule out associated conditions. For example, the presence of anti-Jo antibody in dermatomyositis predicts a superimposed interstitial lung disease. In addition, these patients should also be evaluated for an underlying systemic autoimmune disease with an extensive autoimmune panel and angiotensin-converting enzyme (ACE) levels. In myopathies that are accompanied by polyneuropathy, renal involvement, and a restrictive cardiomyopathy, immunofixation electrophoresis studies in the serum and urine should be considered to rule out the possibility of amyloid disease. Genetic testing is available for some inherited myopathies. These are listed in Table 2.

Ischemic Forearm Test

A traditional test used in the evaluation of a suspected metabolic myopathy is the ischemic forearm test. This is performed by obtaining baseline serum ammonia and lactate levels taken from the forearm. The patient then exercises that arm for 1 minute, after which repeat serum lactate and blood ammonia levels are measured. This is repeated at several intervals (1, 2, 5, and 10 minutes). In normal muscle, the resultant ischemia causes a 3- to 5-fold rise in lactate levels. In contrast, patients with glycogen storage disorders demonstrate no change in lactate levels after exercise.

Electrodiagnostic Studies

The electromyogram (EMG) is an electrical study of the nerves and muscles that plays an important role in confirming the presence, duration, and severity of a myopathy. The study can also disclose special findings such as myotonic potentials. This is the electrical equivalent of clinical myotonia, which is manifested as impaired relaxation of muscles after forceful contraction; for example, patients cannot release objects from their grip. Myotonic potentials have the characteristic sound of a dive bomb on EMG and can help point toward the diagnosis of myotonic dystrophy when found in the appropriate muscles.

Although integral in the evaluation of a myopathy, the EMG can be normal in mild myopathies, steroid myopathies, and a number of

Box 1 Common Causes of Myopathy

Acquired Myopathies

Inflammatory Myopathy
- Polymyositis
- Dermatomyositis
- Inclusion body myositis

Infection
- Viral infections (HIV, influenza virus, Epstein-Barr virus)
- Bacterial pyomyositis (*Staphylococcus aureus* and streptococci are common organisms)
- Spirochete (Lyme disease)
- Parasitic infections such as trichinosis

Toxic Myopathy
- Medications
  - Steroids
  - Cholesterol-lowering medications: statins, fibrates, niacin, and ezetimibe
  - Propofol
  - Amiodarone
  - Colchicine
  - Chloroquine
  - Antivirals and protease inhibitors
  - Omeprazole
  - Tryptophan
- Toxins
  - Alcohol
  - Toluene

Myopathy Associated with Systemic Diseases
- Endocrine disorders
  - Thyroid
  - Parathyroid
  - Pituitary or adrenal dysfunction
- Systemic inflammatory diseases
  - Systemic lupus erythematosus
  - Rheumatoid arthritis
  - Scleroderma
  - Sjögren's syndrome
  - Mixed connective disease
  - Sarcoidosis
- Electrolyte imbalance
  - Potassium or magnesium abnormalities
  - Hypophosphatemia
- Critical illness myopathy
  - Nondepolarizing neuromuscular blocking agents
  - Steroids
- Amyloid myopathy
  - Primary amyloidosis
  - Familial amyloidosis (TTR mutation)

Inherited Myopathies

Muscular Dystrophy
- Dystrophinopathy (Duchenne muscular dystrophy,Becker muscular dystrophy)
- Myotonic dystrophy 1 and 2
- Facioscapulohumeral muscular dystrophy
- Oculopharyngeal muscular dystrophy
- Limb girdle muscular dystrophy

Congenital Myopathy
- Nemaline myopathy
- Central core myopathy

Metabolic Myopathy
- Acid maltase or acid alpha-1,4-glucosidase deficiency (Pompe's disease)
- Glycogen storage disorders 3-11
- Carnitine deficiency
- Fatty acid oxidation defects
- Carnitine palmitoyl transferase deficiency

Mitochondrial Myopathy
- Myoclonic epilepsy and ragged red fibers (MERRF)
- Mitochondrial myopathy, lactic acidosis, and strokes (MELAS)
- Mitochondrial neurogastrointestinal encephalomyopathy (MNGIE)
- Progressive external ophthalmoplegia (PEO)

metabolic myopathies. Therefore, it is important to remember that a normal EMG does not exclude the presence of a myopathy.

Muscle Biopsy

Histopathologic examination of muscle may be helpful in determining the specific type of muscle disease, especially in patients with a suspected inflammatory or infectious myopathy. Selecting the optimal muscle to biopsy is very important because factors such as severe weakness and technical artifacts can hamper an accurate histologic diagnosis. The ideal muscle that should be sampled is one that is clinically involved but still antigravity in strength, because more-severe weakness can lead to unhelpful, nonspecific findings of fibrosis. Also avoid muscles that have been examined by an EMG because the needle portion of the electrical study might have caused local damage, which can result in spurious findings. Common biopsy sites include the biceps and deltoid muscles in the upper extremity and the quadriceps and gastrocnemius muscles in the lower extremity.

TREATMENT

Inherited Myopathies

For most patients with congenital myopathy or muscular dystrophy, the treatment is largely supportive, with physical therapy, occupational therapy, management of contractures, nutrition, and genetic counseling. In patients with Duchenne muscular dystrophy, treatment with prednisone at a dose of 0.75 mg/kg/day has been shown to improve strength and muscle bulk and slow the rate of natural progression of the disease. Patients should also be monitored over time for complications related to kyphoscoliosis or involvement of cardiac, respiratory, or bulbar muscles. In patients with mitochondrial myopathy, small studies have shown some benefit with creatine monohydrate (5-10 g/day), but no consistent benefit was seen with coenzyme Q10 replacement. Finally, genetic counseling should be offered to all patients with inherited myopathy and their family members.

Acquired Myopathies

Myopathies that result from systemic diseases are best treated by correcting the underlying endocrine or electrolyte abnormality. In patients with drug- or toxin-induced rhabdomyolysis, withdrawal of the offending agent is key. Control of the underlying infection is important for bacterial, parasitic, or spirochete-related myopathies as well as postinfectious inflammatory myositis. In HIV-related myositis, treatment with the combination of highly active antiretriviral therapy (HAART) and steroids may be beneficial.

In patients with inflammatory myopathies or those related to underlying autoimmune diseases, a number of immune-modulating medications may be used for treatment. Oral and intravenous steroids are most commonly used, with favorable results in most cases. Regimens of daily prednisone at a dose of 1.5 mg/kg per day or

Table 1 Clinical Features of Common Myopathies

Myopathy	Epidemiology	Distribution of Weakness	Other Systemic Manifestations
Acquired Myopathies			
Dermatomyositis	Female > male Peak incidence: children and ages 40-60 yr	Symmetrical proximal muscle weakness pelvic girdle > shoulder girdle muscles	Skin manifestations: heliotrope rash (purplish discoloration of the eyelids), Gottron's papules (erythematous scaling rash of extensor surfaces of fingers), shawl sign (erythematous rash over the shoulder and exposed areas of the back) Interstitial lung diseases Malignancy GI vasculitis
Polymyositis	Female > male predominance Peak incidence: 20-50 yr	Symmetrical proximal muscle weakness Pelvic girdle > shoulder girdle muscles	Arthralgias
Inclusion body myositis	Men Peak incidence: >50 yr	Asymmetrical quadriceps muscle weakness and finger flexor muscle weakness	Dysphagia
Hypothyroid myopathy	Affects 30%-80% of patients with hypothyroidism	Proximal symmetrical pelvic > shoulder girdle weakness Pseudohypertrophy of muscles	Peripheral neuropathy Delayed relaxation of ankle jerks Myoedema (mounding of muscle when firmly palpated)
Hyperthyroid myopathy	Affects 52%-82 % of patients with hyperthyroidism	Symmetrical proximal weakness, atrophy, some distal muscle involvement	Peripheral neuropathy Graves' ophthalmopathy, extraocular muscle weakness
Sarcoidosis myopathy	Asymptomatic muscle involvement in ≤50% sarcoidosis patients	Symmetrical proximal muscle weakness Focal muscle weakness from sarcoid granuloma	Peripheral neuropathy CNS sarcoidosis Restrictive lung disease Heart failure
Critical illness myopathy	At least as prevalent as critical illness neuropathy Affects approximately 60% of patients with prolonged ICU stay	Symmetrical proximal > distal muscle weakness	Critical illness neuropathy Failure to wean off ventilation
Amyloid myopathy	Rare	Proximal > distal muscle weakness Pseudohypertrophy of muscles Palpable muscle nodules	Macroglossia Peripheral neuropathy Autonomic involvement Restrictive cardiomyopathy
Inherited Myopathies			
Duchenne muscular dystrophy	1 in 3500 male births Age of onset <13 yr	Symmetrical proximal girdle weakness Calf psedohypertrophy Ankle contractures	Cardiomyopathy Kyphoscoliosis Cognitive impairment
Limb girdle muscular dystrophy	1 per 15,000 population	Proximal pelvic > shoulder girdle weakness Calf hypertrophy Scapular winging	Different subtypes may have variable extent of cardiomyopathy or cardiac arrhythmias, respiratory muscle weakness
Myotonic dystrophy 1 and 2 (DM1, DM2)	Approximately 2.5-5.5 per 100,000 population	Distal muscle weakness predominates in DM1; proximal muscle weakness is common in DM2 Clinical myotonia (difficulty relaxing after a forceful muscle contraction)	Cataracts Diabetes mellitus Frontal balding Cardiac arrhythmias Cholecystitis Pregnancy- and labor-related complications Eyelid ptosis without extraocular muscle weakness
Oculopharyngeal muscular dystrophy	Relatively rare	Rarely presents with distal muscle weakness	Mainly manifests with ophthalmoparesis and with bulbar weakness manifesting with dysarthria and dysphagia
Facioscapulohumeral muscular dystrophy	Approximately 4 per 100,000 population	Face and arm weakness, scapular winging, and later distal leg muscle weakness	Hearing loss Retinal telangiectasias
Mitochondrial myopathies	1 per 8000 population	Exercise intolerance Proximal girdle muscle weakness	Extraocular muscle weakness Peripheral neuropathy Migraine headaches Seizures Stroke Diabetes mellitus Cardiac arrhythmias
Acid maltase deficiency or glycogen storage disorder type 2	Approximately 1 in 40,000 newborns	Proximal girdle weakness	Macroglossia, hepatomegaly in infancy Severe ventilatory muscle weakness with adult presentation Cardiomyopathy

CNS, central nervous system; GI, gastrointestinal; ICU, intensive care unit.

Box 2 Laboratory Evaluation for Suspected Myopathy

Confirm the Presence of Muscle Disease
- Creatine phosphokinase
- Aldolase
- Liver function tests
- Lactate dehydrogenase levels

Identify Etiology
- Complete blood count with differential
- Complete metabolic panel
- Thyroid function tests
- Parathyroid hormone level
- Sedimentation rate
- C-reactive protein and antinuclear antibody panel

Suspected Inflammatory Etiology
- Myositis-specific autoantibodies
- Anti–double stranded DNA antibody
- Anti-Scl 70 antibody
- Anti-SSA and SSB antibodies
- Anti-ribonucleoprotein antibody
- Rheumatoid factor
- Anti-PM1 antibody
- Angiotensin-converting enzyme levels

Suspected Mitochondrial or Metabolic Myopathy
- Serum lactate, pyruvate, ammonia, coenzyme Q10 levels
- Ischemic forearm lactate test
- Carnitine levels

Suspected Amyloid Myopathy
- Immunofixation electrophoresis of monoclonal proteins in serum and urine

intravenous methylprednisolone at 500 to 1000 mg for 3 to 5 days are often used. Intravenous immune globulin (IVIg), methotrexate, azathioprine, and cyclophosphamide may also be helpful. Unfortunately, inclusion body myositis, though classified as an inflammatory myopathy, is typically refractory to immunosuppressant treatment and continues to progress, with prominent dysphagia and more generalized weakness over time.

Rhabdomyolysis

For patients who present with rhabdomyolysis, treatment is aimed at preventing kidney failure in the acute setting. Vigorous hydration with close monitoring of kidney function and electrolytes are paramount. In patients with an underlying metabolic myopathy, education about following a more moderate exercise program and avoiding intense exercise and fasting is necessary in preventing recurrent episodes. Measures that have been suggested to be helpful include sucrose loading before exercise in some glycogen storage disorders and a low-fat, high-carbohydrate diet in patients with lipid storage disorders.

SPECIAL CONSIDERATIONS

Statin Myopathy

The incidence of muscle symptoms in patients taking statins has ranged from 5% to 18% in large studies and are reported to be severe in 0.1%. Because statins are one of the most commonly prescribed medications worldwide, these percentages represent a significant number of affected patients. Symptoms can range from mild cramps to more-severe myalgias, pain, and weakness. Rhabdomyolysis has also been reported in rare cases. The exact mechanism by which statins cause myopathy is unknown, but mitochondrial dysfunction and decreased coenyzme Q10 levels have been postulated. Specific risk factors for the development of statin myopathy include higher

Table 2 Commercially Available Genetic Tests in Diagnosis of a Myopathy

Myopathies with Known Genetic Defects	Gene Abnormalities	Pattern of Inheritance
Duchenne muscular dystrophy	Dystrophin gene	X-linked recessive
Becker muscular dystrophy	Dystrophin gene	X-linked recessive
Emery-Dreifuss muscular dystrophy	Emerin gene	X-linked recessive
Limb girdle muscular dystrophy	Lamin A/C Calpain Dysferlin Fukutin related protein	Some are autosomal dominant and others are recessive
Facioscapulohumeral muscular dystrophy	*D4Z4* deletion	Autosomal dominant
Oculopharyngeal muscular dystrophy	GCG repeat expansion in poly A binding protein 2 gene	Autosomal dominant
Myotonic dystrophy 1 and 2	*DMPK* gene for type 1 *CNBP* (ZNF9) gene for type 2	Autosomal dominant
Mitochondrial myopathy	Specific point mutation analysis for diseases like MELAS *POLG1* sequencing for MERRF available Southern blot analysis for mtDNA deletions and mtDNA sequencing	Maternally inherited. But other can be inherited as autosomal dominant or recessive disease
Amyloid myopathy from familial causes	Transthyretin mutation	Autosomal dominant
Statin myopathy (predictor of increased susceptibility)	*SLCO1B1* gene	Unknown

MELAS, mitochondrial myopathy, lactic acidosis, and strokes; MERRF, myoclonic epilepsy and ragged red fibers; mtDNA, mitochondrial DNA.

doses, smaller body frame, liver and kidney disease, diabetes, hypothyroidism, and genetic factors that affect statin metabolism. The use of alcohol or drugs that interfere with statin metabolism, such as gemfibrozil, macrolide antibiotics, antifungals, and HIV protease inhibitors, are also noted risk factors.

Treatment depends on the patient's symptoms and CPK levels. If the CPK is less than five times normal, reassurance will suffice. If CPK levels are between 5 and 10 times normal and the patient is asymptomatic or able to tolerate the symptoms, then the statin can still be continued. However, if the symptoms are intolerable, then the statin should be discontinued until the CPK normalizes. If CPK more than 10 times normal, the statin should be discontinued until levels return to normal. In these cases, once the CPK is again normal, either the same statin can be reintroduced at a lower dosage or on alternate-day dosing, or a different type of statin such as fluvastatin or pravastatin (which have been associated with a lower incidence of myalgias due to their pharmacologic properties) can be tried. But if the CPK ever exceeds 50 times normal, or if kidney failure develops, alternative lipid-lowering strategies like low-density lipoprotein (LDL) apheresis or red yeast rice should be considered. The addition of coenzyme Q10 at a dose of 200 mg/day may also be helpful in reducing the development of statin induced myalgias.

Statins have also been shown to cause an inflammatory myopathy by altering the immune system. This type of myositis does not resolve with statin discontinuation alone and requires immunosuppressive treatments.

Critical Illness Myopathy

Patients with prolonged stays in the intensive care unit (ICU) are at risk for developing critical illness myopathy, which typically results in a flaccid quadriparesis and is often accompanied by critical illness polyneuropathy. As this is a recently coined diagnosis; information on its exact incidence is unknown. A number of studies have shown it to be equal in prevalence to critical illness polyneuropathy, which affects up to 58% of patients with prolonged ICU stays and nearly 80% of patients with multiorgan failure or septic shock. It is thought that critical illness myopathy is the result of a hypercatabolic effect on the muscle or muscle membrane. It has also been associated with the use of high-dose steroids in the ICU setting. For patients with critical illness myopathy, optimization of nutrition and the initiation of intensive physical therapy over a period of several months have shown to be beneficial.

Malignant Hyperthermia

Malignant hyperthermia is a severe reaction to anesthetic agents and depolarizing muscle-blocking agents that manifests as muscle rigidity, fever, muscle necrosis, myoglobinuria, metabolic acidosis, kidney failure, and cardiac arrhythmias. It has been highly associated with central core disease, an inherited myopathy that arises from mutations in the ryanodine receptor gene. Although it is a congenital myopathy, central core disease can manifest in childhood and adulthood. Aggressive treatment with oxygen, intensive body-cooling measures, hydration, hyperkalemia management, and dantrolene can be life saving. Patients with known central core disease and their family members should be warned about the potential risk of malignant hyperthermia preoperatively.

Summary

- Myopathy refers to skeletal and cardiac muscle dysfunction from various inherited, metabolic, inflammatory, infectious, or toxic etiologies.
- Patients typically present with proximal muscle weakness of legs more than arms, with no sensory involvement.
- Age of presentation, duration of illness, and distribution of weakness are helpful in determining the classification and etiology of myopathy.
- Serologic testing, electromyography, muscle biopsy, and genetic testing are helpful tools in identifying the presence of myopathy and determining the etiology.
- Management is largely supportive for an inherited myopathy. In acquired myopathies, treatment is targeted toward the underlying cause.
- Treatment of statin myopathies is dependent on creatine phosphokinase levels and degree of muscle symptoms. Consider lower doses when initiating statin therapy.

Suggested Readings

Ballantyne CM, Corsini A, Davidson MH, et al: Risk for myopathy with statin therapy in high-risk patients. Arch Intern Med 2003;163(5):553-564.

Jacobson TA: Toward "pain-free" statin prescribing: Clinical algorithm for diagnosis and management of myalgia. Mayo Clin Proc 2008;83:687-700.

Limaye VS, Blumbergs P, Roberts-Thomson PJ: Idiopathic inflammatory myopathies. Intern Med J 2009;39(3):179-190.

Manzur AY, Muntoni F: Diagnosis and new treatments in muscular dystrophies. J Neurol Neurosurg Psychiatry 2009;80(7):706-714.

Päivä H, Thelen KM, Van Coster R, et al: High-dose statins and skeletal muscle metabolism in humans: a randomized, controlled trial. Clin Pharmacol Ther 2005;78(1):60-68.

Soni M, Amato AA: Myopathic complications of medical disease. Semin Neurol 2009 ;29(2):163-180.

van Adel BA, Tarnopolsky MA: Metabolic myopathies: update 2009. J Clin Neuromuscul Dis 2009;10(3):97-121.

Venero CV, Thompson PD: Managing statin myopathy. Endocrinol Metab Clin North Am 2009;38(1):121-136.

Headache

Robert S. Kunkel

Many causes of headache have been described in the medical literature. In 1988, the International Headache Society published a long, detailed classification of headache, which has proved helpful for research purposes because it has led to more reproducible and reliable studies in the field of headache. This classification was updated and revised in 2004. For practical clinical purposes, however, all headaches can be classified as one of the primary headache syndromes or as a headache that is caused by or secondary to an underlying disease process or medical condition. Because primary headaches are the most common, this discussion focuses on the diagnosis and management of those syndromes.

DEFINITION

The primary headache syndromes are migraine, tension-type, and cluster headaches. Migraine and cluster headaches are episodic and recurring conditions. Tension-type headache is usually episodic but like migraine, it can become chronic, occurring daily or almost daily for more than 15 days a month.

None of these primary headaches is associated with demonstrable organic disease or structural neurologic abnormality. Laboratory and imaging test results are generally normal. Should an abnormality be found on testing, by definition, it most likely is not the cause of the headache. Similarly, the physical and neurologic examinations are also usually normal, but any abnormalities found are not related to the primary headache. During the headache attack however, cluster and migraine patients might have some abnormal clinical findings, and many patients with tension-type headache have demonstrable tightness in the cervical muscles, with limitation of neck motion, scalp tenderness, or both.

Secondary headaches are usually of recent onset and associated with abnormalities found on clinical examination. Laboratory testing or imaging studies confirm the diagnosis. Recognizing headaches related to an underlying condition or disease is critical not only because treatment of the underlying problem usually eliminates the headache but also because the condition causing the headache may be life-threatening.

PREVALENCE

Primary headaches account for more than 90% of all headache complaints, and of these, episodic tension-type headache is the most common. Almost everyone has had a headache of this type. Although chronic tension-type headache occurs in only slightly more than 2% of the population, it accounts for a large number of visits to the physician's office and missed work days.

Several epidemiologic studies conducted in various areas of the world indicate that the prevalence of migraine headache ranges from 12% to 18% of the population. Migraine is three times more common in female patients.

The prevalence of cluster headache is less certain. This uncommon condition probably affects less than 0.5% of the population but is underdiagnosed and is often believed to be a sinus problem by both patients and physicians. Cluster headache affects men five to eight times more frequently than women.

Because the three primary headache syndromes tend to begin in persons younger than 50 years, anyone older than 50 years with a recent onset of headache should have a thorough examination and testing to look for an underlying cause.

PATHOPHYSIOLOGY

The pathophysiology of migraine, cluster, and tension-type headaches is not well understood. Migraine and cluster headaches are believed to initially begin in the brain as a neurologic dysfunction, with subsequent involvement of the trigeminal nerve and cranial vessels. In cluster headache, most, but not all, sufferers have overactivity of the parasympathetic nervous system. Tension-type headache can be primarily a central neurologic disturbance similar to migraine or can occur as the result of increased cervical and pericranial muscle activity, such as caused by flexion-extension injury of the neck, poor posture, or anxiety with increased clenching or grinding of the teeth.

Migraine is an inherited condition in which there appears to be an episodic instability of the neurovascular system (where serotonin and other neurotransmitters play roles). Available serotonin might be diminished or neuronal receptors for serotonin and other neuroactive substances might at times become less sensitive to these agents. Periodically, the nuclei of the trigeminal nerve appear to become hyperactive and excitable. Efferent impulses over branches of this nerve go to the innervated cranial vessels, causing the release of substances that promote perivascular inflammation and vascular dilation. Dysfunction of other areas of the brainstem and hypothalamus account for the other associated symptoms of migraine, such as nausea, photophobia, phonophobia, and osmophobia.

As the migraine attack progresses, the inflamed perivascular structures irritate nerve endings of the trigeminal nerve and cause afferent stimuli back into the trigeminal neurons of the brain, causing them to become sensitized, and they then continue to fire off. This process is called *central sensitization.* As this cyclic process continues, the scalp becomes sore and tender to ordinary nonpainful touching. This result is called *cutaneous allodynia.*

A few retrospective studies have suggested that closure of a patent foramen ovale is associated with a marked reduction of the frequency of migraine with aura. The foramen ovale does not close at birth in about 20% to 25% of persons. How this septal defect is associated with causing or triggering migraine with aura is unknown. Double-blind studies of catheter closure (or a sham procedure) of patent foramen ovales in migraineurs have been inconclusive.

Cluster headache also is an episodic neuronal dysfunction but more likely involves areas in the hypothalamus rather than the brainstem. There is also a marked increase in blood flow through the internal carotid artery on the headache side during the attack of pain.

SIGNS AND SYMPTOMS

Migraine

Most migraine patients do not have an aura; migraine with aura occurs in only 15% to 20% of sufferers. The aura is a well-defined visual or neurologic deficit lasting less than 1 hour and is followed by the headache within 1 hour. Most auras are visual, with photopsia (flashing lights) being most common. The aura is initially small, then enlarges or moves across the visual field. A typical migraine aura can occur without a headache. This phenomenon tends to occur later in life. Occasionally, a neurologic aura occurs, with a tingling or weakness that slowly spreads up or down an extremity.

Many patients with migraine have prodromal symptoms for many hours or even a day or so before the onset of an attack.

These prodromal symptoms are generally changes in mood or personality. Fatigue also is common, and occasionally hyperactivity occurs.

The migraine attack lasts 6 to 72 hours. The pounding, throbbing pain of moderate to severe intensity is generally unilateral, but some patients experience bilateral pain. Pain caused by migraine worsens with physical activity. Photophobia and phonophobia are very common, and sensitivity to odors is a little less common. Migraine is a sick headache. Nausea occurs in most patients, and vomiting is very common. Dehydration can occur, which increases the pain and disability. Migraineurs want to be quiet, inactive, and in a darkened area during the attack. Approximately 60% of women experience their worst migraine attacks in conjunction with their menstrual period.

Tension-Type Headache

Tension-type headache is characterized by generalized pressure or a sensation of tightness in the head. The discomfort level is usually mild to moderate and does not worsen with activity. Although nausea and photophobia or phonophobia can occur, they generally are not prominent features. Tension-type headache is classified as episodic (<15 days a month) or chronic (>15 days a month).

Some patients with tension-type headache exhibit evidence of increased muscle tension, with prominent scalp tenderness, muscle tenderness in the temporomandibular joint muscles, or tight, tender cervical and trapezius muscles. Poor posture is often evident, which can play a role in causing tension-type headache. If there is no evidence of increased pericranial or cervical muscle tightness (no tenderness or limitation of motion in the neck) found during clinical examination, the pain likely originates centrally or is due to psychological factors.

Cluster Headache

Cluster headache causes intense pain that is generally steady and boring behind one eye. The pain can spread to the temple, face, and even into the upper neck. It is so intense that most sufferers pace the floor or do vigorous exercises during the attack. The attacks are short (usually less than 3 hours in duration) and often last only 30 to 45 minutes. They occur from one to several times a day for a period of several weeks or months, then remit, leaving the patient pain free for several months or years, only to recur.

During a cluster headache cycle, the attacks of pain often occur at the same time each day, most often waking the patient in the early morning hours. Eighty percent of cluster sufferers experience unilateral tearing, with conjunctival injection and ipsilateral nasal congestion. These symptoms clear as the attack leaves. Alcohol brings on an attack within a few minutes in a patient who is in a cluster headache cycle, but it does not induce an attack when the patient is in remission.

Chronic Daily Headache

Daily headache can occur as a chronic tension-type headache, but it is often a combination of tension-type and migraine (the type seen most often in headache clinics). This type of combination headache is not listed in the official classification, so one should diagnose both chronic tension-type headache and migraine in these patients. Most often, this type of combination or mixed headache develops in a person who initially had typical episodic migraine but in whom, over several years, a chronic daily or almost-daily headache develops. Many times, this daily headache seems to occur because of the frequent use of analgesics, especially opiate compounds and those combined with caffeine or butalbital. A daily or near-daily migraine headache can occur from the frequent use of ergotamine tartrate or any of the triptan drugs. This headache pattern has been called rebound headache or medication overuse headache.

Secondary Headache

Secondary headache may be caused by many different diseases. However, neurologic symptoms and signs are almost always present before there is significant headache in patients who have a mass lesion in the brain.

Temporal arteritis generally occurs in persons older than 50 years and may be associated with any type of headache. The pain of temporal arteritis is typically not throbbing and, although it is usually situated in the temples, can be nonlocalized. Fatigue and a low-grade fever are often present. The erythrocyte sedimentation rate is high, usually greater than 60 mm/hour. Diagnosis is confirmed by a temporal artery biopsy, which shows giant cell inflammation. Treatment should begin with 60 to 80 mg of prednisone per day as soon as the diagnosis is suspected, even before the confirmation by biopsy. One study suggested that methotrexate may be effective in allowing treatment with a lower dose of steroids, whereas another study did not show any benefit of adding this drug. If not treated, 20% to 30% of patients with this disease develop permanent partial or complete visual loss in the affected eye. Therefore, prompt treatment is essential.

Aneurysms do not cause chronic recurring headache unless they compress a cranial nerve. They manifest with a severe pain at the time of rupture. Occasionally, an arteriovenous malformation mimics migraine, particularly if it is located in the occipital lobe, but these lesions are more apt to cause seizures or to bleed. Headaches with a postural component need to be evaluated to exclude a lesion in the posterior fossa or a condition with low CSF pressure.

Pericranial inflammation such as a sinus infection, an ear infection, or dental disease should be evident on examination and is usually of a more recent, acute onset. Sleep apnea may be a factor in waking headaches. Systemic conditions such as endocrine disorders, anemia, sepsis, and hypertension can be associated with a non localized headache, but more often such conditions exacerbate an underlying migraine or tension-type headache.

DIAGNOSIS

The diagnosis of one of the primary headache syndromes is based on the history of the condition and the symptoms described by the patient. After talking with the patient, the clinician should have a fairly good idea of what type of headache the person is experiencing and whether it is one of the primary types or due to some underlying neurologic or medical condition.

Any abnormal physical or neurologic examination findings must be investigated. Laboratory studies may be useful in excluding metabolic or endocrine factors that might play a role. A high erythrocyte sedimentation rate in a patient older than 50 years with new headache onset suggests temporal arteritis. This diagnosis must be confirmed by temporal artery biopsy. Scans can be performed to exclude intracranial causes of headache or to rule out lesions that cause neurologic or visual abnormalities associated with headache. Computed tomography scanning of the paranasal sinuses is useful in evaluating the role of acute or chronic sinus infection as a cause of the headache. Magnetic resonance imaging is currently the best scan for viewing the posterior fossa and occipital areas of the brain.

Summary

- The diagnosis of the headache type is most often made by the history of symptoms.
- Headaches caused by disease are usually of recent onset and usually manifest with abnormalities on examination and abnormal tests.
- Look for an underlying condition in a headache that occurs for the first time in a patient older than 40 years.
- Consider temporal arteritis in any new headache beginning after age 50 years.

TREATMENT

Most patients with a primary headache require medication; however, other management methods also may be useful. Secondary headaches usually resolve when the underlying neurologic or systemic problem is treated.

MIGRAINE

Treatment

Some migraine headaches can be relieved with the use of cold packs, pressure on the temple, and sleep. However, most patients require abortive medication, and many are candidates for daily preventive medication.

Educating the migraine patient to recognize and avoid headache triggers helps to reduce the frequency of attacks. Common migraine triggers include weather changes, the estrogen cycle, bright lights, strong odors, stress, "let down" after stress, foods, food additives, and fasting or skipping meals. Migraineurs do better and have fewer headaches by following regular eating and sleeping patterns.

Preventive Medications

Daily prophylactic medication should be considered whenever migraine attacks occur several times a month or are very severe and do not respond well to abortive medication. Essentially six classifications of drugs are useful for migraine prophylaxis: beta blockers, calcium channel blockers, nonsteroidal anti-inflammatory drugs (NSAIDs), antidepressants, antiepileptic drugs, and the serotonin agonist methysergide maleate (Table 1). The beta blockers propranolol and timolol maleate, the anticonvulsants divalproex sodium and topiramate, and methysergide currently are the only drugs approved by the U.S. Food and Drug Administration for migraine prevention. (Methysergide is no longer available in the United States). A few other anticonvulsants such as gabapentin, tiagabine, and pregabalin are useful for neuralgic type of pain and are being evaluated for their effectiveness in preventing migraine but they seem to be less effective in migraine. They have been extensively used off label clinically for migraine prevention. Botulinum toxin type A injected into the scalp muscles has also been found to decrease the frequency and severity of migraine in about 50% of patients so treated. It has not been shown to be very effective in tension-type headaches.

Abortive Medications

All migraine patients with migraine need to take an abortive drug, whether or not they are taking a prophylactic agent (Table 2). For mild attacks, over-the-counter analgesics (especially those containing caffeine) may be useful. A large dose of a rapid-acting NSAID such as meclofenamate, ibuprofen, diclofenac, or naproxen sodium can also prove helpful in mild attacks.

A revolutionary breakthrough in acute migraine treatment occurred with the development of sumatriptan succinate in the late 1980s. The triptan drugs are agonists that affect the 1B and 1D serotonin receptors located in neurons and cerebral vessels. Seven triptan agents are currently available in the United States: sumatriptan succinate (oral, nasal, and injectable), rizatriptan benzoate (oral), zolmitriptan (oral and nasal), naratriptan (oral), almotriptan (oral), frovatriptan (oral), and eletriptan (oral). All are very well tolerated by patients; however, like ergotamine, the triptans should not be used in patients with coronary artery disease, peripheral vascular disease, or uncontrolled hypertension. Triptan drugs are effective in 65% to 70% of patients, completely or significantly relieving migraine pain and associated symptoms within 2 hours of administration. The earlier they are taken in the attack, the more effective they seem to be. Side effects are generally mild, the most common being dizziness,

Table 1 Prophylactic Migraine Drugs

Drug	Usual Daily Dose
Beta Blockers	
Atenolol	50-100 mg
Metoprolol succcinate or tartrate	50-150 mg
Nadolol	20-160 mg
Propranolol	80-240 mg
Timolol maleate	10-20 mg
Calcium Channel Blockers	
Amlodipine besylate	10-20 mg
Diltiazem	80-240 mg
Nimodipine	60-120 mg
Verapamil	180-480 mg
Antiepileptic Drugs	
Divalproex sodium	250-1500 mg
Gabapentin	300-1800 mg
Pregabalin	50-200 mg
Topiramate	25-150 mg
Zonisamide	100-200 mg
Antidepressants	
Amitriptyline	25-150 mg
Citalopram	20-60 mg
Desipramine	25-100 mg
Doxepin	25-150 mg
Duloxetine	30-90 mg
Fluoxetine	20-60 mg
Nortriptyline	25-100 mg
Phenelzine	15-45 mg
Protriptyline	5-10 mg
Sertraline	50-150 mg
Venlafaxine	37.5-150 mg
Nonsteroidal Anti-inflammatory Drugs	
Celecoxib	200-400 mg
Flurbiprofen	100-200 mg
Indomethacin	75-150 mg
Naproxen sodium	500-1000 mg
Serotonin Agonist	
Methysergide maleate	2-8 mg
Antiserotonin/Antihistamine	
Cyproheptadine	4-12 mg

Table 2 Migraine Abortive Agents

Drug	Usual Dosage
Combination Drug	
Isometheptene/ dichloralphenazone/ acetaminophen	Two capsules at onset, then one or two in 1 hr
Anti-inflammatory Drugs	
Ibuprofen	600-800 mg q 4 hr prn
Ketorolac tromethamine oral	10 mg, repeat once in 2 hr prn
Ketorolac tromathamine IV/IM	30 mg, repeat once in 1 to 2 hr prn
Meclofenamate sodium	200 mg, repeat once in 2 hr prn
Naproxen sodium	550 mg, repeat once in 2 hr prn
Triptan Drugs	
Almotriptan	12.5 mg, repeat once in 2 hr prn
Eletriptan	40 mg, repeat once in 2 hr prn
Frovatriptan	2.5 mg, repeat once in 2 hr prn
Naratriptan	2.5 mg, repeat once in 3- 4 hr prn
Rizatriptan	10 mg, repeat once in 2 hrs prn
Sumatriptan, oral	50-100 mg, repeat once in 2 hr prn
Sumatriptan, nasal	20 mg (1 puff), repeat once in 2 hr
Sumatriptan, subcutaneous	6 mg, repeat once in 2 hr prn
Zolmitriptan, oral	2.5 mg or 5 mg, repeat once in 2 hr prn
Zolmitriptan, nasal	2.5 mg or 5 mg (1 puff), repeat in 2 hr prn
Triptan/NSAID	
Sumatriptan/naproxen 85 mg/500mg at onset and repeat in 2 hs prn	
Ergotamine Drugs	
Dihydroergotamine mesylate, nasal	1 puff in each nostril, repeat in 15 min. This is the dose for 1 day
Dihydroergotamine mesylate, IV, IM, and SC	0.5-1 mg, repeat in 1 hr. Maximium dose is 3 mg in 24 hr
Ergotamine tartrate/ caffeine, oral	2 tabs at onset, repeat once every 0.5 hr up to a maximum of 5 tabs
Ergotamine tartrate/ caffeine, suppository	1/2 to 1 at onset, repeat once in 1 hr
Ergotamine tartrate, sublingual	1 at onset, repeat once in 0.5 hr prn

sedation, or mild upper chest tightness that is noncardiac in origin. Unfortunately, headache recurs within 24 hours in up to 30% of users, necessitating an additional dose.

The triptans and other abortive agents are more effective when used early in the migraine attack before central sensitization and the subsequent cutaneous allodynia become established. Combined use of an NSAID with a triptan can offer better headache relief and may be associated with less-frequent recurrence of the migraine. A combination of sumatriptan and naproxen is now available.

Other effective agents available by prescription include a combination of isometheptene mucate, dichloralphenazone, and acetaminophen; ergotamine tartrate (sublingual) or ergotamine tartrate combined with caffeine (oral, suppository) and dihydroergotamine mesylate used parentally or as a nasal spray.

Several parenteral non-narcotic medications have been shown to be very useful in aborting severe migraine attacks. Intravenous dihydroergotamine, prochlorperazine, divalproex, magnesium, ketorolac tromethamine, and steroids can be very effective in stopping a migraine attack without resorting to narcotics.

At times, a rescue medication such as an opiate or a butalbital combination drug may be needed, but with the large number of nonhabituating preparations available, the need to use such drugs is much less now than in the past.

Oral abortive agents, especially the ergotamines, often aggravate nausea and vomiting, which can limit their use. However, taking metoclopramide before taking an abortive agent can control the nausea and enhance the effectiveness of the abortive drug. Other antinausea agents also may be helpful, including prochlorperazine, hydroxyzine pamoate, promethazine, or trimethobenzamide.

Tension-Type Headache

The occasional tension-type headache can be alleviated by a hot shower, massage, sleep, and patient recognition and avoidance of stress factors. Episodic tension-type headache is usually well treated with analgesics such as aspirin, acetaminophen, and NSAIDs or combinations of these agents with caffeine or sedating medications. Some patients, particularly those with tension-type headache caused by stress, benefit from learning relaxation techniques or biofeedback training. An active physical therapy program can decrease chronic neck pain caused by increased cervical muscle spasm or postural abnormalities. When tension-type headache becomes chronic, treatment can be challenging, especially if the patient overuses analgesics and opiates. Treatment will not be effective until the patient stops the frequent use of these acute pain-relieving agents. Patients suffering from chronic tension-type headache often need counselling and psychotherapy to help define and work through long-standing psychological issues.

The most effective group of drugs for the treatment of chronic tension-type headaches is the tricyclic antidepressants. Amitriptyline, doxepin, and nortriptyline are most commonly used. They are usually taken at bedtime because of their sedating effects. Morning sedation, weight gain, dry mouth, and constipation are common side effects. Less-sedating drugs in this group include desipramine and protriptyline. Selective serotonin reuptake inhibitors, such as fluoxetine, sertraline, paroxetine, and citalopram, are better tolerated and have fewer side effects than the tricyclics, but they do not appear to be as effective in easing headache unless the headache is a manifestation of underlying depression. Venlafaxine and duloxetine are both serotonin and norepinephrine uptake inhibitors and may be helpful in chronic pain conditions, including headache. Muscle relaxants such as cyclobenzaprine, orphenadrine citrate, and baclofen may be helpful at times, particularly if increased muscle spasm is present. The central-acting muscle relaxant tizanidine is often quite effective in treating chronic headache, either tension-type or coexisting migraine and tension-type, but it is very sedating.

Cluster Headache

Because the onset of cluster headache attacks is rapid and they can occur several times a day, the best approach to treatment is with daily preventive drugs. Effective prophylactic medications include verapamil, prednisone, lithium carbonate, methysergide, and the antiepileptic drugs divalproex and topiramate. High doses of verapamil

(480-720 mg/day) may be necessary. A pretreatment EKG is recommended prior to starting a large dose of verapamil. Prednisone and methysergide work quickly and often are used with verapamil or lithium initially for a quick response and then tapered while the verapamil or lithium is continued. Prednisone is usually prescribed at 60 mg/day initially and then tapered over 2 to 3 weeks. There are a few reports that topiramate, divalproex, and baclofen are helpful in cluster headache, but no controlled studies have been published, and clinically these drugs do not appear to be effective very often.

Oxygen 100% by mask at a flow rate of 8 to 10 L/min for up to 10 minutes aborts an acute cluster headache in 50% to 60% of patients. Ergotamine tartrate, dihydroergotamine, and any of the triptans usually are very effective, but they are inappropriate in patients who suffer several attacks a day. Fortunately, cluster headache patients do not appear to develop rebound headaches from frequent use of ergotamine tartrate or the triptans, as do migraine sufferers.

Methysergide is the only drug approved in the United States for treating cluster headache, but it is no longer on the market. It is not used very often because of the possible development of retroperitoneal fibrosis or other fibrotic complications. Methysergide should not be used for longer than 4 to 6 months without giving the patient a 4- to 6-week drug holiday. Once the patient is free of cluster attacks for a few weeks, the prophylactic drugs should be tapered and discontinued. They can be restarted at the onset of the next cluster.

Summary

- Help migraine sufferers identify and avoid possible triggers.
- Prophylactic medications are underused in migraine. They can greatly reduce the frequency and severity of migraine attacks.
- Migraine abortive drugs work best when taken early in the attack.
- Cluster patients should take preventive medications early in the cluster.

OUTCOMES

Although few long-term follow-up studies have been conducted, some studies indicate that inpatient treatment of chronic headache sufferers is associated with approximately a 50% improvement rate. Comprehensive outpatient treatment programs are now being used by many headache clinics; however, definitive outcome data are not yet available. Patients in these programs usually are suffering from chronic daily headaches and medication overuse. Most programs include detoxification from analgesics and narcotics and the initiation of preventive medicines as well as psychotherapy, physical therapy, and teaching relaxation and biofeedback techniques, along with educating patients to recognize triggers and be aware of possible factors involved in causing their headaches.

Studies have demonstrated that patients with acute migraine attacks treated with a triptan experience a reduction in visits to the doctor's office and emergency department as well as fewer days lost at work. Treatment of migraine with the newer, more-pecific drugs such as the triptans has greatly reduced the disability associated with this condition.

Comprising representatives of seven organizations, the U.S. Headache Consortium has published evidence-based guidelines for treating migraine headaches based on a review of the literature. These guidelines are an attempt to evaluate the validity of studies done with various abortive and preventive drugs and to rate the effectiveness of these drugs based on those studies in the literature. Non pharmacologic treatments of migraine are also evaluated and rated.

Suggested Readings

American Academy of Neurology: Guideline summary for clinicians: Migraine headache. PDF available at http://www.aan.com/professionals/practice/guidelines/migraine/clinician_summary_migraine.pdf (accessed March 20, 2009).

Diamond S, Freitag FG, Maliszewski M: Inpatient treatment of headache: Long-term results. Headache 1986;26:189-197.

Gillies JD, Lance JW: Pathophysiology of migraine. In Tollison CD, Kunkel RS (eds): Headache: Diagnosis and Treatment. Baltimore, Williams & Wilkins, 1993, pp 77-84.

Hagen K, Zwart JA, Vatten L, et al: Prevalence of migraine and non-migrainous headache-head-HUNT, a large population-based study. Cephalalgia 2000;20:900-906.

Headache Classification Subcommittee of the International Headache Society. The international classification of headache disorders, 2nd ed. Cephalalgia 2004:24(Suppl 1):1-160; PDF available at http://216.25.100.131/ihscommon/guidelines/pdfs/ihc_II_main_no_print.pdf (accessed December 12, 2007).

Jover JA, Hernandez-Garcia C, Morado IC, et al: Combined treatment of giant-cell arteritis with methotrexate and prednisone: A randomized, double-blind, placebo-controlled trial. Ann Intern Med 2001;134:106-114.

Lofland JH, Johnson NE, Batenhorst AS, Nash DB: Changes in resource use and outcomes for patients with migraine treated with sumatriptan: A managed care perspective. Arch Intern Med 1999;159:857-863.

Reisman M, Christofferson RD, Jesurum J, et al: Migraine headache relief after transcatheter closure of patent foramen ovale. J Am Coll Cardiol 2005;45:493-495.

Schwartz BS, Stewart WF, Simon D, Lipton RB: Epidemiology of tension-type headache. JAMA 1998;279:381-383.

Silberstein SD: Migraine pathophysiology and its clinical implications. Cephalalgia 2004:24(Suppl 2):2-7.

Silberstein SD: Practice parameter: Evidence-based guidelines for migraine headache (an evidence-based review): Report of the Quality Standards Subcommittee of the American Academy of Neurology. Neurology 2000;55:754-762.

Silberstein S, Mathew N, Saper J, Jenkins S: Botulinum toxin type A as a migraine preventive treatment. Headache 2000;40:445-450.

Stewart WF, Lipton RB, Celentano DD, Reed ML: Prevalence of migraine headache in the United States. Relation to age, income, race, and other sociodemographic factors. JAMA 1992;267:64-69.

Sleep Disorders

Li Ling Lim and Nancy Foldvary-Schaefer

DEFINITION

Sleep is a normal recurring state of loss of responsiveness to the external environment, now known to be an active physiologic state involving dynamic changes in neural, metabolic, and cardiorespiratory function rather than a passive state that ensues in the absence of wakefulness. Sleep disorders encompass a wide range of conditions that have been most recently categorized in the *International Classification of Sleep Disorders, Second Edition (ICSD-2)*.[1] The ICSD-2 lists more than 80 distinct sleep disorders sorted into eight categories, including the insomnias, sleep-related breathing disorders, hypersomnias of central origin, circadian rhythm sleep disorders, parasomnias, and sleep-related movement disorders.

PATHOPHYSIOLOGY

Normal sleep and wake states are generated by a complex neuronal network in the brain and are regulated by homeostatic and circadian mechanisms. Sleep may be divided into two main stages: rapid eye movement (REM) and non-REM (NREM) sleep. REM sleep is also known as paradoxical sleep, because it resembles wakefulness with desynchronized electroencephalography (EEG) activity, phasic events such as rapid eye movements, and bursts of muscle activity and is characterized by dreaming. NREM sleep is characterized by synchronized EEG activity, muscle relaxation, and decreased heart rate, blood pressure, and tidal volume.

Sleep homeostasis refers to the regulatory mechanism that maintains an overall constancy of sleep intensity and duration. Sleep deprivation creates a sleep debt that must be paid back, resulting in compensatory heightened pressure to sleep and eventual increased sleep intensity and duration. Conversely, excessive sleep reduces sleep propensity and amount of sleep.

Sleep physiology changes with age as the brain matures and eventually degenerates. With advancing age, there is decline in the percentage of deep sleep, more frequent awakenings, and sleep fragmentation. In the elderly, sleep disorders such as obstructive sleep apnea (OSA) occur more frequently. Sleep needs also vary with age, decreasing from 16 hours a day in infancy and stabilizing at 7½ to 8 hours for most normal adults.

SIGNS AND SYMPTOMS

A suggested practical approach when assessing patients with sleep-related disturbances is to elicit symptoms and signs according to the three cardinal clinical presentations of sleep disorders: insomnia, excessive daytime sleepiness, and abnormal movements or behavior in sleep.

Insomnia

Patients with insomnia most commonly describe difficulty with falling asleep and, less commonly, difficulty maintaining sleep or a perception of unrefreshing sleep. Regardless of the cause, insomnia often results in daytime fatigue, general malaise, and in severe cases, cognitive and mood disturbances.

Chronic insomnia often affects social and occupational functioning and diminishes quality of life. In patients with insomnia related to medical and psychiatric conditions, associated symptoms include chronic pain or other physical discomfort, depression, anxiety, and often, psychosocial stressors. Neurodegenerative disorders such as Parkinson's disease and dementia are commonly associated with sleep disturbance. Medications such as steroids, bronchodilators, and some antidepressants can cause insomnia, so a careful drug history is important. Chronic insomnia is often multifactorial, encompassing components related to psychophysiologic issues, drugs, and underlying disease, as well as maladaptive behavioral aspects.

Inadequate sleep hygiene, a common problem of patients with chronic insomnia, is classified in ICSD-2 as a distinct insomnia diagnosis. This term refers to a range of well-recognized sleep-incompatible behavior, which include excessive use of substances that disrupt sleep (e.g., caffeine, nicotine, alcohol), mentally or physically arousing activities close to bedtime, excessive napping or time in bed, irregular sleep-wake times, and preoccupation with sleep difficulty.

Excessive Daytime Sleepiness

Excessive daytime sleepiness refers to the inability to stay alert during the major awake period of the day, resulting in falling asleep at inappropriate times. Excessive daytime sleepiness is more likely to occur in monotonous situations when alerting stimuli are absent, and it is associated with increased risk of accidents, such as when operating motor vehicles or other machinery. The severity of sleepiness can be quantified subjectively using scales such as the Epworth Sleepiness Scale (Box 1) or can be measured objectively in the sleep laboratory using the multiple sleep latency test (MSLT) or maintenance of wakefulness test (MWT).[2] The MSLT measures the physiologic tendency to fall asleep in quiet situations, and the MWT measures the ability to stay awake in quiet situations.

Abnormal Movements or Behavior in Sleep

These encompass the NREM and REM parasomnias, sleep-related movement disorders (mainly restless leg syndrome [RLS] and periodic limb movement disorder [PLMD]), and sleep-related epilepsy. The NREM parasomnias are disorders of arousal seen usually in the pediatric population and include confusional arousals, sleepwalking, and sleep terrors. The REM parasomnias include nightmare disorder and REM sleep behavior disorder (RBD). Although the synchronized state of NREM sleep facilitates epileptic activity in general, some epileptic syndromes have a marked tendency to manifest predominantly during sleep and must be distinguished from the parasomnias, which usually requires EEG documentation of epileptiform discharges. Epileptic phenomena are characterized by repetitive stereotypic behavior, but they can be difficult to distinguish clinically from nonepileptic phenomena.

DIAGNOSIS

Most sleep disorders can be diagnosed by a comprehensive sleep history, which includes a detailed account of routine sleep-related habits (e.g. bedtime, wake time, number of awakenings), sleep duration, sleeping environment, daytime activities, psychosocial stressors, current drug use, and abnormal behavior in sleep. Important collateral information is often provided by a bed partner or other observer or family member regarding behavior that the patient may be unaware of, such as snoring or acting out dreams. Sleep questionnaires detailing pertinent sleep-related information and sleep logs are often useful, especially in documenting sleep-wake patterns in the circadian-rhythm sleep disorders.

The Epworth Sleepiness Scale is often used to assess the level of daytime sleepiness and to monitor the response to therapeutic

Box 1 Epworth Sleepiness Scale

How likely are you to doze off or fall asleep in the following situations, in contrast to feeling just tired? This refers to your usual way of life in recent times. Even if you have not done some of these things recently try to work out how they would have affected you.

Use the following scale to choose the most appropriate number for each situation:

0 = no chance of dozing
1 = slight chance of dozing
2 = moderate chance of dozing
3 = high chance of dozing

Sitting and reading
Watching TV
Sitting inactive in a public place (e.g a theater or a meeting)
As a passenger in a car for an hour without a break
Lying down to rest in the afternoon when circumstances permit
Sitting and talking to someone
Sitting quietly after a lunch without alcohol
In a car, while stopped for a few minutes in traffic

interventions.[2] A score of 10 or more is considered sleepy. Diagnosis of most sleep disorders can be made on the medical history alone, based on pattern recognition of clinical characteristics determined from the comprehensive sleep history and a physical examination.

Sleep Disorders Manifesting with Insomnia

Patients with sleep-onset difficulty might have one of the insomnias as classified in ICSD 2. RLS should be considered, and a careful history should be taken to rule out drugs and underlying medical problems that cause insomnia. The circadian rhythm disorders are less-common causes of sleep-onset insomnia. Also uncommon are sleep-maintenance problems alone causing unrefreshing sleep (without snoring or marked excessive daytime sleepiness) due to OSA or abnormal behavior in sleep. These strikingly abnormal sleep phenomena are usually evident from the history.

Psychophysiologic Insomnia

Psychophysiologic insomnia, also known as primary insomnia, occurs in about 12% to 15% of patients seen at sleep disorders clinics and affects 1% to 2% of the general population. It is characterized by a physiologic heightened arousal state that predisposes to learned sleep-preventing associations, usually in the setting of social and environmental psychosocial stressors. Persons with psychophysiologic insomnia are typically light or poor sleepers and can develop chronic insomnia after an initial episode of acute insomnia that failed to resolve following a precipitating stressful event. A counterproductive overconcern with sleep and the consequences of lack of sleep ensue, leading to a mental hyperarousal state (racing mind) and a form of conditioned insomnia associated with the person's habitual bedtime rituals and sleeping environment. Such patients typically report sleeping better while away from home and their usual routines, such as on vacation or during a business trip. This form of insomnia is often perpetuated because habits incompatible with healthy sleep develop, such as excessive time in bed tossing and turning, watching the clock, intense preoccupation with sleep, and abuse of prescription sleep aids. It is also associated with an increased risk of depression and dependence on hypnotics.

Insomnia Due to Mental Disorder

Insomnia due to underlying psychopathology (usually depression or anxiety) is one of the most frequently encountered problems at sleep disorders clinics, affecting about 3% of the general population, more in women and the middled-aged. Insomnia may be a presenting symptom in a variety of psychiatric conditions, including mood, anxiety, psychotic, and personality disorders.[3]

Insomnia is the most common sleep disturbance associated with major depression, seen in 80% to 85% of patients, usually manifesting as recurrent or early morning awakenings. In anxiety disorders, difficulty falling asleep is more typical and accompanies excessive worrying about a range of activities or events. In contrast to psychophysiologic insomnia, where anxiety is typically focused on sleep difficulty alone, patients with anxiety disorder manifest more pervasive anxiety symptoms attributable to a broader range of reasons. In this diagnostic category, which can closely resemble psychophysiologic insomnia, the underlying mental disorder plays a key role in the insomnia, with greater persistence and severity of the mood or anxiety disorder.

Adjustment Insomnia

Adjustment or acute insomnia refers to sleep disturbance of relatively short duration (<3 months) caused by an identifiable stressor. The 1-year prevalence of adjustment insomnia is estimated to be about 15% to 20% and is more common in women and older adults. The sleep disturbance can occur after positive or negative events, such as getting a new job, an unexpected windfall, work stress, bereavement, or relationship problems, and is expected to resolve once the acute stressor is removed or when the person has adapted to the triggering circumstances.

Jet Lag Disorder

Jet lag disorder is a temporary condition that occurs after air travel across at least two time zones. Symptoms of insomnia (or excessive daytime sleepiness) occur because the endogenous circadian clock is initially misaligned with the external environment. Besides insomnia, associated symptoms can include general malaise and gastrointestinal upset.

Shift-Work Disorder

Shift workers who have to work during the body's usual sleep period as determined by the endogenous circadian clock often complain of sleep-onset insomnia in the morning after the night shift (and conversely, excessive sleepiness when working at night). Shift-work disorder is usually evident from a careful review of the work schedule and typically resolves when the sleep period is restored to a conventional time. Like most circadian rhythm disorders, the diagnosis can be made from history.

Sleep Disorders Manifesting with Excessive Daytime Sleepiness

The most common nonpathologic cause of daytime sleepiness is probably volitional lack of adequate sleep. Habitual sleep duration should be part of the sleep history, and sleeping less than 4 to 5 hours is generally insufficient to maintain normal daytime alertness. The most common cause of excessive daytime sleepiness seen in sleep disorders clinics is OSA. Narcolepsy and the other hypersomnias of central origin are less common.

Obstructive Sleep Apnea

OSA is characterized by recurrent episodes of complete (apneas) or partial (hypopneas) upper airway obstruction during sleep, often associated with oxygen desaturation and recurrent arousals, which are usually quantifiable and confirmed on polysomnography (PSG). The prevalence of OSA syndrome (OSAS, PSG confirmation in the presence of excessive daytime sleepiness) is estimated to be about 4% in men and 2% in women. Risk factors are obesity and craniofacial abnormalities that narrow the upper airway, such as retrognathia or adenotonsillar enlargement. Other risk factors are a large neck circumference, menopause, smoking, and endocrine disorders like hypothyroidism and acromegaly. OSA has been associated with hypertension, ischemic heart disease, stroke, and diabetes. The classic history that often suggests the diagnosis of OSAS includes snoring, excessive daytime sleepiness, witnessed apneas and choking/gasping episodes and unrefreshing sleep regardless of duration, typically (but not always) in an obese or overweight person. Confirmation of diagnosis is by PSG showing at least 5 apneas or hypopneas per hour (an apnea-hypopnea index [AHI] ≥5).

Narcolepsy

Narcolepsy is a rare hypersomnia of central origin affecting 0.02% to 0.18% of Western populations, with onset usually in adolescence or young adulthood (ages 15-25 years). It is characterized by excessive daytime sleepiness, cataplexy, often irresistible sleep attacks, sleep paralysis (transient inability to move or speak) and hypnagogic or hypnopompic hallucinations (usually vivid audiovisual phenomena that occur upon falling to sleep or waking up). Classically, patients with narcolepsy report short, refreshing naps, usually followed by 2 to 3 hours of alertness. Not all narcoleptic patients report cataplexy, the hallmark of narcolepsy, which refers to a sudden loss of muscle tone provoked by strong emotions such as laughter or anger, with preserved consciousness. These patients form a subgroup listed in ICSD-2 as "narcolepsy without cataplexy."

Although a diagnosis can be made by clinical history in typical cases with all the classic features, PSG with MSLT is usually performed to rule out other common causes of excessive daytime sleepiness, like OSA. The MSLT usually shows a short sleep-onset latency (<8 min.) and sleep-onset REM periods (SOREMPs), which refers to the abnormal appearance of REM sleep (usually seen 90 to 120 minutes into sleep) in a 20-minute nap.

Idiopathic Hypersomnia

This form of hypersomnia is characterized by excessive daytime sleepiness which occurs at a young age, usually before age 25 years, and is distinguished from narcolepsy by the absence of cataplexy and other narcolepsy-associated phenomena (e.g., sleep paralysis, hypnagogic hallucinations). Also unlike narcoleptics, who take short refreshing naps, idiopathic hypersomnia patients have long, unrefreshing daytime sleep episodes. On MSLT, such patients also do not have SOREMPs, which are seen in narcolepsy.

Circadian Rhythm Sleep Disorders

In addition to insomnia, this group of disorders, which include shift-work, jet-lag disorders and advanced sleep phase disorder can also manifest with excessive daytime sleepiness. Advanced sleep phase disorder is in seen in about 1% of middle-aged and older adults and is characterized by sleep-wake times that are several hours earlier than conventional or desired times. There is a stable advance of the habitual sleep period, such as sleeping at 6 PM and waking at 2 AM. Such patients complain of excessive daytime sleepiness in the late afternoon and early evening and spontaneous early-morning awakenings.

Sleep Disorders Manifesting with Abnormal Movements or Behavior in Sleep

Restless Legs Syndrome

RLS is a clinical diagnosis based on fulfilling four essential criteria originally proposed in 1995 by the International RLS Study Group and modified in 2002.[4] The four essential criteria for RLS are:

- An urge to move the legs, usually accompanied or caused by uncomfortable and unpleasant sensations in the legs
- The urge to move or unpleasant sensations begin or worsen during periods of rest or inactivity such as lying or sitting
- The urge to move or unpleasant sensations are partially or totally relieved by movement, such as walking or stretching, at least as long as the activity continues
- The urge to move or unpleasant sensations are worse in the evening or at night than during the day or only occur in the evening or at night

RLS affects 5% to 15% of caucasion populations and women more often than men. Sensorimotor symptoms predominate at bedtime and give rise to sleep-onset insomnia. RLS is associated with periodic limb movements in sleep (PLMS) in 80% to 90% of cases, which can contribute to sleep maintenance problems if these are associated with arousals. RLS may be idiopathic or may be related to iron deficiency, peripheral neuropathy, uremia, or pregnancy. The diagnosis is usually straightforward in patients with prominent sensory symptoms (usually in the legs) during wakefulness before sleep onset, which fulfill the clinical diagnostic criteria listed above.

RLS is often confused with periodic limb movement disorder (PLMD), which is a disorder manifesting in sleep rather than wake, causing sleep-maintenance insomnia rather than sleep-onset insomnia as a result of repetitive, stereotyped (triple flexion) leg movements that cause repeated arousals. Whereas RLS is a clinical bedside diagnosis, PLMD requires documentation of frequent PLMS with associated arousals and sleep fragmentation on PSG.

Sleepwalking

Sleepwalking, or somnambulism, consists of complex behavior while in NREM sleep, comprising walking around in an impaired state of consciousness, with or without other actions such as violent behavior, driving a car, or climbing out a window. The prevalence of sleepwalking is higher in children (≤17%) than adults (≤4%). Precipitating factors include sleep deprivation, sleep disorders that precipitate arousals, febrile illness in children, and physical or emotional stress in adults. The main concern of sleepwalking is the risk of self-injury. Any underlying triggers should be identified and treated appropriately.

Sleep Terrors

Sleep terrors, or night terrors, occur in 2% to 3% of children and adults. They consist of arousals from deep NREM sleep and are characterized by intense behavioral manifestations of fear and autonomic hyperactivity (e.g., tachycardia, tachypnea, pupillary dilation, diaphoresis). The episodes are associated with frightening dreams, confusion, disorientation, and amnesia following each episode. They may be difficult to distinguish from other parasomnias or sleep-related epilepsy, which can require PSG for diagnosis.

Nightmare Disorder

Nightmare disorder affects 2% to 8% of the general population, and up to 50% of young children. Recurrent frightening dreams occur in REM sleep, which often result in awakenings and sleep disruption. Patients usually can recall details of their disturbing dream on awakening. In adults, frequent nightmares have been associated with physical or emotional trauma, stress, and psychopathology. Nightmares are characterized by detailed recollection of bad dreams (unlike night terrors, when there is usually amnesia for the event), and should be differentiated from other parasomnias and nocturnal panic attacks. Underlying psychological disturbances should be identified.

REM Sleep Behavior Disorder

RBD affects mainly older men (prevalence of 0.3%-0.5% of the general population). It consists of dream-enactment behavior that causes injury (to self or bed partner) and sleep disruption. Typically such episodes consist of acting out unpleasant or violent dreams with behavior such as shouting, punching, kicking, and running, and they are reported because of sleep-related injury, usually occurring in the last one third of the sleep period. RBD is associated with neurodegenerative disorders, such as Parkinson's disease, and can also be acutely triggered by psychotropic medications or withdrawal from alcohol and sedative-hypnotic agents. As with the other parasomnias, PSG may be required to rule out seizures. Specific treatment is needed to prevent injury.

Testing

Sleep studies are indicated mainly to confirm the nature and severity of sleep-related breathing disorders, help diagnose narcolepsy, and document parasomnias and seizures.

Polysomnography

PSG is the monitoring of physiologic parameters (with EEG, electromyography [EMG], electro-oculography [EOG], electrocardiography [ECG], airflow, respiratory effort, pulse oximetry) and physiologic or pathologic events in sleep. Different NREM and REM sleep stages can be identified based on specific EEG, EMG, and EOG characteristics. Monitoring respiratory parameters and ECG allows simultaneous documentation of sleep-related cardiorespiratory disturbances in conditions such as OSA.

Multiple Sleep Latency Test

The MSLT provides an objective measure of sleepiness. The MSLT is considered the gold standard in the objective evaluation of excessive daytime sleepiness. A mean sleep latency (MSL) of less than 5 minutes is considered pathologic and correlates with severe sleepiness.

The primary indication for the MSLT is to evaluate patients for a diagnosis of narcolepsy. In narcolepsy there is a very short MSL and at least two SOREMPs.

Maintenance of Wakefulness Test

The MWT is a variation of the MSLT and measures the ability of a person to stay awake in the setting of sleep disorders associated with excessive daytime sleepiness, such as narcolepsy and OSA. During nap trials of 20 minutes, a normal MSL is 18 minutes (representing 1 standard deviation below normal). An MSL of less than 11 minutes is considered impaired wakefulness. Values between 11 and 18 minutes are of questionable significance.

Box 2 Sleep Hygiene Instruction

Sleep-Wake Schedule

Get up at about the same time every morning, including weekends.
Maintain a regular schedule of going to bed and waking up.

Stimulus Control

Go to bed only when you are feeling sleepy.
Only use your bed for sleep and sexual activity.
Avoid watching television, working, or reading in bed
If you are not asleep after 20 minutes, get out of the bed. Go back to bed only when you feel sleepy again.

Food and Drink

Avoid heavy meals within 2 hours of bedtime. Try not to go to bed hungry, either.
Try not to drink too much fluid close to bedtime to prevent needing to urinate during the hight.
Avoid using alcohol as a sleep aid.
Limit caffeine use to 1 or 2 beverages a day, no later than 4 hours before bedtime.

Bedtime Routine

Establish a relaxing presleep routine while getting ready to go to bed e.g., reading watching TV, listening to music.
Set aside time to relax and practice natural relaxation techniques e.g., deep breathing, progressive muscle relaxation.

Bedroom Environment

Create an atmosphere conducive to sleep.
Keep a comfortable room temperature.
Avoid loud noises and bright lights in the bedroom.

Napping

Avoid taking long daytime naps unless you are sleep deprived.
Afternoon naps should not exceed 1 hour.

Exercise

Regular physical exercise is encouraged to promote sleep and overall well-being.
Vigorous physical activity should be avoided too close to bedtime.

Worry and Anxiety

Avoid things that can trigger worry or anxiety before bed, like anxiety-provoking, work-related, or other unpleasant tasks, or disturbing television programs.
Reduce the anxiety of anticipation of the following day by making simple preparations like a to-do list or laying out the next day's clothes and shoes.
Some people find writing down a list of worries makes them more manageable.

TREATMENT

Sleep Disorders Manifesting with Insomnia

Lifestyle and Behavioral Modifications

Good sleep hygiene instruction (summarized in Box 2) is helpful for most patients with insomnia because they usually have some component of inadequate sleep hygiene regardless of the primary cause of their insomnia. Especially important are having a fixed wake time and avoiding excessive time in bed engaged in activities other than sleeping. Patients are encouraged to limit their time in bed to achieve a high percentage of actual sleep while in bed (sleep efficiency), principles encompassed in "stimulus control" and "sleep restriction" (Boxes 2 and 3).[5]

Behavioral changes may be sufficient to improve insomnia in many cases. Cognitive behavioral therapy (CBT) refers collectively to the correction of maladaptive attitudes and beliefs regarding sleep and the use of natural relaxation techniques (e.g., deep breathing, progressive muscle relaxation) and includes instruction in good sleep hygiene. CBT and drug therapy may be used in combination for patients with various forms of insomnia, such as psychophysiologic insomnia, idiopathic insomnia, or insomnia due to depression.

Drug Therapy

Sedative-hypnotics are the mainstay of pharmacotherapy for acute and chronic insomnia. Other categories of drugs (e.g., antidepres-

Box 3 Sleep Restriction

Determine the average estimated total sleep time (TST). This information can be obtained from a sleep diary (sleep log), which should be filled out for at least 2 weeks.
Restrict the time in bed (TIB) to the average estimated total sleep time.
Determine the patient's weekly sleep efficiency (TST/TIB × 100%) from the sleep log.
Increase time in bed by 15 to 20 minutes when sleep efficiency exceeds 90%. Decrease it by 15 to 20 minutes when sleep efficiency is below 80%. Keep time in bed the same when sleep efficiency is between 80% and 90%. Adjust time in bed until the ideal sleep duration is obtained.
Do not decrease time in bed to less than 5 hours.
Brief afternoon naps may be allowed in the early phase of treatment.

sants, anxiolytic agents, antiepileptic drugs, antihistamines, melatonin-related drugs) are often used (some off-label) for various types of chronic insomnia. These are listed in Table 1.

Newer drugs for insomnia include the nonbenzodiazepine sedative hypnotics and the melatonin receptor agonist, ramelteon. Generally, shorter-acting drugs are used for insomnias manifesting with sleep-onset difficulty, and longer-acting ones are used for sleep-maintenance insomnia. The choice of drug also is determined by the presence of comorbid conditions e.g., depression [antidepressants], anxiety [anxiolytics], or neuropathic pain [antiepileptic drugs]. For insomnia specifically caused by depression, antidepressants are the initial drugs of choice. For circadian rhythm disorders (e.g., delayed sleep phase disorder), melatonin and melatonin receptor agonists have chronobiotic properties that may be helpful in shifting of the sleep phase. For sleep disturbances related to medical conditions causing pain or respiratory difficulty or related to neurodegenerative disorders, the treatment is that of the underlying condition.

The short-term efficacy of benzodiazepines and nonbenzodiazepine sedative hypnotics such as zolpidem is established, but the longer term use of these agents is controversial because of issues of tolerance and dependence. [6] Studies have supported longer term use with sustained efficacy of the nonbenzodiazepine sedative hypnotics eszopiclone and extended release zolpidem.[7,8] Longer term use of sedative hypnotics should be closely monitored and avoided in patients who already have a history of substance abuse. The lowest effective dose should be used, and intermittent rather than daily use should be encouraged whenever possible to reduce the risk of tolerance. Tapering should be done very slowly over weeks. Patients should be advised of adverse reactions of sedative hypnotics including dependence, tolerance, and abnormal sleep-related behavior (e.g., sleepwalking and sleep eating with zolpidem).

The FDA-approved medications for insomnia include the newer nonbenzodiazepine sedative hypnotics such as zaleplon (Sonata), zolpidem (Ambien), eszopiclone (Lunesta), and ramelteon (Rozerem). With shorter half-lives than the older benzodiazepines, these newer agents are less likely to produce daytime sedation and cognitive disturbance (see Table 1).

Restless Legs Syndrome

The treatment of insomnia related to RLS warrants separate mention and is summarized in Tables 2 and 3. The management of RLS is divided into behavioral and pharmacologic interventions. In general, counterstimulation (rubbing legs, hot or cold baths, ice packs), good sleep hygiene, reduced caffeine and alcohol intake, and avoidance, if possible, of drugs that exacerbate RLS (most antidepressants, neuroleptic agents, and antihistamines) are recommended. Other methods include distracting mental activity (games, hobbies), regular exercise (though not too late in the evening or at night), and avoiding provocative situations (long periods of sitting still). Delaying one's habitual sleep period to the time when symptoms are least troublesome (usually in the late morning) can facilitate sleep, though this is not practical for people with regular office hours. Patients with mild, infrequent RLS might benefit from these behavioral techniques alone, with RLS drugs taken infrequently as needed. Patients with iron deficiency should be investigated for the underlying cause, and oral iron replacement should be initiated. Ferritin levels should be rechecked periodically. A suggested approach to management is given in Table 2.

The main categories of drugs used for the symptomatic treatment of RLS are the dopaminergic agents, antiepileptic drugs (mainly gabapentin), the sedative hypnotics, and the opioid drugs, which are listed in Table 3. Drug therapy should ideally address the distressing limb sensations, as well as associated problems such as insomnia and depression. Most patients with RLS respond to dopaminergic agents.[9,10] However, because of the significant problem of augmentation (about 80% with L-dopa and 30% with dopamine agonists), L-dopa is no longer considered first line and its use is confined to intermittent dosing to provide rapid relief for infrequent symptoms. Augmentation refers to the worsening of RLS symptoms caused by a specific drug, usually the dopaminergic agents, within 6 months of initiating therapy. Typically there is progressively earlier onset of symptoms, with increasing symptom intensity. For patients with severe and frequent symptoms, a dopamine agonist is generally the initial drug of choice.

Circadian Rhythm Sleep Disorders

The mainstays of treatment of these disorders involves planned sleep schedules, timed light exposure, timed melatonin doses, sedative hypnotics, and alerting agents, details of which have been outlined in the 2007 AASM Practice Paremeters.[11] Sedative-hypnotic medications and melatonin improve the quality and duration of daytime sleep of shift workers and sleep in jet lag–induced insomnia. Melatonin reduces sleep-onset latency and shifts circadian rhythms to an earlier time in delayed sleep phase disorder. Melatonin has also been recommended for advanced sleep phase disorder, though there is no reported evidence in support of this.

Sleep Disorders Manifesting with Excessive Daytime Sleepiness

Lifestyle and Behavioral Modifications

Behavioral modifications in sleep disorders causing excessive daytime sleepiness include diet and exercise to promote weight loss, and positional therapy (sleeping in the off-back position) for OSA. Positional therapy has modest benefits in sleep quality, excessive daytime sleepiness, and AHI in positional OSA (defined as a supine AHI at least twice that of the lateral AHI). In narcolepsy, scheduled naps, which are typically refreshing, can help to sustain alertness and reduce the need for stimulant drugs. Planned sleep schedules are also an important part of treating circadian rhythm sleep disorders.

Drug Therapy

Wake-promoting agents that have been used in sleep disorders causing excessive daytime sleepiness include modafinil, methylphenidate, amphetamines, and caffeine. Modafinil (Provigil) can be used to enhance alertness in OSA, narcolepsy, and shift-work disorder. Modafinil promotes wakefulness by an unknown mechanism and is usually given in doses of 100 to 200 mg (maximum 400 mg) daily.

Table 1 Drugs Used In Insomnia

Drug	Half-Life	Dose Range in Adults	Comments
Nonbenzodiazepine Sedative-Hypnotics			
Zaleplon (Sonata)	~1 hr	5-20 mg	
Zolpidem (Ambien)	1.4-4.5 hr	5-10 mg	Adverse effects: Sleepwalking, sleep-eating
Zolpidem CR (Ambien CR)	1.4-4.5 hr	12.5 mg	
Zopiclone (Imovane)	3.5-6.5 hr	3.75-7.5 mg	Not approved for use in the United States
Eszopiclone (Lunesta)	5-7 hr	1-3 mg	Only FDA-approved agent for long-term use
Melatonin and Melatonin-Receptor Agonist			
Melatonin	0.5-2 hr	0.3-40 mg	
Ramelteon (Rozerem)	1-2.6 hr	4-8 mg	Should not be used with fluvoxamine
Benzodiazepines			
FDA-approved for use in insomnia			
Estazolam (Prosom)	10-24 hr	1-2 mg	
Flurazepam (Dalmane)	40-250 hr	15-30 mg	
Quazepam (Doral)	39-73 hr	7.5-30 mg	
Temazepam (Restoril)	8-20 hr	7.5-30 mg	
Triazolam (Halcion)	1.5-5.5 hr	0.125-0.5 mg	
Anxiolytics*			
Alprazolam (Xanax)	6-20 hr	0.25-4 mg (in divided doses)	
Clonazepam (Klonopin)	18-40 hr	0.25-4 mg in divided doses	
Lorazepam (Ativan)	10-20 hr	0.5-6 mg in divided doses	
Sedating Antidepressants†			
Amitriptyline (Elavil)	12-24 hr	10-150 mg (max 300 mg daily)	
Doxepin (Sinequan)	6-8 hr	10-150 mg (max300 mg daily) (divided or once daily)	
Fluvoxamine (Luvox)	15-22 hr	50-300 mg	Also treatment for obsessions and compulsions
Mirtazapine (Remeron)	20-40 hr	7.5-45 mg	
Nefazodone (Serzone)	2-4 hr	50-600 mg (in divided doses)	
Trazodone (Desyrel)	3-6 hr	25-400 mg (in divided doses)	
Antihistamines			
Diphenhydramine (Benadry)	2-8 hr	25-100 mg	
Promethazine (Phenergan)	9-16 hr	12.5-50 mg	
Hydroxyzine (Atarax)	20-25 hr	12.5-100 mg	Also anxiolytic and anti-pruritic
Antiepileptic Drugs			
Insomnia Related to Chronic Pain‡and Epilepsy			
Gabapentin (Neurontin)	5-7 hr	100-1200 mg	Off-label use
Pregabalin (Lyrica)	5-6.5 hr	75-300 mg	Off-label use; also anxiolytic

*Off-label use, not FDA-approved for insomnia.
†Indicated for use in insomnia related to depression. Not FDA-approved for insomnia alone.
‡Examples: neuropathic pain, restless legs syndrome, fibromyalgia.

Table 2 Management of Restless Legs Syndrome

Type	First Choice	Second Choice	Third Choice
Mild			
Intermittent	Behavioral	L-Dopa prn	Sedative hypnotic prn
Persistent	Gabapentin	Dopamine agonist	Sedative hypnotic, opioids
Moderate to Severe			
Intermittent	L-Dopa prn	Sedative hypnotic prn	Opioids Prn
Persistent	Dopamine agonist	Gabapentin	Sedative hypnotic, opioids
Painful	Gabapentin	Opioids	Dopamine agonist

Table 3 Drugs Used In Restless Legs Syndrome

Drug	Dose Range	Half Life	Side Effects
Antiepileptic Drugs			
Gabapentin (Neurontin)	300-2700 mg (max 1200 mg/dose)	5-7 hr	Sedation, dizziness, ataxia
Dopaminergic Agents			
L-dopa (Sinemet)(CR)	50-200 mg	1.5-2 hr	Nausea, vomiting, orthostatic
Pramipexole (Mirapex)*	0.125-1.5 mg	8-10 hr	hypotension, insomnia,
Ropinirole (Requip)*	0.25-3.0 mg	6-8 hr	hallucinations, augmentation
Sedative Hypnotic Agents			
Zaleplon (Sonata)	5-20 mg	~1 hr	Sedation, respiratory
Zolpidem (Ambien)	5-20 mg	1.4-4.5 hr	depression, tolerance,
Clonazepam (Klonopin)	0.25-4 mg	18-40 hr	dependence
Opioids			
Codeine	15-120 mg	2-3 hr	Sedation,
Oxycodone (OxyContin)	5-30 mg	3 hr	constipation, nausea, vomiting,
Hydrocodone	5-30 mg	3 hr	pruritis, dry
Tramadol (Ultram)	50-300 mg	5-8 hr	mouth, dependence
Propoxyphene (Darvon-N)	100-600 mg	6-12 hr	
Methadone	2.5-20 mg	16-22 hr	

*Instructions for patients: Pramipexole 0.25 mg or Ropinirole 0.25 mg: Take ½ tablet 2 hours before bedtime. Increase to 1 tablet after 3 days if no side effects or benefit. Continue to increase by ½ tablet every 3 days until there is benefit or side effects develop.

Methylphenidate (Ritalin) is a central nervous system (CNS) stimulant. The effective dose ranges from 10 to 60 mg daily in divided doses. Sustained-release formulations are available (e.g., Ritalin-LA 10-100 mg once daily, Concerta 18-54 mg once daily). Amphetamines are noncatecholamine sympathomimetic amines with CNS stimulant activity; they have a high potential for abuse. Examples are Adderall (10-60 mg daily in divided doses) and Dexedrine (5-60 mg daily in divided doses). CNS stimulants cause elevations in blood pressure and heart rate and have been associated with arrhythmias and sudden death.

Sleep-Related Breathing Disorders

Positive airway pressure (PAP) is the mainstay of treatment for OSA. This can take the form of continuous, autotitrating, or bilevel positive airway pressure (CPAP, autoPAP, BiPAP). Each has different methods of pressure delivery and all are widely used. Although an effective treatment of choice, CPAP therapy has a high noncompliance rate, ranging from 5% to 50%.[12]

Modafinil is effective in reducing excessive daytime sleepiness and is approved for use in OSA patients with residual excessive daytime sleepiness in spite of adequate CPAP therapy.

Oral appliances are recommended by the American Academy of Sleep Medicine as first-line treatment (as an alternative to CPAP) for mild to moderate OSA and in patients with severe OSA who refuse or fail CPAP.[13]

Surgical options for OSA include bariatric surgery for morbid obesity, which is effective in reducing BMI and AHI, and upper airway surgery.

Narcolepsy

Modafinil and CNS stimulants are used in narcolepsy as alerting agents. Symptoms of cataplexy are treated with REM suppressants such as tricyclic antidepressants e.g., protriptyline (Vivactil 15-40 mg daily) and imipramine (Tofranil 50-150 mg daily) and selective serotonin reuptake inhibitors (SSRIs) such as fluoxetine (Prozac 20-60 mg daily) and sertraline (Zoloft 25-50 mg daily). Sodium oxybate (Xyrem) is a newer drug that some believe has become a first-line agent for treating cataplexy; it also improves sleep quality and excessive daytime sleepiness. The use of sodium oxybate is tightly regulated because of its abuse potential; it is available by prescription only through a restricted distribution program called the "Xyrem Success Program." The effective dose range of Xyrem is 6 to 9 g/night. The recommended initial dose is 4.5 g/night divided into two equal doses of 2.25 g. The starting dosage can be increased in increments of 1.5 g/night (0.75 g/dose) every 1 to 2 weeks to minimize adverse effects.

Sleep Disorders Manifesting with Abnormal Movements or Behavior in Sleep

Parents should be reassured that parasomnias are common and generally benign. Often no specific therapy is required, but sensible safety precautions should be instituted, such as padding the bedroom environment, securing doors and windows, and installing alarm or monitoring systems that track the patient's movements. Parasomnias that pose a risk of injury to the patient or bedpartner and those that are triggered by treatable conditions (e.g., OSA, PLMD) require specific therapy for these conditions. For frequent or potentially injurious parasomnias, benzodiazepines and tricyclic antidepressants may be helpful. Clonazepam has been used successfully, starting at low doses (e.g., 0.25 mg at bedtime) and titrating according to effect and tolerability. It is especially helpful in RBD, which may also be treated with melatonin (dose range 3-12 mg at night) as an alternative monotherapy or add-on for patients who do not tolerate long-acting benzodiazepines.

Summary

- Sleep disorders are common and have a limited range of symptoms. A practical approach to diagnosis is to consider the various diagnoses from the three main symptom categories of insomnia, excessive daytime sleepiness, and abnormal movements in sleep.
- Insomnia is often multifactorial, with specific therapy directed to the cause identified.
- RLS is common cause of sleep disturbance and should be excluded in all patients presenting with sleep-related complaints based on the clinical diagnostic criteria.
- Chronic partial sleep deprivation and OSA are the most commonly encountered causes of excessive daytime sleepiness in practice.
- Sleep studies (PSG) are indicated in the diagnosis of certain conditions such as suspected sleep-related breathing disorders, narcolepsy (PSG with MSLT), injurious parasomnias, and sleep-related epilepsy.
- Many sleep disorders are multifactorial and respond best to a holistic approach, which includes lifestyle modifications, behavioral changes, pharmacotherapy, timed bright light therapy, positive airway pressure therapy, and surgery (for OSA).

Suggested Readings

American Academy of Sleep Medicine: International Classification of Sleep Disorders: Diagnostic & Coding Manual, 2nd ed. Westchester, Ill: American Academy of Sleep Medicine, 2005.

American Academy of Sleep Medicine: Casebook of Sleep Medicine: A Learning Companion to the International Classification of Sleep Disorders, 2nd ed.: Diagnostic & Coding Manual. Westchester, Illinois: American Academy of Sleep Medicine, 2008.

American Psychiatric Association: Diagnostic and Statistical Manual of Mental Disorders, 4th ed. Arlington, Va: American Psychiatric Publishing, 1994.

Iber C, Ancoli-Israel S, Chesson AL, Quan SF: The AASM Manual for the Scoring of Sleep and Associated Events: Rules, Terminology, and Technical Specifications. Westchester, Ill: American Academy of Sleep Medicine, 2007.

Johns MW: A new method for measuring daytime sleepiness: The Epworth sleepiness scale. Sleep 1991;14 (6):540-545.

Kushida CA, Morgenthaler TI, Littner MR, et al. Practice parameters for the treatment of snoring and obstructive sleep apnea with oral appliances: An Update for 2005. Sleep 2006;29(2): 240-243.

Morgenthaler TI, Lee-Chiong T, Alessi C, et al; Standards of Practice Committee of the American Academy of Sleep Medicine: Practice parameters for the clinical evaluation and treatment of circadian rhythm sleep disorders. An American Academy of Sleep Medicine report. Sleep 2007;30(11):1445-1459.

Nowell PD, Mazumdar S, Buysse DJ, et al: Benzodiazepines and zolpidem for chronic insomnia: a meta-analysis of treatment efficacy. JAMA 1997;278(24):2170-2177.

Rechtschaffen A, Kales A (eds): A Manual of Standardized Terminology, Techniques, and Scoring System for Sleep Stages of Human Subjects. US Department of Health, Education, and Welfare Public Health Service, NIH/NIND, 1968.

Restless Legs Syndrome Task Force of the Standards of Practice Committee of the American Academy of Sleep Medicine: An update on the dopaminergic treatment of restless legs syndrome and periodic limb movement disorder. Sleep 2004; 27(3):560-583.

References

For a complete list of references, log onto www.expertconsult.com.

Parkinson's Disease

Patrick Sweeney

James Parkinson (1755-1824), although best remembered for the disease state named after him by Charcot, was a man of many talents and interests. Publishing on chemistry, paleontology, and other diverse topics, early in his career, he was a social activist championing the rights of the disenfranchised and poor. His efforts in this area were enough to result in his arrest and appearance before the Privy Council in London on at least one occasion. In collaboration with his son, who was a surgeon, he also offered the first description, in the English language, of a ruptured appendix.

His small but famous publication, "Essay on the Shaking Palsy," appeared in 1817, seven years before his death in 1824. The clinical descriptions of six patients were a remarkable masterpiece testifying to his prodigious powers of observation because most of the six patients were never actually examined by Parkinson himself; rather, they were simply observed walking on the streets of London.

DEFINITION

Parkinson's disease is a common neurodegenerative disease of the elderly. Typically beginning in the 60s or 70s, it is characterized by the unilateral onset of resting tremor in combination with varying degrees of rigidity and bradykinesia.

PREVALENCE

Parkinson's disease ranks among the most common late-life neurodegenerative diseases, affecting approximately 1.5% to 2.0% of the population older than age 60 years.

PATHOPHYSIOLOGY

Although the etiology of Parkinson's disease is not completely understood, the condition probably results from a confluence of several factors. The first is an age-related attrition and death of the approximately 450,000 dopamine-producing neurons in the pars compacta of the substantia nigra.[1] For every decade of life there is estimated to be a 9% to 13% loss of these dopamine-producing neurons. If carried to its logical extreme, those patients achieving very great age are destined to lose approximately 70% to 80% of these critical neurons before the first signs and symptoms of the disease appear. This age-related attrition may also be the explanation for the subtle extrapyramidal findings that are often found in the octogenarian patient.

Since the early 1980s and the discovery of the potent neurotoxin MPTP/MPP^+ (1-methyl-4-phenyl-1,2,3,6-tetrahydropyridine–1-methyl-4-phenylpyridinium), a byproduct of illicit drug synthesis, the environment has figured prominently in proposed etiologies for Parkinson's disease.[2,3] After the original description of this environmental insult to the dopamine-producing cells of the substantia nigra, a number of other environmental neurotoxins have been described that have led to the parkinsonian state. These discoveries have led to the suggestion that Parkinson's disease might arise as a combined consequence of the ongoing aging process coupled with environmental exposures that accelerate the process of nigral cell death. The unusual clustering of persons, in a Canadian recording studio, who later developed Parkinson's disease (including the actor Michael J. Fox) emphasizes the possible relation of environment to disease development.

The third component of the puzzle is the possibility that some persons might have a predetermined genetic susceptibility to these environmental insults. Although Parkinson's disease has been observed to occur throughout the world and in virtually all ethnic groups, there is a low incidence among Asians and African patients as opposed to white patients. This observation suggests that genetic factors might have an important role in disease production. Other evidence involves twin studies, which initially failed to show a high concordance rate among monozygotic twins but is now being reconsidered in light of new evidence.[4]

In addition, family history appears to be a strong predictor, after age, for development of the disease. A number of families in Greece and Italy with a high penetrance of Parkinson's disease were shown to have a mutation on chromosome 4 for the alpha-synuclein gene.[5] This is a presynaptic protein of unknown function but with the potential, on further study of this mutated gene, to provide insights into the pathogenesis of this form of autosomal dominant Parkinson's disease. Another gene abnormality on the long arm of chromosome 6 has been identified in patients with a peculiar autosomal recessive form of young-onset disease. The protein product of this gene is named Parkin and seems to promote the degradation of certain neuronal proteins. It is closely related to the ubiquitin family of proteins involved in several neurodegenerative disease states.[6] Research continues at a very high level to identify susceptibility genes and to shed additional light on the genetics of Parkinson's disease.

SIGNS, SYMPTOMS, AND DIAGNOSIS

The diagnosis of Parkinson's disease is a clinical exercise. A useful starting point begins first by identifying parkinsonism at definite, probable, and possible levels. Using several clinical extrapyramidal features (resting tremor, rigidity, bradykinesia, postural instability, and freezing) one can confidently say a patient has definite Parkinsonism if he or she has any two of those five features, with one of the two being tremor or bradykinesia.

Once a diagnosis of parkinsonism is made, it is imperative for the physician to exclude pharmacologic causes. Since the recognition, decades ago, that reserpine can produce extrapyramidal side effects, the list of medications that can cause parkinsonism continues to increase each year (Box 1). In addition, unexplained extrapyramidal disease in a young person should always prompt exclusion of Wilson's disease, a metabolic disorder of copper metabolism leading to degenerative changes in the brain.

The asymmetrical and unilateral onset of resting tremor is probably the single best clinical clue that one is dealing with Parkinson's disease, although some of the parkinsonisms can manifest in a similar fashion. A robust response to levodopa is also considered a strong indicator of true Parkinson's disease. Atypical features that may suggest parkinsonism are listed in Box 2. The difficulty in accurately distinguishing between neurodegenerative diseases that have parkinsonian extrapyramidal features (multiple system atrophy, progressive supranuclear palsy [PSP], etc.) is reflected in statistics showing a high rate of misdiagnosis among movement-disorder experts when patients are followed throughout the course of their illness to actual autopsy.[7,8] Both of these series, one from Europe and the other from North America, point out a roughly 24% misdiagnosis rate at autopsy.

There is a growing literature on the usefulness of MRI head imaging in distinguishing parkinsonism from Parkinson's disease. Although there are reports of distinctive features for many of these conditions, perhaps the most reliable and consistent findings are to be found in vascular parkinsonism, wherein the discovery of multiple prior strokes gives the clinician a diagnosis.

Box 1 Medications that Can Produce Parkinsonism

Phenothiazines
Butyrophenones
Selective serotonin reuptake inhibitors
Amiodarone
Diltiazem
Metoclopramide
Valproic acid

Box 2 Features Suggesting Parkinsonism Rather than Parkinson's Disease

Early falling
Early dementia
Early hallucinations
Absence of tremor
Gaze abnormalities

Box 3 Hoehn and Yahr Scale

I: Unilateral disease
II: Bilateral disease
III: Postural instability—mild
IV: Postural instability—marked
V: No independent ambulation

TREATMENT AND OUTCOMES

At least two overriding principles should guide therapy in Parkinson's disease: education and individualization. With regard to education, there are abundant free resources to which the treating physicians can refer patients. The National Parkinson's Disease Foundation and the American Parkinson's Disease Association offer pamphlets, booklets, and resource information to patients and their families simply for the asking. (National Parkinson's Disease Foundation, 800-327-4545; American Parkinson's Disease Association, 800-223-2732). Patient education, as an adjunct to medical therapy of Parkinson's disease, has been studied by Montgomery[9] and has been shown to improve the intermediate-term outcomes.

The second guiding principle should be individualization of treatment based on the specific patient and disease stage. It is useful to conceptualize at least two staging epochs: early versus more advanced disease. The widely used Hoehn and Yahr scale offers some landmarks to help the physician stage a patient (Box 3). In this scheme, purely unilateral disease is designated as stage I. Stage II is represented by bilateral disease no matter how trivial. Stages III and IV add increasing amounts of postural instability and falling. Stage V describes that patient who no longer independently ambulates and is essentially wheelchair confined.

An algorithm has recently been proposed for the symptomatic management of Parkinson's disease. The algorithm suggests the following steps in treating Parkinson's: (1) consider "neuroprotective therapies" immediately following diagnosis, (see later); (2) administer dopamine agonists to control symptoms; (3) add levodopa if agonists alone do not work; (4) use a catechol-*O*-methyltransferase (COMT) inhibitor in conjunction with levodopa for longer-lasting treatment; and (5) consider surgery after exhausting all medical options.[10]

In terms of medical treatment and understanding of basic disease mechanisms, Parkinson's disease has fared better than many of the other well-known neurodegenerative diseases, such as Alzheimer's disease. If one compares past seminal reviews of medical therapy, such as those offered by Yahr[11] and Calne,[12] with the most current

Table 1 Entry-Level Medications

Drug	Dosing
Amantadine	100 mg bid
MAO-B inhibitors	
Zydis selegiline	1.25-2.5 mg qd
Rasagiline	0.5-1.0 mg qd
Anticholinergics	
Trihexyphenidyl	2 mg QD to tid

overview offer by Lang,[13] one can appreciate the state of progress in this area. Comments here are limited to neuroprotective therapy and symptomatic therapy.

With regard to neuroprotective therapy, the hope that the selective MAO-B inhibitor selegiline HCl offered neuroprotection was dashed by the results of the DATATOP study.[14] Although the drug does have some symptomatic benefit, there is no clear evidence from this study that it offers any neuroprotection. Likewise, the antioxidant properties of vitamin E were hoped to be neuroprotective but were shown to be ineffective. Future chapters on neuroprotection in Parkinson's disease will come only with a more complete understanding of the etiology of the disease. Medications that modulate formation of free radicals through oxidative phosphorylation and stabilizing calcium homeostasis will play important roles in this area. A new selective MAO-B?inhibitor, rasagiline (Azilect), is now available for patients. This drug as monotherapy in a dose of 1 mg a day has been found to be effective in early Parkinson's disease.[14] The Adagio study is currently under way to evaluate the neuroprotective potential of rasagiline.

Symptomatic therapy depends on the stage of the disease when it is first diagnosed. For early, mild disease, I prefer using one or more of the triad of amantadine (Symmetrel), one of the two new selective MAO inhibitors (rasagiline or zydis selegiline), and sometimes one of the anticholinergic agents (the last often effective for tremor) that often provide modest relief. Examples and dosing schedules for these medications are listed in Table 1. The use of dopamine agonists in early disease is discussed later.

With advancing disease progressing into the later stages of disability, the main classes of medication are either the dopamine agonists or levodopa itself. Since its introduction into the physicians' armamentarium in the late 1960s, levodopa, the immediate precursor of dopamine, remains the standard in terms of effective treatment for Parkinson symptoms. Levodopa is combined with a peripheral decarboxylase inhibitor (carbidopa); this combination reduces the decarboxylation of levodopa to dopamine outside of the blood-brain barrier, thereby allowing more-efficient dosing of levodopa. Before this drug combination, high doses of levodopa were required because 98% of a given dose of levodopa was converted to dopamine in the periphery, and because dopamine does not cross the blood-brain barrier , it was effectively wasted.

Currently, however, some controversy surrounds just when to initiate levodopa therapy because early use of levodopa (i.e., the patient with minimal symptoms and signs) leads to predictable treatment complications after several years of therapy. These include wearing off, on-off motor fluctuations, and the development of unwanted movements (dyskinesias). The half-life of levodopa is only about 90 minutes, which results in multiple peaks and valleys of drug level during a typical day of therapy. It is now believed that this pulsed stimulation of the dopamine receptors is nonphysiologic when compared with the more constant and tonic physiologically normal state. After several years of treatment (even earlier when the parkinsonian pathology is at a more advanced state), loss of efficacy before the next dose (wearing off), dyskinesias (unwanted

Table 2 Levodopa and Agonist Medications for Advanced Parkinson's Disease

Drug	Size	Dosing (Average)
Levodopa-carbidopa (Sinemet)	25-100 mg	tid-qid
	25-250 mg	tid-qid
Levodopa-carbidopa (Sinemet CR)	25-100 mg	tid-qid
	50-250 mg	tid-qid
Levodopa-carbidopa-entacapone (Stalevo)	50, 100, 150, 200	6-8 day
Ropinirole (Requip)	0.25, 0.5, 1, 2.5 mg	15 mg qd titration
Pramipexole (Mirapex)	0.125, 0.25, 1, 1.5 mg	3-5 mg qd titration

movements of the head, shoulders, or limbs), or on-off periods (radical swings between functioning and nonfunctioning states) appear. Because of this, it is current practice to initiate one of the dopamine agonists, which have longer half-lives than levodopa, when the patient's quality of life demands more-aggressive treatment.

All of the agonists contain a dopamine-like ring moiety, which is believed to be the portion of the molecule that actually stimulates the dopamine receptor. Historically, dopamine agonists were first used only for symptomatic treatment when the patient began to fail traditional therapy. The earlier use of this class of drug represents current theory, which suggests many of the late treatment complications associated with Parkinson's disease treatment are a result of the short half-life of levodopa.

Perhaps the newest application of the agonists involves the issue of neuroprotection. For a number of reasons (one of which is that as a class, agonists do not undergo oxidative metabolism) trials are planned to see if patients treated initially with agonists and levodopa progress in their disease more slowly than patients treated with levodopa alone. At present, of the agonists available in the United States, the new-generation (since 1997) agonists ropinirole (Requip) and pramipexole (Mirapex) are popular.[15] It is believed that the long duration of actions of these drugs, as compared with levodopa, is the seminal reason for the less-frequent development of dyskinesias and fluctuations when these are employed initially as major therapy. Table 2 lists the dopamine agonists as well as levodopa preparations and dosing schedules for these medications.

In mid-2007, the newest dopamine agonist appeared on the market in patch form. Rotigotine (Neupro) allows a constant 24-hour drug level with very stable stimulation of the dopamine receptors. However, the drug was withdrawn (most likely temporarily) from the U.S. market in 2008 due to formulation issues and is only available in Europe at this time. The drug will return to the US market in early 2010.

In recent years, much research has been directed toward inhibiting the other major enzyme system that breaks down levodopa outside of the BBB in the periphery: COMT. At present, two medications are available for this purpose with the most widely used being entacapone (Comtan). When administered (200-mg tablets) with each levodopa-carbidopa dose, it increases the elimination half-life of levodopa and prolongs its action. Thus, the strategy of prolonged and continuous stimulation of the dopamine receptor is maximized by combining levodopa with carbidopa and entacapone. In a large study of 255 patients with fluctuations, the addition of entacapone resulted in a significant increase in on-time of about 1 hour and allowed a reduction of levodopa dosage.[16] In addition, using the controlled-release (CR) preparation early in the course of levodopa therapy might provide additional prolongation. At present, the recommendation for use of entacapone is limited to patients who are experiencing wearing off.

New developments in the mechanism of drug delivery have resulted in a transmucosal form of selegiline. The technique is referred to as the *Zydis formulation* and uses a method that rapidly freezes the drug so that it becomes interlaced as tiny crystals in a medium of gelatin spindles. This allows disintegration of the wafer on the contact with saliva in the mouth. Using this technique, Zydis selegiline (Zelepar) is absorbed directly through the buccal mucosa into the systemic circulation, bypassing the gut and, therefore, first-pass hepatic metabolism. Compared with regular selegiline, this results in higher levels of the medication but with marked reduction in the amphetamine-like metabolites of selegiline. Water is not required to aid in swallowing, because the medication dissolves completely in the saliva in the mouth.

The combination of carbidopa-levidopa and entacapone is now available as a single tablet referred to as *Stalevo.* Each of the four dosage strengths contains 200 mg of entacapone with 50, 100, 150, or 200 mg of carbidopa-levidopa. This convenience allows the patient to take just one pill rather than two. For those who have difficulty swallowing, the physical size of the 50 and 100 mg tablets of Stalevo is actually smaller than the carbidopa-levidopa tablet. Levodopa is also available in a formulation called *Parcopa,* in the same strength as regular carbidopa-levidopa tablets, allowing the convenience of pill dissolution in the mouth so the patient does not have to swallow the pill.

With the use of entacapone, dyskinesias may become more prominent, and a corresponding reduction in levodopa dosing is indicated. About 5% to 10% of patients taking this drug experience a benign urine discoloration (orange tint), which does not require any drug modification.

The benefit of adding folic acid to the drug regimen of patients taking levodopa has been increasingly commented on.[17,18] Administration of levodopa results in hyperhomocysteinemia with resulting potential for vascular endothelial damage. The addition of folic acid lowers the concentration of homocysteine. Finally, last but not least, the value of daily exercise for the Parkinson patient cannot be emphasized enough. A number of exercise programs are available on disk or the Internet. An example is www.delaythedisease.com.

CONCLUSION

Our understanding of the etiology and neurobiology of Parkinson's disease continues to evolve. Matching knowledge gained in these areas with similar progress in neurotherapeutics might one day offer treatments to completely alleviate the burdens of Parkinson's disease.

Summary

- Concepts regarding the cause(s) of Parkinson's disease continue to evolve.
- Effective therapies ranging from education, exercise, and physical therapy, as well as a host of medications exist to manage the symptoms of Parkinson's disease.

In mid to late disease, surgical intervention with deep-brain stimulation rescues many patients from complications that develop in advanced Parkinson's disease.

Suggested Readings

Calne DB: Treatment of Parkinson's disease. N Eng J Med 1993;329:1021-1027.

Fearnley JM, Lees AJ: Ageing and Parkinson's disease: Substantia nigra regional selectivity. Brain 1991;114:2283-2301.

Hughes AJ, Daniel SE, Blankson S, Lees AJ: A clinical pathologic study of 100 cases of Parkinson's disease. Arch Neurol 1993;50:140-148.

Kitada T, Asakawa S, Hattori N, et al: Mutations in the parkin gene cause autosomal recessive juvenile parkinsonism. Nature 1998;392:605-608.

Lang AE, Lozano AM: Parkinson's disease. N Engl J Med 1998;339:1044-1053.

Miller JW, Selhub J, Nadeau MR, et al: Effect of L-Dopa on plasma homocysteine in Parkinson's disease patients. Neurology 2003;60:1125-1129.
Miller T, Woitalla D, Kuhn W: Benefit of folic acid supplementation in Parkinsonian patients treated with levodopa. J Neuro Surg Psychiatry 2003;74:549-551.
Montgomery EB, Lieberman A, Singh G, et al: Patient education and health promotion can be effective in Parkinson's disease: A randomized controlled trial. Am J Med 1994;97:429-435.
Olanow, CW, Watts RL, Koller WC: An algorithm (decision tree) for the management of Parkinson's disease (2001). Neurology 2001;56(Suppl 5):S1-S88.
Parkinson Study Group. Entacapone improves motor fluctuations in levodopa-treated Parkinson's disease patients. Ann Neurol 1997;42:747-755.
Parkinson Study Group: A controlled trial of rasagiline in early Parkinson's disease. Arch Neurol 2002;59:1937-1943.
Polymeropoulos MH, Lavedan C, Leroy E, et al: Mutation in the α-synuclein gene identified in families with Parkinson's disease. Science 1997;276:2045-2047.
Rajput AH, Rozdilsky B, Rajput A: Accuracy of clinical diagnosis in parkinsonism-a prospective study. Can J Neurol Sci 1991;18:275-278.
Shannon KM: New alternatives for the management of early Parkinson's disease. Mov Disord 1996;11:S266.
Tanner CM, Ottman R, Ellenberg JH, et al: Parkinson's disease concordance in elderly male monozygotic and dizygotic twins. Neurology 1997;48:Suppl:A333. (Abstract.)
Vingerhoets FJ, Snow BJ, Tetrud JW, et al: Positron emission tomographic evidence for progression of human MPTP-induced dopaminergic lesions. Ann Neurol 1994; 36:765-770.
Wood N: Genes and parkinsonism. J Neurol Neurosurg Psychiatry 1997;62:305-309.
Yahr MD, Duvoisin RC: Drug therapy of parkinsonism. N Engl J Med 1972;287:20-24.

References

For a complete list of references, log onto www.expertconsult.com.

Dizziness

Neil Cherian

DEFINITION

Dizziness can be described as a sensation or illusion of movement (such as spinning, rotating, tilting, or rocking), unsteadiness, or dysequilibrium. It is commonly accompanied by gait imbalance.

Dizziness is a symptom and not a diagnosis; it can be compared with pain in that respect. It is difficult to quantify because of its subjective nature. Dizziness is not exclusive to the vestibular system. Furthermore, it may be a component of a larger or more diffuse problem.

The nomenclature of dizziness can be divided according to the following list. This breakdown is arbitrary. These descriptions are not quantifiable, are not mutually exclusive, and can lead to further diagnostic dilemmas, yet this approach has persisted probably because of the complex nature of the symptom.

- *Lightheadedness*: a vague sensation of floating or wooziness.
- *Presyncope*: a more extreme form of lightheadedness. It might or might not precede actual syncope and can be accompanied by tachycardia, palpitations, or diaphoresis.
- *Vertigo*: a sensation of movement, often described as a spinning, twisting, or turning.
- *Dysequilibrium*: a sensation of unsteadiness.

Symptoms may be episodic or constant. If they are episodic, they can last anywhere from seconds to minutes or hours to months at a time.

PREVALENCE

Dizziness is a common complaint in the medical environment. It is the third most common symptom presentation (combined with imbalance and falls) for outpatient medical consultation, behind chest pain and fatigue. In the adult population, 42% report dizziness at some time.[1] Dizziness is common in all age groups; however, its frequency does increase with age. Dizziness and related vestibular symptoms are the main reasons for visiting a doctor after 75 years of age. Prevalence rates vary depending on the patient's age and the cause of the dizziness.

PATHOPHYSIOLOGY

Essentially any and every part of the vestibular system can malfunction, potentially providing symptoms of dizziness. Typically, when discussing vestibular symptomatology, the dichotomy of *peripheral vestibular dysfunction* versus *central vestibular dysfunction* is discussed. This method is used here for discussion purposes, although it can be misleading in practice because there is often an overlap between the two. Systemic etiologies, which might or might not act via central vestibular pathways, can also be a helpful way to discuss these issues.

Peripheral Vestibular Disorders

Vestibular Dysfunction

Peripheral vestibular dysfunction refers to dysfunction of the vestibular end-organ (utricle, saccule, semicircular canals) and vestibular nerve.

Vestibular neuronitis (neuritis) can affect one or both vestibular end-organs and can involve them simultaneously or sequentially. The actual portion involved is believed to be the cell bodies of the hair cells that transduce movement within the end-organ and/or the vestibular nerve itself. The neuronitis can occur as a single attack or as multiple attacks. A quantifiable peripheral vestibular loss may be appreciated with caloric testing. The term *neurolabyrinthitis* may be used if there is an associated hearing loss.

Bilateral vestibular hypofunction (partial or complete loss) may be related to bilateral vestibular neuronitis or to toxic or immune mechanisms. Gentamicin and streptomycin are notorious for causing vestibular dysfunction (ototoxicity). In fact, this is exactly why they are used intratympanically to induce vestibular loss, particularly in the treatment of Menière's disease.

Autoimmune ear disease is another cause of peripheral vestibular dysfunction. It is characterized by rapidly progressive, bilateral, sensorineural hearing loss within 3 months.[2] In contrast, ototoxicity can manifest with sudden bilateral loss, whereas age-related and noise-induced hearing loss can develop over many months to years. The most common age at onset of symptoms is 20 to 50 years. Many older patients present with new symptoms when autoimmune ear disease might, in retrospect, have been present for many years. The disease can affect both sexes, but a female preponderance is noted when systemic immune diseases (e.g., rheumatoid arthritis, systemic lupus erythematosus) are present.

Central or systemic vestibular dysfunction includes the vestibular nuclei (superior, inferior, lateral, and medial) where they synapse with numerous pathways including the cerebellar, oculomotor, posterior column, proprioceptive, and vestibulospinal.

Menière's Disease

Menière's disease is a disorder that is often incorrectly diagnosed. It includes the tetrad of vertigo (lasting at least 20 minutes), unilateral tinnitus, low-frequency hearing loss (initial stages with progression to all frequencies), and aural fullness. The symptoms are believed to be associated with a change in fluid pressure within the endolymphatic space. Menière's disease usually starts between the ages of 20 and 60 years (average, 40 years), and women outnumber men by 1.3 to 1. In most patients, only one ear is involved; it is bilateral in about 15% to 20%.

The cause of this disease is not known, although viral injuries of the inner ear and other factors affecting the homeostasis of the inner ear have been proposed. Sodium management is believed to be at the core of the disorder. The vertigo is treatable through either medical or surgical management, although the tinnitus is often difficult to control. Various case series have reported spontaneous resolution rates of up to 30%.

The term *endolymphatic hydrops* is often used to describe Menière's disease. This is actually a misnomer. This term is the pathologic description of the inner ear, which can be seen in Menière's disease. It discusses the physical appearance of the endolymphatic space and the way it is dilated. Other disorders can also lead to endolymphatic hydrops.

Benign Paroxysmal Positional Vertigo

Benign paroxysmal positional vertigo (BPPV) is a common cause of dizziness, particularly in people older than 65 years. Its incidence is estimated at 6000 per million population in those whose illness persists longer than 30 days, although this is probably a gross underestimate. It is easily identifiable with bedside evaluation (Dix-Hallpike testing). All three canals (anterior [superior], posterior, and lateral [horizontal]) may be the source of BPPV, although the posterior semicircular canal is by far the most common source.

Various theories exist regarding the pathogenesis and localization of BPPV. Calcium carbonate is embedded in a proteinaceous matrix on the surface of the utricle, with otoconia as the building block. Through head trauma, infectious or inflammatory processes, or idiopathic mechanisms, the otoconia can dislodge and move to various areas within the endolymphatic space. This pathologic movement of otoconia within the endolymphatic space induces the sensation of movement out of proportion to actual head movement.

Variants of BPPV have been described in the literature, although their existence is controversial. These include cupulolithiasis, in which otoconia are believed to be attached to the cupula; ampullolithiasis, or short-arm BPPV, in which otoconia are within the ampulla of the semicircular canal on the other side of the cupula; and utriculolithiasis, in which otoconia are freely moving within the utricle outside of any of the semicircular canals.

Perilymphatic Fistulas

Perilymphatic fistulas represent a defect of the oval or round window that produces abnormal communication between the fluid surrounding the membranous labyrinth and middle ear space. Fistulas can be spontaneous (implosive or explosive) or acquired.

Implosive fistulas arise from increased pressure in the middle ear resulting from barotrauma; they include rapid airplane descent, external ear trauma, and scuba diving. In these cases, the membranes of the oval or round windows are driven inward to permit escape of perilymph into the middle ear space.

Explosive fistulas arise from increased intracranial pressure such as weight lifting, vigorous coughing, or straining, and it is believed that there is communication with the perilymphatic space by the internal auditory canal. In these cases, the membranes of the oval and round windows are driven outward. Treatment is similar for implosive and explosive fistulas. Acquired fistulas can result from stapes or chronic ear surgery.[3]

Drug-Induced Dizziness

Drug-induced dizziness is common. Given that medication use is ubiquitous and the mechanisms are complex, it is no wonder that so many drugs are implicated in causing dizziness. Certain antiseizure medications (carbamazepine, phenytoin, primidone) and alcohol can cause acute reversible dysequilibrium and chronic irreversible dysequilibrium as a result of cerebellar dysfunction. Sedating drugs (barbiturates, benzodiazepines, and tricyclic antidepressants) can cause a nonspecific dizziness that is believed to be related to diffuse depression of the central nervous system. Antihypertensive medications and diuretics can induce lightheadedness and presyncope by induction of postural hypotension and reduced cerebral blood flow.

A number of drugs can produce a characteristic drug-intoxication syndrome with disorientation, memory and cognitive deficits, gaze-evoked nystagmus, and gait and extremity ataxia. This can be confused with more serious disorders. Alcohol is one example of these drugs; it can cause central nervous system depression and cerebellar toxicity, and it can change the specific gravity of the cupula (motion sensor within the ampulla of the semicircular canal). This change in the cupula explains the positional vertigo and positional nystagmus that are noted with alcohol ingestion.

Drug-induced dizziness or imbalance can be caused by ototoxic drugs such as aminoglycosides (gentamicin, streptomycin) and cisplatin. Vertigo can ensue if hair-cell loss is asymmetrical. If injury is bilateral and symmetrical, oscillopia (the optical illusion that stationary objects are moving back and forth or up and down) and dysequilibrium may be experienced.

Motion-Related Dizziness

Mal de debarquement (MDD) syndrome is a disorder characterized by a persistent sensation of motion after a prolonged period of passive movement.[5] It is commonly experienced after water travel, air travel, or prolonged train rides, although other modes of travel can induce this syndrome, including space flight. The sensation of motion persistence after prolonged travel is physiologic and often short-lived; it is arbitrarily considered pathologic when it remains for at least 1 month. MDD is often incorrectly described as motion sickness; instead, motion, by self-motion or driving, actually often reduces symptoms in MDD. Diagnosis of MDD is essentially made by history: a preceding period of prolonged travel with onset of a similar sensation of motion afterward. Patients often indicate improvement with self-motion (rocking) or while driving. Treatment of MDD is predominantly medical. Vestibular suppressants with diazepam or clonazepam may be helpful in some patients. Spontaneous recovery can occur.

Motion sickness begins with epigastric discomfort and may be accompanied by increased salivation and a feeling of bodily warmth. As discomfort progresses, gastric emptying is inhibited. Symptoms progress to nausea, pallor, sweating, and eventually to vomiting. Some researchers have suggested that there is an additional syndrome of motion sickness that lacks the gastrointestinal complaints and is characterized by drowsiness, headache, apathy, depression, and generalized discomfort. Motion sickness is exacerbated by further activity and movement.

Central Vestibular Disorders

Circulation-Related Causes

Cardiogenic dizziness results from ineffective cerebral or brainstem perfusion. Low cardiac output states include cardiac failure, cardiac tamponade, arrhythmia, and aortic stenosis.

Carotid occlusion rarely causes vertigo because the posterior circulation supplies the brainstem. Only when the posterior and anterior circulations are both severely compromised can carotid disease cause vertigo.

Cerebrovascular conditions such as posterior-circulation ischemia or stroke can cause dizziness because vestibular structures are involved. A number of small- and large-vessel syndromes can include dizziness. Small-vessel syndromes include the following:

- Lateral medullary syndrome (Wallenberg's) with vertigo, dysarthria, Horner's syndrome, and hemiataxia
- Anterior inferior cerebellar artery syndrome, consisting of vertigo and unilateral deafness from labyrinthine artery ischemia; facial weakness; and ataxia
- Labyrinthine (internal auditory) artery syndrome

Large-vessel syndromes include the following:

- Vertebrobasilar insufficiency
- Basilar artery thrombosis
- Vertebral artery thrombosis

Neurocardiogenic dizziness can result from a relative change in the tone of the peripheral vasculature and the heart as the system responds to feedback from the brainstem. Disorders of reduced orthostatic tolerance include neurally mediated syncope, postural tachycardia syndrome,[4] postexercise syndrome, and so on.

Other Causes

Acoustic neuroma (vestibular schwannoma) is a nonmalignant tumor of the eighth cranial nerve and is commonly from the inferior vestibular nerve. Hearing loss is the most common symptom and is often high-frequency and sensorineural in nature. Tinnitus is also very common and tends to be unilateral and on the same side as the tumor. Despite the name *vestibular schwannoma*, dizziness is not common and occurs in less than 20% of patients with this diagnosis. However, unsteadiness may be present in as many as 70% of these patients.

Cervicogenic dizziness is difficult to classify (see discussion later).

Metabolic dizziness can be caused by hypoglycemia and can lead to a spectrum of symptoms that include mild fatigue, tremulousness, diaphoresis, confusion, or lightheadedness, to more-extreme symptoms of lethargy, amnesia, and seizures. It is usually a complication of diabetes mellitus or its treatment, although it can also occur with fasting or after meals. Hypomagnesemia and thyroid dysfunction (hyperthyroid and hypothyroid) can also be culprits of dizziness. Numerous other metabolic conditions can cause similar symptoms.

Migraine-associated dizziness is discussed later.

Psychophysiologic dizziness is the consequence of the integration of various subsystems that pertain to the sense of balance (visual, vestibular, proprioceptive, autonomic), and is not always pathologic. One robust example of this is the sensation of movement that a person might experience when standing at the ledge of a tall building versus just standing on the ground. It is the visual input that fools the brain into thinking that it is moving (visual-vestibular conflict), and the brain must then rely more on ankle proprioception (joint position sense).

Anxiety disorders, panic disorders, and phobias can also interact with disorders of balance and dizziness. Dizziness with anxiety and panic disorders are not related exclusively to hyperventilation. These symptoms may be primary to a psychological or psychiatric disorder or may be exacerbated by a vestibular syndrome. Phobic postural vertigo or phobic dizziness is a morbid fear of falling unassociated with postural or gait instability. It is often associated with panic disorder and agoraphobia, although the patient might focus on the physical symptoms. Patients have a fear of falling while sitting or standing, and this can provoke unpleasant sensations of body acceleration and acceleration of the environment. Neurocardiac disorders, particularly orthostatic intolerance, can mimic or contribute to these disorders. Tachycardia, palpitations, shortness of breath, and presyncope are not limited to disorders of the cardiovascular system.

Vestibular epilepsy may be vague dizziness or true vertigo that may precede the seizure (aura) or actually be or accompany the seizure event.

SYMPTOMS AND SIGNS

Symptoms

On evaluation of the dizzy patient, the following issues should be considered:

- *Hearing:* Reduced acuity, hyperacusis (increased sensitivity to sound), fluctuation, distortion, tinnitus
- *Gait and balance:* Imbalance, falls, ataxia, retropulsion
- *Autonomic symptoms:* Nausea, vomiting, diarrhea, diaphoresis, palpitations, presyncope, or syncope
- *General symptoms:* Headache, neck pain, neck stiffness, state of hydration or dehydration
- *Neurologic symptoms:* Focal weakness, numbness or tingling, visual field reduction or obscuration, mental status changes, photophobia, phonophobia, visual aura

Signs

On evaluation of the dizzy patient, the presence or absence of the following should be assessed:

- *Nystagmus:* Spontaneous, gaze-evoked, post–head-shake, positioning (Dix-Hallpike testing)
- *Auditory:* Rinne and Weber tests
- *Vestibular:* Romberg's sign (regular or sharpened), Fukuda step test, head-thrust test (Halmagyi)
- *Gait:* Base, stability, ataxia, arm-swing
- *Cervical spine:* Range of movement-extension, flexion, total rotation, upper cervical rotation, side bend; tenderness or pain, spasm, weakness

DIAGNOSIS

Benign Paroxysmal Positional Vertigo

The diagnosis of BPPV is made on clinical grounds in a patient with complaints of episodic positional vertigo. It can be confirmed by Dix-Hallpike position testing of the involved ear. This test can be performed at the bedside, by trained physical therapists, or in the vestibular laboratory. Diagnosis is aided by visualization of the eyes, with either Frenzel or infrared video goggles. Both allow diminished visual fixation, although the infrared video goggles allow observation of the eye without light stimulation and allow review of the eye movements at a later time.

The provocation of paroxysmal nystagmus, after a brief delay, in the head-hanging position helps to identify the posterior semicircular canal that is involved. From the patient's frame of reference, stimulation of the right posterior semicircular canal produces a clockwise torsional and upbeat nystagmus, and the left posterior semicircular canal produces a counterclockwise torsional and upbeat nystagmus. On return to a sitting position, the initial nystagmus often reverses. If both responses are seen, the specificity for BPPV is quite high. Dizziness that is out of proportion to the observed nystagmus may also be observed. Caution is advised if the dizziness is reproduced with no observed nystagmus; a diagnosis other than active BPPV should then be considered.[6]

Lateral (horizontal) canal BPPV can also be diagnosed. Symptoms of positional vertigo tend to come with rolling over in bed and are often more intense and more nauseating than posterior-canal BPPV. For diagnosis, the patient can be placed in the supine position with the head up 30 degrees to allow the lateral canal to be placed in the vertical plane. The Lempert, or barbecue roll, procedure may be used to treat this, with the direction of the roll away from the ear that exacerbates symptoms. In other words, if symptoms are produced when the patient rolls to the side that is involved, rolling 360 degrees in the opposite direction might help to reposition the stray otoconiae.

*Menière's Disease**

The following criteria may be used in the diagnosis of Menière's disease.[7]

Vertigo

- Recurrent, discrete episodes of spinning or rotation
- Duration ranging from 20 minutes to 24 hours
- Nystagmus associated with attacks
- Nausea and vomiting possibly accompanying attacks
- Absence of other neurologic symptoms

Deafness

- Fluctuating unilateral hearing deficits
- Sensorineural hearing loss
- Progressive unilateral hearing loss

Tinnitus

- Often low-pitched, and louder with attacks
- Unilateral, on affected side

*Criteria for diagnosing Menière's disease from American Academy of Otolaryngology-Head and Neck Surgery.

Superior Canal Dehiscence

Superior canal dehiscence was first described by Lloyd Minor in 1998.[8] Dehiscence of the bone overlying the superior semicircular canal can result in a syndrome of vertigo and be induced by loud noises (Tullio's phenomenon) or by maneuvers that change middle-ear or intracranial pressure. The symptoms are believed to occur because the dehiscence acts as a third mobile window into the inner ear. Diagnosis is made by high-resolution computed tomography (CT) of the temporal bone demonstrating the dehiscence or thinning of the bone overlying the superior semicircular canal. A low-frequency air-bone gap (at 500 Hz and 1 kHz) with or without a conductive hearing loss may be noted, despite normal middle-ear function. Vestibular-evoked myogenic potential testing may reveal abnormally reduced thresholds. Although both sides are not necessarily symptomatic at the same time, bilateral involvement is common.

Migraine or Migraine-Associated Dizziness

The term *migraine* is synonymous with headache for many people. Its manifestation is not limited to headache, however, and it often occurs without it.

The criteria of Neuhauser and colleagues[9] for migrainous vertigo are:

- Recurrent episodic vestibular symptoms (attacks)
- Migraine headache meeting International Headache Society (1988) criteria[10]
- At least one of the following migrainous symptoms during at least two of these attacks:
  - Migraine-type headache
  - Photophobia
  - Phonophobia
  - Visual or other auras
- Other causes ruled out by appropriate investigations

These criteria should be considered a starting point. Controversy surrounds the issues of migrainous vertigo. Simply the coexistence of dizziness and migraine symptoms does not guarantee that the two are fully related. In many instances, a peripheral vestibular syndrome may actually be exacerbating an underlying migraine disorder.

Cervicogenic Dizziness

Cervicogenic dizziness is a disorder that the literature has alluded to for decades. Basic scientists have suggested for years that stimulation of afferents in the neck chemically, with electrical stimulation, or by ablation can induce a sensation of dizziness, although often not vertigo. The mechanics of the upper cervical spine (particularly C1-C2) and associated distortions of proprioception and kinesthetic function (sensation of relative movement as it pertains to joint function) are believed to be dysfunctional.[11] This can occur with or without neck pain.

Symptoms tend to be vague and are often described as head fullness or heaviness or as lightheadedness. Symptoms may be worsened with computer use, reading, or sustained neck positions, and they are often worse with increased activity and later in the day. Cervicogenic dizziness can manifest in isolation or associated with headache (possibly cervicogenic headache), or it may actually be a factor in precipitating increased migraine activity or orthostatic intolerance. Undiagnosed cervicogenic dizziness can complicate vestibular rehabilitation, and an increase in dizziness with increased head movements is required for vestibular habituation.

Cervicogenic dizziness remains controversial because neck pain, bulging cervical disks, and whiplash remain ubiquitous. The lack of consensus on objective diagnostic criteria and the lack of a sensitive and specific test have only added to the controversy. Neck-vibration testing and vibration-induced nystagmus (nystagmus elicited from neck-vibration testing, which does not always parallel the presence or absence of symptoms) may be beneficial in identifying patients with cervicogenic dizziness.[12] Neck-vibration testing is vibration of various head and neck muscle groups such as the suboccipital, masseter, and sternocleidomastoid, which might reproduce the dizziness; vibration-induced nystagmus is nystagmus elicited from neck-vibration testing, which does not always parallel the presence or absence of symptoms. Apparent risk factors for cervicogenic dizziness include head trauma, neck trauma (commonly whiplash), peripheral vestibular dysfunction, and focal paraspinal muscle weakness. Imaging of the cervical spine with plain films, CT, or magnetic resonance imaging [MRI]) is uninformative. The lack of neck pain does not rule out the possibility of cervicogenic dizziness.

No significant double-blinded studies have been undertaken regarding cervicogenic dizziness. Experience at the Cleveland Clinic Foundation (CCF) and case series in the literature[13] suggest that advanced-level physiotherapy directed toward the upper cervical spine may be beneficial. Therapy modalities should target normalization of biomechanics, range of movement, tone, mitigation of pain or tenderness, strengthening, and resetting of proprioception. Clinical trials at CCF are under way to assess the potential benefit of botulinum toxin combined with neck physiotherapy in the treatment of cervicogenic dizziness. The hypothesis is that botulinum toxin may be beneficial in relieving spasmodic torticollis (neurally sustained spasm), allowing the physiotherapy to progress.

Commonly Performed Tests for Dizziness

Vestibular Test Battery[14]

Rotational chair testing, video nystagmography (infrared video recording of eye movements) to analyze eye movement responses to various maneuvers including Dix-Hallpike test, and supine positional testing with the body supine and head up 30 degrees is helpful in identifying vestibular loss (unilateral and bilateral), active BPPV, otolith dysfunction, and central vestibular disorders (global and focal).

Audiologic Testing

Comprehensive audiometry (behavioral thresholds, pure tone audiometry, acoustic reflexes, tympanometry) and additional testing include auditory brainstem responses, otoacoustic emissions, and electrocochleography. Audiologic testing is helpful in quantifying associated or known audiologic deficits or for surveying for possible auditory pathway involvement.

Imaging

Recommended imaging includes head MRI (internal auditory canal protocol), cervical spine MRI, and temporal bone CT (high-resolution). Temporal bone CT is particularly important for superior canal dehiscence.

Additional Testing

Tilt-table testing is used to assess blood pressure and heart rate function in response to change in position. Head-up tilt (70 degrees) for 10 to 45 minutes can diagnose forms of orthostatic intolerance, vasovagal responses, and postural tachycardia syndrome. Additional testing can assess intravascular volume, autonomic responses, and pulmonary circuit times.

Vestibular-evoked myogenic potentials test vestibular hypersensitivity, and possibly saccular function, by activating sternocleidomastoid muscle contraction. It is helpful in diagnosing Menière's disease and superior canal dehiscence. This test is complementary to conventional vestibular testing.

Fistula testing consists of application of pressure waveforms (positive and negative constant pressure and sinusoidal pressure) to the external auditory canal to elicit nystagmus and vertigo in the absence of middle ear or mastoid disease (Hennebert's sign).

Dynamic platform posturography assesses balance function under conditions in which sensory cues are modified. Conditions include eyes open or closed, visual surround stable or moving, and support surface stable or moving.

TREATMENT AND OUTCOMES

Specific therapies and associated outcomes depend on the diagnosis. A number of modalities are beneficial even when the specific diagnosis is not clear.

Medications

Vestibular suppressants are commonly used. These include antihistamines (e.g., meclizine), anticholinergics (e.g., scopolamine), and benzodiazepines (e.g., lorazepam, diazepam). These medications may be used on a short-term basis or as needed. When used chronically, their benefits can wane, however, and they are commonly used incorrectly. Furthermore, chronic use of these drugs can hamper vestibular adaptation. The side effects may also be deleterious, and they include fatigue, lethargy, and dry mouth.

Antinausea medications (e.g., prochlorperazine, promethazine) may also be prescribed.

Antianxiety medications (benzodiazepines such as alprazolam, diazepam, selective-serotonin reuptake inhibitors) may be provided to patients with associated anxiety.

Assistive devices such as canes and walkers can provide stability to those with balance or orthopedic issues. Canes seem to be carried at certain times, perhaps to provide a sense of security or proprioception (position cues). The use of these devices may be optimized in the hands of an experienced vestibular therapist.

Vestibular rehabilitation (balance therapy) is a discipline within physical therapy that evaluates sensory input (proprioceptive, vestibular, and visual) and how it is used to control static and dynamic balance. Goals are to decrease the risk of falls and increase activities of daily living and functioning at home, as well as managing symptoms, educating patients, and recommending and monitoring the use of assistive devices. In uncontrolled trials of vestibular rehabilitation, improvement in more than 80% of patients has been reported.

Neck physiotherapy is shown to be beneficial managing the vestibular patient (unpublished local experience). A common reason for failure of vestibular rehabilitation is previously unidentified derangements of upper cervical mechanics. Similarly, previously undiagnosed or undertreated migraine disorders have been noted to affect rehabilitation. Active trials of the use of botulinum toxin to manage cervical dysfunction are under way here at the CCF (off-label use).

Treatment for Some Common Causes of Dizziness

Benign Paroxysmal Positional Vertigo

When the involved canal and side have been identified by the Dix-Hallpike maneuver, particle repositioning maneuvers may be performed. Numerous treatments exist, the more common being the Epley canalith repositioning procedure, the Semont liberatory maneuver, and the Brandt-Daroff habituation exercises. The Epley maneuvers were developed by John Epley in the 1970s.[15] Repositioning therapies should be directed to the semicircular canal involved. The goal of the repositioning maneuver is to return the stray otoconia to the utricular macula. The maneuvers may be performed repetitively. Canalith repositioning is more effective than observation alone, despite spontaneous resolution rates of one in three cases after 3 weeks of treatment.[16] This is further supported by current AAN guidelines, which recommend canalith repositioning and the Semont maneuver in the treatment of BPPV; as both have been found to be safe and effective (or possibly effective in the case of the Semont maneuver).[17]

In Menière's disease, medical management is targeted at sodium management. A combination of diuretic therapy and sodium restriction are the mainstays of management. Diuretics such as triamterene and hydrochlorothiazide are commonly used. Sodium restriction may be as simple as not salting foods, counting actual sodium, and adhering to a target sodium amount. Commonly, 1500 to 2000 mg of sodium per day may be recommended.

Symptomatic treatment with sublingual lorazepam (brand preparation only, because the carrier agent is different in the generic preparation and affects absorption) or diazepam may be used as needed to lessen the intensity and sometimes the duration of symptoms.

Numerous surgical approaches exist. The spectrum is wide, ranging from minimally invasive procedures such as endolymphatic sac decompression to vestibular nerve section to cochleosacculotomy to labyrinthectomy. The latter involves the complete removal of the vestibular and auditory apparatus, leaving the patient with deafness and without peripheral vestibular function.

Superior Canal Dehiscence

Surgical treatment is often beneficial. It involves capping the superior aspect of the superior semicircular canal with a foreign material; bone fragments alone may be ineffective because of the constant movement and pressure changes transmitted from the middle ear and the middle cranial fossa. Surgery is performed via a middle fossa approach.

Migraine-Associated Dizziness

Once this diagnosis has been established, treatment is similar to that for migraine headache. Avoidance practices, reduction of systemic medical issues, and abortive and preventive strategies should be used. Certain foods and additives (e.g., aged cheese and meats, red wine, caffeine) as well as hunger, dehydration, and sleep deprivation should be avoided. Reduction of systemic medical issues includes identifying certain disorders such as obstructive sleep apnea, overuse of analgesics (because of increased risk of rebound headaches), and generalized and regional pain syndromes and spine disorders (cervical, thoracic, and lumbar dysfunction). Intravenous infusion treatments with various medications, including metoclopramide, magnesium sulfate, and valproic acid, may be beneficial in managing chronic pain cycles, status migrainosus, and overuse of analgesics.

CONCLUSION

Dizziness is a complex and often multicomponent symptom. Vestibular and nonvestibular etiologies should be considered, and often the two coexist.

Summary

- Dizziness is a symptom and not a diagnosis.
- It is the third most common symptom manifestation (combined with imbalance and falls) for outpatient medical consultation. In the adult population, 42% report dizziness at some time.
- Dizziness is a complex and often multicomponent symptom. Vestibular and nonvestibular etiologies should be considered, and often the two coexist.
- Benign paroxysmal positional vertigo is a common and treatable form of dizziness. Head or ear trauma, viral ear infections, and age are risk factors.
- Migraine-associated dizziness is quite prevalent and may occur without headache.
- The cervical spine might play a role in dizziness (cervicogenic dizziness), although this theory is controversial. Cervicogenic dizziness may be amenable to neck physiotherapy.

Suggested Readings

Baloh RW: Dizziness, hearing loss, and tinnitus. Philadelphia: FA Davis, 1998.

Brown JJ, Baloh RW: Persistent mal de debarquement syndrome: A motion-induced subjective disorder of balance. Am J Otolaryngol 1987;8:219-222.

Epley JM: New dimensions of benign paroxysmal positional vertigo. Otolaryngol Head Neck Surg 1980;88:599-605.

Fife TD, Tusa RJ, Furman JM, et al: Assessment: Vestibular testing techniques in adults and children: Report of the Therapeutics and Technology Assessment Subcommittee of the American Academy of Neurology. Neurology 2000;55:1431-1441.

Fife TD, Iverson DJ, Gronseth GS, et al: Practice parameter: Therapies for benign paroxysmal positional vertigo (and evidence-based review)—Report of the Quality Standards Subcommittee of the American Academy of Neurology. Neurology 2008;70:2067-2074.

Fouad FM, Tadena-Thorne L, Bravo EL, Tarazi RC: Idiopathic hypovolemia. Ann Intern Med 1986;104:298-303.

Furman JM, Cass SP: Balance Disorders: A case-study approach. Philadelphia: FA Davis, 1996.

Goodhill V: Leaking labyrinth lesions, deafness, tinnitus and dizziness. Ann Otol Rhinol Laryngol 1981;90:96-106.

Headache Classification Committee of the International Headache Society: Classification and diagnostic criteria for headache disorders, cranial neuralgias and facial pain. Cephalgia 1988;8(suppl 7):9-96.

Hughes GB, Kinney SE, Hamid MA, et al: Autoimmune vestibular dysfunction: Preliminary report. Laryngoscope 1985;95:893-897.

Minor LB, Solomon D, Zinreich JS, Zee DS: Sound- and/or pressure-induced vertigo due to bone dehiscence of the superior semicircular canal. Arch Otolaryngol Head Neck Surg 1998;124:249-258.

Neuhauser H, Leopold M, von Brevern M, et al: The interrelations of migraine, vertigo, and migrainous vertigo. Neurology 2001;56:436-441.

Oas JG, Cherian N: Vibration-induced nystagmus is not a reliable sign of a unilateral vestibular loss [abstract]. American Academy of Neurology Meeting, April 2001.

Oas JG: Benign paroxysmal positional vertigo: A clinician's perspective. Ann NY Acad Sci 2001;942:201-209.

Pearson BW, Brackmann DE: Committee on Hearing and Equilibrium guidelines for reporting treatment results in Menière's disease [Editorial]. Otolaryngol Head Neck Surg 1985;93:579-581.

Watson MA, Sinclair H: Balancing Act: For people with dizziness and balance disorders. Portland, Ore: Vestibular Disorders Association, 2001.

White J, Savvides P, Cherian N, Oas J: Canalith repositioning for benign paroxysmal positional vertigo. Otol Neurotol 2005;26:704-710.

Wrisley DM, Sparto PJ, Whitney SL, Furma JM: Cervicogenic dizziness: A review of diagnosis and treatment. J Orthop Sports Phys Ther 2000 Dec;30(12):755-766.

References

For a complete list of references, log onto www.expertconsult.com.

Low Back Pain

Kerry H. Levin

DEFINITION

Low back pain can best be described in terms of specific accompanying features. Low back pain is acute if it has a duration of about 1 month or less. Chronic low back pain is usually defined by symptoms of two months or more. Both acute and chronic low back pain can be further defined by the presence or absence of neurologic symptoms and signs. Nonspecific or nonradicular low back pain is not associated with neurologic symptoms or signs. In general, the pain is localized to the spine or paraspinal regions (or both) and does not radiate into the leg. In general, nonspecific low back pain is not associated with spinal nerve root compression. Nonspecific low back pain might or might not be associated with significant pathology on magnetic resonance imaging (MRI) and is often a result of simple soft tissue disorders such as strain, but it can also be caused by serious medical disorders arising in the bony spine, parameningeal, or retroperitoneal regions. See Table 1 for the differential diagnosis for low back pain.

Low back pain accompanied by spinal nerve root damage is usually associated with neurologic signs or symptoms and is described as *radiculopathy.* There is usually pathologic evidence of spinal nerve root compression by disk or arthritic spur, but other intraspinal pathologies may be present and are often apparent on an MRI scan of the lumbosacral spine.

PREVALENCE

Low back pain is second only to upper respiratory illness as a cause for visiting a physician.[1] Up to two thirds of the population has low back symptoms at some time in their lives. In 1995 there were about two worker's compensation claims for low back pain for every 100 workers. Seventy-five percent of patients with acute low back pain are back to work within 1 month of the onset of symptoms, and only 5% are disabled for more than 6 months.[2] However, among those with continuing pain 6 to 10 weeks after onset, most still have some symptoms at 1 year.[3]

Among persons with chronic low back pain without neurologic deficits, a number of factors play a role in the length of disability. Recurrent low back pain and prolonged disability tend to correlate with prior history of low back pain, advancing age, job dissatisfaction, emotional distress, heavy or repetitive lifting and physical work, prolonged sitting or standing, and the presence of a worker's compensation claim or pending litigation.[4]

Lumbosacral radiculopathy and radicular low back pain are less common than nonspecific low back pain. L5 radiculopathy is the most common lumbosacral radiculopathy, usually produced by disk herniation between the fourth and fifth lumbar vertebral bodies. S1 radiculopathy is the next most common, followed by L3 to L4 radiculopathy.

PATHOPHYSIOLOGY

The pathophysiology of nonradicular low back pain is usually indeterminate. In fact, one of the defining features of this disorder is its nonspecific etiology. Pain can arise from a number of sites, including the vertebral column, surrounding muscles, tendons, ligaments, and fascia. Stretching, tearing, or contusion of these tissues can occur after sudden unexpected force applied to the spine from events such as heavy lifting, torsion of the spine, and whiplash injury. Whether muscle spasm is a significant etiology of lumbar spine pain, either as cause or effect of back injury, has not been proved.

The pathophysiology of radicular spine pain and lumbosacral radiculopathy is usually more obvious. Disk herniation through the annulus fibrosis does not in itself produce pain, but compression by disk of the dural lining around the spinal nerve root sleeve is one likely explanation for the back pain associated with acute disk herniation. This is also likely to contribute to the pain from spinal nerve root compression from arthritic spurs at degenerated facet and uncovertebral joints. Compression can directly stretch nociceptors in dura or nerve root sleeve tissues, but ischemia from compression of vascular structures, inflammation, and secondary edema is also likely to play a role in some cases.

SIGNS AND SYMPTOMS

History and physical examination are critical to the diagnosis and thus to the formulation of a rational approach to management. The following briefly summarizes the major points.

History

The medical history should focus on both triggering and alleviating factors, as well as on the character of the pain. Signs and symptoms such as increased pain with Valsalva maneuvers, straight-leg-raising symptoms, the tendency for the pain to radiate into the buttock or leg, the presence of weakness or sensory deficit, and bowel or bladder urgency or incontinence are associated with neurologic causes of low back pain.

The history should also explore factors that increase the likelihood of an underlying systemic disorder as a cause. These include advanced age, history of cancer, unexplained weight loss, use of injected drugs, chronic infection, prolonged duration of pain, pain that does not respond to rest or recumbency, and failure to respond to previous therapy. Box 1 reviews these factors.

Waddell and colleagues have described a number of historical features that point to nonorganic causes for low back pain, predicting delayed recovery and suggesting the need for a multidisciplinary approach to treatment.[5] These are reviewed in Box 2.

Examination

A general examination should be performed to identify potential systemic disorders, such as rheumatologic disease, skin disease, or bone deformities. The spine should be inspected for alignment, curvature, range of motion, focal tenderness, and overlying skin abnormalities such as a tuft of hair or pore. Mechanical maneuvers to elicit radicular and hip-joint symptoms should be considered, including straight-leg raising, reverse straight-leg raising, Patrick's test, and Lasègue's sign.

A careful neurologic examination should be undertaken to exclude motor and sensory deficits. Muscle strength in the L2 through S1 myotomes should be examined. The sensory examination should include soft-touch and pain sensation in the same segmental distributions. Muscle stretch reflexes should be elicited at the knee for the L3 to L4 segment and at the ankle for the S1 segment, and they can also be performed in the posterior thigh at the tendinous insertion of internal hamstrings for the L5 segment.

Waddell and colleagues have also described a number of findings on the physical examination that point to nonorganic causes for low

Table 1 Differential Diagnosis of Low Back Pain

Mechanical Causes	Nonmechanical Causes	Causes of Referred Pain
Idiopathic (sprain, strain)	Malignancy	Pelvic disease (prostatitis, endometriosis, pelvic inflammatory disease)
Spondylosis (disk, annulus, facet)	Infection	Renal disease (kidney stones, pyelonephritis, perinephric abscess)
Compression fracture	Inflammatory spondyloarthropathy (ankylosing spondylitis, psoriatic spondylitis, Reiter's syndrome, inflammatory bowel disease)	Aortic aneurysm
Traumatic fracture	Osteochondrosis	Gastrointestinal disease (pancreatitis, cholecystitis, penetrating ulcer)
Alignment disorders (kyphosis, scoliosis, spondylolisthesis)	Paget's disease of bone	

Box 1 Warning Signals of Systemic Disease Underlying Back Pain

Cancer
Prior history of malignancy
Advanced age
Unexplained weight loss
No pain relief with bed rest
Pain duration greater than 4 to 6 weeks
Failure to respond to standard therapies
Spinal infection
History of intravenous drug use
Urinary tract infection
Skin infection
Compression fracture
Advanced age
Trauma
Prolonged corticosteroid use
Rheumatologic disorders

Box 2 Historical Symptoms Suggesting Nonorganic Causes of Back Pain

Pain at the tip of the tailbone
Whole-leg pain in global distribution
Whole-leg numbness in a global distribution
Sudden give-way weakness of the leg
Absence of even brief periods of relative pain relief
Failure or intolerance of numerous treatments
Numerous urgent care visits or hospitalizations for back pain

Data from Waddell G, Bircher M, Finlayson D, Main CJ: Symptoms and signs: Physical disease or illness behaviour? BMJ (Clin Res Ed) 1984:289:739-741.

back pain, predicting delayed recovery and suggesting the need for a multidisciplinary approach to treatment (Box 3).[6]

DIAGNOSIS

The appropriate evaluation and management of low back pain rest on a few basic principles. First, it is necessary to determine whether the symptoms are caused by nerve root involvement. Second, it is necessary to determine whether the acute or chronic spine pain is related to a serious underlying medical illness that is manifesting itself as spine pain. After an initial assessment of the likely cause of the symptoms, the spine pain can then be treated.

A number of diagnostic tests can help pinpoint the cause of low back pain. Which test is selected depends on a host of factors uncovered during the history and physical examination. The diagnostic tests are described next.

Box 3 Signs on the Physical Examination Indicating Nonorganic Causes of Low Back Pain

Superficial tenderness over the lumbar region to light touch
Nonanatomic tenderness
Exacerbation of pain by applying a few pounds of pressure with the hands to the top of the head
Exacerbation of pain by simulated rotation of the spine
Ability to sit up straight from a supine position, but intolerance of the straight-leg-raising test
Nonanatomic distribution of sensory changes

Data from Waddell G, McCulloch JA, Kummel E, Venner RM: Non-organic physical signs in low-back pain. Spine 1980;5:117-125.

Routine Radiographs of the Spine

Routine spine radiographs are of limited value because they visualize only bony structures. Guidelines from the U.S. Agency for Health Care Policy and Research (AHCPR) indicated value of routine spine radiographs for acute low back pain in the following settings: acute major trauma, minor trauma associated with risk of osteoporosis, risk of spinal infection, pain that does not respond to rest or recumbency, and history of cancer, fever, or unexplained weight loss.[7] They may also be of value in assessing spinal alignment and rheumatologic disorders of bone.

Computed Tomography and Magnetic Resonance Imaging

Computed tomography (CT) and magnetic resonance imaging (MRI) are sensitive tools for evaluating neural structures such as spinal nerve roots and the spinal cord, and they can visualize soft tissue structures within the spinal canal. Of the two modalities, MRI resolution for neural structures is superior to CT. In the absence of motor, sensory, or autonomic deficits, and in the absence of significant trauma, infection, or malignancy, the American Academy of Neurology guideline recommends nonsurgical therapy before these techniques are used in patients with uncomplicated acute low back pain of less than 7 weeks' duration.[8] Patients with acute neurologic deficits associated with low back pain should be considered for MRI or CT of the lumbosacral spine unless surgery and invasive therapeutic options are not indicated.

Computed tomographic Myelography

CT myelography employs traditional myelography (intrathecal instillation of a radiocontrast agent, followed by routine spinal radiographs) followed by CT of the spine. It may be of value when MRI studies are inconclusive, especially in the assessment of the relation between spinal nerve roots and the bony neural foramina. Although this technique involves an invasive procedure, it is the study of choice when there are absolute contraindications to the use of MRI (presence of an implanted electronic device such as cardiac pacemaker or metal object in the inner ear, eye, or brain, such as an aneurysm clip).

Electrodiagnosis

Electrodiagnostic tests assess the neurophysiologic function of peripheral nerves and can identify the presence of various forms of nerve fiber damage. Electrodiagnostic tests (nerve conduction studies and needle electromyography [EMG]) are most useful in the presence of a motor deficit on neurologic examination. Nerve conduction studies are indicated primarily to exclude other neuromuscular disorders that can mimic radiculopathy, such as peripheral polyneuropathy and mononeuropathies. The H-reflex can be a useful nerve conduction study when assessing for the presence of an S1 radiculopathy. The needle electrode examination is most likely to be useful in the presence of clinical weakness. This procedure will help distinguish weakness due to spinal nerve root damage from other causes of weakness identified on the physical examination, such as other neuromuscular disorders, central nervous system disorders, and non-neurologic causes of weakness (pain, malingering). The needle electrode examination should be performed only after at least 3 weeks have passed since the onset of weakness because fibrillation potentials (the major manifestation of acute denervation) do not reliably develop before that time.

Electrodiagnostic testing may be of value in the assessment of patients with postsurgical deficits, multisegmental neurologic deficits, or multilevel intraspinal structural changes. Such patients present with complicated clinical and neuroimaging evidence, and electrodiagnostic testing might clarify issues of the location, activity, and severity of spinal nerve root disease.

TREATMENT

The initial management of acute spine pain must be directed toward determining if a serious neurologic condition exists. If there is a history of recent trauma or serious underlying medical illness, more-aggressive evaluation is warranted. The presence of acute and progressive neurologic dysfunction is an urgent medical problem. This is especially so when there is clinical evidence of bilateral neurologic dysfunction, increasing the likelihood of involvement of the spinal cord or cauda equina. Manifestations include bilateral leg weakness and sensory symptoms, and loss of bowel or bladder control. Such symptoms should trigger an urgent workup that includes MRI studies and possibly neurosurgical consultation.

Acute Low Back Pain

Acute spine pain is very common, and the likelihood of spontaneous recovery is in the range of 80% to 90%. Prolonged inactivity prolongs recovery. Because there is seldom a recognizable structural cause, treatment regimens tend to be nonspecific.

Patient education is important, and part of the therapeutic effort should include patient education about the nature of the condition, the likelihood of a good outcome, and the approach to be taken to speed recovery and minimize the risk of recurrence. Once these approaches to management have been undertaken, if there is no meaningful response to treatment, it is necessary to explore the possibility that psychosocial issues underlie the symptoms.

Acute Nonspecific Back Pain

There is general agreement that patients with acute nonspecific spine pain or nonlocalizable lumbosacral radiculopathy (without neurologic signs or significant neurologic symptoms) require only conservative medical management. Patients should abstain from heavy lifting or other activities that aggravate the pain. Bed rest is not helpful and has been shown to delay recovery.[9] Bed rest may be recommended for the first few days for patients with severe pain with movement. Recommended medications include nonsteroidal anti-inflammatory drugs such as ibuprofen or aspirin. If there are complaints of muscle spasm, muscle relaxants such as cyclobenzaprine may be used in the acute phase of pain. Narcotic analgesia should be avoided, in general, but it can be prescribed in cases of severe acute pain.

A study by Cherkin and coworkers compared standard physical therapy maneuvers and chiropractic spinal manipulation for the treatment of acute low back pain and found that both provide small short-term benefits and improve patient satisfaction, but they increase the cost of medical care and do not decrease the recurrence of back pain.[10] Although patients were somewhat less satisfied with reassurance and an education booklet (the third group in that study), this group fared no worse than the groups receiving therapy.

Acute Lumbosacral Radiculopathy

The initial treatment of the patient with lumbosacral radiculopathy presenting with sensory symptoms and pain without significant neurologic deficits is not different from the approach for the patient with uncomplicated low back pain. However, such patients require observation for possible worsening of their neurologic status.

Acute Radiculopathy with Neurologic Deficits

The treatment plan should fit the severity of the symptoms and signs. The management approach for radiculopathy covers the gamut from avoidance of heavy lifting to laminectomy and fusion. In acute radiculopathy, the goals of treatment should be the reduction of pain and the stabilization or amelioration of neurologic deficits.

Even patients with neurologic deficits such as segmental distributions of weakness, segmental loss of sensation, and reflex changes are likely to have significant spontaneous recovery. The initial approach to their treatment need not be different from that outlined for the patient with radicular sensory symptoms only. Reliable outcome studies that establish guidelines for medical versus surgical treatment in this patient group are not available. However, the risk is clearly greater in this group for progression of the neurologic deficits and residual neurologic impairment if spinal nerve root compression persists.

With a significant motor deficit, it is necessary to identify lesions that are amenable to surgical correction and to exclude the additional (and at times subclinical) presence of spinal cord or cauda equina compression. Thus, MRI studies are appropriate in this setting. With a very large disk protrusion or concomitant spinal cord compression, surgical intervention becomes a more important consideration, especially if neurologic deficits continue to worsen over time or if pain persists.

Management should consist of the avoidance of provocative activities, the use of non-narcotic analgesics, and the use of muscle relaxants if symptoms suggest that spasm is a component. Prolonged inactivity is not beneficial, and mobilization should be encouraged as soon as symptoms stabilize. Gentle exercises, massage, and mobilization are beneficial, but spinal manipulation is not. If there is a strong suspicion of nerve root impingement by disk protrusion or spondylosis, a high-dose, fast-taper course of corticosteroids can be used. A typical course would be prednisone 60 to 80 mg daily for 5 to 7 days, followed by a fast taper to discontinuation over the next 7 to 14 days, but there are no prospective, carefully controlled trials that confirm the value of corticosteroids. Prophylaxis against gastritis is recommended, and special precautions are needed in patients with diabetes; otherwise, the short course of treatment is not likely to produce complications.

Chronic Low Back Pain

When symptoms of spine pain extend beyond 4 to 8 weeks, the condition has moved from the acute to the chronic phase. At this point it is appropriate to reassess the patient's symptoms and examination. If no neuroimaging was performed in the acute phase of the illness, the need for studies at this time should be reassessed. In the face of true radiculopathy with new or worsening neurologic deficits, a surgical opinion should be considered. Depending on the full clinical picture, a number of alternative nonsurgical approaches may be considered at this point, although in general their efficacy has not been proved.

Chronic Nonspecific Back Pain

The standard approach to the patient with nonspecific chronic spine pain is physical therapy. By 3 to 4 weeks after onset of symptoms, unless there is serious underlying structural disease, there is no reason the patient should not be enrolled in an aggressive program of mobilization, postural improvement, and increased endurance. Yoga techniques provide useful stretching maneuvers that the patient can learn by video instruction. In the treatment of subacute and chronic spine pain, osteopathic physicians and chiropractors provide spinal manipulation techniques, such as thrust, muscle energy, counter-strain, articulation, and myofascial release. A study by Andersson and associates in patients with nonradicular lumbar spine pain of 3 to 26 weeks' duration compared a medical program that included physical therapy with a program that included active spinal manipulation.[11] At 12 weeks, there was no significant difference in the degree of improvement between the two groups, although the group that received manipulation required significantly less analgesia, anti-inflammatories, and muscle relaxants, and they used less physical therapy. More than 90% of the patients in both groups were satisfied with their care.

Other treatments have been used with varying results.[12] Transcutaneous electrical nerve stimulation has been used in patients with subacute and chronic spine pain, with varying results. A number of factors appear to influence success, including chronicity of the pain, electrode-pad placement, and prior treatments. Corticosteroid injections in facet joints and epidural locations have been advocated by some clinicians. The value of therapeutic corticosteroid injection in the setting of chronic nonspecific back pain without established radiculopathy has not been proven.

Chronic Lumbosacral Radiculopathy

The long-term outlook is good for significant spontaneous recovery in patients with lumbosacral radiculopathy. However, the pain of acute radiculopathy can persist beyond 3 or 4 weeks, becoming chronic, at which point acute remedies such as rest, analgesics, and cervical traction may be less effective and other therapeutic options must be sought. When the manifestations of radiculopathy are primarily sensory or when the motor deficits are stable, a number of nonsurgical options have come into general use, although their true effectiveness has not yet been proved. The therapies used in patients with chronic nonspecific spine pain may be used in this setting as well, but several other procedures may be considered after conservative maneuvers have failed.

Chronic lumbar radiculopathy can also result from lumbar canal stenosis (LCS). This condition refers to narrowing of the intraspinal (central) canal, which can be associated with narrowing of lateral recesses and neural foramina. The primary symptoms of LCS include discomfort, sensory loss, and weakness in the legs, reflecting dysfunction of multiple spinal nerve roots within the lumbar spinal canal. Lateral recess and neural foraminal stenosis can give rise to lumbar radiculopathy. Neurogenic claudication—the tendency for exacerbation of symptoms due to walking, standing, and maintaining certain postures—is the hallmark of the condition. Neurogenic claudication may be described by patients as discomfort in the buttocks, thighs, or legs on standing or walking, which is relieved by sitting or lying. In one study, 94% of patients with LCS described symptoms of neurogenic claudication.[13] Patients might demonstrate a combination of claudication symptoms and symptoms of more focal lumbar radiculopathy.

Epidural Corticosteroid Injection

Anecdotal reports and retrospective analyses indicate that there is value in epidural corticosteroid injection for chronic radiculopathy, but the few placebo-controlled, prospective studies that have been performed for lumbar procedures have been criticized for design flaws.[14] Of theoretical value, based on the assumption that radiculopathic pain is, at least in part, a result of inflammatory factors such as cytokinins in the vicinity of spinal nerve root compression, epidural corticosteroid injection aims to alleviate pain enough to allow more active physical therapy.

A randomized, double-blind trial performed by Carette and colleagues studied 158 patients with lumbar radiculopathy of 4 to 52 weeks' duration who had evidence of radicular deficits on clinical examination and CT evidence of disk herniation.[15] Six weeks after three epidural injections of either corticosteroids or saline, patients who had received corticosteroids had somewhat more improvement in leg pain, but at 3 months there was no significant difference between the two groups. Twenty-five percent of patients in both groups eventually went on to lumbar spine surgery.

Selective Nerve Root Blocks

Another local injection procedure, selective nerve root block, has been used for diagnostic and therapeutic purposes at the lumbosacral and cervical levels. This diagnostic technique has been used when there is lack of agreement between clinical and neuroimaging findings, when there is atypical limb pain, and when there is a history of failed surgery at the level in question. Nerve root blocks are contraindicated in the presence of systemic infection, local infection, or bleeding diathesis.

For the therapeutic procedure at the cervical level, it is standard practice to use a combination of 0.5 mL of 1% lidocaine and a long-acting corticosteroid. The therapeutic injection is preceded by a localization procedure under fluoroscopic guidance using a nonionic contrast medium to outline the selected nerve root. Pretreatment contrast injection is critical to exclude intravascular needle positioning. The needle may also be misplaced in the epidural space or at the sinuvertebral nerve, in which case selective nerve root block and the selectiveness of the results of injection cannot be verified.

The sinuvertebral nerve (derived from sympathetic fibers from the ramus communicans and fibers from either the primary anterior or posterior ramus) provides innervation over several segments to adjacent dura, posterior longitudinal ligament, and annulus. Although the efficacy of selective nerve root block at the lumbosacral levels has been studied, a further concern regarding the value of this procedure is the placebo response rate, which is reported to be as high as 38%.[16]

Surgical Considerations

Several multicenter trials have compared surgical and medical treatment for lumbar radiculopathy. The Spine Patient Outcomes Research Trial (SPORT) compared surgical and medical therapies for lumbar disk herniation and found that over the short term, surgical patients had fewer symptoms, but over a 2-year period there was no difference between the groups.[17,18] Likewise, in a Dutch study of severe sciatica for 6 to 12 weeks with lumbosacral radiculopathy confirmed by a neurologist, patients were randomized to either conservative treatment (with or without eventual surgery) or early minimal unilateral transflaval surgery with magnification.[19] Patients with severe weakness and cauda equina syndrome were excluded. At 1 year, outcomes were similar for the two groups, although the rates of pain relief and of perceived recovery were faster for those assigned to early surgery.

In another study, patients with lumbar spondylolisthesis, lumbar canal stenosis, and neurogenic claudication with neurologic signs were randomized to conservative treatment or decompressive surgery with spinal fusion.[20] This study demonstrated significantly greater improvement in pain and function among the surgically treated patients, but the analysis was complicated by an unexpectedly high rate of crossover from the conservative treatment group to the surgery group. Back pain did not improve as much as leg pain, indicating that the greatest benefit was likely to have occurred for nerve-root related symptoms.[21] A study of patients with LCS without spondylolisthesis more convincingly demonstrated a benefit for surgically treated patients compared to medically treated patients over a 2-year period.[22]

Factors that should influence the likelihood that surgery will be performed for radiculopathy or LCS include an obvious neurologic deficit, progression of the deficits over time, unresolved pain, and identification of an anatomic lesion that corresponds with the neurologic picture. For patients with a lumbar disk herniation, surgery versus medical treatment may be a lifestyle decision, depending on whether they can alter their lifestyle to accommodate the pain or can obtain surgery to attempt to achieve a faster return to a former lifestyle.[23]

Chronic Pain Syndrome

A small number of patients fail to respond to all the previously discussed therapeutic interventions. Some patients have chronic spine pain without evidence of structural intraspinal pathology, others have had previously treated structural lesions, and some have had multiple previous surgical interventions, a condition described as the failed-back syndrome. The goal in these patients is to improve the ability to perform activities of daily living and to diminish pain perception.

It is well established that a number of nonmedical factors play a role in the triggering and perpetuation of pain behavior. These include psychosocial issues such as job dissatisfaction, family stresses, and underlying psychiatric disorders. In other cases, patients develop a behavior of pain avoidance and fear of pain. Patients with chronic pain are best treated in programs dedicated to the rehabilitation of patients with multifactorial pain syndromes. Functional rehabilitation programs and pain programs concentrate on re-educating the patient to diminish fear of activities of daily living through graded exercise programs, the exploration of psychosocial stressors, and the non-narcotic treatment of pain.[24]

Determination of the degree of impairment and disability is required in patients with chronic disorders who are seeking worker's compensation or permanent disability status. The American Medical Association has published guidelines for the evaluation of permanent impairment, incorporating both an injury model and a range-of-motion model for rating lumbar impairment.[25]

OUTCOMES

Recurrences of low back pain are common. Studies have shown recurrence rates between 30% and 75% within 3 years of the first episode. A Canadian study showed the highest recurrence rate among nurses and truck drivers and the lowest among office workers.[26] Another Canadian study compared two interventions in the rehabilitation of workers who had missed 4 weeks of work. Patients were randomized to occupational intervention (occupational physician, ergonomist, and employer working to improve the work environment and the patient's relation to it) or to clinical intervention (back pain specialist, back school, and functional rehabilitation after 12 weeks off work). The patients fared much better with the occupational intervention.[27]

For patients with radiculopathy, there is less likelihood of early recovery; however, without surgery, about 50% of patients can return to work after 4 to 6 weeks. A study of postal workers who had had lumbar laminectomy showed an almost six-fold greater likelihood for recurrent occupational low back injury.[28]

Summary

- Low back pain is usually caused by mechanical disorders of the spine, with or without involvement of the spinal nerve roots, but it may be a result of nonmechanical causes or may be referred from retroperitoneal sources.
- Diagnosis starts with a careful examination, followed by consideration for neuroimaging studies and electrodiagnostic studies.
- Specific management decisions are based on the duration of symptoms and the presence or absence of neurologic deficits.
- Chronic pain syndromes are often perpetuated by nonmedical factors. Treatment requires a multidisciplinary approach.

Suggested Readings

American Academy of Neurology: Practice parameters: Magnetic resonance imaging in the evaluation of low back syndrome (summary statement). Report of the Quality Standards Committee of the American Academy of Neurology. Neurology 1994;44:767-770.

Andersson GBJ: Epidemiologic features of chronic low-back pain. Lancet 1999;354:581-585.

Bell GR: Implications of the Spie Patient Outcomes Research Trial in the clinical management of lumbar disk herniation. Cleve Clin J Med 2007;74: 572-576.

Carey TS, Garrett J, Jackman A, et al: The outcomes and costs of care for acute low back pain among patients seen by primary care practitioners, chiropractors, and orthopedic surgeons. The North Carolina Back Pain Project. N Engl J Med 1995;333:913-917.

Hall S, Bartleson JD, Onofrio BM, et al: Lumbar spinal stenosis. Clinical features, diagnostic procedures, and results of surgical treatment in 68 patients. Ann Internal Med 1985;103:271-275.

Peul WC, van Houwelingen HC, van den Hout WB, et al: Surgery versus prolonged conservative treatment for sciatica. N Engl J Med 2007;356:2245-2256.

Weinstein JN, Tosteson TD, Lurie JD, et al: Surgical vs nonoperative treatment for lumbar disk herniation. The Spine Patient Outcomes Research Trial (SPORT): A randomised trial. JAMA 2006;296:2441-2450.

Weinstein JN, Lurie JD, Tosteson TD, et al: Surgical vs nonoperative treatment for lumbar disk herniation. The Spine Patient Outcomes Research Trial (SPORT) observational cohort. JAMA 2006;296:2451-2459.

Weinstein JN, Lurie JD, Tosteson TD, et al: Surgical versus nonsurgical treatment for lumbar degenerative spondylolisthesis. N Engl J Med 2007;356:2257-2270.

Weinstein JN, Tosteson TD, Lurie JD, et al: Surgical versus nonsurgical therapy for lumbar spinal stenosis. N Engl J Med 2008;358:794-810.

References

For a complete list of references, log onto www.expertconsult.com.

Section 11

PSYCHIATRY AND PSYCHOLOGY

Behavioral Assessment of the General Medical Patient

George E. Tesar, Joseph Austerman, Leo Pozuelo, and J. Harry Isaacson

Epidemiologic data indicate that over one half of U.S. patients receive mental health care exclusively in the primary care setting.[1] The primary care physician who can readily detect and manage behavior problems will be better equipped to manage this growing demand.

The American Psychiatric Association's *Practice Guideline for Psychiatric Evaluation of Adults* provides a comprehensive overview of elements essential to thorough psychiatric evaluation.[2] Expecting the primary care physician's strict adherence to the *Guideline* is unrealistic and impractical. Time does not permit all areas to be addressed, nor is it necessary in most cases.

The purpose of this chapter, therefore, is to draw on the *Guideline* as well as other resources[3-5] to develop a succinct and targeted summary of elements essential to efficient behavioral assessment by the primary care physician. Developing this skill set is especially important because behavioral disorders are among the most prevalent and treatment-responsive problems encountered in primary care.

EVALUATING THE PRIMARY CARE PATIENT

A behavioral disorder should be included in the differential diagnosis of any patient who presents with repeated complaints, especially fatigue, insomnia, pain, or just feeling overwhelmed. For a variety of reasons, this demands that the primary care physician maintain a high index of suspicion for behavioral disturbance in her or his patients. The patient and physician typically focus on identifying a physical cause for the problem at hand. Failure to find a physical or physiologic basis can leave one or both with the nagging concern that something has been missed. Physicians' time constraints interfere with recognition, thorough assessment, and optimal management of behavioral disturbances.

Patients themselves are also inclined to minimize or ignore behavioral considerations. Psychological symptoms are typically viewed as evidence of weakness or personal failure, so that even under ideal circumstances, patients are unlikely to entertain or accept a behavioral explanation for their distress. The language used to describe symptoms can therefore be problematic, and labeling with psychiatric symptoms or diagnoses can alienate rather than recruit the patient.

The primary care physician must also be aware of and deal with her or his own misgivings about behavioral disorders. The stigma of mental illness is pervasive and originates in each of us. That is, none of us is comfortable with self disclosure, especially when it can result in being labeled crazy or mentally unfit. The primary care physician must overcome her or his own resistance to engage the patient in self revelation that can trigger fear, embarrassment, or shame.

INTERVIEW TECHNIQUES

Ideally, the primary care physician creates an environment that facilitates disclosure of sensitive, personal information. Effective interviewing that achieves this goal also helps maximize data gathering. Effective time management depends on having the skill not only to facilitate but also to tactfully limit patient self-disclosure or somatic preoccupation.

General Approach

The most comprehensive and accurate information is obtained when the examination begins with *open-ended questions* and *active listening* followed by structured inquiry about specific symptoms and events. Open-ended questions give the patient the opportunity to tell things from his or her perspective, and active listening helps verify and enrich the patient's report. Active listening involves periodic feedback to the patient of what the clinician has understood so as to ascertain and clarify what the patient has said. It can also serve to limit and redirect the rambling of an unfocused patient. Active listening facilitates the assimilation of a comprehensive database, and it also conveys to the patient the clinician's sincere effort to understand and to empathize with the patient's circumstances. The clinician's listening attitude helps to establish trust and a collaborative, problem-solving partnership between patient and clinician.

The BATHE Technique

A widely accepted format for organizing the findings of medical examination is the acronym SOAP (subjective, objective, assessment, plan). An alternative that focuses attention on behavior and emotional symptoms occurring in the context of the patient's life circumstances is captured by the acronym BATHE. Proposed by Stuart and Lieberman,[3] the relevant terms and questions are listed in Table 1.

Although the BATHE technique was designed to help primary care physicians integrate effective, time-limited psychotherapy during a brief office visit, it also helps facilitate information gathering during patient evaluation. Once the patient's attention is directed to affect, behavior, and life circumstances, it may be easier to elicit other symptoms potentially relevant to an underlying behavioral disorder. Fundamentally, BATHEing the patient is a way of skillfully drawing attention to the patient's emotional life, reactions to illness and other potential stressors, and the possible relevance of these reactions to the manifesting problem.

DATA GATHERING

The two most important goals of behavioral assessment are accurate formulation of the diagnosis and adequate assessment of risk.

Correct Diagnosis

The *Guideline* lists 16 domains of the clinical evaluation (Table 2). Although thorough psychiatric evaluation demands attention to all domains, targeted assessment by the primary care physician requires attention to history of present illness, past history of similar symptoms and treatment, family history of psychiatric symptoms and diagnosis, substance use, stressors, and level of function. Because most clinically significant behavioral disorders are chronic, recurrent, and familial, attention to the patient's past and family histories can help to confirm suspicion of an underlying behavioral disorder. Also, drug and alcohol abuse commonly accompany primary behavioral illness and cause or mimic secondary behavioral symptoms. Psychiatric diagnostic formulation is discussed more fully later and is summarized in Table 3.

Risk Assessment

Among the most important elements of behavioral evaluation is determination of risk of harm to self or others. Risk assessment has a critical impact on immediate treatment and triage decisions. Failure to assess risk adequately can lead to a potentially devastating outcome. Because of this, some clinicians might underreact by overlooking

Table 1 BATHE Technique

Domain	Recommended Question or Statement	Rationale
Background	"What is going on in your life?"	Elicits life circumstances, potential stresses, etc. Redirects patient from somatic focus
Affect	"How do you feel about that?" or "How has that affected your mood?"	Allows the patient to report feelings, emotions
Trouble	"What about the situation troubles you the most?"	Focuses on the meaning of the circumstances to the patient
Handling	"How are you handling that?"	Provides an assessment of functioning and potentially a connection to the somatic complaint
Empathy	"That must be difficult for you" or "No wonder you're feeling the way you do"	Normalizes the patient's reaction and demonstrates the physician's understanding

Adapted from Stuart MR, Libermann JA: The Fifteen Minute Hour: Applied Psychotherapy for the Primary Care Physician, 2nd ed. Westport, Conn: Praeger, 1993.

Box 1 Referral to Secondary Mental Health Services

Circumstances Warranting Referral

The patient displays signs of suicidal intent or seems to be a risk of harm to others.
The patient is so disabled by the mental disorder that he or she cannot leave the home, look after the children, or fulfill other activities of daily living.
The primary care physician requires the expertise of secondary care to confirm a diagnosis or implement specialist treatment.
The primary care physician feels that the therapeutic relationship with the patient has broken down.
The primary care interventions and voluntary/nonstatutory options have been exhausted.
The patient's physical condition has severely deteriorated.
A particular psychotropic medication is required (e.g., clozapine, lithium).
The patient requests a referral.

Considerations in Making a Referral

The physician should have access to a local resource directory.
The physician should consider coordination issues around the referral (e.g., care program approach, care manager).
The physician should consider implications for the continuing care of the physical health of the patient.

From: World Health Organization: Integrating mental health services into primary health care. Geneva, World Health Organization, 2007. Available at http://www.who.int/mental_health/policy/services/en/index.html (accessed March 15, 2009; Mental Health Policy, Planning and Service Development Information Sheet, Sheet 3.)

behavioral symptoms. Others might overreact by insisting on emergent psychiatric assessment at any mention of suicidal or homicidal thoughts or impulses. Knowing how to assess risk and when and where to seek emergency psychiatric consultation is important. In general, the clinician should determine whether the patient is safe to leave the office, and if so, whether or not return to work is advisable.

The World Health Organization (WHO) has developed guidelines to assist with this process.[4] These are summarized in Box 1. Suicidal and homicidal thoughts, intentions, and planning are addressed in the mental status examination (MSE). More detailed discussion of these issues can be found in the chapter entitled "Management of Office-Based Behavioral Emergencies."

MENTAL STATUS EXAMINATION

Like the physical examination, the MSE is a structured, systematic method for collecting objective data pertinent both to diagnosis and to patient management. The paucity of clinically relevant laboratory, neuroimaging, and other quantifiable markers of psychopathology make effective mental status examination particularly important.

The elements of the MSE performed by psychiatrists are elaborated in the *Guideline*[2]; aspects relevant to the primary care physician are discussed here. Much of the patient's cognitive and emotional status can be inferred during the interview. Attention to important details, however, prevents incorrect inference and facilitates diagnostic accuracy and effective triage. Those interested in developing a more thorough understanding of psychiatric MSE should consult the *Guideline* and other sources.[2,6,7]

Summarized here and in Table 2 are important domains and details of the general mental status examination.

Appearance and General Behavior

Hygiene and attire can help to distinguish a chronic from an acute process, such as chronic paranoid schizophrenia versus acute mania, acute psychosis, or toxic psychoses, delirium, or encephalopathy secondary to drug toxicity, metabolic disturbance, or an acute neurologic event (e.g., stroke, acute hypoglycemia, herpes encephalitis).

Movement and Posture

Look for tics, tremors, and other abnormal movements that suggest primary central nervous system disorders (e.g., Parkinson's disease, Tourette's syndrome, Huntington's disease) or extrapyramidal disorders secondary to antipsychotic drugs (e.g., akathisia, dystonia, parkinsonism, tardive dyskinesia).

Mood and Affect

Mood applies to the prevalent feeling(s) verbalized by the patient, whereas *affect* refers to the current expression of emotion. Affect is described according to its four features: *quality* (e.g., depressed, euphoric, silly, anxious, irritable, angry, flat, euthymic), *intensity* (e.g., bright, blunted), *range* (e.g., labile, constricted, normal), and *congruence* (i.e., with mood and thought content). Examples of incongruent mood and affect include the depressed, hopeless individual who intentionally exhibits a bright affect or the bipolar patient whose underlying depression is masked by manic or hypomanic affect.

Speech and Language

Dysarthria due to substance-induced toxicity or central nervous system pathology is generally easily detected. Be careful to rule out aphasia in the patient whose disorganized verbal production might create a first impression of being psychotic, crazy, or stressed out. Simple tests that screen language function are included in the Mini-Mental State Examination (MMSE).[8]

Pressure of speech describes a person's inability to converse in an appropriate give-and-take fashion, to listen and refrain from speaking while another person speaks. Speech is described as pressured when the listener has difficulty interjecting. Pressured speech is a

Table 2 Domains of the Behavioral Assessment

Domain	Essential*	Details to Explore
Reason for evaluation	×	
Chief complaint	×	
History of present illness	×	Precise time and circumstances at onset of symptom(s) Associated behavioral symptoms with special consideration to diagnostic criteria for psychiatric disorders common in primary care: major depression, bipolar disorder, anxiety disorders, eating disorders, substance use disorders, somatization
Past psychiatric history	×	Similar symptoms in past Unexplained symptoms in past Response to past treatment(s)
Family psychiatric history	×	Actual or suspected psychiatric symptoms or disorders Suicide or suspicious death Substance abuse
Substance abuse (alcohol, drug, tobacco, inhalant)	×	Current and/or past use Consequences (legal, physical, marital, interpersonal, vocational) Last use
General medical history		
Developmental, psychosocial, and sociocultural histories		
Occupational and military histories		
Legal history		
Review of systems		
Physical examination		
Mental status examination	×	Be vigilant and assess for indications of dangerousness: suicide, homicide, psychosis
Functional assessment	×	Can the patient return home, to his or her job? Can the patient perform activities of daily living? Current and baseline global assessments of functioning

*All domains are important. It is recommended, however, that those identified as essential be included in any rapid behavioral assessment by the primary care physician.

Adapted from American Psychiatric Association: Practice Guideline for the Psychiatric Evaluation of Adults, 2nd ed. Washington, DC, American Psychiatric Association, 2006.

hallmark of mania, but should it not be confused for the nonstop ruminative speech of an anxious person or a patient's manipulative efforts to frustrate the examiner's quest for information. Speech that is both pressured and rapid, however, almost certainly indicates mania.

Perceptions

Abnormal perceptions include *hallucinations* (sensory experiences occurring in the absence of an identifiable stimulus), *illusions* (misinterpretation of an identifiable stimulus) and *distortions* (distorted perception of an identifiable stimulus, e.g., micropsia or macropsia). Well-formed, complex auditory hallucinations are more common than visual hallucinations. Both types of hallucinations can occur in schizophrenia and in depression or mania with psychotic features. However, any type of abnormal perception—especially illusions and distortions—should alert the clinician to a toxic, metabolic, structural or epileptic cause.

Thought Process, Flow, and Content

A formal thought disorder (i.e., a disorder of thought process or the form of thought) is thinking that is illogical and hard to follow, or concrete and void of meaningful content. Cognitive disturbances due to frontotemporal pathology (e.g., stroke, dementia, multiple sclerosis) typically produce abnormal form of thought that is concrete, overly detailed, or without clear relationship to other thoughts (loose associations). The literature on schizophrenia, whose hallmark is a formal thought disorder, points to underlying frontal cortical and corticothalamic dysfunction.

Rapid flow (rate) of thought is often described as *flight of ideas* and suggests mania. Psychomotor retardation describes the paucity and slowing of thought (and movement) associated with clinically significant major depression (see elsewhere in this section, "Recognition and Treatment of Depression").

It is especially important, but often difficult, to examine the content of thought, because the validity of findings depends almost exclusively on the patient's openness and cooperation. Suicidal, homicidal, paranoid, and obsessive thoughts are examples of abnormal *thought content* whose disclosure is essential to accurate diagnosis and triage. Any indication that a patient has thoughts of harming himself or herself or someone else requires careful assessment of the intensity and frequency of such thoughts, the degree to which the patient intends to follow through, and the availability of means and circumstances that would permit follow-through (see the later chapter "Psychiatric Emergencies.").

Table 3 Multiaxial System for Formulation of Psychiatric Diagnoses

Axis	Domain	
I	Primary psychiatric disorder	
II	Personality or developmental disorder	
III	Medical disorder(s)	
IV	Psychosocial or environmental problems that contribute to the current problem	Classification of problems: Primary support group Social environment Education Occupation Housing Economic Access to health care Interaction with the legal system; crime Other psychosocial and environmental
V	Global assessment of functioning	Current level (0-100) Highest level in the past year (0-100)

Adapted from American Psychiatric Association: Diagnostic and Statistical Manual, 4th ed, text rev. Washington, DC, American Psychiatric Press, 2000.
Severity rating (based on clinician's judgment):
0 = None
1 = Mild
2 = Mild-to-moderate
3 = Moderate
4 = Moderate-to-severe
5 = Severe
90-100 = Superior functioning
80-89 = Expected response to usual stressors
70-79 = Mild symptoms and/or dysfunction
60-69 = Moderate symptoms and/or dysfunction
50-59 = Severe symptoms and/or dysfunction
40-49 = Elevated risk of harm to self or others
<40 = Acute risk of harm to self or others from psychosis, delirium, or dementia

Cognitive Status

Often used as a synonym for "sensorium," *cognition* technically refers to ability to reason, abstract, and calculate. *Sensorium* includes mental processes that regulate level of consciousness, attention, and memory (orientation, registration, and short- and long-term memory). Tests of attention and memory are included in the Mini-Mental State Examination,[8] as are tests of speech and language (repetition, reading, writing, and comprehension) and constructional ability.

Insight

Level of insight is judged by the patient's ability to recognize whether or not he or she has an illness, and the degree to which it might or might not compromise the patient's function.

Judgment

Judgment is determined by the patient's ability to register, process, manipulate, and act on information in a socially appropriate manner. Abnormalities of cognition, sensorium, behavior (e.g., agitation, combativeness), or affect (severe depression or mania) can interfere with sound judgment.

Intention (Executive Functions)

Although not included in the *Guideline,* executive functions include anticipating, planning, and organizing and executing tasks, functions that depend on an intact dorsolateral prefrontal cortex. Normal impulse control depends on intact orbitofrontal cortex function; high impulsivity can interfere with otherwise normal executive functioning. A quick and effective screen of higher cortical function is clock drawing.[9]

STRUCTURED INTERVIEWS, SCREENING INSTRUMENTS, AND RATING SCALES

Physician-rated behavioral scales and structured interviews[10] are largely relevant to research and not commonly employed in clinical practice. In contrast, patient-rated screening instruments can be a valuable source of data obtained at no cost of physician time (Table 4). Once collected, however, the patient's responses must be reviewed. Failure to review patients' responses can introduce potential liability if, for example, a patient makes a suicide attempt or successfully commits suicide after endorsing "suicidal ideation" on a screening form that was never reviewed by a professional.

Patient-rated screening instruments can be valuable when used on an ad hoc basis to verify a clinical impression and to follow treatment progress. For example, the physician who suspects a clinically significant behavioral disorder can ask the patient to complete a patient-rated questionnaire or survey. The same instrument can be used at subsequent visits as a metric of progress. These instruments can assist with diagnostic verification and symptom measurement, and they provide a time-effective way of collecting and documenting clinically relevant data.

Self-reported behavioral symptoms can also be processed by computer to generate a valid behavioral diagnostic profile. Data that are entered into the computer by the patient manually or by telephone are rapidly analyzed so that valid diagnostic information is available within minutes. Shedler's Quick PsychoDiagnostic Profile[5] and the Patient Health Questionnaire[11] are based on DSM IV diagnostic criteria, have computerized formats, and deliver data analysis on five or more psychiatric disorders commonly seen by primary care physicians (major depression, dysthymia, panic disorder, generalized anxiety disorder, eating disorders, substance-use disorders, and somatization). The Patient Health Questionnaire 9 (see Table 4) is an abridged version of the Patient Health Questionnaire that focuses specifically on criteria for depression.

DIAGNOSIS AND DIAGNOSTIC FORMULATION

The Diagnostic and Statistical Manual of Mental Disorders, fourth edition, text revision (DSM IV-TR)[12] employs a multiaxial system to formulate a diagnosis of behavioral disorders. The five-axis system is depicted in Table 3. It is designed to capture the multiple variables that can contribute to the genesis, severity, and persistence of behavioral symptoms. Although not designed specifically for primary care practice, it is a standard format used by psychiatrists. Familiarity with it can facilitate communication between the primary care physician and mental health professionals.

Axis I codifies the *primary psychiatric disorder* (e.g., major depression, panic disorder, alcohol dependence, conversion disorder). In general, Axis I disorders have a discrete onset, are episodic, and dominate the clinical picture. A patient can have more than one primary psychiatric disorder (e.g., one patient can have major depression, panic disorder, alcohol dependence, and conversion disorder all at once).

Axis II codifies *personality disorders.* Personality is defined by typical, persistent, and predictable patterns of behavior, thinking, and feeling that characterize an individual person. Personality disorder is

Table 4 Self-Report Questionnaires for Common Psychiatric Disorders

Symptom/Behavior	Diagnosis	Instrument	Interpretation
Depressed mood or loss of interest	Major depressive episode (single or recurrent) or Adjustment disorder with depressed mood	Beck Depression Inventory (BDI-II)	≥10 suggests at least mild clinically significant depression Severity correlates positively with score 11-17 = mild 18-23 = moderate ≥24 = severe
		Center for Epidemiologic Studies Depression Scale (CES-D)	≥16 compatible with clinically significant DSM-IV depression Severity correlates positively with score
		Zung Depression Scale	≥50 compatible with clinically significant depression
		Patient Health Questionnaire 9 (PHQ-9)	
		Geriatric Depression Scale (short form)	3 ± 2 = normal 7 ± 3 = mildly depressed 12 ± 2 = very depressed
Depression with history of *mania* or *hypomania*	Bipolar disorder I or II; cyclothymia	Mood Disorder Questionnaire (MDQ)	
Excessive worry/arousal	Generalized anxiety disorder	Zung Self-rating Anxiety Scale	>20 suggests clinically significant anxiety Highest score = 80. Severity correlates positively with score
Anxiety attacks, unexplained episodic pain	Panic disorder	Resources available at http://www.neurotransmitter.net	None validated or normed
Withdrawn, shy	Social anxiety disorder	Liebowitz Social Anxiety Scale*http://www.socialanxietysupport.com/liebowitz.php	
Flashbacks, social withdrawal	Posttraumatic stress disorder	Resources available at http://www.ncptsd.va.gov/ncmain/healthcare/	
Intrusive, unwanted thoughts and/or repetitive or ritualistic activity	Obsessive-compulsive disorder obsessive-compulsive personality disorder	Resources available at http://www.neurotransmitter.net	None validated or normed
Life-long trouble staying focused, getting things done, ± hyperactivity	Attention-deficit/hyperactivity disorder	Wender-Utah Rating Scale http://neurotransmitter.net/adhdscales.html Adult ADHD Self-Report Scale (ASRS) http://neurotransmitter.net/adhdscales.html	

DSM-IV, Diagnostic and Statistical Manual of Mental Disorders, 4th edition, text revision.
*Social phobia scoring scale 55-65 Moderate
65-80 Marked
80-95 Severe
>95 Very Severe

diagnosed when these distinctive patterns are maladaptive and cause significant conflict, distress, or dysfunction. Personality disorders often accompany Axis I disorders and can be difficult to differentiate. A core characteristic of personality disorder is a lack of insight that contributes to ongoing conflict with others and a profound sense of being misunderstood.

Axis III codifies current *medical problems* that may be relevant to the Axis I disorder (e.g., acute myocardial infarction followed by onset of a major depressive episode).

Axis IV codifies categories of *stress* and their severity. Fundamental to accurate formulation of the diagnosis is the recognition that diagnostic criteria (relevant symptoms, duration, and intensity) determine diagnosis—not the stressor(s) that might have triggered the Axis I disorder. For example, a common error is to assume that depressive symptoms and a difficult adjustment constitute a normal reaction in the wake of catastrophic or debilitating medical illness and therefore does not require specific treatment. If the patient meets symptom criteria for a diagnosis of major depression, then regardless of the type and intensity of stress, a diagnosis of major depressive episode is warranted. Symptom burden—not stress—is the principal determinant of diagnosis.

Axis V quantifies the current level of *function* and the highest level in the past year.

SPECIAL POPULATIONS

Difficult Patients

Some patients overuse or misuse the primary care physician's time and services. Many such patients have a behavioral disorder. Occasionally, effective treatment of a previously undiagnosed

Box 2 Illnesses Commonly Associated with Behavioral Comorbidity

Asthma
Cancer (especially pancreatic)
Cardiac arrhythmia
Chronic obstructive pulmonary disease
Congestive heart failure
Diabetes
Epilepsy
Hepatitis C and its treatment with interferon
Human immunodeficiency virus infection or acquired immunodeficiency syndrome
Multiple sclerosis
Myocardial infarction
Parkinson's disease and other movement disorders
Stroke
Transplantation

behavioral disorder solves the problem. In other instances, a multitude of medical and either primary or secondary behavioral disorders can complicate management. Some patients present repeatedly with multiple, often changing somatic complaints, and others manufacture complaints for secondary gain. Many of the most troublesome patients suffer from Axis I disorders (e.g., somatization disorder hypochondriasis, or factitious disorder) or Axis II disorders (e.g., borderline, dependent). These patients require special attention that entails limit-setting and delineation of clear, reasonable expectations. This important topic is discussed further elsewhere.[13]

Chronic Medical Illness

Some chronic debilitating medical illnesses are associated with a high risk of secondary behavioral disorder (Box 2). The primary care physician should be alert to such patients and anticipate their need for specific behavioral treatment or referral.

Dangerous Patients

Patients who make threats or behave in ways that potentially endanger themselves or others must be identified and triaged appropriately. Access to appropriate services is often problematic and requires advance planning.

Pregnant Patients

The pregnant patient with a behavioral disorder might require consultation with a psychiatrist to determine her optimal behavioral treatment program.

Summary

- Primary care physicians are providing a growing fraction of the behavioral health care in the United States.
- Primary care physicians can learn to overcome traditional barriers to detection and effective treatment of their patients' behavioral health problems.
- Detection of behavioral disorders requires that the primary care physician maintain a high index of suspicion.
- The standard psychiatric interview and mental status examination can be modified to accommodate the needs of the primary care physician.

Suggested Readings

American Psychiatric Association: Diagnostic and Statistical Manual of Mental Disorders, 4th ed, text rev. Washington, DC, American Psychiatric Association, 2000.

American Psychiatric Association: Practice Guideline for Psychiatric Evaluation of Adults, 2nd ed. Washington, DC, American Psychiatric Association, 2006. PDF available at www.psych.org/psych_pract/treatg/pg/PsychEval2ePG_04-28-06.pdf (accessed March 15, 2009).

Borson S, Scanlon J, Brush M, et al: The Mini-Cog: a cognitive "vital signs" measure for dementia screening in multilingual elderly. Int J Geriatr Psychiatry 2000;15:1021-1027.

Folstein MF, Folstein SE, McHugh PR: "Mini-mental state." A practical method for grading the cognitive state of patients for the clinician. J Psychiatr Res 1975;12(3):189-198.

Jackson JL, Kroenke K: Difficult patient encounters in the ambulatory clinic: Clinical predictors and outcomes. Arch Int Med 1999;159:1069-1075.

Kroenke K, Spitzer RL: The PHQ-9: A new depression and diagnostic severity measure. Psychiatr Ann 2002;32:509-521.

Rush JA, Pincus HA, First MB, et al: Handbook of Psychiatric Measures. Washington DC, American Psychiatric Association, 2000.

Shedler J, Beck A, Bensen S: Practical mental health assessment in primary care: Validity and utility of the Quick Psycho Diagnostics (QPD) panel. J Fam Practice 2000;49:614-621.

Stuart MR, Libermann JA: The Fifteen Minute Hour: Applied Psychotherapy for the Primary Care Physician, 2nd ed. Westport, Conn, Praeger, 1993.

Strub RL, Black FW: The Mental Status Examination in Neurology, 2nd ed. Philadelphia, FA Davis. 1987.

Trzapacz PT, Baker RW: The Psychiatric Mental Status Examination. New York, Oxford University Press, 1993.

Wang PS, Demler O, Olfson M, et al: Changing profiles of service sectors used for mental health care in the United States. Am J Psychiatry 2006;163:1187-1198.

World Health Organization: Integrating mental health services into primary health care. Geneva, World Health Organization, 2007. Available at http://www.who.int/mental_health/policy/services/en/index.html (accessed March 15, 2009); Mental Health Policy, Planning and Service Development Information Sheet, Sheet3.

References

For a complete list of references, log onto www.expertconsult.com.

Anxiety Disorders

Jess Rowney, Teresa Hermida, and Donald Malone

DEFINITION AND ETIOLOGY

Anxiety is a natural response and a necessary warning adaptation in humans. Anxiety can become a pathologic disorder when it is excessive and uncontrollable, requires no specific external stimulus, and manifests with a wide range of physical and affective symptoms as well as changes in behavior and cognition. As outlined in the *Diagnostic and Statistical Manual of Mental Disorders,* fourth edition, text revision (DSM IV-TR), anxiety disorders include generalized anxiety disorder (GAD), social anxiety disorder (also known as social phobia), specific phobia, panic disorder with and without agoraphobia, obsessive-compulsive disorder (OCD), posttraumatic stress disorder (PTSD), anxiety secondary to medical condition, acute stress disorder (ASD), and substance-induced anxiety disorder.

PREVALENCE AND RISK FACTORS

Anxiety is one of the most prevalent of all psychiatric disorders in the general population. Simple phobia is the most common anxiety disorder, with up to 49% of people reporting an unreasonably strong fear and 25% of those people meeting criteria for simple phobia. Social anxiety disorder is the next most common disorder of anxiety, with roughly 13% of people reporting symptoms that meet the DSM criteria. PTSD, which is often unrecognized, afflicts approximately 7.8% of the overall population and 12% of women, in whom it is significantly more common. In victims of war trauma, PTSD prevalence reaches 20%.

Surprisingly, disorders that are more commonly recognized have lower lifetime prevalence rates; GAD and panic disorder, for example, have lifetime prevalence rates of roughly 5% and 3.5%, respectively. Of the panic sufferers, up to 40% also meet criteria for agoraphobia. Another often underdiagnosed disorder, OCD, is found in 2.5% of the population. Interestingly, a recent study found very little change in the prevalence of mental disorders, including specific anxiety disorders, since 1990.[3]

Genetic risk factors are being studied, and researchers have found genetic predisposition for two broad groups of anxiety disorders: a panic-generalized anxiety-agoraphobia group and a specific phobias group.[4] More clinically important risk factors include comorbid substance abuse and family history. One 20-year study of the offspring of depressed parents found a threefold increase in anxiety disorders, including greater substance abuse, younger onset, and more significant physical health concerns.[5]

PATHOPHYSIOLOGY

Definitive pathophysiologic mechanisms have not yet been determined, but anxiety symptoms and the resulting disorders are believed to be due to disrupted modulation within the central nervous system. Physical and emotional manifestations of this dysregulation are the result of heightened sympathetic arousal of varying degrees. Several neurotransmitter systems have been implicated in one or several of the modulatory steps involved.

The most commonly considered are the serotoninergic and noradrenergic neurotransmitter systems. In very general terms, it is believed that an underactivation of the serotoninergic system and an overactivation of the noradrenergic system are involved. These systems regulate and are regulated by other pathways and neuronal circuits in various regions of the brain, including the locus caeruleus and limbic structures, resulting in dysregulation of physiologic arousal and the emotional experience of this arousal.

Disruption of the gamma-aminobutyric acid (GABA) system has also been implicated because of the response of many of the anxiety-spectrum disorders to treatment with benzodiazepines. There has also been some interest in the role of corticosteroid regulation and its relation to symptoms of fear and anxiety. Corticosteroids might increase or decrease the activity of certain neural pathways, affecting not only behavior under stress but also the brain's processing of fear-inducing stimuli.

Although a genetic predisposition to developing an anxiety disorder is likely,[4] environmental stressors clearly play a role in varying degrees. All of the disorders are affected in some way by external cues and how they are processed and reacted to.

Research has also shown that patients suffering from anxiety are generally more sensitive to physiologic changes than nonanxious patients, and panic disorder sufferers are even more sensitive to these than GAD patients. Objective testing, however, reveals that physiologic changes between anxious and nonanxious patients are comparable. This heightened sensitivity leads to diminished autonomic flexibility, which may be the result of faulty central information processing in anxiety-prone persons.[6]

SIGNS AND SYMPTOMS

A subjective experience of distress with accompanying disturbances of sleep, concentration, and social or occupational functioning are common symptoms in many of the anxiety disorders. Despite their similarities, these disorders often differ in presentation, course, and treatment.

Patients often present with complaints of poor physical health as their primary concern. This can temporarily distract from the underlying anxiety symptoms. This is particularly common in panic attacks (Box 1), which are characterized by a short period of intense fear and a sense of impending doom, with accompanying physical symptoms, such as chest pain, dizziness, and shortness of breath. Very often, these patients first present to an emergency department. When panic disorder is complicated by agoraphobia, the person fears having a panic attack in a place from which escape is perceived to be difficult. The patient then avoids such situations, with subsequent disturbances in functioning.

GAD rarely occurs without a comorbid psychiatric disorder, and the patient experiences consistent worry over multiple areas of his or her life for at least 6 months. Social anxiety disorder describes fear and anxiety in social situations leading to avoidance of social interaction. Specific phobia is characterized by similar symptoms and behavior, but it is triggered by a specific object or situation, such as a fear of certain animals or heights.

Acute stress disorder and PTSD occur after a patient experiences a traumatic event with subsequent physiologic arousal in the face of stimuli that trigger memories of the event, avoidance of such stimuli, and a sense of re-experiencing the event. Acute stress disorder occurs at the time of and shortly after the event, and PTSD is the chronic version of the disorder.

OCD is characterized by repeated actions (compulsions) that serve to reduce anxiety connected to unwanted, intrusive thoughts (obsessions). Commonly seen behaviors are cleaning or washing in response to concerns about contamination or repeatedly checking to see if a stove is turned off in response to concerns over a fire starting. Some people repeatedly check work or seek excessive reassurance due to obsessive self-doubt.

Box 1 DSM IV-TR Criteria for a Panic Attack

A panic attack is a period of intense fear or discomfort, developing abruptly and peaking within 10 minutes, and requiring at least four of the following:

- Chest pain or discomfort
- Chills or hot flushes
- Derealization (feelings of unreality) or depersonalization (being detached from oneself)
- Fear of losing control
- Feeling dizzy, unsteady, lightheaded, or faint
- Feeling of choking
- Nausea or abdominal distress
- Palpitations or tachycardia
- Paresthesias
- Sensations of shortness of breath or smothering
- Sense of impending doom
- Sweating
- Trembling or shaking

Data from American Psychiatric Association: Diagnostic and Statistical Manual of Mental Disorders, 4th ed, text rev. Washington, DC, American Psychiatric Association, 2000.

Box 2 DSM IV-TR Criteria for Generalized Anxiety Disorder

Excessive anxiety about a number of events or activities, occurring more days than not, for at least 6 months.

The person finds it difficult to control the worry.

The anxiety and worry are associated with at least three of the following six symptoms (with at least some symptoms present for more days than not, for the past 6 months):

- Restlessness or feeling keyed up or on edge
- Being easily fatigued
- Difficulty concentrating or mind going blank
- Irritability
- Muscle tension
- Sleep disturbance

The focus of the anxiety and worry is not confined to features of an Axis I disorder, being embarrassed in public (as in social phobia), being contaminated (as in obsessive-compulsive disorder), being away from home or close relatives (as in separation anxiety disorder), gaining weight (as in anorexia nervosa), having multiple physical complaints (as in somatization disorder), or having a serious illness (as in hypochondriasis), and the anxiety and worry do not occur exclusively during posttraumatic stress disorder.

The anxiety, worry, or physical symptoms cause clinically significant distress or impairment in social or occupational functioning.

The disturbance does not occur exclusively during a mood disorder, a psychotic disorder, pervasive developmental disorder, substance use, or general medical condition.

Data from American Psychiatric Association: Diagnostic and Statistical Manual of Mental Disorders, 4th ed, text rev. Washington, DC, American Psychiatric Association, 2000.

DIAGNOSIS

An anxiety disorder can only be diagnosed in a patient who meets DSM IV-TR criteria. Diagnosis is often complicated by other psychiatric disorders. Up to 60% of sufferers of GAD (Box 2) have a comorbid condition; panic disorder and major depressive disorder are the most common. Panic disorder (Box 3) is often comorbid with alcohol abuse, with an increased risk for suicidality. Agoraphobia (Box 4) is commonly connected to panic disorder, and comorbidity rates approach 40%. Many of these disorders have overlapping signs and symptoms, requiring the clinician to explore several lines of questioning to clarify the primary diagnosis.

Box 3 DSM IV-TR Criteria for Panic Disorder

Recurrent unexpected panic attacks

At least one of the attacks has been followed by at least 1 month of one or more of the following:

- Persistent concern about having additional panic attacks
- Worry about the implications of the attack or its consequences
- A significant change in behavior related to the attacks

Presence or absence of agoraphobia

The panic attacks are not due to the direct physiologic effects of a substance (e.g., a drug of abuse, a medication) or a general medical condition (e.g., hyperthyroidism).

The panic attacks are not better accounted for by another mental disorder.

Data from American Psychiatric Association: Diagnostic and Statistical Manual of Mental Disorders, 4th ed, text rev. Washington, DC, American Psychiatric Association, 2000.

Box 4 DSM IV-TR Criteria for Agoraphobia

Fear of being in places or situations from which escape might be difficult (or embarrassing) or in which help might not be available in the event of having unexpected panic-like symptoms.

The situations are typically avoided or require the presence of a companion.

The condition is not better accounted for by another mental disorder.

Data from American Psychiatric Association: Diagnostic and Statistical Manual of Mental Disorders, 4th ed, text rev. Washington, DC, American Psychiatric Association, 2000.

Important in the diagnosis of PTSD (Box 5) is identifying a history of trauma and being sure to ask questions related to avoidance, re-experiencing, and physiologic arousal in the face of triggering stimuli. The most common trauma associated with the disorder is rape. The symptoms of PTSD may be mistaken for depression, other anxiety disorders, or dysfunctional personality traits. Patients might not be able to identify a connection between the symptoms and the trauma history, requiring that the clinician be sensitive to the possibility that a trauma history exists. If the patient presents with complaints within 4 weeks of the trauma (with resolution within 4 weeks of symptom onset) then acute stress disorder (Box 6) should be the diagnosis.

Patients with OCD (Box 7) are often secretive regarding their symptoms. These are secondary to feelings of shame and a sense of isolation. Many are not aware that others suffer from the same constellation of thoughts and behavior. Questions should explore whether certain routines are related to specific phobias (Box 8), thoughts, or images. OCD is often comorbid with major depressive disorder (in two thirds of patients over their lifetime) and panic attacks, with rates of up to 60%. One must also distinguish between OCD and obsessive-compulsive personality disorder (OCPD). Although up to 25% of patients suffering from OCD also suffer from the personality disorder, the two disorders can manifest very differently. Patients with obsessive-compulsive personality disorder have idealized standards often rewarded by others, whereas patients with OCD experience significant distress due to true obsessions and compulsions. If the source of compulsive behavior is kept secret, a patient with OCD can sometimes appear to be suffering from psychosis. The treatment strategy for psychosis differs markedly, making it very important to distinguish between the two when presented with bizarre behavior. Questions should differentiate between voices and intrusive thoughts. The patient suffering from OCD knows his or her thoughts and actions are irrational.

Box 5 DSM IV-TR Criteria for Posttraumatic Stress Disorder

The person has been exposed to a traumatic event in which both of the following were present:

- The person experienced, witnessed, or was confronted with an event that involved actual or threatened death or serious injury or a threat to the physical integrity of others.
- The person's response involved intense fear, helplessness, or horror.

The traumatic event is persistently re-experienced in at least one of the following ways:

- Recurrent and intrusive distressing recollections of the event, including images, thoughts, or perceptions.
- Recurrent distressing dreams of the event.
- Acting or feeling as if the traumatic event were recurring, including a sense of reliving the experience, illusions, hallucinations, and flashback episodes.
- Intense psychological distress at exposure to cues that symbolize an aspect of the traumatic event.
- Physiologic reactivity on exposure to cues that symbolize or resemble an aspect of the traumatic event.

The person persistently avoids stimuli associated with the trauma and has numbing of general responsiveness including at least three of the following:

- Efforts to avoid thoughts, feelings, or conversations associated with the trauma
- Efforts to avoid activities, places, or people that arouse recollections of the trauma
- Inability to recall an important aspect of the trauma
- Markedly diminished interest or participation in significant activities
- Feeling of detachment or estrangement from others
- Restricted range of affect

Persistent symptoms of increased arousal are indicated by at least two of the following:

- Difficulty falling or staying asleep
- Irritability or outbursts of anger
- Difficulty concentrating
- Hypervigilance
- Exaggerated startle response

Duration of the disturbance is more than 1 month.
The disturbance causes clinically significant distress or impairment in social, occupational, or other important areas of functioning.

Data from American Psychiatric Association: Diagnostic and Statistical Manual of Mental Disorders, 4th ed, text rev. Washington, DC, American Psychiatric Association, 2000.

The symptoms of social anxiety disorder (Box 9) can also be confused with psychosis. One must distinguish between paranoia and the fear of being evaluated. Those suffering from social anxiety disorder desire social interaction, but they avoid it to reduce anxiety. When diagnosing specific phobia, the clinician should remember that most patients who meet the criteria have more than one fear-inducing object or situation.

Central to the diagnosis of any of the anxiety disorders is a good history, often requiring collateral from friends and family. Often overlooked is the patient's subjective quality of life.[7] When polled, 59% of PTSD sufferers have an overall quality of life significantly lower than that of the general population, and acknowledging this can increase effective patient care.

It is important to perform a thorough medical workup when initially assessing the patient with anxiety symptoms. The differential diagnosis can include several organic causes, such as endocrine dysfunction, intoxication or withdrawal, hypoxia, metabolic abnormalities, and neurologic disorders. It is also important to rule out other comorbid psychiatric disorders. Severe depression, bipolar disorder, prodromal schizophrenia, delusional disorder, and adjustment disorder can all mimic the signs and symptoms of anxiety. Many organic causes can be ruled out by a thorough history and basic laboratory

Box 6 DSM IV-TR Criteria for Acute Stress Disorder

The person has been exposed to a traumatic event in which both of the following were present:

- The person experienced, witnessed, or was confronted with an event or events that involved actual or threatened death or serious injury.
- The person's response involved intense fear, helplessness, or horror.

Either while experiencing or after experiencing the distressing event, the person has at least three of the following:

- A subjective sense of numbing, detachment, or absence of emotional responsiveness
- A reduction in awareness of his or her surroundings
- Derealization
- Depersonalization
- Dissociative amnesia

The traumatic event is re-experienced in at least one of the following ways: recurrent images, thoughts, dreams, illusions, flashback episodes, or a sense of reliving the experience; or distress on exposure to reminders of the traumatic event.
The patient avoids the stimuli that arouse recollections of the trauma.
The patient has marked symptoms of anxiety or increased arousal.
The disturbance causes clinically significant distress or impairment in social or occupational areas of functioning, or it impairs the person's ability to pursue some necessary task.
The disturbance lasts for a minimum of 2 days and a maximum of 4 weeks and occurs within 4 weeks of the traumatic event.
The disturbance is not better accounted for by brief psychotic disorder and is not merely an exacerbation of a preexisting Axis I or Axis II disorder, substance or general medical condition.

Data from American Psychiatric Association: Diagnostic and Statistical Manual of Mental Disorders, 4th ed, text rev. Washington, DC, American Psychiatric Association, 2000.

Box 7 DSM IV-TR Criteria for Obsessive-Compulsive Disorder

Obsessions

Recurrent and persistent thoughts, impulses, or images that are experienced as intrusive and inappropriate, causing anxiety or distress.
The thoughts, impulses, or images are not simply excessive worries about real-life problems.
The person attempts to ignore or suppress such thoughts, impulses, or images or to neutralize them with some other thought or action.
The person recognizes that the obsessional thoughts, impulses, or images are a product of his or her own mind.

Compulsions

Repetitive behaviors or mental acts that the person feels driven to perform in response to an obsession or according to rules that must be applied rigidly.
The behaviors or mental acts are aimed at preventing or reducing distress or preventing some dreaded event or situation.
These behaviors or mental acts either are not connected in a realistic way with what they are designed to neutralize or prevent, or they are clearly excessive.

Obsessive-Compulsive Disorder

At some point during the course of the disorder, the person has recognized that the obsessions or compulsions are excessive or unreasonable.
The obsessions or compulsions cause marked distress, take up more than 1 hour a day, or significantly interfere with the person's normal routine, occupation, or usual social activities.
If another Axis I disorder, substance use, or general medical condition is present, the content of the obsessions or compulsions is not restricted to it.

Data from American Psychiatric Association: Diagnostic and Statistical Manual of Mental Disorders, 4th ed, text rev. Washington, DC, American Psychiatric Association, 2000.

Box 8 DSM IV-TR Criteria for Specific Phobia

Persistent fear that is excessive or unreasonable, cued by the presence or anticipation of a specific object or situation.
Exposure provokes immediate anxiety, which can take the form of a situationally predisposed panic attack.
Patients recognize that the fear is excessive or unreasonable.
Patients avoid the phobic situation or else endure it with intense anxiety or distress.
The distress in the feared situation interferes significantly with the person's normal routine, occupational functioning, or social activities or relationships.
In persons younger than 18 years, the duration is at least 6 months.
The fear is not better accounted for by another mental disorder.

Data from American Psychiatric Association: Diagnostic and Statistical Manual of Mental Disorders, 4th ed, text rev. Washington, DC, American Psychiatric Association, 2000.

work, including thyroid-stimulating hormone, urine toxicology, electrocardiogram, complete blood count, and metabolic panel. Anxiety disorders are common, however, and finding an underlying medical cause is unusual.

Summary

- Thorough screening history to ensure the patient meets DSM IV-TR criteria for an anxiety disorder.
- Relevant medical examination and laboratory work to rule out organic causes and substance abuse or withdrawal.
- Proper screening of comorbid psychiatric conditions that can mimic or exacerbate anxiety disorders.

TREATMENT

An important part of any intervention with a patient with an anxiety disorder is education. The practice guidelines for panic disorder recommend education of the family as well. Many people are confused by the symptoms and behavior and are reassured to know they are not alone and that there are effective interventions. The patient should receive an appropriate medical workup, such as a physical examination, and studies (e.g., electrocardiogram, thyroid-stimulating hormone) when indicated. After ruling out a medical condition, developing a working alliance with the patient provides a basis for ongoing management and prevents further inappropriate use of the medical system.

A combination of psychotherapy and medication management is recommended in all of the anxiety disorders. Cognitive-behavioral therapy (CBT) has the strongest support of all the psychotherapies, but it requires commitment to treatment on the part of the patient. Its efficacy is also contingent on the ability of the therapist and the length of therapy, with a 78% response rate in panic disorder patients who have committed to 12 to 15 weeks of therapy. Studies show that when compared with patients undergoing treatment as usual, patients treated with a combination of CBT and medication experience nearly twice the remission rate, even when the CBT was administered by someone with minimal to no CBT experience.[8]

The selective serotonin reuptake inhibitors (SSRIs) have been shown to be the best-tolerated medications, and response rates are significantly higher than placebo for panic disorder, OCD, PTSD, social anxiety disorder, and GAD. This class of medication includes fluoxetine (Prozac), fluvoxamine (Luvox), citalopram (Celexa), escitalopram (Lexapro), paroxetine (Paxil), and sertraline (Zoloft). Some improvement should be noted within 3 or 4 weeks, and the dose should be increased if no improvement is seen. In OCD, symptoms

Box 9 DSM IV-TR Criteria for Social Phobia

A fear of one or more social or performance situations in which the person is exposed to unfamiliar people or to possible scrutiny by others and feels he or she will act in an embarrassing manner.
Exposure to the feared social situation provokes anxiety, which can take the form of a panic attack.
The person recognizes that the fear is excessive or unreasonable.
The feared social or performance situations are avoided or are endured with distress.
The avoidance, anxious anticipation, or distress in the feared situation interferes significantly with the person's normal routine, occupational functioning, or social activities or relationships.
The condition is not better accounted for by another mental disorder, substance use, or general medical condition
If a general medical condition or another mental disorder is present, the fear is unrelated to it.
The phobia may be considered generalized if fears include most social situations.

Data from American Psychiatric Association: Diagnostic and Statistical Manual of Mental Disorders, 4th ed, text rev. Washington, DC, American Psychiatric Association, 2000.

can take 8 to 12 weeks to respond to treatment. These patients often require doses at the higher end of the dosage range, so one should not be hesitant to make increases. It is also rare to achieve absolute resolution of symptoms in OCD, and partial reduction is the typical response. In all of the anxiety disorders, SSRIs should be started at low doses and gradually titrated up to therapeutic levels to avoid an initial exacerbation of anxiety.

Benzodiazepines, which have been used commonly in the past to treat anxiety disorders, continue to be useful in the short-term management of symptoms until acceptable reduction of symptoms is achieved with an SSRI or CBT. The tolerability and lack of addiction potential make the SSRIs more desirable for long-term management, but the delay in response makes short-term symptom relief with a benzodiazepine desirable for those with the greatest impairment. Because of the risk for rebound anxiety when withdrawing from benzodiazepines with short half-lives, such as alprazolam (Xanax), many psychiatrists prefer the longer-acting benzodiazepines, such as clonazepam (Klonopin).

If the patient does not respond to the combination of CBT and medication, a re-evaluation of symptoms might reveal a comorbid disorder missed on the first examination. Comorbid psychiatric disorders significantly lower the likelihood of recovery from anxiety and increase recurrence rates.[9] Many clinicians try switching between SSRIs before considering the next step in treatment. A referral to a psychiatrist for further evaluation and management may be necessary if none of these strategies works. Treatment-refractory anxiety can be extremely frustrating for both the patient and clinician. This can lead to increased dependence on benzodiazepines and an escalation of doses required for the same effect.

When approaching the start of therapy, the clinician should reassure the patient that effective treatment is available, but that patience may be necessary until the right combination of modalities is found. Although all of the anxiety disorders display a significant amount of chronicity, most patients have an improved outcome with appropriate treatment. Response rates improve when comorbidity is low. Patients with an earlier onset of symptoms (childhood or adolescence) can generally expect a more chronic course and may by more difficult to treat. In some of the disorders (PTSD, panic disorder), patients sometimes have spontaneous remission or can function despite the symptoms. However, time to resolution of symptoms is shortened and overall functioning can improve with treatment.

Pharmacotherapy often helps to prevent relapse, and rates are improved when effective treatment is continued for 12 months. When considering the terminating pharmacologic treatment, the risk for relapse in all of the disorders should be discussed with the patient. When discontinuing the SSRIs, a slow taper is recommended, with close monitoring for rebound symptoms (headache, gastrointestinal upset, restlessness). If relapse occurs, reinstituting treatment is indicated, and many patients opt for indefinite treatment to maintain remission of symptoms. Lifelong management with pharmacotherapy or psychotherapy, or both, is not unusual for many patients. For many, a maximum reduction of symptoms, rather than a full remission, is an acceptable outcome.

Summary

- Educate the patient and family members about realistic treatment expectations and reassure them of the absence of medical causes.
- First-line treatment is with a selective serotonin reuptake inhibitor, starting at low doses with careful titration so as not to exacerbate anxiety symptoms.
- Initiate cognitive-behavioral therapy along with medication to significantly increase response rates.
- Consider short-term benzodiazepines in more severe cases. Use medications with longer half-lives to minimize withdrawal effects.
- Refer to a mental health professional in difficult cases or for patients with a less-than-expected response to treatment.

PREVENTION AND SCREENING

No biologic markers are specific enough at this time to detect anxiety early, and no research shows that current medications prove efficacious in preventing these disorders. It is therefore important to screen for specific risk factors, such as strong family psychiatric history and concurrent substance abuse. Efforts since the 1990s have improved the diagnosis of these disorders, but the overall quality of care provided to patients remains substandard and CBT continues to be underused.[10] Given the morbidity and mortality due to comorbid conditions, suicide, and higher rates of medical illness, it is essential to complete a comprehensive psychiatric, medical, and substance use history and to treat this disease early and aggressively.

CONSIDERATIONS IN SPECIAL POPULATIONS

Physicians must take precautions when treating certain populations of anxious patients, including patients with substance dependence, chronic obstructive pulmonary disease (COPD) or other respiratory illness, and pregnant or elderly patients. Benzodiazepines are the chief concern in all of these patients. This class of medication can decrease the respiratory rate in many illnesses in which the rate is already compromised (COPD) and can increase the likelihood of delirium in both the elderly and medically ill. Benzodiazepines are also considered generally unsafe for use during pregnancy and have the potential for abuse in patients with substance dependence. In these populations the combined treatment of an SSRI with CBT therapy is preferred. If benzodiazepines are necessary, it is important to start at a low dose, titrate slowly, and plan for only short-term use.

Suggested Readings

American Psychiatric Association: Diagnostic and Statistical Manual of Mental Disorders, 4th ed, text rev. Washington, DC, American Psychiatric Association, 2000.

Bruce S, Yonkers K, Otto M, et al: Influence of psychiatric comorbidity on recovery and recurrence in generalized anxiety disorder, social phobia, and panic disorder: A 12 year prospective study. Am J Psychiatry 2005;162:1179-1187.

Hettema J, Prescott C, Meyers J, et al: The structure of genetic and environmental risk factors for anxiety disorders in men and women. Arch Gen Psychiatry 2005;62:182-189.

Hoehn-Sark R, McLeod D, Funderburk F, et al: Somatic symptoms and physiologic responses in generalized anxiety disorder and panic disorder. Arch Gen Psychiatry 2004;61:913-921.

Kessler R, Demier O, Frank R, et al: Prevalence and treatment of mental disorders 1990-2003. N Engl J Med 2005;352:2515-2523.

Rapaport M, Clary C, Fayyad R, Endicott J: Quality of life impairment in depressive and anxiety disorders. Am J Psychiatry 2005;162:1171-1178.

Roy-Byrne P, Craske M, Stein M, et al: A randomized effectiveness trial of cognitive behavioral therapy and medication for primary care panic disorder. Arch Gen Psychiatry 2005;62:290-298.

Sadock B, Sadock V: Synopsis of Psychiatry, 10th ed. Philadelphia, Lippincott Williams & Wilkins. 2007, pp 579-633.

Stein M, Sherbourne C, Craske M, et al: Quality of care for primary care patients with anxiety disorder. Am J Psychiatry 2004;161:2230-2237.

Stern TA, Herman JB (eds): Massachusetts General Hospital Psychiatry Update and Board Preparation, 2nd ed. McGraw-Hill, 2004, pp 121-126.

Weissman M, Wickramaratne P, Nomura Y, et al: Offspring of depressed parents: 20 years later. Am J Psychiatry 2006;163:1001-1008.

References

For a complete list of references, log onto www.expertconsult.com.

Chronic Nonmalignant Pain

Edward C. Covington and Manu Mathews

DEFINITION

The International Society for the Study of Pain defines pain as an "unpleasant sensory and emotional experience associated with actual or potential tissue damage, or described in terms of such damage."[1] Chronic nonmalignant pain (CNMP) is defined variously as pain lasting 3 months or more, or as pain persisting beyond the time of expected healing. It can begin with trauma (e.g., back strain) or disease (e.g., pancreatitis) or can occur de novo (e.g., fibromyalgia, daily migraine).

PREVALENCE AND RISK FACTORS

One in 10 U.S. adults reports current pain that has lasted a year or more. Reviews have estimated the prevalence of severe chronic pain in the general adult population to be approximately 11%. It is our most common cause of disability.

Risk factors are biologic, sociologic, psychological, and environmental. It is more common in those with depression, anxiety, and substance-use disorders. Pain-associated disability is also more common in those from lower socioeconomic strata and in those who dislike their work or feel underpaid and unsupported at work. Risk is higher in certain vocations (e.g., truck driving), in survivors of overwhelming trauma (e.g., childhood abuse, natural disasters, combat), and in those genetically sensitive to noxious stimulation. Conditions commonly associated with CNMP include spine disease, headache disorders, fibromyalgia, neuropathies, and arthritis.

PATHOPHYSIOLOGY

Pain Biology

Some of the mystery surrounding chronic pain derives from concepts of nociceptive pain, which imply a strong relation between peripheral stimulation and pain perception. Pain is seen as an analogue representation of some event. Because of reliance on this acute pain model, when a patient complains of severe pain and no appropriate pathology is located, it is suspected that the complaints are not valid or that the workup missed something. In fact, excellent health does not preclude severe pain.

Pain is more a creation of the nervous system than a gauge of nociceptor activation.[2,3] Nociceptive afferent signals are subject to marked attenuation and amplification by descending tracts that have their action at the dorsal horn. Further, the presence of prolonged nociceptive stimulation, inflammation, or nerve injury can lead to sensitization of pain transmission fibers, death of inhibitory cells, loss of tonic inhibition, and structural neuroplastic changes. Activation of immune cells, including glia, previously believed to have only structural roles, produces exaggerated, widespread, and mirror image pains.

Pain facilitatory cells in the medulla fire in response to cortical processes, such as vigilance. In animals, simply anticipating a pain and expecting it to be important are sufficient to activate "on" cells, that initiate amplifiers before the pain stimulus has begun. Opioid withdrawal also activates these cells, explaining the associated muscle and bone pain.

Genetic factors modify pain perception and response to endogenous and exogenous opioids. Several single-nucleotide polymorphisms produce greater or lesser pain sensitivity. Imaging shows that persons reporting high or low pain in response to a standard stimulus demonstrate correspondingly high or low activation of the somatosensory cortex, anterior cingulate gyrus (a likely index of affective components of pain), and frontal cortex. The conclusion is that those who report unusual pain actually experience it, absent incentives for misrepresentation.

Patients with idiopathic chronic back pain, whiplash, and fibromyalgia, conditions often believed to be exaggerated or psychogenic, show evidence of central sensitization, again suggesting that their pain is genuine but not due to peripheral structural pathology.

Sensitization also leads to visceral hyperalgesia, which accounts for much obscure abdominal, pelvic, and chest pain. Interestingly, visceral hyperalgesia is easier to elicit in rats made anxious by genetic selection or by early maternal separation. These pain syndromes often respond to agents used for neuropathic pain, such as tricyclics or pregabalin.

Pain Psychology

Although psychological factors are rarely believed to cause pain, they dramatically modulate associated suffering and dysfunction. It has long been known that vigilance, expectation of pain, and reinforcement of pain behavior increase pain behavior, and it has now been demonstrated that these factors increase cortical activation associated with experimental pains. Conversely, distraction reduces pain.

Cognitive Issues

Functional impairment that greatly exceeds pathology is not necessarily psychogenic (Box 1). Patients commonly interpret pain as a sign of fragility, leading to unwarranted self-protection and inactivity. The resulting deconditioning causes minor activities to become painful, creating a cycle of escalating pain and disability.

Maladaptive cognitions play a central role in pain disorders. They tend to be automatic and thus not examined for validity, include such catastrophic interpretations as "the nerves are being crushed" or "these exercises must be tearing something loose," which increase pain and disability.

Personal beliefs in self efficacy versus powerlessness are critical determinants of success in coping with chronic pain. Those who perceive events as a consequence of their own behavior tend to have better mood and function, whereas those who perceive events as due to other people or fate have more depression, anxiety, and dysfunction. The concept of learned helplessness also explains much impairment. A person who perceives himself or herself to be helpless is likely to stop trying entirely, leading to increased disability, depression, and ultimately pain.

Conditioning

Operant conditioning refers to the process by which forms of behavior increase when reinforced and extinguish when not reinforced. Plainly, animal life is contingent on a predisposition to selectively repeat behavior that leads to positive results. Reinforcement influences the extent of pain behavior and sick-role behavior. Although the sick role leads to multiple losses, including income, socialization, sexual function, and self esteem, it also can lead to care from others, a secure income, narcotics, and escape from a noxious work environment. Operant conditioning might explain the generally worse function and therapeutic outcomes seen in patients who are receiving pain-related disability income.

Box 1 Toxic Cognitions in Pain

Physical fragility
Catastrophizing
Personal helplessness
External blame

Box 2 Psychiatric Disorders Commonly Associated with Chronic Nonmalignant Pain

Depression
Anxiety
Addictive disorders
Somatoform disorders
Personality disorders

Box 3 The 3 Cs of Addiction

Loss of Control
Craving or preoccupation
Use despite Consequences

Reinforcers are time dependent, such that immediate weak reinforcers can overcome delayed stronger ones. This explains much maladaptive pain behavior: Actions that initially provided benefit persist after they have become liabilities. Neuroimaging suggests that reinforcing pain behavior can increase its actual perception.

Psychiatric Comorbidity

Although prevalence of comorbidity (Box 2) varies with population, the most common psychiatric disorders in chronic pain are depression, anxiety disorders, substance-use disorders, and somatoform disorders.[4] Conditions such as schizophrenia and mania are relatively uncommon.

Most patients disabled with chronic pain have substantial anxiety, and nearly 30% meet criteria for generalized anxiety disorder. Post-traumatic stress disorder and panic are also common. Anxiety sensitivity characterizes people who misinterpret the normal physiologic changes of anxiety as harbingers of medical catastrophe, such as a stroke. It is associated with chronic pain and with increased response to experimental pain.

The prevalence of depression in pain clinic patients is 30% to 84%. Mood strongly modulates pain, and simply reading sad stories or humorous ones alters pain threshold and tolerance, as does mood induction via hypnosis. In prospective studies, pain predicts the onset of depression, and depression predicts the onset of chronic pain, and they do so to approximately the same degree.

Identifying prescription drug addiction can be challenging, yet critical, because satisfactory management of chronic pain is unlikely in the addict (Box 3). Many hallmarks of addiction to recreational substances (driving citations, cirrhosis, work absenteeism, illegal behavior) are likely to be absent or attributed to pain. Official nomenclature relies heavily on the criteria of tolerance and physical dependence for diagnosing addiction. Although often appropriate for recreational substances, these criteria are not useful for prescribed analgesics. Structured interviews in a rehabilitation hospital identified 23% with active misuse or dependence and 9.4% in remission.

In pain disorder—classified as a somatoform disorder in the Diagnostic and Statistical Manual of Mental Disorders, fourth edition, text revision (DSM IV-TR)—psychological factors are "judged to have important roles in the onset, severity, exacerbation, or maintenance of pain."[5] Other conditions involving physical symptoms or preoccupation with them that cannot be explained medically include somatization disorder, conversion disorder, and hypochondriasis. There is compelling evidence that major traumatic events, including childhood abuse, combat trauma, and natural disasters, often lead to a plethora of physical complaints, including pain, without identifiable medical pathology. Such traumas likely also augment the symptoms of pain that have a medical basis; this, however, is more difficult to establish.

Most studies of personality in CNMP lack pre-pain personality assessment data, and pain changes personality. Those trapped in the sick role often demonstrate inordinate regression and dependence not previously present. Nevertheless, personality disorder impedes coping with the stress of CNMP, thus leading to inordinate dysfunction. Additionally, traumas that damage personality also often lead to functional physical symptoms.

Box 4 Signs and Symptoms in Chronic Nonmalignant Pain

Pain
Function
Mood
Sleep
Consequences ±

SIGNS AND SYMPTOMS

CNMP is not only a perception. CNMP is often associated with impairment in function that encompasses nearly all activities (Box 4). Patients not uncommonly spend upward of 20 hours per day reclining. Such a person reporting a back pain level of 7 of 10 is a far different clinical challenge than is a person whose pain is 7 of 10 but who maintains employment, socialization, and self care.

Sleep disruption is the rule in CNMP patients and is generally attributed to pain. However, counterintuitively, animal and human studies confirm that insomnia is more likely to exacerbate pain than pain is likely to exacerbate insomnia. Consequently, sleep disorder should be addressed specifically, with the expectation that its improvement can reduce pain.

Pain should be quantified (0 = no pain, 10 = the worst pain you can imagine) and characterized as to quality, timing, and relieving and exacerbating factors; however, this is not sufficient to characterize the symptoms. Function must also be assessed, along with emotional status and sleep.

These factors are most economically assessed and monitored over time by a simple self-report scale such as the Pain Disability Index or a similar scale of the clinician's own devising (Fig. 1).

DIAGNOSIS

Diagnostic signs and symptoms of the conditions that underlie CNMP are addressed in their respective chapters. The Institute for Clinical Systems Improvement has prepared guidelines for CNMP assessment and management,[6] a summary of which is available online.[7]

Typical Characteristics

Several characteristics of the diagnostic workup in CNMP are noteworthy. First, it is to be expected that complaints often outweigh physical (and imaging) findings. Laboratory studies are often completely normal. This is because much of the discomfort of CNMP is due to neural sensitization and not peripheral pathology. Thus, after several episodes of pancreatitis, it is common to have persistent pain without laboratory abnormalities. Those with sickle cell disease develop pain between crises. Sciatica persists after diskectomy. Joints hurt when synovitis has resolved and acute-phase reactants have normalized.

Psychogenic pain is often suspected on the basis of nonphysiologic findings, such as Waddell's signs in back pain (Box 5); however, these can be present even when unambiguous pathology explains the complaints. Inconsistencies are of much greater diagnostic import. Symptoms and signs can be inconsistent with anatomy (a patient

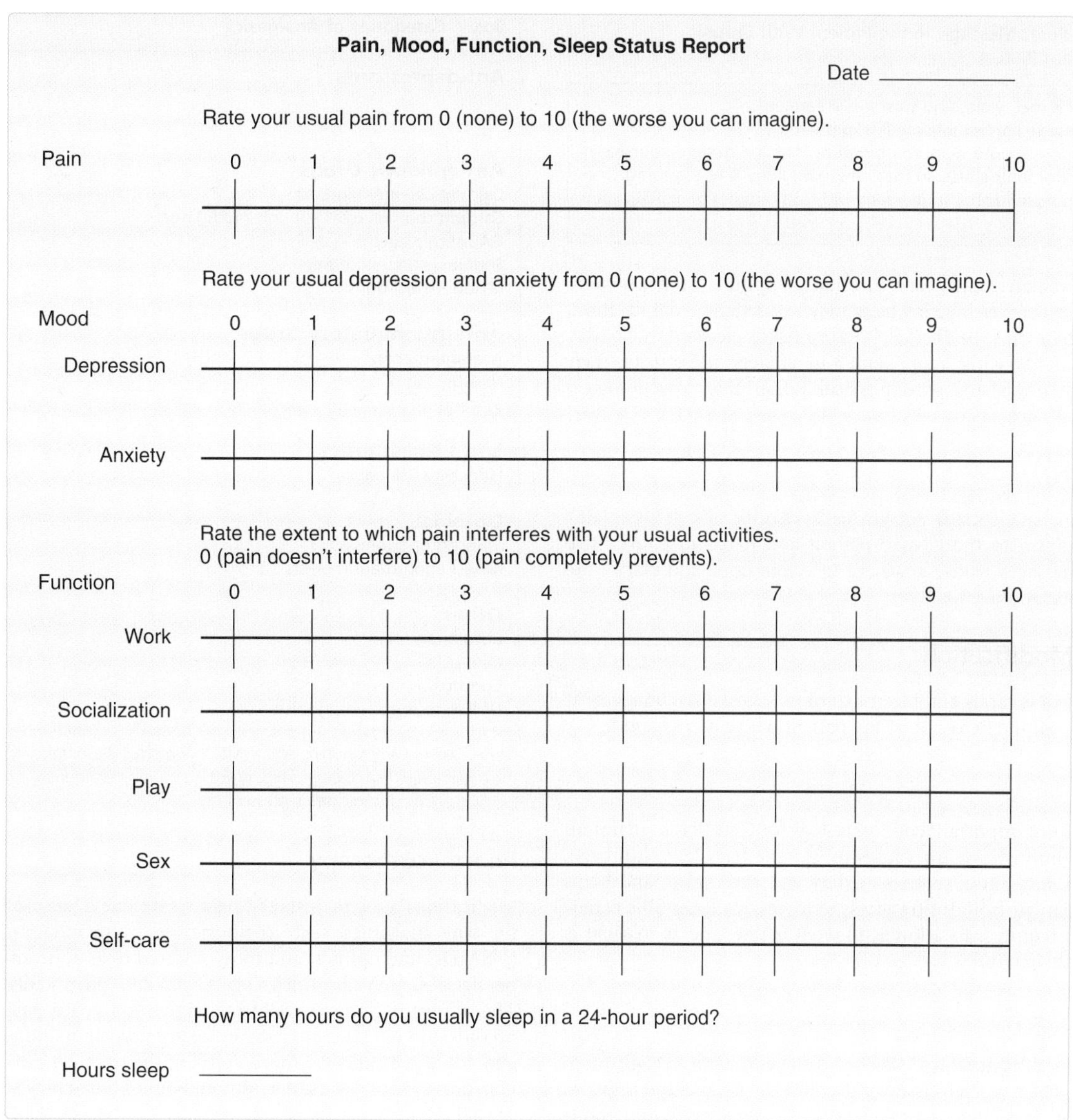

Pain, Mood, Function, Sleep Status Report

Date ____________

Rate your usual pain from 0 (none) to 10 (the worse you can imagine).

Pain 0 1 2 3 4 5 6 7 8 9 10

Rate your usual depression and anxiety from 0 (none) to 10 (the worse you can imagine).

Mood 0 1 2 3 4 5 6 7 8 9 10

Depression

Anxiety

Rate the extent to which pain interferes with your usual activities.
0 (pain doesn't interfere) to 10 (pain completely prevents).

Function 0 1 2 3 4 5 6 7 8 9 10

Work

Socialization

Play

Sex

Self-care

How many hours do you usually sleep in a 24-hour period?

Hours sleep ____________

Figure 1 Status report for pain mood, function, and sleep.

Box 5 Waddell's Signs of Nonphysiologic Pain

- Superficial tenderness
- Nonanatomic tenderness
- Axial loading
- Pain on simulated rotation
- Distracted straight leg raise
- Regional sensory change
- Regional weakness
- Overreaction

presses with the "paralyzed" leg but not with the normal one). They can vary over time or with audience (a patient's limp is much worse in the presence of a spouse).

Somatization is also suggested by preoccupation with somatic or medical issues. Patients with chronic medical problems typically report their symptoms, after which they are easy to distract. The person who cannot be diverted from symptoms, tests, and treatments is likely to be somatizing.

Functional impairment should be congruent with pathology. For example, the antalgic gait of a back patient might or might not be appropriate to the pain experienced, because this is unknowable; however, the same patient has no medical reason for the questionnaire to be in the spouse's handwriting or for the spouse to answer questions regarding the quality of pain or for the spouse to telephone in for prescription refills. These actions suggest inordinate regression, which is a psychological process. Such findings do not rule out organic disease; a person whose limp is dramatically worse in the presence of a spouse might still have a radiculopathy.

In the absence of objective pathology, the organic nature of symptoms is suggested when they are generally congruent with recognized syndromes (postcholecystectomy pain, migraine, fibromyalgia). The more atypical the symptoms, the more likely are psychogenic components.

Lack of consistency in psychological signs can suggest exaggeration, such as a patient whose screening questionnaire suggests severe depression yet is seen animated and laughing with peers in the cafeteria.

Psychological Findings

Patients with CNMP must be screened for psychiatric illness. Self-administered questionnaires (such as Beck's depression inventory) or

Box 6 Five-Point Message to the Patient With Chronic Nonmalignant Pain

- Your pain is real, valid, and warrants treatment.
- It is not due to correctable medical pathology.
- You therefore should work to normalize function despite your pain.
- I will monitor your status so that new pathology is not ignored.
- I will not pursue further unpleasant and costly studies to explain your pain.

a clinical psychiatric interview to elicit symptoms of depression, anxiety, and other psychiatric illness may be used. Suicidal ideation, plan, and intent must be elicited, because risk is elevated in CNMP.

Many patients with depression and anxiety present to their primary care physicians with physical rather than psychological complaints.

TREATMENT

The physician, having made a diagnosis, has a difficult task in explaining the condition to the CNMP patient and needs to convey five important messages whose goals are to create hope and clarify the patient's expectations (Box 6).

Lifestyle Modification

Because CNMP is rarely curable, much of its successful management is contingent on the behavior of the patient who suffers from it.

Exercise

Perhaps the most important coping strategy for CNMP is to maintain fitness. This improves many causes of chronic pain (e.g., lumbago, fibromyalgia, migraine), reduces anxiety and depression, and helps protect the patient from losing access to formerly pleasurable activities. Patients require education as to what is safe, and as to what is harmful versus painful.

Diet

Obesity is a risk factor for CNMP and patients with CNMP often gain weight, which worsens many musculoskeletal pains and impedes rehabilitation. Weight loss programs and Overeaters Anonymous should be recommended, but results are often disappointing. Bariatric surgery may be an option.

Smoking

Smoking is associated with CNMP and impedes rehabilitation. Various nicotine replacement products as well as nicotine receptor agonist therapy are helpful in ending tobacco use, but this often requires education and brief counseling as well.

Daily Activities

A useful sound bite for CNMP patients is, "If your life is empty, pain will fill it up." Distraction reduces pain perception, and even when it does not, a pain of 6 while attending an exciting event is more tolerable than a pain of 6 alone while bored at home. It is appropriate with acute pain and illness to put life on hold while awaiting recovery. This strategy can be devastating in CNMP, so it is critical that patients maintain recreation, hobbies, and social involvement.

Relaxation

Regular practice of such activities as yoga, progressive muscular relaxation, meditation, and even self-hypnosis can reduce pain, stress, and tension, while giving the patient a sense of being back in control.

Box 7 Categories of Analgesics

Antidepressants
SNRIs
TCAs

Antiepileptic Drugs
Calcium channel blockers
Calcium channel $\alpha2\delta1$ subunit modulators
GABAergic agents
Sodium-channel blockers
Mixed medications

Anti-inflammatory Drugs
Acetaminophen
NSAIDs
Steroids

Local Anesthetics
Lidocaine 5% patch

Opioids
μ-Receptor agonists
Mixed agonist/antagonists

Other
Botulinum toxin
Capsaicin
Conotoxin
NMDA receptor antagonists

GABA, gamma-aminobutyric acid; NMDA, **N***-methyl-d-aspartate; NSAIDs, nonsteroidal anti-inflammatory drugs; SNRIs, serotonin-noradrenergic reuptake inhibitors; TCAs, tricyclic antidepressants.*

Pharmacotherapy

Medications are a mainstay of pain treatment. They are divided into the true analgesics, such as nonsteroidal anti-inflammatory drugs (NSAIDs) and opioids, and those referred to as adjuvants or antihyperalgesics, such as antidepressants and antiepileptic drugs (Box 7).[8] The adjuvants are generally ineffective for acute pain. Generally, opioids and NSAIDs are used in nociceptive pain and antiepileptics and antidepressants are more useful in the treatment of neuropathic pain and hyperalgesic states, although opioids can play a role in these as well.

Nonsteroidal Anti-inflammatory Drugs

NSAIDs are useful for mild to moderate pain, especially bone and dental pain. They have opioid-sparing effects. Advantages of NSAIDs include absence of tolerance and psychic dependence. They are relatively safe in short-term use and are therefore often chosen as first-line drugs. Prolonged and high-dose use is more hazardous. Gastrointestinal (GI) complications of NSAIDs are the most prevalent category of adverse drug reactions and approximately 16,500 deaths result from ulcer-related complications in the United States each year.

Opioids

Opioids are appropriate for moderate to severe pain that is unresponsive to nonopioids alone. They are the gold standard for analgesia, and nothing short of conduction block is more effective. They reduce nociceptive and neuropathic pain, although the dose-response curve is shifted to the right in the latter. Opioids are the primary treatment for acute and cancer pain, including recurrent acute pains in sickle cell disease and recurrent pancreatitis.

The appropriateness of opioids for CNMP has been disputed, and its role seemed to evolve from forbidden in the 1970s to mandatory in the 2000s. Currently, opinion is becoming more conservative. Historically it was believed that opioid analgesia for CNMP would

Box 8 The 4 As of Chronic Opioid Analgesia

Aberrant behavior
Activity level
Adverse effects
Analgesia

diminish due to tolerance, leading to a cycle of ever-increasing doses without sustained relief and with ever-increasing risks of toxicity and addiction. These beliefs were based more on theory than on evidence.

In the late 1980s, the tide began to turn. In a seminal article, Melzack[9] held that people suffer not because their discomfort is untreatable but because physicians are reluctant to prescribe morphine. Afraid of turning patients into addicts, physicians deliver amounts that are too small and too infrequent. When patients take morphine for pain, however, addiction is rare. Addiction seems to arise only in those who take it for psychological effects, such as to experience euphoria or to relieve tension. Patients who take morphine for pain do not develop the rapid tolerance that is often a sign of addiction.

Subsequently, controlled studies have compellingly demonstrated the efficacy of opioids in most noncancer chronic pain; however, these studies are almost all short term. Longer-term studies show high drop-out rates and modest (around 30%) pain reduction.[10] Cross-sectional studies demonstrate that patients chronically taking opioids have more pain and less function than those not so treated, but they do not permit conclusions about cause.

Research has helped clarify the question of iatrogenic addiction, and a short term (6 months) trial appears to be very low risk. The risk is higher for inducing relapse of a prior addictive disorder, which is equally disastrous, but essentially unstudied. The key to a trial of chronic opioid analgesia is meticulous monitoring and documentation of drug response and behavior. Passik and Weinreb[11] have proposed four As to identify successful chronic opioid analgesia (Box 8).

When patients are doing well according to these criteria (perhaps with the addition of "affect"), it is likely that opioids are an asset to them. Physicians and patients are at risk when opioids are continued beyond the time of a failed trial. Patients doing poorly on chronic opioids often have improved pain and function when opioids are eliminated.

Many opioid formulations and routes of administration are available. Oral administration is generally as effective as parenteral and is much cheaper. Most opioids are absorbed transmucosally and can be used sublingually, rectally, or vaginally when there are impediments to swallowing or impaired GI absorption. Intrathecal administration might permit more analgesia with some reductions in GI and central nervous system (CNS) side effects; however, after several years, there is likely to be marked dose escalation, diminution of analgesia, and minimal functional improvement, all at considerable cost and risk.

It is generally held, although not conclusively shown, that chronic pain is best treated with agents that maintain a relatively constant blood level, avoiding the peaks and troughs of short-acting agents. Some molecules are intrinsically longer acting (buprenorphine, methadone, levorphanol), and others are made so through transdermal or sustained-release preparations.

The Veterans Health Administration has prepared guidelines for opioid therapy of CNMP.[12]

Antiepileptic Drugs

Antiepileptic drugs (Table 1) are especially useful in neuropathic pain, migraine, and chronic hyperalgesic states. They reduce pain by a number of mechanisms, but the modulators of the $\alpha 2\delta 1$ subunit of the calcium channel have the greatest use, fewest drug interactions, and lowest toxicity.

Antiepileptics are approved for a number of conditions, and randomized controlled trials demonstrate efficacy in several others. They are therefore widely used off-label.

Table 1 Antiepleptic Drugs for Chronic Nonmalignant Pain

Drug	FDA Approved	Evidence for Efficacy (RCTs)
Diabetic Neuropathy		
Pregabalin	×	×
Gabapentin		×
Lamotrigine		×
Fibromyalgia		
Pregabalin		×
Guillain-Barré Syndrome		
Gabapentin		×
Migraine Prophylaxis		
Topiramate	×	×
Valproate	×	×
Neuropathic Cancer Pain		
Gabapentin		
Phantom Limb		
Gabapentin		×
Post-herpetic Neuralgia		
Gabapentin	×	×
Pregabalin	×	×
Spinal Cord Injury		
Gabapentin		×
Lamotrigine (incomplete injury)		×
Trigeminal Neuralgia		
Carbamazepine	×	×
Lamotrigine (add-on refractory)		×

FDA, United States Food and Drug Administration; RCTs, randomized, controlled trials.

Antidepressants

Antidepressants have shown efficacy in a number of types of chronic pain (Box 9). The analgesic and antidepressant actions are independent of each other. Efficacy is primarily shown with agents that inhibit the uptake of serotonin and norepinephrine in the CNS, which potentiates descending spinal inhibitory pathways. Studies typically find little or no analgesic effect of selective serotonin reuptake inhibitors except for (generally weak) benefit from those with some norepinephrine reuptake inhibition as well.[13]

Numerous randomized controlled trials have shown effectiveness in fibromyalgia, functional GI disorders, and headache. Studies in spine pain have largely failed to exclude subjects with depression or sciatica; however, there is some evidence of efficacy of several tricyclics and maprotiline.

Tricyclics have been the most used antidepressants in pain; however, none is approved for such use. The serotonin-norepineph-

Box 9 Antidepressant-Responsive Pains

Arthritis
Central post-stroke pain
Chronic regional pain syndrome
Diabetic neuropathy
Fibromyalgia
Irritable bowel syndrome
Low back pain
Migraine
Neuroma
Phantom pain
Post-herpetic neuralgia
Temporomandibular joint syndrome
Tension headache
Vulvodynia

rine reuptake inhibitors (SNRIs), duloxetine and venlafaxine, are efficacious in some conditions and duloxetine has received FDA approval for treatment of pain of diabetic peripheral neuropathy.

Topical Agents

Local anesthetics applied topically lack systemic effects. Lidocaine 5% patch is indicated for pain from post-herpetic neuralgia and is effective for carpal tunnel syndrome. Open studies suggest possible usefulness in low back pain.

Capsaicin treats pain of post-herpetic neuralgia. It causes persistent activation of the vanilloid receptor, TRPV1, permitting high levels of calcium to enter nociceptors, thereby impairing their function. It is typically not well tolerated, because it produces a burning sensation on initial application that can be painful to regions that are already hyperalgesic. If hand washing is incomplete, capsaicin can later produce considerable pain on contact with mucous membranes and eyes and with other people.

Counterirritants stimulate dermal receptors to produce feelings of heat or cold. They commonly contain such substances as menthol, eucalyptus oil, or salicylates.

A number of other agents have been used topically, including NSAIDs and tricyclic antidepressants. Benefit is generally modest and not well demonstrated.

Rational Polypharmacy

Because psychiatric comorbidity is common in CNMP, many patients receive combinations of psychotropics and analgesics or antihyperalgesics, leading to problems of cost, compliance, drug interactions, and toxicity. Choosing drugs with both psychotropic and analgesic effects helps maximize therapeutic impact and minimize drug burden. For example, several analgesic antiepileptic drugs are also anxiolytic. Evidence supports the use of pregabalin for social phobia and generalized anxiety disorder, gabapentin for social phobia, lamotrigine for posttraumatic stress disorder, and valproic acid for panic disorder.[14] Sedative effects of these drugs can also be used to advantage.

Similarly, tricyclic antidepressants and SNRIs help not only chronic pain and mood but also anxiety. Several have anxiolytic effects comparable with those of diazepam and are effective for sleep.

Psychological Approaches

The profound impact of psychological variables on CNMP requires that these issues be considered in its treatment.[15]

Education

Because misunderstandings and uncertainty exacerbate pain and functional impairment, it is essential to educate patients about their pain, underlying medical conditions, appropriate management strategies, and the critical role of their own actions for pain moderation and successful rehabilitation.

Biofeedback and Relaxation Training

Biofeedback training is based on the fact that control of normally involuntary physiologic functions can be learned if the person (or animal) receives feedback. For example, thermistors provide feedback as to whether a body part (e.g., a finger) is warming or cooling. Most patients rapidly learn to regulate skin temperature, sweating, and superficial muscle tension. Biofeedback is effective in migraine, musculoskeletal pain, and GI pain. It is often combined with such techniques as autogenic training, hypnosis, transcendental meditation, yoga, progressive muscular relaxation, and guided imagery. These have been shown to be beneficial, but there are few studies demonstrating the superiority of any one. They all teach patients to control body responses that they had considered beyond their control, reduce anxiety without the need for drugs, and improve their ability to discriminate the effects of stress on physical function.

Behavior Modification

Rehabilitation is facilitated when others consistently reinforce wellness behavior, such as physical activity and healthy interactions with others, and avoid reinforcing pain behavior and sick role activities. Yet experience with acute illness leads us to attend to CNMP patients when they seem ill and perhaps to leave them alone when they're doing better. Families who learn to reverse these contingencies can help move the patient toward an improved quality of life.

Psychotherapy

Both individual and family therapy may be needed to resolve issues that increase pain, stress, or disability. The best-studied therapies in CNMP pain are cognitive-behavioral therapies, which typically focus on monitoring and correcting automatic negative thoughts, internalization of locus of control, elimination of catastrophizing, and acceptance of pain as an unfortunate problem that needn't control one's life. Numerous studies confirm that cognitive-behavioral therapies improve function and decrease pain in CNMP.

Interventional Pain Management

Interventional pain management strategies[16] in CNMP are listed in Box 10.

Diagnostic blocks may help identify a myofascial or visceral pain component, indicate sympathetically mediated pain, or locate a central pain generator, thereby guiding treatment.

Therapeutic blocks may be temporary or permanent. Permanent is a relative term, because reinnervation occurs after a variable period of time. Even temporary blocks can have a lasting effect because they can facilitate resolution, for example, of radiculitis, or make it easier for patients to engage in rehabilitation exercises they could not otherwise tolerate.

Neuroaugmentation (or neuromodulation) refers to techniques based on stimulation of neural tissues. Spinal cord stimulation involves placement of an electrode, energized by a (usually) implanted programmable generator, against the posterior spinal cord. The most important indications are neuropathic pains. Peripheral nerve stimulators are also used for neuropathic pain and have been efficacious in complex regional pain syndrome. The role of motor cortex stimulation for chronic pain remains to be determined.

Surgical pain management is generally reserved for patients who have failed less aggressive treatments.

Box 10 Pain Interventions

Diagnostic nerve blocks
Intraspinal drug delivery
Neuroaugmentation
Surgical techniques
- Anterolateral cordotomy
- Dorsal root entry zone (DREZ) lesions
- Gasserian ganglion ablations
- Microvascular trigeminal root decompression
- Rhizotomy

Therapeutic blocks

Physical Treatments

Physical therapies play an essential role in the rehabilitation of those with pain-related functional impairment. General reconditioning, focused on endurance, strength, and flexibility, can produce profound effects for a variety of reasons. A significant component of chronic pain is often the deconditioning that results from prolonged inactivity. This leads to weak, shortened muscles that are painful in response to trivial activities. Reconditioning reverses this. Physical reconditioning also markedly reduces patients' sense of helplessness, their ideas that relief can only come from an expert, and their sense of fragility.

A variety of active and passive exercises are useful for specific conditions, such as mechanical low back pain (e.g., McKenzie exercises, Williams exercises), cervicogenic headache, shoulder impingement, piriformis pain, and others.

Massage or myofascial release may be useful for those with muscle pains and trigger points. Identification and treatment of pelvic floor myofascial pains can often produce major benefit for patients with obscure pelvic pain syndromes.

Interdisciplinary Pain Rehabilitation Programs

Interdisciplinary pain rehabilitation programs (IPRPs) provide an approach to management and rehabilitation of CNMP in which professionals with disparate training collaborate to treat patients.[17] Treatment is typically intensive, for as little as 9 hours a week to as long as all day, 5 days a week, for a month or more.

The approach addresses multiple contributors and consequences of pain. Programs typically serve those unresponsive to multiple unimodal therapies, although early treatment is more effective than delayed treatment.

Programs differ in several particulars, but they share the perspectives that when chronic pain does not involve correctable pathology, an endless quest for such is deleterious, and because most chronic pain can be decreased but not eliminated, treatment must be directed toward producing the best possible quality of life despite some persistent pain. Program goals include physical rehabilitation, psychological rehabilitation, and symptom reduction. A number of services are combined to produce these outcomes (Box 11).

Box 11 Interdisciplinary Pain Rehabilitation Program Components

Education
Physical therapy
Occupational therapy
Medications (pain, mood, sleep, anxiety)
Nerve blocks
Biofeedback, relaxation training
Behavior modification
Psychotherapies
Vocational counseling
Chemical dependence treatment
Transcutaneous electrical nerve stimulation (TENS)
Detoxification or weaning
Treatment of psychiatric comorbidity

Studies of IPRP outcomes generally demonstrate improvements in pain, mood, and function. Many patients return to work and decrease their use of health care. Benefits are stable over time. Deconditioning markedly improves, and there are dramatic increases in activity levels, with a substantial decrease in opioid use. From a financial perspective, reductions in surgeries and other use of health care and reduction of disability income demonstrate that IPRP treatment, albeit expensive, is a good investment.

Sanders and colleagues have prepared guidelines for interdisciplinary CNMP rehabilitation.[18]

SPECIAL POPULATIONS

Pain treatment is not evenly distributed in our society. Studies demonstrate that African Americans and Latin Americans are less likely to receive adequate analgesia (e.g., opioids following femoral fracture) than are persons of European descent. The elderly are also at special risk for undertreatment of pain, and those in nursing homes may be sedated when they actually need analgesia. Infants have been believed not to experience pain as do adults, leading to such practices as circumcision without analgesia. Fortunately, these latter misunderstandings have been largely corrected.

GUIDELINES

A search of the National Guideline Clearinghouse[19] revealed 871 guidelines dealing with pain, of which 485 address chronic pain. Some are disease centric (low back pain, sickle cell disease, pelvic pain, osteoarthritis), others drug centric (opioids, NSAIDs), others intervention centric (facet denervation, discography, epidural steroid injections), and others population centric (geriatric, the cognitively impaired).

Summary

- Chronic nonmalignant pain is our leading cause of disability.
- Chronic nonmalignant pain usually results more from sensitization than tissue pathology.
- Management often requires attention to pathology, psychology, and environment.
- Classic and adjuvant analgesics are usually effective but often insufficient.

Suggested Readings

Ballantyne JC: Opioids for chronic nonterminal pain. South Med J 2006;99:1245-1255.

Boswell MV, Shah RV, Everett CR, et al: Interventional techniques in the management of chronic spinal pain: Evidence-based practice guidelines. Pain Physician 2005; 8:1-47.

Costigan M, Woolf CJ: Pain: Molecular mechanisms. J Pain 2000;1(3 Suppl 1):35-44.

Covington EC: The biological basis of pain. Int Rev Psychiatry 2000;12:128-147.

Covington EC, Kotz MK: Psychological approaches to the treatment of pain. In Graham AW, Schultz TK, Mayo-Smith M, et al (eds): Principles of Addiction Medicine, 3rd ed. Washington DC: American Society of Addiction Medicine, 2003, pp 1385-1404.

Dersh J, Polatin PB, Gatchel RJ: Chronic pain and psychopathology: Research findings and theoretical considerations. Psychosom Med 2002;64:773-786.

Gatchel RJ, Okifuji A: Evidence-based scientific data documenting the treatment and cost-effectiveness of comprehensive pain programs for chronic nonmalignant pain. J Pain 2006;7:779-793.

Lynch ME: Antidepressants as analgesics: A review of randomized controlled trials. J Psychiatry Neurosci 2001;26:30-36.

Maizels M, McCarberg B: Antidepressants and antiepileptic drugs for chronic non-cancer pain. Am Fam Physician 2005;71:483-490.

Melzack R: The tragedy of needless pain. Scientific American 1990;262:27-33.

Van Ameringen M, Mancini C, Pipe B, et al: Antiepileptic drugs in the treatment of anxiety disorders. Drugs 2004;64:2200-2220.

References

For a complete list of references, log onto www.expertconsult.com.

Recognition and Treatment of Depression

George E. Tesar

DEFINITION AND ETIOLOGY

Depression is a descriptive term often misused as a diagnostic label. Its misapplication can lead to diagnostic errors and mismanagement. *Depression* is more aptly used to describe a symptom-behavior complex that can be the predominant clinical manifestation of a heterogeneous group of disorders including major depressive disorder (MDD), bipolar disorder (BPD), substance-induced mood disorders, and mood disorder due to a general medical condition.

The symptoms of MDD are nonspecific and are therefore easily confused with a long list of other psychiatric and medical illnesses. Accurate recognition requires that the clinician have a high index of suspicion and know the diagnostic criteria for MDD. In this regard, it is important to distinguish a major depressive episode (MDE) from MDD. An MDE typically represents a single or recurrent episode of MDD, but not necessarily. It could be a consequence of chronic substance abuse, a transient response to life-altering medical illness, or an episode of BPD. In each of these examples, the approach to comprehensive management of an MDE differs from the management of an MDE occurring in the context of MDD. Like other medical illnesses, MDD has significant morbidity and mortality.[1] It often complicates other conditions (e.g., diabetes mellitus, stroke, cancer, heart disease) and makes them more difficult to treat.[2] It also accelerates mortality from these and other medical illnesses.[3]

PREVALENCE AND RISK FACTORS

The National Comorbidity Survey Replication (NCS-R) is the most recent, broad-based assessment of MDD in the community.[4] The NCS-R gathered data on prevalence rates, severity, disability, and rate and quality of treatment for MDD. The 12-month and lifetime prevalence of clinically significant MDD in the NCS-R were 6.6% and 16.2%, respectively. MDD tends not to occur in isolation; 75% to 80% of persons with either 1-year or lifetime MDD had a comorbid anxiety or substance-related disorder. Although 51.6% of patients received some treatment, only 21.7% of the total population of patients with MDD received adequate treatment during a 1-year period.

The first MDE usually occurs during adolescence or early adulthood. There is a bimodal curve of prevalence, with one peak in the late 20s and early 30s and a second peak around 65 to 70 years of age.

Women are affected by MDD two to three times more often than men. This may be explained by psychobiologic risk factors (e.g., menstrual cycle and pregnancy, gender-related vulnerability to interpersonal conflict or loss) and women's tendency to seek health care more than men do.

MDD occurs at higher rates in patients who seek general medical care. Nearly 70% of all antidepressant prescriptions are written by primary care physicians.[5] Depressed patients are high users of medical care, and high users of medical care in general are more likely to have one or more psychiatric disorders. In one study, the 1-month prevalence of MDD in a group of high users was 40.3%.[6]

The risk of developing MDD is manifold and complex.[7] Risk factors include current stress burden; history of early trauma, neglect, abuse, or deprivation; personal and family histories of mood and anxiety disorders; comorbid medical and psychiatric disorders; and personality disorder. Stress is a common, although not invariable, trigger of MDEs, and anyone can develop an MDE. Some, however, especially those with recurrent episodes and family histories of mood, anxiety, or substance abuse disorders, are more likely to develop an MDE even when stress levels are judged to be low. Certain medical disorders (e.g., stroke, neurodegenerative disorders, human immunodeficiency virus [HIV] infection, acquired immunodeficiency syndrome [AIDS], endocrine disorders) are associated with a higher than expected rate of MDD. Diabetes, for example, doubles the odds of comorbid MDD.[8] A meta-analysis of studies that examined the prevalence of MDD in adults with diabetes showed that the prevalence of comorbidity was significantly higher in diabetic women (28%) than in diabetic men (18%) and in clinical (32%) rather than community (20%) samples.[8]

PATHOPHYSIOLOGY AND NATURAL HISTORY

Emerging data support the hypothesis that stress, genetic predisposition, and early life experiences interact to increase the risk of MDD. Our understanding of the precise pathophysiologic mechanisms of MDD continues to evolve.

Family and twin studies suggest that genetic factors predispose to recurrent MDD.[7] There is no one depression gene, nor is depression determined exclusively by genetic factors. Rather, it is more likely that multiple interacting genes code for factors that influence both vulnerability and resilience in the face of stress. One such factor appears to be a polymorphism in the promoter region of the serotonin transporter gene.[9,10]

The timing of stress is also important. Abnormal stress (e.g., neglect, abandonment, physical or sexual abuse) at critical developmental periods can have long-lasting effects on central nervous system development and function.[11]

A variety of studies suggest that brain regions involved in depression include the amygdala, hippocampus, hypothalamus, and prefrontal cortex.[12] The presence of dense projections from the subgenual cingulate to the serotonin-rich brainstem dorsal raphe nucleus suggests that this cortical area plays some role in regulating serotoninergic activity, an activity that may be impaired in depression.[12]

Understanding of the biology of neurotransmission has progressed significantly beyond an appreciation of neurotransmitter synthesis, release, and activation of postsynaptic cell-surface receptors.[13] Signal transduction pathways mediated by second and third messengers (e.g., cyclic adenosine monophosphate [cAMP], protein kinases, and neurotrophic factors) affect gene expression and protein production, with consequent re-regulation of neurotransmission and clinical improvement. The rate of gene expression corresponds more closely to the rate of antidepressant-associated clinical improvement (i.e., weeks) than the more-rapid changes in neurotransmission (i.e., hours to days). Moreover, studies of treatment response suggest a close correlation between antidepressant use and increased levels of proteins, such as brain-derived neurotrophic factor (BDNF).[13] Central hypercortisolemia can mediate stress-induced effects on the brain that are reversed by antidepressant-induced BDNF production.[11,13]

SIGNS AND SYMPTOMS

Most clinicians recognize depression when they see it, or perhaps feel it. The welling up of tears in a patient's eyes, sluggishness, demoralization, or a pessimistic attitude attract the experienced clinician's attention to the possibility of an MDE. Any one symptom of an MDE, however, is not specific and may be present in diverse disorders (see "Differential Diagnosis"). Moreover, even the experienced clinician

Box 1 Signs and Symptoms of a Major Depressive Episode

Depressed or sad mood*
Markedly diminished interest or pleasure in all or almost all activities, especially those the individual normally enjoys*
Sleep disturbance (insomnia or hypersomnia)
Feeling of worthlessness or excessive or inappropriate guilt (not merely self-reproach or guilt about being sick, but rather a firmly held conviction that might in some instances be considered delusional)
Fatigue or loss of energy
Indecisiveness or diminished ability to think or concentrate
A change in appetite (typically decreased, but can be increased in atypical depression), or a significant weight change (>5% of body weight) when not intentionally trying to lose or gain weight
Psychomotor agitation or retardation nearly every day
Recurrent thoughts of death (not just fear of dying), recurrent suicidal ideation without a specific plan, a specific plan for committing suicide, or a suicide attempt

*One or the other of these must be present for a diagnosis of major depressive episode.
Adapted from American Psychiatric Association: Diagnostic and Statistical Manual of Mental Disorders, 4th ed, text rev. Washington, DC, American Psychiatric Association, 2000.

Box 2 Mnemonic Used for Diagnosis of Major Depressive Episode: SIG: E CAPS*

S—*Sleep* disturbance. Typically, difficulty staying asleep; less often, difficulty falling asleep
I—*Interest*, pleasure, or enthusiasm for usual activities is diminished
G—*Guilt*, self-doubt, or loss of self-esteem that is excessive or unwarranted
E—*Energy* level is diminished
C—*Concentration* (or attention) span is poor or worse than usual
A—*Appetite* is impaired. Typically it is diminished and associated with weight loss, but in some cases the patient overeats and gains weight
P—*Psychomotor* activity is abnormal. Typically the patient moves and thinks more slowly; some patients, especially the elderly, can be more restless, explosive, or agitated
S—*Suicidal* thoughts, hopelessness, or thoughts that the patient (and often others) would be better off if the patient were dead

*Signatura (label or let it be printed) for energy capsules.
Adapted from Carey Gross, MD.

Box 3 Diagnostic Criteria for Major Depressive Disorder

Five or more of the 9 symptoms listed in Box 1, at least one of which is either:
Depressed or sad mood
Markedly diminished interest or pleasure in all or almost all activities, especially those the individual normally enjoys
Symptoms are present most of the day, nearly every day for at least 2 weeks
Symptoms cause clinically significant distress or impairment in social, occupational, or other important areas of functioning
Symptoms are not better accounted for by bereavement*
Symptoms do not meet criteria for a mixed episode†

*On average, bereavement lasts 2 months or less. Grief-triggered symptoms lasting longer than 2 months suggest evolution of a major depressive episode.
†A mixed episode is defined by the presence of both depressed and manic symptoms. In addition to having depressive symptoms, the person with a mixed episode is typically irritable, explosive, labile (switches unpredictably from one emotion to another), and pressured (difficult to interrupt). A mixed episode is more consistent with a diagnosis of bipolar disorder rather than major depression and requires different treatment (see the chapter on bipolar disorder).
Adapted from American Psychiatric Association: Diagnostic and Statistical Manual of Mental Disorders, 4th ed, text rev. Washington, DC, American Psychiatric Association, 2000.

who suspects depression must withhold a reflexive impulse to diagnose and treat it. Not all depressive signs and symptoms are diagnostic of MDD.

Symptoms of anxiety (e.g., worry, nervousness, tension, panic attacks) often accompany depression. These can either be secondary to an MDE or represent a comorbid anxiety disorder (see elsewhere in this section, "Anxiety Disorders"). The presence of anxiety often confounds the diagnosis of MDD and encourages treatment with benzodiazepines or other minor tranquilizers rather than antidepressant medication. The clinician must be careful to do a thorough evaluation for MDD when symptoms of anxiety are present.

Other symptoms that are commonly associated with depression and whose presence should trigger concern about underlying, unreported, or masked depression include pain (the more types of pain the patient reports, the greater the likelihood of underlying depression), sexual complaints (problems with sexual functioning or desire), and substance abuse or dependence.

DIAGNOSIS

For a diagnosis of MDD to be considered, a patient must have five or more of the symptoms or signs listed in Box 1, and at least one of those symptoms must be either depressed mood or loss of interest. These symptoms must be present most of the time nearly every day for a period of 2 or more weeks.[14] The well-known mnemonic SIG: E CAPS, developed by Carey Gross (personal communication), can be used to recall these important signs and symptoms (Box 2).

A common error is to regard depressive symptoms as an understandable reaction to grave or disabling medical illness. Neither the severity nor meaning of a precipitating or stressful event is directly relevant to the diagnosis of an MDE. Whether or not a sufficient triggering event has occurred, the diagnosis of an MDE depends instead on the presence of a critical number of signs and symptoms (see "Signs and Symptoms") lasting a sufficient duration. If careful evaluation discloses sufficient number and duration of signs and symptoms, then regardless of the precipitating event the clinician is obliged to make a diagnosis of MDE and recommend appropriate treatment.

MDD is diagnosed (Box 3) exclusively from information obtained at the clinical interview and mental status examination (see elsewhere in this section, "Behavioral Assessment of the General Medical Patient"). Collateral information from family and associates is helpful, particularly when the patient minimizes or ignores psychological features of depression. There are no laboratory findings pathognomonic of MDD. Laboratory testing is useful only to help rule out medical conditions that can mimic MDD (e.g., hypothyroidism, vitamin B_{12} deficiency, sleep apnea).

Symptom clustering is not the only criterion on which the diagnosis is based. The symptoms must also be present for a sufficient period (most of the time nearly every day for at least 2 weeks) and in one way or another must be distressing or disabling.

The term *major* in MDD is potentially misleading because it suggests that severity or seriousness is a diagnostic criterion. In fact, MDEs are rated mild, moderate, or severe depending on how distressing or disabling they are. An MDE can be a first and only lifetime occurrence of depression, or it can be a recurrent episode of MDD. Current protocol is to diagnose MDE as either "MDD, single episode" (DSM IV-TR, 296.20) if there is no past history of MDE, mania, or hypomania, or "MDD, recurrent" (DSM IV-TR, 296.30) if there has been at least one past MDE, and to specify whether the episode is mild, moderate, severe, or associated with psychotic features (the fifth digit of the diagnostic code is rated as 1, 2, 3, or 4, respectively).

Subtypes of MDD include *seasonal, postpartum, atypical,* and *psychotic depressions*. Seasonal depression, or seasonal affective disorder

Table 1 Patient-Rated Screening and Case-Finding Instruments for Major Depressive Disorder

Instrument	Website	Reference
Beck Depression Inventory II*	Harcourt Assessment. www.harcourtassessment.com	Beck AT, Ward CH, Mendelson M, et al: An inventory for measuring depression. Arch Gen Psychiatry 1961;4:53-63.
Zung Self-Rating Depression Scale	http://healthnet.umassmed.edu/mhealth/ZungSelfRatedDepressionScale.pdf	Zung WWK. A rating instrument for anxiety disorders. Psychosomatics 1971;12:371-379
PRIME-MD (self-report format)*	http://www.montana.edu/wwwebm/Archives/PHQ.doc	Spitzer RL, Williams JBW, Kroenke K, et al: Patient Health Questionnaire Study Group. Validity and utility of a self-report version of PRIME-MD: The PH Primary Care Study. JAMA1999;282:1737-1744.
Patient Health Questionnaire-9	http://www.phqscreeners.com/	Kroenke K, Spitzer RL, illiams JB. The PH-9: Validity of a brief depression severity measure. J Gen Int Med. 2002;16:606-613.
Shedler's Quick PsychoDiagnostics Panel†	www.digitaldiagnostics.com	Shedler J, Beck A, Bensen S: Practical mental health assessment in primary care: Validity and utility of the Quick PsychoDiagnostics (QPD) panel. J Fam Practice 2000;49:614-621.

*Copyrighted material for purchase.
†These instruments provide measures of major depressive disorder as well as other behavioral disorders that are common in primary care (e.g., panic disorder, generalized anxiety disorder, eating disorders, alcohol abuse, and somatization).
PRIME-MD, Primary Care Evaluation of Mental Disorders.

(SAD), is diagnosed when depressive episodes occur exclusively during one season or another. Most SAD occurs during autumn and winter (October to March), although a small subset occurs during the summer months. Postpartum depression should be considered when depressive symptoms continue beyond 2 weeks after parturition and satisfy diagnostic criteria for MDD. The designation *atypical* refers to MDEs that are triggered by environmental stresses (especially rejection) and characterized by social withdrawal, hypersomania, and hyperphagia. Finally, psychotic depression is a serious, life-threatening form of MDD associated with a higher rate of suicide and a subsequent dementia rate that is higher than in nonpsychotic MDD. Further discussions of these MDD subtypes appear later.

Detection of an MDE in the context of debilitating medical illness is often difficult. This is because the vegetative symptoms of depression (anorexia, insomnia, fatigue, and impaired attention) can occur as manifestations of severe medical or surgical illness itself. When the cause of these symptoms is ambiguous, the clinician is forced to rely on the presence or absence of typical psychological symptoms or behavior (e.g., crying, expressions of hopelessness or giving up, loss of motivation, excessively low self-esteem). The likelihood of MDD increases significantly when these psychological symptoms accompany the other, nonspecific vegetative symptoms.

Other data that can help confirm or support a clinician's suspicion of MDD include past MDEs (not necessarily detected or formally treated), a family history of mood or anxiety disorders, alcoholism or suicide, and survey tools (Table 1) that screen for depression (see "Screening and Prevention," later).

DIFFERENTIAL DIAGNOSIS

Psychiatric diagnoses that warrant consideration when a patient presents with depressive signs and symptoms are listed in Box 4. Grief is a normal, expected response to loss or the threat of loss and is not a diagnosis. Prolonged (unresolved) grieving, however, can become an MDE. Adjustment disorder with depressed mood is a transient, dysfunctional, but generally self-resolving response to stress that lacks sufficient diagnostic criteria for a diagnosis of MDE. The recommended treatment for adjustment disorder with depressed mood is psychotherapy and not antidepressant medication.

Box 4 Differential Diagnosis of Major Depressive Disorder: Psychiatric Disorders

Mood
Bipolar disorder
Cyclothymia
Dysthymia

Anxiety
Agoraphobia
Generalized anxiety disorder
Posttraumatic stress disorder
Social anxiety disorder

Substance-Related
Alcohol- or drug-induced mood disorder
Amphetamine or cocaine withdrawal

Somatoform
Hypochondriasis
Somatization disorder

Personality
Avoidant
Borderline
Histrionic
Narcissistic

Organic Mental
Delirium (hypoactive)
Dementias (subcortical)
Mild cognitive impairment

Other
Adjustment disorder with depressed mood
Attention deficit disorder

MDD is one of a number of mood disorders including dysthymia, BPD, and cyclothymia.[14] Dysthymia and cyclothymia are considered subsyndromal variants of MDD and BPD, respectively. Dysthymia is diagnosed when chronic low-grade depressive symptoms (insufficient number and intensity to qualify as MDE) are present 50% of the time or more for 2 or more years. Dysthymia often accompanies chronic, disabling medical illness and is less responsive to antidepressant treatments than MDD. This may be explained in part by the continuing stress of enduring medical symptoms and disability, or it may be due to the ineffective coping of a patient with a personality disorder.

Bipolar disorder (BPD) is an essential consideration in the differential diagnosis of MDD. An MDE—not mania or hypomania—is the most common clinical presentation in patients with BPD. Correct identification of bipolar depression (MDE in the context of BPD) depends on eliciting a history of manic or hypomanic episodes. This can be difficult and time-consuming for even the most astute clinician. However, making the correct diagnosis has important implications for treatment selection and prognosis (see elsewhere in this section, "Bipolar Disorder").

Diagnoses that resemble but by definition are not mood disorders include *adjustment disorder with depressed mood*, *depression secondary to a general medical condition*, and *substance-related mood disorder*.[14] The causes of these are different from those of MDD, and they therefore warrant a different approach to management. In most instances the diagnosis of adjustment disorder with depressed mood is relevant to persons who do not have a personal or family history of mood disorder. Depression secondary to a general medical condition and substance-related mood disorder imply that the MDE has been triggered by and will resolve with treatment of the underlying medical condition or chemical dependency.

Because depressive symptoms are nonspecific, both patient and primary care specialist generally feel obliged first to rule out other medical conditions (Box 5). When a full constellation of signs and symptoms that meet diagnostic criteria for an MDE is present, however, MDD should be handled as a diagnosis of inclusion rather than exclusion. Early and effective treatment with antidepressant medication need not interfere with a thorough medical workup. Moreover, a successful response to antidepressant medication could forestall unnecessary laboratory testing and repeat office visits.

Box 5 Differential Diagnosis of Major Depressive Disorder: General Medical Conditions

Collagen
Fibromyalgia
Polymyalgia rheumatica

Endocrine
Adrenal insufficiency
Cushing's syndrome
Diabetes
Hyperparathyroidism
Testosterone deficiency
Thyroid dysfunction

Infection
AIDS/HIV
Infectious mononucleosis
Influenza
Tertiary syphilis
Tuberculosis
Viral hepatitis

Neoplastic
Disseminated carcinomatosis
Pancreatic cancer

Neurologic
Dementias
Frontal lobe syndrome
Huntington's disease
Mild cognitive impairment
Parkinson's disease
Periventricular small vessel disease
Postconcussive syndrome
Sleep apneas

Toxicity
Anticholinesterases (donepezil)
Beta blockers (especially propranolol)
Corticosteroids
Contraceptives
Cyclosporine
H_2 Blockers (cimetidine, famotidine, ranitidine)
Interferon
Methyldopa
Metoclopramide
Reserpine
Vincristine
Vinblastine

Vitamin Deficiency
B_{12}
C
Folate
Niacin
Thiamine

AIDS/HIV, acquired immunodeficiency syndrome or human immunodeficiency virus infection.

TREATMENT

General Approach

The standard of care for a moderate to severe MDE (*not* an MDE occurring in the context of BPD or ongoing substance abuse) combines antidepressant medication with patient education, psychotherapy, or other nondrug treatments. Because a mild MDE is often self-limited, the best approach in any given patient may be to withhold treatment and monitor. This should not be viewed as permission to ignore or overlook mild depression. Instead, the clinician should put depression—whatever its intensity—on the problem list and recommend treatment if symptoms persist and cause significant distress or dysfunction.

Suicide Risk Assessment

The workup of a patient with depressive symptoms must include an assessment of suicide risk (see elsewhere in this section, "Psychiatric Emergencies"). Most patients with mood disorders do not make suicide attempts or commit suicide. However, at least 50% of suicides are committed by patients with a mood disorder. If the patient does not spontaneously mention or allude to suicidal thoughts or thoughts of death, the clinician must ask. Contrary to the beliefs of some, asking does not sow the seed of suicidal thinking. Although patients are typically reluctant to talk about such issues, they generally experience relief when given the opportunity to do so.

The patient who has risk factors for suicide (e.g., personal or family history of attempts or completions, alcoholism, drug abuse, severe anxiety, violence, or impulsivity) and asserts intent or plan should be referred for urgent or emergent evaluation. Clinician skill, judgment, and experience as well as resource availability influence disposition and whether a routine (within 2 weeks), urgent (within 24-48 hours), or emergent (within 12 hours on site or at another site—emergency department or psychiatrist's office—to which the patient's transport is assured) referral is made.

Patient Education

Patients are often relieved when a diagnosis has been identified that accounts for their symptoms. The stigma of a diagnosis of MDD can be dispelled with information about its medical underpinnings and the availability of effective treatments. Educating the patient helps foster a strong therapeutic alliance and adherence to treatment.

Table 2 Phases of Treatment with Antidepressant Medication

Phase of Treatment	Typical Duration	Indication(s)	Goals	Strategy
Acute	4-12 wk	Single or recurrent episode of major depression	Remission of index episode	Select antidepressant. Start at subtherapeutic dose to minimize risk of side effects Increase at roughly weekly intervals to therapeutic dose Refer to psychiatrist instead or after two unsuccessful medication trials
Continuation	4-6 mo	Goal of acute phase treatment achieved	Continued remission Prevent relapse (return of the index episode)	Continue same dose required to achieve remission during acute phase Monitor for relapse If relapse occurs, increase dose, initiate augmentation strategy, or switch to new agent
Maintenance	>9-12 mo Optimal duration is uncertain	Three prior episodes of depression *or* Two prior episodes *plus* First-degree relative with major mood disorder; Recurrence within 1 yr of prior effective treatment; Onset of first episode before age 20 yr; Both episodes were severe, sudden, or life-threatening in the past 3 yr	Prevent recurrence of depression	Continue same dose used successfully during continuation phase Monitor for recurrence Increase dose, initiate augmentation strategy, or switch to a new agent if there is a recurrent episode

Adapted from Agency for Health Care Policy and Research: Clinical Practice Guideline: Depression in Primary Care, vols. I and II. Washington, DC, U.S. Government Printing Office, 1993.

In addition to medication, a variety of treatments are indicated for MDD and include psychotherapy, exercise, light therapy, and a growing number of neuromodulation techniques, the most established of which is electroconvulsive therapy (ECT) (discussed later).

Antidepressant Medications

General Approach

The pharmacologic treatment of MDD is generally divided into three phases: *acute, continuation*, and *maintenance*. The indications, goals, duration, and strategies of treatment during these phases are presented in Table 2 and can also be reviewed by consulting the Agency for Healthcare Research and Quality (formerly the Association for Health Care Policy and Research).[15]

Antidepressant medication should be considered for moderate to severe MDD.[16] A large variety of antidepressants is available (see Table 2). There is no single best agent, and selection depends on the patient's antidepressant treatment history, potential drug interactions, and desired side-effect profile (Tables 2, 3, and 4).

There is no test available that predicts individual response to antidepressant medication in general or to any single agent in particular. Empirical trial and error are necessary, with a favorable response in roughly one half and remission in nearly one third of patients with a single therapeutic medication trial.[17] If the first agent is ineffective, the diagnosis should be reviewed for accuracy and then, if depression is still present, another antidepressant should be tried. At least one within-class alternative should be tried before switching to an agent from a different class (see Table 2).[17]

Many patients who initially respond favorably still have residual symptoms. Increasing the antidepressant dosage, using augmentation strategies, or switching to another medication are treatment options for such patients. Referral to a psychiatrist should be considered for persistent depression that has not responded to one or at most two trials of antidepressant medication.

Selecting Antidepressants

Familiarity with antidepressant classes and side-effect profiles helps inform treatment selection (see Tables 2 and 3). In an antidepressant-naïve patient, virtually any antidepressant qualifies as a first-line agent. Selective serotonin reuptake inhibitors (SSRIs), including fluoxetine (Prozac), sertraline (Zoloft), paroxetine (Paxil), citalopram (Celexa), and escitalopram (Lexapro), enjoy the widest prescription in the United States and are generally the first to be prescribed. Compared with SSRIs, bupropion (Wellbutrin), mirtazapine (Remeron), and the norepinephrine-serotonin reuptake inhibitors (NSRIs) such as venlafaxine (Effexor) and duloxetine (Cymbalta) have similar efficacy and favorable side-effect profiles. Many clinicians consider venlafaxine and duloxetine superior to SSRIs, but the database is insufficient to verify this impression.

Unlike the monoamine oxidase inhibitors (MAOIs) and tricyclic antidepressants (TCAs), all of these newer antidepressants have a lower risk of cardiovascular side effects and are comparatively safe in overdose. SSRIs and NSRIs can cause sexual dysfunction (delayed or inhibited sexual climax) in 25% to 40%, whereas bupropion, mirtazapine, and nefazodone are much less likely to do so. The risk of hypertension increases with daily doses of venlafaxine greater than 225 mg. Mirtazapine, like TCAs (e.g., amitriptyline, imipramine, doxepin), can cause unacceptable weight gain, and it also increases the risk of orthostatic hypotension. The U.S. manufacturer of Serzone (nefazodone) discontinued the product in 2004 because of reports of fatal liver toxicity. Generic nefazodone, however, continues to be manufactured. Like maprotaline and amoxapine (see Table 2), it should be reserved for treatment-resistant MDD when other agents have failed.

After remission has been achieved in the acute phase, the antidepressant dosage used to achieve remission should be continued for another 4 to 6 months.[15] Thereafter, the decision to prescribe maintenance therapy depends on the number and severity of past MDEs.

Table 3 Antidepressant Drugs Approved by the FDA*

Generic	Trade	Drug Class	Date of Approval (m/d/y)	Starting Dose† (mg/d)	Therapeutic Range‡ (mg/d)	Half-Life§ (h)	Schedule
Amitriptyline	Elavil	TCA	4/7/1961	25	150-300	12-24	qhs
Amoxapine¶	Asendin	NSRI	9/22/1980	100	200-300	8-30	bid
Bupropion	Wellbutrin	NDRI	12/30/1985	75	300-450	20	tid
	Wellbutrin SR	NDRI	10/4/1996	100	300-450	20	bid
	Wellbutrin XL	NDRI	8/29/2003	150	300-450	20	qd
Citalopram	Celexa	SSRI	7/17/1998	10	20-40	35	qd
Desipramine	Norpramin	TCA	11/20/1964	25	150-300	21-23	qd
Doxepin	Sinequan	TCA	9/23/1969	25	150-300	17-51	qhs
Duloxetine	Cymbalta	NSRI	8/3/2004	20	30-60	12	bid
Escitalopram	Lexapro	SSRI	8/14/2002	10	10-20	27-32	qd
Fluoxetine	Prozac, Serafem	SSRI	12/29/1987	10	20	4-16 d	qd
Imipramine	Tofranil	TCA	4/16/1959	25	150-300	11-25	qhs
	Tofranil PM	TCA	3/11/1973	75			qhs
L-Deprenyl¶	Emsam (Selegiline)	MAOI	2/27/2006	6	12	10	qd**
Maprotiline¶	Ludiomil	NRI/TetraCA	12/1/1980	25	150	43-90	qhs
Mirtazapine	Remeron	Other	6/14/1996	15	15-45	20-40	qhs
Nefazodone‡‡		Other	9/16/2003	200	600	2-4	bid-tid
Nortriptyline	Pamelor	TCA	8/1/1977	10	75-150	16-44	qd
Paroxetine	Paxil	SSRI	12/29/1992	10	20-40	24	qd
	Paxil-CR	SSRI	2/16/1999	12.5	25-62.5	21	qd
Phenelzine	Nardil	MAOI	6/9/1961	15	45-90	12	bid-tid
Protriptyline	Vivactyl	TCA	9/27/1967	5	15-30	60-90	tid
Sertraline	Zoloft	SSRI	12/30/1991	50	50-200	26	qd
Tranylcypromine	Parnate	MAOI	2/21/1961	10	20-60	4-8	bid-tid
Trazodone††	Desyrel	Other	12/24/1981	100	300-600	3-9	bid-tid
Trimipramine	Surmontil	TCA	6/12/1979	25		11-23	qhs
Venlafaxine	Effexor	NSRI	12/28/1993	25	225-375	5-11	tid
	Effexor XR	NSRI	10/20/1997	37.5	225-375	5-11	qd

*Obtained from FDA website on January 1, 2007.

†Elderly, debilitated, or anxious patients might need to start treatment at lower doses than these.

‡Increase dose until either therapeutic or adverse effects occur.

§The wide ranges reported are a function of active metabolites or individual metabolic rates.

¶Still in production but have limited usefulness because of the adverse effect profiles. Therefore, use is relegated to severe, treatment-resistant depression. Amoxapine and maprotaline can cause severe extrapyramidal side effects and have low toxic-to-therapeutic ratios, leading to elevated risks of seizures and cardiac arrhythmias at high-normal doses. The U.S. manufacturer discontinued production of Serzone when a small number of reports of fatal hepatitis appeared in the literature. Several generic manufacturers, however, continue to produce it.

¶The levo-isomer and therefore a close chemical relative of citalopram, escitalopram has distinctive activity that distinguishes it clinically from citalopram.

**Administered transdermally from a patch that must be changed daily.

††In low doses (50-150 mg) it is effective for promoting and maintaining sleep.

‡‡No longer manufactured.

FDA, United States Food and Drug Administration; MAOI, monoamine oxidase inhibitor; NDRI, norepinephrine-dopamine reuptake inhibitor; NRI/TetraCA, norepinephrine reuptake inhibitor/tetracyclic antidepressant; NSRI, norepinephrine-serotonin reuptake inhibitor; SSRI, serotonin selective reuptake inhibitor; TCA, tricyclic antidepressant.

Table 4 Antidepressant Drug Side Effects

Drug	Anticholinergic Effects*	Sedation	Activation†	Postural Hypotension	Hypertension	Sexual Dysfunction††	Seizures§	Weight Gain	Comments
Amitriptyline	+++	++++	+	+++		++	++	++++	
Amoxapine		+++		+++		++	++++	+++	Loxapine, an antipsychotic, is an active metabolite that accounts for reports of amoxapine-associated extrapyramidal effects, including movement disorders, tardive dyskinesia, and neuroleptic malignant syndrome
Bupropion			+++				+++		Seizure risk is elevated at therapeutic doses, and the risk of seizures increases dramatically at doses >450 mg qd
Citalopram						+++	+	+	
Desipramine	++	+	++	++	++		++	++	Quinidine-like effects that can prolong the QTc and lead to heart block
Doxepin	+++	+++		+++		++	++	++++	Quinidine-like effects that can prolong the QTc and lead to heart block
Duloxetine			+++		++	+++	+	++	Risk of medication-induced hypertension is dose related
Escitalopram						++	+	+	
Fluoxetine			+++			+++	+	+	
Imipramine	+++	+++		+++		++	++	+++	Quinidine-like effects that can prolong the QTc and lead to heart block
L-Deprenyl			++						Patients taking MAOIs must adhere to a low-tyramine diet and avoid medications that can result in life-threatening hypertensive crisis or serotonin syndrome Doses ≤9 mg are much less likely than other MAOI drugs to cause harmful interactions with tyramine and drugs
Maprotiline		+++		+++		++	+++	+++	Quinidine-like effects that can prolong the QTc and lead to heart block
Mirtazapine		++++		+++				++++	

Table 4 Antidepressant Drug Side Effects—cont'd

Drug	Anticholinergic Effects*	Sedation	Activation†	Postural Hypotension	Hypertension	Sexual Dysfunction††	Seizures§	Weight Gain	Comments
Nefazodone		++++		+++				++	Risk of medication-induced hypertension is dose related
Nortriptyline	++	+	++	+		+++	++	++	Quinidine-like effects that can prolong the QTc and lead to heart block This is the TCA least likely to cause postural hypotension
Paroxetine	+	++	++	+		+++	+	++	Minor withdrawal symptoms (flulike) can occur with sudden discontinuation
Phenelzine		++	++	++++		++		++++	Risk of medication-induced hypertension is dose related
Protriptyline	++++		+++	++			++	+	Quinidine-like effects that can prolong the QTc and lead to heart block
Sertraline			+++			+++	+	+	
Tranylcypromine			+++	++					Patients taking MAOIs must adhere to a low-tyramine diet and avoid a wide variety of medications that can result in life-threatening hypertensive crisis or serotonin syndrome
Trazodone		++++		+++		++		+++	Associated with non–dose-related priapism
Trimipramine	+++	+++	++	+++		++	++	+++	Quinidine-like effects that can prolong the QTc and lead to heart block
Venlafaxine			+++		+++	+++	+	+	Risk of medication-induced hypertension is dose related Minor withdrawal symptoms (flulike) can occur with sudden discontinuation

*Clinical manifestations include dry mouth, blurred vision, mydriasis, tachycardia, constipation, and confusion.
†Headache, tremor, restlessness.
††Impotence, delayed ejaculation, anorgasmia. Bupropion, mirtazapine, and nefazodone are the antidepressants least likely to cause sexual side effects.
§Nearly all antidepressants reduce seizure threshold. SSRIs, however, are unlikely to have a clinically significant effect on seizure threshold, even in overdose.
MAOI, monoamine oxidase inhibitor; SSRI, selective serotonin reuptake inhibitor; TCA, tricyclic antidepressant.

Any decision to discontinue medication should be followed by gradually tapering medication. This involves reducing the total daily dosage by approximately 30% weekly, or more slowly if the patient develops withdrawal symptoms (e.g., tremulousness, excitability, vertigo, nausea, or other nonspecific discomfort). Attempts to discontinue antidepressant medication may be thwarted either by the patient's intolerance of withdrawal or by recurrence of depressive symptoms. Distinguishing drug withdrawal from symptom recurrence can be difficult but is best accomplished by prolonging the taper.

Therapeutic Trial

Fundamental to all successful antidepressant therapy is a *therapeutic trial* of adequate dosage and adequate duration of treatment.[15] There is substantial evidence that a majority of patients with MDD do not receive adequate treatment trials.[4] The clinician must arrange for follow-up to ensure that the maximum recommended dosage of medication has been taken daily for at least 4 to 6 weeks. If some response is evident within the first 4 weeks, treatment should be continued for at least 6 weeks. No response to a therapeutic dose of medication by week 4, however, is an almost certain indication that another agent should be tried.[15]

Psychotherapy

Psychotherapy alone may be effective for mild to moderate MDD or as an adjunct to antidepressant medication for moderate to severe MDD.[15] Most primary care physicians are unlikely to provide psychotherapy, but knowledge about this treatment modality should facilitate selection and referral of appropriate patients. Commonly used models of psychotherapy include cognitive-behavioral therapy (CBT), interpersonal therapy (IPT), and insight-oriented approaches such as psychodynamic and client-centered therapies. Formats in which psychotherapies are delivered include individual, group, marital (or couples), family, and intensive outpatient programs. The goal of psychotherapy is to relieve depressive symptoms by exploring for and resolving issues such as grief, cognitive distortions, role changes, interpersonal disputes, and impaired coping.

Exercise

Exercise should be recommended to all depressed patients. Numerous studies substantiate its positive effect on mood. If nothing else, exercise provides a structured activity that, when performed regularly, can enhance the depressed patient's sense of competence and self-esteem.

Light Therapy for Seasonal Affective Disorder

Light therapy has been used effectively to treat seasonal depression. SAD (or seasonal mood disorder) is a subtype of MDD that occurs annually, usually starting in fall or winter and ending in spring or early summer. It is more than just "winter blues" or "cabin fever." Morning light therapy for at least 30 minutes every day is the most effective treatment. Improvement can occur within 2 to 4 days and reach full benefits within 2 to 4 weeks. An appliance that delivers at least 10,000 lux is recommended. Companies that manufacture lamps with the appropriate specifications include SunBox and Northern Light Technologies.

An unusual form of SAD that occurs during the summer months appears to be triggered by unusual heat sensitivity. Not surprisingly, the treatment involves minimizing heat exposure.

Electroconvulsive Therapy and Other Neuromodulation Technologies

Electroconvulsive therapy (ECT) is perhaps the most effective antidepressant treatment available.[15] It is typically used only as a last resort because of the need for hospital-level care and general anesthesia. A significant number of patients who are resistant to antidepressant medication, however, benefit from ECT. Maintenance ECT is indicated for those whose recurrent depressions do not respond to maintenance antidepressant medication.

Vagus nerve stimulation (VNS) received Food and Drug Administration approval in 2005 for treatment of refractory depression. Its special value may be in reducing the need for ECT and medication therapies in the maintenance phase of treatment.

Other novel neuromodulation techniques that are still under investigation include repetitive transcranial magnetic stimulation (rTMS) and deep brain stimulation (DBS). The efficacy of rTMS remains controversial, and the need for daily treatments administered by a technician presents logistic challenges. The use of DBS for treatment-refractory depression has produced some exciting results, but the scope of its application has yet to be determined.

PREVENTION AND SCREENING

The primary prevention of MDD depends on socioeconomic and biologic strategies that alter risk factors, such as economic deprivation, child abuse and neglect, and genetic predisposition. Probably the most that can be done at present, however, is in the realm of secondary and tertiary prevention. This involves overcoming barriers to timely recognition and treatment of MDD. Education, universal access to treatment, and provision of uniformly effective treatments are important and as-yet-unachieved goals.

Survey instruments can be used to assist in diagnosing MDD (see Table 1). They have been used either to screen for depression and other common psychiatric disorders or to verify and reinforce the diagnosis of clinical impression. Survey instruments can be completed by hand, telephone, or computer without requiring the clinician's valuable time. An important incidental finding in studies using computer-driven technologies is that patients are more likely to reveal personal information to a computer than they are in a face-to-face clinical encounter.

Once sensitive information surfaces, it must be dealt with. The clinician's response to information about hopelessness or suicidal ideation, for example, has important clinical and potential legal ramifications. Rather than ignoring or avoiding such information, a more effective measure is to delegate responsibility for follow-up to another clinician in the practice (e.g., physician's assistant, clinical nurse specialist). On-site collaboration with one or more mental health specialists (nurse clinician, psychiatrist, psychologist, social worker) has been found to offer the most effective means of dealing with the problem of depression in primary care.[18]

SPECIAL POPULATIONS

Geriatric Age Group

In general, geriatric depression responds well to traditional therapies, but it takes longer to respond to antidepressant medications, and elderly patients can exhibit greater sensitivity to potentially activating agents (e.g., fluoxetine, sertraline, and bupropion). Use of TCAs and other agents that cause postural hypotension should be reserved for second- or third-line use. Use of venlafaxine in the elderly is associated with a higher-than-average risk of urinary hesitancy or retention. Patients with periventricular small-vessel disease and those with multiple lacunar infarcts can present with signs and symptoms that resemble depression (e.g., apathy, psychomotor retardation, lack of initiative), and for these reasons might respond to antidepressant medication suboptimally or not at all.

Children and Adolescents

All patients treated with antidepressants should be carefully monitored at all times for intensification of suicidal thinking, but especially following initiation of treatment. There appears to be a greater risk of antidepressant-induced suicidal ideation shortly after starting antidepressant medication in children and adolescents. It is believed that undiagnosed BPD may be an important variable that accounts for this finding.

Pregnant Women

All antidepressant medications are classified as Class C by the Food and Drug Administration. Although all antidepressant medications pose an unsubstantiated risk to the developing fetus, withholding of antidepressant medication in cases of moderate to severe depression can also pose substantial risk to both the mother and fetus. Therefore, any woman who becomes pregnant and is either taking antidepressant medication or might require it should be referred for consultation to a psychiatrist, preferably one with specialty knowledge in this area.

Substance Abusers

Detection of substance abuse, like MDD, often requires a high index of suspicion. When both occur simultaneously, the standard of care is to require cessation of substance abuse followed by reassessment to determine continuing indication for antidepressant treatment. Many MDEs that occur in the context of substance abuse resolve with cessation of the abused substance, particularly alcohol. Cessation of cocaine dependence, however, is typically followed by severe depression that requires aggressive antidepressant treatment. Treatment with antidepressant medication is necessary when MDD is comorbid with substance abuse, but timing is important to avoid implying to the patient that antidepressant treatment is compatible with continued substance use.

Suicidal Patients and Others at Risk

Not all patients who voice suicidal thinking are at imminent risk of self harm. Because of the difficulty of accessing specialty services it behooves the generalist to develop some sophistication in risk assessment (see elsewhere in this section, "Psychiatric Emergencies").

Psychotic Patients

Patients with MDD and psychosis require aggressive antidepressant and antipsychotic treatment. If oral medication is ineffective, then ECT is indicated. In general, the first priority in the treatment of psychotic depression is control of psychotic thinking and behavior. Administration of an atypical antipsychotic usually serves this purpose. Olanzapine (Zyprexa) 2.5 to 5 mg or quetiapine (Seroquel) 25 to 100 mg daily are recommended starting doses. Referral to a psychiatrist is recommended if improvement is not rapid.

Summary

- Major depressive disorder, a common medical disorder with clinically significant morbidity and mortality, is often undiagnosed and undertreated.
- Detection of a major depressive episode in the primary care setting often requires a high index of suspicion.
- Case-finding (or screening) instruments can be used for early detection, verification of clinical impression, or data collection and documentation.
- Optimal treatment of a major depressive episode depends on whether it represents an episode of recurrent major depressive disorder or bipolar disorder or if it is a consequence of medical illness or substance abuse.
- A therapeutic trial of antidepressant medication constitutes a sufficient dosage taken for a sufficient period of time.
- Nonpharmacologic antidepressant therapies include brief psychotherapy, exercise, and light therapy; these are effective either alone or in combination with antidepressant medication.

Suggested Readings

Agency for Health Care Policy and Research (AHCPR): Clinical Practice Guideline: Depression in Primary Care, Volumes I & II. Washington, DC: U.S. Government Printing Office, 1993.

American Psychiatric Association: Diagnostic and Statistical Manual of Mental Disorders, 4th ed, text rev. Washington, DC: American Psychiatric Association, 2000.

Anderson RJ, Freedland KE, Clouse RE, Lustman PJ: The prevalence of comorbid depression in adults with diabetes: A meta-analysis. Diabetes Care 2001;24:1069-1078.

Barrett JE, Barrett JA, Oxman TE, Gerber PD: The prevalence of psychiatric disorders in a primary care practice. Arch Gen Psychiatry 1988;45:1100-1106.

DeBattista C, Schatzberg AF: Psychotropic dosing and monitoring guidelines. Primary Psychiatry 2006;13:61-81.

Duman RS, Malberg J, Thome J: Neural plasticity to stress and antidepressant treatment. Biol Psychiatry 1999;46:1181-1191.

Heim C, Newport DJ, Bonsall R, et al: Altered pituitary-adrenal axis responses to provocative challenge tests in adult survivors of childhood abuse. Am J Psychiatry 2001;158:575-581.

Kendler KS, Gardner CO, Prescott CA: Toward a comprehensive developmental model for major depression in women. Am J Psychiatry 2002;159:1133-1145.

Kessler RC, Berglund P, Demler O, et al: The epidemiology of major depressive disorder. Results from the National Comorbidity Survey Replication (NCS-R). JAMA 2003;289:3095-3105.

References

For a complete list of references, log onto www.expertconsult.com.

Bipolar Disorder

Sami Khalife, Vivek Singh, and David J. Muzina

DEFINITION AND ETIOLOGY

Bipolar affective disorder (BPD), classified as a mood disorder,[1] is a chronic, recurrent illness associated with high rates of morbidity, disability, and premature death from suicide. The disturbance of mood in BPD is episodic and recurrent, cycling at varying intervals from one mood state to another. Current classification schemes are based on the predominant pattern of mood (i.e., depression, mania, hypomania, or mixed states), the intensity of mood, and the rate of cycling from one mood to another (Fig. 1). Disturbed mood in BPD is typically accompanied by reckless and impulsive behavior, psychotic symptoms (e.g., delusions, hallucinations, and disorganized thinking), and cognitive disturbances.

PREVALENCE AND RISK FACTORS

Epidemiologic studies report a lifetime prevalence of BPD ranging from 1% to 10% of the U.S population. This broad range is due at least in part to inconsistent inclusion of BPD subtypes from one study to the next. Although much debate exists regarding the true prevalence of BPD, most experts agree that it is higher than the traditionally accepted rate of 0.5% to 1.5%.

The prevalence of BPD is the same in males and females, although male patients have more manic episodes and female patients have more depressive episodes. The first lifetime manifestation of BPD is typically a major depressive episode (MDE), with onset during late adolescence or early adulthood. The first episode of mania or hypomania might not occur until several years later, and until that time a diagnosis of BPD cannot be made. It is uncommon for the first manic episode to occur after age 30 years, although onset after age 60 years has been reported. In general, late-onset mania suggests drug toxicity or an underlying medical disorder until proved otherwise.

BPD is a familial disorder with genetic underpinnings. A higher rate of mood and anxiety disorders exists in the first-degree relatives of persons with BPD than in the general population. The primary risk factor for the development of BPD is a family history of BPD. A family history of BPD in a patient who presents with an MDE should alert the clinician to the possibility of an underlying bipolar diathesis and the corresponding treatment guidelines this entails.[2]

Factors that increase the risk of relapse or recurrence following a period of euthymic mood include not taking maintenance medication, abrupt discontinuation or rapid tapering of mood-stabilizing medication, the postpartum period, season, abnormal levels of psychosocial stress, serious medical illness (e.g., depression following myocardial infarction), and endogenous hormone fluctuations (e.g., thyroid dysfunction, menstrual cycle, menopause).

PATHOPHYSIOLOGY AND NATURAL HISTORY

The pathophysiology of BPD is under active investigation. Neuroimaging studies point to involvement of cortical, limbic, basal ganglia, and cerebellar structures in BPD. Genetic research has identified various loci that might contribute to the genesis of BPD. Lines of evidence point consistently to one or more defects in mitochondrial energy production as a basis for BPD.[3] DNA microarray technology used to analyze gene expression in postmortem brain has disclosed abnormalities related to the electron transport chain and G-protein coupled receptor signaling.[4,5] Lithium treatment, continued until the time of death, has been associated with evidence in postmortem brain of enhanced neuroprotection.[5] These and other findings underscore the biologic basis of BPD and suggest directions for future targeted drug development.

The natural history of BPD is depicted in Figure 2. In addition to episodes of either full-blown mania or major depression, patients can have episodes of subsyndromal depression, hypomania, or mixed states characterized by simultaneous occurrence of both depressive and manic features. Traditionally, classic BPD has been depicted as mood episodes alternating from mania to depression and back, but the variable course depicted in Figure 3 is more common. The natural course of bipolar disorder is for episode frequency to gradually increase and for an ever-increasing percentage of episodes to be characterized by depression.

In addition to the adverse psychosocial, vocational, and societal impacts of BPD, the lifetime suicide rate associated with BPD (15.6%) is higher than corresponding rates in any other psychiatric disorder. The risk of suicide by persons with BPD is highest during depressed or mixed states. Hopelessness can help to predict suicidal behavior during depression. Younger age and patients' subjective rating of depression severity can predict an elevated risk of suicide in mixed episodes.[6,7]

SIGNS, SYMPTOMS, AND DIAGNOSIS

The hallmark and distinguishing feature of BPD is episodic abnormally elevated mood. Classic mood elevation in BPD is characterized by euphoria and excitement. In practice, the predominant mood is often irritability rather than euphoria. In addition to mood elevation, the symptoms of mania include inflated self-esteem, decreased need for sleep, pressured and often loud speech, flight of ideas, distractibility, and increased goal-directed behavior often focused on pleasurable activities that have a high potential for becoming reckless and self destructive. Hypomania is a lesser form of mania, that is, mania minus the grossly impaired judgment that results in damaging, irresponsible behavior (e.g., excessive and indiscriminate sexual activity, spending, or traveling without heed to their consequences). Boxes 1 through 3 feature the diagnostic criteria for mania, hypomania, and mixed states as described in the *Diagnostic and Statistical Manual of Mental Disorders*, fourth edition, text revision (DSM IV-TR).[1] The diagnostic criteria for a major depressive episode can be found in the chapter on depression.

Diagnostic criteria for BPD require a history of at least one manic or hypomanic episode.[1] BPD is subdivided into types I and II to reflect the type of manic episodes the patient reports. A diagnosis of bipolar I disorder is given if there has been at least one lifetime episode of mania or a true mixed episode; a diagnosis of bipolar II disorder depends on at least one lifetime episode of hypomania, with none of the episodes achieving criteria for mania. The significance of this distinction continues to be debated. Recurrent MDEs typify both BPD types I and II. The complete diagnostic criteria for BPD types I and II are listed in Boxes 4 and 5.

Figures 4 through 6 graphically illustrate common courses of mood episodes in patients with different subtypes of BPD. Current thinking questions the adherence to strict diagnostic criteria for BPD episodes. This may have led to an overdiagnosis of BPD, which until recently was underdetected or misdiagnosed as recurrent major depressive disorder (MDD). This is an error that is easily committed even by experienced clinicians, because MDEs and dysthymia constitute the predominant mood disturbance in BPD, especially BPD type II. Inquiry about a personal or family history of manic or

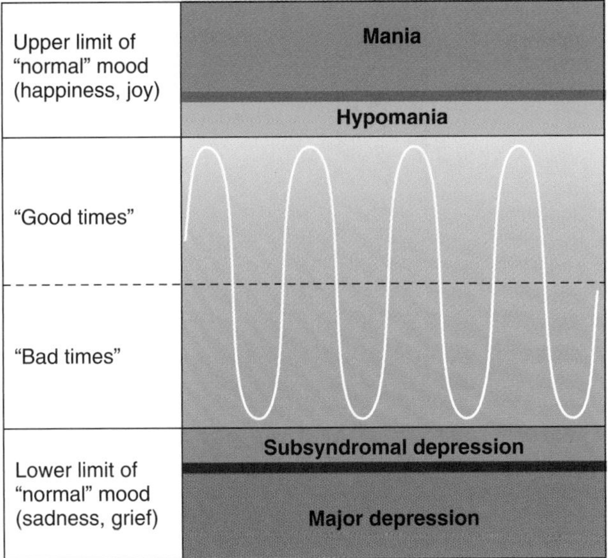

Figure 1 Normal mood cycles.

Symptom Domains of Bipolar Disorder

Manic Mood and Behavior
- Euphoria
- Grandiosity
- Pressured speech
- Impulsivity
- Excessive libido
- Recklessness
- Social intrusiveness
- Diminished need for sleep

Dysphoric or Negative Mood and Behavior
- Depression
- Anxiety
- Irritability
- Hostility
- Violence or suicide

Bipolar Disorder

Psychotic Symptoms
- Delusions
- Hallucinations
- Formal thought disorder

Cognitive Symptoms
- Racing thoughts
- Distractibility
- Disorganization
- Inattentiveness

Figure 2 Symptom domains of bipolar disorder.

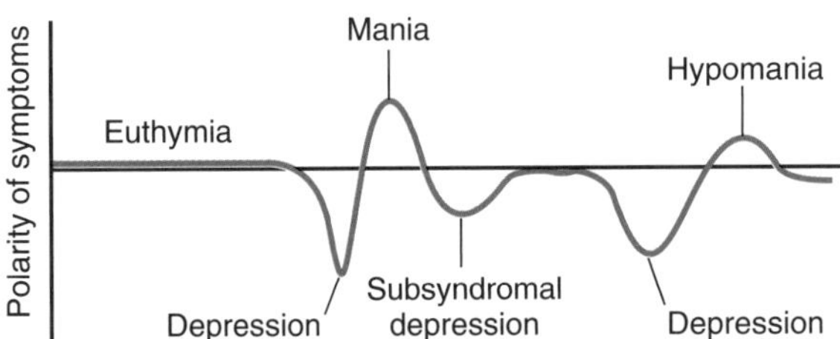

Figure 3 Natural history of bipolar disorder.

Box 1 DSM IV-TR Criteria for a Manic Episode

A distinct period of abnormally and persistently elevated, expansive, or irritable mood, lasting throughout at least *1 week* (or any duration if hospitalization is necessary).

During the period of mood disturbance, three (or more) of the following symptoms have persisted (four if the mood is only irritable) and have been present to a significant degree:
- Inflated self-esteem or grandiosity
- Decreased need for sleep (e.g., feels rested after only 3 hours of sleep)
- More talkative than usual or pressure to keep talking
- Flight of ideas or subjective experience that thoughts are racing
- Distractibility (attention too easily drawn to unimportant or irrelevant external stimuli)
- Increase in goal-directed activity (either socially, at work or school, or sexually) or psychomotor agitation
- Excessive involvement in pleasurable activities that have a high potential for painful consequences (e.g., unrestrained buying sprees, sexual indiscretions, or foolish business investments)

The symptoms do not meet criteria for a mixed episode (see Box 3).

The mood disturbance is sufficiently severe to cause marked impairment in occupational functioning or in usual social activities or relationships with others or to necessitate hospitalization to prevent harm to self or others, or the mood disturbance has psychotic features.

The symptoms are not due to the direct physiologic effects of a substance (e.g., a drug of abuse, medication, or other treatment) or a general medical condition (e.g., hyperthyroidism)

Note: Features in italics distinguish a manic from a hypomanic episode. Features of hypomanic episodes are listed in Box 2.

DSM IV-TR, Diagnostic and Statistical Manual of Mental Disorders, fourth edition, text revision (DSM IV-TR).

Adapted from American Psychiatric Association: Diagnostic and Statistical Manual of Mental Disorders, 4th ed, text rev. Washington, DC, American Psychiatric Association, 2000.

Box 2 DSM IV-TR Criteria for a Hypomanic Episode

A distinct period of persistently elevated, expansive, or irritable mood, lasting throughout at least 4 days, that is clearly different from the usual nondepressed mood.

During the period of mood disturbance, three (or more) of the following symptoms have persisted (four if the mood is only irritable) and have been present to a significant degree:
- Inflated self-esteem or grandiosity
- Decreased need for sleep (e.g., feels rested after only 3 hours of sleep)
- More talkative than usual or pressure to keep talking
- Flight of ideas or subjective experience that thoughts are racing
- Distractibility (i.e., attention too easily drawn to unimportant or irrelevant external stimuli)
- Increase in goal-directed activity (socially, at work or school, or sexually) or psychomotor agitation
- Excessive involvement in pleasurable activities that have a high potential for painful consequences (e.g., unrestrained buying sprees, sexual indiscretions, or foolish business investments)

The episode is associated with an unequivocal change in functioning that is uncharacteristic of the person when not symptomatic.

The disturbance in mood and the change in functioning are observable by others.

The episode is not severe enough to cause marked impairment in social or occupational functioning, or to necessitate hospitalization, and there are no psychotic features.

The symptoms are not due to the direct physiologic effects of a substance (e.g., a drug of abuse, medication, or other treatment) or a general medical condition (e.g., hyperthyroidism)

Note: Features in italics distinguish a manic from a hypomanic episode. Features of manic episodes are listed in Box 1.

DSM IV-TR, Diagnostic and Statistical Manual of Mental Disorders, fourth edition, text revision (DSM IV-TR).

Adapted from American Psychiatric Association: Diagnostic and Statistical Manual of Mental Disorders, 4th ed, text rev. Washington, DC, American Psychiatric Association, 2000.

Box 3 DSM IV-TR Criteria for a Mixed Episode

The criteria are met both for a manic episode (Box 1) and for a major depressive episode (see Box 3 in the chapter on depression) (except for duration) nearly every day for at least 1 week.
The mood disturbance is sufficiently severe to cause marked impairment in occupational functioning or in usual social activities or relationships with others or to necessitate hospitalization to prevent harm to self or others, or the mood disturbance has psychotic features.
The symptoms are not due to the direct physiologic effects of a substance (e.g., a drug of abuse, medication, or other treatment) or a general medical condition (e.g., hyperthyroidism).

DSM IV-TR, Diagnostic and Statistical Manual of Mental Disorders, fourth edition, text revision (DSM IV-TR).
Adapted from American Psychiatric Association: Diagnostic and Statistical Manual of Mental Disorders, 4th ed, text rev. Washington, DC, American Psychiatric Association, 2000.

Box 4 DSM IV-TR Criteria for Bipolar Type I Disorder Not Otherwise Specified

Criteria, except for duration, are currently (or most recently) met for a manic, a hypomanic, a mixed, or a major depressive episode.
There has previously been at least one manic episode or mixed episode.
The mood symptoms cause clinically significant distress or impairment in social, occupational, or other important areas of functioning.
The mood symptoms in the first two criteria are not better accounted for as schizoaffective disorder and are not superimposed on schizophrenia, schizophreniform disorder, delusional disorder, or psychotic disorder not otherwise specified.
The mood symptoms in the first two criteria are not due to the direct physiologic effects of a substance (e.g., a drug of abuse, medication, or other treatment) or a general medical condition (e.g., hyperthyroidism).

Adapted from American Psychiatric Association: Diagnostic and Statistical Manual of Mental Disorders, 4th ed, text rev. Washington, DC, American Psychiatric Association, 2000.

Box 5 DSM IV-TR Criteria for Bipolar Type II Disorder

Presence (or history) of one or more major depressive episodes.
Presence (or history of at least one hypomanic episode.
There has never been a manic episode or a mixed episode.
The mood symptoms in the first two criteria are not better accounted for as schizoaffective disorder and are not superimposed on schizophrenia, schizophreniform disorder, delusional disorder, or psychotic disorder not otherwise specified.
The symptoms cause clinically significant distress or impairment in social, occupational, or other important areas of functioning.

Adapted from American Psychiatric Association: Diagnostic and Statistical Manual of Mental Disorders, 4th ed, text rev. Washington, DC, American Psychiatric Association, 2000.

hypomanic episodes is therefore crucial when evaluating a patient who presents with an MDE. Other features of BPD that distinguish it from MDD include earlier age at onset; more frequent mood episodes, rapid onset of symptoms; shorter symptom-free intervals; chaotic interpersonal, social, and vocational adjustments; and response to antidepressant treatment characterized by unusual sensitivity to standard antidepressant doses or rapid loss of initial therapeutic response.

Figure 3 depicts four separate symptom domains that can be seen in various combinations with BPD.

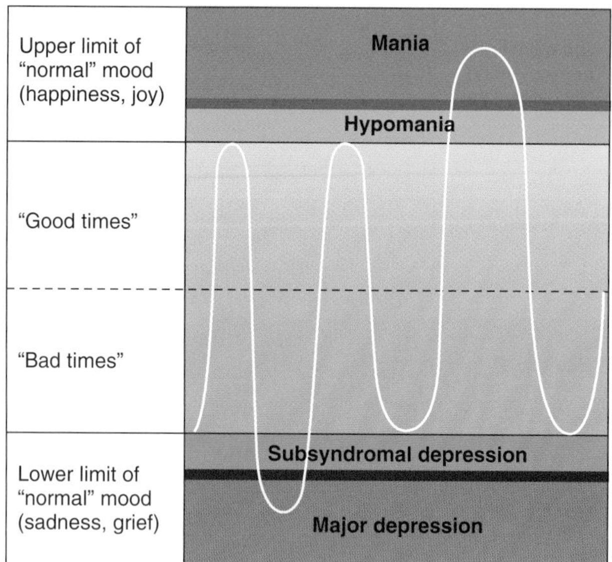

Figure 4 Bipolar type I disorder.

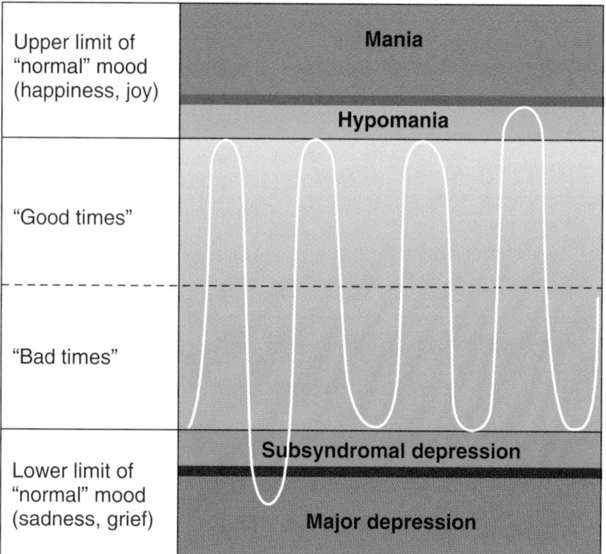

Figure 5 Bipolar type II disorder.

Summary

- If an active mood episode is identified, rule out mood disorder due to a general medical condition or one that is substance-related.
- If psychosis accompanies a mood episode, rule out schizophrenia, schizoaffective disorder, delusional disorder, or psychosis due to a general medical condition.
- BPD is an important consideration in the differential diagnosis of a major depressive episode.
- Definitive diagnosis is not always possible after a first visit. When available, obtain collateral information from family or other associates as well as medical records that document previous treatment trials.

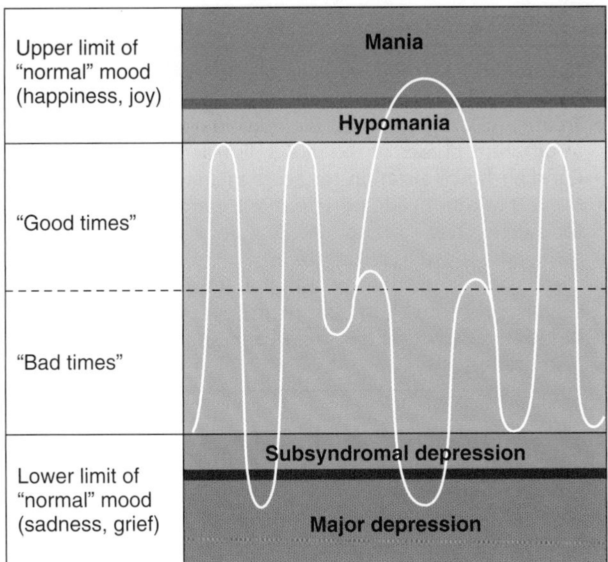

Figure 6 Bipolar type I mixed state.

Box 6 Basic Principles of Managing the Bipolar Patient

Create and foster a therapeutic alliance

- Take extra time to listen and communicate with patients and their families
- Encourage peer-to-peer support

Offer education about the diagnosis and treatment

- Educate patient and family about the seriousness of the illness and benefits of appropriate therapy
- Provide the patient with patient-education materials

Enhance adherence with treatment

- Educate the patient and family about medication treatment options, therapeutic effects, possible adverse effects, and the likely need for long-term medication
- Encourage the patient and family to express their treatment preferences

Monitor and manage symptoms and risk

- Encourage the patient to permit ongoing involvement of one or more trusted family members or friends in the patient's treatment
- Solicit information from family and other third parties when assessing risk, especially suicide risk, substance use, and social isolation
- Encourage open discussion about the need to recognize and manage risky behavior (e.g., limit access to dangerous machinery, credit cards)
- During times the patient is well, engage the patient and family (or partner) to develop interventions that target reckless or dangerous behavior during future illness episodes
- Encourage self monitoring of mood and medication use and of sleep patterns
- Encourage regularity of sleep, daily activities, and medication use

TREATMENT

Patients who are agitated or irrational or who present a danger to themselves or others require urgent (next day) or emergent (same day) evaluation by a psychiatrist, unless the primary physician is comfortable with acute stabilization. For less-pressing cases of suspected BPD, appropriate treatment may be started while awaiting completion of the referral process to a psychiatrist. Occasionally, the primary care physician who is familiar with the assessment and treatment of BPD may accept full responsibility for the BPD patient's management, although this typically happens after consultation with a psychiatrist.

The basic principles of managing the bipolar patient are listed in Box 6. United States Food and Drug Administration (FDA)-approved agents for treating BPD are listed in Table 1.

Mania is generally more easily managed than depression, although it requires hospitalization more often. Many more FDA-approved options exist for mania than for bipolar depression. There are no FDA-approved treatments for hypomania. Clinical experience suggests, however, that agents approved for mania are generally effective for hypomania, sometimes at lower doses. Mild mania and hypomania often respond to one antimanic drug, whereas acute manic crises often require two or more agents to stabilize the mood.

Mixed depressive and manic episodes present a difficult treatment challenge best met by first stabilizing manic behavior and then addressing depression. An atypical antipsychotic or a mood stabilizer is typically administered to stabilize the manic behavior, and depression is addressed with standard antidepressant treatment. An alternative is to initiate treatment with a combined pharmacologic approach. These include simultaneously administering an antidepressant and an antipsychotic, administering mood-stabilizing medication, or administering the combination formulation of olanzapine and fluoxetine (OFC, Symbyax).

OFC is the only FDA-approved treatment for acute bipolar depression and delivers both antidepressant and antipsychotic medications simultaneously in one preparation. Antidepressants, when prescribed alone, are not effective for bipolar depression and are not formally indicated for such use by the FDA. Olanzapine, used either alone or as OFC has been associated with weight gain and hyperglycemia, and there are published case reports of diabetic ketoacidosis. Because these potential adverse outcomes are not unique to olanzapine and are regarded as an effect of the atypical antipsychotic class, OFC should be considered as a first-line treatment for bipolar depression. OFC is for oral use only. Dosing can be started with OFC 6/25 (olanzapine 6 mg and fluoxetine 25 mg) daily and adjusted as necessary to OFC 12/50 (olanzapine 12 mg and fluoxetine 50 mg) daily.

Other atypical antipsychotics continue to receive attention as potential antidepressant agents in BPD. Investigation of quetiapine (Seroquel) as monotherapy for bipolar depression has produced promising results and might receive FDA approval in the near future. A dosage range of 300 to 600 mg daily is recommended for treating depression associated with acute BPD type I or II.[8]

Recent evidence-based practice guidelines also recommend the mood stabilizers lithium or lamotrigine (Lamictal), or both, as first-line agents for acute bipolar depression.[7] Neither is currently FDA approved for this indication, and the strength of the data supporting their use for bipolar depression is modest at best. Their off-label use is nevertheless recommended, given the paucity of effective treatments for bipolar depression. Lithium is most effective at doses that achieve serum blood levels of 0.8 to 1.5 mEq/L. Lamotrigine should be started at 25 mg daily and increased every 1 to 2 weeks to a therapeutic dose, typically in the range of 50 to 200 mg daily. Titration of both agents should be monitored closely to avoid lithium toxicity (tremor, nausea, diarrhea) or lamotrigine-induced rash that, if unchecked, can progress to toxic epidermal necrolysis or Stevens-Johnson syndrome.

Table 2 outlines the initial steps recommended for treating acutely depressed versus manic states in patients with bipolar disorder.[9]

Electroconvulsive therapy can effectively be used to treat either manic or depressive episodes, although it is generally reserved for medication-refractory cases.

Table 1 FDA-Approved Drugs for Bipolar Type I Disorder

Drug	Mania	Depression	Maintenance
Aripiprazole	x	x	x
Carbamazepine ER	x		
Chlorpromazine	x		
Lamotrigine			x
Lithium	x		x
Olanzapine	x		x
Olanzapine-fluoxetine combination		x	
Quetiapine	x		
Risperidone	x		
Valproate, Divalproex ER	x		
Ziprasidone	x		

FDA, United States Food and Drug Administration.

Summary

- Maintaining a strong working alliance with the bipolar patient typically requires additional time, effort, and skill.
- Treatment strategies must be individualized and adjusted at different phases of the mood disorder.
- Consider hospitalization for acute mania.
- Numerous approved and effective treatments are available for mania. They are also effective, but not FDA approved, for hypomania and mixed states.
- Olanzapine-fluoxetine combination (OFC) and mood stabilizers are first-line treatments for bipolar depression. Monotherapy with a traditional antidepressant is discouraged.

PREVENTION AND SCREENING

BPD cannot be prevented. Once this mood disorder has declared itself, the patient should be counseled regarding the chronic risk for relapse and recurrence; lifetime treatment is recommended. Periodic medical monitoring for complications is crucial in preventing unwanted outcomes, such as the metabolic syndrome.

Table 2 Initial Treatment Guidelines for Bipolar Disorder

Step 1			Step 2		Step 3 and Beyond
Drug	**Starting Dose**	**Target**	**Drug**	**Starting Dose**	**Options**
Depression					
Lithium	300-450 mg bid	Serum level > 0.8 mEq/L	OFC*	6 mg/25 mg hs	Combinations of lithium, lamotrigine, OFC, quetiapine
Lamotrigine	25 mg qd Initial and target doses may be affected by concomitant meds (see prescribing information)	Dose 50-200 mg/day	Quetiapine†	100 mg hs; increase to 300 mg hs by day 3	Add traditional antidepressant‡ to one or more of these ECT
Mania§					
Lithium	300-450 mg tid	Serum level generally 1.0-1.5 mEq/L	Choose 2 of the following in combination:		Other 2-drug combinations (choose from lithium, VPA, AAPs, carbamazepine, oxcarbamazepine, topiramate)
Valproic acid	500 mg tid				ECT
Divalproex	750 mg hs		Lithium		Clozapine
Atypical antipsychotic¶	Initial dosing varies, refer to prescribing information		VPA or divalproex		Triple drug therapy
			AAP¶		

*FDA approved for BPD type I depression.
†Pending FDA approval for BPD types I and II depression
‡Selective serotonin reuptake inhibitor, serotonin and norepinephrine uptake inhibitor, buproprion, venlafaxine, mirtazapine.
§For moderate to severe manic episodes, two-drug combination therapy is recommended as first step.
¶Excluding clozapine and aripiprazole.
¶Excluding olanzapine and clozapine. These are less than ideal initial choices because of tolerability issues, primarily metabolic and/or hematologic.
AAP, atypical antipsychotic; BPD, bipolar disorder; ECT, electroconvulsive therapy; FDA, United States Food and Drug Administration; meds, medications; OFC, olanzapine-fluoxetine combination; VPA, valproic acid.
Based on Suppes T, Dennehy EB, Hirschfeld RM, et al: The Texas implementation of medication algorithms: Update to the algorithms for treatment of bipolar I disorder. J Clin Psychiatry 2005;66:870-886.

Screening tools are available, although they should not be viewed as an alternative to thorough diagnostic evaluation. The Mood Disorder Questionnaire (MDQ) is a validated screening instrument for BPD.[10] It can be found online (search "MDQ download") in both English and Spanish versions. The Bipolar Spectrum Diagnostic Scale (BSDS) involves an easy-to-read, one-page story that depicts typical mood swing experiences. The patient places a check mark at the end of each sentence that conforms with the patient's own experience.[11] The BSDS is also available online (search "bipolar diagnostic spectrum scale").[12]

SPECIAL POPULATIONS

Children and Adolescents

The literature regarding medication treatment for children and adolescents with BPD is limited, and many of the current recommendations are based on studies of adults.

Pregnant Women

Pregnancy does not affect the risk of bipolar relapse. In contrast, the postpartum period is associated with increased risk for bipolar relapse and illness onset. Treatment of acute mood episodes during pregnancy requires a careful consideration of the potential teratogenic effects of medications versus the harmful effects of an ill mother on the unborn child. Many women require maintenance treatment during pregnancy. Many strategies have been advanced, therefore, to reduce the risk potential of pharmacologic treatment of BPD in the pregnant woman. These have included monotherapy with the lowest effective dose of a drug for the shortest period, preconception coadministration of multivitamins with folate, and avoidance of antimanic agents during the first trimester.

Human Immunodeficiency Virus–Seropositive Patients

Mania can be seen early in the course of human immunodeficiency virus (HIV) infection but is more common as the illness progresses. Irritability is more common than euphoria. Manic episodes appear to be more common in the setting of opportunistic infections (e.g., cryptococcal meningitis) associated with acquired immunodeficiency syndrome (AIDS) and also in association with drugs used to treat patients with HIV and AIDS (e.g., zidovudine, efavirenz, steroids). Treatment of mania secondary to HIV-related illness should be directed toward symptoms and underlying causes. Pharmacologic management of mania in HIV-infected persons often includes a combination of an anticonvulsant mood stabilizer plus an antipsychotic. Patients with primary BPD who are also HIV seropositive should receive recommended treatment for acute mood episodes, although careful attention must be paid to an increased risk for drug interactions in this population.

Suggested Readings

American Psychiatric Association: Practice Guideline for the Treatment of Patients with Bipolar Disorder, 2nd ed. Washington, DC, American Psychiatric Association, 2002, pp 525-612.

American Psychiatric Association: Diagnostic and Statistical Manual of Mental Disorders, 4th ed, text rev. Washington, DC, American Psychiatric Association, 2000.

Baldessarini RJ, Pompili M, Tondo L: Suicide in bipolar disorder: Risks and management. CNS Spectrums 2006;11:465-471.

Calabrese JR, Keck PE Jr, Macfadden W, et al: A randomized, double-blind, placebo-controlled trial of quetiapine in the treatment of bipolar I or II depression. Am J Psychiatry 2005;162:1351-1360.

Fattal O, Budur K, Vaughan AJ, Franco K: Review of the literature on major mental disorders in adult patients with mitochondrial diseases. Psychosomatics 2006;47:1-7.

Ghaemi SN, Miller CJ, Berv DA, et al: Sensitivity and specificity of a new bipolar spectrum diagnostic scale. J Affect Disord 2005;84:273-277.

Hirschfeld RM, Williams JB, Spitzer RL, et al: Development and validation of a screening instrument for bipolar spectrum disorder: the Mood Disorder Questionnaire. Am J Psychiatry 2000;157:1873-1875.

Muzina DJ, Calabrese JR: Guidelines for the treatment of bipolar disorder. In Stein DJ, Schatzberg A, Kupfer DJ (eds): Textbook of Mood Disorders. Washington, DC, American Psychiatric Association, 2005, pp 463-483.

Ryan MM, Lockstone HE, Huffaker SJ, et al: Gene expression analysis of bipolar disorder reveals downregulation of the ubiquitin cycle and alterations in synaptic genes. Mol Psychiatry 2006;11:965-978.

Suppes T, Dennehy EB, Hirschfeld RM, et al: The Texas implementation of medication algorithms: Update to the algorithms for treatment of bipolar I disorder. J Clin Psychiatry 2005;66:870-886.

Sun X, Wang JF, Tseng M, Young LT: Downregulation in components of the mitochondrial electron transport chain in the postmortem frontal cortex of subjects with bipolar disorder. J Psychiatry Neurosci 2006;31(3):189-196.

Valtonen HM, Suominen K, Mantere O, et al: Suicidal behaviour during different phases of bipolar disorder. J Affect Disord 2007; 97:101-107.

References

For a complete list of references, log onto www.expertconsult.com.

Eating Disorders

Kathleen N. Franco

DEFINITION AND ETOLOGY

Eating disorders are syndromes characterized by severe disturbances in eating behavior and by distress or excessive concern about body shape or weight. Presentation varies, but eating disorders often occur with severe medical or psychiatric comorbidity. Denial of symptoms and reluctance to seek treatment make treatment especially challenging.

CLASSIFICATION

Major eating disorders can be classified as anorexia nervosa (Box 1), bulimia nervosa (Box 2), and eating disorder not otherwise specified (Box 3). Although criteria of the *Diagnostic and Statistical Manual of Mental Disorders*, fourth edition, text revision (DSM IV-TR1), allow diagnosis of a specific eating disorder, many patients demonstrate a mixture of both anorexia and bulimia. Up to 50% of patients with anorexia nervosa develop bulimic symptoms, and a smaller percentage of patients who are initially bulimic develop anorexic symptoms.[2]

Anorexia nervosa has two subtypes: restrictive eating and binge eating alternating with restrictive eating at different periods of the illness. Patients with bulimia nervosa can be subclassified into purging and nonpurging. Many patients have a combination of eating disorder symptoms that cannot be strictly categorized as either anorexia nervosa or bulimia nervosa and are technically diagnosed as eating disorder not otherwise specified. Obesity alone is not considered an eating disorder.

Listed in the DSM IV-TR appendix, binge eating disorder is defined as uncontrolled binge eating without emesis or laxative abuse. It is often, but not always, associated with obesity symptoms. Night eating syndrome includes morning anorexia, increased appetite in the evening, and insomnia. Often obese, these patients can have complete or partial amnesia for eating during the night.

Eating disorders before puberty include food avoidance emotional disorder, which is similar to anorexia; selective eating of only a few foods; pervasive refusal syndrome, with reduced intake and added behavioral problems; and functional dysphagia with no organic etiology. Unpleasant mealtimes and conflicts over eating can precede these conditions of childhood. Pica and rumination are not considered eating disorders, but rather are feeding disorders of infancy and childhood.

RISK FACTORS AND PREVALENCE

Eating disorders have been reported in up to 4% of adolescents and young adults. The most common age at onset for anorexia nervosa is the mid teens; in 5% of the patients, the onset of the disorder is in the early twenties. The onset of bulimia nervosa is usually in adolescence but may be as late as early adulthood.[2-3]

Gender Prevalence

Both anorexia nervosa and bulimia nervosa are more commonly seen in girls and women. Estimates of female-to-male ratio range from 6:1 to 10:1.

Lifetime Prevalence

The reported lifetime prevalence of anorexia nervosa among women has ranged from 0.5% when narrowly defined to 3.7% for more broadly defined anorexia nervosa. With regard to bulimia nervosa, estimates of lifetime prevalence among women range from 1.1% to 4.2%. Prevalence of eating disorders in young children is unknown. However, children as young as 5 years have reported awareness of dieting and know that inducing vomiting can produce weight loss. Eating disorder not otherwise specified is the most prevalent eating disorder.

Cultural Considerations

Eating disorders are more common in industrialized societies where there is an abundance of food and being thin, especially for women, is considered attractive.[3] Eating disorders are most common in the United States, Canada, Europe, Australia, New Zealand, and South Africa. However, rates are increasing in Asia, especially in Japan and China, where women are exposed to cultural change and modernization. In the United States, eating disorders are common in young Latin American, Native American, and African American women, but the rates are still lower than in white women. African American women are more likely to develop bulimia and more likely to purge. Female athletes involved in running, gymnastics, or ballet and male body builders or wrestlers are at increased risk.

PATHOPHYSIOLOGY AND NATURAL HISTORY

Biologic and psychosocial factors are implicated in the pathophysiology, but the causes and mechanisms underlying eating disorders remain uncertain.[2-4]

Biologic Factors

First-degree female relatives and monozygotic twin offspring of patients with anorexia nervosa have higher rates of anorexia nervosa and bulimia nervosa. Children of patients with anorexia nervosa have a lifetime risk for anorexia nervosa that is tenfold that of the general population (5%). Families of patients with bulimia nervosa have higher rates of substance abuse, particularly alcoholism, affective disorders, and obesity.

Endogenous opioids might contribute to denial of hunger in patients with anorexia nervosa. Some hypothesize that dieting can increase the risk for developing an eating disorder. Increased endorphin levels have been described in patients with bulimia nervosa after purging and may be likely to induce feelings of well being. Diminished norepinephrine turnover and activity are suggested by reduced levels of 3-methoxy-4-hydroxyphenylglycol in the urine and cerebrospinal fluid of some patients with anorexia nervosa. Antidepressants often benefit patients with bulimia nervosa and support a pathophysiologic role for serotonin and norepinephrine.

Starvation results in many biochemical changes such as hypercortisolemia, nonsuppression of dexamethasone, suppression of thyroid function, and amenorrhea. Several computed tomography (CT) studies of the brain have revealed enlarged sulci and ventricles, a finding that is reversed with weight gain. In one study using positron emission tomography (PET), metabolism was higher in the caudate nucleus during the anorectic state than after hyperalimentation.

Anorexia risk may increase with a polymorphism of the promoter region of serotonin 2a receptor. The melanocortin 4 receptor gene is hypothesized to regulate weight and appetite. Polymorphism in the gene for agouti-related peptide might also play a role at the melan-

Box 1* DSM IV-TR Criteria for Anorexia Nervosa

Criteria

Refusal to maintain body weight at or above a minimally normal weight for age and height: Weight loss leading to maintenance of body weight <85% of that expected or failure to make expected weight gain during period of growth, leading to body weight less than 85% of that expected.

Intense fear of gaining weight or becoming fat, even though under weight.

Disturbance in the way one's body weight or shape are experienced, undue influence of body weight or shape on self evaluation, or denial of the seriousness of the current low body weight.

Amenorrhea (at least three consecutive cycles) in postmenarchal girls and women. Amenorrhea is defined as periods occurring only following hormone (e.g., estrogen) administration.

Type

Restricting type: During the current episode of anorexia nervosa, the person *has not* regularly engaged in binge-eating or purging behavior (self-induced vomiting or misuse of laxatives, diuretics, or enemas).

Binge-eating-purging type: During the current episode of anorexia nervosa, the person *has* regularly engaged in binge-eating or purging behavior (self-induced vomiting or the misuse of laxatives, diuretics, or enemas).

**See also Box 3.*

Adapted from American Psychiatric Association: Diagnostic and Statistical Manual of Mental Disorders, 4th ed, text rev. Washington, DC, American Psychiatric Association, 2000.

Box 2* DSM IV-TR Criteria for Bulimia Nervosa

Criteria

Recurrent episodes of binge eating characterized by both:

Eating, in a discrete period of time (e.g., within any 2-hour period), an amount of food that is definitely larger than most people would eat during a similar period of time and under similar circumstances

A sense of lack of control over eating during the episode, defined by a feeling that one cannot stop eating or control what or how much one is eating

Recurrent inappropriate compensatory behavior to prevent weight gain

Self-induced vomiting

Misuse of laxatives, diuretics, enemas, or other medications

Fasting

Excessive exercise

The binge eating and inappropriate compensatory behavior both occur, on average, at least twice a week for 3 months.

Self evaluation is unduly influenced by body shape and weight.

The disturbance does not occur exclusively during episodes of anorexia nervosa.

Type

Purging type: During the current episode of bulimia nervosa, the person has regularly engaged in self-induced vomiting or the misuse of laxatives, diuretics, or enemas.

Nonpurging type: During the current episode of bulimia nervosa, the person has used inappropriate compensatory behavior but has not regularly engaged in self-induced vomiting or misused laxatives, diuretics, or enemas.

**See also Box 3.*

Adapted from American Psychiatric Association: Diagnostic and Statistical Manual of Mental Disorders, 4th ed, text rev. Washington, DC, American Psychiatric Association, 2000.

cortin receptor. In bulimia nervosa there is excessive secretion of ghrelin. Ghrelin receptor gene polymorphism is associated with both hyperphagia of bulimia and Prader-Willi syndrome.

Perhaps some of the most fascinating new research addresses the overlap between uncontrolled compulsive eating and compulsive drug seeking in drug addiction.[4] Reduction in ventral striatal dopamine is found in both of these groups. The lower the frequency of dopamine D_2 receptors, the higher the body mass index. Obese persons might eat to temporarily increase activity in these reward circuits. Frequent visual food stimuli paired with increased sensitivity of right orbitofrontal brain activity is likely to initiate eating behavior. Marijuana's well-known appetite stimulant effect is likely due to its agonist activity at cannabinoid receptors, and cannabinoid receptor antagonism has been associated with reduced binge eating (Fig. 1).

Box 3* DSM IV-TR Criteria for Eating Disorder Not Otherwise Specified

Eating disorder not otherwise specified includes disorders of eating that do not meet the criteria for any specific eating disorder.

For female patients, all of the criteria for anorexia nervosa are met except that the patient has regular menses.

All of the criteria for anorexia nervosa are met except that, despite significant weight loss, the patient's current weight is in the normal range.

All of the criteria for bulimia nervosa are met except that the binge eating and inappropriate compensatory mechanisms occur less than twice a week or for less than 3 months.

The patient has normal body weight and regularly uses inappropriate compensatory behavior after eating small amounts of food (e.g., self-induced vomiting after consuming two cookies).

Repeatedly chewing and spitting out, but not swallowing, large amounts of food.

Binge-eating disorder is recurrent episodes of binge eating in the absence if regular inappropriate compensatory behavior characteristic of bulimia nervosa.

**See also Boxes 1 and 2.*

Adapted from American Psychiatric Association: Diagnostic and Statistical Manual of Mental Disorders, 4th ed, text rev. Washington, DC, American Psychiatric Association, 2000.

Psychosocial Factors

High levels of hostility, chaos, and isolation and low levels of nurturance and empathy are reported in families of children presenting with eating disorders.[1-3] Anorexia has been postulated as a reaction to demands on adolescents to behave more independently or to respond to societal pressures to be slender. Anorexia nervosa patients are usually high achievers, and two thirds live at home with parents. Many consider their bodies to be under the control of their parents. Family dynamics alone, however, do not cause anorexia nervosa. Self-starvation may be an effort to gain validation as a unique person. Patients with bulimia nervosa have been described as having difficulties with impulse regulation.

Course and Prognosis

As a general guideline, it appears that one third of patients fully recover, one third retain subthreshold symptoms, and one third maintain a chronic eating disorder.[1-3]

Anorexia Nervosa

Long-term follow-up shows recovery rates ranging from 44% to 76%, with prolonged recovery time (57 to 59 months). Mortality (up to 20%) is primarily from cardiac arrest or suicide. Good prognostic factors are admission of hunger, lessening of denial, and improved self esteem. Poorer prognostic factors are initial lower minimum weight, presence of vomiting or laxative abuse, failure to respond to previous treatment, disturbed family relationships, and conflicts with parents.

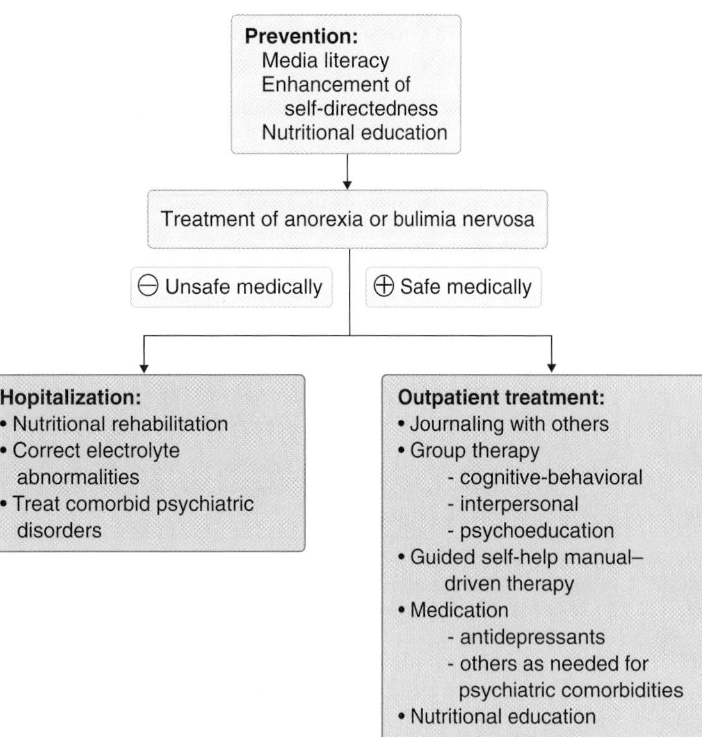

Figure 1 **Comprehensive treatment plan for the patient with an eating disorder.**

Bulimia Nervosa

Little long-term follow-up data exist. Short-term success is 50% to 70%, with relapse rates between 30% and 50% after 6 months. These patients have an overall better prognosis as compared with anorexia nervosa patients. Poor prognostic factors are hospitalization, higher frequency of vomiting, poor social and occupational functioning, poor motivation for recovery, severity of purging, presence of medical complications, high levels of impulsivity, longer duration of illness, delayed treatment, and premorbid history of obesity and substance abuse.

SIGNS AND SYMPTOMS

Anorexia Nervosa

The essential features of anorexia nervosa are refusal to maintain a minimally normal body weight, intense fear of gaining weight, and significant disturbance in the perception of the shape or size of one's body.[1-3] Patients commonly lack insight into the problem and are brought to professional attention by a family member. DSM IV-TR identifies two subtypes of anorexia nervosa: restricting type and binge eating–purging type. Comorbid psychiatric symptoms include depressive symptoms such as depressed mood, social withdrawal, irritability, insomnia, and decreased sexual interest. Many depressive features may be secondary to the physiologic sequelae of semistarvation. Symptoms of mood disturbances need to be reassessed after partial or complete weight restoration. Obsessive-compulsive features—thoughts of food, hoarding food, picking or pulling apart small portions of food, or collecting recipes—are common. Anxiety symptoms and concerns of eating in public are also common.

Bulimia Nervosa

The essential features are binge eating and inappropriate compensatory behavior such as fasting, vomiting, using laxatives, or exercising to prevent weight gain. Binge eating is typically triggered by dysphoric mood states, interpersonal stressors, intense hunger following dietary restraints, or negative feelings related to body weight, shape, and food. Patients are typically ashamed of their eating problems, and binge eating usually occurs in secrecy. Unlike anorexia nervosa, bulimia nervosa patients are typically within normal weight range and restrict their total caloric consumption between binges.

DIAGNOSIS

Rating Instruments

In addition to the clinical interview, the Eating Attitudes Test, Eating Disorders Inventory, Body Shape Questionnaire, and others can be used to assess eating disorders.[5]

Comorbidity of Eating Disorders

Psychiatric

Common comorbid conditions include major depressive disorder or dysthymia (50%-75%), sexual abuse (20%-50%), obsessive-compulsive disorder (25% with anorexia nervosa), substance abuse (12%-18% with anorexia nervosa, especially the binge-purge subtype, and 30%-37% with bulimia nervosa), and bipolar disorder (4%-13%).[1-4]

Medical

There are many complications related to weight loss, purging and vomiting, and laxative abuse (Box 4). When obesity is associated with the eating disorder, hyperlipidemia, diabetes mellitus, sleep apnea, joint injury, hypertension, and cardiac and respiratory disorders can result.

DIFFERENTIAL DIAGNOSIS

Anorexia Nervosa

Medical illnesses include brain tumors and other malignancies, gastrointestinal disease, and acquired immunodeficiency syndrome (AIDS).

Box 4 Medical Complications of Eating Disorders

Weight Loss
Amenorrhea
Bradycardia
Cold intolerance
Constipation
Cyanosis
Edema
Hypoglycemia
Low albumin
Orthostatic blood pressure drop
Osteoporosis, stress fractures
Structural and functional brain changes
Thyroid dysfunction

Appetite Suppressant Abuse
Anxiety
Hypertension
Tachyarrhythmia
Tremors

Purging (Abuse of Laxatives, Ipecac, or Diuretics)
Abnormal colonic motility
Arrhythmias
Cardiac and other myopathies
Dehydration
Dental caries
Electrolyte abnormalities
Gastrointestinal irritation, bleeding, or reflux
Parotid abnormalities
Secondary renal failure

Other psychiatric disorders with disturbed appetite or food intake include depression, somatization disorder, and schizophrenia. Patients with depressive disorder generally do not have an intense fear of obesity or body image disturbance. Depressed patients usually have a decreased appetite, whereas anorexia nervosa patients claim to have a normal appetite and to feel hungry. Patients with somatization disorder do not generally express a morbid fear of obesity. Severe weight loss and amenorrhea longer than 3 months are unusual in somatization disorder. Schizophrenic patients might have delusions about food being poisoned but rarely are they concerned with caloric content. They also do not express a fear of gaining weight.

Bulimia nervosa patients usually maintain their weight within a normal range.

Bulimia Nervosa

General medical conditions of central nervous system pathology, such as brain tumors, can simulate bulimia nervosa. Kluver-Bucy syndrome is a rare condition characterized by hyperphagia, hypersexuality, and compulsive licking and biting. Klein-Levin syndrome, also rare, is more common in men and consists of hyperphagia and periodic hypersomnia.

Patients with the binge-purge subtype of anorexia nervosa fail to maintain their weight within a normal range. Patients with borderline personality disorder sometimes binge eat but do not have other criteria for bulimia nervosa.

TREATMENT

A comprehensive treatment plan including a combination of nutritional rehabilitation, psychotherapy, and medication is recommended (see Fig. 1).[6-10] The patient's weight and cardiac and metabolic status determines the acuteness of the illness and the need for hospitalization (Box 5). Treatment guidelines are well documented by the American Psychiatric Association in its practice guideline for treating eating disorders.[6]

Box 5 Indications for Hospitalization

Weight <75% of individually estimated healthy weight
Rapid, persistent decline in oral intake or weight despite maximally intensive outpatient interventions
Prior knowledge of weight at which physical instability is likely to occur in the particular patient
Serious physical abnormalities
Electrolyte or metabolic abnormalities
Hematemesis
Vital sign changes including orthostatic hypotension and heart rate <40 bpm or >110 bpm
Inability to sustain body core temperature
Comorbid psychiatric illness (suicidal, depressed, unable to care for self, etc.)

Aims of treatment are to restore the patient's nutritional status and establish healthy eating patterns, treat medical complications, correct core dysfunctional thoughts related to the eating disorder, enlist family support, and provide family counseling.

Nutritional Rehabilitation

Expected rates of controlled weight gain should be 2 to 3 pounds per week for inpatients and 0.5 to 1 pound per week for outpatients. Intake levels should start at 30 to 40 kcal/kg per day (1000-1600 kcal/day) in divided meals. If oral feeding is not possible, progressive nocturnal nasogastric feeding can lessen distress (physical and psychological) during early weight gain.

Daily morning weights, vital signs, fluid intake, and urine output should be measured. Frequent physical examinations should be performed to detect circulatory overload, refeeding edema, and bloating. Monitor serum electrolyte levels (low potassium or phosphorus), and get an electrocardiogram if needed.

Stool softeners, not laxatives, should be used to treat constipation. The diet should be supplemented with vitamins and minerals.

Patients should be given positive reinforcement (praise) and negative reinforcement (restrictions of exercise and purging). They should be closely supervised, and access to bathrooms should be restricted for at least 2 hours after meals. After weight restoration has progressed, stretching can begin, followed by gradual reintroduction of aerobic exercise.

Psychosocial Treatment

Psychosocial treatments are required during hospitalization as well as after discharge.[6-9] Commonly used models include dynamic expressive-supportive therapy and cognitive-behavioral techniques (planned meals and self-monitoring, exposure, and response prevention). Research data more strongly support the efficacy of cognitive-behavioral and interpersonal therapies. Although cognitive-behavioral therapy is important, its benefits increase with the addition of a nutritional component.

Group therapy, support groups, and 12-step programs like Overeaters Anonymous may be useful as adjunctive treatment and for relapse prevention. Family therapy and marital therapy are helpful in cases of dysfunctional family patterns and interpersonal distress.

Guided self-help manuals can reduce the number of binge-purge episodes in at least some patients with bulimia nervosa. In fact, a manual-driven self-help approach incorporating cognitive-behavioral principles combined with keeping contact with a general practice physician in one study did as well as specialist-based treatment in reducing bulimic episodes. Computer-based health education can improve knowledge and attitudes as a patient-friendly adjunct to therapy.[7]

One unique approach is a behavioral family-based therapy for elementary school-age children with behavioral problems, disordered eating, and obesity. Children and parents were examined and tested before and after the intervention and all lost weight. Although eating disorders did not resolve, other behavioral problems did. There was less parental dissatisfaction as children developed better awareness and behavior patterns.

Higher self-directedness at baseline is a good predictor of improvement at the end of a variety of interventions, as well as follow-up 6 to 12 months later. This might help explain why manual-driven self-help and psychoeducational programs that emphasize improvement of self-esteem and reassessment of body image have achieved some success.

Medication

Anorexia Nervosa

The evidence for significant efficacy is lacking, with very few methodologically sound studies.[2,3,6,10] Although medication is less successful in anorexia nervosa than in bulimia nervosa, it is most often used in anorexia nervosa after weight has been restored but may begin earlier when indicated. Medication helps maintain weight and normal eating behavior and can treat associated psychiatric symptoms.

Selective serotonin reuptake inhibitors (SSRIs) (e.g., fluoxetine) are commonly considered for patients with anorexia nervosa who have depressive, obsessive, or compulsive symptoms that persist in spite of or in the absence of weight gain. Tricyclic antidepressants are also effective in treating eating disorders. However, they should be used with caution, because they have greater risks of cardiac complications, including arrhythmias and hypotension.

Low doses of antipsychotics may be used for marked agitation and psychotic thinking, but they can frighten patients by increasing appetite dramatically, particularly if the patient is not psychotic. Antianxiety medications, such as benzodiazepines, may be used for extreme anticipatory anxiety concerning eating.

Estrogen replacement alone does not generally appear to reverse osteoporosis or osteopenia, and unless there is weight gain, it does not prevent further bone loss. There is very limited evidence of bisphosphonate's efficacy in treating associated osteoporosis.

Promotility agents such as metoclopramide are commonly used for bloating and abdominal pains due to gastroparesis and premature satiety, but they require monitoring for drug-related extrapyramidal side effects.

Recombinant human growth hormone has helped stabilize patients medically in shorter hospital stays.

Bulimia Nervosa

Antidepressants are used primarily to reduce the frequency of disturbed eating and treat comorbid depression, anxiety, obsessions, and certain impulse-disorder symptoms. Medication can reduce binge episodes, but is not sufficient to be the sole treatment. The only medication approved by the U.S. Food and Drug Administration for bulimia nervosa is the SSRI fluoxetine (Prozac). Several studies have demonstrated efficacy of other SSRIs including sertraline (Zoloft), paroxetine (Paxil), and citalopram (Celexa); tricyclic antidepressants including imipramine (Tofranil), nortryptyline (Pamelor), and desipramine (Norpramin); and monoamine oxidase inhibitors (MAOIs) including tranylcypromine (Parnate). Doses of tricyclic antidepressants and MAOIs parallel those used to treat depression, but higher doses of fluoxetine (≤80 mg/day) may be needed to treat bulimia nervosa. Bupropion (Wellbutrin) has been associated with seizures in purging bulimic patients and its use is not recommended.

Other psychotropic drugs are sometimes used. Lithium continues to be used occasionally as an adjunct for comorbid disorders. Various anticonvulsants have successfully reduced binge eating for some patients, but they can also increase appetite. Topiramate lowers appetite but has been associated with cognitive side effects. Sibutramine has also been used to reduce appetite in bulimia nervosa and binge-eating disorder.

SCREENING AND PREVENTION

Prevention programs presented in schools to both genders or through organizations like the Girl Scouts have been successful in reducing risk factors for eating disorders. Often focusing on media literacy and interactive discussion, there are increasing reports of short-term and longer-term benefits in body satisfaction and acceptance of normal growth.[9]

Summary

- The lifetime prevalence of anorexia and bulimia combined may be as high as 5% or more of the general population.
- Bulimia nervosa is more common than anorexia nervosa and has a better prognosis.
- The rate of mood, anxiety, and substance use disorders is higher in the families of bulimic than anorectic patients.
- Hospitalization is indicated when body weight drops below 75% of ideal body weight, in the presence of significant fluid and electrolyte imbalance, and when heart rate falls below 40 bpm or rises above 110 bpm when the patient stands.
- Antidepressant medication is more effective for bulimia nervosa than for anorexia nervosa.
- Anorexia nervosa and bulimia nervosa respond well to a combination of individual, family, and group psychotherapy interventions that focus on the recovery of normal eating behavior.

Suggested Readings

American Psychiatric Association: Diagnostic and Statistical Manual of Mental Disorders, 4th ed, text rev. Washington, DC: American Psychiatric Association, 2000.

American Psychiatric Association: Eating disorders measures. In American Psychiatric Association: Handbook of Psychiatric Measures. Washington, DC: American Psychiatric Association, 2000, pp 647-673.

American Psychiatric Association Work Group on Eating Disorders: Practice guideline for the treatment of patients with eating disorders. Am J Psychiatry 2000;157(1Suppl):1-39.

Bailer V, de Zwaan M, Leisch F, et al: Guided self-help versus cognitive-behavioral group therapy in the treatment of bulimia nervosa. Int J Eating Disorders 2004;35:522-537.

Claudino AM, Hay P, Lima MS, et al: Antidepressants for anorexia nervosa. Cochrane Database Syst Rev 2006;(1):CD004365.

Devlin M, Jahraus J, Dobrow I: Eating disorders. In J Levenson (ed): Textbook of Psychosomatic Medicine. Washington, DC: American Psychiatric Association, 2005, pp 311-334.

Durand M, King M: Specialist treatment versus self-help for bulimia nervosa: A randomized, controlled trial in general practice. Br J Gen Prac 2003;53:371-377.

Fairburn C, Harrison PJ, Brownell K: Eating disorders. Lancet 2003;361:407-416.

Volkow ND, Wise RA: How can drug addiction help us understand obesity? Nature Neurosci 2005;8:555-560.

Wade TD, Davidson S, O'Dea JA: A preliminary controlled evaluation of a school-based media literacy program and self-esteem program for reducing eating disorder risk factors. Int J Eating Disorders 2003;33:371-383.

References

For a complete list of references, log onto www.expertconsult.com.

Smoking Cessation

Kathleen Ashton and *David Streem*

Tobacco use is the leading preventable cause of morbidity and mortality in the United States. Approximately 440,000 deaths each year are attributed to smoking. It is the most common cause of cancer-related deaths in this country, including deaths from lung cancer, laryngeal cancer, esophageal cancer, oral cancer, and bladder cancer. Tobacco use is also a leading cause of *heart disease*, *stroke*, and *chronic obstructive pulmonary disease*. Research suggests that tobacco use results in more than $157 billion in annual health-related costs.

DEFINITION

Nicotine dependence is characterized by both tolerance and withdrawal symptoms in relation to nicotine use. Nicotine dependence can occur with cigarette smoking, smokeless tobacco use, or cigar or pipe smoking. For the purposes of this chapter, the phrases "quitting smoking" will be used to represent complete abstinence from tobacco products, and "success" will be used to represent lifetime abstinence.

PREVALENCE AND RISK FACTORS

Fifty-five percent of Americans have tried smoking. Approximately 22.8% of Americans are current smokers and 30% are ex-smokers. The rates of smoking in the general U.S. population decreased from nearly 42% in 1965 to just over 25% in 1990, but the rate of decline has slowed markedly since 1990. Approximately 20% of all Americans meet criteria for nicotine dependence at some point in their lives. Among smokers, 50% to 80% are estimated to meet criteria for nicotine dependence.

Nicotine dependence is more prevalent in persons with mental disorders, especially mood disorders and schizophrenia. According to DSM-IV-TR, 55% to 90% of those with a mental disorder smoke compared with 22% of the general population.

In 2001, 25.2% of U.S. males and 20.7% of females were smokers. There appear to be genetic factors that contribute to nicotine dependence; the risk for those with a first-degree relative who smokes is three times that of those in a family of nonsmokers. In children, depressed mood, poor grades, and antisocial behavior correlate with smoking rates, but the effects of modeling by peers and family are also likely to be critical factors.

PATHOPHYSIOLOGY

From the first use of nicotine, physical effects increase the likelihood of repeated nicotine consumption. Nicotine binds to cholinergic receptors in the central nervous system. In response to repeated nicotine use, the receptors rapidly desensitize and increase in number, and both these phenomena conspire to increase the addictive power of nicotine. Dopaminergic neurons within the nucleus accumbens (a brain structure associated with rewards and reinforcement) are activated by projections from nicotine-stimulated neurons. Cell bodies in the ventral tegmental area (a structure associated with perception and modulation of pleasure) are stimulated directly by nicotine, and these neurons project directly to the nucleus accumbens (NAcc). As a result of the widespread neuronal activation, nicotine users experience pleasure, reduced fatigue, increased information-processing ability, reduced anxiety, and other reinforcing effects.

Tolerance develops as the frequency and dose of nicotine use increase. Increasingly desensitized cholinergic receptors on neurons projecting to the NAcc are quickly produced (upregulated) to compensate for the actions of nicotine on the brain. The release of dopamine in the NAcc falls as these desensitized neurons fail to produce the necessary baseline stimulation without the presence of sufficient concentrations of nicotine. Withdrawal symptoms occur when the concentration of nicotine fails to maintain stimulation of the ventral tegmental area and the NAcc. These effects are mediated by increases in noradrenergic outflow from the locus coeruleus and other areas.

Smoking increases the metabolism of several medications, including cyclobenzaprine, naproxen, verapamil, propranolol, and warfarin. Conversely, the blood levels of these medications can increase when smoking cessation is attempted.

SIGNS, SYMPTOMS, AND DIAGNOSIS

The first step in treating nicotine dependence is identifying tobacco users. Practice guidelines for nicotine dependence include those from the U.S. Department of Health and Human Services and the American Psychiatric Association. These guidelines suggest asking patients systematically at each visit whether they use tobacco. This question should be part of an expanded vital signs assessment or in a computer reminder system that is part of the electronic medical record. There is strong evidence that documenting smoking status at every visit increases clinician recognition of nicotine dependence and intervention. The criteria for diagnosis of nicotine dependence follow those for other forms of substance dependence.

The following are DSM-IV-TR criteria for diagnosis of nicotine dependence. The user must demonstrate at least three of the following criteria occurring at the same time during a 12-month period:

- Tolerance; signs of tolerance are a need for a markedly increased amount of nicotine to produce the desired effect or a diminished effect with continued use of the same amount of nicotine.
- Withdrawal, as manifested by either the characteristic nicotine withdrawal syndrome, or nicotine (or a closely related substance) is taken to relieve or avoid withdrawal symptoms.
- Nicotine is used in larger amounts or over a longer period than intended.
- The user has a persistent desire or makes unsuccessful attempts to cut down on tobacco.
- A great deal of time is spent in obtaining or using the substance (e.g., chain smoking).
- Important social, occupational, or recreational activities are reduced because of tobacco use.
- Use of the substance continues despite recurrent physical or psychological problems caused or exacerbated by tobacco: for example, continuing to smoke despite diagnoses such as hypertension, heart disease, cancer, bronchitis, and chronic obstructive lung disease.

Nicotine withdrawal is defined by the DSM-IV-TR as a condition in which a person, after using nicotine daily for at least several weeks, exhibits at least four of the following symptoms within 24 hours after reduction or cessation of nicotine use:

- Dysphoric or depressed mood
- Insomnia
- Irritability, frustration, or anger
- Anxiety
- Difficulty concentrating
- Restlessness
- Decreased heart rate

Once a diagnosis of nicotine dependence is made, it is useful to characterize the degree to which the patient is physically dependent on smoking. The Fagerström Test for Nicotine Dependence (FTND) (Table 1), can be helpful in determining whether nicotine replacement will be necessary and to what degree. The six-question FTND deals with total tobacco intake and craving severity.

Table 1 Fagerstrom Test for Nicotine Dependence

Question	0 Points	1 Point	2 Points	3 Points
How soon after you wake up do you smoke your first cigarette?	>60 min	31-60 min	6-30 min	<5 min
Do you find it difficult to refrain from smoking in places where it is forbidden, eg, church, library, cinema?	No	Yes		
Which cigarette would you hate most to give up?	Any other	First one in the morning		
How many cigarettes per day do you smoke?	<10	11-20	21-30	>30
Do you smoke more frequently during the first hours of waking than during the rest of the day?	No	Yes		
Do you still smoke if you are so ill that you are in bed most of the day?	No	Yes		
Classification of Dependence				
0-2	Very low			
3-4	Low			
5	Moderate			
6-7	High			
8-10	Very high			

Adapted with permission from Heatherton TF, Kozlowski LT, Frecker RC, et al: The Fagerström Test for Nicotine Dependence: A revision of the Fagerström Tolerance Questionnaire. Br J Addict 1991;86:1119-1127.

TREATMENT

Primary care providers are likely to be most effective in using brief interventions and providing advice and/or prescriptions for pharmacologic interventions. They may also be an important link in providing patients with referrals to more intensive counseling programs and additional education.

Brief Interventions for a Primary Care Setting

Minimal or brief interventions require little cost or time from the provider. There is strong evidence that patients who are consistently advised by health care providers to quit smoking are more likely to take steps to stop. Decision trees (Fig. 1) can be helpful in guiding clinicians through smoking-cessation counseling with patients.

Interventions as short as 3 minutes can substantially increase cessation rates. One common brief intervention designed for health care providers is the five-A method, which involves the following:

- Asking about tobacco status at each visit
- Advising all tobacco users to quit
- Assessing the patient's willingness to quit
- Assisting the patient in quitting
- Arranging for follow-up contact

Providers can assess a patient's readiness to quit using the transtheoretical model of behavior change. If the patient has not thought about quitting or is considering quitting but not in the next few months, they are in the precontemplation or contemplation stage. At this stage, the provider can use motivational interviewing skills to help increase readiness for cessation.

Health care providers can use the five Rs to help enhance a patient's motivation to quit:

- Discuss why quitting is personally *r*elevant.
- Identify potential *r*isks associated with smoking.
- Identify potential *r*ewards and benefits related to quitting.
- Identify potential barriers or *r*oadblocks that might impede the quitting process.
- *R*epeat motivational interventions at each visit.

In general, patients at this stage are unlikely to benefit from advice-giving as much as a nonthreatening discussion of what is keeping them from quitting at this time.

Patients who have made plans to quit or who are in the process of quitting are in the preparation or action stage. These are the patients who will most benefit from brief interventions such as:

- Helping the patient identify a "quit date"
- Asking the patient to elicit support from friends and family
- Having the patient write down the reasons for quitting or coping strategies
- Having patients remove tobacco products from their environment
- Discussing coping strategies such as replacements (sugar-free gum, water) and distraction (keeping busy, exercising)
- Referring the patient to an intensive smoking cessation counseling program
- Providing the patient with advice about nicotine replacement and/or discussing use of bupropion or varenicline as a cessation aid

Preventing relapse is important for patients in the maintenance stage (those who have quit smoking). Providers at this stage can educate patients in issues important in preventing relapse, such as being aware of the potential impact of stressful events. In patients who have never smoked, providing reinforcement and encouraging continued abstinence can be effective strategies for prevention. In patients who have relapsed, it is important to deflect guilt and self-doubt with reminders about the frequency of relapse and the need for a renewed commitment to abstinence. Consistently working with patients on smoking cessation increases the chances of success.

Primary care providers may also choose to refer their patients to *intensive counseling* programs for smoking cessation. Intensive interventions are recommended by national guidelines as first-line treatments and refer to specifically tailored educational programs involving repeated face-to-face contact in an individual or group setting and including a psychotherapy component. More-intensive programs appear to generate better outcomes. Intensive programs help patients cope with nicotine withdrawal through a number of behavioral strategies including using social supports, relaxation training, and cognitive restructuring.

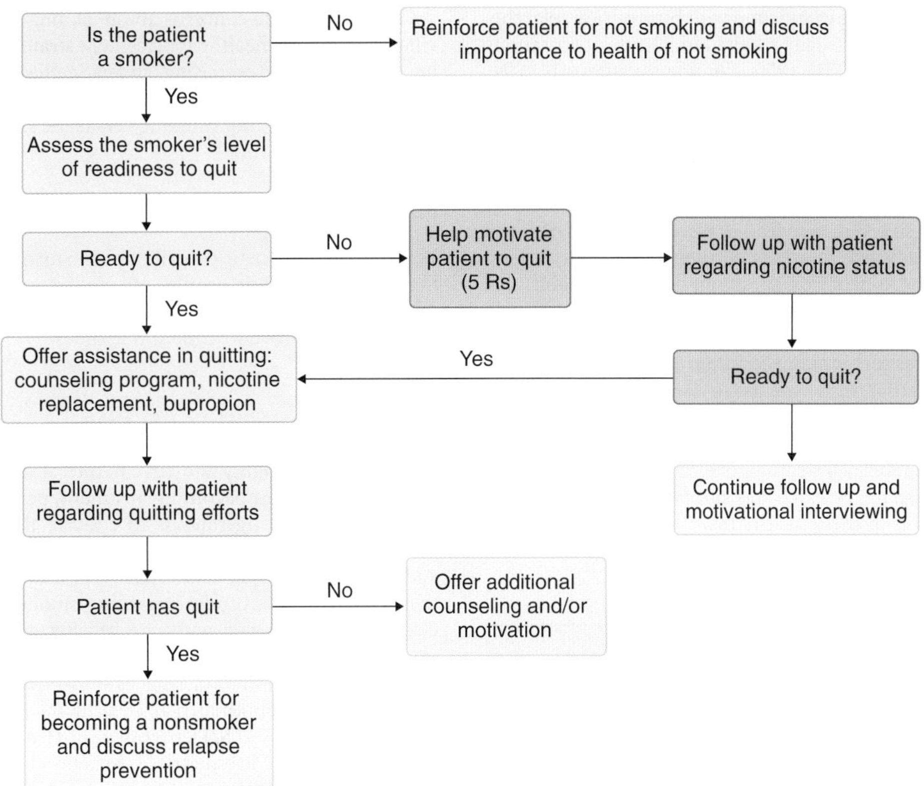

Figure 1 **Algorithm for counseling patients with nicotine dependence.**

Pharmacologic Options

National guidelines recommend that pharmacologic therapy be considered for all smokers attempting to quit unless the drug is medically contraindicated. Research suggests that pharmacologic interventions are most effective in the context of a behavioral counseling program.

Nicotine Replacement Therapies

Nicotine replacement therapies (NRTs) work by delivering nicotine into the body to ease withdrawal while allowing the smoker to break the behavioral habits associated with the cigarette itself. The fact that 50% of all quitters report withdrawal symptoms makes clear the value in reducing or eliminating the likelihood that these symptoms will impair a quitter's ability to remain abstinent. Behavioral counseling (either brief or intensive) is an important adjunct to any pharmacologic intervention for smoking cessation.

Nicotine gum is available in 2-mg and 4-mg pieces and is sold without a prescription. Patients must be instructed to soften the gum and park it between the cheek and gum rather than chew it. Chewing the gum continuously or drinking acidic beverages reduces nicotine absorption. Advantages include rapid absorption of nicotine, with resultant reduction in withdrawal symptoms.

Nicotine patches have the advantage of a delivery system that maintains nicotine levels throughout a longer period than any other system. Patches are designed to deliver nicotine transdermally over a 16- or 24-hour period. The most common side effects are rash and insomnia. Switching from 24-hour to 16-hour release systems can often solve sleep problems associated with longer-release patches. Patients usually use patches at a steady dose daily for 6 to 12 weeks, then taper slowly over an additional 6 to 12 weeks. Nicotine nasal sprays, inhalers, and lozenges are also available.

Non-Nicotine Medications

Bupropion hydrochloride (Zyban) also has demonstrated efficacy in smoking cessation. Bupropion is an atypical antidepressant with noradrenergic and dopaminergic effects. Numerous studies have shown that bupropion therapy, given in the context of a comprehensive smoking cessation program, doubled the number of subjects reporting no nicotine use in the week before the follow-up contact. The recommended and maximum dose of bupropion is 300 mg a day, given as 150 mg twice daily. Dosing should begin at 150 mg a day—given every day for the first 3 days—followed by a dose increase for most patients to the recommended usual dose of 300 mg a day.

Therapy is typically begun 1 to 2 weeks before the patient's predetermined smoking quit date. Treatment should continue for 12 weeks. Bupropion is contraindicated in those with a seizure disorder, those with anorexia or bulimia, or those who have used a monoamine oxidase inhibitor (e.g., selegiline [Eldepryl], tranylcypromine [Parnate], or phenelzine [Nardil]) within the previous 14 days. Health care providers interested in prescribing bupropion should thoroughly review the manufacturer's product information before deciding to initiate therapy.

Varenicline was approved by the FDA in 2006 for the treatment of nicotine dependence and is recommended by the treatment guidelines as first-line treatment. This medication appears to represent a partial agonist that binds with high affinity to the neuronal nicotinic acetylcholine receptor. Nicotine stimulation of this particular receptor, with which varenicline binds with high specificity, is associated with significant mesolimbic dopamine release, which serves to reinforce nicotine ingestion. The high affinity with which varenicline binds to this receptor prevents nicotine itself from stimulating the receptor, thereby reducing the reinforcing properties of nicotine ingestion.

In three studies comparing varenicline with buproprion, placebo, or both, varenicline 1 mg twice daily resulted in 52-week continuous abstinence rates of 21% to 23% (95% confidence intervals [CIs] ranging from 17% to 28%), whereas buproprion and placebo produced rates of 14% to 16% (95% CI, 11%-20%) and 4% to 10% (95% CI, 1%-13%), respectively.[1-3] The most commonly reported side effects have been nausea, insomnia, and headache. Disturbing or bizarre dreams have been reported at higher rates than placebo, but these have rarely been so severe as to lead to discontinuation of treatment. The FDA has advised clinicians to monitor patients taking varenicline for changes in behavior, agitation, depressed mood, suicidal thoughts or behavior, and worsening of preexisting psychiatric illnesses.

Alternative therapies for smoking cessation include a wide range of strategies from herbal supplements to laser treatments. Two popular alternative therapies include hypnosis and acupuncture. Currently, both acupuncture and hypnosis should be considered as supplements to well-established treatments rather than first-line recommendations because the research has not been conclusive concerning the effectiveness of these treatments.

Summary

- Ask every patient about tobacco use.
- Engage patients in brief counseling.
- Discuss pharmacologic options including nicotine replacement, varenicline, and bupropion therapy.
- Consider referral to intensive smoking cessation treatments.

TREATMENT OUTCOMES

Abstinence Rates

Fully 70% of smokers report wanting to quit, and 46% attempt to quit each year. Only 5% to 7% of them are abstinent from smoking for an entire year after quitting. Several factors appear to affect rates of abstinence in different groups. Women have less success with quitting smoking and higher rates of relapse. Patients with higher levels of nicotine dependence (as evidenced by higher FTND scores) and those with a history of depression also have lower abstinence rates. African Americans and Chinese Americans have lower smoking cessation numbers than European Americans. The primary care provider should consider referring patients in these groups to a more-intensive smoking cessation program and adding nicotine replacement or bupropion (or both) to increase the likelihood of successful abstinence.

Meta-analysis of multiple research studies suggests that intensive counseling programs significantly increase cessation rates. Research suggests that more is better, with more frequent counseling leading to better cessation rates. Bupropion and nicotine gum have been shown to double the rate of abstinence.

Weight Gain

Weight gain is a common problem that can negatively affect rates of successful smoking cessation. Weight gain in patients following smoking cessation can be attributable to replacing the oral nicotine habit with another oral habit: consuming food. Patients undergoing cessation are also likely to be able to taste and smell food better following smoking cessation, which may contribute to overeating. Other mechanisms contributing to weight gain after smoking cessation include increased caloric intake, decreased resting metabolic rate, and decreased physical activity. Estimated average weight gain as a result of smoking cessation is approximately 4 pounds for both men and women.

To help alleviate concerns about gaining weight, health care providers can discuss healthy replacement strategies for nicotine including drinking water, exercising, and eating healthful foods such as raw fruits and vegetables. Many patients also benefit from a discussion of the benefits of quitting smoking versus the risks of the small amount of actual weight gain.

Future Directions

Research on the genetic contributions to nicotine dependence suggest that someday, genetic profiles of smokers may be used by providers to choose the type, duration, and dose of treatments for individual smokers to improve treatment outcomes.

PREVENTION AND SCREENING

Considering the highly addictive nature of nicotine and the difficulties smokers face in becoming abstinent, perhaps the best approach to reducing smoking rates is to educate the public regarding the dangers of smoking and to prevent exposure to nicotine before an addictive pattern establishes itself. Clinicians can have an effect on the formation of attitudes regarding smoking in young people by clearly explaining the negative health effects and costs of exposure to cigarettes. Health care providers should also consider supporting tobacco control legislation, such as smoke-free laws. Reviewing available practice guidelines such as *Treating Tobacco Use and Dependence: 2008 Update* by the U.S. Department of Health and Human Services and the American Psychiatric Association's 2006 *Practice Guideline for the Treatment of Patients with Nicotine Dependence* can help clinicians stay up to date on the current state of understanding of this significant public health problem.

Suggested Readings

American Psychiatric Association: Diagnostic and Statistical Manual of Mental Disorders, 4th ed., text rev. Washington DC: American Psychiatric Association, 2000.

American Psychiatric Association: Practice Guideline for the Treatment of Patients with Nicotine Dependence. American Psychiatric Association, 2006. Available at http://www.psychiatryonline.com/content.aspx?aID=141810 (accessed March 20, 2009).

Baillie AJ, Mattick RP, Hall W, et al: Meta-analytic review of the efficacy of smoking cessation interventions. Drug Alcohol Rev 1994;13:157-170.

Carpenter MJ, Hughes JR, Solomon LJ, et al: Both smoking reduction with nicotine replacement therapy and motivational advice increase future cessation among smokers unmotivated to quit. J Consult Clin Psychol 2004;72:371-381.

Cofta-Woerpel L, Wright KL, Wetter DW: Smoking cessation 3: Multicomponent Interventions. Behav Med 2007;32:135-149.

Fiore MC, Novotny TE, Pierce JP, et al: Methods used to quit smoking in the United States: Do smoking cessation programs help? JAMA 1990;263:2760-2765.

Heatherton TF, Kozlowski LT, Frecker RC, et al: The Fagerström test for nicotine dependence: A revision of the Fagerström tolerance questionnaire. Br J Addict 1991;86:1119-1127.

Hughes JR: Nicotine-related disorders. In Sadock B, Sadock A (eds): Kaplan and Sadock's Comprehensive Textbook of Psychiatry, 8th ed. Philadelphia: Lippincott Williams & Wilkins, 2005, pp 1257-1264.

Jain A: Treating nicotine addiction. BMJ 2003;327:1394-1395.

Lerman CE, Schnoll RA, Munafo MR: Genetics and smoking cessation: Improving outcomes in smokers at risk. Am J Prev Med 2007;33(6 Suppl):S398-S405.

Office of the Surgeon General: Clinical guidelines: Treating Tobacco Use and Dependence: 2008 Update, U.S. Department of Health and Human Services, 2008: available at: www.surgeongeneral.gov/tobacco/default.htm (accessed March 20, 2009).

Office of the Surgeon General: The health benefits of smoking cessation: A report of the Surgeon General. DHHS pub. (CDC) 90–8416. Washington, DC: U.S. Government Printing Office, 1990.

Stapleton JA, Watson L, Spirling LI et al: Varenicline in the routine treatment of tobacco dependence: A pre-post comparison with nicotine replacement therapy and an evaluation in those with mental illness. Addiction 2007;103:146-154.

West R, Baker CL, Cappelleri JC, Bushmakin AG: Effect of varenicline and buproprion SR on craving, nicotine withdrawal symptoms, and rewarding effects of smoking during a quit attempt. Psychopharmacology 2008;197:371-377.

References

For a complete list of references, log onto www.expertconsult.com.

Psychiatric Emergencies

George E. Tesar

DEFINITION AND ETIOLOGY

Behavioral emergencies include any patient-initiated threat of harm to self, health care personnel, or others in the patient's sphere of influence. Among the difficulties a primary care physician faces in dealing with behavioral emergencies is their infrequency and unpredictability. Periodic review of the principles of recognizing and managing these problems is therefore recommended.

Suicide, homicide, and other forms of violence are considered together and, unless otherwise specified, are referred to collectively as *aggression*. In fact, each is a form of potentially destructive aggression with only the targeted object differing. Each shares with the others their cause, risk, clinical presentation, and management. The primary goal in office-based primary care is rapid recognition of potential or actual aggression, reduction of potential for danger, timely triage, and effective disposition of the potentially dangerous patient.

Effective management of potential or actual danger depends on accurate risk assessment. All forms and appearances of threat must be taken seriously and not ignored; not all, however, require emergent action. Underreaction to threat can have devastating consequences, and overreaction can lead to frustration and dissatisfaction on the parts of the patient, family, physician, and those whose emergent assistance is being demanded.

All forms of aggression exist along a continuum from thought to action. It helps to remind patients—and perhaps oneself—that thoughts, feelings, and images (all collectively referred to as *ideation*) are *not* actions or behavior. Many persons are frightened by their own impulses and fantasies. Although ideation increases the risk of action, it does not necessarily constitute imminent risk of action. The level of risk increases as *ideation* develops into *intent*, especially when a *plan* has been devised that employs potentially lethal *means* to which the patient has *access*.

PREVALENCE AND RISK FACTORS

Homicide in the workplace is an unusual event.[1,2] A study of U.S. workplace violence from 1993 through 1999 identified an average annual homicide rate of 1 per 100,000 workers.[2] Shooting was the most common method used, and the offender was more often a stranger than known to the victim. These findings are especially relevant to the medical field, whose personnel, particularly nurses, are exposed to comparatively high rates of assault. The same study showed an overall average annual rate of 904 simple assaults per 100,000 U.S. workers, with 1140 per 100,000 workers occurring in medical settings. Drugs or alcohol were known to be involved in 35%, and the offender was unknown to the victim in nearly 60% of assaults.

Factors that increase risk of aggression (Box 1) also result in higher group-related rates of aggression. For example, the annual incidence of suicide in the United States is 10.7 suicides for every 100,000 persons, and the estimated lifetime rate is 0.72%. In persons with a mood disorder, the lifetime rate is 14.6% to 15.5%, and in those with previous suicide attempts it is 27.5%.[1] The estimated lifetime rate of suicide in schizophrenia is 6%.

Women make many more unsuccessful suicide attempts than men, and men complete suicide more often and do so by more violent means (e.g., shooting, jumping, hanging). The suicide death rate among men peaks in the 40- to 44-year-old age group. The rate of completed suicide in men begins to increase starting at age 65 years and peaks at age 85 years or older when the rate has been documented to be as high as 60 per 100,000.[1] Among those in the 14- to 25-year-old age group, suicide is the third leading cause of death, whereas it is the ninth leading cause of death in the general population.

Aggressive impulses, whether suicidal or homicidal, are often triggered by frustration, anger, fear, or hopelessness; the circumstances—real or perceived—that fostered those feelings; and any type of intoxicant that intensifies distressing feelings or perceptions and increases impulsivity.

PATHOPHYSIOLOGY AND NATURAL COURSE

The evidence base for the pathophysiology of aggression and violence is large. Postmortem cerebrospinal fluid levels of serotonin and its metabolites are significantly lower in victims of homicide or suicide than in those whose death was nonviolent. Provocation of aggressive ideation and imagery has been associated with positron-emission tomography (PET) scan evidence of metabolic hyperactivity in the amygdala and subgenual prefrontal cortex, areas also involved in the pathogenesis of major depressive disorder.

SIGNS AND SYMPTOMS

In Samuel Shem's classic, *The House of God*, the character known as Fat Man laid down "13 Laws of the House." Law Number Three was, "At a cardiac arrest, the first procedure is to take your own pulse."[3] Intended humorously, this maxim serves also as serious advice to the clinician faced with a potentially violent, impulsive, or suicidal patient. A clinician's sense of discomfort, apprehension, or irritability can be a clue to similar distress in the patient. These feelings, often vague and not immediately evident, can serve as both barometer and alerting device, drawing the examiner's attention to patient characteristics that point to a violent lifestyle or violence potential. Signs of traumatic injury (e.g., facial scars), jailhouse tattoos, fixed gaze, or a clenched jaw also point to violence potential. These and other signs of impending violence or suicidal behavior are listed in Box 2.

Accurate assessment of the patient's symptoms is often difficult, because most such patients have trouble verbalizing their feelings or are prone to withhold or distort relevant information. Symptoms associated with a high risk of suicide are often difficult to disclose (e.g., hopelessness, profound guilt, shame or humiliation, despair, anxiety, panic, intense anger, or intractable psychic or physical pain). In these situations, using oneself as a barometer, as described above, becomes an essential evaluative tool. A patient's threats can arouse fear, anger, and a defensive response, especially by a physician who is caught off guard. It is important that the physician monitor his or her subjective response to avoid reacting to the patient in a fashion that induces guilt or shame.

DIAGNOSIS

Careful diagnostic assessment during a behavioral emergency must await crisis stabilization and assurance of everyone's safety (see "Treatment"). In fact, diagnostic assessment often occurs simultaneously as the clinician quickly surveys observable diagnostic clues (e.g., general appearance, hygiene, and gross motor activity).

Aggression directed at oneself or others is often the manifesting feature of psychiatric illness that has not yet been identified or whose

Box 1 Risk Factors for Aggression

Current or Past Suicidal or Homicidal Thoughts and Behavior
Suicidal or homicidal *ideas*
Suicidal or homicidal *plans*
Suicidal or homicidal *attempts* (including aborted or interrupted attempts)
Lethality of suicidal or homicidal plans or attempts
Suicidal or homicidal *intent*

Psychiatric Diagnoses
See Box 3

Physical Illnesses
See Box 4

Psychosocial Issues
Recent lack or loss of social support
Unemployment
Drop in socioeconomic status
Poor relationship with family
Domestic partner violence
Any recent stressful life event

Childhood Traumas
Sexual abuse
Physical abuse

Genetic and Familial Factors
Family history of suicide or homicide
Family history of mental illness, including substance-use disorders

Psychological Symptoms
Hopelessness
Psychic pain
Severe or unremitting anxiety
Panic attacks
Shame or humiliation
Psychological turmoil
Decreased self-esteem
Extreme narcissistic vulnerability

Behavioral Features
Impulsiveness
Aggression, including violence against others
Agitation

Cognitive Features
Loss of executive function
Thought constriction (tunnel vision)
Polarized thinking (all-or-nothing)
Closed-mindedness

Demographic Features
Male gender
Widowed, divorced, or single marital status, particularly for men
Elderly age group
Adolescent and young adult age groups
White race
Homosexual or bisexual orientation

Additional Features
Access to firearms
Substance intoxication
Unstable or poor relationship with one's psychotherapist

Adapted from American Psychiatric Association: Assessment and treatment of patients with suicidal behaviors. American Psychiatric Association Practice Guidelines for the Treatment of Psychiatric Disorders. Washington DC: American Psychiatric Association, 2004.

Box 2 Signs of Impending Violence

Scars or wounds on the face, arms, or torso suggesting past violent altercations
Jailhouse tattoos (e.g., primitive figures, crosses, "LOVE" printed across the knuckles)
Abnormal pupil size (either increased or decreased), suggesting substance intoxication or withdrawal
Speech that is threatening, loud, or profane
Increased muscle tension, such as sitting on the edge of the chair or gripping the arms
Tremor
Hyperactivity, such as pacing
Slamming doors or knocking over furniture

Adapted from Duhart, DT: Violence in the Workplace,1993-99. Bureau of Justice Statistics. NCJ 190076, December 2001. Available at http://www.ojp.usdoj.gov/bjs/pub/pdf/vw99.pdf (accessed March 20, 2009).

Box 3 Psychiatric Disorders Associated with Increased Risk of Suicide or Other Forms of Violence

Major depressive disorder
Bipolar disorder (especially depressive or mixed states)
Schizophrenia
Anorexia nervosa
Alcohol use disorder (acute intoxication or withdrawal)
Other substance use disorders (cocaine, amphetamines, phencyclidine)
Substance withdrawal (opiates, cocaine, amphetamines)
Personality disorders (especially borderline and antisocial)
Comorbidity of Axis I and/or Axis II disorders

Adapted from American Psychiatric Association: Assessment and treatment of patients with suicidal behaviors. American Psychiatric Association Practice Guidelines for the Treatment of Psychiatric Disorders. Washington DC: American Psychiatric Association, 2004.

Box 4 General Medical Conditions Associated with Increased Risk of Suicide or Other Forms of Violence

Diseases of the central nervous system
- Multiple sclerosis
- Huntington's disease
- Brain and spinal cord injuries
- Seizure disorders

Malignant neoplasms
HIV/AIDS
Peptic ulcer disease
COPD, especially in men
Chronic hemodialysis-treated renal failure
Systemic lupus erythematosus
Pain syndromes
Disability or functional impairment

AIDS, autoimmune deficiency syndrome; COPD, chronic obstructive pulmonary disease; HIV, human immunodeficiency virus.
Adapted from American Psychiatric Association: Assessment and treatment of patients with suicidal behaviors. American Psychiatric Association Practice Guidelines for the Treatment of Psychiatric Disorders. Washington DC: American Psychiatric Association, 2004.

treatment has failed (Box 3). Acute psychosis in the context of schizophrenia, a mood disorder, or substance abuse can develop explosively and unpredictably. Acute medical illness (e.g., diabetes, cancer, HIV) can also manifest with violent or aggressive behavior or with hopelessness and suicidal ideation (Box 4). Substance abuse and substance-related conditions (e.g., acute intoxication or withdrawal) must always be considered when a patient presents with signs or symptoms of aggression. Although each of these disorders is associated with a statistically higher risk of suicide or other dangerous aggression, none by itself is highly predictive of dangerous conduct.

Box 5 Factors that Reduce Risk of Aggression

Children in the home
Sense of responsibility to family
Pregnancy (except among those with postpartum psychosis or mood disorder)
Religiosity
Life satisfaction
Reality testing ability
Positive coping skills
Positive problem-solving skills
Positive social support
Positive relationship with one's psychotherapist

Adapted from American Psychiatric Association: Assessment and treatment of patients with suicidal behaviors. American Psychiatric Association Practice Guidelines for the Treatment of Psychiatric Disorders. Washington DC: American Psychiatric Association, 2004.

DIFFERENTIAL DIAGNOSIS

Perhaps the most important consideration in the differential diagnosis is distinguishing nonpsychotic disorders from those in which the patient's actions are influenced by psychosis, delirium, or dementia. When the patient's capacity to make reasonable and sound judgments is grossly impaired, the risk of harm to oneself or others increases, and responsibility for ensuring safety shifts exclusively to the health care professional in charge. The emergency imperative—as determined by a patient's diminished capacity to learn new information and make sound judgments—gives the clinician the right to make necessary decisions, to access information without the patient's approval, and to violate patient confidentiality if necessary.

TREATMENT

Effective management of the potentially dangerous patient depends on accurate assessment of intensity and cause of dangerous conduct. Triage and disposition are more easily effected by accurate assessment and by advance knowledge of one's institutional policies and resources. Even under the best of circumstances, dangerous patients and the clinicians who care for them often face obstacles to efficient patient disposition.

Patient Assessment

Accurate assessment of potential dangerous action depends on the clinician's ability to gather data on the current manifestation of risk-related behavior, psychiatric illness, history of aggression, psychosocial stressors, and individual strengths or vulnerabilities.[1] It is also useful to ask about factors associated with protective effects against suicide and other forms of violence (Box 5).

Rapport building is crucial. Focus on the patient's needs, wishes, and well-being by conveying a desire to help while always keeping the patient's best interests in mind. "What do you need (want)? Don't worry; we're here to do what's in your best interest." Confronting the patient or asserting one's authority is not recommended. Rather, speaking in a measured tone of voice, adopting a calm posture with hands visible (especially with paranoid, visibly angry, or threatening patients), and attending to the patient's level of comfort (e.g., offering water) maximize the likelihood that the patient will choose to speak openly and honestly.

The clinician who suspects suicidal (or homicidal) ideation should begin with questions that address the patient's feelings about living: "Have you ever felt that life was not worth living?" or "Did you ever wish you could go to sleep and just not wake up?" If the patient endorses these thoughts, important follow-up questions include, "Is death something that you have thought about recently?" or "Have things ever reached the point that you've thought of harming yourself?" If the patient has had thoughts of suicide (or homicide), "When did you first notice such thoughts?" "How close have you come to acting on those thoughts?" "How likely do you think it is that you will act on them in the future?" "Have you made a specific plan to harm or kill yourself (or someone else), and if so, what does that plan involve?" "Are you able to carry out your plan?" "Are guns or other weapons available to you?"

Other important areas of investigation and attention include signs and symptoms of psychiatric disorders, with particular attention to mood disorders, schizophrenia, substance-use disorders, anxiety disorders, and personality disorders (particularly, borderline and antisocial personality disorders). Past episodes of illness and both current and past treatments should be addressed, as well as family history of psychiatric disorders, suicide, homicide, and other forms of violence.

Acute Intervention

If rapport building fails and the patient cannot be engaged in honest self-disclosure, the clinician should endeavor to involve significant others, friends, associates, or family with the dual goals of collecting relevant collateral information and sharing responsibility for protection and safety. The patient who exhibits signs and symptoms of psychosis (e.g., paranoia or auditory hallucinations that are encouraging destructive actions) requires immediate medical evaluation and, if medically cleared, might require involuntary psychiatric hospitalization.

When the clinician concludes that the safety of others is endangered, safety measures must be taken. This might involve stepping out of the office to call security personnel or having a secretary or associate make the call. Ultimately, responsibility rests with the clinician to notify a seriously threatened party.[4] Before notifying a threatened person, however, the clinician should weigh the risk of harm to the threatened party against the risk of unnecessarily arousing worry and distress in that person.

Access to Means

The clinician is faced with a challenging situation when the patient presents with a weapon (e.g., handgun or knife). Rather than asking the patient to hand over the weapon, take advantage of the opportunity to establish rapport by asking why the patient feels it necessary to carry a weapon. The question allows the clinician to show concern and a desire to understand, and the patient's answer provides clues to the nature and risk of the threat. If it is appropriate, then ask the patient to relinquish the weapon. If the request meets resistance, it is best to demur. Above all, never take a weapon directly from the patient.

Whenever a patient threatens harm to him- or herself or someone else, it is essential to inquire about the imagined method of aggression and about access to weapons or other means to enact the threat. In addition to firearms, other means used to commit suicide or homicide include medications, poisons, exhaust from a car or truck, gas from a stove or heater, a pipe or girder around which to hang a noose, or a balcony from which to jump. It is helpful to determine not just whether the patient has access but exactly *how* and *where* the patient imagines using the weapon or other means to accomplish the act. "What kind of gun do you have? Where is the weapon? Have you ever used it? Do you have ammunition? Where would you point the gun?" "What kind of rope would you use; around what would you secure it; and do you have one strong enough to hold you?" "From where would you jump?" Probing in this fashion allows one to determine the probability that the patient would actually follow through with the threat. Family or others close to the patient should be informed and encouraged to confiscate any and all means.

Potential for Rescue

Another important variable to consider when assessing risk is *where* the patient intends to perpetrate the threatened behavior. The more isolated the location and distant from other people, the greater the likelihood that the patient will succeed.

Triage and Disposition

Often the most difficult component of effective patient management is the process of referral, especially when urgent or emergent evaluation by a behavioral specialist is deemed necessary. If clinical evaluation reveals no cause for significant concern, then the clinician may elect to begin treatment for the disorder that best accounts for suicidal or homicidal ideation. Otherwise, referral to a behavioral health practitioner or the nearest emergency facility is recommended. It pays to have set up efficient lines of referral in advance. This is often difficult given the access problems faced by many psychiatric services. The resource of last resort is the closest emergency facility.

SCREENING AND PREVENTION

Every effort should be made to organize office space so that the clinician can access the door at least as easily as the patient can. Also, offices should be outfitted with alarm systems placed strategically (e.g., under a desk, on a portable device carried by the practitioner) to alert security personnel in the event of an emergency.

Hospital organizations have tried in some instances to flag the charts of patients who have previously exhibited suicidal or violent behavior in the hospital. This has been associated with a reduction in episodes of violence or self-destructive behavior.

On the whole, it is difficult to screen for or predict low-frequency, impulsive behavior. Although implementing measures that reduce access to weapons and other instruments of violence is important, even the most sophisticated efforts are imperfect. Metal-detecting devices fail to identify nonmetal objects that can be used to harm oneself or others (e.g., plastic or wooden utensils), and they have little usefulness in outpatient office practice.

In addition to the measures identified, the most important prevention technique is clinician training, avoidance of high-risk situations, and a high index of suspicion for concealed threat. Clinicians are warned never to see potentially violent or disruptive patients in isolated circumstances where help is not available.

SPECIAL POPULATIONS

Geriatric Patients

Suicide rates are higher in older adults than in persons in any other age group. This burden is carried exclusively by men.

Substance Abusers

Many acts of suicide or homicide occur in the context of intoxication from alcohol or other substances. Patients who make a suicide attempt while intoxicated often retract all thoughts of suicide once they are sober.

Patients with Intractable Pain

Chronic, persistent pain from any cause increases the risk of suicide in part because of the unremitting distress. However, risk is also increased when a frustrated, beleaguered clinician either dismisses the patient or projects disappointment onto the patient.

Certain Ethnic Groups

In contrast to elderly white men, the highest suicide rates among Native and African Americans occur in adolescent boys and men in early adulthood.

Patients with Borderline and Antisocial Personality Disorders

Among the most challenging clinical problems is the management of patients with borderline or antisocial personality disorders who contemplate suicide chronically or make frequent gestures or attempts. Their impulsive, demanding, and manipulative behavior can make accurate risk assessment nearly impossible. Referral to a psychiatrist or other behavioral health care professional is essential. Crisis intervention in the nearest facility that offers this option, referral to emergency facilities, and judicious use of psychiatric inpatient facilities are often necessary to manage these patients.

Summary

- Behavioral emergencies include any threat to the safety of the patient, staff, or others in the patient's sphere.
- Be prepared. Plan for resources and personnel who can ensure safety and effect rapid disposition in the event of a behavioral emergency.
- The physician who encounters a potentially violent patient is advised to heed his or her own subjective response to the patient.
- Every effort should be made to develop rapport with the potentially dangerous patient.
- Diagnostic assessment and specific treatment can be administered once safety is ensured.

Suggested Readings

American Psychiatric Association: Assessment and treatment of patients with suicidal behaviors. In American Psychiatric Association: Practice Guidelines for the Treatment of Psychiatric Disorders. Washington DC: American Psychiatric Association, 2004.

Duhart DT: Violence in the Workplace, 1993-99. Bureau of Justice Statistics. NCJ 190076, December 2001. Available at http://www.ojp.usdoj.gov/bjs/pub/pdf/vw99.pdf (accessed March 20, 2009).

Hyman SE: The violent patient. In SE Hyman, GE Tesar (eds): Manual of Psychiatric Emergencies, 3rd ed. Boston: Little, Brown, 1994, pp 28-37.

Shem S: The House of God: The Classic Novel of Life and Death in an American Hospital. New York: Dell Publishing, 1978, p 3.

References

For a complete list of references, log onto www.expertconsult.com.

Schizophrenia and Acute Psychosis

Manu Mathews, George E. Tesar, Omar Fattal, and David J. Muzina

DEFINITION AND ETIOLOGY

Schizophrenia is a chronic and disabling neuropsychiatric illness possibly best characterized as a syndrome rather than as a single disease entity. The abnormal, often bizarre behavior that typifies schizophrenia is a product of disturbances in cognition, perception, and volition. Clinical manifestations are believed to result from incompletely understood dysregulation of frontotemporal and limbic neurocircuitry. The National Alliance for Mental Illness (NAMI), a patient- and family-oriented self-help group, has designated schizophrenia a brain disorder, emphasizing that schizophrenia is not simply a product of dysfunctional parenting or other psychosocial stressors. Studies have consistently shown, however, that both genetic and nongenetic factors play a role in the origin of schizophrenia.

PREVALENCE AND RISK FACTORS

The point prevalence of schizophrenia is 1% to 1.5%, a finding that has been fairly constant across time, cultures, races, and continents. It is equally prevalent in men and women. In the United States, about 2.5% of total annual health care expenditures are for schizophrenia. Globally, schizophrenia is a leading cause of disease burden and disability. The lifetime risk of suicide is nearly 7% compared with 14% to 15% for mood disorders such as major depression and bipolar disorder.[1]

The familial nature of the illness has long been recognized. Mounting evidence supports a strong genetic contribution, but genetic factors alone do not fully account for the variance in cause. As with other common illnesses such as hypertension, the risk of developing schizophrenia is a product of multiple genes interacting not only with one another but also with environmental factors. It is also possible that specific risk factors predict occurrence of specific schizophrenia subtypes.

Genetic Risk Factors

Accumulating evidence shows that genetic and neurodevelopmental factors are associated with greater susceptibility to schizophrenia. According to twin and adoption studies, up to 50% of identical (monozygotic) twins share a diagnosis of schizophrenia, compared with about 12% of nonidentical (dizygotic) twins. The strength of genetic factors varies across families, but approximately 10% of a patient's first-degree relatives (parents, siblings, and children) are also schizophrenic, as are 50% of the children of two schizophrenic parents. Reports indicate suggestive linkage on chromosomes 1, 3, 5, and 11 and on the X chromosome.

Season of Birth

The birth rate of patients with schizophrenia is 5% to 8% higher worldwide than the birthrate of the general population in the winter and spring months. No proven explanation exists for this phenomenon. A greater likelihood of viral exposure during winter months has been proposed.

Early Developmental Insults

A comparatively high rate of peripartum infant hypoxia has been associated with structural brain abnormalities (e.g., increased ventricular and decreased hippocampal volumes) in schizophrenic patients and their nonschizophrenic siblings.

Other Factors

Population density, industrialization, emigration, and low socioeconomic status at birth have been proposed as possible influences on the development of schizophrenia.

PATHOPHYSIOLOGY AND NATURAL HISTORY

Gross inspection of the schizophrenic brain reveals no abnormalities. Modern neuroimaging techniques, however, including computed tomography (CT), magnetic resonance imaging (MRI), functional MRI (fMRI), and positron emission tomography (PET), demonstrate evidence of nonspecific structural and metabolic abnormalities in the frontotemporal cortices and periventricular limbic structures of the schizophrenic brain. Detailed postmortem analysis of protein profiles and metabolic patterns in the brains of schizophrenic patients point to mitochondrial dysfunction as a distinctive feature.[2]

Neural transmission has long been an object of investigation in schizophrenia. The first agents to demonstrate promise in the pharmacologic control of schizophrenia were recognized to have dopamine-blocking properties. Several neurotransmitter systems have been implicated, but the primary focus has been on dopamine and the brain structures that are high in its content (substantia nigra, ventral tegmentum, mesolimbic structures, and the tuberoinfindibular system). Five dopamine receptor subtypes (D_1 through D_5) have been identified. Blockade of the D_2 receptor appears to have the greatest relevance to the antipsychotic efficacy as well as adverse effects of neuroleptic drugs. The site of D_2-receptor blockade is also relevant to its benefits and adverse effects. Extrapyramidal symptoms can be attributed to D_2-receptor blockade in the substantia nigra and ventral tegmentum, positive symptom suppression to D_2 blockade in mesolimbic structures, and hyperprolactinemia to D_2 blockade in the tuberoinfindibular structures (dopamine is a prolactin-inhibiting factor). The relationship to schizophrenia of serotonin, glutamate, gamma-aminobutyrate, neurotensin, and their relevant receptors is also under investigation.

SIGNS AND SYMPTOMS

The median age at onset for the first psychotic episode of schizophrenia is in the early to mid-20s for men and in the late 20s for women. A prodromal phase that lasts months to years can precede the first psychotic episode. Acute psychosis, the hallmark of the acute phase, follows the prodrome insidiously or occurs abruptly and sometimes explosively. The natural history without treatment (and sometimes with) is for symptoms to wax and wane, punctuated by recurrent episodes of acute psychosis. The pattern of symptoms can change

Box 1 Schizophrenia Symptoms and Symptom Dimensions

Positive*
Hallucinations (typically auditory but also visual)
Delusions (paranoid delusions, nihilistic delusions, delusions of control)
Unusual behavior (stereotypies, mannerisms)

Negative[†]
Reduced emotional (affective[‡]) range
Diminished speech production (poverty of speech)
Loss of interest (anhedonia[‡])
Loss of drive, initiative (apathy, abulia[‡])
Indecisiveness (ambivalence[‡])

Cognitive[†]
Poor attention
Working memory impairment
Formal thought disorder (tangential thinking, loose associations)[§]
Concrete thinking and impaired abstraction
Executive function deficits[¶]

**Typically bizarre (i.e., unreal, other-worldly, or impossible).*
[†]*Negative and cognitive symptoms of schizophrenia correlate with neuroimaging evidence of dorsolateral prefrontal cortex dysfunction.*
[‡]*These are the 4 As of Bleuler.*
[§]*Formal thought disorder (a disorder of the form of thought) is also considered a positive symptom.*
[¶]*Executive functions are the ability to initiate, regulate, plan, and sequence activities. The negative symptoms (apathy, indecision) can represent impaired executive functions.*

over time, with progressive deterioration of function and cognition in some instances and progressive improvement of psychotic symptoms and function in others. Full recovery is uncommon, especially if the illness has been present for some years. Comorbid substance abuse is common, prolongs the illness, and contributes to treatment resistance.

The prodomal phase of schizophrenia is characterized by social avoidance, emotional flattening, eccentricity or magical thinking, idiosyncratic speech, and peculiarities of attitude and behavior that fail to meet criteria for a specific psychiatric illness. Prodromal symptoms that suggest social anxiety, panic, obsessive-compulsive or major depressive disorder, and antisocial behavior or substance misuse often lead to early misdiagnosis and unsuccessful treatment efforts.

Factor analysis has identified three main psychotic symptom dimensions in schizophrenia: positive, negative, and cognitive. The acute phase of the illness features a predominance of positive psychotic symptoms, whereas the chronic phase is typified by negative and cognitive symptoms. Unlike other types of psychosis, the positive symptoms of schizophrenia are complex and bizarre (i.e., having to do with unreal or unearthly events). Negative symptoms are believed to reflect neuroimaging evidence of reduced metabolic activity in the dorsolateral prefrontal cortex. Positive symptoms might represent abnormal temporal lobe activity. Characteristic features of positive, negative, and cognitive symptoms are outlined in Box 1.

Box 2 DSM IV-TR Criteria for the Diagnosis of Schizophrenia

Characteristic Symptoms
At least two of the following symptoms must be present, and each must be present for a significant portion of time during a 1-month period (or less if successfully treated):

- Delusions
- Hallucinations
- Disorganized speech (e.g., frequent derailment or incoherence)
- Grossly disorganized or catatonic behavior
- Negative symptoms (e.g., affective flattening, alogia, avolition)

Only one symptom is required if:

- Delusions are bizarre
- Hallucinations consist of a voice keeping up a running commentary on the person's behavior or thoughts
- Two or more voices are conversing with each other

Social and Occupational Dysfunction
For a significant portion of the time since the onset of the disturbance, one or more major areas of functioning such as work, interpersonal relations, or self-care are markedly below the level achieved before the onset

When the onset is in childhood or adolescence, failure to achieve expected level of interpersonal, academic, or occupational achievement

Duration
Continuous signs of the disturbance persist for at least 6 months

This 6-month period must include at least 1 month of characteristic symptoms (i.e., active-phase symptoms), or less than 1 month if successfully treated, and can include periods of prodromal or residual symptoms

During these prodromal or residual periods, the signs of the disturbance may be manifested by only negative symptoms or two or more characteristic symptoms present in an attenuated form (e.g., odd beliefs, unusual perceptual experiences)

Schizoaffective and Mood Disorder Exclusion
Schizoaffective disorder and mood disorder with psychotic features have been ruled out because either

- No major depressive, manic, or mixed episodes have occurred concurrently with the active-phase symptoms
- Mood episodes have occurred during active-phase symptoms, but their total duration has been brief relative to the duration of the active and residual periods

Exclusion of Substance Use and General Medical Conditions
The disturbance is not due to the direct physiologic effects of a substance (e.g., drug of abuse, a medication)

The disturbance is not due to the direct physiologic effects of a general medical condition

Relation to a Pervasive Developmental Disorder
If there is a history of autistic disorder or another pervasive developmental disorder, the additional diagnosis of schizophrenia is made only if prominent delusions or hallucinations are also present for at least 1 month (or less if successfully treated).

DIAGNOSIS

Accurate diagnosis of schizophrenia is often challenging because symptoms are nonspecific and because progression to full illness is gradual. Relevant signs and symptoms must be present for at least 6 months before a diagnosis of schizophrenia can be made. Acute psychosis is a necessary but insufficient criterion for diagnosing schizophrenia. The diagnostic criteria for schizophrenia are symptomatic, functional, and time based, and they require exclusion of both medical and other psychiatric disorders that can mimic schizophrenia. Schizophrenia is largely a diagnosis of exclusion. The diagnostic criteria for schizophrenia specified by the *Diagnostic and Statistical Manual of Mental Disorders,* fourth edition, text revision (DSM IV-TR)[2] are presented in Box 2.

Schizophrenia also has subtypes (Box 3) defined exclusively by symptom predominance. Their validity remains controversial.

DIFFERENTIAL DIAGNOSIS

If symptoms are not specific and signs and symptoms do not last for 6 months as required for diagnosing schizophrenia, the clinician is obliged to eliminate other important diagnostic considerations. These include psychiatric disorders, substance use, and general medical disorders (Boxes 4 and 5).

Box 3 Subtypes of Schizophrenia

Paranoid
Preoccupation with one or more delusions or frequent auditory hallucinations
None of the following is prominent:

- Disorganized speech
- Disorganized or catatonic behavior
- Flat or inappropriate affect.

Disorganized
Disorganized speech and behavior and flat or inappropriate affect are prominent
Criteria are not met for catatonic type

Catatonic
Motor immobility, catalepsy, stupor
Excessive motor activity that appears to be purposeless
Extreme negativisim or mutism
Peculiarities of voluntary movement (inappropriate or bizarre posturing), stereotyped movements, prominent mannerisms, or prominent grimacing
Echolalia or echopraxia (repeating the examiner's verbalizations or movements)

Undifferentiated
Characteristic symptoms (see Box 2) are present, but the criteria are not met for the other subtypes listed here

Residual
Absence of prominent delusions, hallucinations, disorganized speech, and grossly disorganized or catatonic behavior
Continuing evidence of negative symptoms (see Box 1) or two or more characteristic symptoms (see Box 2) in an attenuated form (e.g., odd beliefs, unusual perceptual experiences)

Adapted from Markowitz JS, Brown CS, Moore TR: Atypical antipsychotics Part I: Pharmacology, pharmacokinetics and efficacy. Ann Pharmacotherapy 1999;33:73-85.

Box 4 Psychiatric and Substance Use Disorders that Can Cause Acute Psychosis

Psychiatric
Bipolar disorder
Major depression with psychotic features
Schizophrenia
Schizoaffective disorder
Schizophreniform disorders
Brief psychotic disorder
Factitious disorder with psychological signs and symptoms
Side effect of antidepressant medications

Drug Abuse
Drug use

- Hallucinogens (PCP, LSD, LSD flashbacks)
- Amphetamine psychosis
- Marijuana use (with panic reactions)

Drug withdrawal

- Alcohol
- Opiates
- Sedative-hypnotic agents (barbiturates, benzodiazepines).

LSD, lysergic acid diethylamide; PCP, phencyclidine.
Adapted and modified from Hyman SE: Acute psychoses and catatonia. Hyman SE, Tesar GE (eds): Manual of Psychiatric Emergencies, 3rd ed. Boston, Little, Brown, 1994, p 145.

Box 5 General Medical Conditions that Can Cause Acute Psychosis

Industrial Exposures
Acute intermittent porphyria
Carbon disulfide
Cushing's syndrome
Heavy metals
Hypocalcemia and hypercalcemia
Hypoglycemia
Hypothyroidism and hyperthyroidism

Neurologic Disorders
Central nervous system neoplasm
Early Alzheimer's disease
Encephalitis, meningitis, brain abscess
Huntington's disease
Neurosyphilis
Seizure disorder (temporal lobe epilepsy, postictal psychosis)
Stroke (right thalamic, Wernicke's aphasia)
Wilson's disease

Nutritional Deficiencies
Korsakoff's psychosis (thiamine deficiency)
Pellagra (niacin deficiency)
Vitamin B_{12} deficiency
Wernicke's encephalopathy (thiamine deficiency)

Systemic Illness with Central Nervous System Effects
Hepatic encephalopathy
HIV/AIDS encephalopathy
Hypoxic encephalopathy
Lupus cerebritis
Pancreatic encephalopathy
Paraneoplastic syndrome

Toxic Reactions to Medications
ACE inhibitors
Anticholinergic agents
Antihistamines
Digitalis
Dopaminergic agents (bromocriptine, levodopa, ropinirole, mirapex)
Glucocorticoids
Isoniazid
NSAIDs (indomethacin, sulindac)
Over-the-counter sleep aids
Stimulants (methylphenidate [Concerta, Focalin, Metadate, Ritalin], dextroamphetamine [Dexedrine, Adderall])

ACE, angiotensin-converting enzyme; AIDS, autoimmune deficiency syndrome; HIV, human immunodeficiency virus; NSAID, nonsteroidal anti-inflammatory drug.
Adapted and modified from Hyman SE: Acute psychoses and catatonia. Hyman SE, Tesar GE (eds): Manual of Psychiatric Emergencies, 3rd ed. Boston, Little, Brown, 1994, p 145.

Acute psychosis, although not recognized as a diagnostic term in the DSM IV-TR, is commonly used to describe a rapid deterioration of behavior associated with hallucinations and delusions. Schizophreniform disorder, brief psychotic disorder, and organic psychoses fall under this rubric. The DSM IV-TR diagnosis of schizophreniform disorder depends on the persistence of schizophrenia-like symptoms for at least 1 month and exclusion of other causes of acute psychosis. Brief psychotic disorder (often referred to as brief reactive psychosis) lasts less than 1 month, but more than 1 day. It is typically regarded as a reaction to marked stress in persons with borderline or antisocial personality disorders.

Schizoaffective disorder is a chronic mental illness that includes prominent features of both schizophrenia and a mood disorder. The diagnostic criteria for schizoaffective disorder are characteristic symptoms of schizophrenia (see Box 2) concurrent with a major mood disturbance (major depressive or manic episode). Although mood symptoms and episodes must be present for a substantial portion of the total course of the illness, a diagnosis of schizoaffective disorder also requires that psychotic symptoms, such as delusions or hallucinations, have been present for a minimum of 2 weeks in the absence of an active mood disturbance.

Delusional disorder is distinguished from schizophrenia by delusions (e.g., erotomanic, grandiose, jealous, persecutory, somatic, mixed) that are not bizarre and functioning that is not markedly impaired. Hallucinations are generally not present.

A diagnosis of mood disorder with psychotic features is made if psychotic symptoms occur solely during episodes of mood disturbance.

Acute psychosis caused by substance use or medication toxicity is distinguished from schizophrenia by clear-cut evidence of substance-use leading to symptoms.

TREATMENT

General Approach

The successful treatment of schizophrenia requires simultaneous attention to medical variables and others not traditionally considered in the medical domain. A multimodal approach encompassing biologic and psychosocial therapies as well as programs that offer rehabilitation and social reintegration has been found to be most effective. Schizophrenia generally does not occur in isolation but rather with other comorbid conditions, commonly alcohol or drug abuse, or both. Failure to recognize and treat comorbid substance abuse is a common cause of treatment resistance in schizophrenia. Comprehensive management of schizophrenia, therefore, typically requires the involvement of a multidisciplinary team including a psychiatrist, social worker, case manager, individual or family therapist, and one or more family members. Episodes of illness can require treatment in multiple settings, including outpatient, intensive outpatient, hospital, and residential.

The primary care physician's principal role involves recognizing the illness, initiating treatment, and referring to a psychiatrist.

Treatment of schizophrenia is divided into three phases: acute, stabilization, and stable.[3] Generally, the illness first comes to medical attention with the presentation of an acute psychotic episode. Acute psychosis, like schizophrenia, has a differential diagnosis that includes general medical, psychiatric, and substance-use disorders, (see Boxes 4 and 5). At this point the primary care physician's role may be to ensure safe transfer of the acutely psychotic patient to an emergency facility where appropriate evaluation and stabilization can be conducted. Once the proper treatment regimen for a schizophrenic patient has been identified, the primary care physician may be called on to prescribe maintenance medication, with specialist referral for assistance in managing recurrent illness episodes.

Proper medical care is another important consideration in the comprehensive management of the schizophrenic patient. The patient's idiosyncratic behavior, poor hygiene, or nonadherence to medical recommendations often interferes with attention to and successful management of medical problems. Schizophrenic patients have a high incidence of cardiovascular problems such as hypertension and coronary artery disease, diabetes, and tobacco-related disorders. Given that many schizophrenics are homeless, higher rates of tuberculosis, HIV infection, and problems associated with poor foot care are also common in this population.

Box 6 Life-Endangering Causes of Acute Psychosis or Delirium: WWHHHIMPS

Withdrawal from alcohol or barbiturates
Wernicke's encephalopathy
Hypertensive crisis
Hypoglycemia
Hypoxemia (cerebral)
Intracranial process (tumor, stroke)
Meningitis or encephalitis
Poisoning (overdose, heavy metal toxicity)
Seizures (postictal state, temporal lobe epilepsy)

Table 1 Laboratory Investigation in Acute Psychosis and Chronic Schizophrenia

Test	Acute Psychosis*	Chronic Schizophrenia†
Blood glucose	×	‡
Blood glucose, fasting		×
Brain MRI or CT	×	‡
BUN	×	‡
CBC	×	‡
Creatinine	×	‡
ECG	×	‡
EEG	‡	
Electrolytes	×	‡
Hepatitis B and C	‡	‡
HIV	‡	‡
Lipid profile		×
Liver function	×	‡
Pregnancy (women with childbearing potential)	×	‡
Syphilis (RPR, VDRL)	×	‡
Toxicology (serum and urine)	×	‡
Vitamin B_{12} and folic acid blood levels	×	

BUN, blood urea nitrogen; CBC, complete blood count; CT, computed tomography; EEG, electroencephalogram; ECG, electrocardiogram; HIV, human immunodeficiency virus; MRI, magnetic resonance imaging; RPR, rapid plasma reagin; VDRL, Venereal Disease Research Laboratory.

*For all first-episode psychoses or acute psychoses in which the patient's history is unknown.

†Patients who have an existing diagnosis of schizophrenia and require regular monitoring of medical status.

‡Order only if the clinical situation warrants it or if the test result is considered important for routine monitoring of physical status.

Acute Phase: Treatment of Acute Psychosis

The first priority in management of acute psychosis is the safety of patient and staff (see elsewhere in this section, "Psychiatric Emergencies"). This includes simultaneous attention to potentially life-endangering causes of acute psychosis or delirium (Box 6) and other psychiatric, substance-use (see Box 4), and general medical (see Box 5) causes. Identification of the underlying cause of the acute psychosis requires a thorough evaluation that includes the patient's psychiatric and medical histories; collateral information from the family, workplace, school, and other sources; physical and mental status examinations; and laboratory investigation. Typically, much of this information either is not available or is difficult to obtain, and the clinician is forced to rely on rapid observation, clinical intuition, and laboratory measures (Table 1). A commonly raised question is

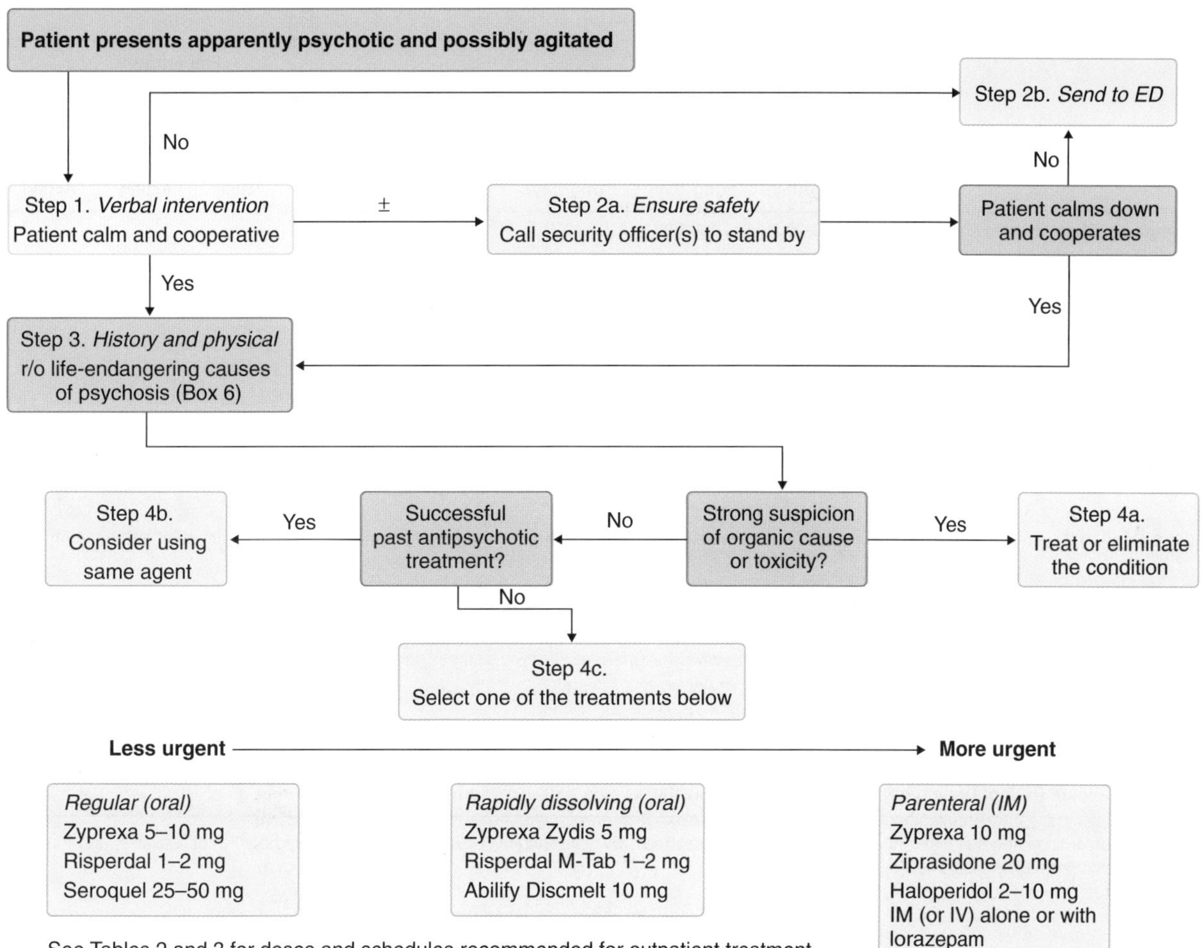

Figure 1 **Algorithm for managing acute psychosis.** ED, emergency department; r/o, rule out.

whether or not to obtain brain neuroimaging. Most experts recommend CT scanning or MRI during a first psychotic episode. An electroencephalogram should be obtained if one suspects organic psychosis such as delirium (encephalopathy). If an underlying cause of psychosis is discovered, it should be corrected (e.g., hypoglycemia, cerebral vasculitis, seizures). In the absence of a definitive cause, the focus can shift to pharmacologic intervention. Voluntary or involuntary hospitalization is often necessary for the first episode of psychosis in schizophrenia.

The traditionally accepted regimen for rapid control of agitation associated with acute psychosis is oral or intramuscular lorazepam (Ativan) 1-2 mg, alone or in combination with haloperdidol (Haldol) 2-5 mg. Rapidly acting alternatives include oral or intramuscular olanzapine (Zyprexa) 5-10 mg or oral ziprasidone 20 mg IM or 60-80 mg. Oral dispersible forms of olanzapine (Zyprexa Zydis) 5-10 mg and risperidone (Risperdal M-Tabs) 1-2 mg are useful when rapid absorption is desired and for noncompliant patients who cheek medication. Simultaneous intramuscular olanzapine and lorazepam is not recommended because it has been associated with respiratory failure. An algorithm for treating acute psychosis is presented in Figure 1.

Pharmacologic Treatment of Schizophrenia

Antipsychotics are considered to be the first line of therapy in the pharmacologic treatment of schizophrenia. They are generally categorized as first-generation (typical) antipsychotics (FGAs) or second-generation (atypical) antipsychotics (SGAs). Typical starting and therapeutic doses of FGAs and SGAs are listed in Tables 2 and 3.

A guideline for the pharmacologic management of schizophrenia is presented in Figure 2. The choice of antipsychotic drug, dosage, and desired route of administration is based on phase of treatment, intensity of agitation, adherence to treatment recommendations, history of response to antipsychotic medications, and antipsychotic side-effect profile.

The FGAs are broadly classified into the phenothiazines (e.g., chlorpromazine) and butyrophenones (e.g., haloperidol). The phenothiazines are more anticholinergic, cause more weight gain, and are more likely than butyrophenones to cause postural hypotension. Overdose is more likely to be fatal with phenothiazines than with butyrophenones. Haloperidol, the most widely prescribed butyrophenone, is associated with a high risk of all types of extrapyramidal symptoms (EPS). Although effective, the FGAs have fallen out of favor because of their side-effect profiles, especially their propensity to cause EPS (Box 7).

The SGAs affect several receptor types—serotonin, histamine, noraderenergic, and muscarinic—in addition to the D_2 receptors.[4] The multiplicity of receptors targeted by SGAs contributes to their efficacy and side-effect profiles. The results of the oft-cited Clinical Antipsychotic Trials of Intervention Effectiveness (CATIE) study demonstrated that FGAs and SGAs have similar efficacy, but both groups have potentially troublesome side effects that warrant careful

Table 2 First-Generation (Atypical) Antipsychotics

	Daily Dosage				Preparations				
							IM		
Drug	Starting (mg/day)	Range (mg/day)	Maximum (mg/day)	Schedule	Pill, Capsule	Elixir	Short Acting	Long Acting	IV
Chlorpromazine (Thorazine)*	50-100	400-800	1000	bid	×				
Thioridazine (Mellaril)*	50-100	150-300	800	bid-qid	×				
Trifluoperazine (Stelazine)*	2-4	5-10	40	bid	×				
Fluphenazine (Prolixin)*	0.5-1	5-10		bid	×				
Fluphenazine decanoate	12.5	25-50	100	q 3-6 wk				×	
Perphenazine (Trilafon)*	12-24	32-64	64	tid-qid	×				
Molindone (Moban)	50-75	50-200	225	tid-qid	×	×			
Loxapine (Loxitane)	10-20	60-100	250	bid	×				
Thiothixene (Navane)	6-10	5-15	60	bid-tid	×				
Haloperidol (Haldol)*	2-10	5-15	100	bid-tid	×				
Haloperidol lactate	1-5	5-10	100	bid-tid			×		×†
Haloperidol decanoate (Haldol Decanoate)	25	50-100	450	q mo				×	

Note: First-generation antipsychotics are no longer considered first-line treatment for schizophrenia unless an atypical antipsychotic is not available, and then either haloperdiol or chlorpromazine should be considered.

*The U.S. manufacturer discontinued use. Production of the generic form continues.

†Not approved by U.S. Food and Drug Administration for IV use, but off-label use is common when IV access is available.

Table 3 Second-Generation (Atypical) Antipsychotics

	Daily Dosage				Preparations				
								IM	
Drug	Starting (mg/day)	Range (mg/day)	Maximum (mg/day)	Schedule	Pill, Capsule	Rapidly Dissolving	Elixir	Short Acting	Long Acting
Clozapine (Clozaril)	25	300-600	900	bid	×				
Risperidone (Risperdal)	1-2	4-8	16	qd-bid	×	×			
Risperidone (Risperdal M-Tab)	1-2	4-8	16	qd-bid		×			
Risperidone (Risperdal Consta)	12.5	25	50	q 2 wk					×
Olanzapine (Zyprexa)	5-10	15-20	20	qd-bid	×			×	
Olanzapine (Zyprexa Zydis)	5-10	15-20	20	qd-bid		×			
Ziprasidone (Geodon)	40-80	80-160	160	bid	×			×	
Quetiapine (Seroquel)	50-100	400-800	800	bid	×				
Aripiprazole (Abilify)	5-10	15-30	40	qd	×				

Note: All second-generation (atypical) antipsychotics have U.S. Food and Drug Administration approval for use in schizophrenia.

*Not considered a first-line agent. Requires weekly monitoring of white blood cell count (WBC) for the first 6 months of treatment and then biweekly thereafter for the duration of use.

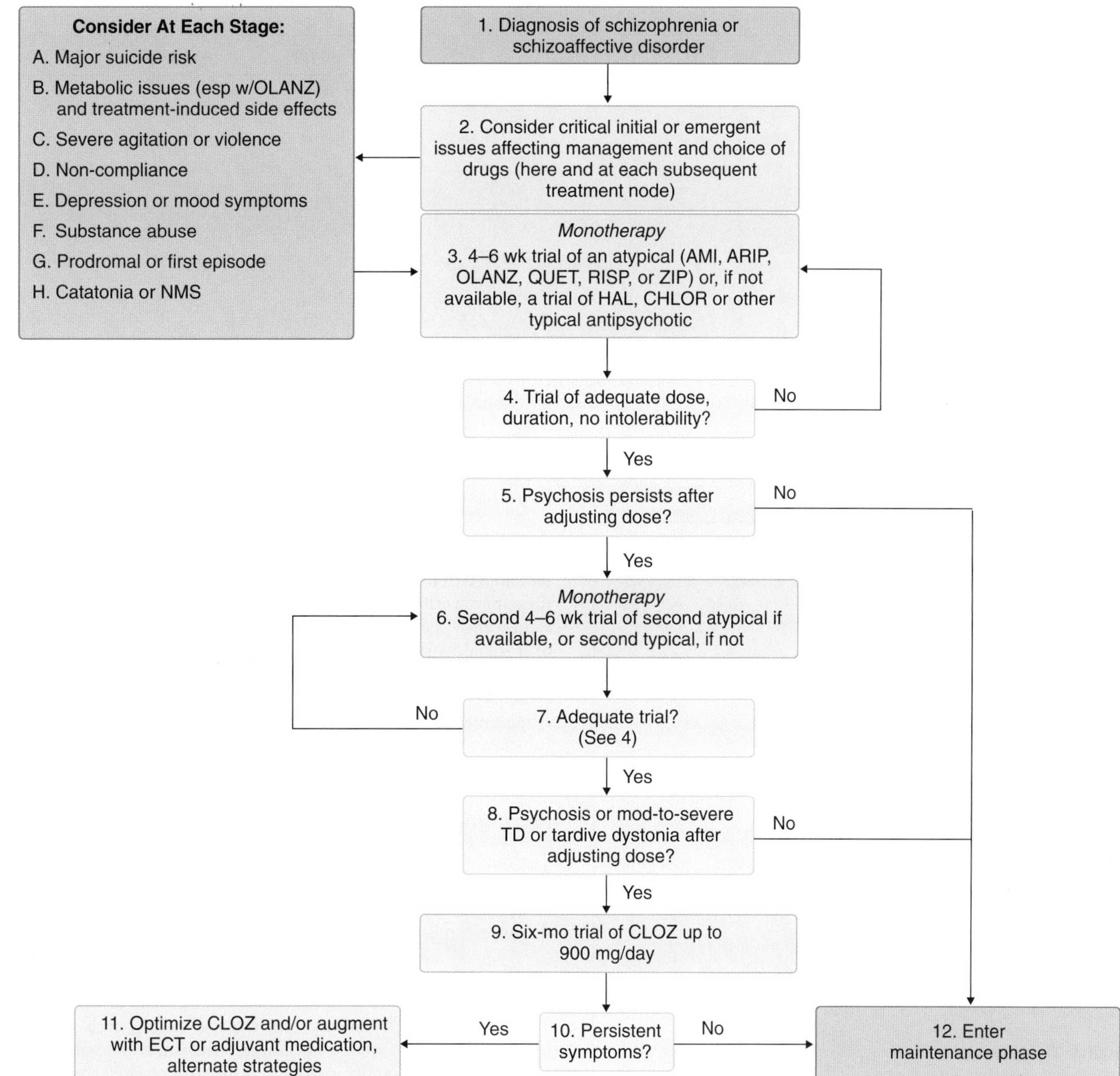

Figure 2 **International Psychopharmacology Algorithm Project algorithm for schizophrenia.** For descriptive not prescriptive purposes. AMI, amisulpride; ARIP, aripiprazole; CHLOR, chlorpromazine; CLOZ, clozipine; ECT, electroconvulsive therapy; esp, especially; HAL, haloperidol; NMS, neuroleptic malignant syndrome; OLANZ, olanzapine; QUET, quetiapine; RISP, risperidone; TD, tardive dyskinesia; ZIP, ziprasidone. *© 2004-2006 International Psychopharmacology Algorithm Project (IPAP) www.ipap.org.*

monitoring and can disrupt otherwise effective treatment.[4-6] Although SGAs are less likely to cause EPS, they are not risk free. Quetiapine is the least likely to cause EPS. The risk of other adverse effects varies among individual SGAs. Their relative risk profiles for different side effects are presented in Table 4. Clozapine (Clozaril), the first SGA to be developed and marketed, has retained its reputation for being the most effective of all antipsychotics at treating negative symptoms. Unfortunately, its tendency to cause bone marrow suppression, weight gain, and the metabolic syndrome also distinguishes it from the other SGAs. It is therefore used only selectively.

Stabilization Phase

The dosage of medication used to achieve remission or optimal control in the acute phase should be continued for at least 6 months to prevent relapse. Psychotherapeutic interventions remain supportive. Patients should be helped with the transition to life in the community and helped to adjust to their lives outside the hospital through realistic goal setting.

Stable Phase

The goals of the stable phase are sustained symptom control or remission. Monthly to semiannual monitoring for treatment adherence, relapse, and intolerance to medications is recommended. Signs and symptoms of weight gain, increasing waist circumference, hyperlipidemia, and hyperglycemia should be monitored, as well as evidence of abnormal involuntary movements.[7] The Abnormal Involuntary Movement Scale (AIMS) (Table 5) should be used serially to rate presence and intensity of movement disorder.

Continued antipsychotic treatment reduces the risk of symptom relapse. There are no strict guidelines for the minimum antipsychotic

Table 4 Monitoring Parameters for Patients on Second-Generation Antipsychotics

Parameter	Baseline	4 wk	8 wk	12 wk	Quarterly	Annually	5 Yearly
Personal and family history	×					×	
Weight and BMI	×	×	×	×	×		
Waist circumference	×					×	
Blood pressure	×			×		×	
Fasting plasma glucose	×			×		×	
Fasting lipid profile	×			×			×

Note: More frequent assessments may be warranted based on clinical status.

Based on American Diabetes Association 2004 consensus guidelines. American Diabetes Association, American Psychiatric Association, American Association of Clinical Endocrinologists, North American Association for the Study of Obesity: Consensus development conference on antipsychotic drugs and obesity and diabetes. Diabetes care 2004;27:596-601.

BMI, body mass index.

Box 7 Treatment of Extrapyramidal Symptoms

Acute Dystonia
Benzotropine mesylate (Cogentin) 2 mg PO/IM/IV bid
Diphenhydramine (Benadryl) 25-50 mg IM/IV
Trihexyphenidyl (Artane) 2-5 mg PO bid-tid

Akathisia
Clonazepam 0.5 mg PO bid
Lorazepam 1 mg PO tid
Pramipexole 0.125-0.5 mg PO qd
Propranolol 10-30 mg tid
Ropinirole 1-4 mg PO qd

Neuroleptic Malignant Syndrome
Anticholinergics (benztropine, trihxyphenidyl)
Dantrolene sodium
Dopamine agonists (amantadine, bromocriptine, ropinirole, pramipexole)

Parkinsonism
Amantadine 100 mg PO bid
Anticholinergics (benztropine, trihexyphenidyl)
Pramipexole 0.125-0.5 mg PO qd
Ropinirole 1-4 mg PO qd

Tardive Dyskinesia
No uniformly effective treatment

Tardive Dystonia
Anticholinergics are sometimes helpful

Withdrawal Dyskinesia
Resume same antipsychotic agent

Neuroleptic-induced catatonia
Anticholinergics (benztropine, trihexyphenidyl)
Bromocriptine 10 mg PO tid
Dopamine agonists (amantadine, bromocriptine, ropinirole, pramipexole)

dose required for preventing relapse. For FGAs, the optimal dose is regarded as the minimum dose at which mild EPS are detectable on physical examination. SGAs can be administered at therapeutic doses well below their EPS threshold.

Pharmacologic treatment of schizophrenia is essential but insufficient. Optimal outcome requires additional use of psychosocial therapies and programs that foster recovery through vocational rehabilitation and social reintegration.

Psychosocial Interventions

Assertive Community Treatment

Developed in the late 1960s, assertive community treatment provides the patient with around-the-clock support in the community, thereby significantly reducing the time spent in hospitals. A team composed of a social worker, nurse, and case manager provides treatment in community settings. Services delivered include case management, initial and ongoing assessments, access to psychiatric services, employment and housing assistance, family support and education, substance-abuse services, and any other services and supports critical to successful adaptation in the community.

Psychotherapy

The quality of the therapeutic alliance may be the best predictor of compliance and outcome. The emphasis is on education, support, and problem-solving, rather than on developing insight. Therapy of this type can be provided on an individual or group basis.

Family Therapy

The schizophrenic's behavior can trigger a vicious cycle of conflict between the patient and family. Anger, criticism, and devaluing comments directed by family members at the patient—referred to in the literature as high expressed emotion—are associated with a greater increase of relapse even when pharmacologic management is optimal. A therapist works with the family to reduce expressed emotion by educating about schizophrenia and helping to modify the behaviors and attitudes that undermine the patient.

Social Skills Training

The principles of learning theory are used to improve social skills such as interpersonal relationships, employment, and leisure. Behaviors such as odd facial expressions, lack of spontaneity, and inappropriate perception of others' emotional states are targeted and modified.

Vocational Rehabilitation

Workshops and part-time employment programs help the patient acquire greater functionality.

SCREENING AND PREVENTION

Most prevention efforts are in the realm of secondary and tertiary prevention, that is, reducing the number and severity of episodes.

Table 5 Abnormal Involuntary Movement Scale

Assessment

1. Observe the patient's gait on the way into the room.
2. Have the patient remove gum or dentures if they do not fit properly.
3. Determine if the patient is aware of any abnormal movements.
4. Have the patient sit on a firm, armless chair with hands on knees, legs slightly apart, and feet flat on the floor. Now and throughout the examination, look at the entire body for movements.
5. Have the patient sit with hands unsupported, dangling over the knees.
6. Ask the patient to open the mouth twice. Look for tongue movements.
7. Ask the patient to protrude the tongue twice.
8. Ask the patient to tap the thumb against each finger for 15 sec with each hand. Observe face and legs.
9. Have the patient stand with arms extended forward.

Rating

Rate each item on a 0 to 4 scale for the greatest severity observed. Movements that occur only on activation merit 1 point less than those that occur spontaneously.

Score					
Movement	**None**	**Minimal***	**Mild**	**Moderate**	**Severe**
Face and Mouth					
Muscles of facial expression	0	1	2	3	4
Lips and perioral area	0	1	2	3	4
Jaw	0	1	2	3	4
Tongue	0	1	2	3	4
Extremities					
Arms	0	1	2	3	4
Legs	0	1	2	3	4
Trunk					
Neck	0	1	2	3	4
Shoulders	0	1	2	3	4
Hips	0	1	2	3	4
Global					
Severity of abnormal movements	0	1	2	3	4
Incapacitation due to abnormal movements	0	1	2	3	4
Patient's awareness of abnormal movements (0 = unaware; 4 = severe distress)	0	1	2	3	4

*May be the extreme of normal.
Modified from Guy W: ECDEU Assessment Manual for Psychopharmacology. Rockville, Md, U.S. Department of Health, Education and Welfare, 1976.

Public health efforts to educate about schizophrenia help to reduce stigma and resistance to seeking treatment. Family history of schizophrenia is an important indicator of risk that should increase vigilance for early detection and treatment of prodromal symptoms. Once the diagnosis is made, the team should develop a comprehensive treatment plan that includes family involvement with goals of adhering to treatment and reducing symptoms. Assertive community treatment has been very effective at maintaining community and keeping patients out of the hospital. Assiduous attention to substance abuse and abstinence is a key to a good outcome in schizophrenia.

CONSIDERATIONS IN SPECIAL POPULATIONS

Populations with special needs include patients with pervasive developmental disorders and mental retardation, women with childbearing potential, and the homeless.

Summary

- Schizophrenia is a treatable neuropsychiatric disorder present in approximately 1% of the general population.
- The etiology is multifactorial and includes genetic, developmental, and possibly environmental causes.
- The signs and symptoms of schizophrenia are nonspecific, warranting a thorough evaluation for other medical and psychiatric disorders that can manifest with psychosis.
- The general physician should be familiar with the use, benefits, and potential adverse effects of antipsychotic medications used to treat schizophrenia.
- The metabolic syndrome is a common comorbidity, especially since the introduction of atypical (second-generation) antipsychotics.

Suggested Readings

American Diabetes Association, American Psychiatric Association, American Association of Clinical Endocrinologists, North American Association for the Study of Obesity: Consensus development conference on antipsychotic drugs and obesity and diabetes. Diabetes Care 2004;27:596-601.

American Psychiatric Association: Practice guideline for the treatment of patients with schizophrenia, 2nd ed. Available at http://www.psychiatryonline.com/pracGuide/pracGuideTopic_6.aspx (accessed March 20, 2009).

Kaplan HI, Sadock BJ (eds): Comprehensive Textbook of Psychiatry, 6th ed, vol 1. Baltimore: Williams & Wilkins, 1995, pp 984-987.

Kessler RC, McGonagle KA, Zhao S, et al: Lifetime and 12-month prevalence of DSM-III-R psychiatric disorders in the United States. Results from the National Comorbidity Survey. Arch Gen Psychiatry 1994;51:8-19.

Lieberman JA, Stroup TS, McEvoy JP, et al: Clinical Antipsychotic Trials of Intervention Effectiveness (CATIE) Investigators. Effectiveness of antipsychotic drugs in patients with chronic schizophrenia. N Engl J Med 2005;353(12):1209-1223.

Markowitz JS, Brown CS, Moore TR: Atypical antipsychotics Part I: Pharmacology, pharmacokinetics and efficacy. Ann Pharmacotherapy 1999;33:73-85.

Newcomer JW: Second generation antipsychotics and metabolic effects: A comprehensive literature review. CNS Drugs 2005;19(Suppl):1-93.

Rossler W, Salize HJ, van Os J, Riecher-Rossler A: Size of burden of schizophrenia and psychotic disorders. Eur Neuropsychopharmacol 2005;15(4):399-409.

References

For a complete list of references, log onto www.expertconsult.com.

Drug Abuse and Addiction

Gregory B. Collins, Mark S. McAllister, and Kamala Adury

DEFINITION AND ETIOLOGY

A diagnosis of either substance abuse or addiction is made when symptoms indicate a maladaptive pattern of substance use resulting in clinically significant impairment or distress. Substance abuse manifests with social, interpersonal, physical, and legal problems, whereas addiction is characterized by (1) physical dependence, manifested through tolerance and withdrawal, and (2) behavioral manifestations, evidenced by an inability to control use, continued use despite adverse consequences, and social dysfunction (Boxes 1 and 2).[1] Current thinking favors the view that chemical dependency is a result of complex genetic, environmental, psychological, physical, and social factors.

PREVALENCE AND RISK FACTORS

The Substance Abuse and Mental Health Services Administration indicated that 22.5 million Americans, or 9.4% of the population older than 12 years, met criteria for substance abuse or dependence in 2004.[2] Although alcohol-related disorders account for the majority of these individuals, illicit drug use or a combination of alcohol and illicit drug use is responsible for a significant proportion. Despite recent declines in use, marijuana remains the most commonly used illicit drug. There has been a significant increase in the nonmedical use of prescription opioids among young adults in recent years. Over this same period, the use of other illicit drugs by young adults has either decreased or remained stable. From 1993 to 2003, the number of substance abuse treatment admissions increased by almost 14%.[3] Increases in the number of admissions for marijuana, opioid, and stimulant use are largely responsible for this finding. In 1993, the largest proportion of admissions was in the 25- to 34-year-old age group (40%).[3] By 2003, that age group accounted for only 25% of admissions. In the same time period, the proportion of admissions increased for all other age groups, with the largest increase seen among admissions older than 45 years. Substance abuse often starts in adolescence. Several factors have been identified that may be of predictive value in determining risk for the development of substance-related disorders.[4] These risk factors fit into four categories, or domains, that consist of community, family, school, and individual/peer (Table 1).

SIGNS AND SYMPTOMS

Drug addiction can be regarded as having psychological and physical components, but the exact pathophysiology has not yet been entirely elucidated. Currently, the only practical way to diagnose drug addiction is to observe its consequences or symptoms. Usually, these symptoms are reflected in the deterioration of marital, occupational, emotional, spiritual, legal, financial, or physical well being. If the drug use repeatedly causes problems in one or more of these areas, the diagnosis of chemical dependency can be made, even though the patient may believe that he or she can stop using drugs. Because of the complex nature of the etiology of chemical dependency, most professionals pay little attention to how the chemically dependent person came to be addicted. Looking for underlying problems or causes before a period of stable abstinence has been achieved may at times be fruitless and even detrimental. Often, a better approach is to direct treatment at eliminating the use of psychoactive substances, while recognizing that the patient is suffering from a compulsion to return to active substance use.

Chemical dependency is a great masquerader, often disguising itself as a medical or psychiatric complaint. Patients rarely seek treatment for substance-related disorders. Usually they are in the physician's office for one or more secondary disorders, such as seizures, systemic or local infections, accidents, trauma, burns, or other organ pathology. The presenting complaint also may be psychiatric with the appearance of anxiety, depression, personality disorder, or paranoid ideation. Complaints of chronic pain may be present, such as fibromyalgia, arthritis, disk disease, or other painful conditions "requiring" opioid medication. The role of the physician is to see through the manifesting symptoms and diagnose the chemical problem. If drugs have anything to do with the problem, the possibility of chemical abuse should be investigated further.

Problems often arise because physicians tend to recognize only late-stage physical complications and withdrawal symptoms as indicative of chemical dependency. They should, however, cultivate the skill of diagnosing substance dependence at a much earlier point in this progressive disability, when manifestations are subtle. The earliest symptoms are generally adverse effects on marriage and job, which often antedate by many years any detectable physical consequences. It is, therefore, a good idea to ask, "Did this problem have anything to do with your drug use?" or "Were you using drugs when the problem occurred?" If the answer is yes, the physician should explore the possibility of a chronic, serious, or incipient problem with substance abuse.

DIAGNOSIS

The diagnosis of chemical dependency is usually made on the basis of information obtained from the medical history, physical examination, psychological assessment, laboratory tests, and reports of concerned others. In addition, several empirically validated screening tools are available that require little time or training to use during an initial assessment. Examples include the CAGE[5] screen for alcohol abuse or the Drug Abuse Screening Test[6] for other commonly abused substances.

The medical history should survey recent drug use, including alcohol, tobacco, analgesics, sedatives, tranquilizers, cocaine, marijuana, and any others. Has there been a pattern of increasing the dosage or frequency of these drugs? Has the patient received treatment from numerous doctors or hospitals? Is the patient unwilling to reveal the names or places of the previous treatment? Does the individual have a vague physical problem such as back pain without radiologic changes, or conversely, does he or she present with an exotic chronic disease that causes intermittent bouts of pain? Is there any deception or major omission in the medical or psychiatric history? Does the patient acknowledge an earlier alcohol problem or previous drug treatment? Are other risk factors present such as easy access to drugs (e.g., with health care professionals) or peer pressure (e.g., in sports or entertainment figures)? Has the patient been arrested for driving while intoxicated or under the influence? Have there been any other drug- or alcohol-related arrests? Is there a history of drug-involved marital discord or job trouble? Has there been any drug-related trauma, violence, explosion, or burns? Is there a history of any drug withdrawal symptoms, such as sweating, nausea, vomiting, or seizures?

Any elicited acknowledgment of substance use deserves further inquiry including the onset, quantity, frequency, and duration of use. Patterns of escalating use including the most recent dose of each substance used and the time elapsed since last use should be ascer-

Box 1 DSM-IV-TR Criteria for Substance Abuse

A maladaptive pattern of substance use leading to clinically significant impairment or distress, as manifested by one (or more) of the following, occurring within a 12-month period:

- Recurrent substance use resulting in a failure to fulfill major role obligations at work, school, or home (e.g., repeated absences or poor work performance related to substance use, substance-related absences, suspensions, or expulsions from school; neglect of children or household)
- Recurrent substance use in situations in which it is physically hazardous (e.g., driving an automobile or operating a machine when impaired by substance use)
- Recurrent substance-related legal problems (e.g., arrests for substance-related disorderly conduct)
- Continued substance use despite having persistent or recurrent social or interpersonal problems caused by or exacerbated by the effects of the substance (e.g., arguments with spouse about consequences of intoxication, physical fights)

The symptoms have never met the criteria for substance dependence for this class of substance.

Adapted from American Psychiatric Association. Diagnostic and Statistical Manual of Mental Disorders, Fourth Edition, Text Revision. Washington, DC. American Psychiatric Association, 2000.

Box 2 DSM-IV-TR Criteria for Substance Dependence

A maladaptive pattern of substance use, leading to clinically significant impairment or distress, as manifested by three (or more) of the following, occurring at any time in the same 12-month period:

- Tolerance, as defined by either of the following:
- A need for markedly increased amounts of the substance to achieve intoxication or desired effect
- Markedly diminished effect with continued use of the same amount of the substance
- Withdrawal, as manifested by either of the following:
- The characteristic withdrawal syndrome is demonstrated for the substance.
- The same (or a closely related) substance is taken to relieve or avoid withdrawal symptoms.
- The substance is often taken in larger amounts or over a longer period than was intended.
- There is a persistent desire or unsuccessful efforts to cut down or control substance use.
- A great deal of time is spent in activities necessary to obtain the substance (e.g., visiting multiple doctors or driving long distances), use the substance (e.g., chain smoking), or recover from its effects.
- Important social, occupational, or recreational activities are given up or reduced because of substance use.
- The substance use is continued despite knowledge of having a persistent or recurrent physical or psychological problem that is likely to have been caused or exacerbated by the substance (e.g., current cocaine use despite recognition of cocaine-induced depression, or continued drinking despite recognition that an ulcer was made worse by alcohol consumption).

The diagnosis should specify "With Physiologic Dependence" (either item 1 or 2 is present) or "Without Physiologic Dependence" (neither item 1 nor item 2 is present).

Adapted from American Psychiatric Association. Diagnostic and Statistical Manual of Mental Disorders, Fourth Edition, Text Revision. Washington, DC. American Psychiatric Association, 2000.

Table 1 Risk Factors for Adolescent Drug Use

Individual	Community
Alienation and rebelliousness	Availability of drugs
Friends who engage in the problem behavior	Community laws and norms favorable toward drug use
Favorable attitudes toward the problem behavior	Transitions and mobility
Early initiation of the problem behavior	Low neighborhood attachment and community disorganization
Constitutional factors	Extreme economic deprivation
Family	**School**
Family history of the problem behavior	Early and persistent antisocial behavior
Family management problems	Academic failure beginning in late elementary school
Family conflict	Lack of commitment to school
Favorable parental attitudes and involvement in the problem behavior	

tained. Because many patients are using more than one substance, the history should routinely include questions regarding the use of substances other than the patient's drug of choice. Specifically, use of over-the-counter medications and prescription medications should be examined because many patients do not consider these agents to be prone to abuse. Any attempts to limit, control, or cease substance use are also important to discuss as well as the circumstances surrounding relapse.

The physical examination should be comprehensive because chronic substance abuse can adversely affect virtually any organ system. The physician should look for signs of drug use, such as residual white powdery substance (cocaine or heroin) around the nares or alcohol on the breath. Clothing and personal effects may reveal an interest in drugs or the drug culture. Check for the presence of medications or drugs, as well as administering paraphernalia including syringes, needles, cellophane bags, paper wrappers, crack pipes, volatile ether, sodium bicarbonate, quinine, razor blades, and tiny spoons. The patient may wear drug-related insignias on belts, shirts, and rings. Physical signs of chronic drug administration may be present (Table 2).

Psychological manifestations may include a recent drug-related personality change of any type. There may be evidence of intoxication: staggering gait, slurred speech, nodding off, nonsensical conversing, or forgetfulness. Anxiety and nervousness may be present with anger, irritability, and impatience. Agitation or even hostility may require emergency protective precautions. The patient may be confused or disoriented and may have evidence of hallucinations or paranoid delusions. Conversely, behavior may be dull, apathetic, and listless. Drug seeking may be in evidence. It is also important to ascertain the presence of any coexisting psychiatric disorders because management of such disorders may profoundly affect the success of substance-related treatment. The evaluation of psychiatric symptoms may be aided by repeated, longitudinal assessments taking into account the presence or absence of concurrent substance use.

Laboratory testing may help to confirm the presence of alcohol or drugs, may establish evidence of organ damage, or may suggest the presence of a drug or alcohol problem. Negative or normal laboratory studies, however, do not rule out a substantial drug problem. A toxicology screen for substance abuse is warranted in any suspicious circumstance. A supervised urine collection is best for drugs. Alcohol requires testing of the blood or breath. Blood studies may indicate effects on internal organs, toxicity, or related infections. A tuberculosis (TB) skin test is advisable. The electrocardiogram may

Table 2 Physical Findings and Complications of Chronic Drug Addiction

Organ or Organ System	Complication
Skin	Needle marks, injection "tracks" over veins, scars, ulcerations, cellulitis, necrotic tissue, jaundice
Eyes	Pupillary constriction (opiates) or dilation (stimulant, opiate or benzodiazepine withdrawal), scleral icterus
Respiratory	Nasal mucosal inflammation or septal perforation, coarsened voice or chronic bronchitis from cocaine freebasing or marijuana smoking
Cardiovascular	"No veins" limiting intravenous access and blood for laboratory sampling, bacterial endocarditis
Autonomic nervous system	Elevated blood pressure, abnormal heart rate (bradycardia or tachycardia), tremor, diaphoresis, brisk reflexes
Liver	Tenderness or enlargement
Neuromuscular	Seizures, aseptic necrosis of large muscle masses causing scarring, fibrosis, and boardlike rigidity of affected muscles

reflect arrhythmia or ischemia (cocaine), and a chest radiograph may show infectious granulomas, diffuse fibrosis, TB, or pneumonia.

It is always helpful for a physician to receive confirmation about a patient's substance abuse from concerned others, such as the spouse or persons close to the patient. In this regard, physicians must be discreet in their inquiries so as not to reveal privileged information or jeopardize the patient's reputation. Generally, eliciting information from the family is the best way to proceed. If family members reveal serious concerns because of substance use, the physician can support these concerns and assist the family to motivate the patient to accept help. It is equally as important to discern whether household members or friends may interfere with the patient's efforts at abstinence. In this regard, the substance use status of those close to the patient should be considered and their willingness to quit at the same time or refrain from use around the individual should be assessed.

Summary

- Substance abuse is often diagnosed by observing its consequences or symptoms.
- Continued use of drugs in spite of serious consequences is a hallmark of addiction.
- Chronic substance abuse can adversely affect virtually any organ system.
- Assessment and treatment of coexisting psychiatric disorders profoundly affect the success of substance abuse treatment.
- Collateral information obtained from individuals close to the patient can aid in the assessment and diagnosis.

TREATMENT

Physician management of drug abuse consists of two fairly distinct processes that should be implemented concurrently for optimal benefit. These are detoxification, where a patient withdrawing from the effects of illicit drugs is stabilized, and the psychological component, which generates motivation to maintain abstinence. These processes vary with the specific drugs of abuse and the patterns of behavior exhibited by the substance abuser.

Detoxification

Opioids

Treatment for opioid dependence has two alternative approaches: detoxification or maintenance therapy. Detoxification involves the short-term pharmacologic management of the physical symptoms of opioid withdrawal and is designed to bring patients to an opioid-free state while engaging them into drug-free, relapse prevention therapy. Symptoms of withdrawal from opioids can be quite severe, depending on the potency of the abused opioid, route of administration, and duration of use. Manifestations of opioid withdrawal include muscle and joint pains, restlessness, irritability, nausea, vomiting, diarrhea, insomnia, mydriasis, diaphoresis, rhinorrhea, piloerection, tachycardia, and hypertension. In general, seizures are not associated with opioid withdrawal, but can be present during withdrawal from meperidine (Demerol) or propoxyphene (Darvon).

Management of the opioid withdrawal syndrome can be accomplished through various pharmacologic methods. One approach is to use long-acting opioid agonists, such as methadone or buprenorphine (Subutex). For cases of street heroin use, usually 20 to 30 mg/day of methadone, in divided doses four times daily, will suffice to start. For recently acquired addictions or for patients abusing less potent opioids such as codeine or propoxyphene, 2 to 10 mg of methadone per day in divided doses will usually suffice. Addicts tolerant to large daily doses of potent pharmaceutical opioids such as hydrocodone and oxycodone may need 40 to 100 mg/day or more of methadone, usually given in divided doses, with respiratory status closely monitored. Naloxone should be kept on hand in the event of inadvertent methadone overdose. Once stabilized on a consistent dose, methadone can be tapered while titrating for the patient's comfort level. Federal law restricts use of methadone for opioid dependence to specially licensed hospitals and clinics. Physicians may not prescribe methadone or other opioids for the treatment of opioid dependence outside of these specially licensed settings.

At times, α_2-adrenergic agonists, such as clonidine, are used with or without methadone detoxification. Clonidine helps to ameliorate withdrawal symptoms, particularly anxiety, by reducing secretion of norepinephrine from the locus coeruleus, but this drug is often an inadequate replacement for potent opioids. One should observe for any hypotensive episodes with clonidine. The initial dose of clonidine is 0.1 mg one to four times daily, and the dose is tapered as tolerated.

Buprenorphine is a partial agonist at the mu opioid receptor and an antagonist at the kappa receptor and has been used for opioid detoxification and initial stabilization in recent years.[7] Slow dissociation from the receptor sites results in a long duration of action. Although buprenorphine produces mild subjective reinforcement, a ceiling effect exists because of its partial agonist activity so that increasing doses do not produce similarly increasing euphoria or respiratory depression. This offers a distinct advantage over methadone, which at higher doses produces not only greater euphoric effect, but also greater abuse liability and more intense withdrawal symptoms as well as higher risks for respiratory depression and death by overdose. Like methadone, however, buprenorphine has abuse potential if used parenterally. Because of this liability, a combination tablet of buprenorphine and naloxone (Suboxone) was developed to deter the possibility of diversion and improper use. The combination product is currently marketed in a buprenorphine to naloxone ratio of 4 : 1.

It is advisable that patients be experiencing mild to moderate withdrawal symptoms before initiating therapy with buprenorphine. This may occur as little as four hours from the time of last use if the patient is abusing short-acting opioids such as street heroin, or significantly longer, 48 hours or more, for patients on long-acting opioids such as methadone or oxycodone. It is recommended that patients taking long-acting opioids reduce their dose to a methadone-equivalent dose of 30 mg/day or less before changing to buprenorphine.

Start-up doses of buprenorphine are typically 2 to 4 mg every 6 hours, with supplemental doses of 2 mg given every 2 to 4 hours as needed. When the patient is comfortable, the dosage can be tapered down over ensuing days or weeks. Physicians who prescribe buprenorphine in the treatment of opioid addiction must obtain a waiver from federal methadone regulations through the Substance Abuse and Mental Health Services Administration. Physicians obtaining such a waiver may prescribe buprenorphine for inpatient or outpatient management and no special hospital license is required. It should be noted that all opioid detoxification and drug-free approaches enjoy limited success in terms of treatment retention and prevention of relapse.[8]

Maintenance therapy for opioid dependence, on the other hand, involves the replacement of abused opioids with medically prescribed slow-onset, long-acting opioids that have reduced abuse potential. Such medications exhibit cross-tolerance at the opioid receptor thus preventing opioid withdrawal and they compete with opioid receptor binding sites, thereby blocking the effects of self-administered exogenous opioids such as heroin. Contrary to the detoxification process, no attempt at weaning the medication is performed once stabilization is achieved. Maintenance treatment is sustained as long as the patient continues to benefit, is at continued risk of relapse, has no serious side effects, and the clinician believes such treatment is still required. In contrast to detoxification therapy, multiple controlled studies clearly support the effectiveness of maintenance therapy on treatment retention[9] as well as on reduction of illicit opioid use, criminal activities, and human immunodeficiency virus seroconversion.[10] We prefer to use either methadone (available to outpatients only through federally regulated methadone clinics), buprenorphine, or the combination of buprenorphine and naloxone for maintenance therapy. As noted above, physicians obtaining a waiver from federal methadone regulations can prescribe both preparations of buprenorphine for opioid dependence.

Initial maintenance dosing of buprenorphine is 4 mg or buprenorphine/naloxone 4/1 mg. Subsequent daily dosing should be increased by 2 to 4 mg to achieve a maintenance dose in the range of 12 to 16 mg of buprenorphine. Rarely do patients require dosages exceeding 32 mg. It should be noted that because of the partial agonist nature of the drug, increases in dose are not necessarily reflected by increases in subjective effect. Higher doses do, however, provide more effective blockade of the effects of illicit opioids. All patients, unless they have significant contraindications such as pregnancy or hypersensitivity to naloxone, should be maintained on the combination product to minimize the possibility of diversion and abuse.[11] Switching from buprenorphine alone to the combination product is done maintaining the same dosage of buprenorphine. Usually buprenorphine can be administered once daily, although many patients prefer divided doses.

Tramadol (Ultram) is an analgesic that works through modulation of the GABAergic, noradrenergic, and serotonergic systems. Its analgesic and dependence properties stem from its action at the mu opioid receptor. Even though it has liability for dependence, it is not currently scheduled by the U.S. Drug Enforcement Administration. It may cause seizures while being abused in doses of more than 500 mg (10 tablets) daily but not in the withdrawal phase. Signs and symptoms of withdrawal may include typical opioid withdrawal and/or atypical withdrawal symptoms such as severe anxiety and panic attacks, confusion, delusions, hallucinations, depersonalization, derealization, paranoia, and unusual sensory phenomena such as numbness, tingling, paresthesia, and tinnitus. Detoxification consists of gradual dose reduction, low-dose benzodiazepines, or both, especially in the case of atypical withdrawal.

Table 3 Benzodiazepine Dose Equivalency

Generic Drug	Brand Name	Equivalent Dose (mg)
Alprazolam	Xanax	1
Chlordiazepoxide	Librium	25
Clonazepam	Klonopin	2
Diazepam	Valium	10
Flurazepam	Dalmane	15
Lorazepam	Ativan	1
Oxazepam	Serax	10
Temazepam	Restoril	15

Benzodiazepines

Signs and symptoms of benzodiazepine withdrawal are more or less similar to alcohol withdrawal. In milder forms these include anxiety, insomnia, tremors, brisk reflexes, dilated pupils, progressive weakness, dizziness, and nausea or vomiting. A more severe form may also include tonic-clonic seizures, delirium, confusion, disorientation, agitation, hypertension, tachycardia, and visual hallucinations.

Generally, a longer-acting benzodiazepine such as chlordiazepoxide (Librium) is used for detoxification because it can be tapered more easily without risk of abrupt withdrawal. Also, it is less likely to be used illicitly. Chlordiazepoxide must be used cautiously in individuals with liver dysfunction because its psychoactive metabolites can build up quickly to toxic levels. The initial dosage depends on the pattern of illicit use and manifestation of symptoms, such as elevation of blood pressure or pulse rate, temperature, tremor, and hyper-reflexiveness. Patients with delirium or with a history of seizures associated with benzodiazepine withdrawal should be treated with a much slower taper. Antipsychotics may be helpful for agitation and psychotic symptoms associated with delirium. Anticonvulsant medications such as phenytoin in addition to the benzodiazepine should be used if deemed necessary for seizures or seizure prophylaxis.

Withdrawal from benzodiazepines may last several weeks and often requires a gradual taper of medication. The dosage of chlordiazepoxide is anywhere between 10 and 100 mg orally every 6 hours plus additional doses of 10 to 50 mg every 6 hours as needed. The total requirement in the initial 24 hours is the starting dose, which is tapered subsequently. Many physicians outside of the setting of addiction medicine are not familiar with chlordiazepoxide and prefer to use the same benzodiazepine that the patient used illicitly for detoxification. This approach works well for mild addiction but the longer-acting benzodiazepines are still preferable for more severe forms. Dosage conversions for benzodiazepines are shown in Table 3.

Some physicians avoid medications with abuse potential for detoxification and rely on gabapentin (Neurontin) because it acts on the GABA receptors similar to the benzodiazepines and has anticonvulsant properties. The dosage range of gabapentin is between 300 and 3600 mg daily in three divided doses. The initial dosing depends on the extent of daily benzodiazepine use and manifestations of withdrawal. Neurontin is tapered as tolerated.

Barbiturates and Sedative-Hypnotics

The recognition of sedative addiction comes about by observing a pattern of increasingly heavy use of sedatives, such as carisoprodol (Soma), whose breakdown product, meprobamate, is a powerful sedative, or barbiturate analgesics, such as butalbital (Fiorinal).

Barbiturates tend to produce rapid sedation and tolerance. These drugs can cause withdrawal convulsions if the dosage is reduced too rapidly. Because of this, the detoxification process should be done on an inpatient basis. For barbiturate detoxification, an initial challenge dose of 200 mg of pentobarbital sodium (Nembutal) is used to assess patient tolerance. If the patient becomes drowsy or ataxic or presents with nystagmus, tolerance is mild and only a modest dosage schedule is indicated, such as 100 to 200 mg of pentobarbital by mouth four times daily. If no effect is seen 2 hours after the initial challenge dose, a stronger regimen may be required, such as 300 to 400 mg by mouth four times daily. A slow taper of the dosage from these starting levels and supplementation with anticonvulsants such as phenytoin, should then be undertaken.

Cocaine

Cocaine withdrawal causes symptoms of autonomic arousal such as palpitations and sweating along with anxiety and dysphoria. It also causes intense craving, which has been postulated to be due to the β-adrenergic system, involved in augmenting the memory related to emotionally arousing systems. Propranolol, which is a nonselective β-adrenergic antagonist, has been shown to reduce the anxiety and symptoms of autonomic arousal associated with cocaine craving. Also, propranolol may decrease the reinforcing effects of cocaine and reduce cocaine desirability. This may lead to improved treatment adherence and abstinence. In a recent 10-week double-blind study, 199 patients dependent on cocaine with severe withdrawal symptoms were assigned to propranolol, amantadine, or placebo. It was found that, among patients who were highly compliant with treatment medication, propranolol treatment was associated with better treatment retention and higher rates of cocaine abstinence compared with placebo.[12] These data are consistent with previous studies with propranolol on similar subsets of cocaine addicts.

Some studies have involved the use of antidepressants for cocaine dependence, especially for dysphoria associated with cocaine withdrawal, with varying results. These studies indicate that tricyclic antidepressants, such as imipramine or desipramine may reduce craving for cocaine and at the same time exert antidepressant action for general dysphoria. We recommend the use of a combination of propranolol and imipramine. The dosing of propranolol is 20 mg three times daily and that of imipramine is 25 mg three times daily.

Cocaine-induced delusions, which mostly occur during intoxication, usually cease in a few hours without the use of pharmacotherapy. It may be helpful to use antipsychotics or benzodiazepines if the delusions are severe or causing distress to the patient. For cocaine-induced vasospasm, which may involve the coronary arteries producing angina or cerebral vasculature producing stroke, appropriate treatment should be given, preferably in the intensive care setting.

Amphetamines

After prolonged heavy use of amphetamines, a withdrawal syndrome may occur. Often referred to as "crashing," this phenomenon is characterized by depressed mood, fatigue, disturbed sleep, and pronounced dreaming. Amphetamines suppress REM sleep and can cause a rebound increase in REM sleep after the drug is withdrawn. Beginning within 24 hours after the last dose, the patient may sleep for increasing periods, up to 18 to 20 hours per day for the next 72 hours. Other symptoms include irritability, impulsivity, insatiable hunger, headaches, profuse sweating, and muscle or stomach cramps. The depression generally peaks 48 to 72 hours after the last dose and persists for several weeks. Suicidal ideation occasionally occurs during this period. If depression persists longer, an underlying disorder should be considered and antidepressant therapy should be instituted. There is no generally accepted detoxification agent, although dextroamphetamine, methylphenidate, imipramine, and bupropion have been used.[13-15]

Treatment of patients presenting with amphetamine-induced psychosis, in an acutely intoxicated, agitated, or delusional state requires inpatient supervision. These patients should be placed in a quiet room and provided with reassurance. Intramuscular haloperidol (Haldol) 1 to 5 mg three times daily for the first day, and as needed thereafter, should be started if necessary for the control of agitation. Diazepam (Valium) 10 to 20 mg orally or intramuscularly may be substituted, especially if the patient has seizures. It is also vital to establish a follow-up relationship with the patient, explaining that episodes of depression, apathy, and lack of initiative may occur over the next 2 to 4 months and that this may tempt the patient to resume amphetamine use.

Behavioral Approach

Treatment Setting

There are three kinds of treatment settings available to patients, depending on the severity of their addiction.[16] The first is inpatient hospitalization, wherein patients who are intoxicated or withdrawing from drugs have serious medical or psychiatric comorbid conditions or uncontrolled drug use with previous failed treatments. The second one is residential treatment, wherein people having significant deficits in social or vocational skills are placed and specially trained in such areas and other strategies to help them stay sober. The third option involves either partial hospitalization, where patients are not at risk for withdrawal or other clinical comorbid conditions, or intensive outpatient programs that meet three to five times weekly for a few months. Outpatient aftercare visits on a weekly basis in individual or group settings are strongly advised.

Follow-up

During hospitalization for detoxification, the patient and physician should establish a plan for a long-term follow-up program and other specialized treatments. Appropriateness for a residential chemical dependency rehabilitation program should be considered. Such programs provide an intense educational and motivational experience, overcoming denial and resistance in a supportive milieu. Outpatient aftercare programs are appropriate when reasonable abstinence and emotional and physical stability are achieved.

Urine Monitoring

We suggest frequent randomized urine testing for a minimum of 1 to 2 years for most patients. Most of these urine checks are obtained randomly, approximately once a week, and are collected under supervision.

Self-Help Groups

These include Alcoholic Anonymous (AA), Narcotic Anonymous (NA), Cocaine Anonymous (CA), and others. Such groups provide frequent and powerful therapeutic reinforcement for recovering patients. As a rule, patients are mandated to attend these self-help groups, and attendance usually begins during the initial treatment episode.

Psychotherapy

There have been much data to suggest that psychotherapy is an important tool in promoting sobriety. It includes cognitive-behavioral therapy, individual therapy, interpersonal therapy, group therapy, and other modalities. The main goal of any of these modalities is to motivate the patient to remain abstinent from drugs, to teach coping mechanisms, to improve interpersonal and social skills, to build a support system, and to teach stress management. All of these assist the patient in forgoing perceived rewards of resuming substance use as well as tolerating the withdrawal symptoms which can be prolonged in some cases.

Recovering patients need to be given respect and praise for maintaining an abstinence program and for participating in treatment modalities. They have to sacrifice much in the way of time, energy, and expense to conquer this illness. Understanding, praise, and firm support are a physician's most important tools.

Aftercare

It is important to continue the physician-patient relationship following the detoxification period. Patients should be encouraged to bring all their requests for medications and other medical consultations to the treating physician's attention first. We recommend prohibiting the ingestion of any medication other than ibuprofen without prior approval. We also check periodically for intravenous injection tracks on our needle-using patients. Urine toxicology screens should be performed regularly. It is important to avoid prescribing any psychoactive drugs especially sedatives, analgesics, and tranquilizers. These medications carry a substantial risk of inducing medical dependency. One should strongly recommend to medication-dependent patients that they abstain from drinking alcohol. In many such patients, drinking escalates rapidly to full-blown alcoholism, whereas in other people, drinking leads to relapse of drug use. It is important to maintain close contact with patient's spouse or family for at least 1 to 2 years.

It is best to regard addiction as a chronic, relapsing condition that is never cured, only held in remission. It requires lifelong commitment on the part of the patient and appropriate support from the physician to treat this potentially fatal illness.

Summary

Pharmacotherapy

- *Opiates*: Although complete abstinence is desirable, maintenance therapy with methadone or buprenorphine is of proven benefit.
- *Benzodiazepines*: Withdrawal may be prolonged and detoxification with long-acting agents is preferred.
- *Barbiturates*: Detoxification should be performed on an inpatient basis because of a risk of seizures.
- *Cocaine*: Combination of propranolol and imipramine might be helpful for dysphoria and craving.
- *Amphetamines*: Depressive symptoms accompany withdrawal and require ongoing support and occasionally medication to prevent relapse.

Behavioral Approach

- Behavior modification should be used early on in the treatment process to help teach skills needed for long-term sobriety.

PREVENTION

Effective prevention of substance-related disorders begins with an appreciation that abuse can easily become dependence and that patients who are chemically dependent are addicted to the substance that is destroying their lives. Primary prevention for physicians involves premorbid educational efforts, particularly those directed at adolescents, as well as cautious prescribing practices when administering addictive medications. Medication abuse can be difficult to detect because the addicted person often offers plausible reasons for needing the medications. The clinician should be wary of the signs of addiction and always obtain a substance abuse history before prescribing controlled drugs. It is important to remember that dependence is chronic and lifelong, and that patients with a history of drug dependence are always at high risk of addictive relapse if mood-altering drugs are reintroduced to them. Secondary prevention involves early recognition and treatment of developing cases and very often depends on the physician's awareness of the prevalence of substance abuse in any patient population, recognition of classic behavioral signs and patterns suggesting addiction, and discretion and judgment in refusing to prescribe addictive medications. Substance-related behaviors, including noncompliance, denial, or even hostility can place formidable obstacles in the path of the treating physician and challenge even the most experienced clinicians.

Suggested Readings

American Psychiatric Association. Diagnostic and Statistical Manual of Mental Disorders, 4th ed, text rev. Washington, DC: American Psychiatric Association, 2000.

American Psychiatric Association. Practice Guideline for the Treatment of Patients with Substance Use Disorders, 2nd ed. Washington, DC: American Psychiatric Association, 2006.

Chan-OB T, Kuntawongse N, Boonyanaruthee V: Bupropion for amphetamine withdrawal syndrome. J Med Assoc Thai 2001;84(12):1763-1765.

Collins GB, McAllister MS: Buprenorphine in the management of opioid dependence. Cleve Clin J Med 2007;74:514-520.

Fiellin DA, Kleber H, Trumble-Hejduk JG, et al: Consensus statement on office-based treatment of opioid dependence using buprenorphine. J Subst Abuse Treat 2004;27(2):153-159.

Fleming PM, Roberts D: Is the prescription of amphetamine justified as harm reduction measure? J R Soc Health 1994;114(3):127-131.

Galloway G, Newmeyer J, Knapp T, et al: Imipramine for the treatment of cocaine and methamphetamine dependence. J Addict Dis 1994;13(4):201-216.

Kampman KM, Dackis C, Lynch KG, et al: A double-blind, placebo-controlled trial of amantadine, propranolol, and their combination for the treatment of cocaine dependence in patients with severe cocaine withdrawal symptoms. Drug Alcohol Depend 2006;85:129-137.

Marsch LA: The efficacy of methadone maintenance interventions in reducing illicit opiate use, HIV risk behavior, and criminality: A meta-analysis. Addiction 1998;93(4):515-532.

Mayfield D, McLeod G, Hall P: The CAGE questionnaire: Validation of a new alcoholism screening instrument. Am J Psychiatry 1974;131:1121-1123.

O'Connor PG: Methods of detoxification and their role in treating patients with opioid dependence. JAMA 2005;294(8):961-963.

Skinner HA: The Drug Abuse Screening Test. Addict Behav 1982;7:363-371.

Strain EC, Bigelow GE, Liebson IA, et al: Moderate- vs high-dose methadone in the treatment of opioid dependence: a randomized trial. JAMA 1999;281(11):1000-1005.

Substance Abuse and Mental Health Services Administration, Office of Applied Studies. Results from the 2004 National Survey on Drug Use and Health: National Findings (NSDUH Series H-28, DHHS Publication No. SMA 05-4062). Rockville, Md, Department of Health and Human Services, 2005.

Substance Abuse and Mental Health Services Administration, Office of Applied Studies. Treatment Episode Data Set (TEDS): 1993-2003. National Admissions to Substance Abuse Treatment Services (DASIS Series: S-29, DHHS Publication No. SMA 05-4118). Rockville, Md, Department of Health and Human Services, 2005.

Substance Abuse and Mental Health Services Administration, Office of Applied Studies. Risk and Protective Factors for Adolescent Drug Use: Findings from the 1999 National Household Survey on Drug Abuse (Analytic Series A-19, DHHS Publication No. SMA 04-3874). Rockville, Md, Department of Health and Human Services, 2004.

References

For a complete list of references, log onto www.expertconsult.com.

Alcohol Abuse and Dependence

David Streem

The *Diagnostic and Statistical Manual of Mental Disorders*, fourth edition, text revision (DSM IV-TR) lists diagnostic criteria for substance abuse and substance dependence. The criteria are applied to all potentially habit-forming substances, of which alcohol is only one. Taken as a whole, however, the underlying problem in substance-use disorders is an inability to control substance intake with resulting social, occupational, and medical consequences.

PREVALENCE AND RISK FACTORS

Alcohol dependence affects 10% to 15% of men and 3% to 8% of women at some point in their lifetime. This translates into a point prevalence of about 4% and 5% for alcohol dependence and abuse, respectively. Meanwhile, it has been reported that 30% of the American populace engage in risky or unhealthy drinking patterns, defined as at least five standard drinks per day or 15 standard drinks per week for men, or at least four standard drinks per day or eight standard drinks per week for women. A standard drink in the United States is defined as a drink containing about 14 grams of pure alcohol, the content of alcohol in 12 ounces of beer, 5 ounces of table wine, or 1.5 ounces of 80-proof whiskey (http://www.niaaa.nih.gov/NR/rdonlyres/1D2BE3DF-18D7-47EE-98C5-E907C7611929/0/StandardDrink.pdf). The prevalence of alcohol dependence in primary care settings ranges from 20% to 36%, pointing to the medical comorbidity suffered by alcohol-dependent patients and the value of screening for the disorder. Currently, it is estimated that only about 10% of patients with alcohol dependence are recognized and receive proper intervention in primary care settings.

The role of family and genetic history in increasing the risk of alcohol-use disorders cannot be overstated. Many studies have demonstrated that the presence of a first-degree relative with alcohol dependence increases the risk of the disorder from 8% to 25%. There appears to be special transmissibility of alcohol dependence when the relationship is between an alcohol-dependent father and a son. This relationship increases the risk to the son even more dramatically. A pattern of early onset (before age 25 years) and the presence of antisocial personality disorder in the alcohol-dependent parent can increase the risk even further. Children of nonalcoholics raised in adoptive alcoholic homes do not exhibit increased risk of alcohol dependence, whereas children of alcoholic parents suffer an elevated risk even if adopted by nonalcoholics at a young age.

Other significant risk factors include other psychiatric disorders, such as major depression, bipolar disorder, panic disorder, generalized anxiety disorder, attention-deficit disorder, and schizophrenia. No protection is provided by high educational level or socioeconomic status.

PATHOPHYSIOLOGY AND NATURAL HISTORY

Particular behaviors are associated with a higher risk of addiction. Children displaying low levels of harm avoidance and reward dependence and a high potential for novelty seeking are at high risk for alcohol dependence later in life. These children are apparently relatively less fearful of potentially dangerous activities, less interested in reward or approval from others, and attracted to unfamiliar experiences.

First exposure to alcohol seems to have less impact on a person's risk of developing alcohol-use disorders than the age at first intoxication. However, these differences are small compared with what commonly happens in young adults developing alcohol use disorders. During this time, most persons experience moderation in alcohol intake in response to negative feedback from social systems (peers, family, work, legal) and a personal recognition of transient physical and emotional consequences of drinking excessively such as depressed mood, nausea, and headache.

Many persons with a genetic predisposition to alcohol-use disorders are insensitive to the unpleasant effects of alcohol intoxication such as sedation, ataxia, and incoordination. They seem to function better than their peers after an equal intake of alcohol. As their frequency and amount of drinking per occasion increase, activity in the reward centers of the brain declines. Without alcohol present, stimulation of the nucleus accumbens and activity of the prefrontal cortex are low enough to produce dysphoria and cravings. The effects of other life consequences (either positive or negative) on reward circuit functioning are diminished, so that only changes in brain alcohol concentration have reinforcing value. Eventually, the person becomes unable to function at all without constantly maintaining brain alcohol concentrations within an increasingly narrow range. Levels just below this range cause dysphoria and cravings, and levels just above this range result in unconsciousness, gait abnormalities, incontinence, or inability to function in the person's particular environment.

SIGNS AND SYMPTOMS

Box 1 lists some of the symptoms of which patients complain that should lead a health care provider to consider alcohol dependence.

The development of tolerance is also a feature of alcohol dependence. *Tolerance* is defined by DSM IV-TR as "either a need for markedly increased amounts of [alcohol] to achieve intoxication or desired effect, [or] markedly diminished effect with continued use of the same amount of [alcohol]." An additional consideration when the substance abused is alcohol is switching one's drink of choice to accommodate increasing alcohol intake. For example, a change from beer or wine as the alcoholic beverage of choice to whiskey or vodka, or a change from consuming mixed drinks to unmixed liquor suggests progression of the disease.

Early signs of excessive drinking, even legal activities like driving under the influence (DUI), domestic violence, assault and battery, or drunk and disorderly conduct are often ignored, minimized, or rationalized by patients. Although legal charges, job failures, or marital strain lead a person to cut down on his or her drinking temporarily, many struggle to convince themselves they still can control their drinking by restricting the settings, times, or amounts they drink. For example, they might try restricting drinking to family settings, drink only in the evening, or abstain from "hard" liquor such as whiskey or vodka.

Well-intentioned attempts to cut down or control use are often *illusory* and unsuccessful. Typically, after struggling to maintain previously set limits on alcohol use, persons begin violating those limits by drinking alone or in secret; hiding alcohol around the house, in the car, or at work; coming up with other reasons to explain absences from home and from work, or resorting to cough syrup or mouthwash that contains alcohol.

DIAGNOSIS

A variety of instruments are available for detecting alcohol dependence. Perhaps the simplest and most familiar is the CAGE questionnaire. Box 2 reviews the components of the CAGE questionnaire.

Box 1 Problems that Can Suggest Alcohol Dependence

Tremors
Insomnia
Depressed mood
Generalized anxiety
Panic attacks
Weight or appetite change
Falls, dizziness, or poor balance
Memory loss
Poor concentration
Fatigue
Cardiomyopathy
Elevated liver enzymes
Thrombocytopenia
Anemia
Headache
Nausea or vomiting
Abdominal pain
Hematemesis
Hypertension not responding to treatment

Box 2 CAGE Questionnaire

Have you ever felt you should **C**ut down your alcohol intake?
Have you ever felt **A**nnoyed by criticism of your drinking?
Have you ever felt **G**uilty about your drinking?
Have you ever taken a drink first thing in the morning (**E**ye-opener) to steady your nerves?

Answering "yes" to one of the four questions in the CAGE increases the likelihood of an alcohol-use disorder to at least 90%. Although the CAGE is fast and easy to administer and score, it does suffer from some limitations. Its sensitivity varies among different cultures and it is less sensitive in women. Also, some questions are more sensitive to a diagnosis of alcohol dependence than others.

Developed by the World Health Organization, the Alcohol Use Disorders Identification Test (AUDIT) has been validated in several cultures and provides good sensitivity in both genders. The test is a 10-item multiple-choice questionnaire that takes 5 minutes to complete and is easily scored. Scoring has been tied to intervention recommendations with several different levels of intensity. If certain questions with higher sensitivity are answered in the scored direction, it will increase the intensity of the intervention recommendation. A free AUDIT manual with guidelines for use in primary care is available online (http://whqlibdoc.who.int/hq/2001/WHO_MSD_MSB_01.6a.pdf).

When either the CAGE or the AUDIT raises the suspicion of an alcohol-use disorder, a full alcohol and drug history should be obtained from the patient and confirmed (if possible) by a knowledgable third party such as a spouse or parent. Especially important data are peak alcohol use, frequency and amount of alcohol use over the last month, and time and amount of last alcohol use. Also important are past consequences (legal, social, occupational), medical complications such as delirium tremens, withdrawal tremors or seizures, and longest period of abstinence from alcohol.

The DSM IV-TR criteria for the diagnosis of substance (in this case alcohol) abuse include whether any recurrent social, legal, or interpersonal problems related to alcohol use have occurred in the last 12 months. Any recurrent failure of major role obligations, recurrent legal problems, or social or interpersonal problems related to alcohol satisfy the criteria listed in Box 3. In the case of alcohol dependence, the criteria are more exclusive and are listed in Box 4. In the case of a person who meets criteria for both conditions, only the diagnosis of substance dependence is made.

Box 3 DSM IV-TR Diagnostic Criteria for Substance Abuse

Substance abuse is a maladaptive pattern of substance use leading to clinically significant impairment or distress as manifested by at least one of the following and occurring within a 12-month period:

- Recurrent substance use, resulting in a failure to fulfill major role obligations at work, school, or home (e.g., repeated absences or poor work performance related to substance use; substance-related absences, suspensions, or expulsions from school; neglect of children or household)
- Recurrent substance use in situations in which it is potentially hazardous (e.g., driving an automobile or operating a machine when impaired by substance use)
- Recurrent substance-related legal problems (e.g., arrests for substance-related disorderly conduct)
- Continued substance use despite having persistent or recurrent social or interpersonal problems caused or exacerbated by the effects of the substance (e.g., arguments with spouse about consequences of intoxication, physical fights)

The symptoms have never met the criteria for substance dependence for this class of substance.

DSM-IV-TR, Diagnostic and Statistical Manual of Mental Disorders, fourth edition, text revision.

Box 4 DSM IV-TR Diagnostic Criteria for Substance Dependence

Substance dependence is a maladaptive pattern of substance use leading to clinically significant impairment or distress as manifested by at least three of the following and occurring at any time in the same 12-month period:

- Tolerance, as defined by either of the following:
  - A need for markedly increased amounts of the substance to achieve intoxication or desired effect
  - Markedly diminished effect with continued use of the same amount of the substance
- Withdrawal, as manifested by either of the following:
  - The characteristic withdrawal syndrome for the substance
  - The same (or a closely related) substance is taken to relieve or avoid withdrawal symptoms
- The substance is often taken in larger amounts or over a longer period than was intended.
- There is a persistent desire or unsuccessful efforts to cut down or control substance use.
- A great deal of time is spent in activities necessary to obtain the substance (e.g., visiting multiple doctors or driving long distances), use the substance (e.g., chain-smoking), or recover from its effects.
- Important social, occupational, or recreational activities are given up or reduced because of substance use.
- The substance use is continued even though a persistent or recurrent physical or psychological problem is likely caused or exacerbated by the substance (e.g., current cocaine use despite recognition of cocaine-induced depression, or continued drinking despite recognition that an ulcer was made worse by alcohol consumption).

DSM-IV-TR, Diagnostic and Statistical Manual of Mental Disorders, fourth edition, text revision.

Laboratory Tests

Detecting acute ingestion of alcohol is a relatively simple matter. For \$100 to \$400, an outpatient clinic can purchase a breathalyzer that is easy to use and reasonably accurate. Confirmatory testing can be obtained through a blood alcohol level. Other procedures are rapidly gaining popularity, such as saliva test strips and sweat patch testing.

Certain blood tests can detect chronic alcohol consumption. Elevations in the level of γ-glutamyl transferase (GGT) can be caused by consuming four or more drinks per day for 4 to 8 weeks before the test. At least 4 weeks of abstinence may be required to return the GGT to the normal range. The most significant limitation of relying on the GGT is that it is elevated in other illnesses (e.g., viral

Box 5 Typical Initial Laboratory Examination of Patients with Alcohol-Use Disorders

Blood alcohol level
Complete blood count (CBC), including mean corpuscular volume (MCV)
Complete metabolic panel
Electrocardiogram
γ-Glutamyl transferase (GGT)
Human immunodeficiency virus (HIV)
Tuberculosis purified protein derivative (PPD)
Remote viral hepatitis panel
Thyroid-stimulating hormone (TSH)
Urine drug screen

hepatitis, certain prescription medications). Patients with severe liver damage might not have enough viable hepatic tissue for alcohol consumption to generate an elevated GGT. In known alcoholics without significant nonalcoholic liver disease, however, an elevated GGT should raise suspicion of relapse.

Measurement of carbohydrate-deficient transferrin (CDT) is being used more often to screen for excessive drinking. Although it may be currently less available and usually cannot be completed as quickly as a GGT, the CDT does offer some advantages. The CDT becomes elevated within 1 to 2 weeks of heavy drinking, identifying excessive drinking patterns possibly more quickly than GGT. Also, the CDT is not affected by cirrhosis or viral hepatitis.

Red blood cell mean corpuscular volume (MCV), aspartate aminotransferase (AST), and alanine aminotransferase (ALT) also may be elevated in patients engaging in heavy alcohol consumption; however, these tend only to provide supporting evidence. The sensitivity and specificity of these tests are simply too low for proof of alcohol consumption without other, more reliable evidence.

These biochemical markers of alcohol consumption cannot assess one of the key features needed for the diagnosis of alcohol-use disorders: consequences. For this reason, research groups have assessed the increased sensitivity and specificity of combining self-report questionnaires with biochemical markers. For example, the combined finding of an AUDIT score greater than 8 with at least two abnormal biologic markers of heavy alcohol consumption resulted in a combined test with sensitivity and specificity greater than 90%, and it improved the positive predictive value over the AUDIT used alone.

Once a diagnosis of an alcohol-use disorder is made, several tests should be performed to assess for other conditions that either commonly exist with alcohol dependence or can exacerbate the damage caused by heavy alcohol consumption. These are listed in Box 5.

Practice Guidelines

The National Institute on Alcohol Abuse and Alcoholism has published a practice guideline for primary care physicians. The guide (and other useful information for physicians and patients) can be downloaded from the NIAAA website.

Summary

- Patients with a family history of addiction are at high risk themselves.
- Patients with any of a number of common psychiatric disorders are also at risk.
- CAGE and AUDIT are useful screening tools.
- γ-Glutamyl transferase (GGT) and carbohydrate-deficient transferrin (CDT) can be useful markers of excessive alcohol use.

TREATMENT

Intervention and Lifestyle Modifications

Once an alcohol-use disorder is identified, the next step is presenting the diagnosis and recommendations to the patient. Because denial and minimization are common in addiction, the initial intervention is especially important. Depending on the situation, family members can help by reinforcing a physician's concerns and recommendations.

The physician should start by expressing his or her concerns based on as many hard facts, specifically applicable to the patient, as are available. Next, the physician should frame the problem as a disease and absolve the patient of any sense of responsibility for the development of the disease. It should be emphasized, however, that responsibility for proper management of this disease rests with the patient. The physician should convey confidence that change is possible, and then present clear advice on what choices the patient has for addressing the problem.

Without enlisting the patient's motivation to change the situation, treatment outcome will likely suffer. The patient must assert some control over the decision to enter treatment, but it is perfectly appropriate for that decision to be influenced by family, occupational, legal, or medical consequences if positive steps toward recovery do not occur. The goal of an intervening person (personal physician, employer, spouse, or someone else) is not to shield the patient from such consequences but to point them out and to empathize with and support the patient.

What specific recommendations should be made? In actively drinking patients with a history of withdrawal seizures or delirium tremens, immediate referral to a hospital-based chemical dependency treatment center is essential. Similarly, patients with signs of active withdrawal, such as tremor, hyperreflexia, palmar diaphoresis, tachycardia, or hypertension, are at risk for withdrawal complications and should be referred for inpatient management. Patients who have consumed alcohol in the 72 hours before assessment might still be at risk for developing withdrawal or delirium tremens and should be monitored carefully. Thiamine prophylaxis for Wernicke's encephalopathy should begin immediately.

For patients meeting the criteria for alcohol dependence but not in danger of developing withdrawal, a strong recommendation for abstinence from alcohol should be made. All alcohol should be removed from the home. If the home environment does not facilitate sobriety, referral should be made to a residential chemical dependency treatment center where the patient can focus on recovery without distraction. Because social isolation can be a relapse trigger for many alcoholics, living alone outside the controlled environment of a residential treatment center should be discouraged. Alternatively, the patient can move to a residence with a sober, stable support system while participating in outpatient treatment.

Patients meeting criteria for alcohol abuse but not alcohol dependence should remove alcohol from the home and avoid situations potentially associated with alcohol-related consequences. Abstinence from alcohol should be recommended, especially if the patient has comorbid psychiatric disorders or a family history of addiction. Attending self-help meetings should also be recommended.

The presence of complicating medical conditions (e.g., a preexisting seizure disorder, hepatic encephalopathy) can lead the physician to encourage a higher level of care than would be indicated without such a comorbid condition. Similarly, complex psychiatric comorbidity, limited acceptance of addiction diagnosis, nonsupportive home environment, or recent failure to maintain abstinence at a lower level of care should also lead to placing a patient at the partial hospital or inpatient levels of care. The American Society of Addiction Medicine patient placement criteria include recommendations for the correct treatment level in a particular situation.

In a patient who has agreed to enter treatment and abstain from alcohol, a critical step in early recovery is identification of triggers.

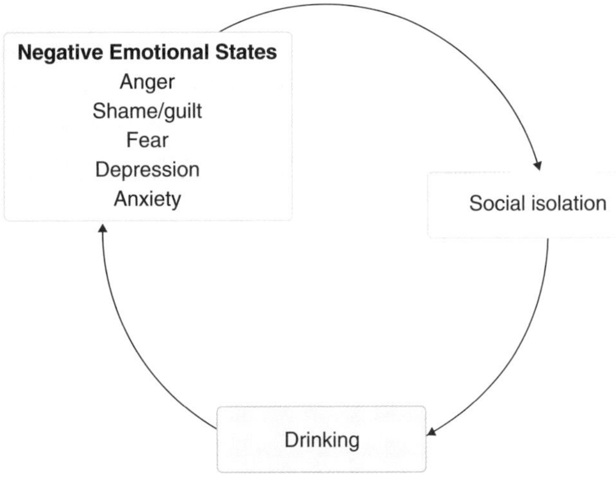

Figure 1 The self-reinforcing addictive cycle.

Box 6 Common Relapse Triggers

- Negative emotional states (e.g., anger, shame, guilt, depression, loneliness, fear)
- Negative physical states (e.g., insomnia, fatigue, chronic pain)
- Positive emotional states
- Intimacy
- Social drinking
- Interpersonal conflicts in family or at work
- Social pressure
- Urge to drink

Triggers are situations, people, emotions, or problems that can place a person at high risk for relapse. In the brain, the potential for reactivation of abnormal activity in reward circuitry can last many years into recovery. Common triggers are listed in Box 6. When potential triggers are identified, a relapse prevention plan particular to that trigger can be quickly developed in the office. For example, a patient identifies as a trigger the local bar where he or she engaged in after-work drinking. With the help of a physician, nurse, or counselor, the patient can develop a relapse prevention plan to attend a self-help meeting each day immediately after work instead of heading home along the usual route past the bar. A list of after-work meetings can be developed and kept in the patient's car, purse, or briefcase.

By far the most common trigger leading to relapse is the failure to cope effectively with negative emotional states. As seen in Figure 1, negative emotional states lead to social isolation and eventual drinking. Twelve-step programs (e.g., Alcoholics Anonymous) spend a great deal of time discussing healthier coping strategies for negative emotional states. In fact, only step 1 of the 12 steps mentions alcohol at all. The other 11 steps concentrate mainly on managing anger, guilt, shame, anxiety, and social isolation.

Alcoholics Anonymous and other 12-step programs attempt to create a fellowship of recovering people who support each other through the recovery process and who provide validation, a sense of social connectedness, and mentorship. The mentorship component of the program is provided by a sponsor. A sponsor is a member of the 12-step program with several years of sobriety who assists new members in finding appropriate meetings, identifying triggers, and working through the steps. Sponsors often have a great deal of contact with persons who are early in recovery or experiencing difficulty staying sober. Sponsors, always of the same gender, should have limited or no direct connection to the newly recovering person before the decision to join the program. Persons often obtain a sponsor by informing the leaders of a recovery meeting that they need a sponsor.

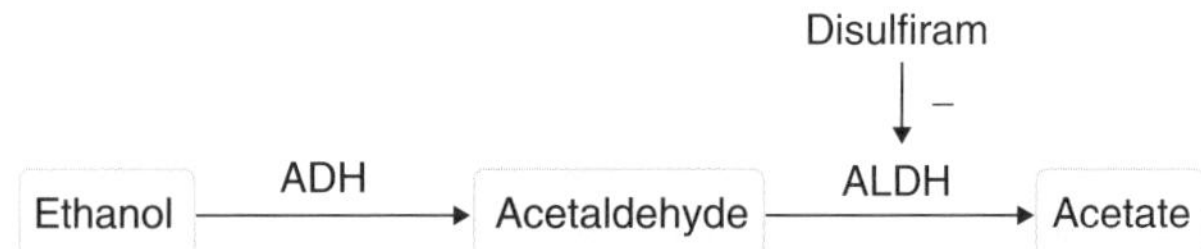

Figure 2 **Mechanism of action of disulfiram.** ADH, alcohol dehydrogenase; ALDH, aldehyde dehydrognase.

As a newly recovering person begins changing his or her behavior, regular medical management interventions during early recovery can improve treatment outcomes. A typical brief intervention after an initial decision to engage in treatment includes a review of exposure to triggers and asking about any exposure to alcohol between visits. Identification of triggers associated with any relapses should lead to a relapse prevention plan to reduce the likelihood of future relapse. Recovery meeting attendance and intensity of sponsor contact should be logged. The patient is strongly encouraged to obtain a sponsor as soon as possible if he or she has not yet identified one. Adherence with medication prescribed is discussed and side effects noted. Family members are encouraged to attend family support meetings through organizations such as Al-Anon and Alateen.

Medical Options

An increasing number of medications have been approved by the U.S. Food and Drug Administration (FDA) for the treatment of alcohol dependence.

The first FDA approval was granted to disulfiram, an aversive therapy that interferes with the enzyme aldehyde dehydrogenase (ALDH), as shown in Figure 2. When alcohol is ingested, alcohol dehydrogenase metabolizes ethyl alcohol into acetaldehyde. In the presence of disulfiram, ALDH is blocked and acetaldehyde levels rise, causing tachycardia, hypertension, headache, nausea, vomiting, and in rare cases, death. Disulfiram continues to interfere with ALDH functioning up to 2 weeks after the last administered dose. Because of the potential serious consequences of drinking while ALDH is blocked, disulfiram prescription is typically restricted to alcohol-dependent physicians and others who are highly motivated, display low impulsivity, and understand the risks of such a medication in the presence of even tiny amounts of alcohol.

In 1994, the FDA approved naltrexone, an opiate-receptor antagonist, for treating alcohol dependence. In 2006, the FDA approved a depot form of the drug for once-per-month intramuscular administration. Naltrexone's exact mechanism of action in alcohol dependence is unclear, but it might interrupt reinforcement of drinking behavior, which is mediated by the binding of endogenous opioids to receptors in central reward circuitry. Reports of hepatotoxicity warrant regular monitoring of liver function tests.

In 2004, the FDA approved acamprosate, a medication used in Europe for treating alcohol dependence since the early 1990s. Its mechanism of action is unknown, but is believed to involve modulation of the *N*-methyl-D-aspartate (NMDA) glutamate receptor activity. Glutamate binds to NMDA in several areas of the reward circuitry of the brain, opening a calcium channel that results in neuronal excitation. Acamprosate might reduce glutamate-mediated neuronal excitation to overexcite neurons in the most critical brain structures involved in addiction, the nucleus accumbens and the ventral tegmental area. Compared with disulfiram and naltrexone, there are fewer adverse effects and precautions associated with acamprosate. It may be taken by patients with liver dysfunction. It should not be used in patients with severe renal dysfunction.

There are no particular drug-drug interactions that would prevent otherwise healthy people from tolerating combinations of these three medications. However, evidence of added benefit conferred by coadministration of two or all three of the medications is scant.

Treatment Outcomes

At 1 year of sobriety, the factors most associated with good outcome are AA participation, high treatment motivation, and an absence of comorbid psychiatric conditions. *AA participation* implies regular recovery meeting attendance, regular sponsor contact, and actively working through the 12 steps. Treatment of comorbid psychiatric disorders at the start of addiction treatment increases the likelihood of better addiction treatment outcomes.

The effect of available medications on long-term treatment outcomes is unclear. Most current studies of pharmacologic treatment followed patients for a period of 1 year or less. In a recent large study of alcoholism treatment options including oral naltrexone, acamprosate, brief medical follow-ups, or combined behavioral intervention, only acamprosate showed no evidence of improved drinking outcomes at the 1-year follow-up point. Regardless of whether any longer-term treatment effect is demonstrated, currently available medications might still provide benefits in early recovery. The FDA is currently assessing the premarket approval applications for several medications claiming a benefit in treating alcohol dependence.

Summary

- Provide patients with clear but empathic feedback on your concerns, diagnosis, and recommendations.
- Follow-up frequently during the first 6 to 12 months of recovery.
- Medication options may improve outcomes, especially in the short term.
- Long-term outcome is best in motivated patients who participate in 12-step recovery programs and are free from other psychiatric disorders.
- Patients at risk for alcohol withdrawal should be referred to an inpatient chemical dependency program.

PREVENTION AND SCREENING

The key to preventing the development of alcohol-use disorders lies in identifying and educating persons most susceptible to the condition. Because of the high risk suffered by persons with a family history of addiction, family education during addiction treatment is essential. Patients in addiction treatment who have children or are planning to have children should be counseled to discourage alcohol exposure in their children. Patients struggling with other psychiatric disorders that place them at risk for developing an alcohol-use disorder should be advised to abstain from alcohol for the duration of their psychiatric treatment.

SPECIAL POPULATIONS

Pregnant women have the potential to cause the most far-reaching adverse outcomes from drinking alcohol. Beyond the specific risks to the mother, alcohol ingestion in any amount can lead to harmful effects on the developing fetus. It is very important to stress to pregnant women that there is no proven safe level of alcohol use during pregnancy.

Women in general require special attention in addiction treatment for two reasons. First, women in addiction treatment suffer a higher prevalence of comorbid psychiatric disorders than men. Careful evaluation for disorders such as depression, panic disorder, bipolar disorder, and eating disorders is especially important in women. Untreated (or ineffectively treated) comorbid psychiatric disorders will have a negative impact on treatment outcome. Second, because women make up only about one third of the population in addiction treatment, most mixed-gender treatment populations (and mixed self-help groups) contain a majority of men, and as a result tend to focus on men's issues. It is important that women involve themselves in at least some women-only self-help meetings to ensure proper attention to their particular challenges in addiction recovery.

Suggested Readings

American Psychiatric Association: Diagnostic and Statistical Manual of Mental Disorders, 4th ed, text rev. Washington, DC: American Psychiatric Association, 2000.

American Society of Addiction Medicine: Patient Placement Criteria, 2nd rev ed. Philadelphia: Lippincott Williams & Wilkins, 2001.

Anton RF, O'Malley SS, Ciraulo DA, et al: Combined pharmacotherapies and behavioral interventions for alcohol dependence: The COMBINE study: A randomized controlled trial. JAMA 2006 295;17:2003-2017.

Babor TF, Higgins-Biddle JC, Saunders JB, Monteiro MG: The Alcohol Use Disorders Identification Test: Guidelines for use in primary care, 2nd ed. Geneva: World Health Organization, 2001. PDF available at http://whqlibdoc.who.int/hq/2001/WHO_MSD_MSB_01.6a.pdf (accessed March 20, 2009).

Collins GB: Treatment of alcoholism: The role of the primary care physician. Postgrad Med 2003 69;1:145-149.

Dolman JM, Hawkes ND: Combining the AUDIT questionnaire and biochemical markers to assess alcohol use and risk of alcohol withdrawal in medical inpatients. Alcohol Alcohol 40;6:515-519.

Fuller RK, Branchey L, Brightwell DR, et al: Disulfiram treatment of alcoholism: A Veterans Administration cooperative study. JAMA 256;11:1149-1155.

Garbutt JC, Kranzler HR, O'Malley SS, et al: Efficacy and tolerability of long-acting injectable naltrexone for alcohol dependence. JAMA 293;13:1617-1625.

National Institute on Alcohol Abuse and Alcoholism: Helping Patients Who Drink Too Much: A Clinician's Guide, updated 2005 edition. Bethesda, Md, National Institute on Alcohol Abuse and Alcoholism, 2005. Available at http://pubs.niaaa.nih.gov/publications/Practitioner/CliniciansGuide2005/clinicians_guide.htm (accessed March 20, 2009).

Saitz R: Unhealthy alcohol use. N Engl J Med 352;6:596-607.

Shuckit MA, Tapert S: Alcohol. In Galanter M, Kleber HD (eds): The American Psychiatric Association Textbook of Substance Abuse Treatment, 3rd ed. Washington, DC: American Psychiatric Association, 2004, pp 151-166.

Yip L: Ethanol. In Goldfrank LR, Flomenbaum NE, Lewin NA, et al (eds): Goldfrank's Toxicologic Emergencies, 7th ed. New York: McGraw-Hill, 2002, pp 952-965.

Attention-Deficit/Hyperactivity Disorder in Adults

George E. Tesar and Raul J. Seballos

DEFINITION AND ETIOLOGY

Attention-deficit/hyperactivity disorder (ADHD) is the current diagnosis for what was previously labeled *minimal brain damage, minimal brain dysfunction, hyperkinetic impulse disorder,* and *hyperactive child syndrome.*[1] Contrary to popular belief, at least 60% of children with ADHD continue to exhibit features of the disorder during adulthood. ADHD in adults is associated with significant psychiatric morbidity and higher than average rates of divorce, unemployment, substance abuse, and motor vehicle accidents.[2] Poor adjustment and performance can have an erosive effect on self-esteem, leading to clinically significant anxiety or depression, or both, which are often the presenting features of adult ADHD in the primary care setting.

PREVALENCE AND RISK FACTORS

ADHD is a neurobiologic disorder with strong genetic determinants. Strict application of diagnostic criteria has been associated with a mean prevalence of 5% to 7% across studies of children and adolescents.[3] Approximately 60% to 70% of affected children transition into adulthood with some or all of the signs and symptoms of the disorder.[3]

Family and genetic studies have shown ADHD to be the most heritable of psychiatric disorders.[4] Results from the National Comorbidity Survey Replication estimated a 4.4% prevalence of current ADHD in the U.S. adult population.[5] There was a high rate of psychiatric comorbidity in ADHD adults: 38% had a mood disorder, 47% had an anxiety disorder, 15% had a substance-use disorder, and nearly 20% had an impulse-control disorder. The odds of having both ADHD and another disorder were highest for drug dependence (odds ratio [OR], 7.9), dysthymia (OR, 7.5), and bipolar disorder (OR, 7.4).[5]

PATHOPHYSIOLOGY AND NATURAL HISTORY

A variety of neurochemical and neuroanatomic deficits have been associated with ADHD.[1,6,7] Studies employing structural neuroimaging point to an absence, in persons with ADHD, of the frontal lobe asymmetry seen in normal controls[1]; in control subjects (no ADHD), the right frontal lobe tends to be larger than the left. Structural and functional neuroimaging studies have demonstrated decreased function and size of the prefrontal cortex, anterior cingulate, caudate nucleus, and cerebellar vermis in ADHD children, and most (but not all) studies demonstrate this deficit on the right.[6-8]

Candidate gene selection is based on the hypothesis that deficient dopamine availability contributes to ADHD. Genes studied include those relevant to production of proteins involved in dopamine *synthesis* (dopa decarboxylase, the enzyme responsible for conversion of L-dopa to dopamine), *inactivation* (the dopamine and norepinephrine transporters), and *degradation* (catechol-*O*-methyltransferase) and in dopamine receptor activity (especially the dopamine D_4 receptor).[7] No one gene or its protein derivatives has been found to have a consistent relation with ADHD, which suggests that like most psychiatric disorders, ADHD is the consequence of polygenetic influences.

SIGNS AND SYMPTOMS

The manifestations of ADHD in adults are generally less obvious than in children. Adults tend not to exhibit the impulsive, overactive behavior distinctive of many ADHD children and adolescents.[1,2] Common dysfunctional behavioral patterns in adults with ADHD include task avoidance, waiting until the last moment to complete a task, completing all but the most important tasks, and taking on new tasks before finishing others (Table 1).[2] Impatience, irritability, and explosiveness are common as well. Common comorbidities complicate the array of signs and symptoms that ADHD adults can present with. Abnormal mood, vocational and interpersonal problems, and substance abuse are often the problems that patients present with when the underlying primary diagnosis is ADHD.

DIAGNOSIS

Diagnostic criteria have been developed for children and adolescents (Box 1)[9] but not specifically for adults. Despite having clinically significant ADHD, many adults do not fulfill the threshold of six or more criteria defined for children and adolescents. This points to the fundamental problem of employing a descriptive nosology to define clinical disorders. Future editions of the *Diagnostic and Statistical Manual of Mental Disorders* (DSM) will struggle with this dilemma until the pathophysiologic mechanisms of specific psychiatric disorders such as ADHD are better understood.

Figure 1 is an algorithm for diagnosing ADHD in the adult patient. The core criteria for the diagnosis of adult ADHD is the evidence of the disorder during childhood, symptom persistence, and functional impairment.[3] Determining whether the patient fulfilled these criteria depends almost exclusively on the patient's knowledge of his or her childhood behavior and school performance. Most adults with ADHD recall some evidence of problems related to either inattention or hyperactivity during childhood. Trouble sitting still, frequent fighting, temper outbursts, tendency to daydream, or suboptimal school performance is typical. Those with clinically significant ADHD who report successful school performance may have compensated with higher-than-average intellectual strengths, had an insufficiently challenging curriculum, or simply do not remember accurately. School performance records or collateral information from parents can be very helpful. Published questionnaires can be used to capture the necessary information and can assist with (but not confirm) the diagnosis (Box 2). Ultimately, however, the clinician must rely on the patient's veracity and accuracy of recall.

There is no diagnostic laboratory test for ADHD. Neuropsychological testing can be used to determine whether or not a learning disability is present (e.g., dyslexia), but it cannot confirm the diagnosis of ADHD (by definition, not a learning disability). Although neuroimaging and genetic testing offer attractive diagnostic potential, they are not sufficiently specific or sensitive for routine clinical use.

The difficulty of diagnosing ADHD in adults results largely from the nonspecificity of this behavior-symptom complex. Compounding the lack of specificity, many adults with long-standing undiagnosed and untreated ADHD develop secondary mood, anxiety, or

Table 1 Common Dysfunctional Behavior Patterns in Adults with ADHD

Behavior	Description	Short-Term Gain and Long-Term Loss
Anticipatory avoidance	Magnifying the difficulty of a pending task and doubts about being able to complete it Results in rationalizations to justify procrastination	Defers short-term stress but often creates a self-fulfilling prophecy because the task looms ahead and can seem overwhelming when facing a deadline
Brinkmanship	Waiting until the last moment (e.g., the night before) to complete a task, often when facing an impending deadline	Deadline-associated stress can be focusing, but this tactic leaves little room for error and can yield a substantial result
Pseudoefficiency	Completing several low-priority, manageable tasks (e.g., checking e-mail) but avoiding high-priority tasks (e.g., a project for work)	Creates sense of productivity by reducing items on a to-do list but defers a more difficult project
Juggling	Taking on new, exciting projects and feeling busy without completing projects already started	It is easier to become motivated to start a novel project than to complete an ongoing one Pattern usually results in several incomplete projects

ADHD, attention-deficit/hyperactivity disorder.
Adapted with permission from Rostain AL, Ramsay JL: Adults with ADHD? Try medication and psychotherapy. Curr Psychiatry 2006;5:13-27.

Box 1 Diagnostic Criteria for Attention-Deficit/Hyperactivity Disorder

Diagnostic Criteria
- Meets symptom criteria
- Some inattention or hyperactivity-impulse symptoms causing impairment are present before age 7 years
- Some impairment from symptoms present in two or more settings (e.g., home, school or work, social)
- Clear evidence of clinically significant impairment in social, academic, or occupational functioning

Symptom Criteria
At least six symptoms of inattention or at least six symptoms of hyperactivity or impulsivity have persisted for at least 6 months and occur often enough to be maladaptive and inconsistent with developmental level.

Inattention
- Fails to pay close attention to details or makes careless mistakes in schoolwork, work, or other activities
- Has difficulty sustaining attention in tasks or play activities
- Does not seem to listen when spoken to directly
- Does not follow through on instructions and fails to finish schoolwork, chores, or work duties (not due to oppositional behavior or failure to understand)
- Has difficulty organizing tasks and activities
- Avoids, dislikes, or is reluctant to engage in tasks requiring mental effort (e.g., schoolwork, homework)
- Loses things necessary for tasks or activities (e.g., written instructions, school assignments, textbooks, pencils, tools, toys)
- Is easily distracted by extraneous stimuli
- Is forgetful in daily activities

Hyperactivity
- Fidgets with hands or feet and squirms in seat
- Leaves seat in classroom or other situations where remaining seated is expected
- Runs about or climbs excessively in situations where these activities are considered inappropriate; in adolescents or adults, this feature may be limited to subjective feelings of restlessness
- Has difficulty in playing or engaging in leisure activities quietly
- Is on the go or acts as if driven by a motor
- Talks excessively

Impulsivity
- Blurts out answers before questions are completed
- Has difficulty awaiting turn (impatient)
- Interrupts or intrudes on others (e.g., butts in on conversations, games)

Exclusion Criteria
- Symptoms do not occur exclusively during course of a pervasive developmental disorder, schizophrenia, or psychotic disorder.
- Symptoms are not better accounted for by another mental disorder (e.g., mood disorder, anxiety disorder, dissociative disorder, personality disorder).

Situational Notes
Symptoms might not be observable when the patient is in highly structured or novel settings, engages in interesting activity, receives one-on-one attention or supervision, or is in a situation with frequent rewards for appropriate behavior.

Symptoms typically worsen in situations that are unstructured, minimally supervised, or boring or that require sustained attention or mental effort.

In adolescents *(or adults)*, symptoms include restlessness (rather than hyperactivity, as seen in children), impaired academic performance, low self esteem, poor peer relations, and erratic work record.

Adapted from American Psychiatric Association: Diagnostic and Statistical Manual of Mental Disorders, 4th ed, text rev. Washington, DC: American Psychiatric Association, 2000.

substance-use disorders, alone or in combination, that become the focus of clinical attention and obscure detection of the more fundamental problem with attention. The National Comorbidity Survey Replication showed that many adults with ADHD are receiving treatment for other comorbid mental or substance-use disorders but not for ADHD.[5]

DIFFERENTIAL DIAGNOSIS

Virtually any type of distress, regardless of the cause, can interfere with normal attention. Therefore, the feature that distinguishes ADHD from other causes of inattention is a lifelong pattern of the behavior-symptom complex. When this criterion is not met,

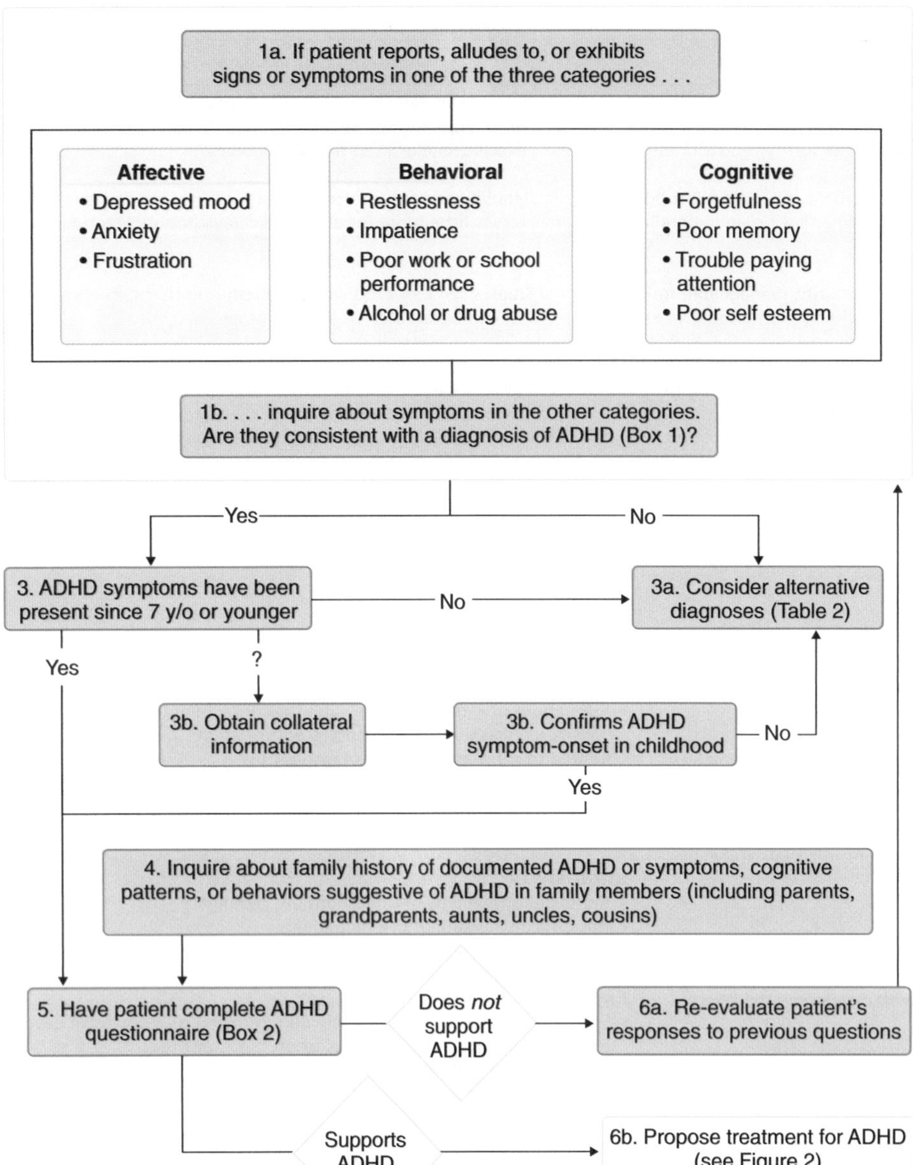

Figure 1 **Algorithm for assessing and treating attention-deficit/hyperactivity disorder (ADHD).** y/o, years old.

Box 2 Rating Scales Used in Diagnosing Attention-Deficit/Hyperactivity Disorder

Adult ADHD Self-Report Scale (AASRS) Symptom Checklist
PDF available at http://www.med.nyu.edu/psych/assets/adhdscreen18.pdf (accessed March 20, 2009).

Barkley ADHD Behavior Checklist for Adults
In Barkley RA (ed): Attention-Deficit Hyperactivity Disorder: A Handbook for Diagnosis and Treatment, 3rd ed. New York, Guilford Press, 2006.

Conners' Adult ADHD Rating Scales (CAARS)Available for purchase from http://www3.parinc.com/products/product.aspx?Productid=CAARS# (accessed March 20, 2009).

Wender-Utah Rating Scale (WURS)Available at http://168.144.150.122/Wender%20Utah%20Rating%20Scale%20checklist.pdf (accessed March 20, 2009).

ADHD, attention-deficit/hyperactivity disorder.

other diagnoses must be considered (Table 2). Adults with ADHD are at greater risk for having or developing mood, anxiety, and substance-use disorders.[5] Accurate diagnosis of these disorders and determining whether they are comorbid or secondary to ADHD have important implications for treatment selection and prognosis. Successful treatment of a comorbid disorder reduces symptom burden, but it does not affect the symptoms and behavior of ADHD. On the other hand, successful treatment of ADHD can result in improvement of secondary anxiety, depression, or substance abuse. Certain disorders that are commonly associated with or have features that can mimic ADHD are listed in Table 2.

Table 2 Differential Diagnosis of Attention-Deficit/Hyperactivity Disorder

Diagnosis	DSM IV-TR	Feature(s) Shared with ADHD
Mood Disorders		
Major depression	296.2-3	Trouble concentrating; trouble initiating and completing tasks
Dysthymia	300.4	Trouble concentrating; trouble initiating and completing tasks
Depression NOS	311	Trouble concentrating; trouble initiating and completing tasks
Bipolar disorder	296.4-6	Distractability, hyperactive behavior
Cyclothymia		Distractability, hyperactive behavior
Anxiety Disorders		
Generalized anxiety disorder	300.02	Inattention, distractability
Social anxiety disorder	300.23	Performance anxiety, task avoidance (especially tasks performed in front of others), unsatisfying social interaction
Obsessive-compulsive disorder	300.3	Repetitious activity
Anxiety disorder NOS	300.00	Inattention, distractability
Substance-Use Disorders		
Nicotine dependence	305.10	Poor job performance and socialization
		Commonly comorbid with ADHD
Alcohol abuse or dependence	305.0/303.90	Poor job performance and socialization
		Commonly comorbid with ADHD
Cannabis abuse or dependence	305.20/304.30	Poor job performance and socialization
		Commonly comorbid with ADHD
Impulse-Control Disorders		
Intermittent explosive disorder	312.34	Impulsivity, aggression
Impulse control disorder NOS	312.30	Impulsivity, trouble with task completion
Learning Disorders		
Learning disorder NOS	315.9	History of poor school and job performance
Early onset dementia	290.10	Poor attention, forgetfulness
Mild MR	317	Trouble with learning, reading, attention
Personality Disorders		
Borderline personality disorder	301.83	Impulsivity, aggression
Antisocial personality disorder	301.7	Impulsivity, aggression, history of poor school and job performance

ADHD, attention-deficit/hyperactivity disorder; DSM IV-TR, Diagnostic and Statistical Manual of Mental Disorders, 4th edition, text revision; MR, mental retardation; NOS, not otherwise specified.

TREATMENT

Figure 2 is a management algorithm. Optimal treatment of adult ADHD invariably requires pharmacotherapy. Adding life-skills coaching or cognitive-behavioral therapy, or both, in either individual or group settings can further improve outcome, but by themselves they are generally insufficient. Partners and family members can benefit from better understanding of the impact of ADHD on the patient's behavior and interpersonal style.[2]

Baseline measures of weight, heart rate, and blood pressure should be obtained before starting stimulant or nonstimulant medication. The patient with a history of cardiovascular abnormalities, in particular structural heart disease (e.g., idiopathic hypertrophic subaortic stenosis) should avoid stimulant medication in favor of a nonstimulant agent such as atomoxetine, bupropion, or modafanil. Treatment of such patients should involve close collaboration with an internist or cardiologist.

Medications

The standard of care for adults has evolved largely from studies in children, and the medications used in adults are the same as those used in children and adolescents with ADHD (Table 3).

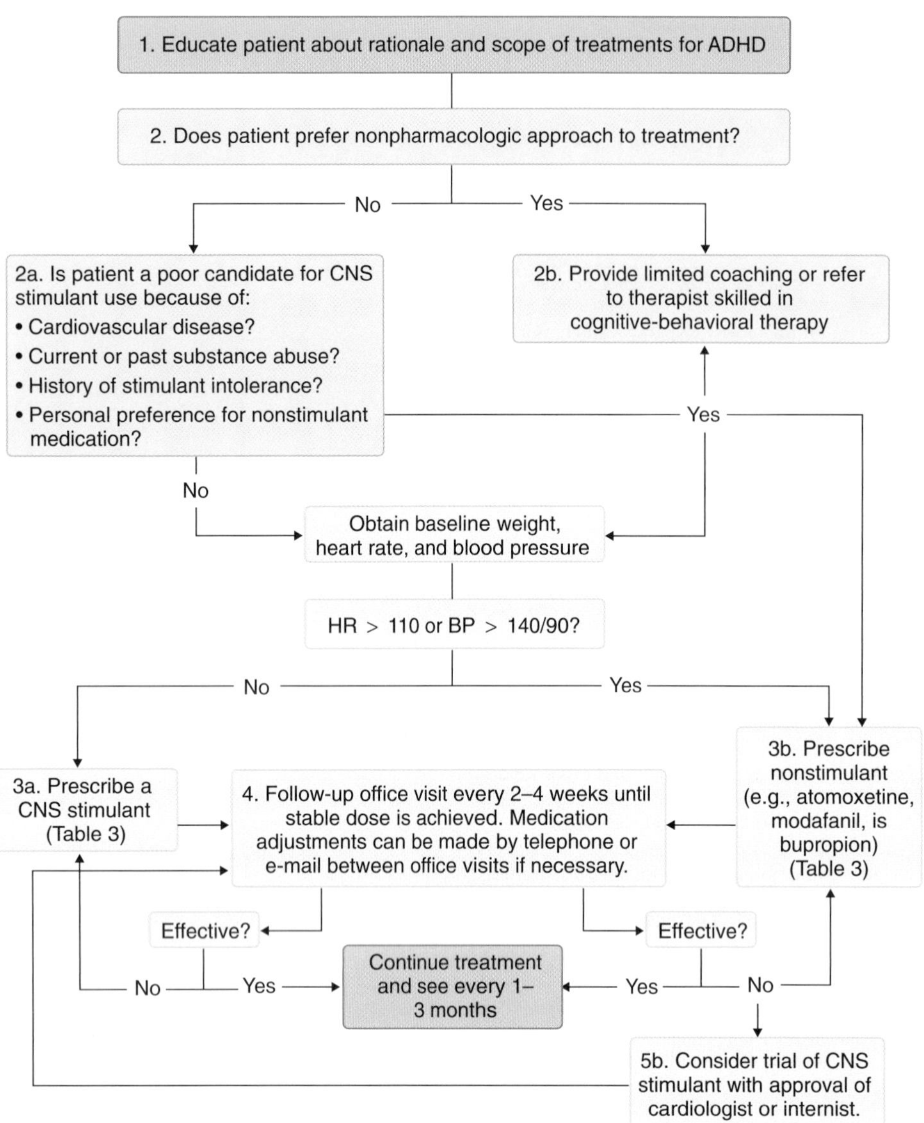

Figure 2 **Treatment algorithm for patients who meet diagnostic criteria for attention-deficit/hyperactivity disorder (ADHD).** CNS, central nervous system; BP, blood pressure; CNS, central nervous system; HR, heart rate.

Central nervous system (CNS) stimulants such as dextroamphetamine, methyphenidate, and dexmethylphenidate are the drugs of choice for ADHD in both children and adults. Their therapeutic effect is associated with enhancement of central dopaminergic and noradrenergic activity.[1] CNS stimulant compounds augment synaptic catecholamine concentrations by triggering presynaptic release of dopamine (and to a lesser extent norepinephrine) and also by blocking their reuptake.[7] Drugs that influence both dopaminergic and noradrenergic function (e.g., dextroamphetamine, methylphenidate, dexmethylphenidate) are *stimulants*, and those that have less or no impact on dopamine and more on norepinephrine are *nonstimulants*, such as atomoxetine (Strattera). Other nonstimulant agents whose mechanism of action in ADHD is not fully understood include bupropion and imipramine.

Dose

The dosage of medication must be individualized by increasing gradually to maximal benefit while avoiding side effects. These principles hold for both stimulant and nonstimulant drugs. Clinical experience suggests a fine line between too little and too much medication.

Onset of Effect

Stimulant drugs have a rapid onset of effect. Clinical effects are felt within 15 to 30 minutes of oral administration, and peak blood levels are achieved within approximately 2 hours. It can take a week or more, however, to achieve full therapeutic effect. Assessing the patient's response to medication must account for exposure to circumstances that affect attention (e.g., comorbid disorders, environmental stress) and how effectively the patient monitors his or her response to medication. The nonstimulants work more gradually and can take days to weeks to achieve a full therapeutic effect.

The stimulants come in immediate-release and sustained-release forms (see Table 3). Immediate-release forms last anywhere from 2 to 6 hours, necessitating 2 to 4 doses daily. Sustained-release forms last 8 to 12 hours, permitting once- or twice-daily dosing.

Side Effects

Stimulant side effects are typically dose related and include nausea, headache, jitteriness, tics, high blood pressure, and high heart rate. They also have potential for abuse. Patients with baseline tachyarrhythmia, hypertension, or structural heart disease are at high risk

Table 3 Medications for Attention-Deficit/Hyperactivity Disorder

Drug	Trade Name	Dosage Form (mg)	Dose* (mg)	Duration (h)	Frequency	Comments
CNS Stimulants						
Dexmethylphenidate	Focalin	2.5, 5, 10	5-20	3-6	tid-qid	Dextroisomer of methylphenidate Start at 50% of current daily dose to convert from methylphenidate
	Focalin XR	2.5, 5, 10	10-20	8-10	qd-bid	Dextroisomer of methylphenidate Start at 50% of current daily dose to convert from methylphenidate
Dextroamphetamine	Dexedrine	5	10-30	3-6	bid-tid	
	Dexedrine spansule	5, 10, 15	10-30	6-8	qd-bid	Dexedrine spansule
Methylphenidate	Concerta	18, 27, 36, 54	18-54	10-12	qd	The FDA-approved max dosage in children and adolescents is 54 mg qd, but doses of 108 mg qd have been used successfully in children and adults
	Metadate ER†	10, 20	20-60	6-8	qd-bid	
	Metadate CD	10, 20, 30, 40, 50, 60		8-10	qd-bid	
	Methylin	5, 10, 20 5/5 mL, 10/5 mL solution	15-45	3-6	tid-qid	
	Methylin ER†			6-8	qd-bid	
	Ritalin	5, 10, 20	10-40	3-6	tid-qid	
	Ritalin SR	20		6-8	qd-bid	
	Ritalin LA	20, 30, 40		6-8	qd-bid	Lasts longer than SR
Mixed-amphetamine salts	Adderall	5, 7.5, 10, 12.5, 15, 20, 30		6-8	qd-bid	
	Adderall XR	5, 10, 15, 20, 25, 30	20-60	8-10	qd-bid	
	Vyvanse	30, 50, 70	30-100	12	qd-bid	Pro-drug
Selective Norepinephrine Reuptake Inhibitor						
Atomoxetine	Strattera	10, 18, 25, 40, 60	40-100	24	qd-bid	Better than placebo, but not as effective as CNS stimulants in controlled trials for ADHD
Alternative Medications‡						
Bupropion	Wellbutrin	75, 100	150-450	24	tid	
	Wellbutrin SR	100, 150, 200	150-450	24	bid	
	Wellbutrin XL	150, 300	150-450	24	qd	
Desipramine	Norpramin	10, 25, 50, 75, 100, 150	100-200	24	qd	
Modafinil	Provigil	100, 200	100-400		qd	

ADHD, attention-deficit/hyperactivity disorder; CNS, central nervous system; FDA, U.S. Food and Drug Administration.
*The last dose is the FDA-approved maximum daily dosage in children.
†There is no obvious difference between these two products in terms of dosage, duration, and efficacy.
‡These agents may be effective in some instances of ADHD but have not been shown in controlled trials to be more effective than placebo. They are not approved by the FDA for treating ADHD.

for stimulant-induced aggravation of these abnormalities. The nonstimulant atomoxetine can cause increases in heart rate and blood pressure, but it is far less likely to do so than stimulants are. Its most common side effects include dry mouth, nausea, and sexual difficulties. Nonstimulants have no abuse potential.

PREVENTION AND SCREENING

It is reasonable to expect that timely and effective treatment should reduce the risk of psychosocial morbidity associated with ADHD. A small but growing body of evidence suggests that patients with ADHD who are treated for it have less substance abuse, better work and academic performance, and better outcomes in general than those who are not treated.[10]

If the extensive psychosocial morbidity of ADHD can be prevented, then it stands to reason that it should be identified and treated as early as possible. In fact, many adults go through life without recognizing they have ADHD. This, as well as the complex comorbidities (e.g., depression, anxiety, substance abuse) that often trigger a request for help, make it difficult to detect ADHD.

Three validated patient self-report instruments are available to screen for ADHD in adults; alternatively, they can be used to substantiate a physician's clinical impression. The World Health Organization (WHO) Adult Self-Report Screener (ASRS) for Adult Attention Deficit Disorder (ADD) includes six questions rated on a scale from 0 to 4 (0 = never, 1 = rarely, 2 = sometimes, 3 = often, 4 = very often). The maximum score is 24; the higher the score, the more likely that ADHD is present. The Wender Utah Rating Scale

(WURS) was originally used as a research instrument and validated as a screener subsequently. A score of 46 or more obtained from adding the ratings on items 3-7, 9-12, 15-17, 20, 21, 24-29, 40, 41, 51, 56, and 59 is highly predictive of a diagnosis of ADHD. The Conner Adult ADHD Rating Scales (CAARS) elicit self reports and observer ratings. Further information about these scales and their acquisition is available in Box 2.

SPECIAL POPULATIONS

Geriatric Patients

There is no age limit for the diagnosis of ADHD. Geriatric-age patients with a diagnosis of ADHD can benefit considerably from appropriate treatment. Older patients are more likely, however, to have coexisting cardiovascular abnormalities that warrant careful monitoring during treatment with stimulant medication.

Potential Substance Abusers

The challenge for the prescribing physician is to keep stimulant medications out of the hands of persons prone to drug or alcohol addiction. The risk of stimulant-induced substance abuse in uncomplicated adult ADHD is minimal. This risk liability is further reduced by the use of long-acting agents (see Table 3). Effective treatment of ADHD should reduce the risk of substance abuse, especially when substance abuse is secondary to ADHD. For persons with ADHD and comorbid substance abuse or dependence, the treatment of choice includes a nonstimulant agent such as atomoxetine, buproprion, or imipramine. A blanket policy of refusal to prescribe CNS stimulants to patients with a history of drug abuse, however, is ill advised. In all cases, substance abuse must be stabilized first, and ADHD treatment can be initiated as soon as the substance abuse is stabilized.

Patients with Cardiovascular Disease

CNS stimulant medications are relatively contraindicated in patients with hypertension, cardiac arrhythmia, tachycardia, coronary artery disease, and structural heart disease (e.g., idiopathic hypertrophic subaortic stenosis). Nonpharmacologic therapies or nonstimulant medications should be tried first in such patients. If these are ineffective, however, and the fully informed patient desires a trial of stimulant medication, it should be prescribed with careful monitoring in conjunction with the supervision of a cardiologist or internist to minimize the risk of adverse outcome.

Epileptic Patients

CNS stimulants do not cause a clinically significant reduction in seizure threshold and therefore can be used safely in patients with epilepsy.

Pregnant Women

All CNS stimulant drugs are listed as class C and should therefore be avoided if possible during pregnancy.

Summary

- Adult attention-deficit/hyperactivity disorder (ADHD) is a familial disorder with first manifestations before age 7 years.
- At least 60% of children with ADHD continue to exhibit clinically significant features of the disorder as adults.
- ADHD is among the most heritable of psychiatric disorders.
- Undiagnosed or untreated ADHD is associated with significant morbidity, including higher-than-expected rates of maladaptive behavior, family problems including divorce, problematic employment, substance abuse, motor vehicle accidents, and secondary mood and anxiety disorders.
- The primary treatment for adult ADHD is a methylphenidate- or amphetamine-based compound supplemented when necessary with structured, skills-based cognitive-behavioral therapy.

Suggested Readings

American Psychiatric Association: Diagnostic and Statistical Manual of Mental Disorders, 4th ed, text rev. Washington, DC: American Psychiatric Association, 2000.

Barkley RA: Attention-Deficit Hyperactivity Disorder: A Handbook for Diagnosis and Treatment, 2nd ed. New York: Guilford Press, 1998, pp 3-55.

Biederman J, Safren SA, Seidman LJ, et al: ADHD: Applying practice guidelines to improve patient outcome and executive function. J Clin Psychiatry 2006;67:2014-2025.

Hudziak JJ, Derks EM, Althoff RR, et al: The genetic and environmental contributions to attention deficit hyperactivity disorder as measured by the Conners' Rating Scales-Revised. Am J Psychiatry 2005;162:1614-1620.

Kessler RC, Adler L, Barkley R, et al: The prevalence and correlates of adult ADHD in the United States: Results from the national comorbidity survey replication. Am J Psychiatry 2006;163:716-723.

Lamberg L: ADHD often undiagnosed in adults. Appropriate treatment may benefit work family social life. JAMA 2003;290:1565-1597.

McGough JJ, Barkley RA: Diagnostic controversies in adult attention deficit hyperactivity disorder. Am J Psychiatry 2004;161:1948-1956.

Pliszka SR: Neuroscience for the Mental Health Clinician. New York: Guilford Press, 2003, pp 147-150.

Rostain AL, Ramsay JL: Adults with ADHD? Try medication and psychotherapy. Curr Psychiatry 2006;5:13-27.

Vaidya CJ, Bunge SA, Dudukovic NM, et al: Altered neural substrates of cognitive control in childhood ADHD: Evidence from functional magnetic resonance imaging. Am J Psychiatry 2005;162:1605-1613.

References

For a complete list of references, log onto www.expertconsult.com.

Coping with Chronic Medical Illness

Tatiana Falcone and *Kathleen N. Franco*

DEFINITION AND ETIOLOGY

Distressing or disabling chronic medical illness challenges effective coping. Faced with a growing population of aging patients who endure chronic medical illness, the primary care physician must have strategies that accurately assess patient coping skills and facilitate more-effective coping when necessary. Knowledge of the patient's baseline coping skills and a high index of suspicion for factors that threaten effective coping are essential to accurate assessment and achievement of optimal patient coping. In addition to effective listening and empathy, the primary care physician can call on a variety of sources to help facilitate patient coping.

PREVALENCE AND RISK FACTORS

Eighty percent of elders have at least one chronic illness. In 2000, 4.2 million Americans were 85 years or older; by 2030, this group is expected to more than double. Life expectancy has consistently increased since the 1980s.[1] Improved treatment of illnesses that previously led to premature mortality (e.g., diabetes, cancer, HIV, stroke) has contributed to this trend. This growing elderly population is faced with the new challenge of effective coping. Many factors, in addition to the burden caused by the illness, influence coping. These include the patient's age, ethnic background, cultural values, gender, diagnosis, support systems, prior experiences, understanding of illness, and personality traits.[2]

Having strong support systems enhances coping ability. Access to community agencies, family, and friends eases the burden of coping with chronic illness, as do prayer and strong religious faith.

Social withdrawal or isolation, in contrast, make coping more difficult. In the United States, widowed women are less likely than their male counterparts to remarry, and therefore they must find alternatives to partner affection and communication for continued support. However, even beyond that associated with depression, general dysfunction from chronic illness is greater if marital distress or punishing verbal responses about symptoms from the spouse is ongoing.[3] Comorbid psychiatric illness (e.g., mood disorders, panic disorder, schizophrenia) or neurologic illnesses that causes cognitive, affective, or behavioral disturbances (e.g., Parkinson's disease, stroke, dementia) compounds the difficulties of effective coping. Acute illness, especially when perceived as life threatening (e.g., acute myocardial infarction), can trigger clinically significant anxiety, demoralization, or even depression that compromise effective coping.[4]

SIGNS AND SYMPTOMS

Each individual patient has a unique style of coping. Kahana and Bibring's classic treatise on personality and response to medical illness provides a useful heuristic for identifying typical coping patterns (Table 1).[5] Recognition of the differing patterns helps to inform caregiver responses that, if tailored appropriately, will be perceived as supportive rather than confrontational. Breakdown of coping is suggested by maladaptive behaviors such as nonadherence to treatment recommendations, missing medical appointments, not taking prescribed medication, or avoiding laboratory testing. Anger, rigidity, and unprovoked irritability or hostility also suggest poor coping and should trigger further investigation for underlying depression, anxiety, or psychosis.[5]

Emotional Responses to Medical Illness

Response to medical illness is governed to a large degree by the meaning of the illness to the patient. The belief that a diagnosis of cancer is synonymous with a death sentence or that diabetes signals inevitable blindness can trigger panic, depression, or anger. Careful attention to the patient's point of view is essential to identifying catastrophic thinking, core beliefs, and associated core emotions.[1] Lazarus lists some core emotions in coping with medical illness including anger, anxiety, guilt, fright, shame, sadness, happiness, envy, relief, and hope.[2] Either acute or chronic medical illness is likely to trigger anxiety and depression in patients with mood or anxiety disorders.[2] Psychological variables are often more powerful predictors of poor quality of life than physical symptoms.[6]

Coping Styles

Patients tend to exhibit typical coping patterns consistent with their personality traits. As described by Kahana and Bibring (see Table 1), specific traits respond best to particular management strategies. Recognition of these traits and appropriate responses to them by health care personnel increase the likelihood that the patient will respond optimally to care management. Failure to recognize and respond to characteristic behavioral patterns risks conflict with the patient, who feels misunderstood and mistreated (see Table 1).[7]

Adaptive and Maladaptive Responses

Coping styles are often described in terms of predominant defenses used by the patient. Defenses are mental (intrapsychic) maneuvers—generally unconscious—that protect one from distress caused by unacceptable thoughts or feelings. Vaillant has proposed a hierarchical organization of defenses from psychotic to immature, neurotic, and mature. Studies of the relation between defenses and coping styles indicate that high-functioning persons use predominantly mature and neurotic defenses, whereas less-resilient persons (generally those with personality disorders) exhibit more primitive (immature and psychotic) defense mechanisms.[8] Examples of defense mechanisms include suppression (mature), repression (neurotic), passive-aggressive behavior (immature), and denial (psychotic).

Each defense represents a way one might respond when receiving unwelcome news, for example, a diagnosis of myocardial infarction. A mature, adaptive response involves suppression of fear in the service of compliance with further evaluation and testing. Forgetting to pick up prescribed medication at the pharmacy is an example of repression. Passive-aggressive behavior might manifest as repeated failure to follow through with recommended exercise and dietary management. Denial might manifest as refusing to accept the diagnosis of myocardial infarction and threatening to leave the emergency department against medical advice.[8]

Even generally high-functioning persons can regress in the face of life-threatening illness. Such regression can resemble the behavior of a dependent child or an angry adolescent. Hypersexual behavior in the male whose masculinity has been threatened by disabling illness is another example of regressive behavior.

As many as 50% of patients do not take medications as prescribed. Physicians are often unaware that their patients are not taking their medication. Side effects, cost, stigma, poor

Table 1 Personality Profiles and Reactions to Illness

Personality	Patients who ...	Often feel ...	Are helped by ...
Dependent	Ask lots of questions Make it hard for you to end the conversation or leave the room	Afraid that you won't find them worthy Afraid you won't want to care for them	Offering regular, brief sessions Setting tactful limits that reassure the patient and do not annoy staff
Obsessive	Are insistent Are detail oriented	Are angry when they can't control their illness, the staff, and the schedule	Offering detailed explanations Providing choices whenever possible Trying to use patient input collaboratively
Narcissistic	Are self-centered Criticize others Believe no one is qualified	Are fearful, threatened, and vulnerable	Avoiding confrontation, but emphasizing they deserve the best care we can provide Keeping them informed (same message from all staff)
Suffering victim	Always have symptoms and request much attention Might not follow recommendations	Suffering is their role; illness punishes them (and sometimes physician) but hopes doctor will keep trying	Regular visits, no matter how varying the complaints Encouraging them to "suffer" through treatments
Paranoid	Do not trust Refuse to participate in plans Threaten to sign out of the hospital against medical advice	They are being taken advantage of by others or purposefully neglected or harmed	Staying calm Not arguing Offering understanding of their position Making clear recommendations
Histrionic	Are flirtatious Want to call the doctor by his or her first name	They want to be special in the eyes of the physician Illness will invalidate them or make them unattractive	Encouraging the patient to verbalize concerns Setting boundaries for the relationship Remaining courteous and objective
Schizoid	Are very lonely Tend to avoid medical care	Doctors are invading their privacy	Engaging them in helping to make medical decisions

understanding, poor rapport with the prescribing physician, and treatment complexity contribute to nonadherence.

Perry and Viderman discussed psychological underpinnings leading to nonadherence. Patients might do this to defend against humiliation or counteract a feeling of helplessness. They also may be expressing anger toward the physical disorder or toward the physician for not being able to eradicate the illness.[9]

Signing out against medical advice is another maladaptive response that occurs in about 2% of all hospital discharges. Different factors can play roles, including anger toward the medical team or the caregiver, anxiety, withdrawal from abused substances, or intense denial of the illness. Some patients may be psychotic from a primary psychiatric disorder such as schizophrenia or a bipolar condition or secondarily from delirium or dementia.[10]

DIAGNOSIS

If the patient's coping strategies are ineffective or causing trouble, the patient should be screened for a major psychiatric disturbance (Axis I), particularly when there is poor adherence to treatment. Depressed patients with low energy and little motivation might not be able to follow the treatment, and bipolar hypomanic patients might believe they don't need treatment. Psychotic, paranoid patients can feel threatened by the treatment or the doctor. Fearing they will not be taken seriously due to the stigma of mental illness, some omit telling their general practitioner about their psychiatric diagnosis. Patients avoid taking newly recommended medications if they fear side effects or interactions with their current psychiatric medications.[4]

If the major diagnosis is Axis II (personality disorder), psychotherapy, patience, and defining boundaries can reduce the wear and tear on the patient and the physician.

Stressors with social, economic, or emotional valence can affect coping behavior.

Dependency on alcohol and other substances of abuse can easily become the preferred way for some patients to cope, particularly when they have inadequate interpersonal support. The physician must carefully screen to be certain pain control is truly adequate, because the patient might simply be trying to self-medicate.

There are some differences among the psychiatric factors that affect coping. A patient who has a major Axis I diagnosis often needs pharmacologic treatment. Often, a consultation with a psychiatrist is a good idea to make sure the patient is receiving the optimal combination of medications and that drug interactions are avoided. If the major diagnosis is Axis II, the essential treatment is psychotherapy. The physician must keep in mind that these patients struggle with basic coping skills. Axis III refers to the patient's medical conditions that can affect the psychiatric presentation, and vice versa. Reviewing all the social, economic, emotional, and family situations that might be affecting the patient's coping behavior provides important data for Axis IV. Axis V is a scale from 0 to 100 that provides an overview of how the patient is functioning and if the patient will be able to manage outside of the hospital.[11]

If the primary physician is not certain a psychiatric disorder exists and is causing maladaptive coping or requires treatment, a psychiatric consultation is recommended.

TREATMENT

The physician can gather the patient's emotional reactions and cognitive interpretations about the illness to identify patient strengths and to discern ways the patient has handled stressful situations in the past. A practical approach that is helpful to any physician is to attempt to choose a setting conducive to communicating with and understanding the patient. In particular, the doctor should allow adequate time for questions from the patient and the family. Explore the patient's current understanding of their current medical problems and how the patient is using available support. Inquire about the emotional reaction, how the patient is feeling, and how the family is coping with the medical illness. Assess how spirituality or religion plays a role in the patient's life.

Determine what sources of support are available for the patient, such as church, community, friends, or family. High social support of patients in heart failure reduced anxiety and depression in a 9 month longitudinal study.[12] The physician can recommend seeking out such support persons and groups or ask if the patient would like additional help. Make sure the patient hears your support and understands that there is always hope. Many resources are available that can be very beneficial for patients. A nurse practitioner can make extra visits to educate the patient about the medical condition; a home health aide can assist a patient having problems dealing with disability, lacking assistance with medications, or even accessing care. Social services can identify local or nationally sponsored support groups or other community resources. Not only can multidisciplinary teams provide support and improve compliance,[13] they can also build affirming, open dialogue and enhance confidence when patients truly participate with their team.[14] Family members are always a great resource because they often know how the patient is doing at home. Self-help manuals and leaflets can benefit motivated patients and families. Scholten and colleagues[15] demonstrated functional and social benefits for patients with rheumatoid arthritis lasting up to 5 years after an intensive 9-day multidisciplinary program that included education, gym exercises, use of devices, counselling, dietetics, and discussion of social assistance.

If the physician notices the patient has difficulties adjusting, such as with medication noncompliance or contradictory answers, the assistance of a mental health professional can be very helpful. Patients with increased isolation, hopelessness, serious nonadherence to treatment, or irrational behavior should be referred early to a psychiatrist.[16]

A few groups are trying diverse programs that might save time or money or simply have more appeal for some patients. Researchers compared a standard support group with an educational group learning about imagery, meditation, rituals, and affirmation. Breast cancer patients randomized for 12 weeks to either found participation improved quality of life and reduced anxiety and depression.[17]

Self-regulation interventions help patients balance problem focused input with emotional regulation to cope with illness related distress.[18] It is interesting that pure problem-focused interventions have not always been successful and even occasionally have had negative outcomes. More recent research describes how, through writing, talking, or thinking, patients can be taught to regulate their emotions, conferring benefits for their physical health conditions.

For most chronic medical conditions, a healthy lifestyle would benefit patients physically and mentally, if they were able to follow one. Physicians have told patients about the advantages of weight loss, cessation of smoking, reducing alcohol, exercising, and others. Both patient and physician set goals, but the unhealthy habits return. The patient returns to status quo, or potentially even feelings of hopelessness.

Physicians of all specialties can learn motivational interviewing.[19] Steps to this approach are effective and can hold feelings of hopelessness significant rewards for patients. (Box 1).

PREVENTION AND SCREENING

There are no well-accepted guidelines that work in every patient with any chronic medical illness. There are some recommended guidelines for certain diseases, such as cancer or cardiopulmonary disease that are easily accessed through organizational websites.

Patients with previously diagnosed psychiatric disorders are at higher risk for problematic coping when confronted with a life-threatening condition or a worsening of their chronic medical illness. Some psychotropic medications can interfere with the treatment of medical illness.[7] Fortunately, there are guidelines and options for treating all the major Axis I disorders. Certainly improving a patient's mental health can benefit the patient's efforts to cope with the medical condition.[11]

Box 1 Motivational Interviewing

Asking permission to discuss with the patient
Begin with an open-ended question
Reflect back the patient's opinion
Explore the importance of this topic from the patient's point of view
What would make that increase or decrease
How confident is the patient that if they wanted to make a change, they could
What would make that rise or fall
Expose the ambivalence
Reflect to them
When they are ready, work out a plan together

SPECIAL POPULATIONS

Compared to 50 years ago, the stigma of having cancer has been reduced. However, many cancer patients still feel stigmatized. If depression coexists, it produces an extra barrier to treatment.

Patients with cancer have a 1.5-fold increased suicide risk over that of the general population. Passive suicidal thoughts are common (8% in terminal phases).

Men are at increased risk for suicide. Other risk factors include advanced stage of disease, poor prognosis, delirium with poor impulse control, inadequately controlled pain, family history of suicide, previous suicide attempts, physical and emotional exhaustion, and social isolation. Hopelessness and extreme need for control also increase risk. Patients with cancer in the head, neck, or gastrointestinal system have a higher risk of suicide and alcohol disorders.[16]

Summary

- Chronic medical illness challenges patient's coping skills.
- The effectiveness of coping is determined by premorbid (baseline) coping strategies, current illness burden including comorbid psychiatric disorder(s), and availability of support mechanisms.
- Common indicators of ineffective coping include nonadherence to treatment, denial or minimization of illness, substance abuse, and high use of health care.
- In addition to empathic listening and support, the physician should mobilize other sources of support including ancillary medical staff, family, religious, and illness-oriented support groups.
- Motivational interviewing holds promise for primary care specialists aspiring to help patients discover their own ambivalence and who have a desire to change unhealthy ways.

Suggested Readings

Baile W, Buckman R, Lenzi R, et al: SPIKES-a six-step protocol for delivering bad news: Application to the patient with cancer. Oncologist 2000;5:302-311.

Felton B, Revenson T: Age differences in coping with chronic illness. Psychol Aging 1987;2(2):164-170.

Gazzola L, Muskin PR: The impact of stress and the objective of psychosocial interventions. In Schein LA, Bernard HS, Spitz HI, Muskin PR (eds): On Psychosocial Interventions in Psychosocial Treatment for Medical Conditions: Principles and Techniques. New York: Brunner-Routledge, 2003, pp 373-406.

Green S: Principles of medical psychotherapy. In Stoudemire A, Fogel BS, Greenberg D (eds): Psychiatric Care of the Medical Patient, 2nd ed. New York: Oxford University Press, 2000, pp 17-30.

Groves M, Muskin P: Psychological responses to illness. In Levinson J (ed): The American Psychiatric Publishing Textbook of Psychosomatic Medicine. Washington, DC: American Psychiatric Association, 2005, pp 68-88.

Kahana RJ, Bibring G: Personality types in medical management. In Zinberg NE (ed): Psychiatry and Medical Practice in a General Hospital. New York: International Universities Press, 1964, pp 108-123.

Lazarus RS, Folkman S: Stress, Appraisal and Coping. New York: Springer, 1984.

Perry S, Viederman M: Management of emotional reactions to acute medical illness. Med Clin North Am 1981;65:3-14.

Penley JA, Tomaka J, Wiebe JS: The association of coping to physical and psychological health outcomes: A meta-analytic review. J Behav Med 2002;25:551-603.

Robinson R, Jorge R, Moser D, et al: Escitalopram and problem-solving therapy for prevention of post-stroke depression. JAMA 2008;299(20):2391-2400.

Valliant GE: Ego Mechanisms of Defense: A Guide for Clinicians and Researchers. Washington DC, American Psychiatric Association, 1992, pp 29-42.

References

For a complete list of references, log onto www.expertconsult.com.

Section 12

PULMONARY

Bronchitis

Marie M. Budev and *Herbert P. Wiedemann*

Based on Laennec's work,[1] the CIBA symposium proposed that chronic bronchitis was to be defined as "chronic or recurrent excessive mucus secretion in the bronchial tree" manifested clinically by cough and expectoration of no other origin, and that bronchitis found in chronic obstructive pulmonary disease (COPD) should be distinguished from that of nuisance bronchitis or Laennec's catarrh by the presence of airflow limitation.[2,3] Chronic bronchitis and emphysema often have similar causes (tobacco use) and often occur together. As a result, the umbrella term of chronic obstructive pulmonary disease is often used synonymously to describe both clinical entities.[4,5] The disabling and debilitating nature of COPD is often punctuated by intermittent acute bacterial exacerbations of chronic bronchitis (ABECB) that contribute greatly to the morbidity and the overall diminished quality of life in these patients. In fact, bacterial exacerbations are the leading cause of death in COPD.[6]

DEFINITION

The definition of bronchitis is one that remains largely subjective and has few rare objective correlates. The American Thoracic Society defines chronic bronchitis as the presence of chronic productive cough for 3 months in each of the 2 successive years in a patient in whom other disease states that can cause similar symptoms have been excluded.[7] The most commonly used definition of an ABECB is a subjective increase in dyspnea, increased sputum volume, or increased sputum purulence. Anthonisen and colleagues attempted to stratify the severity of an ABECB based on these very symptoms.[8] According to the Anthonisen severity scale, type I (severe) episodes of ABECB have all three clinical findings, and type II (moderate) exhibit two clinical findings. Type III exacerbations (mild) have one of the clinical findings plus one of the following: an upper respiratory tract infection in the past 5 days, fever without any other apparent cause, increased cough or wheezing, or a 20% increase in the respiratory rate or heart rate above baseline.[9] In many guidelines, this scale is used to assess the severity of an exacerbation and direct management.

PREVALENCE AND EPIDEMIOLOGY

The worldwide prevalence of chronic bronchitis and ABECB is likely to be underestimated due to the variability in the definition of COPD. Traditionally, it has been believed that chronic bronchitis is a major component in 85% of patients with COPD.[10] In the United States alone, more than 16 million people are affected with COPD, and it is estimated that more than 12 million of those suffer from chronic bronchitis symptoms.[7] Acute exacerbations in more than 50% of cases of chronic bronchitis and COPD, particularly those meeting the Anthonisen criteria, are likely the result of infectious pathogenic bacteria. Overall, these exacerbations occur more often in smokers than in nonsmokers. After an acute exacerbation, many patients experience a decrease in quality of life, and subsequently more than 50% of patients are readmitted with an ABECB more than once in the following 6 months. Therefore, one of the main goals of therapy in managing COPD is to reduce the number and severity of exacerbations.

Acute exacerbations of chronic bronchitis and COPD are the main causes of medical visits and hospitalizations, resulting in economic costs in excess of $5 billion yearly. In one prospective series, the costs of treating COPD and ABECB were found to be almost twice those reported for asthma. The prevalence of COPD, and thus the prevalence of ABECB, continues to rise as the population ages, and it is the only leading cause of death for which the mortality rate is currently increasing.[5,7]

PATHOLOGY AND PATHOPHYSIOLOGY

The pathologic lesions of chronic bronchitis involve morphologic changes in both the large and small airways. In patients with chronic bronchitis, these airways contain a marked presence of inflammatory cells with a predominance of monocytes, lymphocytes, and $CD8^+$ cells as well as neutrophils in the airway lumen. In the large airways, inflammation leads to metaplasia of both the columnar and goblet cells that line the epithelium. In addition, there is an increase in the size of the mucus-secreting glands in smooth muscle, connective tissue in the bronchial wall, and degeneration of the airway cartilage.

Evidence is emerging that ABECBs are associated with increased airway inflammation. There appears to be a clear association between the degree of inflammation and the severity and frequency of the exacerbations. Bronchoalveolar lavage (BAL) specimens taken during ABECB show increases in the absolute number and percentage of neutrophils. Levels of interleukin 8 (IL-8), a potent neutrophil chemotactic factor, leukotriene B4, and myeloperoxidase (MPO) all have been found to be increased during ABECB. In addition, cytokine levels in BAL fluid have been noted to be higher during ABECB.

In a normal patient, the respiratory tree is sterile. In a stable chronic bronchitis patient, the sputum produced is usually mucoid and scant. Even in this quiescent period, however, cultures of sputum can yield potentially pathogenic bacteria in 25% to 50% of cases. Organisms including nontypeable *Haemophilus influenzae, Moraxella catarrhalis,* and *Streptococcus pneumoniae* have been found to be the predominant organisms in early studies. Once these bacteria colonize the lower airway, they can directly cause airway inflammation and impaired mucociliary clearance, perpetuating a vicious circle of impairing local defenses.

Bacteria have been isolated from the sputum in approximately 60% of ABECB cases. The most common organisms isolated include *H. influenzae, Haemophilus parainfluenzae, S. pneumoniae,* and *M. catarrhalis* (Box 1). The contributions of these four organisms can depend on the severity of underlying airway disease. A number of studies have found more virulent organisms in the airways of severe chronic bronchitis patients with acute exacerbations, including *Staphylococcus aureus, Pseudomonas* species, and members of the Enterobacteriaceae family. In general, during ABECB, many of the same bacteria that are found in the airways during clinically stable periods are present but at higher colony counts. The role of atypical pathogens such as *Mycoplasma* and *Chlamydia* species seem to follow three separate mechanisms in ABECB. First, infection with Chlamydia pneumoniae infection at an early age can make airways more susceptible to effects of irritants such as cigarette smoke and can increase the risk of chronic bronchitis later in life. Second, both these species can cause ABECB themselves. Last, atypical organisms and viruses can cause a primary infection that can lead to severe lower airway inflammation, enabling a secondary increase in bacterial proliferation that can lead to an exacerbation.

DIAGNOSIS

The clinical diagnosis of ABECB traditionally uses some combination of the original three Anthonisen criteria: increased cough, dyspnea, or increased sputum purulence from baseline. There are no

Box 1 Responsible Bacteria in Acute Exacerbations of Chronic Bronchitis

Common Bacterial Pathogens (30%-50%)
Haemophilus influenza
Haemophilus parainfluenzae
Streptococcus pneumoniae
Moraxella catarrhalis

Less-Common Bacterial Pathogens (10%-15%)
Pseudomonas aeruginosa
Enterobacteriaceae
Other gram-negative bacilli
Staphylocccus aureus
Other gram-positive cocci

Atypical Pathogens (<5%-15%)
Chlamydia pneumoniae
Mycoplasma pneumoniae

characteristic laboratory or radiographic tests that can confirm the diagnosis of ABECB.

Some clinicians have proposed major and minor criteria; the major criteria consist of the original Anthonisen criteria and the minor criteria consist of wheezing, sore throat, cough, and symptoms of the common cold, including nasal congestion or discharge. They define an ABECB as the presence of at least two major symptoms or one major symptom and one minor symptom for at least 2 consecutive days.

There are no characteristic physical findings in ABECB. Some have suggested that severe exacerbations may be associated with body temperatures greater than 38.5° C, although this is highly controversial. Chest radiographs are not helpful in making the diagnosis of ABECB, but they can indicate pneumonia or other diagnoses, such as congestive heart failure. The exception to this is a patient presenting to the emergency department or being hospitalized where routing chest x-rays have revealed abnormalities that led to changes in management (16% to 21% of cases). Sputum Gram stain and culture have a limited role in diagnosing ABECB due to frequent colonization of airways in chronic bronchitis patients. Sputum analysis should be reserved for patients with frequent exacerbations or in patients with purulent sputum in whom there is a suspicion of more virulent or resistant bacteria. Spirometry during an acute exacerbation has little value, but it is important to know the pre-exacerbation state forced expiratory volume in 1 second (FEV_1) as a predictor of an adverse outcome of ABECB.

TREATMENT

Therapy should be directed toward three major goals: relief of symptoms, prevention of transient loss of pulmonary function (can lead to hospitalization), and reassessment of the disease in an attempt to reduce the risk of any further exacerbations. Patients should be removed from any further airway irritants including dust, pollutants, and cigarette smoke. Pharmacologic therapy should be aimed at decreasing the work of breathing, decreasing airway inflammation, lowering the bacterial burden of the lower airways, and treating resulting hypoxia.

The role of antimicrobial therapy in the treatment of ABECB remains controversial despite numerous therapeutic trials of antibiotics for more than 50 years. Most comparative trials have found equivalence in the use of antimicrobials. Differences in study end points, differences in patient groups studied, and variations in antibiotics used have made the comparison of these studies difficult. Not all antibiotics used to treat ABECB have the same spectrum of activity or pharmacokinetic properties. Therefore, numerous factors should be considered when selecting an antimicrobial agent.

Antibiotics should have both in vitro and in vivo activities against the most commonly associated pathogens implicated in ABECB, including *H. influenzae, S. pneumoniae,* and *M. catarrhalis.* In certain subgroups of patients with severe obstructive disease, coverage might need to be extended to include other pathogens such as *S. aureus, Pseudomonas aeruginosa,* species in the family Enterobacteriaceae, and atypical pathogens. Special attention should be paid to local and regional resistance profiles for the major bacterial pathogens. For example, at the Cleveland Clinic Foundation, the resistance rate of *S. pneumoniae* to penicillin is 42%; in Detroit, it is as low as 5.2%.[9]

The major oral antimicrobials used to treat ABECB are listed in Table 1. Antimicrobial therapy is appropriate for patients with an ABECB if they fall into the Anthonisen type I or type II categories but is not warranted in patients with a type III exacerbation. High-risk patients, including patients who have significant pulmonary impairment (FEV_1 < 50% or lower than predicted), who have four or more exacerbations per year, or who use supplemental oxygen or chronic oral corticosteroids, should be treated with antibiotics during ABECB. Due to emerging antimicrobial resistance, second-generation macrolides and some second- and third-generation cephalosporins may be used to treat ABECB rather than traditional first-line agents (aminopenicillins, doxycycline, trimethoprim-sulfamethoxazole [TMP-SMX]). A failure rate of 13% to 25% can be expected after treatment of ABECB with a traditional first-line antibiotic (amoxicillin, TMP-SMX, tetracycline, erythromycin). Patients who have structural lung disease, who chronically use corticosteroids, and who frequently use antimicrobials are at higher risk for P. aeruginosa infection and should be treated with antipseudomonal agents such as the fluoroquinolones. Patients who have been treated in the past 3 months for ABECB and who present with a relapse or reoccurrence of ABECB should be treated with a different class of antibiotics.

Bronchodilator therapy, including inhaled β-adrenergic agonists (albuterol, fenoterol, metaproterenol, terbutaline) and anticholinergic agents (ipratropium bromide), might improve airflow during acute exacerbation. Although long-acting β agonists in theory provide longer symptomatic relief, these agents have not been studied in ABECB and are not recommend at present. The choice of delivery system-metered dose inhaler (MDI) versus nebulized bronchodilators-should be determined based on cost and the patient's ability to use an MDI with a spacer. For patients already taking an oral methylxanthine, it is acceptable to continue this medication, keeping in mind that drug interactions with certain antibiotics (ciprofloxacin, clarithromycin) can occur and dosages need to be adjusted accordingly. In patients with moderate to severe exacerbations , good evidence supports treatment with oral or parenteral steroids for 5 to 14 days in general but not beyond 2 weeks. A number of randomized, placebo-controlled trials have demonstrated that systemic steroids lead to decreased treatment failure and shorten hospitalization rates. The mechanism by which steroids increase recovery in ABECB is not clear. Steroids are effective in decreasing airway edema and mucus hypersecretion and in increasing secretory leukoproteinase inhibitor (SLPI) in airway epithelial cells, which can have antiviral and antibacterial activities. There is no defined role for inhaled steroids in ABECB.

Supplemental oxygen should be provided carefully during an acute exacerbation to avoid hypoxemia, with the goal of maintaining a partial pressure of oxygen in arterial gas at or just above 60 mm Hg. The decision regarding long-term need for oxygen should not be made during an acute exacerbation, but patients should have an ambulatory desaturation study performed before discharge from the hospital to determine if supplemental home oxygen is needed. Expectorants or cough suppressants can provide subjective relief, but no evidence shows that these agents improve lung function or hasten clinical recovery in ABECB. There is no beneficial effect of chest physiotherapy in recovery from an ABECB. Instead, patients should be kept adequately hydrated to decrease viscosity of mucus. There is no evidence supporting the use of leukotriene receptor antagonists

Table 1 Oral Antibiotics Used in the Treatment of Acute Exacerbations of Chronic Bronchitis

Antibiotic	Spectrum of Activity and Resistance Pattern	Comments
Penicillins		
Amoxicillin	No activity against atypical and beta-lactamase-producing bacteria Penicillin resistance concerning with *Streptococcus pneumoniae* Limited activity against Enterobacteriaceae	Resistance limits use
Amoxicillin-clavulanate	Activity against major pathogens No activity against atypical bacteria Penicillin resistance concerning with *S. pneumoniae* Moderate activity against Enterobacteriaceae	More costly Gastrointestinal side effects
Cephalosporins		
General	Activity against major pathogens No activity against atypical bacteria Resistance concerning with *S. pneumoniae* Moderate activity against Enterobacteriaceae	Alternative to beta-lactam agents and generally as effective
Second Generation		
Cefaclor	Can be destroyed by *Haemophilus influenzae* and *Moraxella catarrhalis* enzymes	Associated with failure in patients with severe disease
Cefprozil	Moderate *H. influenzae activity*	
Cefuroxime		
Loracarbef	Moderate *H. influenzae* activity	
Third Generation		
Cefdinir		
Cefibuten	No activity against *Staphylococcus aureus* Marginal activity against *S. pneumoniae*	Poor gram-positive activity limits use
Cefixime	Poor activity against *S. aureus*	
Cefpodoxime		
Macrolides		
General	Macrolide resistance concerning with S. pneumoniae Active against atypical organisms Not active against Enterobacteriaceae	
Azithromycin	Greatest activity against *H. influenzae*	Short course of 3-5 days may be used
Clarithromycin	Greatest activity against *S. pneumoniae*	Alteration of taste may be an issue with bid dosing
Erythromycin	Poor activity against *H. influenzae*	Limited spectrum of activity
Tetracyclines		
Doxycycline	Covers major pathogens and atypical organisms *S. pneumoniae* resistance is common	Maybe an alternative to quinolones and macrolides when atypical coverage is needed
Minocycline	Similar to doxycycline	Limited spectrum of activity
Tetracycline	Limited activity against major pathogens Active against atypical bacteria	

Table 1 Oral Antibiotics Used in the Treatment of Acute Exacerbations of Chronic Bronchitis—cont'd

Antibiotic	Spectrum of Activity and Resistance Pattern	Comments
Fluoroquinolones		
General	Active against all major pathogens, atypical pathogens, Enterobacteriaceae, and *Pseudomonas aeruginosa*	
Ciprofloxacin	Least active against *S. pneumoniae* Greatest activity against *P. aeruginosa*	Use if P. *aeruginosa* coverage is required
Gatifloxacin	Enhanced gram-positive activity	
Levofloxacin		
Moxifloxacin	Greatest activity against *S. pneumoniae*	
Other		
Trimethoprim-sulfamethoxazole	Covers major pathogens No atypical coverage *S. pneumoniae resistance is common*	Resistance limits use

Adapted from Dever LL, Shashikumar K, Johanson WG: Antibiotics in the treatment of acute exacerbations of chronic bronchitis. Expert Opin Investig Drugs 2002;11:911-925.

in ABECB. In appropriate patients, noninvasive ventilation in acute exacerbations of COPD has been shown to reduce mortality, decrease the need for intubation and mechanical ventilation, and decrease the length of hospital and intensive care unit stay.

OUTCOMES

Hospitalization due to ABECB carries a short-term mortality rate of approximately 4% in patients with mild to moderate disease. The 1-year mortality rate for patients with severe disease can be as high as 46%. Many of the patients hospitalized for ABECB require subsequent readmissions because of persistent symptoms and often experience a temporary decrease in their functional abilities. Overall, ABECB contributes significantly to the morbidity and the diminished quality of life experienced by people with COPD.

Summary

- AABECBs are characterized by an increase in cough, sputum production, and dyspnea.
- Bacterial exacerbations of chronic bronchitis are the leading cause of death in patients with chronic obstructive pulmonary disease.
- After an ABECB, most patients experience a decrease in quality of life, and more than one half of patients require rehospitalization in the following 6 months.
- The most common bacteria isolated from the sputum in approximately 60% of ABECBs are Haemophilus influenza, Haemophilus parainfluenza, Streptococcus pneumoniae, and Moraxella catarrhalis.
- The role of antimicrobial therapy in the treatment of mild ABECBs remains controversial.

Suggested Readings

The COPD Guidelines Group of the Standards of Care Committee of the BTS. BTS guidelines for the management of chronic obstructive pulmonary disease. Thorax 1997;52(Suppl 5):S1-S28.

Pauwels RA, Buist AS, Calverly PM, et al, for the GOLD Scientific Committee: Global strategy for the diagnosis, management, and prevention of chronic obstructive pulmonary disease: NHLBI/WHO Global Initiative for Chronic Obstructive Lung Disease (GOLD) Workshop summary. Am J Respir Crit Care Med 2001;163:1256-1276.

References

For a complete list of references, log onto www.expertconsult.com.

Chronic Obstructive Pulmonary Disease

Georges Juvelekian and James K. Stoller

Recently, chronic obstructive pulmonary disease (COPD) has gained interest as a major public health concern and is currently the focus of intense research because of its persistently increasing prevalence, mortality, and disease burden. COPD was responsible for more than 2.5 million deaths worldwide in 2000 alone,[1] and it currently ranks as the fourth leading cause of death in the United States, surpassed only by heart disease, cancer, and cerebrovascular disease.[2,3] COPD is projected to have the fifth leading burden of disease worldwide by the year 2020.[4] COPD is one of the leading causes of disability worldwide and is the only disease for which the prevalence and mortality rates continue to rise.

This chapter presents a concise overview of COPD. We address its definition, prevalence and epidemiology, pathology and pathophysiology, diagnosis, therapy, and outcomes. Also, because of recent insights regarding the relation between COPD and sleep disorders, we include a discussion on sleep and COPD.

DEFINITIONS

COPD is broadly defined and encompasses several clinical and pathologic entities, primarily emphysema and chronic bronchitis. Evidence of airflow obstruction that is chronic, progressive, and for the most part fixed characterizes COPD. Notwithstanding the presence of irreversible airflow obstruction in COPD, most persons (~60%-70%) demonstrate a reversible component of airflow obstruction when tested repeatedly.[5-8]

Emphysema is specifically defined[5-8] in pathologic terms as "alveolar wall destruction with irreversible enlargement of the air spaces distal to the terminal bronchioles and without evidence of fibrosis." *Chronic bronchitis* is defined as "productive cough that is present for a period of three months in each of two consecutive years in the absence of another identifiable cause of excessive sputum production."

The American Thoracic Society (ATS), British Thoracic Society (BTS), and European Respiratory Society (ERS) definitions of COPD emphasize chronic bronchitis and emphysema, but the Global Initiative for Chronic Obstructive Lung Disease (GOLD) proposes a definition of COPD that focuses on the progressive nature of airflow limitation and its association with abnormal inflammatory response of the lungs to various noxious particles or gases.[5-8] According to the GOLD document, COPD is defined as "a disease state characterized by airflow limitation that is not fully reversible. The airflow limitation is usually both progressive and associated with an abnormal inflammatory response of the lungs to noxious particles or gases."[8]

PREVALENCE AND EPIDEMIOLOGY

The prevalence of COPD is increasing. In 1994, there were approximately 16.2 million men and women suffering from COPD in the United States and more than 52 million persons around the world.[1,2,8] The worldwide prevalence is likely to be underestimated for several reasons, including the delay in establishing the diagnosis, the variability in defining COPD, and the lack of age-adjusted estimates. Age adjustment is important because the prevalence of COPD in persons younger than 45 years is low, and the prevalence is highest in patients older than 65 years. In 1995, 553,000 patients were treated for COPD in the United States, and two thirds of those were older than 65 years. The prevalence in those older than 65 years was four times that in the 45- to 64-year-old group.[9,10] The gender distribution of COPD is also changing, and as of 2000, COPD deaths in women exceeded the number in men.[2]

Because of its chronic and progressive nature, COPD represents a massive and growing burden in direct and indirect costs. In developing countries where smoking continues to be extremely prevalent, the health and economic burdens are higher than in developed nations. Because people constitute an essential role in the economy of developing countries, the disability caused by COPD further magnifies the problem.

Although it has been difficult to estimate the costs associated with COPD, they include direct costs pertaining to outpatient and inpatient care expenses, the indirect costs resulting from the loss of productivity caused by premature death and disability, and the additional cost of disability. In the United States, for instance, hospitalization constitutes the bulk of all COPD-related health costs. In 1993, direct health costs of COPD were $14.7 billion, and the overall burden was estimated at more than $30 billion.[1,2,10]

PATHOGENESIS AND PATHOLOGY

As indicated in the definition of emphysema, the pathologic hallmark is elastin breakdown with resultant loss of alveolar wall integrity. This process is triggered by the exposure of a susceptible person to noxious particles and gases. Cigarette smoke remains the main causative agent, involved in more than 90% of cases. However, other gases and particles have been shown to play a role in pathogenesis, which is a result of an inflammatory process. In contrast to the eosinophilic inflammation seen in asthma, the predominant inflammatory cell is the neutrophil. Macrophages and $CD8^+$ T lymphocytes are increased in the various parts of the lungs, and several mediators, including leukotriene B_4, interleukin 8, and tumor necrosis factor, contribute to the inflammatory process.[6]

Oxidative stress is regarded as another important process in the pathogenesis of COPD, and altered protease-antiprotease balance, at least in persons with severe deficiency of α_1-antitrypsin, has been shown to predispose to a panacinar form of emphysema. Persons with severe deficiency of α_1-antitrypsin can develop emphysema at an early age (e.g., by the fourth decade), in contrast to the "usual" emphysema, which typically begins in the sixth decade.

The pathologic hallmark of chronic bronchitis is an increase in goblet cell size and number that leads to excessive mucus secretion. Airflow obstruction and emphysematous change are common but not universal accompaniments. When COPD is complicated by hypoxemia, intimal and vascular smooth muscle thickening can cause pulmonary hypertension, which is a late and poor prognostic development in COPD.[5-8,11,12]

DIAGNOSIS

The diagnosis of COPD is suggested by findings on history or physical examination, or both, and is confirmed by laboratory tests, usually with a supportive risk factor (e.g., familial COPD or cigarette exposure, or both). Spirometry is indispensable in establishing the diagnosis because it is a standardized and reproducible test that objectively confirms the presence of airflow obstruction. Character-

Table 1 Staging of Disease Severity

Disease Severity FEV_1 Predicted	ATS	ERS	BTS	GOLD
Stage 0: at risk	—	—	—	Normal Chronic symptoms (cough, sputum production)
Stage I: mild	≥50%	≥70%	≥60%	≥80% With or without chronic symptoms
Stage II: moderate	35-49%	50-69%	40-59%	50%-79% With or without chronic symptoms
Stage III: severe	<35%	<50%	<40%	30%-49% With or without chronic symptoms
Stage IV: very severe	—	—	—	<30% or <50% with chronic respiratory failure

ATS, American Thoracic Society; BTS, British Thoracic Society; ERS, European Respiratory Society; FEV_1, forced expiratory volume in 1 second; FVC, forced vital capacity; GOLD, Global Initiative for Chronic Obstructive Lung Disease.

istically, spirometry shows a decreased forced expiratory volume in 1 second (FEV_1) and a decreased FEV_1/FVC (forced vital capacity) ratio.[5-8] Evidence of reversible airflow obstruction, defined as a post-bronchodilator rise of FEV_1 and/or FVC by 12% and 200 mL, is present in up to two thirds of patients with serial testing. Measurement of the diffusing capacity for carbon monoxide (D_LCO) can help differentiate between emphysema and chronic bronchitis. Specifically, in the context of fixed airflow obstruction, a decreased diffusing capacity indicates a loss of alveolar-capillary units, which suggests emphysema.

Deficiency of α_1-antitrypsin is an uncommon cause of emphysema that continues to be under-recognized by practicing clinicians.[13-15] The clinical recognition of patients with this condition is also based on clinical suspicion, but as outlined in the American Thoracic Society/European Respiratory Society (ATS/ERS) evidence-based standards document, specific circumstances should prompt suspicion of α_1-antitrypsin deficiency. They include emphysema occurring in a young person (age ≤45 years) or without obvious risk factors (e.g., smoking or occupational exposure) or with prominent basilar emphysema on imaging, necrotizing panniculitis, antineutrophil cytoplasmic antibody (C-ANCA)-positive vasculitis, bronchiectasis of undetermined etiology, otherwise unexplained liver disease, or a family history of any one of these conditions, especially siblings of *PI*ZZ* individuals.[13]

The most common symptoms and signs include cough, dyspnea on exertion, and increased phlegm production. Additional signs and symptoms include wheezing, prolonged expiration with pursed-lip breathing, barrel chest, use of accessory muscles of breathing and, in advanced cases, cyanosis, evidence of right heart failure, and peripheral edema. A chest radiograph is usually obtained to exclude other etiologies but might show hyperinflation and flattening of the diaphragm with increased retrosternal space on the lateral view and hyperlucency reflecting oligemia. The chest radiograph is an insensitive test for diagnosing emphysema and is abnormal only when emphysema is relatively advanced. In contrast, high-resolution computed tomography (CT) scanning is far more sensitive and specific than chest x-ray for diagnosing emphysema and readily identifies bullae and blebs that are the consequences of alveolar breakdown. However, save for its role in selecting the proper candidate for lung volume reduction surgery, the additional data from CT rarely alter therapy, making CT scanning not currently indicated for routine clinical use.[5-8]

Classification of Severity

Because the degree of FEV_1 reduction has prognostic implications and correlates with mortality and morbidity, a staging system based on the degree of airflow obstruction has been proposed by the different societal guidelines. As reviewed in Table 1, four groups—the ATS, the ERS, the British Thoracic Society (BTS), and GOLD—have developed staging systems for COPD based on the value of FEV_1 percent predicted. All systems propose three- or four-stage classifications of COPD, although the FEV_1 criteria vary among systems.[5-8]

In the context that one major purpose of staging systems is to establish prognosis, attention has focused on the value of including weight (i.e., body mass index [BMI]), dyspnea, and exercise capacity (i.e., the 6-minute walk distance), with FEV_1 in staging COPD.[16] Indeed, the resultant index, called BODE (for *B*MI, *o*bstruction, *d*yspnea, and *e*xercise capacity) has been shown to better predict survival in COPD than FEV_1 alone. BODE scores of 0 to 10 (most impaired) are stratified into four quartiles, which discriminate mortality risk better than FEV_1 alone.

Natural History and Prognosis

Several factors influence the natural history and affect survival in patients with COPD. These factors include age, smoking status, pulmonary artery pressure, resting heart rate, BMI, airway responsiveness, hypoxemia, dyspnea, exercise capacity, and most importantly, the level of FEV_1, which remains the single best indicator of prognosis.

Few interventions have been shown to change the natural history of COPD. For persons hypoxemic in room air, survival can be improved by use of supplemental oxygen.[17] Smoking cessation can improve survival in smokers,[18,19] and lung volume reduction surgery can improve survival in selected patients.[20]

Acute exacerbations of COPD (AECOPD) are a significant contributor to mortality. For example, in the SUPPORT study[21] of patients with AECOPD admitted to the hospital, of 1016 inpatients admitted with hypercapnic respiratory failure, 89% survived the acute hospitalization, but only 51% were alive at 2 years. Patient characteristics associated with mortality at 6 months included increased severity of illness, lower body mass index, older age, poor prior functional status, lower PaO_2/FIO_2 (inspired fraction of oxygen), and lower serum albumin. However, congestive heart failure and cor pulmonale were associated with longer survival time at 6 months, and this was attributed to the effective therapy available for the management of these conditions. The overall severity of illness on the third day of hospitalization, as measured by the Apache III score, was the most important independent predictor of survival at 6 months.[21]

Notably, in another study of patients with AECOPD, the development of hypercapnia during an acute exacerbation of COPD appeared not to affect the risk of death with AECOPD.[22] Specifically, in a prospective study involving 85 patients admitted with acute exacerbation and followed for 5 years, the mortality rate was not significantly different between hypercapnic and eucapnic persons. In contrast, patients with chronic hypercapnia demonstrated a much poorer outcome, with only an 11% 5-year survival rate.[23] Notwithstanding these insights, well-designed studies and controlled trials are necessary to improve our ability to predict the outcomes for patients with this disease.

SLEEP AND COPD

In the context of a growing understanding of sleep and the interactions between disorders of sleep and COPD, this section reviews the mechanism of hypoxemia in sleep and the overlap between COPD and obstructive sleep apnea syndrome (OSAS).

Hypoxemia During Sleep in COPD

Under normal circumstances, sleep results in a decrease in ventilation and in chemo-responsiveness to the arterial partial pressure of carbon dioxide ($Paco_2$).[24,25] The decreased ventilation appears to be almost entirely related to a drop in tidal volume. Normally, this decrease in tidal volume does not result in hypoxemia, because the drop in the arterial partial pressure of oxygen (Pao_2) occurs on the flat portion of the oxyhemoglobin dissociation curve, thereby preserving the oxygen saturation (Sao_2). However, in patients with COPD, whose oxygenation during wakefulness may already be on the steep portion of the oxyhemoglobin dissociation curve, hypoxemia during sleep can occur as tidal volume falls.

The most pronounced hypoxemia occurs during the rapid eye movement (REM) stage of sleep because of the generalized muscle hypotonia that accompanies REM sleep. REM-associated hypoxemia can reach critically low levels, especially in patients with already borderline waking oxygenation, with potentially deleterious clinical consequences such as cardiac dysrhythmias, pulmonary hypertension, and polycythemia.

Hypoxemia during sleep in COPD is primarily a result of hypoventilation, but it is also caused by a decrease in functional residual capacity (FRC) and a worsening ventilation/perfusion ($\dot{V}/\dot{Q}$) mismatch.

COPD and Obstructive Sleep Apnea Syndrome

The co-occurrence of COPD and OSAS, also referred to as the *overlap syndrome,* involves a minority of COPD patients, but identifying these patients is important because their nocturnal hypoxemia tends to be more pronounced, leading to a greater likelihood of adverse clinical events. It follows that in patients with the overlap syndrome, therapy must be directed at their COPD *and* at the OSAS.

TREATMENT

Stable COPD

Once the diagnosis of COPD is established and the stage of the disease is determined, attention turns to patient education and modification of risk factors, to pharmacologic and nonpharmacologic methods needed to ameliorate the signs and symptoms of COPD, and to optimizing patients' longevity and functional status.[26,27]

Patient education is an essential component of treatment because it facilitates reduction of risk factors and improves the individual patient's ability to cope with the disease. Education requires a team approach that includes, in addition to the physician and the patient, home health nurses, social workers, physical therapists, occupational therapists, and others. In addition to risk-factor reduction, education should provide a basic, simple-to-understand overview of COPD, its pathophysiology, medications and their proper use, and instructions on when to seek help. Discussing end-of-life issues and establishing advance directives are facilitated by the educational process, especially when applied in the setting of pulmonary rehabilitation.[28,29]

Smoking cessation is a cornerstone of patient education and confers many benefits, including slowing the accelerated rate of FEV_1 decline among smokers, improvements in symptoms, and lessening the risk of lung cancer. For example, data from the Lung Health Study (LHS) show that in the sustained nonsmokers over that 11-year study, the rate of FEV_1 decline slowed to 30 mL per year in men and 22 mL per year in women compared with the 66 mL per year and 54 mL per year decline in continuing male and female smokers, respectively. The result was that 38% of continuing smokers had an FEV_1 less than 60% of predicted normal at 11 years compared with only 10% of sustained quitters. Aggressive smoking cessation intervention with counseling and nicotine patch allowed 22% of LHS participants to achieve sustained smoking cessation over 5 years, and 93% of these participants were still abstinent at 11 years.[18,19,26]

Available strategies for smoking cessation include nicotine replacement (available in gum, patch, inhaler or nasal spray), bupropion (an antidepressant), smoking-cessation programs, varenicline,[30] counseling, and combinations of these. Randomized, controlled trials suggest that the combination of nicotine replacement and bupropion confers greater likelihood of achieving smoke-free status than either therapy alone.[31] Use of the partial acetylcholine receptor agonist varenicline appears to allow higher rates of smoking cessation than does buproprion.[30]

Beyond education and smoking cessation, the goals of pharmacologic and nonpharmacologic treatments are to enhance survival, quality of life, and functional status and to lessen mortality. As reviewed in Table 2, available treatments include bronchodilators, corticosteroids, immunizations, antibiotics, mucokinetics, and others.

Bronchodilators

Bronchodilators are a mainstay of COPD treatment and include β-adrenergic agonists, anticholinergics, and methylxanthines. β-Adrenergic agonists are effective in alleviating symptoms and improving exercise capacity, and they can produce significant increases in FEV_1.[5,6] Their effect is achieved through smooth-muscle relaxation, resulting in improved lung emptying, reduced thoracic gas volume and residual volume, and lessened dynamic hyperinflation. It is believed that the increase in exercise tolerance and reduction in symptoms of breathlessness are primarily a result of an improvement in inspiratory capacity rather than an increase in FEV_1. Oral theophylline has been shown to lessen dyspnea and improve the health-related quality of life despite lack of significant rise in FEV_1, with improvements believed to be a result of increased respiratory muscle performance. However, the narrow therapeutic index of methylxanthines and their potential for adverse drug-drug interactions have hindered their widespread use. Long-acting formulations have allowed more-consistent and stable plasma levels, thereby mitigating the problem.

Phosphodiesterase Inhibitors

Newly developed oral, highly selective phosphodiesterase 4 (PDE4) inhibitors roflumilast[32] and cilomilast,[33] have shown promise in the management of stable COPD. Specifically, a randomized, double-blind study involving more than 1400 patients with moderate-to-severe COPD compared patients assigned to receive 250 μg of roflumilast, 500 μg of roflumilast, or placebo over a period of 24 weeks. The primary end points were post-bronchodilator FEV_1 and health-related quality of life. Secondary end points included the rate of COPD exacerbations. Although there was no significant difference in the post-bronchodilator FEV_1 in the treatment arms, both were superior to placebo ($P < .0001$). Similar findings were reported in the health-related quality of life and rate of exacerbations with an acceptable safety profile.[32]

Similarly, cilomilast was compared with placebo in a double-blind, placebo-controlled, parallel group trial. Here, patients were

Table 2 Recommendations by Professional Societies for Management of Stable COPD

American Thoracic Society 1995 Consensus	European Respiratory Society 1995 Consensus	British Thoracic Society 1997 Consensus	Global Initiative for Chronic Obstructive Lung Disease 2005 Evidence-Based Review
Diagnostic Testing			
Recommended:	Recommended:	Recommended:	Recommended:
Spirometry	Spirometry	Spirometry	Spirometry
Pre- and post BD	Pre- and post-BD	Pre- and post-BD	Pre- and post-BD
Pre- and post-corticosteroids only if inadequate response to treatment	Pre- and post-corticosteroids in stages 2 and 3	Pre- and post-corticosteroids in stages 2 and 3	Pre- and post-corticosteroids in stages 2 and 3
CXR	CXR	CXR in moderate or severe disease	CXR to exclude alternative Dx
CT: not routinely, but helpful in predicting the benefit of pulmonary resection for giant bullous disease	CT assessment of bullae	Restricted to assessment of bullous emphysema	CT when Dx is in doubt or if LVRS is contemplated
ABG in stages 2 and 3	ABG in stages 2 and 3 or $Sao_2 < 92\%$	ABG in severe disease	ABG if FEV_1 is <40% or with symptoms suggestive of RHF or in respiratory failure
α_1-AT deficiency in early, severe disease	α_1-AT deficiency in early, severe disease	Not discussed	α_1-AT deficiency in early COPD (age <45) or strong family history
Bronchodilator Therapy			
β_2 Agonist first line PRN use; anticholinergic first line for regular use; theophylline and/or sustained release albuterol for persistent symptoms	β_2 Agonist or anticholinergic as needed; combination if needed; theophylline if no response to other BD; long-acting inhaled β_2 agonist or oral if needed	Short-acting β_2 agonist or inhaled anticholinergic as needed; regular β_2 agonist and/or anticholinergics and/or combination for advanced stages; long-acting β_2 agonist if evidence of improvement; theophylline is of limited value	Short-acting BD as needed Regular treatment with one or more BD in advanced stages; long-acting inhaled BD more convenient; combination BD and anticholinergics is better than either agent alone
Corticosteroids			
If corticosteroid response established: Lowest effective oral dose used Insufficient data to support use of aerosolized steroid	If corticosteroid response established: Inhaled steroids Inhaled steroids in patients with mild disease but "fast decline" of FEV_1 (>50 mL per yr)	If corticosteroid response established: Inhaled steroids	If corticosteroid response established: Inhaled steroids Inhaled steroids in stages 2 and 3 Long-term oral steroids not recommended
Antibiotics			
Not recommended	Not recommended	Not recommended	Not recommended
Mucokinetics			
Not recommended	Not recommended	Not recommended	Not recommended
α_1-Antitrypsin Augmentation Therapy			
In appropriate patients	Not recommended	Not discussed	In appropriate patients
Vaccinations			
Influenza recommended; pneumococcal recommended	Influenza recommended; pneumococcal, insufficient data	Influenza recommended; pneumococcal, insufficient data	Influenza recommended pneumococcal, insufficient data
Smoking Cessation			
Recommended; smoking cessation protocol	Recommended	Recommended	Recommended
Lung Volume Reduction Surgery			
In appropriately selected patients	In appropriately selected patients	In appropriately selected patients	Not recommended, insufficient data

Table 2 Recommendations by Professional Societies for Management of Stable COPD—cont'd

American Thoracic Society 1995 Consensus	European Respiratory Society 1995 Consensus	British Thoracic Society 1997 Consensus	Global Initiative for Chronic Obstructive Lung Disease 2005 Evidence-Based Review
Lung Transplantation			
In appropriately selected patients	In appropriately selected patients	In appropriately selected patients	In appropriately selected patients
Home Mechanical Ventilation			
Non-elective ventilation supported; elective ventilation not supported	No recommendation provided	Elective and non-elective ventilation modestly supported	Not supported
Long-Term Oxygen Therapy			
Recommended in patients with chronic hypoxemia	Recommended in patients with chronic hypoxemia	Recommended in patients with chronic hypoxemia	Recommended in patients with chronic hypoxemia
Pulmonary Rehabilitation			
Recommended; upper extremity training and breathing retraining supported	Recommended	Recommended	Recommended along with nutritional counseling, and education

ABG, arterial blood gas; α_1-AT, α_1-antitrypsin; BD, bronchodilator; COPD, chronic obstructive pulmonary disease; CXR, chest radiograph; CT, computed tomography; Dx, diagnosis; FEV_1, forced expiratory volume in 1 second; LVRS, lung volume reduction surgery; RHF, right heart failure.

assigned to cilomilast 15 mg orally twice daily versus placebo, and followed for 24 weeks. Change from baseline FEV_1 and St. George's Respiratory Questionnaire (SGRQ) scores were the primary end points, with the rate of COPD exacerbations as the main secondary end point. Again, cilomilast was statistically superior to placebo in all study end points, with mild-to-moderate adverse events that were self-limited.[33] As promising as these studies seem, more studies are needed before these new PDE4 inhibitors become part of standard therapy for the stable COPD patient.[5,33]

β-Adrenergic Agonists

In the early stages of COPD (e.g., stage I), a short-acting β-adrenergic agonist (e.g., albuterol, terbutaline) or an anticholinergic is used on an as-needed basis. As the disease progresses (e.g., stages II and III), regular use of one or more bronchodilators is often recommended. Some data suggest that a combination of albuterol and ipratropium bromide provides better bronchodilation than either agent alone.[5,34-36]

In 2004, the United States Food and Drug Administration approved a new anticholinergic agent, tiotropium, for the long-term, once daily, maintenance treatment of bronchospasm associated with stable COPD, including chronic bronchitis and emphysema.[37] Although this is the same indication granted to ipratropium, tiotropium has shown significant advantages over ipratropium, both pharmacologically and clinically. Specifically, tiotropium blocks the M_1 to M_5 muscarinic receptors with a 6- to 20-fold greater affinity than ipratropium and for a longer period[38-40] and dissociates more rapidly from the M_2 receptor associated with acetylcholine release, thereby conferring theoretical advantages over ipratropium.

These advantages were shown in clinical trials comparing the two agents. Specifically, tiotropium demonstrated significantly greater bronchodilation than ipratropium, and users experienced less dyspnea, fewer acute exacerbations, reduced albuterol use, and improved nocturnal oxygen saturation.[39-42] When compared with long-acting β_2-agonists, tiotropium provided greater bronchodilation and more-reduced dyspnea than salmeterol. A large double-blind, placebo-controlled trial showed a significantly greater reduction in yearly incidence as well as delay to first COPD exacerbation compared with either salmeterol or placebo.[42]

Results of a large randomized, controlled trial (called UPLIFT) comparing the efficacy of tiotropium have shown that tiotropium conferred benefits of a lower exacerbation frequency but neither slowing of FEU_1 decline nor a lower mortality rate.[43]

Corticosteroids

Although widely used, oral and inhaled corticosteroids have a limited role in managing patients with stable COPD. Several groups suggest brief trials of oral corticosteroids for patients with stable COPD. For example, the BTS suggests a course of oral prednisone (e.g., 30 mg daily) taken for 2 weeks, or a course of inhaled steroid (e.g., beclomethasone 500 μg twice daily or the equivalent) taken for 6 weeks.[7] Similarly, the ERS suggests a trial of corticosteroids (e.g., 0.4-0.6 mg/kg/day) taken for 2 to 4 weeks. Patients with significant FEV_1 responses are considered candidates for long-term inhaled corticosteroids.[6] At the same time, four randomized, placebo-controlled trials of inhaled corticosteroids in patients with COPD have shown no effect on the rate of FEV_1 decline,[27,44-47] although one study suggested that steroid recipients experienced fewer COPD exacerbations than nonrecipients.[46]

A more-recent trial was conducted comparing the effect of the salmeterol-fluticasone combination with either agent alone and with placebo. It found that the combination therapy was significantly more effective than sole therapy with the long-acting bronchodilator, or fluticasone, or placebo in patients with COPD. The TRISTAN study, a 52-week, randomized, placebo-controlled study involving 1465 patients with moderate-to-severe COPD, showed significant improvement in FEV_1 in the salmeterol-fluticasone combination versus salmeterol (treatment difference of 73 mL, $P < 0.0001$), fluticasone (treatment difference of 95 mL, $P < 0.0001$),[48] and placebo (treatment difference of 133 mL, $P < 0.0001$). Other benefits included a decrease in the use of rescue medications in the combination group and a significant improvement in health status as defined by the St. George's Respiratory Questionnaire compared with the fluticasone group but not the salmeterol group. The rate of moderate and severe exacerbations was reduced by 25% in the combination group compared with placebo.[48]

This finding becomes all the more significant in the context that severe acute exacerbations have an independent negative impact on prognosis, with increased mortality associated with the frequency of severe exacerbations.[49] In a prospective cohort of 304 men with severe COPD (mean FEV_1, 46% of predicted), older age, Pco_2, and acute exacerbation of COPD represented independent indicators of poor prognosis, and patients with three or more exacerbations showed the greatest mortality risk.[49] Whether the combination of an inhaled corticosteroid and long-term bronchodilator enhances survival in patients with COPD is the subject of ongoing research.[50]

Several randomized, controlled clinical trials have assessed the role of inhaled corticosteroids (e.g., called Euroscop, ISOLDE, Copenhagen City, Lung Health Study, and OPTIMAL) and of inhaled steroids combined with long-acting β agonists in exacerbation frequency, quality of life, rate of change of FEV_1, and, in one study (TORCH), mortality. The weight of evidence suggests that inhaled corticosteroids can lessen the frequency of acute exacerbations of COPD, but (with the exception of the TORCH trial) inhaled steroids do not appear to affect the rate of FEV_1 decline. The combination of inhaled fluticasone and salmeterol appears better than placebo in enhancing health-related quality of life and lessening exacerbation frequency. The one trial (TORCH) that examined mortality as a primary outcome measure showed that the combination of inhaled fluticasone and salmeterol (500 μg/50 μg, respectively, twice daily) conferred a 2.6% absolute reduction in mortality (15.2%-12.6%; 17.5% relative reduction), although this difference missed statistical significance ($P = 0.052$).

Currently, inhaled corticosteroids are widely used, especially for patients with frequent exacerbations of COPD, although recent concerns about excess pneumonia risk in users of inhaled steroids have spurred some controversy and will certainly receive prospective scrutiny.

Immunizations

Yearly prophylactic immunization with the influenza vaccine has been shown to reduce the incidence of influenza by 76% and is strongly recommended.[51-53] Immunization once with the 23-polyvalent pneumococcal vaccine in patients with COPD or, in the special case of patients with immunodeficiency or those with splenectomy, every 5 years, is also recommended.[53] The role of different pneumococcal vaccine preparations is being examined as part of the COPD Network, a multicenter consortium sponsored by the National Institutes of Health.

Antibiotics

Prophylactic antibiotics have not shown benefit in the management of stable COPD and are not recommended,[5-8] although forthcoming trials regarding daily azithromycin and periodic moxifloxacin might affect current understanding and recommendations.

Mucokinetic Agents

Mucoactive agents are varied and include ambroxol, erdosteine, carbocysteine, iodinated glycerol, *N*-acetylcysteine, surfactant, and others, all of which have been studied with conflicting results. However, a Cochrane systematic review of 23 randomized, controlled trials in Europe and the United States associates the long-term use (>2 months) of oral mucolytics with a reduction in acute COPD exacerbations and days of illness and suggests considering these agents in patients with recurrent, prolonged, severe COPD exacerbations.[54] Still, the latest guidelines by the ATS and BTS do not recommend the routine use of mucoactive agents in the management of chronic COPD.[5-8]

Others

Antitussives containing narcotics and other therapies, such as inhaled nitric oxide, may be harmful. Their use in COPD is contraindicated.[5-8] In the specific case of α_1-antitrypsin deficiency, intravenous augmentation therapy with pooled human plasma antiprotease can raise serum levels of α_1-antitrypsin above a protective threshold value (11 micromolar).[13] Available evidence suggests that augmentation therapy can slow the rate of FEV_1 decline in persons with severe deficiency of α_1-antitrypsin (e.g., with the *PI*ZZ* phenotype) and established airflow obstruction of moderate severity (e.g., FEV_1 30%-65% of predicted). Currently available α_1-proteinase inhibitors in the United States include Prolastin (Talecris, Research Triangle, NC), Aralast (Baxter Healthcare, Deerfield, Ill), and Zemaira (CSL Behring, King of Prussia, Penn).

Nonpharmacologic treatment of COPD includes pulmonary rehabilitation, long-term oxygen therapy, ventilatory support, and lung volume reduction surgery (LVRS). Pulmonary rehabilitation is recommended at all stages by all available guidelines (see Table 2).[5-8,55] Aerobic lower extremity training can improve exercise endurance, dyspnea, use of health care, and overall quality of life. Upper extremity-exercise and respiratory muscle training also appear helpful.[5,54]

Long-term oxygen therapy for patients with hypoxemia has been shown to improve survival in eligible patients with COPD.[17] Criteria for prescribing long-term oxygen therapy include a Pao_2 less than 55 mm Hg or Sao_2 less than 88% with or without increased $Paco_2$, or Pao_2 between 55 and 59 mm Hg or Sao_2 less than 89%, with right-sided failure reflected by evidence of pulmonary hypertension or polycythemia (e.g., hematocrit >55%).

Nocturnal noninvasive ventilatory support still has an unproven role in managing patients with stable COPD. LVRS involves resecting 20% to 35% of the emphysematous lung to improve lung mechanics. The procedure was first proposed by Brantigan and Mueller in the late 1940s,[55] but it was abandoned then because of unacceptably high associated mortality. More recently, randomized, controlled trials show that LVRS is contraindicated in patients with severely impaired lung function (e.g., FEV_1 <20% predicted, homogeneous emphysema and/or lung diffusing capacity for carbon monoxide <20% predicted)[20-56] but that patients with moderate degrees of airflow obstruction who undergo LVRS might experience an improved FEV_1, walking distance, and quality of life.[20,57-59] In the results of the National Emphysema Treatment Trial (NETT), a randomized, controlled trial of LVRS versus medical therapy (including rehabilitation) in which 1218 subjects with moderate COPD (FEV_1 <45% predicted) were enrolled, the LVRS group overall experienced improved disease-specific quality of life and exercise capacity compared with the medically managed group.[20] On the other hand, the LVRS group had rates of survival similar to those of the medically managed group. In subsets defined by prespecified exploration, a survival advantage was observed in the subgroup of patients with predominantly upper lobe emphysema and low baseline (i.e., postrehabilitation) exercise capacity (defined as a maximal workload at <25 watts for women and 40 watts for men).[20] A longer-term overall survival benefit was demonstrated in those allocated to LVRS.

Lung transplantation is an option for patients with severe airflow obstruction and functional impairment. The 5-year actuarial survival rate for patients undergoing single-lung transplantation for COPD is 43.2%.[60-62] Selection criteria include an FEV_1 less than 25% predicted or a $Paco_2$ greater than 55 mm Hg or cor pulmonale, or both. A large multicenter controlled trial of oxygen versus no oxygen sponsored by the National Institutes of Health (Long-term Oxygen Treatment Trial [LOTT]) is examining the survival benefits of supplemental oxygen for patients with COPD and moderate hypoxemia

Table 3 Recommendations by Professional Societies for Management of Acute Exacerbations of COPD

American Thoracic Society	European Respiratory Society	British Thoracic Society	Global Initiative for Chronic Obstructive Lung Disease
Bronchodilators			
Recommended: β_2 agonists ± anticholinergics; IV aminophylline if inadequate response	Recommended: β_2 agonists ± anticholinergics; methylxanthines if needed as second-line therapy in severe exacerbations	Recommended: β_2 agonists ± anticholinergics; IV aminophylline if inadequate response	Recommended: β_2 agonist dose increase ± anticholinergics ± IV aminophylline depending on disease severity
Corticosteroids			
Oral or systemic	Oral or systemic empirically	7-14 days of systemic steroids	Systemic steroids
Antibiotics			
Narrow-spectrum antibiotic; broad spectrum if no response	Inexpensive antibiotic empirically for 7-14 days; if ineffective, choice guided by sputum culture	Common oral antibiotics usually adequate Broader spectrum if no response or if more severe exacerbation	Empirically with increased sputum volume and purulence based on local sensitivity patterns to usual pathogens
Oxygen Therapy			
Raise Pao_2>60 mm Hg	Keep Sao_2≥90% and/or Pao_2≥60 mm Hg. Avoid $Paco_2$ *rise* by >10 mm Hg or pH *drop* to <7.25	Raise Pao_2 to ≥50 mm Hg while avoiding pH <7.26	Keep Sao_2>90% and Pao_2>60 mm Hg
Ventilatory Support			
NIPPV or invasive mechanical ventilation based on criteria	NIPPV in appropriate patients	NIPPV or invasive mechanical ventilation if pH <7.26 with rising $Paco_2$ despite controlled oxygen therapy	NIPPV or invasive mechanical ventilation based on selection and exclusion criteria.
Chest Physiotherapy			
Only if sputum volume is >25 mL/day	Help in clearance of secretions	Not recommended	May be beneficial in certain circumstances

COPD, chronic obstructive pulmonary disease; NIPPV, noninvasive positive pressure ventilation.

(pulse oximetry saturation of 89%-92% on room air at rest). Results are forthcoming.

Acute Exacerbations of COPD

Acute exacerbation of COPD (AECOPD) represents an acute worsening of the patient's baseline condition, generally characterized by worsened dyspnea and increased volume and purulence of sputum.[5-8,63,64] Depending on the severity of baseline COPD, additional derangements can occur, including hypoxemia, worsening hypercapnia, cor pulmonale with worsening lower extremity edema, or altered mental status.

The main goals of treating AECOPD are to restore the patient to his or her previous stable baseline and to prevent or reduce the likelihood of recurrence. This requires identifying the precipitating factor or condition and reversing or ameliorating it while optimizing gas exchange and improving the patient's symptoms. Treatment modalities similar to the ones used in stable COPD are used in managing acute exacerbations (Table 3). These include oxygen therapy, bronchodilators, antibiotics, corticosteroids, mechanical ventilation, and others.

Oxygen Therapy

The role of oxygen therapy is to correct the hypoxemia that usually accompanies the AECOPD. The end point is to maintain oxygen tension at approximately 60 to 65 mm Hg, thereby assuring near-maximal hemoglobin saturation while minimizing the potential for deleterious hypercapnia. Hypercapnia complicating supplemental oxygen is mainly a result of ventilation-perfusion mismatch, with generally smaller contributions of depression of the respiratory drive and the Haldane effect.

Bronchodilators

Bronchodilators are widely used in AECOPD, and β-adrenergic agonists and anticholinergics are first-line therapies. As in stable COPD, both can improve airflow in AECOPD, and although recommendations vary, combined therapy is often recommended. β-Adrenergic agonists have a quicker onset of action, whereas anticholinergics have a more favorable side-effect profile. Because of their potential side effects, as well as their limited benefit, methylxanthines are used mostly as second-line therapy.[5-8]

Antibiotics

Antibiotics play a favorable role in treating AECOPD, especially in the setting of increased volume and purulence of phlegm.[64-66] A narrow-spectrum antibiotic (e.g., amoxicillin, trimethoprim-sulfamethoxazole, doxycycline) is often recommended as first-line therapy, although use of a beta-lactam/beta-lactamase combination has been recommended in patients with severe AECOPD, and fluoroquinolones have been used in patients suspected to be colonized with *Pseudomonas aeruginosa*.[8] The optimal duration of treatment is still unclear, although most guidelines recommend treating for between 7 and 14 days.[63]

Corticosteroids

Randomized clinical trials generally support the use of systemic corticosteroids to enhance airflow and to lessen treatment failure in AECOPD. Prolonged therapy beyond 2 weeks confers no additional benefits, with 5 to 10 days being the likeliest optimal duration.[67-69]

Noninvasive Positive Pressure Ventilation and Mechanical Ventilation

Noninvasive positive pressure ventilation (NIPPV) is emerging as a preferred method of ventilation in adequately selected patients with acute respiratory acidemia.[70-72] This mode is used in the treatment of acute respiratory failure of many causes, including COPD. Appropriate patient selection is critical to ensure the success of NIPPV. Poor candidates are those with acute respiratory arrest, altered mental status with agitation or lack of cooperation, distorted facial anatomy preventing proper application of the mask, cardiovascular instability, or excessive secretions. NIPPV improves symptomatic and physiologic variables; reduces the need for intubation, hospital stay, and mortality[71]; and does not use additional resources.[72]

For patients who do not qualify for NIPPV or who show evidence of worsening respiratory failure and life-threatening acidemia despite NIPPV, intubation and mechanical ventilation are indicated. This method of ventilation carries numerous risks and complications, including ventilator-acquired pneumonia and barotrauma. Adequate ventilator management is necessary, and every effort should be undertaken to minimize the duration of mechanical ventilation.

Others

Mucolytics, expectorants, and chest physiotherapy have not been shown to improve the outcome and are not recommended.[5-8]

CONCLUSIONS

Overall, COPD poses a common and significant clinical challenge for patients and clinicians alike. Clinicians' expert knowledge regarding diagnosis and management can enhance patients' longevity and quality of life. Results of emerging studies will likely lead to enhancements in current management and new paradigms in managing patients with COPD.

Summary

- COPD is emerging as a major cause of morbidity and mortality in the United States. COPD currently is the fourth leading cause of death among Americans.
- COPD is under-recognized overall, as is α_1-antitrypsin deficiency, a genetic predisposition to COPD.
- Among the available therapies for COPD, many can improve symptoms (e.g., bronchodilators, pulmonary rehabilitation). Three treatments—smoking cessation, supplemental oxygen used 24 hours a day, and lung volume reduction surgery—have been shown to prolong life in appropriately selected COPD patients.

Suggested Readings

AACP/AACVPR Pulmonary Rehabilitation Guidelines Panel. Pulmonary rehabilitation: Joint ACCP/AACVPR evidence-based guidelines. Chest 1997;112:1363-1396.

American Thoracic Society. Standards for the diagnosis and care of patients with chronic obstructive pulmonary disease.www.thoracic.org, accessed May 30, 2008

American Thoracic Society/European Respiratory Society Statement: Standards for the diagnosis and management of individuals with α_1-antitrypsin deficiency. Am J Respir Crit Care Med 2003;168:818-900.

Anthonisen NR, Connett JE, Murray RP: Smoking and lung function of Lung Health Study participants after 11 years. The Lung Health Study Research Group. Am J Respir Crit Care Med 2002;166:675-679.

Maurer JR, Frost AE, Estenne M, et al: International guidelines for the selection of lung transplant candidates. The International Society for Heart and Lung Transplantation, the American Thoracic Society, the American Society of Transplant Physicians, the European Respiratory Society. Transplantation 1998;66:951-956.

Calverley PM, Anderson JA, Celli B, et al. Salmeterol and fluticasone propionate and survival in chronic obstructive pulmonary disease. N Engl J Med 2007; 356: 775-789.

Aaron SD, Vandemheen KL, Ferguson D, et al. Tiotropium in combination with placebo, salmeterol, or fluticasone-salmeterol for treatment of chronic obstructive pulmonary disease: a randomized trial. Ann Intern Med 2007; 146: 545-555.

National Emphysema Treatment Trial Research Group. A randomized trial comparing lung-volume-reduction surgery with medical therapy for severe emphysema. N Engl J Med 2003;348:2059-2073.

Pauwels RA, Buist AS, Calverley PM, et al: GOLD Scientific Committee. Global strategy for the diagnosis, management, and prevention of chronic obstructive pulmonary disease: NHLBI/WHO Global Initiative for Chronic Obstructive Lung Disease (GOLD) Workshop summary. Am J Respir Crit Care Med 2001;163:1256-1276. www.goldcopd.com

Pauwels RA, Lofdahl CG, Laitinen LA, et al: Long-term treatment with inhaled budesonide in persons with mild chronic obstructive pulmonary disease who continue smoking. European Respiratory Society Study on Chronic Obstructive Pulmonary Disease. N Engl J Med 1999;340:1948-1953.

Sutherland ER, Cherniack RM: Management of chronic obstructive pulmonary disease. N Engl J Med 2004;350:2689-2697.

The Lung Health Study Research Group. Effect of inhaled triamcinolone on the decline in pulmonary function in chronic obstructive pulmonary disease. N Engl J Med 2000;343:1902-1909.

References

For a complete list of references, log onto www.expertconsult.com.

Cough

Rachel M. Taliercio and Daniel A. Culver

Cough is the most common single reason for primary care physician visits and is a common source of referrals to pulmonologists.[1] In otherwise healthy persons, self-limited cough can occur as part of local irritation due to a viral rhinitis or respiratory infection. Chronic or persistent cough, defined as lasting more than 8 weeks, is also usually not caused by a life-threatening disorder. However, the frequency of this complaint, its effect on quality of life, and the potential for distress and concern about an underlying cause make chronic cough an important problem.

Because cough is a symptom that is a common pathway for a variety of diverse conditions and has no reliable objective monitoring tools, physicians' management of cough is actually quite variable. A common situation that clinicians face is the presence of a cough of unclear cause in the setting of a normal chest x-ray and normal spirometry. A number of studies suggest that in addition to a history and physical, a systematic diagnostic approach including a chest x-ray, spirometry, bronchoprovocation study in a pulmonary laboratory, sinus imaging, and esophageal pH monitoring yield a specific diagnosis in the vast majority of patients (>95%) with chronic cough.[2] However, routinely obtaining all these tests is cumbersome and expensive in clinical practice, and some might not be readily available. Thus, it remains unclear whether most patients should undergo a trial of empirical therapy (either sequential or concurrent) or an aggressive and targeted diagnostic evaluation. In clinical practice, it is likely that both of these approaches are used in conjunction.

For a symptom such as cough, simply excluding certain serious causes can go a long way to reassuring the patient as well as the clinician and allowing a period of observation. An optimal, cost-effective approach to the management of chronic cough remains controversial. Because chronic cough is rarely progressive, often self-limited, and due to a benign cause in most cases, we recommend a stepwise approach employing empirical therapy targeted at the most common diagnoses, without extensive initial diagnostic testing (Fig. 1).

DEFINITION AND PATHOPHYSIOLOGY

Cough is a protective physiologic reflex that augments mucociliary clearance of airway secretions. The cough reflex is characterized by the generation of high intrathoracic pressures against a closed glottis, followed by forceful expulsion of air and secretions on glottic opening. Intrathoracic pressures of up to 300 mm Hg and expiratory velocities approaching 500 miles per hour may be achieved.[2] These high velocities serve to tear off mucus from the airway walls so the cough can effectively expel droplets into the air.[3] Although it often serves a protective role, cough can become harmful when it is excessive and nonproductive. The high intrathoracic pressures and velocities generated during vigorous coughing produce hemodynamic changes analogous to chest compressions.[4]

Although a typical cough has a characteristic acoustic profile and is universally recognizable, there is no clinical test that can document and confirm the presence of cough. This has hampered progress in the study of cough, and most of our understanding of the neuronal regulation of cough is derived from animal studies. The role of vagal afferent nerves in initiating the cough reflex is undisputed; however, the function of the various afferent neuronal subtypes in the regulation of cough is not well understood. The symptom of cough involves a reflex arc originating in peripheral cough receptors. Afferent nerves are most concentrated in the epithelia of the upper and lower respiratory tracts, but they are also located in the external auditory meatus, tympanic membrane, esophagus, stomach, pericardium, and diaphragm. For example, in a small percentage of patients, mechanical stimulation of the ear can evoke cough by stimulating afferent nerves carried by the auricular branch of the vagus nerve.[5]

Rapidly adapting receptors and C fibers are two afferent nerve subtypes that have been extensively studied and are theorized to play important roles in the regulation of cough. Rapidly adapting receptors are activated by mechanical forces such as lung inflation and deflation, whereas C fibers are much more sensitive to chemical stimuli, primarily bradykinin. Signals from the receptors are carried by vagal afferents to a medullary cough center, which then trigger cough activation via efferents mediated by the vagal, phrenic, and spinal motor nerves. Irritation anywhere along the reflex arc by a disease process can cause cough. The exact role of each of the various subtypes in the mediation of cough remains to be fully elucidated.[5]

PREVALENCE

Cough is the single most common symptom prompting outpatient medical visits in the United States.[6] Persistent cough is a common reason for referral to a pulmonologist or allergist. The population point-prevalence of chronic cough depends on smoking status, ranging from 5% to 40%. Although cough can cause a variety of anatomic and physiologic complications, 98% of patients in one series listed the suspicion of underlying disease to be the major factor prompting them to seek medical attention. The aggregate cost of treatment for cough exceeds several billion dollars in the United States alone. This estimate does not include resources expended for repeated diagnostic studies.

SIGNS AND SYMPTOMS

Most patients seek medical attention because of complications of cough, either psychological or physical. The most common complications include feeling that something is wrong (98%), exhaustion (57%), feeling self-conscious (55%), insomnia (45%), lifestyle change (45%), musculoskeletal pain (45%), hoarseness (43%), excessive perspiration (42%), and urinary incontinence (39%).[2] A host of other physiologic symptoms occur occasionally due to the high intrathoracic and intra-abdominal pressures achieved. The most prevalent symptoms include cough syncope, cardiac dysrhythmias, headache, subconjuctival hemorrhage, inguinal herniation, and gastroesophageal reflux. It is important to elicit which specific cough-related symptoms are bothersome for the patient as a guide to the pace and scope of diagnostic testing.

ETIOLOGY

Although the character of the cough has been shown to be of no diagnostic value, it is useful to classify cough by duration as a means of narrowing the differential diagnosis. Acute cough has been defined as one with a duration of less than 3 weeks at presentation.[1] Some clinicians have proposed a category of subacute cough, with a duration of 3 to 8 weeks. Although this classification system is widely used and accepted by most experts, there are no case series assessing the relative frequency of causes in either the acute or subacute categories.

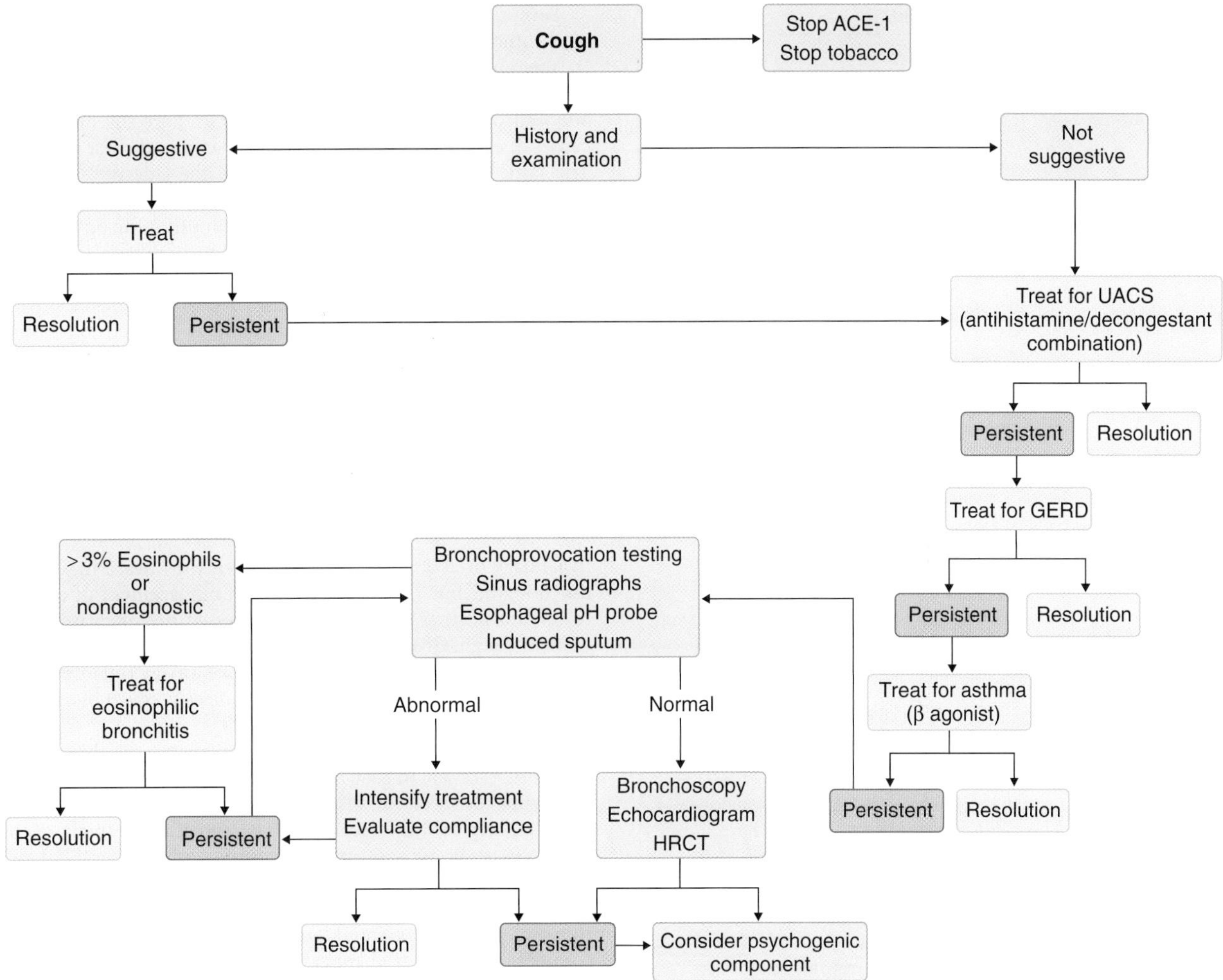

Figure 1 **An algorithm employing empirical therapy targeted at the most common diagnoses of chronic cough.** ACE, angiotensin-converting enzyme; GERD, gastroesophageal reflux disease; HRCT, high-resolution computed tomography; UACS, upper airway cough syndrome.

Chronic cough is defined as lasting longer than 8 weeks. Most of the attention by clinicians is devoted to chronic or persistent cough because this is the variety that usually prompts patients to seek medical care.

Acute and Subacute Cough

The most common cause of acute cough, as defined by a time course of less than 3 weeks, is overwhelmingly considered to be the common cold. Although there are no case series addressing the frequency of the common cold as a cause of acute cough, epidemiologic data support the relation. Acute cough is, by definition, self-limited. Cough that lasts longer than 3 weeks but does not become chronic falls into the subacute category. Postinfectious cough due to irritation of cough receptors accounts for most of these cases. Most commonly, persistent inflammation caused by a preceding viral upper respiratory infection is the culprit.

Acute bronchitis, as the term implies, is a lower respiratory tract syndrome and another common source of acute cough. It manifests as a persistent cough, with or without sputum production, in patients with a normal chest radiograph. Although it is much less prevalent than the common cold, acute bronchitis is the most common diagnosis given to patients presenting to a physician with acute cough. It is caused by a respiratory virus more than 90% of the time. Viral cultures and serologic assays are not routinely ordered; hence, the organism responsible is rarely identified.

Distinction between the common cold and acute bronchitis is often impossible to make and usually clinically irrelevant in otherwise healthy persons. Bacterial infections are implicated in less than 10% of cases of acute bronchitis. Despite this, reports have indicated that more than two thirds of patients receive antibiotic therapy for acute bronchitis. Elderly patients are more likely to receive broad-spectrum antibiotics, and nine out of ten smokers receive antibiotics despite the lack of evidence that smoking itself is a risk factor for bacterial infection. Treatment of self-limited bronchitis with antibiotics is often fueled by public expectation. In this circumstance, the descriptors a physician uses can make a difference. Patients are less likely to feel that antibiotics are necessary when the term "chest cold" is used as opposed to "bronchitis."[7]

A common diagnostic challenge encountered in the outpatient setting is determining the need for a chest radiograph. Pneumonia can also manifest with acute cough, and its manifestation can be more subtle in the elderly. Prospective studies have shown that the history and physical examination alone can predict the likelihood of pneumonia and therefore the need for a chest radiograph. A diagnosis of pneumonia is unlikely in the absence of tachycardia, tachypnea, fever, and evidence of focal consolidation on chest examination. The presence of purulent sputum does not distinguish between acute bronchitis and pneumonia.[7]

Table 1 Common Causes of Acute Cough

Cause	Recommended Treatments	Comments
Viral rhinosinusitis	Antitussives Decongestants First-generation antihistamines Ibuprofen	Difficult to distinguish from acute sinusitis Neuraminidase antagonists may be helpful if started early
Acute bronchitis	Antitussives	Antibiotics are not routinely indicated
Acute sinusitis	Antibiotics Decongestants First-generation antihistamines	Treatment duration is 2-3 wk
Allergic or irritant rhinitis	Irritant avoidance Nonsedating antihistamines	Nasal corticosteroids are useful for maintenance therapy
Acute exacerbation of COPD	β Agonist or anticholinergic MDI with spacer Antibiotics Systemic corticosteroids	
Pertussis	Macrolides (if started within 8 days of symptom onset) TMP-SMX (macrolide allergy)	Diagnosis is difficult (serologic or nasopharyngeal culture)
Mycoplasma	Macrolides Alternative: tetracyclines	

COPD, chronic obstructive pulmonary disease; MDI, metered-dose inhaler; TMP-SMX, trimethoprim-sulfamethoxazole.

The most common causes of acute cough are listed in Table 1. In the presence of a compatible history and examination, further diagnostic testing is usually not necessary. Under-recognized causes of acute or subacute cough include pertussis and mycoplasma infection. Rarely, life-threatening illnesses manifest primarily with acute cough. Examples include pulmonary embolus, cardiogenic pulmonary edema, and pneumonia. The mainstay of treatment includes nonspecific antitussive therapy. Newer generation nonsedating antihistamines are not as effective in reducing cough compared with the older, first-generation antihistamine-plus-decongestant preparations. Bronchodilators are not recommended as adjunctive treatment unless baseline airflow obstruction is present. Expectorants and mucolytics, although commonly used, have not been proved beneficial.[8]

Chronic Cough

Determining the cause of chronic cough is often very challenging. As a general principle, the positive and negative predictive values of tests for the cause of chronic cough are poor, implying that attribution of cause depends on a response to specific therapy. Additionally, in 18% to 62% of patients, there are two significant causes, and in up to 42% there are three.[9-11] In studies from cough clinics, the data suggest that there is little or no diagnostic value in descriptive features such as cough frequency, character, or sputum production. In addition, the most common causes of chronic cough can manifest with cough as the sole presenting symptom.

Several prospective studies have attempted to delineate the causes of chronic persistent cough and have reached the same conclusion. In the absence of smoking and angiotensin-converting enzyme (ACE) inhibitors, upper airway cough syndrome (UACS), asthma, and gastroesophageal reflux disease (GERD) are the most common causes of chronic cough in patients with a normal chest radiograph.[12] The same triad applies in children and the elderly.[2,13] Outside the United States, nonasthmatic eosinophilic bronchitis (NAEB) is a recognized cause of chronic cough, accounting for up to one third of cases in some series. Even in immunocompromised hosts and areas where tuberculosis is endemic, UACS, asthma, GERD, and NAEB are the most common causes reported. Chronic bronchitis, usually resulting from cigarette smoking, is believed to be the most common overall cause of chronic cough, but most smokers with cough typically do not seek medical attention. All of these data are derived from studies of patients referred to pulmonologists or cough clinics; however, it is likely that a similar spectrum of causes accounts for most patients seen by primary care providers.

Upper Airway Cough Syndrome

In January of 2006, the American College of Chest Physicians published a guideline on the diagnosis and management of cough. The review on postnasal drip (PND) addressed the unclear relation of PND to cough. Given the lack of understanding about whether PND is the cause of cough or a consequence of airway inflammation that is producing cough, the term *upper airway cough syndrome* was adopted as a more accurate descriptor.

UACS is the single most common cause of chronic cough, accounting for 8% to 87% of cases, either exclusively or in combination with other factors.[2,13] Categories of UACS-induced cough include allergic rhinitis (seasonal or perennial), perennial nonallergic rhinitis (vasomotor or nonallergic rhinitis with eosinophilia), postinfectious UACS, bacterial sinusitis, allergic fungal rhinitis, occupational rhinitis, rhinitis medicamentosa, and pregnancy-associated rhinitis. All patients should undergo evaluation for exposure to common allergens or chemical irritants. An episodic rhinitis might suggest that an occupational factor is involved.[14]

The pathogenesis of cough in UACS involves stimulation of afferent receptors in the upper airway, rather than run-off of secretions into the lower airway. Associated symptoms include rhinorrhea, nasal congestion, a sensation of drainage or tickle in the oropharynx, and throat clearing. Physical examination can reveal nasal congestion or discharge, nasal mucosal bogginess, mucous in the oropharynx, or a cobblestone appearance of the oropharyngeal mucosa. The examination findings are nonspecific, however, and may be present in any of the other major causes of chronic cough. Although most patients have at least one symptom or sign, UACS can manifest as cough alone up to 20% of the time.[12] Because it is highly prevalent and may be otherwise clinically unapparent, it is reasonable to employ a brief trial of empirical treatment in the approach to diagnosis. Ultimately, UACS is a syndrome without a clear definition, and its role in chronic cough is best proven by a response to therapy.

The presence of copious sputum is associated with an increased likelihood of chronic sinusitis, but neither the clinical examination nor historical features reliably differentiate it from other causes of UACS.[11,13] Excessive sputum production, defined as greater than 30 mL per day, can be a manifestation of asthma, GERD, and bronchiectasis. Patients with chronic sinusitis can present with a nonproductive cough as their sole symptom.

Among patients with chronic cough, up to 38% have some radiologic sinus abnormality.[15] Thus, a finding of sinus mucosal thickening on radiographs has only a 29% to 81% positive predictive value (PPV) for chronic sinusitis that is responsible for cough.[2,15] Additionally, mucosal thickening is seen in bacterial and viral infections and cannot be used to distinguish between the two. The presence of air-fluid levels on four-view sinus x-rays is more specific for diagnosing sinusitis, and one report documented a 100% PPV.[15] Commonly, sinusitis is evaluated by computed tomography (CT) scan.

Asthma

In most series, asthma is the second most common cause of chronic cough in adult nonsmokers, present in 14% to 55% of cases.[16,17] Historical features of wheezing, chest tightness, or exertional dyspnea in response to triggers such as strong odors or perfumes, cold air, or allergens should suggest the diagnosis. However, the PPV of a suggestive history is only 56%.[18]

Cough is a feature in nearly all cases of asthma. In a subset of asthmatic patients, cough is the primary or sole symptom, a condition termed *cough-variant asthma* (CVA). Cough-variant asthma accounts for 6.5% to 57% of all asthmatic patients.[2] Many of these patients later develop classic asthma symptoms.[18]

The physical examination and spirometry can be entirely normal in patients with chronic cough due to asthma. The most useful test to support the diagnosis is a bronchoprovocation test with inhaled methacholine. The methacholine challenge test (MCT) is highly sensitive, and a negative test virtually excludes the diagnosis of asthma. A 20% decrement in forced expiratory volume in 1 second (FEV_1) after methacholine inhalation, although indicating bronchial hyperresponsiveness, can have a positive predictive value as low as 74% for diagnosing the cause of cough.[19] Even detailed analysis of MCT characteristics cannot reliably enhance specificity. Thus, proof that asthma is the inciting factor in chronic cough requires demonstration of a response to directed therapy.

Gastroesophageal Reflux Disease

Gastroesophageal reflux disease (GERD), alone or in combination with other conditions, accounts for up to 40% of cases of chronic cough around the world.[16] It has been recognized as a contributor to cough with increasing frequency in observational studies; in some series it has surpassed other etiologies as a cause for chronic cough.[2,16] Recognition, diagnosis, and treatment of GERD are among the most challenging of all cough etiologies, with a number of unclarified issues. Patients with GERD are commonly asymptomatic, and it can be assumed that the condition is therefore underrecognized.

In a minority of cases, reflux-mediated irritation of laryngeal receptors or episodic microaspiration underlie GERD-induced cough. The cough is usually attributable to a reflex loop involving vagal afferents in the distal esophagus, and proximal reflux is unnecessary in the pathogenesis.[20] Reflux into the distal esophagus alone can stimulate the esophageal-bronchial cough reflex. It is important to recognize that nonacid reflux can cause chronic cough, and these patients do not respond to acid-suppression therapy. Coughing itself can induce reflux by an unknown mechanism and create a vicious self-perpetuating cycle, making identification and treatment of GERD crucial in the integrated management of all cough syndromes.[21]

Symptomatic heartburn or water brash occurs in only a minority (25%-50%) of patients.[2] Other historical features such as exacerbation at night, in the supine position, or after eating do not reliably differentiate GERD-induced cough from other causes.[16] GERD also commonly accompanies other causes of cough; up to 80% of asthmatic patients have abnormal 24-hour pH probe findings.[2] Recurrent elevations in abdominal pressure can contribute to this phenomenon.

Ambulatory 24-hour esophageal pH monitoring is the most reliable test for GERD. It is important to include a temporal symptom log when conducting pH monitoring so as to document the causality of reflux events vis-à-vis cough. Often, close examination reveals that cough preceded the reflux event. A temporal symptom log can also substantiate GERD as a cause of cough even when pH probe scores lie within the normal range. In untreated patients, the pH probe carries a 90% to 100% sensitivity, but the positive predictive value may be as low as 35% when using therapeutic response as a gold standard.[2,22]

The esophageal pH monitoring study will be negative in patients with nonacid reflux, and if this condition is suspected, barium esophagography may be helpful. A newer test, impedance plethysmography using an esophageal probe, may also be able to identify patients with nonacid reflux. However, there are no published data to suggest that outcomes are improved with this device.

Most patients with GERD do not have endoscopic findings that suggest acid reflux, such as esophagitis or Barrett's epithelium, and a normal endoscopy does not rule out GERD as a source of cough. It is reasonable to empirically treat patients who fit the clinical profile before testing. Similar to other causes of chronic cough, a definitive diagnosis is established only when the cough resolves with treatment.

Nonasthmatic Eosinophilic Bronchitis

A subset of patients has been recognized with increased sputum eosinophils in the absence of demonstrable bronchial hyper-responsiveness. These patients are typically nonsmokers and have a chronic cough that responds to corticosteroids. The frequency of this syndrome has been reported to be as high as 10% to 30% in patients with chronic cough who are referred to a specialist.[23] Diagnosis is usually made by demonstration of induced sputum eosinophilia (>3%). If induced sputum cannot be obtained or is nondiagnostic, bronchoscopy with bronchial wash can provide useful information. The pathogenesis of NAEB is not well understood, although, similar to asthma, an inhaled allergen or environmental agent is theorized to play a role. Persistent eosinophilic airway inflammation can lead to progressive airflow obstruction, and NAEB may be implicated as a causative factor in COPD.[24] The frequency and significance of NAEB remain incompletely understood.

Chronic Bronchitis

Chronic bronchitis is characterized by a productive cough on most days for 3 months in 2 consecutive years. It may be caused by irritant-induced inflammation or by the need to mobilize excessive secretions. Although chronic bronchitis is a common cause of cough in the population, it is present in only 5% of those seeking medical attention for cough.[9,10] Cigarette smoke is the most common irritant associated with chronic bronchitis. There is a direct relation between the incidence of chronic bronchitis and the number of cigarettes smoked. As the airflow obstruction becomes more severe, the incidence of cough increases. Clinicians should also inquire about passive smoke exposure because it is linked to chronic productive cough. Occupational exposures or inflammatory bowel disease can also trigger this syndrome.[25]

The cause of cough in chronic bronchitis is multifactorial, with bronchial secretions and airway inflammation playing a primary role. Patients with airflow obstruction cannot generate an effective cough to clear secretions. Retained secretions can worsen cough and incite a self-perpetuating cycle. Acute respiratory infections, whether viral or bacterial, are a common cause of exacerbations in chronic bronchitis. Patients typically present with increased cough, sputum production, and worsening dyspnea.[25]

The mainstay of treatment is avoiding the offending agent(s). Cough completely resolves or significantly decreases in 90% of patients after smoking cessation. In contrast to acute bronchitis, exacerbation of chronic bronchitis should be treated with antibiotics. Particular vigilance is warranted when there is a change in the character of the cough or sputum, because this may be the manifesting feature of a superimposed bronchogenic carcinoma.

Bronchiectasis

The prevalence of bronchiectasis has decreased considerably, and it is now present in <4% of persons with chronic cough.[9-11] It develops when chronic inflammation or infection leads to progressive airway damage. Bronchi become dilated, with chronic inflammatory cells in the mucosa and mucous pooling within the airway lumen. Bronchial artery proliferation and arteriovenous malformation can be associated with bronchiectasis, and patients can present with recurrent hemoptysis. The most common cause of bronchiectasis in the United States is cystic fibrosis. Focal bronchiectasis can occur when a larger airway is obstructed; this is seen with endobronchial tumors, enlarged lymph nodes, foreign bodies, and broncholiths.

Most patients with bronchiectasis produce large volumes of sputum, for example, 30 mL/day. However, a history of excessive mucoid sputum production is not specific for the diagnosis, and a few patients have dry bronchiectasis, in which there is no sputum production. Chest x-ray might reveal evidence of tubular or cystic structures representing dilated, mucus-filled bronchi. High-resolution chest CT scanning is a more sensitive tool to evaluate patients with equivocal or negative chest x-ray findings. Nearly all patients in published series with bronchiectasis as the cause of chronic cough had suggestive chest x-ray findings.[9,10]

Postinfectious Cough

Airway inflammation can follow any respiratory tract infection; up to one quarter of such infections may be complicated by persistent cough.[2] Increased cough receptor sensitivity or temporary bronchial hyperresponsiveness, probably related to epithelial damage, likely account for this phenomenon. Postinfectious cough is a diagnosis of exclusion, and by definition it eventually resolves, but its duration may be prolonged. For this reason, 8 weeks is a more clinically useful working definition of chronic cough than 3 weeks. Postinfectious cough is usually caused by respiratory viruses, *Mycoplasma* spp, *Chlamydia pneumoniae* (strain TWAR), or *Bordatella pertussis*. Vigorous coughing can stimulate esophageal reflux, which has been implicated as a cause of postinfectious cough.[26]

Pertussis, or whooping cough, is a severe and debilitating cough illness that can last for weeks to months. A common misconception is that pertussis is a disease of infants and children. Active pertussis infection in adolescents and adults is an under-recognized cause of chronic cough. One investigation found a 21% incidence of pertussis in a group of patients with a cough duration of 2 weeks to 3 months.[27] In recent years, the incidence of pertussis has increased, most likely due to a combination of waning immunity and increased detection of the illness. Patients experience periodic episodes of violent coughing, and post-tussive emesis is common. The inspiratory whooping sound typical in children is generally not heard in adults.[26,28]

Angiotensin-Converting Enzyme Inhibitors

ACE normally degrades proinflammatory mediators, such as bradykinins and substance P. Inhibition of this action lowers the threshold for cough sensitivity. Cough due to ACE inhibitors is a class effect and has been documented with all ACE inhibitors. Switching to another agent will not ameliorate the symptoms. Usually, cough begins within 1 week of starting the medication, but it can begin as late as 1 year later. Approximately 10% to 20% of patients develop cough, but in many it is not bothersome. Asthmatic patients are not at increased risk. Cough resolution may be delayed for up to 1 month after discontinuing the drug. Angiotensin II receptor blockers do not cause cough and therefore are useful therapeutic alternatives.

Cancer

Bronchogenic carcinoma is an infrequent cause of chronic cough (≤2%), although most patients with intrathoracic malignancies develop cough at some point in the course of their disease. Cough receptors are more highly concentrated in the larger airways; thus, cough is more common in malignancies with a predilection for central airways, such as squamous cell and small cell cancers. A history of tobacco use or new-onset cough or hemoptysis in a heavy cigarette smoker should heighten clinical suspicion. Prospective trials of chronic cough have found a 100% negative predictive value for a normal or unchanged chest x-ray, but the numbers in these studies were small.[2] In patients with a normal chest x-ray who have persistent cough and hemoptysis after antibiotic treatment, a fiberoptic bronchoscopic examination may be indicated to exclude the diagnosis.

Psychosomatic Cough

Psychosomatic cough is rare, especially in adults. It is a diagnosis of exclusion and should not be entertained until all other potential causes have been investigated, with therapeutic trials of adequate intensity and duration. There are no distinguishing historical features to reliably differentiate it from other etiologies.[16] Habit cough is a syndrome of persistent, habitual throat clearing that might respond to biofeedback. In distinction, psychogenic cough usually implies an underlying psychiatric disorder. Most patients with psychogenic cough harbor an intractable fear of a serious underlying medical disease.

Rare Causes of Chronic Cough

Rare causes of chronic cough include interstitial lung disease (e.g., idiopathic pulmonary fibrosis, sarcoidosis), occult aspiration, pulmonary abscess, foreign body, occult congestive heart failure, occult pulmonary emboli, and nasal polyps. Disorders of any of the locations of cough receptors (external auditory canal, tracheobronchial tree, pleura, pericardium, diaphragm, esophagus, stomach) can also cause chronic cough.

DIAGNOSIS

The management of chronic cough typically involves some combination of simple screening studies (chest x-ray and spirometry), additional specific diagnostic studies (methacholine provocation, sinus imaging, or a pH probe), and empirical therapy for the three most common entities (rhinitis, asthma, GERD) (see Fig. 1). Patients who lack specific clues by history and examination and who have a normal chest x-ray and spirogram represent the most common management dilemma for the clinician. A major decision involves the extent of specific diagnostic testing as opposed to trials of empirical therapy. Randomized clinical trials do not provide adequate guidance to help the clinician choose between these two strategies. The approach is usually negotiated with the patient, partly based on the level of subjective distress and on the level of exasperation by the patient and the clinician.

Pinpointing the cause of chronic cough is often difficult. Cough may be the sole manifestation of disorders such as asthma, GERD, or UACS, with a paucity of other historical features to suggest the correct diagnosis. Features of cough, such as timing, associated sputum production, and cough character (e.g., brassy), are not helpful in distinguishing causes.[16] A high percentage of patients have two or more responsible causes. Finally, there are no diagnostic tests with a sufficiently high positive predictive value to reliably implicate any particular cause of cough. Thus, diagnosis hinges on demonstration of a response to a specific therapy.

Evaluation and treatment using our algorithm (see Fig. 1) assume that failure to remedy the cough using trials of empirical therapy will precipitate appropriate diagnostic testing. A significant fraction of nonresponders fail treatment due to inadequate intensity or duration of treatment. One study found that the diagnosis was correct in 14% of referred patients, but the treatment regimens were insufficient.[10] In these cases, diagnostic testing facilitates appropriate narrowing and intensification of treatment. Because the overwhelming majority

Table 2 Treatment for Postnasal Drainage Syndromes

Syndrome	Treatment	Examples	Comments
Generic rhinitis	First-generation antihistamine plus decongestant combination	Dexbrompheniramine maleate 6 mg plus pseudoephedrine 120 mg bid	Nasal corticosteroids are useful for maintenance therapy Ipratropium nasal MDI is also effective
Allergic rhinitis	Second-generation antihistamine Nasal corticosteroid Allergen avoidance	Loratidine 10 mg/day Beclomethasone nasal 42 μg each nostril qid	Cromolyn, azelastine, leukotrine inhibitors are also useful Consider allergy testing
Vasomotor rhinitis	Anticholinergic nasal spray	Ipratropium 0.06% 2 puffs/nostril 4-6 times/day	Mediated by autonomic instability
Chronic sinusitis	First-generation antihistamine plus decongestant (3 wk) Nasal decongestant (5 days) Appropriate antibiotics (≥3 wk)	Dexbrompheniramine Pseudoephedrine as above Oxymetazoline 2 sprays bid	Use antibiotic active against *H. influenzae, S. pneumoniae*, oral anaerobes Nasal corticosteroids after cough resolves

MDI, metered-dose inhaler.

of patients have UACS, asthma, or GERD, it is crucial to assiduously investigate the roles of each before further investigations.

Common causes for diagnostic frustration include inadequate diagnosis and inadequate treatment. All tests used for evaluating chronic cough have a poor positive predictive value. Over-reliance on historical features or cough characteristics can thwart accurate diagnosis because these are often misleading. The cause of cough may be otherwise clinically silent, and 18% to 62% of chronic coughs are due to two or more causes. Diagnostic testing that suggests an underlying cause does not ensure that cough is caused by that etiology. Inadequate treatment regimens are a common reason for failure to alleviate symptoms, and eradication of related symptoms (heartburn, nasal congestion) does not ensure that an underlying cause is sufficiently treated. Treatments themselves can frustrate the search. Central cough suppressants, such as dextromethorphan and codeine, should generally be avoided; they might serve as a temporizing measure but can distract from the search for a specific cause. Pressurized metered-dose inhalers (MDIs) can exacerbate cough-variant asthma.

The American College of Chest Physicians and the British Thoracic Society advise obtaining a chest x-ray before starting empirical therapy.[29] Although most investigators recommend chest x-ray early in the evaluation of chronic cough, only 4% to 11% of nonsmokers have culpable abnormalities.[9,10] The yield of fiberoptic bronchoscopy is similarly low, and only 4% of patients with normal chest x-rays have endobronchial abnormalities. Even with a finding of endobronchial pathology, the positive predictive value is only 50% to 89%.[2] In assessing for the presence of uncommon causes of chronic cough, chest CT scanning has a relatively higher diagnostic yield (abnormal in up to 42% of patients with a normal chest radiograph) and should be performed before cardiac tests in the absence of cardiac symptoms.[29]

Some situations merit special consideration. Consider foreign body inhalation in patients who present with sudden-onset cough. Consider sinus imaging if a patient suspected of having rhinitis or UACS does not respond to empirical therapy; chronic sinusitis can be otherwise clinically silent.[14] In patients who do not respond to empirical treatment for UACS and GERD and who have a normal chest x-ray, normal spirometry, and negative methacholine challenge test, it is reasonable to empirically treat with a short course of inhaled corticosteroids. Resolution of cough would support the diagnosis of NAEB. Occupational and environmental exposures should be considered as exacerbating factors in all patients who present with cough. Indoor allergens, such as pets and dust mites, and secondhand exposure to cigarette smoke are common environmental causes that are easily modifiable.[27]

TREATMENT

Rhinitis and Upper Airway Cough Syndrome

Initial therapy for most postnasal drainage syndromes should include an antihistamine-decongestant combination (Table 2). First-generation antihistamines, such as dexbrompheniramine maleate or azatadine maleate, have been demonstrated to be superior to second-generation (nonsedating) drugs, due to their additional anticholinergic activity.[2] If drowsiness is problematic, therapy may be initiated with bedtime dosing before instituting twice-daily dosing. Second-generation antihistamines are useful primarily in allergic rhinitis syndromes. The role of bacteria in perpetuating chronic sinusitis is controversial, and treatment regimens are not well defined. Except for chronic sinusitis, in most patients symptoms respond within 1 week. Long-term use of topical decongestants should be discouraged to avoid rebound nasal congestion (rhinitis medicamentosa).

Initial empirical therapy with an antihistamine-decongestant has been shown to be effective in a large percentage of patients who present with chronic cough. This reflects the prevalence of UACS among patients with chronic cough.[19]

Asthma

Most patients respond favorably to β-agonist inhalers, usually within 1 week. However, maximal responses may be delayed for 6 to 8 weeks.[2,9] Using a pressurized MDI can aggravate cough, and we recommend a dry powder device or addition of a spacer. Inhaled corticosteroids might also be required to optimize therapy for most patients. Mast cell stabilizers, such as cromolyn sodium, are also effective. A few patients require oral corticosteroids for symptom control. Zafirlukast, a leukotriene inhibitor, has been shown to have an antitussive effect in patients with cough variant asthma.

The presence of bronchial hyperresponsiveness should be demonstrated by provocation testing or reliable history before initiating oral steroids and when bronchodilators alone are ineffective in the presence of high clinical suspicion. Caution is warranted when interpreting the results of empirical therapeutic success with asthma therapy; NAEB and postinfectious cough might respond similarly. For this reason, we recommend at least one attempt to taper therapy. Steroids should also be tapered in patients whose MCT was obtained in the setting of a postinfectious cough.

Gastroesophageal Reflux Disease

Treatment of GER should begin with maximal therapy. Patients should avoid reflux-predisposing foods (fatty foods, chocolate, caffeine, alcohol), give up tobacco, elevate the head of the bed, and not eat within 2 or 3 hours before lying down. These are important lifestyle adaptations that can significantly diminish cough. Proton pump inhibitors (PPIs) should be used as the mainstay of medical therapy. In nonsmokers with a normal chest x-ray in whom asthma, UACS, and NAEB have been ruled out, empirical treatment has been shown to be cost effective.[21] We recommend commencing treatment with twice-daily PPIs, dosed just before the morning and evening meals; later, therapy may be de-escalated if proven effective. Onset of response can take up to 3 months, with maximal effects of treatment delayed for up to 6 months.[2] Response rates of 70% to 100% have been reported when the end point is improvement in cough.[2] However, the true response rate is unknown, because therapeutic response is the only indication; there is no objective gold standard to prove GERD is the cause of cough. The role of nonacid reflux in cough pathogenesis is also currently unknown, but it probably accounts for some percentage of nonresponders.

Ambulatory pH monitoring should be considered in patients who fail maximal therapy. Unfortunately, this test is usually only available in larger academic centers. Treatment response in patients with GERD can be prolonged and even take up to 6 months. Intensive treatment for at least several months should be attempted before referral for further diagnostic testing. Documentation of persistent symptomatic acid reflux should prompt consideration of esophageal fundoplication. The operative risk and morbidity of fundoplication have diminished considerably due to the expanding use of laparoscopy. Success rates approaching 85% may be expected for improvement of cough after surgical management.[30]

Eosinophilic Bronchitis

Inhaled corticosteroids are usually effective, but a few patients require a short course of oral steroid therapy.[23] A 2- to 3-week course of prednisone at 30 mg/day is sufficient; a small percentage of patients require maintenance therapy, generally with inhaled corticosteroids.

Chronic Bronchitis

Smoking cessation markedly reduces symptoms in more than 50% of patients within a month. Cough frequency and sputum production are most effectively decreased by ipratropium MDI (2 puffs qid). Mucolytics are not helpful, and the symptomatic benefit of ICS has not been demonstrated.

Bronchiectasis

The excessive secretions of bronchiectasis mandate persistent cough for mobilization. Complete cough suppression is neither achievable nor desirable. Chest physiotherapy techniques are useful for patients who produce large volumes of sputum and during disease flares. Flares might also require prolonged antibiotic courses. A beneficial role for β agonists or theophylline has not been demonstrated in treating chronic cough.

Postinfectious Cough

Postinfectious cough usually responds to treatment analogous to asthma. Alternatively, ipratropium has proven efficacy. Ongoing infections should be treated with appropriate antibiotic therapy (see Table 1).

CONCLUSION

Evaluation of cough depends on a systematic review of potential causes. The balance between empiricism and testing is often dictated by the patient's clinical course and quality of life. In most cases, empirical therapy targeted at the most common diagnoses leads to significant improvement or resolution of cough, obviating the need for extensive diagnostic testing. A chest radiograph and spirometry are recommended before referring a patient to a specialist.

The cause of chronic cough may be otherwise clinically silent, and it is not uncommon for there to be more than one contributing factor. Ultimately, delineation of the underlying cause can be accomplished only by demonstrating a response to therapy. Complete resolution of chronic cough can take weeks to months, and both the physician and patient need to set realistic treatment goals. Inadequate length of treatment, insufficient medication intensity, and patient nonadherence are common reasons for treatment failure. For this reason, a combination of systematic empiricism and limited adjunctive diagnostic testing are appropriate for most patients.

Summary

- In the absence of smoking and angiotensin-converting enzyme inhibitors, upper airway cough syndrome, asthma, and gastroesophageal reflux disease are the most common causes of chronic cough in patients with a normal chest radiograph.
- In most cases, empirical therapy targeted at the most common diagnoses leads to significant improvement or resolution of cough, obviating the need for extensive diagnostic testing.
- Inadequate length of treatment, insufficient medication intensity, and patient nonadherence are common reasons for treatment failure.
- Ultimately, determining the underlying cause of cough is accomplished by demonstrating a response to therapy.

Suggested Readings

Braman SS: Chronic cough due to acute bronchitis: ACCP evidence-based clinical practice guidelines. Chest 2006;129:95S-103S.

Braman SS: Chronic cough due to chronic bronchitis: ACCP evidence-based clinical practice guidelines. Chest 2006;129:104S-115S.

Brightling CE, Ward R, Goh KL, et al: Eosinophilic bronchitis is an important cause of chronic cough. Am J Respir Crit Care Med 1999;160:406-410.

Canning BJ: Anatomy and physiology of the cough reflex: ACCP evidence-based clinical practice guidelines. Chest 2006;129:33S-47S.

Irwin RS: Chronic cough due to gastroesophageal reflux disease: ACCP evidence-based clinical practice guidelines. Chest 2006;129:80S-94S.

Irwin RS, Boulet LP, Cloutier MM, et al: Managing cough as a defense mechanism and as a symptom. A consensus panel report of the American College of Chest Physicians. Chest 1998;114:133S-181S.

Irwin RS, Curley FJ, French CL: Chronic cough. The spectrum and frequency of causes, key components of the diagnostic evaluation, and outcome of specific therapy. Am Rev Respir Dis 1990;141:640-647.

Mello CJ, Irwin RS, Curley FJ: Predictive values of the character, timing, and complications of chronic cough in diagnosing its cause. Arch Intern Med 1996;156:997-1003.

Pratter MR: Chronic upper airway cough syndrome secondary to rhinosinus diseases (previously referred to as postnasal drip syndrome): ACCP evidence-based clinical practice guidelines. Chest 2006;129:63S-71S.

Pratter MR: An empiric integrative approach to the management of cough: ACCP evidence-based clinical practice guidelines. Chest 2006;129:222S-231S.

References

For a complete list of references, log onto www.expertconsult.com.

Cystic Fibrosis

Marie M. Budev and Atul C. Mehta

Cystic fibrosis (CF) is the most common, classic mendelian autosomal recessive, life-limiting disease among the white population.[1,2] It is a multisystem disease that results from loss of function in the CF transmembrane conductance regulator (*CFTR*) gene, classically leading to respiratory tract, gastrointestinal (GI), pancreatic, and reproductive abnormalities.[2] CF was recognized as a distinct clinical entity in 1938 and was believed to be invariably fatal during infancy.[3]

Since the 1970s, the life spans of CF patients have been prolonged, with advances in early diagnosis, care, and disease therapy. Early diagnosis has been improved by newborn screening. Advances in care include management of meconium ileus and improved methods of sputum clearance and managing respiratory failure. Improvements in disease therapy include better antibiotics, especially macrolides, and better pancreatic enzymes. With current management, almost 80% of patients with CF will reach adulthood; thus, CF is no longer a purely pediatric disease.[4-6] For patients born in the 1990s, the median survival is predicted to be greater than 40 years.[5] As more CF patients are surviving longer, adult issues including careers, relationships, and family are becoming important.[6] A range of comorbid conditions that are more prevalent in adult CF patients are also being encountered with increasing frequency as this population matures, including osteoporosis, diabetes, joint diseases, malnutrition, severe lung disease with bronchiectasis, colonization by resistant pathogens, severe gastric reflux, chronic sinusitis, and periportal fibrosis.[7]

Delivery of health care to the CF patient is now relevant to the nonpediatric physician. In fact, the multifaceted needs of the adult CF patient have led to the development of a nationwide network of more than 83 adult CF care programs in conjunction with the Cystic Fibrosis Foundation.[8] These comprehensive CF centers provide patients with a multidisciplinary approach based on the original pediatric CF centers. The aims of adult CF care include delivery of optimum care, access to pertinent medical resources, coordination of care among specialists and primary care providers, and a strong emphasis on independence and improving the quality of life of the patient who has CF.[5] The physician is also faced with another challenge, in which the adult CF patient presents with atypical features that might have gone unrecognized. In this chapter, we cover the salient features of CF, including prevalence and the issues surrounding neonatal screening, pathophysiology, diagnosis, and new and emerging therapies for this complex multisystem disease.

DEFINITION

CF is a genetic disease affecting approximately 30,000 children and adults in the United States. A defective gene causes the body to produce an abnormally thick, sticky mucus that leads to airway obstruction, subsequent life-threatening lung infections, end-stage lung disease, and bronchiectasis. These thick secretions also obstruct the pancreas, preventing digestive enzymes from reaching the intestines, leading to pancreatic insufficiency, malabsorption, and, in extreme cases, malnutrition.

PREVALENCE

Ethnicity

CF is a disease that occurs predominantly in the white population, with a rate of one in 2500 live births. Two percent to 5% of whites are carriers of the *CFTR* gene mutation (having one normal and one abnormal gene) but have no overt clinical signs of disease. CF is not rare in African American populations, but it occurs at the much lower frequency of approximately one in 17,000 live births.[9] In general, mutations of the CF gene are most prevalent in persons of northern and central European ancestries or of Ashkenazi Jewish descent, and they are rarely found in Native Americans, Asians, or native Africans.[10] Although the prevalence of CF is lower in the African American population, the mean age at diagnosis is younger in black patients than in white patients. Overall, the clinical manifestations are similar in both racial groups except that black patients tend to have more severe GI issues, including poor nutritional status.[10] There are more than 23,000 patients with CF in the United States.[6]

Gender

CF occurs equally often in male and female patients. In general, female patients with CF fare significantly worse than male patients. Female patients become infected with *Pseudomonas aeruginosa* earlier and have worse pulmonary function, worse nutritional status, and earlier mortality.[11-13] A Cystic Fibrosis Registry analysis from the University of Wisconsin[14] demonstrated that CF is diagnosed in girls at a later age than boys by at least 4 months, or even later when the analysis was limited to children presenting with only respiratory symptoms (40.7 months for diagnosis in girls vs. 22.3 months for diagnosis in boys). Implications for disease outcomes caused by delayed diagnosis of CF in girls may be present based on this recent analysis, but the reason for this delay is not clear or obvious.[15]

PATHOPHYSIOLOGY

CF is an autosomal recessive trait caused by mutations at a single gene locus on the long arm of chromosome 7. The gene product cystic fibrosis transmembrane conductance regulator (CFTR) is a 1480-amino acid polypeptide.[16,17] CF reflects the loss of function of the CFTR protein. The CFTR protein normally regulates the transport of electrolytes and chloride across epithelial cell membranes.[18]

More than 1000 mutations of the *CFTR* gene have been described.[19] The most common mutations of *CFTR* can be classified into six groups based on their known functional consequences.[20] This classification allows categorization of *CFTR* mutations based on molecular mechanisms, but phenotypic appearance depends on the type of mutation (class), location of the gene, molecular mechanism, and interaction with other mutations, as well as genetic and environmental influences.[21]

The most common mutation of the *CFTR* gene is caused by deletion of phenylalanine at position 508 (ΔF508) and occurs with varying frequency in different ethnic groups.[22] Worldwide, this allele is responsible for approximately 66% of all CF chromosomes.[23]

SCREENING

About 1000 infants are born with CF every year. CF is diagnosed in most of these children at a mean age of 3 to 4 years.[24] Nearly 10% of CF patients receive their diagnosis when they are older than 18 years.

Newborn screening for CF has been instituted in eight states, but national screening plans have not been mandated. In all, CF is diagnosed in 10% of infants in the United States either by prenatal diagnosis (3%) or by newborn screening (7%).[25] Newborn CF screening has been advocated by clinicians and CF groups as an early means of identifying asymptomatic patients so as to initiate early therapy to prevent long-term sequelae of the disease.[26] The currently available genetic screening tools for CF include the Guthrie test, in which measurements of the immunoreactive trypsinogen in dried blood are taken, and measurement of the most common CF mutations, including ΔF508.[26] ΔF508 is the most commonly reported gene mutation and is responsible for 70% of the mutated alleles in white patients. It is caused by a 3-bp deletion in the *CFTR* gene, resulting in the loss of the amino acid at position 508 of the CFTR protein. Homozygosity of this mutation is severe, resulting in both pulmonary and pancreatic disease.[27]

Recommendations for carrier screening or population screening have been proposed by the American College of Obstetricians and Gynecologists, the National Institutes of Health, and the American College of Medical Genetics; they are designed to identify at-risk couples before the birth of a child with CF.[28] Screening should be *offered to* adults with a family history of CF, reproductive partners of persons with CF, and white (including Ashkenazi Jewish) patients who are planning pregnancy. Screening should be *made available to* persons of color.

The efficacy of CF screening program is based on a multitude of factors. One factor is identification of the CF carrier status of each partner, which helps to determine the risk to the fetus. Issues to keep in mind include the gestational age at which the couple presents for prenatal care and the feasibility of pregnancy termination. These factors should be included in the CF screening discussion with parents. The screening of couples can follow two approaches: The female partner is screened first, and if she tests positive for CF carrier status, then the male partner is tested; or both partners are screened concurrently to use time efficiently for decision making, especially if more than one recessive disorder is being considered. Important information to discuss with patients before screening include the aim of screening, the voluntary nature of screening, medical and genetic issues surrounding CF, the prevalence of CF, the interpretation of the test results, and individual values.[29]

Carrier screening neither detects all mutations that could be present nor estimates the residual risk (the chance that the patient still carries a copy of a *CFTR* mutation despite negative testing). CF is an autosomal recessive disorder, and persons with CF typically have inherited one mutated allele from each parent. It is very rare to inherit two mutated alleles from one parent and none from the other.[29,30]

For couples who have one child with CF or who are known to be carriers, prenatal diagnosis of CF is available through chorionic villus sampling in the first trimester or by amniocentesis in the second or third trimester. Some patients undergo prenatal testing to help in deciding to terminate or continue the pregnancy.

Box 1 Signs and Symptoms of Cystic Fibrosis

Respiratory
Airway colonization
Asthma
Bronchitis
Chronic productive cough
Clubbing
Nasal polyps
Pansinusitis
Pseudomonas aeruginosa infection
Staphylococcal pneumonia

Gastrointestinal
Biliary cirrhosis
Diabetes
Distal intestinal obstructive syndrome
Failure to thrive
Fat-soluble vitamin deficiency (vitamins A, D, E, and K)
Meconium ileus
Portal hypertension
Recurrent right lower quadrant pain
Recurrent pancreatitis

Genitourinary
Absence of bilateral vas deferens
Cervical plugging
Female urinary incontinence
Infertility
Recurrent vaginal yeast infections

Adapted from Welsh MJ, Tsui L-C, Boat TF, et al: Cystic fibrosis. In Scriver CR, Beaudet AL, Sly WS, et al (eds): The Metabolic and Molecular Basis of Inherited Disease. New York: McGraw-Hill, 1995, p 3801.

SIGNS AND SYMPTOMS

Signs and symptoms of CF are listed in Box 1.

Respiratory Inflammation and Infections

Because the epithelial cells of an organ are affected by a variety of *CFTR* mutations, the consequences of the mutation vary depending on the organ involved. The pathologic changes differ in the secretory cells, sinuses, lungs, pancreas, liver, or reproductive tract. The hallmark of CF and the cause of death in more than 90% of patients is chronic pulmonary disease caused by bacterial and viral pathogens and leading to a host inflammatory response. The most profound changes occur in the lungs and airways, where chronic infections involve a limited number of organisms including *P. aeruginosa*, which is implicated most often, followed by *Staphylococcus aureus*, *Haemophilus influenzae*, and *Stenotrophomonas maltophilia*.[6] Children with CF are first infected with *Staphylococcus* and *Haemophilus* species and later with *Pseudomonas* species.

Several theories have been proposed to explain the limited number of organisms involved in CF pulmonary infections, including the *inflammation-first hypothesis*,[31] the *infection-first hypothesis*,[32] the *cell-receptor hypothesis*,[17] and the *salt defensins hypothesis*.[33] The salt defensins hypothesis proposes that CF airway cells have properties similar to those of sweat glands that inactivate substances called defensins, leading to bacterial multiplication and infections. These theories, however, do not explain the presence of mucoid *S. aureus* or mucoid-type *P. aeruginosa*.

The *isotonic fluid depletion and anoxic mucus theory* proposes that water- and volume-depleted airway fluid leads to mucus viscosity, subsequent defective ciliary clearance, and a cough that is inadequate to clear the airways. Thus, bacteria in the CF lung are trapped within this viscous airway fluid and multiply within anaerobic growth conditions by changing from a nonmucoid to a mucoid type of organism.[34-36] The transformation of these bacteria to a biofilm-encased form is a means of protection from normal host defenses and antibiotics, making eradication difficult.[37] A neutrophil-dominated airway inflammation is certainly present in CF lung disease, even in clinically stable patients.[31,38]

It seems that early pediatric colonization with either *P. aeruginosa* or *S. aureus* has a significant impact on CF lung disease in adulthood. Another organism unique to CF with a significant impact on adult CF lung disease is *Burkholderia cepacia*. Earlier, this organism was uniformly associated with poor clinical outcomes, but now it is recognized that outcomes might depend on the actual genotype of the organism.[39]

Clinically, CF pulmonary exacerbations are manifested as an increase in respiratory symptoms including cough and sputum production, with associated systemic symptoms that include malaise and anorexia.[40] Patients rarely have fever and leukocytosis, and in most cases radiographic changes are minimal during an exacerbation.[9] An exacerbation can be documented by a decrease in pulmonary function, which usually returns to normal after the acute exacerbation resolves. As the lung disease progresses, bronchiolitis and bronchitis become evident, with bronchiectasis as a consequence of the persistent obstruction-infection insult. Overall, bronchiectasis in CF is more severe in the upper lobes than in the lower lobes. Pathologic examinations have demonstrated bronchiectatic cysts in more than 50% of end-stage CF lung on autopsy studies.[41] Subpleural cysts often occur in the upper lobes and can contribute to the frequent occurrence of pneumothorax in patients with late-stage CF. The reported incidence of spontaneous pneumothorax in CF ranges between 2.8% and 18.9%.[42] The patient with spontaneous pneumothorax usually presents with acute onset of chest pain or dyspnea. In one study, chest pain was the manifesting symptom in more than 50% of patients. Dyspnea occurred in more than 65% of patients.[43] In the same study, hemoptysis was present in 19% of patients, probably as a result of bronchial artery enlargement, and subsequent tortuosity within ectatic airways made vessels delicate and more prone to bleed.[44]

Children without a prior, established diagnosis of CF often present with cough and upper respiratory tract infections that persist longer than expected. Patients whose CF is diagnosed when they are older often do not have the underlying pancreatic insufficiency that is typical of the younger patient with classic CF. Patients with CF diagnosed in adulthood usually present with chronic respiratory infections, but these are usually milder and less likely to be pseudomonal.[42]

Several interstitial lung diseases have been described during autopsy of the CF lung, including the usual interstitial pneumonitis, bronchiolitis obliterans organizing pneumonia, and diffuse alveolar damage.[45] The upper respiratory tract is also involved in CF, most patients suffer from acute and chronic sinusitis caused by hypertrophy and hyperplasia of the secretory components of the sinus tract.[46] Another common feature is the presence of pedunculated nasal polyps.[47] Sleep-disordered breathing and nocturnal hypoxia, mainly during rapid-eye-movement (REM) sleep and hypoventilation, have also been described in CF patients.[48]

Gastrointestinal Tract

GI symptoms in CF manifest early and continue throughout the life span of a CF patient. Because of defects in *CFTR*, meconium ileus can occur at birth, and distal intestinal obstruction syndrome (the meconium ileus equivalent) occurs in 40% of older CF patients. The distal intestinal obstruction syndrome has been associated with inadequate use of pancreatic enzyme and dietary indiscretion without appropriate use of pancreatic enzyme.[9] CF patients with obstruction can present with abdominal pain and often a palpable mass in the right lower quadrant on physical examination. Associated symptoms include anorexia, nausea, vomiting, and obstipation. With more frequent events, adhesions can develop due to inflammation, leading to a mechanically dysfunctional intestine that can eventually require surgical resection.

As a result of the *CFTR* defect, the biliary ducts can become plugged and clogged, leading to liver involvement and biliary cirrhosis in 25% of patients with CF. Hepatic steatosis can result from malnutrition, and congestion can result from hypoxia-induced cor pulmonale.[2] Symptomatic liver disease with the sequelae of cirrhosis, including esophageal varices, is uncommon. Fecal loss of bile acids is increased in CF, leading to a reduction in the bile salt pool and a propensity for cholelithiasis. Approximately 30% of adult CF patients present with a hypoplastic, poorly functioning gallbladder, and about one third of that population develops gallstones.[49,50]

About 90% of patients with CF have pancreatic insufficiency. It is believed to be related to reduced volumes of pancreatic secretions and reduced concentrations of bicarbonate excretion. As a result, digestive proenzymes are retained when the pancreatic duct is blocked, leading to organ tissue destruction and fibrosis. Lipids and fat-soluble vitamins (D, E, K, and A) are therefore malabsorbed, and the malabsorption can eventually lead to a hypermetabolic state and increased endobronchial infections because of an inverse relation between metabolic states and lung function in CF patients.[51] Patients with no evidence of pancreatic insufficiency usually manifest milder disease and are less likely to have the ΔF508 mutation.[9]

CF-related diabetes usually develops after the second decade of life and rarely before the age of 10 years, due to sparing of Langerhans cells. Over time, pancreatic destruction and fibrosis occur, caused by obstruction of the pancreatic ducts and later leading to amyloid deposition, and diabetes ensues.[52,53] Patients with CF-related diabetes experience more severe lung disease and nutritional deficiencies than CF patients without diabetes. Bone disease, including osteoporosis and osteopenia, is multifactorial in CF because of malnutrition, cytokines, and hormonal disorders in androgen (hypogonadism) and estrogen production and because of glucocorticoid therapy.[54]

Fertility and Reproduction

Now that many more CF patients are surviving into their 40s, issues of family and children have gained more attention. Most male CF patients are infertile because of aspermia secondary to atretic or bilateral absence of the vas deferens or seminal vesicle abnormalities.[55] It is believed that during fetal life, the vas deferens becomes plugged with mucoid secretions and subsequently gets reabsorbed. Libido and sexual performance are not affected. Artificial insemination may be used for couples desiring offspring by obtaining microscopic epididymal sperm sampling. Female CF patients usually have normal reproductive tracts, although the cervical mucus may be tenacious as a result of *CFTR* mutation, thus blocking the cervical canal and possibly interfering with fertility. Overall, women with CF are not as infertile as their male counterparts, and birth control must be discussed with female patients reaching sexual maturity.[56] The endometrium and fallopian tubes contain very small amounts of *CFTR* and usually remain normal.[57] Onset of menarche is usually normal except in girls who are severely ill and undernourished.

Since the 1960s, the prognosis for CF and pregnancy has improved greatly. Maternal deaths usually occur in women with the most severe lung disease. It appears from multiple case studies that the decline of lung function and the absolute value of the FEV_1 may be more important in determining fetal outcome.[58,59] One study, by Canny and colleagues, recommended an FEV_1 of greater than 70% as a requirement for a successful pregnancy outcome.[59] Normal lung function leads to a normal pregnancy. Pulmonary status can worsen in women with poor lung function during pregnancy, but this is still debated. Termination of pregnancy has been recommended if the FEV_1 is less than 50%; however, reports do exist of successful pregnancies with low FEV_1.[60] Extremes of low body weight have resulted in terminations and premature deliveries and may be a relative contraindication.[61] In terms of infant health, it should be kept in mind that all infants will be carriers of a maternal gene for CF. Case reports have reported fetal anomalies caused either by treatment, by maternal complications, or by chance itself.[57]

Vaginal yeast infections and urinary incontinence have now become major issues in female CF patients as they mature. Many patients have persistent yeast infections as a result of frequent antibiotic therapy. Suppression of cough in an attempt to prevent urinary leak can prevent women from aggressively continuing chest physiotherapy.[62,63]

Sweat Glands

During the great summer heat wave of 1939 it was discovered that patients with CF were especially susceptible to heat prostration and associated cardiovascular collapse and death after initial symptoms. This sweat defect was discovered by Di Sant'Agnese and eventually led to the modern day sweat test used in the diagnosis of CF. In the sweat duct, *CFTR* is the only channel by which chloride can be reabsorbed from sweat.[63,64]

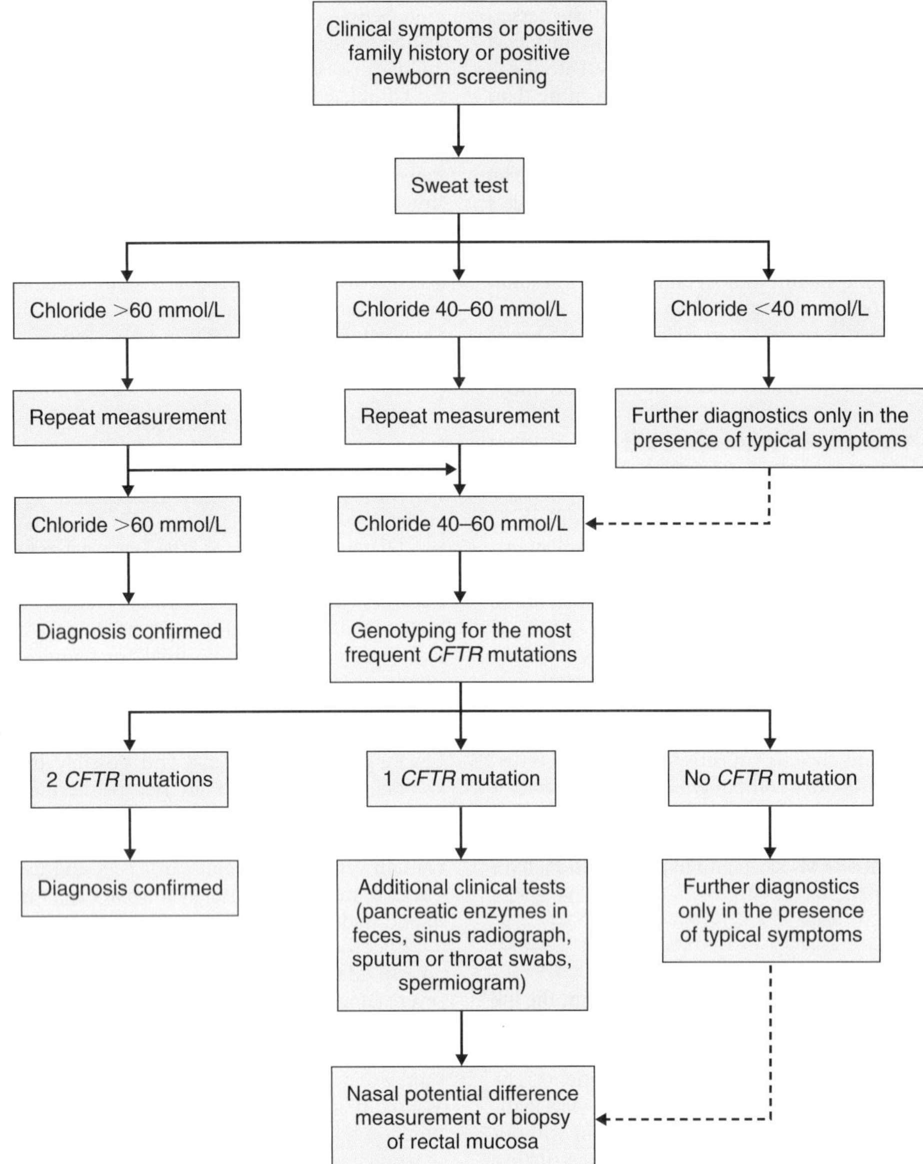

Figure 1 **Algorithm for diagnosing cystic fibrosis.** *Adapted from Ratjen F, Doring G: Cystic fibrosis. Lancet 2003;361:681-689.*

DIAGNOSIS

In 1998, the Cystic Fibrosis Foundation issued a consensus statement regarding the diagnosis of CF.[1] According to the panel, the diagnosis of CF should be made on the basis of one or more characteristic phenotypic features: history of a CF sibling, presence of a positive newborn screening test, and laboratory confirmation of a *CFTR* abnormality by an abnormal sweat chloride test, identification of mutations in a gene known to cause CF, or in vivo demonstration of an ion transport abnormality across the nasal epithelium (Fig. 1). However, if these classic criteria as described by the committee are not present, CF still cannot be ruled out in its entirety. In patients who present later in childhood or in early adulthood, these classic criteria might not be present. In these patients, typical pulmonary symptoms or GI symptoms may be absent, and instead pancreatitis, male infertility, or sinusitis or nasal polyps may be present.[18]

Sweat Testing

Sweat testing, in which a minimally acceptable volume or weight of sweat (≥50 mg) must be collected during a 30-minute period to ensure an average sweat rate of 1 g/m^2 per minute, using the Gibson and Cooke method.[63,64] A sweat chloride reading of more than 60 mmol/L on repeated analysis is consistent with a diagnosis of CF but must be interpreted in the context of the patient's history, clinical presentation, and age.[1] Approximately 5% of patients with CF have normal sweat test results.[7] A negative sweat test does not rule out the possibility of CF in the presence of appropriate symptoms and clinical signs (pancreatitis, sinus disease, and azoospermia) and should be repeated. False positives can result for many reasons, but poor technique and patient nutritional status, including anorexia, can yield false results.

Nasal Potential Measurements Voltage

Nasal potential measurements measure the voltage difference and correlate with the movement of sodium across the cell membrane. In CF, the *CFTR* mutation renders this physiologic function abnormal, leading to a large drop in the potential in patients with CF. The presence of nasal polyps or irritated nasal mucosa can yield a false-negative result. Overall, testing using this method is complicated and time consuming.[65]

Genotyping

Because of the more than 1000 *CFTR* mutations associated with CF, commercially available probes test only for a limited number of mutations, which constitute more than 90% of the most common mutations known to cause CF but which can vary from region to region. A mutation can be found in most symptomatic patients, but in a small percentage the mutation can be absent.[66] Therefore, clinical manifestations or family history are important to the diagnosis. If an abnormality does exist, the combination of two CF mutations plus an abnormal sweat chloride test is accepted for diagnosis. Mutation analysis can be used not only to confirm diagnosis but also to provide genetic information for family members, predict certain phenotypic features, and possibly help in allocating patients for research trials.

Ancillary Testing

In patients with atypical features, a number of clinical and radiologic tests may be performed to assess for a CF phenotype, including assessment of respiratory tract microbiology, chest radiographs, computed tomography of the chest, sinus evaluation, genital tract evaluation, semen analysis, and pancreatic functional assessment. The hallmarks of CF are pancreatic insufficiency and malabsorption, which can lend themselves to laboratory examination such as measurement of serum trypsinogen or pancreas-specific elastase, and fecal fat analysis or reduced fecal concentration of chymotrypsin.[67,68] In addition, pansinusitis is so common in CF patients and generally uncommon in non-CF children that the presence of this entity on examination and sinus radiographs should prompt a suspicion of CF.[69] In a male patient with obstructive azoospermia confirmed with testicular biopsy, CF should be strongly considered, although other diseases, such as Young's syndrome, can cause pulmonary disease and azoospermia.[70]

Airway inflammation, even in the absence of active infection, is present in young and older patients with CF. Therefore, bronchoalveolar lavage (BAL) can show a predominance of neutrophils in patients with CF. In atypical presentations, with no evidence of pulmonary disease, a BAL with evidence of a high neutrophil count can provide further support for the diagnosis of CF in the presence of azoospermia or pancreatic disease.[47] Isolation of the mucoid type of *P. aeruginosa* by BAL or sputum analysis, oropharyngeal swab, or sinus culture is highly suggestive of CF.[1]

TREATMENT

Gene Treatment

The cure for CF is to restore the function of *CFTR*. This has been attempted with in vivo gene therapy in CF patients using adenoviral vectors and cationic liposome transfer, although lasting physiologic effects have not been noted.[71,72] Although it is still far from being a standard treatment, gene therapy for CF has been making significant strides.

Protein modification is based on the concept that the abnormal CFTR protein can be taught to transport water and electrolytes. The CFTR ΔF508 protein mutation is the most common mutation responsible for CF. This abnormal mutation is recognized by the endoplasmic reticulum and degraded rather than glycosylated and transported to the cell surface. Aminoglycosides, including gentamicin, allow few of the *CFTR* mutations to reach the respiratory epithelial cells in patients with CF. Other compounds, including phenylbutyrate, phenybutyrate, and genistein, have been tested to act as similar chaperones to the *CFTR* mutation.[73-76]

Another ongoing approach includes gene transfer, in which both endogenous stem cells in the lung and mouse-derived cells have been noted to transform into airway and epithelial cells after systemic adminstration.[77]

Table 1 Cystic Fibrosis Foundation Guidelines for Cystic Fibrosis Care

Care	Frequency
Outpatient visits	4/yr
Pulmonary function tests	≥2/yr
Respiratory cultures	≥1/yr
Creatinine level	1/yr
Glucose	1/yr for patients >13 yr
Liver enzymes	1/yr

Adapted from Cystic Fibrosis Foundation: Cystic Fibrosis Foundation Patient Registry Annual Data Report 2002. Bethesda, Md, Cystic Fibrosis Foundation, 2003.

Symptomatic Treatment

Since the early 1990s, the Cystic Fibrosis Foundation has developed guidelines to help guide the care of patients with this complex disease (Table 1).[1]

Respiratory Care

Respiratory disease is the major cause of mortality and morbidity in CF. All patients with CF should be monitored for changes in respiratory disease. A persistent cough in a CF patient is not normal, and the cause should be aggressively pursued.

Spirometry is a useful tool for monitoring pulmonary status. Initial lung function in most CF patients is normal. Later, the small peripheral airways become obstructed, leading to changes on spirometry at low lung volumes. Later still, decreased flow occurs at larger lung volumes. CF usually produces an obstructive pattern on spirometry, but a restrictive pattern can indicate substantial gas trapping. In general, a 10% decrease in FEV_1 is considered a sign of worsening lung function and possibly a sign of a respiratory infection.[78] Patients with an FEV_1 of less than 30% of predicted are at higher risks for nocturnal hypoxia and hypercapnia and should be evaluated for nocturnal desaturation.

Oxygen saturation should be monitored routinely to assess the need for supplemental oxygen in patients with moderate to severe disease. Structural changes can also be noted using radiographic studies. Annual chest radiographs are recommended for unstable CF patients and may be useful in documenting the progression of disease or response to treatment. In patients with stable clinical states, chest radiographs should be performed every 2 to 4 years instead of annually. If bronchiectasis is suspected, high-resolution computed tomography is indicated (see Fig. 1).[78]

Inhaled Bronchodilators. Inhaled bronchodilators, specifically β agonists, can be administered by nebulizer, metered-dose inhaler, or oral inhaler in CF patients with a documented drop in FEV1 by 12% or 200 mL, indicating bronchodilator response in the effort to treat airway hyperreactivity.[79] Few studies show significant improvement in clinical pulmonary function with routine use of bronchodilator therapy. Long-term use of β agonists should be approached with caution, because animal studies have shown submucosal gland hypertrophy and a possible hypersecretory state with prolonged use, although no human studies have duplicated this finding.[80] Salmeterol, a long-acting β agonist, is effective in decreasing nocturnal hypoxia in patients with CF.[81] Hypertonic saline, either a 6% or a 3% solution, has been shown to reduce sputum viscoelasticity and to increase cough clearance in CF patients.[82]

Dornase alfa (recombinant human deoxyribonuclease I; Pulmozyme) in addition to hypertonic saline is believed to improve mucociliary clearance by hydrolyzing extracellular DNA, which is present at high levels in CF patients. Improved lung function has been noted with the use of this drug. In a multicenter placebo-controlled study, patients treated with dornase alfa had a 12.4% improvement in FEV_1 above baseline and a 2.1% increase compared with those receiving placebo ($P < 0.01$).[83,84] Side effects of dornase alfa include hoarseness, changes in phonation, and mild pharyngitis.[5] A mucolytic agent such as *N*-acetylcysteine (NAC) can be used for airway clearance, although few data exist to support the use of NAC.[85] Given its unpleasant side effects, including noxious odor and potential for bronchospasm, NAC has a limited role in CF.

Airway Clearance. Airway clearance techniques should be routinely performed on a daily basis by all CF patients[86] before eating, and usually bronchodilators are used during or before airway clearance treatment. Inhaled corticosteroids and antibiotics should usually be reserved until the airway clearance technique is completed so that airways have fewer secretions, allowing greater penetration of medications. In selecting a particular treatment, the patient's age, preference, and lifestyle should be taken into account, because no one technique is superior.

Chest physiotherapy consisting of chest percussion and postural drainage (chest clapping) is the primary method of secretion clearance. The patient is usually positioned so that gravity assists in draining mucus from areas of the lung while avoiding the head-down position. Using cupped hands or a clapping device, the chest wall is vibrated or percussed to clear mucus. The therapy can be used on patients of all ages and can be concentrated in certain areas of the lungs that need more attention. Usually, an additional caregiver is needed to provide this treatment, but patients who are independent may be able to perform their own percussion on the front and sides of the chest.[87] Assisting the cough of a CF patient through external application of pressure to the epigastric or thoracic cage can assist in the clearance.[87]

A forced exhalation, or *huff*, during mid or low lung volumes can improve mucus clearance. A technique called *forced expiration* consists of two huffs followed by relaxed breathing. Unlike postural drainage, the active cycle of breathing treatment improves lung function without decreasing oxygenation and does not need an assistant.[88] This airway clearance technique is a combination of breathing control, thoracic expansion, and the forced expiration technique. It improves oxygen delivery to the alveoli and distal airways and promotes clearance of mucus to the proximal airways, to be cleared by huffing.[89]

Autogenic drainage is a method of breathing performed at three different lung volumes to augment airflow in the different divisions of the airways. Air needs to be moved in rapidly to unstick mucus and avoid airway collapse. No desaturations occur during this technique, but it does require concentration and might not be appropriate for young CF patients.[88]

The application of positive expiratory pressure (PEP) by mechanical ventilation or by intermittent positive pressure breathing devices can assist in airway collapse in CF. Bronchiectasis resulting in wall weakness can lead to collapse and retained secretions. Low-pressure PEP, high-pressure PEP, and oscillation PEP are three methods to help reduce airway collapse, all using a device that provides expiratory lengthening and manometric measurements at the mouth.[87] Oscillating PEP can enhance clearance of secretions in a way that is relatively easy for the patient. It is low cost, and it is easily movable.[90]

High-frequency chest wall compression is performed using a compression vest that allows therapy to large chest-wall areas simultaneously. No assistance is needed with this therapy, and it may be ideal for the independent CF patient.[91]

Intrapulmonary percussive ventilation provides frequent, small, low-pressure breaths to the airways in an oscillatory manner. This method is limited by its high cost and lack of portability, but unlike some other devices it can be used to deliver medications.[78]

The effect of exercise in CF is not clear. Whether it enhances mucus clearance is debatable, but quality of life improves and there is a lower mortality rate among CF patients who exercise regularly.[78] Regular exercise enhances cardiovascular fitness, improves functional capacity, and improves quality of life; therefore, exercise should be advocated strongly in the adult CF patient.[5]

Some of the contraindications to airway therapy include poorly controlled reflux disease, massive hemoptysis, and the presence of an untreated pneumothorax.

Antibiotics. Improved antibiotics against bacterial infections, especially P. aeruginosa, have resulted in an increased life span for the CF patient. The aim of CF therapy should be prevention of bacterial lung infections. Environmental hygiene measures, including cohorting patients according to infection status, can limit cross-reaction.[92] The most important bacterial organisms in CF are *S. aureus, P. aeruginosa,* and *B. cepacia,* but others have also emerged including S. maltophilia, Achromobacter xylosoxidans, and nontuberculous bacteria.[93] Intravenous antibiotics are the mainstay of therapy for acute exacerbations. The choice of antibiotic is difficult in CF because of resistance patterns; therefore, the choice should be based on the most recent sensitivities of the surveillance sputum cultures. If a recent culture is not available, antibiotic coverage should include treatment for both *Staphylococcus* and *Pseudomonas* species. Most centers typically choose a third-generation cephalosporin and an aminoglycoside, given for 2 to 3 weeks intravenously at higher doses because of the volume of distribution in CF patients.

Inhaled antibiotic aerosols can effectively minimize toxicity and allow certain aminoglycosides to be administered at ome. Limiting factors include cost, taste, and distribution in severe disease and acute exacerbations.[9] Many CF centers have adopted the Copenhagen Protocol in dealing with infection when, with the first isolation of *Pseudomonas* species, oral ciprofloxacin and inhaled colistin are started, with intravenous antibiotics given every 4 months to prevent reinfection. Cohorting and environmental and nutritional issues are monitored as well, leading to a significant reduction of chronic infection with *Pseudomonas* species and better pulmonary function.[76]

Several large randomized studies have demonstrated a benefit of macrolides in CF patients. The results of these investigations seem to indicate that the immunomodulatory effect of these medications and not the antibacterial effect is responsible for the outcomes of the medication. Experts have suggested using macrolides for 6 months (azithromycin or clarithromycin) in CF children or in adults not improving on conventional therapy.[94] Azithromycin has been shown to be highly effective in improving pulmonary function over a 6-month period in CF patients homozygous for ΔF508 and not receiving dornase alfa.[95]

Other Treatments. In patients with allergic bronchopulmonary aspergillosis or asthma, oral corticosteroids can be used. Although alternate-day steroids have been used in the past for CF exacerbations to reduce airway inflammation, experts agree that this method should be used more cautiously. Ibuprofen has been used as an anti-inflammatory agent, and in one trial lung function declined more slowly in ibuprofen users.[96] Other therapies currently undergoing trials include surfactant to reduce sputum adhesiveness, gelsolin to sever F-actin bonds in sputum (thus reducing the tenacity of sputum), and thymosin B 4 to improve sputum transport.[76]

Lung Transplantation

In advanced lung disease resulting from CF, the options for treatment are limited. Lung transplantation is the only effective therapeutic option not only to prolong survival (1 year survival >80%; 5-year survival, 60%[97]) but also to improve quality of life. The International Lung Transplant Committee issued guidelines in 1998 for the selection of lung transplantation candidates.[98] Based on these criteria, CF patients should be referred for transplantation when the FEV_1 is less

Box 2 Indications for Lung Transplantation in Cystic Fibrosis

FEV$_1$ predicted < 30%
Rapidly progressive respiratory deterioration
Increasing number of hospital admissions
Massive hemoptysis
Recurrent pneumothorax
Pao$_2$ < 55 mm Hg
Paco$_2$ > 50 mm Hg
Multiresistant organisms
Wasting

Note: Young female patients should be referred earlier due to overall poor prognosis.
Adapted from Boehler A: Update on cystic fibrosis selected aspects related to lung transplantation. Swiss Med Wkly 2003;133:111-117.

than 30% of predicted, if hypoxia or hypercapnia is present, if hospitalizations increase in frequency, or if hemoptysis or cachexia is an issue (Box 2). Early in the history of lung transplantation, CF patients colonized with *B. cepacia* were not candidates for transplantation, but recent advances in careful, specific taxonomic testing of *B. cepacia* have allowed this patient population to be eligible for transplantation at many centers, including our own.[99]

Severe liver disease, including portal hypertension, is present in 3% of the CF population. In this population, combined liver and lung transplantation should be considered. Overall survival in combined liver and lung transplantation is 64% at 1 year and 56% after 5 years.[100] Patients with severe cachexia and a low body mass index (<18 kg/m^2) are at an increased risk of death while on the waiting list for lung transplantation, and interventions for nutritional support should be instituted to prevent further weight loss.[101]

Pleural adhesion and previous pleurodesis are not contraindications to transplantation. If pleurodesis is indicated, we recommend that it be performed in conjunction with a transplantation center to minimize any complications that can occur at the time of transplantation.

Unstable CF patients requiring mechanical ventilation are not candidates for lung transplantation at any transplant center. Meyers and colleagues reported 1-year outcomes in stable, mechanically ventilated patients who underwent transplantation.[102] Currently, only a limited number of centers perform lung transplantation in ventilator-dependent patients.

Recent attention has focused on living lobar transplantation, which involves the removal of a lower lobe from each of two donors and subsequent transplant into a child or small adult.[103] Short-term outcomes have been comparable with those using cadaveric transplants. This procedure involves three patients and thus a possible increase in the potential morbidity and mortality, although no donor deaths have been reported.[104]

For more information on identifying which patients are more likely to benefit from receiving a lung transplant, contact the Cleveland Clinic Foundation Lung Transplant Center or the Cystic Fibrosis Foundation's website. More than 1400 people have received lung transplants since 1988.[6]

Nutritional Care and Supplementation

CF patients should eat a well-balanced diet (a standard North American diet with 35%-40% fat calories) without fat restriction, always given with enteric-coated pancreatic enzymes. Anthropomorphic measurements should be made every 3 to 4 months, and CF patients should be educated regarding their ideal body weight range. Annual complete blood cell count, albumin, retinol, and tocopherol measurements are recommended. Pancreatic enzymes should be given with each meal and snack, along with vitamin A 10,000 IU/day, vitamin E 200-400 IU/day, vitamin D 400-800 IU/day with adequate sunlight exposure, and vitamin K 2.5 to 5.0 mg/week. If the body mass index decreases, enteral feeding should be considered through gastrostomy tubes or jejunostomy tubes.

For CF patients with partial obstructions or distal intestinal obstructive syndrome, early recognition is vital to avoid surgical intervention. In addition, aggressive hydration, addition of pancreatic enzymes, H$_2$ blockers, and agents to thin bowel contents (including the radiographic contrast solution diatrizoate) may be used. Complete obstructions should be treated with enemas, oral mineral oil, and oral polyethylene glycol-3350 solutions.[9]

PROGNOSIS

Overall, the life expectancy in CF has risen since the 1980s. Recent figures show the median age of survival increased by 14 years in 2000 compared with figures from 1980; the predicted mean survival age was 31.6 years in 2000.[6] In 1990, 30% of patients in the CF Registry were older than 18 years. This has continued to rise: 40.2% of patients in 2002 were older than 18 years. Although overall survival rates have improved, female patients have had consistently poorer survival rates than male CF patients in the age range from 2 to 20 years. It is not clear why this is the case.[105]

Lung function predictions over time are difficult to estimate, but CF patients often have extended periods of stabilized lung function that can last for 5 years or more. Most patients have full-time or part-time jobs, and many are married and have children. In the patient registry,[6] more than 185 women who had CF were pregnant in 2002.[8]

Many patients have normal life spans, and end-of-life options need to be addressed with patients and their families. Advance-care planning should be done early in the disease course. The goal of advance-care planning is to respect the patient's wishes.[5]

Summary

- CF is the most common autosomal recessive, life-limiting disease among the white population.
- With current management, almost 80% of patients with CF will reach adulthood. The delivery of health care to the adult CF patient has thus become relevant to the nonpediatric physician.
- CF is caused by a defective gene that causes the body to produce an abnormally thick, sticky mucus that leads to airway obstruction, subsequent life-threatening lung infections, and end-stage lung disease.
- CF is an autosomal recessive trait; the most common mutation in the *CFTR* gene is caused by the deletion of phenylalanine at position 508 (ΔF508).
- Newborn screening for CF has been instituted in eight states, although national screening plans have not been mandated.
- The most profound changes from CF occur in the lungs and airways, where chronic infections involve a limited number of organisms including *P. aeruginosa*, which is implicated most often, followed by *S. aureus*, *H. influenzae*, and *S. maltophilia*.
- Gastrointestinal symptoms in CF occur early and continue throughout the life of a CF patient. Problems include intestinal obstruction and various aspects of pancreatic insufficiency.
- Female patients with CF are not as infertile as their male counterparts, and birth control must be discussed with female patients reaching sexual maturity.
- The Cystic Fibrosis Foundation has guidelines to help guide the care of patients with this complex disease.

Suggested Readings

Cystic Fibrosis Foundation: Going the distance to a cure: 2002 Annual Report. Bethesda, Md: Cystic Fibrosis Foundation, 2003.

Elborn JS: How can we prevent multisystem complications of cystic fibrosis? Sem Res Crit Care Med 2007;28:303-311.

Rosenstein BJ, Cutting GR: The diagnosis of cystic fibrosis: A consensus statement. Cystic Fibrosis Foundation Consensus Panel. J Pediatr 1998;132:589-595.

Rubin BK: Overview of cystic fibrosis and non-CF bronchiectasis. Semin Respir Crit Care Med 2003;24:619-627.

Yankaskas JR, Marshall BC, Sufian B, et al: Cystic fibrosis adult care: Consensus conference report. Chest 2004;125:1S-39S.

References

For a complete list of references, log onto www.expertconsult.com.

Interstitial Lung Disease

Jeffrey T. Chapman

The term *interstitial lung disease* (ILD) refers to a broad category of lung diseases rather than a specific disease entity.[1,2] It includes a variety of illnesses with diverse causes, treatments, and prognoses. These disorders are grouped together because of similarities in their clinical presentations, plain chest radiographic appearance, and physiologic features.

Because there are more than 100 separate disorders, it is helpful to group them based on cause, disease associations, or pathology. An organizational scheme is presented in Figure 1. First, the diseases are broken down into those with known causes or associations and those of unknown cause. Diseases with known causes are further classified based on specific exposure, association with systemic disease, or association with a known genetic disorder. These groups are further divided into specific disease entities. Using this organizational scheme, one can perform a careful and complete history, working toward an accurate diagnosis and appropriate therapy.

PATHOPHYSIOLOGY

As the name implies, the histologic abnormalities that characterize ILD generally involve the pulmonary interstitium to a greater extent than the alveolar spaces or airways, although exceptions exist. The interstitium is the area between the capillaries and the alveolar space. In the normal state, this space allows close apposition of gas and capillaries with minimal connective tissue matrix, fibroblasts, and inflammatory cells such as macrophages. The interstitium supports the delicate relation between the alveoli and capillaries, allowing efficient gas exchange. When responding to any injury, whether from a specific exposure (e.g., asbestos, nitrofurantoin, moldy hay), an autoimmune-mediated inflammation from a systemic connective tissue disease (e.g., rheumatoid arthritis), or unknown injury (e.g., idiopathic pulmonary fibrosis), the lung must respond to the damage and repair itself. If the exposure persists or if the repair process is imperfect, the lung may be permanently damaged, with increased interstitial tissue replacing the normal capillaries, alveoli, and healthy interstitium.

These pathologic abnormalities can lead to profound impairment in lung physiology. Gas exchange is impaired due to ventilation-perfusion ($\dot{V}/\dot{Q}$) mismatching, shunt, and decreased diffusion across the abnormal interstitium. Work of breathing is markedly increased because of decreased lung compliance. Together, these physiologic impairments lead to the exercise intolerance seen in all of the ILDs. Unfortunately, if the initiating injury or abnormal repair from injury is not halted, progressive tissue damage can lead to worsening physiologic impairment and even death.

CHARACTERISTICS

Clinical Signs and Symptoms

Many of the ILDs have similar clinical features and are not easily distinguished on examination. Symptoms are generally limited to the respiratory tract. Exertional breathlessness (dyspnea) and a nonproductive cough are the most common reasons patients seek medical attention. However, sputum production, hemoptysis, or wheezing are helpful in classifying the disease. If the patient also has prominent nonrespiratory symptoms, such as myalgia, arthralgia, or sclerodactyly, ILD might be the result of underlying connective tissue disease.

Physical Examination

Most patients with ILD have bilateral inspiratory fine crackles, which usually are most prominent at the lung bases. However, some diseases, such as sarcoidosis and lymphangioleiomyomatosis, have only decreased breath sounds without adventitious sounds despite markedly abnormal chest radiographs. Expiratory wheezing is relatively uncommon, and its presence suggests either airway involvement as part of the primary disease process or concomitant airways disease such as emphysema or asthma. Occasionally, wheezing is a clue to a particular diagnosis, such as sarcoidosis, which can involve the airways as well as the interstitium.

Signs of pulmonary arterial hypertension with right ventricular dysfunction, such as lower-extremity edema or jugular venous distention, can occur late in the course of any ILD and are not helpful in diagnosing a specific ILD.

Examination also can disclose features of underlying connective tissue disease, including active joint inflammation (synovitis), joint deformities, or skin rash.

Radiographic Features

There is considerable variability among the specific diseases in the character and distribution of radiographic abnormalities. However, for most ILDs, the plain chest radiograph reveals reduced lung volumes with bilateral reticular or reticulonodular opacities. The ready availability of high-resolution computed tomography (HRCT) has highlighted significant radiographic differences between diseases that have similar plain chest radiographic patterns.[3] HRCT has the ability to better define the specific characteristics of lung parenchyma seen in each disease, increasing the chance of making a confident diagnosis.[4]

The plain chest radiograph and HRCT features of idiopathic pulmonary fibrosis (IPF) are important patterns to recognize because, next to sarcoidosis, IPF is the most common ILD, several other ILDs have a similar appearance, and IPF images are the prototypic pattern of fibrotic injury response in the lung. The plain radiograph and HRCT in IPF reveal bilateral, peripheral and basilar predominant disease with reticulonodular infiltrates, often with honeycomb, cystic changes. Figure 2 shows a plain radiograph with bibasilar reticulonodular infiltrates. Note the overall volume loss and poorly demarcated pleural-parenchymal borders along the hemidiaphragms and heart, indicating parenchymal abnormalities extending to the pleura. Figure 3 shows an HRCT image of IPF, with distortion of the lung architecture and traction bronchiectasis, especially at the lung bases. As predicted by the plain radiograph, the abnormalities are strikingly located in the subpleural and dependent areas of the lung. Ground glass abnormalities, increased attenuation of the lung tissue without distortion of the underlying blood vessels or bronchi, are absent or minimal in classic IPF. Pleural disease and significant lymphadenopathy are not seen, although up to two thirds of IPF patients have mild mediastinal adenopathy.[5] As the burden of disease increases, the chest x-ray examination can reveal multiple tiny cysts in the most markedly involved regions. This cystic pattern, called honeycombing, reflects end-stage fibrosis and is a feature of many end-stage ILDs.

In contrast to the fibrotic type of injury, some diseases cause an inflammatory abnormality with a much different radiographic

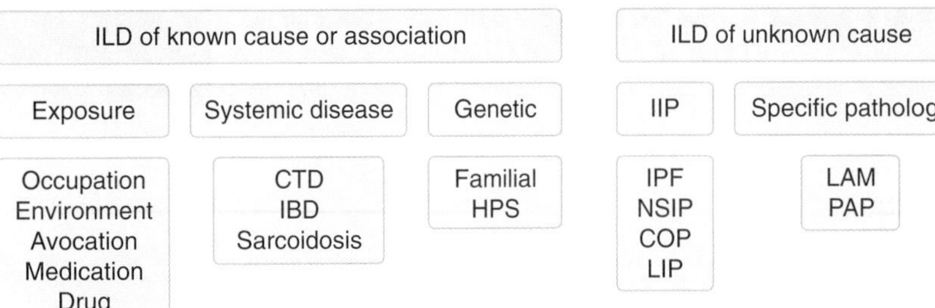

Figure 1 Current organization of interstitial lung disease (ILD). COP, cryptogenic organizing pneumonia; CTD, connective tissue disease; HPS, Hermansky-Pudlak syndrome; IBD, inflammatory bowel disease; IIP, idiopathic interstitial pneumonia; IPF, idiopathic pulmonary fibrosis; LAM, lymphangioleiomyomatosis; LIP, lymphocytic interstitial pneumonia; NSIP, nonspecific interstitial pneumonitis; PAP, pulmonary alveolar proteinosis.

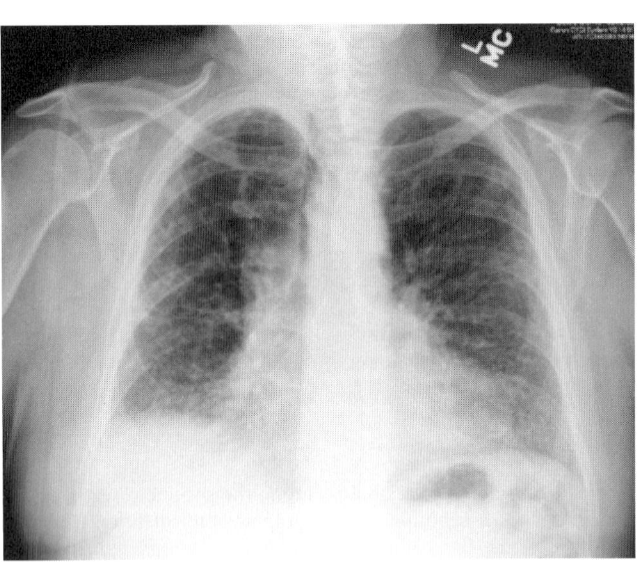

Figure 2 Plain chest radiograph of idiopathic pulmonary fibrosis.

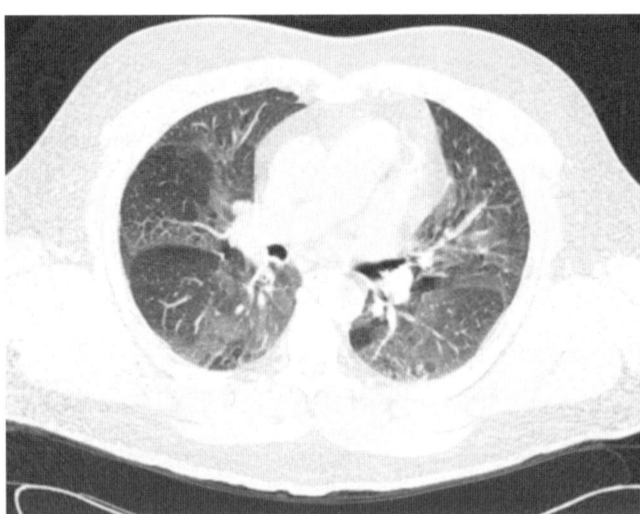

Figure 4 High-resolution computed tomography scan of ground glass opacity infiltrates.

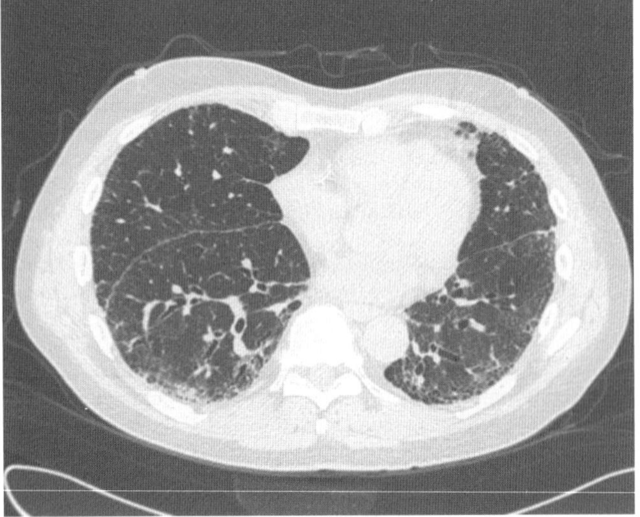

Figure 3 High-resolution computed tomography scan of idiopathic pulmonary fibrosis.

image. In cellular nonspecific interstitial pneumonia, the predominant abnormality is ground glass without distortion of the lung architecture or loss of volume, as seen in Figure 4. In addition, the central and mid lung zone locations of abnormalities are distinct from IPF. Understanding these two patterns as ends of an extreme, we shall see how the clinician is able to evaluate other diseases in a similar context.

Physiologic Features

Similar to the radiographic findings, among the specific diseases there can be considerable variability in the physiologic abnormalities seen. However, a restrictive physiologic impairment is the common finding.[6] Thus, both forced expiratory volume in one second (FEV_1) and forced vital capacity (FVC) are diminished, and the FEV_1/FVC ratio is preserved or even supranormal. Lung volumes are reduced, as is the diffusing capacity of the lung for carbon monoxide (D_LCO). This reduction in diffusing capacity reflects a pathologic disturbance of the alveolar-capillary interface.

Although not commonly pursued, the compliance characteristics of the lungs can be evaluated with an esophageal balloon to measure intrathoracic pressure at various lung volumes. In almost all of the ILDs, the lungs have reduced compliance and require supranormal transpleural pressures to ventilate. This lack of compliance results in small lung volumes and increased work of breathing.

Less often, physiologic obstruction may be the pattern seen. This can be the result of the primary disease process (e.g., lymphangioleiomyomatosis, pulmonary Langerhans cell histiocytosis; some sarcoid patients) or concomitant emphysema or asthma.[7] Thus, if ILD develops in a patient with significant emphysema, the opposing physiologic effects of the two diseases can result in deceptively normal spirometry and lung volume measurements, as well as apparently normally compliant lungs. However, because both emphysema and ILD result in impaired gas exchange, the D_LCO is significantly decreased.

SELECT SPECIFIC TYPES

Exposure-Related Interstitial Lung Disease

Occupational Exposure

The three most common types of occupational ILD are asbestosis, chronic silicosis, and coal worker's pneumoconiosis (CWP). Predictable clinical and radiographic abnormalities occur in susceptible patients who have been exposed to asbestos.[8] These abnormalities include pleural changes (plaques, fibrosis, effusions, atelectasis, and mesothelioma), parenchymal scarring, and lung cancer. Asbestos exposure alone increases the risk of lung cancer only minimally (1.5-3.0 times). Asbestos exposure and cigarette smoking, however, act synergistically to greatly increase the risk of cancer.

Asbestos exposure also can result in benign asbestos pleural effusions (BAPE) or an entity known as rounded atelectasis. BAPE may be asymptomatic or may be associated with acute chest pain, fever, and dyspnea. Generally, lag time is shorter between the initial asbestos exposure and the development of BAPE (<15 years) than that seen with other manifestations of asbestos exposure. The effusions are characteristically exudative and are often bloody. In a patient with a history of asbestos exposure and a bloody pleural effusion, the major differential diagnostic concern is malignant pleural effusion, particularly associated with mesothelioma, another asbestos-related disease. The clinical course of BAPE is that of spontaneous resolution, often with recurrences, and treatment is drainage to alleviate symptoms. Rounded atelectasis typically manifests as a pleural-based parenchymal mass that may be mistaken for carcinoma. The characteristic computed tomography (CT) features, however, such as evidence of local volume loss, pleural thickening, and the comet tail appearance of bronchi and vessels curving into the lesion may be used to help distinguish rounded atelectasis from carcinoma.

The term *asbestos-related pulmonary disease* may be used to encompass all of these entities, and asbestosis is reserved for patients who have evidence of parenchymal fibrosis. Most patients with asbestosis have had considerable asbestos exposure many years before manifestation of the lung disease. Exposure is often associated with occupations such as shipbuilding or insulation work. Patients report very slowly progressive dyspnea on exertion[9] and have crackles on lung examination. Physiologic testing shows restrictive impairment, with reduced D_LCO. The chest x-ray examination reveals bilateral lower-zone reticulonodular infiltrates similar to those seen in IPF. With an appropriate exposure history, the presence of radiographic pleural plaques or rounded atelectasis can indicate asbestos as the cause of the ILD, although neither of these findings is required for establishing the diagnosis.

No medical therapy has been demonstrated to improve or decrease the progression of asbestosis. Unfortunately, severe impairment typically occurs 30 to 40 years after exposure, making almost all patients ineligible for lung transplantation because of age. Management of asbestosis is therefore supportive.

Chronic silicosis results from chronic exposure to inhaled silica particles. Occupations that commonly entail exposure to silica include mining, tunneling, sandblasting, and foundry work. The chest radiograph commonly shows upper lung zone–predominant abnormalities characterized by multiple small nodular opacities in the central lung tissue. These nodules can slowly coalesce into large masses known as progressive massive fibrosis (PMF). Enlargement and eggshell calcification of the hilar lymph nodes are common. Functional and physiologic impairments in chronic silicosis are quite variable. Some patients with abnormal chest radiographs report few, if any, symptoms and can have normal lung examination and pulmonary function tests. Unfortunately many patients are impaired and have mixed restrictive and obstructive impairments with reduced diffusion capacity. The physiologic impairment can remain stable or, if PMF occurs, can progress even in the absence of continued exposure. Symptoms are typically exertional dyspnea and variable mucus production.

It is important to recognize the association of silicosis with lung cancer and active tuberculosis.[10] Patients with silicosis are at increased risk for lung cancer, and the risk is increased when combined with exposure to tobacco smoke, diesel exhaust, or radon gas. Silicosis patients develop active tuberculosis 2- to 30-fold more often than coworkers without silicosis. This association is especially important in societies with a high incidence of human immunodeficiency virus (HIV) infection, which markedly increases the risk of silicosis-associated active tuberculosis.

CWP develops as the result of chronic inhalation of coal dust. In the past, it was assumed that silica dust was responsible for the pulmonary disease seen among coal miners because the clinical and radiographic features are quite similar to those of chronic silicosis. However, it is now recognized that CWP and silicosis are the results of distinct exposures. Simple CWP, characterized by multiple small nodular opacities on the chest x-ray film, is asymptomatic. Cough and shortness of breath do not develop unless the disease progresses to PMF similar to that seen in silicosis.

There are no proven therapies for either silicosis or CWP other than eliminating future exposure. In patients with significant obstructive impairment or mucus production, inhaled bronchodilators and corticosteroids might relieve some symptoms. Exacerbations can be frequent and are treated with antibiotics and systemic corticosteroids.

Medication, Drug, and Radiation Exposure

Many drugs have been associated with pulmonary complications of various types, including interstitial inflammation and fibrosis, bronchospasm, pulmonary edema, and pleural effusions.[11] Drugs from many different therapeutic classes can cause ILD, including chemotherapeutic agents, antibiotics, antiarrhythmic drugs, and immunosuppressive agents (Box 1). There are no distinct physiologic, radiographic, or pathologic patterns of drug-induced ILD, and the diagnosis is usually made when a patient with ILD is exposed to a medication known to result in lung disease, the timing of the exposure is appropriate for the development of the disease, and other causes of ILD have been eliminated. Treatment is avoidance of further exposure and systemic corticosteroids in markedly impaired or declining patients.

Exposure to therapeutic radiation in the management of cancer can result in ILD. Patients presenting within 6 months of radiation therapy generally have ground glass abnormalities believed to represent acute inflammation. The ground glass abnormalities can occur in both radiation-exposed and unexposed tissue. Short-term systemic corticosteroid treatment can improve lung function. In contrast, dyspnea that develops more than 6 months after therapy typically appears as densely fibrotic tissue within the radiation port. On CT examination, a straight line indicating the margin of radiation is often evident, as seen in Figure 5. These patients do not improve with corticosteroid therapy, and treatment is supportive.

Hypersensitivity Pneumonitis

Hypersensitivity pneumonitis is a cell-mediated immune reaction to inhaled antigens in susceptible persons.[12] Patients must be sensitized by an initial exposure, with subsequent re-exposure leading to acute hypersensitivity pneumonitis or chronic hypersensitivity pneumonitis. Patients with acute hypersensitivity pneumonitis usually present with sudden shortness of breath, chest pain, fever, chills, malaise, and a cough that may be productive of purulent sputum. In comparison, patients who are chronically exposed to low levels of inhaled antigens can develop subtle interstitial inflammatory reactions in the lung that do not result in noticeable symptoms for months to years; these patients present with severe, impairing disease, which can be very difficult to distinguish from IPF.

Box 1 Drugs Associated with the Development of Interstitial Lung Disease

Antibiotics
Nitrofurantoin
Sulfasalazine

Anti-inflammatory Agents
Aspirin
Etanercept
Gold
Infliximab
Methotrexate
Penicillamine

Cardiovascular Agents
Amiodarone
Tocainide

Chemotherapeutic Agents
Azathioprine
Bleomycin
Busulfan
Carmustine
Chlorambucil
Cyclophosphamide
Cytosine arabinoside
Etoposide
Flutamide
Imatinib
Lomustine
Melphalan
Methotrexate
Methyl-CCNU
Mitomycin-C
Procarbazine
Vinblastine
Zinostatin

Drugs Inducing Systemic Lupus Erythematosus
Hydantoin
Hydralazine
Isoniazid
Penicillamine
Procainamide

Illicit Drugs
Heroin
Methadone
Propoxyphene
Talc as an IV contaminant

Miscellaneous agents
Drugs inducing pulmonary infiltrate and eosinophilia
Hydrochlorothiazide
Oxygen
Radiation
l-Tryptophan

CCNU, 1-(2-chloroethyl)-3-(4-methylcyclohexyl)-1-nitrosourea.
Data from Camus P: Drug induced infiltrative lung diseases. In Schwarz MI, King TE (eds): Interstitial lung disease, 4th ed. Hamilton, Ontario, BC Decker, 2003, pp 485-534.

Common organic antigens known to cause hypersensitivity pneumonitis include bacteria and fungi, which may be found in moldy hay (farmer's lung) or in the home environment, particularly in association with central humidification systems (humidifier lung), indoor hot tubs, and animal proteins (e.g., bird fancier's lung). Inorganic antigens from vaporized paints and plastics can also lead to hypersensitivity pneumonitis. Numerous established antigens are listed in Table 1, along with the typical source of exposure and the associated syndrome.

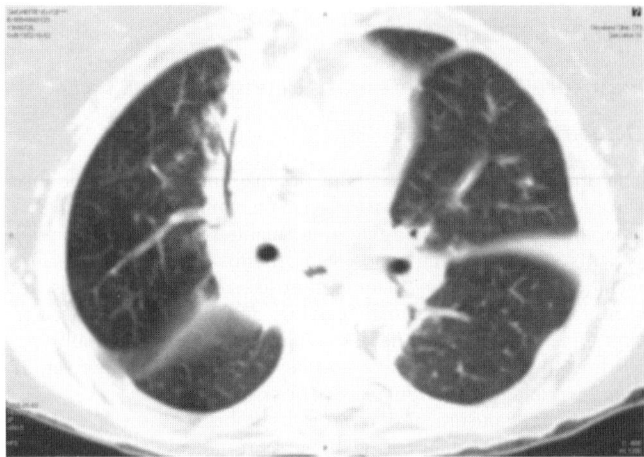

Figure 5 **High-resolution computed tomography slice demonstrating dense fibrosis with a nonanatomic straight line boundary.**

Because the relation between an exposure and the lung disease might not be obvious, a careful systematic occupational, environmental, and avocational history is critical in evaluating patients with ILD. Elements that strongly suggest a diagnosis of hypersensitivity pneumonitis are exposure to an appropriate antigen and the correct temporal relation of symptoms to the exposure. Blood samples may be obtained to determine whether there has been an antibody response to certain antigens associated with hypersensitivity pneumonitis (serum precipitins); however, the presence of such antibodies is not sufficient to establish the diagnosis of hypersensitivity pneumonitis because many persons develop antibodies in the absence of disease. Likewise, the absence of detectable antibodies does not rule out the diagnosis of hypersensitivity pneumonitis because the culprit may be an antigen that is not included in the blood analysis.

Specific therapies for hypersensitivity pneumonitis are strict antigen avoidance and immunosuppression with corticosteroids in patients with symptomatic or physiologically impairing disease. In acute hypersensitivity pneumonitis, corticosteroids appear to hasten recovery but do not improve ultimate lung function.[13] In chronic hypersensitivity pneumonitis, patients with fibrosis on CT scan have shorter survival, and it is unknown if long-term immunosuppression is beneficial.[14]

Tobacco Exposure

Although the association between tobacco use and COPD is well known, the relation with ILD is less well appreciated. It is a risk factor for the development of IPF, but it is not the sole cause. However, three types of ILD have a strong association with cigarette smoking: desquamative interstitial pneumonitis, respiratory bronchiolitis associated-interstitial lung disease (RB-ILD), and pulmonary Langerhans cell histiocytosis (PLCH).

Approximately 90% of patients with desquamative interstitial pneumonitis and RB-ILD are current or former tobacco smokers. HRCT usually demonstrates micronodular central infiltrates in RB-ILD and diffuse ground glass in desquamative interstitial pneumonitis. Spirometry is variable; most patients have significant restriction and variable amounts of obstruction. As with other toxic exposures, complete avoidance of all smoke is important for these patients. In RB-ILD, physiologic stabilization and occasionally even improvement can occur after abstinence from tobacco. In desquamative interstitial pneumonitis, the benefits of smoking cessation are unclear.

PLCH is an interstitial lung disease found in adult smokers. Patients usually have a significant smoking history and develop cough and progressive dyspnea on exertion. Chest examination is

Table 1 Causes of Hypersensitivity Pneumonitis

Antigen	Exposure	Syndrome
Amoebae		
Acanthamoeba castellani	Contaminated water	Humidifier lung
Acanthamoeba polyphaga	Contaminated water	Humidifier lung
Naegleria gruberi	Contaminated water	Humidifier lung
Animal Proteins		
Avian proteins	Bird droppings, feathers	Bird-breeder's lung
Urine, serum, pelts	Rats, gerbils	Animal handler's lung
Bacteria		
Thermophilic Bacteria		
Saccharopolyspora rectivirgula	Moldy hay	Farmer's lung
Thermoactinomyces vulgaris	Moldy sugarcane	Bagassosis
Thermoactinomyces sacchari	Mushroom compost	Mushroom worker's lung
Thermoactinomyces candidus	Heated water reservoirs	Humidifier lung, air conditioner lung
Nonthermophilic Bacteria		
Bacillus subtilis, Bacillus cereus	Water, detergent	Humidifier lung, washing powder lung
Chemicals		
Isocyanates, trimellitic anhydride	Paints, resins, plastics	Chemical worker's lung
Copper sulfate	Bordeaux mixture	Vineyard sprayer's lung
Phthalic anhydride	Heated epoxy resin	Epoxy resin lung
Sodium diazobenzene sulfate	Chromatography reagent	Pauli's reagent alveolitis
Pyrethrum	Pesticide	Pyrethrum hypersensitivity pneumonitis
Fungi		
Aspergillus spp	Moldy hay	Farmer's lung
	Water	Ventilation pneumonitis
Aspergillus clavatus	Barley	Malt worker's lung
Alternaria spp.	Wood pulp	Woodworker's lung
Aureobasidium pullulans	Water	Humidifier lung
Cladosporium sp.	Hot-tub mists	Hot-tub hypersensitivity pneumonitis
Merulius lacrymans	Rotten wood	Dry rot lung
Penicillium casei, P. roqueforti	Cheese	Cheese washer's lung
Penicillium frequentans	Cork dust	Suberosis
Trichosporon cutaneum	Damp wood and mats	Japanese summer-type hypersensitivity pneumonitis

Data from Selman M: Hypersensitivity pneumonitis. In Schwarz MI, King TE (eds): Interstitial Lung Disease, 4th ed. Hamilton, BC Decker, 2003.

notable for diffuse inspiratory crackles. HRCT demonstrates central mid lung zone stellate nodules with adjacent thin-walled cysts. Pulmonary physiology generally reveals obstructive impairment with a decreased D_LCO. The pathologic pattern is unique; the hallmark Langerhans histiocytes are seen in groups of star-shaped nodules, with destruction of adjacent lung tissue. Although PLCH is pathologically similar to childhood LCH, the adult form does not typically involve bone and is not proven to respond to chemotherapy, as the childhood form does. The relation of these two disorders has yet to be defined.

Primary treatment is abstinence from all tobacco exposure, either primary or secondhand. In patients with mild or moderate disease, lung function can stabilize after smoking cessation, but some patients progressively decline. Stabilization or improvement with oral corticosteroids is described, but overall benefit is unproven. Patients with progressive disease despite avoidance of all smoke exposure may be offered lung transplantation.

Systemic Disease–Associated Interstitial Lung Disease

Connective Tissue Disease

ILD is a well-known complication of various connective tissue diseases.[15] The most commonly implicated disorders are scleroderma, rheumatoid arthritis, Sjögren's syndrome, polymyositis or dermatomyositis, and systemic lupus erythematosus.

In any of these disorders, pulmonary involvement can remain undetected until significant impairment is present, because these patients may be inactive because of the underlying connective tissue disease. However, there is generally poor correlation between the severity of the pulmonary and nonpulmonary manifestations of these diseases. In some instances, the lung disease overshadows or even predates the other symptoms of the underlying disease. When symptoms develop, dyspnea and cough are common. On chest examination, rales, wheezing, or even a pleural rub may be heard because of the varied patterns of lung involvement in these disorders. Physiology is usually restrictive, with decreased D_LCO, but it may be obstructive, depending on the anatomic location of the disease, especially with Sjögren's disease.

Unsurprisingly, HRCT findings are variable, and range from normal lung architecture to ground glass abnormalities to reticular and fibrotic changes.[16] The pathologic pattern of injury with these diseases is as equally diverse and correlates with the HRCT findings. Nonspecific interstitial pneumonitis (NSIP) is an inflammatory injury pattern associated with ground glass on HRCT scan, and organizing pneumonia is seen with patchy consolidated lung on air bronchograms. Both of these pathologic patterns can improve with aggressive immunosuppression. At the other end of the pathologic response spectrum is usual interstitial pneumonitis, which is associated with reticular opacities and honeycomb cystic fibrosis on HRCT scan. It appears to respond little to immunosuppression, although long-term controlled studies are lacking.

Specific treatment of these systemic inflammatory diseases is highly individualized. Patients with evidence of systemic inflammation, an inflammatory pathologic pattern such as NSIP or organizing pneumonia, or rapidly progressive symptoms are usually treated with prolonged immunosuppressive agents such as cyclophosphamide, azathioprine, mycophenolate, or tacrolimus.[17,18]

Recent studies have begun to provide evidenced-based therapy for these diverse patients. The Scleroderma Lung Study demonstrated that one year of oral cyclophosphamide modestly improved lung function compared with a modest decline in the control group. Curiously, those with the highest degree of fibrosis on HRCT improved most, and ground glass or an inflammatory pattern on bronchoalveolar lavage did not predict benefit. Unfortunately, after one year off immunosuppressive therapy, the cyclophosphamide-treated patients worsened and were indistinguishable from the untreated control group. Many hypothesize that to preserve any lung function gained by cyclophosphamide, continued immunosuppression, usually with mycophenolate, is necessary.

PM-ILD is being increasingly recognized as a common disease entity. Patients usually present with mechanics hands, consisting of thickened skin and painful fingertip fissures; 50% have Jo-1 antibodies on antinuclear antibody testing. Lung pathology is typically fibrotic NSIP or organizing pneumonia. As would be expected with these inflammatory patterns of injury, patients usually benefit from immunosuppression. Classic treatment is with cyclophosphamide, but tacrolimus is emerging as a salvage agent.

Sarcoidosis

Sarcoidosis is an idiopathic multisystem inflammatory disorder that commonly involves the lungs.[19] In fact, it is the most common of the ILDs in the United States. The tissue inflammation that occurs in sarcoidosis has a characteristic pattern in which the inflammatory cells collect in microscopic nodules called granulomas. Unlike IPF, sarcoidosis is more common among young adults than it is among older persons. Sarcoidosis often follows a benign course without symptoms or long-term consequences, and it can spontaneously remit.

The most common manifestation of sarcoidosis is asymptomatic hilar adenopathy. Less often, the chest x-ray demonstrates parenchymal opacities in the mid lung zone; these may be nodular, reticulonodular, or alveolar. When symptoms occur, cough, chest pain, dyspnea, and wheezing are most common. Pulmonary physiology may be normal, restrictive, obstructive, or mixed and can include a reduced D_LCO. Obstructive impairment may be related to endobronchial granulomatous inflammation or scarring.[20]

Corticosteroids are commonly used in managing sarcoidosis, but treatment usually is reserved for patients with marked symptoms or physiologic impairment attributable to the disease.[21] Other organs that can require corticosteroid therapy include the heart, uvea (uveitis), and central nervous system (cranial nerve abnormalities). Measurement of disease activity remains difficult in many patients. Serum angiotensin-converting enzyme levels and gallium scans are not well correlated with disease activity, and their routine use is discouraged. When there is active disease, acutely ill patients are treated with prednisone, and long-term immunosuppression is with methotrexate and cyclophosphamide, although infliximab is emerging as a useful agent in some patients.

Interstitial Lung Disease of Unknown Cause

Idiopathic Interstitial Pneumonia

Unfortunately, even after a comprehensive evaluation many patients with ILD do not have a well-defined specific exposure, a systemic illness, or an underlying genetic cause. Their ILD belongs to either the idiopathic interstitial pneumonia (IIP) group or to the group consisting of unique pathologic patterns as described by surgical lung biopsy.

Idiopathic Pulmonary Fibrosis

Idiopathic pulmonary fibrosis (IPF) is the most common IIP and is defined as a progressive fibrotic lung disease isolated to the lung.[22] The majority of patients are older than 60 years, and IPF is extremely unusual in persons younger than 40 years. Risk factors for developing IPF include exposure to smoke, metal dust, farming dust, and hairdressing chemicals. Patients present with chronic cough and exertional dyspnea, and HRCT demonstrates bibasilar, peripheral reticular abnormalities with focal honeycomb cystic change.

Usual interstitial pneumonitis is the pathologic pattern of injury seen in IPF patients. Usual interstitial pneumonitis is characterized by heterogeneous fibrosis most prominent in the peripheral areas, with minimal inflammation. Patients other than those with IPF can have usual interstitial pneumonitis on surgical lung biopsy (e.g., connective tissue disease), so this pattern of injury and repair is not unique to IPF.

Patients with an IIP and a classic presentation of age older than 60 years, progressive dyspnea and cough, basilar lung crackles, and HRCT findings of bibasilar, subpleural fibrosis and honeycomb cyst formation might not require a surgical lung biopsy for diagnosis.[23,24] Transbronchial lung biopsies are often obtained at bronchoscopy during the evaluation of ILD and to identify mimics of IPF such as sarcoidosis and chronic hypersensitivity pneumonitis. The small biopsies obtained by this route may be able to identify granulomatous inflammation but cannot provide a definitive diagnosis of usual interstitial pneumonitis because this diagnosis requires a piece of tissue much larger than that obtained by transbronchial biopsy.

The majority of patients die of progressive fibrosing lung disease within 4 years of diagnosis. Emerging data show that approximately one half of patients die following disease that gradually progresses over several years.[25] The other one half experience stable lung function or minimal decline for months to years, only to have sudden worsening over a few weeks or months leading to death. Baseline parameters that predict an increased risk of death include severity of dyspnea, severity of restrictive physiologic defect, reduced D_LCO, pulmonary arterial hypertension, degree of fibrosis on HRCT, and SaO_2 desaturation on exertion.[26] Serial parameters that predict poor survival include worsening dyspnea, FVC, and D_LCO.

No medical therapy has proved beneficial for IPF. Trials have demonstrated no benefit with interferon gamma and etanercept. Several medications are currently under investigation, including bosentan, imatinib, and pirfenidone. Oral corticosteroids and cytotoxic agents such as azathioprine are most commonly used for immunosuppression, although they appear to benefit only a minority of patients and are the subjects of a current IPFnet trial.[27-29]

Studies have highlighted the importance of pulmonary arterial hypertension (PAH) in IPF.[30] The degree of PAH does not always correlate with the burden of fibrosis on CT scan or FVC, implying that a vascular process other than obliteration of the capillary bed from fibrosis occurs.[31] Significant PAH is suggested in patients with markedly impaired diffusion capacity but relatively preserved FVC. Several PAH agents are under investigation in IPF, but their use outside of trials is not recommended.

Nonspecific Interstitial Pneumonia

Nonspecific interstitial pneumonitis (NSIP) is an IIP with diffuse inflammation seen on surgical lung biopsy.[32] These patients are on average 7 to 10 years younger than those with IPF, but considerable overlap exists. The degree of accompanying interstitial fibrosis varies between patients. The combination of fibrosis and inflammation (fibrotic NSIP) is most common. Pure cellular NSIP is less common. Patients present with chronic or subacute cough and dyspnea. HRCT demonstrates predominant ground glass abnormalities in cellular NSIP and both ground glass and fibrotic changes in fibrotic NSIP. Given that there are significant clinical and radiographic overlaps between fibrotic NSIP and IPF, surgical lung biopsy is often required to distinguish these two.

The prognosis is much better for NSIP than for IPF, and most patients survive 7 to 10 years. Immunosuppression with oral corticosteroids and cytotoxic immunosuppressive agents is the primary therapy. Type and duration of therapy are guided by disease activity and degree of inflammation on biopsy and ground glass on HRCT. Pathologic NSIP is not a unique pattern and can often be seen in connective tissue disease or hypersensitivity pneumonitis; a thorough investigation for these should be undertaken to rule out these alternative diagnoses.

Cryptogenic Organizing Pneumonia

Cryptogenic organizing pneumonia (COP), is the revised nomenclature for bronchiolitis obliterans organizing pneumonia (BOOP). Patients are younger than those with IPF, and they present with acute or subacute dyspnea and cough. About one third describe an antecedent viral illness; however, no other risk factors are known. HRCT demonstrates alveolar filling, with air bronchograms mimicking acute pneumonia. The classic COP patient presents after having failed to improve despite several courses of antibiotics. Diagnosis occasionally requires surgical lung biopsy, especially if the clinical and radiographic features are uncertain, because small areas of organizing pneumonia can be seen in a variety of inflammatory and fibrotic disorders on transbronchial lung biopsy.

Most patients improve with oral corticosteroids (0.5-1.0 mg/kg for 6-12 weeks). However, many patients have recrudescence after corticosteroid withdrawal and require long-term immunosuppression with cytotoxic immunosuppressive agents. A minority of patients develop progressive fibrosis despite aggressive immunosuppression and can be offered lung transplantation. Organizing pneumonia is not a unique pathologic pattern and is often associated with connective tissue disease. A thorough investigation must be undertaken to eliminate alternative diagnoses.

Lymphocytic Interstitial Pneumonia

Lymphocytic interstitial pneumonia is a rare disorder of polyclonal lymphocyte aggregates that accumulate diffusely in the interstitium.[33] The diagnosis almost always requires surgical lung biopsy. Patients are typically younger than IPF patients and present with subacute dyspnea and cough. Pulmonary function testing can show a mixed picture. HRCT typically shows diffuse ground glass attenuation with varying amounts of fibrosis. Most patients respond well to oral corticosteroids; a minority require long-term immunosuppression. Lymphocytic interstitial pneumonia is often associated with connective tissue diseases, especially Sjögren's syndrome and in patients with immunodeficiency, and these possibilities should be investigated in all patients with lymphocytic interstitial pneumonia.

Interstitial Lung Disease with Distinct Pathology

Lymphangioleiomyomatosis (LAM) is a rare disorder of abnormal smooth muscle tissue proliferating around small airways leading to severe obstruction and destruction of alveoli with resultant thin-walled cyst formation.[34] All patients are women, although both male and female patients with tuberous sclerosis complex can develop lung pathology identical to LAM termed tuberous sclerosis complex lymphangioleiomyomatosis (TSC-LAM).

Dyspnea on exertion and an obstructive ventilatory impairment with a reduced D_LCO are almost always present except in very early disease. Disease progression is quite variable; some women have steadily worsening lung function during midlife, and some elderly women experience extremely slow decline over many years. Risk factors for worsening lung function include a significant bronchodilator response and possibly childbearing. Other important disease manifestations include pneumothorax from a ruptured subpleural cyst, occasionally associated with air travel. Unilateral or, less commonly, bilateral chylothorax is seen in about one third of patients. This results from lymphatic obstruction by abnormal smooth muscle tissue. Treatment with a low-fat diet or blocking gut fat absorption is usually ineffective, and pleurodesis is required. Importantly, pleurodesis does not preclude subsequent lung transplantation.

Treatment is with inhaled bronchodilators and inhaled corticosteroids. Younger patients might ultimately require lung transplantation. Early studies with the immunosuppressant rapamycin, which also inhibits LAM cell proliferation, have been promising, and larger trials are under way.

TREATMENT

Oxygen Therapy

Because hypoxemia is common in ILD, supplemental oxygen therapy is often prescribed, although it has not been studied as extensively as in chronic obstructive pulmonary disease. Patients with ILD should have arterial oxygen saturation determined at rest and especially during exertion, because many patients with only mild disease desaturate with exertion despite normal saturation at rest. Although studies are limited, supplemental oxygen delivered via nasal cannula can prevent resting hypoxemia and allow greater exertion before desaturation. These benefits can improve quality of life and potentially ward off development of pulmonary arterial hypertension, although further studies are needed.

We favor continuous rather than pulse delivery because the desaturation with activity seen in most patients is not rectified with pulse therapy. For most patients, liquid oxygen is the best source to provide adequate flow rates. In motivated patients, transtracheal delivery of supplemental oxygen increases the efficiency of delivery and improves cosmesis. However, patients must be chosen carefully because of the need for frequent care and the risk of mucus desiccation and rare hemorrhage.

Pulmonary Rehabilitation and Exercise Therapy

As with supplemental oxygen therapy, pulmonary rehabilitation in the management of ILD has not been as well studied as it has in obstructive lung disease. Pulmonary rehabilitation is important in building aerobic fitness, maintaining physical activity, and improving quality of life. We encourage all of our patients to enroll in outpatient pulmonary rehabilitation and to continue maintenance therapy.

Vaccinations and Infection Avoidance

Because many ILD patients are treated with immunosuppressive medications and are at some modest increased risk for the development of infections, patients with ILD should receive a pneumococcal vaccine per the Centers for Disease Control and Prevention (CDC) guidelines and a yearly influenza virus vaccine. Additionally, we recommend that patients practice good hand hygiene (e.g., frequent hand washing). We do not recommend the use of masks or special antibacterial products. Patients treated with certain specific immunosuppressive regimens should receive Pneumocystis prophylaxis.

Transplantation

The only therapy shown to prolong life in patients with end-stage, particularly fibrotic, ILD is lung transplantation.[35] Transplantation has been performed successfully in the management of most ILDs. Enthusiasm for the procedure is tempered by the significant risk of mortality at 1 year (10%-25%) and 5 years (50%-60%). Many patients with ILD are older than the upper age limit of 65 years. Comorbidities such as gastroesophageal reflux disease, common in a number of ILDs, preclude lung transplantation due to the increased risk of chronic rejection and death.

CONCLUSION

The entities grouped as ILDs are a diverse group of illnesses of varied causation, treatment, and prognosis. In general, these diseases manifest as chronic, progressive dyspnea on exertion and cough. Findings on examination are often limited to the chest in the form of fine inspiratory crackles. The most common chest radiograph finding is diffuse reticular or reticulonodular infiltrates with reduced lung volumes. Pulmonary function testing usually reveals restrictive physiology and decreased diffusion capacity; however, other patterns can be seen. Therapy depends on the underlying disease and may consist of immunosuppressive drugs and avoidance of disease-inducing exposures.

Summary

- Chronic nonmalignant pain (CNMP) is our leading cause of disability.
- The interstitial lung diseases are a diverse group of disorders organized by cause.
- A careful history, paying attention to exposures and systemic diseases, is required to arrive at a correct diagnosis.
- High-resolution computed tomography scanning and pulmonary function testing are integral to diagnosing and monitoring disease progression.
- Treatment depends entirely on the disease cause and may include observation, exposure avoidance, or immunosuppression.

Suggested Readings

Baughman RP: Pulmonary sarcoidosis. Clin Chest Med 2004;25:521-530, vi.

Chetta A, Marangio E, Olivieri D: Pulmonary function testing in interstitial lung diseases. Respiration 2004;71:209-213.

Collard HR, King TE Jr, Bartelson BB, et al: Changes in clinical and physiologic variables predict survival in idiopathic pulmonary fibrosis. Am J Respir Crit Care Med 2003;168:538-542.

Davies HR, Richeldi L, Walters EH: Immunomodulatory agents for idiopathic pulmonary fibrosis. Cochrane Database Syst Rev 2003;(3):CD003134.

Hunninghake GW, Lynch DA, Galvin JR, et al: Radiologic findings are strongly associated with a pathologic diagnosis of usual interstitial pneumonia. Chest 2003;124:1215-1223.

King TE Jr: Clinical advances in the diagnosis and therapy of the interstitial lung diseases. Am J Respir Crit Care Med 2005;172:268-279.

Orens JB, Estenne M, Arcasoy S, et al: International guidelines for the selection of lung transplant candidates: 2006 update—A consensus report from the Pulmonary Scientific Council of the International Society for Heart and Lung Transplantation. J Heart Lung Transplant 2006;25:745-755.

Raghu G, Brown KK: Interstitial lung disease: Clinical evaluation and keys to an accurate diagnosis. Clin Chest Med 2004;25:409-419, v.

Selman M: Hypersensitivity pneumonitis: A multifaceted deceiving disorder. Clin Chest Med 2004;25:531-547, vi.

Strange C, Highland KB: Interstitial lung disease in the patient who has connective tissue disease. Clin Chest Med 2004;25:549-559, vii.

References

For a complete list of references, log onto www.expertconsult.com.

Lung Cancer

Peter J. Mazzone

DEFINITION

Lung cancer is a major public health problem. In the United States, 31% of cancer deaths in men and 26% of cancer deaths in women are secondary to lung cancer. Efforts at early detection and treatment have been frustrating, and hence the overall prognosis remains poor. Just over one in eight lung cancer patients will be living 5 years after their diagnosis. Most cases of lung cancer would be prevented if people did not smoke tobacco products. Unfortunately, data on worldwide tobacco consumption suggest that lung cancer will remain an epidemic for years to come. Advances in understanding the pathogenesis, early detection, and therapy of lung cancer are in progress.

PREVALENCE

In 2007, approximately 213,380 new cases of lung cancer were diagnosed in the United States. Lung cancer is the second most frequently diagnosed cancer in both men and women; prostate and breast cancers are the most frequent in men and women, respectively (Fig. 1). The incidence of lung cancer peaked in men in 1984 (86.5/100,000 men) and has subsequently been declining (69.1/100,000 men in 1997). In women, the incidence increased during the 1990s, with a leveling off toward the end of the decade (43.1/100,000 women). These trends parallel the smoking patterns of these two groups.

Lung cancer is the leading cause of cancer-related mortality in both men and women. It surpassed colon cancer in the early 1950s in men and breast cancer in the late 1980s in women. Mortality rates in men declined significantly in the 1990s, whereas a slow increase occurred in women. These rates again parallel the smoking patterns of these two groups (Figs. 2 and 3). There were an estimated 160,390 deaths in 2007 in the United States secondary to lung cancer. This means that lung cancer accounts for approximately 29% of all cancer deaths. In men, lung cancer becomes the leading cause of cancer-related mortality from age 40 onward. In women, lung cancer surpasses breast cancer in those 60 years and older.[1]

RISK FACTORS

About 85% to 90% of patients with lung cancer have had direct exposure to tobacco. Many tobacco-related carcinogens have been identified; the two major classes are the *N*-nitrosamines and polycyclic aromatic hydrocarbons. A dose-response relation exists between the degree of exposure to cigarette smoke and the development of lung cancer. The age at which smoking began, the number of cigarettes smoked per day, and the duration of smoking all influence the likelihood of developing lung cancer. Also, the intensity of smoking, the depth of inhalation, and the composition of the cigarette influence the risk.

All cell types of lung cancer are associated with smoking. The strongest associations are with small cell and squamous cell carcinomas. The risk of developing lung cancer decreases over time after smoking cessation, although it never reaches that of a lifelong nonsmoker. Cigar smoking is also an independent risk factor for developing lung cancer.[2]

Exposure to sidestream smoke, or passive smoking, might lead to an increased risk of lung cancer. The risk varies with the level and duration of exposure. It is generally a much lower risk than is active smoking.[3] Some suggest the risk is negligible.[4]

Many other risk factors have been identified (Box 1). Occupational agents are known to act as lung cancer carcinogens. Arsenic, asbestos, and chromium have the highest risk. An estimated 2% to 9% of lung cancers are related to occupational exposures. An inherited genetic predisposition has epidemiologic support as a risk factor, but the mechanisms are theoretical at this time.[5] Women appear to have a higher baseline risk of developing lung cancer as well as a greater susceptibility to the effects of smoking. Differences in the metabolism of tobacco-related carcinogens and their metabolites or an effect of hormone differences are believed to account for the increased susceptibility.[6]

Dietary factors can modify risks. Higher consumption of fruits and vegetables is associated with a reduced lung cancer risk, and an increased dietary fat intake might lead to a higher risk. Supplementation with vitamins A and E, and beta carotene has not positively influenced risk.[7]

Chronic obstructive pulmonary disease is an independent risk factor. This risk increases as the forced expiratory volume in 1 second (FEV_1) decreases.[8,9]

CLASSIFICATION

Pathologic features, visible on light microscopy, are used to categorize lung cancers. Lung cancers are divided into two major groups, small cell and non–small cell. These groups guide current evaluation and therapeutic decisions. The non–small cell cancer category consists of adenocarcinoma, squamous cell carcinoma, large cell carcinoma, and variants (Fig. 4).

Since the 1980s, the proportions of lung cancers that are adenocarcinomas and squamous cell carcinomas have changed. In North America, approximately 40% of all lung cancers are adenocarcinomas, and 20% to 25% are squamous cell. These figures were reversed in the past. The increased incidence of lung cancer in women (who are more likely to have adenocarcinomas) and changes in smoking habits are believed to account for this change.

PATHOPHYSIOLOGY

The pathophysiology of lung cancer development is complex and incompletely understood. The genes influenced in the pathogenesis of lung cancer produce proteins involved in cell growth and differentiation, cell cycle processes, apoptosis, angiogenesis, tumor progression, and immune regulation. Unveiling these mechanisms should translate into novel means of risk stratification, prevention, early detection, and therapy.

SIGNS AND SYMPTOMS

The clinical manifestations of lung cancer result from the effects of local growth of the tumor, regional growth or spread through the lymphatic system, hematogenous distant metastatic spread, and remote paraneoplastic effects from tumor products or immune cross-reaction with tumor antigens (Box 2).

Local growth in a central location can cause cough, hemoptysis, or features of large-airway obstruction. Peripheral growth can also cause cough and dyspnea. If the pleura or chest wall becomes involved, pain can occur. Regional growth can lead to esophageal compression (dysphagia), recurrent laryngeal nerve paralysis (hoarseness), phrenic nerve paralysis with an elevated

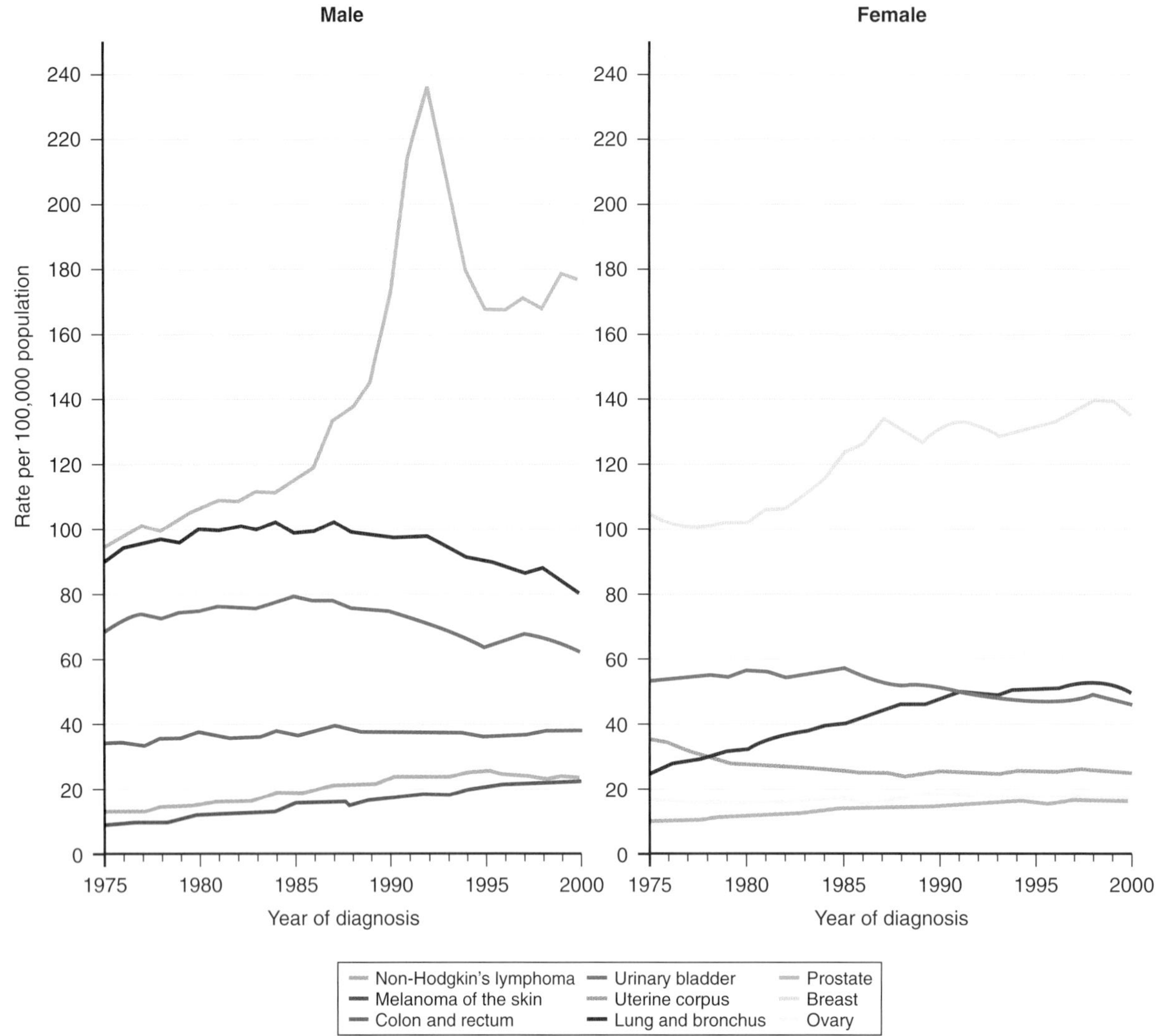

Figure 1 Age-adjusted cancer incidence rates for male and female population, United States, 1975-2003. Rates are per 100,000 population, adjusted to the 2000 U.S. standard population. The incidence of lung cancer in men and women has paralleled smoking habits. *(From Jemal A, Siegel R, Ward E, et al: Cancer statistics, 2007. CA Cancer J Clin 2007;57:43-66.)*

Box 1 Lung Cancer Risk Factors

Tobacco Smoke Exposure
- Active (mainstream)
- Cigarette
- Cigar
- Passive (sidestream)

Occupational and Environmental Exposures
- Arsenic
- Asbestos
- Beryllium
- Bis(chloromethyl)ether
- Cadmium
- Chromium
- Nickel
- Polycyclic aromatic hydrocarbons
- Radon
- Vinyl chloride

Other Factors
- Chronic obstructive pulmonary disease
- Dietary factors
- Gender
- Genetic predisposition

hemidiaphragm (dyspnea), and sympathetic nerve paralysis leading to Horner's syndrome (ptosis, miosis, anhidrosis, and enophthalmos). Apical growth can lead to Pancoast's syndrome, with shoulder pain radiating in an ulnar distribution. The superior vena cava can become obstructed and the heart and pericardium can become involved. Lymphatic obstruction and spread can lead to dyspnea, hypoxia, and pleural effusions.

Distant metastatic disease can affect most organs. Neurologic symptoms can suggest brain metastases or spinal cord compression, and pain could indicate bone metastases. Laboratory abnormalities can point to bone marrow or liver involvement. Imaging might detect adrenal involvement.

Paraneoplastic syndromes can occur before the primary tumor appears and thus can be the first sign of disease or an indication of tumor recurrence. Paraneoplastic endocrine syndromes occur when the tumor produces hormones. The three most common are ectopic Cushing's syndrome, the syndrome of inappropriate antidiuretic hormone (SIADH), and humoral hypercalcemia of malignancy. Ectopic Cushing's syndrome occurs in 2% to 10% of patients with small cell carcinoma. The clinical manifestations are less prominent than in Cushing's disease; biochemical abnormalities predominate, whereas the physical changes are less prominent. The SIADH is also more common in small cell carcinoma, occurring in 7% to 11% of

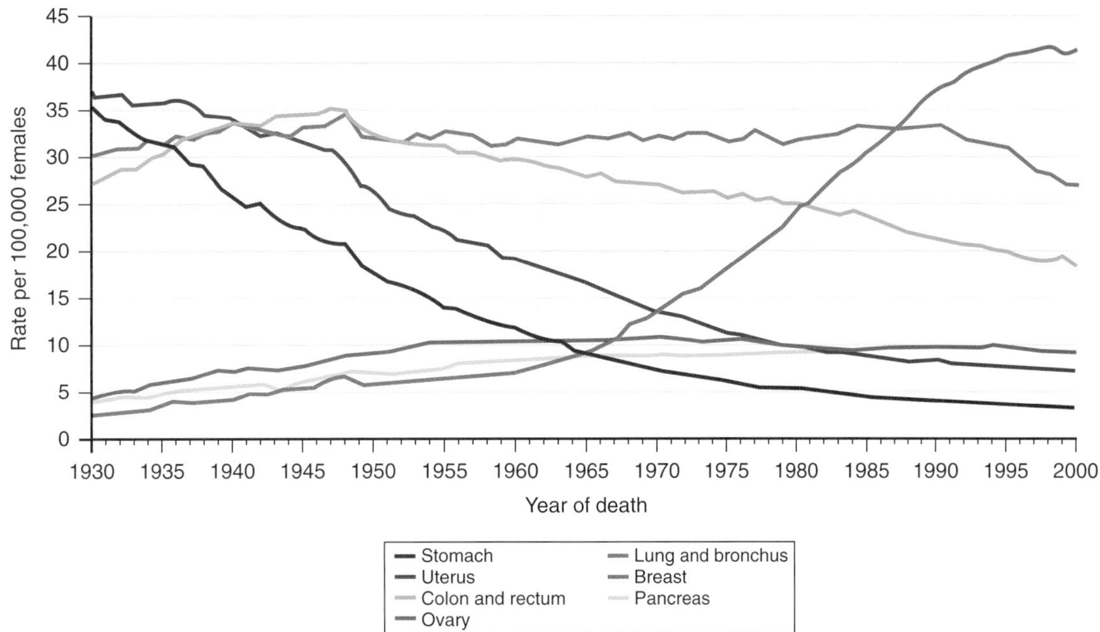

Figure 2 Age-adjusted cancer death rates for female population, United States, 1930-2003. Rates are per 100,000 female population, adjusted to the 2000 U.S. standard population. Lung cancer surpassed breast cancer as the leading cause of cancer-related mortality in women in the late 1980s. *(From Jemal A, Siegel R, Ward E, et al: Cancer statistics, 2007. CA Cancer J Clin 2007;57:43-66.)*

patients. The manifestations of hyponatremia (mental status changes, lethargy, or seizures) are often absent despite very low sodium levels, because the rate of decline is typically prolonged. Humoral hypercalcemia of malignancy, resulting from the production of parathyroid hormone-related protein by the tumor, is most commonly associated with squamous cell carcinoma. Fatigue, mental status changes, weakness, gastrointestinal symptoms, polyuria, and electrocardiogram changes may occur.

Paraneoplastic neurologic syndromes affect all parts of the nervous system. An immune response to tumor antigens that cross-react with common antigens expressed in the nervous system seems to take place. This leads to manifestations that vary depending on where in the nervous system these antigens are expressed. Paraneoplastic limbic encephalitis is characterized by mood and behavior changes, memory problems, and seizures; paraneoplastic cerebellar degeneration manifests with ataxia, nystagmus, dysarthria, and diplopia; and paraneoplastic opsoclonus-myoclonus manifests with involuntary eye movements, myoclonus, truncal ataxia, dysarthria, and encephalopathy. Each of these is more common with small cell carcinoma, can occur in the presence of anti-Hu antibodies, and can occur as part of a more diffuse anti-Hu syndrome (the encephalomyelitis and subacute sensory neuropathy syndrome).

Other paraneoplastic neurologic syndromes include cancer-associated retinopathy and the Lambert-Eaton myasthenic syndrome. In cancer-associated retinopathy (most common with small cell carcinoma), rapid vision loss, ring scotomata, photosensitivity, night blindness, and color vision loss can occur in association with autoantibodies directed against retinal proteins. Lambert-Eaton myasthenic syndrome is the most common of the neurologic paraneoplastic syndromes and is present in 3% of small cell carcinomas. Proximal muscle weakness (which might improve with exercise) is most prominent in the lower extremities, and autonomic features predominate. Autoantibodies directed against P/Q type voltage-gated calcium channels are believed to be responsible.

Other paraneoplastic syndromes include skeletal and connective tissue syndromes (clubbing, hypertrophic pulmonary osteoarthropathy), coagulation and hematologic disorders, cutaneous and renal manifestations, and systemic symptoms (anorexia, cachexia, and weight loss).[10]

DIAGNOSIS

Approximately 85% of patients with lung cancer are symptomatic at presentation. In the remainder, lung cancer is detected by radiographic evaluation initiated for an unrelated problem. This proportion might change in the future if currently investigated screening techniques prove beneficial. Chest radiography and computed tomography (CT) are performed at most patients' initial evaluation. Clinical and radiographic features of the presentation dictate further evaluation.

Clinical features that suggest malignancy on initial evaluation include older age, current or past history of tobacco abuse, hemoptysis, and the presence of a previous malignancy. Radiographic features suggesting malignancy include the absence of a benign pattern of calcification in the detected lesion, a nodule or mass that is growing, a nodule with a spiculated or lobulated border, a larger lesion (>3 cm is considered malignant unless proven otherwise), and a cavitary lesion that is thick walled. Modern imaging techniques are used to alter the clinical probability of malignancy and hence influence biopsy decisions. Positron emission tomography (PET) using ^{18}F fluorodeoxyglucose is the most-studied ancillary imaging technique. It has a sensitivity of 97% and a specificity of 78% as used in clinical practice.[11] Single-photon emission CT and lung nodule enhancement with contrast-enhanced CT are less well established.

Ultimately, tissue needs to be obtained to confirm the diagnosis of lung cancer. Flexible bronchoscopy and transthoracic needle biopsy are the invasive, nonsurgical approaches used to obtain tissue. If they fail or are deemed unnecessary, a surgical approach is used.

Flexible bronchoscopy has a high diagnostic yield for endoscopically visible lesions. The addition of endobronchial needle aspiration to conventional sampling techniques (washing, brushing, and endobronchial biopsy) improves this yield. The diagnostic yield from peripheral lesions is lower. Conventional sampling techniques and peripheral transbronchial needle aspiration complement each other. Factors that influence the diagnostic yield of flexible bronchoscopy

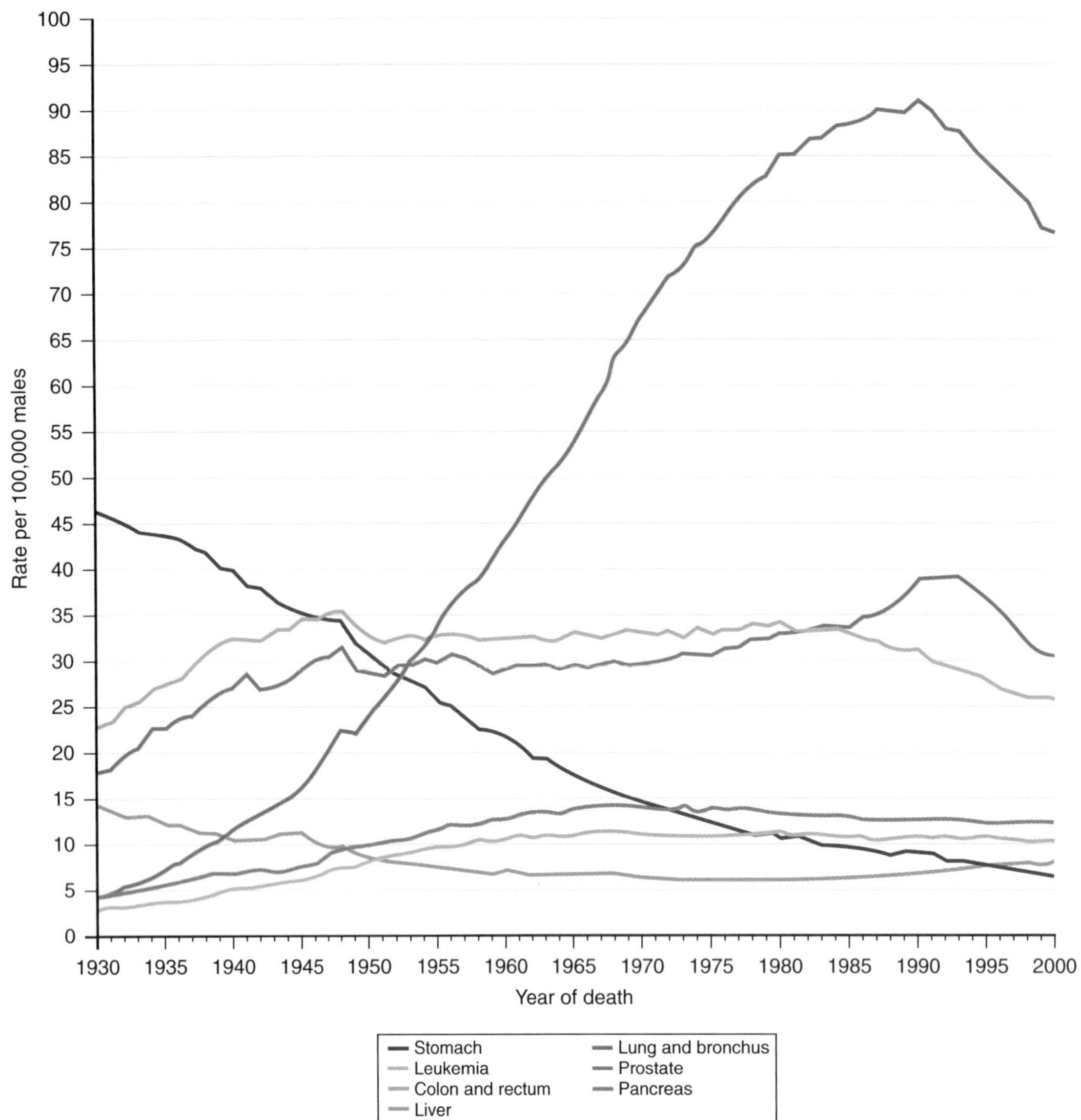

Figure 3 Age-adjusted cancer death rates for male population, United States, 1930-2003. Rates are per 100,000 male population, adjusted to the 2000 U.S. standard population. Lung cancer has been the leading cause of cancer-related mortality in men since the early 1950s. Mortality rates began to decline in the 1990s. *(From Jemal A, Siegel R, Ward E, et al: Cancer statistics, 2007. CA Cancer J Clin 2007;57:43-66.)*

for peripheral lesions include the size of the lesion, its location, and a bronchus sign on CT. Smaller, more peripheral lesions, without a visible bronchus within or leading directly to them, are unlikely to be diagnosed by flexible bronchoscopy.

Transthoracic needle biopsy, using fluoroscopic or CT guidance, can be used to obtain tissue. The positive predictive value of this procedure is high, the negative predictive value is modest, and the rate of establishing a specific benign diagnosis is low. Smaller nodules in central locations have lower diagnostic rates. A higher rate of pneumothorax occurs with transthoracic needle biopsy; thus, flexible bronchoscopy is often attempted first.[12]

STAGING

Accurately characterizing the anatomic extent of disease in a patient with lung cancer guides the treatment and prognosis. Non–small cell lung cancer is staged using the TNM system (T for extent of primary tumor, N for regional lymph node involvement, and M for metastasis). The most recent revision[13] to this staging system occurred in 2009 (Tables 1 and 2). Small cell lung cancer is staged as limited or extensive disease. Limited-stage disease is indicated when the tumor is confined to a hemithorax (including ipsilateral mediastinal and supraclavicular lymph nodes), and thus can be encompassed in a radiotherapy port. Extensive-stage disease is indicated when the tumor extends beyond these boundaries. The overall condition of the patient should be considered as well as the anatomic extent of the tumor. The history and physical examination are important in guiding testing.

The proper use of testing to stage a patient with lung cancer is addressed in a set of guidelines.[14]

Local and Regional Disease

The extent of locoregional spread is best evaluated using CT of the chest extending to the upper abdomen to include the liver and adrenals. This should be ordered in all patients. The detection of parietal pleural, chest wall, and mediastinal invasion by the primary tumor is limited with CT. Magnetic resonance imaging (MRI) is not more accurate except in the setting of a Pancoast tumor. The sensitivity and specificity of CT for evaluating regional lymph node involvement are modest, commonly noted to be as low as 60% and rarely greater than 75%. PET seems to have better test characteristics for staging mediastinal nodes, with sensitivities and specificities greater than 90%.[15] Integrated PET-CT scanning appears to have better test characteristics than PET and CT used alone or in conjunction.[16]

Because noninvasive tests have false-positive results, tissue confirmation is necessary. Bronchoscopy with transbronchial needle aspiration is useful to stage the mediastinum. Endobronchial and endoscopic ultrasound-guided needle sampling of the mediastinum has been reported to accurately stage the mediastinum.[17] If sampling is negative, then mediastinoscopy, mediastinotomy, or thoracoscopy will confirm the nodal status. Debate exists about mediastinal sampling in the face of negative imaging. Despite the advances in imaging technology and sampling techniques, definitive surgical resection and mediastinal dissection remains the gold standard. The assigned clinical stage (determined by testing, including mediastinoscopy) is often lower than the pathologic staging (assigned after surgery).

Metastasis

The evaluation of metastatic disease also takes into consideration the history, physical examination, laboratory results (electrolytes, calcium, alkaline phosphatase, liver profile, and creatinine), and pathology results. All patients should have their chest CT scanning extended through the adrenals, because metastatic disease to these glands is usually asymptomatic, and often no alterations are seen in routine laboratory tests. A contrast-enhanced CT scan, ultrasound, or MRI of the liver should be performed if the chest CT, laboratory results, or clinical evaluation suggests metastatic disease to this organ.

A head CT should be performed if symptoms or signs of metastatic disease are present or when evaluating what appears to be stage IIIA or B disease. Head CTs are often performed despite a lack of symptoms, in deference to the published guidelines. This is probably justifiable in small cell carcinoma, but it is debatable in other lung cancers. Many choose to use MR imaging of the brain because it has greater sensitivity to detect metastatic disease.

PET is used to stage all but brain metastases. The rate of detection of distant metastases using PET is higher than previously used approaches.[18]

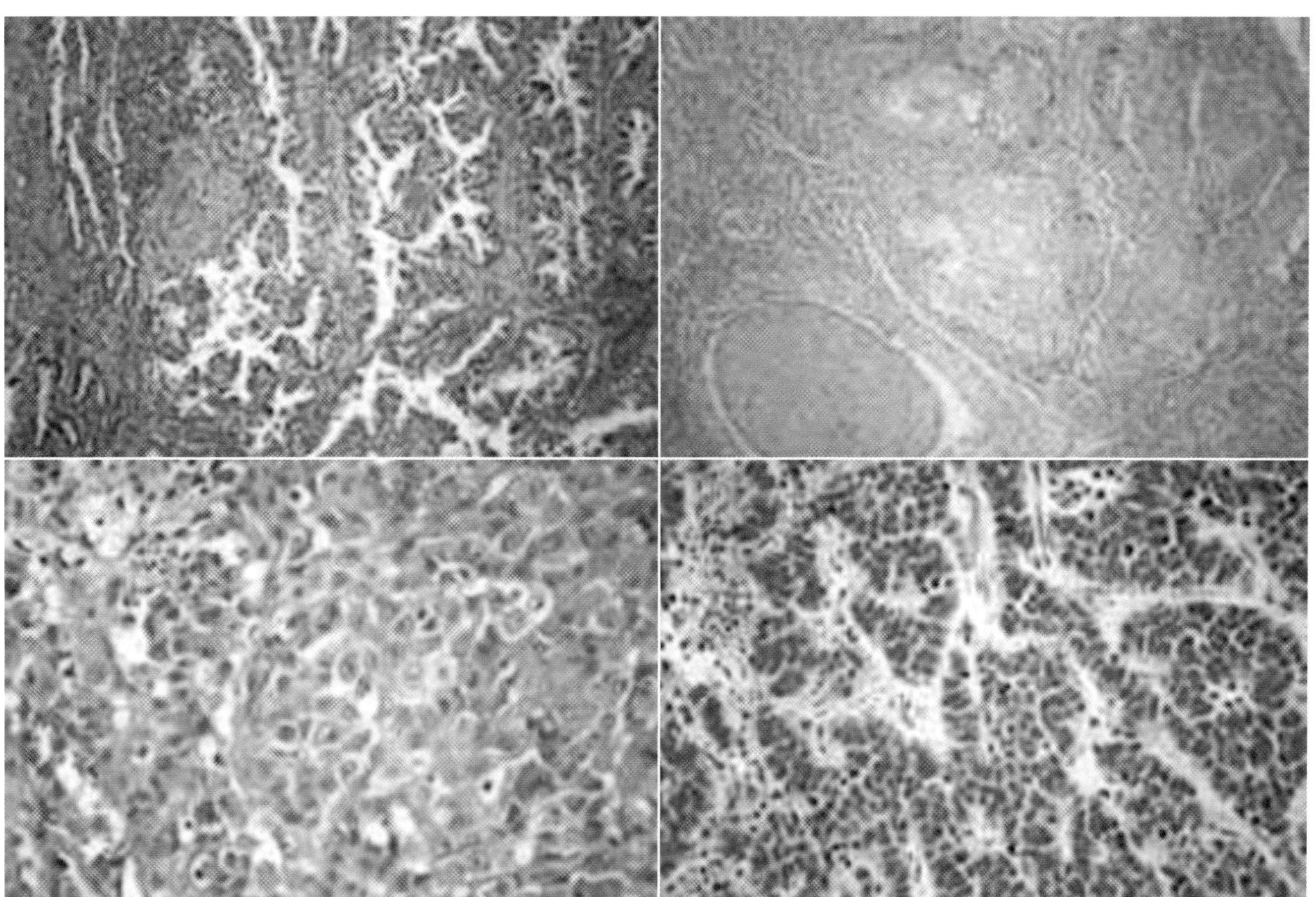

Figure 4 Lung cancer histology. *Top left,* Adenocarcinoma characterized by heterogeneous differentiation in the same tumor. *Top right,* Squamous cell carcinoma characterized by the presence of cytokeratin differentiation with keratinization and intercellular bridges. *Bottom left,* Large cell carcinoma characterized by sheets and nests with extensive necrosis, large nuclei with prominent nucleoli, and lack of definitive evidence of squamous or glandular differentiation. *Bottom right,* Small cell carcinoma characterized by round to fusiform nuclei, nuclear molding, faint or absent nucleoli, and scant cytoplasm.

Box 2 Lung Cancer Manifestations

Neoplastic

Local Growth
Cough
Dyspnea
Hemoptysis
Pain

Regional Growth
Dysphagia
Dyspnea
Hoarseness
Horner's syndrome
Hypoxia
Pancoast's syndrome
Pericardial or pleural effusions
Superior vena cava syndrome

Metastatic Disease
Headache
Hepatomegaly
Mental status change
Pain
Papilledema
Seizures
Skin or soft tissue mass
Syncope
Weakness

Paraneoplastic

Cutaneous, Skeletal
Acanthosis nigricans
Clubbing
Dermatomyositis
Hypertrophic osteoarthropathy

Endocrine
Cushing's syndrome
Humoral hypercalcemia
SIADH
Tumor necrosis factor (cachexia)

Hematologic
Anemia
Polycythemia
DIC
Eosinophilia
Granulocytosis
Thrombophlebitis

Neurologic
Cancer-associated retinopathy
Encephalomyelitis
Lambert-Eaton syndrome
Neuropathies
Cerebellar degeneration

Renal
Glomerulonephritis
Nephrotic syndrome

DIC, disseminated intravascular coagulation; SIADH, secretion of inappropriate diuretic hormone.

Performance Status

Coincident with the evaluation of the anatomic stage of disease should be an evaluation of the patient's performance status. This is important in determining an individual patient's ability to tolerate any proposed treatment. Like anatomic staging, performance status is a predictor of outcome. The two most commonly employed scales of performance status are the Zubrod scale and the Karnofsky scale. Although their definitions differ, their general principles are the same, with ratings based on activity level, independence in daily activities, and severity of symptoms.

Further evaluation of performance status may be necessary in those for whom surgical resection is indicated. To determine if a patient will tolerate lung resectional surgery, reports of activity tolerance and pulmonary function testing are used. Although no one pulmonary function study or absolute cutoff has proved ideal, the FEV_1 and diffusing capacity for carbon monoxide (D_LCO) are the most commonly used measures.

Traditional preoperative cutoff values are being replaced by percent predicted postoperative values. Percent predicted postoperative values of FEV_1 and D_LCO can be calculated by multiplying the percent predicted preoperative value by the fraction of the total number of lung segments that will remain postoperatively. Alternatively, quantitative perfusion imaging can be used to guide the calculation. If the percent predicted postoperative FEV_1 and D_LCO are greater than 40%, then the patient should be able to tolerate surgery. Thus, as would be expected, a pneumonectomy requires better preoperative lung function than does a lobectomy.

When doubt remains, or when measured values and predictions seem discordant with a patient's reported activity tolerance, a cardiopulmonary exercise study should be performed. If the maximum oxygen consumption is greater than 15 mL/kg/min, a lobectomy should be reasonably well tolerated. If it is less than 10 mL/kg/min, conventional surgery should not be performed. Values between these two should be considered on a case-by-case basis. Patients with marginal lung function might tolerate resection if a lesser resection is possible (wedge resection or segmentectomy) or if resection can be combined with a lung volume reduction procedure.[19]

SCREENING FOR LUNG CANCER

Given the poor prognosis for advanced-stage lung cancer and the high percentage of patients who present in an advanced stage, there has been great interest in screening for lung cancer. The earliest efforts at radiographic screening were from the analysis of mass chest x-ray screenings from the population of one city. This was followed by large efforts in the 1970s to use chest x-ray or sputum, or a combination of the two, as screening tools. Despite considerable ongoing debate about the design and analysis of these randomized studies, they have been interpreted as not showing that screening with plain chest x-ray or sputum examination (or both) has a beneficial effect on mortality from lung cancer.

Given the somewhat disappointing overall results from chest x-ray as a screening technique, more recent efforts have centered on the use of low-dose CT scanning as a screening tool. Important highlights of several available CT studies include the ability to find many early-stage lung cancers and the long survival times of patients with lung cancer diagnosed at an early stage. Difficulties with CT as a screening test and limitations of the trial designs that have been identified in these studies include an inability to comment on mortality specific to lung cancer, a large number of benign nodules being identified (5%-50% of participants on the initial scan), intense testing protocols required to follow the identified nodules to ensure they are not cancerous, invasive procedures performed on some benign nodules, and questionable cost effectiveness. Recent major publications highlight the contentious nature of this topic. One report suggests a survival of 80% for all patients with screen-detected lung cancers, and the other suggests that lung cancer is found and treated in more persons who are screened, but the mortality rate from lung cancer is not lower.[20,21]

Because it is still to be proved whether CT screening will reduce overall and disease-specific mortality rates, current guidelines do not recommend lung cancer screening for asymptomatic persons at risk for lung cancer. Individual patients at risk for lung cancer are being

Table 1 TNM Descriptors

Descriptor	Description	Criteria
Primary Tumor (T)		
T1	A small tumor that is not locally advanced or invasive	<3 cm in diameter; T1a ≤ 2 cm; T1b > 2 cm ≤ 3 cm Surrounded by lung or visceral pleura Does not extend into the main bronchus
T2	A larger tumor that is minimally advanced or invasive	>3 cm in diameter, ≤7 cm; T2a > 3 cm ≤ 5 cm; T2b > 5 cm ≤ 7 cm Might invade the visceral pleura Might extend into the main bronchus but remains >2 cm from the main carina Might cause segmental or lobar atelectasis
T3	Any size tumor that is locally advanced or invasive up to but not including the major intrathoracic structures	> 7 cm or Might involve the chest wall, diaphragm, mediastinal pleura, parietal pericardium, main bronchus within 2 cm of the main carina (not involving the main carina) Might cause atelectasis of the entire lung Presence of satellite tumor nodule(s) within the primary tumor lobe
T4	Any size tumor that is advanced or invasive into the major intrathoracic structures	Any size Invades the mediastinum, heart, great vessels, trachea, esophagus, vertebral body, main carina Presence of satellite tumor nodule(s) in a different ipsilateral tumor lobe
Regional Lymph Node Involvement (N)		
N1	Metastatic disease to nodes within the ipsilateral lung	Direct extension to intrapulmonary nodes Metastasis to ipsilateral peribronchial and/or hilar nodes (nodal stations 10 through 14)
N2	Metastatic disease to nodes beyond the ipsilateral lung but not contralateral to the primary tumor	Metastasis to the ipsilateral mediastinal and/or subcarinal nodes (nodal stations 1 through 9)
N3	Metastatic disease to nodes distant to those included in N2	Metastasis to contralateral mediastinal and/or hilar nodes ipsilateral or contralateral scalene and/or supraclavicular nodes
Metastases (M)		
M0	Local or regional disease No distant metastases	
M1	Disseminated disease m1a – Presence of satellite tumor nodule(s) in contralateral lung malignant pleural or paranodal effusion m1b – Distant metastases present	

advised of their risk and educated about the current state of early detection. If testing is to occur, it should be in a trial setting involving multidisciplinary specialty groups.[22,23]

TREATMENTS AND OUTCOMES

Treatments and outcomes for lung cancer are shown in Box 3 and Tables 2 and 3.

Non–Small Cell Lung Cancer

Surgical resection offers the best chance of cure for early-stage non–small cell lung cancer (stages I and II). Survival after resection in pathologic stage IA approaches 73% at 5 years, and in pathologic stage IB it is closer to 50%. Vascular invasion and tumor differentiation may be prognostic factors. There does not seem to be a difference in survival in patients who have adenocarcinoma and those who have squamous cell carcinoma. Recurrence usually involves distant metastases. Limited resections in persons unable to tolerate lobectomy produce slightly lower survival rates, with higher rates of local recurrence when broadly applied.[24] In an elderly population, limited resection may perform as well as traditional anatomic resection.

Survival after resection in pathologic stage IIA is 46% at 5 years, and that in pathologic stage IIB is around 37%. Patients with adenocarcinoma may have poorer survival rates than those with squamous cell carcinoma. Again, most recurrences involve distant metastases.

Traditional radiotherapy has been used with curative intent in early-stage non–small cell lung cancer, either in patients who cannot tolerate surgery or in those who elect not to undergo surgery. A 5-year survival rate in combined stages I and II disease approaches 15% with radiotherapy alone. There is a high rate of local recurrence, and most deaths are due to lung cancer. Advances in stereotactic body radiotherapy have provided an additional tool for treating this group. This tool gives us the ability to target the tumor with minimal effect on surrounding normal lung tissue. Impressive response rates are being reported.[25]

Adjuvant therapy has been attempted in early-stage non–small cell lung cancer patients who have undergone surgical resection. Adjuvant radiotherapy might improve local control but it does not improve survival (with the possible exception of those who have undergone incomplete resection). Adjuvant chemotherapy has shown benefit in select patients with completely resected stages IB to IIIA lung cancers, and so it should be strongly considered.[26]

Locally advanced tumors (T3) can often be completely resected, although central T3 tumors are somewhat less resectable than those involving the chest wall. The survival rates in T3 patients with chest-wall involvement and negative nodes approximates those of

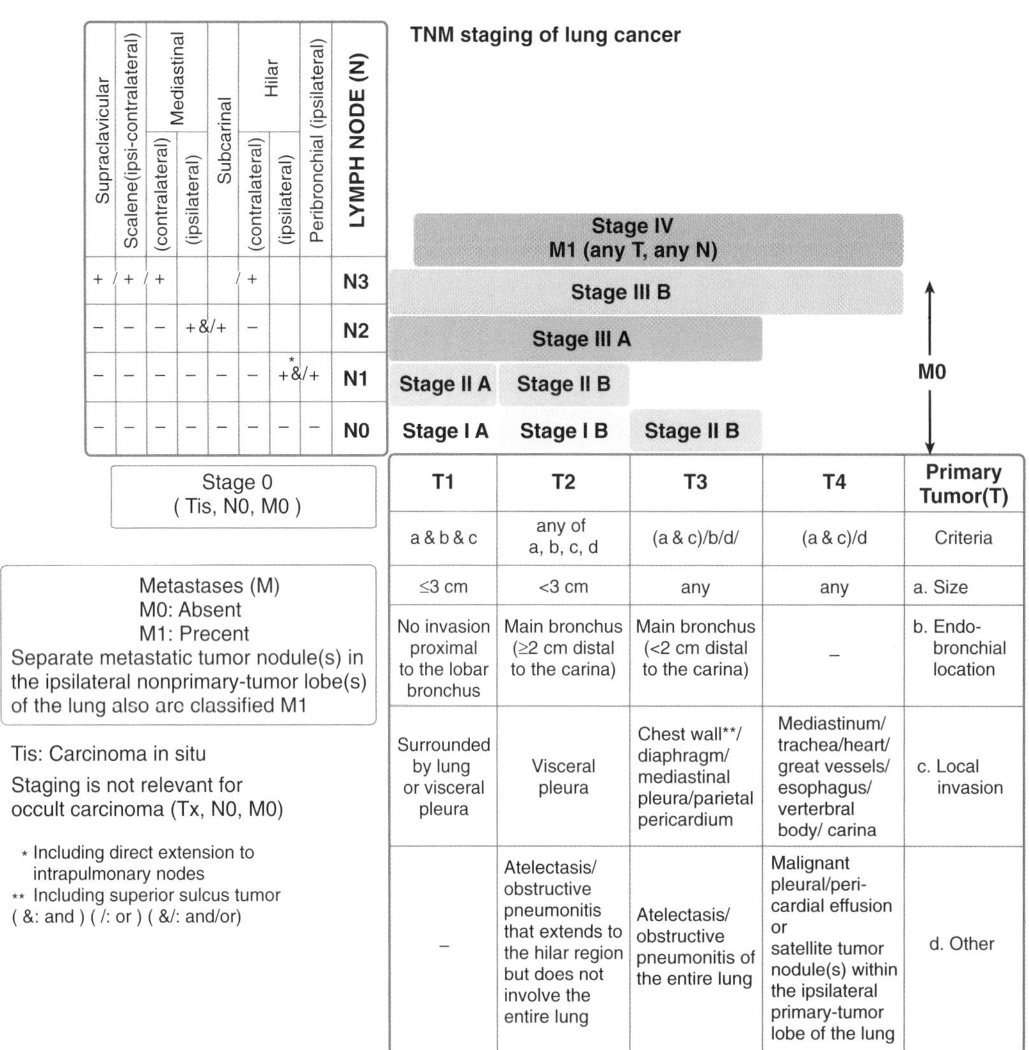

Figure 5 **Reference chart for tumor, node, and metastasis (TNM) staging of lung cancer.** *(From Lababede O, Meziane MA, Rice TW: TNM staging of lung cancer: a quick reference chart. Chest 1999;115:233-235.)*

other stage IIB patients. The best results occur when complete resection is possible. With nodal involvement at any level, survival falls dramatically and thus is classified in a higher stage. T3 involvement of the mediastinum or mainstem bronchus portends a poorer prognosis, with 5-year survival rates of less than 30%.

When a Pancoast tumor is present, chemoradiotherapy followed by surgical resection (lobectomy and chest-wall resection) are performed if possible. The invasion of local structures (rib, vertebral body, subclavian artery, or sympathetic chain) is a poor prognostic sign. Two thirds of patients have a recurrence, and two thirds of these are local.

The approach to N2 (stage IIIA) disease varies somewhat from place to place. Unselect patients have a low rate of complete resection with primary surgery, and patients with incompletely resected lesions do poorly. Patients without radiographic evidence of N2 disease but who are found at surgery to have N2 disease do better than those with preoperative evidence of N2 disease. The more advanced the node involvement (number, extension, or location), the poorer the prognosis. Given this, protocols using multimodal therapy are being investigated. Induction with chemotherapy with or without radiotherapy leads to objective responses in most patients, many of whom are downstaged. Downstaging predicts survival. A greater percentage of patients treated with induction therapy are able to undergo complete resection. Although multimodality therapy is often offered to those who can tolerate it, the selection of patients and therapy is best served in the setting of a study. Advances in each of the modes of therapy will lead to evolution of treatment over time.

T4 disease without advanced nodal status (stage IIIB) may be considered surgical in a few settings. T4 disease involving the main carina may be considered for resection at centers with expertise. The role of induction therapy in this setting is yet to be defined. Disease at the N3 level (stage IIIB) is generally considered nonsurgical. Advances in induction therapy might alter this notion in time, and trials of multimodality therapy are ongoing. When surgery is not considered in stage IIIA or IIIB disease, concurrent chemoradiotherapy, using a platinum-based regimen, is the standard of care in a patient with a reasonable performance status. Survival is in the 9% to 24% range at 5 years. There is a suggestion that newer agents may be as effective with less toxicity.[27] Further studies are ongoing.

In stage IV lung cancer, platinum-based chemotherapy regimens have been shown to improve survival and enhance quality of life, and they are also cost effective. This treatment is most appropriate for patients with a good performance status. The addition of a VEGF inhibitor to treatment in those without squamous cell carcinoma, hemoptysis, or brain metastases, has led to improved outcomes. EGFR inhibitors are used as second or third line therapy. They are most effective for women, those who have never smoked, or those with adenocarcinoma. Studies of other novel agents and non–

Box 3 Options for Treating Lung Cancer

Non–Small Cell Lung Cancer

Stages IA, IB, IIA, and IIB

Surgical resection is the standard of care if the patient is deemed able to tolerate it

Limited resection is used if the patient is unable to tolerate larger resection

Radiotherapy is used if the patient is unable to tolerate resection or chooses not to undergo resection

Adjuvant radiotherapy is possibly of use if incomplete resection was performed

Consider adjuvant chemotherapy

Stage IIIA

Concurrent chemoradiotherapy using a platinum-based regimen if performance status is reasonable

Induction chemoradiotherapy followed by resection in select patients, ideally as part of a study protocol

Stage IIIB

Concurrent chemoradiotherapy using a platinum-based regimen if performance status is reasonable

Induction chemoradiotherapy followed by resection in highly select patients, only as part of a study protocol

Stage IV

Platinum-based chemotherapy regimen in patients with adequate performance status

Small Cell Lung Cancer

Limited-Stage

Combination chemotherapy with concurrent hyperfractionated radiotherapy if performance status is adequate

Prophylactic cranial radiation for those with a complete response to chemoradiotherapy

Extensive-Stage

Combination chemotherapy if performance status is adequate

Table 2 Non–Small Cell Lung Cancer Staging

Stage	Description
IA	T1a, b N0 M0
IB	T2a N0 M0
IIA	T1a, b N1 M0; T2a N1 M0; T2b N0 M0
IIB	T2b N1 M0, T3 N0 M0
IIIA	T3 N1 M0, T(1-3) N2 M0, T4N(0-1) M0
IIIB	T4 N(2-3) M0, T(1-4) N3 M0
IV	T(any) N(any) M1a, b

Table 3 Non–Small Cell Lung Cancer

	Five-Year Survival (%)	
Stage	Clinical	Pathologic
IA	50	73
IB	43	58
IIA	36	46
IIB	25	36
IIIA	19	24
IIIB	7	9
IV	2	—

Data from Goldstraw P. J Thorac Oncol 2007;2:706-714.

platinum-based regimens are ongoing. Resection of an isolated brain metastasis in patients with a good performance status can improve survival. Molecular markers may guide the choice of therapies in the near future.

Small Cell Lung Cancer

Treatment of small cell lung cancer is based on its staging (limited versus extensive). In limited-stage disease, combination chemotherapy with concurrent hyperfractionated radiotherapy is recommended. Etoposide and a platinum agent are standard, but trials with newer agents are ongoing. Prophylactic cranial radiation is generally recommended for patients who have a complete response to chemoradiotherapy. Surgery is limited to cases in which the diagnosis is in doubt or in cases that have not responded to chemoradiotherapy but remain resectable. In patients with extensive-stage disease, combination chemotherapy improves the quality of life and median survival. Etoposide and a platinum agent are standard, although we are awaiting trials of newer agents. A poor performance status and an elevated lactate dehydrogenase level portend a poor prognosis. Radiotherapy to the chest may be used in patients who have a complete response to chemotherapy in disease residing outside the chest.[28]

Palliation

Palliation of symptoms related to lung cancer is an important aspect of the overall management. The judicious use of analgesic agents for pain, antiemetics for nausea, and antidepressants can improve quality of life. Radiotherapy can be used to palliate bone pain related to metastatic disease, hemoptysis, or symptoms of airway obstruction. Invasive bronchoscopic procedures (e.g., laser ablation, electrocautery, stent placement) can palliate patients with airway obstruction.

Summary

- Lung cancer causes more cancer-related deaths in the United States than the next four causes of cancer-related mortality combined.
- The most important and easily modifiable risk factor for lung cancer is cigarette smoking.
- Symptoms are often absent until lung cancer has advanced; thus, only 15% of lung cancer patients live for 5 years after their diagnosis.
- The stage of lung cancer and the patient's performance status guide treatment decisions and influence the prognosis.
- Surgery is the treatment of choice for early stage non–small cell lung cancer. Chemotherapy is the modality of choice for advanced non–small cell lung cancer. Chemotherapy with or without radiation therapy is used to treat small cell lung cancer.

Suggested Readings

Bach PB, Niewoehner DE, Black WC: Screening for lung cancer. The guidelines. Chest 2003;123:83S-88S.

Georgoulias V, Papadakis E, Alexopoulos A, et al: Platinum-based and non–platinum-based chemotherapy in advanced non–small-cell lung cancer: A randomised multicentre trial. Lancet 2001;357:1478-1484.

Ginsberg RJ, Rubenstein LV: Randomized trial of lobectomy versus limited resection for T1N0 non–small cell lung cancer. Lung cancer study group. Annals Thorac Surg 1995;60:615-622.

Gould MK, Maclean CC, Kuschner WG, et al: Accuracy of positron emission tomography for diagnosis of pulmonary nodules and mass lesions: A meta-analysis. JAMA 2001;285:914-924.

Jemal A, Siegel R, Ward E, et al: Cancer statistics, 2007. CA Cancer J Clin 2007;57:43-66.

Mazzone PJ, Arroliga AC: Lung cancer: Preoperative pulmonary evaluation of the lung resection candidate. Am J Med 2005;118:578-583.

Mazzone P, Jain P, Arroliga AC, Matthay RA: Bronchoscopy and needle biopsy techniques for the diagnosis and staging of lung cancer. Clin Chest Med 2002;23(1):137-158, ix.

Goldstraw P, Crowley J, Chansky K, et al: The IASLC Lung cancer staging project: Proposals for the revision of the TNM stage groupings in the forthcoming (seventh) edition of the TNM classification of malignant tumors. J Thorac Oncol 2007;2:706-714.

Silvestri GA, Gould MK, Margolis ML, et al: Noninvasive staging of non-small cell lung cancer: ACCP evidence-based clinical practice guidelines (2nd edition). Chest 2007;132:178S-201S.

Spira A, Ettinger DS: Multidisciplinary management of lung cancer. N Engl J Med 2004;350:379-392.

References

For a complete list of references, log onto www.expertconsult.com.

Occupational Lung Disease

Raed A. Dweik and Peter J. Mazzone

Exposure to dust in the workplace is associated with a variety of pulmonary and systemic illnesses. The term *pneumoconiosis* is derived from Greek and simply means "dusty lungs." In current medical practice, the term is reserved for the permanent alteration of lung structure caused by inhalation of a mineral dust and the reaction of the lung tissue to this dust. The reactions that occur within the lungs vary with the size of the dust particle and its biologic activity. Some dusts (e.g., barium, tin, iron) do not result in a fibrogenic reaction in the lungs, but others can evoke a variety of tissue responses. Such responses include nodular fibrosis (silicosis), diffuse fibrosis (asbestosis), and macule formation with focal emphysema (coal worker's disease). Still others (e.g., beryllium) can evoke a systemic response and induce a granulomatous reaction in the lungs. Pneumoconioses can appear and progress after the exposure has ceased. Regression does not occur, and treatment is mostly symptomatic and supportive.

As we move well into the 21st century, and due to improvements in industrial hygiene practices and dust control measures, we will probably be seeing less of the traditional pneumoconioses in the industrialized countries. We will, however, start seeing more of the immunologically mediated disorders related to more modern technologies, such as hard metal disease and chronic beryllium disease. In this chapter, we discuss a few of the traditional dust exposures (asbestos, silica, coal, and hard metals) and the illnesses they produce. Special emphasis is given to beryllium-induced lung disease because of its emerging role and the need for increased awareness to recognize persons at risk based on recent advances in the understanding of its pathophysiology.

ASBESTOS-RELATED LUNG DISEASE

Exposure to asbestos occurs during its mining, milling, and transporting, as well as during the manufacture and application of asbestos-containing products. The most common industries in which exposure occurs are the construction and shipbuilding industries. The most common occupations are plumbing, pipefitting, insulating, and electrical work. This exposure can lead to a variety of lung diseases including pleural diseases and the pneumoconiosis asbestosis. Asbestos is also a known carcinogen.[1-4]

Pleural Diseases

Four forms of *pleural disease* related to asbestos exposure have been described: pleural plaques, benign asbestos pleural effusions, pleural fibrosis, and malignant mesotheliomas.

Pleural plaques are the most common manifestation of asbestos exposure. They are smooth, white, raised, irregular lesions found on the parietal pleura, commonly located in the lateral and posterior midzones and over the diaphragms (Fig. 1). They are commonly asymptomatic and are recognized only on chest imaging. Macroscopic calcification is common. Plaques are not associated with the development of a malignant mesothelioma. They are, however, markers of asbestos exposure, and thus persons with pleural plaques are at risk for developing pulmonary fibrosis, mesothelioma, and lung cancer.

Benign asbestos pleural effusions may be silent or can manifest with pain, fever, and shortness of breath. They are an early manifestation of asbestos exposure, occurring within 15 years of the initial exposure. The diagnosis of this condition is one of exclusion. It requires known asbestos exposure; an exudative, bloodstained, lymphocyte-predominant effusion; lack of tumor development over a 3-year follow-up; and no evidence of another cause of the effusion. Often a thoracoscopy with biopsy is performed to exclude other causes. A benign asbestos pleural effusion is usually transient but requires close follow-up. It is not associated with the development of a malignant mesothelioma.

Pleural fibrosis typically occurs in persons who have had a remote exposure to asbestos (>20 years before) that was short lived and heavy in intensity. It can occur as a focal or diffuse process. The fibrosed pleura can surround the lung, leading to a trapped lung, or can fold in on itself, encasing a portion of the parenchyma. The masslike lesion that results is known as *rounded atelectasis.* All forms of pleural fibrosis are difficult to distinguish from malignancy, and they usually require biopsies to ensure benignity. The presence of pleural fibrosis indicates an increased risk of pulmonary fibrosis.

Asbestos exposure is responsible for most cases of malignant mesothelioma. The presentation is typically the insidious onset of nonpleuritic chest wall pain 20 to 40 years after the initial exposure. The pain can radiate to the upper abdomen or shoulder and is often associated with dyspnea and systemic symptoms. The mass typically involves both the parietal and visceral pleura. Local invasion is common, with symptoms stemming from the organs invaded. Chest imaging typically reveals an effusion ipsilateral to the pleural disease and might show pleural plaques in the contralateral hemithorax. Open biopsy is required for the diagnosis. Treatment options are unsatisfactory. There is no synergy between smoking and asbestos exposure for the development of a malignant mesothelioma.

Asbestosis

The term *asbestosis* refers to pulmonary fibrosis secondary to asbestos exposure. Risk factors for the development of asbestosis include increased levels and duration of exposure, younger age at initial exposure, and exposure to the amphibole fiber type. It is not associated with smoking.

Common symptoms include progressive shortness of breath and a nonproductive cough. Chest pain may be reported. On examination, inspiratory crackles on lung auscultation and digital clubbing are present with varying frequency.

The parenchymal fibrotic changes are most prominent in the lower lobes and subpleural areas. *Pulmonary function testing* reveals restrictive lung disease with a decreased diffusing capacity for carbon monoxide. Thus, radiographic and physiologic testing findings can be indistinguishable from those of other causes of pulmonary fibrosis. The presence of concomitant pleural disease and the finding of asbestos or ferruginous bodies (Fig. 2) in pathologic samples help to support the diagnosis.

Asbestosis can appear and progress long after exposure has ceased. It can remain static or can progress over time. There is no known effective therapy. The number of reported deaths from asbestosis has increased over time, related to the use of asbestos in a time-delayed manner (Fig. 3).

Asbestos as a Carcinogen

Asbestos is a known carcinogen. The risk of developing lung cancer in a person exposed to asbestos is enhanced in a multiplicative fashion by concomitant cigarette smoking. *Lung cancer* more commonly occurs in persons who also have asbestosis. All cell types are associated with exposure. The lag time to the development of lung

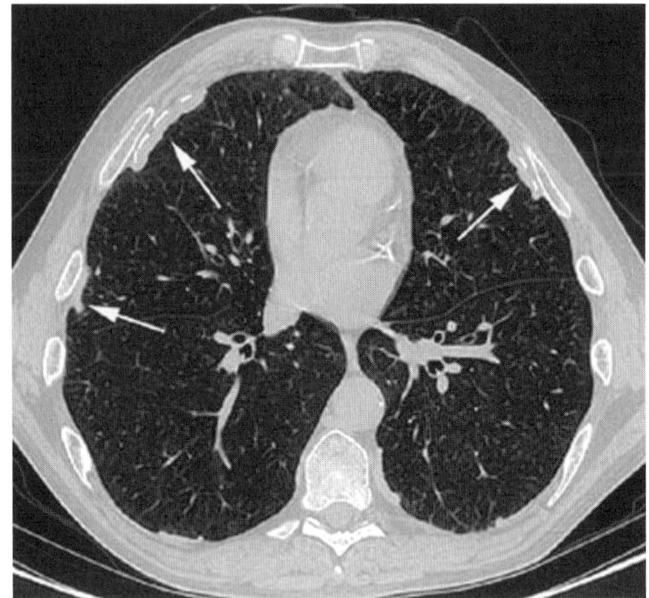

Figure 1 Computed tomography of the chest demonstrating pleural plaques *(arrows)* resulting from asbestos exposure. *(Courtesy of Dr. Omar Lababede.)*

cancer is usually more than 20 years. Treatment follows the principles of lung cancer therapy in persons without prior asbestos exposure. Comorbid lung disease can limit the treatment options.

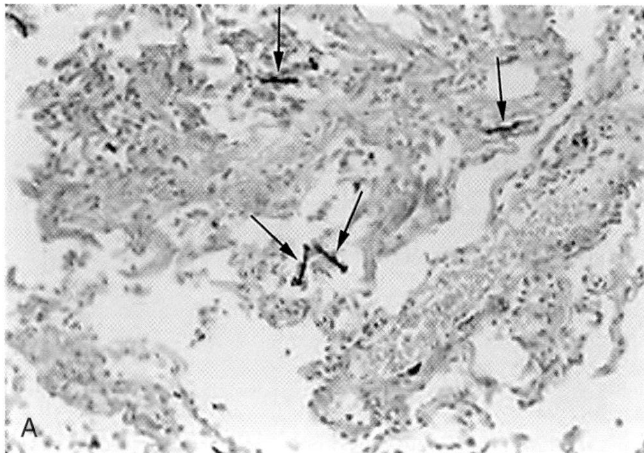

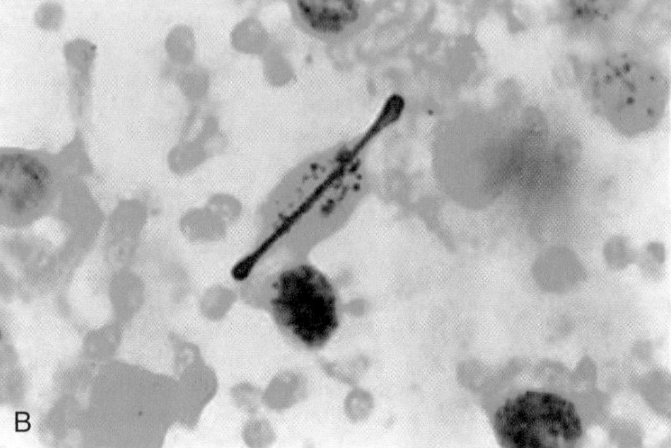

Figure 2 **Pleural disease concomitant with asbestos or ferruginous bodies in pathologic samples. A,** Asbestos ferruginous bodies *(arrows)* (hematoxylin and eosin ×100). **B,** Ferruginous body (hematoxylin and eosin ×250). *(Courtesy of Dr. Carol Farver.)*

SILICA EXPOSURE

Exposure to crystalline silica occurs when silica-containing rock and sand are encountered. This most commonly occurs in occupations associated with construction, mining, quarrying, drilling, and foundry work. A variety of conditions have been associated with inhalation of crystalline silica, including silicosis, tuberculosis, obstructive lung disease, and lung cancer.[1,3-6]

Silicosis

Inhalation of crystalline silica can lead to a fibronodular parenchymal lung disease known as *silicosis.* This most commonly occurs in a form known as *chronic* or *simple silicosis.* Persons with chronic silicosis typically have had more than 20 years of silica exposure. They are usually without symptoms, although shortness of breath and cough can develop. Their disease is thus recognized radiographically with multiple small nodules with an upper lobe predominance (Fig. 4). Hilar adenopathy with eggshell calcification can be seen. Pulmonary function abnormalities do not invariably occur. Pathologically, the nodules are recognized as silicotic nodules.

The pulmonary nodules seen with chronic silicosis can progressively conglomerate and be accompanied by fibrosis, a state that has been termed *conglomerate silicosis and progressive massive fibrosis.* Shortness of breath and cough can become debilitating. Pulmonary function testing often shows a mixed obstructive and restrictive defect, with a reduction in the diffusing capacity. Death due to silicosis continues to occur (Fig. 5).

Acute and accelerated forms of silicosis are more rapidly progressive, typically associated with intense exposure to silica. Acute silicosis can develop within months of exposure and resembles acute airspace disease on radiographs. Pathology mimics alveolar proteinosis, with proteinaceous material in the alveoli, but interstitial involvement and early nodule formation can be seen. Rapid progression to acute respiratory failure is common. Accelerated silicosis occurs after 5 to 15 years of exposure. Patients are usually symptomatic and often progress to respiratory failure and death. They are recognized by the development of upper zone nodules and fibrosis on radiographs and numerous nodules with interstitial fibrosis on pathology.

Mycobacterial Disease

Mycobacterial disease is known to occur with increased frequency in persons with silicosis. Persons with chronic silicosis have an incidence of mycobacterial tuberculosis that is three times greater than that of age-matched controls. Those with acute and accelerated silicosis have the highest incidence of mycobacterial disease. Others exposed to silica but without silicosis might have an excess risk of developing tuberculosis.

Given the high incidence of tuberculosis in these patients, it is recommended that persons with silicosis or long-term exposure to crystalline silica should receive a tuberculin skin test. If the reaction is 10 mm or greater and there is no evidence of active tuberculosis, tuberculosis chemoprophylaxis should be administered. If symptoms or radiographic changes suggest the possibility of mycobacterial disease, routine or induced sputum should be obtained and bronchoscopy considered. If active tuberculosis is confirmed, standard tuberculosis therapy, with a regimen containing rifampin, should be administered. Similarly, if a nontuberculous mycobacterium is identified, standard therapy for that organism should be administered.

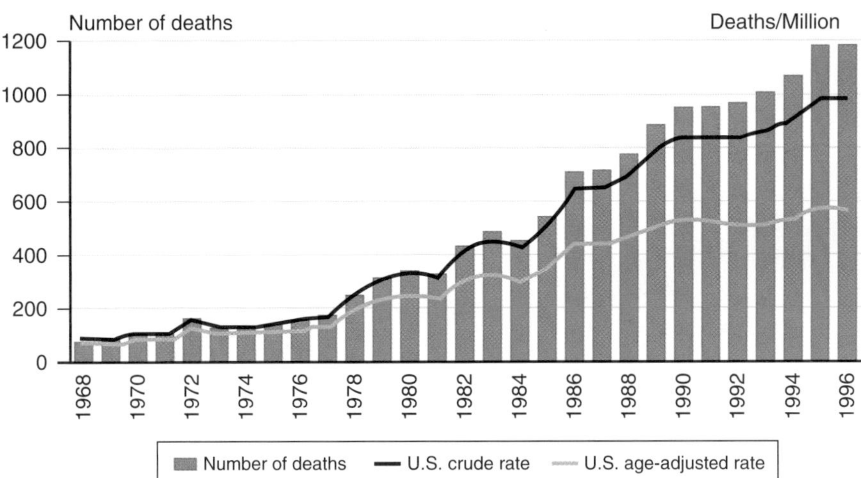

Figure 3 The number of deaths from asbestosis has increased through the years, related to asbestos use in a time-delayed fashion. *(From National Institute for Occupational Safety and Health (NIOSH): Work-Related Lung Disease Surveillance Report, 1999, publication no. 2003-111. Morgantown, WV, Division of Respiratory Disease Studies, NIOSH, 2000.)*

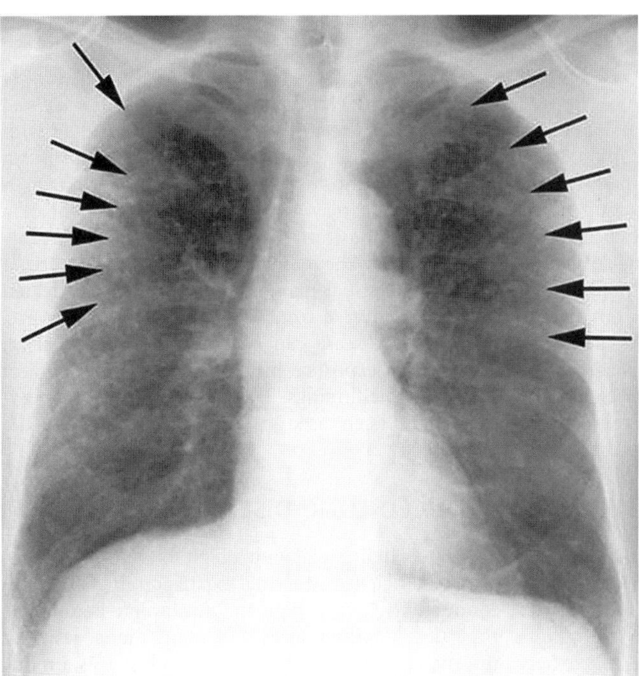

Figure 4 This chest radiograph shows the multiple small nodules *(arrows)* with upper lobe predominance characteristics. *(Courtesy of Dr. Omar Lababede.)*

Obstructive Lung Disease and Lung Cancer

Exposure to crystalline silica has been associated with the development of obstructive lung disease, chronic bronchitis, and emphysema. These associations are more prominent in those with silicosis. The intensity of dust exposure appears to affect the development of obstructive lung diseases. Tobacco smoking can have an additive effect.

According to the International Agency for Research on Cancer, there is sufficient evidence to classify silica as carcinogenic in humans. Available studies are complicated by multiple confounders and selection biases. Despite this, the bulk of the evidence supports an increased risk of lung cancer in tobacco smokers with silicosis. The relation is less clear for never-smokers and for persons exposed to silica who do not have silicosis.

Other Associations

Evidence suggests a relation between appreciable silica exposure and the development of scleroderma. Less evidence is available to support an association with rheumatoid arthritis or systemic lupus erythematosus. Similarly, reports of renal disease associated with silica exposure require further evidence to confirm a link.

COAL DUST EXPOSURE

Deposition of coal dust in the lungs can lead to lung disease. Coal mining is the major source of exposure. The tissue reaction to coal dust inhalation is the development of a coal macule. Focal emphysema can form around the macule. This combination is termed a *coal nodule* and is the characteristic lesion of simple coal worker's pneumoconiosis (CWP). In addition to CWP, coal dust exposure is also related to the development of airflow limitation, chronic bronchitis, and emphysema. Silica exposure often occurs in combination with coal dust exposure; thus, the previously described silica-related illness might also be seen.[1,3]

Simple CWP is usually without symptoms. Shortness of breath or a productive cough is often related to chronic bronchitis or airflow obstruction. Progressive massive fibrosis (PMF) can occur, more commonly when there has also been exposure to silica. Symptoms advance as the PMF worsens (Fig. 6). Deaths from CWP continue to occur (Fig. 7).

Given the common absence of symptoms, simple CWP is often a radiographic diagnosis. Chest imaging reveals small nodules with upper and posterior zone predominance. Hilar lymph node enlargement is not uncommon, although eggshell calcification does not generally occur. When PMF occurs, these small nodules coalesce, forming opacities larger than 1 cm. These lesions are odd-shaped, usually bilateral, and progressive, and they can cavitate or become calcified. Care must be taken because lesions diagnosed radiographically as PMF are often shown later to have been tumors, tuberculosis scars, or Caplan's nodules (see later).

Simple CWP tends to have little effect on lung function. Airflow limitation, restriction, and a reduction in diffusing capacity can all be seen when PMF develops. Pulmonary hypertension can develop in advanced disease.

Complications of CWP include a higher incidence of mycobacterial disease (although not as high as with silicosis), and an increased risk of stomach cancer. Tuberculin skin testing, chemoprophylaxis, and treatment of active tuberculosis are as recommended in silicosis. Caplan's syndrome is a nodular form of CWP seen in persons with rheumatoid arthritis. The nodules are multiple, tend to be larger than typical coal nodules, develop over short periods of time, and cavitate

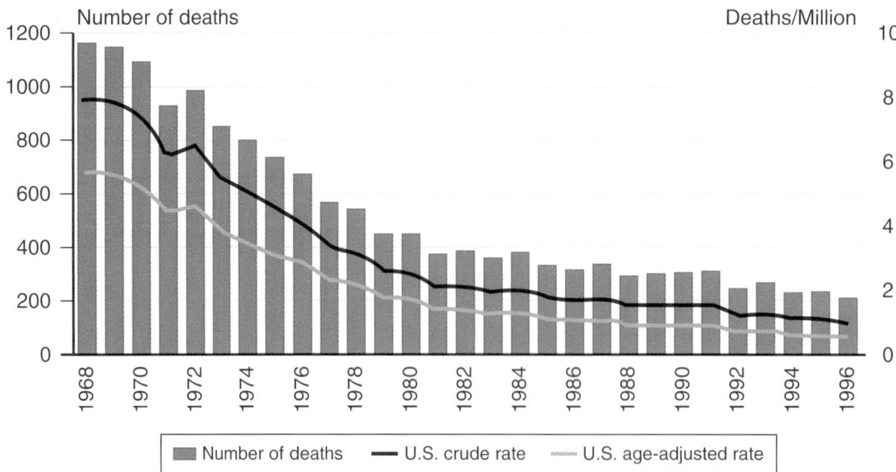

Figure 5 The number of deaths and death rates from silicosis have declined but not disappeared over time. *(From National Institute for Occupational Safety and Health (NIOSH): Work-Related Lung Disease Surveillance Report, 1999, publication no. 2003-111. Morgantown, WV, Division of Respiratory Disease Studies, NIOSH, 2000.)*

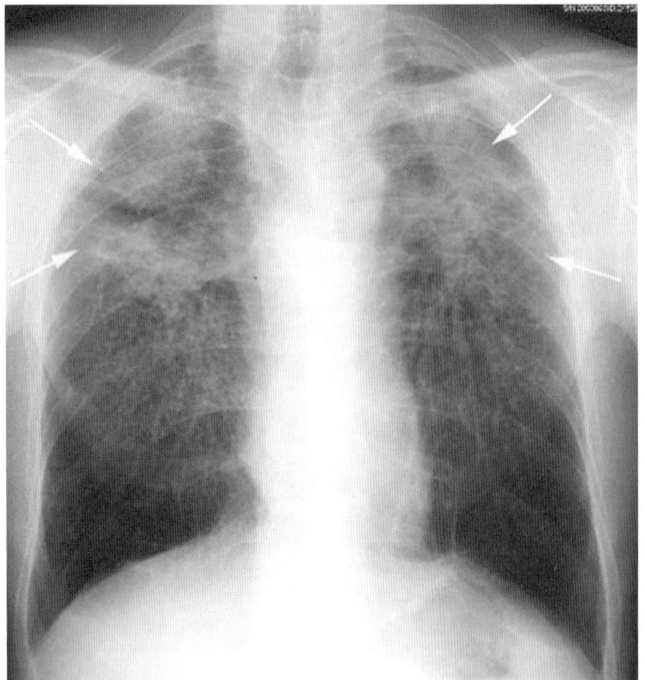

Figure 6 Progressive massive fibrosis *(arrows)*. *(Courtesy of Dr. Omar Lababede.)*

more often. These findings usually occur concomitantly with the joint manifestations, active arthritis, and the presence of circulating rheumatoid factor.

HARD METAL DISEASE

Hard metal, or cemented tungsten carbide, is found in tools for high-speed cutting, drilling, grinding, or polishing of other metals or hard materials. The consensus is that the agent responsible for the disease is the cobalt used as a catalyst to promote the binding of tungsten to carbon rather than the tungsten carbide itself. Workers in industries that manufacture cutting tools, drills, and the like are at highest risk. However, users of such tools (e.g., dental laboratories, sharpeners of saws, and diamond polishers) can also be exposed.

Work-related illness in hard metal disease includes *asthma* and *interstitial lung disease*. The disease can manifest acutely with rapidly progressing dyspnea after relatively short exposure, or it can manifest more insidiously and usually after long exposure. An acquired hypersensitivity can play a role in the development of a hypersensitivity bronchitis or asthma-like picture in a small percentage of workers in hard metal. The interstitial fibrosis is characterized by fibrosing alveolitis, interstitial pneumonitis, and multinucleated giant cells (Fig. 8) also recovered from the bronchoalveolar lavage. Both interstitial and area disease can occur in the same patient. Diagnosis is based on an exposure history, a compatible clinical presentation, and pathologic findings. Treatment is mostly supportive. Corticosteroids have been used to treat patients with acute presentation.[7,8]

BERYLLIUM-INDUCED LUNG DISEASE

Beryllium is an extremely light metal with a high modulus of elasticity (stiffness), a low coefficient of thermal expansion, high thermal and electrical conductivity, and a high melting point. Because of these unique properties, beryllium is used in many industries (Box 1). Pure beryllium metal is useful in the nuclear industry as a moderator of neutrons, increasing the effectiveness of the chain reaction. More often, it is formulated as an alloy or an oxide.[9,10]

Prevalence and Risk Factors

Historically, acute toxicity was associated with occupational exposures to concentrations of soluble beryllium salts greater than 100 $\mu g/m^3$. With the advent of industrial control measures to minimize air levels, acute pulmonary syndromes have virtually disappeared.

Persons who work with beryllium continue to be at risk for developing chronic beryllium disease (CBD or berylliosis). This is a granulomatous lung disease similar to sarcoidosis that is caused by a delayed-type hypersensitivity reaction in which there is a proliferation of beryllium-specific T cells.[11] About 10% of exposed persons develop beryllium hypersensitivity, and about 5% of those exposed develop CBD (Fig. 9). The most significant exposure is in the occupational setting. Occupations with the highest potential for exposure are those involved with primary production, metal machining, and reclaiming scrap alloys. Other high-exposure areas are in the nuclear power, aerospace, and electronic industries (Box 2).[12,13]

In addition to environmental exposure, genetic predisposition seems to have a major role in the development of CBD. A variant of

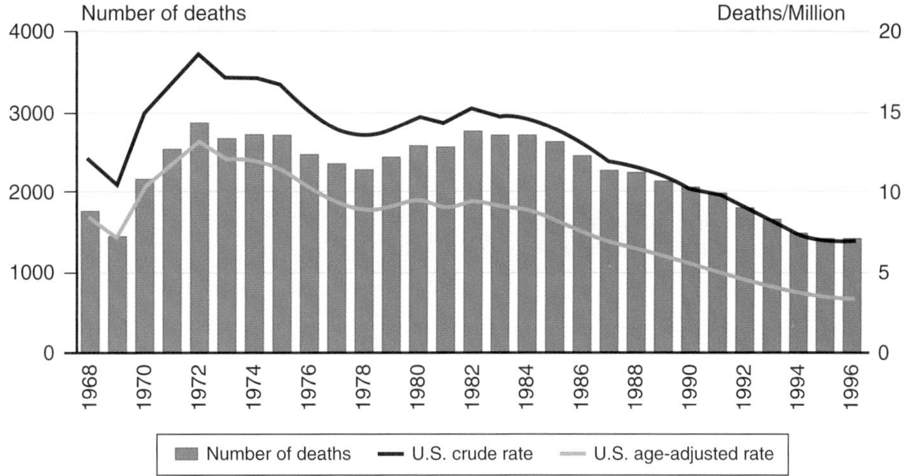

Figure 7 Death rates from coal-worker's pneumoconiosis have decreased modestly over time. *(From National Institute for Occupational Safety and Health (NIOSH): Work-Related Lung Disease Surveillance Report, 1999, publication no. 2003-111. Morgantown, WV, Division of Respiratory Disease Studies, NIOSH, 2000.)*

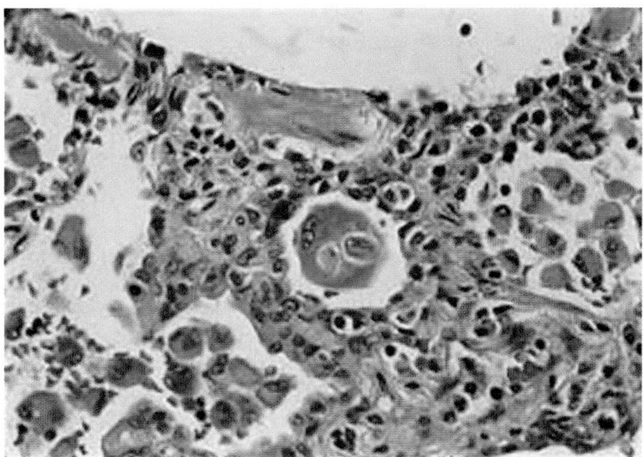

Figure 8 Multinucleated giant cells. *(Courtesy of Dr. Carol Farver.)*

the human leukocyte antigen (HLA-DPb1 [Glu69]) is found in 80% to 97% of patients with CBD and in only 30% of controls.[14,15]

Signs and Symptoms

The lung is the primary organ affected by CBD. Other organs can also be affected, including the extrapulmonary lymph nodes, skin, salivary glands, liver, spleen, kidneys, bone, myocardium, and skeletal muscle. Symptoms are usually nonspecific and occur late in the course of the disease. Dyspnea is the most common symptom, but some patients also present with cough, chest pain, arthralgia, fatigue, and weight loss. Physical signs, like symptoms, occur late in the course of disease and include inspiratory crackles on pulmonary auscultation, lymphadenopathy, skin lesions, and hepatosplenomegaly. Pulmonary function testing reveals an obstructive pattern in 39% and a restrictive pattern in 20% of patients with CBD. DL_{CO} (the lung diffusion capacity for carbon monoxide) also declines over time in 36% of persons. However, the most sensitive test is abnormalities in gas exchange during exercise.

A chest radiograph is normal in about one half the patients with documented CBD. Abnormal findings in the other one half include hilar adenopathy or increased interstitial markings, or both. High-resolution CT (HRCT) of the chest is more sensitive than chest

Box 1 Common Uses of Beryllium

Applications
Aircraft brakes and landing gear
Aircraft engines
Automotive electronics
Ball bearings
Ceramic applications
Computer electronics
Electrical components
Electrical contacts
Gears
Golf clubs
Inertial guidance systems
Injection and blow mold tooling
Laser tubes
Rocket engine liners
Spark plugs
Springs
Turbine rotor blades
Welding electrodes
X-ray tube windows

Industries
Gas industry
Oil industry

Box 2 Industries that Use Beryllium

Industries that Use Beryllium Heavily
Beryllium and beryllium alloy machine shops
Beryllium extraction
Electronics
Nuclear weapons manufacturing

Industries that Use Beryllium Less Heavily
Aerospace
Automotive
Ceramics
Computers
Dental appliances

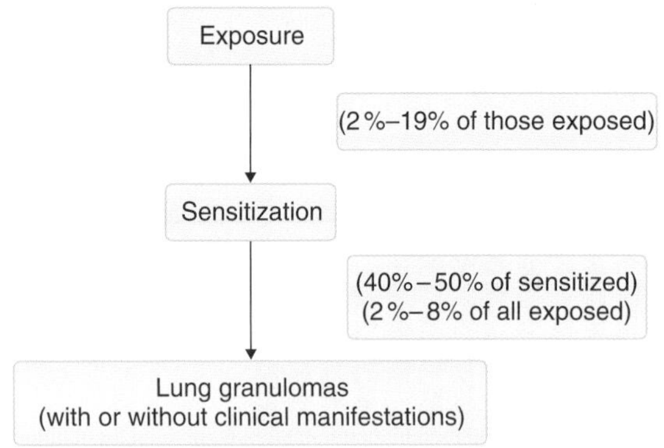

Figure 9 Epidemiology of chronic beryllium disease.

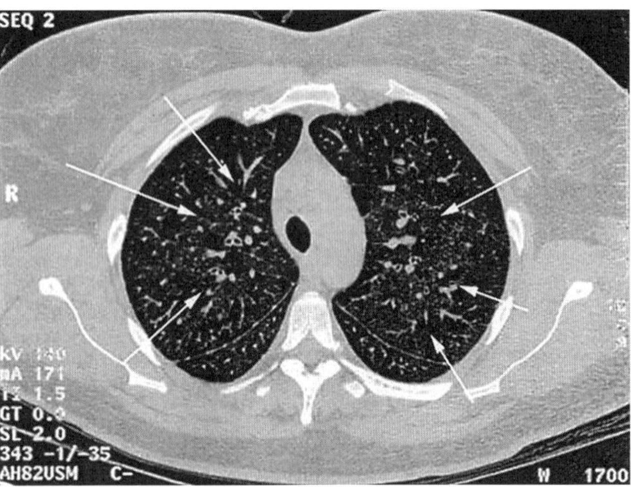

Figure 10 High-resolution computed tomography scan of the chest showing ground-glass attenuation *(arrows).*

radiography. Typical findings on HRCT are ground-glass opacification (Fig. 10), parenchymal nodules, or septal lines. HRCT, however, can show negative results in up to 25% of patients with documented CBD.[9,10,16,17]

Diagnosis

The diagnosis of CBD is based on the presence of a positive blood test or bronchoalveolar lavage beryllium-specific lymphocyte proliferation test (BeLPT) and the presence of non-necrotizing granuloma on lung biopsy.

The blood BeLPT is the screening test of choice to identify beryllium workers who develop beryllium sensitization or CBD. It involves exposing peripheral blood mononuclear cells in vitro to beryllium salts at varying concentrations for varying time intervals, looking for cell proliferation. This test is performed only in select, specialized laboratories around the country (Box 3).[18,19] Patients who have a positive blood BeLPT but no lung pathology are considered to be sensitized to beryllium but do not have CBD. They remain, however, at a lifelong risk for developing CBD.

There are many similarities between CBD and sarcoidosis (Table 1). Without a suspicion of beryllium exposure, almost all cases of CBD are diagnosed as sarcoidosis. For the same reason, all patients with sarcoidosis should have a detailed occupational history to exclude history of exposure to beryllium.[9,10]

Flexible fiberoptic bronchoscopy with bronchoalveolar lavage and transbronchial biopsy usually necessary to confirm a suspected diagnosis of CBD. Bronchoscopy is also helpful in excluding other possible causes with similar presentations, such as hypersensitivity pneumonitis or mycobacterial or fungal infection. The presence of non-necrotizing granulomas on transbronchial biopsy is the hallmark of CBD and is diagnostic in the appropriate clinical and epidemiologic settings. The granulomas in CBD are indistinguishable from sarcoid granulomas (Fig. 11). This is why exposure to beryllium (confirmed by occupational history, a positive BeLPT test, or beryllium in the tissue) is an integral part of the diagnosis of CBD. Patients with CBD usually have lymphocytosis (>20% lymphocytes in fluid from bronchoalveolar lavage). The BeLPT can also be performed on mononuclear cells from bronchoalveolar lavage fluid. An open lung biopsy is rarely needed but could be resorted to if the transbronchial biopsy is negative and the suspicion for CBD remaines high. Although the diagnostic yield is slightly higher than in transbronchial biopsy, the risk is also significantly higher. Serum levels of angiotensin-converting enzyme inhibitors may be high in CBD as in other granulomatous diseases, but this has no diagnostic value.[9,10,12,18]

Box 3 Select Locations for Beryllium Lymphocyte Proliferation Testing in the United States

Cleveland Clinic Foundation
Department of Clinical Pathology, L40
9500 Euclid Avenue
Cleveland, OH 44195-0001
Phone: (216) 444-2200 or 1-800-223-2273, ext 48844 or 55763
Fax: (216) 445-8160

Hospital of the University of Pennsylvania
Pulmonary Immunology Laboratory
833 BRB II/III
421 Curie Boulevard
Philadelphia, PA 19104-4283
Phone: (215) 573-9906
Fax: (215) 349-5172

National Jewish Center for Immunology and Respiratory Medicine
Cellular Immunology Tests
Pulmonary Division and Occupational/
Environmental Medicine Division
1400 Jackson Street
Denver, CO 80206
Phone: (303) 388-4461

Specialty Laboratories, Inc.
OncQuest
2211 Michigan Avenue
Santa Monica, CA 90404-3900
Phone: (310) 828-6543 or 1-800-421-4449

Treatment

All patients with CBD should be advised to avoid any further beryllium exposure. Although there is no proof that cessation of exposure to beryllium will improve the disease or halt its progression, it is prudent to avoid further exposure due to the immune-mediated nature of the disease. There is currently no cure for CBD, and no controlled studies for CBD are available. However, based on anecdotal reports and on the pathogenesis of the disease (immune mediated), and because of the similarities with sarcoidosis, CBD is treated with corticosteroids. Because therapy is not curative and has significant side effects, it is recommended only in patients who are symptomatic or demonstrate decline in their pulmonary function. In patients in whom corticosteroids fail or who develop significant side effects, methotrexate may be considered. In end-stage cases, lung transplantation may be considered.[9,10]

Table 1 Clinical and Laboratory Features of Chronic Beryllium Disease and Sarcoidosis

Feature	Chronic Beryllium Disease	Sarcoidosis
Occupational exposure to beryllium	Yes	No
Onset	Acute or insidious	Acute or insidious
Respiratory symptoms	Predominant organ affected	Predominant organ affected
Erythyma nodosum	No	Yes
Dermatitis	Yes	No
Cardiac	Rare	Common
Pulmonary physiology	Gas exchange abnormalities are common Obstruction early Mixed obstruction and restriction, or pure restriction, late	Gas exchange abnormalities are common Restriction, obstruction, or mixed pattern
Bilateral hilar adenopathy	Uncommon	Common
Infiltrates	Diffuse nodular or linear opacities Can be absent	Nodular and/or linear opacities May be more focal than in CBD
Computed tomography	Small nodules, septal lines, ground-glass appearance, adenopathy	Small nodules, septal lines, adenopathy
Beryllium lymphocyte proliferation test	Positive	Negative
Granulomas	Noncaseating granuloma	Noncaseating granuloma
Other histology	Diffuse mononuclear cell infiltrate is common Bronchial submucosa is involved occasionally	Diffuse mononuclear cell infiltrate is common Bronchial submucosa is involved occasionally
Beryllium in tissues	Yes	No
Tuberculin skin test	Negative	Negative
Kveim skin test	Negative	Positive
Beryllium patch skin test	Positive	Negative
Elevated serum ACE	Uncommon	Common
Response to steroid therapy	Often stabilizes disease, can improve pulmonary physiology and symptoms, usually requires continuous therapy	Often stabilizes disease that has not spontaneously remitted, can require continuous therapy
Prognosis	Variable; cor pulmonale and progressive fibrosis in some patients, more benign in others	Good prognosis for approximately 80% of patients, may progress to end-stage fibrosis and cor pulmonale

ACE, angiotensin-converting enzyme; CBD, chronic beryllium disease.

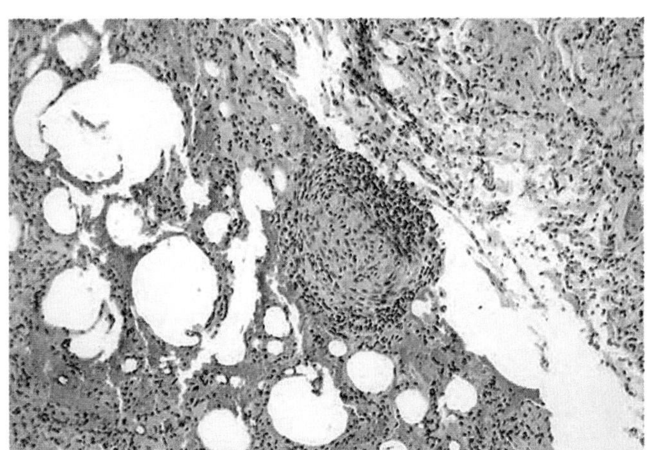

Figure 11 The granulomas in chronic beryllium disease are indistinguishable from sarcoid granulomas.

In summary, chronic beryllium disease (CBD, berylliosis) is an occupationally acquired granulomatous lung disease similar to sarcoidosis. It is caused by exposure to beryllium in genetically susceptible persons. CBD should be suspected in persons with beryllium exposure who present with pulmonary symptoms or have a positive screening blood BeLPT.

Summary

- Exposure to dust in the workplace is associated with a variety of pulmonary and systemic illnesses (pneumoconiosis).
- Pneumoconioses can appear and progress after the exposure has ceased. Regression does not occur, and treatment is mostly symptomatic and supportive.
- Asbestos exposure can lead to a variety of lung diseases including pleural diseases and asbestosis. Asbestos is also a known carcinogen.
- Many conditions have been associated with inhalation of crystalline silica, including silicosis, tuberculosis, obstructive lung disease, and lung cancer.
- Simple coal worker's pneumoconiosis tends to have little effect on lung function. Airflow limitation, restriction, and a reduction in diffusing capacity can all be seen when progressive massive fibrosis develops.
- Chronic beryllium disease (berylliosis) is an occupationally acquired granulomatous lung disease similar to sarcoidosis. It is caused by exposure to beryllium. Chronic beryllium disease should be suspected in patients with beryllium exposure who present with pulmonary symptoms or have a positive screening blood beryllium-specific lymphocyte proliferation test.

Suggested Readings

Beckett WS: Occupational respiratory diseases. N Engl J Med 2000;342:406-413.

Beckett WS, Abraham J, Becklake M, et al: Adverse effects of crystalline silica exposure. Official statement of the American Thoracic Society Committee of the Scientific Assembly on Environmental and Occupational Health. Am J Respir Crit Care Med 1997;155:761-768.

Berlin JM, Taylor JS, Sigel JE, et al: Beryllium dermatitis. J Am Acad Dermatol 2003;49:939-941.

Cullen MR: Respiratory diseases from hard metal exposure. A continuing enigma. Chest 1984;86:513-514.

Culver DA, Dweik RA: Chronic beryllium disease. Clin Pulm Med 2003;10:72-79.

Diagnosis and initial management of nonmalignant diseases related to asbestos. Am J Respir Crit Care Med Sep 15 2004;170(6):691-715.

Dweik RA: Berylliosis. Available at http://www.emedicine.com/med/topic222.htm (accessed March 20, 2009).

National Institute for Occupational Safety and Health (NIOSH): Work-Related Lung Disease Surveillance Report, 1999, publication no. 2003–111. Morgantown, WV, Division of Respiratory Disease Studies, NIOSH, 2000. PDF available at http://www.cdc.gov/niosh/docs/2000-105/2000-105.html (accessed March 20, 2009).

National Institute for Occupational Safety and Health (NIOSH): NIOSH Hazard Review: Health effects of occupational exposure to respirable crystalline silica. DHHS (NIOSH) publication no. 2002-129, April 2002. Available at http://www.cdc.gov/niosh/docs/2002-129/02-129a.html (accessed March 20, 2009).

Wagner GR: Asbestosis and silicosis. Lancet 1997;349:1311-1315.

References

For a complete list of references, log onto www.expertconsult.com.

Pleural Disease

Raed A. Dweik

DEFINITION

The pleural cavity contains a relatively small amount of fluid, approximately 10 mL on each side.[1] Pleural fluid volume is maintained by a balance between fluid production and removal, and changes in the rates of either can result in the presence of excess fluid, traditionally known as a *pleural effusion*.

The classic work of Light and colleagues in 1972 demonstrated that 99% of pleural effusions could be classified into two general categories: transudative or exudative (see Light's criteria under "Diagnosis").[2] A basic difference is that transudates, in general, reflect a systemic perturbation, whereas exudates usually signify underlying local (pleuropulmonary) disease.

PREVALENCE

Pleural disease, specifically pleural effusions, is one of the more common clinical problems encountered by the internist. Estimates of the incidence of pleural effusions vary, with some estimating an annual incidence of up to 1 million in the United States. The more common causes of transudative effusions are congestive heart failure and hypoalbuminemic states (e.g., cirrhosis), and those of exudative effusions are malignancy, infection (e.g., pneumonia), and pulmonary embolism.

PATHOPHYSIOLOGY

The accumulation of pleural fluid can usually be explained by increased pleural fluid formation or decreased pleural fluid absorption, or both. Increased pleural fluid formation can result from elevation of hydrostatic pressure (e.g., congestive heart failure), decreased colloid osmotic pressure (e.g., cirrhosis, nephrotic syndrome), increased capillary permeability (e.g., infection, neoplasm), passage of fluid through openings in the diaphragm (e.g., cirrhosis with ascites), or reduction of pleural space pressures (e.g., atelectasis). Decreased pleural fluid absorption can result from lymphatic obstruction or from elevation of systemic venous pressures resulting in impaired lymphatic drainage (e.g., superior vena cava [SVC] syndrome).

The presence of fluid in the normally negative-pressure environment of the pleural space has a number of consequences for respiratory physiology. Pleural effusions produce a restrictive ventilatory defect and also decrease the total lung capacity, functional residual capacity, and forced vital capacity.[3] They can cause ventilation-perfusion mismatches and, when large enough, compromise cardiac output.

The differential diagnosis of pleural effusions is briefly summarized in Boxes 1 and 2.

SIGNS AND SYMPTOMS

Many patients are asymptomatic on the discovery of a pleural effusion. When present, symptoms are usually due to the underlying disease process. Pleuritic chest pain indicates inflammation of the parietal pleura (because the visceral pleura is not innervated and thus not sensitive to pain). Other symptoms include dry, nonproductive cough and dyspnea. Physical examination findings that can reveal the presence of an effusion are reduced tactile fremitus, dull or flat note on percussion, and diminished or absent breath sounds on auscultation. It is also important to note the presence of other clues that can point to the cause of the effusion (e.g., signs of heart failure, breast masses).

DIAGNOSIS

Imaging Studies

Chest Radiography

The posteroanterior and lateral chest radiographs are still the most important initial tools in diagnosing a pleural effusion (Fig. 1). Free pleural fluid gravitates to the more dependent portions of the space; thus, most fluid collects around the inferior surface of the lung posteriorly, spilling out laterally and anteriorly as the amounts increase. About 50 mL of fluid is needed to be visible on the lateral radiograph as a meniscus posteriorly, and when more than 500 mL is present, the meniscus usually obscures the entire hemidiaphragm.[4] The lateral decubitus films help in differentiating free fluid from loculated fluid (that which is confined by fibrous pleural adhesions).

Ultrasound

Ultrasound is useful both as a diagnostic tool and as an aid in performing thoracentesis. Its major advantage over conventional radiography is its ability to differentiate between solid and liquid components and thus assist in identifying pleural fluid loculations. It is also valuable in detecting subpulmonic or subphrenic pathology.

Computed Tomography

Cross-sectional computed tomography (CT) (Fig. 2) helps distinguish anatomic compartments more clearly (e.g., the pleural space from lung parenchyma). This modality is useful as well in distinguishing empyema (split pleura sign) from lung abscess, in detecting pleural masses, and in outlining loculated fluid collections.[5]

Laboratory Studies

Ideally, the workup of a pleural effusion begins with a diagnostic thoracentesis followed by classification of the pleural fluid into either a transudate or an exudate. In 1972, Light and coworkers developed the currently accepted benchmark in classifying pleural fluid[2]:

- Ratio of pleural fluid protein to serum protein greater than 0.5
- Ratio of pleural fluid lactate dehydrogenase (LDH) to serum LDH greater than 0.6
- Pleural fluid LDH greater than two thirds the upper limit of normal for serum LDH (a cutoff value of 200 IU/L was used previously)

Pleural fluid is classified as an exudate if it meets *any one* of the aforementioned criteria. Conversely, if all three characteristics are not met, then the fluid is classified as a transudate. Following these guidelines, the original study of Light and colleagues[2] had a diagnostic sensitivity of 99% and specificity of 98% for an exudate. In more recent years, as noted by Tarn and Lapworth,[6] a number of studies used modifications to Light's criteria but had poorer diagnostic accuracy.

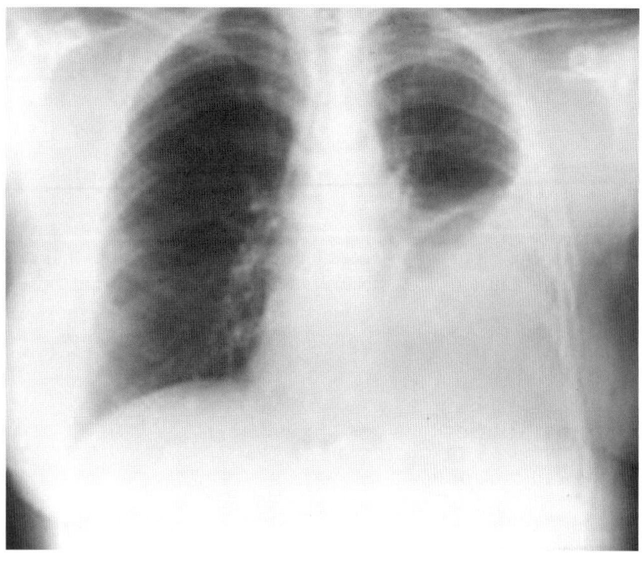

Figure 1 Posteroanterior chest radiograph showing pleural effusion in the left lung. The fluid fills about half of the left hemithorax.

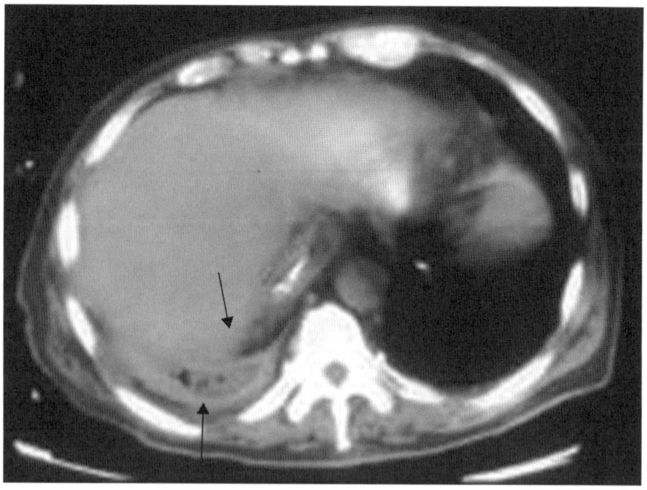

Figure 2 Computed tomography scan showing pleural effusion in the right lung. Notice the split pleura *(arrows)* characteristic of empyema. *Courtesy of Dr. Peter O'Donovan.*

Box 1 Select Causes of Transudates

- Atelectasis (early)
- Cirrhosis
- Congestive heart failure
- Hypoalbuminemia
- Nephrotic syndrome
- Peritoneal dialysis
- Urinothorax

Box 2 Select Causes of Exudates

- Asbestos exposure
- Atelectasis (chronic)
- Chylothorax
- Connective tissue disease
- Drugs (e.g., amiodarone)
- Esophageal rupture
- Hemothorax
- Infection (bacteria, viruses, fungi, tuberculosis, or parasites)
- Malignancy
- Pancreatitis
- Postcardiotomy syndrome
- Pulmonary embolism
- Subdiaphragmatic abscess
- Uremia

Additional Markers

Cholesterol

Although the reason is unclear, cholesterol concentration is higher in exudates than in transudates. Various studies have looked at the usefulness of cholesterol measurements alone, as a fluid-to-serum ratio, or in combination with LDH, with cutoffs ranging from 45 to 60 mg/dL. Currently, pleural fluid cholesterol measurements, on their own, probably reduce misclassifications but cannot be used as a substitute to measurements of protein and LDH.

Serum–Pleural Fluid Albumin Gradient

One of the limitations of the Light criteria is that they can misidentify some transudates as exudative effusions (e.g., in patients with heart failure who undergo diuretic treatment). Roth and colleagues used the serum-effusion albumin gradient (serum albumin concentration minus effusion albumin concentration) with a cutoff of 12 g/L (exudates if below that level, transudates if above), and obtained a specificity of 100% as compared with 72% with Light's criteria.[7] However, use of this marker alone can result in misclassification of many exudates as well.

Glucose

Very low glucose levels (<25 mg/100 mL), although not pathognomonic, are seen in a few diseases. Rheumatoid arthritis, tuberculosis, empyema, and tumors or malignancy with extensive involvement of the pleura are most commonly associated with very low glucose levels.

Amylase

Elevated pleural fluid amylase is seen with pancreatitis and esophageal rupture and in approximately 10% of malignant effusions.

pH

Normal pleural fluid pH has been estimated to be around 7.64. Good and colleagues noted that a pH of less than 7.30 suggests the presence of an inflammatory or infiltrative process.[8] These processes can include parapneumonic effusions, empyema, malignancy, connective tissue diseases, tuberculosis, and esophageal rupture. Urinothorax is peculiar in that it is the only cause of a low pH transudative effusion. According to the current American College of Chest Physicians (ACCP) consensus statement on the treatment of parapneumonic effusions,[9] pH is the preferred pleural fluid chemistry test (determined using a blood gas analyzer) for classifying the category of a parapneumonic effusion for subsequent management (See "Treatment and Outcomes" and Table 1).

Table 1 Management of Patients with Parapneumonic Effusions

Pleural Anatomy	Pleural Fluid Bacteriology	Pleural Fluid Chemistry	Need for Drainage
Minimal effusion (<10 mm on lateral decubitus view); free-flowing	Cx and GS unknown	pH unknown	No
Small to moderate effusion (>10 mm to <one half of hemithorax on lateral decubitus view); free-flowing	Negative Cx and GS	pH > 7.20	No
Large effusion (>one half of hemithorax on lateral decubitus view) *or* loculated fluid *or* thickened pleura	Positive Cx or GS	pH < 7.20	Yes
Any	Pus	pH < 7.0	Yes

Cx, culture; GS, Gram stain.

Adenosine Deaminase

Adenosine deaminase levels tend to be higher in tuberculous pleural effusions than in other exudates. A level greater than 70 U/L is highly suggestive of tuberculous pleuritis, whereas a level less than 40 U/L virtually rules out this diagnosis. Other pleural diseases where high adenosine deaminase levels may be seen are rheumatoid pleuritis and empyema.[10]

Other Diagnostic Modalities

Pleural Biopsy

The use of an Abrams needle to obtain specimens from the parietal pleura has become less common with the increasing availability of improved serum markers and thoracoscopy. At present, a needle biopsy of the pleura is used mainly to diagnose tuberculous pleuritis when other markers (e.g., adenosine deaminase) are negative.

Thoracoscopy

Invasive techniques for the diagnosis of pleural effusions have gained more popularity with the advent of video-assisted technology. Thoracoscopy offers the advantages of visual evaluation of the pleura, direct tissue sampling, and therapeutic intervention (e.g., dissecting loculations and pleurodesis). Medical thoracoscopy (performed by pulmonologists under conscious sedation) and video-assisted thoracoscopic surgery (VATS), which is performed by surgeons under general anesthesia, are indicated for diagnosing pleural effusions that have remained undiagnosed despite previous, less-invasive tests (e.g., thoracentesis).[10]

TREATMENT AND OUTCOMES

Therapeutic Thoracentesis

Drainage of a pleural effusion is indicated in complicated parapneumonic effusions or empyema (see Table 1), for symptomatic relief of dyspnea, and to evaluate underlying lung parenchyma. The current guidelines proposed by the ACCP for the treatment of parapneumonic effusions[9] categorize the risk of poor outcome as well as the need to drain the effusion based on the pleural space anatomy, pleural fluid bacteriology (culture and Gram stain), and pleural fluid chemistry (pH).

Therapeutic thoracentesis may be repeated if indicated; however, more definitive therapy (e.g., pleural sclerosis; see following) is usually needed to treat recurrent symptomatic pleural effusions. At any one time, no more than 1 L to 1.5 L of fluid should be removed (unless pleural space pressure is monitored) to avoid re-expansion pulmonary edema and post-thoracentesis shock. Supplemental oxygen is probably of benefit as well, because post-thoracentesis decreases in arterial oxygenation have also been reported, the magnitude and duration of which roughly correlate with the amount of fluid removed.

Pleural Sclerosis and Fibrinolytics

The use of a sclerosing agent to produce a chemical serositis and subsequent fibrosis of the pleura is indicated in recurrent symptomatic malignant effusions. Agents such as talc, doxycycline, bleomycin, and quinacrine have been used. All fluid must be drained initially and that full expansion of the underlying lung (usually via a tube thoracostomy) is essential before proceeding with sclerosis. Failure of treatment is usually due to the inability to approximate the pleural surfaces during administration of the agent. With proper technique, however, doxycycline sclerosis has been reported to be 80% to 90% effective.

Randomized, controlled trials have shown that fibrinolytics (urokinase or streptokinase instilled via a tube thoracostomy) improved fluid drainage and chest radiograph findings significantly, and it was an effective treatment for managing parapneumonic effusions.[11,12]

Surgery

The inadequacy of conventional drainage strategies has led the ACCP consensus panel to recommend video-assisted thoracoscopic surgery (VATS) and thoracotomy as acceptable approaches to managing patients with complicated pleural effusions. Parietal pleurectomy and decortication of the visceral pleura are definitive procedures with excellent response rates. Morbidity and mortality rates remain high, however, and the patient's general medical condition, expected long-term prognosis, and baseline lung function should be considered before proceeding with surgery.[13]

Pleural Effusions in Specific Diseases

Collagen Vascular Diseases

The pleura is involved in a majority of patients with systemic lupus erythematosus (SLE) at some time during the course of their disease. These pleural effusions are usually small and bilateral, and the most common symptom is chest pain. Previous studies have shown that the finding of lupus erythematosus cells and high antinuclear antibody titers in pleural fluid have a high specificity but are not particularly sensitive in diagnosing this condition. Therefore, routine use of these tests is not currently recommended. SLE effusions are usually responsive to corticosteroids.

Pleural effusions occur less commonly in patients with rheumatoid arthritis and, in contrast to SLE effusions, they occur more commonly in men. A striking characteristic of rheumatoid effusions is their low glucose level (<25 mg/dL). The measurement of rheumatoid factor in pleural fluid is also not useful, because this can be elevated in other inflammatory states. In contrast to SLE, there is little evidence that corticosteroids are beneficial in treating rheumatoid pleurisy, probably because the natural history of this disease is much more variable.

Malignancy

The pleura is involved in neoplastic disease more commonly through metastasis than through primary tumors. Lung and breast cancers

Box 3 Common Causes of Chylothorax

Filariasis
Idiopathic
Intestinal lymphangiectasia
Lymphangiomyomatosis
Subclavian venous thrombosis
Trauma (including surgery)
Tumors

are the leading causes of metastatic disease to the pleura. Other less common causes are hematologic (e.g., lymphoma, leukemia), ovarian, and gastrointestinal tumors. Cytologic examination of the pleural fluid is positive in more than 50% of cases with pleural involvement. Tumor markers (e.g., carcinoembryonic antigen [CEA] are not specific enough to be recommended routinely in establishing the diagnosis. Immunocytometry has been used to establish the diagnosis of lymphoma and has been helpful in cases of idiopathic effusions when conventional techniques were nondiagnostic.[14]

Chylothorax

Leakage of chyle from a disruption of the thoracic duct leads to a chylothorax. Common causes of this condition are listed in Box 3. Although the gross appearance of milky fluid usually indicates the diagnosis, the best way to ascertain this diagnosis is by measuring pleural fluid triglyceride levels (Fig. 3). A triglyceride level greater than 110 mg/dL confirms the diagnosis, whereas a level less than 40 mg/dL excludes the diagnosis. The finding of chylomicrons in the effusion (using electrophoresis) also establishes the diagnosis.

Treatment of a chylous effusion is aimed at preventing the complications of malnutrition due to the continuous loss of protein, fat, and electrolytes. Conservative measures include shifting to a medium-chain triglyceride diet to minimize the accumulation of fluid and total parenteral nutrition. Definitive treatment modalities include thoracic duct ligation or pleuroperitoneal shunt implantation. Pleurodesis is not very effective due to the anti-inflammatory characteristics of chyle.

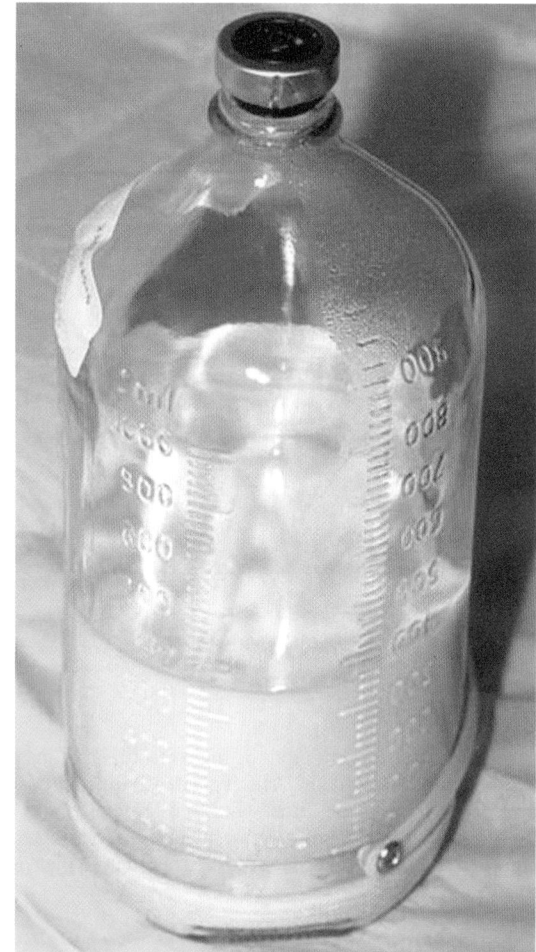

Figure 3 **Chylothorax.** Notice the white milky color of the fluid.

Hemothorax

Whenever the gross appearance of pleural fluid is bloody, a hematocrit level should be determined. Hemothorax is considered present when the pleural fluid hematocrit is greater than 50% of the peripheral blood hematocrit. Hemothorax most commonly results from chest trauma. Nontraumatic hemothorax, although uncommon, must alert the clinician to the possibility of malignancy or pulmonary embolism. Treatment of this condition requires immediate chest tube thoracostomy and, if bleeding persists (drainage >200 mL/hr), subsequent thoracotomy.

Coronary Artery Bypass Graft

Approximately one half of patients who undergo coronary artery bypass grafting develop pleural effusions. The precise pathophysiology of this postoperative occurrence is unclear, but it is probably related to pleural trauma during surgery or bleeding into the pleural space. Light and coworkers[15] divided these large effusions into two categories: those that occur within 30 days of surgery and those that occur after. Within 30 days of surgery, the fluid is bloody, eosinophilic, and easily resolvable with drainage (thoracentesis). After 30 days, the fluid is clear yellow and predominantly lymphocytic, but these effusions are difficult to manage because they often recur. In either case, it is easy to distinguish these effusions from those caused by congestive heart failure, because the former are usually exudative.

Other Pleural Diseases

Pneumothorax

Air between the right lung and chest wall (in the pleural space) is termed *pneumothorax* (Fig. 4). Box 4 lists the classification of pneumothoraces. Common causes of pneumothorax include trauma, iatrogenic factors (e.g., thoracentesis, mechanical ventilation), chronic obstructive pulmonary disease, infection, and malignancy.

The incidence of primary spontaneous pneumothorax is higher in men younger than 40 years, and the relative risk rises with heavy smoking. Secondary spontaneous pneumothorax is a more serious condition, because it further compromises an already abnormal lung function. Most secondary spontaneous pneumothoraces are related to chronic obstructive pulmonary disease or infection (e.g., *Pneumocystis jiroveci*). Trauma-related pneumothorax can result either in an open (to the atmosphere) pneumothorax or a closed (tension) pneumothorax, in which intrapleural pressures commonly exceed atmospheric pressures.

Box 5 summarizes the currently adopted ACCP guidelines for the treatment of spontaneous pneumothorax.[16] Traumatic pneumothorax usually requires placement of a thoracostomy tube until the air leak resolves. The ACCP consensus statement also recommends surgical intervention (thoracoscopy with bullectomy and a procedure to produce pleural symphysis) in preventing the recurrence of secondary pneumothoraces.[16]

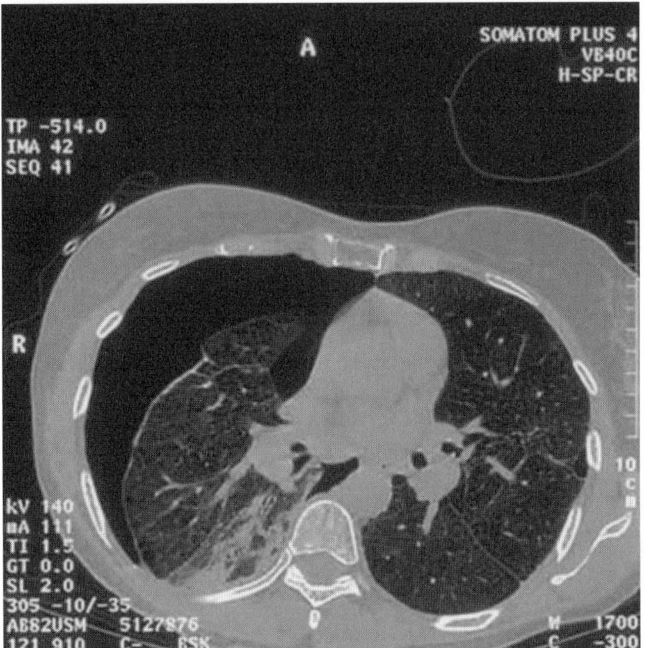

Figure 4 **Pneumothorax.** Air between the right lung and chest wall (in the pleural space).

Box 4 Classification of Pneumothorax

Traumatic or iatrogenic
Spontaneous (without antecedent cause):
- Primary (no underlying lung pathology)
- Secondary (underlying lung pathology)

Asbestos-Related Pleural Disease

The spectrum of pleural diseases with asbestos exposure ranges from the classic pleural plaques to effusions and malignancy. Pleural plaques are fibrous lesions found mostly on the parietal pleura after more than 20 years of exposure. They are considered markers of clinically relevant asbestos exposure and can occur without any evidence of asbestos-related lung disease[17]; furthermore, they are not considered to be premalignant lesions. Small, benign effusions are common and are often the earliest manifestations (within the first 20 years) of exposure, and the pathologic findings are nonspecific. On examination of the pleural fluid, however, the presence of mesothelial cells with atypical features makes it difficult to distinguish these benign effusions from effusions due to mesothelioma. Therefore, benign asbestos pleural effusions are exudates that can represent a diagnostic problem when other signs of asbestos exposure have not yet appeared.

Wagner and associates recognized the association of mesothelioma and asbestos in 1960.[18] Most patients are middle-aged and have a significant history of asbestos exposure. The diagnosis is often suggested by the history of cough and pleuritic chest pain as well as chest CT results and findings of elevated hyaluronic acid levels in pleural fluid. The diagnosis is confirmed by tissue biopsy through thoracoscopy or thoracotomy. The prognosis of patients with mesothelioma is generally poor (<1 year survival after diagnosis), and the management involves multimodality therapy.

AIDS-Related Pleural Disease

The immunologic impairment in AIDS leads to a variety of infectious and neoplastic processes. Infectious complications include the development of bacterial parapneumonic effusions and empyema. In developing countries, tuberculous involvement of the pleura is common. *P. jiroveci*, although a common cause of pneumonia in patients with AIDS, is rarely a cause of pleural effusions. However, *P. jiroveci* has been associated with pneumothorax in this patient population, so much so that the development of an unexplained spontaneous pneumothorax in a person infected with human immunodeficiency virus should prompt a search for *P. jiroveci* infection.[19] Pleural effusions can also occur with Kaposi's sarcoma and non-Hodgkin's lymphoma, and responses to treatment for these disease entities have been poor.

Box 5 Management of Spontaneous Pneumothorax

Primary Spontaneous Pneumothorax

Stable Patients with Small Pneumothoraces

Observation in the emergency department for 3 to 6 hours
Discharge home if a repeat chest radiograph excludes progression
Follow up within 12-48 hours with repeat chest radiograph to document resolution

Stable Patients with Large Pneumothoraces

Hospitalization
Re-expansion of lung using a small-bore catheter or placing a 16-22 F chest tube
Suction if lung fails to re-expand

Unstable Patients with Large Pneumothoraces

Hospitalization
Chest tube placement with 16-22 F standard chest tube
Use 24-28 F chest tube if the patient has a large air leak or requires positive-pressure ventilation

Secondary Spontaneous Pneumothorax

Hospitalization
Observation or treatment with a chest tube, depending on the extent of the symptoms and the course of the pneumothorax

Summary

- Pleural effusion is usually the result of an imbalance between fluid production and removal.
- Light's criteria help differentiate transudative pleural effusions, which usually reflect a systemic disease, from exudative effusions, which usually signify underlying local (pleuropulmonary) disease.
- The more common causes of transudative effusions are congestive heart failure and hypoalbuminemic states (e.g., cirrhosis); common causes of exudative effusions are malignancy, infections (e.g., pneumonia), and pulmonary embolism.
- Ideally, the workup of a new pleural effusion begins with a diagnostic thoracentesis unless the amount of fluid is too small.
- The management of pleural effusions associated with pneumonia (parapneumonic effusions) is based on the pleural space anatomy, pleural fluid bacteriology (culture and Gram stain), and pleural fluid chemistry (pH).
- Medical or surgical thoracoscopy offers the advantages of visual evaluation of the pleura and direct tissue sampling, and it can be helpful for the diagnosis of unknown pleural effusions and in the management of complicated effusions.

Suggested Readings

Baumann MH, Strange C, Heffner JE, et al; AACP Pneumothorax Consensus Group. Management of spontaneous pneumothorax: An American College of Chest Physicians Delphi consensus statement. Chest 2001;119:590-602.

Bouros D, Schiza S, Patsourakis G, et al: Intrapleural streptokinase versus urokinase in the treatment of complicated parapneumonic effusions: A prospective, double-blind study. Am J Respir Crit Care Med 1997;155:291-295.

Colice GL, Curtis A, Deslauriers J, et al: Medical and surgical treatment of parapneumonic effusions: An evidence-based guideline [AACP consensus statement]. Chest 2000;118:1158-1171.

Light RW: The undiagnosed pleural effusion. Clin Chest Med 2006;27(2):309-319.

Light RW, MacGregor MI, Luchsinger PC, et al: Pleural effusions: The diagnostic separation of transudates and exudates. Ann Intern Med 1972;77:507-513.

Mehta AC, Dweik RA: Pleural diseases. In Stoller JK, Michota FA, Mandell BF (eds): Cleveland Clinic Intensive Review of Internal Medicine, 4th ed. Philadelphia: Lippincott Williams & Wilkins, 2005, pp 452-466.

Rodriguez-Panadero F, Janssen JP, Astoul P: Thoracoscopy: General overview and place in the diagnosis and management of pleural effusion. Eur Respir J 2006;28(2):409-422.

Sahn SA: State of the art-the pleura. Am Rev Respiratory Dis 1988;138:184-234.

Tarn AC, Lapworth R: Biochemical analysis of pleural fluid: What should we measure? Ann Clin Biochem 2001;38:311-322.

Wagner JC, Sleggs CA, Marchand P: Diffuse pleural mesothelioma and asbestos exposure in northwestern Cape Province. Br J Industrial Med 1960;17:260-271.

References

For a complete list of references, log onto www.expertconsult.com.

Pulmonary Embolism

Anil Gopinath and Thomas R. Gildea

DEFINITION AND ETIOLOGY

Pulmonary embolism (PE) refers to the presence of endogenous or exogenous substances within the pulmonary vascular bed that result in partial or complete hindrance to blood flow. Among all causes for PE, deep venous thrombosis is the most common (Box 1).

PREVALENCE AND RISK FACTORS

Pulmonary embolism is, in the overwhelming majority, a consequence of deep venous thrombosis (DVT); the two together constitute venous thromboembolism (VTE). The incidence of PE thus reflects the presence of risk factors for VTE in a given population (Box 2).

A brief recap of venous anatomy may be helpful. The deep venous system of the lower extremities includes the anterior tibial, posterior tibial, and peroneal veins. The anterior and posterior tibial veins join to form a common trunk: the popliteal vein. The peroneal vein either joins the anterior and posterior tibial veins to form the popliteal vein or joins a variable length after its formation. The soleal and gastrocnemius veins, which lie within the eponymous muscles, drain into the popliteal vein.

There are many known risk factors for VTE and PE (see Box 2). These seemingly disparate risk factors may be easier to comprehend if Virchow's triad (venous stasis, hypercoagulability, and endothelial injury) is remembered. The pathogenic mechanisms underlying the risk factors for VTE are either the de novo development or an accentuation of pre-existing elements of Virchow's triad. Thus, trauma can result in immobility (venous stasis), tissue injury (leading to hypercoagulability), and endothelial injury. Patients who have pre-existing risk factors for VTE (e.g., hypercoagulability) may be more at risk for developing VTE after a predisposing event (e.g., surgery or trauma) than another person who experiences similar events but is free from risk factors. The presence of several risk factors in a patient results in a synergistic increase in the risk for VTE.

A subset of patients with DVT will develop pulmonary embolism. The location of the thrombus within the deep venous system is a key factor in this progression. Proximal (knee and above) deep vein involvement portends an increased risk of pulmonary embolism. A high probability ventilation/perfusion ($\dot{V}/\dot{Q}$) scan (suggestive of PE) was seen in 40% to 50% of patients with symptomatic proximal DVT but with no symptoms of PE.[1] The real incidence of PE is probably higher, even when false-positive high-probability $\dot{V}/\dot{Q}$ scans are accounted for, because the sensitivity of a high-probability scan is only about 50%. Quantifying symptomatic PE in untreated proximal DVT is understandably difficult; one review suggested an incidence of 50% over a 3-month period in this group.[1]

In contrast, progression with distal (calf) DVT is less common. Asymptomatic distal (calf) DVT progresses in only about one sixth of patients to involve more-proximal veins.[1] Symptomatic distal DVT extends proximally in up to one third of such episodes.

DIAGNOSIS

There is no clinical feature and no single diagnostic test that reliably distinguishes patients with and without PE. In any patient, the presence of multiple signs, symptoms, and historical features that are known to occur with a higher frequency in patients with PE increases the likelihood of PE. This rationale underlies the development of clinical prediction models for PE (Tables 1 and 2) and, in turn, implies that excessive reliance on any one element for diagnosing PE can be misleading. This approach has been formally evaluated for clinical prediction models for DVT where individual elements of the Wells clinical prediction rule for DVT were less helpful for diagnosing DVT than when combined in a prediction model.[2] It is likely that a similar situation exists for clinical prediction rules for PE as well.

Efforts to identify modalities (e.g., helical computed tomography [CT]) that have a high negative predictive value independent of clinical assessment have not been entirely successful. In particular, there are concerns about selection bias in studies on helical CT, the modality on which most attention has been focused in the search for a context-independent test.[3] At present, diagnostic algorithms that include clinical prediction rules, laboratory tests, and imaging are the most reliable ways to diagnose PE.

CLINICAL FEATURES

Symptoms commonly associated with pulmonary embolism include dyspnea, chest pain, cough, hemoptysis, apprehension, palpitations, syncope, and sweating. Pleuritic chest pain and sudden dyspnea are significantly more common in patients with pulmonary embolism but are not pathognomonic.[4] Signs commonly associated with PE include tachypnea, tachycardia, neck vein distention, a fourth heart sound, a loud pulmonary component of the second heart sound, inspiratory crackles, pleural rub, and low-grade fever (<38.0° C). Tachypnea and tachycardia are more common in patients with PE, but the other signs are not helpful in distinguishing between patients with and without PE.[4]

Clinical Prediction Rules

The Prospective Investigation of Pulmonary Embolism Diagnosis (PIOPED) study results suggested that the clinical impression of an experienced physician, arrived at by the synthesis of clinical symptoms, signs, laboratory data, and imaging, had reasonable correlation with the actual incidence of pulmonary embolism in each of the incidence categories (low, intermediate, and high).[5] Clinical prediction rules thus evolved in a milieu of accumulating data that underscored the unreliability of individual signs or symptoms or a syndromic approach to the diagnosis of PE and the possibility of improved diagnostic performance from a systematic evaluation of a group of key factors (risk factors, signs, symptoms, imaging) that were helpful in discriminating between patients with and without PE.

Many different clinical prediction rules have been proposed.[6] The simplified (or modified) Wells prediction rule[7] has been used in most prospective validation studies (see Table 1). It evaluates seven factors and categorizes patients into three risk categories: low, intermediate, and high. In a prospective study that used the simplified Wells prediction rule, the incidence of PE was 1.3%, 16.2%, and 40.6% in the low-, intermediate-, and high-risk categories, respectively.[8]

Wells and colleagues,[7] in the same study, included alternative cutoff values for the clinical prediction rule that yielded a dichotomous outcome ("PE likely" and "PE unlikely") instead of the three risk categories (see Table 1). This was done to help dichotomize the patient population into those who did not need further investigations (those who were in the "PE unlikely" group and had negative D-dimer tests) and all others who would need further workup. With this dichotomous model and additional D-dimer testing, 46% of the patients in their validation cohort were categorized as "PE unlikely" and had negative D dimers.[7] In this subgroup (PE unlikely and

Box 1 Causes of Pulmonary Embolism

Most Common
Lower limb deep venous thrombosis (majority of cases)

Less Common
Air embolism
Amniotic fluid embolism
Cement (polymethylmethacrylate) embolism
Fat embolism
Hydatid embolism
Iodinated oil
Metallic mercury embolism
Septic pulmonary embolism (infective endocarditis, catheter, infected pacemaker leads)
Talc embolism
Tumor embolism
Miscellaneous (catheter fragments, cotton fibers)

Adapted from Han D, Lee KS, Franquet T, et al: Thrombotic and nonthrombotic pulmonary arterial embolism: Spectrum of imaging findings. Radiographics 2003;23:1521-1539.

Box 2 Risk Factors for Venous Thromboembolism

Strong Risk Factors (Odds Ratio >10)
Fracture (hip or leg)
Hip or knee replacement
Major general surgery
Major trauma
Spinal cord injury

Other Risk Factors
Immobility
Cancer therapy
Previous venous thromboembolism
Malignancy
Increasing age
Pregnancy and the postpartum period
Estrogen-containing oral contraception or hormone replacement therapy
Selective estrogen receptor modulators
Acute medical illness
Heart or respiratory failure
Inflammatory bowel disease
Nephrotic syndrome
Myeloproliferative disorders
Paroxysmal nocturnal hemoglobinuria
Obesity
Smoking
Varicose veins
Central venous catheterization
Inherited or acquired thrombophilia

Adapted from Geerts WH, Pineo GF, Heit JA, et al: Prevention of venous thromboembolism: The Seventh ACCP Conference on Antithrombotic and Thrombolytic Therapy. Chest 2004;126:338S-400S; and Anderson FA Jr, Spencer FA: Risk factors for venous thromboembolism. Circulation 2003;107:I9-I16.

negative D dimer), the rate of PE was only 1.7%. In comparison, only 27% of patients had a combination of low risk and negative D dimer as assessed by the three-category model in the same study.[7] The dichotomous model was thus able to limit further investigations in 46% of patients, with no increase in the incidence of PE on follow-up. A prospective study has confirmed the safety of the two-category approach along with CT angiography and D-dimer testing.[9]

At present, sufficient data support the use of the Wells prediction rule (either the two- or three-category modification) in conjunction with a sensitive D-dimer test in patient populations known to have a relatively low incidence of PE.[7,9]

Table 1 Clinical Prediction Rules (Wells Score)

Variable	Points
Clinical signs and symptoms of DVT (minimum of leg swelling and pain with palpation of the deep veins)	3
Alternative diagnosis is less likely than PE	3
Heart rate >100 bpm	1.5
Immobilization or surgery in the previous 4 wk	1.5
Previous DVT or PE	1.5
Hemoptysis	1
Malignancy (on treatment, treated in the last 6 mo or palliative)	1

DVT, deep venous thrombosis; PE, pulmonary embolism.

Table 2 Risk Categories Based on Wells Score

Cumulative Score	Risk Category
Version Used in PIOPED II	
<2	Low
2-6	Intermediate
>6	High
Version Used in CHRISTOPHER Study	
≤4	PE unlikely
>4	PE likely

PE, pulmonary embolism; PIOPED, Prospective Investigation of Pulmonary Embolism Diagnosis.
Adapted from Wells PS, Anderson DR, Rodger M, et al: Derivation of a simple clinical model to categorize patients probability of pulmonary embolism: Increasing the model's utility with the SimpliRED D-dimer. Thromb Haemost 2000;83:416-420.

Any score not validated prospectively or developed in a patient population that is distinctly different (ethnicity, encounter setting, high vs. low incidence of PE, pre-screened patient population with a low incidence of alternative diagnosis) from the one the score is being applied to might not categorize patients as well as in the original study. In a retrospective study of PIOPED patients, the Wells score performed poorly in specific subgroups (surgical, ICU and CCU groups), but its diagnostic accuracy was acceptable for outpatients.[10]

It is unlikely that a particular schema will suffice for all clinical situations, and therefore it is difficult to recommend a particular prediction rule for universal use. The rigid application of clinical scores is not advocated; in the modified Wells score, this is explicitly avoided by the inclusion of a high scoring criterion that reminds the clinician to judge whether an alternative diagnosis is less likely than PE (see Table 1).[4] Thus, with due diligence, clinical assessment models (modified Wells score, Geneva score) can be used by physicians of varying levels of experience to classify patients into low-, intermediate-, and high-risk categories as accurately as experienced physicians can by their clinical gestalt.[3]

D Dimer

D dimer is produced by the breakdown of cross-linked fibrin by the fibrinolytic system. D-dimer levels are elevated in acute thromboembolism and result from the lysis of cross-linked fibrin within the thrombus. D-dimer levels are, however, elevated in other conditions (e.g., postoperative state, cancer, pregnancy) and thus are not pathognomonic for thromboembolic disease. Because elevated D-dimer levels are nonspecific and are not diagnostic for PE, the value of D-dimer testing rests on the ability of a negative test (a low value) to predict the absence of PE.

A highly sensitive D-dimer test would ensure levels above the chosen threshold for nearly all patients with PE. However, such high sensitivity often comes at the cost of low specificity (high false-positive rates). Even if elevated levels are not taken as evidence of PE, positive D-dimer tests usually result in further investigations, each with its adverse effects and inherent false-positive and false-negative rates. If more patients are directed toward further investigations after a highly sensitive D-dimer test, the advantage of detecting a higher number of true positives will be offset to a greater or lesser degree by the cost and adverse effects associated with investigating a greater absolute number of patients. As is evident, a balance between high sensitivities (ensuring that no patients with PE are missed) and high specificity (ensuring that no normal patient receives anticoagulation for an erroneous diagnosis of PE) is essential. A false-negative rate of 1% to 2% is considered acceptable for a diagnostic protocol (not each individual test) in view of similar numbers encountered with pulmonary angiography, which is considered the gold standard.[4]

An appropriate protocol categorizes a patient into differing risk categories with a clinical prediction rule (e.g., low, intermediate, and high risk for the Wells score), thus estimating the pretest probability based on incidence rates for similar patients in historical validation studies (e.g., 1%-3% for the low-risk category in the Wells score). An appropriate protocol also selects a test with an appropriate likelihood ratio (e.g., negative likelihood ratio of 0.13 for the ELISA assay) and yields a post-test probability (<1% for this example). Thus, an adequate match between the patient population and the selected clinical prediction rule is necessary to ensure a reasonably accurate estimation of the pretest probability. Similarly, a test with an appropriate likelihood ratio is necessary to ensure that it significantly changes the pretest probability.[4]

These considerations have a direct bearing on D-dimer tests used in diagnosing PE. Many different assays are used for D-dimer assessment. A meta-analysis by Stein[11] demonstrated better sensitivity and likelihood ratios for enzyme-linked immunosorbent assay (ELISA)-based methods than for other assays. The sensitivity of the quantitative rapid ELISA assay was 95%, with a negative likelihood ratio of 0.13 (cutoff value <500 ng/mL). A negative test thus effectively excludes patients who have a low pretest probability. These variations underscore the importance of knowing the particular assay used locally.

The results of a D-dimer test, irrespective of the sensitivity of the assay, cannot be interpreted in isolation. The diagnostic accuracy of D-dimer test is less in hospitalized patients than in outpatients.[12] The incidence of a false-negative D-dimer result in patients categorized as "PE likely" or high probability for PE was considerable (10.3% and 20%, respectively) in one study, although a less-sensitive whole-blood assay was used.[7] Even when sensitive assays are used, the false-negative rate rises as the pretest probability rises. These considerations reiterate the necessity for interpreting results from diagnostic studies as well from clinical prediction rules in the context of the various factors that can influence the manifestations and sequelae of PE.

Helical Computed Tomography

There has been a profusion of studies evaluating the role of spiral CT in suspected PE. One issue that has been examined is whether the pulmonary angiogram can still be considered the gold standard in the current era of multidetector CT (MDCT) given the substantial interobserver variation with angiography.[13,14] However, although interobserver agreement improves with thinner-collimation MDCT scanners,[15] there is no conclusive proof that agreement rates are significantly greater than with pulmonary angiogram in studies that directly compare these modalities.[16,17] In addition, there is no conclusive proof that MDCT has greater sensitivity than pulmonary angiography in detecting subsegmental emboli; two studies produced discordant results.[16,17] Thus, there is no reason, at present, to believe that prior studies with pulmonary angiograms need to be re-examined in light of the improvements in CT technology.

More importantly, it may well be that subsegmental emboli do not have the same implications as larger proximal emboli. In the original PIOPED study, 20 patients were inadvertently left untreated as a result of missed diagnosis on initial pulmonary angiograms that were later reclassified as positive angiograms by the central panel of angiogram readers.[18] The overwhelming majority of the patients (84%) had segmental or more distal clots. There were no differences in mortality or recurrent PE (fatal or nonfatal) between the treated and untreated groups. The absence of a detrimental effect with small subsegmental PE might explain why clinical outcomes do not differ significantly in untreated patients with negative CT angiograms (single detector or multiple detector) even though the sensitivity for subsegmental PE is less for single-detector CT when compared with multidetector CT.[19,20] In addition, the mortality and recurrence rates are not significantly different from those for patients with negative pulmonary angiogram.[20] As an editorial pointed out, outcome studies and accuracy studies might not yield similar results.[21] As it pertains to subsegmental PE, it may be that beyond some threshold, increasing accuracy in diagnosis does not translate into better outcomes; that is, all clots might not have equal significance. However, these conclusions do not apply to all patient populations; subsegmental emboli can be significant in patients with prior cardiopulmonary disease and may be important as a marker of a prothrombotic state and increased risk of recurrence in those who have persistent risk factors.

These observations tie in neatly with two studies that evaluated the use of multidetector CT within a diagnostic algorithm.[9,22] The Christopher study[9] used a modified Wells score and a sensitive D-dimer assay. Patients who were in the "PE unlikely" group and had a negative D-dimer result had no further investigations. All other patients had a CT, either multidetector or single detector. Patients in the "PE likely" group who had negative CT scans had rates of fatal or nonfatal PE that were no different from rates in the "PE unlikely" group who had negative D-dimer rates and were not different from rates in historical controls with negative pulmonary angiograms.[9] The majority were outpatients, and the incidence of PE and the prevalence of persistent risk factors (e.g., malignancy, paralysis) were low.[9]

The PIOPED II study classified patients into low-, intermediate-, and high-risk categories using modified Wells criteria.[7] There was an interaction among CT angiogram results (with or without CT venography), the risk category, and PE location such that a positive CT angiogram (CTA) and CT venogram (CTV) was more likely to reflect the presence of an actual thrombus (positive predictive value) when the pretest probability was high and when the thrombus was proximally located. CTA plus CTV had higher sensitivity than CTA alone, but it had equivalent sensitivity to CTA assessment in conjunction with risk category. When the clinical assessment was discordant with the CTA results, the negative predictive value was lower and further investigations (USG, pulmonary angiogram, $\dot{V}/\dot{Q}$ scan) were necessary to exclude PE.[22]

At present, single-detector or multidetector CT scan results need to be assessed in light of the pretest probability. Proximal thrombi are detected well across all risk categories, whereas false-positive and false-negative rates for subsegmental clots are high when the risk category and CT scan results are discordant. Because there is no consensus on the management of subsegmental clots, further workup is recommended when such discordant results are seen. A recent article by the PIOPED II investigators outlines one such algorithm.[23]

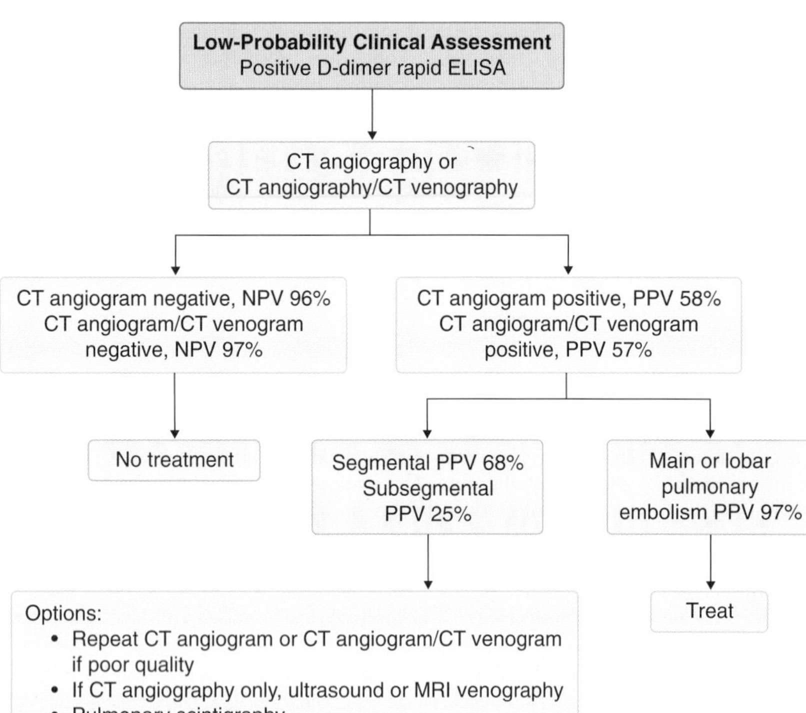

Figure 1 Diagnostic algorithm for investigating pulmonary embolism when the pretest probability is low. Pretest probability is assessed by the modified Wells score (see Table 1). CT, computed tomography; MRI, magnetic resonance imaging; NPV, negative predictive value; PPV, positive predictive value. *Reproduced from Stein PD, Woodard PK, Weg JG, et al: Diagnostic pathways in acute pulmonary embolism: Recommendations of the PIOPED II investigators. Am J Med 2006;119:1048-1055.*

Ventilation-Perfusion Scanning

$\dot{V}/\dot{Q}$ scanning was the first-line imaging test study until the advent of helical CT. The performance characteristics of $\dot{V}/\dot{Q}$ scanning have been documented meticulously in the landmark PIOPED study.[5] The combination of high or low pretest clinical probability and concordant $\dot{V}/\dot{Q}$ scan results predicts the presence or absence of PE with a high degree of accuracy. The traditional problem with $\dot{V}/\dot{Q}$ scanning has been the high incidence of nondiagnostic tests and indeterminate results and consequently the inability to definitively categorize a majority of the tested patients.

A randomized. controlled trial sought to determine whether CTPA was noninferior to $\dot{V}/\dot{Q}$ scanning in ruling out PE in acutely symptomatic patients.[24] The primary endpoint was met, demonstrating that CTPA was not inferior to $\dot{V}/\dot{Q}$ scanning in ruling out PE. The study also demonstrated that if the group of patients with nonhigh probability $\dot{V}/\dot{Q}$ scan results and PE unlikely by Wells score also had negative D-dimer tests and negative leg ultrasonography, the outcomes at 3 months were similar to those of patients who had negative CTPA and negative leg USG. This suggests that indeterminate results on $\dot{V}/\dot{Q}$ scans are not dead ends but can be clinically useful if incorporated into an appropriate algorithm.

Echocardiography

Echocardiography is usually not considered a diagnostic modality for pulmonary embolism, although a sensitivity of 60% to 80% and a specificity of 95% to 100% have been reported with transesophageal echocardiogram.[25] Transthoracic echocardiography is more commonly used during workup of pulmonary embolism and is mainly used to detect the presence of right ventricular dysfunction. In hemodynamically unstable patients who are believed to have a PE, this finding defines the PE as massive and is an indication for thrombolysis.

Diagnostic Algorithms

The diagnostic algorithms used in two prospective studies, the Christopher study[9] and the PIOPED II study,[22] have been validated by the favorable outcomes observed in these studies. However, these algorithms might not be universally applicable. Both strategies were validated in studies that were primarily composed of outpatients, had a low-to-moderate incidence of PE, and had a low incidence of persistent thrombogenic risk factors. This might not be appropriate in the hospitalized, the critically ill, and other groups not represented in the study. The PIOPED II investigators synthesized available evidence and expert opinion to recommend an algorithm organized by the pretest clinical risk category (Figs. 1 to 3).[23]

TREATMENT

Lifestyle Modification

Patients with PE and those with lower-limb DVT are often advised bed rest for the initial few days of therapy. For patients with DVT, there is no evidence of a beneficial effect of absolute bed rest or increased risk of adverse events with mobilization.[26] Early mobilization with compression stockings may be helpful in decreasing the incidence of post-thrombotic syndrome.[26] Absolute bed rest might not be mandatory for every patient with PE as well, given data from historical cohort studies in patients with PE and the large fraction of patients with symptomatic DVT who have occult PE. However, the effect of PE on the patient's cardiopulmonary status needs to be assessed while making the decision for mobilization given the increased incidence of VTE in older patients who often have preexisting cardiopulmonary disease.

Medical Options

Current treatment regimens in PE are derived from trials evaluating different anticoagulation drugs and regimens in patients with DVT.

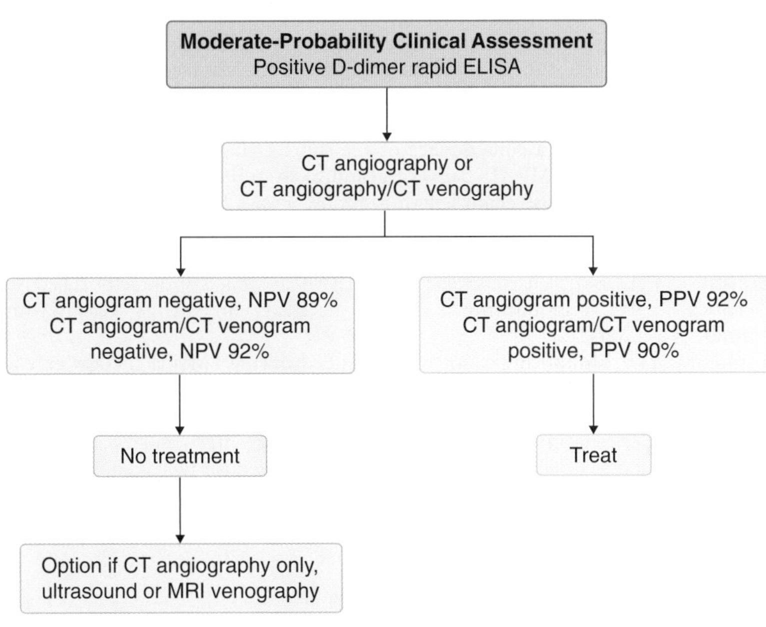

Figure 2 Diagnostic algorithm for investigation of pulmonary embolism when the pretest probability is moderate. Pretest probability is assessed by modified Wells score (see Table 1). CT, computed tomography; MRI, magnetic resonance imaging; NPV, negative predictive value; PPV, positive predictive value. *Reproduced from Stein PD, Woodard PK, Weg JG, et al: Diagnostic pathways in acute pulmonary embolism: Recommendations of the PIOPED II investigators. Am J Med 2006;119:1048-1055.*

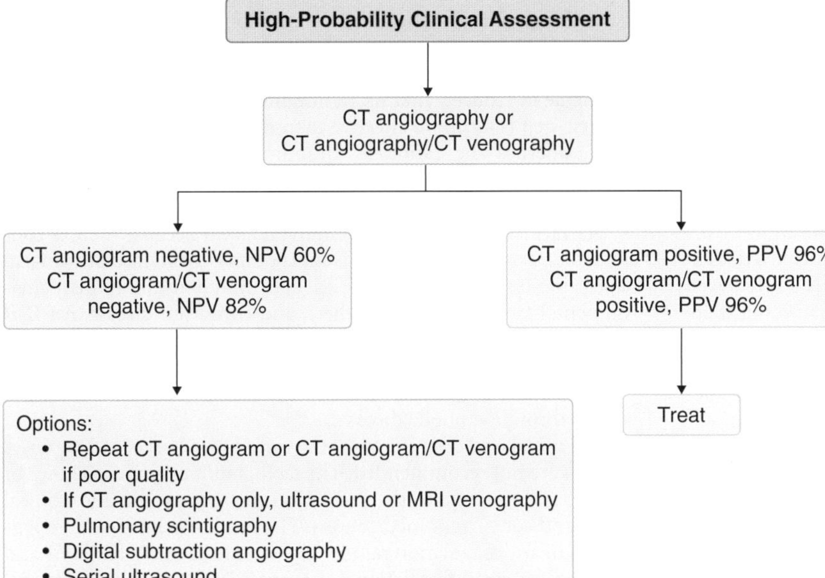

Figure 3 Diagnostic algorithm for investigation of pulmonary embolism when the pretest probability is high. Pretest probability is assessed by modified Wells score (see Table 1). CT, computed tomography; MRI, magnetic resonance imaging; NPV, negative predictive value; PPV, positive predictive value. *Reproduced from Stein PD, Woodard PK, Weg JG, et al: Diagnostic pathways in acute pulmonary embolism: Recommendations of the PIOPED II investigators. Am J Med 2006;119:1048-1055.*

This approach is appropriate because both DVT and PE are parts of the spectrum of VTE. However, regardless of the similarity in the pathogenic mechanisms, the occurrence of PE is still a signal event. Patients who present with PE are more likely to die of recurrent VTE than patients who present with DVT. Whether this is because of an intrinsic difference in disease mechanisms or a difference in the comorbidities inherent in patient populations with PE is unknown.[27]

Treatment should be started promptly in VTE disease. Failure to achieve rapid and full anticoagulation in the first 24 hours is associated with an increase in long-term (months) recurrence rates for VTE.[28] Thus, treatment regimens for PE, except in special circumstances (e.g., renal failure, pregnancy), should include prompt administration of an adequate dose of unfractionated heparin (UFH) or low-molecular-weight heparin (LMWH) and concurrent administration of oral warfarin. Monitoring activated partial thromboplastin time (aPTT) for UFH and prothrombin time (usually expressed as the international normalized ratio [INR]) for the anticoagulant activity of warfarin is essential for achieving and maintaining safe and effective anticoagulation. Because of the predictable pharmacokinetics of LMWH, and consequently the ability to give weight-based doses without having to monitor coagulation parameters, LMWH is advocated as first-line therapy for DVT and nonmassive PE in current guidelines.

Heparin

Heparin acts mainly through enhancing the activity of antithrombin III (ATIII). Heparin binding to ATIII induces conformational changes that accelerate the intrinsic slow thrombin inhibitory activity of ATIII. The transformed ATIII then binds and inhibits factors within the coagulation cascade, including thrombin, as well as other activated factors including Xa, IXa, XIa, and XIIa. Inhibition of thrombin activity also results in inhibition of thrombin-induced platelet activation and factors V and VIII.

Heparin is a heterogeneous mixture of different chain lengths, and only about one third of the chains possess the binding site, a specific pentasaccharide sequence, for ATIII. The remainder of the chain length, irrespective of the presence of the pentasaccharide sequence, binds nonspecifically to various proteins in the coagulation cascade. The inhibition of factor Xa differs in that the only requirement for factor Xa inhibition is the presence of the pentasaccharide sequence that binds to ATIII. These binding characteristics have led to the development of drugs that are effective in Xa inhibition but that do not inhibit other factors (fondaparinaux) or inhibit them weakly (LMWH). Inhibition of other clotting factors requires, in addition to the pentasaccharide sequence, the bridging action resulting from nonspecific interaction of the remainder of the heparin chain with domains on the clotting factors. The nonspecific charge-dependent interactions of heparin are responsible for most of the limitations and adverse effects of heparin.

Unfractionated heparin (UFH) is typically used in venous thromboembolic disease in an inpatient setting to achieve rapid anticoagulation. The rapid achievement of adequate anticoagulation during the acute phase of VTE prevents recurrent DVT and also averts the potential prothrombotic effects of warfarin during the first few days of administration. LMWH is recommended over UFH for patients with VTE except for patients with submassive PE or renal failure, patients scheduled for invasive procedures, and patients who are critically ill and in whom rapid, reliable cessation of the anticoagulant effect is important.

Intravenous administration of a weight-based loading dose (80 U/kg) and maintenance dose (18 U/kg) of UFH is recommended for achieving adequate anticoagulation rapidly. UFH can also be administered subcutaneously for full therapeutic anticoagulation, although this route is much less commonly used. Adequate anticoagulation with heparin results when a plasma concentration of 0.3 to 0.7 IU/L (as measured by factor Xa inhibition) is achieved. Historically, an aPTT level 1.5 to 2.5 times the control value was believed to represent adequate anticoagulation with heparin. However, there is wide variability in the actual level of anticoagulation achieved for a given aPTT range depending on the reagent used for the aPTT test. This makes it imperative that aPTT values that correlate with adequate anticoagulation (as defined by factor Xa inhibition) be established for the particular reagent used in the local laboratory, and the heparin protocol used in any institution must be tailored to reflect variations in aPTT. aPTT reflects the level of factor IIa inhibition more closely than the level of factor Xa inhibition.

aPTT values are obtained 6 hours after initiation of therapy and 6 hours after dose changes. These values are best used in conjunction with a protocol to adjust heparin dosage until aPTT values are in the desired range (as described earlier). Values are obtained daily thereafter unless warranted otherwise by the clinical status.

Adverse effects of heparin include bleeding and heparin-induced thrombocytopenia, Osteoporosis can occur with long-term use. Skin lesions, hypoaldosteronism, and hypersensitivity reactions are rare complications. Bleeding while on UFH is usually managed by discontinuing heparin administration; protamine reverses the anticoagulant effect of heparin, but it is infrequently used except in special settings.

Low-Molecular-Weight Heparins

LMWHs are derived from heparin by enzymatic or chemical depolymerization; different methods yield different mixtures of heparin chains. The different LMWHs are therefore not interchangeable. Depolymerization yields shorter chain lengths with reduced binding to specific proteins (coagulation factors, plasma proteins), macrophages, endothelial cells, platelets, and osteoblasts and is responsible for the superior pharmacokinetic and adverse-effect profile of LMWH as compared with UFH. As for UFH, a third of the LMWH chains contain the specific pentasaccharide sequence that binds to ATIII. As a consequence of the shorter chain length, only 25% to 50% of LMWH chains can bind to thrombin, in comparison with UFH, whose chain length is almost always long enough to bind to thrombin. This results in a greater anti-Xa to anti-IIa activity for LMWH, as compared with UFH, where the ratio is 1 : 1. Anti–factor Xa assay is used instead of aPTT (which reflects anti–factor IIa activity) if monitoring is deemed necessary in patients treated with LMWH.

Monitoring is not recommended during LMWH therapy except in special circumstances such as renal failure and in obese patients. Anti–factor Xa activity usually peaks 4 hours after administration. The optimum level of anti–factor Xa activity is not established; a range of 0.6 to 1.0 IU/L has been advocated for twice-daily administration with enoxaparin and nadroparin (cf. therapeutic range for UFH: 0.3-0.7 IU/L) for treatment of venous thromboembolism.

Warfarin

Warfarin is the drug most commonly used for long term-anticoagulation. Vitamin K is reduced in a two-step process from an epoxide form to a reduced form (vitamin KH_2), which then takes part in a reaction that carboxylates (γ-carboxylation) clotting factors and yields the epoxide form again. Carboxylation is necessary for optimal activity of clotting factors II, VII, IX, and X and of protein C and protein S. Warfarin inhibits both of the enzymes that convert vitamin K epoxide to reduced vitamin K; inhibition of the enzyme catalyzing the first step is far more effective than inhibition of the second step. This underlies the rationale for administering vitamin K_1 (the product of the first step) exogenously to counter excessive anticoagulation produced by warfarin.

Warfarin dosage needs to be individualized because there is considerable variation in the effectiveness of any given dose of warfarin depending on genetic factors (race and inherited mutations), environmental factors (drugs and diet), and comorbid disease. An INR of 2.0 to 3.0 is recommended as the target for anticoagulation with warfarin for VTE. Higher INR ranges result in more bleeding complications, and lower INR targets result in greater recurrences of venous thromboembolic disease.

The initial oral dose is 5 to 10 mg once a day. Large loading doses (20 mg) are not recommended. The factors influencing the choice of the initial dose include the indication, patient profile and clinical status, and concurrent medications. The need to achieve a therapeutic level of anticoagulation rapidly is greater for acute VTE (DVT and PE) than for atrial fibrillation, because the risk for short-term and long-term recurrences increases with delay in appropriate therapy. Initiating anticoagulation with a warfarin dose of less than 5 mg may be optimal for inpatients, the elderly, and patients with organ failure.[29] Irrespective of the initial dose, dosing algorithms, if applicable to the patient population in question, are useful in achieving early and stable anticoagulation.[30]

Length of Anticoagulation

The duration of anticoagulation depends mainly on the inciting risk factor. When the risk factor is transient, anticoagulation is recommended for 3 months after a first episode of PE. When the PE is believed to be secondary to idiopathic DVT, anticoagulation is recommended for 6 to 12 months, and indefinite anticoagulation may be considered depending on cardiopulmonary status and patient characteristics. For patients with PE in the context of malignancy, LMWH is recommended for 3 to 6 months and probably indefinitely or until resolution of the malignancy.

Thrombolytics

Thrombolytics are used to lyse existing thrombi and relieve the hemodynamic effects of PE. Massive PE is an accepted indication for thrombolytics. Thrombolytics are not indicated in patients with PE without evidence of RV dysfunction. Other indications (submassive PE) are controversial and under study.

Thrombolectomy

Nonmedical interventions for PE include catheter-based embolectomy and surgical embolectomy. These are limited to those who are hemodynamically compromised and are not able to receive standard treatment (thrombolysis). Experiences with these modalities are limited, and there is no consensus on indications or on patient groups who would benefit.

Guidelines

The American College of Chest Physicians issued a revised version of evidence-based guidelines for the management and diagnosis of venous thromboembolic disease in 2008. The guidelines provide summary recommendations, a comprehensive review of the evidence base for these recommendations, and the areas of uncertainty that remain. The material presented in this chapter draws on this excellent resource in many areas, especially in areas relating to drug pharmacology and pharmacokinetics. There are no substantial deviations from the management perspectives outlined in the guidelines.

Summary

- Pulmonary embolism is one manifestation of venous thromboembolic disease and usually develops from a venous thrombus involving the proximal lower-limb veins.
- The systematic use of clinical prediction rules in conjunction with D-dimer testing and computed tomography helps in the diagnosis of PE.
- Rapid and effective anticoagulation is the mainstay in the management of PE.
- Low-molecular-weight heparin (for rapid short-term anticoagulation) and warfarin (for oral long-term anticoagulation) are currently recommended. A target INR of 2.0 to 3.0 is recommended. The duration of anticoagulation depends on the underlying risk factors.

Suggested Readings

American College of Chest Physicians Consensus Committee on Pulmonary Embolism: Opinions regarding the diagnosis and management of venous thromboembolic disease. Chest 1998;113;499-504.

Anderson FA Jr, Spencer FA: Risk factors for venous thromboembolism. Circulation 2003;107:I9-I16.

Antithrombotic Therapy for Venous Thromboembolic Disease: American College of Chest Physicians evidence-based clinical practice guidelines (8th edition) Chest 2008;133:454S-545S. Individual guidelines available for download from http://www.chestjournal.org/cgi/content/abstract/133/6_suppl/454S (accessed March 20, 2009).

Chunilal SD, Eikelboom JW, Attia J, et al: Does this patient have pulmonary embolism? JAMA 2003;290:2849-2858.

Goldhaber SZ: Pulmonary embolism. N Engl J Med 1998;339:93-104.

Goodacre S, Sutton AJ, Sampson FC: Meta-analysis: The value of clinical assessment in the diagnosis of deep venous thrombosis. Ann Intern Med 2005;143:129-139.

Kearon C: Natural history of venous thromboembolism. Circulation 2003;107:I22-I30.

Stein PD, Fowler SE, Goodman LR, et al: Multidetector computed tomography for acute pulmonary embolism. N Engl J Med 2006;354:2317-2327.

Stein PD, Woodard PK, Weg JG, et al: Diagnostic pathways in acute pulmonary embolism: Recommendations of the PIOPED II Investigators. Radiology 2007;242:15-21.

Wells PS, Rodger M: Diagnosis of pulmonary embolism: When is imaging needed? Clin Chest Med 2003;24:13-28.

References

For a complete list of references, log onto www.expertconsult.com.

Pulmonary Function Testing

Thomas R. Gildea and *Kevin McCarthy*

Pulmonary function testing has come into widespread use since the 1970s. This has been facilitated by several developments.[1,2] Because of miniaturization and advances in computer technology, microprocessor devices have become portable and automated with fewer moving parts. Testing equipment, patient maneuvers, and testing techniques have become widely standardized throughout the world through the efforts of professional societies. Widely accepted normative parameters have been established.

DEFINITION

Pulmonary function testing is a valuable tool for evaluating the respiratory system, representing an important adjunct to the patient history, various lung imaging studies, and invasive testing such as bronchoscopy and open-lung biopsy. Insight into underlying pathophysiology can often be gained by comparing the measured values for pulmonary function tests obtained on a patient at any particular point with normative values derived from population studies. The *percentage of predicted normal* is used to grade the severity of the abnormality. Practicing clinicians must become familiar with pulmonary function testing because it is often used in clinical medicine for evaluating respiratory symptoms such as dyspnea and cough, for stratifying preoperative risk, and for diagnosing common diseases such as asthma and chronic obstructive pulmonary disease.

Pulmonary function tests (PFTs) is a generic term used to indicate a battery of studies or maneuvers that may be performed using standardized equipment to measure lung function. PFTs can include simple screening spirometry, formal lung volume measurement, diffusing capacity for carbon monoxide, and arterial blood gases. These studies may collectively be referred to as a *complete pulmonary function survey*.

Before a spirogram can be meaningfully interpreted, one needs to inspect the graphic data (the volume-time curve and the flow-volume loop) to ascertain whether the study meets certain well-defined acceptability and reproducibility standards. Tests that fail to meet these standards can provide useful information about minimum levels of lung function, but, in general, they should be interpreted cautiously. The interpretive strategy usually involves establishing a pattern of abnormality (obstructive, restrictive, or mixed), grading the severity of the abnormality, and assessing trends over time. Various algorithms are available. Automated spirometry systems usually have built-in software that can generate a preliminary interpretation, especially for spirometry; however, algorithms for other pulmonary function studies are not as well established and necessitate appropriate clinical correlation and physician oversight.

PHYSIOLOGY

Basic concepts of normal pulmonary physiology that are involved in pulmonary function testing include mechanics (airflows and lung volumes), the ventilation-perfusion interrelationship, diffusion and gas exchange, and respiratory muscle or bellows strength. Ventilation is the process of generating the forces necessary to move the appropriate volumes of air from the atmosphere to the alveoli to meet the metabolic needs of the body under a variety of conditions. Simply, the contraction of the diaphragm and other inspiratory muscles expands the thorax, generating negative pressure in the pleural space. One component of pleural pressure, known as *transpulmonary pressure,* causes a flow of air into the airways and lungs (inspiration). When the transpulmonary and alveolar pressures equilibrate, airflow stops, the inspiratory muscles relax, and the lungs and chest wall elastic recoil raise pleural pressure, forcing air out of the lungs (expiration).

With a forced exhalation, the early portion of the spirometry maneuver is characterized by high flows, mostly from large airways, and the latter portion is characterized by low flows with a larger contribution from the smaller airways.[3] Forced inspiration is generally not flow limited and is a function of overall muscular effort. In contrast, a variety of factors affect expiratory flow, including the overall driving pressure, airway diameter, overall distensibility of the lungs and chest wall, dynamic airway collapse (from a flow-limiting segment), and muscular effort. The overall driving pressure is the pressure head at the alveolus, or P_{ALV}, which is the difference between pleural pressure (P_{PL}) and negative transpulmonary pressure (P_{TP}). So:

$$P_{ALV} = P_{PL} + P_{TP}$$

The mechanism for the maximal expiratory airflow limitation seen in normal airways results from the gradual drop in pressure inside the conducting airways from the alveoli to the mouth, creating a transmural pressure gradient with the pleural pressure. This can cause dynamic airway compression and narrowing or closure of airways that have lost elastic recoil support from the lung parenchyma.

BATTERY OF MANEUVERS

Pulmonary function studies use a variety of maneuvers to measure and record the properties of four lung components. These include the airways (large and small), lung parenchyma (alveoli, interstitium), pulmonary vasculature, and the bellows-pump mechanism. Various diseases can affect each of these components.

Spirometry

Spirometry is the most commonly used lung function screening study. It generally should be the clinician's first option, with other studies being reserved for specific indications. Most patients can easily perform spirometry when coached by an appropriately trained technician or other health care provider. The test can be administered in the ambulatory setting, physician's office, emergency department, or inpatient setting. The indications for spirometry are diverse (Box 1). It can be used for diagnosing and monitoring respiratory symptoms and disease, for preoperative risk stratification, and as a tool in epidemiologic and other research studies.

Spirometry requires a voluntary maneuver in which a seated patient inhales maximally from tidal respiration to total lung capacity and then rapidly exhales to the fullest extent until no further volume is exhaled at residual volume[3] (Figs. 1 and 2). The maneuver may be performed in a forceful manner to generate a forced vital capacity (FVC) or in a more relaxed manner to generate a slow vital capacity (SVC). In normal persons, the inspiratory vital capacity, the expiratory SVC, and expiratory FVC are essentially equal. However, in patients with obstructive small airways disease, the expiratory SVC is generally higher than the FVC. This difference might, however, be due partly to the difficulty in maintaining a *maximum* expiratory

Box 1 Indications for Spirometry

Diagnostic

To evaluate symptoms

- Chest pain
- Cough
- Dyspnea
- Orthopnea
- Phlegm production
- Wheezing

To evaluate signs

- Chest deformity
- Cyanosis
- Diminished breath sounds
- Expiratory slowing
- Overinflation
- Unexplained crackles

To evaluate abnormal laboratory tests

- Abnormal chest radiographs
- Hypercapnia
- Hypoxemia
- Polycythemia

To measure the effect of disease on pulmonary function

To screen persons at risk for pulmonary diseases

- Smokers
- Persons in occupations with exposures to injurious substances

  Some routine physical examinations
- To assess preoperative risk
- To assess prognosis (lung transplant, etc.)
- To assess health status before enrollment in strenuous physical activity programs

Monitoring

To assess therapeutic interventions

- Bronchodilator therapy
- Steroid treatment for asthma, interstitial lung disease, etc.
- Management of congestive heart failure
- Other (antibiotics in cystic fibrosis, etc.)

To describe the course of diseases affecting lung function

- Pulmonary diseases
- Obstructive small airway diseases
- Interstitial lung diseases
- Cardiac diseases
- Congestive heart failure
- Neuromuscular diseases
- Guillain-Barré syndrome

To monitor persons in occupations with exposure to injurious agents

To monitor for adverse reactions to drugs with known pulmonary toxicity

Evaluation of Disability or Impairment

To assess patients as part of a rehabilitation program

- Medical
- Industrial
- Vocational

To assess risks as part of an insurance evaluation

To assess persons for legal reasons

- Social Security or other government compensation programs
- Personal injury lawsuits
- Other

Public Health

Epidemiologic surveys

Comparison of health status of populations living in different environments

Validation of subjective complaints in occupational or environmental settings

Derivation of reference equations

Box 2 Types of Spirometers

Volume

Bellows
Rolling seal
Water
Dry

Flow Sensing (Pneumotach)

Fleisch
Screen
Hot-wire
Turbine

Adapted from Miller WF, Scacci R, Gast LR: Laboratory Evaluation of Pulmonary Function. Philadelphia, JB Lippincott, 1987.

effort for an extended time period without experiencing dizziness or lightheadedness.

A spirometer, including the waterless, rolling seal type, and Stead-Wells water seal type is an instrument that directly measures the volume of air displaced or measures airflow by a flow-sensing device, such as a pneumotachometer or a tube containing a fixed resistance to flow (Box 2).[2] Today, most clinical pulmonary function testing laboratories use a microprocessor-driven pneumotachometer to measure air flow directly and then to mathematically derive volume.

A spirogram is a graphic representation of bulk air movement depicted as a volume-time tracing or as a flow-volume tracing. Values generated from a simple spirogram provide important graphic and numeric data regarding the mechanical properties of the lungs, including airflow (forced expiratory volume in 1 second [FEV_1] along with other timed volumes) and exhaled lung volume (FVC or SVC). The measurement is typically expressed in liters for volumes or in liters per second for flows and is corrected for body temperature and pressure of gas that is saturated with water vapor. Data from a spirogram provide important clues to help distinguish obstructive pulmonary disorders that typically reduce airflow, such as asthma and emphysema, from restrictive disorders that typically reduce total lung volumes, including pulmonary fibrosis and neuromuscular disease.

A number of spirometry standards have been developed over the years. The American Thoracic Society standardization guidelines for acceptability and reproducibility criteria are shown in Box 3.[4] A well-trained pulmonary function technician usually coaches the patient through the session until the demonstrated reproducibility of key parameters suggests the results represent the best possible measure of lung function at that time.

Forced Expiratory Volume in 1 Second

The FEV_1 is the most widely used parameter to measure the mechanical properties of the lungs. In normal persons, the FEV_1 accounts for the greatest part of the exhaled volume from a spirometric maneuver and reflects mechanical properties of the large and the medium-sized airways. In a normal flow-volume loop, the FEV_1 occurs at about 75% to 85% of the FVC. This parameter is reduced in obstructive and restrictive disorders. In obstructive diseases, FEV_1 is reduced disproportionately to the FVC, reducing the FEV_1/FVC ratio below the lower limit of normal and indicates airflow limitation. In restrictive disorders, the FEV_1, FVC, and total lung capacity are all reduced, and the FEV_1/FVC ratio is normal or even elevated.

Forced Vital Capacity

FVC is a measure of lung volume and is usually reduced in diseases that cause the lungs to be smaller. Such processes are generally termed *restrictive* and can include disorders of the lung parenchyma, such as pulmonary fibrosis, or of the bellows, including kyphosco-

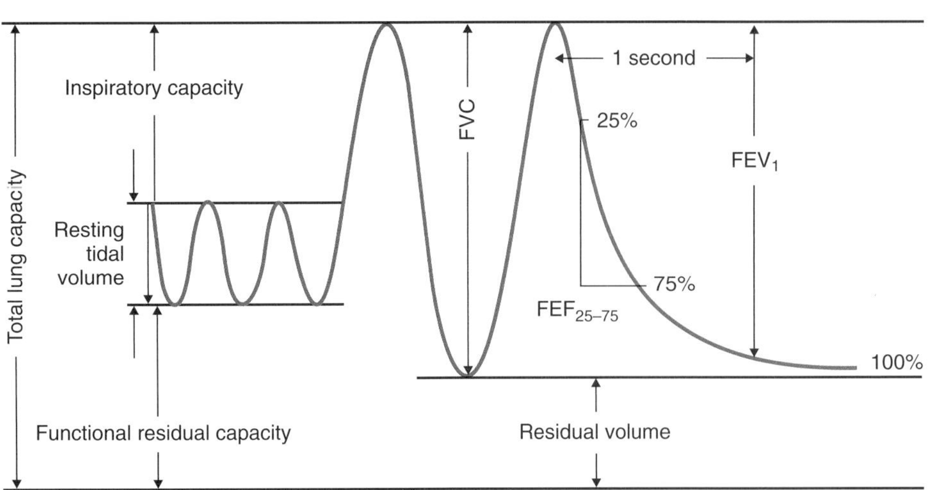

Figure 1 **Spirogram with volumes and measurements.** FEF_{25-75}, forced expiratory flow at 25%-75% vital capacity; FEV_1, forced expiratory volume in 1 second; FVC, forced vital capacity. *(Adapted from Siberry GK, Iannone R (eds) The Johns Hopkins Hospital Harriet Lane Handbook, 15th ed. St. Louis: Mosby, 1999.)*

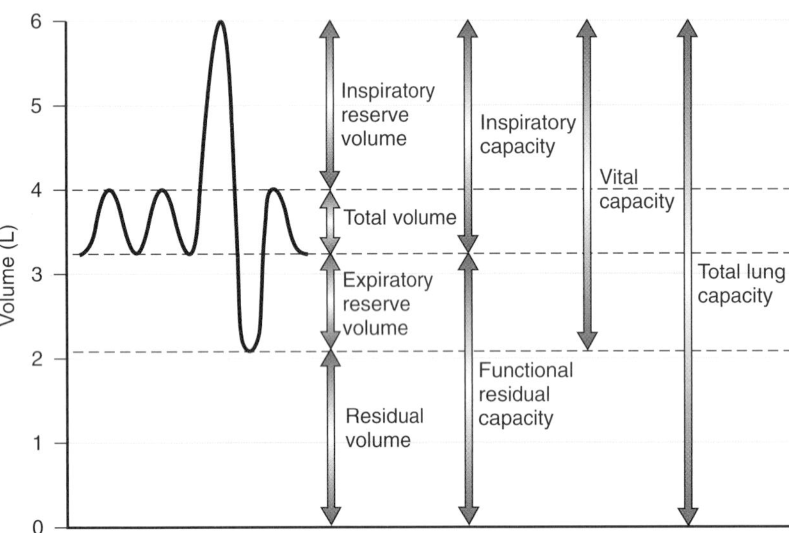

Figure 2 **Normal spirogram and subdivisions of lung volume.** Volume describes the smallest subdivisions that do not overlap, and capacity describes the combinations of these volumes. *(Adapted from Albert RK, Spiro SG, Jett JR (eds): Comprehensive Respiratory Medicine. St Louis: Mosby, 1999, p 43.)*

liosis, neuromuscular disease, and pleural effusion. However, a reduction in FVC is not always due to reduced total volumes and can occur in the setting of large lungs hyperinflated due to severe airflow obstruction and air trapping, as in emphysema. In this setting, the FVC is decreased due to reduced airflow, air trapping, and increased residual volume, a phenomenon referred to as *pseudorestriction.* Reduced FVC can occur despite a normal or increased total lung volume. Therefore, FVC is not a reliable indicator of total lung capacity or restriction, especially in the setting of airflow obstruction. The overall accuracy of the FVC for restriction is about 60%.[5]

Volume-Time Tracing and Flow-Volume Loop

The volume-time tracing and flow-volume loop ascertain the technical adequacy of a maneuver and therefore the quality of the data (see Box 3) as well as identifying the anatomic location of airflow obstruction. The volume-time tracing is most useful in assessing whether the end-of-test criteria have been met, whereas the flow-volume loop is most valuable in evaluating the start-of-test criteria. The technique of back-extrapolation of the start of the test to establish a zero time point on the volume-time tracing has been carefully defined and provides a uniform start point for timed measurements. It corrects for delayed or hesitant starts that might otherwise be mistaken for a falsely reduced FEV_1. Standards for acceptability define limits for the degree of hesitation that can still yield an acceptable FEV_1 (see Box 3). The loss of elastic recoil characteristic of emphysema results in airflow limitation during the maximal forced exhalation that may be grossly underestimated if the patient applies less than maximal expiratory force. Such efforts may still be deemed acceptable using the criteria of extrapolated volume. The time to peak flow appears to have excellent usefulness in identifying such efforts in this population (time to peak flow will be greater than 120 msec when effort is submaximal), but it is not yet a recommended acceptability criterion (Fig. 3).

The shape of the flow-volume loop can indicate the location of airflow limitation, such as the large upper airways or smaller distal airways (Fig. 4). With common obstructive airflow disorders, such as asthma or emphysema, the disease generally affects the expiratory limb and can reduce the effort-dependent peak expiratory flow as well as subsequent airflows that are independent of effort. The descending limb of the expiratory loop is typically concave. In contrast, several unusual anatomic disorders that narrow the large airways can produce a variety of patterns of truncation or flattening of either one limb of the loop (variable upper airway obstruction) or both limbs of the loop (fixed upper airway obstruction).

Additional Tests

A variety of parameters selectively reflect small airways.[6] These include measures of flow from a spirogram, such as the maximal

Box 3 Acceptability and Reproducibility Criteria for Spirograms

Acceptability Criteria

Free from artifacts

- Cough or glottis closure during the first second of exhalation
- Early termination or cutoff
- Variable effort
- Leak
- Obstructed mouthpiece

Good start

- Extrapolated volume is <5% of FVC or 0.15 L, whichever is greater

  or

- Time to PEF is <120 ms (optional until further information is available)

Satisfactory exhalation

- 6 sec of exhalation and/or a plateau in the volume-time curve

  or

- Reasonable duration or a plateau in the volume-time curve

  or

- The subject cannot or should not continue to exhale

Repeatability Criteria

After three acceptable spirograms have been obtained, apply the following tests.

- Are the two largest FVCs within 0.2 L of each other?
- Are the two largest FEV_1s within 0.2 L of each other?

If both of these criteria are met, the test session may be concluded.
If both of these criteria are not met, continue testing until:

- Both of the criteria are met with analysis of additional acceptable spirograms

  or

- A total of eight tests have been performed

  or

- Save a minimum of three best maneuvers

Adapted from American Thoracic Society: Single-breath carbon monoxide diffusing capacity (transfer factor). Recommendations for a standard technique—1995 update. Am J Respir Crit Care Med 1995;152:2185-2198.

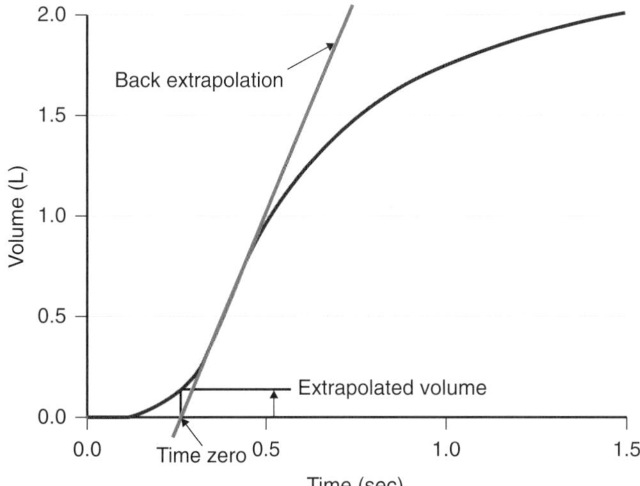

Figure 3 Spirogram illustrating the back extrapolation method of determining time zero. *(Adapted from Miller MR, Hankinson J, Brusasco V, et al: American Thoracic Society/European Respiratory Society Task Force: Standardization of spirometry. Eur Resp J 2005;26:319-338.)*

midexpiratory flow (MMEF) or forced expiratory flow at 25% to 75% vital capacity (FEF_{25-75}). The FEF_{25-75} is the slope of the spirogram between the 25th and the 75th percentiles of an FVC maneuver. Normal values and lower limits of normal for the FEF_{25-75}% have been published.[7] Care must be taken to use the statistically defined lower limit of normal and avoid assessing this parameter using the percentage of predicted normal value because the lower limit of normal falls significantly with age.

The closing volume from a single-breath N_2 test and frequency-dependent dynamic lung compliance also can be used to detect small airways disease. It is believed that small airways dysfunction can precede and exist separately in the setting of a normal FEV_1 and FVC. The hypothesis is that smokers might have isolated small airways dysfunction and that there is an obligatory passage through a silent period during which only sensitive tests are impaired. However, there is a greater coefficient of variation for these tests of small airways function. In addition, because these measures are vitally influenced by lung volumes, they cannot be interpreted separately without volume correction. Therefore, in practice, these tests have not been particularly helpful to practicing clinicians, and the American Thoracic Society does not recommend their use for detecting small airways disease.[6] Normal values for a new parameter to assess small airways function, the FEV_3/FVC ratio, are available, but this parameter has not yet been sufficiently validated.[8]

Bronchoprovocation

To define whether nonspecific airway hyperreactivity is a mechanism for atypical chest symptoms of unclear origin, inhalational challenge tests are often used in the pulmonary function laboratory.[9-11] Methacholine and histamine are the agents most often used with this procedure, although other agents may also be useful. Methacholine is considered safe, can be used in outpatient clinics, and has no systemic side effects.

When the baseline spirogram is relatively normal, inhalational challenge may be performed by aerosolizing progressive concentrations of methacholine by a dosimeter. This is typically performed as a five-stage procedure with five different increasing concentrations. After each stage, the patient performs a spirometry. When there is a 20% reduction in the FEV_1, the test is terminated and is considered positive for airway hyperreactivity. The provocative concentration dosage level of the inhalational agent required to produce a 20% reduction in the FEV_1 is labeled PC_{20FEV1}. If the drop in FEV_1 is less than 20% after five stages of this procedure, the challenge test is considered negative for airway hyperreactivity. A PC_{20FEV1} of less than 8 mg/mL suggests clinically important airway hyperreactivity.

Bronchial hyperreactivity, as assessed by this inhalational challenge procedure, is very sensitive for the presence of active or current asthma. A positive test strongly suggests bronchial asthma. However, this test may be falsely positive in a variety of conditions, including chronic obstructive pulmonary disease, parenchymal respiratory disorders, congestive heart failure, recent upper respiratory tract infection, and allergic rhinitis. A negative inhalational challenge with methacholine or histamine has been believed to exclude active symptomatic asthma as a cause for the patient's chest symptoms; however, a recent study suggests that significant changes in another measure of airway function, specific airways conductance (SGaw), can occur during a methacholine challenge in the absence of a significant change in FEV_1. This study was duplicated in our laboratory with the same results (unpublished).

Lung Volumes

Because spirometry is an expiratory maneuver, it measures exhaled volume or vital capacity but does not measure residual volume, functional residual capacity (resting lung volume), or total lung capacity. Vital capacity is a simple measure of lung volume that is usually reduced in restrictive disorders; however, reduction in the

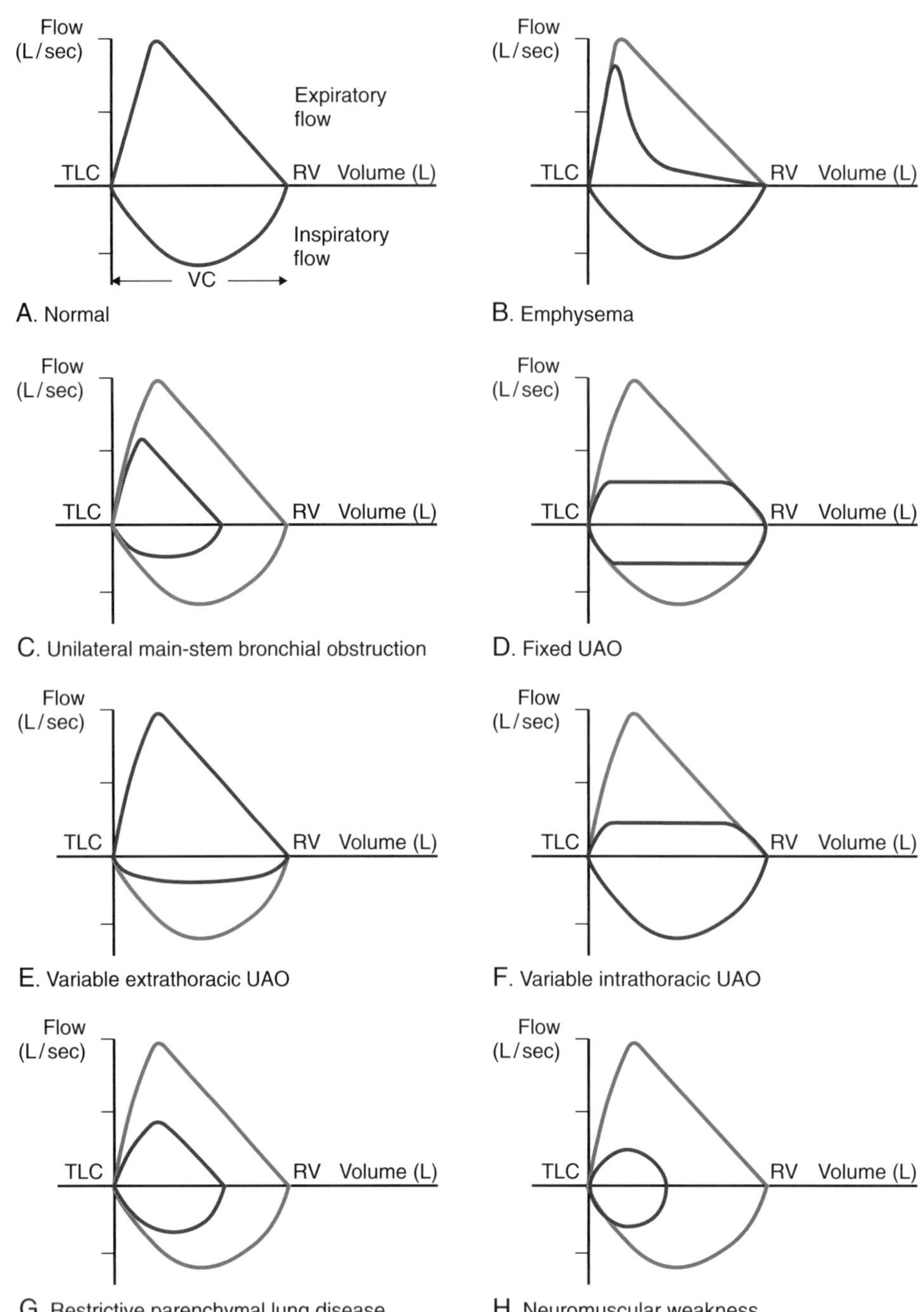

Figure 4 Appearance of flow-volume loops of various pulmonary disorders compared with normal (A). RV, residual volume; TLC, total lung capacity; UAO, upper airway obstruction;voc.

vital capacity measured during spirometry should prompt measurement of lung volumes to confirm the presence or absence of a true restrictive ventilatory disorder.

Other pulmonary function methodology is required to formally measure total lung capacity, which is derived from the addition of functional residual capacity (FRC) to inspiratory capacity obtained from spirometry.[2] FRC is usually measured by a gas dilution technique or body plethysmography. Gas dilution techniques are based on a simple principle, are widely used, and provide a good measurement of all air in the lungs that communicates with the airways. A limitation of this technique is that it does not measure air in noncommunicating bullae, and therefore it can underestimate total lung capacity, especially in patients with severe emphysema.

Gas dilution techniques use either closed-circuit helium dilution or open-circuit nitrogen washout. They are based on the inhalation of a known concentration and volume of an inert tracer gas, such as helium, followed by equilibration of 7 to 10 minutes in the closed-circuit helium dilution technique. The final exhaled helium concentration is diluted in proportion to the unknown volume of air in the patient's chest (residual volume). Usually, the patient is connected at the end-tidal position of the spirometer; therefore, the lung volume measured is FRC. In the nitrogen-washout technique, the patient breathes 100% oxygen, and all the nitrogen in the lungs is washed out. The exhaled volume and the nitrogen concentration in that volume are measured. The difference in nitrogen volume at the initial concentration and at the final exhaled concentration allows a calculation of intrathoracic volume, usually FRC.

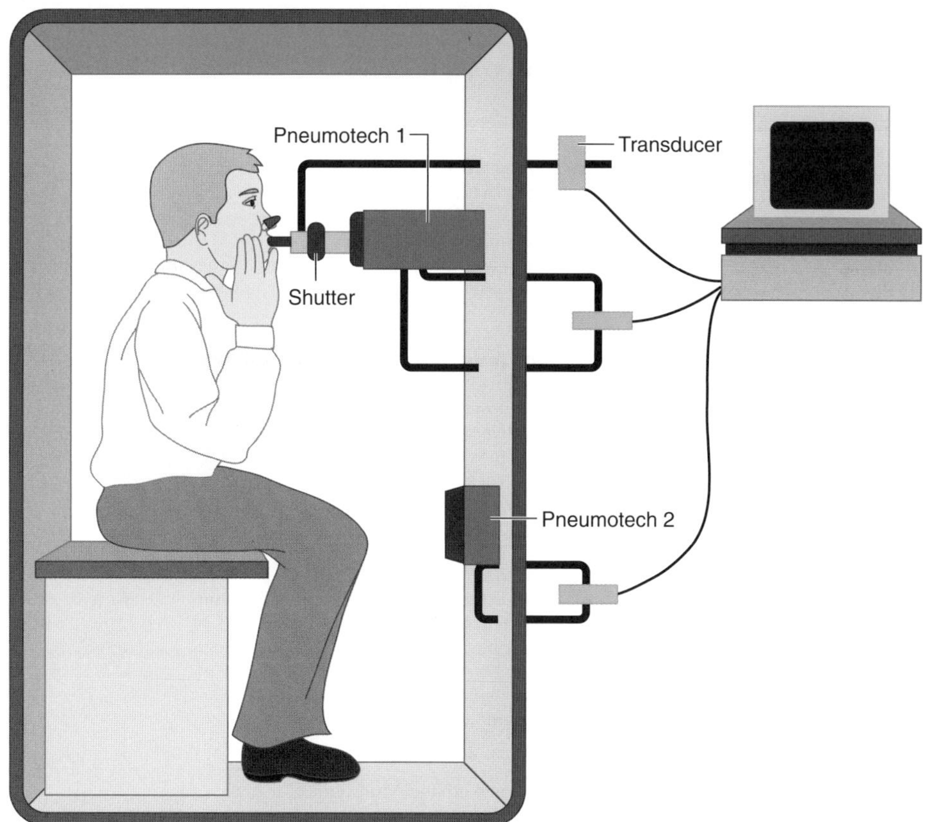

Figure 5 Schematic of a plethysmograph (body box). *(Adapted from Murray JF, Nadel JA (eds): Murray and Nadel's Textbook of Respiratory Medicine, 3rd ed. Philadelphia: WB Saunders, 2000, p 795.)*

Body plethysmography is an alterative method of measuring lung volume that takes advantage of the principle of Boyle's law, which states that the volume of gas at a constant temperature varies inversely with the pressure applied to it. The primary advantage of body plethysmography is that it can measure the total volume of air in the chest, including gas trapped in bullae. Another advantage is that this test can be performed quickly. Drawbacks include the complexity of the equipment as well as the need for a patient to sit in a small enclosed space. A patient is placed in a sitting position in a closed body box with a known volume (Fig. 5). From the FRC, the patient pants with an open glottis against a closed shutter to produce changes in the box pressure proportionate to the volume of air in the chest. The volume measured by this technique is referred to as *thoracic gas volume* (TGV) and represents the lung volume at which the shutter was closed, typically FRC.

After the FRC is measured by any of these techniques, measurement of lung subdivisions (inspiratory capacity, expiratory reserve volume, vital capacity) ensues, ideally while the patient is still on the mouthpiece. From these volumes and capacities, the residual volume and total lung capacity can be calculated.

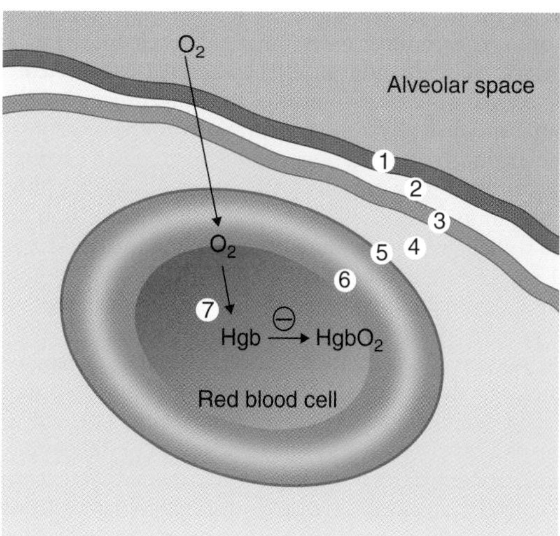

Figure 6 Schematic illustrating barriers to oxygen transport from the alveolus to the hemoglobin molecule. 1, Alveolar epithelium; 2, tissue interstitium; 3, capillary epithelium; 4, plasma layer; 5, red cell membrane; 6, red cell cytoplasm; 7, hemoglobin binding forces. Hgb, hemoglobin; $HgbO_2$, oxyhemoglobin. *(Adapted from Miller WF, Scacci R, Gast LR: Laboratory Evaluation of Pulmonary Function. Philadelphia: JB Lippincott, 1987.)*

Diffusing Capacity

Understanding gas diffusion through the lungs requires recognizing the basics of the gas exchange interface and of the various forces at work by which oxygen and carbon dioxide move by molecular diffusion. Diffusion is limited by the surface area in which diffusion occurs, capillary blood volume, hemoglobin concentration, and the properties of the lung parenchyma that separate the alveolar gas from the red blood cell with the capillary (alveolar-capillary membrane thickness and/or the presence of excess fluid in the alveoli) (Fig. 6).[2]

Because all lung volume is not exchanged, most gas exchange occurs as a function of diffusion independent of bulk flow. The role of ventilation is to reset concentration of the bulk flow of gas with the ambient air and to provide a constant gradient for oxygen and carbon dioxide. As spirometry measures the components of this bulk flow exchange, diffusing capacity measures the forces at work in molecular movement with its concentration gradient from the alveolar surface through to the hemoglobin molecule.[12] The clinical test diffusing capacity of the lung most commonly uses carbon monoxide as the tracer gas for measurement because of its high affinity for binding to the hemoglobin molecule. This property allows a better measurement of pure diffusion, such that the movement of the carbon monoxide in essence only depends on the properties of the diffusion barrier and the amount of hemoglobin. The properties of oxygen and its relatively lower affinity for hemoglobin compared with carbon monoxide also make it more perfusion dependent; thus, cardiac output can influence actual measurement of oxygen diffusion measurements.[12]

Diffusing capacity of the lung for carbon monoxide (D_LCO) is the measure of carbon monoxide transfer. In Europe, it is often called the *transfer factor of carbon monoxide,* which describes the process more accurately. D_LCO is a measure of the interaction of alveolar surface area, alveolar capillary perfusion, the physical properties of the alveolar capillary interface, capillary volume, hemoglobin concentration, and the reaction rate of carbon monoxide and hemoglobin. After a number of simplifications, the commonly used clinical tests to measure D_LCO are based on a ratio between the uptake of carbon monoxide in milliliters per minute divided by the average alveolar pressure of carbon monoxide.[13] Overall, D_LCO is expressed as the uptake of carbon monoxide in milliliters of gas at standard temperature and pressure, dry, per minute, and per millimeter of mercury driving pressure of carbon monoxide. In principle, the total diffusing capacity of the whole lung is the sum of the diffusing capacity of the pulmonary membrane component and the capacity of the pulmonary capillary blood volume.[12,13]

All methods for measuring diffusing capacity in clinical practice rely on measuring the rate of carbon monoxide uptake and estimating carbon monoxide driving pressure.[12] The most widely used and standardized technique is the single-breath breath-holding technique. In this technique, a subject inhales a known volume of test gas that usually contains 10% helium, 0.3% carbon monoxide, 21% oxygen, and the remainder nitrogen. The patient inhales the test gas and holds his or her breath for 10 seconds. The patient exhales to wash out a conservative overestimate of mechanical and anatomic dead space. Subsequently, an alveolar sample is collected. D_LCO is calculated from the total volume of the lung, breath-hold time, and the initial and final alveolar concentrations of carbon monoxide. The exhaled helium concentration is used to calculate a single-breath estimate of total lung capacity and the initial alveolar concentration of carbon monoxide. The driving pressure is assumed to be the calculated initial alveolar pressure of carbon monoxide. The calculated D_LCO is a product of the patient's single-breath estimate of total lung capacity multiplied by the rate of carbon monoxide uptake during the 10-second breath hold.

Hemoglobin concentration is a very important measurement in interpreting reductions in D_LCO. Because the hemoglobin present in the alveolar capillaries serves as a carbon monoxide sink such that oxygen and carbon monoxide are removed from dissolved gases, the concentration gradient from alveolar to arterial blood remains relatively constant in favor of dissolved gas flow toward the arterial circulation. In this way, a D_LCO may be decreased when the patient is anemic. Because the level of hemoglobin present in the blood and diffusing capacity are directly related, a correction for anemic patients (D_LCOc) is used to further delineate whether a D_LCO is decreased due to anemia or due to parenchymal or interface limitation. Recent work suggests strongly that the practice of dividing the calculated D_LCO by the single-breath estimate of total lung capacity (VA) to correct for low lung volumes (the D_L/VA ratio) can yield a large number of false-negative results, and this practice should be used cautiously if at all.

A list of conditions associated with abnormal D_LCO is listed in Box 4.[6] Diseases such as interstitial pulmonary fibrosis or any interstitial lung disease can make the D_LCO abnormal long before spirometry or volume abnormalities are present. Low D_LCO is not only an abnormality of restrictive interstitial lung disease but also can occur in the presence of emphysema. In emphysema, the lung volumes may be normal or hyperinflated; therefore, the D_L/VA is not useful. Additionally, the loss of alveolar surface area, the pathologic lesion of emphysema, is not proportionate to volume. Thus, one can understand that other obstructive entities that predominantly affect the airways can have similar spirometry, but a low D_LCO implies a loss of alveolar surface area consistent with emphysema. Unfortunately, it is not always this simple. Some forms of interstitial lung disease can have components of restrictive physiologies, such as low lung volume and clear evidence of decreased diffusion but also can have airway flow limitation. Sarcoidosis and Wegener's granulomatosis can produce an endobronchial component of airway webs or strictures, limiting flow before overt volume loss, and sufficient interstitial granulomatous inflammation to reduce the D_LCO.

On the other end of the spectrum, alveolar hemorrhage or congested capillary beds can actually increase the D_LCO. Hemoglobin trapped in proximity to alveolar gas will absorb carbon monoxide despite the actual severe limitation of gas exchange and oxygen delivery.

As for spirometry, predicted formulas have been established for D_LCO and D_L/VA. Differences in race have been observed in normal

Box 4 Processes Associated with Alterations in D_LCO

Obstructive Lung Diseases
Cystic fibrosis
Emphysema

Parenchymal Lung Diseases
Drug reactions (e.g., amiodarone, bleomycin)
Idiopathic
Interstitial lung disease
Lung disease caused by fibrogenic dusts (e.g., asbestosis)
Lung disease caused by biologic dusts (e.g., allergic alveolitis)
Sarcoidosis

Pulmonary Involvement in Systemic Diseases
Dermatomyositis-polymyositis
Inflammatory bowel disease
Mixed connective tissue disease
Progressive systemic sclerosis
Rheumatoid arthritis
Systemic lupus erythematosus
Wegener's granulomatosis

Cardiovascular Diseases
Acute and recurrent pulmonary thromboembolism
Acute myocardial infarction
Fat embolization
Mitral stenosis
Primary pulmonary hypertension
Pulmonary edema

Other
Acute and chronic ethanol ingestion
Bronchiolitis obliterans with organizing pneumonia (BOOP)
Chronic hemodialysis
Chronic renal failure
Ciagarette smoking
Cocaine freebasing
Diseases associated with anemia
Marijuana smoking

Increases In D_LCO
Diseases associated with increased pulmonary blood flow (e.g., left-to-right intracardiac shunts)
Diseases associated with polycythemia
Exercise
Pulmonary hemorrhage
D_LCO, diffusing capacity of carbon monoxide.

Table 1 Exhaled Oral Nitric Oxide

Category	Volume (ppb)		Interpretation
	Adult	Child	
Normal	5-20	5-15	Normal
High normal or increased	20-35	15-25	Moderately raised exhaled nitric oxide can indicate underlying airway inflammation Colds and influenza can transiently raise exhaled nitric oxide, and some patients have higher baseline exhaled nitric oxide levels than others
Elevated	>35	>25	Indicates ongoing eosinophilic inflammation Symptomatic patients are likely to respond to steroids Possible causes (if already on steroids) include poor compliance, recent allergen exposure, inadequate steroid dose, and poor steroid response Not all patients with high exhaled nitric oxide levels experience symptoms

subjects, and a race correction of 7% is allowed for African American patients.[6]

Exhaled Nitric Oxide

The measurement of exhaled nitric oxide as a reflection of airway inflammation is gaining rapid acceptance as a pulmonary function test. Normal values have been shown to depend on the exhaled flow rate during the measurement. The test is repeated until three reproducible results are obtained. The mean value is reported. Patients are asked to inspire to total lung capacity and then exhale into an analyzer using a steady, controlled exhaled flow rate. The test is rapid and safe and can be performed by most patients. The normal values shown in Table 1 are for a measurement flow rate of 50 mL/sec.[14]

EQUIPMENT

A detailed discussion of equipment is beyond the scope of this chapter. The American Thoracic Society has gone to great lengths to standardize and publish detailed recommendations regarding spirometry, lung volumes, and diffusing capacity.[4,12] These guidelines include the selection of equipment, important technical considerations for variability, and standardization between laboratories for the maneuver. Box 3 lists the acceptability and reproducibility criteria for an adequate spirogram. Table 2 summarizes equipment quality control as recommended by the American Thoracic Society,[4] and Box 5 lists the suggested performance standards for an office spirometer.

NORMALITY AND PREDICTED EQUATIONS

Studies from a healthy population indicate that parameters of lung function, such as FEV_1 or FVC, are affected most significantly by standing height, age, gender, race, and, to a lesser extent, weight.[7,15-21]

Table 2 Equipment Quality Control Summary

Test	Minimum Interval	Action
Volume	Daily	3-L syringe check
Leak	Daily	3 cm H_2O constant pressure for 1 min
Linearity	Quarterly Weekly (flow spirometers)	1-L increments with a calibrating syringe measured over the entire volume range (flow spirometers simulate several different flow ranges)
Time	Quarterly	Mechanical recorder check with stopwatch
Software	New versions	Log installation date and perform test using known subject

Adapted from American Thoracic Society: Single-breath carbon monoxide diffusing capacity (transfer factor). Recommendations for a standard technique—1995 update. Am J Respir Crit Care Med 1995;152:2185-2198.

Box 5 Performance Standards for an Office Spirometer

A volume spirometer should:

- Accumulate volume for greater than 30 sec
- Accommodate volumes of up to 7 L
- Be accurate to within 3% or 50 mL of a test volume

A flow-sensing spirometer should:

- Be able to measure flows up to 12 L/sec
- Be accurate to within 5% or 0.2 L/sec

Both need:

- Regular maintenance
- Routine checks of accuracy of the spirometer and the computer

Adapted from American Thoracic Society: Single-breath carbon monoxide diffusing capacity (transfer factor). Recommendations for a standard technique—1995 update. Am J Respir Crit Care Med 1995;152:2185-2198.

If we assume that lung function has a normal gaussian distribution, then a wide range of values may be considered normal.[1] Because there is no absolute cut-off point for what is normal in biologic systems, an arbitrary statistical approach is widely used to define the lowest 5% of the population as abnormal. Over the years, many regression equations have been generated by several investigators using different methodologies to study a variety of populations.[7,15,17] The recommendation is for clinical laboratories to choose a published reference standard that is most similar to the typical patient population at a given institution as well as the testing methods used. The most commonly used standards are those of Morris and colleagues,[19] Crapo and colleagues,[20] Knudson and colleagues,[21] and the National Health and Nutrition Examination Survey (NHANES III).[7] These reference standards are based on a cohort of normal subjects of similar age, height, and race, with *normal* being defined as persons without a history of smoking or disease that can affect lung function.

Many approaches have been developed to determine the normal range of spirometry.[6] These approaches have included using a fixed percentage of predicted (75%) and a fixed FEV_1-to-FVC ratio, (<0.70), both of these approaches have no statistical basis and are not recommended.

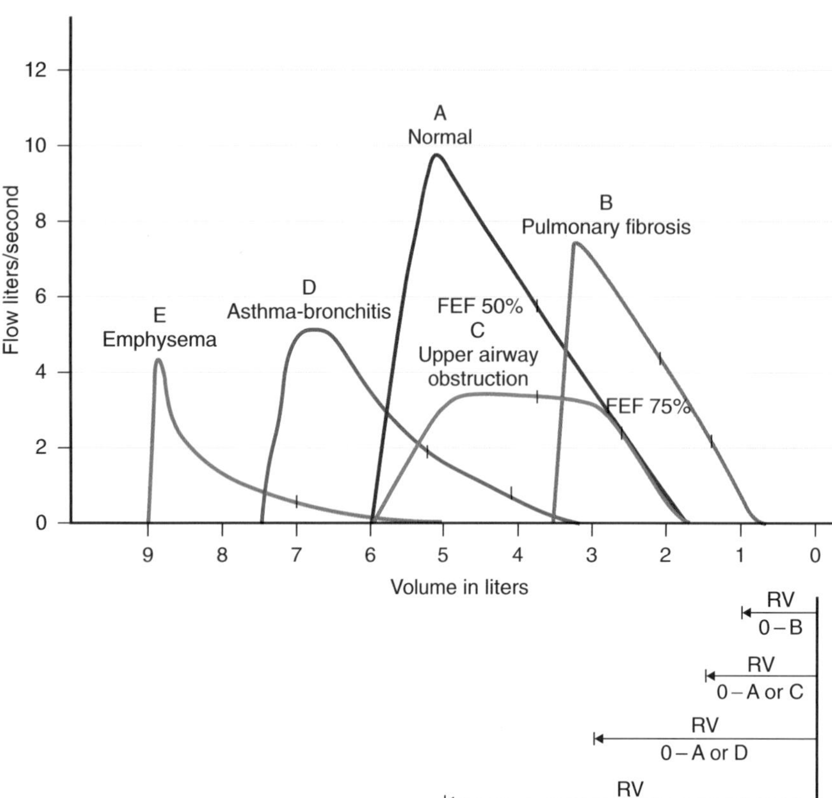

Figure 7 Flow volume profile for obstructive and restrictive respiratory disorders. FEF, forced expiratory flow. *(Adapted from Miller WF, Scacci R, Gast LR: Laboratory Evaluation of Pulmonary Function. Philadelphia: JB Lippincott, 1987.)*

The American Thoracic Society recommends using the concept of lower limit of normal by identifying the lowest 5% of a population, or patients that fall outside the limits of 1.645 standard deviations from the mean.[6] This value may be calculated by multiplying 1.645 times the standard error of estimate (1.645 × SEE).

Weight is less important as a predictor of lung function. Obese patients might have abnormal spirometry (decrease in FVC) based on the diaphragm's ability to displace the intra-abdominal fat. Body weight has little impact on intrathoracic volume.

Race plays an important role in determining normal lung function; it has been recognized that persons of different races for any given height and age have proportionately different lung volumes. Specifically, based on anthropometric differences, the lung function for African Americans is systematically lower compared with whites.[6] The American Thoracic Society recommends a 12% correction for African Americans for FEV_1, FVC, and total lung capacity. The FEV_1-to-FVC ratio in African Americans may be slightly higher compared with whites. A 7% correction for lower values is recommended for FRC and residual volume. However, race-specific reference standards are preferred.

Over time, the NHANES III reference equations will likely become the standard in most pulmonary function testing laboratories around the country.[7] The methodologies and the sample size are most robust for this dataset, as well as being representative of the American population.

CLINICAL INTERPRETIVE STRATEGIES

Spirometry

In 1991, the American Thoracic Society issued a position statement regarding interpretive strategies, which forms the basis for PFT interpretation in practice.[6] As previously discussed, spirometry is the most widely used screening test of lung function or pulmonary function studies. It is usually the first test to be performed and interpreted. Supplemental studies may be conducted as needed, such as a formal lung volume measurement, diffusing capacity, methacholine provocation test, or cardiopulmonary exercise studies. Spirometry is usually adequate for preoperative risk assessment and stratification. It is also often adequate for rotated obstructive lung disease, such as emphysema or asthma. However, when a patient's symptoms or clinical history cannot be explained by findings on spirometry or when multiple coexisting processes (e.g., dyspnea with both heart and lung disease) are present, then further testing is usually warranted.

In a simplistic way, respiratory disease can be classified as *obstructive* or *restrictive* processes. Obstructive disorders, such as emphysema or asthma, are characterized by airflow limitation, have increased lung volumes with air trapping, and have normal or increased compliance (based on pressure volume profile). In contrast, restrictive disorders such as pulmonary fibrosis are characterized by reduced lung volumes and an increase in overall stiffness of the lungs (with reduced compliance) (Fig. 7). Box 6 summarizes the common obstructive and restrictive lung diseases.

Once the technical adequacy of the spirogram has been established, the next step is to classify whether the study is normal or has an obstructive pattern, a restrictive pattern, or a mixed obstructive and restrictive pattern. Figure 8 summarizes this algorithm. In general, the measured values are compared with the lower limits of normal predicted values from one of the published studies. Airflow obstruction exists, by definition, when the ratio of FEV_1 to FVC is below the lower limits of normal. When this ratio is above the lower limits of normal, obstruction is usually excluded. However, occasionally, early termination or short expiratory time can artifactually reduce FVC and falsely normalize the FEV_1/FVC ratio to mask obstruction.

Box 6 Common Restrictive and Obstructive Lung Diseases

Common Obstructive Lung Diseases
Asthma
Asthmatic bronchitis
Chronic obstructive bronchitis
Chronic obstructive pulmonary disease (includes asthmatic bronchitis, chronic bronchitis, emphysema, and the overlap between them)
Cystic fibrosis
Emphysema

Common Restrictive Lung Diseases
Beryllium disease
Congestive heart failure
Idiopathic pulmonary fibrosis
Infectious inflammation (e.g., histoplasmosis, mycobacterium infection)
Interstitial pneumonitis
Neuromuscular diseases
Sarcoidosis
Thoracic deformities

Once the presence of airflow obstruction is established, then a typical approach in the laboratory is to administer two puffs of inhaled albuterol and repeat the spirogram after 15 minutes to establish bronchodilator responsiveness. Lack of bronchodilator response certainly does not exclude asthma, and the result needs to be used in the context of a patient's clinical history.

Lung Volumes

Because the FVC is not a reliable measure of total lung capacity, spirometry can only suggest a restrictive process and, in general, should be followed up by lung volume measurement. The algorithm for lung volume interpretation is shown in Figure 9. When spirometry suggests a restrictive process or when the abnormalities seen on the spirogram do not adequately explain a patient's clinical history, then formal measurements of lung volume are helpful. Box 7 summarizes the American Thoracic Society's criteria for grading the severity of lung function abnormalities. Total lung capacity can be particularly helpful when a patient has severe airflow obstruction and has a reduction in FVC. In this case, a normal or increased total lung capacity excludes an associated restrictive process, and the reduction in FVC is actually a pseudorestriction.

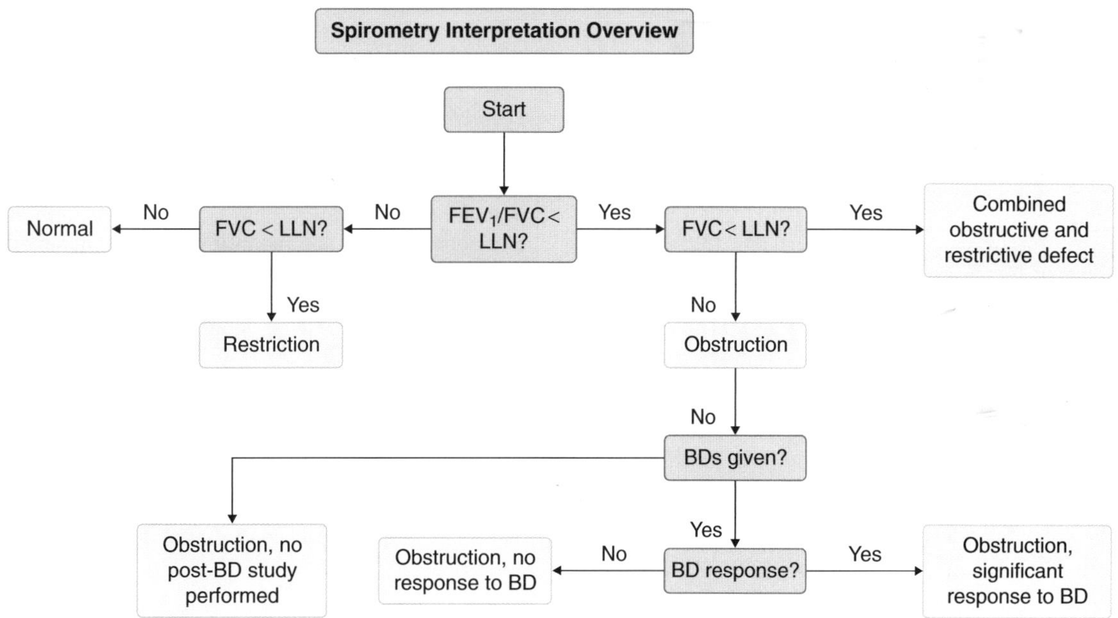

Figure 8 Algorithm for spirometry interpretation. BD, bronchodilator; FEV_1, forced expiratory volume in 1 second; FVC, forced vital capacity; LLN, lower limit of normal.

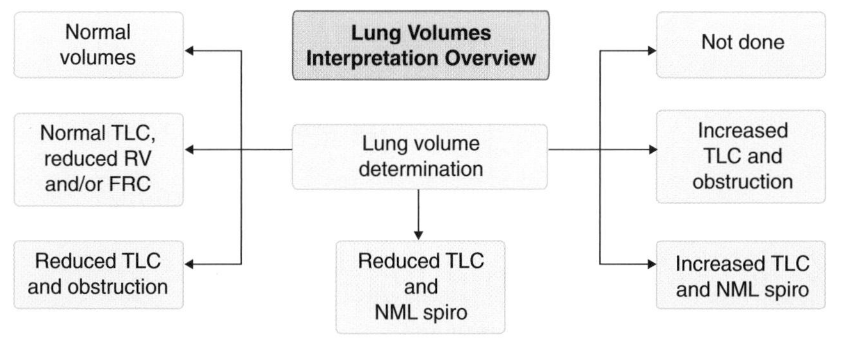

Figure 9 Algorithm for interpreting lung volume. FRC, functional residual capacity; NML, normal; RV, residual volume; spiro, spirometry; TLC, total lung capacity.

Box 7 Example of Criteria for Assessing the Severity of Abnormalities

Normal

The test is interpreted as within normal limits if both the VC and the FEV_1/VC ratio are in the normal ranges.

Obstructive Abnormality

The test is interpreted as showing obstructive abnormality when the FEV_1/VC ratio is below the normal range. The severity of the abnormality might be graded as follows:

May be a physiologic variant: Predicted FEV_1 ≥100%
Mild: Predicted FEV_1 <100% and ≥70%
Moderate: Predicted FEV_1 <70% and ≥60%
Moderately severe: Predicted FEV_1 <60% and ≥50%
Severe: Predicted FEV_1 <50% and ≥34%

Restrictive Abnormality

The test is most reliably interpreted as showing restrictive abnormality on the basis of total lung capacity. If this total lung capacity not available, one may interpret a reduction in the VC without a reduction of the FEV_1/VC ratio as a restriction of the volume excursion of the lung. The severity of the abnormality might be graded as follows:

Based on the TLC

Mild: Predicted TLC < LLN but ≥70%
Moderate: Predicted TLC <70% and ≥60%
Moderately severe: Predicted TLC <60%

Based on Spirometry

Mild: Predicted VC < LLN but ≥70%
Moderate: Predicted VC <70% and ≥60%
Moderately severe: Predicted VC <60% and ≥50%
Severe: Predicted VC <50% and ≥34%
Very severe: Predicted VC <34%

FEV_1, forced expiratory volume in 1 second; LLN, lower limit of normal; TLC, total lung capacity; VC, vital capacity.

Adapted from American Thoracic Society: Lung function testing: Selection of reference values and interpretative strategies. Am Rev Respir Dis 1991;144:1202-1218.

Diffusing Capacity of Carbon Monoxide

Diffusing capacity is a pulmonary function test that is commonly performed to help further characterize abnormalities in spirometry or lung volume measurements. The D_LCO has greater degrees of variability between laboratories and requires some level of expertise to perform reliably.

Several processes can affect diffusing capacity (see Box 4). Our proposed approach to the interpretation of diffusing capacity is shown in Figures 10 and 11. A pattern of diffusing capacity reduced proportionate to airflow obstruction (a proportionate reduction in FEV_1 and D_LCO) is typical for emphysema. A D_LCO is reduced proportionately to a reduction in total lung capacity in the context of restrictive abnormalities suggests a parenchymal process such as pulmonary fibrosis. An isolated or disproportionate reduction in diffusing capacity along with either normal or fairly well preserved mechanics suggests predominantly a pulmonary vascular process such as primary pulmonary hypertension or thromboembolic disease.

Anemia or carboxyhemoglobinemia (from smoking) could affect the measured D_LCO.[10] The concept of a reduced D_LCO that normalizes after correction for a lung volume measurement is often used to describe an extrathoracic or extraparenchymal disease process such as resection, obesity, or neuromuscular disease.[2] However, as noted previously, this approach has many limitations.

Summary

- Lung function testing helps us to understand the physiologic working of the lungs and chest mechanics.
- Pulmonary function testing is the primary method used to diagnose, stage, and monitor various pulmonary diseases.
- Lung function testing requires operators to follow published guidelines for administering and interpreting tests.

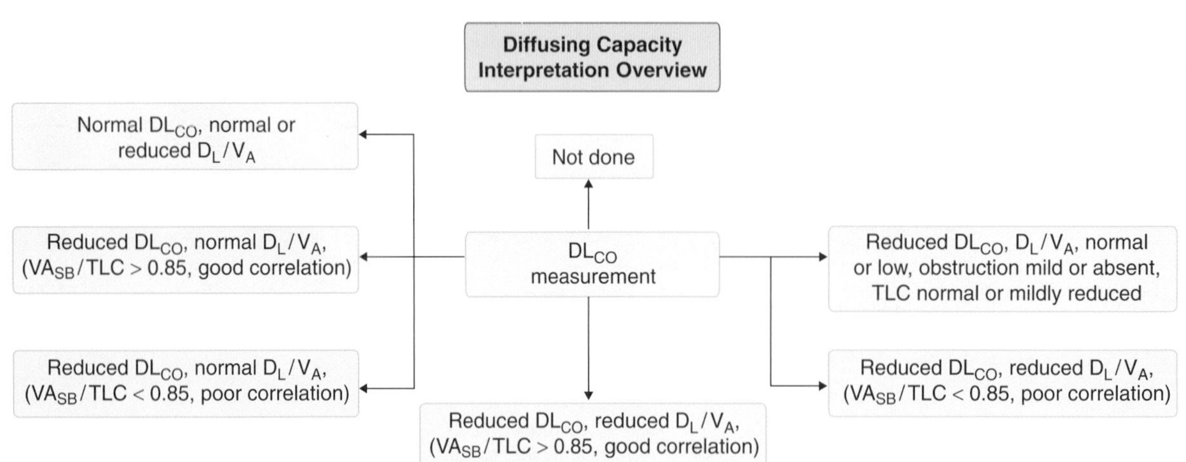

Figure 10 Overview of interpretation of diffusing capacity.

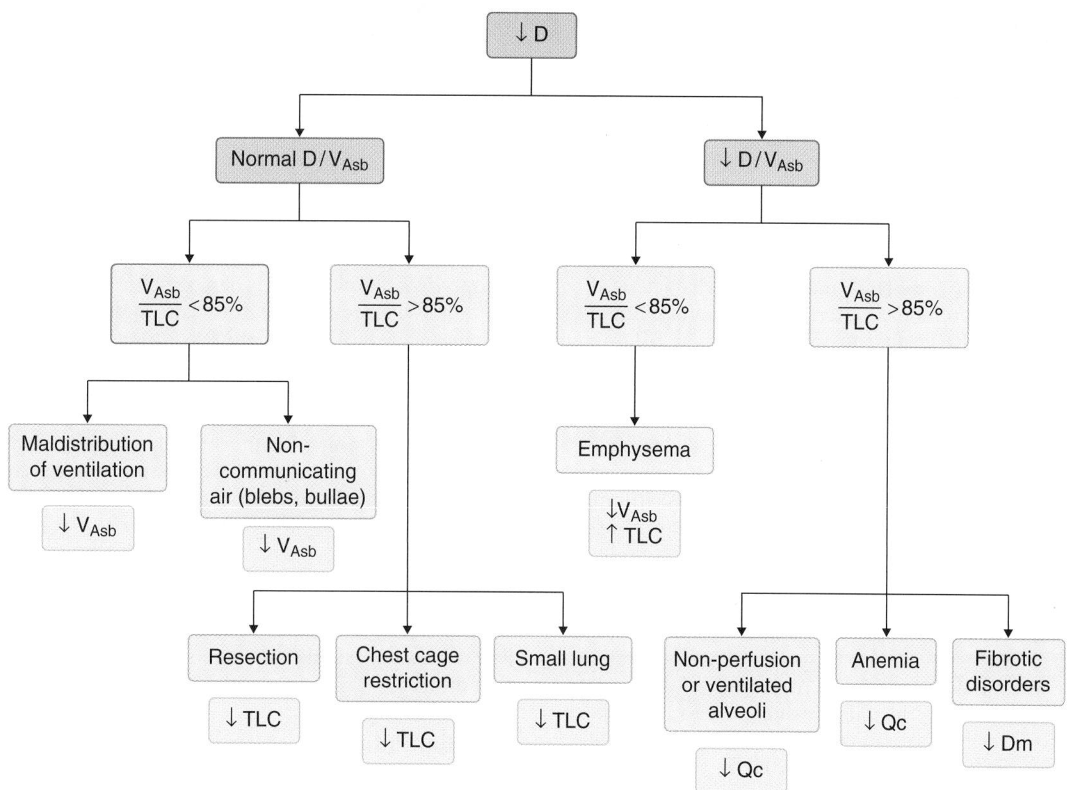

Figure 11 Algorithm for interpreting diffusing capacity. D_LCO, diffusing capacity of the lung for carbon monoxide; D_L/VA, diffusing capacity adjusted for alveolar volume; TLC, total lung capacity; VASB, alveolar volume in a single breath. *(Adapted from Miller WF, Scacci R, Gast LR: Laboratory Evaluation of Pulmonary Function. Philadelphia: JB Lippincott, 1987.)*

Suggested Readings

American Thoracic Society: Single-breath carbon monoxide diffusing capacity (transfer factor). Recommendations for a standard technique-1995 update. Am J Respir Crit Care Med 1995;152:2185-2198.

Becklake M, Crapo RO, Buist S, et al: Lung function testing: Selection of reference values and interpretative strategies. Am Rev Respir Dis 1991;144:1202-1218.

Crapo RO, Casaburi R, Coates AL, et al: Guidelines for methacholine and exercise challenge testing, 1999. This official statement of the American Thoracic Society was adopted by the ATS Board of Directors, July 1999. Am J Respir Crit Care Med 2000;161:309-329.

Hankinson JL, Odencrantz JR, Fedan KB: Spirometric reference values from a sample of the general U.S. population. Am J Respir Crit Care Med 1999;159:179-187.

Miller MR, Hankinson J, Brusasco V, et al; American Thoracic Society/European Respiratory Society Task Force: Standardization of spirometry. Eur Resp J 2005;26:319-338.

Miller WF, Scacci R, Gast LR: Laboratory Evaluation of Pulmonary Function. Philadelphia: JB Lippincott, 1987.

References

For a complete list of references, log onto www.expertconsult.com.

Pulmonary Hypertension

Raed A. Dweik

DEFINITION AND ETIOLOGY

Pulmonary hypertension is a hemodynamic state characterized by elevations in the mean pulmonary arterial pressure and pulmonary vascular resistance (PVR) leading to right ventricular failure and premature death. Pulmonary hypertension is defined by an increase in the mean pulmonary artery pressure above 25 mm Hg at rest or 30 mm Hg with exercise. Because this definition is based on hemodynamic criteria, pulmonary hypertension can be the result of a variety of diseases of different causes. Pulmonary arterial hypertension (PAH), however, should be distinctly differentiated from pulmonary venous hypertension resulting in left heart disease. Thus, the definition of PAH also requires normal pulmonary artery occlusion (or wedge) pressure to exclude elevations of pulmonary artery pressure simply as a compensation for elevated pressures in the left heart. PAH is commonly caused by or associated with an underlying pulmonary, cardiac, or systemic disease (associated PAH [APAH], previously known as secondary pulmonary hypertension). Rarely, PAH is present in the absence of an identifiable cause or associated underlying disease and is referred to as idiopathic PAH (IPAH) or primary PAH (PPH). A familial form of IPAH (FPAH) accounts for about 6% of cases.[1,2]

The small case series on elevated pulmonary artery pressures in otherwise healthy young individuals in the 1950s and 1960s and the epidemic of anorexigenic-associated PAH in Europe led to the first World Health Organization (WHO) conference on PPH in 1973.[3] The 1973 conference provided a pathology-based classification of the disease. Pulmonary hypertension was previously classified into two categories: primary or secondary, depending on the absence or presence of identifiable causes or risk factors. The diagnosis of PPH was one of exclusion after ruling out all causes of pulmonary hypertension. The second WHO conference on pulmonary hypertension, held in Evian, France, in 1998,[4] classified pulmonary hypertension based on similarities in the clinical features[4] and was revised in Venice, Italy, in 2003[5] to reflect the current treatment-based approach to pulmonary hypertension classification[5] (Box 1). PAH can be associated with a variety of known diseases, such as connective tissue diseases, portal hypertension, and human immunodeficiency virus (HIV) infection, in addition to the classic idiopathic form (see Box 1). All these conditions are believed to share equivalent obstructive pathologic changes of the pulmonary microcirculation, suggesting shared pathobiologic processes among the different processes leading to PAH.[5]

Parts of this review pertain to some but not all forms of pulmonary hypertension. The terms *pulmonary hypertension, PAH, APAH, FPAH*, and *IPAH* are used carefully as they are defined here, and they should not be viewed as interchangeable. Although the old term *primary pulmonary hypertension* is currently not in common use, it will still be used here when historically appropriate and for practical purposes can be considered interchangeable with the more current term IPAH. Much of the discussion of pathophysiology focuses on IPAH because it is the most carefully defined and studied form. The etiology, classification, and therapy sections pertain to PAH in general, reflecting the direction in the field. Pulmonary venous hypertension is a separate entity and is not discussed further.

PREVALENCE AND RISK FACTORS

As part of an international effort to better understand this rare condition, the Division of Lung Disease of the National Heart, Lung, and Blood Institute initiated in 1981 the national registry for PPH. Through 1985, 187 patients from 32 referral centers nationwide were prospectively enrolled. Their demographic characteristics constitute the best available information to date on the epidemiology of PPH. The mean age (±SD) of the population was 36.4 (±15) years, with a range of 1 to 81 years. There were 1.7 female patients for each male patient in the registry, and female patients tended to present with more severe symptoms. The mean time from onset of symptoms to diagnosis was 2 years. Right ventricular hypertrophy was found in 87% of patients and right atrial pressure was elevated in 72% of patients. The estimated median survival was 2.8 years, with single-year survival rates of 68% at 1 year, 48% at 3 years, and 34% at 5 years.[6,7]

No studies on the incidence of IPAH have been performed as of early 2008, but estimates of 1 to 2 cases per million inhabitants per year have been made. The underdiagnosis or underreporting of this rare disease with subtle presentation makes a true incidence calculation difficult.

Familial Pulmonary Hypertension

In the national registry for PPH, 12 (6%) of the 187 enrolled patients had a first-degree relative affected by the same disease process. Familial PPH appears to be inherited as an autosomal dominant trait with a variable but low genetic penetrance, and some persons inherit the trait without exhibiting the phenotype. Furthermore, genetic anticipation affects the gene penetrance, with subsequent generations developing PPH at an earlier age. In 1997, the gene for familial IPAH was mapped to chromosome 2q31-32. In 2000, the bone morphogenetic protein receptor 2 *(BMPR2)* gene was identified as the actual gene for familial IPAH and its product was recognized as being a transforming growth factor β (TGF-β) receptor. Mutations in BMPR2 were also found in 13 (26%) of 50 patients with sporadic or nonfamilial IPAH in one series, suggesting a role of this receptor in the disease. Those discoveries in the genetics of familial IPAH have opened the way to a better understanding of the pathogenesis of IPAH.[8-11]

Hospitalization and Death

Although the idiopathic form (IPAH/PPH) is rare, other forms of pulmonary hypertension are fairly common. Death rates for primary pulmonary hypertension as the underlying cause of death have increased since 1979, and the number of all cases is likely higher than that reported because of difficulties in detecting the disease. A report by the Centers for Disease Control and Prevention (CDC) published in November 2005 described trends between 1980 and 2002 in diagnosed pulmonary hypertension-related deaths and hospitalizations. These are the only national surveillance data available for pulmonary hypertension. Because pulmonary hypertension might be more likely to be reported secondary to other diseases, the report presented data for pulmonary hypertension as any contributing cause of death or as any-listed hospital diagnosis. The report compiled mortality data from the National Vital Statistics System (NVSS) and hospital discharge data from the National Hospital Discharge Survey (NHDS) for 1980 to 2002 and Medicare hospital claims data for 1990 to 2002.

Since 1980, the numbers of deaths and hospitalizations and the rates of death and hospitalization have increased for pulmonary hypertension, particularly among women and older adults. Between 1980 and 2000, death rates were higher for men than women;

Box 1 Clinical Classification of Pulmonary Hypertension, Venice 2003

1. Pulmonary arterial hypertension (PAH)
   1.1. Idiopathic (IPAH)
   1.2. Familial (FPAH)
   1.3. Associated with (APAH):
      1.3.1. Connective tissue disease
      1.3.2. Congenital systemic-to-pulmonary shunts
      1.3.3. Portal hypertension
      1.3.4. HIV infection
      1.3.5. Drugs and toxins
      1.3.6. Other (thyroid disorders, glycogen storage disease, Gaucher's disease, hereditary hemorrhagic telangiectasia, hemoglobinopathies, myeloproliferative disorders, splenectomy)
   1.4. Significant venous or capillary involvement
      1.4.1. Pulmonary veno-occlusive disease (PVOD)
      1.4.2. Pulmonary capillary hemangiomatosis (PCH)
   1.5. Persistent pulmonary hypertension of the newborn (PPHN)
2. Pulmonary hypertension associated with left heart diseases
   2.1. Left-sided atrial or ventricular heart disease
   2.2. Left-sided valvular heart disease
3. Pulmonary hypertension associated with lung respiratory diseases and/or hypoxia
   3.1. Chronic obstructive pulmonary disease
   3.2. Interstitial lung disease
   3.3. Sleep-disordered breathing
   3.4. Alveolar hypoventilation disorders
   3.5. Chronic exposure to high altitude
   3.6. Developmental abnormalities
4. Pulmonary hypertension due to chronic thrombotic and/or embolic disease
   4.1. Thromboembolic obstruction of proximal pulmonary arteries
   4.2. Thromboembolic obstruction of distal pulmonary arteries
   4.3. Nonthrombotic pulmonary embolism (tumor, parasites, foreign material)
5. Miscellaneous

Compression of pulmonary vessels (adenopathy, tumor, fibrosing mediastinitis)
Histiocytosis X
Lymphangiomatosis
Sarcoidosis

HIV, human immunodeficiency virus.
Adapted from Simonneau G, Galiè N, Rubin LJ, et al: Clinical classification of pulmonary hypertension. J Am Coll Cardiol 2004;43:5-12.

however, by 2002, no difference in rate was observed because of increasing death rates among women and declining death rates among men. Hospitalization rates were higher for men than for women until 1995; after 1995, higher rates were observed among women. Death rates since 1985 and Medicare hospitalization rates throughout the reporting period between 1990 and 2002 have been higher for blacks than for whites. In addition, two distinct geographic clusters were observed for the highest hospitalization rates in the Medicare population, and the highest death rates for pulmonary hypertension were in the western United States and in the Appalachian region.

The report concluded that although pulmonary hypertension historically has been considered a disease of women of childbearing age, it affects all ages and racial populations. Older women represent the majority of patients and decedents with this condition.[12]

PATHOPHYSIOLOGY AND NATURAL HISTORY

Pulmonary arterial hypertension affects the small muscular arteries and arterioles and is histologically characterized by endothelial and smooth muscle cell proliferation, medial hypertrophy, and thrombosis in situ. The hypertensive pulmonary arteriopathy seen in patients with IPAH affects the muscular arteries and arterioles and probably represents a combination of injury and repair. Several different histopathologic patterns can be seen, none of which is pathognomonic, however, because the diagnosis of IPAH still relies on excluding secondary causes.

Plexigenic pulmonary arteriopathy is the most common lesion seen in IPAH. It is characterized by medial hypertrophy, fibrotic intimal lesions that can compose organized thrombi, and destructive lesions involving the entire arterial wall. Another lesion is thrombotic pulmonary arteriopathy defined by the presence of organized mural thrombi resulting from thrombosis in situ in the setting of an intact arterial wall and a nondilated vessel. The pattern of an increased thickness of the medial smooth muscle wall, the duplication of the elastic laminae in muscular arteries, and the muscularization of the arterioles form the third type of histopathologic lesion in IPAH, referred to as *isolated medial hypertrophy*. This rare pattern can actually precede the formation of the plexigenic lesions and is believed to be reversible with treatment.

The pathogenesis of IPAH remains speculative and involves a combination of noxious stimuli affecting a predisposed vasculature. Until recently, the prevailing understanding about the pathogenesis of pulmonary hypertension was that the elevated pulmonary vascular resistance seems to result from an imbalance between locally produced vasodilators such as nitric oxide and prostacyclin and vasoconstrictors such as endothelin and thromboxane (vasoconstriction theory). Based on more recent evidence, however, our current understanding of the disease is changing to reflect the role of vascular wall remodeling in the form of proliferating endothelial and smooth muscle cells and abnormalities in the extracellular matrix that contribute to the increased pulmonary vascular resistance. The most obvious predisposing factors are the mutations in the *BMPR2* gene that result in FPAH and some cases of sporadic IPAH. The epidemic of PAH that developed in users of appetite-suppressant drugs, probably through the drug's serotoninergic effect, is an example of a noxious stimulus causing PAH. However, because only 0.1% of aminorex users were actually affected, other predisposing factors must exist for IPAH in exposed persons.

PAH is also associated with connective tissue diseases without any obvious pathophysiologic link. The possibility of an autoimmune injury leading to the vasculopathy has been proposed. Deficiency of thyroid hormone, either through a shared autoimmune insult to both the thyroid gland and the pulmonary vasculature, or the loss of a vasomotor role of the thyroid hormone has also been found to be associated with IPAH. Furthermore, the paracrine actions of the vascular endothelium appear dysfunctional in PAH, resulting in abnormal proliferation of vascular smooth muscle and endothelial cells, which might contribute to the observed increased pulmonary vascular resistance in this disease.[2]

Many advances have been made in revealing the pathogenesis of PAH. In many instances, however, the cause or effect explanation for the observed abnormalities remain blurred, because initial diagnosis in most patients is at advanced stages of pulmonary hypertension.

PATHOBIOLOGIC BASIS OF THERAPY

The median life expectancy from the time of diagnosis in patients with IPAH before the availability of disease-specific therapy was 2.8 years. Discoveries in three main pathobiologic pathways (nitric oxide, endothelin, and prostacyclin) have revolutionized our approach to the treatment of PAH and allowed the development of effective therapies that have changed the course of this previously uniformly fatal disease. Newer and probably more effective therapies are likely to develop as our understanding of remodeling and thrombosis improves.[2]

Nitric Oxide

The endothelium-derived relaxing factor nitric oxide (NO) has been shown to play a pivotal role in the pathobiology of IPAH. As a potent pulmonary vasodilator, NO that is produced locally in the lungs has profound effects on smooth muscle relaxation and proliferation, maintaining the normal pulmonary vascular tone. The unique lung anatomy with the close proximity of the airways to the blood vessels allows NO that is produced in high levels in the upper and lower airways by nitric oxide synthase II (NOSII) to affect the pulmonary vascular tone in concert with the low NO levels that are produced by nitric oxide synthase III (NOSIII) in the vascular endothelium. Patients with IPAH have low levels of NO in their exhaled breath, and the severity of the disease inversely correlates with NO reaction products in bronchoalveolar lavage fluid.[13-15] Exogenous administration of NO gas by inhalation is probably the most effective and specific therapy for IPAH, but cost and unresolved technical difficulties in the delivery system of inhaled NO have limited the use of NO gas to testing for vasoreactivity during pulmonary artery catheterization.

Endothelin-1

Endothelin-1 is a peptide produced by the vascular endothelium that has potent vasoconstrictive and proliferative paracrine actions on the vascular smooth muscle cells. The pulmonary circulation plays an important role in the production and clearance of endothelin-1, and this physiologic balance is reflected in the circulating levels of endothelin-1. Patients with pulmonary hypertension, IPAH in particular, have an increased expression of endothelin-1 in pulmonary vascular endothelial cells, and serum endothelin-1 levels are increased in patients with pulmonary hypertension.[16,17]

Prostacyclin

The endothelium also produces prostacyclin (PGI_2) by cyclooxygenase metabolism of arachidonic acid. Prostacyclin causes vasodilation throughout the human circulation and is an inhibitor of platelet aggregation by its action on platelet adenylate cyclase. The final enzyme in the production of PGI_2 is prostacyclin synthase. The remodeled pulmonary vasculature in lung tissue obtained from patients with severe IPAH expresses low levels of prostacyclin synthase when compared with normal lung tissue. In addition, PGI_2 metabolites are diminished in the urine of patients with pulmonary hypertension, further emphasizing the role of prostacyclin in this disease.[18,19]

Remodeling

In addition to the pulmonary vasoconstriction that results from the dysregulation of the local endothelial mediators as discussed above, pulmonary vascular remodeling seems to play a major role in the increased vascular resistance seen in IPAH. An abnormal proliferation of endothelial cells occurs in the irreversible plexogenic lesion. Those proliferating endothelial cells are monoclonal in origin, raising the possibility that a random somatic mutation may be one of the initial steps leading to sporadic IPAH. In addition, pulmonary vascular smooth muscle cells that normally have a low rate of multiplication undergo proliferation and hypertrophy. Those smooth cell changes arise from the loss of the antimitogenic endothelial substances (e.g., PGI_2 and NO) and an increase in mitogenic substances (e.g., endothelin-1). Other stimuli arise from locally activated platelets, which release thromboxane A_2 and serotonin; thromboxane A_2 and serotonin act as growth-promoting substances on the vascular smooth muscle cells. In fact, elevated blood levels of serotonin are found in patients with IPAH; the source of serotonin may be an abnormality in the platelets, which is the main source of this substance in the human circulation. Pulmonary vascular smooth cell hyperplasia also correlates with polymorphism and overexpression of a serotonin transporter, which might constitute an additional factor in a person's genetic susceptibility to developing IPAH. On the other hand, the pulmonary artery smooth muscle cells in IPAH appear to be in an abnormally depolarized state. This abnormal resting potential results in a heightened state of vasoconstriction secondary to increased levels of cytosolic Ca^{2+} and seems to relate to a primary dysfunction or downregulation of the voltage-gated K^+ channels.

In addition to the smooth muscle cell proliferation, abnormalities in extracellular matrix contribute to the medial hypertrophy in PAH. Through a dynamic process of matrix protein degradation and synthesis triggered by the high flow and pressure in the pulmonary vasculature, the extracellular matrix is remodeled, contributing to the obliterative changes seen in the pulmonary arteries.[2,20]

Thrombosis

In a large retrospective series that looked at lung tissue obtained from autopsy material from patients with IPAH, 22 out of 56 pathologic specimens had evidence of thrombi confined to the small muscular arteries. This was atypical for the classic appearance of venous thromboembolism, and the concept of thrombosis in situ in IPAH emerged. Whether the prothrombotic milieu is a consequence or a cause of the vasculopathy, pulmonary arterial hypertension remains debatable. The determinants of this increased propensity for thrombosis arise at the microvasculature level, where the dysfunctional endothelium loses the anticoagulant properties that usually prevent intravascular clotting of blood material. Instead, the procoagulation mediators that are usually inhibited under physiologic conditions seem to be activated. In fact, blood thrombin activity is increased in patients with pulmonary hypertension, indicating activation of intravascular coagulation, whereas soluble thrombomodulin, a cell membrane protein that acts as an important site of thrombin binding and coagulation inactivation, is decreased. In addition, PGI_2 and NO, both inhibitors of platelet aggregation, are decreased at the level of the injured endothelial cell, as discussed earlier. Circulating platelets in patients with PAH seem to be in a continuous state of activation and contribute to the prothrombotic milieu by aggregating at the level of the injured endothelial cells.[2,20]

SIGNS AND SYMPTOMS

The manifestation of pulmonary hypertension is nonspecific, leading to delays in evaluation and diagnosis. The clinical suspicion of pulmonary hypertension should arise in any case of dyspnea without overt signs of specific heart or lung disease or in patients with underlying lung or heart disease whenever there is increasing dyspnea unexplained by the underlying disease itself. The symptoms of pulmonary hypertension can also include fatigue, weakness, angina, syncope, and abdominal distention. Symptoms at rest are reported only in very advanced cases.[1]

The physical signs of pulmonary hypertension include left parasternal lift, loud pulmonary component of the second heart sound (P_2), pansystolic murmur of tricuspid regurgitation, diastolic murmur of pulmonary insufficiency, and right ventricular S_3. Jugular vein distention, hepatomegaly, peripheral edema, ascites, and cool extremities may be seen in patients with advanced disease. Central cyanosis might also be present. The lung examination is usually normal.

The clinical suspicion is also raised when symptoms and signs are present in subjects with conditions that can be associated with PAH, such as connective tissue diseases, cirrhosis of the liver, HIV infection, and congenital heart diseases. Pulmonary hypertension can sometimes be suspected when abnormal electrocardiographic, chest radiograph, or echocardiographic findings are detected in the course of procedures performed for other clinical reasons.[1]

DIAGNOSIS

The diagnosis is now more clearly defined and follows the currently accepted clinical classification.[1] Algorithms are available for various

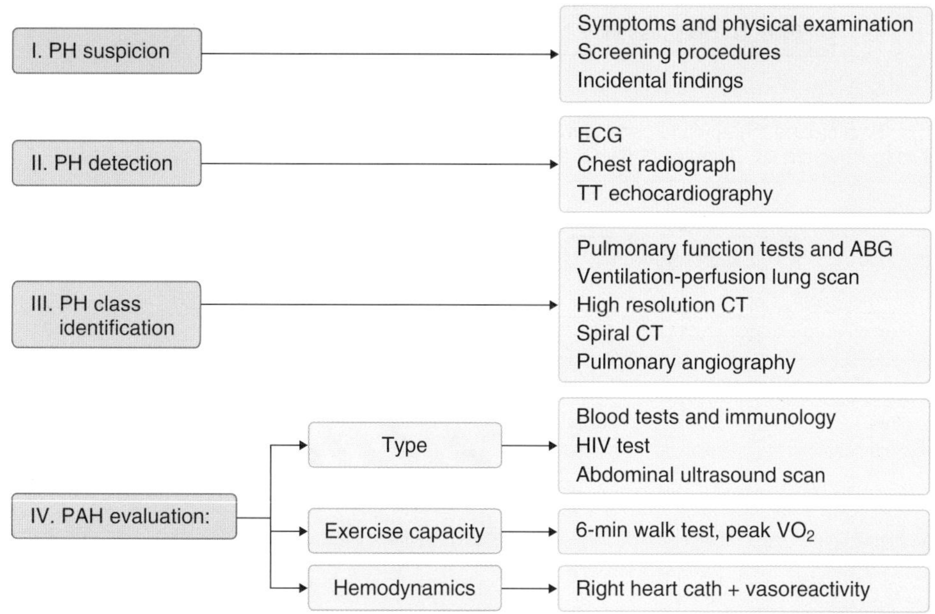

Figure 1 Simplified diagnostic approach to pulmonary hypertension. ABG, arterial blood gases; cath, catheterization; CT, computed tomography; ECG, electrocardiogram; HIV, human immunodeficiency virus; PH, pulmonary hypertension; PAH, pulmonary arterial hypertension; TT, transthoracic; VO_2, oxygen consumption. *(From Galie N, Torbicki A, Barst R, et al: Guidelines on diagnosis and treatment of pulmonary arterial hypertension. The Task Force on Diagnosis and Treatment of Pulmonary Arterial Hypertension of the European Society of Cardiology. Eur Heart J 2004;25(24):2243-2278.)*

investigative tests and procedures that exclude other causes and ensure an accurate diagnosis of PAH. The diagnostic process of pulmonary hypertension requires a series of investigations that are intended to make the diagnosis, to clarify the clinical class of pulmonary hypertension and the type of PAH, and to evaluate the functional and hemodynamic impairments. For practical purposes a sequential approach is recommended that starts with clinical suspicion of pulmonary hypertension leading to detection of the disease followed by confirmation and determination of severity. Due to the nonspecific manifestation of pulmonary hypertension, awareness by health care professionals in primary care settings is crucial for early detection and appropriate referral. Once pulmonary hypertension is detected, further evaluation should be performed at a specialized center. This typically includes testing to identify the clinical class and the functional capacity, which are essential to planning appropriate therapy. Figure 1 outlines the recommend approach.

The electrocardiogram might show right ventricular hypertrophy, right-axis deviation, or right atrial enlargement. Radiographic signs of pulmonary hypertension include enlarged main and hilar pulmonary arterial shadows (>17 mm) with attenuation of peripheral pulmonary vascular markings (pruning) and right ventricular enlargement. Although these findings may be helpful in advanced cases, they are neither specific nor sensitive enough by themselves. Echocardiography is usually the first test to suggest pulmonary hypertension. Pulmonary artery catheterization is usually required to confirm the presence and severity of pulmonary hypertension. It may also be useful in establishing the cause and determining the severity.

The rest of the workup is directed at excluding or confirming the presence of underlying diseases and assessing the degree of functional impairment. Pulmonary function testing is needed to exclude underlying lung disease. Ventilation-perfusion lung scanning or spiral computed tomography (CT) scans of the chest are obtained to rule out chronic thromboembolic pulmonary hypertension (CTEPH), a potentially curable cause of pulmonary hypertension. Normal scans essentially exclude surgically accessible chronic thromboembolic disease, but abnormal or indeterminate scans need to be followed by pulmonary angiography, which is the definitive test for diagnosing CTEPH. High-resolution CT scans of the chest are useful in looking for parenchymal lung diseases. Serologic testing is useful in looking for an underlying associated connective tissue disease. Overnight oximetry or polysomnography is useful in detecting obstructive sleep apnea contributing to pulmonary hypertension. A cardiopulmonary exercise test or the simpler and more widely available 6-minute walk test is used to assess functional capacity. Vasoreactivity testing during pulmonary artery catheterization may be helpful in determining prognosis and can help guide therapeutic decisions. Short-acting agents used for determining vasoreactivity include intravenous epoprostenol, adenosine, and inhaled nitric oxide.[1,3,21-33]

TREATMENT

Medical Treatment

General Measures

Oral anticoagulation improves survival in IPAH and is recommended in all these patients unless there is a contraindication. The recommended target international normalized ratio (INR) is approximately 1.5 to 2.5. The role of anticoagulation in other forms of PAH is less clear. Supplemental oxygen should be used to maintain oxygen saturation greater than 90%, especially because hypoxemia is a major cause of pulmonary vasoconstriction. Diuretics are indicated for right ventricular volume overload, and digoxin is reserved for patients with refractory right ventricular failure and for rate control in atrial flutter or fibrillation.[1,28] Specific vasodilator therapy is discussed later. The choice of a specific agent depends on the severity of the disease based on patient symptoms (per New York Heart Association classification) and hemodynamics (Fig. 2).

Calcium Channel Blockers

Patients with IPAH who respond to vasodilators in the short term have improved survival with long-term use of calcium channel blockers. Thus, these agents should be considered in all patients who have significant and definite responses to a short-acting vasodilator. Unfortunately, only a fraction of IPAH patients qualify for and benefit from long-term therapy with oral calcium channel blockers.[22,31]

Prostanoids

Epoprostenol delivered by continuous intravenous infusion improves exercise capacity, hemodynamic variables, and survival in IPAH

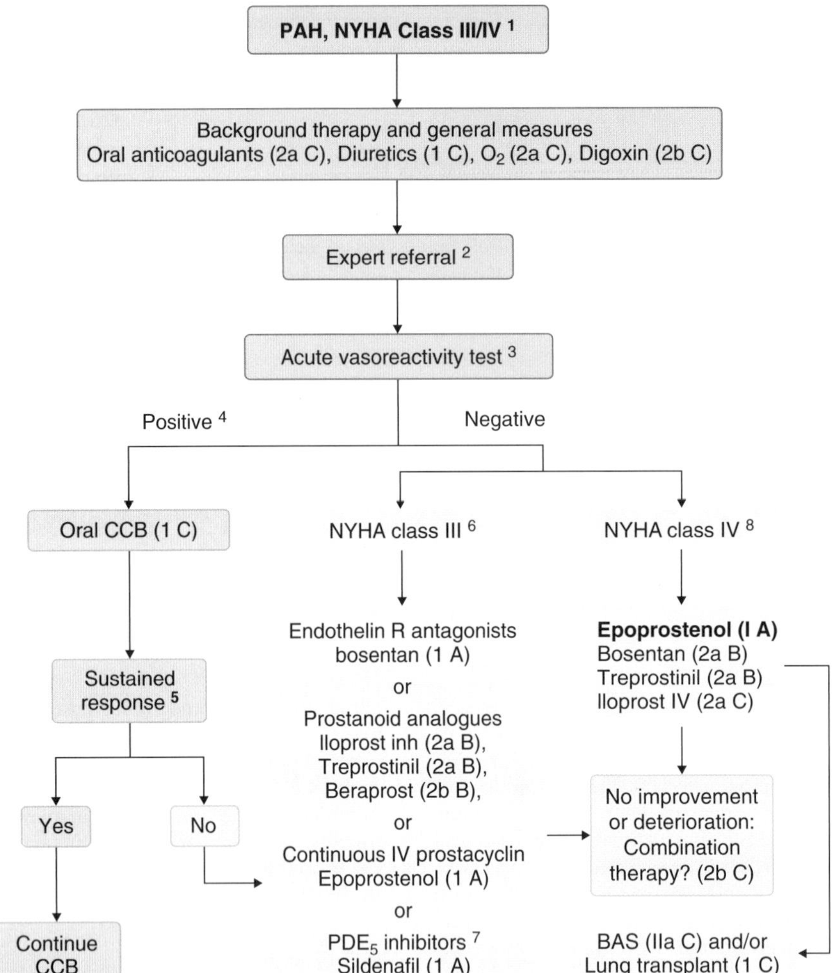

Figure 2 Evidence-based treatment algorithm for diagnosing and treating pulmonary arterial hypertension. 1. The algorithm is restricted to patients in NYHA functional class III or IV because they represent the largest population included in controlled clinical trials. For NYHA class I or II, very few data are available. In addition, the different treatments have been evaluated mainly in patients with sporadic IPAH and in PAH associated with scleroderma or anorexigen use. These recommendations should be extrapolated to the other PAH subgroups with caution. 2. Because of the complexity of the acute vasoreactivity tests and because of the treatment options available, it is strongly recommended that consideration be given to referring patients with PAH to a specialized center. 3. An acute vasoreactivity test should be performed in all patients with PAH, even if the greater incidence of positive response is achieved in patients with IPAH and PAH associated with anorexigen use. 4. A positive acute response to vasodilators is defined as a fall in mean pulmonary artery pressure of ≥10 mm Hg to ≤40 mm Hg, with an increase or unchanged cardiac output during acute challenge with inhaled nitric oxide, IV epoprostenol, or IV adenosine. 5. Sustained response to CCBs is defined as patients being in NYHA functional class I or II with near-normal hemodynamics after several months of treatment. 6. In patients in NYHA functional class III, first-line therapy may include oral endothelin receptor antagonists, chronic IV epoprostenol, or prostanoid analogues. 7. Currently, sildenafil is approved for PAH by the FDA. 8. Most experts consider that NYHA functional class IV patients in unstable condition should be treated with IV epoprostenol because it improves survival, its action is rapid, and there is worldwide experience using it. BAS, balloon atrial septostomy; CCB, calcium channel blocker; inh, inhaled; IPAH, idiopathic pulmonary arterial hypertension; IV, continuous intravenous; NYHA, New York Heart Association; PAH, pulmonary arterial hypertension; PDE, phosphodiesterase; R, receptor. Evidence-based medicine grades: A, randomized controlled trials (RCTs), meta-analyses, well-designed systematic reviews; B, case-control or cohort studies, retrospective studies, certain uncontrolled studies; C, consensus statements, expert guidelines, unusual practice, opinion. Levels of evidence: 1, Evidence and/or general agreement that a given diagnostic procedure/treatment is beneficial, useful and effective; 2a, Weight of evidence/opinion is in favor of usefulness/efficacy; 2b, Usefulness/efficacy is less well established by evidence/opinion. *(From Galie N, Torbicki A, Barst R, et al: Guidelines on diagnosis and treatment of pulmonary arterial hypertension. The Task Force on Diagnosis and Treatment of Pulmonary Arterial Hypertension of the European Society of Cardiology. Eur Heart J 2004;25(24):2243-2278.)*

patients and is the treatment of choice for severely ill patients. Epoprostenol therapy, however, is complicated by the instability of the drug at room temperature and the need for continuous intravenous infusion because of the drug's short half-life. Common side effects include headache, flushing, jaw pain, diarrhea, nausea, skin rash, and musculoskeletal pain. Catheter-related complications include infection and thrombosis.

Treprostinil is a stable prostacyclin analogue with a longer half-life, which allows subcutaneous or intravenous administration. In addition to side effects seen with epoprostenol, patients receiving treprostinil subcutaneously might also experience pain at the infusion site. An inhaled form of the drug has recently been approved as well.

Iloprost is a stable prostacyclin analogue that can be delivered by inhalation. Due to the relatively short duration of action of inhaled iloprost, it needs to be taken six to nine times a day. Common side effects include cough, flushing, and headache. Inhaled iloprost may be useful as an adjunct to oral therapy.

The main impediment to the use of prostanoids has been the route of delivery. Orally administered prostanoids are under development.[22,31]

Endothelin-Receptor Antagonists

Bosentan, an orally administered endothelin receptor antagonist, improves walking distance, hemodynamic variables, and functional class in patients with PAH. The main side effect is the asymptomatic increase in liver enzyme levels, which necessitates monitoring liver function at least monthly in all patients receiving the medication. Other potential side effects include anemia, edema, teratogenicity, testicular atrophy, and male infertility. Several other endothelin antagonists are currently in clinical trials, and some have already been approved in Europe.[22,31]

Phosphodiesterase-5 Inhibitors

Sildenafil, a phosphodiesterase (PDE) type 5 inhibitor, reduces pulmonary arterial pressure and is effective in the treatment of pulmonary hypertension. By inhibiting PDE_5, sildenafil stabilizes cyclic guanosine monophosphate (cGMP, the second messenger of nitric oxide), allowing a more sustained effect of endogenous nitric oxide, an indirect but effective and practical way of using the NO-cGMP pathway. Sildenafil has been approved by the U.S. Food and Drug Administration for use in PAH. Other longer-acting PDE_5 inhibitors are being evaluated in clinical trials.[22,31] Tadalafil is a long-acting PDEs inhibitor that was recently approved by FDA for use in PAH.

Surgery

Atrial Septostomy

The role of balloon atrial septostomy in the treatment of PAH patients is uncertain but might be beneficial in the setting of severe disease with recurrent syncope or right heart failure (or both) despite maximal medical therapy. The procedure can also be used as a bridge to lung transplantation. The rationale for its use is that the controlled creation of an atrial septal defect would allow right-to-left shunting, leading to increased systemic output and systemic oxygen transport despite the accompanying fall in systemic arterial oxygen saturation. The shunt at the atrial level would also allow decompression of the right atrium and right ventricle, alleviating signs and symptoms of right heart failure. Balloon atrial septostomy is a high-risk procedure and should be performed only in experienced centers to reduce the procedural risks.[1,23]

Lung Transplantation

Lung transplantation has been used in treatment for pulmonary hypertension since the 1980s, even before current medical therapies were available. It is indicated in PAH patients with advanced disease that is refractory to available medical therapy. Single and bilateral lung transplantations have been performed for IPAH, but most transplant centers currently perform bilateral lung transplantation to minimize postoperative complications. The 3- and 5- year survival rates after lung and heart-lung transplantation are approximately 55% and 45%, respectively.[1,23]

Pulmonary Thromboendarterectomy

Pulmonary thromboendarterectomy provides a potential surgical cure and should be considered in all patients with chronic thromboembolic PAH (CTEPH) affecting central pulmonary arteries. Pulmonary angiography is required to confirm surgical accessibility of chronic thromboemboli. The procedure requires cardiopulmonary bypass and involves dissecting well-organized thromboembolic material as well as part of the intimal layer of the pulmonary arterial bed. Patients with suspected CTEPH should be referred to centers experienced in the procedure for consideration of this procedure. In patients with operable CTEPH, pulmonary thromboendarterectomy is the treatment of choice because it improves hemodynamics, functional status, and survival.[1,23]

SPECIAL POPULATIONS

Portopulmonary Hypertension

PAH is a well-recognized complication of chronic liver diseases. Portal hypertension rather than the liver disease itself seems to be the main determining risk factor for developing pulmonary hypertension. The mechanism remains unknown but the presence of portosystemic shunt might allow vasoconstrictive and vasoproliferative substances, normally cleared by the liver, to reach the pulmonary circulation. The fraction of patients with portopulmonary hypertension in the National Institutes of Health (NIH) registry was 8%, and it can be seen in up to 10% of patients evaluated for liver transplantation. Thus, echocardiographic screening for detecting pulmonary hypertension in patients with liver disease is appropriate in symptomatic patients and is recommended in candidates for liver transplantation.

Pulmonary artery catheterization should be performed in all patients with increased right ventricular pressure on echocardiography. Hemodynamically, patients with portopulmonary hypertension might have a significantly higher cardiac output and significantly lower systemic vascular resistance and pulmonary vascular resistance than patients with other forms of PAH.

The treatment of portopulmonary hypertension can be challenging and is not well standardized. The general approach is similar to that in IPAH, except that anticoagulation is not recommended because of the risk of bleeding, and bosentan is avoided because of the potential for hepatoxicity.[34,35]

Pulmonary Arterial Hypertension in Hypoxic Lung Disease

Pulmonary hypertension in the setting of chronic hypoxia due to underlying lung disease represents a challenging area for evaluation and management. Although chronic hypoxia is a recognized cause of pulmonary hypertension, it would rarely lead to severe pulmonary hypertension. Nonetheless, patients with advanced chronic obstructive pulmonary disease (COPD) and interstitial lung disease who develop pulmonary hypertension tend to have a worse outcome. Thus, patients with chronic hypoxia who have a marked elevation in pulmonary pressure should be evaluated for other causes of the pulmonary hypertension.

The questions of when the pulmonary hypertension is disproportionate to the underlying lung disease and whether vasodilator therapy would be of any benefit remain unanswered. The current opinion suggests that, in general, mean pulmonary artery pressures greater than 50 mm Hg are out of proportion to underlying lung disease. The first-line and most important therapy in these cases is supplemental oxygen. Unfortunately, none of the medical treatments developed for pulmonary arterial hypertension has been shown to be effective in these patients.

This situation may be different for sleep apnea because effective therapy is available for the underlying disease. When mild pulmonary hypertension is associated with the sleep apnea, the first line of therapy should be directed at treating the sleep apnea followed by re-evaluation for pulmonary hypertension. If pulmonary hypertension persists despite adequate therapy for sleep apnea, consideration should be given to treating the pulmonary hypertension as a separate disease.[21]

Surgery

Elective surgery involves an increased risk in patients with PAH. The increased risk is proportionate to the severity of the disease. It is not clear which type of anesthesia is advisable, but probably local and regional anesthesia are better tolerated than general anesthesia. Surgery preferably is performed at referral centers with experienced anesthesia and pulmonary hypertension teams that can deal with potential complications. Anticoagulant treatment should be interrupted for as short a period as possible. In patients with CTEPH, bridging with heparin is recommended to minimize the time off anticoagulation.[1]

Pregnancy

Although successful pregnancies have been reported in IPAH patients, pregnancy and delivery in PAH patients are associated with an increased mortality rate of 30% to 50%, and pregnancy should be avoided or terminated. An appropriate method of birth control is highly recommended in all women with pulmonary hypertension who have childbearing potential. Unfortunately, there is no current consensus on the most appropriate birth control method in PAH patients. Because of the increased risk of thrombosis with estrogen-based contraception, some experts suggest the use of estrogen-free products, surgical sterilization, or barrier methods.[1]

Air Travel

Because hypoxia can worsen vasoconstriction in PAH patients, it is best to avoid or prepare for hypoxic situations such as going to high altitude or flying. Supplemental oxygen should be considered in all PAH patients planning to travel by air. A flight simulation test before the flight can help determine oxygen needs at altitude.[1]

Summary

- *Pulmonary arterial hypertension* (PAH) refers to a group of diseases characterized by high pulmonary artery pressure that can be the end results of a variety of disease states and underlying conditions. Idiopathic PAH (IPAH) affects a predominantly young and productive population and is more common in female patients than male patients.
- The workup of a patient with suspected pulmonary hypertension is designed to confirm the diagnosis, exclude or confirm the presence of an underlying cause, and assess the severity of the disease.
- IPAH is histologically characterized by endothelial and smooth muscle cell proliferation, medial hypertrophy, and thrombosis in situ.
- The pathogenesis of PAH remains speculative. An elevated pulmonary vascular resistance seems to result from an imbalance between locally produced vasodilators and vasoconstrictors, in addition to vascular wall remodeling. Several mediators, including nitric oxide, prostacyclin, and endothelin, appear to play a central role in the pathobiology of PAH.
- Currently available specific therapies for pulmonary hypertension are based on our understanding of the metabolic pathways of these mediators. Future therapies will likely reflect our improved understanding of the proliferative and vascular remodeling pathways.

Suggested Readings

Badesch DB, Abman SH, Ahearn GS, et al: Medical therapy for pulmonary arterial hypertension: ACCP evidence-based clinical practice guidelines. Chest 2004;126(1 Suppl):35S-62S.

D'Alonzo GE, Barst RJ, Ayres SM, et al: Survival in patients with primary pulmonary hypertension: Results from a national prospective registry. Ann Intern Med 1991;115(5):343-349.

Galie N, Branzi A: Pulmonary arterial hypertension: Therapeutic algorithm. Ital Heart J 2005;6(10):856-860.

Galie N, Torbicki A, Barst R, et al: Guidelines on diagnosis and treatment of pulmonary arterial hypertension. The Task Force on Diagnosis and Treatment of Pulmonary Arterial Hypertension of the European Society of Cardiology. Eur Heart J 2004;25(24):2243-2278.

Ghamra ZW, Dweik RA: Primary pulmonary hypertension: An overview of epidemiology and pathogenesis. Cleve Clin J Med Apr 2003;70(Suppl 1):S2-S8.

Hoeper MM, Krowka MJ, Strassburg CP: Portopulmonary hypertension and hepatopulmonary syndrome. Lancet 2004;363(9419):1461-1468.

Hyduk A, Croft JB, Ayala C, Zheng K, Zheng ZJ, Mensah GA. Pulmonary hypertension surveillance-United States, 1980-2002. MMWR Surveill Summ 2005;54(SS05):1-28.

Kaneko FT, Arroliga AC, Dweik RA, et al: Biochemical reaction products of nitric oxide as quantitative markers of primary pulmonary hypertension. Am J Respir Crit Care Med 1998;158(3):917-923.

McGoon M, Gutterman D, Steen V, et al: Screening, early detection, and diagnosis of pulmonary arterial hypertension: ACCP evidence-based clinical practice guidelines. Chest 2004;126(1 Suppl):14S-34S.

Rubin LJ: Diagnosis and management of pulmonary arterial hypertension: ACCP evidence-based clinical practice guidelines. Chest 2004;126(1 Suppl):7S-10S.

Simonneau G, Galiè N, Rubin LJ, et al: Clinical classification of pulmonary hypertension. J Am Coll Cardiol 2004;43:5-12.

References

For a complete list of references, log onto www.expertconsult.com.

Sarcoidosis

Daniel A. Culver

DEFINITION AND CAUSES

Sarcoidosis is a systemic disorder characterized by non-necrotizing granulomatous inflammation, with varying degrees of concomitant fibrosis. It predominantly affects the lungs, eyes, and skin. A transmissible cause has long been suspected based on epidemiologic studies, transmission via organ transplantation, and experimental data.[1,2] However, the causative agent(s) remain(s) unknown at present (Box 1).

PREVALENCE AND RISK FACTORS

Epidemiologic characterization of sarcoidosis is problematic due to variability in case definitions, ascertainment bias, and lack of precise diagnostic methods. Population-based chest x-ray screening programs in Scandinavia and the United Kingdom have suggested that there are a sizeable number of asymptomatic patients whose disease never becomes overt.[3,4]

Demographic factors, including race, ethnicity, age, and gender, markedly influence incidence. In the United States, the incidence in African Americans is 3.8-fold higher than in whites, conferring an overall lifetime risk of 2.4% versus 0.85%.[5] Most patients present between the ages of 20 and 40 years, although a number of studies have suggested a second peak after 50 years, especially in women.[6,7]

Familial clustering of sarcoidosis was first recognized 80 years ago. In A Case-Control Etiologic Study of Sarcoidosis (ACCESS), a recently completed descriptive U.S. study, the familial relative risk of sarcoidosis was estimated using 736 patients, who were matched for age, gender, and geographic location with 10,862 first-degree and 17,047 second-degree relatives.[8] The relative risk for development of disease in a first- or second-degree relative was 4.7 after adjustments for age, gender, relative class, and shared environment.

Disease presentation and natural history are also influenced by epidemiologic factors. White patients tend to present more often without symptoms, whereas severe multisystem disease occurs more often in blacks.[9,10] Black race has been described as conferring added mortality; however, data from population-based settings have suggested that at least part of the differential outcome may be related more to access to medical care than to inherent differences in disease behavior.[11-13] The ACCESS study systematically characterized 736 newly diagnosed patients at ten U.S. centers.[14] Organ involvement was significantly influenced by demographic variables, including age, sex, and race (Fig. 1).[15]

PATHOPHYSIOLOGY AND NATURAL HISTORY

Sarcoid inflammation is characterized by non-necrotizing granulomas (Figs. 2 and 3). The granuloma is a compact mass of cells that walls off foreign antigens, typically microbes. Epithelioid histiocytes, together with a few multinucleated giant cells, compose the core, surrounded by an outer rim of T lymphocytes. The lymphocyte population is oligoclonal, with restricted T cell receptor repertoires, consistent with an antigen-driven process. Inflammation in sarcoidosis is dependent on persistent stimulation by $CD4^+$ T cells.[16] Thus, polymorphisms of the major histocompatibility complex and the T cell receptor that modulate affinity for the antigen may be responsible for development or course of the disease.[17] Granulomatous inflammation that is widespread or at critical locations (e.g. A-V node) can lead to functional organ impairment. However, it is not uncommon for organ involvement to be clinically silent.

The search for a causative agent has spanned more than a century. It is still unknown whether a single agent triggers the disease or if sarcoidosis represents a stereotyped immune response to diverse etiologies. A large number of infectious and noninfectious agents have been proposed (see Box 1). Recent attention has focused most prominently on *Mycobacteria* spp.[18,19] and *Propionibacterium acnes*,[20] but the evidence to date has been inconclusive and sometimes contradictory.

The natural history of disease is variable. Spontaneous resolution occurs within 5 years in approximately two thirds of patients[10]; over a 2-year follow-up period in ACCESS, 80% demonstrated either improvement or stability, with no requirement for treatment.[15] Features believed to predict poor prognosis vary among studies (Box 2); of all the putative risk factors, no study to date has comprehensively ascertained which are independently associated with disease chronicity or progression.

Staging of pulmonary disease based on the chest x-ray (Fig. 4) allows a general prediction of outcome. For chronic sarcoidosis, there is a striking degree of heterogeneity between patients: Some have persistent inflammation, and others shift to a fibrotic phenotype. This shift is not seen in all patients, and the onset and pace of the fibrosis are likewise highly variable. Large-scale epidemiologic surveys have suggested that between 5.4% and 10% of cases are fibrotic at presentation alone. In the United States, pulmonary fibrosis is the leading cause of death in sarcoidosis, which carries a mortality rate of 1% to 5%. Other complications of pulmonary sarcoidosis include mycetomas, pleural effusions, bronchiectasis, pulmonary hypertension, endobronchial stenosis, and, rarely, bullous lung disease. Depression, chronic pain syndromes resembling fibromyalgia, and sleep apnea are prevalent in sarcoidosis patients.

SIGNS AND SYMPTOMS

Sarcoidosis can affect any organ, although the lungs are involved in up to 95% of patients (Fig. 5). Other organ systems commonly affected include the skin, eyes, and lymphoreticular system. Estimates of organ involvement are confounded by the method of discovery, referral bias, and the sensitivity of diagnostic modalities. Why different organs are differentially affected in various patients is unclear. Manifesting symptoms are organ dependent, but the most common ones include fatigue, arthralgias, diffuse pain syndromes, cough, dyspnea, wheezing, chest discomfort, rash, photophobia, scleritis, decreased visual acuity, weight loss, and fever.

In the lungs, important differential diagnostic possibilities include granulomatous infections, idiopathic interstitial pneumonias, hypersensitivity pneumonitis, and asthma. Cutaneous manifestations are protean.[21] Ultimately, one quarter of patients develop at least one dermatologic feature. Erythema nodosum is associated with acute onset of disease and confers a good prognosis. Lupus pernio is a chronic plaquelike induration of the face, usually appearing with

Box 1 Suspected Causes of Sarcoidosis

Infectious
Mycobacteria
Tuberculous
Nontuberculous*
Cell-wall deficient (L-forms)*
Bacteria
Corynebacterium spp.
*Propionibacterium acnes**
Tropheryma whippleii
Others
Fungi
Cryptococcus spp.
Endemic fungi
Viruses
Cytomegalovirus
Epstein-Barr virus
Herpes simplex virus
Others

Noninfectious
Dusts
Clay
Pine
Pollen
Talc
Mixed*
Metals
Aluminum
Beryllium†
Zirconium

*These organisms have been the focus of most recent studies, but no single agent is confirmed. It is very possible that several disparate agents induce similar reactions leading to sarcoidosis.
†Beryllium causes a histologically identical pulmonary reaction, but berylliosis can be differentiated from sarcoidosis by exposure history and lymphocyte proliferation testing.
Note: Many of these are no longer considered relevant suspects as triggers for sarcoidosis.

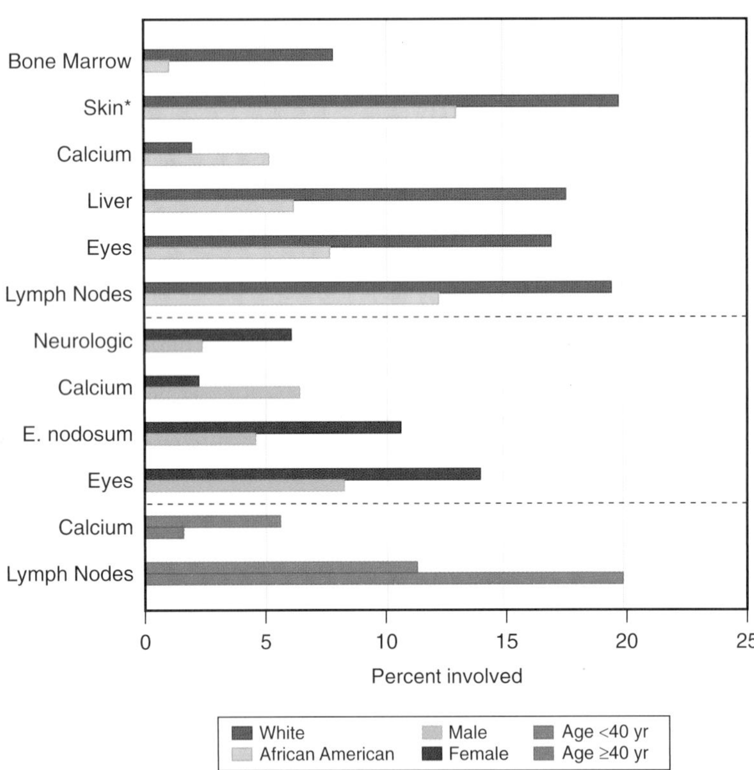

Figure 1 Demographic predictors of organ involvement in sarcoidosis. E. nodosum, erythema nodosum. *Not including erythema nodosum. *Adapted from Baughman RP, Teirstein AS, Judson MA, et al: Clinical characteristics of patients in a case control study of sarcoidosis. Am J Respir Crit Care Med 2001:164:1885-1889, with permission.*

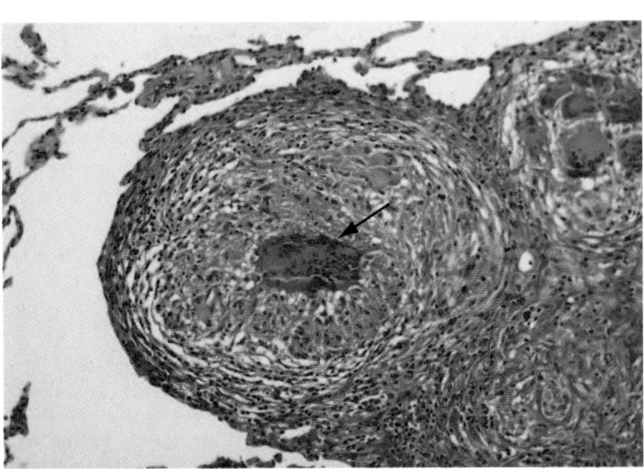

Figure 2 Non-necrotizing pulmonary granuloma. Well-formed non-necrotizing pulmonary granuloma characteristic of sarcoidosis. The granuloma is composed of a core of epithelioid histiocytes surrounded by a rim of lymphocytes. There is a large multinucleate giant cell in the center *(arrow). Image courtesy of Carol Farver, MD.*

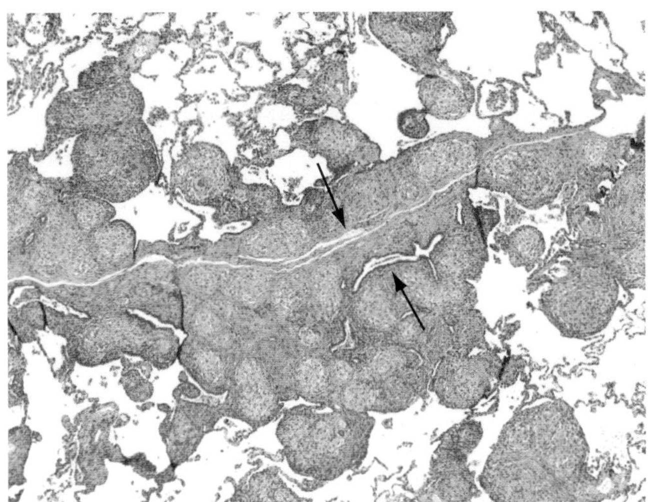

Figure 3 Distribution of granulomas in pulmonary sarcoidosis. The granulomas are typically found in a lymphatic distribution, coursing along the pulmonary veins *(upper arrow)* and the airways *(lower arrow)*. *Image courtesy of Carol Farver, MD.*

Box 2 Proposed Clinical Prognostic Factors for the Outcome of Sarcoidosis

No study to date has comprehensively ascertained which factors are independently associated with disease chronicity or progression.

Favorable	**Unfavorable**
White race	Black race
Löfgren's syndrome	Age >40 years
Scadding stage I chest radiograph	Organomegaly
	Lupus pernio
	Cardiac disease
	Nephrocalcinosis
	Sinus involvement
	Bone involvement

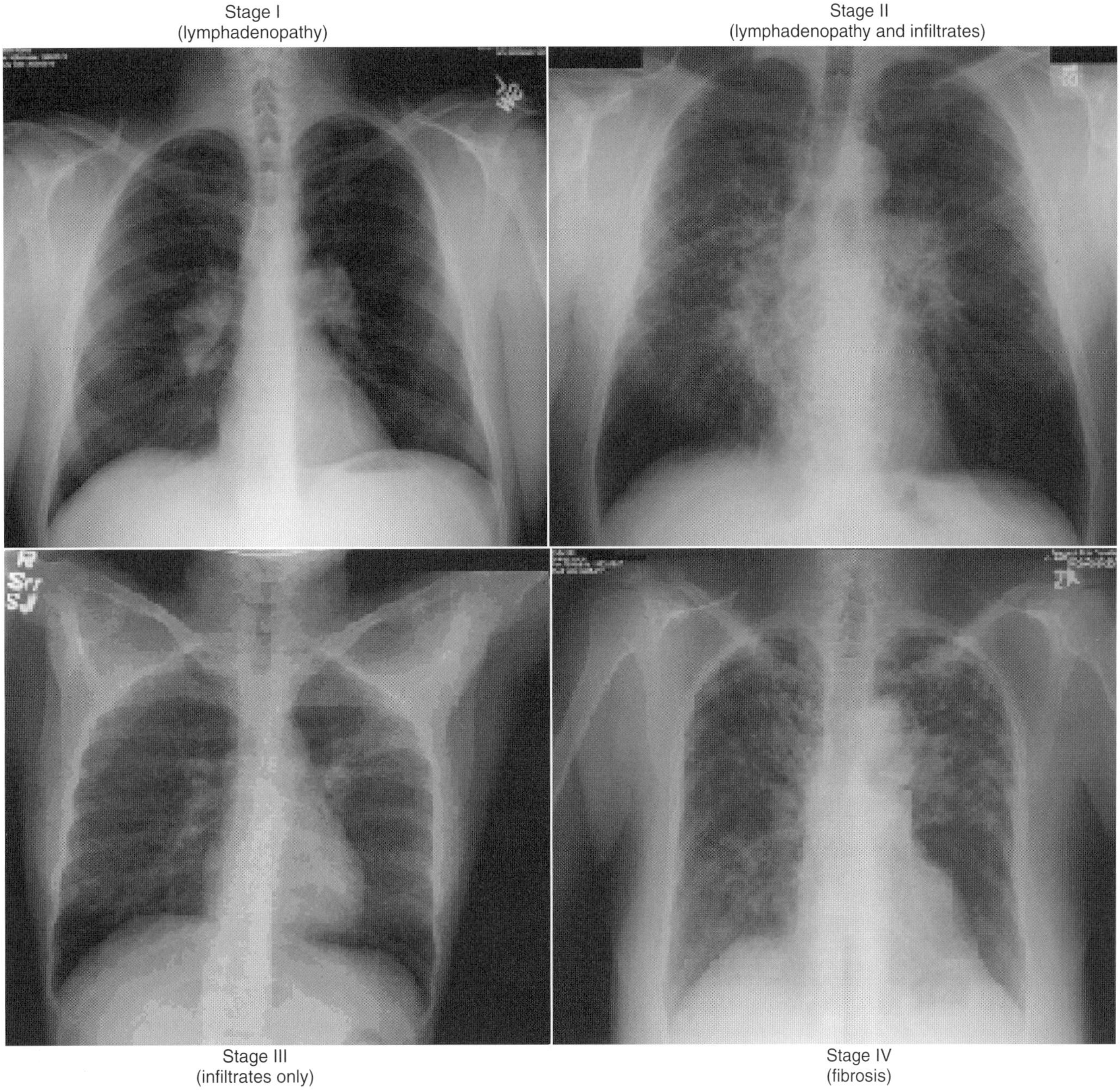

Stage I
(lymphadenopathy)

Stage II
(lymphadenopathy and infiltrates)

Stage III
(infiltrates only)

Stage IV
(fibrosis)

Figure 4 Common chest radiograph stages of sarcoidosis, as classified by the Scadding method (see text).

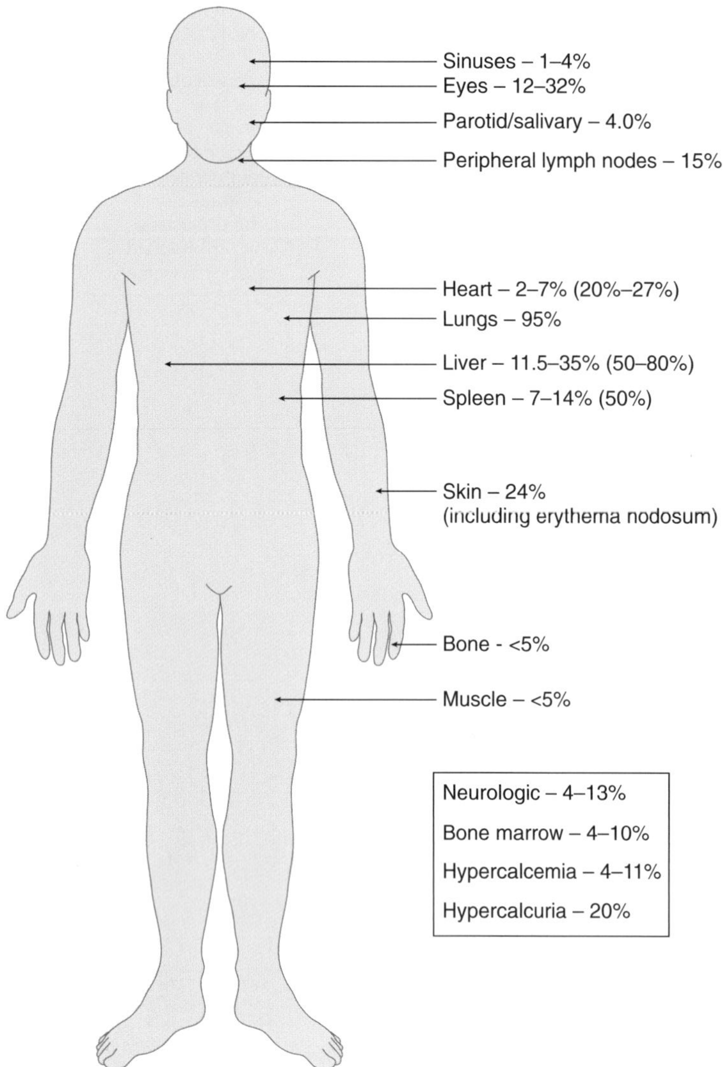

Figure 5 Percentage of overt organ involvement. Occult involvement is in parentheses.

violaceous discoloration of the cheeks, lips, nose, and ears (Fig. 6). It can erode into cartilage or bone, causing permanent disfigurement. Lupus pernio generally portends chronic, multisystem sarcoidosis, is more common in older African-American and West Indian women, and is notoriously difficult to treat. Other skin lesions include plaques, maculopapular eruptions, hypo- or hyperpigmented patches, subcutaneous nodules, and alopecia (Fig. 7).

Any ocular structure can be affected. In acute disease, anterior uveitis (iritis) causes photophobia, conjunctivitis, tearing, pain, and blurred vision (Fig. 8). It is usually easily treated with topical therapy. Chronic inflammation is typically more insidious and can affect the anterior and posterior structures. Retinal involvement, with characteristic candle-wax dripping exudates (Fig. 9), multifocal choroiditis (Fig. 10), macular edema, and neovascularization may be asymptomatic but always requires treatment.

Other commonly affected organs include the liver and spleen, with elevated liver enzymes or radiologic organomegaly in approximately 50% of patients.[22,23] However, these rarely cause symptoms or functional impairment. Uncommon manifestations include neurologic, cardiac, bone marrow, renal, exocrine gland, sinonasal, and bone disease. Clinically relevant presence of these uncommon manifestations is often associated with chronic or progressive sarcoidosis. When they are discovered as incidental findings on imaging studies or biopsies, they do not usually portend significant organ dysfunction.

DIAGNOSIS

Sarcoidosis is a diagnosis of exclusion. In an appropriate clinical setting, the presence of non-necrotizing granulomas, without evidence for infection, is the usual criterion to suggest the diagnosis. Sarcoidosis mimics and nonspecific granulomatous reactions should be excluded by a careful examination and by medical, occupational, and medication histories. Box 3 lists pulmonary diseases that are often confused with sarcoidosis. In practice, the disease is most often diagnosed by biopsy of accessible tissues,

Box 3 Pulmonary Mimics of Sarcoidosis

- Granulomatous diseases
- Infections (fungal, mycobacterial, others)
- Chronic beryllium disease
- Hypersensitivity pneumonitis
- Other exposures (methotrexate, metals)
- Rheumatologic syndromes (Wegener's granulomatosis, Churg-Strauss syndrome)
- Lymphoma
- Tumor-associated granulomas
- Other parenchymal lung diseases (e.g. pulmonary fibrosis)
- Asthma

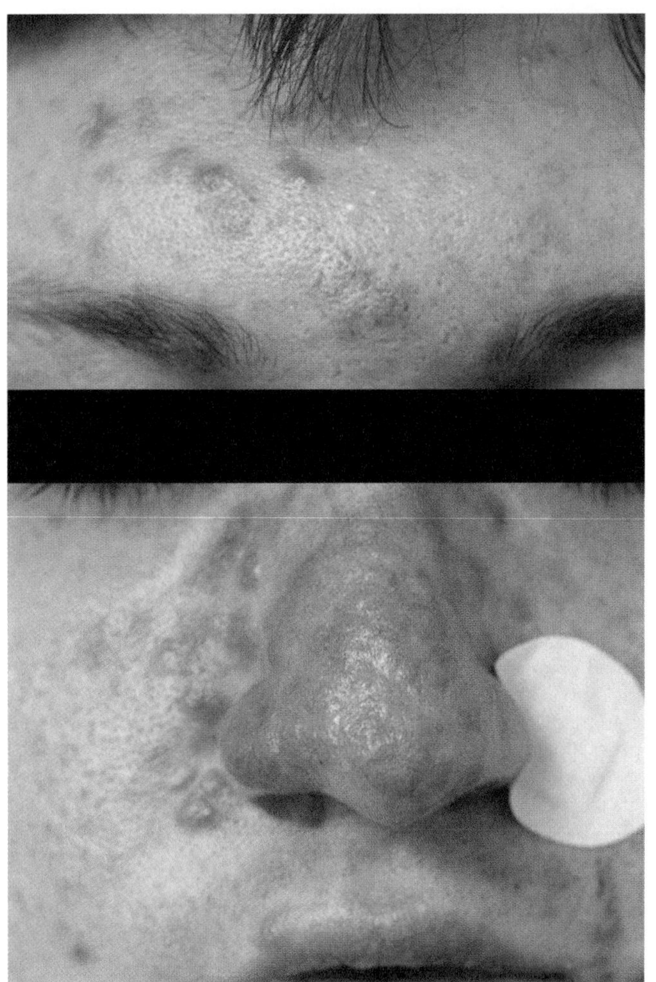

Figure 6 Usual skin lesions in lupus pernio.

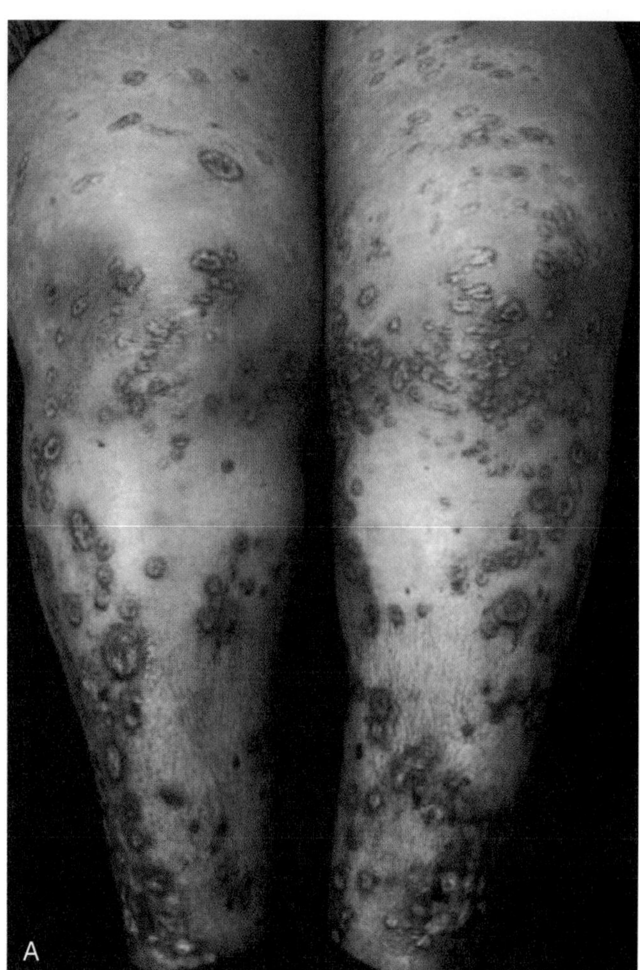

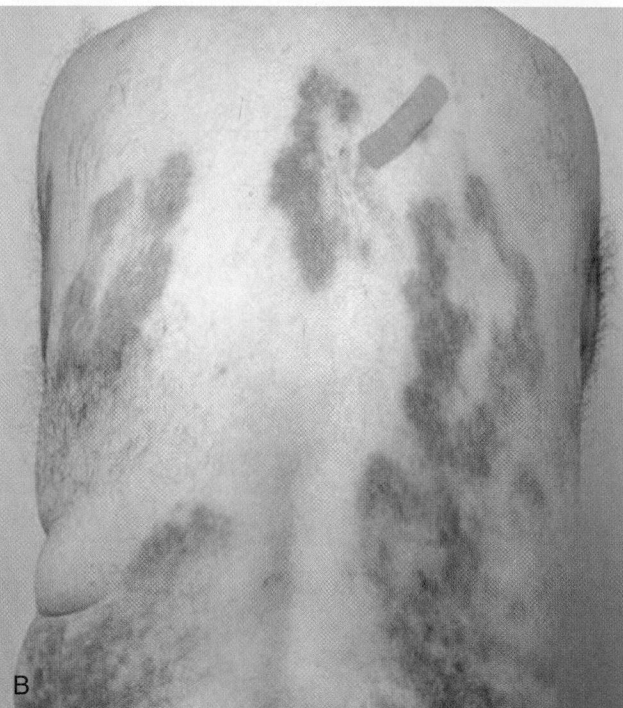

Figure 7 Other skin lesions in lupus pernio include plaques (A) and erthythematous patches (B).

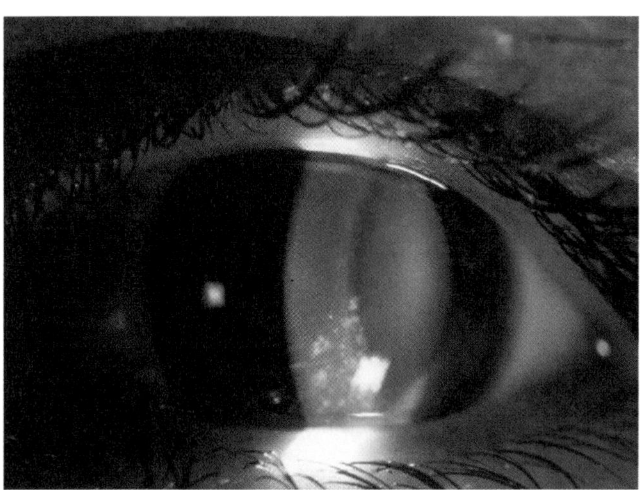

Figure 8 Keratitic precipitates from acute anterior uveitis.

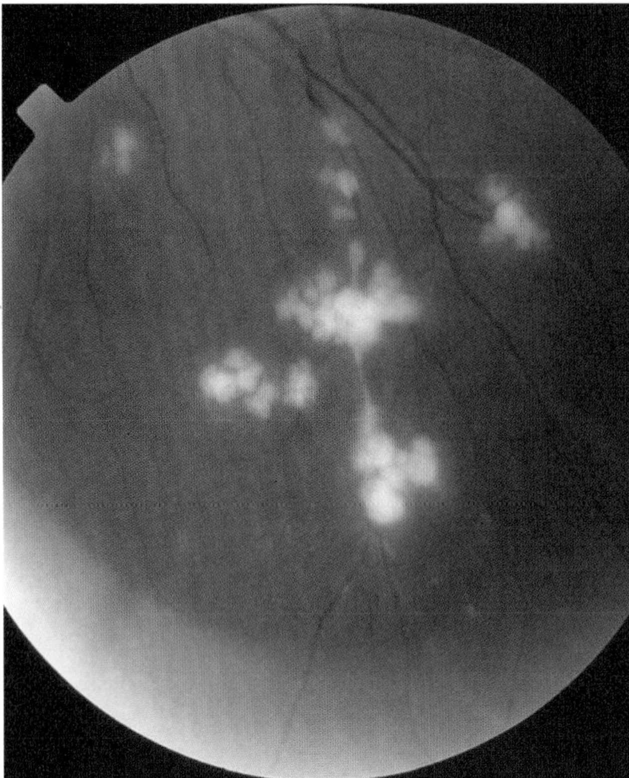

Figure 9 **Candle-wax-drippings appearance of retinal vasculitis in posterior chamber ocular sarcoidosis.**

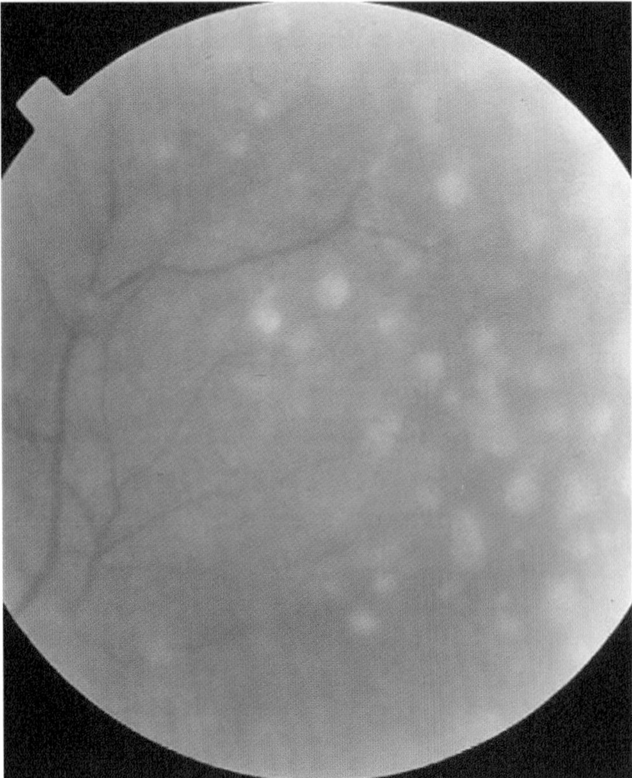

Figure 10 **Multifocal choroiditis.**

usually skin, lungs, or peripheral lymph nodes. We recommend a histologic diagnosis before commencing any treatment, in the presence of any atypical clinical features, or when there is suspicion that an alternative diagnosis (e.g., lymphoma) could be present. When sarcoidosis is suspected in extrapulmonary organs, chest imaging or random transbronchial biopsy may be useful to help confirm the diagnosis.[24]

Bronchoscopy is a reliable, minimally invasive technique to diagnose the disease. Combination of transbronchial biopsy with endobronchial (mucosal) biopsy or transbronchial needle aspiration of enlarged lymph nodes increases the sensitivity of the technique to as much as 91%. Endobronchial ultrasonography has been used more recently to further improve diagnostic yield. Samples should be analyzed for infectious agents by appropriate stains, including stains for mycobacteria and fungus, as well as by culture.

The Scadding scale, a descriptive schema that allows a loose characterization of the chance for disease remission, is used widely to describe chest x-ray findings.[25] Use of the scale entails several caveats: The stages of the Scadding scale do not represent sequential or temporal disease states, the predictive ability of the scale allows an approximation of outcome only, there are no data correlating stages of the scale with treatment response, the scale was developed more than 50 years ago from only 136 British patients, and the usefulness of the scale has not been validated in comparison with chest computed tomography (CT). The most common radiologic findings include bilateral hilar and mediastinal lymphadenopathy and bilateral nodular or reticulonodular infiltrates. Features that should prompt consideration of an alternative diagnosis include pleural effusion, unilateral abnormalities, and the presence of calcification in the lymph nodes. Chest CT usually shows typical micronodular infiltrates distributed in a bronchovascular pattern, and often predominating in the mid to upper lung zones.

Other diagnostic testing may be appropriate as guided by the initial symptoms and examination findings. Routine testing for elevated liver enzymes, hypercalcemia, renal dysfunction, ophthalmologic involvement, and electrocardiogram (ECG) abnormalities is standard at baseline. Other common tests to assess for organ involvement demonstrate various sensitivity and specificity, depending on the population studied.

Magnetic resonance imaging (MRI) with gadolinium or gallium is useful for diagnosing neurologic involvement, but nonspecific.[26] However, leptomeningeal enhancement after gadolinium has been shown to predict reversibility of sarcoid lesions.[27] Lumbar puncture should be performed in the appropriate clinical context to exclude mycobacterial or fungal infections. CSF analysis might reveal lymphocytosis, elevated protein, oligoclonal bands, and elevated angiotensin converting enzyme levels.[28]

Thallium or sestamibi scintigraphy is useful to identify areas of active or inactive myocardial involvement.[29] It is more sensitive than gallium scan. In the presence of unremarkable coronary angiograms, abnormal thallium scans in patients with known sarcoidosis are highly suggestive of myocardial involvement.[30] However, asymptomatic patients with abnormal thallium scans are unlikely to have clinically bothersome long-term disease.[31] Newer imaging techniques, such as fluorodeoxyglucose positron emission tomography (FDG-PET) and gadolinium-enhanced MRI are promising modalities for diagnosis and for monitoring treatment response.

ECG, Holter monitoring, and event monitoring can identify patients with dysrhythmias, and a baseline ECG is recommended for all patients with newly diagnosed sarcoidosis. Endomyocardial biopsy is rarely useful, due to poor sensitivity.[32] Therefore, a nondiagnostic biopsy should not preclude treatment when clinical suspicion is high.

The initial evaluation should include an assessment accounting for the common manifestations. Other assays of disease activity have been the subject of intense investigation, including serum angiotensin-converting enzyme level, gallium-67 scan, bronchoalveolar lavage fluid characteristics (CD4/CD8 ratio, total lymphocyte count), and numerous other biomarkers; unfortunately, none has consistently predicted disease course in multiple populations. Recent data have demonstrated that the presence of certain human leukocyte antigen (HLA) haplotypes (e.g., HLA-DR17 and HLA-DQB1) confer good prognosis in certain European populations.[33] However, the usefulness of HLA typing in other populations has not been confirmed. For now, chest x-ray stage, demographic features, clinical involvement, and serial pulmonary function testing remain the best indicators in assessing prognosis and therapeutic decisions.

TREATMENT

Several situations warrant aggressive systemic treatment. The most commonly accepted indications include active neurologic or cardiac involvement of any degree (except Bell's palsy), severe hypercalcemia, ocular disease refractory to topical therapy, lupus pernio, significant hepatic involvement, symptomatic splenic disease, and bulky lymphadenopathy resulting in symptomatic compression of surrounding structures. Other scenarios that require case-by-case decisions include sarcoid myositis; sinonasal, gastrointestinal, exocrine gland, or skin involvement; granulomatous nephritis; and bone disease. Constitutional symptoms, such as fatigue and achiness, are clinically bothersome for a large percentage of patients; they are best approached with nonsteroidal anti-inflammatory medications and careful assessment for the presence of depression, reserving the toxicities of steroids for patients with potentially life-threatening progressing disease. Neuropathic symptoms, often manifesting as paresthesias or pain syndromes, may be due to small-fiber neuropathy that can be present in some patients.

Several principles guide treatment strategy: Corticosteroids prevent granuloma formation in most patients, and they reverse immunologic derangements. Granuloma formation proceeds at varying rates between patients, necessitating individualized treatment strategies. A threshold dose of medication is usually required for effectiveness. Different tissues respond differently to various medications.[16] For example, antimalarial medications are effective for hypercalcemia and skin disease but have little effect on pulmonary disease.

Decisions to treat pulmonary sarcoidosis should be framed in the context of the lack of evidence that treatment significantly changes the natural history of the disease. The likelihood of spontaneous remission, degree of physiologic impairment, magnitude of symptoms and chronicity of disease must be considered. For patients with acute (<2 years) disease, systemic treatment is generally withheld unless there are significant symptoms, moderate to severe physiologic impairment, or rapid progression and chest imaging suggesting the presence of reversible disease (e.g., infiltrates that are not wholly fibrosis). For patients with chronic disease (≥2 years), the chances of spontaneous remission are low. The general goal of therapy in this group is to define the lowest dose of medication needed to maintain stability. Significant pulmonary symptoms might also be due to pulmonary vascular involvement, a diagnosis that should be considered in patients whose symptoms are disproportionate to the degree of parenchymal involvement.

Corticosteroids are the current first-line agents for treatment because clinical experience is greatest with them, they generally have acceptable (and reversible) side-effect profiles, and the time to onset of effect is quicker than for most alternatives. For pulmonary disease, initial doses of 20 to 30 mg/day of prednisone are probably sufficient. Although some clinicians have advocated higher doses (1 mg/kg per day), the ratio between benefit and toxicity of such doses is usually unfavorable. Improvements in symptoms, chest radiographs, and lung function tests are typical; failure to respond within 2 to 3 months suggests the presence of steroid-refractory disease. Although some clinicians have advocated every-other-day dosing regimens, this approach might not be sufficient to control active granuloma formation. In general, I suggest that systemic treatment of pulmonary disease should entail at least weeks to months of therapy.

Inhaled corticosteroids may be useful for symptoms of bronchospasm and cough in conjunction with bronchodilators. Numerous trials have assessed their usefulness in treating parenchymal disease, with the net result suggesting that they have very modest to no benefits. However, for patients with mild disease, a trial of inhaled corticosteroids is generally well tolerated and may be helpful.

Steroid-sparing agents are used when steroids are ineffective or cause unacceptable side effects. Methotrexate, a folic acid analogue with anti-inflammatory and antiproliferative properties, is generally used as a second-line agent, but it has not been subjected to rigorous controlled studies. In small trials, it has been effective for controlling disease and reducing corticosteroid dose for acute and chronic disease.[34,35] Doses of 10 to 20 mg per week are typically used, and treatment response can require 3 to 6 months of therapy. The purine analogue azathioprine is also effective as a steroid-sparing agent, but its use is limited due to its potential for substantial toxicity.[36] One series suggested that leflunomide might be useful in conjunction with methotrexate.[37] For severe or refractory disease, agents with greater potential for toxicity may be necessary, including cyclophosphamide and chlorambucil. Antimalarial agents are often efficacious for treating dermatologic disease, sinonasal sarcoid, osseous disease, and hypercalcemia.

Newer approaches include antagonists of tumor necrosis factor α (TNF-α), including thalidomide and monoclonal antibodies such as infliximab or adalimumab.[38,39] The largest randomized controlled double-blind study of therapy in sarcoidosis included 138 patients with pulmonary disease of more than 1 year's duration.[40] Use of infliximab resulted in a modest net gain of 2.5% from baseline in FVC at 24 weeks, compared with no change for placebo. The clinical importance of this finding is questionable; however, it is evident that a portion of patients treated with this medication experience substantial benefits after failing other medical approaches. A major challenge for treatment decision-making in sarcoidosis is the lack of head-to-head studies between agents. For now, toxicity profile, clinician comfort, and experience are likely to be important factors guiding therapeutic choices. As additional biologic agents become available for use in other diseases, their application to sarcoidosis will be best elucidated by development of controlled trials. Due to the heterogeneity of the disease, designing these trials will be challenging.

Summary

- Sarcoidosis is a systemic granulomatous disease, of unknown etiology, which most often affects the lungs, skin, and eyes.
- In the United States, sarcoidosis is more prevalent and more severe in blacks than in whites. The prevalence has been estimated at 35/100,000 in blacks and 11/100,000 in whites.
- Approximately two thirds of patients experience resolution of their disease without specific therapy.
- Treatment of sarcoidosis relies on a combination of immunosuppressive medications and realistic appraisal of therapeutic goals.

Suggested Readings

Baughman RP, Drent M, Kavuru M, et al: Infliximab therapy in patients with chronic sarcoidosis and pulmonary involvement. Am J Respir Crit Care Med 2006:174:795-802.

Baughman RP, Teirstein AS, Judson MA, et al: Clinical characteristics of patients in a case control study of sarcoidosis. Am J Respir Crit Care Med 2001:164:1885-1889.

Hillerdal G, Nou E, Osterman K, Schmekel B: Sarcoidosis: Epidemiology and prognosis. A 15-year European study. Am Rev Respir Dis 1984:130:29-32.

Hunninghake GW, Costabel U, Ando M, et al: ATS/ERS/WASOG statement on sarcoidosis. American Thoracic Society/European Respiratory Society/World Association of Sarcoidosis and other Granulomatous Disorders. Sarcoidosis Vasc Diffuse Lung Dis 1999:16:149-173.

Judson MA, Baughman RP, Thompson BW, et al: Two year prognosis of sarcoidosis: The ACCESS experience. Sarcoidosis Vasc Diffuse Lung Dis 2003:20:204-211.

Moller DR: Treatment of sarcoidosis—from a basic science point of view. J Intern Med 2003;253:31-40.

Rybicki BA, Iannuzzi MC, Frederick MM, et al: Familial aggregation of sarcoidosis. A Case-Control Etiologic Study of Sarcoidosis (ACCESS). Am J Respir Crit Care Med 2001:164:2085-2091.

Rybicki BA, Major M, Popovich J Jr, et al: Racial differences in sarcoidosis incidence: A 5-year study in a health maintenance organization. Am J Epidemiol 1997:145:234-241.

Song Z, Marzilli L, Greenlee BM, et al: Mycobacterial catalase-peroxidase is a tissue antigen and target of the adaptive immune response in systemic sarcoidosis. J Exp Med 2005:201:755-767.

Ziegenhagen MW, Muller-Quernheim J: The cytokine network in sarcoidosis and its clinical relevance. J Intern Med 2003;253:18-30.

References

For a complete list of references, log onto www.expertconsult.com.

Sleep-Disordered Breathing

Marie M. Budev and *Joseph A. Golish*

Humans spend almost 30% of their lives sleeping. Since the 1970s, physicians have begun to recognize many of the detrimental consequences of sleep disturbances produced by abnormal breathing patterns, termed *sleep-disordered breathing* (SDB).[1] Sleep apnea and other sleep-related breathing disorders constitute the greatest number of sleep disorders seen by pulmonologists and general practitioners in the outpatient setting. SDB has been associated with considerable morbidity.

SDB comprises a wide spectrum of sleep-related breathing abnormalities; those related to increased upper airway resistance include snoring, upper airway resistance syndrome (UARS), and obstructive sleep apnea-hypopnea syndrome (OSAHS).[2] Many clinicians regard SDB as a spectrum of diseases.[3] This concept suggests that a person who snores may be exhibiting the first manifestation of SDB and that snoring should not be viewed as normal. A patient can move gradually through the continuum, for example, with weight gain and eventual development of pickwickian syndrome or with alcohol or sedative use, which can cause a person who snores to turn into a snorer with obstructive sleep apnea (OSA). Continuous positive airway pressure (CPAP) can be effective in treating apnea, but the patient may be left with continued residual UARS or snoring.[4] Therefore, the clinician must recognize the continuum state of this disease entity because patients can continue to suffer from symptoms caused by one aspect of SDB while being treated for another aspect of SDB.

SNORING

Snoring is one of the most common aspects of SDB and has been described throughout history. In the past, snoring generally had been considered a social nuisance without no consequences for the snorer, only for the suffering bed partner. After sleep apnea syndrome was recognized, snoring began being viewed as an important clinical symptom. Although it is by far the most common symptom of sleep apnea and is usually the main reason for a patient visit, not all patients who snore have sleep apnea.

Definition

Although the definition of snoring may differ depending on the "ear of the beholder," it is defined by the *Random House Dictionary of the English Language* as "breathing during sleep with hoarse or harsh sounds as caused by the vibrating of the soft palate."[5] The International Classification of Sleep Disorders: Diagnostic and Coding Manual defines *primary snoring* (ICSD 786.09) as "loud upper airway breathing sounds in sleep, without episodes of apnea or hypoventilation."[6]

Prevalence

It is clearly recognized that snoring is common in the general population, but estimates vary widely of its prevalence in different populations. These differences mainly are due to subjective perception, depending on who is reporting the snoring (the snorer or the bed partner) and how the question is asked by the clinician. Overall, snoring is reported to affect 19% to 37% of the general population and more than 50% of middle-aged men.[7] Male predominance has been noted in all snoring epidemiologic studies, possibly due to the differences in perception of snoring by men and women. Other possible reasons for increased male predominance include differences in pharyngeal anatomy and function, hormonal differences and their effects on upper airway muscles, and differences in body fat distribution.

Pathophysiology

Snoring is a result of the changes in the configuration and properties of the upper airway (from the nasopharynx to the laryngopharynx) that occurs during sleep. This sound can be produced by any membranous portion of the airway that lacks cartilaginous support, including the soft palate, uvula, and the pharyngeal walls. Snoring is usually an inspiratory sound, but it can also occur in expiration.[8] Snoring can occur during any stage of sleep but is more common during stages 2, 3, and 4. This is because airway elastance and muscle tone due to sympathetic activity and neural output to the upper airway walls are different during rapid eye movement (REM) and non-REM sleep. Multiple predisposing factors can lead to a snoring abnormality, including age (middle or advanced), regional obesity, body posture, use of alcohol and muscle relaxants, retrognathia, nasal blockage, and smoking.[9]

Signs and Symptoms

A primary snorer is usually asymptomatic and does not suffer from cardiovascular disease. Snoring in this population is usually an annoyance to the bed partner, and the snorer might deny any symptoms of daytime somnolence or difficulty with concentration. In contrast, snoring also can occur in conjunction with a disordered sleep pattern and may be associated with a range of symptoms, including overt OSAHS.

Bed partners, family members, or friends who have shared a room with the sleeping patient initially might complain of loud or disruptive noises. Patients sometimes complain of snoring themselves, a feeling of tiredness on waking, excessive sleepiness during the day, poor work performance, and difficulty with concentration.

Diagnosis

A complete history and careful physical examination are paramount in assessing whether sleep apnea is present in a patient with snoring symptoms. The history and examination results also guide the clinician in deciding whether a nocturnal polysomnogram is necessary and in determining appropriate treatment.

The history should be obtained in the presence of the bed partner, who usually initiates the visit, because the snorer often is unaware of snoring. The clinician also should assess the degree of social disruption caused by the snoring. He or she should ask the bed partner the number of years' duration of the snoring, frequency of snoring (every night or intermittent), postural dependence (lying on side or back), and the association of posture with cessation of breathing.

The patient's risk factors should be assessed, including male gender, increase in weight, ingestion of alcohol, allergies, nasal obstruction, trauma, use of muscle-relaxing medications, and smoking. An assessment of daytime functioning, including concentration levels, work performance, and sleepiness, should be documented. The Epworth Sleepiness Scale (Table 1), which assesses the level of daytime sleepiness, has been used to distinguish primary snoring from OSAHS.[10] A history should be sought of previous surgery or trauma to the upper airways (any site between the nose and the larynx) because the compliance of the airways may be affected. A family predisposition to snoring has been described, and

Table 1 The Epworth Sleepiness Scale

How likely are you to doze off or fall asleep in the following situations, in contrast to feeling just tired? This refers to your usual way of life in recent times. Even if you have not done some of these things recently, try to work out how they would have affected you. Use the following scale to choose the most appropriate number for each situation:

0 = Would never doze

1 = Slight chance of dozing

2 = Moderate chance of dozing

3 = High chance of dozing

Situation	Score 0	1	2	3
Sitting and reading				
Watching television				
Sitting inactive in a public place (theater, meeting)				
Lying down to rest in the afternoon when circumstances allow				
Sitting and talking to someone				
Sitting quietly after lunch without alcohol				
In a car, while stopped for a few minutes in traffic				
Total score				

many snorers admit to other family members of having a history of snoring if asked.[11]

Laboratory tests for hypothyroidism or acromegaly are indicated only if clinical signs suggest the presence of these disorders. The decision to order other laboratory investigations should be based on the possible medical consequences of the patient's snoring, the probability that apnea is present, and factors that can influence successful treatment.

The two main studies usually used to evaluate snoring are nocturnal polysomnography and an airway assessment. In a position statement, the American College of Chest Physicians and the Association of Sleep Disorders Centers have declared that only snorers suspected of having sleep apnea syndrome should undergo polysomnography.[12] The American Thoracic Society has declared in its position statement that snoring alone is not an indication for a sleep study.[13]

In symptomatic snorers with daytime somnolence, reduced performance, reduced attention, and tiredness, a full nocturnal polysomnogram is needed to establish a diagnosis of sleep apnea or UARS. Nocturnal polysomnography with a recording of sleep architecture and arousals is necessary.

Polysomnography remains the gold standard for diagnosing SDB. A complete polysomnography is often termed a *full sleep study*. Sleep is recorded from a number of electrophysiologic signals as well as from breathing and limb movement electrodes. This includes an electroencephalogram (EEG) with two leads, electromyography, electro-oculography, respiratory signals from airflow measurements from nasal pressure, nasal temperature, expired carbon dioxide, ventilation from thoracoabdominal movements or nasal pressure, oxygenation levels, and possibly esophageal balloon pressures. Other signals include an electrocardiogram tracing during sleep, pulse rate, position, esophageal pH, and video recording. A detailed airway assessment of upper airway volume and area is not done routinely because it does not predict successful surgical outcomes in a nonapneic snorer. If surgery is being considered, further radiographic imaging can provide an airway assessment and may include cephalometric measurements, computed tomography, or magnetic resonance imaging.

Treatment

Because snoring and sleep apnea are contained within a spectrum of disease states, the treatment of snoring and sleep apnea can overlap. Treatment of snoring should be directed at improving sleep apnea or UARS. In the snorer without sleep apnea or in the primary snorer, initiation of treatment can improve quality of life. Lifestyle modification should be addressed in all patients who snore, including reduction of risk factors such as obesity, alcohol consumption, and use of muscle relaxants.

Noninvasive treatments should be recommended initially, including nasal dilators, tongue-retaining devices, and mandibular advancement appliances that can be fixed or adjusted. Used to treat apneic snorers, tongue-retaining devices hold the tongue in a forward position by applying negative pressure. Subsequently, obstruction at the base of the tongue is relieved and nasal breathing is promoted. In 1995, the Task Force for the Standards of Practice Committee of the American Sleep Disorders Association recommended offering oral appliances to all nonapneic snorers.[14]

Nonsurgical methods such as treating coexisting allergies or nasal congestion, reducing weight, changing sleeping positions, and using ear plugs have met with limited success. Although many of these modalities are anecdotally successful, their efficacy has not been demonstrated in a randomized controlled setting.[15]

Patients should be counseled that CPAP carries the greatest guarantee that snoring will be abolished. Application of nasal CPAP via a nasal mask has significantly altered the medical treatment of sleep apnea, because CPAP can almost completely eliminate snoring. Most nonapneic snorers are reluctant to commit to nasal CPAP, and compliance can become an issue that leads to limited efficacy in this population.

Surgical approaches should be discussed only with patients who suffer from obvious anatomic abnormalities, including nasal or pharyngeal obstruction. Discussions in conjunction with a surgical team should focus on improvement of symptoms; patients should not expect complete resolution of snoring through surgical techniques. Nasal surgery for the relief of nasal obstruction due to septal deviation or polyps may be associated with improvement in snoring in up to 75% of patients.[16] It is believed that nasal surgery alone is unlikely to cure snoring, but it can improve breathing, allowing patients to better tolerate therapies such as nasal CPAP. Uvulopalatopharyngoplasty (UPPP) (Fig. 1) and laser-assisted palatal surgery each have reported success rates of greater than 70% for primary snoring.[17]

Laser-assisted uvulopalatoplasty (LAUP) is similar to conventional UPPP but is performed in an outpatient setting under local anesthesia. Less adjacent palatal tissue is resected and only partial uvulectomy is performed. LAUP is a sequential procedure that usually takes three or four outpatient visits to complete.[18]

Outcomes

The best ways to assess snoring treatment outcomes are through the subjective method (by asking the bed partner or the snorer about the effects of therapy) and through the objective method, which is also problematic because no standardized measurement techniques and data analysis protocols exist. With these limitations, it is more appropriate to assess treatment outcomes subjectively using a well-designed

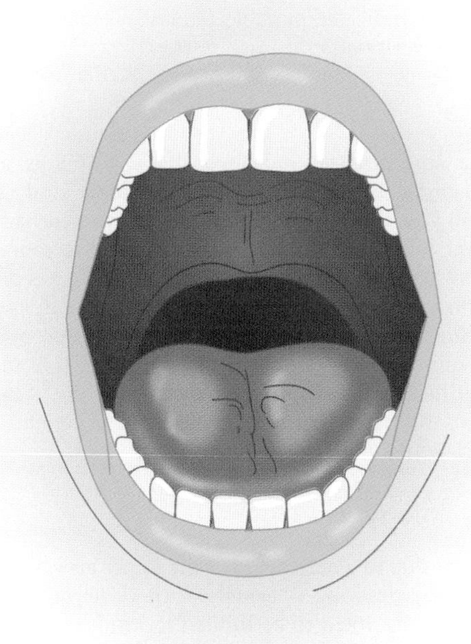

Figure 1 **Reduction in posterior pharyngeal tissue and absence of the uvula are seen following uvulopalatopharyngoplasty.** © *Cleveland Clinic Foundation, 2003.*

questionnaire answered by the person who can best assess the state of snoring before and after the intervention.

UPPER AIRWAY RESISTANCE SYNDROME

UARS can cause symptoms similar to those found in OSA, yet this syndrome is considerably different due to the lack of oxygen desaturation found during sleep studies. *Upper airway resistance syndrome* was a term first applied to patients who were found to have excessive daytime sleepiness without a clear cause on a multiple sleep latency test, which was further documented by an overnight polysomnogram. These patients were often said to have idiopathic hypersomnia. After many of these patients were further tested with invasive polysomnography (including an esophageal balloon transducer and full pneumotachograph), they were found to have increased upper airway resistance. Resistance was indicated by increased negative esophageal inspiratory pressure.[2]

Definition

UARS is characterized by repeated arousals, due to upper airway resistance, that lead to excessive daytime sleepiness. This disorder often produces a snoring pattern termed *crescendo snoring*. When the crescendo snoring episode ends, an arousal occurs with rapid decrease in upper airway resistance; the snoring then disappears and stops for a period. UARS events are noted to be typically short: one to three breaths in duration. These events have been termed *respiratory effort-related arousals* (RERAs). In UARS, unlike in OSAHS, there is no evidence of oxygen desaturation.[2] For the measurement criteria to be classified as a RERA, there must be a pattern of progressively increased negative esophageal pressure that is terminated by a sudden change in the pressure to a less-negative level and a sleep arousal. Furthermore, the event must last 10 seconds or longer.

Prevalence

The prevalence of UARS in the general adult population is unknown, yet it has been estimated to be as high as 10% to 15% when the definition is applied to adults who suffer from snoring and excessive daytime sleepiness.[19] It has been suggested that UARS occurs in a less-obese younger population and more commonly in women than does OSAHS.[2]

Pathophysiology

Guilleminault and coworkers[20] demonstrated that many nonapneic patients show a reduction in cross-sectional area of the pharynx during sleep. Reduction in airway area is sufficient to avoid hypopneas and apnea but enough to increase upper airway resistance. Patients with UARS suffer from increased airway resistance, which generates snoring and then leads to arousal episodes and ultimately to excessive daytime sleepiness.

Signs and Symptoms

Although patients with UARS share no standard clinical presentation, the cardinal symptom of UARS is excessive daytime sleepiness or fatigue. Some patients also complain of difficulty with concentration, morning headaches, impotence, difficulty sleeping, or restless sleep. They often report having repetitive nightmares, such as choking or being buried alive, which can suggest difficulty with breathing. Again, snoring is not a necessary feature of this syndrome because the upper airway resistance is due to a partial decrease in airway cross-sectional area; therefore, the airway walls do not have to vibrate and produce a snoring sound.[3]

Diagnosis

UARS should not be overdiagnosed. Three essential clinical features consistently have been used by investigators and authors to diagnose UARS: excessive daytime somnolence; an elevated EEG arousal index, with the arousal related to increased respiratory efforts; and a normal respiratory disturbance index (RDI) of less than five events per hour of sleep.[21]

UARS is present only if there are documented elevations in upper airway resistance, sleep fragmentation, and daytime dysfunction or excessive daytime sleepiness. The clinical complaint of fatigue or daytime sleepiness can be documented by an abnormal increase in the Epworth Sleepiness Scale (see Table 1) score to a value greater than 10 or by use of another validated sleep questionnaire. A low RDI is also needed to distinguish UARS from OSAHS. The elevated EEG arousal index related to increased respiratory efforts is the specific measurement that distinguishes UARS from idiopathic hypersomnolence.[22] The clinical complaint of snoring (including crescendo snoring), increase in snoring intensity before EEG arousals, and clinical improvement with a short-term trial of nasal CPAP can be regarded as supporting a diagnosis of UARS.

The diagnosis of UARS requires full polysomnography. Although measurements of upper airway resistance were first used, based on the original definition of UARS, substitute measurements of effort and ventilation may be used as long as there is no evidence of hypopneas or apneas. A normal apnea-hypopnea index (AHI) of less than five events per hour of sleep should be seen on the polysomnograph. Additionally, EEG arousals should occur at a rate of more than 10 per hour of sleep and must be associated with increased respiratory effort (usually made by nocturnal esophageal pressure monitoring).

Current literature supports that esophageal pressures greater than −10 cm H_2O are abnormal. The measurement of esophageal pressure is the gold standard for measuring respiratory effort and is the only consistent measurement reported for the diagnosis of UARS. Substitute measurements can include inductive plethysmography, strain gauges, oronasal temperature measurements, nasal pressures, and the carbon monoxide levels in exhaled gas. Arousals are documented from the EEG tracings and electromyography, although changes in heart rate, ventilation, and other measurements of autonomic activity may play some role in the future.[3]

Treatment

CPAP, surgery, oral appliances, and weight loss are possible treatment options for UARS. Ideally, the recommended treatment of UARS should be effective, relieve symptoms, and produce normalized studies after therapy. These therapies also should be covered by health insurance and have long-term effectiveness. Thus far, however, none of the proposed treatments has fully met these criteria.

Outcomes

Data in the sleep literature are not clear-cut regarding the efficacy, safety, and compliance of UARS treatment modalities, including weight loss, nasal CPAP, oral appliances, and surgery.

OBSTRUCTIVE SLEEP APNEA–HYPOPNEA SYNDROME

OSAHS is not a new clinical entity but is one that has been recognized only recently. Evolving from the historical accounts of sleep apnea to the present day, the most significant development in the diagnosis of sleep-disordered breathing is the publication of the American Academy of Sleep Medicine's report on recommendations for syndrome definition and measurement techniques in clinical research. Within this report, the older term *obstructive sleep apnea* was appropriately changed to the newer term *obstructive sleep apnea–hypopnea syndrome*.[22] The complications and potential consequences of OSAHS include increased risks of hypertension and cardiovascular events as well as cerebrovascular events. OSAHS affects not only the health of the sufferer but also the bed partner's sleep state.[23]

Definition

OSAHS is characterized by recurrent episodes of partial or complete airway obstruction during sleep due to repetitive collapse of the pharynx, necessitating recurrent awakenings or arousals to re-establish airway patency. This airway obstruction or partial obstruction manifests in a reduction in airflow, termed *hypopnea*, or in a complete cessation of airflow, termed *apnea*, despite ongoing inspiratory effort. Hypopnea is defined in adults as a 10-second event during which there is continued breathing but in which ventilation during sleep is reduced by at least 50% from baseline. Apnea is total cessation of airflow for at least 10 seconds. Apnea can be obstructive or central. Obstructive apnea is defined as cessation of airflow but with continued respiratory effort, whereas central apnea is a state in which airflow and respiratory effort are both absent. Apnea also can be both central and obstructive, although obstructive apnea is more common. Hypopnea can produce clinical sequelae similar to those of apnea, but in general, apnea is associated with a greater fall in oxygen saturations.

For sleep-disordered breathing to be diagnosed as OSAHS, the patient must have at least five obstructed breathing events per hour (or 30 events per 6 hours of sleep). These events can be a combination of OSA, hypopnea, or respiratory effort–related arousals. The patient must also have either excessive daytime sleepiness or at least two of choking or gasping from sleep, recurrent awakenings from sleep, feeling unrefreshed after sleep, daytime fatigue, or poor concentration. This second group of signs and symptoms must not be better explained by other factors.[2]

The RDI (or AHI) is the number of apneas plus hypopneas per hour of sleep. This index has now become the standard by which to define and quantify the severity of OSAHS. An RDI of more than 15 events per hour indicates possible OSAHS. Generally, as the RDI increases, the severity of apnea increases.

Prevalence

Most apnea studies have indicated that OSAHS is a relatively common disorder. In a large U.S. epidemiologic study in subjects ages 30 to 60 years, 24% of men and 9% of women had abnormal AHI indices.[2] Overall, it has been estimated that more than 158 million adults ages 25 years and older suffer from sleep apnea and that more than 10 million men and women currently go untreated for the disorder in the United States. Currently, the prevalence of OSAHS is conservatively estimated to be 1% to 2% in middle-aged men and one half that, or approximately 0.5% to 1%, in middle-aged women.[24] It is estimated that only 1% of OSAHS patients are receiving appropriate treatment for their disease.[25]

Pathophysiology

OSAHS occurs due to a narrowing of the upper airway during sleep. The site of the narrowing is usually at the level of the pharynx.[26] Airway occlusion is noted to be limited to inspiration, which exerts negative pharyngeal pressure and reduces the tone of the genioglossus muscle. This theory remains the cornerstone of understanding OSAHS.

Upper airway size in OSAHS patients is smaller than in normal subjects, as assessed by CT scan and resistance measurements. Patients with OSAHS also have been noted to have a more elliptical upper airway shape than normal subjects, but this may be due to increased body mass as well. The difference in airway size in OSAHS patients is due to fat deposition and facial bone structure. Obese patients with OSAHS have fat deposits lateral to the pharynx. Although this fat deposit might not be substantial, it can predispose patients to OSAHS.[27] Retroposition of the maxilla and mandible predisposes patients to OSAHS due to a narrowing of the pharynx caused by posterior displacement of the tongue and palate. These facial traits also are more common in families with OSAHS.[28] Patients with OSAHS also have increased palatal muscle bulk, which usually responds to positive pressure.

Genetics might play an important role in the pathophysiology of OSAHS. The disorder is more common among family members suffering from OSAHS than in the general population. This relation seems to be independent of familial obesity tendencies.[8]

Signs and Symptoms

The dominant symptoms of OSAHS are sleepiness and daytime somnolence. Other symptoms include difficulty with concentration, fatigue, unrefreshing sleep, nocturnal choking, nocturia, depression, and decreased libido. Bed partners might report snoring, apneas, restless sleep, or irritability. In investigating sleepiness, note whether the patient falls asleep frequently against his or her will or in a dangerous situation, such as when driving.

Although there is no gold standard definition for sleepiness, the Epworth Sleepiness Scale can assist the clinician in documenting this symptom. A score of greater than 12 of 24 points on the Epworth scale is defined as abnormally sleepy (see Table 1). Morning headache was initially reported as a feature of OSAHS, but its true association is debatable.[29] Patients should also be asked about weight gain and the relation of developing symptoms to any gain in weight.

Although physical examination has not proved helpful in identifying patients with SDB, BMI and neck circumference (indicators of obesity) appear to be good clinical predictors for OSAHS. BMI (weight in kg/height in meters) is the most commonly used clinical predictor for OSAHS. Obesity is defined as a BMI greater than 30 kg/m^2. Upper body obesity also may be associated with a higher risk for OSAHS.

Physical findings of OSAHS can include obesity, increased neck circumference, crowding of the upper airway, macroglossia, enlarged tonsils, nasal obstruction, retrognathia, hypertension, lower limb edema, and signs of cor pulmonale. Laboratory investigations can include secondary polycythemia, proteinuria respiratory failure, nocturnal cardiac arrhythmia, and gastroesophageal reflux disease.

Diagnosis

Because many of the symptoms of OSA are nonspecific, the index of clinical suspicion for OSAHS needs to be high to make the diagnosis. The differential diagnosis for OSAHS should include primary snoring, chronic hypoventilation syndrome, and central sleep apnea and Cheyne-Stokes respiration.

Patients suspected to have OSAHS should undergo polysomnography. Because night-to-night variability can occur in mild cases of the disorder, misdiagnosis can occur. Therefore, a negative first-night test is insufficient to rule out OSAHS in patients in whom there is a high clinical suspicion of the disease.

Many other types of sleep studies are available, with varying settings and parameters measured. A complete level I study is performed in the laboratory; partial and limited studies can be conducted in the home. However, the American Sleep Disorders Association advises that standard polysomnography is the accepted test for diagnosing and determining the severity and treatment of OSA. The association recommends that portable or unattended recordings are an acceptable alternative only when clinical symptoms are severe and indicate sleep apnea, initiation of treatment is urgent and a standard polysomnography is not readily available, the patient cannot be studied in a sleep laboratory, or follow-up studies are needed to evaluate therapy response.

Treatment

Adequate treatment of OSAHS results in improvement of symptoms and can alter morbidity and mortality outcomes. Current therapies in the treatment of sleep apnea are aimed at widening the pharyngeal airway, making it less apt to collapse, or at pneumatically splinting the airway open using CPAP. CPAP is very effective in eliminating pharyngeal collapse, improving overall symptoms, and reducing cardiovascular sequelae, making it the treatment of choice for OSAHS.

Bilevel positive airway pressure (BiPAP) allows the clinician to set different pressures for inspiratory and expiratory breaths. This may be beneficial for patients who occasionally complain of feeling excessive air pressure or of having the sensation of exhaling against positive pressure. The routine use of BiPAP has not been shown to increase compliance, but in patients who have high CPAP requirements, BiPAP may be a more comfortable option.

Oral appliances can enlarge the pharyngeal airway during sleep by moving either the tongue or the mandible anteriorly, partially relieving apnea. Such appliances are probably more useful in patients with mild apnea than in those with severe apnea.

Upper airway surgery, including radiofrequency ablation of the tongue or soft palate (somnoplasty), LAUP, UPPP, or genioglossal advancement with hypoid myotomy, bimaxillary advancement, or maxillomandibular advancement, aims to enlarge the pharyngeal space and prevent airway collapse. Success rates range from 30% for the less aggressive interventions to 90% for the more aggressive procedures. Common side effects include pain, alteration in taste, and nasal regurgitation.

The role of pharmacotherapy for sleep apnea remains controversial. Experimental evidence suggests that serotoninergics at certain doses improve sleep efficiency; however, sufficient data are not available to support their routine use.

Outcomes

OSAHS outcomes, including feelings of vitality, energy, and mental summary scores, all improve with treatment. Significant study data have accumulated demonstrating reductions in cardiovascular morbidity and mortality with CPAP therapy for OSAHS. In fact, health care use is significantly reduced when patients adhere to CPAP therapy, resulting in fewer physician claims and hospital stays.

Summary

- *Sleep-disordered breathing* refers to a wide spectrum of sleep-related breathing abnormalities; those related to increased upper airway resistance include snoring, upper airway resistance syndrome, and obstructive sleep apnea-hypopnea syndrome.
- Polysomnography remains the gold standard for diagnosing sleep-disordered breathing.
- Lifestyle modifications should be addressed in all patients suffering from snoring, including reduction of risk factors such as obesity and use of alcohol and muscle relaxants.
- Patients should be counseled that continuous positive airway pressure carries the greatest assurance that snoring will be abolished.
- Surgical approaches should be discussed with only a limited number of patients, mainly those who suffer from obvious anatomic abnormalities

Suggested Readings

American Academy of Sleep Medicine: International Classification of Sleep Disorders, revised: Diagnostic and Coding Manual. Chicago, American Academy of Sleep Medicine, 2001, p 195. PDF available at http://www.esst.org/adds/ICSD.pdf (accessed March 20, 2009).

Bloom JW, Kaltenborn WT, Quan SF: Risk factors in a general population for snoring. Importance of cigarette smoking and obesity. Chest 1988;93:678-683.

Callop N, Cassel DK: Snoring and sleep disordered breathing. In Lee-Chiong T Jr, Sateia M, Carskadon M (eds): Sleep Medicine. Philadelphia: Hanley & Belfus, 2002, pp 349-355.

Gavriely N, Jensen O: Theory and measurements of snores. J Appl Physiol 1993;74:2828-2837.

Lugaresi E, Cirignotta F, Coccagna G, Piana C: Some epidemiological data on snoring and cardiocirculatory disturbances. Sleep 1980;3:221-224.

Lugaresi E, Cirignotta F, Montagna P, et al: Snoring: Pathogenic, clinical, and therapeutic aspects. In Kryger M, Roth T, Dement W (eds): Principles and Practice of Sleep Medicine, 2nd ed. Philadelphia: WB Saunders, 1994, pp 621-629.

Phillipson EA, Remmers JE: American Thoracic Society Consensus Conference on indications and standards for cardiopulmonary sleep studies. Am Rev Respir Dis 1989;139:559-568.

The Random House Dictionary of the English Language. New York: Random House; 2001.

Schwab RJ, Goldberg AN, Pack AJ: Sleep apnea syndromes. In Fishman AP (ed): Fishman's Pulmonary Diseases and Disorders, 3rd ed. New York: McGraw-Hill, 1998, pp 1617-1646.

Slutsky A: The impact of sleep disordered breathing on other diseases. Presented at 98th International Conference of the American Thoracic Society, Atlanta, May 17-22, 2002. Available at http://www.medscape.com/viewarticle/437261 (accessed March 20, 2009).

References

For a complete list of references, log onto www.expertconsult.com.

Section 13

RHEUMATOLOGY AND IMMUNOLOGY

Laboratory Evaluation of Rheumatic Diseases

Marina Magrey and Abby Abelson

The diagnosis of rheumatologic diseases is based on clinical information, blood and imaging tests, and in some cases on histology. Blood tests are useful in confirming clinically suspected diagnosis and monitoring the disease activity. The tests should be used as adjuncts to a comprehensive history and physical examination.

The value of a test in diagnosing a certain condition depends on its pretest probability. A positive test result with high pretest probability helps to make a diagnosis, but a negative test result with low pretest probability helps to rule out the diagnosis. However, clinicians cannot rely heavily on blood tests in making the diagnosis of rheumatologic diseases, except for certain tests that are highly specific for certain diseases. Improper application of these tests leads to misdiagnosis, inappropriate therapy, and unnecessary health care expenses. This chapter discusses blood tests that are useful in evaluating various rheumatologic diseases.

ACUTE-PHASE REACTANTS

Acute-phase reactants are proteins whose plasma concentration increases (positive acute-phase proteins) or decreases (negative acute-phase proteins) by at least 25% during inflammatory states.[1] Box 1 lists positive and negative acute-phase reactants. The effect of inflammatory molecules such as interleukin (IL)-6, IL-1, tumor necrosis factor α (TNF-α), interferon gamma (IFN-γ), and transforming growth factor β (TGF-β) causes a change in hepatic protein synthesis collectively known as acute-phase response. Erythrocyte sedimentation rate (ESR) and C-reactive protein (CRP) are the most widely measured acute-phase reactants in clinical practice.

ESR is a measure of the height of erythrocytes that fall through plasma in a Westergen or a Wintrobe tube over a period of 1 hour. ESR can be greatly influenced by the shape and number of red blood cells as well as other plasma constituents like fibrinogen, globulins, and albumins. It can be spuriously high in the absence of inflammation, as in anemia, nephritic syndrome, and hypergammaglobulinemia, and it can be spuriously normal in cryoglobulinemia and hemoglobinopathy. ESR increases steadily with age, and the upper limit varies with sex; hence, ESR is difficult to interpret compared to CRP.

The concentration of CRP in serum is more sensitive than ESR to evaluate and monitor inflammation, and it is independent of factors that affect ESR. It correlates better with disease activity, and the rise in CPR level is seen much earlier than that of other acute-phase reactants, usually 4 to 6 hours after tissue injury.

Both ESR and CRP levels can be elevated in a wide variety of conditions including trauma, infection, infarction, neoplasms, and inflammatory arthritis. Usually ESR and CRP levels correlate well, but in some patients levels may be discordant for reasons that are unclear. They are very useful in monitoring disease activity in rheumatologic conditions such as rheumatoid arthritis, polymyalgia rheumatica,[2] and giant cell arteritis. Some studies have shown that the pretreatment ESR value is of some prognostic value in polymyalgia rheumatica. Most patients with active lupus have normal or minimally elevated CRP levels, and markedly elevated concentrations of CRP in SLE should raise a suspicion of bacterial infection. Other causes for elevated CRP in SLE patients include serositis, synovitis, and vasculitis.

ANTINUCLEAR ANTIBODIES

Antinuclear antibodies (ANAs) directed against a variety of nuclear antigens have been detected in the serum of patients with many rheumatic and nonrheumatic diseases as well as in healthy persons. Various immunochemistry techniques are used to detect and characterize these ANAs. These methods include immunofluorescence microscopy, hemagglutination, immunodiffusion, complement fixation, and enzyme-linked immunosorbent assay (ELISA).

Immunofluorescent microscopy performed on human epithelial-2 (Hep-2) cells is widely used for initial screening. It is a highly sensitive test and is often abnormal in patients with ANA-associated diseases, but the specificity is low and the test has many false-positive results. It is reported as positive or negative and includes a titer. ANA testing performed using ELISA technology is very sensitive and has a high incidence of false-positive results (Fig. 1).

Clinical Applications

ANA testing is very useful in establishing a diagnosis of systemic lupus erythematosus (SLE). Nearly all patients with SLE have a positive ANA test, with a sensitivity of 93% to 95% and a specificity of 57%.[3] However, even healthy persons can have a positive ANA test at lower titers. About 25% to 30% of healthy persons have a positive test with a titer of 1:40, 10% to 15% at a titer of 1:80, and 5% at a titer of 1:160 or greater. The frequency increases with age, particularly in women. ANA titer of 1:40 is seen in 25% to 30% of relatives of patients with rheumatologic disorders.[3]

A positive ANA in a patient with low pretest probability is often of unclear significance. Due to the low prevalence of SLE (40-50/100,000), most people with positive ANA do not have lupus (positive predictive value [PPV], 11%). However, a high ANA titer (>1:640) should increase the suspicion for an autoimmune disorder, although not diagnostic of a disease, and patients with high titers should be carefully followed for the development of connective tissue disorder. ANA titer is not routinely used for assessing the disease activity in lupus, and serial ANA testing is therefore not useful.

In addition to lupus, ANA testing is helpful in diagnosing other rheumatic diseases such as systemic sclerosis and Sjögren's syndrome (Table 1). The sensitivity of ANA in diagnosing systemic sclerosis is 85% and the specificity is 54%.[3] Although ANA is not included in the 2002 classification criteria for Sjögren's syndrome, it is found in 80% of patients with primary Sjögren's syndrome and at high titers (>1:320) in nearly one half of the patients.[4] Patients presenting with Raynaud's phenomenon should also have ANA testing because a positive ANA test indicates an increased risk of developing an associated systemic rheumatic disease from 19% to 30%, whereas a negative test indicates a risk of 7%.[5] Additionally, ANA testing helps to stratify the risk of uveitis in patients with juvenile idiopathic arthritis.

Antinuclear Antibodies in Other Diseases

ANA can also be positive in many autoimmune disease states not associated with connective tissue diseases, such as autoimmune hepatitis, primary autoimmune cholangitis, primary biliary cirrhosis, and Crohn's disease. Other disorders associated with positive ANA titer include such chronic infectious diseases as mononucleosis, subacute bacterial endocarditis, tuberculosis, and lymphoproliferative diseases. Hence, ANA testing should be reserved for patients with high suspicion for systemic autoimmune disease, such as young women with fatigue, joint pain, and rash, and should not be used as a screening test in patients complaining of generalized fatigue and musculoskeletal pain, particularly elderly patients.

Types

There are different types of ANAs based on their target antigen, including single-stranded DNA (ssDNA) and double-stranded DNA (dsDNA), nuclear histone and nonhistone nuclear proteins, and RNA protein complexes. The staining pattern seen on indirect immunofluorescence (IIF) gives some indication of the specificity of the antibodies in the sample (Table 2 and see Fig. 1). Identification of the specificity for extractable nuclear antigens (ENA) is warranted because this can further differentiate between the distinct types of autoimmune connective tissue diseases. Hence, a positive ANA test should be followed by an anti-DNA antibodies assay.

Box 1 Positive and Negative Acute-Phase Reactants

Positive Acute-Phase Reactants
Alpha$_1$-antitrypsin
Ceruloplasmin
Complement components
C-reactive protein
Ferritin
Fibrinogen
Haptoglobin
Serum amyloid A

Negative Acute-Phase Reactants
Albumin
Transferrin
Transthyretin

Table 1 Sensitivity and Specificity of Antinuclear Antibody in Various Connective Tissue Diseases

Disease	Sensitivity (%)	Specificity (%)
Systemic lupus erythematosus	93-95	57
Scleroderma	85	54
Polymyositis, dermatomyositis	61	63
Rheumatoid arthritis	41	56
Sjögren's syndrome	48	52
Raynaud's phenomenon	64	41
Juvenile chronic arthritis	57	39
Juvenile chronic arthritis with uveitis	80	53

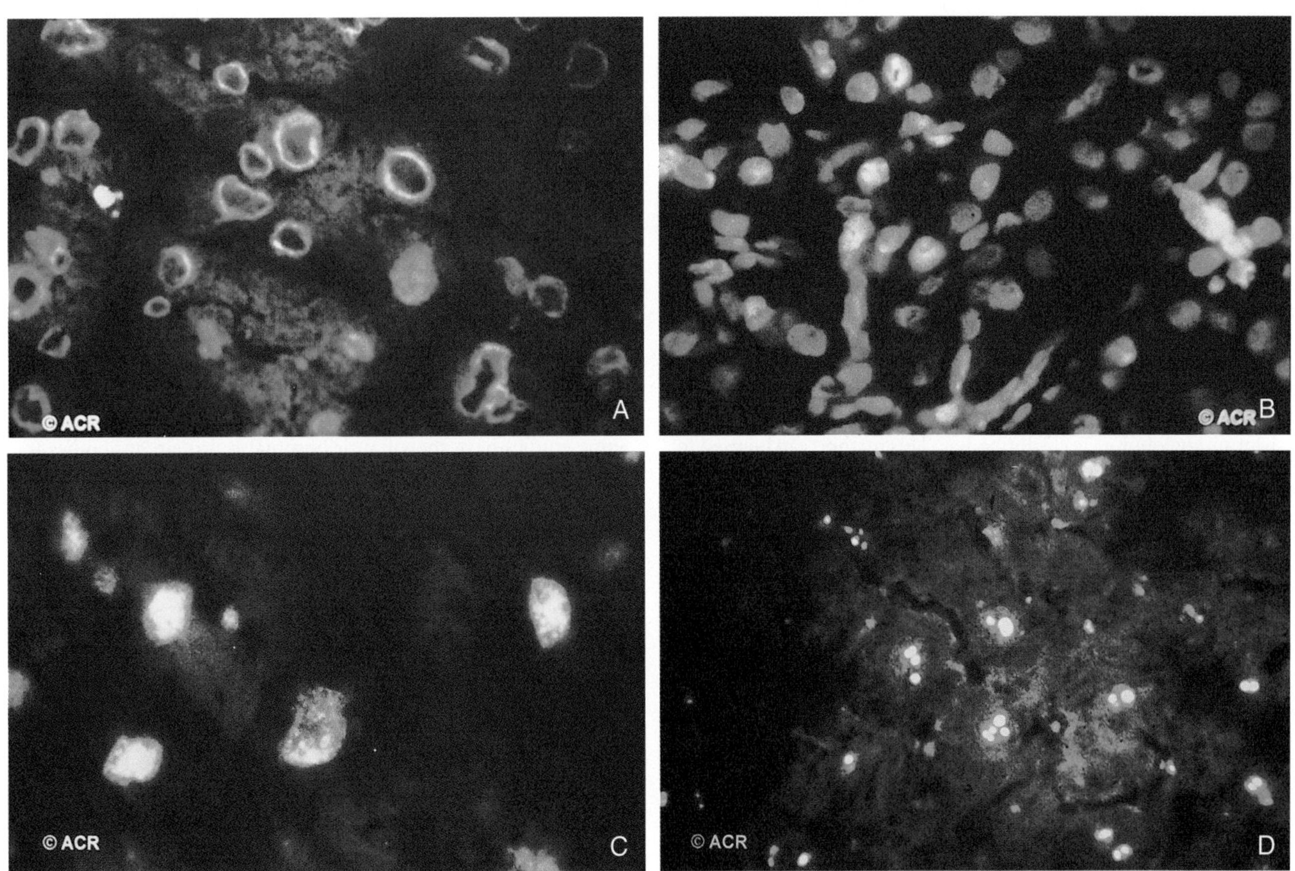

Figure 1 Antinuclear antibody pattern in mouse liver. A, Peripheral (rim) pattern. **B,** Homogenous (diffuse) pattern. **C,** Speckled pattern. **D,** Nucleolar. *(From Schur PH, Shmerling RH: Laboratory Tests in Rheumatic Diseases. In Hochberg MC, Silman AJ, Smolen JS, et al (eds): Practical Rheumatology. St. Louis, Mosby, 2004, pp 60. Courtesy of Dr. Peter Schur and UpToDate.)*

SECTION 13 RHEUMATOLOGY AND IMMUNOLOGY

Table 2 Identifying Antinuclear Antibodies

Antigen	Disease Association
Homogenous and Diffuse	
DNA-histone complex (nucleosome)	SLE (60%) Drug-induced lupus (95%)
Peripheral Rim	
dsDNA	SLE
Speckled	
RNA polymerase types II and III	Systemic sclerosis
RNP	MCTD (100%)
Scl-70	Systemic sclerosis (15%-70%)
Sm	SLE (25%-30%)
SS-A	Sjögren's syndrome (8%-70%) SLE (35%-40%)
SS-B	Sjögren's syndrome (14%-60%) SLE (15%)
Nucleolar	
Nucleolar RNA, RNA polymerase 1	Systemic sclerosis
Pm-scl	Polymyositis
Centromere	
CENP	Limited scleroderma

MCTD, mixed connective tissue disease; SLE, systemic lupus erythematosus.

Anti-DNA Antibodies

Antibodies to dsDNA are often measured in SLE and are commonly referred to as anti-DNA antibodies. They are very useful in the diagnosis of SLE and assessment of disease activity, and they are associated with lupus nephritis.

The most commonly used techniques for measuring anti-dsDNA antibodies are ELISA and immunofluorescence (e.g., using *Crithidia luciliae* as substrate). Radioimmunoassay (e.g., the Farr assay) is still available but its use has declined. The hemoflagellate *Crithidia luciliae* contains in its kinetoplast pure dsDNA, not complexed to proteins. Serially diluted serum samples are added to the slide carrying *Crithidia* cells. Binding of antibodies is visualized by fluoresceinated anti-immunoglobulin (Ig) G antibodies. This method can be used to confirm the presence of anti-dsDNA antibodies when the ELISA results are discrepant.

The sensitivity of anti-dsDNA antibody for diagnosis of SLE is 57.3% and the specificity is 97.4%.[6] These antibodies are present at some time in the course of the disease as the levels fluctuate and may be absent at times. Anti-DNA antibodies have been reported in patients with a variety of other rheumatologic and nonrheumatologic diseases including rheumatoid arthritis, Sjögren's syndrome, scleroderma, drug-induced lupus, Raynaud's phenomenon, mixed connective tissue disease, discoid lupus, myositis, chronic active hepatitis, uveitis, Graves' disease, and anticardiolipin antibody syndrome and in women with silicone breast implants. Not all patients with SLE have positive anti-dsDNA antibodies; therefore, a negative test does not exclude the diagnosis of SLE. The prevalence of patients with a positive anti-DNA assay despite a negative ANA has been reported to be 0% to 0.8%. Therefore, unless there is a reasonable suspicion that the ANA is falsely negative, anti-DNA antibody testing is not generally indicated in ANA-negative patients.

Anti-Smith and Antiribonucleoprotein Antibodies

Antibodies directed against small nuclear riboprotein include anti-Smith (anti-Sm) antibody and antiribonuclear protein (anti-RNP) antibodies. They bind to related but distinct antibodies.

Anti-Sm antibodies are very useful for confirming the diagnosis of SLE. A positive test result strongly supports the diagnosis, although a negative test result cannot exclude it. The sensitivity of anti-SM antibody for diagnosis of lupus ranges from 24% to 30%, and specificity ranges from 96% to 98%.[7]

Anti-RNP antibodies bind to protein containing U1-RNA. They coexist with anti-Sm antibodies in many patients with SLE. They have a very low sensitivity and moderate specificity for diagnosing SLE, but they are very useful in diagnosing mixed connective tissue disease. The sensitivity of anti-RNP antibodies for diagnosing mixed connective tissue disease is 71% to 100% and the specificity is 84% to 100%.

Sjögren's Syndrome Antibodies

The Sjögren's syndrome A antigen (anti-SSA/Ro) consists of 52- and 60-kDa proteins (called Ro52 and Ro60) complexed with Y1-Y5 RNAs. Anti-SSA/Ro and anti-SSB/La antibodies are detected by counterimmunoelectrophoresis, ELISA, and Western blot. ELISA and Western blot are the most sensitive assays but are less specific.

Anti-SSA antibodies are seen in 50% to 60% of patients with primary Sjögren's syndrome and rarely in healthy persons.[8] These antibodies are also detected in other autoimmune diseases including rheumatoid arthritis, SLE, and polymyositis. About 10% to 15% of patients with secondary Sjögren's syndrome and 35% to 40% of patients with SLE have anti-SSA antibodies. Moreover, their presence is associated with development of extraglandular features including vasculitis, lymphadenopathy, nephritis, and leukopenia in patients with Sjögren's syndrome[4] and with features including photosensitivity, subacute cutaneous lupus, cutaneous vasculitis, neonatal lupus, and congenital heart block.

Anti-SSB antibodies are present in 40% to 50% of patients with primary Sjögren's syndrome and in 15% of patients with SLE but rarely in other connective tissue diseases. These antibodies are sometimes seen in patients with autoimmune hepatitis.

Antibodies to both SSA and SSB antibodies should be checked in patients with sicca symptoms. Patients with primary Sjögren's syndrome and positive SSA and SSB antibodies represent a subset of patients who have more active disease and who need very close follow-up to watch for the development of extraglandular features.[4]

Antiribosomal P Protein Antibodies

Some studies have shown antiribosomal P protein antibodies to be highly specific for lupus and associated with neuropsychiatric lupus. They are detected in 10% to 20% of patients with SLE. However, the diagnosis of neuropsychiatric lupus is still based on clinical grounds.

Antihistone Antibodies

Antihistone antibodies are present in more than 95% patients with drug-induced lupus and up to 80% of patients with idiopathic lupus. However, the mere presence of antihistone antibodies does not indicate drug-induced lupus. Up to 80% of patients taking procainamide for 1 to 2 years develop positive ANAs, but most do not develop drug-induced lupus.

Anticentromere, Anti-Scl-70, and Anti-U3-Ribonuclearprotein Antibodies

Anticentromere antibodies are associated with limited cutaneous systemic sclerosis, previously called CREST (*c*alcinosis, *R*aynaud's phenomenon, *e*sophageal dysmotility, *s*clerodactyly, *t*elangectasia] syndrome).They are rarely found in patients with other connective tissue diseases or in healthy persons, making them highly specific for diagnosing systemic sclerosis. The sensitivity of anticentromere antibodies for the diagnosis of limitied cutaneous systemic sclerosis is 31%, and specificity is 97%.[9] They are very useful in distinguishing patients with limited systemic sclerosis from patients with diffuse systemic sclerosis or with primary Raynaud's phenomenon. Anticentromes antibodies are predictive of limited cutaneous involvement or decreased likelihood of investital being displayed in systemic sclerosis.

Anti-Scl-70 antibody is also very useful in diagnosing systemic sclerosis. This antibody is seen in 20.2 % of patients with systemic sclerosis and is highly specific (100%) for diffuse disease.[9] Anti Scl-70 and anticentromere antibodies rarely coexist in the same person. The presence of anti-Scl-70 antibodies is useful in predicting a greater likelihood for the development of diffuse cutaneous involvement and radiographic pulmonary fibrosis with an abnormal pulmonary function test.

The antinucleolar antibodies (such as RNA-polymerase I, II, and III; anti-PM Scl; and anti-Th/To) are infrequently present in patients with systemic sclerosis, which limits their predictive value in the diagnosis. However, they are highly specific for the diagnosis of systemic sclerosis.

Miscellaneous Antinuclear Antibodies

Polymyositis and dermatomyositis are associated with autoantibodies against a group of aminoacyl tRNA synthetases. These include Jo1,PL-7,PL-12,EJ, and OJ. The anti-Jo1 antibodies are present in 20% to 25% of adult myositis patients and are highly specific for myositis associated with a constellation of symptoms including skin involvement, lung disease, Raynaud's phenomenon, inflammatory arthritis, and fever. Anti-Mi-2 antibodies are more specific for dermatomyositis and are associated with a favorable long-term prognosis.

RHEUMATOID FACTOR

Rheumatoid factor (RF) autoantibodies are directed against the Fc portion of IgG. The most commonly measured RF is IgM. The other RFs include IgG, IgE, and IgA. Box 2 shows RF positivity in different diseases.

RF is detected in a wide variety of rheumatic and nonrheumatic conditions, as shown in Box 2. It is commonly used in diagnosing rheumatoid arthritis. The sensitivity of RF for diagnosing rheumatoid arthritis is around 50% to 80%, and specificity is 85% to 90%, as reported by some studies where patients with advanced disease were tested. RF may be negative in the early stages of rheumatoid arthritis, and positivity increases over time.

RF alone cannot be used for diagnosis of rheumatoid arthritis. Around 15% to 20% of patients with rheumatoid arthritis never have RF positivity, and 2% to 10% of healthy persons are RF positive. Hence, positive RF alone does not confirm rheumatoid arthritis and negative RF does not exclude it.[10] RF testing must be ordered more selectively, and the best time to obtain the test may be when the suspicion of rheumatoid arthritis is low and a negative test would provide significant reassurance.[10] There is a correlation between higher RF concentrations and more-severe disease and poor prognosis, but the use of RF in monitoring disease activity is unclear.

ANTI–CYCLIC CITRULLINATED PEPTIDE ANTIBODIES

Anti–cyclic citrullinated peptide (anti-CCP) antibodies are directed against citrulline residues formed in post-translational modification of arginine. They are often elevated in patients with rheumatoid arthritis. They have a reported sensitivity of 30% to 60% and a specificity of 95% to 98% among patients meeting the criteria for rheumatoid arthritis.

Two of the most important clinical uses of this test are its high specificity for the disease and the presence of anti-CCP antibodies in early-phase rheumatoid arthritis. Some studies have shown that anti-CCP antibodies can appear in the circulation several years before the onset of rheumatoid arthritis. The presence of anti-CCP antibodies in early disease is highly predictive for more-rapid radiographic progression of disease, meaning patients with anti-CCP antibodies have significantly more joint damage than patients without this antibody.[11] Hence, anti-CCP antibody should be checked in patients in whom rheumatoid arthritis is suspected on clinical grounds.

Patients with chronic hepatitis C virus infection sometimes have high titers of RF and a variety of rheumatic symptoms, but anti-CCP antibody is rarely found in these patients.[12] Presence of anti-CCP antibody in such cases supports the diagnosis of concomitant rheumatoid arthritis, although a negative test does not exclude it.

Box 2 Rheumatoid Factor Positivity in Different Diseases

Rheumatic Conditions (Sensitivity)
Cryoglobulinemia (40%-100%)
Polymyositis and dermatomyositis (5%-10%)
Rheumatoid arthritis (50%-90%)
Sjögren's syndrome (75%-95%)
Systemic lupus erythematosus (15%-35%)
Systemic sclerosis (20%-30%)

Nonrheumatic Conditions
Bacterial endocarditis
Infections

- Hepatitis
- Leprosy
- Parasites
- Syphilis
- Tuberculosis

Malignancy
Pulmonary disease

- Interstitial pulmonary fibrosis
- Sarcodosis
- Silicosis

Primary biliary cirrhosis

ANTINEUTROPHIL CYTOPLASMIC ANTIBODIES

Antineutrophil cytoplasmic antibodies (ANCAs) are useful adjuncts to the clinical diagnosis of certain specific diseases, such as Wegener's granulomatosis and microscopic polyangiitis. These antibodies are directed against several neutrophilic cytoplasmic components. The two main techniques for detecting ANCAs are IIF and ELISA.

IIF assay does not identify the specific antigen responsible for the immunofluorescence. ELISA is more specific and helps to identify the specific target antigen. The two relevant target antigens are proteinase 3 (PR3) and myeloperoxidase (MPO). Both PR3 and MPO are located in the azurophilic granules of neutrophils and peroxidase-positive lysosomes of monocytes. Antibodies with target specificities for PR3 and MPO are called PR3-ANCA and MPO-ANCA. IIF without identification of MPO and PR3 antigen is incomplete and of no value.

Pattern

When serum from patients with vasculitis is incubated with ethanol-fixed human neutrophils, two major immunofluorescence patterns are observed: the c-ANCA pattern and the p-ANCA pattern

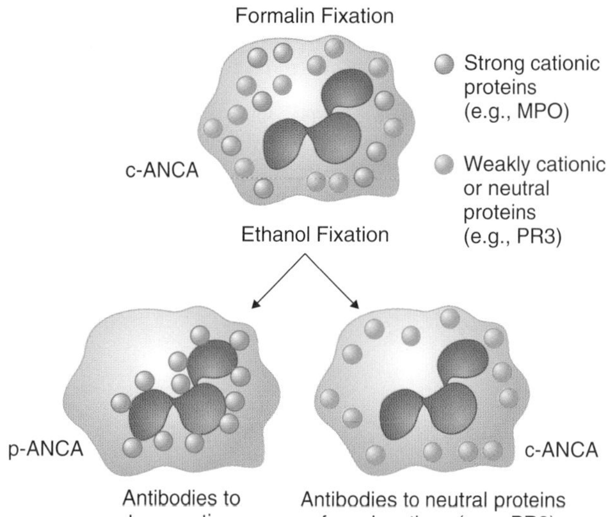

Figure 2 Pattern of antineutrophil cytoplasmic antibodies. Demonstration of cytoplasmic and perinuclear antineutrophilic antibodies by indirect immunofluorescence within normal neutrophils. ANCA, antineutrophil cytoplasmic antibody; c-ANCA, cytoplasmic-staining antineutrophil cytoplasmic antibody; MPO, myeloperoxidase; p-ANCA, perinuclear-staining antineutrophil cytoplasmic antibody; PR3, proteinase 3. *(From Hoffman GS, Specks U: Antineutrophil cytoplasmic antibodies. Arthritis Rheum 1998;41:1521-1537.)*

(Fig. 2). The accuracy of the results is based on the experience of the laboratory personnel interpreting ANCA immunofluorescence results.[13]

The c-ANCA pattern indicates diffuse staining throughout the cytoplasm, and in most cases the antibodies responsible for this pattern are directed against PR3. However, autoantibodies against other defined and undefined cytoplasmic agents, including bactericidal/permeability-increasing protein (BPI) and, rarely, MPO, can cause cytoplasmic fluorescence.

The p-ANCA pattern indicates staining around the nucleus, and the antibody responsible for this pattern is usually against MPO. However, autoantibodies against elastase, cathepsin G, lactoferrin, lysozyme, and azurocidin have also been identified as causing the p-ANCA pattern.

Atypical ANCA patterns are sometimes observed on immunofluorescence in patients with immune-mediated conditions other than systemic vasculitis, such as inflammatory bowel disease, autoimmune liver disease, malignancies, and other rheumatic diseases. Such patterns are often confused with the p-ANCA pattern.

Interpretation

Clinicians interpreting ANCA results should bear in mind that the results can vary from laboratory to laboratory, and hence serial determinations should be performed by the same laboratory.[13] The predictive value of ANCA testing depends heavily on the clinical presentation of the patient in whom the test is performed. ANCA assays should be ordered only when the pretest probability for Wegener's granulomatosis and microscopic polyangiitis is very high.

Clinical Utility

Wegener's granulomatosis is almost always associated with ANCA positivity. Between 70% and 90% of patients with Wegener's granulomatosis are ANCA positive, with the c-ANCA pattern and antibodies directed against PR3. About 5% to 20% of patients with Wegener's granulomatosis have the p-ANCA pattern, with antibodies directed against MPO. The sensitivity of c-ANCA and PR3-ANCA is related to the extent, severity, and activity of disease at the time of testing. Patients with mild Wegener's granulomatosis may be ANCA negative. Diagnosis of Wegener's granulomatosis is based on the clinical picture; PR3-ANCA just assists in diagnosis.

Between 40% and 80% of patients with microscopic polyangiitis are ANCA positive. These patients usually have the p-ANCA pattern with MPO specificity.

ANCAs, both with PR3 and MPO specificity, have been detected in Churg-Strauss syndrome, but MPO specificity is more common. Antiglomerular basement membrane (anti-GBM) antibody disease may be associated with ANCAs. The clinical significance of anti-GBM antibodies and ANCA is uncertain.

Drug-Induced Vasculitis

Certain drugs are reported to induce ANCA reactivity with varying symptoms. Minocycline-associated arthritis, fever, and livedo reticularis can be ANCA positive, with anti-MPO antibodies. Propylthiouracil-induced vasculitis is also ANCA positive, with specificity to several different target antigens including PR3, MPO, and elastase. Hydralazine-associated vasculitis may be ANCA positive, with anti-MPO antibodies.

Monitoring

A rise in ANCA titers may be associated with relapses, but not always. Elevated ANCA titer should not be used as a sole parameter for preemptive therapy.[14] Therapy should only be based on clinical or pathologic evidence of relapse. The role of sequential ANCA titers after the diagnosis is established is unclear. One study showed a weak association between disease activity and ANCA levels.

COMPLEMENT

The complement system consists of plasma and membrane proteins that provide innate defense against microbial pathogens. Complement activation is usually assessed by determining the levels of individual complement components such as C3 and C4 and by quantifying the CH50 (total hemolytic complement) activity. Complement levels are measured by either functional or antigenic assays. CH50 is a useful tool for assessing all nine components of the classic pathway (C1, C2, C3, C4, C5, C6, C7, C8, and C9). CH50 is undetectable when there is complete deficiency of any individual complement component. Classic pathway activation is indicated by low levels of C3 and C4. Alternate pathway activation is indicated by low levels of C3 but normal C4.

Complement measurement is an important diagnostic tool in many connective tissue disorders. Hypocomplementemia is present in disorders associated with excessive levels of immune complexes such as SLE and cryoglobulinemia. There is a significant association between low complement levels and lupus nephropathy.[15] The utility of low complement levels as predictors of lupus flares is controversial; some studies have found a clear association with lupus activity and others show no correlation. A high frequency of positive ANA and anti-dsDNA in patients with primary antiphospholipid antibody syndrome with hypocomplementemia probably suggests that these patients might develop a lupus-like illness.

Low complement levels are also seen in inherited complement deficiency. Inherited complement deficiencies of C1, C2, and C4 predispose to SLE. Complete deficiency of C3 is rare and manifests in childhood as severe recurrent infections with pyogenic organisms. Complete deficiency of C4 is rare because four genes encode the C4 protein. Partial deficiency due to the presence of one, two, or three null alleles can produce persistently low levels of C4 and predispose to SLE. Deficiency of C1 esterase inhibitor leads to unregulated C1 esterase and to depression of C4 levels.

ANTIPHOSPHOLIPID ANTIBODIES

Antiphospholipid antibodies include antibodies directed against phospholipid-associated proteins such as cardiolipin, β_2-glycoprotein 1, and prothrombin. These antibodies are usually measured in patients with SLE, recurrent thrombosis, and recurrent fetal loss, raising the possibility of antiphospholipid antibody syndrome. The antiphospholipid syndrome is characterized by venous thrombolism, arterial thrombosis, or pregnancy morbidity (individually or in combination), together with antiphospholipid antibodies and lupus anticoagulant.

The anticardiolipin antibodies are measured by ELISA and usually include three serotypes: IgG, IgM, and IgA. International criteria for negative, low, medium, and high levels have been set, and standards are available for laboratory calibrations. These antibodies should be present in medium to high concentrations on at least two occasions about 12 weeks apart to establish a diagnosis of antiphospholipid antibody syndrome, along with some clinical criteria. A number of studies have shown that acute medical illness and infections can lead to a transient increase of the antibodies.

Summary

- ESR and CRP are markers of inflammation and are elevated in inflammation. ESR can be elevated without inflammation in hypergammaglobulinemia or anemia.
- CRP is a more sensitive marker of inflammation and is independent of factors affecting ESR.
- Many patients with active lupus do not have elevated CRP levels; elevated CRP can suggest bacterial infection.
- ANA testing is very useful in establishing a diagnosis of SLE. Nearly all patients with lupus have a positive ANA (sensitivity is 93%-95%, but specificity is 57%). However, most patients with positive ANA do not have lupus, because the prevalence of lupus is low in the general population.
- ANA titer is not used for assessing the disease activity in lupus. Thus, serial ANA testing is of unknown value.
- Anti-DNA antibody testing is very useful in the diagnosis of SLE and is also a useful biomarker of SLE disease activity.
- Anti-Scl 70 antibody is very useful in diagnosing systemic sclerosis and anticentromere antibody in diagnosing limited scleroderma. Anti-Scl 70 and anticentromere antibodies rarely coexist in the same patient.
- SSA and SSB antibodies should be checked in patients with sicca symptoms. Patients with primary Sjögren's syndrome with SSA or SSB antibodies represent the most clinically and immunologically active subset. These patients need very close follow-up for development of extraglandular features.
- The sensitivity of rheumatoid factor for rheumatoid arthritis is around 50% to 80% and specificity is 85% to 90%. It may be negative in the early stages of rheumatoid arthritis, and positivity increases over time.
- Between 70% and 90% of patients with Wegener's granulomatosis test positive for ANCAs in the c-ANCA pattern, with antibodies directed against PR3. A negative ANCA assay does not exclude Wegener's granulomatosis.
- Between 40% and 80% of patients with microscopic polyangiitis are ANCA positive and usually have the p-ANCA pattern with MPO specificity.
- The role of sequential ANCA titers after the diagnosis is established is unclear. A recent study showed a weak association between disease activity and ANCA levels.
- Inherited deficiencies of complements C1, C2, and C4 predispose to SLE.

Suggested Readings

Blumenthal DE: Tired, aching, ANA-positive: Does your patient have lupus or fibromyalgia? Cleve Clin J Med 2002;69(2):143-146, 151-152.

Hoffman GS, Specks U: Antineutrophil cytoplasmic antibodies. Arthritis Rheum 1998;41:1521-1537.

Kerr GS, Fleisher TA, Hallahan CW, et al: Limited prognostic value of changes in antineutrophil cytoplasmic antibody titer in patients with Wegener's granulomatosis. Arthritis Rheum 1993;36:365-371.

Kushner I: Acute phase proteins. UpToDate (requires paid subscription).

Nardi N, Brito-Zerón P, Ramos-Casals M, et al: Circulating auto-antibodies against nuclear and non-nuclear antigens in primary Sjögren's syndrome: Prevalance and clinical significance in 335 patients. Clin Rheumatol 2006;25:341-346.

Nishimura K, Sugiyama D, Kogata Y, et al: Meta-analysis: Diagnostic accuracy of anticyclic citrullinated peptide antibody and rheumatoid factor for rheumatoid arthritis. Ann Intern Med 2007;146(11):816-817.

Shmerling RH, Delbanco TL: How useful is the rheumatoid factor? An analysis of sensitivity, specificity, and predictive value. Arch Intern Med 1992;152:2417-2420.

Sibley J: Laboratory tests. Rheum Dis Clin North Am 1995;21:407-428.

Slater CA, Davis RB, Shmerling RH: Antinuclear antibody testing. A study of clinical utility. Arch Intern Med 1996;156(13):1421-1425.

Tedeschi A, Baratè C, Minola E, Morra E: Cryoglobulinemia. Blood Rev 2007;21(4):183-200.

References

For a complete list of references, log onto www.expertconsult.com.

Fibromyalgia

William S. Wilke, Abby Abelson, and Ravindran Padmanabhan

Primary care physicians are often faced with the challenge of caring for patients with fibromyalgia syndrome (FMS). FMS is a complex condition characterized by pain amplification, musculoskeletal discomfort, and systemic symptoms. In the United States, it is the third or fourth most common reason for a rheumatology referral.

DEFINITION

Approximately 10% to 12% of the general population has widespread chronic pain. FMS is a concept designed to account for such generalized chronic and idiopathic pain. The 1990 classification criteria of the American College of Rheumatology (ACR) is based on the analysis of more than 300 variables such as symptoms, physical findings, and laboratory and radiologic studies by a study committee.[1] The mandatory defining symptom is widespread pain not explained by an inflammatory or degenerative musculoskeletal disorder.

The ACR criteria for diagnosis of FMS have two components. The first is widespread pain for at least 3 months (pain in the left side of the body, *plus* right side of the body, *plus* pain above the waist, *plus* pain below the waist, *plus* axial pain; axial pain includes pain in the cervical spine, or thoracic pain, or pain in the low back or anterior chest wall). The second is the presence of 11 tender points among 18 specified sites as shown in Figure 1. Pressure of 4 kg/cm (enough to whiten the examiner's fingernail) should be applied to each point for a few seconds.[2]

It is important to remember that there are more than 600 muscles in the human body, each of which might theoretically contain a tender point. The 18 tender points recommended by the ACR represent only a sample of widespread pain in any given patient. If a patient has widespread pain in many other areas, it is entirely possible that he or she has fibromyalgia.[3]

The presence of many tender points on digital palpation validates the diagnosis. According to the ACR criteria, the finding of 11 of 18 specified tender points provided a sensitivity of 88% and a specificity of 81% in distinguishing fibromyalgia from other chronic causes of musculoskeletal pain.[1] In addition, the criteria committee found that several other disorders are often associated with FMS, including sleep disturbance, fatigue, paresthesias, anxiety, and headache or irritable bowel syndrome. Frederick Wolfe, the chairman of the criteria committee, later wrote that the presence of seven (40%) of the tender points and at least three of the six features mentioned earlier are highly suggestive of FMS.

It is now widely accepted that numerous other conditions can overlap with FMS (Box 1). These include irritable bowel syndrome, tension-type headaches, migraine, temporomandibular dysfunction, myofascial pain syndrome, chronic fatigue syndrome, restless legs syndrome, and multiple chemical sensitivities, to name just a few.

PREVALENCE

The prevalence of FMS in the general community is 2% for both sexes. Women are affected more than men; the prevalence is 3.4% for women and 0.5 % for men. The prevalence increases with age, reaching 7% in women ages 60 to 79 years.[4]

PATHOPHYSIOLOGY

A heightened pain response is present in patients with FMS. This is now known to be caused by altered processing of nociceptive stimuli by the central nervous system.[5,6] Levels of substance P and abnormal antinociceptive peptides are elevated in the cerebrospinal fluid of patients with FMS.[7] FMS might be best understood as a heightened response of the entire nervous system, as if the volume has been turned up.[8,9] Inheritance of a short allele of the serotonin transporter promoter gene has taken serotonin metabolism to center stage and suggests a possible heritable mechanism in the pathogenesis of FMS.[10] Other studies have postulated serotonin deficiency as a pathophysiologic mechanism in FMS.[11] A group of excitatory amino acids-L-tryptophan, alanine, histidine, lysine, proline and serine, to name a few-are also decreased in the spinal fluid in patients with FMS.[12]

Although some reports have suggested that muscle tissue is normal in FMS, others have found increased moth-eaten and ragged red type I and type II fiber atrophy on light microscopy.[13,14] Other clinicians have found myofibril lysis or swollen abnormal mitochondria on electron microscopy.[13,14] However, it is unclear whether these changes are due to deconditioning or to FMS itself.[2]

Slow-wave sleep abnormalities are also present, and a significantly increased amount of alpha-wave intrusion into delta-wave sleep during non–rapid eye movement (non-REM) sleep is responsible for more awakenings and other symptoms of nonrestorative sleep. Sleep apnea and restless legs syndrome, nocturnal myoclonus, and bruxism have been reported in some studies.[2] Severe dysautonomia, or reflex sympathetic dystrophy, coexists with FMS and is believed by some clinicians to be a subtype of FMS.[2]

PREDISPOSING FACTORS

One half of all FMS cases have no apparent cause. The most common cause of secondary FMS is trauma. Even trivial trauma can act as the inciting agent and lead to the development of widespread pain within 3 months. Numerous infectious agents such as herpes viruses, parvovirus, *Borrelia burgdorferi*, human immunodeficiency virus, and *Brucella* species have been implicated as the causes of a postinfectious fatigue-like syndrome.[2] To date, however, no clinical or serologic studies have proved an etiologic role for Epstein-Barr virus, parvovirus or, indeed, any virus. Heavy lifting and bending, or prolonged sitting at word processing stations, might induce secondary FMS. Heroin, cocaine, and alcohol withdrawal can also induce a FM-like syndrome, as can administration of interferon alfa or interleukin-2. Life-altering events such as death of a loved one, loss of a job, or divorce in the presence of poor coping mechanisms can bring out FMS.[2] Emotional trauma such as physical or sexual abuse or post-traumatic stress disorder can act as triggers.

CLINICAL MANIFESTATIONS

All patients have widespread pain and tender points. Although stiffness may be present in the early hours, pain is worse in the late afternoon and early evening. Most patients report that symptoms are worsened by cold and humid weather, winter months, poor sleep, mental stress, or physical inactivity and are improved by warm and dry weather, summer months, rest, moderate physical activity, good sleep, and relaxation.[15] Approximately 80% of patients experience fatigue, poor sleep, and complaints of weakness with normal muscle strength. Most persons with FMS have anxiety or depression, often related to pain. A sense of bloatedness, numbness, or tingling may also be present. Dysautonomia may be the cause of dry eyes, skin hyperemia, skin tenderness to touch, and bloating. Some patients

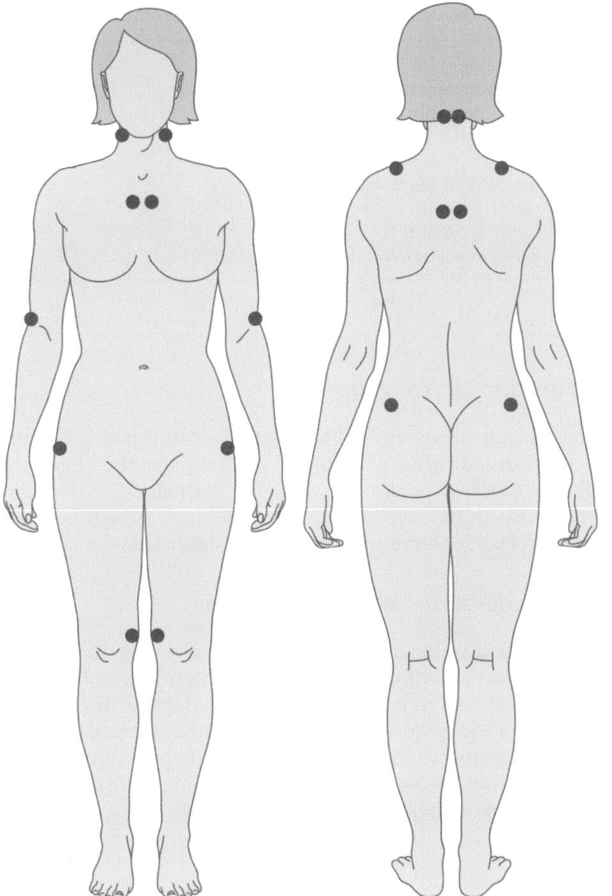

Figure 1 Pain on digital palpation must be present in 11 of 18 tender point sites as follows: occiput: bilateral, at the suboccipital muscle insertions; low cervical: bilateral, at the intertransverse spaces of C5-C7; trapezius: bilateral, at the midpoint of the upper border; supraspinatus: bilateral, at origins, above the scapular spine near the medial border; second rib: bilateral, just lateral to the costochondral junctions; lateral epicondyle: bilateral, 2 cm distal to the epicondyles; gluteal: bilateral, in upper outer quadrants in the anterior fold of the muscle; greater trochanter: bilateral, posterior to the trochanteric prominence; knee: bilateral, at the medial fat pad, proximal to the joint line. *(Adapted from Wallace DJ: The fibromyalgia syndrome. Ann Med 1997;29:9-21.)*

Box 1 Conditions Commonly Associated with Fibromyalgia

- Cognitive dysfunction
- Cold intolerance
- Dizziness
- Dysautonomia
- Endocrine dysfunction
- Interstitial cystitis
- Irritable bladder syndrome
- Irritable bowel syndrome
- Migraine headaches
- Multiple chemical sensitivities
- Myofascial pain syndrome
- Sicca symptoms
- Temporomandibular joint dysfunction

complain of fever and swollen glands. Indeed, if these are present, alternative diagnoses should be entertained. In the elderly, fewer functional symptoms such as anxiety, stress, and unrefreshed sleep are present. However, the elderly have more musculoskeletal complaints than their younger counterparts. FMS can be confused with polymyalgia rheumatica, primary Sjögren's syndrome, or rheumatoid arthritis in the elderly.

WORKUP

The physical examination should be a fibromyalgia-focused approach. Routine vital signs should be taken, with special attention paid to blood pressure measurements in the recumbent and standing positions. Several findings relevant to FMS should be noted during the first few minutes of the encounter (e.g., posture and mood). Lymphadenopathy and thyroid swellings should be sought. Often, what was first believed to be a tender lymph node is, on re-examination, in fact a tender carotid artery.

Tender points should be sought and other systems examined as suggested by the history. Diagrams can be used by the patient to highlight tender points. A fibromyalgia patient can have osteoarthritis, inflammatory arthritis, bursitis, tendinitis, or adhesive capsulitis. However, these diagnoses are not justified in the absence of a history of trauma, presence of calcification, or a swollen bursa on radiograph or magnetic resonance imaging. Paresthesias in the presence of objective weakness should warrant a full neurologic examination because conditions such as cervical spinal stenosis and Chiari malformations can mimic some of the symptoms of FMS. A patient with a Chiari malformation has worsening of radicular symptoms on neck flexion or abnormal neurologic signs such as brisk lower-limb reflexes or weakness in the upper extremities. Instruments such as the Beck Depression Index, the Fibromyalgia Impact Questionnaire, and the Epworth Sleep Scale can provide valuable insights.

No special laboratory or radiologic testing is necessary to make a diagnosis of FMS. A reasonable initial workup should include a complete blood cell count, complete metabolic panel, and a urinalysis. Tests of creatine kinase and thyroid-stimulating hormone may be performed if clinically indicated. One of the common referrals to the rheumatology clinic is a positive antinuclear antibody (ANA) test. This test should not be ordered unless there is a clinical suspicion of connective tissue disease. In a study by Yunus and colleagues, 11% of female patients with FMS had positive findings on ANA tests. Importantly, 10% of healthy female controls also had a positive ANA.[16] Sleep studies may be indicated if the history suggests heavy snoring, daytime sleepiness, or leg movements.

DIAGNOSIS AND DIFFERENTIAL DIAGNOSIS

Classification criteria are not designed to diagnose disease in an individual patient. Rather, a careful history and physical examination should remain the cornerstones of diagnosis, as with any disease or syndrome. To meet the criteria for FMS, patients with FMS must have chronic widespread pain, fatigue, and associated symptoms such as sleep disturbances and headaches to begin with. FMS should be differentiated from rheumatoid arthritis, osteoarthritis, and other systemic illnesses.

The differential diagnosis of FMS includes hypothyroidism, polymyalgia rheumatica, osteomalacia, metabolic and inflammatory polyarthropathies, spondyloarthropathy, radiculopathy, pleuritic or cardiac pain syndromes, and extrapyramidal disease.

Common pitfalls in dealing with FMS patients include concurrent medical or psychiatric illnesses. Spondyloarthropathy can have very subtle clinical findings and can be misdiagnosed as having FMS. FMS may be misdiagnosed as osteoarthritis in elderly patients, the pertinent clinical findings being pain on movement and a more localized pain in osteoarthritis. FMS is present in 40% of patients with systemic lupus erythematosus and in 10% to 30% of patients with rheumatoid arthritis. FMS can also be misdiagnosed as Lyme disease or systemic lupus erythematosus. Approximately 25% to 50% of patients referred to Lyme disease clinics turned out to have FMS,[17,18] and 25% of patients referred to rheumatology clinics based on positive ANA test results had FMS.[19]

TREATMENT

If the diagnosis is made early enough, patients with FMS tend to do well with simple management techniques.[20] FMS as a syndrome is poorly understood in the primary care setting. In one study, patients received a diagnosis of FMS after seeing an average of three doctors with the same complaints.[21] Patients might undergo unnecessary and extensive workups including myelograms, cancer workups, adrenal evaluations, and even laparotomies in some cases.

Patient education remains a cornerstone in the management of FMS. Providing patients with literature regarding their illness and explaining to them that they are indeed dealing with a real disorder is an ideal starting point. At the same time, patients need to be reassured that they are dealing with a nondestructive, although not necessarily benign, illness.

Response to treatment can be assessed in a variety of ways as suggested in a review by Bennett.[3] Questionnaires that provide information about quality of life give the best details from a patient's perspective about overall self-assessment of change. The Short Form 36 (SF 36) is one of the health questionnaires that can be used. Pain can be assessed using the visual analogue scale (VAS). If depression is an issue, this can be monitored using a daily diary or the Beck Depression Inventory.[3] A questionnaire that provides an overall view of the many problems a patient experiences in fibromyalgia can be assessed using the Fibromyalgia Impact Questionnaire (FIQ).[22] The FIQ is currently the most widely used questionnaire and by one survey the most useful.[3]

Treatment in FMS can be divided into nonpharmacologic and pharmacologic means. It is important that a multidisciplinary program use both strategies.[23]

Nonpharmacologic Treatments

Nonpharmacologic treatments include cardiovascular fitness training, electromyogram biofeedback, hypnotherapy, acupuncture, and cognitive-behavioral therapy.

Exercise is often recommended as a treatment for FMS. Many trials have now proved that aerobic exercise produces significant positive changes in experimental groups of FMS patients.[24] The aerobic exercise recommended should be of low impact, such as isometric exercises, swimming, or aerobic walking. Ferraccioli and colleagues found improvements lasting up to 6 months in patients treated with electromyographic biofeedback.[25] Improvement was defined in this study as decreases in tender point counts, decrease in early morning stiffness (measured in minutes) and decrease in pain as measured by the visual analogue scale (VAS).

Buckelew and colleagues found that biofeedback in conjunction with low-impact exercise produced better results than each of the modalities on its own.[26]

Deluze and colleagues found that that significant improvements in pain occur when patients with FMS are treated with real electroacupuncture as opposed to sham treatment.[27] However, because patients still continued with cotreatments during this study, confounding results were always possible. Assefi and colleagues compared real acupuncture with a sham procedure in 100 FMS patients.[28] Patients experienced 20% improvement with both procedures, demonstrating that real acupuncture was no better than sham acupuncture.

Haanen and colleagues showed significant improvement in five outcome measures in a group treated with hypnotherapy as compared with a physical therapy program.[29] However, there was a lack of standardization of physical therapy in this study.

In a systematic review evaluating the evidence from randomized controlled trials for nonpharmacologic treatments in FMS, Sim and Adams concluded that few studies tested comparable interventions, the methodologic quality of such studies was generally poor, the statistical power was low, and statistical analyses were insufficient.[30]

Box 2 Classes of Drugs Used in Fibromyalgia Syndrome

- Anxiolytics
- Growth hormone injections
- Nonselective serotonin reuptake inhibitors
- Nonsteroidal anti-inflammatory drugs
- Opioids
- Selective serotonin reuptake inhibitors
- Sleep aids
- Tricyclic antidepressants
- Trigger-point injections with lidocaine

Pharmacologic Treatments

Pharmacologic treatment for FMS (Box 2) remains largely empirical and aimed at individual symptoms. Pain is the symptom most amenable to pharmacologic intervention. Pharmacologic treatment should also be used for coexisting conditions in FMS such as irritable bowel and bladder syndromes or migraine headaches.

Nonsteroidal Anti-inflammatory Drugs

Nonsteroidal anti-inflammatory drugs (NSAIDs) act on peripheral pain generators and can address issues such as myofascial pain, bursitis, and tendinitis in patients with FMS. Patients with FMS at the severe end of the spectrum do not respond to simple analgesics and need more aggressive interventions. Central pain is not responsive to NSAIDs, and in these cases, centrally acting analgesics are the preferred mode of treatment.

Opioids

Opioids are effective in acute and chronic pain states. The use of opioid analgesics in FMS is a widely debated issue. True addiction develops in 0.5% of patients prescribed opioids for treatment of chronic pain.[31] The more problematic issues of long-term opioid use are effects on cognition, reduced motivation to pursue nonpharmacologic approaches in FMS, aggravation of depression, and stigmatization by society and physicians.

All patients are expected to develop dependency; that is, these drugs cannot be abruptly withdrawn without causing unpleasant side effects such as pruritus, nausea, and drowsiness. It is important to screen patients for previous problems with opioid use and benzodiazepine dependence before embarking on this route in the treatment of FMS. Frequent re-evaluation of the patient is especially important in this setting, with the goal being improved function rather than mere pain relief. If improved function is not achieved, if severe side effects are encountered, or if maladaptive behavior develops, patients should be weaned from these agents and not restarted on them.[32]

Tramadol is also effective in FMS patients with mild to moderate pain and may be the only centrally acting analgesic necessary in an office setting. Abuse has been documented in less than one case per 100,000 patients.[33] If tramadol is chosen, the dose should be low to begin with and then increased gradually to avoid nausea and dizziness. Seizures have been reported, especially when this agent is combined with antidepressants.[34]

Activation of *N*-methyl-D-aspartate (NMDA) receptors can lead to abnormal modulation of nociceptive impulses. Good experimental evidence exists that pain in FMS can be ameliorated by blocking NMDA receptors. A Swedish group was able to abolish pain by infusing ketamine in patients with FMS.[35]

Antidepressants

Antidepressants have been crucial in the management of many chronic pain states including FMS. Antidepressants improve sleep, fatigue, pain, and well-being. They do not specifically improve tender points.[32]

Three classes of antidepressants were evaluated in a large meta-analysis of antidepressants in FMS[36]: tricyclic antidepressants (TCAs, nine trials), selective serotonin reuptake inhibitors (SSRIs, three trials), and *S*-adenosylmethionine (SAMe, two trials). The odds ratio for improvement with therapy in this meta-analysis was 4:2. The efficacy of TCAs is short lived, at least in the tertiary care setting. The SSRIs have disappointing analgesic effects in FMS, although these agents help improve concomitant mood disorders. A combination of fluoxetine and amitriptyline was found to be more effective than either agent alone or placebo.[37] Controlled trials of duloxetine and milnacipram have documented benefit versus placebo.[38,39]

Experts in FMS have found that nonselective serotonin reuptake inhibitors, especially those with a noradrenergic component (venlafaxine, nefazadone, or bupropion) seem to be more effective for treating fatigue, which is the most difficult symptom in FMS to treat pharmacologically.

Miscellaneous Agents

α_2-Adrenergic agonists such as tizanidine have been used successfully in chronic pain disorders. There have been no trials of these agents in FMS. Tizanidine has antinociceptive, antispasmodic, and sedating effects, which might explain its anecdotal benefit in FMS.

Serotonin antagonists have been the subject of many recent trials in FMS. These drugs have been used in the control of nausea and vomiting in patients who have received chemotherapy or radiation. Tropisetron was evaluated in a short-term, double-blinded study involving 418 patients with FMS. In that study, 40% of patients reported a 55% reduction in pain scores.[40] Preliminary results of studies using serotonin antagonists in FMS have been encouraging, and results of long-term placebo-controlled studies are awaited.

Pregabalin, an anticonvulsant with analgesic properties, has been shown to produce global improvement in a large (459 patient) placebo-controlled trial at a dose of 450 mg a day. A high incidence of dizziness (49.2%) and somnolence (28%) limits its usefulness.[41]

Sodium oxibate is chemically related to the naturally occurring metabolite of the human central nervous system that promotes stages three and four non-REM sleep, γ-hydroxybutyrate. Sodium oxibate has been shown to reduce pain in FMS when taken at a nightly divided dose of 6 g in a small controlled trial.[42] Because it is also known as the "date rape" drug, it is only available in a prescription from physicians who enroll in a special program sponsored by the makers.

Treatment of Specific Symptoms

Sleep

Before pharmacologic treatment is initiated, certain measures must be tried. Caffeinated beverages should be avoided 4 to 6 hours before the patient goes to bed. The bedroom should be used only for sleep and sexual activities. Relaxation techniques such as yoga, gentle stretching, or listening to soothing music are all helpful. Pure sedatives such as benzodiazepines, antihistamines, and antidepressants are the pharmacologic therapies available. Restless legs syndrome often responds to low-dose clonazepam (0.5 to 1 mg at bedtime), carbidopa/levodopa (10/100 mg at the evening meal), or low-dose narcotics at bedtime. Care should be taken when clonazepam is used on a long-term basis because it causes prominent withdrawal symptoms when discontinued abruptly. Patients with sleep apnea require continuous positive airway pressure. Specific symptoms should be sought in the history that point to a diagnosis of sleep apnea, because this diagnosis is often missed.[32]

Mood Disturbances

Patients with FMS often suffer from dysphoria or frank clinical depression. Although antidepressants are used in the treatment of FMS itself, the doses used are often suboptimal for the treatment of depression. SSRIs, which have fewer side effects than TCAs, are useful in managing depression in the FMS patient. The nonselective serotonin reuptake inhibitors with a noradrenergic component, such as venlafaxine, nefazadone, and bupropion, are better tolerated in this group of patients.[32]

Fatigue

The pathophysiology of fatigue is poorly understood, which makes it one of the most difficult symptoms to treat in FMS. Nonselective serotonin reuptake inhibitors show encouraging results. Also, the serotonin-receptor antagonist tropisetron shows a beneficial effect in FMS-related fatigue and in chronic fatigue syndrome.[32]

FUTURE DIRECTIONS

Controversy regarding the very existence of FMS persists today, as it did a century ago. Medical professionals and patients in one camp believe that FMS is not a true syndrome per se because it does not fit into a biomedical cause-and-effect model. In another camp are those who believe that FMS is a nonentity defined by physicians' and society's perceptions of psychosocial stress. However, an infective or immune cause cannot always explain a disease process. Rarely does a costly evaluation of FMS find a cause or suggest a definitive diagnosis. There is no clear evidence that FMS is a disease of muscle. There is also no evidence of pathologic abnormalities at tender points or trigger points.

In reviews by Goldenberg,[19,43] the author suggests that future research should focus on how FMS ties in with other poorly understood syndromes such as irritable bowel syndrome and migraine headaches. Genetic factors, physical or sexual abuse, and chronic psychological stress might provide a premorbid susceptibility to FMS. Neurohormonal dysregulation might result in abnormal blood flow to some areas of the brain that regulate pain perception, such as the thalamus and caudate nucleus.

As has been mentioned, randomized clinical trials in FMS suffer from methodologic weaknesses. In trials evaluating the impact of medical treatments on FMS, cointerventions such as exercise or education have not been measured. The long-term outcome in FMS has been evaluated in very few studies. Natural history reports indicate that complete remissions are unusual and that patients continue to be symptomatic, but gradual and modest improvement with time is common.[43] It may be said that a single cause for syndromes such as FMS, irritable bowel syndrome, chronic fatigue syndrome, or irritable bladder syndrome might never be found. Each of these entities might fit into a psychosocial rather than a biomedical model.

Summary

- Fibromyalgia syndrome is the muscle pain component of altered central nervous system processing, and because of this it is associated with many other symptoms.
- The pathophysiology of fibromyalgia syndrome is intimately related to the effects of psychological distress and disordered sleep on the central nervous system.
- The simple, effective approach to treatment employs the combination of patient education, improved mood and sleep, and aerobic exercise.

Suggested Readings

Bennett RM: Emerging concepts in the neurobiology of chronic pain: Evidence of abnormal sensory processing in fibromyalgia. Mayo Clin Proc 1999;74:385-398.

Goldenberg D: Fibromyalgia syndrome a decade later: What have we learned? Arch Intern Med 1999;159:777-785.

Goldenberg DL, Burckhardt C, Crofford L: Management of fibromyalgia syndrome. JAMA 2004:292:2388-2395.

Goldenberg D, Mayskiy M, Mossey C, et al: A randomized, double-blind crossover trial of fluoxetine and amitriptyline in the treatment of fibromyalgia. Arthritis Rheum 1996;39:1852-1859.

Mease P: Fibromyalgia syndrome: Review of clinical presentation, pathogenesis, outcome measures, and treatment. J Rheumatol 2005;32(Suppl 75):6-21.

Russell IJ, Vaereroy H, Javors M, Nyberg F: Cerebrospinal fluid biogenic amine metabolites in fibromyalgia/fibrositis syndrome and rheumatoid arthritis. Arthritis Rheum 1992;35;550-556.

Sorensen J, Bengtsson A, Backman E, et al: Pain analysis in patients with fibromyalgia: Effects of intravenous morphine, lidocaine, and ketamine. Scand J Rheumatol 1995;24:360-365.

Wilke, WS: The clinical utility of fibromyalgia. J Clin Rheumatol 1999;5:97-102.

Wolfe F, Smythe HA, Yunus MB, et al: The American College of Rheumatology 1990 criteria for the classification of fibromyalgia: REPORT of the Multicenter Criteria Committee. Arthritis Rheum 1990;33:160-172.

References

For a complete list of references, log onto www.expertconsult.com.

Gout and Pseudogout

Feyrouz Al-Ashkar

Crystal-induced arthropathies are a group of disorders that involve deposition of crystals into joints and soft tissues, resulting in articular and periarticular inflammation and injury. Examples of such crystals are monosodium urate (MSU), calcium pyrophosphate dehydrate (CPPD), hydroxyapatite, and calcium oxalate. The crystals most commonly involved in joint inflammation and seen in synovial fluid analysis are the MSU crystals involved in gout and the CPPD crystals involved in pseudogout.

GOUT

Definition

Gout is a crystal deposition disease characterized by the supersaturation and precipitation of MSU crystals in tissues resulting in inflammation and, consequently, tissue damage. Gout is characterized by acute or subacute attacks of joint or soft tissue inflammation resulting from MSU crystal deposition. The clinical course of gout can be summarized into the stages of acute intermittent gout and chronic tophaceous gout.

Hyperuricemia is the underlying metabolic aberrancy in gout and is defined as the serum urate level, in body fluids, above which urate precipitates into monosodium urate crystals. A urate level greater than 6.8 mg/dL is considered hyperuricemia.

Prevalence

Gout is a fairly common disease, more common in men than women, and rare in premenopausal women. There have been few studies on the incidence or prevalence of gout and even fewer on CPPD arthropathy. In a population of medical students with a median age of 22 years, the cumulative incidence of gout was reported as 8.6%.[1] In this same study, body mass index (relative risk [RR], 1.12), excessive weight gain (RR, 2.07), and hypertension (RR, 3.26) were identified as risk factors for developing gout.[1]

Overall, the prevalence of gout in the U.S. population increased between 1990 and 1999,[2] and factors such as lifestyle habits, obesity, diet, alcohol intake, comorbid diseases such as hypertension, and the use of diuretics were identified as potential contributing factors.[3] A study done in the United Kingdom, examining the epidemiology of gout, reported the prevalence of gout to be 1.4% in 1999 and as high as 7% in men older than 65 years.[4] Reviews have found that epidemiologic investigations suggest that incidence of gout is on the rise worldwide.[5]

The annual incidence of gouty arthritis is about 5% at serum urate levels of 9.0 mg/dL or higher and less than 1% at urate levels of 7 mg/dL and lower.[6]

Pathophysiology

Gout is an inflammatory crystal arthropathy that results from the pathogenic effect of MSU crystals in the joints and soft tissue. Uric acid in body fluid, at pH 7.4, exists in the urate form. Thus, when referring to uric acid in physiologic fluid it is preferable to use the term *urate.*

Uric acid comes from the metabolism of purine nucleotides. Purine metabolism leads to inosine then hypoxanthine. Hypoxanthine is metabolized to xanthine and xanthine to uric acid. These two last steps are catalyzed by the enzyme xanthine oxidase, which is the major site for pharmacologic intervention by allopurinol. Uric acid, in humans, is the final product. Human beings lack the ability to degrade urate further.[7]

Minimal amounts of urate are eliminated through the urinary and intestinal tracts. Therefore, when the human body is unable to eliminate large burdens of urate, hyperuricemia develops. As urate levels increase and saturate the synovial fluid or soft tissues, crystals precipitate, leading to tissue damage and the development of tophi. After urate crystals deposit in soft tissues and joints, monocytes and macrophages are activated in an attempt to clear the crystals by phagocytosis. This then leads to the release of proinflammatory cytokines and chemokines into the surrounding area, triggering a cascade of acute inflammatory reaction and influx of neutrophils into the joint, for example.[7,8]

The mechanism leading to the self-limited inflammatory process is not fully unveiled. The innate anti-inflammatory processes, mediated by anti-inflammatory cytokines, possibly are called into action and interrupt the inflammatory process.[8] Thus, the natural course of gout is one that would resolve spontaneously in 1 to 2 weeks on average.[7]

An additional proposed mechanism has been elucidated in research work indicating the role of an inflammasome and interleukin 1 (IL-1) in the pathogenesis of inflammation induced by monosodium urate (the crystal in gout) and calcium pyrophosphate dehydrate (the crystal in pseudogout). Cryopyrin inflammasome detects MSU and CPPD crystals, resulting in an inflammatory cascade by activation of IL-1.[9] These IL-1–mediated inflammatory effects of MSU crystals could potentially be blocked by IL-1 inhibitors, such as anakinra. This presents opportunities for the management of patients with gouty arthritis who are otherwise intolerant of or inadequate responders to standard anti-inflammatory therapies. Large randomized, controlled trials are required to assess the benefit and safety of blocking IL-1 in the management of polyarticular gouty arthritis.

Clinical Manifestations

The cascade of pathologic events leads to acute inflammation of the joint or soft tissue. The clinical manifestations of gout include arthritis, direct soft tissue damage, and accumulation of MSU crystals, known as tophi, in soft tissue and bones. Hyperuricemia can also result in uric acid nephrolithiasis and possible nephropathy if uric acid accumulates in the renal interstitium and tubules.

The arthritis in acute gout usually manifests as asymmetric monoarticular or oligoarticular inflammation, lasts 3 to 10 days, and resolves spontaneously. Eventually the attacks occur more frequently, last longer, and do not resolve completely, leading to chronic gouty arthropathy. Gouty arthropathy can lead to erosions and joint destruction, but it is distinguished from rheumatoid arthritis by the absence of joint space narrowing and absence of periarticular osteopenia.

In general, joints involved in gout include the lower extremity joints as well as those of the upper extremities. Inflammation in joints such as the first metatarsophalangeal (MTP) joints is termed *podagra* and is highly suggestive of gout. Any joint in the feet, ankles, knees, hands, wrists, or elbows may be involved. Acute gout can occur in bursae, such as the olecranon or prepatellar bursae, causing bursitis.

Occasionally, a gout attack triggers a systemic inflammatory response manifesting with fevers, leukocytosis, elevated sedimentation rates, and elevated C-reactive protein (CRP).

Acute attacks can be precipitated by several factors, such as increased alcohol consumption (especially beer), trauma, use of diuretics, dehydration, cyclosporine, diet (organ meat, shellfish), and any drug that can lead to sudden changes (increase or decrease) in urate levels, such as hypouricemic agents.[10,11]

When urate accumulates in a supersaturated medium, it can deposit in soft tissue or bones and form a tophus. Tophi can be present over the helices of the ears, extensor areas of the limbs, pressure areas such as the finger pads, and over the Achilles tendons. Occasionally, they are not seen on physical examination but are noted on x-ray films as cystic or masslike lesions. In general, a tophus on radiographic films is radiolucent, but when it occurs over a calcified nodule it may be seen as radioopaque.[12]

Diagnosis

Analysis of Synovial Fluid

Synovial fluid analysis is the gold standard for diagnosis ,and one should attempt a synovial aspiration for microscopic analysis whenever feasible.

Synovial fluid analysis offers a valuable diagnostic tool for evaluating patients with gout or pseudogout. Once the fluid is aspirated, it can be examined grossly for color and turbidity. In general, transparent synovial fluid in the syringe is more suggestive of a noninflammatory condition, whereas fluid that appears turbid or purulent is more suggestive of inflammation or infection (e.g., rheumatoid arthritis, gout, septic arthritis). However, gross appearance alone is by no means diagnostic.

To confirm or rule out infection, the fluid needs to be processed for Gram stain and culture. It is possible to have concomitant gout and septic arthritis at the same time. On microscopic examination, the number of white blood cells (WBCs) per high-power field can be estimated. The WBC count may be a useful adjunct in estimating the degree of inflammation present.[13] With gout, synovial fluid analysis reveals leukocytosis, a nonspecific finding of inflammatory arthritis including infectious and crystalline causes.

Crystal analysis is done with compensated polarized light. An accurate diagnosis can be made by a trained observer by detecting and identifying MSU crystals or CPPD crystals.[14]

MSU crystals are birefringent, with strong negative elongation when viewed under compensated polarized light. CPPD crystals are weakly birefringent and rhomboid or rod shaped. CPPD crystals might not be as evident and thus possibly missed, especially if the analysis is not done by a trained examiner.[13-15] In addition to shape and birefringence, MSU and CPPD differ in color depending on the axis of orientation with respect to the polarizer. When the axis of the MSU crystal is parallel to the polarizer it appears yellow, and when it is perpendicular it appears blue. The CPPD crystal is the reverse of that, so when the CPPD crystal is parallel it appears blue and when perpendicular it appears yellow (Table 1).[13]

Table 1 Differences Between Monosodium Urate and Calcium Pyrophosphate Dehydrate Crystals with Synovial Analysis

Characteristic	MSU	CPPD
Birefringence	Strong	Weak
Shape	Needle-like, sharp edges	Rhomboid, rod-like
Color parallel to polarizer	Yellow	Blue
Color perpendicular to polarizer	Blue	Yellow

CPPD, calcium pyrophosphate dehydrate; MSU, monosodium urate.

Blood Tests

Urate levels are not helpful in the acute gouty attack because they fluctuate and may be normal, low, or elevated. In chronic gout, a urate level is helpful in determining hypouricemic therapy. Once a hypouricemic agent is started, the dose should be adjusted according to urate blood levels (see later).

Other blood tests, such as a complete blood count, a creatinine, and transaminases are useful for assessing contraindications to a drug, to evaluate for other comorbid diseases, and for monitoring drug toxicity after initiating therapy. For example, colchicine is not indicated if the patient has evidence of bone marrow suppression. If there is any evidence of renal insufficiency, therapy with uricosuric medications (such as probenecid or sulfinpyrazone) would not be effective because they require functional renal apparatus to excrete excess urate. In addition, the dose of allopurinol will have to be decreased, and colchicine should be avoided.

Urine Tests

A 24-hour urine test for uric acid levels is necessary when considering a uricosuric agent, such as probenecid or sulfinpyrazone. Because results are partly affected by diet, it is best to repeat the test twice on two separate occasions. If the 24-hour urine levels are abnormally elevated, then uricosuric agents should not be used so as to avoid an increased risk of urate stones.

Radiography

Changes of arthropathy take years to develop, but findings of erosions can appear sooner. Distributions of affected areas include most commonly the feet, ankles, hands, wrists, and elbows. Well-defined erosions with sclerotic margins and overhanging edges are classic in gout. Little or no joint space narrowing and no periarticular osteopenia can differentiate gout from rheumatoid arthritis.[12]

Comorbid Conditions

Once the diagnosis of gout has been made, other associated medical conditions need to be considered, such as alcoholism, the metabolic syndrome, myeloproliferative disorders, and possible medication triggers (diuretics, cyclosporine). Any comorbid disease should be appropriately managed as clinically indicated.

Differential Diagnosis

Differential diagnosis of monoarticular arthritis includes infection, pseudogout, atypical rheumatoid arthritis, trauma, and fracture. The differential diagnosis should be considered based on the history and clinical presentation. Thus, the best approach starts with a good history and physical examination. If the history and clinical examination do not indicate a history of trauma or fracture, then a synovial aspiration, as discussed earlier, is performed, rather than an x-ray of the joint.

Erosive gouty arthropathy can mimic rheumatoid arthritis or CPPD arthropathy. Often, patients with advanced gouty arthropathy, especially of the hands, are mistakenly treated for rheumatoid arthritis.

Treatment

Treatment depends on the clinical presentation and findings. The aim in treating gout is to treat the acute attack, prevent future attacks, and prevent chronic joint and soft tissue mutilation from chronic tophaceous gouty arthropathy. As discussed earlier, gout is characterized by the acute or subacute attacks of joint or soft tissue inflammation resulting from deposit of MSU crystals. Hyperuricemia and gout may be divided into three stages: asymptomatic hyperuricemia, acute intermittent gout, and chronic tophaceous gout.

Asymptomatic Hyperuricemia

There are no sufficient data to support treatment of asymptomatic hyperuricemia with hypouricemic agents. In general, initiating such therapy in asymptomatic persons is not recommended, but one should consider investigating the underlying comorbid conditions and treating those conditions as clinically indicated.

Acute Intermittent Gout

The acute attack can be managed with colchicine, nonsteroidal anti-inflammatory drugs (NSAIDs), or corticosteroids (intra-articular injection or systemic). The choice of agent is dictated by the patient's tolerance of those medications and the presence of any comorbid diseases that prevent the use of such drugs. Younger, otherwise healthy patients who can tolerate NSAIDs or colchicine may be treated with either. NSAIDs should be avoided in patients who are intolerant of such drugs or in whom such drugs are contraindicated. NSAIDs are contraindicated in renal disease, insufficiency, or failure; gastrointestinal bleeding, ulcers, or gastritis; high risk of cardiovascular disease; and history of allergy to the drug. Occasionally, in an acute gouty attack, when all of these medications are contraindicated, narcotics may be used to relieve pain until the acute attack has resolved.

Nonsteroidal Anti-inflammatory Drugs. Although indomethacin has been traditionally used for acute gout, most other NSAIDs can be used as well. NSAIDs provide rapid symptomatic relief within the first 24 hours. Indomethacin can be given at a dose of 150 mg (in three divided doses) daily for the first 3 days then 100 mg (in two divided doses) for 4 to 7 days.[16]

NSAIDs should be avoided in patients who are intolerant of such medications or who have other comorbid conditions contraindicating their use. Avoid NSAIDs in patients at risk for gastrointestinal (GI) bleeding, GI intolerance, or gastropathy; renal failure; hepatic failure; congestive heart failure; asthma; or hypersensitivity to NSAIDs. Avoid NSAIDs in the third trimester of pregnancy.

Adverse effects of NSAIDs should be discussed with the patient. These include potential GI intolerance, GI bleeding,[17] GI ulceration or perforation, nephrotoxicity, prolonged bleeding, fluid retention, risk of cardiovascular events, Stevens-Johnson syndrome, and others.

Colchicine. Colchicine originates from the autumn crocus plant; it works as an anti-inflammatory agent.[18] Early on, colchicine blocks microtubule assembly in neutrophils, which attenuates phagocytosis and the transport of MSU crystals to the lysosome.[6] Colchicine impedes the activation of neutrophils in the vicinity of MSU crystals by blocking the release of chemotactic factors, thus diminishing recruitment of polymorphonuclear leukocytes to the inflamed joint.[18]

Colchicine offers the best response when initiated within the first 48 hours of acute gout. Patients usually notice improvement within 48 hours of therapy. During acute gout, oral colchicine can be started at 0.6 mg three or four times daily (taken preferably every 8 hours or in doses separated by at least 1 hour) for 2 days, then decreased to twice daily. Colchicine should not be prescribed to be taken until diarrhea develops, because this will only add more ailment to the patient already suffering from marked pain. Once symptoms resolve, colchicine may be stopped. However, colchicine may be continued at a dose of 0.6 mg every 12 hours to prevent further attacks.

Intravenous colchicine should be used only by experienced rheumatologists and reserved for hospitalized patients, if absolutely necessary, who are unable to take oral colchicine. Caution must be used with dosing, which must not exceed 3 mg per dose. Intravenous colchicine carries a high risk of myelosuppression, can be caustic, and has been associated with fatalities.

Onset of action (pain relief) is 24 hours after the first oral dose. Colchicine requires dose adjustment with decreased renal function and should not be used in dialysis patients because it is not dialyzable.

Adverse effects of colchicine include diarrhea, abdominal cramping, bone marrow suppression, axon-loss neuropathy, myopathy (especially in renal insufficiency), potential liver toxicity, arrhythmia, shock, and skin rash (uncommon). Use caution in patients with biliary obstruction, hepatic failure, or renal insufficiency or end-stage renal disease and in pregnant women, neutropenic patients, and transplant patients on cyclosporine. Concomitant use of colchicine with cyclosporine can lead to rapid-onset myopathy and increased myelosuppression.[16,18]

Corticosteroids. It is best to consider steroids in the absence of concomitant infection. In the case of systemic infections or septic arthritis, steroids should be avoided if possible. Corticosteroids may be used locally as an injection or systemically (orally, intramuscularly, or intravenously). Corticosteroids are usually very effective, and response is noticed within 24 hours of beginning therapy.

Oral corticosteroids can be used in the form of a methylprednisolone pack or prednisone starting at 40 mg or less, with a gradually tapering dose.[6,16,18] Systemic steroids are the preferred agents in patients with renal failure in whom NSAIDs and colchicine are contraindicated. Local steroid injections may be the best alternative route of administration in patients who are unable to tolerate systemic therapy with steroids, NSAIDs, or colchicine. Steroids, however, are not usually the first line of therapy because of their potential adverse effects such as hyperglycemia, gastrointestinal diseases, weight gain and fluid retention, muscle weakness, immune suppression, and long-term effects such as those on bone resorption. The potential adverse effects need to be considered when making the decision of treating acute gout.

Chronic Tophaceous Gout

The main goal of treatment is to decrease urate levels to less than the level of precipitation, which is 6.8 mg/dL. The therapeutic target level should be less than 6 mg/dL, at which level risk of gout attack is decreased and so is the formation of tophi (for which urate levels of <5 mg/dL are preferred).

The decision to start a hypouricemic agent needs to be considered on a patient-by-patient basis, taking into consideration factors such as the absence of definite reversible causes of hyperuricemia, the number of attacks (two or more acute gouty attacks), the degree of hyperuricemia, and the presence of tophi. The decision should be clearly discussed with the patient, because treatment with a hypouricemic agent is usually lifelong and compliance is crucial.[16] Hypouricemic therapy should be started only after the acute attack has completely resolved so as to avoid exacerbation of the attack. Prophylactic agents (colchicine, NSAIDs, or systemic steroids) should be initiated concurrently with hypouricemic drugs to decrease the risk of an acute gouty attack. Hypouricemic drugs include xanthine oxidase inhibitors (e.g., allopurinol), uricosuric agents (e.g., probenecid, sulfinpyrazone, benzbromarone), and new agents (febuxostat and PEG-uricase).

Allopurinol. Allopurinol inhibits xanthine oxidase, the enzyme responsible for the conversion of hypoxanthine to xanthine to uric acid. Steady doses of this drug thus result in decreases in the serum urate levels and dissolution of tophi. Before starting allopurinol, a thorough discussion with the patient is necessary regarding potential adverse effects. The patient must be cautioned about early signs and symptoms of hypersensitivity reactions.

Potential adverse effects of allopurinol include rash, nausea, vomiting, renal failure or impairment, and, less commonly, nephrolithiasis, bone marrow suppression, angioedema, bronchospasm, exfoliative dermatitis, pancreatitis, hepatitis, peripheral neuropathy,

Stevens-Johnson syndrome, and toxic epidermal necrolysis.[19] Allopurinol hypersensitivity syndrome can manifest with erythematous rash, fever, hepatitis, eosinophilia, or acute renal failure. Allopurinol hypersensitivity is a serious and potentially life-threatening reaction to allopurinol. If hypersensitivity is suspected, the drug should be discontinued immediately and the patient should be followed closely for failure of symptoms to resolve and for any progression of symptoms. Hypersensitivity can occur in patients with renal insufficiency; therefore, a low starting dose, 25 to 50 mg, is recommended in this patient population.

Drug interactions occur with oral anticoagulation (such as warfarin), azathioprine, mercaptopurine, cyclophosphamide, cyclsoporine, and iron supplements. Allopurinol, azathioprine, and mercaptopurine share the same enzyme, xanthine oxidase, and could therefore increase the levels of those drugs, leading to exaggerated marrow suppression. Caution is necessary with the use of allopurinol in patients treated with cyclosporine, because this combination can lead to an increase in the serum levels of cyclosporine.

The recommended starting dose is 100 mg a day, increasing gradually every 2 weeks to reach a target serum uric acid level of less than 6 mg/dL. In patients with renal impairment, it is safer to start at 25 to 50 mg a day.

Uricosuric Drugs. Uricosuric agents available in the United States are probenecid and sulfinpyrazone; benzbromarone is not available in the United States. These agents inhibit the urate-anion exchanger in the proximal tubule that mediates urate reabsorption, leading to increased urate excretion through the kidneys. It is advisable to maintain good urine volume and avoid dehydration in patients taking those agents.

Before starting uricosuric agents, a 24-hour urine excretion of uric acid should be checked. These drugs are avoided in patients who have overproduction of urate. In addition, these drugs should be avoided in patients with a history of urate nephrolithiasis.

For probenecid, as with all hypouricemic drugs, it is advisable to start at a low dose and increase gradually to the target serum urate level. The starting dose is 250 mg twice a day. The maintenance dose varies and on average is 500 to 1000 mg two or three times a day. The maximum effective dose is 3000 mg a day.

For sulfinpyrazone, the starting dose is 50 mg twice a day, and the average dose varies, depending on serum urate levels, from 100 to 200 mg three or four times a day. The maximum effective dose is 800 mg a day.

Adverse effects include rash, precipitation of acute gouty arthritis, GI intolerance, and uric acid stones. Probenecid, in particular, increases urinary calcium excretion in gouty patients and thus is contraindicated in patients with a history of calcium or urate nephrolithiasis.

Drug interactions with probenecid include interference with penicillin and ampicillin excretion and autoimmune hemolytic anemia.

Febuxostat and PEG-Uricase. Febuxostat and PEG-uricase (Puricase) might have an advantage with their potential role in patients who are allergic or refractory to treatment with allopurinol. However, this specific indication has not been fully investigated.

Febuxostat is a nonpurine selective inhibitor of xanthine oxidase[20] that has undergone phase I, II, and III trials for treating hyperuricemia in patients with gout.[21] It earned approval from the U.S. Food and Drug Administration (FDA) in February 2009. Current data indicate that it is a potent inhibitor of the enzyme that leads to significant urate reduction and is comparable with allopurinol.[22]

In a study comparing febuxostat with allopurinol in patients with gout and urate levels of at least 8 mg/dL, urate levels dropped to less than 6 mg/dL in 53% of patients who received 80 mg of febuxostat, whereas this level was achieved in only 21% in the allopurinol group.[22] The response was more impressive in the group taking 120 mg of febuxostat. This response was also consistent with reduction in tophus size in both groups.

This study proves the superiority of febuxostat to 300 mg of allopurinol, and it also emphasizes the importance of titrating the dose to reach target levels instead of using a standard dose of 300 mg in all patients. Furthermore, after cessation of prophylaxis (colchicine or naproxen was used), after week eight of starting febuxostat or allopurinol, the incidence of gout flares doubled in the group taking 120 mg of febuxostat and tripled in the group taking 80 mg of febuxostat and 300 mg of allopurinol.[22] This result supports the concept of necessary long-term prophylaxis for acute gout attacks when hypouricemic therapy is initiated.

Febuxostat is well tolerated, even in patients with mild renal impairment, without the need for dosage adjustment.

The most frequently reported adverse effects are diarrhea, back pain, headaches, and arthralgias and patients should monitored for thromboembolic events and increase in hepatic transaminases. Adverse effects were not increased in subjects with moderate renal insufficiency (creatinine 1.6-2.0 mg/dL). The doses used in trials were 40, 80, and 120 mg orally daily; however the dose to be used in clinical practice may be closer to 80 mg.[22a]

PEG-uricase is the pegylated form of uricase, the enzyme that catalyzes conversion of urate to allantoin. This enzyme is naturally lacking in human beings, and thus we are unable to catabolize urate naturally. The enzyme itself is highly immunogenic.

This drug has been used in the past, as Rasburicase, to treat tumor lysis syndrome. However, serious allergic reactions resulted after repeated infusions of this drug, which has limited its use to a one-time infusion. To make the drug less immunogenic, it was pegylated. Pegylation prevented production of antibodies to the uricase protein.

It has been given intravenously or subcutaneously in the studies and has been shown to be safe so far; larger studies are under way. Puricase is promising, and it is probably the most impressive drug used in decreasing tophi burden. However, more data are needed to assess its long-term safety and tolerability.[23]

Prophylaxis during Hypouricemic Treatment

During treatment with a urate-lowering agent, urate levels fluctuate, leading to increased risk of gout attacks. The best prevention is caution using prophylaxis therapy. Colchicine is the most popular prophylaxis. However, in patients who are unable to take colchicine, NSAID therapy or low-dose steroids may be helpful.

Colchicine prophylaxis helps decrease the risk of recurrent flares. Ample data suggest benefit from treating patients with colchicine during initiation of allopurinol therapy. Prophylactic therapy should continue for 6 months to 1 year, if possible.[22,24]

Foods and beverages have long been known to cause gout and gouty attacks. Diet can have some influence on hyperuricemia and gouty attacks, but dietary factors are not sufficient to explain the majority of gout attacks. Patients are encouraged to follow healthy diets sufficient in dairy products; to avoid excessive consumption of alcohol (especially beer), shellfish, and organ meats; and to consume other protein-rich foods in moderation.[10,11] Patients whose diets are poor in dairy products have a higher risk of developing gout attacks than those who consume more dairy products.[11,25]

Special Considerations

Gout in the Young

Gout or hyperuricemia in an adolescent or child is invariably a manifestation of an underlying metabolic or inherited enzyme deficiency. Therefore, gout in the young, although rare, should trigger a workup for such diseases.

Gout in Postmenopausal Women

Gout is not uncommon in postmenopausal women. Estrogen has natural uricosuric effects in premenopausal women. However, after menopause the uricosuric effect is lost and risk of developing gout is increased. Therefore gout in postmenopausal women is more common and tends to involve the upper extremities more often.[26]

Transplant Recipients

Use allopurinol with caution in patients taking azathioprine (in the cases of transplant patients and patients with systemic inflammatory diseases who require azathioprine). The combination of azathioprine and allopurinol increases the levels of azathioprine in the blood, and this increases the risk of bone marrow suppression.[27] Moreover, cyclosporine, another agent used commonly in transplant patients, can increase urate levels.

Metabolic Syndrome

The metabolic syndrome needs to be considered and identified in patients with hyperuricemia. In this case, it is essential to treat the underlying conditions, such as hypertension, overweight, dyslipidemia, and insulin resistance, in addition to treating gout. When an antihypertensive is being considered, losartan offers an advantage because it has mild hypouricemic properties. Prevention of obesity and hypertension might decrease the incidence of gout and morbidity.[1]

PSEUDOGOUT

Definition

Pseudogout is a clinical syndrome in which calcium pyrophosphate dehydrate (CPPD) crystals deposit in joints and soft tissue, resulting in inflammation and tissue damage. The clinical presentation resembles gout in its acute attacks of crystal synovitis, thus the term *pseudogout.* When calcification of cartilage is apparent under radiographic examination of joints, the syndrome is called *chondrocalcinosis.* Although CPPD crystal deposition and chondrocalcinosis are seen in pseudogout, not all patients with chondrocalcinosis or CPPD crystal deposition present with pseudogout.

Prevalence

Limited studies published in the literature have specifically addressed the epidemiology of pseudogout. Epidemiologic studies regarding pseudogout or CPPD arthropathy have not been consistent in using universal investigative methods. Some looked at the prevalence of CPPD arthropathy described radiographically by the finding of chondrocalcinosis in degenerative joint diseases,[28] and others looked at synovial fluid analysis.

This discrepancy creates limitations in extrapolating these data to patients with the clinical constellation of symptoms of pseudogout. A study that looked at age distribution of patients with CPPD by radiographic examination reported the prevalence to be 15% between the ages of 65 and 74 years and higher than 40% after the age of 84 years.[28]

Genetic factors have been investigated and are believed to cause familial autosomal dominant CPPD chondrocalcinosis. Studies are looking at mutations of the chondrocalcinosis ANKH gene, but its functional role is not fully understood.[29]

This disease is not commonly encountered at a younger age without a previous history of trauma or surgery. The disease is seen more commonly after age 50 years, and it has no definite ethnic or gender predilection.[30]

Pathophysiology

Although the pathogenesis of CPPD deposition and pseudogout is not as well understood as the pathogenesis of gout, there is probably excessive pyrophosphate production in cartilage resulting in calcium pyrophosphate supersaturation and the formation of CPPD crystals.[31,32]

Chondrocalcinosis and pseudogout may be associated with certain underlying diseases such as trauma to the joint, hyperparathyroidism, hypomagnesemia, hypophosphatasia, hypothyroidism, and hemochromatosis.[33] This highlights the importance of addressing other possible underlying diseases when evaluating the patient with pseudogout and chondrocalcinosis.

Clinical Manifestations

Although CPPD crystal deposition disease encompasses a variety of clinical manifestations ranging from asymptomatic to goutlike (pseudogout), rheumatoid arthritis–like (pseudo-rheumatoid arthritis) or osteoarthritis-like (pseudo-osteoarthritis), pseudogout is distinguished by acute attacks of synovitis mimicking gout. These acute or subacute attacks can involve one or multiple joints, commonly not more than four or five joints at one time.[34] Pseudogout, like gout, however, can manifest with more systemic features such as fevers, malaise, leukocytosis, and elevated acute phase reactants (sedimentation rate and CRP). Acute attacks may be indistinguishable from acute gout. In fact, it is often difficult to differentiate both without a synovial fluid analysis. Patients have joint pain, synovitis with joint tenderness, and swelling. Pseudogout and gout can share similar joint predilection, but pseudogout affects larger joints more commonly than gout (knee joints) and less so the smaller joints (first metatarsophalangeal joints). It also affects the elbow, shoulder, wrist, and metacarpophalangeal joints.

Diagnosis and Differential Diagnosis

Because pseudogout closely resembles gout, the definite diagnosis of pseudogout often necessitates synovial fluid analysis. Synovial fluid should be microscopically analyzed for cell count and crystal analysis under compensated polarizing microscopy. In addition, fluid should be examined for Gram stain and culture, especially if crystals are not found.[35] On synovial fluid polarization, CPPD crystals might not be as evident as MSU crystals. They are weakly birefringent under polarized light and have a rhomboid or rod-shaped appearance. They are seen either intracellularly or extracellularly, and detection might not be as accurate if fluid analysis is delayed.[15] In addition, because pseudogout and gout can coexist, MSU crystals might also be observed. White cell counts can range from a few thousand cells up to 80,000 to 100,000 per high-power field.

Radiographs can show chondrocalcinosis in the joint involved and other more typical joints even if pseudogout is not clinically active at the time of presentation. They are helpful in confirming the clinical impression (especially the knee joints, wrists, and anteroposterior view of the pelvis) and extent of joint degeneration; however, radiographs are not required to make the diagnosis once CPPD crystals are seen under polarized light. Chondrocalcinosis is seen in the knees (hyaline cartilage and menisci), the wrists (fibrocartilage), and other joints such as intervertebral discs and symphysis pubis. Other radiographic features include joint space narrowing, subchondral new bone formation, normal mineralization, cysts more prominent than in osteoarthritis, bilateral preponderance, and osteophyte formation.[12,36] Certain metabolic conditions associated with CPPD disease, such as in hemochromatosis, have characteristic findings such as joint narrowing of the metacarpophalangeal joint spaces, squaring of the bone ends, subchondral cysts, and hook-like osteophytes on the radial aspects of the metacarpal heads, especially the second and third metacarpophalangeal joints.[37]

Most of the differentials mentioned with gout can be considered here. Infection is always a major differential, especially in the patient presenting with new acute monoarticular arthritis. In addition, septic arthritis can coexist in the joint that has been or is involved in an acute pseudogout attack. Thus, it is important to aspirate the involved joint whenever possible for microscopic examination of the synovial fluid and Gram stain and culture. Other differentials include trauma, bleeding, and other crystal-deposit diseases. Calcium pyrophosphate deposition disease mimics polymyalgia rheumatica.[38]

Treatment

The optimal therapy is one that promptly treats an acute attack, prevents further attacks, and prevents or reverses the degenerative joint disease associated with CPPD arthropathy. Unfortunately, there is no proven therapy that fits this description.

The treatment of pseudogout is mostly tailored to the manifesting symptoms. In patients presenting with one or two points of acute synovitis, rapid relief of pain and inflammation is accomplished with joint aspiration and steroid injection, if no infection is present. In fact, patients often find relief from the joint aspiration itself. When more than two joints are involved it is not feasible to inject all the joints, so treatment is directed more toward systemic therapy. The side effects and toxicities of NSAIDs, colchicine, or systemic glucocorticoids are similar to those discussed for gout. Colchicine at a dose of 0.6 mg once or twice daily may be effective as a prophylactic measure to reduce the number of attacks in a year,[39] especially in patients who experience three or more attacks a year. Unlike gout, however, there are no hypouricemic equivalents to improve the long-term control of pseudogout and to prevent or reverse CPPD crystal deposit disease.

The outcome of patients with pseudogout is influenced by genetic predisposition, extent of crystal deposition and joint degeneration, and aggravating factors from the underlying associated diseases. A study looked at the outcomes of 104 patients with pyrophosphate arthropathy for a mean of 4.6 years and found that patients presenting with acute attacks have a good prognosis, and some patients might not have a progressive disease.[40]

Special Considerations

Because CPPD deposition disease is associated with variety of underlying conditions,[33,41] I recommend screening for hyperparathyroidism, hypothyroidism, hypomagnesemia, hypophosphatasia, and hemochromatosis. Blood should be tested for intact parathyroid hormone, calcium, phosphorous, thyroid-stimulating hormone, magnesium, ferritin, iron transferrin, and alkaline phosphatase. Treatment of associated diseases is recommended. However, it is unclear if treatment of comorbid conditions would decrease the chondrocalcinosis or reverse joint degeneration.

CONCLUSIONS

Crystal deposition disease is a fairly common condition. It is encountered by rheumatologists and other physicians. Gout and pseudogout are the most commonly encountered, but one needs to be aware of the presence of other types of crystal arthropathy, such as hydroxyapatite crystal deposition disease. In this case, crystals might not be seen on classic synovial analysis.

Gout and pseudogout can manifest with similar symptoms, and their signs might not be distinguishable; thus, it is essential to aspirate the affected joint or bursa for synovial fluid and crystal analysis whenever possible. Cell count, Gram stain, and culture, in the right clinical setting, should be sought.

Once the diagnosis is made, treatment for acute attack should be commenced using the least-toxic agent. Treatment should be initiated while taking into consideration other comorbid conditions, such as renal disease, gastric disease, organ transplant, drug interactions, and others, because these will dictate the choice of therapy. In the case of gout, once the acute disease has resolved, the patient should be followed to assess for indications and need for hypouricemic therapy.

New drugs are on the horizon for managing chronic tophaceous gout. Febuxostat has been approved by the FDA, and PEG-uricase could soon earn FDA approval. Keeping on the lookout for new research data, indications, contraindications, and criteria for use of these drugs is essential, because these drugs might come with different criteria for initiating therapy.

Summary

- In patients presenting with acute joint swelling, the differential diagnosis should include evaluation for infection.
- Joint aspiration should be considered in acute swollen joints if possible, and fluid should be analyzed for cell count, cultures, and crystals.
- The gold standard for diagnosing gout or pseudogout is synovial fluid analysis using polarized light microscopy.
- The examiner should be familiar with and trained in crystal identification using polarized light microscopy.
- Monosodium urate crystals appear yellow when parallel to the axis and blue when perpendicular; calcium pyrophosphate dehydrate crystals appear blue when parallel to the axis and yellow when perpendicular.
- Choice of therapy for the treatment of acute gout or pseudogout should take into consideration the patient's comorbidities and risk of medication of choice.
- Acute gout and pseudogout may be treated with colchicine, nonsteroidal anti-inflammatory drugs, or corticosteroids (systemic or intra-articular).
- Treatment of chronic gout and hyperuricemia requires a hypouricemic agent.
- Newer drugs are on the horizon for the management of gout offering additional alternatives to allopurinol and probenacid.

Suggested Readings

Baker DG, Schumacher HR Jr: Acute monoarthritis. N Engl J Med 1993;329:1013-1020.

Becker MA, Schumacher HR Jr, Wortmann RL, et al: Febuxostat, a novel nonpurine selective inhibitor of xanthine oxidase: A twenty-eight-day, multicenter, phase II, randomized, double-blind, placebo-controlled, dose-response clinical trial examining safety and efficacy in patients with gout. Arthritis Rheum 2005;52:916-923.

Borstad GC, Bryant LR, Abel MP, et al: Colchicine for prophylaxis of acute flares when initiating allopurinol for chronic gouty arthritis. J Rheumatol 2004;31:2429-2432.

Choi HK, Atkinson K, Karlson EW, et al: Alcohol intake and risk of incident gout in men: A prospective study. Lancet 2004;363:1277-1281.

Choi HK, Atkinson K, Karlson EW, et al: Purine-rich foods, dairy and protein intake, and the risk of gout in men. N Engl J Med 2004;350:1093-1103.

Choi MH, MacKenzie JD, Dalinka MK: Imaging features of crystal-induced arthropathy. Rheum Dis Clin North Am 2006;32:427-446.

Choi HK, Mount DB, Reginato AM; American College of Physicians; American Physiological Society: Pathogenesis of gout. Ann Intern Med 2005;143:499-516.

Martinon F, Glimcher LH: Gout: New insights into an old disease. J Clin Invest 2006;116:2073-2075.

Martinon F, Petrilli V, Mayor A, et al: Gout-associated uric acid crystals activate the NALP3 inflammasome. Nature 2006;440:237-241.

Pascual E, Jovani V: Synovial fluid analysis. Best Pract Res Clin Rheumatol 2005;19:371-386.

Schlesinger N: Management of acute and chronic gouty arthritis: Present state-of-the-art. Drugs 2004;64:2399-2416.

References

For a complete list of references, log onto www.expertconsult.com.

Paget's Disease of Bone

Elizabeth File and *Abby Abelson*

DEFINITION

Paget's disease of bone (PDB) is a focal, chronic skeletal disorder characterized by enhanced resorption of bone as a result of overactivity of osteoclasts followed by the formation of bone by osteoblasts. This process results in a disorganized, mosaic pattern of woven and lamellar bone that is associated with increased vascularity, marrow fibrosis, and mechanical weakness. The affected bones can become enlarged, less able to resist stress, and deformed. PDB can affect one bone, termed *monostotic* PDB; however, it is more commonly *polyostotic*. The axial skeleton is primarily affected and typically includes the pelvis (72%), lumbar spine (58%), femur (55%), thoracic spine (45%), skull (42%), and tibia (35%), whereas the feet, hands, and facial bones are rarely affected.[1] The most common locations for monostotic disease include the tibia and iliac bones.

EPIDEMIOLOGY

It is difficult to estimate the incidence of PDB because most patients are asymptomatic. The global prevalence varies from 1.5% to 8.3% depending on factors such as age, country of residence, and sex.[2,3] Incidence increases after age 50 years.[2] The prevalence is higher in the United Kingdom, France, Germany, Australia, New Zealand, and North America.[2] It is rare in Asia, India, and Scandinavia. PDB is slightly more prevalent in men than in women.[3]

ETIOLOGY

The exact cause of PDB is uncertain. However, available data suggest that genetic factors or viral infection, or both, might play a pathogenic role. PDB tends to aggregate in families, and between 14% and 25% of family members of patients with Paget's disease eventually contract the disease.[4,5] First-degree relatives of patients with PDB have a 7- to 10-fold increase in risk of developing the condition.[4,5] Other studies have also suggested that a viral infection might play a role in the etiology of PDB.

The theory for a viral basis originated from a study showing that both the nuclei and cytoplasm of osteoclasts from patients with PDB contained uncharacterized viral particles not found in normal osteoclasts.[6] A subsequent study using electron microscopy confirmed the presence of nuclear and cytoplasmic virus-like inclusion bodies in pagetic osteoclasts that resembled paramyxoviral nucleocapsids.[7] Proteins derived from the respiratory syncytial virus and measles virus are present in pagetic osteoclasts and in cells obtained from pagetic bone cultures.[8,9] Although supported by some studies, this viral hypothesis remains controversial, but it does suggest that the development of PDB might result from a latent viral infection of osteoclasts in a genetically susceptible person.

CLINICAL PRESENTATION

Approximately 70% of patients with PDB are asymptomatic.[10] The diagnosis is usually made by an incidental finding on radiograph or by routine chemistry screen showing an elevated serum alkaline phosphatase concentration. However, some patients present with a wide range of symptoms. The classic clinical manifestation of PBD is local bone pain that is usually continuous and present at rest.[10] The temperature of the skin over the affected long bone or skull can be elevated, which is probably caused by increased vascularization of the surrounding tissue and bone.[11] PBD can cause skeletal deformities, such as bowing of long bones, enlarged skull, pelvic alterations, and osteoarthritis if the afflicted area of bone is located in proximity to a joint. The bowing deformities, particularly in the tibia and femur, can cause gait changes and mechanical stresses.

PDB can lead to several comorbid conditions. Traumatic and pathologic fractures can occur.[11] Fractures of long bones may be a serious complication, because excessive blood loss can occur as a result of the increased vascularity of pagetic bone. In less than 1% of patients with PDB, osteosarcomas can develop.[2] These tumors have a poor prognosis, with a 5-year survival rate of approximately 10%.[12] PDB is also associated with neurologic complications including deafness, facial nerve palsies, radiculopathies, and spinal cord compression.[10] These neurologic symptoms generally result from nerve compression by enlarging bone or by interference with the blood supply. Vascular steal syndromes affecting the spinal cord and cerebral supply have been observed.[10] Compression of the base of the skull, known as *platybasia*, can occur, leading to hydrocephalus, nerve entrapment, and cerebellar dysfunction.[13] This can lead to symptoms of nausea, ataxia, incontinence, gait disturbance, or dementia.[13]

PDB is associated with high cardiac output, hypercalcemia, and hyperparathyroidism. High-output heart failure is rare and is a result of increased vascularization of metabolically active pagetic bone. Hypercalcemia is also rare and is normally seen in patients with severe disease who are immobile. Some studies have found an association between PDB and hyperparathyroidism, which could also account for the increase in calcium.[14]

DIAGNOSIS

As previously mentioned, asymptomatic patients with PDB are usually initially identified incidentally by radiograph or by an elevated bone-specific alkaline phosphatase obtained on routine chemistry panels.

The principal mode of diagnosis of PDB is radiographic examination of the skeleton. Plain radiographs of an affected bone reveal osteolytic, osteoblastic, or mixed lesions. Other characteristic radiologic findings include transverse lucent areas, enlargement of bones, expanding lytic changes, thickened cortices, or osteoporosis circumscripta, which refers to extensive lytic involvement in the skull.[10]

Although the radiograph is a powerful diagnostic tool for PDB, bone scanning is a more sensitive test in identifying pagetic lesions.[15] Bone scanning detects up to 50% more lesions than can be observed on radiographs.[15] Thus, bone scans are particularly useful when a patient first presents with symptoms of PDB. As soon as abnormalities are identified by bone scan, they should be confirmed by conventional radiography in at least one site of bone.[15] Repeat bone scans and radiographs are not needed unless the patient has new or progressive symptoms.

Bone biopsy may be necessary if malignant transformation of the bone is suspected.[15] The most important feature of malignant change of the bone is cortical destruction and the presence of a soft tissue mass outside of the bone.[12]

PDB is characterized by accelerated bone turnover. Therefore, elevated levels of biochemical markers of bone turnover provide a general indication of the extent of disease activity. Total serum alkaline phosphatase activity, which is a reflection of increased bone formation, is elevated in 85% of untreated PDB patients.[15] In studies that compare various markers of bone turnover in patients with PDB, bone-specific alkaline phosphatase has a diagnostic sensitivity of 84%, and total serum alkaline phosphatase has a diagnostic sensitivity of 74%.[16] The alkaline phosphatase is a useful marker of disease activity, extent and severity of disease, and treatment efficacy. Accelerated bone resorption also occurs in PDB. Thus, increased urinary excretion of pyridinoline and hydroxyproline, markers of bone resorption, are observed.[16]

TREATMENT

The indications for treatment of PDB include bone pain, bone deformity, extensive skull involvement, hypercalcemia, fractures, neurologic compromise, monostotic disease of a tibia or femur in whom progression is likely, and high-output heart failure.[2,15] Treatment is also indicated in the presence of moderately active asymptomatic disease, with serum alkaline phosphatase at least three to four times the upper limit of normal, in patients with disease at sites where complications could occur. These sites include weight-bearing bones, areas near major joints, and vertebral bodies. For patients with moderately active disease before elective surgery on the affected bone(s), prophylactic therapy is also used to reduce hypervascularity and blood loss.[2] Some studies indicate that antipagetic treatment is valuable for symptomatic as well as asymptomatic patients, with the goal of reducing local disease progression and the risk of future complications.[2] In general, because therapy is effective and safe, treatment should be withheld only in asymptomatic patients whose disease is located only in areas with no risk of complications.[17]

The drugs used to treat PDB suppress osteoclastic activity. The medications that are currently approved by the Food and Drug Administration in the United States are salmon and human calcitonin, given subcutaneously, and various bisphosphonates.

The most commonly used agents are the bisphosphonates, which are pyrophosphate analogues that inhibit bone resorption. Etidronate was the first clinically available agent for the treatment of PDB. It is administered at a dose of 5 mg/kg/day orally for 6 months. Although etidronate has been shown to be effective for treating PDB, the newer generation of bisphosphonates is superior at achieving normalization of biochemical indices of bone turnover.[18] Tiludronate can be used for treatment at a dose of 400 mg/day orally for 3 months. Alendronate is given at 40 mg/day orally for 6 months, and risedronate is given at a dose of 30 mg/day orally for 2 months.

The oral bisphosphonates have the drawback of gastrointestinal side effects, especially esophagitis. They should be taken with 6 to 8 ounces of water and the patient should be in the upright position for at least 30 minutes without other oral intake. In the United States, pamidronate is given as an intravenous infusion.

Although several different treatment paradigms have been evaluated, one recommended treatment regimen consists of either three infusions of 60 mg at intervals of 2 weeks or six infusions of 30 mg at intervals of 2 weeks.[15] However, the dose and number of treatments depend on the individual patient and the severity of the disease.[15]

The FDA has approved another medication that looks promising for PDB, zoledronic acid. It was shown that a single infusion of zoledronic acid 5 mg produced a more-rapid, more-complete, and more-sustained response in Paget's disease than did daily treatment with risedronate.[19]

Treatment efficacy can be monitored via clinical and biochemical responses. Effective therapy for PDB results in a reduction in bone turnover, with a substantial decrease in the serum alkaline phosphatase. It is recommended to check the alkaline phosphatase every 3 months for the first 6 months of therapy and thereafter at intervals of every 6 months.[15]

Summary

- PDB is a focal, chronic skeletal disorder characterized by enhanced bone resorption and formation.
- Many patients with PDB are asymptomatic; however, the classic clinical manifestation is local bone pain.
- An elevated bone-specific alkaline phosphatase and characteristic radiographic findings help to diagnose PDB.
- Zoledronic acid was recently approved by the FDA for the treatment of PDB.

Suggested Readings

Alvarez L, Guanabens N, Peris P, et al: Discriminative value of biochemical markers of bone turnover in assessing the activity of Paget's disease. J Bone Miner Res 1995;10:458-465.

Ankrom MA, Shapiro JR: Paget's disease of bone (osteitis deformans). J Am Geriatr Soc 1998;46:1025-1033.

Delmas PD, Meunier PJ: The management of Paget's disease of bone. N Engl J Med 1997;336:558.

Drake WM, Kendler DL, Brown JP: Consensus statement on the modern therapy of Paget's disease of bone from a Western Osteoporosis Alliance symposium. Biannual Foothills Meeting on Osteoporosis, Calgary, Alberta, Canada, September 9–10, 2000. Clin Ther 2001;23:620-626.

Frassica FJ, Sim FH, Frassica DA, Wold LE: Survival and management considerations in post irradiation osteosarcoma and Paget's osteosarcoma. Clin Orthop 1991;270:120.

Kanis JA: Clinical features and complications. In Kanis JA (ed): Pathophysiology and Treatment of Paget's Disease of Bone. London: Martin Duntz Ltd, 1998, pp 110-138.

Lyles KW, Siris ES, Singer FR, Meunier PJ: A clinical approach to diagnosis and management of Paget's disease of bone. J Bone Miner Res 2001;16:1379-1387.

Meunier PJ, Salson C, Mathieu L, et al: Skeletal distribution and biochemical parameters of Paget's disease. Clin Orthop 1987;217:37-44.

Mii Y, Miyauchi Y, Honoki K, et al: Electron microscopic evidence of a viral nature for osteoclast inclusions in Paget's disease of bone. Virchows Arch 1994;424;99-104.

Mills BG, Singer FR, Weiner LP, et al: Evidence for both respiratory syncytial virus and measles virus antigens in the osteoclasts of patients with Paget's disease of bone. Clin Orthop 1984;303-311.

Ooi CG, Fraser WD: Paget's disease of bone. Postgrad Med J 1997;73:69-74.

Posen S, Clifton Bligh P, Wilkinson M: Paget's disease of bone and hyperparathyroidism: Coincidence or causal relationship? Calcif Tissue Res 1978;26:107.

Rebel A, Baslé M, Pouplard A, et al: Bone tissue in Paget's disease of bone. Ultrastructure and Immunocytology. Arthritis Rheum 1980;23:1104-1114.

Rebel A, Malkani K, Baslé M, Bregeon C: Nuclear inclusions in osteoclasts in Paget's bone disease. Calcif Tissue Res 1976;21 Suppl 113.

Reid IR, Miller P, Lyles K, et al: Comparison of a single infusion of zoledronic acid with risedronate for Paget's disease. N Engl J Med 2005;353:898.

Rousiere M, Michou L, Cornelis F, Orcel P: Paget's disease of bone. Best Pract Res Clin Rheumatol 2003;17:1019-1041.

Selby PL, Davie MWJ, Ralston SH, Stone MD: Guidelines on the management of Paget's disease of bone. Bone 2002;31:366-373.

Siris ES: Epidemiologic aspects of Paget's disease: Family history and relationship to other medical conditions. Semin Arthritis Rheum 1994;23:222.

Siris ES, Ottoman R, Flaster E, Kelsey JL: Familial aggregation of Paget's disease of bone. J Bone Miner Res 1991;6:495.

References

For a complete list of references, log onto www.expertconsult.com.

Osteoarthritis

William S. Wilke and John Carey

Osteoarthritis, which is the most common form of arthritis in the United States and other Western countries, is increasing in incidence as the population ages, and it is likely to rise further with the obesity epidemic. Significant disability and loss of function are associated with this disease, and its management is an enormous cost to the health care system. Progress in prevention and treatment has been slow, related in part to the insidious onset and generally slow progression of the disease.[1-3] As a result, clinical trials can take many years to show a significant disease benefit. Therefore, despite its being the most prevalent form of arthritis, few long-term clinical trials have studied the therapeutic outcomes.

DEFINITION

Osteoarthritis (also known as *degenerative arthritis, hypertrophic arthritis*, or *age-related arthritis*) implies an inflamed joint by its very name, but for a long time the role of inflammation in osteoarthritis has been somewhat controversial. The pathology reflects the result of joint disease, with loss and erosion of articular cartilage, subchondral sclerosis, and bone overgrowth (osteophytes).

Rather than one uniform disease, osteoarthritis may be a primary or an idiopathic phenomenon, or it may be secondary to some other disorder. Osteoarthritis is also commonly seen as a secondary form of arthritis in patients with other inflammatory arthritides, such as rheumatoid arthritis. Mechanical and genetic factors play roles in the development of this disease as well. Histologic evidence clearly shows ongoing inflammation and cartilage destruction in osteoarthritis, although not to the same degree as in other arthritides, such as rheumatoid arthritis.[1,4,5]

PREVALENCE AND INCIDENCE

Osteoarthritis is the most prevalent form of arthritis in the United States, affecting more than 70% of adults between 55 and 78 years of age.[5] Women are affected more than men.[5,6] Hip osteoarthritis is more common in Western populations, suggesting that race and environmental factors might also be important.[5] The incidence of symptomatic knee osteoarthritis is 1% per year, with a radiographic incidence of 2% per year. The rate of radiographic progression has been estimated at about 4% per year.[6]

PATHOPHYSIOLOGY

Understanding the metabolic pathways at the molecular level has greatly enhanced our understanding of the tissue factors involved.[7]

Although the role of inflammation in osteoarthritis has been unclear for a long time, significant progress has been made in more recent years. The molecular pathways involved are being more clearly defined, and this is an area of intense ongoing research. Studies also show that there are ongoing inflammation and synovitis that result in permanent joint damage.[1,5,8] At times, this may be more striking, with flares of symptoms or joint effusions. Effusions can be very large at times, and we have aspirated more than 100 mL of fluid from an acutely swollen knee on more than one occasion. Biopsies of synovium from patients with osteoarthritis show more inflammatory infiltrates than normal controls do.

Some patients appear to have a more hereditary form of this disease. The striking features are usually seen in women who, shortly after menopause, develop distal (Heberden's nodes) and proximal (Bouchard's nodes) interphalangeal joint involvement in their hands, which eventually leads to the characteristic bony swelling and correlates with the presence of radiographic knee involvement.[8] Previous trauma or other prior joint insults, such as inflammation, infection, or avascular necrosis, increase the risk of developing osteoarthritis at that anatomic site.[1,8]

Histologically, articular cartilage comprises chondrocytes and their extracellular matrices. Three distinct zones are recognizable: superficial, middle, and deep. Mechanical or inflammatory injury that disrupts these zones can lead to irreparable damage and to further inflammation and cartilage degradation as the body attempts to heal itself. In essence, there is a defective repair mechanism, resulting in scarring, thinning, and erosion of the articular cartilage in the joints of subjects with osteoarthritis.[9] Several cytokines, such as interleukin-1β and transforming growth factor β, proteases (the most important of which is matrix metalloprotease), and nitric oxide synthetase all appear to be essential for cartilage degradation in the pathogenesis of osteoarthritis. It was previously believed that bone changes occur later in this disease, but newer evidence suggests that subchondral bone changes might take place earlier than previously suspected.[10] Increased production of bone and cartilage degradation products has been shown to herald more rapid disease progression.[4]

SYMPTOMS, SIGNS, AND DIAGNOSIS

Stiffness, joint pain, and swelling are the earliest symptoms of osteoarthritis. In contrast to inflammatory arthritis, the pain of osteoarthritis is often exacerbated by activity or weight bearing and relieved by rest. Early symptoms are usually of an insidious nature and often do not correlate well with radiographic abnormalities. Later, extensive bone changes, muscle weakness, and loss of joint integrity can lead to more-dramatic joint deformity and disability. Physical findings include painful limitation of movement, bony crepitus, and, occasionally, joint effusions and joint line or bone tenderness. As the disease progresses, more permanent joint deformities can occur in the forms of contractures, osteophytes, and loss of joint function.

Synovial fluid analyses and laboratory investigations are generally not diagnostic. Their utility lies mainly in excluding other causes for the patient's symptoms or other common forms of arthritis such as crystal deposition diseases. Newer studies using markers of bone, cartilage, and synovium turnover might help identify patients who have a more rapidly progressive form of joint disease, but they are not recommended in routine clinical practice. Data on high-sensitivity C-reactive protein have been reported, with somewhat conflicting findings. Elevated levels of C-reactive protein appear to correlate best with symptoms of pain and stiffness rather than extent or progression of disease.[11]

Radiographic studies are reserved for patients with symptoms. They are useful in excluding other causes of the patient's symptoms and in evaluating the extent of joint pathology. However, although radiographs might show osteoid changes such as joint-space narrowing, effusions, bone cysts, and osteophytes, radiographs are limited in sensitivity and in their ability to show nonosseous structures.

Ultrasound, computed tomography, and magnetic resonance imaging (MRI) might show more extensive joint detail. Although changes in soft tissue and cartilage are better visualized by MRI than by radiographs, and MRI is more sensitive for picking up early bone changes, this is generally unhelpful to the practicing physician. Felson and colleagues have shown that men with osteoarthritis of the knee who have MRI evidence of subchondral bone bruising or marrow edema experience a more rapid progression of their disease than men who do not have these signs. Joint malalignment correlates strongly with the presence of the bone marrow lesions.[10] In addition, asymptomatic patients with osteoarthritis might have significant abnormalities on MR imaging, making abnormal findings even harder to interpret.[12] These more-expensive imaging modalities are usually reserved for evaluating other possible causes of symptoms, such as meniscal tears and tumors. Until it can be shown that a therapeutic intervention can significantly prevent or retard the progression of this disease, the role of these imaging modalities in osteoarthritis is of limited value.

TREATMENT

Treatments have not been shown to reverse this disease, although some treatments can halt its progression. The goal of treatment is adequate pain relief and preservation of function. The American College of Rheumatology[2] (ACR) and the European League Against Rheumatism (EULAR) have published guidelines for managing hip and knee osteoarthritis.

Weight loss, even small amounts, can significantly benefit overweight arthritis patients. Relaxation programs and moderate exercise, good nutrition, and education can all help relieve suffering in arthritis patients. Caring health care professionals can alleviate worry and help a patient to achieve realistic goals. Devices such as canes, supports, and braces can take some stress off the affected joint. Avoiding aggravating factors such as trauma, excessive weight gain, or overly strenuous exercise is essential. Other analgesic therapies, such as heating pads or ice packs, also alleviate suffering. Care should be taken, as in all pain-related illnesses, to treat concomitant aggravating factors, such as psychosocial stress or other painful maladies, such as secondary bursitis.[2,3,5]

Analgesics and Anti-Inflammatories

Acetaminophen (paracetamol in Europe) is generally recommended as first-line pharmacologic therapy. Acetaminophen is a relatively safe treatment and has significantly lower gastrointestinal (GI), renal, and cardiovascular toxicities than other medications. When taken on a regular basis, doses of 500 to 750 mg three to four times daily can provide substantial relief. Care should be taken not to exceed 4 g/day.[2,3]

Nonsteroidal anti-inflammatory drugs (NSAIDs) can provide significant acute relief in patients with osteoarthritis. However, because osteoarthritis occurs more commonly in older patients who often have other comorbidities, the use of NSAIDs is limited by their potential for or actual side effects. Notably, they can cause or worsen GI hemorrhage, renal insufficiency, congestive heart failure, and hypertension.

Several agents (e.g., rofecoxib, celecoxib) that specifically inhibit cyclooxygenase-2 (COX-2) are approved in the United States (by the U.S. Food and Drug Administration [FDA]) and in Europe for use in arthritis patients. Although they are more expensive than over-the-counter generic drugs, they have a better GI safety profile. The concern with these newer agents, as for the older NSAIDs, is that there may be an increased risk of cardiovascular events for patients taking these medications.[13] Indeed, one of these agents (rofecoxib [Vioxx]) was withdrawn from the market because of evidence documenting such side effects. Whether these findings are specific to rofecoxib or represent a class effect remains to be determined. They should be used with extreme caution or not at all in patients with renal or cardiovascular disease.

Topical aspirin or NSAID preparations, which are more widely available in Europe, are an alternative to oral medications. However, the incidence of side effects from NSAIDs is often dose related, and thus they should probably be reserved for acute flares or more recalcitrant disease.

Nonacetylated Salicylates

Nonacetylated salicylate compounds such as choline magnesium trisalicylate (Trilisate) 500 to 750 mg two or three times daily are effective therapies for many patients, and we have had success using this group of drugs. These medications have fewer adverse GI effects than regular aspirin compounds or NSAIDs and provide a less-expensive alternative to the COX-2 inhibitors. Salicylate levels can also be measured relatively easily in serum, similar to other pharmaceutical compounds, although this is not routine practice.

Steroids

Systemic steroids are not indicated in the management of osteoarthritis. However, local intra-articular injection of corticosteroids can provide significant relief of pain and stiffness, and despite the evidence in randomized trials, clearly some patients have very long-lasting pain relief from a single injection. This should be performed in a sterile manner by physicians experienced with this technique; side effects such as infection, bruising, lipodystrophy, and osteonecrosis are rare with careful technique. Most of the benefit in randomized, double-blind, placebo-controlled trials seems to have occurred soon after the injection, and improvement of symptoms may be greatest in those with joint effusion.[14,15] Intra-articular triamcinolone 40 mg injections every 3 months for 1 to 2 years showed no effect on radiographic progression.[15]

Synovial fluid should be aspirated, if possible, with an aseptic technique before injection. The fluid should be sent for the usual studies such as Gram stain, culture, cell count, and differential, and an extensive examination for crystals should be performed by a person familiar with this technique. Other studies may be performed as the situation dictates. Studies such as fluid pH, viscosity, glucose, antinuclear antibody, and rheumatoid factor are unhelpful in most circumstances.

Alternative Treatments

Viscosupplements, although approved by the FDA, appear to provide little more relief than sham injections. Despite the promise for these drugs, well-performed placebo-controlled trials have had disappointing results.[16,17] Thus, we do not recommend routine use of intra-articular hyaluronate or its derivatives until there is stronger evidence that they are clearly beneficial.

Many patients with osteoarthritis use alternative therapies in an attempt to relieve their suffering. Natraceuticals have shown some promise in this regard. Glucosamine and chondroitin sulfate are by far the most-studied agents in this category and have been shown in several studies to be as effective as acetaminophen and NSAIDs, with significantly fewer adverse effects. These agents appear to significantly alleviate pain and suffering by an unknown mechanism. They have a slow onset of action (placebo-controlled trials show that it takes several weeks to see an effect in the treated groups), and they appear to have a more sustained post-treatment effect than NSAIDs or analgesics.[1,3,18,19] A 3-year placebo-controlled trial showed that glucosamine might retard radiographic progression.[19] We recommend trying glucosamine and chondroitin sulfate at a dose of 1200 to 1500 mg daily in most patients with osteoarthritis, given that the safety profile and efficacy are similar to those of NSAIDs and acetaminophen.

Acupuncture, although used by many patients, appears to be no better than sham needling in controlled trials,[5] and it is not without its own risks, which include reports of hepatitis transmission and pneumothoraces.

Narcotic Analgesics

Narcotic analgesics should be reserved for patients with severe joint disease and intolerable suffering who are not candidates for other therapeutic interventions or for whom other therapeutic interventions have failed. Short courses, however, can be used effectively. Less-potent medications, such as the new combination tramadol/acetaminophen, should be tried first, reserving narcotic medications for those who still have severe pain. Usual precautions should be taken when prescribing these, such as counseling patients about their correct use and addictive potential.

Antidepressants

Depression and arthritis are common and often coexist. Treatment of depressive symptoms in older adults with arthritis resulted in significantly less pain and depression and overall improvement in health and quality of life.[20] Thus, care should be taken to evaluate and treat patients for concomitant depression when managing their arthritis.

Surgery

The efficacy of arthroscopy for osteoarthritis remains controversial. It is under review by the ACR and is not recommended in the 2003 EULAR guidelines.[2,3] Progress in joint replacement surgery has been remarkable in the past few decades, particularly for knee and hip arthritis. Arthroplasty is now used to treat many patients with severe osteoarthritis, especially those who are appropriate surgical candidates and for whom more-conservative measures have failed.

Joint replacements can wear out after an average of 10 to 15 years, although some patients do well for much longer. Newer components and improved techniques might increase the longevity of these replacements in the future. Reoperation after the original replacement surgery may be more complex and can have higher failure and infection rates.

CONCLUSIONS

Osteoarthritis is the most common form of arthritis in the United States. The incidence increases with advancing age. Many patients can achieve significant relief of their symptoms with appropriate care. Current therapies are being investigated to see if they improve the long-term outcomes of this disease. Ongoing research is aiming to identify patients who have a more rapidly progressive illness, and it is evaluating disease-specific molecular pathways as potential new targets for intervention. Advances in joint replacement surgery have made this an excellent treatment for many patients with more-severe disease.

Summary

- Whether it is primary or secondary, osteoarthritis is characterized by loss and erosion of cartilage, subchondral sclerosis, and overgrowth of bone.
- The pathogenesis of osteoarthritis is driven by heredity, prior insults to the joint, and mild-to-moderate local inflammation.
- The diagnosis of osteoarthritis is made on the basis of signs and symptoms of joint swelling, pain, and hypertrophy in characteristic joints and is confirmed by x-ray.
- Primary treatment of osteoarthritis includes joint protection, strengthening the muscles around the joint, weight loss for hip and knee osteoarthritis, and acetaminophen.
- Nonsteroidal anti-inflammatory drugs are safest when used intermittently.

Suggested Readings

Altman RD, Hochberg MC, Moskowitcz RW, Schnitzer TJ: Recommendations for the medical management of osteoarthritis of the hip and knee: 2000 update. American College of Rheumatology Subcommittee on Osteoarthritis Guidelines. Arthritis Rheum 2000;43:1905-1915.

Brooks P: Inflammation as an important feature of osteoarthritis. Bull World Health Organ 2003;81:689-690.

Felson DT, Anderson JJ: Hyaluronate sodium injections for osteoarthritis: Hope, hype, and hard truths. Arch Intern Med 2002;162:245-247.

Gaffney K, Ledingham J, Perry JD: Intra-articular triamcinolone hexacetonide in knee osteoarthritis: Factors influencing the clinical response. Ann Rheum Dis 1995;54:379-381.

Jordan KM, Arden NK, Doherty M, et al: EULAR recommendations 2003: An evidence based approach to the management of knee osteoarthritis: Report of a task force of the Standing Committee for International Clinical Studies Including Therapeutic Trials (ESCISIT). Ann Rheum Dis 2003;62:1145-1155.

Lin EHB, Katon W, Von Korff M, et al: Effect of improving depression care on pain and functional outcomes among older adults with arthritis: A randomized, controlled trial. JAMA 2003;290:2428-2434.

Mainil-Varlet P, Aigner T, Brittberg M, et al: Histological assessment of cartilage repair: A report by the Histology Endpoint Committee of the International Cartilage Repair Society (ICRS). J Bone J Surg Am 2003;85A(suppl 2):45-57.

Mandell BF: COX-2 inhibitors: Balancing the hope, the hype, and the concern. Cleve Clin J Med 2001;68:899.

Richy F, Bruyere O, Ethgen O, et al: Structural and symptomatic efficacy of glucosamine and chondroitin in knee osteoarthritis: A comprehensive meta-analysis. Arch Intern Med 2003;163:1514-1522.

Sturmer T, Brenner H, Koenig W, Gunther KP: Severity and extent of osteoarthritis and low grade systemic inflammation as assessed by high sensitivity C reactive protein. Ann Rheum Dis 2004;63:200-205.

References

For a complete list of references, log onto www.expertconsult.com.

Primary Angiitis of the Central Nervous System

Rula A. Hajj-Ali and Leonard H. Calabrese

Vasculitis that affects the central nervous system (CNS) is one of the most formidable diagnostic and therapeutic challenges for physicians because the clinical manifestations of CNS vasculitis are highly variable, the CNS is a common target of many forms of systemic vasculitis and may also be the sole target of vasculitis, and specific noninvasive tests are lacking and material for pathophysiologic investigation is limited. Correct diagnosis requires a high degree of suspicion coupled with knowledge of other diseases that can masquerade as vasculitis.

DEFINITION

A primary vasculitis limited to the CNS is referred to as *primary angiitis* of the central nervous system (PACNS). A generalized systemic vasculitic process can also involve the CNS, and in such cases, it is referred to as *secondary vasculitis* of the CNS. Secondary vasculitis is not discussed in this chapter.

The earliest reports of PACNS described the disease as fatal and progressive, limited to the CNS, and characterized by rich granulomatous vasculitis. The disease was named *granulomatous angiitis* of the CNS (GACNS), and it remained a rare diagnostic entity until the 1980s. Increasing reports of successful treatment with cyclophosphamide and glucocorticoids as well as the use of angiography for the diagnosis of PACNS heightened the interest in the diagnosis. In 1988, Calabrese and Mallek proposed criteria for the diagnosis of PACNS (Box 1).[1]

In the 1990s, we and others began to question whether PACNS is a homogeneous disease or whether different clinical subsets exist. A subset angiitis diagnosed on the basis of angiography and with a predictably more benign outcome requiring less-intensive therapy was identified and originally named *benign angiopathy* of the central nervous system (BACNS). Because BACNS is now recognized to be characterized by vasospasm and closely resembles other vasospastic disorders such as Call-Fleming syndrome, postpartum angiopathy, migrainous vasospasm, and drug-induced arteritis, all of these disorders have been grouped under the term *reversible cerebral vasoconstriction syndromes* (RCVS).

Most cases of either angiographically or histopathologically documented PACNS do not fall distinctly within the categories of either GACNS or RCVS and are thus considered atypical. Most atypical cases of PACNS have clinical features that preclude a ready diagnosis of RCVS: They have a GACNS-like presentation, but their biopsies reveal nongranulomatous pathology or they have unusual clinical presentations.

PREVALENCE

PACNS was first described in the mid-1950s. By 1986, only 46 cases had been reported in the English-language medical literature. Since 1975, an increasing number of cases have been described, and 99 cases were reported through 1990. Today, although PACNS is still uncommon, its specter is often raised in patients with neurologic problems of obscure origin, making its diagnostic approach a relevant clinical issue.

PATHOPHYSIOLOGY

PACNS is a heterogeneous disease with different clinical subsets of unknown etiology and pathogenesis. The pathologically defined entity (GACNS) is primarily a leptomeningeal and cortical vasculitis involving the small and medium leptomeningeal and cortical arteries. Pathologic findings include classic granulomatous angiitis with Langhans' or foreign body giant cells, necrotizing vasculitis, or a lymphocytic vasculitis. The initial event that primes the inflammatory cells is not known. However, the final pathway of inflammation leads to occlusion of the involved blood vessel, thrombosis, and, ultimately, ischemia and necrosis of the territories of the involved vessels. Limited data suggest an association with systemic viral illnesses or a state of altered host defense and PACNS. Duna and colleagues[2] analyzed 168 reported cases of PACNS and found that 29 of these were associated with an illness characterized by an immunosuppressive state, including corticosteroid therapy, lymphoproliferative or myeloproliferative disorders, and human immunodeficiency virus (HIV) infection. In addition, a variety of pathogens have been documented in association with CNS arteritis, including varicella-zoster virus (VZV), HIV, and cytomegalovirus.[3-5]

It is likely that in the setting of altered host defense mechanisms or in a predisposed patient, a pathogen escapes immune defense mechanisms and induces arteritis. In support of this hypothesis is the well-defined clinical syndrome of post–herpes zoster ophthalmicus contralateral hemiplegia. In this syndrome, a contralateral hemiplegia occurs weeks to months after VZV infection of the trigeminal ganglion and nerve, apparently resulting from the retrograde spread of VZV to intracranial vessels. Viral particles have been identified in the cytoplasm and nuclei of smooth muscle cells within the walls of affected vessels. HIV infection has been similarly described in such a setting.[6,7]

Alternatively, RCVS is diagnosed solely by angiopathy and has been dubbed *angiopathy* rather than *angiitis*, reflecting the uncertainty of the underlying pathology. By virtue of its angiographic diagnosis, few cases have included brain biopsies, and these have been uniformly unrevealing. It has been proposed that RCVS represents a form of reversible vasoconstriction or spasm rather than true arteritis. Supporting this contention, the clinical and angiographic presentations of patients with RCVS is often identical to those of the cerebral vascular syndromes seen after exposure to sympathomimetic drugs, to those found in the setting of complex headaches and pheochromocytoma, and, rarely, to those in the postpartum period. In addition, data from our recent cohort of patients with BACNS imply that cerebral artery vasospasm may be the underlying pathology.[8] In this series, 10 of 16 patients underwent follow-up cerebral angiography over 4 weeks to 8 months, which revealed total or near-total resolution of the angiographic findings in all patients. The reversibility of the angiographic findings suggests a vasospastic process rather than a true arteritis. However, it is also possible that some patients presenting with the diagnostic criteria of RCVS have true angiitis, although the few biopsies performed in such patients have been unrevealing.

SIGNS AND SYMPTOMS

The clinical features of patients with PACNS differ according to their subset or clinical variant. Three different subsets have been described: GACNS, RCVS, and atypical PACNS.[9] Their frequency of distribution is shown in Figure 1.

Granulomatous Angiitis of the Central Nervous System

GACNS represents about 20% of all patients with PACNS. Epidemiologic data for this disease are limited, but it appears to be male-

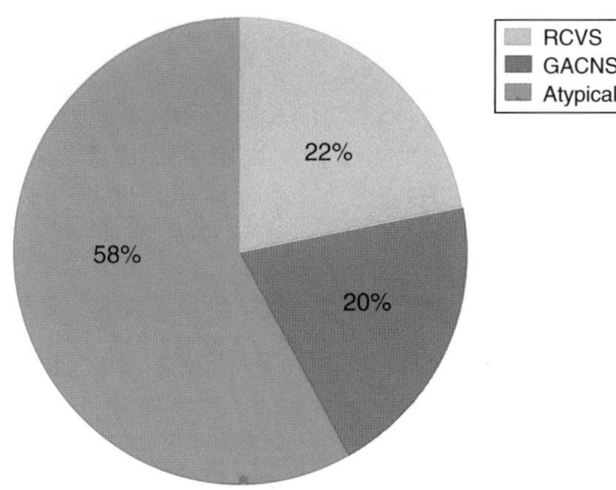

Figure 1 **Clinical subsets of patients with PACNS.** Frequency of nosologic subsets of PACNS at the Cleveland Clinic Foundation. GACNS, granulomatous angiitis of the central nervous system; PACNS, primary angiitis of the central nervous system; RCVS, reversible cerebral vasoconstrictive syndrome.

Box 1 Proposed Criteria for Primary Angiitis of the Central Nervous System

The presence of an acquired and otherwise unexplained neurologic deficit

- *With* presence of either classic angiographic or histopathologic features of angiitis within the CNS
- *And* no evidence of systemic vasculitis or any condition that could elicit the angiographic or pathologic features

Adapted from Calabrese LH, Mallek JA: Primary angiitis of the central nervous system: Report of 8 new cases, review of the literature, and proposal for diagnostic criteria. Medicine (Baltimore). 1988;67:20-39.

Box 2 Clinical Features of Primary Angiitis of the Central Nervous System

- Headaches
- Encephalopathy
- Strokes/transient ischemic attack
- Seizures
- Behavioral changes
- Focal motor/sensory abnormalities
- Ataxia
- Cranial neuropathies
- Visual changes
- Myelopathy
- Radiculopathy

predominant and occurs at any age. It is characterized by a long prodromal period, usually of 6 months or longer, and few patients present acutely.

The most common manifesting signs and symptoms are headaches and mental status changes. Transient ischemic attacks, strokes, seizures, ataxia, visual changes, aphasia and, rarely, coma can develop in patients with GACNS (Box 2). Alteration of level of consciousness is common. Signs and symptoms of systemic vasculitis, such as peripheral neuropathy, fever, weight loss, or rash are usually lacking. Because the vasculitis can affect any area of the CNS, presentation varies widely, and no set of clinical signs is specific for the diagnosis. GACNS may be suspected in the setting of chronic meningitis, recurrent focal neurologic symptoms, unexplained diffuse neurologic dysfunction, or unexplained spinal cord dysfunction not associated with systemic disease or any other process.

Table 1 Reversible Cerebral Vasoconstrictive Syndrome

Feature	Number (%)
Demographic and Clinical Symptoms	
Mean age, years (range)	40 (10-66)
Female/male, *n*	13/3
Mean prodrome, days (range)	25 (0-155)
Mean follow-up, months (range)	35 (0-128)
Headaches, *n* (%)	14 (88)
Focal symptoms, *n* (%)	10 (63)
Diffuse symptoms, *n* (%)	7 (44)
Constitutional symptoms, *n* (%)	1 (6)
Diagnostic Studies	
Severe CSF abnormalities,**n* (%)	1 (7)
Abnormal MRI, *n* (%)	10 (77)
Positive brain biopsy, *n* (%)	0 (0)
Positive cerebral angiography, *n* (%)	16 (100)
Reversibility of angiographic finding	100%

*Protein >70 mg/dL or white blood cell count >10/mm^3.
CSF, cerebrospinal fluid; MRI, magnetic resonance imaging.
Adapted from Hajj-Ali RA, Furlan A, Abou-Chebel A, Calabrese LH: Benign angiopathy of the central nervous system: Cohort of 16 patients with clinical course and long-term follow-up. Arthritis Rheum 2002;47:662-669. With permission.

Reversible Cerebral Vasoconstrictive Syndrome

BACNS is a subset of PACNS diagnosed on the basis of a characteristic set of clinical findings and a classic or high-probability angiogram. In 1993, we proposed the term "benign angiopathy of the CNS" to define case reports and clinical series of cases diagnosed on the basis of angiography alone that had far more benign outcomes than those described for GACNS. This nomenclature has evolved further into RCVS.[10] RCVS is a distinct nosologic subset (Table 1) characterized by clearly distinguishable clinical features, treatments, and outcomes, in contradistinction to GACNS. Patients with RCVS are more likely to be female; they generally present with an acute onset of headache or neurologic event, and their clinical course is more often monophasic and benign than that of patients with GACNS. The distinction between the two subsets is generally not difficult to recognize because signs and symptoms are sharply different (Table 2).

We have described a large series of patients with RCVS that included the clinical, laboratory, and radiologic features of 16 patients as well as their treatments and outcomes.[8] In this cohort, the mean age was 40 years, with female predominance (female-to-male ratio, 4.3 : 1). The most common manifesting symptom was headache, which occurred in 14 of the 16 (88%), followed by focal symptoms in 10 (63%), and diffuse symptoms in 7 (44%) (see Table 1). Cerebral angiography studies were highly abnormal in all patients. Abnormalities on magnetic resonance imaging (MRI) were found in 10 out of 13 (77%) patients. Cerebrospinal fluid (CSF) analysis showed mild or normal results in most patients. Follow-up cerebral angiography, performed in 10 out of 16 (63%) of the patients, revealed total and near-total resolution of changes in all patients (Fig. 2). This suggests that reversibility of the angiographic findings at the follow-up study is essential to securing the diagnosis.

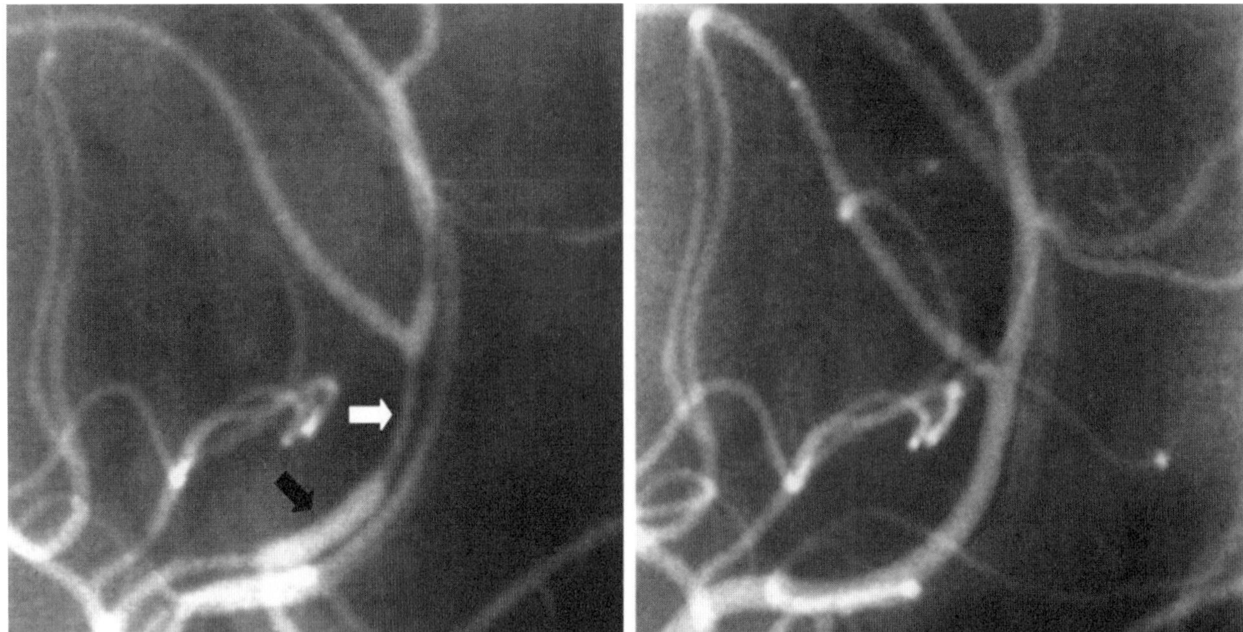

Figure 2 Cerebral angiography of a patient with reversible cerebral vasoconstrictive syndrome at diagnosis *(left)* and after 1 month of therapy *(right)*. Note the multiple areas of stenosis *(white arrow)* and dilation *(black arrow)* in multiple vessels of the M2 branch of the middle cerebral artery, and their resolution after treatment. *(Adapted with permission from Hajj-Ali RA, Furlan A, Abou-Chebel A, Calabrese LH: Benign angiopathy of the central nervous system: Cohort of 16 patients with clinical course and long-term followup. Arthritis Rheum 2002;47:662-669.)*

Table 2 Clinical and Diagnostic Characteristics of RCVS and GACNS

	RCVS	GACNS
Patients	Female-predominant	Male-predominant
Disease onset	Acute	Chronic
Clinical course	Monophasic	Recurrent
CSF findings	Normal	Abnormal
Abnormal angiography	100%	15%
Diagnostic modality	Angiography	CNS biopsy
Treatment	GC and CCBs	GC and CYC
Outcomes	Excellent*	Good†

*100% of RCVS patients had mild-to-no disability on the Barthel Index[15] at follow-up.

†86% of GACNS patients showed mild to no disability and 14% moderate to severe disability on the Barthel Index[15] at follow-up.

BACNS, benign angiopathy of the central nervous system; CCBs, calcium channel blockers; CNS, central nervous system; CSF, cerebrospinal fluid; CYC, cyclophosphamide; GC, glucocorticoids; GACNS, granulomatous angiitis of the central nervous system; RCVS, reversible cerebral vasoconstriction syndrome.

Primary Angiitis of the Central Nervous System: Atypical Cases

Most PACNS patients present with atypical PACNS. This category does not fit the diagnostic criteria for either GACNS or RCVS, yet these patients demonstrate angiographic or histopathologic evidence of PACNS. Included in this group are patients with abnormal CSF findings that preclude a diagnosis of RCVS, or patients with GACNS-like presentation but without granulomatous features on CNS biopsies. In addition, patients presenting with PACNS at unusual anatomic sites such as the spinal cord or those presenting with mass lesions are included in this category.

DIAGNOSIS

The approach to patients with suspected PACNS is not uniform and varies depending on the clinical presentations and subsets described earlier. In most instances, and depending on the clinical setting, the diagnosis of CNS vasculitis is secured by either a positive biopsy or high-probability vascular imaging, such as angiography, while excluding other conditions that can mimic the disease (Fig. 3). Important conditions that can manifest as PACNS and that should be excluded before making any definitive diagnosis include infections, neoplasms, drug exposure, vasospastic disorders, systemic vasculitides, and vasculopathies (Box 3).

Laboratory Tests

No blood studies are diagnostic for CNS vasculitis. Acute-phase reactants, such as sedimentation rate and C-reactive protein, are usually normal in patients with PACNS. If serum markers of inflammation are elevated, secondary forms of CNS vasculitis should be evaluated. If the history and physical examination point to a systemic vasculitis, testing should proceed accordingly. Testing for a variety of infectious organisms, such as mycobacteria, fungi, and HIV, is warranted in patients presenting with chronic meningitis. Other serologic tests are indicated if there is a history of exposure, such as tick bites in Lyme disease. Evaluation for hypercoagulable states and emboli and investigation of drug exposure, including over-the-counter medications, are essential in patients who present with acute focal or multifocal disease.

Cerebrospinal Fluid Analysis

Analysis of the CSF is essential. It is a helpful tool in patients with suspected CNS vasculitis and is of great value in ruling out infectious

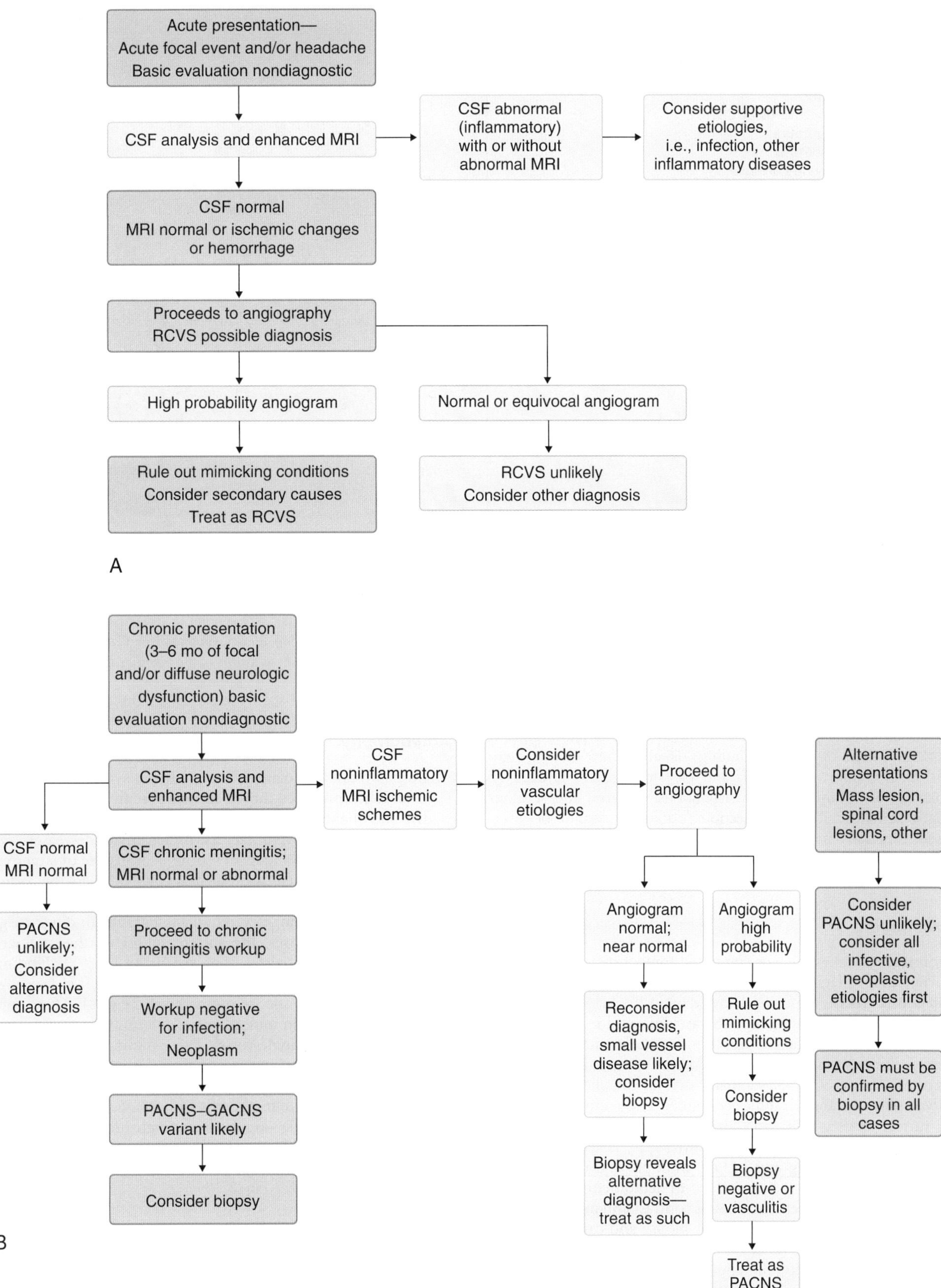

Figure 3 **Clinical algorithm: the approach to primary angiitis of the central nervous system. A,** Acute presentation. **B,** Chronic presentation. CNS, central nervous system; CSF, cerebrospinal fluid; GACNS, granulomatous angiitis of the central nervous system; PACNS, primary angiitis of the central nervous system; MRI, magnetic resonance imaging; RCVS, reversible cerebral vasoconstrictive syndrome.

Box 3 Mimics of Primary Angiitis of the Central Nervous System

Systemic Vasculitides and Connective Tissue Diseases
- Polyarteritis nodosa
- Allergic granulomatosis
- Vasculitis with connective tissue disease
- Henoch-Schönlein purpura
- Wegener's granulomatosis
- Temporal and Takayasu's arteritis
- Behçet's syndrome
- Systemic lupus erythematosus
- Sarcoidosis
- Lymphomatoid granulomatosis

Infection
- Viral
- Bacterial
- Fungal
- Rickettsial

Neoplasm
- Hodgkin's and non-Hodgkin's lymphomas
- Leukemia
- Atrial myxoma
- Malignant angioendotheliomatosis

Miscellaneous
- Fibromuscular dysplasia
- Moyamoya disease
- Thrombotic thrombocytopenic purpura
- Cerebrovascular atherosclerosis
- Embolic disease
- Antiphospholipid syndrome
- Drug exposure (sympathomimetic drugs)

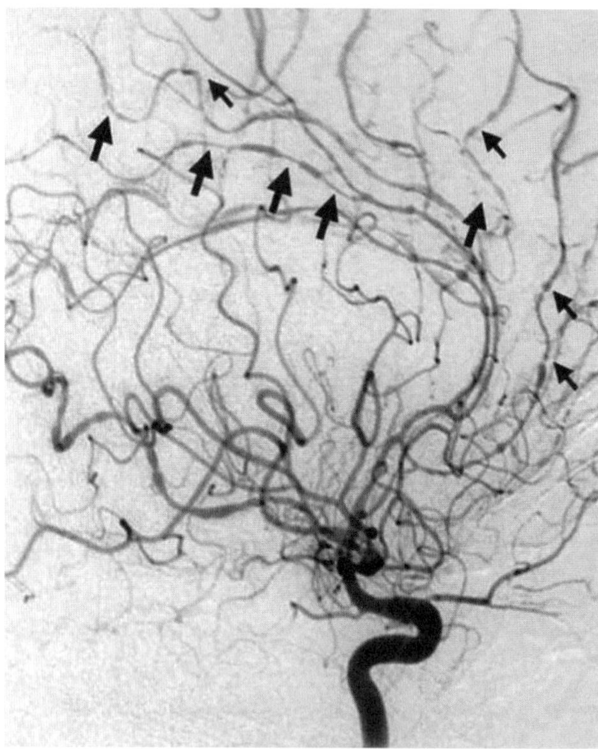

Figure 4 **Typical angiographic findings in a patient with central nervous system vasculitis.** *Arrows* point to areas of alternating stenosis and ectasia. *(Adapted from Hajj-Ali RA, Ghamande S, Calabrese LH, Arroliga AC: Central nervous system vasculitis in the intensive care unit. Crit Care Clin 2002;18:897-914.)*

mimics. CSF findings are abnormal in 80% to 90% of pathologically documented cases of PACNS. Findings usually reflect aseptic meningitis, with modest pleocytosis and elevated protein levels. The importance of obtaining appropriate stains, cultures, and serology evaluations to exclude any infectious etiologies cannot be overstressed, especially in patients presenting with chronic meningitis. Patients with RCVS typically have a normal or near-normal CSF analysis.

Neuroimaging

Neuroimaging studies, such as computed tomography and MRI, are important in the diagnosis of PACNS but are not specific or sufficient for diagnosis. MRI is a more sensitive diagnostic imaging technique than computed tomography in CNS vasculitis, and it should be the initial study of choice when approaching a patient with unexplained ischemia, except when cerebral hemorrhage is suspected. The sensitivity of MRI varies with the standard used for the final diagnosis of CNS vasculitis. In angiographically defined cases, the sensitivity of MRI varies between 77% and 100%.[8,11] In our experience with biopsy-proven cases, the sensitivity of MRI approaches 100%. Findings on MRI are varying and include multiple and often bilateral infarcts in cortex, deep white matter, or leptomeninges, with or without contrast enhancement. Sites of contrast enhancement in the leptomeninges provide ideal places for biopsy and can increase the yield of this technique. Advanced neuroradiographic techniques such as the inclusion of diffusion- and fluid-attenuated inversion recovery MRI sequences, single photon emission computed tomography (SPECT), or positron emission tomography (PET) increase the sensitivity of finding abnormalities but not the specificity for diagnosis. Combining neuroimaging with lumbar puncture increases the overall sensitivity; a normal MRI and lumbar puncture have a high negative predictive value against a diagnosis of GACNS.

Angiography

Angiography is a vital diagnostic modality in evaluating patients with CNS vasculitis provided that its limited specificity and lack of quantitative and qualitative codification are appreciated. Cerebral angiography is limited by several factors. Its sensitivity decreases with the caliber of the vessel, being most sensitive for disease of larger vessels. In pathologically proven cases, such as GACNS where the pathologic involvement is predominantly in the small penetrating vessels beneath the leptomeninges, cerebral angiography findings are generally normal.[12] Moreover, the interpretation of the angiographic findings is often limited by poor specificity (26%).[13] Findings on angiography include alteration of the vessel caliber (i.e., beading) and absence or cutoff of one or more vessels (Fig. 4). These types of changes may be seen in multiple vessels in multiple vascular beds or may be limited to a single vessel. These findings are not diagnostic and can be encountered in vasospastic, infectious, embolic, and atherosclerotic diseases and in hypercoagulable states, and they should be carefully interpreted. In patients with RCVS, involvement of multiple vessels in multiple vascular beds (high-probability angiogram) is characteristic, and documentation of reversibility of the angiographic abnormalities, along the course of the disease, is essential to secure the diagnosis (see Fig. 2).

Pathologic Examination of the Central Nervous System

Histologic confirmation of vasculitis is considered the standard for the diagnosis of CNS vasculitis, but this procedure is also limited by several factors. First, the procedure is highly invasive and requires the skills of an experienced neurosurgeon, who might not always be available. Second, the technical aspects of the procedures should be tailored to the individual patient. In patients with suspected GACNS, the procedure of choice is open-wedge biopsy of the tip of the nondominant temporal lobe with sampling of the overlying leptomeninges and underlying cortex. Alternatively, directing the biopsy to an area of leptomeningeal enhancement, when present, might increase the sensitivity.[14] CNS vasculitis is a notoriously patchy disease, which limits the sensitivity of the procedure, and as many as 25% of the biopsies are falsely negative.[12] Finally, the presence of vasculitis in the biopsy specimen should not preclude performing special stains and cultures for occult infections that can produce secondary vascular inflammation.

TREATMENT

Several issues emerge when treating CNS vasculitis. An accurate diagnosis, the most important initial step, is hampered by the protean manifestations of the disease and the lack of specific and sensitive noninvasive studies coupled with the low specificity and test efficiency of the invasive studies, such as biopsy and angiography. At the same time, diagnosis and treatment are urgent if permanent neurologic damage is to be avoided. A major problem for clinicians is how to monitor disease activity and not confuse irreversible target-organ damage with treatment-resistant disease.

Granulomatous Angiitis of the Central Nervous System: Treatment

There are no controlled studies of therapy for GACNS, and therapeutic guidelines are based largely on experts' consensus opinion. On the basis of the historical literature, GACNS is a progressive and highly lethal disorder; thus, patients are treated with a combination regimen of cyclophosphamide and glucocorticoids. Originally, cyclophosphamide treatment was continued for approximately 1 year after remission. More recently, and similar to the treatment of antineutrophilic cytoplasmic antibody–associated vasculitis, the goal is to limit exposure to alkylating agents by treating with oral cyclophosphamide for 3 to 6 months and, once the patient is in remission, to switch to an antimetabolite such as azathioprine or methotrexate for the duration of therapy. Oral glucocorticoids are used, as in Wegener's granulomatosis, starting with 1 mg/kg/day of oral prednisone and gradually tapering to a small daily dose over 8 to 12 weeks. Assessment of disease activity includes monitoring of any new neurologic event, serial MRI examinations at 3- to 4-month intervals, and evaluation and documentation of clearance of CSF abnormalities. Serial MRI examinations are performed primarily to search for silent progression during tapering of therapy rather than to look for radiographic resolution. Adjunctive therapies, such as prophylaxis for *Pneumocystis carinii* infection and adequate prophylaxis for osteoporosis, should be implemented to avoid treatment-related toxicities.

Reversible Cerebral Vasoconstrictive Syndrome: Treatment

As in GACNS, there are no controlled therapeutic studies in patients with RCVS. In general, RCVS patients are treated less aggressively than patients with GACNS. In our experience,[8] patients are generally treated with glucocorticoids for not more than 6 months, and most patients were treated with adjunctive calcium channel blockers. We usually initiate therapy with prednisone 1 mg/kg/day in divided doses in addition to verapamil 240 mg/day. The dose of verapamil is increased if symptoms are not controlled, particularly headaches. In patients with more-catastrophic presentation (e.g., strokes or major focal neurologic deficits), intravenous methylprednisolone pulse therapy is initiated. Occasional patients with mild disease burden are treated with calcium channel blockers alone. When clinical remission is achieved, a follow-up angiography is performed at 6 to 12 weeks to document total or near-total resolution of the underlying abnormalities. When improvement cannot be documented on angiography or when there is angiographic progression, the diagnosis of RCVS should be re-evaluated and other entities should be considered. The absence of dynamic angiographic changes after therapy suggests atherosclerotic disease, embolic disease, a hypercoagulable state or, rarely, that this is an aggressive form of true angiitis that is being undertreated.

Atypical Primary Angiitis of the Central Nervous System: Treatment

Most cases of PACNS in the atypical category can be initially treated with glucocorticoids alone, with tailoring of treatment according to severity and/or progression of the disease. For patients with an RCVS-like presentation, the addition of a calcium channel blocker is warranted. Cyclophosphamide might need to be added in patients with a severe presentation.

OUTCOMES

Earlier descriptions characterized PACNS as a fatal disease, and most cases were diagnosed postmortem. In the early 1980s, reports of successful treatment emerged and physicians became more interested in the diagnosis of CNS vasculitis. With better understanding of the subsets of the disease, the advancing therapy, and treatment-related toxicities as well as the advent of neuroradiology, more favorable outcomes and improving mortality rate have been reported.

We have studied the long-term outcomes of the PACNS cohort at the Cleveland Clinic Foundation (total of 54 patients). Forty-one PACNS patients were interviewed and their outcomes were analyzed using the Barthel Index, a validated scale used for patients with stroke, as well as a new scale developed expressly for this investigation (cognitive index).[15] Overall, the outcome was favorable, with a 29% (16 of 54 patients) relapse rate and 10% mortality rate (5/54). Eighty percent (33/41) of the interviewed patients demonstrated mild to no impairment on the Barthel Index. Using the cognitive index, mild deficits of concentration and memory and decreased energy level were the most common symptoms. The benign outcome of RCVS patients was documented by this series, with 94% (15/16) of these patients experiencing significant recovery and 71% (5/7) showing no evidence of long-term disability.[8]

Summary

- A primary vasculitis limited to the central nervous system is referred to as *primary angiitis* of the central nervous system (PACNS) and is one of the most formidable diagnostic and therapeutic challenges to physicians.
- Correct diagnosis requires a high degree of suspicion coupled with knowledge of other diseases that can masquerade as PACNS.
- PACNS is a rare disease but has been increasingly recognized in recent years.
- Prompt diagnosis either by biopsy of CNS tissues or by angiography with rigorous exclusions is essential.
- PACNS is best approached by an organized team with expertise in neurovascular disease, immunology or rheumatology, neuroradiology, and neuropathology.
- RCVS is a subset of PACNS diagnosed on the basis of angiography and with a predictably more benign outcome requiring less intensive therapy.
- RCVS is a form of reversible cerebral vasoconstrictive disorder. The diagnosis of this variant is critical to optimal patient care.
- GACNS is a clinical subset of PACNS that is a pathologically defined entity characterized by vasculitis involving the small and medium leptomeningeal and cortical arteries.
- Distinction among the different entities is essential given the diverse therapeutic implications.

Suggested Readings

Calabrese LH: Primary angiitis of the central nervous system. In Hochberg MC, Silman AJ, Smolen JS, et al (eds): Rheumatology, 3rd ed. New York: Mosby, 2003, pp 1705-1714.

Calabrese LH: Vasculitis of the central nervous system. Rheum Dis Clin North Am 1995;21:1059-1076.

Calabrese LH, Gragg LA, Furlan AJ: Benign andiopathy: A distinct subset of angiographically defined primary angiitis of the central nervous systems. J Rheumatol 1993;20:2046-2050.

Calabrese LH, Furlan AJ, Gragg LA, Ropos TJ: Primary angiitis of the central nervous system: Diagnostic criteria and clinical approach. Cleve Clin J Med 1992;59:293-306.

Calabrese LH, Mallek JA: Primary angiitis of the central nervous system. Report of 8 new cases, review of the literature, and proposal for diagnostic criteria. Medicine (Baltimore) 1988;67:20-39.

Duna GF, Calabrese LH: Limitations of invasive modalities in the diagnosis of primary angiitis of the central nervous system. J Rheumatol 1995;22:662-667.

Duna GF, George T, Rybicki L, Calabrese LH: Primary angiitis of the central nervous system (PACNS): An analysis of unusual presentations [abstract]. Arthritis Rheum 1995;38:S340.

Gilden DH, Kleinschmidt-DeMasters BK, LaGuardia JJ, et al: Neurologic complications of the reactivation of varicella-zoster virus. N Engl J Med 2000;342:635-645; erratum 2000;342:1063.

Hajj-Ali RA, Furlan A, Abou-Chebel A, Calabrese LH: Benign angiopathy of the central nervous system: Cohort of 16 patients with clinical course and long-term follow-up. Arthritis Rheum 2002;47:662-669.

Hajj-Ali RA, Villa-Forte A, Abou-Chebel A, et al: Long-term outcomes of patients with primary angiitis of the central nervous system (PACNS) [abstract]. Arthritis Rheum 2000;43:S162.

Linnemann CC, Alvira MM: Pathogenesis of varicella zoster angiitis in the CNS. Arch Neurol 1980;37:239-240.

Parisi JE, Moore PM: The role of biopsy in vasculitis of the central nervous system. Semin Neurol 1994;14:341-348.

Pomper MG, Miller TJ, Stone JH, et al: CNS vasculitis in autoimmune disease: MR imaging findings and correlation with angiography. Am J Neuroradiol 1999;20:75-85.

Yankner BA, Skolnik PR, Shoukimas GM, et al: Cerebral granulomatous angiitis associated with isolation of human T-lymphotrophic virus type III from the central nervous system. Ann Neurol 1986;20:362-364.

Yankner BA, Skolnik PR, Shoukimas GM, et al: Cerebral granulomatous angiitis associated with isolation of human T-lymphotrohic virus type III from the central nervous systems. Ann Neurol 1986;20:362-364.

References

For a complete list of references, log onto www.expertconsult.com.

Polymyalgia Rheumatica and Giant Cell Arteritis

Molloy Eamonn, Curry L. Koening, and Gary S. Hoffman

Polymyalgia rheumatica (PMR) and giant cell arteritis (GCA) are two related, immune-mediated, inflammatory conditions that occur in the elderly. PMR coexists in 40% of patients with GCA. Similarly, 10% of PMR patients develop GCA at some point during their disease course. The relation between PMR and GCA is further demonstrated by their preference for similar patient populations, linkage to the same HLA haplotypes, similar cytokine patterns in temporal artery biopsies, and similarities in anatomic involvement on PET imaging.[1-3] PMR and GCA represent two extremes of a disease spectrum.

POLYMYALGIA RHEUMATICA

Definition

Bruce is credited with the first description in 1888 of PMR, which he described as "senile rheumatic gout."[4] However, Barber coined the term polymyalgia rheumatica in 1957, and it has become the universally accepted name for this condition.[5]

PMR is characterized by proximal, symmetrical musculoskeletal pain and stiffness. Symptoms of systemic inflammation are also common. A dramatic response to low-dose corticosteroids can be a valuable diagnostic tool in patients for whom the diagnosis is uncertain. The lack of response to prednisone raises the possibility of a paraneoplastic process manifesting with proximal pain and stiffness. In patients who have a dramatic response to treatment there is still a need for caution because some patients (~11%) with an initial PMR-like presentation evolve into a phenotype that is more that of rheumatoid arthritis and, less often, other systemic rheumatic illnesses.[6]

Epidemiology

PMR has a predilection for patients older than 50 years. The mean age at onset is 73 years, and women are affected more often than men. Its annual incidence in Olmstead County, Minnesota, a population with mostly Scandinavian heritage, is 59 per 100,000. The annual incidence of the disease increases with age.[7] Whites of northern European descent have a higher incidence of disease than people of African American or Latin American descent.[8,9]

Pathophysiology

Much has been learned about PMR and GCA, but their cause remains unknown. Their cause is likely multifactorial, resulting in the interplay of age, environment, and genetic susceptibility. The suggestion that PMR may be a forme fruste of GCA was first advanced in the 1950s and 1960s.[5] The pathophysiology for both diseases is similar, with abnormalities of cellular immunity leading to vessel and systemic inflammation. Sixteen percent to at least 20% or more of PMR patients demonstrate arteritis on histologic examination, requiring the diagnosis to be changed to GCA.[10] Cytokines such as interleukin (IL)-1, IL-6, and tumor necrosis factor (TNF)-α are important in the development of inflammation in GCA.[11] Messenger RNA (mRNA) for interferon-gamma (IFN-γ) and IFN-γ protein, a product of Th1 lymphocytes, is found in the arterial wall of GCA patients. This suggests that IFN-γ may be a necessary element in the development of vasculitis. The classic histologic features of GCA, which include inflammatory cells involving the adventitia of a muscular artery and migrating toward the media and intima, consist of Th1 cells, dendritic cells, and macrophages.[9]

Signs and Symptoms

Most patients describe subacute onset of symptoms that remain persistent over time. Seventy percent to 95% of patients report symmetrical shoulder girdle pain and stiffness. Fifty percent to 70% report neck and pelvic girdle pain. Concurrent pain in the upper arms and thighs is common and is usually worse in the morning. Shoulder and leg discomfort can lead to difficulty dressing, hair grooming, and rising from a chair. One third of patients have flulike symptoms described as fever, malaise, anorexia, or weight loss.[12]

Physical examination findings may reveal pain that limits active range of motion in the shoulders and hips. Passive range of motion should be normal. Despite subjective symptoms of muscle weakness, muscle strength testing should be normal unless it is affected by examination discomfort or by another condition.[12] Approximately 50% of patients have been said to present with distal extremity abnormalities including swelling of the knees, wrists, or metacarpophalangeal joints. Other reported findings include soft-tissue swelling; pitting edema of the hands, ankles, and feet; and median nerve compression. However, these findings are typical of inflammatory joint disease and not PMR. The examiner should direct the evaluation along other lines in attempting to define another diagnosis. Frank synovitis of the hands or feet should suggest rheumatoid arthritis or another inflammatory arthropathy. Thus, further laboratory and imaging may be needed to differentiate the two. (See the chapter "Rheumatoid Arthritis").

Diagnosis

The diagnosis of PMR is based primarily on clinical features. Elevated acute phase reactants provide secondary support for the diagnosis. The erythrocyte sedimentation rate (ESR) is greater than 40 mm/hr in 90% of cases. Other laboratory findings include an elevated C-reactive protein (CRP), normocytic normochromic anemia, thrombocytosis, and elevated alkaline phosphatase. Elevation of muscle enzymes, such as creatine kinase and aldolase, is not a feature of PMR and should prompt consideration of an alternative diagnosis.

In 1979, Bird and colleagues proposed diagnostic criteria for PMR (Table 1). Patients who fulfilled any three criteria or had one criterion along with vasculitis on a temporal artery biopsy were considered to have PMR.[13] In 1984, Healy proposed that patients older than 50 years, seronegative for rheumatoid factor, and any three clinical features (neck, shoulder, or pelvic girdle pain, morning stiffness, elevated ESR, or rapid response to low-dose steroids) have PMR.[14] Although these criteria should serve as guidelines for the diagnosis of PMR, most authorities agree that no single feature is necessary to diagnose it in all cases. The features noted in these criteria are common enough that if patients present without these symptoms or have a suboptimal response to corticosteroids, the diagnosis should be reconsidered. Conditions that can mimic PMR include malignancies, chronic infections, drug reactions, and other rheumatic conditions such as seronegative rheumatoid arthritis or polymyositis.[6]

Table 1 Often-Cited Diagnostic Criteria for Polymyalgia Rheumatica

Authors and Year Proposed	Proposed Criteria	Requirement for Making Diagnosis
Bird et al. (1979)	Age ≥65 yr Bilateral shoulder pain and stiffness Acute or subacute onset (<2 wk) ESR >40 mm/hr Depression and/or weight loss Bilateral tenderness in upper arm muscles Morning stiffness >1 hr	Any three of these criteria, or any one plus positive temporal artery biopsy
Jones and Hazelman (1981)	ESR >30 mm/hr or CRP >6 mg/L Shoulder and pelvic girdle pain Exclusion of rheumatoid arthritis or other inflammatory arthropathy, myopathy, malignancy Morning stiffness >1 hr Rapid response to corticosteroids	All criteria must be met
Chuang et al. (1982)	Age ≥50 ESR >40 mm/hr >1 mo bilateral aching and stiffness of at least two of the following areas: Neck or torso, shoulders or proximal arms, hips or proximal thighs Exclusion of other causes	All criteria must be met
Healey (1984)	>1 mo of neck, shoulder, or pelvic girdle pain (any two areas) Morning stiffness >1 hr Elevated ESR (≤40 mm/hr) Exclusion of other diagnoses Rapid response to daily, low-dose steroid therapy (e.g., prednisolone ≤20 mg)	All criteria must be met

CRP, C-reactive protein; ESR, erythrocyte sedimentation rate.

Treatment

The first successful use of corticosteroids in patients with PMR was reported by Kersley in 1951.[5] Since that time, it has remained the cornerstone of therapy for PMR. Prednisone or prednisolone is the most commonly used corticosteroids. Starting doses range from 15 to 20 mg per day. A dramatic response to therapy with near-total relief of symptoms should occur within 1 to 5 days. Lack of a dramatic response to corticosteroids should prompt physicians to reconsider the diagnosis. A gradual decline of the acute phase reactants should be expected but should never be the sole gauge of therapy. After an adequate response to corticosteroids has been achieved, the initial dose should be maintained for 1 month before beginning a slow taper to the lowest effective dose. One to 2 years of treatment with corticosteroids should be expected, and a few patients require low-dose prednisone for several years.[15]

Disease flares during the corticosteroid taper are common and often require temporary increases in therapy. Disease flares can occur in the presence of normal acute-phase reactants. Increases in acute phase reactants mandate an evaluation to be sure that comorbid conditions are not responsible for such changes. Isolated increases in acute-phase reactants should lead to more careful monitoring and not to reflexive increases in corticosteroids doses.[16]

Corticosteroids are the cornerstone of therapy, but they are not without side effects. Most patients have at least one relapse as corticosteroids are tapered, and adverse events occur in almost every patient. The role of immunosuppressive agents other than corticosteroids in PMR is controversial. Methotrexate has been studied in two randomized, double-blind, controlled trials. Van der Veen and colleagues reported that patients randomized to take oral methotrexate (10 mg/week) had the same number of relapses and received the same total cumulative prednisone dose compared with patients who received placebo.[17] Caporali and colleagues reported that patients randomized to oral methotrexate (10 mg/week) for 48 weeks had fewer relapses and required lower cumulative prednisone doses than patients who took placebo.[18] However, further review of the patients who received methotrexate revealed that they had the same number of relapses while they were taking prednisone as did patients who received placebo. Furthermore, the number of corticosteroid-related adverse events was equal in both treatment groups and the total cumulative prednisone dose reduction achieved by taking methotrexate in place of placebo equaled only about 1 mg/day.[19]

TNF-α, a cytokine produced by macrophages and T-lymphocytes, appears to play a significant role in the inflammatory process of PMR and GCA. In one pilot study, 3 mg/kg of intravenous infliximab was administered as adjunctive therapy to patients on corticosteroids. This therapy allowed 12 months of remission in three out of four patients treated with the drug.[20] These results were not seen in a recent double-blind, randomized, placebo-controlled study by the same author. Patients who received 3 mg/kg of infliximab at the same dosing intervals as used for rheumatoid arthritis over 22 weeks experienced the same number of weeks in remission as those who received placebo. No difference was seen in the duration of corticosteroid therapy or in the total number of patients who were able to discontinue corticosteroids between the groups.[21]

Outcomes

Adequate treatment with corticosteroids allows most patients to remain symptom free. Patients who have PMR need continued follow-up to monitor for drug-related toxicities and for possible progression to GCA. The development of a new headache or visual changes should prompt immediate medical evaluation and institution of higher doses of corticosteroids. Bilateral upper- and lower-extremity blood pressures should be obtained periodically. Differences between contralateral extremity pressures of 10 mm Hg or more should be considered abnormal. Bruits over carotid, subclavian, or femoral arteries may be due to either atheromatous disease or GCA and require further evaluation by vascular imaging.

GIANT CELL ARTERITIS

Definition

GCA is a vasculitis characterized by granulomatous inflammation of medium-sized and large arteries. Inflammation is seen more commonly in the extracranial branches of the carotid arteries and other primary branch vessels of the aortic arch. Less often, internal branches of the carotid are affected, most notably the ophthalmic and posterior ciliary arteries; stenosis or occlusion of these arteries can cause loss of vision. At least one out of five patients develop large-vessel inflammation that can lead to branch vessel (e.g., most often subclavian) stenosis and less often aneurysmal dilation of the aorta (especially aortic root) or branch vessels.[22] GCA is the most common vasculitis in whites older than 50 years. It has a predilection for people of northern European heritage. Women are affected at least twice as often as men.[9]

Prevalence

In the United States, GCA affects about 18 of 100,000 people older than 50 years. The epidemiologic characteristics of GCA are similar to those of PMR. The incidence of GCA is much higher in the northern latitudes, with a mean age at onset of 74 years. GCA and PMR might represent opposite ends of a disease spectrum, with many patients presenting features of both diseases. Approximately 40% of GCA patients have concurrent features of PMR at some point during their disease course.[23]

Pathophysiology

The cause of GCA is unknown, but vessel inflammation is cell mediated and not autoantibody induced. Dendritic cells, macrophages, and Th1-lymphocytes enter the vessel wall via the vasa vasorum and spread through the arterial adventitia.[24] A small fraction of activated T lymphocytes in the artery wall become clonally expanded. The cause for the clonal expansion is unknown but may be from a yet-unidentified neoantigen present in the arterial wall.[25] A broad range of proinflammatory cytokines, growth factors, and metalloproteinases are associated with inflammatory cell migration throughout the arterial media and intima. This panarterial inflammation leads to arterial damage, intimal proliferation, and ultimately luminal narrowing (Fig. 1). The luminal narrowing is responsible for ischemic events (loss of vision, stroke, and claudication). Understanding how these cytokines participate in inflammation will lead to better-targeted therapies in both GCA and PMR.[26]

Signs and Symptoms

Headache is the most common symptom in GCA and occurs in 63% to 87% of patients. Systemic symptoms including fever, weight loss, and myalgias occur in 50% of patients.[27] Other symptoms include scalp pain, jaw pain while chewing, and arm or leg claudication. Vision loss, the most dreaded complication of GCA, occurs in more than 30% of patients.[28] Anterior ischemic optic neuropathy is the most common cause of blindness. Twenty-seven percent of patients develop either an aortic aneurysm or large artery stenosis at some point during their disease course. Six percent of patients who develop an aortic aneurysm present with symptoms consistent with a dissection of the aneurysm.[22] Extremity claudication occurs when aortic branch vessels, such as the subclavian artery, become critically narrow. Stroke and vision loss can occur without any preceding symptoms; however, patients can present with insidious nonspecific symptoms before the diagnosis of GCA is made. Forty percent of patients present with symptoms not considered classic for GCA. These symptoms can include cough, throat pain, or tongue pain.

A thorough physical examination may reveal a prominent, tender temporal artery. Evaluation of the artery may reveal a decreased pulse and a nodular appearance. Asymmetrical extremity blood pressures or pulses, bruits over subclavian or carotid arteries, or a murmur of aortic insufficiency suggests aortic or primary aortic branch involvement.

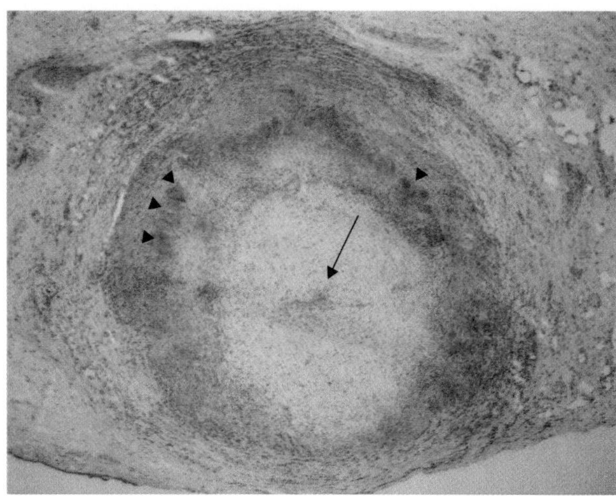

Figure 1 Cross-section of a temporal artery from a patient with GCA (stained with hematoxylin/eosin). Inflammatory cells are shown infiltrating the entire arterial wall. The *short arrows* point to areas of granulomatous inflammation with multinucleated giant cells located at the intima-medial junction of the artery. The *long arrow* shows complete arterial luminal occlusion caused by intimal hyperplasia. GCA, giant cell arteritis. *(Courtesy of Jose Hernandez-Rodriguez MD.)*

Diagnosis

Similar to PMR, no serologic test is diagnostic for GCA. Diagnosis is based on clinical symptoms in the presence of abnormal acute-phase reactants. More than 90% of patients have an elevated ESR. An elevated CRP, alkaline phosphatase, and platelets are not uncommon. Temporal artery biopsy is considered the standard diagnostic test for GCA. The sensitivity of biopsy, in series from medical practitioners, in detecting GCA is about 50%.[29] The yield of biopsy is a function of pretest probability, which might explain why some ophthalmology and other series, in which visual abnormalities were common, have yields as high as 80%.[30] Biopsy of the contralateral temporal artery adds very little to the sensitivity of the test.[31]

Imaging of the vessel lumen with arteriography or magnetic resonance arteriography (MRA) may reveal aortic or arterial branches with stenoses or aneurysms (Fig. 2). The subclavian arteries, carotid arteries, and ascending aorta are the most commonly affected areas. Other arterial branches, such as the mesenteric and renal arteries, can also be affected. Vascular PET imaging with ^{18}F-fluorodeoxyglucose may reveal vessel uptake in GCA as well as PMR. It is a more sensitive marker for disease than biopsy, but its diagnostic specificity is still in the process of being defined.[32]

Treatment

Corticosteroids are the drug of choice for the treatment of GCA. They quickly reduce symptoms and decrease risk of visual complications from 60% to 14%.[33] Therapy with corticosteroids should start when GCA is first suspected. Waiting to start corticosteroids until after a temporal artery biopsy could result in irreversible loss of vision.

The optimal initial dose of prednisone is unclear, but most authorities agree that the initial dose should be between 40 and 60 mg/day. Doses of at least 60 mg are preferred when presenting features include ophthalmic or neurologic complications. Some

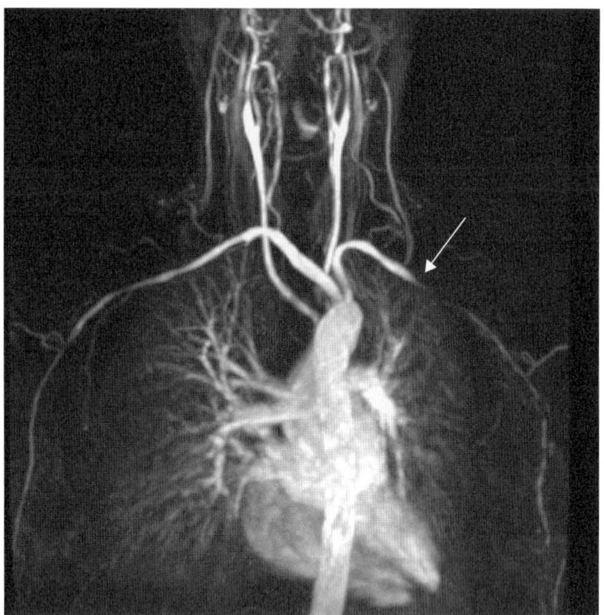

Figure 2 MRA of the aorta and its primary branches in a patient with GCA. The *arrow* shows a left subclavian artery stenosis. GCA, giant cell arteritis; MRA, magnetic resonance arteriography. *(Courtesy of Jose Hernandez-Rodriguez MD.)*

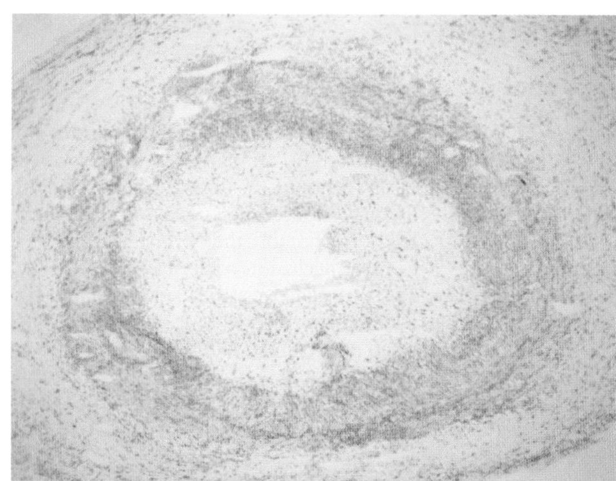

Figure 3 Cross-section of a temporal artery in a patient with giant cell arteritis (GCA). Inflammatory cells containing tumor necrosis factor α are noted to stain brown by immunohistochemistry. *(Courtesy of Jose Hernandez-Rodriguez MD.)*

authorities advocate intravenous methylprednisolone at doses of 1000 mg a day for 3 to 5 days in patients presenting with blindness.[33-35] The initial oral dose of corticosteroids should continue for 1 month before taper is considered. Many tapering schedules exist but few have been studied in clinical trials. One general rule is to taper by 10% to 20% every 2 weeks.[9] Treatment duration is different for each patient. Long-term therapy is required in most patients. It is not unusual for corticosteroid therapy to extend beyond 4 years.[36-38]

The efficacy of methotrexate in Wegener's granulomatosis and Takayasu's arteritis has led to its use in three randomized, double-blind, placebo-controlled trials for GCA. Jover and colleagues reported that patients randomized to methotrexate doses of 10 mg/week had fewer relapses and lower cumulative steroid doses compared with those who received placebo. However, a difference in relapse rates was only noted after 1 year of disease. There was no advantage to methotrexate in the first year. In addition, patients who received methotrexate had the same number of steroid-related side effects as those who received placebo.[39] Hoffman and colleagues conducted the only multicenter, randomized, double-blind, placebo-controlled trial of methotrexate at doses of 15 mg each week. Their conclusions did not support the use of methotrexate as adjunctive therapy with corticosteroids. Patients who were randomized to receive methotrexate did not have reduced disease activity, cumulative corticosteroid doses, or corticosteroid-related toxicities.[40] Spiera and colleagues reported similar results.[41] The use of adjunctive methotrexate as a steroid-sparing agent in patients with GCA remains a controversial issue.

The finding of abundant TNF-α in GCA arteries (Fig. 3) has led investigators to study TNF-α inhibition as a potential disease modulator in GCA. Hoffman and colleagues reported results of a multicenter, randomized, double-blind, placebo-controlled trial of intravenous infliximab as adjunctive therapy to corticosteroids in patients with newly diagnosed GCA.[42] The study was stopped at 22 weeks when infliximab was shown to not improve durability of remission or reduce cumulative steroid doses. The results of this study suggest that although TNF is found in abundance in affected vessels, it might not play a critical role in the pathogenesis of GCA. Other mediators might play more important roles in disease propagation.

Aspirin (ASA) is known to reduce the risks of ischemic stroke and myocardial infarction.[43,44] No prospective trial has ever been done to see if antiplatelet therapy reduces the risk of cranial ischemic complications in patients with GCA. A recent review of 175 GCA patients by Nesher and colleagues observed that patients who took low-dose ASA (100 mg/day) were five times less likely to present with visual complications or stroke.[45] A second report by Lee and colleagues showed similar results in patients on antiplatelet or anticoagulant therapy.[46] Sixteen percent of GCA patients taking ASA, warfarin, or clopidogrel developed an ischemic event compared with 48% of patients not on this therapy ($P < 0.0005$). Bleeding complications were not increased in the patients on antiplatelet or anticoagulant therapy. The authors concluded that adjunctive low-dose ASA should be considered in all patients with GCA who have no contraindications for its use.

Outcomes

Some studies have found that the overall mortality in patients with GCA is similar to that of age- and gender-matched controls. Other studies have noted an increase in mortality, particularly from cardiovascular events. There is agreement that patients with GCA are at higher risk of death from the complications of aortic aneurysms. Thoracic aneurysms are 17 times more likely to occur in GCA patients and can occur at any time during the disease course. Fifty percent of patients with aortic aneurysms experience dissection or rupture of their aneurysm.[22,47-49] Cost-benefit data are not available. Because the risks of aortic catastrophes are well documented, we recommend careful auscultation for aortic valve murmurs or bruits, which should be followed by MRA or CT angiography to determine the nature and seriousness of the aortic lesion. Size of the lesion, hemodynamic consequences, and change over time per sequential imaging determine the need for surgical interventions.

Nearly every patient treated with long-term corticosteroids develops complications related to therapy. Sixty percent develop severe adverse events such as corticosteroid-induced diabetes, avascular necrosis, glaucoma, or vertebral fractures.[50] Corticosteroid-induced osteoporosis is a well-known complication of long-term steroid use. Medications such as calcium, vitamin D, and anti-resorptive agents should be considered in every patient who will receive corticosteroids for more than 3 months. Screening for osteoporosis with bone densitometry at the induction of corticosteroid therapy (and at regular intervals) is as important an intervention as prescribing steroids to prevent blindness.

Summary

- Clinicians should inquire about headache, jaw pain, and vision loss in all PMR patients at every clinic visit because 10% will develop GCA at some point during their disease course.
- Lack of a response to corticosteroids or the inability to taper below 20 mg/day should raise the possibility of a paraneoplastic process in patients with GCA.
- Isolated increases in acute phase reactants in GCA and PMR should never lead to reflexive increases in corticosteroids doses but lead to more careful monitoring for a disease flare.
- Aortic aneurysms occur in about one of five patients with GCA and should be periodically screened for in every patient.
- Corticosteroids remain the standard of care for the treatment of GCA and PMR.

Suggested Readings

Aiello PD, Trautmann JC, McPhee TJ, et al: Visual prognosis in giant cell arteritis. Ophthalmology 1993;100:550-555.

Doran MF, Crowson CS, O'Fallon WM, et al: Trends in the incidence of polymyalgia rheumatica over a 30 year period in Olmsted County, Minnesota, USA. J Rheumatol 2002;29:1694-1697.

Evans JM, O'Fallon WM, Hunder GG: Increased incidence of aortic aneurysm and dissection in giant cell (temporal) arteritis. A population-based study. Ann Intern Med 1995;122:502-507.

Gonzalez-Gay MA, Garcia-Porrua C, Salvarani C, et al: The spectrum of conditions mimicking polymyalgia rheumatica in northwestern Spain. J Rheumatol 2000;27:2179-2184.

Hoffman GS, Cid MC, Hellmann DB, et al: A multicenter, randomized, double-blind, placebo-controlled trial of adjuvant methotrexate treatment for giant cell arteritis. Arthritis Rheum 2002;46:1309-1318.

Hunder GG: The early history of giant cell arteritis and polymyalgia rheumatica: First descriptions to 1970. Mayo Clin Proc 2006;81:1071-1083.

Nesher G, Berkun Y, Mates M, et al: Risk factors for cranial ischemic complications in giant cell arteritis. Medicine (Baltimore) 2004;83:114-122.

Nuenninghoff DM, Hunder GG, Christianson TJ, et al: Mortality of large-artery complication (aortic aneurysm, aortic dissection, and/or large-artery stenosis) in patients with giant cell arteritis: A population-based study over 50 years. Arthritis Rheum 2003;48:3532-3537.

Weyand CM, Goronzy JJ: Giant-cell arteritis and polymyalgia rheumatica. Ann Intern Med 2003;139:505-515.

Wilke WS, Hoffman GS: Treatment of corticosteroid-resistant giant cell arteritis. Rheum Dis Clin North Am 1995;21:59-71.

References

For a complete list of references, log onto www.expertconsult.com.

Rheumatoid Arthritis

William S. Wilke

DEFINITION

Rheumatoid arthritis (RA) is the most common form of chronic inflammatory arthritis. Although most readily recognized by its articular manifestations, RA can affect any organ system. The presentation and disease course are distinct for any individual patient, making diagnosis and management a thoughtful, complex, and dynamic process. The diagnostic criteria for RA (Box 1)[1] may be used to classify disease in patients in the appropriate clinical setting, but in early disease the criteria may be less helpful in establishing the diagnosis. Whether disease expression is confined to mild articular manifestations or manifests as severe, multisystem disease, our current understanding demands that patients receive early and aggressive therapy. Achieving prompt control of local and systemic inflammatory processes minimizes damage of articular structures, preserves function, and reduces early mortality.

PREVALENCE

RA affects about 1% of the world's population[2] when defined by either the presence of serum rheumatoid factor (RF) or erosive changes on radiographs in a patient with a compatible clinical presentation. Its incidence is two to three times greater in women, and this disparity is most pronounced in patients younger than 50 years.[3] The incidence of RA continues to increase with age until about the seventh decade of life.[4]

PATHOPHYSIOLOGY

The cause of RA is unknown. The combination of genetic susceptibility with an as-yet-unidentified inciting event (or events) leads to disease expression. The concordance of RA in identical twins is reported as 15% to 30%, suggesting that nongenetic factors have a predominant impact on disease expression.[2,5] However, the association of HLA-DR with RA is well established. There is an increased relative risk of RA of about 4 to 5 in patients with this allele.[6] Whether shared alleles contribute to disease severity is controversial. More data are needed to establish the precise role of genetic factors.

Infectious agents have long been suspected as potential triggers of RA. Although investigations have failed to identify any one organism in synovial tissue or fluid, polymerase chain reaction techniques have detected bacterial nucleotide sequences in synovial tissues in RA patients. Viral pathogens are also under study, with the Epstein-Barr virus (EBV) targeted for several reasons. RA patients have been found to have higher levels of virus-infected B cells and higher levels of EBV antibody titers than the general population. In addition, the ability of the virus to activate B cells to produce RF has generated interest in this virus as a potential trigger.[7] Other viruses of interest include parvovirus B19 and the retroviruses, but conclusive data definitely identifying any viral pathogen as a causative agent are lacking. In fact, bacterial and viral antigenic particles may be carried to sites of inflammation by gut-associated macrophages.[8]

Rheumatoid factor, an immunoglobulin (Ig)M antiglobulin against the Fc portion of human IgG, is detected in about 70% of patients with RA. Evidence suggests its participation in disease pathogenesis. The presence of RF in RA is associated with extra-articular manifestations of disease, and its absence is generally associated with milder disease. Its proposed mechanisms include enhanced presentation of immune-complexed antigens, cross-linkage and stabilization of low-avidity IgG antibodies, and cryoprecipitation.[4] RF is not specific for RA, despite its name, and it may be found in other conditions including bacterial infection, lymphoproliferative disorders, liver disease, and other autoimmune disorders.

Although inciting factors have yet to be identified, the presence and activity of a number of proinflammatory chemokines and cytokines have established roles in disease pathogenesis. The activation and infiltration of T cells and macrophages in the synovium result in production of interleukin-1, -2, -6, -8, -10, -17; tumor necrosis factor-α (TNF-α); platelet-derived growth factor; insulin-like growth factor; and transforming growth factor β.[9] These effector molecules are implicated in synovial tissue inflammation and proliferation, cartilage and bone destruction, and systemic effects. B cells also infiltrate the synovium and differentiate into plasma cells, producing polyclonal immunoglobulin and RF. In addition, synovial fibroblasts are activated, releasing collagenases and activating metalloproteinase gene expression, which leads to destruction of matrix tissues. The net result of these activities is pannus formation with articular cartilage invasion, periarticular erosions and osteoporosis, and joint swelling with destruction of periarticular structures. Cigarette smoking increases the risk of developing RA and negatively influences disease course.[10,11]

CLINICAL MANIFESTATIONS

Generally, signs and symptoms of RA begin insidiously and are additive over weeks to months. They commonly include fatigue, malaise, generalized stiffness, and generalized arthralgias or myalgias. Synovitis usually develops gradually, often involving the hands, wrists, knees, or feet, often symmetrically. However, in 10% to 15% of patients, the onset of disease is explosive, with polyarthritis, fever, lymphadenopathy, and splenomegaly developing over days to weeks.[2,8] It is imperative in patients with the latter manifestation to consider other common causes of acute polyarthritis, such as parvovirus infection.

Evidence of articular disease in RA can appear as swelling, tenderness, warmth, and painful motion. The outward appearance of the joints does not necessarily correlate with the amount of active synovitis or pain expressed by the patient. Patients often complain of morning stiffness, a characteristic of inflammatory arthritis. Stiffness, known as *gelling,* can also manifest after brief periods of inactivity. The joints most often involved in RA include the proximal interphalangeal (PIP) and metacarpophalangeal (MCP) joints, wrists, elbows, shoulders, knees, ankles, and subtalar and metatarsophalangeal (MTP) joints. The cervical spine is the only characteristic axial location, and atlantoaxial subluxation is a known complication. Inadequately treated articular inflammation progresses to weakening or destruction of supportive structures, including the associated joint ligaments, tendons, cartilage, and bone. In addition, the pain associated with ongoing synovitis often leads to decreased motion at the affected joints. This, in addition to the ongoing pathologic tissue changes, results in loss of range of motion or, at its most extreme, soft-tissue contractures, fibrosis, and bony ankylosis.

One of the most common extra-articular manifestations of RA is the formation of rheumatoid nodules. This is usually associated with the presence of RF, and it occurs most often in patients with high titers of RF. Rheumatoid nodules develop in 20% to 35% of patients, most often on extensor surfaces and often in response to repetitive trauma.[2] However, they can develop at any location and have rarely been identified within the pleura or meninges. Rheumatoid nodules are identified definitively by biopsy, which reveals an outer zone of

Box 1 Criteria for the Classification of Rheumatoid Arthritis

For classification purposes, a patient has rheumatoid arthritis if he or she has satisfied at least four of these seven criteria. Criteria 1 through 4 must have been present for at least 6 weeks. Patients with two clinical diagnoses are not excluded. Designation as classic, definite, or probable rheumatoid arthritis is not to be made.

1. Morning stiffness
   Morning stiffness in and around the joints
   Lasting at least 1 hour before maximal improvement
2. Arthritis of three or more joint areas
   At least three joint areas simultaneously have had soft tissue swelling or fluid (not bony overgrowth alone) observed by a physician
   The 14 possible areas are right or left PIP, MCP, wrist, elbow, knee, ankle, and MTP joints.
3. Arthritis of hand joints
   At least one area swollen (as defined in 2) in a wrist or in an MCP or PIP joint
4. Symmetrical arthritis
   Simultaneous involvement of the same joint areas (as defined in 2) on both sides of the body
   Bilateral involvement of PIPs, MCPs, or MTPs is acceptable without absolute symmetry
5. Rheumatoid nodules
   Subcutaneous nodules over bony prominences, or extensor surfaces, or in juxta-articular regions, observed by a physician
6. Serum rheumatoid factor
   Demonstration of abnormal amounts of serum rheumatoid factor by any method for which the result has been positive in <5% of normal control subjects
7. Radiographic changes
   Radiographic changes typical of rheumatoid arthritis on posteroanterior hand and wrist radiographs, which must include erosions or unequivocal bony decalcification localized in, or most marked adjacent to, the involved joints
   Osteoarthritis changes alone do not qualify

MCP, metacarpophalangeal; MTP, metatarsophalangeal; PIP, proximal interphalangeal.

Adapted with permission from Kirkham BW, Lassere MN, Edmonds JP, et al: Synovial membrane cytokine expression is predictive of joint damage progression in rheumatoid arthritis: a two-year prospective study (the DAMAGE study cohort). Arthritis Rheum 2006;54:1122-1131.

granulation tissue, a mid-zone of palisading macrophages, and a central zone of necrotic material.[9]

Vasculitis can also occur as an extra-articular manifestation of RA. This most often manifests as leukocytoclastic vasculitis, which may be an isolated skin finding. With involvement of medium-sized vessels, which is less common, any organ system may be involved, and the disorder may be organ or life threatening. Patients should be carefully assessed for other possible causes (such as infection) before vasculitis is attributed solely to RA. Rheumatoid vasculitis has been associated with a variety of predisposing factors including male sex, high RF titers, erosive joint disease, other extra-articular disease, and glucocorticoid (GC) therapy.[2]

Ocular manifestations of RA are diverse and range from mild, asymptomatic findings to aggressive, vision-threatening disease. RA is often associated with secondary Sjögren's syndrome (keratoconjunctivitis sicca), which can manifest with eye dryness, foreign-body sensation in the eye, or photophobia. Both scleritis and episcleritis are associated with RA. Scleritis may be associated with severe corneal inflammation, leading to a corneal melt, or with scleromalacia perforans. Chronic inflammation, resulting in perturbation of the intraocular anatomy, can lead to glaucoma. Corticosteroid therapy can be an important factor in cataract formation.

The most common manifestation of pulmonary disease in RA is interstitial lung disease (ILD). The manifestation of RA-associated ILD often parallels that of idiopathic pulmonary fibrosis, often with similar imaging and histopathologic findings. Patients with severe RA or those who smoke are more likely to develop RA-associated ILD. Bronchiolitis obliterans organizing pneumonia has also been described in association with RA. Patients can present with cough, fever, dyspnea, and fatigue. This is a nonspecific entity that could also result from an unrelated process, such as infection. Biopsy is required to exclude other underlying causes. Nodular lung disease in RA can occur in both the pleura and lung parenchyma, with solitary or multiple lesions that can coalesce or cavitate. Diagnosis of RA-associated nodular lung disease requires biopsy. The histopathologic appearance of the lesion is that of a rheumatoid nodule. Evidence of pleural inflammation in RA patients is often noted at autopsy, but it is usually subclinical in life.[12] Effusions are often exudative and characteristically have a low glucose concentration. It is important to remember that effusions associated with infectious processes often share these characteristics, mandating cultures to exclude infection.

Rheumatoid pericarditis, as with rheumatoid pleuritis, is often diagnosed at autopsy. Pericardial disease is seen most often in RF-positive patients and is more common in patients with nodular disease.[13] Although pericardial tamponade and constrictive pericarditis are very rare, this can result in hemodynamic compromise that requires intervention. Myocarditis can occur in RA, either in the form of nodular granulomatous disease or as diffuse interstitial inflammation. Nodular disease in the conduction system can cause atrioventricular block. Granulomatous disease of the heart valves can lead to valvular insufficiency. Coronary arteritis in RA is rare and can result in myocardial infarction, but most events from ischemic coronary disease in RA patients are caused by atherosclerosis. Patients with RA have an increased atherosclerotic burden (as demonstrated by increased carotid intima-medial thickness and plaque scores) and increased risk of cardiovascular events compared with age- and sex-matched controls.[14,15] Although the exact mechanisms of increased atherogenesis in RA are not understood, RA activity has been associated with increased arterial stiffness and endothelial dysfunction that correlate with cardiovascular risk.[16,17]

Renal disease associated with RA is rare. Manifestations include renal vasculitis, glomerulonephritis and, in patients with sustained inflammation, secondary renal amyloidosis.[13] The most common hematologic manifestation of RA is a mild normocytic hypochromic anemia, which occurs in most patients, representing the anemia of chronic disease. Felty's syndrome is characterized by neutropenia, often with associated anemia and thrombocytosis, with splenomegaly and occasionally with leg ulcers. This closely resembles the large granular lymphocyte (LGL) syndrome in RA. Although it is likely that these disorders are related and represent different points on a spectrum of hematologic disease in RA, it is important to differentiate the two, because LGL may be associated with transformation to leukemia. In addition, patients with RA have a risk of lymphoma (both Hodgkin's and non-Hodgkin's) and leukemia two to three times greater than that of the general population.[13]

DIAGNOSIS

There is no unique test or feature that is pathognomonic for RA. Rather, the diagnosis is made by recognizing a pattern of signs and symptoms. The classification criteria listed in Box 1 are helpful in classifying patients for the purpose of clinical research studies, but they might not clearly establish the diagnosis in any individual patient.

A history consistent with the diagnosis of RA includes prolonged morning stiffness that may be improved by activity, polyarthralgias or polyarthritis (or both), joint gelling, and fatigue. Examination findings that suggest RA include symmetrical polyarthritis and rheumatoid nodules. Serologic and imaging studies may be helpful in excluding mimics of RA and confirming the diagnosis when pretest probability is high. Arthrocentesis is not diagnostic but is useful in excluding infection. Radiographic changes include periarticular osteopenia, joint space loss, and erosions. Although most serologic studies are not sensitive or specific for RA in general, the use of antibodies to cyclic citrullinated peptides (anti-CCP antibodies) has been demonstrated[18] to be more than 90% specific for RA. In patients with an atypical presentation or when another diagnosis is equally likely (e.g., hepatitis C), anti-CCP antibodies may be useful in confirming a diagnosis of RA.

Differential Diagnosis

The list of RA mimics is extensive. RA can resemble any disorder causing acute or chronic polyarthritis. A thorough history and examination are often helpful in the differential diagnosis in the individual patient.

Infectious arthropathies are an important consideration in the setting of fever and polyarthritis. Infections often result in a transiently positive RF, so this is not helpful in differentiation. If bacterial arthritis is suspected, joint aspiration and synovial fluid cultures and blood cultures are often helpful in establishing the diagnosis. One exception is gonococcal arthritis, in which synovial cultures are often negative. Lyme disease is also associated with negative synovial fluid cultures, and it should be considered when a patient has been in an endemic region where tick exposure was likely. Viral infections, both acute and chronic, can result in a polyarthritis that is clinically indistinguishable from RA. Acute viral infections, such as parvovirus B19 infection, often distinguish themselves by a history of exposure, an accompanying rash, and their self-limited course. Even when disease is well established, it is essential to exclude chronic hepatitis infection or human immunodeficiency virus, especially when considering instituting immunosuppressive therapy.

Other connective-tissue diseases can manifest similarly to RA. Patients with systemic lupus erythematosus (SLE) can have a similar distribution of joint involvement but rarely have erosive disease. Jaccoud's arthropathy often leads to deformities that are similar in appearance to those in RA, but these changes result not from joint destruction but from tendon and ligament laxity. These deformities, unlike those in RA, are readily reducible on examination. In most cases, the other clinical manifestations of SLE and serologic findings are helpful in establishing the diagnosis. Psoriatic arthritis, when present without rash, may be difficult to distinguish from RA. Involvement of the sacroiliac joints or the distal interphalangeal joints of the hands can provide a clue to diagnosis. Fortunately, their treatment regimens have significant overlap, so even when differentiation is not possible, instituting effective and appropriate treatment is not hampered.

The other seronegative spondyloarthropathies (reactive arthritis, ankylosing spondylitis, inflammatory bowel disease–associated arthropathy) can also closely resemble RA. Asymmetrical joint involvement, the absence of small-joint disease, sausage-like appearance of digits, and involvement of the lumbosacral spine all favor the seronegative arthropathies. Polymyositis and dermatomyositis can manifest with arthralgias, arthritis, and joint stiffness, similar to RA. Muscle weakness and antibodies associated with these disorders most often readily distinguish these disorders from RA.

Polyarticular crystal arthropathies can also mimic RA. Radiographs might also show joint erosions, but in calcium pyrophosphate dihydrate deposition disease, chondrocalcinosis is often apparent. Synovial fluid analysis is diagnostic of crystal arthropathy.

Polymyalgia rheumatica and giant cell arteritis can manifest with symmetrical polyarthritis. In these patients, a detailed history can help identify the characteristics of these disorders (e.g., a new, unrelenting headache, predominant shoulder and hip girdle involvement). In cases where history does not make the distinction, careful observation of the evolution of the disease over time is key, because the clinical courses and potential serious complications associated with these disorders are quite different.

Systemic vasculitis can manifest with polyarthritis, and, in the case of Wegener's granulomatosis, it can also be RF positive. A thorough history and examination with directed serologic and imaging evaluation aid in differentiating these disorders.

Fibromyalgia (FMS) can manifest with diffuse symmetrical arthralgias and stiffness at rest, but the absence of synovitis, the lack of pain on motion, and normal laboratory and imaging studies confirm the diagnosis of FMS. It is important to remember that FMS is present in 10% to 15% of patients with rheumatic diseases such as SLE and RA; hence, its diagnosis does not exclude other concomitant disease.[19,20]

Sarcoidosis can manifest with polysynovitis and is not infrequently RF-positive, but it has other distinguishing characteristics that often help to differentiate it from RA. In Löfgren's syndrome, the acute onset of polyarthritis is accompanied by erythema nodosum and hilar adenopathy. Chronic sarcoid arthropathy may clinically closely mimic RA, and on radiographs it can show bony destruction similar to that in RA. Tissue biopsy may be necessary in these instances if no other manifestations of sarcoidosis are present to establish the diagnosis.

Osteoarthritis is best differentiated from RA by a careful history and examination. The absence of systemic inflammatory signs and symptoms, onset in later life, and the pattern of joint involvement are often enough to distinguish the two disorders. Erosive osteoarthritis can have an inflammatory appearance on examination, but it tends to involve the PIP joints primarily, is not associated with proliferative synovitis, is not RF positive, and has a distinct radiographic appearance.

Malignant diseases are uncommon RA mimics. Local bone or joint involvement from cancer usually manifests as monoarticular arthritis. However, lymphoproliferative or myeloproliferative disorders can occur with polyarthralgias or polyarthritis. In addition, paraneoplastic syndromes can manifest with polyarticular symptoms designated as *hypertrophic osteoarthropathy.* Digital clubbing, bone pain on palpation or percussion, and periosteal reaction on radiography help to establish this diagnosis.

Imaging

Characteristic radiographic findings of RA include periarticular osteopenia, joint space loss, and marginal joint erosions. These changes are often not seen in early disease; only 15% to 30% of patients have erosions visible on radiographs during the first year of the disease.[21] Because erosions most often appear first on the hands, wrists, or feet, these are the areas that should be initially imaged when the diagnosis is suspected.

Magnetic resonance imaging (MRI) is useful in detecting RA before radiographic changes can be detected. MRI is more sensitive in detecting erosions, and it is capable of identifying bone marrow edema and synovial hypertrophy.[22] Both of these findings predict the development of erosive disease.

Ultrasonography is used infrequently in establishing a diagnosis of RA, and it is more sensitive in detecting synovial and tendon inflammation than clinical examination alone.[23,24] Ultrasonography might also be useful in guided joint aspiration and injection.

Monitoring Disease Activity

It cannot be overemphasized that the timely institution of therapy in RA has a significant impact on preserving joint structure and function and has implications for the patient's long-term overall health and function. If control of disease is achieved early (e.g., within the first several months), the rate of radiographic progression and joint destruction is minimized. Although the best outcomes are obtained with early aggressive control of disease, it is never too late to intervene if ongoing inflammation is present.

Disease activity and response to therapy are best followed clinically by the use of scaled measurements that are assessed at each visit. A number of instruments have been validated for use in RA. The ACR preliminary definition of improvement in rheumatoid arthritis (ACR 20, 50, and 70, with the numbers referring to percentage of improvement) is commonly used in assessment for

Box 2 American College of Rheumatology Preliminary Definition of Improvement in Rheumatoid Arthritis (ACR 20)

Required
- ≥20% improvement in tender joint count
- ≥20% improvement in swollen joint count

In addition to >20% improvement in three of the following five categories:
- Patient pain assessment
- Patient global assessment
- Physician global assessment
- Patient self-assessed disability
- Acute-phase reactant (erythrocyte sedimentation rate or C-reactive protein)

Adapted from Felson DT, Anderson JJ, Boers M, et al: American College of Rheumatology. Preliminary definition of improvement in rheumatoid arthritis. Arthritis Rheum 1995;38:727-735.

clinical trials and includes serologic and physical assessments (Box 2).[25]

However, the dichotomous ACR criteria are less sensitive for overall changes than are continuous measures such as the Disease Activity Score or the Simple Disease Activity Index. For this reason, these continuous scales are recommended for monitoring disease activity and response to therapy. The Stanford Health Assessment Questionnaire is another often-used tool that provides much useful information regarding the ability of the patient to carry out the activities of daily living and is a practical means of tracking the efficacy of therapy. The common coexistence of depression in chronic disease and its impact on emotional and physical health should not be overlooked.

Failure to treat depression in patients with RA significantly affects their well-being no matter how well their disease is controlled. The Beck Depression Index is a useful questionnaire to screen for clinical depression in patients with RA and other chronic diseases.

TREATMENT

The mainstays of therapy in RA are the disease-modifying antirheumatic drugs (DMARDs). These medications prevent or reduce joint destruction, maintain or improve function, and, in some cases, improve other aspects of the patient's general health.

Glucocorticoids

Glucocorticoids (GCs) are used to suppress inflammation and preserve joint structure and thus may be considered DMARDs. They are often used at disease onset or with disease flares as a temporary aid in obtaining disease control. Because of their long-term side effects, it is desirable to obtain disease control without chronic use of GCs whenever possible and to use the lowest doses necessary. In a long-acting form, they are also useful for intra-articular injection when only one or two joints are active. GCs in high doses are an essential part of treating organ-threatening disease in RA, such as in rheumatoid vasculitis. They are also useful in maintaining disease control during pregnancy when most other DMARDs are contraindicated.

Methotrexate

Methotrexate (MTX) should be considered first-line therapy for the treatment of RA. MTX is a folic acid antagonist, but its precise mechanism of action in RA treatment is unknown. MTX acts within weeks to diminish disease activity. It has also been shown to decrease radiographic progression of disease.[26] MTX can be used in combination with other DMARDs to achieve and maintain disease remission.

Although initially the potential hepatotoxicity of MTX caused concern, long-term follow-up of patients on chronic MTX therapy has alleviated many of these worries. Serious irreversible liver damage is rare in patients who do not have hepatitis and who consume minimal amounts of alcohol and have regular laboratory monitoring. Generally, liver enzymes are measured after 1 month of therapy, and are repeated at 8- to 12-week intervals after a stable dose is established.

MTX can result in a hypersensitivity-type reaction, MTX-associated pneumonitis, that can manifest with nonspecific symptoms such as fever, fatigue, cough, or dyspnea. When this diagnosis is suggested, MTX should be discontinued immediately. This manifestation can be indistinguishable from infection, and appropriate investigations and treatment for both should be initiated immediately. Biopsy may be necessary to establish the diagnosis.

Because the half-life of MTX primarily depends on renal function, patients with chronic renal insufficiency should not be treated with this agent. To minimize alopecia, mouth ulcers, nausea, and hepatic toxicity, folic acid (1-2 mg/day) should be given to all MTX-treated patients.

Hydroxychloroquine, Sulfasalazine, and Leflunomide

Hydroxychloroquine and sulfasalazine are DMARDs that provide mild anti-inflammatory activity in most patients. They are used as single agents (only in patients with very mild, nonerosive disease) or in combination. They are both well tolerated and have few side effects. Their major application in RA is as a supplement to MTX or other DMARD therapy. Leflunomide, a pyrimidine synthesis inhibitor, is also used as add-on therapy with MTX or other agents. Leflunomide can cause liver enzyme elevation and requires regular liver enzyme monitoring.[27]

Two important combination strategies have been tested and reported. Triple therapy combining sulfasalazine, hydroxychloroquine, and MTX is more effective than monotherapy and not more toxic.[28] The BeSt trial demonstrated that initial treatment with MTX combined with an anti–tumor necrosis factor (anti-TNF) agent was the safest and most effective therapy when compared with three less-aggressive strategies.[29]

Anti–Tumor Necrosis Factor Agents

The anti-TNF agents are highly effective DMARDs. Etanercept, infliximab, and adalimumab are all in use as second-line therapy for RA. They are most often added to MTX or other ongoing therapy. A bonus effect of the anti-TNF agents in RA is their impact on vascular function. Endothelium-dependent vasodilation, a marker of endothelial function, is improved by anti-TNF therapy, suggesting a potential protective effect on vascular function.[30] Further studies are needed to determine the impact of anti-TNF agents on the accelerated atherogenesis associated with RA. Infliximab should be administered with MTX to prevent the development of neutralizing antibodies that can render infliximab less effective.

Before therapy with an anti-TNF agent is initiated, patients should be screened by skin test and chest radiograph for the presence of tuberculosis. TNF has an important role in the formation of granulomas; this was recognized when reactivation tuberculosis emerged as a complication of anti-TNF therapy.

The anti-TNF agents also have other significant immunosuppressive effects. Infections in patients being treated with these agents can progress more rapidly and follow a more fulminant course. Signs and symptoms of any significant infectious process (e.g., anything requiring antibiotic, antiviral, or antifungal therapy) mandate the temporary discontinuation of any of these agents until the infection is resolved.

The role of these agents in the development of hematologic malignancies is unclear. Although the development of lymphomas during therapy with these agents has been documented, as previously discussed, these occur de novo at higher rates in patients with RA.[13] No further malignancy evaluation outside of routine health screening is advised for patients on anti-TNF therapies. The development of a malignancy, however, is an indication to discontinue anti-TNF therapy.

The significance of the induction of antinuclear and other autoantibodies by anti-TNF agents is unclear because most patients with this phenomenon do not phenotypically express autoimmune syndromes associated with these antibodies.[31]

The relation of anti-TNF therapy to congestive heart failure is unclear. Studies of anti-TNF therapy for the treatment of heart failure were discontinued because of lack of efficacy, and a few studies have associated high doses of infliximab with exacerbation of congestive heart failure in patients with preexisting cardiovascular disease.[32,33] However, this finding is controversial. A study by Wolfe and Michaud[34] found that patients with RA, when compared with patients with OA, have an increased incidence of heart failure at baseline. However, patients with RA in this study who were treated with an anti-TNF agent had a decreased incidence of heart failure. The standard of care is avoidance of anti-TNF therapy in decompensated heart failure.

A rare but potentially devastating adverse effect of anti-TNF therapies is demyelinating disease. New-onset multiple sclerosis, optic neuritis, and transverse myelitis have been reported with anti-TNF therapy.[35-37]

Other DMARDs

Two new biologic agents have been approved for the treatment of RA. The first is abatacept, a fully humanized fusion protein that binds to CD80/86 on the lymphocyte, thereby preventing interaction with CD on the macrophage. This interaction prevents T cell activation. The second, rituximab, is a chimeric IgG1 monoclonal antibody, which depletes circulating B lymphocytes. Both are demonstrated to be safe and effective when combined with MTX and to provide a significant response in patients who had previously failed anti-TNF therapy.[38,39] They appear to be equally safe when compared with anti-TNF therapy with similar infusion reactions. Abatacept should not be given to patients with chronic obstructive pulmonary disease because of a small but significant increase of pulmonary infection encountered in early trials.

Several other agents are used as second- and third-line therapies in RA. There is evidence that minocycline, cyclosporine, mycophenolate mofetil, and azathioprine have some efficacy in patients with RA. Fewer data exist for their use than for the other DMARDs. Since the advent of anti-TNF agents, these agents are used less often.

Nonsteroidal Anti-inflammatory Drugs

Nonsteroidal anti-inflammatory drugs (NSAIDs) and analgesics should be used as symptomatic therapy only in combination with DMARD therapy in RA. These agents do not have any significant positive impact on disease progression or function. They should never be the primary or sole therapy in patients with RA. Therapy with these drugs can result in gastritis, peptic ulcer disease, hypertension, edema, or renal insufficiency. Selective cyclooxygenase-2 inhibitors, such as celecoxib and rofecoxib, confer a lower risk of gastrointestinal erosions and ulcerations, but they are otherwise as toxic as their predecessors. The concern with these newer agents, as for the older NSAIDs, is that there may be an increased risk of cardiovascular events for patients taking these medications. Indeed, one of these agents, rofecoxib (Vioxx), was withdrawn from the market because of evidence documenting such side effects. Whether these findings are specific to rofecoxib or represent a class effect remains to be determined. They should be used with extreme caution or not at all in people with renal or cardiovascular disease.

Preservation of bone integrity in RA is an important component of therapy. Osteopenia and osteoporosis are common comorbid conditions of RA, which can be accelerated by episodic or chronic GC therapy. Patients with RA who are receiving GCs should have regular bone density measurements, independent of age.

Physical and occupational therapy are important in maintaining joint mobility and function. Goals of therapy include restoring and preserving function, decreasing pain, improving strength and endurance, and enhancing cardiovascular fitness. Therapy also provides patient education regarding the use of assistive devices, joint protection, and rest.

Surgical intervention is indicated in RA when medical therapy fails to adequately preserve joint function or achieve acceptable pain control. Preoperative evaluation of the patient with RA is key in reducing surgery-related morbidity and mortality. Patients should be evaluated with flexion and extension radiographs for cervical spine instability. Cervical spine instability with significant subluxation places the patient at risk for impingement of the spinal cord with routine procedures such as endotracheal intubation. Patients with cervical spine instability should undergo neurosurgical evaluation before any surgical intervention. Hoarseness or pain with phonation should alert the clinician to possible cricoarytenoid joint involvement, which can complicate intubation. The increased prevalence of atherosclerotic cardiovascular disease in patients with RA warrants cardiac clearance before surgery. Active joint or systemic infection is a contraindication to elective surgical intervention.

Perioperative DMARD therapy remains a topic of debate. Studies have demonstrated conflicting data; both increased and decreased incidence of infectious complications have been reported when MTX is continued perioperatively. However, it is clear that postoperative flares increase when MTX therapy is withheld for 1 month.[40] A dialogue with the surgical team is often helpful in assessing perioperative infection risk to determine how best to minimize complications while decreasing the risk of disease flare. As a compromise, we recommend withholding MTX for one dose before and after surgery. Anti-TNF agents are generally discontinued for several weeks before and after surgery, even for limited procedures.

GC therapy should not be abruptly discontinued under any circumstances. Patients should be receiving the minimum required dose of steroids preoperatively to lessen adverse effects on wound healing. There is no general consensus on stress-dose steroids (administered as 50 to 100 mg intravenous hydrocortisone every 8 hours on the day of surgery). When this therapy is used, the steroid dose should be quickly tapered over several days to the preoperative dose.

NSAIDs are usually withheld 1 to 2 weeks before any surgical procedure because of their effect on platelet function.

SPECIAL CONSIDERATIONS

There should be little delay in initiating DMARD therapy, including combinations, in patients with RA after the diagnosis is established. The goal of complete suppression of disease activity as determined by clinical and serologic assessments should be continuously pursued, as allowed by potential and experienced adverse medication effects.

Patients with inactive RA can suffer progressive degenerative joint structural damage as a consequence of prior inflammatory disease, leading to significant pain and disability. DMARD therapy should not be initiated or modified based on these changes if no active inflammation is ongoing. Treatment should address pain control and improvement of function by other medical or surgical means, as appropriate.

In patients with monoarticular arthritis or flare of just one joint, even in established RA, it is critical to assess for posttraumatic, crystal-induced, and septic arthritis by joint aspiration with synovial fluid examination and cultures.

In the setting of acute infection, most DMARDs (except for GC and hydroxychloroquine) should be discontinued until treatment has been completed and the infectious process has resolved.

Summary

- The clinical diagnosis of RA is made by the history and physical examination and depends on the insidious onset of symmetrical pain and swelling in mostly small peripheral joints.
- Rheumatoid factor is not necessary to confirm the diagnosis, but when present it is associated with more-severe joint disease and extra-articular manifestations.
- MRI can be used to facilitate diagnosis in occult or early cases because it is more sensitive for synovitis and changes in bone than radiographic studies.
- Prompt treatment with disease-modifying agents to normalize C-reactive protein and minimize the swollen joint count represents the standard of care.
- Measures of disease activity, such as the Disease Activity Index, and measures of outcome, such as the Health Assessment Questionnaire, should be recorded at every outpatient visit.

Suggested Readings

Goekoop-Ruiterman YP, de Vries-Bouwstra JK, Allaart CF, et al: Clinical and radiographic outcomes of four different strategies in patients with early rheumatoid arthritis (the BeSt study): A randomized, controlled trial. Arthritis Rheum 2005;52:3381-3390.

Gonzalez-Juanatey C, Llorca J, Testa A, et al: Increased prevalence of severe subclinical atherosclerotic findings in long-term treated rheumatoid arthritis patients without clinically evident atherosclerotic disease. Medicine 2003;82:407-413.

Hoving JL, Buchbinder R, Hall S, et al: A comparison of magnetic resonance imaging, sonography, and radiography of the hand in patients with early rheumatoid arthritis. J Rheumatol 2004;31:663-675.

Kirkham BW, Lassere MN, Edmonds JP, et al: Synovial membrane cytokine expression is predictive of joint damage progression in rheumatoid arthritis: A Two-Year Prospective Study (the DAMAGE Study Cohort). Arthritis Rheum 2006;54:1122-1131.

O'Dell JR, Leff R, Paulson G, et al: Treatment of rheumatoid arthritis with methotrexate and hydroxychloroquine, methotrexate and sulfasalazine, or the combination of the three medications: Results of a two-year randomized, double-blind, placebo-controlled trial. Arthritis Rheum 2002;46:1164-1170.

Saraux A, Berthelot JM, Devauchelle V, et al: Value of antibodies to citrulline-containing peptides for diagnosing early rheumatoid arthritis. J Rheumatol 2003;30:2535-2539.

Stolt P, Bengtsson C, Nordmark B, et al: Quantification of the influence of cigarette smoking on rheumatoid arthritis: Results from a population-based case-control study, using incident cases. Ann Rheum Dis 2003;62:835-841.

Vaudo G, Marchesi S, Gerli R, et al: Endothelial dysfunction in young patients with rheumatoid arthritis and low disease activity. Ann Rheum Dis 2004;63:31-35.

Wolfe F, Michaud K: Heart failure in rheumatoid arthritis: Rates, predictors, and the effect of anti–tumor necrosis factor therapy. Am J Med 2004;116:305-311.

Wolfe F, Michaud K: Severe rheumatoid arthritis (RA), worse outcomes, comorbid illness, and socio-demographic disadvantage characterize RA patients with fibromyalgia. J Rheumatol 2004;31:695-700.

References

For a complete list of references, log onto www.expertconsult.com.

Septic Arthritis

Abby Abelson

DEFINITION

Septic arthritis is infection, usually bacterial, in the joint cavity. Since septic arthritis can lead to rapid joint destruction, immediate accurate diagnosis is essential. The joint cavity is normally sterile, with synovial fluid and cellular matter, including a few white blood cells. The majority of patients with bacterial septic arthritis will present with acute monoarthritis.

PREVALENCE

The incidence of septic arthritis has been estimated at 2 to 10 cases per 100,000 in the general population and as high as 30 to 70 cases per 100,000 in patients with rheumatoid arthritis.[1,2] The most common mode of spread is hematogenous, with predisposing factors including intravenous drug use, presence of indwelling catheters, and underlying immunocompromised states. Other potential predisposing conditions include preexisting arthritis such as rheumatoid arthritis, gout, or osteoarthritis. The knee is the most commonly involved joint, accounting for about 50% of the cases.[3]

PATHOPHYSIOLOGY

The most common route of spread is hematogenous; other routes include trauma or inoculation, as during steroid injections. On entering the joint space, the bacteria initially deposit in the synovial membrane and produce an inflammatory reaction, usually with polymorphonuclear and synovial cells, which readily migrate into the synovial fluid. Synovial membrane hyperplasia develops in 5 to 7 days, and the release of cytokines leads to hydrolysis of proteoglycans and collagen, cartilage destruction, and eventually bone loss.[4] Direct pressure necrosis due to large synovial effusion results in further cartilage damage. Antigen-specific and polyclonal B-cell activation are seen in *Staphylococcus aureus* experimental arthritis.

The presence of the *cna* gene in *S. aureus* causes a higher incidence of septic arthritis in mouse experiments. This suggests that the cna gene product, a collagen adhesion factor, plays an important role in the development of septic arthritis.[5]

Most septic arthritides are monomicrobial infections, but polymicrobial infections may be seen in patients with direct inoculation of the joint space. The most common bacterial isolates in native joints include gram-positive cocci, with *S. aureus* found in 40% to 50% of the cases. Other isolates include *Neisseria gonorrhoeae*, streptococci, and gram-negative cocci, each in about 10% to 20% of cases. Other organisms less commonly isolated include mycobacteria and fungi.[3,6] Gram-negative bacilli are often present in neonates, the elderly, and patients with immune deficiency disorders. *N. gonorrhoeae* is seen in sexually active young adults, usually with associated dermatitis and tenosynovitis. Mycobacterial infections should be suspected in patients from endemic areas, and fungal arthritides are seen in immunocompromised patients. *Haemophilus influenzae* was a common cause of bacterial arthritis in young children, but the incidence has decreased almost 70% to 80% since the widespread use of *H. influenzae* b vaccine.[7]

SIGNS AND SYMPTOMS

Patients with septic arthritis usually present with a single swollen joint with pain on active or passive movement. The knee is involved in about 50% of the cases, but wrists, ankles, and hips are also commonly affected. Septic arthritis manifests as polyarticular arthritis in about 10% to 19% of patients and is more common in patients with prior joint damage, as in rheumatoid arthritis, gout, and systemic connective tissue disorders.[8]

Pertinent history in any patient with suspected septic arthritis includes joint disease, immunosuppressive states, intravenous drug use, recent steroid injection, history of sexually transmitted disease, and any constitutional symptoms. Physical examination should include a careful assessment of the pattern of joint involvement and inflammation of the eyes, skin, or mucosa and other sites of potential infection. Figure 1 gives a suggested algorithm for the workup of a single inflamed joint.

A classic presentation for septic arthritis is a febrile patient who has rigors, an increased leukocyte count, and elevated sedimentation rate. However, none of these is highly sensitive or specific for septic arthritis. In one series, only 40% to 60% of patients with septic arthritis were febrile, only 25% to 60% had an elevated leukocyte count, and only 60% to 80% had a sedimentation rate greater than 50 mm/hr.[4,9]

DIAGNOSIS

Synovial fluid analysis is of paramount importance in diagnosing and managing septic arthritis. It should include Gram stain, culture, leukocyte count with differential, and crystal examination under a polarized microscope. Controversy exists as to whether synovial fluid culture yield is increased by the inoculation of blood culture bottles at the bedside as compared with using conventional agar plate culture in the laboratory. A study has shown no difference in the rate of isolation of bacteria by either of these methods.[10]

A synovial fluid leukocyte count of greater than 50,000 with a polymorphonuclear leukocyte predominance is usually seen in septic arthritis. This can, however, also be seen in crystal arthropathies, which can complicate the clinical picture. A history of gout in the same joint or the presence of crystals in the synovial fluid can indicate an episode of gout or pseudogout rather than septic arthritis.

Gram stain is positive in 11% to 80% of cases, but an occasional false positive is seen due to precipitated mucin in the synovial fluid. Synovial fluid culture is positive in up to 90% of nongonococcal bacterial arthritides.[4]

Synovial fluid glucose, protein, and lactic acid concentration are not well standardized and hence are not useful in the diagnosis of septic arthritis. Synovial polymerase chain reaction (PCR) has been used to diagnose *Yersinia* species, *Chlamydia* species, *Ureaplasma urealyticum*, *N. gonorrhoeae*, and *Borrelia burgdorferi*.[4] It may be useful in the diagnosis of a fastidious organism and assist in the diagnosis of partially treated cases. Counterimmunoelectrophoresis has not been well studied in diagnosing synovial fluid infection and is not used for diagnosis of septic arthritis.

DIFFERENTIAL DIAGNOSIS

Other Rheumatic Diseases

In patients with chronic joint disease who present with one or more inflamed joints, septic arthritis should always be considered. These patients are inherently at a higher risk for infection due to their damaged joints. Septic arthritis in rheumatoid arthritis is associated with a higher mortality rate of 25% to 30% due to delays in diagno-

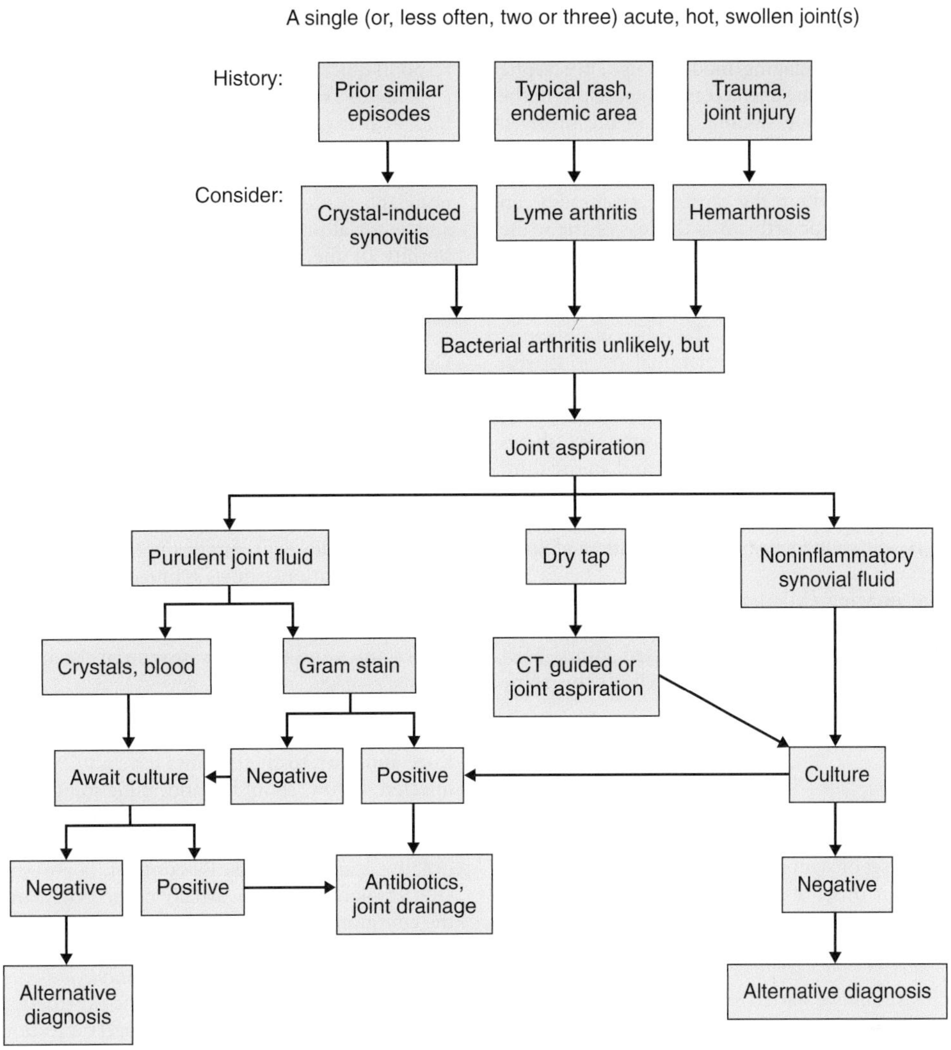

A single (or, less often, two or three) acute, hot, swollen joint(s)

History: Prior similar episodes → Consider: Crystal-induced synovitis
History: Typical rash, endemic area → Consider: Lyme arthritis
History: Trauma, joint injury → Consider: Hemarthrosis

Bacterial arthritis unlikely, but

Joint aspiration

Purulent joint fluid
Dry tap
Noninflammatory synovial fluid

Crystals, blood
Gram stain
CT guided or joint aspiration

Await culture
Negative
Positive
Culture

Negative
Positive
Antibiotics, joint drainage
Negative

Alternative diagnosis
Alternative diagnosis

Figure 1 **Algorithm for evaluating a hot, swollen joint.** CT, computed tomography. *(Adapted from Ruddy S, Harris ED Jr, Sledge CB (eds): Kelley's Textbook of Rheumatology, 6th ed. Philadelphia, WB Saunders, 2001, p 1472.)*

sis and initiation of treatment, because it can mimic an acute flare-up of the disease.[11]

Gout and pseudogout usually manifest similarly to septic arthritis, with pain, inflammation, and occasional constitutional symptoms. The presence of crystals on synovial fluid analysis is imperative to making the diagnosis of crystal arthropathy. In all patients with acute effusion of unknown cause, synovial fluid should be sent for Gram stain and culture.

Viral Arthritis

Acute polyarthritis with a fever and rash can be the initial manifestation of many viral infections including rubella, hepatitis B and C, and parvovirus. Human immunodeficiency virus (HIV) infection has also been associated with a subacute monoarthritis or oligoarthritis.

Lyme Disease

Lyme disease should be suspected in patients with a history of tick exposure or travel to endemic areas who present with typical erythema chronicum migrans, transient polyarthalgias, and other systemic symptoms. Chronic monoarthritis, especially of the knee, can be seen, and chronic persistent synovitis develops in 20% of the patients with untreated Lyme disease.[3] Serologic tests can be confirmatory in certain patients, and treatment with oral or intravenous antibiotics is curative in most cases.

Reactive Arthritis

Seronegative spondyloarthropathies associated with HLA B27 antigens, including Reiter's syndrome, psoriatic arthritis, ankylosing spondylitis, and arthritis associated with inflammatory bowel disease, can manifest as an acute inflamed joint. These patients usually have other manifestations of the disease including gastrointestinal or genitourinary symptoms, skin lesions, or uveitis, which can suggest the diagnosis. These joint inflammations are sterile and are reactive to infection or inflammation elsewhere in the body. Post-streptococcal infection can also mimic septic arthritis. Persistent microbial antigens have been demonstrated with PCR studies in the synovial fluid of patients with reactive arthritis.[3]

Infective Endocarditis

About 15% of patients with infective endocarditis have septic arthritis or bone infection. These patients can also present with sterile synovitis or arthralgias mimicking septic arthritis.

IMAGING

Radiography should be the first imaging modality used for septic arthritis. The inflamed synovial tissue and accompanying fluid in the joint cause a symmetrical soft-tissue swelling around the involved joint, as manifested by a widened joint space or displacement of the fat pads around the joint. Marginal erosions or erosion of bone that sits uncovered by cartilage but within the capsular attachment can also be seen. The hallmark of septic arthritis is the loss of the white cortical line over a long contiguous segment, unlike the segmental disruption seen in inflammatory arthropathies. Bacterial infection of a joint usually causes rapid joint space loss, with aggressive erosive changes and preservation of mineralization. The tuberculous septic joint tends to preserve the joint and causes marginal erosions with extensive demineralization and little repair.[12]

Bone scintigraphy may be used if radiographs are normal. A three-phase scan using Tc 99m methylene diphosphonate shows increased uptake in the synovium of the septic joint and, in the third phase, increased uptake in the articular ends of the bone. Gallium-67 citrate can be used in conjunction for additional information. However, it still may be difficult to distinguish an inflamed joint from an infected joint.

Magnetic resonance imaging (MRI) is highly sensitive for the diagnosis of septic arthritis, although it still lacks specificity because it cannot reliably distinguish inflamed from infected joints. MRI has been considered the diagnostic modality of choice by some clinicians.[12]

TREATMENT

One of the most important predictors of a good outcome in septic arthritis is the rapidity with which treatment is instituted. Patients treated within 7 days of onset of symptoms tend to do well, and those treated after 1 month of the onset of symptoms usually do poorly.[13]

Antibiotics

Initial antibiotic therapy should be started empirically without awaiting the final results of culture. Choice of antibiotic is based on the patient's age, presumed source of infection, patient's own infection profile, presence of immunosuppression including history of diabetes, and the suspected pathogenic organism. Parenteral antibiotics should always be used, at least in the initial part of the treatment regimen. Initial empiric therapy for septic arthritis should be vancomycin to cover gram-positive cocci, including staphylococci and gonococcus. Directed therapy with oxacillin, cephazolin for staph aureus should be given for 4 weeks. Direct instillation of the antibiotic into the joint is not necessary and has not been shown to be more effective than parenteral antibiotics.

Duration of antibiotic treatment is more controversial and depends on the organism isolated at final culture and its response to the given antibiotic. In uncomplicated cases, 2 weeks of therapy for *H. influenzae*, streptococci, or gram-negative cocci and 4 weeks of therapy for staphylococci and gram-negative bacilli may be adequate.[14] Directed therapy for gonococcus with cephtriaxone should be given for 2 weeks. With the advent of home intravenous antibiotic therapy, these patients can be treated with parenteral antibiotics on an outpatient basis.

A decrease in the white blood cell count in serial synovial fluid samples between 5 and 7 days of therapy reflects a control of infection.[9]

Drainage of Infected Joints

Most uncomplicated cases can be drained with needle aspiration. Some infected joints, including the hip, shoulder, and sacroiliac joints, might not be easily aspirated. In these cases, an open arthrotomy may be considered as an initial approach. Any joint with limited accessibility, including the sternoclavicular or the sternomanubrial joints, should also be managed surgically.[13,15] Any joint that does not respond quickly to antibiotic therapy must also be treated surgically.

Patients with underlying diseases, including diabetes, rheumatoid arthritis, immunosuppression, or other systemic symptoms, should be treated more aggressively with earlier surgical intervention. The goal of surgery is to remove all purulent material and nonviable tissue and to determine the need for synovectomy. Culture and synovial biopsies can be obtained after débridement to ensure sterility of the joint.[15,16] The knee, shoulder, and ankle joints are especially amenable to arthroscopic débridement in adult and pediatric patients.

After arthrotomy, joints—especially hips—should be closed. Drainage of the joints with closed suction systems is recommended; there are no standards for how long drains should remain in place.

Repeated irrigation and distention of a joint at the bedside under local anesthetic have been described to be effective in certain cases. This approach, called *tidal irrigation*, may be a useful adjunct to medical therapy in certain patients.[13,15]

Any infected limb should be splinted in the position of function, with knees splinted in extension, hips placed in balanced suspension in neutral rotation, elbows splinted at 90 degrees, and wrists splinted in neutral to slight extension. Once an infection is under control, immediate joint mobilization should be started slowly. This prevents contractures and promotes healing of the articular cartilage.[17]

Infection of Prosthetic Joints

Knee and hip prosthetic joints have a 0.5% to 2% risk of becoming infected. Elbow, shoulder, and ankle joints have a higher infection rate of up to 6% to 9%.[18] Early infections (<12 weeks after implantation) are usually from a skin pathogen, most likely a coagulase-negative staphylococcus. By contrast, late-onset infections (>1 year after implantation) are usually caused by hematogenous spread of the common organisms, including such gram-negative organisms as *Escherichia coli*, *Proteus mirabilis*, and *Pseudomonas aeruginosa* and gram-positive organisms, with *Staphylococcus epidermidis* being more common than *S. aureus*.[19] The prosthesis and binding cement provide an avascular region for bacteria to flourish away from the immunologic defenses of the body. Adherent bacteria multiply and elaborate glycocalyx, eventually forming thick biofilms that further impair host defenses. Also, in the biofilm, bacteria older than 7 days have been shown to have higher resistance to antibiotics.[20] Empiric therapy with vancomycin should be given to cover staph aureus, staph epidermidis, and streptococcus. Directed therapy with oxacillin or cefazolin (staph aureus), vancomycin (staph epidermidis), or penicillin G or ampicillin (streptococcus) should be continued for 4 weeks.

Patients with rheumatoid arthritis, prior joint infection, prolonged surgical time, postoperative bleeding, urinary tract infection, and advanced age have a higher risk of infection. Pain, wound drainage, erythema, and induration at the site of the incision in early-onset infection, and fever and increased C-reactive protein in late-onset infection, are the usual signs of prosthetic joint infection. The sensitivity and specificity of scintigraphy including technetium-colloid scan, gallium-67 scan, or indium-labeled autologous white blood cell scan are low.[13] Joint space fluid or tissue is required for definite diagnosis. Surgical biopsy or arthroscopy is sometimes required, especially in late-onset infection with minimal symptoms.

Removal of the prosthetic joint is necessary in an overwhelming majority of cases. This may be done by excision arthroplasty or by reimplantation of the joint. Reimplantation may be a one-stage procedure or a two-stage procedure, with 4 to 6 weeks of antibiotic therapy between the removal and reimplantation of a new prosthesis. The success rates for reimplantation range from 39% to 91% for a one-stage procedure and 73% to 100% for a two-stage procedure.[21] Long-term suppressive antibiotics without removal of the prosthetic joint may be considered in patients in whom surgical removal is not possible, with an avirulent pathogen sensitive to oral antibiotics, and if the prosthesis is not loose.

Dental prophylaxis is not routinely recommended in patients with a prosthetic joint, but it may be considered in patients with diabetes, immunosuppressive therapy, or rheumatoid arthritis.[22]

Neisseria gonorrhoeae Septic Arthritis

Disseminated gonococcal infection is the most common cause of infection in young adults, particularly pregnant and perimenstrual women. It accounts for 3% to 7.5% of all culture-positive septic arthritis reported. Women are four times more likely to be affected and usually have associated asymptomatic genital, anal, or pharyngeal gonococcal infections. These can manifest as monoarticular, polyarticular, or disseminated infections.

Gram stain is positive in 25% and culture in 50% of the cases.[23] Thus, the diagnosis is often made from signs and symptoms, such as the presence of a rash with positive *N. gonorrhoeae* culture from a genitourinary source. Synovial PCR may be useful in detecting gonococcal DNA from the joints. Third-generation cephalosporins, such as ceftriaxone, are the agents of choice because of increasing penicillin resistance.

SPECIAL CONSIDERATIONS

Polyarticular Septic Arthritis

Polyarticular septic arthritis is seen in 10% to 19% of nongonococcal infections, usually due to staphylococcal infection of large joints in patients with underlying rheumatoid arthritis.[8,11] The mean number of joints infected is four, and extra-articular signs of infection are often seen. The prognosis is poor, with a mortality rate up to 32% noted in certain series. Poor prognosis is conferred by older age (>50 years), rheumatoid arthritis, and staphylococcal infection, but the overall mortality has remained unchanged since the 1990s.[8,13]

Septic Arthritis Following Arthrocentesis

The incidence of septic arthritis following arthrocentesis is low, ranging between 1 per 1000 and 1 per 16,000; this may be increased if corticosteroids are instilled.[24] Most cases of infection usually occur when transient bacteremia colonizes the needle track and causes seeding of the joint. Skin flora are rarely found to be the cause, but aseptic technique during the procedure is imperative. The presentation is similar to that of septic arthritis from other causes, and one should have a high level of clinical suspicion.

Septic Arthritis with Crystal-Induced Arthritis

Crystal-induced arthritis can mimic septic arthritis, with fever, constitutional symptoms, and high synovial white cell count. The coexistence of gout and septic arthritis is rare, although well-documented cases have been reported in the literature.[25] This should be suspected in patients with worsening synovitis despite treatment of gout, fever accompanying polyarthritis, acute arthritis after treatment of infection at a different site, and new joint involvement in a patient with gout. Synovial fluid analysis with Gram stain and culture is critical in making the diagnosis in such patients. In a series from the Mayo Clinic, five of the 314 patients with pseudogout had concomitant septic arthritis.

Septic Arthritis with Rheumatoid Arthritis

Septic arthritis in patients with rheumatoid arthritis can manifest very similarly to an acute flare of the disease. Septic arthritis in these patients can also be insidious in presentation because some of these patients may be taking corticosteroids. In one series, fever and constitutional symptoms were often absent, and only 56% of cases had an elevated peripheral leukocyte count. Use of corticosteroids, cytotoxic drugs, and impaired host defenses including decreased chemotaxis and complement levels predispose patients with rheumatoid arthritis to infection.[13] *S. aureus* is the main pathogen (76% of patients), and gram-negative bacilli are responsible for the remaining cases. Polyarticular infection can occur in 25% of cases.[13] These patients should be managed aggressively, and early surgical exploration and drainage of the joints are indicated.[15]

Septic Arthritis in HIV Patients

Septic arthritis may be seen more often in patients with HIV infection. Its occurrence is usually associated with parenteral drug use or behavioral risk factors. *N. gonorrhoeae* is the most common organism reported in homosexual men. In advanced HIV infection, atypical mycobacterial species including *Mycobacterium avium-intracellulare* and *Mycobacterium kansasii* have been implicated in joint infections. At CD4 counts of less than 100, HIV-infected patients are also at risk for fungal infections, particularly *Candida albicans* and *Sporothrix schenckii*.[26]

Septic Arthritis in Intravenous Drug Users

Knee and wrist joints are the most common joints involved in intravenous drug users. *Staphylococcus* species and gram-negative bacteria, including *P. aeruginosa*, *Enterobacter* species, and *Serratia* species are the common pathogens. These patients usually have a very favorable outcome despite infection with virulent organisms.[27]

Specific Associations

Certain pathogens have been associated with specific patient subgroups, such as *Salmonella* species in patients with systemic lupus erythematosus or in sickle cell disease patients.[4] *U. urealyticum* infection has been described in hypogammaglobulinemic patients; PCR can aid in diagnosis. *Pasteurella multocida* rarely causes septic arthritis following a penetrating bite, particularly from cats and dogs. Metacarpophalangeal and proximal interphalangeal joints can be involved with *Mycobacterium marinum* infection acquired through exposure to fresh water or marine life.[4]

Summary

- Acute monoarthritis should be evaluated emergently to rule out the possibility of septic arthritis.
- Untreated septic arthritis can lead to rapid joint space destruction and systemic sepsis, so early diagnosis is imperative.
- Consider septic arthritis in patients with underlying inflammatory arthritis if one joint is more acutely inflamed than others.
- Aspiration of the involved joint is critical to identifying the organism.
- Therapy with empirical antibiotics should immediately follow aspiration, with subsequent narrower coverage only after culture results are obtained.
- Risk factors including old age, trauma, limb ulceration, and prior hospitalization can predict the likely organism infecting the joint.
- Patients receiving immunosuppressive medications, steroids, and chemotherapy are at greater risk for developing septic arthritis.
- Treatment includes appropriate joint drainage and surgical options depending on the joint involved.

Suggested Readings

Dubost JJ, Soubrier M, De Champs C, et al: No changes in the distribution of organisms responsible for septic arthritis over a 20 year period. Ann Rheum Dis 2002;61:267-269.

Faraj AA, Omonbude OD, Godwin P: Gram staining in the diagnosis of acute septic arthritis. Acta Orthop Belg 2002;68:388-391.

Goldenberg DL: Septic arthritis. Lancet 1998;351:197-202.

Gupta MN, Sturrock RD, Field M: Prospective comparative study of patients with culture proven and high suspicion of adult onset septic arthritis. Ann Rheum Dis 2003;62:327-331.

Gupta MN, Sturrock RD, Field M: A prospective 2-year study of 75 patients with adult-onset septic arthritis. Rheumatology (Oxford) 2001;40:24-30.

Li SF, Henderson J, Dickman E, Darzynkiewicz R: Laboratory tests in adults with monoarticular arthritis: Can they rule out a septic joint? Acad Emerg Med 2004;11:276-280.

Margaretten M, Kohlwes J, Moore D, Bent S: Does this patient have septic arthritis? JAMA 2007;297:1478-1488.

Mathews CJ, Kingsley G, Field M, et al: Management of septic arthritis: A systematic review. Ann Rheum Dis 2007; 66:440-445.

Ross JJ, Shamsuddin H: Sternoclavicular septic arthritis: Review of 180 cases. Medicine (Baltimore) 2004;83:139-148.

Swan A, Am H, Dieppe P: The value of synovial fluid assays in the diagnosis of joint disease: A literature survey. Ann Rheum Dis 2002;61:493-498.

Yu KH, Luo SF, Liou LB, et al: Concomitant septic and gouty arthritis: An analysis of 30 cases. Rheumatology (Oxford) 2003;42:1062-1066.

References

For a complete list of references, log onto www.expertconsult.com.

Soft-Tissue Rheumatic Conditions

Judith Manzon and Raymond Scheetz

Soft-tissue rheumatic disorders are painful conditions arising from periarticular musculoskeletal structures. This discussion focuses on regional soft tissue disorders that are commonly encountered in the primary care setting. When evaluating musculoskeletal complaints, an intra-articular process (arthritis) should first be excluded.

SHOULDER

Rotator Cuff Disorders

The rotator cuff is composed of four muscles: the subscapularis anteriorly (internal rotator), supraspinatus superiorly (elevator), and the infraspinatus and teres minor posteriorly (external rotators). Together they provide dynamic stability to the shoulder joint (Fig. 1).

Rotator cuff disorders range from impingement syndrome to tendon rupture. Impingement syndrome includes rotator cuff tears, tendinitis, and subacromial bursitis. The supraspinatus and infraspinatus tendons are particularly susceptible to impingement or tearing given their location beneath the coracoacromial arch. Because of their proximity, secondary involvement of the subdeltoid and subcoracoid bursae can also occur.

Although pain is the most common symptom of rotator cuff disorders, patients might also complain of weakness and loss of motion. The pain is usually localized to the lateral arm and shoulder and can awaken the patient during the night. Pain is worsened with overhead activities such as using a hair dryer and combing hair. Painful weakness, atrophy, and inability to abduct and elevate the arm are seen in more advanced conditions.[1]

The age of the patient can also provide clinical clues to the diagnosis. Underlying instability is more likely in a younger patient, and a mechanical or degenerative cause is more likely in an older patient (Table 1).

On physical examination, there is tenderness to palpation of the proximal humerus at the insertion site of the rotator cuff. Tenderness of the shoulder anteriorly suggests biceps tendinitis, whereas more lateral tenderness suggests supraspinatus tendinitis or subdeltoid bursitis. Passive ROM is greater than active ROM, with a painful arc between 60 and 120 degrees of abduction. The Neer and Hawkins impingement tests can be done to evaluate for rotator cuff disorders. With the Neer impingement test, the examiner forcibly flexes the patient's arm forward with one hand while stabilizing the patient's shoulder with the other hand. The Hawkins impingement test involves forward flexion of the shoulder to 90 degrees and internal rotation of the shoulder. Pain with these maneuvers suggests an impingement syndrome.[2]

When evaluating periarticular shoulder disorders, it is also important to test the strength of the rotator cuff muscles. The subscapularis is tested with resisted internal rotation, the supraspinatus is tested with resisted abduction in the plane of the scapula, and the infraspinatus and teres minor are tested with resisted external rotation. Weakness may be the result of pain inhibition or may be true weakness. The impingement test may be helpful in these cases. Approximately 5 to 10 mL of 1% lidocaine is injected into the subacromial bursa, and if the pain is relieved by at least 50%, then impingement is the more likely cause. Weakness that persists despite pain relief is probably true weakness.

Imaging of the shoulder is usually not necessary unless symptoms persist for more than 3 to 4 months despite conservative therapy. Other indications for imaging include features suggesting a need for surgery or if the diagnosis is in doubt. Findings on plain radiographs that can be associated with impingement include arthritic changes of the glenohumeral joint, subacromial space calcifications, acromial spurs, or decreased distance between the acromion and the humeral head. Arthrography was formerly the gold-standard imaging study for full-thickness rotator cuff tears, but it is now largely replaced by magnetic resonance imaging (MRI). The finding of a rotator cuff irregularity on imaging, however, does not necessarily imply causality of symptoms, because up to 26% of asymptomatic people have a rotator cuff tear on MRI.[3]

Rotator cuff tendinitis and subacromial bursitis are initially managed with a short period of rest (up to a week) and nonsteroidal anti-inflammatory drugs (NSAIDs). If this approach fails, a subacromial corticosteroid injection may be tried (Fig. 2 and Box 1). Once the pain is improved and normal shoulder movement has returned, a supervised therapy program should be instituted to strengthen the rotator cuff muscles and preserve range of motion. If symptoms persist despite an adequate trial of these measures, surgery may be indicated.

Rotator cuff tears are treated in a manner similar to that for rotator cuff tendinitis. However, corticosteroid injection is not advised within 4 to 6 weeks of an acute injury. Indications for surgical intervention of complete tears are controversial. Earlier surgery for acute ruptures in young or active patients has been advocated.

Biceps Tendinitis

Biceps tendinitis usually occurs in association with rotator cuff impingement rather than in isolation. Pain is localized over the anterior shoulder and can radiate to the biceps muscle. Palpation of the bicipital groove reproduces the pain. Yergason's maneuver can be used to isolate and stress the bicipital tendon. The elbow is flexed to 90 degrees, and the forearm is pronated while keeping the arm against the body to prevent shoulder motion. The patient then supinates the forearm while the examiner resists this motion. Pain with this maneuver suggests bicipital tendinitis.[4] Pain may also be reproduced with Speed's test, which requires the patient, with the elbow in extension, to flex the shoulder against resistance.

Biceps tendinitis is managed conservatively with a short period of rest followed by physical therapy, NSAIDs, and local corticosteroid injections (Fig. 3). The examiner should evaluate for underlying rotator cuff disorders; failure to do so can result in recurrence of symptoms. For refractory cases, surgery may be considered.

Adhesive Capsulitis

Adhesive capsulitis, also known as frozen shoulder, is characterized by pain and global restriction of both active and passive glenohumeral joint motion. The joint capsule adheres to the anatomic neck and becomes thickened and contracted. It can be idiopathic (primary adhesive capsulitis) or related to other conditions such as diabetes mellitus, thyroid disease, hyperlipidemia, pulmonary disorders, and trauma (secondary adhesive capsulitis). Women in their sixth decade are most commonly affected.[5]

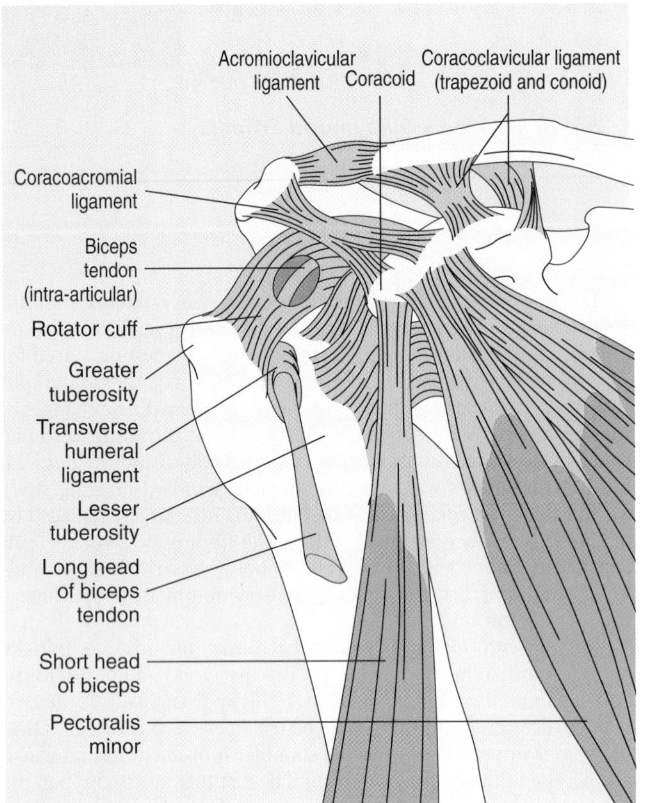

Figure 1 Ligamentous and musculotendinous attachments about the shoulder joint. *From Hochberg MC, Silman Aj, Smolen JS et al (eds): Practical Rheumatology, 3rd ed. Philadelphia: Mosby, 2004.*

There are three phases in the natural history of this condition. The shoulder is initially painful, then it is painful and stiff, and eventually it becomes more stiff than painful. Patients complain of pain without any precipitating event; pain is brought on by movement of the shoulder. Night pain is common. On examination, the shoulder is tender and there is loss of active and passive range of motion in all planes. Radiographic films of the shoulder and laboratory testing are usually unrevealing. The diagnosis is predominantly made on clinical grounds.

Gradual spontaneous improvement of the pain occurs 1 to 3 years after onset, but there is often some residual limitation of shoulder motion. Because prolonged immobility of the glenohumeral joint allows adhesions to form, early mobilization is key. Physical therapy, NSAIDs, and local injections of glucocorticosteroids can be used for pain relief. Although less common, other methods to improve range of motion include manipulation under anesthesia, arthroscopic capsulotomy, and hydrodistention of the joint to lyse adhesions and stretch the capsule.

ELBOW

Medial and Lateral Epicondylitis

Both medial and lateral epicondylitis are due to repetitive microtrauma from work or sports activities that involve repetitive twisting or gripping movements. Examples include tennis, golf, carpentry, gardening, and dentistry.

Medial epicondylitis, also known as golfer's elbow, is the result of repetitive flexion and pronation of the wrist. Tenderness over the medial epicondyle can be elicited with palpation over the medial epicondyle. Pain is reproduced with resisted wrist flexion and pronation. On the other hand, lateral epicondylitis, often referred to as tennis elbow, is seen with repetitive extension and supination of the wrist. It causes pain over the lateral epicondyle with palpation and is reproduced with resisted wrist extension and supination.[6]

The initial treatment for epicondylitis is splinting of the elbow at 90 degrees of flexion for 3 to 5 days. If symptoms persist, other conservative measures such as nonsteroidal anti-inflammatory drugs (NSAIDs), ice, or local glucocorticosteroid injections may be tried (Fig. 4). For chronic cases of epicondylitis, a compression band may be used for symptomatic relief. Pain that is refractory to these measures should raise suspicion for medial or ulnar nerve entrapment, which might require surgical intervention.

Olecranon Bursitis

The bursa is a synovial tissue–lined sac that provides a gliding surface to reduce friction between tendons and muscles over bony structures. Inflammation of this structure resulting from overuse, infection, trauma, or systemic inflammatory disease is known as *bursitis.*

Patients with olecranon bursitis complain of swelling over the posterior elbow and tenderness with pressure, but they have normal elbow range of motion. Pain may be minimal. When localized erythema is present, infection or gout should be excluded by aspiration. Drainage and protective measures against trauma are usually sufficient. A compression bandage might provide enough pressure to prevent reaccumulation of fluid in the bursa. In some instances, the bursa can be excised if there is persistent infection or recurrent bursitis.[7]

WRIST

de Quervain's Tenosynovitis

de Quervain's tenosynovitis is inflammation and stenosis of the tendon sheath enveloping the abductor pollicis longus and the extensor pollicis brevis as they course through the sheath at the level of the radial styloid process. It can be seen in pregnancy and in new mothers, the latter possibly related to lifting or holding their babies with an outstretched thumb. It might result from repetitive motions that involve pinching with the thumb and twisting the wrist.

There is pain and occasionally swelling over the radial styloid. Pain is associated with movement of the thumb and wrist. The Finklestein maneuver can elicit pain in patients with de Quervain's tenosynovitis. The thumb is folded across the palm and the other fingers form a fist around the thumb. The wrist is passively deviated toward the ulnar side. It should be noted, however, that this maneuver can also cause pain in persons with osteoarthritis of the first carpometacarpal joint. Thus, the presence of first carpometacarpal joint osteoarthritis should also be evaluated if the Finklestein test is positive.

This condition is treated initially with wrist splinting and NSAIDs. If symptoms persist, a local corticosteroid injection can be given. In rare cases, surgical decompression with or without tenosynovectomy is necessary.[8]

KNEE

Anserine Bursitis

The anserine bursa lies beneath the pes anserinus, which comprises the conjoined tendons of the sartorius, gracilis, and semitendinosus muscles. This bursa is situated between these tendons and the tibial collateral ligament.

Anserine bursitis is most common in obese, middle-aged to elderly women with knee osteoarthritis. Other predisposing factors

Table 1 Differential Diagnosis of Shoulder Pain

Diagnosis	Age	Type of Onset	Location of Pain	Night Pain	Active Range of Motion	Passive Range of Motion	Impingement Signs	Radiation of Pain	Parasthesias	Weakness	Instability	Radiographic Changes	Special Features
Rotator cuff tendinitis	Any	Acute or chronic	Deltoid region	+	↓↓ Guarding	Normal	+++	–	–	Only due to pain	Look for	In chronic cases	Painful arc of abduction
Rotator cuff tears (chronic)	>40 yr	Often chronic	Deltoid region	++	↓↓↓	Normal (can ↓ later)	++	–	–	++	–	+	Wasting of cuff muscles
Bicipital tendinitis	Any	Overuse	Anterior	–	↓ Guarding	Normal	+	Occasionally into biceps	–	Only due to pain	Look for	None	Special examination tests
Calcific tendinitis	30-60 yr	Acute	Point of shoulder	++	↓↓↓ Guarding	Normal except for pain	+++	–	–	Only due to pain	–	++	Tenderness ++
Capsulitis (frozen shoulder)	>40 yr	Insidious	Deep in shoulder	++	↓↓	↓↓	+	–	–	–	–	–	Global range of motion ↓
Acromioclavicular joint	Any	Acute or chronic	Over joint	Lying on side	↓ Full elevation	Normal	–	–	–	–	–	In chronic cases	Local tenderness
Osteoarthrosis of glenohumeral joint	>40 yr	Insidious	Deep in shoulder	++	↓↓	↓↓	–	–	–	May have mild	–	+++	Crepitus
Glenohumeral instability	Usually <25 yr	Episodic	Anterior or posterior	–	Only apprehension	Only apprehension	Possible	–	+ With acute episodes	+ With acute episodes	+++	Often	Stress tests
Cervical spondylosis	>40 yr	Insidious	Suprascapular	Often	Normal	Normal	–	++	+++	+	–	In cervical spine	Pain with neck movement
Thoracic outlet syndrome	Any	Usually with activity	Neck, shoulder, arm	–	Normal	Normal	–	++	++	++	–	–	Special examination tests

From Hochberg MC, Silman Aj, Smolen JS et al (eds): Practical Rheumatology, 3rd edition. Philadelphia: Mosby, 2004.

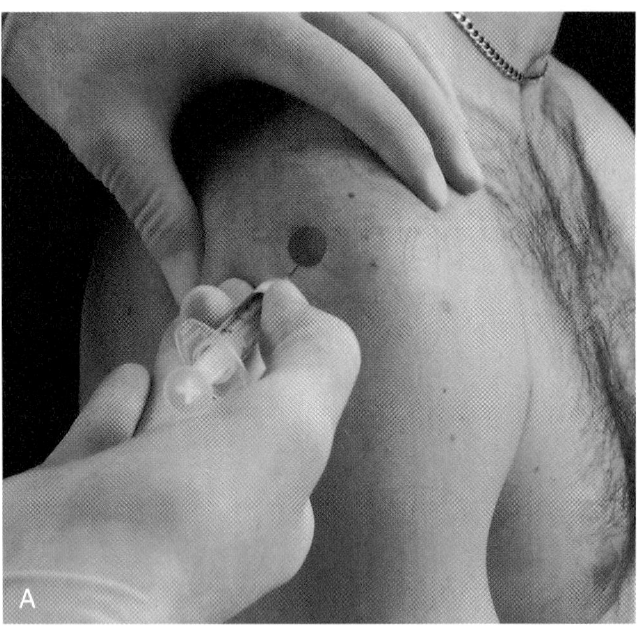

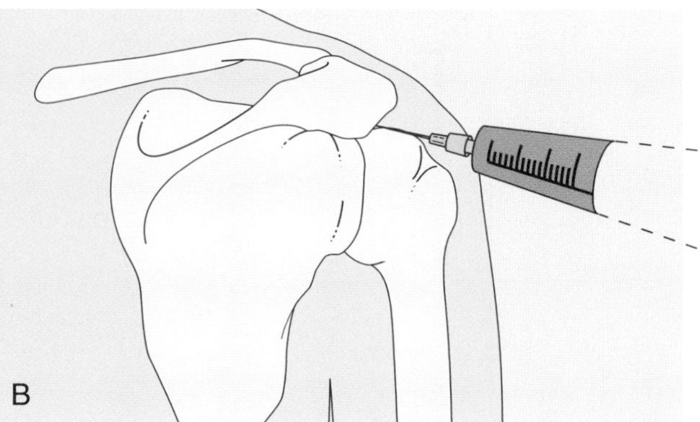

Figure 2 **A** and **B**, Posterolateral approach to the subacromial bursa. *From Hochberg MC, Silman Aj, Smolen JS et al (eds): Practical Rheumatology, 3rd ed. Philadelphia: Mosby, 2004.*

Box 1 Equipment Required for Joint and Soft-Tissue Injections

Skin Preparation
Alcohol swabs
Antiseptic solution (povidone-iodine)
4 × 4 gauze pads

Local Anesthetic
1% lidocaine

Needles
23- to 27-gauge needles for local anesthetic
18-gauge needles for large to moderate sized joints (e.g., knees, shoulders, ankles)
23- to 25-gauge needles for small joints (e.g., wrists, metacarpophalangeal joints)

Syringes
3-mL or 5-mL syringe for anesthetic-steroid injection
10-mL to 50-mL syringe for joint aspiration

Miscellaneous
Gloves
Forceps for removing needles from syringe
Specimen tubes or plates for cultures and fluid studies

From Hochberg MC, Silman Aj, Smolen JS et al (eds): Practical Rheumatology, 3rd edition. Philadelphia: Mosby, 2004.

include genu valgum, hamstring contractures, and an out-toeing gait. Patients complain of medial knee pain that can sometimes radiate to the posterior medial thigh. It is accentuated with stair climbing. On examination, pain and tenderness are localized to approximately 3 to 5 inches below the medial knee joint line. Treatment consists of NSAIDs, stretching exercises of the adductor and quadriceps muscles, and corticosteroid injection into the bursa.[9]

HIP

Trochanteric Bursitis

Trochanteric bursitis is the most common cause of pain around the hip joint. It can be associated with hip osteoarthritis, leg-length discrepancy, and scoliosis. It is more commonly seen in women.

Trochanteric bursitis is manifested as a deep, aching pain on the lateral aspect of the hip and thigh. It is brought on by activities that involve hip flexion such as walking, squatting, and climbing stairs. Pain improves with rest and is exacerbated by applying pressure to the affected side. The pain may be so severe that it causes a limping gait.

It is clinically diagnosed by noting point tenderness over the greater trochanteric region. Tenderness may also be seen along the lateral aspect of the thigh. Additionally, pain can be elicited by hip flexion, external rotation, and resisted abduction.

Trochanteric bursitis is treated with a local injection of corticosteroid into the bursa (Fig. 5). Weight loss, rest, stretching and strengthening exercises of the gluteus medius muscle, and NSAIDs can also be helpful.

Summary

- When evaluating musculoskeletal complaints, an intra-articular process (arthritis) should first be excluded.
- Soft-tissue rheumatic disorders are diagnosed based on clinical grounds. Imaging and laboratory testing is usually not necessary unless the diagnosis is in question or the symptoms fail to respond to conservative management.
- Most soft-tissue rheumatic disorders can be managed conservatively. Rarely is surgical intervention necessary.

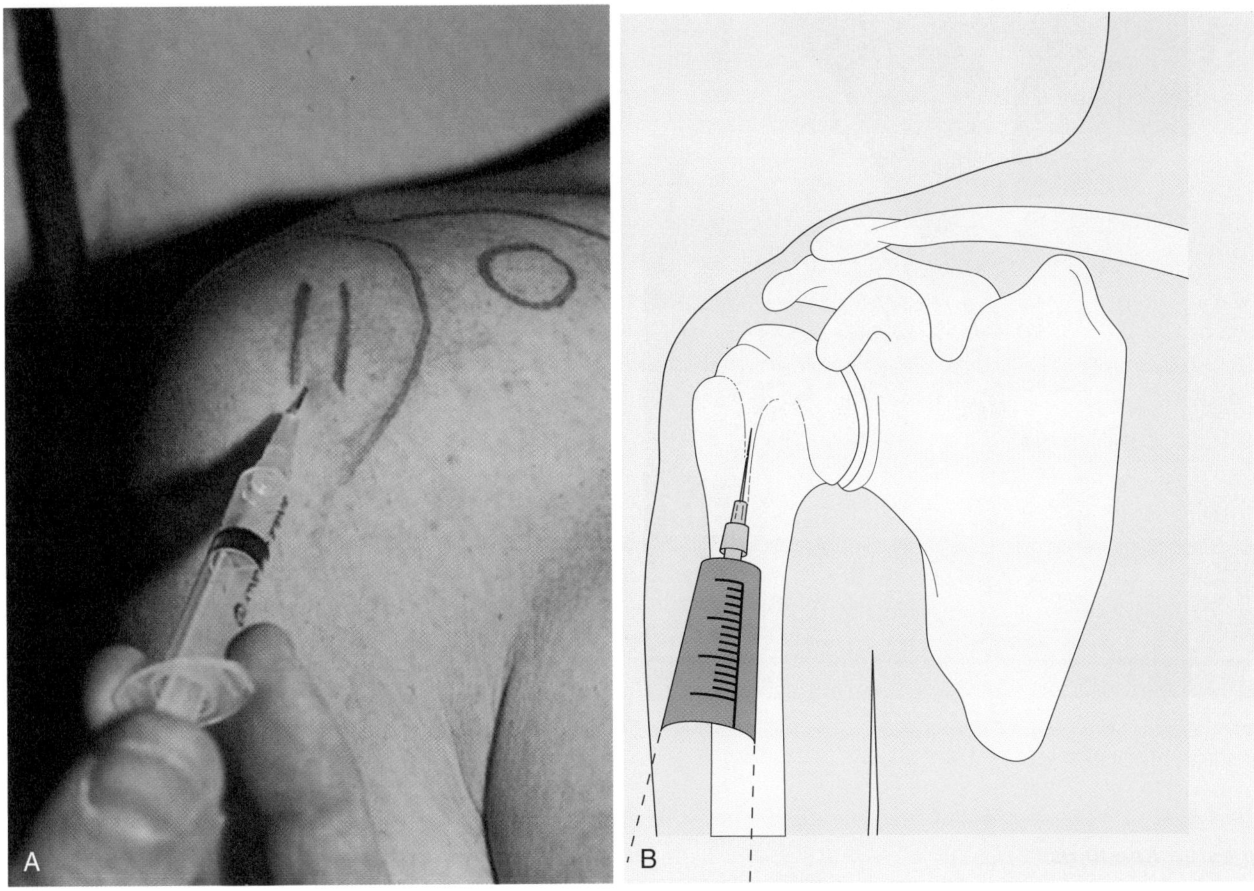

Figure 3 **A** and **B**, Injection into the bicipital groove. *From Hochberg MC, Silman Aj, Smolen JS et al (eds): Practical Rheumatology, 3rd ed. Philadelphia: Mosby, 2004.*

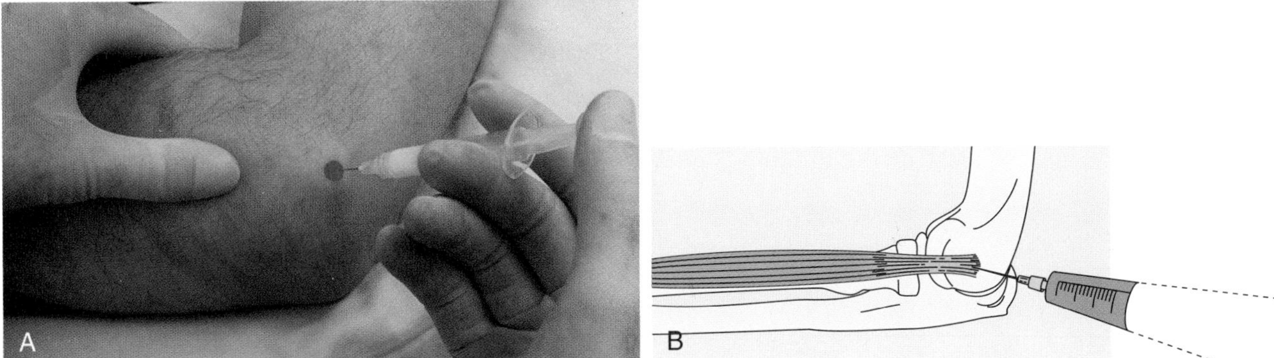

Figure 4 **A** and **B**, Injection into the lateral epicondyle. *From Hochberg MC, Silman Aj, Smolen JS et al (eds): Practical Rheumatology, 3rd ed. Philadelphia: Mosby, 2004.*

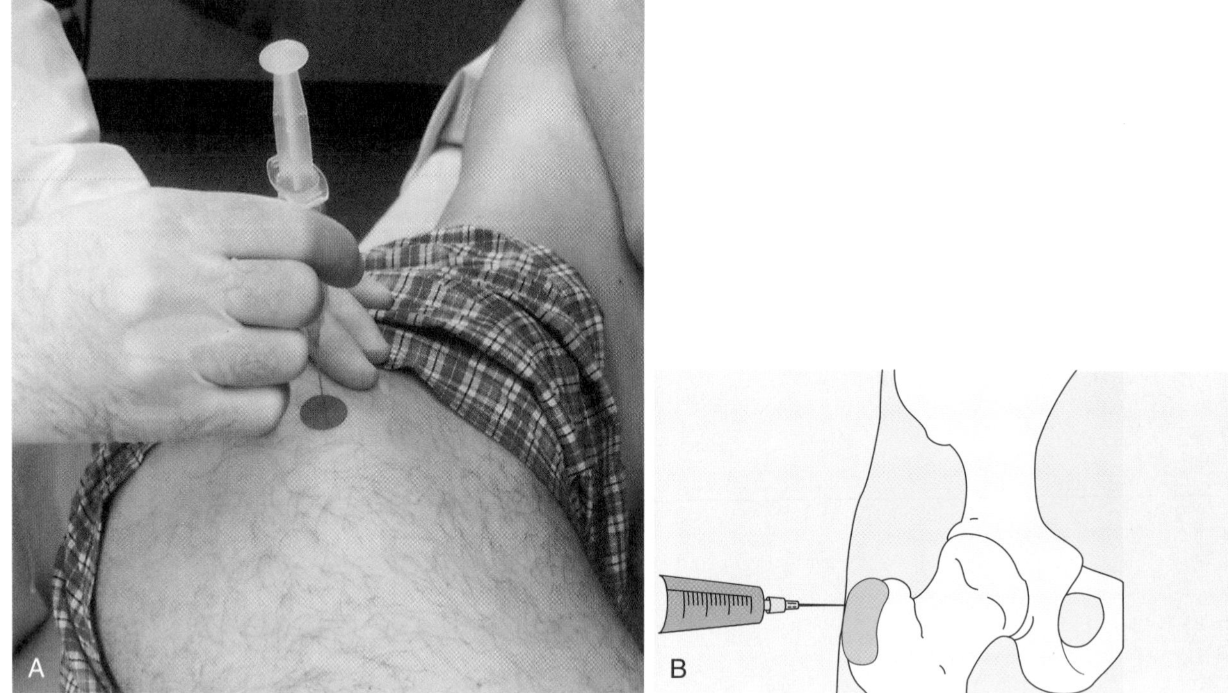

Figure 5 **A** and **B**, Injection of the trochanteric bursa. *From Hochberg MC, Silman Aj, Smolen JS et al (eds): Practical Rheumatology, 3rd ed. Philadelphia: Mosby, 2004.*

Suggested Readings

Alvarez-Nemegyei J, Canoso JJ: Evidence-based soft tissue rheumatology: Epicondylitis and hand stenosing tendinopathy. J Clin Rheumatol 2004;10:33-40.

Alvarez-Nemegyei J, Canoso JJ: Evidence-based soft tissue rheumatology IV: Anserine bursitis. J Clin Rheumatol 2004;10:205-206.

Belzer JP, Durkin RC: Common disorders of the shoulder. Prim Care 1996;23:365-388.

Botstein GR: Soft tissue rheumatism of the upper extremities: Diagnosis and management. Geriatrics 1990;45:30-43.

Chard MD: The elbow. In Hochberg MC, Silman Aj, Smolen JS et al (eds): Practical Rheumatology, 3rd ed. Philadelphia: Mosby, 2004, pp 205-213.

Gomoll AH, Katz JN, Warner JJP, et al: Rotator cuff disorders: Recognition and management among patients with shoulder pain. Arthritis Rheum 2004;50:3751-3761.

McFarland EG, Sanguanjit P, Tasaki A, et al: Shoulder examination: Established and evolving concepts. J Musculoskel Med 2006;23:57-64.

Reilly P, Macleod I, Macfarlane R, et al: Dead men and radiologists don't lie: A review of cadaveric and radiological studies of rotator cuff tear prevalence. Ann R Coll Surg Engl 2006;88:116-121.

Reveille JD: Soft-tissue rheumatism: Diagnosis and treatment. Am J Med 1997;102:23S-29S.

References

For a complete list of references, log onto www.expertconsult.com.

Systemic Lupus Erythematosus

Bridget Wright, Swati Bharadwaj, and Abby Abelson

DEFINITION

Systemic lupus erythematosus (SLE) is a prototypic autoimmune disease that has a broad range of clinical manifestations. In SLE, tissue damage in multiple organs is caused by autoantibodies and immune complexes. Because other autoimmune diseases, infectious diseases, central nervous system diseases, and fibromyalgia can also manifest with multisystem disease involvement, these other conditions need to be considered when considering a diagnosis of SLE.

EPIDEMIOLOGY

SLE is a disease that can affect persons of all ages and ethnic groups and both sexes, but more than 90% of new patients presenting with SLE are women in the childbearing years. The reported prevalence of SLE is 20-150 per 100,000. In the United States, data from states with large urban populations indicated the prevalence was 104-170 per 100,000 women.[1] This gender disparity is not as prominent in early life (<20 years of age) and later in life (>40 years of age).[2]

The LUMINA (Lupus in Minority population, Nature versus nurture) cohort is providing a more generalizable database for the epidemiology of SLE. LUMINA is a longitudinal outcome study of patients with SLE. This study does not include patients younger than 17 years. Among the LUMINA cohort, 90% of SLE patients are female, 44% are African American, 23% are Latin American, and 32% are white.[3] Based on 2004 data from the National Health and Nutrition Examination Survey (NHANES), the prevalence of SLE patients receiving treatment was 100 per 100,000 among American women.[4]

Although patients with SLE almost uniformly present with a positive antinuclear antibody (ANA) test, other conditions exhibit positive ANAs as well. Craig and colleagues found an ANA titer of 1:64 or greater in 15% of healthy women younger than 40 years and in 24% of women older than 40 years.[5] The American College of Rheumatology criteria for SLE ensure uniformity of patients in research studies.

PATHOPHYSIOLOGY

Patients with SLE have a complex array of abnormalities involving their immune system. Twin studies and genetic linkage studies suggest that heredity plays a role in the development of lupus.[6] Many biochemical studies have revealed abnormalities in T cell function, B cell function, programmed cell death (apoptosis), immune complex clearance, complement function and deficiencies, and nucleosome processing.[7,8] In general, these studies support an abnormal functioning immune system. It is still not clear exactly what starts the immune dysregulation, but it does appear to require a genetically susceptible host affected by either a exogenous trigger or an endogenous metabolic disturbance that causes the loss of tolerance to self antigen.[9,10]

Different ethnic groups have different genetic abnormalities; for example, east Asians with SLE have more cytotoxic T lymphocyte antigen-4 (CTLA-4), and whites with lupus nephritis have more abnormalities in Fc-γ receptors.[11,12] In the future, a specific genetic and immunity-based diagnosis may be given, such as T cell protein kinase type I deficiency.[13]

The majority of the pathology in lupus is related to deposits of immune complex. The immune complexes deposit in various organs, which triggers complement and other mediators of inflammation. Autoantibodies in SLE are directed against a wide variety of self antigens. Autoantibodies directed against nuclear self antigen (ANA) are the most characteristic of SLE.[13] Commonly found target nuclear antigens in SLE include native DNA, denatured DNA, histone, Smith, U1 ribonuclear protein (RNP), SSA, SSB, and ribosomal RNP. Among these, double-stranded DNA (dsDNA) and Smith appear to be unique to SLE. Therefore, it can be helpful, in diagnosing SLE, to look for these more-specific autoantibodies to help in establishing the diagnosis.

CLINICAL PRESENTATION

Constitutional

SLE can affect any of the major organ systems. As its name implies, SLE can also have systemic or constitutional symptoms. These symptoms can mimic other autoimmune diseases, infectious diseases, endocrine abnormalities, chronic fatigue, and fibromyalgia. Because the general symptoms are not specific, it is important to use them along with more organ-specific symptoms that can help differentiate lupus from other diseases. Common symptoms elicited by history include fever, fatigue, weight loss, myalgia, and arthralgia. There are many reports of these nonspecific symptoms with or without rash occurring after sun exposure.

Dermatologic

Lupus was first described as a dermatologic condition. The SLE patient often presents to a physician when the cutaneous manifestations occur. Because of the photosensitive nature of the rash, the prevalence of rash in SLE depends on the region of the world in which the patient lives. It is also important to remember that lupus can be limited to the integumentary system. Box 1 lists the common forms of lupus when it involves the skin.

Red plaques that occur on sun-exposed areas of the body characterize acute cutaneous lupus. Acute cutaneous lupus can have associated alopecia, but the rash and hair loss do not lead to scarring. The malar or butterfly rash is the best-known manifestation of acute cutaneous lupus. The malar rash spares the nasolabial folds; the body of the butterfly is separate from its wings.

Discoid lesions can also occur in systemic lupus but are not as common as the acute cutaneous lupus rash. Discoid lesions are often scarring. The rash of subacute cutaneous lupus often appears as annular rings with crusted margins and spares the mid face. Lupus panniculitis manifests as a deeper rash that is often tender; it can look like erythema nodosum, which is another type of panniculitis. SLE can manifest with a vasculitic type of rash: palpable purpura or pernio. Pernio is an erythematous, often painful area at the tip of a digit seen after cold exposure.

The oral and nasal ulcers of systemic lupus are classically described as painless; however, these lesions may be quite painful. Oral involve-

Box 1 Common Forms of Cutaneous Lupus

Acute cutaneous lupus
Chronic or discoid lupus
Lupus panniculitis
Lupus pernio
Subacute cutaneous lupus
Tumid lupus

ment most commonly affects the posterior aspect of the hard palate. The nasal and oral ulcers usually are recurrent or chronic. Mucous membrane involvement can also involve the vagina. Young sexually active women should be evaluated with this in mind.

Musculoskeletal

The most common initial manifestation of SLE is arthralgia or arthritis,[14] with a frequency of 48% in patients followed for 10 years.[15] Arthralgia, expressed by the patient as pain and stiffness, is more common than objective arthritis. The arthritis in SLE can be migratory and transient; it may be present at the time the patient makes the appointment but resolved by the time of the evaluation. Arthritis in SLE tends to have fewer erosions and fixed deformities compared with rheumatoid arthritis.

There is a clinical condition described as "rhupus." These patients have a rheumatoid arthritis-like presentation along with other characteristics of lupus; this is a rare entity, but one that should be kept in mind. Periarticular inflammation is more common in lupus. This periarticular inflammation often involves the tendon sheaths and can lead to Jaccoud's arthropathy. Jaccoud's arthropathy involves swan-neck deformities of the fingers, which are reducible.[16,17]

Muscle disease is fairly common in SLE. These patients often present with myalgia complaints, and the cause of these muscle pains is not always clear. Again, it is important to recognize that SLE patients often have coexisting fibromyalgia complaints related to chronic disease, poor sleep, inactivity, and depression or mood problems. Some SLE patients have myositis that can be proved by biopsy. The frequency of myositis in lupus patients is approximately 4%. The biopsy is often similar to polymyositis. If myositis is suspected by elevations in the creatine kinase without specific muscle weakness, magnetic resonance imaging (MRI) of the gluteal and upper thigh muscles can be used to look for an abnormal signal, which might lead to a potential biopsy site. It is important to distinguish nonspecific myalgia from myositis, because treatment could be affected.

Osteonecrosis is an important musculoskeletal component of SLE. It can manifest as acute joint pain in patients with advanced disease or during periods of high-dose corticosteroid use. Retrospective studies have shown that higher doses of corticosteroids in the first 6 to 18 months of treatment are associated with osteonecrosis.[18,19] Duration of treatment or disease severity does not correlate with the onset of osteonecrosis.[18] It is important to investigate large joint pain, particularly hip or knee pain, in a patient with SLE. Because the beginning stages of osteonecrosis do not show changes on plain film, MRI should be considered in patients with negative plain films and persistent or unexplained pain. Osteonecrosis can be debilitating, however, and early diagnosis with limited weight bearing can prevent subsequent joint replacement in some.

Pulmonary

Serositis can affect both the cardiac and pulmonary systems, and cardiac and pulmonary serositis often coexist. Most large studies on the outcomes and frequency of particular manifestations of lupus assess for serositis but not for specific types. In patients with lupus followed for 10 years, pleural effusions occur in as many as 50% of patients. These effusions are often small and bilateral but occasionally can be unilateral and quite large. Effusions are often accompanied by pleuritic chest pain. It is important to consider infection in patients with newly diagnosed or longstanding SLE presenting with pleural effusions. Box 2 reviews the results of pleural effusion evaluation in SLE.

Box 2 Findings in Patients with SLE-Related Pleural Effusion

Lupus pleuritis or pleural effusions
Exudate
Normal glucose (low in rheumatoid arthritis)
White blood cell count moderately increased
Polymorphonuclear predominance early
Lymphocyte predominance late
Antinuclear antibodies
Negative cultures

SLE, systemic lupus erythematosus.

Lupus patients can develop other forms of pulmonary disease including shrinking lung, acute pneumonitis, chronic or fibrotic pneumonitis, alveolar hemorrhage, pulmonary hypertension, and thromboembolic-related disease. Shrinking lung is believed to be related to diaphragmatic weakness and decreased chest wall compliance.[20,21] Pulmonary function tests in these patients do not explain the patient's complaints of dyspnea, but chest radiographs reveal bibasilar atelectasis and upward deviation of the diaphragm.

Acute pneumonitis has an abrupt onset with fever, cough, pleuritic chest pain, hemoptysis, and dyspnea. Pulmonary function tests might reveal severe restriction, and pulmonary infiltrates are seen on chest radiography.[22] The incidence of acute pneumonitis is not clear, but Matthay observed an incidence of 11.7% in his SLE population.[22] Infectious causes must always be ruled out in these patients before the diagnosis of acute lupus pneumonitis is entertained. This workup usually requires bronchoscopy with cultures. Biopsies consistent with lupus pneumonitis reveal acute alveolar injury with edema, hyaline membrane formation, and perivascular inflammation.[23] It has been noted that a higher-than-expected percentage of lupus patients with pneumonitis are positive for SSA.[24]

Chronic pneumonitis is an insidious form of lung involvement with progressive dyspnea and diffuse interstitial lung infiltrates on plain chest radiography. Pulmonary function testing shows a restrictive pattern with decreased diffusion capacity. The incidence of chronic lung involvement in lupus is less than 10%.[25]

Pulmonary vascular involvement in lupus is also observed. This includes diffuse alveolar hemorrhage, thromboembolic disease, and pulmonary hypertension. Diffuse alveolar hemorrhage is an emergency manifesting with sudden-onset shortness of breath, dropping hemoglobin, and diffuse infiltrates on chest radiography. Although hemoptysis generally occurs at some point in this illness, less than one half of patients presenting with lupus-related alveolar hemorrhage have this symptom. Bronchoscopy can demonstrate red blood cells and hemosiderin-laden macrophages. These patients require high-dose corticosteroids.

Thromboembolic disease associated with antiphospholipid antibodies can lead to acute pulmonary embolism with acute pulmonary hypertension. Chronic small pulmonary embolisms can be associated with this disease and lead to slowly worsening pulmonary hypertension. Pulmonary hypertension can develop as a sequela from thromboembolic lung disease, but it can also be primary (cor pulmonale). It is important to keep this in mind, especially in patients with breathlessness, normal oximetry, and normal chest radiography, because an echocardiogram can indicate the diagnosis.

Cardiac

Cardiac involvement occurs in 20% to 30% of patients with SLE. It is most common in Latin Americans, followed by African Americans, then whites.[26] Pericardial effusions are seen in about 20% of patients with SLE; however, more than 50% are found to have effusions on autopsy. When symptoms do occur, they include precordial chest pain, which is worse with lying down and relieved with leaning forward. A pericardial rub can often be heard on clinical examination. Many patients with clinically silent disease are found to have pericardial effusions when enlarged cardiac silhouette is seen on chest radiography, fluid is found on computed tomography (CT) of the chest, or echocardiogram obtained for other reasons reveals effusion. It is unusual (<1%) for pericardial effusions related to lupus to progress to tamponade.[27] However, when pericardiocentesis has been necessary, the fluid reveals leukocytosis with neutrophil predominance, low glucose, reduced complement levels, low complement activity, and positive ANA.[27] Pericardial and pleural effusions usually respond to corticosteroid therapy.

Valvular involvement in lupus is common and often asymptomatic. The mitral valve is involved most often. Mitral valve prolapse has been observed in 25% of lupus patients as opposed to 9% of controls.[28] Valvular abnormalities in lupus include vegetations, regurgitation, and valvular stenosis. Because stroke, peripheral embolism, heart failure, death, and infective endocarditis can be associated with valvular abnormalities, cardiac auscultation and palpation should be done routinely. If abnormalities or changes from previous examination are noted, further investigation with echocardiography should be pursued.

Verrucous endocarditis is also common in SLE. Verrucae consist of immune complexes, mononuclear cells, fibrin, and platelet thrombi. In a study using transesophageal echocardiography, 43% of SLE patients were found to have verrucous lesions. Scarring and valve deformation can occur subsequent to the healing of these lesions. These lesions are often asymptomatic; however, awareness of these lesions is important because they can produce emboli or become secondarily infected.

Myocarditis also can occur in SLE but is uncommon. It should be suspected if there is resting tachycardia. Myocarditis can lead to global cardiac dysfunction as well as electrophysiologic abnormalities. Myocardial biopsy may be needed in cases where acute myocarditis is suspected versus fibrosis or myocardial infarction. Treatment for acute myocarditis requires high-dose glucocorticoids plus additional immunosuppression.

Coronary artery disease (CAD) has been recognized in several studies to be increased in patients with SLE compared with the general population, even when traditional cardiac risk factors are eliminated. Important risk factors in lupus patients include use of glucocorticoids, chronic nephritis, antiphospholipid antibodies,[29] and increased oxidative stress.[30] It is important to be aware of the increased incidence of CAD, especially because SLE often affects young women who are traditionally not thought to be at high risk for CAD. Any traditional risk factors for CAD such as smoking, inactivity, obesity, and elevated cholesterol should be addressed in this population. Hypertension should be aggressively controlled, which can be difficult in patients with underlying renal disease. In addition, since women with SLE have a 7- to 50-fold increased risk of CAD, which can lead to significant morbidity and premature death, a high index of suspicion is warranted when SLE patients present with dyspnea, chest pain, chest pressure, decreased exercise tolerance, or atypical symptoms.

Vascular

Raynaud's phenomenon occurs in one third of patients at the onset of SLE, and more than one half develop it during the course of their disease. Unlike Raynaud's phenomenon in systemic sclerosis, patients with lupus rarely develop ischemic digits or digital ulcers. Raynaud's phenomenon can affect the fingers, toes, ears, nose, and even the tongue. It is often triggered by cold, cigarette smoke, caffeine, over-the-counter cold medications, and stress. Livedo reticularis also is commonly seen in lupus patients and is due to spasm of the dermal ascending arterioles.

Venous thromboembolism is known to be associated with antiphospholipid antibody syndrome, which can coexist with SLE. However, venous thromboembolism is also increased in lupus patients who have a history of smoking at the time of diagnosis, increased disease activity over time, increased mean dose of glucocorticoids, shorter disease duration at the time of diagnosis, and presence of lupus anticoagulant.[31]

Lupus patients can also develop inflammatory vascular disease in the form of vasculitis. It is difficult to estimate the incidence of vasculitis in lupus because reporting has been mainly in the form of case reports or series, and the diagnosis of vasculitis is often based on clinical acumen without biopsy-proven vasculitis. Vasculitis in SLE is due to a complex interplay between immune cells, endothelial cells, deposition of autoantibodies, and immune complex deposition. In addition to reports of small- and medium-vessel vasculitis involving all the major organs including the skin, gastrointestinal (GI), pulmonary, cardiac, and genitourinary systems, there are reports of vasculitis affecting the placenta, leading to fetal mortality. There have also been case reports of SLE and Takaysu's arteritis.

Renal

Lupus nephritis is a common and potentially devastating manifestation of lupus. Renal disease in lupus is associated with significant morbidity and mortality. In general, lupus nephritis occurs in more than half of SLE patients. However, there is a disparity between nephritis in Latin Americans and African Americans compared with whites. The incidence of nephritis is 60% for Latin Americans, 69% for African Americans, and 29% for whites.[32]

Although nephritis can occur during a flare of SLE with skin manifestations or other organ system involvement, it often occurs without other clinical signs of active lupus. Thus, it is of key importance that patients with lupus have routine urine analysis with microscopy looking for protein, blood, and cellular casts. Patients can present with constitutional symptoms including fatigue, weight loss, and fever, as well as hypertension and edema, but generally patients do not develop symptoms until late in the disease process of nephritis.

Lupus nephritis is primarily caused by the deposition of immune complexes. The size of the complexes determines the location of deposition and therefore leads to differences in classification (mesangial, focal, diffuse).[33] Once deposited, the immune complexes can set off the complement cascade, producing cellular damage and chemoattractants (C3a and C5a), leading to further recruitment of inflammatory cells. Immune complexes also can lead to upregulation of adhesion molecules on endothelial cells, leading to recruitment of immune cells such as macrophages and T cells, which in turn produce cytokines. Damaged glomerular cells also can produce cytokines that lead to further increase in the inflammatory infiltration.[33-35]

The classification of lupus nephritis is based on renal biopsy. The specific class does give helpful information regarding outcomes and specific therapeutic regimens. If possible, a biopsy should be obtained on any patient in whom renal involvement in suspected. Although there are studies looking at the presence of renal abnormalities in patients with no suspected renal involvement, renal biopsy need not be done routinely on patients with normal creatinine values and normal urine analysis. The 2003 revision of the classification of glomerulonephritis in SLE divides the disease process into six classes, with subdivisions of classes III and IV (Box 3).

The primary complication of lupus nephritis is permanent renal damage. This damage may be severe enough that it leads to renal failure and dependence on dialysis. All of the complications associated with renal failure apply to these patients, such as hypertension, fluid overload, premature vascular calcifications, hyperlipidemia, and premature coronary artery disease.

Gastrointestinal

GI effects from SLE are not clearly defined. SLE can involve any part of the GI tract as a result of disease activity or side effects of medications.[36]

Box 3 International Society of Nephrology/Renal Pathology Society (ISN/RPS) 2003 Classification of Lupus Nephritis

Class I: Minimal mesangial lupus nephritis
Class II: Mesangial proliferative lupus nephritis
Class III: Focal lupus nephritis

- III (A): active lesions
- III (A/C): active and chronic lesions
- III (C): chronic lesions

Class IV: Diffuse lupus nephritis (≥50% of glomeruli)

- Diffuse segmental (IV-S) or global (IV-G) lupus nephritis
- IV (A): active lesions
- IV (A/C): active and chronic lesions
- IV (C): chronic lesions

Class V: Membranous lupus nephritis
Class VI: Advanced sclerosing lupus nephritis (≥90% globally sclerosed glomeruli without residual activity)

Oral Cavity

About one half of patients with systemic lupus have oral ulcers that are usually painful if discoid and painless if erythematous. They tend to be located on the hard palate, on the buccal mucosa, or along the vermilion border.[37] Oral ulcers are one of the nonspecific findings in lupus and are by no means diagnostic of the disease itself. They can support a diagnosis of lupus when present with other lupus symptoms and serologies. In a setting of established lupus they could represent a disease flare, side effects of medications such as methotrexate, or an opportunistic infection. Treatment of oral ulcers is directed at the cause and consists of controlling the disease activity, administering folic or folinic acid (if they are caused by methotrexate), or treating the infection. Symptomatic treatment is directed at relieving the pain with pain medications or local application of crushed 1-mg prednisone tablets.

Esophagus

Lupus patients occasionally complain of dysphagia or odynophagia. This can be multifactorial from hypomotility,[38] from reflux disease, or from candidiasis from immunosuppression. If the symptoms are severe, they deserve a regular dysphagia evaluation with motility studies, x-rays, and maybe an endoscopy. Although treatment is directed at the cause, motility drugs are no longer favored due to their arrythmogenic potential. Antireflux medications or antifungals are used when appropriate.

Abdomen

Abdominal pain is a diagnostic challenge in SLE and is probably one of the most clinically threatening GI manifestation to be aware of. Min and colleagues looked at causes of acute abdominal pain in SLE patients in emergency departments (EDs). They documented that 59.1% of visits to the ED by SLE patients were from pain due to ischemic bowel disease.[39] The other causes were splenic infarcts, renal venous thrombosis, pancreatitis, serositis, upper GI bleeds, pelvic inflammatory disease, and ectopic pregnancy. Peptic ulcer disease with perforation also manifested as an acute abdomen in a small number of patients with SLE and concomitant NSAID use.[37] Medina and colleagues emphasized the importance of early laparotomy in SLE patients with higher SLE disease activity index (SLEDAI) scores and acute abdominal pain. They studied the relation between SLEDAI scores and sources of an acute abdomen in 51 SLE patients and found that patients with intra-abdominal vasculitis (19) or thrombosis (3) had higher SLEDAI scores than 14 patients who had active SLE with non-SLE-related acute abdomen. Fifteen patients with inactive SLE had intra-abdominal pathology unrelated to SLE.[40] Treatment of acute abdominal pain is directed at the cause, with appropriate medical or surgical management of the presenting manifestation.

Intestines

In the bowel, SLE can manifest with vasculitis, malabsorption, or dysmotility.[37] Mesenteric vasculitis in lupus can manifest as an acute abdomen with fever, nausea, vomiting, diarrhea, and rectal bleeding or with the characteristic mesenteric ischemic pain related to meals. The mesenteric involvement can be attributed to either a lupus flare or antiphospholipid antibodies. Suspicion based on a clinical, angiographic, or CT examination of mesenteric vasculitis without bowel perforation warrants an evaluation by a rheumatologist and a possible aggressive therapeutic approach with intravenous steroids with or without other cytotoxic agents, besides the routine treatments with nothing by mouth, IV fluids, cultures, and broad-spectrum antibiotics.[41] If there is intestinal perforation from vasculitis, surgery is the first option followed by cautious start of steroids and cytotoxic agents in the postoperative period. Malabsorption in the form of a protein-losing enteropathy in lupus is uncommon and manifests with diarrhea, abdominal pain, and anasarca. The enteropathy might respond to steroids with or without cytotoxic drugs.

Pancreas

Pancreatitis in lupus is uncommon and could occur in a setting of high SLEDAI scores, antiphospholipid antibody syndrome, and probable steroid use.[37] The more likely causes, as in any other setting, are gallstones, alcohol, and hypertriglyceridemia. Treatment is the same as for pancreatitis from any other cause and includes nothing by mouth, IV fluids, withholding causal drugs, and, rarely, use of steroids if the cause is established by exclusion.

Liver

Drugs, viruses, fatty infiltration, or congestion have been implicated as more common causes of liver enzyme abnormalities in SLE patients.[37] Hepatitis from lupus (lupus hepatitis), although uncommon, manifests as a mild elevation in liver enzymes (aspartate transaminase [AST], alanine transaminase [ALT)], lactate dehydrogenase [LDH], alkaline phosphatase), usually in a setting of active lupus. Such biochemical liver abnormalities from an SLE flare have a tendency to reverse with steroids. Lupoid hepatitis is a separate entity and is considered a subset of chronic active autoimmune hepatitis, where the liver is the main organ of involvement. Patients with lupus hepatitis and lupoid hepatitis can have arthralgias, hypergammaglobulinemia, and positive ANAs.[37] Serologic differentiation may be possible at times and in general involves the presence of anti–ribosomal P and dsDNA autoantibodies in lupus hepatitis versus anti–smooth muscle and auto–liver-kidney-mitochondrial (LKM) antibodies in lupoid hepatitis. Definite differentiation is only possible on histology, which shows a lobular involvement in lupus hepatitis versus rosetting of liver cells and dense lymphoid infiltrate in lupoid hepatitis.

Neuropsychiatric

Neuropsychiatric SLE (NPSLE) could be defined as the neurologic syndromes of the central, peripheral, and autonomic nervous systems and the psychiatric syndromes observed in patients with SLE in which other causes have been excluded.[42,43] NPSLE has many diagnostic and prognostic implications. The American College of Rheumatology (ACR) committee has developed 19 NPSLE case definitions with diagnostic criteria, exclusions, associations, and ascertainment, as well as reporting standards. The complete case definitions are on the ACR website (http://www.rheumatology.org). The proposed pathologic mechanisms of NPSLE are highly complex and poorly understood. They could be vasculopathic (injury, infarcts, accelerated atherosclerosis, perivascular inflammation), occasionally vasculitic, autoantibody mediated (antiphospholipid, antineuronal, anti-RNP), steroid mediated, or biochemically mediated.

Neurologic Manifestations

Neurologic manifestations can be primary (from SLE) or secondary (due to disease complications and treatment). They can then be either organic or functional (psychosis).

Seizures occur in one third of the cases and portend a poor overall prognosis.[44] They could be generalized or partial and simple or complex and can be acute or from chronic scarring. For seizures, treatment data are scarce, and appropriate antiseizure medications are used along with a short course of steroids if there is an SLE flare.

CNS vasculitis tends to manifest with fevers, headaches, cognitive deficits, and confusion in the setting of serologic and radiologic markers of a lupus flare and can rapidly progress to seizures, loss of consciousness, and psychosis. Evaluation requires a brain MRI, magnetic resonance angiogram (MRA), and a spinal tap. Treatment is intravenous pulse steroids followed by oral steroids and cyclophosphamide.

Headaches in lupus are very common, but they have been reported to have no causal relation, no association with disease severity, and no particular mechanisms and require the regular headache evaluation, unless there are sudden headaches in a person who was previously free of headache and who has neurologic and psychiatric changes.[45] SLE headaches are managed as usual headaches unless there is a definite lupus flare.

Stroke can occur in 19% of patients either from a lupus flare or from secondary antiphospholipid antibody syndrome.[46] Treatment for stroke is empirical and is tailored to each patient based on the presentation. General principles of aggressive primary and secondary stroke prevention also apply in a lupus patient. If a stroke is from high antiphospholipid antibody (APLA) titers, chronic anticoagulation is recommended if there is no concomitant danger of intracranial hemorrhage. If this is catastrophic APLA syndrome, plasmapheresis, pulse steroids, and cytoxan are also considered. If the stroke is from a lupus flare (i.e., is not thrombotic), steroids with or without cytoxan traditionally have been used.[47]

Neuropathies can be peripheral, autonomic, or cranial.[48] Wrist drops and foot drops occasionally result from peripheral nerve vasculitis. Besides an electromyogram (EMG), a nerve biopsy could also be obtained. For EMG-positive peripheral neuropathy, initial treatment is typically higher doses of prednisone, especially in patients with sensorimotor loss, along with neurontin or tricyclic antidepressants. Steroid-sparing agents such as imuran may be used thereafter. If the EMG is negative, neurontin or a tricyclic antidepressant should suffice. With cranial neuropathies, the mainstay of treatment is higher doses of prednisone.

Movement disorders (chorea and ataxia) tend to be self-limited without treatment.

Transverse myelitis is coincident with a lupus flare and is a rheumatologic emergency. This manifests with a sudden onset of lower extremity weakness or sensory loss plus loss of rectal and urinary bladder sphincter control, usually with clinical symptoms of a lupus flare.[49] Transverse myelitis needs to be aggressively treated with pulse steroids followed by 1 mg/kg oral prednisone, cytoxan, and, sometimes, plasmapheresis.[50]

Ophthalmic involvement can occur as a rash on the eyelids, keratoconjuctivitis, retinal vasculitis, retrobulbar optic neuritis, or retinal vein or artery occlusions.[51] Eye involvement can result from SLE or concomitant APLA. Ophthalmic treatment options are prednisone, plaquenil, and occasionally cytoxan for optic neuritis that does not respond to prednisone. If there is retinal artery or vein involvement from APLA, anticoagulation should be considered.

Meningitis in SLE is rare and has a CSF picture of aseptic meningitis.

Psychiatric Manifestations

Psychiatric manifestations of SLE can be either primary and organic (psychosis, cognitive dysfunction, dementia) or secondary and functional (depression, anxiety, mania, personality disorders). The distinction should be based on psychological testing and on diagnostic studies such as CT, MRI, electroencephalography, evoked potential studies, cerebrospinal fluid studies, and single-photon emission CT (SPECT).[52]

Psychosis occurs in about 5% of SLE patients either from the lupus itself or from steroids and is a diagnosis of exclusion. Besides antipsychotic medications and a strong social support system, high doses of intravenous steroids have been used for a few weeks in divided doses. Cytoxan or azathioprine can also be tried if there has been no improvement with steroids in a couple of weeks.

Cognitive disorders are common and occur in 20% to 80% of patients. Treatment is based on the cause (drug or disease) and should also involve cognitive retraining. Dementia is severe cognitive dysfunction from multiple small ischemic strokes that may be worsened by high doses of steroids; therefore social support and antidepressants are key.[53]

Neonatal Lupus

Neonatal lupus occurs in 1% to 2% of babies.[54] At-risk babies are those born to mothers with SLE, anti-Ro/SSA, and anti-La/SSB. These babies are at risk for neonatal heart blocks, AV nodal damage due to binding of antibodies, and, rarely, sinoatrial node damage. They can have partial or complete heart blocks, bradycardia, and a self-limited erythematous annular rash on the scalp and periorbital area. Fetal bradycardia during routine fetal auscultation, ultrasound, or echocardiogram in a high-risk mother should raise suspicion of neonatal heart block. Other uncommon manifestations are transposition of the great vessels, ostium primum atrial septal defect, ventricular septal defect, endocardial fibroelastosis, and myocarditis. Other systemic manifestations reported are hepatobiliary and hematologic.

Prenatal screening in high-risk mothers is important and guides the use of fetal echocardiograms. Fetal echocardiograms are routinely done once a week in the second trimester and then every other week until 32 weeks' gestation.

A pediatric rheumatologist should be involved early. Fetal monitoring in high-risk pregnancies and postnatal monitoring in affected babies are important. Incomplete heart block in the fetus tends to respond to fluorinated glucocorticoids if started immediately and continued until delivery. It is usually stopped if there is no response in 4 to 6 weeks. A baby with complete heart block might need a pacemaker.

Drug-Induced Lupus

Drug-induced lupus is epidemiologically, clinically, and serologically different from SLE. The male-to-female distribution is equal and the average age is 50 years. The most common drugs implicated are isoniazid, hydralazine, and procainamide. Other drugs implicated include minocycline, aldomet, diltiazem, penicillamine, infliximab, etanercept, rifampin, quinidine, captopril, beta blockers, anticonvulsants, sulfa, and amiodarone.

Most patients present with arthralgias or arthritis, and about one half of the patients have serositis. Organ involvement is uncommon in drug-induced lupus. Serologically, 95% of patients are antihistone positive, and the Sm and dsDNA are rarely positive. In comparison, in SLE, most patients are dsDNA positive and 80% are antihistone positive.[55]

Diagnosis should be suspected with acute lupus-like clinical signs and symptoms not involving a major organ and antihistone antibodies without dsDNA antibodies in the setting of an offending drug. Besides stopping the implicated medication, other treatment options are NSAIDs, antimalarials, and sometimes steroids and cytotoxic agents for drug-induced vasculitis or serositis. The disease tends to resolve within 6 months of discontinuing the drug.

Antiphospholipid Antibody Syndrome

APLA syndrome can be primary (idiopathic) or secondary (e.g., from SLE, infection, drugs). It causes arterial and venous thromboses leading to strokes, myocardial infarction, pulmonary embolism, deep venous thrombosis, fetal loss, anemia, thrombocytopenia, and livedo reticularis–like skin rash. In the clinical setting of lupus, an elevated partial thromboplastin time (PTT) should raise the suspicion of the presence of APLAs. Suspicion should be higher in an SLE patient who suffers a thrombotic event.

Besides a rapid plasma reagin, which gives a false-positive lupus anticoagulant test result, evaluation should involve a detailed lupus anticoagulant panel, which should ideally include prothrombin time (PT), activated PTT, dRVVT/KCT (dilute Russell's viper venom time and kaolin clotting time), mixing study, hex phase screen, hex phase confirm, platelet neutralization, and circulating anticoagulant. Lupus anticoagulant can be present in healthy subjects and can be transient in infections, and its presence should be interpreted in the right clinical and serologic settings. High-titer immunoglobulin (Ig) G/IgM cardiolipin antibodies and β2 glycoprotein have been associated with higher risk of thrombotic events and should also be tested.

For a definite diagnosis of APLA, the ACR has criteria. Briefly, frequent miscarriages and stillbirths or one or more clinical episodes of arterial or venous thrombosis confirmed by imaging or histology and the presence of lupus anticoagulant or medium to high titer IgG/IgM cardiolipin antibody or β2 glycoprotein antibody on at least two occasions 6 weeks apart is confirmatory for APLA syndrome.

Treatment is mainly anticoagulation and must be tailored to the clinical setting.[56] In a patient with thrombosis and positive ALPA, heparin initially followed by long-term warfarin therapy is recommended. In a patient with positive ALPA but no thrombotic events, a trial of prophylactic aspirin 81 mg daily (clopidogrel for patients allergic to aspirin) or aspirin with plaquenil have been tried. In catastrophic APLA with organ damage, anticoagulation and high-dose intravenous steroids for 3 days followed by 1 to 2 mg/kg of prednisone daily have been used with or without plasmapheresis. Cyclophosphamide may be added and is most useful in a concomitant acute lupus flare. The traditional belief has been that primary APLA syndrome might not respond to cytotoxic therapy; however, cyclophosphamide is sometimes lifesaving in catastrophic APLA syndrome by an unknown mechanism. Intravenous immune globulin has also been tried in APLA-associated microangiopathies.

DIAGNOSIS

Diagnosis of SLE is made on clinical criteria supported by serologic data and appropriate imaging studies and biopsies as indicated. The ACR criteria for SLE are available on the ACR website. Four of 11 criteria are required to make a diagnosis of SLE. Although the criteria are helpful, not all patients fulfill these criteria clinically, and criteria have to be used with caution in clinical settings.

Tests

A patient referred for incidental positive ANA should have a careful history and physical examination to look for clinical findings of SLE. Not all patients with a positive ANA have SLE or a connective tissue disease. Two percent to 5% of healthy persons carry a low to moderate positive ANA. On the other hand, if there is a clinical suspicion of SLE, a detailed workup should be initiated with appropriate blood tests, urine tests, x-rays, and other studies that may be required based on the presentation.

In an outpatient setting, most rheumatologists order a white blood cell count (WBC) with differential, comprehensive metabolic panel (CMP), erythrocyte sedimentation rate (ESR), C-reactive protein (CRP), ANA panel, Smith, RNP, SSA and SSB, complements C3 and C4, dsDNA, and a urine analysis. Most rheumatologists also screen their patients for tuberculosis, hepatitis, thyroid diseases, and pregnancy, because a positive test affects the choice of immunosuppression and future follow-up. It is also worthwhile to check for APLAs (lupus anticoagulant, cardiolipin antibodies, and β2 microglobulin) because SLE and APLA commonly coexist and are often found together in patients with prior thrombotic events or frequent miscarriages.

If one suspects primary Sjögren's syndrome, rheumatoid factor (RF), cryoglobulin levels, and β2 microglobulins should be checked. Primary Sjögren's syndrome patients tend to have a positive ANA, rheumatoid factor, and SSA or SSB. Occasionally these patients have sicca symptoms and negative laboratory results, in which case a lip biopsy with a focus score is required to prove or disprove the diagnosis of primary Sjögren's syndrome. Sjögren's syndrome, however, can also be secondary to any underlying connective tissue disease, especially SLE and rheumatoid arthritis.

Other diagnostic tests are ordered as indicated and consist of joint x-rays and chest x-ray; renal ultrasound; CT scans of the chest, abdomen, and pelvis; echocardiograms; CT angiograms; electromyography and nerve conduction tests; neuropsychiatric testing; vascular studies; and biopsies of the skin, kidneys, nerves, and lungs.

Diagnosis

In the right clinical setting, leukopenia or lymphopenia, anemia, or thrombocytopenia with a positive ANA of 1:60 or higher suggests a diagnosis of SLE. The ANA panel might exhibit antibody patterns such as dsDNA, RNP, Smith, SSA, SSB, or histones. If it does, other multisystem diseases should be considered in addition to SLE, including Sjögren's syndrome, myositis, or drug-induced lupus, depending on the clinical features and autoantibodies isolated.

Table 1 lists some of the common tests and expected abnormalities, the possible mechanisms, clinical features, autoantibodies, and suggested specificities.[57] This table is not a standardized guideline, and tests can vary in different clinical settings. The clinical assessment and tests must be combined to make an appropriate diagnosis of SLE.

Assessing Organ Risk and Activity

If the SLE is active, the ESR and CRP are usually elevated, although sometimes they are normal. The complements C3 and C4 are usually low, especially in the setting of organ involvement such as the kidneys, but they can also be normal. A urine analysis is very important, and one must look for evidence of microscopic blood and proteinuria. If there is proteinuria, a 24-hour urine protein-to-creatinine ratio should be checked. If the dipstick is positive for blood, the urine should be manually spun in a centrifuge to look for dysmorphic red cells, granular casts, hyaline casts, and red blood cell or mixed casts to rule out renal involvement from SLE. Red cell casts and mixed casts tend to suggest inflammatory activity in the glomeruli and usually indicate the need for a kidney biopsy and referral to a nephrologist. If other organs are involved, such as the brain, lungs, or GI tract, appropriate laboratory, imaging, and biopsy studies may be required.

Follow-up Data

If immunosuppressive treatment is started with methotrexate, azathioprine, or mycophenolate mofetil, the complete blood count (CBC), basic metabolic profile, liver function tests, ESR, and CRP are usually monitored every month for the first 3 months and every 2 months for the next 6 months, and then the intervals are gradually

Table 1 Diagnostic Tests for Systemic Lupus Erythematosus

Test	Possible Abnormalities	Mechanism	Significance and Use
CBC plus differential	Anemia, thrombocytopenia, leukopenia, lymphopenia, occasional neutropenia	Autoantibodies to RBCs (Coombs), lymphocytes, platelets	Disease activity markers for SLE and APLA Monitor drug side effects
Basic metabolic panel	Elevated BUN/Cr ratio	Immune complex glomerulonephritis in SLE Renal artery thrombosis from APLA	Diagnosis Follow SLE nephritis Monitor drug side effects
ESR and CRP	Elevated	Inflammatory markers	Disease activity marker for follow-up if elevated at diagnosis
Complements (C3, C4)	Low	Immune complex consumption	Disease activity marker Low C3 and C4 can also be seen in some primary complement deficiencies
Urine chemistry	Proteinuria, hematuria, RBCs, red cell and mixed casts	Glomerulonephritis or glomerular damage	SLE nephritis and/or nephrotic syndrome
LFTs	Elevated transaminases and/or alkaline phosphatase Low protein or albumin	Unknown mechanism or concomitant NSAID use	Lupus hepatitis, nephrotic syndrome (low albumin), drug side effects
ANA (IFA + EIA)	Useful as a screening test +ANA > 1:80 or ≥1:60 in right clinical setting are suggestive, although not diagnostic, of SLE Titers > 1:640: look harder for ANA+ diseases if no obvious symptoms		ANA-negative lupus is rare (manifests with photosensitivity, Raynaud's syndrome, rash, serositis) ANA+ can be present in 2%-5% of healthy people and in other CTDs some of which are RA, JIA, scleroderma, MCTD, Sjögren's syndrome, dermatomyositis, polymyositis, Hashimoto's thyroiditis, lupoid hepatitis, and (occasionally) as an epiphenomenon in cancer, hepatitis, or transient infections ANA is not a disease activity marker and is mainly diagnostic
ENA panel	Anti-Sm, anti-RNP, antihistone, anti-SSA/Ro, anti-SSB/La, antiribosomal P, SCL-70, and anticentromere These are not disease activity markers and are purely diagnostic	Antibodies to specific nuclear proteins	Anti-Sm: Highly specific for SLE Anti-histone: drug-induced lupus (95%) and SLE (80%) Anti-SSA/SSB: primary Sjögren's syndrome, SCLE, neonatal lupus and SLE with secondary Sjögren's syndrome Anti-RNP: SLE (musculoskeletal, Raynaud's phenomenon), MCTD Antiribosomal P: SLE (psychiatric and CNS) SCL-70: systemic sclerosis Anticentromere: CREST syndrome
dsDNA antibody	Positive Higher titers seem to predict disease severity at times	Antibodies to the dsDNA	Diagnostic of SLE May be used as a disease activity marker Absent in drug-induced lupus Higher titers in renal involvement
APLAs	Lupus anticoagulant panel, cardiolipin antibody panel, β2 glycoprotein	Antibodies to membrane phospholipids	Moderate to high titers of IgG and IgM in primary or secondary APLA syndrome

APLA, antiphospholipid antibody; BUN, blood urea nitrogen; CBC, complete blood count; CNS, central nervous system; Cr, creatinine; CREST, calcinosis, Raynaud's syndrome, esophageal involvement, sclerodactyly, telangiectasia; CRP, C-reactive protein; CTD, connective tissue disease; dsDNA, double-stranded DNA; EIA, enzyme immunoassay; ENA, extractable nuclear antigens; ESR, erythrocyte sedimentation rate; IFA, immunofluorescent antibody; Ig, immunoglobulin; JIA, juvenile idiopathic arthritis; LFTs, liver function tests; MCTD, mixed connective tissue disease; NSAID, nonsteroidal anti-inflammatory drug; RA, rheumatoid arthritis; RBC, red blood cell count; RNP, ribonuclear protein; SCLE, subacute cutaneous lupus erythematosus; SLE, systemic lupus erythematosus; SS, Sjögren's syndrome.

increased if the results are acceptable. The frequency of blood tests depends on the choice of immunosuppressive medications. Cyclophosphamide requires more frequent monitoring than the other cytotoxic agents and should be done by a rheumatologist on a regular basis. Use of hydroxychloroquine requires only annual eye examinations and is usually used in mild SLE with mucocutaneous, skin, joint, or serosal symptoms without organ involvement.

The dsDNA, C3, C4, ESR, CRP, CBC, basic metabolic profile, liver function tests, and urine sediment can all be used as markers of disease activity. When there is more systemic involvement, such as the lungs and brain, appropriate imaging studies should also be followed periodically.

TREATMENT

Treatment options include steroids, hydroxychloroquine, dapsone, azathioprine, methotrexate, mycophenolate mofetil, cyclophosphamide, and rituximab. Two studies of lupus treatment of randomized controlled trials (RCTs) were recently published. The EXPLORER (Efficacy and Safety of Rituximab in Patients with SLE) was a phase II/III randomized, double-blind, placebo-controlled multicenter trial evaluated treatment with rituximab in patients with active SLE but excluded patients with active nephritis, or who were being treated with high-dose prednisone or cytoxan. Preliminary results concluded that rituximab was not superior to rituximab in these patients. The

LUNAR Study (Efficacy and Safety of Rituximab in patients with ISN/PRS Class II or III lupus nephritis was a phase III randomized, double-blind, placebo-controlled trial that compared the efficacy and safety of rituximab plus mycophenylate with placebo plus mycophenylate in SLE patients with proliferative nephritis. Preliminary results showed that rituximab plus mycophenylate was *not* superior to mycophenylate. Treatments have been discussed briefly with each section separately. Because SLE has a wide spectrum of symptoms and organ involvement, treatment strategies must be individualized for each patient, the organ system involved, and the severity of involvement. Immunosuppressive agents should be used only after infection and malignancy have been ruled out. In patients undergoing immunosuppressive treatment, physicians must continue to be vigilant for infections, both common and opportunistic, and for malignancies. Care of patients with SLE involves ongoing assessment of the patient's lupus activity and other comorbid conditions.

Osteoporosis prevention and treatment (especially in patients taking steroids), lipid and blood pressure control, antibiotic prophylaxis, and vigilant ongoing age-appropriate malignancy screenings are all treatment measures that are essential for the care of patients with SLE.

Standardized measures of disease activity such as SLICC (Systemic Lupus International Collaborating Clinics), BILAG (British Isles Lupus Assessment Group), and SLE activity scales are usually used in research settings. The SLICC/ACR damage index for SLE encompasses net damage from disease, treatment, or other events. A full history, physical examination, and serologic data such as complements, dsDNA, inflammatory markers, and a urine analysis can be used as markers of disease activity.

OUTCOME AND PROGNOSIS

Even with better survival rates, the mortality rate from SLE is still three times higher than the general population. Prognosis is worse in African American patients, in patients with early-onset disease, and in patients with renal, cardiopulmonary, and CNS involvement. Treatment of SLE with immunosuppressive drugs and cytotoxic agents can result in significant morbidity and mortality from concomitant infections. However, the prognosis for SLE patients in the United States has improved dramatically since the 1950s due to improved diagnostic methods, vigilant follow-up, and newer treatment options. Ongoing research and clinical progress will help improve prognosis and the future quality of life of patients with SLE.

Summary

- SLE is a prototypic autoimmune disease that can manifest with symptoms involving multiple organ systems in all ages and both sexes, but most initially presenting patients are women of childbearing age.
- The diagnosis of SLE is based on clinical features and the presence of autoantibodies. High-titer IgG antibodies to dsDNA and antibodies to the Smith antigen are both specific for SLE.
- ANAs are positive in more than 95% of patients with SLE, so repeated negative tests make the diagnosis unlikely. Positive ANAs, especially in low titers, can be seen in up to 30% of healthy persons.
- Lupus manifestations of nephritis, cardiovascular disease, neurologic disease, pulmonary disease and hematologic syndromes can require urgent intervention with immunosuppressive therapies.
- Patients with SLE are at higher risk for some malignancies.
- Patients with SLE are at higher risk of cardiovascular disease and stroke, and the excess risk is not explained by traditional risk factors.
- When patients with SLE taking immunosuppressive therapy present with additional symptoms that could result from flares of their disease, they must be evaluated to rule out infection before increasing their immunosuppression.

Suggested Readings

Buyon JP, Clancy RM: Neonatal lupus syndromes. Curr Opin Rheumatol 2003;15:535-541.

Buyon JP, Petri MA, Kim MY, et al: The effect of combined estrogen and progesterone hormone replacement therapy on disease activity in systemic lupus erythematosus: A randomized trial. Ann Intern Med 2005;142(12 Pt 1):953-962.

Calvo-Alen J, Toloza SM, Fernandez M, et al: Systemic lupus erythematosus in a multiethnic US cohort (LUMINA). XXV. Smoking, older age, disease activity, lupus anticoagulant, and glucocorticoid dose as risk factors for the occurrence of venous thrombosis in lupus patients. Arthritis Rheum 2005; 52(7):2060-2068.

Cervera R, Khamashta MA, Font J, et al: Morbidity and mortality in systemic lupus erythematosus during a 10-year period: A comparison of early and late manifestations in a cohort of 1,000 patients. Medicine (Baltimore) 2003;82(5):299-308.

D'Cruz DP, Khamashta MA, Hughes GR: Systemic lupus erythematosus. Lancet 2007;369(9561):587-596.

Greco TP, Conti-Kelly AM, Matsuura E, et al: Antiphospholipid antibodies in patients with coronary artery disease: New cardiac risk factors? Ann N Y Acad Sci 2007;1108:466-474.

Hanly JG: ACR classification criteria for systemic lupus erythematosus: Limitations and revisions to neuropsychiatric variables. Lupus 2004;13(11):861-864.

Jennekens FG, Kater L: The central nervous system in systemic lupus erythematosus. Part 1. Clinical syndromes: A literature investigation. Rheumatology (Oxford) 2002;41(6):605-618.

Joseph G, Lammie, GA, Scolding, NJ: CNS lupus: A study of 41 patients. Neurology 2007;69:644-654.

Lockshin MD, Erkan D: Treatment of the antiphospholipid syndrome. N Engl J Med 2003;349:1177-1179.

Maksimowicz-McKinnon K, Magder LS, Petri M: Predictors of carotid atherosclerosis in systemic lupus erythematosus. J Rheumatol 2006;33(12):2458-2463.

Oelke K, Richardson B: Pathogenesis of lupus. Arthritis Rheum 2002;47(3):343-345.

Peponis V, Kyttaris VC, Tyradellis C, et al: Ocular manifestations of systemic lupus erythematosus: A clinical review. Lupus 2006;15(1):3-12.

Petri M: Monitoring systemic lupus erythematosus in standard clinical care. Best Pract Res Clin Rheumatol 2007;21(4):687-697.

Uribe AG, McGwin G Jr, Reveille JD, Alarcon GS: What have we learned from a 10-year experience with the LUMINA (Lupus in Minorities; Nature vs. Nurture) cohort? Where are we heading? Autoimmun Rev 2004;3(4):321-329.

Zoma A. Musculoskeletal involvement in systemic lupus erythematosus. Lupus 2004;13(11):851-853.

References

For a complete list of references, log onto www.expertconsult.com.

Systemic Scleroderma

Soumya Chatterjee

DEFINITION AND ETIOLOGY

Scleroderma, or systemic sclerosis (SSc), is a chronic multisystem autoimmune disease characterized by a vasculopathy, diffuse fibrosis of skin and various internal organs, and immune abnormalities. The clinical manifestations of this disease are extremely heterogeneous and depend on the presence and degree of various internal organ involvement.

CLASSIFICATION

There are two major forms of scleroderma, localized scleroderma and systemic scleroderma (sclerosis). Diffuse (dcSSc) and limited (lcSSc) scleroderma are the two main types of systemic sclerosis.

Localized Scleroderma

The more common form of the disease, localized scleroderma, only affects the skin without any internal organ involvement. It often appears in the form of waxy patches (morphea) (Fig. 1A), or streaks on the skin (linear scleroderma). It is not uncommon for this less-severe form of scleroderma to regress or stop progressing without treatment (Box 1). Localized scleroderma can be disfiguring and sometimes requires systemic therapy to control disease activity.

Systemic Scleroderma

Systemic scleroderma always leads to some internal organ involvement. It is further divided into two subsets of disease, limited or diffuse (see Box 1). According to LeRoy and colleagues, limited or diffuse disease is based on the extent of skin tightening.[1] In limited disease (formerly called CREST [*c*alcinosis, *R*aynaud's phenomenon, *e*sophageal dysmotility, *s*clerodactyly, and *t*elangiectasias] syndrome), skin tightening is confined to the fingers, hands, and forearms distal to the elbows, with or without tightening of skin of the feet and of the legs distal to the knees. Proximal extremities and the trunk are not involved. In diffuse disease or diffuse cutaneous systemic sclerosis (dcSSc), the skin of the proximal extremities and trunk is also involved. Both dcSSc and lcSSc are associated with internal organ involvement; however, patients with dcSSc are at greater risk for clinically significant major organ dysfunction (Box 2). Systemic sclerosis sine scleroderma (ssSSc) is a rare disorder in which patients develop vascular and fibrotic damage to internal organs (phenotypically similar to that in limited scleroderma), in the absence of cutaneous sclerosis.

EPIDEMIOLOGY

Systemic scleroderma is a rare disorder, with an annual incidence in the United States of about 20 cases per 1 million adults.[2] Several studies have estimated the prevalence of systemic sclerosis in the United States to be around 240 cases per 1 million adults.[3] International reports from Britain and Japan suggest a lower prevalence of around 35 cases per 1 million adults.[3] Women are roughly four times more likely than men to develop systemic scleroderma. African Americans are at greater risk for diffuse disease.[2,3] Most patients with systemic scleroderma present in the third or fourth decade of life.

Age- and gender-adjusted mortality rates for patients with dcSSc are approximately five to eight times greater than those of the general population.[3] Survival, which is strongly dependent on the degree of internal organ involvement, has improved over the past few decades due to the advent of newer classes of drugs. The average 10-year survival rate is now 70% to 80%.[4] Diffuse disease has a variable disease course, but it still carries a relatively poor prognosis. Progressive pulmonary fibrosis, pulmonary hypertension, severe gastrointestinal involvement, and scleroderma heart disease are the main causes of death. Limited disease has a relatively better prognosis except when pulmonary hypertension develops as a late complication. In a large cohort of patients in metropolitan Detroit, the poor prognostic markers were found to be older age at onset, male gender, African American race, and involvement of certain organ systems (heart, interstitial lung disease, pulmonary hypertension, and severe gastrointestinal disease).[2]

PATHOPHYSIOLOGY AND PATHOGENESIS

Scleroderma is characterized by immune system activation, endothelial dysfunction, and enhanced fibroblast activity.[5]

The earliest stage in the development of the scleroderma lesion is endothelial cell activation and vascular damage, the precise inciting events of which are unknown. This is followed by the extravasation of inflammatory cells, which initially are of the monocytic lineage. Later, there is a lymphocyte-predominant infiltrate. Eventually, a population of fibroblasts is activated. The autonomous activated fibroblasts continue to produce the excessive extracellular matrix that underlies the ultimate fibrotic pathology of scleroderma. Within the advanced lesional skin, there is very little visible evidence of ongoing inflammation, suggesting that this is a self-perpetuating fibrotic process.

The endothelium contributes to the regulation of the contraction and relaxation of vascular smooth muscle cells through the production and release of endothelium-derived vasoactive substances including prostacyclin (prostaglandin [PG]I_2), endothelium-derived relaxing factor (EDRF or nitric oxide), and endothelin. The impairment of endothelium-dependent vascular smooth muscle relaxation has been confirmed by the evidence of reduced serum levels of nitric oxide and prostacyclin in scleroderma. This state is probably worsened by increased endothelin levels that contribute to vasospasm and smooth muscle hypertrophy.

Vascular injury occurs before clinically evident fibrosis. There is an altered functional state of the endothelium characterized by increased permeability, enhanced vasoreactivity, enhanced expression of adhesion molecules, altered balance between hemostatic and fibrinolytic factors, platelet activation, and altered vascular wall growth. Most damage occurs at the level of the cutaneous circulation and in the microvasculature of various internal organs.[4] Small arteries and capillaries constrict. Fibroproliferative changes in the vasculature ensue later, eventually leading to obliteration of the vascular lumen, resulting in ischemia.

Endothelin-1 plays an important role in the pathogenesis of scleroderma. Elevated plasma endothelin is seen in scleroderma-associated pulmonary hypertension. During an episode of Raynaud's phenomenon, endothelin release is augmented. Increased endothelin-1 is also found in the bronchoalveolar lavage fluid from scleroderma patients and in prescleroderma skin and early diffuse skin lesions. Scleroderma lung fibroblasts shows elevated endothelin-1 expression and increases in endothelin-1 binding sites.

There are many other potent mediators of tissue fibrosis that are believed to play an important role in the pathogenesis of sclero-

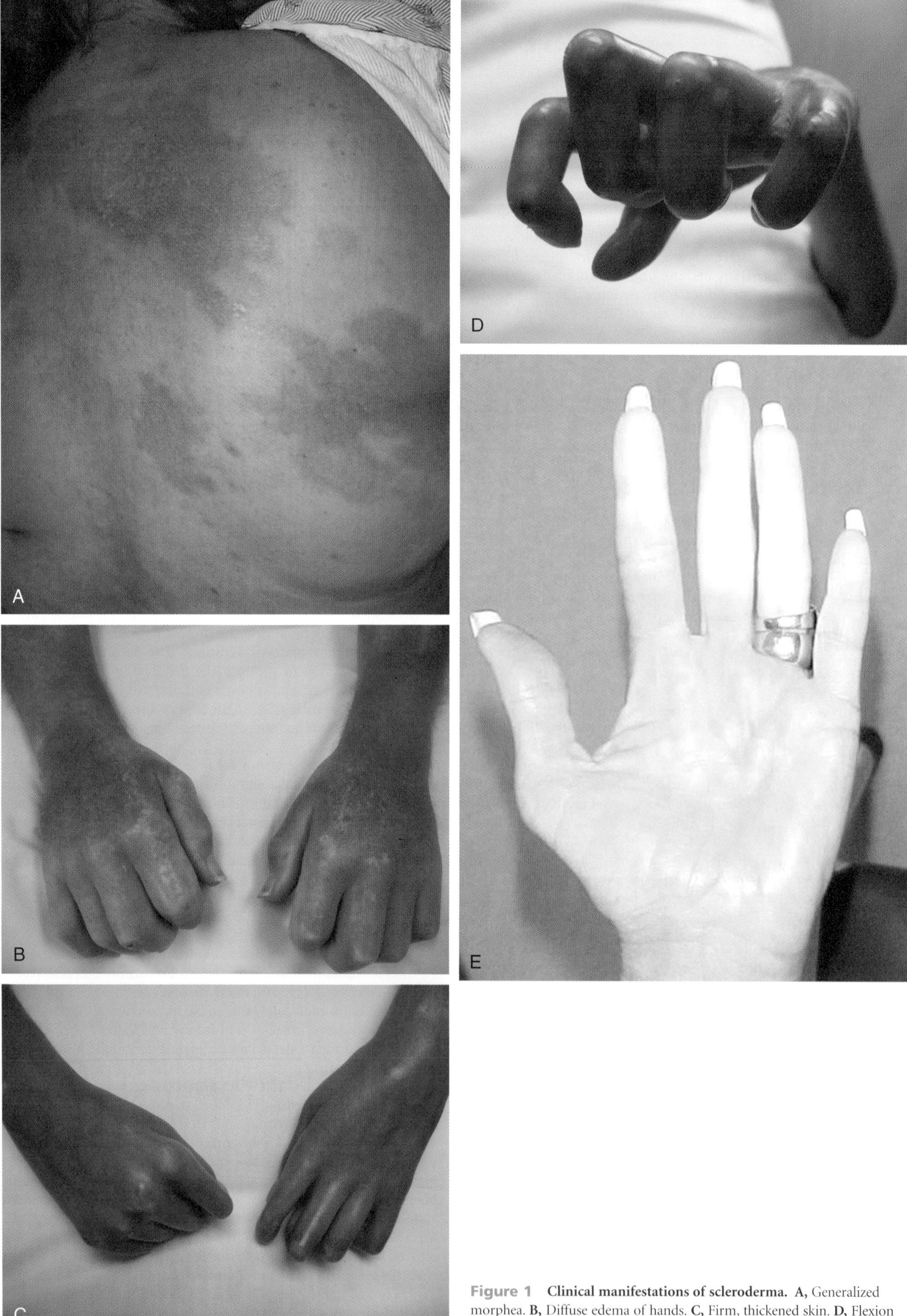

Figure 1 Clinical manifestations of scleroderma. A, Generalized morphea. **B,** Diffuse edema of hands. **C,** Firm, thickened skin. **D,** Flexion contractures of fingers. **E,** Raynaud's phenomenon (pallor phase).

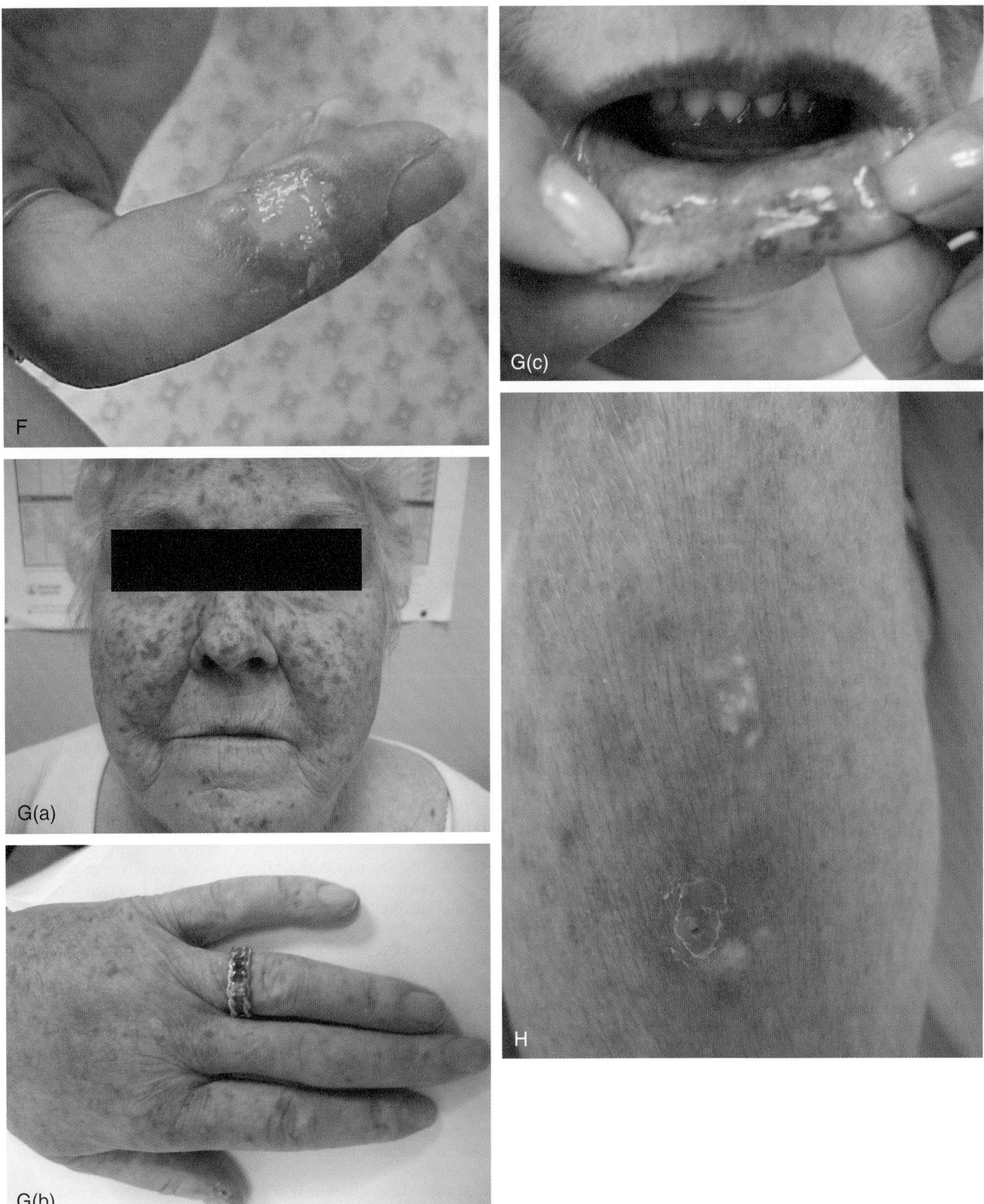

Figure 1, cont'd **F,** Ischemic digital ulcer. **G,** Telangectasias on the face *(a)*, dorsum of the hand *(b)*, mucosa *(c)*. **H,** Calcinosis cutis.

Box 1 Classification of Scleroderma

Localized Scleroderma (Localized cutaneous fibrosis)
Limited or generalized morphea: Circumscribed patches of sclerosis
Linear scleroderma: Linear lesions seen in childhood
En coup de sabre: Linear lesions of the scalp or face

Systemic Scleroderma (Cutaneous and noncutaneous involvement)
Limited cutaneous systemic sclerosis (lcSSc), formerly called CREST syndrome (calcinosis of the digits, *R*aynaud's phenomenon, esophageal dysmotility, sclerodactyly, and *t*elangiectasias)
Diffuse cutaneous systemic sclerosis (dcSSc): Sclerosis of proximal extremities, trunk, and face
Systemic sclerosis sine scleroderma (ssSSc): Organ fibrosis only; no skin thickening

Box 2 Subsets of Systemic Sclerosis

Diffuse Cutaneous Systemic Sclerosis (dcSSc)
Onset of Raynaud's within 1 year of onset of skin changes (puffy or hidebound skin)
Truncal and acral skin involvement
Presence of tendon friction rubs
Early and significant incidence of interstitial lung disease, oliguric renal failure, diffuse gastrointestinal disease, and myocardial involvement
Absence of anticentromere antibodies
Nailfold capillary dilation and capillary destruction
Antitopoisomerase antibodies (30% of patients)

Limited Cutaneous Systemic Sclerosis (LcSSc)
Raynaud's phenomenon for years (occasionally decades)
Skin involvement limited to hands, face, feet, and forearms (acral) or absent
A significant late incidence of pulmonary hypertension, with or without interstitial lung disease, trigeminal neuralgia, skin calcifications, telangiectasias
A high incidence of anticentromere antibodies (70%-80%)
Dilated nailfold capillary loops, usually without capillary dropout

Adapted from LeRoy EC, Black C, Fleischmajer R, et al: Scleroderma (systemic sclerosis): Classification, subsets and pathogenesis. J Rheumatol 1988;15:202-205.

derma. One of the key factors that has received the most attention as a very potent profibrotic factor, indirectly implicated very strongly in the pathogenesis of systemic sclerosis, is transforming growth factor (TGF)-β1. A number of studies have shown that TGF-β1 is a potent profibrotic factor in vitro and that TGF-β1 ligand expression is upregulated in the skin and the lungs of scleroderma patients. In very early lesional skin, immunostaining shows TGF-β1 ligand expression. There is also disruption of TGF-β1 receptor expression leading to modulation of TGF-β activity.

Other key growth factors that have also been implicated in the pathogenesis are connective tissue growth factor (CTGF), platelet-derived growth factor (PDGF) and the beta chemokines monocyte chemoattractant protein (MCP)-1 and MCP-3. There may be a sequential interplay between these growth factors as the disease develops. Chemokine expression is an early feature of skin sclerosis, and fibroblasts are producers of these chemokines. Data suggest that PDGF receptor and ligand expression, and tumor necrosis factor (TNF)-α expression also occur. All of these factors are considered to be important early in the pathogenesis of scleroderma. Connective tissue growth factor was originally speculated to be an important downstream mediator of TGF-β1, but now it seems more likely to be a cofactor in TGF-β1–mediated activation of fibroblasts.

CLINICAL MANIFESTATIONS

Clinical manifestations of systemic sclerosis are heterogeneous and vary as a result of type of disease (limited or diffuse) and organ involvement (Box 3). Patients with diffuse disease (dcSSc) are at risk of developing rapidly progressive skin fibrosis and widespread, severe, internal organ involvement. Patients with lcSSc have a disease course characterized by slowly progressive skin changes not extending beyond the elbows and knees into the proximal extremities or trunk, along with varying degrees of internal organ involvement.

Raynaud's phenomenon is present in most patients with systemic sclerosis and is often the earliest manifestation of disease. In patients with limited disease, it may be present for years before clinically significant skin changes or internal organ involvement develops. Although some patients with Raynaud's phenomenon may not develop the entire spectrum of triphasic color changes (pallor, dusky cyanosis, and red engorgement),[4] most have digital pallor in response to cold or stress.

Cutaneous changes usually begin with an early phase of skin edema, manifested as swollen fingers and hands (see Fig. 1B). In dcSSc, these changes are followed by the development of firm, thickened skin over the extremities (see Fig. 1C), trunk, and face. The patients in whom these changes develop more rapidly are at greater risk for serious internal organ involvement such as pulmonary fibrosis and renal failure. Skin thickening typically peaks in the first 3 to 5 years.[6] As a result of skin thickening, flexion contractures can develop over joints (see Fig. 1D). Skin thickening may then begin to regress slowly over time. In patients with lcSSc, early symptoms include Raynaud's phenomenon (see Fig. 1E) and ischemic digital ulceration (see Fig. 1F). Skin thickening and digital edema are confined to the distal extremities (distal to the elbows and the knees). As the disease progresses, there may be an increase in cutaneous telangiectasias on the face and hands (see Fig. 1G[a] and [b]), calcinosis cutis (see Fig. 1H), and ischemic digital ulcers. Sometimes mucosal telangiectasias also develop (see Fig. 1G[c]).

Patients may complain of dyspnea or a nonproductive cough as a manifestation of underlying pulmonary disease. Some patients may be asymptomatic but have changes on physical examination (basilar rales) or on chest radiography (lower-lobe interstitial infiltrates). Shortness of breath, fatigue, chest pain, and occasionally syncope may be warning signs of pulmonary arterial hypertension. In this situation, physical examination can reveal a loud pulmonary second sound (P_2), left parasternal heave, lower-extremity edema, and other signs of right-sided heart failure. Pulmonary function tests may be abnormal and can reveal restrictive changes even in the absence of radiographic changes or exertional dyspnea. Patients with dcSSc often develop interstitial lung disease, and about 20% to 30% of patients with lcSSc later develop pulmonary arterial hypertension without interstitial lung disease. Patients with dcSSc and rapidly progressive skin changes or those with antitopoisomerase-1 antibodies (anti-Scl-70) are at risk for earlier onset of severe pulmonary disease.[7]

Scleroderma renal crisis is characterized by the development of severe hypertension, renal failure, and microangiopathic hemolytic anemia. A small subset (10%) of patients develop normotensive renal crisis.[8] Patients with rapidly progressive diffuse skin fibrosis, antecedent use of glucocorticoids, presence of RNA polymerase III antibody, or those with a new onset pericardial effusion are at greatest risk. The development of renal crisis is not seen in patients with lcSSc. Most cases occur in the first few years of dcSSc. Renal failure can follow a rapidly progressive course, and early recognition and control of hypertension with angiotensin-converting enzyme inhibitors are critical.

Gastrointestinal involvement is common in both forms of systemic sclerosis. Atrophy of the muscularis mucosa and submucosal fibrosis result in varying degrees of esophageal and other gastrointestinal dysfunction. Complaints of dysphagia and heartburn are common and often signal the development of esophageal dysmotil-

Box 3 Major Clinical Manifestations of Systemic Sclerosis

Cutaneous
Diffuse edema of hands and feet (early stages)
Progressive skin tightening
Sclerodactyly
Calcinosis
Telangiectasias
Digital ulcers and pits
Contractures
Hyperpigmentation, hypopigmentation, salt and pepper skin
Characteristic facies

Vascular
Raynaud's phenomenon
Nailfold capillary changes
Digital ischemia and ulcers
Vasculitic leg ulcers (rare)

Pulmonary
Interstitial lung disease, including alveolitis and interstitial fibrosis
Pulmonary hypertension
Recurrent aspiration pneumonitis caused by esophageal reflux and dysmotility
Chest wall restriction (decreased thoracic compliance)
Respiratory muscle weakness

Cardiac
Cardiomyopathy (systolic and diastolic dysfunction): Congestive heart failure
Conduction defects

- Septal infarction pattern
- Ventricular conduction abnormalities
- Arrhythmias
- Heart blocks

Pericarditis or pericardial effusion (impending renal crisis)

Renal
Scleroderma renal crisis (hypertension, renal failure MAHA)

Musculoskeletal and Rheumatologic
Arthralgia
Tendon friction rubs (relatively specific for diffuse scleroderma)
Inflammatory arthritis, erosive arthropathy (rare)
Myopathy, myositis

Gastrointestinal
Gastroesophageal reflux
Esophageal dysmotility, aperistaltic esophagus
Esophageal stricture
Adenocarcinoma arising in Barrett's esophagus (occasionally)
Watermelon stomach (gastric antral vascular ectasias [GAVE]): Iron-deficiency anemia
Decreased peristalsis throughout the GI tract, leading to bloating, early satiety, stasis, and pseudo-obstruction
Bacterial overgrowth and malabsorptive diarrhea, alternating diarrhea and constipation
Megacolon (rare)
Colonic wide-mouth diverticuli (usually asymptomatic)
Pneumatosis cystoides intestinales
Primary biliary cirrhosis
Anal incontinence

Endocrine
Hypothyroidism

Neurologic
Carpal tunnel syndrome
Trigeminal neuralgia

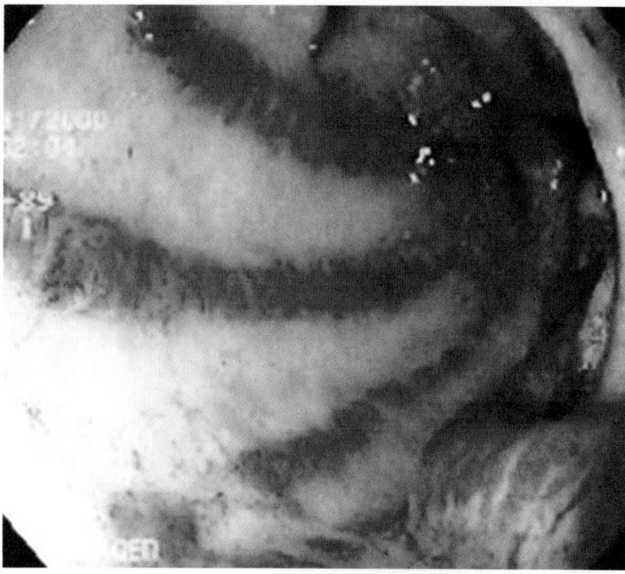

Figure 2 Watermelon stomach (gastric antral vascular ectasias [GAVE]). *From Miller ML: Winners of the 2002 American College of Rheumatology Annual Slide Competition [submitted by April Chang-Miller and Mark V. Larson]. Arthritis Rheum 2003;48(10):2737-2738. © 2003 American College of Rheumatology.*

ity. Esophageal disease results in reflux esophagitis, esophageal strictures, and eventual development of an atonic esophagus. Gastric antral vascular ectasias (GAVE or watermelon stomach) can lead to chronic upper gastrointestinal bleeding and iron-deficiency anemia (Fig. 2). Gastric dysmotility is not rare and can lead to postprandial bloating and early satiety. Small intestinal motility may also be affected, resulting in constipation, varying degrees of malabsorption, and bacterial overgrowth (causing episodes of diarrhea). Severe constipation may develop from colonic hypomotility. Gastrointestinal bleeding is infrequent, but may occur from erosive esophagitis, GAVE, and wide-mouth diverticula in the colon. Pneumatosis cystoides intestinalis can manifest as an acute abdomen, leading to unnecessary laparotomy. Fecal incontinence may develop due to fibrosis of the anal sphincter. Patients with lcSSc sometimes develop primary biliary cirrhosis.

Although subclinical cardiac involvement is common (in autopsy studies), clinical manifestations of cardiac involvement are fortunately rare. Myocardial fibrosis may develop in patients with dcSSc, resulting in cardiac failure, arrhythmias, and conduction defects. Other features of systemic scleroderma include dry eyes and mouth (due to secondary Sjögren's syndrome) and hypothyroidism. Musculoskeletal involvement is common and can manifest as nonspecific myalgias and arthralgias. True arthritis is rare. Muscle weakness may also occur, associated with elevation of serum levels of muscle enzymes. A true scleroderma-polymyositis overlap syndrome occurs in some cases, and is more commonly seen in children. Erectile dysfunction in men is common and is partly attributed to impaired local circulation.

DIAGNOSIS

The diagnosis of systemic scleroderma is usually made on the basis of the characteristic cutaneous finding of skin thickening, in association with Raynaud's phenomenon and varying degrees of internal organ involvement. In early disease, Raynaud's phenomenon may be the only manifestation. Nailfold capillaroscopy (Fig. 3) may be helpful in determining whether Raynaud's phenomenon is primary (Raynaud's disease) (see Fig. 3A) or is secondary to a systemic autoimmune disorder such as scleroderma (see Fig. 3B to D).[9] Other

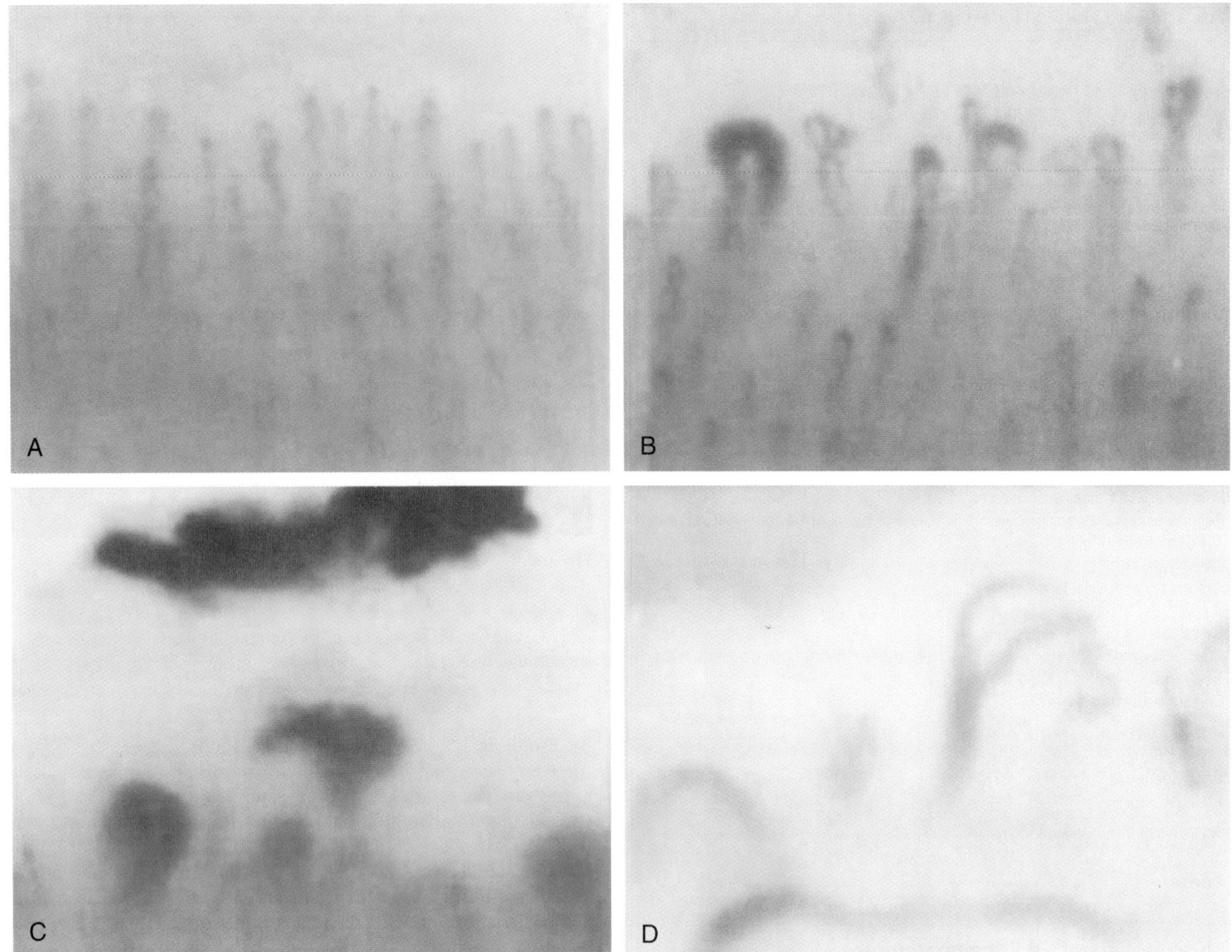

Figure 3 **Nailfold capillaroscopy (×200). A,** Normal nailfold capillaroscopy pattern. **B,** Early scleroderma pattern shows well-preserved capillary architecture and density and presence of dilated and giant capillaries. **C,** Active scleroderma pattern shows frequent giant capillaries and hemorrhages, moderate loss of capillaries, and disorganization of capillary architecture. **D,** Late scleroderma pattern shows severe capillary architecture disorganization with dropouts, presence of arborized capillaries, and absence of giant capillaries.

Box 4 American College of Rheumatology Diagnostic Criteria for Systemic Sclerosis

Major Criterion

Proximal sclerodermatous skin changes (proximal to the metacarpophalangeal joints)

Minor Criteria*

Sclerodactyly

Digital pitting scars of fingertips or loss of substance of the distal finger pads

Bibasilar pulmonary fibrosis

**The patient should fulfill the major criterion or two of the three minor criteria.*

Adapted from Preliminary criteria for the classification of systemic sclerosis (scleroderma). Subcommittee for scleroderma criteria of the American Rheumatism Association Diagnostic and Therapeutic Criteria Committee. Arthritis Rheum 1980;23:581-590.

disorders associated with scleroderma-like skin changes, such as eosinophilic fasciitis and nephrogenic systemic fibrosis, are not associated with Raynaud's phenomenon or nailfold vascular changes.

Diagnostic criteria for scleroderma have been proposed by the American College of Rheumatology (Box 4).[10] However, there are limitations regarding their usefulness, especially for lcSSc, and experts have recommended some modifications to the original criteria.[9]

A complete blood count, complete metabolic panel, muscle enzymes, thyroid function test, and urinalysis are indicated in all patients. Serologic testing for autoantibodies can be helpful in diagnosing and classifying systemic sclerosis.[11] However, none of the serologic tests is sensitive enough to independently exclude disease. Antinuclear antibody (ANA) is positive in 60% to 80% of patients with scleroderma. Anticentromere antibodies (ACAs) are found in roughly 60% to 80% of patients with lcSSc and only rarely in patients with dcSSc. Antibodies to topoisomerase-1 (Scl-70 antibodies) are present in about 30% of patients with dcSSc. The presence of either ACA or anti-Scl-70 is highly specific (95%-99%) for the diagnosis of lcSSc and dcSSc, respectively. These antibodies are only rarely present in healthy subjects and in patients with other rheumatologic diseases. The presence of ACA or anti-Scl-70 antibodies is also highly specific for underlying systemic sclerosis in patients presenting initially with isolated Raynaud's phenomenon and therefore may be helpful when Raynaud's phenomenon is the initial manifestation.[12]

Once the diagnosis has been established, the clinician must determine whether the disease is diffuse or limited, based on the extent of skin tightening. The initial evaluation on the physical examination

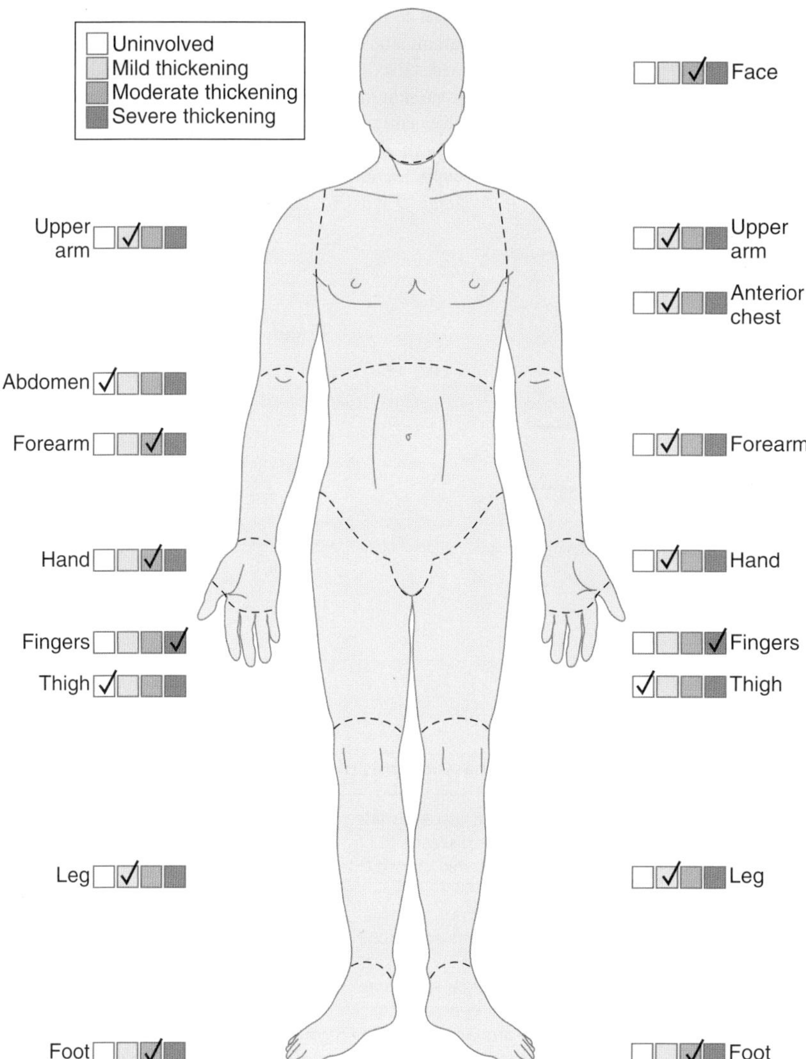

Figure 4 Clinical assessment of skin thickening (modified Rodnan skin scoring). *From Wigley FM: Systemic sclerosis: Clinical features. In Klippel JH, Dieppe PA (eds): Rheumatology, vol. 2, 2nd ed. St Louis, Mosby, 2000, pp 9.1-9.14.*

should include a skin score. The modified Rodnan skin score (MRSS) is the most widely used. The total skin surface area is arbitrarily divided into 17 different areas: fingers, hands, forearms, arms, feet, legs, and thighs (in pairs), and face, chest, and abdomen (Fig. 4). In each of these areas, the skin score is evaluated by manual palpation. The skin score is 0 for uninvolved skin, 1 for mild thickening, 2 for moderate thickening, and 3 for severe thickening (hidebound skin). The total skin score is the sum of the skin scores of the individual areas, the maximum possible score being 51. The skin score tends to correlate with the extent of dermal fibrosis, which in turn correlates with the extent of fibrosis and dysfunction of the internal organs, such as pulmonary fibrosis, scleroderma heart disease, renal disease, and gastrointestinal involvement. With the onset of diffuse scleroderma, the skin score tends to rise rapidly, but it usually reaches a plateau in the first 3 to 5 years and then may start regressing slowly over the years (Fig. 5). The skin score in limited scleroderma, on the other hand, does not progress that fast, and the total skin score is never as high as in diffuse disease (see Fig. 5). The extent of skin thickening must be carefully documented in all follow-up visits. The degree of organ involvement must also be determined by history, physical examination, laboratory markers, and various other studies as appropriate.

Complaints of dysphagia, heartburn, early satiety, nausea and vomiting can be investigated with endoscopy and esophageal manometry (although in practice these invasive studies are often not routinely performed unless there is a reason to suspect esophageal stricture, Barrett's esophagus, or adenocarcinoma). Pulmonary function studies, including spirometry for forced vital capacity (FVC) and diffusion capacity for carbon monoxide (D_LCO), may suggest the presence of interstitial lung disease (ILD), when both FVC and D_LCO are reduced. Chest radiography and high-resolution computed tomography of the chest may suggest the presence of ILD and help differentiate active alveolitis (ground-glass opacification) from established pulmonary fibrosis (coarse reticulation and honeycombing) (Fig. 6).

Bronchoscopy with bronchoalveolar lavage (BAL) may be indicated to evaluate for alveolitis (>3% neutrophils, >2% eosinophils, or both, in BAL fluid). Transbronchial or open lung biopsy may rarely be necessary to characterize the nature of the ILD histologically. Nonspecific interstitial pneumonitis (NSIP) is the most common histologic subtype of ILD in scleroderma; less common types are usual interstitial pneumonitis (UIP) or cryptogenic organizing pneumonia (COP).

An isolated or disproportionate reduction in D_LCO relative to the forced vital capacity and total lung capacity can raise the suspicion of pulmonary hypertension. Surface echocardiography followed by right-heart catheterization are necessary to evaluate and confirm the presence of pulmonary hypertension.

In all newly diagnosed patients with scleroderma, a baseline pulmonary function test (spirometry and D_LCO) and an echocardiogram are recommended, for early diagnosis of ILD and pulmonary hypertension. These tests should be repeated at least annually, even

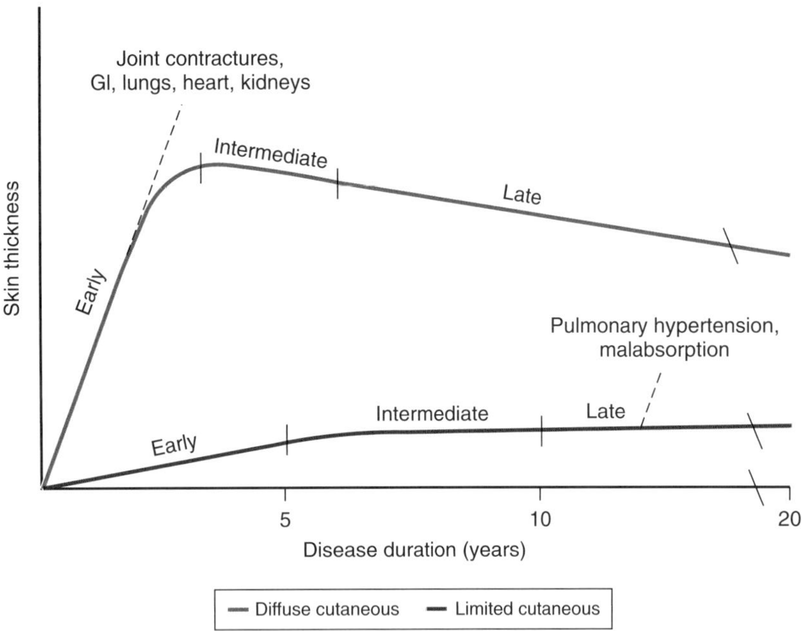

Figure 5 Diffuse and limited scleroderma. Diagrammatic representation of the stages of diffuse and limited scleroderma over time, including the usual relation between skin thickening and various organ system involvements. GI, gastrointestinal. *From Medsger TA Jr: Classification, prognosis. In Clements PJ, Furst DE (eds): Systemic Sclerosis, 2nd ed. Philadelphia: Lippincott Williams & Wilkins, 2004, pp 17-28.*

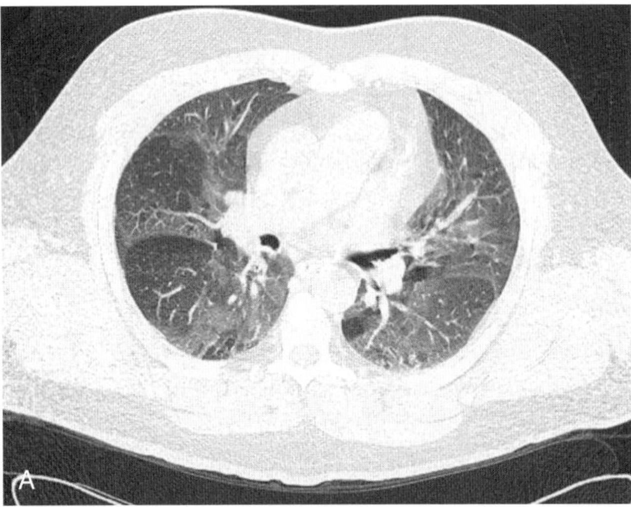

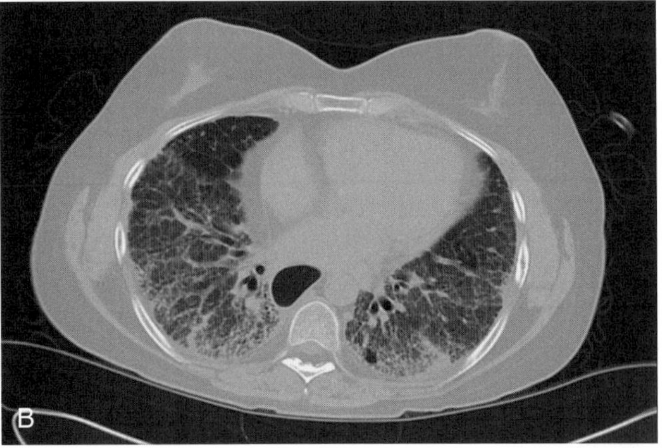

Figure 6 High-resolution computed tomography scan of the chest. **A,** Ground-glass opacification. **B,** Coarse reticulation and honeycombing.

Box 5 Differential Diagnosis of Systemic Sclerosis

- Mixed connective tissue disease
- Graft-versus-host disease
- Nephrogenic systemic fibrosis (formerly known as nephrogenic fibrosing dermopathy)
- Diabetic scleredema
- Diffuse fasciitis with eosinophilia (Shulman's syndrome)
- Toxic oil syndrome
- Eosinophilia-myalgia syndrome
- Lichen sclerosus et atrophicus
- Sclerodermiform acrodermatitis chronica atrophicans (Lyme disease)
- Scleromyxedema (lichen myxedematosus) associated with paraproteinemia
- Drugs and toxins (L-tryptophan, bleomycin, pentazocine, carbidopa, vinyl chloride, silica)

in asymptomatic patients. An annual 6-minute walk distance assessment is also recommended in all patients. This is a simple way of evaluating severity and response to therapy in patients with pulmonary hypertension and is found to correlate with survival.

To investigate the possibility of renal crisis, monitoring of blood pressure, tests of renal function, urinalysis, and peripheral blood smear are necessary in all patients with new onset or worsening hypertension, renal insufficiency, or new anemia (microangiopathic hemolytic anemia) in the absence of blood loss.

DIFFERENTIAL DIAGNOSIS

Some conditions associated with scleroderma-like skin changes and included in the differential diagnosis of systemic sclerosis are listed in Box 5. Readers can refer to appropriate texts for detailed descriptions of these entities.

TREATMENT

In addition to taking prescribed medications correctly and regularly, a person with scleroderma can take many steps to better manage the disease.

Exercise

Regular exercise not only helps improve overall physical and spiritual well-being but it also helps keep the joints flexible and improves circulation. Physical therapy is often helpful in patients with diffuse disease with widespread skin involvement, muscle weakness, and joint contractures.

Skin Protection

Taking proper precautions and care of the skin can be beneficial for symptoms of Raynaud's phenomenon and for the dry, thick patches of skin that result from localized scleroderma. During the colder months, patients should dress appropriately. Keeping the body warm and protected from the cold weather with a hat, gloves, and a scarf will help keep the blood vessels in the extremities open and the circulation flowing. Patients should be advised to wear multiple thin layers and wear loose-fitting boots or shoes to keep the blood supply moving to the feet. A humidifier in the house helps keep the air moist. Patients should use soaps and creams that are designed especially for dry skin.

Diet

Aside from eating healthy foods to get the proper amounts of vitamins and nutrients, it is important to eat foods that do not aggravate existing stomach problems. Patients should avoid excess alcohol use, smoking, and foods that cause heartburn. Water or another liquid helps soften food further. High-fiber foods decrease constipation. Eating frequent, smaller meals as opposed to three large meals enables the body to digest the food more easily. After a large meal, patients should wait at least 4 hours before lying down. Raising the head end of the bed about 15 cm (6 in) by placing wooden blocks underneath it helps reduce acid reflux while sleeping.

Dental Care

For patients with scleroderma who also have Sjögren's syndrome, proper dental care is essential. Sjögren's syndrome increases the risk of developing cavities and tooth decay.

Stress Management

Because the effects of stress can play a part in reducing blood flow and can affect many other aspects of emotions and health, it is important to learn to manage or reduce stress. This can be done by getting proper sleep and rest, avoiding stressful situations when possible, eating a healthy diet, learning methods to control anxiety, and exercising regularly.

ASSESSMENT OF DISEASE ACTIVITY AND TREATMENT

Institution of therapy is predicated on proper assessment of disease activity and organ involvement. The extent of skin thickening is useful for assessing overall disease activity, disease subset (lcSSc or dcSSc), prognosis, and risk of internal organ involvement.[6]

Although no therapy is proved to reverse the vascular and fibrotic damage in patients with scleroderma, several therapies are available in an effort to slow down disease progression, improve vascular function, limit mortality, and provide supportive symptomatic care.

Patients with Raynaud's phenomenon are advised to stop smoking, avoid cold exposure, wear warm clothing and gloves, and avoid vasoconstrictive substances (clonidine, sympathomimetics, cocaine, ergot alkaloids). Various pharmacologic agents are aimed at reversing digital vasospasm. The dihydropyridine calcium channel blockers (amlodipine and long-acting preparations of nifedipine) are first-line agents for the treatment of scleroderma-associated Raynaud's phenomenon.[13] Sustained-release preparations are preferred, and the dose should be adjusted to reduce the severity and frequency of attacks. Patients should be monitored for dose-limiting side effects such as worsening of acid reflux symptoms, lower extremity edema, headache, flushing, and hypotension. For patients who do not respond to calcium channel blockers, other drugs such as topical nitrates, and α-adrenergic blockers (such as prazosin or tamsulosin) may be tried.

The role of antiplatelet and anticoagulant therapy is unclear, although in the absence of contraindications, most experts would recommend low dose aspirin to patients with Raynaud's phenomenon. Phosphodiesterase-5 (PDE_5) inhibitors like sildenafil, tadalafil or vardenafil, have been found to be particularly useful in ameliorating refractory digital ischemia and ulceration, presumably because of their vasodilative properties, although they have not yet received regulatory approval for this indication.[14] Endothelin receptor antagonists (such as bosentan) are proved effective for the prevention of ischemic digital ulcers.[13,15] Intravenous prostanoids (e.g., epoprostenol, alprostadil, or iloprost) have also been shown to ameliorate severe digital ischemia and improve digital ulceration. Patients with critical digital ischemia require hospitalization, pain relief, intravenous prostanoid therapy,[13] and, in the presence of concomitant infection, systemic antibiotics. Angiographic assessment may be necessary to evaluate the extent of vascular disease. When medical therapy fails, digital sympathectomy may be tried to inhibit sympathetic-mediated vasoconstriction.

Because of its anticollagen and immune-modulating effects, D-penicillamine has been used in patients with dcSSc in an effort to slow skin fibrosis. Although small observational studies had demonstrated a small benefit in 5-year mortality and a decrease in development of visceral disease, the role of D-penicillamine remains unclear. Clements and colleagues did not show an advantage of high-dose D-penicillamine over low-dose D-penicillamine therapy, and patients in the high-dose arm had a higher withdrawal rate as a result of adverse events.[16]

Cyclophosphamide may be beneficial in patients with interstitial lung disease associated with scleroderma.[4] Multiple uncontrolled studies had suggested that cyclophosphamide might slow the loss of, or even improve, lung function (specifically FVC) in the setting of early scleroderma with declining FVC and progressive dyspnea.[17] Based on these earlier studies, the NIH conducted a randomized double-blind, placebo controlled, multicenter study to determine the effects of oral cyclophosphamide on lung function and health-related symptoms in patients with evidence of active alveolitis from scleroderma-related interstitial lung disease. The results showed that 1 year of oral cyclophosphamide had a statistically significant but clinically modest beneficial effect on the FVC. There were improvements in the dyspnea score, skin score, and health-related quality of life. More toxicity (especially leukopenia) was seen in the cyclophosphamide arm. The effects on lung function were maintained through the 24 months of the study.[18] Follow-up was continued in these patients for the second year, and the results were published recently.[19] It was found that although the dyspnea scores remained better in the cyclophosphamide arm, the benefit from cyclophosphamide on pulmonary function, health status, and skin score was not sustained until the end of the 24 months of follow-up.

Methotrexate has been shown to improve skin scores, but the effects were modest.[19] Corticosteroids may be useful in the treatment of myositis and alveolitis, but their use is limited by the observation that high doses can precipitate renal crisis.[8] Immunoablation combined with autologous stem cell rescue is still considered experimental, but one report documented improved skin scores.[20] However, 1-year mortality was high after transplantation.[21]

Gastroesophageal reflux usually responds to proton pump inhibitors, and motility disorders are treated with prokinetic agents such as metoclopramide and domperidone. For significant small bowel hypomotility and intestinal pseudo-obstruction, octreotide 50 to 100 μg subcutaneous injection daily may be beneficial.[22,23] Small bowel malabsorption and diarrhea caused by bacterial overgrowth might respond to chronic, alternating regimens of antibiotics (e.g., doxycycline, metronidazole, or ciprofloxacin). Endoscopy-directed dilation may be necessary in cases of esophageal stricture leading to dysphagia, and argon plasma coagulation (APC) may be indicated for gastric bleeding from ectatic vessels (GAVE).

Angiotensin-converting enzyme inhibitors should be used at the first sign of renal crisis (severe hypertension, renal failure, and microangiopathic hemolytic anemia). Their early use is critical in preserving renal function, controlling hypertension, and improving survival during renal crisis. In the hope that control of reninmediated hypertension can result in renal recovery, therapy with angiotensin-converting enzyme inhibitors should be continued even in the face of renal insufficiency requiring dialysis.[24]

Hypoxia from pulmonary hypertension is treated with oxygen. Epoprostenol is an intravenous prostacyclin analogue delivered by continuous central infusion. In clinical trials, it has been shown to improve functional status.[25] Iloprost and treprostinil are synthetic prostacyclins; iloprost is delivered by inhalation, and treprostinil is delivered subcutaneously or intravenously. Bosentan is an oral endothelin receptor antagonist that can improve functional status in patients with pulmonary arterial hypertension associated with systemic sclerosis.[26] Ambrisentan, an endothelin-A receptor antagonist,[27] and sildenafil, a PDE_5 inhibitor,[28] have also received FDA approvals for the treatment of pulmonary hypertension. Long-term anticoagulation is preferably avoided for patients with scleroderma-associated pulmonary hypertension because of the risk of serious bleeding from ulcerative esophagitis or GAVE.

FUTURE DIRECTIONS

The central role of TGF-β in inducing endothelial damage and fibroblast activation has led investigators to target this molecule as a promising site for future therapies. Indeed, anti–TGF-β drugs and other cytokine-based therapies could theoretically provide true disease modification, especially in patients with early disease, before cutaneous and internal fibroses result in significant irreversible damage.[29]

CONCLUSION

Although no cure has been found for scleroderma, the disease is often slowly progressive and manageable, and people who have it can lead healthy and productive lives. Like many other conditions, education about scleroderma and local support groups can be the greatest tools for managing the disease and reducing the risk of further complications.

Summary

- The initial presentation in most scleroderma patients is Raynaud's phenomenon.
- Nailfold capillary microscopy can help differentiate primary Raynaud's phenomenon from that secondary to an underlying connective tissue disease.
- Although not specific, ANA has high sensitivity in scleroderma (60%-80%) and is useful as a screening test.
- Limited and diffuse diseases have different disease courses and prognoses. The nature and extent of organ system involvement also determine the prognosis.
- Therapeutic modalities now include ACE inhibitors for scleroderma renal crisis; parenteral prostanoids, oral endothelin receptor antagonists, and PDE_5 inhibitors for pulmonary hypertension; cyclophosphamide for interstitial lung disease in early scleroderma; and octreotide for intestinal pseudo-obstruction.

Suggested Readings

Badesch DB, Tapson VF, McGoon MD, et al: Continuous intravenous epoprostenol for pulmonary hypertension due to the scleroderma spectrum of disease. A randomized, controlled trial. Ann Intern Med 2000;132:425-434.

Clements PJ, Furst DE (eds): Systemic Sclerosis, 2nd ed. Philadelphia: Lippincott Williams & Wilkins, 2004.

Korn JH, Mayes M, Matucci CM, et al: Digital ulcers in systemic sclerosis: Prevention by treatment with bosentan, an oral endothelin receptor antagonist. Arthritis Rheum 2004;50:3985-3993.

LeRoy EC, Black C, Fleischmajer R, et al: Scleroderma (systemic sclerosis): Classification, subsets and pathogenesis. J Rheumatol 1988;15:202-205.

Mayes MD, Lacey JV Jr, Beebe-Dimmer J, et al: Prevalence, incidence, survival, and disease characteristics of systemic sclerosis in a large U.S. population. Arthritis Rheum 2003;48:2246-2255.

Medsger TA Jr: Natural history of systemic sclerosis and the assessment of disease activity, severity, functional status, and psychologic well-being. Rheum Dis Clin North Am 2003;29:255-273, vi.

Preliminary criteria for the classification of systemic sclerosis (scleroderma). Subcommittee for scleroderma criteria of the American Rheumatism Association Diagnostic and Therapeutic Criteria Committee. Arthritis Rheum 1980;23:581-590.

Rubin LJ, Badesch DB, Barst RJ, et al: Bosentan therapy for pulmonary arterial hypertension. N Engl J Med 2002;346:896-903.

Simms RW, Korn JH: Cytokine directed therapy in scleroderma: Rationale, current status, and the future. Curr Opin Rheumatol 2002;14:717-722.

Tashkin DP, Elashoff R, Clements PJ, et al: Cyclophosphamide versus placebo in scleroderma lung disease. N Engl JMed 2006;354:2655-2666.

References

For a complete list of references, log onto www.expertconsult.com.

Psoriatic Arthritis

M. Elaine Husni

Psoriatic arthritis (PsA) is a unique type of inflammatory arthritis that is associated with skin psoriasis. There is increasing evidence on molecular, cellular, and tissue levels that PsA is a distinctive form of inflammatory arthritis compared with rheumatoid arthritis (RA), the most common form of inflammatory arthritis. Psoriatic arthritis can affect the joints and surrounding structures such as the tendons and ligaments, specifically as dactylitis and enthesitis. In addition to the psoriatic skin changes, it can affect the scalp and nails, causing pitting, ridging, and distal onycholysis. Prompt diagnosis and treatment can relieve pain and inflammation and possibly help prevent progressive joint involvement and damage.

SIGNS AND SYMPTOMS

PsA causes, pain, swelling, stiffness, and tenderness of the joints, which limits motion. The disease has a heterogenous presentation including monoarthritis, oligoarthritis, or polyarthritis. The most common peripheral joint involvement is in the distal interphalangeal joints; this is commonly associated with nail changes of that digit. PsA can also affect the lower back, knees, ankles, and wrists. It can be associated with fatigue and morning stiffness. This disease can also involve the spine and the sacroiliac joint either alone or in combination with peripheral disease.

The psoriatic skin disease usually precedes the joint symptoms. More than 60% to 70% of psoriasis patients present many years before joint symptoms occur, and about 10% to 15% of patients present with concomitant skin and joint symptoms. Skin psoriasis typically manifests with silvery or gray scaly patches on the extensor surfaces (elbows and knees), torso, lower spine, and scalp. Therefore, a careful patient history can also provide important diagnostic clues to this heterogeneous presentation. For example, a family history of psoriasis or prior history of skin rash might warrant greater scrutiny of hidden areas such as scalp, umbilicus, ears, and perianal areas.

Because the clinical presentation can be varied, five different subtypes of PsA have been described and can overlap (Box 1). These include distal interphalangeal joint–predominant arthritis, symmetric polyarthritis-predominant arthritis, asymmetric oligoarthritis or monoarthritis, axial disease predominant spondylitis and/or sacroiliitis, and arthritis mutilans. Arthritis mutilans is a very rare, painful, and rapidly destructive type of PsA. This condition is characterized by deforming arthritis especially of the hands and by resorption of phalangeal bones (Figs. 1 and 2).

Other distinctive clinical features include sausage-like swelling of the fingers and toes, called *dactylitis.* This can also be seen in patients with reactive arthritis conditions. Inflammation of the tendon sheath (tenosynovitis) or inflammation of the entheses (enthesitis) is also seen. Inflammation of the eye, such as conjunctivitis, can also be associated with PsA.

PREVALENCE, RISK FACTORS, AND NATURAL HISTORY

The exact prevalence of PsA is unknown, but estimates vary from 0.3% to 1% of the U.S. population, with a reported prevalence of 7% to 42% in patients with psoriasis.[1] Psoriatic arthritis can develop at any time, but it appears most often between the ages of 30 and 50. Unlike other types of inflammatory arthritis, which have a large female predominance, PsA seems to affect men at about the same or slightly higher rate compared to women.

The onset of PsA symptoms may vary. Typically, PsA manifests as a mild, oligoarticular disease, but it can become polyarticular with time and progresses to a severe, erosive condition in at least 20% of patients. Aggressive disease is seen more commonly in those who exhibit polyarticular or erosive PsA at presentation. Additional factors can predictive a worse prognosis for psoriatic patients. These include extensive skin involvement, strong family history of psoriasis, and disease onset before 20 years of age (Box 2).

PATHOPHYSIOLOGY

There appear to be multiple factors contributing to the pathogenesis of PsA, including genetic, environmental, and immunologic. The exact cause of PsA has not been identified, and the concomitant pathogenic connection between the skin and joints is not clear.

Genetic Factors

As many as 40% of people with PsA have a family history of skin or joint disease.[2] Interestingly, children of parents with psoriasis are three times more likely to have psoriasis and are at greater risk for developing PsA than children born to parents without psoriasis. There are proposed major histocompatibility complex (MHC) and non-MHC loci that may be associated with increased susceptibility to PsA.

Environmental Factors

Bacterial and viral infections have been implicated as a cause or trigger in PsA. Some studies on psoriatic plaque have suggested enhanced humoral and cellular immunity to gram-positive bacteria; however, no direct relationship between bacteria and psoriasis has been proved. Another environmental trigger has been proposed in relation to the Koebner phenomenon, whereby arthritis can develop at sites of traumatized skin.[3]

Immunologic Factors

The most compelling pathogenic factors are the similar immunopathology of psoriasis and PsA. There is evidence that activated T cells are present in both skin and joint tissue. The success of anti–tumor necrosis factor α (TNF-α) therapy for both skin and joint symptoms of PsA patients has also provided new insights into the pathogenesis of PsA. It is likely that cytokines such as TNF-α are critically involved in guiding the inflammatory process, leading to cartilage and bone degradation as well skin inflammation.

DIAGNOSIS

Diagnosing PsA is necessarily complex; the most critical factor is the absence of validated criteria for identifying and classifying cases and for diagnosing the disease. The standard rheumatologic laboratory tests such as rheumatoid factor and anti–cyclic citrullinated peptide (anti-CCP) and radiographic changes may be negative, adding to the difficulty of diagnosis.

PsA is mainly diagnosed by establishing the presence of characteristic signs and symptoms associated in both the skin and joints and by ruling out more common inflammatory arthritis. However, these clinical features are not confined to PsA, and PsA and RA share many common characteristics. Diagnosis may be easier to confirm if

Box 1 Subtypes of Psoriatic Arthritis

Distal interphalangeal joint–predominant arthritis (10%)
Symmetric polyarthritis-predominant arthritis (5%-20%)
Asymmetric oligoarthritis or monoarthritis (70%-80%)
Axial disease predominant spondylitis and/or sacroiliitis (5%-20%)
Arthritis mutilans (rare)

Box 2 Predictors of Worse Prognosis

Polyarticular or erosive disease at presentation
Association with extensive skin involvement
Strong family history of skin disease
Disease onset at younger than 20 years of age

psoriasis coexists with symptoms of arthritis. However, in as many as 15% of cases, symptoms of PsA appear before symptoms of psoriasis (psoriatic arthritis sine psoriasis). A careful medical history, physical examination, blood tests, magnetic resonance imaging (MRI), and x-rays of the involved joints along with a dermatologic evaluation may be used to diagnose PsA.

It is important diagnose PsA early so that treatment can quickly relieve pain and inflammation and prevent irreversible joint damage. Without treatment, PsA is potentially disabling and crippling. In the very early stages of the disease, x-rays usually do not reveal signs of arthritis and might not help in making a diagnosis. In the later stages, x-rays can show changes that are characteristic of PsA, such as the pencil-in-cup sign, where the end of the bone gets whittled down to a sharp point. The most typical radiographic changes include erosive changes similar to those seen in RA (in the paramarginal rather than marginal areas) and new bone formation in the distal peripheral joints and at the enthesial sites. Additional x-ray changes include fluffy periostitis, ankylosis, and loss of bone at the distal phalanges. MRI can be more sensitive in detecting soft tissue inflammation as well as changes in the sacroiliac joints. However, most of the changes can occur in the later stages of the disease where clinical signs and symptoms for PsA have already been established.

Initially, most patients with PsA were thought to have mild, short-lived form of arthritis. However, it is now known that PsA can affect joints early in the disease course with irreversible joint damage, and skin psoriasis can severely decrease in a patient's quality of life.

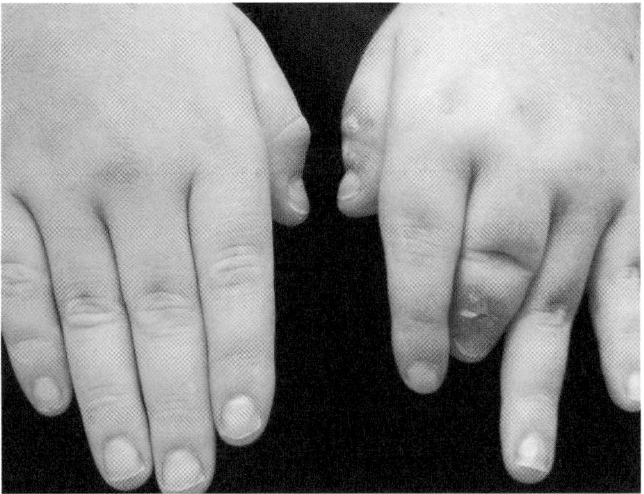

Figure 1 **Destructive arthritis of the third digit.** This patient has arthritis mutilans affecting his third digit, along with nail changes of the same digit. Psoriasis is noted on his thumb. *Courtesy of Dr. A. Qureshi, Brigham and Women's Hospital, Boston.*

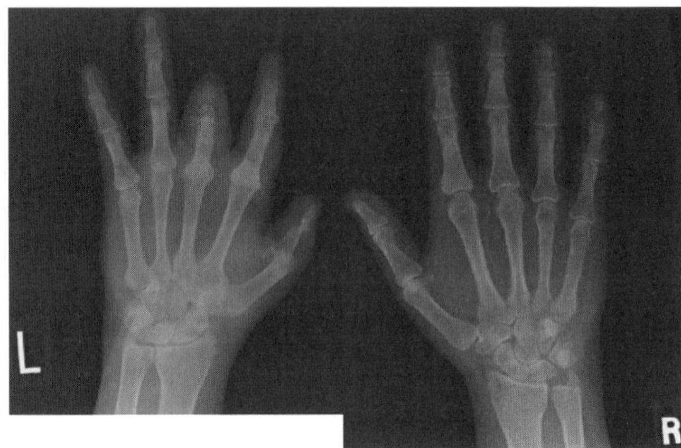

Figure 2 **Destructive arthritis of the third digit.** These radiographs are from the same patient as in Figure 1 and show distal bone resorption. *Courtesy of Dr. A. Qureshi, Brigham and Women's Hospital, Boston.*

TREATMENT

The goals of treatment for PsA should include early diagnosis, with early aggressive treatment aimed at halting or minimizing joint damage and clearing the skin psoriasis. The treatment recommendations for PsA have been largely borrowed from other inflammatory arthritis treatment protocols such as RA trials. Thus, the use of nonsteroidal anti-inflammatory drugs (NSAIDs) and traditional disease-modifying antirheumatic drugs (DMARDs) have been based upon expert consensus among rheumatologists and dermatologists; only a limited number of evidence-based clinical trials exist for PsA patients. Optimal treatment of PsA should be targeted to both skin and joint disease, In addition, a subset of PsA patients require additional treatment for nail and scalp involvement and for dactylitis and enthesis involvement. There has been great interest in newer agents (such as biologic therapies) that may be used as monotherapy or in combination with traditional DMARDs to treat both the skin and joint symptoms of this condition.

Because PsA has such a heterogeneous presentation, treatment can usually be tailored to the predominant arthritis presentation. In general, treatment can be aimed at peripheral or axial predominance, skin and nail predominance, or dactylitis and enthesitis. Mild or limited joint disease might respond to initial treatment with NSAIDs; however, DMARDs are indicated in patients with more-aggressive and erosive disease.

Steroidal and Nonsteroidal Anti-inflammatory Therapy

Initial therapy for PsA involving peripheral and axial disease is NSAIDs. However, with limited studies in this population, it is also important to note that NSAIDs have not demonstrated disease modification but rather are shown to decrease pain scores and joint symptoms compared to placebo. There has also been some concern that NSAID therapy can exacerbate the skin disease,[4] with the potential mechanism of shunting of arachidonic acid metabolites down the leukotriene pathway. Other studies have concluded this is not a substantial clinical problem.[5]

In general, steroid therapy has not been a mainstay of treatment because of the risk of provoking a pustular flare of the skin disease upon withdrawal. Occasionally, rheuamtologists have found intra-articular injections of corticosteroid very useful in the management of monoarthritis or oligoarthritis.

Traditional DMARD Therapy

The most widely used first-line DMARD agent that has demonstrated efficacy in a randomized clinical trial for both joint and skin disease for PsA is methotrexate. Although this drug is more widely studied in RA patients, methotrexate does have the longest duration of clinical experience in PsA patients. Overall, dosages of methotrexate can average a low weekly dosage of 5-10 mg, which can be increased as needed up to 20-25 mg per week. Patients on methotrexate do need to avoid alcohol because of the potential for liver abnormalities that can be associated with its use. Rheumatologists and dermatologists commonly use methotrexate for these conditions; however, the guidelines on long-erm monitoring and proper patient selection to minimize toxicity of this therapy differ among the subspecialties specifically in regard to the need for liver biopsy during treatment with methotrexate. Female patients attempting to conceive must avoid methotrexate as it has been demonstrated to cause birth defects.

Sulfasalazine has also been shown to be effective in treating peripheral joint symptoms, although it has less effect on skin and axial disease symptoms in PsA.

Other traditional disease-modifying agents for inflammatory arthritis have been used in PsA patients, such as azathioprine, leflunomide, and cyclosporine. However, only very small controlled trials with limited numbers of PsA patients have been completed with these agents. These treatments have been generally reserved for patients who appear to be intolerant of the better-studied DMARDs, such as methotrexate or sulfasalazine.

Biological Response Modifiers

More-targeted biological therapy for autoimmune disease has made a significant improvement in the way we can treat PsA. With advancing knowledge in immunology and molecular biology, bioengineered proteins or small molecules have been developed to block very specific targets; these are called *biologic response modifiers.* The most efficacious biologic response modifiers specifically inhibit TNF-α, which has been implicated as the critical molecule responsible for mediating the progression of joint and skin damage in these patients.

Three TNF inhibitors are approved by the U.S. Food and Drug Administration (FDA) for PsA: etanercept (a soluble fusion protein of TNF-α p75 receptor domains and an immunoglobulin (Ig)G Fc region), infliximab (a chimeric monoclonal anti–TNF-α antibody), and adalimumab (a fully human anti-TNF monoclonal antibody). These agents have been studied extensively in RA patients and demonstrate great clinical improvement in the signs and symptoms of inflammatory arthritis as well as improved functional status and quality of life.

The efficacy of etanercept has been confirmed in a large randomized, controlled trial of 205 PsA patients; improved America College of Rheumatology (ACR) clinical responses were seen at week 24.[6] ACR responses are clinical composite response criteria developed by the ACR. For example, ACR 20 response would necessitate that a patient have a 20% reduction in the number of swollen and tender joints, and a reduction of 20% in three of the following five indices: physician global assessment of disease, patient global assessment of disease, pain, CRP/ESR, and HAQ. ACR 50 and ACR 70 require 50% and 70% reduction respectively in the same measures. The standard measure used in psoriasis—PASI75 (psoriasis activity and severity index, 75% improvement of a psoriatic lesion)—was achieved in 23% of subjects with etanercept compared with 3% with placebo.

The efficacy of infliximab has been confirmed in several studies. The largest of these is IMPACT II (Infliximab Multinational Psoriatic Arthritis Controlled Trial) with 200 PsA patients. Improved ACR clinical responses and PASI scores were improved in subjects in IMPACT.[7] Adalimumab was also shown to be effective in PsA in one of the largest double-blind, placebo-controlled phase III trials, studying 313 PsA patients using ACR20/50/70 and PASI scores.[8]

Overall, anti-TNF therapy has been most effective in alleviating symptoms of axial disease, which methotrexate and sulfasalazine have been less likely to mitigate. Other biologic agents have been studied for PsA but were found to be more efficacious for the skin psoriasis than for the joint disease, including alefacept (fully humanized fusion protein, which binds to CD2 on memory T cells) and efalizumab (humanized antibody to the CD11 subunit of lymphocyte function-associated antigen 1 [LFA-1]).

The safety of anti-TNF agents has been studied in the above-mentioned clinical trials as well as postmarketing surveillance databases in both RA and PsA populations. Common adverse events of these agents include injection site reactions (usually self-limiting), increases upper respiratory illness, and, less commonly, a lupus-like syndrome. Additional rare but significant adverse effects have been found including the development of serious opportunistic infections such as tuberculosis. There have also been reports of new demyelinating disease, blood disorders, and the initiation and relapse of lymphoma. These adverse side effects must be carefully weighed against the potential benefits of slower disease progression in each patient.

Treatment with anti-TNF inhibitors has been a remarkable breakthrough in the treatment of PsA. In addition to improvement in the peripheral joint disease and skin psoriasis, there is a significant benefit in alleviating symptoms of axial disease, dactylitis, and enthesitis compared to traditional therapy. Because these agents have been highly successful in both skin and joint disease, it is important to build collaborative approaches with both rheumatologic and dermatologic specialties to optimize management of this disease.

Despite the success of biologic response modifiers, a limited number of patients do not respond to this treatment. Thus, additional targets are being studied where higher standards of clinical remission or arresting radiographic progression may be achieved. In certain cases, surgical options may be needed to correct severe joint destruction with joint replacement surgery.

Summary

- Presentation is heterogeneous; PsA is easily confused with rheumatoid arthritis or gout.
- Disease can affect both the skin and joints but not necessarily at the same time.
- It can affect any joint in the body.
- Up to 40% of patients can have a positive family history of psoriasis or arthritis.
- Up to 20% of patients with psoriasis develop PsA.
- There is no definitive laboratory or x-ray evidence for definitive diagnosis.

Suggested Readings

Gelfand JM, Gladman DD, Mease PJ, et al: Epidemiology of psoriatic arthritis in the population of the United States. J Am Acad Dermatol 2005;53(4):573.

Gladman DD: Mortality in psoriatic arthritis. Clin Exp Rheumatol 2008;26(5 Suppl 5):S62-S65.

Gladman DD, Mease PJ, Strand V, et al: Consensus on a core set of domains for psoriatic arthritis. J Rheumatol 2007;34(5):1167-1170.

Mease P: Current treatment for psoriatic arthritis and other spondyloarthritides. Rheum Dis Clin North Am. 2006;32(Suppl 1):11-20.

Mease P: Psoriatic arthritis therapy. Curr Opin Rheumatol 2005;17:426-432.

Qureshi AA, Dominguez P, Duffin KC, et al: Psoriatic arthritis screening tools. J Rheumatol 2008;35(7):1423-1425.

References

For a complete list of references, log onto www.expertconsult.com.

Ankylosing Spondylitis

Matthew P. Bunyard

DEFINITION

Ankylosing spondylitis is classified along with the seronegative spondyloarthritic diseases. Ankylosing spondylitis is a chronic, systemic, inflammatory disease that affects primarily the sacroiliac joints and spine. Certain peripheral joints and tendons can also be affected, and extra-articular manifestations may be present. The disease typically affects young adults, and there are strong genetic features.

The spondyloarthritides, as a subset, have several distinguishing features that are shared among them. The diseases are seronegative by definition. There are common genetic factors including the human leukocyte antigen (HLA) B27 gene. Axial involvement, including sacroiliitis, can be seen in all and is essential for the diagnosis of ankylosing spondylitis. Enthesitis, or inflammatory changes of the tendon and ligament attachment to bone, is the primary pathologic phenomenon. The spondyloarthritides share many extra-articular features including uveitis, dermatitis, and colitis.

ETIOLOGY

The etiology of ankylosing spondylitis remains unclear. There is solid evidence pointing to a genetic component and risk. The HLA B27 gene is commonly present, and there is a strong familial association. Infective mechanisms have been proposed but seem less evident than in the reactive arthritides.

PREVALENCE AND RISK FACTORS

The prevalence of ankylosing spondylitis is 0.1% to 1.4%, depending on the population studied.[1] The disease is more common in Caucasians than in other races. Typically, but not universally, the prevalence reflects the associated prevalence of the HLA B27 gene in that population.[2] Ankylosing spondylitis is discovered to be the etiology in 4% to 5 % of patients with chronic low back pain.[3]

In North American Caucasians, the HLA B27 gene is found in 7% of the normal population and in more than 90% of patients with ankylosing spondylitis.[2] A person who is HLA B27 positive has a 5% to 6% chance of developing the disease.[4] There is a fivefold to 16-fold increase in having ankylosing spondylitis if a first-degree relative has the disease.[5] The HLA B27 factor makes up about a third of the overall genetic risk.

In the past, ankylosing spondylitis was thought to be an overwhelmingly male disease, but the actual male-to-female ratio is closer to 3:1. The median age of onset is 23 years. Ankylosing spondylitis rarely has its initial manifestation after age 40 years; however, there can be a delay in diagnosis.

PATHOPHYSIOLOGY AND NATURAL HISTORY

Pathogenesis

The pathogenesis of ankylosing spondylitis remains unclear to date. It is assumed to be immune mediated. There is an obvious cytokine role, because patients show improvement with anti–tumor necrosis factor α (anti–TNF-α) agents. As discussed earlier, there is also a genetic component, and the HLA B27 gene is found in more than 90% of patients with ankylosing spondylitis, although the incidence varies some depending on the population studied. Familial aggregation is seen even without the HLA B27 gene. An infectious trigger for the disease remains an intriguing hypothesis. Studies with animal models show that rodents that have HLA B27 and are raised in a germ-free environment do not develop disease; however, in a regular environment, they develop a disease similar to ankylosing spondylitis.[6] To date however, no infectious trigger has been unequivocally established, as with reactive arthritis.

Pathology

Enthesitis, in both the axial and the appendicular skeleton, is the primary pathologic feature of the spondyloarthritides.[7] The enthesis is where the tendon or ligament attaches to bone. The progression is typically edema of bone followed by erosion, then ossification, then finally ankylosis. The sacroiliac joints exhibit inflammation followed by ankylosis. In the spine, one can see inflammation at the junction of the annulus fibrosis of the disk cartilage with the margin of vertebral bone. Ultimately, this leads to formation of syndesmophytes, with bridging that leads to the radiographic appearance of a bamboo spine (see the discussion of imaging, later). The spinal facet joint can exhibit synovitis followed by ankylosis. In the peripheral skeleton, one sees synovitis and enthesitis.

SIGNS AND SYMPTOMS

Symptoms

Spinal and sacroiliac symptoms are typically early and the most prominent. Low back pain is the first symptom in more than 75% of patients. In some patients, the symptoms are more in the buttock. Over time, the patient experiences limited spinal mobility. One of the keys to the diagnosis of ankylosing spondylitis is identifying features of inflammatory low back pain.[3,8] This includes onset before the age of 40 years, insidious onset, chronic (>3 months) pain, morning stiffness for longer than 30 minutes, improvement with exercise, awakening with pain in the second half of the night, and alternating buttock pain (Box 1).

Enthesopathic symptoms can be spinal or peripheral. Axial enthesitis includes costovertebral, manubriosternal, sternal clavicular, and costochondral. Some patients experience decreased chest expansion. Examples of extraspinal enthesisits include dactylitis (sausage digit), Achilles tendinitis, and plantar fasciitis.

Inflammatory arthritis likewise can be axial or appendicular. The hips and shoulders are commonly involved. In the peripheral skeleton, patients typically experience lower extremity and asymmetric patterns of involvement.

Finally, extra-articular manifestations may be present (Box 2). Eye involvement is the most common, with anterior uveitis (or iritis) seen in 25% to 40% of patients who have ankylosing spondylitis.[9] This precedes the spinal symptoms in some cases.

Cardiovascular involvement includes valvular heart disease, aortitis (almost always ascending thoracic), and conduction disturbances. Pulmonary manifestations include decreased chest expansion with extrathoracic restrictive lung disease and fibrotic upper lobe disease.[10] The bowel can be involved even in cases without frank inflammatory bowel disease. Mild colitis can be seen in upwards of 50% to 60% of cases, and it can be asymptomatic.[11] A small percentage of patients progress to inflammatory bowel disease. Conversely, one can see an ankylosing spondylitis type of picture with frank inflammatory bowel disease. Neurologically, one can see cord compression and, rarely, cauda equina syndrome.[12] Although there is syndesmophyte formation, the bone itself becomes osteoporotic.

Box 1 Diagnosing Inflammatory Low Back Pain

Onset before the age of 40 years
Insidious onset
Greater than 3 months in duration (chronic)
Morning stiffness >30 minutes
Improvement with exercise but not with rest
Awakening with pain in the second half of the night
Alternating buttock pain

Box 2 Extra-articular Manifestations of Ankylosing Spondylitis

Ocular

- Iritis
- Conjunctivitis (reactive arthritis)

Cardiovascular

- Valvular heart disease
- Aortitis
- Conduction disturbance

Pulmonary

- Restrictive lung disease
- Upper lobe fibrosis

Gastrointestinal

- Colitis

Neurologic

- Cauda equina syndrome
- C1-C2 subluxation

One should be vigilant for compression fractures and subluxation with even minimal trauma. Atlantoaxial instability and subluxation, similar to that seen with rheumatoid arthritis, has been demonstrated with ankylosing spondylitis.[13]

Ankylosing spondylitis is a systemic disease, and fatigue and malaise are not uncommon. Fever and weight loss are rarely seen, however.

Physical Findings

On the physical examination of the spine, in general, there is decreased range of motion and tenderness. When examining the neck, one sees decreased range of motion and increased occiput-to-wall distance. In the thoracic spine, one sees decreased chest expansion, kyphosis, and costochondral tenderness. In the lumbar spine, a decreased Schober's index is seen (Fig. 1).

Several maneuvers elicit pain in the sacroiliac joints: the FABER (*f*lexion *ab*duction *e*xternal *r*otation), or Patrick's, test; Gaenslen's test; anteroposterior and lateral pelvic compression; and tenderness of the sacroiliac joint with direct pressure (Fig. 2).

Enthesitis can be demonstrated on the axial and peripheral examination. Common locations are the costochondral and Achilles regions.

Peripheral arthritis can be observed. The hip joints are most common, but one can also see an asymmetric arthritis, which is more common in the lower extremities.

DIAGNOSIS

The diagnosis of ankylosing spondylitis is made on the basis of a combination of suggestive symptoms, physical examination findings, and imaging. The most common classification system is the modified New York criteria[14] (Box 3); however, these have never been validated for clinical use. A common dilemma in making the diagnosis arises in early cases with normal plain radiographs (see the discussion of imaging, later). From a more practical standpoint, a useful strategy for diagnosisng ankylosing spondylitis is identifying features of inflammatory low back pain as noted previously (see Box 1).[3,8]

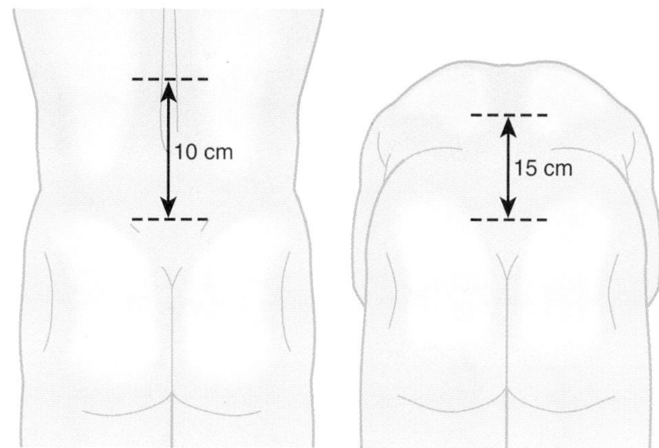

Figure 1 **Schober's index.** With the patient standing erect, mark the first line at the sacral dimples and then the second line 10 cm above this point. The patient flexes forward. The measured increased expansion should be more than 5 cm in the normal person.

Box 3 Modified New York Criteria (1984) for Diagnosing Ankylosing Spondylitis

Clinical Criteria

Low back pain and stiffness for >3 months that improves with exercise but not with rest
Limitation of lumbar spine mobility in both the sagittal and frontal planes
Limitation in chest expansion as compared with normal range for age and sex

Radiologic Criteria

Unilateral sacroiliitis of grade 3-4 *or*
Bilateral sacroiliitis of grade ≥2

Grading

Definite ankylosing spondylitis if the radiological criterion is associated with at least one clinical criterion
Probable ankylosing spondylitis if

- Three clinical criteria are present *or*
- The radiologic criterion is present without any signs or symptoms satisfying the clinical criteria

From van der Linden S, Valkenburg H, Cats A: Evaluation of diagnostic criteria for ankylosing spondylitis. A proposal for modification of the New York criteria. Arthritis Rheum 1984;27:361-368.

Although there are several formal tools for assessing the activity and severity of disease, these can be cumbersome in clinical practice.[15] For functional, in-office clinical purposes, a minimal set of indicators includes global pain, axial pain, degree and duration of morning stiffness, limitation of activities, and the physician's global assessment.

Laboratory Tests

The HLA B27 gene is not a diagnostic test. The sensitivity and specificity vary depending on race or ethnicity.[2] For example, in the Caucasian population, about 90% of ankylosing spondylitis patients and 6% to 10% of the entire population have the HLA B27 gene. In certain cases, testing for the HLA B27 gene may be useful in determining the need for further evaluation. Acute-phase reactants,

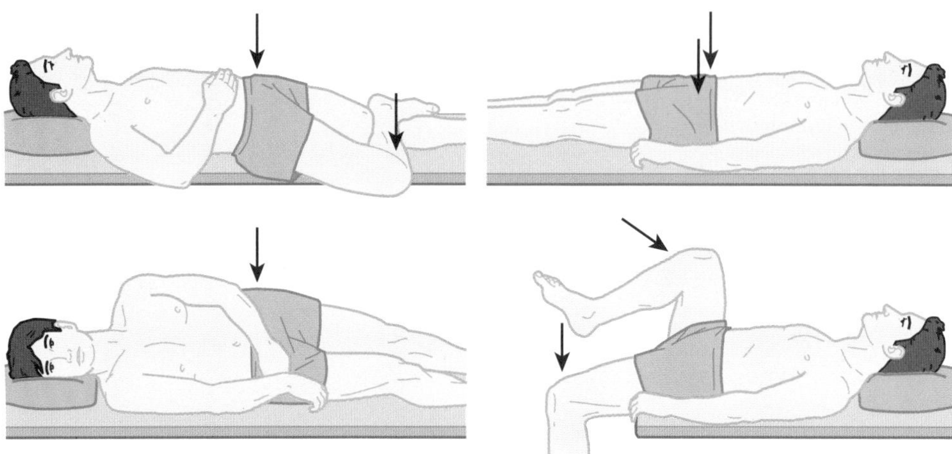

Figure 2 Maneuvers to elicit sacroiliac joint tenderness. *Upper left:* FABER (*f*lexion *ab*duction *e*xternal *r*otation), or Patrick's, test. *Upper right:* Anteroposterior pelvic compression. *Lower left:* Lateral pelvic compression. *Lower right:* Gaenslen's test.

including erythrocyte sedimentation rate (ESR) and C-reactive protein (CRP), may be variably elevated. This may be more highly associated with peripheral arthritic activity. The rheumatoid factor and antinuclear antibody are negative because the spondyloarthritides are seronegative by definition.

Imaging

Plain films of the sacroiliac joints are the standard initial test for diagnosing ankylosing spondylitis (Figs. 3 and 4). Sacroiliitis is the cardinal feature and is essential for diagnosis based on the 1984 modified New York criteria.[14] The findings are classically symmetric and radiographicaly graded as 1 through 4: suspicious, minimal, moderate, ankylosis. Plain films of the lumbar, thoracic, and cervical spine can demonstrate syndesmophytes, squaring of vertebral bodies, ossification of ligament, and disease of the facet joints (Figs. 5 and 6). Radiographic damage may be assessed using the modified Stokes Ankylosing Spondylitis Spine Score [SASSS].[16] Sacroiliitis identified by plain x-rays of the sacroiliac joints is still the gold standard for diagnosis and is a relatively fast and cheap test. However, the findings of sacroiliitis on plain x-ray can lag for years behind symptoms and are subject to varied interpretation.[17]

Because of this, other imaging modalities have been suggested as being superior, especially with earlier disease.[18] Nuclear medicine bone scanning is not favored at this time. With this modality, the sacroiliac joints are sometimes difficult to assess, especially if there is bilateral disease. It is typically a sensitive, but highly nonspecific tool. Computed tomography (CT) scanning of the sacroiliac joints can identify the margins of the bony cortex, and therefore one might be able to see erosions better.[19] Chronic changes may be easier to identify by CT, but this tool is less helpful in identifying inflammatory joint and bone changes. There is also the risk of significant radiation exposure.

Magnetic resonance imaging (MRI) of the sacroiliac joints and bony pelvis includes T1- and T2-weighted images taken in coronal and axial planes. T1 with gadolinium or fat-suppressed T2 images are the most helpful for seeing inflammatory features (Figs. 7 and 8). With active, inflammatory sacroiliitis, one sees increased T1 gadolinium-enhanced or fat-suppressed T2 signal from the adjacent bone and bone marrow, suggesting edema.[20] Synovitis and erosions can also be visualized. Although standard radiographs are still considered the image of first choice, MRI may be most useful in the case of high clinical suspicion and normal or equivocal radiographs.[21] MRI has the highest sensitivity and specificity of all imaging techniques for

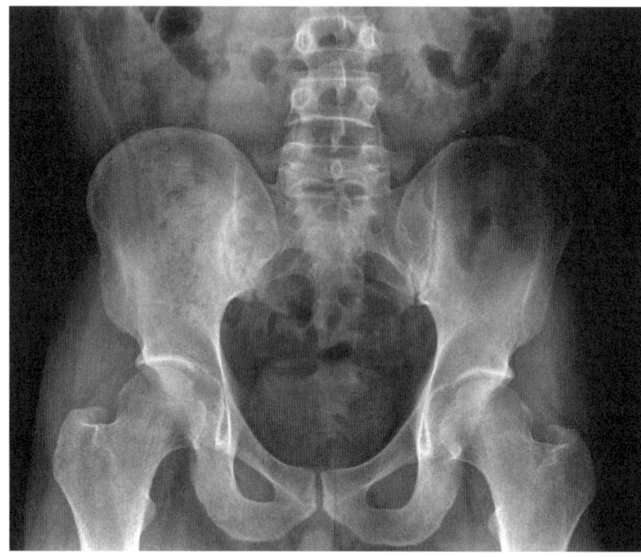

Figure 3 Early radiographic evidence of sacroiliitis in ankylosing spondylitis. *(Courtesy of Jean Schils, MD, Cleveland Clinic.)*

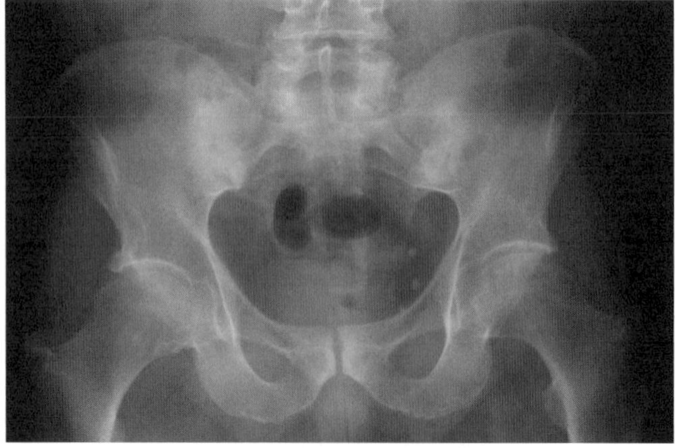

Figure 4 Late stage sacroiliitis with extensive sclerosis and early ankylosis. *(Courtesy of Jean Schils, MD, Cleveland Clinic.)*

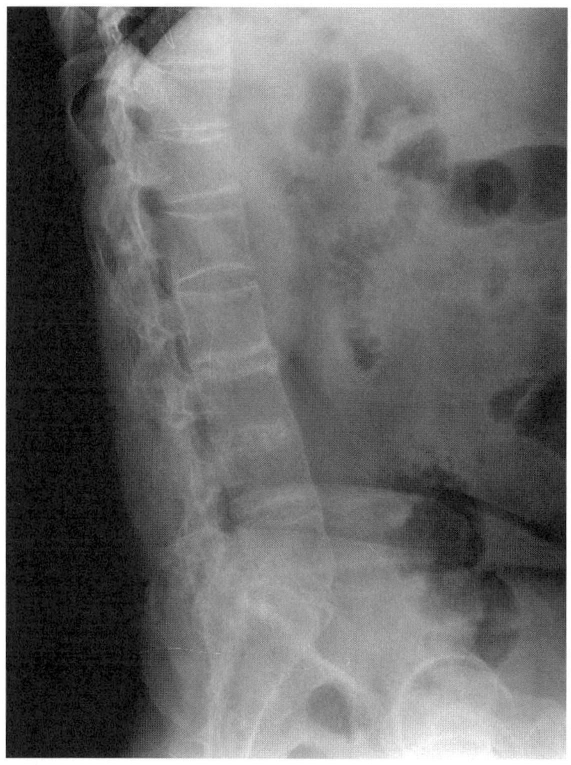

Figure 5 **Lateral lumbar x-ray demonstrating bridging syndesmophytes and the classic "bamboo spine" appearance in later stages of ankylosing spondylitis.** *(Courtesy of Jean Schils, MD, Cleveland Clinic.)*

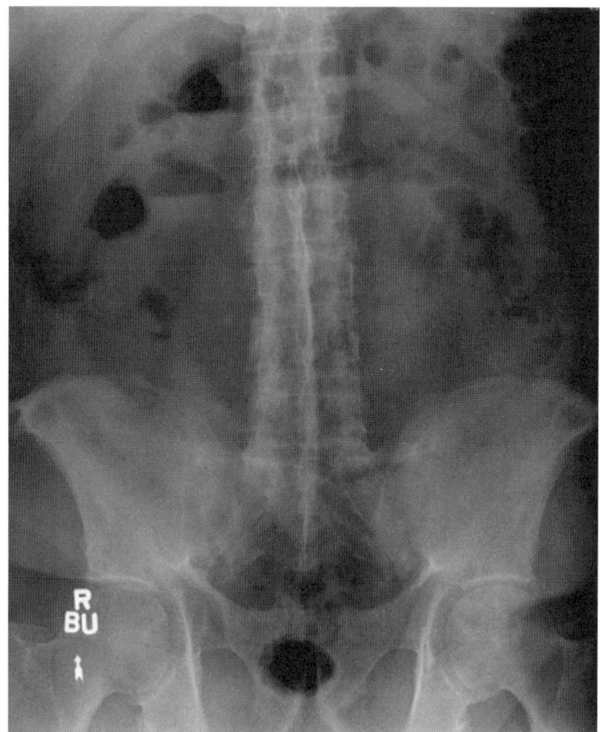

Figure 6 **Anteroposterior lumbar x-ray of the same patient as in Figure 5.** *(Courtesy of Jean Schils, MD, Cleveland Clinic.)*

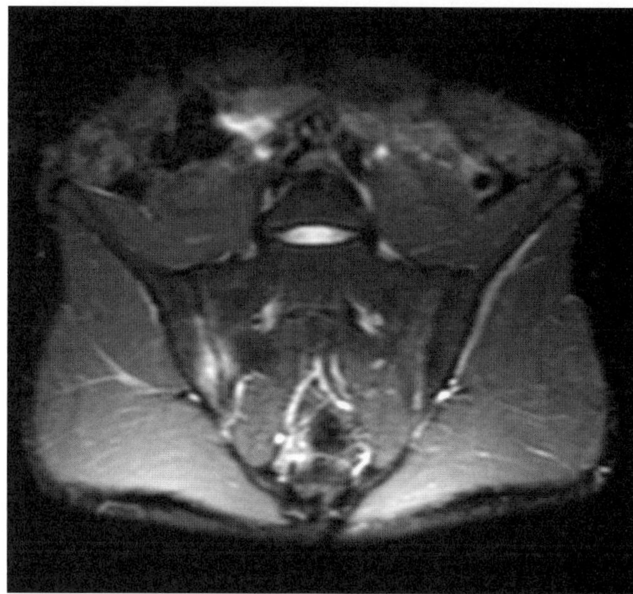

Figure 7 **MRI of the sacroiliac joints.** Axial fat-suppressed T2 image demonstrating early sacroiliitis on the *right* (note bright signal in bone surrounding the joint). *(Courtesy of Jean Schils, MD, Cleveland Clinic.)*

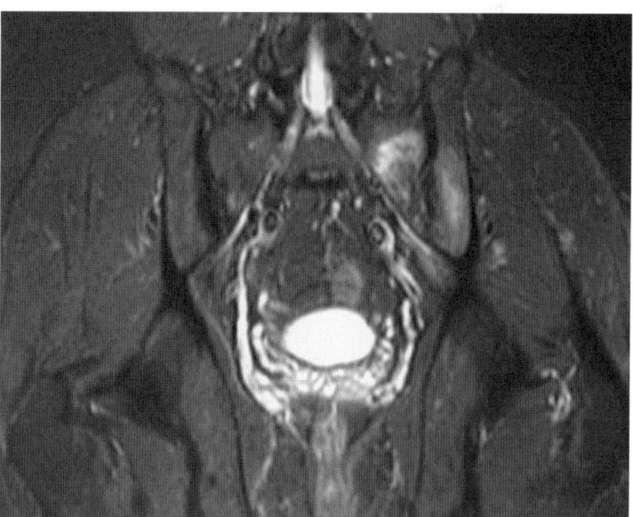

Figure 8 **MRI of the sacroiliac joints.** Coronal fat-suppressed T2 image demonstrating sacroiliitis on the left sacroiliac joint (note bright signal in bone surrounding the joint). *(Courtesy of Jean Schils, MD, Cleveland Clinic.)*

sacroiliac joint inflammation.[22] One can assess both acute and chronic changes at once, and there are no radiation concerns. MRI can also be used to assess spinal inflammation. MRI has several disadvantages: it is expensive, it is time consuming, and it requires specialized interpretation.

Summary

- Historical features of inflammatory low back pain
- Physical examination findings of decreased range of motion in the spine or limited chest expansion, or both
- Laboratory testing (relatively unhelpful)
- Plain radiograph findings of sacroiliitis
- MRI findings of sacroiliitis in the appropriate historical setting with plain films normal

TREATMENT

At this time, there is no known curative treatment for ankylosing spondylitis. Goals of treatment are to reduce pain and stiffness, slow progression of the disease, prevent deformity, maintain posture, and preserve function. Physical therapy, exercise, and medications are the main forms of treatment. There are rare opportunities for surgical intervention.

Lifestyle Modification

Physical therapy and exercise regimens are prescribed for all patients with ankylosing spondylitis. This has been shown to improve measures of pain, spinal mobility, patient functioning, and well-being. Supervised programs have been found to be better than at-home versions.[23] Patient education programs can increase understanding and compliance. Cigarette smoking has been associated with a poor functional outcome,[24] and patients should be encouraged to quit.

Medical Options

Nonsteroidal anti-inflammatory drugs (NSAIDs) should be prescribed for all patients unless contraindicated. They appear to provide benefits in both pain and function. Generally, regardless of the NSAID used, the maximum approved dosage is required for efficacy. In a pooled analysis of NSAIDs versus placebo over 6 weeks, NSAIDs significantly improved spinal pain, peripheral joint pain, and function. Cyclooxygenase-2 inhibitors were equally effective, although effect on peripheral arthritis was not investigated.[25] Their disease-modifying properties remain unclear. Possible radiographic slowing has been demonstrated with continuous versus on-demand use.[26] Side effects are common, typically mild, and mainly gastrointestinal. Rarely, there can be more significant gastrointestinal, renal, hepatic, and cardiovascular toxicities.

Systemic corticosteroids are typically not necessary and have only a limited role. However, injectable steroid preparations can be used for enthesitis and peripheral arthritis. Injection of long-acting steroids into the sacroiliac joints has been found to be beneficial in some.[27]

The use of disease-modifying antirheumatic drugs (DMARDs) has been adapted mainly from use in rheumatoid arthritis. Several agents have been employed, including gold salts, methotrexate, sulfasalazine, hydroxychloroquine, and leflunomide.

In a Cochrane meta-analysis of 11 randomized, controlled trials, sulfasalazine demonstrated some benefit in reducing ESR, morning stiffness and peripheral arthritis (two trials) and no benefit in improving physical function, pain, spinal mobility, enthesitis, or patient and physician global assessment.[28] Patients with early disease, elevated ESR, and peripheral arthritis might benefit from a trial of sulfasalazine. Side effects are typically dose related, mild, and mainly gastrointestinal. Rarely there are more serious allergic, hematologic, and renal toxicities.

A similar meta-analysis of two trials with methotrexate versus naproxen demonstrated no difference in outcomes of pain, function, peripheral arthritis, enthesitis, morning stiffness, patient and physician global assessement, ESR, or CRP.[29] Additional randomized, controlled studies with higher dosages for longer periods of time are necessary.

Four anti–TNF-α agents in the United States (infliximab, golimumab, etanercept, and adalimumab) have been evaluated and approved by the U.S. Food and Drug Administration (FDA) for use in ankylosing spondylitis. 80% of patients respond to at least one of the agents, and the response is typically rapid and sustainable.[30] The larger clinical trials data for all four drugs demonstrate relatively similar results. Using standard clinical assessment tools, 50% to 60% of patients achieved more than 20% clinical trial response (Ankylosing Spondylitis Assessment Study Group [ASAS 20]) at 24 weeks.[31,32,33,41] Observational studies have demonstrated continued response at 2 years.[34,35] In a pooled analysis of six of the studies, TNF antagonists have demonstrated moderate to large effects on spinal pain, peripheral joint pain, and function.[25] Lack of response to one of the agents does not predict response to another. Predictors of positive response include shorter disease duration, better functional index, higher disease activity, and higher CRP.[36] These drugs are not available in oral form and are quite expensive. Side effects include infections (re-activation of latent tuberculosis or fungi), demyelination, and injection or infusion reactions. The disease-modifying capabilities of these agents are still being assessed. In infliximab-treated patients, the MRI activity score was significantly reduced.[37] However, in another study, radiographic progression continued, but at a slower rate than in traditional cohorts.[38]

Surgical Options

Total hip replacement is the most common surgery performed in patients with ankylosing spondylitis.[39,40] Revision surgery may be necessary, because these patients typically present at a young age and when they are still active. Heterotopic ossification following joint replacement is a well-described but still unusual complication following hip replacement. Cervical fusion is indicated for the rare patient with neurologic complications of atlantoaxial subluxation. This is managed similarly to rheumatoid arthritis.

Ultimately, each patient's treatment must be individualized. Considerations must be made for the level of disease activity, degree of functional impairment, concomitant illnesses, tolerance of medications, and patient and physician expectations.

Summary

- Education, physical therapy, and exercise is essential for all patients.
- All patients should take NSAIDs patients unless they are contraindicated.
- Local cortisone injections should be given for enthesitis or peripheral arthritis.
- Consider sulfasalazine for peripheral arthritis unresponsive to NSAIDs.
- Consider anti–TNF-α treatment for peripheral arthritis unresponsive to these treatments or spinal disease unresponsive to physical therapy and NSAIDs.

Suggested Readings

Khan M: Ankylosing spondylitis: Burden of illness, diagnosis and effective treatment. J Rheumatol 2006;33:S 78 & 1-31.

Rudwaleit M: How to diagnose axial spondyloarthritis early. Ann Rheu Dis 2004;63:535-543.

Zochling J: Current evidence for the management of ankylosing spondylitis: a systemic literature review for the ASAA/EULAR management recommendations in AS. Ann Rhem Dis 2006;65:423-432.

van der Heijde D, Landewe R: Imaging in Spondylitis. Curr Opin Rheumatol 2005;17: 413-417.

Braun J: International ASAA consensus statement for the use of anti-tumour necrosis factor agents in patients with AS. Ann Rheum Dis 2003;62:817-824.

References

For a complete list of references, log onto www.expertconsult.com.

Takayasu's Arteritis

José Hernández-Rodríguez, Kathleen Maksimowicz-McKinnon, and Gary S. Hoffman

DEFINITION AND ETIOLOGY

Takayasu's arteritis (TA) is a large-vessel vasculitis of unknown etiology that has a predilection for the aorta and its primary branches. Sustained inflammation of involved vessels leads most often to stenotic or occlusive lesions and can also result in development of aneurysms.[1]

EPIDEMIOLOGY

TA is a rare disorder that has been described in patients of all races, but it occurs most often in Asian countries. The estimated annual incidence in North America is only 2.6 cases per million population.[2] Female patients are affected up to 10 times more often than male patients, and the peak incidence is in the third decade of life.[1]

PATHOPHYSIOLOGY

Vascular injury is mediated by the actions of macrophages, cytotoxic T cells, γδ T cells, and natural killer cells,[3,4] which are the main constituents within the inflammatory infiltrates. The inflammatory process leads to myointimal proliferation, with subsequent vessel wall thickening and luminal stenosis, the most common lesion of TA. Lesions that predominantly cause destruction of the muscularis and the elastica can result in vascular dilatation or aneurysms. Such abnormalities most commonly occur in the aortic root and arch.

Cytokines (such as tumor necrosis factor-α [TNF-α], interleukin-6 ([IL-6], and interferon gamma [IFN-γ]), a variety of chemokines, and other proteins (including perforin and matrix metalloproteinases) are involved in induction and amplification of the inflammatory response and tissue injury.[3-5] IL-6 and chemokine (C-C motif) ligand 5 (CCL5 or RANTES) serum levels correlate with disease activity in TA patients.[6] On the other hand, it is well known that TNF-α plays an important role in granuloma formation and TNF-α can be demonstrated within the vessel wall in large vessel vasculitis.[7] Compared to normal controls, messenger RNA (mRNA) for TNF is increased in peripheral blood mononuclear cells of TA patients.[5,8,9] Serum TNF-α[5,8,9] is similarly increased in TA patients compared to healthy persons. A potential role for TNF-α in the pathogenesis of TA is suggested by the efficacy of anti–TNF-α therapies in patients with refractory TA.[10]

SIGNS AND SYMPTOMS

One of the difficulties in making a diagnosis of TA lies in the heterogeneity of presentations. TA manifests with clinically nonspecific signs and symptoms of systemic inflammation in about 50% of patients.[11] These include fever, weight loss, malaise, and generalized arthralgias and myalgias. The most common symptoms and signs of TA in different cohorts of patients (Americans,[1,11] Italians,[12] Mexicans,[13] and Indians[14]) have been reviewed.[11] Diminishing or absence of pulse or blood pressure, asymmetry of blood pressure in upper or lower extremities, bruits (most often found over the carotid, subclavian, abdominal, and femoral arteries), claudication of extremities, fatigue, and headache are present at the time of disease onset in about half of patients.[11] The most commonly involved arterial territories in American cohorts are the aorta and subclavian arteries, followed by carotid, mesenteric, iliofemoral, and vertebral arteries.[11]

Symptomatic involvement of coronary and pulmonary arteries is less commonly detected.[11] However, in asymptomatic TA patients, imaging of pulmonary vasculature has shown evidence of involvement in more than 50% of cases.[15,16] Stenotic vascular lesions are found in more than 90% of patients; dilatation or aneurysm formation makes up 17% to 25% of lesions.[11,12] The aortic root is the most common location for aneurysmal disease and can lead to clinically apparent valvular regurgitation, which occurs in a quarter of patients.[11] Rupture of an aortic arch aneurysm and congestive cardiac failure due to aortic insufficiency or hypertension are two of main causes of death in TA patients.[1,11,12]

Hypertension is a major source of disease-related morbidity and is present in at least 40% of U.S. and European patients.[11,12] It has been noted in up to 80% of patients from India, Japan, Mexico, and Korea.[11] Renal artery stenosis (Fig. 1) is present in 25% to 80% of patients and is the most common cause of hypertension,[11] which can also result from suprarenal aortic stenosis or decreased aortic compliance.[17]

Neurologic symptoms are present in more than 50% of patients.[11] These can result from stenosis of carotid or vertebral arteries (Fig. 2), which leads to dizziness, syncope, vertigo, and orthostatic symptoms. More-severe manifestations, such as transient ischemic attack or stroke, are seen in up to 5% to 10% of patients and are more often experienced by patients with carotid or vertebral disease. Headache occurs in 40% to 57% of patients.[11]

Although visual disturbances, including amaurosis fugax and permanent blindness, have been described in 12% to 30% of some TA series,[1,11,18] permanent loss of vision is quite uncommon in North American patients.[1,11] Hypoperfusion of retinal and choroidal vessels due to stenosis of carotid arteries is responsible for TA retinopathy, which is characterized by dilation of small vessels, formation of microaneurysms and arteriovenous anastomoses, and neovascularization of the retina. Its reported incidence is 14% to 33% in Asian patients.[18] Hypertensive retinopathy and glucocorticoid adverse events affecting eyes (e.g., glaucoma, cataracts) are common in TA and also need to be considered in these patients.

Pulmonary involvement in TA is characterized by vasculitis affecting the large or medium-sized pulmonary arteries. These abnormalities (occlusion, stenosis, and post-stenotic dilatation) are detected in more than 55% of TA patients on imaging studies,[15,16] but most are asymptomatic. Manifestations of pulmonary vascular involvement can become apparent years before the systemic arterial disease has been suspected. Clinical symptoms such as hemoptysis, dyspnea, cough, or chest pain occur in about 25% of patients. Shortness of breath, not clinically attributable to cardiac or pulmonary disease, affects almost 20% of patients.[17] Rare cases of TA with interstitial pneumonitis, pleural effusion, massive hemoptysis, and thrombosis of pulmonary arteries have been reported.[16,19] Perfusion lung scans can be abnormal in 76% of patients[20] and mimic chronic thromboembolic disease. In these cases, the differential diagnosis of both entities needs to be considered.[19]

Visceral artery involvement is described in 20 to 40% of cases.[11] Lesions of the celiac trunk or mesenteric arteries can result in ischemia of the abdominal viscera. However, clinical symptoms are infrequent and many lesions do not cause gastrointestinal ischemic symptoms.

Dermatologic manifestations are noted in up to 28% of patients. Although rare cases of cutaneous necrotizing and granulomatous vasculitis have been described, more common associations

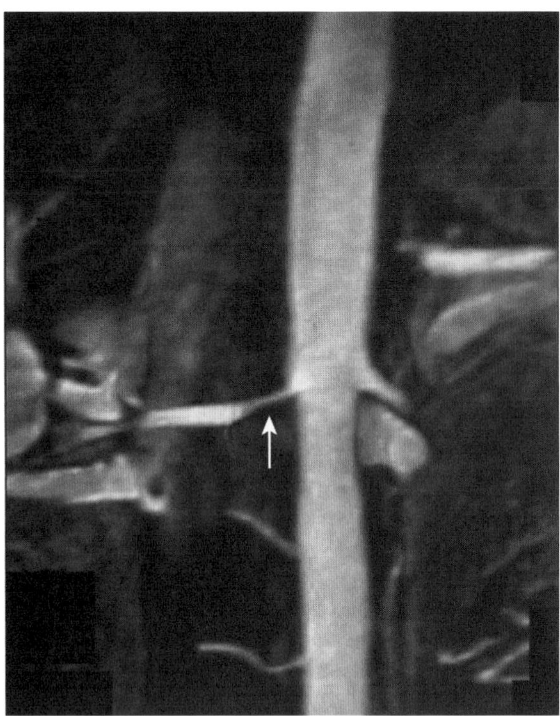

Figure 1 **Stenosis of the right renal artery.**

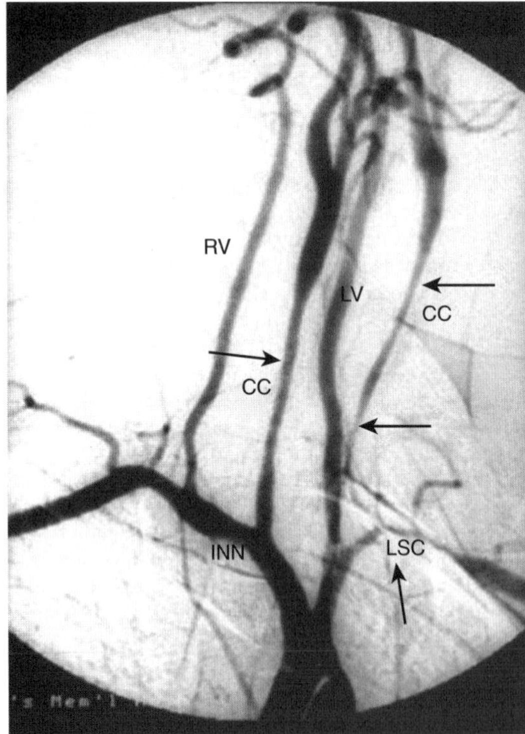

Figure 2 **Stenotic lesions of the left subclavian (LSC) and bilateral common carotid (CC) arteries.**

are erythema nodosum, erythema induratum, and pyoderma gangrenosum.[21]

DIAGNOSIS

The diagnosis of TA relies on clinical findings in the setting of compatible vascular imaging abnormalities.

Laboratory Tests

No serologic tests have sufficient sensitivity and specificity to be considered a gold standard for diagnosis.[22] Although acute-phase reactants may be helpful in assessing disease activity, in many patients they may not correlate with systemic symptoms or progressive change on imaging studies. Normal acute-phase reactants also do not ensure disease remission.[22] Sequential imaging evaluations have revealed disease progression (as determined by the presence of new vascular lesions in new territories) in more than 50% of patients with clinically stable profiles and normal erythrocyte sedimentation rate (ESR).[11,23] Clinical evaluation also underestimates the presence of subclinical disease activity; 44% of patients with TA with apparent clinically quiescent disease undergoing bypass have histopathologic evidence of vascular inflammation.[1]

Vascular Imaging Techniques

Hitherto, the gold standard for supporting the diagnosis of TA has been contrast angiography imaging. It provides information about vessel lumen caliber, permits recording of intravascular pressure measurements, and, when necessary, provides opportunities for intervention (e.g. angioplasty).[1] Catheter-directed angiography, however, has limitations, including its inability to provide information about vessel wall thickness. It also carries risks related to arterial invasiveness and rarely injury, intravascular contrast reactions, and renal toxicity. Cardiovascular magnetic resonance (C-MR) with its two components, contrast-enhanced MRI and MR angiography (MRA, conventional or three-dimensional), is now considered by some to have diagnostic accuracy almost as good as conventional catheter-directed angiography for large-vessel vasculitis. Although measurements of intravascular pressure or intravascular interventions are not possible with C-MR, images can be provided with a good safety profile and without the use of nephrotoxic contrast agents. For these reasons, C-MR overall is advantageous for initial diagnosis and for routine sequential follow-up for vasculitis involving large vessels.[24]

Although MRI can provide additional information on the inflammatory status of the vessel wall, the value of the data regarding prediction of vascular anatomic change is uncertain.[25,26] Positron emission tomography (PET) imaging using labeled fluorodeoxyglucose has been demonstrated to be useful in identifying the presence or absence of inflammation within large vessels.[26,27]

Combinations of some of these techniques, such as MRI/MRA or computed tomography–angiography with PET, are being used with promising results. However, additional studies are needed to more clearly define the performance characteristics of each technique, especially in regard to imaging enhancement, and how imaging findings correlate with disease progression when studied longitudinally. Although enhancement usually suggests inflammation, this remains an assumption and it is uncertain whether vessel repair and remodeling also produce similar findings. The accuracy of persistent enhancement in predicting later vessel anatomic change (stenoses or aneurysms) is also uncertain.

Histologic Diagnosis

Biopsies of large vessels are usually not practical. However, when a patient undergoes surgery for a vascular complication, it is recommended that a specimen of an involved artery be obtained for histologic examination.[28] Lesions can reveal granulomatous arteritis, with lymphoplasmacytic infiltrates, multinucleated giant cells, and cytotoxic and γδ T lymphocytes,[28-30] as well as patchy destruction of medial musculoelastic lamina and different degrees of fibrosis and myointimal proliferation.[30]

Differential Diagnosis

TA can mimic other conditions. Diseases such as Marfan's syndrome, type IV Ehlers-Danlos syndrome, and other congenital disorders of connective tissue can manifest with aneurysmal disease and aortic valve insufficiency. However, these diseases are not associated with large-vessel stenoses, the hallmark of TA. Signs and symptoms of systemic inflammation are absent in genetic vascular disorders of collagen and fibrillin synthesis, for which the histologic finding is cystic medial degeneration.

Infectious etiologies should be considered in all patients with large-vessel aneurysms. Agents known to cause aortic aneurysms include bacterial, syphilitic, mycobacterial, and mycotic pathogens. Stenotic disease in the setting of infection is uncommon.

Atherosclerotic vascular disease can manifest similarly to TA, but the setting in which these disorders occur helps to distinguish each. TA is more prevalent in young female patients and preferentially affects the large vessels of the upper extremities and the aortic root. Atherosclerosis more often occurs in older persons and is more common in the vessels of the lower extremities and abdominal aorta.

Rarely TA initially exhibits pulmonary perfusion scan abnormalities similar to those of chronic thromboembolic disease. TA needs to be ruled out when insidious progressive or episodic dyspnea occurs, in conjunction with multiple segmental pulmonary perfusion defects in a young patient.

Other vasculitides, such as Cogan's syndrome, Behçet's syndrome, systemic lupus erythematosus (SLE), sarcoidosis, and the spondyloarthropathies, may be associated with large-vessel vasculitis. Fortunately, in most cases their other disease manifestations help to distinguish them from TA.

The overlap between TA and giant cell arteritis is generally underappreciated. For example, patients with TA might have musculoskeletal features that are similar to those of polymyalgia rheumatica, or they might experience amaurosis, blindness, jaw claudication, or headaches. In patients presenting between the ages of 45 and 55 years, distinguishing between the two disorders may be merely a matter of semantics.

Summary

- It is important to be mindful of the heterogeneity of presentations of TA.
- The diagnosis of TA should be entertained in the setting of symptoms of ischemia or claudication or with findings of hypertension, absent pulse(s), or asymmetry of blood pressures in a younger patient.
- In many TA patients, normal acute-phase reactants can be misleading because progressive abnormalities in vascular anatomy can occur in spite of such "reassuring" data.
- Cardiovascular MR can be used in routine care in TA in the initial diagnosis and during the follow-up. Sequential imaging of the entire large-vessel anatomy might detect new lesions or the evolution of previously noted abnormalities.
- Other diseases, especially congenital and infectious, can mimic large-vessel vasculitis and should be considered in the differential diagnosis.

TREATMENT

Assessment of Disease Activity

One of the challenges in managing TA is determining disease activity. Kerr and colleagues[1] defined active disease according to the existence of new or worsening of any two or more of the following parameters, signs or symptoms of vascular ischemia or inflammation, increase in sedimentation rate, new angiographic features in new territories, and systemic symptoms not attributable to another disease.

Although these features have been demonstrated to be helpful when present, their absence does not ensure disease remission; that is, they are not adequately sensitive. These criteria have been used in studies of TA patients,[12,31] and when used in conjunction with serial imaging, they are the most effective means available for monitoring of TA activity and guiding treatment decision making.

Pharmacologic Therapy

Glucocorticoids are the baseline for treatment of active disease. Initial therapy generally consists of prednisone in dosages of 0.5 to 1 mg/kg/day. High doses of glucocorticoids result in clinical improvement in almost all patients and lead to remission in about 60%. However, when prednisone is tapered to less than 20 mg/day, most patients suffer relapse.[11,23] The high rate of relapse and the development of new arterial lesions while receiving glucocorticoid therapy mandates addition of another immunosuppressive agent, such as methotrexate (15-25 mg/week), for better control of disease remission and reduction of disease and glucocorticoid-associated morbidity.[28] However, when glucocorticoid discontinuation is attempted with the aid of methotrexate or other cytotoxic agents, relapses still occur in most patients. Azathioprine added to glucocorticoids may be effective in controlling systemic symptoms and disease progression.[32] Mycophenolate mofetil is of uncertain efficacy.[32] Cyclophosphamide (1-2 mg/kg/day orally) when added to glucocorticoids, can help achieve and maintain disease remission. Because of the risk of severe toxicity with long-term therapy (>3-6 months), this drug is only recommended for patients with severe TA refractory to other immunosuppressive therapy.[28,32] When remission has been induced with cyclophosphamide over 3 to 4 months, long-term maintenance of remission should be attempted with methotrexate.[28]

Minocycline, besides having antimicrobial activity, also suppresses production of metalloproteinases. It has been used in addition to glucocorticoids in a series of 11 patients with TA. Results were encouraging in regard to reducing levels of acute-phase reactants and improving control of disease activity. However, randomized studies must be done to establish the value of this agent in TA.[33]

In a study performed at the Cleveland Clinic, Hoffman and coworkers showed anti–TNF-α agents to be efficacious in sustaining glucocorticoid-free remissions in more than 60% of patients with previously refractory TA.[10] In an extended study, the same authors have documented the sustainability of anti–TNF-α therapy in maintaining disease remission for a longer follow-up period in most, although not all, patients (mean follow-up, >2 years).[34] Supporting these findings are several case reports of relapsing TA that have been successfully treated with anti-TNF agents[35-38] Further randomized, controlled studies are required to accurately establish the efficacy and safety of anti–TNF-α therapy in TA patients.

Other biologic therapies are beginning to be tested in TA. In this regard, anti–IL-6 receptor antibody (tocilizumab) has shown successful control in a single case of a 20-year-old woman with TA and ulcerative colitis.[39]

Endovascular and Surgical Treatment

Surgical interventions for revascularization in TA patients are indicated for ischemia-related symptoms of cervicocranial artery stenosis, coronary artery ischemia, renal artery stenosis leading to renovascular hypertension, severe extremity claudication, moderate to severe aortic valve regurgitation or stenosis of the descending or abdominal aorta, and aortic aneurysm at risk of rupture or dissection.[28] Procedures to re-establish flow in stenotic or occluded vessels include surgical use of synthetic grafts or autologous vessel bypass, endarterectomy, and percutaneous transluminal angioplasty (PTA). Aortic root replacement or repair is employed for aortic insufficiency, which is usually associated with aortic valve replacement for regurgitant flow.[28]

In two American longitudinal cohorts, intervention for either vessel stenosis or aortic regurgitation was required in one half to two thirds of TA patients over mean periods of 3 to 5 years.[1,11] PTA and stenting used alone or as a combined treatment in TA have been reviewed in a study that included 11 series of TA patients and 224 vascular lesions. Patency rate was variable among series.[11] In our experience at the Cleveland Clinic, a cohort of 30 TA patients were followed for a mean of 3 years and re-evaluated with sequential imaging studies (mean interval between studies, 4.8 months). A total of 64 revascularization procedures were carried out. All patients had stenotic vascular lesions. Angioplasty and vascular bypass and reconstruction procedures were performed in 20 and 44 instances, respectively. Overall, bypass grafts had better sustained patency than angioplasty or stent-treated vessels. Restenosis or occlusion after intervention occurred in 78% of angioplasty and 36% of bypass procedures. Bypass was especially successful when it was feasible to use autologous donor vessels.[1,40]

Revascularization procedures in TA ideally should be performed during disease remission. In one series of 42 TA patients undergoing surgical revascularization, all of the five patients with quiescent disease, who were not receiving glucocorticoids at the time of surgery, and 20 of 24 (83%) patients with quiescent disease, who were receiving glucocorticoids at the time of surgery, did not require a new revascularization procedure after 10 years follow-up. However, four of seven (57%) patients with active disease and on glucocorticoid therapy at the time of surgical repair required new operation to maintain or re-establish vascular patency.[41] At the time of bypass procedures, tissue should be obtained from the origin or insertion of grafts whenever possible to help determine disease activity. This is particularly important because clinical symptoms and acute-phase reactants might not accurately reflect disease activity.[11,28]

Although some cases of aortic branch vessel and coronary artery stenosis have been treated with endarterectomy, this procedure is technically difficult or impossible to perform effectively, and it can even be dangerous in TA because arterial lesions can be rigid and often involve the entire thickness of the vessel wall.[28]

Surgical risk is increased in patients with TA. One series, following 106 patients over a mean period of 19.8 years, stratified postoperative mortality into early and late deaths. Early deaths, defined as death occurring during hospitalization, occurred in 11% of patients.[42] Death occurred in most as a result of cardiovascular complications including congestive heart failure, aneurysm rupture, stroke, or hemorrhage. However, another series of 33 patients reported only one perioperative death (resulting from infection) over a mean follow-up period of 3 years.[43] In general, perioperative mortality is influenced by a number of factors, and the experience of the surgical team and medical center in caring for TA patients is a crucial element of surgical success.[28]

Treatment of Hypertension

Detection and treatment of hypertension in TA is critical in achieving good long-term outcomes. Recognition of hypertension is often delayed because of the high incidence of subclavian and innominate artery stenoses, which can cause falsely low peripheral blood pressure readings in reference to pressure in the aortic root. When stenoses affect all extremities, there might not be any peripheral extremity where blood pressure measurements reflect central aortic pressures. Thus, it is crucial for the clinician to have a map of the entire large-vessel anatomy to identify potential territories at risk and to provide proper care for patients with TA and central hypertension. The importance of complete vascular imaging at the time of diagnosis cannot be overemphasized. When stenoses make reliability of extremity blood pressure recordings questionable, invasive angiography with measurement of central aortic pressure and determination of gradients is critical. In these cases, even when the accuracy of peripheral measurements has been established, identifying a target pressure range that minimizes end-organ damage while allowing vital organ perfusion in the setting of arterial stenoses can be challenging. Close monitoring with avoidance of abrupt decreases in mean pressures is critically important.

Preventive Cardiology and Lifestyle Modification

Persistent inflammation, per se, may be a risk factor for premature atherosclerosis in a variety of chronic illnesses such as rheumatoid arthritis and SLE. Indeed, when compared with healthy controls, TA patients have increased carotid intima medial thickness[44] and increased arterial stiffness,[45] which are surrogate markers for coronary atherosclerosis. Furthermore, intima medial thickness is increased even in patients with angiographically normal carotid arteries in the setting of active disease.[44] Additionally, stenotic and dilated lesions of large and medium-sized arteries in TA become sites of unusually high turbulence and consequent vascular stress. Areas of turbulent flow have been recognized as foci for arterial atherosclerotic lesions in animal and human studies. Although not yet carefully studied in TA and in other vasculitides, these experiences emphasize the importance of identifying, treating, and monitoring all modifiable cardiovascular risk factors in these patients. Therefore, in addition to vigilant monitoring and control of hypertension, a preventive cardiology consultation to address additional screening for cardiovascular risk factors and management of them is recommended in all TA patients.

Summary

- Disease activity should be assessed with the combination of clinical manifestations, ESR, and vascular imaging techniques. Better surrogate markers of disease status are needed.
- Prednisone is the gold standard for initial therapy, but additional agents are needed in most cases. Methotrexate, if not contraindicated, is the preferred second agent.
- The use of anti-TNF agents in the treatment of TA remains under investigation. Based on initial encouraging results, these agents may be considered when prednisone in combination with other immunosuppressive agents has failed to control disease.
- Among revascularization procedures, bypass with autologous vessel grafts has shown better long-term patency than other procedures. However, in many circumstances (e.g. aortic reconstruction) autologous donor vessels are not feasible. When possible, revascularization should be performed when disease is quiescent.
- Diagnosis and control of hypertension is critically important. Hypertension is often unrecognized because of stenosis of large vessels supplying blood to the extremities. Hence, comprehensive arterial imaging needs to be performed at the time of diagnosis and sequentially as part of disease surveillance.

MORBIDITY AND MORTALITY

Chronic morbidity and disability is common in TA[1,11] and is directly correlated with the vascular territories involved, frequency of disease relapse, and extent of disease. In addition, there is considerable morbidity associated with immunosuppressive therapies (e.g. infections, hypertension, diabetes, osteoporosis, or cataracts related to use of corticosteroids). Patients with hypertension, aortic aneurysms, aortic valve insufficiency, coronary artery involvement or severe functional disability have a greater risk of premature death.[17] Although death from TA is uncommon, when it does occur, in most cases it is the result of cardiovascular complications including congestive heart failure, aneurysm rupture, stroke, or hemorrhage.[28,43] Postoperative mortality, defined as death occurring during hospitalization, has been observed in up to 11% of patients.[42] Other series have reported few postoperative mortalities.[1,11] Low all-cause mortality rates (3%-4%) have been reported in American cohorts over median follow-up periods of 3 to 5 years,[1,11] and 5- to 10-year survival rates are achieved in 74% to 90% of patients.[17,28,31]

NEW PERSPECTIVES AND SPECIAL CONSIDERATIONS

Systemic therapies with immunosuppressive and antiproliferative agents (e.g. sirolimus, everolimus) are currently in use in cardiac transplant protocols. These agents target the maladaptive response of intimal hyperplasia that leads to allograft vasculopathy. New stents, impregnated with slow-release forms of these agents, are being used to decrease intimal proliferation and restenosis. Sirolimus-eluting stents have demonstrated higher efficacy than conventional stents in patients with atherosclerotic coronary artery disease. It would be of interest to determine if there may be a role for such stents in large-vessel vasculitis.

Anti-TNF strategies and other biologic therapies that have shown benefit in other rheumatic diseases deserve to be investigated in randomized, controlled trials in TA. The use of platelet antiaggregation or anticoagulant treatment in patients with giant-cell arteritis seems to protect from the development of ischemic complications.[46] Although antiplatelet therapy might be recommended in TA patients, however, its value in this disease has not yet been investigated in a controlled trial.

Patients with TA require a multidisciplinary approach for optimal care. The team should include rheumatology, imaging, cardiovascular, and surgical specialists.

Suggested Readings

Hoffman GS: Takayasu arteritis: Lessons from the American National Institutes of Health experience. Int J Cardiol 1996;54(Suppl):S99-S102.

Hoffman GS, Merkel PA, Brasington RD, et al: Anti–tumor necrosis factor therapy in patients with difficult to treat Takayasu arteritis. Arthritis Rheum 2004;50:2296-2304.

Kerr GS, Hallahan CW, Giordano J, et al: Takayasu arteritis. Ann Intern Med 1994;120:919-929.

Koening CL, Langford CA: Novel therapeutic strategies for large vessel vasculitis. Rheum Dis Clin North Am 2006;32:173-186, xi.

Liang P, Hoffman GS: Advances in the medical and surgical treatment of Takayasu arteritis. Curr Opin Rheumatol 2005;17:16-24.

Maksimowicz-McKinnon K, Clark TM, Hoffman GS: Limitations of therapy and a guarded prognosis in an American cohort of Takayasu arteritis patients. Arthritis Rheum 2007;56:1000-1009.

Miyata T, Sato O, Koyama H, et al: Long-term survival after surgical treatment of patients with Takayasu's arteritis. Circulation 2003;108:1474-1480.

Park MC, Lee SW, Park YB, et al: Clinical characteristics and outcomes of Takayasu's arteritis: Analysis of 108 patients using standardized criteria for diagnosis, activity assessment, and angiographic classification. Scand J Rheumatol 2005;34:284-292.

Pipitone N, Versari A, Salvarani C: Role of imaging studies in the diagnosis and follow-up of large-vessel vasculitis: An update. Rheumatology (Oxford) 2008;47:403-408.

References

For a complete list of references, log onto www.expertconsult.com.

Cardiovascular Risk and Prevention in Rheumatic Diseases

Elaine Husni and Atul Khasnis

We now recognize coronary artery disease (CAD) as a significant contributor to morbidity and mortality in various rheumatic diseases. This enlightenment has stemmed from clinical observations in patients as well as from basic research that is providing a better understanding of this connection. Improved understanding of the underlying mechanisms, better ability to assess the cardiovascular risk in these patients, and institution of timely intervention can result in improved outcomes. An ideal risk-assessment model is still needed, and an alliance between preventive cardiology and rheumatology can be immensely useful in comprehensive delivery of care to patients with rheumatic diseases.

CONNECTION BETWEEN CORONARY ARTERY DISEASE AND RHEUMATIC DISEASE

What is the connection between CAD and rheumatic diseases?

The inflammatory nature of atherosclerosis has been proved beyond doubt.[1] Atherosclerotic affliction of the endothelium and rheumatoid affliction of the synovium can be envisioned as similar inflammatory processes that affect single-cell-thick layers and result from infiltration by cells of the immune system (macrophages, T-cells) as well as transformation and dysfunction of resident cells (endothelial and synovial fibroblasts, respectively). Abnormalities in cadherins, which are transmembrane adhesion proteins, have been proposed to play a role in synovial fibroblast proliferation in rheumatoid arthritis (RA)[2] and smooth muscle proliferation in atherosclerosis.[3] Identical clonal T-cell subset ($CD4^+$ $CD28^-$) expansion has been observed in the synovium of patients with RA and in the atherosclerotic plaques of patients with unstable angina.[4] The initial inciting event in either process is unknown, but ultimately the earliest observed pathology is cellular dysfunction that creates an imbalance in a host of cellular processes that are finely regulated at various levels. Most systemic autoimmune diseases are characterized by inflammation, and this is hypothesized to be the driver fueling accelerated atherosclerosis observed in these diseases (Box 1).

Endothelial dysfunction is the earliest event that signals the development of atherosclerosis. Circulating cytokines that cause endothelial dysfunction accompany systemic inflammation. The normal endothelium is a single-cell-thick semipermeable membrane that has myriad balanced functions (antithrombotic, vasodilator, anti-inflammatory, nonadhesive for platelets, semipermeable). Inflammatory processes disrupt many of these functions. In addition to causing direct effects on the endothelium, inflammation can promote atherosclerosis by indirect mechanisms such as unfavorable alteration of the lipid profile, arterial wall stiffening, and alteration of body-mass index. Tumor necrosis factor α (TNF-α) is a key cytokine in many inflammatory rheumatic diseases such as RA and psoriatic arthritis.

One of the earliest actions of TNF-α discovered was its ability to cause dyslipidemia (hypertriglyceridemia) in patients with *Trypanosoma brucei* infection.[5] This dyslipidemic action of TNF-α is mediated by suppression of lipoprotein lipase in adipocytes[6] and also by release of the most active form of the enzyme from the endothelial cell surface.[7] TNF-α directly affects endothelium, rendering it a promoter of coagulation and inflammation by altered cell morphology and altered surface expression of molecules.[8] Other cytokines commonly released during inflammatory diseases such as interferon-γ (INF-γ), interleukin-1 (IL-1), and IL-6 also have an adverse effect on the lipid profile, rendering it proatherogenic.

INF-γ is also known to inhibit lipoprotein lipase (similar to TNF-α), but it might have an antiatherogenic role as well.[9] The resulting lipid profile is hypertriglyceridemia, low total cholesterol, low high-density cholesterol (HDL), and increased oxidized low-density cholesterol (ox-LDL). The dyslipidemia also correlates with the degree of inflammation in various diseases with improvement in atherogenic profile seen after treatment.[10]

Other mechanisms of accelerated atherosclerosis include hyperhomocysteinemia[11] and dysfunctional HDL cholesterol observed in diseases such as systemic lupus erythematosus (SLE) and RA. C-reactive protein (CRP), which is a commonly elevated acute phase reactant in systemic inflammatory autoimmune diseases, might serve as a marker for underlying inflammation, but it also might play a pathogenic role in endothelial damage via complement activation.[12] (see Box 1)

Studies of plaque histology in patients with RA have shown extensive involvement of cells of the immune system in plaque formation and potential destabilization resulting in plaque rupture that often underlies precipitation of clinical acute coronary syndromes.[13] The presence of T and B lymphocytes in the atherosclerotic plaque might also be the missing link that implicates infection as a causative factor in this disease. In a study of atherosclerotic plaques from two patients who were dying of ischemic heart disease, prominent B lymphocytes were described in the adventitia and within the plaque, suggesting different immune alterations than those observed in traditional atherosclerosis.[14]

Circulating immune complexes abound in SLE, and these might have a role in myocardial infarction.[15] Studies have shown that IFN-γ and immune complexes bound to C1q reduce expression of the enzyme cholesterol 27-hydroxylase in human aortic endothelial cells, peripheral blood mononuclear cells, and monocyte-derived macrophages. Immune complexes down-regulate the enzyme only after complement fixation via interaction with the 126-kD C1qRp protein on endothelial cells.[16] The CD40 ligand (CD40L) on the T cell that binds CD40 on the macrophage as a costimulatory interaction has also received a lot of attention in atherosclerotic mechanisms in SLE; T cell activation via this mechanism is common to both.[17,18] Interestingly, although CD40L plays a role in atherosclerotic plaques, soluble CD40L does not correlate with measures of subclinical atherosclerosis in SLE.[19] The presence and titers of antibodies to oxidized LDL (oxLDL) have been shown to be specific for SLE.[20] but their exact role in pathogenesis remains to be determined. Insulin resistance as measured by the Homeostasis Model Assessment (HOMA) has been found to be more elevated in patients with RA (correlating with IL-6 and TNF-α levels) than in SLE (correlating with body mass index).[21]

There is ongoing research to unravel other mechanistic connections between atherosclerosis and systemic autoimmune disease. The main difficulty lies in determining whether the discovered molecule or cell is truly pathogenic, an innocent bystander, or merely an epiphenomenon. To this end, applying principles similar to Koch's postulates in whole or part may be necessary.

Box 1 Mechanisms of Accelerated Atherosclerosis in Systemic Inflammatory Autoimmune Disease

Direct Effects
Endothelial dysfunction

- Antibody mediated endothelial cell damage
- Immune complex mediated endothelial cell damage
- Cytokine mediated

Prothrombotic milieu
Dysfunctional high-density lipoprotein
Autoantibodies

Indirect Effects
Hypertension
Diabetes/insulin resistance
Renal dysfunction
Increased body mass index
Dyslipidemia
Hyperhomocystinemia

SPECIFIC DISEASE STATES

Rheumatoid Arthritis

In a prospective cohort study of 114,342 women participating in the Nurses' Health Study who were free of cardiovascular disease and RA at baseline in 1976, 527 incident cases of RA and 3622 myocardial infarctions and strokes were confirmed during 2.4 million person-years of follow-up. The adjusted relative risk in women with RA was 2.0 for myocardial infarction and 1.48 for stroke. Women with at least 10-year duration of RA had a threefold risk for myocardial infarction.[22] In a British cohort study, the mere presence of rheumatoid factor (RF) has been associated with a threefold risk of ischemic heart disease in men, independent of traditional cardiovascular risk factors.[23] This has also been shown in a Finnish study of more than 4000 patients who were followed for 15 years. The presence of moderate titer RF (>1:28) predicted worse survival even in patients who did not develop RA (false-positive RF).[24] This raises the question about what RF positivity might actually represent in terms of being a marker for other systemic processes that ultimately accelerate senescence.

In a study of 606 seropositive RA patients over 15 years from North Sweden, the standardized mortality ratio in both sexes for cardiovascular disease was 1.46 and for ischemic heart disease was 1.54 compared to the reference population. Using multiple Cox regression analyses, male sex, higher age at disease onset, and former cardiovascular event increased the death rate. Male sex, high age at disease onset, and hypertension increased the risk of cardiovascular events. Interestingly, traditional risk factors such as diabetes mellitus or treatment with corticosteroids, DMARD, or hormone replacement therapy did not influence the risks of death or first cardiovascular event.[25] The combination of positivity for RF and anti–cyclic citrullinated peptide (anti-CCP) antibodies with smoking carries the highest risk (eightfold) of cardiovascular mortality.[26] An older age of onset of RA is also associated with more-severe CAD.[27] Because inflammation is a major determinant of accelerated atherosclerosis in RA, it is not surprising that more severe and extra-articular disease is associated with onset of coronary artery disease and the first-ever clinical cardiovascular event.[28] Patients with RA also have a more-severe quality of atherosclerosis that is characterized by inflammatory plaques that are more unstable and prone to rupture.[29] The increased cardiovascular risk in RA stems from risk factors directly related to disease as well as worsening traditional cardiovascular risk factors.

An increased incidence of the metabolic syndrome has been observed in patients with RA. In a study of 154 patients with RA, the metabolic syndrome was present in 42% of patients with long-standing RA, 30% with early RA, and 22% of controls ($P = 0.03$). Patients with the metabolic syndrome had a twofold increase in coronary-artery calcification scores on electron beam computed tomography (EBCT) independent of age and sex.[30] The role of TNF-α and its downstream signaling molecule nuclear factor κB (NF-κB) are well established in RA. Osteoprotegerin is a decoy receptor for the NF-κB ligand. Patients with RA have been found to have elevated osteoprotegerin levels that correlate with coronary-artery calcification independently of cardiovascular risk factors and disease activity.[31] Osteoprotegerin is being studied as a biomarker for heart failure and long-term outcomes after acute coronary syndromes, but it has not been studied in RA.[32]

Significant subclinical atherosclerosis exists in patients with RA. If subclinical atherosclerosis is detected, risk factors, including inflammation, will have to be modified more aggressively. Subclinical atherosclerosis has been assessed using EBCT,[33] and carotid artery plaque has been assessed by measuring intima-medial thickness (IMT) using B-mode ultrasound.[34] Other measures for assessing vascular disease include measurement of pulse wave velocity and augmentation index (measures of arterial stiffness)[35] and echocardiographic assessment of coronary flow reserve (for coronary microcirculation).[36] Abnormalities in all these measures have been reported in patients with RA and correlate with duration of disease. These alterations reflect the multilevel cardiac and vascular dysfunction associated with RA. Silent myocardial ischemia is common in patients with RA.[37] When patients develop clinical acute coronary syndromes, their presentation is more likely to be atypical.[38] The Framingham score is useful and correlates with the duration of disease and presence of coronary calcification.[39]

Controlling disease activity is key to improving survival in these patients. Methotrexate, one of the most commonly used drugs for RA, has been shown to reduce cardiovascular mortality in these patients (hazard ratio 0.3 for cardiovascular death and 0.6 for non-cardiovascular death).[40] However, hyperhomocysteinemia has been reported in patients on methotrexate and sulfasalazine and in patients with a mutation in the methylene tetrahydrofolate reductase (MHTFR) gene.[41] A study of the British Biologics Register comparing rates of myocardial infarction (MI) in 8670 RA patients treated with anti–TNF-α agents and 2170 patients with active RA treated with traditional disease-modifying antirheumatic drugs (DMARDs) found that RA patients treated with anti–TNF-α did not have a lower incidence of MI, but the risk of MI was significantly lower in those who responded to therapy by 6 months compared with nonresponders (3.5 vs. 9.4 per 1000 person-years).[42] This reflects better control of inflammation in these patients.

Statins are now well known to have immunomodulating properties. In patients with RA treated with atorvastatin (40 mg), significant improvement in disease activity scores for RA were observed at 6 months, with a clinically meaningful response achieved in patients on atorvastatin compared to placebo (31% vs. 10%). C-reactive protein, erythrocyte sedimentation rate, and swollen joint count all improved in the atorvastatin group.[43]

One of the largest trials, the QUEST-RA study conducted in 15 countries and including more than 4000 patients, echoes the previous findings of male susceptibility to cardiovascular disease and myocardial infarction, the association of cardiovascular disease with extra-articular RA disease, and reduction in mortality with use of disease-modifying therapy.[44]

The search for understanding the pathophysiology of atherosclerosis in patients with RA aspires to provide a better explanation for the observed but unaccounted-for increased cardiovascular risk and possible therapeutic targets for intervention. One of the breakthroughs in this area has been the discovery of proinflammatory HDL.[45] This is observed in 20% of patients with RA and is dysfunctional in that it does not protect LDL against oxidation, thereby removing this intrinsic protective mechanism against atherosclerosis. Another molecule of interest has been the receptor for advanced glycosylation end products (RAGE), which might influence the response to inflammation.[46]

Systemic Lupus Erythematosus

The bimodal distribution of mortality in lupus was recognized three decades ago; the first peak results from the disease, and the second peak is an effect of premature cardiovascular mortality. Patients with SLE have a 4- to 10-fold greater risk of atherosclerotic cardiovascular disease and a 50-fold increase in myocardial infarction compared with the general population.[47] The mean age of first myocardial infarction among SLE patients is approximately 49 years.[48] Among SLE patients younger than 35 years, acute myocardial infarction is the most common initial clinical presentation of CAD, followed by congestive heart failure, sudden death, and angina.[49] Coronary artery affliction from SLE can result from myriad mechanisms, including but not limited to accelerated atherosclerosis, dyslipidemia, hyperhomocystinemia, hypercoagulability related to antiphospholipid antibodies, and vasculitis.

In 1975, Bulkley and Roberts noted coronary atherosclerosis in 8 of 36 young SLE patients at autopsy and first implicated corticosteroids in its etiology.[50] Similar to RA, subclinical atherosclerosis has been well documented in patients with SLE using IMT,[51] pulse wave velocity,[52] and determination of coronary flow reserve[53]; accelerated atherosclerosis has been reported despite good disease control in long-standing SLE, underlining subclinical inflammation.[54] Subclinical atherosclerosis on EBCT also correlates with cardiac risk scores such as the Framingham Risk calculator and the Pathobiological Determinants of Atherosclerosis in Youth (PDAY) score.[55] Similar to patients with RA, this well-appreciated increased cardiovascular risk is based on a combination of traditional cardiovascular risk factors, systemic inflammation, and yet-unknown drivers of the atherosclerotic process. Older age at diagnosis, longer disease duration, higher cumulative corticosteroid dose, hypertension, and hypercholesterolemia, have all been shown to predict cardiovascular mortality.[56] The relationship with corticosteroid use may be direct from ensuing dyslipidemia or diabetes, but the need to use of corticosteroids could also reflect greater underlying inflammation. Other risk factors include male sex, elevated homocysteine, and renal insufficiency.[57] Hydroxycholoroquine has a beneficial effect on the lipid profile in patients with SLE.[58] Increased IMT in patients with SLE has been correlated with hypertension, systematic coronary risk evaluation index, CRP, vascular cell adhesion molecule-1 (VCAM-1), von Willebrand's factor, matrix metalloproteinase 3 (MMP-3), and tissue inhibitor of metalloproteinase 1 (TIMP-1) and inversely correlated with MMP-9.[59] This has an impact on arterial remodeling in patients with SLE. We now know from studies of coronary artery disease that arterial remodeling is as important a determinant of luminal narrowing as plaque progression. Negative or constrictive remodeling is detrimental to maintaining arterial patency.

Compared to patients with primary antiphospholipid syndrome (APS), carotid plaque was more prevalent and appeared earlier in patients with SLE. SLE patients with secondary APS had a higher prevalence of carotid plaque than patients with primary APS (37.5% vs. 8%, $P = 0.03$). The presence of plaque in SLE patients correlated with higher disease activity scores and older age.[60] However a clear pathogenic role for antiphospholipid antibodies (APLAs) in atherosclerosis in patients with SLE has not been borne out by other studies.[61] The presence of antiphospholipid antibodies is linked more directly to acute coronary events such as myocardial infarction rather than stable coronary artery disease. APLAs predispose to thrombosis over plaques, probably resulting in acute worsening of myocardial ischemia.[62] Some newer risk factors that could contribute to development of atherosclerosis include CRP and antibodies to β2 glycoprotein I (anti-β2GPI), oxidized low-density lipoprotein (anti-oxLDL), and heat shock protein (anti-HSP) 60/65 antibodies.[63] The long-term use of corticosteroids is also associated with accelerated atherosclerosis, probably through worsening dyslipidemia.[64,65] Atorvastatin use over an 8-week period has produced improved endothelial function in patients with SLE.[66] Proinflammatory (dysfunctional) HDL has been reported in 45% of patients with SLE, which is twice the number of patients with RA and 10 times the number of control patients.[45] Antibodies to lipoprotein lipase have been reported in patients with SLE.

In a study using myocardial perfusion scintigraphy with single photon emission computed tomography (SPECT) using technetium-sestamibi scanning in 90 female SLE patients (20-55 years old, with disease duration >5 years and current or previous steroid treatment for >1 year), 30 of the 90 had myocardial perfusion defects. Angiography in 21 of these 30 patients showed plaques in 8 of the 21 patients (38%). Abnormal angiographic findings were associated with higher number of CAD risk factors, higher SLE disease activity scores, presence of hypertension, and postmenopausal status. In patients with more than four risk factors for CAD, coronary stenosis was present in 67%. Based on this study, myocardial scintigraphy appears to be a reasonable tool to screen SLE patients for CAD. Patients with abnormal scintigraphy results and more than four risk factors for CAD should undergo coronary angiography.[67] Intravascular ultrasound of the coronary arteries in a patient with SLE showed diffuse plaque formation, intimal thickening, partial calcification, and partial eccentric lipid-rich plaque, which reflects the observed histopathology in these patients.[68]

Large-scale studies regarding outcomes of therapeutic coronary interventions are not available due to the rare nature of the underlying disease. Coronary artery bypass grafting has been successfully reported in two patients with SLE.[69] Studies involving greater numbers of patients are needed in order to study the outcomes of coronary intervention in these patients. This is especially true in an era of advances in cardiovascular technology, where recognition of possible adverse outcomes (complications or reintervention) can allow early recognition and treatment.

Systemic Sclerosis

Systemic sclerosis (SSc) is a unique autoimmune disease that has a significant microvasculopathy component. Endothelial dysfunction is a key abnormality in this disease. However, it is an exceedingly rare disease. Cardiac involvement in SSc is characterized by patchy myocardial fibrosis (from repeated microvascular ischemia and inflammation), diastolic dysfunction, and pulmonary hypertension. Cardiac arrhythmias and conduction disturbances are a hallmark of cardiac involvement, especially worsened by autonomic dysfunction. Renal involvement often leads to hypertension, which exacerbates the diastolic dysfunction. Chest pain can occur from a mismatch of perfusion and oxygen supply to the right ventricular musculature in patients with pulmonary hypertension, but the coronary angiographic picture may be completely normal.

Subclinical atherosclerosis and associated elevated proinflammatory HDL have been reported in patients with SSc.[70] Increased lipoprotein(a), oxLDL, inflammation, vasospasm, and endothelial dysfunction are well known in SSc. Generalized premature atherosclerosis has not been detected in SSc.[71] Noninvasive strategies such as strain rate imaging, transthoracic coronary flow reserve, and brachial artery flow-mediated dilatation are noninvasive modalities for detecting left ventricular myocardial and vascular involvement caused by SSc.

In an angiographic study of 172 patients with SSc, the prevalence of CAD was found to be similar to that in the population without SSc. There was no association between SSc subsets, duration of the disease, duration of Raynaud's phenomenon, skin sclerosis score, autoantibody profile, and CAD.[72] However, SSc is characterized by microvascular dysfunction, an entity that cannot be evaluated by conventional coronary angiography.

Measures of diastolic dysfunction such as impaired ventricular relaxation times and abnormal ratios of early to late diastolic filling (E/A ratios) can be quantitated using modalities such as Doppler myocardial imaging.[73] Early microvascular dysfunction, which is common in diffuse SSc, can be evaluated using coronary flow reserve measurements on echocardiography before and after pharmacologic stress and by sestamibi SPECT scanning.[74,75]

On angiography, patients with SSc are 34 times more likely to have normal coronary arteries.[76] This underlines the microvascular dysfunction seen in this disease. In 14 asymptomatic female patients with SSc, the angiographic abnormalities observed were ectasia, slow flow, spasm, stenosis, tortuosity, and calcification of the coronary arteries.[77] This suggests that angiographic abnormalities do not correlate with clinical symptoms. Increased arterial stiffness has also been reported in these patients.[78] Statins, by virtue of their effects on endothelial dysfunction and inflammation, might have some benefit in patients with SSc.[79]

There remains much to be desired in exploring the mechanisms of microvascular ischemia, injury, and consequences thereof that define SSc. Owing to the rarity of this disease, large-scale studies are difficult to perform. It would be useful to remember that because there exists microvascular insufficiency, in some patients it may be unrealistic to expect that correction of macroscopic obstructive epicardial coronary disease will lead to abatement of symptoms. We still need better means to quantitate the microvascular disease, the real target in these patients. There is no large body of data available on surgical or percutaneous intervention for CAD in these patients.

Spondyloarthropathies

The spondyloarthropathy family is also a group of inflammatory disorders that is not exempt from its accompanying burden of the cardiovascular consequences of chronic inflammation. Endothelial dysfunction has been observed in patients with ankylosing spondylitis and psoriatic arthritis.[80,81] Patients with psoriasis have been found to have a higher incidence of multiple cardiovascular risk factors, especially those characterizing the metabolic syndrome.[82] Patients with psoriatic arthritis have higher subclinical atherosclerosis measured by carotid IMT even in the absence of clinically obvious cardiovascular risk factors.[83] However, other studies have failed to show subclinical atherosclerosis in patients treated for psoriatic arthritis in the absence of traditional cardiovascular risk factors,[84] again highlighting the importance of treatment in controlling inflammation in this disease.

In a cross-sectional study of prevalence and risk factors for RA, psoriatic arthritis and ankylosing spondylitis, the prevalence ratios of IHD, atherosclerosis, peripheral vascular disease, congestive heart failure, cerebrovascular disease, type 2 diabetes mellitus, hyperlipidemia, and hypertension were higher in patients than controls.[85] A proatherogenic milieu is reported in patients with psoriatic arthritis.[86] Although large studies on coronary artery involvement in reactive arthritis have not been done, there is one case report of coronary ostial narrowing as a complication of aortitis.[87] Improvement in microvascular dysfunction after treatment of ankylosing spondylitis with etanercept has been documented.[88] Aortic valve involvement occurs in ankylosing spondylitis and reactive arthritis, and the ensuing aortic regurgitation might have consequences on coronary blood flow as well.

Primary Vasculitides

The vasculitides are characterized by histopathologic evidence of inflammation of blood vessels. Because inflammation of blood vessels is the hallmark, endothelial dysfunction is inherent in these diseases. Atherosclerosis is now increasingly recognized in patients with primary vasculitides. The mechanisms include direct endothelial dysfunction including increased expression of adhesion molecules, circulating CRP and cytokines, antibodies to endothelial cells, thrombosis, and heightened traditional cardiovascular risk factors.[89]

Giant cell arteritis typically occurs in patients older than 50 years, a population that has accumulated traditional cardiovascular risk factors for atherosclerotic disease, so it is not surprising to find an increased incidence of cardiovascular disease. In a retrospective Canadian study of 1141 patients with GCA, the composite end point of subsequent diagnosis or surgical treatment for CAD, stroke, peripheral arterial disease, or aneurysm or dissection of the aorta was more common in patients with GCA than in patients with osteoarthritis (12.1 vs. 7.3/1000 person-years). The adjusted hazard ratio for cardiovascular disease was 1.6 in patients with GCA compared to patients with osteoarthritis and 2.1 in patients with GCA versus unaffected control patients.[90]

In a study of 50 patients with small-vessel vasculitis, subclinical atherosclerosis as measured by IMT in the carotid, aorta, and femoral arteries was greater than in the control group.[91] This finding was independent of traditional cardiovascular risk factors and CRP levels, suggesting direct endothelial abnormalities separate from systemic inflammation.

Coronary artery involvement in Takayasu's arteritis is often ostial from the arteritis rather than from atherosclerotic disease.

ASSESSING THE RISK

The first step to risk assessment is to acknowledge the risk. Most patients with systemic inflammatory autoimmune diseases are seen at regular intervals, and this provides an opportunity to assess them for premature cardiovascular disease. The Framingham risk score is still a useful score that has been validated in patients with RA to assess cardiovascular risk. Higher Framingham scores correlate with longer disease duration and coronary calcium scores.[39]

The evaluation of these patients is similar to other patients without these conditions but with a lower clinical threshold and increased awareness on the part of the physician. A composite assessment of history, physical examination, laboratory studies, and imaging can provide a good baseline estimate of the patient's cardiovascular health. The history should include questions about angina or angina equivalents, symptoms of cerebrovascular insufficiency, and claudication in pertinent patients. A good physical examination can reveal signs of hyperlipidemia, diagnose hypertension, and clinically assess large-vessel status and valvular heart disease in these patients. Laboratory tests should include a lipid profile, creatinine, and markers of inflammation at regular intervals as needed and guided by therapy. Checking homocysteine levels may be necessary in specific cases.

Patients with symptoms or abnormalities on screening should be referred to specialist colleagues for further detailed evaluation and therapy as deemed indicated. A collaborative effort with preventive cardiology can go a long way in optimizing the cardiovascular health of these patients. This has been shown and recommended based on the experience of patients with SLE in the Pittsburgh cohort.[92] This also offers the potential to build a combined rheumatology and cardiology database of these patients that can help evaluate, design, and infer meaningful data about clinical and basic science queries related to cardiovascular disease in this population.

Routine imaging for subclinical atherosclerosis is not standard of care or recommended at this time. However, the development of risk score tools such as SHAPE (Screening for Heart Attack Prevention and Education) are the first step toward measuring the burden of subclinical atherosclerosis.[93] The need to assess peripheral arterial disease in these patients as a significant component of the vascular disease burden cannot be overemphasized.

TREATMENT

Therapy in these patients is not much different in terms of managing traditional cardiovascular risk factors such as controlling blood pressure, reducing hyperlipidemia, quitting smoking, taking regular exercise and improving diet. Because inflammation is the common thread that runs through all systemic autoimmune diseases and atherosclerosis, it is key to control systemic inflammation. This is evident from trials that demonstrate improved cardiovascular outcomes from the use of various immunosuppressive medications in the treatment of systemic rheumatic diseases.

Hydroxychloroquine is a unique medication that has lipid-lowering and antithrombotic properties. This medication should be used regularly in patients with SLE. Cardiologists regularly use statins owing their multiple beneficial effects for patients with hyperlipidemia and CAD. Statins have now been shown to have anti-inflammatory actions, which might serve the dual purpose of cardioprotection and rheumatic disease modification. Low-dose aspirin should also be used for these patients in the absence of contraindications to its use. Because a larger cumulative dose of corticosteroids has been shown to contribute to accelerated atherosclerosis, trying to achieve disease control with other DMARDs while trying to minimize prednisone use should be one of the goals of therapy.

Folate supplementation in patients taking methotrexate might reduce the consequent hyperhomocystinemia and provide added cardiovascular protection.[94] The use of newer medications, such as anticytokine therapies, might result in better cardiovascular outcomes than before. This remains to be studied, because some of the newer therapies have been available only in recent years.

THE FUTURE

Where do we go from here? The future holds a lot of hope. With increasing awareness and literature regarding the cardiovascular risk in systemic autoimmune diseases, new mechanistic insights are being gained each day with the ultimate goal being their translation into therapeutic targets. The alliance between cardiology and rheumatology has to grow stronger, especially because there are multiple shared mechanisms in atherosclerosis and systemic rheumatic diseases. Newer medications will be available in both specialties in the future, and their effects on atherosclerosis progression remain to be seen.

The development of a composite cardiovascular score to assess this risk is imperative. The integration of clinical information, laboratory data, and imaging information will equip us to provide the most clinically meaningful therapies for our patients. There are ongoing studies to assess the utility of available imaging modalities such as multirow detector CT (MDCT) and cardiac MRI in measuring atherosclerotic burden of disease.

The role of systemic inflammation in promoting atherosclerosis as it is understood today is still an oversimplification of myriad processes at work. A number of mechanistic explanations will come from the research bench; strong clinical research will be necessary to transform these basic science insights into strategies for better risk modification and management. Diabetes mellitus is well accepted as a CAD equivalent due to the risk it portends for outcomes in ischemic heart disease. Rheumatoid arthritis has a risk comparable to that in diabetes for myocardial infarction (odds ratio, ~ 3.0). Lipid-lowering guidelines recommend specific targets for lipid lowering in patients with diabetes; no such recommendations exist for systemic rheumatic diseases, most likely due to lack of well-done trials.

In the future, the availability of pharmacogenomic data could refine the approach to drug selection for individual patients, with the ability to confidently predict a therapeutic response. Until then, we must use our heightened awareness and clinical judgment to produce the best cardiovascular outcomes in our patients with systemic inflammatory autoimmune diseases.

Summary

- Risk of coronary artery disease is increased in patients with systemic rheumatic diseases.
- Increased risk occurs as a consequence of traditional and nontraditional risk factors.
- Collaborate with preventive cardiology.
- Controlling inflammation (disease activity) at all costs is central to management.
- Minimize prednisone use; use DMARDs for disease control.
- Use hydroxychloroquine for its anti-inflammatory, lipid lowering, and antithrombotic properties.
- Treat traditional cardiovascular risk factors as well.

Selected Readings

Bruce IN, Gladman DD, Urowitz MB: Premature atherosclerosis in systemic lupus erythematosus. Rheum Dis Clin North Am 2000;26:257-278.

Choi HK, Herman MA, Seeger JD, et al: Methotrexate and mortality in patients with rheumatoid arthritis: A prospective study. Lancet 2002;359:1173-1177.

Chung CP, Oeser A, Avalos I, et al: Utility of the Framingham risk score to predict the presence of coronary atherosclerosis in patients with rheumatoid arthritis. Arthritis Res Ther 2006;8(6):R186.

Elliott JR, Manzi S, Edmundowicz D: The role of preventive cardiology in systemic lupus erythematosus. Curr Rheumatol Rep. 2007;9(2):125-130.

Gonzalez-Juanatey C, Llorca J, Amigo-Diaz E, et al: High prevalence of subclinical atherosclerosis in psoriatic arthritis patients without clinically evident cardiovascular disease or classic atherosclerosis risk factors. Arthritis Rheum 2007;57(6): 1074-1080.

Khurma V, Meyer C, Park GS, et al: A pilot study of subclinical coronary atherosclerosis in systemic sclerosis: Coronary artery calcification in cases and controls. Arthritis Rheum 2008;59(4):591-597.

Libby P: Inflammation in atherosclerosis. Nature 2002;420(6917):868-874.

Manzi S, Meilahn EN, Rairie JE, et al: Age-specific incidence rates of myocardial infarction and angina in women with systemic lupus erythematosus: Comparison with the Framingham Study. Am J Epidemiol 1997;145:408-415.

McMahon M, Grossman J, FitzGerald J, et al: Proinflammatory high-density lipoprotein as a biomarker for atherosclerosis in patients with systemic lupus erythematosus and rheumatoid arthritis. Arthritis Rheum 2006;54(8):2541-2549.

Naranjo A, Sokka T, Descalzo MA, et al: Cardiovascular disease in patients with rheumatoid arthritis: Results from the QUEST-RA study. Arthritis Res Ther 2008; 10(2):R30.

Solomon DH, Karlson EW, Rimm EB, et al: Cardiovascular morbidity and mortality in women diagnosed with rheumatoid arthritis. Circulation 2003;107:1303-1307.

References

For a complete list of references, log onto www.expertconsult.com.

Section 14

WOMEN'S HEALTH

Breast Disorders and Breast Cancer Screening

Mark Mayer, Pelin Batur, and Halle Moore

DEFINITION

Evaluation of breast complaints and screening for breast cancer account for a significant part of primary care practice and are the dual roles of the primary physician. Complaints most commonly presented include breast pain, breast lumps, and nipple discharge. These symptoms often arise from benign conditions, but accurate evaluation is essential.

PREVALENCE

In one study, 16% of women between ages 40 and 69 years came to the doctor with breast complaints over a 10-year period.[1] Estimates of the number of insured women between ages 50 and 64 years getting screening mammography at least every 2 years vary from 72% to 81%[2]; uninsured women clearly obtain less preventive care. Breast cancer is diagnosed in about 213,000 women in the United States each year. The breast cancer mortality rate has declined gradually since 1990 to about 41,000 per year.

PATHOPHYSIOLOGY

Most breast lumps and other breast complaints are due to benign conditions. Breast pain can be produced by fibrocystic changes, mastitis, pendulous breasts, or hidradenitis suppurativa. Chest wall pain, which may be felt as breast pain, can have many causes that do not originate in the breast. These include gallbladder disease, ischemic heart disease, trauma, intercostal neuralgia, costochondritis, and thoracic spine arthritis. Many breast lumps are due to fibrocystic changes. Most lumps are benign, but of all complaints, they constitute the greatest percentage of symptoms leading to a diagnosis of cancer. Nipple discharge is usually benign, especially if nonbloody, bilateral, and not spontaneous. Discharge can be due to medications, hormonal factors, prior nursing or pregnancy, or, less commonly, cancer.

Risk factors for the development of breast cancer include increased age, genetic predisposition, and increased exposure to estrogen.[3] Breast cancer risk is increased even if the nearest relative with breast cancer is a third-degree relative.[4] Among women with a positive family history of breast cancer, having multiple first-degree relatives with premenopausal breast cancer confers the highest risk; a small minority of these are associated with *BRCA1* or *BRCA2* mutations. A number of models for assessing risk of carrying a mutation have been proposed. All account for early-onset breast cancer in the family, and most give weight to the number of affected relatives.[5]

Increased exposure to estrogen modestly raises the risk of breast cancer. Early menarche (before age 12 years) and late menopause (after age 55 years), both markers of increased estrogen exposure, confer some increased risk. The role of hormone therapy (HT) is controversial. The Women's Health Initiative, the first large-scale randomized placebo-controlled trial of postmenopausal hormone use, showed a 26% increased risk of breast cancer. However, this was after 5.2 years of use and only in women who used combination estrogen and progestin in the form of Prempro.[6] In contrast, women in the estrogen-only arm of this trial, using Premarin, did not have any increased risk of breast cancer. The Million Women Study in the United Kingdom is the largest nonrandomized study of hormone use. This study concluded that all types of hormone use, including estrogen-only forms, increased the risk of breast cancer compared with never users. The risk increased with increasing duration of use.[7]

SIGNS AND SYMPTOMS

Breast pain, breast lumps, and nipple discharge are the most common complaints presented to the physician. Screening is performed in the absence of symptoms; when symptoms exist, the evaluation may dictate going beyond screening procedures. In addition to a history and examination directed by the complaint, any benign disorders identified may need to be treated. If cancer is considered once the history and physical examination are completed, discussions about diagnostic modalities such as imaging, aspiration, or biopsy may need to be addressed at the time of the office visit. Depending on the clinical evaluation, referral may be suggested even with pending imaging studies.

DIAGNOSIS

History

History should include the characteristics of symptoms and their timing in relation to menstrual cycles. Breast pain is most commonly caused by fibrocystic changes. Other causes include mastitis, which usually produces sudden pain, with signs of inflammation. Pendulous breasts can cause pain. Hidradenitis suppurativa can manifest as breast nodules and pain; signs of infection and possible concomitant involvement of the axilla should be evaluated. One should be alert for history suggesting thoracic arthritis, chest wall inflammation, breast or axillary infection, cholecystitis, or cardiac ischemia.

The presence or absence of *lumps* should be ascertained, and whether they wax and wane with the menstrual cycle (suggesting fibrocystic changes). Lumps associated with nipple discharge, particularly unilateral bloody discharge, are worrisome.

Symptoms of *nipple discharge* should be elicited. The overall rate of malignancy is low (probably around 1%). If the discharge is nonbloody, the risk of cancer is lower. Purulent discharge may be caused by mastitis or a breast abscess. Milky discharge may persist after childbearing and can occur with some medications (see "Treatment"). An endocrine workup (for prolactin excess) may be needed if symptoms are sustained or are associated with menstrual problems. Prior biopsies, prior treatments, and use of hormones should be ascertained.

Risk factors for cancer should be assessed whether symptoms are present or the visit is for screening only. These include age, menarche before age 12 years, menopause after age 55 years, and first live birth at age 30 years or older. Information should be obtained about previous biopsies (whether ductal hyperplasia and, if so, whether atypical), and the number of first-degree relatives with breast cancer (and at what age their cancer was detected). The Gail Model Risk Assessment Tool may be used to help calculate risk from these history questions.[8] A computer disk for use of the Gail model is available from the National Cancer Institute to use in calculating this. Such estimates can aid in decision making, particularly about chemoprevention.

Physical Examination

There is an overall consensus that clinical breast examination (CBE) is useful in screening as well as in evaluation of a lump, although there has been debate on this issue. Four screening clinical trials included both mammography and CBE, four others evaluated mammography only, but no trial studied CBE alone without mammography. In a comparison of studies including both screening modalities, the range of cancers detected by CBE but not by mammography was 3% to 45%. Although the sensitivity of mammography is greater than that of CBE, there is a residual diagnostic value of CBE that favors its continued use in screening.[9]

Careful, systematic palpation has been shown to increase detection of breast lumps. Patient position, palpation of breast boundaries, and examination pattern and technique are important variables in CBE.[9]

The physical examination should include inspection and palpation. Inspection of the breasts can be done with the woman sitting with hands on her hips; some advocate inspection also with the patient sitting with her hands on top of her head, pushing downward. The examiner looks for lumps, asymmetry, or skin dimpling.

The breasts should be palpated for evaluation of texture and detection of masses. The supine patient position is preferable because CBE requires flattening breast tissue against the patient's chest, and the distance from skin to chest wall is minimized with the patient supine. The patient's ipsilateral hand should be brought up to head level for examination of the lateral aspect of the breast; the elbow should be at shoulder level for examination of the medial part of the breast.

The examination pattern should be systematic. It is important to include the area bordering the clavicle, and laterally toward the axilla, so as to ensure examination of all breast tissue. One preferred method is to start at the axilla in the midaxillary line and then cover the breast by palpating in parallel lines, in vertical strips to the sternum. A rectangular area bordered by the clavicle, the midsternum, the midaxillary line, and the bra line should be covered (Fig. 1). Small circular motions should be made at each step using the pads of the index, third, and fourth fingers, with gradated pressure (Fig. 2).

Examination of the axillae for lymph nodes should follow breast examination. Examination along the chest wall is especially important. The position and size of any nodes should be recorded. The presence of lymphadenopathy should prompt referral to a breast specialist, although the significance of shotty nodes is unclear.

The character of breast lumps is particularly important. Characteristics that suggest cancer include a hard or gritty texture, immobility, an irregular border, and a size greater than 2 cm. A new dominant mass or a gritty or growing lump deserves evaluation by a breast specialist. Unfortunately, likelihood ratios for these signs indicating cancer are not very large, except for the presence of fixed lesions and lump size greater than 2 cm.[9]

After the history and physical examination, further assessment of breast lumps may include careful clinical follow-up, ultrasound, mammography, and biopsy. Guidelines for screening mammography are reviewed in the "National Guidelines" section.

Mammography

Mammography may be performed as an adjunct to the physical examination in evaluating breast lumps or as a screening tool. Mammography is not generally useful in women younger than 35 years who present with a lump.[10] Ultrasonography may be useful in evaluating lumps in these younger women, although it is important to refer to a breast specialist for any lesion in doubt.

Evaluating Symptoms

Mammography is usually recommended as part of the evaluation in women older than 35 years who have a breast mass, to help evaluate the mass and to search for other lesions. It is an error to rely on negative mammogram results when there is a *clinically suspicious* lump. In such cases, the mammogram is a diagnostic adjunct to the surgeon, and negative findings should not preclude referral.

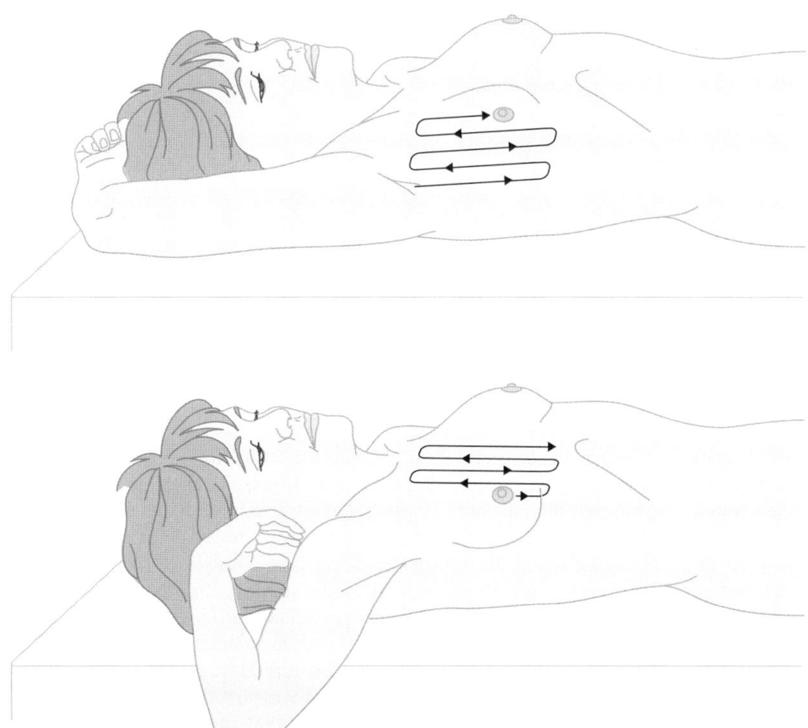

Figure 1 Position of the patient and direction of palpation for clinical breast examination. Palpation is on the lateral *(top)* and medial *(bottom)* portions of the breasts. *Arrows* indicate vertical strip pattern of examination. *(From Barton MB, Harris R, Fletcher SW: Does this patient have breast cancer? The screening clinical breast examination: Should it be done? How? JAMA 1999;282:1270-1280.)*

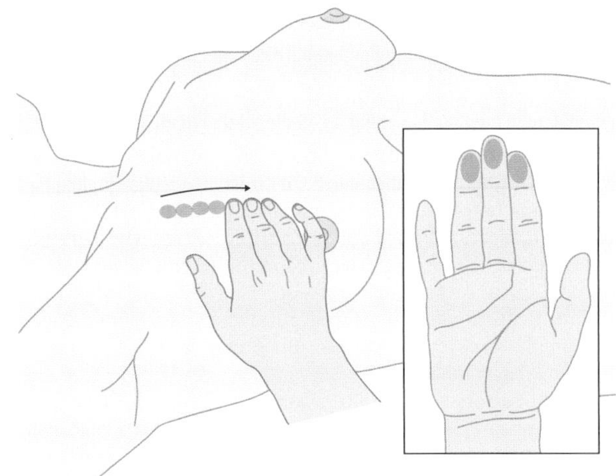

Figure 2 **Pads of the index, third, and fourth fingers *(inset)* make small circular motions, as if tracing the outer edge of a dime.** *(From Barton MB, Harris R, Fletchér SW: Does this patient have breast cancer? The screening clinical breast examination: Should it be done? How? JAMA 1999;282:1270-1280.)*

Mammographic findings that suggest cancer include increased density, irregular border, spiculation, and clustered irregular microcalcifications. Round, dense lesions on mammography might represent cystic fluid. Ultrasonography can often suggest a cystic lesion, and needle aspiration can confirm this.

Mammography findings are usually negative when mammography is used to evaluate breast pain, although it may be of reassurance value in this setting.

Screening

The age at which to begin mammography for screening is controversial. There have been eight major trials of mammography screening. The observed change in breast cancer mortality has varied widely among these studies. Differences in randomization techniques, quality of the mammograms, duration of follow-up, and evolving treatments for breast cancer during the trials have made it difficult to draw conclusions about mammographic screening. There have been several meta-analyses of the effect of mammographic screening. Differences in these derive from the time they were done, the presence or absence of follow-up data from individual trials, and the exclusion of certain trials in some meta-analyses.

A consensus has emerged that women between 50 and 69 years should be screened by mammography. Results of a meta-analysis[11] of breast cancer screening trials found a 26% reduction in breast cancer mortality over 7 to 9 years among women screened at ages 50 to 74 years.

For women first screened in their 40s, the magnitude of breast cancer mortality reduction is at best 18% after 10 to 18 years of follow-up.[12] Although some guidelines discuss starting mammographic screening earlier in women with a family history of breast cancer, data on the sensitivity of mammograms show no better cancer detection rates in this group.[13] However, due to a higher pretest probability of breast cancer in those with a family history, the positive predictive value of mammograms is higher for those women (and therefore the false-positive rate is lower for them).

The number needed to be screened to prevent one death from breast cancer is estimated at between 1500 and 2500 for women screened in their 40s.[14] In addition, nearly one half of women screened starting at age 40 years have at least one abnormal screening mammogram during the subsequent 10-year period, leading to additional mammographic views and biopsies for a significant number. Many of these abnormal screening studies prove to be false positives.

If the patient or physician finds a palpable lump, a diagnostic (four-view) mammogram, with or without ultrasound, may be used to help guide diagnosis. Again, mammography is not sufficient to exclude cancer in the evaluation of a palpable mass (see the discussions of ultrasonography and triple diagnosis).

Ultrasonography

Ultrasonography does not have a role as a single or initial study in screening for breast cancer. However, it is very useful for evaluating breast lumps and in further defining mammographic abnormalities. It is especially useful in women younger than 35 years, when a mass is noted on screening mammography but is not palpable, when a patient declines aspiration of a mass, and if a mass is too small or too deep for aspiration.

The risk of cancer is low if a simple cyst is found on ultrasound. One study found no cancers in 223 cysts.[15] However, some experts recommend moving directly to fine-needle aspiration if a simple cyst is found at the site of a palpable mass.[16] In our experience, we have found only one cancer in a "simple cyst" noted by ultrasound; the "cyst" was 2 cm in size, new, and palpable by patient and physician, and it warranted aspiration based on its size.

Fine-Needle Aspiration

Fine-needle aspiration can be performed to aspirate a palpable suspected cyst. A 22- or 24-gauge needle is inserted into a cyst that has been stabilized with the other hand. If nonbloody fluid is obtained, it can be discarded, because no cancer was found in nonbloody cyst fluid in a large series.[17] A clinical recheck should be performed in 4 to 6 weeks; recurrence of the lump should prompt surgical referral. Bloody fluid should be sent for pathologic analysis. Cancer is found in approximately 1% of bloody aspirates.[17] When no fluid is obtained, cells can be obtained for cytologic evaluation with fine-needle aspiration biopsy.

Core Needle Biopsy

A larger needle (14- to 18-gauge) is used for core needle biopsy. It is mostly used for evaluating nonpalpable breast masses (those found on mammography only), with ultrasound or mammographic guidance. Agreement between core needle biopsy and surgical biopsy was 94% in seven studies.[18]

Triple Diagnosis

The combination of the physical examination, mammography, and fine-needle aspiration biopsy for diagnosing palpable lumps is referred to as *triple diagnosis.* There is excellent sensitivity (99%) and specificity (99%) with this approach.[19] If any of these three modalities suggests cancer, excisional biopsy is warranted.

TREATMENT

Breast Pain

Treatment for breast pain depends on an accurate diagnosis. Antibiotics may be required for some infections; abscesses or hidradenitis can require surgical drainage. Breast reduction surgery may be helpful for those with pendulous breasts and resultant pain.

Treatment of fibrocystic disease is aimed at relieving pain. Wearing a soft brassiere with good support may be helpful. Acetaminophen or a nonsteroidal anti-inflammatory drug can also help. Some patients note relief of pain with avoidance of caffeine, but this has not been proved by controlled studies. Use of vitamin E (400 U) is supported by some studies. Other possibly helpful remedies include evening primrose oil (1500-3000 mg/day) or vitamin B_6. Optimal doses of vitamin B_6 are unclear, although it is prudent to avoid doses greater than 50 mg/day, due to risk of neuropathy. Oral contraceptives have shown some promise, and those containing progestins with androgenic properties (e.g., 19-norprogestins) may be more beneficial. Danazol inhibits estrogen secretion and can behelpful; side effects include weight gain, acne, hirsutism, and amenorrhea.

Lumps and Discharge

Treatment of a breast lump or nipple discharge depends on the results of history, physical examination, and sometimes diagnostic studies. Characteristics of lumps suggesting malignancy include size (>2 cm), firmness, immobility, and irregularity. The triple diagnosis protocol outlined in the previous section is helpful in sorting out whether lumps are benign or malignant. Benign lumps should be followed up clinically.

Nipple discharge can be caused by several factors. Some medications (e.g., phenothiazines) can cause increased prolactin levels and thus nipple discharge; change in medication may be needed. Pituitary adenomas can lead to increased prolactin. Endocrine studies, starting with a prolactin level, should be obtained if discharge is persistent. Medical or surgical therapy may be warranted if a prolactinoma is identified. Nipple stimulation can sometimes cause discharge, and cessation may be required to stop symptoms. Cytology of suspect nipple discharge (especially bloody discharge) can be obtained, and galactography can also be performed. Fiberoptic ductography is available in some centers and should improve our ability to find papillary lesions. If nipple discharge is associated with a palpable mass, referral to a breast surgeon is mandatory.

Breast Cancer

Once breast cancer is discovered—because of a palpable lump, nipple discharge, or screening—it is best treated by a multidisciplinary team, including surgeons and a medical oncologist. Ongoing involvement of the primary physician is helpful for maintaining emotional support and to monitor the overall health of the patient. A recent guideline for breast cancer treatment can be found on the Institute for Clinical Systems Improvement (ICSI) website.

Treatment of early-stage breast cancer generally includes local therapy to treat the breast and regional lymph nodes as well as systemic therapy aimed at eradicating any occult disseminated cancer cells that have the potential to develop into overt metastatic disease over time.

Local Treatment

Local therapy for breast cancer generally consists of surgery with or without radiation therapy. The primary tumor in the breast can be removed with a mastectomy or with breast-conserving surgery, also known as *lumpectomy* or *partial mastectomy*. An axillary dissection allows for pathologic evaluation of the axillary lymph nodes for regional spread of disease. This procedure is often replaced by the more limited sentinel lymph node procedures, which limit the extent of surgery required in the axilla by using a blue dye and a radioactive tracer to identify the lymph nodes that are first to drain the affected area and, therefore, believed most likely to contain metastases if present. The term *modified radical mastectomy* refers to a mastectomy with axillary lymph node dissection. Radiation therapy is included to reduce the risk of local recurrence following breast-conserving surgery or following mastectomy when local recurrence risk is believed to be high based on tumor and patient characteristics.

Systemic Treatment

Systemic treatment for early stage breast cancer includes endocrine therapy such as tamoxifen or aromatase inhibitors, chemotherapy, and the monoclonal antibody trastuzumab (Herceptin). Endocrine treatment is indicated for most breast cancers that express the estrogen receptor or progesterone receptor, or both. Aromatase inhibitors, such as anastrozole, letrozole, and exemestane, are effective only in postmenopausal women, whereas tamoxifen can be used in postmenopausal and premenopausal women as well as in men with breast cancer. Endocrine therapy is generally given for a minimum of 5 years in the adjuvant (postoperative) setting.

Adjuvant or neoadjuvant (preoperative) chemotherapy is administered when the patient is at significant risk for distant recurrence. The benefit of chemotherapy is greatest in younger patients, those with lymph node involvement, and when estrogen receptors are absent. Most other subsets of patients, however, also derive some benefit from chemotherapy that must be weighed against the potential for toxicity.

Trastuzumab is a monoclonal antibody that targets Her2neu, a protein overexpressed in approximately one fourth of breast cancers. In conjunction with chemotherapy, one year of trastuzumab therapy further reduces recurrence risk in patients with Her2neu overexpressing breast cancer.

Palliative Treatment

When breast cancer does recur in the form of metastatic disease, life expectancy is limited. Treatment may prolong life and offer palliation of symptoms. Management often involves sequential use of a variety of treatments including endocrine therapy, chemotherapy, and biologic therapies either alone or in specific combinations. Radiation treatment can provide effective palliation for painful bone lesions or for brain metastases. Adjunctive treatments include analgesics, antiemetics, antidepressants, and bisphosphonates that reduce complications related to bone metastases.

OUTCOMES

It is estimated that there were 213,000 cases of breast cancer diagnosed in the United States in 2006. The breast cancer mortality rate has been decreasing since 1991, with an estimated 40,970 fatalities in 2006.[20] A similar decrease has been noted since the late 1980s in the United Kingdom. Breast cancer mortality has been decreasing even among women excluded from screening protocols by age, and there is evidence that adjuvant hormonal and cytotoxic treatments reduce mortality.[21,22] The reduction has probably been multifactorial, with screening, prompt evaluation of palpable lumps, chemotherapy, and hormone therapy all contributing.[23]

GUIDELINES

National Guidelines

There are a number of breast cancer screening guidelines in North America. Each organization making recommendations has a publication or website with its guidelines. A comparison of the guidelines can be found at http://www.guidelines.gov.

The American Cancer Society (ACS) recommends CBE every 3 years between ages 20 and 39 years. The National Cancer Institute recommends against screening mammography in women younger than 40 years, because there are no data showing benefit in this age group. The recommendation for a baseline mammogram has likewise disappeared from the American Cancer Society recommendations.

The ACS and the American College of Radiology recommend yearly screening with mammography and CBE starting at age 40 years. The Canadian Task Force recommends screening with CBE and mammography from ages 50 to 69 years and recommends against screening from ages 40 to 49 years. The U.S. Preventive Services Task Force (USPSTF) recommends screening with mammography with or without CBE every 1 to 2 years from age 40 years. They note that the age at which screening should be stopped is unclear, although women with a comorbidity limiting life expectancy have

Table 1 Recommendations for Breast Cancer Screening

Age (years)	American Cancer Society	U.S. Preventive Services Task Force	National Cancer Institute	Canadian Task Force on Preventive Health Care	American College of Radiology
20-39	Clinical breast exam every 3 yr		No data for benefit or for performing baseline mammogram		
40-49	Clinical breast exam and mammogram yearly	Mammogram with or without clinical breast exam every 1-2 yr	Screening mammogram and clinical breast exam decrease breast cancer mortality	Recommend against screening	Mammogram and clinical breast exam yearly
50-69	Clinical breast exam and mammogram yearly	Mammogram with or without clinical breast exam every 1-2 yr	Screening mammogram and clinical breast exam decrease breast cancer mortality	Clinical breast exam and mammogram during periodic health examination	Mammogram and clinical breast exam yearly
70+	Cessation of screening is not age related but due to comorbidity	When to discontinue mammogram is unclear; those with comorbidities are less likely to benefit	Screening might or might not be helpful		

less benefit. The National Cancer Institute of the National Institutes of Health notes that screening mammography in women ages 40 to 70 years decreases breast cancer mortality and that screening by CBE reduces breast cancer mortality. These statements are tempered by a discussion of the harms of screening (Table 1).

As noted in the diagnosis section, it is estimated that the number of women needed to be screened with mammography to avoid one breast cancer death would be 1500 to 2500 for women screened in their 40s. Because of the high false-positive rate in this population, with a lower pretest probability of disease, about one half of women screened annually starting at age 40 years would require a follow-up diagnostic mammogram during the subsequent 10-year period.

Common-Sense Approach

In the absence of consensus in national guidelines, we favor the following approach to screening. In women younger than 40 years who are concerned because of a family history of breast cancer, we review with them the data for apparent lack of efficacy of mammography.[10] The sensitivity of mammograms is known to be less for young women, and to gradually rise with age.[13] The relative contribution of the physical examination to diagnosis is probably greater in young women, so careful CBE on a yearly basis is probably useful. We also offer to calculate breast cancer diagnosis percentage risk using the Gail model.[8] If there is a family history of more than one first-degree relative with breast cancer or a family history of bilateral premenopausal breast cancer, it is reasonable to discuss genetic testing.

For women in their 40s, we briefly review the data from clinical trials and the recommendations of the ACS and USPSTF. The public tends to be most familiar with the ACS guidelines. Many women want a straightforward recommendation. If a woman seeks more information, we try to inform her about some of the subtle issues.

We offer mammograms to women who are 40 years or older, but we emphasize that, due to the lower sensitivity of mammography in younger women, in our opinion CBE is especially important.

The approach to women 50 to 69 years old is easier because of the consensus among guidelines. We recommend CBE and mammography annually. Of course, risk assessment may be important at any age. It is sometimes sought due to a new family history or a benign biopsy.

In women older than 70 years, although the incidence of breast cancer mortality is high, it represents a stable portion of all deaths because other causes of mortality are also rising. Screening mammography trials that have included older women have not reported significant breast cancer mortality reduction in this group, although there are fewer women in this age range studied overall.

Summary

- The reduction in breast cancer mortality since 1990 has probably been multifactorial, with screening, prompt evaluation of palpable lumps, chemotherapy, and hormonal therapy all contributing.
- Risk factors for developing breast cancer include increased age, genetic predisposition, and increased exposure to estrogen.
- The Gail Model Risk Assessment Tool may be used to help calculate breast cancer risk from a patient's history and is available from the National Cancer Institute (NCI).
- There are a number of breast cancer screening guidelines in North America but most recommend screening yearly starting at age 40 years. A comparison of the guidelines can be found at http://www.guidelines.gov.
- Due to the lower sensitivity of mammography in younger women, the clinical breast examination is especially important.
- Characteristics of breast lumps that suggest cancer include a hard or gritty texture, immobility, an irregular border, and a size greater than 2 cm.
- The combination of the physical examination, mammography, and fine-needle aspiration biopsy for diagnosing palpable lumps is referred to as *triple diagnosis;* there are excellent sensitivity and specificity with this approach. If any of these three modalities suggests cancer, excisional biopsy is warranted.
- There have been attempts to identify women with the most to gain from continuing mammography. One suggestion is to target women with higher bone mineral density for biennial screening from ages 70 to 79 years, because case finding is more fruitful in this group.[24] Others have suggested that the overall health of the woman be assessed, and those with greater residual life expectancy be targeted for screening. The latter is the basic approach we take. If the woman is in good health, we continue to offer CBE and mammography.

Suggested Readings

American Cancer Society: Breast Cancer Facts & Figures 2009. PDF available for download at http://www.cancer.org/docroot/stt/stt_0.asp (accessed March 20, 2009).

Armstrong K, Eisen A, Weber B: Assessing the risk of breast cancer. N Engl J Med 2000;342:564-571.

Barton MB, Harris R, Fletcher SW: Does this patient have breast cancer? The screening clinical breast examination: Should it be done? How? JAMA 1999;282:1270-1280.

Beral V; Million Women Study Collaborators: Breast cancer and hormone-replacement therapy in the Million Women Study. Lancet 2003;362:419-427.

Berry DA: Benefits and risks of screening mammography for women in their forties: A statistical appraisal. J Natl Cancer Inst 1998;90:1431-1439.

Early Breast Cancer Trialists' Collaborative Group: Tamoxifen for early breast cancer: An overview of the randomised trials. Lancet 1998;351:1451-1467.

Gail MH, Brinton LA, Byar DP, et al: Projecting individualized probabilities of developing breast cancer for white females who are being examined annually. J Natl Cancer Inst 1989;81:1879-1886.

Kerlikowske K, Grady D, Rubin SM, et al: Efficacy of screening mammography. A meta-analysis. JAMA 1995;273:149-154.

Kerlikowske K, Salzmann P, Phillips KA, et al: Continuing screening mammography in women aged 70 to 79 years: Impact on life expectancy and cost-effectiveness. JAMA 1999;282:2156-2163.

Peto R, Boreham J, Clarke M, et al: UK and USA breast cancer deaths down 25% in year 2000 at ages 20-69 years. Lancet 2000;355:1822.

Rossouw JE, Anderson GL, Prentice RL, et al: Risks and benefits of estrogen plus progestin in healthy postmenopausal women: Principal results From the Women's Health Initiative randomized controlled trial. JAMA 2002;288:321-333.

References

For a complete list of references, log onto www.expertconsult.com.

Cervical Cancer Screening and Prevention

Xian Wen Jin

This chapter provides a concise review of the definition, prevalence, and contemporary concepts of the pathogenesis of cervical cancer. In addition, the new standard of care and the current practice guideline in screening and prevention are highlighted.

DEFINITION

Cervical carcinoma originates from the endocervical squamocolumnar epithelial junction. Squamous cell carcinoma represents 90% of cervical carcinomas and develops from precancerous lesions and cervical dysplasia.[1]

PREVALENCE

Cervical cancer is the second leading cause of death from cancer in women worldwide. It is the third most common gynecologic malignancy in the United States and ranks 13th in cancer deaths for American women.[2] In the United States, an estimated 13,000 new cases of invasive cervical cancer were diagnosed each year, with 4100 deaths.[3,4] Cervical cancer mortality in the United States has decreased over the last five decades by 70%, largely as a result of the introduction of the Papanicolaou (Pap) test.

PATHOPHYSIOLOGY

Invasive cervical cancer develops from a preinvasive state termed *cervical intraepithelial neoplasia* (CIN). CIN 1 represents mild dysplasia and is now classified as low-grade squamous intraepithelial lesions (LSILs), CINs 2 and 3 encompass moderate-to-severe dysplasia and are classified as high-grade squamous intraepithelial lesions (HSILs) based on the Bethesda cervical cytology reporting system.[5] Most LSILs spontaneously resolve, whereas high-grade squamous intraepithelial lesions (HSILs) are more likely to progress to invasive cervical cancer. HSILs are typically detected at an average of 10 to 15 years younger than for invasive cervical cancer. For example, the typical age range for diagnosis of carcinoma in situ is 25 to 35 years, whereas that for invasive cancer is older than 40 years.[6]

Infection of the cervical epithelium with oncogenic types of human papillomavirus (HPV) is essential to the development of cervical cancer and its precursor lesions (Fig. 1).[7,8] Early epidemiologic studies found that at least 76% of cases of CIN could be attributed to HPV infection.[9] Women with CIN lesions in the study exhibited the typical epidemiologic profile of sexually transmitted infection: more sexual partners, earlier age at first sexual intercourse, and lower socioeconomic status.

Evidence supporting the association between infection by carcinogenic HPVs and the subsequent development of virtually all cervical cancer is conclusive. Cervical squamous intraepithelial lesions demonstrate the classic morphologic changes of HPV infection, such as epithelial hyperplasia (acanthosis) and degenerative cytoplasmic vacuolization (koilocytosis) in terminally differentiated keratinocytes with atypical nuclei.[10] HPV has been observed in these lesions using electron microscopy.[11] In addition, HPV structural proteins have been detected in surgical specimens using immunohistochemical staining with antibodies that specifically detect HPV viral antigens.[12] Large serial studies from 22 countries have shown that more than 90% of cervical squamous cell carcinomas contain DNA from high-risk HPV types, presumably transmitted during sexual activity.[7] A more recent study[13] indicated the worldwide HPV prevalence in cervical cancer is as high as 99.7%. Furthermore, HPV DNA has been extracted from metastatic cervical cancer tissues and cervical cancer tumor cell lines in culture.[14,15]

Eighty types of HPV have been sequenced, and approximately 30 of these infect the female and male genital tracts.[16] Eighteen genital HPV subtypes (16, 18, 26, 31, 33, 35, 39, 45, 51, 52, 53, 56, 58, 59, 66, 68, 73, and 82) are classified as high risk because of their close causative association with cervical cancer.[17]

Research in the last decade has provided a better understanding of the molecular carcinogenesis of HPV. In vitro infection of human epithelial cells by carcinogenic HPV subtypes induces indefinite cell growth, or cell immortalization.[18,19] Two HPV viral proteins, E6 and E7 proteins, are required for cell immortalization.[20-22]

Further studies[23-25] revealed that E6 proteins from high-risk HPV interact with the cellular tumor suppressor protein p53. The p53 suppresses cell proliferation by arresting growth in the G1 phase of the cell cycle. E6 proteins from high-risk HPV complexes with p53 and results in the rapid proteolytic degradation of p53 proteins.[23,24] The decreased level of p53 protein abolishes the cell's ability to suppress uncontrolled cell proliferation.[25] On the other hand, E7 proteins from high-risk HPV bind to another cellular tumor suppressor, the retinoblastoma protein (pRB), and disrupt the complex between the cellular transcription factors E2F-1 and pRB. The free E2F-1 stimulates cellular DNA synthesis and uncontrolled cell proliferation.[26] E6 and E7 proteins from HPV-16 can also cooperate to induce centrosome-related mitotic defects and genomic instability.[27] It is clear that persistent infection by oncogenic HPVs is a prerequisite for the development of cervical cancer and its precursor lesions, although only a few women infected with HPV eventually develop cervical cancer.

SCREENING

The conventional Pap test has been the mainstay of cervical cancer screening since its inception in the 1950s. Screening protocols remained unchanged for the first four of the last five decades. Standardization of cervical cytology and reporting terminology was accomplished in 1988 with the implementation of the Bethesda system.

Remarkable new advances in the last decade have transformed our screening protocol. Cervical cytology specimen adequacy and more accurate interpretations of cervical cancer precursors have been achieved by using new liquid-based cervical cytologic smear technology (ThinPrep).[28-30] Using the revised Bethesda cytology reporting system (2001), clinicians can better triage patients with abnormal cervical cytology based on less ambiguous terminology.[31,32] Data from the National Cancer Institute-sponsored multicenter randomized clinical trial (ALTS trial, 2001) have demonstrated the clinical value of HPV testing in triaging women with atypical squamous cells of undetermined significance (ASC-US).[31-33] After a diagnosis of ASC-US, clinicians can determine on the basis of HPV testing results whether a woman requires colposcopic examination or needs only to repeat Pap tests 1 year later. More recently, multiple large-scale, cross-sectional studies from several countries have compelled the U.S. Food and Drug Administration (FDA) to approve the hybrid capture 2 test for HPV as an adjunct to the Pap test in primary screening (March, 2003).[34-38] It is now evident that virtually all squa-

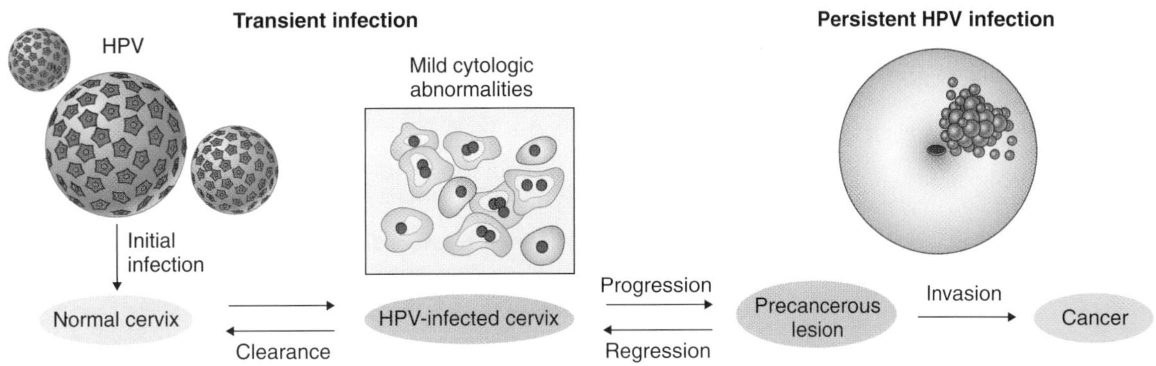

Figure 1 **Role of human papillomavirus infection in the development of cervical cancer.** *(Adapted with permission from Wright TC Jr, Schiffman M: Adding a test for human papillomavirus DNA to cervical-cancer screening. N Engl J Med 2003;348:489-490.)*

mous-cell cervical cancers are caused by one of the 18 types of oncogenic HPV.[39] As a result, many groups, including the American Cancer Society, the American College of Obstetricians and Gynecologists, the American Society for Colposcopy and Cervical Pathology, and the U.S. Preventive Services Task Force have issued new screening guidelines since 2002.[40-42] The following discussions will highlight the consensus recommendations from these organizations and provide clinicians with updates in screening protocols.

CURRENT PRACTICE GUIDELINES

Initiation of Screening

Because of the uncommon occurrence of cervical cancer in women younger than 21 years the high regression rate of LSIL, and the transient nature of HPV infection in sexually active young women, the American Cancer Society, the American College of Obstetricians and Gynecologists, and the U.S. Preventive Services Task Force unanimously recommend that screening begins approximately 3 years after a woman begins having vaginal intercourse, but no later than age 21.

The basis of the above recommendation is that cervical cancer and its precursor lesions are almost always related to acquisition of oncogenic HPV infection through vaginal intercourse. It usually takes 3 to 5 years to develop these lesions after the first exposure to HPV infection, and cervical cancer in patients younger than 19 years is rare.[43-46]

The incidence of invasive cervical cancer was 0/100,000/year for ages 10 to 19 years and 1.7/100,000/year for ages 20 to 24 years, according to the data from the National Cancer Institute's Surveillance, Epidemiology and End Results (SEER) program.[47] In addition, studies on the natural history of LSILs and HPV infection in young women aged 13 to 22 years have shown that most HPV infections are transient, with a 70% regression rate within 3 years. Ninety percent of LSILs in this age group spontaneously regress.[48-50] Furthermore, the average time of progression for HSILs to a carcinoma in situ or cancer for women younger than 25 years was approximately 5 years.[51]

Adding HPV DNA Testing to Screening

HPV DNA testing is now included in screening as an adjunct to the Pap test for women 30 years and older. This new screening protocol takes advantage of the high sensitivity and high negative predictive value of HPV DNA testing and the high specificity of cervical cytology. Multiple large-scale studies from several countries, evaluating the role of HPV testing in primary screening, have shown that the combination of a negative Pap test and a negative HPV DNA test indicates the absence of CIN 3 or cancer with almost 100% certainty.[34-38] These studies demonstrate that 80% to 100% of cases of histologically confirmed CIN 2 or cancer were found to be positive for high-risk HPV. The sensitivity of HPV DNA testing to detect CIN 2 or a higher-grade lesion is higher than that of a single Pap test. The sensitivity is even higher than that of HPV DNA testing alone, when HPV DNA testing is combined with Pap testing.

The rationale for recommending HPV testing in women 30 years and older is based on the finding that the prevalence of high-risk HPV infection declines with age. Among women older than 29 years who have ASC-US, only 31.2% have a high risk for HPV positivity, whereas in women age 28 or younger, high-risk HPV positivity rises to 65%.[52] Although HPV infections are extremely common in sexually active younger women, most of these infections will resolve spontaneously or cause only transient, minor lesions. It is very likely that HPV DNA positivity with increased age may reflect the persistence of HPV. This group of older women is at increased risk for development of cervical cancer. Therefore, the specificity and the positive predictive value of an HPV DNA test increases with the age of the woman.

The American Cancer Society and American College of Obstetricians and Gynecologists endorse combined Pap and HPV DNA testing in primary screening. Traditional annual screening with a Pap test is still an acceptable option. However, the U.S. Preventive Services Task Force found insufficient evidence to recommend for or against the routine use of HPV DNA testing in a primary screening protocol.

Screening Interval

Women Younger Than 30 Years

The American Cancer Society recommends that cervical screening be performed annually with conventional Pap tests or every 2 years using liquid-based cytology after initiation of screening.[40] The American College of Obstetricians and Gynecologists recommends that women in this age group should undergo annual screening.[41] The recent guideline of the U.S. Preventive Services Task Force calls for screening every 3 years.[42] The rationale for this screening interval was based on relative-risk data on invasive cervical cancer after a negative Pap test result.

The difference in risk for progression to invasive cancer in the intervals between screenings is very small when 1-, 2-, and 3-year screening intervals are compared by using conventional Pap tests. Most studies suggest that the relative risk with a 2-year screening interval is 1 to 2 above annual screening, and the relative risk with a 3-year screening interval is in the range of 2 to 3 above annual screening. Longer screening intervals of 4 to 10 years correlate with increased risk of invasive cervical cancer during the interval.[53-59] A large, prospective cohort study of more than 120,000 women in the United States found no significant statistical difference in the age-adjusted incidence rate of HSILs, carcinoma in situ, or invasive carcinoma among women screened at 1, 2, or 3 years after a normal Pap test.[60] In addition, the absolute risks of cervical cancer after one, two, and three or more consecutive negative Pap tests was estimated as 3.09, 2.56, and 1.43 per 100,000 women, respectively, based on long-term follow-up data from 2.4 million women belonging to a prepaid health plan.[61]

It is the consensus recommendation from the American Cancer Society and the American College of Obstetricians and Gynecologists that younger women (younger than age 30) be screened at a shorter interval: 1 year rather than 2 to 3 years, because the sensitivity of the Pap test alone is less than ideal.

Women Older than 30 Years

If the Pap test and the HPV DNA test are both negative in a woman at or after age 30, screening should be performed every 3 years, according to the latest guideline from the American Cancer Society and the American College of Obstetricians and Gynecologists. This recommendation is based primarily on the following key evidence: high-risk HPV infection is required for the development of virtually all cervical cancer,[39] and the time from initial HPV infection to development of cervical cancer usually exceeds 10 years.[62] A similarly effective screening model exists in colon cancer screening. In a person age 50 years or older who has average risk and a negative colonoscopy, the next colonoscopy should be performed in 10 years. In contrast, because of the lack of definitive prospective data, the U.S. Preventive Services Task Force does not recommend for or against the routine use of HPV testing as a primary screening test.

Discontinuing Screening

Current American Cancer Society guidelines recommend that women older than 70 years who have had three or more normal Pap tests and no abnormal Pap tests in the last 10 years may choose to stop Pap test screening. The guidelines of the U.S. Preventive Services Task Force call for discontinuing screening at age 65. The guidelines issued by the American College of Obstetricians and Gynecologists suggest that physicians should determine on an individual basis when to discontinue screening.

There is very low risk of developing cervical cancer for women older than 50 years in the screened population.[63-68] In women older than 65 years with at least one negative Pap test within the last 3 years, there is a low rate of LSIL and HSIL. In addition, it is also difficult to obtain satisfactory samples for interpretation from older women because of cervical atrophy and stenosis. However, it is probably reasonable to screen women age 70 and older who have not been screened previously and have new sexual partners.

Screening After Hysterectomy

According to the guidelines issued by the American Cancer Society, the American College of Obstetricians and Gynecologists, and the U.S. Preventive Services Task Force, screening after total hysterectomy for benign gynecologic disease is not indicated when there is no history of prior CIN, the cervix has been completely removed, and there is no histologic evidence for CIN in the hysterectomy specimen. The incidence of vaginal carcinoma is 1 to 2/100,000/year, far lower than that for cervical carcinoma.[69] Thus, the diagnostic yield of vaginal cytology to screen for this cancer after a hysterectomy that includes cervix removal is quite low. Two hundred and twenty women randomly selected from 2066 women who had had a hysterectomy for benign conditions and were followed for an average of more than 7 years in a retrospective study identified only seven patients who had intraepithelial cytologic abnormalities but no vaginal cancer.[70] In addition, a cross-sectional study of more than 5000 screening cytology tests in women who had had hysterectomy for benign reasons found only one case of dysplasia and no cancer.[71] However, a recent study indicated that almost 10 million women

Box 1 Current Practice Guidelines for Screening

Recommendations for Cervical Cancer Screening 43-45

HPV DNA testing for primary screening

ACS: Yes, in combination with the Papanicolaou (Pap) test in women 30 years and older

ACOG: Same as ACS recommendation

USPSTF: Insufficient evidence to recommend for or against routine use

When to Start Screening

ACS: Approximately 3 years after the onset of vaginal intercourse; no later than age 21

ACOG: Same as ACS

USPSTF: Same as ACS

Screening Interval

ACS: Annual with conventional Pap test or every 2 years using liquid-based ThinPrep until age 30. At or after age 30, Pap combined with HPV testing; if both negative, every 3 years

ACOG: Annually in women <30 years; in women >30 years, same as ACS

USPSTF: Every 3 years

When to Stop Screening

ACS: Age 70 and older who have had three or more consecutive normal Pap tests

ACOG: Individual basis

USPSTF: Age 65 if patient had adequate recent screening with normal Pap smears

Screening after Hysterectomy

ACS: If hysterectomy for a benign condition: no more screening; if hysterectomy was for precancer: continue screening for 10 years to achieve three consecutive negative Pap tests; if hysterectomy was for cancer, continue screening as long as the patient is in reasonably good health

ACOG: If hysterectomy was for grade 2 or 3 cervical intraepithelial neoplasia, continue annual screening until three consecutive Pap smears are negative

USPSTF: Same as ACS

ACOG, American College of Obstetricians and Gynecologists; ACS, American Cancer Society; USPSTF, United States Preventive Services Task Force.

who had had a hysterectomy are being screened even though they are not at risk of developing cervical cancer.[72] Education for clinicians and patients is critical in following cervical cancer screening guidelines (Box 1).

Management of Women with Abnormal Cervical Cytology

Every year approximately 3.5 million women receive a diagnosis of abnormal cervical cytology requiring further evaluation or follow-up. Ignoring this low-grade abnormal cervical cytology is clearly dangerous, yet performing immediate colposcopy for 3.5 million women is definitely not cost-effective and is unnecessary. To help physicians make appropriate evidence-based clinical decisions, the American Society for Colposcopy and Cervical Pathology issued a consensus guideline for the management of women who had an abnormal Pap test in 2002.[73] The recommendations are outlined in Figure 2.

Guidelines for Women with Specific Combinations of Combined HPV and Pap Test Results

Following the recent approval by the FDA of HPV testing as an adjunct in primary cervical screening, many more women will

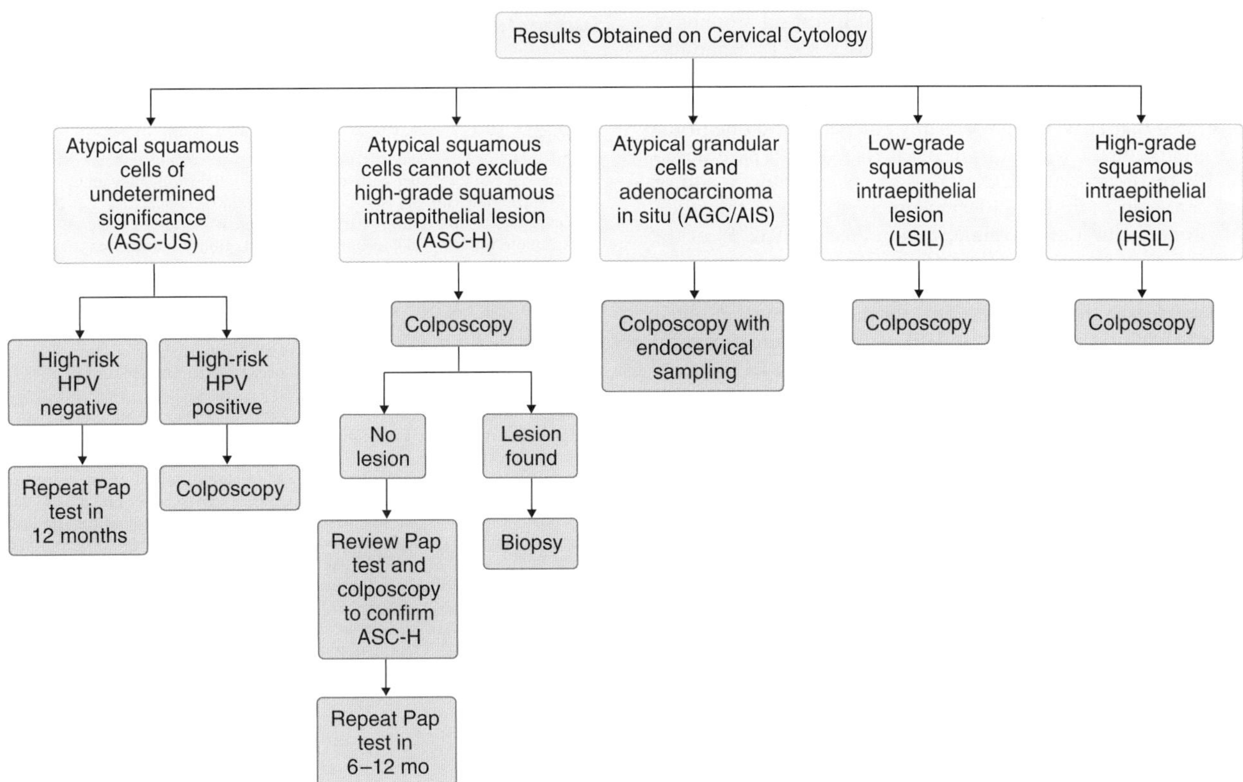

Figure 2 **Management guideline for women with abnormal Pap tests.** *(Reprinted with permission from Jin XW, Zanotti K, Yen-Lieberman: New cervical cancer screening strategy: Combined Pap and HPV testing. Cleve Clin J Med 2005;72[2]:141-148. © 2005 The Cleveland Clinic Foundation. All rights reserved.)*

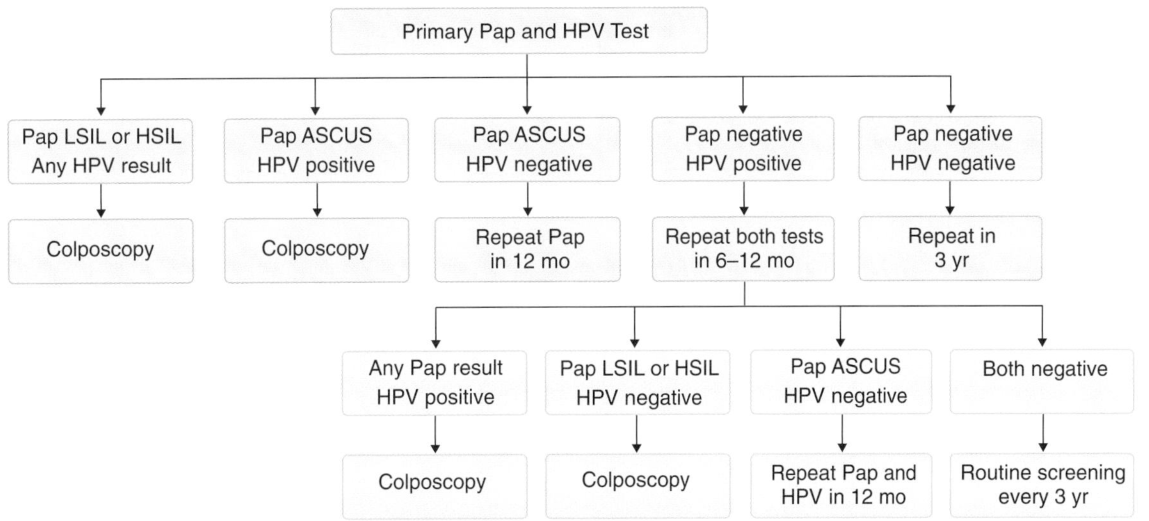

Figure 3 **Management algorithm for women with combinations of test results from combined human papillomavirus and Pap testing.** ASCUS, atypical squamous cells of undetermined significance; HSIL, high-grade squamous intraepithelial lesion; LSIL, low-grade squamous intraepithelial lesion. *(Adapted with permission from Wright, et al. Interim guidance for the use of human papillomavirus DNA testing as an adjunct to cervical cytology for screening. Obstet Gynecol 2004;103[2]:304-309.)*

undergo combined HPV and Pap tests each year. Clinicians will need to effectively manage women with different combinations of test results. Therefore, the National Cancer Institute, the American Cancer Society, and the American Society of Colposcopy and Cervical Pathology cosponsored a workshop in 2003 and issued an interim guideline to assist clinicians in using HPV testing in primary screening.[74] This interim guidance is summarized in Figure 3.

PREVENTION

One of the most exciting advances in cervical cancer prevention is the successful development of the HPV-16 vaccine and its efficacy in preventing HPV-16/18-associated preinvasive cervical lesions and persistent HPV-16/18 infection.[75-77] The FDA approved Merck's Gardasil, a quadrivalent HPV 6.11.16, 18 recombinant vaccine, in June of 2006. This vaccine consists of recombinant L1 capsid proteins of specific HPV types that form "viral-like particles" (VLP). It induces type-specific neutralizing antibody and is given as intramuscular injections at 0, 2, and 6 months. Data from a large clinical trial have demonstrated that HPV vaccine is highly efficacious. No one in the vaccine group and 21 women from the placebo group have developed HPV-16/18-associated CIN 2/3 or adenocarcinoma in situ or cervical cancer in more than 10,000 women enrolled in the study. The Advisory Committee on Immunization Practices (ACIP) of the Center for Disease Control and Prevention (CDC) has recommended immunization for cervical cancer prevention in females 9 to 26 years of age. This elegant study demonstrated for the first time that cervical cancer could be prevented by an HPV vaccine. Future successful development of an HPV vaccine against all oncogenic HPV strains could make the dream of cervical cancer eradication a reality.

CONCLUSION

Screening for cervical cancer reduces invasive cervical cancer incidence and mortality. New knowledge of the development of cervical cancer, new technologies such as the liquid-based cervical cytologic smear, and HPV DNA testing have transformed cervical cancer screening. Clinicians should be aware of the current concepts and practice guidelines and make decisions based on the most current evidence.

Summary

- Cervical cancer is one of the few highly preventable cancers. The early detection and removal of precancerous cervical lesions effectively abolish the development of invasive cervical cancer.
- The Pap test has been the standard screening test in the Western world for the last five decades. Cervical cancer incidence and mortality have been reduced dramatically as a result of successful screening in many countries.
- Tremendous advances in newer cytologic techniques and in our in-depth understanding of cervical cancer pathogenesis have led to many updates of our screening strategy since the turn of this century.

Suggested Readings

ACOG Committee on Practice Bulletins. ACOG Practice Bulletin: Clinical management guidelines for obstetrician-gynecologists. Number 45, August 2003. Cervical cytology screening (replaces committee opinion 152, March 1995). Obstet Gynecol 2003;102:417-427.

Bosch FX, Manos MM, Munoz N, et al: Prevalence of human papillomavirus in cervical cancer: A worldwide perspective. International Biological Study on Cervical Cancer (IBSCC) Study Group. J Natl Cancer Inst 1995;87:796-802.

Human papillomavirus testing for triage of women with cytologic evidence of low-grade squamous intraepithelial lesions: Baseline data from a randomized trial. The Atypical Squamous Cells of Undetermined Significance/Low-Grade Squamous Intraepithelial Lesions Triage Study (ALTS) Group. J Natl Cancer Inst 2000;92:397-402.

Koutsky LA, Ault KA, Wheeler CM, et al: A controlled trial of a human papillomavirus type 16 vaccine. N Engl J Med 2002;347:1645-1651.

Koutsky LA, Holmes KK, Critchlow CW, et al: A cohort study of the risk of cervical intraepithelial neoplasia grade 2 or 3 in relation to papillomavirus infection. N Engl J Med 1992;327:1272-1278.

Munoz N, Bosch FX, de Sanjose S, et al: Epidemiologic classification of human papillomavirus types associated with cervical cancer. N Engl J Med 2003;348:518-527.

Solomon D, Schiffman M, Tarone R, ALTS Study Group. Comparison of three management strategies for patients with atypical squamous cells of undetermined significance: Baseline results from a randomized trial. J Natl Cancer Inst 2001;93:293-299.

Walboomers JM, Jacobs MV, Manos MM, et al: Human papillomavirus is a necessary cause of invasive cervical cancer worldwide. J Pathol 1999;189:12-19.

Wright TC Jr, Cox JT, Massad LS, et al: ASCEP-Sponsored Consensus Conference. 2001 Consensus Guidelines for the management of women with cervical cytological abnormalities. JAMA 2002;287:2120-2129.

Wright TC Jr, Schiffman M, Solomon D, et al: Interim guidance for the use of human papillomavirus DNA testing as an adjunct to cervical cytology for screening. Obstet Gynecol 2004;103:304-309.

References

For a complete list of references, log onto www.expertconsult.com.

Female Contraception

Shakuntala Kothari

Unintended pregnancy is a major women's health problem. In the United States, about 50% of all pregnancies are unplanned. This article covers female contraceptive methods, sterilization, and emergency contraception approved for use in the United States

PRESCRIBING CONTRACEPTIVES

The choice of contraceptive method is determined by the woman's health, frequency of sexual activity, number of sexual partners, and desire for permanence, as well as the efficacy of the contraceptive method (Table 1).[1] There are several contraindications for combination hormonal contraceptives. They include previous thromboembolic event or stroke, liver disease, history of estrogen-dependent tumor, undiagnosed abnormal uterine bleeding, hypertriglyceridemia, and smoking in women older than 35 years.[2]

Women with one or more contraindications should not be prescribed combination hormonal contraceptives. Use of combination contraceptives by diabetic women should be limited to those who do not smoke, are younger than 35 years, and are otherwise healthy. Progesterone injections are safer in women who suffer from migraines, headaches, lupus, sickle cell anemia, hypertension, or diabetes with vascular disease and in those older than 35 years.

Specific screening before prescribing contraceptives is not mandatory. However, patients at risk for high blood pressure should undergo screening before initiating contraception. At the initial visit, a 3-month follow-up is suggested for counseling and reinforcement and then yearly thereafter. Women should be counseled about the efficacy, side effects, and correct methods of use; about the signs and symptoms that require return to the physician; and about protection against sexually transmitted diseases (STDs).

MECHANISM OF ACTION OF HORMONAL CONTRACEPTIVES

Hormonal contraceptives include combination estrogen and progestin and progestin only. Estrogen effects include inhibition of ovulation and prevention of follicular maturation through suppression of ovarian steroid production and possibly decreased responsiveness to gonadotropin-releasing hormone. Conversely, progestin leads to changes in the endometrium that make implantation less likely, increased thickness of cervical mucus that makes sperm penetration difficult, and impairment of normal tubal mobility.[2] Most progestins are derivatives of testosterone and thus have residual androgenic activity. It is this androgenic aspect of progestins that causes many of the side effects and metabolic complications.

ORAL CONTRACEPTIVES

Combination Pills

Regimens

The first hormonal agents contained high doses of estrogen and progestin. Lower doses are as effective and cause fewer side effects, which include headache, breast tenderness, nausea, and hypertension. In particular, lower doses of ethinyl estradiol are associated with less risk of thrombosis. Nowadays, contraceptive pills contain less than 50 μg of ethinyl estradiol; most contain 30 or 35 μg, and the newer ones contain 20 or 25 μg.

Newer progestins with fewer androgenic effects include desogestrel and norgestimate.

In some newer regimens, the patient takes placebo pills for fewer days per month than with older regimens, or the placebo pills have been replaced by low-dose hormone pills. These regimens reduce the number of days of withdrawal bleeding, with the intent of improving contraceptive effectiveness, patient adherence, and patient tolerance and reducing side effects. In other newer regimens, hormonal contraceptives are taken in longer cycles to lengthen the intervals between withdrawal bleeding, or continuously, so that the patient has no bleeding at all.

Ethinyl estradiol/norethindrone (Femcon Fe) has the same active ingredients as Ovcon 35. The difference is that Ovcon 35 pill must be swallowed, whereas Femcon Fe is a spearmint-flavored, chewable tablet. In addition, the placebo pill contains iron.

Ethinyl estradiol/drospirenone (Yasmin) is a combined oral contraceptive containing drospirenone and ethinyl estradiol. Yaz has the same dose of drosperinone as Yasmin but a lower dose of ethinyl estradiol. It contains 24 days of active medication and 4 days of placebo. Drospirenone is a spironolactone analogue with antiandrogenic and antimineralocorticoid properties. The antimineralocorticoid effect of drospirenone reduces water retention and bloating. These agents should not be used in women with hepatic failure, renal insufficiency, or adrenal insufficiency. Women taking nonsteroidal anti-inflammatory agents, potassium-sparing diuretics, angiotensin-converting enzyme inhibitors, angiotensin II receptor antagonists, or potassium supplements should have their serum potassium levels checked during the first treatment cycle. Yaz is the first and only hormonal contraceptive that has been shown to be effective for the treatment of premenstrual dysphoric disorder.

Loestrin 24 Fe provides 3 more days of active hormonal pills than Loestrin for a total 24 days of active medication followed by 4 days of iron-containing placebo pills.

Levonorgestrel/ethinyl estradiol (Seasonale) is a 91-day oral contraceptive regimen that contains levonorgestrel (progestin) and ethinyl estradiol for 12 weeks (84 days), followed by 1 week of placebo. Women have only four menses per year. Seasonique is the same formulation as Seasonale but with the addition of ethinyl estradiol in a lower dose during the 13th week, without levonorgestrel. This addition may reduce the hormonal withdrawal symptoms such as menstrual migraine and dysmenorrhea that can occur during the placebo week with long-cycle hormonal contraceptives. Women on continuous long-cycle hormonal contraception tend to have more unscheduled bleeding than do women on shorter-cycle regimens.

Ethinyl estradiol/levonorgestrel (Lybrel) is taken in a continuous, noncyclic, 365-day regimen. There is no hormone-free period with this regimen. Therefore, hormone levels remain constant, ovulation is suppressed, and women have no menstrual bleeding. It was recently approved by the U.S. Food and Drug Administration (FDA).

Side Effects, Advantages, and Precautions

Dizziness, weight gain, nausea, spotting, amenorrhea, and breast tenderness are among the most common side effects. There is no inhibition of spontaneity, and the contraceptive effects end after 3 months of stopping the pill. Pills must be taken the same time each day, require a prescription, provide no protection against STDs, and need a barrier method for the first 7 days of use. Certain drugs such as rifampin, amoxicillin, metronidazole, tetracyclines, and cephalexin can decrease the effectiveness of the pills.

Table 1 Effectiveness of Contraceptive Methods

Contraceptive Method	Pregnancies per 100 Women in First 12 Months of Use	
	As Commonly Used	Perfect Use
Combined oral contraceptives	5	0.1
Progestin-only pills	5	0.5
Depot medroxyprogesterone acetate	0.3	0.3
Female sterilization	0.5	0.5
Levonorgestrel IUD (Mirena)	0.1	0.1
Copper IUD (ParaGard T 380A)	0.8	0.6
Lactation amenorrhea method	2	0.5
Male condoms	14	3
Diaphragm with spermicide	20	6
Female condoms	21	5
Spermicides	26	6
Cervical cap		
Nulliparous women	20	9
Parous women	40	26
Coitus interruptus	19	4
Symptothermal	—	2
Ovulation method	—	3
Rhythm method	—	9
No method	85	85

Similar data are not yet available for newer methods including the shield, patch, or hormonal ring.

Adapted from Gallo MF, Grimes DA, Schulz KF: Cervical cap versus diaphragm for contraception. Cochrane Database Syst Rev 2002, I:CD003551.

Progestin-Only Pills

Progestin-only pills (or minipills) are associated with more breakthrough bleeding than combination pills and have slightly higher failure rates. Irregular bleeding, weight gain, and breast tenderness are the most common side effects. Progestin-only pills are a good option for patients who need to avoid estrogen (Fig. 1). Precautions are similar to those for combined oral contraceptives. Minipills offer less protection against ectopic pregnancy.

Noncontraceptive Benefits of Oral Contraceptives

Oral contraceptives have been successfully used in the treatment of hyperandrogenism, including idiopathic hirsutism and polycystic ovary syndrome. Levonorgestrel-containing preparations can aggravate these problems and should, therefore, be avoided in these cases. Oral contraceptives are also used in the treatment of dysmenorrhea, menorrhagia, hypothalamic amenorrhea, hormone replacement in women with primary hypogonadism, and premenstrual syndrome. They lead to lower risk of iron deficiency anemia caused by increased menstrual flow; ectopic pregnancy in the case of combination contraceptives; ovarian cysts; postmenopausal hip fractures in women who used combined contraceptives in their 30s; benign breast disease; ovarian cancer; and endometrial cancer. Preparations containing low doses of estrogen (20 μg) are often used in perimenopausal women. They help to relieve vasomotor flushing, but symptoms recur during the placebo period.

INJECTABLE CONTRACEPTION

Depot Medroxyprogesterone Acetate

Depot medroxyprogesterone acetate (DMPA; Depo-Provera) is a progesterone that prevents ovulation in addition to causing changes in cervical mucus and the endometrium. It is given as an injection in the buttocks or upper arm within 5 days after the beginning of the normal menstrual cycle and is repeated every 3 months. It is more effective than oral contraceptives.

Side effects include irregular bleeding, weight gain, headache, mood change, abdominal pain, dizziness, weakness or fatigue, and breast tenderness. After 1 year of use, 50% of women have amenorrhea.[3] This is not harmful,[3] and periods return shortly after the drug is stopped. Studies released in 2004 show that DMPA is associated with a loss of bone density, resulting in an increased risk of osteoporosis. The bone loss appears not to be reversed when the woman stops taking DMPA. DMPA is not recommended for long-term use and is especially not recommended when patients are still growing.

DMPA is safe, is reversible, maintains spontaneity, and has noncontraceptive benefits similar to those of oral contraceptives. Ovulation is suppressed for at least 14 weeks, so delay of up to 2 weeks in the next injection is acceptable. Women with a lapse of more than 14 weeks should have pregnancy ruled out. There is reduced menstrual cramping and pain, fewer periods, and lower chance of anemia.

Precautions include spotting, especially during the first 3 months, and lack of protection against STDs. Fertility usually returns within 6 to 9 months after stopping but can take up to 18 months.[3] Patients on DMPA are advised to exercise and take adequate amounts of calcium. A bone density test may be prudent if DMPA is used for more than 2 years.

IMPLANTABLE CONTRACEPTION

As of 2002, Norplant is no longer being manufactured. Women should be encouraged to contact their physician near the end of the 5-year expiration date of their Norplant system.

Single-rod progestin implant (Implanon) is placed subdermally in the inner arm. Contraception is provided by slow release of 68 mg of the progestin etonogestrel, which is initially released at 60 to 70 μg/day, decreasing to 35 to 45 μg/day at the end of the first year, to 30 to 40 μg/day at the end of the second year, and then to 25 to 30 μg/day at the end of the third year.

Side effects include spotting, irregular bleeding, and amenorrhea. Irregular bleeding is the primary reason for discontinuation. Fluid retention, weight gain, and breast tenderness are less common. Potential complications of insertion include infection, hematoma formation, local irritation or rash, expulsion, and allergic reactions. A single case of injury to the branches of the medial antebrachial cutaneous nerve during insertion has been reported. Nerve injury can result in impaired sensibility, severe localized pain, or the formation of painful neuroma.

Insertion is on office procedure done with or without local anesthesia. The rod can be removed at any time, but it must be removed at the end of 3 years. Ovulation resumes shortly after removal.

Correct insertion technique and timing of insertion play major roles in the effectiveness of Implanon. The FDA has mandated that providers undergo special training to place and remove Implanon.

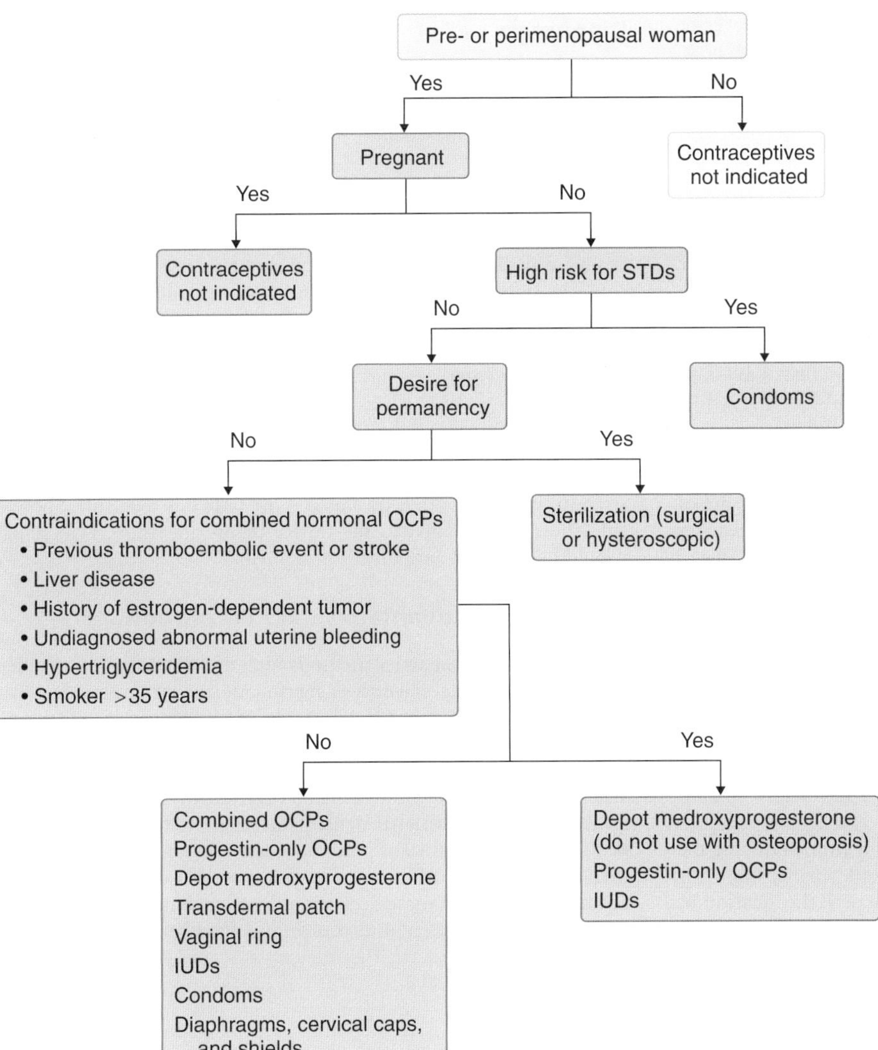

Figure 1 Progestin-only pills are a good option for patients who need to avoid estrogen. IUDs, intrauterine devices; OCPs, oral contraceptive pills; STDs, sexually transmitted diseases.

Implanon should be inserted between day 1 and day 5 of the menstrual cycle. If done during other days of the menstrual cycle, a pregnancy test must be done. The patient should be advised to use another method of contraception for at least 1 week after insertion.

TRANSDERMAL CONTRACEPTION

The transdermal patch (Ortho Evra) consists of three layers. The middle layer contains norelgestromin and ethinyl estradiol. The inner layer is an adhesive and the outer is a protective cover. The patch contains 150 μg of norelgestromin and 20 μg of ethinyl estradiol. The first patch should be applied within the first 5 days of the menstrual cycle, and backup contraceptives should be used concomitantly for 7 days. A new patch should be applied every week for 3 weeks, followed by 1 patch-free week.

The patch exposes women to higher levels of estrogen than most oral hormonal contraceptive pills. The FDA has added new warnings that users could have twice the risk of blood clots than users oral hormonal contraceptives due to higher levels of estrogen exposure.

Application sites include the buttocks, abdomen, outer arms, and torso, except the breasts. The patch may be a good option for women who have difficulty adhering to other hormonal contraceptive regimens.

Physicians must balance the higher estrogen exposure against the chance of pregnancy. The patch completely detaches in 2% to 6% of cases. If it is replaced within 48 hours, no backup contraception is needed. If the patch-free interval exceeds 2 days, pregnancy should be ruled out, a new patch should be placed, and a backup contraceptive method should be used for 7 days. In case of skin irritation, the patch should be removed and a new patch applied to another site. Women weighing more than 198 pounds should not use the patch because its effectiveness is reduced. Ortho Evra offers no protection against STDs.

HORMONAL RING

The NuvaRing is a nonbiodegradable, flexible vaginal ring made of a polymer of ethylene vinyl acetate and magnesium stearate. The outer diameter of the ring is 54 mm, and the cross-sectional diameter is 4 mm. It releases 120 μg of etonogestrel and 15 μg of ethinyl estradiol daily. The ring is left in place for 3 weeks, followed by 1 ring-free week.

Vaginal discharge, vaginitis, and irritation can occur. Side effects are otherwise similar to those of oral combination pills.

The ring can be inserted at any time during the first 5 days of the menstrual cycle. A new ring should be inserted each month. The hormonal ring provides good cycle control.

If the ring is expelled during the first 3 weeks of use, it should be washed with lukewarm water and then replaced. If the ring-free interval is longer than 3 hours, a backup contraceptive method should be used concomitantly for 7 days. The ring should never be left in place for more than 4 weeks. If the ring is left in place, pregnancy should be ruled out before a new ring is inserted, and a backup method should be used for 7 days after inserting a new ring. It provides no protection against STDs.

INTRAUTERINE DEVICES

There are currently two intrauterine devices (IUDs) on the market, the copper ParaGard T 380A and the levonorgestrel system, Mirena. Today's IUDs are safe and slightly more effective than oral contraceptives (see Table 1). The copper IUD is a T-shaped device made of soft, flexible plastic with threads on the end that extend from the cervix and into the upper vagina. Copper IUDs induce a foreign-body reaction in the endometrium, leading to inflammation that prevents viable sperm from reaching the fallopian tubes.

The levonorgestrel-releasing IUD is a T-shaped polyethylene device. The frame is 32 mm in both horizontal and vertical directions. The vertical stem contains a mixture of silicone and 52 mg of levonorgestrel surrounded by a Silastic capsule. The device releases 25 µg of levonorgestrel daily. It has an effective life of 5 years. It can be inserted within the first 7 days of onset of menstruation. This device causes changes in the lining of the uterus so that the fertilized egg cannot implant, and it thickens the cervical mucus to make sperm entry difficult.

Side effects include cramping during insertion, bleeding, pelvic inflammatory disease, and perforation of the uterus.

Spontaneity is maintained, and there are marked reductions in menstrual blood loss and dysmenorrhea. Copper IUDs last for 10 years; the Mirena system is effective for 5 years. Fertility returns rapidly after discontinuation of IUDs.

Expulsion of the copper IUD occurs in 5% of women during the first year. Expulsion rates for Mirena are a little higher than for copper IUDs. Each month, the woman should check the location of the threads of the copper IUD with her finger and she should notify the physician if she does not feel them. There is a mildly increased risk of ectopic pregnancy. Ovarian cysts are three times more common in users of this device. Twenty percent of women develop amenorrhea by the end of the first year of use. The risk of pelvic infection is higher during the first 20 days of Mirena insertion. There is also no protection against STDs.

BARRIER CONTRACEPTIVES

Prescription barrier methods include the diaphragm, cervical caps, and shields (Table 2). They cover the cervix and prevent sperm entry into the cervix. These devices are less effective than hormonal forms of contraception. The female condom and spermicides are nonprescription barrier methods. Female condoms are similar in efficacy to other barrier methods but have the benefit of some protection against STDs. Spermicides should be used in combination with other barrier methods.

Table 2 Select Barrier Contraception Methods

Method	Left in Place After Intercourse (Hours)	Remove Within (Hours)
Diaphragm	6	24
Prentif (latex) cervical cap	8	48
FemCap (silicone) cervical cap	6	48
Lea's shield	8	48

Diaphragm

The diaphragm is a dome-shaped rubber disk with a flexible rim. The effectiveness depends on the proper fit as determined by the physician.

Cervical Cap

The cervical cap is smaller than a diaphragm. It fits securely in the vagina, covering the cervix, and must be fitted by a physician. Two types are available. The latex cervical cap (Prentif) has a firm, flexible rim. The silicone FemCap comes in three sizes, ranging from 22 mm to 30 mm. It is reusable for 2 years.

Cervical Shield

The cervical shield is a dome-shaped disk made of silicone. It has a one-way valve that creates suction by venting trapped air between the shield and cervix. It acts by preventing sperm entry. It also has a strap for easy removal. Lea's shield is the only one available. Spermicide should be applied to the device before insertion. Lea's shield should be replaced annually.

Side Effects, Advantages, and Precautions

Side effects of these barrier methods include vaginal irritation; allergic reactions to latex, silicone, or spermicide; urinary tract infections; and the rare risk of toxic shock syndrome if left in place too long. They are safe, effective, reusable, and have no effect on the menstrual cycle. These methods are less effective than hormonal contraception and provide no protection against STDs. Use of cervical shields can lead to falsely abnormal Papanicolaou (Pap) tests. Resizing should be done after abdominal or pelvic surgery, after any pregnancy longer than 14 weeks, and after any significant weight change. To protect against pregnancy, the devices should be left in place for a certain minimum of time after intercourse and then removed to decrease risk of infection.

Spermicides

Spermicides contain chemicals that kill or damage sperm. They come in the forms of creams, gels, films, suppositories, and tablets. Side effects include irritation, allergic reaction, and urinary tract infections. Spermicides are inexpensive and do not require a prescription. They offer no STD protection, and they are less effective and should supplement other barrier methods.

Contraceptive Sponge

The Today Sponge, a nonhormonal contraceptive spermicidal sponge is now back on the market for over-the-counter purchase. The effectiveness of the Today sponge when used appropriately and consistently is 89% to 91%. This is a nonhormonal contraceptive and lacks hormonal side effects. It requires no special fitting, becomes effective immediately after insertion, and protects against pregnancy for the next 24 hours without the need of additional spermicide. It mimics the feel of vaginal tissue and is therefore not detected by partners. The Today sponge should be kept in place for 6 hours after intercourse to ensure effective contraception. However, it should not be left in place for more than 30 hours after insertion.

Female Condoms

The Reality female condom consists of a lubricated polyurethane sheath with a flexible polyurethane ring on each end. One ring is inserted into the vagina much like a diaphragm, while the other remains outside, covering the labia. Side effects include irritation and allergic reactions. The female condom might offer some protection against STDs, but for highly effective protection, male latex condoms should be used instead. The male and female condoms should not be used at the same time because they will not both stay in place.

FEMALE STERILIZATION

Hysteroscopic Sterilization

Hysteroscopic sterilization (Essure) is a new method of sterilization that uses a transcervical approach. The micro-insert consists of a stainless-steel inner coil, an elastic outer coil, and polyethylene fibers. The coil is inserted into the uterine end of the fallopian tube using a hysteroscopic technique. The outer coil expands to anchor the insert. The polyethylene fibers expand and cause inflammation and extensive fibrosis, resulting in permanent occlusion of the fallopian tubes by 12 weeks. Women should use a backup method for 12 weeks.

Side effects include pain after insertion and a small increased risk of ectopic pregnancy. Because this is a permanent method of contraception, women do not have to worry about pregnancy and the side effects of contraceptives.

Hysterosalpingography should be done at the end of 12 weeks to confirm tubal occlusion. Failure to correctly place the micro-inserts can lead to expulsion.

Tubal Ligation

Tubal ligation is a surgical procedure requiring anesthesia in which the fallopian tubes are cut or tied. The surgery takes about 30 minutes. The procedure does not affect sexual activity or the menstrual cycle. There is a risk of bleeding from the site, infection side effects from anesthesia, bowel or bladder injury, and injury to the skin. There is a slightly increased risk of ectopic pregnancy.

NATURAL FAMILY PLANNING

Sperm can live in the female reproductive tract for up to 7 days, whereas the egg lives for 1 day. Safe days occur 2 days after ovulation and continue until the next menses. This knowledge forms the basis for natural family planning.

In the ovulation method, the days just before and after ovulation are determined by checking cervical mucus. Mucus is stretchy and clear at the time of ovulation.

In the symptothermal method, daily temperature is recorded on a chart. Body temperature rises 2 days before ovulation. Consistency of cervical mucus is also monitored.

The rhythm method is based on calendar calculations of previous menstrual cycles. This method does not allow for normal changes in the menstrual cycle and is not as reliable as the ovulation or symptothermal method. This method is not recommended. Women who have no variation in the length of their menstrual cycle can use the rhythm method to know when they are ovulating (14 days before the start of menses).

The lactation amenorrhea method is a contraceptive method based on natural postpartum infertility, when a woman is amenorrheic and exclusively breastfeeding. The infant's suckling suppresses production of hormones. All three criteria—exclusive or near-exclusive breast-feeding, no menses since delivery, and less than 6 months postpartum—must be satisfied to effectively use this method.

EMERGENCY ORAL CONTRACEPTION

Plan B, or the levonorgestrel regimen, is the only emergency contraceptive pill regimen currently approved in the United States. It consists of two 0.75-mg levonorgestrel pills taken 12 hours apart. The first pill should be taken as soon as possible within 72 hours of unprotected intercourse.[4] It has been approved for sale by pharmacists to women age 18 and older presenting photo identification. The Yuzpe regimen, marketed as Preven, is no longer available in the United States.

Emergency contraceptive pills are not teratogenic. Thus, a pregnancy test is not required before treatment. The only indication for emergency contraception is unprotected intercourse. Failure rate is 0.4% when treatment is initiated within 24 hours and 2.7% when treatment is initiated 48 to 72 hours after intercourse.

Plan B should not be used in cases of known or suspected pregnancy, hypersensitivity to components, or undiagnosed abnormal vaginal bleeding. Major side effects include nausea and vomiting.

CONCLUSION

The range of available contraceptive options has increased markedly over the past 5 years. This progress is likely to continue as consumers seek safer, more-effective contraceptive methods. Improved counseling and knowledge should lead to more consistent and correct use of contraceptives and decreased numbers of unplanned pregnancies.

Summary

- Unintended pregnancy is a major health problem; 50% of pregnancies are unplanned.
- The most effective and reversible contraceptive methods include the oral contraceptive, injectable contraceptive, implantable contraceptive, hormonal ring, and intrauterine devices.
- Barrier methods of contraception are less effective than hormonal forms of contraception.
- Natural family planning methods are not reliable and are not recommended.
- Levonorgestrel (brand name Plan B) is the only emergency contraceptive pill approved in the United States.

Suggested Readings

Burkman RT: Oral contraceptives: Current status. Clin Obstet Gynecol 2001;44:62-72.

Gallo MF, Grimes DA, Schulz KF: Cervical cap versus diaphragm for contraception. Cochrane Database Syst Rev 2002, I:CD003551.

Kaunitz AM: Injectable long-acting contraceptives. Clin Obstet Gynecol 2001;44:73-91.

Rawlins S, Smith D: Innovative contraception: New options in hormonal contraception. Am J Nurse Practitioners 2002;6:9-28.

Thomas MA: Postcoital contraception. Clin Obstet Gynecol 2001;44:101-105.

References

For a complete list of references, log onto www.expertconsult.com.

Female Sexual Dysfunction

Julie A. Elder and *Yvonne Braver*

DEFINITIONS

Sexual dysfunction is defined as a disturbance in, or pain during, the sexual response. This problem is more difficult to diagnose and treat in women than it is in men because of the intricacy of the female sexual response. In 1998, the Sexual Function Health Council of the American Foundation of Urologic Disease revised the preexisting definitions and classifications of FSD.[1] Medical risk factors, etiologies, and psychological aspects were classified into four categories of FSD: hypoactive sexual desire, arousal, orgasmic disorders, and sexual pain disorders.

- *Hypoactive sexual desire* is the persistent or recurrent deficiency (or absence) of sexual fantasies or thoughts and/or the lack of receptivity to sexual activity.
- *Sexual arousal disorder* is the persistent or recurrent inability to achieve or maintain sufficient sexual excitement, expressed as a lack of excitement or a lack of genital or other somatic re-sponses.
- *Orgasmic disorder* is the persistent or recurrent difficulty, delay, or absence of attaining orgasm after sufficient sexual stimulation and arousal.
- *Sexual pain disorder* includes dyspareunia (genital pain associated with sexual intercourse); vaginismus (involuntary spasm of the vaginal musculature that causes interference with vaginal penetration), and noncoital sexual pain disorder (genital pain induced by noncoital sexual stimulation).

Each of these definitions has three additional subtypes: lifelong versus acquired; generalized versus situational; and of organic, psychogenic, mixed, or unknown causative origin.

PREVALENCE

Approximately 40 million American women are affected by FSD.[2] The National Health and Social Life Survey, a probability sample study of sexual behavior in a demographically representative cohort of U.S. adults ages 18 to 59, found that sexual dysfunction is more prevalent in women (43%) than in men (31%), and increases as women age.[3] Married women have a lower risk of sexual dysfunction than unmarried women. Hispanic women consistently report lower rates of sexual problems, whereas African American women have higher rates of decreased sexual desire and pleasure than do white women. Sexual pain, however, is more likely to occur in white women. This survey was limited by its cross-sectional design and age restrictions, because women older than 60 years were excluded. Also, no adjustments were made for the effects of menopausal status or medical risk factors. Despite these limitations, the survey clearly indicates that sexual dysfunction affects many women.

PATHOPHYSIOLOGY

FSD has both physiologic and psychological components. It is important to first understand the normal female sexual response to understand sexual dysfunction. Physiologically, sexual arousal begins in the medial preoptic, anterior hypothalamic, and limbic-hippocampal structures within the central nervous system. Electrical signals are then transmitted through the parasympathetic and sympathetic nervous systems.[2]

Physiologic and biochemical mediators that modulate vaginal and clitoral smooth-muscle tone and relaxation are currently under investigation. Neuropeptide Y, vasoactive intestinal polypeptide, nitric oxide synthase, cyclic guanosine monophosphate, and substance P have been found in vaginal-tissue nerve fibers. Nitric oxide is believed to mediate clitoral and labial engorgement, whereas vasoactive intestinal polypeptide, a nonadrenergic/noncholinergic neurotransmitter, may enhance vaginal blood flow, lubrication, and secretions.[4]

Many changes occur in the female genitalia during sexual arousal. Increased blood flow promotes vasocongestion of the genitalia. Secretions from uterine and Bartholin glands lubricate the vaginal canal. Vaginal smooth muscle relaxation allows for lengthening and dilation of the vagina. As the clitoris is stimulated, its length and diameter increase and engorgement occurs. In addition, the labia minora promote engorgement because of increased blood flow.

FSD is psychologically complex. The female sexual response cycle was first characterized by Masters and Johnson in 1966 and included four phases: excitement, plateau, orgasm, and resolution.[5] In 1974, Kaplan modified this theory and characterized it as a three-phase model that included desire, arousal, and orgasm.[6] Basson proposed a different theory for the female sexual response cycle,[7] suggesting that the sexual response is driven by the desire to enhance intimacy (Fig. 1). The cycle begins with sexual neutrality. As a woman seeks a sexual stimulus and responds to it, she becomes sexually aroused. Arousal leads to desire, thus stimulating a woman's willingness to receive or provide additional stimuli. Emotional and physical satisfaction is gained by an increase in sexual desire and arousal. Emotional intimacy is then ultimately achieved. Various biologic and psychological factors can negatively affect this cycle, thereby leading to FSD.

SIGNS AND SYMPTOMS

Sexual dysfunction manifests in a variety of ways. It is important to elicit specific signs and symptoms because many women make generalizations about their sexual problems-describing the trouble as a decrease in libido or overall dissatisfaction. Other women may be more specific and recount pain with sexual stimulation or intercourse, anorgasmia, delayed orgasm, and decreased arousal. Postmenopausal women with estrogen deficiency and vaginal atrophy may also describe a decrease in vaginal lubrication.

DIAGNOSIS

History

An accurate diagnosis of FSD requires a thorough medical and sexual history. Issues such as sexual preference, domestic violence, fears of pregnancy, human immunodeficiency virus, and sexually transmitted diseases must be discussed. In addition, specific details of the actual dysfunction, identifying causes, medical or gynecologic conditions, and psychosocial information must be obtained.[8] FSD is often multifactorial, and the presence of more than one dysfunction should be ascertained. Patients may be able to provide insight into the cause or causes of the problem; however, various tools are available to assist with obtaining a good sexual history. The Female Sexual Function Index (FSFI) is one such example.[9] This questionnaire contains 19 questions and categorizes sexual dysfunction in the domains of desire, arousal, lubrication, orgasm, satisfaction, and pain. The FSFI and other similar questionnaires can be filled out before the appointment time to expedite the process.

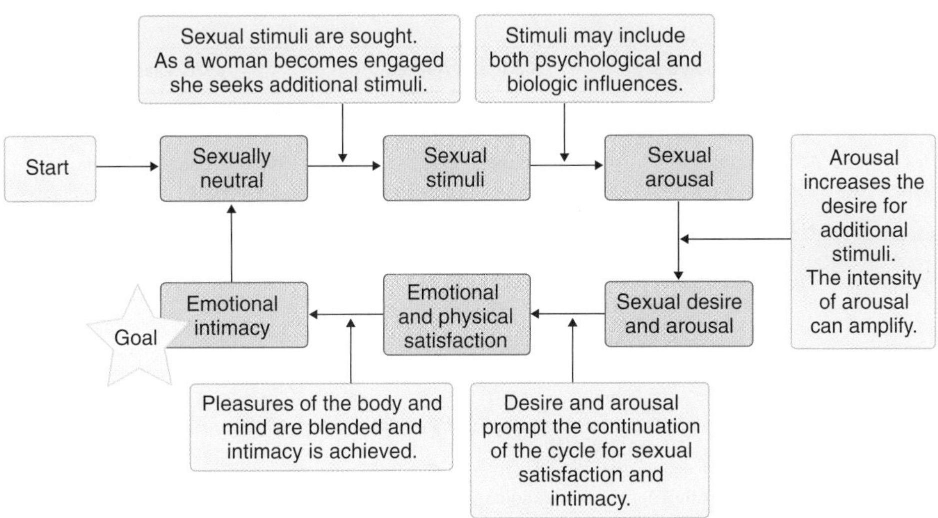

Figure 1 Basson proposed a different theory for the female sexual response cycle, suggesting that the sexual response is driven by the desire to enhance intimacy. *(From Basson R: Human sex-response cycles. J Sex Marital Ther 2001;27:33-43.)*

Table 1 Medical Causes of Female Sexual Dysfunction

Cardiovascular	Gastrointestinal	Neurologic	Rheumatologic	Endocrine	Psychological
Hypertension	Cancer	Paralysis	Fibromyalgia	Diabetes	Depression
Coronary artery disease	Irritable bowel	Multiple sclerosis	Arthritis	Thyroid disease	Intra- or interpersonal conflicts
Myocardial infarction	Colostomy	Neuropathies	Autoimmune disorders	Adrenal disorders	Life stressors
Peripheral vascular disease		Stroke		Prolactinomas	Anxiety

Data from Bachman GA, Phillips NA. Sexual dysfunction. In Steege JF, Metzger DA, Levy BS (eds): Chronic Pelvic Pain: An Integrated Approach. Philadelphia, WB Saunders, 1998, pp 77-90.

FSD needs to be categorized according to the onset and duration of symptoms. It is also imperative to determine whether the symptoms are situational or global. Situational symptoms occur with a specific partner or in a particular setting, whereas global symptoms relate to an assortment of partners and circumstances.

A variety of medical problems can contribute to FSD (Table 1).[10] Vascular disease, for example, may lead to decreased blood flow to the genitalia, causing decreased arousal and delayed orgasm. Diabetic neuropathy may also contribute to the problem. Arthritis may make intercourse uncomfortable and even painful. It is essential to aggressively treat these diseases and inform patients of how they can affect sexuality.

There are many gynecologic causes of FSD, contributing to physical, psychological, and sexual difficulties (Box 1).[8] Women who have undergone gynecologic surgeries (i.e., hysterectomies and excisions of vulvar malignancies) may experience feelings of decreased sexuality because of alterations in or loss of psychological symbols of femininity. Women with vaginismus may find vaginal penetration painful and virtually impossible. Alterations in hormones during pregnancy or the postpartum period may lead to a decrease in sexual activity, desire, and satisfaction, which may be prolonged by lactation.[11]

Prescription and over-the-counter medications should be reviewed to identify any contributing agents (Table 2).[12,13] Consideration should be given to dosage adjustments, medication alterations, and even drug discontinuation, if possible. In addition, use of recreational drugs, alcohol, and alternative therapies should be discussed.

Psychosocial and psychological factors should also be identified. For example, a woman with a strict religious upbringing may have feelings of guilt that decrease sexual pleasure. A history of rape or sexual abuse may contribute to vaginismus. Financial struggles may preclude a woman's desire for intimacy.

Box 1 Gynecologic Etiologies of Female Sexual Dysfunction

- Bartholin gland cysts
- Cancer
- Clitoral adhesions
- Cystocele or rectocele
- Dermatitis
- Endometriosis
- Episiotomy scars
- Lichen sclerosis
- Myalgias
- Pelvic inflammatory disease
- Uterine fibroids
- Uterine prolapse
- Vaginal tissue atrophy
- Vaginismus
- Vaginitis
- Vestibulitis
- Vulvar dystrophy

Physical Examination

A thorough physical examination is required to identify disease. The entire body and genitalia should be examined. The genital examination can be used to reproduce and localize pain that is encountered during sexual activity and vaginal penetration.[14] External genitalia should be inspected. Skin color, texture, thickness, turgor, and the amount and distribution of pubic hair should be assessed. Internal mucosa and anatomy should then be examined and cultures taken if indicated. Attention should be given to muscle tone, location of episiotomy scars and strictures, tissue atrophy, and the presence of

Table 2 Medications That May Cause Female Sexual Dysfunction

Antihypertensives	Antidepressants	Anxiolytics	Illicit and Abused Drugs	Miscellaneous
Benazepril (Lotensin)	Amoxapine (Asendin)	Alprazolam (Xanax)	Alcohol	Acetazolamide (Diamox)
Clonidine (Catapres)	Bupropion (Wellbutrin, Zyban, Wellbutrin SR)	Barbiturates	Amphetamines	Amiodarone (Cordarone, Pacerone)
Lisinopril (Prinivil, Zestril)	Buspirone (BuSpar)	Clomipramine (Anafranil)	Amyl nitrate	Bromocriptine (Parlodel)
Methyldopa (Aldomet)	Fluoxetine (Prozac, Seraphim)	Clonazepam (Klonopin)	Barbiturates	Cimetidine (Tagamet)
Metoprolol (Lopressor, Toprol XL)	Imipramine (Tofranil)	Diazepam (Valium, Diastat)	Cocaine	Danazol (Danocrine)
Propranolol (Inderal, Inderal LA)	Paroxetine (Paxil)	Lithium (Eskalith, Eskalith CR, Lithobid, Lithonate)	Diazepam (Valium, Diastat)	Digoxin (Lanoxin, Digitek, Lanoxicaps)
Reserpine (Serpasil)	Phenelzine (Nardil)	Lorazepam (Ativan)	Marijuana	Diphenhydramine (Benadryl)
Spironolactone (Aldactone)	Sertraline (Zoloft)	Perphenazine (Trilafon)	MDMA (ecstasy, methyl-methylene dexamphetamine)	Ethinyl estradiol (Estinyl, FEMHRT, various oral contraceptives)
Timolol (Blocadren)	Trazodone (Desyrel) Venlafaxine (Effexor)	Prochlorperazine (Compazine)	Morphine Tobacco	Gemfibrozil (Lopid) Medroxyprogesterone (Amen, Cycrin, Depo-Provera, Provera) Metronidazole (Flagyl) Niacin (Niacor, Niaspan) Phenytoin (Dilantin) Ranitidine (Zantac)

Data from Drugs that cause sexual dysfunction: an update. Med Lett Drugs Ther 1992;34:73-78; Finger WW, Lund M, Slagle MA: Medications that may contribute to sexual disorders. A guide to assessment and treatment in family practice. J Fam Pract 1997;44:33-43.

discharge in the vaginal vault. Some women with vaginismus and severe dyspareunia may not endure a normal speculum and bimanual examination—a "monomanual" examination using one to two fingers may be better tolerated.[8] The bimanual or monomanual examination can give information about rectal disease, uterine size and position, cervical motion tenderness, internal muscle tone, vaginal depth, prolapse, ovarian and adnexal size and location, and vaginismus.

Laboratory Tests

Although no specific laboratory tests are universally recommended for the diagnosis of FSD, routine Pap smears and stool guaiac tests should not be overlooked. Baseline hormone levels may be helpful when indicated, including thyroid-stimulating hormone, follicle-stimulating hormone (FSH), luteinizing hormone (LH), total and free testosterone levels, sex hormone-binding globulin (SHBG), estradiol, and prolactin.

The diagnosis of primary and secondary hypogonadism can be assessed with FSH and LH. An elevation of FSH and LH may suggest primary gonadal failure, whereas lower levels suggest impairment of the hypothalamic-pituitary axis. Decreased estrogen levels can lead to decreased libido, vaginal dryness, and dyspareunia. Testosterone deficiencies can also cause FSD, including decreased libido, arousal, and sensation. SHBG levels increase with age but decrease with the use of exogenous estrogens.[15] Hyperprolactinemia may also be associated with decreased libido.

Other Tests

Some medical centers have the capacity to perform additional testing, although many of these tests are still investigational. The genital blood flow test uses duplex Doppler ultrasonography to determine peak systolic and diastolic velocities of blood flow to the clitoris, labia, urethra, and vagina. Vaginal pH can serve as an indirect measurement of lubrication. Pressure-volume changes can identify dysfunction of vaginal tissue compliance and elasticity. Vibratory perception thresholds and temperature perception thresholds may offer information regarding genital sensation.[2] Clitoral electromyography may also be beneficial in evaluating the autonomic innervation of the corpus clitoris.[16] These tests may be helpful in guiding medical therapy.

TREATMENT AND OUTCOMES

Once a diagnosis is made, suspected causes should be addressed. For example, diseases such as diabetes or hypothyroidism must be aggressively treated. Consideration should also be given to changes in medications or dosages.

Patients should be educated about sexual function and dysfunction. Information about basic anatomy and the physiologic changes associated with hormonal fluctuations may help a woman better understand the problem. There are many good books, videos, websites, and organizations available that can be recommended to patients (Table 3).

If no exact cause can be identified, basic treatment strategies should be applied. Patients should be encouraged to enhance stimulation and avoid a mundane routine. Specifically, the use of videos, books, and masturbation can help maximize pleasure. Patients should also be encouraged to make time for sexual activity and communicate with their partners about sexual needs. Pelvic muscle contraction during intercourse, background music, and the use of fantasy may help eliminate anxiety and increase relaxation. Noncoital behaviors, such as massage and oral or noncoital stimulation, should also be recommended, especially if the partner has erectile dysfunction. Vaginal lubricants and moisturizers, positional

Table 3 Resources for Patients

The Kinsey Institute Morrison 313 Indiana University Bloomington, IN 47405 Phone: 812-855-7686 www.indiana.edu/~kinsey	*For Women Only: A Revolutionary Guide to Overcoming Sexual Dysfunction and Reclaiming Your Sex Life* by L. Berman, J. Berman, et al. New York, Henry Holt, 2001	www.tantra.com Resource for books, tapes, music and general information on sexuality and spirituality
American Association of Sex Educators, Counselors, and Therapists (AASECT) P.O. Box 5488 Richmond, VA 23220-0488 www.aasect.org	*Sex Information, May I Help You?* by I. Alman Burlingame, CA: Down There Press, 1992	www.sexologist.org The American Board of Sexology website. Provides list of board-certified sex therapists in each state
Sexuality Information and Education Council of the United States (SIECUS) 130 West 42nd Street, Suite 350 New York, NY 10036-7802 Phone: 212/819-9770 www.siecus.org	*How to Have Magnificent Sex: The 7 Dimensions of a Vital Sexual Connection* by L. Holstein New York, Harmony Books, 2001	

changes, and nonsteroidal anti-inflammatory drugs may reduce dyspareunia.[17]

Hypoactive Sexual Desire

Desire disorders are often multifactorial and may be difficult to treat effectively. For many women, lifestyle issues such as finances, careers, and family commitments may greatly contribute to the problem. In addition, medications or another type of sexual dysfunction (i.e., pain) may contribute to the dysfunction. Individual or couple counseling may be of benefit because there is no medical treatment geared toward this specific disorder.

Hormone replacement therapy can affect sexual desire. Estrogen may benefit menopausal or perimenopausal women. It can enhance clitoral sensitivity, increase libido, improve vaginal atrophy, and decrease dyspareunia. In addition, estrogen can improve vasomotor symptoms, mood disorders, and symptoms of urinary frequency and urgency.[18] Progesterone is necessary for women with intact uteri using estrogen; however, it may negatively affect mood and contribute to decreased sexual desire.

Testosterone appears to directly influence sexual desire, but data are controversial regarding its replacement in androgen-deficient premenopausal women. Indications for testosterone replacement include premature ovarian failure, symptomatic premenopausal testosterone deficiency, and symptomatic postmenopausal testosterone deficiency (includes natural, surgical, or chemotherapy-induced deficiency).[18] Currently, however, there is no national guideline for testosterone replacement in women with sexual dysfunction. In addition, there is no consensus regarding what are considered normal or therapeutic levels of testosterone therapy for women.[14]

Before initiating therapy, potential side effects and risks of treatment should be discussed. Androgenic side effects can occur in 5% to 35% of women taking testosterone and they include acne, weight gain, hirsutism, clitorimegaly, deepening of the voice, and lowering of high-density lipoprotein cholesterol.[19] Baseline levels of lipids, testosterone (free and total), and liver function enzymes should be obtained in addition to a mammogram and Pap smear if indicated.

Postmenopausal women may benefit from 0.25 to 2.5 mg of methyltestosterone (Android, Methitest, Testred, Virilon) or up to 10 mg of micronized oral testosterone. Doses are adjusted according to symptom control and side effects. Methyltestosterone is also available in combination with estrogen (Estratest, Estratest HS). Some women may benefit from topical methyltestosterone or testosterone propionate compounded with petroleum jelly in a 1% to 2% formula. This ointment can be applied up to three times per week.[8,18] It is important to periodically monitor liver function, lipids, testosterone levels, and androgenic side effects during treatment.

There are various over-the-counter herbal products that advertise improvement in female sexual dysfunction and restoration of hormone levels. Although evidence is conflicting, many of these products lack sufficient scientific studies required to support the manufacturer's claims of efficacy and safety.[20,21] Patients should be cautioned about the potential for side effects and drug-to-drug interactions with these products.

Tibolone is a synthetic steroid with tissue-specific estrogenic, progestogenic and androgenic properties. It has been used in Europe for the past 20 years in the prevention of postmenopausal osteoporosis and in the treatment of menopausal symptoms, including sexual dysfunction. It is not yet available in the United States, but is actively being studied.[22]

Sexual Arousal Disorder

Inadequate stimulation, anxiety, and urogenital atrophy may contribute to arousal disorder. A pilot study of 48 women with arousal disorder showed that sildenafil (Viagra) significantly improved subjective and physiologic parameters of the female sexual response.[23] Other treatment options for arousal disorder include lubricants, vitamin E and mineral oils, increased foreplay, relaxation, and distraction techniques. Estrogen replacement may benefit postmenopausal women, because urogenital atrophy is one of the most common causes of arousal disorder in this age group.

Orgasmic Disorder

Women with orgasmic disorders often respond well to therapy. Sex therapists encourage women to enhance stimulation and minimize inhibition. Pelvic muscle exercises can improve muscle control and sexual tension, whereas the use of masturbation and vibrators can increase stimulation. The use of distraction (i.e., background music, fantasy, and so forth, can also help minimize inhibition).[8]

Sexual Pain Disorder

Sexual pain can be classified as superficial, vaginal, or deep. Superficial pain is often caused by vaginismus, anatomic abnormalities, or irritative conditions of the vaginal mucosa. Vaginal pain can be caused by friction as a result of inadequate lubrication. Deep pain can be muscular in nature or associated with pelvic disease.[14] The type(s) of pain a woman experiences can dictate therapy, thereby making an aggressive approach to an accurate diagnosis imperative. The use of lubricants, vaginal estrogens, topical lidocaine, moist heat to the genital area, NSAIDs, physical therapy, and positional changes may help to minimize discomfort during intercourse. Sex therapy may benefit women with vaginismus because it is often triggered by a history of sexual abuse or trauma.

CONCLUSION

The complexity of sexual dysfunction in women makes the diagnosis and treatment difficult. Disorders of desire, for example, are difficult to treat, whereas disorders such as vaginismus and orgasmic dysfunction easily respond to therapy. Numerous women suffer from FSD; however, it is unknown how many women are successfully treated.

Until recently, there has been limited clinical or scientific research in the field of FSD. Although some progress has been made, additional research is needed to assess treatment efficacy and establish national treatment guidelines.

Summary

- Physicians must encourage patients to discuss Female Sexual Dysfunction (FSD).
- The Sexual Function Health Council of the American Foundation of Urologic Disease has classified FSD into four categories: desire, arousal, orgasmic, and sexual pain disorders.
- An accurate diagnosis of FSD requires a thorough medical and sexual history including issues of sexual preference, domestic violence and fears of pregnancy, human immunodeficiency virus and sexually transmitted disease.
- Even if no exact cause can be identified, basic treatment strategies such as enhancing stimulation, avoiding mundane routines, making time for sexual activities, communicating with their partners about sexual needs, and using noncoital behaviors can be applied.
- Patients want to talk about sexual problems with physicians, but often fail to do so, thinking their physicians are too busy, the topic is too embarrassing, or there is no treatment available.[24] FSD is a serious problem in the United States and unfortunately it often goes untreated. It is a difficult and complex problem to address in the medical setting, but it must not be neglected. Physicians must encourage patients to discuss FSD, and then aggressively treat the underlying disease or condition.

Suggested Readings

Aschenbrenner D: Avlimil taken for female sexual dysfunction. A J Nurs 2004;104:27-29.

Bachman GA, Phillips NA: Sexual dysfunction. In Steege JF, Metzger DA, Levy BS (eds): Chronic Pelvic Pain: An Integrated Approach. Philadelphia: WB Saunders, 1998, pp 77-90.

Basson R: Human sex-response cycles. J Sex Marital Ther 2001;27:33-43.

Basson R, Berman JR, Burnett A, et al: Report of the international consensus development conference on female sexual dysfunction: Definitions and classifications. J Urol 2000;163:888-893.

Berman JR, Berman L, Goldstein I: Female sexual dysfunction: Incidence, pathophysiology, evaluation, and treatment options. Urology 1999;54:385-391.

Berman JR, Berman LA, Lin A, et al: Effect of sildenafil on subjective and physiologic parameters of the female sexual response in women with sexual arousal disorder. J Sex Marital Ther 2001;27:411-420.

Berman JR, Goldstein I: Female sexual dysfunction. Urol Clin North Am 2001;28:405-416.

Byrd JE, Hyde JS, DeLamater JD, Plant EA: Sexuality during pregnancy and the year postpartum. J Fam Pract 1998;47:305-308.

Drugs that cause sexual dysfunction: An update. Med Lett Drugs Ther 1992;34:73-78.

Finger WW, Lund M, Slagle MA: Medications that may contribute to sexual disorders. A guide to assessment and treatment in family practice. J Fam Pract 1997;44:33-43.

Kang BJ, Lee SJ, Kim MD, Cho MJ: A placebo-controlled, double-blind trial of Ginkgo biloba for antidepressant-induced sexual dysfunction. Human Psychopharmacology. 2002;17:279-284.

Kaplan HS: The New Sex Therapy: Active Treatment of Sexual Disorders. London: Bailliere Tindall, 1974.

Laumann EO, Paik A, Rosen RC: Sexual dysfunction in the United States: Prevalence and predictors. JAMA 1999;281:537-544.

Marwick C: Survey says patients expect little physician help on sex. JAMA 1999;281:2173-2174.

Masters EH, Johnson VE: Human Sexual Response. Boston: Little, Brown, 1966.

Messinger-Rapport BJ, Thacker HL: Prevention for the older woman. A practical guide to hormone replacement therapy and urogynecologic health. Geriatrics 2001;56:32-34, 37-38, 40-42.

Modelska K, Cummings S: Female sexual dysfunction in postmenopausal women: Systematic review of placebo-controlled trials. Am J Obstet Gynecol 2003;188:286-293.

Park K, Moreland RB, Goldstein I, et al: Sildenafil inhibits phosphodiesterase type 5 in human clitoral corpus cavernosum smooth muscle. Biochem Biophys Res Commun 1998;249:612-617.

Phillips NA: Female sexual dysfunction: Evaluation and treatment. Am Fam Physician 2000;62:127-136, 141-142.

Phillips NA: The clinical evaluation of dyspareunia. Int J Impot Res 1998;10(Suppl 2):S117-S120.

Rosen R: The Female Sexual Function Index (FSFI): A multidimensional self-report instrument for the assessment of female sexual function. J Sex Marital Ther 2000; 26:191-208.

Slayden SM: Risks of menopausal androgen supplementation. Semin Reprod Endocrinol 1998;16:145-152.

Striar S, Bartlik B: Stimulation of the libido: The use of erotica in sex therapy. Psychiatr Ann 1999;29:60-62.

Yilmaz U, Soylu A, Ozcan C, Caliskan O: Clitoral electromyography. J Urol 2002;167:616-620.

References

For a complete list of references, log onto www.expertconsult.com.

Endometrial, Ovarian, and Cervical Cancer

Kristine Zanotti

CARCINOMA OF THE ENDOMETRIUM

Definition

Endometrial cancer arises from the glandular tissue within the uterine lining.

Prevalence

Endometrial cancer is the most common of the gynecologic malignancies. Approximately 2% to 3% of women in the United States will develop cancer of the endometrium at some point during their lives. With an estimated 37,000 new cases last year, it is the fourth most common malignancy among women. It predominantly affects older women, with 75% of cases occurring in the postmenopausal years.

Pathophysiology

Endometrial cancer is a heterogeneous disease that is believed to have two biologically different subtypes, implying two different mechanisms for its origin.

Low-Risk Subtype

The most common subtype is a well-differentiated carcinoma (grade 1 or 2 endometrioid histology) that behaves in an indolent fashion, causes bleeding symptoms in its early stages, and is curable in most cases. Risk factors for this low-risk subtype are well known and are related to an increase in circulating estrogens: obesity, chronic anovulation and nulliparity, estrogen replacement therapy (unopposed by progesterone), and tamoxifen use.

High-Risk Subtype

The high-risk subtype accounts for a minority of endometrial malignancies. These poorly differentiated tumors (grade 3 endometrioid, clear cell, and papillary serous carcinoma) are not associated with increased circulating estrogens. Rather, they appear to occur spontaneously in postmenopausal women without clearly defined risk factors. These tumors metastasize early and account for a disproportionate number of mortalities from endometrial malignancy. Modes of spread include local invasion and lymphatic and vascular embolization. The most common metastatic sites include the cervix, adnexa, and retroperitoneal lymph nodes.

Signs and Symptoms

Endometrial cancer usually manifests with abnormal uterine bleeding. It should be suspected in any postmenopausal woman with bleeding symptoms. Pre- or perimenopausal women might have bleeding abnormalities such as menorrhagia or metrorrhagia.

Less commonly, asymptomatic women can present with an abnormal Papanicolaou (Pap) smear revealing atypical or malignant endometrial cells. A normal Pap smear in a symptomatic woman, however, must never be relied on to exclude endometrial pathology.

Diagnosis

A complete physical examination is the first step in the evaluation of a woman with suspected endometrial cancer. Inspection of the vulva, anus, vagina, and cervix is necessary to evaluate for metastatic lesions. A biopsy should be done for any suspicious genital tract lesions detected on examination. Bimanual and rectovaginal examination to evaluate the uterus, cervix, adnexa, parametria, and rectum is essential. Palpation of the inguinal and supraclavicular nodes may reveal enlargement in advanced cases with metastatic disease.

Histologic evaluation of endometrial tissue is necessary. An endometrial biopsy can be performed safely and easily in the office setting in most symptomatic patients. The sensitivity for detecting endometrial carcinoma approaches that of a dilation and curettage (D&C) and avoids the expense and morbidity of an operative procedure. Several biopsy instruments are available for use, including the Pipelle sampler and Novak curette.

Occasionally, D&C is necessary to obtain tissue for histologic evaluation. Cervical stenosis and patient discomfort are common indications for D&C. This outpatient surgical procedure may be performed using a paracervical block with sedation; however, in some cases, general or regional anesthesia may be preferred. Hysteroscopy and saline infusion sonography visualize endometrial lesions, such as polyps, within the uterine cavity and can be useful adjuncts to endometrial sampling techniques.

If endometrial cancer is confirmed, further studies are needed to optimize treatment planning, including a chest x-ray to rule out metastatic disease. Other studies may be performed based on a patient's risk factors and symptoms at presentation. These include computed tomography (CT) scans of the abdomen and pelvis with oral and intravenous contrast (for preoperative assessment of extrauterine tumor spread in high-grade endometrial malignancies); sigmoidoscopy, colonoscopy, or barium enema; intravenous pyelogram; and serum cancer antigen 125 (CA 125) assay for papillary serous carcinoma.

Treatment

Treatment is based on the surgically determined disease stage and on assessment of prognostic features.[1] Staging of endometrial cancer is defined by the International Federation of Gynecology and Obstetrics (FIGO) criteria outlined in Table 1. Surgical staging by exploratory laparotomy requires a peritoneal cytology assessment, intraoperative inspection of the abdominal and pelvic organs (diaphragm, liver, omentum, pelvic and aortic lymph nodes, peritoneal surfaces) for evaluation of metastatic disease, hysterectomy with bilateral salpingo-oophorectomy, and retroperitoneal lymph node sampling.[2]

Surgery

Although endometrial cancer is traditionally managed by laparotomy, increasing evidence supports the safety and efficacy of laparoscopic hysterectomy in appropriately selected patients at low risk for extrauterine tumor spread.

Adjuvant Treatment

The need for adjuvant therapy is based on disease stage and on risk factors for tumor recurrence.

Stage I Disease. For disease confined to the uterus, patients are placed in low-, intermediate-, and high-risk categories, and adjuvant therapies are based on pathologic features. In general, stage I tumors

Table 1 FIGO Staging for Endometrial Carcinoma

Stage	Definition
I	Carcinoma confined to the corpus uteri
II	Carcinoma that involves the corpus and the cervix but has not extended outside the uterus
III	Carcinoma that extends outside the uterus but is confined to the true pelvis and/or retroperitoneal lymph nodes
IV	Carcinoma that involves the bladder or bowel mucosa or that has metastasized to distant sites

FIGO, International Federation of Gynecology and Obstetrics.

Table 2 Endometrial Carcinoma: Stage at Presentation and 5-year Relative Survival Rate

Disease Extent	Stage Distribution (%)	Survival (%)
All stages	—	84
Localized	73	96
Regional	13	66
Distant	9	27
Unstaged	4	53

Adapted from Ries LAG, Kosary CL, Hankey BF, et al (eds): SEER Cancer Statistics Review, 1973-1995. Bethesda, National Cancer Institute, 1998.

that are higher grade and more deeply invasive into the myometrium have a greater risk for recurrence and benefit from adjuvant therapy postoperatively.

Whole-pelvis radiotherapy, with or without vaginal cuff brachytherapy, is the most commonly used adjuvant postoperative treatment modality. Patients with the histologic variant papillary serous carcinoma, an aggressive endometrial lesion with a high risk for extrapelvic recurrence, are generally offered chemotherapy to reduce postoperative recurrence risk, although this treatment is controversial.

Stage II Disease. For disease involving the uterine cervix, there are several treatment options. When unsuspected cervical stromal involvement is found during surgery, postoperative external-beam radiotherapy with vaginal cuff brachytherapy is indicated. If cervical involvement is known preoperatively, various combinations of surgery and radiotherapy have been used:

- Hysterectomy, bilateral salpingo-oophorectomy, and node sampling followed by postoperative irradiation
- Preoperative intracavitary and external-beam radiation therapy followed by hysterectomy and bilateral salpingo-oophorectomy
- Radical hysterectomy and pelvic lymphadenectomy

Unfortunately, there is no standard treatment for stage II endometrial cancer, and the equivalence of these strategies has not been assessed in comparative randomized trials.

Stage III Disease. In general, postoperative whole-pelvis radiotherapy (vaginal cuff brachytherapy) is indicated when disease involves adnexal structures or retroperitoneal nodes. Patients with para-aortic involvement might benefit from extended-field radiotherapy.

Stage IV Disease. The site of metastatic disease and associated symptoms dictate the appropriate treatment of stage IV endometrial cancer. For bulky pelvic disease, radiation therapy consisting of a combination of intracavitary and external beam irradiation is used. When distant metastases are present, systemic therapy is indicated. Satisfactory tumor responses to hormonal treatment with progestational agents can often be achieved in well-differentiated (grades 1 and 2) tumors. Useful chemotherapeutic agents include doxorubicin and paclitaxel.

Outcomes

Endometrial cancer is one of the most curable of the gynecologic cancers because most patients have well-differentiated tumors and present with symptoms early in the disease process (Table 2). Five-year survival rates are much poorer in patients with the less common and poorly differentiated tumor histologies. These patients often present with metastatic disease and account for a disproportionate number of endometrial cancer deaths.

CANCER OF THE OVARY

Definition

Ovarian cancer is a heterogeneous group of malignancies that arises from the various cell types that compose the organ.

Epithelial

Nearly 90% of ovarian malignancies are classified as epithelial ovarian carcinomas. These cancers arise from the germinal epithelium lining the ovary. Epithelial ovarian cancer can be further subdivided into several histologic cell types: serous, mucinous, endometrioid, clear cell, transitional, and undifferentiated carcinomas. The risk of epithelial ovarian cancer increases with age and is found predominantly in postmenopausal women. Epithelial tumors of low malignant potential (borderline ovarian carcinoma) are a histologic variant that is less aggressive than their invasive epithelial counterparts, are found in younger women, and are often confined to the ovary at diagnosis.

Germ Cell

Germ cell tumors account for approximately 5% of all ovarian cancers and recapitulate the developing embryo or placental structures. Histologic subtypes include dysgerminoma (most common), endodermal sinus tumor, immature teratoma, choriocarcinoma, and embryonal carcinoma. Germ cell ovarian cancer can occur in women of any age, but approximately 80% of these are diagnosed in women younger than 30 years.

Sex Cord–Stromal

Sex cord–stromal tumors, which account for approximately 5% of all ovarian cancers, develop in the connective tissue and supporting ovarian stroma. These tumors are generally less aggressive and often produce steroid hormones, including estrogen, progesterone, and testosterone. Some patients with hormone-producing tumors present with signs and symptoms of steroid excess, such as vaginal bleeding or hyperandrogenism.

Prevalence

According to the American Cancer Society, there were more than 23,000 new cases of ovarian cancer and 14,000 deaths from the disease in the United States in 2001. It is estimated that a woman has a 1% to 2% lifetime risk for developing ovarian cancer.

Ovarian carcinoma is the fifth most frequent cause of cancer death in women, and one half of all cases occur in women older than 65 years.

Pathophysiology

The cause of ovarian cancer is poorly understood; however, risk factors and mode of spread have been well described.

Risk Factors

The most significant risk factor for ovarian cancer is a positive family history. When two or more first-degree relatives have or have had ovarian cancer, a woman's lifetime risk for developing this cancer is 7%. If a heritable cancer syndrome is identified, this lifetime risk can increase 17- to 50-fold. Three dominantly inherited mutations are known to be associated with the development of approximately 10% of all ovarian carcinomas: breast-ovarian cancer syndrome, which is associated with mutations in *BRCA-1* and *BRCA-2* genes; site-specific ovarian carcinoma; and hereditary nonpolyposis colorectal cancer (Lynch syndrome II), which is associated with mutations in mismatch repair genes. Advanced age is also associated with increased risk, whereas high parity, oral contraceptive use, tubal ligation, and hysterectomy decrease one's risk.

Mode of Spread

Ovarian cancer usually spreads via cellular shedding into the peritoneal cavity followed by implantation on the peritoneal surface. Local invasion of the bowel and bladder is common in advanced cases. Tumor cells also may block diaphragmatic lymphatics. The resulting impairment of lymphatic drainage of the peritoneum is believed to play a role in development of ascites in ovarian cancer. Transdiaphragmatic spread and seeding of the pleura with pleural effusion are also common in advanced cases.

Signs and Symptoms

Unfortunately, most patients with epithelial ovarian cancer experience few or no symptoms until the disease has widely metastatasized. Manifesting symptoms usually relate to an increasing intra-abdominal tumor burden and ascites and are often vague, mimicking other more common diseases. Symptoms include fatigue; bloating or a feeling of fullness; abdominal swelling or pain; early satiety; vague but persistent gastrointestinal complaints, such as gas, nausea, and indigestion; frequency or urgency of urination; change in bowel habits; unexplained weight loss or gain; shortness of breath; and obstructive symptoms, such as nausea, vomiting, and constipation or obstipation.

On the other hand, borderline, germ cell, and sex cord–stromal tumors are often confined to the ovary at the time of diagnosis. They may be quite large at presentation, and associated symptoms may be related to their large size. These masses are occasionally detected during the screening pelvic examination. More commonly, patients feel the mass themselves or present with symptoms of acute abdomen due to torsion of the adnexa or rupture of the tumor.

Diagnosis

A complete physical examination is the first step in the diagnosis of ovarian cancer. Although pelvic examination is notoriously inefficient at detecting presymptomatic early ovarian cancer, a pelvic mass can often be palpated on examination in symptomatic patients. The finding of a unilateral or bilateral nonmobile (fixed) mass is characteristic of epithelial ovarian carcinoma. Cul-de-sac masses may also be palpated with rectovaginal examination. Impingement of the rectum and compromise of lumen diameter can also be appreciated on this examination. Abdominal distention due to ascites is another common finding. The distended abdomen is dull to percussion and an omental cake may be palpated in the upper abdomen. Further diagnostic workup is necessary to establish extent of disease and exclude other causes of an adnexal mass, carcinomatosis, or ascites.

Imaging Studies

Transvaginal ultrasound uses higher-frequency sound waves to image the ovaries, allowing improved morphologic characterization. The addition of color flow Doppler can further characterize the mass. A vascular mass with low resistive indices supports a diagnosis of malignancy. Chest x-ray might indicate pleural effusion, which is common in patients with ovarian carcinomatosis. CT scans of the abdomen and pelvis with intravenous and oral contrast characterize tumor burden and assist in evaluating other causes of adnexal mass, carcinomatosis, or ascites. Other studies may be performed based on a patient's risk factors and symptoms at presentation. These include sigmoidoscopy, colonoscopy, or barium enema; upper gastrointestinal endoscopy; and intravenous pyelogram.

Serum Tumor Markers

Serum tumor markers can assist in preoperative evaluation; however, their limitations must be understood so they are not misinterpreted or obtained inappropriately. Serum testing is essential to monitoring treatment response for ovarian cancer, but its usefulness as a diagnostic tool is hindered by poor sensitivity and specificity. CA 125 is a high-molecular-weight glycoprotein that is expressed by more than 80% of nonmucinous epithelial ovarian cancers. Although elevated in most women with advanced ovarian cancer, only 50% of patients with early-stage disease have an elevated CA 125, and mucinous epithelial ovarian cancers express this antigen poorly. Furthermore, an elevated CA 125 is not specific for ovarian cancer. Many nongynecologic and benign gynecologic conditions also are associated with elevations in this serum antigen.

If nonepithelial ovarian cancer is suspected, other tumor markers may be useful to assist in diagnosis. Alpha fetoprotein, human chorionic gonadotropin, and lactic dehydrogenase may be expressed by germ cell malignancies. If metastatic colon or pancreatic carcinoma is suspected, serum carcinoembryonic antigen and CA 19-9 might also be elevated. Limitations in the sensitivity and specificity of these tests must be understood so they can be interpreted appropriately for each patient.

Paracentesis

Malignant ascites is common in patients with metastatic epithelial ovarian carcinoma. However, ascites due to other conditions such as congestive heart failure and cirrhosis must be ruled out by careful history and, if necessary, diagnostic testing.

Although paracentesis may be performed for cytologic examination, diagnostic paracentesis is not necessary for most patients if they have already been deemed appropriate for exploratory surgery and operative management. Furthermore, a negative cytology from preoperative paracentesis does not exclude the possibility of malignancy, and differentiating the site of tumor origin is rarely possible on cytologic examination. Large-volume therapeutic paracentesis, however, may be useful for palliation of symptoms of abdominal distention and associated respiratory compromise due to diaphragmatic elevation.

Consultation

If a reasonably high probability for ovarian malignancy exists, consultation with a gynecologic oncologist is essential to ensure appropriate preoperative counseling and preparation, operative management, and postoperative care.

Table 3 FIGO Staging for Ovarian Cancer

Stage	Definition
I	Growth limited to the ovaries
II	Growth involves one or both ovaries with pelvic extension
III	Tumor with peritoneal implants outside the pelvis, or positive retroperitoneal or inguinal nodes, or both
IV	Tumor involves one or both ovaries with distant metastasis

FIGO, International Federation of Gynecology and Obstetrics.

Treatment

Ovarian cancer is initially managed with exploratory laparotomy to confirm the diagnosis and determine the extent of disease (surgical staging) and for tumor cytoreduction.

Histologic Identification

The availability of reliable intraoperative frozen section is essential for optimal surgical decision making and management. For example, fertility-sparing surgery may be an option in select ovarian malignancies, such as germ cell tumors. In addition, although tumor debulking appears to have survival benefit in patients with ovarian malignancies, carcinomatosis related to an extraovarian primary tumor does not necessarily benefit from such measures.

Surgical Staging

Accurate staging determines both treatment and prognosis. Inadequate surgical staging is a common problem in patients with presumed early-stage disease when the operating surgeon does not perform the necessary procedures for adequate staging. Therefore, it is imperative that the operating surgeon is familiar with staging criteria and has the surgical skills necessary to perform all the necessary steps of the staging procedure. FIGO staging criteria are described in Table 3.

Cytoreduction

Metastatic implants of ovarian cancer typically involve the peritoneal surfaces and are often amenable to resection along with the primary tumor mass. Although not documented by any randomized clinical trial, optimal tumor cytoreduction (defined as removal of the primary tumor and all gross metastatic implants to less than 1 cm residual in largest diameter) is believed to improve chemotherapy response and disease-free survival.[3] To achieve these goals, surgical techniques such as en bloc hysterectomy with resection of the rectosigmoid, small bowel, total omentum, spleen, and possibly more may be necessary.

Aggressive resection of tumor does not appear to have any clinical advantage unless all metastatic implants also can be optimally reduced. The operating surgeon must exercise judgment as to whether optimal tumor reduction is possible and can be safely achieved without incurring significant complications that would delay chemotherapy.

Adjuvant Treatment

Most, but not all, ovarian cancer patients require adjuvant chemotherapy after surgery. The importance of adequate surgical staging is evident when making decisions regarding adjuvant therapy in stage I disease. Most chemotherapy can be given on an outpatient basis, although some regimens are given over a period of several days, requiring hospitalization.

For epithelial ovarian cancer, platinum-based therapy-either cisplatin or carboplatin-in combination with paclitaxel has demonstrated the highest activity of all agents studied.[4] These agents are generally given intravenously every 3 weeks for a total of six courses. One study, however, suggests that continuation of single-agent paclitaxel for 12 courses is associated with an improved disease-free survival. Although its impact on overall survival is uncertain, these findings have the potential to significantly affect recommended adjuvant therapy for this disease.

Stage I Disease. Patients with stage Ia or Ib tumors that are well-differentiated (grade 1) have an excellent prognosis, and the addition of adjuvant chemotherapy has not been demonstrated to improve survival in these patients. However, caution must be exercised when considering withholding adjuvant therapy in patients with presumed stage I disease who have not had the benefit of adequate surgical staging. Reoperation for staging purposes is an option in these patients. Patients with grades 2 and 3 tumors are at increased risk for recurrence and appear to benefit from adjuvant chemotherapy.

Stages II to IV Disease. The use of adjuvant chemotherapy has survival and palliative benefits in patients with metastatic ovarian carcinoma and a larger tumor burden. Adjuvant therapy for tumors of borderline histology is generally not indicated. Little evidence exists that postoperative chemotherapy or radiation therapy alters the course of these tumors in any beneficial way.

All patients with germ cell tumors, except those with stage I, grade 1 immature teratoma and stage IA dysgerminoma, require postoperative chemotherapy.[5] With platinum-based combination chemotherapy, the prognosis for patients with endodermal sinus tumors, immature teratomas, embryonal carcinomas, choriocarcinomas, and mixed tumors containing one or more of these elements has improved dramatically.

Most patients with advanced ovarian cancer ultimately develop progressive or recurrent disease after initial surgery and adjuvant chemotherapy and require some form of palliative therapy. Patients with recurrent ovarian carcinoma are considered either platinum sensitive or platinum resistant, depending on whether the response duration was less than or longer than 6 months from prior therapy with a platinum-based agent. Potentially platinum-sensitive patients often benefit from re-treatment with a platinum-based agent. Owing to its favorable toxicity profile, carboplatin is ideally suited for palliative therapy in the appropriate patient.

Platinum-resistant patients, on the other hand, generally have more limited responses to alternative chemotherapeutic agents. A number of second-line chemotherapeutic agents might have palliative benefit, including paclitaxel, liposomal doxorubicin, topotecan, and gemcitabine. Because of poorer response rates in most patients with platinum-resistant disease, participation in clinical trials evaluating new therapies is also appropriate.

When disease-related symptoms can be palliated, such as the reversal of intestinal obstruction, surgical intervention might improve the quality of life. However, palliation is rarely achieved in advanced disease when there are multiple areas of partial or complete obstruction or when the transit time is prolonged due to diffuse peritoneal carcinomatosis.

Outcomes

Survival in ovarian cancer is related to surgical stage and tumor histology (Table 4). Patients with borderline tumors, germ cell malignancies, and sex cord–stromal tumors often present with earlier-stage disease and generally have improved prognoses.

Table 4 Ovarian Carcinoma: Stage at Presentation and 5-Year Relative Survival Rate

Disease Extent	Stage Distribution (%)	Survival (%)
All stages	—	50
Localized	25	95
Regional	9	79
Distant	61	28
Unstaged	6	29

Adapted from Ries LAG, Kosary CL, Hankey BF, et al (eds): SEER Cancer Statistics Review, 1973-1995. Bethesda: National Cancer Institute, 1998.

Table 5 FIGO Staging for Cervical Cancer

Stage	Definition
0	Preinvasive disease (carcinoma in situ)
I	Carcinoma strictly confined to the cervix
II	Carcinoma that extends into the parametrium (but not onto the pelvic sidewall) or the upper two thirds of the vagina
III	Carcinoma that has extended onto the pelvic sidewall or involves the lower one third of the vagina. All cases with a hydronephrosis or nonfunctioning kidney should be included, unless they are known to be due to other causes.
IV	Carcinoma that has extended beyond the true pelvis to distant organs or has clinically involved the mucosa of the bladder, rectum, or both

FIGO, International Federation of Gynecology and Obstetrics.

CANCER OF THE CERVIX

Definition

Cervical carcinoma has its origins at the squamocolumnar junction or the cervix. The precursor lesion is dysplasia or carcinoma in situ (cervical intraepithelial neoplasia III). Squamous cell carcinoma accounts for 90% and adenocarcinoma accounts for 10% of cervical cancers.

Prevalence

Last year, cervical cancer was diagnosed in approximately 14,000 women in the United States, and there were 4,700 deaths from the disease. Peak incidence of cervical carcinoma is at 51 years of age, whereas that for carcinoma in situ is approximately 10 years younger.

Pathophysiology

Epidemiologic studies convincingly demonstrate that the major risk factor for preinvasive or invasive cervical carcinoma is infection with the human papillomavirus (HPV). HPV DNA is detected in virtually all cervical cancers, with HPV subtypes 16, 18, and 31 identified most commonly. Other known risk factors include early age at first intercourse, number of sexual partners, and a positive smoking history.

Cervical carcinoma spreads predominantly by local invasion and lymphatic metastasis. The most common metastatic sites include the vagina, parametrium, and pelvic lymph nodes.

Signs and Symptoms

Precancerous changes of the cervix rarely cause symptoms and are generally detected by pelvic examination and Pap smear screening. Symptoms usually do not appear until lesions become cancerous and invade underlying cervical stroma. Postcoital vaginal spotting may be one of the first symptoms of the disease. Ultimately, an enlarging and vascular tumor mass can become ulcerated, leading to frank vaginal bleeding, heavy vaginal discharge, or both. As the tumor invades locally or spreads into the regional lymphatics, patients develop pain, lower extremity edema, and lower extremity deep venous thrombosis.

Diagnosis

Cervical cancer may be detected in its early stages by the screening Pap smear or by identification of larger lesions in the symptomatic patient. The Pap smear is a screening test only. Patients whose Pap smears indicate cytologic abnormalities suggestive of high-grade lesions are at risk for invasive cancer and warrant further diagnostic testing with colposcopy. Ablative procedures should not be performed without a thorough colposcopic examination.

Colposcopy is a technique of visually evaluating the cervix for abnormalities. The colposcope is a magnifying device that aids the examination of the cervix. Light filters and staining solutions are used in combination to identify cervical dysplasia. If an abnormality is identified, a biopsy may be recommended. Treatment is usually based on the results of the biopsy. Referral to an expert familiar with the colposcopy technique and the treatment of cervical dysplasia is recommended.

When a colposcopic abnormality or a grossly visible cervical lesion is identified, a biopsy is necessary for histologic evaluation. Pap smear cytology is not adequate for diagnosis. Cervical biopsy may be accomplished in an office setting using any number of instruments, such as the Tischler-Morgan, Kevorkian, and mini-Townsend biopsy instruments or even a loop electrode.

With documented invasive cervical carcinoma, further diagnostic workup is necessary to establish the extent of disease. Cervical cancer staging is defined clinically by FIGO criteria using physical examination and a limited number of diagnostic studies (Table 5).

A pelvic examination is necessary to assess tumor size and configuration and to identify possible vaginal metastasis and parametrial or pelvic sidewall involvement. Additionally, lymphatic metastasis is common in advanced cervical cancer. Assessment of groin and supraclavicular lymph nodes might reveal enlargement. Lower extremity edema might also be present with an expanded tumor diameter, significant pelvic lymphadenopathy, or both. Homans' sign or a palpable cord may be identified if there is an associated deep venous thrombosis.

Chest x-ray can identify pulmonary metastasis. Computed tomography of the abdomen and pelvis (with oral, rectal, and intravenous contrast) allows for more complete assessment of tumor extent within the abdomen and pelvis. Although not part of FIGO clinical stage criteria, it is useful for treatment planning. An intravenous pyelogram may be obtained if ureteral obstruction or bladder involvement is suspected. Cystoscopy or sigmoidoscopy may be obtained if bladder involvement, rectal involvement, or both are suspected.

Treatment

Treatment and prognosis of cervical cancer are greatly affected by the extent of disease at the time of diagnosis.

Stage 0 Disease (Carcinoma in Situ)

Invasive cervical carcinoma must be excluded with confidence before therapy for preinvasive disease is undertaken. Standard treatment options include excisional and ablative therapy. In general, excisional therapies are preferred because they are associated with a lower failure rate and provide tissue for histologic evaluation to assess margins and exclude invasion. Excisional therapies include the loop electrosurgical excision procedure (LEEP), laser conization, cold knife conization, and extrafascial hysterectomy. Ablative therapies include cryotherapy and laser ablation therapy.

In most cases, outpatient LEEP is preferred.[6] LEEP uses a fine wire loop with electrical energy flowing through it to remove the transformation zone of the cervix or focal areas of dysplasia. It can quickly and easily be performed in an office setting and generally requires only local anesthesia, thus avoiding the risks associated with general anesthesia. Cold knife or laser conization require general anesthesia.

Stage Ia1 (Microinvasive Cervical Cancer)

Cervical cancer in its earliest stages of invasion is termed microinvasive carcinoma. It is defined as invasion of the stroma no greater than 3 mm deep and no wider than 7 mm in diameter with no lymph-vascular space involvement.

Disease meeting this strictly defined criteria has a very limited risk for lymphatic metastasis, and outcome is excellent with less-radical therapies. Expert pathology review is essential when considering less radical therapies for disease qualifying as microinvasive. Equivalent treatment options include extrafascial hysterectomy, cervical conization, and intracavitary radiation alone (without external beam radiotherapy).

All Other Stage I and Stage IIa Disease

Risk for lymphatic metastasis is increased with larger and more deeply invasive lesions. For this reason, radical therapies are necessary, and referral to a qualified gynecologic oncologist is appropriate and recommended.

Therapy selection depends on patient factors, tumor factors, and surgical expertise. Radical hysterectomy with bilateral pelvic lymphadenectomy is one option; combined external beam radiotherapy and brachytherapy with concurrent chemotherapy is an equivalent option.

Several randomized phase III trials have shown an overall survival advantage for cisplatin-based therapy given concurrently with radiation therapy. As a result of these findings, the National Cancer Institute issued a clinical announcement suggesting that "strong consideration should be given to the incorporation of concurrent cisplatin-based chemotherapy with radiation therapy in women who require radiation therapy for treatment of cervical cancer."[7]

Stages IIb to IVa Disease

With tumor spread beyond the cervix and upper vagina, cure rates for radical surgery decline. Stages IIb to IVa cervical cancer are best treated by radiation therapy using combined external beam pelvic radiation and concurrent cisplatin-based chemotherapy with intracavitary brachytherapy or interstitial therapy.

Stage IVb Disease

Patients with distant metastasis are no longer amenable to cure by radiation therapy. Unfortunately, response rates to standard chemotherapy are generally less than 20% and are typically brief. All patients with distant metastasis or recurrent disease should be considered appropriate candidates for phases I and II clinical trials investigating new treatments.

Palliative treatment options include radiation therapy to relieve pelvic disease and chemotherapy with agents such as cisplatin, ifosfamide, paclitaxel, gemcitabine, and irinotecan.[8]

Table 6 Cervical Carcinoma: 5-Year Relative Survival Rate

Disease Extent	Survival (%)
All stages	84
Localized	96
Regional	66
Distant	27

Adapted from Ries LAG, Kosary CL, Hankey BF, et al (eds): SEER Cancer Statistics Review, 1973-1995. Bethesda, National Cancer Institute, 1998.

Outcomes

If not diagnosed in its early stages, cervical cancer carries high mortality (Table 6). Properly diagnosed and managed, tumor control of in situ cervical carcinoma should be nearly 100%.

Summary

- Endometrial cancer is one of the most curable of the gynecologic cancers because most patients have well-differentiated tumors and present with symptoms early in the disease process.
- A woman's lifetime risk for developing ovarian cancer is 7% when two or more first-degree relatives have this cancer. This lifetime risk can increase 17- to 50-fold if a heritable cancer syndrome is identified.
- Unfortunately, most patients with epithelial ovarian cancer experience few or no symptoms until the occurrence of widespread metastatic disease.
- Serum tumor markers can assist in the preoperative evaluation of ovarian cancer; however, their limitations must be understood so they are not misinterpreted or obtained inappropriately.
- Epidemiologic studies convincingly demonstrate that the major risk factor for preinvasive or invasive cervical carcinoma is infection with the human papillomavirus (HPV).

Suggested Readings

Creasman WT, Morrow CP, Bundy BN, et al: Surgical pathologic spread patterns of endometrial cancer. A Gynecologic Oncology Group Study. Cancer 1987;60(Suppl 8):2035-2041.

Ferenczy A, Choukroun D, Arseneau J: Loop electrosurgical excision procedure for squamous intraepithelial lesions of the cervix: Advantages and potential pitfalls. Obstet Gynecol 1996;87:332-337.

Gershenson DM, Morris M, Cangir A, et al: Treatment of malignant germ cell tumors of the ovary with bleomycin, etoposide, and cisplatin. J Clin Oncol 1990;8:715-720.

Hoskins WJ, Bundy BN, Thigpen JT, Omura GA: The influence of cytoreductive surgery on recurrence-free interval and survival in small-volume stage III epithelial ovarian cancer: A Gynecologic Oncology Group study. Gynecol Oncol 1992;47:159-166.

McGuire WP, Hoskins WJ, Brady MF, et al: Cyclophosphamide and cisplatin compared with paclitaxel and cisplatin in patients with stage III and stage IV ovarian cancer. N Engl J Med 1996;334:1-6.

National Cancer Institute: Long-term data support cisplatin-based chemoradiation for cervical cancer. Available at http://www.cancer.gov/clinicaltrials/results/cisplatin-cervical0507 (accessed March 20, 2009).

Omura GA: Chemotherapy for cervix cancer. Semin Oncol 1994;21:54-62.

Ries LAG, Kosary CL, Hankey BF, et al (eds): SEER Cancer Statistics Review, 1973-1995. Bethesda: National Cancer Institute, 1998.

References

For a complete list of references, log onto www.expertconsult.com.

Hormone Therapy and the Risk of Venous Thromboembolism

Holly L. Thacker

Exogenous hormone therapy (HT) is used by millions of women yearly as hormone contraception (HC) or postmenopausal hormone therapy (PHT). Because these drugs are usually prescribed to healthy women, the issue of the risks of therapy has received considerable attention. This chapter reviews the risks of venous thromboembolism (VTE) associated with HT, including hormonal contraceptive preparations, postmenopausal HT, and selected estrogen receptor modulator (SERM) therapy. The chapter on venous thromboembolism covers pathophysiology, diagnosis, treatment, and outcomes.

Retrospective and prospective studies have shown a twofold to fourfold increase in the relative risk of VTE with the use of either HC, PHT, or SERM treatments. Prospective randomized controlled trials have shown an increase in VTE with the use of PHT and the SERM raloxifene.[1] Yet clinical thrombotic events are rare in the general population, and overall they are more of a rare side effect than the main effect of exogenous hormone use and should not in general be a contraindication to initiating therapy in healthy women who have indications for therapy.

Whether to prescribe HT depends on the net benefit for the woman after any additive risk factors are taken into account. Risk factors include differences in the thrombotic potential of various preparations, specifically oral versus transdermal, as well as a family and especially personal history of VTE. The presence of additive factors such as immobility, obesity, surgery, anesthesia, and varicose veins increase the risk of VTE.

HORMONE CONTRACEPTION

The introduction of the hormonal contraceptive pill in 1959 was a major medical achievement that changed the way women could control reproduction and thereby achieve a greater life expectancy and better health status. HC remains the most popular form of reversible contraception worldwide.

Definition

The term *hormonal contraception* for many physicians is synonymous with the oral contraceptive pill (OCP). Millions of women rely on OCPs as their contraceptive method of choice. The U.S. Food and Drug Administration (FDA) has reported that no other medication in the history of medical science has been studied more extensively than the OCP. Newer forms of HC include one transdermal patch,[2] one vaginal ring (Nuvaring), and one long-acting progestin-only 3-year implant. The risks of VTE may be greater with transdermal HC and less with transdermal PHT. The risk is affected not only by estrogenic dosage but also by the type of progestin combined with estrogen.

Most HCs are a combination of estrogen in the form of ethinyl estradiol and an androgen-derived progestin. In an effort to improve options and adherence to contraception, HC has expanded to include a weekly dermal patch (Ortho Evra), a hormonal vaginal contraceptive ring (NuvaRing), and less-androgenic progestins such as desogestrel and drospirenone. Also available are progestin-only HC agents: the progestin-only minipill including norethindrone acetate (Micronor), injectable medroxyprogesterone (Depo-Provera), a subdermal implantable norelgestromin device (Implanon), and a levonorgestrel-releasing intrauterine system (Mirena). Relatively few thrombotic occurrences have been reported for progestin-only HC, and progestin-only therapy is generally presumed to have less risk than estrogen-progestin HC, just as estrogen-alone PHT has been shown to have less VTE risk than estrogen-progestin PHT.

Hormone Contraception and Venous Thromboembolism

The first case of thrombosis associated with HC occurred in 1961 when a nurse taking a high-dose estrogen OCP developed a pulmonary embolism. Myocardial infarction and stroke were reported in OCP users during the following years and were associated with older women who smoke and use HC. These early reports seemed to suggest that the thrombotic potential of the OCP was related to its relatively high estrogen content of 50 μg or more.

By the 1970s, the low-dose OCP, containing 35 μg ethinyl estradiol, was introduced. In the 1990s, less-androgenic progestins (desogestrel, gestodene, and norgestimate) were developed, containing even lower formulations of ethinyl estradiol (20-25 μg ethinyl estradiol). The newer progestins have fewer androgenic effects than the traditional progestins (norethindrone acetate and levonorgestrel). Yet some of these newer progestins, such as desogestrel, have been found, in a number of European epidemiologic studies, to be associated with an increase in VTE compared with the older contraceptive preparations despite the lower overall estrogen content.[3]

Clinical trials designed to compare thrombogenic risks of HC have been observational and comparable. HC and the risk of VTE have mainly been investigated in case-control studies followed by a series of cohort analytic studies. The first case-control study, in 1967 by the Royal College of General Practitioners, reported that users of oral contraceptives had a threefold increased risk of venous thrombosis compared with nonusers. Most of these studies indicated that the risk was immediate, in the early phases of use, and did not further increase with a longer duration of use.

More recent studies have found a twofold to sixfold increased risk for venous thrombosis for OCP users. In the landmark Leiden Thrombophilia Study, the absolute risk for VTE was estimated at 0.8 per 10,000 per year among nonusers and 3.0 per 10,000 per year among HC users. Overall, these numbers seem to indicate a low absolute risk, translating into thousands of women needing to abstain from HC use to prevent one case of thrombosis a year.

Although HC may be associated with a significant portion of VTE events in young women, it does not account for all VTE events. Many other risk factors need to be considered in deciding whether some women have a higher risk of thrombosis when using HC, including obesity, age, a personal or family history of a VTE event, or the presence of a familial hypercoagulable state (including factor V Leiden, prothrombin 20210A, or deficiencies of protein C, protein S, or antithrombin). With the familial thrombophilic states, including protein C, protein S, and antithrombin deficiencies, the risk of first thrombosis is significantly increased. In addition, reports of mild hyperhomocysteinemia (homocysteine >18.5 μmol/L) is a common risk factor for VTE. Most importantly, a past history of a VTE event is the strongest indicator for recurrence in the future. Furthermore, pregnancy itself increases the risk of VTE.

Pathophysiology

The factors and mechanism by which female hormones lead to a prothrombotic state are complex and not fully understood. Procoagulant factors include modest increases in the levels of factor VII, factor VIII, factor X, prothrombin, and fibrinogen, with associated decreases in the anticoagulant proteins including antithrombin and protein S. Using a thrombin-generation assay, it has been noted that women taking HC actually develop activated protein C resistance, which might provide an explanation for the increased thrombotic risk associated with HC users who are carriers of factor V Leiden mutation. It appears that the newer progestins, such as desogestrel, might further activate protein C resistence.

Factor V Leiden Mutation

Of all the inherited thrombophilias, the factor V Leiden mutation is believed to be the most common cause of congenital hypercoagulability states today and may be responsible for about one half of all cases of familial venous thrombosis. Approximately 5% of all white women carry the factor V Leiden mutation. Women who are heterozygous and especially homozygous for the factor V Leiden mutation have a greater thrombotic risk when using any HC preparation. In women who carry the factor V Leiden mutation, the frequency of puerperal death from pulmonary embolism ranges from 1 in 2000 women to 1 in 15,000 women. One of the great benefits of HC is the prevention of pregnancy and pregnancy-associated morbidity and mortality.

Carriers of the factor V Leiden mutation had an eightfold increased risk of VTE in the landmark Leiden Thrombophilia Study. The study also suggested that the incidence of VTE was multiplied in a heterozygotic carrier of factor V Leiden who was also an HC user compared with a woman not carrying the mutation and not using HC. Higher risks have been reported for patients homozygous for the factor V Leiden mutation, with a marked increase in homozygous carriers using HC compared with noncarriers who were not users. Other investigations have confirmed the increased relative risk of VTE for users of HC who are also factor V Leiden carriers. The VTE risk for women with the factor V Leiden mutation is estimated to be increased twofold to fourfold. The adjusted risk estimate for a heterozygotic factor V Leiden carrier using HC is increased to 10-fold to 15-fold. However, the factor V Leiden mutation is not a reason for withholding HC from carriers of the mutation who have not themselves experienced a VTE.[4]

Benefits of Hormone Contraception

HCs have benefits beyond contraception. Limiting HC therapy can actually lead to an increase in the rate of unintended pregnancies, which themselves increase the rate of VTE compared with the nonpregnant state. HCs have an excellent risk-to-benefit balance compared with other contraceptive methods currently available. They are one of the most effective reversible means of preventing pregnancy. Discouraging the use of such an effective means of contraception could result in unwanted and unplanned pregnancies, leading to a greater risk of VTE or possibly contributing to the development of preeclampsia, abruptio placentae, fetal growth retardation, stillbirth, and miscarriage.

HC also has noncontraceptive benefits, including decreased dysfunctional uterine bleeding, reduction of dysmenorrhea, and treatment of endometriosis, acne, premenstrual dysphoric disorder, and functional ovarian cysts. HC also provides significant protection from ovarian and endometrial cancers. Carriers of the *BRCA1* and *BRCA2* mutations who use HC have a reduced incidence of ovarian cancer. The incidence and mortality associated with ovarian cancer (lifetime risk, 1 in 57) are greater than the attributable risk of developing VTE disease in a woman with factor V Leiden mutation and using HC (risk, 1 in 9259 women). Denying these carriers HC might actually be harmful.

POSTMENOPAUSAL HORMONE THERAPY

Definition

The primary role for PHT is relief of postmenopausal symptoms including vasomotor instability, genitourinary atrophy, quality-of-life issues, and bone protection. The chapter on menopause covers this in detail.[5] Although the thrombogenicity of HC has been recognized since the 1960s, convincing evidence for the thrombogenic potential of PHT has emerged only since the 1990s and after the initial recruitment for the Women's Health Initiative (WHI).

Most PHT preparations contain an estrogen and a progestin to avoid endometrial hyperplasia or stimulation. In women who have a uterus, progestin therapy is included with estrogen; estrogen-only therapy is used in women without a uterus. Common combined, continuous hormone preparations in North America include conjugated estrogens plus medroxyprogesterone (which were used in the WHI). Micronized estradiol is also available in a transdermal patch, a gel, vaginal tablets, transdermal lotion, and vaginal rings.

POSTMENOPAUSAL HORMONE THERAPY AND VENOUS THROMBOEMBOLISM

Some of the most recent evidence regarding the risk of VTE and PHT came from the terminated estrogen-progestin arm and estrogen-only arm of the WHI. Although the development of VTE was not one of the primary outcomes of this trial, multivariate analysis showed it to be the most significant risk. The use of PHT increased the risk of VTE twofold, which means PHT users have 34 VTE events annually per 10,000 women versus 16 VTE events per 10,000 women who are not PHT users. The risk of VTE with PHT persisted throughout the 5-year study and was notably less in the estrogen-only arm (women with hysterectomy not needing a progestin).[6]

The ESTHER (EStrogen and THromboEmbolism Risk) study group, a French case-controlled study, reported that oral but *not* trandermal PHT estrogen was associated with increased risk of VTE in postmenopausal women.[7] Their data suggest but do not confirm that transdermal estrogen may be safer than oral estrogen with respect to VTE risk. The original publication from the WHI indicated an increased risk for cardiovascular disease in PHT users. However, after central adjudication, these data did not show any significant increased risk for cardiovascular disease in PHT users.[8]

The estrogen formulations used in the postmenopausal state are used at a much lower dose than those used in HC and appear to have significantly lower biologic potency than HC. Although transdermal PHT is reported to be safer with respect to VTE, transdermal HC is reported to increase the risk of VTE at 4 to 8 per 10,000 women compared with 2 to 5 per 10,000 women using oral HC. This increase may be related to the higher total estrogen exposure. The SERM raloxifene (Evista), which is approved to prevent and treat postmenopausal osteoporosis, has been reported to increase the risk VTE twofold.

Early studies of PHT showed a slight increase in the risk of venous thrombosis, but subsequent studies did not repeat those findings. Only since the 1990s has a series of studies demonstrated that PHT users have a twofold to fourfold increased risk of venous thrombosis, and that PHT, regardless of duration of use, increases thrombosis risk. As with HC, studies have shown that the risk of VTE is highest during the first year of use.

Pathophysiology

The hemostatic effects of estrogens in oral PHT are similar to those in HC. All estrogens (oral or transdermal) seem to increase the levels of procoagulant factors VII, X, XII, and XIII and to decrease anticoagulant factors such as protein S and antithrombin, leading to a more procoagulant state not balanced by fibrinolytic activity.

Factor V Leiden Mutation

The factor V Leiden mutation and prothrombin 20210A mutation are the two most common prothrombotic mutations. Women who are taking PHT and who have the factor V Leiden mutation have a 15-fold increase in the risk of VTE compared with women who do not have the mutation and do not use PHT, suggesting that with PHT, as with HC and factor V Leiden, the risk is more than additive. The Heart and Estrogen/Progestin Replacement Study and the Estrogen Replacement and Atherosclerosis trial, two randomized controlled trials that looked at PHT and secondary cardiovascular outcomes, found a 1.7% and 2.6% respective increase in VTE in women using PHT. Further investigation, through genotyping of blood samples, found that 16.7% of women with VTE carried the factor V Leiden mutation, versus 6.3% of controls.

SELECTIVE ESTROGEN RECEPTOR MODULATORS

Tamoxifen, raloxifene, and other SERMs have apparent antiestrogenic effects on the breast and varying effects on the endometrial tissue. Tamoxifen is used for breast cancer treatment and prevention, and raloxifene is used to prevent and treat osteoporosis. But there is an estrogenic effect on blood clotting by these agents, and in general they confer the same risks of VTE as does PHT. In a controlled trial of tamoxifen versus placebo, an increase was observed in the relative risk of deep venous thrombosis (relative risk, 1.6) in women with breast cancer. The MORE (Multiple Outcomes for Raloxifene Evaluation) trial has not reported any increased risk of arterial thrombotic events or early cardiovascular harm, but it has a reported a twofold or greater risk of VTE in the raloxifene-treated group.

PRACTICAL RECOMMENDATIONS

Any woman with a personal or family history of VTE who is contemplating starting HC, PHT, or a SERM should be screened for a hereditary thrombophilia; however, screening of the general population without a personal or family history of VTE before starting hormone therapy is not recommended. The most challenging subset of women are those with known thrombophilia who have pressing indications for HC, PHT, or SERM therapy. Aromatase inhibitors (anastrozole, exemestane, letrozole) are favored in women with breast cancer who have a history of VTE because there has been no reported increased risk of VTE with these agents. There are other options for osteoporosis treatment, including bisphosphonates (risedronate, alendronate, and ibrandronate). These women are also candidates for nonhormonal contraception, such as barrier contraception or the copper T380A IUD, as well as the progestin-only HC.

Summary

- Any hormonal therapy, including hormonal contraception, postmenopausal hormone therapy, and selective estrogen receptor modulators, increases the risk for venous thromboembolism.
- Factor V Leiden mutation, the most common cause of congenital hypercoagulability, increases the risk of venous thromboembolism. Factor V Leiden mutation with any hormone therapy increases the risk of VTE in a multiplicative fashion. However, most women with factor V Leiden who use hormone therapy do not suffer from venous thromboembolism.
- Careful and individual risk-to-benefit analysis is needed in any woman needing hormone therapy.

Suggested Readings

Barrett-Connor E, Mosca L, Collins P, et al: Effects of raloxifene on cardiovascular events and breast cancer in postmenopausal women. N Engl J Med 2006;33:125-137.

Canonico M, Oger E, Plu-Bureau G, et al: Hormone therapy and venous thromboembolism among postmenopausal women: Impact of the route of estrogen administraion and progestagens: The ESTHER Study. Circulation 2007;115:840-845.

Cole JA, Norman H, Doherty M, et al: Venous thromboembolism, myocardial infarction, and stroke among transdermal contraceptive system users. Obstet Gynecol 2007;109:339-346.

Curb JD, Prentice RL, Bray PF, et al: Venous thrombosis and conjugated equine estrogen in women without a uterus. Arch Intern Med 2006;166(7):772-780.

Jick H, Kaye JA, Vasilakis-Scaramozza C, et al: Risk of venous thromboembolism among users of third generation oral contraceptives compared with users of oral contraceptives with levonorgestrel before and after 1995: Cohort and case-control analysis. BMJ 2000;321:1190-1195.

Manson JE, Hsia J, Johnson KC, et al: Estrogen plus progestin and the risk of coronary heart disease. N Engl J Med 2003:349:523-534.

North American Menopause Society: Estrogen and progestogen use in peri- and postmenopausal women: March 2007 position statement of The North American Menopause Society. Menopause 2007:14(2);168-182.

Vandenbroucke JP, Koster T, Briet E, et al: Increased risk of venous thrombosis in oral-contraceptive users who are carriers of factor V Leiden mutation. Lancet 1994;344:1453-1457.

References

For a complete list of references, log onto www.expertconsult.com.

Infertility

Tommaso Falcone

DEFINITION

Infertility, the inability to conceive after a year of trying, has resulted in an increasing number of physician visits since the 1980s.

PREVALENCE

The Centers for Disease Control and Prevention (CDC) reported that in 1995, 15% of women (>9 million) between the ages of 15 and 44 years received an infertility service.[1] Two thirds of these patients consulted for advice or investigation. Only one third of the patients consulted a physician for infertility treatment such as ovulation induction, surgery, or assisted reproductive technology (ART). Therefore, the primary care physician has a significant role to play in providing infertility services to women. Furthermore, many causes of infertility are associated with significant medical problems that a primary care physician should manage.

PATHOPHYSIOLOGY

Lifestyle

The trend of delayed marriage and childbirth is the main social cause of infertility. Twenty percent of women have their first child after the age of 35 years.

Smoking, alcohol, and stress are clearly associated with diminished fertility. Smoking accelerates the natural loss of oocytes and is associated with decreased pregnancy rates from all ART. Passive smoking has also been demonstrated to have an effect on fertility.

It is not clear if a low weekly alcohol intake in women (<5 drinks per week) is associated with decreased fertility. This intake level is generally indicated to encourage women who are trying to conceive to avoid or limit alcohol intake. Heavy alcohol intake is associated with reproductive abnormalities in men (such as testicular atrophy), but minimal to moderate alcohol intake does not seem to have an effect.

Stress is an independent risk factor that is associated with poorer results from ART.[2] This effect is seen even if there is no disruption of the menstrual cycle.

Heavy use of marijuana decreases fertility in men and women. The effect is clear and reproducible in women, whereas it is equivocal in men. Box 1 shows a partial list of other potential toxins associated with decreased fertility. Some studies have linked high caffeine intake with delayed conception.[3] Saliva and most lubricants sold in pharmacies are spermicidal.

Fertility and Age

Increasing age is an independent risk factor for decreased fertility. Reproductive aging is attributed mostly to the ovaries.[4] Recipients of donated oocytes have pregnancy and live birth rates close to those of the age group of the donor. After age 30 years, there is a substantial decline in fertility and an increase in spontaneous pregnancy loss.

Follicular loss is a progressive process that depletes the germ cell pool by menopause. This loss is independent of hormonal therapy, such as birth control pills, and accelerates in the last decade before menopause. Observational studies of U.S. populations that have high birth rates and that condemn the use of contraception demonstrate decreasing fertility with age. By the age of 35 years, a woman has one half the chance of becoming pregnant that a 25-year-old woman has. The age of the male partner does not affect the ability of the sperm to fertilize an oocyte.

The most common causes of infertility are listed in Box 2.

Tubal Disease and Pelvic Adhesions

Tubal disease is still the most common cause of infertility in United States. The most common cause of tubal disease is previous pelvic inflammatory disease (PID). Most cases of PID in the United States are caused by sexually transmitted disease. Westrom demonstrated that subsequent tubal infertility developed in 12% of women after one episode of PID, in 23% of women after two episodes of PID, and in 54% of women after three episodes of PID.[5]

Endometriosis

Endometriosis is another common cause of pelvic disease that is associated with significant pelvic pain and infertility. It is characterized by the presence of endometrial glands and stroma outside of the uterus. The disease process is associated with reflux of menstrual debris into the peritoneal cavity. However, because this reflux occurs in the majority of women, there must be an associated immunologic or genetic abnormality that allows the disease to develop. A variety of cellular and humoral abnormalities have been reported in these patients. The peritoneal cavity has an increased number of activated macrophages. These macrophages secrete a variety of cytokines that might be associated with the observed peritoneal inflammatory reaction. The peritoneal cavity might have a wide spectrum of lesions ranging from a few peritoneal implants to severe adhesive disease that involves all pelvic organs.

Anovulation

The most common cause of anovulation in North America is polycystic ovary syndrome (PCOS). PCOS is a metabolic disorder with a primary reproductive manifestation. The term PCOS is a misnomer because there are no cysts in the classic gynecologic sense. Many subcapsular follicles of less than 10 mm with increased thecal and stromal tissue characterize the morphology of the PCOS ovary.[6]

Most women with PCOS have insulin resistance that is independent of weight.[7] Fasting and postprandial hyperglycemia are uncommon at this stage of the disease process when patients present with infertility. However, these patients are at greater risk for developing type 2 diabetes. There usually is a strong family history of diabetes or abnormal glucose tolerance. PCOS patients who achieve pregnancy often have gestational diabetes. Obesity is an independent disorder with associated endocrine changes that influence the phenotypic expression of PCOS patients.

Hyperprolactinemia is another common cause of anovulation. The elevated serum prolactin is due to a primary pituitary abnormality such as hyperplasia or an adenoma of the prolactin-secreting cells. Uncommonly, serum prolactin levels are elevated secondary to hypothyroidism. These patients usually have a disruption of the menstrual cycle. The most common nonmenstrual symptoms are headaches and galactorrhea.

Other causes of anovulation are listed in Box 3.

Box 1 Reproductive Toxins

Dry Cleaning
Perchloroethylene

Medical and Dental Offices
Anesthesia
Ethylene oxide
Nitrous oxide

Painting
Ethylene glycol

Printing, Painting, and Hairstyling
Solvents (e.g., toluene)

Box 2 Common Causes of Infertility

Disorders of ovulation
Idiopathic infertility
Male factor infertility
Pelvic pathology (tubal disease and endometriosis)

Box 3 Common Causes of Anovulation

Competitive exercise
Eating disorders
Hypo- or hyperthyroidism
Menopause
Polycystic ovary syndrome
Primary pituitary hyperprolactinemia
Stress and anxiety

Male Factor Infertility

A significant part of infertility is due to the male factor. Environmental toxins, drugs such as cimetidine, and heavy tobacco, marijuana, and alcohol use can be associated with decreased sperm parameters and reduced fertility. Chemotherapy and radiotherapy for the treatment of malignancies are associated with severely depressed sperm counts that are sometimes irreversible. Counseling these patients to cryopreserve sperm before initiating treatment is important. Excellent success rates have been reported with the use of this sperm.

Increased scrotal temperature as a result of a febrile illness can cause a temporary alteration of semen parameters that is only identified 2 to 3 months after the episode.[8] This is the time required for a germ cell to develop into a mature spermatozoon. Radiant heat, such as that experienced by welders or foundry workers, can also affect semen quality. However, conditions that result in a minor increase in scrotal temperature only, such as tight underwear, have not been shown to alter sperm function.

A varicocele, a dilation of the veins that ascend from the testes, is associated with abnormal semen parameters.

Several genetic abnormalities are associated with male factor infertility. Congenital bilateral absence of the vasa deferentia (CBAVD) is associated with mutations of the cystic fibrosis transmembrane regulator gene. Chromosomal abnormalities have been detected in about 10% to 15% of azoospermic men and about 5% of oligospermic men. Sex chromosome aneuploidies such as Klinefelter's syndrome are the most commonly reported.

Microdeletions of the long arm of the Y chromosome are also associated with severe oligospermia or azoospermia. The AZF (azoospermia factor) locus has three regions: AZFa, AZFb, AZFc. A deletion in any one of these regions can lead to complete absence of sperm. If sperm are found and pregnancy is achieved through ART, these deletions may be passed on to the male offspring. There is a high prevalence of altered integrity of the genetic material in the sperm in the infertile males. This is reflected by the degree of high levels of DNA fragmentation, which is associated with male infertility.

Box 4 Key Questions on the History

General
Age
Duration of infertility
Previous pregnancies with the current partner

Ovulatory Disorders
Alcohol or cigarette consumption
Menstrual cycle abnormalities
Weight problems (overweight or underweight)

Tubal Disease
History of sexually transmitted disease, pelvic inflammatory disease
Previous pelvic or tubal surgery

Endometriosis
Dysmenorrhea
Dyspareunia
Pelvic pain

Male Disorders
Family history of male infertility
Infections
Operative procedures related to the genital tract

SIGNS AND SYMPTOMS

A detailed history usually gives a general idea of the possible causes of infertility. Box 4 outlines the key questions on the history that might point to a particular cause. A discussion with the patient should include environmental factors that might affect fertility.

Deep dyspareunia and dysmenorrhea are the most common symptoms reported in patients with endometriosis. Pelvic examination is best carried out during a menstrual period. During this time, specific areas of tenderness and modularity can be more easily identified.

PCOS should be suspected if there is a history of a menstrual disorder such as amenorrhea or oligomenorrhea associated with androgen excess. PCOS usually starts at puberty and is associated with irregular periods and some manifestation of hyperandrogenism. The androgen excess could be a clinical manifestation, such as acne or hirsutism, or a laboratory finding of an elevated androgen level (Box 5). Increasing weight influences the expression of the disease. A variety of medical problems are associated with PCOS (Box 6).

DIAGNOSIS

A semen analysis, a hysterosalpingogram (HSG), and assessment of ovulation should be included in the initial investigation of all infertile couples (Box 7).

Male Partner

The initial screening evaluation for the male partner is a detailed history and two semen analyses taken at least 1 month apart. However if the abnormal result is due to an acute insult such as a viral infection, it will take 2 to 3 months before sperm parameters change. Therefore, the test should be repeated after an appropriate period of time.

Box 5 Manifestations of Polycystic Ovary Syndrome

Clinical
Acanthosis nigricans
Androgen excess
Infertility
Menstrual disorder
Obesity

Biochemical
Abnormal LH/FSH ratio
Abnormal lipoprotein profile (increased triglycerides, low-density lipoprotein cholesterol and total cholesterol and decreased high-density lipoprotein cholesterol)
Decreased sex hormone-binding globulin
Elevated serum androgens (testosterone, androstenedione, DHEAS)
Insulin resistance (abnormal fasting glucose-to-insulin ratio)
Mildly elevated prolactin

Imaging Studies
Ultrasound appearance of polycystic ovary syndrome

Note: Not all manifestations are present in all patients.
DHEAS, Dehydroepiandrosterone sulfate; FSH, follicle-stimulating hormone; LH, luteinizing hormone.

Box 6 Medical Problems Associated with Polycystic Ovary Syndrome

Cardiovascular disease
Diabetes mellitus
Abnormal uterine bleeding
Endometrial cancer
Hyperandrogenic states such as acne and hirsutism
Lipid disorders

Box 7 Basic Infertility Investigation

Assessment of ovarian reserve
Confirmation of ovulation
Hysterosalpingogram
Semen analysis

A history of testicular injury, viral infection, or surgery in a man with an abnormal semen analysis requires a urologic evaluation. The World Health Organization's recommended normal values are given in Box 8. If any of the results are out of the normal range, the test is considered abnormal.

Most semen parameters reported on a routine semen analysis have a large coefficient of variation (CV). For example, a recent proficiency testing report by the American Association of Bioanalysts (Brownsville, Tex) reported a CV of 20% for sperm count and 39% for morphology. Kruger Strict Criteria rather than the WHO standard are sometimes used to evaluate the morphology of the sperm. Normal is considered to be any result greater than 14%. If the semen analysis is abnormal, the male partner should be referred for evaluation to a specialist in male reproduction.

Endocrine evaluation is indicated for patients with low sperm counts or a history of sexual dysfunction. The initial screening tests are a serum FSH and testosterone. Antisperm antibody testing is considered by some infertility specialists to be part of the standard semen analysis. Others assess the presence of these antibodies only if the semen analysis results demonstrate an isolated decrease in motility or increased agglutination. A history of testicular trauma, surgery of the testes or vas deferens (such as a vasectomy reversal), or infection requires assessment of these antibodies. Antisperm antibodies that are clinically significant are those that occur on the surface of the sperm. Cystic fibrosis genetic screening, karyotyping, and microdeletion analysis of the Y chromosome should be offered in appropriate cases of male factor infertility. The extent of sperm DNA fragmentation can be determined by a variety of sperm chromatin structure assays.

Box 8 Prevalence of Abnormal Clomiphene Challenge Test in a General Infertile Population

<30 years of age: 3%
30-34 years of age: 7%
35-39 years of age: 10%
>40 years of age: 26%

From Scott RT, Leonardi MR, Hofmann GE, et al: A prospective evaluation of clomiphene citrate challenge test screening of the general infertility population. Obstet Gynecol 1993;82:539-544.

Female Partner

Ovarian Reserve

Many reproductive endocrinologists think that an assessment of ovarian reserve should be performed in all infertile patients older than 34 years. Younger patients should be assessed if there is a history of ovarian surgery, a poor response to previous infertility treatment, or a family history of early menopause. Patients who have received gonadotoxic drugs and with idiopathic infertility should also have this assessment. All patients should be screened before beginning intensive infertility treatment such as in vitro fertilization (IVF).

Two commonly used tests measure ovarian reserve. Both measure serum follicle-stimulating hormone (FSH) levels. If the levels are increased above a specified level, the probability of achieving pregnancy is reduced. Many laboratories report a level above 10 mIU/mL in the early follicular phase as abnormal. The prognostic significance of this test depends on the assay used by the laboratory. Therefore, it is important to validate that the laboratory meets published criteria. Increased FSH levels appear to be related to decreasing production of inhibin by the granulosa cells.

A serum FSH and estradiol is obtained on the third day of the menstrual cycle. In practice, the test is equally valid when performed on day 2, 3, or 4 of the cycle. Numerous studies have shown that an abnormal test result, an elevated level of FSH, is associated with 95% to 100% failure to conceive with IVF. Upper limits used range from 11 to 14 IU/L. The test has been validated in patients who will be undergoing superovulation for IVF or insemination and in a general infertile population.[9] The prevalence of an abnormal test depends on age. An abnormal test result is associated with a poor pregnancy rate irrespective of age. An elevated day 3 estradiol (>80 pg/mL) is also associated with a poor response to medical treatment of infertility. A normal test result does not mean that a patient will achieve pregnancy with IVF.

A more sensitive test for ovarian reserve is the clomiphene challenge test (CCT). Twice as many patients were identified as poor responders with the CCT than with a day 3 FSH level alone. Clomiphene citrate 100 mg daily is prescribed from days 5 to 9 of the cycle, and a day 3 and a day 10 FSH are drawn. Any level more than 10 mIU/mL is considered an abnormal test. Alternatively, the day 3 and day 10 serum FSH levels can be added. In a series by Loumaye and colleagues, a summed FSH level of more than 26 was associated with a zero pregnancy rate.[10] The test was validated in a general infertility population as well as in patients undergoing ovarian stimulation with gonadotropins. The incidence of abnormal tests increases with age (Box 8). Although the CCT has a predictive value of 95% to 100% for not achieving a pregnancy, it still has a poor sensitivity for identifying patients who will not succeed with infertility treatment.

The abnormally high serum levels in FSH seen with these tests have been attributed to a decreased production of inhibin. Serum inhibin is a peptide heterodimer secreted by granulosa cells. Although serum inhibin might prove to be a better assessment of ovarian reserve, the assay is not available in many centers. Other tests that are currently under investigation are antimüllerian hormone, a peptide secreted by the granulosa cells, and an antral follicle count. Antral follicles are follicles 2 to 6 mm in diameter. An ultrasound performed in the follicular phase can determine a total number of these follicles. A lower number is associated with a poorer outcome from ART.

National practice guidelines can be found at the official website for the American Society for Reproductive Medicine. Essentially all the recommendations have been covered in this chapter.[11]

Tubal Patency

HSG assesses tubal morphology and patency. It is usually performed in the follicular phase after the end of the menses. If a history suggests PID, an erythrocyte sedimentation rate (ESR) should be obtained, and the HSG should be postponed if the ESR is elevated. If the ESR is normal, give doxycycline 100 mg twice a day for 5 days starting 2 days before the procedure. Patients with dilated tubes on HSG are at significant risk for developing acute PID after the procedure. If dilated tubes are found on HSG, doxycycline 100 mg twice a day for 5 days should be given. Evidence of tubal disease requires referral for laparoscopy. Patients with a documented history of PID should be referred for laparoscopy.

Ovulation

There are several methods to evaluate ovulation. Women with regular monthly periods are unlikely to be anovulatory. Basal body temperature charts are inexpensive and sometimes useful, but they are cumbersome and time consuming. They should not be overinterpreted. If there is a biphasic pattern, the patient is most likely ovulating.

We prefer to measure a single serum progesterone level in the luteal phase. This could be timed on the basis of a home urinary luteinizing hormone (LH) test kit. The onset of the LH surge occurs 34 to 36 hours before ovulation. Most LH kits detect this surge. Urine is collected between 10 AM and 8 PM. It should not be the first urine after waking. In an ideal 28-day cycle, testing is started on the 10th day of the cycle. A serum progesterone level is drawn approximately 5 to 7 days later. Levels greater than 3 ng/mL indicate the luteal phase. A serum level greater than 10 ng/mL is usually associated with an ovulatory cycle with a normal luteal phase.

Anovulation or a history of irregular menstrual periods should be investigated with serum thyroid-stimulating hormone (TSH), FSH, and prolactin levels. If the patient presents with amenorrhea, serum estradiol levels should also be assessed.

If the signs and symptoms suggest PCOS, then serum levels of androgens and 17-hydroxyprogesterone should be obtained as well. The serum androgens are usually in the upper range of normal or higher. Serum levels for TSH, prolactin, FSH, and LH should also be obtained. Other disorders that can cause a similar phenotype are 21-hydroxylase deficiency, Cushing's syndrome, and an androgen-secreting adrenal or ovarian tumor. A consensus group from the European Society for Human Reproduction and Embryology and the American Society for Reproductive Medicine has determined that to make a diagnosis of PCOS, the patient must have two out of three indicators: oligo- or anovulation, clinical or biochemical signs (or both) of hyperandrogenism, and polycystic ovaries seen on ultrasound (Fig. 1).

Ultrasonography and endometrial biopsy are not considered parts of the basic infertility investigation. No blood tests or imaging studies can correctly diagnose endometriosis. Although ultrasound might identify an ovarian cyst that includes an endometrioma in the differential diagnosis, it is not conclusive. All serum markers are nonspecific. Laparoscopy is still required to make a definitive diagnosis.

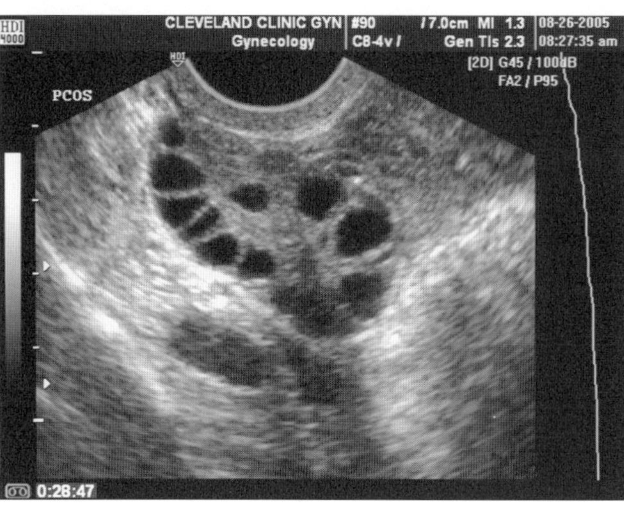

Figure 1 Ultrasound of the ovaries of a woman with polycystic ovary syndrome.

Although traditionally evaluation of sperm and mucus interaction has been performed with a postcoital test, it is no longer considered a part of routine testing. Intrauterine inseminations are used so frequently with many infertility treatments that we are treating any subtle cervical abnormality.

TREATMENT

Standard textbooks of reproductive medicine define infertility as the inability to conceive after 1 year of unprotected intercourse. This does not mean that we would not treat a patient with an obvious problem of anovulation or obstructed fallopian tubes if she has attempted to achieve pregnancy for less than 1 year. In patients older than 35 years, earlier investigation may be considered.

Anovulation

Once the diagnosis of PCOS is made, treatment should focus on modifying insulin resistance. Decreasing insulin levels with metformin will decrease androgen levels and result in ovulatory cycles. Diet and exercise will have the same effect. The primary approach is diet, weight loss, and exercise. In one study, 60 of 67 anovulatory patients with a body mass index (BMI) of 30 kg/m^2 or more resumed spontaneous ovulation after losing 10 kg. Of these patients, 77% achieved pregnancy spontaneously (35%) or with the help of medication. The miscarriage rate was significantly reduced.[12]

If diet and exercise are not successful, then a trial of metformin should be offered. However, it is generally accepted that metformin or other drugs that modify insulin resistance are inferior to clomiphene therapy for induction of ovulation.[13,14] Clomiphene citrate, an antiestrogen drug, is the only FDA-approved drug for inducing ovulation. This drug is started at 50 mg/day from cycle days 5 through 9. The drug can be used for 5 days starting on day 3, 4, or 5. If ovulation is not detected, the dose is increased in increments of 50 mg to a maximum dose of 200 mg. If maximum doses of clomiphene do not induce ovulation, additional medication can be given.

Metformin 1500 mg/day in divided doses has been shown to be effective in cases of clomiphene citrate failure. It can be added to the clomiphene protocol. Typically, metformin is given for several months and clomiphene is added. Side effects are mostly gastrointestinal. Low-dose corticosteroids with clomiphene might help if the adrenal androgens are elevated.

If ovulation is still not induced, the patient should be referred for ovulation induction with gonadotropins. These patients have a high rate of ovarian hyperstimulation syndrome. Aromatase inhibitors such as letrozole can be tried in patients who fail clomiphene and metformin before attempting injectable medication. Letrozole is not FDA approved for this indication but has been shown in numerous case series to be an effective ovulation-induction drug.

Tubal Disease

Mild cases of tubal disease can be treated with laparoscopic surgery. In moderate and severe cases of tubal disease, IVF is associated with better pregnancy rates with a smaller incidence of ectopic pregnancy. The most recent data for IVF success rates (2004) are available through the CDC.[15] The live birth rates per 100 cycles initiated are 36.9% for women younger than 35 years, 29.3% for women between 35 and 37 years, 19.5% for women between 38 and 40 years, and 10.7% for women older than 40 years. Severely damaged tubes (hydrosalpinx) are associated with decreased IVF pregnancy rates and should be removed before starting an IVF cycle.

The main complications associated with IVF are the potential for ovarian hyperstimulation syndrome and multiple births. Multiple births are associated with a higher incidence of prematurity and low birth weight. There do not appear to be any developmental problems with the offspring. There may be a slight increase in sex chromosome abnormalities and congenital malformations.

Endometriosis

Treatment of endometriosis can be surgical or medical. Hormone treatments with drugs that suppress the menstrual cycle, such as gonadotropin-releasing hormone (GnRH) agonists, danazol, or progestins, have clearly been shown *not* to improve fertility. Although there is some controversy as to the success of surgical treatment of early disease, there are clear data to show that surgery is quite effective in treating advanced endometriosis.

Surgical treatment of endometriosis can usually be accomplished by laparoscopy, especially at early stages of the disease. Advanced endometriosis with severe adhesive disease can also be managed laparoscopically, but many gynecologists prefer to approach the disease by laparotomy. These cases often have rectal involvement and require extensive pelvic dissection. Pregnancy rates are similar with either approach. None of the different energy forms, such as lasers, has been shown to be associated with a higher pregnancy rate than conventional laparoscopic techniques.

If surgery fails or is not an option, then ART provides an excellent outcome.

Male Factor Infertility

Mild male factor infertility can be treated with intrauterine insemination. However, most moderate to severe male factor infertility requires IVF with intracytoplasmic sperm injection (ICSI). This procedure consists of a direct injection of a single spermatozoon or spermatid into the oocyte. Success rates have been equivalent to those of IVF cycles with normal sperm. In our experience, the pregnancy rate per embryo transfer is 41%, a rate similar to that in patients with normal sperm.

The management of men with no sperm in the ejaculate, azoospermia, is complex. If there is no obstruction of the ejaculatory ducts, it is called *non-obstructive azoospermia* (NOA). NOA can be due to a primary hypothalamic or pituitary problem. In these cases, treatment is aimed at the cause, such as hyperprolactinemia. Most cases are due to a primary testicular disorder and are usually idiopathic or the result of some genetic disorder, as discussed earlier. Some of these patients have testicular sperm and therefore require a procedure to extract the sperm. The extracted sperm can then be used with IVF to achieve fertilization.

Other patients with azoospermia have an obstruction of the ejaculatory ducts, termed *obstructive azoospermia*. The most common duct obstructed is the vas. If the cause of the obstruction was a previous vasectomy, then a vasectomy reversal is possible. This procedure is associated with a high pregnancy rate. A congenital obstruction is usually bilateral. The treatment is microsurgical epididymal sperm extraction followed by IVF.

In Vitro Fertilization

IVF is the most commonly used ART procedure for infertility.[16] Tens of thousands of babies have been born around the world with this procedure. Success rates have improved dramatically because of improvements in laboratory methods for handling gametes and early embryos.[15] The general principles of IVF have not changed. The patients are given gonadotropins to stimulate the ovaries, and oocyte maturation is assessed by ultrasonography and blood levels of estradiol. The oocytes are retrieved by transvaginal aspiration under conscious sedation. After fertilization, the embryos are grown to either a cleaved stage of 6 or 7 cells (day 3 after fertilization) or a blastocyst stage (day 5 after fertilization). An embryo transfer is then performed. Extra embryos can be cryopreserved effectively and with a high pregnancy rate.

CONCLUSION

Infertility is a medical problem of the couple. There is a natural decrease in fertility with age, and therefore investigation and management are initiated earlier in some couples. There are many environmental and medical problems that might cause infertility in either partner. Some disorders that cause infertility have a long-term impact on the patient's health.

Most patients consult physicians for advice and investigation. Therefore, the primary care physician should be aware of the most common causes of infertility. A few basic investigations can be performed before referral to an infertility specialist. Basic treatment of anovulation is straightforward.

Summary

- Basic investigation of the infertile couple requires an assessment of the male partner with a semen analysis and documentation of ovulation and tubal patency in the female partner.
- Polycystic ovary syndrome (PCOS) is the most common cause of anovulation, and sexually transmitted disease is the most common cause of tubal disease.
- Clomiphene citrate is the drug therapy of choice for treating anovulation associated with infertility.
- Severe male factor infertility is associated with genetic disorders such as mutations in the cystic fibrosis genes and is treated effectively only with in vitro fertilization.

Suggested Readings

Abma JC, Chandra A, Mosher WD, et al: Fertility, Family Planning, and Women's Health: New Data from the 1995 National Survey of Family Growth. Vital and Health Statistics 23(19), May 1997. Hyattsville, MD: National Center for Health Statistics, 1997, pp 65-66.

American Society for Reproductive Medicine: Practice committee reports: Guidelines, statements and opinions of the ASRM Practice Committee. Available at http://www.asrm.org/Media/Practice/practice.html#Guidelines (accessed March 20, 2009).

Centers for Disease Control and Prevention: 2004 Assisted Reproductive Technology (ART) Report. Available at http://www.cdc.gov/art/ART2004/index.htm (accessed March 20, 2009).

Clark AM, Thornley B, Tomlinson L, et al: Weight loss in obese infertile women results in improvement in reproductive outcome for all forms of fertility treatment. Hum Reprod. 1998;13:1502-1505.

Falcone T, Finegood DT, Fantus IG, Morris D: Androgen response to endogenous insulin secretion during the frequently sampled intravenous glucose tolerance test in normal and hyperandrogenic women. J Clin Endocrinol Metab 1990;71:1653-1657.

Gallardo E, Simon C, Levy M, et al: Effect of age on sperm fertility potential: Oocyte donation as a model. Fertil Steril 1996;66:260-264.

Goldberg J, Falcone T, Attaran M: In vitro fertilization update. Clev Clin J Med 2007;74:329-338.

Hatch EE, Bracken MB: Association of delayed conception with caffeine consumption. Am J Epidemiol 1993;138:1082-1092.

Legro RS, Barnhart HX, Schlaff WD, et al: Clomiphene, metformin, or both for infertility in the polycystic ovary syndrome. N Engl J Med 2007;356:551-566.

Loumaye E, Billion JM, Mine JM, et al: Predication of individual response to controlled ovarian hyperstimulation by means of a clomiphene citrate challenge test. Fertil Steril 1990;53:295-301.

Manheimer E, Zhang G, Udoff L, et al: Effects of acupuncture on rates of pregnancy and live birth among women undergoing in vitro fertilisation: systematic review and meta analysis. Br Med J 2008;336:545-549.

Palomba S, Orio F Jr, Falbo A, et al: Prospective parallel randomized, double-blind, double dummy controlled clinical trial comparing clomiphene citrate and metformin as the first-line treatment for ovulation induction in nonobese anovulatory women with polycystic ovary syndrome. J Clin Endocril Metab 2005;90:4068-4074.

Rotterdam ESHRE/ASRM-Sponsored PCOS Consensus Workshop Group: Revised 2003 consensus on diagnostic criteria and long-term health risks related to polycystic ovary syndrome. Fertil Steril 2004;81:19-25.

Scott RT, Leonardi MR, Hofmann GE, et al: A prospective evaluation of clomiphene citrate challenge test screening of the general infertility population. Obstet Gynecol 1993;82:539-544.

Wang C, McDonald V, Leung A, et al: Effect of increased scrotal temperature on sperm production in normal men. Fertil Steril 1997;68:334-339.

Westrom L, Joesoef R, Reynolds G, et al: Pelvic inflammatory disease and fertility. A cohort study of 1,844 women with laparoscopically verified disease and 657 control women with normal laparoscopic results. Sex Transm Dis 1992;19:185-192.

References

For a complete list of references, log onto www.expertconsult.com.

Menopause

Julie A. Elder and *Holly L. Thacker*

DEFINITION

Menopause is defined as the absence of menses for 1 year. Women usually experience menopause between 40 and 55 years of age, with the median age being 51. Smokers and women with chronic illnesses tend to experience menopause at an earlier age (Box 1).

Menopause transition consists of fluctuating ovarian function and occurs 2 to 8 years before menopause and up to 1 year after the final menses. It is a progressive process that eventually leads to persistent ovarian failure. The change in hormones during this period is often responsible for the clinical signs and symptoms that many women experience. Systems affected by the perimenopausal phase include skin and hair, genitourinary (GU), neuroendocrine, cardiovascular, and skeletal. The North American Menopause Society has published a comprehensive online study guide related to menopause and offers testing to credential menopause practitioners.

Premature ovarian insufficiency (POI) is the cessation of ovarian function before the age of 40. It occurs in less than 1% of all women. There are many reasons for secondary amenorrhea in addition to primary ovarian failure. Secondary causes of POI include chromosomal abnormalities (e.g., fragile X syndrome), autoimmune disorders, physical insults to the ovaries, isolated ovarian antibodies, and gonadotropic receptor defects. Pregnancy must always be considered in the differential diagnosis of secondary amenorrhea.

PATHOPHYSIOLOGY

A female ovary has the greatest number of oocytes during the fifth month of gestation and has about 1 to 2 million oocytes at birth. As a woman ages, the process of atresia reduces the number of oocytes, so that at the time of menopause a woman may have only a few hundred to a few thousand oocytes left. The ovary primarily produces estrogen, progesterone, and androgens.

Estrogen

Estrone (E_1), estradiol (E_2), and estriol (E_3) are three endogenously produced estrogens. Estradiol (E_2) is produced by the dominant ovarian follicle during the monthly menstrual cycle and is the most potent natural estrogen. Estrone (E_1) is the dominant form of estrogen during menopause. It is produced in small quantities by the ovary and the adrenal glands, and is principally derived by the peripheral conversion of androstenedione in adipose tissue.

Progesterone

Progesterone is produced by the corpus luteum and promotes thickening of the endometrium in preparation for a fertilized ovum. Progesterone also inhibits the actions of estrogen on certain tissues. In an anovulatory woman, no corpus luteum is formed. Therefore, estrogen often goes unopposed. This can lead to a buildup of the endometrium, causing irregular menstrual bleeding in the perimenopausal phase.

Menstruation

Menarche, or the first menses, usually begins around the age of 12 years. It is divided into three phases: follicular, ovulatory, and secretory. The follicular, or proliferative, phase is marked by the first day of menses. Estradiol (E_2) is produced during this phase by a dominant ovarian follicle and causes proliferation of the endometrium. Through a negative feedback system, follicle-stimulating hormone (FSH) production is decreased. Luteinizing hormone (LH), however, increases and eventually triggers ovulation. When LH peaks, ovulation occurs. During this ovulatory phase, progesterone levels increase, whereas estrogen levels decrease.

Formation of a corpus luteum begins the secretory phase in which estrogen, progesterone, and androgens are secreted. Estrogen promotes cellular proliferation, whereas progesterone causes swelling and secretory development of the endometrium. If pregnancy does not occur, estrogen and progesterone levels fall and the endometrium is shed during menses.

Menopause

The menopausal ovary no longer produces estradiol (E_2) or inhibin. Therefore, FSH and LH are no longer inhibited by estrogen's negative feedback mechanism. Fluctuations and deficiencies in estrogen levels cause many of the menopausal signs and symptoms.

SIGNS AND SYMPTOMS

Various tissues throughout the body are rich in estrogen receptors. When estrogen levels decrease or fluctuate, a number of systems can be directly affected (Box 2).

Vasomotor and neuroendocrine hot flashes are common among women in the menopause transition. They are usually self limited but can continue for years. Hot flashes involve a sensation of warmth throughout the body, often accompanied by flushing. In addition, some women experience cephalalgia, nausea, or diaphoresis. Palpitations, dizziness, and "skin crawling" sensations are other vasomotor symptoms that women might encounter. Women with known depression or panic disorders might have exacerbations of their disease if they have associated menopausal symptoms.

Skin and hair estrogen deficiency leads to mucosal dryness, particularly in the eyes, nose, mouth, and vagina. Some women might also notice a loss of skin elasticity associated with decreased collagen and elastin production. Decreased estrogen levels are associated with a relative surplus of androgens. Androgen excess can cause male-pattern alopecia, hirsutism, and a deepening of the upper register of the voice.

Urogenital estrogen receptors are located on many tissues, including the urethra and bladder. During the estrogen deficiency state of menopause, urethral tissue can become thin, ultimately causing dysuria, urinary incontinence, and increased urinary frequency. In addition, changes in the vulva and vagina can occur, including vaginal atrophy, cervical atrophy, and vaginal dryness. Dyspareunia may result, as well as postcoital bleeding, pruritus vulvae, and discomfort during routine pelvic examinations. Women may also experience sexual dysfunction and a decreased libido.

Skeletal bone mass peaks at 30 years of age and starts to decline thereafter. This decline accelerates throughout the menopause transition and menopausal years. Genetics, estrogen status, exercise, and calcium and vitamin D intake all play significant roles in bone mass. Estrogen has a protective effect on bones by inhibiting overall bone loss. Postmenopausal women can lose up to 4% to 5% of their bone density annually due to the loss of estrogen. Bone loss is especially prominent in the trabecular spine.

Box 1 Factors that Affect the Onset of Menopause

Earlier Onset
Current smoking
Nulliparity
Pelvic radiation and chemotherapy
Medical treatment for depression
Familial

Later Onset
Multiparity
Increased body mass index
Higher cognitive scores in childhood
Familial

Box 2 Effects of Estrogen Loss

Symptoms (Earlier Onset)
Hot flashes/vasomotor symptoms
Minor mood disturbances
Sleep disturbances
Urogenital symptoms

Physical Signs (Intermediate Onset)
Vaginal atrophy
Osteopenia/low bone density
Scalp hair loss or hirsutism

Potential Disease Related to Hormonal Status (Later Onset)
Osteoporosis

Cardiovascular Disease

The incidence of cardiovascular disease increases after menopause. Specifically, the risk of coronary heart disease is two to three times higher for postmenopausal women compared with premenopausal women of the same age. Alarmingly, after the age of 65, one out of every three women has some form of cardiovascular disease (CVD). Hormone therapy (HT) is no longer used to prevent CVD based on the Heart and Estrogen-Progestin Replacement Study (HERS) trial and Women's Health Initiative (WHI) results; however the effects of the timing of HT initiation are being investigated.

DIAGNOSIS

Women undergoing the menopause transition or menopausal changes seek medical counsel for a variety of reasons. Absent or irregular menses, insomnia, depression, cephalalgia, and vasomotor instability are just a few of the reasons women visit their physicians. Many women access information about menopause through a variety of sources including friends, family, Internet sources, television and other forms of media, which may not be accurate sources of information.

The initial evaluation by the health care provider should include a comprehensive history and physical examination accompanied by select laboratory studies and patient education. In addition, family, social, sexual, and medication histories are imperative. A complete physical examination might provide diagnostic clues to a woman's menopausal state. For example, a loss of height might suggest osteoporosis and a pelvic examination might reveal vaginal atrophy from lack of estrogen.

Baseline laboratory studies should also be performed including a screening thyroid stimulating hormone (TSH). During the menopause transition, FSH levels fluctuate, making a serum level unreliable for diagnostic purposes. In the face of prolonged amenorrhea with or without menopausal symptoms, an FSH level >40 mIU/mL is considered diagnostic of menopause. Although in this setting, a FSH evaluation is rarely needed to confirm the postmenopausal state. If a woman has taken oral contraceptives during the perimenopausal period, she must be taken off them for several months before an accurate FSH level can be determined. Serum estradiol levels fluctuate in perimenopausal women, making it a test that is seldom useful in diagnosing menopause. Testosterone and dehydroepiandrosterone (DHEA) levels are indicated only if a woman has symptoms of hyperandrogenism or if she is taking over-the-counter hormones that may contain these potent androgens.

TREATMENT

Various organizations provide recommendations regarding the treatment of menopause. The North American Menopause Society guidelines contain some of the most accurate and clinically relevant information. Women should be educated about the risks and benefits of HT and consider it based on personal risk assessment and quality of life issues. There are certain situations during which the use of HT is not recommended.

Contraindications to Hormone Therapy

Absolute contraindications to HT include pregnancy, an active venous thrombosis or embolism, undiagnosed vaginal bleeding, active liver disease, active breast or endometrial cancer, and active cardiovascular disease.

Relative contraindications to HT include a history of previously treated breast or uterine cancer, previous thromboembolism, gall bladder disease, uncontrolled hypertension, migraine headaches, uterine fibroids, seizure disorders, hypertriglyceridemia, and a history of CVD. When considering the use of HT, risks and benefits must be individualized.

Risks of Hormone Therapy

Thromboembolism

There is an increased risk of developing thromboembolism associated with HT use. It is estimated that the incidence of deep venous thrombosis (DVT) or pulmonary embolus (PE) occurs in 3 of 10,000 HRT users annually, especially during the first year of therapy. This risk is present regardless of the form of hormonal or transdermal estrogen used. Based on the conjugated equine estrogen/medroxyprogesterone (CEE/MPA) arm of the WHI, the risk of venous thromboembolism (VTE) persisted in subsequent years. A more recent randomized trial revealed a higher incidence of VTE in HT users, specifically in women who were older in age and overweight or obese, or both. In the estrogen-only arm of the WHI, conjugated equine estrogens had less risk for VTE than the combination estrogen-progestin regimen. The type of estrogen a woman takes may also influence her risk for VTE. However, the U.S. Food and Drug Administration (FDA) classifies all estrogen as having the same risks.

Gallbladder Disease

An increase in the incidence of gallbladder disease is noticed in women on HT. The HERS trial revealed that women with coronary artery disease had a 40% increased risk for developing symptomatic gallbladder disease while on HT.

Endometrial Cancer

The risk of developing endometrial adenomatous hyperplasia, a precursor for endometrial cancer, occurs in women with a uterus who are on estrogen therapy alone (unopposed estrogen). Current therapeutic regimens recommend that women on HT with intact uteri receive combinations of estrogen and progestin. This decreases the risk of endometrial cancer to baseline.

Breast Cancer

The increase in the relative risk of developing breast cancer associated with long-term use (>5 years) HT is a major reason that some women choose not to take it. The CEE/MPA arm of the WHI showed a hazard ratio of 1.26 (confidence interval [CI], 1.0-1.56). The degree of risk, however, is quite controversial. Various studies have shown that HT is associated with an increased risk of breast cancer, but others have not concurred. Short-term HT, used to treat menopausal symptoms, appears not to increase a woman's chance of developing breast cancer. However, women on HT for more than 5 to 10 years are calculated to have less than one extra occurrence of breast cancer per 1000 women. There are no prospective, randomized controlled studies showing that women on HT are more likely to die of breast cancer. The estrogen only arm of the WHI showed no increased risk of breast cancer in women with a hysterectomy in taking estrogen alone. In fact, women adherent to conjugated estrogen showed a reduced risk of breast cancer.

The Boston Nurses Healthy Study showed no increase in breast cancer in women using estrogen therapy (ET) for up to 15 years. After 15 years of use, however, ET was associated with an increased risk for breast cancer.

Benefits of Hormone Therapy

Vasomotor Symptoms

HT is effective in the treatment of hot flashes and is currently the only FDA-approved therapy. Many women only need vasomotor control for short periods of time (<5 years). HT has also been shown to improve symptoms of anxiety, irritability, and depression associated with menopause.

Osteoporosis

Hormone therapy is FDA-approved for the prevention and management of osteoporosis. A woman must continue HT indefinitely to sustain the bone protective benefits. In the WHI, impressive reductions in all types of fractures were seen. Most women take HT for less than 2 years; therefore, women with osteoporosis, low bone density, or both need alternative treatments. In addition to taking estrogen, it is recommended that women take 1200 mg of calcium a day. If a woman is not on HT, or is older than 65 years, 1500 mg of calcium daily is recommended. A clinical practice guideline for osteoporosis appears on the National Osteoporosis Foundation website. Vitamin D deficiency is widespread in North America and at least 400 to 800 IU of vitamin D are recommended daily.

Vaginal Atrophy

HT has been shown to improve the symptoms of vaginal atrophy in the intravaginal, oral, and transdermal forms.

Cognition

The effects of HT have been controversial in the literature. Observational studies have suggested a decreased risk of developing Alzheimer's dementia; however, HERS data found that older women with coronary artery disease on HT scored worse on verbal fluency tests and had worse cognition than women taking placebo. In addition, the WHI memory study revealed that HT did not prevent mild cognitive impairment and, in fact, doubled the relative risk of dementia, suggesting that, like cardiovascular disease, timing is important.

Table 1 Vaginal Estrogens

Drug	Dosing
Premarin cream (conjugated equine estrogen)	2 g daily (intravaginally) × 2 wk, then 1 g 1-3 × per wk
Estrace cream (estradiol)	2 g daily (intravaginally) × 2 wk, then 7 g weekly
Vagifem tablets (estradiol)	25 μg daily (intravaginally) × 2 wk, then 25 μg 2 × per wk
Estring (intravaginal ring) (estradiol)	Delivers 7.5 μg daily (intravaginally) locally for 90 days
Femring (intravaginal ring) (estradiol)	Delivers 50 μg or 100 μg (locally and systemically) daily for 90 days

Other Benefits

The WHI showed less risk of colon cancer with HT, hazard ratio 0.63 (CI, 0.43-0.92); however, ET did not show a reduction in colon cancer. HT and ET have no effect on ovarian cancer risk.

Types of Hormone Therapy

Estrogen

Estrogen is given orally, vaginally, or transdermally. Women with GU atrophy may benefit from intravaginal estrogen therapy, used with or without standard HT (Table 1). Signs and symptoms of urogenital or vaginal atrophy can be assessed by visual inspection at the routine pelvic examination every 1 to 2 years.

Women should be queried regarding complaints of sexual dysfunction, vaginal dryness, and dyspareunia. Intravaginal estrogen comes in various forms, including creams, tablets, and an intravaginal ring (Estring) that the woman herself can insert every 3 months. A health care provider can also insert and remove the ring, but generally the woman accomplishes this easily. The Estring vaginal ring has the added benefit of no significant systemic effects or endometrial stimulation, which is an advantage to women with uteri/endometria who are not using progestins and for women who are suffering from local GU symptoms. The Femring gives both local and systemic estrogen to women without uteri who have vasomotor symptoms.

The use of intravaginal estrogen creams and tablets may periodically necessitate evaluation of the endometrium with an outpatient endometrial pipelle biopsy because some of this estrogen is systemically absorbed and may stimulate endometrial growth. Estrogen therapy in a woman with an intact uterus must be accompanied by a progestin to prevent endometrial hyperplasia. Many oral forms of estrogen are available (Table 2). Transdermal estradiol in patch form may be beneficial for women who do not tolerate or cannot take oral forms because of nausea (Table 3). The patch may also be clinically beneficial to women with syndrome X, or insulin resistance accompanied by elevated triglycerides. Transdermal estradiol does not increase triglyceride levels, whereas oral estrogen does. Menostar is an ultra, ultra low-dose estrogen patch (0.014 mg/day) that has recently been approved for unopposed estrogen use in postmenopausal women. It is indicated for bone protection only and does not offer any vasomotor symptom relief. Estrasorb lotion (0.05 mg/day) has been approved for vasomotor symptom control, and Estrogel (0.06% topical gel) has been approved for vasomotor symptoms and vulvar/vaginal atrophy.

Oral estrogen doses vary. The standard starting dose of oral conjugated equine estrogen (CEE) or synthetic conjugated estrogen is no longer 0.625 mg daily, although lower doses (e.g., 0.45 mg or

Table 2 Oral Estrogens

Drug	Low and Starting Dose	Standard Dose	Intermediate Dose	High Dose	Highest Dose
Premarin (CEE)	0.3 mg 0.45 mg	0.625 mg	0.9 mg	1.25 mg	2.5 mg
Estrace (E_2)	0.5 mg	1 mg	—	2 mg	—
Ogen (E_1)	—	0.625 mg	—	1.25 mg	2.5 mg
Ortho-Est	—	0.625 mg	—	1.25 mg	—
Menest (esterified E)	0.3 mg	0.625 mg	—	1.25 mg	2.5 mg
Enjuvia (synthetic CE)	0.3 mg 0.45 mg	0.625 mg	0.9 mg	1.25 mg	—
Femtrace (estradiol acetate)	0.45 mg	—	0.9 mg	1.8 mg	—

Table 3 Transdermal Estrogens

Drug	Low Dose	Medium Dose	High Dose	Higher Dose	Change Patch
Estraderm	—	0.05 mg	—	0.10 mg	Every 3.5 days
Esclim (reservoir patch)	0.025 mg, 0.0375 mg	0.05 mg	0.075 mg	—	Every 3.5 days
Vivelle Dot	0.025 mg, 0.0375 mg	0.05 mg	0.075 mg	0.10 mg	Every 3.5 days
Alora	0.025 mg	0.05 mg	0.075 mg	0.10 mg	Every 3.5 days
Climara	0.025 mg	0.05 mg	0.075 mg	0.10 mg	Weekly

0.3 mg) may suffice. The dose can be adjusted higher or lower according to the woman's symptoms after 1 month of therapy. Higher doses of estrogen are often required in younger women who have undergone hysterectomy Based on the women's HOPE trial results, ultra-low doses of HT, such as 0.3 or 0.45 mg of CEE combined with ultra-low doses of medroxyprogesterone acetate (MPA, 1.5 mg), are effective for symptom control.

Some women favor estrogens such as conjugated equine estrogen (Premarin) that have been used clinically for more than 60 years. Other women, however, prefer "synthetic" forms of conjugated estrogens (e.g., Enjuvia) that are not derived from animal products. Women who cannot tolerate conjugated estrogens may do better with other forms of estrogen, such as bioidentical estrone (E_1), micronized estradiol (E_2), or transdermal estradiol (E_2). Other women prefer oral estradiol (E_2) (the most potent form of estrogen) that is found in Femtrace (doses of 0.45 mg, 0.9 mg, and 1.8 mg).

It is important to note that although all postmenopausal estrogens have been FDA approved to treat vasomotor and local GU atrophy, only some estrogens have been FDA approved to prevent postmenopausal osteoporosis (PMOP). Examples of ET and HT products that are FDA approved to prevent PMOP include Premarin, Prempro, Estrace, Ogen, Vivelle, Climara, femhrt, and Activella. The newest low-dose HT is femhrtLo; it may afford symptom control, but it does not necessarily provide bone protection-so women on low doses of HT should have their bone density monitored periodically.

Progesterone

Progesterone is produced naturally in the body from the corpus luteum after ovulation and functions to down-regulate estrogen receptors. Progestagens include progesterone and progestins, which are synthetic formulations that are better absorbed than is progesterone. (Although oral absorption is improved with micronized progesterone in oil.) Oral progestins can be taken on the first 12 days of each month (cyclic) or taken continuously throughout the entire month (Box 3). For cyclic therapy, 5 to 10 mg of medroxyprogesterone acetate (MPA) or 200 mg of micronized progesterone (Prometrium) is taken orally with food, in the evenings of days 1 through 12. Younger and heavier women may require more progestins. Generally cyclic therapy is used for recently menopausal women because the goal is to switch to "continuous combined" (daily estrogen and progestin) therapy to promote amenorrhea, which is favored in older women and in women who do not want any monthly bleeding. For continuous estrogen-progestin therapy, 2.5 to 5 mg of MPA is taken orally every day. If ultra-low doses of estrogen are used, then lower doses of daily PA can be used, such as 1.5 mg of MPA or 100 mg of Prometrium or 4% Prochieve vaginal gel. The NIH and NAMS recommend using the lowest effective dose of hormone therapy for the shortest duration of time consistent with the reason the woman is using hormone therapy, with periodic reassessments recommended.

Box 3 Oral Progestins

Provera: MPA 5-10 mg on days 1-12 or 2.5 mg daily or 1.5 mg daily
Amen: MPA 10 mg on days 1-12
MPA: MPA 1.5 mg may be combined with 0.3 or 0.45 mg of conjugated equine estrogen
Prometrium: Progesterone USP 100 mg daily or 200 mg on days 1-12, taken at night with food

MPA, medroxyprogesterone acetate.

Cyclic regimens often cause withdrawal bleeding, whereas continuous use over 6 months induces amenorrhea in the majority of users. If amenorrhea is not induced after 6 months of continuous

Table 4 Combined Regimens

Activella	1 mg 17 β-estradiol + 0.5 mg norethindrone acetate (NA)
Femhrt	5 μg ethinyl estadiol (EE) + 1 mg NA
Femhrt low dose	2.5 μg EE + 0.5 mg NA
Prefest	1 mg 17 β-estradiol for 3 days, alternating with 1 mg 17 β-estradiol + 0.09 mg NA for 3 days
Prempro	0.625 mg conjugated equine estrogen (CEE) + 5 mg medroxyprogesterone acetate (MPA) or 0.625 mg CEE + 2.5 mg MPA
Prempro low dose	0.45 mg CEE +1.5 mg MPA or 0.3 mg CEE +1.5 mg MPA
Premphase	0.625 mg CEE (alone days 1-14) followed by 0.625 mg CEE + 5.0 mg MPA (days 15-28)
CombiPatch	0.05 mg 17 β-estradiol + 0.25 or 0.14 mg NA every 3.5 days
ClimaraPro	0.045 mg 17 β-estradiol with 0.015 mg of levonorgestrel (weekly patch)

therapy, an endometrial biopsy or at the least a transvaginal ultrasound should be strongly considered to assess the endometrial thickness. Endometrial stripes of over 5 mm in postmenopausal women are suspect. Heavy bleeding persisting for more than 1 week per month also warrants an endometrial biopsy. Progestins are also combined with estrogen in a transdermal patch (CombiPatch) or weekly Climara-Pro or in an oral pill formulation (Table 4). Newer progestins, such as drospirenone, which have been used in the oral contraceptives Yasmin and Yaz, are now available in combination with estradiol for postmenopausal women (Angeliq 1 mg of estradiol and 0.5 mg DSP) for HT.

Other Treatment Options

In addition to standard HT, many women prefer alternative therapies such as herbal medicines and vitamin therapies.

Some of the more popular therapies for hot flashes include black cohosh, dong quai, and evening primrose oil. Black cohosh (Remifemin) is approved by the German Commission E for only 6 months of use. This agent may help with menopausal vasomotor symptoms; however, no studies on long-term benefits or risks are available. In general, "alternative" or "natural" therapies appeal to many women. However, they are not well studied, and their long-term outcomes are unknown and none has been shown to be salutary to the skeleton or GU tract. Their long-term use cannot be safely recommended. Women need to be informed that "natural" or bio-identical does not necessarily equate with "safe and free from problems." Therapeutic options are covered in The North American Menopause Society online study guide and their consensus panel on the treatment of menopausal vasomotor symptoms. Future options for vasomotor symptom control may include norepinephrine serotonin reuptake inhibitors and combinations of estrogen or selective estrogen receptor modulators.

Summary

- Menopause is a normal life cycle event that may or may not be accompanied by symptoms and medical consequences.
- The skeleton and the GU tract (vagina and base of the bladder) are the most likely organ systems to be affected by lowered estrogen levels.
- The severity of menopausal symptoms varies, and the need for hormone therapy (HT) needs to be individualized and periodically assessed for risks and benefits to the individual woman.
- There are a multitude of estrogen and progestagens with various doses and routes of administration.

Suggested Readings

American Society for Reproductive Medicine: www.asrm.org. Includes information regarding reproductive medicine and biology.

Anderson GL, Limacher M, Assaf AR, et al: Effects of conjugated equine estrogen in postmenopausal women with hysterectomy: The Women's Health Initiative randomized controlled trial. JAMA 2004;291:1701-1712.

Grady D: Effect of postmenopausal hormonal therapy on cognitive function: The hormone therapy and estrogen/progesterone replacement study. Amer J Med 2002;113:543-548.

Grodstein F, Manson JE, Stampfer MJ: Hormonal therapy and coronary heart disease: The role of time since menopause and age at hormone initiation. J Women's Health 2006;15:35-44.

National Institutes of Health, the National Heart, Lung, and Blood Institute, and the Women's Health Initiative: www.nhlbi.nih.gov. Provides comprehensive information regarding the Women's Health Initiative, one of the largest preventive health studies in the United States.

National Osteoporosis Foundation: www.nof.org. Includes comprehensive information about osteoporosis evaluation, diagnosis, and treatment.

North American Menopause Society: www.menopause.org. Includes comprehensive information about menopause.

Stefanick ML, Anderson GL, Margolis KL, et al, for WHI Investigators. Effects of CEE on breast cancer and breast cancer screening in postmenopausal women with hysterectomy: WHI. JAMA 2006;295:1647-1657.

Menstrual Dysfunction

Linda Bradley

DEFINITION

Dysfunctional uterine bleeding (DUB) is defined as abnormal bleeding in the absence of intracavitary or uterine pathology.

Most menstrual cycles occur every 22 to 35 days. Normal menstrual flow lasts 3 to 7 days, with most blood loss occurring within the first 3 days. The menstrual flow amounts to 35 mL and consists of effluent debris and blood. Patients with menorrhagia lose more than 80 mL of blood with each menstrual cycle and often develop anemia. In general, most normal menstruating women use five or six pads or tampons per day. Although approximately 16 mg of iron are lost with each menstrual cycle, this rarely results in anemia in women with adequate intake of dietary iron.

More than 50% of women who complain of menorrhagia might not actually have heavy menses. Some patients change their sanitary products more often for hygienic reasons or because of personal preference or concern for toxic shock syndrome than because of heavy flow. Social obligations, sexual activity, hobbies, work, and travel are not interrupted with normal menstrual function.

Menstrual patterns associated with abnormal uterine bleeding are defined in Box 1.

PREVALENCE

Approximately 9% to 30% of reproductive-age women have menstrual irregularities requiring medical evaluation.[1] Approximately 15% to 20% of scheduled office gynecologic visits are for evaluation of abnormal uterine bleeding, exceeded only by vaginitis as a chief complaint.

PATHOPHYSIOLOGY

Simplistically, normal menstrual bleeding results from fluctuations in the hypothalamic-pituitary-adrenal-ovarian axis, leading to predictable denudation and sloughing of the endometrium. Hemorrhage followed by prompt hemostasis and repair causes stabilization and regrowth of the endometrium. Physiologically, constant low levels of estrogen prime the endometrium. Normal secretion of progesterone from the corpus luteum stabilizes the endometrium, decreases vascular fragility, and supports the endometrial stroma. Patients with menorrhagia typically have an imbalance of prostaglandin levels and increased fibrinolytic activity.

Abnormal uterine bleeding generally can be categorized as anovulatory bleeding or ovulatory dysfunctional bleeding. Anovulatory DUB is caused by failure of the corpus luteum to sustain the developing endometrium. Patients with anovulatory cycles typically do not experience premenstrual syndrome—breast discomfort, increased mucoid vaginal discharge, or premenstrual cramping and bloating—characteristic of ovulatory cycles. Anovulatory cycles can coexist with intracavitary lesions. The most common causes of anovulatory cycles include polycystic ovary syndrome (PCOS), hypothalamic amenorrhea, premature ovarian failure, and hyperprolactinemia.[2] Bleeding is often noncyclic, variable in amount and volume, and unpredictable. Ovulatory cycles are predictable but might coexist with intracavitary lesions, including polyps or fibroids, and cause erratic bleeding.

DIAGNOSIS

History and Examination

The diagnosis has three main components. The physician should note the presence of galactorrhea, weight gain, acanthosis nigricans, evidence of hypothyroidism or hyperthyroidism, virilization, and acne. First, a detailed medical history and thorough review of systems must be obtained. Eliciting a detailed clinical history alerts the astute physician to systemic and medical conditions that cause menstrual dysfunction (Box 2). Inherited and acquired coagulation disorders and liver and renal diseases often manifest with symptoms of abnormal uterine bleeding. Second, the physical examination must be detailed and complete, even in the presence of heavy bleeding. The gynecologic examination must be performed with specific attention to the vagina, cervix, uterus, and adnexa to exclude pathology. Finally, appropriate laboratory studies should be ordered based on the clinical history obtained. Following the American College of Obstetrics and Gynecology (ACOG) guidelines eliminates costly and unnecessary laboratory testing.[3]

Pregnancy testing must always be performed in sexually active women. Women with profuse menorrhagia and a normal-size uterus should be screened for von Willebrand's disease because 13% to 20% of women who are candidates for surgical intervention have the subtle form (type 1 disease). Successful medical options for treatment of women with von Willebrand's disease include oral contraceptive therapy (88% successful), desmopressin acetate, antifibrinolytic agents, and plasma-derived concentrates rich in the high-molecular-weight multimers of von Willebrand's factor (vWF).[4]

Liberal use of endometrial biopsy is encouraged in women older than 35 years who have increased risk factors for endometrial hyperplasia and endometrial cancer. Risk factors include diabetes, prolonged steroid use, obesity, long history of irregular cycles, unopposed estrogen therapy, and suspected polycystic ovary syndrome.

Special Categories of Abnormal Uterine Bleeding

Adolescence

The adolescent patient with irregular and heavy menses should be evaluated more thoroughly for coagulopathies because 20% to 30% might have a major bleeding diathesis.[5] Specifically, adolescents need to be evaluated for von Willebrand's disease with a ristocetin cofactor assay for vWF before hormonal therapy is initiated to prevent false-negative results. This assay is the best single screening test for von Willebrand's disease. Laboratory testing in the adolescent should include serum human chorionic gonadotropin level (hCG), bleeding time, prothrombin time and partial thromboplastin time, complete blood count (CBC) with platelets, and vWF.

Perimenopause

Women entering the perimenopause might have recurrent bouts of DUB and associated physical complaints due to changes in the hypothalamic-pituitary axis. The hormonal milieu is associated with decreased inhibin levels and variable estradiol levels, normal follicle-stimulating hormone (FSH), and menstrual cycles that can be episodically ovulatory.[6] Myriad menstrual complaints occur during the perimenopause, including menometrorrhagia, amenorrhea, and oligomenorrheic cycles. Additionally, decreased mental clarity, diminished concentration, vaginal dryness, decreased libido, hot flushes, and night sweats are classic hallmarks of perimenopause.

Oral contraceptive therapy is quite useful during the perimenopause and should be the first line of therapy rather than conventional hormone replacement therapy.[7] Traditional doses of postmenopausal hormone replacement therapy do not suppress ovulation or prevent pregnancy as do traditional oral contraceptive pills. In healthy nonsmoking women older than 35 years, oral contraceptive

Box 1 Definitions of Abnormal Menstrual Bleeding

Amenorrhea: Absence of menses for 6 months or absence of menstrual cycle for three cycles
Menorrhagia: Heavier and increased amount of flow occurring at regular intervals or loss of >80 mL of blood
Metrorrhagia: Irregular episodes of bleeding
Menometrorrhagia: Longer duration of flow occurring at unpredictable intervals
Oligomenorrhea: Cycle length >35 days
Polymenorrhea: Cycle length >21 days
Postmenopausal bleeding: Bleeding that occurs more than 12 months after the last menstrual cycle

Box 2 Causes of Menstrual Dysfunction

Anatomic
Adenomyosis
Endometriosis
Endometritis
Fibroids
Hyperplasia
Malignancy
Polyps
Retained products of conception

Endocrine
Adrenal gland dysfunction
Elevated prolactin level
Estrogen-producing tumors
Hypothalamic or pituitary gland dysfunction
Thyroid dysfunction

Hematologic
Anemia
Coagulopathy
Idiopathic thrombocytopenic purpura
Leukemia
Prothrombin deficiency
von Willenbrand's disease

Systemic Disease
Anorexia
Chronic illness
Hypersplenism
Liver disorders
Obesity
Rapid fluctuations in weight
Renal impairment

Medications
Anticoagulants
Herbal and soy products
Steroids

Miscellaneous
Depression
Excessive alcohol intake
Sexually transmitted diseases
Smoking

pills regulate menstrual cycles, decrease vasomotor symptoms, improve bone mineral density, and decrease the need for surgical intervention for DUB.

Menopausal Bleeding

Bleeding occurring more than 1 year after cessation of menses or during hormone replacement therapy or tamoxifen use requires thorough evaluation. Although the most common cause of postmenopausal bleeding is atrophy, intracavitary pathology and cancer must be excluded. Approximately 10% of women with postmenopausal bleeding have endometrial cancer. The likelihood of endometrial cancer increases with each decade and must be aggressively excluded.

TREATMENT

Once the cause of DUB is identified, appropriate therapy can be instituted. Medical therapy with oral contraceptives or progesterone is a mainstay in the treatment of anovulatory menstrual cycles. Patients with ovulatory DUB must be evaluated for intracavitary uterine pathology because hormonal dysfunction is not likely the cause of bleeding. Patients with anatomic causes associated with abnormal bleeding can be treated surgically.

Operative Hysteroscopy

Submucosal Fibroids and Endometrial Polyps

Submucosal fibroids and endometrial polyps vary in number, location, and size. When patients have intracavitary pathology, an altered endometrial surface area, increased endometrial fragility and vascularity, endometrial irregularities, and abnormal prostaglandin levels contribute to DUB. Intracavitary lesions can coexist with anovulatory and ovulatory cycles. Office hysteroscopy and saline infusion sonography (SIS) are the most accurate methods to detect intracavitary lesions. Outpatient hysteroscopic myomectomy and polypectomy are quick, safe, and effective treatment modalities and are associated with a high level of patient satisfaction.[8]

Intramural Fibroids

Intramural fibroids also can cause disturbances in menstrual flow. The mechanisms are unclear but may be attributable to topographic endometrial abnormalities, endometrial glandular atrophy overlying the fibroid, venous congestion, increased endometrial surface area, and alteration in prostaglandin levels.

Several treatment options are available for symptomatic intramural fibroids. The treatment decision depends on whether the patient desires to become pregnant or to preserve the uterus. When a woman wishes to remain fertile, an abdominal or laparoscopic myomectomy may be recommended. The surgical route for myomectomy depends on the number, size, and location of the fibroids as well as on the physician's surgical skill.

When pregnancy is not desired and fibroids contribute to heavy menstrual bleeding, the patient can be offered a minimally invasive outpatient procedure called *uterine artery embolization.* Transcutaneous insertion of a catheter through the femoral artery and subsequent occlusion of the uterine artery with Embospheres (Biosphere Medical, Rockland, Mass), polyvinyl alcohol beads, polyvinyl alcohol coils, or Gelfoam causes cessation of blood flow to the fibroid. Shortly thereafter, the fibroid necroses and shrinks. Menorrhagia-related symptoms resolve in 85% to 95% of menorrhagia patients treated with uterine artery embolization.[9]

Hysterectomy offers definitive therapy for patients with uterine fibroids who have completed childbearing and who do not desire to preserve the uterus. Laparoscopic, vaginal, or abdominal hysterectomy are surgical options. Factors influencing the surgical route include the number, sizes, and locations of fibroids; concomitant pelvic pathology; and surgical skill of the physician.

Dilation and curettage is no longer acceptable as the single surgical treatment for menorrhagia or DUB. In the past, this procedure was commonly used to treat menstrual aberrations; however, its inaccuracy often resulted in missed diagnoses, incomplete removal of intracavitary pathology, failure to treat DUB, and high false-negative rates.[10] Operative hysteroscopy coupled with directed hysteroscopic endometrial sampling is the gold standard to evaluate the uterine cavity in the surgical suite. This evaluation can be performed in the presence of heavy bleeding, and coexisting intrauterine pathology can be removed.

Endometrial Ablation

Endometrial ablation is an alternative to hysterectomy for women with DUB. It usually is recommended after unsuccessful medical therapy for women with a normal uterine cavity who have completed childbearing and have a negative laboratory workup. Hysteroscopic and global endometrial ablation procedures destroy the basalis layer of the endometrium, preventing regeneration and thereby altering menstrual flow. This results in Asherman's syndrome, which is characterized by hypomenorrhea, eumenorrhea, or amenorrhea. Endometrial ablation is an outpatient procedure associated with a rapid return to work, minimal complications, and high patient satisfaction rates. Approximately 20% to 30% of patients who undergo endometrial ablation become amenorrheic, 65% to 70% become hypomenorrheic, and 5% to 10% do not respond to treatment.

Medical Treatment

DUB due to anovulatory cycles is best treated medically. Surgery should be reserved for patients who do not respond to medical therapy or for whom medical therapy is contraindicated.

Several medical strategies are effective in treating this disabling condition. Therapy should be individually tailored after a review of the risks, benefits, concerns, and contraindications. Generally, oral contraceptives and progesterone therapy are the mainstays of medical treatment for women who do not desire children.

Danazol therapy creates a hypoestrogenic state and decreases menstrual blood loss by 70% to 80%. A conventional dosing schedule of 400 to 800 mg daily as well as a less-traditional schedule of 50 to 100 mg daily is helpful. Typical side effects of danazol therapy include weight gain, acne, and potential alteration of lipid levels.[11]

Treatment with gonadotropin-releasing hormone (GnRH) (Depo Lupron or Synarel) creates a hypoestrogenic, menopause-like condition. Cessation of menstruation usually occurs within 3 months of initiating therapy. Menopausal symptoms, including hot flushes, night sweats, vaginal dryness, bone loss, joint pain, decreased concentration, and diminished libido, can occur with therapy. Compliance with therapy is generally good, despite these symptoms. Because osteoporosis is the biggest risk of prolonged therapy, treatment is limited to 6 months unless estrogen is added. GnRH is a great option for the woman in late perimenopause who has significant contraindications to other medical therapy. Halting menses is a relief to these patients, and after therapy, many women spontaneously transition into menopause. Additionally, intermittent depot leuprolide (Lupron) therapy in women with uterine fibroids provides a mean additional 9 months of symptom control (range, 2 to >25 mo).[12]

The levonorgestrel-releasing intrauterine system (Mirena) provides another effective treatment option for DUB. This intrauterine device produces a dramatic decline in menstrual blood loss (65%-98%) within 12 months of use. There is little systemic absorption of progesterone. The device, imbedded with 20 μg of levonorgestrel, causes pseudodecidual changes and amenorrhea. It can play an important role in women who have menorrhagia but who also need contraception, have a normal-size uterus, and wish to avoid surgery.[13]

Nonsteroidal anti-inflammatory drugs (NSAIDs) decrease rates of dysmenorrhea and significantly reduce clotting and menstrual blood loss. Some studies have demonstrated a 50% to 80% reduction in blood loss with proper use of NSAIDs.[14] Patients are advised to begin therapy 1 to 2 days before expected menstruation and to continue therapy throughout the menses. NSAID therapy also can be combined with oral contraceptives, if needed.

Oral contraceptives clearly play many roles in the treatment of menorrhagia and DUB. Short-term high-dose therapy is used when excessive bleeding results in an emergency. It successfully stops heavy menstrual bleeding in adolescents and perimenopausal women. Any low-dose (30-35 μg) ethinyl estradiol product can be taken every 6 hours for 5 days to rapidly stop heavy menstrual bleeding. Once bleeding has stabilized, a single daily maintenance dose provides a regular menstrual cycle as well as contraception.

Progesterone therapy is effective in women with anovulatory menstrual cycles. It stabilizes the proliferative endometrium and induces regular sloughing. Cyclic progesterone therapy is useful in women with contraindications to estrogen therapy (women older than 35 years who smoke, have a history of deep venous thrombosis, or have high risk factors for cardiovascular disease). Generally, medroxyprogesterone acetate 10 mg for 10 to 14 days each month induces a regular withdrawal bleed. This dosage does not provide contraception.

Long-acting progesterone therapy in the form of medroxyprogesterone acetate (MDPA) SR (Depo-Provera) stops menses in most patients. Standard dosing involves MDPA 150 mg administered intramuscularly every 3 months. Approximately, 80% to 90% of patients completing 12 months of MDPA therapy become amenorrheic. Side effects can include weight gain, irregular bleeding, and depression.

ACOG practice bulletin guidelines mandate thorough evaluation and medical treatment of noncyclic uterine bleeding. Treatment depends on desire for future fertility, tolerance of medical therapy, age, and severity of symptoms. When medical therapy fails, more-aggressive surgical options are considered.[3]

Clinical Tools to Evaluate the Endometrium

Historically, medical therapy is instituted for 3 months; when response to therapy is unsuccessful, additional evaluation is warranted. These ACOG guidelines are appropriate for hemodynamically stable patients with normal laboratory evaluation. Increasingly, an imaging evaluation is being used with the initial workup.[15]

Endometrial biopsy is generally performed in the office with a pipelle. The procedure can be performed quickly, is associated with few complications, and is generally well tolerated by the patient. Biopsy has a high sensitivity for detecting endometrial cancer and hyperplasia but a low sensitivity for detecting intracavitary lesions, including polyps and submucosal fibroids. Lesions encompassing a small surface area are likely to be missed. The biopsy instrument samples only 10% to 25% of the endometrial cavity. Patients with persistent symptoms despite normal biopsy results need further evaluation.

Transvaginal Ultrasound

Transvaginal ultrasound (TVUS) is extremely helpful in evaluating women with postmenopausal bleeding. TVUS permits rapid assessment of size, position, and presence of uterine fibroids. Adnexal pathology can be assessed. The endometrial echo measurement is critical in evaluating the health of the endometrium. If uterine size is greater than 12 gestational weeks, then transabdominal scanning is preferred. Measurement of the endometrial echo in the postmenopausal woman is very helpful in determining whether endometrial biopsy or further imaging studies are necessary. Normally, the endometrial echo measures less than 5 mm. Increased endometrial thickness is associated with endometrial hyperplasia, endometrial polyps, fibroids, and endometrial cancer. When the endometrial echo is greater than 5 mm or is indistinct or indeterminate, an enhanced view is required with SIS or hysteroscopy. An endometrial echo of less than 5 mm is associated with malignancy in less than 0.5% of cases.

Saline-Infusion Sonography

SIS infuses saline into the endometrial cavity during TVUS to enhance the image. (This technique is also called echohysteroscopy, hydrosonography, sonohysterography, sonohysterogram, sonohysterosalinogography, and sonoendovaginal ultrasound. The term *saline-infusion sonography* provides a more exact definition of the technique.[15]) SIS allows the clinician to evaluate the uterus for intracavitary lesions more accurately than TVUS. Causes of increased endometrial thickness can be clearly differentiated with saline infusion.

Current indications for SIS include abnormal bleeding in premenopausal or postmenopausal patients; evaluation of an endometrium that is thickened, irregular, immeasurable, or poorly defined on conventional TVUS; irregular-appearing endometrium with TVUS in women using tamoxifen; the need to differentiate between sessile and pedunculated masses of the endometrium; and presurgical evaluation of intracavitary fibroids.

Hysteroscopy

Thin operative hysteroscopes with outer diameter sizes ranging from 3 to 5 mm can easily and comfortably be used in the office. Hysteroscopy permits full visualization of the endometrial cavity and endocervix. Rapid visual inspection permits accurate diagnosis of atrophy, endometrial hyperplasia, polyps, fibroids, and endometrial cancer. Direct endometrial biopsies are possible with some hysteroscopes. When the endometrial cavity is normal, aggressive medical therapy can be considered.

OUTCOMES

DUB is usually well categorized after the initial history, physical examination, and laboratory evaluation. Medical management is the mainstay unless uterine pathology is present. Patients with intrauterine polyps and submucosal fibroids have excellent relief of symptoms following operative hysteroscopy. Surgical therapy with endometrial ablation offers 90% success for treating menorrhagia and dysfunctional bleeding in women with a normal uterine cavity who do not desire children but have negative workup results. Fortunately, hysterectomy is the last resort for DUB in this era of many alternative medical and surgical treatments.

Summary

- The evaluation of abnormal uterine bleeding requires a complete physical examination, detailed medical history, and laboratory testing.
- The endometrial cavity can be evaluated with office hysteroscopy or saline infusion sonography.
- Uterine fibroid embolization is an excellent alternative to hysterectomy in appropriately triaged patients.
- Dilation and curettage is no longer the first choice for evaluating the endometrial cavity.
- The levonorgestrel intrauterine system provides an excellent means to control abnormal uterine bleeding in patients with a normal uterine cavity.

Suggested Readings

American College of Obstetricians and Gynecologists: ACOG Practice Bulletin. Clinical management guidelines for obstetrician-gynecologists number 34, February 2002. Management of infertility caused by ovulatory dysfunction. Obstet Gynecol 2002;99(2):347-358.

American College of Obstetricians and Gynecologists: ACOG Practice Bulletin. Management of anovulatory bleeding. Int J Gynaecol Obstet 2001;72(3):263-271.

American College of Obstetricians and Gynecologists Committee on Gynecologic Practice: Committee Opinion: no. 263, December 2001. von Willebrand's disease in gynecologic practice. Obstet Gynecol 2001;98:1185-1186.

Bettocchi S, Ceci O, Vicino M, et al: Diagnostic inadequacy of dilatation and curettage. Fertil Steril 2001;75:803-805.

Carlson KJ, Nichols DH, Schiff I: Indications for hysterectomy. N Engl J Med 1993;328:856-860.

Claessens EA, Cowell CA: Acute adolescent menorrhagia. Am J Obstet Gynecol 1981;139:277-280.

Hurskainen R, Teperi J, Rissanen P, et al: Quality of life and cost-effectiveness of levonorgestrel-releasing intrauterine system versus hysterectomy for treatment of menorrhagia: A randomised trial. Lancet 2001;357:273-277.

Hurst BS, Stackhouse DJ, Matthews ML, Marshburn PB: Uterine artery embolization for symptomatic uterine myomas. Fertil Steril 2000;74:855-869.

Jones H: Clinical pathway for evaluating women with abnormal uterine bleeding. Obstet Gynecol Surv 2002;57:22-24.

Pasqualotto EB, Margossian H, Price LL, Bradley LD: Accuracy of preoperative diagnostic tools and outcome of hysteroscopic management of menstrual dysfunction. J Am Assoc Gynecol Laparosc 2000;7:201-209.

Scialli AR, Levi AJ: Intermittent leuprolide acetate for the nonsurgical management of women with leiomyomata uteri. Fertil Steril 2000;74:540-546.

Stabinsky SA, Einstein M, Breen JL: Modern treatments of menorrhagia attributable to dysfunctional uterine bleeding. Obstet Gynecol Surv 1999;54:61-72.

Vargyas JM, Campeau JD, Mishell DR Jr: Treatment of menorrhagia with meclofenamate sodium. Am J Obstet Gynecol 1987;157:944-950.

Widrich T, Bradley LD, Mitchinson AR, Collins RL: Comparison of saline infusion sonography with office hysteroscopy for the evaluation of the endometrium. Am J Obstet Gynecol 1996;174:1327-1334.

References

For a complete list of references, log onto www.expertconsult.com.

Polycystic Ovary Syndrome

Marjan Attaran

Polycystic ovary syndrome (PCOS) is the most commonly encountered endocrinopathy in women of reproductive age. It has significant reproductive and nonreproductive consequences.[1] Women of any ethnic background can present with PCOS. In a prospective study of 400 women of reproductive age, 4% to 4.7% of white women and 3.4% of African American women had PCOS.[2] A similar rate of 4% to 6% has been found in other populations. Because patients with PCOS can present with an assortment of complaints such as menstrual disturbances, infertility, hirsutism, and acne, their point of entry into the medical system may be by way of a primary care physician, gynecologist, endocrinologist, or dermatologist. Thus, all these disciplines need to be familiar with this syndrome and its long-term consequences.

DEFINITION AND DIAGNOSIS

Historically, there has been a lack of consensus regarding the features that define PCOS. A meeting convened by the National Institutes of Health (NIH) in 1990 stressed three key features necessary for the diagnosis of PCOS: The patient must exhibit ovulatory dysfunction; there must be evidence of clinical hyperandrogenism or biochemical hyperandrogenemia; and other disorders must be excluded, such as nonclassic congenital adrenal hyperplasia, androgen-secreting tumors, and hyperprolactinemia or thyroid disorders.

Because 16% to 25% of the normal population has polycystic-appearing ovaries on ultrasound,[3] the presence of polycystic ovaries was considered to be suggestive but not diagnostic of PCOS. However, the Rotterdam European Society of Human Reproduction/American Society for Reproductive Medicine (ESHRE/ASRM)-Sponsored PCOS Consensus Workshop Group that convened in 2003 now requires the existence of two of the following three criteria to make the diagnosis of PCOS[4]: oligo-ovulation or anovulation, clinical or biochemical signs of hyperandrogenism, and polycystic ovaries.

Even after these criteria have been met, other potential causes of hyperandrogenism must be excluded. To exclude congenital adrenal hyperplasia, a basal early-morning level of 17-α hydroxyprogesterone is performed in the follicular phase. Total testosterone level may be evaluated to rule out an androgen-secreting tumor. Although luteinizing hormone (LH) levels are high in most women with PCOS, the Rotterdam consensus panel considered it unnecessary to assess the LH level routinely. Free testosterone and dehydroepiandrosterone sulfate (DHEAS) levels may be checked when clinical suspicion is high for PCOS but the patient does not exhibit clinical signs of hyperandrogenism.

PATHOPHYSIOLOGY

The basic pathophysiologic defect is unknown in PCOS; however, because this disorder tends to cluster in families, a genetic cause is believed likely. Hyperandrogenism is a common finding in first-degree relatives of women with PCOS. The rates of PCOS in mothers and sisters of patients with PCOS were 24% and 32%, respectively.[5] Increased insulin resistance has been noted in mothers and sisters of women with PCOS.[6] Several large research groups are actively searching for a genetic cause of this syndrome. The mode of inheritance is uncertain at this point, and the role of shared environmental factors such as diet and lifestyle in the manifestation of the disease is unknown. Loci proposed and investigated as possible PCOS genes include *CYP11A*, the insulin gene, and a region near the insulin-receptor gene.[7] The wide range of PCOS symptoms likely plays a significant role in the inability thus far to identify a specific gene mutation.

Although the pathophysiology of PCOS is not clear, a variety of biochemical abnormalities have been described with this syndrome. Hyperinsulinemia is noted in 50% to 70% of PCOS patients. It is defined as impaired action of insulin on glucose transport and antilipolysis in adipocytes in the presence of normal insulin binding. Hyperinsulinemia causes or exacerbates hyperandrogenemia. Increased insulin levels at the ovarian level lead to increased androgen production from the ovarian thecal cells. In an in vitro model, Nestler and colleagues[8] demonstrated increased testosterone production by theca cells of women with PCOS exposed to insulin compared with testosterone production from the theca cells of normal women. Also, by suppressing hepatic production of sex hormone binding globulin (SHBG), insulin increases unbound levels of testosterone. At the level of the granulosa cell, insulin amplifies the response of granulosa cells to LH. Thus, these cells undergo abnormal differentiation and premature arrest of follicular growth, and thus anovulation.

Elevated androgen levels also lead to decreased levels of SHBG. Greater unbound androgen levels are likely to produce a greater clinical response, such as hirsutism and acne. Most patients with PCOS show evidence of clinical hyperandrogenism. However, a small fraction does not, which might warrant a biochemical investigation. In such cases, measurement of free testosterone should be considered, although most direct assays for free testosterone have limited value for evaluating the hyperandrogenic woman. The methods recommended at the consensus meeting to determine free testosterone are by equilibrium dialysis, by calculation of free testosterone from measurement of SHBG and total testosterone, or by ammonium sulfate precipitation. DHEAS may be measured, because a small percentage of patients with PCOS have isolated elevations in this hormone. However, there were not enough data for the consensus meeting to support the routine measurement of androstenedione.

Another key feature of PCOS is altered gonadotropin dynamics. Several studies have shown higher LH pulse and amplitude in women with PCOS.[9] Although a higher LH level drives the ovarian theca cells to produce more androgens, insufficient follicle-stimulating hormone (FSH) may be the more immediate cause of anovulation. In most women with PCOS, LH levels are elevated or the LH/FSH ratio is high; however, the mean LH pulse amplitude is attenuated in obese women with PCOS.[10] Thus, the LH value or LH/FSH ratio is not helpful in establishing this diagnosis in such patients.

SIGNS AND SYMPTOMS

PCOS symptoms have a gradual onset. Although symptoms of PCOS can exist at the time of menarche, most patients do not seek help until their early to mid 20s.

Menstrual Irregularities and Reproductive Issues

Abnormal vaginal bleeding is a typical complaint that ranges from amenorrhea to oligomenorrhea to menorrhagia and metrorrhagia. Because patients with PCOS experience irregular and incomplete endometrial shedding, endometrial hyperplasia and cancer must be aggressively ruled out; thus, an endometrial biopsy should be considered. Adults with prolonged episodes of bleeding unresponsive to treatment and those with irregular bleeding and long durations of amenorrhea should undergo endometrial biopsy regardless of their age. Other studies, such as ultrasound of the uterus and endometrial lining, can assist with this decision. About 15% to 30% of women with PCOS claim to have regular periods despite documented anovulation.

Because these patients are anovulatory, they present with infertility issues. They can also have increased incidence of pregnancy loss and pregnancy complications.[11,12] Spontaneous abortion occurs in one third of all pregnancies in women with PCOS, which is double the rate of normal women. After pregnancy is established, perinatal mortality is increased at least 1.5 times.[13] Pregnancy complications can include gestational diabetes, pregnancy-induced hypertension, and increased rate of intrauterine fetal demise. Currently, it is unclear whether PCOS independent of obesity leads to poor obstetric outcome. In a case-control study, Haakova and colleagues compared the pregnancy outcomes of a group of women with PCOS with those of a group of healthy weight-matched women. The investigators were unable to show a higher rate of pregnancy complications in the PCOS group.[14]

Skin Manifestations

Depending on ethnic background, skin manifestations vary. Compared with Asian women, Middle Eastern or Mediterranean women are more likely to complain of hirsutism. Other women's primary skin complaint may be acne. Excessive growth of terminal hair is noted on the upper lip, sideburn areas, chin, and periareolar, abdominal, back, and buttock areas. Signs of virilization are lacking. In some cases, there is evidence of alopecia, which can be extremely disturbing to patients. Other dermatologic findings include acanthosis nigricans and skin tags, which may be manifestations of insulin resistance.

Obesity and Metabolic Abnormalities

Although the prevalence of obesity is high in patients with PCOS, in large series the rate varies. Depending on the series, the rate of obesity in the PCOS population ranges from 38% to 87%.[15] Variables that can influence this number include diagnostic criteria and geographic and environmental factors. Because obesity is associated with insulin resistance, many women with PCOS have insulin resistance, but insulin resistance in PCOS is independent of obesity. Dunaif and colleagues showed that the insulin sensitivity of nonobese women with PCOS approached that of obese controls. Obese women with PCOS had higher insulin resistance than cycling obese women in the control group.[16]

PCOS patients are at higher risk for the metabolic syndrome, which is a group of cardiovascular risk factors that include dyslipidemia, type 2 diabetes mellitus, hypertension, and obesity. In a study of 254 women with PCOS, the prevalence of impaired glucose tolerance was 31% compared with 10.3% in controls, and the prevalence of type 2 diabetes was 7.5 % compared with 1.5% in controls.[17] At the Rotterdam PCOS consensus workshop, three of the five criteria in Table 1 were considered necessary for a diagnosis of the metabolic syndrome.

Table 1 Criteria for the Diagnosis of Metabolic Syndrome

Risk Factor	Cutoff
Abdominal obesity	>88 cm
Triglycerides	≥150 mg/dL
High-density lipoprotein cholesterol	<50 mg/dL
Blood pressure	≥130/≥85 mm Hg
Fasting and 2-h glucose levels from oral glucose tolerance test	110-126 mg/dL and/or 2-hr glucose 140-199 mg/dL

Adapted from Rotterdam ESHRE/ASRM-Sponsored PCOS Consensus Workshop Group: Revised 2003 consensus on diagnostic criteria and long-term health risks related to polycystic ovary syndrome. Fertil Steril 2004;81:19-25.

TREATMENT

Treatment is typically directed at the manifesting symptoms of PCOS. Several treatment options are available, but few randomized trials exist to help provide a clear treatment guideline.

Lifestyle Modification

In conjunction with medical therapy, focus should be directed at lifestyle modification by diet and exercise if the patient is overweight. Even small amounts of weight loss have established menstrual cyclicity, increased spontaneous ovulation and pregnancy rates, and increased sensitivity to ovulation-induction medications.[18] Also, the rate of miscarriages decreased and live births increased.[19] A significant impact on the metabolic consequences of PCOS is also expected with weight loss, because insulin and triglyceride levels decrease and high-density lipoprotein cholesterol increases.

Oral Contraceptive Pills

Oral contraceptive pills are typically the first line of therapy for management of irregular bleeding in women with PCOS who are not interested in conception. Cyclic withdrawal of estrogen and progesterone leads to complete endometrial shedding and resolution of most abnormal bleeding. Exposure to the progestin in oral contraceptives leads to reduction in the risk of endometrial cancer and hyperplasia. In addition, the steroids cause a decrease in LH levels and a subsequent decrease in androgen production. Finally, they also increase SHBG production, and the resulting decreased free testosterone levels lead to diminished hirsutism and acne.

Antiandrogens

If the degrees of hirsutism and acne are significant, antiandrogens are used. Although they are slow to show results (a minimum of 6-9 mo), a significant change in thickness of the hair shaft and reduction of sexual hair growth can be seen. Spironolactone, up to 200 mg/day, is the most common antiandrogen used in PCOS patients in the United States. Moghetti and colleagues[20] demonstrated that there is no difference in the effectiveness of spironolactone, flutamide, or finasteride. Because of their possible impact on the development of a male fetus, they are rarely used alone. Usually they are given in conjunction with oral contraceptive pills.

Ovulation-Induction Agents

Ovulation can be induced with clomiphene citrate in more than 80% of anovulatory patients. This drug is typically the first line of therapy, although pregnancy rates are only about 40%. Other agents that may be used to induce follicular growth and subsequent ovulation include insulin-sensitizing agents, exogenous gonadotropins, and aromatase inhibitors.

Insulin-Sensitizing Agents

These agents increase tissue sensitivity to insulin action. Metformin is a biguanide drug that has traditionally been used to manage frank diabetes. It is believed to increase peripheral glucose uptake, and because it does not precipitate hyperinsulinemia, it does not cause hypoglycemia. A review of the literature[21] shows that on average, body mass index decreased by 4% and androgen levels decreased by 20% with metformin compared with placebo. However, this does not translate into a significant impact on hirsutism.

Metformin regularizes menstrual cyclicity, typically within 3 months of initiating the drug. If ovulation has not been induced within 3 months of initiating metformin in anovulatory infertile women, clomiphene citrate is typically added to the regimen. Several studies show higher ovulation rates in patients on metformin and clomiphene citrate than rates achieved with placebo or with clomiphene citrate alone.[22,23] Currently, there is no clear consensus on whether all patients with PCOS should initially undergo a trial of metformin to induce ovulation or whether they should take metformin only after clomiphene citrate has failed to induce ovulation. A 2003 Cochrane review on the use of insulin-sensitizing agents in patients with PCOS concludes that metformin is justified as first-line therapy for ovulation induction.[24]

Another area of potential controversy is the use of metformin solely for restoring menstrual cyclicity. Because metformin does not consistently lead to regular periods, it cannot be recommended as the first line of therapy for this symptom; oral contraceptives are still considered the first line of therapy for cyclic endometrial shedding. However, because oral contraceptives can exacerbate insulin resistance, metformin may be considered for morbidly obese women who are at significant risk for insulin resistance.

A review of the literature indicates that use of metformin in women with PCOS decreased fasting insulin levels, low-density lipoprotein, and blood pressure.[24] However, because of the lack of long-term data, it is unknown whether these changes translate into a decreased likelihood of cardiovascular disease and diabetes. Hence other pharmacologic interventions may be necessary, as directed by an internist, to address the specific metabolic abnormality. Finally, metformin cannot be advocated as a replacement for exercise and diet modification. The Diabetes Prevention Program Research Group demonstrated that although metformin significantly reduces the frequency of type 2 diabetes in nondiabetic patients who have high serum glucose concentrations, exercise has a greater impact in reducing the incidence of diabetes.[25]

Metformin is used in doses of 1500 to 2000 mg/day. Gastrointestinal symptoms are its main side effects and include nausea, vomiting, diarrhea, and flatulence. These symptoms are typically transient. Gradual increase of the dose can decrease these side effects. This medication is contraindicated in women with hepatic or renal impairment and in those with conditions that increase the risk of lactic acidosis.

LAPAROSCOPIC OVARIAN DRILLING

Laparoscopic ovarian drilling is the modern version of the ovarian wedge resection. The premise is destruction of stromal tissue leading to decreased androgen production and subsequent change in the hormonal profile. Testosterone levels decrease and LH levels seem to drop after ovarian drilling. Hirsutism has been noted to improve for up to 9 years. Ovulatory rates of up to 74% and pregnancy rates of 50% to 70% have been reported.[26] Because these results are similar to those noted with metformin, it may be more prudent to proceed with metformin therapy initially in anovulatory women not at risk for tubal factor infertility. Laparoscopy carries the inherent risks associated with surgery. In addition, this procedure may be associated with subsequent periadnexal adhesions.

OUTCOMES

Awareness has developed of some of the long-term implications of PCOS that extend well into the postmenopausal years. The physician is responsible not only for offering medical treatment options but also for educating the patient regarding the possible long-term consequences of the syndrome.

Endometrial Cancer

Women with PCOS have chronic anovulation. The endometrial lining is exposed to unopposed estrogen for long durations. These patients are believed to be at increased risk for endometrial cancer. However, there is minimal epidemiologic evidence to support this theory.[27]

Diabetes

There is clear evidence that women with PCOS have an increased likelihood of impaired glucose tolerance and are at increased risk for type 2 diabetes mellitus.[17] Women with PCOS who have a family history or are obese are at even greater risk for developing diabetes. Unfortunately, fasting glucose concentration is a poor predictor of diabetes in this population. However, impaired glucose tolerance is known to be a risk factor for the development of frank diabetes. Because the prevalence of impaired glucose tolerance and diabetes is high in obese PCOS patients,[7] the Rotterdam PCOS consensus group advises performing a screening 2-hour oral glucose tolerance test in obese women.

Cardiovascular Disease

Cardiovascular risk factors are increased in patients with PCOS when compared with weight-matched controls.[28] High-density lipoprotein cholesterol levels are lower and triglyceride levels and very-low-density lipoprotein cholesterol are higher.[29] Several studies on women with PCOS seem to demonstrate an increase in blood pressure. However, blood pressure is affected by a variety of factors that include weight, genetics, and stress. Thus, it is not clear whether lean insulin-resistant women with PCOS are also at higher risk for developing hypertension. An increase in coronary artery calcification has also been reported in women with PCOS.[30]

It has been very difficult to sort out the individual effects of PCOS and obesity on cardiovascular risk factors, because obesity can negatively affect blood pressure, the lipid profile, and insulin resistance. All these factors are believed to lead to a higher incidence of cardiac events in women with PCOS. However, despite these risk factors, there is no consistent epidemiologic evidence that these patients in fact do have an increased incidence of coronary heart disease.[31,32]

Summary

- Patients with PCOS can present with an assortment of complaints such as menstrual disturbances, infertility, hirsutism, and acne. Their point of entry into the medical system may be from their primary care physician, gynecologist, endocrinologist, or dermatologist.
- Between 15% and 30% of women with PCOS claim to have regular periods despite documented anovulation.
- Even small amounts of weight loss have established menstrual cyclicity, increased spontaneous ovulation and pregnancy rates, and increased sensitivity to ovulation-induction medications.
- Oral contraceptive pills are typically the first line of therapy for managing irregular bleeding in women with PCOS who are not interested in conception.
- The physician is responsible for educating the patient regarding the possible long-term consequences of the syndrome. These include endometrial cancer, diabetes, and cardiovascular disease.

Suggested Readings

Carmina E, Lobo RA: Polycystic ovary syndrome (PCOS): Arguably the most common endocrinopathy is associated with significant morbidity in women. J Clin Endocrinol Metab 1999;84:1897-1899.

Franks S: Polycystic ovary syndrome. N Engl J Med 1995;333:853-861.

Hardiman P, Pillay OC, Atiomo W: Polycystic ovary syndrome and endometrial carcinoma. Lancet 2003;361:1810-1812.

Heard MJ, Pierce A, Carson SA, Buster JE: Pregnancies following use of metformin for ovulation induction in patients with polycystic ovary syndrome. Fertil Steril 2002;77:669-673.

Hoeger K: Obesity and weight loss in polycystic ovary syndrome. Obstet Gynecol Clin North Am 2001;28:85-97.

Knowler WC, Barrett-Connor E, Fowler SE, et al; Diabetes Prevention Program Research Group: Reduction in the incidence of type 2 diabetes with lifestyle intervention or metformin. N Engl J Med 2002;346:393-403.

Polson DW, Wadsworth J, Adams J, et al: Polycystic ovaries: A common finding in normal women. Lancet 1988;1:870-872.

Rotterdam ESHRE/ASRM-Sponsored PCOS Consensus Workshop Group: Revised 2003 consensus on diagnostic criteria and long-term health risks related to polycystic ovary syndrome. Fertil Steril 2004;81:19-25.

Talbott E, Guzick D, Clerici A, et al: Coronary heart disease risk factors in women with polycystic ovary syndrome. Arterioscler Thromb Vasc Biol 1995;15:821-826.

Wild RA: Long-term health consequences of PCOS. Hum Reprod Update 2002;8:231-241.

References

For a complete list of references, log onto www.expertconsult.com.

Premenstrual Dysphoric Disorder

Gurjit Kaur

DEFINITION AND ETIOLOGY

Premenstrual dysphoric disorder (PMDD) is a severe form of premenstrual syndrome (PMS) that causes marked social impairment in approximately 5 of 100 women. Women present with multiple physical and behavioral symptoms including fatigue, irritability, bloating, anxiety, breast tenderness, and mood lability which occur exclusively in the 10 to 14 days before menses. The exact cause of PMDD is unknown, but it is believed that the normal cyclic fluctuation of hormone levels in the menstrual cycle leads to symptoms.

PREVALENCE AND RISK FACTORS

PMS is a common condition that affects as many as 75% of menstruating women. It is characterized by a myriad of physical and behavioral symptoms that occur repetitively in the luteal phase of the menstrual cycle. Women with PMS often describe feelings of anger, fatigue, abdominal bloating, irritability, anxiety, breast tenderness, changes in appetite and sleep, and headaches. These symptoms usually do not preclude a woman from performing her day-to-day activities.

On the other hand, a very small subgroup of women (3%-8%)[1] in their late 20s to mid-30s suffer from a severe form of PMS that is serious enough to interfere with their daily functioning and personal relationships. These women suffer from PMDD, a condition first defined in 1987 in the *Diagnostic and Statistical Manual of Mental Disorders* (DSM-III-R) and subsequently modified in 2000 in the manual's fourth revised text edition (DSM IV-TR).

Some women are more prone to PMDD, including women in their 20s to mid-30s,[2] women with a prior history of mood disorders[3] and women with low parity (fewer pregnancies lead to additional hormone exposure from more menstrual cycles).[4] Genetic and psychosocial factors may also cause increased risk to develop PMDD.[3]

PATHOPHYSIOLOGY

A number of theories have been suggested to explain PMDD, but the most current theory suggests that cyclic changes in ovarian steroids interact with central neurotransmitters to create symptoms of PMDD.[3] In other words, normal ovarian function rather than hormone imbalance is the inciting factor for PMDD-related biochemical events in the central nervous system.[3,5] Serotonin is the neurotransmitter most studied in PMDD, although there is likely a role for gamma-aminobutyric acid (GABA) and β-endorphin. Deficiencies of trace elements may also be implicated.

Ovarian Steroids

In 1984, Muse and associates[6] studied the effects of medical ovariectomy using the gonadotropin-releasing hormone (GnRH) agonist leuprolide, which led to resolution of symptoms by eliminating the fluctuation of ovarian hormones. In the 6-month study of eight patients, symptoms resolved with GnRH treatment, but recurred when the medication was withdrawn.[6] However, cyclic changes in ovarian steroids may not be the sole explanation for symptoms in PMDD. Estrogen and progesterone levels of control subjects and women with premenstrual symptoms have been shown to be the same, suggesting that affected women may have an abnormal response to normal hormone levels.[6]

Neurotransmitters

The three main neurotransmitters implicated in PMDD are serotonin, GABA, and β-endorphin. Evidence currently suggests a leading role for altered serotonin levels in the etiology of PMDD. Central serotonin levels are typically low in women with PMDD, and symptoms worsen with depletion of the serotonin precursor tryptophan.[7,8] Notably, many women report benefiting from selective serotonin reuptake inhibitors (SSRIs). The role of GABA has not been clearly defined, but some women improve with the GABA agonist alprazolam. Differences in β-endorphin levels between the periovulatory and premenstrual phases remain unconfirmed.

Vitamins and Minerals

Several attempts to link vitamin and mineral deficiencies with PMDD have been inconclusive. No observable differences have been found in levels of vitamin A, vitamin E, or vitamin B_6 in affected or unaffected women. Treatment with vitamin B_6 supplements has shown inconsistent results. Additionally, initial studies suggested that women with PMDD may have lower levels of magnesium,[9] although subsequent studies have not confirmed this finding.[10] Calcium levels may also be low in the premenstrual phase.[11]

DIAGNOSIS

PMDD is accurately diagnosed with a thorough history and physical examination and by excluding other causes for the patient's symptoms. The history must review psychiatric disorders in the patient and her family. The clinician should distinguish PMDD from other psychiatric disorders with premenstrual exacerbation. Symptoms should be limited to the luteal phase (second half) of the menstrual cycle, and the patient must be symptom free in the follicular phase (first half). Symptoms also must be of such magnitude that they markedly impair the woman's day-to-day functioning. Women must also not be on hormones, including oral contraceptives.

DSM-IV Criteria

The DSM-IV criteria published in 2000 by the American Psychiatric Association are most commonly used for the diagnosis of PMDD. The presence of five or more of the following symptoms, which must be documented by the patient in most menstrual cycles during the past 12 months, is required to make the diagnosis of PMDD. These symptoms must be present most of the time in the week before menses and resolve in the first few days after menses begins. Also, one of the five symptoms must be one of the first four listed.[12]

- Marked depression with feelings of hopelessness
- Marked anxiety or tension (patient feels wound up or on edge)
- Marked affective lability (patient gets tearful suddenly or becomes more sensitive)
- Irritability, anger, and increased interpersonal conflicts
- Decreased interest in activities of daily living, which may include social withdrawal (work, school, friends, or family)
- Fatigue and decreased energy level
- Appetite changes (overeating or cravings)

Box 1 Criteria for the Diagnosis of Premenstrual Dysphoric Disorder

Symptoms begin 1 wk before menses and resolve in the first few days after menses begins (must occur during most menstrual cycles in the past 1 year).

One of the five symptoms must be one of the first four on the following list:

- Depressed mood with feelings of hopelessness
- Anxiety or tension
- Affective lability
- Irritability and anger
- Decreased interest in usual activities and social withdrawal
- Lack of energy (fatigue)
- Appetite changes (overeating/undereating)
- Changes in sleep pattern (hypersomnia/insomnia)
- Feeling out of control or overwhelmed
- Difficulty with concentration
- Somatic symptoms such as bloating, mastalgia, or headaches

Symptoms must be severe enough to interfere with work, school, usual activities, or interpersonal relationships.

Symptoms may be superimposed on an underlying psychiatric disorder, although they may not be an exacerbation of another condition.

Criteria A, B, C, and D must be confirmed by prospective daily charting for a minimum of two consecutive symptomatic menstrual cycles.

Modified with permission from Diagnostic and Statistical Manual of Mental Disorders: DSM IV-TR, 4th ed. Washington, DC, American Psychiatric Association, 2000.

- Hypersomnia or insomnia
- Feeling out of control or overwhelmed
- Difficulty with concentration
- Somatic symptoms such as abdominal bloating, breast tenderness, headaches, or joint pain

Additionally, symptoms must be severe enough to interfere with one's usual activities and relationships and should be confirmed by prospective daily charting for at least two to three menstrual cycles. The clinician should also be aware that symptoms may be superimposed on an underlying psychiatric disorder, although the symptoms may not be an exacerbation of another disorder (Box 1).[12]

Symptom Inventory

Several questionnaires can be used to record symptoms of PMDD, such as the Calendar of Premenstrual Experiences (COPE), the Moos Menstrual Distress Questionnaire (MDQ), the Premenstrual Assessment Form (PAF), and the Prospective Record of the Impact and Severity of Menstruation (PRISM). These forms are similar and are all cited in the literature. The patient should be advised to record her symptoms for at least 2 to 3 months using one of the symptom inventory forms to observe fluctuation of symptoms during the menstrual cycle. It has been suggested that there must be at least a 30% worsening of symptoms between the follicular and luteal phases in each cycle to diagnose PMDD, regardless of which assessment tool is used. The percentage of worsening is calculated by the formula.[3]

$$(\text{luteal score} - \text{follicular score})/\text{luteal score} \times 100 = \%\ \text{change}$$

If no symptom-free period is present, it may be useful to refer the patient to a women's health psychiatrist to evaluate for a mood or anxiety disorder.

Differential Diagnosis

Because PMDD is a diagnosis of exclusion, the clinician should rule out other conditions that may manifest similar signs or symptoms (Box 2).

Box 2 Differential Diagnosis of PMDD

Thyroid disorders
Migraines
Chronic fatigue syndrome
Irritable bowel syndrome (IBS)
Seizures
Anemia
Endometriosis
Psychiatric disorders
Substance abuse, including drugs and alcohol

Diagnostic Testing

No objective testing exists, but laboratory testing should include a complete blood count, chemistry profile, and thyroid-stimulating hormone to evaluate for anemia, electrolyte abnormalities, and thyroid problems, respectively.

Summary

- PMDD is a clinical diagnosis made after excluding other conditions.
- DSM-IV criteria are used for diagnosis.
- A symptom diary for at least 2 to 3 months is necessary to determine when symptoms occur (follicular or luteal phase of the menstrual cycle).
- Laboratory testing is useful to exclude anemia, electrolyte abnormalities, and thyroid problems.

TREATMENT

Multiple treatment options are available for PMDD; however, no single intervention is effective for all women. Initial treatment should begin with lifestyle changes and then proceed to medications such as SSRIs (standard); anxiolytics (alprazolam and buspirone); ovulation suppressants (GnRH agonists, danazol, and oral contraceptive pills [OCPs]); and diuretics (Box 3). Radical treatment such as ovariectomy may be indicated in women refractory to medical treatment. Three studies have demonstrated complete resolution of symptoms in PMDD-affected patients after ovariectomy.[13-15] When considering ovariectomy in women of childbearing age, the clinician should remember that this drastic measure can increase the risks of cardiovascular disease and osteoporosis in the absence of adequate estrogen replacement therapy.

Lifestyle Modifications

Treatment should begin with a 2- to 3-month trial of lifestyle changes while the patient charts her symptoms. Dietary changes, such as reducing salt, sugar, caffeine, dairy products, and alcohol, often aid in decreasing fluid retention, irritability, and bloating. Eating frequent and small portions high in carbohydrates may improve symptoms; this is believed to occur by increasing relative tryptophan levels (a precursor in the serotonin pathway). Exercise, relaxation, and stress management also are recommended for a general state of well-being. Some women also benefit from yoga, which improves muscle flexibility and alleviates stress. If possible, women also can try to schedule their more challenging and stressful events during the follicular phase (as opposed to the luteal phase).

Selective Serotonin Reuptake Inhibitors

SSRIs are considered first-line pharmacologic treatment for PMDD. Studies have shown that intermittent luteal-phase dosing has

Box 3 Medications for Premenstrual Dysphoric Disorder

Selective serotonin reuptake inhibitors (first line)

- Fluoxetine (Prozac, Sarafem) 10 to 20 mg/day or 90 mg once a wk for 2 wk in the luteal phase
- Sertraline (Zoloft) 50 to 150 mg/day
- Paroxetine CR (Paxil CR) 12.5 to 37.5 mg/day

Other serotoninergic antidepressants

- Venlafaxine (Effexor) 50 to 150 mg/day
- Clomipramine (Anafranil) 25 to 75 mg/day

Other agents
Alprazolam (Xanax) 0.25 mg three to four times daily in the luteal phase, taper at the onset of menses
Buspirone (BuSpar) 5 to 10 mg three times daily during the luteal phase
Leuprolide (Lupron) depot 3.75 mg IM/mo
Danazol (Danocrine) 600 to 800 mg/day in divided doses
Bromocriptine (Parlodel) 2.5 mg once daily just before ovulation until the onset of menses
Spironolactone (Aldactone) 50 to 100 mg/day for 7 to 10 days during the luteal phase
Drospirenone (Yasmin)
Meclofenamate (Meclomen) 100 mg twice a day at the onset of menses

fewer adverse effects and is just as effective as full-cycle dosing.[16-18] SSRIs have proved to be effective in more than 60% of treated patients.[19]

FDA-approved options for daily luteal-phase dosing include fluoxetine 10 to 20 mg/day, sertraline 50 to 150 mg/day, and paroxetine CR 12.5 to 37.5 mg/day. A recent study showed that fluoxetine may be efficacious when given at a dose of 90 mg once weekly for two weeks in the luteal phase.[20]

Side effects of SSRIs include sexual dysfunction, insomnia, fatigue, nervousness, headache, nausea, and diarrhea. These agents have a fast onset of action: 1 to 2 days in the treatment of PMDD as compared with their onset of action for depression.

Alprazolam

Alprazolam, a GABA agonist, is a benzodiazepine anxiolytic that is effective for symptoms such as tension, anxiety, irritability, and hostility. Treatment can be initiated at 0.25 mg three to four times daily in the luteal phase and tapered one to two times daily at the onset of menses, finally stopping 1 to 2 days after menses begin. It is considered a second-line treatment because of its addictive potential.

Buspirone

Buspirone, a partial 5-HT_1 receptor agonist, has also been shown to be effective because of its anxiolytic properties. Unlike alprazolam, it is not addictive. Dosing may be given at 5 to 10 mg three times daily during the luteal phase.

GnRH Agonists

GnRH agonists are also effective in reducing PMDD symptoms. They downregulate GnRH receptors, causing a decrease in luteinizing hormone and follicle-stimulating hormone levels. This subsequently inhibits ovulation, which decreases estrogen and progesterone levels, thereby creating pharmacologic menopause. Treatment-limiting side effects include hot flashes, headaches, muscle aches, vaginal dryness, and irritability; therefore, this class of medication is reserved for patients with severe symptoms unresponsive to other medical treatment measures. GnRH agonists are expensive; they also have hypoestrogenic side effects, which cause concern for the development of osteoporosis. For this reason, they are not recommended for use longer than 6 months. If a GnRH agonist needs to be used for longer than 6 months, continued symptom relief can be provided by using add-back therapy with estrogen and progesterone.[21]

Danazol

Danazol is a weak synthetic androgen that suppresses ovarian steroid production by inhibiting luteinizing hormone and follicle-stimulating hormone secretion. It is given at 600 to 800 mg/day in divided doses. Danazol's use is limited because of multiple androgenic and antiestrogenic side effects, including amenorrhea, weight gain, acne, fluid retention, hirsutism, hot flushes, vaginal dryness, and emotional lability.

Oral Contraceptives

The efficacy of OCPs for the treatment of PMDD has not been established because of conflicting data, and more studies are indicated. Freeman and colleagues[22] showed that a unique OCP consisting of 30 μg ethinyl estradiol and 3 mg drospirenone (Yasmin) was beneficial for a number of symptoms, including bloating, breast tenderness and swelling. The combination agent also has antiandrogenic properties that may relieve acne and hirsutism.

Bromocriptine

Bromocriptine, a dopamine agonist, is useful in decreasing mastalgia by lowering prolactin levels. It is dosed as 2.5 mg once daily just before ovulation until the onset of menses. Side effects may include dizziness and nausea.

Diuretics

Spironolactone is the diuretic most studied because of its antimineralocorticoid and antiandrogenic properties. Symptoms most likely to improve include bloating, swelling, breast tenderness, and acne. It may be tried in dosages of 50 to 100 mg/day for 7 to 10 days during the luteal phase. Side effects, including lethargy, headache, and irregular menses, are more common during continuous dosing. Serum potassium levels should be monitored periodically because spironolactone can cause hyperkalemia.

Other Medications

Nonsteroidal anti-inflammatory drugs (NSAIDs) are available over the counter and are effective for dysmenorrhea. Generic names include ibuprofen and naproxen. Meclofenamate (Meclomen), an NSAID available by prescription, can reduce menstrual cramps and flow. The typical dose is 100 mg twice daily. Acetaminophen may also be beneficial for pain.

Alternative Therapies

Today, women are more likely to seek other integrative therapies for PMDD. One large trial has shown that 1200 mg of elemental calcium daily is effective in alleviating tension, anxiety, fluid retention, and food cravings.[23] Physicians are most often asked about vitamin supplementation; controlled studies with vitamin A, vitamin E, and vitamin B_6 have failed to consistently show a benefit. Although popular, herbal products are not FDA approved, and some have caused significant toxicities as well as drug-herb interactions. Other innovative therapies include acupuncture, biofeedback, homeopathy, massage, reflexology, and light therapy.[24]

Suggested Readings

Casper RF, Hearn MT: The effect of hysterectomy and bilateral oophorectomy in women with severe premenstrual syndrome. Am J Obstet Gynecol 1990;162:105-109.

Casson P, Hahn PM, Van Vugt DA, et al: Lasting response to ovariectomy in severe intractable premenstrual syndrome. Am J Obstet Gynecol 1990;162:99-105.

Cronje WH, Vashisht A, Studd JW: Hysterectomy and bilateral oophorectomy for severe premenstrual syndrome. Hum Reprod 2004;19:2152-2155.

Diagnostic and Statistical Manual of Mental Disorders, 4th ed., Text Revision: Washington, DC, American Psychiatric Association, 2000:771-773 and Appendix B.

Eriksson E: Serotonin reuptake inhibitors for the treatment of premenstrual dysphoria. Clin Psychopharmacol 1999;14 (Suppl 2):S27-S33.

Facchinetti F, Borella P, Fioroni L, et al: Reduction of monocyte's magnesium in patients affected by premenstrual syndrome. J Psychosom Obstet Gynaecol 1990;11:221.

Frackiewicz EJ, Shiovitz TM: Evaluation and management of premenstrual syndrome and premenstrual dysphoric disorder. J Am Pharm Assoc (Wash) 2001;41:437-447.

Freeman EW, Kroll R, Rapkin A, et al: Evaluation of a unique oral contraceptive in the treatment of premenstrual dysphoric disorder. J Womens Health Gend Based Med 2001;10:561-569.

Freeman EW, Rickels K, Schweizer E, et al: Relationships between age and symptom severity among women seeking medical treatment for premenstrual symptoms. Psychol Med 1995;25:309-315.

Halbreich U, Bergeron R, Yonkers KA, et al: Efficacy of intermittent, luteal phase sertraline treatment of premenstrual dysphoric disorder. Obstet Gynecol 2002;100: 1219-1229.

Kaur G, Gonsalves L, Thacker HL: Premenstrual dysphoric disorder: A review for the treating practitioner. Cleve Clin J Med 2004;71:303-321.

Menkes DB, Coates DC, Fawcett JP: Acute tryptophan depletion aggravates premenstrual syndrome. J Affect Disord 1994;32:37-44.

Miner C, Brown E, McCray S, et al: Weekly luteal-phase dosing with enteric-coated fluoxetine 90 mg in premenstrual dysphoric disorder: A randomized, double-blind, placebo-controlled clinical trial. Clin Ther 2002;24:417-433.

Mortola JF, Girton L, Fischer U: Successful treatment of severe premenstrual syndrome by combined use of gonadotropin-releasing hormone agonist and estrogen/progestin. J Clin Endocrinol Metab 1991;72:252A-252F.

Muse KN, Cetel NS, Futterman LA, et al: The premenstrual syndrome. Effects of "medical ovariectomy." N Engl J Med 1984;311:1345-1349.

Okey R, Stewart J, Greenwood M: Studies in the metabolism of women. IV. The calcium and inorganic phosphorus in the blood of normal women at the various stages of the monthly cycle. J Biol Chem 1930;87:91-102.

Rivera-Tovar AD, Frank E: Late luteal phase dysphoric disorder in young women. Am J Psychiatry 1990;147:1634-1636.

Rosenstein DL, Elin RJ, Hosseini JM, et al: Magnesium measures across the menstrual cycle in premenstrual syndrome. Biol Psychiatry 1994;35:557-561.

Schmidt PJ, Neiman LK, Danaceau MA, et al: Differential behavioral effects of gonadal steroids in women with and in those without premenstrual syndrome. N Engl J Med 1998;338:209-216.

Steiner M, Born L: Diagnosis and treatment of premenstrual dysphoric disorder: An update. Int Clin Psychopharmacol 2000;15 (Suppl 3):S5-S17.

Taylor DL, Matthew RJ, Ho BT, et al: Serotonin levels and platelet uptake during premenstrual tension. Neuropsychobiology 1984;12:16-18.

Thys-Jacobs S, Starkey P, Bernstein D, et al: Calcium carbonate and the premenstrual syndrome: Effects on premenstrual and menstrual symptoms. Premenstrual Syndrome Study Group. Am J Obstet Gynecol 1998;179:444-452.

Wikander I, Sundblad C, Andersch B, et al: Citalopram in premenstrual dysphoria: Is intermittent treatment during luteal phases more effective than continuous medication throughout the menstrual cycle? J Clin Psychopharmacol 1998;18:390-398.

Young SA, Hurt PH, Benedek DM, et al: Treatment of premenstrual dysphoric disorder with sertraline during the luteal phase: A randomized, double-blind, placebo-controlled crossover trial. J Clin Psychiatry 1998;59:76-80.

References

For a complete list of references, log onto www.expertconsult.com.

Vaginitis

Anita Shivadas

DEFINITION AND ETIOLOGY

Vaginitis is a term that is applied to vulvovaginal symptoms of varying causes. Symptoms of vaginitis are common and account for about 10 million office visits a year. However, the symptoms are nonspecific and multifactorial. Infection is the most common cause; some of the other causes are listed in Box 1. Careful history taking combined with physical examination and simple microscopic analysis can help ascertain a diagnosis and tailor a treatment. This can help avoid misdiagnosis and treatment failure as well as symptom recurrence.

EPIDEMIOLOGY

The exact incidence of vaginitis is unknown, but it is estimated that most women experience at least one episode in their lifetime. The associated distress and discomfort often lead women to self-diagnose vaginitis and use over-the-counter preparations improperly. The three most common causes of vaginitis include bacterial vaginosis, candidal vulvovaginitis, and trichomonas vaginitis.

SYMPTOMS AND SIGNS

Clinical Signs and Symptoms

Symptoms of vaginitis include vaginal discharge, irritation, pruritus, odor, and, occasionally, dyspareunia, vaginal bleeding, and dysuria. Symptoms tend to be nonspecific and overlap among the different etiologic factors. Some historical clues can help suggest a diagnosis.

Bacterial vaginosis manifests with a scant, homogenous, sometimes malodorous discharge with limited symptoms of inflammation, such as pruritus and soreness. Women often admit to a recent change in sex partner. Bacterial vaginosis is also associated with vaginal douching.

Candida classically manifests with a scant, curdy, white discharge associated with marked pruritus and soreness. Medications that can be associated with vulvovaginal candidiasis include systemic antibiotics, oral contraceptive pills (especially those containing higher estrogen levels), oral steroids, and other immunosuppressive agents. Diabetes can cause sporadic as well as recurrent vulvovaginal candidiasis.

Trichomonas vaginitis manifests with frothy green discharge and inflammatory signs. The patient might give a history of a recent change in sex partner.

Atrophic vaginitis occurs in postmenopausal women and manifests with vaginal dryness, dyspareunia, and dysuria.

Physical Examination

Physical examination should mainly be used to evaluate for the presence of cervical inflammation (suggesting an alternative etiology) and to exclude the clinical presence of pelvic inflammatory disease.

On physical examination, the vaginal discharge is thick, white, and adherent in candidiasis; thin and fishy-smelling in bacterial vaginosis, and greenish-yellow and purulent in trichomoniasis. Candidiasis and trichomoniasis (but not bacterial vaginosis) are also associated with vulvar and vaginal erythema. Atrophic vaginitis is associated with scant, thin vaginal discharge and atrophic changes, such as thinning and loss of rugae in the vaginal mucosa.

Cervical inflammation suggests cervicitis contributing to vaginal discharge. Cervical motion tenderness suggests pelvic inflammatory disease.

Vaginal pH should be obtained at the time of the physical examination and is probably the most important diagnostic clue.

DIAGNOSIS

Due to the nonspecific nature of the symptoms and physical examination findings, the diagnosis of vaginitis is mainly made by using a combination of vaginal pH, amine test, microscopy findings, and, sometimes, vaginal cultures. Table 1 provides a summary of the differential diagnosis of vaginal discharge.

Vaginal pH

Vaginal pH is obtained by placing a drop of the vaginal discharge on a pH strip. It must be remembered that the pH can be altered by vaginal lubricants as well as other factors such as blood or urine. Vulvovaginal candidiasis is associated with a normal vaginal pH between 4.0 and 4.5. A vaginal pH greater than 4.5 suggests infections such as bacterial vaginosis and trichomonal vaginitis.

Amine Test

The amine or whiff test is done by placing a drop of the vaginal discharge on a slide and adding a drop of 10% KOH. A fishy amine odor indicates bacterial vaginosis. The odor is caused by volatilization of amines, a by-product of anaerobic metabolism. The amine test is occasionally positive with trichomoniasis.

Microscopy

Microscopy should be performed using saline and 10% KOH mounts. Figure 1 provides an illustration of various saline microscopic findings.

Saline Mount

Cells that can be seen in the saline mount include vaginal epithelial cells, rods and cocci, polymorphonuclear cells (PMNs), clue cells, motile trichomonads, and candidal hyphae. Normal vaginal epithelial cells are squamous. Parabasal cells appear in postmenopausal women and are associated with atrophic vaginitis.

Rods are the predominant microorganisms in normal vaginal discharge and with candidiasis. Loss of rods and increased coccobacilli occur with bacterial vaginosis and atrophic vaginitis.

Abundant PMNs are seen with the purulent discharge associated with trichomoniasis. Motile trichomonads, which are slightly larger than PMNs, are only seen in 60% to 70% of culture-confirmed cases of trichomoniasis.

Clue cells are the single most reliable predictor of bacterial vaginosis. These are epithelial cells studded with adherent coccobacilli and represent between 5% and 50% of the epithelial cells seen in bacterial vaginosis.

Potassium Hydroxide Mount

The KOH mount is particularly useful for diagnosing candidal vaginitis. Branching hyphae of *Candida albicans* can be seen.

Vaginal Cultures

Due to the low sensitivity of microscopic tests, vaginal cultures can be obtained in microscopy-negative cases. Vaginal candidiasis often manifests with a compatible history and normal pH and negative microscopy. In these cases, hypersensitivity, contact dermatitis, and allergic or chemical vaginitis can be excluded by obtaining a vaginal culture. Similarly, culture techniques have a high sensitivity in trichomonas vaginitis (95%) and should be considered in patients with an elevated vaginal pH, increased numbers of PMNs, and absence of motile trichomonads and clue cells or when microscopy is unavailable or yields unreliable results.

Box 1 Causes of Vaginitis

Infectious Vaginitis

Common Causes

Bacterial vaginosis (40%-50% of cases)
Vulvovaginal candidiasis (20%-25% of cases)
Trichomoniasis (15%-20% of cases)

Less-Common Causes

Atrophic vaginitis with secondary bacterial infection
Foreign body with secondary infection
Desquamative inflammatory vaginitis (clindamycin responsive)
Streptococcal vaginitis (group A)
Ulcerative vaginitis associated with *Staphylococcus aureus* and toxic shock syndrome
Idiopathic vulvovaginal ulceration associated with HIV infection

Noninfectious Vaginitis

Chemical or other irritant
Allergic, hypersensitivity, and contact dermatitis (lichen simplex)
Traumatic vaginitis
Atrophic vaginitis
Postpuerperal atrophic vaginitis
Desquamative inflammatory vaginitis (steroid responsive)
Erosive lichen planus
Collagen vascular disease, Behçet's syndrome, pemphigus syndromes
Idiopathic vaginitis

Cervical Cultures

Cervical cultures for DNA amplification and diagnosis of *Chlamydia trachomatis* and *Neisseria gonorrhoeae* infection should be obtained in women with a history of high-risk sexual behavior, symptomatic sexual partners, and cervical motion tenderness on physical examination (suggesting pelvic inflammatory disease).

The Amsel criteria are used to diagnose bacterial vaginosis. The diagnosis requires three of the following four characteristics:

- Homogenous, thin discharge
- pH >4.5
- Positive whiff test
- Clue cells on microscopy

The prevalence of bacterial vaginosis and trichomoniasis is high in HIV-seropositive women and in seronegative controls matched for high-risk behavior. Hence, identification of these infections should prompt screening for HIV and other sexually transmitted diseases.

TREATMENT

Bacterial Vaginosis

Standard regimens can achieve cure rates between 70% and 90% for confirmed cases of bacterial vaginosis (Table 2). Oral and topical routes have equal efficacy, and nitroimidazole and clindamycin reg-

Table 1 Differential Diagnosis of Vaginitis

Variable	Normal	Vulvovaginal Candidiasis	Bacterial Vaginosis*	Trichomoniasis	Atrophic Vaginitis
Symptoms	None or mild, transient	Pruritus, soreness, change in discharge, dyspareunia	Malodorous discharge, no dyspareunia	Malodorous, purulent discharge, dyspareunia	Dyspareunia, vaginal dryness
Signs	—	Vulvar erythema, edema, fissure	Adherent discharge	Purulent discharge, vulvovaginal erythema	Vestibular and vaginal thinning
pH	4.0-4.5	4.0-4.5	>4.5	5.0-6.0	>6.0
Amine test	Negative	Negative	Positive (~70%-80%)	Often positive	Negative
Saline microscopy	PMN:EC ratio <1; rods dominate; squames +++	PMN:EC ratio <1; rods dominate; squames +++; pseudohyphae (~40%)	PMN:EC ratio <1; loss of rods; increased coccobacilli; clue cells (>90%)	PMN ++++; mixed flora; motile trichomonads (60%)	PMN + to ++; loss of rods; increased cocci and coliforms; parabasal cells
10% KOH examination	Negative	Pseudohyphae (~70%)	Negative	Negative	Negative
Miscellaneous	—	Culture if microscopy is negative	Culture of no value	Culture if microscopy is negative	—
Differential diagnosis	Physiologic leukorrhea	Contact irritant or allergic vulvitis, chemical irritation, focal vulvitis (vulvodynia)		Purulent vaginitis, desquamative inflammatory vaginitis, atrophic vaginitis plus secondary infection, erosive lichen planus	

*For bacterial diagnosis, the Amsel criteria require the presence of three of four clinical signs for diagnosis: homogeneous discharge, a positive whiff-amine test, pH >4.5, and the presence of clue cells.

EC, epithelial cells; PMN, polymorphonuclear leukocytes.

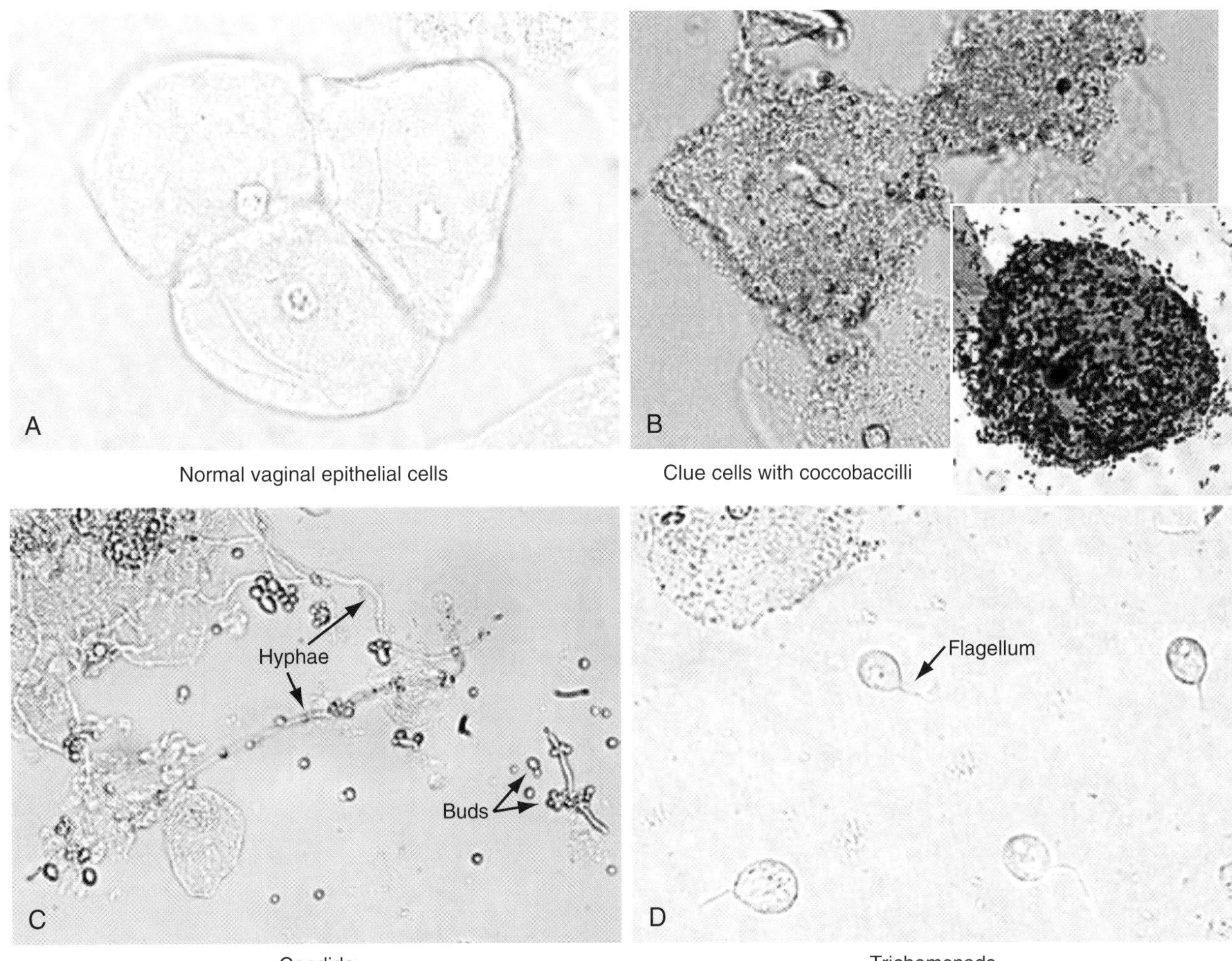

Figure 1 Microscopic examination of vaginal samples. A, Normal saline wet mount showing a clump of three normal vaginal epithelial cells (original magnification ×600). **B,** Normal saline wet mount showing two clue cells (original magnification ×400). *Inset,* Gram stain demonstrating how coccobaccilli on the surfaces of vaginal epithelial cells create the characteristic granular appearance and indistinct borders of clue cells (original magnification ×1000). **C,** Normal saline wet mount showing numerous *Candida* hyphae *(arrows)* and buds (original magnification ×400). **D,** Normal saline wet mount showing four trichomonads. Trichomonads can often be identified easily because of their characteristic jerky motility (original magnification ×600). *(**A** reproduced with permission from William L. Thelmo, MD. **B** and **C** reproduced with permission from Lorna Rabe, Magee-Women's Research Institute, Pittsburgh, Pa. **D** reproduced with permission from the Medical Laboratory Evaluation proficiency testing program of the American College of Physicians Services, Inc. From Anderson MR, Klink K, Cohrssen A: Evaluation of vaginal complaints. JAMA 2004;291:1368-1379.)*

Table 2 Treatments for Bacterial Vaginosis

Drug	Formulation	Dosage Regimen
Oral		
Clindamycin	75-mg, 150-mg, 300-mg caps	300mg bid × 7 days
Metronidazole (Flagyl)	250-mg, 500-mg tabs	500mg bid × 7 days
		750mg bid × 7 days 2g as a one-time dose
Vaginal		
Clindamycin	2% cream	1 app (100mg drug) qd × 7 days
Metronidazole	0.75% gel	1 app (37.5mg drug) qd × 5 days

app, applicator; cap, capsule; tab, tablet.

imens are also equally efficacious. Vaginal routes have the main advantage of reduced gastrointestinal symptoms, but they have the disadvantage of being inconvenient and being associated with a high risk of vaginal candidiasis.

Asymptomatic bacterial vaginosis should only be treated in pregnant women and before elective gynecologic surgery. Bacterial vaginosis in pregnant women is associated with an increased risk of preterm prelabor rupture of membranes and preterm delivery as well as endometritis and wound infections after cesarean delivery. Bacterial vaginosis has also been implicated in post-hysterectomy vaginal-cuff cellulitis. Despite the association between bacterial vaginosis and preterm birth, most studies in general obstetric populations have not found that treatment of asymptomatic infection reduced the incidence of preterm labor or delivery. Based on these data, screening and treating all pregnant women who have asymptomatic bacterial vaginosis to prevent preterm birth and its consequences are not recommended by the United States Preventive Services Task Force (USPSTF). Screening and treatment of bacterial vaginosis could be considered in women with a previous preterm birth so as to lower the rate of preterm prelabor rupture of membranes and low birth weight, because these conditions are associated with maternal and neonatal morbidity.

After therapy, approximately 30% of patients with initial responses have a recurrence of symptoms within 3 months. The reasons include reinfection or, more likely, relapse due to failure to eradicate the organism or failure to re-establish the normal protective vaginal flora dominated by lactobacilli. Resistance has been seen with clindamycin, but metronidazole resistance has not yet been reported. Management of symptomatic relapsed patients should involve prolonged therapy for 10 to 14 days. Vaginal lactobacillus replacement is still considered a research endeavor, and commercially available lactobacillus preparations are not recommended. Maintenance regimen of vaginal metronidazole gel, 0.75%, has shown efficacy in excess of 70% but has a high rate of relapse on cessation of the suppressive therapy.

Despite evidence of sexual transmission, no study has demonstrated prevention of recurrence with treatment of male sexual partners.

Candida Vulvovaginitis

Candida albicans is the major yeast implicated in most cases of vaginitis (80%-90%). Other candidal species, including *Candida torulopsis* and *Candida glabrata,* can also be associated with vaginitis. Azoles, which are fungistatic and act by inhibiting cell wall metabolism, are the mainstay of treatment for vaginal candidiasis. They are available over the counter and by prescription. They are available in topical and oral forms. Table 3 provides a list of available formulations.

Cure rates of 80% to 90% can be achieved with all the azole agents listed in Table 3. Topical nystatin is less effective, with cure rates of 50% to 80%. The choice between oral and topical therapies should be based on patient preference as well as factors such as compliance, cost, ability to insert vaginal preparations, history of response or adverse reactions to prior treatments, and duration of therapy. The main disadvantage of the topical route is localized burning due to irritant or allergic reactions. Oral therapy with a single dose of fluconazole is as effective as a 3-day course of topical terconazole and a 7-day course of clotrimazole. Systemic side effects are mild, infrequent, and self-limited. They include gastrointestinal intolerance, headache, and rash. Persistent symptoms should be re-evaluated and vaginal yeast cultures should be obtained.

C. glabrata is less likely to respond to azole medications. Boric acid 600 mg topically daily for 14 days is an effective treatment option.

During pregnancy, topical therapy is preferred to limit drug exposure in the fetus. Fluconazole has been categorized as class C during pregnancy.

Table 3 Treatments for Vaginal Candidiasis

Drug	Formulation	Dosage Regimen
Over the Counter		
Butoconazole (Femstat)	2% cream	5 g/day × 3 days
Clotrimazole (Gyne-lotrimin, Mycelex)	1% cream	5 g/day × 7-14 days
	100-mg vaginal tab	1 tab/day × 7 days *or* 2 tabs/day × 3 days
	500-mg vaginal tab	1 tab
Miconazole (Monistat)	2% cream	5 g/day × 7 days
	100-mg vaginal sup	1 sup/day × 7 days
	200-mg vaginal sup	1 sup/day × 3 days
	1200-mg vaginal sup	1 sup
Tioconazole (Vagistat)	2% cream	5 g/day × 3 days
	6.5% cream	5 g in a single dose
Prescription		
Terconazole (Terazol)	0.4% cream	5 g/day × 7 days
	0.8% cream	5 g/day × 3 days
Nystatin (Mycostatin)*	1,000,000-U vaginal tab	1 tab/day × 14 days
Ketoconazole (Nizoral)	400-mg oral tab	1 tab bid × 5 days
Itraconazole (Sporanox)	200-mg oral tab	1 tab id × 1 day *or* 1 tab qd × 3 days
Fluconazole (Diflucan)	150-mg oral tab	Single dose

Note: There are no significant differences in efficacy among topical and systemic azoles. Cure rates are >80% for uncomplicated vulvovaginal candidiasis.
*The cure rate with nystatin is 70%-80%.
sup, suppository; tab, tablet.

Recurrent Vulvovaginal Candidiasis

Recurrent vulvovaginal candidiasis (RVVC) is defined as four or more episodes of candidal infection per year. Less than 5% of healthy women are affected by this condition. Pathogenetic factors contributing to RVVC include infection with *C. glabrata* and other non-*albicans Candida* species, persistence of *C. albicans* due to inadequate treatment, diabetes mellitus and impaired glucose tolerance, recent antibiotic use, estrogen use, immunosuppressive therapy, and behavioral factors. Behavioral factors associated with RVVC include vaginal douching as well as contraceptive practices associated with a higher risk of candidiasis, such as diaphragm use, spermicide use, and intrauterine devices. However, in approximately one half of women with RVVC, there are no identifiable risk factors and the pathogenesis remains unknown. Sexual intercourse has not been associated with an increased incidence of *Candida* colonization. Hypotheses regarding *Lactobacillus* deficiency in women with RVVC have not been substantiated.

Before treatment for RVVC, a vaginal culture to confirm the diagnosis and determine the species is strongly advisable. Maintenance antifungal suppressive therapy for 6 months with either ketoconazole 100 mg orally daily, itraconazole 50 to 100 mg orally daily, clotrimazole 500-mg vaginal suppositories weekly, or fluconazole 150 mg orally weekly for 6 months is recommended. Approximately 50% of women have no symptoms after 6 months of treatment. Those who have recurrent symptoms after 6 months of therapy might need longer courses of maintenance therapy. Recurrent infections with *C. glabrata* can be treated with topical boric acid 600 mg daily for 2 weeks. Topical flucytosine can be used for resistant *C. glabrata* and *C. tropicalis* species. However, it is expensive, and prolonged use is associated with resistance. The use of combination therapy has not been studied. Studies have also failed to demonstrate a benefit to treating a woman's partner. Other approaches, such as hormonal manipulation with depot medroxyprogesterone, eating yogurt, and desensitization to candida antigen, lack sufficient data to support recommending their use.

Trichomoniasis

The 5-nitroimidazole group of drugs, which includes metronidazole and tinidazole, are effective treatment choices for trichomoniasis. Oral therapy is preferred because infections of urethra and periurethral glands, which are not eradicated by vaginal therapy, are sources for endogenous recurrence. The recommended treatment choice of the Centers for Disease Control and Prevention (CDC) guidelines is a single 2-g oral dose of metronidazole. The alternative regimen is metronidazole 500 mg twice a day for 7 days. Treatment of all sexual partners is necessary to avoid recurrence. Cure rates approach 90% with either regimen. The side effects of metronidazole therapy are nausea, headache, metallic taste in the mouth, and disulfiram-like effect with alcohol. The advantages of single-dose therapy include better compliance, a lower total dose, a shorter period of alcohol avoidance, and possibly decreased candida superinfection.

Metronidazole resistance in *T. vaginalis* isolates is uncommon. Most *T. vaginalis* strains are usually susceptible to metronidazole with a minimum inhibitory concentration (MIC) of 1 µg/mL. Low-level resistance, defined as a MIC of 50 to 100 µg/mL, occurs in 1% to 3% of isolates. These strains manifest with early relapse or failure to respond to single-dose 2-g therapy. Conventional therapy with metronidazole 500 mg twice a day for 7 days can achieve adequate treatment of low-level resistant strains. Higher levels of metronidazole resistance require oral metronidazole 2 g per day for 3 to 5 days according to the CDC guidelines. However, failure of this high-dose regimen has also been reported. Tinidazole, which is now available in the United States, is an alternative for metronidazole-resistant strains of *T. vaginalis*. Tinidazole has been approved at a dose of 2-g single dose orally as first-line therapy for trichomoniasis. The optimal dose and duration of therapy for metronidazole-resistant *T. vaginalis* infections are as yet to be determined. For metronidazole-resistant strains, a more prolonged course may be necessary. Tinidazole is better tolerated than metronidazole in terms of both gastrointestinal and central nervous system side effects, especially at higher doses. Tinidazole should also be prescribed to the partner of the woman harboring the resistant *T. vaginalis*.

Trichomoniasis treatment during pregnancy is controversial. Metronidazole readily crosses the placenta; however, it is unclear if it is teratogenic. Most physicians prefer to avoid it in the first trimester of pregnancy. Clotrimazole can temporarily relieve the symptoms of trichomoniasis. Treatment may be delayed until after the first trimester of pregnancy. Breast-feeding should be delayed or withheld for 24 hours after taking metronidazole.

Other Causes of Vaginitis

The treatment for other types of vaginitis depends on the cause. Atrophic vaginitis can be treated with local or systemic estrogens. Desquamative inflammatory vaginitis is a chronic purulent vaginitis with negative cultures, which responds to topical 2% clindamycin. Bacterial vaginitis complicating atrophic vaginitis or a foreign body superinfection can be treated with antibiotics and foreign body removal, when appropriate. Noninfectious causes of vaginitis include irritants and allergens. Management includes removing the offending agent, applying topical corticosteroids (used cautiously to avoid local burning), taking sodium bicarbonate sitz baths, and applying vegetable oil topically.

Summary

- A careful history, physical examination, and simple microscopy can help ascertain a diagnosis and tailor treatment while avoiding misdiagnosis, treatment failure, and symptom recurrence.
- The three most common causes of vaginitis are bacterial vaginitis, candidal vulvovaginitis, and trichomonal vaginitis.
- Physical examination should mainly be used to evaluate for cervical inflammation (suggesting an alternative cause) and to exclude pelvic inflammatory disease.
- The diagnosis of vaginitis is mainly made by using a combination of vaginal pH, amine test, microscopy findings, and, sometimes, vaginal cultures.
- Other causes of vaginitis include atrophic vaginitis, desquamative inflammatory vaginitis, a foreign body infection, and irritants and allergens.

Suggested Reading

Amsel R, Totten PA, Spiegel CA, et al: Nonspecific vaginitis. Diagnostic criteria and microbial and epidemiologic associations. Am J Med 1983;74(1):14-22.

References

For a complete list of references, log onto www.expertconsult.com.

Section 15

PREVENTIVE MEDICINE

Principles of Screening

Raul J. Seballos

Preventive medicine encompasses primary, secondary, and tertiary preventive measures such as screening, counseling, immunization, and prophylaxis. The goal of primary prevention is to prevent new disease cases by reducing risk factors. Primary preventive measures are designed to prevent the onset of a targeted condition; they are activities that help avoid a specific health care problem. For example, smoking cessation can reduce the incidence of lung cancer. Other examples of primary prevention practices include immunization and prophylaxis.

The goal of secondary prevention is to detect disease or cancer, thereby leading to early treatment and improved prognosis. Secondary preventive measures identify and treat asymptomatic persons who already have certain risk factors or in whom the condition is not yet clinically apparent. Screening tests are examples of secondary preventive measures. With early case diagnosis, a disease's natural course, or how an illness unfolds over time without treatment, can often be altered to maximize a patient's well-being and minimize suffering. For example, a mammogram that detects an early-stage breast cancer can lead to a more definitive and curative procedure.

Tertiary prevention manages an existing disease, with the goal to restore a patient to highest function, minimize the negative consequences of the disease, and prevent disease-related complications. Examples include eliminating offending allergens from an asthmatic patient's environment and routinely screening for and managing early renal, eye, and foot problems in a diabetic patient.

An ideal screening test would be a reasonably priced, noninvasive procedure. This screening test must identify a disease that is clinically significant and that, if left untreated, will cause significant morbidity and mortality. In addition, the ideal screening test must be for a disease that has a preclinical phase, a presymptomatic stage for which the disease is detectable. Finally, the disease must have an acceptable treatment course.

The ideal screening test must also be sensitive and specific. Table 1 illustrates these principles. The test must be able to correctly identify patients who have the disease (sensitivity) and those who do not have the disease (specificity). For example, for a medical test to determine if a person has a certain disease, the sensitivity to the disease is the probability that if the person has the disease, the test will be positive. The sensitivity is the ratio of true positive (TP) results to all diseased cases in the population. The specificity to the disease is the probability that if the person does not have the disease, the test will be negative. That is, the specificity is the ratio of true negative results to all negative cases in the population.

The positive predictive value (PPV) is the ratio of patients with positive test results who are correctly identified to all patients who tested positive for the disease [PPV = TP/(TP + FP)] (where FP stands for *false positive*). A negative predictive value (NPV) is the ratio of patients with negative test results who are correctly identified to all patients who test negative for the disease [NPV = TN/(TN + FN)] (where TN stands for *true negative* and FN stands for *false negative*).

Prevalence of a disease in a statistical population is defined as the total number of cases of a given disease in a specified population at a specified time and/or the ratio of the number of cases of a disease present in a statistical population at a specified time and the number of persons in the population at that specified time. For example, in 2007, according to the U.S. Centers for Disease Control and Prevention (CDC), obesity prevalence was 33.3% among men and 35.3% among women.[1,2]

Incidence of a disease is defined as the number of new cases of the disease occurring in a population during a defined time interval. It is a measure of the risk of disease. In short, prevalence is a proportion, and incidence is a rate. Prevalence involves all affected persons, regardless of the date of contracting the disease. To illustrate, diabetes mellitus is becoming a major health issue in the United States. The number of existing cases (prevalent cases) and the number of new cases (incident cases) of diabetes are increasing, and most of this increase is not a result of the aging of the U.S. population. Between 1980 and 1996, the number of persons with diagnosed diabetes increased by 2.7 million. In 1996, about 8.5 million persons in the United States (3.2% of the population) reported that they had diabetes mellitus.[3] The incidence of diabetes increased in the early 1980s but leveled off in the middle of the decade. It then increased in the 1990s. In 1996, the age-adjusted incidence of diabetes (2.79 per 1000 population) was 18% higher than the incidence in 1980 (2.36 per 1000 population). In the 1990s, the number of new cases of diabetes averaged more than 760,000 per year.[3]

PERIODIC HEALTH EXAMINATION

Since the 1980s, the American College of Physicians, the American Medical Association, the U.S. Preventive Services Task Force (USPSTF), and the U.S. Public Health Service have all agreed that routine annual checkups for healthy adults should be abandoned in favor of a more selective approach to preventing and detecting health problems. Nevertheless, the public expects to be given a comprehensive annual physical examination and extensive routine testing.[4] Table 2 is the 2006 USPSTF Guide to Clinical Preventive Services.[5] As Dr. Reinhart indicated in his letter to the editor, there are "probably very few of us, at any age, who would not be candidates for at least some health advice, such as on diet, exercise, or substance use or abuse. It also seems logical to believe that at least to some degree, repetition of health advice may have cumulative value."[6] Lastly, better patient adherence to a healthy lifestyle can lead to better health outcomes. A major factor promoting such adherence is the doctor-patient relationship or rapport with a physician. The annual physician examination is an extremely valuable building block in achieving such rapport.[6]

ADULT IMMUNIZATIONS

Immunization is an example of a primary preventive practice. The current Adult Immunization Schedule is available on the CDC's website.[7] Detailed discussion of each of the recommended immunizations is discussed in the Infectious Disease section of this book.

Summary

- Preventive medicine encompasses primary, secondary, and tertiary preventive measures such as screening, counseling, immunization, and prophylaxis.
- An ideal screening test would be a reasonably priced, noninvasive procedure that is highly sensitive and specific.
- Numerous medical organizations have agreed that routine annual checkups for healthy adults should be abandoned in favor of a more selective approach to preventing and detecting health problems.

Table 1 Predictive Value of Test

Result	Disease	No Disease	Total
Positive test	True positive (TP)	False positive (FP)	Total patients with positive test (TP + FP)
Negative test	False negative (FN) Total patients with disease	True negative (TN) Total patients without disease	Total patients with negative test (TN + FN) Total patients
Sensitivity = TP/(TP + FP)	Positive predictive value = TP/(TP + FP)		
Specificity = TN/(TN + FP)	Negative predictive value = TN/(TN + FN)		

Table 2 Preventive Services Recommended by the USPSTF

					Adults		Special Populations	
Condition	Intervention	Recommendations	Adults	Special Populations	Men	Women	Pregnant Women	Children
Abdominal aortic aneurysm	Screening	One-time screening by ultrasonography in men aged 65 to 75 who have ever smoked	x					
Alcohol misuse	Screening and behavioral counseling		x	x	x			
Aspirin for primary prevention of cardiovascular events	Prevention	Adults at increased risk for coronary heart disease	x	x				
Bacteriuria	Screening for symptomatic infection				x			
Breast cancer	Chemoprevention	Discuss with women at high risk for breast cancer and at low risk for adverse effects of chemoprevention		x				
Breast cancer	Screening	Mammography every 1-2 yr for women ≥40 yr		x				
Breast and ovarian cancer susceptibility	Genetic risk assessment and *BRCA* gene mutation testing	Refer women whose family history is associated with an increased risk for deleterious mutations in *BRCA1* or *BRCA2* genes for genetic counseling and evaluation for *BRCA* gene testing		x				
Breast-feeding	Behavioral interventions to promote	Structured education and behavioral counseling programs		x	x			
Cervical cancer	Screening	Women who have been sexually active and have a cervix		x				
Chlamydial infection	Screening	Sexually active women ≤25 yr and other asymptomatic women at increased risk for infection Asymptomatic pregnant women ≤25 yr and others at increased risk						
Colorectal cancer	Screening	Men and women ≥50 yr	x	x				
Dental caries in preschool children	Prevention	Prescribe oral fluoride supplementation at currently recommended doses to preschool children >6 mo whose primary water source is deficient in fluoride				x		
Depression	Screening	In clinical practices with systems to ensure accurate diagnoses, effective treatments, and follow-ups	x	x				

Continued

Table 2 Preventive Services Recommended by the USPSTF—cont'd

					Adults		Special Populations	
Condition	**Intervention**	**Recommendations**	**Adults**	**Special Populations**	**Men**	**Women**	**Pregnant Women**	**Children**
Diabetes mellitus in adults, type 2	Screening	Adults with hypertension or hyperlipidemia	x	x				
Diet	Behavioral counseling in primary care to promote a healthy diet	Adults with hyperlipidemia and other known risk factors for cardiovascular and diet-related chronic diseases	x	x				
Gonorrhea	Screening	All sexually active women, including those who are pregnant, at increased risk for infection (i.e., are young or have other individual or population risk factors)		x	x			
Gonorrhea	Prophylactic medication	Prophylactic ocular topical medication for all newborns against gonococcal ophthalmia neonatorum				x		
Hepatitis B virus infection	Screening	Pregnant women at first prenatal visit			x			
High blood pressure	Screening		x	x				
HIV	Screening	All adolescents and adults at increased risk for HIV infection and all pregnant women	x	x	x	x		
Lipid disorders	Screening	Men ≥35 yr and women ≥45 yr Younger adults with other risk factors for coronary disease Screening for lipid disorders to include measurement of total cholesterol and HDL cholesterol						
Obesity in adults	Screening	Intensive counseling and behavioral interventions to promote sustained weight loss for obese adults	x	x				
Osteoporosis in postmenopausal women	Screening	Women ≥65 yr and women ≥60 yr at increased risk for osteoporotic fractures		x				
Rh(D) incompatibility	Screening	Blood typing and antibody testing at first pregnancy-related visit Repeated antibody testing for unsensitized Rh(D)-negative women at 24-28 wk gestation unless the biologic father is known to be Rh(D) negative						
Syphilis infection	Screening	Persons at increased risk and all pregnant women	x	x	x			
Tobacco use and tobacco-caused disease	Counseling to prevent	Tobacco cessation interventions for those who use tobacco Augmented pregnancy-tailored counseling to pregnant women who smoke						
Visual impairment in children <age 5 yr	Screening	To detect amblyopia, strabismus, and defects in visual acuity				x		

Note: The USPSTF recommends that clinicians discuss these preventive services with eligible patients and offer them as a priority. All these services have received an "A" (strongly recommended) or a "B" (recommended) grade from the Task Force.

HDL, high-density lipoprotein; HIV, human immunodeficiency virus; USPSTF, United States Preventive Services Task Force.

Adapted from Agency for Healthcare Research and Quality: The Guide to Clinical Preventive Services, 2006: Recommendations of the U.S. Preventive Services Task Force. Available at http://www.ahrq.gov/clinic/pocketgd.pdf (accessed March 20, 2009).

Suggested Readings

Agency for Healthcare Research and Quality: The Guide to Clinical Preventive Services, 2006: Recommendations of the U.S. Preventive Services Task Force. Available at http://www.ahrq.gov/clinic/pocketgd.pdf (accessed March 20, 2009).

Centers for Disease Control and Prevention: State-specific prevalence of obesity among adults-United States, 2005. MMWR Morb Mortal Wkly Rep 2006;55(36);985-988.

Centers for Disease Control and Prevention: Data & Trends: Diabetes Surveillance System. 1999 Surveillance Report. Chapter 1: The Public Health Burden of Diabetes Mellitus in the United States. Available at http://www.cdc.gov/diabetes/statistics/survl99/chap1/prevalence.htm (accessed March 20, 2009).

Centers for Disease Control and Prevention: Recommendations and guidelines: Adult immunization schedule. Available at http://www.cdc.gov/vaccines/recs/schedules/default.htm#adult (accessed March 20, 2009).

Oboler SK, Prochazka AV, Gonzales R, et al: Public expectations and attitudes for annual physical examinations and testing. Ann Intern Med 2002;136:652-659.

Reinhart D. Annual physical examination: Necessary or needless? Ann Intern Med 2003;138(5):W-W48.

References

For a complete list of references, log onto www.expertconsult.com.

Cancer Screening

Raul J. Seballos

Early diagnosis and detection of cancer profoundly affect survival rates and maximize positive outcomes. Major screening guidelines exist for the most common cancers: colon, breast, cervical, and prostate. Advanced imaging techniques, biomarkers, and multimodal approaches are providing promising strategies for detecting and diagnosing cancer at its earliest and most treatable stages. However, a large fraction of the population does not undergo appropriate screening or is screened inconsistently. For example, in 2004, among adults older than 50 years, the prevalence of having an endoscopic procedure within the past 5 years for colorectal cancer screening was 52.1%, and the prevalence of doing an at-home fecal occult blood test (FOBT) within the past year was only 19%. Overall, among adults older than 50 years, the prevalence of having had either an FOBT or endoscopic procedure was 52.1%. In addition, compared with persons with health insurance, the uninsured nonelderly group was significantly less likely to have had a colorectal cancer screening.[1] Access, insurance coverage, and patient discomfort are all barriers to obtaining these preventive procedures. Physicians should discuss these cancer screening guidelines and recommend which test is most appropriate to increase patient awareness and follow-through and in turn promote long-term health.

As of 2008, prostate cancer, lung and bronchus cancer, and colon cancer remain the top three leading new cancer cases in men. Breast, lung and bronchus, and colon cancers remain the top three cancers in women. Lung and bronchus cancer remains the leading cause of cancer-related deaths in both men and women, with the 5-year survival rate averaging 15%.[2]

COLON CANCER

In 2008, about 10% of new cancer cases in both men and women in the United States were colorectal cancer. The diagnosis will be made in approximately 77,250 men and 71,560 women in the United States, and approximately 49,960 will die from it.[1]

Screening measures for colorectal cancer include colonoscopy, flexible sigmoidoscopy, and FOBT. Most organizations recommend that screening start at age 50 years. The standard screening procedure is the colonoscopy every 10 years, which allows a complete examination of the entire colon. The procedure is both diagnostic and preventive, especially when an adenomatous polyp or precancerous polyp is removed. Flexible sigmoidoscopy and double-contrast barium enemas (DCBEs) should be done at 5-year intervals.

A thorough discussion of the specific modalities of colon cancer screening is discussed in "Treatment of Colorectal Cancer," elswhere in this text. The role of the primary care physician is to educate and provide reassurance that these cancer-screening procedures are relatively safe. Newer technologies, such as computed tomography (CT) colonography and stool DNA testing, need further study before being accepted as part of the preventive approach to detect colon cancer in the average-risk patient.

BREAST CANCER

Breast cancer is the leading cause of new cancer in women in the United States (approximately 26% of all new cancer cases).[1] In 2008, approximately 182,460 women in the United States learned they had breast cancer, and 40,480 died from it. Most organizations agree that breast cancer screening should start at age 40 years for the average-risk woman.

Physicians should discuss with their patients the benefits of regular screening, the limitations of mammography, and the need for further testing, including breast biopsy, for false-positive results. The U.S. Preventive Services Task Force (USPSTF)[3] recommends a mammography every 1 to 2 years, and the American Cancer Society (ACS) recommends one annually. Decisions on when to stop mammography screening should be individualized and based on a patient's life expectancy and comorbid conditions.

Advanced screening modalities such as breast ultrasound, full-field digital mammography, and breast magnetic resonance imaging (MRI) may be more appropriate for women who are at higher risk for breast cancer. The breast MRI procedure has been found to be highly sensitive but less specific than conventional mammography. Breast MRI may be most useful in women with a family history of breast cancer or those who test positive for the breast cancer gene *(BRCA)*. Protein biomarkers for breast cancer, which include inflammatory markers, cell-cell contact, and tissue repair processes, a re still under investigation but might be able to differentiate normal breast tissue from malignant breast tissue.

The USPSTF currently recommends against routine use of tamoxifen or raloxifene for the primary prevention of breast cancer in women at low or average risk for breast cancer. They recommend that physicians discuss chemoprevention with women at high risk for breast cancer and at low risk for adverse effects of such treatment. A more detailed discussion on breast disorders and breast cancer screening is found in the "Women's Health" section of this text.

CERVICAL CANCER

Recommendations for cervical cancer screening have changed because of advances in cervical cancer screening that uses liquid-based cytology and advances in human papillomavirus (HPV) testing. The American College of Obstetricians and Gynecologists (ACOG) and the USPSTF recommend initial testing with either the traditional Papanicolaou (Pap) smear or liquid-based cytology starting by age 21 years or approximately 3 years after the first sexual intercourse.[4,5] Future screenings should occur every year with a traditional Pap smear or every 2 years with liquid-based cytology. At or after age 30 years and with three normal test results, intervals can be increased to every 2 to 3 years with traditional Pap smear or every 3 years with HPV assay testing plus cervical cytology. Screening can be discontinued at age 70 years for women who have had three or more normal Pap test results in the previous 10 years or who have had a total hysterectomy. A more detailed discussion, including the new HPV vaccination and management of abnormal Pap smears, is found in the chapter "Cervical Cancer Screening and Prevention."

PROSTATE CANCER

Prostate cancer is the leading type of new cancer cases in men in the United States and accounts for about 25% of all new cancers. In 2008, prostate cancer was diagnosed in approximately 186,320 men, and about 28,660 died as a result of it. If prostate-specific antigen (PSA) testing and digital rectal examination (DRE) can diagnose early stages of moderate- to high-grade prostate cancer, then mortality rates from prostate cancer can be reduced. No major medical organization in the United States endorses universal screening for average-risk men. In August 2008, the USPSTF concluded that the current evidence is insufficient for screening men younger than 75 years. For the first time, the task force recommended against routine prostate screening in men 75 years or older. However, all organizations recommend that for men, starting at age 50 years, physicians should discuss the risks and potential benefits of PSA testing, consider patient preferences, and individualize the decision to test.[6]

The controversy of PSA testing lies in its poor specificity (high false-positive findings), which leads to unnecessary biopsy. There are no specific guidelines regarding cutoff values to recommend prostate biopsy. An increase of more than 0.75 ng/mL per year (PSA velocity) can indicate the need for a prostate biopsy. It is generally accepted to stop screening for prostate cancer if the man's life expectancy is less than 10 years. A more extensive discussion of prostate cancer takes place in the chapter "Prostate Cancer."

LUNG CANCER

In 2008, approximately 161,840 people died from lung cancer–related causes. This is greater than colorectal, breast, and prostate cancers combined.[2] To date, no screening modalities have been shown to reduce mortality rates. The benefit of screening for lung cancer with sputum cytology, chest x-rays, or low-dose CT has not been established in any group, including asymptomatic high-risk populations such as older smokers. Although sensitivity of low-dose CT for detecting lung cancer is four times greater than the sensitivity of chest x-ray, the low-dose CT is associated with higher false-positive results, more radiation exposure, and increased costs compared with chest x-ray.[3]

Current large randomized, controlled trials to evaluate the effect of lung cancer screening on mortality, such as the Prostate, Lung, Colorectal and Ovarian Cancer Screening Trial (PLCO), are ongoing. This is a large-scale clinical trial to determine whether certain cancer screening tests reduce deaths from prostate, lung, colorectal, and ovarian cancers.[7] The underlying rationale for the trial is that screening for cancer might allow doctors to discover and treat the disease earlier. Numerous epidemiologic and ancillary studies are included to answer related crucial questions. A more detailed discussion on lung cancer occurs in the chapter "Lung Cancer."

CONCLUSIONS

Several organizations recommend a number of cancer screening guidelines. However, recommendations for screening for colon, breast, cervical, and prostate cancers are very similar. Table 1 depicts

Table 1 Cancer Screening Recommendations for the Average-Risk Adult

American Cancer Society[1]	U.S. Preventive Services Task Force[3]
Breast	
Age ≥20 yr	Age ≥40 yr
BSE optional	Mammography every 1-2 yr ± CBE
Age 20-30 yr	
CBE every 3 yr	
Age≥40 yr	
Mammography annually	
Cervix	
Age ≥18 yr	Recommendations
Conventional Pap test annually, *or*	Screening for cervical cancer in women who have been sexually active and have a cervix
Liquid-based cytology every 2 yr after first sexual intercourse or by age 21 yr	Optimal age to begin screening is unknown
Age ≥30 yr with 3 normal consecutive Pap tests	No routine screening for cervical cancer in women >65 yr who have had adequate recent screening with normal Pap smears and are not otherwise at high risk for cervical cancer
Conventional Pap test or liquid-based prep every 2-3 yr, *or*	No routine Pap smear screening in women who have had a total hysterectomy for benign disease
Conventional Pap test or liquid-based prep with HPV assay every 3 yr	Conclusions
Age ≥70 yr with ≥3 normal Pap tests and no abnormal Pap tests in the past 10 yr	The evidence is insufficient to recommend for or against routine use of new technologies to screen for cervical cancer
May stop	The evidence is insufficient to recommend for or against routine use of HPV testing as a primary screening test for cervical cancer
Women with hysterectomy	
May stop	
Colon	
Age ≥50 yr:	Age ≥50 yr
FOBT or FIT annually, *or*	FOBT annually, *or*

Continued

Table 1 Cancer Screening Recommendations for the Average-Risk Adult—cont'd

American Cancer Society[1]	U.S. Preventive Services Task Force[3]
Flex sig every 5 yr, *or*	Flex sig every 5 yr, *or*
FOBT or FIT annually plus flex sig every 5 yr, *or*	FOBT annually plus flex sig every 5 yr, *or*
DBCE every 5 yr, *or*	DBCE every 5 yr, *or*
Colonoscopy every 10 yr	Colonoscopy every 10 yr
Endometrial Women at menopause	No mention
Inform about risks and symptoms of endometrial cancer and strongly encouraged to report any unexpected bleeding or spotting	
Prostate Age ≥50 yr	
PSA blood test plus DRE offered annually	Evidence is insufficient to recommend for or against routine screening for prostate cancer using PSA or DRE for men <75 yr. Recommend against screening for men ≥75 yr.
Cancer-Related Checkup Include examination for cancers of the thyroid, testicles, ovaries, lymph nodes, oral cavity, and skin cancer	Evidence is insufficient to recommend for or against routine screening for lung, oral, and skin cancers
Health counseling about tobacco, sun exposure, diet and nutrition, risk factors, sexual practices, and environmental and occupational exposures	Recommends against screening for bladder, ovarian, pancreatic, and testicular cancers in asymptomatic adults

BSE, breast self-examination; CBE, Clinical breast examination; DBCE, Double contrast barium enema; DRE, Digital rectal examination; FIT, fecal immunochemical test; flex sig, flexible sigmoidoscopy; FOBT, Fecal occult blood test (at-home procedure for collecting two samples from three consecutive specimens); HPV, human papilloma virus; Pap, Papanicolaou; prep, preparation; PSA, prostate-specific antigen test.

an overall summary of screening guidelines for these four most common cancers. Every effort should be made to educate and reduce the barriers to screening. Physicians need to take a more proactive approach. They should discuss these cancer screening guidelines and recommend which test is most appropriate to increase patient awareness and promote long-term health. Patients must also take greater responsibility for their own proper nutrition and exercise to lower their risk for cancer.[8]

Summary

- Early diagnosis and detection of cancer profoundly affect survival rates and maximize positive outcomes.
- Breast cancer in women and prostate cancer in men are the leading causes of new cancers in the United States.
- Lung and bronchus cancer remains the leading cause of cancer-related death in men and women, and the 5-year survival rate averages 15%.
- Several organizations recommend a number of cancer screening guidelines. However, recommendations for screening for colon, breast, cervical, and prostate cancers are very similar.

Suggested Readings

Agency for Healthcare Research and Quality: The Guide to Clinical Preventive Services, 2007: Recommendations of the U.S. Preventive Services Task Force. Available at http://www.ahrq.gov/clinic/pocketgd08/pocketgd08.pdf (accessed March 20, 2009).

American College of Obstetrics and Gynecology: ACOG practice bulletin. Cervical cytology screening. Number 45, August 2003. Int J Gynaecol Obstet 2003;83(2):237-247.

American Urological Association: Prostate-specific antigen best practice policy. Oncology 2000;14(2):267-286.

Gohagan JK, Prorok PC, Hayes RB, Kramer BS, for the PLCO Project Team. The Prostate, Lung, Colorectal and Ovarian (PLCO) Cancer Screening Trial of the National Cancer Institute: History, organization, and status. Controlled Clinical Trials 2000;21:251S-272S.

Jemal A, Siegel R, Ward E, et al: Cancer statistics 2008. CA Cancer J Clin 2008;58:71-96.

Kushi LH, Byers T, Doyle C, et al: American Cancer Society guidelines on nutrition and physical activity for cancer prevention: Reducing the risk of cancer with healthy food choices and physical activity. CA Cancer J Clin 2006;56:254-281. Available at http://caonline.amcancersoc.org/cgi/reprint/56/5/254 (accessed March 20, 2009).

Smith RA, Cokkinides V, Eyre HJ: American Cancer Society guidelines for the early detection of cancer, 2006. CA Cancer J Clin 2006;56:11-25. Available at http://caonline.amcancersoc.org/cgi/reprint/56/1/11 (accessed March 20, 2009).

U.S. Preventive Services Task Force: Screening for cervical cancer. January 2003. Available at http://www.ahrq.gov/clinic/uspstf/uspscerv.htm (accessed March 20, 2009).

References

For a complete list of references, log onto www.expertconsult.com.

Preventive Measures and Screening for Ophthalmic Problems

Jeffrey Y. Chung and Rishi P. Singh

Vision is essential to the patient's quality of life and has a significant impact on morbidity. Myriad activities, from reading medication labels to using visual cues to ambulate in a room, arguably make vision one of the most important systems in the body. Declines in the visual system can lead to the inability to live independently, economic hardship, and psychological difficulties.[1,2] In fact, recent research has shown that certain eye disorders are associated with declines in quality of life measures regardless of measured visual acuity. This may be because the visual system is multifaceted, and impairment can cause changes in other aspects such as contrast sensitivity, peripheral vision, color vision, dark and light adaptation, glare, and depth perception.[3]

The prevalence and disabling effects of eye-related illness such as cataract, glaucoma, age-related macular degeneration, and diabetic retinopathy increase as the population ages. An estimated 3.3 million Americans ages 40 years and older have some visual impairment (best corrected vision between 20/40 to 20/200 in the better-seeing eye). It is estimated that 937,000 Americans are legally blind, with a best corrected vision of less than 20/200 in the better-seeing eye.[4] Formalized research reports have validated the significance of vision in the physical well-being of the geriatric patient. For example, the Blue Mountain Eye Study found that visual impairment was strongly associated with two or more falls in elderly adults.[5] The Beaver Dam study confirmed these findings, showing that patients older than 60 years who had impaired vision had an increased rate of hip fractures and decreased mobility.[6]

The leading cause of blindness and visual impairment differs among race categories. Age-related macular degeneration is the most prevalent cause of blindness of among whites, and glaucoma and cataract are the leading causes among African American and Latin American patients. Table 1 summarizes the important causes among these groups. Cataract was the most common contributor of low vision, accounting for approximately one half of the patients with low vision in each category. Overall, the age-adjusted blindness prevalence was higher for African Americans (odds ratio [OR], 2.77) and Latin Americans (OR, 3.13) as compared with whites (OR, 1.00). African American male patients had a significantly higher prevalence of blindness than female patients. The prevalence of visual impairment increases with age, and it incrases dramatically after the age of 75 years.[7] Applying the prevalence in race and age category to U.S. census projections for 2020, the number of blind persons older than 40 years in the United States is expected to increase by approximately 70% to 1.6 million, with an additional 3.9 million persons making a total of 5.5 million visually impaired Americans.[7]

Screening for ophthalmic issues has been shown to have a significant benefit in the elderly population. In a 5-year study of Medicare beneficiaries, those who had regular eye examinations experienced less decline of vision and functional status than those who had less-frequent examinations.[8] Ophthalmologists are best qualified to perform comprehensive ophthalmic screening and evaluation for cataracts. The frequency of screenings depends on the patient's clinical history as well as the findings during the most recent examination. Because the primary line of defense is prevention of these pathologic conditions, this chapter explores the screening measures and the current literature on the prevention of these disorders.

CATARACTS

The development of cataracts is a lifelong process involving a change in the chemical composition and disarrangement of lens fibrils. Only when the opacification causes significant visual loss and symptoms should the cataractous lens be removed and replaced with an artificial lens.

Cataract is the leading preventable cause of blindness in the United States and the world today.[9] It is responsible for 60% of all Medicare costs related to vision.[10] In the United States, an estimated 20.5 million (17.2%) Americans older than 40 years have a cataract in either eye. Women have a significantly higher age-adjusted prevalence of cataract than men in the United States. The number of Americans affected by cataract and undergoing cataract surgery will dramatically increase by 2020 as the U.S. population ages. The total number of persons who have cataract is estimated to rise to 30.1 million by 2020, and those who are expected to undergo cataract surgery will rise to 9.5 million by 2020.[11]

There are several different types of cataracts, each with its own pathology, anatomic location, and risk factors. Numerous potential risk factors have been associated with cataract formation. However, most of these studies are observational, and a true cause-and-effect relation cannot be proved. Furthermore, many of these studies are limited in their power because they failed to correlate cataract exposure to the risk factor in a standardized fashion.[12] The causes of cataracts are multifactorial and include age, diabetes, inflammation, trauma, and drugs such as steroids. Studies of potential risk factors for cataract formation are summarized in Box 1.

The prevention of cataracts has been studied in numerous clinical trials evaluating nutritional or vitamin supplementation. Thus far, no study has shown a significant benefit in delaying the onset and progression of cataract formation.[13-15] The Roche European American Cataract trial showed some protective effect from the use of vitamins C and E and beta-carotene, but this was not found in the European arm.[16] The American Academy of Ophthalmology (AAO) has no recommendations for nutritional supplements to prevent cataracts or delay progression.

Smoking has been directly linked to cataract formation and shows a dose-response effect. Several studies have shown decreased cataract formation in past smokers as compared with current smokers, illustrating a significant benefit from smoking cessation.[17-20] Cumulative exposure to ultraviolet (UV) B radiation has been associated with the development of cataracts, and therefore reduced sun exposure, UVB-protective sunglasses, and brimmed hats should be recommended to patients.[21-23] Long-term use of inhaled and oral corticosteroids has demonstrated a higher risk of formation.[24,25] Many studies have also found that diabetes mellitus is a risk factor for cataract formation and that tight glucose control can reduce the progression to cataract formation.[26]

For screening, patients can be stratified into those without risk factors, those with risk factors, and those with conditions that require intervention. The AAO recommends that patients ages 65 years and older have ophthalmic examinations every 1 to 2 years in the absence of risk factors and those 55 to 64 years have an examination every 1 to 3 years. Patients with risk factors or those with conditions that

Table 1 Leading Causes of Visual Impairment in the United States

Disease	African Americans		European Americans		Latin Americans	
	Blindness (%)	Low Vision (%)	Blindness (%)	Low Vision (%)	Blindness (%)	Low Vision (%)
AMD	4.4	3.2	54.4	22.9	14.3	14.1
Cataract	36.8	50.9	8.7	59.2	14.3	46.7
Diabetic retinopathy	7.3	14.5	5.4	4.9	14.3	13.0
Glaucoma	26.0	14.3	6.4	3.3	28.6	7.6

Blindness is defined as visual acuity less than 20/200 best corrected in the better-seeing eye.
Visual impairment is defined as one-eye vision less than 20/200.
AMD, age-related macular degeneration.

Box 1 Risk factors for Developing Cataracts

Increased Risk
Diabetes
Family history
Hypertension
Inhaled corticosteroids
Myopia
Obesity
Ocular trauma
Smoking
Systemic corticosteroids
UVB light exposure

Decreased Risk
Statin use

No Benefit or Unknown
Aspirin

Adapted from American Academy of Ophthalmology: Preferred practice pattern: Cataract in the Adult Eye. Available at http://www.guideline.gov/summary/summary.aspx?doc_id=10173 (accessed March 20, 2009).

might require interventions should have more frequent follow-ups, depending on the nature of the cataract and the functional visual impairment it causes.

GLAUCOMA

Glaucoma is a group of diseases with the common characteristic of optic neuropathy associated with visual field loss, with elevated intraocular pressure as the primary risk factor. The two major forms of glaucoma are open-angle glaucoma (OAG) and angle-closure glaucoma (ACG). ACG refers to closure of the angle formed between the iris and cornea, thereby restricting the outflow of aqueous fluid through the trabecular meshwork at the apex of the angle. OAG includes glaucoma conditions where the angle appears normal, with outflow obstruction likely at the level of trabecular meshwork or beyond. Both processes of aqueous outflow restriction lead to buildup of fluid and pressure in the eye, with associated optic neuropathy and visual field loss.

Between 1991 and 1999, the prevalence of glaucoma among Medicare recipients increased from 8.4% to 25.4%. Among patients with glaucoma, those with primary OAG increased from 4.6% to 13.8%, and those with ACG also increased from 0.7% to 2.7%.[27] The overall prevalence of OAG in the U.S. population 40 years and older in 2000 was estimated to be 1.86%, with 1.57 million white and 398,000 African American persons affected. After applying race-, age-, and gender-specific rates to the U.S. population as determined in the 2000 U.S. census, it is estimated that OAG affects 2.22 million U.S. citizens. Owing to the rapidly aging population, the number with OAG will increase by 50% to 3.6 million in 2020. African American patients had almost three times the age-adjusted prevalence of glaucoma as white patients.[28] Risk factors for OAG include elevated intraocular pressure, older age, positive family history, African or Latin American descent, and thinner central corneal thickness. Other possible risk factors include low diastolic perfusion pressures, diabetes, myopia, and systemic hypertension.[29]

Screening for OAG can be attempted by intraocular pressure measurement, optic nerve and nerve fiber layer appearance, and visual field testing, all cumbersome approaches to screening. Measuring intraocular pressure alone is not an effective screening tool because many population-based studies have shown persons with primary OAG and an intraocular pressure of less than 22 mm Hg, the usual screening cutoff.[30] Another method of attempted screening is to test visual fields. Perimetry based on frequency-doubling technology shows promise as a screening tool to detect moderately glaucomatous eyes. The positive predictive value found in a retrospective series was 32.6% to 45.1%, and the negative predictive value was 98.7%.[31]

Thus far, no effective screening process has been identified from extensive review of the literature.[32] Screening by a combination of positive family history and elevated intraocular pressure showed an 82% sensitivity for OAG.[29,33,34] The more likely scenario for screening larger populations will be a combination of intraocular pressure measurement, visual field testing, and optic nerve head cupping evaluation.

AGE-RELATED MACULAR DEGENERATION

Age-related macular degeneration (AMD) involves the destruction of the retina and commonly affects central vision or the macula and its supportive tissue underneath. Early manifestations include the appearance of drusen, waste products of metabolism underneath the retina. Vision loss is manifested in the dry, non-neovascular, form with progressive atrophy of the retina and retinal pigment epithelium in a geographic pattern. In the wet or neovascular form, more-rapid visual loss occurs secondary to leakage, bleeding, and fibrotic scarring from neovascular tissue proliferating under the retina.

The overall prevalence of neovascular AMD and geographic atrophy in the U.S. population older than 40 years is estimated to be 1.47%, with 1.75 million Americans having AMD. A survey of Medicare beneficiaries between 1994 and 1998 showed a prevalence of wet macular degeneration of between 0.37% and 1.14%, compared with 1.48% obtained from the Beaver Dam Eye Study.[35] The prevalence of AMD increases dramatically with age, with more than 15% of the white women older than 80 years having neovascular AMD or geographic atrophy, or both. More than 7 million persons had drusen measuring 125 μm or larger and were, therefore, at substantial risk for developing AMD. Owing to the rapidly aging population, the number of Medicare recipients with AMD increased from 5.0% to 27.1% between 1991 and 1999. The percentage of patients with AMD is expected to increase by 50% to 2.95 million in 2020.[36]

Although an estimated 80% of AMD patients have the non-neovascular form, the neovascular form may be responsible for almost 90% of the severe visual loss from AMD.[37,38] Advancing age is a major risk factor for AMD. In the Framingham Eye Study, 6.4% of patients ages 65 to 74 years had signs of macular degeneration. This rate increases to 19.7% in patients older than 75 years.[39]

Antioxidant vitamin and mineral supplementation of vitamins C and E, beta-carotene, zinc, and copper has been shown by the Age-Related Eye Disease Study (AREDS) to reduce the rate of development of advanced AMD from those with intermediate stage or unilateral advanced AMD. In this patient population, the AREDS vitamin and mineral formula reduced the 5-year risk of progression to advanced AMD by 25% and reduced moderate visual loss by 19%. However, beta-carotene administration has been associated with increased risk for lung cancer in heavy smokers and in persons with asbestos exposure.[40]

Other risk factors for AMD include cigarette smoking, hyperopia, light iris color, hypertension, hypercholesterolemia, female gender, cardiovascular disease, and low level of dietary antioxidants and other dietary factors.[41] Recent studies have highlighted the possible relation between complement factor H mutations and AMD. Homozygous patients with the risk allele have a 7.4-fold increased risk of AMD development and progression.[42] Finally, the role of heredity has been supported by many studies.[43]

Persons without any risk factors for AMD should be evaluated by the standard age criteria set by the AAO. Patients older than 65 years should have yearly examinations, and patients aged 40 to 64 years should have an examination every 1 to 2 years. Patients with early or intermediate retinal changes from AMD should be seen annually. They should also be educated about the symptoms indicating advancement of AMD and the need to contact the ophthalmologist when new changes arise. Follow-up examinations in patients with advanced AMD are also helpful because they can permit evaluation of signs in the contralateral eye, provide an opportunity for the patient to discuss new preventive measures, and reinforce self-monitoring.

DIABETIC RETINOPATHY

Like AMD, diabetic retinopathy manifests itself in two forms, nonproliferative and proliferative (neovascular). Early diabetic retinopathy involves abnormality of existing retinal vessels seen by vascular leakage, retinal hemorrhage, tissue infarction, and nonperfusion. Macular edema, a result of leaking microaneurysms causing fluid accumulation in the macula, represents a visually significant entity in nonproliferative retinopathy. In the proliferative forms, abnormal vessels grow secondary to signals from the ischemic retina. Bleeding into the vitreous (secondary to abnormal neovascularization) causes vision loss. Neovascular proliferation also causes tractional retinal detachment and severe loss of vision when left untreated.

The duration of diabetes is a major risk factor for development of diabetic retinopathy. According to the Wisconsin Epidemiologic Study of Diabetic Retinopathy, 25% of patients with type 1 diabetes develop retinopathy after 5 years, 60% after 10 years, and 80% after 15 years. In patients with type 2 diabetes, 40% of those taking insulin and 24% not taking insulin develop retinopathy within 5 years of diagnosis. After 19 years, these rates increase to 84% and 53%, respectively.[44,45]

Although the development of retinopathy in diabetic patients is difficult to prevent, tight glucose control can reduce progression to visually significant diabetic retinopathy. Intensive glucose control has been shown to reduce development of retinopathy by 76% in patients with type 1 diabetes within 3 years. The risk of retinopathy progression is reduced by 54%, and the risk of progression to proliferative disease is reduced by 47%.[46] In patients with type 2 diabetes, tighter blood glucose control reduced the need for laser surgery by 29%. Concurrent control of hypertension resulted in a 47% reduction of vision decrease.[47] A recent (ACCORD) study on the effects of even more intense glucose control with a goal of hemoglobin A_{1c} of below 6% (vs. 7%) found an increased relative mortality of 22% in the tightly controlled group after a 3.5-year follow up. The question of increased benefit with even tighter glycemic control may be clarified as more data emerge.[48]

In patients with poorly controlled diabetes, vision fluctuations can occur as changes in serum osmolality affect the refractive qualities of human lenses. This acute phenomenon does not necessarily correlate with the presence of diabetic retinopathy. A stable blood glucose level can ensure proper vision testing as well as proper refraction measurement if corrective lenses are needed.

Regular ophthalmologic examination for patients with diabetes should be emphasized. With treatments for diabetic retinopathy effective in preventing vision loss in 90% of the patients, the numbers of patients referred by primary care physicians are far below those recommended by the American Diabetes Association guideline.[49] Between 50% and 60% of Medicare beneficiaries with diabetes were found to receive annual eye examinations within a 15-month survey period.[50] The Wisconsin Epidemiologic Study of Diabetic Retinopathy found 11% of patients with type I diabetes and 7% of patients with high-risk proliferative retinopathy had no examination by an ophthalmologist within 2 years.[51]

Routine medical eye examinations are beneficial to patients, because many changes due to diabetic retinopathy may be visually subtle or affect peripheral visual areas not commonly noticed. For patients with diabetes, the AAO recommends a comprehensive eye examination schedule of initial examination within 5 years after onset of type 1 diabetes, with yearly follow-ups; initial examination at diagnosis of type 2 diabetes, with yearly follow-ups; and examination before pregnancy for all women with diabetes, before conception or early in the first trimester, with follow-ups every 1 to 3 months for severe nonproliferative diabetic retinopathy and every 3 to 12 months if retinopathy is milder.

Routine eye examinations allow patients to receive advice about self-protective activities for disease prevention. Closer monitoring can be planned for patients with worrisome findings on the initial examination such as nonperfusion of the retina without formation of proliferative disease, or edema adjacent to the macula but not clinically significant for laser treatment. Good glucose control should be maintained in conjunction with primary care physicians and possible nutritional consultation.

Summary

- Age-related macular degeneration is the most prevalent cause of blindness among whites.
- Glaucoma and cataract are the leading causes of blindness among African American and Latin American patients.
- Smoking, ultraviolet B radiation, inhaled or oral corticosteroids, and diabetes are risk factors for cataract progression.
- Risk factors for glaucoma include elevated intraocular pressure, age, positive family history, and African or Latin American ancestry.
- Development of age-related macular degeneration has been linked to cigarette smoking, hereditary factors, and age.
- Tight glucose control in diabetes can reduce progression in diabetic retinopathy.

Suggested Readings

Age-Related Eye Disease Study Research Group: A randomized, placebo-controlled, clinical trial of high-dose supplementation with vitamins C and E, beta carotene, and zinc for age-related macular degeneration and vision loss: AREDS report no. 8. Arch Ophthalmol 2001;119:1417-1436.

Age-Related Eye Disease Study Research Group: A randomized, placebo-controlled, clinical trial of high-dose supplementation with vitamins C and E and beta carotene for age-related cataract and vision loss: AREDS report no. 9. Arch Ophthalmol 2001;119:1439-1452.

Congdon N, O'Colmain B, Klaver CC, et al: Causes and prevalence of visual impairment among adults in the United States. Arch Ophthalmol 2004;122:477-485.

Congdon N, Vingerling JR, Klein BE, et al: Prevalence of cataract and pseudophakia/aphakia among adults in the United States. Arch Ophthalmol 2004;122:487-494.

Diabetes Control and Complications Trial Research Group: The effect of intensive treatment of diabetes on the development and progression of long-term complications in insulin-dependent diabetes mellitus. N Engl J Med 1993;329:977-986.

Kahn HA, Leibowitz HM, Ganley JP, et al: The Framingham Eye Study. II. Association of ophthalmic pathology with single variables previously measured in the Framingham Heart Study. Am J Epidemiol 1977;106:33-41.

Lee PP, Feldman ZW, Ostermann J, et al: Longitudinal rates of annual eye examinations of persons with diabetes and chronic eye diseases. Ophthalmology 2003;110:1952-1959.

Lee PP, Feldman ZW, Ostermann J, et al: Longitudinal prevalence of major eye diseases. Arch Ophthalmol 2003;121:1303-1310.

Pollack AL, Brodie SE: Diagnostic yield of the routine dilated fundus examination. Ophthalmology 1998;105:382-386.

West SK, Valmadrid CT: Epidemiology of risk factors for age-related cataract. Surv Ophthalmol 1995;39:323-334.

References

For a complete list of references, log onto www.expertconsult.com.

Perioperative Evaluation

Christopher M. Whinney

Operative treatment of disease has a tremendous yet unrecognized impact on modern medical systems. An estimated 26 million patients underwent surgery in the United States in 2005. Serious adverse events occur in more than 1 million of these patients, at an estimated cost of $25 billion annually. With the aging population, it is anticipated that surgical referrals will increase by 25%, costs by 50%, and costs of perioperative complications by 100%. Given these staggering numbers, it is imperative that clinicians involved with patients undergoing surgery know the basics of perioperative diagnosis and management.

CARDIOVASCULAR EVALUATION AND MANAGEMENT

Cardiovascular complications are one of the most common perioperative adverse events in patients undergoing noncardiac surgery. Although in absolute numbers they are rare, they are associated with a mortality rate as high as 70%. It is essential for clinicians to be familiar with current cardiac risk evaluation and preventive strategies for patients undergoing noncardiac surgery.

PREOPERATIVE CARDIAC ASSESSMENT

The core goals of preoperative cardiac assessment are to determine the status of the patient's cardiac conditions, to provide an estimate of risk, to determine if further testing is warranted, and to determine if interventions are warranted to reduce perioperative cardiac risk.

Prior History

The prior cardiovascular history of the patient is the foundation of the perioperative assessment. Because the incidence of perioperative cardiovascular events varies according to the patient risk profile, risk of the proposed surgery, and the patient's functional capacity, all of these elements should be part of the preoperative history.

The clinician should inquire about prior myocardial infarction, congestive heart failure, valvular disease, angina, or arrhythmia. If the patient has had prior diagnostic testing or therapeutic interventions, inquire about when and where these were done and the results of such procedures. Traditional risk factors, such as hypertension, dyslipidemia, tobacco use, and diabetes, are essential elements, as well as comorbid conditions that might limit functional capacity such as peripheral vascular disease, chronic obstructive pulmonary disease, cerebrovascular disease, and renal insufficiency. Current symptoms such as chest pain at rest or on exertion, shortness of breath, claudication, syncope or presyncope, or anginal equivalent symptoms should be noted.

Functional capacity is vital information, because exercise capacity is a reliable predictor of future cardiac events. This is usually expressed in metabolic equivalents (METs), where one MET is defined as the oxygen consumption of a 70-kg man at rest. Greater than 7 METs of activity tolerance is considered excellent, whereas less than 4 METs is considered poor activity tolerance. The Duke Activity Status Index suggests questions that correlate with METs levels; for example, walking on level ground at about 4 miles per hour or carrying a bag of groceries up a flight of stairs expends approximately 4 METs of activity. Patients limited in their activity from noncardiac causes, such as severe osteoarthritis or general debility, are categorized as having poor functional capacity, because one cannot discern if significant cardiac conditions exist without the benefit of noninvasive cardiac testing.

The degree of surgical risk contributes to a patient's risk for cardiac complications. In general, procedures that are longer and have greater potential for blood loss, hemodynamic instability, and intravascular fluid shifts carry greater risk. Procedural risk is stratified into high (estimated mortality >5%), intermediate (mortality 1%-5%), and low (<1%) risk categories. Vascular surgery procedures are considered high risk procedures, with the exception of carotid endarterectomy; the literature cites an event rate between 1 and 5% for this procedure, categorizing it as an intermediate-risk operation.

The physical examination serves to confirm the above information and can reveal information of importance unknown to the patient. Vital signs can detect hypertension or hypotension, tachycardia or bradycardia, significant arrhythmias, or hypoxia if pulse oximetry is used. Jugular venous distension, the presence of an S_3 gallop, or rales suggest decompensated heart failure. Cardiac murmurs should be noted, especially if aortic stenosis is suspected. Carotid, femoral, or abdominal bruits suggest the presence of peripheral vascular or cerebrovascular disease.

The electrocardiogram is a commonly used tool in traditional preoperative cardiac assessment, although its role in the asymptomatic patient is unclear. Incidental findings that might be significant include evidence of prior myocardial infarction (MI), conduction abnormalities such as second- or third-degree heart block, bundle branch block, and left ventricular hypertrophy suggesting hypertensive heart disease. Although the current literature notes no evidence that asymptomatic findings on the preoperative EKG affect postoperative cardiac risk, clinicians often obtain this test as a preoperative baseline for comparison in the patient with prior heart disease or with significant clinical predictors for cardiovascular events.

Risk Stratification

Since Goldman and colleagues created the first risk-stratification tool in the late 1970s, several risk indices have been published, each with their own benefits and limitations. The most prominent in use are the guidelines published jointly by the American College of Cardiology and the American Heart Association, (the ACC/AHA guidelines), most recently revised in September 2007. The stepwise risk assessment recommended by the ACC/AHA is demonstrated in Figure 1. This revision incorporates a simple, validated assessment tool called the Revised Cardiac Risk Index (RCRI). The RCRI discerns the presence of six independent predictors of major cardiovascular complications (Box 1). The authors of this tool did not make recommendations for risk reduction, but subsequent studies suggest the use of beta blockers based on RCRI score results.

Noninvasive Testing

In patients with suspicion for occult coronary artery disease or with risk factors and limited functional capacity, noninvasive cardiac testing can further unveil the presence of significant coronary artery disease and assess the patient's functional capacity. Treadmill stress testing, with and without thallium imaging, has been assessed in the literature and found to have excellent negative predictive value for perioperative cardiac events. Dipyridamole or adenosine thallium imaging can be used in patients unable to reach an adequate heart rate with physical activity and also has a comparable negative predictive value. In addition, dobutamine echocardiography has similar efficacy in risk stratification, with the added advantage of lower cost;

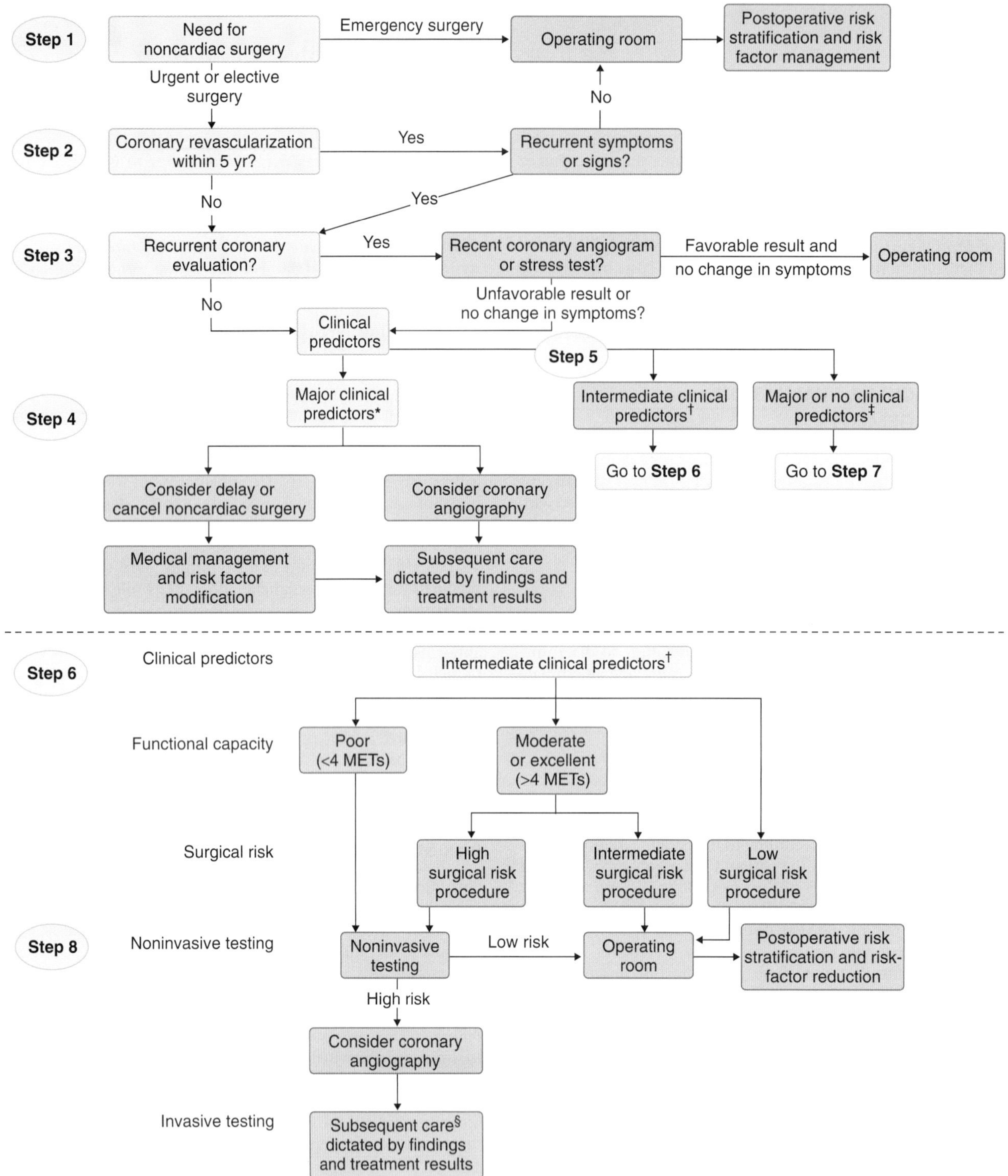

Figure 1 Cardiac evaluation and care algorithm for noncardiac surgery based on active clinical conditions, known cardiovascular disease, or cardiac risk factors for patients 50 years of age or older. Consider perioperative beta blockade for populations in which this has been shown to reduce cardiac morbidity/mortality. *Clinical risk factors include ischemic heart disease, compensated or prior heart failure, diabetes mellitus, renal insufficiency, and cerebrovascular disease. ACC/AHA, American College of Cardiology/American Heart Association; HR, heart rate; LOE, level of evidence; MET, metabolic equivalent. *(Reproduced with permission from Fleisher LA, Beckman JA, Brown KA, et al: ACC/AHA 2007 guidelines on perioperative cardiovascular evaluation and care for noncardiac surgery: A report of the American College of Cardiology/American Heart Association Task Force on Practice Guidelines (Writing Committee to Revise the 2002 Guidelines on Perioperative Cardiovascular Evaluation for Noncardiac Surgery). Circulation 2007;116:e418-e499.)*

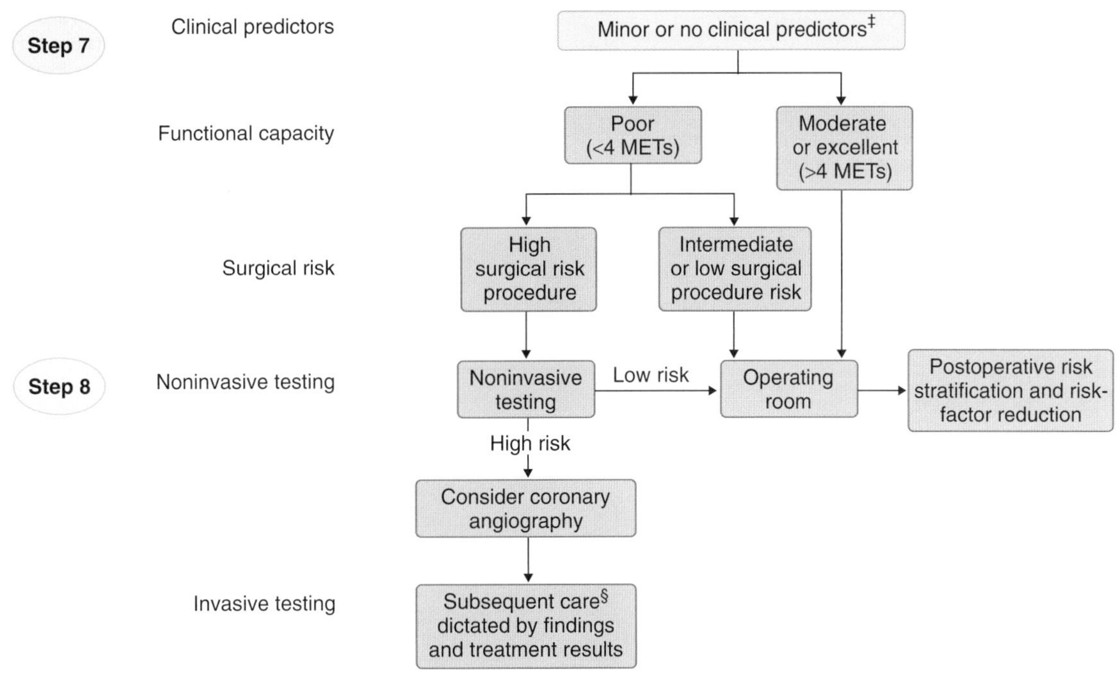

Figure 1, cont'd.

Box 1 Revised Cardiac Risk Index Criteria

High-risk surgical procedure, defined as intraperitoneal, intrathoracic, or suprainguinal vascular procedure

Ischemic heart disease, defined as the following:

- History of myocardial infarction
- History of or current angina
- Use of sublingual nitroglycerine
- Positive exercise test results
- Q waves on electrocardiogram
- Patients who have undergone percutaneous transluminal coronary angioplasty or coronary artery bypass graft surgery and who have chest pain presumed to be of ischemic origin

Cerebrovascular disease, defined as the following:

- History of transient ischemic attack
- History of cerebrovascular accident

Diabetes mellitus requiring insulin therapy

Chronic renal insufficiency, defined as a baseline creatinine level of at least 2.0 mg/dL (177 μmol/L)

Adapted from Lee TH, Marcantonio ER, Mangione CM, et al: Derivation and prospective validation of a simple index for prediction of cardiac risk of major noncardiac surgery. Circulation 1999;100(10):1043-1049.

this test is more limited in patients with preexisting wall motion abnormalities or in the presence of bundle branch blocks. Transthoracic echocardiography may be helpful if congestive heart failure (CHF) or significant valvular disease is suspected (ejection fraction <35% has been shown to predict postoperative CHF), but this should not be pursued for screening purposes. Although these tests have good negative-predictive value, they have poor positive-predictive value for perioperative cardiac events; thus, a positive test is more limited in its value.

Coronary Artery Revascularization

If significant coronary artery disease is seen by noninvasive testing or by cardiac catheterization, options for management include medical optimization or revascularization. Asymptomatic patients with prior coronary artery bypass graft (CABG) surgery or percutaneous coronary interventions have lower rates of perioperative mortality and nonfatal myocardial infarction (MI) compared with historical controls; this protective effect lasts approximately 4 to 6 years. However, studies such as the CARP and DECREASE-V trials suggest that prophylactic revascularization, even in high-risk surgeries, provide no risk reduction in patients without unstable symptoms. This may in part be due to the risks of the revascularization itself (CABG surgery complications or stent thrombosis). If patients have an independent indication for revascularization, this should be pursued and elective surgery should be postponed; otherwise, medical optimization should be considered as the primary means of risk reduction.

Perioperative Risk Reduction

Medical means of perioperative cardiac risk reduction in recent times have predominantly focused on two classes of medications: selective β_1 antagonists (beta blockers) and 3-hydroxy-3-methylglutaryl coenzyme A (HMG-CoA) reductase inhibitors (statins).

Beta blockers are well established to reduce cardiac mortality, MI, and ischemia in ambulatory settings; four studies between 1996 and 2001 found that perioperative beta blockade reduced the risk of death, MI, or both between 50% and 90% at postoperative intervals from 28 days to up to 2 years. Subsequent randomized, controlled trials of vascular surgery patients showed no clear benefit from metoprolol on major cardiac events; a meta-analysis by Devereaux and colleagues of the trials showed a small benefit on 30-day adverse outcomes that failed to reach statistical significance. A retrospective review by Lindenauer and coworkers that evaluated data on more than 600,000 patients extracted from Medicare databases used the RCRI score and found that low-risk patients (RCRI = 0) did not benefit and might actually have been harmed by beta blockade, but higher risk patients (RCRI ≥3) had significant risk reductions for in-hospital death.

The recently published POISE trial was a randomized, controlled trial of more than 8000 patients spanning 21 countries comparing extended-release metoprolol with placebo. Metoprolol administra-

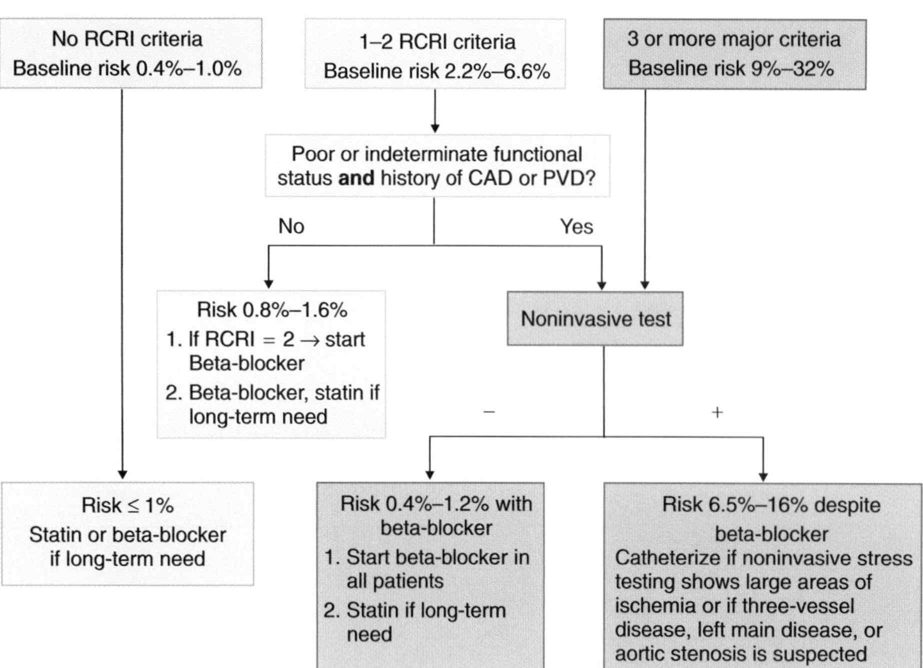

Figure 2 Suggested algorithm for perioperative of beta blockers. CAD, coronary artery disease; PVD, peripheral vascular disease; RCRI, Revised Cardiac Risk Index. *(From Auerbach AD, Goldman L: β-Blockers and reduction of cardiac events in noncardiac surgery: Clinical applications. JAMA 2002;287[11]:1445-1447.)*

tion reduced the risk of nonfatal myocardial infarction, cardiac revascularization, and clinically significant atrial fibrillation 30 days after randomization compared with placebo. However, the beta-blocker group suffered a significantly higher risk of overall mortality, stroke, and clinically significant hypotension and bradycardia. Criticisms of the trial methodology included the high dose of beta blocker used (100 mg preoperatively followed by 200 mg daily postoperatively as tolerated hemodynamically) and the lack of dose titration; however, this is the largest randomized trial of perioperative beta blockade to date, and it suggests that harm might outweigh benefit. Further studies are needed to define more clearly the population who will benefit from prophylactic beta blockade, as well as the optimal regimen in both dose and timing. The algorithm suggested by Auerbach and Goldman for selecting patients for beta blockade (Fig. 2) is still a reasonable method to use until further trial data are available.

Statin therapy has been evaluated in the perioperative setting by observational studies by Poldermans and colleagues and by Kertai and colleagues and by a small randomized trial by Durazzo and coworkers. These studies consistently reveal 60% to 70% reduction in mortality in patients taking statins. Because patients at risk for postoperative MI and cardiac events often have indications for statins, the perioperative period may be an opportunity to start appropriate statin therapy in these patients.

PREOPERATIVE PULMONARY ASSESSMENT

In contrast to cardiovascular risk assessment and management, the literature on perioperative pulmonary assessment and intervention is less robust. However, the American College of Physicians has published a summary of the literature and guidelines for evaluation and management.

Postoperative pulmonary complications (PPCs) are equally prevalent compared with cardiac complications and contribute similarly to morbidity, mortality, and length of postoperative hospital stay. Patient factors increasing risk for PPCs include the presence of chronic obstructive pulmonary disease, age older than 60 years, American Society of Anesthesiologists (ASA) class II or greater, functional dependence, and congestive heart failure. However, obesity and mild to moderate asthma have not been consistently shown to predict PPCs. A low serum albumin level (<35 g/dL) has been found to be a powerful predictor of PPCs, likely as a reflection of impaired general health or immune compromise.

Surgical factors increasing PPC risk include thoracic or abdominal surgical site (which can lead to splinting due to pain and impaired diaphragmatic excursion; neurosurgery; head and neck procedures; vascular procedures, especially abdominal aortic aneurysm repair; any emergent procedures; use of general anesthesia, and prolonged (>3 hours) procedures.

Routine pulmonary function testing and chest radiography are not indicated preoperatively because they do not predict PPCs; obtain these only if the patient is symptomatic, has unexplained dyspnea, or is undergoing lung volume reduction surgery or other intrathoracic procedures.

Interventions that have been found successful for reducing PPCs in high-risk patients include incentive spirometry or deep breathing exercises, and selective use of nasogastric tube decompression only if needed. Neither right heart catheterization nor total enteral or parenteral nutrition demonstrate benefit in reducing PPCs.

Until recently, no scoring systems existed for predicting PPCs akin to those used for cardiovascular risk stratification. Researchers with the Veterans' Administration National Surgical Quality Improvement Project (NSQIP) developed and prospectively validated scoring systems for predicting postoperative pneumonia and respiratory failure that includes many of these predictors in a numeric scoring system. Although these tools have prognostic value, guidance of preventive therapy based on these tools is limited.

Other ongoing avenues of research include the effect of obstructive sleep apnea on PPCs and the role of continuous positive airway pressure (CPAP) or bilevel positive airway pressure (BiPAP) in preventing or treating postoperative respiratory failure and PPCs.

MANAGEMENT OF ANTICOAGULATION

Venous Thromboembolism

Venous thromboembolism (VTE), which includes deep vein thrombosis (DVT) and pulmonary embolism (PE), are quite common causes of morbidity and mortality that are largely preventable in the postoperative patient. Several national quality improvement organizations have cited VTE prophylaxis for patients at risk as a priority for both individual physicians and for hospitals, because this intervention reduces both adverse patient outcomes and hospital costs.

Surgical patients in particular have significantly increased risks for VTE due to advanced age, multiple medical comorbidities, and prolonged procedure times, in addition to the hypercoagulable state of surgery and immobility. Thus, clinicians must consider VTE risk and risk-reduction strategies in all patients undergoing surgery.

Postoperative DVT is typically asymptomatic, and fatal PE can often be the first sign of VTE; screening modalities (such as with venous duplex imaging) in asymptomatic patients have low sensitivity to detect clot, so it is not appropriate to use these unless clinical suspicion is present. Therefore, the approach of choice is to systematically apply prevention strategies to all patients undergoing surgery, with treatment choices based on patient-related and procedure-related risks.

Patient-related risk factors for VTE include age older than 40 years, malignancy, immobilization, varicose veins, severe cardiopulmonary disease (prior MI, congestive heart failure [CHF], chronic obstructive pulmonary disease [COPD]), prior stroke, paralysis or spinal cord injury, prior VTE events, hyperviscosity syndromes (polycythemia vera or malignancy related), and major vascular injury.

VTE risks also vary with the type of procedure; patients who have had orthopedic procedures or spinal cord injuries have the highest reported rates in the literature in the absence of prophylaxis (as high as 60%-80%). These patients require the most aggressive approach, often combining pharmacologic and nonpharmacologic means. In contrast, outpatient procedures such as cataract surgery and laparoscopic procedures have quite a low risk for perioperative VTE and do not require preventive means other than early ambulation unless other VTE risks are present. Other surgery types, including general, vascular, gynecologic, and neurosurgical, have similar risks for VTE and may be stratified based on patient age, preexisting risk factors, and length of operation.

Prevention of Postoperative Venous Thromboembolism

Modalities to prevent VTE events are categorized into nonpharmacologic and pharmacologic means. Nonpharmacologic methods include early ambulation, graduated compression stockings, and intermittent pneumatic compression devices. Pharmacologic methods routinely evaluated include aspirin, low-dose unfractionated heparin (LDUH), low-molecular-weight heparin (LMWH), warfarin, and factor Xa inhibitors such as fondaparinux. Several new classes of antithrombotic agents are being evaluated, including direct Xa and IXa inhibitors, and agents that are active through antithrombin, heparin cofactor II, and protein C.

The American College of Chest Physicians (ACCP) recommendations for antithrombotic prevention of perioperative VTE is highlighted in Table 1 based on the risk for thromboembolism. Note that aspirin alone is not recommended by the ACCP guidelines, due to data showing limited effectiveness compared with other modalities and increased bleeding risk, mostly gastrointestinal in origin.

The use of inferior vena cava (IVC) filters has increased significantly over the past several decades, and an increasing number are being placed for prophylaxis in high-risk patients. Retrievable IVC filters have been developed that can be removed up to 180 days after placement. However, placing retrievable IVC filters appeared to be cost prohibitive in studies of multisystem trauma patients. Because it is not clear that they improve outcomes, are costly, and have a high rate of complications (29%, including improper placement, migration, caval occlusion or wall penetration, and venous stasis), current ACCP guidelines do not support prophylactic placement of IVC filters. However, patients who cannot tolerate pharmacologic prophylaxis, who have a complication of anticoagulation, or who have a temporary contraindication are reasonable candidates for temporary IVC filter placement for protection from fatal or disabling PE.

Bridging Therapy

More than 2 million Americans currently take anticoagulant agents for prevention or treatment of thromboembolic events. As the population ages, so will the frequency of surgical procedures, and consequently clinicians will need to manage perioperative anticoagulation more often. Discontinuation of anticoagulation leaves patients unprotected from thromboembolic risk for several days around the time of surgery. However, aggressive anticoagulation in the postop-

Table 1 Levels of Thromboembolism Risk and Recommended Thromboprophylaxis in Hospital Patients*

Levels of Risk	Approximate DVT Risk without Thromboprophylaxis (%)†	Suggested Thromboprophylaxis Options‡
Low Risk		
Minor surgery in mobile patients	<10	No specific thromboprophylaxis
Medical patients who are fully mobile		
Moderate Risk		
Most general, open gynecologic or urologic surgery patients	10-40	LMWH (at recommended doses), LDUH bid or tid, fondaparinux
Medical patients, bed rest or sick		
Moderate VTE risk plus high bleeding risk		Mechanical thromboprophylaxis§
High Risk		
Hip or knee arthroplasty, HFS	40-80	LMWH (at recommended doses), fondaparinux, oral vitamin K antagonist (INR 2-3)
Major trauma, SCI		
High VTE risk plus high bleeding risk		Mechanical thromboprophylaxis§

*The descriptive terms are purposely left undefined to allow individual clinician interpretation.

†Rates based on objective diagnostic screening for asymptomatic DVT in patients not receiving thromboprophylaxis.

‡See the relevant section in this chapter for specific recommendations.

§Mechanical thromboprophylaxis includes IPC or VFP and/or GCS; consider switch to anticoagulant thromboprophylaxis when high bleeding risk decreases.

DVT, deep vein thrombosis; GCS, graduated compression stockings; HFS, hip fracture surgery; INR, international normalized ratio; IPC, intermittent pneumatic compression; LDUH, low-dose unfractionated heparin; LMWH, low-molecular-weight heparin; SCI, spinal cord injury; VFP, venous foot pump; VTE, venous thromboembolism.

Adapted from Table 5 in Geerts WH, Bergqvist D, Pineo GF: Prevention of venous thromboembolism: American College of Chest Physicians evidence-based clinical practice guidelines (8th edition). Chest 2008;133:381S-453S.

Box 2 Bridging and Risk for Thromboembolism

High Risk for Thrombolism: Bridging Advised

Known hypercoagulable state as documented by a thromboembolic event and one of the following:

- Protein C deficiency
- Protein S deficiency
- Antithrombin III deiciency
- Homozygous factor V Leiden mutation
- Antiphospholipid-antibody syndrome

Hypercoagulable state suggested by recurrent (≥2) arterial or idiopathic venous thromboemoblic events*

Venous or arterial thromboembolism in prior 1-3 months

Rheumatic atrial fibrillation

Acute intracardiac thrombus visualized by echocardiogram

Atrial fibrillation plus mechanical heart valve in any position

Older mechanical valve model (single-disk or ball-in-cage) in mitral position

Recently placed mechanical valve (<3 mo)

Atrial fibrillation with history of cardioembolism

Intermediate Risk for Thromboembolism: Bridging on a Case-by-Case Basis

Cerebrovasscular disease with multiple (≥2) strokes or transient ischemic attacks without risk factors for cardiac embolism

Newer mechanical valve model (e.g., St. Jude) in mitral position

Older mechanical valve model in aortic position

Atrial fibrillation without a history of cardiac embolism but with multiple risks for cardiac embolism†

Venous thromboembolism >3-6 months ago‡

Low Risk for Thromboembolism: Bridging Not Advised

One remote venous thrombolism (>6 months ago)‡

Intrinsic cerebrovascular disease (e.g., carotid atherosclerosis) without recurrent strokes or transient ischemic attacks

Atrial fibrillation without multiple risks for cardiac embolism

Newer-model prosthetic valve in aortic position

**Not including primary atherosclerotic events, such as stroke or myocardial infarction due to cerebrovascular or coronary disease*

†For example, ejection fraction <40%, diabetes, hypertension, nonrheumatic valvular heart disease, transmural myocardial infarction within preceding month.

‡For patients with a history of venous thromboembolism undergoing major surgery, consideration can be given to postoperative bridging therapy only (without preoperative bridging).

From Jaffer AK, Brotman DJ, Chukwumerije N: When patients on warfarin need surgery. Cleve Clin J Med 2003;70:973-984.

erative period can increase bleeding risk. Thus, clinicians must consider the indication for long-term anticoagulation and extrapolate the risk for thrombotic events compared to the risk for bleeding events (Box 2).

High-risk patients have up to a 10% rate of thromboembolism per year, and the concern for a thromboembolic event outweighs the perceived bleeding risk. The ACCP guidelines suggest bridging anticoagulation in this patient population, which involves discontinuing warfarin 5 or 6 days before surgery and initiating subcutaneous LMWH or intravenous unfractionated heparin at a therapeutic dose when the patient's INR falls below the therapeutic range. The bridging agent is stopped immediately before surgery (from 6 to 24 hours prior), and anticoagulation is resumed as soon as possible after surgery.

Low-risk patients have an annual arterial thromboembolic risk of less than 5%, or a monthly VTE risk of less than 2%. Because the perioperative bleeding risk with bridging therapy outweighs the thromboembolic risk in these patients, bridging therapy is not indicated. Warfarin can be discontinued approximately 5 days before surgery and resumed after surgery when the bleeding risk related to surgery is minimal.

Moderate-risk patients have an annual arterial event risk of between 5% and 10% and a monthly VTE risk between 2% and 10%. These patients might have comparable risks of bleeding and thromboembolism, so individual patient and procedure factors must be assessed on a case-by-case basis in these patients.

Assessment of perioperative thromboembolic risk is not simply achieved by taking the yearly risks and dividing by 365 to obtain a daily risk. Surgery creates a prothrombotic milleu that can increase VTE risk by 100-fold. In addition, discontinuation of warfarin has been associated with biochemical evidence of rebound hypercoagulability, although this phenomenon has not been demonstrated clinically. Therefore, even in low- and intermediate-risk patients, appropriate VTE prophylaxis measures should still be applied, even if bridging therapy is not indicated.

In addition, consider the consequences of the thromboembolic event being averted by bridging. While arterial events are less frequent, they cause significantly more death and disability when they do occur (20%-30% mortality and 30%-40% rate of disability, compared with combined rates of 5%-10% for VTE and 3%-13% for bleeding events).

Intravenous unfractionated heparin and LMWH are typically used for bridging therapy, although the use of LMWH in patients with mechanical heart valves is controversial.

The prescribing information for enoxaparin states that its use for "thromboprophylaxis in pregnant women with mechanical prosthetic heart valves has not been adequately studied." This refers to the study where two of eight pregnant women receiving enoxaparin developed clots resulting in blockage of the valve and leading to maternal and fetal death, whereas none of four patients receiving unfractionated heparin developed valve thrombosis.

In the two deaths, anti-Xa levels were subtherapeutic at some points during treatment; subsequent studies note that the physiology of pregnancy can affect the pharmacokinetics of enoxaparin, leading to lower anti-Xa levels. Therefore, if enoxaparin is to be used in pregnant patients for any reason, anti-Xa levels should be checked frequently and kept between 0.5 and 1.2 anti-Xa units. Nevertheless, unfractionated heparin should be used for any pregnant patients who have mechanical heart valves and require bridging therapy.

However, several studies document the safety of use of LMWH for bridging in patients with mechanical heart valves; in a review of data on 461 patients from 10 studies, three patients had transient ischemic attacks and no patients had strokes or valve thromboses.

PERIOPERATIVE MANAGEMENT OF MEDICATION

Stopping and restarting medications in the perioperative period is an essential component of perioperative care. Appropriate management of medications helps maintain stability of chronic conditions, prevent medication withdrawal, avoid interactions with anesthetic agents, and facilitate transition to discharge. Although published clinical trial data in this area are limited, management strategies are extrapolated based on case reports, expert consensus, in vitro studies, and drug manufacturer's recommendations.

Postoperatively, patients manifest a significant stress response, including an increase in pituitary, adrenal, thyroid, and hypothalamic activity, which leads to heightened sympathetic nervous system activity. This can affect the activity and metabolism of medications for chronic conditions. Also, gut motility and absorption may be diminished by factors such as villous atrophy, splanchnic blood flow changes, ileus, and narcotics use. In one study of general surgery patients, patients taking chronic medications had 2.5 times the likelihood of developing postoperative complications.

Several general principles can be applied in managing perioperative medications. First, medications with significant withdrawal potential that do not negatively affect the procedure or administration of anesthesia should be continued during the perioperative period. Examples of this include beta blockers and alpha blockers such as clonidine. Second, medications that increase surgical risk and are not essential for short-term quality of life should be discontinued during the perioperative period. If a medication does not fall clearly into one of these categories, then one must rely on physician judgement, based on the stability of the condition being treated and concerns about the anesthetic and surgery.

Cardiovascular medications in general should be continued throughout the perioperative period because they treat and stabilize conditions such as coronary artery disease, CHF, and cardiac arrhythmias. Some notable exceptions include anticoagulants and antiplatelet agents (discussed later) and diuretics. Angiotensin-converting enzyme (ACE) inhibitors and angiotensin receptor antagonists are associated with hypotension with induction of anesthesia, often requiring intraoperative pressor therapy. The literature notes a lower mortality with perioperative ACE inhibition, but these studies do not note whether these agents were stopped before surgery, how far in advance they were stopped, and how quickly they were restarted after surgery if they were stopped. More studies are needed in this area, but given the available data, it seems prudent to discontinue ACE inhibitors or ARBs on the morning of surgery.

Statins (HMG-CoA reductase inhibitors) have clear associations with perioperative mortality benefit by data from randomized trials and epidemiology. They might prevent vascular events by other mechanisms besides cholesterol lowering, such as stabilizing plaque, reducing inflammation, and decreasing thrombogenesis. Previous concerns for increased risk of rhabdomyolysis are not well founded, because these were based on scant individual case reports with marked confounding. Because no studies have evaluated their prophylactic use in the perioperative setting, our recommendation is to continue statins if patients take them for established indications, or consider starting statin therapy if these indications are present.

Antiplatelet agents include aspirin, nonsteroidal anti-inflammatory drugs (NSAIDs), and thienopyridines, such as clopidogrel. Although aspirin and clopidogrel are typically used for patients with preexisting coronary, cerebral, or peripheral vascular disease for maintaining vessel patency and reducing risk of these events, they also increase the risk of postoperative bleeding. For most patients, short-term discontinuation of these agents perioperatively does not lead to increased adverse outcomes; therefore, it is reasonable to discontinue them 7 to 10 days before elective surgery. One important exception to this risk equation is when patients have a recently placed drug-eluting stent (DES) in a coronary artery or arteries. Premature discontinuation of antiplatelet agents tremendously increases the risk for early and late stent thrombosis, which has a case fatality rate of 45% and a 70% rate of myocardial infarction. A science advisory from a multisociety panel recommends deferring elective surgery at least 12 months in this patient population, if at all possible, and continuing both agents throughout the perioperative period if surgery within 12 months of DES implantation is necessary. If bleeding risk is high, then continuation of aspirin without thienopyridine therapy is warranted. For bare metal stents, uninterrupted dual antiplatelet therapy for a minimum of 6 weeks is recommended, because these stents endothelialize more quickly than DESs.

PERIOPERATIVE MANAGEMENT OF DIABETES

Tight glycemic control in the perioperative period is clearly associated with reductions in mortality and length of stay in the critical care unit, as well as reductions in wound infections and complications in cardiac surgery patients. However, many clinicians fear the possibility of perioperative hypoglycemic events given the variable caloric intake and disruption of anabolic and catabolic processes surrounding major surgery.

Patients on intermediate-acting insulin should take at least one half to two thirds of their evening dose the night before and on the morning of surgery, because approximately one half of insulin is used for non-nutrient metabolic needs. Full dose of intermediate or long-acting insulin (such as glargine) should be considered. Insulin coverage should be anticipatory and dosed for basal coverage (with long-acting and intermediate-acting agents) and mealtime doses, with additional units for coverage as needed (with short-acting or ultrashort-acting insulin). Sliding-scale insulin alone is insufficient and has been shown to lead to unacceptable rates of hyperglycemia and hypoglycemia. Insulin administration should also mirror the route and frequency of nutrient intake; continuous feedings require more continuous insulin administration (such as with an insulin drip or long-acting subcutaneous agent), whereas intermittent feedings require intermittent insulin doses for mealtimes or bolus feedings.

Herbal medications are used by up to one third of patients undergoing surgery. These agents are often perceived by the public as being natural and therefore completely safe; however, they have no FDA regulation because they are considered food supplements, and they can contain variable amounts of the active ingredient, among other compounds. On the other hand, prescription medicines are often perceived as artificial and therefore less safe, despite rigorous standards from the FDA for dosing and safety. Clinicians must be mindful to specifically inquire about herbal preparations and over-the-counter medications, because many patients might not even consider these to be medications. These agents should be discontinued at least 1 week before surgery, preferably 2 weeks.

Psychiatric medications should be continued perioperatively, because decompensation of psychiatric conditions should be avoided if possible. Agents such as selective serotonin reuptake inhibitors, serotonin-norepinephrine reuptake inhibitors, and benzodiazepines are safe to continue. Some concern exists for perioperative arrhythmias in conjunction with tricyclic antidepressants, but the literature does not support this concern. Monoamine oxidase inhibitors are used much less often today, but they still are used for refractory depressive disorders. These agents lead to an accumulation of biogenic amines in the central nervous system, which can lead to a hypertensive crisis if used with indirect sympathomimetics or to a serotonin-like syndrome when used with meperidine or dextromethorphan. However, anesthesia may be performed safely if meperidine is avoided, and only direct-acting sympathomimetics such as phenylephrine are used.

Suggested Readings

Ansell J: The perioperative management of warfarin therapy. Arch Intern Med 2003;163:881-883.

Arozullah AM, Khuri SF, Henderson WG, et al: Development and validation of a multifactorial risk index for predicting postoperative pneumonia after major noncardiac surgery. Ann Intern Med 2001;135(10):847-857.

Arozullah AM, Daley J, Henderson WG, et al: Multifactorial risk index for predicting postoperative respiratory failure in men after major noncardiac surgery. The National Veterans Administration Surgical Quality Improvement Program. Ann Surg 2000;232(2):242-253.

DeFrances CJ, Cullen KA, Kozak LJ, et al: National Hospital Discharge Survey: 2005 annual summary with detailed diagnosis and procedure data. National Center for Health Statistics. Vital Health Stat 13 2007;(165):1-209.

Fleisher LA, Beckman JA, Brown KA, et al: ACC/AHA 2007 guidelines on perioperative cardiovascular evaluation and care for noncardiac surgery: Executive summary: A report of the American College of Cardiology/American Heart Association Task Force on Practice Guidelines (Writing Committee to Revise the 2002 Guidelines on Perioperative Cardiovascular Evaluation for Noncardiac Surgery). Circulation 2007;116;1971-1996.

Geerts WH, Bergqvist D, Pineo GF: Prevention of venous thromboembolism: American College of Chest Physicians evidence-based clinical practice guidelines (8th edition). Chest 2008;133:381S-453S.

Hlatky MA, Boineau RE, Higginbotham MB, et al: A brief self-administered questionnaire to determine functional capacity (the Duke Activity Status Index). Am J Cardiol 1989;64: 651-654.

Jaffer AK: Anticoagulation management strategies for patients on warfare who need surgery. Cleve Clin J Med 2006;73(Suppl 1):S100-S105.

Lee TH, Marcantonio ER, Mangione CM, et al: Derivation and prospective validation of a simple index for prediction of cardiac risk of major noncardiac surgery. Circulation 1999;100(10):1043-1049.

Michota FA Jr: Preventing venous thromboembolism in surgical patients. Cleve Clin J Med 2006;73(Suppl 1):S88-S94.

Pass SE, Simpson RW: Discontinuation and reinstitution of medications during the perioperative period. Am J Health Syst Pharm 2004;61(9):899-912.

POISE Study Group: Effects of extended-release metoprolol succinate in patients undergoing non-cardiac surgery (POISE trial): A randomized controlled trial. Lancet 2008;371(9627):1839-1847.

Qaseem A, Snow V, Fitterman N, et al: Risk assessment for and strategies to reduce perioperative pulmonary complications for patients undergoing noncardiothoracic surgery: A guideline from the American College of Physicians. Ann Intern Med 2006;144(8):575-580.

Wesorick DH, Eagle KA: The preoperative cardiovascular evaluation of the intermediate-risk patient: New data, changing strategies. Am J Med 2005;118(12):1413.e1-e9.

Aging and Preventive Health

Ronan Factora

ROLE OF FRAILTY IN PREVENTIVE HEALTH

Health maintenance and preventive measures contribute to the maintenance of independent function and quality of life in the elderly individual. As with younger adults, optimization of management of chronic and acute disease processes helps to maintain optimal health in elderly patients. Numerous chapters in this text are devoted to management of specific disease processes pertinent to this population. These include the following:

- Cardiology: Atrial Fibrillation, Cardiac Arrhythmias, Heart Failure, Peripheral Arterial Disease, Preventative Cardiology, Syncope
- Dermatology: Photo Aging
- Endocrinology: Erectile Dysfunction, Diabetes, Osteoporosis, Male Hypogonadism
- Gastroenterology: Colorectal Neoplasia
- Hematology/Oncology: Anemia, Multiple Myeloma, Breast Cancer Screening, Prostate Cancer
- Infectious Disease: Immunization for Adults
- Nephrology: Slowing Progression of Renal Disease
- Neurology: Alzheimer's Disease, Antiplatelet Agents in Secondary Stroke Prevention, Carotid Vascular Disease, Dizziness, Low Back Pain, Parkinson's Disease, Stroke, Tremors
- Psychiatry and Psychology: Delirium, Depression, and Other Mood Disorders
- Pulmonary Disease: Chronic Obstructive Pulmonary Disease
- Rheumatology: Gout, Osteoarthritis
- Women's Health: Breast Cancer Risk Assessment and Prevention, Cervical Cancer Screening and Prevention, Menopause, Osteoporosis, Urinary Tract Infections in Adults

Beyond this, other factors contribute to this goal: physical activity, nutritional status, and cognitive and social stimulation. The idea of modifying these factors to foster the process of successful aging has been discussed in detail, and continues to be the focus of research.[1] In the elderly population, addressing these issues helps to maintain physical health, independence, and quality of life.

The concept and definition of frailty continue to evolve. Despite recent conventions and definitions, physicians usually say "they know frailty when they see it." Frailty has been characterized as an interaction between loss of muscle mass (sarcopenia), presence of multiple chronic illnesses, and loss of functional independence (Fig. 1).[2] Factors that have been identified as comprising the frailty phenotype include the loss of muscle mass, muscle weakness, poor endurance or energy, slowness, and low physical activity.

With normal aging and accumulation of chronic diseases, the risks for functional decline and loss of independence increase. Decline is especially marked in individuals with multiple chronic illnesses who experience multiple exacerbations of chronic illness or acute illnesses. Typically, these individuals tend to be less physically active. Lean muscle mass declines as a result of inactivity. This leads to a reduction in resting energy expenditure, reduction in caloric intake, and weight loss (lean muscle mass along with fat). Sarcopenia increases, tolerance of physical activity decreases, and the cycle repeats itself.

Homeostatic reserve is defined as the redundancy of physiologic functions present in human systems that is used to overcome acute and chronic health insults. The frailty phenotype can be used as a marker indicating a critical threshold in decline of homeostatic reserve. It also has been hypothesized to be a contributing factor to progression of chronic disease states, development and worsening of geriatric syndromes, and decline in ability to perform activities of daily living (see Fig. 1).

Decline in cognitive abilities contributes to decline in functional independence. With normal aging, processing speed of the brain declines and recall time increases. Risk of developing Alzheimer's disease increases each year after age 60. Comorbid illnesses such as stroke, diabetes, hypertension, and hyperlipidemia may also increase the risk of dementia. Current research has been focused on treating the consequences of dementia, but no treatment modality is currently available to reverse the process or halt its progression. Loss of cognitive reserve and the development of dementia have been associated with a greater risk of developing delirium, which is associated with increased morbidity and mortality in the context of acute illness.

Loss of homeostatic reserve puts the individual in a vulnerable position, whereby acute health events may lead to loss of function and independence and reduction in quality of life. An example of such an outcome is the admission of an elderly person into the hospital for a urinary tract infection. The patient, already having problems maintaining independent function at home (because of mobility issues and cognitive impairment), experiences various hospitalization insults, including delirium related to medications, immobility (from restraints and bed rest), and deconditioning. Such individuals are typically discharged to a rehabilitation facility. Delirium and underlying cognitive impairment lead to poor recovery of independent ambulatory function; eventually this patient is transferred to a nursing home. The patient never regains independence to a level that is safe to be at home.

The loss of homeostatic reserve and the development of frailty can be manifested in the myriad of syndromes encountered in the elderly. Geriatric syndromes include falls, delirium, malnutrition, urinary incontinence, and deconditioning. These syndromes typically arise out of several contributing factors. Identification of specific risk factors related to these syndromes has been shown to reduce the risk of their development.

Arguably, through interventions to maintain physical and cognitive reserves, it may be possible to prevent, slow, or reverse the development of the frailty phenotype and cognitive decline in healthy elderly individuals, even for those who have already developed loss of homeostatic reserve. As understanding of these relations grows, randomized trials of targeted interventions may more accurately determine the efficacy of therapies to these end points. In the interim, it is worthwhile to look at the available literature and examine which interventions may be of benefit.

PHYSICAL ACTIVITY

Engagement in physical activity often declines with increasing age. Benefits of regular exercise have been studied extensively and are myriad, including reduction in risk of heart attack and stroke, improvement of diabetic control, stress reduction, improvement of pulmonary function, reduction of osteoarthritic pain and stiffness, and reduction of depressive symptoms. Beyond the benefits associated with chronic disease processes, physical activity in and of itself helps to maintain pulmonary and cardiac function, as well as musculoskeletal mass and tone.

There is a clear connection between maintenance of muscle strength, cardiovascular tone, and the ability to perform activities of

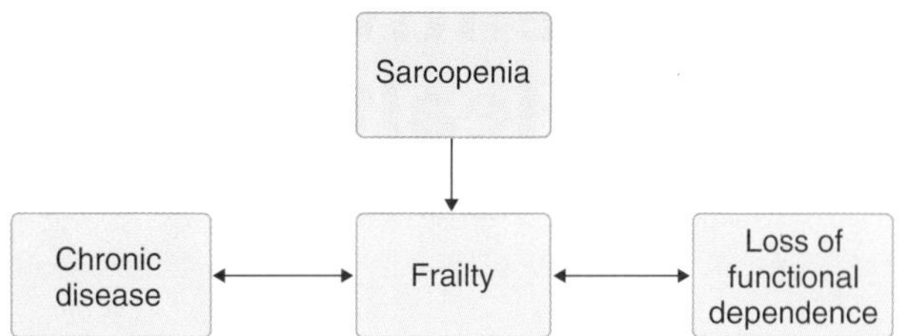

Figure 1 The interaction of the frailty phenotype with its proposed constituents.

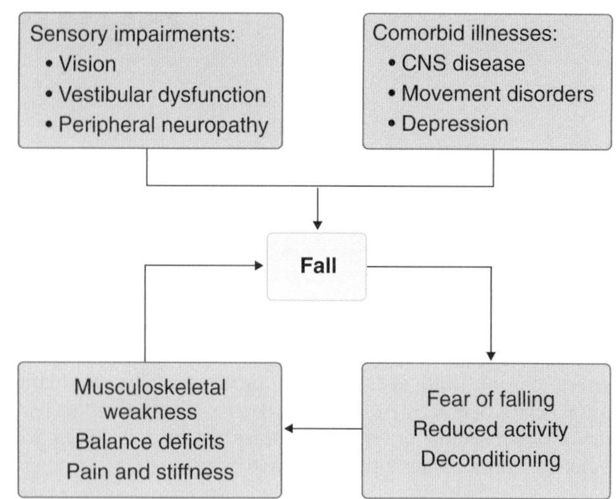

Figure 2 The cycle of falls. Several factors contribute to the risk of falls; after the sentinel event of a fall, development of fear of falling also increases risk.

daily living, to engage in leisure activities, and maintain quality of life. Intensity of physical activity and appropriate nutrition contribute to the maintenance of muscle mass. With normal aging, a reduction in muscle mass does occur. Participating in a regular exercise program can help reduce the risk of developing sarcopenia and its consequences.[3]

Targeted exercise types may also help specific areas of weakness and reduce the risk of functional decline. Exercise types include weight training, cardiovascular fitness, balance training, and flexibility training. Each type has its benefits. Strength training through use of resistance exercises helps to maintain muscle bulk and tone. Exercise of large muscle groups used in weight bearing helps to maintain mobility (for example, quadriceps strength is needed to maintain the ability to stand and properly ambulate). An example of this is in maintaining arm and leg strength to be able to perform light and heavy lifting needed to do housework. Such exercises can also be beneficial in maintaining the ability to participate in leisure (gardening, golfing) and social activities (dancing). With reduced use, slow twitch fibers eventually atrophy and convert to fatty tissue, with consequent reduction in muscle bulk, function, and potential decline in physical functional capacity.

Cardiovascular exercise is beneficial in maintaining physical activity tolerance. Even a simple regimen of walking for at least 30 minutes daily for three or more days of the week has demonstrated benefit. Reduced cardiovascular tone can result from a sedentary lifestyle, but may also be a consequence of comorbid illnesses that affect physical activity (congestive heart failure, peripheral vascular disease, osteoarthritis). Prolonged inactivity leads to a reduction in physical activity tolerance. The individual can become more limited in his or her ability to engage in activities that require some level of physical exertion. Thus, activities previously performed with no difficulty become burdensome. This can potentially lead to social isolation, further inactivity, and a cycle of declining quality of life and depression. One example could be loss of ability to volunteer at a community center because of significant exertional dyspnea related to walking; this can lead to reduction in volunteerism, less time spent socializing, potentially more time spent at home, and greater inactivity.

Along with cardiovascular tone, adequate balance and flexibility contribute to ambulatory ability. Several disease processes can affect these factors, including cerebrovascular disease, osteoarthritis, peripheral neuropathy, joint replacement surgeries, visual impairment, and vestibular dysfunction. A reduction in balance or flexibility because of these factors can increase the risk of falls in the individual (Fig. 2).

A fall is a sentinel event signaling a decline in an individual's physical homeostatic reserve, marking a point of greatest risk for loss of independence. Typically, several factors contribute to this end point and punctuate the multifactorial nature of the development of frailty and loss of functional capacity. Risk of falls is greatest after acute illness. These periods are associated with bed rest, inactivity, and inadequate nutritional intake. The consequence is development of deconditioning. Many hospitalized elderly patients who were initially able to ambulate on admission end up being discharged requiring a walker or wheelchair, all as a result of weakness that developed during acute hospitalization. A decline in the ability to ambulate can lead to a decline in ability to perform activities of daily living independently, increased reliance on others for assistance, and increased risk of social isolation.

Falls themselves are risk factors for future falls. Development of fear of falling because of feelings of unsteadiness or a fall can prompt an individual to limit physical activity. This may further perpetuate the cycle of inactivity, further reductions in muscular and cardiovascular tone, reduced oral intake, impaired nutritional status, and further decline. Several studies have been conducted confirming the benefit of the exercise Tai Chi in improving balance and reducing the risk of falls.[4] Engaging in this or similar activities may improve or enhance balance and flexibility.

With greater amounts of exercise, greater benefits can be derived from it. The maintenance and increase of reserve functional capacity are important concepts in the elderly population. Homeostatic reserve allows an individual to overcome the results of acute insults to health. The presence of a greater amount of homeostatic reserve allows an individual to recover more quickly and more completely from acute declines in health. Decline in homeostatic reserve in all systems as a part of the aging process is generally recognized. This is accelerated by chronic disease processes and acute illness. The consequence is an impaired ability to recover from acute illness, the potential for permanent impairment, and development of a new functional baseline.

Ultimately, the goal in participation of physical activity in the healthy elderly population is maintenance and development of physical functional reserve capacity. For individuals suffering acute illness, appropriate physical activity in the form of physical therapy, rehabilitation, and scheduled exercise can accelerate recovery to a functional baseline.

INTERVENTIONS FOR NUTRITION

Normal aging is associated with changes in body composition. Lean muscle mass declines and percentage of body fat increases. Caloric intake has been demonstrated to decline with increasing age in several observational studies. Several factors associated with normal aging contribute to this decline. These include a reduction in the senses of smell and taste, increased cholecystokinin production leading to earlier and more pronounced satiety with small meals, and reduced gastric motility (Box 1).[5]

Although many of these factors occur as an inexorable process of normal aging, many other risk factors for nutritional decline and

Box 1 Age-Related Changes That Affect Appetite

Sensory Changes
Decreased odor perception
Increase in taste thresholds
Decline in taste sensitivity

Gastrointestinal Tract Changes
Earlier satiation
Reduced fundal compliance
Delayed gastric emptying

Hormonal Changes
Increased serum leptin
Decreased serum testosterone
Increased serum cholecystokinin
Increased inflammation-mediated cytokines
IL-1, TNF-α, IL-6, and ciliary neurotrophic factor

Central Nervous System Changes
Decreased opioid receptor activity
Reduction in physical activity
Decline in resting metabolic rate

IL, interleukin; TNF, tumor necrosis factor.
From Morley JE: Decreased food intake with aging. J GerontolA Biol Sci Med Sci 2001;56(Spec No 2):81-88.

subsequent weight loss can be identified. Several observational studies have demonstrated that significant weight loss, low BMI, and protein energy undernutrition are associated with increased morbidity and mortality in the elderly. In many circumstances, presence of any of these problems is under-recognized.

A full discussion regarding diagnosis of malnutrition and evaluation of weight loss is beyond the scope of this chapter. A pattern of significant weight loss (loss of ≥10 lbs or 10% of baseline body weight within a 6-month period) should prompt evaluation. If a cause, or contributing factors, is identified, intervention may be able to reverse the decline.

Nutritional status and levels of physical activity are inexorably linked. Decreases in physical activity are associated with a reduction in caloric needs, reduction in appetite, and subsequent weight loss. Muscle mass tends to decline in this scenario. With greater levels of activity, caloric needs increase, and a stimulation of appetite develops. In this circumstance, lean muscle mass may also increase as a result of increased physical activity.

Identification of risk factors for undernutrition and malnutrition may provide the opportunity for intervention for those at risk. The "DETERMINE Your Nutritional Status" checklist is useful in identifying these risk factors (Box 2).[6] Especially common problems that contribute to weight loss in the elderly include dental problems, social isolation, economic issues, and the presence of depression and cognitive impairment. Timely interventions may prevent development of protein-calorie undernutrition and maintain proper nutrition and weight.

Chronic diseases, specifically disease processes associated with chronic inflammation, affect appetite and accelerate reduction in caloric intake. Cytokines and other inflammatory factors have been identified as contributing factors to the development of anorexia. Additionally, commonly used medications have side effects that reduce appetite, palatability and flavor of food, or cause nausea, diarrhea, or headaches that may affect an individual's ability to eat (Box 3). Many of the chapters in this text address chronic diseases commonly encountered in the elderly population. Optimal management of these conditions can be beneficial in reducing their potential impact on morbidity associated with malnutrition.

When the underlying condition cannot be quickly or adequately treated (i.e., progressive dementia, depression, dentition issues), boosting caloric intake through dietary modifications can prevent

Box 2 DETERMINE Checklist of Risk Factors for Malnutrition

***D*isease**
Chronic diseases impairing appetite or ability to eat
Mood and cognitive disorders

***E*ating Poorly**
Inadequate food or poor food quality/caloric intake
Skipping meals; drinking too much alcohol

***T*ooth Loss or Mouth Pain**
Missing or rotting teeth
Missing or poorly fitting dentures

***E*conomic Hardship**
Inadequate income to buy food

***R*educed Social Contact**
Single, widowed
No family or community supports

***M*ultiple Medicines**
Causing nausea, taste alterations, constipation, or anorexia
Includes dietary supplements, over-the-counter medications, and herbal products

***I*nvoluntary Weight Loss or Gain**
Due to undiagnosed medical conditions such as cancer, malabsorption syndromes, metabolism-altering states

***N*eeds**
Assistance with self care
Problems with transportation for shopping
Problems with ambulation or cooking

***E*lder Years**
Older than age 80

From Posner BM, Jette AM, Smith KW, Miller DR: Nutrition and health risks in the elderly: The nutrition screening initiative. Am J Public Health 1993;83(7):972-978.

Box 3 Commonly Prescribed Medication Classes Associated with Anorexia in the Older Patient

Antidepressants: selective serotonin reuptake inhibitors
Antibiotics
Ferrous sulfate
Furosemide and sulfa medications
Nonsteroidal anti-inflammatory drugs
Angiotensin-converting enzyme inhibitors
Antihistamines
Digoxin

further weight loss. Such interventions may include reduction in size but increased frequency of meals, discontinuation of dietary restrictions, addition of high calorie–content foods to the mealtime regimen, additional of snacks, and provision of dietary supplements. Box 4 lists other simple recommendations that can be made to increase caloric intake of food.

Normal aging is associated with physiologic changes that alter eating habits. Risk factors for malnutrition can be easily identified using widely disseminated screening tools. Interventions in at-risk patients or those patients with malnutrition or observed weight loss may help to reverse these conditions.

INTERVENTIONS FOR COGNITIVE FUNCTION

Cognitive impairment and dementia occur commonly in the elderly population, and increases in incidence with in those older than 65

Box 4 Recommendations for Enhancing Caloric Content of Foods

Make an effort to eat regularly; more frequent small meals are an appropriate substitute for fewer larger meals during the day
Provide snacks throughout the day

- Cheese and crackers
- Canned, fresh, or dried fruits
- Cereals, breads, muffins
- Nuts, peanut butter
- Yogurt

Eat fresh vegetables such as carrots, broccoli, or celery as a snack; use a dip to increase the calories.
Adjust flavors and textures of foods to increase appeal.
Drink a nutritional supplement such as Boost, Ensure, or Carnation Instant Breakfast cold or add a scoop of ice cream for a great-tasting shake.
Add nonfat powdered milk to foods such as creamed soups, mashed potatoes, gravies, sauces, hot cereal, scrambled eggs, beverages such as milk or Boost, puddings, and custards. (add 2 or more tablespoons (tbl) to each serving; 1 tbl = 25 kcal and 3 g protein).
Add honey, corn syrup, maple syrup, brown sugar (provided you are not diabetic) to foods such as hot or cold cereal, fruit, sweet potatoes, coffee, and winter squash. (1 tbl = 50 kcal)
Add combinations of grated cheese, margarine, gravies, sauces, and cream cheese (depending on your medical condition) to starchy foods, eggs, vegetables, and creamy soups. (1 tbl = 25-100 kcal)

years. Several studies have analyzed risk factors for development of dementia, specifically Alzheimer's disease. Beyond health risk factors such as diabetes, hypertension, and hyperlipidemia, several lifestyle factors such as economic background, level of education, physical activity, and leisure activities have been studied to determine a link between them and risk for cognitive decline.[7]

Investigators have long hypothesized the link between leisure activities and risk of developing dementia. One recent observational study did identify links between a reduced risk of developing Alzheimer's disease and participation in specific types of leisure activities.[8] The leisure activities associated with a reduced risk included reading, playing board games, playing musical instruments, and dancing. Increased frequency of participation in these activities was also noted to be associated with an increased level of protection.

Ongoing clinical trials continue to evaluate the value of such activities in the prevention of cognitive impairment. Even in patients who already have some level of cognitive impairment, benefit can still be garnered by encouraging participation in cognitively stimulating activities.

Despite encouragement to participate in such activities, barriers preventing the individual to do so may exist. Identifying these may lead to interventions and greater participation. Simple screening for visual and hearing impairments may lead to correction of previously unidentified deficits. Even if medical management is optimized and visual deficits can no longer be corrected, adaptive equipment to assist in performing activities of daily living or participating in leisure activities can be made available and consequently increase the patient's quality of life. Referral to a local sight center or blindness clinic may be useful in achieving this goal. Hearing aids are expensive (the individual is typically left to cover the entire cost) and can be unobtainable because of financial constraints for many elderly individuals. Less costly but still effective hearing augmentative devices may be more readily available; contacting an audiologist may be helpful. These devices may improve an individual's ability to engage in social activities.

Assessment of gait may reveal previously unreported pain issues and instability. Appropriate evaluation and management, including analgesic therapy (when indicated), may increase the individual's willingness to ambulate. A physical therapy evaluation can be useful in assessing reasons for gait instability and recommending appropriate assistive devices to improve the patient's safety and promote greater independence with walking.

Physical and cognitive limitations may also limit the individual's ability to drive or arrange alternative modes of transportation. Social isolation further limits available options for travel. Enlisting the assistance of available family and friends of the patient may be a way to overcome this. By contacting the local Alzheimer's Association or community agency on aging, nearby adult daycare facilities, senior centers, and community centers may be identified that may be able to provide transportation; they may also be able to provide listings for transportation services that could be made available for a nominal fee. Local churches or religious organizations as well as the Veterans Administration facilities may also be able to provide appropriate services.

Optimization of chronic illnesses associated with increased risk of developing dementia, and increased participation in leisure activities can be protective against the development of dementia (specifically Alzheimer's disease). A dose relation exists between amount of participation in leisure activities and reduction in risk of developing dementia. Encouraging elderly individuals to participate in such activities and addressing barriers that may impair their participation can be beneficial.

Summary

- Frailty as a syndrome occurs in the elderly and is a result of several contributing factors. This phenotype has been described in detail, and interventions addressing the hypothesized risk factors for frailty continue to be studied. By addressing the specific components related to frailty, functional decline may be prevented to some degree.
- Promotion of physical activity has been demonstrated to be helpful in maintaining physical functioning in the areas of strength, flexibility, and balance. Monitoring nutritional intake and avoiding or reversing significant weight loss can also reduce associated morbidity and mortality and may lead to maintenance of independence.
- Management of chronic comorbid illnesses should focus on limiting their impact on function (especially sensory impairments).
- Elderly individuals should also be encouraged to participate in social and cognitively stimulating activities to help maintain cognition and physical functioning.

Suggested Readings

Fried LP, Tangen CM, Walston J, et al: Frailty in older adults: Evidence for a phenotype. J Gerontol A Biol Sci Med Sci 2001;56(3):M146-M156.
Morley JE: Decreased food intake with aging. J Gerontol A Biol Sci Med Sci 2001;56(Spec No 2):81-88.
Posner BM, Jette AM, Smith KW, Miller DR: Nutrition and health risks in the elderly: The nutrition screening initiative. Am J Public Health 1993;83(7):972-978.
Province MA, Hadley EC, Hornbrook MC, et al: The effects of exercise on falls in elderly patients. A preplanned meta-analysis of the FICSIT Trials. Frailty and Injuries: Cooperative Studies of Intervention Techniques. JAMA 1995;273(17):1341-1347.
Rowe JW, Kahn RL: Human aging: Usual and successful. Science 1987;237(4811):143-149.
Singh MA: Exercise comes of age: Rationale and recommendations for a geriatric exercise prescription. [see comment]. J Gerontol A Biol Sci Med Sci 2002;57(5):M262-M282.
Snowdon DA, Nun S: Healthy aging and dementia: Findings from the Nun Study. Ann Int Med 2003;139(5 Pt 2):450-454.
Verghese J, Lipton RB, Katz MJ, et al: Leisure activities and the risk of dementia in the elderly. N Engl J Med 2003;348(25):2508-2516.

References

For a complete list of references, log onto www.expertconsult.com.

Introduction to Integrative Medicine

Thomas J. Morledge

Integrative medicine refers to the integration of alternative and complementary medicine with traditional allopathic medicine. I have found that having knowledge and tools in both areas allows me to provide the best care for my patients. It is clear that allopathic medicine provides many powerful lifesaving treatments to our patients. However, we need to offer our patients with chronic medical disorders an integrated approach, taking into account their individual situations, the interactions between the environment, and their particular genetic uniqueness. It is estimated that there are more than 2 million polymorphisms that can potentially affect the way a person experiences health or disease.

Because the breadth of alternative medicine cannot be summarized in a single writing, this chapter focuses on one field in integrative medicine, functional medicine.[1] Functional medicine is an individualized approach to patient care that focuses on restoring balance to the dysfunctional systems by strengthening the fundamental physiologic processes that underlie them, and by adjusting the environmental inputs that nurture or impair them. Functional medicine looks at the triggers and mediators that lead to a particular clinical state. This takes into account the environmental factors that wash over a patient's particular genetic uniqueness that then can result in either vitality or dysfunction. The environmental effect can be as broad as the mind's influence on the psychoneuroendocrine system or as narrow as a conditionally essential nutrient in a metabolic pathway that has been affected by an environmental toxin.

Functional medicine uses a matrix of core clinical imbalances (Fig. 1) to organize a structural framework around a patient's complex presentation. These core imbalances include:

- Neurotransmitter and hormonal imbalances
- Oxidation-reduction imbalances and mitochondropathy
- Detoxification and biotransformational imbalances
- Immune and inflammatory imbalances
- Digestive, absorptive, and microbiologic imbalances
- Structural imbalances from cellular membrane function to the musculoskeletal system

Biochemical individuality is the rule rather than the exception and is the result of having thousands of genetic polymorphisms. One of the exciting frontiers that is emerging in functional medicine is the application of genetic analysis in areas such as inflammation and detoxification. It is the role of the clinician to examine this complex web of interactions and develop a treatment plan to help our patients. Functional medicine provides a robust paradigm to explore each patient's story in the context of the environment's influence on his or her particular spiritual, emotional, and biochemical uniqueness.

OXIDATIVE STRESS

Processes

Proposed mechanisms of aging as well as neurodegenerative and other organ-specific degenerative diseases have focused on the susceptibility of the cell to oxidative stress. Research in this area has demonstrated the role of oxidative stress-induced mitochondrial dysfunction and the subsequent cascade of mitochondria-initiated cellular apoptosis. Oxidative stress is also related to the development of certain cancers.

Oxidative stress occurs when either endogenously metabolic generated reactive molecules or exogenous reactive substances in the environment interact with biologic structures, resulting in altered cellular physiology. Endogenously produced reactive oxygen species (ROS) include molecules such as superoxide, peroxynitrite, peroxyl radicals, hydroxyl, hydroxyl radicals, and singlet oxygen. Most ROS originate intracellularly in the mitochondria, which converts the energy potential from macronutrients from the diet into cellular energy currency that includes adenosine triphosphate (ATP), reduced nicotinamide adenine dinucleotide (NADH), and reduced flavin adenine dinucleotide ($FADH_2$). Through the process of oxidative phosphorylation in the mitochondria, molecular oxygen is consumed and reduced to water. However, about 1% of the oxygen is converted to superoxide anion (O_2^-). These ROS molecules, if left unchecked, damage cellular structures such as mitochondrial membranes, proteins, and DNA. Mitochondrial DNA is especially vulnerable to oxidative damage because it lacks the protective and repair mechanisms found in nuclear DNA. Repeated injury to DNA results in a cumulative loss of function. After enough hits, the mitochondria and the bioenergetics of the cell are altered in ways that can result in cellular apoptosis and loss of organ function.

Cells have developed antioxidant defenses to protect cellular proteins, membranes, and nucleic acids. These molecules include coenzyme Q10 (CoQ_{10}), lipoic acid, and glutathione. Enzymatic processes that also contribute to antioxidant defense include superoxide dismutase, catalase, glutathione reductase, and glutathione peroxidase.

Oxidative stress can be assessed in the laboratory by measuring oxidized products from cellular damage. The unsaturated component of lipid membranes undergoing oxidative damage releases lipid peroxides. Oxidative injury to arachidonic acid results in the production of isoprostanes. Oxidation of guanosine molecules in DNA produces 8-hydroxydeoxyguanosine (8OHdG), which has a close relation with neuronal oxidative stress. Methods of measuring these products of oxidation are commercially available.

The production of ATP from oxidative phosphorylation depends on organic acids generated from the Krebs cycle. To function correctly, the enzymatic processes in the Krebs cycle depend on cofactors that include nicotinamide dinucleotide derived from niacin, FAD derived from riboflavin, and thiamine pyrophosphate derived from thiamine. The production of energy from fatty acids depends on the transport of free fatty acids across the mitochondrial membrane, which requires conjugation to carnitine by the enzyme carnitine palmitoyltransferase I. The free fatty acids are then deconjugated for use in energy production.

Antioxidants

Today's standard American diet is poor in nutrients, rich in calories, high in glycemic load, and deficient in antioxidants. These processed foods lack the phytonutrients that provide our cells with the information to orchestrate a balanced cellular physiology to prevent cancer and inflammatory conditions. Antioxidant-rich foods in the diet are the major sources of supplemental antioxidants. The richly pigmented phytochemicals in vegetables and fruits serve antioxidant functions, and intake of vegetables and fruits has been associated with a decreased risk of some cancers. The antioxidant activity produced by whole foods, as measured by products of oxidative stress in humans, outperforms antioxidants taken as supplements.[2]

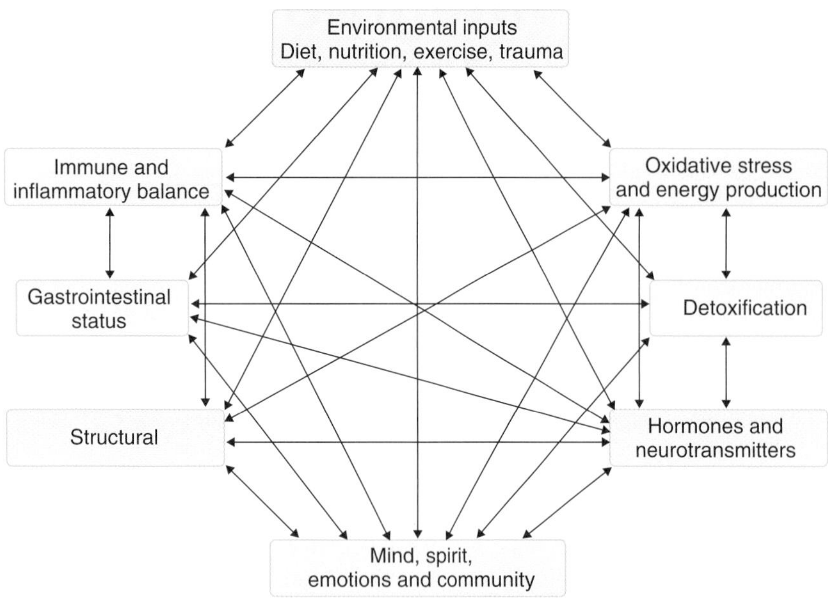

Figure 1 Institute for Functional Medicine Clinical Matrix for Core Imbalance. *(From the Institute for Functional Medicine: Textbook of Functional Medicine. Gig Harbor, Wash: The Institute for Functional Medicine, 2005, p 100. © 2005 The Institute of Functional Medicine.)*

Although many substances in vegetables and fruits have been identified, many remain unidentified, and the biologic effect of a particular herb or plant could be related to effects of the particular plant's various phytochemicals on multiple-cell-signaling biochemical pathways.

Green tea, rich in catechins, has demonstrated antioxidant properties related to the combination of aromatic and hydroxyl groups that make up the structure of these polyphenols. Other biologic effects of green tea include inhibition of arachidonic acid metabolites, thus reducing inflammatory responses; activation of hepatic enzymes that promote the detoxification of xenobiotic compounds; and positive effects on intestinal microflora by raising levels of Lactobacillus and Bifidobacterium while lowering levels of potential pathogenic bacteria. One of the major polyphenols in green tea, (−)-epigallocatechin-3-gallate (ECGC), has been shown to decrease lipopolysaccharide-induced tumor necrosis factor (TNF) production in a dose-dependent manner.

Curcumin (derived from turmeric, the yellow spice in curries) has been shown to have a broad range of cellular effects in addition to its potent antioxidant activity. It has potent anti-inflammatory effects that may be related to its ability to inhibit biosynthesis of inflammatory prostaglandins from arachidonic acid and also its inhibitory effect on neutrophil aggregation. Molecular targets include the inhibition of cell-signaling pathways associated with inflammation that includes nuclear factor-κB (NF-κB), cyclooxygenase-2 (COX-2), and 5-lipoxygenase (5-LOX). It also affects many pathways associated with cancer.[3]

Lycopene, a red carotenoid pigment, is found in a variety of plants including guava, pink grapefruit, watermelon, and tomatoes. Lycopene is a potent antioxidant that might protect vulnerable cellular components from reactive oxygen damage. Epidemiologic data show lycopene to be associated with a reduced risk of prostate cancer. Clinical trials have also demonstrated a prevention or reduction of the progression of high-grade prostate intraepithelial neoplasms into prostate cancer. Serum lycopene levels are inversely related to prostate-specific antigen (PSA) levels. Mechanisms in addition to the antioxidant effects can include inhibition of insulin-like growth factor-1 and other cell-signaling effects.[4]

In addition to whole foods, dietary supplements used to support these processes include those directed at facilitating energy production at the level of the Krebs cycle and oxidative phosphorylation. They can serve as cofactors in the processes for the generation of ATP and as antioxidants to quench aberrant ROS. Many of the substrates used in these processes are conditionally essential, which implies that under certain conditions, optimal function cannot be maintained through endogenous synthesis alone.

CoQ_{10} (ubiquinone) is a potent antioxidant and also a bioenergetic enzyme that participates in electron transport during oxidative phosphorylation. CoQ_{10} biosynthesis is impaired by statin medications that inhibit the enzyme 3-hydroxy-3-methylglutaryl coenzyme A (HMG-CoA) reductase, thus producing lower tissue levels of CoQ_{10}. CoQ_{10} supplementation has been shown to potentially benefit a number of neurodegenerative diseases, including Parkinson's disease, Alzheimer's disease, and Huntington's disease.[4] Additionally, it has shown benefit in prophylaxis for migraine headache and in treating congestive heart failure, periodontal disease, and hypertension. It has also been shown to reduce doxorubicin-induced myocardial toxicity in patients receiving chemotherapy without compromising the chemotherapeutic effectiveness. Dosages as high as 1200 mg/day have been successfully used in clinical studies in patients with Parkinson's disease.

α-Lipoic acid (ALA) is a molecule that serves as a coenzyme in several complexes in the mitochondria, including pyruvate dehydrogenase in the Krebs cycle. ALA is also a potent antioxidant in water and in lipophilic solvents. In its reduced form, dihydrolipoic acid has been demonstrated to have distinct antioxidant actions that include free radical-scavenging activity; it also can regenerate endogenous antioxidants such as glutathione, CoQ_{10}, and vitamins E and C. Studies in patients with diabetes have shown improvement in measurements of oxidative stress.[5] ALA has also resulted in significant clinical improvement in symptom scores in patients with diabetic polyneuropathy.[6] ALA supplementation in animal models has resulted in improvement in outcomes following central nervous system reperfusion injury and protects against cataract formation in animals with induced diabetes.[7] ALA has also been used successfully to prevent liver failure in patients with amanita mushroom poisoning. Besides its direct antioxidant effects, ALA might also influence clinical outcomes through other important mechanisms and pathways such as by modulating inflammation through its inhibitory affect on NF-κB activation.[8] Therapeutic doses of ALA are in the range of 600 mg daily.

Many foods and supplements that have primarily been believed to have antioxidant properties also play a role in modulating inflammation, have anticancer properties through cell-signaling pathways, and can influence many physiologic effects through a plethora of other mechanisms and processes. Primary prevention of cancer and

Box 1 Herbal Supplements and Nutraceuticals

Nutraceuticals and herbal preparations can be used to functionally:
Support a balanced detoxification process
Decrease inflammation through a variety of pathways in either arachidonic acid production or through inhibition of cytokines of NF-κB
Provide antioxidant support to quench ROS formation
Support gastrointestinal function to prevent downstream inflammatory processes

NF-κB, nuclear factor-κB; ROS, reactive oxygen species.

Box 2 Resources About Antioxidant Foods and Supplements

Education

The Institute for Functional Medicine: http://www.functionalmedicine.org/

Laboratory Testing

Genova Diagnostics

- http://www.genovations.com/home/index.html (genetic testing for polymorphisms related to detoxification and inflammation)
- http://www.gdx.net/home/ (digestive and metabolic function)

Metametrix Clinical Laboratory: www.metametrix.com (nutritional and metabolic function)
Spectracell Laboratories: www.spectracell.com (functional analysis of essential micronutrients)

Evaluations of Supplement and Herb Quality

Consumer Lab: http://www.consumerlab.com/

degenerative diseases through the intake of a whole-foods diet seems prudent. We are beginning to have the tools available to identify persons at increased risk for oxidative damage and development of degenerative disease due to their specific genetic polymorphisms. Targeted dietary and nutraceutical supplemental therapy is possible for these people based on sound scientific data and inferences (Box 1). The ideal of having outcome studies for many of these proposed treatments is a story in progress. Resources are listed in Box 2.

DETOXIFICATION AND BIOTRANSFORMATION

Toxins that are present in our bodies originate from environmental exposures including the air we breathe, water we drink, food we eat, and the complex array of molecules we produce in our bodies that are metabolites of physiologic processes. The greatest amount of energy that our bodies use outside of our growing years pertains to detoxifying these toxic molecules to prevent oxidative damage to vital intracellular proteins, DNA, and lipid membranes. This complex process has to be able to recognize thousands of diverse molecules and perform a highly orchestrated synchronous detoxification process that includes molecular modification by phase I enzymes, conjugation to water soluble molecules by phase II enzymes, and then efflux out of the cells by phase III proteins. Hundreds of proteins participate in these processes, which are highly dependent on having the necessary substrate available to complete these processes.

Detoxification begins at the intestinal epithelium. High concentrations of CYP 3A4 (a major cytochrome P-450 enzyme involved in metabolism of many drugs) and phase III antiporter activities are found at the tips of intestinal villi. Other tissues with significant detoxification systems include the lungs, kidneys, reproductive tissues, and nasal epithelium. The ability of the nasal epithelium to detoxify xenobiotics is important so that loss of our ability to detect scents due to habituation does not occur. The fragrance produced by a rose must be metabolized by our detoxification system to allow the system to become resensitized so we can to continue to perceive the fragrance.

Each person has a unique biochemistry to detoxify substrate, which depends on individual genetic makeup, the load of environmental or endogenous toxins, and the substrate available to accomplish this task. Because single nucleotide polymorphisms (SNPs) can occur in any combination of the enzymes involved in these processes, some persons present with signs and symptoms of toxicity such as fatigue, neurologic complaints, and cancer whereas others with similar exposures do not present with any problems. Laboratory testing is currently available for gene panels that are involved in detoxification and biotransformation. Obtaining gene panels on our patients might help us determine this aspect of their risk for developing diseases related to detoxification. Specific minimally processed whole foods or nutritional supplements can be prescribed to optimize the function of these processes.

A classic example of the detoxification process is metabolism of acetaminophen (Fig. 2). Acetaminophen is primarily metabolized through a phase II process that includes sulfation to form acetaminophen sulfate and glucuronidation to form acetaminophen glucuronide. These compounds are then safely eliminated. If these pathways are impaired or compromised by depletion of essential cofactors, acetaminophen undergoes phase I biotransformation to *N*-acetyl-*p*-benzoquinone imine (NAPQI). NAPQI is a highly reactive molecule, and if it is not rapidly conjugated with glutathione, it will cause cellular toxicity. If the phase I cytochrome P-450 enzyme CYP 2E1 is induced to promote biotransformation to NAPQI, or if essential cofactors for phase II conjugation are lacking, the outcome favors production of this reactive intermediate, which can cause cellular damage and possibly liver failure.

Phase I biotransformation can be induced by various substrates or can be competitively inhibited. Genetic variations through SNPs also occur that can result in either increased or decreased enzyme kinetics. Phase II conjugation may be affected by individual polymorphisms and is also subject to available substrate for conjugation and elimination. For optimal biotransformation, phase I and phase II need to function in a balanced manner. Reactive intermediates produced through phase I processes are conjugated by phase II processes. In the case of acetaminophen toxicity, ethanol induction of CYP 2E1 results in increased production of NAPQI. At the same time, a fasting state can deplete the limited supply of sulfur-containing amino acids used as phase II substrates. This imbalanced state can result in liver toxicity at what we would consider normal doses of acetaminophen.

Although there are many likely processes that ultimately result in altered cellular physiology and the development of malignancies, detoxification and biotransformation play critical roles as a link to make persons either more susceptible or less susceptible to the environmental mediators of cancer development. Our diet can have either a positive or negative effect in this cascade of nutragenomic-influenced events. As an example, estrogen metabolism is influenced by both phase I and phase II processes. A study of the expression of estrogen-metabolizing enzymes in human breast tissue has found increased levels of CYP 1B1(increased enzyme activity) and decreased levels of catechol-*O*-methyl-transferase (COMT) in patients with breast cancer.[9] Both of these are common polymorphisms found in the general population. These changes favor the metabolism of estrogen to its carcinogenic metabolites. Similar findings have been demonstrated in men with prostate cancer, thus suggesting the importance of estrogen metabolism in the development of this malignancy.[10]

Diet and nutritional supplements can be used to help balance the biotransformation of estrogen metabolites toward less-carcinogenic precursors. In general, fruits and vegetables contribute to the upregulation of hepatic detoxification enzymes. Phytonutrients can potentially affect hormone response or metabolism through a variety of mechanisms that include competitive inhibition at receptor sites, induction or inhibition of phase I processes, or upregulation of phase

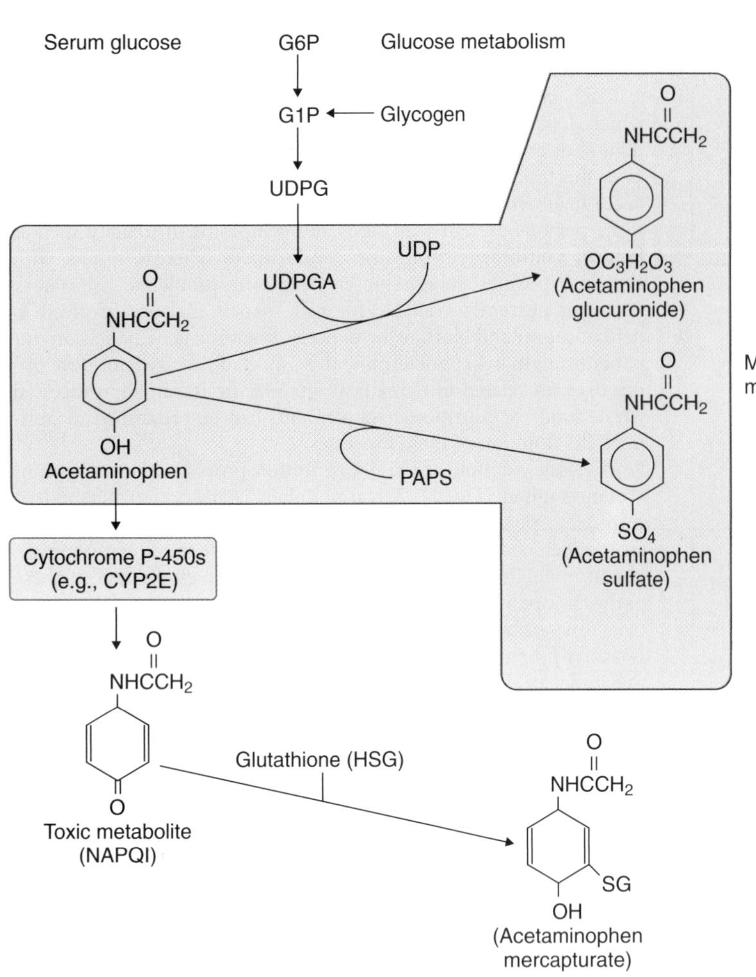

Figure 2 Acetaminophen metabolism. G1P, glucose-1-phosphate; G6P, glucose-6-phosphate; HSG, glutathione; NAPQI, *N*-acetyl-*p*-benzoquinone imine; PAPS, adenosine 3′-phosphate 5′-phosphosulfate; UDP, uridine diphosphate; UDPG, uridine 5′-diphospho-α-D-glucose; UDPGA, uridine 5′-diphospho-α-D-glucuronic acid. *(From the Institute for Functional Medicine: Textbook of Functional Medicine. Gig Harbor, Wash: The Institute for Functional Medicine, 2005, p 289. © 2005 The Institute of Functional Medicine.)*

II processes. It remains to be seen through clinical trials whether whole food or supplement use can influence clinical outcomes.

Indol-3-carbinol (I3C) is a compound found in cruciferous vegetables such as broccoli, cauliflower, cabbage, and Brussels sprouts. I3C can shift the metabolism of estrogen to the protective 2-hydroxy estrogens by upregulating the expression of CYP 1A1 that increases the 2-hydroxylation of estradiol and estrone. Research has also shown that I3C induces in vitro tumor cell death by regulating the apoptotic pathway and through selective stimulation of a tumor-suppressor gene.

As mentioned, patients with breast cancer express lower levels of COMT. COMT is important in the metabolism of estrogen to products that have lower potential for oxidative DNA damage and reduced inflammatory properties. *S*-adenosylmethionine (SAMe) is a substrate for COMT methylation, and availability of SAMe depends on its own set of factors, which include polymorphisms for methylenetetrahydrofolate reductase (MTHFR), nutritional status, and environmental factors. Supplementation with SAMe in patients who have COMT polymorphisms, in addition to folic acid, and vitamins B_{12}, and vitamins B_2 and B_6 for those with MTHFR polymorphisms, can supply the needed substrate to favor the metabolism of estrogen to noncarcinogenic molecules. Moreover, the flora of the colon can influence detoxification and estrogen metabolism through the bacterial production of β-glucuronidase, which deconjugates glucuronyl side chains, resulting in enterohepatic recirculation of the transformed molecule, leading to increased toxic load. This example illustrates the weblike interaction of molecular processes that is the rule rather than the exception in biologic systems.

Curcumin (the principal curcuminoid of turmeric) is another herb that influences detoxification. In vitro and animal studies have shown that curcumin inhibits phase I CYP 1A1 and increases activity of phase II reactions. Curcumin has been shown in animal models to induce apoptosis in colon and breast cancers. It also downs regulates molecules in the inflammatory pathway, including COX-2, 5-LOX, NF-κB, and TNF. Green tea also affects detoxification by affecting phase I and phase II enzyme activity, has anti-inflammatory effects. Green tea polyphenols have been studied as cardiovascular disease and chemopreventive agents.[11-13] Many phytonutrients have been demonstrated to have a broad range of effects on a variety of cellular physiologies including detoxification, inflammation, and oxidative stress (Fig. 3).

Depending on the clinical presentation of the patient and our underlying knowledge of the various detoxification pathways, we have the opportunity to improve the function of these pathways through nutritional supplementation. This can be illustrated through the following case history. A 50-year-old patient who is a laboratory technician in an area hospital presents with episodic extreme fatigue that would last for several days following the landing of life flight helicopters at the heliport near his laboratory. His physical examination and routine laboratory tests to evaluate the fatigue were unremarkable. Symptoms suggesting a detoxification issue included a perceived heightened olfactory sensitivity to exhaust and diesel fumes (this may be related to enhanced elimination of these substances through phase I detoxification in the nasal epithelium, thus increasing sensitivity due to a reduction of neuronal habituation). Genomic testing on this patient revealed polymorphisms in the phase I enzymes CYP 1B1 and CYP 2E1. Polymorphisms for phase II enzymes included a null genetic expression (no gene present) for hepatic glutathione-*S*-transferase. This combination of environmental and genetic interactions could result in the rapid conversion of

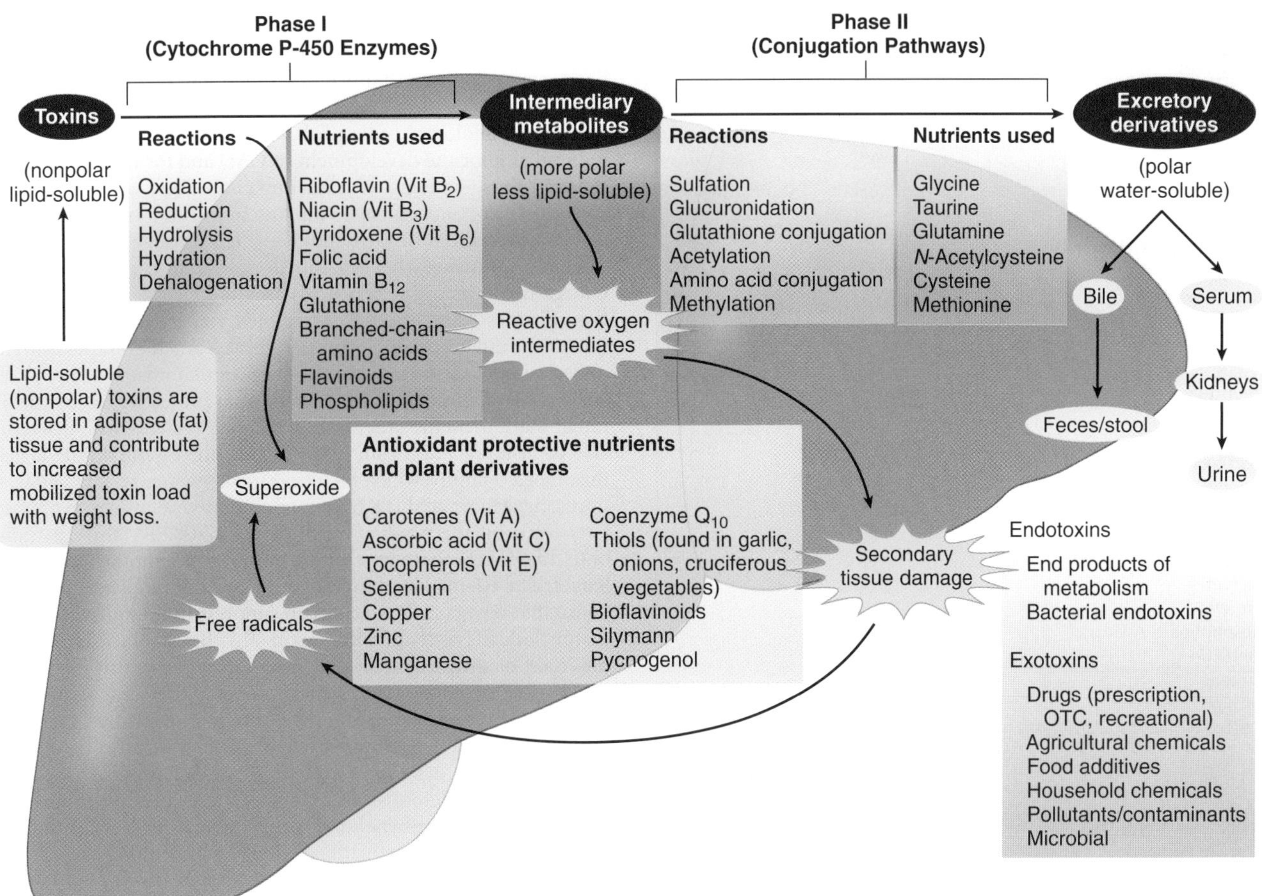

Figure 3 Nutrient and herbal supplements to support detoxification. OTC, over the counter; Vit, vitamin. *(From the Institute for Functional Medicine: Textbook of Functional Medicine. Gig Harbor, Wash: The Institute for Functional Medicine, 2005, p 278.© 2005 The Institute of Functional Medicine.)*

hydrocarbons to reactive intermediates by phase I that could not be optimally conjugated by phase II, resulting in toxic metabolites and the manifestation of his symptoms. Treatment was initiated with a combination of supplements and herbs that supported phase II detoxification through the addition of antioxidants and cofactors. Within weeks, his clinical symptoms resolved completely after years of intermittent fatigue due to environmental exposures. As an additional preventive strategy, this patient should also include in his diet cruciferous vegetables and phytonutrients to favor the conversion of estrogen to safer metabolites, which could also result in a lower risk of prostate and other cancers.

Detoxification and biotransformation illustrate the individual approach we need to take with our patients given their unique genetic determinants that are influenced by powerful environmental factors. This web of complex interactions examined in the functional medicine paradigm gives us an opportunity to offer our patients additional options in their quest for health and wellness.

IMMUNE AND INFLAMMATORY IMBALANCES

Immune and inflammatory imbalances can affect every organ system and can manifest as common clinical disorders that include neurodegenerative disorders, coronary heart and peripheral vascular disease, asthma, eczema, inflammatory bowel disease, connective tissue disease, and many other disorders. Being able to mount an immune response is critical to our survival, but when the response is perpetuated after the insult has been eliminated or as a result of disordered regulation, destruction to the host occurs and results in chronic inflammatory disease processes. This state of dysfunction was likely present long before the manifestation of the disease process. In many instances, this dysfunction occurs decades before the clinical presentation. The host's susceptibility to inflammatory processes can be related to genetic uniqueness as manifested by cell membrane proteins involved in antigen presentation and cytokine polymorphisms. Triggers and mediators of inflammatory responses include infections, dietary factors, environmental toxins, and even the bacterial composition of the digestive tract. We again begin to appreciate the weblike interactions that the mediators of inflammation have on virtually all the organ systems of the patient.

Advances in genetics and molecular biology have provided us with many new tools to examine the pathogenesis and propagation of immune and inflammatory disorders. Functional medicine provides a paradigm to examine and to modulate these states of dysfunction by applying our understanding of the underlying pathophysiology and the factors that support optimal function. Factors that support optimal function can be as specific as a nutritional supplement that modulates the inflammatory response or as broad as the mind-body influence on the mediators of inflammation (Box 3).

Inflammation can be identified on the physical examination by the classic signs and symptoms including redness, increased temperature, swelling, and pain. The molecular mediators of inflammation interact in a complex and synchronous array of events that either serve to destroy invading organisms or that hover in an anticipatory mode in ongoing vigilance that serves to protect the host. When this balance is tipped in the direction of activation by any one of a variety

Box 3 Nutritional and Botanical Inhibitors of Inflammation

Cyclooxygenase
EPA
Feverfew
Ginger
Green tea
Turmeric

Cytokines and/or NF-κB
Boswellia
Cat's Claw
Devil's Claw
Feverfew
Ginger
Green tea
Turmeric

Lipooxygenase
Boswellia
EPA
Feverfew
Garlic
Quercetin
Turmeric
Phospholipase A_2Licorice
Quercetin
Turmeric

EPA, eicosapentaenoic acid; NF-κB, nuclear factor-κB.

of triggers, these processes can then become perpetuated and result in disease processes.

Coronary artery disease (CAD) has evolved from the concept that atherosclerosis was a localized lipid storage disease that resulted in mechanical obstruction of blood flow to a dynamic process. It is now characterized as an inflammatory disorder from its earliest stage in atheroma formation to the clinical hallmark of acute myocardial infarction related to inflammatory-mediated plaque rupture. This process of inflammation has a number of potential triggers and mediators. Modification of unhealthy lifestyle habits remains the single most powerful strategy for preventing CAD. Several studies have shown the positive effect of aerobic exercise on various cytokines that are associated with inflammation. Healthy diets, such as a Mediterranean diet, reduce the intake of saturated fats and thus lower the precursor intake of arachidonic acid and affect the cascade of proinflammatory prostaglandins and leukotrienes.[14] Whole foods, especially those rich in phytonutrients, have beneficial effects due to their antioxidant and anti-inflammatory properties. Meals with high glycemic loads (which include highly processed or quickly digested macronutrients) can induce an inflammatory response as monitored by levels of C-reactive protein (CRP). A whole-food diet has a lower glycemic index, because foods are digested slowly and the fluctuations of blood glucose levels are less pronounced.

Mind-body interventions, such as meditation, result in modulation of the autonomic nervous system, which in turn influences endothelial function. There is strong evidence of reduced adverse events in patients who have established coronary heart disease and who use stress-reduction techniques. Heart rate variability represents a beat-to-beat variation in the sinoatrial node activation and can be noninvasively measured to determine output of the autonomic nervous system. Patients who have low heart rate variability have increased risks for sudden death as well as recurrent coronary events.[15] Specific meditative and biofeedback techniques can modulate heart rate variability in subjects who are skilled in using these techniques.[16]

CRP is a marker and possibly a mediator of systemic inflammation. Serum levels of this protein have been shown to be independently correlated with an increased risk of adverse cardiovascular events. Association of elevated CRP levels with stress has also been demonstrated.[17] There is also evidence of a relation between reduced heart rate variability and subclinical inflammation in patients without apparent heart disease.[18]

In epidemiologic studies, fish intake has been associated with a reduced risk for the development of CAD and for the risk of sudden death in those patients with existing CAD. Fatty acids are essential constituents of and influence the function of cell membranes. They are also precursors of eicosanoids, which through their messenger functions influence the inflammatory response of the organism. Omega-6 and omega-3 fatty acids are the substrates for the production of series 1 and series 3 eicosanoids, respectively, which serve to inhibit the inflammatory response, whereas arachidonic acid-derived eicosanoids of the series 2 family are proinflammatory (Fig. 4).

Acute inflammation often serves a protective role. Chronic inflammation, on the other hand, is often associated with deleterious affects. Fish oils are mostly composed of the essential fatty acids in the omega-3 family, which includes eicosapentaenoic acid (EPA) and docosahexaenoic acid (DHA). In addition to the influence of omega fatty acids on the production of eicosanoids, EPA also can inhibit both the 5-LOX pathway in neutrophils and monocytes and the leukotriene B4-mediated function in neutrophils.[19] There is also evidence that omega-3 fatty acids can suppress mononuclear cytokines that includes TNF-α and interleukin (IL) 1β. Like the thiazolidinedione class of drugs used in diabetes management, fish oils are also peroxisome proliferator-activated receptor (PPAR) γ agonists that can modulate the expression of this family of genes. An example of this effect is the lowering of triglyceride levels through fish oil supplementation.

Fish oils have demonstrated clinical efficacy in chronic inflammatory conditions. The benefits of supplemental fish oils in the treatment of rheumatoid arthritis are well documented. A diet low in arachidonic acid and the addition of fish oil has been shown to produce a superior result to that of diet alone.[20] Other inflammatory conditions, including inflammatory bowel disease, immunoglobulin (Ig) A nephropathy, psoriasis, and coronary artery disease, are modified by fish oils. In the Gruppo Italiano per lo Studio della Sopravvivenza nell'infarto miocardio (GISSI)-Prevenzione clinical trial, supplementation with only 1 g of omega-3 fatty acids per day resulted in an approximate 20% decrease in cardiovascular mortality.[21]

Laboratory testing is available to determine the contents and ratios of fatty acids from serum samples. It is important to make sure that the fish oil supplement has been purified and tested for heavy metals and other contaminants. Manufacturers should supply third-party testing results when requested to confirm this. It is also important to review the concentrations of the actual omega-3 components (EPA and DHA) because the potency varies from product to product. Dosing recommendations for specific conditions are varied and range from 1 to 9 g of omega-3 fatty acids. It can take several months to notice a clinical response in patients with active inflammatory disorders. Although omega-3 fatty acids can affect platelet aggregation, no data suggest any increased risk of hemorrhagic events. However, caution is suggested when adding omega-3 fatty acids to the diet of patients who are taking anticoagulants or antiplatelet therapy. Fish oils should be discontinued one week before surgical procedures to decrease the risk of hemorrhage.

With the recent clinical concerns related to the prostacyclin-mediated adverse effect of COX-2 inhibitors and concern over similar issues with COX-1 inhibition, natural anti-inflammatory agents represent another possible treatment modality for inflammatory conditions such as osteoarthritis and rheumatoid arthritis. These herbal preparations might modulate inflammation at various points in the inflammatory pathways, including modulation of cytokine production or production of arachidonic acid proinflammatory products (see Box 3). Clinical trials for specific conditions have been performed with herbal preparations and can help direct the clinician in the use of these agents. An excellent resource to review the quality of supplements can be found at www.consumerlabs.com.

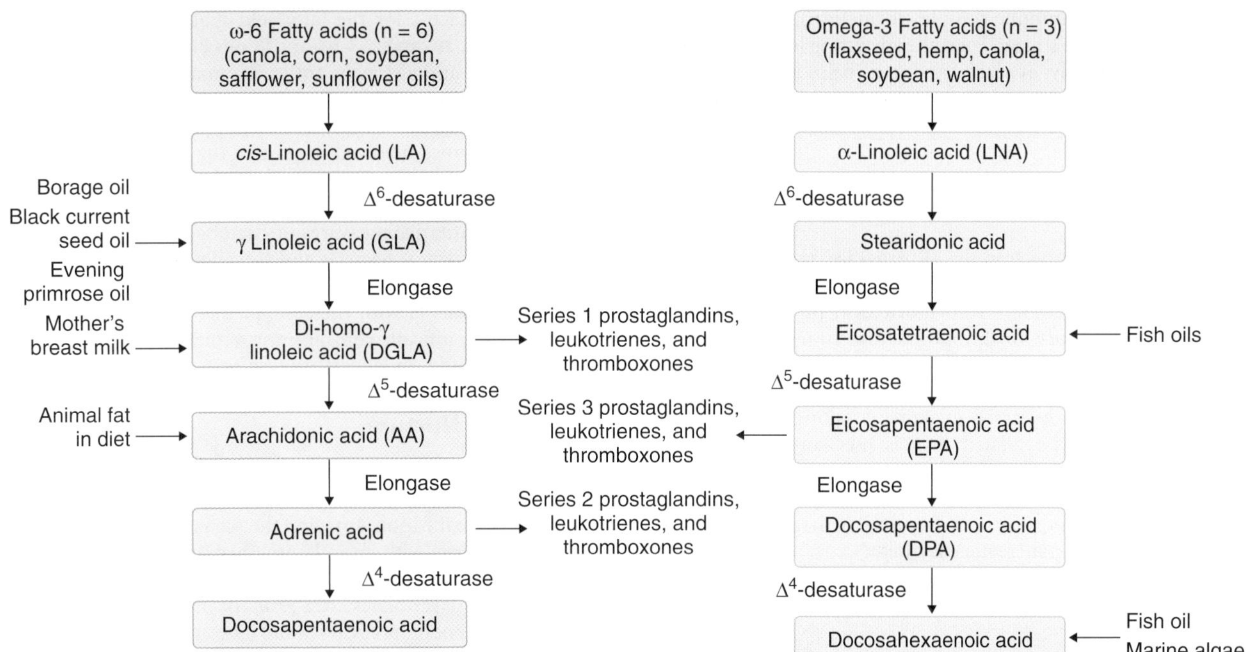

Figure 4 **Prostaglandin precursors of omega-6 and omega-3 fatty acid metabolism.** *(From the Institute for Functional Medicine: Textbook of Functional Medicine. Gig Harbor, Wash: The Institute for Functional Medicine, 2005, p 420. © 2005 The Institute of Functional Medicine.)*

GASTROINTESTINAL IMBALANCES

We consume approximately 30 to 60 tons of food in our lifetime. This food intake is composed of macromolecules, micronutrients that include vitamins and minerals, toxins, and other organisms capable of invasion. The gastrointestinal (GI) tract must function in an optimal fashion to be able to process and absorb these molecules and to keep invading organisms or toxins from entering the host. The microflora of the colon, which is composed of approximately 100 billion bacteria, is also intimately involved in intestinal health and generates metabolic byproducts that support the health of the host in a symbiotic fashion. Disruption of this flora (dysbiosis) can result in the production of toxic bacterial metabolites or the reduction in beneficial byproducts. Approximately 60% of the immune system is located in the GI tract and is referred to as the gastrointestinal associated lymphoid tissue (GALT). Activation of GALT can have far-reaching downstream effects, as can be seen in the peripheral manifestations of inflammatory bowel syndrome or gluten sensitivity. The GI system can have large effects on either keeping physiologic processes in balance or initiating and perpetuating imbalances in inflammation, oxidation, and detoxification, which are often manifest in organ systems that seem far removed from the GI system.

Macromolecules must be processed to their basic building blocks to be absorbed via transport mechanisms in the small intestine. Potential disruptions can occur in this process at any of a number of sites. Hydrochloric acid production in the stomach, pancreatic enzyme production, loss of tight junctions of the small bowel intestinal epithelium (causing leaky gut), and dysbiosis can all result in GI dysfunction and downstream effects. Functional disorders such as irritable bowel syndrome can occur as a result of this disordered physiology.

The 4R Model

Remove

One clinical paradigm used extensively in functional medicine is referred to as the 4R model. The first approach in the 4R model, remove, refers to the elimination of pathogenic organisms including fungi, pathogenic bacteria, parasites, and other ingested substances that include environmental toxins and foods. Food allergy is believed to be mediated by the passage of incompletely digested proteins across the intestinal epithelium, where it stimulates an immune response with the production of IgG antibodies. With continued ingestion of these proteins and translocation across the intestinal epithelium due to leaky gut, immune complexes are formed that result in immune activation. This is in contrast to the traditional concept of food allergy, which is IgE mediated and can represent a life-threatening, immediate type of immune reaction.

Infants have been shown to have impaired tight junctions of the enterocytes, and introduction of antigenic foods within the first 6 to 12 months is associated with the development of inflammatory skin conditions. Symptoms suggesting IgG-mediated food allergies include irritable bowel syndrome, apthous ulcers in the oral mucosa, serous otitis media, migraine headaches, asthma, chronic sinusitis, nasal congestion (without rhinorrhea), eczema, and memory loss. IgG-mediated food allergy might trigger other disorders (through stimulation of the immune system via immune complexes) such as rheumatoid arthritis and inflammatory bowel disorders. Peptides produced through the partial hydrolysis of gluten and casein that leak across an impaired GI mucosa have opioid properties and can result in neurobehavioral symptoms.

Leaky gut can be related to infections, use of NSAIDs, and the development of dysbiosis related to antibiotic use. One study has demonstrated a higher incidence of functional GI complaints in patients who had received antibiotics months before the development of symptoms.[22] Studies have also suggested that antibiotics can increase the risk of Crohn's disease.[23] Leaky gut can be tested for by ingesting lactulose and mannitol and measuring urinary ratios of these substances in the urine. Lactulose is not normally absorbed, and an elevated ratio might suggest impaired mucosal integrity.

Removal of offending foods by following an oligoantigenic diet and observing clinical improvement is the gold standard for assessing food allergies. Elimination diets are typically continued for approximately 1 month, and then food groups are reintroduced every 4 days or so. If symptoms recur with re-introduction (it can take a week of continued ingestion to develop clinical symptoms due to the delayed type of response from immune complex formation), then that food is identified as a possible trigger. Food allergy testing for IgG antibodies is also commercially available and can help guide decisions regarding dietary modifications. The results from these tests seem to be quite variable, so proceeding straight to the elimination diet is a better practice if possible.

Replace

Replace, the second approach in the 4R program, refers to the supplementation of digestive factors that may be reduced, therefore preventing optimal function. Hydrochloric acid production in the gastric mucosa is necessary for the optimal digestion of proteins and for the absorption of nutrients such as calcium. With increasing age, impairment in the production of HCl becomes more common. Osteoporosis has been described in patients taking proton pump inhibitors, which may be related to this mechanism. Pancreatic enzymes may be functionally deficient in a variety of clinical conditions including eczema and steatorrhea. The symptoms in patients with irritable bowel syndrome can improve with the addition of empirical supplemental pancreatic enzymes.

Reinoculate

Reinoculate is the third step. This refers to the supplementation of desirable microorganisms (probiotics) into the GI tract. This balance, involving hundreds of species of bacteria, can be impaired through the use of antibiotics and through exposure to environmental toxins. The environmental influence on the colonization of the intestinal microflora begins at the time of delivery and continues for the first 2 years of life. The maternal microflora inoculates the infant and influences the development of this symbiotic relationship and eventual milieu of the GI tract. Commonly prescribed probiotics include *Lactobacillus* and *Bifidobacteria.* Within each of these groups of bacteria, there are many species, and each has its unique characteristics and produces different effects in clinical trials.

Probiotics can inhibit pathogenic bacteria through a variety of proposed mechanisms that include competition for bacterial adhesion sites and bactericidal activity against pathogenic bacteria. Probiotics produce metabolites, such as butyric acid, that are beneficial to barrier function and colonocyte health. Studies have demonstrated the effectiveness of probiotics in children with viral diarrhea illness. Use of probiotics shortened the course of diarrhea and reduced hospitalization.[24] Probiotics have also been shown to modulate the course of ulcerative colitis[23] Saccharomyces boulardii, when given in conjunction with vancomycin, has been demonstrated to reduce the likelihood of recurrent *Clostridium difficile* enterocolitis.[25] Caution must be exercised in extremely ill patients because the use of this normally nonpathogenic organism has resulted in fungemia. The use of probiotics together (synbiotics) has been shown to be beneficial in specific clinical situations.

In addition to reinoculation, the addition of prebiotics can provide nutritional substrate for the beneficial bacteria that in turn results in the production of short-chain fatty acids (SCFAs), which are believed to provide up to 70% of the nutritional energy used by colonic cells. Examples of prebiotics include fructans, fructo-oligossaccharides, inulin, and arabinogalactans. Soluble fiber is also an important nutritive source for probiotics.

Repair

Repair is the final step in the 4R program. Nutrients that have been shown to support the repair process of the intestinal epithelium include glutamine, zinc, pantothenic acid, and essential fatty acids. Glutamine represents the major metabolic fuel for the epithelial cells in the small intestine. Pantothenic acid (vitamin B_5) is needed for the production of coenzyme A (CoA) and acyl carrier proteins (ACP). CoA is a cofactor in more than 70 enzymatic pathways, and ACP is an essential cofactor for the fatty acid synthase complex. Essential fatty acids such as omega-3 from fish oils are involved in cell membrane function and also have anti-inflammatory properties.

Laboratory testing to support the clinician is commercially available. Stool testing for meat fibers can imply adequacy of HCl and pancreatic enzymes involved in protein digestion. Stool fat analysis can suggest adequacy of lipase production. SCFA levels can suggest the amount and composition of the beneficial bacteria. Stool cultures can assess quantitative measures of Lactobacillus and Bifidobacteria along with pathogenic bacteria and yeast. Stool should also be examined for ova and parasites. In patients with irritable bowel syndrome, empirical treatments with these supplements in a stepwise fashion can result in significant clinical improvements that might not have been evident based on laboratory results.

Nature and Nurture

The web of interactions expands as we consider the influence of the GI tract on downstream processes such as inflammation, oxidative stress, and detoxification. Imagine the scenario where the patient in our office presents with an inflammatory condition such as eczema or rheumatoid arthritis. We know that approximately 70% of cancers and other disease processes are a result of the environment and 30% are related to genetic predisposition. The environment washes over the genes to result in either an inhibition or potentiation of genetic expression. Our hypothetical patient then received antibiotics or had some other insult that favored the development of a dysbiosis and leaky gut that in turn resulted in immune complex formation and activation of cytokines. He also inherited an SNP that results in the enhanced production of an inflammatory cytokine, which in turn is expressed in this inflammatory condition for which he is now being evaluated. His diet consists of highly processed inflammatory foods, which is the usual complement of the standard American diet. The trigger for this clinical condition occurred years before the presentation. It was potentiated and mediated through diet, obesity, and genetic predisposition. Understanding these interconnections gives us additional tools to evaluate and treat our patients in a more comprehensive manner.

CONCLUSION

The quest of people is to live a long, healthy, and fulfilling life. Since the mid-19th century, the average American lifespan has increased by approximately 2.5 years per decade. Healthy lifestyle activities are associated with decreased disability, illness, and a more functional status. The lifestyle factors that have the highest correlation to health are smoking, body mass index, and exercise. The greatest focus of prevention by allopathic and integrative medicine practitioners should be geared toward smoking cessation, consuming a healthy diet, achieving a healthy body weight, and regular exercise. As our knowledge in molecular medicine advances, we can now demonstrate that these activities have associated biologic markers that show improvement in cellular function, decreased inflammatory mediators, and a reduction in oxidative stress. Thus, we can now look for a molecular basis for what we have shown to be either a beneficial or detrimental lifestyle. Before disease becomes apparent, considerable dysfunction has occurred. If it is possible to intervene in this state of dysfunction and supply the needed nutrients or achieve lifestyle changes, then disease could be prevented.

The sobering reality is that our youngest generation is predicted to have a shorter lifespan than their parents due to obesity and the development of type 2 diabetes. The prevalence of type 2 diabetes is expected to reach 50% in some minorities. The Pima Indians have a rate of diabetes that reaches 90%. Traditionally they survived in a hostile environment where the next meal was not necessarily around the corner. To survive in this environment, they needed to develop thrifty genes so that in times when food was available they could store it efficiently. When their environment changed and highly processed, nutrient-poor, calorie-dense food became immediately available in the convenience store or at the fast-food establishment, their genotype continued in its thrifty mode and resulted in the development of obesity and type 2 diabetes with its myriad of complications, human suffering, and health care costs.

As health care providers we need to be mindful and vocal to promote positive lifestyle changes through education for our own families, patients, employees, school systems, and other institutions. There are many different starting points to accomplish this in our patients, including stress reduction, healthy whole-food diets, and exercise. We may be that ripple in a pond and touch many lives in the future through our work. We have the opportunity to affect the children, grandchildren, and future generations of the patients we serve.

Summary

- Many patients take supplements or nutraceuticals.
- The clinician must understand the scientific rationale for the use of particular herbs and supplements and must have resources to help guide patients and to prevent drug interactions.
- The science supporting the use of supplements is robust, although clinical outcome studies are lacking for various reasons.

Suggested Readings

Alternative Medicine Review Monographs, vol 1. Dover, Idaho, Thorne Research, 2002.

Davidson GP, Butler RN: Probiotics in pediatric gastrointestinal disorders. Curr Opin Pediatr 2000;12(5):477-481.

Institute for Functional Medicine: Textbook of Functional Medicine. Gig Harbor, Wash: The Institute for Functional Medicine, 2005.

Maxwell PR, Rink E, Kumar D, Mendall MA: Antibiotics increase functional abdominal symptoms. Am J Gastroenterol 2002;97(1):104-108.

Mohanty NK, Saxena S, Singh UP, et al: Lycopene as a chemopreventive agent in the treatment of high-grade prostate intraepithelial neoplasia. Urol Oncol 2005;23(6):383-385.

Singh S, Chakravarti D, Edney JA, et al: Relative imbalances in the expression of estrogen-metabolizing enzymes in the breast tissue of women with breast carcinoma. Oncol Rep 2005;14(4):1091-1096.

References

For a complete list of references, log onto www.expertconsult.com.

Preventing Toxic Drug Interactions and Exposures

Donald A. Moffa, Jr.

As practicing physicians, we are charged with caring for our patients with compassion and rigor. Our prescribing privilege is a powerful tool to help heal our patients and a toxic means to harm them if we are careless, lack knowledge of potential drug interactions, or disregard this knowledge.

More than 3200 prescription drugs, 300 dietary supplements, and 600 herbal products occupy pharmacy shelves in the United States,[1] and more than one half of our patients cannot recite an accurate list of their medications.[2] This creates a regrettable scenario when we write prescriptions for patients with whom we have little history, we see in our partners' absence, or we rush to treat in a busy emergency department with the goal of easing *dis*ease while assuring safety in our treatment methods.

We do our best to avoid adverse drug interactions. However, for patients taking two medications, the risk of a drug interaction is 15%. This risk rises to 40% for those taking five medications and to an alarming 80% for patients taking seven or more.[3] The risk of a toxic medication interaction is real considering that more than one half of noninstitutionalized adults older than 65 years take five or more different medications, and 12% use 10 or more.[4] In hospitalized patients, adverse drug interactions are estimated to be as high as the fourth leading cause of death.[5]

EPIDEMIOLOGY

The most dangerous drug combinations in the nursing home population involve warfarin interactions with nonsteroidal anti-inflammatory drugs (NSAIDs), sulfonamides, macrolides, or quinolones; angiotensin-converting enzyme (ACE) inhibitor interactions with potassium supplements or spironolactone; digoxin interactions with amiodarone; and theophylline interactions with quinolones.[6] Toxic drug interactions can occur any time two or more medications compete is such a way that their pharmacologic interaction causes a detrimental physiologic response, when a medication is prescribed in excessive amounts, or when one medication produces untoward consequences although it is prescribed according to established guidelines. This last effect is often the most difficult to predict because drug absorption and metabolism can vary with age, concomitant illness, gastric motility, pH of the gastrointestinal milieu, genetic variation, smoking, or some other obscure physiologic parameter.

THE CYTOCHROME P-450 MONOOXYGENASE SYSTEM

The system responsible for most drug metabolism in the human body is the cytochrome P-450 monooxygenase system (CYP-450). Composed of more than 30 heme-containing isoenzymes, the CYP-450 is embedded in the lipid bilayer of the endoplasmic reticulum of hepatocytes, enterocytes of the small intestines, and, in lesser quantities, in other tissues including the kidneys, lungs, and brain.[2] The major isoenzymes responsible for drug metabolism in humans are CYP3A4, CYP2D6, CYP1A2, and CYP2C; CYP3A4 and CYP2D6 account for the bulk of drug metabolism. CYP3A4 is the most abundant CYP-450 isoenzyme in the small intestine (responsible for much first-pass drug metabolism) and in the liver[7] and accounts for more than 50% of drug metabolism.[2]

Some drugs are metabolized by more than one CYP isoenzyme, so that inhibition in its metabolism by one pathway can lead to a compensatory increase in its metabolism by another. Moreover, a drug that is metabolized by one CYP pathway can, at the same time, inhibit another CYP isoenzyme such that the inhibition of the second pathway leads to the toxic accumulation of a drug that is normally metabolized by the second pathway.[2]

Genetic polymorphism affects drug metabolism such that some persons are *extensive metabolizers* and others are *poor metabolizers* of medications. From 5% to 10% of whites and 1% to 3% of Asians and African Americans are poor metabolizers by the CYP2D6 isoenzyme, and poor metabolizers by this pathway are at risk for tricyclic antidepressant (TCA)-induced cardiotoxicity and neuroleptic-induced side effects.[8] Prodrugs that are normally converted to their active metabolites (e.g., codeine requires biotransformation to morphine) may be ineffective in poor metabolizers. CYP2C9, CYP2C10, and CYP2C19 make up the metabolically active CYP2C isoenzyme subfamily, and the CYP2C10 isoenzyme exhibits genetic polymorphism, and 20% of African Americans and Asians and up to 5% of whites are poor metabolizers. Of course, whether or not your patient is a poor metabolizer is not apparent, nor may it be clinically relevant. Measuring the *O*-demethylated metabolite of dextromethorphan in the urine will help determine who is an extensive metabolizer and who is a poor metabolizer.[7]

Cytochrome P-450 Isoenzyme Induction and Inhibition

Drug metabolism by the CYP-450 system is important to prevent accumulation of medications and substances toxic to the body, but the ability to induce the CYP-450 system can decrease with age or with organ dysfunction (e.g., cirrhosis, hepatitis).[7] Isoenzyme inhibition by compounds that compete with the primary drug for the isoenzyme binding site can last several days, and the rate-limiting step in reversal of the inhibition can depend on isoenzyme turnover itself. The CYP-450 isoenzyme half-life ranges from 1 to 6 days[7] and may be inhibited or induced by secondary medications.

Isoenzymes can also be affected by the consequences of other isoenzyme interference. For example, warfarin is a compound of *R*- and *S*-enantiomers, and the *S*-warfarin enantiomer has a significantly greater anticoagulant effect. CYP1A2 metabolizes *R*-warfarin and CYP2C9 metabolizes *S*-warfarin, and *R*-warfarin inhibits CYP2C9. It is not a long stretch to imagine that any drug inhibiting CYP1A2, the isoenzyme that hydrolyzes the *R*-warfarin enantiomer, can secondarily inhibit *S*-warfarin metabolism by the accumulation of *R*-warfarin, increasing the anticoagulation effect of a seemingly stable warfarin dose. In this example, a medication such as ciprofloxacin enhances warfarin's own ability to anticoagulate.

CYP-450 enzyme synthesis may be stimulated by increases in hepatic blood flow (such as with hepatic enlargement by phenytoin therapy), and isoenzyme function may be enhanced for more rapid drug metabolism by induction from other substances (such as CYP1A2 induction by cigarette smoke or charcoal-broiled foods).[7] Notwithstanding isoenzyme inhibition or induction, many commonly prescribed medications pose challenges for the physician to avoid causing toxicity when given in combination with other medications.

WARFARIN

Warfarin combined with other medications accounts for the most common dangerous drug interactions.[6] Warfarin is prescribed with increasing frequency in patients with vascular stagnation states (e.g., atrial fibrillation, ventricular aneurysm), peripheral vascular disease leading to limb ischemia and stroke, and hypercoagulable conditions causing venous thromboembolic events (e.g., deep venous thrombosis, pulmonary embolism). Warfarin toxicity can lead to life-threatening intracranial and gastrointestinal hemorrhages, and the physician should pause to think about medication interactions when prescribing any drug, especially antibiotics and anti-inflammatories, to a patient taking warfarin.

Among the list of medications that inhibit warfarin metabolism and enhance its anticoagulation effects are cimetidine, selective serotonin reuptake inhibitors (SSRIs), antifungals (fluconazole, itraconazole, ketoconazole), erythromycin, (possibly clarithromycin), omeprazole, ciprofloxacin, norfloxacin, trimethoprim-sulfamethoxazole (TMP-SMX), and amiodarone.[2,7] Cimetidine is a potent CYP-450 inhibitor, confounding the metabolism of many medications including warfarin by CYP1A2 inhibition of *R*-warfarin metabolism. Omeprazole inhibits *R*-warfarin metabolism and can increase anticoagulation, but lansoprazole does not and may be considered an alternative treatment in the appropriate patient needing a proton pump inhibitor.[7]

Of the antibiotics that enhance warfarin's anticoagulation effect, erythromycin, ciprofloxacin, and TMP-SMX appear to have the most predictable interaction. Concomitant erythromycin use can cause a twofold increase in the international normalized ratio (INR) after 7 days of treatment. Azithromycin does not appear to increase warfarin's anticoagulant effect, but clarithromycin should be prescribed with caution because it can increase the risk of bleeding.[7] Quinolones can interact with warfarin after 2 to 16 days,[7] and ciprofloxacin can cause life-threatening hemorrhage in patients formerly stable on warfarin therapy.[9] Ofloxacin is less likely than ciprofloxacin to cause a dangerous interaction with warfarin, and levofloxacin and lomefloxacin are alternative quinolones with little or no effect on warfarin metabolism.[7] TMP-SMX enhances anticoagulation by inhibiting CYP2C9, which metabolizes *S*-warfarin and can cause serious bleeding in combination with warfarin.[2] Nonetheless, consider checking the INR more frequently, perhaps every other day, in patients for whom these antibiotic combinations with warfarin cannot be avoided.

Prescribing warfarin with other medications that inhibit coagulation or platelet function is risky and should only proceed when a well-defined end point supersedes the chance of causing hemorrhage, such as when low-molecular-weight heparin is given concurrently as a bridge to full anticoagulation therapy with warfarin. Synergy from the antiplatelet effect of NSAIDs and the anticoagulant effect of warfarin increases the risk of bleeding and usually occurs from the accidental combination of the two classes of medications, and although the risk of bleeding is less with cyclooxygenase (COX)-2 inhibitors than with traditional NSAIDs, the risk remains significant. Celecoxib competitively inhibits CYP2C9, the isoenzyme that metabolizes *S*-warfarin, and significantly increases INR and bleeding risk.[10,11]

Amiodarone, which is metabolized by CYP2C9 and decreases the total body clearance of both *R*- and *S*-warfarin, can increase bleeding. The increased anticoagulation effect begins 1 to 2 weeks after starting amiodarone and can last up to 3 weeks after discontinuing the antiarrhythmic. Consider reducing the warfarin dose by 25% when giving it in combination with amiodarone.[7]

Some medications can induce warfarin metabolism, thereby reducing the risk of bleeding. Failed anticoagulation has been observed when rifampin, carbamazepine, phenobarbital, or phenytoin is given in combination with warfarin. These medications induce *S*-warfarin metabolism.[7]

DIGOXIN

Digoxin serum concentration has a narrow therapeutic range. Its absorption is affected by gastrointestinal pH, intestinal contents, motility, and blood flow. The kidneys excrete digoxin. Any medication with anticholinergic properties that slows gastrointestinal motility or any condition that impairs digoxin excretion can increase digoxin's concentration and the risk of digoxin toxicity. Patients at highest risk for digoxin toxicity are those who have renal insufficiency, congestive heart failure, and dehydration. Antibiotics such as clarithromycin, erythromycin, and tetracycline can alter the gut flora and increase digoxin levels, as can other medications that reduce renal clearance, such as quinidine, amiodarone, and verapamil.[2] Consider reducing digoxin dosing by 50% when giving it with amiodarone, and monitor levels.

PHENYTOIN

Medications that inhibit phenytoin metabolism (CYP2C) and can favor phenytoin toxicity include cimetidine, omeprazole (impairs phenytoin elimination after 8 days), fluconazole, isoniazid, topiramate, and fluvoxamine.[7] In a similar fashion of isoenzyme induction with warfarin, rifampin induces phenytoin metabolism by the CYP2C isoenzyme and can cause therapeutic failure. It sometimes seems, however, that the most likely cause for phenytoin failure is not its interactions with other medications but our patients' failure to take the anticonvulsant in the first place.

THEOPHYLLINE

Theophylline is metabolized by CYP1A2. Cimetidine decreases theophylline clearance by 30%, and it takes approximately 2 days for theophylline to reach its new steady state when given in combination with cimetidine.[12] Other medications that interfere with theophylline metabolism and increase its serum concentration are erythromycin and clarithromycin (which decrease theophylline clearance by approximately 25% after 7 days), the quinolones ciprofloxacin and norfloxacin, isoniazid (after at least 6 days of coadministration), fluvoxamine (increases theophylline concentrations two- to threefold), and oral contraceptives (which decrease theophylline clearance by 30%). As an alternative to reducing theophylline dosing and diligently measuring its serum concentration, consider prescribing other antibiotics (azithromycin, dirithromycin, oflaxacin, levofloxacin, lomefloxacin, other tuberculosis therapy), other psychiatric medications, and alternative means of contraception.[7] Rifampin, carbamazepine, phenobarbital, phenytoin, and cigarette smoke induce theophylline metabolism, thereby decreasing theophylline's serum concentration. Cigarette smokers might need twice the usual theophylline dose to achieve a therapeutic concentration; the enzyme induction effect can last for several months after smoking cessation.[7]

ANTIDEPRESSANTS, ANTIPSYCHOTICS, BENZODIAZEPINES, AND NARCOTICS

Although little is known about the true mechanisms by which antidepressant and antipsychotic medications work, many interactions among them and other drugs are characterized, and toxicity of one or another substance occurs by affecting the CYP-450 system. Fluoxetine, paroxetine, and sertraline, to a lesser extent, inhibit the CYP2D6 isoenzyme. Coadministration of any of these can increase the plasma concentrations of each, perhaps to toxic levels.[7] Fluvoxamine inhibits CYP1A2 and increases the plasma concentrations (with accompanying clinical symptoms) of amitriptyline, clomipramine, clozapine, desipramine, imipramine, and haloperidol.[7] Fluoxetine can cause delirium when given in combination with clarithromycin.[7] Avoid giving SSRIs to patients taking class Ic antiarrhythmics.[7]

Interactions with benzodiazepines are often unexpected but may be predictable, because benzodiazepines have a significant inhibitory effect on CYP-450 isoenzymes, and other substances that induce the isoenzymes can diminish the benzodiazepine's intended effect. Smokers experience less drowsiness than nonsmokers when taking chlordiazepoxide or diazepam due to CYP1A2 isoenzyme induction from cigarette smoke. Rifampin induces benzodiazepine metabolism (CYP3A4) and can decrease its effect. Omeprazole inhibits diazepam metabolism (CYP2C) and increases its elimination half-life by 130%.[7] Fluoxetine and fluvoxamine increase the serum concentration of alprazolam, midazolam, and triazolam (CYP3A4 inhibition) and can potentiate psychomotor effects.[7] Grapefruit juice increases midazolam peak serum concentrations by 50%,[13] whereas nefazodone increases alprazolam and triazolam serum concentrations.[7] Consider decreasing dosages by as much as 75% of the usual dose when giving benzodiazepines in these combinations.

Similar to concurrent benzodiazepine use, rifampin increases the rate of opioid metabolism (CYP2D6) and may induce narcotic withdrawal symptoms.[7] Codeine is a prodrug that requires demethylation to its active form. Demethylation by the CYP-450 system is impaired in poor metabolizers and may be inhibited in extensive metabolizers who are taking drugs that compete for the same metabolic pathway, thereby reducing codeine's analgesic effect.[7] However, inhibition of the CYP3A4 metabolic pathway can enhance the effects of some narcotics. For example, surgical patients taking erythromycin who are also given alfentanil might experience prolonged respiratory depression.[14] Cimetidine doubles fentanyl's elimination half-life (CYP3A4 inhibition) and decreases meperidine clearance (CYP2D6 inhibition).[7] Meperidine's metabolite, normeperidine, is renally excreted and lowers the seizure threshold in patients with seizures. This can prove troublesome for some patients with renal insufficiency who are given meperidine for analgesia.

CARDIOVASCULAR DRUGS AND STATINS

Erythromycin, itraconazole, and cimetidine inhibit the metabolism of many cardiovascular medications and can increase serum concentrations to toxic levels, causing clinically significant effects. Itraconazole and erythromycin increase felodipine levels (CYP3A4 inhibition) and cause clinically significant changes in systolic and diastolic blood pressures and heart rate. Rifampin given with verapamil causes a tremendous increase in verapamil clearance by inducing the CYP3A4 isoenzyme responsible for its metabolism. Other calcium channel blockers may be similarly affected. Quinidine inhibits CYP2D6 (affecting flecainide, mexilitine, propafenone, and propranolol metabolism) and is metabolized by CYP3A4. CYP3A4 interactions are well documented with cimetidine, phenytoin, phenobarbital, rifampin, metronidazole, and ciprofloxacin. Consider alternative therapy. HMG-CoA reductase inhibitors can cause a diffuse myopathy, and the greatest risk is when they are prescribed with other medications such as cyclosporine, gemfibrozil, niacin, itraconazole, and erythromycin that compete with the CYP3A4 isoenzyme pathway.[7]

CHEMOTHERAPEUTIC MEDICATIONS

CYP3A4 metabolizes several chemotherapeutic medications including epipodophylotoxins, tamoxifen, paclitaxel, vinca alkaloids, and ifosfamide,[7] the last of which requires biotransformation to its cytoxic metabolite and an inactive metabolite that, incidentally, is neurotoxic. Drugs that induce CYP3A4 (rifampin, carbamazepine, phenobarbital, phenytoin) can promote ifosfamide metabolism and, hence, neurotoxicity.[7] CYP3A4 inhibitors including ketoconazole, itraconazole, diltiazem, verapamil, and cyclosporine can interfere with ifosfamide metabolism, but the clinical significance is not known.[7]

Vinblastine metabolism is inhibited by doxorubicin, etoposide, ketoconazole, and erythromycin, although the clinical significance is not known.[7] Nifedipine increases vincristine's elimination half-life fourfold, and toxicity is possible. Itraconazole (but not fluconazole) reduces busulfan clearance, making fluconazole an attractive choice for treating fungal infections in patients taking busulfan.[7] Phenobarbital and phenytoin increase etoposide's metabolism, and its metabolism is inhibited by cyclosporine.[7] Tamoxifen metabolism is inhibited by erythromycin, cyclosporine, nifedipine, and diltiazem. Cyclosporine decreases doxorubicin clearance by one half, increasing the likelihood of toxicity with signs including nausea, vomiting, and myelosuppression.[7]

Cyclosporine undergoes premetabolism in the small intestine, with further metabolism in the liver by CYP3A4 isoenzymes. Drugs (e.g., ketoconazole, verapamil, nicardipine, fluconazole, itraconazole, erythromycin, clarithromycin, tacrolimus) that inhibit CYP3A4 can increase cyclosporine serum concentrations. Cyclosporine degradation is increased by the CYP3A4 inducers rifampin, phenytoin, carbamazepine, and phenobarbital.[7]

PROTEASE INHIBITORS

Significant interactions occur with saquinavir, ritonavir, indinavir, and nelfinavir, all of which inhibit CYP3A4 isoenzyme. Ritonavir also inhibits CYP2D6 and reduces the clearance of medications metabolized by that isoenzyme, including benzodiazepines, calcium channel blockers, antidepressants, antiarrhythmics, corticosteroids, anticoagulants, opiates, and clarithromycin.[7]

Rifampin decreases saquinavir concentrations by isoenzyme induction so that patients concurrently treated for tuberculosis might require alternative antimycobacterial regimens.[15] Other CYP3A4 inducers that can decrease protease inhibitor serum concentrations include phenobarbital, phenytoin, carbamazepine, dexamethasone, and tobacco.[7]

ESTROGENS AND CORTICOSTEROIDS

Clinically significant interactions with oral contraceptive pills (OCPs) from CYP3A4 isoenzyme induction that reduce OCP effectiveness are reported with carbamazepine, ethosuximide, phenobarbital, phenytoin, primidone, and rifampin. Antibiotic therapy can interfere with OCP effectiveness. In these cases, one may consider alternative contraception, medroxyprogesterone, or higher OCP doses.[7] OCPs reduce prednisolone clearance and increase phenytoin concentrations.[7] Therefore, consider frequent phenytoin concentration monitoring to avoid toxicity.

ANGIOTENSIN-CONVERTING ENZYME INHIBITORS, POTASSIUM-SPARING DIURETICS, AND POTASSIUM SUPPLEMENTS

Other toxicities can occur aside from involving the CYP-450 system. Life-threatening hyperkalemia can occur when patients take excessive potassium supplementation (especially in renal failure), when they are prescribed the combination of ACE inhibitors and spironolactone (a common regimen in treating congestive heart failure), or from other medications that either increase potassium absorption or decrease potassium clearance. Medications that can cause life-threatening hyperkalemia include amiloride, ACE inhibitors, beta blockers, cyclosporine, digoxin, heparin, NSAIDs, intravenous penicillin G potassium, pentamidine, potassium-sparing diuretics, spironolactone, succinylcholine, triamterene, and trimethaprim.[2] Consider alternative medications in any patient who may be at risk for hyperkalemia.

SEROTONINERGIC AGENTS

Patients taking serotoninergic medications are at risk for the potentially life-threatening complication of serotonin syndrome when taking any other medication that can increase serotoninergic activity. Serotonin syndrome involves excessive serotonin stimulation at the 5-HT_{1A} receptor, both centrally and peripherally. Minor clinical features include neuromuscular, autonomic, and cognitive and behavioral excitation. More-severe cases can include seizure, coma, hyperthermia, rhabdomyolysis, organ failure, and cardiac arrest, and serotonin syndrome may be confused with neuroleptic malignant syndrome (NMS) or overdose.[2] Medications that inherently increase serotoninergic activity include SSRIs, monoamine oxidase inhibitors (MAOIs), MDMA (3,4-methylenedioxymethamphetamine), cocaine, and tramadol. Dextromethorphan, SSRIs, and meperidine block serotonin reuptake, MAOIs inhibit serotonin breakdown, and buspirone and lithium act as serotonin precursors.[2] All can contribute to serotonin toxicity, especially if given in combination or if taken surreptitiously.

NONSTEROIDAL ANTI-INFLAMMATORY DRUGS

NSAID use is not benign, and serious toxicity can occur even when taken in commonly advised doses. Adverse gastrointestinal effects, including bleeding from NSAID use, is estimated to account for the 15th most common cause of death in the United States.[16] NSAIDs are on the Beers list of drugs to avoid in the elderly. One should prescribe NSAIDs for the elderly with extreme caution and understand the risk of significant hemorrhage when NSAIDs are concurrently taken with warfarin, other NSAIDs or antiplatelet agents, and sulfonylurea agents.[2]

MEDICATIONS THAT PROLONG THE QT INTERVAL

Medications that prolong the QT interval of the cardiac conduction cycle increase the risk of ventricular dysrythmias such as torsades de pointes. Notwithstanding their intended benefit, several culprit drugs have been withdrawn from the market because of their arrhythmogenic potential. These include terfenadine, astemizole, cisapride, and sparfloxacin. It is fortunate that similar medications within the same drug classes are available in their place. However, other medications can prolong the QT interval, including antiarrhythmics (amiodarone, disopyramide, procainamide, quinidine), calcium channel blockers (diltiazem, verapamil), antibiotics (gatifloxacin, levofloxacin, moxifloxacin, azithromycin, clarithromycin, erythromycin), antifungals (fluconazole, itraconazole, ketoconazole), antidepressants (amitriptyline, desipramine, imipramine, fluvoxamine, nefazodone), antipsychotics (droperidal, haloperidol, pimozide, thioridazine, ziprasidone), and protease inhibitors (delavirdine, indinavir, saquinavir, nelfinavir, ritonavir).[2] Although there are no strict warnings against using these medications (except, perhaps, the black box warning for droperidol), it is reasonable to suggest avoiding them in combination to the allowable extent and to check baseline and subsequent electrocardiograms to follow the QT interval for signs of toxicity and the potential for dysrhythmia.

MEDICATIONS IN THE ELDERLY AND IN CHILDREN

Prescribing medications to patients at the extremes of age is often troublesome for the physician. Children might not have developed the necessary metabolic pathways. The elderly, whose metabolism has slowed, might have confounding medical conditions that prevent drug absorption or elimination.

Considering the most common drug classes of medications dispensed to children (analgesics, antibiotics, antiepileptics, asthma and allergy medications, and psychotropic medications), approximately 15% of medications have a potential dosing error (including overdosing and underdosing with respect to dosing guidelines).[17] This could have toxic consequences. The most common medication errors for children are in prescribing analgesics; oxycodone is most commonly overdosed 15% of the time. Antiepileptics are the most commonly underdosed medication class (20% of the time). The potential for prescribing error for amoxicillin is 3% and 12% for cephalexin but 33% for azithromycin.[17] It is, also, ill-advised to prescribe topical diphenhydramine to children because the large surface area on the skin for absorption and the unchecked distribution of the medication can lead to high serum levels, sedation, and obtundation.[18-20]

An estimated 30% of hospital admissions for the elderly are linked to drug-related problems or toxic drug effects.[21] This might cost $85 billion and 106,000 deaths annually.[21] Medication-related deaths, if categorized as such, may be the fifth leading cause of death in the United States.[21] According to the National Healthcare Quality Report for 2005, the percentage of elderly Americans who take at least one of the 33 drugs considered to be potentially inappropriate for the elderly according to the Beers criteria[21] dropped from 21.3% in 1996 to 18.4% in 2002.[22] This shows improvement in physicians' prescribing practices, but clearly there is more improvement to be made. Box 1 lists drugs at highest risk for causing adverse reactions when given to the elderly.

GRAPEFRUIT JUICE

Grapefruit juice contains furanocoumarin derivatives that can inhibit the CYP3A isoenzymes. It appears that only the CYP3A isoenzymes in the mucosal enterocytes of the small intestine are affected and not those of the liver. The isoenzymes are both reversibly and irreversibly inhibited, and it can take up to 72 hours to regenerate them after ingesting only a small amount grapefruit juice. For grapefruit juice to significantly affect a medication's metabolism, the drug must be a substrate of the CYP3A isoenzyme, have poor oral bioavailability because of extensive presystemic metabolism, and undergo extensive biotransformation by CYP3A in enterocytes. Significant interactions that raise circulating drug levels are unlikely, but the medications with the largest possibility for interaction are lovastatin, simvastatin, buspirone, and amiodarone.[23]

PREVENTION

Knowledge of adverse drug interactions and toxic combinations is the framework for preventing iatrogenic harm. Knowing one's patient is integral to avoiding prescribing errors. Nutritional state, alcohol consumption, cigarette smoking, herbal medications, even grapefruit juice can affect drug metabolism, leading to the possibility of drug toxicity. Several resources including personal digital assistant (PDA) formularies and online drug formularies are available to help the physician check medication interactions. Using electronic medical records with integral prescription-writing software makes it easier to document a patient's adverse medication history and can alert the physician about potential medication interactions for future prescriptions. Physician order entry can help reduce medication conflicts for our patients. The most immediate solutions in avoiding medication interactions are to avoid prescribing redundant medications and similar classes of medications, to advise patients against taking competing over-the-counter medications, to control patients' chronic medical conditions, to counsel against alcoholism, and to assist them with smoking cessation.

Box 1 Medications with Potentially High Risk of Adverse Effects in the Elderly

Amphetamines and Anorexic Agents
All except methylphenidate hydrochloride

Antiarrhythmics
Amiodarone
Disopyramide

Antibiotic
Nitrofurantoin

Anticholinergics and Antihistamines
Chlorpheniramine
Cyproheptadine
Dexchlorpheniramine
Diphenhydramine
Hydroxyzine
Promethazine
Tirpelennamine

Antidepressants
Amitriptyline
Fluoxetine, daily

Antiemetic
Tirmethobenzamide

Barbiturates
All except phenobarbital or when used to control seizures

Benzodiazepines
Chlorazepate
Chlordiazepoxide
Chlordiazepoxide-amitriptyline
Clidinium-chlordiazepoxide
Diazepam
Flurazepam
Halazepam
Quazepam
Short-acting doses greater than:

- Alprazolam (2 mg)
- Lorazepam (3 mg)
- Oxazepam (60 mg)
- Temazepam (15 mg)
- Triazolam (0.25 mg)

Gastrointestinal Antispasmotics
Belladonna alkaloids
Dicyclomine
Hyscyamine
Clidinium-chlordiazepoxide
Propantheline

Hypoglycemic
Chlorpropamide

Laxatives (Long-term Use)
Bisacodyl
Cascara sagrada
Neoloid (except in combination with opiods)

Miscellaneous
Guanadrel
Guanethidine
Meprobamate
Mesoridazine
Methyldopa
Methyltestosterone
Mineral oil
Nifedipine
Thioridazine
Thyroid, dessicated
Ticlopidine

Muscle Relaxants
Carisoprodol
Chlorzoxazone
Cyclobenzaprine
Metaxalone
Methocarbamol
Orphenadrine
Oxybutynin

Narcotic Analgesics
Meperidine
Pentazocine

Nonsteroidal Anti-inflammatory Drugs
Indomethacin
Ketorolac
Long-term use of:

- Naproxen
- Oxaprozin
- Piroxicam

Adapted Fick DM, Cooper JW, Wade WE, et al: Updating the Beers criteria for potentially inappropriate medication use in older adults: Results of a US consensus panel of experts. Arch Intern Med 2003;163(22):2716-2724 (table 1).

Summary

- The risk of a drug interaction is more likely the more medications a patient takes.
- Warfarin, angiotensin-converting enzyme (ACE) inhibitors, digoxin, and theophylline are often associated with the most dangerous drug interactions.
- So many drug interactions are possible with warfarin that prescribing any medication to the patient taking warfarin should give the physician pause to consider the potential for drug toxicity or to consult a prescribing formulary.
- Consider lifestyle choices when prescribing medications that require therapeutic serum concentrations and are metabolized by cytochrome pathways affected by cigarette smoking and diet, for example.
- Rifampin, phenytoin, carbamazepine, phenobarbital, and tobacco are potent inducers of the cytochrome P-450 system.
- The risk of myopathy attributed to statins is increased when they are taken in combination with cyclosporine, gemfibrozil, niacin, itraconazole, or erythromycin.
- Life-threatening hyperkalemia is possible in patients taking amiloride, ACE inhibitors, beta blockers, cyclosporine, digoxin, heparin, nonsteroidal anti-inflammatory drugs, intravenous penicillin G potassium, pentamidine, potassium-sparing diuretics, spironolactone, succinylcholine, triamterene, or trimethoprim.
- Many commonly prescribed medications from various classes can prolong the QT interval.
- Children are often underdosed or overdosed with medications, and the elderly can experience untoward effects from medications that younger adults might not.

Suggested Readings

Agency for Healthcare Research and Quality: National Healthcare Quality Report 2005. PDF available at http://www.ahrq.gov/qual/nhqr05/nhqr05.pdf (accessed January 23, 2008).

Fick DM, Cooper JW, Wade WE, et al: Updating the Beers criteria for potentially inappropriate medication use in older adults: Results of a US consensus panel of experts. Arch Intern Med 2003;163(22):2716-2724.

Gaeta TJ, Fiorini M, Ender K, et al: Potential drug-drug interactions in elderly patients presenting with syncope. J Emerg Med 2002;22(2):159-162.

Greenblatt DJ, Patki KC, von Moltke LL, Shader RI: Drug interactions with grapefruit juice: An update. J Clin Psychopharmacol 2001;21(4):357-359.

Gurwitz JH, Field TS, Avorn J, et al: Incidence and preventability of adverse drug events in nursing homes. Am J Med 2000;109(2):87-94.

Kaufman DW, Kelly FP, Rosenberg L, et al: Recent patterns of medication use in the ambulatory adult population of the United States: The Slone survey. JAMA 2002;287(3):337-344.

McPhillips HA, Stille CJ, Smith D, et al: Potential medication dosing errors in outpatient pediatrics. J Pediatr 2005;147:761-767.

Michalets EL: Update: Clinically significant cytochrome P-450 drug interactions. Pharmacotherapy 1998;18(1):84-112.

Prybys KM: Deadly drug interactions in emergency medicine. Emerg Med Clin North Am 2004;22:845-863.

Wolfe MM, Lichtenstein DR, Singh G: Gastrointestinal toxicity of anti-inflammatory drugs. N Engl J Med 1999;340:1888-1899.

References

For a complete list of references, log onto www.expertconsult.com.

Index

A

Page numbers followed by *f*, indicate figures; *t*, tables; *b*, boxes.

B

D

E

G

N

Q

S

U